REQUIRED FOR ACCESS TO ONLINE COURSE MATERIALS

NAVIGATE 2 FLIPPED ACCE

Nancy Caroline's Emergency C
Eighth Edition

Subscription Length: 365 Days

GETTING STARTED

Getting started is easy. Before you begin, you will need:

1. A valid email address
2. A new Access Code (found beneath the foil below)

NOTE: If the Access Code has already been used, new Access Codes are available at www.psglearning.com, bookstores, and retailers everywhere.

If you are enrolling in an instructor-led course, your instructor may provide you with a Course ID. A Course ID is a unique code that connects you to your instructor's course. Before enrolling, please contact your instructor for your Course ID.

For a complete listing of Navigate 2 system requirements, go to: www.psglearning.com/techsupport.

REVEAL YOUR ACCESS CODE

Beneath the foil below, you will find your unique 10-digit Access Code. Scratch off the foil to reveal your unique 10-digit Access Code.

NOTE: This Access Code is valid for one account setup only.

REDEEM YOUR ACCESS CODE

Go to www.psglearning.com and click *Redeem an Access Code*. Read and accept the terms and conditions, enter your 10-digit Access Code, click *Redeem*, and confirm your selection.

Next, follow the onscreen instructions to set up your account with Jones & Bartlett Learning. As part of this process, you will be asked for your email address and a password. You will use this email address and password combination each time you log in to Navigate 2.

LOG IN TO YOUR ACCOUNT

After you complete the account setup process, you will be asked to validate your email address and password. Once validated, your Navigate 2 product will be listed on your Products tab. Click on the Navigate 2 product name to begin learning.

To return to Navigate 2, go to www.psglearning.com and click *Log In to Your Account.*

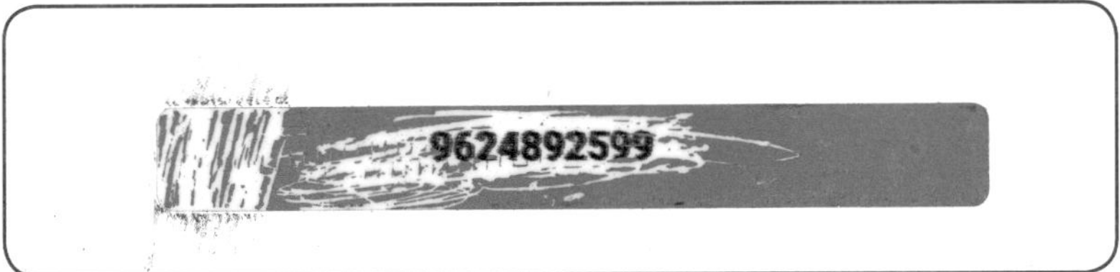

TECHNICAL SUPPORT

If you need help creating your account or technical support along the way, please:

- Visit www.psglearning.com/techsupport
- Email *support@psglearning.com*
- Call Monday through Friday from 8:30 a.m. to 8:00 p.m. Eastern Standard Time at 1-978-443-5000

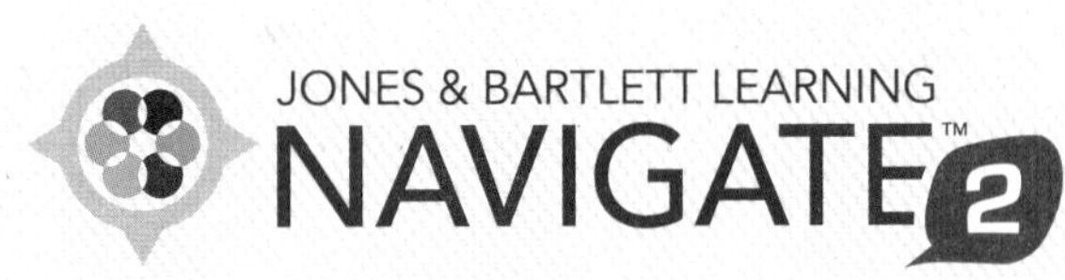

ACCESS CODE ALREADY USED? Individual Access Codes are available at www.psglearning.com, bookstores, and retailers everywhere.

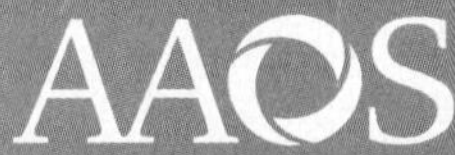

Eighth Edition

Nancy Caroline's Emergency Care in the Streets

Volume 1

Preparatory
The Human Body and Human Systems
Patient Assessment
Pharmacology
Airway Management
Medical

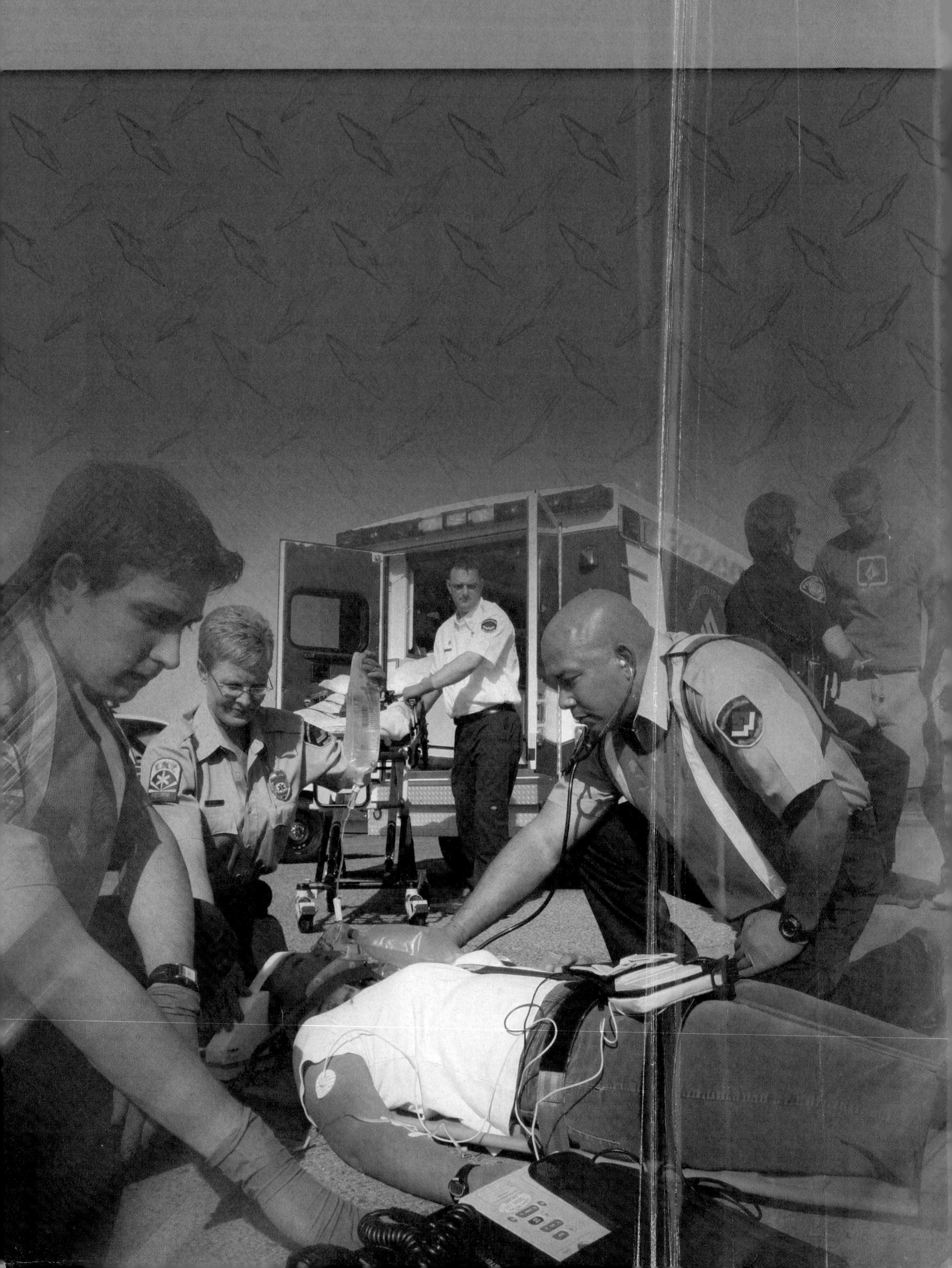

Eighth Edition

Nancy Caroline's Emergency Care in the Streets

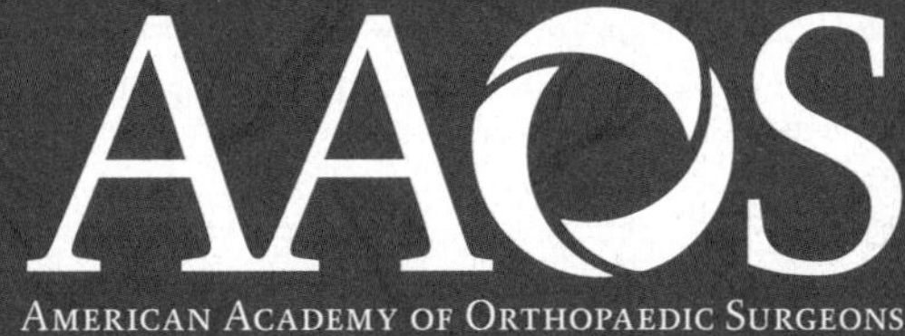

Series Editor:
Andrew N. Pollak, MD, FAAOS

Lead Editors:
Barbara Aehlert, MSEd, BSPA, RN
Bob Elling, MPA, EMT-P

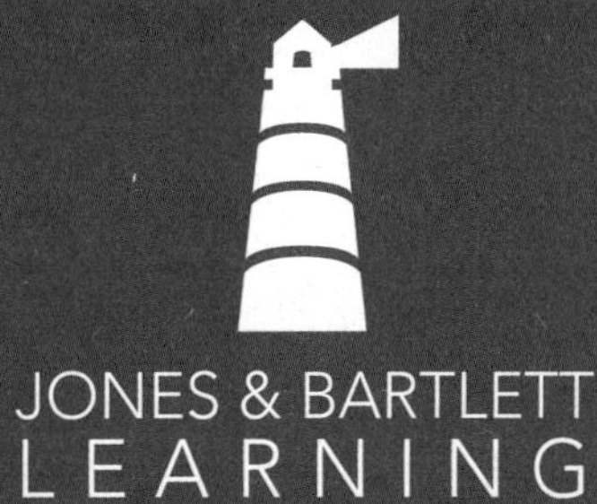

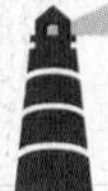

World Headquarters
Jones & Bartlett Learning
5 Wall Street
Burlington, MA 01803
978-443-5000
info@jblearning.com
www.jblearning.com

Jones & Bartlett Learning books and products are available through most bookstores and online booksellers. To contact Jones & Bartlett Learning directly, call 800-832-0034, fax 978-443-8000, or visit our website, www.jblearning.com.

Substantial discounts on bulk quantities of Jones & Bartlett Learning publications are available to corporations, professional associations, and other qualified organizations. For details and specific discount information, contact the special sales department at Jones & Bartlett Learning via the above contact information or send an email to specialsales@jblearning.com.

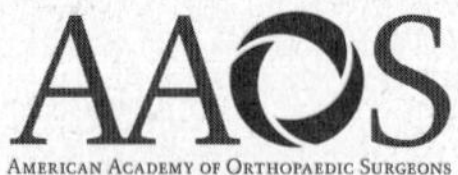

Editorial Credits:
Chief Education Officer: Ellen C. Moore
Director, Department of Publications: Hans J. Koelsch, PhD
Senior Manager, Book Program: Lisa Claxton Moore
Managing Editor: Kimberly D. Hooker
Senior Editor, Publications: Steven Kellert

13720-0

Production Credits
General Manager, Professional Certification and Licensure: Doug Kaplan
General Manager and Executive Publisher: Kimberly Brophy
VP, Product Development: Christine Emerton
Senior Acquisitions Editor: Tiffany Sliter
Product Development Manager: Jennifer Deforge-Kling
Senior Editor: Carol B. Guerrero
Senior Editor: Janet Morris
Senior Editor: Alison Lozeau
Senior Editor: Amanda Mitchell
Senior Editor: Barbara Scotese
Development Editor: Carly Mahoney
Editorial Assistant: Jessica Sturtevant
Editorial Assistant: Ashley Procum
Director of Production: Jenny L. Corriveau
Production Editor: Kristen Rogers
Director of Sales, Public Safety Group: Patricia Einstein
Director of Marketing Operations: Brian Rooney
VP, Manufacturing and Inventory Control: Therese Connell
Composition: S4Carlisle Publishing Services
Cover Design: Kristin E. Parker
Director of Rights & Media: Joanna Gallant
Rights & Media Specialist: Robert Boder
Media Development Editor: Troy Liston
Cover Image (Title Page, Part Opener, Chapter Opener): © Jones & Bartlett Learning. Courtesy of MIEMSS. Background: © Photos.com/Getty.
Printing and Binding: LSC Communications
Cover Printing: LSC Communications

Library of Congress Cataloging-in-Publication Data
Names: American Academy of Orthopaedic Surgeons, author. | Pollak, Andrew N., editor. | Elling, Bob, editor. | Aehlert, Barbara, editor.
Title: Nancy Caroline's emergency care in the streets / American Academy of Orthopaedic Surgeons ; series editor: Andrew N. Pollak ; lead editors: Bob Elling, Barbara Aehlert.
Other titles: Emergency care in the streets
Description: Eighth edition. | Burlington, MA : Jones & Bartlett Learning, [2018] | Preceded by Nancy Caroline's emergency care in the streets. 7th ed. 2013. | Includes bibliographical references and index.
Identifiers: LCCN 2017024835 | ISBN 9781284457278 (casebound)
Subjects: | MESH: Emergency Treatment | Emergency Medical Services | Emergency Medical Technicians
Classification: LCC RC86.7 | NLM WB 105 | DDC 616.02/5--dc23
LC record available at https://lccn.loc.gov/2017024835

6048

Printed in the United States of America
24 23 22 21 20 10 9 8 7 6 5

Brief Contents

Contents: Volume 1

Section 6: Medical 901

Skill Drills: Volume 1

Prepare for Class with Navigate 2 Digital Curriculum Solution Packages

Navigate 2 resources offer unbeatable value with mobile-ready course materials to help you prepare for your paramedic class.

Purchase access to the Advantage, Preferred, or Premier option at 25% off!*

ADVANTAGE PACKAGE

Navigate 2 Advantage Access Includes:

- eBook
- Study Center
- Assessments
- Analytics
- Fisdap Internship Scheduler
- Fisdap Skills Tracker

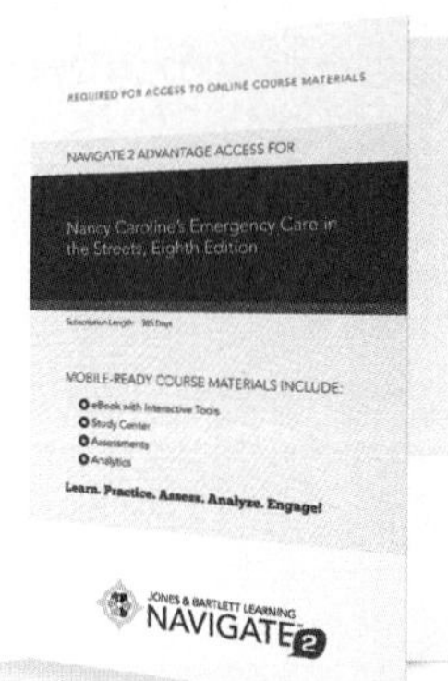

ISBN: 978-1-284-45702-5

PREFERRED PACKAGE

Navigate 2 Preferred Access Includes:

- eBook
- Study Center
- Assessments
- Analytics
- TestPrep
- Fisdap Internship Scheduler
- Fisdap Skills Tracker

ISBN: 978-1-284-13723-1

PREMIER PACKAGE

Navigate 2 Premier Access Includes:

- eBook
- Study Center
- Assessments
- Analytics
- TestPrep
- Lectures
- Simulations
- Fisdap Internship Scheduler
- Fisdap Skills Tracker

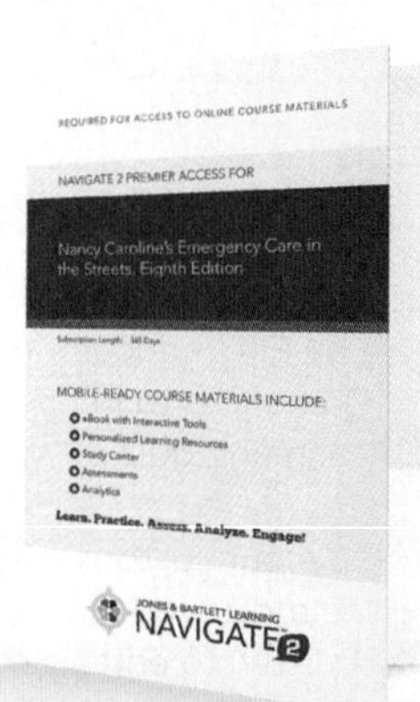

ISBN: 978-1-284-13727-9

Order today at www.psglearning.com

*Prices subject to change. Access codes to Navigate 2 course materials are available at 25% off the cost of the textbook.

Acknowledgments

The American Academy of Orthopaedic Surgeons and the Public Safety Group would like to acknowledge the editors, authors, and reviewers of previous editions of *Nancy Caroline's Emergency Care in the Streets* who were involved in the development of this textbook.

Series Editor

Andrew N. Pollak, MD, FAAOS
The James Lawrence Kernan Professor and Chairman, Department of Orthopaedics, University of Maryland School of Medicine
Chief of Orthopaedics, University of Maryland Medical System
Medical Director, Baltimore County Fire Department
Director, Shock Trauma Go Team
Special Deputy US Marshal

Series Editor Designee

Alfonso Mejia, MD, MPH
Program Director, Orthopedic Surgery Residency Program
Vice Head, Department of Orthopedic Surgery
University of Illinois College of Medicine
Medical Director
Tactical Emergency Medical Support Physician
South Suburban Emergency Response Team
Chicago, Illinois

Lead Editors

Barbara Aehlert, MSEd, BSPA, RN

Bob Elling, MPA, EMT-P
Educator, Author, and Advocate
High Quality Endeavors, Ltd.
Lake Placid, New York
SMG Events Medic
Albany, New York
Olympic Regional Development Authority Medic
Lake Placid, New York

Authors

Matthew Adams, AAS, FP-C, NRP
Chapters 27, 47, 49, 52
Duke Life Flight
Durham, North Carolina

Barbara Aehlert, MSEd, BSPA, RN
Chapters 8, 17, 19, 22, 26, 36, 43, 53, Appendix
President, Southwest EMS Education, Inc.

Leaugeay Barnes, MS, NRP, NCEE
Chapter 23
Tulsa Community College
Tulsa, Oklahoma

Andrew Bartkus, RN, MSN, JD, CEN, CCRN, CFRN, NREMT-P, FP-C
Chapters 13, 45
Sandoval Regional Medical Center
Rio Rancho, New Mexico

Ann Bellows, RN, NR-P, EdD
Chapter 25
Eastern New Mexico University, Ruidoso
Central New Mexico Community College
Outreach Education Opportunities
Las Cruces, New Mexico

Dave Bledsoe, RN, NREMT-P, LNC
Chapter 4
Orlando, Florida

Charles D. Bortle, EdD, NRP, RRT-NPS, CHSE
Chapters 16, 32
Director, Center for Clinical Competency
Einstein Medical Center Philadelphia
Philadelphia, Pennsylvania

Chad E. Brocato, DHSc, JD, REMT-P
Chapter 31
Division Chief
Pompano Beach Fire-Rescue
Pompano Beach, Florida

Bruce Butterfras, MSEd, LP
Chapter 29
Assistant Professor, Director of Bachelor Degree Program
Department of Emergency Health Sciences
The University of Texas Health Science Center at San Antonio
San Antonio, Texas

Derya Caglar, MD
Chapter 43
Associate Professor, Pediatrics
University of Washington School of Medicine
Seattle, Washington
Attending Physician, Emergency Medicine
Seattle Children's Hospital
Seattle, Washington

Julie Chase, MSEd, FAWM, TP-C
Chapter 34
Program Director
Immersion EMS Academy LLC
Berryville, Virginia

Patricia R. Chess, MD
Chapter 42
Professor of Pediatrics (Neonatology) and Biomedical Engineering
Director, Neonatal-Perinatal Medicine Fellowship Program
Vice-Chair for Education, Pediatrics
University of Rochester Medical Center
Golisano Children's Hospital at Strong
Rochester, New York

Stephen John Cico, MD, MEd
Chapter 43
Assistant Dean for Educational Affairs & Faculty Development
Dean's Offices of Educational Affairs and Faculty Affairs & Professional Development (OFAPD)
Associate Professor of Clinical Emergency Medicine & Pediatrics
Fellowship Director for Pediatric Emergency Medicine
Division of Emergency Pediatrics
Department of Emergency Medicine
Indiana University School of Medicine
Indianapolis, Indiana

David L. Dalton, BS, Paramedic
Chapter 3
Captain, Training Officer & AHA TC Coordinator
St. Charles County Ambulance District
St Peters, Missouri

Rommie L. Duckworth, LP
Chapters 30, 48, 50, 51
Founder, Director
New England Center for Rescue and Emergency Medicine
Sherman, Connecticut

Anne Austin Ellerbee, NRP, AAS
Chapter 46
H.E.R.O. Training Company
Thomaston, Georgia

Bob Elling, MPA, EMT-P
Chapters 11, 12, 39, 40
Educator, Author, and Advocate
High Quality Endeavors, Ltd.
Lake Placid, New York
SMG Events Medic
Albany, New York
Olympic Regional Development Authority Medic
Lake Placid, New York

Wm. Travis Engel, MSc, OMS-IV, NRP, FP-C
Chapters 41, 42, 45
Liberty University College of Osteopathic Medicine
Lynchburg, Virginia

John Farris, EMT-P, CP-C
Chapter 53
Mobile Integrated Health Paramedic, MedStar Mobile Healthcare
Chair, Fort Worth Safe Communities Elder Abuse Prevention Task Force
President, Tarrant County Adult Protective Services Community Board
Adjunct Clinical Instructor, UNTHSC Texas College of Osteopathic Medicine
Fort Worth, Texas

Cullen K. Griffith, MD
Chapter 37
Orthopaedic Trauma
Orthopaedic Specialty Group
Fairfield, Connecticut

Carol Gupton, NRP, BSEMS
Chapter 22
Papillion Fire Department
Papillion, Nebraska

Seth C. Hawkins, MD, FACEP, FAEMS, MFAWM
Chapter 38
Burke County EMS
Wake Forest University Department of Emergency Medicine
Morganton, North Carolina

Rhonda J. Hunt, BAS, NRP
Chapter 7
Albany State University
Albany, Georgia

Howard E. Huth III, BA, EMT-P
Chapter 10
Director, SUNY Cobleskill Paramedic Program
NYS DOH Bureau of EMS Regional Faculty
Cobleskill, New York

Don Kimlicka, NRP, CCEMT-P
Chapters 1, 2
Executive Director/Critical Care Paramedic
Clintonville Area Ambulance Service
Clintonville, Wisconsin
State of Wisconsin EMS Advisory Board
Adjunct Faculty, MidState Technical College
Wisconsin Rapids, Wisconsin
Adjunct Faculty, Nicolet Technical College
Rhinelander, Wisconsin

Sean M. Kivlehan, MD, MPH, NREMT-P
Chapter 21
Brigham and Women's Hospital
Harvard Medical School
Boston, Massachusetts

Deborah Lardner, DO, DTM&H, FACOEP
Chapter 51
Boarded Emergency Medicine/Family Medicine
CityMD—Corporate Offices
New York, New York

Nirupama Laroia, MD
Chapter 42
Professor of Pediatrics/Neonatology
University of Rochester Medical Center
Golisano Children's Hospital
Section Chief, Neonatology & Medical Director, Special Care Nursery
Rochester General Hospital
Rochester, New York

Edward "Ted" H. Lee, EdS, NRP, CCEMT-P
Chapter 35
Associate Professor/Program Chair Emergency Medical Services
Missouri Southern State University
Joplin, Missouri

Yogangi Malhotra, MD, FAAP
Chapter 42
Assistant Professor of Pediatrics
Division of Neonatology
Albert Einstein College of Medicine
Children's Hospital at Montefiore
Montefiore New Rochelle
New Rochelle, New York

Astra P. Paro, AS, CCEMT-P
Chapter 36
Charleston, South Carolina

Michael D. Passafaro, DO, DTM&H, FACEP, FACOEP
Chapter 51
CarePoint Health
Jersey City, New Jersey

Jason C. Perry, RN, CEN, CFRN
Appendix
Sandoval Regional Medical Center
Rio Rancho, New Mexico

Stephen J. Rahm, NRP
Chapter 15
Deputy Chief, Office of Clinical Direction
Co-Chair, Centre for Emergency Health Sciences
Bulverde Spring Branch Emergency Services
Spring Branch, Texas

Becky Ridenhour, PharmD
Appendix
Progress West Hospital
O'Fallon, Missouri

Rob Schnepp
Chapter 49
Division Chief, Special Operations (retired)
Alameda County Fire Department
California

Shadrach Smith, BS Bio, LP, NRP
Chapters 24, 30
Paramedic Advantage
Anaheim, California

Chuck Sowerbrower, MEd, NRP, NCEE, CCP-C
Chapters 18, 20
Sinclair Community College
Dayton, Ohio

Bryan L. Spangler, DHSc, NRP, NCEE, CMTE
Chapter 19
EMS Program Director
Central Ohio Technical College
Newark, Ohio

Chris Stratford, MS, BSN, RN, NRP
Chapter 28
University of Utah Center for Emergency Programs
Salt Lake City, Utah

John vonRosenberg, MA, FP-C, NRP
Chapter 9
Air Methods
Edenton, North Carolina

Robert Vroman, MEd, BSNRP
Chapters 33, 34
Associate Professor of EMS
Red Rocks Community College
Lakewood, Colorado

Bryan Ware, EMTP, Fire Chief
Chapters 4, 6, 30, 31, 32, 33, 35, 36, 41, 43, 44
Beulah Fire Protection District
Beulah, Colorado

Katherine H. West, RN, BSN, MSEd
Chapter 26
Infection Control Consultant
Infection Control/Emerging Concepts, Inc.
Manassas, Virginia

Keith Widmeier, BA, NRP, FP-C
Chapters 14, 44, Appendix
Director of Education
Good Fellowship Ambulance & EMS Training Institute
West Chester, Pennsylvania

Gordon H. Worley, RN, MSN, FNP, EMT-P, CFRN
Chapter 5
Sutter Amador Hospital
Jackson, California

Matt Zavadsky, MS-HSA, EMT
Chapter 53
Chief Strategic Integration Officer
MedStar Mobile Healthcare
Fort Worth, Texas

Contributors

Elyse K. Lavine, MD
Mount Sinai St. Luke's/Mount Sinai West
New York, New York

Jeffrey S. Rabrich, DO, FACEP, EMT-P
Medical Director
Mount Sinai St. Luke's Emergency Department
Assistant Professor of Emergency Medicine
Icahn School of Medicine at Mount Sinai
New York, New York

Ancillary Authors

Kimberly Bailey, MA, NRP, CHSE, SCCEM
Emerging Infectious Disease Planner
SC DHEC Office of Public Health Preparedness
Columbia, South Carolina

Sharon F. Chiumento, BSN, EMT-P
Lead Instructor, Monroe Ambulance, University of Rochester
Guest Instructor, Monroe Community College
Rochester, New York

Stephen J. Rahm, NRP
Deputy Chief, Office of Clinical Direction
Co-Chair, Centre for Emergency Health Sciences
Bulverde Spring Branch Emergency Services
Spring Branch, Texas

Brittany Ann Williams, DHSc, RRT-NPS, NREMT-P
Professor, Respiratory Care
Director, Clinical Education
Santa Fe College
Gainesville, Florida

Reviewers

J. Adam Alford, BS, NRP
Old Dominion EMS Alliance
Richmond, Virginia

Robert Jay Alley, MS, Paramedic
Blue Ridge Community College
Flat Rock, North Carolina

Hector D. Arroyo Jr, EMT-P, CIC
Senior EMT/Paramedic Instructor
FDNY-EMS—Borough of Manhattan Community College
New York, New York

Alan M. Batt, MSc, GradCert ICP, CCP
Fanshawe College
Ontario, Canada

Edward Bays, BS, NRP
EMS Education Director
Mountwest Community & Technical College
Huntington, West Virginia

Shawn Bjarnson
Advanced Emergency Medical Technician and Law Enforcement Officer
Gunnison Valley Hospital
Gunnison, Utah

Mark A. Boisclair, MPA, NRP, US Army (retired)
Chattahoochee Valley Community College
Phenix City, Alabama

Phillip J. Borum, MPA, RN, CPEN, Paramedic
Assistant Professor/Lead Paramedic Instructor
Santa Fe College Emergency Medical Services Programs
Gainesville, Florida

Jason L. Brooks, MA, NRP
University of South Alabama
Mobile, Alabama

Wayne D. Burdette Jr, MS, NRP
Gwinnett County Fire & Emergency Services
Lawrenceville, Georgia

Karen Burns
Clovis Fire Department
Clovis, New Mexico

Aaron R. Byington, MA, NRP
Battalion Chief/Paramedic
Layton City Fire Department
Layton, Utah

Elliot Carhart, EdD, RRT, NRP
Jefferson College of Health Sciences
Largo, Florida

Joshua Chan, BA, NRP, FP-C
Life Link III, Flight Paramedic
Minneapolis, Minnesota
Glacial Ridge Health Systems, EMS Educator
Glenwood, Minnesota

Julie Chase, MSEd, FAWM, TP-C
Program Director
Immersion EMS Academy LLC
Berryville, Virginia

Ted Chialtas
Fire Captain/Paramedic, Paramedic Program Coordinator
San Diego Fire-Rescue Department
San Diego, California

Sharon F. Chiumento, BSN, EMT-P
Lead Instructor, Monroe Ambulance, University of Rochester
Guest Instructor, Monroe Community College
Rochester, New York

Glenn Coffin
EMTS-Emergency Medical Teaching Services, Inc.
Pembroke, Massachusetts

Jason Lee Collins, BS, NRP
Rockingham Community College
Wentworth, North Carolina

Kevin T. Collopy, BA, FP-C, CCEMT-P, NR-P, CMTE
Clinical Outcomes Manager
AirLink/VitaLink Critical Care Transport
New Hanover Regional Medical Center
Wilmington, North Carolina

Hiram Colon
Paramedic
FDNY EMS Bureau of Training
Bayside, New York

Helen Compton, NRP
Lifestar Ambulance
Emporia, Virginia
Mecklenburg County Rescue
Clarksville, Virginia

George W. Contreras, MPH, MS, MEP, CEM, EMTP
Associate Professor and Director of Allied Health
Kingsborough Community College
Brooklyn, New York

Scott Cook, MS, CCEMTP
Southern Maine Community College
South Portland, Maine

Bob Coschignano
Lieutenant/Hazmat Technician
City of Orlando Fire Department
Orlando, Florida

Kent Courtney, NREMT-P
EMS Educator, Emergency Specialist
Peabody Western Coal Company
Essential Safety Training and Consulting
Northern Arizona Healthcare
Rimrock, Arizona

Matthew A. Crawford, NREMT-P, UMBC-CCT
CAMC
Sutton, West Virginia

Mark Cromer, MS, MBA, NRP
Jefferson College of Health Sciences
Roanoke, Virginia

Mike Cronin, EMT-P, EMI
Director of Public Safety
Knox Technical Center
Mount Vernon, Ohio

Anthony Cuda, NRP
ALS Program Coordinator
Community College of Allegheny County
Pittsburgh, Pennsylvania

Kevin Curry, AS, NRP, CCEMTP, I/C
United Training Center
Lewiston, Maine

Lyndal M. Curry, MS, NRP
Southern Union State Community College
Opelika, Alabama

Andrew J. Davis, NREMT-P
Gwinnett County Fire Academy
Dacula, Georgia

Lynne Dees, PhD, NRP
UCLA Center for Prehospital Care
David Geffen School of Medicine
Los Angeles, California

James DiClemente, MBA, NRP
Pro EMS Center for MEDICS
Cambridge, Massachusetts

Thomas Dobrzynski, BS, NRP
Sanford Health EMS Education
Fargo, North Dakota

Jeannett Edwards-Banks, NRP, BS, MEd
James City County Fire Department
Williamsburg, Virginia

Wm. Travis Engel, MSc, OMS-IV, NRP, FP-C
Liberty University College of Osteopathic Medicine
Lynchburg, Virginia

Reuben Farnsworth, CCP-C, NRP
RockStar Education & Consulting
Cedaredge, Colorado

Jason Ferguson, BPA, NRP
Central Virginia Community College
Lynchburg, Virginia

David Fifer, NRP
Lecturer, Emergency Medical Care
Eastern Kentucky University
Department of Fire Protection and Paramedic Science
Richmond, Kentucky

Darrell Wayne Fixler, RRT, NRP
Fort Rucker Fire & EMS
Fort Rucker, Alabama

John A. Flora, Paramedic, EMS-I
Columbus Division of Fire
Columbus, Ohio

Charles Foat, PhD, Paramedic
Johnson County Community College
Overland Park, Kansas

Jeffrey L. Foster, CCEMTP, NRP, I/C, EMD
CarolinaEast Health System
New Bern, North Carolina

Lori Gallian, BS, EMT-P
Cascade Training Center
Roseville, California

Scott A. Gano, BS, NRP, FP-C, CCEMT-P
Assistant Professor
Paramedic Program Director
Columbus State Community College
Columbus, Ohio

Fidel O. Garcia, Paramedic
President, Owner
Professional EMS Education
Grand Junction, Colorado

Rodney Geilenfeldt II, BS, EMT-P
Paramedic Coordinator
EMSTA College
Santee, California

Jeffery D. Gilliard, NRP, CCEMTP, FPC, BS
EMETSEEI Institute
Rockledge, Florida

Jamie O. Gray, BS, AAS, FF, NRP (NAEMT/NAEMSE)
Alabama Office of EMS
Montgomery, Alabama
Captain, Elmore Fire Department
Elmore, Alabama

Bill Grayson, NRP
Oklahoma City Community College
Oklahoma City, Oklahoma

James E. Gretz, NRP
Education Center Manager
JeffSTAT—Thomas Jefferson University Hospitals
Philadelphia, Pennsylvania

Jeffrey R. Grunow, MSN, NRP, NCEE
Associate Professor - EMT/Clinical Coordinator
Emergency Care & Rescue Department
Weber State University
Ogden, Utah

Kevin M. Gurney, MS, CCEPT-P, I/C
Delta Ambulance
Waterville, Maine

Jason Haag, CCEMT-P, CIC
Finger Lakes Ambulance
Finger Lakes Regional EMS Council
Wayne County ALS
Geneva, New York

Steven E. Hall Jr, EMT-P
Dabney S. Lancaster Community College
Clifton Forge, Virginia

Kirk Hallett, NREMT-P, CCT
Vital Knowledge Group
Richmond, Virginia

Joseph J. Hamilton, PA-C, NRP
Mt. Nebo Training
Provo, Utah

Jennifer Hannigan, MEd, Paramedic, CLI
Fire Department of the City of New York
Emergency Medical Services Bureau of Training
Bayside, New York

Anthony S. Harbour, BSN, MEd, RN, NRP
Director
Southern Virginia EMS
Roanoke, Virginia

Charles Phillip Head III, BHS, NRP, FP-C, CP-C
Manager of EMS Education
Greenville Health System
Greenville, South Carolina

Greg Helmuth, BA, NREMT-P
Hawkeye Community College
Waterloo, Iowa

Thomas Herron
Roane State Community College
Knoxville, Tennessee

Paul Hitchcock, NRP
Department of Homeland Security
Reston, Virginia

Henry 'Butch' Hoffmann, BA, EMT-P (retired)

Michele M. Hoffman, MSEd, RN, NREMT, AMWAc
James City Volunteer Rescue Squad
Toano, Virginia

James Hood, Paramedic
Lenoir County Emergency Services
Kinston, North Carolina

Troy Hoover, NRP, CCP-C, FP-C
Guardian Flight
Price, Utah

Mark A. Huckaby, NRP
OhioHealth Emergency Medical Services
Columbus, Ohio

James B. Huettenmueller, BSEd, NRP
Tulsa Tech
Tulsa, Oklahoma

Sandra Hultz, NRP
EMS Instructor
Holmes Community College
Ridgeland, Mississippi

Joseph Hurlburt, BS, NREMT-P, EMT-P I/C
Instructor Coordinator/Training Officer
Rapid Response EMS
Romulus, Michigan

Gene Iannuzzi, RN, MPA, CEN, EMT-P
Assistant Professor and EMS Program Director
Borough of Manhattan Community College
New York, NY

Darin Jackson, MDiv, Paramedic
Asheville-Buncombe Technical Community College
Asheville, North Carolina

Adam Johnson, NRP
Rhinelander Fire Department
Nicolet Area Technical College
Northcentral Technical College
Rhinelander, Wisconsin

Travis Karicofe, EMS Training Officer
Harrisonburg Fire Department
Harrisonburg, Virginia

Jared Kimball, NREMT-P
Tulane Trauma Education
New Orleans, Louisiana

Timothy M. Kimble, AAS, NRP
Carilion Clinic Life Support Training Center
Craig Co Emergency Services
Roanoke, Virginia

Don Kimlicka, NRP, CCEMT-P
Executive Director/Critical Care Paramedic
Clintonville Area Ambulance Service
Clintonville, Wisconsin
State of Wisconsin EMS Advisory Board
Adjunct Faculty, MidState Technical College
Wisconsin Rapids, Wisconsin
Adjunct Faculty, Nicolet Technical College
Rhinelander, Wisconsin

Mark A. King, MA, EMT-P, MEMS
Instructor Coordinator Paramedic
Kennebec Valley Community College
Fairfield, Maine

Blake Klingle, MS, RN, CCEMT-P
EMS Instructor/Coordinator
Waukesha County Technical College
Pewaukee, Wisconsin

Jim Ladle, BS, EMT-P, FP-C, CCP-C
South Jordan Fire Department
South Jordan, Utah

John F. LeBlanc Jr, AHS, NRP
Greenville Technical College
Greenville, South Carolina

William J. Leggio Jr, EdD, NRP
Creighton University EMS Education
Omaha, Nebraska

Daniel W. Linkins, BHS, NRP, NCEE
John Tyler Community College
Chester, Virginia

Tony Lipari, NREMTP
Operations Administrator
Bolton EMS
Bolton Landing, New York

Joshua Lopez, BS-EMS, NRP, I/C
University of New Mexico School of Medicine
Emergency Medical Services Academy
Kirtland Air Force Base Pararescue Paramedic Program
Albuquerque, New Mexico

Ricky Lyles, NRP
Southside Virginia Community College
Victoria, Virginia

Patty Maher, MPA, EMTP
Daytona State College
Daytona Beach, Florida

Richard Main, MEd, NRP
College of Southern Nevada
Las Vegas, Nevada

Jeanette S. Mann, BSN, RN, NRP
Director of EMS Program
Dabney S. Lancaster Community College
Clifton Forge, Virginia

Scotty A. McArthur, BS, NRP
University of South Alabama
Mobile, Alabama

Rod McGinnes, Paramedic, MPH
College of Central Florida
Ocala, Florida

Lucian Mirra, MEd, NRP
University of Virginia
Charlottesville, Virginia

Keith A. Monosky, PhD, MPM, EMT-P
Director, EMS Paramedicine Program
Professor, Department of Health Sciences
Central Washington University
Ellensburg, Washington

Nicholas J. Montelauro, BS, NRP, FP-C, NCEE
MHP Education and Training
Terre Haute, Indiana

John Morrissey, NREMT-P
NYS Department of Health Bureau of Emergency Medical Services and Trauma Systems
Albany, New York

Gregory S. Neiman, MS, NRP, NCEE, CEMA (VA)
Virginia Office of EMS
Richmond, Virginia

C. Jill Oblak, MA, MBA, NRP
Penn State University
Fayette, the Eberly Campus
Uniontown, Pennsylvania

Jim O'Connor, EMTP
Columbus Division of Fire
Columbus, Ohio
Hocking College
Nelsonville, Ohio

Laurie Oelslager, EdD, NRP, CMPA, AHA Regional Faculty
South Central College
Mankato, Minnesota

Danny K. Opperman Jr, MICP, NRP, BS
EMS Educator/Clinical Coordinator
Atlantic Cape Community College
Health Professions Institute
Atlantic City, New Jersey

Kate Passow, NRP
Physicians Transport Service
Herndon, Virginia

Nancy Peifer, PhD, MSN, RN
Palm Beach State College
Loxahatchee, Florida

Jose A. Perez, Paramedic, CLI
Fire Department of New York
New York City, New York

Timothy J. Petreit, MBA, NRP
Montgomery Fire/Rescue
Montgomery, Alabama

Joyce Pettengill
Department Chair EMS
Fayetteville Technical Community College
Fayetteville, North Carolina

Ian Pleet
MedStar/SITEL
Washington, District of Columbia

Jonathan R. Powell, BS, NRP
Department of EMS Education
University of South Alabama
Mobile, Alabama

Lionel Powell, EMT-P, MHEd
An Act of Caring
West Valley, Utah

Dr. Ernest K. Ralston, PG, EMT-P
Center of Asymmetric Emergency Medicine and Training, Inc.
Centreville, Virginia

Kevin Ramdayal, NREMT-P
FDNY EMS Academy
Bayside, New York

Kenneth D. Raynor, BS, NRP
Primary Instructor Emergency Medicine
Joint Special Operations Medical Training Center, USASWCS
Fort Bragg, North Carolina

William Raynovich, NREMTP, EdD, MPH
Creighton University
Omaha, Nebraska

Curtis A. Rhodes, AAS, NRP, CCEMT-P
Gordon Cooper Technology Center
Shawnee, Oklahoma

Chris Rock, RN, MSN
Paramedic Program Director
City of Tacoma Fire Department
Tacoma, Washington

Hector Roman, RN, EMT-P, TP-C
Reva Air Ambulance
Fort Lauderdale, Florida

Jamie Rossborough, NRP, CCEMT-P, FP-C
Captain/Paramedic
Sunset Fire Department
Sunset, Utah
University of Utah
Salt Lake City, Utah

Jose V. Salazar, MPH, CEMSO, CTO, NRP
Loudoun County Fire and Rescue
Leesburg, Virginia

Keith A. Sharisky, NRP
Aberdeen Fire/Rescue
Aberdeen, South Dakota

Jeb Sheidler, MPAS, PA-C, ATC, NRP
Executive Director, Trauma Services
Lutheran Hospital
Fort Wayne, Indiana
Training Officer Bath Township Fire Department
Tactical Paramedic, Allen County Sheriff's Office
Lima, Ohio

Karla Short, EMT-P, BBA, MEd
Columbus State Community College
Columbus, Ohio

Warren Short Jr, BS, NRP
Virginia Department of Health, Office of EMS
Glen Allen, Virginia

Douglas P. Skinner, MPA, NRP, NCEE
SCS Safety, Health and Security Associates LLC
Leesburg, Virginia
Prince George's Community College
Largo, Maryland

Jason P. Smith, MS
Barry University
Miami Shores, Florida

Jeremy Smith, Instructor, NRP
Joint Special Operations Medical Training Center
Fort Bragg, North Carolina

Scott A. Smith, MSN, APRN-CNP, ACNP-BC, CEN, NRP, I/C
Yarmouth, Maine

Andrew Snodgrass, NREMT-P, EMSI
Creighton University EMS Education
Omaha, Nebraska

Sandra A. Sokol
Monroe Technology Center/Loudoun County Fire Rescue Training Academy
Leesburg, Virginia
Captain, Battalion 4 Station 18
Dale City Volunteer Fire Department
Dale City, Virginia

Mark Spangenberg, CCEMTP/IC
Milwaukee Area Technical College
Milwaukee, Wisconsin

Sara Sproule, NRP, CCEMT-P
Prince William County Department of Fire and Rescue
Prince William County, Virginia

Nathan Stanaway, BS, NRP
Greenville Technical College
Greenville, South Carolina

Lieutenant Bruce J. Stark, NRP, TP-C
Fairfax County Fire and Rescue Department
Fairfax, Virginia

Andrew W. Stern, NRP, CCEMT-P, MPA, MA
Clinical Instructor
Hudson Valley Community College
Rensselaer, New York

Melissa J. Stoddard, NRP, MPH
Tacoma Community College
Tacoma, Washington

Jonathan C. Stone, MPA, NRP, FP-C
Herriman, Utah

Holly Ann Sturdevant, NRP, CC
Old Dominion EMS Alliance
Richmond, Virginia

Bruce Swanson, Paramedic, EMS Captain
Huntsville Fire & Rescue
Huntsville Fire & Rescue Training Academy
Huntsville, Alabama

Benjamin D. Symonds, BA, NRP
Kirkwood Community College
Cedar Rapids, Iowa

Justin G. Tilghman, MS, CEM, EMTP
Lenoir Community College
Kinston, North Carolina

Scott Tomek, MA, Paramedic
Manager, Quality/Safety/Risk
Allina Health EMS
Risk Manager-Allina Corporate Security
St. Paul, Minnesota
Clinical Skills Instructor
University of Minnesota School of Medicine
Emergency Medicine Program
Minneapolis, Minnesota
Paramedic
Woodbury Public Safety
Woodbury, Minnesota

Stephen Trala, MPH, BSN, RN, NRP
The University of Vermont Medical Center Health Net Transport
Burlington, Vermont

Amy E. Trujillo, NREMT-P, BS
Montana Medical Transport
Helena, Montana

Brian Turner, CCEMT-P, RN
Trinity Medical Center
Rock Island, Illinois

William H. (Bill) Turner, MS, NRP
Program Director-Emergency Medical Technology
Shawnee State University
Portsmouth, Ohio

Micheal D. Vance Jr, NRP, LP, BA
Education Coordinator
MedStar Training Academy
Fort Worth, Texas

Scott Vanderkooi, BS, NRP
University of South Alabama
Department of EMS Education
Mobile, Alabama

Leo Vanderpool, EMT-P
Fire Department of the City of New York
New York, New York

Athanasios T. Viglis, NRP
Fire Fighter
Henrico County Division of Fire
Henrico, Virginia

Jimmy Walker, NREMT-P
Midlands EMS
West Columbia, South Carolina

Jon Walker, NRP
Upper Valley Ambulance (retired)
Fairlee, Vermont

Kelly Walsh, RN, BSN, PHRN
Advanced Medical Transport
Peoria, Illinois

Tom Watson, AS, AAS, Paramedic
Adjunct Instructor
Texas A&M University System, Texas Engineering Extension Service, EMS/Public Health Grant Program
College Station, Texas

Gregory West, EdD, JD, NRP
Waukesha County Technical College
Pewaukee, Wisconsin

Monette Wiedlebacher, BA, EI, Paramedic
Stark State College
North Canton, Ohio

Michael H. Wilhelm, CRNA, APRN
Integrated Anesthesia Associates, School of Nurse Anesthesia
Hartford, Connecticut

Dustin Williams, BS, NRP
Deputy Chief
Christiansburg Rescue
Christiansburg, Virginia

Karen "Keri" Wydner Krause, RN, CCRN, EMT-P
Lakeshore Technical College
Cleveland, Wisconsin

David Yarmesch, BSOL, CSSGB, AAS-EMS, Paramedic, EMSI
EMS Coordinator
The MetroHealth System
Adjunct Faculty
Cuyahoga Community College
Cleveland, Ohio

▶ Photoshoot Acknowledgments

We would like to thank the following people and institutions for their collaboration on the photoshoots for this project. Their assistance was greatly appreciated.

Technical Consultants and Institutions

UMass Memorial Paramedics—Worcester EMS
Worcester, Massachusetts

Centre for Emergency Health Sciences
Bulverde Spring Branch Emergency Services
Spring Branch, Texas

Richard A. Nydam, AS, NREMT-P
Training and Education Specialist, EMS
UMassMemorial Paramedics—Worcester EMS
Worcester, Massachusetts

Stephen J. Rahm, NRP
Deputy Chief, Office of Clinical Direction
Co-Chair, Centre for Emergency Health Sciences
Bulverde Spring Branch Emergency Services
Spring Branch, Texas

Scotty Bolleter, BS, EMT-P
Chief, Office of Clinical Direction
Chair, Centre for Emergency Health Sciences
Bulverde Spring Branch Emergency Services
Spring Branch, Texas

Equipment

Jerry Flanagan
Account Manager
BoundTree Medical
Dublin, Ohio

Rachel Jackson, NREMT-P
Paramedic
UMass Memorial Paramedics—Worcester EMS
Worcester, Massachusetts

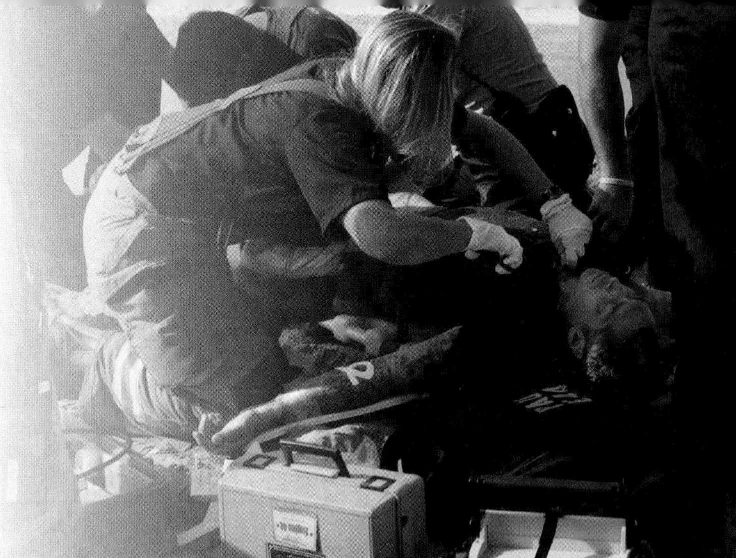

SECTION 1

Preparatory

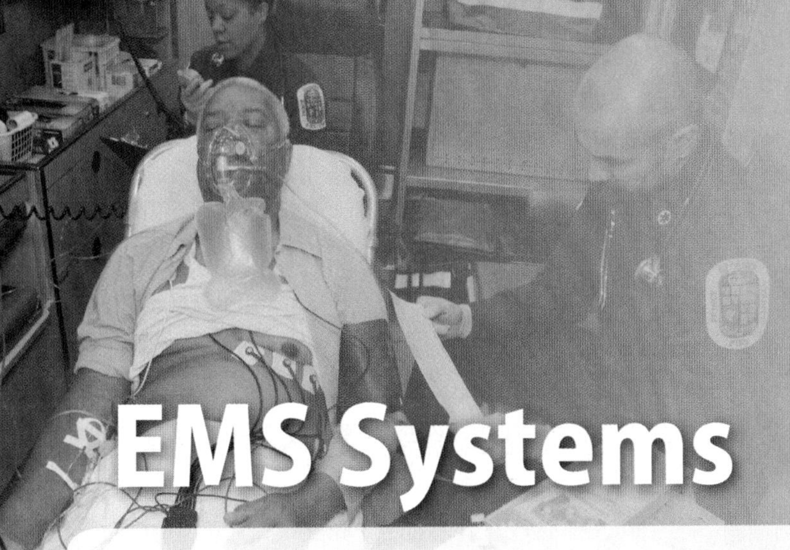

CHAPTER 1

EMS Systems

National EMS Education Standard Competencies

Preparatory

Integrates comprehensive knowledge of the EMS system, safety/well-being of the paramedic, and medical/legal and ethical issues which is intended to improve the health of EMS personnel, patients, and the community.

Emergency Medical Services (EMS) Systems

- EMS systems (p 4, 11-12)
- History of EMS (pp 4-9)
- Roles/responsibilities/professionalism of EMS personnel (pp 17-21)
- Quality improvement (p 22-24)
- Patient safety (pp 4, 9, 18-20, 22-23)

Research

- Impact of research on emergency medical responder (EMR) care (pp 24-25)
- Data collection (pp 25-27)
- Evidence-based decision making (pp 29-30)
- Research principles to interpret literature and advocate evidence-based practice (pp 28-30)

Knowledge Objectives

1. List key developments in the history of emergency medical services (EMS). (pp 4-9)
2. Discuss the processes of licensure and certification. (pp 9-10)
3. Define reciprocity, including its relevance to the practice of emergency medical care. (p 10)
4. List the five main types of services that provide emergency medical care. (pp 10-11)
5. Discuss the critical points, required components, and system elements of EMS. (pp 11-12)
6. Describe the levels of EMS education in terms of skill sets needed for each of the following: emergency medical responder, emergency medical technician, advanced emergency medical technician, and paramedic. (pp 12-13)
7. Discuss the role of the National Scope of Practice and the *National EMS Education Standards* as they relate to the levels of EMS education. (pp 13-14)
8. Discuss initial paramedic education and the importance of continuing education. (pp 13-14)
9. Describe various types of transports the paramedic may perform, including transports to specialty centers and interfacility transports. (pp 14-15)
10. Discuss the paramedic's role in working with other health care providers and public safety agencies. (pp 15-16)
11. Characterize the EMS system's role in prevention and public education in the community. (pp 16, 18, 20, 26)
12. Describe the attributes that a paramedic is expected to possess. (pp 17-18)
13. Describe the roles and responsibilities of the paramedic. (pp 19-21)
14. Discuss issues relating to the appropriate method of transport, as well as non-transport situations. (pp 20, 22)
15. Describe how medical direction of an EMS system works and the paramedic's role in the process. (pp 21-22)
16. Discuss the purpose of the EMS continuous quality improvement (CQI) process. (pp 22-24)
17. Discuss examples of how errors can be prevented when providing EMS care. (pp 23-24)
18. Discuss the importance of medical research and its role in refining EMS practices. (p 24)
19. List the types of research and subtypes within each category. (pp 26-27)
20. Discuss ethical considerations related to conducting medical research. (pp 27-28)
21. Define peer-reviewed literature and describe how this relates to a practicing paramedic. (p 29)
22. Discuss evidence-based medicine and how to incorporate this concept into everyday paramedic practice. (pp 29-30)

Skills Objectives

There are no skills objectives for this chapter.

Introduction

The **emergency medical services (EMS)** system is no longer considered to be in its infancy; nonetheless, it continues to evolve. When it was initially established, a responder was called to a location for people who were ill or injured and simply transported them rapidly to a medical facility; this was often called "load and go." As awareness of EMS capabilities grew, the need for improved systems in various, primarily rural, locations became evident. This awareness, along with research and guidelines from national organizations, has led to the advancement of EMS. As a paramedic, you will encounter many different situations. The most important thing to remember is your call is a true emergency in the eyes of the callers or patients, so do not judge them if you feel it is not. In reality, the majority of your calls will not entail true life threats, but they are to your patients **Figure 1-1**. The public's perception of you will often be compared with what is seen on television, read in published articles, and patients' previous experiences; it will also be based on your treatment of their loved ones. As you move forward in your education and career, always be ready for change as EMS continually evolves. Regardless of whether you will be a volunteer or serve with a paid career department, continued education is a must; some of what you learn today may not be applicable tomorrow. Whenever you are in uniform or representing your profession, whether on duty or off, treat all people you encounter with respect and dignity.

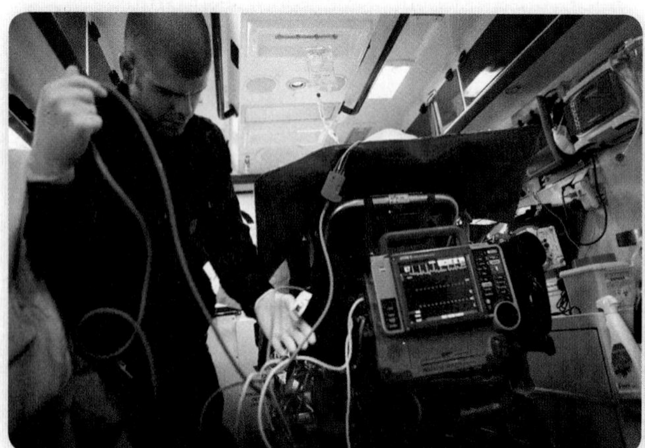

Figure 1-1 Today's prehospital care professionals are highly trained to provide a wide variety of emergency medical services to the public.

Patient Safety

Rescuer safety is extremely important, but so is the patient's safety! Why all this emphasis on patient safety? A patient's care process is very complex, with many separate components (prehospital care, emergency department providers, radiology, laboratory, transport, etc). These groups must coordinate their actions as part of the joint effort that makes up the patient's overall health care experience. In an ideal world, a patient moves seamlessly from the field through the various departments and from initial presentation to disposition. Of course, we do not live in such an ideal world, and the complexity of all this provides many opportunities for process failures, errors, and adverse outcomes.

EMS System Development

The History of EMS

Much of the prehospital emergency medical care you will deliver as a paramedic can be attributed directly or indirectly to the visionary advances of pioneers in the field including Drs. Peter Safar and Nancy Caroline. You will read more about them later in this chapter. If you research the history of EMS, you may be surprised to learn how long organized systems have been in place. For example, the first recorded use of an ambulance was by the military during the Siege of Málaga in 1487. This was strictly for

YOU are the Paramedic **PART 1**

At 1618 hours you are dispatched to the 300 block of Hunt Road for a report of a collision between a car and a motorcycle; you notify dispatch that you are en route. Three minutes later as you are nearing the crash scene, you notice a car parked diagonally across the road and a motorcycle lying on its side about 20 feet (6 m) farther up from the car. You note fluid leaking from underneath the car and it appears no one is inside the car. A crowd of bystanders is gathered at a driveway and you notice a man holding a motorcycle helmet. You think this may be the rider until the man steps to the side of the crowd and you see someone lying supine on the ground. You also note two women who are trying to talk to a young woman; she is screaming hysterically. No other public safety agencies have arrived on scene. You do not notice any hazards at this time.

As you exit the ambulance and approach the scene, you see there is damage to the right front fender and the passenger door of the car. The man holding the helmet turns and calls to you to hurry. He tells you he was driving the car and that he is fine, but the motorcycle rider is "hurt bad."

1. What is your first action as you are approaching the scene and conducting a scene size-up?
2. What role(s) does the emergency medical services system play in this call?

transport, and there was no documentation that any actual medical care was provided. It was during the 1800s when EMS started to make some headway with the following key developments:

- 1800–Baron Dominique-Jean Larrey, chief physician in Napoleon's army, is credited with establishing the first prehospital system for triaging and transporting patients.
- 1860 to 1870–Civilian ambulance services began in Cincinnati, Ohio in 1865 and in New York, New York in 1869. In New York City, ambulances (horse-drawn carriages) were dispatched by telegraph from Bellevue Hospital's Centre Street branch. In the first year alone, the ambulances responded to more than 1,800 calls for help throughout the city.

Words of Wisdom

Nancy Lee Caroline was born in a Boston suburb to Leo and Zelda Caroline in 1944. Nancy had a strong social conscience and devoted her life to medicine, teaching, and her patients—and she had a superb sense of humor. She has often been rightly called the "Mother of Paramedics" because of her dedication to paramedic education **Figure 1-2**. She died of multiple myeloma at age 58 in 2002.

Nancy's medical career began at the young age of 15 in the pathology laboratory of the famous Benjamin Castleman, MD, at Massachusetts General Hospital, where she conducted medical research long before she entered college. Nancy majored in linguistics at Radcliffe College, and received her MD degree from Case Western Reserve University in 1977. Thereafter, she took a fellowship in critical care medicine at the University of Pittsburgh. It was here that she began her groundbreaking work in paramedicine.

Around that time, the late Peter Safar, MD, was overseeing a US Department of Transportation grant to create a curriculum for paramedics. Dr. Safar offered Nancy an opportunity, as medical director of Freedom House Enterprises Ambulance Service, to train paramedics chosen from a group of African-American men who did not have a chance to complete their high school educations. Nancy was extremely successful—so successful that she was asked to write a curriculum for paramedic training, a curriculum that was published as the first edition of the textbook you are reading—*Emergency Care in the Streets.*

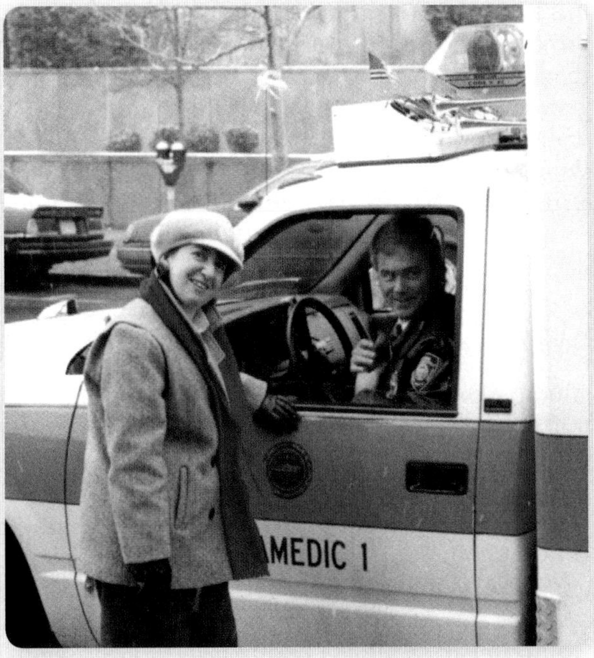

The list of Nancy's other accomplishments is long. She served as the first medical director of Israel's Red Cross society (Magen David Adom) where, in addition to training the first Israeli paramedics, she took extensive Hebrew lessons (it was a point of pride for her to develop a knowledge of the languages in whatever country she was working). After her tenure there ended in 1981, Nancy relocated to Nairobi, Kenya, to become Senior Medical Officer of the African Medical and Research Foundation (AMREF), the foundation that oversees the famous Flying Doctors service. When she became aware of the devastating famine that overtook Ethiopia in the early 1980s, Nancy became a consultant for the League of Red Cross Societies, writing a handbook on basic life support and running classes on first aid for African nations. Nancy worked with the Ethiopian Orthodox Church to provide better nourishment and health care to children in over 600 orphanages. In addition, Nancy served as director of medical programs for the American Jewish Joint Distribution Committee in Addis Ababa.

In 1987, she returned to Israel to serve as medical consultant for the Center for Educational Technology and for AMREF, developing training materials in emergency medicine and writing correspondence courses for rural health workers in Africa. She also served as an adjunct professor at the University of Pittsburgh's medical school, and, while volunteering in the Department of Oncology in Tel Hashomer, Nancy collaborated with Alexander Waller, MD, on the *Handbook of Palliative Care in Cancer.*

Nancy settled in Metula, Israel. She realized there was a need for special care in north Israel for people with advanced cancer. In 1995, she founded the Hospice of the Upper Galilee (HUG). In 2002, she married geneticist and molecular biologist Lazarus Astrachan.

Nancy left the world too soon, but unquestionably left the world a better place. Despite all her accomplishments, the compliment that meant the most to her was to be called the Mother of Paramedics. Nancy was, no doubt, the best mother paramedics could have.

Figure 1-2 Nancy L. Caroline with an ambulance from the Boston Department of Health and Hospitals.

Photo of Nancy L. Caroline provided in loving memory of her mother, Zelda Caroline.

- 1899–The first operated automobile-type ambulance came out of Michael Reese Hospital in Chicago, Illinois.

The 1900s continued to see the evolution of EMS with changes occurring between World Wars I and II. During this time, a major shift occurred; however, due to the lack of manpower resulting from the wars, many hospital-based ambulance services did not survive. Some key developments in EMS before 1950 included the following:

- 1926–Phoenix Fire Department added service similar to present-day EMS.
- 1928–Julian Stanley Wise launched the first rescue squad out of Roanoke, Virginia called Roanoke Life Saving and First Aid Crew. Soon after, numerous other rescue squad organizations were developed along the East Coast, primarily in New Jersey.
- 1940s–Because of a shortage of medical personnel, the role of EMS was turned over to fire and police departments. Unfortunately, there were no minimum training standards set. Also, the role of providing emergency medical care was not always immediately accepted or welcomed.

The 20th Century and Modern Technology

During World Wars I and II, battlefield corps—systems for field treatment and transport—continuously evolved as new techniques were learned that improved field care. In the 1950s and 1960s, EMS began to make major strides forward. During the 1950s and the Korean War, military medical researchers recognized that bringing hospital-type services closer to the field might give patients a better chance of survival. Helicopters were first used in 1951 during the Korean War. They brought patients to Mobile Army Surgical Hospitals (MASH units), which helped thousands of soldiers and civilians survive Figure 1-3. In 1956, Drs. James Elan and Safar developed mouth-to-mouth resuscitation. The first portable defibrillator was developed by Frank Pantridge in 1959.

In the late 1950s and early 1960s, however, the focus moved back to bringing the hospital to the patient in some European countries. **Mobile intensive care units (MICUs)** were developed and staffed by specially trained physicians. This concept quickly spread to the United States, but US physicians were in short supply, and physicians who were interested had minimal expertise outside of the hospital. Physicians were then asked, "Can a person who is not a physician be trained to perform advanced medical skills?" Many answered "Yes."

In 1965 the National Academy of Sciences and the National Research Council released "The White Paper" or *Accidental Death and Disability: The Neglected Disease of Modern Society*; the paper was subsequently published in 1966. Some of the findings in this paper include the following:

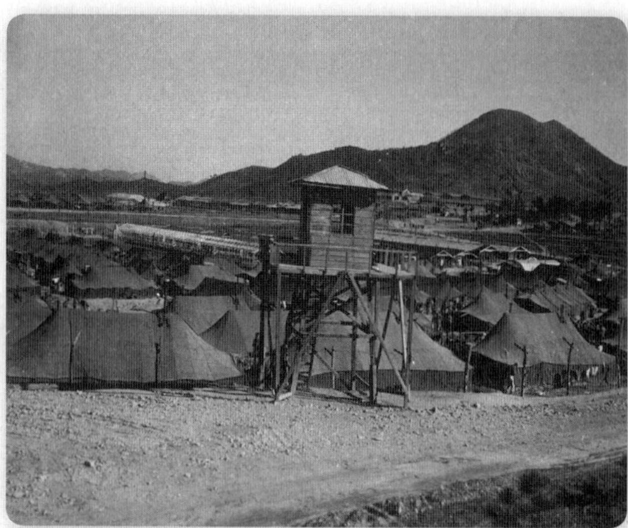

Figure 1-3 Temporary hospitals, such as this one in use during the Korean War, were set up to provide more rapid care for the injured.

- A lack of uniform laws and standards
- Ambulances and equipment were of poor quality or nonexistent
- Lack of communication between EMS and hospitals
- Lack of personnel training
- Hospitals only had part-time staff
- More people died in motor vehicle crashes than in the Vietnam war

Through these findings, The White Paper outlined 10 critical points to establish a functioning system. As a result, the National Highway Safety Act of 1966 was enacted. In this act, the US Department of Transportation (US DOT) was created to provide authority and financial support for the development of basic and advanced life support programs. In 1968, the Task Force of the Committee of EMS drafted basic training standards, and the principles of a 9-1-1 system to provide universal access to emergency services were created. Table 1-1 lists the critical points, required components, and system elements of EMS that ultimately developed as a result of publication of The White Paper.

In 1969, a year after basic training standards were developed, Dr. Eugene Nagel, then of Miami, Florida, began training firefighters from the Miami Fire Department with advanced emergency medical skills, thus creating the first true paramedic program Figure 1-4. Dr. Nagel took the use of advanced emergency medical treatment one step further. He developed a telemetry system that enabled firefighters to transmit a patient's electrocardiogram (ECG) to physicians at Jackson Memorial Hospital and to receive radio instructions from the physicians regarding what measures to take. Dr. Nagel is often called the "Father of Paramedicine." Additionally in 1969, standards for ambulance design and equipment were published.

During the 1970s, advancements in EMS continued, helicopters became more available, and the National Registry of Emergency Medical Technicians (NREMT) began.

The first EMT textbook, *Emergency Care and Transportation of the Sick and Injured*, was published by the American Academy of Orthopaedic Surgeons (AAOS) in 1971. In that same year, the AAOS began training EMTs nationwide through a national workshop. In the following year, the first television series focused on EMS, *Emergency!*, started a very successful 8-year run. The lead characters, John Gage and Roy DeSoto, became household names. Many EMS providers still reflect on this series because of its realistic depiction of modern day EMS. In 1973, the Emergency Medical Services Systems Act defined 15 required components of an EMS system, listed in Table 1-1, with emphasis on regional development and trauma care. The act provided a structure and uniformity to the EMS system that came out of pioneering programs in Miami, Seattle, Pittsburgh, and the Illinois Trauma System (Dr. David Boyd).

Table 1-1 Critical Points, Required Components, and System Elements of EMS

Year	Source	Item
1966	*Accidental Death and Disability: The Neglected Disease of Modern Society* (The White Paper)	Critical points for establishing a functioning EMS system: **1.** Develop collaborative strategies to identify and address community health and safety issues. **2.** Align the financial incentives of EMS and other health care providers and payers. **3.** Participate in community-based prevention efforts. **4.** Develop and pursue a national EMS research agenda. **5.** Pass EMS legislation in each state to support innovation and integration. **6.** Allocate adequate resources for medical direction. **7.** Develop information systems that link EMS across its continuum. **8.** Determine the costs and benefits of EMS to the community. **9.** Designate a single nationwide emergency telephone number. **10.** Ensure all calls for emergency help are automatically accompanied by location-identifying information.
1973	The Emergency Medical Services Systems Act	Required components of an EMS system: **1.** Integration of health services **2.** EMS research **3.** Legislation and regulation **4.** System finance **5.** Human resources **6.** Medical direction **7.** Education and training systems **8.** Public access and education **9.** Prevention **10.** Transportation **11.** Communication systems **12.** Clinical care facilities **13.** Patient information and education systems **14.** Mutual aid agreements **15.** Evaluation
1988	The National Highway Traffic and Safety Administration	NHTSA's essential EMS elements: **1.** Regulation and policy **2.** Resource management **3.** Human resources and training **4.** Transportation **5.** Facilities **6.** Communication **7.** Public information and education **8.** Medical direction **9.** Trauma systems **10.** Evaluation

(continued)

Table 1-1 Critical Points, Required Components, and System Elements of EMS *(Continued)*

Year	Source	Item
1996	The National Highway Traffic and Safety Administration	System attributes from the *EMS Agenda for the Future*: **1.** Integration of health services **2.** EMS research **3.** Legislation and regulation **4.** System finance **5.** Human resources **6.** Medical direction **7.** Education systems **8.** Public education **9.** Prevention **10.** Public access **11.** Communication systems **12.** Clinical care **13.** Information systems **14.** Evaluation

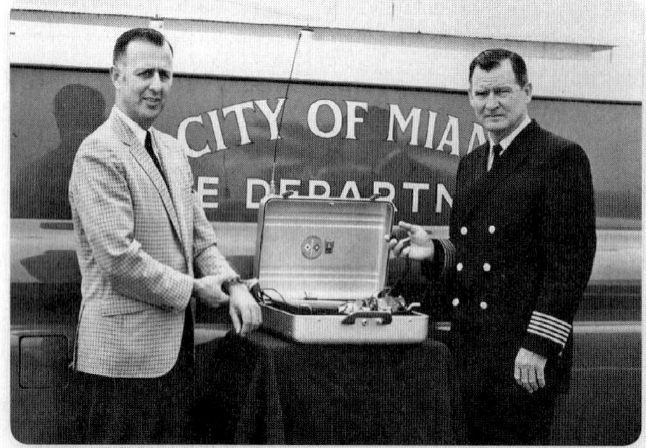

Figure 1-4 Dr. Eugene Nagel, widely considered the Father of Paramedicine, provided much-needed leadership to the developing field of EMS training. Here he is shown (at left) in 1967 with Chief Larry Kenney of the Miami Fire Department, with the first telemetry package to be used by paramedics.

In 1974, after a federal report disclosed that less than half of ambulance personnel completed sufficient training, guidelines were published for the development and implementation of EMS systems. In 1975, the American Medical Association recognized emergency medicine as its own specialty branch within medicine. Many cities set up individual advanced EMS training, and regions added their own spin to what they thought was the essential standard of care, but it was not until 1977 that the first National Standard Curriculum for paramedics was developed by the US DOT. This first paramedic curriculum was based on the work of Dr. Nancy Caroline.

Through the 1980s and 1990s, changes continued in EMS and the number of trained personnel grew significantly. The National Highway Traffic Safety Administration (NHTSA) developed 10 system elements, listed in Table 1-1, in an effort to sustain EMS systems. Unfortunately, federal funding and staff were reduced, and the responsibility for EMS was transferred to the states. Although it was made clear that the federal funding being provided was just "seed money" and that long-term local funding strategies needed to be developed, many states apparently believed the federal dollars would not go away. Unfortunately, they did and to this day, funding is still a major roadblock for local governments as well as states.

Several other major legislative initiatives also came about during this time, such as the Emergency Medical Services for Children (EMSC) program grant funding that was implemented in 1985.[1] In 1986, an amendment was made to the Public Safety Officers' Benefits Program in which families of firefighters, members of a rescue squad, and members of an ambulance crew were compensated if the provider was killed in the line of duty. As progress continued into the 1990s, **trauma systems** started making headway. Some of these secondary programs received federal funding, but in present day they are still struggling to prove necessity and maintain this funding. Their expertise is vital to further advancement in EMS, but some of the advancements are held back because of this lack of funding.

EMS continues to evolve and change in the 21st century. Numerous initiatives are appearing, such as EMS Compass. This organization measures performance in EMS. The goal of tracking performance is to help identify best care practices and eventually help establish performance benchmarks throughout the country.[2] The idea that EMS training can be used in many other areas of health care instead of strictly in an ambulance is also being recognized. Paramedics are being used in hospital emergency departments, health care clinics, and physicians' offices. Community paramedicine, a health care model in which experienced paramedics receive advanced training to

Patient Safety

Each hospital and emergency medical services system manages its safety culture locally; they choose the programs to implement to manage safety concerns. A **safety culture** has several key features:

- Acknowledges organizations that engage in high-risk activities and determines the importance of consistent safe operations to counteract these risks
- Supports a blame-free environment where errors can be reported without fear of punishment
- Maintains organizational commitment to address reported errors and safety concerns

An organization's safety culture can be measured using validated surveys given to providers, such as the Patient Safety Culture Survey and the Safety Attitudes Questionnaire developed by the Agency for Healthcare Research and Quality (AHRQ). These surveys ask providers to rate the safety culture of their workplace and the organization in its entirety. The AHRQ provides yearly updates benchmarking data from the hospital survey. Specific activities, such as teamwork training, executive walk-rounds, and established safety teams, have been associated with some improvements in safety culture measurements but are not yet linked to lower error rates.

provide additional services in the prehospital environment, is becoming a reality, and you will see continuing strides in this area. You will learn more about this later in Chapter 53, *Career Development*. It is important to note that these additional capabilities are not being developed to replace current health care modalities, but rather to utilize the capabilities of paramedics in areas not served previously, for example, assisting a home health nurse.

Licensure, Certification, and Registration

Throughout this section, we may refer to licensure and/or registration uniformly. Depending on your state or location, you may be licensed or you may be registered. **Registration** means that records of your education, state, or local licensure, and recertification will be held by a recognized board of registration. **Licensure** is how states control who is allowed to practice as a health care provider. Once you complete your initial paramedic education, depending on your state, you will be eligible to take your state's certification examination. Some states require you to test and establish licensure through a registry system such as the National Registry of EMTs (NREMT). A **certification** examination is used to ensure health care providers have at least the same basic level of knowledge and skill. Once you have passed the required examinations, your state and/or NREMT will give you a certificate or license. Different states refer to the authority granted to you to function as

YOU are the Paramedic PART 2

As you acquire a general impression of the patient, you observe he is a young man and appears to be unresponsive. It appears he was not wearing any protective clothing and some of the bystanders tell you they took off his helmet "so he could breathe." You note that your patient is breathing, but his breaths are very shallow and he has some minor bleeding from an obvious fracture of his left lower leg. Before you reach the patient, the hysterical woman runs to you and begs you to hurry up and do something because her "boyfriend is dying!" She does not think you are moving fast enough. The two women try again to console her, but she is frantic. You have been told she was not involved in the crash.

Recording Time: 1 Minute	
Appearance	Pale, not moving, obvious deformity of left lower leg
Level of consciousness	Unresponsive to all stimuli
Airway	Patent
Breathing	Rapid and shallow, with what appears an asymmetrical pattern
Circulation	Rapid and weak radial pulses

3. What aspects of professionalism must be employed in this situation?
4. Aside from those noted in the previous question, what other roles and responsibilities are vital as a prehospital health care professional?

a paramedic as licensure, certification, or credentialing. For the purposes of this text, *licensure* will be used. It is unlawful to perform the functions of a paramedic prior to licensure, or to be more specific, it is considered practicing medicine without a license unless you are directly supervised by a paramedic program internship preceptor as a part of your training program. Although holding a license shows you have successfully completed the education and testing requirements to achieve such a license, it does not mean that you can perform as a paramedic without or outside the supervision of your service's physician medical director. Agencies (state, local, and national) still require that paramedics receive **medical direction** (both online and off-line). The concept and principles of medical control will be discussed later in the chapter.

If your state requires you to pass the NREMT cognitive and psychomotor examinations to become licensed, you will have to pass a written exam as well as numerous practical skills. To be eligible, first you must successfully complete initial paramedic education through an accredited program. Your school is required to verify your course completion before you can sit for the exam. The National Registry exam tests to the Paramedic Psychomotor Competency Portfolio, a comprehensive collection of skills and scenarios crucial to paramedic practice. Detailed information on the examination requirements can be found at the NREMT website, nremt.org.

The Committee on Accreditation of Educational Programs for the EMS Professions (CoAEMSP) is the only accrediting body for paramedic programs to date. The mission of the CoAEMSP is to continuously improve the quality of EMS education through accreditation and recognition services for the full range of EMS professions. Because of changes to the National Scope of Practice, the need to expand the professional image of EMS, and the desire to establish consistent guidelines for paramedicine, the number of accredited paramedic training facilities will grow significantly over the next few years.

Reciprocity

Each state has different licensing or certification requirements and procedures regardless of whether they follow the National Scope of Practice model. Granting certification to a provider from another state or agency is known as **reciprocity**. If you are planning to relocate to another state or country, investigate the licensure process beforehand. Keep in mind, many other countries will not accept the training provided in the United States and reciprocity will not be automatically accepted. Many states recognize National Registry certification as part of their reciprocity process. In many cases, as a paramedic, you will be required to hold current state licensure, to be in good standing, and to have National Registry certification. Some states will still require you to challenge their requirements; in other words, you may still be required to go through that state's written and/or practical evaluations prior to reciprocity being granted. Others may request your education transcript and continuing education hours. You will also likely be required to provide information for a criminal background check. Because you will be an integral part of the health care system, most states want to ensure you do not have previous issues that could call into question your integrity or professionalism. Finally, some states will require a fee to process your reciprocity application and provide a license.

Traditional EMS Employment

Once you become a licensed paramedic, you will have a variety of different career options available to you. Although, in general, your scope of practice will remain the same, there may be slight modifications of what will be expected of you. Working hours can vary greatly from 24-hour to 12-hour to 8-hour shifts, or any number of schedule shifts. Some career possibilities include the following:

- **Fire-based EMS.** In general, most EMS that are integrated into a fire department are paid and operated by the municipal government. Depending on your state, this may not always be the case. Some locations operate fully with non-paid volunteers, while others use providers who are paid per call; they do not receive compensation until a call comes in. EMS may have a separate management system within these organizations and operate independently from the fire side of the organization. Due to the numerous expectations of both areas, depending on the specific situation in any one agency, separate management systems of operations may or may not be valuable. If there is separate management, the managers often still report to a main chief or director to ensure consistency in department operations. Fire and EMS personnel may respond together to major incidents when additional manpower is required; you may have a dual role working with both fire and EMS providers. There has been an increase in fire-based EMS roles, since, due to the incidence of fires being low thanks to prevention efforts, fire departments can better justify keeping a staffed in-house department if they add EMS.
- **Third-service EMS (municipalities) (single and shared).** Depending on financial capability, some municipalities establish and operate their own ambulance services independent of fire, police, and other public safety entities. In some cases, independent ambulance agencies offer their services under contract to municipalities who can't afford their own services. Some states allow multiple municipalities to share services under agreements with each being an equal owner. These shared services reduce the cost to all, which allows them to cover the cost of providing paramedic service. Normally, third-service systems function completely

independent of fire service; therefore, if you need fire or rescue assistance, you may need to request response; they may not be sent automatically. This works both ways. The fire department may need to request EMS response for medical support, unless the agencies have established a prearranged response process.

- **Private EMS agency (both for profit and nonprofit).** In general, private services operate similarly to third-service EMS agencies. The major difference is they contract their services to municipalities. The contract can include anything from managing an existing service to providing full service to the communities. Operations of private service vary greatly. Some follow standard 24-hour shift practices, while others follow a "status systems management" structure. What this means is providers report to a central location at the beginning of the shift, pick up an ambulance, and are sent to a staging area within the service area. The location of the staging area is often established depending on past requests for service. Although in most cases, this functions well, since emergencies cannot be predicted, there is the potential that a serious call may have to wait a significant length of time for a unit to arrive.
- **Hospital-based EMS.** These services can vary greatly, but, in most cases, hospital-based services tend to offer interfacility-type transports, as well as aeromedical services, which are offered in larger and remote organizations. Some hospitals also offer 9-1-1 response and paramedic intercept service in some locations. Often times, as a paramedic working in a hospital-based system, you will be required to assist with patient care in other areas of the hospital during your down time. Typically you will function in an emergency department (ED), but you may be part of an internal emergency response team. One benefit of being part of a hospital-based team is the access to information you have from various medical providers, especially in complex cases.
- **Hybrid or other.** As paramedicine continues to grow, so will the various expectations and jobs you may encounter. Many large companies, such as oil drilling platforms and factories with hundreds or thousands of employees, have their own medical response and care facilities. In some areas, paramedics work in conjunction with primary care providers, physician assistants, and nurse practitioners. There are numerous companies whose business is to hire personnel to fill medical positions at specific locations, such as national parks, amusement parks, and other venues. Regardless of where you work as a paramedic, keep your training and skills current to ensure you are ready at all times.

The EMS System

Today's EMS system is a complex network of coordinated services providing various levels of care to a community. These services work in unison to meet both the growing and standing needs of the citizens in the community in which they reside. As a paramedic, you are part of this network; therefore, you must stay active in your community to be able to meet the ever-changing needs.

The EMS network begins with citizen involvement in the complex EMS system. In most cases, the public does not understand EMS and knows only what is seen in newspapers, television, and movies. Be prepared; they may consider the inappropriate behaviors of actors on EMS TV series to be a reflection of reality; you will also have the task to educate them on the truth. They may need to be taught what is an emergency and what is not, how to activate the EMS system, and how basic care can be provided before EMS arrives. Remember, the public usually does not have medical training or knowledge and in their eyes a simple cut may be an emergency.

When you are called to a "sick person" at 0200 hours who has only a common cold and cannot sleep, you must avoid becoming angry with the patient, your career, or your EMS system. You will find in your education there are many general symptoms that could cause you to overlook a serious problem. Be compassionate and caring with your patient; this will build the patient's trust of both you and the EMS system. Factors that play a role in determining the outcome or likelihood of your patient's survival include the following:

- Bystander care
- Dispatch (including prearrival directions)
- Response (both mode and distance)
- Prehospital assessment and care provided (level of EMS-trained personnel)
- Transportation (ground ambulances, critical care units, air transport)
- Emergency department care (on-duty trained emergency physicians and staff)
- Definitive care (including trauma, pediatric, and neurologic specialists)
- Rehabilitation

When the members of the public activate the EMS system, their first contact is usually a dispatcher. Requirements for dispatcher training vary greatly from state to state, and oftentimes dispatchers have to cover police and fire communications as well as all general department phone calls. Dispatchers must interpret the caller's needs to determine if it is an emergency by extracting appropriate information, and then decide what resources need to be sent. Scene findings do not always exactly reflect the information received by dispatch and relayed to you. You must remember that dispatch is only able to provide you the information that the caller provides to them; never under- or overestimate that information or get angry with dispatch if their information is completely different from what you encounter on scene.

Words of Wisdom

A patient may experience only once what you as a paramedic may experience hundreds of times. Understand the patient's anxiety and lack of knowledge.

Being active in your community keeps you on top of the best local resources and enables you to answer questions regarding your patient care plan. Ask yourself, "Does the receiving facility have the resources needed for this patient?" If the answer is no, your next question may be, "Is there an appropriate facility within a reasonable distance?" And, of course, remember, in some regions competent adult patients may be able to request the facility to which they wish to be transported. However, if it is different from the facility you feel would be most appropriate, this is the time once again for you to educate your patient but not to argue. If ultimately you cannot talk the patient into going to the facility you feel is best, consider assistance from online (direct) medical control. If that fails, document the patient's choice and your efforts to educate on your prehospital care report.

Special Populations

EMS systems must be capable of handling many different situations including obstetric, pediatric, and geriatric emergencies. Proper procedures, drug dosages, and even assessment techniques may vary depending on the age, gender, or even race of the patient.

Levels of Education

Licensure of EMS personnel is usually a state function, subject to the laws and regulations of the state in which the EMS provider practices. For this reason, there are variations from state to state in the scope of practice and in education and relicensure requirements. The following information explains how the system is supposed to work from the federal level to the local level.

At the federal level, NHTSA brought in experts from around the country to create the *National EMS Scope of Practice Model*. This document provides overarching guidelines as to what skills each level of EMS provider should be able to accomplish. The next step is the state level. Because licensure is usually a state function, laws and regulations are enacted to specify how EMS providers will operate. These laws are then executed by the state EMS administrative offices, which control licensure. Many states have a set of statutes or rules to be followed as well as a scope of practice for every EMS level. Finally, the service's, local, or regional medical director normally develops a set of patient care guidelines that outline the approved skills and treatments for each level. For example, the medications that will be carried on your ambulance or where patients are transported are day-to-day operational concerns in which the medical director may have direct input. Keep in mind, every state varies on the role of the medical director, so ensure you understand and follow your state's processes.

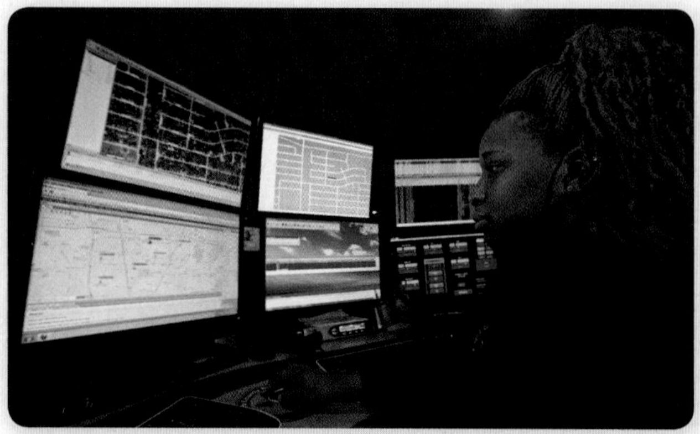

Figure 1-5 The dispatcher coordinates the entire rescue effort. He or she interprets a caller's information and then sends appropriate personnel and resources to the scene.

The national guidelines are intended to create more consistent delivery of EMS across the country. The medical director can limit the scope of practice but cannot expand it beyond state law. Expanding the scope of practice requires state approval.

In 2009, the National Standard Curricula for all levels of EMS providers were revised to a new format and renamed the *National EMS Education Standards*. In the United States, NHTSA is the federal administrative source for these standards and related documents. The *National EMS Education Standards* for the four levels of EMS providers can be downloaded from the NHTSA website at ems.gov.

▶ The Dispatcher

The dispatcher plays a key role in an EMS call. He or she receives and enters all information on the call, interprets the information, and in turn, relays it to the appropriate resources Figure 1-5. In some locations, the dispatcher may be trained as an emergency medical dispatcher. This person will have the added task of giving simple prearrival instructions (ie, cardiopulmonary resuscitation [CPR], bleeding control) after asking a series of call-related questions from the caller in hopes that this care may benefit the patient until you arrive on scene.

▶ Emergency Medical Responder

Until recently, this level was known as the "first responder." Not all states have this as a certification and/or licensing level, and for those states that do, there can be considerable variability in requirements and allowed skills. In the generic use of the term, an emergency medical responder (EMR) is usually a person trained in CPR and/or first aid. In some states, EMRs can function only as part of an organized group and that group must be affiliated with a transporting ambulance service. As a paramedic, you will

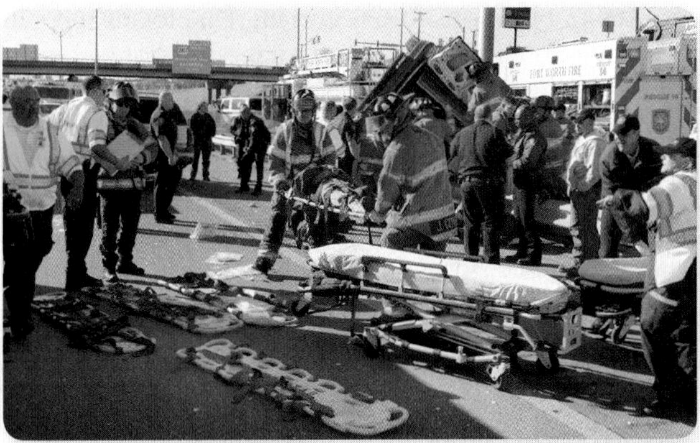

Figure 1-6 The emergency medical responder is critical for providing the initial emergency patient care, particularly when medical personnel must travel long distances to a scene.

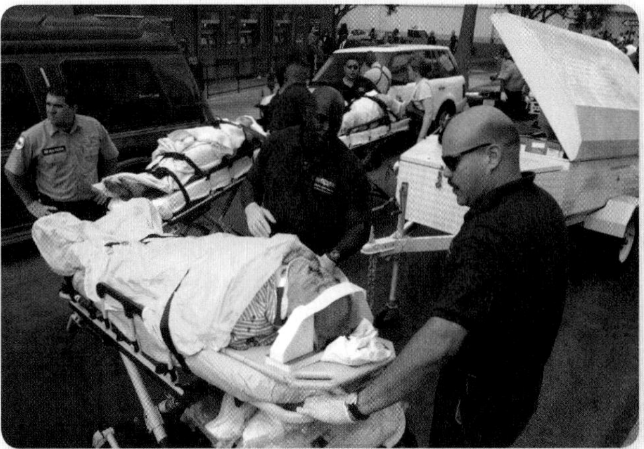

Figure 1-7 Emergency medical technicians constitute the majority of EMS providers.

need to familiarize yourself with the level of training of the EMRs in your system.

From an EMS point of view, an EMR has completed a course that covers the *National EMS Education Standards* for the EMR level. This training will help the EMR recognize the seriousness of a patient's condition, administer appropriate basic care, and relay information to the paramedic. EMRs are an essential level of provider to the EMS system, especially in rural areas **Figure 1-6**.

EMT

Historically called the EMT-Basic (EMT-B), the EMT is the backbone and primary provider level in many EMS systems. This is also the level of certification required before being able to enter a paramedic education program. Much lifesaving care is provided at this level.

Skills and treatments vary from state to state. EMTs may be trained in advanced airway intervention, limited medication administration, and intravenous (IV) fluid therapy; however, EMTs with this expanded scope of practice are not recognized at a different certification level per the *National EMS Education Standards*. In EMS, there are more providers trained and certified at the EMT level than at any other level **Figure 1-7**.

Advanced EMT

The level formerly called EMT-Intermediate (EMT-I) has gone through numerous changes over the years. It was initially developed in 1985 and was known as the EMT-I 85 level. The skill level for the EMT-I saw a significant change in 1999, when a major revision of the 1985 curriculum took place. More recently, changes made within the National Scope of Practice have eliminated the intermediate level, and it has been replaced with the Advanced EMT (AEMT) level in most states. AEMTs are trained in more advanced pathophysiology, as well as some advanced procedures such as establishing IV access, administering IV fluids, performing blood glucose monitoring, administering several medications, and performing some advanced airway management.

Controversies

Some argue all that is needed in an urban setting are AEMTs rather than paramedics, whereas others argue AEMTs perform ALS skills without having adequate academic preparation and should be phased out. The jury is still out on whether this particular level of training will become an attractive option for jurisdictions and EMS providers.

Paramedic

Currently, paramedic is the highest EMS skill level you can be certified or licensed at the national level. In 1998, the US DOT paramedic curriculum underwent major revisions and the level of training and skills increased greatly. In 2009, when the *National EMS Education Standards* were completed, the skills allowed at the paramedic level changed to some extent. Starting in 2013, to test through NREMT, a paramedic student must have attended and successfully completed training at an accredited institution. States that do not employ NREMT as their testing mechanism may not require institutions to be accredited. Although you may hold a license or certification independently, states require paramedics to function directly under the guidance of a licensed physician and to be affiliated with a paramedic-level service. In some states, paramedics are allowed to complete further education and earn the title of critical care paramedic. This varies widely from state to state, so research your state's laws to see if this is allowed.

Paramedic Education

Initial Education

Education may vary from state to state, but for the most part all states base their paramedic education programs on the *National EMS Education Standards* for the paramedic. As mentioned, significant changes were made to these standards, formerly called curricula, in 2009. A major recommendation was the inclusion of a college-level anatomy and physiology course. Some training institutions offer this as part of a paramedic training program; others require it as a prerequisite. The *National EMS Education Standards* outline the minimum of what a paramedic must know to practice. States require varying hours of education, but the national average falls between 1,000 and 1,500 hours of combined classroom, clinical, and field education. Some leaders want to structure education so the paramedic designation is achieved through an associate or bachelor's degree accredited program. A distinct benefit of this is it can give paramedics credits that could be used in achieving higher-level college degrees.

Words of Wisdom

The number of calls you go on is not the deciding factor on how much more education you need.

▶ Continuing Education

Most states require paramedics to complete a certain number of continuing education hours and/or a refresher program. Such programs keep you up-to-date on new research findings, new techniques, and skills, and help prevent degradation of those skills used less frequently **Figure 1-8**. Continuing education can also showcase current issues in your state that impact you and your system's ability to provide quality emergency medical care. Continuing education can be enjoyable, and it should be. Whenever possible, you should attend conferences and seminars, ideally, with some of them being out of your region and/or state, which helps broaden your knowledge base and EMS network. Consider attending conferences that may not be designed for paramedics, such as those targeted at nurses or physicians. Read EMS journals and research publications to stay current. Due to advances in technology, Internet-based continuing education resources have expanded greatly; however, ensure these programs meet your state or national requirements. When you seek continuing education options, consider those organizations that have made the effort to become accredited through the **Commission on Accreditation for Pre-Hospital Continuing Education (CAPCE)**, formerly called the Continuing Education Coordinating Board for EMS (CECBEMS). This organization develops continuing education standards and is involved in setting accreditation standards for prehospital providers.[3]

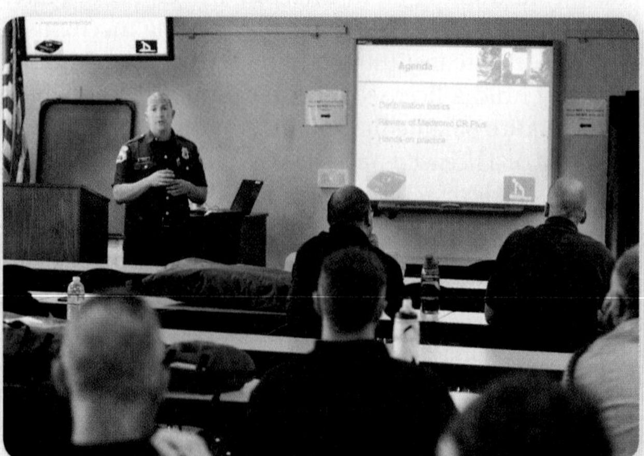

Figure 1-8 Continuing education can keep you up-to-date on technologic improvements that are continually made available to paramedics.

Get everyone in your service involved in postrun critiques—they can be beneficial in identifying problem areas in your practice. Postrun critiques are considered to be a form of continuing education in some states.

No matter what requirements are mandated by your state licensing agency, responsibility for continuing medical education ultimately rests with you. You know which areas of your knowledge have diminished and which skills require additional refresher efforts. You are the only person who will have to live with the questions and doubts that inevitably arise after something goes wrong in the field. If something does go wrong, after the call is not the time to realize you should have done something different or attended extra training. Continuing medical education is a way to help ensure you are following the latest best practices and will build confidence in your skills.

Additional Types of Transports

▶ Transport to Specialty Centers

In addition to hospital emergency departments, many EMS systems include specialty centers that focus on specific types of care (such as trauma, burns, poisoning, and cardiac or psychiatric conditions) or specific types of patients (for example, children). Specialty centers normally have in-house specialists, while other facilities must page operating teams, surgeons, or other specialists from outside the hospital. Typically, only a few hospitals in a region are designated as specialty centers. Transport time to a specialty center may be slightly longer than the time to an emergency department, but patients will receive definitive care more quickly at a specialty center.

Know the location of the centers in your area and when you should transport the patient directly to one. Sometimes, air medical transport will be necessary. Local, regional, and state protocols may guide your decision in these instances.

▶ Interfacility Transports

Many EMS agencies provide interfacility transportation for nonambulatory patients or patients with acute and chronic medical conditions requiring medical monitoring. This transportation may include transferring patients to and from hospitals, skilled nursing facilities, board and care homes, or even their home residence.

During ambulance transportation, the health and well-being of the patient is your responsibility. If medical control is required during transport, it comes from the transporting facility until you arrive at the receiving facility and hand off care with a report. Obtain the patient's medical history, chief complaint, and latest vital signs and provide ongoing patient assessment. In certain rare circumstances, a nurse, physician, respiratory therapist, or other medical team will accompany you with the patient, especially when the patient requires care that extends beyond your scope of practice.

Working With Other Professionals

▶ Working With Hospital Staff

Become familiar with the receiving hospitals you will transport to, the functions of staff members, and their normal operating procedures in all areas of the hospital, especially the emergency department. Also, learn about advances in emergency medical care and how to interact with hospital personnel. This experience will help you to understand how your care influences a patient's recovery and will emphasize the importance and benefits of proper prehospital care. It will also show you the consequences of delay, inadequate care, or poor judgment. You are an integral part of a patient's care plan; therefore, interact professionally with all hospital personnel who will be part of your patient's care. Never ridicule or undermine any member of the hospital staff. Always remember that the care a patient receives in the hospital may differ from what you do in the field.

Physicians are not likely to be in the field with you to provide personal, on-the-spot instructions. However, you may consult with appropriate medical staff by using the radio through established (online) medical control procedures. A physician or nurse may serve as an instructor for medical subjects in your education program. Through these experiences, you will become more comfortable using medical terms, interpreting patient signs and symptoms, and developing patient management skills.

YOU are the Paramedic PART 3

An initial assessment reveals that the patient is unresponsive and the only visible injury is the patient's leg. You note damage to the left side of the helmet. While your partner is gathering immobilization equipment, fire department rescue personnel arrive and you ask one of them to talk with the girlfriend and find out as much information about the patient as possible.

Further assessment reveals diminished breath sounds on the left side and distended neck veins. His radial pulses are weakening and increasing in rate. Your partner inserts an oral airway and begins ventilating the patient with a bag-mask device and 100% oxygen while rescue personnel assist you in packaging the patient on the long backboard. His left leg is secured to his right leg and bleeding is controlled with direct pressure and a dressing. He is loaded into the ambulance and you quickly obtain vital signs. The rescuer who was talking to the girlfriend tells you the patient is 22 years old, has no medical history, and takes no medications. The girlfriend does not think he is allergic to anything. He has a blood glucose level of 102 mg/dL and you note asymmetric movement of his left chest. The cardiac monitor shows a sinus tachycardia without ectopy.

Your partner tells you it is becoming difficult to ventilate the patient. On the basis of your findings, you recognize that the patient may have a tension pneumothorax. The only definitive treatment is a needle thoracostomy (decompression). Even though you have had training for performing this procedure, your standing orders do not allow it.

Recording Time: 6 Minutes	
Respirations	12 breaths/min assisted with ventilations
Pulse	138 beats/min, weak radials
Skin	Pale, cool, diaphoretic
Blood pressure	96/54 mm Hg
Oxygen saturation (Spo_2)	92% with ventilations by a bag-mask device and 100% oxygen
Pupils	Equal but sluggish to react

5. Even though you do not have standing orders to perform a needle decompression, you know this is what the patient needs. How will you handle getting approval to perform this procedure?

6. How will you make the determination of how and where to transport this patient?

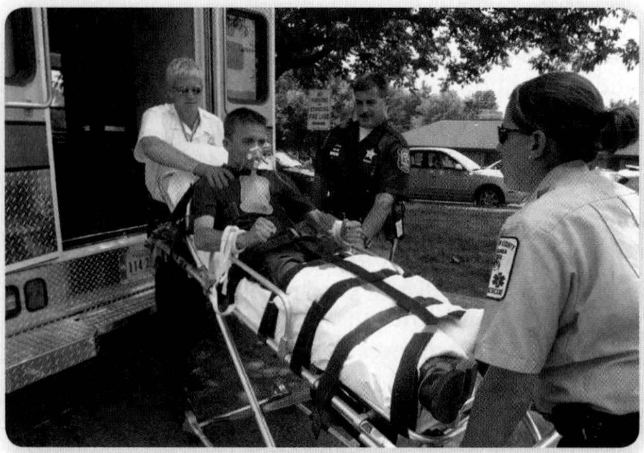

Figure 1-9 You will work with law enforcement personnel when dealing with violent patients.

▶ Working With Public Safety Agencies

Some public safety personnel have EMS training. Become familiar with the roles and responsibilities of these workers. Personnel from certain agencies are better prepared than you are to perform certain functions. For example, employees of a utility company are better equipped to control downed power lines than are you or your partner. Law enforcement personnel are better able to handle violent scenes and traffic control, while you and your partner are better able to provide emergency medical care Figure 1-9. If you work together, recognizing that each person has special training and a job to do at the scene, effective scene and patient management will prevail. Remember, the best, most efficient patient care is achieved through cooperation among agencies.

▶ Continuity of Care

In addition to responding to EMS calls, taking care of the patient, transporting, and returning to service, EMS providers have responsibilities to the community. The community has expectations of EMS providers and, as health care providers and public servants, you must project confidence to the community you serve. As previously mentioned, the general public usually has no idea what EMS truly does, so this is your ultimate opportunity to educate them.

Whether you are working in the public or private sector, encourage people in the community to become involved in your service to some level. Present-day medicine focuses on prevention—getting involved in community efforts is your opportunity to use your medical expertise to help the people you serve. For example, review the types of calls you respond to most commonly. Then, use this information to develop a variety of prevention strategies or activities within your community to reduce those types of calls. For example, perhaps your community has many calls relating to accidental falls. There are training programs available to help identify possible causes of falls known as "fall prevention programs." You can visit homes in your community to offer suggestions for prevention.

As a new paramedic, you will be considered part of the health care and emergency services community. You will work side by side with other professionals and groups. For example, you will integrate your work with other medical professionals, law enforcement, emergency management and disaster services, home health groups, such as hospice, and of course emergency responders. It is vital that you understand your role as well as the roles of those with whom you interact to ensure calls run as smoothly as possible. You must also be prepared for any number of situations, and establish expectations for each role.

Words of Wisdom

The best paramedics will continually seek out education and refresh their basic life support skills as well as advanced life support skills.

National EMS Group Involvement

Many national and state organizations exist, and many invite paramedic membership. These organizations have an impact on the future direction of EMS, so it is very important for you to identify and become involved in them. You will also have access to many valuable resources to help you develop yourself and your service area and to improve your problem-solving skills. One of the common goals of many national and state organizations is to promote uniformity of EMS standards and practices. Some of these organizations are listed in Table 1-2.

Table 1-2 National EMS Organizations

- National Highway Traffic Safety Administration (NHTSA)
- National Association of Emergency Medical Service Physicians (NAEMSP)
- National Association of State EMS Officials (NAEMSO)
- National Association of EMS Educators (NAEMSE)
- National Registry of EMTs (NREMT)
- National Association of EMTs (NAEMT)
- Emergency Medical Services for Children (EMSC)
- American College of Emergency Physicians (ACEP)
- American Ambulance Association (AAA)
- Committee on Accreditation of Educational Programs for the Emergency Medical Services Professions (CoAEMSP)
- International Association of Flight and Critical Care Paramedics (IAFCCP)

Evidence-Based Medicine

Evidence-based research can be found in the following publications: *Journal of Trauma and Acute Care Surgery, New England Journal of Medicine, Journal of the American Medical Association, Prehospital Emergency Care, Circulation,* and the *Annals of Emergency Medicine.*

Professionalism

During your paramedic education, you will learn a vast amount of information designed to make you a **health care professional**, practicing at the paramedic level. A **profession** is a field of endeavor that requires a specialized set of knowledge, skills, and expertise, often gained after lengthy education.

A health care professional has the following attributes:

- Conforms to the same standards of other health care professions
- Provides quality patient care
- Instills pride in the profession
- Strives continuously for high standards
- Earns respect from others in the profession
- Meets high societal expectations of the profession whether on or off duty

You must meet standards, competencies, and continuing education requirements. The paramedic profession has expected standards and performance parameters as well as a code of ethics. Collectively, these are the standards by which you will be measured.

It is imperative that you remember you are in a highly visible role in your community **Figure 1-10**. Professional image and behavior must be a top priority whether you are in uniform on duty, or off duty in street clothes. You represent the agency, city, county, district, or state you work in. It is said people will make an initial judgment of you within the first 10 seconds of meeting you, even if you say nothing. A positive impression will usually instill complete trust from your patients and their family; however, a negative impression will not only reflect on you, but also your service, and a negative image is very hard to change. As a paramedic, you will meet new people every day as part of your career. To provide the best possible care, you must instill confidence, plus establish and maintain credibility. Whenever you walk into a situation, remember that a significant part of your job is to continually show your concern for the well-being of your patients and their families. Your appearance is also of utmost importance—it has more impact than you may think. It is not appropriate to arrive at a call in dirty clothes, with dirty hands, and smelling offensively. Appear and act like a professional at all times. Professionalism holds no boundaries; saying you are only a volunteer or a part-time worker is not an excuse.

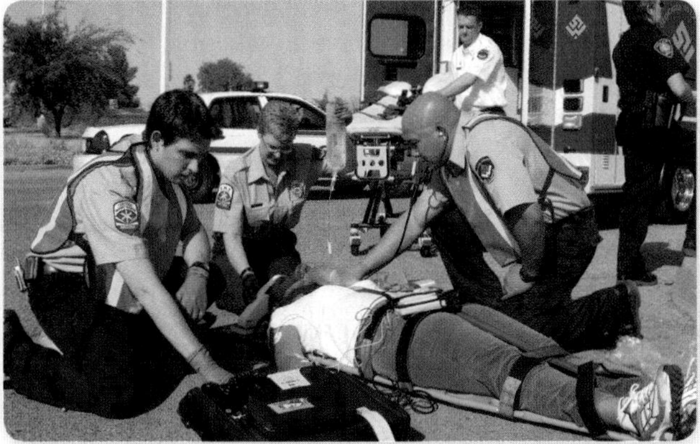

Figure 1-10 Adopting a professional attitude and appearance is a critical part of working with the public and earning their trust.

Words of Wisdom

Earning paramedic licensure entails new prestige, but it also imposes new responsibilities. Paramedics are entrusted with the lives of other people and, although some calls will be terrifying and challenging to you, there is no more awesome or sacred responsibility than that. Your education as a paramedic must not stop with this textbook. Continue to read and study and ask questions. Refine your knowledge and skills, so you may give to each patient the best of which you are capable. Realize that having a wealth of knowledge and skills does not mean you can and must use them on every call. Like a physician, you have a wealth of capabilities, so learn when and when not to use them and how to do so appropriately. Learn to conduct yourself with humility, to accept criticism, to learn from mistakes as well as from triumphs, and to demand of yourself and your colleagues nothing less than the best. Only then will the title of paramedic signify what it is meant to signify: a commitment to other people.

You are an integral part of the entire health care system; therefore, present a professional image and treat others in the profession with the respect you would want to be treated with. It is inappropriate to argue with other health care providers or hospital staff, but there is an appropriate circumstance to have professional discussions regarding patient care. Remember, you are a patient advocate and it is appropriate for you to raise concerns about patient care professionally at appropriate times and locations. There may be occasions where differences of opinion exist; these are best addressed by contacting a supervisor. Such conversations may identify instances when other branches of health care do not follow the same practices as EMS, due to different expectations or requirements.

Other attributes of professionalism as a paramedic include the following:

- **Integrity.** The single most important attribute. Be open, honest, and truthful with your patients and coworkers.

- **Empathy.** Show your patients, their families, and other health care professionals that you identify and understand their feelings. It is okay to show emotions to some extent.
- **Self-motivation.** Have an internal drive for excellence, which is often a driving force to ensure you always behave in a professional manner. Continuously educate yourself, accept negative or constructive feedback, and perform with minimal supervision.
- **Confidence.** Show you are confident in your abilities and skills, so you instill confidence in your patients and colleagues. Continually strive to be the best paramedic you can; attend educational sessions and perform self critiques. These measures are only a few of the items available that will build confidence, and thus, help you to run your calls smoothly and effectively.
- **Communications.** Express and exchange your ideas, thoughts, and findings with other professional colleagues. Make conscious reminders to yourself to listen well and speak directly, without using confusing medical terms, when you interact with patients and their families. Clear, professional written documentation is also important. Record keeping and reporting is a responsibility of all EMS providers.
- **Teamwork and respect.** Teamwork is required in EMS. On every call, everyone must work together to achieve a common goal—to provide the best possible prehospital care to ensure the overall well-being of your patient. Most often in the field, you as the paramedic are considered the team leader. Being the team leader does not entitle you to undermine other team members, regardless of their level; instead, you must help guide and support the team. Remain flexible and open for change at any moment and communicate at an appropriate place and time with other members of the team to resolve problems. Always be as respectful of others as you would expect them to be with you.
- **Patient advocacy.** Advocacy includes advocating for the patients you treat, and advocating for changes in the EMS system that will improve care or save lives. Always act in the best interest of your patients while respecting their wishes and beliefs, regardless of your own. This includes patients with special needs and those with different lifestyles, values, and cultures from your own. Never allow your personal feelings about a patient to impact the care you provide. Respect those you serve. While you need to communicate to do your job, be sure you maintain a high level of confidentiality. Whatever details you have to communicate about your patient, ensure your communication about the patient does not occur in front of anyone who is not on your team. This will be discussed in greater detail in Chapter 4, *Medical, Legal, and Ethical Issues*. When you talk to members of your team, do so in private and away from the public's ear, quietly and with appropriate respect. Your role as a patient advocate means you should always be on the lookout for spousal abuse, child abuse or neglect, and elder abuse or neglect. If abuse is suspected, report and communicate your findings to the appropriate authorities or as outlined in your state's law.
- **Injury prevention.** As a paramedic, you are in the unique position of seeing the patient's surroundings prior to transport. If you spot a potential hazard (such as a loose rug at the top of the stairs), use your diplomatic skills and talk about your findings to the patient or a family member. Get involved with training programs such as those on the topics of fall prevention or child passenger safety. You may prevent a potential injury. Discuss the importance of using bike helmets, safety belts, and child car seats whenever you can. It is another way of preventing injuries.
- **Careful delivery of service.** Paramedics must deliver the highest quality patient care. Pay careful attention to detail and continuously evaluate and reevaluate your performance. Use other medical professionals as resources, not adversaries. Follow policies, protocols, and procedures as well as the orders of your superiors.
- **Time management.** Time management is an important skill in any profession. Use your time wisely; for example, prioritize your patient's needs, always keep your ambulance ready to go, and ensure you document each emergency call as soon as it has concluded. Each is a component of professional delivery of service. Use down time to research and retrain yourself on rarely used skills or topic areas.
- **Administration.** Part of your role as a paramedic will be administrative. In addition to documenting each call thoroughly and professionally, you may be asked to take on special projects or station duties. As you advance in your career, you may play a role in working with other agencies and forging partnerships with other public safety resources. You may be appointed to a leadership position within your organization; this is your opportunity to shine and to help others achieve their goals within your service.

As the health care industry gains a better understanding of a paramedic's skills and abilities, more health care locations are using paramedic services within their organizations. For example, many hospitals now incorporate paramedics in their emergency departments and clinics. Physician offices also are identifying the benefits of using paramedic services within their organizations. With the recent advent of the emerging forms of influenza, some clinics and local public health departments used paramedics to administer vaccines, while in other locations paramedics help home health organizations. You will perform special types of transports beyond your standard 9-1-1 emergency calls. Your service may provide transfers between health care locations; these may include specialty services such as critical care, neonatal, or high-risk obstetric transfers. The expertise that a paramedic acquires is a very important part of the entire emergency medical environment; offer your abilities in all ways possible.

Roles and Responsibilities

So what does it actually mean to be a paramedic? What are your roles? What are your responsibilities? These are the questions you should ask yourself throughout your career. The EMS system continues to grow and mature, and with those changes will come new roles and additional responsibilities. Some of the primary responsibilities are shown in Figure 1-11 and include the following:

- **Preparation.** Be prepared physically, mentally, and emotionally. Keep up your knowledge and skill abilities. Ensure you have the appropriate equipment for your call and that it is in good working order. When the call comes in, your chance to prepare has ended.
- **Response.** Responding to the event in a timely, safe manner is very important. High speed—running "hot" without due regard for your safety, your partner's, your patient's, and that of other people on the highway (even if they should get out of your way but do not)—is not acceptable. In most cases, running "hot" offers no measurable benefit to patient outcome.
- **Scene management.** Your first priority is to ensure your safety and the safety of your team. Then you must ensure the patient is safe, as well as any bystanders. Part of your preparation before you reach the scene should include considering all possibilities from dispatch information; however, never set your mind on a single possibility based on dispatch information. Once you are at the scene, assess the situation as the nature of the call may give valuable information. Scene safety includes but is not limited to wearing personal protective equipment (PPE) such as gloves, masks, or

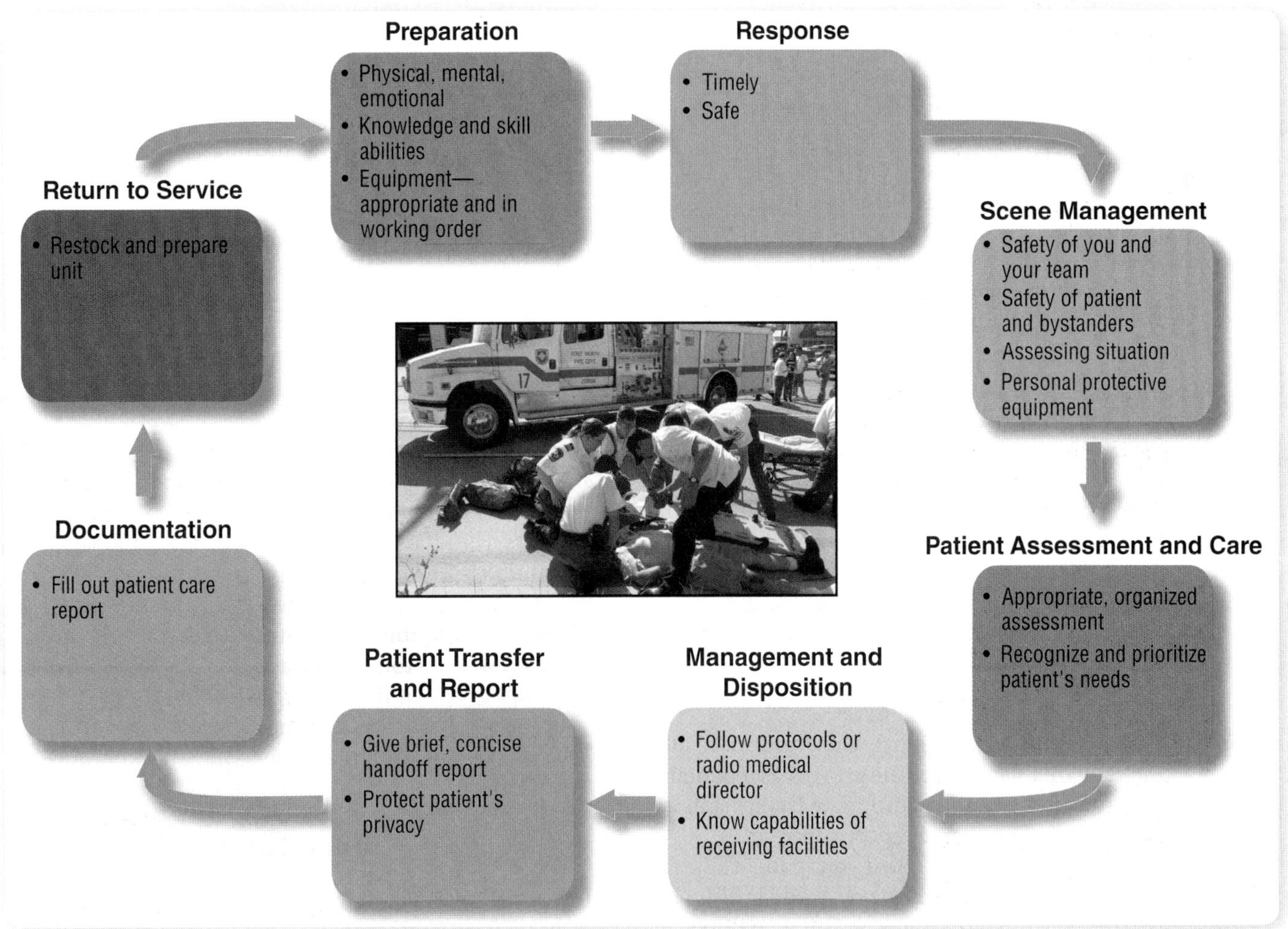

Figure 1-11 Paramedics follow an important sequence of procedures for each emergency call.

goggles. The paramedic often sets the example for safety to the members of the EMS team.

- **Patient assessment and care.** Perform an organized assessment of all patients. Although a patient assessment is similar at all EMS levels, you will learn additional concepts about assessment in this textbook. Recognize and prioritize the patient's needs on the basis of the injuries or the illness most in need of urgent treatment.
- **Management and disposition.** Follow medical guidelines or protocols approved by your medical director and possibly your state. However, sometimes, when you are in the field, you will discover that the protocols or guidelines might not cover the situation you are in. This is the time to make online contact with your medical control physician and use critical thinking skills. Having a good working relationship with your medical director is critical. You are the eyes, ears, and touch for the medical director. Situations that require a protocol or guideline variance or a decision that may be outside of your scope of practice need to be communicated with your medical director. If you are unable to make contact, you must closely weigh your decisions before any intervention and communicate to your medical director as soon as possible. Although most calls will require transport to an emergency department, you must also be aware of other transport and destination decisions. For example, a patient with carbon monoxide poisoning may need to be transported to a hospital with a hyperbaric chamber—would you know where it is and how to access it? Your local receiving facilities may not keep you apprised of their capabilities; therefore, it is your responsibility to know your area's local health care abilities. Know which facilities have specialty cardiac programs, and which are capable of handling trauma or pediatric emergencies. Know the capabilities of all receiving facilities you may interact with before a call; this will assist you in making the right decision or providing information to your patient and his or her family. You may also respond to calls where the patient refuses your care; this will be covered further in Chapter 4, *Medical, Legal, and Ethical Issues*.
- **Patient transfer and report.** Once you arrive at the receiving facility, continue to act as a patient advocate and give the appropriate facility staff a brief, concise handoff report. Once again, use discretion so you protect your patient's privacy. Keep in mind, if the receiving facility is extremely busy, they may not offer you the time you prefer to do a handoff report. Do not become frustrated or angry; do your best to get as much pertinent information to them as possible and ensure the facility is aware and ready to take over patient care.
- **Documentation.** After you transfer the patient, it is extremely important that a patient care report be filled out, preferably immediately. Many states require some sort of written report be left at the facility. If this is not possible or required, inform the facility how to reach you in case they have a question. Also, the report serves as a legal record of all aspects of the call. Physicians must document their care of patients—so must you. Guidelines for documentation will be covered in Chapter 6, *Documentation*.
- **Return to service.** Every person on the EMS team is responsible for restocking and preparing the unit as quickly as possible for the next call. Preparing for the next call should be the first item you complete when you return from a call. Failure to do so can bring about serious legal consequences if another call comes in and the unit is not fully restocked and ready to respond.

Words of Wisdom

One of your responsibilities as an EMS professional is to provide emotional support. Remember, calming and reassuring the patient, the family, and other responders can go a long way in making you an effective paramedic.

You are looked upon as a health care professional, so take advantage of this role. Educate the public about what you do and its importance. Get involved with prevention, community, and leadership activities whenever possible Figure 1-12. Never miss an opportunity to teach the community about prevention of injury and illness. Explain

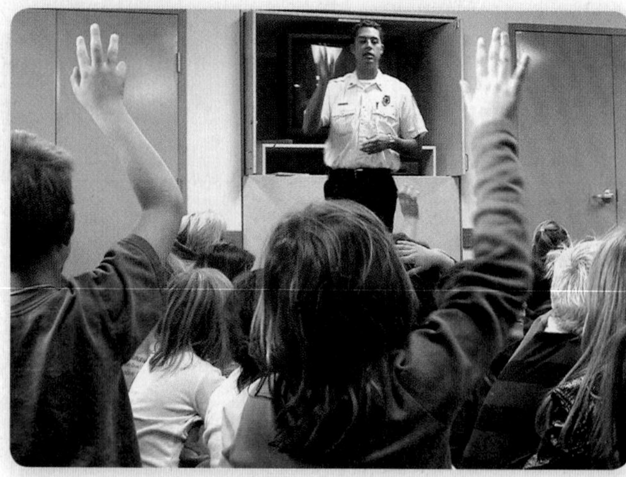

Figure 1-12 Part of your role as a public servant is to interact with and educate the public.

Courtesy of Captain David Jackson, Saginaw Township Fire Department to people how to appropriately use your services. In the areas where trained EMS staff are limited, use your abilities to promote programs that get the public involved such as CPR and AED training, one of the proven determinants of whether or not a person in cardiac arrest will live or die.

Paramedics may have other health care responsibilities such as working in clinics, free-standing emergency facilities, and hospitals. Home visits by paramedics under direct medical control (Mobile Integrated Healthcare) are also in the early stages of development; this is discussed in more depth in Chapter 53, *Career Development*. In recent years with the rise in influenza and possible pandemic issues, paramedics along with home health nurses are being used to evaluate people at home and provide some immunization and medication administration.

Providers at all levels of EMS need to be advocates for prehospital health care, which often means setting well-thought-out campaigns for EMS. Research your community, look at the strengths and weaknesses of the system, and develop plans for initiatives to improve the system. Many people lack an understanding of the role of EMS and do not recognize how vital EMS is until a loved one becomes ill unexpectedly. By involving yourself in your communities, you can both educate and advocate. It is up to all EMS personnel to educate the media and public. Strive to stay at the top of your profession. Continue your education and become a mentor for new EMS professionals.

Documentation & Communication

Documentation of equipment repairs and checks is nearly as important as documenting patient care.

Medical Direction

One important difference between providers with different levels of EMS education is that paramedics carry out advanced cardiologic, pharmacologic, and trauma care skills. However, paramedics do not have independent authority to act. Physicians who are educated about the levels and the extent of the education of EMS personnel play a vital role in medical direction of a service. The best medical director is one who is active in all aspects of the service he or she is overseeing, a role far beyond signing forms. The role of an EMS medical director may include the following:

- Educate and train personnel.
- Participate in the recommendation or selection of new personnel.
- Participate in the recommendation or selection of equipment.
- Develop clinical protocols or guidelines in collaboration with other EMS personnel who are considered experts in the field.
- Develop and assist in a quality improvement program.
- Provide input into patient care.
- Interface between EMS systems and other health care agencies.
- Serve as an EMS advocate to the community.
- Serve as the "medical conscience" of the EMS system.

The medical director provides online and off-line medical control. **Online (direct) medical control** is medical direction given in real time to an EMS service or provider (either by radio or other electronic communication). It is typically provided by an emergency physician working in a hospital emergency department that serves as a base station for EMS units in the area and not directly by your medical director. **Off-line (indirect) medical control** is medical direction given through a set of protocols, policies, and/or standards developed by or with the approval of your medical director. The benefit to online medical control is it provides immediate and specific patient care resources, allows telemetry transmission, allows for continuous quality improvement, and can offer on-scene assistance. In some locations, video telemetry is available that allows the medical control physician to see exactly what the EMS team is seeing. Off-line medical control allows for the development of protocols or guidelines, standing orders, procedures, and training. A **protocol** or guideline is a treatment plan for a specific illness or injury. A **standing order** is a type of protocol or guideline that is a written document signed by the EMS system's medical director that outlines specific directions, permissions, and sometimes prohibitions regarding patient care that is rendered prior to contacting medical control (for example,

Words of Wisdom

In some cases, you may encounter a physician on scene. If the physician is familiar with EMS protocols or happens to be your medical director, it can be a great help. But you may be caught between what the physician on the scene wants to do and the protocols that your medical director has given your service. Remember, you work with your physician medical director and you must adhere to the local protocols and standing orders.

Remain calm and composed should the physician on the scene demand medical control of the situation.

Politely explain all your actions must be in accordance with your EMS medical director's protocols. Point out that you can transfer care of the patient only to an onsite physician if that physician is now taking full responsibility for the patient and will be present during transport, riding with the patient in your ambulance to the emergency department, as well as signing for any orders given. Most states and services have rules that EMS must follow in these cases. They also require release forms to be signed by the onsite physician. The only exception to this is if the onsite physician happens to be the service's medical director.

chest decompression). Protocols or guidelines are usually developed in conjunction with national standards. For example, EMS personnel often use the American Heart Association advanced cardiac life support algorithms as a guide for developing a treatment protocol for cardiac patients (discussed in detail in Chapter 17, *Cardiovascular Emergencies*). Protocols dictate what type of equipment and supplies are approved and needed as well as minimum expectations of personnel. The medical director also plays a role after the ambulance run. Medical directors help with patient care report review or even personally perform such reviews to ensure continuous quality improvement.

Patient Safety

Paramedics sometimes perform interfacility transfers. Recent adverse events associated with interfacility transfers have drawn closer scrutiny. A recent Canadian study suggests that the event rate is lower when transports are staffed with specially trained critical care transport providers.[4] Overall, the data indicate that 1 in 15 patients experienced one of several adverse events during transport, including hypotension, initiation of vasopressor therapy, and respiratory events. An analysis showed that hemodynamic instability requiring intervention such as fluids or vasopressors was by far the most common adverse event, followed by respiratory instability or hypoxia. Additionally, in-transit critical care events were independently associated with mechanical ventilation and baseline hemodynamic instability.

Some problematic events have been identified in relation to specific types of transports. For pediatric transports, the most common adverse events noted were hypothermia, medication errors, tachycardia, procedure error, loss of IV access, and cyanosis. Of interest, the adverse event rate was lower in this population when specialized teams performed the transport.

The value of employing specialty-trained teams in interfacility transport of complex cases is increasing as newer and more advanced therapies become more widely employed during transport, such as inhaled nitric oxide and extracorporeal membrane oxygenation.

In a review of adult transports, one group of authors found that 70% of adverse events could have been avoided by better preparation prior to transport, communication between the sending and receiving facilities, and the use of checklists and protocols.[5]

Improving System Quality

Making a good thing better should always be part of your paramedic career. A tool often used to continually evaluate your care is called **continuous quality improvement (CQI)**. **Quality control** is another process that evaluates problems and finds solutions. CQI is a process of assessing current practices and looking for ways to create ongoing improvement, thus reducing the chance of a problem arising in the first place. When properly developed and followed, a CQI program can help you and your service.

The process of CQI is dynamic, and your EMS system should develop a structure before a CQI assessment program is launched. Also, check with your state or region to identify any requirements they may have for CQI. A good CQI process should include the following:

- Identify any departmental or system-wide issues.
- Identify specific items that need to be measured.
- Conduct an in-depth review of the issue(s).
- Evaluate the issue(s) and develop a list of remedies.
- Develop an action plan for correction of issue(s).
- Enforce a plan of action, including time frames.
- Reexamine the issue.
- Identify and promote excellence found in patient care during the evaluation.
- Identify modifications that may be needed to protocols and standing orders.
- Identify situations that are currently not addressed by protocols and standing orders.

Although it may not be feasible, all ambulance runs should be reviewed. Ultimately, the focus of CQI needs to be on improving patient care. Often providers show hesitation with a CQI process because of fear of being ridiculed or reprimanded. To avoid this, it is important to use your CQI process not as a punitive tool, but as a constructive tool for continuous improvement.

Some services will choose to perform quality control as peer review **Figure 1-13**. Peer review is a good learning experience if the people performing the reviews have proper and consistent guidelines to follow and keep an open mind. No matter how good your education, you will still make mistakes and miss things from time to time. When a peer reviewer finds things you can improve, you should look at it as an educational tool. In an ideal system, the members of the peer review team rotate on and off, meaning, at some point you will also serve as a reviewer. Caution: never use this process as a tool to

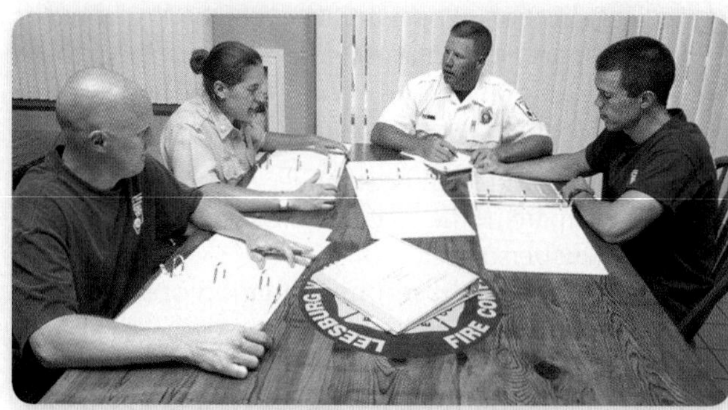

Figure 1-13 Peer reviews should be seen as a constructive part of paramedic practice.

demean or belittle a fellow paramedic. Nor should you discuss your findings with anyone who is not identified as part of the review process. Be professional.

A comprehensive CQI program can help prevent problems from arising by evaluating day-to-day operations and identifying possible stress points in these operations. These may include the following:

- Medical direction issues
- Education
- Communications
- Prehospital treatment
- Transportation issues
- Financial issues
- Receiving facility review
- Dispatch
- Public information and education
- Disaster planning
- Mutual aid

A function of the evaluation process for ensuring quality control is to determine ways to eliminate human error. To cut down on the potential for errors, ensure adequate lighting when handling medications and keep interruptions to a minimum. Keep medications in a specific location and in their original packaging to reduce the potential for errors.

High-risk activities include handing off patients. You must deal with the issues not only of the physical transfer of the patient from your stretcher, but also communication with the next caregiver in line. Provide a written copy of your assessment and treatment along with the verbal report to help to ensure the continuum of care. It is imperative that you give a report of your care of the patient and any changes that may have occurred since you took over care. Other safety issues revolve around advanced airway management, medication administration, and safe transport (such as avoiding ambulance crashes and providing proper immobilization) of patients who may have potential traumatic injuries.

It is important that you strive to identify potential errors and eliminate them as much as possible. Understand the circumstances that cause errors to help you identify those that can be prevented. There are three main sources of errors. They can occur as a result of a rules-based failure, a knowledge-based failure, or a skills-based failure (or any combination of these). For example, does a paramedic

YOU are the Paramedic — PART 4

Due to the urgency of the situation, you ask one of the rescue personnel who has been cleared to drive your unit to drive the ambulance and to start transport to the Mayfield Medical Center, a trauma center that is 9 miles (14 km) away. It is 1628 hours. You call medical control and give a thorough description of the mechanism of injury, signs and symptoms, presentation, and vital signs and request orders to perform a needle decompression. The physician tells you to go ahead with the procedure and to advise him of any changes.

As soon as you complete the procedure, your partner states there is less resistance as he ventilates the patient. You note that chest rise is almost symmetrical and his blood pressure and pulses improve. He is still unresponsive.

You arrive at the trauma center at 1638 hours. You give a verbal and a written report to the receiving facility. You and your partner clean and ready the ambulance in case you receive another call before you get back to your station. You save a copy of the report for your supervisor to add to a study being done on the benefits of prehospital needle decompression. Ten minutes later you are in service and dispatched immediately to another call.

Recording Time: 13 Minutes	
Respirations	12 breaths/min assisted with bag-mask ventilations
Pulse	118 beats/min
Skin	Pale, slightly diaphoretic
Blood pressure	104/62 mm Hg
Oxygen saturation (Spo_2)	98% on oxygen via bag-mask
Pupils	Equal but sluggish to react

7. Explain why this situation is a good example of how EMS research may help future patients through evidence-based practice.
8. How is retrospective research beneficial for educating EMS personnel?

have the legal right to administer the particular medication needed by the patient? If not, a rules-based failure has occurred if a paramedic assists with the administration. Does a paramedic know all of the pertinent information about the medication being delivered? If not, a breakdown at this point, such as the administration of the wrong medication, would be referred to as a knowledge-based failure. Finally, is the equipment operating and being used properly? If not, a skills-based error has occurred. Any error can come from multiple sources.

Agencies need to have clear protocols, which are detailed plans that describe how certain patient issues, such as chest pain or shortness of breath, are to be managed. In some states, guidelines are used instead of protocols. Each has a different meaning. Services that have active medical directors will offer guidelines which describe allowable treatment plans that you as a paramedic can use to determine what you need to do and when, without contacting medical control first. Protocols normally outline a care plan in a specific order and do not allow you to flex outside of the medical director's treatment plan without contacting him or her first. Protocols and guidelines need to be understood by all paramedics within the service. You may fail if you follow a protocol or guideline to exactness, but you may also fail if you do not. Be prepared to make modifications and use the best resource you have available: online (direct) medical control.

The environment can be part of the reason for errors. Are there ways to limit distractions? Can paramedics find what they need in a timely manner? Sometimes the solution is as easy as ensuring flashlights are available on all ambulances. Make sure all drugs and equipment are properly labeled and organized.

When you are about to perform a skill, ask yourself, "Why am I doing this?" Consider the reason for your actions to allow you time to reflect and make a more informed decision. Just because you have the ability to perform a large variety of procedures, does not mean you should. It should be clear in your mind why you are using a skill or administering a medication. If you cannot come up with a solution to the patient's problem, ask for help. Talk with your partner, contact medical control, or call your EMS supervisor.

Another way for you to help limit medical errors is to use "cheat sheets." Have a copy of your protocol book with you. Although some may suggest that reviewing a protocol during a call is admitting you do not know what you are doing, in actuality you cannot memorize all aspects of your protocols. Choosing to review and confirm that your decision is correct shows true professionalism and concern for your patient. Emergency physicians have many reference materials available to them. Physicians recognize that they cannot memorize everything, so referencing a book or other reliable resources helps ensure the use of accurate information.

Preventing errors requires being conscientious of protocols and not allowing interruptions while providing patient care. Use decision-making aids, such as algorithms, and reflect on what has been done as an informal critique for future improvement of your performance. Finally, after a troublesome call, sit down and talk. Talk with your partner and/or your supervisor. Discussing events that recently happened provides an excellent avenue for learning. Your discussions can help lead to changes in protocol, changes in how equipment is stocked, or even the purchase of new equipment.

EMS Research

As medicine has increasingly been drawn toward **evidence-based practice**, so has the EMS system. Although EMS systems have been used for more than 40 years, minimal research has been conducted to prove what you will do as a paramedic will truly improve patient outcome. Due to emphasis by numerous organizations and the public's eye, patient care protocols must be based on scientific findings as often as possible. An important step in the effort to link scientific findings to patient care was taken in 2001 with the publication of the *National EMS Research Agenda,* a document commissioned by the Department of Transportation and the Department of Health and Human Services, which has described processes and set goals for the optimization of prehospital emergency medical care. A publication at the ems.gov website titled *Progress on Evidence-Based Guidelines for Prehospital Emergency Care* outlines some of the progress in relation to research findings. Research can force a dramatic departure from the standardized, non-evidence-based method of operation historically used in EMS. For example, studies have continued to show that a "hands only" CPR technique by bystanders, along with early use of an AED, greatly improves the chances that a victim of sudden cardiac arrest will survive to release from the hospital. Previously, the treatment protocol dictated care for airway and breathing first for all patients and then care for circulation (the ABCs). However, research has shown that to provide the best outcome for patients in cardiac arrest, circulation should be addressed first, changing the ABCDE acronym in the context of cardiac arrest to CABDE. Similar studies are planned or in progress to either change or reaffirm the standards of care provided in prehospital medicine.

It is important to ensure that research is performed by properly educated researchers, and although the majority of researchers have a PhD or MD degree and vested interest in EMS research, anyone can be part of research if properly trained. The National Registry of EMTs and the Robert Wood Johnson Foundation continue to research various topics that relate to emergency medical care and emergency services in general.

An increase in the number of accredited colleges and universities that provide an EMS track for paramedics is a tremendous benefit to the EMS system and research. You can now enter the EMS field not only trained as a paramedic, but also holding a bachelor's degree. Although the EMS field is currently primarily composed of providers who hold a license or certification, paramedic students who have bachelor's degrees will further enhance the professional image within the medical community. Many of these learning institutions also produce high-quality research, which then feeds back into the educational system and practice. As a paramedic student, you may have the opportunity to assist in a research project geared toward your career; this is an opportunity you should not pass up. You may be part of something that will eventually change the future of EMS.

▶ The Research Process

The first step in conducting research is to identify the specific problem, procedure, or question to be investigated. In general, a research topic usually arises when a certain practice is questioned. You may identify items during your paramedic calls that could initiate valid research projects. For example, the efficacy of endotracheal intubation and rapid sequence intubation in the field has been a popular research topic as well as "lights and siren" responses. Even if the topic has been investigated before, it can often be revisited. Research findings can be flawed and a new study may identify flaws or enhance previous research findings. Some research topics are driven by a product manufacturer or an entity that is strictly out to prove something right or wrong regardless of its importance in EMS. Therefore, carefully reviewing the research—in its entirety and not just the summary—is very important. Once the question has been determined, a **research agenda** is developed. This agenda specifies the questions to be answered, the specific aims to be addressed, and the precise methods by which the study will be carried out and the data will be gathered. Although numerous additional questions may arise from results during the study, the researcher must adhere to the research agenda and answer the specific questions at hand. Other items of interest encountered during the course of the research may themselves become topics of research in a separate study.

Once a qualified researcher has decided on a specific question to be answered, the next step is to determine the **research domain** in which the study should be conducted. A research domain is the area of research (clinical, basic science, systems, or education). A clinical domain, for example, would include stroke research involving clinical trials that would lead to improved patient care. An example of basic science research is a study of the effectiveness of a new drug in limiting carbon monoxide poisoning in an animal model. A systems domain in EMS research would focus on operations, such as the effects of sleep-deprived EMS providers on patient care. An education domain would focus on how programs are taught, such as a study of the components that make up high-performing paramedic programs. These may also include research on education competency standards.

EMS research may be performed by EMS providers, but it is usually performed by people who are studying a particular branch of medicine or science. EMS research may be performed within a **research consortium**; this is a group of agencies working together to study a particular topic. Paramedics may be involved in collaborative research by gathering data. For example, you may be part of a study to determine the outcome of a STEMI (ST-segment elevation myocardial infarction) patient if transported to a facility that does not offer cardiac specialty services such as a cardiac catheterization lab, or whether time saved in helicopter transport truly improves outcomes. In some cases, you may be asked to identify certain populations for research or even gather volunteers from calls you are on. If you are asked to identify patients, have some information with you regarding the research. If a patient agrees to become part of the research, obtain informed consent from the patient specifically for the research; the informed consent the patient gives you to treat him or her during the emergency is not the same as authorization to use the data in research. *It is important that initiatives associated with research never take priority over care the patient may need.* If the patient agrees to participate, note this in your patient care report. Your job is to ensure you accurately gather and report data about the patients you encounter who fit within the study's parameters. The information gathered will then be analyzed by the researchers to answer the question at hand. The results could then be shared with the rest of the EMS and scientific community to, hopefully, improve patient care practices. Evidence-based medical practice is based on such research.

▶ Funding

Before a research project involving any human research subjects can begin, approval of an **institutional review board (IRB)** is required in order to ensure that the rights of study subjects are protected throughout the study. An institutional review board involves a group or institution that reviews the research. The requirements for review, which makes research legal, ethical, and potentially eligible for federal funding, were devised in 1966 by the US Public Health Service.

Major research requires specific funding. In particular, large clinical trials or systems research can carry a significant fiscal cost. This cost is funded through a variety of sources, such as local or federal government, nonprofit foundation grants, and industry or corporate funding. To qualify for a federal or public grant, the study must first go through a rigorous evaluation process to ensure it will answer a question within the domain covered by the grant. The methods and results are then subject to stipulations placed on them by the grantor. Similarly, nonprofit organizations or foundations will fund research in their specific areas of interest, and typically will have some control over the methods used. Corporate support can be in the form of a grant to a nonprofit research organization, or more commonly as a chartered research project to validate a product manufactured by the corporation, such as a new medication or piece of medical equipment. When you are seeking funding, keep in mind, there may be some grants that have stipulations that may be perceived as trying to alter outcomes in favor of the grantor. Before applying for a grant, ensure you meet all the criteria and can adhere to the expectations throughout the entire project.

Any type of support given to a researcher is considered funding, including free lab space, travel, or assistants to help with the research. To prevent the appearance of bias or potential conflicts of interest, researchers should disclose all sources of funding and support and maintain total transparency with regard to their research methods.

▶ Types of Research

There are different types of research, including quantitative and qualitative. The type of research that will yield the best results may depend on the research topic and what the researcher wishes to learn.

Qualitative research focuses on questions within a context of surrounding events and concurrent processes and attempts to build a more complete, holistic picture. In other words, qualitative research takes into account the real-world factors that may have influenced the results of a study and may attempt to interpret the results to account for these factors. Oftentimes, qualitative research is used when specific answers cannot be identified in quantitative research. Qualitative research often involves the interpretation of previously published data by the researcher and making a statement of the findings. Qualitative methods investigate the why and how of decision making, not just what, where, and when. It is difficult to evaluate qualitative studies using set guidelines. Rather, each study must have a set of parameters specific to the question. Some medical research falls into the qualitative category.

Quantitative research is based on numeric data. Types of quantitative research include the following:

- **Experimental research.** A scientific approach to research in which a researcher controls, manipulates, and then measures one or more variables to ascertain how manipulating the variables affects the subjects. Experimental research is concerned with cause-and-effect relationships.
- **Nonexperimental research.** Descriptive research that does not involve experimentation using patients and manipulating variables to reach a conclusion. For example, a study on the effectiveness of different levels of pain management would be unethical or even difficult to conduct on humans; therefore, data would be gathered through interviewing patients and watching vital sign parameters.
- **Survey research.** In this type of research, conclusions are based on survey results. To be valid, researchers must identify what is being measured and determine the appropriate sample size. Additionally, the sample population must reflect the composition of the population being researched. For example, if a study of the incidence of cancer were conducted in an area that had a particularly high incidence of cancer, the results of that study would not be indicative of the whole country. Therefore, it is imperative that when you review a research paper you identify whether the outcome would be similar in your location.

Retrospective research uses available data, for example, from medical records or patient care reports. Research may involve examining those records to determine the types of calls that occur at night versus daytime or, the number of calls where substance abuse was the cause of the patient's complaint. This information is then used to develop educational sessions for EMS personnel or can be used to plan public education and public prevention strategies. It may be necessary for the researcher to collaborate with a hospital or group of hospitals in gathering the necessary patient outcome information. To comply with federal laws such as the Health Insurance Portability and Accountability Act (HIPAA), patient identification information may have to be deleted from records prior to the change of hands between agencies. However, in some states governmental or municipal agencies have rules that supersede HIPAA requirements and establish all information as public record.

Many large retrospective studies collect and analyze data from widespread, sometimes nationwide, databases. Such databases may link EMS, hospitals, and even post-hospitalization providers into the system and allow for a broad, total picture of the patient population in question. Nationwide databases for cardiac arrest patients, patients requiring extracorporeal membrane oxygenation, children, and trauma registries exist within the United States. Nationwide databases are typically overseen by a centralized agency, for example, within the federal government; data are usually collected by state or local governments to populate the databases. The same techniques of data collection and analysis can be used at the local level for smaller research projects; data from various hospitals and EMS agencies can be entered into a centralized database that can then be used to study specific patient populations. For accurate research results, however, there must be clear-cut guidelines for data entry so that comparisons of data can be made.

In addition to retrospective research, other types of research include prospective research, cohort research, and case studies. **Prospective research** studies gather information as events occur in real time. A **cohort research** examines patterns of change, a sequence of events, or trends over time within a certain population or "cohort" of study subjects. Inversely, a **case study** method is the investigation and documentation of a single case over a period of time.

Additionally, these categories can be subgrouped as cross-sectional or longitudinal. The **cross-sectional design** collects all data at one point in time, essentially serving as a "snapshot" of events and information. The

longitudinal design collects information at various set time intervals. Therefore, a prospective study must have, by design, a longitudinal data-gathering method, whereas retrospective, cohort, or case study research can utilize either a cross-sectional or longitudinal data collection technique.

Finally, a **literature review** is a form of research in which the existing literature is reviewed, and the researcher analyzes the collection of research to draw a conclusion.

Research Methods

A beginning step in conducting research is to identify the group or groups of people necessary for the research. Once the group(s) is identified, it may be refined further, such as limiting the research to people in a specific age bracket, with a certain medical condition, or of a specific gender. As an example, a researcher may wish to study men over the age of 50 who have high blood pressure. Once the list of eligible subjects is identified, researchers randomly choose who will be part of the research. There are many different ways to achieve this. A list of subjects or groups can be computer-generated (**systematic sampling**) or time frame parameters can be set (**alternative time sampling**). Finally, the least preferred method is when subjects are manually assigned to a specific researcher (**convenience sampling**), rather than being randomly assigned. Even in the best cases, **sampling errors** can occur. For example, a study may fail to include all of the needed subjects, or there may be people in the study who meet criteria but still are not the best representation. Also, consider the number of people you wish to participate. It is recommended you select a much higher number than you need, so you allow for those who will not complete the study or will fall out of the research parameters. For example, if you need 500 participants, you may want to consider searching for 600 candidates.

Parameters should be identified in research. Parameters outline the type of people who are appropriate for the study. Another tool to consider is **blinding**, in which investigators are unaware of the study arm into which the subject being interviewed has been enrolled. There are single-, double-, and triple-blinded studies where one, two, or all parties are blinded, respectively. When participants of the research project are advised of all aspects of the project, it is known as an **unblinded study**.

As research continues, data will be acquired. The gathered statistics can be either in a **descriptive** or **inferential** format. In a descriptive format, observations are made, but no attempts are made to alter or change an event. In an inferential format, a hypothesis is used to prove one finding over another. Descriptive statistics can also be performed in either a qualitative or quantitative style. The quantitative approach covers additional variables, such as the mean, median, and mode. For example, in a study on diabetes in women who are between 30 and 40 years old, the mean age of study participants equals the average age of the subjects, the median age is the midpoint age of the subjects, and the mode is the most frequent age of the subjects. Finally, **standard deviation** outlines how much the values in a set of data differ from the mean.

Ethical Considerations

As in many aspects of a profession, there are **ethical** items to consider when conducting research. One entity that monitors whether a study is conducted ethically is the organization's institutional review board (IRB), whose primary purpose is to ensure the protection of study participants and to ensure appropriate conduct. Researchers must ensure any risks to study subjects will not outweigh the potential benefits. They must acquire consent from all subjects and be certain their rights and welfare are adequately protected. Any potential conflicts of interest to the study should be identified. For example, if a person is involved in a similar study, or is employed by the person or company sponsoring the study, this would be considered a conflict of interest and that person should be removed from the study. Subjects must be allowed to participate voluntarily without being coerced. Subjects must also be informed of all potential risks that may occur and be allowed to withdraw from the research at any time **Figure 1-14**. At a minimum, the subjects should be advised they are protected by the Office of Human Research Protections. This office offers materials to those involved in research. The Food and Drug Administration also offers guidance for researchers on a variety of topic areas. To ensure the research is not flawed, the potential of subject withdrawal or any other possible variable that may affect the outcome should be identified before the study begins.

Patients who are potential participants in a clinical domain research trial must be informed about the study protocols prior to participating in the study. For example, a pharmaceutical corporation may have introduced a new respiratory medication. To validate the effectiveness of the medication, patients are entered into a trial,

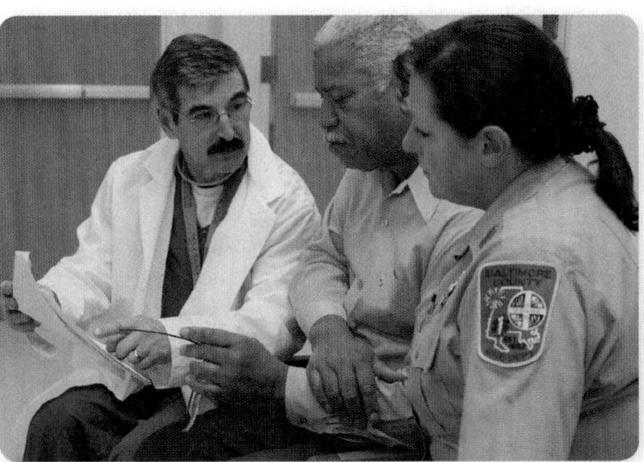

Figure 1-14 Any person who participates in a research study should be well-informed of the study's goals as well as the potential risks and any potential benefits associated with participation.

in which they will either receive the new medication, a more well-studied medication, or perhaps a placebo. The patient would have to be informed of the potential effects (positive or adverse) of participating in the study and sign a waiver to be entered into the program. In some cases, a treatment that is being studied may be administered in emergency situations under waiver of informed consent; it is assumed the patient would want the treatment to be given because of its lifesaving potential.

Evidence-Based Medicine

It is important to ensure that the research you are using for decisions is credible and follows proper research processes.

For example, a supposedly well-designed and conducted study submitted in 1998 on the topic of a potential link between vaccines and autism did not outline a control group or actual studies.[6] It was devised through personal recollection of people and vague conclusions that offered no statistical proof.

Extensive research ensued over the following years. Although the original 1998 "study" claimed there was a direct link, as of 2005, over 31 validated studies had been performed including studies involving more than 10 million children, clearly demonstrating no link between vaccination and autism.[7]

Similarly, many research papers on the efficacy of vaccines have been performed. Valid research shows that vaccines greatly reduce the risk of death and disability, with no link to autism.

This example shows the importance of reviewing research papers referenced in a current study.

▶ Evaluating Medical Research

Paramedics must know how to evaluate what is true medical research and what is a printed personal preference. When you are evaluating a research article, look for certain criteria to determine the quality of the research. Table 1-3 provides 15 questions to answer when evaluating and interpreting research. Once you have identified the type of study, its methods, and its strengths, it is time to actually look at the body of the study itself. Most important, you must avoid the temptation to skim through the study and look at only a couple of findings. If you do not read the entire study, you may miss key points that will alter your understanding of the information presented. To start, determine what the hypothesis of the study is, and whether the population base matches your region. For example, if you work in an area where environmental temperatures are high, such as Arizona, how relevant would a study on hyperthermia be if it is performed in a normally cold environment such as Alaska? Valid studies have a clearly stated hypothesis and clearly defined outcome measurements. Avoid studies with vague hypotheses or outcome measurements, as those are frequently subject to manipulation. The more subjects involved in a study, the more relevant the data is likely to be. For example, if you were reading two studies on the validity of aspirin for active chest pain, and one study includes a patient base of 1,000 while the other has a patient base of 15,000, the information gathered from the latter study will likely be more relevant.

Next, look at the patient and selection criteria. How were they decided upon and were they selected at random? What inclusion criteria existed for entry into the study? For a study to be valid, all subjects need to be accounted for, even if they did not make it into the final outcome. If subjects were dropped from the study, there should be clear reasons as to why. Then, consider the number of subjects. Is the number the same at the beginning and at the end, including any patients who dropped out? If the numbers do not match, the data is essentially invalid and should not be considered. Basically, any discrepancies during a study should be reported and explained.

Determine how the data was analyzed. Ensure the methods of analysis are appropriate for what the study is designed to measure.

Identify the authors of the study and their conclusions; be certain their conclusions are not biased in any way based on financial or other conflicts of interest that may sway the final analysis. Finally, determine whether the outcome and results are significant, both statistically and clinically. Statistical significance describes how often

Table 1-3 Fifteen Questions to Answer When Evaluating and Interpreting Research

1. Was the research peer reviewed?
2. What was the research hypothesis?
3. Was the study approved by an institutional review board and conducted ethically?
4. What was the population being studied?
5. What were the inclusion and exclusion criteria?
6. What method was used to acquire a sample of patients?
7. How many groups were the patients divided into?
8. How were the study subjects assigned to the groups?
9. What type of data was gathered?
10. Did the study have enough subjects involved?
11. Are there any confounding variables unaccounted for?
12. Were the data analyzed correctly?
13. Is your conclusion logically supported by the data?
14. Will it apply in your local EMS systems?
15. Were the subjects similar to the patients in your local EMS systems?

the results of a study may happen by chance. For example, if the likelihood that different outcomes between different groups of subjects is due to chance alone is less than 5%, the difference is said to be statistically significant. Of equal importance is the clinical significance. For example, if the finding is effective in enough patients to make it a useful treatment for the majority? For example, if a new medication resulted in a benefit for only 1 of every 1,000 patients and costs $5,000 per dose, would this be considered statistically significant? Would that medication be worth it? However, if that same medication resulted in an 80% likelihood of a positive outcome, therefore, showing clinically significant results, would that be worth it?

The type of journal in which the research is published is also an important part of determining quality and validity. One method of ensuring quality and validity is through the **peer review** process. Many medical journals accept research studies from a wide variety of sources. Prior to publication, these studies are sent to other subject matter experts (the author's "peers") for review of the content and research methods. The research and its conclusions are then accepted, revised, or rejected based on the findings of the peer review. This method allows for greater checks and balances in ensuring quality of the research methods and validity of research conclusions. Many EMS and medical peer-reviewed journals are available in print.

Additionally, the widespread proliferation of medical information on the Internet has resulted in specific Internet sites becoming valid tools for accessing research. Sources range from a wide source such as Google Scholar, to more medically specific sources such as Medscape and PubMed, which contain a substantial number of published articles from various journals and publications. When you are reviewing the research available on a particular topic, this is a useful tool for finding peer-reviewed research.

As discussed, a research study must follow a structured process. A good study will define exactly what it is intended to be measured, the population affected, and the goal of the research. A good research article will have adequate data; for example, 5,000 people were identified and followed over a 5-year period, with data available from all people involved. With any research topic, there are limitations as to what can be measured and how accurately. If in reviewing a research article, you find that some people backed out, died, or were omitted for any reason not originally anticipated or outlined, then the results may be flawed.

Essentially, as a new paramedic it is extremely important that you review research carefully. You owe it to yourself as well as your patients to thoroughly read and understand relevant studies.

▶ Evidence-Based Practice

Evidence-based practice is becoming an integral part of functioning as a paramedic. Your patient care should be focused on the procedures that have proven useful in improving patient outcomes. There is a limited amount of prehospital EMS research in relation to other areas of medical research; however, as EMS research continues, evidence-based practice will have a correspondingly greater role in EMS. High-quality patient care should focus on procedures useful in improving patient outcomes through sound research. It is important for EMS providers to stay up-to-date on the latest advances in health care. Roughly every 5 years or more frequently as needed, the International Liaison Committee on Resuscitation (ILCOR) revises CPR and other resuscitation guidelines based on review of new evidence published throughout the world; these revised guidelines are then published by the American Heart Association (AHA). This is an excellent example of use of medical evidence to develop specific treatment guidelines for use in the prehospital care environment. To learn more about the science of developing consensus guidelines for resuscitation, refer to the ILCOR website. One word of caution: When reading new research results, make sure you understand what the results mean. Ask questions, and critically evaluate published studies. Conclusions that seem too good to be true may very well be.

Evidence-Based Medicine

In 2015, ILCOR, along with its member the AHA, released an updated consensus document on the science of resuscitation which supports the 2015 Guidelines for Cardiopulmonary Resuscitation and Emergency Cardiovascular Care. Those Guidelines are referenced throughout this book, especially in the sections related to cardiology, neurology, pediatrics, and resuscitation. Some highlights of these Guidelines include:

- Revised recommendation that in adults, chest compressions should be delivered at a rate of 100 to 120 per minute and at a depth between 2 to 2.4 inches (5 to 6 cm).
- Differentiation of in-hospital and out-of-hospital chains of survival.
- Addition of life-threatening opioid overdose algorithm.
- Recommendation to consider the value of emergent response notification by cell phone to off-duty rescuers.
- Recommendation that high-risk venues develop community public access defibrillation programs.
- Strengthen the value of lay rescuer compression-only CPR even without dispatcher guidance.
- Establish a goal of compressions performed at least 60% of the time (compression ratio) with as few interruptions as possible.

These are only some of the important changes. Several minor changes to medications and postresuscitation procedures are also noted in the summary of changes available on the AHA website.

Table 1-4 American Heart Association Classes of Recommendations and Levels of Evidence

Class (Strength) of Recommendation	Level (Quality) of Evidence
Class I (Strong)	Level A (Highest quality evidence)
Class IIa (Moderate)	Level B-R (Randomized)
Class IIb (Weak)	Level B-NR (Nonrandomized)
Class III (No Benefit – Moderate)	Level C-LD (Limited Data)
Class III (Harm – Strong)	Level C-EO (Expert Opinion)

Data from: American Heart Association. Highlights of the 2015 American Heart Association guidelines update for CPR and ECC. https://eccguidelines.heart.org/index.php/circulation/cpr-ecc-guidelines-2/. Published October 15, 2015. Accessed September 26, 2016.

To link medical research and evidence to patient care, you must ensure that the quality of the evidence is sufficient to justify changing patient care protocols. To ensure quality evidence, researchers often rate the quality of a study. There are many different rating systems. For example, the American Heart Association assigns class (strength) of recommendation and levels (quality) of evidence Table 1-4.

Quality EMS research has many benefits for the future. In all health care fields, research determines the effectiveness of treatment—what works and what does not work. Because funding for EMS continues to be a challenge and many aspects of what you will do are coming under scrutiny, it will be important that you and EMS in general are able to prove that your actions make a difference. Proper research achieves this when it is outcome-based, which means the topic generates thoughts on improving the overall patient outcome. Research can help identify which procedures, medications, and treatments work and which do not. Once a study is released and your medical director has decided to follow its recommendations, your service should measure the results of these new practices in your CQI program. These can be as simple as changing jump kit design to providing for a faster door-to-drug administration time for cardiac patients, to adding equipment such as transport ventilators or devices to providing therapeutic hypothermia. These combined efforts eventually will lead to a higher professional image to the community of the services that you provide, regardless of whether you are volunteer or a paid career paramedic.

YOU are the Paramedic SUMMARY

1. What is your first action as you are approaching the scene and conducting a scene size-up?

As you are approaching the scene, do not only look for hazards, but also for the need for any additional resources. Have the fire department dispatched for scene hazards, extrication (for example, from a vehicle), and additional help. Request law enforcement personnel for traffic control and/or crowd control. Are there any other hazards requiring specialized care such as downed power lines or spilled hazardous materials such as oil or gasoline? Do a quick visual inspection to determine the mechanism of injury. How many patients do you see? Call for additional units as soon as possible to minimize scene time and the length of time it will take for all patients to reach definitive care.

2. What role(s) does the EMS system play in this call?

The role of the EMS system at this call will be the same as for all calls: to provide high-quality patient care and transport within the scope of practice for level of licensure. The EMS network begins with citizen involvement. The public must recognize a need and be aware of how to access the EMS system in their community. The public must also be educated on what to do and what not to do to patients prior to your arrival. Once the EMS system has been activated, a dispatcher receives the information, processes or interprets the information, identifies whether this is an actual emergency, and then dispatches appropriate units.

The role of the EMS system continues when providers, such as paramedics, arrive on scene. Roles at the scene will

YOU are the Paramedic SUMMARY (continued)

include determining what is happening at the scene and developing a plan of care for the patients, including deciding on the appropriate transport method and receiving facility.

3. What aspects of professionalism must be employed in this situation?

As a health care professional, you must provide care appropriate for your level of licensure and do so in a manner that builds confidence in your patient as well as others on scene. You are in a highly visible role and will be judged on your level of professionalism and your overall appearance. You are a representative of your profession as well as agency. You must continually show that you are truly concerned for the well-being of your patient and his or her family.

In this situation, you must employ integrity as well as empathy when dealing with the patient's girlfriend. She is scared and upset, as most people are when faced with a traumatic situation they are not familiar with. Communicating with her should not take precedence over patient care, but a kind word can make all the difference. Be aware the girlfriend may be a valuable source of information regarding the patient's history. If you deem the situation serious enough that the patient needs your immediate care, ask another responder to gather this information from her. Work as a team with your partner and, in this case, rescue personnel to help assess, treat, and transport this patient. Ask one of the rescue personnel to talk with the girlfriend and let her know you are doing everything possible to help the patient. Also, let her know which hospital you are transporting him to. You should act as an advocate for this patient because he is unable to speak for himself and advise the hospital of any information received from the girlfriend on scene.

4. Aside from those noted in the previous question, what other roles and responsibilities are vital as a prehospital health care professional?

Educating the public is a large part of your responsibility as a paramedic. You should involve yourself in prevention, community, and leadership activities whenever possible. The public should know how to appropriately use your services, and promotion of public involvement in activities such as cardiopulmonary resuscitation (CPR) training is vital in areas where EMS resources are limited.

5. Even though you do not have standing orders to perform a needle decompression, you know this is what the patient needs. How will you handle getting approval to perform this procedure?

If protocols or care guidelines do not cover the situation you are in, contact online (direct) medical control for guidance. It is imperative that you have a good working relationship with your medical director and the physicians at the hospitals where you frequently transport patients. You are their eyes and ears on the scene and you must provide a clear picture of the circumstances for medical control when requesting orders for actions that fall outside of your protocols. Explain the situation, including your findings, pertinent negatives and vital signs, and your estimated time of arrival, to the physician and provide the reason you are requesting your order. Once the order is given, repeat it back to the physician. Perform the procedure, and then contact medical control with an update.

6. How will you make the determination of how and where to transport this patient?

Appropriate transport and destination decisions are often made through cooperation with other medical professionals. The patient's injuries and presentation should dictate whether he is taken to the closest facility (ie, cardiac arrest) or to a more appropriate location that may be farther away (ie, a trauma center in the case of this patient).

The patient in this scenario has an altered mental status and respiratory compromise, making this an emergency transport. If definitive care is a great distance, air transport may be a better option. Know the capabilities of your local hospitals; many can provide lifesaving and stabilizing care in the emergency department and then arrange to transfer the patient to a more definitive location. However, if the patient potentially needs surgical intervention for stabilization, then transporting him to a facility other than a trauma center may only delay definitive care and increase the risk of morbidity or mortality.

YOU are the Paramedic SUMMARY (continued)

7. Explain why this situation is a good example of how EMS research may help future patients through evidence-based practice.

Through evidence-based practice, patient care is focused on the procedures that have proven useful in improving patient outcomes—needle decompression in this instance. Documenting procedures that have benefited patients in the past helps provide information so research may lead to establishing protocols or standing orders for similar patients in the future.

8. How is retrospective research beneficial for educating EMS personnel?

Retrospective research uses currently available information. Continuous quality improvement (CQI) is a form of retrospective research; examining patient care records helps determine opportunities for improvement and provides information to guide the educational needs for EMS personnel. It can also be used to plan public education and prevention strategies.

EMS Patient Care Report (PCR)

Date: 04-20-18	**Incident No.:** 0457832	**Nature of Call:** MVC	**Location:** 300 block of Hunt Road		
Dispatched: 1618	**En Route:** 1618	**At Scene:** 1621	**Transport:** 1628	**At Hospital:** 1638	**In Service:** 1648

Patient Information

Age: 22 **Sex:** M **Weight (in kg [lb]):** 78 kg (172 lb)	**Allergies:** None known **Medications:** None **Past Medical History:** None **Chief Complaint:** AMS, possible pneumothorax, possible open fx of L lower leg

Vital Signs

Time: 1627	**BP:** 96/54	**Pulse:** 138	**Respirations:** 12	**Spo_2:** 92% on O_2 via bag-mask
Time: 1634	**BP:** 104/62	**Pulse:** 118	**Respirations:** 12	**Spo_2:** 98% on O_2 via bag-mask
Time:	**BP:**	**Pulse:**	**Respirations:**	**Spo_2:**

EMS Treatment (circle all that apply)

Oxygen @ 15 L/min via (circle one): NC NRM (**Bag-mask device**)		(**Assisted Ventilation**)	(**Airway Adjunct:** Oral)	**CPR**
Defibrillation	(**Bleeding Control**)	(**Bandaging**)	(**Splinting**)	(**Other:** Cardiac monitor)

Narrative

22-year-old man involved in an MVC—motorcycle rider who hit car, unresponsive, possible tension pneumothorax, and open fx of L lower leg with minor bleeding. Helmet removed by bystanders prior to EMS arrival. On arrival pt supine on ground unresponsive, pupils equal but sluggish to react, presents with very diminished breath sounds on the left, hyperresonance to percussion, JVD, cardiac monitor showing sinus tach without ectopy, glucose 102 mg/dL. Skin pale, cool, diaphoretic. Inserted oropharyngeal airway, assisted ventilations with bag-mask, splinted L leg to R leg—bleeding controlled with direct pressure and bandaging, full spine immobilized on scoop stretcher with c-collar and blocks, circulation grossly intact in all extremities before and after immobilization. Ventilations became increasingly difficult. Obtained orders from medical control for needle decompression. After performing in 3rd intercostal space midclavicular, ventilations improved, neck veins now flat, Spo_2 increased to 98%, radial pulses stronger and increase in BP, no change in mental status. Transported to Mayfield Medical Center without incident.**End of report**

Prep Kit

▶ Ready for Review

- World Wars I and II saw the development of ambulance corps to rapidly care for and remove injured soldiers from the battlefields.
- During the Korean and Vietnam Wars, wounded soldiers could be saved by using helicopters to rapidly move them from the battlefield to a medical unit.
- In 1966 the National Academy of Sciences and the National Research Council published "The White Paper" outlining 10 critical points.
  - From these points the National Highway Safety Act was instituted in 1966.
  - The US Department of Transportation was also created.
- Paramedics are required to be licensed. This may also be called certification or credentialing. Performing functions as a paramedic prior to licensure is unlawful.
- The standards for prehospital emergency medical care and the people who provide it are governed by the laws in each state and are typically regulated by a state office of EMS.
- A paramedic has a variety of career options. Traditional employment options include fire-based EMS, third-service EMS, private EMS agencies, hospital-based EMS, and hybrid models in which paramedics work alongside other providers or for specific venues.
- There are generally four levels of training: emergency medical responder, emergency medical technician, advanced emergency medical technician, and paramedic. Variations exist from state to state. At the advanced life support levels (paramedic and AEMT), personnel may perform invasive procedures through standing orders or guidance from online (direct) medical control.
- Paramedics may be involved in a variety of types of transports, including transports to specialty centers that focus on specific types of care of specific populations. They may also perform interfacility transports.
- Paramedics work with other health care providers and other public safety agencies. Becoming familiar with their roles and responsibilities is beneficial when on EMS calls.
- Continuing education programs expose paramedics to new research findings and refresh their skills and knowledge; consider those accredited through the Commission on Accreditation for Pre-Hospital Continuing Education (CAPCE).
- Each EMS system has a physician medical director who authorizes the providers in the service to provide medical care in the field. Medical control is typically both off-line (indirect) and online (direct).
- The paramedic profession contains expected standards and performance parameters as well as a code of ethics.
- Professional attributes that a paramedic is expected to have include integrity, empathy, self-motivation, confidence, communication skills, teamwork, respect, patient advocacy, injury prevention efforts, careful delivery of service, time management skills, and administrative skills.
- Some of the primary paramedic responsibilities include preparation, response, scene management, patient assessment and care, management and disposition, patient transfer and report, documentation, and return to service.
- Quality control and continuous quality improvement are tools paramedics use to evaluate the care they provide to patients.
- Research helps bring together the findings of many professionals involved in EMS and brings forth a consensus of what EMS personnel should or should not do. Types of research include quantitative and qualitative research.
- There are many ethical considerations in conducting medical research. Researchers must obtain consent from study subjects, fully inform them of the research parameters, and ensure that the rights and welfare of subjects are protected.
- Paramedics must know how to evaluate medical research. Become familiar with criteria for determining the quality of the research, including how to recognize peer-reviewed literature, and how to use the Internet for finding quality research articles.
- Evidence-based practice is becoming an integral part of functioning as an EMS provider. Engage in reviewing medical literature as it becomes available, and make efforts to stay on top of changing guidelines related to your practice of paramedicine.

▶ Vital Vocabulary

alternative time sampling Time parameters that are set during a research project.

blinding The method of not giving the specifics of a project to the people participating in a research or study.

case study A type of research in which a single case is investigated and documented over a period of time.

Prep Kit *(continued)*

certification A process in which a person, an institution, or a program is evaluated and recognized as meeting certain predetermined standards to provide safe and ethical care.

cohort research A type of research that examines patterns of change, a sequence of events, or trends over time within a certain population of study subjects.

Commission on Accreditation for Pre-Hospital Continuing Education (CAPCE); An organization that develops continuing education standards and is involved in setting accreditation standards for prehospital providers; formerly called the Continuing Education Coordinating Board for Emergency Medical Service (CECBEMS).

continuous quality improvement (CQI) A system of internal and external reviews and audits of all aspects of an EMS system.

convenience sampling A type of research in which subjects are manually assigned to a specific person or crew, rather than being randomly assigned; the least-preferred component of research.

cross-sectional design A data collection method in which all data at one point in time is collected, essentially serving as a "snapshot" of events and information.

descriptive A research format in which an observation of an event is made, but without attempts to alter or change it.

emergency medical services (EMS) A health care system designed to bring immediate on-scene care to those in need along with transport to a definitive medical care facility.

ethical A behavior expected by a person or group following a set of rules.

evidence-based practice The use of practices that have been proven to be effective in improving patient outcomes.

health care professional A person who follows specific professional attributes that are outlined in this profession.

inferential A research format that uses a hypothesis to prove one finding from another.

institutional review board (IRB) A group or institution that follows a set of requirements for review that were devised by the US Public Health Service.

licensure The process whereby a state allows qualified people to perform a regulated act.

literature review A form of research in which the existing literature is reviewed, and the researcher analyzes the collection of research to draw a conclusion.

longitudinal design A data collection method in which information is collected at various set time intervals, and not just at one time.

medical direction Direction given to an EMS system or provider by a physician.

mobile intensive care units (MICUs) An early title given to an ambulance-style unit.

off-line (indirect) medical control Medical direction given through a set of protocols, policies, and/or standards.

online (direct) medical control Medical direction given in real time to an EMS service or provider.

parameters Outlined measures that may be difficult to obtain in a research project.

peer review The process used by medical magazines, journals, and other publications to ensure the quality and validity of an article before it is published, and which involves sending the article to subject matter experts for review of the content and research methods.

profession A specialized set of knowledge, skills, and/or expertise.

prospective research A type of research that gathers information as events occur in real time.

protocol A treatment plan developed for a specific illness or injury.

qualitative A type of descriptive statistic in research that does not use numeric information.

quality control The responsibility of the medical director to ensure the appropriate medical care standards are met by EMS personnel on each call.

quantitative A type of measurement in research that uses a mean, median, and mode.

reciprocity The process of granting licensure or certification to a provider from another state or agency.

registration Providing information to an entity that stores it in some form of record book. In the context of EMS, records of your education, state or local licensure, and recertification are held by a recognized board.

research agenda The specific questions that a study aims to answer, and the precise methods in which the data will be gathered.

research consortium A group of agencies working together to study a particular topic.

research domain The area (clinical, basic science, systems, or education) that will be impacted by a study.

retrospective research Research performed from current available information.

Prep Kit *(continued)*

safety culture In an EMS organization, a system of beliefs and practices that: (1) acknowledge that organizations engage in high-risk activities, (2) determine the importance of consistent safe operations to counteract these activities, (3) support a blame-free environment where errors can be reported without fear of punishment, and (4) maintain organizational commitment to address reported errors and safety concerns.

sampling errors Expected errors that occur in the sampling phase of research.

standard deviation A measure of the range of scores in a set of data relative to the mean score.

standing order A type of protocol that is a written document signed by the EMS system's medical director that outlines specific directions, permissions, and sometimes prohibitions regarding patient care that is rendered prior to contacting medical control.

systematic sampling A computer-generated list of subjects or groups for research.

trauma systems The collaboration of prehospital and in-hospital medicine that focuses on optimizing the use of resources and assets of each with a primary goal of reducing the mortality and morbidity of trauma patients.

unblinded study A type of study in which the subjects are advised of all aspects of the study.

▶ References

1. EMSC IIC. Emergency Medical Services for Children Innovation & Improvement Center website. https://emscimprovement.center. Accessed August 8, 2016.
2. About EMS Compass. EMS Compass website. http://www.emscompass.org/about-ems-compass/. Accessed April 21, 2016.
3. About CAPCE. Commission on Accreditation for Pre-Hospital Continuing Education website. https://www.cecbems.org/About.aspx. Accessed September 26, 2016.
4. Singh JM, MacDonald RD, Ahghari M. Critical events during land-based interfacility transport. *Ann Emerg Med*. 2014:64(1):9–15.
5. Ligtenberg JM, Arnold LG, Stienstra, et al. Quality of interhospital transport of critically ill patients: a prospectiveaudit. *Crit Care*. 2005;9(4):R446–R451.
6. Federman RS. Understanding Vaccines: A Public Imperative. *Yale J Biol Med*. 2014;87(4):417–422.
7. Taylor LE, Swerdfeger AL, Eslick GD. Vaccines are not associated with autism: an evidence-based meta-analysis of case-control and cohort studies. *Vaccine*. 2014;32(29):3623–3629.

Assessment *in Action*

While on shift, you and your partner are dispatched to a call for a 57-year-old man having chest pain. On arrival, his wife tells you he has an extensive cardiac history and hands you a bag full of medications. The patient is pale, diaphoretic, and clutching his chest. He says the pain is on the left side of his chest and radiating up into his jaw and down his left arm. He has not experienced relief from the nitroglycerin he took prior to your arrival.

During the primary survey, you notice that he is breathing at 22 breaths/min with adequate tidal volume and his oxygen saturation is 97% on room air. His radial pulse is rapid and irregular. He tells you that his pain is a "10" on a 1 to 10 scale. He is placed on the stretcher in a position of comfort and quickly loaded into the ambulance for further evaluation, treatment, and transport.

Assessment *in Action* *(continued)*

1. What part of the initial report on this patient is most important?

A. He has left-sided chest pain.
B. He has a cardiac history.
C. His pain is not relieved with nitroglycerin.
D. He has many medications.

2. Why is the patient experiencing pale, diaphoretic skin?

A. The patient has a perfusion problem.
B. The patient is in a cold environment.
C. This is common with all cardiac patients.
D. The patient is anxious.

3. Which paramedic-level skill is essential for assessing this patient?

A. IV therapy
B. Oxygen administration
C. 12-lead ECG
D. Administration of nitroglycerin

4. Which of the following interventions would be the best for this patient?

A. Intravenous line
B. Oxygen by nonrebreathing mask
C. Chewable baby aspirin
D. Nitroglycerin infusion

5. As a licensed paramedic, you may be called on to perform advanced cardiology and pharmacologic skills that are otherwise performed only by physicians or other advanced practitioners. What gives the paramedic the authority to act?

A. A medical director
B. Protocols
C. Standing orders
D. Reciprocity

6. You are caring for a patient at the scene of an accident, when a man steps forward and tells you he is a physician and he wants to assist in taking care of your patient. You do not recognize him, but he shows you his physician credentials. How should you handle this situation?

7. Why has aspirin been found to be so important in acute myocardial infarction?

8. Explain the purpose of EMS research and how to determine if a research article is high quality.

9. Describe traditional avenues of EMS employment.

10. Explain the concept of reciprocity.

CHAPTER 2

Workforce Safety and Wellness

National EMS Education Standard Competencies

Preparatory

Integrates comprehensive knowledge of the EMS system, safety/well-being of the paramedic, and medical/legal and ethical issues which is intended to improve the health of EMS personnel, patients, and the community.

Workforce Safety and Wellness

- Provider safety and well-being (pp 39-46)
- Standard safety precautions (pp 46-51)
- Personal protective equipment (pp 46-49)
- Stress management (pp 53-60)
  - Understanding and dealing with death and dying (pp 60-63)
- Prevention of response-related injuries (pp 39-40, 44)
- Prevention of work-related injuries (pp 39-40, 44)
- Lifting and moving patients (pp 43-44)
- Disease transmission (p 46)
- Wellness principles (pp 39-46)

Medicine

Integrates assessment findings with principles of epidemiology and pathophysiology to formulate a field impression and implement a comprehensive treatment/disposition plan for a patient with a medical complaint.

Infectious Diseases

Awareness of

- A patient who may have an infectious disease (pp 46-48)
- How to decontaminate equipment after treating a patient (Chapter 46, *Transport Operations*)

Assessment and management of

- A patient who may have an infectious disease (Chapter 26, *Infectious Diseases*)
- How to decontaminate the ambulance and equipment after treating a patient (Chapter 46, *Transport Operations*)
- A patient who may be infected with a bloodborne pathogen (Chapter 26, *Infectious Diseases*)
  - Human immunodeficiency virus (HIV) (Chapter 26, *Infectious Diseases*)
  - Hepatitis B (Chapter 26, *Infectious Diseases*)
- Antibiotic-resistant infections (Chapter 26, *Infectious Diseases*)
- Current infectious diseases prevalent in the community (Chapter 26, *Infectious Diseases*)

Anatomy, physiology, epidemiology, pathophysiology, psychosocial impact, presentations, prognosis, and management of

- HIV-related disease (Chapter 26, *Infectious Diseases*)
- Hepatitis (Chapter 26, *Infectious Diseases*)
- Pneumonia (Chapter 16, *Respiratory Emergencies*)
- Meningococcal meningitis (Chapter 26, *Infectious Diseases*)
- Tuberculosis (Chapter 26, *Infectious Diseases*)
- Tetanus (Chapter 26, *Infectious Diseases*)
- Viral diseases (see Chapter 16, *Respiratory Emergencies,* Chapter 26, *Infectious Diseases*, and Chapter 43, *Pediatric Emergencies*)
- Sexually transmitted disease (Chapter 26, *Infectious Diseases*)
- Gastroenteritis (Chapter 20, *Abdominal and Gastrointestinal Emergencies*, and Chapter 26, *Infectious Diseases*)
- Fungal infections (Chapter 26, *Infectious Diseases*)
- Rabies (Chapter 26, *Infectious Diseases*)
- Scabies and lice (Chapter 26, *Infectious Diseases*)
- Lyme disease (Chapter 26, *Infectious Diseases*)
- Rocky Mountain Spotted Fever (Chapter 26, *Infectious Diseases*)
- Antibiotic-resistant infections (Chapter 26, *Infectious Diseases*)

Knowledge Objectives

1. Describe the components of personal well-being and their importance in managing stress. (pp 39-46)
2. List the seven factors that have been found to improve heart health, according to the American Heart Association. (pp 39-40)
3. Explain how mental, emotional, and spiritual well-being pertain to your paramedic career. (pp 44-46)

4. Define infectious disease and communicable disease. (p 46)
5. Discuss the various routes of disease transmission. (p 46)
6. Describe the standard precautions that are used to prevent infection when treating patients. (pp 47-48)
7. Explain the importance of immunizations. (pp 47-48)
8. Describe the various types of personal protective equipment used to protect against airborne and bloodborne pathogens. (pp 47-50)
9. Discuss the importance of ambulance cleaning and disinfection. (p 50)
10. Explain postexposure management when exposed to patient blood or body fluids, including completing a postexposure report. (p 51)
11. Recognize the possibility of hostile situations and the steps to take to deal with them. (p 51)
12. Discuss how to determine scene safety and prevent work-related injuries at the scene of a traffic incident. (pp 51-52)
13. Describe the physiologic, physical, and psychological responses to stress. (pp 55-57)
14. Describe reactions to expect from ill and injured patients, including how you can effectively work with people exhibiting a range of stress-related behaviors. (pp 55-58)
15. Discuss techniques for working at particularly stressful situations, including mass-casualty incidents or the death of a child. (pp 58-63)
16. Describe issues concerning care of the dying patient, death, and the grieving process of family members. (pp 60-63)
17. Describe posttraumatic stress disorder (PTSD) and steps that can be taken, including critical incident stress management, to decrease the likelihood that PTSD will develop. (p 63)

Skills Objectives

1. Demonstrate the necessary steps to manage a potential exposure situation. (p 51)

Introduction

As a paramedic, you have taken steps to provide a higher level of care to the community. You are dedicated to providing prehospital emergency care and transport for those in need, which not only makes your job gratifying, but also very demanding. You will learn many skills to assist with the delivery of emergency medical care, but do not lose sight of the most important factor—your personal wellness and safety, both on scene and off. Because of the existence of scene hazards, environmental conditions, human-made threats, and infectious diseases, scene safety is crucial. The demands placed on you as a paramedic can be either minimal or extreme. For example, you may find yourself working a double shift or holding more than one job, which can compromise your safety because of the lack of rest. Even a single shift may be so busy that you never get time to sit down. Add to that the challenge of making sure you have a proper meal, and you can easily find yourself overworked, undernourished, and at risk for numerous health issues.

With the increasing demands placed on paramedics, your preparation is of the upmost importance. As you begin your career, you may be assigned to a veteran paramedic who will serve as your mentor. Many veterans may have been trained before wellness and safety training were given such high importance in emergency medical

YOU are the Paramedic PART 1

You are performing your morning ambulance check when a call comes in at 0712 hours for a possible cardiac arrest at 984 Solomon Street. You are en route 1 minute later. The traffic is very heavy at this time, and you become agitated as you try to navigate through it. The frustration builds as you think about the dispatch information and the potential of running a field code. You have not had much rest, because you just came from another EMS job where you were busy all night. Besides the lack of rest, you have not been eating well lately, frequently relying on a drive-through meal. You also have been slacking on your workout routine; you have gained a few pounds and notice that you get winded more easily than before. Your coworkers have noted this change and have brought it to your attention, but you tell them you are young and can handle it.

1. The decline of your physical well-being will eventually affect your attitude and, in turn, put your job at risk. What steps can you take to avoid this outcome?
2. Why is it so important to also find ways to enhance your mental, emotional, and spiritual well-being?

Words of Wisdom

New diseases garner media attention, as occurred with Zika virus and Ebola virus when they emerged in the United States. See Chapter 26, *Infectious Diseases*, for a discussion of these diseases and others.

Some diseases may result in a patient being isolated or quarantined. These practices are not the same. According to the Centers for Disease Control and Prevention (CDC), isolation separates a sick person with a contagious disease from people who are not sick, whereas quarantine refers to the restriction of the movements of a person who may have been exposed to a contagious disease to monitor him or her for signs of illness.[1]

services (EMS). Regardless of whom you will work with, this chapter is designed to highlight current suggestions for wellness and how to keep yourself ready for any emergency. Maintaining your health from the beginning will help to ensure a long, healthy, and satisfying career when you become that veteran in 20 or more years.

Several recent studies have assessed injury, illness, and death among EMS workers. One 2013 study entitled *Injuries and Fatalities Among Emergency Medical Technicians and Paramedics in the United States* found that EMS has one of the lowest overall fatality rates compared with other emergency services, such as law enforcement and the fire service.[2] Fatalities tended to be linked to transportation crashes, with ambulance crashes resulting in the highest number of deaths. These ambulance crashes primarily occurred during emergent responses.

The same study reported that in nonfatal injuries, EMS also beat out all other emergency professions. The common injuries were strains and sprains, usually sustained on initial scene response and while moving a patient. The most common injury site was the back. The authors concluded that injuries are not only costly; they tax the system with the loss of available providers. Finally, the authors found that fatigue and sleep deprivation were the major contributing factors to injuries and fatalities. The study revealed that being awake for 21 hours is equal to being legally intoxicated.

Data from the National Highway Traffic Safety Administration shows an annual estimate of 1,500 ambulance crashes in the United States. Fifty nine percent occurred during emergent response, while 34% occurred while non-emergent. From 2007 to 2011 there were over 3,000 crashes involving ambulances, causing 1,400 injuries. Of this number, 29 crashes were fatal, with 33 total fatalities.[3] Additional information about the safe operation of EMS vehicles can be found in the EMS Vehicle Operator Safety course, sponsored by the National Association of Emergency Medical Technicians.

These findings emphasize that, as a new paramedic, you must be aware of your health and well-being while also being aware of your limitations. Never push yourself beyond your normal limits, and seek assistance whenever possible. Finally, always be aware of hazards and other traffic.

Components of Well-Being

Wellness was first defined in 1654 as the quality or state of being in good health, especially as an actively sought goal. A focus on wellness is indeed an important component of any EMS training program because it will enable providers to have a long, rewarding career in patient care.

Wellness is often considered to have three components: physical, mental, and emotional. Some believe that a fourth component, spiritual, is also essential.

Physical Well-Being

If you are in top physical condition and become injured, then you will tend to heal more quickly and with fewer complications than if you were in poor physical condition. Muscle strength, flexibility, cardiac endurance, emotional equilibrium, posture (both sitting and standing), state of hydration, the foods you eat, and the amount of sleep you get will have an effect on your quality of life. Each of these factors may directly impact your chances of avoiding injury or illness on the job. For example, the Life's Simple 7 list from the American Heart Association (AHA) includes seven factors that have been found to improve heart health **Figure 2-1**. Factors include: get active, control cholesterol, eat better, manage blood pressure, lose weight, reduce blood sugar, and stop smoking. Taking these steps can improve your overall physical and mental well-being.

Nutrition

As a paramedic, you will encounter many patients who are in poor health as a result of poor nutrition—yet some EMS providers practice extremely poor nutritional habits themselves. Even though nutritional information changes regularly, current nutritional guidelines are readily available. Research often points out the consequences of poor nutrition, including heart disease, type 2 diabetes, obesity, and a variety of medical conditions. Although EMS providers are strongly encouraged to maintain good health, many services still require providers to work 24-hour shifts, often without meals or rest breaks. Situations like this will clearly challenge you as you try to live a healthy lifestyle.

The US Department of Agriculture (USDA) *Dietary Guidelines for Americans 2015-2020* (available online) suggest eating foods from six categories—fruits, vegetables, proteins, grains, dairy products, and oils—in suggested portions. Research has shown that each person's nutritional requirements are different; therefore, tailor your eating style for your individual needs. For example, a

Manage blood pressure
Control cholesterol
Get active
Lose weight
Reduce blood sugar
Eat better
Stop smoking

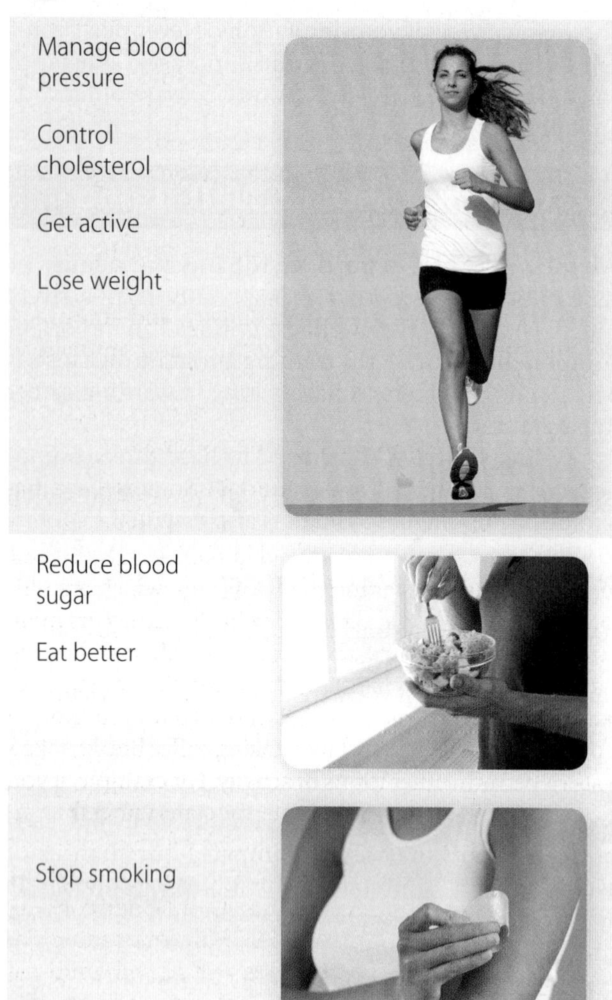

Figure 2-1 The Life's Simple 7 list from the AHA includes seven factors that have been found to improve heart health.

© Antonio Guillem/Shutterstock; © Prostock-studio/Shutterstock; © bikeriderlondon/Shutterstock.

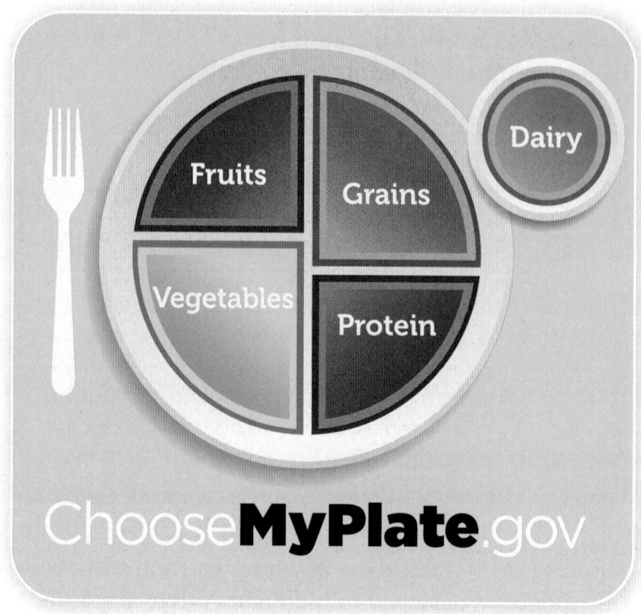

Figure 2-2 The USDA's MyPlate icon emphasizes healthy portions of vegetables, fruits, grains, proteins, and dairy.

Courtesy of USDA.

moderately active woman age 19 to 30 years requires around 2,000 calories per day. This same calorie level is also suggested for sedentary men older than 50 years. On the Choose MyPlate website produced by the USDA (ChooseMyPlate.gov), the MyPlate icon provides a quick look at the recommended relative portion sizes of five of the food groups Figure 2-2 .[4] The amount you need from each of these groups is directly dependent on your age, sex, and level of physical activity.[5] Follow these guidelines to get the nutrients you need:

- **Fruits.** Any fruit or 100% fruit juice counts as part of the Fruit Group. Fruits may be fresh, canned, frozen, or dried, and may be whole, cut-up, or pureed.
- **Vegetables.** Any vegetable or 100% vegetable juice counts as a member of the Vegetable Group. Vegetables may be raw or cooked; fresh, frozen, canned, or dried/dehydrated; and may be whole, cut-up, or mashed. Vary the vegetables you eat; eat more dark green vegetables and orange vegetables, as well as beans and peas. It is suggested that half of your plate should be fruits and vegetables.
- **Grains.** Any food made from wheat, rice, oats, cornmeal, barley or another cereal grain is a grain product. Bread, pasta, oatmeal, breakfast cereals, tortillas, and grits are examples of grain products. Make half your grains whole. Whole grains are healthier because they contain important nutrients that reduce the risk of disease. They also contain more protein and more fiber.
- **Protein foods.** All foods made from meat, poultry, seafood, beans and peas, eggs, processed soy products, nuts, and seeds are considered part of the Protein Foods Group. Beans and peas are also part of the Vegetable Group. Go lean on protein; choose low-fat or lean meats and poultry. Bake, broil, or grill. Vary your choices with more fish, beans, peas, nuts, and seeds.
- **Dairy.** All fluid milk products and many foods made from milk are considered part of this food group. Most Dairy Group choices should be fat-free or low-fat. Foods made from milk that retain their calcium content are part of the group. Foods made from milk that have little to no calcium, such as cream cheese, cream, and butter, are not. Calcium-fortified soymilk (soy beverage) is also part of the Dairy Group.

- **Oils.** Oils are fats that are liquid at room temperature, like the vegetable oils used in cooking. Oils come from many different plants and from fish. Oils are *not* a food group, but they provide essential nutrients. Therefore, oils are included in USDA food patterns. Know your fats; make most fat sources from fish, nuts, and vegetable oils. Limit solid fats, like butter, stick margarine, shortening, and lard; avoid trans fats such as partially hydrogenated oils **Figure 2-3**.

Finally, it is important to read the nutrition label of prepared or processed foods. Many such foods include sodium as a preservative and will have sodium levels that can reach 50% of your daily allowance with one meal. Look at the amount and type of fat, as well as the make-up of the carbohydrates (starches, sugars, and fiber). Remember, even though a food product may be advertised as "fat free," it is not necessarily healthy for you. Look for foods with high fiber content; fiber helps you feel full longer, keeps digestive bacteria healthy, and lowers blood pressure and cholesterol.

Because of the nature of your job, planning healthy, full-course meals will be challenging. Plan for your shift as if you will get minimal time to rest or to eat a meal. Bring bottles of water and various healthy snack bars or fruit with you. When you are hungry, fast food will be tempting—try to avoid it, because the high amount of fat found in much fast food will not be enough to sustain your energy level. Also avoid candy bars, caffeine, and energy drinks; they may give you an instant burst of energy, but after that initial rush of caffeine and sugars runs out, you will feel even more exhausted.[5]

Weight Control

As a paramedic, you will have to act quickly and appropriately. Each day you must observe, assess, access, cope with, and control chaotic situations; therefore, staying fit is an important component for all people who work in the areas of public service. Many of the habits you practice as an adult were formed during your youth. Often, the activities that made you the happiest as a child are the ones that drive you later in life—including eating well and staying active. Although it may be challenging, you can change habits developed in childhood.

The USDA's dietary guidelines include the following key principles:

- Follow a healthy eating pattern across the lifespan.
- Focus on variety, nutrient density, and amount.
- Limit calories from added sugars and saturated fats and reduce sodium intake.
- Shift to healthier food and beverage choices.
- Support healthy eating patterns for all.[5]

The dietary guidelines further define a healthy eating pattern, and deemphasize dieting.[5] Diets are generally not as effective as making healthy food choices. The typical American consumes far too many calories, which are ultimately stored as fat. As you age, this fat storage occurs more readily and becomes much harder to eliminate. The goal should be gradual weight reduction, which is much safer than crash dieting. Gradual weight loss requires you to make a plan and stick to it. Rather than taking coffee breaks, take a walk or perform other forms of activity. For example, if you work in a multi-level building, take the stairs rather than an elevator. Stand up and move around as much as you can; avoid sitting for hours while watching TV, browsing the Internet, or using social media. If you must eat out, consider smaller meals or even sharing a meal with your partner. Eat oatmeal or cold cereal for breakfast, a salad with minimal or no dressing and half a sandwich for lunch, and a sensible dinner that consists of baked or broiled foods.

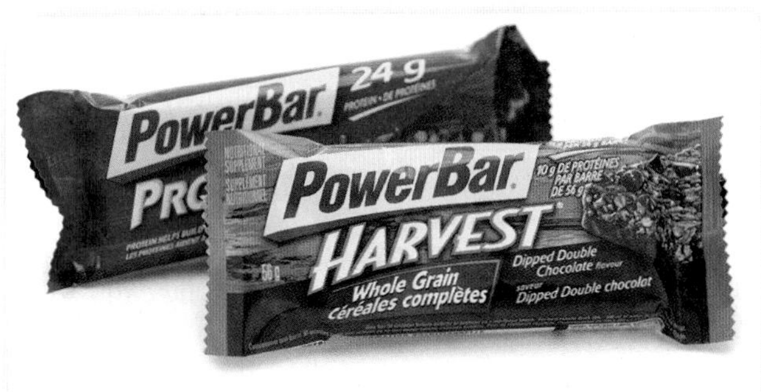

Figure 2-3 Health bars (pictured above) are a quick, healthy alternative to fast food.

Exercise

Regular exercise is associated with overall body weight, nutritional status, and hydration. It has been shown to improve sleep, mental capacity, ability to cope with stress, sex life, and overall long-term health. The exercise program you choose depends on your personal preferences and fitness goals. You are more likely to stick with an exercise program if it is something you enjoy. Aim to maintain, or improve, three areas: your cardiovascular endurance, your flexibility, and your overall physical strength. If you are just beginning an exercise program, then it is recommended that you consult with your primary care physician. Although you may be eager to achieve weight loss and get in shape, you must take it slowly to avoid injury. Remember, you did not gain weight overnight.

In general, it is recommended that adults engage in at least 30 minutes of moderate to vigorous physical activity every day to help build optimal cardiovascular endurance. However, any planned physical activity is helpful. Although you may feel you get enough of a workout during your shift at a busy department, the activity on

Words of Wisdom

Tips for healthy eating include:

- Avoid oversized portions, eat slowly, and allow your body time to identify fullness.
- Focus on fruits and vegetables.
- Vary the types of foods you eat. For example, alternate between seafood, meat, and beans as your protein sources.
- Drink water instead of soda (including diet soda) or other sugary drinks.
- Read food labels closely. Choose foods with lower calories, and lower amounts of fat, sugar, and sodium, as well as high amounts of fiber.

an EMS call is not sufficient to meet the suggested activity requirements for wellness. To stay in good physical condition, you need to find a healthy balance between full-out physical activity (when you are "running hot") and no activity at all Figure 2-4. Many departments are realizing peak physical condition is important and may provide their employees with workout equipment to use both on and off duty.

Depending on your level of health, you should attempt to reach your target heart rate every time you exercise; however, this should not be the goal if you are just beginning an exercise program. The goal is to gradually increase your activity to meet your target heart rate. The AHA suggests that your target be between 50% and 69%

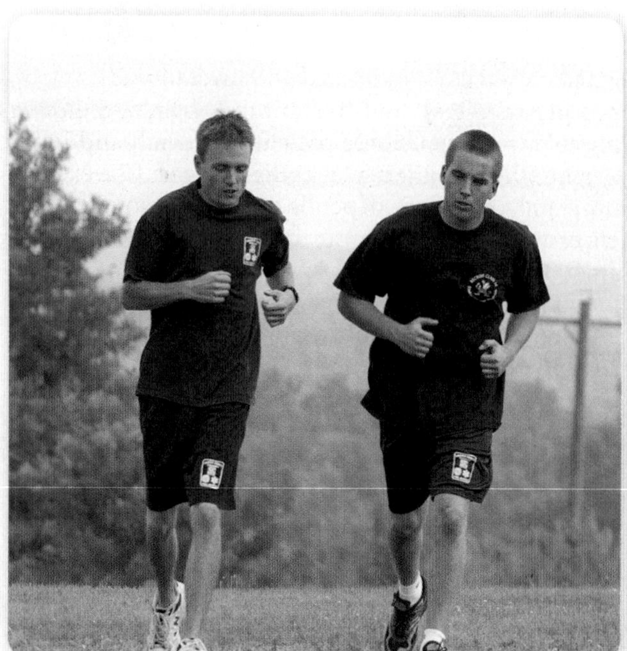

Figure 2-4 Regular exercise—apart from the work you do on EMS calls—should be part of your daily or weekly routine.

of your maximum heart rate.[6] The method to find your target heart rate is as follows:

1. Take 220 and subtract your age in years to find your estimated maximum heart rate (not target range). For example, if you are 40 years old, then your maximum heart rate would be 180 beats/min.
2. Multiply your maximum heart rate by 0.5 and 0.69 to find your target range. In this case, it would be 90 to 124 beats/min.

If you know your resting heart rate, which would be your pulse upon first waking up in the morning and before you get out of bed, then calculate your target heart rate as follows:

1. Subtract your age in years from 220. Next, subtract your resting heart rate.
2. Multiply this number by 0.5 to 0.8, and then add your resting heart rate to find your target range.

For example, a 40-year-old has a resting heart rate of 60 beats/min. Calculations would be as follows:

1. **Resting heart rate**
   60 beats/min
2. **Maximum heart rate**
   220 − 40 = 180 beats/min
3. **Maximum heart rate minus resting heart rate**
   180 − 60 = 120 beats/min
   120 × 0.5 = 60 beats/min
   120 × 0.8 = 96 beats/min
4. **Target heart rate**
   60 + 60 = 120 beats/min
   96 + 60 = 156 beats/min
   Range: 120 to 156 beats/min

Smoking and Tobacco

The negative effects of smoking in relation to health continues to grow. As mentioned earlier, our behavior as adults is often linked to our youth, and some studies suggest that the presence of smokers in the family increases your likelihood to smoke. If you do not smoke, then do not start! With the numerous regulations that have been placed on smoking and advertising, the number of smokers dropped. But now with the vapor-type smoking devices, this habit has seen a resurgence, especially among the Millennial generation. These are banned on airplanes and in many public spaces. Research is underway on the effects of these new devices. You must also understand that everyone responds differently to smoke, and some of your patients may be highly sensitive to its odor. If you smoke right before a call, then the smell on your uniform may be enough to cause serious effects in an already sick patient.

If you do smoke and are trying to quit, then first understand that smoking is truly an addiction and quitting may not be easy. Seek help. Many services now offer smoking cessation classes. Talk to your primary care physician. A variety of programs exist that help to reduce a smoker's psychological dependency. These programs may include instructions, electronic media (for example, DVDs), medications, and counseling to provide ongoing support. Other options include psychotherapy, hypnotism, and acupuncture. The effectiveness of these options appears to be dependent on the individual.

In recent years, electronic cigarettes (e-cigarettes) have become a popular alternative to tobacco cigarettes. Also called electronic nicotine delivery systems or personal vaporizers, these devices simulate smoking tobacco by producing an aerosol made by vaporizing a flavored liquid solution. Though studies indicate that e-cigarettes are less dangerous than other tobacco products, the extent of the danger has not yet been determined.[7] Consequently, these devices should be avoided.

Alcohol Use

As a paramedic, you may notice some people express the common idea that drinking alcohol can alleviate stress, particularly after a "bad call." Alcohol is a drug that can modify how the brain perceives stress. Unfortunately, alcohol cannot alleviate stress, and the uncomfortable nature of stress persists beyond the duration of the effects of the alcohol. Be aware that using alcohol to cope with stress can lead to dependence and result in a magnification of the impact of the stressful situation on your life.

Words of Wisdom

Being a paramedic in the field is physically and mentally demanding. Following simple guidelines for nutrition, exercise, and mental health will greatly enhance and prolong your career. Consider establishing a group of coworkers who share ideas for wellness, or start a friendly weight-loss or activity-level competition. Remember, the only way to benefit from these wellness goals is to commit to them for the long haul.

Circadian Rhythms and Shift Work

Your job as a paramedic will often conflict with your body's circadian rhythm, or natural timing system. Your circadian rhythm is controlled by special areas of your brain, called the suprachiasmatic nuclei, which govern your so-called internal clock. Ignoring your circadian rhythm can cause you to experience consistent difficulties with sleep, higher thought functions, physical coordination, and even social functions. Try to determine what your natural rhythms are and design a schedule that is best for you. Research on circadian rhythms is only beginning to appear in medical journals, suggesting that someday a person might be able to alter his or her internal clock.

Some tips for dealing with shift work are as follows:

- Avoid caffeine.
- Eat healthy meals and try to eat at the same times every day.
- Keep a regular sleep schedule.

Most important, do not overlook the need for rest, whatever your individual rhythm may be. Current research and literature have shown that inadequate sleep has the same effect on your body and mind as intoxication. Inadequate sleep can result in serious consequences while operating an emergency vehicle or determining and administering medications.

Periodic Health Risk Assessments

Besides sleep, diet, exercise, hydration, and all the other things that make up a healthy lifestyle, you need to understand that hereditary factors may also have an effect on your overall health. Research your family's health history. Alzheimer disease, chemical addiction, cancer, cardiac illness, hypertension, migraine, mental illness, and stroke all feature prominent hereditary factors. The most common of all heredity health risk factors are heart disease and cancer. Although family history cannot be changed, you can modify your lifestyle to help you deal with any hereditary issues that arise.

Share this information with your personal physician. Work with him or her to set up a schedule for health assessments, building them into your routine physical checkups. Your physician should be your ally in screening for these diseases and in assessing your lifestyle as well as your heredity.

Body Mechanics

As a paramedic, you will be required to lift and move a variety of patients. Some patients are small and lightweight, whereas others may have significant obesity. You can develop a number of habits to prepare yourself to safely lift most weight ranges, including the following actions:

- **Minimize the number of total body lifts you have to perform.** When patients need to be lifted, be prepared and plan the lift. In many cases, patients do not need to be lifted to a cot or any other location. For example, a patient with an isolated arm laceration and no other issues can walk to the ambulance. Evaluate every situation to identify the easiest and safest way to lift or move a patient.
- **Coordinate every lift prior to performing the lift.** Advise your patients regarding what they may experience during the lift so they do not panic. Once the lift is planned, use clear communication to execute it, such as, "On the count of three, lift." Be sure to plan and clarify

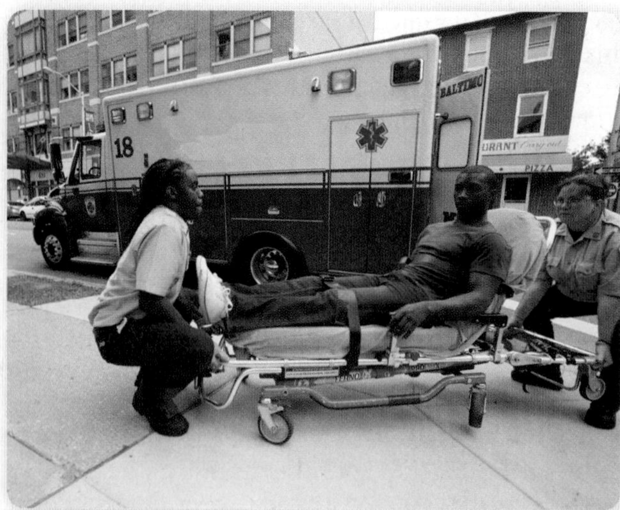

Figure 2-5 If your body is properly aligned when you lift, then the line of force exerted against the spine occurs in an essentially straight line down the vertebrae. In this way, the vertebrae support the lift.

with your team members, in advance, whether the lift will occur on three, or after you say "three."

- **Minimize the total amount of weight you have to lift.** If you have extra people available, then ask for assistance. In some cases, your patient might be able to offer some assistance with moving. If possible, remove any unneeded equipment from the cot.
- **Never lift with your back.** A back injury can be career ending, but you can prevent issues if you do not lift with your back. To help protect your back, follow these precautions **Figure 2-5**:
  - Always keep your back in a straight, upright position and lift without twisting.
  - When lifting, spread your legs about 15 inches (38 cm) apart (shoulder width) and place your feet so your center of gravity is properly balanced. Keep your head upright and facing forward.
  - Hold your back upright as you bring your upper body down by bending your knees.
  - Lift by raising your upper body and arms and by straightening your legs until you are standing.
  - Always lift with your legs, not with your back!
  - Remember to breathe while lifting; do not hold your breath.
  - If you are working with a partner while lifting, then be sure to plan your counting style and exactly how the lift will be performed.
- **Do not carry what you can put on wheels.** Position the ambulance, and the cot, as close to the patient as you can. Most stair chairs now have tracks to make going down stairs easier and safer.
- **Ask for help.** Any time you need to move a patient who cannot or should not walk, consider the possibility of asking an extra person to help you **Figure 2-6**.

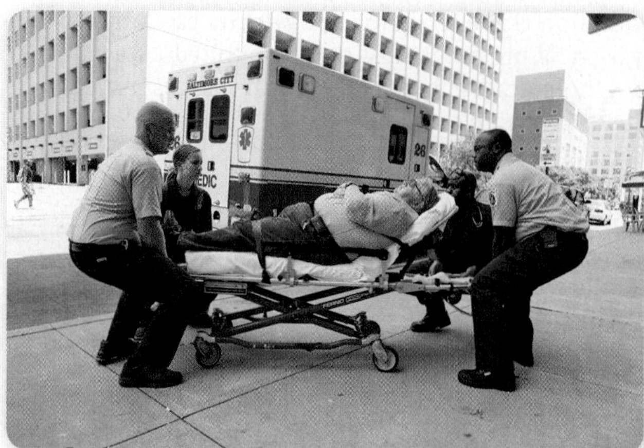

Figure 2-6 Never hesitate to ask for help from your coworkers, or to provide it when you are asked.

▶ Mental Well-Being

As a paramedic, you will not only be exposed to diseases and injuries, but also to stress. When you are subjected to stress, your **fight-or-flight response** is activated. This is the same system that is activated when you exercise or do something fun to promote the feeling of well-being (known as positive stress). It is crucial that you prepare yourself for how you will react when the fight-or-flight response activates. If you are unconditioned or unprepared for stress, then you will not adapt as well to the physiologic responses to your stressor, including increased sympathetic tone, which results in dilation of the pupils, increased heart rate, dilation of the bronchi, mobilization of glucose, shunting of blood away from the gastrointestinal tract and cerebrum, and increased blood flow to the skeletal muscles. These physiologic responses help you deal with the stressful situation immediately, during which you should rely on preplanning and gut instinct as your main resources. However, to maintain your mental well-being for the long term, you need to be able to balance stressful situations with the use of appropriate coping skills.

As a paramedic, you will need to be in control of your emotions at all times, regardless of the situation. Remember, a professional is someone who can remain calm and think clearly when everything else is in disarray. The most important step you can take to control your fight-or-flight response is to plan for it. Many resources are available to help you prepare for stressful situations, such as a physical exercise program or counseling. Stress management is discussed in more detail later in this chapter.

▶ Emotional Well-Being

Paramedics have a natural interest in helping people. To remain healthy throughout your career in EMS, you need to make a deliberate effort to create a healthy balance between your work and home life. Although you may become dedicated to your work, you must separate yourself from your career from time to time—regardless of how much you enjoy it—and focus on your personal life and family. Family members may not understand your EMS life and may feel neglected, or may be otherwise impacted by the effects of your stress. Even if you share the same career as family members and friends, it is still extremely unhealthy to live the lifestyle every day without taking time to step back and reassess.

As an EMS practitioner, you will pour a large amount of energy into EMS, and although this is admirable, you still need to be able to deal with the stress that you are exposed to on the job. A common stressor in EMS is how to deal with patient disability and death. Another common stressor is the "frequent flyer," and the combative and/or belligerent patient. Remember, many of these patients have medical conditions or traumatic injuries that cause their behaviors, but nonetheless, such situations will be stressful for you. As a new paramedic, you may feel that you can or must save every life or have a positive effect on every patient, but in reality, outcomes with some patients will be negative, even with your best efforts. It is important to learn not to take such situations personally.

Good paramedics are strong, sensitive people Figure 2-7. However, these traits are also intertwined with normal emotional reactions to stressors of the job; therefore, you need to develop strategies for coping with stress. If you are approached by a coworker or leader who has noticed changes in your behavior, then take his or her concerns seriously; these could be warning signs that indicate you need to seek assistance. If you note changes in your coworkers, then do not ignore them; pick the appropriate time and, in a calm manner, express to them what you are noticing. Put aside any discomfort you may have about expressing your observations or fear of their reaction, because the action you are taking may be the first step in moving someone back to emotional and physical well-being.

▶ Spiritual Well-Being

Spirituality is an unseen dimension of human experience. Some people address it with formal religion. Medical care supports the dignity and value of life and the sacredness

YOU are the Paramedic PART 2

You arrive on scene 7 minutes later, only to realize you have been to this residence before, and you recall that a 23-year-old man with a history of leukemia lives here. When you arrive, family members inform you it is the same man and his condition has deteriorated rapidly over the past few weeks. Your heart drops as you remember the times you transported him and the conversations you had. You remember thinking to yourself how lucky you are to be healthy and have a good job. This courageous young man has always remained positive about his condition, making you and everyone around him feel better. You feel guilty for the way you have reacted while responding to this call—obviously your frustrations are nothing compared with the magnitude of this family's emotions.

His mother allows you into the house and tells you he began feeling ill yesterday and would not eat last night. She just came in to check on him and found him not breathing.

Recording Time: 0 Minutes	
Appearance	Pale, cyanotic, appears lifeless
Level of consciousness	Unresponsive
Airway	Open and clear
Breathing	Apneic
Circulation	Pulseless
Skin	Cold to touch

3. According to the report from his mother, the patient has been apneic for an unknown amount of time. What should be your next action(s)?

4. On the basis of your previous interactions with the patient, which stage of the grieving process do you feel he reached?

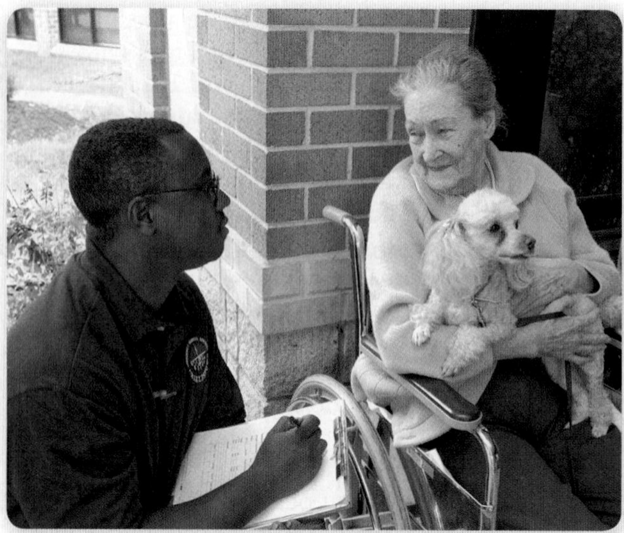

Figure 2-7 One thing that draws people to work as a paramedic is the pleasure of interacting closely with people.

of all people. Your respect for the beliefs of patients or families will help in providing effective patient care.

Disease Transmission

As a paramedic, you will be called on to treat and transport patients with a variety of infectious or communicable diseases. At times, you may have to transport a chronically ill patient without knowing that he or she has an infectious or contagious disease until well after the call. Therefore, make every attempt to identify the disease if you have a good indication that one may be present. An **infectious disease** is a medical condition caused by the growth and spread of small, harmful organisms within the body. A **communicable disease** is a disease that can be spread from one person or species to another. Chapter 26, *Infectious Diseases*, covers the emergency medical care of patients with infectious diseases and protection from specific diseases in greater depth, whereas this chapter covers general protection of the paramedic against such diseases.

Many people confuse the terms *infectious* and *contagious*. In fact, all contagious diseases are infectious, but only some infectious diseases are contagious. For example, pneumonia caused by pneumococcus bacteria is an infectious process, but it is not contagious. In other words, it will not be transmitted from one person to another. However, other infectious agents, such as the hepatitis B virus (HBV), are contagious because they can be transmitted from one person to another.

Immunizations, personal protective equipment (PPE), and simple handwashing can dramatically minimize your risk of **infection**. When you use these protective measures, your risk of contracting a serious infectious or communicable disease is greatly reduced. Proper cleaning and disinfecting of the ambulance and equipment after each call will also help to prevent transfer of diseases to other patients.

When you come in contact with a patient who poses a potential risk of infection to you, discretion is imperative while communicating with other health care providers and your coworkers. Do not give out sensitive patient history over the radio during your patient care report or to anyone who is not directly involved with the patient's care. However, during your transfer of care, provide a complete patient history for the receiving facility. Also include all patient history in your written documentation.

Whereas all infections result from an invasion of body spaces and tissues by germs, different germs use different means of attack. These means are known as the mechanisms of transmission. **Transmission** is the way an infectious agent is spread. Infectious diseases can be transmitted in several ways, consisting of contact (direct or indirect), airborne, foodborne, and vector-borne (transmitted through insects or parasitic worms) transmission.

Contact transmission is the movement of an organism from one person to another through physical touch. The two types of contact transmission are direct and indirect. **Direct contact** occurs when an organism is moved from one person to another through touching without any intermediary. For example, **bloodborne pathogens** are microorganisms that are present in human blood and can cause disease in humans if blood containing the pathogen enters the bloodstream. Another example of direct contact is sexual transmission. Patients who are infected with the human immunodeficiency virus can transfer the virus to their partners during sex.

Indirect contact involves the spread of infection between the patient with an infection to another person through a contaminated, inanimate object. The object that transmits the infection is called a fomite. A needlestick is an example of the spread of infection through indirect contact. In this case, the virus moves from the patient to the needle to the health care provider. This route of transmission was common many years ago before the advent of safety equipment such as needleless intravenous (IV) systems.

Airborne transmission involves spreading an infectious agent through mechanisms such as droplets or dust. The common cold is moved from person to person by coughing and sneezing. Because of airborne transmission, it is unsanitary to use your hands to cover a cough or sneeze because the organism travels onto your hands. Using a tissue when coughing or sneezing is better for controlling the spread of organisms, but you then have a piece of tissue full of organisms. One of the best techniques to avoid contaminating your hands is to cough or sneeze into your inner arm or sleeve. Because you do not touch objects with your inner arms, the risk of moving the organism to an object or person is reduced. The organisms are trapped in the fabric and will eventually die.

Protecting Yourself

Much has changed in EMS since its inception. The use of PPE was uncommon in the early years. It was a status symbol to show how much blood and dirt you were coated with. Surgeons in the 1800s took similar pride in their messy operating aprons, but they were transmitting infectious diseases. Present-day EMS is changing continuously, and new suggestions for protection are made frequently.

Thanks to the research and reporting done by the CDC, EMS providers are now more aware that biohazards are an integral part of their profession and can have long-term effects on the health care worker if certain precautions are not adhered to.[8,9] EMS follows **standard precautions.** Standard precautions approach all body fluids as being potentially infectious. Table 2-1 summarizes the CDC recommendations.

▶ Immunizations

As a paramedic, you are at risk for acquiring an infectious or communicable disease. Using basic protective measures can minimize the risk.

Prevention begins by maintaining your personal health. You should receive annual health exams. A history of all your childhood infectious diseases should be recorded and kept on file. Childhood infectious diseases include chickenpox, mumps, measles, rubella, and whooping cough. If you have not had one of these diseases, then you must be immunized.

Table 2-1 Standard Precautions for the Care of All Patients in All Health Care Settings

Component	Recommendation
Hand hygiene	▪ After touching blood, body fluids, secretions, excretions, or contaminated items ▪ Immediately after removing gloves ▪ Between patient contacts
Personal Protective Equipment	
Gloves	▪ For touching blood, body fluids, secretions, excretions, or contaminated items ▪ For touching mucous membranes and nonintact skin
Gown	▪ During procedures and patient care activities when contact of the health care provider's clothing/exposed skin to copious amounts of blood, body fluids, secretions, excretions, or contaminated items is anticipated
Mask, eye protection, face shield	▪ During procedures and patient care activities likely to generate splashes or sprays of blood, body fluids, secretions, or excretions. Examples include suctioning or ET intubation
HEPA respirator or N95 mask	▪ When working with a patient with TB
Patient Care Environment	
Soiled patient care equipment	▪ Handle in a manner that prevents transfer of microorganisms to others and to the environment ▪ Wear gloves if visibly contaminated ▪ Hand hygiene
Environmental controls	▪ Have procedures for the routine care, cleaning, and disinfection of environmental surfaces ▪ Special attention to frequently touched surfaces within the ambulance (handrails, seats, cabinets, doors) ▪ Have patients with TB wear a surgical mask
Textiles and laundry	▪ Handle in a manner that prevents transfer of microorganisms to others and to the environment
Needles and other sharp objects	▪ Do not recap, bend, break, or hand-manipulate used needles ▪ Use safety features when available (needleless IV systems) ▪ Place sharps in puncture-resistant containers

(continued)

Table 2-1 Standard Precautions for the Care of All Patients in All Health Care Settings *(Continued)*

Component	Recommendation
Special Circumstances	
Patient resuscitation	▪ Use mouthpiece, resuscitation bag, or other ventilation devices to prevent contact with mouth and oral secretions
Respiratory hygiene/cough etiquette	▪ Instruct symptomatic patients to cover mouth/nose when sneezing or coughing ▪ Use tissues and dispose in no-touch receptacle ▪ Perform hand hygiene after touching tissues ▪ Place surgical mask on patient/provider ▪ If mask cannot be used, then maintain special separation distance (more than 3 ft [about 1 m]) if possible

Abbreviations: ET, endotracheal; HEPA, high-efficiency particulate air; IV, intravenous; TB, tuberculosis

Data from: Centers for Disease Control and Prevention. Guideline for Hand Hygiene in Health-Care Settings: Recommendations of the Healthcare Infection Control Practices Advisory Committee and the HICPAC/SHEA/APIC/IDSA Hand Hygiene Task Force. MMWR 2002;51(No. RR-16). Siegel JD, Rhinehart E, Jackson M, Chiarello L, and the Healthcare Infection Control Practices Advisory Committee, 2007 Guideline for Isolation Precautions: Preventing Transmission of Infectious Agents in Healthcare Settings. http://www.cdc.gov/hicpac/pdf/Isolation/Isolation2007.pdf.

The CDC and the Occupational Safety and Health Administration (OSHA) have developed requirements for protection from bloodborne pathogens such as HBV.[10] Your EMS system should have an immunization program in place. Immunizations should be kept up-to-date and recorded in your file. Recommended immunizations include the following:

- Tetanus-diphtheria boosters (every 10 years)
- Measles, mumps, rubella (MMR) vaccine
- Influenza vaccine (yearly)
- HBV vaccine and, if applicable, hepatitis C screening
- Varicella (chickenpox) vaccine or having chickenpox

You should also have a skin test for TB before you begin working as a paramedic. The purpose of the test is to identify anyone who has been exposed to tuberculosis in the past. Testing should be repeated every year if you have been exposed to the disease. Be aware that routine testing may cause an individual to build up a reactive tolerant level, resulting in signs of a positive skin test even if he or she is not infected. It is important to know that a positive skin test does not mean you have TB; it indicates you may have been exposed. Additional follow-up will be needed to determine whether the disease is active, such as radiologic or even blood tests to confirm or clear the results. Other vaccines that are now being suggested include pertussis (whooping cough) and *Staphylococcus aureus*.[11]

If you know you will be transporting a patient who has a communicable disease, then you have a definite advantage. In this situation, your health record will be valuable. If you have already had the disease or been vaccinated, then your risk is significantly reduced or eliminated. However, you will not always know whether a patient has a communicable disease. Therefore, always take standard precautions if the possibility of exposure to blood or other body fluids exists.

▶ Personal Protective Equipment and Practices

At a minimum, each ambulance should be equipped with certain PPE, not just because it is the law under OSHA, but because it is an important part of ensuring your safety. At a minimum, you should have access to gloves, facial protection (masks and eyewear), gowns, and N95 or N100 respirators. The following paragraphs explain the importance of using **infection control** practices.

Wear Gloves

Gloves are absolutely essential on any EMS call, and some patient encounters warrant more than one set of gloves for a provider, depending on the procedure, the patient's history, and the environment **Figure 2-8**. Any time you could be exposed to a patient's body fluids, consider donning a new set of gloves before loading the patient in the ambulance. Be sure to take off your gloves before you drive or leave the ambulance. Use nitrile (nonlatex) gloves if possible to avoid developing a sensitivity to latex or exposing a patient who may have a latex allergy.

Words of Wisdom

If you do not have access to soap and water, then carry waterless hand wipes in your ambulance and use them instead. Isopropyl alcohol, the active ingredient they contain, is a very effective bactericide.

Whatever else you do, wash your hands.

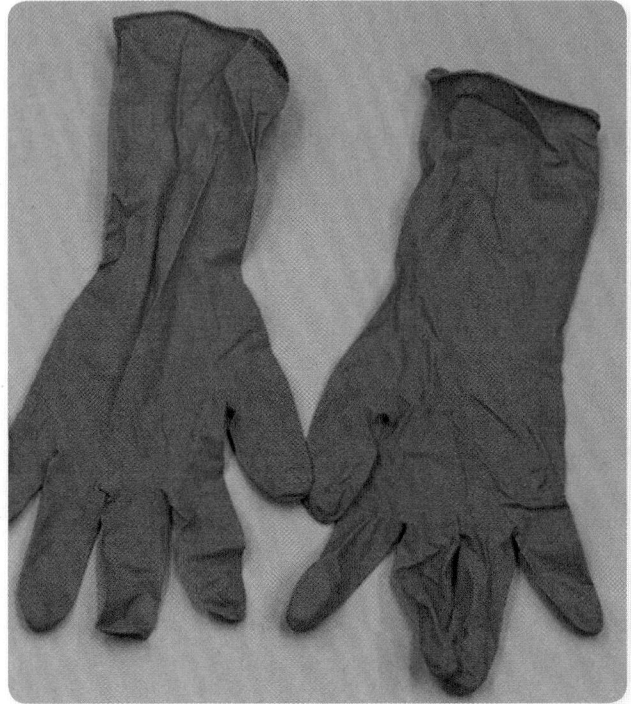

Figure 2-8 Use nitrile gloves on every EMS call.

Wash Your Hands

Get used to washing your hands before and after using the bathroom, before ingesting anything by mouth, before getting into your personal vehicle after a call or shift, and before and after any physical contact between you and a patient or an instrument. Also wash your hands after you remove your gloves.

When you do wash your hands, wash them vigorously with antimicrobial foam or gel for at least 20 seconds before rinsing with clean water.[12] Wash your hands routinely and often. Turn handwashing into a habit. Habits are reliable, even when you are stressed.

Use Hand Lotion

Because of the need for frequent handwashing, your hands will begin cracking because the natural oils are also washed off your skin. Use hand lotion several times a day both on and off duty. Your skin is a very effective barrier to pathogens, as long as it has not been breached by the drying effects of frequent washing.

Use Eye Protection

Many seasoned paramedics make it their standard practice to wear anti-splash eyewear throughout any patient contact. That is a good idea. Eye protection is an absolute necessity during suctioning or intubation procedures. In fact, during intubation, a face shield may offer better protection. Prescription eyeglasses do not offer the same level of protection; use goggles or shields to cover them.

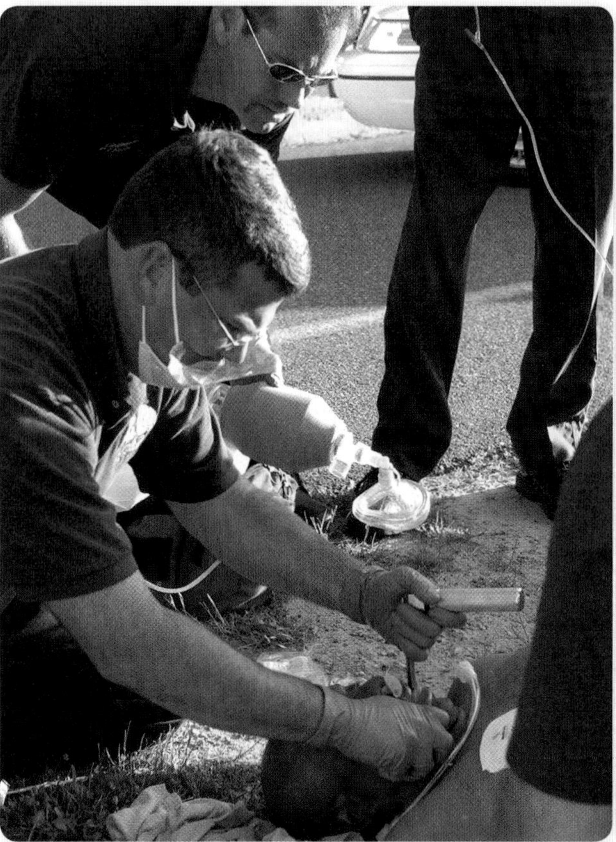

Figure 2-9 You always need to protect yourself from contact with any type of body fluids.

Consider Wearing a Mask

If either you or your patient has an airborne disease, then protect yourself with a surgical mask at the minimum. A surgical mask protects against additional infections during a weakened state. If you are sick, then stay at home; this step is the best prevention to avoid illness. In particular, you should not respond to calls involving patients with compromised immune systems when you are sick.

Protect Your Body

Masks and gowns are appropriate whenever you care for a patient who is extremely messy or bloody Figure 2-9. A 30-gallon (114-L) trash bag can be used as a two-armed glove to slide a patient from a couch or bed onto an ambulance cot if the patient is covered with feces, urine, or blood. After the patient has been moved, you can simply turn the bag inside-out, squeeze the air out of it, tie a knot in its open end, and place it in a hazardous materials (HazMat) bag.

Incontinence barriers should be laid out on a surface if the patient is leaking any type of fluid or has skin lesions.

N95 or N100 Respirators

Read some of the recent statistics by the CDC regarding TB and you will realize this is one of the most common diseases contracted. In 2014, the CDC and world public health associations estimated that 9.6 million people are affected with TB worldwide, with 1.5 million deaths a year.[13] The chance of getting the TB bacillus makes it that much more important to wear the N95 or N100 respirator Figure 2-10 and not just a simple surgical mask. These respirators often require fit testing, which may be offered at your service.

Clean Your Ambulance and Equipment

Sanitize your patient compartment surfaces frequently, but especially the ambulance cot, the bench seat, the grab rails, the deck and deck hardware, and the interior and exterior areas around the door handles. Clean these surfaces daily and after every call. Remove the cot mounts at least once a week to get rid of the dried blood and vomit that tend to accumulate there. Clean this area more often if you have had messy calls. Routinely sanitize the telephones and microphones—especially the ones in the patient compartment, which you may have handled while wearing contaminated gloves.

Sanitize or replace your pen often. You typically handle it several times during every call, with your gloves on. Then, you handle it after the call, after you have washed your hands. Likewise, sanitize your stethoscope with alcohol or disinfectant wipes after every call.

Discard any piece of equipment that is intended for single use in an appropriate HazMat bag. For any reusable piece of equipment that has had direct contact with the patient or patient's body fluids, use a commercial disinfecting agent for decontamination. You can also use bleach diluted in water (1:10) as a disinfecting agent. Disinfection kills many of the microorganisms on the surface of your equipment. Be aware of the type of disinfecting agent you use. Not all disinfectants can be used on every surface, and some are harmful if they come in contact with your skin. Depending on the agent, you may need to keep the surface wet with the disinfectant for 5 minutes or more.

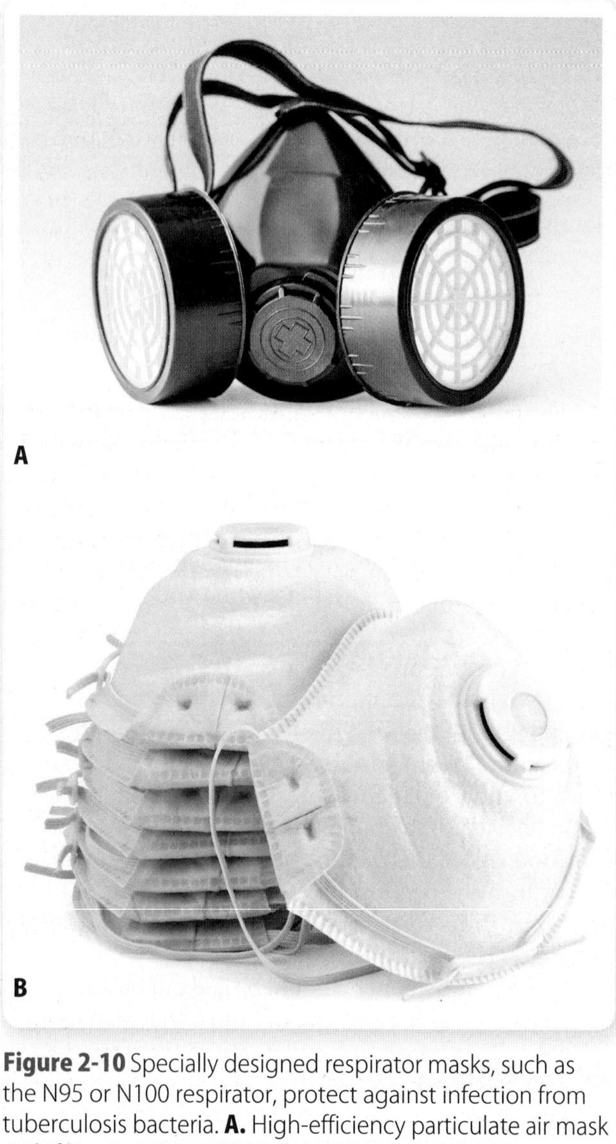

A

B

Figure 2-10 Specially designed respirator masks, such as the N95 or N100 respirator, protect against infection from tuberculosis bacteria. **A.** High-efficiency particulate air mask with filter cannisters. **B.** N95 mask.

Properly Dispose of Sharps

Disposal containers (large for the ambulance and small for carry-in gear) for sharps, such as needles and blades, are essential to protect crews against needlesticks or cuts Figure 2-11.

Consider Wearing Turnout Gear

Turnout gear can be bulky, expensive, and uncomfortable. It does not protect against bullets or knives, but it can protect you from many kinds of chest and abdominal trauma, such as those that occur during extrications and in emergency vehicle crashes. If your service does not have turnout gear, then any scene where turnout gear would be appropriate (such as vehicle crashes) should be handled by properly equipped rescue personnel. Also keep

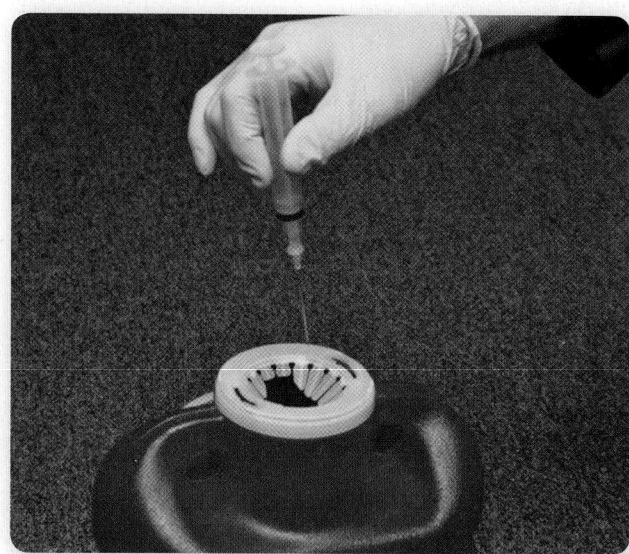

Figure 2-11 Any needles or blades must be disposed of in a sharps container.

in mind that turnout gear is hard to clean; avoid using it in situations that will likely expose you to a patient's blood or body fluids.

▶ Management of an Exposure

In the event that you have been exposed to a patient's blood or body fluids, follow your local EMS guidelines. Generally, any EMS provider who has had significant exposure should do the following:

- Turn patient care over to another EMS provider.
- Wash the affected area immediately with soap and water.
- If your eyes were exposed, then rinse them with water for at least 20 minutes as soon as possible.
- Follow your department's infection control plan.
- Comply with all reporting requirements.
- Get a medical evaluation.
- Obtain proper immunization boosters.
- Document the incident, including the actions taken to reduce chances of infection.

▶ Hostile Situations

As a paramedic, you may be involved with or asked to assist during hostile situations. Potential hostile situations can often be identified using dispatch information, such as a report that "The patient is uncooperative," or "The patient is making verbal threats." In December 2003, the National Association of EMS Physicians released a position statement that, for the first time, offered an official endorsement of the rights to safety not only of patients but also of EMS providers. If you must respond to a hostile situation, then it is best to stage a safe distance away and wait for law enforcement to secure the scene. Specifically, beware of any call dispatched as a fight, stabbing, shooting, domestic disturbance, "person down," or "unknown medical aid." Every one of these calls is suspicious and warrants an initial response by police. In addition, you should request law enforcement to any call that your gut instincts suggest could be violent.

It is imperative that you seek any necessary training to help you understand how to safely handle hostile situations. Numerous resources are available, including Tactical Emergency Medical Services or Rescue Task Force programs. Many law enforcement agencies have used these courses to develop their own systems that fit their regions. If you are going to be routinely involved in hostile situations, then your EMS agency should first work with your local law enforcement and identify needs, then fill those needs preferably by their recommendations.

Never enter the scene first if the element of hostility is known or can be anticipated in advance. Discipline yourself to scrutinize all information that comes to you from others, and keep yourself on "yellow alert" any time you are on duty. Remember, waiting for law enforcement to arrive does not make you an uncaring provider. If you get hurt, then you will be unable to help other patients.

Before you come in contact with a hostile patient, carefully review your surroundings. First identify the fastest way to exit the area, then look for potential weapons in the general area and within reach of the patient. After you make contact with a hostile patient, listen more than you talk, and do not argue with or ridicule the patient. Concentrate on de-escalating the patient's emotions. Many hostile patients who start out unwilling to go to the hospital will agree to transport as a result of your patience, tactful reasoning, and reassurance.

Remember that anytime you are on someone else's turf, he or she has a clear advantage. You can expect him or her to know everything about the environment while you know nothing (including the location of any weapons). Hostile patients in their home environments are much more dangerous there than anywhere else—especially in poor lighting.

> **Words of Wisdom**
>
> Some of the most dangerous calls are those with limited or vague information. If a 9-1-1 caller refuses to give adequate information to a dispatcher, then the dispatcher should communicate that fact to you. Ensure law enforcement has been dispatched or request law enforcement to respond to the scene first or with you to ascertain safety.

Finally, show empathy and understanding on the scene, and you will earn the trust of your patients. Knowledge of diverse cultures plays a major role in effective communication. The more you know about the people you serve, the more likely you will know their customs and expectations. Be diligent in your pursuit of treating all patients with respect and dignity, putting your personal prejudices aside. By doing so, you can potentially lessen the stress of the emergency situation.

▶ Traffic Incidents

Regardless of where you live or work, motor vehicles may move at high speeds, may carry hazardous substances, and may collide with one another in locations that are

> **Words of Wisdom**
>
> If you are the first unit to arrive on the scene, then perform a scene size-up and notify other responding units of any actual or potential hazards that may be present. Your first job is to ensure your safety as well as the safety of your crew and any bystanders.

dangerous for you and all involved. It is important to stay aware of your surroundings, even the familiar ones that you see day in and day out. With the widespread use of various technologies such as smartphones and global positioning systems, distracted driving is becoming as problematic at driving under the influence of drugs or alcohol. At many scenes, bystanders or other motorists want to see what the action is all about. In focusing on the traffic incident, they may not pay attention to you; therefore, you always need to be aware of other vehicles and onlookers.

Like any scene, your approach at a traffic incident should include a visual assessment of your entire surroundings. Look for hazards before you enter the scene. Hazards include downed power lines or poles, leaking fuel, and potential for fire. Become familiar with your response area to determine your best and safest route. This is critical information, because it also alerts those who might be available to help you with traffic control, air support, HazMat, terrain issues, and potential destinations. Some states have programs in place that help with traffic incident management. For example, the state of Wisconsin initiated the TIME Program, which stands for Traffic Incident Management Enhancement. This program teaches all emergency responders the safest way to set up a scene and how to identify hazards. As a new paramedic, seek out any programs and resources your state or location may offer—your life could depend on it.

Traffic may be only one of the many hazards at the scene of a motor vehicle crash **Figure 2-12**. For example, parking a hot, running ambulance over dry grass may initiate a grass or vehicle fire. Remember, your primary concern at any scene is safety; safety for yourself as well as for those around you. Identify as many hazards as possible while you drive up and before leaving your unit.

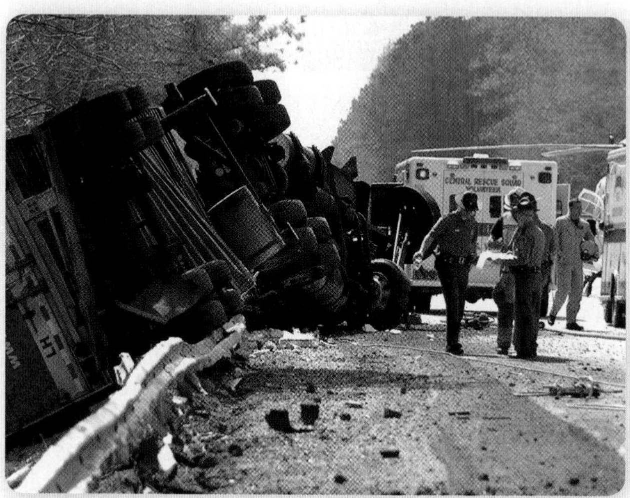

Figure 2-12 To minimize the risk of any additional incidents at a busy crash scene, it is important to place your vehicle in a safe, visible location from which you can easily exit and one that is not too close to potential hazards.

Begin making physical observations a mile or so before you approach the scene. Watch the traffic, pay attention to the wind direction, look for smoke, and begin planning for lighting and weather-related issues. As you get closer, note the kinds of vehicles and obstacles involved. If traffic is not yet handled, then determine the flow of traffic and how to control it initially.

Important considerations include the following: How big an incident do you have, both in size and scope? Are you dealing with commercial carriers of industrial products? What resources will you need immediately? What is the topography? Where will leaking fluids drain naturally (if evident)? Where do you eventually want to park the ambulance? What will your working space be?

Words of Wisdom

The safe operation of emergency vehicles is an important part of any EMS provider's job. Principles of properly and safely operating an emergency vehicle include judicious use of lights and siren, proceeding cautiously through intersections, always remaining calm, and never assuming that other drivers will yield. These and other principles are covered in greater detail in Chapter 46, *Transport Operations*.

Driving with lights and siren does not authorize you to ignore due regard for other motorists on the roadway or to drive at excessive speeds. Remember that ambulances do not handle the same as other motor vehicles. They require significantly more time and distance to stop, and you can more easily lose control of the ambulance. Most states have specific rules or statutes on use of lights and siren.

Words of Wisdom

Scene safety begins with preparation. As you and your partner or crew prepare to respond to the scene, make sure you fasten your seat belts and shoulder harnesses before you move the ambulance.

Patient Safety

Human errors often occur in the context of a poorly designed system. For example, lapses in human tasks may occur secondary to long work hours, and predictable mistakes occur when inexperienced staff members face complex cognitive decisions. Instead of punishing the person, the systems approach to EMS seeks to identify the situations that give rise to human error and change the underlying problem.

Stress

As discussed previously, EMS is a high-stress job. Understanding the causes of stress and knowing how to deal with stress is crucial to your job performance, health, and interpersonal relationships. To prevent stress from negatively affecting your life, you need to understand what stress is, its physiologic effects, what you can do to minimize these effects, and how to deal with stress on an emotional level.

Any event that causes you to react physically, emotionally, or mentally is considered **stress**. Stress events may be pleasant, unpleasant, mild, or intense. Hans Selye, MD, PhD, considered the so-called father of stress theory, has defined biologic stress as the "nonspecific response of the body to any demand made upon it."

Stress is a reaction of the body to any agent or situation (**stressor**) that requires the person to adapt. Adaptation is necessary for meeting the demands of everyday life. By itself, stress is neither a good thing nor a bad thing; nor should stress be avoided. Selye classified stress into two categories: eustress (positive stress), the kind of stress that motivates a person to achieve; and distress (negative stress), the stress that a person finds overwhelming and debilitating **Figure 2-13**.

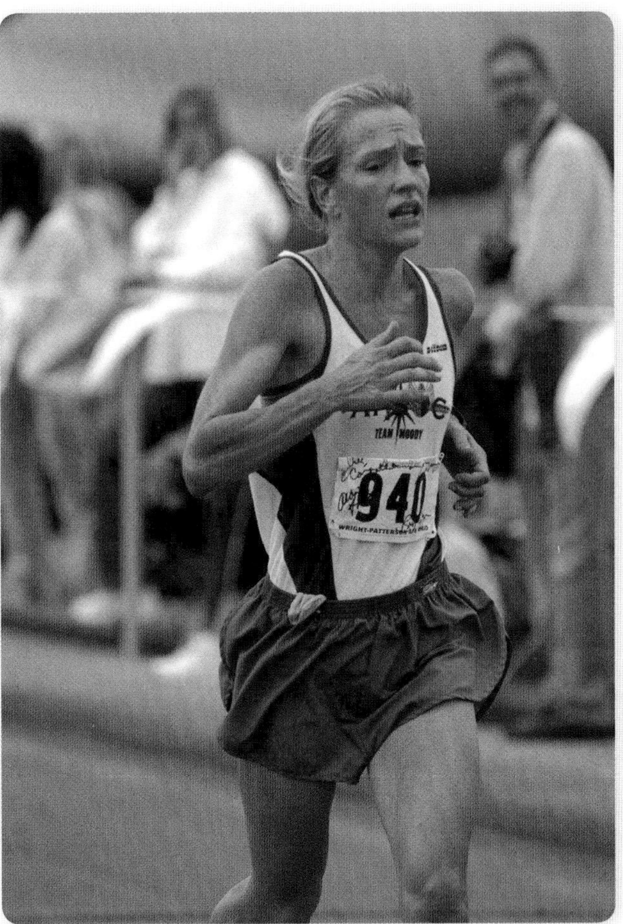

Figure 2-13 Positive stress (eustress) can push you to greater achievements.

Courtesy of Island Photography/U.S. Air Force.

Words of Wisdom

As a paramedic, you may be led to believe that showing emotion is a sign of weakness. However, showing appropriate emotions in certain situations can actually help a grieving family or patient. Everyone reacts differently to stressful events. Some people may get angry, whereas others may laugh or be silent. Do not assume that people are not affected by stress because they do not react in a way you feel they should.

What Triggers Stress

A stress response often begins with events that are perceived as threatening or demanding, but the specific events that trigger the reaction vary enormously from person to person. The following factors are the most common stress triggers in most people:

- Loss of a loved one (death of a spouse, family member, close friend, or colleague) or of a valued possession
- Personal injury or illness
- A major life event (starting or finishing school, marriage, divorce, pregnancy, or having children leave home)
- Job-related stress (conflicts with others, excessive responsibility, the possibility of losing a job, or changing a job)

YOU are the Paramedic PART 3

Your partner attaches the cardiac monitor to the patient and you note asystole in two leads. As you were lifting his shirt for your partner to attach the electrodes, you also noticed some lividity. Family members are starting to arrive. The patient's mother is becoming hysterical and asks you to do something. She tells you her son cannot be dead because she asked God to give him just a few more months. Your partner steps outside to call the dispatcher, law enforcement, and the coroner, and leaves you to talk with the family.

5. How will you explain the situation to the family, and what is your responsibility to them?
6. Which stage of the grieving process is the patient's mother exhibiting?

During the past three decades, a number of studies have assessed the psychological stress levels in paramedics. The studies that seek to evaluate stress levels and compare them usually examine life-change units, or LCUs. These LCUs were originally described in the Life Change Theory by Adolph Meyer and further explored by researchers Thomas Holmes and Richard Rahe.[14] The researchers used the "Social Readjustment Rating Scale" that ranks 43 stress-producing events in a person's life and provides a weighted score for each event Table 2-2.[14] The authors

Table 2-2 Social Readjustment Rating Scale

Rank	Life Event	LCU	Rank	Life Event	LCU
1	Death of a spouse	100	23	Son or daughter leaving home	29
2	Divorce	73	24	Trouble with in-laws	29
3	Marital separation	65	25	Outstanding personal achievement	28
4	Jail term	63	26	Spouse begins or stops work	26
5	Death of close family member	63	27	Begin or end school	26
6	Personal injury or illness	53	28	Change in living conditions	25
7	Marriage	50	29	Revision of personal habits	24
8	Fired at work	47	30	Trouble with boss	23
9	Marital reconciliation	45	31	Change in work hours or conditions	20
10	Retirement	45	32	Change in residence	20
11	Change in health of family member	44	33	Change in schools	20
12	Pregnancy	40	34	Change in recreation	19
13	Sexual dysfunction	39	35	Change in church activities	19
14	Gain of new family member	39	36	Change in social activities	19
15	Business readjustment	39	37	Mortgage or loan of less than $10,000	17
16	Change in financial status	38	38	Change in sleeping habits	16
17	Death of close friend	37	39	Change in number of family get-togethers	15
18	Change to different line of work	36	40	Change in eating habits	13
19	Change in number of arguments with spouse	35	41	Vacation	13
20	Mortgage over $100,000	31	42	Christmas	12
21	Foreclosure of mortgage or loan	30	43	Minor violation of the law	11
22	Change in responsibilities at work	29			

Check off those events that currently apply to your life and add up the corresponding points. A score below 150 is thought to be within the range of normal stress. A score between 150 and 199 suggests a mild stress; between 200 and 299 points suggests a moderate stress; above 300 points is indicative of a major stress.

Abbreviation: LCU, life-change unit

predicted that a score above 150 LCU could cause or be associated with the development of disease and illness (eg, heart attack, stroke).[14]

To deal effectively with stress, as a paramedic, you need to make a personal appraisal of the stress triggers in your life and take or plan appropriate actions to minimize their effects.

▶ The Physiology of Acute Stress

One of the fundamental models for stress evolved from studies of how humans responded to threats. It was observed that when a person perceived an event as threatening, a standard series of physiologic reactions was triggered, whatever the threat (this is why Selye referred to stress as a nonspecific response).

Typically, these physiologic reactions prepare the body for the fight-or-flight response by activating the sympathetic nervous system (discussed further in Chapter 8, *Anatomy and Physiology*). The fight-or-flight response was a very useful survival mechanism for early humans, mobilizing the person to either defend (fight) or to run away (flight) in the face of possible danger. In the modern world, however, the automatic fight-or-flight response to stressful circumstances is not as useful as it was once thought to be. Most of the stressors that you face today should not be solved by fighting or running away. In fact, most negative stress responses are the result of an accumulation of smaller stress events, thereby placing the body in a continuous, unrelieved state of alert. Chronic exhaustion and ill health can result. Therefore, you should evaluate and handle every stress event immediately, especially if it is negative in nature. Running away or ignoring the problem will not make it go away.

Reactions to stress can be categorized as acute, delayed, or cumulative. **Acute stress reactions** occur during stressful situations. As a paramedic, you may feel nervous and excited, and your ability to focus may increase. If the stress of the situation becomes too great, however, then you may experience negative emotional and physical reactions.

Delayed stress reactions manifest after the stressful event. During a crisis, you will be able to focus and function, but afterwards, you may be left with nervous, excited energy that continues to build. As a new paramedic, you must identify events that may cause a delayed stress reaction in you and learn stress management techniques to improve your ability to effectively manage stress when it occurs.

Cumulative stress reactions can occur when you are exposed to prolonged or excessive stress. After the stressful event is over, you may be unable to shake off its effects—even with the aid of stress management techniques. Inevitably, another stressful situation occurs and then another. Each time, you may find it harder to recover from the event, and you become more exhausted and overwhelmed. Cumulative stress can result in physical symptoms, which are your body's way of saying there is a problem. These symptoms include fatigue, changes in appetite, gastrointestinal problems, or headaches. Stress may cause insomnia or hypersomnia, irritability, inability to concentrate, and hyperactivity or underactivity. In addition, stress may manifest itself through psychological reactions such as fear, dull or nonresponsive behavior, depression, oversensitivity, anger, irritability, frustration, isolation, inability to concentrate, alcohol or drug abuse, and loss of interest in work or sexual activity. Your fast-paced lifestyle as a paramedic compounds these effects by not allowing you to rest and recover after periods of stress. Prolonged or excessive stress has been proven to be a strong contributor to heart disease, hypertension, cancer, alcoholism, and depression. Additionally, cumulative stress can eventually lead to job burnout, which is discussed later in this chapter.

▶ How People React to Stressful Situations

Anyone—the patient, the family, bystanders, or health care professionals—who confronts critical illness or injury responds in some way to the stresses of each emergency.

Words of Wisdom

Learn to look for or recognize signs of stress in yourself, your coworkers, and your patients. Early discovery can often allow you to practice techniques to prevent the stress from worsening.

Responses of Patients to Illness and Injury

Patients' responses to emergencies are determined by their personal methods of adapting to stress. As a paramedic, it will help you to recognize certain common patterns of coping. A common response by many patients is anxiety. Some people will exhibit their anxiety by denying it; others become irritable or angry and may direct this hostility towards you. It is important to not take such behavior personally. Remaining calm and reassuring is one of the best de-escalation techniques. Several common reactions to illness and injury include the following:

- **Fear.** Patients may have realistic fears, such as fear of pain, disability, or death (or fear of their economic effects). Patients may also fear the actions you need to take to care for them, such as using needles to start an IV line or give medications.
- **Depression.** Depression is a common and natural response to loss. The patient who has had a stroke, for example, may have lost the ability to move an arm or leg on one side of the body and even the ability to speak, but can understand everything you say and do. Depression may also be evident when you are

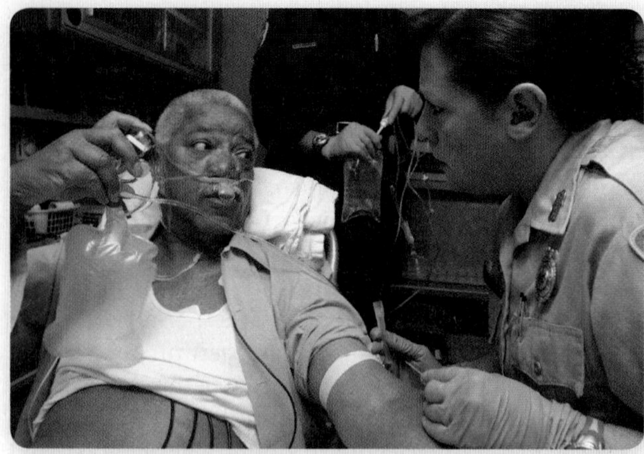

Figure 2-14 The sudden loss of control a patient feels when being treated during an emergency can lead to unexpected and sometimes extreme reactions.

on a scene where you have just ceased efforts to resuscitate a loved one.

- **Anxiety.** Patients may exhibit diffuse anxiety, a feeling of helplessness or a loss of control. People whose self-esteem depends on being active, independent, and aggressive are particularly vulnerable to anxiety when they become ill or injured. At times, anxiety may appear similar to anger; it is imperative that you recognize the difference. If you incorrectly identify someone as angry, then this may put you in a defensive position and may prevent you from addressing the patient's anxiety and individual care needs.
- **Anger.** Anger is one of the most difficult problems for many EMS providers to deal with Figure 2-14. You may have a natural tendency to think, "I am trying to help this person, so why is he taking it out on me?" It is crucial to remember that some patients often respond to fear, discomfort or limitation of function through anger, and their extreme reactions are not the fault of either you or your team.
- **Confusion.** Confusion can occur with anyone, but more commonly among older patients in whom illness or injury may cause disorientation. Confusion is furthered by the presence of unfamiliar people and equipment, which may seem overwhelming. If a patient appears confused, then it is important that you explain carefully at the outset who you are and what you plan to do. Allow the patient enough time (within reason) to gather his or her thoughts and become comfortable with the situation.

In addition to experiencing the reactions just described, some patients may show one or more of the following psychological **defense mechanisms**:

- **Denial.** Patients often ignore or diminish the seriousness of the emergency situation. Some patients may downplay their symptoms with words such as "only" or "a little," whereas others may dismiss their symptoms altogether only to describe them to hospital staff after arrival at the emergency department. You may have to seek out others for reliable information in these cases.
- **Regression.** Regression is a return to an earlier age level of behavior or emotional adjustment. Children often exhibit this defense mechanism when under stress because of the fear of "getting in trouble." Adults may also revert to childlike behaviors when under stress. Patients with other psychological disorders may exhibit regression normally.
- **Projection.** Projection is attributing personal (sometimes unacceptable) feelings, motives, desires, or behavior to others. Patients who express vehement indignation or anger can unconsciously be denying their own "bad" behavior by attributing it to other people.
- **Displacement.** Displacement occurs when someone redirects an emotion from the original cause of the emotion (such as a cardiac condition) to a more immediate substitute (such as a paramedic). Displacement is often the operative mechanism when patients express anger towards you, but in reality, patients are angry at someone else—themselves, a family member, fate, or just the situation.

As noted, most of the psychological stress responses are not under your patients' conscious control. It is not uncommon for ill or injured patients to respond angrily toward EMS providers, only to forget about it after the situation has passed.

Often, reactions to illness or injury are rooted in the patient's culture. Modern society is becoming more multicultural, and people of some cultures may openly exhibit behavior that might be considered inappropriate in another culture. It is important for you to respect the cultural background of your patient. Never attempt to change someone's behavior just because it is different from your own.

Many Americans place great emphasis on making eye contact, having a firm handshake, and respecting personal space. Some patients may not make eye contact because their culture believes that lowered eyes shows deference to your authority and uniform. When making physical contact, obtain permission, if possible, beforehand. Identify and understand the cultural differences of the populations you serve Figure 2-15.

Responses of Family, Friends, and Bystanders

Bystanders and family members may exhibit responses that are similar to those exhibited by patients. Family members may be anxious, panicky, or—especially if they

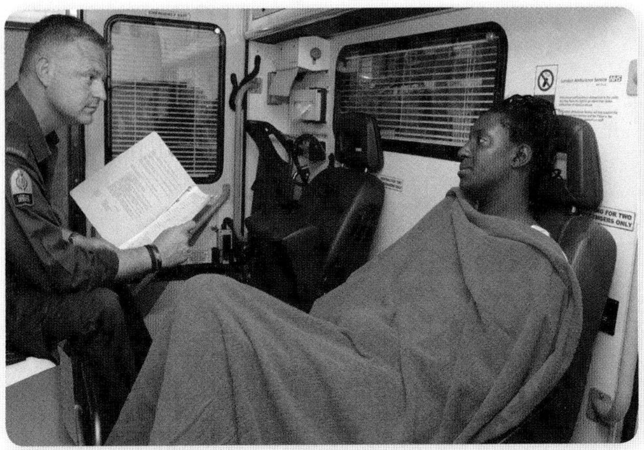

Figure 2-15 Particularly when serving people whose backgrounds are different from your own, you must always maintain an open, nonjudgmental attitude.

are struggling with guilt—angry. Consciously or unconsciously, family members may feel responsible for what has happened; for instance, they may believe that if they had kept a closer eye on a child, for instance, he or she would not have run out into the street and become injured. Some family members may insist that you do something differently or act more quickly during an emergency.

As a paramedic, you must recognize that the patient's family and friends have concerns too and that their behavior, however unpleasant, is a result of distress. Do not take it personally, and remain calm. Reassure family members that you are doing everything you can and that you have physician guidance available at all times. You will often enter situations in which everyone is under stress, and you have no guarantee that people are going to behave appropriately.

In a situation involving mass casualties, such as a multiple-vehicle collision, building collapse, or natural disaster (such as a tornado, flood, or earthquake), both patients and bystanders may react by becoming dazed, disorganized, or overwhelmed. Reactions to stress are defined differently depending on the organization or resource; below are five of the most common reactions. In general, people with these reactions (including your coworkers) should be removed from the scene, but not left alone—find someone who is capable of handling them.

- **Anxiety.** Signs of anxiety include sweating, trembling, weakness, nausea, and sometimes vomiting. People experiencing this response can recover fully within a few minutes and provide useful assistance if properly directed. You are also not immune to anxiety. It is important you are able to identify this response and accept assistance as needed.
- **Blind panic.** A more worrisome reaction is blind panic, in which a person's judgment seems to disappear entirely. He or she may not fully understand the situation at hand or its dangers. Blind panic is particularly dangerous because it may cause mass panic among others present.
- **Depression.** Depression is seen in the people who sit or stand in a numbed, dazed state. Depressed bystanders need to be brought back to reality as soon as possible; do not leave them to sit and dwell on the situation.
- **Overreaction.** People who overreact to stress tend to talk compulsively, joke inappropriately, become overly active, and race from one task to another without accomplishing anything useful.
- **Conversion hysteria.** In conversion hysteria, the patient subconsciously converts anxiety into a bodily dysfunction; he or she may be unable to see or hear or may become paralyzed in an extremity.

More details on how to cope with bystanders are found in Chapter 47, *Incident Management and Mass-Casualty Incidents*.

Special Populations

When children are seriously ill or injured, family members and other people at the scene may become frantic. You need to remain calm and confident in your skills because this may be all that is needed to provide reassurance to everyone at the scene. Children will often respond better to people who are calm, even if their illnesses or injuries are significant.

Responses of the Paramedic

As discussed, you are not immune to the stresses of emergency situations. Expect that you will sometimes experience a multitude of feelings, not all of them pleasant. Even unpleasant feelings are natural, and although it may be difficult, you must keep control of them during an emergency or when dealing with patients and their loved ones. An attitude of outward calm and confidence on your part will do much to relieve the anxieties of others at the scene—and that, too, is part of a paramedic's therapeutic role.

One common reaction among health care professionals is a feeling of irritation at the patient who does not appear to be particularly ill or injured. Consider the possibility that people who call 9-1-1 with seemingly minor complaints are calling because in their eyes, it is an emergency—for example, imagine a woman who calls 9-1-1 because she cannot get to sleep. Her problem is that it is her first night back home after the funeral of her husband. She is scared to death of her first night alone in the house and she did not know who else to call. Remember, laypeople do not have the training and understanding that you have. You can take advantage of situations like the above example to educate and politely remind people that their nonemergent issue can prevent you from being available for someone who may truly need you.

> **Words of Wisdom**
>
> Do not assume that seemingly nonemergency complaints are not a sign of something wrong. Tunnel vision can cause many mistakes in patient assessments and ultimately in patient outcomes.

▶ Coping With Your Own Stress

Some early warning signs of your own stress may include heart palpitations, rapid breathing, chest tightness, and sweating. You may find that you no longer enjoy your career or that you lack the energy or the desires you once had. It is important that you identify your body's reaction to the fight-or-flight response. You may notice rapid breathing and breathlessness, unnecessary shouting, and perhaps the use of inappropriate language that you would not normally use. As discussed previously, others may notice signs of stress and alert you; do not become offended because this observation can help you take appropriate and immediate action. You can prepare for or handle stress in many different ways. Remember that once you enter fight-or-flight mode, you are primarily functioning by instinct. Consider the following stress management techniques:

- **Controlled deep breathing.** Take deep breaths in through the nose and out through the mouth. Controlled deep breathing may flood the body and brain with oxygen just prior to activation of the fight-or-flight response and may help prevent it from engaging.
- **Progressive relaxation.** Progressive relaxation is a strategy in which you tighten and then relax specific muscle groups to initiate muscle relaxation throughout the body. This technique may be performed before, during, or after a call.
- **Professional assistance.** Even the best paramedic may not be able to handle the continuous onslaught of stressful events. Seek out professional services such as employee assistance programs or critical incident stress management services described later in this chapter Figure 2-16.

Other coping strategies include focusing on the immediate situation while on duty. Remind yourself, "I will do my very best, even if the situation does not turn out well."

As discussed previously, avoid excessive amounts of stimulants such as caffeine or the urge to use alcohol, cigarettes, or sleeping aids after a stressful event. Attempt to get enough natural rest. Exercise vigorously and regularly (although not right before bedtime). Identify people and activities that make you laugh or feel good, or befriend a coworker who can relate to you and offer support when needed.

▶ Burnout

Another sign of stress is job burnout. Why should you start worrying now about something that may not ever happen? You must understand that the beginning of your EMS career is the right time for you to start developing attitudes and habits that will help prevent burnout.

Burnout is the exhaustion of physical or emotional strength. You may find that you no longer enjoy your career or that you lack the energy or the desires you once had. Burnout, in fact, may be a consequence of chronic, unrelieved stress. Your job as a paramedic is full of potential stressors. Of course, EMS professionals are not the only people susceptible to burnout; it can happen to anyone in any field. Burnout develops because of the way a person reacts to stress, but it does not occur solely because of stress. EMS-related stress is often associated with interpersonal relationships, pay, prestige, fringe benefits, and other legitimate issues. The timeline for burnout will vary among people; a situation that burns out one paramedic in a year may take 10 years for the next paramedic, or not at all. A paramedic who never takes a vacation may experience burnout more quickly than colleagues who do. One technique to prevent burnout is

YOU are the Paramedic PART 4

You hold the patient's mother and tell her and the family that he has been down too long, that there is nothing that can be done, and that he has died. You explain he has no cardiac activity and blood has started to pool in the dependent areas of his body. The mother is hysterical and begs you to do something. You calmly repeat that there is nothing you can do, and ask her if there is someone you can call to help with her grieving. You also ask if her son was a hospice patient. She tells you that they did not think it was time for that. Her 19-year-old nephew steps in and accuses you of not knowing your job. He is becoming increasingly hostile. You know that law enforcement personnel are en route, but it may be a few minutes before they arrive.

7. How should you deal with the nephew's hostility?
8. How will you deal with your own feelings and stress related to this call?

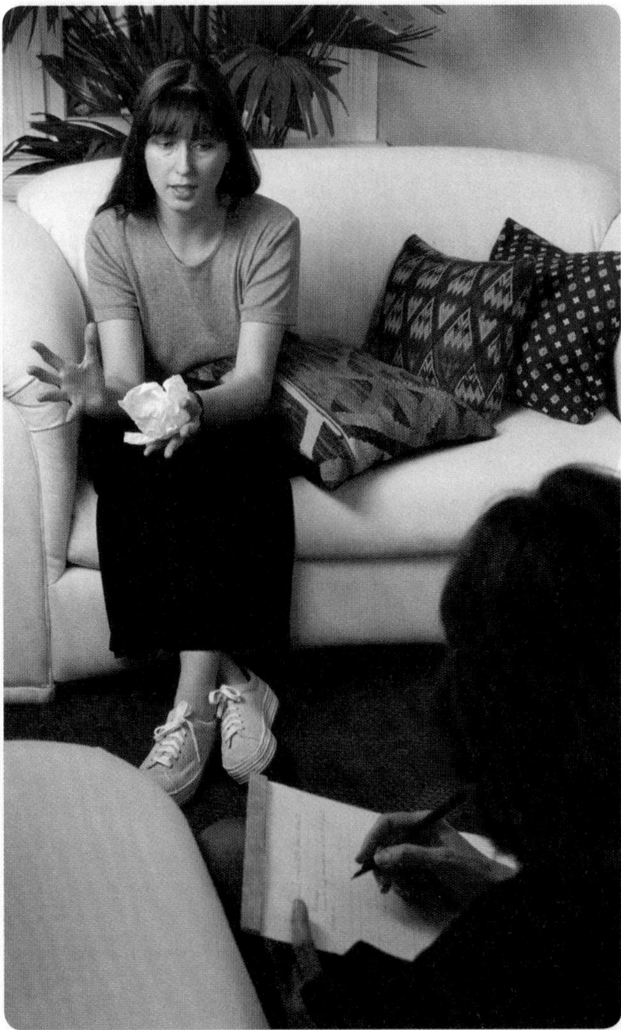

Figure 2-16 Consulting with a professional counselor or therapist can be an important part of dealing with stress and maintaining your emotional well-being. Consulting a professional does not mean you are weak and unable to handle stress; every professional, including you, has a breaking point.

to turn off your pager when off duty and make yourself unavailable from time to time.

One person's eustress may be another's distress. The reason is that distress is a learned reaction, based on the way a person perceives and interprets the world around him or her. In other words, distress is nearly always the result of what a person believes. Here are some beliefs that are common among EMS personnel:

- I have to be perfect all the time.
- My safety depends on being able to anticipate every possible danger.
- I am totally responsible for what happens to patients; if they die, then it is my fault.
- If there is something I do not know, then people will think less of me.
- If I show emotions, then I am weak and unable to handle stress.
- A good paramedic never makes mistakes.

These are all false beliefs and can lead to burnout. Prevention and relief of stress among EMS personnel begin with the recognition that such beliefs are unrealistic and invalid.

Words of Wisdom

Dealing with stress as a paramedic requires the ability to emotionally distance yourself from the situation, and accepting the limits of what you can personally do.

Like many of the medical conditions you will study in this textbook, burnout is a type of illness and it has signs and symptoms. The signs and symptoms may seem trivial at first, but when ignored the illness grows in nature until it becomes debilitating. Symptoms of impending burnout include the following:

- Chronic fatigue and irritability
- Cynical, negative attitude
- Lack of desire to report to work
- Emotional instability (crying easily, losing your temper without provocation, laughing inappropriately)
- Changes in sleep patterns (insomnia or sleeping more than usual), and waking without feeling refreshed
- Feelings of being overwhelmed or being helpless or hopeless
- Loss of interest in hobbies
- Decreased ability to concentrate
- Declining health (having frequent colds, stomach upsets, and muscle aches and pains, especially headaches or backaches)
- Constant tightness in your muscles
- Overeating, smoking, or abusing drugs or alcohol

Some paramedics have been in the field for 20 years and show no signs of burnout, reporting to work every day with the same enthusiasm they did as rookies. What is their secret? In general, the paramedics who do not experience burnout are those who have learned to respect and value themselves. These paramedics have also identified and dealt with the causes of burnout and taken actions to prevent it. It is truly not as easy as it sounds, but as a new paramedic, you should learn from them. Practically speaking, what does it mean to respect and value yourself? How can you translate that attitude into concrete action? Some of the steps you can take to protect yourself from burnout are summarized in Table 2-3.

Table 2-3 Dr. Caroline's Guidelines for Preventing Burnout

1. Paramedic heal thyself! Take care of your own health.
   - Get enough rest.
   - Eat a balanced diet.
   - Get regular physical exercise—at least 30 minutes of aerobic activity (walking, running, or swimming) three to four times a week.
   - Do not abuse your body. Smoking, overindulgence in alcohol, taking recreational drugs, or self-prescribing any other drugs are all forms of self-abuse.
2. Give yourself some "me" time every day. Some of the most stress-resistant paramedics are those who have learned the techniques of meditation and can thereby escape now and then to a quiet place within themselves. Try different methods of meditation or relaxation and see which one works best for you.
3. Learn how to relax Figure 2-17.
   - Take time for hobbies.
   - Engage in social activities with people not involved in EMS.
   - Leave your job behind when your shift is over.
4. Do not make unreasonable demands on yourself.
   - Forget the idea that you have to be perfect. No one is perfect. If you do the best job you can, then that is good enough.
   - You do not have to be right all the time. Accept the fact that now and then you will make a mistake—and that the world will not come to an end on account of it.
5. Do not make unreasonable demands on others.
6. Stay in touch with your feelings.
   - Find someone you can talk to. Share the stress.
   - Cry when you need to. There is no shame in being sad sometimes.
7. Learn techniques for managing stress while on duty. Do not let stress accumulate.
8. Debrief after tough calls.

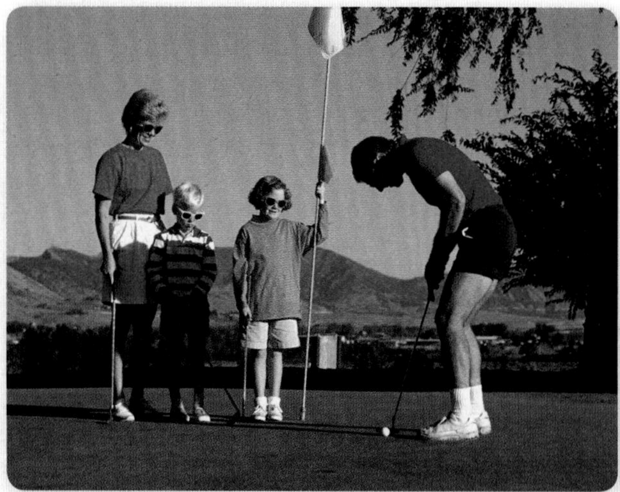

Figure 2-17 One of the best ways of dealing with the stress of working as a paramedic is to invest in relationships and activities outside of work that are meaningful to you. Make the most of your time off; it is an opportunity to refresh yourself.

Coping With Death and Dying

As a paramedic, you will deal with death sometime in your career. What do you say to people who know they are dying? What do you say to a bereaved parent, spouse, or other family member? How do you deal with your own feelings when a patient has died while under your care? These are all questions you need to be able to answer for yourself eventually, and it may take a lifetime to sort them out.

Death in the Western hemisphere is generally regarded as a traumatic experience, something to be feared and postponed as long as possible. Think about it—an average person's only experience with death is through the death of another. As a paramedic, you will be there when people are born and you will be there when many of them die. Every one of these encounters is an honor—a most private moment in someone's life, to which you and a small number of your coworkers are invited. In some cultures, these moments are a holy time, and regardless of culture, it is likely one of the most important moments in a person's life. Many patients will exhibit great dignity while they are dying, which may show you how to die with dignity someday.

As a paramedic, remember you will have the opportunity to help a great many people, but few resuscitations will be successful, no matter how long your career. Yours may be the last face a dying person sees, so make it count; show compassion and concern for the individual as well as for his or her family and friends. What follows are some general guidelines and techniques for dealing with the dying, their families, and your own stress.

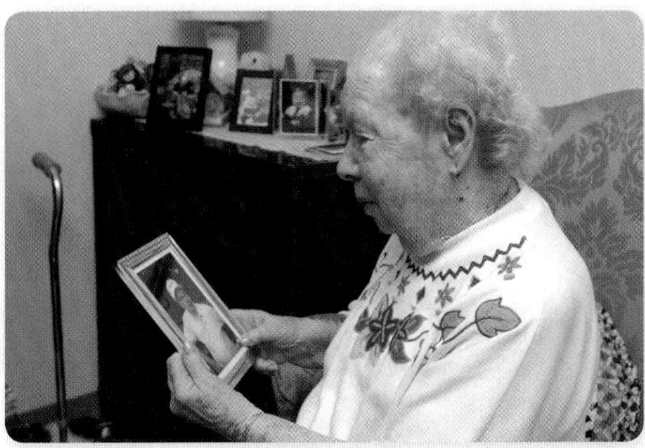

Figure 2-18 People usually go through a lengthy process of grieving before fully accepting the death of a loved one.

▶ Stages of the Grieving Process

In her classic study, *On Death and Dying*, Elisabeth Kübler-Ross, MD, defined five stages through which grieving people—usually the dying, but sometimes their survivors—often proceed **Figure 2-18**.[15] Each of these stages in some way helps the dying or their family members adapt to their own reality. It helps to be aware of these stages, and to consider the behavior of dying patients or their families in the context of the grieving process. Be aware that all people do not follow the stages in order and that you may arrive after a certain stage has already passed.

- **Stage 1: Denial.** It has already been discussed that denial is a mechanism by which people attempt to ignore a problem or pretend it does not exist. Denial is a way of buffering bad news until the person can mobilize the resources to deal with that news more effectively. Allow people enough time to work through this stage and offer assistance only if they ask for it.
- **Stage 2: Anger.** When people can no longer deny the reality of a situation, anger over the loss may replace denial. They may ask, "Why me?" and displace their anger randomly to those around them. As mentioned earlier, such anger may be very difficult for you to deal with. Some people may exhibit their anger through physical actions; be prepared for that reaction and keep yourself and others safe.
- **Stage 3: Bargaining**. When anger does not change the painful reality of a situation, people may resort to bargaining, that is, trying to make some sort of deal in hopes of postponing the inevitable ("If I can just live long enough to see my daughter's wedding, then I'll die in peace.").
- **Stage 4: Depression.** When bargaining fails to change the reality of a loss and people must come to terms with dying, a sudden and enormous sense of loss occurs. They may become very quiet. Depression is especially common among couples who have been married or together for most of their lives and have rarely spent time apart. People may want permission to express their sorrow—in words, in tears, or in what Kübler-Ross calls "the silence that goes beyond words." Acknowledge their loss and sadness, and if they act like they want to cry, offer some tissues, a towel, or a shoulder to cry on. If they seem to want a hug, then offer it. If they seem to just want to be quiet by themselves, then do what you can to accommodate that as well. It is not wrong for you to appropriately exhibit emotions to the grieving person.
- **Stage 5: Acceptance.** In the final stage of grief, people who are dying prepare to disengage from the world around them. They shed their fears and most of their other feelings as well, and begin to loosen the ties that bind them to the living. When the dying person enters the acceptance stage, it is often the family that is in need of the most help. Although families may know of an upcoming death, when that time actually comes, their emotions and reactions may change completely. The process of dying is not pleasant and it may be shocking when death occurs.[15]

▶ Dealing With the Dying Patient

People who are dying generally know, at the very least, that their situation is serious; they may be well aware that they are dying and may want to talk about it. Some health care professionals are reluctant to discuss death with patients, so they try to maintain an attitude of reassurance by saying "Everything will be alright." Perhaps the most important thing you can do for dying patients is to let them know that you understand and will talk about death if they wish. Do not give a false sense of hope to the situation; do not say the patient will recover when he or she may not. You do not need to come right out and ask, "Do you want to talk about dying?" You can simply say "If there is anything you would like to talk about, then I will listen."

Let patients talk as much as they wish **Figure 2-19**. Make some appropriate physical contact. Hold their hand, put a hand on their shoulder, or make some other unmistakable gesture of empathy.

What if patients come straight out and ask you, "Am I going to die?" Your answer should acknowledge the seriousness of their condition without taking away all hope. For example, you might say, "Your illness is serious, but we will give you the best care available."

Dying patients also need to feel that they still have some control over their lives. When people lose all control over their lives, they may lose a large measure of their dignity and self-respect. As much as possible, explain to them what you are doing and allow them to participate in their treatment. Ask them if there is anyone they would

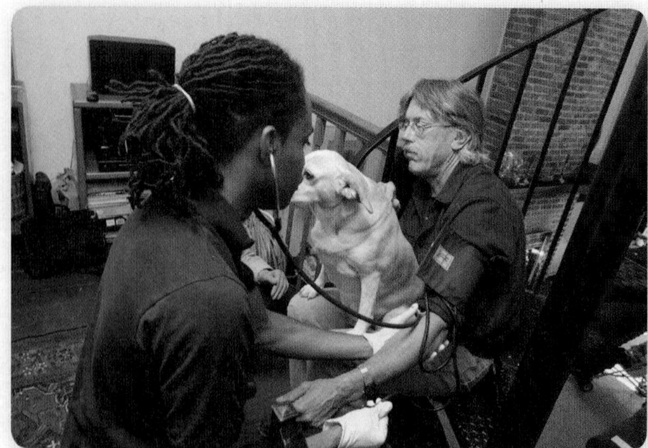

Figure 2-19 Be aware that each patient will have different ways of dealing with his or her immediate situation. Some patients may be relieved to talk openly about how they feel, whereas others may have a greater sense of privacy or stoicism.

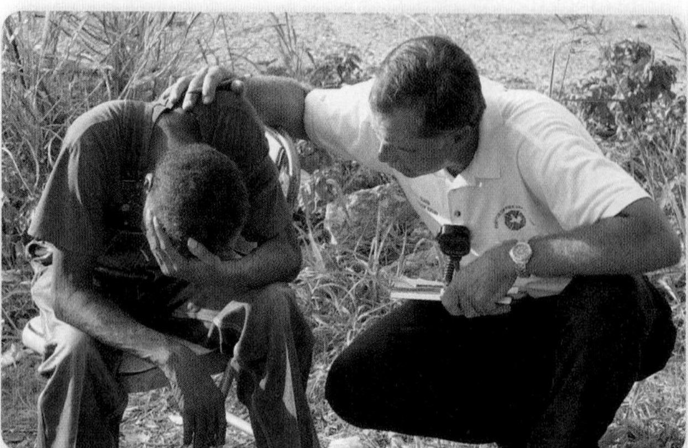

Figure 2-20 While on the scene, one of your responsibilities is to help family members through the initial period after the death of a loved one.

like you to contact or if they have any special instructions they want conveyed to someone. If they do ask you to convey a message, then write it down word-for-word as they state it to you. Also, throughout your career you will find that people who know they are going to die will often look you in the eye and say, "I think I am going to die." Regardless of the situation, always provide the best emergency medical care you can.

Dealing With a Grieving Family

Suppose you are called to the scene where a child has been run over by a truck. You can see at a glance that the child is dead. Two police officers are with the child's mother, who is crying hysterically. The fact that there is nothing you can do for the child does not mean that the call is over. There is another patient at the scene—the child's mother—and the call is not over until you have done all you can for her Figure 2-20.

Your local protocol may state that you have to verify death by cardiac monitor strip. Be aware that by doing so in a case like this, the action may give the mother false hope that you can or are going to resuscitate the child.

What kinds of things can you do for a grieving family? How can you help them begin the process of dealing with their loss? Here are a few guidelines:

- Do not try to hide the body of the deceased patient from the family, even if the body has been badly mutilated. In situations where the deceased patient's appearance may be disfigured, attempt to warn or educate the family beforehand about what they may see. People who are prevented from seeing the body of a loved one may later have enormous difficulty working through their grief because they may be unable to get beyond their denial. Seeing the body therefore helps the person achieve closure of the situation.
- For similar reasons, do not use euphemisms for death, such as "expired" or "passed away." The family needs to hear the word "dead."
- Do not hurry to clear away all your resuscitation equipment. Let the family see the equipment before you start tidying up and packing away your gear, so that they will know that everything possible was done.
- Give the family some time with their loved one, especially when the deceased patient is a child. If the death occurred in a public place, then move the deceased into the ambulance or protect the scene from onlookers, and let the family say goodbye in their own way.
- Try to arrange for further emotional support. Offer to contact a neighbor, friend, or the family's clergy.
- Accept the family's right to experience a variety of feelings—guilt, shock, denial, or anger.

Dealing With a Grieving Child

You need to be particularly sensitive to the emotional needs of children and how they differ depending on their age group. Children up to age 3 years will be aware that something has happened and people are sad. Children age 3 to 6 years of age believe that death is temporary and may continually ask when the person will return. The family should emphasize to the child that he or she was not responsible for the death, that the family member will not be coming home, and also that it is OK to cry when you are sad.

Children age 6 to 9 years may mask their feelings in an effort to not look babylike. Family members should discuss the normal feelings of grieving with the child. Also, they should not hesitate to cry in front of the child.

Children age 9 to 12 years may want to know details surrounding the incident. Family members should encourage the sharing of feelings and memories to facilitate the grieving process.

Patient Safety

Shortly after a serious adverse event or sentinel event happens, a debriefing may occur. The debriefing is a powerful inquiry tool in which a concise exchange occurs to identify what happened, what was learned, and what can be done better in the future. A member of senior leadership usually leads the debriefing. The senior leadership should also use the debriefing to provide emotional support to staff and/or family, determine reporting obligations, and perhaps visit the event site. The debriefing does not focus on system changes and it should not be used for disciplinary purposes.

▶ After the Call Is Over

Many calls can be shocking. In those cases, everyone involved in the call is likely to experience some intense feelings. If these feelings stay bottled up, then all types of problems may result later. Therefore, every ambulance service needs to develop routine procedures for debriefing after any call, especially those that involve the death of a patient. All those who participated in the call need a chance to sit down together, in an atmosphere of confidentiality, and air their feelings about what happened.

Most calls should not disrupt your normal life functions. But, depending on a number of variables, some especially traumatic calls can preoccupy even well-adjusted providers for weeks or even months afterward. This type of delayed stress reaction is called **posttraumatic stress disorder (PTSD)**. A **critical incident** is one that overwhelms the ability of an EMS worker or an EMS system to cope with the experience, either at the scene or later.

Most paramedics never experience PTSD, but it can occur. Let your superiors know if you or a coworker is experiencing one or more of the following signs of PTSD:

- You have trouble getting an incident out of your thoughts.
- You keep having flashbacks of an incident.
- You have nightmares or other sleep disturbances after an incident.
- Your appetite is not the same after an incident.
- After an incident, you laugh or cry for no good reason.
- You find yourself withdrawing from coworkers and family members after an incident.
- You rely on alcohol or cigarettes, or make other unhealthy choices to calm you down.

Critical incident stress management (CISM) is a resource available for emergency personnel who have been involved in particularly traumatic calls or incidents. CISM is a process that was developed to address acute stress situations and potentially decrease the likelihood that PTSD will develop after such an incident. Although public safety organizations have used CISM for more than 30 years, no concrete evidence exists on the efficacy of CISM to prevent PTSD or burnout. The following are suggested events where some sort of debriefing or management may be considered:

- Serious injury or death of a fellow worker in the line of duty
- Suicide of a fellow worker
- Mass-casualty incidents, such as an airliner crash or train wreck
- Serious injury or death of a child
- Intense media attention to an incident

It is impossible to predict how any given person will react. People should be offered opportunities to debrief, but it should never be forced on them or made mandatory.

Some EMS systems still have CISM teams or a form thereof to provide support after a traumatic call—but sometimes even during the incident itself. The intervention may take the form of a brief (usually about 30 minutes) defusing session right after the call, in which all who were involved in the incident are offered an opportunity to express their feelings about what happened. A formal debriefing is usually coordinated and should be handled by one or more professional counselors 24 to 72 hours after an incident, when it becomes clear that the incident has had a serious impact and is causing persistent symptoms among the crew. Again, this process should be optional.

Some services may offer an **employee assistance program (EAP)**. This resource is normally provided by a trained, professional counselor who works outside of the service and is off duty. Successful EAPs should not focus only on work-related issues, because some personal events may lead to poor work choices and unacceptable behaviors. The EAP is successful only if those who attend do so by their own choice and are willing to share every issue that may bother them. If you or your coworkers note changes in your behavior at work and an EAP is available, then it is a worthwhile venture to pursue for the betterment of your health and career.

Controversies

Psychology professionals and EMS professionals alike have debated the effectiveness of CISM for some time. Be open-minded about the experience and then draw your own conclusion.

Peer Support and Suicide Prevention

As with all populations, EMS providers are not immune to thoughts of suicide or suicide attempts. Because prolonged stress is a risk factor for suicide, prevention starts with recognizing that you or your colleagues are becoming overwhelmed. Even if you do not identify suicidal tendencies in yourself, you may receive input from colleagues. Do not disregard what you recognize or what others note to you. A survey showed that 37% of EMS respondents contemplated suicide and 6.6% attempted it.[16] Although the attempt number may seem relatively low, in comparison, the CDC showed levels for the general population to be 3.7% and 0.5% respectively.[16] The study suggests that emergency workers are at higher risk for suicidal thoughts and attempts than non-emergency workers.[16] As discussed throughout this chapter, it is important for you to be aware of the signs of stress and burnout in yourself as well as in coworkers. Any suicidal thoughts or attempts must be taken seriously.

YOU are the Paramedic SUMMARY

1. The decline of your physical well-being will eventually affect your attitude and, in turn, put your job at risk. What steps can you take to avoid this outcome?

The components of physical well-being include proper nutrition, exercise, adequate sleep, and the avoidance of unhealthy habits or substances. Eat healthy meals, preferably at the same time each day. Plan meals in advance and account for the possibility that you may not be near a microwave or refrigerator. Follow the USDA MyPlate dietary guidelines. Carry bottled water and snacks with you like raisins, nuts, and fruits.

Exercise is important for weight management and stress management. Choose an activity you enjoy because you will be more likely to stick with it. Your exercise regimen should be focused on three areas: cardiovascular endurance, flexibility, and physical strength. Try to engage in at least 30 minutes of moderate to vigorous physical activity most days of the week. Avoid caffeine, tobacco use, and excessive alcohol consumption.

It is also important to keep a regular sleep schedule, even though this is virtually impossible when working shift work. Get as much sleep as possible as time permits.

2. Why is it so important to also find ways to enhance your mental, emotional, and spiritual well-being?

The ability to think clearly and react properly is strongest when your mental well-being is in check. Practice techniques for coping with the fight-or-flight response before they are needed to help guide you when an emergency situation arises. To maintain your emotional health, you need a balance between your life at work and life away from work. When you are off duty, try to stay off duty.

Maintain your skills and education and accept the fact that patients may not do well or die. This reality is not something that you can control (unless you are directly responsible for that death through negligence). Strive to do your best and remember that you are valuable and what you do does make a difference.

You may not be a member of an organized religious group, but if you are, then you may find comfort in these beliefs. Medical care supports the dignity and value of life, and the sacredness of individuals. Having a rich sense of your own spirituality will help to keep your life in good perspective.

3. According to the report from his mother, the patient has been apneic for an unknown amount of time. What should be your next action?

The first step is to ensure that the patient cannot be resuscitated. Attach the cardiac monitor and check for asystole in two leads. If there is electrical activity, then consider proceeding with cardiopulmonary resuscitation and follow local protocols for the presenting rhythm. If the patient presents with asystole, or if other signs of obvious death are present, then refrain from disturbing the body and tell the family that your findings clearly show the person has died and it is not possible to change the situation.

Also notify the dispatcher, who should send law enforcement personnel if not already done, and contact the coroner. In most states, the coroner or medical examiner will make decisions on death scenes (for example, whether an autopsy is needed, where to transport the deceased person, and who will sign the death certificate). If you note anything of a suspicious nature, then do not attempt to address your concerns with anyone related to the deceased. Note your findings and address your concerns with law enforcement or the coroner. In most areas it is also standard for law enforcement personnel to write a report, even for instances of death from obvious natural causes—such as an older person with a long history of cancer, etc.

4. On the basis of your previous interactions with the patient, which stage of the grieving process do you feel he reached?

The patient had reached the acceptance stage of grief. During your previous interactions with the patient, you observed that he appeared to be prepared for his inevitable death, yet maintained a positive outlook despite this.

5. How will you explain the situation to the family, and what is your responsibility to them?

Telling the family that a loved one has died is never easy. Be direct. Do not "sugarcoat" the situation and do not use

YOU are the Paramedic SUMMARY *(continued)*

euphemisms for death. It is important to use the word "dead" or "died" to help the family move past their denial. Allow the family to see the body if they choose, unless it is a potential crime scene. Give the family some time with the patient to allow them the chance to say goodbye. Try to arrange for further support as needed. If they request it, then call a neighbor, religious person, or other family members to come over. Never contact people on behalf of the family without their request.

Probably the hardest part is to remind yourself not to take things personally if the family becomes upset with you. They may experience guilt, shock, denial, or anger, and you have to recognize that these are coping mechanisms that are not directed at you. Treat them with respect and empathy and allow them to work through their grief while offering to assist with whatever they may need. Often, after the family members become accustomed to the situation, they will realize how they treated you and offer apologies. If that occurs, then accept the apology without recourse.

6. Which stage of the grieving process is the patient's mother exhibiting?

She appears to be in two stages. She is still in denial, but is also trying to bargain. She understands that her son is terminally ill, but is still hopeful that the problem can be fixed. Her son's death, however, is reality, and she may move rapidly into the depression stage.

The loss of a child is a traumatic experience, no matter what the child's age. The patient you can help in this situation is the mother. Ask her what you can do to help. If she asks you for help, then suggest support groups that may be offered through the local hospital or other agencies. Each situation is different and should be handled based on the needs of the bereaved.

7. How should you deal with the nephew's hostility?

The first step is to make sure that you remove yourself from a dangerous situation and request law enforcement personnel if they are not already en route or on scene. Removing yourself from a dangerous situation does not mean that you are abandoning your patient.

A person's behavior can change at the blink of an eye during critical situations or when faced with death. Use your intuition or gut instincts to help predict when a hostile situation is developing. If you are in contact with an aggressive person, then listen without arguing. Concentrate on de-escalating his or her emotions. An upset person does not listen or reason well; often his or her fight-or flight-response has been activated. It is important to build a rapport with the person. Rapport is based on empathy and understanding. Although you do not want to say, "I know how you feel," it is important to stress, "I will help you if you would like. Let me know how I can help you." Remember to put aside any personal prejudices and do your best to be understanding and accepting.

8. How will you deal with your own feelings and stress related to this call?

As a new paramedic, understand that you cannot save every patient. You need to frequently remind yourself, "I will always provide the best care possible in all situations, but not all patients will have a positive outcome in spite of that." Dealing with stress is part of being a paramedic. When the situation involves a child, coworker, or family member, it can be much more difficult to handle.

This call could be particularly stressful because of your frustrated frame of mind en route to the call, followed by your sudden change of emotions when you arrived on scene. Although death can be stressful, this situation could very easily be a trigger for acute stress. Talking with your partner should be the first step and possibly all that will be needed. However, if you find yourself becoming more irritable, losing sleep, drinking more, or recognize any other signs that indicate you are not coping well, then it is imperative that you seek professional assistance. Most calls should not disrupt your normal daily functions, but if you find yourself preoccupied for weeks or months afterwards, then you may be experiencing posttraumatic stress disorder. Report any concerns to your supervisor immediately and follow departmental policies for seeking help.

EMS Patient Care Report (PCR)					
Date: 01-12-18	**Incident No.:** 1101034	**Nature of Call:** Possible cardiac arrest		**Location:** 984 Solomon Street	
Dispatched: 0712	**En Route:** 0713	**At Scene:** 0720	**Transport:**	**At Hospital:**	**In Service:** 0755
Patient Information					
Age: 23 **Sex:** M **Weight (in kg [lb]):** 70 kg (154 lb)			**Allergies:** No known drug allergies **Medications:** See list (attached to report) **Past Medical History:** Leukemia **Chief Complaint:** Cardiac arrest		

YOU are the Paramedic SUMMARY *(continued)*

Vital Signs				
Time: 0721	**BP:** 0	**Pulse:** 0	**Respirations:** 0	**Spo_2:**
Time:	**BP:**	**Pulse:**	**Respirations:**	**Spo_2:**
Time:	**BP:**	**Pulse:**	**Respirations:**	**Spo_2:**
EMS Treatment (circle all that apply)				
Oxygen @ ______ L/min via (circle one): **NC NRM Bag-mask device**		**Assisted Ventilation**	**Airway Adjunct**	**CPR**
Defibrillation	**Bleeding Control**	**Bandaging**	**Splinting**	**Other:** Cardiac monitor
Narrative				

Dispatched to a possible cardiac arrest. Arrived on scene to find a 23-year-old man lying supine in bed apneic and pulseless. Mother states that pt refused to eat last night and she found him "not breathing" just prior to calling EMS. Pt cold to touch, no obvious signs of injury, presents with dependent lividity. Cardiac monitor shows asystole in two leads. Pt has history of leukemia and mother states "he has been getting worse over the past month." He was not a hospice pt. Mother also stated that he was not "feeling well" last night. Patient has been down for an unknown amount of time. Contacted Medical Control with information and were given approval to withhold resuscitation @ 0722. Advised dispatch to notify law enforcement and coroner of death. Stayed on scene with pt and family until turned over to coroner.**End of report**

Prep Kit

▶ Ready for Review

- As a paramedic, you need to know how to ensure your own well-being.
- Wellness has at least four dimensions: physical, mental, emotional, and spiritual. It is important to keep all four dimensions healthy and balanced.
- The Life's Simple 7 list from the American Heart Association feature seven factors that have been found to improve heart health: get active, control cholesterol, eat better, manage blood pressure, lose weight, reduce blood sugar, and stop smoking.
- Nutrition plays a key role in maintaining day-to-day energy and maintaining a healthy body for life. The *Dietary Guidelines for Americans, 2015-2020* from the US Department of Agriculture outlines guidelines for nutrition.
- Practice proper lifting and moving techniques to protect your body and lengthen your career.
  - Minimize the number of total body lifts you have to perform.
  - Coordinate every lift prior to performing the lift.
  - Minimize the total amount of weight you have to lift.
  - Never lift with your back.
  - Do not carry what you can put on wheels.
  - Ask for help anytime.
- A communicable disease is any disease that can be spread from person to person or animal to person. Infectious diseases can be transmitted by contact (direct or indirect), or they are airborne, foodborne, or vector-borne.
- Even if you are exposed to an infectious disease, your risk of becoming ill is low. Whether or not an acute infection occurs depends on several factors,

Prep Kit *(continued)*

including the amount and type of infectious organism and your resistance to that infection.

- You can take several steps to protect yourself against exposure to infectious diseases, including remaining up-to-date with recommended vaccinations, taking standard precautions at all times, and handling all needles and other sharp objects with great care.
- Because it is often impossible to tell which patients have infectious diseases, avoid direct contact with the blood and body fluids of all patients whenever possible.
- Standard precautions are protective measures designed to prevent health care workers from coming into contact with germs carried by patients. One extremely effective step is properly washing your hands. Also use the proper personal protective equipment for the situation, including gloves, gowns, eye protection, masks, and possibly other specialized equipment.
- Infection control should be an important part of your daily routine. Be sure to follow the proper steps when dealing with potential exposure situations. Know what to do if you are exposed to an airborne or bloodborne disease.
- Cleaning your ambulance and equipment is part of protecting yourself and your patients. Decontamination of equipment and supplies that have been potentially exposed to body substances requires a different cleansing routine than just soap and water; disinfectant may be required.
- Keep yourself on alert while you are on duty. Do not be afraid to ask for the police to respond to or enter a scene first.
- During your career, you will be exposed to many hazards. Some situations will be dangerous to you or your crew. In these cases, you should be properly protected, or you must avoid the situation altogether.
- Scene hazards include traffic hazards, unstable vehicles, other traffic, bystanders, potential exposure to hazardous materials, electricity, and fire. Your safety is the most important consideration. Never approach a scene without first observing it from a safe distance.
- The most dangerous calls are your everyday ones because you become comfortable with them and may let down your guard.
- Your primary concern at any scene is safety—safety for yourself as well as those around you.
- Safe emergency vehicle operation is crucial to the safety of the paramedic, crew, patient, and other motorists.
- Stress reactions can be acute, delayed, or cumulative. Posttraumatic stress disorder is a syndrome with onset following a traumatic, usually life-threatening event. Critical incident stress management is a process developed to address acute stress situations. You may also seek help through an employee assistance program.
- Learn how to effectively control stress so that it does not affect your wellness. Take appropriate action. Initial stress management techniques include the following:
  - Controlled deep breathing
  - Progressive relaxation
  - Professional assistance
- A patient's reaction to stress may include fear, anxiety, depression, anger, confusion, denial, regression, projection, and displacement.
- You are not immune to the stresses of emergency situations and may experience a multitude of feelings; not all of them will be pleasant.
- Burnout is a consequence of chronic, unrelieved stress.
- As a paramedic, you will be present when people are born and you will be there when people die. The patient who is dying may be aware of that fact and may want to talk about it. Be prepared to listen and provide empathy; you may be the last person he or she sees or talks to.
- Be aware of behavioral changes in yourself as well as in your coworkers, which may indicate a risk for suicide. Reach out to professionals who are specifically trained to assist, and take advantage of resources such as employee assistance programs and the critical incident stress management process.

▶ Vital Vocabulary

acute stress reaction Reaction to stress that occurs during a stressful situation.

airborne transmission The spread of an organism in aerosol form, such as droplets or dust.

blind panic A fear reaction in which a person's judgment seems to disappear entirely; it is particularly dangerous because it may cause mass panic among others.

bloodborne pathogens Pathogenic microorganisms that are present in human blood and can cause disease in humans; include, but are not limited to, hepatitis B virus, and human immunodeficiency virus.

Prep Kit *(continued)*

burnout The exhaustion of physical or emotional strength.

communicable disease Any disease that can be spread from person to person or from animal to person.

conversion hysteria A reaction in which a person subconsciously transforms his or her anxiety into a bodily dysfunction; the person may be unable to see or hear or may become partially paralyzed.

critical incident An event that overwhelms the ability to cope with the experience, either at the scene or later.

critical incident stress management (CISM) A process which utilizes trained counselors who confront responses to critical incidents and help to defuse them, directing emergency services personnel toward physical and emotional equilibrium.

cumulative stress reaction Prolonged or excessive stress.

defense mechanisms Psychological ways to relieve stress; they are usually automatic or subconscious; they include denial, regression, projection, and displacement.

delayed stress reaction Reaction to stress that occurs after a stressful situation.

denial An early response to a serious medical emergency, in which the severity of the emergency is diminished or minimized. Denial is the first coping mechanism for people who believe they are going to die.

direct contact Exposure to or transmission of a communicable disease from one person to another by physical contact.

displacement A defense mechanism characterized by the redirection of an emotion from one person to another.

employee assistance program (EAP) A counseling program to help with situations that may affect the health and well-being of emergency medical services professionals.

fight-or-flight response A physiologic response to a profound stressor that helps a person deal with the situation at hand; features increased sympathetic tone and results in dilation of the pupils, increased heart rate, dilation of the bronchi, mobilization of glucose, shunting of blood away from the gastrointestinal tract and cerebrum, and increased blood flow to the skeletal muscles.

indirect contact Exposure or transmission of disease from one person to another by contact with a contaminated, inanimate object.

infection The invasion of a host or host tissues by organisms such as bacteria, viruses, or parasites, with or without signs or symptoms of disease.

infection control Procedures to reduce transmission of infection among patients and health care personnel.

infectious disease A disease that is caused by the growth and spread of small, harmful organisms within the body. or one that is capable of being transmitted with or without direct contact.

posttraumatic stress disorder (PTSD) A delayed stress reaction to a previous incident, often the result of one or more unresolved issues concerning the incident.

projection A defense mechanism characterized by blaming unacceptable feelings, motives, or desires on others.

regression A defense mechanism characterized by a return to more childlike behavior while under stress.

standard precautions Protective measures that have traditionally been developed by the Centers for Disease Control and Prevention for use in dealing with objects, blood, body fluids, or other potential exposure risks of communicable disease.

stress A reaction of the body to any agent or situation that requires the person to adapt.

stressor Any agent or situation that causes stress, whether good or bad.

transmission The way in which an infectious agent is spread: contact (direct or indirect), airborne, foodborne, or vector-borne.

▶ References

1. Quarantine and isolation. Centers for Disease Control and Prevention website. https://www.cdc.gov/quarantine/. Updated August 15, 2016. Accessed October 5, 2016.
2. Maguire BJ, Smith S. Injuries and fatalities among emergency medical technicians and paramedics in the United States. *Prehosp Disaster Med.* 2013;28(4):376–382.
3. The National Highway Traffic Safety Administration. *The National Highway Traffic Safety Administration and Ground Ambulance Crashes. April 2014.* https://www.naemt.org/Files/HealthSafety/2014%20NHTSA%20Ground%20Amublance%20Crash%20Data.pdf. Accessed September 13, 2016.
4. Choose MyPlate. U.S. Department of Agriculture. https://www.choosemyplate.gov/. Accessed September 29, 2016.

Prep Kit *(continued)*

5. U.S. Department of Health and Human Services and U.S. Department of Agriculture. *2015–2020 Dietary Guidelines for Americans*. 8th Edition. December 2015. Available at http://health.gov/dietaryguidelines/2015/guidelines/.
6. Target heart rates. American Heart Association website. http://www.heart.org/HEARTORG/HealthyLiving/PhysicalActivity/FitnessBasics/Target-Heart-Rates_UCM_434341_Article.jsp#.V9q9TpgrKhc. Updated October 12, 2016. Accessed September 29, 2016.
7. Raloff J. Health risks of e-cigarettes emerge. *Science News*. https://www.sciencenews.org/article/health-risks-e-cigarettes-emerge. Published June 3, 2014. Accessed September 1, 2014.
8. Centers for Disease Control and Prevention. Guideline for Hand Hygiene in Health-Care Settings: Recommendations of the Healthcare Infection Control Practices Advisory Committee and the HICPAC/SHEA/APIC/IDSA Hand Hygiene Task Force. *MMWR*. 2002;51(No. RR-16).
9. Siegel JD, Rhinehart E, Jackson M, Chiarello L, and the Healthcare Infection Control Practices Advisory Committee, 2007 Guideline for Isolation Precautions: Preventing Transmission of Infectious Agents in Healthcare Settings. http://www.cdc.gov/hicpac/pdf/Isolation/Isolation2007.pdf.
10. Bloodborne infectious diseases: HIV/AIDS, hepatitis B, hepatitis C. Centers for Disease Control and Prevention website. The National Institute for Occupational Safety and Health (NIOSH). http://www.cdc.gov/niosh/topics/bbp/default.html. Updated September 7, 2016. Accessed October 14, 2016.
11. Vaccines & immunizations. Centers for Disease Control and Prevention website. http://www.cdc.gov/vaccines/index.html. Updated August 31, 2016. Accessed May 27, 2016.
12. Handwashing: clean hands save lives. Centers for Disease Control and Prevention website. http://www.cdc.gov/handwashing/when-how-handwashing.html. Updated September 4, 2015. Accessed October 14, 2016.
13. Tuberculosis (TB) data and statistics. Centers for Disease Control and Prevention website. http://www.cdc.gov/tb/statistics/default.htm. Updated September 24, 2015. Accessed October 14, 2016.
14. Holmes TH, Rahe RH. The social readjustment rating scale. *J Psychosom Res*. 1967;11(2):213-218.
15. Kübler-Ross E. *On Death and Dying*. New York, NY: Macmillan Company; 1969.
16. Newland C, Barber E, Rose M, Young A. Survey reveals alarming rates of EMS provider stress and thoughts of suicide. *JEMS*. 2015;40(10):30-4. http://www.jems.com/articles/print/volume-40/issue-10/features/survey-reveals-alarming-rates-of-ems-provider-stress-and-thoughts-of-suicide.html. Accessed October 14, 2016.

Assessment *in Action*

It is near dark and you are dispatched to the scene of a single-vehicle crash. As you approach the scene, you see a small pickup truck at the bottom of a ravine. Rescue personnel on scene tell you one person is inside and no signs of life have been observed. You are safely assisted down the treacherous embankment by rescue personnel; you can barely see what appears to be a young man in the driver's seat. The rescue personnel also state that it will take an extended period to extricate the patient.

You reach in through a shattered window and note the patient is not breathing; you cannot feel a carotid pulse. He also has brain matter exposed from a depressed skull fracture and blood is draining from his ear on the side you can see. You have no access to the rest of his body because the crumpled metal of the vehicle is encompassing him, so CPR is not an option. You contact medical control to report your findings and agree to withhold resuscitation.

Assessment in Action (continued)

1. While viewing the wreckage at the bottom of the ravine, it is natural for you to be bombarded with adrenaline and rush into an unsafe situation in an attempt to help the patient. It is critical that you remain calm in emergency situations by controlling the fight-or-flight response. All of the following are methods of coping with stress EXCEPT:

A. controlled deep breathing.
B. professional assistance.
C. increased caffeine consumption.
D. progressive relaxation.

2. If it were possible to untangle this patient from the vehicle, then he would then have to be carried back up a significant grade to reach the ambulance. To reduce your exposure to damage when lifting your maximum weight, which of the following statements expresses the proper technique for lifting?

A. Always lift with your back.
B. Keep the feet and knees together for proper balance.
C. Place all equipment on the stretcher so you will only have to make one lift.
D. Keep your back in a straight, upright position and lift without twisting.

3. You realize that you are extremely agitated and that your pulse rate is elevated. You also note an overwhelming sense of helplessness. Your patient that you were supposed to save is beyond your help. This sense of helplessness, along with the other issues that have been building for weeks, can lead to a condition that is a consequence of chronic, unrelieved stress called:

A. conversion hysteria.
B. distress.
C. burnout.
D. anxiety.

4. Very traumatic calls, such as this one, can preoccupy even well-adjusted providers for weeks or even months afterward. This condition is known as:

A. a critical incident.
B. posttraumatic stress disorder.
C. burnout.
D. denial.

5. Motor vehicle crashes such as this have the potential for exposure to body fluids because of open injuries caused by broken glass and jagged metal. What personal protective equipment should be used for this situation?

A. Gloves, goggles, mask, N95 respirator, and turnout gear
B. Mask or N95 respirator
C. Turnout gear and N95 respirator,
D. Turnout gear and self-contained breathing apparatus

6. The death of the patient, along with the lack of ability to help, can trigger a stress response for you and it is natural to subconsciously attempt to relieve it. Regression and projection are types of:

A. denial.
B. defense mechanisms.
C. displacement.
D. professional assistance.

7. Situations such as this require that you be physically fit and well to access the patient. Along with the components of a healthy lifestyle, you should be aware of hereditary factors. The most common of all health risk factors are cancer and:

A. heart disease.
B. Alzheimer disease.
C. chemical addiction.
D. hypertension.

8. One definition of _______________ is the "nonspecific response of the body to any demand made on it."

A. adaptation
B. stress
C. eustress
D. distress

9. Traffic may be only one of the many hazards at the scene of a motor vehicle crash. What type of problems might you encounter en route to and after arrival at the scene?

10. When responding to a mass-casualty incident, both patients and bystanders may react by becoming dazed, disorganized, or overwhelmed. What reactions in this circumstance may present a problem requiring that these people be removed from the scene?

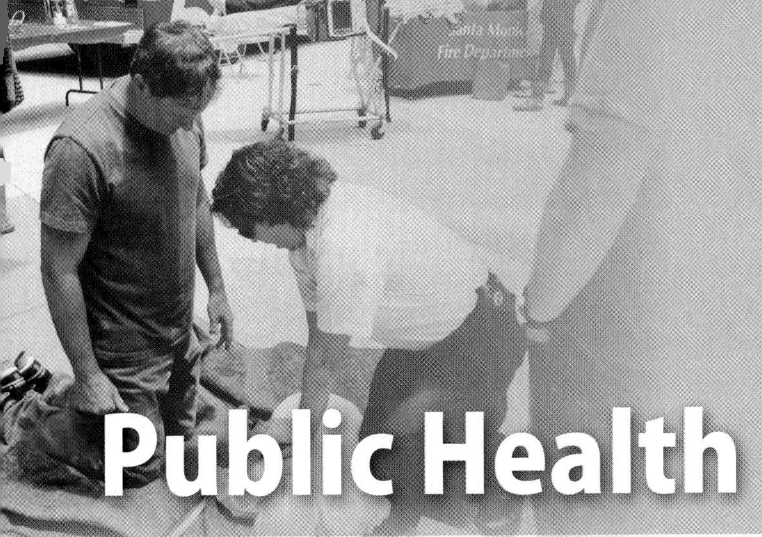

CHAPTER 3

Public Health

National EMS Education Standard Competencies

Public Health

Applies fundamental knowledge of principles of public health and epidemiology including public health emergencies, health promotion, and illness and injury prevention.

Knowledge Objectives

1. Define public health and its role in the health care system. (p 72)
2. Define intentional injuries and unintentional injuries. (p 72)
3. Discuss the detrimental effects of injuries as related to public health. (pp 72-74)
4. Discuss pediatric injuries and risk factors for them. (pp 73-74)
5. Discuss the detrimental effects of chronic and acute illness as related to public health. (p 74)
6. Explain the concept of years of potential life lost. (pp 74-75)
7. Explain the relevance of a teachable moment in EMS. (pp 75-77)
8. Discuss the principles of injury prevention, including education, enforcement, engineering/environment, and economic incentives. (pp 77-79)
9. List the major public health laws, regulations, and guidelines in place in the United States, including the purpose of each. (p 80)
10. Explain the paramedic's unique role in promoting public health, both in terms of illness and injury. (p 81)
11. Define primary prevention and secondary prevention; include examples of each. (pp 81-82)
12. Define morbidity and mortality. (p 83)
13. Discuss the concept of injury surveillance and how it relates to EMS. (p 83)
14. Explain the Haddon Matrix and how it can be used in the understanding and prevention of injury. (pp 83-84)
15. List ways a paramedic can promote injury prevention in his or her community. (pp 85-88)
16. Describe the steps involved in organizing a community prevention program. (pp 86-88)

Skills Objectives

There are no skills objectives for this chapter.

YOU are the Paramedic PART 1

You are dispatched to the scene of a motor vehicle crash reportedly involving two patients and a possible ejection. You are very familiar with this stretch of roadway, as you have responded to many other crashes there. A sharp curve in the road has a reputation for leaving drivers in a ditch or worse; thus, you suspect the injuries may be serious, and you request an additional unit be dispatched.

1. What is the most appropriate way to respond to this scene?
2. Based on the information provided, what potential injuries and complications should you anticipate?

Introduction

Several years ago, San Diego paramedic Paul Maxwell responded to a call for a possible drowning.[1] A 2-year-old boy had wandered away from a day care facility and fallen into a neighbor's backyard pool. Despite everyone's best efforts, he could not be resuscitated. The mother was inconsolable and her cries haunted the paramedic.

Maxwell wondered how such tragedies could be prevented—if he could help it, he never wanted to go on another call like that again. Doing a little investigation, and looking up incidents on his emergency medical services (EMS) system's database, he discovered a pattern of increased drownings in his region. Maxwell made the decision to get involved. In cooperation with his EMS agency, he contacted other groups in his community with an interest in child safety. Using his system's data and motivated by his firsthand knowledge of the suffering that such deaths inflict, Maxwell began a coordinated effort to reduce backyard pool drownings in his community. In time, through the development of legislation and education, Maxwell's program successfully contributed to a significant reduction in drownings.

This story illustrates the important and powerful role that an EMS provider can have in injury or illness prevention. This chapter discusses injury and illness prevention as they relate to public health, and defines the EMS provider's role in promoting public health in his or her community.

Role of Public Health

For decades, the health care system in the United States concentrated on treating illnesses and injuries as opposed to preventing them. However, due in part to skyrocketing health care costs, the incidence of chronic disease, and health care reform, there has been a shift in focus toward greater emphasis on prevention.

According to the American Public Health Association, **public health** is defined as "the practice of preventing disease and promoting good health within groups of people."[2] A common misconception regarding public health agencies is the notion that their primary mission is to provide clinical services for those who are otherwise unable to access health care services elsewhere. In reality, public health professionals examine the overall needs of the population at large to determine the best use of health resources to enhance the quality of life for the public in general. Traditionally, this has included efforts to prevent and control communicable disease and promote health within a community. Examples include immunization and nutrition programs for children; environmental health monitoring, regulation, and remediation; community planning; and exploration of the social determinants of health.

Public Health Threats

Table 3-1 shows the top 10 causes of death in the United States in 2014. That year, almost 74% of all deaths were caused by something in this list.[3] This information is extremely important in understanding the impact that injuries and illnesses have on different age groups.

Injuries

Intentional injuries include any injury or death that is self-inflicted or perpetrated by another person, usually in the context of violence. Examples of intentional injuries include assault, self-harm behavior, intentional overdose, and suicide Figure 3-1. By contrast, **unintentional injuries** occur without intent to cause harm; these are events that might be called accidents. Unintentional injuries account for the vast majority of all injuries Figure 3-2. An injury or illness **risk** is a potentially hazardous situation in which the well-being of people can be harmed. **Risk factors** are characteristics that increase the likelihood that a person will suffer a particular disease or injury.

Referring to Table 3-1, additional research gives crucial information that can aid in recognizing and perhaps even preventing certain kinds of injuries.

When you combine fatal unintentional and intentional injuries, injury becomes the third leading cause of death for all age groups.[4,5] Thus, injury is one of the greatest threats to public health in the United States. Table 3-2 shows the top five causes of death from unintentional injury in 2016. Does anything about the list surprise you?

Table 3-1 Top 10 Causes of Death in 2014

1. Heart disease
2. Cancer
3. Chronic, lower respiratory disease[a]
4. Unintentional injuries[a]
5. Stroke (cerebrovascular diseases)
6. Alzheimer disease
7. Diabetes
8. Influenza and pneumonia
9. Kidney disease (ie, nephritis, nephrotic syndrome, and nephrosis)
10. Intentional self-harm (eg, suicide)

[a]Though listed separately, these two listings caused an equal number of deaths in 2014.

Data from: Centers for Disease Control and Prevention, National Center for Health Statistics. Underlying Cause of Death 1999-2014 on CDC WONDER Online Database, released 2015. Data are from the Multiple Cause of Death Files, 1999-2014, as compiled from data provided by the 57 vital statistics jurisdictions through the Vital Statistics Cooperative Program. Accessed at http://wonder.cdc.gov/ucd-icd10.html. Accessed September 1, 2016; Heron M. Deaths: Leading causes for 2014. *National Vital Statistics Reports*. 2016;65(5):9. http://www.cdc.gov/nchs/data/nvsr/nvsr65/nvsr65_05.pdf. Accessed August 30, 2016; and Murphy S, Kochanek K, Xu J, Arias E. Mortality in the United States, 2014. National Center for Health Statistics Data Brief. 2015;229:1-8. http://www.cdc.gov/nchs/data/databriefs/db229.htm. Accessed September 1, 2016.

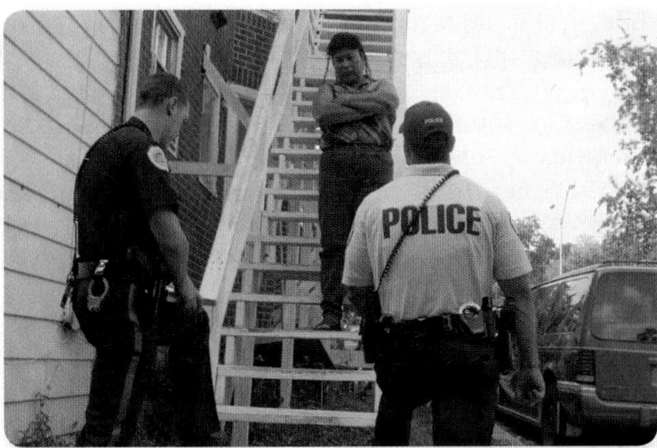

Figure 3-1 Intentional injuries include all cases of abuse of a spouse, child, or older adult. As a medical professional, you have an ethical, professional, and—in most states—a legal obligation to report these cases.

© Mikael Karlsson/On Scene Photography.

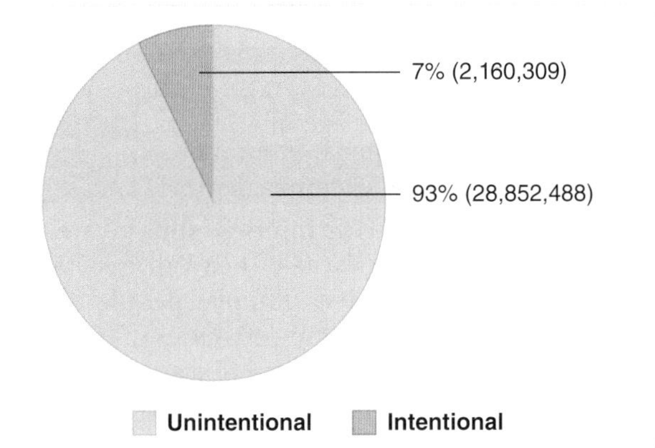

Figure 3-2 The majority of all injuries are unintentional.

Data from: NEISS All Injury Program operated by the Consumer Product Safety Commission for numbers of injuries. Bureau of Census for population estimates. National Center for Injury Prevention and Control, Centers for Disease Control and Prevention, 2014. http://webappa.cdc.gov/cgi-bin/broker.exe. Accessed August 30, 2016.

Unintentional Injuries in Children

In the United States, injury is the leading cause of death in children ages 19 and younger.[6] In 2009 and 2010, children and teens accounted for an estimated 33.7 million annual average emergency department (ED) visits, with almost 12 million of these involving injuries.[7] Compared to adults, children have thinner skin, a smaller airway, a larger head in proportion to their bodies, and lesser ability to protect themselves from harm **Figure 3-3**. Such differing characteristics put them at greater risk for sustaining injuries or being more seriously affected by them.

Risk Factors for Children

Injury patterns vary widely depending upon a child's age, gender, socioeconomic status, developmental stage, family environment, and a whole host of other factors.[8] Thus, it is imperative for parents, teachers, and health care providers to be aware of the threats and to remain vigilant in order to take preventive measures.

Many people believe that schools are becoming increasingly more violent, making the risk of *intentional* injuries an ever-present and growing threat to the safety of students. Certainly, the very real tragedies that have occurred—from school shootings to bullying and suicide—have captured our attention on multiple occasions. However, despite these

Table 3-2 Top Five Causes of Death by Unintentional Injury, 2016

1. Poisoning
2. Motor vehicle collision
3. Falls
4. Choking and suffocation
5. Drowning

Data from: Top causes of unintentional injury and death in homes and communities. The National Safety Council. 2016. http://www.nsc.org/learn/safety-knowledge/Pages/safety-at-home.aspx. Accessed November 8, 2016.

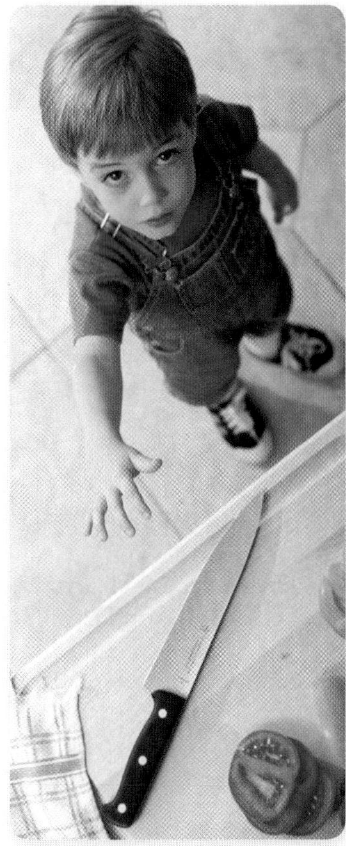

Figure 3-3 Children are at higher risk of sustaining serious injuries from an accident. Parents should always be on the alert for potential dangers within reach of a child.

© SuperStock/age fotostock.

distressing stories, *unintentional* injuries—accidents—are much more common and therefore represent a much greater threat.

Most frequently, injuries received at school occur during sports activities, industrial arts classes, and playground activities. Each year about 200,000 children 14 years of age and younger sustain injuries while playing on playgrounds, with more than 20,000 of these children suffering traumatic brain injuries.[9] The CDC also reports that more than 2.6 million children and teenagers are evaluated in the ED each year for sports-related injuries.[10]

▶ Chronic Illness

Chronic illnesses and diseases also represent a significant threat to public health in the United States. Annually, 7 out of 10 Americans die from chronic diseases, with cancer, heart disease, and stroke causing more than 50% of the deaths.[3] In 2012, about one-half of all adults—117 million Americans—had at least one chronic illness.[11] One in four had two or more chronic diseases.[11] **Table 3-3** summarizes US chronic illness statistics.

In 2011, asthma, a common chronic illness, was the primary diagnosis in 1,781,000 visits to the ED.[12] Among these, 611,000 occurred in patients less than 15 years of age.[12] Another 772,000 cases occurred in patients between 15 and 64 years of age.[12]

▶ Acute Illness

In April of 2009, the H1N1 influenza virus was first detected in a 10-year-old patient in California. As an outbreak unfolded, the CDC declared a US Public Health Emergency for H1N1 influenza, which eventually became a global pandemic as defined by the World Health Organization (WHO) in June of 2009. In September of that year, the Food and Drug Administration approved four vaccines for children and adults to try to prevent the disease. Through vaccination and ongoing communication from the CDC, prevention efforts targeted those people most susceptible to acquiring the illness. The WHO declared an end to the emergency in August 2010.[13]

Other health threats include contamination of the water supply, contamination of seafood (eg, from oil leaks), radiation leaks, lack of sanitary conditions after natural disasters, and increased incidence of cancer after major incidents.

The Cost of Public Health Threats

Beyond the unquestionable physical and emotional pain and suffering for patients and their families, the costs of injury and illness are far-reaching. The financial impact on families and communities cannot be understated, as the costs of health care, insurance, and additional governmental assistance programs rise in response.

Societal costs of injuries can be measured using the concept of **years of potential life lost (YPLL)**. This method assumes that, on average, most people live a productive life until the age of 65 years. For example, if a 22-year-old is killed in a bicycle crash, 43 years of potential life are lost (YPLL = 65 – Age at death). The YPLL associated with injuries is far greater than the YPLL linked with cancer or heart disease. Several reasons exist for this. First, younger people typically participate in more risk-taking activities than do older generations and as a result are more susceptible to fatal injuries. Older people do die from injuries, but when they do, fewer YPLL are lost than in a younger patient. In the preceding example, the 22-year-old patient had 43 YPLL. Suppose that the patient were 64 years old

Table 3-3 Chronic Illnesses in the United States

- 7 of 10 Americans die each year from chronic diseases.
- In 2012, approximately 117 million American adults had at least one chronic condition.
- Diabetes is the leading cause of kidney failure, blindness, and amputations of the lower extremities in Americans 20 years of age and older.
- Arthritis is the most common cause of disability, significantly impairing the lives of over 22 million Americans.
- 1 in every 3 adults is obese.
- 1 in 5 children and young adults between the ages of 2 and 19 years is obese.
- One-third of people with a chronic illness encounter basic or social problems that impair daily life.

Data from: Murphy S, Kochanek K, Xu J, Arias E. Mortality in the United States, 2014. National Center for Health Statistics Data Brief. 2015;229:1-8. http://www.cdc.gov/nchs/data/databriefs/db229.htm. Accessed September 1, 2016; Ward B, Schiller J, Goodman R. Multiple chronic conditions among US adults: a 2012 update. *Prev Chronic Dis*. 2014;11:130389. Accessed September 1, 2016; National diabetes statistics report: estimates of diabetes and its burden in the United States. Centers for Disease Control and Prevention. 2014. https://www.cdc.gov/diabetes/pubs/statsreport14/national-diabetes-report-web.pdf. Accessed September 9, 2016; Chronic diseases: the leading causes of death and disability in the United States. Centers for Disease Control and Prevention website. http://www.cdc.gov/chronicdisease/overview/. Updated February 23, 2016. Accessed September 1, 2016; Hootman J, Brault M, Helmick C, Theis K, Armour B. Prevalence and most common causes of disability among adults—United States, 2005. *MMWR*. 2009;58(16):421-426; Ogden C, Carroll M, Fryar C, Flegal K. Prevalence of obesity among adults and youth: United States, 2011–2014. NCHS data brief. 219: 2015. https://www.cdc.gov/nchs/data/databriefs/db219.pdf. Accessed August 31, 2016; and Houtum L, Rijken M, Groenewegen P. Do everyday problems of people with chronic illness interfere with their disease management? Biomed Central website. http://bmcpublichealth.biomedcentral.com/articles/10.1186/s12889-015-2303-3. Accessed August 31, 2016.

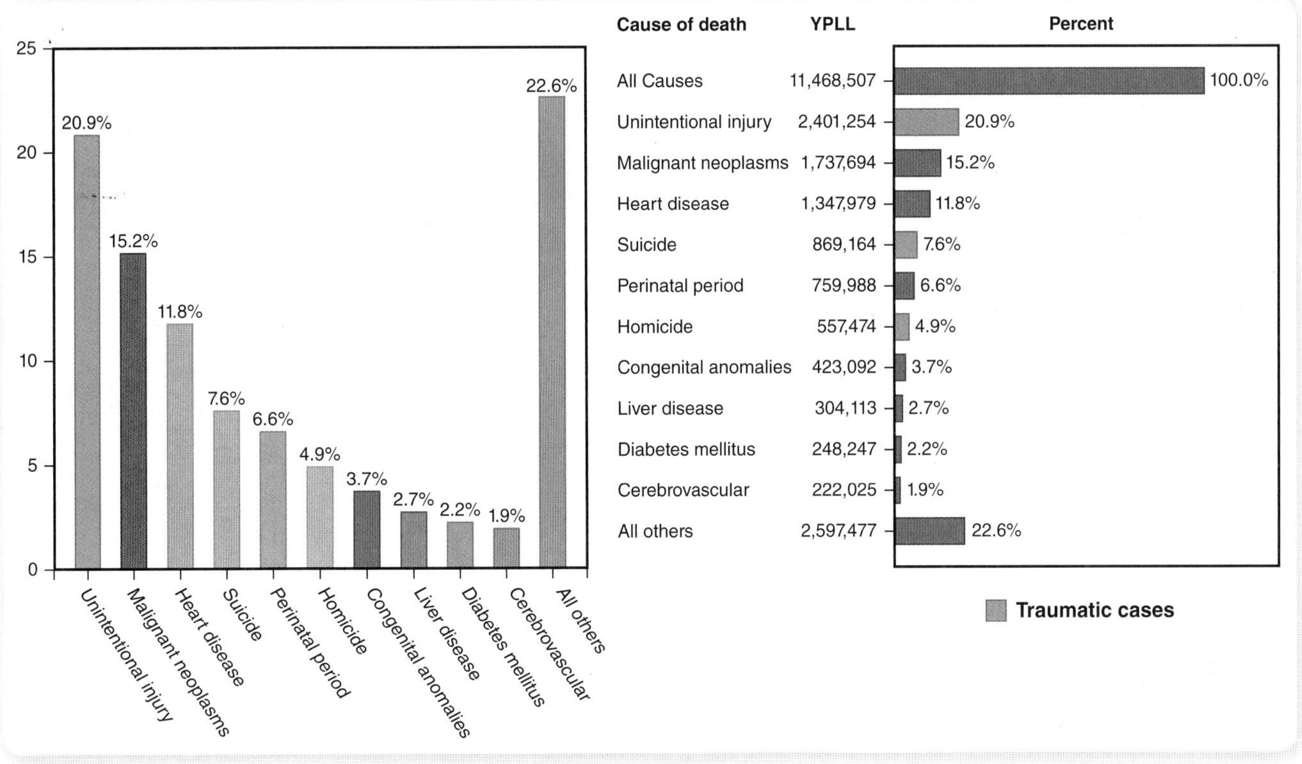

Figure 3-4 Years of potential life lost before age 65, categorized by cause of death (all races, both sexes, all deaths).

Data from: National Center for Injury Prevention and Control, 2014, United States.

when he was struck on the bicycle; in this case, only 1 year would be lost.

Because medical conditions such as heart disease and cancer cause death at a later age, they typically result in a lower YPLL than trauma. However, in some instances, such as congenital heart disease, a medical condition can cause significant YPLL. Finally, years of life lost are associated with death secondary to injury or illness as well as disability. Consider again the 22-year-old in a bicycle crash. If the patient did not die, but rather remained in a comatose state for the rest of his life, the term *YPLL* could still be applied. Although the patient did not lose potential life, he did lose years in which he would be earning income, paying taxes, and making other contributions to society.

Who pays for these costs? Unfortunately, *everyone* does. Through higher taxes and higher insurance premiums, we *all* pay the price.

Figure 3-4 compares years of potential productive work life lost by injury with other causes of death.

The Teachable Moment

You are on the scene of a motor vehicle collision (MVC). No one is seriously injured, but the driver admits he was not wearing his seat belt. As you prepare for transport, you look your patient in the eye and say, "You were very lucky this time. I've seen a lot of very severe injuries and even deaths caused by crashes much less serious than this one. You really need to wear your seat belt *every* time you get into a vehicle. It could save your life."

Near misses like these cause people to realize just how vulnerable they truly are and how perilous their actions could have been; thus, the lesson is more likely to stick. This is an example of a *teachable moment*, the time immediately following an event, when the sense of distress and danger is still very real and everyone concerned is perhaps more receptive to instruction on how the event or illness could have been prevented. In that moment, the role of the EMS provider as a caregiver and protector is perhaps at its strongest, giving you an optimal position to convey and reinforce the message. Understand that the concept of the teachable moment extends well beyond the realm of trauma to include frightening and potentially devastating medical incidents such as a diabetic who develops coma after missing breakfast. The coma is easily reversed with medication, but it could easily have resulted in death if not discovered in time and could easily have been prevented with more diligent attention to meal timing.

During a teachable moment, you can penetrate an individual's usual facade and reach his or her core values. However, when you do so, tread carefully. Lecturing a mother immediately after her child has been seriously injured is unlikely to be effective; in fact, it might cause her to become defensive or even hostile toward you. Therefore, it's crucial that you choose your moment wisely. Use good judgment, be nonjudgmental, and be sensitive to the emotionally charged nature of the situation Figure 3-5. Factors that constitute a teachable moment include:

- The injuries or illnesses are such that the parents, companions, or the patients themselves will be receptive to the message; you are aware of how ethnic and religious differences must temper the message.
- The scene is conducive to delivering such a message in a nonthreatening, nonjudgmental way. You are not intruding inappropriately or causing embarrassment that could lead to the opposite reaction.
- There is a definitive prevention measure that could have helped, such as using a seat belt, getting a flu shot, installing a car seat correctly, stopping smoking, wearing a helmet, or keeping firearms locked and safe. Vague advice is less likely to have a lasting effect.

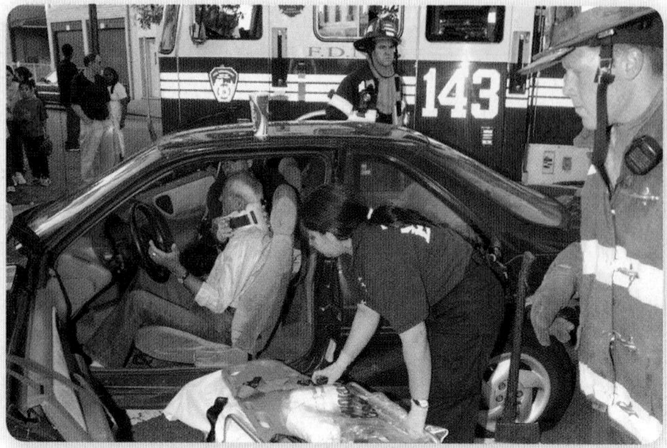

Figure 3-5 When injuries are not apparently serious, consider reinforcing the need for safety to prevent future injuries. Remind vehicle drivers and occupants of the importance of compliance with seat belt laws.

Sometimes, a teachable moment can be preemptive, taking place well before a tragic event occurs. For example, imagine you are providing a wellness check in the home of an older patient when you notice a potential tripping

YOU are the Paramedic PART 2

Upon arrival, you find a single vehicle angled downward in a ditch, with severe front-end damage that apparently resulted from a high-speed impact with a tree. You can see a woman sitting in the driver's seat with a volunteer firefighter holding her cervical spine neutral and in-line. Several feet away from the vehicle, another woman stands holding a crying infant with several obvious abrasions and blood on his face. The woman holding the infant states she was not involved in the crash, but she and her husband saw it happen. She says that, upon impact with the tree, the infant, still in his car seat, was thrown from the vehicle, landing in the ditch. She then raced across the street and removed the child from the car seat. At the same time, her husband hurried over to check on the driver and then called 9-1-1.

Your partner is speaking with the driver, who is crying uncontrollably and shouting, "I'm fine. Please just take care of my baby!" She had been wearing her seat belt and her only complaint is mild ankle pain. The second unit arrives and assumes care for the mother, at which time you and your partner focus on the infant, an 8-month-old boy. Immediately, you see he has a 1-inch-long laceration surrounded by a 2-inch-diameter hematoma on the right side of his forehead (the bleeding was controlled prior to your arrival). Additionally, you observe a slight degree of angulation in the infant's left forearm.

Recording Time: 0 Minutes	
Appearance	Agitated and crying
Level of consciousness	Awake and age appropriate
Airway	Open, clear, and patent
Breathing	Rapid rate, frequent gasping while crying
Circulation	Brachial pulse is strong, rapid, and regular. Skin is pink, warm, and dry. Bleeding from head laceration has been controlled.

3. What are the risk factors associated with the infant's injuries?
4. Is this a teachable moment?

hazard in the living room. Taking the time to inform the patient of the danger and then giving advice as to how this threat can be averted may very well save the patient from a fall and injury in the future. The informal nature of this education makes it perhaps the most effective kind you can provide.

Words of Wisdom

The concept of the teachable moment is important and valuable, but it must be used correctly. It is important to avoid communication that could be perceived as belittling, condescending, pedantic, or otherwise disrespectful. For example, in a situation where the paramedic is relatively young (in his or her 20s) and the patient is perhaps older (in his or her 50s or older), if the patient perceives the paramedic to be lecturing or scolding, the paramedic's efforts will be counterproductive. Use good communications skills, be culturally sensitive, and be nonjudgmental at all times.

The best teachable moments are those that convey positive reinforcement. If people are wearing seat belts properly and survive a crash with little or no injury, tell them, "It's a good thing you had your seat belts on." You will notice smiles on their faces and they will likely remember your statement forever.

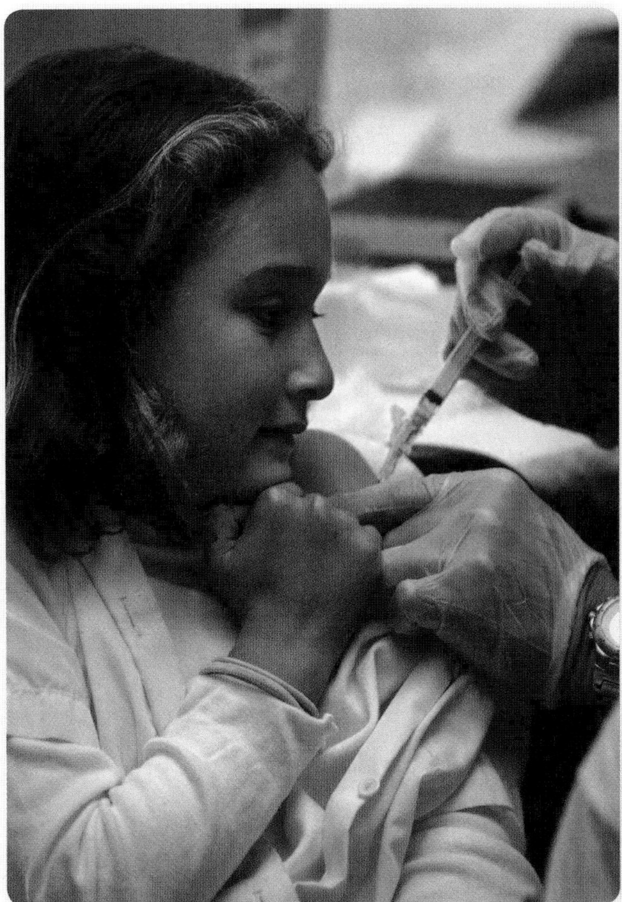

Figure 3-6 Vaccination programs allow the general public to receive flu vaccinations, helping to reduce the overall incidence of the flu.

Prevention

Public health efforts aim to have an impact on people within an entire city, community, state, or country. For example, a vaccination program conducted by a local health department may provide flu vaccines to children and adults in its community **Figure 3-6**. Through these efforts, people stay well during flu season, use health care resources less, continue going to school, and remain productive in their jobs. The quality of life improves for the whole community, the economy is more stable with its workforce intact, and health care costs are lowered.

▶ The 4 Es of Prevention

Interventions—specific actions intended to improve health and safety outcomes—need to combine *education* with three other types of interventions: *enforcement, engineering/environment*, and *economic incentives*. These are commonly referred to as the "4 Es of prevention" **Figure 3-7**. The most effective prevention efforts reflect a combination of these interventions.

Education

Most paramedics know that people can behave in ways that cause them to become injured, ill, or put others at risk. Many people do not know and therefore cannot assess the risk of doing something—"I didn't know it was unsafe to put my baby's seat in the front passenger seat" or "I didn't think I needed a flu shot." Or people know the risk—"I won't wear seat belts, they are too uncomfortable" or "I don't believe in giving my baby all of those shots"—and disregard it anyway. Through education you can often inform people about potential dangers and then act to persuade them to change risky behavior. Show moms and dads how to use an infant car seat. Tell people about the horrors of being thrown from a vehicle. Relate general information about people you have treated who were at risk of death from the flu. Explain how pertussis, which was once nonexistent in the United States due to adequate vaccinations, is once again being seen in this country and why childhood immunizations are so important. **Table 3-4** lists several additional health and safety tips that anyone can put to use if they are made aware.

To be effective, messages need to be tailored to very specific groups and reinforced with meaningful rewards. Educational techniques that seem to be particularly promising include the use of contracts or participant commitment, incentives, behavioral feedback, and modeling.

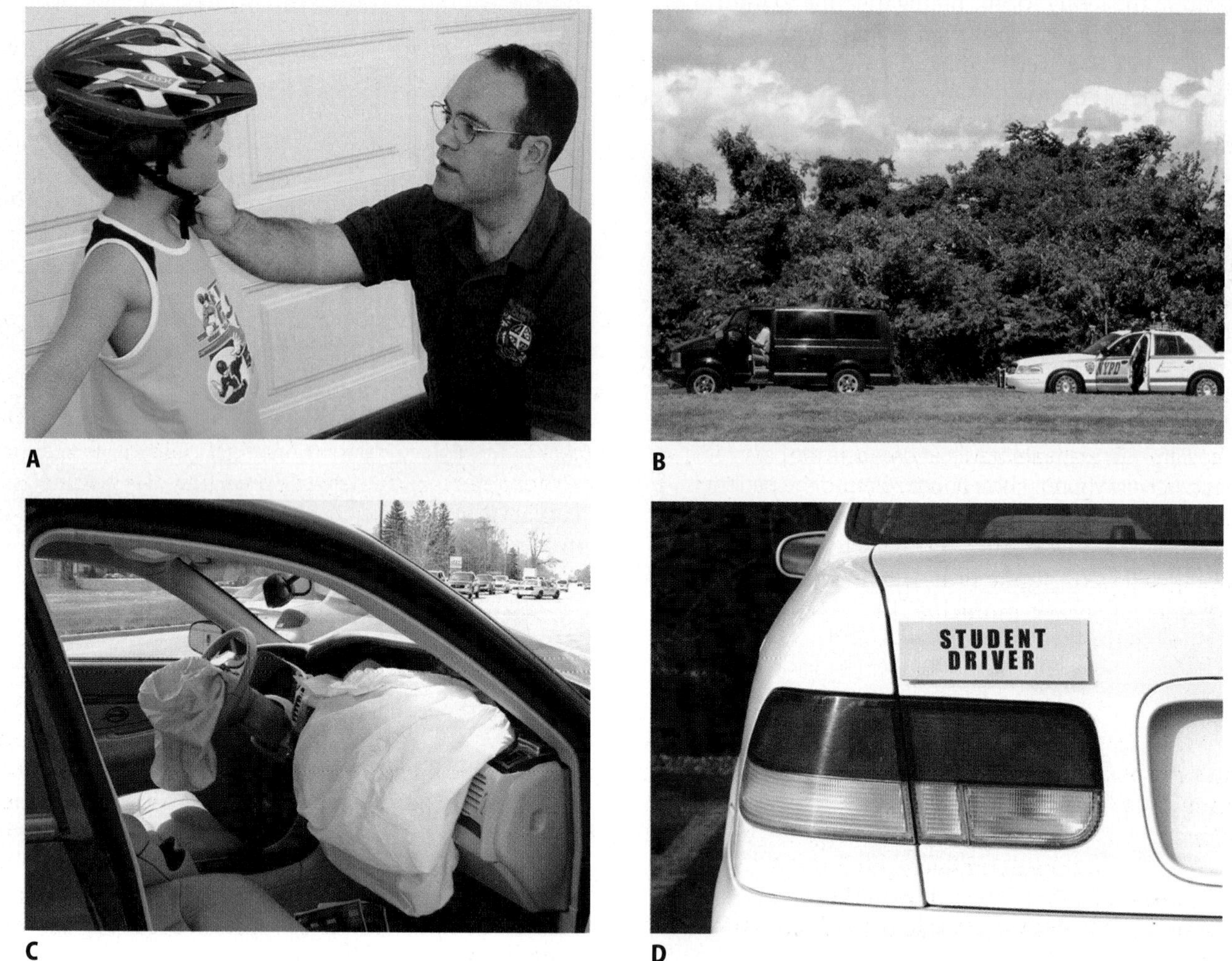

Figure 3-7 The 4 Es of prevention include education **(A)**, enforcement **(B)**, engineering/environment **(C)**, and economic incentives **(D)**. Examples of economic incentives include lower insurance rates for young drivers who have taken approved driver education programs or for adults who do not smoke.

A: Courtesy of Henry Pollak; B: © Vladimir Korostyshevskiy/Shutterstock.; C: Courtesy of Captain David Jackson, Saginaw Township Fire Department; D: © Jones & Bartlett Learning. Photographed by Kimberly Potvin.

Table 3-4 Tips for Promoting Safety and Health

- Teach children about safety measures, such as never inserting their fingers into a wall socket, avoiding the oven and stove, and avoiding the pool when adults are not directly supervising.
- Supervise children at all times.
- Once they are old enough to understand, teach children how to dial 9-1-1, and teach them when it is appropriate to do so.
- Program emergency phone numbers into your telephone. Include numbers for the local police department, fire department, EMS, and poison control. If your phone is not programmable, post these phone numbers in a nearby visible location such as on the refrigerator.
- Ensure your home and its exterior are well lit and that surfaces are even.
- Ensure all electrical cords are placed out of the flow of traffic.
- Avoid small rugs or runners that are not slip-resistant.
- Install and maintain smoke alarms.
- If your home uses gas heat, install and maintain carbon monoxide detectors.
- Use safety latches to prevent children opening drawers or cabinets that contain potentially dangerous substances, such as medicines or cleaning products.
- Install safety gates around stairs and swimming pools.
- Keep your hot water heater adjusted to less than 120°F (48.9°C) to prevent burns.
- Teach hands-only CPR to your family and friends.

Abbreviations: CPR, cardiopulmonary resuscitation; EMS, emergency medical services

Modified from National Public Health Week April 4–10, 2011. American Public Health Association. http://www.nphw.org/nphw11/tips_home.htm. Accessed April 20, 2011.

Enforcement

Sometimes, despite your best efforts, even though some members of your community may understand the risks, their behavior will not necessarily change. However, one advantage to any educational effort is that it can occasionally pave the way to legislative and environmental/technological changes.

Sometimes behavior change can be facilitated by changes in the law. Legislation/regulation formulates rules that require people, manufacturers, and governments to comply with certain safety practices. Elected government bodies legislate, or enact laws, that require safe practices. Bureaucracies or agencies that set policies and establish procedures create regulations that control the manufacture, sale, and/or use of products. All these measures have been shown to be helpful in enforcement of safety regulations.

There are many rules, regulations, guidelines, and laws that govern public health. Some are federal while individual states or municipalities promulgate others. A few examples are provided in Table 3-5.

Economic Incentives

Saving money by receiving a reduction in your insurance rates for being a careful driver or a nonsmoker is one example of how monetary incentives can reinforce safe behavior. Also, organizations often recognize the value of offering free or subsidized safety products (bike helmets, fire extinguishers, safety locks, smoking cessation kits, contraceptives), which may lead to a reduction in certain threats to public health.

Engineering/Environment

Most EMS providers can think of spots on the road where environmental changes such as adding guardrails or smoothing out dangerous curves could prevent crashes. Indeed, making environmental changes or changing the way certain products are designed (eg, adding a new safety feature to vehicles) can offer automatic protection from injury, often without any conscious change in a person's behavior. These are called **passive interventions**. One example of this is the development of child-resistant medication bottles, a passive intervention that reduces poisonings and can be more effective and reliable than simply trying to keep the bottle out of a child's reach.

Strategies to modify environmental factors are often expensive and can include social, legal, political, and cultural approaches. Thus, they typically occur only after public awareness has been increased, thereby motivating the community to take responsibility for seeing positive changes made.

▶ The Value of Passive Interventions

Passive interventions—those preventive measures that do not require conscious effort on the part of a potential victim—are often the most successful. Also referred to as automatic protection, passive interventions include such things as the use of sprinkler systems in commercial buildings, airbags in automobiles, and softer, yielding materials as playground surfaces. These measures can provide 24-hour protection without requiring any real effort on the part of the user.

YOU are the Paramedic — PART 3

Following your local protocol, you take measures to protect the infant's spine. Your partner informs you that, according to his mother, the child has no significant medical history, has no known allergies, and does not take any medications. The woman holding the infant tells you that she found him face down, still strapped into his car seat, and crying when she got to him. However, no one on the scene can say with certainty whether the child lost consciousness.

Recording Time: 3 Minutes	
Respirations	42 breaths/min
Pulse	138 beats/min
Skin	Pink, warm, and dry
Oxygen saturation (Spo_2)	99% on room air
Pupils	PERRLA

5. What primary prevention measures might have helped to circumvent this traumatic incident? List any passive interventions that could have made a positive impact.

Table 3-5 Public Health Laws, Regulations, and Guidelines to Improve Safety and Prevention

Law	Date	Description
Motorcycle helmets	As of June 2015	No federal law. State laws vary widely. 19 states, the District of Columbia, Puerto Rico, and the US Virgin and Northern Mariana Islands had laws requiring *all* riders to wear a helmet. Most other states and territories required *some* riders to wear a helmet (usually based upon the rider's age). 3 states (Illinois, Iowa, and New Hampshire) did not have a motorcycle helmet law.
Bicycle helmets	As of July 2012	No federal law. 22 states, the District of Columbia, and over 200 municipalities and counties had child helmet laws. Most of these laws only cover bicyclists less than 18 years of age. 13 states had no state or local bicycle helmet laws.
Seat belts	As of November 2016	34 states and the District of Columbia had laws allowing law enforcement to stop and cite violators independent of any other traffic violations. 15 states had laws that only permitted law enforcement to give citations to violators who had initially been stopped for some other violation. New Hampshire had no seat belt law for adults.
Smoking and tobacco laws (federal)	2009	The 2009 Family Smoking Prevention and Tobacco Control Act, Food and Drug Administration, restricted the sale, distribution, and marketing of cigarettes and smokeless tobacco products to youth in the United States.
Smoking and tobacco laws (state and local)	As of October 2016	Highly variable from one state or municipality to another. Of all states, along with the District of Columbia, Puerto Rico, and the US Virgin Islands, 25 had "comprehensive" laws that require non-hospitality workplaces, bars, and restaurants to be 100% smoke-free. In 30 others, similar laws apply only to restaurants and bars, but not workplaces. And 21 have laws that only regulate smoking in gambling establishments.
State of New York regarding AEDs	2002	Law passed that required at least one AED in each school and that at least one staff member be trained in its use. Saved at least 95 lives as of February 2017.
State of Connecticut regarding AEDs	2009	Law that made AEDs available in public schools; ensured that at least two staff members are trained to use them; prompted by the death of a 15-year-old student who died after collapsing during a run at school. Companion bill reduced liability issues for AED users.

Abbreviation: AED, automated external defibrillator

Data from: Motorcycle helmet use. Insurance Institute for Highway Safety Highway Loss Data Institute website. www.iihs.org/iihs/topics/laws/helmetuse?topicName=motorcycles. Accessed August 2, 2016; Bicycle Helmet Safety Institute. Helmets.org website. http://www.helmets.org/mandator.htm. Accessed August 4, 2016; Seatbelt laws. Governors Highway Safety Association website. http://www.ghsa.org/html/stateinfo/laws/seatbelt_laws.html. Accessed November 29, 2016; Overview List - how many smokefree laws? Americans for Nonsmokers' Rights website. www.no-smoke.org/pdf/mediaordlist.pdf from http://www.no-smoke.org/goingsmokefree.php?id=519. Published October 1, 2016. Accessed October 19, 2016; and Success stories. LA12.org: Taking Our Children Out of Harm's Way website. http://la12.org/success-stories/. Accessed February 24, 2017.

Comparing education to automatic protection strategies, consider how each might aid in the prevention of head and chest injuries in MVCs:

- **Option 1.** Educate people on the importance of wearing their seat belts.
- **Option 2.** Mandate that all new vehicles be manufactured with automatic seat belts and airbags installed.

The automatic protection offered by Option 2 is more likely to reduce injuries, because people do not have to do anything to make it work. However, the most effective strategies include a combination of education, enforcement, engineering/environmental modifications, and/or economic incentive programs. Education, in particular, is always a factor. Motor vehicle passengers need to know that airbags do not replace the need for seat belts.

Why EMS Should Be Involved

In the historic National Academy of Sciences/National Research Council's 1966 study, *Accidental Death and Disability: The Neglected Disease of Modern Society*, the commission noted that just as EMS could help with trauma *after* an event, injury prevention initiatives could help *before* an accident happened.[14]

In 1996, representing every imaginable EMS constituency, the *Consensus Statement on the EMS Role in Primary Injury Prevention* contended that working toward this level of prevention should be seen as an "essential" activity "that must be undertaken by the leaders, decision-makers, and providers of every EMS system."[15]

Primary prevention is the name given to actions that stop injuries or illnesses before they begin. **Secondary prevention** measures take place after a patient has sustained an injury or developed an illness, in which case the goal is to "prevent" the problem from getting worse (eg, stabilizing a fractured extremity to prevent further tissue, nerve, or vascular damage; or administering epinephrine to a patient having an allergic reaction to a bee sting).

Historically, EMS has focused almost exclusively on *secondary* prevention. Fortunately, however, EMS culture has changed in recent years, and providers are now more involved in *primary* prevention efforts within their communities (Figure 3-8).

Unlike other medical professionals, EMS providers see citizens in their homes and environments and during activities of daily life. As a result, EMS providers have more opportunities for prevention education than do other health care professionals. As previously stated, both the community and the health care system benefit more from preventing injuries and illness than from trying to treat them after they occur. Additional advantages of EMS involvement in prevention education follow:

- EMS providers are widely distributed among the population.
- In a remote setting, EMS providers may be the most medically educated people available. EMS providers may be the only source of help, whether they are a 1-hour drive down the mountain to the nearest ED or 200 miles offshore on an oil platform.
- There are more than 826,111 credentialed EMS providers in the United States at the EMT, advanced, and paramedic levels.[16]
- EMS providers are considered advocates of the health care consumer. EMS providers work in concert with their patients and their patients' families.
- EMS providers are welcome in schools and other environments.
- EMS providers are considered authorities on injury and prevention.

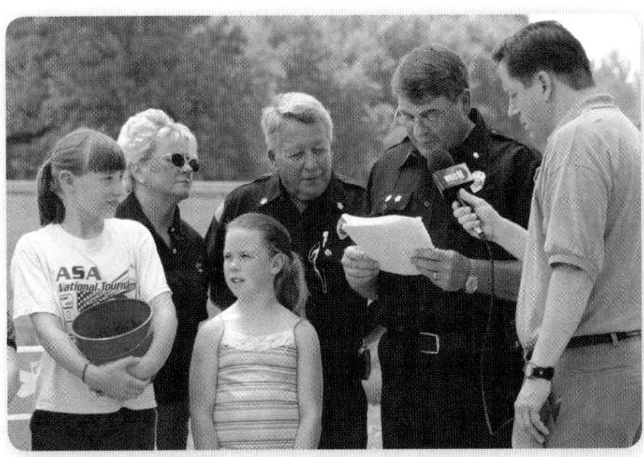

Figure 3-8 Embracing the full role of a paramedic means being involved in the concerns of your community.

How EMS Can Get Involved

Motivated by their field experiences, EMS providers have emerged as strong advocates—and practitioners—of injury and illness prevention. A number of paramedics have taken a more proactive role in new prevention programs, sometimes taking the lead in developing these programs.

For example, in 2016, paramedic Lisa Cassidy of the St. Charles County Ambulance District in Missouri lead the charge in an awareness campaign called "Stop Heroin." Emboldened by a rising problem of heroin abuse in the community and the tragic deaths of many young users, Cassidy and over 200 of her colleagues began every shift by donning "Stop Heroin" uniforms. Every day across the county, the public saw paramedics on calls, at schools, and at other community events, wearing shirts that boldly proclaimed "Stop Heroin." This sparked a public awareness campaign ultimately featured in local and national publications. When asked why she became involved in the initiative, Cassidy said, "When it comes to drug use and overdoses, EMS has always been 'reactive.' Someone overdoses, we give Narcan, transport . . . the end. Since Narcan does not always work, I and the rest of my colleagues are all too often forced to deliver the worst news that a

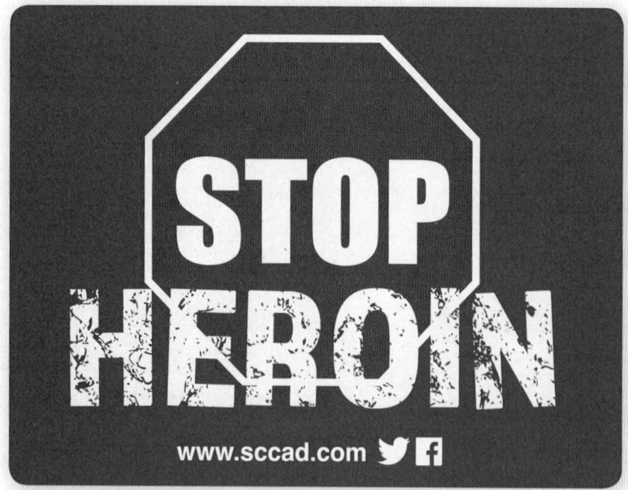

Figure 3-9 Inspired by the passionate convictions of paramedic Lisa Cassidy, the St. Charles County Ambulance District began an aggressive awareness and prevention campaign targeting heroin abuse in their community.

Courtesy of St. Charles County Ambulance District.

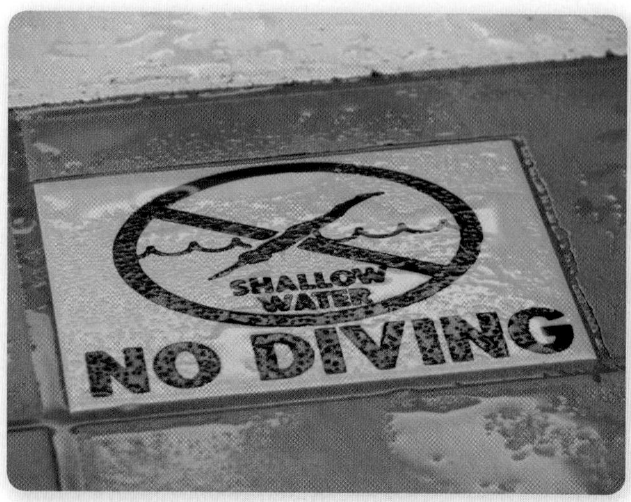

Figure 3-10 Many rules of public safety exist because of the persistent efforts of medical professionals and other involved citizens.

© Dewitt/Shutterstock.

mother or father will ever receive: that we did everything we could, but their child is dead. This conversation was happening over and over, and with increasing frequency in our community. I decided that, as the organization that sees these situations firsthand, we should be part of the conversation, and hopefully, have a hand in developing a meaningful solution to the problem that is plaguing our county" Figure 3-9.

Strategies that promote interventions might include fundraisers to purchase and distribute free bicycle helmets to children, car seat checks and installations, appearing at health fairs, giving speeches to community groups and schoolchildren, blood pressure checks, fall prevention services for older adults, or swimming safety education Figure 3-10.

One of the most visible ways in which EMS professionals have interacted with public health agencies is through the provision of immunizations. Consider how EMS professionals are ideally suited to reach at-risk populations. Their inherent mobility allows them to reach widely dispersed populations, an advantage that might be especially helpful in rural areas where vaccination sites are either scarce, too far away, or impractical for people without a reliable means of transportation. One other benefit may be the typically positive perception of EMS in small communities; this puts providers in an ideal position to bring aid to patients and families who are unable or unwilling to use private or governmental health care services.

Many EMS providers have the requisite clinical training in medication security, aseptic technique, medication administration, postinjection care, documentation of such things as informed consent for treatment, and how to discuss risks, benefits, and possible side effects with the patient. Combined with the routine tasks performed by paramedics on the ambulance, this training makes them excellent candidates for the administration of vaccines to adults and children.

Of course, for such a program to work, EMS must work closely with the local public health agency to develop a plan that addresses all logistical matters, clearly defines each person's role and responsibilities, identifies and resolves any issues pertaining to the need for additional training, clearly explains the procedures for procuring the vaccine, and forestalls potential liability issues. Most of the time, these challenges are nowhere near as complicated as they may sound.

The Pennsylvania MEDICVAX project demonstrated the efficacy of EMS agencies in providing more than 2,000 adult influenza vaccinations. Most likely, nearly one-third of the clients would not have received vaccinations otherwise.[17]

As the health care landscape continues to change in response to legislation like the Affordable Care Act, paramedics across the United States have begun to witness the next evolution in the field of EMS. The terms *community paramedic* and *mobile integrated health care* have garnered nationwide attention over the past several years. In fact, several states have already implemented education requirements and legislation that recognizes the legitimacy of community paramedicine. Other states are already doing the same.

The concept of community paramedicine, discussed in Chapter 53, *Career Development*, gives providers many new and expanded avenues for preventing illnesses and injuries as part of their regular daily duties. Conducting home health visits and well-being checks, providing wound

Words of Wisdom

In addition to being a health care provider, you—like any other health professional—must also be a health educator and advocate. Teaching helps keep your skills sharp; at the same time, it identifies you as a resource person in the community.

care and other in-home therapies, ensuring medication compliance—the possibilities seem endless. EMS agencies that offer community paramedic services may eventually be recognized as a cost-effective supplement or alternative to ED visits and hospital admissions.

By offering these expanded services, EMS agencies could take a more proactive approach in decreasing the **morbidity** (number of nonfatal injuries and subsequent disability) and **mortality** (death rate) of their patients. Providers could also play a significant role in reducing unnecessary hospital readmission, wherein patients who were recently discharged from the hospital return only days later for conditions that could have been managed or prevented at home. These readmissions are not only expensive for the patient but also for hospitals (which may be at risk for the additional financial exposure under certain circumstances) and society at large, which will ultimately bear the financial burden through increases in insurance premiums and health care costs.

As for the financial benefits for EMS systems, opportunities for reimbursement could exist through creative contracting with hospitals, managed care agencies, or other third-party payers who recognize the significant financial savings they could realize through a partnership with the EMS agency.

The Canadian province of Nova Scotia has taken this idea one step further and introduced the concept of primary care paramedic. By providing nontransport preventive and primary care services as part of a paramedic-based integrated care model on two remote islands in the province, hospitalizations of residents of the islands were reduced 23% over a 3-year study period.[18]

Documentation & Communication

Do not forget special population groups in your safety and prevention programs. For instance, you may find different illness and injury patterns related to ethnicity and can present these topics through your programs. Have printed materials available in all languages throughout your community. Do not neglect people with physical and developmental disabilities. Do your best to get the word out in every way possible.

Special Populations

With a growing geriatric population, a good flu prevention program may be one of the keys to preventing an overload of the health care system. Evaluate all community options available to the older population in your area and bridge any gaps with programs to meet their needs and prevent illnesses related to the flu.

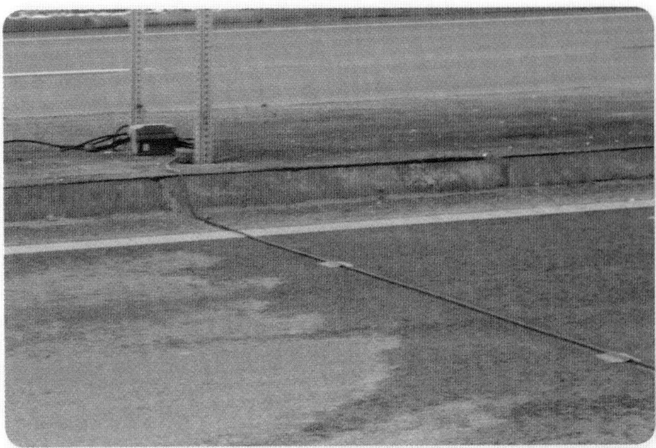

Figure 3-11 One type of surveillance that is familiar to anyone who drives is the use of technology that can tally the number of cars using a particular roadway.

Injury and Illness Surveillance

In prevention, **surveillance** involves watching over society, and collecting and analyzing data. It is the ongoing, systematic collection, analysis, and interpretation of data essential to the planning, implementation, and evaluation of public health practice **Figure 3-11**.

Once the data have been carefully analyzed and interpreted by **epidemiologists**, scientists who study the causes, patterns, prevalence, and control of disease in groups of people—a field of study referred to as **epidemiology**—the information can be employed in the development of interventions intended to prevent further injury or illness.

Words of Wisdom

One manner in which EMS can assist public health efforts is through the use of dispatch data as **syndromic surveillance**. In a syndromic surveillance system, information regarding the number and nature of medical cases is compared with an expected volume of calls for the community at a given time and place. If cases exceed the expected volumes, epidemiologists are alerted to the possibility of an outbreak of disease.

A strong surveillance system is fundamental to creating an effective prevention program. In the case of injury surveillance, you need to know *who* is being injured, *where*, *by what* mechanism, and—if readily discernable—*why*. For the most effective injury and disease surveillance program, begin by becoming familiar with the injuries and diseases common within your community.

The Haddon Matrix

William Haddon, Jr, MD, the National Highway Traffic Safety Administration's first director, was given a mandate: to find ways to prevent people from being killed and

Documentation & Communication

In the setting of a possible public health threat, the patient care reports that paramedics write following every call may be read and analyzed by epidemiologists to identify leading causes of injury or illness and how to correct them. To guarantee "clean" data, you must completely fill out all the required fields in an EMS report no matter how minute the details may seem. Information such as a patient's gender or whether he or she was restrained during a motor vehicle collision is imperative for accurate analysis. Your narrative section is equally important, if not more so. Be as accurate and detailed as possible when reporting the circumstances behind an injury or illness. Although you may have checked the appropriate box in your care report, do not forget to describe the details. Narratives tell the story of what happened, helping the reader see the incident through his or her mind's eye. This firsthand information is often lost in hospital and police reports that rely on third- and fourth-hand information hours or days later; thus, it is crucial that your reports be clear and concise, yet thorough and detailed.

injured on the nation's highways. Haddon created a matrix that identified several principles of injury prevention.[19,20] The matrix proved so successful in helping researchers think about injuries, that it was named after Haddon: the **Haddon matrix**. Haddon added the factor of *time* to the previous models used to address the causes of injury. The host, agent, and environment are seen as factors that interact over time to cause injury. These factors correspond to three phases of the event: pre-event, event, and post-event. The matrix uses nine separate components to analyze the injury. The Haddon matrix encourages creative thinking in understanding the causes of and potential interventions for injury. Table 3-6 shows a Haddon matrix for the example of bicycle–motor vehicle collisions.

Most EMS providers are trained to respond in the *post-event* phase, after an injury or illness has taken place. This is *reactive*, not preventive. However, the post-event phase may be the optimal time to reflect on the event and apply your firsthand knowledge, asking, "*Why* did this happen?" and "*How* might this be prevented in the future?"

If you are willing to expend the extra effort, truly fulfilling your role as your patients' advocate, you might be surprised at the difference you can make, motivating other medical professionals and organizations, your local

Table 3-6 Childhood Motor Vehicle Occupant Injuries Using the Haddon Matrix

	Host (Human)	Agent (Car Seat/Vehicle)	Environment
Pre-event	▪ Wear seat belts and use car seats at all times. ▪ Ensure the babysitter, day care, and extended family members use car seat. ▪ Drive defensively. ▪ Reduce driving during high-risk times, such as rush hour, holiday weekends, or high-speed long-distance travel.	▪ Maintain up-to-date recall information on car seats. ▪ Manufacture easy-to-use car seats. ▪ Provide 3-point seat belts in rear seating positions. ▪ Regulate good maintenance and safety features of vehicle.	▪ Enforce seat belt and car seat laws. ▪ Encourage safer roads with lower speeds, breakaway poles, and medians. ▪ Encourage low-cost car seat programs. ▪ Conduct media and education campaigns about seat belts, car seats, drunk driving, and enforcement.
Event	▪ Driver maintains control of vehicle. ▪ Driver is belted. ▪ Child is restrained.	▪ Seat belts and correctly used car seats restrain and protect. ▪ Vehicle design provides crash protection.	▪ Breakaway signs and light poles are in place. ▪ Guardrails and medians are in place.
Post-event	▪ Bystanders are trained in first response. ▪ EMS personnel are expertly trained in treating pediatric injuries as well as car seat and seat belt extrications.	▪ Ambulances are outfitted with up-to-date supplies and equipment designed for children.	▪ Roadside call boxes are in place. ▪ 9-1-1 and emergency medical dispatch systems are in place. ▪ Adequate road shoulders for emergency use are in place. ▪ There is quality EMS response and transport. ▪ The patient is transported to a trauma center per protocol.

government, and other members of your community to get involved. Through your eyes—the eyes of someone uniquely qualified to speak to the problem—perhaps they will be compelled to examine the problem more closely and ultimately to pursue and implement strategic solutions in the *pre-event* phase, sparing someone's son or daughter, or mother or father from experiencing an event in the first place. Prevention is always better than crisis management.[21]

Getting Started in Your Community

Every community has its own unique problems, many of which have a negative impact on the well-being of its residents. Trying to address all of these issues would be an overwhelming task. It would divide attentions in so many different directions that it would be nearly impossible to research, develop, and implement any meaningful and effective interventions for every problem. Therefore, the most effective prevention programs elect to focus on problems that impair the health and well-being of the greatest number of people, thereby potentially *helping* the greatest number of people.

In time, perhaps you'll get the opportunity to target other problems you want to address, even though they may only impact a minority of the population. However, by first tackling those issues that affect the greatest number of citizens, you and your community will feel a sense of pride at accomplishing a task that has had maximum impact on the community's well-being.

Words of Wisdom

Start your project with small, realistic goals. Contact other communities that have addressed similar problems. Learn from them, and perhaps you will avoid wasting time and energy creating something that already exists.

Recognizing Injury and Illness Patterns in Your Community

To be effective in prevention, you need to understand the specific and perhaps unique patterns of injuries and illnesses that occur in your community. Examine the characteristics of your community's population, environment, and the types of risks present. Your regional or state EMS department or public health office would be an excellent place to start, because they will likely have the most data, statistics, and other resources with relevant information. Many state organizations even make this information available on the Internet.

As an EMS provider, you can make a difference by being diligent in your documentation. Your firsthand observations may be relevant to other agencies such as law enforcement, the legal system, and social services seeking to intercede in settings of intentional violence. Paramedic training prepares you to recognize and report the signs and risk factors associated with, for example, intentional violence and empowers you to be proactive

YOU are the Paramedic PART 4

Once the infant is immobilized and loaded into the ambulance, you decide the mechanism of injury alone is reason to commence rapid transport to the closest trauma center. En route, you start an intravenous (IV) line, clean and dress the wound on his head, and splint his left arm. Upon arrival at the trauma center, you find the pediatric trauma team awaiting your report.

Recording Time: 10 Minutes	
Respirations	42 breaths/min
Pulse	126 beats/min
Skin	Pink, warm, and dry
Cardiac monitor	Sinus tachycardia without ectopy
Oxygen saturation (Spo_2)	99% on room air
Pupils	PERRLA

6. Apply the Haddon Matrix to this scenario.
7. What steps have you taken that would be considered secondary injury prevention?
8. What steps could you take to develop a prevention program to reduce similar incidents in the future?

Documentation & Communication

The importance of collecting data in measuring trends, validating interventions, assessing resources, and ultimately, persuading others to act, cannot be overstated. For the EMS provider, this process begins with the prehospital care report. By accurately describing the details of the scene, the mechanism of injury, the nature of the injury or illness, status of the patient's immunizations, and the use or absence of protective devices, you are providing important evidence demonstrating the scope of the problem.

in the fight against suicide, domestic violence, and child abuse. This medical training and the unique perspective of being present at the scene makes you among the few professionals able to provide this invaluable service.

As you make the journey from rookie paramedic to seasoned EMS veteran, never forget that your actions or inactions will influence other members of your crew, as well as the next generation of paramedics. The example you set will have an impact long after you retire.

Words of Wisdom

As an EMS provider, you are continually taught to use personal protective equipment such as a helmet, reflective vest, and gloves and to observe traffic and other safety laws while on the job. The need for personal safety doesn't stop when your shift is over though. Wear a seat belt and observe safety laws in everything you do. Practice a safe lifestyle both on and off the job.

▶ Prevention Programs for Children

Many prevention programs focus on children. There are various government and private grants, commercial sponsors, and nonprofit groups that will support car seat inspections, helmet donations, fundraising events, and more, because they recognize the serious threat that injury poses to children. One such resource is Safe Kids Worldwide, a nonprofit organization made up of more than 400 coalitions in the United States and partners in over 30 countries. This organization's goal is to reduce the prevalence of preventable childhood injuries.[22] Its website is filled with helpful information, including examples of how other groups have addressed challenges similar to yours and resources that can assist you as you formulate new ideas.

Sometimes, our focus on children's issues can have other unintended benefits. One of these is the "pass-along effect," wherein other members of a child's family benefit from the message originally intended solely for the welfare of the child. An example of this phenomenon occurs when a third-grader is educated on the importance of wearing a seat belt and later insists that Daddy buckle up, too.

With the wide array of injuries affecting children, how should you prioritize your prevention efforts? Experts in public health suggest focusing on injuries associated with a high rate of mortality, hospitalizations frequently accompanied by long-term disability, or those known to have highly effective countermeasures. In other words, give priority to injuries that are common, severe, and readily preventable.

▶ The Five Steps to Developing a Prevention Program

This step-by-step approach to establishing an injury prevention program, as advocated by the Emergency Medical Services for Children (EMSC) program, emphasizes the need to carefully establish goals and objectives with measurable outcomes.[23] (Although the following discusses childhood prevention programs, the methods can be applied to other age groups as well.)

1. **Conduct a community assessment.** Bring people and groups together to assess what is already being accomplished in your region and to establish what resources (expertise, time, money) are potentially available. Ensure you invite people who represent the community at large, in all its diversity, including survivors of injuries or major illnesses and their families Figure 3-12. Recognize that there may be members who have had a loved one die as a result of a preventable injury or illness; these people can be powerful advocates. Potential partners include:
   - EMS groups (private and public ground and air ambulance services, fire departments and firefighter unions, volunteer services, rescue squads, lifeguards)

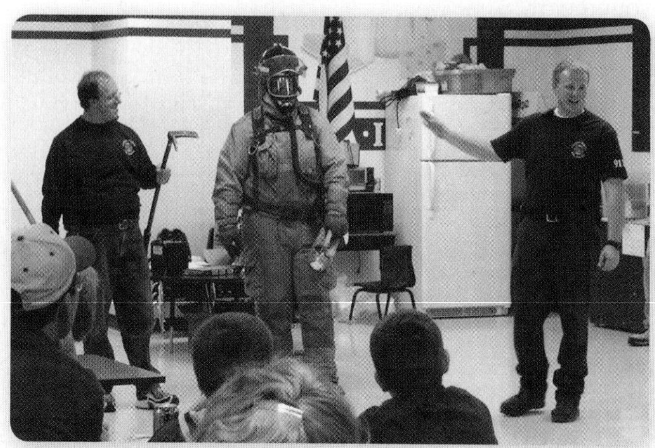

Figure 3-12 Fire safety training is an example of ways in which public safety agencies engage in injury prevention activities.

- Law enforcement (police departments and police officers, unions, sheriff's office, highway patrol, training academies)
- School groups (parent-teacher associations, student clubs, school boards, faculty)
- The media (management, editorial board members, staff reporters)
- Public health officials and health care providers (groups representing emergency physicians and nurses, pediatricians, managed care organizations, hospitals, clinics)
- Members of the business community (including those related to insurance, cars, sports, home improvements, safety equipment, local chambers of commerce)
- Religious organizations, civic groups, and service clubs (such as the Kiwanis and the Boy Scouts and Girl Scouts)
- Sports-related organizations (such as Little Leagues or YMCAs)
- Local chapters of nonprofit groups (such as Safe Kids coalitions, Mothers Against Drunk Driving, the American Red Cross, the Alzheimer's Association) **Figure 3-13**
- Local and national celebrities, community leaders, and elected officials
- Research groups (such as those at state universities, private colleges, community colleges)

2. **Define the problem.** On the basis of the community assessment and the data you have been able to gather, define the problem in specific, quantifiable terms. For example, you should be able to answer the following questions for your community:
   - What are the most frequent causes of fatal and nonfatal childhood injuries?
   - What are the most frequent diseases and chronic illnesses in the community?
   - What populations (by age, location, and other characteristics) are at highest risk of these injuries or illnesses? When and where are they occurring?
   - What, if anything, is already being done to prevent these injuries or illnesses?
   - Is an effective intervention available? What resources do you have to develop, implement, and evaluate different interventions?
3. **Set goals and objectives.**
   - **Goals.** Make this a broad, general statement about the long-term changes the prevention initiatives are designed to make. (For example, a goal can be to decrease preventable injuries to children on the community's roadways.)
   - **Objectives.** Make these specific, time-limited, and quantifiable. There are two types: **process objectives** (eg, 1,000 child safety seats will be distributed to low-income families within the next 18 months, or 500 older adult community members will receive the flu vaccine) and **outcome (impact) objectives** (eg, the bicycle safety program will increase the rate of helmet use by children younger than 18 years from 30% to 50% within the next 18 months, or the flu clinic will increase the number of flu vaccinations by 25% during the next year).
4. **Plan and test interventions.** Interventions are the actions you take to accomplish your goals and objectives. Using the 4 Es of prevention, brainstorm about options. Consider the resources you have available, and consider what other communities have done in similar situations. You may discover an intervention that proved successful for them, in which case you might be able to duplicate their actions. Experienced prevention specialists also suggest that you consider timing and cultural elements as you plan your intervention. Finally, getting a sample group together and testing the intervention before actually initiating the full program often helps to improve your chances of success.
5. **Implement and evaluate interventions.** There is a science to planning, implementing, and evaluating an intervention. To be credible, the results of your intervention must be measurable. A formal **evaluation** will definitively tell you whether you have met your goals and objectives. You want to spend your time and resources on efforts that you can *show* make a difference. For example, if your goal is to increase the usage of seat belts, you could establish a measurable objective such as, "seat belt usage in the community will increase by 50%." To

LAMAR
Designate A Driver,
Or One Will Be
Designated For You.
MADD
800-444-6233

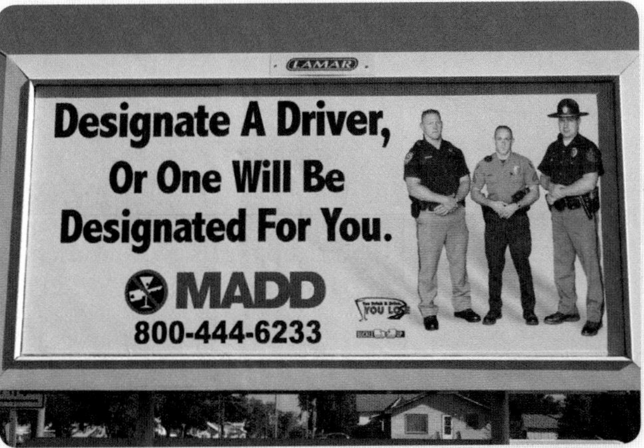

Figure 3-13 There are many organizations that can serve as potential partners in an injury prevention campaign.

measure the effectiveness of your interventions, you could place volunteers at intersections throughout the city. These volunteers would then count every belted and non-belted motorist who stops in front of them, allowing you to measure the results of your interventions.

Finally, be aware that many, if not most, interventions demand ongoing attention to remain effective. The EMS service which had initial success in reducing backyard drownings saw the numbers go back up a few years after rolling out the program, as public interest and enthusiasm began to wane. Legislation to fence pools had a positive effect, but alone, without the continuation of other interventions like education, it was insufficient. The service had to redouble their efforts to reestablish the educational pieces that had worked so well in the beginning. This case illustrates why you should consider building a long-term maintenance plan into any intervention program, if you wish to see it keep its momentum.

Community Organizing

Those in EMS who have created successful prevention programs give the following advice as you build your team and create an implementation plan:

- Identify a lead person to coordinate the effort.
- Build as broad a base of support as possible.
- Create a realistic time line for any project, keeping in mind that most must be ongoing to be effective.
- Gather data and facts that pinpoint who is being injured where, with what, and how frequently, or data on what types of diseases are most common in your community.
- Choose goals and objectives that are SMART—Simple, Measurable, Accurate, Reportable, and Trackable; build consensus in the community on the need for action.
- Ensure you understand the religious, ethnic, cultural, and language challenges that you may face in implementing an intervention.
- Do not reinvent the wheel—seek out others who have had success with similar interventions or who have expertise in public health.
- Anticipate opposition and expect some losses; turf battles are common but not inevitable.
- As you lobby to legislators, be brief in phone calls, visits, and testimony.
- Set up your program so that you can measure results and make changes as needed.
- Establish self-sustaining funding sources.
- Keep a sense of humor and persist—change does not happen overnight.

Funding a Prevention Program

Ideally, emergency services should have the resources to incorporate primary prevention activities into their normal operating budget. But as a relatively new expansion of the EMS mission, this will take time. However, highly motivated and creative people have found a number of innovative ways to secure the resources they need, including:

- Partnering with the local media to create prevention messages, especially related to seasonal injuries or hazards.
- Seeking grants from regional, state, or national sources, such as the EMSC program. (Contacting your state EMS office about grant programs is a good place to start.)
- Seeking sponsorships from local nonprofit service organizations or commercial firms.

Networking with other organizations interested in prevention often provides greater leverage in seeking grants or sponsorships. Perhaps the EMS provider donates the time of volunteers and is a credible voice in the community, whereas the partner provides organizational resources and knowledge about establishing a scientifically credible injury intervention.

Summary

Today, the field of medicine continues to dedicate more and more attention and resources to the mission of public health, promoting health and wellness and *preventing* injury and illness, rather than merely treating them after the fact. Efforts such as vaccine programs, helmet safety education, and disease screening keep people well and decrease health care costs.

However, prevention is not a goal reserved solely for public health specialists. We can all play a part. There have been many EMS providers who have embraced leadership roles in primary prevention after witnessing too many horrific examples of needless suffering. These leaders have recognized the unique opportunities afforded to them as first responders. How can *you* make a difference in your community?

YOU are the Paramedic SUMMARY

1. What is the most appropriate way to respond to this scene?

As with any call, you should wear your seat belt, stop at all red lights and stop signs, and operate with due regard for others. Keep in mind that despite the use of lights and sirens, other drivers may not be able to hear or see your ambulance coming. A good rule of thumb is to perceive your lights and siren as a means of *requesting* the right-of-way. Other considerations include weather, road construction, traffic control, the presence of bystanders or children, and the need for additional specialty resources.

2. Based on the information provided, what potential injuries and complications should you anticipate?

Because there have been multiple crashes in this location, the environment may be a part of the problem. The negative bank of the curve, combined with the potential for excessive speed, increases the likelihood of an accident and serious injury. Any time an ejection occurs, the assumption is that restraints were not used properly, and subsequently, the threat of life-threatening trauma is greatly increased (eg, head and spine, severe external or internal blood loss, etc). One other consideration is the possibility that drugs and/or alcohol contributed to the crash, in which case further scene safety issues arise.

3. What are the risk factors associated with the infant's injuries?

Having been ejected from the vehicle, the infant is at risk for significant injuries that could result in permanent disability or death. Beyond the visible injuries of a head hematoma/laceration and a forearm fracture, you should maintain a high index of suspicion for occult injuries—those not readily seen. Consider the mechanism of injury. Because the car seat was thrown from the vehicle, the patient may have come into contact with surfaces within the vehicle (eg, a window or windshield), and any object outside the vehicle, including the ground, trees, etc.

4. Is this a teachable moment?

No. Because of the potentially critical status of the infant and the mother's level of distress over her baby's welfare, this is not the appropriate time for a teachable moment. Under less severe circumstances, the improperly secured car seat would meet the criteria for a teachable moment.

5. What primary prevention measures might have helped to circumvent this traumatic incident? List any passive interventions that could have made a positive impact.

Some primary prevention measures in this scenario might include: *environmental* changes such as improved warning systems (eg, reflective signs with flashing lights to alert drivers to the sharp curve ahead); installation of safety equipment such as reflective guardrails or other *engineering* projects such as reconstructing the roadway to eliminate the sharp degree of the problematic curve; greater enforcement of traffic laws, with higher fines for exceeding the speed limit (*economic incentives*) along with stronger law enforcement presence in the area; and/or *educating* parents on the proper installation of infant car seats, perhaps even offering free car seat inspections at fire and ambulance bases.

6. Apply the Haddon Matrix to this scenario.

In this call you may view the event in the following manner:

- Pre-event:
  - Ensure a car seat is used and properly secured.
  - Drive defensively.
  - Car seat manufacturers must ensure that their products meet standards.
  - Vehicle should provide for easy installation.
  - Maintain vehicle in proper working order.
  - Enforce car seat laws.
  - Install guardrails, traffic lights, and stop signs.
  - Provide patrol in the area to enforce speed laws.
  - Offer education on the proper use of car seats.
- Event:
  - Child is properly restrained.
  - Driver maintains control of the vehicle.
  - Car seat is used correctly.
  - Vehicle design provides crash protection.
  - Guardrails, stop signs, traffic lights in place.
- Post-event:
  - First responders are trained and available.
  - Paramedics are up-to-date with pediatric certifications.
  - Ambulance is stocked with pediatric supplies.
  - Enhanced 9-1-1 is available.
  - Road shoulder is sufficient for emergency use.
  - Trauma center is nearby.

7. What steps have you taken that would be considered secondary injury prevention?

The mechanism of injury indicates the need for spinal precautions. Following your local protocol to ensure the spine is protected and gaining IV access are secondary preventive measures you have taken to be prepared in the event that the infant's status deteriorates en route. Monitoring the infant's vital signs and electrocardiogram, and providing rapid transport to the closest, most appropriate facility are all crucial elements for secondary prevention in this case.

YOU are the Paramedic SUMMARY (continued)

8. What steps could you take to develop a prevention program to reduce similar incidents in the future?

As part of your community assessment (your first step), researching call volume from this area would be a good place to start, as would retrieving information from local law enforcement and fire departments. Use these data to seek out identifiable patterns, then formulate a definition for the problem. Next, set a measurable and reasonable goal for reducing crashes and serious injuries in the designated area, and then define your objectives. Your objectives might involve such interventions as offering free workshops for car seat installation and lobbying to have the roadway reconstructed and guardrails installed. Look for similar locales that have experienced similar problems under similar circumstances and learn how those communities addressed the matter. Was it effective? What did they learn along the way? Can they offer any helpful suggestions? Finally, put your plan into action, and after a predetermined period of time, evaluate the effectiveness of the interventions. Compare new data to the old data to see whether there have been any positive changes. Regardless of the outcome, use your findings to alter your goals and objectives as needed to become even more effective.

EMS Patient Care Report (PCR)					
Date: 01-02-18	**Incident No.:** 1101234		**Nature of Call:** MVC		**Location:** Hwy 232 @ Needle Road
Dispatched: 1420	**En Route:** 1422	**At Scene:** 1437	**Transport:** 1449	**At Hospital:** 1504	**In Service:** 1511
Patient Information					
Age: 8 months **Sex:** M **Weight (in kg [lb]):** 10 kg (22 lb)			**Allergies:** No known drug allergies **Medications:** None **Past Medical History:** None **Chief Complaint:** Lac/hematoma to R forehead, possible fx to L forearm		
Vital Signs					
Time: 1440	**BP:**	**Pulse:** 138	**Respirations:** 42	**Spo_2:** 99% on room air	
Time: 1447	**BP:**	**Pulse:** 126	**Respirations:** 42	**Spo_2:** 99% on room air	
Time:	**BP:**	**Pulse:**	**Respirations:**	**Spo_2:**	
EMS Treatment (circle all that apply)					
Oxygen @ _____ L/min via (circle one): **NC NRM Bag-mask device**		**Assisted Ventilation**	**Airway Adjunct**	**CPR**	
Defibrillation	**Bleeding Control**	**Bandaging**	**Splinting**	**Other:** Cardiac monitor (circled)	
Narrative					

Unit 1 responded to a single-vehicle MVC with ejection. En route, EMS contacted dispatch to request an additional unit. Upon arrival, EMS found the vehicle in a ditch with moderate to severe damage, including a shattered window. A bystander stood several feet away from the vehicle, holding a crying 8-month-old infant. According to the bystander, the infant was thrown from the vehicle, along with his car seat, landing face down in the ditch, still secured in the car seat. The bystander removed the patient from the car seat prior to EMS arrival. The patient's mother was still in the vehicle's driver seat, AAOx4 and denying injury. The second unit arrived soon after Unit 1 made patient contact, at which time they assumed care of the mother.

The infant patient presented with blood on his face from an approximately 3 cm lac superior to the right orbit with a hematoma surrounding the lac. Bleeding was controlled prior to arrival. The patient also presented with angulation to the L forearm. Skin was pink/warm/dry, eyes were PERRLA; however, it is unknown whether the patient experienced any loss of consciousness. The patient's spine was secured according to local protocol. Vital signs were normal for patient's age (see vitals section). EMS initiated an IV, monitored ECG, dressed and bandaged the wound, and splinted the L forearm. Rapid transport to Midland Trauma Center due to MOI. No changes en route.**End of report**

Prep Kit

▶ Ready for Review

- Public health is a field that encompasses health promotion and disease prevention for *groups* of people. Public health professionals examine the overall needs of the population to determine the best use of health resources and enhance quality of life for the public in general.
- Public health threats include both injuries and illnesses. Years of potential life lost (YPLL) is a way to measure the cost of unintentional injury to society. It assumes that an average productive work life continues for 65 years. The age of death is deducted from 65, leaving the YPLL.
- A teachable moment is an opportunity to convey and reinforce a message. Certain factors must be present for a teachable moment to exist. The best teachable moments are those that utilize positive reinforcement.
- The 4 Es of prevention are education, enforcement, engineering/environment, and economic incentives.
- Passive interventions are measures that do not require a conscious decision to act. An example is airbags in automobiles.
- The 1966 National Academy of Sciences/National Research Council study, *Accidental Death and Disability: The Neglected Disease of Modern Society*, noted that EMS could be a great asset in the post-event phase (secondary prevention) and that pre-event prevention (primary prevention) could significantly reduce the prevalence of injury or illness before it develops.
- The 1996 *Consensus Statement on the EMS Role in Primary Injury Prevention* emphasized that primary injury prevention is an essential activity of EMS.
- EMS providers can work with public health agencies on prevention efforts, such as providing immunizations. In the subfields of community paramedicine and mobile integrated health care, paramedics work in the community to prevent illness and injury as part of their regular daily duties.
- Surveillance is the ongoing systematic collection, analysis, and interpretation of data essential to the planning, implementation, and evaluation of public health practice. Data are then analyzed and interpreted by epidemiologists. Surveillance is crucial to an effective prevention program.
- The Haddon Matrix uses nine separate components to analyze injury. The host, agent, and environment are factors that interact over time to cause injury during the pre-event, event, and post-event phases. The matrix encourages creative thinking in understanding the causes and potential interventions for injury.
- The most effective prevention programs focus on problems that impair the health and well-being of the greatest number of people. To get started in your community, examine the population, environment, and types of risks present.
- Diligence in documentation is one way you can make a difference, especially in relation to cases involving intentional violence. Learn to recognize signs and risk factors associated with intentional violence, and include these in accurate, thorough documentation.
- Prevention programs often focus on children. Injury patterns in children vary widely depending on a range of factors, some of which include the child's age, gender, socioeconomic status, development stage, and family environment.
- There are five main steps to developing a prevention program:
  - Conduct a community assessment.
  - Define the problem.
  - Set goals and objectives.
  - Plan and test interventions.
  - Implement and evaluate interventions.
- Creating a successful prevention program includes drafting an implementation plan that covers aspects such as data, goals, timelines, and funding sources. To fund a prevention program, consider partnering with local media, obtaining grants, or seeking sponsorship from local organizations or firms.

▶ Vital Vocabulary

epidemiologist Public health professional who investigates patterns and causes of disease and injury in a given population, and seeks to reduce the risk, occurrence, and negative impacts of these threats through research, public education, and legislative change.

epidemiology The study of the causes, patterns, prevalence, and control of disease in groups of people.

evaluation Collection of the methods, skills, and activities necessary to determine whether a service or program is needed, likely to be used, conducted as planned, and actually helps people.

Haddon matrix A framework developed by William Haddon, Jr, MD, as a method to generate ideas about injury prevention that address the host, agent, and environment and their impact in the pre-event, event, and post-event phases of the injury process.

Prep Kit *(continued)*

intentional injuries Injuries that are purposefully inflicted by a person on himself or herself or on another person; examples include suicide or attempted suicide, homicide, rape, assault, domestic abuse, elder abuse, and child abuse.

interventions In the context of prevention, specific measures or activities designed to meet a program objective; categories include education/behavior change, enforcement/legislation, engineering/technology, and economic incentives.

morbidity Number of nonfatally injured or disabled people; usually expressed as a rate, meaning the number of nonfatal injuries in a certain population in a given time period divided by the size of the population.

mortality Deaths caused by injury and disease; usually expressed as a rate, meaning the number of deaths in a certain population in a given time period divided by the size of the population.

outcome (impact) objectives State the intended effect of the program on participants or on the community in such terms as the participants' increased knowledge, changed behaviors or attitudes, or decreased injury rates.

passive interventions Something that offers automatic protection from injury or illness, often without requiring any conscious change of behavior by the person; child-resistant bottles and airbags are examples.

primary prevention Keeping an injury or illness from occurring.

process objectives State how a program will be implemented, describing the service to be provided, the nature of the service, and to whom it will be directed.

public health An industry whose mission is to prevent disease and promote good health within groups of people.

risk A potentially hazardous situation that puts people in a position in which they could be harmed.

risk factors Characteristics of people, behaviors, or environments that increase the chances of disease or injury; some examples are alcohol use, poverty, smoking, or gender.

secondary prevention Reducing the effects of an injury or illness that has already happened.

surveillance The ongoing systematic collection, analysis, and interpretation of injury data essential to the planning, implementation, and evaluation of public health practice.

syndromic surveillance Monitoring and comparing the current number and nature of medical cases against the expected volume of these cases at a given time and place in the community.

unintentional injuries Injuries that occur without intent to harm (commonly called accidents); some examples are motor vehicle collisions, poisonings, drownings, falls, and most burns.

years of potential life lost (YPLL) A way of measuring and comparing the overall impact of deaths resulting from different causes; calculated based on a fixed age minus the age at death.

References

1. Goodwin J. Annual award recognizes excellence in prevention. American College of Emergency Physicians website. https://www.acep.org/_ems-week-microsofte/annual-award-recognizes-excellence-in-prevention/. Accessed August 31, 2016.
2. American Public Health Association. Get the facts. What is public health? Our commitment to safe, healthy communities. https://www.apha.org/~/media/files/pdf/factsheets/whatisph.ashx. Accessed December 7, 2016.
3. Murphy S, Kochanek K, Xu J, Arias E. Mortality in the United States, 2014. National Center for Health Statistics Data Brief. 2015;229:1-8. http://www.cdc.gov/nchs/data/databriefs/db229.htm. Accessed September 1, 2016.
4. All injuries. Centers for Disease Control and Prevention website. http://www.cdc.gov/nchs/fastats/injury.htm. Accessed August 29, 2016.
5. NEISS all injury program operated by the Consumer Product Safety Commission for numbers of injuries. Bureau of Census for Population Estimates. National Center for Injury Prevention and Control, Centers for Disease Control and Prevention, 2014. http://webappa.cdc.gov/cgi-bin/broker.exe. Accessed August 30, 2016.
6. Injury prevention and control: protect the ones you love—child injuries are preventable. Centers for Disease Control and Prevention website. https://www.cdc.gov/safechild/. Updated May 2, 2016. Accessed February 4, 2017.
7. Albert M, McCaig F. Injury-related emergency department visits by children and adolescents: United States, 2009–2010. NCHS data brief, no. 150. Hyattsville, MD: National Center for Health Statistics. 2014. https://www.cdc.gov/nchs/data/databriefs/db150.htm. Accessed February 4, 2017.
8. Liller K. Unintentional injuries in children. *Pediatr Rev.* 2011;32(10):431-438; quiz 439.
9. Playground safety. Injury prevention and control: protect the ones you love—child injuries are preventable. Centers for Disease Control and Prevention website. https://www.cdc.gov/safechild/playground/index.html. Updated May 2, 2016. Accessed February 4, 2017.

Prep Kit *(continued)*

10. Sports safety. Injury prevention and control: protect the ones you love—child injuries are preventable. Centers for Disease Control and Prevention website. https://www.cdc.gov/safechild/sports_injuries/index.html. Updated April 30, 2016. Accessed February 4, 2017.
11. Ward B, Schiller J, Goodman R. Multiple chronic conditions among US adults: a 2012 update. *Prev Chronic Dis.* 2014;11:E62.
12. National Hospital Ambulatory Medical Care Survey: 2011 emergency department summary tables. Centers for Disease Control and Prevention website. http://www.cdc.gov/nchs/data/ahcd/nhamcs_emergency/2011_ed_web_tables.pdf. Accessed February 27, 2017.
13. WHO Director-General declares H1N1 pandemic over. World Health Organization website. http://www.euro.who.int/en/health-topics/communicable-diseases/influenza/news/news/2010/08/who-director-general-declares-h1n1-pandemic-over. Published August 10, 2010. Accessed February 7, 2017.
14. Committee on Trauma and Committee on Shock. *Accidental Death and Disability: The Neglected Disease of Modern Society*. Washington, DC: National Academy of Sciences; 1966:10.
15. National Highway Traffic Safety Administration (NHTSA), U.S. Department of Transportation. *Consensus Statement on the EMS Role in Primary Injury Prevention*. Washington, DC: NHTSA; 1996.
16. McCallion T. NASEMSO survey provides snapshot of EMS industry. Journal of Emergency Medical Services website. http://www.jems.com/articles/2011/11/nasemso-survey-provides-snapshot-ems-ind.html. Published November 15, 2011. Accessed February 7, 2017.
17. Mosesso V, Packer C, McMahon J, Auble T, Paris P. Influenza immunizations provided by EMS agencies: the MEDICVAX Project. *Prehosp Emerg Care.* 2003;7(1):74-78.
18. Misner D. Community paramedicine: a part of an integrated health care system. The Community Paramedic website, developed by Premergency. http://communityparamedic.ca/site/media/download_gallery/Community%20Paramedicine%20Article%20NS.pdf. Published 2004. Accessed December 7, 2016.
19. The facts. National Highway Traffic Safety Administration website. https://one.nhtsa.gov/nhtsa/Safety1nNum3ers/june2015/S1N_June15_ChangeTrafficSafety_3.html. Accessed February 4, 2017.
20. Runyan C. Using the Haddon matrix: introducing the third dimension. *Inj Prev.* 1998;4(4):302-307.
21. Dalton D. *Enough Is Enough: Finding Balance in an Imbalanced World.* Bloomington, IN: Xlibris Publishing; 2003.
22. Who we are. Safe Kids Worldwide website. https://www.safekids.org/who-we-are. Accessed February 4, 2017.
23. McNeil M, Dieckmann RA, Westlake D, Salaber S. EMSC recommendations for illness and injury prevention. www.emsa.ca.gov/media/default/pdf/emsa190.pdf. Accessed February 7, 2017.

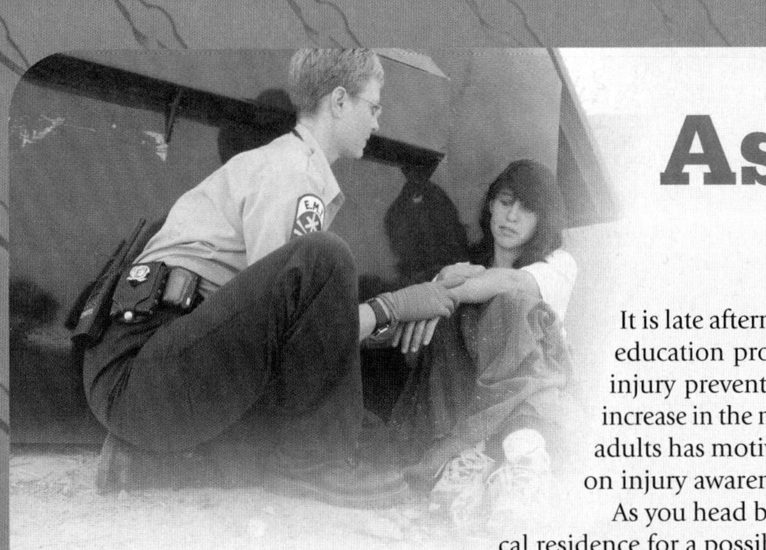

Assessment *in Action*

It is late afternoon and you have just attended a continuing education program on the importance of participating in injury prevention activities in your community. A sudden increase in the number of injuries involving children and older adults has motivated your department to launch a campaign on injury awareness and prevention.

As you head back to the station you are dispatched to a local residence for a possible burn victim. The dispatcher tells you that

Assessment *in Action* *(continued)*

the caller is hysterical, repeating, "My baby is burned!" You respond that you are en route and approximately 5 minutes from the scene. On arrival a woman who is holding a 3-year-old boy meets you. She tells you that her son pulled a pot of hot water off the stove down onto his arms. He has superficial burns to both forearms and the back of his left hand. He has stopped crying and does not appear to be in a lot of distress.

1. During your prevention class, you learned that ______ are specific prevention measures or activities designed to increase positive health and safety outcomes.

A. interventions
B. passive interventions
C. primary injury preventions
D. secondary injury preventions

2. This incident was easily preventable by turning the pot handle inward on the stove to keep it out of the child's reach. This is an example of a:

A. pre-event precaution.
B. passive intervention.
C. primary injury prevention.
D. secondary injury prevention.

3. The child was curious and reached for the pot, pulling it down onto himself. Such events are referred to as ______ injuries.

A. intentional
B. unintentional
C. passive
D. primary

4. The ______ in this situation was the pot being turned so that it was in reach of the child.

A. injury
B. intervention
C. incentive
D. injury risk

5. As you are examining the child and dressing his injuries, you take a moment to politely emphasize to his mother the importance of having pot handles turned inward, toward the stove, so handles are out of a child's reach. This is known as a(n):

A. teachable moment.
B. evaluation.
C. implementation plan.
D. injury surveillance.

6. Even though most traumatic injuries involving children (such as the one in this scenario) are unintentional, there are others that are ______, such as child abuse.

A. preventable
B. intentional
C. teachable
D. passive

7. You provide the mother with suggestions for how she can make her home safer for her child, perhaps preventing future injuries. However, in general, for education to be truly effective, it should be accompanied by:

A. enforcement, engineering/environment, and economic incentives.
B. surveillance, goals, and objectives.
C. implementation, evaluation, and data analysis.
D. enforcement, process objectives, and passive interventions.

8. Because there has been an obvious increase in call volume for falls and other unintentional injuries, your department has decided to design and implement an injury prevention program. Your supervisor asks you to head up the program. How will you proceed?

9. Getting involved in injury prevention is an important part of a paramedic's job. This should start with preventing your own injuries. List some precautions you can take to prevent injuries.

10. Your community has experienced a sharp increase in 9-1-1 calls involving children who have overdosed on prescription pain medications. In addition to your department, what local agencies, businesses, and organizations might be able to provide you with resources, partnerships, and other assistance in developing and implementing an intervention program?

CHAPTER 4

Medical, Legal, and Ethical Issues

National EMS Education Standard Competencies

Preparatory

Integrates comprehensive knowledge of the EMS system, safety/well-being of the paramedic, and medical/legal and ethical issues, which is intended to improve the health of EMS personnel, patients, and the community.

Medical/Legal and Ethics

- Consent/refusal of care (pp 109-112)
- Confidentiality (pp 98, 104-106)
- Advance directives (pp 117-120)
- Tort and criminal actions (pp 100-102)
- Evidence preservation (pp 107-108)
- Statutory responsibilities (pp 103-104, 113-116)
- Mandatory reporting (p 108)
- Health care regulation (pp 103-107)
- Patient rights/advocacy (pp 97, 99, 112, 116-117)
- End-of-life issues (pp 117-120)
- Ethical principles/moral obligations (pp 97-99)
- Ethical tests and decision making (pp 97-99, 109-111, 120)

Knowledge Objectives

1. Differentiate between laws and ethics. (pp 96-102)
2. Describe medical ethics, including the implications for paramedics. (pp 97-99)
3. Discuss the legal system in the United States and how it affects paramedics. (pp 100-102)
4. Differentiate between civil and criminal law relevant to paramedics. (pp 100-101)
5. Describe the process of a typical lawsuit against emergency medical services. (p 102)
6. Discuss the legal and ethical accountability of paramedics. (p 103)
7. Discuss legislation that affects paramedic practice. (pp 103-107)
8. Differentiate between licensure and certification as they apply to paramedic practice. (p 104)
9. Explain the importance and necessity of patient confidentiality and the standards for maintaining patient confidentiality that apply to paramedic practice. (pp 104-106)
10. Discuss the legal and ethical issues surrounding patient transport. (pp 106-107)
11. Describe the actions that you should take to preserve evidence at a crime or motor vehicle crash scene. (pp 107-108)
12. Explain the mandatory reporting requirements for special situations, including abuse or neglect, drug-related injuries, childbirth, suicide, and crime scenes. (p 108)
13. Differentiate between expressed, informed, implied, and involuntary consent. (p 109)
14. Describe the processes you should use to determine consent or valid refusal, especially relative to the patient's decision-making capacity. (pp 109-111)
15. Identify the steps to take if a patient refuses care, and when to transport a patient against his or her will. (pp 110-112)
16. Identify methods for obtaining consent for minors, including exceptions for emancipated minors. (p 112)
17. Discuss the legal ramifications of patient restraint, both physical and chemical, for patient and practitioner safety. (p 113)
18. Define the four elements that must be present to prove negligence: duty, breach of duty, proximate cause, and damage (harm). (pp 113-116)
19. Discuss abandonment as it relates to paramedic practice. (p 116)
20. Discuss patient rights, including autonomy, end-of-life decisions, and the moral and ethical implications of do not resuscitate orders and other advance directives. (pp 116-120)
21. Identify situations in which it would be appropriate for you to cease resuscitation efforts or to not initiate resuscitation efforts in the field. (pp 119-120)
22. Discuss your responsibilities relative to resuscitation efforts for patients who are potential organ donors. (pp 120-121)

23. Discuss common defenses to litigation, including contributory negligence. (p 121)
24. Describe forms of legal immunity that can apply to you as a paramedic. (pp 121-122)
25. Discuss employment legislation regarding sexual harassment, discrimination, disabilities, the Family and Medical Leave Act, Occupational Safety and Health Administration law, and other legislation that applies to paramedic practice. (pp 122-125)

Skills Objectives

There are no skills objectives for this chapter.

Introduction

All medical professionals provide care under laws—like many human activities in a democracy. As a paramedic, you too will be governed by a set of laws affecting how you treat patients. Laws define our obligations and protect our rights and the rights of others. **Ethics** are principles, either personal or societal, that determine what is right and wrong. One of the major differences between laws and ethics is that laws have sanctions for violations that are enforceable **Figure 4-1**. As a paramedic responding to an emergency, you work within a framework of several types of laws that are set down by the federal government and/or the state government, including:

- Motor vehicle laws for the operation of an emergency vehicle
- Emergency medical services (EMS) legislation
- Medical licensing statutes and regulations
- Civil and criminal statutes about touching, treating, transporting, and possibly injuring another person
- Confidentiality laws such as the Health Insurance Portability and Accountability Act (HIPAA)

It is essential, therefore, that you have a basic understanding of laws and ethics applicable to prehospital emergency care. Failure to perform your job within the law can result in civil liability or even criminal liability. Indeed, malpractice lawsuits against EMS providers are increasing.[1] Practicing outside the law may also result in regulatory action within your state—a disciplinary hearing, for example—or action by your agency and medical director. An EMS provider can be prosecuted in any or all of the above jurisdictions for the same case.

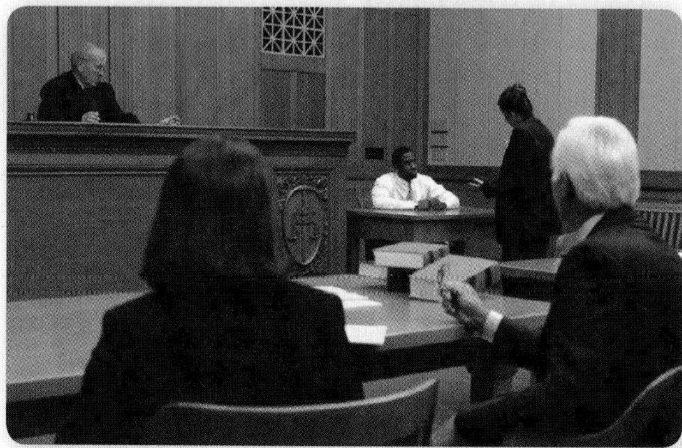

Figure 4-1 Unlike ethics, laws are enforceable rules that all citizens are obliged to follow. Paramedics are sometimes called into court to testify and provide evidence regarding cases under investigation or that are being litigated.

YOU are the Paramedic PART 1

You are eating breakfast at 0737 hours when you are dispatched to 487 Lenore Street for an unresponsive person. While you are en route, you and your partner discuss what could possibly be wrong with this patient—cardiac arrest, hypoglycemia, or stroke.

You arrive on scene at 0742 hours and are met at the ambulance by a woman who tells you that her 64-year-old mother is "acting strangely" this morning. She says that she would not respond to her at all and then she started "talking out of her head." She also says her mother does not want to go to the hospital.

1. What type of consent is required to treat a patient with altered mental status?
2. What information must you determine prior to allowing a patient to refuse care?

Ethics is the branch of philosophy that deals with the study and understanding of the distinction between right and wrong and the manner in which people apply concepts of right and wrong to their personal and professional lives. *Applied ethics* refers to the use of ethical values. In the past, the terms *ethics* and **morality** (pertaining to conscience, conduct, or character) were sometimes distinguished from one another, but today, the two words are commonly used interchangeably and little, if any, meaningful difference exists between the two. A moral paramedic is an ethical paramedic.

This chapter reviews important legal and ethical concepts affecting paramedic practice. However, this text is only a framework to help you understand these issues. It cannot substitute for competent legal advice because many laws and legal obligations differ from state to state. Contact an attorney who specializes in the representation of medical professionals if you need legal advice related to your practice.

Words of Wisdom

Without question, your best legal protection is to provide a careful, detailed patient assessment and appropriate emergency medical care, followed by complete and accurate documentation. Be a strong patient advocate. Practice within your scope of practice and be respectful to patients, their property, and their privacy.

Words of Wisdom

Many state EMS offices have websites with information on laws that affect emergency medical responders, emergency medical technicians, and paramedics. It is a good idea for you to review the laws of the state in which you work.

Medical Ethics

It is important to understand the difference between your personal ethics and the ethics of your profession. Personal ethics are the product of your upbringing, family and community influences, your religious background, and your conscience. Professional ethics, on the other hand, arise out of the standards and practices of your profession, the Code of Professional Conduct, and in certain cases, various state and federal laws such as HIPAA (discussed later in this chapter). Situations may arise in which your personal ethical beliefs may come into conflict with the professional ethical standards. In almost every such case, you will be bound by professional ethics and must understand that your personal ethics must be temporarily set aside.

As a paramedic, always be ethical in your practice and be aware of your own moral standards in your daily work. The interests of your patient must always take precedence over personal beliefs and standards Figure 4-2.

Ethics related to the practice and delivery of health care is known as medical ethics (sometimes called bioethics). Your understanding of medical ethics must be formed as a part of, and consistent with, the general codes of the health care professional Figure 4-3. Throughout history, many codes of ethics for health professionals have been published. The Declaration of Geneva, first drafted by the World Medical Association in 1948, provides a good example; it is the oath taken by many medical students on completion of their studies, at the time of being admitted to the medical profession:

> "I solemnly pledge myself to consecrate my life to the service of humanity; I will give to my teachers the respect and gratitude that is their due; I will practice my profession with conscience and dignity; the health of my patient will be my first consideration; I will respect the secrets which are confided in me, even after the patient has died; I will maintain by all the means in my power the honor and noble traditions of the medical profession; my colleagues will be my sisters and brothers; I will not permit considerations of age, disease or disability, creed, ethnic origin, gender, nationality, political affiliation, race, sexual orientation, social standing or any other factor to intervene between my duty and my patient; I will maintain the utmost respect for human life; I will not use my medical knowledge to violate human rights and civil liberties, even under threat; I make these promises solemnly, freely and upon my honor."[2]

Similar principles underlie the more detailed *Code of Ethics for EMS Practitioners*, which was issued by the

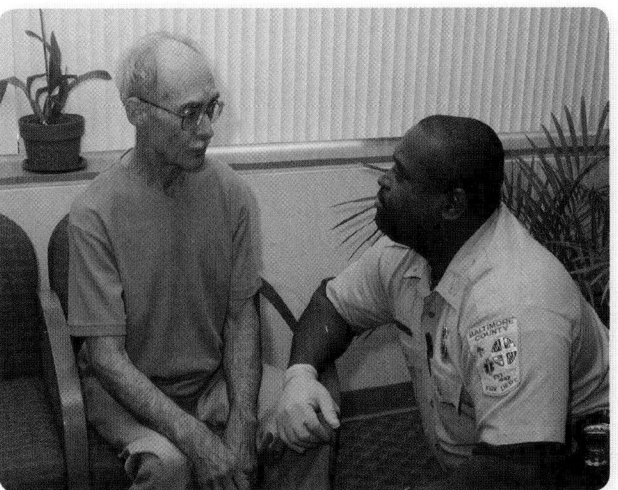

Figure 4-2 As a paramedic serving a diverse public, you will frequently work with people who have cultural backgrounds that are different from your own. Work to set aside your own personal beliefs when making decisions on the patient's behalf.

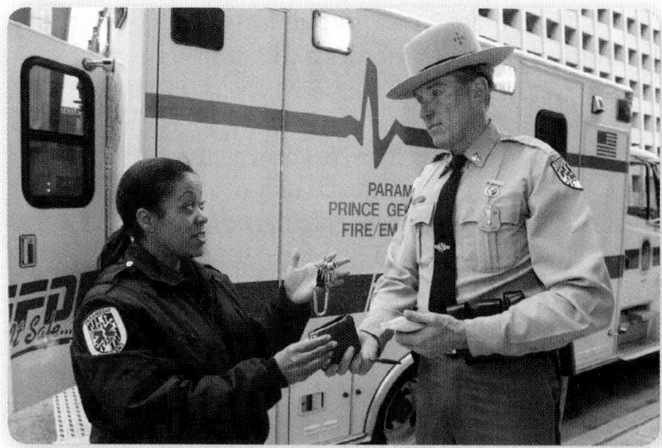

Figure 4-3 When people call 9-1-1, they trust you not only to provide proper emergency medical care, but also to use sound ethical judgment—which includes the safeguarding of their personal possessions.

National Association of Emergency Medical Technicians (NAEMT) in 1978 and is still in effect today:

"Professional status as an Emergency Medical Services (EMS) Practitioner is maintained and enriched by the willingness of the individual practitioner to accept and fulfill obligations to society, other medical professionals, and the EMS profession. As an EMS practitioner, I solemnly pledge myself to the following code of professional ethics:

- To conserve life, alleviate suffering, promote health, do no harm, and encourage the quality and equal availability of emergency medical care.
- To provide services based on human need, with compassion and respect for human dignity, unrestricted by considerations of nationality, race, creed, color, or status; to not judge the merits of the patient's request for service, nor allow the patient's socioeconomic status to influence our demeanor or the care that we provide.
- To not use professional knowledge and skills in any enterprise detrimental to the public well being.
- To respect and hold in confidence all information of a confidential nature obtained in the course of professional service unless required by law to divulge such information.
- To use social media in a responsible and professional manner that does not discredit, dishonor, or embarrass an EMS organization, co-workers, other health care practitioners, patients, individuals or the community at large.
- To maintain professional competence, striving always for clinical excellence in the delivery of patient care.
- To assume responsibility in upholding standards of professional practice and education.
- To assume responsibility for individual professional actions and judgment, both in dependent and independent emergency functions, and to know and uphold the laws which affect the practice of EMS.
- To be aware of and participate in matters of legislation and regulation affecting EMS.
- To work cooperatively with EMS associates and other allied healthcare professionals in the best interest of our patients.
- To refuse participation in unethical procedures, and assume the responsibility to expose incompetence or unethical conduct in others to the appropriate authority in a proper and professional manner.[3]

In addition to the foregoing, your state may have its own code of ethics for EMS professionals and it is possible that the service or company you work for has its own set of policies, rules, or regulations that will provide guidance regarding ethical expectations of its employees. The ICARE program, developed by a group of EMS students and educators, incorporates many of the finest qualities of EMS professionals.[4] ICARE (which stands for integrity, compassion, accountability, respect, and empathy) is an excellent concept for you to remember and incorporate into the emergency medical care that you provide to your patients.[4] All of the various codes and rules of right and wrong ultimately stem from a concern for the welfare of the patient, and it is a safe generalization that if you place the welfare of the patient ahead of all other considerations, then you will rarely (if ever) commit an unethical act in the practice of emergency medical care.

It would be impossible to list all the ethical dilemmas potentially encountered in your work as a paramedic. Regardless of the ethical circumstances you may encounter, you should always apply three basic ethical concepts, considered an inherent part of health care for centuries, when making a decision. These ethical principles are: (1) to do no harm, (2) to act in good faith, and (3) to always act in the patient's best interest.

The principle of "First, do no harm" (Latin: *primum non nocere*) essentially means that you should take all due care in ensuring that your patient receives the best possible care and that your actions do nothing to harm the patient. It requires you to take care in the way you assess, treat, and transport your patients so that you do nothing to exacerbate their medical condition or to cause an additional injury or medical condition.

The two principles of acting in good faith and acting in the best interest of your patient go hand in hand. These principles are simply a reinforcement of your commitment to always place the interests of the patient above all else and to make decisions that are motivated by a clear desire to benefit your patient. You may at times make decisions on behalf of an unconscious or otherwise incompetent patient that the patient or a family member will later question. In such circumstances, you should be able to state confidently that the decision you made was motivated by your desire to benefit the patient.

As a paramedic, you must be accountable for your actions at all times. How you handle teamwork, your personal attitude on the job, justice and respect for patient autonomy, and cultural or lifestyle diversity will ultimately shape your career. Consider what type of a paramedic you want to become **Figure 4-4**. It is helpful for you, as a new paramedic, to choose a mentor whose style and professionalism you wish to emulate.

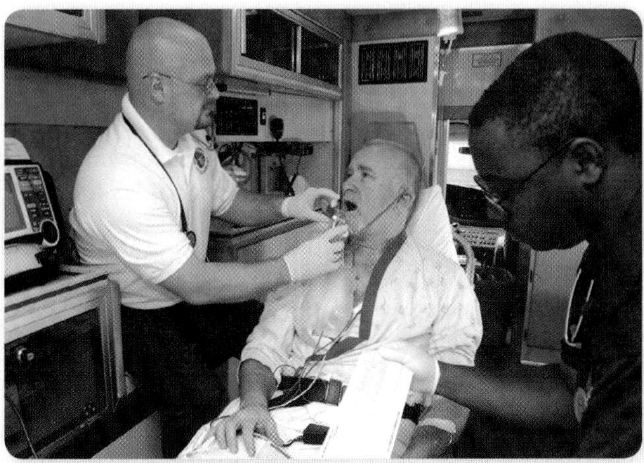

Figure 4-4 One of the best ways to hone your skills as a paramedic is to find a good mentor whose work ethic and attitude you admire.

Controversies

Some religious beliefs influence a patient's decision about treatment and may be different from what you think is best for a patient. For example, patients sometimes refuse standard lifesaving therapies and treatments based on their religious convictions.

Professional ethics are extremely important as the EMS profession continues its pursuit of being recognized and funded in the same manner as the other medical professions. Immature, unprofessional behavior is unethical and has no place in this profession. Criminal acts, such as sexual misconduct, substance abuse, patient abuse, and harassment or stalking of coworkers, are both unethical and illegal. Off-duty misconduct can, and does, affect your reputation and may affect your employment status as well. News stories that depict EMS personnel engaged in any immature or illegal activities serve to lessen the public's confidence in the services you provide. Inappropriate use of emergency vehicles, inappropriate visitors entertained at the station, and use of alcohol on duty are strictly forbidden. Unfortunately, another significant ethical and legal problem that has occurred in EMS is the falsification of training and certification; for example, falsely representing one's level of certification or falsifying training records.[5,6] The practitioner who falsely represents himself or herself will face charges; any EMS instructor who signs off on such a falsification will face similar charges as well. These charges can range from suspensions and revocations of licensure, but could also extend to criminal and civil charges based on the patient's outcome.

Always be respectful of patients and never do anything to violate the trust that patients have placed in you. As a paramedic, you are expected to honor the trust that has been bestowed on you as a member of the health care profession, to act ethically and professionally in every circumstance, and to avoid any misconduct that could call into question your ethics or integrity. Regrettably, some paramedics have violated the ethical standards of their profession and have mistreated patients in a variety of ways. Such misconduct has included discriminatory and abusive treatment, embellishing the patient assessment finding over the radio in an effort to obtain drug orders from the physician, and even sexual abuse. These violations of ethical standards have a negative impact on the profession itself, not just on those involved. Fortunately, these cases of misconduct are rare. The ethics of your profession require total commitment to acting in the best interest of your patient, and to otherwise conduct yourself in a professional and ethical manner at all times—that is, caring about your patients, coworkers, and the EMS system as a whole. Therefore, you should not overlook other EMS providers engaging in misbehavior. Promptly report any misconduct to the appropriate chain of command. Similarly, you are obligated to report medical errors you either make or witness to the medical director as soon as possible.

Paramedics who choose to become patient advocates, who participate in and actively seek out the best in training and professional development, and who put the good of the team above their own personal aspirations will ultimately succeed and be rewarded with a fulfilling career in EMS. Good ethics can be instilled by good mentors. People seem to perform best when they share themselves and work toward an end much greater than themselves. EMS is an evolving specialty, and the future of it lies in your hands.

▶ Ethics and EMS Research

EMS practices have largely evolved like the rest of EMS—with grassroots effort and precious little research to confirm the effectiveness of the procedures used in the prehospital setting. Properly randomized, controlled studies in EMS are uncommon, but they are emerging. Remember that the first principle of medical practice is to do no harm, and therefore you must continue to seek further education about the effectiveness of EMS practice. Some of EMS care still relies on anecdotal experience that is unsupported by research. Some EMS procedures, however well-intentioned, prove not to be helpful to patients. As a health care provider, you must be aware of procedures that are not recommended, even if anecdotally those procedures worked for you or your colleagues in the past. Conducting EMS studies on critically ill or injured patients without their **consent** (agreement to accept a medical intervention) is a true ethical dilemma. These patients are usually unable to give consent, and their physical state is so compromised that even if they are conscious, they may be unable to absorb information to give informed consent (discussed later in this chapter). Continue to make yourself aware of how researchers are handling this issue and other ethical debates concerning patients in research.

The Legal System in the United States

Federal and state governments make, administer, and interpret laws that affect paramedics. Each level of government has three branches Figure 4-5. The legislative branch, made up of elected officials (Congress at the federal level; state legislatures at the state level), makes the laws. The judicial branch (consisting of the court system) enforces and interprets laws and resolves disputes based on interpretation of laws. Common law can also affect EMS. **Common law** (case law) is defined as a decision that has been made by a judge through a court case based on his or her interpretation of the statutes and constitutions. A common law can be overturned either by another court with a higher authority or the issuing court at a later time.

Courts have a number of levels, including trial courts and appellate courts. Although many people believe that all law comes from statutes passed by the legislative branch, this notion is not true. Court decisions, especially those issued by appellate courts, establish precedent and become the law of the state in which you live and practice as a paramedic. In most cases, these court decisions establish the standards of negligence (discussed later in this chapter) that will apply if you are sued by a patient.

The third branch—the executive or administrative branch—reports to the president (in Washington, DC) or the governor (in your state capital) and is made up of various cabinets and agencies (the bureaucrats) that carry out and administer the laws. The agencies often use regulations to establish how things should be done. Agencies such as the Occupational Safety and Health Administration and the US Department of Transportation at the federal level, and the Department of Health at the state level, are examples of parts of the administrative branch.

All states now have some type of legislation that sets out the framework for the EMS system. In addition, administrative regulations may be set forth by state agencies or county governments that regulate the practice of paramedics. It is vital for you to know and understand the laws and administrative regulations that affect your practice in your home state.

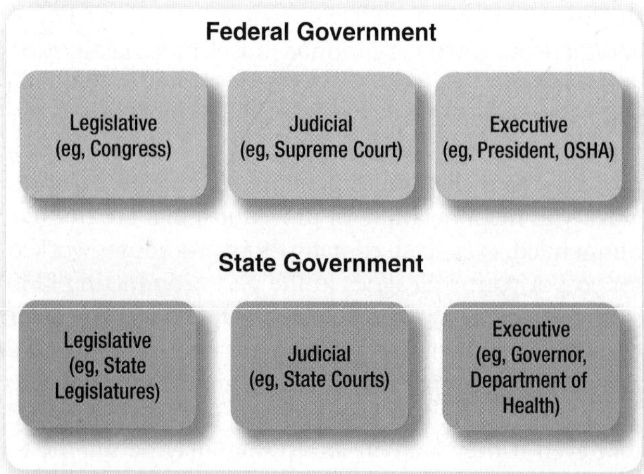

Figure 4-5 Both federal and state governments enact and review legislation that is specific to paramedics.

Types of Law

Two kinds of law govern paramedics in court: civil law, under which a patient can sue you for a perceived injury, and criminal law, in which the state can prosecute you for breaking a legal statute. Malpractice lawsuits are tried under civil law. Although some lawsuits may be based on state statutes, most claims will arise out of principles of negligence established by prior court decisions. Many cases of medication misuse will be tried under criminal law.

A substantial part of civil law is concerned with establishing **liability**, or responsibility. When a person experiences an injury and seeks redress for that injury, the judicial process must determine who was responsible. For example, a patient or (if the patient died) a surviving relative may be dissatisfied with the medical care the patient received. The patient or surviving relative may feel that inadequate medical care led to a bad outcome. People have a constitutional right to take legal action against the physician, nurse, paramedic, or other involved parties. However, the person who is suing must prove that the medical providers he or she is suing caused harm by failing to provide medical care that met the accepted standards. A bad outcome alone does not necessarily mean the medical provider was negligent; the patient or surviving relative has to prove all of the elements of negligence before a lawsuit will be successful. A claim that contains all of the foregoing elements is sometimes referred to as an actionable cause.

A legal action of that sort is called a **civil lawsuit**—that is, an action instituted by a private person or entity (the **plaintiff**) against another private person or entity (the **defendant**)—and the wrongful act that gives rise to a civil lawsuit is called a **tort**. The law recognizes two classifications of torts: unintentional torts (commonly referred to as negligence) and intentional torts (those that describe an intent to cause harm). The objective of a civil lawsuit is usually some sort of compensation (**damages**) for the injury the plaintiff sustained.

In cases of medical liability, the plaintiff usually seeks monetary compensation for physical suffering, mental anguish, hospital and medical bills, and sometimes loss of earnings or earning capacity. In certain cases, the court may also award **punitive damages** (usually monetary compensation) if the misconduct of the EMS provider was intentional or constituted a reckless disregard for the safety of the public. To succeed in a civil lawsuit, the plaintiff needs to show that a majority of the believable evidence favors his or her position, and then convince the jury of this position.

Lawsuits against EMS providers most often result from emergency vehicle crashes. In Chapter 3, *Public Health*, you learned about the importance of safe driving to your personal health and well-being. Safe driving is a key to preventing lawsuits. Vehicle crashes are all too common and

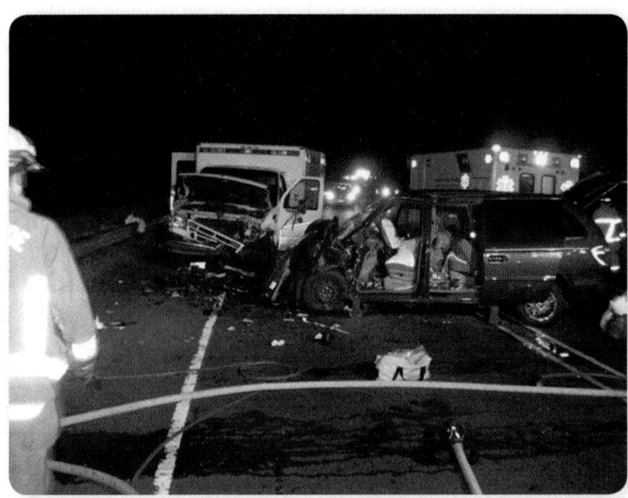

Figure 4-6 Civil lawsuits against paramedics often arise from emergency vehicle crashes.

Courtesy of Oregon State Police.

cause expensive property damage as well as serious harm to patients, bystanders, and EMS providers Figure 4-6.

Other kinds of lawsuits against EMS providers are on the rise each year.[1] Many of these lawsuits involve dispatch and transport issues, such as those involving a delayed transport response or patient deterioration after not being transported. Other lawsuits address the quality of the emergency medical care provided by the EMS providers, especially paramedics.

Sometimes the same allegedly wrongful or harmful act that gave rise to a civil lawsuit may also result in criminal prosecution. A **criminal prosecution** is an action taken by the government against a person the prosecutors feel has violated criminal laws. In a criminal case, the government must prove guilt beyond all reasonable doubt to a jury. If the government succeeds, then the defendant can be fined or imprisoned or both.

The criminal laws most likely to apply to prehospital care include **assault**, **battery**, and **false imprisonment**.

- Assault occurs when a person (the EMS provider) instills the fear of immediate bodily harm or breach of bodily security (including loss of freedom) to another (the patient)—regardless of whether the threat of harm is actually carried out. Threatening to restrain a patient who does not want to be transported could be considered assault.
- Battery occurs when the defendant (the EMS provider) touches another person (the patient) in a harmful or offensive way without his or her consent. Charges of battery may arise if you make physical contact with a patient before asking if you may touch him or her.
- False imprisonment occurs when a person (the patient) is intentionally and unjustifiably detained against his or her will by another (the EMS provider). Charges of false imprisonment may arise if you transport a patient without the patient's consent or use restraints in a wrongful manner.

The difference between assault and battery can be summarized with the following example. Saying, "I'm going to kick your teeth in!" is assault; actually kicking the person's teeth in is battery. Just about any act of medical treatment performed without consent may be considered assault or battery or both, because such acts constitute a threat to the patient's bodily security ("Now I'm going to stick you with this needle. . .") and unauthorized contact with the patient's body.

To prosecute a criminal charge of assault or battery, the prosecution generally needs to prove the intent to cause harm. In a civil case, the plaintiff need only establish that the conduct took place without his or her consent.

Though the charge of false imprisonment is extremely rare in EMS, occasionally EMS providers may be charged with battery when physically forcing someone to be transported, especially with the use of restraints, in the absence of just cause. In essence, your best protection against these charges is to obtain informed consent for almost everything you do, or clearly document the need to restrain the patient for his or her own protection Figure 4-7. All medical care providers need to get informed consent, but you will need some guidelines and tips (presented later in this chapter) that may not apply to most hospital-based personnel.

EMS providers used to be taught that they should be aware of kidnapping and possible criminal or civil charges being brought against them in cases in which a patient was transported against his or her will; however, no successful prosecution has ever been achieved against a paramedic for this action. As with kidnapping, no successful criminal prosecution has ever been achieved against a paramedic for false imprisonment. Successful civil prosecutions for false imprisonment are extremely rare.

As a paramedic, you may also be sued for **defamation**, which is intentionally making a false statement through written or verbal communication that injures a person's

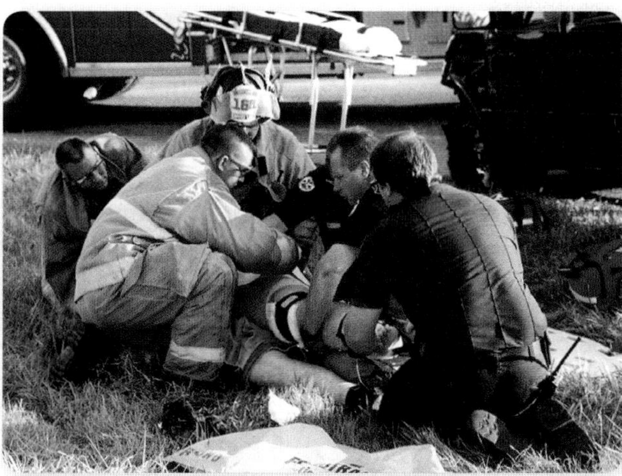

Figure 4-7 Your best prevention against any legal action is to obtain informed consent whenever possible, and to keep the needs of your patient as your top priority.

© Dan Myers.

good name or reputation. It must be emphasized that this must be a *false statement*. Truth is an absolute defense against any type of defamation claim. As a paramedic, you are encouraged to always make absolutely truthful statements. **Libel** is making a false statement in the written form that injures a person's good name. When you write your patient care report (PCR), avoid using terms that may be considered judgmental or offensive, such as "the patient appears to be drunk." Instead, you may write, "The patient smelled of ETOH." Whatever your personal views, think about the way in which your PCR would read in court. Do not let thoughtless comments become evidence against you.

Slander is making a false oral statement that injures a person's good name. Once again, avoid using terms that could be considered judgmental or offensive to the patient when you are passing along prehospital care information to emergency department (ED) personnel. Always keep in mind that your patient is someone's son or daughter, husband or wife, brother or sister, or father or mother. How would you like information about members of your own family to be treated when information is relayed to the hospital?

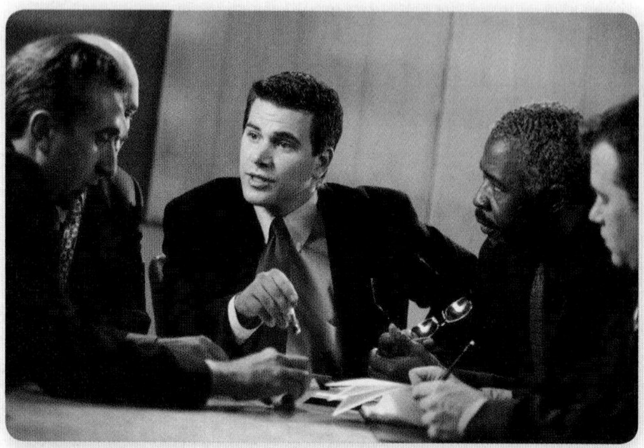

Figure 4-8 The process of a lawsuit can take years, and because of expenses associated with a trial, can result in out-of-court settlements.

Words of Wisdom

Being courteous, honest, and professional will prevent most patients from complaining or filing lawsuits.

▶ The Legal Process

A civil lawsuit begins when a dissatisfied patient contacts an attorney, who then files a document for a lawsuit (called a complaint) on behalf of the patient with a local court. The court where the action is first filed is generally referred to as the court of original jurisdiction. In the context of EMS, the complaint will contain the general allegations against you and the EMS system, but may not contain much specific information about what the patient thinks went wrong. The patient's attorney (or the attorney's staff) must hand-deliver a copy of the complaint and a notice called a summons to all people or agencies named in the lawsuit, notifying them of the complaint and the need to respond. From start to finish, a lawsuit may take several years. Because the lawsuit may not begin until several years after you see the patient, good documentation is essential to defending a lawsuit.

Your attorney will usually be assigned to you by the insurance company that handles claims for your employer, whether the employer is a government or private agency. The response, or answer to the complaint, will be filed by your attorney. After the complaint is filed and you (through your attorney) have answered, a period known as the discovery period begins. The discovery period can last anywhere from a few months to more than 2 years **Figure 4-8**. During the discovery period, the attorneys on both sides seek to find out as much about the case as possible. They will exchange written questions that must be answered by the parties under oath, exchange documents such as the patient's medical record, and take depositions (statements taken under oath). Stay in touch with your attorney during this time and ask for a full explanation of everything that is happening. Your attorney will also prepare you for a deposition, instructing you where to go, what to wear, and how to respond to certain types of questions.

Attorneys may also file motions (requests for the court to take an action) and argue them before the judge. Your attorney will seek to have the lawsuit dismissed by filing motions. The plaintiff's attorney may ask the court to rule on certain portions of the claim by filing other motions. Either side may file motions asking the court to compel the other side to produce documents or information that is being withheld.

Most civil cases are resolved during a settlement process because it is expensive and time-consuming to take a case through trial. Settlement processes involve the parties and their attorneys in mediation, which is a conference set up to see if the parties can agree on a dollar amount that will resolve the case, or an arbitration, which is a mini-trial in which a single arbitrator or a panel of arbitrators will make a decision based on the evidence presented by both sides.

If the case does not resolve during the settlement process, then it will proceed to trial. During a trial, the judge rules on what the law is and the jury decides what the facts are. Trial juries can be unpredictable; if they perceive that the EMS system has failed to meet community standards, then large monetary damages can be rewarded. In most cases, the trial will be the final step in the judicial process, but the party that loses at trial always has the right to have the decision reviewed by an appellate court. Appeals are costly and time consuming, however, and only a small percentage of cases are ever appealed.

Legal Accountability of the Paramedic

The Paramedic and the Medical Director

The relationship between the paramedic and the medical director is complex and often not well understood. Ultimately, you have three lines of authority to answer to within the EMS system: the medical director, the licensing agency, and the employer. Although some overlap exists, it is important to keep these distinctions in mind. State EMS legislation usually requires that you perform advanced procedures and skills only under the supervision of a physician. Legislation may also require the EMS system to have a medical director. Although the medical director is in a supervisory relationship with the paramedic, legally speaking, the paramedic is not the agent of the physician.

Your actions as a paramedic, therefore, are not the actions of the physician, and you will be held accountable for your own actions. However, the medical director can be held legally accountable for failing to supervise you closely enough, or for failing to take action if your performance is not up to standard. The medical director may restrict your practice, or even withdraw supervision entirely, if he or she does not believe you are performing as you should be. The medical director may also require certain remedial training if you are weak in some areas of practice. Although the medical director's remedial requirements may ultimately result in employment actions, medical directors are generally not held legally responsible for disciplinary actions taken by employers.

Many of your activities as a paramedic require an order from a licensed physician. Orders may be given by radio or mobile phone (online medical control) or instead may be defined by protocols, or standing orders (off-line medical control), but in any case, you are not at liberty to disregard or reverse a physician's order unless you truly believe that carrying out the order will harm the patient. That fact may give rise to difficult situations, such as instances in which you find yourself at the scene of an emergency together with a physician who may not be knowledgeable in prehospital emergency care. Under those circumstances, you may feel that the orders of the on-scene physician are inappropriate. However, you are on questionable legal ground if you choose to disregard a physician's orders, assuming the physician is licensed in that state and the order is appropriate. To avoid conflicts in such situations, it is best to ask the service medical director to develop protocols ahead of time defining the paramedic's relationship with the medical director of the service and with other physicians in the community, including bystander physicians. A physician is not required to ride to the hospital with EMS personnel unless he or she has performed procedures above the level of the EMS providers or has otherwise assumed responsibility for patient care. Always be sure that the physician is licensed in your state, and document the physician's name and contact information, before allowing him or her to provide patient care. If conflicts do arise between you and physician bystanders in the field, then online medical control should resolve them. Do not follow a physician's order that falls outside of your scope of practice. Such action would fall under the **borrowed servant doctrine**, a principle which absolves your institution from liability when you act beyond your scope of certification or training by following someone else's orders.

Documentation & Communication

If you must deviate from your protocols because of unusual circumstances, then consult with online medical control and make sure you document it well on your PCR.

EMS-Enabling Legislation

Most states have what is called EMS-enabling legislation, which defines how EMS is structured and designates responsibilities to government agencies. These laws also provide the state-based framework for the paramedic's actual practice—what you are permitted to do in the field. For example, EMS legislation may define the need for a medical director, and may also define the scope of practice for the different levels of EMS personnel. Familiarize yourself with the EMS legislation in your state and any regulations that flow from those statutes.

Administrative Regulations

Administrative regulations—set forth by bureaucracies at the state and federal levels—affect and define the specific rules under which paramedics practice. For example, regulations may set out the precise skills and medications to be used by each level of EMS provider. Regulations—usually developed by either the state's Department of Health or the county agency responsible for regulating EMS practice—may further define your role in the emergency medical care of patients. Regulations may also define the requirements for licensure or certification, renewal requirements, continuing education requirements, and a list of behaviors that may subject you to suspension or revocation of your license or certification.

If you provide less than adequate care, or fail to meet the requirements for recertification, then the administrative agency may also take action against your paramedic license. A license is not a right, but rather a privilege, granted by a government agency, allowing you to provide care to its citizens. Failure to abide by the regulations can have serious consequences.

Licensure and Certification

The terms *licensure* and *certification* are often confused because, in some states, paramedics are considered licensed but in others they are considered certified. Certification generally refers to a certain level of credentials based on hours of training and assessment exams, and addresses criteria met for minimum competency. Certification may be granted by a governmental agency or by a private organization such as the American Heart Association or the American Red Cross. The fact that you have received certification from a private organization does not necessarily mean that you have authority to practice the skills included in that certification. Licensure refers to a carefully defined level of practice, usually granted by a government agency or local authority such as a state health department or county EMS authority. Often, these agencies themselves create and administer the licensing exams. A license itself is a privilege granted by a government authority on certain conditions. You must comply with the government's requirements for professional behavior, continuing education, and licensure renewal, or risk losing that privilege. The rights and privileges conferred by licensing in one state may not be conferred in other states that certify, rather than license, paramedics.

Another concept that you may encounter is that of credentialing. Credentialing may be adopted by a specific EMS agency as part of its employment requirements. For example, although you may be licensed as a paramedic by your state, the service for which you are seeking work may impose additional requirements as part of its eligibility standards. Typically, this may include things such as certification in cardiopulmonary resuscitation (CPR), trauma, or advanced cardiac life support, or passing a regional protocol examination.

Discipline and Due Process

If you commit an infraction of the rules pertaining to licensure, then the agency that granted the license may seek to restrict, suspend, or even revoke the privilege to practice.

When an administrative agency proposes a licensing action, you have a right to **due process**. Due process is a right to a fair procedure for the action the agency proposes to take. Due process has two components: Notice and the Opportunity to be heard. Notice means that the agency must notify you of the actions that allegedly constitute the infraction, usually by receipt of a certified letter containing a Notice of Contemplated Action. The letter informs you of the proposed action to be taken and the sections of the regulations the agency is alleging were violated. The letter also informs you of your right to a hearing and the procedure for requesting a hearing. The hearing provides an opportunity for you to tell your side of the story. If the licensing agency still believes licensure action is warranted after the hearing, then it will send a Notice of Final Action. You may have appeal rights if a final licensure action is taken.

▶ Medical Practice Act

In most states, physicians and other health care practitioners are enabled to function through the provisions of a **Medical Practice Act**. This act usually defines the minimum qualifications of those who may perform various health services, defines the skills that each type of practitioner is legally permitted to use, and establishes a means of licensure or certification for different categories of health care professionals. Requirements for relicensure or recertification based on continuing education and other factors may also be included in the Medical Practice Act. In some cases, Medical Practice Acts may require that a physician assume responsibility for competency of the paramedic through mandatory training, skill competency testing, and run review. Become familiar with the terms of the Medical Practice Act in your state.

▶ Scope of Practice

The **scope of practice** for paramedics may be spelled out in the EMS legislation or regulations of your state. The scope of practice is emergency medical care that you are permitted to perform according to the state under its license or certification; however, a local medical director may limit the skills you may perform under his or her supervision (for example, rapid sequence intubation).

If you carry out a procedure for which you are not authorized under the enabling legislation, then you are practicing outside your scope of practice, which may be considered negligence or, in some states, even a criminal offense (considered practicing medicine without a license). Do not confuse the scope of practice with the standard of care, which is what a reasonable paramedic in a similar situation would do. This topic is discussed later in this chapter.

▶ Health Insurance Portability and Accountability Act

The **Health Insurance Portability and Accountability Act (HIPAA)** provides stringent privacy requirements for patient information. The act was enacted in 1996 and provides for criminal sanctions as well as civil penalties for releasing a patient's private medical information in an unauthorized manner. The HIPAA Privacy Rule, which is the most relevant part of HIPAA for health care providers, is enforced by the Office for Civil Rights at the US Department of Health and Human Services. The HIPAA Privacy Rule protects a person's protected health information (PHI). Additionally, the HIPAA Security Rule is the portion of HIPAA that pertains to protecting electronic health information.

Medical information can be disclosed only if it is necessary for a patient's treatment, for payment or medical billing operations, or when the release has been authorized in writing by the patient or a lawful patient representative. HIPAA was created not to stop the flow and continuity of a patient's health care information, but to control the distribution of information to ensure the patient's privacy. In

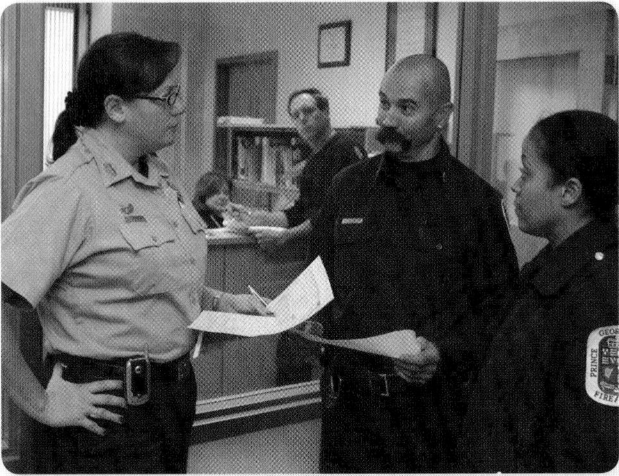

Figure 4-9 Remember that the Health Insurance Portability and Accountability Act guarantees a patient's confidentiality at all times. Be careful never to discuss a patient's condition in public.

essence, HIPAA mandates that patient information should not be shared with entities or people not involved in the care of the patient. Several special situations exist that may require the release of patient information without the patient's authorization (discussed next). HIPAA requires each EMS agency to have a privacy officer responsible for ensuring that all PHI that the service deals with, in either written, electronic, or oral/verbal form, is not released in an unauthorized manner. Be aware of where written patient information is at all times, and you cannot casually discuss a patient where you might be overheard—such as in an elevator Figure 4-9. Use caution when you are giving reports or discussing patient information in other public places such as crash scenes or common areas in the ED. Sharing patient stories with other paramedics may subject you to liability. Similarly, use caution when members of the media or the public are riding with your service to ensure PHI is not disclosed without the patient's consent.

HIPAA requires you to provide patients with a copy of your service's privacy policies. Although this step can often be difficult to perform in an emergency setting, it is your obligation to do the best that you can to comply with the law. Most services create multipage leaflets that can be handed out to patients.

Some states also have laws pertaining to patient confidentiality; a breach of that confidentiality may allow patients to sue for unauthorized release of their medical information Figure 4-10. Confidentiality is also a part of the Code of Ethics for Emergency Medical Technicians issued by the NAEMT. If your service receives a subpoena for a patient's PHI, then be sure to notify legal counsel before releasing a patient's medical record to anyone.

Special HIPAA Circumstances

Many EMS providers are confused about the legal issues surrounding HIPAA and feel that any release of a patient's

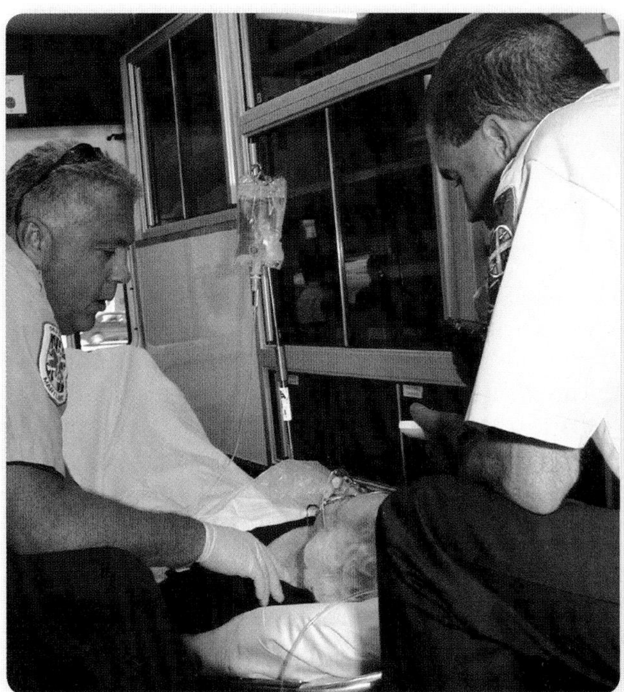

Figure 4-10 When you communicate with a patient, be sensitive to his or her point of view, and the environment in which you choose to communicate.

private medical information may result in penalties. The HIPAA Privacy Rule acknowledges that patient information must sometimes be shared for the betterment of society as a whole. The Privacy Rule permits covered entities to disclose PHI to public health authorities who are legally authorized to receive such reports for the purpose of preventing or controlling disease, injury, or disability. These exceptions include legally mandated reporting (eg, dog bites, gunshot wounds, alleged child abuse or neglect), authorized data collection and research by public health agencies (eg, births, deaths, diseases that are being investigated or are at risk of causing a public epidemic), authorized requests by law enforcement agencies, and information required to be disclosed pursuant to a valid subpoena.

Exchange of health information for a medical need is allowed under HIPAA, and is in fact ethical and necessary. For example, the electronic transfer of health information from your electronic PCR to the receiving hospital is perfectly appropriate. It is also appropriate for a physician to dictate patient information into a dictation machine, which is then transcribed into the patient's medical record. Furthermore, it is permissible under HIPAA for hospitals to share information with EMS providers about patient outcome for the purposes of quality assurance, quality improvement, and education. For example, when you treat and transport a patient to the receiving facility, you may follow up to inquire about what further care your patient required after you transferred care. It is clearly important and necessary for you to understand the outcome of your interventions so that you can learn. Finally, the exchange of health information for the purposes of insurance and billing is appropriate, although in most cases the billing agency must sign an agreement indicating that the health information will be used for billing purposes only, and will not be shared with outside parties.

HIPAA Implications for Electronic Communications

Because of the popularity of social media networks, many EMS agencies have created policies to address issues associated with the sharing of patient care information over the Internet. Some agencies have gone as far as prohibiting EMS providers from carrying camera-enabled mobile phones while on duty. You must ensure that everyone on your call understands that patient information should never be posted (eg, in the form of photos, videos, comments, or other data) on any social media network due to HIPAA regulations.

As a paramedic, you have a unique view from where you treat patients. Many times, recordings of emergency scenes are captured by camera—for example, the camera of an EMS vehicle, or a photograph taken by EMS responders to illustrate the mechanism of injury at a crash scene. Make certain that if a camera is used on scene or during patient treatment, then no patient identifiers are present that could allow someone who was not involved in patient care to identify the patient.

HIPAA also regulates the manner in which you and your service transmit PHI electronically. The widespread use of Bluetooth and other wireless technologies also increases the potential for patient information to be stolen by hackers. The Safeguards Principle of HIPAA requires that reasonable administrative, technical, and physical safeguards be put in place to aid in the protection of patient information. If you are unsure whether the equipment you may be using is safeguarded, then seek the advice of the administrators in your organization.

HIPAA Training

HIPAA rules and regulations should be taught to all entities involved. Each agency in the United States that is a covered entity defined by the US Department of Health and Human Services should follow HIPAA guidelines to help protect the patient and the provider. As mentioned previously, each agency must have a designated privacy officer who can help you better understand all of the rules and regulations associated with HIPAA and your role in EMS. Your employer is required to provide you with HIPAA training at the time you are hired and then again on an annual basis.

▶ Emergency Medical Treatment and Active Labor Act

The **Emergency Medical Treatment and Active Labor Act (EMTALA)** was enacted in 1986 to combat the practice of so-called patient dumping and pays particular attention to the practice of sending women in labor to distant hospitals. Patient dumping occurs when hospital ED staff deny medical screening or stabilizing treatment, or when staff inappropriately transfers a person whose condition is unstable. Historically, most patient dumping occurred when hospital staff discovered that the patient did not have health insurance or was otherwise unable to pay. In recent years, *economic triage* has been introduced. This term refers to the practice of making health care decisions based on the ability of the patient or the insurance carrier to provide payment for services. Although such considerations may have a place in certain aspects of the health care field, an EMS provider should never make a decision to treat or transport based on financial considerations, regardless of the current financial state of the EMS employer. As a paramedic, your only consideration should be the needs of the patient; reimbursement issues should be addressed by billing personnel. Paramedics have occasionally been accused of providing a lower standard of care for indigent people or those on public assistance; therefore, make sure that financial status never becomes a deciding factor in your practice. Always provide the highest possible quality of emergency medical care to all patients, regardless of their financial status.

As a paramedic, it is also important that you have a clear understanding of local protocols regarding the choice of hospitals to which you may transfer your patient. In some rural areas, only one hospital may be available, but in other places several options may be available. Some EMS systems simply require you to transfer the patient to the nearest hospital. In other systems, however, protocols dictate that hospital selection be based on the specific needs of the patient. For example, some patients may require the services of a trauma center, a children's hospital, or a hospital with cardiac catheterization capabilities. Depending on local protocols, you may be able to make the choice of destination alone, whereas in others you may be required to consult with medical control in making such decisions. It is important to become familiar with the protocols in your area of practice.

EMTALA issues are regulated by the Centers for Medicare and Medicaid Services (CMS) and carry severe monetary penalties—up to and including loss of Medicare funding—for hospitals that fail to comply. The CMS also issues severe fines for hospitals and physicians who violate EMTALA provisions. In addition, EMTALA further allows private citizens to sue for violations of the act. Under most circumstances, neither an ambulance service nor a paramedic can be sued or charged with a violation under EMTALA. An ambulance service that is owned by a hospital, however, may be subject to a claim under EMTALA in certain cases.

EMTALA has complex language that appears to be medical language but is actually legal language. For example, an *emergency medical condition* under EMTALA refers to what most paramedics would call an *acute situation*. EMTALA guarantees a medical screening exam, and treatment to stabilize any emergency medical conditions

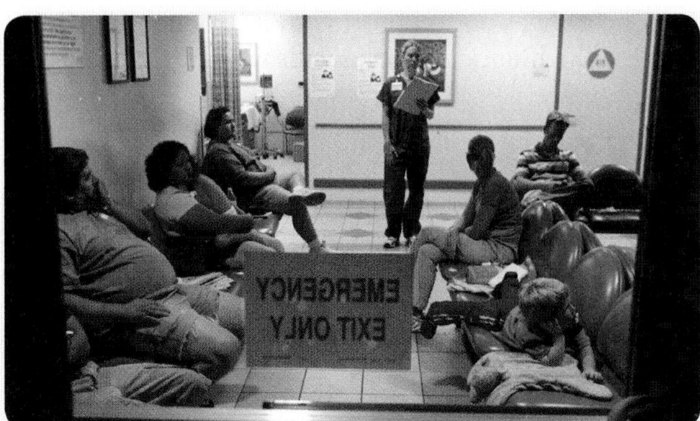

Figure 4-11 Emergency Medical Treatment and Active Labor Act legislation requires that every patient who presents to a hospital receive emergency medical treatment—regardless of his or her ability to pay for medical treatment when it is received.

found, to any patient presenting to a hospital that has an ED Figure 4-11. It prohibits discrimination for any reason, including the ability to pay. Some urgent care centers may also be covered by EMTALA. Although EMTALA does not directly regulate paramedics, EMS is often the vehicle—both figuratively and literally—by which patient dumping takes place.

EMTALA also regulates patient transfers and applies to both the sending and receiving facilities. As a paramedic, you should never transfer a patient between facilities who needs emergency medical care that falls outside your scope of practice, and you must feel comfortable that the patient is stable enough to transfer. A transferring hospital staff has an obligation to ensure the transferring ambulance and crew are capable of meeting the needs of the patient during transfer and should request an ambulance that is appropriately staffed and equipped. It would be a potential EMTALA violation if hospital staff requested a basic life support (BLS) ambulance and crew to transport a patient with a serious cardiac condition who required cardiac monitoring and the administration of medication during the transport. Should a patient need a higher level of care, it is the responsibility of the transferring hospital staff to provide someone to ride along (a nurse, respiratory therapist, or even a physician). Make sure you have received all appropriate paperwork before leaving on a patient transfer, including all pertinent medical records, laboratory results, x-rays, and other documents. When you arrive at the receiving hospital, that hospital staff should have a bed ready for the patient, after agreeing to accept the patient.

▶ Emergency Vehicle Laws

Most states have specific statutes that define an emergency vehicle and what traffic should do when an emergency vehicle approaches. Although these laws vary somewhat from state to state, it is important to remember that these statutes still require emergency vehicles to be operated in a safe and prudent manner. Laws governing emergency vehicle operation do not authorize speeding, running red lights, or driving the vehicle in an unsafe manner if any of those activities put the public at unreasonable risk. Most state laws establish a higher standard for the emergency vehicle operator by making him or her responsible for operating the vehicle with *due regard* (proper consideration and attention) for the safety of all others.[7] If a crash occurs, then EMS providers will often be found at fault in civil cases brought against the drivers. Worse, if you are the driver, then you might also be charged criminally for such situations. Although it is important to know the laws of your state about emergency vehicle operation, remember that the blue Star of Life on the side of your vehicle and the flashing red lights on top do not exempt you from defensive driving and common courtesy; you will be held responsible for your actions.

Emergency vehicle operators are professionals trained to operate their vehicle safely at all times, and to anticipate reactions from other drivers in stressful situations. Remember, a collision could not only result in injuries to innocent people, but also could injure or delay treatment of the original patient who needs your help. Collisions involving emergency vehicles are by far the most common cause of paramedics facing legal action, be it criminal, civil, or administrative.

▶ Transportation

You should transport patients to the hospital of their choice when possible and reasonable; however, most EMS systems have protocols that direct paramedics to transport certain types of patients to particular hospitals. Examples of these patients include those who have experienced trauma, stroke, and cardiac events; homeless patients; mentally ill patients; and patients with obesity. The capability of each hospital to care for particular kinds of patients should guide the EMS system in developing transport protocols. Transportation of patients to a facility that does not have the ability to care for their particular illness or injury can result in liability for the paramedic.

Decisions made by paramedics not to transport patients at all have been the subject of litigation. A number of studies have demonstrated that paramedics should not be compelled to decide which patients need to be transported to the hospital for any health conditions. The whole EMS system, including paramedics, does not have access to sophisticated diagnostic tools or radiography in the prehospital setting. Failure to transport a patient whose condition later deteriorates can bring about a lawsuit that is difficult to defend. Again, most EMS systems have protocols outlining when it is acceptable not to transport a patient, and many require consultation with online medical control.

▶ Crime Scene and Emergency Scene Responsibilities

When you handle a situation involving a death, or any potential crime scene, remember that it may take law enforcement officials some time to figure out whether the scene involved a suicide, homicide, or some other form of criminal activity. It is important for you to use extreme caution and not disturb or destroy potential evidence.

If the scene is a vehicle crash, then do not move anything unless you have to—including broken glass, pieces of metal, or even a beer can. Leave deceased people where they are until a coroner or medical examiner arrives to investigate.

If the incident scene is indoors, then do not touch anything you do not have to touch, such as telephones or doorknobs, because of the risk of eliminating fingerprints. Carefully document any statements made by witnesses and get their contact information. Limit the number of EMS personnel who enter the scene because each person who enters the scene further contaminates what may later turn out to be a crime scene. If it is necessary to move furniture or other objects, then notify law enforcement personnel that you have done so. Preserve any clothing that you remove from the patient, and make every attempt not to alter evidence on the clothing (eg, do not cut through bullet or knife holes).

Remember that in cases of sexual assault, the patient may carry vital pieces of evidence such as fiber, hair, sperm, or blood on his or her body—take care to protect this evidence.

If the scene involves a death, then stay with the body until the police arrive, and protect the scene from contamination by bystanders, family members, media, or additional EMS personnel.

If you have any doubt about the possibility of saving the patient, then initiate resuscitation and transport him or her to the hospital.

Patient Safety

Be aware that the perpetrator may still be at or near the crime scene and could be a factor in when and how you care for your patient.

▶ Mandatory Reporting

Each state has its own requirements regarding categories of cases that must be reported to the appropriate authorities. These cases include some of the most difficult ones you will see as a paramedic.

Virtually every state has laws requiring EMS providers to report suspected child and elder abuse. It is essential for you to be familiar with the reporting requirements of your own state. In most states, reporting laws also contain **immunity** provisions that protect the health care provider who files reports from legal liability, provided the report was not made with malicious intent. Failure to report is a crime and in many states has very serious implications. If your state requires you to report, then complete the reporting yourself; do not pass along the information expecting someone else will make the report.

The obligation to report is most frequently applied to the following categories of cases:

- Neglect or abuse of children
- Neglect or abuse of older people
- Domestic violence
- Injury sustained during the commission of a felony, or specific injuries considered to be of suspicious origin (such as gunshot wounds or stab wounds)
- Drug-related injuries
- Childbirth occurring outside a licensed medical facility
- Rape
- Animal bites
- Certain communicable diseases

Because reporting requirements vary widely from state to state, learn the laws of your state and observe the reporting obligations that apply to you.

Words of Wisdom

Be observant and report any suspicious signs or symptoms to the proper authorities.

▶ Coroner and Medical Examiner Cases

Every EMS system should have a list of procedures for cases that involve the coroner and medical examiner Figure 4-12. Although coroner laws vary somewhat from state to state, generally you should notify the police of all coroner cases, including the following situations:

- Obvious or suspected homicide
- Obvious or suspected suicide
- Any other violent or sudden, unexpected death
- Death of a prison inmate

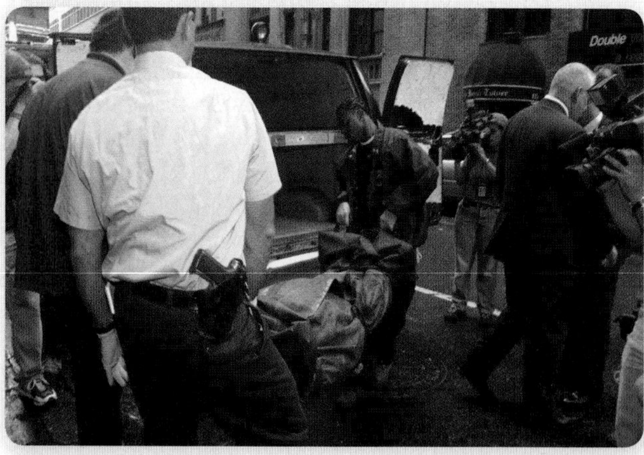

Figure 4-12 In any situation involving the death of a person, contact the police or coroner with pertinent details, depending on local protocols.

Paramedic–Patient Relationships

The most important premise affecting paramedics is one that does not appear in any of the statute books; it is the rule of doing what is best for the patient. You are trained in emergency medical care, not law. Every decision regarding patient care that you make, therefore, should be based on the standards of good medical care—not on the possible legal consequences. When you do what is best for the patient within your scope of practice, it is unlikely you will run afoul of the law—and in the event a lawsuit is initiated, your defense will be greatly enhanced if you have always kept the patient's best interest in mind.

Consent and Refusal

Prior to providing emergency medical care, you must obtain the consent of the patient. Any touching of a patient's body without consent may give rise to charges of assault and battery. The concept of consent refers to patients who are of legal age and who possess **decision-making capacity** (the capacity to make appropriate medical care decisions for themselves). Patients with decision-making capacity have the right to refuse all or part of the emergency medical care offered to them. Be familiar with the two types of consent: informed consent and implied consent.

Informed consent is a patient's voluntary agreement to be treated after being told about the nature of the disease, the risks and benefits of the proposed treatment, alternative treatments, or the choice of no treatment at all. You must obtain informed consent from every adult patient who has decision-making capacity. To obtain informed consent, use the following four steps:

1. Describe the suspected injury or illness to the patient.
2. Describe the treatment you would like to administer, and list potential risks associated with the proposed treatment.
3. Discuss any alternative types of treatment available.
4. Advise the patient regarding potential consequences of refusing treatment.

A number of things such as language barriers, emotional states, and mental abilities may impede your ability to give patients the information they need to make informed decisions. The key is to ensure your patient understands what you are trying to do and grants you permission to treat. Although informed consent under emergency conditions may lack the formality seen in a hospital, you must document the patient's consent in your PCR to protect you against potential legal action.

Informed patient consent is routinely obtained verbally but may also be communicated through patient conduct, such as the patient rolling up a sleeve to allow you to take his or her blood pressure. **Expressed consent** is a type of informed consent that occurs when the patient does something, either by telling you or by taking some sort of action, that demonstrates he or she is giving you permission to provide emergency medical care.

Implied consent is a form of consent assumed to be given by unconscious adults or by adults who are too ill or injured to consent verbally to emergency lifesaving treatment. In those cases, you assume that the patients would want care because of the severity of their condition, but the patients do not have decision-making capacity at the time that treatment is necessary. If a patient shows convincing evidence that his or her decision-making capacity is altered, such as signs of mental illness, shock, stress, confusion, head injury, etc, then you may treat the patient under implied consent, because treatment is in his or her best interest.

Some EMS personnel incorrectly use the term **involuntary consent** to refer to situations in which a law enforcement officer or a legal guardian grants permission to treat someone who is under arrest (or otherwise in custody), incapacitated, a minor, or for other reasons. Involuntary consent is an oxymoron because consent can never be involuntary. People under arrest or in prison do not necessarily lose their right to be involved in medical treatment decisions. It is not uncommon for a law enforcement officer to direct EMS personnel to treat a person under arrest, but you should continue to follow informed consent guidelines. If a prisoner refuses treatment, then involve medical control. Likewise, do not assume that a law enforcement officer—or anyone else—has the right to refuse treatment for a patient. If the patient desires treatment, then do all in your power to treat the patient and document accordingly.

Decision-Making Capacity

Refusals, like consent, must be informed refusals, and all the same prerequisites apply. Patients must have decision-making capacity to be able to refuse care. Decision-making capacity is the ability of patients to understand the information you are providing to them, coupled with the ability to process that information and make a choice regarding medical care that is appropriate for them. You have a number of tools you can use to evaluate a patient's decision-making capacity, but the best one is your ability to talk to the patient to find out whether the patient understands what is happening to him or her. In addition, if pulse oximetry and blood glucose measurements are outside normal ranges, then these readings can provide measurable information regarding your patient's ability to understand and communicate. Detailed documentation of decision-making capacity is important to include in your PCR to show that the patient was able to understand your proposed treatment plan.

If a conscious patient with decision-making capacity refuses to consent to treatment, that person may not be treated without a court order Figure 4-13. In such instances, consult with medical control for instructions.

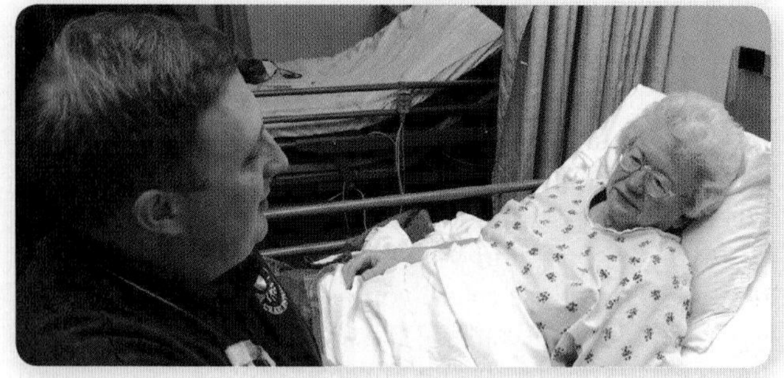

Figure 4-13 When a conscious patient with decision-making capacity makes a decision, you must respect that decision.

The most prudent approach is for you to inform the person in a calm and sympathetic manner of the possible consequences of refusing treatment. Keep in mind that many people who refuse medical treatment do so out of fear and emotional distress, and you need to recognize and manage the patient's distress in an understanding way. It is not uncommon for patients to refuse treatment and transportation to the hospital because of a concern for the costs associated with the ambulance and hospital treatment. Addressing these concerns can be challenging for you and may require all of your "people skills."

Be wary of situations when a patient refuses treatment and/or transport, but you believe that treatment and/or transport is in his or her best interest. The patient may be alert and oriented, but may be incapable of making an informed decision even after you have communicated with him or her to the best of your ability. A number of factors may prevent the patient from making an informed refusal. Some of these factors include:

- Head injury
- Altered mental status
- Unstable vital signs
- Abnormal blood glucose levels
- Abnormal oxygen saturation levels
- Cerebral ischemia
- Mental illness
- Drug or alcohol intoxication
- Urinary tract infection
- Suicidal or homicidal ideation
- Inability to cope with emotional distress
- Developmental disability

If you reasonably suspect that a patient has an issue that impedes his or her ability to give either informed consent or informed refusal, then take aggressive steps in the best interest of the patient. If you have the ability to contact medical control for direction, then immediately inform medical control of your concerns, and your basis for these concerns. Ask for guidance in transporting the patient against his or her will, and the best way to accomplish this. If you do not have access to medical control, then it is usually best to follow your instincts and transport the patient against his or her will if forcible transport can be accomplished reasonably and safely. Consider calling for assistance from your EMS agency or law enforcement, and be keenly aware of your local protocols and resources in this regard. Use whatever resources you have available.

In particular, psychiatric emergencies present challenges with respect to consent. When a person's life is not in danger, a police officer is generally the only person given the authority to restrain and transport that person against his or her will. EMS providers should not do so except at the express request of the police. Notably, neither a physician nor the patient's family may authorize such transport in most regions; they may authorize involuntary commitment, but their authority does not extend to the forcible transport of a patient against his or her will. Therefore, it is essential for every EMS system to establish protocols, based on local laws, for dealing with the mentally impaired patient who refuses transport. In many instances, the participation of the police will be required, and the role of each agency involved should be clearly defined beforehand.

Courts have given EMS personnel substantial leeway in the decisions to transport patients against their will whenever the on-scene paramedics have acted in the best interest of the patient and have proper documentation. The vast majority of court rulings reflect the belief of the court that the duty of the paramedic is to act in the best interest of the patient and suspect the worst. As a paramedic, you are not expected to diagnose the patient's condition in the field, and you are not held to the standard of a medical professional with a higher degree. It is generally assumed that no harm is done to the patient if he or she is treated and transported against his or her will when the paramedic has used his or her best judgment on the patient's behalf. If the patient is taken to the hospital and the physician determines that he or she has adequate mental capacity to refuse further treatment, then the patient has only lost time.

It is very challenging to decide when to transport a patient against his or her will. If you believe that the patient is not competent to make a reasonable decision regarding his or her care, and that treatment is necessary, then it is better to treat the patient. You are less likely to face legal consequences for treating a patient who should be treated—even against his or her will—than abandoning that patient. (Abandonment is discussed later in this chapter.) Individual state statutes provide more guidance in this situation. Check the state statutes where you practice, and become familiar with them.

Consider that some patients refuse treatment as a way of denying that they have a problem—such as the middle-aged man with chest pain who refuses treatment to deny the possibility that he may be experiencing a heart attack. A sympathetic ear and a little reassurance on your part will often convert an unconvinced patient into someone you can help. Remember the phrase: "It never hurts to have these things checked out."

Having a patient speak with medical control by radio or telephone may be helpful at times. If the patient is still declining emergency medical care after your explanation of the medical situation and the possible consequences of refusing treatment, and no evidence exists that the patient is impaired in any way that would prohibit an informed refusal, then there is not much further that you can do. However, even at that point, you must maintain a courteous, sympathetic attitude. It is inappropriate for you to consider the person who refuses treatment a "bad patient" and/or to behave in a hostile or aggressive manner toward him or her. Remember, you are at the scene to help the patient, so try to find out what is bothering the patient and why he or she is rejecting help. Always respect the patient's rights.

Let patients know that your chief concern is their well-being, and tell them that it is all right to change their mind. Urge patients to seek further medical evaluation from the physician of their choice. Help them make concrete plans for follow-up. Some patients will consent to transport but will not consent to treatment; others may consent to treatment but refuse transport. If patients refuse transport, then try to make sure that someone will be with them after you leave and always advise them to call 9-1-1 again for help if needed.

Never threaten a patient in any way. Some examples include telling a patient that he or she will be taken forcefully to the hospital if they call 9-1-1 again; threatening to cause pain to the patient if he or she is uncooperative (for example, intravenous [IV] injection, nasogastric tube insertion); or threatening to restrain the patient. All of these actions would not only be highly unprofessional and inappropriate, but would also constitute assault. Remember, following through on these actions would constitute battery.

▶ Documenting Informed Refusal

Your documentation of patient refusals is critically important should litigation arise in which the patient claims you committed abandonment. The documentation of refusals is covered in detail in Chapter 6, *Documentation*. Document all findings of your assessment and mental status exam carefully, including the patient's history, the patient's stated reasons for refusing care, and all instructions and explanations given to the patient. Note how much time you spent attempting to provide emergency medical care. The report should be signed by the patient and by an impartial observer (eg, a police officer, if available). The purpose of a witness or observer is to hear the exchange of the information, not just to sign a piece of paper with his or her name. Soliciting for signatures from others at the scene who may not have been paying attention to your conversation or the information exchanged with the patient may pose legal issues.

YOU are the Paramedic — PART 2

You are led into the kitchen and see an older woman sitting at the kitchen table drinking coffee. She looks up as you walk in and starts to yell at her daughter. "I told you not to call them! I'm not going!" She is pale, frail-looking, and obviously very agitated. Her daughter tells you that her mother has had small strokes in the past as the result of a small brain tumor. She also tells you her mother does not have a do not resuscitate order, but she does have an advance directive. She also takes medication for high blood pressure, hypothyroidism, and elevated cholesterol levels.

Recording Time: 0 Minutes	
Appearance	Pale, agitated
Level of consciousness	Appears alert
Airway	Open and clear
Breathing	Appears normal
Circulation	Pale, but her nail beds are pink

3. What are the possible consequences of treating this patient without her consent?
4. On the basis of her history, what might be her problem?

Words of Wisdom

Prehospital refusal of treatment forms must be supported with action. Legally, you must have undertaken the process of attempting to obtain informed consent to treat the patient. Just because a patient has signed a refusal form does not mean that the patient has given you an informed refusal. You must have informed the patient of what you propose to do to care for him or her, and the potential risks of refusing that care, and provide that information in a manner he or she is capable of understanding.

It can be frustrating and difficult to accept the fact that a patient may refuse all or part of emergency medical care. However, it is important to respect a patient's rights, regardless of whether it is contrary to your beliefs or what you think you should be doing. Courts have upheld patient refusals when paramedics carefully documented a patient's decision-making capacity, and their explanation of the possible consequences of refusing care.

▶ Minors

Minors present special issues for the paramedic. Because minors have no legal status, they can neither refuse nor consent to emergency medical care. In the case of children and adults who have legal guardians, consent must be obtained, if possible, from a parent or legal guardian of the patient. If the parent or guardian is unavailable, then emergency treatment to sustain life may be undertaken without direct consent under the doctrine of implied consent. Also be aware of the legal principle known as **in loco parentis**. This term literally means "in the place of the parent." This principle may also apply in school, day care, or summer camp if a parent is unavailable. The school administrator or day care director may make treatment and transportation decisions on behalf of the minor.

A particularly difficult circumstance can arise if a parent or legal guardian refuses to grant consent to treat a minor who clearly requires lifesaving or limb-saving treatment. Although adults clearly have the right to refuse treatment for themselves, state laws generally do not permit a parent or guardian to deny treatment to a minor. In fact, the failure of a parent or guardian to allow such treatment may constitute neglect. If confronted with such a circumstance, then notify law enforcement and medical control. State law may permit the state to assume custody of the minor for purposes of ensuring that necessary emergency treatment be provided.

Emancipated minors are under the legal age (generally 18 years) in a given state but can be treated as legal adults because of qualifying circumstances. Individual state law determines what circumstances qualify a minor as emancipated, although most states recognize any minor who has been emancipated by court order. Other states add criteria such as marriage, pregnancy, or active military service. Emancipated minors may be treated as adults when obtaining consent or refusal.

As with adult patients who refuse transport, if you reasonably suspect the patient is a minor and the patient has no proof that he or she is not, then be prepared to transport. Legally speaking, you are better off erring on the side of caution—that is, in favor of transport and acting in the best interest of the patient— rather than abandoning the patient.

Special Populations

Although legislation varies in different areas, in most states, a pregnant teenager is considered emancipated during her pregnancy and can make all legal and medical decisions for herself and her unborn baby. However, the minute she delivers the baby, she once again assumes the status of a minor, and her parents or legal guardians make all of her medical and legal decisions. She does, however, remain the legal guardian for her baby and can make all medical and legal decisions for him or her (even though she cannot make them for herself).

Overall, obtaining consent for medical treatment may be one of the more difficult skills to acquire as a new paramedic; however, you will find that your expertise will build over time. A patient or even a child's guardian may not want you to assess and treat for a variety of reasons Figure 4-14. Therefore, keep in mind that as a patient advocate, you must anticipate potential challenges for obtaining permission and be prepared to discuss the need for emergency medical care.

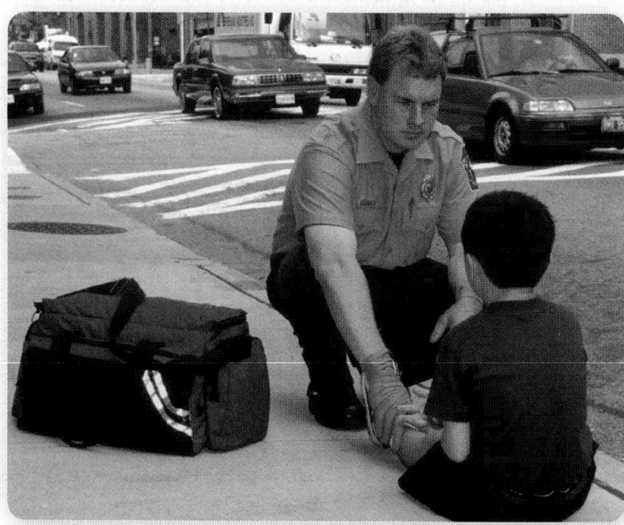

Figure 4-14 When you are dealing with a young child, explain to him or her the need for treatment, and consult his or her parent or guardian.

> **Words of Wisdom**
>
> Never tell patients that you are going to do a procedure. Instead, ask them if you can perform the procedure and explain to them why they need it.

▶ Violent Patients and Restraints

The use of force by paramedics against patients has been the cause of numerous lawsuits in recent years. However, in the reality of today's EMS practice, you will encounter violent patients who must be restrained to protect the patients themselves and to protect those who are trying to care for them.

Under the law, you can use force only in response to a patient's use of force against you. If you are attacked, then you may defend yourself against the attack. However, the use of temporary disabling sprays, knives, or firearms are generally outside the scope of paramedic practice and are usually prohibited by the EMS agency. The amount of force that you are allowed to use under the law is either equal to or slightly greater than the force offered by the patient, and must be in response to the patient's actions. Violence against EMS providers is on the rise. For your own personal safety, do not enter a scene that is unsafe until law enforcement personnel can secure the scene and make it safe for you to enter.

In situations requiring patient restraint for medical reasons, it is important to understand that you may restrain patients only when the patients are a danger to themselves or to others Figure 4-15. Violence can be the result of hypoxia, hypoglycemia, mental illness, brain injury, drug abuse or overdose, alcohol, or a variety of other underlying medical and psychiatric causes. Specific medical protocols should cover what is considered appropriate in your EMS system for restraining patients, and should spell out what medications or devices are allowed for use in restraining patients. Many EMS systems use medications (ie, chemical restraints), such as benzodiazepines or antipsychotics, to calm patients who are violent and need transportation to a hospital to discover the underlying medical or psychiatric cause of their outbursts.

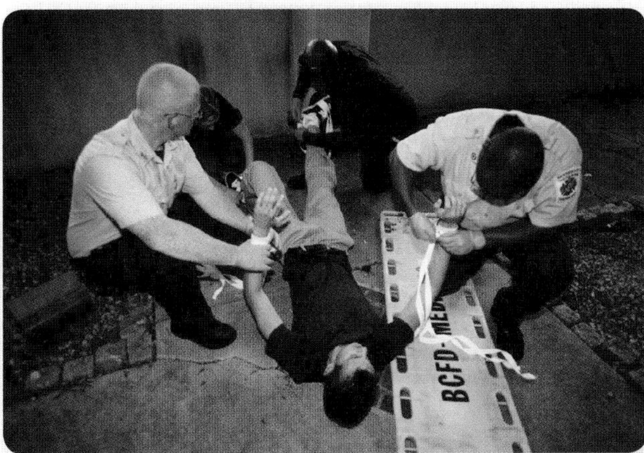

Figure 4-15 Use restraint only when absolutely necessary to ensure your own safety and that of the patient. It will most likely take several strong people to fully restrain a patient. Never use restraint as a form of punishment.

Negligence and Protection Against Negligence Claims

Unless some type of immunity is present, nothing can protect the paramedic from liability for **negligence**, a serious charge. Negligence occurs when a series of events happens:

1. The paramedic—or, in some cases, the EMS system—had a legal duty to the patient (duty to act). For example, a paramedic hired to serve a community has a legal duty to the citizens of that community.
2. A breach of duty occurred; that is, the person accused of negligence failed to act as another person with similar training would have acted under the same or similar circumstances. Breach of duty may involve doing less than the person was trained to do (an error of omission; ie, a paramedic who fails to splint an injured extremity) or doing more than the person was trained to do (an error of commission; ie, a paramedic who sutures a laceration when doing so is not within the scope of practice).
3. The failure to act appropriately was the proximate cause (the first event in a chain of events) of the plaintiff's injury.
4. Harm resulted.

As a paramedic, you and the EMS system in which you work are protected from liability as long as you perform according to the standards for paramedics and EMS systems. Your best protection is to behave in all circumstances according to established procedures and standards set by national agencies, such as the guidelines for ambulance design and equipment from the National Highway Traffic Safety Administration. Although those standards are not law, they can be introduced as evidence in litigation and may affect the outcome of a lawsuit. It is therefore in your best interest to make sure that your emergency vehicle is maintained in optimal condition and equipped according to prevailing standards.

Paramedics frequently ask if they should obtain their own insurance coverage despite the fact that they generally will be covered by the insurance provided by their employers. Although the insurance carried by your employer will generally cover you in any situation related to your employment, having additional insurance is often a good idea. Having your own liability policy will provide you with protection in several possible circumstances:

- If your employer's insurance carrier is required to pay out on a claim based on wrongdoing for which you are responsible, then it is possible (though rare) that the carrier will try to recover against you personally.
- If you are sued as a result of having provided off-duty emergency assistance.
- If you are an instructor teaching EMS-related classes outside the scope of your employment and are sued by a student or other party.

Insurance of this type is generally reasonably priced and may be a wise investment.

One aspect of negligence is the presence of *foreseeability*. This concept implies that the injury, or harm, could have been predicted and therefore avoided if the proper precautions had been taken. For example, giving an incorrect dosage of a drug will foreseeably result in harm to a patient, just as running a red light while en route to a call may foreseeably result in a motor vehicle crash.

Negligence is commonly divided into three categories: (1) malfeasance, (2) misfeasance, and (3) nonfeasance. **Malfeasance** occurs if you perform an act that you were never authorized to do, such as a medical intervention that is outside of the scope of practice. **Misfeasance** occurs if you perform an act that you are legally permitted to do, but you do so in an improper manner. For example, you administer a medication that is clearly within the scope of practice but accidentally calculate an incorrect dose. **Nonfeasance** occurs if you fail to perform an act that you are required or expected to perform. Failure to perform CPR when a patient goes into cardiac arrest would be an example of nonfeasance.

▶ Elements of Negligence

Duty

Duty is prescribed by the law: it is what you, as a paramedic, must do and how you must do it. Without question, your first duty as a paramedic is to do no further harm to a patient.

The first element of negligence a patient must prove for a lawsuit to be successful is that of **duty**. Duty relevant to medical negligence is defined as "an obligation, to which law will give recognition and effect; to conform to a particular standard of conduct toward another."[8] If a person fails to perform according to that standard, and this failure caused the injury, then he or she may be considered legally liable.

Much confusion surrounds the concept of legal duty in EMS. For example, many paramedics think that they have a legal obligation to stop at roadside crashes simply because they are paramedics. However, in all but a few states, this is not the case. Although you may feel an ethical obligation to stop and assist, the law in most states does not require it. You are obligated to respond to calls when working a shift or while volunteering for a squad. Most services have a policy addressing the discovery of another incident while en route to a call or en route to the hospital with a patient. The key to legal duty is to make sure the appropriate personnel are dispatched if you cannot stop to render assistance due to the severity of the patient you are currently treating.

Another misconception is the idea that if you put a sticker that says "paramedic" on your personal vehicle, this identification somehow invokes a **legal obligation** (a duty enforceable in a court of law) to stop at all emergencies.[9] This is not true. However, you do have a legal obligation to perform within the standard of care if you decide to stop and provide assistance. In addition, you have a further legal duty not to abandon the patient after treatment has begun. It is important to understand your legal obligations when you are off duty. Learn your state laws, and educate your peers regarding these off-duty obligations.

The concept of duty extends to maintaining licensure or certification, attending continuing education courses, and maintaining your skills. Maintaining your health and psychological well-being so that you will be prepared for the rigors of prehospital patient care is essential. In addition, you have a duty to check your equipment at the beginning of each shift and ensure all equipment is functioning properly. Finally, you have a duty to honor your patient's rights to privacy and their rights to refuse or limit the care you provide.

EMS agencies—and even entire EMS systems—can be held to a legal duty. EMS agencies have a duty to respond to calls for aid and to use mutual aid resources appropriately if call volume is too heavy to allow response within an appropriate time frame. Some EMS agencies may operate with formal contracts that specify legal duties, such as minimum response times.

Legal duty is a concept in the law that tells you what your standards of practice are. It is an unpredictable legal concept, often defined in the context of a case tried in a court of law. But the concept of legal duty is used by attorneys defending EMS providers. For example, in a lawsuit against an off-duty paramedic who stopped at a crash to render aid, the paramedic's attorney may attempt to show that the paramedic had no duty to the patient, but instead provided assistance he or she was not required by law to provide.

Remember, attorneys are often trained to work from the most general defense to the most specific elements of the case. Lack of legal duty is a general defense; however general it is, it may still be true.

Breach of Duty

The second element a patient must prove for a lawsuit to be successful is that the paramedic failed to perform within the **standard of care**. The standard of care is what a reasonable paramedic, in the same or similar situation, would have done. In a lawsuit, a jury will listen to the testimony of expert

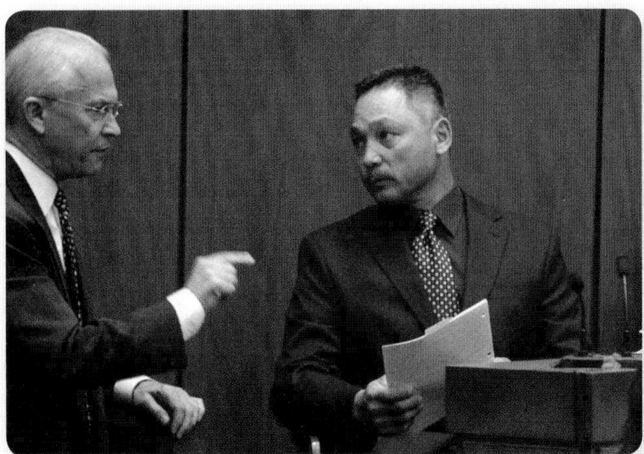

Figure 4-16 Court discussions will be based on your documentation and testimony. Make sure your documentation is neat, thorough, and accurate.

witnesses on both sides and ultimately decide whether your care was reasonable or not. These expert witnesses will provide a number of sources on which to base their testimony about whether your care was reasonable. Those sources will include their own training and experience; your training, experience, and continuing education; textbooks; protocols; national standards; standard operating procedures; and the PCR. Good documentation will go a long way to prove your high standards of care **Figure 4-16**.

Some states differentiate between **ordinary negligence** and **gross negligence**. How high a standard of care you will be held to varies from one state to another. Some states provide immunity for all but the poorest emergency medical care given by the paramedic. This immunity often comes in the form of a **Good Samaritan law** (discussed later in this chapter) in those cases in which the paramedic was off duty and no compensation was paid for the assistance provided.

In states that follow a gross negligence standard, a lawsuit against a paramedic will not be successful unless that paramedic has seriously departed from the accepted standards. Actions are grossly negligent if they are found to be willful or wanton (malicious) under the law. This standard is difficult for a plaintiff to meet. Usually, either intentional conduct or recklessness is essential to a finding of willful or wanton conduct. For example, *Black's Law Dictionary* defines willful misconduct as "intentional disregard to safety of others,"[10] and wanton misconduct as "the reckless disregard for the safety and rights of others while knowing harm or injury may result."[11] Some states have defined wanton misconduct as "reckless disregard," "utter indifference," or "conscious disregard" for the safety of others. If you can convince the jury that you acted in good faith, then you will usually not be found negligent.

In other states, a plaintiff will have to show only ordinary negligence, which can be a failure to act or a simple mistake that causes harm to a patient. It is much easier for a plaintiff to prove negligence under the ordinary negligence standard.

In certain circumstances, a special theory of negligence known as **res ipsa loquitur** may apply even though the plaintiff is unable to demonstrate clearly the exact manner by which an injury occurred. *Res ipsa loquitur* means "the thing speaks for itself." Under this theory, you could be held liable upon a showing that the plaintiff was injured, that the instrumentality causing the injury was in your control, and that such injuries do not ordinarily occur unless negligence is present. For example, you and your partner are called to the home of a patient who had a loss of consciousness as a result of an apparent drug overdose. While loading the patient into the ambulance, your partner slips, causing the stretcher to tip over; the patient strikes the ground and sustains a large laceration to his head. The patient later sues for negligence. Because the patient was unconscious at the time of the incident, he is unable to describe how the fall took place. Under the doctrine of *res ipsa loquitur*, the patient can prevail in his lawsuit by showing that he was under your care, that he sustained an injury, and that his injury would not have occurred unless negligence was present.

Another type of negligence is known as **negligence per se**. The principle of negligence per se is generally applied in those circumstances in which a paramedic inexcusably violates a statute. An example might be when you treat a patient even though your license is expired. A finding that a statute has been violated can sometimes lead to an automatic finding of negligence.

Proximate Cause

Even in cases in which the paramedic had a legal duty to the patient, and the paramedic breached the standard of care, a plaintiff must still link the act that fell below the standard of care directly to his or her injury by showing that the act (or failure to act) proximately caused the harm. *Black's Law Dictionary* defines **proximate cause** as "that which, in a natural and continuous sequence, unbroken by any intervening cause, produces injury, and without which the result would not have occurred."[12] Simply stated, a plaintiff will have to prove that your improper action, or failure to act, was the cause of the injury.

Failure to secure a patient on a backboard can be the proximate cause of severing the spinal cord. Proving that an act or a failure to act caused an injury is the most difficult part of a lawsuit. For example, imagine that you are treating a patient from a motor vehicle crash who has a spinal cord injury and you drop the stretcher during patient care. The patient may try to show that his or her injury resulted from the dropped stretcher and not from the crash itself. In such a case, careful documentation of the patient's neurologic status at the time you first encountered the patient would be essential to your defense.

Harm

The final element plaintiffs must prove in a negligence lawsuit is that they were harmed. Although physical injury is usually part of any lawsuit for medical negligence, patients may also claim damages for emotional distress, loss of income, loss of enjoyment of life, loss of spousal consortium, loss of household services, and loss of future earning capacity. They will have to show that your actions as a paramedic were proximate causes of each of these losses.

Words of Wisdom

As a paramedic, you may sometimes face ethical conflict regarding the allocation of limited resources during triage situations. For example, would you give special consideration to an injured person whom you knew personally? Would you be more likely to provide prompt emergency medical care for an innocent patient while delaying care to a more seriously injured perpetrator? Would you be able to apply triage protocols objectively to a person who is abusive toward you? Triage requires you to be professional and ethical in every respect because decisions made during triage can affect life and death. Triage procedures are discussed in Chapter 47, *Incident Management and Mass-Casualty Incidents*.

▶ Abandonment

Abandonment is a form of negligence that involves the termination of medical care without the patient's consent. The term also implies that the patient had a continuing need for medical treatment and that the abrupt termination of treatment was the cause of subsequent injury or death. Therefore, after you have responded to an emergency, you may not leave a patient in need of medical treatment until another competent health care professional with an equal or higher level of training has taken responsibility for that patient's care. Notify an appropriate health care professional of the patient's presence in the ED, and that you are transferring responsibility for patient care to that person.

It is also important that you complete a written report, which is often submitted electronically and frequently arrives after the call. It is important that the ED physician or nurse who is taking over care of your patient receives this report. The written report will permit the ED physician and staff to review your findings in the field, the medications you gave the patient, and the procedures you performed.

Some situations may not require transport and are not considered abandonment. EMS systems frequently receive calls for service for patients who may not really need treatment or transportation. A patient may have fallen and needs help getting up from the floor or may want your help administering his medication. Or, a patient who has a legitimate medical emergency, such as hypoglycemia, may feel fine after treatment and may not require transport to a hospital. Your local medical director should provide protocols for these situations. However, in general, it is a good idea to encourage transport.

In addition, some ambulance services, particularly in rural areas, may employ providers of various levels of training and may not have a full staff of paramedics at all times. In those areas, even if you make the initial response, you may not need to be part of the transport crew if the patient does not need advanced care. If in doubt, then contact your medical control.

Many EMS systems provide a tiered response, with BLS providers reaching the patient quickly, followed by advanced life support (ALS) providers. If a BLS crew responds and makes an improper determination that a patient does not need ALS care, then the system may be exposed to liability. Your service needs to work with every provider involved to set up protocols that provide guidance for the situations in which a BLS crew may cancel the response of an incoming ALS crew.

Patient Autonomy

It is well-established fact that patients have the right to direct their own care and to decide how they want their end-of-life medical care provided to them. This right, known as **patient autonomy**, has come to the forefront of medical ethics. In almost every case, except where the patient is a minor or lacks decision-making capacity, you must respect and honor the patient's right to make medical decisions, however irrational or unsound those decisions may appear.

Patients' decisions may not be accepted by other members of the public or other members of the patient's family, but it is important for you to remember that the courts, including the United States Supreme Court, have clearly recognized the right of patients to make decisions about their own medical care, even if that decision will bring about the patient's death. Ethics has become the subject of many discussions between paramedics who find themselves in the unique position of being accountable to more systems than the average health care provider in trying to respect the wishes of the patient. The EMS system, your medical director, the EMS agency for which you work, and your community's standard of care can compete with the wishes of the patient. These competing interests can create an ethical conflict that you will need to resolve through communication with all parties involved.

Occasionally, a physician will give an order that you feel is detrimental to the patient's best interests. It is important for you to immediately discuss with the physician why you feel that way. Remember, you are often in a better position to see what is going on with the patient, and a big part of your job is to communicate fully with the physician. Never perform a procedure or administer a medication that you believe will be detrimental to the patient. For example, if a physician asks you to perform a procedure in which you are not trained or asks you to administer a medication in a dose that is well outside the range of your protocols, then it is essential to obtain clarification from the physician and communicate your objections. You could discuss your current standing orders and offer a feasible alternative within your scope of practice, or you could request that the physician speak with your medical director. In all circumstances, act in the patient's best interest as his or her advocate.

▶ Advance Directives

An **advance directive** is usually a written document (but can also be an oral statement) that expresses the wants, needs, and desires of a patient in reference to his or her future medical care. Advance directives state what medical care the patient wants or does not want when the patient is unable to express his or her wishes. Living wills, do not resuscitate (DNR) orders, and organ donation orders are all advance directives.

Advance directives differ from state to state. In some states, a DNR order (also known as a resuscitation directive) may restrict any ALS care, whereas others provide for comfort care, including pain medications and oxygen therapy. In Colorado, a person designated as the medical durable power of attorney (discussed next) can revoke a resuscitation directive. However, in Montana, the patient or physician is the only one who can revoke a resuscitation directive.

Whether EMS personnel are bound by advance directives is a function of state law—and such laws, like those that cover DNR orders, are usually strict, often limited to terminal patients in nursing homes or hospice care. Learning and following the laws of your state will provide a framework for decisions regarding advance directives.

Living Will and Health Care Power of Attorney

The **living will** and the **health care power of attorney** are types of advance directives in which a patient can express wishes regarding end-of-life medical care. These directives are sometimes called health care "durable" powers of attorney because they remain in effect after a patient loses decision-making capacity. The issue of dealing with powers of attorney can sometimes be confusing. First of all, various types of powers of attorney exist and not all of them authorize the designated agent to make decisions regarding health care. Older patients commonly execute powers of attorney that enable others to conduct financial affairs on their behalf and which have no effect on health care whatsoever. It is also possible that a power of attorney may have been executed outside the state in which the patient now resides and its effect within your state may be questionable. As a paramedic, you should ask to see the power of attorney and then carefully review it to determine whether it authorizes the agent to make health care decisions. Most states recognize that advanced directives, except for DNR

YOU are the Paramedic PART 3

The patient's daughter brings you a list of her mother's medications and you quickly review it— carvedilol (Coreg), lisinopril (Prinivil), levothyroxine (Synthroid), and simvastatin (Zocor). She also hands you a copy of the advance directive that states the patient wishes no heroic measures be taken if she is not breathing and does not have a pulse.

The patient tells you her name is Mary, but cannot tell you what day of the week it is or how old she is. She agrees to let you take her vital signs, but still says she will not go to the hospital. Measurement of her blood glucose level shows a reading of 138 mg/dL.

Her daughter tells you that her mother's symptoms have been going on for several days, but today she is worse. She keeps forgetting basic things and is now refusing to eat. She thinks her mother might be having "ministrokes" and her confusion is getting worse.

Recording Time: 4 Minutes	
Respirations	20 breaths/min, regular
Pulse	108 beats/min, strong radials
Skin	Cool and dry
Blood pressure	152/98 mm Hg
Oxygen saturation (Spo_2)	97% on room air
Pupils	PERRLA

5. Would it be considered abandonment if you left the scene at this point?
6. Does the patient's advance directive take precedence over her current wishes?

orders, probably will not apply in emergency situations because the paramedic is unable to take the time to read and interpret a legal document on the scene. When you are in doubt, contact medical control for assistance.

Living wills generally require some kind of precondition to activate, such as a terminal illness or an irreversible coma. The living will should spell out exactly what kind of treatment a patient wishes to be given should he or she become incapacitated. A living will often contains a health care power of attorney, which designates another person (eg, a spouse, partner, adult sibling, or parent) to make health care decisions for the patient at any time the patient is unable to make those decisions. The person designated to make decisions does not have to be a relative, but may be someone close to the patient who understands his or her wishes. In those cases where the living will does not contain a health care power of attorney, its use in the field will be limited and once again, you should consult medical control.

The person who carries the health care power of attorney is often called the **surrogate decision maker** Figure 4-17. The surrogate decision maker is legally obligated to make decisions as the patient would want, and has presumably discussed these decisions with the patient. It is important to bear in mind that the surrogate decision maker has no authority until the patient becomes incapable of making decisions. If you arrive on scene and find that a surrogate decision maker is attempting to make decisions that conflict with a competent patient's decisions, then always follow the patient's decisions. Do not refuse emergency medical care to a patient who desires it.

Words of Wisdom

Do not be confused: A living will is not the same as a DNR order. The living will allows for decisions to be made regarding DNR orders if a patient becomes incapacitated or unable to make his or her own decisions.

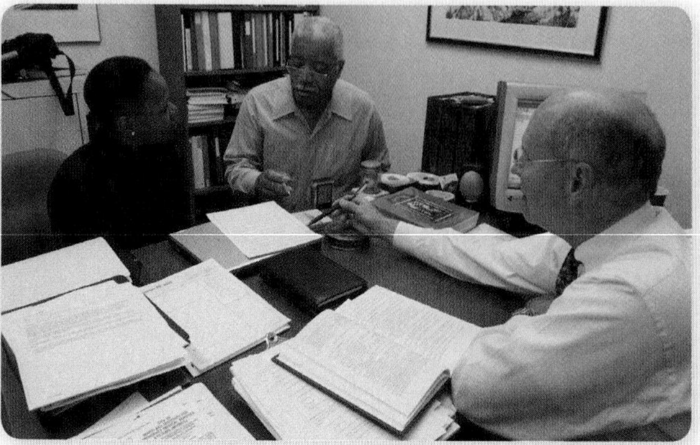

Figure 4-17 A surrogate decision maker (often a child or other close relative) is frequently designated when a person draws up a living will.

DNR Orders

As mentioned previously, a **do not resuscitate (DNR) order** (also referred to as *do not attempt resuscitation [DNAR]*) is an advance directive that describes which life-sustaining procedures, if any, should be performed if a patient's medical condition suddenly deteriorates. During the last 20 years, DNR orders were finally recognized in the prehospital setting Figure 4-18. EMS has now joined the

A

PREHOSPITAL MEDICAL CARE DIRECTIVE
(side one)

IN THE EVENT OF CARDIAC OR RESPIRATORY ARREST, I REFUSE ANY RESUSCITATION MEASURES INCLUDING CARDIAC COMPRESSION, ENDOTRACHEAL INTUBATION AND OTHER ADVANCED AIRWAY MANAGEMENT, ARTIFICIAL VENTILATION, DEFIBRILLATION, ADMINISTRATION OF ADVANCED CARDIAC LIFE SUPPORT DRUGS AND RELATED EMERGENCY MEDICAL PROCEDURES.

Patient: ______________________ Date: __________
(Signature or mark)

Attach recent photograph here or provide all of the following information below:
Date of Birth __________
Sex ______ Race ______
Eye Color __________
Hair Color __________

PHOTO

Hospice Program (if any) __________
Name and telephone number of patient's physician __________

(side two)

I have explained this form and its consequences to the signer and obtained assurance that the signer understands that death may result from any refused care listed above (on reverse side).

______________________ Date__________
(Licensed health care provider)

I was present when this was signed (or marked). The patient then appeared to be of sound mind and free from duress.

______________________ Date__________
(Witness)

B

Outside the Hospital Do - Not - Resuscitate Identification Card

Patient's Full Name__________

I affirm that I have authorized an Outside the Hospital Do - Not - Resuscitate Order for this patient and have documented the grounds for the order in this patient's medical file.

Attending Physician Signature__________

Attending Physician (print)__________

Address__________ **Phone**__________

Date__________

I, ______________________,
(name)
authorize emergency medical services personnel to withhold or withdraw cardiopulmonary resuscitation from me in the event I suffer cardiac or respiratory arrest.

I understand this means that if my heart stops beating or I stop breathing, no medical procedure to restart heart function or breathing will be instituted.

I understand that I may revoke this order at anytime.

Patient or Patient's Representative

Signature__________

Date__________

Figure 4-18 A. An example of a wallet-sized do not resuscitate (DNR) order. **B.** An example of a pocket-sized DNR order.

medical community in recognizing that patients have the same rights to direct and refuse care outside the hospital that they do inside the hospital. Many states now have DNR forms specific to EMS, and most states have laws that govern the natural process of dying and what rights patients have to direct that process.

States have their own procedure for how to recognize a valid DNR order. Some states rely on a written physician order (which might not be available to the EMS provider), while others may require the patient to wear an identification bracelet or necklace. In some cases, such jewelry indicates that the patient has consented to the release of stored information, such as the patient's DNR status, to medical personnel Figure 4-19. In some states, DNR orders expire within a specified time frame and must be renewed to remain valid, whereas others may have no expiration date. It may also be a requirement that the DNR order be executed within your state by a physician licensed to practice medicine within the state. Be familiar with the documents used in your state and what you are expected to do if the documents are unavailable.

Although laws might differ from state to state, generally speaking, DNR orders must meet the following requirements to be valid:

- Clearly state the patient's medical condition(s)
- Signature of the patient or legal guardian
- Signature of one or more physicians
- In some states, DNR orders contain expiration dates, whereas in others, no expiration date is included. DNR orders with expiration dates must be dated in the preceding 12 months to be valid.

However, even in the presence of a DNR order, you are still obligated to provide supportive measures if indicated (oxygen, pain relief, and comfort) to a patient who is not in cardiac arrest, whenever possible. Each ambulance service, in consultation with its medical director and legal counsel, must develop a protocol to follow in these circumstances.

Withholding or Withdrawing Resuscitation

Current bioethical guidelines rely on the use of common sense and reasonable judgment in deciding when to stop CPR and resuscitation efforts, or to decline to initiate them at all. The National Association of EMS Physicians has published data and guidelines for the termination of resuscitation of nontraumatic cardiopulmonary arrest that demonstrates the benefits of on-scene resuscitation, along with when to terminate resuscitation.[13] These guidelines have been adopted by a multitude of EMS organizations across the United States, allowing for field personnel to make a clinical decision regarding resuscitation based on downtime, poor outcome analysis, and family input. For some organizations, these guidelines represent a paradigm shift from previous resuscitation modalities that has caused hesitation in implementing such practices, yet sufficient studies document the benefit of adopting such practices.[13] Each resuscitation should be based on the futility of such efforts. Futile resuscitation efforts—interventions that studies have shown do not benefit patients—are not medically or ethically indicated Figure 4-20.

If you are unsure of the time of a cardiac arrest, begin care and immediately contact medical control to discuss termination of the resuscitative effort.

You will need to consider the time it will take for a patient to reach definitive care at the hospital and the likelihood of survival—especially if you work in rural and wilderness areas. Occasionally, you will hear a story about a patient who has recovered from what appeared to be a hopeless situation, thus, providing motivation for you to attempt to save a patient under the most impossible circumstances. Remember that rare survival cases should not be the guide to your decisions about resuscitation efforts, even though terminating lifesaving efforts in the field may seem contrary to your instincts as a health care provider.

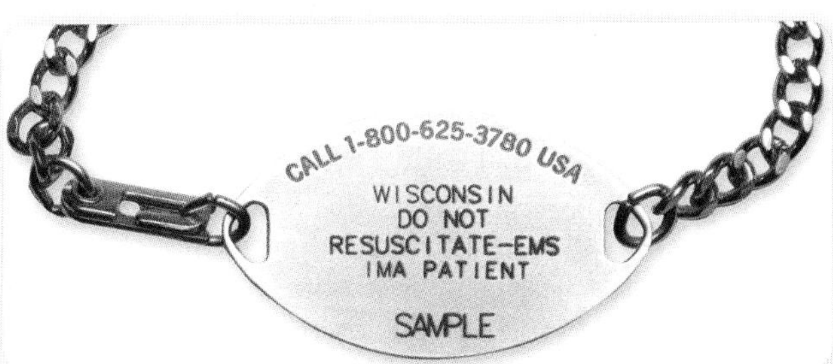

Figure 4-19 Medical identification bracelets can provide access to vital information about a patient, including important medical conditions and possible do not resuscitate orders. In the case of Medic Alert bracelet, the EMS provider can obtain stored patient information from the Medic Alert Foundation.

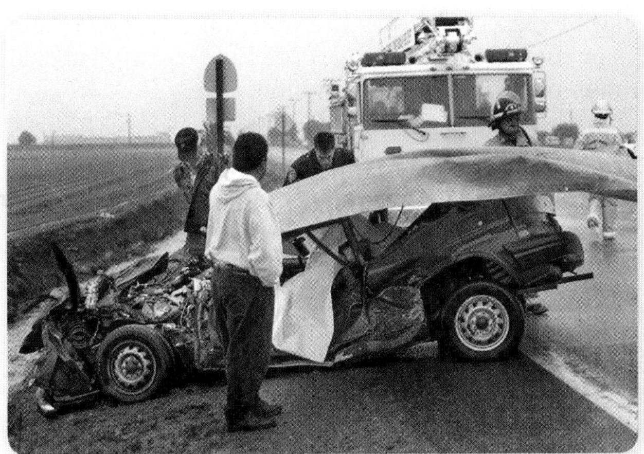

Figure 4-20 Although your instincts are always to try to sustain life at whatever cost, sometimes it is clear that resuscitation efforts will be futile, and should be withheld per local protocols.

Termination of resuscitative efforts is discussed in Chapter 39, *Responding to the Field Code*. Each state has different laws that may define the role of the paramedic in resuscitation issues. In some jurisdictions, you may be able to pronounce death, while in others only a medical investigator or physician may do so. State laws continue to govern your practice even if the patient is clinically deceased. Some of these laws include guidelines concerning situations in which even BLS measures are inappropriate. For example, do not attempt resuscitation for patients who are obviously dead (eg, livor or rigor mortis or putrefaction), or who have injuries incompatible with life (eg, decapitation). If resuscitation has already begun, then cessation of these efforts in the field may be appropriate in cases of blunt trauma arrest, a prolonged rescue or response time, or other lengthy medical resuscitation efforts.

The decision to halt resuscitation is particularly difficult and emotional when you are caring for a pediatric patient. Studies have shown that paramedics feel particularly uncomfortable about terminating resuscitation in children. Paramedics and other medical professionals tend to be action-oriented people who feel that they must "do something" (as part of their moral code). However, in some situations, you can do more for the grieving family than for the child who has died. Ethically, you should be prepared to support the family, which can be the hardest part of the job.

Training, literature reviews, and open discussions about what actions are medically appropriate within EMS protocols should provide you guidance and ease concerns about difficult resuscitation situations. Continuing education regarding resuscitation issues may provide alternative viewpoints and a broader picture that allow you to make appropriate decisions in the field.

Acquire a thorough understanding of the basic consequences of typical EMS interventions. Ultimately, medical interventions and lifesaving attempts may prolong suffering or fail to return a patient to a meaningful life. When in doubt, do not hesitate to consult medical control. If communication is hindered because of terrain or wilderness conditions, then your judgment will benefit from knowing about interventions and consequences of those interventions ahead of time.

▶ End-of-Life Decisions

You will often deal with patients at the very end of their lives. These patients and their families should be treated with the utmost respect and empathy. You should never think: "Why did they bother to call 9-1-1 if they don't want us to do anything?" (This example represents the paramedic's moral code getting in the way of the paramedic's medical ethics.) Instead, understand that the family of a dying patient, even one under hospice care, may not know how to check a pulse, and may not understand that difficult, agonal gasps may continue for hours before a patient dies. Furthermore, a loved one, despite knowing that death is near, may call for an ambulance, not knowing what else to do at the moment of death. Many people have never been with someone at the moment of death. If information and emotional support is what they need, then provide it—it is part of your job.

Also, remember to avoid imposing your own moral code on a patient whose value system may be different from your own. You will encounter dying patients with varied cultural beliefs; thus, be prepared to respect a patient's wishes even if the patient's lifestyle or religious beliefs differ greatly from your own.

You are likely to encounter confusing scenarios when the DNR paperwork may not be immediately available. It is permissible, if not obligatory, that you begin resuscitation efforts and then discontinue them (with agreement from online medical control) if and when the paperwork is confirmed. In other situations, the paperwork may be present, but family members may disagree with the DNR order and insist that you begin resuscitation. In these situations, avoid any hostile encounters while carrying out the patient's wishes to the best of your ability. Contact medical control in confusing situations involving resuscitation questions. The medical control physician can be a valuable resource in such circumstances.

Medical Orders for Life-Sustaining Treatment (MOLST)

An end-of-life document has emerged in recent years and is known as Medical Orders for Life-Sustaining Treatment (MOLST) or Physician Orders for Life-Sustaining Treatment (POLST). Although similar to a DNR in many respects, the MOLST is more expansive. It is intended to be followed by all health care providers, not just EMS personnel. The DNR generally applies to patients who are in cardiac arrest, whereas MOLST may apply to patients with impending pulmonary failure who are not in cardiac arrest. MOLST orders typically contain provisions that address the initiation of CPR, intubation, feeding tubes, the use of antibiotics, and **palliative care** (intended to provide comfort and relief from pain). They apply only when the patient has lost decision-making capacity. MOLST orders are not used in all states, and it is important that you check to see if your state has adopted such provisions.

Organ Donation

A major issue in medical ethics involves the potential for patients with mortal injuries to donate organs. Donor organs are badly needed within the medical system, with patients waiting years for a match.

In specific circumstances, a patient who is not successfully resuscitated may be a potential organ donor. Certain centers can procure organs, including the kidneys and liver, in certain situations. These situations typically occur after in-hospital cardiac arrest but may be associated with certain specific out-of-hospital cardiac arrest situations that occur in close proximity to specialized centers. Be aware of your local centers and the respective protocols and capabilities.

Whether or not a patient should be kept alive for the sole purpose of organ donation is an issue that you

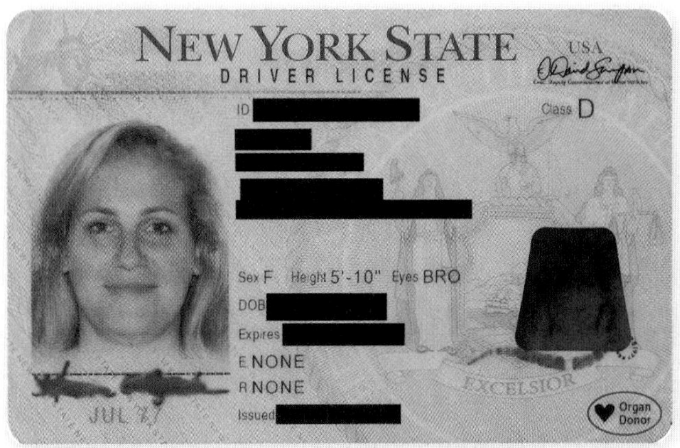

Figure 4-21 Most states have an organ donation designation on the driver's license, either on the front or reverse side (here, it is shown at lower right).

should discuss with your medical director and local hospital system. The parameters for viable organs should be clearly spelled out within the individual EMS system. Also understand the state law concerning organ donation: in many cases, a patient must have witnessed, informed consent (usually in writing).

In general, major organs such as the kidneys and liver are not appropriate for organ donation after prolonged hypotension or CPR. However, other tissue such as the corneas and skin may be valuable. Many states have programs that allow patients to agree to organ donation by making a notation on their driver's licenses Figure 4-21. If the patient's wishes regarding organ donation are unknown, then consent should be obtained from a family member before any arrangements are made to keep a patient alive solely for purposes of organ donation.

Another resource that might be available to your EMS system are continuing education workshops offered by organ transplant teams and EMS leaders to increase awareness of the vital role of EMS in securing transplants.

Defenses to Litigation

Over the last 10 years, the media and public education have made the public more aware of what to expect from the local EMS system. If citizens perceive your response as delayed or your efforts as incompetent, then they will often file lawsuits seeking compensation for injuries they believe were caused by inadequate EMS care. If you do not explain to your patients why you were delayed, or why a procedure is difficult, then you leave yourself open to the consequences of unanswered questions that can lead a patient to seek legal action. In essence, your first defense to litigation is an open, informative, trust-based relationship with your patients. When this relationship is not possible or fails in its intent, and litigation occurs, several legal defenses may be used in the courtroom.

If a lawsuit is filed against you, then you and the agency with which you are employed may implement one of two commonly used defenses: statute of limitations and contributory negligence. Every state has laws that limit the time within which a lawsuit may be filed. Such laws are called **statutes of limitations**. The time to file may be as short as 1 year in some states, whereas in other states the time may be as long as 5 or 6 years. A lawsuit that is filed beyond these statutory periods can be dismissed as untimely. However, these statutory periods are typically extended for minors until the minor reaches the age of majority.

Another potential defense is known as **contributory negligence**. This defense will apply when the plaintiff has done something that contributes to his or her own injuries. For example, you encounter a patient with chest pain that appears to be cardiac in nature. Prior to administering nitroglycerin, you inquire about any recent use of erectile dysfunction medications. The patient denies the use of any such medication despite the fact that he used one of the medications several hours earlier. Shortly following the administration of nitroglycerin, the patient experiences a severe drop in blood pressure and almost dies as a result of the interaction between the nitroglycerin and erectile dysfunction medication. In the lawsuit that follows, you are able to assert the defense of contributory negligence because the patient failed to state that he had used the medication several hours earlier, and that usage clearly contributed to his adverse reaction to the nitroglycerin.

Good Samaritan Legislation

Although every state has some form of a Good Samaritan law, not every state extends such protection to all citizens and off-duty EMS personnel. As an EMS provider, you should contact your state legislators to determine which level of Good Samaritan protection is offered.[14] Although the laws were initially passed to encourage the public to help at emergency scenes, many of these statutes also operate to provide some protection for EMS personnel who are off duty and assist at an emergency. The laws of most states limit the legal protection provided: the emergency care must be given free of charge (gratuitously). As a general rule, if you are on duty and have a legal duty to a patient, then the Good Samaritan law will not protect you. Good Samaritan laws may help cover you if you render assistance in another state, but they do not supersede the laws of the licensing agency in your own state.

Most Good Samaritan laws also require that people responding to an emergency do all that they can, within their knowledge, to support and sustain life and to prevent further injury. As a paramedic, you are not expected to function as a physician; however, you are expected to deploy those skills that any other paramedic with similar training would use under the same or similar circumstances.

Courts have not been generous in applying the Good Samaritan law during routine EMS work. Courts have been applying the concept of immunity only during emergencies.

Governmental Immunity

An abiding principle of English law is that you cannot sue the queen (or king) because "the queen can do no wrong." In the United States, this concept, called sovereign immunity, has taken the form of legislation that identifies only limited types of lawsuits that can be filed against government agencies. Paramedics working for government agencies, such as a fire department, also have some governmental immunity for their actions. The immunity statutes may also set limited time frames in which lawsuits can be filed, and may limit the amount of money a plaintiff can recover.

Qualified Immunity

Governmental immunity does not cover civil rights violations, and attorneys can file lawsuits against paramedics in the public sector for violating the civil rights of their patients. The most common complaint occurs when EMS personnel either improperly restrain a violent patient or use excessive force to restrain a patient. Civil rights lawsuits may also be filed if your conduct as a paramedic deviates so far from the standard of care that a civil rights violation is said to occur.

Paramedics who work or volunteer for public agencies (such as fire departments), who are sued by patients alleging civil rights violations, may have another type of immunity called **qualified immunity**. Under this doctrine, you are held liable only when the plaintiff can show that you violated a clearly established law of which you should have known. This kind of immunity does not apply to tort cases.

Employment Law and the Paramedic

In addition to the legal issues that arise out of your role as a paramedic providing patient care, there are a number of important laws that affect your relationship with your employer. In fact, over the course of your career as a paramedic, the chances of becoming involved in a legal issue regarding your employment are probably as great, if not greater, than your chances of being sued by a patient. The relationship between employer and employee involves an ever-increasing complexity of state and federal laws and regulations with which you should have a basic understanding.

YOU are the Paramedic — PART 4

You talk to Mary and explain to her that she needs to be evaluated. She starts to cry and tells you, "They are just sending me to that hospital to die." You convince her that this is not true and that she needs to see a physician so that she will feel better. She reluctantly agrees to go with you and says that she has a slight headache but otherwise feels fine. You perform a stroke assessment and see no signs of deficits.

At 0752 hours, the patient is on a stretcher in the ambulance and you are en route to the hospital. You start a 20-gauge IV line in her left antecubital fossa and draw blood. You administer normal saline at a TKO (to keep open) flow rate. She will not tolerate a nasal cannula, so you monitor her oxygen saturation level. The cardiac monitor shows sinus tachycardia without ectopy.

You reassess her vital signs en route and transport her to Cedar's Medical Center. You arrive at the hospital at 0804 hours. You give a report to the receiving nurse and are back in service at 0810 hours.

Recording Time: 14 Minutes	
Respirations	18 breaths/min, regular
Pulse	102 beats/min, strong radials
Skin	Cool and dry
Blood pressure	162/94 mm Hg
Oxygen saturation (Spo_2)	98% on room air
Pupils	PERRLA

7. If the patient had continued to refuse treatment and transport, then what options might you have exercised?
8. Under which type of consent was this patient treated?

▶ Americans With Disabilities Act

The Americans With Disabilities Act (ADA) is a federal law that was adopted in 1990 to protect qualified people with disabilities from being discriminated against in employment. The law generally applies to all employers with a minimum of 15 employees, but state laws providing similar protection may include employers with even fewer employees. The law applies to all aspects of employment including hiring, promotions, training, salary, benefits, and termination. A common misconception about the ADA is that it requires employers to hire employees with disabilities who may not be qualified for the job. This notion, of course, is not true. To be protected by the ADA, a person must meet the following two basic qualifications:

1. He or she must have a physical or mental disability that limits one or more major life activities such as hearing, seeing, walking, or speaking; and
2. He or she must possess the basic qualifications of the job and be able to perform the essential functions of the job adequately, with or without reasonable accommodations.

An employer may not inquire about an applicant's disability or require a medical exam until after a job offer has been made. If a person with a disability would be able to perform the essential functions of the job using reasonable accommodations, then the employer may be required to provide and pay for the cost of these accommodations. The law does not require an employer to provide accommodations that would result in an undue hardship to the employer or to other employees.

The ADA does not require an employer to give preference to a person with a disability. It simply requires that an employer make employment decisions based on reasons that are unrelated to the disability in which the applicant or employee is capable of performing the essential functions of the job.

▶ Title VII of the Civil Rights Act

Title VII is the section of the Civil Rights Act of 1964 that prohibits discrimination in employment based on race, color, religion, sex, or national origin. In addition, this section of the law provides protection against sexual harassment in the workplace. The antidiscrimination provisions of Title VII apply to all aspects of employment including recruiting, hiring, promotions, benefits, and termination. Like the ADA, Title VII applies only to businesses with more than 15 employees.

Today it is unusual for an employer to blatantly refuse to hire or promote someone based on race, sex, religion, color, or national origin. Successful claims of discrimination often involve the identification of a discriminatory hiring pattern that develops over time and that demonstrates that a particular class of people, such as women or African Americans, are rarely hired or promoted and are vastly under-represented in the overall workforce.

Certain hiring practices violate Title VII even when these practices appear neutral. For example, imagine that an employer places a classified ad seeking to hire paramedics and states that one of the qualifications for the job is a minimum height of 5 feet 9 inches (175 cm). Although this qualification might seem neutral with respect to sex, it would have an obvious negative impact on the ability of women to be considered for the job because only a small percentage of women would meet the minimum height requirement. The burden would be on the employer to prove that it was necessary for a paramedic to be at least 5 feet 9 inches (175 cm) to perform the functions of the job effectively. Clearly, the employer could not meet this burden.

▶ Sexual Harassment

Sexual harassment litigation is one of the most common claims filed under Title VII, and it has seen its share of claims in EMS. Two types of sexual harassment claims exist: (1) **quid pro quo** ("this for that") claims, in which a person in authority attempts to exchange some work-related benefit such as a raise or promotion for inappropriate employee actions (eg, sexual favors); and (2) **hostile environment** claims. These are claims in which the employer or an agent of the employer either creates or allows to continue an offensive practice related to sex that makes it uncomfortable or impossible for an employee to continue working. Sexual harassment can occur between any combination of sexes, sexual orientations, or gender identities.[15] Most sexual harassment claims fall into the category of hostile environment. No precise definition exists in the law of the types of conduct that would constitute sexual harassment, but court decisions over the years have identified a number of circumstances that can be considered harassment. These include the following:

- Sexual jokes or comments
- Display of sexually offensive photographs or other material
- Unwelcome sexual advances
- Inappropriate and unwelcome touching or kissing
- Inappropriate inquiry into an employee's sex life

All employers have an obligation to prevent sexual harassment from occurring and to investigate any and all claims of sexual harassment promptly. As part of their obligation under the law, employers should provide training in sexual harassment for all newly hired employees and for all employees on an annual basis. As an employee, promptly report any conduct that you feel constitutes sexual harassment to your supervisor or to the human resources department of your organization.

▶ Additional Federal Laws Dealing With Discrimination

Several other federal laws prohibit various types of discrimination in the workplace. These include the following:

1. The *Pregnancy Discrimination Act* makes it illegal to discriminate in all areas of employment

based on pregnancy, childbirth, or any medical condition related to pregnancy. This law was adopted in 1978 as an amendment to Title VII. Prior to the enactment of this law, it was not uncommon for employers to refuse to hire women who were pregnant or to terminate women after they became pregnant. The law also requires employers to provide health benefits and medical leave for pregnancy and childbirth equal to those provided for other medical conditions.

2. The *Equal Pay Act of 1963* makes it illegal to pay different rates of pay to men and women if they perform equal work in the same workplace. Executives and managers are generally exempt from the provisions of the law.
3. The *Age Discrimination in Employment Act of 1967* protects people who are age 40 years or older from discrimination in all aspects of employment based on age. The law applies to businesses with 15 or more employees.

▶ State Laws

Many states have also passed laws that deal with discrimination in the workplace. For the most part, these laws address the same issues covered under federal law. In some cases, these laws provide more rights than the federal laws. For example, some state laws prohibit discrimination based on sexual orientation, marital status, or gender identity, which may not all be covered under federal law.[16] Also, many discrimination protections under federal law do not apply to employers with fewer than 15 employees, whereas many state laws do apply. It is important to become familiar with the laws of your state.

▶ Family and Medical Leave Act

The Family and Medical Leave Act (FMLA) of 1993 is a federal law that grants eligible employees the right to take up to 12 weeks of unpaid leave per year under certain circumstances. To be eligible under the law, an employee must work for an employer with at least 50 employees and have worked for that employer for at least 12 months. Leave may be taken to deal with a medical condition of the employee or a family member, or the birth or adoption of a child.

Some states have passed their own Family Leave Acts that may provide the employee with more rights than the federal law or which may apply to employers with fewer than 50 employees.

▶ Occupational Safety and Health Administration

The Occupational Safety and Health Administration (OSHA) is the federal agency that regulates safety in the workplace. States may enforce regulations tighter than those set by OSHA but may not make regulations more lenient. All employers are covered either by OSHA or an OSHA-approved safety plan. Under the OSHA Act of 1970, all employers have several basic responsibilities including the following:

- To comply with all OSHA standards, rules, and regulations that are applicable to his or her business
- To provide all employees with a workplace that is free from hazards
- To warn employees of potential hazards
- To ensure all employees are provided with appropriate safety equipment
- To establish and maintain a reporting system for all workplace injuries or illnesses
- To provide training for all employees

Health care employers have some additional responsibilities that are unique to the industry, including the following:

- Development of an exposure control plan to assist employees who may have been exposed to certain bloodborne pathogens
- Development of training programs for all newly hired employees as well as annual refresher training for all employees that address issues related to bloodborne pathogens
- Making the hepatitis B vaccine available at no charge to all employees
- Development of guidelines regarding the use of standard precautions

OSHA regulations and standards are often changing, and as a paramedic, you should do your best to be as familiar as possible with these changes. In the EMS environment, thousands of EMS employees sustain injuries and illnesses each year. You share an obligation, along with your employer, to do all that you can to avoid injuries.

▶ Ryan White Act

The Ryan White Act is a federal law that provides certain safeguards and protections for health care workers who are exposed or potentially exposed to certain designated diseases. The diseases that are covered have been established by the Centers for Disease Control and Prevention and include human immunodeficiency virus, acquired immunodeficiency syndrome, tuberculosis, hepatitis B, meningitis, diphtheria, hemorrhagic fevers, plague, and rabies.

The Ryan White Act contains several important provisions, which include the following:

- Hospitals and emergency response employers are required to establish a notification system to be used when an exposure occurs.
- Employers must appoint a designated infection control officer to handle exposures and to assist all employees who may have been exposed.
- Access to the medical records of the patient who is the source of the exposure may be obtained to determine whether the patient has tested positively for, or is exhibiting signs and symptoms of, a covered infectious disease.

If you believe that you have been exposed to an infectious disease, then promptly notify the infection control officer within your service. The infection control officer will be aware of any state-specific laws related to infectious disease exposure.

▶ National Labor Relations Act

Many paramedics are employed by EMS agencies that are unionized. Unionization means that at some point, the employees have elected to have a union represent them as their collective bargaining agent for purposes of negotiating issues such as compensation, benefits, and work conditions. The National Labor Relations Act, also known as the Wagner Act, is the primary law that establishes the rights of unions and union workers and regulates unfair labor practices by employers. Under this law, employees have a wide variety of rights with which they should become familiar. In addition to the provisions of the National Labor Relations Act, each state has its own set of laws that affect the rights of union members. In some states, so-called right to work laws do not allow an employer or a union to require you to join a union as a condition to being hired or retained on the job. In other states, you may be required to join the union within a certain time period after you are hired.

YOU are the Paramedic SUMMARY

1. What type of consent is required to treat a patient with altered mental status?

Any patient who is incapacitated and unable to make a decision for himself or herself is treated under implied consent. This principle applies to any patient who is too ill or injured to consent to emergency lifesaving treatment. It is assumed that the patient would want emergency medical care because of the severity of his or her condition. Implied consent is also applied to minors or those adults who have guardians when a serious illness or injury has occurred and a parent or guardian is not present.

2. What information must you determine prior to allowing a patient to refuse care?

First determine the patient's decision-making capacity by talking with her. Factors that will help you include her orientation to person, place, and time; use of drugs or alcohol; potential head trauma; the patient's medical history; vital signs; blood glucose levels, and oxygen saturation level. Remember, for a patient to refuse treatment and/or transport, he or she must be able to understand the information given regarding their condition and care and make a decision based on that information. As a general rule, a patient with an altered mental status or unstable vital signs probably cannot be considered able to refuse transport. To avoid potential legal action, follow the protocols of your service.

3. What are the possible consequences of treating this patient without her consent?

Touching and/or treating a patient without his or her consent may be grounds for charges of assault, battery, and possibly false imprisonment. These charges may be the result of using improper methods of restraint, failing to ask for permission prior to touching or making physical contact, or transporting a patient without his or her consent. However, the patient must be of legal age and demonstrate the ability to make informed decisions and refuse emergency medical care.

4. On the basis of her history, what might be her problem?

The patient has a history of transient ischemic attacks (TIAs), a brain tumor, hypothyroidism, hypertension, and hyperlipidemia. Any or all of these conditions could be the problem or could be contributing factors. She is exhibiting symptoms similar to TIAs with the periods of unresponsiveness. However, because the confusion is lasting for more than 24 hours, another or an additional cause is likely. The brain tumor could also be a major factor. It may be growing or pressing on certain areas of the brain that are causing the signs and symptoms. Hypertension may be a contributing factor for TIAs, or could exacerbate the brain tumor. Hypothyroidism causes a myriad of signs and symptoms, and taking too much or too little of her medication may result in the changes in mental status. Hyperlipidemia indicates that she already has an excess of cholesterol. If any blockages in major vessels supplying the brain are present, then hypoxia and an altered mental status may be the result.

5. Would it be considered abandonment if you left the scene at this point?

Yes. The patient obviously has an altered mental status and abiding by her wishes not to be transported would be abandonment. A patient with an altered mental status does not have decision-making capacity and cannot refuse. After you respond to a call and make contact with a patient, you cannot legally release care of that patient unless the patient is competent to refuse care or you have turned care over to someone of an equal or higher level of training.

6. Does the patient's advance directive take precedence over her current wishes?

If she is capable of making informed decisions, then she can override the advance directive. In this situation, the patient is not in cardiac arrest so it is not an issue because her advance directive is specific to a cardiac arrest.

YOU are the Paramedic SUMMARY *(continued)*

7. If the patient had continued to refuse treatment and transport, then what options might you have exercised?

Having her daughter talk to her may have helped, but if all else failed, then it would have become necessary to contact medical control for direction. She has proven to have an altered mental status and cannot refuse care because of her impaired decision-making capacity. In such a situation, follow local protocols, and prior to contacting medical control, ensure you have all of the information concerning the patient—vital signs, blood glucose level, medical history, medications, and any findings—readily available.

Not only can medical control direct you in the proper handling of the patient, but also having the patient speak directly to the physician on the phone may be enough to convince her that transport is necessary. Continue to be patient but firm in expressing to the patient why she needs to be transported for emergency medical care.

8. Under which type of consent was this patient treated?

The patient was treated under informed consent as well as implied consent. She has an altered mental status, which technically means that she can be treated under implied consent.

She was also treated under informed consent. She is not completely disoriented and understands most of what you are telling her. She agrees initially to allow you to take vital signs. She understands what you are about to do and gives you permission to do it. These actions constitute informed consent.

EMS Patient Care Report (PCR)					
Date: 02-02-18	**Incident No.:** 02110985		**Nature of Call:** Unresponsive person	**Location:** 487 Lenore Street	
Dispatched: 0737	**En Route:** 0738	**At Scene:** 0742	**Transport:** 0752	**At Hospital:** 0804	**In Service:** 0810

Patient Information	
Age: 64 **Sex:** F **Weight (in kg [lb]):** 69 kg (152 lb)	**Allergies:** Penicillin **Medications:** Coreg, Synthroid, Zocor, Prinivil **Past Medical History:** HTN, brain tumor, TIAs, hyperlipidemia, hypothyroidism **Chief Complaint:** Slight headache, acting strangely, altered mental status

Vital Signs				
Time: 0746	**BP:** 152/98	**Pulse:** 108	**Respirations:** 20	**Spo_2:** 97% on room air
Time: 0756	**BP:** 162/94	**Pulse:** 102	**Respirations:** 18	**Spo_2:** 98% on room air
Time:	**BP:**	**Pulse:**	**Respirations:**	**Spo_2:**

EMS Treatment (circle all that apply)				
Oxygen @ ______ L/min via (circle one): **NC NRM Bag-mask device**		**Assisted Ventilation**	**Airway Adjunct**	**CPR**
Defibrillation	**Bleeding Control**	**Bandaging**	**Splinting**	(circled) **Other:** Cardiac monitor

Narrative
EMS responded to a possible unresponsive person to find a 64 y/o woman reporting "slight" headache and altered mental status. Pt alert, but confused, oriented to person, place, and event, but not time. Daughter states that she has been this way for several days and has periods of not responding at all. Pt is ambulatory, no apparent distress noted, and no neuro deficits. PERRLA, glucose level is 138 mg/dL, heart monitor showing sinus tach without ectopy. Nothing else significant noted. Pt refused oxygen, but maintaining Spo_2 level on room air within normal limits. 20-gauge IV L antecubital fossa with blood drawn for labs and NS at TKO. Transported to Cedar's Medical Center, no changes en route.**End of report**

Prep Kit

▶ Ready for Review

- As a paramedic, you operate in a community that exposes you to professional liability and that requires you to have a solid understanding of law and ethics. Failing to perform your job as expected within the medical community, the legal community, and the regulations of the jurisdiction in which you function will expose you to civil and/or criminal liability.
- When personal ethics conflict with professional ethics, you usually will be bound by professional ethics and must temporarily set aside personal ethics.
- Three primary ethical principles to apply to your practice are: (1) to do no harm, (2) to act in good faith, and (3) to always act in the patient's best interest.
- EMS research, while important, presents unique ethical dilemmas regarding informed patient consent. Staying aware of the issues and the latest research is the best way to promote the development of evidence-based practice for paramedics.
- The foundation of the legal system in the United States is the federal government. The three branches of government are the executive, judicial, and legislative branches.
- The two types of law are civil and criminal.
  - Civil cases result in monetary damages.
  - Criminal cases result in incarceration of a person.
- As a paramedic, you are particularly susceptible to charges of assault and battery. Assault is when you instill the fear of bodily harm in a person. Battery is when you unlawfully touch another person without his or her consent.
- Charges of false imprisonment, although extremely rare, can occur if you restrain a patient against his or her will. Protection against this charge can exist only if appropriate documentation and policy exist regarding the specific call.
- Defamation, slander, and libel present risks to you if you make statements, either verbal or written, that injure a person's good name.
- Lawsuits follow a general process that starts with a complaint or notice of complaint, a response or answer by the defendant, discovery, settlement discussions, and trial process.
- You are subject to multiple legal jurisdictions, including state law, state regulations, local medical protocol, and departmental policy.
- Medical directors have a supervisory relationship over paramedics, but you are held personally responsible for your own actions.
- Your actions function as an extension of a series of medical directions from the medical director that are either online or off-line. These directives are binding unless you believe that your actions will cause harm to the patient.
- State legislation enables paramedics to practice in every state. It is your responsibility to understand the statutes of the state in which you practice.
- State jurisdictions issue paramedics either licenses or certificates. You must understand that the licensure or certification is a privilege—not a right—extended by the governing authority that allows you to practice within the enacting legislation.
- You have a right to due process, a fair procedure that includes appropriate legal notice of the action to be taken against you, and the opportunity to be heard before the licensing or certifying agency.
- State laws define scope of practice for the paramedic, which specifies your limits of practice allowed under the Medical Practice Act.
- HIPAA was first enacted in 1996 to protect a person's private health information, but permits disclosure when necessary for the betterment of society as a whole, such as when data are used to protect or improve public health.
- EMTALA is another federal law designed to prevent hospital emergency departments from turning patients away for any reason, including the ability to pay for care.
- Emergency vehicle operations must be performed in a manner that protects the public from further injury. No call can justify driving in a manner that endangers the public.
- Transportation to a certain medical facility should be determined by taking into account the patient's preference and the medical needs of the patient.
- Crime scenes present the intersection between EMS and law enforcement. You have an obligation to assist the law enforcement community in preservation of evidence and documentation of scenes or actions that may later be introduced on behalf of a criminal prosecution.
- You can be held legally responsible if you fail to report cases such as suspected abuse or neglect, domestic violence, gunshot or stab wounds, childbirth outside a medical facility, rape, infectious diseases, or animal bites.
- Immediately report suspected homicides, suicides, prison inmate deaths, and other violent or unexpected deaths to local law enforcement personnel to allow a coroner or medical examiner to examine the body.
- All patients of sound mind have the legal right under the Constitution of the United States of America to privacy, consent, and refusal. You cannot infringe

Prep Kit *(continued)*

on these inalienable rights unless you believe that patients are not of sound mind and pose a detriment to themselves or others.

- Patient refusals pose a large potential legal liability to paramedics. Your only protection against a civil lawsuit over a refusal will be the documentation at the time of the incident.
  - A refusal signature without narrative and evidence of a physical assessment is worthless.
- Obtain informed consent from patients prior to any medical process, including the physical exam.
- Obtain expressed consent—action demonstrating permission to provide care—from patients before initiating treatment.
- Implied consent is a form of consent assumed to be given by unconscious adults or by adults who are too ill or injured to consent verbally to emergency lifesaving treatment. In those cases, you assume that the patients would want care because of the severity of their condition.
- Determining the decision-making capacity of a patient can be tricky. Tools such as pulse oximetry and blood glucose measurements can provide factual documentation of patient awareness and ability to make clear decisions regarding his or her medical care. If you reasonably suspect that a patient has an issue that impedes his or her ability to give either informed consent or informed refusal, then take aggressive steps in the best interest of the patient. In any questionable circumstance, thorough documentation and consultation with medical control will provide the best protection against lawsuits.
- Minors pose challenges that local jurisdictions must address before a call occurs. In general, if the patient is a minor, then the minor has neither the right to consent to care nor the right to refuse it, although exceptions for emancipated minors exist.
- Violent patients may be restrained using physical or chemical means if they are a danger to themselves or others. Always follow local medical and law enforcement protocols when addressing the needs of violent or potentially violent patients.
- Negligence occurs only when the following four processes have occurred:
  - Duty to act. The paramedic must have had a legal duty to the patient.
  - Breach of duty. The paramedic did not fulfill that duty.
  - Proximate cause. The paramedic's breach of duty caused the plaintiff's injury.
  - Injury resulted. An injury occurred as a result of the above.
- Negligence can be categorized as acts of commission (malfeasance and misfeasance) or acts of omission (nonfeasance).
- As the highest level of prehospital emergency care provider, you must ensure you do not abandon your patients. Abandonment can occur anytime you turn over patient care inappropriately or to a person with level of training lesser than your own.
- Documentation is the only methodology to prevent the appearance of abandonment.
- Patients have the right to determine their own care. You must understand your legal limitations based on any advance directives issued by the patient.
- DNR orders are a specific form of advance directive that generally define the care a patient wants when lifesaving procedures are required. A DNR order is *not* a "do-not-care-for-the-patient" order.
- Patients often decide on medical care and treatment issues prior to an emergency. Be familiar with DNR orders, living wills, health care powers of attorney, surrogate decisions, and organ donation orders.
- Futile resuscitation efforts, which you may encounter, need to be addressed and considered prior to an emergency event. Weighing various ethical issues prior to their occurrence can help prevent and reduce suffering in your patient population.
- You may provide care when off duty and, in most jurisdictions, be protected under the Good Samaritan laws. Remember that you are only protected if you perform within your training and education and if you do not receive any compensation.
- You can be protected under certain governmental immunity clauses. These protections may be invalid if you have committed negligence or if you are deemed to be personally liable.
- Two common legal defenses are the statute of limitations (time in which to file a lawsuit) and contributory negligence, when a plaintiff has contributed to the negative outcome by committing an act or failing to disclose relevant information to medical practitioners.
- Several federal and state laws affect the relationship between you and your employer. These laws promote a healthier, safer workplace by addressing topics such as discrimination, sexual harassment, family leave, and occupational safety regulations.

Prep Kit *(continued)*

▶ Vital Vocabulary

abandonment Termination of medical care for the patient without giving the patient sufficient opportunity to find another suitable health care professional to take over his or her medical treatment.

advance directive A written document or oral statement that expresses the wants, needs, and desires of a patient in reference to future medical care; examples include living wills, do not resuscitate orders, and organ donation orders.

assault To create in another person a fear of immediate bodily harm or invasion of bodily security (including loss of freedom).

battery The unlawful physical acting upon a threat—the use of force against another, resulting in harmful, offensive, or sexual contact.

borrowed servant doctrine A principle which absolves an institution of liability when one of its members acts beyond his or her scope of certification or training by following someone else's orders.

civil lawsuit An action instituted by a person or entity against another person or entity.

common law A decision that has been made by a judge through a court case based on his or her interpretation of the statutes and constitutions; can be overturned either by another court with a higher authority or the issuing court at a later time; also called case law.

consent Agreement by the patient to accept a medical intervention.

contributory negligence Act(s) committed by plaintiff that contributes to adverse outcomes.

criminal prosecution An action instituted by the government against a person for violation of criminal law.

damages Compensation for injury awarded by a court.

decision-making capacity The patient's ability to understand and process the information given to him or her and the proposed treatment plan.

defamation Intentionally making a false statement, through written or verbal communication, which injures a person's good name or reputation.

defendant In a civil lawsuit, the person against whom a legal action is brought.

do not resuscitate (DNR) order A type of advance directive that describes which life-sustaining procedures should be performed in the event of a sudden deterioration in a patient's medical condition.

due process A right to a fair procedure for a legal action against a person or agency; has two components: Notice and Opportunity to be Heard.

duty Legal obligation of public and certain other ambulance services to respond to a call for help in their jurisdiction.

emancipated minor A person who is under the legal age (generally 18 years) in a given state, but is legally considered an adult because of other circumstances.

Emergency Medical Treatment and Active Labor Act (EMTALA) A federal law enacted in 1986 to combat the practice of patient dumping (hospitals refusing to admit seriously ill patients or women in labor who could not pay, forcing emergency medical services providers to dump the patients at another hospital). Issues are regulated by the Centers for Medicare and Medicaid Services and the law carries severe monetary penalties—up to and including loss of Medicare funding—for hospitals and physicians that fail to comply.

ethics A set of values in society that differentiates right from wrong.

expressed consent A type of informed consent that occurs when the patient does something, either through words (verbal or written) or by taking some sort of action, that demonstrates permission to provide emergency medical care.

false imprisonment Intentionally or unjustifiably detaining a person against his or her will. Some examples include transporting a patient without his or her consent, or using restraints in a wrongful manner.

Good Samaritan law A statute providing limited immunity from liability to people responding voluntarily and in good faith to the aid of an injured person outside the hospital.

gross negligence Negligence that is willful, wanton, intentional, or reckless; a serious departure from the accepted standards.

health care power of attorney A legal document that allows another person to make health care decisions for the patient, including withdrawal or withholding of care, when the patient is incapacitated.

Health Insurance Portability and Accountability Act (HIPAA) The law enacted in 1996 that provides for criminal sanctions as well as for civil penalties for releasing a patient's protected health information in a way not authorized by the patient.

hostile environment Situation in which an employer or an employer's agent either creates or allows to

Prep Kit (continued)

continue an offensive practice related to sex that makes it uncomfortable or impossible for an employee to continue working.

immunity Legal protection from penalties that could normally be incurred under the law.

implied consent Assumption on behalf of a person unable to give consent that he or she would have done so.

in loco parentis Phrase meaning "in the place of the parent" that is used to describe situations in which a designated authority figure makes medical treatment and transport decisions for a minor child when a parent or guardian is unavailable.

informed consent A patient's voluntary agreement to be treated after being told about the nature of the disease, the risks and benefits of the proposed treatment, alternative treatments, or the choice of no treatment at all.

involuntary consent An oxymoron, because consent is never involuntary; often used to describe a figure of authority dictating medical care be given to someone in custody, incapacitated, or a minor.

legal obligation A duty that is enforceable in a court of law.

liability A finding in civil cases that the majority of the evidence shows the defendant was responsible for the plaintiff's injuries.

libel Making a false statement in written form that injures a person's good name.

living will A type of advance directive, generally requiring a precondition for withholding resuscitation when the patient is incapacitated.

malfeasance Unauthorized act committed outside the scope of medical practice defined by law.

Medical Practice Act An act that usually defines the minimum qualifications of those who may perform various health services, defines the skills that each type of practitioner is legally permitted to use, and establishes a means of licensure or certification for different categories of health care professionals.

misfeasance Appropriate act performed in an improper manner, such as a medication administered at the wrong dose.

morality Pertaining to conscience, conduct, and character.

negligence Professional action or inaction on the part of the health care practitioner that does not meet the standard of ordinary care expected of similarly trained and prudent health care practitioners and that results in injury to the patient.

negligence per se Inexcusable violation of a statute, such as practicing paramedicine without a valid license or certification.

nonfeasance Failing to perform a required or expected act.

ordinary negligence Negligence that is a failure to act, or a simple mistake that causes harm to a patient.

palliative care A type of medical care intended to provide comfort and relief from pain.

patient autonomy The right to direct one's own medical care, and to decide how end-of-life medical care should be provided.

plaintiff In a civil lawsuit, the person who brings a legal action against another person.

proximate cause The specific reason that an injury occurred; one of the items that must be proven in order for a paramedic to be held liable for negligence.

punitive damages Compensation, usually monetary, awarded to a plaintiff for intentional or reckless acts committed by the defendant.

qualified immunity Protection in which the paramedic is only held liable when the plaintiff can show that the paramedic violated clearly established law of which he or she should have known.

quid pro quo Circumstance in which a person in authority attempts to exchange some work-related benefit, such as a raise or promotion, for an inappropriate employee action (eg, sexual favors); literal translation from Latin is "this for that."

res ipsa loquitur Theory of negligence that assumes an injury can only occur when a negligent act occurs.

scope of practice Describes what a state permits a paramedic practicing under a license or certification to do.

slander Making a false oral statement that injures a person's good name.

standard of care Describes what a reasonable paramedic with training would do in the same or a similar situation.

statutes of limitations Laws that limit the time period within which a lawsuit may be filed.

surrogate decision maker A person designated by a patient to make health care decisions as the patient would want when the patient becomes incapable of making decisions.

tort A wrongful act that gives rise to a civil lawsuit.

Prep Kit *(continued)*

▶ References

1. National Practitioner Data Bank. Statistics for National Practitioner Data Bank medical malpractice payment reports and adverse action reports. https://www.npdb.hrsa.gov/resources/npdbstats/npdbStatistics.jsp. Accessed January 10, 2017.
2. WMA declaration of Geneva. World Medical Association, Inc. website. http://www.wma.net/en/30publications/10policies/g1/. Accessed December 21, 2016.
3. Code of ethics and EMT oath. National Association of Emergency Medical Technicians website. https://www.naemt.org/about_us/emtoath.aspx. Accessed December 21, 2016.
4. Smith M. Do you care enough to ICARE? *EMS Mag.* 2008;37(7):26-27. http://www.icarevalues.org/EMS_Mag.pdf. Accessed December 20, 2016.
5. Maggiore WA. Problem of fraudulent EMT certification growing. *J Emerg Med Serv.* 2010;35(8). http://www.jems.com/articles/2010/07/problem-fraudulent-emt-certifi.html. Accessed January 12, 2017.
6. A matter of integrity. *J Emerg Med Serv.* 2010;35(9). http://www.jems.com/articles/print/volume-35/issue-9/patient-care/matter-integrity.html. Accessed January 12, 2017.
7. "Due regard." *Black's Law Dictionary.* 2nd ed. http://thelawdictionary.org/due-regard/. Accessed January 12, 2017.
8. Keeton WP, Dobbs D, Keeton RE, Owen DG. *Prosser and Keeton on Torts.* 5th ed. St. Paul, MN: West Group; 1984.
9. "Legal obligation." *Black's Law Dictionary.* 2nd ed. http://thelawdictionary.org/legal-obligation/. Accessed January 12, 2017.
10. "Willful misconduct." *Black's Law Dictionary.* 2nd ed. http://thelawdictionary.org/willful-misconduct/. Accessed January 12, 2017.
11. "Wanton misconduct." *Black's Law Dictionary.* 2nd ed. http://thelawdictionary.org/wanton-misconduct/. Accessed January 12, 2017.
12. "Proximate cause." *Black's Law Dictionary.* 2nd ed. http://thelawdictionary.org/proximate-cause/. Accessed February 9, 2017.
13. Millin MG, Khandker SR, Malki A. Termination of resuscitation of nontraumatic cardiopulmonary arrest: resource document for the National Association of EMS Physicians position statement. *Prehosp Emerg Care.* 2011;15(4):547-554. https://www.ncbi.nlm.nih.gov/pubmed/21843074. Accessed January 19, 2017.
14. Emergency volunteer toolkit: volunteer protection acts and Good Samaritan laws fact sheet. Association of State and Territorial Health Officials website. http://www.astho.org/Programs/Preparedness/Public-Health-Emergency-Law/Emergency-Volunteer-Toolkit/Volunteer-Protection-Acts-and-Good-Samaritan-Laws-Fact-Sheet/. Accessed January 12, 2017.
15. Sex-based discrimination. U.S. Equal Employment Opportunity Commission website. https://www.eeoc.gov/laws/types/sex.cfm. Accessed December 21, 2016.
16. What you should know about EEOC and the enforcement protections for LGBT workers. U.S. Equal Employment Opportunity Commission website. https://www.eeoc.gov/eeoc/newsroom/wysk/enforcement_protections_lgbt_workers.cfm. Accessed December 21, 2016.

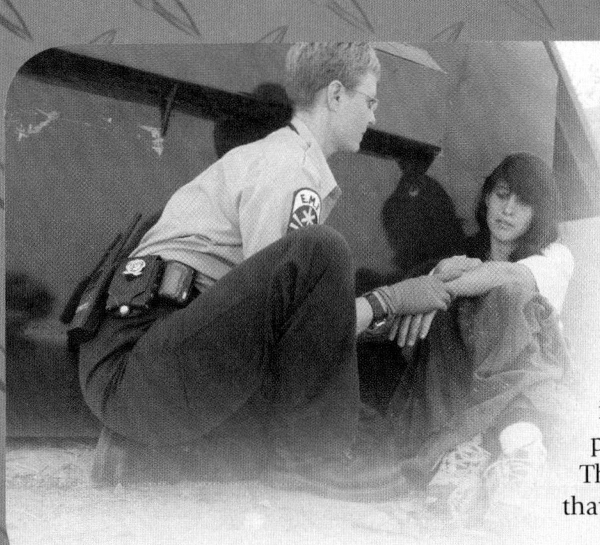

Assessment *in Action*

You are dispatched to 745 Reader Street for a possible suicide attempt. This home is a residential neighborhood and the dispatcher tells you that the patient is a man with a shotgun in the rear bedroom. A police officer is on the phone with the patient, who says he will kill anyone who tries to stop him. The police have set up a perimeter around the house and ask that you stand by at a nearby intersection.

Assessment *in Action* (continued)

You are staging at the intersection when the dispatcher notifies you that shots have been fired. Police are requesting that you come inside—the subject has shot himself and the scene is secure. As you reach the house, a police officer asks that only one paramedic enter the scene to determine whether anything can be done to save the patient.

You follow the police officer to the bedroom and are presented with a middle-aged man lying supine across the bed with his legs hanging off the end. The shotgun has fallen to the side and it is obvious that he had the barrel in his mouth when he pulled the trigger. The top of his head is missing and brain matter is visible on the wall and ceiling. He has no pulse and you determine that he has injuries that are incompatible with life.

1. How should you respond in situations when you are unsure whether to attempt resuscitation?

A. Contact medical control.
B. Wait for your partner to make a decision.
C. Start resuscitation if you are unsure.
D. Consult law enforcement personnel.

2. As you are leaving the scene, you are approached by a reporter who asks that you give him only the patient's age and sex and to tell him if he is still alive. He has been listening to a scanner and knows most of the story. To give him this information would be a(n) ____ violation.

A. ethical
B. HIPAA
C. civil
D. EMTALA

3. If you make the decision to treat this patient, then which type of consent would be used?

A. Implied consent
B. Informed consent
C. Consent as an emancipated minor
D. Expressed consent

4. You have determined that the patient has injuries that are incompatible with life. How should you proceed?

A. Cover him with a sheet.
B. Immediately leave the scene.
C. Preserve the crime scene.
D. Roll the patient to look for any other injuries.

5. Your best protection in court is thorough and accurate documentation. Which characteristic of an effective PCR describes your assessment for justifying your actions for this patient?

A. Date and times
B. History
C. Physical exam
D. Treatment

6. Four components are required to prove negligence. If you have not met the standard of care in treating this patient, then which requirement for proving negligence does this fulfill?

A. Duty
B. Breach of duty
C. Proximate cause
D. Harm

7. The family has decided to sue for lack of care because they feel the patient may have had a chance had he received prompt care. This sort of legal action is known as:

A. a civil lawsuit.
B. slander.
C. defamation.
D. a tort.

8. Prior to accepting a patient's consent or refusal of treatment, you must evaluate the patient's decision-making capacity. How is this step accomplished?

9. You are called to the scene of a violent patient with diabetes who is hypoglycemic. His wife tells you that she was able to check his blood glucose level just prior to calling and it was 34 mg/dL. He is refusing to allow anyone near him and will not eat anything. How will you proceed?

10. You are called to the scene of a middle-aged man reporting chest pain. The location of this call is approximately equidistant between two certified hospitals with catheterization labs. The wife asks you, "Which hospital would be the best option for my husband?" Because of your recent experience at Hospital A, during which you felt a patient with an acute myocardial infarction received improper treatment, you tell the wife, "Hospital A does not know what they are doing with cardiac patients. We should go to Hospital B." Which legal concept does this statement violate and why?

CHAPTER 5

Communications

National EMS Education Standard Competencies

Preparatory

Integrates comprehensive knowledge of the EMS system, safety/well-being of the paramedic, and medical/legal and ethical issues which is intended to improve the health of EMS personnel, patients, and the community.

EMS System Communication

Communication needed to

- Call for resources (p 138)
- Transfer care of the patient (pp 149-150)
- Interact within the team structure (pp 135, 146-150)
- EMS communication system (pp 138-144)
- Communication with other health care professionals (pp 146-150)
- Team communication and dynamics (pp 135-136, 150)

Therapeutic Communication

Principles of communicating with patients in a manner that achieves a positive relationship

- Interviewing techniques (pp 152-154)
- Adjusting communication strategies for age, stage of development, patients with special needs, and differing cultures (pp 155-160)
- Verbal defusing strategies (pp 152-153, 155)
- Family presence issues (pp 134, 135, 149-152)
- Dealing with difficult patients (p 155)
- Factors that affect communication (pp 134-135)

Medical Terminology

Integrates comprehensive anatomic and medical terminology and abbreviations into written and oral communication with colleagues and other health care professionals.

Knowledge Objectives

1. Discuss the importance of effective communication while providing emergency medical care. (p 134)
2. Describe the communication loop and how it is used to communicate effectively. (p 135)
3. List barriers to effective verbal communication. (p 135)
4. Explain the importance of emergency medical dispatch (EMD) and prearrival instructions in a typical emergency medical services (EMS) response. (pp 136-138)
5. Explain the role of the emergency medical dispatcher in a typical EMS response. (pp 136-138)
6. Describe the components, function, and use of the local dispatch communications system. (pp 137-138)
7. List the phases of EMD. (p 138)
8. Explain basic concepts of radio communications. (p 139)
9. List the components of communications systems. (pp 139-141)
10. Differentiate between the following types of communications technologies:
    - Simplex radio systems (p 140)
    - Duplex radio systems (p 140)
    - Multiplex radio systems (p 140)
    - Digital radio systems (p 140)
    - Repeaters (p 140)
    - Digital trunked radio systems (p 141)
    - Cellular technology (p 142)
    - Biotelemetry (pp 143-144)
    - Computer networks (pp 142-144)
11. Define interoperability, including its importance during large-scale events. (pp 141-142)
12. Recognize the protected legal status of patient health information. (pp 142, 145, 149)
13. Describe the functions and responsibilities of the Federal Communications Commission. (p 144)
14. Describe the phases of communication necessary to complete a typical EMS response. (pp 146-148)
15. Describe the format for reporting essential patient assessment information to medical control. (pp 148-149)

16. Describe the importance of effective verbal communication of patient information to the hospital. (pp 149-150)
17. List factors that may enhance verbal communication. (pp 150-152)
18. Identify internal and external factors that affect your patient/bystander interview. (pp 150-152)
19. Discuss the strategies for developing patient rapport. (pp 151-152)
20. Provide examples of open-ended and closed-ended questions. (p 152)
21. Discuss interviewing strategies to obtain useful information from a patient. (pp 152-154)
22. Discuss common errors to avoid when interviewing a patient. (p 154)
23. Identify the nonverbal skills that are used when interviewing a patient. (p 154)
24. Describe the strategies that are used when interviewing a patient who is hostile or potentially violent. (pp 154-155)
25. Summarize developmental considerations of various age groups that influence patient interviewing. (pp 155-156)
26. Discuss the techniques that are used when interviewing patients with special challenges. (pp 156-157)
27. Define cultural competence. (p 157)
28. Discuss interviewing considerations used in cross-cultural communications. (pp 157-158, 160)
29. Provide examples of traditional folk medicine, including why it is important to understand those practices. (pp 158-159)

Skills Objectives

There are no skills objectives for this chapter.

Introduction

This chapter will discuss communication, how to effectively communicate, and how to use communications technologies. The ability to communicate clearly is a core emergency medical services (EMS) skill, and is one of the most important factors in EMS operations. You must be able to communicate with the dispatch center to receive the information you need to respond to an emergency call. You will need to communicate with other members of the EMS system, including your partner, other responders, and hospital personnel. You must also be able to communicate effectively with patients, family members, and bystanders, often when they are under considerable stress.

Many factors can influence how effectively you are able to communicate, including your communication style, knowledge level, ability to listen and comprehend, ability to accurately convey information, and life experience. Communication can also be affected by your tone of voice (especially important on the radio or over a telephone), body language (important in face-to-face interactions), and your ability to use technology.

Documentation & Communication

Communicate (intransitive verb): To transmit information, thought, or feeling so that it is satisfactorily received or understood
Communication (noun): A process by which information is exchanged between individuals
Communications (noun): The technology of the transmission of information[1]

YOU are the Paramedic PART 1

An older man is not feeling well. His family becomes concerned and activates the EMS system by calling 9-1-1.

1. As a paramedic in the EMS system, how will you be notified about the location and nature of the incident?
2. What will the dispatcher be doing while you are en route to the call?
3. How will you communicate with the other responders and agencies involved in the emergency response?

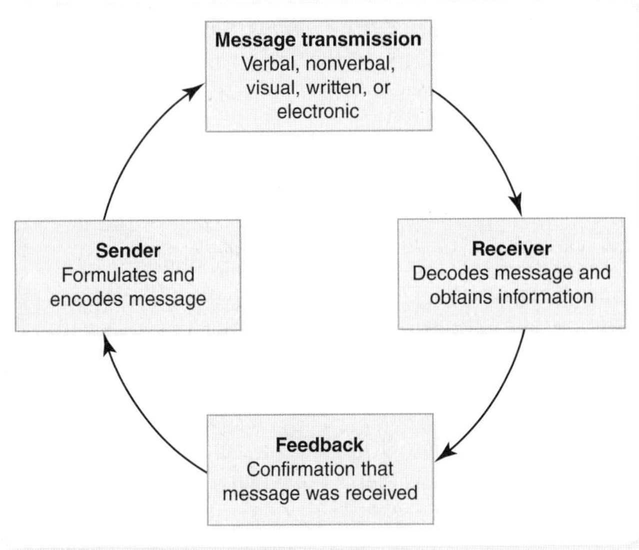

Figure 5-1 The communication loop.

▶ Communication Theory

Communication is both an interactive and a circular process or loop **Figure 5-1**. It begins with the sender, who formulates and encodes the message to be sent. *Encoding* involves determining the words or ideas to be sent and formatting the information for transmission. The message is then transmitted to the receiver. The receiver receives and decodes the message to get the information being relayed. Many methods of transmitting information are available, the most common of which are:

- Verbal
- Nonverbal (body language, facial expressions, etc)
- Written
- Visual (photographs, images, charts, electrocardiogram [ECG] tracings, etc)
- Electronic (voice, data, text, images, and video)

The final step in effective communication is feedback, which is the confirmation by the receiver that the message was accurately received. Feedback also permits clarification of the message if it was unclear. This step completes the communication loop. A simple example of the communication loop in action might be:

- **Dispatcher:** *Medic 1, Central Dispatch, traffic collision, respond Priority 1 to the intersection of West Main and Third Street.* (Information is encoded and transmitted.)
- **Paramedic:** *Central Dispatch, Medic 1 copies, responding Priority 1 to West Main and Third.* (Information is received, decoded, understood, and confirmed.)

> **Words of Wisdom**
>
> Think of it as an honor to be asked into a patient's home.

▶ Barriers to Effective Communication

You will encounter a wide range of potential barriers to communication in your interactions with patients, family members, and bystanders. These challenges can include language barriers, vision or hearing impairment, impaired cognition or confusion, psychiatric conditions, substance abuse, preexisting medical conditions, lack of ability to comprehend, stress, and preconceptions.

To minimize these barriers, it is important to adjust how you communicate. If you are working with a patient who speaks another language and have only a limited vocabulary in that language, then use a qualified interpreter whenever possible. This practice helps to minimize the risk of missing critical information or of using the wrong word, which could cause confusion or be insulting to the patient.

You may experience communication barriers when interacting with coworkers or other members of the EMS system, such as the use of different terminology or definitions by other agencies or jurisdictions, interoperability (technology compatibility) issues, and communications system failures. This chapter will address how to deal with each of these challenges.

Your attitude and demeanor can also affect communication. For example, the message that you send (either intentionally or unintentionally) when caring for a patient who is homeless may be different from the message you send to a well-dressed resident of an upscale neighborhood. Treat every patient you encounter professionally and to the best of your ability, regardless of his or her circumstances.

Response to the Call for Emergency Medical Services

▶ Phases of EMS Dispatch

All EMS calls originate when someone, generally a member of the public, recognizes that a potential medical emergency exists and reports it to the local emergency response system. In most parts of the United States, this step is accomplished by calling 9-1-1. This telephone call is automatically routed to a **public safety answering point (PSAP)**. A primary PSAP may either dispatch resources directly or route the call to a secondary PSAP, such as a specialized EMS dispatch center.

Patient Safety

During the 1980s, several catastrophic airline crashes led the airline industry to examine what went wrong. One of the biggest issues identified was a lack of communication between the pilots and other crew members. Copilots and others often recognized the developing problems, but were unwilling to speak up or question the pilot's judgment due to the prevailing cockpit culture, or were ignored when they reported a hazardous situation. This lack of communication led to bad decisions by the pilots in command, which resulted in crashes that cost many lives.

Crew resource management (CRM) is an operational practice developed by the US Air Force and the airline industry. CRM is designed to enhance teamwork and reduce preventable errors, and involves all members of the flight crew in decision making and flight safety. It encourages all fight crew members to pay attention, voice concerns, and participate in the decision-making process. They are expected to question any decisions they feel are unsafe or unwise. The essence of CRM is teamwork, based on effective communication. It utilizes all available resources to maximize safety. CRM principles have been adapted by the military and in many health care settings, including the air medical (helicopter and fixed-wing) industry.

Many of the characteristics of these high-stakes environments may also be found in EMS. The use of CRM in EMS involves teamwork and effective communication between all members of the response team. It keeps everyone on the same page and reduces the risk of errors that would stem from a lack of awareness of real or possible risks to the patient or responders.[2]

In practice, CRM begins with a pre-briefing while en route to the call. When responding to a traffic collision with a report of multiple patients, for example, pre-planning can involve designating who will be in charge, who will perform triage, and who will begin treatment. After EMS providers arrive on scene, CRM involves frequent check-ins and updates, reassessments of the situation, and fine-tuning of the plan as necessary. Crew members should cross-check each other when a high risk of errors exists; for example, double-checking medication doses when treating a pediatric patient. Every member of the team is responsible for maintaining a wide awareness and letting others know if a potential problem or risky situation is identified. Concerns voiced by any member of the team need to be taken seriously by the rest of the team.

CRM training and practice should be a part of EMS education. It is being incorporated into the National Registry of Emergency Medical Technicians Paramedic Psychomotor Competency Portfolio.[3]

Calls to 9-1-1 for emergency medical assistance are answered in most EMS systems by a program called **emergency medical dispatch (EMD)**. This program is specifically designed to meet the unique needs of EMS response and of callers reporting a medical emergency. The term **dispatch** means to send to a specific destination or to send on a task; however, the emergency medical dispatcher does much more than simply send ambulances to emergencies. The dispatcher functions as a vital part of the EMS team. The dispatcher obtains as much information as possible about the emergency, determines which resources are needed, and dispatches the appropriate vehicles and personnel to the scene. In some systems, the EMD process also includes emergency medical care instructions to the 9-1-1 caller. The dispatcher monitors and coordinates communication with responders in the field during all phases of the response, locates and sends additional resources as needed, and maintains written and electronic records of the call.[4]

Emergency dispatch of EMS calls is a component of the overall public safety system. An EMS response will almost always include an ambulance, but may also include fire service, rescue, or law enforcement units. As a paramedic, it is important for you to understand how the ambulance and overall dispatch systems in your area operate.

Information Gathering

When someone calls for an ambulance, he or she is often in distress. This emotional state can interfere with his or her ability to convey information. The most effective method of gathering information from a caller who is under stress is to use a series of short questions. When a 9-1-1 call comes in, the dispatcher will try to elicit the following information:

- **The exact location of the patient or patients.** This information includes the street name and number, the proper geographic designation (such as whether the street is East Maple or West Maple), and the name of the community (because adjacent towns may have streets with the same name). If the call comes from a rural area, then the dispatcher will try to establish landmarks (such as the nearest cross street or business establishment, water tower, or antenna).
- **The telephone number of the caller.** This information is important if the call is disconnected or the dispatcher needs to call back for more information. It is common for responders to be unable to find the address and to need to ask for help from the original

caller. Asking for the caller's telephone number also helps discourage nuisance calls, because prank callers are reluctant to supply their phone numbers.
  - Many areas have **enhanced 9-1-1 systems** in which much of this information, such as the phone number and address of the caller, is determined and displayed automatically by the computer dispatch terminal.
  - In areas with enhanced wireless (cellular) 9-1-1 systems, dispatchers are able to see the number of the wireless (mobile) phone from which the call was placed, and in many cases, the latitude and longitude of the caller's location from the global positioning system (GPS) receiver of the phone. This technology can be especially useful for wireless calls from remote locations.
- **Why EMS was called.** This information is the caller's perception of the nature of the emergency.
- **Information about the patient's condition.** More specific information will help the dispatcher evaluate the urgency of the situation and decide whether he or she needs to provide the caller with prearrival instructions by phone. The dispatcher should ask:
  - Is the patient conscious?
  - If not, then is the patient breathing?
  - Is the patient bleeding badly?
- **Details about the location.** Additional information that will help responders access the scene as quickly and safely as possible, such as whether the residence door is locked or whether any pets are present.
- **Information about the situation.** This information will enable the dispatcher to estimate the magnitude of the emergency, and identify which resources will be required. For example, if the emergency is a motor vehicle crash, then the dispatcher should ask about:
  - The types of vehicles involved (sedans, trucks, motorcycles, buses, etc).
  - If a commercial truck is involved, then does the caller have any indication of what sort of cargo it is carrying? A truck carrying hazardous materials (hazmat) requires a different approach from one carrying bananas.
  - The number of people injured and an estimate of the extent of injuries.
  - Apparent hazards at the scene, such as heavy traffic, downed power lines, fire, spilled chemicals, and peculiar odors. Information about such hazards enables the dispatcher to contact other agencies that may need to be involved, such as utility workers to manage downed wires or hazmat teams to deal with spilled fuel or chemicals.

Dispatch

As soon as the dispatcher has obtained the address of the emergency, the telephone number of the caller, and the nature of the emergency, he or she will ask the caller to wait on the line. Based on the nature and location of the call and the resources that are available, the dispatcher determines which resources need to be dispatched. The dispatcher then notifies these resources and informs them about the nature of the call and its exact location. Dispatch may be performed using a radio, telephone, push-to-talk (PTT) cellular device, pager, or computer terminal.

After the ambulance is dispatched, the dispatcher will return to the caller to obtain the rest of the information described earlier. Further questioning may reveal special circumstances that might affect the response. The dispatcher will relay this information while the responding unit is en route. This process permits the EMS crew to determine whether to respond using the lights and siren (based on local protocols), and to anticipate and prepare for any tasks that may need to be performed at the scene.

Computer Assisted Dispatch

Most EMS systems utilize **computer assisted dispatch (CAD)** systems, which make use of linked dispatch center computer consoles and vehicle-mounted mobile data terminals (MDT). The CAD system enables the dispatcher to view all information about the call, including information received from the caller, times of events, and visual prompts that list the key questions to ask the caller. The CAD system may also display additional information provided by the enhanced 9-1-1 system, such as maps, the fastest route to the location of the call, prior calls to the same address, and known hazards at the call location (such as toxic chemicals stored at a business, potentially dangerous pets, etc). The CAD system may make recommendations about which EMS units to dispatch based on location and response times. Using the CAD system, the dispatcher is able to send all of this information to the responding EMS crew via the MDT, permitting the crew to see what is displayed on the CAD terminal.

Advice to the Caller

After directing the necessary resources (ambulance, fire, rescue, law enforcement, etc) to the scene and alerting responders to any special circumstances, the dispatcher will return to the telephone and inform the caller what is being done (eg, "An ambulance is on the way and should be there in about 5 minutes.") If the dispatcher suspects the patient has a life-threatening emergency, then he or she may be able to provide prearrival medical instructions to the caller through the EMD program. These instructions can include a range of emergency medical care techniques, such as airway maintenance,

Table 5-1 Phases of Emergency Medical Dispatch

Phases of Dispatch/ Information Gathered	Dispatcher Action
▪ Initial receipt of 9-1-1 call	▪ Answers telephone promptly ▪ Identifies agency
▪ Information gathering • Address/location of incident • Call-back number • Perceived emergency • Patient's name and condition • For traffic incidents: ♦ Number of vehicles ♦ Types of vehicles ♦ Number of patients • Hazards at the scene	▪ Obtains as much information as possible about the emergency
▪ Dispatch	▪ Dispatches ambulances and other resources (fire, law enforcement, etc) as needed ▪ Notifies responding units of special situations ▪ Contacts hazmat teams and other agencies as needed ▪ Monitors communications from the field
▪ Advice to the caller	▪ Informs the caller what is being done ▪ Gives patient care instructions by phone, if required
▪ Ongoing communications with responding units in the field	▪ Logs response and arrival times ▪ Coordinates requests for additional resources ▪ Facilitates communications with other agencies or medical facilities ▪ Remains aware of the location and status of all units in the field

Data from: Association of Public-Safety Communications Officials. Minimum training standards for public safety telecommunicators. APCO ANS 3.103.2.2015. https://www.apcointl.org/doc/911-resources/apco-standards/75-minimum-training-standards-for-public-safety-telecommunicators/file.html. Accessed December 6, 2016.

the Heimlich maneuver, hands-only cardiopulmonary resuscitation, or hemorrhage control. The caller is likely to be in an agitated state, so the dispatcher's instructions must be clear and simple.

Ongoing Communications With Responding Units in the Field

It is important for the dispatcher to remain aware of what is occurring in the field and to stay in contact with the ambulance and other responders. As mentioned previously, the dispatcher is your resource for contacting other agencies, such as fire, rescue, and law enforcement, whose presence may be required at the scene. The dispatcher can also request any specialized resources that may needed, such as heavy extrication or air medical transport. The dispatcher can coordinate communications between the ambulance and medical control (discussed later in this chapter), or provide assistance in determining the appropriate destination facility. The phases of the emergency medical dispatch process and the roles of the dispatcher are summarized in Table 5-1. It is routine practice to use 24-hour (standard military) time in EMS dispatch and documentation (24-hour time is discussed in Chapter 6, *Documentation*).

EMS Communications Systems

During an emergency response, you will use a variety of communications equipment. Some EMS systems utilize basic two-way radio systems, whereas others use sophisticated, computerized radio systems. The use of cellular technology is becoming increasingly common. All of these communications systems and devices use radio signals to send and receive information, and it is important for you to understand basic radio communications theory and how radio equipment operates.

EMS and public safety communications systems are generally dependable, but anything based on technology can (and at some point will) fail. Having backup communications systems is essential. Backup systems may include independent radio frequencies and systems, cell phones, satellite telephones, or MDTs. Backup systems are discussed in more detail later in this chapter.

▶ Basic Radio Communications Theory

Radio Waves

Radio waves are a type of electromagnetic radiation that may be encoded to carry a wide variety of information. The basic radio wave onto which a signal is encoded is called a carrier wave.[5,6]

Radio Frequencies

The radio **frequency** is the number of oscillations (or cycles) per second of the carrier wave, typically measured in **hertz (Hz)**. One hertz equals one cycle per second, one megahertz (MHz) equals one million cycles per second, and one gigahertz (GHz) equals 1,000 MHz, or 1 billion cycles per second. A radio wave with a frequency of 156.075 MHz is oscillating 156,075,000 times per second.[5,6]

Frequencies are grouped into bands by the **Federal Communications Commission (FCC)**. Each band is assigned by the FCC for a specific purpose. EMS and public safety communications systems typically operate in the **very high frequency (VHF) band**, from 30 MHz to 300 MHz, and in the **ultra high frequency (UHF) band**, from 300 MHz to 3.0 GHz. The higher frequency bands generally have less interference, but also have a shorter transmission range.[5,6]

FCC Narrow-Band Standards

The number of agencies using radio systems has expanded over the years, and new technologies have been developed. The FCC recognized that a need existed to allocate more frequencies for public safety and EMS use. Under previous standards, individual frequency assignments were spaced 25 KHz (0.025 MHz) apart. Effective January 1, 2013, frequencies in the public safety radio spectrum between 150 to 174 MHz and 421 to 470 MHz were reassigned with a spacing of 12.5 KHz, referred to as **narrow-band** technology. Radios that use the older 25 kHz technology may no longer be used. The narrow-band system has effectively doubled the number of frequencies available for public safety and EMS use. It also supports newer, more sophisticated digital radio systems.[7] Narrow-band radio standards are discussed further in the *Interoperability* section of this chapter.

Radio Signals

Radio communications require two types of devices. The transmitter takes data or sound, converts it into a radio signal, and transmits it on the designated frequency. The receiver collects the radio signal and translates it back into data or sound. Most radios used in EMS communications contain both a transmitter and a receiver, and are referred to as **transceivers** (two-way radios).[5,6]

A limiting factor affecting all radio signals is range. The range of a transmitter depends on its output power, the frequency being used, the location and size of its antenna, and whether or not an uninterrupted "line of sight" (path) to the receiver exists. The farther the receiver is from the antenna of the transmitter, the weaker the signal becomes. Anything that interrupts the radio signal, such as buildings, mountains, or other large objects, can reduce the effective range of the radio.[5,6]

A constant level of static or background **noise** is present on all radio frequencies. To prevent having to listen to static when a radio signal is not being transmitted, radio receivers are equipped with a filtering system known as **squelch**. The squelch setting can be adjusted to block out the background noise, but still allow radio signals to be heard.[5,6]

▶ Communications Systems Components

Base Stations

Base station radios are the most powerful radios in the communications system, with a transmitter output power of up to 275 watts. They have a fixed location, such as a dispatch center or hospital. Base stations have large antennas, which are usually placed on top of buildings or tall masts, giving them a longer range than mobile or portable radios. They are often capable of operating on multiple frequencies and bands. Some hospitals and dispatch centers have access to multiple radio systems.

YOU are the Paramedic — PART 2

Your unit arrives at the residence. An older woman meets your crew at the door. She tells you that her husband has cancer and that he is not feeling well. After ensuring that the scene is safe, you enter the residence. You see a frail-looking older man sitting in a recliner. The room is immaculately clean. A television is playing loudly in the corner of the room. The wife tells you her husband does not hear well.

4. How will you initiate communication with this patient?
5. Is the television noise a consideration in your assessment?

Mobile Transceivers

Mobile transceivers are mounted in vehicles and aircraft, and operate by using the power system of the vehicle. They use an antenna that is externally mounted on the vehicle. The transmitter output power can vary from 5 to 50 watts, and they can have a line-of-sight range of up to 15 miles (24 km).

Portable Transceivers

Portable transceivers are small, battery-powered units (sometimes called "handhelds" or "walkie-talkies"). The transmitter output power is low, typically between 1 and 5 watts, and small, radio-mounted antennas typically limit the range to 3 to 5 miles (5 to 8 km). Most portable radios operate on one band and have either single- or multiple-channel capabilities. Portable, handheld radios are useful when you must work at a distance from your vehicle but need to stay in communication with the dispatch center, medical control, or with other EMS providers **Figure 5-2**.

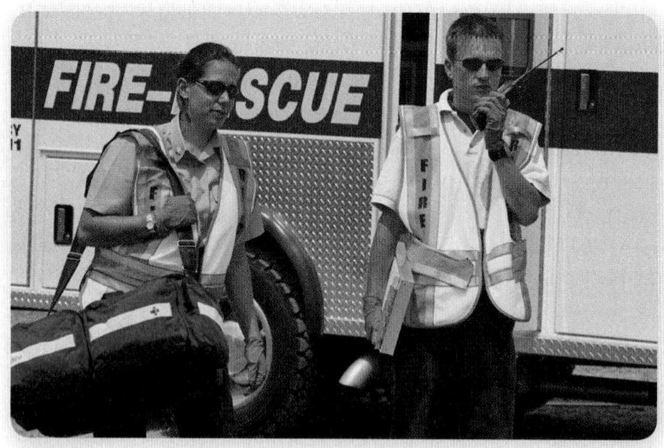

Figure 5-2 A portable radio is essential if you need to communicate with the dispatcher, other units on scene or responding to the scene, or medical control when you are away from the ambulance.

Radio Systems

Simplex is the most basic type of radio system, with all radio transmissions occurring on the same frequency. Simplex radios allow multiple users to communicate with each other using one common frequency. Simplex systems are normally restricted to line of sight. In public safety and EMS communications, simplex radios are usually used only for short-range communications, such as for tactical use at an incident scene.

Duplex radio systems utilize a pair of frequencies. Radio signals are transmitted on one frequency and received on a second frequency. Semi-duplex systems allow communication in only one direction at a time and the use of repeaters (discussed next), whereas full-duplex systems allow continuous communication in both directions at the same time (similar to a telephone).

Multiplex radio systems utilize radio signals to carry multiple streams of audio and/or data at the same time. Commercial frequency modulation (FM) radio uses a multiplex signal to carry stereo sound. The most common use of multiplex technology in EMS communications systems is to transmit both voice and ECG tracings (biotelemetry). This topic is discussed later in this chapter.

Digital radio systems allow the transmission of digital signals (computer, etc) or analog (voice) signals that have been digitized and compressed by a computer. Digital signals are clearer than analog signals and allow the transmission of a greater volume of data in the same bandwidth. Digital radios can communicate with other digital radios and with analog radios.[6]

Repeaters

Repeaters are used in most semi-duplex radio systems. A **repeater** is a specialized base station transceiver with a powerful transmitter and a large antenna, typically located on a high spot such as a tower, mountaintop, or tall building **Figure 5-3**. It receives the radio signal on the transmit (input) frequency and rebroadcasts it at a higher power level on the receive (output) frequency. The

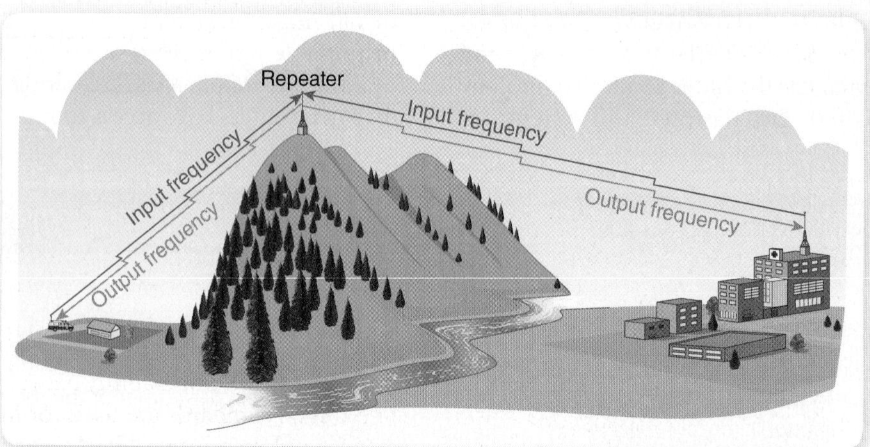

Figure 5-3 Repeaters utilize paired radio frequencies to bypass obstacles such as hills, and extend the range of portable transceivers.

use of repeaters allows the radio system to cover a much larger geographic area and to bypass obstructions such as hills, canyons, or buildings. It also permits lower powered transceivers, such as portable units, to communicate over greater distances. Vehicles may also have repeaters to retransmit signals from a portable unit using the vehicle radio. Most radio systems have multiple repeaters placed in different locations throughout the service area.[6]

Encoded radio signals allow multiple users to share frequencies and repeaters. The most common type of encoding used in public safety and EMS radio systems is the Continuous Tone-Coded Squelch System (CTCSS), also known as the "PL" (short for private line) system. The CTCSS transmits a continuous, inaudible tone along with the regular radio signal. Receivers that have a CTCSS decoder set to that tone will be able to receive the transmission, whereas receivers without it will not. Encoding allows the use of multiple repeaters on the same frequencies. The CTCSS encoding specifies which repeater will "open" to receive and retransmit the signal.

Another encoding system used in some regions is the Dual-Tone Multi-Frequency (DTMF) system. DTMF tones are encoded using a keypad on the transmitter. These tones then "dial-in" and activate the designated remote receiver, permitting it to receive the transmission. Systems using UHF-band MED channels frequently make use of this type of encoding.[8]

Digital Trunked Radio Systems

Trunked radio systems are sophisticated digital communications networks, usually operating in the 800 and 900 MHz UHF bands. They utilize multiple repeaters and computers to route radio traffic within the system. Trunked radio systems can carry voice or data, such as CAD system information. In a trunked system, the transceiver is set to a channel or mode, rather than to a specific frequency. Each mode is designated for a particular purpose, such as dispatch, tactical operations, or hospital communications. The frequencies of the network are "pooled" by the computer and when a transceiver in the system needs to transmit on a selected mode, the network assigns that transmission to the next available frequency. When the transmission is completed, the frequency goes back into the pool.[6]

Radio Dead Spots

Radio dead spots are areas where mobile or portable radios are unable to communicate with a repeater or each other. These radio dead spots may be caused by distance, such as in rural areas, or by obstructions such as mountains, buildings, or other tall objects. It is important that you learn the locations of radio dead spots in your service area.

There are many ways to establish or maintain communications in radio dead spots. One method is to use alternative communications systems, such as cell or **landline** (wired) phones. In rural areas, additional repeaters can be installed, or agreements can be established with federal or state agencies to use their radio systems as backup. Use of another agency's radio frequencies and/or repeaters should only occur with prior permission, or in the event of an emergency during which no other option exists.

In urban settings, radio dead spots often occur in areas with tall buildings, inside large buildings, and in underground locations such as subways or basements. In locations where radio communications are used frequently, small local repeaters can be installed in building lobbies or subway stations. If a local repeater is unavailable, then a temporary relay station may be created by positioning an emergency responder with a portable radio at the top of the subway stairs or near a building exit, where he or she can establish direct communications with both responders on the inside and with the incident commander or a local repeater on the outside.

▶ Interoperability

During your career as a paramedic, you will likely be involved in one or more large-scale events, such as natural disasters or mass-casualty incidents (MCIs). Such incidents may overwhelm available resources and may require help from outside agencies. This assistance is typically referred to as **mutual aid**. Local agencies enter into mutual aid agreements with neighboring or regional jurisdictions to back up each other in the event of a large-scale incident.

Mutual aid requests can range from requesting additional ambulances from nearby communities to a large-scale disaster that necessitates a state or national-level response. These events will require members of multiple agencies to work together under high-stress and high-stakes conditions. To achieve cooperation, each agency's communications system must be compatible with that of the other agency. This principle is referred to as **interoperability**.

The current drive for interoperability stems from a number of large-scale incidents in which mutual aid responders with incompatible radio systems were unable to communicate with local agencies or with one another. To address this situation, the US Department of Homeland Security developed the SAFECOM communications program. These national interoperability standards were released in 2006 and are intended to develop "a system of interoperable public safety communications across all local, tribal, state, and federal 'first responder' communications systems."[9]

An important part of these interoperability standards is the use of nationally standardized frequencies for disasters and other communications. These frequencies have been established as a part of the FCC's narrow-band system. Each state has also established its own internal standards for interoperability between local jurisdictions. These state standards are used for MCIs and other local mutual aid responses, whereas national standards are used for interstate and national events. State standards often also include designated statewide frequencies for specific purposes, such as air-to-ground communications.

The Association of Public-Safety Communications Officials has established digital radio hardware standards, known as the Project 25 (P25) standards. These standards ensure the digital radio equipment supplied by different manufacturers to the public safety communications community are compatible with one another.[10] Radios that are P25 compliant meet these national standards for hardware design, narrow-band compliance, and interoperability. They are capable of communicating with both analog (legacy) radio systems and newer digital radio systems. This characteristic is referred to as "backwards compatibility."

▶ Cellular Technology

Cell phones have been used in EMS communications for many years. As the technology of smartphones and tablet computers has advanced, the use of cellular technology has become a more important component of EMS and public safety communications systems **Figure 5-4**. A cell phone is a low-power, portable radio that communicates through a series of interconnected repeaters called cells. These cells are linked by a sophisticated computer system and connected to the telephone network.

Cell phones should be programmed with important and commonly used telephone numbers such as medical control, local hospital emergency departments (EDs), and dispatch centers. Cell phones can provide direct access to hospitals, poison control centers, and other services that may not have direct radio communications capabilities. Telephone calls may be patched into radio networks through dispatch centers or base stations, enabling direct communication between a paramedic using a radio in the field and another party using a telephone, such as a medical control physician.

Smartphones have brought previously unheard-of capabilities to the EMS provider. Smartphones allow users to communicate wirelessly using voice, text, and video, and to take and send photographs or videos to other devices.

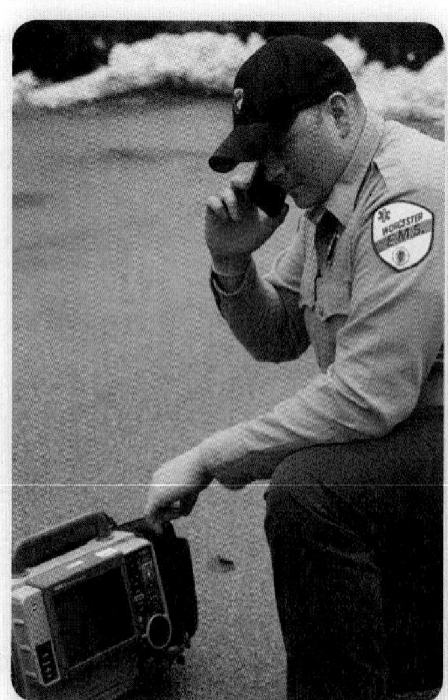

Figure 5-4 Cell phones are a common adjunct to the communications infrastructure of many EMS systems.

They frequently have built-in GPS receivers with mapping software and are able to access a huge range of medical applications (software), including local EMS protocols, pharmaceutical references, and medical reference books. Other types of cellular devices that may be used in EMS and public safety communications systems include PTT devices and tablet computers that may be used for patient care reports and billing.

As a paramedic, it is important that you be aware of the privacy implications of taking photographs or videos using smartphones or tablets. Although the ability to document the appearance of a wrecked vehicle to show to the receiving trauma surgeon may seem harmless, you need to protect the patient's right to privacy as outlined in the Health Information Portability and Accountability Act (HIPAA). Use of these types of images must be done only in a secure fashion, following local EMS guidelines or protocols. Some EMS systems use mobile applications that capture the image and send it directly to secure medical charting software, so that the image is not stored on the individual phone or tablet. It is always inappropriate to post images, video, or other individually identifiable patient information on social media. Paramedics and other health care providers have lost their jobs and faced other significant penalties for doing so.[11]

Another evolving use of cellular technology that is important for EMS is **automatic crash notification (ACN)**, also known as advanced automatic crash notification. ACN systems utilize specialized onboard computers in motor vehicles to send data to a monitoring station in the event of a crash. That information can include the following:

- Geographic location of the crash
- Vehicle type
- Severity of the crash
- Principle direction of force at the point of impact
- Whether seat belts were in use
- Whether airbags were deployed

ACN may also allow direct two-way voice communication with the occupants of the vehicle. This data has been shown to provide an accurate prediction of the severity of potential injuries to the occupants of the vehicle, and can help to determine transport decisions (such as whether a patient should be transported to a trauma center, or whether a helicopter should be dispatched to a remote motor vehicle crash scene).[12]

▶ Satellite Communications

Satellite telephones can be valuable in rural and remote areas with unreliable or absent radio and cell phone coverage. They are also an invaluable resource in disaster situations. This technology is expensive, which can limit its use when other alternatives exist.

The global positioning system (GPS) is a satellite network that utilizes handheld or vehicle-mounted receivers to locate the user's position and provide directions to other locations, such as an emergency scene. GPS data may be used to track the location of ambulances, other emergency vehicles, and aircraft. **Geographic information system (GIS)** technology utilizes computerized GPS mapping systems to perform the following functions:

- Track and predict ambulance response times
- Determine the distance to the closest trauma center or other hospitals from specific locations
- Track the frequency of motor vehicle crashes and the severity of injuries from different geographic locations
- Determine the location of emergency helipads
- Provide other information useful in EMS system operations and planning.

GIS data can be used to improve ambulance response and transport times by having resources located where and when they are most likely to be needed, and to guide what resources may need to be sent to a given location, based on past responses.

Satellite distress beacons and messengers can be a worthwhile safety technology for ambulances and emergency medical personnel who operate in rural or remote locations, or during search and rescue or disaster operations. Most beacons and messengers have built-in GPS receivers that will transmit the location of the beacon to the satellite. All such beacons are capable of sending emergency distress messages, and some are also able to send tracking data and text messages via the satellite system.

▶ Backup Communications Systems

Any system that relies on technology has the potential to fail. The higher the consequences of such a failure, the more important it is to have an effective backup system. As mentioned previously, all EMS and public safety communications systems need to have some type of backup plan. The most commonly used backup system is an alternate radio system, typically one that relies on basic technology such as VHF or UHF simplex and duplex radios and redundant repeaters, and which can be easily accessed by base, portable, and mobile radios. Almost every EMS system uses landline and cell phone networks as a backup to other communications technologies. Backup systems should also include generators at dispatch centers and hospitals to maintain radio communications in the event of power outages. Backup systems may be shared between several local agencies (EMS, fire, law enforcement, etc).

In disaster situations, the primary methods of communication may be out of service. Towers and repeaters may be damaged, cell sites may be disabled, and computer networks may be down. In these circumstances, having redundant or backup systems is essential. Local and regional disaster plans often make use of amateur radio groups such as the Amateur Radio Emergency Service (ARES) and the Radio Amateur Civil Emergency Service (RACES) as additional backup systems.[13] It is important that you understand how to access and use ARES, RACES, and/or all of the backup communications systems utilized in your service area.

▶ Biotelemetry

Biotelemetry is the measurement and transmission of vital signs and other physiologic data to a **remote terminal**. Biotelemetry, often referred to simply as telemetry, is used to monitor the health of astronauts in space and NASCAR drivers during a race.[14,15] In EMS, it is mostly used to send ECG data to the medical control physician or a hospital ED. ECG telemetry originated in Miami, Florida during the early 1970s, and had an important role in establishing the paramedic profession. Telemetry made it possible for physicians to supervise paramedics caring for patients in the field. It was the technical feasibility of such supervision that convinced the medical community and the public to accept the idea of paramedics performing advanced procedures such as defibrillation. As EMS systems have matured and paramedics have become more and more skilled, the use of ECG telemetry to confirm cardiac rhythms before treatment has become much less common. Most EMS systems now rely on the paramedic to assess the patient's cardiac rhythm and make independent treatment decisions.

In recent years, advances in medicine and communications technology have again made ECG telemetry a valuable EMS tool. The current national standard of care for patients with an acute ST-segment elevation myocardial infarction (STEMI) is percutaneous coronary intervention (PCI), also known as cardiac catheterization. Rapid transport of patients directly to the closest primary PCI hospital/STEMI receiving center and short "door-to-balloon" times have been shown to result in much better patient outcomes.[16] Many EMS systems now have policies in place to bypass non-PCI hospitals and transport patients directly to a primary PCI center, if such a facility is readily available.[17] (See Chapter 17, *Cardiovascular Emergencies*, for more information on care of patients with STEMI.)

Cell phone networks, broadband networks, and digital radio systems have the capability to directly transmit 12-lead ECG tracings and other data from the field to the hospital.[16] New, secure systems can send the ECG tracing to anyone with access to an Internet connection. This practice permits the medical control physician to diagnose STEMI before the patient reaches the hospital, and to make appropriate destination and treatment decisions, such as to transport directly to the cardiac catheterization lab. In some EMS systems, paramedics are responsible for interpreting the ECG tracing and making the destination decision.

Another exciting area of advancement in EMS and other areas of health care is **telemedicine**. Telemedicine technology uses specialized computer terminals and networks that permit secure two-way transmission of sound, video, vital signs, ECG tracings, and other diagnostic data. This technology allows the interactive exchange of information between the paramedic and the medical control physician.[18] Telemedicine technology can facilitate rapid assessment and treatment of a wide range of conditions and patients in the prehospital setting, including patients with stroke and STEMI, as well as pediatric and trauma patients.

New technology is constantly being introduced, and what was once new and cutting edge quickly becomes the standard. Ambulances are now being outfitted with internal wireless networks that can communicate with onboard devices and multiple outside computer networks using broadband, cellular, wireless (Wi-Fi), and other communications networks.[19] It is crucial to familiarize yourself with the telemetry, telemedicine, and other communications technologies used in your area. EMS systems must keep up with advances in technology that can improve the communication of information and the quality of emergency medical care.

Communicating by Radio

The effectiveness of an EMS communications system depends on both the hardware/software in use and the people who use it. Communicating by radio under emergency conditions requires a knowledge of the process of communication and an understanding of the technical operations of radios and other devices described earlier, as well as an appreciation of the conventions and etiquette of radio communications. Keep your communications simple, brief, and direct.

FCC Regulations

All radio and television communications in the United States are regulated by the FCC.[20] The FCC issues radio station licenses, allocates frequencies, develops technical standards, and establishes and enforces rules and regulations for the operation of radio equipment. FCC officials monitor transmissions on various frequencies and conduct spot checks of base stations to ensure they are properly licensed. Fines and other penalties can be imposed on agencies and individual providers for failing to follow the rules and regulations of the FCC.

The FCC requires that frequencies allocated for public safety and EMS communications be used only for that purpose. The transmission of messages unrelated to the provision of EMS and the use of obscene language are forbidden. If it is necessary for a dispatcher to communicate a personal message to you, then he or she should call your personal cell phone, or notify you by radio to contact the base or dispatch center by phone. If you have a personal request of the dispatcher, then you should use a telephone.

Clarity of Transmission

Below are some basic guidelines that can help you improve the clarity of your radio communications:

- Know what you want to say before beginning your transmission.
  - Make notes (or use the run sheet).
  - Anticipate what questions you may be asked.

YOU are the Paramedic — PART 3

You bend down to the patient's eye level and introduce yourself and your partner. The patient looks at you and smiles. You ask the patient for his name. The patient continues to smile and looks to his wife. The wife states her husband's name is John Smith. She leans over to her husband's left ear and yells, "They wanted to know your name, John!" Mr. Smith nods in acknowledgment. You continue with your assessment and ask, "May we call you John?" Mrs. Smith answers the question for her husband, "Yes, he goes by John."

Recording Time: 2 Minutes	
Appearance	Frail
Level of consciousness	Responds to voice
Airway	Open
Breathing	Adequate
Circulation	Adequate

6. What does it mean to "get on the same level as the patient"? What is the importance of this action?
7. How can you address the problem of a family member answering questions for the patient?

- Before you begin to transmit, make sure the radio is turned on. Check the volume setting and listen to make sure the channel is clear.
  - If another transmission is in progress, then wait until both parties have finished transmitting before you transmit.
- Keep your mouth close to the microphone, but not too close. About 2 to 3 inches (5 to 7 cm) is usually ideal.
- After the channel is clear, press the PTT key on the microphone or the side of the handheld radio for at least 1 second before you start speaking, which ensures the beginning of your message is not cut off.
- Start your transmission with the identifier (number or name) of the unit being called, then your own identifier (*"Mercy Hospital, this is Medic 3."*).
  - This practice ensures the unit being called is alerted and will be listening when you give your own identification, thereby avoiding unnecessary delays.
  - If you initially say, *"Medic 3 calling Mercy Hospital,"* the recipients may not pay attention until you have mentioned their identifier and will miss who is calling. They would then respond, *"This is Mercy Hospital, what unit is calling?"*
  - This practice is a general radio convention. Some EMS systems may use a different format. Learn and use the accepted radio format for your area.
- Wait for a response to ensure the other station is listening.
- Speak slowly, clearly, and distinctly, pronouncing each word carefully.
- Do not shout, speaking at too high a volume distorts the signal. Speak in a normal pitch.
- Remain calm and speak in a normal and conversational tone. Keep your voice free of emotion.
- Use clear text (plain language), and only use radio codes that are specifically approved by your system and that everyone will understand. When in doubt, avoid using radio codes in your transmissions. Clear text communications and codes are discussed in more detail later.
- If you have a lot of information to convey, then break your transmission into short (30-second) chunks.
  - Pause periodically for questions, etc.
  - Say "break" to signify a pause.
- When speaking a word or name that might be misunderstood, spell it using the International Radiotelephony Phonetic Alphabet Table 5-2 or a similar system.
- When speaking numbers that might be misunderstood, first transmit the number as a whole, then digit by digit. For example, if the patient's respirations are 16 breaths per minute, then you would say, "Respirations are sixteen, that is, one-six."
- Confirm receipt of all replies.
  - Repeat information back to ensure accuracy ("parroting").
- Indicate when your transmission is completed.

Table 5-2 International Radiotelephony Phonetic Alphabet

A	Alfa (or Alpha)	**J**	Juliett (or Juliet)	**S**	Sierra
				T	Tango
B	Bravo	**K**	Kilo	**U**	Uniform
C	Charlie	**L**	Lima	**V**	Victor
D	Delta	**M**	Mike	**W**	Whiskey
E	Echo	**N**	November	**X**	X-ray
F	Foxtrot	**O**	Oscar	**Y**	Yankee
G	Golf	**P**	Papa	**Z**	Zulu
H	Hotel	**Q**	Quebec		
I	India	**R**	Romeo		

Data from: International Civilian Aviation Organization. Alphabet—Radiotelephony. http://www.icao.int/Pages/AlphabetRadiotelephony.aspx. Accessed January 13, 2017.

▶ Content of Transmissions

The content of your radio communications need to be accurate and concise Figure 5-5 . Here are some other guidelines about the content of EMS radio communications:

- Consider that everything you say over the radio is being said in public. A patient or visitor in the hallway of the ED, a 12-year-old radio enthusiast playing with a scanner, or a local reporter may be listening to your transmission. This consideration also applies to communications over cell phones or digital trunked systems. Do not say anything on the radio you do not want others to hear.
- It is essential to protect the privacy of the patient at all times. As mentioned previously, this confidentiality is required by HIPAA regulations. Do not use the patient's name on the air, and do not unnecessarily transmit personal information about the patient. Sensitive information is usually best given face to face to the receiving facility staff.
- Be impersonal. Use "we," not "I," to refer to yourself, and use proper names and titles ("Paramedic Smith") to refer to others.
- Use proper and correct medical terminology.
- Avoid using words that are difficult to hear. The words "yes" and "no" may be easily missed in

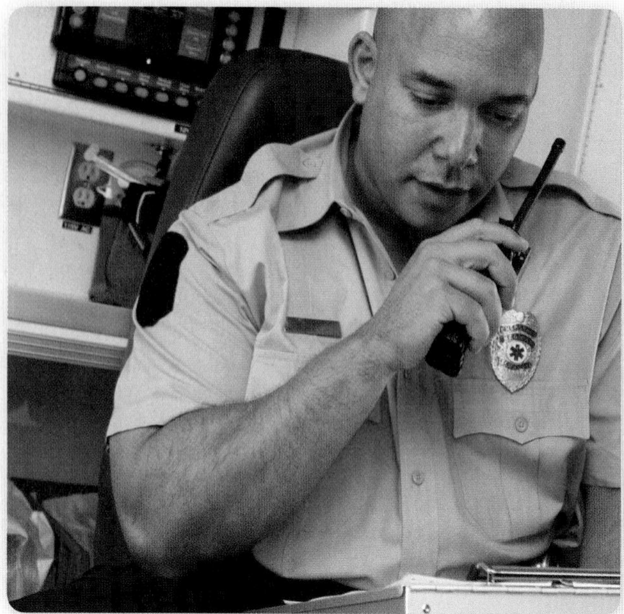

Figure 5-5 Give the radio report in an objective, accurate, and professional manner.

transmission; use "affirmative" and "negative" instead.

- Act professionally. Do not try to be a comedian or a critic. The radio is not the place for sarcasm or other poor conduct. Use standard formats agreed on by your EMS agency for transmission of information. When the listeners know what they are listening for, they are less likely to miss parts of the transmission.
- When you receive instructions by radio from dispatch or medical control, "parrot" the order back to make certain you have understood it correctly. If the physician instructs you to "Administer lidocaine 75 milligrams slowly IV", then you would respond, "Copy lidocaine, 75 milligrams slowly IV."
- Question any orders you did not hear clearly or did not understand.
- If you have a long message to transmit, then break the message into 30-second segments, checking at the end of each segment to determine whether it was received and understood. The accepted way to signify a pause is to say "break," which lets the receiver know you are pausing and permits them to ask questions, if necessary.
- When you finish transmitting, notify the receiver that the transmission is finished by saying "over," "end of transmission," or "clear."

Codes

The **ten-code** system and other radio codes were once in common use, but have been phased out in most EMS systems. One of the biggest drawbacks of using radio codes is that the same code often has different meanings in different jurisdictions. For example, the code "10-55" can mean an intoxicated driver, a coroner's case (deceased person), or a bomb threat, depending on the jurisdiction.

A code system used by dispatchers in many EMS systems is the **medical priority dispatch system (MPDS)**. The MPDS uses a specific format to indicate the nature of the emergency (EMD protocol) and the priority (determinant level/number). The dispatcher uses this information to decide the priority and response mode when assigning the responding units. These codes may or may not be relayed to the responding units, based on local system protocol. The general format is standardized, but the specific priority codes may vary between jurisdictions.

The National Incident Management System (NIMS) discourages the use of all radio codes. The preferred format is clear text, which is discussed below. For radio codes to be of any use, everyone using the radio system must know the meaning of the code words. If codes or other specific terminology are used in your agency, then learn and use them correctly. The NIMS is discussed further in Chapter 47, *Incident Management and Mass-Casualty Incidents*.

Clear Text Communications

There is no room for misunderstandings and miscommunication during the response to an emergency incident. The larger the incident, the more important it is that responders, dispatchers, and incident commanders all use common terminology. For these reasons, the preferred communications format in many systems is **clear text** (also called plain language). This practice simply means using regular language and accepted terms to communicate. For example, to request additional resources, you would say: "Dispatch, this is Medic 17. We will require two additional advanced life support ambulances. Request that they approach from the south."

Clear text is the format recommended by the NIMS interoperability standards.[21] Having interoperable radio equipment is of limited value if those using the equipment are essentially speaking different languages.

▶ Communications Formats Used During the Different Phases of the Response

Each agency or region will have its own format for radio and other communications. The details will vary between different regions and agencies, but the basics are common to all systems. This section will review the basic format for each phase of an EMS response, but it is important for you to familiarize yourself with the expected format or formats used in your area.

Dispatch Communications

When you are alerted by dispatch about an EMS call, record the location and call information as it is provided. This step is important to ensure you fully understand the dispatch. After the call is dispatched and you have recorded the details, respond back to the dispatcher that you have received the information. A basic sequence is as follows:

- **Dispatch:** *Medic 2, Regional Dispatch. Priority 1: Motor vehicle collision, Second Street at Main Street. Possibly two patients. Time 2104.*
- **Medic 2:** *Regional Dispatch, Medic 2 copies, Priority 1: motor vehicle collision, Second Street at Main Street, two patients.*

Your response to dispatch confirms that you have received the message and are preparing to respond to the appropriate location, ensures that an effective and accurate transfer of information has occurred, and establishes your dispatch time.

Response to the Scene Communications

After receiving the information and acknowledging the call, you need to determine how to get to the location of the call. This process may involve using the crew's knowledge of the area, paper maps, or a GPS-based electronic navigation system. As you begin to travel toward the scene, you need to notify dispatch. This step lets them know you are on the way and establishes your en-route time. This exchange could be as follows:

- **Medic 2:** *Regional Dispatch, Medic 2 en route to Second Street at Main Street.*
- **Dispatch:** *Medic 2, en route at 2105.*

Your next transmission should be your arrival on scene. This step allows you to update dispatch and establishes your arrival time. Your notification can be as follows:

- **Medic 2:** *Medic 2, on scene. Confirm two vehicles, moderate damage; both occupants are still in vehicles. Notify any other responders that access to Second Street is blocked and they need to approach from the north side of the street.*
- **Dispatch:** *Medic 2, arrived. Two vehicles, occupants inside, approach to Second Street is blocked. On scene time is 2110.*

With this exchange, you have confirmed arrival, the number of vehicles and patients, and the location of the patients. You have also provided important prearrival instructions for the other responding units. This is an appropriate time to request additional resources, if any are needed.

You may find that you need additional resources (more ambulances, a heavy rescue unit, a hazmat team, a helicopter, etc) at any point during a response. Any time that you determine that additional resources are needed is an appropriate time to request them. Other times to consider making such a request include while you are en route to the scene (based on either what you know or can anticipate about the scene), and after you have had the opportunity to determine the number of patients and the nature of their injuries, and the presence or absence of any physical entrapment.

Patient Safety

The **universal timeout** is a planned pause before the beginning of a procedure that improves safety and communication among all personnel, and helps prevent human errors. It allows time for everyone to silently review important aspects of the procedure with minimal distraction, ensure all preparations and equipment are in place, and confirm the correct procedure is being performed on the correct site. This concept is used in aviation (silent, or "sterile," cockpit during takeoff and landing) and is required in hospitals before surgical or other procedures. The timeout has been shown to reduce preventable errors, even under high-stress conditions.[22]

The use of the timeout has value in the EMS environment as well. Examples include performing a timeout prior to critical decisions or procedures in the field, and on EMS arrival to the receiving facility for trauma and other critical patients so that no key information is lost during the transfer of patient care. Many procedures that need to be performed during a 9-1-1 call are emergent and time critical, and a group pause may not always be possible. In these situations, you can perform a quick internal timeout to ensure you are ready. A version of this approach has been taught in EMS training programs for years, with the advice to "Stop, take a deep breath, think, and then act." In a situation such as an interfacility transport, more time may be available, making a general timeout more feasible.

On-Scene and Tactical Communications

While you are operating at the scene of an emergency medical call, you need to stay in contact with other responders at the scene. This contact is typically accomplished using a portable radio on an assigned tactical channel. Use of a tactical channel or frequency takes on-scene communications off of the main dispatch channel, leaving it open for other radio traffic. In the event of a large-scale incident, a more involved communications plan may be implemented, using different frequencies or channels for different purposes (triage, rescue operations, air medical, etc).

Patient Transport Communications

After you have assessed your patient and begun treatment, you need to prepare for transport. This process involves two further phases of communication. The first is advising dispatch of the transport, and the second is contacting medical control and/or the receiving facility.

You must inform dispatch that you are transporting. This information lets them know your status and establishes a time stamp for departing the scene. When contacting dispatch, your radio report may be as follows:

- **Medic 2:** *Medic 2, leaving Second and Main, en route to Municipal Hospital, two patients on board, nonemergency traffic.*

- **Dispatch:** *Medic 2, received. I show you en route to Municipal Hospital, nonemergency traffic with two patients. Time 2134.*

This transmission documents the fact that you have completed operations at the scene and are on the way to the hospital, and that the response is nonemergent. The next radio transmission to dispatch is to notify them of your arrival at the medical facility. This radio report can be as follows:

- **Medic 2:** *Medic 2, arrived at Municipal Hospital, out of service.*
- **Dispatch**: *Medic 2 received. I have you out at Municipal Hospital and unavailable for service. Time 2145.*

In this exchange, the EMS unit confirms arrival at the hospital and establishes its status. This step is important because it documents your unit is unavailable for further responses at this time. You may not be available for service while you turn over patient care, give your report, and restock your ambulance.

After you have completed these tasks and are ready for another call, you need to update dispatch that you are back in service. Never assume that dispatch knows your status. For example:

- **Medic 2:** *Medic 2, we are clear of Municipal Hospital and available.*
- **Dispatch**: *Medic 2 received. I show you back in service and available. Time 2159.*

▶ Relaying Information to Medical Control

The legal basis for paramedic practice is supervision by a physician. This supervision may take the form of **off-line medical control**, in which you may perform certain procedures or treatments based on protocols or standing orders without physician contact, and **online medical control**, in which the physician gives patient-specific orders and instructions directly to you by radio or telephone. Many EMS systems operate on a hybrid of these two models. Routine emergency medical care is covered by protocols, but more complex situations require physician contact and guidance.

When you are in the field, your radio communications with the medical control physician need to be clear, concise, and accurate. Using a standard format for communicating patient information over the radio will ensure significant information is relayed in a consistent manner and that nothing is omitted **Figure 5-6**.

The following section discusses the essential patient assessment information that needs to be contained in your radio report to the medical control facility. It is common in larger EMS systems for the paramedic to need to transport to hospitals other than the assigned medical control facility. In these cases, always follow local protocol and notify both facilities of your destination. When the patient is being transported to a different facility, advise medical control of the reason for this destination choice, and the name of the receiving facility.

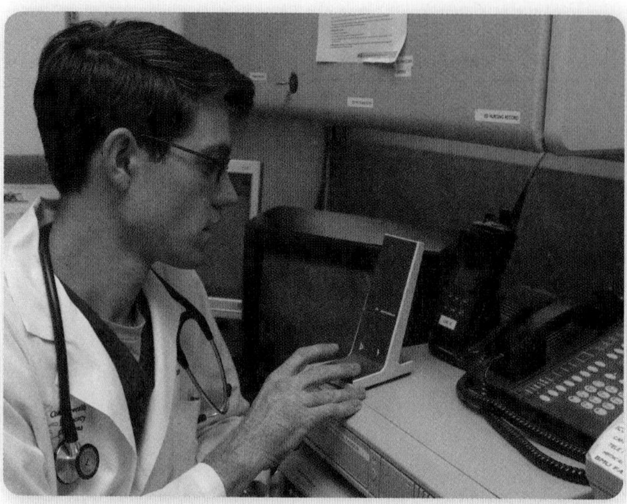

Figure 5-6 Use a standard format for communicating patient information to medical control.

Format for Reporting Medical Information

The two keys to a good radio report are being organized and knowing what you want to say before beginning your transmission. It is important that you include all required information. It is a good idea to write your reporting format on a notecard and affix the notecard to your handheld transmitter or in the ambulance near the radio so you may refer to it while making your report. The exact format will vary between EMS systems, but the following information needs to be included in all medical radio reports:

- Destination facility and estimated time of arrival (ETA)
- The patient's age and sex
- The patient's chief complaint
- A brief, pertinent history of the present illness or injury
- Medications and important allergies
- Anything the physician needs to know about the patient's past medical history relative to the current situation, including major underlying medical conditions
- The patient's level of consciousness and degree of distress
- The patient's mental status
- The patient's vital signs
- The pertinent physical findings in head-to-toe order
- ECG findings
- Treatment given so far and response to treatment

Here is a clear, concise, and accurate medical control transmission regarding a patient in congestive heart failure:

- **Paramedic:** *Memorial Hospital, this is Medic 8.*
- **Hospital:** *Medic 8 go ahead, this is Dr. McCalla, time is 1643.*
- **Paramedic:** *Memorial Hospital, this is Paramedic Garcia on Medic 8, we are en route to your facility*

with an ETA of 11 minutes. Onboard we have a 53-year-old male patient reporting severe shortness of breath, which awakened him from sleep and is worse when he is lying down. He has a history of hypertension and takes hydrochlorothiazide. He is alert, denies chest pain, and is in significant respiratory distress. Cardiac monitor shows a sinus tachycardia at 130 with a corresponding pulse, respirations of 36 and labored, BP of 190/120, and pulse oximetry is up from 88% to 96%. He has crackles and wheezes in both lung fields. There is no jugular vein distention. He has 2+ pitting ankle edema. We have him on low-concentration oxygen and have established a saline lock. Do you have any questions or orders?

The preceding transmission was organized and to the point. The physician hearing it would easily recognize that this is a hypertensive patient in left-sided heart failure, and would be able to make a good decision about treatment orders. When paramedics call in without using a standard reporting format, the physician might have to spend time gleaning the information to know what is going on. In contrast, consider the following dialogue:

- **Paramedic:** *Memorial Hospital, we have a patient with a pulse of 130, a blood pressure of 190/120, and respirations of 30. We're sending you a strip.*
- **Physician:** *Who is this calling?*
- **Paramedic**: *This is Medic 8.*
- **Physician:** *Medic 8, what's the patient's problem?*
- **Paramedic**: *He's short of breath.*
- **Physician:** *How long has this been going on?*
- **Paramedic:** *Just a minute* (pause). *He says it woke him up from sleep about an hour ago.*
- **Physician:** *Does he have any underlying medical conditions?*
- **Paramedic:** *He takes medicine for hypertension.*
- **Physician:** *Is he in any distress?*
- **Paramedic:** *Yes, he's having a hard time breathing.*
- **Physician:** *What do his lungs sound like?*
- **Paramedic:** *He has crackles and wheezes all over.*
- **Physician:** *Where are you taking him?*
- **Paramedic:** *To your hospital.*
- **Physician:** *What is your ETA?*
- **Paramedic:** *11 minutes.*

This exchange was disorganized, incomplete, and inefficient. This type of exchange wastes time, causes frustration, and creates a high risk of important information being missed or not clearly communicated. To avoid ineffective conversations, first gather your information thoroughly at the scene, organize it clearly in your mind, and only then pick up the microphone. Listening to recorded medical control calls can be an effective way to learn the format of your system.

It is important to continue your assessment of the patient. After your radio report is completed, reassess your patient and be alert for any changes. All patients have the potential to get worse rapidly. Report any changes in an update to the receiving facility.

Patient Safety

Breakdowns in communication that almost led to errors or harm are referred to as near misses or close calls. A near miss is any event that could have led to an adverse patient consequence but did not; it is indistinguishable from a full-fledged adverse event in all but the outcome.

An example of a near miss would be if a medical control physician ordered a medication without considering the patient's allergies, but you checked for allergies and spoke with the physician before administering the medication. Thus, the physician's error was caught and you did not give the contraindicated medication.

In-Person Report and Transfer of Care Communications

The final phase of your patient care communication is your bedside report to the receiving facility medical and nursing staff. This is the point where you transfer (hand off) patient care to the receiving facility staff. It is important that you relay all pertinent information. Use the same format as your radio report, but with additional detail as required, and include any updates to the information provided in your radio report.

Keep in mind that the patient, and possibly the family, will also be listening **Figure 5-7**. If you need to communicate sensitive information, it may be more appropriate to step outside the patient care room or to speak in a softer tone to the receiving staff. Always respect the patient's right to privacy. See Chapter 4, *Medical, Legal, and Ethical Issues* for more on patient confidentiality and HIPAA.

The final step is to make sure that you have answered all questions from the medical and nursing staff. Patient

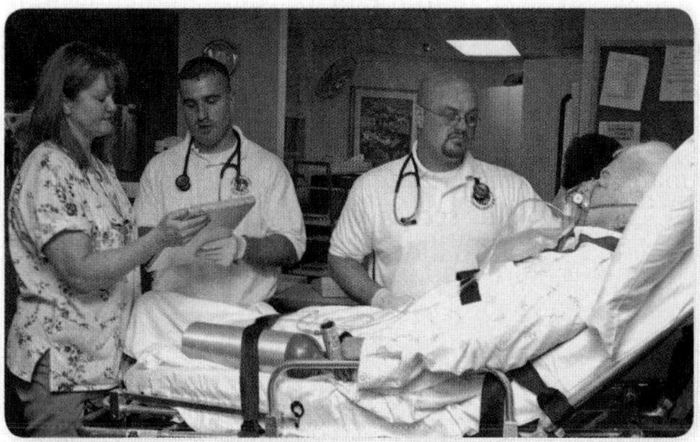

Figure 5-7 Be mindful of how you provide your report when the patient or family members are present.

handoff also involves written documentation. Your charting needs to reflect the emergency medical care you provided and be consistent with your verbal report. See Chapter 6, *Documentation*, for more information on documentation.

Patient Safety

Transfer of patient care, or handoff, is one of the highest risk aspects of emergency (or any) medical care. Multiple handoffs may occur between various providers, including physicians, nurses, paramedics, emergency medical technicians, and other responders. It is easy for errors or omissions to occur during handoffs. Numerous studies of prehospital communications have examined the handoff between EMS and ED or hospital staff.[23] Studies have demonstrated a loss of key clinical information during handoff, such as changes in vital signs (eg, transient hypotension), medications administered, and changes in ventilator settings—all of which may directly lead to patient harm. To help prevent such errors, you are strongly encouraged to use a standardized approach.

One method used by many health systems is the **situation, background, assessment, and recommendation (SBAR)** technique. This technique has become a best practice in health care to accurately relay critical information. The SBAR technique allows for a brief, yet complete and expected, handoff of information. Everyone involved in the handoff has a shared mental model, improving the safety of the transition of care. The elements of the SBAR technique are as follows[24]:

- **Situation.** Briefly describe the current situation. Give a clear, succinct overview of the pertinent issues.
- **Background.** Briefly state the pertinent history. What got us to this point?
- **Assessment.** Summarize the facts and give your best assessment. What is going on? Use your best judgment.
- **Recommendation.** Which actions are you asking for? What do you want to happen next?

Medical Terminology. As mentioned previously, using medical terminology correctly is essential for effective EMS communication. It improves the accuracy of your communication. Familiarize yourself with the accepted or approved medical terminology and abbreviations used in your EMS system. Medical terminology may seem to be a foreign language, and in fact it is. Most medical terminology comes from Greek and Latin. A review of Chapter 7, *Medical Terminology*, can help you become proficient in medical terminology.

Words of Wisdom

As a paramedic, you can be your own worst enemy when communicating with others on the health care team. Paramedics sometimes use big words to try to impress the person listening to or reading their reports. Some medical terminology can be misunderstood, especially over a radio or telephone. Words that contain *hyper-*, *hypo-*, *inter-*, or *intra-* tend to sound the same when a person is excited or in a hurry. As a result, orders for medications or procedures can be incorrect. In some cases, the orders may not be received at all. To avoid errors, remember to keep your communication simple and to the point. Moreover, make sure you use proper terminology, grammar, and spelling.

Therapeutic Communication

As a paramedic, your job will involve daily interactions with people, often when they are at their worst or most vulnerable. At least half of the calls you will run as a paramedic will take you into people's homes, day and night, and in the most private moments of their lives. Try to see every invitation into the home of someone else as a personal honor in a time and place where no one else would be welcome Figure 5-8.

You will often work in noisy, chaotic, bizarre, and sometimes dangerous environments. Under these

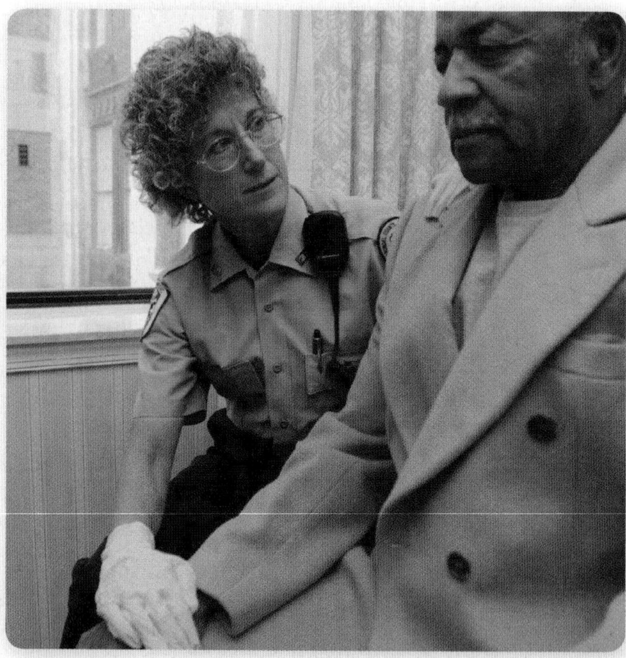

Figure 5-8 Think of it as an honor to be asked into a patient's home. Always be respectful and kind.

circumstances, communicating with patients (and their family members) can be particularly challenging. In these types of situations, other responders will look to you for leadership. If the scene is noisy, then do not shout. When you shout, so does everyone else. When people are shouting, they tend to get excited. If you remain calm and in control, then so will others.

If you are answering a call in a dark, noisy place such as a bar, then ask the bartender to turn off the music, turn up the lights, and keep an eye on the other patrons. If you must use a noisy compressor or run a diesel engine on the scene, then shut it off as soon as you can. Talk close to your patient's ears in a calm voice. This technique lets him or her know that you have your emotions under control. This technique will help the patient stay calm as well.

Therapeutic communication involves the use of specific strategies to encourage the patient to express ideas and feelings. It is also a way to convey your respect, acceptance, and genuine concern for someone you have never met before. If you want people to tell you about their problems, then you need first to convince them you want to hear what they have to say. Give patients your undivided attention, listen and pay attention to what they say, and always carry a notepad and write things down. It is inefficient and erodes patient confidence to repeat questions because you did not record the answer the first time you asked.

An excellent way to demonstrate that you are really listening is a technique called active listening. Active listening involves repeating back the key parts of a patient's responses to questions. Repeating this information back helps to assure the patient that you are really listening, and confirms the information the patient is providing.

▶ Developing Rapport

An important first step in every patient encounter is to develop a good rapport. To be able to treat a patient effectively, you need to obtain accurate information about the patient's condition and medical history. This process is much easier if the patient is calm and trusts you. Start by trying to put the patient in crisis at ease.

Information gathering is a learned skill. Even under the best circumstances, getting necessary information can be a challenging task. Some patients are resistant to giving details about themselves. Others may have trouble focusing on you because of the chaos of the emergency scene, or they may be distracted by their physical or emotional conditions, or they may feel threatened by you or others at the scene.

For a patient who is reluctant to share personal information, start by explaining why you need his or her name and date of birth. Reassure him or her that all the information is confidential and will be protected as mandated by federal law. Moving the patient to the ambulance can help create a calmer atmosphere for the patient and make talking and listening easier. Ask personal questions quietly and in private whenever possible. Even if you have earned a patient's trust, many people just do not want to talk about certain things in front of others.

If the patient is reluctant to communicate because he or she feels threatened, then cautiously approach the patient and use open posturing (eg, stand with your palms facing out). Smile and be calm. Reassure the patient, and if possible, move a little slower than usual. All of these actions can promote a less threatening environment.

Words of Wisdom

Patients will notice how you treat or are treated by other EMS personnel at the scene. If you are treated with respect, and if you treat others with respect, then the patient will have more confidence in you as well.

Introductions

The first step in promoting open communication is the introduction. As soon as is reasonably possible, introduce yourself. A simple greeting will usually suffice; for example: "Good afternoon, sir. My name is Erica. I am a paramedic with the fire department. What is your name?" Establishing eye contact can reassure the patient and help you begin your neurologic exam. Lack of a response may indicate altered mental status. A far-off stare may suggest substance abuse or a psychiatric condition. The eyes may also signal that someone is becoming hostile or potentially violent.

If no threat is evident, then get on the same level as the patient. Sit on a chair or squat next to him or her. This technique promotes trust and helps alleviate anxiety. Getting on the same level is especially helpful when dealing with children. Position yourself where the patient can easily see you, and so that those with hearing impairment may better observe your lips and facial expressions. Be aware of your own body language, which can either put the patient at ease or make him or her uncomfortable. Use open-handed gestures, do not cross your arms, and do not react to the patient's responses with skepticism. Body language is discussed in more detail later in this chapter.

Use the patient's name in all interactions. A good rule of thumb is if the patient is your age or younger, then call the patient by his or her first name. If the patient is older than you, then address them as "sir," "ma'am," "mister," "missus," or "miss." Speak slowly and calmly, and always be honest, because a falsehood can permanently damage the patient's trust in you.

Respect and Protect People's Modesty

Modesty matters—no matter how acute the medical condition or injury may be. It is especially important to older adults, adolescents, and young children. If the

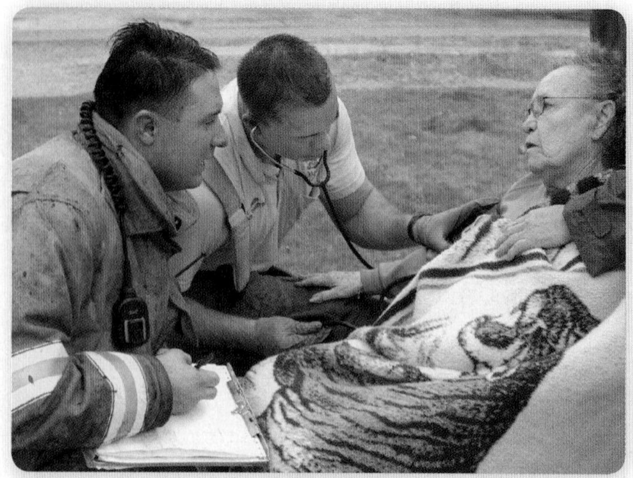

Figure 5-9 Show your patient the same respect you would want others to show your father, brother, mother, or sister. Protect a patient's modesty with a blanket or towel.

patient is not personally sensitive to modesty, then his or her family members most certainly will be Figure 5-9.

▶ Conducting the Interview

Two types of questions are used in effective interviewing. The first is the **open-ended question**. Always start with open-ended questions when interviewing your patients. This technique allows the patient to freely give you information and allows you to begin to assess his or her mentation. Examples of open-ended questions are "How are you feeling right now?" and "Can you tell me what happened?" Ask one question at a time and do not rush the patient; let him or her answer at his or her own pace.

The second type of question is the **closed-ended question** or direct question. This type of question is meant to elicit a specific answer. Examples of closed-ended questions are "What year were you born?" and "Does your arm hurt here?" (while you palpate the injured area). It is a good idea to develop a standard set of medical history questions that you ask almost all patients. Use simple language that people without medical training can understand, but avoid talking down to them.

▶ Strategies to Elicit Useful Reponses to Questions

When people are in crisis, they may experience a breakdown in their ability to communicate. It can be almost impossible to think and organize your thoughts when you are terrified or in pain. Asking simple open- and close-ended questions may not yield the information you need to get a clear picture of what is going on. In such a situation, you can utilize a variety of interviewing tools to get the answers you need.

Reflection

Reflection is the repetition of a word or phrase that a patient has used in previous statements to encourage more detail. For example, the patient may have said, "I could not catch my breath."

- **Paramedic:** *You say you could not catch your breath, ma'am?*

YOU are the Paramedic PART 4

Your partner asks Mrs. Smith to please take her to John's medications so she can make note of them. Mrs. Smith willingly complies. You are still on the same level as John and you slowly ask in a slightly louder voice, "Can you understand me, John?" After a pause, John answers, "Yes."

Recording Time: 5 Minutes	
Respirations	14 breaths/min
Pulse	76 beats/min, strong and regular
Skin	Pale, cool, dry
Blood pressure	110/66 mm Hg
Oxygen saturation (Spo_2)	93% room air
Pupils	PERRLA

8. Give some examples of effective communication techniques for people with hearing impairment.
9. How can your body language affect your assessment of this patient?

- **Ms. Williams:** *Well, my chest felt tight, and I could not breathe fully.*
- **Paramedic:** *What were you doing when this episode occurred?*
- **Ms. Williams:** *I was in my chair, and it started all of a sudden.*

This technique has given you vital information. Now you are aware that the onset was sudden and did not result from exertion, which is more information than was originally communicated by the patient.

Empathy

Empathy can be described as putting yourself in the patient's position.

- **Paramedic:** *Why did you call us tonight, Mr. Smith?*
- **Mr. Smith:** *I feel so sad and depressed. I cannot seem to function.*
- **Paramedic:** *What do you think is making you feel this way, sir?*
- **Mr. Smith:** *I have not been normal since my wife died of cancer last week. I just do not have the spirit to continue.*
- **Paramedic:** *I am sorry to hear about your wife, Mr. Smith. I understand how difficult this time must be. I am here to help you.*

This patient may or may not have other issues affecting his health, but he is in need of help.

Confrontation

Confrontation is the technique of making the patient aware that something is not consistent with his or her story. Always consider whether using this technique could provoke the patient. The key is to remain professional and nonjudgmental. Consider a patient who has been involved in a traffic incident who is in your ambulance:

- **Paramedic:** *What caused you to lose control of your vehicle?*
- **Mr. Jones:** *I was just driving along when I skidded on something.*
- **Paramedic:** *Have you been drinking alcohol tonight?*
- **Mr. Jones:** *No, nothing tonight.*
- **Paramedic:** *Anything you tell me is confidential, and I detect the smell of alcohol on your breath. There were also some empty bottles in your vehicle. It is important you tell me the truth so I can make sure that we and the hospital staff can take proper care of you.*
- **Mr. Jones:** *Yes, I had four beers tonight.*

Interpretation

If you are not sure what a patient is trying to tell you, then sometimes it can be helpful to restate what you think he or she said. Then invite the patient to correct you. Interpretation can also be used when a patient refuses to give information that you need to determine a course of treatment.

With this method, you begin by diplomatically telling the patient what you think is going on, and then asking him or her if you are right. For example, you are with a patient who is 16 years old. Her parents have called you because she was "acting depressed and we think she is on drugs." You remove her to the ambulance for transport, and she says, "I don't know how I got in this mess."

- **Paramedic:** "What mess?"
- **Patient:** "I can't say. I don't want to hurt my parents."
- **Paramedic:** "Why do you think you are hurting your parents?"
- **Patient:** "They never liked my boyfriend, and now I'm in trouble."
- **Paramedic:** "Did your boyfriend hurt you?"
- **Patient:** "No, but I can't tell my parents what is wrong."
- **Paramedic:** "This may be totally wrong, but I must ask this question so I can inform the physician for your well-being. Do you think you are pregnant?"
- **Patient:** (starting to cry) "I don't know, but I think I may be."

The skill of interpretation requires you to use your best intuition and diplomatic skills. One of the best phrases to begin with is, "So, if I understand what you are saying correctly . . ."

Facilitation

If patients hesitate to answer questions completely, then encourage them to provide you with more information. One useful expression is simply, "Please say more." Another is, "Please feel free to tell me about that."

Silence

If you sense that patients are trying to put something into words but are having trouble expressing themselves, then remember this famous advice: "Never miss a good opportunity to shut up." Be patient. Do not say anything at all for a few seconds. Let the patient talk.

Clarification

If you do not understand what patients have told you, then ask them to explain what they mean. This method communicates that you are listening and taking their comments seriously. It may also help you understand what they are trying to tell you.

Redirection

Sometimes patients will mention something in passing or will avoid answering a specific question. You can politely redirect their attention to that question (several times, if necessary) until you get them to answer it.

Simplification and Summarization

Some patients have a hard time speaking plainly, no matter how hard they try. It can be difficult to communicate with people who have psychiatric conditions, who fabricate their diseases, and who are afraid or upset. If patients give you a confusing or disorganized response, then try putting their comments into simpler terms and see if they agree with your synopsis. This method can help them focus their thoughts and help you as an interviewer.

▶ Common Interviewing Errors

In addition to good interviewing techniques, the following are some common errors that should be avoided:

- **Never provide false assurance or make unlikely claims.** Your job is to be neutral and objective. Assuring someone that he or she will be fine seems like a simple and caring statement, but never make promises you cannot keep.
- **Do not offer a diagnosis or medical advice that is beyond your scope of practice.** It is appropriate to give your medical opinion and offer advice based on your individual scope of practice and your best judgment, such as the following: "I do not know if the pain in your chest is from your heart or from indigestion, but I am concerned that it may be your heart. I think we should take you to the hospital so that you can be fully evaluated."
- **Do not ask leading questions.** You may not get a reliable answer from a question such as, "You have not been having any blurry vision, have you?"
- **Avoid interrupting the patient or talking too much.** You need to hear what the patient has to say.

▶ Nonverbal Skills

Consider the following nonverbal communication skills that you need to master. Always keep in mind the adage, "You only get one chance to make a first impression." People often form opinions of others at the first observation. If you look sloppy and unkempt, then the patient may form the impression that your knowledge and skills are also inferior. A professional appearance and demeanor is likely to instill confidence in patients.

Be patient and calm, because acting impatient will make the patient feel uncomfortable and stressed. It is understood that most emergencies require quick action; however, you can still be efficient and fast while displaying an air of patience and calm.

Avoid a closed posture (such as crossing your arms) because this type of body language sends negative signals. Be aware of your facial expressions and gestures. Do not frown or smirk at the patient's answers. Do not roll your eyes at your partner. Maintain constant, nonjudgmental eye contact. Keep your tone of voice neutral, and encourage answers; do not demand them.

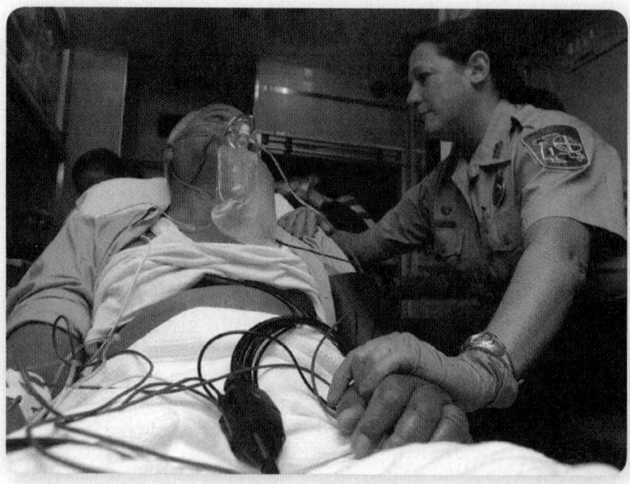

Figure 5-10 A gentle touch on the hand, arm, or shoulder can comfort someone who is sick or hurt and scared.

Some people do not like to be touched at all, whereas other people feel it is a valuable demonstration that someone cares about them. Try gently touching the patient on a neutral part of the body, such as a shoulder or arm. This technique can reassure him or her and reduce anxiety (Figure 5-10). If the patient pulls away from you, it is likely that touch may not be a valuable strategy in this instance. If the patient reacts positively by leaning toward you or seeming to relax, then a therapeutic touch will work with him or her.

Patient Safety

Some interesting research has been performed on how patients who have been involved in a physically or psychologically traumatic event are affected by the actions and perceived attitude of those caring for them, including EMS personnel. Studies have demonstrated that showing empathy; explaining what is going on, what you need to do, and why you need to do it (eg, start an intravenous [IV] line); involving patients in their care; and giving patients choices when possible are actions that can reduce the potential severity of post-traumatic stress experienced by these patients. Do not underestimate the positive effect you can have by being emotionally supportive and caring for your patients.[25]

▶ Special Interview Situations

Certain situations in your paramedic practice may require special communication techniques. Some of these situations may include uncommunicative patients, hostile or violent patients, older patients, young children, and patients with special challenges. Avoid stereotyping any of these groups of patients, which will impair effective communication.

People Who Are Hostile or Violent

Emergency situations can be emotional for the people involved, particularly patients and their loved ones. This heightened emotion may cause some people to become hostile, even toward you. Pay attention and always act in a manner to ensure your own safety and the safety of others.

It is important to acknowledge the hostile person's concerns and to empathize with him or her. Remain calm and try to understand the person's arguments. Use interpretation, clarification, and summarization to help the person feel heard and understood. Consider the possibility that you may be unable to defuse a situation involving a hostile person, in which case you may have to defer to law enforcement personnel.

During your career as a paramedic, you are guaranteed to receive some insults from people who are in crisis, and that will probably happen on a near-daily basis. It is especially predictable when you are dealing with people who are chemically impaired. Discipline yourself to never respond in kind. Nothing escalates a situation faster than trading insults with people—especially when witnesses are present. Not only does this type of behavior make no sense, but also it is unprofessional and can be dangerous. In this day of smartphone cameras and social media, you do not want to lose your temper and have it show up minutes later on the Internet.

Hostile or angry patients may present a threat to you and others. They may be under the influence of drugs or alcohol, or they may have behavioral or mental health issues. These factors can make the patient's behavior unpredictable. Always approach a hostile or angry patient with caution and maintain eye contact. Avoid interviewing him or her by yourself. It is a good idea for your partner to be present, but have him or her stay a little farther back to prevent the patient from feeling crowded. Have additional backup units, either law enforcement personnel or other EMS responders, close by when dealing with a potentially violent individual. The following are some additional tips for dealing with potentially violent patients:

- As you enter the scene, identify escape routes. Do not permit the patient to get between you and the only way out of the room.
- Approach the patient from the front, with your hands visible and palms open.
- Begin by introducing yourself, explaining your role, and asking for the patient's name.
- If safe to do so, then get on the same level as the patient.
- Ask permission to ask questions and touch the patient.
- Always be honest.
- Be wary for signs of impending attack such as clenched fists, hostile language, tensed neck and face muscles, and threatening gestures.

Words of Wisdom

Make it part of your routine to look for aggressive body language that signals increased anger and a possible attack. These signs include clenched fists, intense staring directed at you, and breathing heavily through clenched teeth.

Sexually Aggressive Patients

Occasionally, you will encounter a patient who is sexually aggressive towards you or other responders. This situation can occur with both male and female patients and male and female responders. Begin by making sure you have someone else present at all times when you are with the patient. Communicate professionally and politely. Make sure your words are not sexually ambiguous. Most of all, maintain professionalism at all times. Follow your agency's policies, document your encounter meticulously, and get witness names and signatures on the patient notes or run report. This topic is covered in further detail in Chapter 11, *Patient Assessment*.

Special Considerations of Age

Do not presume that older people are harder to communicate with than young people just because of their age. When sick, their illnesses do tend to be more complex than those of younger people. They may have more than one disease process, and they may be taking several kinds of medications. Members of the older adult population have a wide range of individual differences in hearing, eyesight, mentation, and mobility, to which you may need to adapt. Each patient is an individual, and you need to base your assessment and treatment on his or her individual needs, not on a blanket set of assumptions.

Children can pose communication challenges even to the best paramedics. They tend to protest pain vigorously, they may be afraid of strangers, they may panic when separated from their parents or caregivers, and their bodies may seem unfamiliar to you. Many paramedics are not as experienced or as comfortable with taking children's vital signs, starting IV lines, or intubating children as they are with adults. This hesitance is common, but with a little practice, you can become comfortable with these skills.

The most important aspect of your initial contact with children is friendly eye contact; a reassuring smile; and calm, patient explanations geared to match the child's age and level of understanding. Minimize your movements, lower your voice, and touch as gently as you can. Start by talking with the patient's parent or caregiver. This step will show the child that his or her parent or caregiver trusts you, which can improve his or her trust in you as well.

Try keeping your eye level at or below the child's level. You may try sitting on the floor and placing the child on the cot or on a parent or caregiver's lap **Figure 5-11**. When you examine a toddler (age 1 to 3 years) or young child, follow the reverse order of your normal exam by starting at the feet and move towards the head. This process is often less intimidating for the child. Whenever possible, involve a parent or caregiver in the hands-on care of a conscious young child. This technique is more important with infants and toddlers and less helpful with older children.

When parents or caregivers are unavailable or in other stressful situations, toys may be useful for bridging the gap between paramedics and some children **Figure 5-12**. Many EMS programs stock their ambulances with teddy bears for toddlers. Local public service groups or clubs often donate stuffed toys to hospitals and EMS agencies.

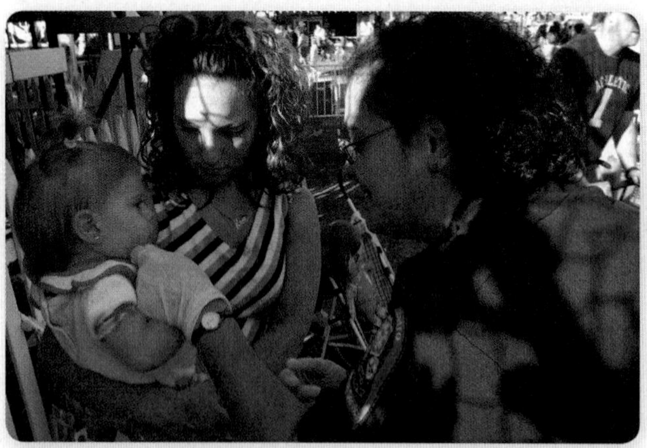

Figure 5-11 When you examine a young child, involve the parents or caregivers. Have a parent hold the child on his or her lap, or ask the parent to keep the child occupied while you work.

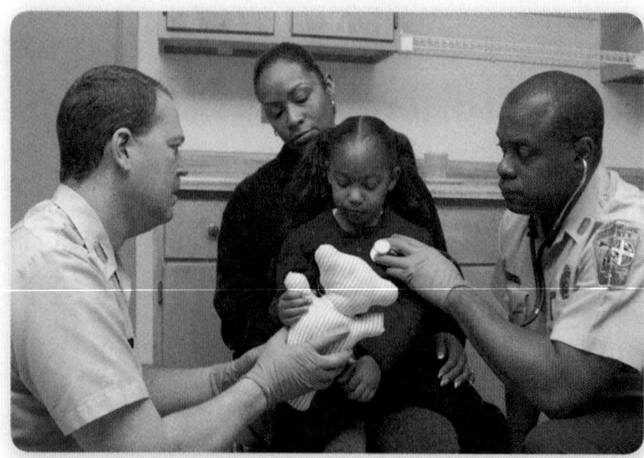

Figure 5-12 A stuffed animal or toy can put a young child at ease.

Adolescents (beginning at around age 13 years) may not want their parents or caregivers present during questioning or the physical exam. If an adult insists on monitoring your conversation with an adolescent, then this fact should raise concern in your mind. Do not refuse this prerogative of a parent, but be sure you communicate the situation to the ED physician or staff. Generally, it is a good idea to treat adolescents as adults. You may gain more cooperation by offering adolescents options and honoring their choices, but never offer an option you know you cannot honor.

Make special efforts to protect the modesty of patients older than age 2 years, and of adolescents in particular. Patients in this age grouping are becoming more aware of their bodies and may be especially embarrassed during a physical exam. Avoid disrobing the patient unless necessary.

People With Special Challenges

Do not overlook the needs of people with difficulties with speech, hearing, sight, and/or other kinds of communication disorders. When you encounter a patient who has trouble communicating, remember that family members or primary caregivers who know these patients well can facilitate your efforts. For example, many caregivers enroll in classes for sign language and lip reading to facilitate communication with these patients. They can also help you alleviate the patient's fear and anxiety. If a patient wears eyeglasses or a hearing aid, then ensure those items are available and functional.

Many caregivers find that therapeutic touch and eye contact are helpful bridging mechanisms when caring for patients with special challenges. For example, a light touch on a patient's shoulder can convey kindness, whereas a firm grasp can express reassurance. Some patients respond well to brief, one-armed hugging.

A particularly challenging group of patients are those with autism. Autism can vary in severity and falls under a broader category known as **pervasive developmental disorders (PDDs)**. PDDs cause delays in many areas of childhood development, such as the development of skills to communicate and interact socially, and the effects can be lifelong.

Children with autism may have difficulty developing language skills and understanding what others say to them. They also may have difficulty communicating nonverbally, such as through hand gestures, eye contact, and facial expressions. Not every person with autism will have difficulty with language. Some people with autism may be unable to speak, whereas others may have rich vocabularies and be able to talk about specific subjects in great detail. Most children with autism have little or no problem pronouncing words. The majority will have difficulty using language effectively, especially when they talk to other people. They also may be unable to understand body language and the nuances of vocal tones.

Children with autism who can speak will often say things that have no meaning or that seem out of context in conversations with others. One example is the use of continuous repetition of words or phrases. When you communicate with a patient with autism, it may be best to address questions to the parent or caregiver. They are often your best resource for communicating with the patient.

For additional information about communicating with and caring for these patients, refer to Chapter 45, *Patients with Special Challenges*.

Cross-Cultural Communication

Cultural Competence

When faced with a stressful situation, different people will react differently. Often this response is driven by the individual's cultural background and upbringing. The reactions of those in some cultures to injury, illness, or death may seem strange (and sometimes even unsettling) to members of other cultures. As a health care provider, it is very important that you avoid viewing others from an ethnocentric perspective. **Ethnocentrism** is the belief that one's own culture or ethnic group is inherently superior to others, or that one's own cultural viewpoint is always "right," while the viewpoints of others are "wrong." An ethnocentric viewpoint interprets the actions and beliefs of those from different cultural or ethnic groups based solely upon the standards and values of one's own culture.

An ethnocentric viewpoint can lead to incorrect assumptions, and may interfere with your ability to provide appropriate emergency medical care because you have misinterpreted key information. An example may be an Ethiopian patient with shortness of breath. If you apply oxygen, then the patient and his or her family may become agitated and fearful. The dominant American cultural belief is that oxygen use is routine and comforting, but the Ethiopian cultural belief is that the use of oxygen signifies grave or near-fatal disease.[26] The ethnocentric response to this situation would be to assume that the patient and family are "being stupid" or behaving in an irrational manner, whereas the culturally competent response is to try to understand why the patient is reacting in a manner you did not anticipate. The reactions of those from different backgrounds may be unfamiliar to you, but they are not wrong. They are simply different, and are dictated by the expectations of the individual's culture. It is important for you to understand these differences.

Culture can be defined as the system of beliefs, attitudes, and behaviors that are learned and shared by members of a group. The group may be defined by a shared ethnic background, language, or religion; or the group may be based on another shared identity, such as the military or the gay community. Health care and EMS have their own distinctive cultures, with their own languages, traditions, rituals, and rites of initiation.

Human beings are not born with a sense of culture; it is learned from others. Your first introduction to your culture was provided by your parents and family. As time goes by, people learn other aspects of culture from friends, social and religious groups, the media, and many other sources. As an individual, you are a blend of many cultural influences. You may be a member of a cultural group that is based on ethnicity, language, or religion, but you are also a member of the cultures of your city or region, your circle of friends, and your profession. People switch their cultural identities and practices depending on the circumstances. How you interact with your aging relatives is different from how you relate to your friends, your coworkers, or your patients.

Every person you encounter has a similar mixture of cultural influences that will impact how they behave and how they will react when stressful situations arise. It is your responsibility as a paramedic to recognize these differences, and to understand how they may affect your interactions with the diverse population you serve. This understanding is referred to as **cultural competence**. In EMS, cultural competence may be defined as an understanding of the predominant cultures that exist in the geographic area in which you provide patient care.

The rest of this section will focus on developing your awareness of how cultural beliefs and practices affect people's views of health, illness, and health care. It will also explore how to effectively interact and communicate with patients and families from different cultures. This discussion will primarily examine ethnic and traditional cultural groups and their health beliefs and practices. It is not possible in this limited space to provide detailed descriptions of all cultural health practices that you may encounter. This section will highlight some examples that illustrate the wide range of cultural beliefs and practices, but it is important for you to identify the primary cultural groups in your area and to learn about their specific cultural and health care practices.

Cultural Awareness

Body Language

Body language and gestures are common, but may be interpreted differently by members of different cultures. The intended meaning may not be recognized and lead to confusion, or an innocent gesture in one culture may be considered rude in another. Perhaps the most universal cross-cultural gesture is the smile. A smile is readily understood by most every culture and conveys goodwill.

Every culture has its own social norms, religious practices, and interpretation of body language. What may be perceived as rude or odd may simply be a difference of cultural standards. It is not possible in this chapter to cover all of the possible cultural norms you may encounter, but the following list illustrates a few cultural practices that you should be aware of:

- **Eye contact.** Members of some cultures may avoid making direct eye contact. Avoiding eye contact is a sign of respect in many Native

American cultural groups, and in some Asian, African, Latin American, and Caribbean cultures. Prolonged eye contact is acceptable in the Arab world, Somalia, Brazil, and most European cultures.

- **Touching with the left hand.** Islamic and Hindu cultures avoid touching with the left hand because traditionally this hand was used for unclean functions. It is considered rude to use the left hand in greeting.
- **Touching the head.** Members of many Asian cultures do not touch the head. The head is considered to be the most sacred part of the body and is the residence of the soul. Touching the head may put the soul in jeopardy.
- **Feet.** Showing the bottom of the feet is considered offensive in many Muslim nations as well as most of Thailand.
- **Hands on hips.** This posture can be a sign of hostility in Mexico and Argentina.
- **Nodding.** Members of Indian and Arabic cultures may signal agreement by moving the head from side to side (the Western "no"). Some members of Asian cultures will nod to indicate "I acknowledge you are speaking to me," but it does not necessarily indicate agreement.
- **Hand gestures.** Hand gestures can have very different meanings in different cultures. Some gestures may be innocuous to one cultural group, but insulting to another. Learn about and be cautious with your use of hand gestures with those from different cultures in your community.

Words of Wisdom

It is important to become familiar with the cultural groups that live in your service area. Some areas have organized cultural awareness training programs. If no such programs are available in your community, then consider organizing one. Invite representatives from local religious or cultural organizations to meet with your EMS agency and develop training classes. Other resources may include local hospitals, colleges, and community groups.

Traditional Folk Medicine and Understanding of Illness

Not every culture views health and illness in the same way. Most of the patients you will encounter will subscribe to the western biomedical model, which emphasizes a biologic understanding of disease and injury, and the use of scientifically proven diagnostic tests and treatments. It views illness as a battle to be won by using tools such as laboratory tests, x-rays, medications, and surgical procedures.

Many immigrants to the United States follow the traditional folk medicine practices of their culture or homeland. Traditional models of illness typically involve a belief that health is the result of a balance of forces. If an imbalance occurs, then the individual becomes ill. Treatments and remedies are aimed at restoring the balance. Other beliefs may view illness as a result of the loss of one's spirit or of magical influences Table 5-3. Humoral medicine practices were followed by western medicine well into the 1800s, and some practices have regained popularity among followers of the so-called New Age movement. It is not uncommon for immigrants, and the children of immigrants, to practice a blend of western and traditional health practices, and they may alternate between their traditional healer and their western medical provider.

Two folk medicine practices that are important for you to be aware of are "cupping" and "coining," because they may be easily misinterpreted as signs of physical abuse. These practices are further discussed in Chapter 43, *Pediatric Emergencies*.[27] An important part of your history taking is to ask if any traditional healing practices have been used.

Another area of traditional folk medicine is the use of herbal medications. Many pharmaceuticals in common use today were derived from older folk remedies. These herbal medications include aspirin from birch bark used to reduce pain or fever, and quinine from the cinchona tree used to treat malaria. The use of traditional remedies is widespread, and an awareness of what the patient is taking is important. Many herbal medications have significant pharmacologic effects that may be a source of the patient's symptoms, or they may interact with other prescribed medications.

Patients may also be taking medications brought from their native country or supplied by family members back home. These medications often have different brand or generic names than their North American equivalents, or they may not be approved for use in the United States. The best practice is to collect all of the patient's medications (over the counter, prescribed, herbal, and those from foreign pharmacies) and bring them to the hospital with the patient so they can be identified, and so that the receiving staff are aware of everything the patient is taking.

Finally, consider that the patient may not share the beliefs of his or her family or cultural background and therefore may disagree with family members regarding his or her condition and treatment. Always remain sensitive to the patient's individual religious, cultural, and sociological beliefs.

Language Interpretation

Probably the biggest communication challenge with members of other cultures is a situation in which no common language exists. This challenge makes it difficult, if not impossible, to perform a good history and assessment.

Table 5-3 Traditional Beliefs About Health, Illnesses, and Folk Treatments

Beliefs	Examples	Folk Treatments
Humoral balance	▪ Balance between humors: blood, yellow bile, black bile, phlegm ▪ Each humor is associated with a season, element, organ, and/or specific qualities of heating/cooling and moisture/dryness	▪ "Feed a cold, starve a fever." • Foods thought to be heating or cooling ▪ Imitative magic (drawing the sickness [poison] from the body): • Coining: heated oil is applied to the skin, then coins are rubbed on the skin, creating red welts • Cupping: heated glass jars or cups are placed on skin; as cups cool, they create suction, red marks, and sometimes bruises • Ear candles: waxed paper cones are inserted into the ear canal and burned to remove earwax ▪ Bleeding and blistering as treatments to restore the balance
Illness as a loss of spirit	▪ The individual's spirit may flee the body because of: • Sudden noises • Physical trauma or injury • Spiritual or emotional trauma	▪ Rituals to return the wandering spirit to the body
Illness as the result of magical forces	▪ The evil eye	▪ As with loss of spirit (listed above), rituals to return the wandering spirit to the body ▪ Charms or amulets meant to ward off the evil eye or other curses

Data from: Juckett J. Cross-cultural medicine. American Family Physician. 2005: 72(11): 2267-2274. Lipson JG, Dibble SL. Culture & Clinical Care. San Francisco, CA: UCSF Nursing Press; 2005.

YOU are the Paramedic PART 5

You find that John is able to hear you with some minor adjustments on your part. He tells you he feels weak. He states his physician put him on a new "heart pill" within the last week. He thinks it is making him sick and he cannot remember the name of it. You assemble oxygen via nasal cannula for the patient. When you go to put the cannula on the patient, he pushes your hand away and turns his head. You state, "John, it is just a cannula." He reluctantly lets you apply it.

Recording Time: 10 Minutes	
Respirations	14 breaths/min
Pulse	78 beats/min
Skin	Pale, cool, dry
Blood pressure	110/64 mm Hg
Oxygen saturation (Spo_2)	98% on 4 L/min via nasal cannula
Pupils	PERRLA

10. How could you have prevented the patient's reaction to the nasal cannula?

Table 5-4 Language Interpretation Resources

Option	Advantages	Disadvantages
Interpreters provided by the hospital or dispatch center	▪ Qualified medical interpreters ▪ May be available by telephone or radio	▪ Not present with you in the field ▪ Selection of languages may be limited ▪ Hours of availability may be limited
Other responders as interpreters (other EMS personnel, firefighters, law enforcement, etc)	▪ Easy access	▪ May or may not be fluent, or may not have knowledge of medical terminology ▪ May be unable to accompany the patient to the hospital
Interpretation services via telephone	▪ Easy access from anywhere ▪ Qualified medical interpreters	▪ Requires telephone access ▪ Usually involves a subscription or other fee
Electronic translation applications (smartphones, etc)	▪ Easy access from tablet or smartphone ▪ Many are inexpensive	▪ Not specific to medical interpretation ▪ May not meet legal requirements
Family members or friends as interpreters	▪ Often present with the patient at the scene ▪ Patient may be more comfortable with a family member or friend	▪ May have limited fluency ▪ May have limited understanding of the questions being asked, or of medical concepts ▪ Accuracy of interpretation may be questionable (eg, they may edit what the patient says or give their own opinion, not what the patient has said)
Minors acting as interpreters	▪ Immediately available ▪ May have good bilingual ability	▪ Seldom a good idea ▪ May have limited fluency ▪ Often will have limited understanding ▪ Accuracy of interpretation may be questionable ▪ Ethics of using young children in this role are questionable

Abbreviation: EMS, emergency medical services

Language interpretation is vital when caring for a patient who speaks a different language, including people with hearing impairment who use sign language.

Unless you are fluent in the other language, it is always best to make use of a qualified interpreter. Health facilities are legally required to provide interpretation services, and patients in the prehospital setting deserve the same level of service. Obtaining qualified medical interpretation is more challenging in the field, but it is possible. A list of the types of interpretation services that may be available to you is listed in Table 5-4. When dealing with a patient who speaks another language, you should always assume you are missing something important in your history and assessment, and act accordingly.

YOU are the Paramedic SUMMARY

1. As a paramedic in the EMS system, how will you be notified about the location and nature of the incident?

A call for emergency medical assistance will be placed through 9-1-1 to the PSAP, where a dispatcher will obtain the information and direct the appropriate resources (you) to the scene.

2. What will the dispatcher be doing while you are en route to the call?

The dispatcher will obtain more information from the caller and provide any necessary prearrival medical instructions to the caller. The dispatcher will update the ambulance crew with any new information.

YOU are the Paramedic SUMMARY *(continued)*

3. How will you communicate with the other responders and agencies involved in the emergency response?

Communication between responders will use the emergency communications system, which may make use of radio, cellular devices, or computer terminals. The most common method of on-scene communications will be on a simplex channel using portable and mobile radios.

4. How will you initiate communication with this patient?

As soon as is reasonably possible, begin by introducing yourself. This introduction does not entail any special social skills or societal standards. For example, say: "Good morning, my name is Mark. I am a paramedic with the fire department. What is your name?" This simple exchange offers comfort and promotes a feeling of togetherness and goodwill.

Be sure you make eye contact and maintain it. This action reinforces trust and honesty. It also allows you to evaluate the patient's neurologic status, because certain conditions can cause an altered mental status that is evident through the person's gaze. A vague, far-off stare may suggest the presence of physical issues or substance abuse. The eyes may also signal agitation, hostility, or possible violence.

5. Is the television noise a consideration in your assessment?

Sometimes, even with the best communication techniques, it is difficult to communicate with the patient. External factors such as noise, disruptive scenes, language barriers, and sensory impairment can make communication difficult. In this situation, the noise of the television may interfere with effective communication with the patient. Resist the urge to walk over and simply turn it off. Whenever possible, ask permission before moving furniture or turning off appliances. The respect you demonstrate will go a long way to improving overall communications with your patient.

6. What does it mean to "get on the same level as the patient"? What is the importance of this action?

If no threat is evident, then physically get on the same level as the patient. This practice means placing yourself in a position in which the patient will not have to look up at you, which promotes trust and alleviates anxiety. This technique is especially useful when dealing with children. In essence, you are demonstrating a stance of equality through physical orientation.

7. How can you address the problem of a family member answering questions for the patient?

If this type of problem occurs, then do not become irritated with the family member. This specific method of communication may work well for this couple because the patient has a hearing impairment. You have a number of options available to you. You can politely ask the family member to allow the patient to speak so you can hear his or her voice. You can also ask the family member to perform another function, like gathering medications, which will allow you to speak one-on-one with the patient. Whatever you choose to do, do it tactfully.

8. Give some examples of effective communication techniques for people with hearing impairment.

Differing levels of hearing impairment exist. These range from minimal deficits to total deafness. Do not yell, because the patient may not have hearing impairment. Take your cues from family members. In this case, Mrs. Smith leaned close to the patient's left ear and spoke to him. Alternately, position yourself so the patient can clearly see you; speak slowly and clearly to the patient. Many people who are deaf or hard of hearing are able to read lips and facial expressions. You may also try writing down your questions and allowing the patient to write his or her answer. It may be necessary to utilize an American Sign Language interpreter when working with people who are deaf.

9. How can your body language affect your assessment of this patient?

Avoid a closed posture (such as crossing your arms) because this type of body language sends negative signals. Be mindful of your facial expressions and gestures. Do not frown or smirk at the patient's answers. Rolling your eyes at your partner is also not appropriate because it is rude, and could provoke a fight from a patient with a behavioral issue. Maintain constant, nonjudgmental eye contact. Demonstrate patience to the patient. Use open-handed gestures to demonstrate openness.

10. How could you have prevented the patient's reaction to the nasal cannula?

It can be frightening when someone reaches over your face with a piece of equipment. You told the patient, "It is just a cannula." Does the patient know what a cannula is and what it is designed to do? Before touching a patient, you need to educate and communicate what you are trying to do for a patient. Explain what an oxygen cannula does, how it is worn, and how it will help before placing it on the patient's face. The same is true for any item you place on the patient.

YOU are the Paramedic SUMMARY *(continued)*

EMS Patient Care Report (PCR)					
Date: 07-01-18	**Incident No.:** 876		**Nature of Call:** General medical		**Location:** 450 Maple Street
Dispatched: 0810	**En Route:** 0812	**At Scene:** 0816	**Transport:** 0836	**At Hospital:** 0845	**In Service:** 0855
Patient Information					
Age: 86 **Sex:** M **Weight (in kg [lb]):** 59 kg (130 lb)			**Allergies:** No known drug allergies **Medications:** Numerous—see attached list **Past Medical History:** Pancreatic cancer, A-fib **Chief Complaint:** General weakness		
Vital Signs					
Time: 0821	**BP:** 110/66	**Pulse:** 76	**Respirations:** 14	**Spo$_2$:** 93% on room air	
Time: 0826	**BP:** 110/64	**Pulse:** 78	**Respirations:** 14	**Spo$_2$:** 98% on 4 L/min NC	
Time:	**BP:**	**Pulse:**	**Respirations:**	**Spo$_2$:**	
EMS Treatment (circle all that apply)					
Oxygen @ 4 **L/min via (circle one):** (**NC**) **NRM** **Bag-mask device**		**Assisted Ventilation**	**Airway Adjunct**	**CPR**	
Defibrillation	**Bleeding Control**	**Bandaging**	**Splinting**	**Other:**	
Narrative					
Pt is an 86-year-old man with a history of cancer who reports general weakness and difficulty breathing for the past 2-3 days. Pt states his physician changed a cardiac medication within the last week and pt believes this may be causing the weakness, but he does not know the name of the medication. Pt is alert and oriented x4, sitting in a recliner. Breath sounds are equal but diminished in all fields, with no wheezing. Pt denies chest pain, dizziness, and nausea/vomiting. Cardiac monitor shows atrial fibrillation. Extensive medication list attached to this report. Pt placed on 4 L/min O_2 NC prior to transport. Pt lifted from recliner to stretcher and secured. Medical control report to Dr. Brown, no orders. Pt transported without change to Regional Hospital. Report to Shari, RN upon arrival.**End of report**					

Prep Kit

▶ Ready for Review

- To fulfill your role as a paramedic, you must be able to communicate rapidly, efficiently, and effectively when responding to an emergency call.
- The phases of communication during an EMS call include notification, information gathering, dispatch, response, potential prearrival instructions for the caller, communication during on-scene care, transport, and communication with medical control or the receiving facility while en route.
- Dispatchers communicate with people who call 9-1-1 in an emergency, and with the EMS responders being sent to the scene. The dispatcher identifies the exact location of the patient, the telephone number, the nature of the emergency, and specific

Prep Kit (continued)

information about the patient's condition and emergency, such as the types of vehicles involved in a motor vehicle crash or hazards at the scene.

- Dispatchers are also responsible for monitoring communications with the ambulance, coordinating communication with medical control and other agencies, and recording the times when the various phases of the call occurred.
- Emergency medical dispatch requires special training that teaches dispatchers to provide basic medical instructions to emergency callers over the phone. Updates resulting from this prearrival care can be communicated to the EMS crew as they are en route.
- Radio is one of the main methods of communication in EMS. The most commonly used bands for medical communications are the VHF band and UHF band. The higher the frequency, the less interference there is, but the shorter the transmission range.
- Systems used for radio transmission include simplex, duplex, and multiplex.
  - Simplex operates on one frequency and allows the transmission to go one way.
  - Duplex utilizes two paired frequencies which may allow simultaneous transmission and reception or the use of repeaters to boost range.
  - Multiplex allows for the transmission of multiple data streams simultaneously.
- An EMS communications system consists of a base station, mobile and portable transceivers, repeaters, and a backup communications system.
- Digital trunked radio systems utilize sophisticated computer systems to manage frequency and channel use for multiple users, and permit communication between a wide range of users.
- Interoperability is the capability of radio communications systems to communicate with each other, and with equipment from different manufacturers and systems.
- The FCC controls frequency allocation and licensing in the United States. It also establishes technical standards for radio equipment, establishes and enforces rules and regulations for the operation of radio equipment, and monitors transmissions. Communications over frequencies assigned for medical purposes are to be used strictly for that purpose.
- Cell phones are becoming more common in EMS communications systems. Many newer cell phones (smartphones) have GPS systems built in, which aid the enhanced 9-1-1 operator to determine exactly where the call is being made.
- Biotelemetry (or telemetry) is used to transmit patient data to a distant terminal. In EMS, it is most often used to transmit 12-lead ECGs. This technology can be useful in diagnosing STEMI and can allow medical control or you to make appropriate treatment and destination decisions.
- Keep radio communication clear, accurate, and concise. One of the main goals is clarity. Use the international radiotelephony phonetic alphabet to aid transmission of spellings.
- Remember that your words can be heard by anyone who is listening. Keep your communications professional at all times. Do not transmit a patient's name or personal information over the radio, which would be in violation of HIPAA.
- Most EMS systems use clear text or plain language in radio communications, but some still use radio codes. If your agency uses codes, then be sure to learn them.
- When you report medical information, include the destination facility and ETA; patient's age and sex; chief complaint; brief history; medications and important allergies; level of consciousness and degree of distress; mental status; vital signs; physical findings in head-to-toe order; ECG findings; treatment; and response to treatment.
- Many of the calls you will run as a paramedic will take you into people's homes, day and night, and in the most private moments of their lives. Try to see every invitation into the home of someone else as a personal honor in a time and place where no one else would be welcome. Give your patients your undivided attention.
- Active listening is repeating the key parts of a patient's responses to questions. It helps confirm the information the patient is providing and avoids any misunderstanding.
- As a therapeutic communicator, your most essential challenge is to convey calm, genuine concern for someone you have never met.
- When you first meet a patient, introduce yourself and ask for his or her name. This technique communicates your respect.
- Patient modesty matters, no matter how acute the medical condition. If the patient is not personally sensitive to it, then family members most certainly are.
- When you need to know how patients feel, try asking open-ended questions—questions that do not have a yes or no answer, and which do not give them specific options from which to choose. When you are trying to find specific facts (for example, a medical history), use closed-ended or direct questions.

Prep Kit (continued)

- If you sense that patients are trying to put something into words, but are having trouble, be patient. Do not say anything at all for a few seconds. Let them talk.
- If you have tried clarification and you are still not sure what patients are trying to tell you, then sometimes it helps to vocalize what you think they have said and invite them to correct you.
- Nonverbal communication can be as powerful as words.
- Direct eye contact generally communicates honesty and concern, but this technique may not be the case in some cultures.
- Posture is important. Try to position your eyes at the same level or below the level of the patient's eyes.
- Some people do not like to be touched at all. To others, it is a valuable assurance that someone cares about them. Try gently touching the patient on a neutral part of the body, such as a shoulder or arm, especially when you are trying to reassure him or her or to reduce fear.
- Hostile or angry patients may present a threat to you and others. Always approach with caution and maintain eye contact. Do not interview hostile or potentially violent patients or bystanders by yourself.
- Do not presume that older people are harder to communicate with than younger people, just because of their age.
- Children can pose treatment and communication challenges even to the most experienced EMS personnel. Minimize your movements, lower your voice, and touch them as gently as you can. Try keeping your eye level with or below the child's eye level by sitting on the floor and placing the child on the cot or on a parent or caregiver's lap.
- When you encounter a patient who has trouble communicating, remember that family members or primary caregivers who know these patients well can facilitate your efforts. They can also help you alleviate the patient's fear and anxiety.
- Interacting with people of cultures different from your own can be challenging. Learn about the different cultural groups that exist in your service area. It is considered respectful if you make an effort to learn about another person's language and culture.
- Manners, hand gestures, and body language may differ among cultures. Remember that another person's culture may have different rules for polite behavior than your own.
- You may encounter traditional or folk medicine practices that seem strange to you. If you encounter something you do not understand, then consider that the patient or family may be trying to manage the illness using traditional health practices from their native culture.
- Make use of qualified medical interpreters whenever possible for patients who speak a different language. Be cautious when using family members to interpret, and avoid using young children unless no other option is available.

▶ Vital Vocabulary

automatic crash notification (ACN) On-board computer systems in motor vehicles that automatically send telemetry data to a monitoring service in the event of a crash, which then relays the data to emergency responders; also called advanced automatic crash notification.

base station A radio at a fixed location (such as a hospital or dispatch center) consisting of a transmitter, receiver, and antenna.

biotelemetry Transmission of physiologic data, such as an electrocardiogram, from the patient to a distant point of reception (commonly referred to in emergency medical services as telemetry).

cell phones Wireless telephones that communicate via radio waves with the telephone system through an interconnected network of repeater stations called cells.

clear text Using regular language (plain English) and accepted terms to enhance clarity of communication, rather than using ten-codes or other code systems.

closed-ended question A question that is specific and focused, requiring either a yes or no answer, or an answer chosen from specific options.

computer assisted dispatch (CAD) Linked dispatch center computer consoles and vehicle-mounted mobile data terminals

crew resource management (CRM) An operational practice designed to enhance communication and teamwork, and to thereby reduce preventable errors.

cultural competence An understanding of the predominant cultures that exist in the geographic area in which the paramedic provides patient care.

culture The system of beliefs, attitudes, and behaviors that are learned and shared by members of a group.

digital radio The transmission of information via radio waves using native digital (computer) data or analog (voice) signals that have been converted to a digital signal and compressed.

dispatch To send to a specific destination or to send on a task.

Prep Kit *(continued)*

duplex Radio system using paired frequencies to permit the use of remote repeaters or simultaneous transmission and reception.

emergency medical dispatch (EMD) A program specifically designed to meet the unique needs of emergency medical services response and of callers reporting a medical emergency, including first aid instructions given by specially trained dispatchers to callers over the telephone while an ambulance is en route to the call.

encoded radio signals An embedded signal that permits controlled access to the radio transmission.

enhanced 9-1-1 system An emergency communications system that collects information about 9-1-1 calls from the telephone network, such as the phone number and location of the caller, and displays this information on the dispatcher's computer terminal.

ethnocentrism Viewing other cultures based solely upon the standards and values of one's own culture; a belief in the inherent superiority of one's own cultural or ethnic group.

Federal Communications Commission (FCC) The independent government agency that regulates interstate and international communications by radio, television, wire, satellite and cable in all 50 states, the District of Columbia, and US territories.

frequency The number of cycles (oscillations) per second of a radio signal.

geographic information system (GIS) Technology that uses global positioning system and other data to map the locations of objects and events.

hertz (Hz) Unit of measure of a frequency equal to 1 cycle per second; 1 million Hz equals one megahertz and 1000 megahertz equals one gigahertz.

interoperability Public safety communications systems which are compatible across all local, tribal, state, and federal agencies.

landline Communications system linked by wires, usually in reference to a conventional telephone system.

medical priority dispatch system (MPDS) A dispatch system using a specific format to indicate the nature of the emergency and its priority.

mutual aid Assistance to other nearby agencies when local resources are overwhelmed.

multiplex Simultaneous transmission of multiple data streams, most often voice and electrocardiogram signals.

narrow band Reassignment of frequencies by the Federal Communications Commission to a 12.5 megahertz spacing, now required for all emergency medical services and public safety radio systems.

noise Interference in a radio signal.

off-line medical control Patient care orders in the form of protocols or standing orders that do not require direct contact with the medical control physician.

online medical control Patient care orders provided directly to the paramedic by the medical control physician by radio or telephone.

open-ended question A question that does not have a yes or no answer, and that does not give the patient specific options from which to choose.

pervasive developmental disorders (PDDs) A group of disorders that cause delays in many areas of childhood development, such as the development of skills to communicate and interact socially, and may include repetitive body movements and difficulty with changes in routine; includes autism and Asperger syndrome, among others.

public safety answering point (PSAP) The location to which 9-1-1 calls are routed, which may or may not serve as the dispatch center.

radio dead spots Areas where mobile or portable radios are unable to communicate with a repeater.

remote terminal A terminal that receives transmissions of telemetry and voice from the field and transmits messages back, usually through the base station.

repeater Remote radio transceiver that receives radio signals and rebroadcasts them at a higher power, extending the range of a radio communications system.

simplex Radio communication using a single frequency.

situation, background, assessment, and recommendation (SBAR) A structured patient report format designed to convey important information in a concise manner.

squelch Filtering system to block background noise when a radio is on but not receiving a signal.

telemedicine Computer-based system permitting real-time two-way audio, video, and data communication between the paramedic and medical control physician.

ten-code A radio code system using the number 10 plus another number. No longer used in many emergency medical services systems.

therapeutic communication Communicating with the patient using specific strategies to encourage the patient to express ideas and feelings, and to convey respect and acceptance.

transceiver A radio containing both a transmitter and a receiver, a two-way radio.

Prep Kit *(continued)*

trunked radio system Computerized sharing of radio frequencies by multiple units, agencies, or systems.

ultra high frequency (UHF) band The portion of the radio frequency spectrum between 300 and 3,000 megahertz.

universal timeout A planned pause before the beginning of a procedure that improves communication among all personnel involved and reduces preventable errors.

very high frequency (VHF) band The portion of the radio frequency spectrum between 30 and 300 megahertz.

▶ References

1. "Communicate." *Merriam-Webster: Dictionary and Thesaurus*. http://www.merriam-webster.com. Accessed March 25, 2016.
2. Trembley AL, Page D. EMS improves with crew resource management training. *J Emerg Med Serv.* http://www.jems.com/articles/print/volume-40/issue-4/departments/research-review/ems-improves-with-crew-resource-management-training.html. April 6, 2015. Accessed November 6, 2016.
3. Page D. New psychomotor exam for nationally registered paramedics begins in January. *J Emerg Med Serv*. http://www.jems.com/articles/print/volume-41/issue-10/departments-columns/priority-traffic/new-psychomotor-exam-for-nationally-registered-paramedics-begins-in-january.html. Published October 1, 2016. Accessed December 6, 2016.
4. APCO International. *Minimum Training Standards for Public Safety Telecommunicators.* APCO ANS 3.103.2.2015. https://www.apcointl.org/doc/911-resources/apco-standards/75-minimum-training-standards-for-public-safety-telecommunicators/file.html. Accessed December 6, 2016.
5. Wilson MJ. *The ARRL Operating Manual*. 9th edition. Newington, CT: The Amateur Radio Relay League; 2007:2-1–4-28.
6. U.S. Fire Administration, Federal Emergency Management Agency. *Voice Radio Communications Guide for the Fire Service: June 2016.* https://www.usfa.fema.gov/downloads/pdf/publications/voice_radio_communications_guide_for_the_fire_service.pdf. Accessed December 8, 2016.
7. Federal Communications Commission. Narrowbanding Overview. https://www.fcc.gov/general/narrowbanding-overview. Updated February 3, 2016. Accessed April 4, 2016.
8. Office of Emergency Communications, U.S. Department of Homeland Security. *National Interoperability Field Operations Guide, Version 1.4.* January 2011. https://www.dhs.gov/xlibrary/assets/nifog-v1-4-resized-for-pda-viewing.pdf. Accessed January 13, 2017.
9. U.S. Department of Homeland Security. Statement of Requirements for Public Safety Wireless Communications and Interoperability. The SAFECOM Program. Ver. 1.1. January 26, 2006. http://www.emsa.ca.gov/Media/Default/PDF/sorv1.pdf. Accessed February 22, 2017.
10. APCO Project 25 Steering Committee. APCO Project 25 Statement of Requirements. http://project25.org/images/stories/ptig/docs/Technical_Documents/12131211_Approved_P25_SoR_12-11-13.pdf. Published December 11, 2013. Accessed March 30, 2016.
11. Ludwig G. What are you posting on Facebook? *Firehouse*. December 3, 2010. http://www.firehouse.com/article/10465142/firefighters-and-paramedics-getting-in-trouble-over-posts. Accessed December 6, 2016.
12. Wang SC, Kohoyda-Inglis CJ, MacWilliams JB, et al. Results of first field test of telemetry based injury severity prediction. Abstract presented at: 24th International Technical Conference on the Enhanced Safety of Vehicles (ESV); June 8-11, 2015; Gothenburg, Sweden. https://www.acep.org/globalassets/support/innovatED_supportfiles/results-of-first-field-test-of-elemetry-based-injury-severity-predictio.pdf. Accessed January 13, 2017.
13. Amateur Radio Relay League. Two flavors of amateur radio emergency operation. http://www.arrl.org/ares-races-faq. Accessed May 2, 2016.
14. Grigoriev AI, Orlov OI. Telemedicine and spaceflight. *Aviat Space Environ Med*. 2002; 73(7):688-93.
15. Grose T. Speed is the drug. *Newsweek*. http://www.newsweek.com/2014/05/02/speed-drug-248536.html. Published April 24, 2014. Accessed March 18, 2016.
16. Rao A, Kardouh Y, Darda S, et al. Impact of the prehospital ECG on door-to-balloon time in ST elevation myocardial infarction. *Catheter Cardiovasc Interv*. 2010 Feb;75(2):174-8. doi:10.1002/ccd.22257.
17. American Heart Association. Recommendations for Criteria for STEMI Systems of Care. http://www.heart.org/HEARTORG/HealthcareResearch/MissionLifelineHomePage/EMS/Recommendations-for-Criteria-for-STEMI-Systems-of-Care_UCM_312070_Article.jsp#.VxBY_mNQGlA. Published August 23, 2013. Updated October 4, 2016. Accessed May 15, 2016.
18. Bashford C. Telemedicine today: part 1—getting started. http://www.emsworld.com/article/12184039/telemedicine-today-part-1-getting-started. *EMSWorld*. Published March 21, 2016. Accessed March 28, 2016.
19. Sierra Wireless. The "firstnet-ready" mobile office: top considerations for connecting first

Prep Kit *(continued)*

responders [White paper]. http://www.jems.com/whitepapers/2015/12/the-firstnet-ready-mobile-office-top-considerations-for-connecting-first-responders.whitepaperpdf.render.pdf. Published November 10, 2015. Accessed March 25, 2016.

20. e-CFR Title 47, Chapter 1, Subchapter D, Part 90, Subpart B, §90.15. Electronic Code of Federal Regulations. U.S. Government Publishing Office. http://www.ecfr.gov/cgi-bin/text-idx?SID=b41258b0691d3b0b98a9ff13931e8597&mc=true&node=pt47.5.90&rgn=div5#se47.5.90_115. Accessed March 28, 2016.
21. Federal Emergency Management Agency. NIMS and use of plain language [FEMA publication no. NA: 023-06]. https://www.fema.gov/pdf/emergency/nims/plain_lang.pdf. Updated December 19, 2006. Accessed April 10, 2016.
22. Harrington JW. Surgical time outs in a combat zone. *AORN J.* 2009; (89)3:535-537.
23. American College of Emergency Physicians. Transfer of patient care between EMS providers and receiving facilities [Policy statement]. *Ann Emerg Med.* 2013;63(4):503. doi:10.1016/j.annemergmed.2013.12.023.
24. SBAR toolkit. Institute for Healthcare Improvement website. http://www.ihi.org/resources/pages/tools/sbartoolkit.aspx. Accessed January 13, 2017.
25. Masters R. Preventing invisible wounds. *EMSWorld*. http://www.emsworld.com/article/12223916/preventing-invisible-wounds. Published August 1, 2016. Accessed December 6, 2016.
26. Beyene Y. Ethiopians and Eritreans. In: Lipson JG, Dibble SL, eds. *Culture & Clinical Care*. San Francisco, CA: UCSF Nursing Press; 2008:163-176.
27. Galanti G-A. *Caring for Patients from Different Cultures.* 4th ed. Philadelphia, PA: University of Pennsylvania Press; 2008:197-200.

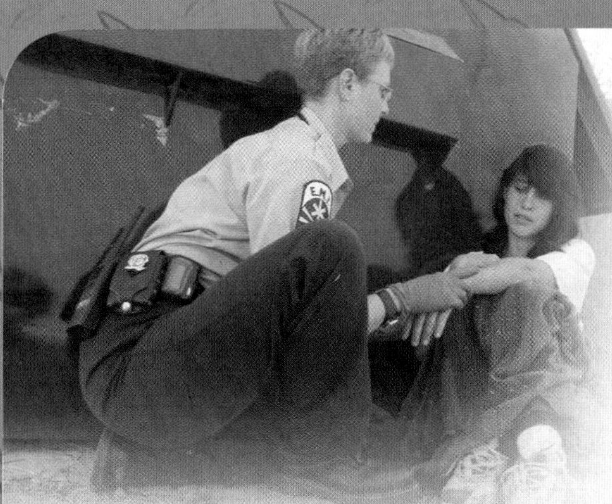

Assessment *in Action*

You are dispatched to a motor vehicle collision at a busy intersection. Initial reports indicate that several vehicles are involved with an unknown number of patients, and some patients may be entrapped. Your response time to the scene is approximately 2 minutes.

1. The 9-1-1 caller reporting the collision is agitated and yelling. What should the dispatcher do to obtain the necessary information from the caller?

- **A.** Ask the caller to put someone else on the phone.
- **B.** Ignore the caller and attempt to determine the location of the call using the GPS data from the cellular signal.
- **C.** Ask specific questions in a calm voice, such as the exact location of the incident and the number of vehicles involved.
- **D.** Send a law enforcement officer to the location to confirm the collision before dispatching the ambulance.

2. Which of the following factors would you NOT discuss with your team during your response to this call?

- **A.** The duties of each team member on initial arrival to the scene
- **B.** The location and capabilities of the closest hospital
- **C.** Where to locate a helicopter landing zone
- **D.** What additional resources may be needed

Assessment *in Action* *(continued)*

3. When would it be appropriate to post photographs of patients at the incident scene or other identifiable patient information on social media?

- **A.** When you believe that the event is newsworthy
- **B.** When requested to do so by coworkers or supervisors who were not present at the scene
- **C.** When the patient is a well-known public figure
- **D.** It is never appropriate to post photographs or identifiable patient information on social media.

4. Dispatch assigns a single tactical frequency to be used by all responders for on-scene communications. This type of communication system is called a ___________ system.

- **A.** duplex
- **B.** simplex
- **C.** mono-frequency
- **D.** primary

5. An EMS supervisor unit arrives and establishes a triage area. You are assigned to transport a critically injured patient to the local trauma center. What information should you transmit to your dispatch center on leaving the scene?

- **A.** Patient's name, ambulance number, and the number of patients in your ambulance
- **B.** Destination facility, mode of transport, and the nature of the patient's injuries
- **C.** Unit number, destination facility, and the number of patients in your ambulance
- **D.** Unit number, destination facility, and the nature of the patient's injuries

6. You are transporting with the lights and siren activated, and the ambulance cabin is noisy. Your patient is awake and alert. Which of the following methods is the best example of how to obtain a medical history from this patient?

- **A.** Postpone obtaining the patient's medical history or medications; this information can be determined at the hospital.
- **B.** Lean close and calmly say, "I know you are scared and in pain, but it is important that I ask you some questions."
- **C.** Write notes on a dry erase board and hold it in front of the patient.
- **D.** Look in his wallet for a medical information card or for a medical ID bracelet, because it is too noisy to communicate.

7. You contact the destination trauma center by radio and provide a report to medical control. Which of the following is the best example of a well-organized radio report?

- **A.** Destination facility, estimated time of arrival, a brief history of the present illness or injury, pertinent physical findings in head-to-toe order, treatment performed
- **B.** Treatment performed, estimated time of arrival, physical findings in head-to-toe order, a description of the crash scene and vehicle damage, patient's personal physician
- **C.** Destination facility, patient's insurance information, a brief history of the present illness or injury, pertinent physical findings in head-to-toe order, treatment performed
- **D.** Medical control facility, comprehensive medical history, physical exam findings in order of severity, treatment performed, location of call

8. You send a 12-lead ECG to the medical control physician. The technology used to send this tracing is called:

- **A.** biotelemetry.
- **B.** biophysics.
- **C.** telecardiology.
- **D.** direct medical control.

9. Should you treat patients from different cultures the same way you would a member of your own culture?

10. How can you handle a hostile patient more effectively?

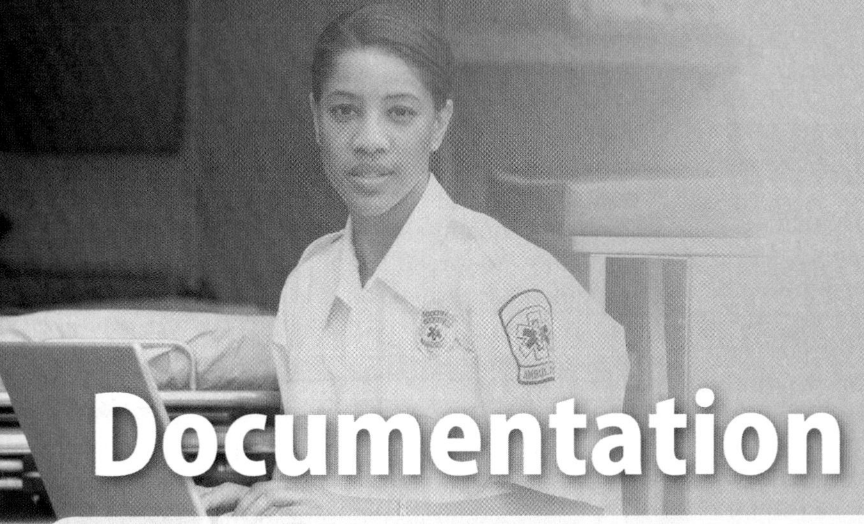

CHAPTER 6

Documentation

National EMS Education Standard Competencies

Preparatory

Integrates comprehensive knowledge of EMS systems, the safety/well-being of the paramedic, and medical/legal and ethical issues, which is intended to improve the health of EMS personnel, patients, and the community.

Documentation

- Recording patient findings (pp 170, 173-174, 179-183)
- Principles of medical documentation and report writing (pp 170-179)

Knowledge Objectives

1. Explain the legal implications of the patient care report (PCR). (pp 170-171)
2. Discuss the implications of the Health Insurance Portability and Accountability Act of 1996 as they relate to documentation. (pp 171, 182, 185)
3. Describe the purposes of documentation. (pp 171-172)
4. Compare handwritten PCRs with electronic PCRs, and discuss the pros and cons of each type. (pp 172-173)
5. Identify the information required in a PCR, including the standard items that must be documented for every emergency call. (p 173)
6. Discuss the process for documenting transfer of care and care prior to arrival. (pp 173-174)
7. Discuss the process for documenting refusal of care, including the legal implications. (pp 174-178)
8. Discuss state and/or local reporting requirements for special circumstances, including workplace injuries and illnesses, mass-casualty incidents, occupational exposures, cases of alleged abuse or neglect, and involvement of on-scene physicians or other agencies. (pp 175, 178-179)
9. Discuss various formats for the narrative portion of the PCR. (pp 179-181)
10. Discuss why it is important that documentation be accurate, legible, and professional. (pp 181-184)
11. Explain the procedure to follow should an error occur during or after creating a PCR. (pp 184-185)
12. Discuss the consequences of intentional falsification of documentation. (p 185)
13. Discuss why it is important to accurately document incident times. (pp 185-186)

Skills Objectives

1. Demonstrate completion of a PCR. (pp 179-186)

YOU are the Paramedic PART 1

Your unit has been dispatched to a single-vehicle collision involving a pole near the county courthouse at approximately 1300 hours on a weekday. On arrival, you ensure the scene is safe before you exit the ambulance. The vehicle appears to have light damage to the front bumper and hood. You don your personal protective equipment and approach the vehicle. As you are walking up, a man opens the door of the vehicle and attempts unsuccessfully to stand up. The man falls back down on the seat and exclaims in a loud, slurred voice, "I need my lawyer." You look past the patient into the passenger compartment and see that the air bags have deployed.

1. What is your first consideration in regard to this patient?
2. What is your first consideration in regard to the scene?

Introduction

Although documentation may not be the first item that comes to mind when you are thinking of pursuing a career in emergency medical services (EMS), it is an important part of the patient care process. Thorough documentation pulls together the run for all parties involved. The adage, "No job is finished until the paperwork is done" is especially true in EMS. Your report, most commonly referred to as the **patient care report (PCR)** or sometimes called the prehospital care report, is the only written record of the events that transpired during the call for service. The ability to write an effective, accurate, and proper PCR is one of the most important skills you will learn as a paramedic. The PCR is the legal record for the call, and it will be a part of the patient's medical record and the patient's chart in the emergency department (ED) of the hospital. A complete PCR will not only allow other health care providers to obtain information about what occurred from the start of the call to its conclusion, but will also help guide future patient care via research and quality assurance **Figure 6-1**. As a paramedic, you must be able to create a PCR thoroughly and efficiently.

You need to know what constitutes a PCR, what information must be included, who might read the PCR, when the PCR must be completed, and what terminology may be used. The information in your report may be categorized as either objective or subjective. **Objective information** includes the measurable signs that you observe and record, such as blood pressure. **Subjective information** includes information that is told to you, but which cannot be seen, such as the symptoms patients describe—the degree of pain, for example. When you write your PCR, try to utilize the patient's own words as much as possible. Place quotation marks around any direct statements; for example, "The patient rates the pain an '8' on a 0 to 10 scale." You must record both objective *and* subjective information and the details of patient care for every call. The PCR needs to be complete, accurate, and legible because it can provide the basis of defense in legal proceedings. The PCR is vitally important to your service or agency for many other reasons, including the facilitation of quality care, continuity of care, and billing to insurance. Your report should paint a picture of the entire call that is accurate and clear to the reader.

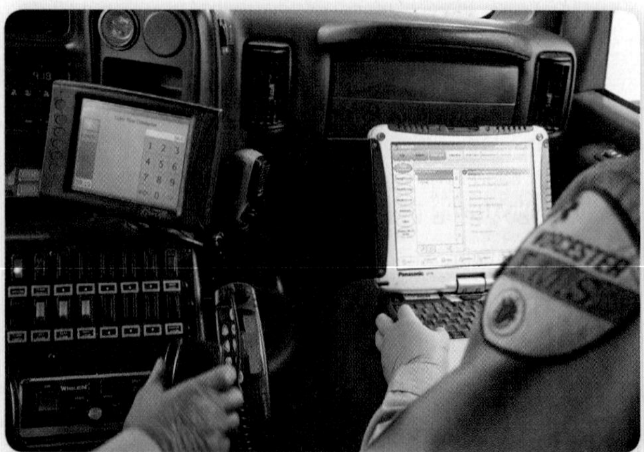

Figure 6-1 Electronic patient care reports, shown here, are becoming the standard in EMS documentation.

Legal Implications of a PCR

Although you may include subjective information from the patient in your report (such as statements from him or her about symptoms), do not include any personal bias or your opinions. For example, avoid subjective statements such as, "The patient was drunk and out of control." Instead, use objective statements such as, "The patient had an altered mental status and stated he had 'eight beers' today." Poorly written, inappropriately documented PCRs could have adverse implications for patient care and for your career. Omissions or errors in your report could lead to further errors in care. Improper and inadequate reports also could result in litigation, loss of job or position, a negative reflection on your reputation as an EMS professional, and more.

The US court system has found paramedics guilty of neglect based on the failure to perform patient exams and submit completed paperwork. In one such example, a crew responded to the scene of a motor vehicle crash and the patient declined medical transport after a brief discussion with the paramedics. The crew cleared the scene without evaluating the patient. Later, the paramedics were called back for the same patient who had collapsed at the scene. The paramedics claimed that they owed no duty to act because they never initiated patient care. The judge did not accept this claim and found the paramedics to be negligent. Proper patient assessment should have been conducted and associated with a complete PCR. Even if the patient had refused any contact by the paramedics, they should have documented the refusal to help defend why they were unable to assess the patient.

No matter your particular writing style, your report should be complete, well written, legible, professional, and your sole source of information about the call. Your report may also be used in legal proceedings against you or someone else. In some cases, it may be your only defense against a complaint about a call—if you document what happened, then you will have solid evidence of your conduct and what transpired on the call. Your memory may not serve you well 5 to 7 years from now, but your written report will remain as the only record of why you performed a certain procedure or why you administered a particular medication to a patient. If it is well written, it will jog your memory and should provide a clear picture of the events of the call to all who read it. As discussed in Chapter 7, *Medical Terminology*, it is important that you use correct spelling, proper grammar, and accurate terminology in your report. Improper documentation could result in patient care errors and leave your professional character at stake if the report is called into question. The consequences of poor documentation will be discussed later in this chapter.

Finally, the Health Insurance Portability and Accountability Act (HIPAA) has ramifications related to patient care reporting. Refer to Chapter 4, *Medical, Legal, and Ethical Issues* for a discussion of HIPAA.

Words of Wisdom

HIPAA requires that reasonable administrative, technical, and physical safeguards be in place to aid in the protection of patient information. If you are unsure whether the equipment you may be using is safeguarded, then seek the advice of the administrators in your organization.

Documentation & Communication

To help protect patient information, do not leave paper PCRs or assessment cards on counters or any other area that is not secured. Always sign out of any computer systems that you may be using to create your ePCR after completing it. Many agencies use lockboxes as the location where completed paper PCRs should be placed.

Purposes of Documentation

Continuity of Care

The PCR serves as a record of the patient's condition on your arrival at the scene, the care that was provided, any changes in the patient's condition en route, and condition on arrival at the hospital. It is crucial that you document the incident as clearly as possible because the PCR will help other health care providers at the hospital understand the particular emergency and assessments and treatments performed thus far. Accurate reporting helps paint a picture of the environment the patient was taken out of, the mechanism of injury (MOI) or nature of illness (NOI), and ultimately leads to better patient care.

Minimum Requirements and Billing

Billing and administration are significant reasons why your PCR needs to be accurate and complete. Most EMS agencies bill for services to recover the costs of providing patient care. For complete and accurate revenue recovery, you must document all procedures performed, obtain the correct diagnosis codes (ICD-10 codes), and obtain the appropriate **medical necessity** signature (where required). Medicare, a national insurance program, sets the standard for medical necessity. The chart shown in Table 6-1 gives some of the significant findings that are required to show that the patient needed to be transported by an ambulance rather than by other means of transportation.

Table 6-1 Significant Findings That Indicate Medical Necessity for Ambulance Transport

- Patient is transported in an emergency mode (Code 3).
- Patient is in shock.
- Patient needs to be restrained.
- Patient requires emergency treatment while being transported (eg, oxygen therapy, intravenous therapy).
- Patient must be immobilized for transport or fracture management.
- Patient is experiencing an acute myocardial infarction or stroke.
- Patient has uncontrollable hemorrhage.
- Patient is able to be moved only by a stretcher because of a condition.

Data from Superseded Local Coverage Determination for Ambulance Services (Ground Ambulance…). Centers for Medicare & Medicaid Services. https://www.cms.gov/medicare-coverage-database/details/lcd-details.aspx?LCDId=35162. Accessed July 18, 2016.

In the narrative portion of your PCR (the section that allows for free-form writing), be as specific as you can. Include information such as which quadrant the abdominal pain may be in, what supplies you utilized, what rhythm the cardiac monitor showed, and if it was a diabetes-related condition, whether it was hypo- or hyperglycemia. Some insurance companies will deny charges for anything that is not documented in the narrative statement. (Narrative writing is discussed later in this chapter.) You need to document why a patient may have needed emergency care, especially in the case of private or scheduled transports, to ensure your service's billing information will result in payment from the responsible insurer, agency, or private payer. It is imperative for you to be accurate and complete in your documentation so that time is not spent correcting the documentation, thus delaying billing processing. You will often be trained by your agency and its billing company about what additional forms you need to complete as a part of each EMS response. You must understand that completing billing paperwork and supplying the most accurate and defensible information to the EMS agency are necessary portions of the call.

EMS Research

Just as billing has become necessary in EMS, so has research. As mentioned in Chapter 1, *EMS Systems*, proper documentation done by all EMS providers results in compiled data that are reviewed by researchers who then use that data to justify innovative, lifesaving techniques. Many states now require EMS agencies to submit data to the state EMS office to verify call volumes and skills used. This data may include the number of calls an agency responds to, the types of calls, care provided, and patient outcomes. Such patient care data collection can lead to improvement of the EMS system as a whole.

The National Emergency Medical Services Information System (NEMSIS) stores standardized EMS data from each individual state. This central repository will help assist states in collecting comparable data elements so the entire nation can benefit from research and use the trends for future curriculum development. The goal of NEMSIS is to define EMS care by collecting data to improve patient care, indicating equipment needs, and defining a standard of care across the nation.

▶ Incident Review and Quality Assurance

On occasion, PCRs may be requested for medical audits and other educational activities. Run reviews, or sessions in which peers and other medical professionals review PCRs for adherence to local protocols, quality assurance, and quality monitoring, should take place regularly. Peer review sessions not only support a healthy quality assurance process, but also allow the reviewers to learn from the patient care techniques used by others. Your reports may be used to calculate the number of times you have performed a specific skill, such as medication administration or oral intubation. Always accurately document all skills attempted and performed during patient care.

Documentation & Communication

EMS agencies and departments should have a process to ensure that all reports are well written, as well as a quality assurance program to ensure that no discrepancies exist between what was written in the PCR and what actually occurred on the call.

Types of PCRs

EMS has entered an age in which electronic documentation has become the standard. Although some services still use paper documentation, you will most likely document your emergency calls and other reports electronically. The many benefits of electronic documentation are discussed later in this section. Perhaps the most significant benefit is the ability for electronic data to be shared—not only between the facilities and personnel involved in a patient's care, thereby improving continuity and efficiency, but also among state and national databases to improve national data collection and further the advancement of evidence-based practice.

A multitude of PCR designs exist throughout the United States and range from half-page notes to complete and thorough reports. EMS patient care reporting has evolved over the years because the field of medicine has recognized the necessity for information about the patient's condition and interventions performed in the field. Some services have developed PCRs that nearly eliminate the narrative section and replace the space with either check boxes or dropdown menus with predetermined terms. You may encounter some reports that have hundreds of check boxes allowing for you to mark every action you took. The problem with these types of reports is that the format increases the risk of errors that may occur when your eyes become overwhelmed by so many check boxes and you accidentally select the wrong box. Regardless of what form of patient reporting your service may use, it is important that you obtain the proper information.

In most areas of the country, paper reporting has become a thing of the past because it is a duplication of work in the health care system. To fulfill EMS data collection requirements, handwritten reports must be entered into an electronic system, either by health care agencies or by outsourcing to third-party companies. Along with the additional data entry needs, a paper system also requires space to store the records, possibly for a lengthy period depending on state laws. The final reason for a shift away from paper reporting systems is error reduction. Too often, poor penmanship and spelling mistakes lead to medical errors related to medication doses and orders; an electronic system minimizes these errors. However, unless your ambulance has a printer in the unit, you most likely will be using a written refusal form when it is necessary to obtain a signature from the patient. You should then leave him or her with a copy of the refusal form. Patient refusals are discussed later in this chapter.

Many companies have created a variety of options for ePCRs. These services range from the scanning of paper forms to the creation of computer-based programs and applications for desktops, laptops, tablets, and smartphones that allow for more accurate and legible reports Figure 6-2.

Modern data systems can incorporate data from various sources, such as multiple facilities. This feature is in line with the major effort on the part of hospitals and physicians to improve the quality of cardiac, stroke, and diabetic care, and improve the success of resuscitation efforts. Such cutting-edge systems will ultimately include EMS documentation so that the PCR contains both information from the field and further data from the hospitals or facilities where the patient was treated. The result will be one comprehensive record of the care the patient received.

To ensure that data can be shared on a national level, electronic documentation systems should be NEMSIS-compliant. As mentioned, data submission to NEMSIS is important for EMS research, and to assess and improve EMS care throughout the country. The goal of NEMSIS is to facilitate submission of EMS data from all states, and part of that process is to implement electronic documentation systems in all states. Today, the majority of states and territories of the United States are either submitting electronic data to NEMSIS, or are actively working toward achieving this goal in the near future.

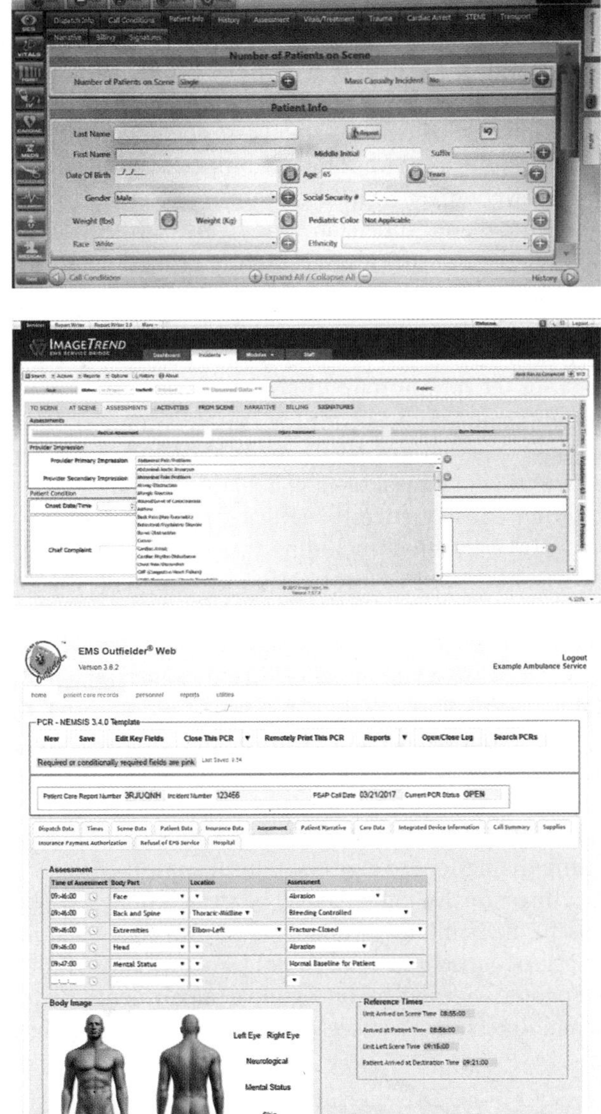

Figure 6-2 A variety of software programs exist for creating electronic patient care reports, allowing EMS personnel to clearly document details of the call.

Documentation for Every EMS Call

Every EMS call requires documentation. The **minimum data set** is the clinical assessment standard information that must be documented on every emergency call as set by Medicare and Medicaid, and per the National Highway Traffic Safety Administration for the purpose of the national data system. The minimum data set is divided into two sections: run data and patient data. Run data consist of such information as incident times, locations, responding units, and the names of crew members working at the incident. Patient data includes the following basic patient information:

- Chief complaint
- Level of consciousness (according to the AVPU [Awake and alert, responsive to Verbal stimuli, responsive to Pain, Unresponsive] scale) or mental status
- Vital signs
- Assessment
- Patient demographics (age, sex, ethnic background)

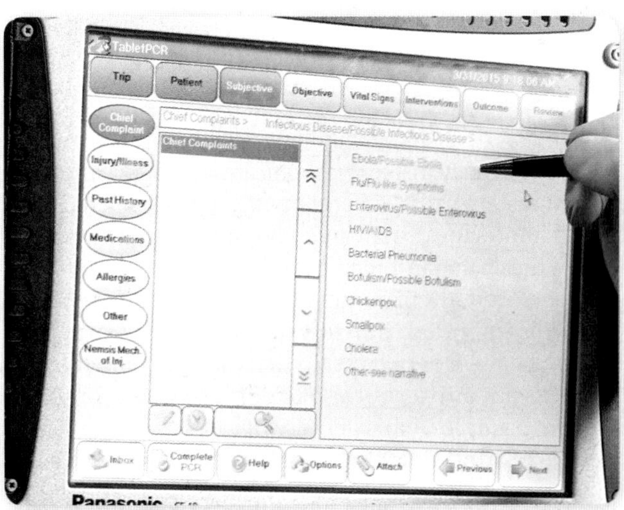

Figure 6-3 The minimum data set includes both patient information and administrative information.

The PCR should contain your objective observations of the scene, as well as the treatments provided, the effects of those treatments, and any changes that occurred in the patient's condition during the emergency call Figure 6-3. Your objective observations of the scene need to reflect such factors as the living conditions of the home, the MOI in a motor vehicle crash, or other areas of concern that you might have but which do not meet the reporting criteria. Depending on the type of your transport service, you may need to differentiate the treatments between those that were scheduled, such as in a transfer transport, and those that were unexpected because of changes in a patient's condition.

Transfer of Care

As the growing need for medical care begins to exceed that which is available, EMS personnel are seeing overwhelmed EDs and often find themselves leaving patients in hallways waiting to be seen. In your PCR, it is important that you are able to show in whose care you left the patient; otherwise, you could face allegations of abandonment (as discussed in Chapter 4, *Medical, Legal, and Ethical Issues*). Some agencies have begun to require signatures from physicians or nurses to verify that the patient was left with a medical professional with a higher level of training. Another situation that may require you to document a transfer of care is when you hand over your patient to another agency, such as an air medical team.

▶ Care Prior to Arrival

More emergency dispatch centers are shifting to a sophisticated system called **emergency medical dispatch (EMD)**, which allows the dispatcher to provide simple directions for medical care and medication administration via the phone. You may encounter such cases in your response area. It is important not only to obtain the information from the patient or caller as to what care they have received prior to your arrival, but also to document such findings. A good example of this delivery of care is when a person calls 9-1-1 and tells the dispatcher at an EMD center that he or she is experiencing chest pain. After detailed questioning, the dispatcher may have the patient chew 324 mg of aspirin, for example. If you fail to obtain such information from the patient, then that information is not relayed to the hospital via your PCR. As a result, the patient could accidentally receive another dose of the same medication, increasing the risk of complications.

You may also encounter off-duty health care providers and/or lay people providing emergency care prior to EMS arrival. Be sure to include their names and procedures in your report with specific notations that this emergency medical care was provided prior to your arrival.

Situations Requiring Additional Documentation

Certain special situations require additional or different reporting procedures. These situations are discussed in the next sections.

▶ Refusal of Care

Legal aspects of patient care were discussed in Chapter 4, *Medical, Legal, and Ethical Issues*, but this section will cover the necessary documentation in more depth. With the increase in malpractice lawsuits, refusal of care is one of the most difficult elements of patient care documentation, but also one of the most important. Competent adult patients have the right to refuse medical care or to consent to treatment. Know and understand the rights of your patients. Familiarize yourself with the applicable laws in your state about patient care and who has the right to refuse such care. For a person to refuse care, the decision must be based on the patient's sufficient knowledge of his or her situation.

Your most important job is to ensure your patient is fully informed about his or her current situation, his or her right to receive or refuse medical care, and the consequences of a refusal of care. Explain in great detail the potential consequences of refusing medical care when it may be warranted, including the possibility of death. You must convey this information in a language that the person understands, and then document this information on the PCR. In some agencies, the EMS provider will have a witness observe him or her reading the refusal statement to the patient, and will then ask the patient to initial the statement followed by a signature on the refusal section of the PCR. The refusal documentation should clearly show the process you went through, how was it was documented, and who witnessed it. The process is not merely about getting the patient to sign the refusal section.

Unresponsive patients may be treated under implied consent. Be familiar with the laws of your state regarding the age of consent, care of minors, emancipated minors, and people with mental or cognitive impairments, such as mental illness or the effects of drug or alcohol use. Above

YOU are the Paramedic — PART 2

The engine company that was dispatched with you arrives on scene, and they park their vehicle to ensure scene safety. Your crew directs the engine company to make sure the crashed vehicle is secure while you and your partner attempt to speak to the patient. The patient yells at you to leave him alone. Your partner taps your shoulder and asks you if you smell alcohol and you reply that you do. She also points to an empty vodka bottle on the floor of the vehicle. The patient yells, "You don't know who I am, do you? You're going to pay!" You hear a bystander say, "Isn't that Assemblyman Taylor?"

Recording Time: 0 Minutes	
Appearance	Awake
Level of consciousness	Alert
Airway	Open
Breathing	Adequate
Circulation	Appears normal

3. Why is it unacceptable to document the patient's appearance as "drunk" on a PCR?

4. Would it be acceptable to document that the patient is "yelling" for the breathing description on a PCR?

all else, you need to confirm that every reasonable effort has been made to ensure the patient's welfare and best interests.

If the person refusing care has an obvious injury or medical condition that requires immediate medical attention, then involve online medical control for further guidance and assistance. In such cases where you do not agree with the refusal, your agency should have a protocol or policy in place to guide your next steps—for example, contact your supervisor, involve law enforcement, or involve medical control. If contact is made with any of those parties, then document it on the PCR, including the events that transpired.

It is essential that you have a witness to the refusal process to ensure that your patient has sufficient knowledge of the situation to make an informed choice. If the patient refuses to sign the refusal form, then your witness should also be present. Document the observations of the witness, and include his or her name and contact information as well.

Perform or attempt a complete medical history and patient assessment when possible and practical. This process includes obtaining a full set of baseline vital signs. If a patient refuses to allow such an assessment, then document this carefully on the PCR. Be sure to evaluate the patient's mental status using the AVPU scale. You may consider a person's mental status to be impaired if the person makes nonsensical statements or is not oriented to person, place, or time. The impairment can be a result of an injury, a medical condition (such as electrolyte imbalance or hypoglycemia), mental illness, or use of drugs or alcohol.

Always politely and tactfully explain to patients that they have the right to change their mind and may contact EMS later. Such an exchange of information should be witnessed and documented with signatures. Include identifying information such as phone numbers of the witnesses involved, who frequently may be law enforcement personnel or others at the scene. Clearly document the emergency medical care that you intended to provide if the patient had not refused care. You should also document in whose care you left the patient, such as self, law enforcement personnel, or family member.

Also, be sure that you have proposed all potential methods of care, including alternative options, even if they are not your first choice of treatment. For example, you could suggest that the patient be taken to the hospital for further care by a family member. Although that situation may not be ideal, the patient will ultimately be seen at the hospital. Always encourage transport via ambulance because a patient's condition can change at any time, and without medical personnel available to assist, the change could have serious consequences.

At times, patients may agree to transport but refuse a particular procedure, such as intravenous therapy or immobilization. In such cases, handle the refusal of the specific procedure(s) as if it is a complete refusal of care. Include an explanation of any associated risks and complications of refusal, a signature from the patient acknowledging refusal of a portion of care, and a signature from a witness. Ensure complete and accurate documentation **Figure 6-4**.

Table 6-2 provides a reasonable list of items to include when documenting a refusal of care within the PCR.

▶ Workplace Injuries and Illnesses

With the growing budgetary restrictions in many workplaces, a paramedic often provides medical care in the workplace rather than a traditional nurse. According to guidelines from the Occupational Safety and Health Administration (OSHA), workplace injuries must be logged. Institutions may also have specific forms and requirements for documenting workplace injuries. Many injuries are minor, requiring only basic first aid and thus do not require an OSHA record; however, local documentation may still be required by the employer. When you document a workplace injury or illness, be sure to document what precautions were taken and what protective equipment was being worn by the person involved. Companies can be fined heavily for safety violations, so proper documentation is important from the perspective of both the employer and OSHA. Note that reporting regulations vary from state to state. Familiarize yourself with the requirements of your state. As a paramedic, you may also perform medical monitoring for hazardous materials teams, may respond to the workplace injuries of other public employees, or may experience on-the-job injuries or illnesses yourself, which you will need to appropriately document and report to supervisors to receive workers' compensation.

▶ Special Circumstances

You may encounter many circumstances during your career that puzzle you with the documentation requirements. Some of those situations could be mass-casualty incidents (MCIs), occupational exposures, cases of alleged abuse or neglect, and instances when a physician arrives or is already present on the scene of a call. Each of these situations may require specialized forms per your state or local agency, so become familiar with these local forms of documentation and the requirements for use.

During an MCI, the patient load can easily overwhelm providers and, in the best interest of patient care, documentation often occurs initially on triage tags. Do not wait until an MCI occurs to become familiar with triage tags. Learn where they are stored, the information needed on the tags, and situations that may warrant use in your agency or department. Triage tags and procedures are discussed in Chapter 47, *Incident Management and Mass-Casualty Incidents*. Although the triage tag is designed to relay information, it is important for each emergency responder completing the tags to supply as much information as possible on them. When the time comes to transport the patient, the crew in the ambulance should complete a PCR on each patient. Although the information will be limited on the PCR, it is still imperative to complete the report to the best of your ability.

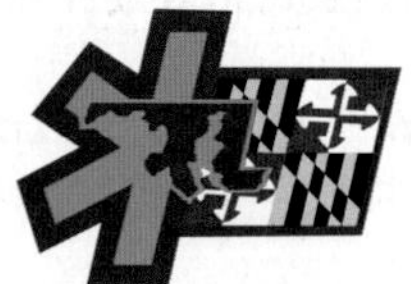

Patient Initiated Refusal of EMS

Patient Name: Doe, John	Primary Care Giver: John Smith, NREMT-P	
Agency: BALTIMORE COUNTY FIRE DEPARTMENT	Incident#: 1122141	eMEDS#: 00314105399
Unit #: Medic 14	Inc Date Entered: 11/22/2016	Inc Time Entered: 1824 hrs

I (or my guardian) have been informed regarding the state of my present physical condition to the extent I allowed an examination, and I (or my guardian) hereby refuse to accept such medical care and/or transportation as recommended by representatives of the EMS System above.

I (or my guardian) do hereby for myself, my heirs, executors, and administrators and assigns forever release and fully discharge said EMS system, its officers, employees, medical consultants, hospitals, borrowed servants or agents from any and all conceivable liability that might arise from this refusal of care and/or transportation, and I (and my guardian) therefore agree to hold them completely harmless. I (or my guardian) have been informed that a refusal of care and/or transportation for an evaluation may cause me to suffer PAIN, DISABILITY, LOSS of FUNCTION, WORSENING of my CONDITION, or even DEATH as a result of my illness/injury. As a competent adult, I (or my guardian) fully understand all of the above, and am/is capable of determining a rational decision on my own behalf.

Providers: When encountering a patient who is attempting to refuse EMS treatment or transport, access his or her condition, and record whether the patient screening reveals any lack of medical decision-making capability (1-3,4a or b) or high risk criteria (5-8).

1) Medical Capacity: Was the patient disoriented to person? If yes, transport	☐ Yes ☑ No
2) Medical Capacity: Was the patient disoriented to place? If yes, transport	☐ Yes ☑ No
3) Medical Capacity: Was the patient disoriented to time? If yes, transport	☐ Yes ☑ No
4) Medical Capacity: Was the patient disoriented to situation? If yes, transport	☐ Yes ☑ No
5) Medical Capacity: Did the patient show altered level of consciousness? If yes, transport	☐ Yes ☑ No
6) Medical Capacity: Alcohol or drug ingestion by history or exam with slurred speech? If yes, transport	☐ Yes ☑ No
7) Medical Capacity: Alcohol or drug ingestion by history or exam with unsteady gait? If yes, transport	☐ Yes ☑ No
8) Medical Capacity: Patient does not understand the nature of illness and potential for bad outcome? If yes, transport	☐ Yes ☑ No
9) At Risk Criteria (Abnormal vital signs): For adults. Pulse greater than 120 or less than 60? If yes, consult	☐ Yes ☑ No
10) At Risk Criteria (Abnormal vital signs): For adults. Systolic BP less than 90? If yes, consult	☐ Yes ☑ No
11) At Risk Criteria (Abnormal vital signs): For adults. Respirations greater than 30 or less than 10? If yes, consult	☐ Yes ☑ No
12) At Risk Criteria (Abnormal vital signs): For minor/pediatric patients. Age inappropriate HR? If yes, consult	☐ Yes ☑ No
13) At Risk Criteria (Abnormal vital signs): For minor/pediatric patients. Age inappropriate RR? If yes, consult	☐ Yes ☑ No
14) At Risk Criteria (Abnormal vital signs): For minor/pediatric patients. Age inappropriate BP? If yes, consult	☐ Yes ☑ No
15) At Risk Criteria: Serious chief complaint (chest pain, SOB, syncope)? If yes, consult	☐ Yes ☑ No
16) At Risk Criteria: Head injury with history of loss of consciousness? If yes, consult	☐ Yes ☑ No
17) At Risk Criteria: Significant MOI or high suspicion of injury? If yes, consult	☐ Yes ☑ No

Inc. Date: 11/22/2016 Patient Name: Doe, John BALTIMORE COUNTY FIRE DEPARTMENT Page: 1
Incident #: 1122141 Date Printed: 11/24/2016 18:24

18) At Risk Criteria: For minor/pediatric patients. ALTE, significant past medical history, or suspected intentional injury? If yes, consult	☐ Yes ☑ No
19) At Risk Criteria: Provider impression is that the patient requires hospital evaluation? If yes, consult	☐ Yes ☑ No
20) Providers: Did you perform an assessment (including exam) on this patient? If yes to # 20, skip to # 22	☐ Yes ☑ No
21) Providers: If unable to examine, did you attempt vital signs?	☐ Yes ☑ No
22) Providers: Did you attempt to convince the patient or guardian to accept transport?	☐ Yes ☑ No
23) Providers: Did you contact medical direction for patient still refusing service?	☐ Yes ☑ No
24) Patient: The patient or his or her representative refuses EMS examination.	☐ Yes ☑ No
25) Patient: The patient or his or her representative refuses EMS treatment.	☐ Yes ☑ No
26) Patient: The patient or his or her representative refuses EMS transport.	☐ Yes ☑ No

Patient Signature: **Printed Name:**

Patient Phone: **Date:** 18:24 11/24/2016

Patient Address:

Initial Disposition

PatientRefusedExam ☑	PatientRefusedTreatment ☑	PatientRefusedTransport ☑
PatientAcceptedExam ☐	PatientAcceptedTreatment ☐	PatientAcceptedTransport ☐
Auth.DecisionMaker(ADM)RefusedExam ☐	Auth.DecisionMaker(ADM)RefusedTreatment ☐	Auth.DecisionMaker(ADM)RefusedTransport ☐

Intervention

Attempt to Convince Patient ☑ Attempt to Convince Family Member/Auth. Decision Maker (ADM) ☐ Contact Medical Direction ☑ Contact Law Enforcement ☐ None of the Above Available ☐

AMA Contact Medical Direction Facility St Elsewhere Hospital

Final Disposition

Patient Refused Exam ☐	Patient Refused Treatment ☐	Patient Refused Transport ☑
Patient Accepted Exam ☑	Patient Accepted Treatment ☑	Patient Accepted Transport ☐
Auth. Decision Maker (ADM) Refused Exam ☐	Auth. Decision Maker (ADM) Refused Treatment ☐	Auth. Decision Maker (ADM) Refused Transport ☐

Provide in the patient's own words why he/she refused the above care/service:

"Patient reports that despite the damage to his vehicle, he has only a small laceration on his finger and no other symptoms. He eventually agreed to allow EMS to evaluate him and provide a bandage for a small finger laceration (index finger, right hand). He agreed to follow-up with his primary care MD later today. When offered transport to the hospital he indicated, "No. thanks. I will be fine." Discussed plan with Dr Smith at St Elsewhere ED who agreed with plan and recommended reiterating to Mr Smith the importance of close follow-up with his primary care MD for tetanus prophylaxis and consideration of laceration care to include sutures.

Inc. Date: 11/22/2016 Patient Name: Doe, John BALTIMORE COUNTY FIRE DEPARTMENT Page: 2

Incident #: 1122141 Date Printed: 11/24/2016 18:24

Figure 6-4 A competent adult patient has the right to refuse medical treatment, but it is essential that you fully inform the patient of potential consequences.

Table 6-2 Components of a Thorough Patient Refusal Document
Evidence the patient is able to make a rational, informed decision.
Documentation of complete assessment. If the patient refuses care or does not allow a complete assessment, then document that the patient did not allow for proper assessment and document whatever assessments were completed.
Discussion with the patient as to what care/transportation you would like to provide.
Discussion with the patient as to what may happen if he or she does not allow care or transportation. (You should list these consequences clearly and include the possibility of severe illness/injury or death if care or transportation is refused.)
Discussion with family members/friend/bystanders to encourage the patient to allow care.
Discussion with medical direction according to local protocol.
Discussion with the patient regarding other alternatives (such as going to see his or her family physician, or having a family member drive him or her to the hospital).
Discussion with the patient regarding the willingness of EMS to return if the patient changes his or her mind.
Signatures: Have a family member, police officer, or bystander sign the form as a witness. If the patient refuses to sign the refusal form, then have a family member, police officer, or bystander sign the form verifying that the patient refused to sign.

During the course of your work as a paramedic, you will be exposed to body fluids or other potentially toxic or infectious agents. If your barrier devices fail or do not offer enough protection, then complete an occupational exposure report. In states where it is now legal to use marijuana for medical or recreational purposes, some agencies consider marijuana smoke to be an occupational exposure. If you are exposed to marijuana smoke on a call, then include this information in your narrative report. Because each agency or state creates their own forms for these exposures, it is important that you familiarize yourself with the requirements. If you treat and/or transport a coworker for an occupational exposure, then complete a full PCR along with the occupational exposure form.

You may encounter additional specialized documentation when you are called to scenes of alleged neglect or abuse. It is imperative that you supply as much detail as possible about these circumstances because your initial findings may be the focus of a criminal investigation. Some providers do not document their suspicions of abuse and neglect for fear of allegations from the patient or the abuser of **slander**

YOU are the Paramedic PART 3

You and your partner attempt to reason with the patient to allow you to do an assessment for injuries. The patient tries to push you away and slurs, "Keep your hands off me! I have rights!" You contact your dispatcher to confirm that law enforcement officers are en route to your location.

Recording Time: 5 Minutes	
Respirations	Unable to measure; appear adequate, approximately 20 to 24 breaths/min
Pulse	Unable to measure
Skin	Unable to measure; appears pink
Blood pressure	Unable to measure
Oxygen saturation (Spo_2)	Unable to measure
Pupils	Unable to measure

5. How should you document that the patient has directed you to "keep your hands off," as well as account for your inability to obtain the patient's vital signs?
6. Does this patient have the right to refuse treatment?

(a false verbal statement that injures a person's good name). Document your objective findings and allow the legal system to investigate and make the ultimate determination of abuse or neglect.

When a physician of any specialty arrives or is present on the scene of your call, he or she may have the authority under local protocol to interject with patient care and give directives. Once a physician begins care that is beyond the paramedic's scope, most protocols require that he or she accompany the patient to the hospital to avoid being accused of abandonment. When you complete your documentation of such a run, document all orders and actions given by the physician.

Also document the use of mutual aid services such as helicopters, specialized rescue teams, and other agencies called in to assist. Document unusual occurrences as well, including the need to secure the patient with restraining devices for safe transport. If you need to summon an additional crew or specialty vehicle for lifting a heavy patient or if you will have an extended scene time owing to a prolonged extrication, then clearly document this information to explain why something out of the ordinary occurred. In the event that severe weather conditions delay your response, document this information as well.

Another special circumstance includes the appropriate documentation, as defined by medical control and the laws of your state, concerning the drawing of a blood sample as evidence for law enforcement personnel who have a driver suspected of being under the influence in their custody. Always follow the policy of your medical director in these special circumstances.

Community paramedicine programs are increasing in number across the United States. Paramedics in these programs may need to provide documentation beyond what is typically included under the prehospital model. If you operate within such a program, then ensure you understand and follow your state and local guidelines.

Finally, the presence of controlled substances in the field of EMS is increasing. As a paramedic, you are responsible for the security and accountability of these medications. Most services require a double-signature system any time a controlled substance is checked, used, discarded, or replaced. In your PCR, document the date and time, the amount of substance used versus the amount wasted, the patient to whom it was given, and by whom it was given, along with any specialized accountability forms your agency uses.

Completing a PCR

You must understand that EMS documentation is a required and necessary element of patient care. Just as you take pride in your patient care skills, you should take pride in your documentation skills. Now that you have been given an overview of the various aspects of the PCR along with special situations to document, you will learn how to complete the PCR.

The PCR Narrative

As mentioned earlier, the PCR contains check boxes as well as a narrative portion. The narrative portion of the PCR should be a detailed segment indicating the elements of the call. It should be written in a format accepted by your agency and should be accurate and complete. Simply writing "Followed ACLS protocols" may not be sufficient documentation for your agency or medical director. Record specifics of the call, such as "The patient was intubated with a 7.5 ET tube and ventilatory assistance provided with supplementary oxygen at 15 L/min. ET tube placement was confirmed by breath sounds, chest rise, and a tube check, before securing the ET tube at the mark of 22 at the teeth. The end-tidal CO_2 detector and pulse oximeter were placed immediately and their readings were: SpO_2 94% and $ETCO_2$ 35 mm Hg." (Always be sure to clarify which is which.) Also, some services will attach a copy of the reading to the documentation; you may wish to do this. Table 6-3 provides guidelines on how to write the narrative portion of your report.

In the narrative section, document any medical control orders and/or medical advice that you received. In some EMS systems, you must also document items such as consultations, orders requested or received from medical control, and any refusal situations in which medical control has been consulted. Simply writing "See refusal on back" is not an effective method of patient care documentation.

Many methods for narrative documentation exist. Your EMS agency or medical director may prefer a specific method to be used when documenting PCRs. Be familiar with the approved methods and all required elements for report writing for your agency. Some examples of narrative writing styles for PCRs are as follows:

- **Chronological order.** This method allows you to explain the call in a story format from start (time of the initial dispatch) to finish (completion of the call) Figure 6-5.
- SOAP method: **Subjective information, Objective information, Assessment, and Plan (for treatment).** This simple and logical method allows you to document various aspects of the patient care encounter Figure 6-6.
- CHARTE method: **Chief complaint, History, Assessment, Treatment, Transport, and Exceptions.** This method is similar to the SOAP method, but allows you to break down the narrative into logical sections similar to that of your patient assessment Figure 6-7.
- **Body systems/parts approach.** In this format, your assessment of each body system is documented from head to toe. This method of report writing may be difficult to apply in EMS and may be too time-consuming for paramedics.

Although the CHARTE and SOAP methods are widely used in EMS, the chronological method paints the clearest picture and might provide your best legal defense if you need to defend your report in court.

Table 6-3 How to Write a Narrative

Topic	Items to Include
Standard precautions	State which precautions you used and why.
Scene safety	Did you have to make your scene safe? If so, then state what you did and why you did it. Did this step create a delay of patient care?
MOI/NOI	Simply state. For example, "motor vehicle crash" or "difficulty breathing."
Number of patients	Record only when more than one patient is present. For example, "This is patient 2 of 3."
Additional resources	Did you call for help? If so, then state why, at what time, and what time the help arrived. Was transport delayed?
Cervical spine	State whether you applied manual stabilization or full spinal immobilization. You may want to include the reason why. For example, "Because of the significant MOI . . ."
Initial general impression	Simply state, if not already documented on the PCR.
LOC	Report LOC, any changes in LOC, and at what time changes occurred.
Chief complaint	Note and quote pertinent statements made by the patient and/or bystanders, including any pertinent negatives. For example: "Patient denies chest pain . . ."
Life threats	List all interventions and how the patient responded. For example, "Assisted ventilations with oxygen (15 L/min) at 20 breaths/min with no change in LOC."
ABCDE	Document what you found, and any interventions performed.
Oxygen	Record whether you administered oxygen, how you applied it, and how much you administered.
Primary survey, patient history, secondary assessment, or reassessment	State the type of assessment you used and any pertinent findings. For example, "Secondary assessment revealed unequal pupils, crepitus to right ribs, and an apparent closed fracture of the left tibia." Note the time each assessment was made and the findings.
SAMPLE/OPQRST	Note and quote any pertinent answers.
Vital signs	Record the times when you took the patient's vital signs and the findings. (Your service may want you to record vital signs in the narrative portion, as well as other places in the PCR.)
Medical direction	Quote any orders given to you by medical control and state who gave them.
Management of secondary injuries/treat for shock	Report all interventions, at what time they were completed, and how the patient responded.

Abbreviations: ABCDE, Airway, Breathing, Circulation, Disability, and Exposure; LOC, level of consciousness; MOI, mechanism of injury; NOI, nature of illness; OPQRST, Onset, Provocation/palliation, Quality, Region/radiation, Severity, Timing; PCR, patient care report; SAMPLE, Signs and symptoms, Allergies, Medications, Past pertinent medical history, Last oral intake, Events leading up to the illness or injury

Squad called to residence for ill man. On arrival found an alert and oriented 78 yo man sitting on the couch reporting CP. Pt sts this began approximately 30 min prior when he was mowing the lawn. Pt denies any radiation of the pain and rates it at a "7" out of 10 on pain scale. Pt has a known cardiac history with an MI 2 years prior. Pt is compliant with all meds as listed above. Pt denies any SOB or N/V with this episode. V/S stable, lungs CTA, Spo_2 93% RA, Skin pale/warm/dry to touch, PEARRL 4 mm, GCS 15. Pt placed on O_2 @ 15 L/min via NRB. Monitor showed RSR @ 88 bpm without ectopy. IV of NS was established in L AC with 18 g @ TKO (medic 785). 4 × 81 mg ASA were given PO @ 1501 (medic 785). Pt was given 1 SL 0.4 mg nitro @ 1503 with relief down to a "4" on scale (medic 785). V/S still stable. Secondary exam showed negative new findings. Med control contacted with negative orders. Left pt in care of ED staff with report in room 7.

Figure 6-5 Example of a narrative written in chronological order.

Note: In this example, "(medic 785)" identifies which provider performed the intervention. His or her initials may also be used. It is important to document who performed the procedure, because the person who is writing the narrative may not have been the crew member who performed the procedure or administered the medication.

(S) Called to scene for 78 yo man complaining of chest pain. Pt states pain began approximately 30 min prior to arrival when he was mowing the lawn. Pt denies any radiation of pain. States pain is "7" out of 10 on pain scale. Pt has known cardiac hx with an MI 2 yrs prior. Pt denies SOB or N/V. Pt has no allergies and is compliant with all meds listed above.

(O) U/A found Pt sitting on the couch. Pt alert and oriented with NARD and strong radial pulse. Pt calm and cooperative. Skin: Pale/warm/dry. Pupils PEARRL 4 mm, GSC 15. Lungs CTA. No noted JVD. Abd soft and nontender. PMS × 4. Secondary exam unremarkable.

(A) Possible MI.

(P) Primary, secondary Hx, V/S as listed above. Assisted pt to cot. Cardiac monitor: showed RSR @ 88 bpm without ectopy. IV: NS 18 g in L AC @ TKO (BW); Spo_2 93% RA, O_2 @ 15 L/min via NRB 100%; 4 × 81 mg ASA given PO, 1 SL 0.4 mg nitro (BW) pain down to "4". Transported to ________. Pt care transferred to ED with report.

Figure 6-6 Example of a narrative written with the SOAP method.

(C) 78 yo man complaining of chest pain without radiation. Pt sts pain is a "7" out of 10 on pain scale.

(H) Pt has a known cardiac history with an MI 2 years prior.

(A) Pt denies any SOB or nausea/vomiting with this episode. Vital signs stable, lungs clear to auscultation, Spo_2 93% RA, skin pale/warm/dry to touch, PEARRL 4 mm, GCS 15. Monitor showed RSR @ 88 bpm without ectopy.

(R) Pt placed on O_2 @ 15 L/min via NRB. IV of NS was established in L AC with 18 g @ TKO (medic 785). 4 × 81 mg ASA were given PO @ 1501 (medic 785). Pt was given 1 SL 0.4 mg nitro @ 1503 (medic 785).

(T) Pt improved during transport, pain went down to a "4" on the scale, V/S remained stable, and patient care was transferred to ED staff.

(E) None.

Figure 6-7 Example of a narrative written with the CHARTE method.

Regardless of the style of narrative report writing you and your service agree on, be sure to follow it routinely. If you switch from one format to another or attempt to change formats during report writing, then you may forget certain elements or essential details. Proper grammar and spelling are essential when writing reports. Consider carrying a pocket guide, reference manual, or medical terminology book in your ambulance to avoid spelling errors.

When you write your PCR, be sure to document any **pertinent negatives**—a record of negative findings that warrant no care or intervention but indicate that a thorough exam and history were performed. For example, "The patient denies any shortness of breath with his chest pain, patient denies any radiation of the chest pain to other parts of the body." This statement indicates that you not only obtained the information about the chest pain, but also inquired about shortness of breath and radiation of the pain.

The use of pertinent spoken accounts made by your patient and others on scene may be essential to the continuum of patient care. If you reference any spoken accounts made by the patient or others in your PCR, then be sure to indicate who made the statement and place his or her exact words in quotation marks.

Pertinent spoken accounts may include statements about the patient's behavior, the MOI, and safety-related information such as the use of weapons. It can also be helpful to list information that may be useful to criminal investigators as a part of their investigation, disposition of valuables, admissions of suicidal intentions made by a patient, or any first aid interventions provided by bystanders before the arrival of EMS.

▶ Elements of a Properly Written PCR

The accuracy of documentation depends on the completeness and precision of the report. You must provide all information, such as incident times and narrative information. Complete all sections of the report, even if a section was not applicable to the call. For example, if your PCR has a section of check boxes for specific information for cardiac arrest calls but the call you are documenting was not a cardiac arrest call, then note that on the report in a manner that is approved by your agency. Simply leaving the check boxes blank may raise questions about the completeness of the report.

When you handwrite a report, write legibly in ink. The color of ink used may be determined by your EMS agency.

Standard ink colors of black and blue are most commonly selected. Handwriting, especially in the narrative portion of the report, needs to be neat and easily read by others. In addition, take great care to not contaminate your written reports with any liquids found in the field. Place all your completed reports in a secure location agreed on by you and your partner that protects the patient's privacy, until they can be secured in the proper place at your EMS agency office or headquarters.

The PCR needs to be timely, even in EMS systems where call volume is high. If you respond to multiple calls without accurately completing PCRs before proceeding to the next call, then you may forget details and/or omit important information. Even worse, you may record inaccurate information. Your EMS agency should allow you a reasonable amount of time to complete your reports, replenish supplies, and clean and disinfect vehicles before returning them to service. Many paramedics use assessment cards during their calls to take notes, and use the electrocardiogram (ECG) monitor to note times and vital signs. They then complete the PCR after the call, rather than on the bumpy ride to the hospital. Set aside time at the hospital to neatly complete all documentation. If you do not have enough time to complete the full PCR while at the hospital, then you must still leave a written record with the patient. In these cases, most EMS systems will have a so-called drop report or transfer report **Figure 6-8**. These single-page, abbreviated forms are used as a memory aid during an EMS call. If you are unable to remain at the hospital to complete the PCR, then copy these documents and leave them with the nurse or physician. Some states require that copies of written reports be supplied to the receiving facility or hospital within a specific time frame, such as 24 hours. Know the applicable laws and requirements of your state and EMS system. In some systems, EMS providers fax the completed form to the ED because the hospital has a secure fax location that meets HIPAA requirements.

As mentioned previously, all PCRs should be free of jargon, slang, and personal opinions. Be certain that your documentation is not libelous. **Libel** is a false statement in written form that could be harmful to a person's current or future reputation. Document true and accurate statements only. If quotes from bystanders or statements made by the patient are used, then be sure to indicate who made them and place the exact words in quotation marks on the report.

Carefully review all reports before submitting them to the receiving medical facility and to your EMS agency. Always review your PCR for completeness, accuracy, and the proper use of grammar, spelling, medical terminology, and abbreviations. Your goal is to file a complete, accurate, professional, and legible report.

Documentation & Communication

Remember to document problems encountered when responding to or during the call (eg, an infectious disease exposure, a delayed response, a conflict at the scene with family or other response agencies, an MCI, an injury to an EMS provider that happened while providing care to the patient, etc).

YOU are the Paramedic PART 4

Law enforcement officers arrive on scene. At about that time the patient yells, "Great! Officers, arrest these people. They're harassing me!" One officer tells the patient to relax and do what the EMS crew asks, saying, "All they are trying to do is make sure you're OK." The officer asks the patient, "Have you been drinking today?" The patient replies, "I had a few at lunch is all. I'm just fine." The officer asks for, and receives, the patient's driver's license. He says to the patient, "I'm sure you are aware, Assemblyman Taylor, that there are laws you have to obey and it would look much better to your constituents if you cooperated. Going to the hospital in an ambulance is much better than in a police car." The patient agrees and you can finally assess the patient and prepare for transport.

Recording Time: 15 Minutes	
Respirations	16 breaths/min with adequate tidal volume
Pulse	100 beats/min, strong and regular
Skin	Warm, dry, pink
Blood pressure	130/80 mm Hg
Oxygen saturation (Spo_2)	97% on ambient air
Pupils	PERRLA

7. Is it important to document the interaction between the patient and law enforcement officers when no patient care is involved?

8. What is the legal basis to determine whether a patient is competent to refuse care?

Maryland Institute For
Emergency Medical Services Systems

Short Form Patient Information Sheet 2012

Jurisdiction: ________ Date: ________
Incident #________ Time Arrived at Hospital: ________
Unit #: ________
Age: ____ DOB: ________ Wt: ____ Kg Gender: ❑M ❑F
Priority: ❑1 ❑2 ❑3 ❑4 Trauma Category: ❑A ❑B ❑C ❑D
Patient's Name: ________
Patient's Address: ________
City: ________ State: ________
Point of Contact: ________ Phone Number: ________
Chief Complaint: ________
Time of Onset: ________ Past Medical History: (DNR/MOLST ❑A1 ❑A2 ❑B)
Cardiac ❑ CHF ❑ Hypertension ❑ Seizure ❑ Diabetes ❑ COPD ❑ Asthma ❑
Other: ________
Current Meds: ________
Allergies: Latex ❑ Penicillin/Ceph ❑ Sulfa ❑ Other: ________

Assessments

Vitals	Respiration	Skin	GCS
Time: ____	Left / Right	❑ Warm	Eyes (4): ____
B/P: ____ / ____	❑ Clear ❑	❑ Hot	Verbal (5): ____
Pulse: ____	❑ Rales ❑	❑ Cool	Motor (6): ____
Respirations: ____	❑ Labored ❑	❑ Dry	TOTAL: ____
SAO2: ____ %	❑ Stridor ❑	❑ Clammy	
Capnography: ____	❑ Rhonchi ❑	❑ Diaphoretic	**Pupils**
Carbon Monoxide: ____	❑ Wheezes ❑	❑ Cyanotic	❑ PERRL
Repeat Vitals	❑ Decreased ❑		❑ Unequal
Time: ____	❑ Agonal ❑		❑ Fixed/Dilated
B/P: ____ / ____	❑ Absent ❑		
Pulse: ____			**Neuro**
Respirations: ____	**Pulse**		❑ A ❑ V
SAO2: ____ %	❑ Regular ❑ Irregular		❑ P ❑ U
Capnography: ____	❑ JVD ❑ Peripheral Edema		
Carbon Monoxide: ____	Cap Refill: ____ seconds		

Assessment

Procedures

Cardiac Rhythm:	Cincinnati Stroke Scale
________	*Normal/Abnormal*
12 Lead Transmit Yes ❑ No ❑	Facial Droop Normal ❑ Abnormal ❑
Perform 12 Lead Yes ❑ No ❑	Arm Drift Normal ❑ Abnormal ❑
Glucometer:	Speech Normal ❑ Abnormal ❑
________	Last Known Well Time/Date: ________
❑IV1 ❑IV2	**Oxygen**
❑IO ❑EJ	❑ NRB Mask ❑ King Airway
Amount Infused:	❑ Nasal Cannula ❑ CPAP
________	❑ NPA/OPA ❑ NDT
CPR Performed Yes ❑ No ❑	❑ BVM ❑ Ventilator
ROSC Yes ❑ No ❑	❑ ET ❑ NT ❑ NGT
Induced Hypothermia Yes ❑ No ❑	❑ Easy Tube

Treatment:

Jurisdictional Additions:

Print Provider Name: ________

Figure 6-8 Prehospital notepad/drop report (transfer report).

Too often, the importance of report writing and documentation in EMS is ignored. Always remember that the report that you write reflects directly on you. Remember, your call is incomplete until you have completed the documentation process.

▶ The Consequences of Poor Documentation

Inappropriate, inaccurate, and poor documentation can adversely affect the quality of care received by patients after arrival at the hospital. For example, imagine that you administered a breathing treatment en route to the hospital but forgot to document the medication, procedure, and the time of administration. The hospital would not be aware of the medication administration, and the patient could be treated inappropriately because of your failure to document the care you provided. When you document what the patient or family members tell you and your findings from examining the patient, you enhance the quality of patient care. For example, do not forget to document the specific time that a suspected stroke patient was last seen "normal" by family members; this information is important to the window of time for treatment using fibrinolytics. As another example, if hospital personnel know that a patient has a seizure disorder or that a patient who has had transient ischemic attacks in the past had symptoms of stroke en route to the hospital, then proper care can be planned.

As mentioned previously, the legal implications of documentation can be significant. Poorly written, inaccurate, or illegible reports might lead a judge or jury to decide in favor of the plaintiff. Conversely, a lawyer may decide not to pursue a case when the documentation reveals a correctly written and well-documented report.

The following is an example that illustrates the importance of neat and accurate documentation. The EMS agency in a town was being sued for providing inappropriate care to a patient with a spine injury. During the discovery phase of the lawsuit, the attorney for the town decided to settle the case out of court based on the fact that the PCR was sloppy (because sloppy documentation implies sloppy care) and incomplete (because the providers did not clearly document whether distal pulses and motor and sensory functions were assessed before and after immobilization of the patient).

Another example of poor documentation was a case where a 15-year-old boy had been involved in a motor vehicle crash and the paramedic crew had to secure his airway because of head trauma. The patient was transferred to a trauma center, where the ED physician found the patient to be extubated. The patient survived but sustained a significant brain injury. The family sued the paramedic crew, claiming that their son was brain damaged from the hypoxia caused by the failed intubation and not the significant head trauma. The crew testified that they had continuous capnography indicating a secured airway throughout transport, yet they had failed to document such readings in their narrative. Although it was likely that the patient was extubated while being moved to the exam bed in the ED, the crew's failure to document their readings resulted in a ruling for the family. The agency lost a significant monetary amount as a result.

Poor documentation skills can also affect your reputation as a paramedic. Poorly written, inappropriate, or inaccurate reports might make others question the care provided, whereas a well-written report shows organizational skills, knowledge of patient conditions and needs, and respect for organizational policies and procedures. Part of being a good paramedic is completing the paperwork and reports as required. If you find it difficult to write reports, then seek additional classes or study report writing skills to enhance your abilities. Your agency or service might have an educational program to assist you with such education and training.

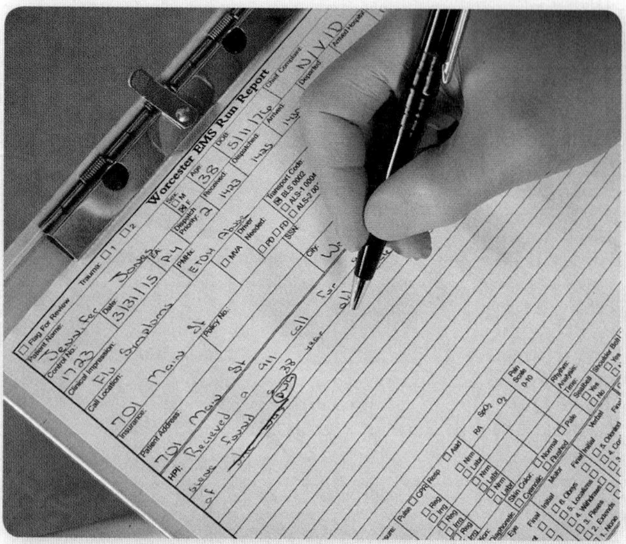

Figure 6-9 If you make a mistake while handwriting your report, the proper way to correct it is to draw a single horizontal line through the error, initial it, and write the correct information next to it.

Patient Safety

To Err Is Human reported in 1999 that almost 100,000 Americans die each year secondary to medical errors (ie, the eighth leading cause of death in the United States). The major revelation in this report was the concept that failures or errors in care were frequently not the result of individual behavior or decisions, but rather were often related to the intrinsic processes of care in the health care system. Thus, the IOM suggested, efforts to improve safety should focus on improving process errors rather than targeting people. Slowly over time, the idea of "system failure" rather than "human error" has gained credence. Organizations, such as the National Quality Forum, the Institute for Healthcare Improvement, the Agency for Healthcare Research and Quality, and others are invested in decreasing the frequency of medical errors. An analysis published in 2016 suggests medical errors may now be the third leading cause of death, annually claiming some 251,000 lives in the United States.[1]

Errors and Falsification

Although you should make every attempt to create an accurate and legible initial report, it may be necessary to revise or correct your PCR at times. If a report has to be revised or corrected, then note the date and time of the revised report and the purpose for writing the revision or making the correction. Never discard or destroy the original PCR.

Only the person who wrote the original report can revise it. Additions or notations added by others after the completion of the report may raise questions about the authenticity of the report and the confidentiality practices of your agency. Routine administrative report handling and reviews are necessary for entering information into computer databases, billing for services, and quality assurance monitoring. At no time should administrative activities involve altering or rewriting the report or portions of it.

If you make an error when handwriting your report, place a single, horizontal line through the error and initial and date the line, preferably in a different color ink. Write the corrected information next to it (Figure 6-9). Do not erase information, scribble through errors, or use correction fluid or tape. Remember, the PCR is a legal document.

If you discover an error after submitting an ePCR, then most systems will allow for amendments but will prevent erasure in a completed document. Refer to the operating directions as to how to make an amendment to the original ePCR. If it is not possible to electronically change the report, then print a copy of the ePCR and follow the same procedure used for a written document. When it is possible to make corrections electronically, keep in mind that the system records a so-called change history, even though the end product does not show it. Therefore, once a run has been posted, it is essential that you document the reason why any amendments to an ePCR were made. Most ePCR systems keep a record of who made an alteration to the report and when it was made.

Patient Safety

It is widely believed that near miss events are heavily underreported. A near miss is an unplanned event that did not cause an injury, illness, or damage, but had the potential to do so. Often staff will not report these events for fear of discipline, a perceived a lack of support or caring by supervisors, or belief that it is unnecessary to report the incident if no patient harm occurred. In fact, near miss events are among the most important to report, because they provide the organization with an opportunity to analyze its processes and improve safety. Moreover, talking about near misses can be easier for staff because there are fewer liability concerns when no one was actually harmed.

Patient Safety

The EMS Voluntary Event Notification Tool (EVENT) is an anonymous, nonpunitive, and confidential system that was launched by the National Association of Emergency Medical Technicians (NAEMT) in 2012. The goals of such systems are to identify flawed processes and systems that require improvement.

If you forgot to include important information, then you may need to write an addendum to your original report. You may also need to write an addendum if you are asked to write statements of events for matters related to quality assurance or risk management and to answer complaints. In your addendum, note that it was added to your original report and the reason for the late entry. Include the date of entry, the time of entry, and your signature.

Supplemental narratives may also be needed if additional information becomes available after the original report has been written. Document such reports with the date, the time, the reason for the added information, and your signature. Some EMS agencies use a supplemental report to write lengthy information when space on the original report is limited. Follow the policies of your service for using supplemental reports and the procedures for writing them. Regardless of when the supplemental reports are added, they should be attached in some way to the original report for record-keeping purposes.

You may be required to obtain and document billing information for the service(s) provided. You need to understand the sensitive and confidential nature of such information and the laws and regulations pertaining to billing and documentation security under HIPAA. EMS agencies should take care not to add additional information provided by billing clerks or others after the report has been submitted. Doing so might be in violation of local, state, or federal laws. If you have additional information to document after handing in the form, then follow the policy of your agency regarding whether a supplementary form is needed. Always be honest and thorough in your documentation process.

Controversies

Because of strict guidelines for what is considered a medical necessity for emergency ambulance transportation, some agency leaders urge providers not to document certain findings with the patient, such as the patient's ability to ambulate. Other leaders have urged providers to document findings that meet the medical necessity standards to help bring in revenue. Intentionally documenting inaccurate or fraudulent information is unethical, as well as illegal, and could lead to the loss of your certification.

Lost reports pose huge legal implications for paramedics, EMS agencies and departments, and medical directors. Remember, you are responsible for ensuring that your reports are completed and turned in as required by policy or procedure. (Do not keep copies of your reports. If you need to document numbers of procedures or ages of patients for your paramedic internship, then follow the specific policy of your training center.) If lost reports are an ongoing concern for an agency or provider, then steps should be taken to correct the problem. Know that attempting to recreate PCRs is irresponsible and possibly illegal. Also, record keeping may be a legal requirement in your state, and there may also be a specified time requirement for submission of reports.

Documentation & Communication

Reports should be complete to the point that people reviewing them, whether your medical director or the administrative office clerk billing for the service provided, can read them and understand exactly what transpired on the EMS call. If your report does not paint a clear picture of what happened, then it is not written well. Remember, your report is a reflection of your actions and your professionalism.

Documenting Incident Times

Accurate timekeeping is essential to all EMS operations. The role of timekeeper falls to dispatchers. You must also keep track of time during your documentation of the incident. Compare your times with those of the dispatcher to ensure accuracy and proper timekeeping, and ensure that your and your dispatcher's clocks are synchronized. For example, if your ECG monitor reports or documentation times are not in sync with those of the dispatcher, then this discrepancy could create a controversy in the courtroom.

In particular, it is critically important that you track and document the following incident times:

1. **Time of call.** Time when the call for help is placed or requested
2. **Time of dispatch.** Time when call is toned or alerted for a response
3. **Time of arrival at the scene.** Time when EMS unit arrives on scene
4. **Time with patient.** Time recorded when patient contact is made (which may not be the same as time of arrival. For example, when responding to a patient on the 17th floor of a high-rise building, you should include the time it takes to physically get to the patient.)
5. **Time of medication administration.** Time when medications are administered for adherence to protocols (Example: 1 × 0.4 mg of nitroglycerin was given SL at 1804 without relief [medic 785])
6. **Time of medical procedure.** Time when a procedure is conducted on the patient, such as when vital signs are taken, when a patient is intubated, or when a child is delivered. (Example: Pt was intubated with a 7.5 fr endotracheal tube with confirmation of negative epigastric sounds, clear bilateral lung sounds in all fields, and a waveform capnography reading of 35 mm Hg at 1807 [medic 785])
7. **Time of departure from scene.** Time recorded when EMS unit leaves the scene
8. **Time of arrival at medical facility.** Time when arriving at the medical facility (if a patient is transported)
9. **Time of transfer of care.** Time when care was transferred to another health care professional at the receiving facility (if a patient is transported)
10. **Time back in service.** Time when EMS unit and crew are ready for return to service

It is standard procedure to use 24-hour (military) time in EMS documentation. This format ensures that each time is unique; for example, 1:00 AM cannot be confused with 1:00 PM. Military times are shown in Table 6-4.

Table 6-4 Military Time

Standard Time	Military Time	Standard Time	Military Time
Midnight	0000	Noon	1200
1:00 AM	0100	1:00 PM	1300
2:00 AM	0200	2:00 PM	1400
3:00 AM	0300	3:00 PM	1500
4:00 AM	0400	4:00 PM	1600
5:00 AM	0500	5:00 PM	1700
6:00 AM	0600	6:00 PM	1800
7:00 AM	0700	7:00 PM	1900
8:00 AM	0800	8:00 PM	2000
9:00 AM	0900	9:00 PM	2100
10:00 AM	1000	10:00 PM	2200
11:00 AM	1100	11:00 PM	2300

YOU are the Paramedic SUMMARY

1. What is your first consideration in regard to this patient?

The patient is not well enough to stand up when he attempts to exit the vehicle under his own power and appears to have inadequate balance. At this point, you do not know whether the patient has been drinking. The patient's behavior could be the result of medical conditions such as diabetes, an allergic reaction, or cardiac insufficiency. Trauma may also be present. The patient may have struck his head, which could be affecting his balance. He may also have something as simple as a foot injury that is painful to stand on. Slurred speech may be caused by loose teeth or dentures from the crash. Do not assume a patient has been drinking. You must obtain more information in order to make the determination.

2. What is your first consideration in regard to the scene?

Although the visible damage to the vehicle appears to be minor, hazards ranging from leaking fluids to sharp, torn metal may still be present. Because of potential hazards, it is essential that you wear personal protective equipment to ensure your safety, even if the scene initially appears to be safe. The county courthouse would be a busy place at 1300 hours on a weekday, and you should be concerned with traffic control as well as crowd control. Ensure that law enforcement personnel have been dispatched to the incident.

3. Why is it unacceptable to document the patient's appearance as "drunk" on a PCR?

Document only the facts. Do not describe the situation according to your first suspicions, such as describing

YOU are the Paramedic SUMMARY *(continued)*

the patient as "Awake and appears drunk." Subjective statements such as this will come back to haunt you in a courtroom as you try to define how you determined the patient was "drunk." Include objective findings, such as, "has an altered mental status," or "smells of alcohol." Perform a thorough assessment before determining whether a patient is intoxicated.

4. Would it be acceptable to document that the patient is "yelling" for the breathing description on a PCR?

The patient is obviously breathing because he is attempting to extricate himself from the vehicle. You do not have the other points of direct assessment to determine respiratory rate, rhythm, and quality. You are directly witnessing the patient yelling, which is an accurate description of your initial observation, so you could document this.

5. How should you document that the patient has directed you to "keep your hands off," as well as account for your inability to obtain the patient's vital signs?

Use the patient's own words as much as possible. It would be acceptable to write, "When attempting to approach the patient to begin an assessment, the patient stated, 'Keep your hands off of me.' We were unable to assess pulse, respiration, blood pressure, pupils, Spo_2 level, or skin signs other than visually until after the intervention of law enforcement." Review Chapter 4, *Medical, Legal, and Ethical Issues,* for information on the concepts of patient consent and refusal.

6. Does this patient have the right to refuse treatment?

The patient is exhibiting signs associated with being intoxicated. The patient told the officer that he had had a few drinks at lunch. You also saw an empty bottle of alcohol on the floor of the vehicle. Because the patient's decision-making ability has been impaired, you should not accept a refusal request. You also need to further assess the patient's mental status (orientation to person, place, and time).

7. Is it important to document the interaction between the patient and law enforcement officers when there is no patient care involved?

It is essential that you document the interaction between the law enforcement officer and the patient. State laws usually allow officers to detain people if they are a "danger to themselves or others." Please review the rights of law enforcement officers in relation to patients for your area. In this case, the officer appealed to the patient's sense of self to convince him of the better of two courses of action, so detaining the patient was not necessary. When you document interaction between law enforcement personnel and a patient, make sure to document the officer's name, badge number, and agency on your form. This information will help you and your agency if you should need more information on the call.

8. What is the legal basis to determine whether a patient is competent to refuse care?

As a paramedic, you should be familiar with the laws of your state regarding the age of consent, care of minors, emancipated minors, and people with mental or cognitive impairments, such as mental illness or the effects of drug or alcohol use. Above all else, you need to ensure that every reasonable effort has been made for the patient's welfare and best interests. Do not assume the patient is "just drunk," and always provide the highest level of care.

EMS Patient Care Report (PCR)					
Date: 06-01-18	**Incident No.:** 890		**Nature of Call:** MVC	**Location:** 200 First Street	
Dispatched: 1300	**En Route:** 1301	**At Scene:** 1305	**Transport:** 1335	**At Hospital:** 1345	**In Service:** 1350
Patient Information					
Age: 60 **Sex:** M **Weight (in kg [lb]):** 113 kg (250 lb)			**Allergies:** No known drug allergies **Medications:** None **Past Medical History:** None **Chief Complaint:** MVC		

YOU are the Paramedic SUMMARY *(continued)*

Vital Signs				
Time: 1320	**BP:** 130/80	**Pulse:** 100	**Respirations:** 16	**Spo_2:** 97%
Time:	**BP:**	**Pulse:**	**Respirations:**	**Spo_2:**
Time:	**BP:**	**Pulse:**	**Respirations:**	**Spo_2:**
EMS Treatment (circle all that apply)				
Oxygen @ ______ L/min via (circle one): **NC NRM Bag-mask device**		**Assisted Ventilation**	**Airway Adjunct**	**CPR**
Defibrillation	**Bleeding Control**	**Bandaging**	**Splinting**	**Other:**
Narrative				

Arrived on scene to find a single-vehicle collision involving a pole in front of the county courthouse. On exiting our unit, we witnessed a man open the driver's door of the vehicle involved in the crash and attempt to exit the vehicle without assistance. He could not keep his balance and sat back down on the driver's seat. Once we approached the vehicle, we determined that the air bag system had deployed on impact. There is minimal visible damage to the front of the vehicle. Pt contact was made with a 60 yo male who was awake but disoriented. When attempting assessment of the pt's blood pressure, pulse, respiration, and Spo_2 level, the pt, in slurred speech, stated "I need my lawyer" and "Keep your hands off me." The pt exhibited signs associated with being intoxicated. Open empty vodka bottle was clearly visible on the floor of the vehicle. Confirmed that law enforcement was en route. Officer B.D. Smith, Badge 1345, Downtown Police Dept, and Officer R.H. Jenkins, Badge 1429, also from Downtown, arrived to assist. Officer Smith was able to convince the pt to allow our assessment, treatment, immobilization, and transport without further incident. This accounts for the initial delay in obtaining vital signs on this pt. Pt was cooperative and his condition remained unchanged during transport. V/S stable as listed, Spo_2 97% RA, lungs CTA, skin pink/warm/dry to touch, PEARRL 5mm. Primary survey and secondary assessment findings were unremarkable. Downtown Hospital med control was contacted with negative orders. Pt was transported and verbal report given to Shelley RN on pt transfer.**End of report**

Prep Kit

▶ Ready for Review

- For each emergency medical services (EMS) call, you must complete a formal written report before you leave the hospital. This action is a vital part of providing emergency medical care and ensuring the continuity of patient care. This information guarantees the proper transfer of responsibility, complies with the requirements of health departments and law enforcement agencies, and fulfills administrative needs.
- Your written or electronic patient care report (PCR) serves as a legal record. It should be complete, well-written, legible, and professional.
- Your report may be used in legal proceedings against you or someone else, and it is the only record of the care you provided and why.
- When you document what a patient said, use the patient's actual words and enclose them in quotation marks.
- Billing and administration are significant reasons why your PCR needs to be accurate and complete. Be sure to document all procedures performed, obtain the correct diagnosis codes (ICD-10 codes), and

Prep Kit (continued)

obtain the appropriate medical necessity signature (where required).

- The PCR may be handwritten or electronically written. Either way, it will include a checklist and a narrative portion. The report should be objective, accurate, and neat; this reflects good patient care.
- If a patient refuses care, then ensure that you have obtained vital signs and a complete history, fully inform the patient of the situation, involve medical control if needed, and thoroughly document the situation. Also document in whose care the patient was left.
- Special situations that may require filling out different or additional forms include injuries that occur in the workplace, mass-casualty incidents, exposure to potentially infectious diseases, cases that involve alleged abuse or neglect, transfer of care to an on-scene physician, interfacility transports, calls involving controlled substances, cancelled emergency calls, and calls involving other agencies. Reporting regulations vary from state to state, and you should familiarize yourself with the requirements of your state.
- Many methods exist for recording the narrative in your patient care report. Use the chronological method unless your agency requires another format. Examples of other methods are the SOAP method, the CHARTE method, and the body systems approach.
- The PCR needs to be filled out in a timely manner. Be sure to fill it out directly after the call.
- If you must revise or correct your PCR, then note the date, time, and purpose for the correction. Use your system's protocol for amending electronic reports. If you must correct a handwritten report, then place a single, horizontal line through the error and write the correct information next to it. Write down what did or did not happen and the steps that were taken to correct the situation.
- Falsifying information on the PCR may result in suspension and/or revocation of your certification/license.
- Inaccurate or poor documentation could lead to subsequent health care providers providing inappropriate care to the patient. It could also be detrimental for you if a lawsuit is initiated, and could negatively affect your reputation.
- Accurate timekeeping is essential to all EMS operations. The use of 24-hour (military time) is standard in EMS documentation.

▶ Vital Vocabulary

CHARTE method A narrative writing method that allows the narrative to be broken down into logical sections similar to the steps of the patient assessment; components include chief complaint, history, assessment, treatment, transport, and exceptions.

emergency medical dispatch (EMD) A system that assists dispatchers in selecting appropriate units to respond to a particular call for assistance and provides callers with vital instructions until the arrival of EMS crews.

libel A false statement in written form that defames a person's good name.

medical necessity A standard used by Medicare to determine whether a patient's condition requires ambulance transport in a particular situation.

minimum data set The mandatory clinical assessment standard information that must be documented on every emergency call as set by Medicare and Medicaid, and per the National Highway Traffic Safety Administration for the purpose of the national data system.

objective information Information that is observable and measurable, such as a patient's blood pressure.

patient care report (PCR) A legal document used to record all patient care activities during an incident; a handwritten or electronic report that describes the nature of the patient's injuries or illness at the scene and the treatment provided; also known as the prehospital care report.

pertinent negatives Findings that warrant no medical care or intervention, but which show evidence of the thoroughness of the patient exam and history.

slander A false verbal statement that injures a person's good name.

SOAP method A narrative writing method in which information is organized into four categories: Subjective information, Objective information, Assessment, and Plan (for treatment).

subjective information Information that is obtained from the patient, but which cannot be seen, such as the symptoms a patient describes.

▶ References

1. Makary MA, Daniel M. Medical error—the third leading cause of death in the US. *BMJ* 2016;353:i2139.

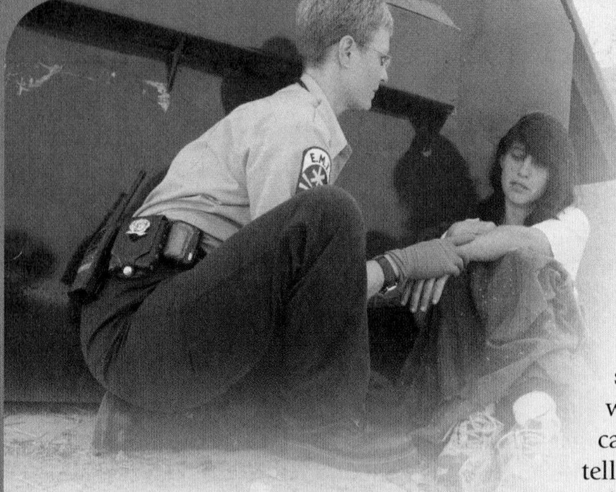

Assessment *in Action*

You and your partner are dispatched to a local stadium where a football game is in progress. A player is unresponsive after being tackled. On arrival, your unit is directed onto the field by security. As your vehicle approaches the area where the player went down, you see numerous flashes apparently coming from cameras. A law enforcement officer walks up to your vehicle and tells you that the scene is safe and the crowds and press members are under the control of law enforcement personnel. You exit the vehicle and wade into the press to get to the patient. The athletic team trainers as well as the team physician are taking care of the patient by placing him in full spinal immobilization. As you bend down to the patient, a reporter sticks a microphone in front of you and asks, "Is this kid's career over?" You look over your shoulder for your partner, who is making his way toward you through the reporters.

1. Which of the following actions would be MOST appropriate upon your arrival?

- **A.** Obtain information from the athletic trainers and team physician regarding any care administered prior to your arrival.
- **B.** Determine how many reporters have had access to the patient since his injury.
- **C.** Confirm the patient signed a HIPAA release for the athletic trainers and team physician.
- **D.** Contact the team's public information officer to handle the questions from the reporters.

2. What is the term used to describe a false verbal statement that injures a person's reputation?

- **A.** Slander
- **B.** Ethics violation
- **C.** Verbal assault
- **D.** Libel

3. Which of the following pieces of information would be critical to obtain from the team physician and athletic trainers?

- **A.** Whether any HIPAA violations occurred with the media prior to your arrival
- **B.** A detailed description of the mechanism of injury
- **C.** Whether the patient's emergency contacts have been notified
- **D.** A detailed list of the personal items that may have been removed from the patient prior to your arrival

4. Which of the following terms describes what the patient tells you is bothering him or her?

- **A.** Objective information
- **B.** Chief complaint information
- **C.** Subjective information
- **D.** Minimum data set

5. Documentation of the chief complaint, vital signs, level of consciousness, patient demographics, and assessment information is referred to as the:

- **A.** minimum data set.
- **B.** maximum data set.
- **C.** HIPAA data set.
- **D.** patient care report.

6. After you have completed and submitted your electronic report, you realize you had made an error. Which of the following actions would be the MOST appropriate to take?

- **A.** Do nothing, because the report has already been submitted.
- **B.** Re-open your electronic report and correct the error without notifying anyone of the change.
- **C.** Notify the appropriate supervisor of the mistake and ask to make a change to the report.
- **D.** Notify the appropriate supervisor of the error and complete a supplemental report.

7. Which form of consent allows you to treat an unresponsive patient?

- **A.** Informed consent
- **B.** Implied consent
- **C.** Expressed consent
- **D.** Involuntary consent

8. Imagine you answered the reporter about the future of the patient's sports career. Are you in violation of HIPAA?

9. How is the right of the press to cover stories balanced with the patient's right to privacy?

10. To ensure proper documentation and continuity of care, list the information you should obtain from the athletic trainers and/or team physician prior to departing with the patient.

CHAPTER 7

Medical Terminology

National EMS Education Standard Competencies

Medical Terminology

Uses foundational anatomic and medical terms and abbreviations in written and oral communication with colleagues and other health care professionals.

Knowledge Objectives

1. Explain the purpose of medical terminology and the importance of being familiar with it. (pp 191-192)
2. Explain the Greek and Latin origins of medical terms. (pp 192-193)
3. Define medical eponyms, homonyms, antonyms, and synonyms; include examples for each. (pp 193-194)
4. Name the four word parts or components used to build medical terms; include examples of each. (pp 194-198)
5. Describe how compound words are created and how the plural is formed when using medical terminology; include examples of each. (p 198)
6. Describe the anatomic position and why it is used. (pp 198-199)
7. List the three planes of the human body. (p 199)
8. List medical terms associated with regional anatomy. (pp 200-201)
9. Explain the importance of using accurate medical terminology for direction, movement, and position in your documentation and other communication. (pp 201-205)
10. Describe the topography of the abdominal region, including the four abdominal quadrants and the nine abdominal regions. (pp 204-205)
11. Identify specialized prefixes used to indicate position, direction, and location. (pp 205-206)
12. Define specific terms used to indicate the patient's position on the scene or prior to transport: prone, supine, Fowler position, and recovery (left lateral recumbent) position. (pp 206-207)
13. Interpret standardly accepted medical abbreviations, acronyms, and symbols. (pp 207-208)
14. Identify error-prone medical abbreviations, acronyms, and symbols. (p 208)
15. Know appropriate terminology related to pharmacology. (pp 209-210)

Skills Objectives

There are no skills objectives for this chapter.

Introduction

As a paramedic, it is imperative that you develop a strong working knowledge of medical terminology, the international language of medicine and health care. Medical terminology is used to describe and record every aspect of patient care, including medical history, assessment results, treatment, and outcomes. The language of medicine is derived primarily from Greek and Latin terms. If you understand the origin of medical terms (words), the components (parts), and the guidelines for forming words, you'll be able to identify and use medical terminology correctly and communicate effectively with other health care providers.

Consider what could happen if you, as a paramedic, used medical terminology incorrectly:

- A term used incorrectly in a radio report or documented improperly in the patient care report could lead to the patient being given an ineffective or even harmful treatment at the hospital.
- The patient could lose trust in the paramedic's ability to care appropriately for him or her.

Your comprehension of key terms, acronyms, symbols, and abbreviations is important for effective communication and documentation. Understanding medical terminology requires you to break down each word into its separate components—prefix, suffix, and root—and to have a good working knowledge of those parts. Learn the established and accepted medical terms and abbreviations for your local area. Some emergency medical services (EMS) systems have specific lists of approved medical abbreviations and terms you must use.

In addition to accepted terminology, you'll undoubtedly hear some common slang terms used in EMS, such as "boarding a patient" for transport or "bagging" or "tubing" the patient during airway management. The more extensive your vocabulary is, the more competent you'll be seen to the rest of the medical community and the better the patient care you'll be able to deliver. Download a medical terminology app or carry a field guide or documentation handbook, so you can quickly and easily look up any unfamiliar terms without memorizing page after page of terms Figure 7-1.

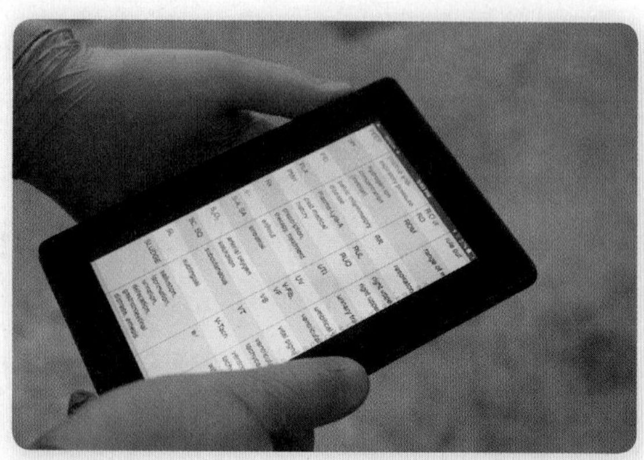

Figure 7-1 Medical terminology apps are an excellent resource to reference terms while working in the field.

Words of Wisdom

Never use a medical term if you're uncertain of its meaning. If you can't remember *femur*, it's better to say "thigh bone" than to risk using an incorrect term.

Origins

Understanding the origins of medical terms helps you decipher the meanings of terms. Most medical terms have Greek or Latin origins Table 7-1. In general, medical terms that refer to disease are derived from Greek words. Words that refer to anatomic structures are usually derived from Latin words. The original word and the meaning are often interesting. For example, the word *muscle* comes from a Latin word for mouse, because the movement of a muscle under the skin was thought to resemble the scampering of a mouse. The word coccyx, the lower end of the spine, originated from the Greek word for cuckoo because it resembles a cuckoo's bill.

YOU are the Paramedic PART 1

You and your partner are dispatched to a local elementary school to help a person who has fallen. Upon arrival, you are directed to the playground where a young boy is lying beneath a set of playground climbing bars on his left side, curled into a fetal position, sniffling and holding his abdomen. His second-grade teacher, Miss Hawthorne, tells you he fell from the top, approximately 5 feet (2 m), and has a bump on the right side of his head just above his eye. She says she has been trying to keep him still and has not let him try to get up.

Recording Time: 0 Minutes	
Appearance	Awake
Level of consciousness	Alert
Airway	Open
Breathing	Adequate
Circulation	Appears normal

1. What is the correct medical term for the position in which the child is lying?
2. How can knowledge of medical terminology assist in your documentation of care for this patient?

Table 7-1 Selected Medical Terms With Greek or Latin Origins

Greek	Disease	Latin	Anatomic
burs/o	bursitis	dors/o, dors/i	back/dorsal
cholecyst/o	cholecystitis	faci/o	face/ facioplegic
gloss/o	glossitis	lingua	tongue/ linguistic
hepat/ic	hepatitis	mamm/o	breast/ mammogram
nephr/o	nephritis	ren	kidney/renal

Eponyms

The language used in medicine also comes from eponyms and terms that have resulted from advances in modern medicine, such as *fiberoptic* and *pacemaker*. An **eponym** is the name of a disease, device, procedure, or drug that is based on the person who invented, discovered, or first described it. You use eponyms every day and may not even be aware of where they originated. For example, the diesel engine is named for its German inventor, Rudolf Diesel. The word *denim* is derived from the French *serge de Nîmes*, a serge fabric from the town of Nîmes in France. Medical eponyms sometimes appear in the possessive form (such as Hodgkin's disease) and sometimes not (Hodgkin disease). (Note: This text does not include the possessive form.) As in this example, they often include the name of the physician or surgeon who discovered, described, developed, identified, or invented a particular anatomic part or region, physiologic function or process, disease or syndrome, diagnostic or surgical procedure, treatment protocol, or instrument:

- McBurney point
- Foley catheter
- Babinski reflex
- Crohn disease
- Cesarean section
- Levine sign
- Apgar score

In medical terminology, we can often use a single word to express a concept that might otherwise require many words of explanation. For example, you can say "arthritis" faster than you can say "inflammation of the joint." In the next section, we'll take a more in-depth look at commonly used medical terms and their meanings.

Homonyms

Incorrect pronunciation of medical terms can lead to misdiagnosis or other serious medical errors. Correct pronunciation and spelling are especially important with certain words known as **homonyms**—pairs of words that are pronounced almost the same way. For instance, *ileum* (il'e-um) is the last anatomic portion of the small intestine, while *ilium* is the largest bone of the pelvis. Or compare *dysphagia* with *dysphasia*. These two words may be spelled similarly and sound almost identical, but they have very different meanings. The word root *-phasia* means speaking, whereas *-phagia* means eating or swallowing. The prefix *dys*-means difficult or painful. *Dysphasia*, then, means difficulty speaking, while *dysphagia* means difficulty eating or swallowing.

Patient Safety

One type of medication error involves prescribing and dispensing "look alike, sound alike" (LASA) medications (eg, magnesium sulfate and morphine [MS and MS04]). The Joint Commission recommends focusing on prescription legibility through improved handwriting or the use of electronic prescriptions. Other solutions include physically separating LASA medications into different storages areas and using "tall man" or mixed-case lettering to emphasize the differences in drug names (ie, DOPamine versus DoBUTamine).

Words of Wisdom

A thorough knowledge of anatomy and an understanding of the context in which each term is typically used can help you determine (and spell) which word is the correct one to use in a given situation.

Antonyms

Different word parts perform different functions. **Antonyms** are pairs of word roots, prefixes, or suffixes that have the opposite meaning of another word Table 7-2.

Synonyms

Synonyms are pairs of word roots, prefixes, or suffixes that have the same or almost the same meaning. For example, the prefixes of the words pneumonologist and pulmonologist both mean lung, yet these words are not interchangeable. The reasons for this are more historical than logical; the term *pneumonologist* simply has not gained acceptance, but the term *pulmonologist* has. Table 7-3 shows more synonyms you're likely to encounter in your work.

Table 7-2 Selected Antonyms Used in Medical Terminology

Antonyms		Examples			
		Word Part and Meaning		Opposite Word Part and Meaning	
Antonyms	Pairs of word roots, prefixes, or suffixes that have opposite meanings	eu-	good	mal-	bad
		dextro-	right	sinistr/o	left
		ad-	toward	ab-	away from

Table 7-3 Selected Synonyms Used in Medical Terminology

Synonyms		Examples			
		Word Part and Meaning		Similar Word Part and Meaning	
Synonyms	Pairs of word roots, prefixes, or suffixes that have the same or almost the same meaning	pulmon/o	lung (as in pulmonologist)	pneum/o	lung (as in pneumonia)
		mammo/o	breast (as in mammogram)	mast/o	breast (as in mastectomy)
		cardi/o	heart (as in cardiology)	coron/o	heart (as in coronary)
		nephr/o	kidney (as in nephritis)	ren/o	kidney (as in renal)
		angi/o	vessel (as in angiogram)	vas/o	vessel (as in vascular)

Components of a Medical Term

When you encounter a new word, break it up into its component parts. Some medical terms are quite long, consisting of three or four parts. If you know the meaning of each part, you can combine the definitions to determine the broader meaning of the word. Medical terms are composed of distinct parts that perform specific functions:

- **Prefix.** The portion that appears before the word root
- **Suffix.** The portion that appears after the word root
- **Word root.** The foundation of the term
- **Combining vowel.** Vowel that links one or more word roots to an other component of a term

The way in which the parts of a word are combined determines its meaning. Changing or deleting any portion of a term can significantly alter its content. For example, hyperglycemia (hi'per-gli-se'me-ah) is too much blood glucose, and hypoglycemia (hi'po-gli-se'me-ah) is too little blood glucose. Thus, accurate spelling is essential in medical terminology.

▶ Prefixes

Prefixes are often found in general language (for instance, *auto*pilot, *sub*marine, *tri*cycle),and they are common in medical and scientific terminology. A prefix appears at the beginning of a word and generally describes the location or intensity of the word root that follows. Of course, not all medical terms have prefixes. A prefix does not change the meaning of the word root—*cutaneous* means skin regardless of what precedes it, for example. However, the prefix does change the meaning of the medical term as a whole by describing the what, how, why, or when of the root. To expand on our previous example, the prefix *sub-* means below; therefore, *subcutaneous* means "below the skin." Another word, *atypical,* which means "not typical," can easily be understood when you know it's formed from the prefix *a-*, which means not, and the word root *typical.*

By learning to recognize a few commonly used medical prefixes, you can determine the meaning of terms that may not be immediately familiar to you. *Hypo-*, for instance, is a prefix that means low. We can add it to the word root *volumen*, meaning "volume," and the suffix *-emia*, meaning "blood," to figure out what hypovolemia means:

- Hypovolemia = Low blood volume

Likewise, we can add *hypo-* to the word root *glyc/o*, meaning glucose, and the suffix *-emia*:

- Hypoglycemia = Low blood glucose

Sometimes we have just two word parts to work with. In the following example, we can define "hypotension" by adding *hypo-* to the word root *tensio*, which means "to stretch":

- Hypotension = Low blood pressure

Master tables at the end of this chapter list medical terminology, including prefixes, suffixes, word roots, and abbreviations, you'll use most every day in your work.

▶ Numerical Prefixes

Many prefixes are used to indicate the number of sides, limbs, or sensory organs affected ("monocular vision," for example). Other numerical prefixes are used to specify time, such as "octogenarian" (a person between 80 and 89 years of age) or to indicate quantities that are uncountable (semicomatose, for instance). Common numerical prefixes are listed in Table 7-4.

▶ Suffixes

A *suffix* is a component added to the end of a word root. It changes or adds to the word's meaning or provides further definition. In medical terminology, a suffix usually specifies a procedure, condition, disease, or part of speech. For example, the suffix *-ase* indicates an enzyme. Lipase (*lip-*, which means fat, plus *-ase*) is an enzyme that digests fats. Gastritis, which means inflammation of the stomach, is a combination of the word root *gastr-*, which means stomach, and the suffix *-itis*, which means inflammation. Suffixes are able to change the medical term to a noun or adjective as needed.

▶ Word Roots

The *word root* establishes the basic meaning of the word and frequently indicates a body part. Some books use the term *word root*; others use *root word*. The terms are synonymous. Prefixes are added to the beginning of a word root, and suffixes are added to the end of a word root. Changing the prefix or suffix will change the meaning of the term. Some word roots are complete words by themselves, but not all are. Furthermore, the same word root may have

YOU are the Paramedic PART 2

After briefly speaking with the teacher, you kneel down to get eye level with the child. "Hi, I'm a paramedic, and we're here to take care of you. My partner, Matt, is going to hold your head really still while we talk for a minute. Does your head or your tummy hurt?"

He says his name is Tommy and his stomach hurts more than his head does. He is alert and oriented to person, place, time, and event. His respiratory rate is 22 breaths/min and normal, and his radial pulse is strong and regular, with a rate of 104 beats/min. He says he's been dizzy all morning, and it made him fall. Miss Hawthorne tells you that Tommy has type 1 diabetes. The school nurse has arrived and indicates that his mother reported that his glucose level was 183 mg/dL when he arrived at school this morning. The nurse also states that he's not allergic to any medications.

Recording Time: 3 Minutes	
Respirations	22 breaths/min
Pulse	104 beats/min
Skin	Cool and dry
Oxygen saturation (Spo_2)	98%
Pupils	PERRLA

3. Why would you want to avoid using medical terminology when talking to this patient?
4. What are the correct medical terms to describe Tommy's mental status and blood glucose level?
5. How would you document that the patient has no medication allergies?

Table 7-4 Common Numerical Prefixes

Prefix	Meaning	Example	Definition
un-	one	unilateral	Affecting one side of the body
dipl-	double or in pairs	diplopia	Double vision
null-	none	nullipara	A woman who has never given birth
primi-	first	primigravida	A woman pregnant for the first time
multi-	many	multipara	A woman who has given birth to more than one child
bi-	two	bilateral	Pertaining to both sides of the body
tri-	three	trigeminy	Irregular heart rhythm consisting of two normal beats followed by one premature beat
quad-	four	quadriplegia	Paralysis of all four extremities
tetra-	four	tetralogy of Fallot	A congenital anomaly involving four anatomic abnormalities of the heart
quint-	five	quintipara	A woman who has had five pregnancies resulting in five live births
sexti-	six	sextuplets	Six offspring of the same pregnancy
septi-	seven	septuplets	Seven offspring of the same pregnancy
octo- or octi-	eight	octigravida	A woman pregnant for the eighth time
nona-	nine	nonan	Occurring on the ninth day
deca-	ten	decagram	Measurement of ten grams
semi-	half; part	semiconscious	Partially conscious
hemi-	half; one sided	hemiplegia	Weakness on one side of the body
ambi-	both	ambidextrous	Able to use right and left hands equally
pan-	all, entire	pandemic	An epidemic over a wide area

different meanings in different fields of study. You may have to consider the context of a word before assigning its meaning.

▶ Colors

Several word roots are used to describe color. The most common include those listed in Table 7-5.

▶ Combining Forms and Vowels

Some word roots, prefixes, and suffixes cannot combine with other word forms without help Table 7-6. To make pronunciation easier, sometimes it's necessary to change the last letter or the last few letters of a word root or prefix when a suffix is added. These letters, called combining vowels, facilitate the formation of new, more complex terms. They often consist of a vowel, most commonly *o*, added to a word root to create a combining form. A **combining form** is a word root, prefix, or suffix with an added vowel, known as a *combining vowel*. For example, in *osteopathic*, the first word root is *osteon* (Greek for bone). The "n" is dropped and the combining vowel *o* added to create the combining form *oste/o*. Thus, adding the "o" facilitates the addition of a second combining form, *-pathy* (from the word root *patho-*, meaning disease).

Let's take another example. The word root *gastr-*, which means stomach, cannot combine gracefully with *megaly*, which means enlargement. The resulting term

Table 7-5 Word Roots That Describe Color

Root	Definition	Example	Definition
cyan/o	blue	cyanosis	Blue discoloration of the skin
leuk/o	white	leukocyte	White blood cell that fights infection
erythr/o	red	erythrocyte	Red blood cell that contains hemoglobin to carry oxygen
cirrh/o	yellow-orange	cirrhosis	Inflammation of an organ, such as cirrhosis of the liver, which causes yellow-orange pigmentation of the skin
melan/o	black	melena	Black, tarry stool caused by upper GI bleeding
poli/o	gray	poliomyelitis	An acute viral disease that attacks the gray matter of the brain
alb-	white	albinism	Condition in which a person's skin, hair, and eyes lack pigmentation (white hair, very pale skin, and a nonpigmented iris)
chlor/o	green	chlorophyll	Green pigment in leaves that is necessary for the plant to carry out photosynthesis

Abbreviation: GI, gastrointestinal

Table 7-6 Selected Combining Forms

Combining Form	Meaning	Combining Form	Meaning
brachi/o	arm	pil/o	hair
cardi/o	heart	steth/o	chest
carp/o	wrist	thorac/o	chest, thorax
cephal/o	head	thyr/o	thyroid gland
cervic/o	neck	trache/o	trachea
encephal/o	brain	ureter/o	ureter
faci/o	face	vas/o	vessel
gloss/o	tongue	vesic/o	bladder, blister
nas/o	nose	viscer/o	viscera
ot/o	ear		

"gastrmegaly," would be awkward to pronounce and would have an odd spelling. A hyphen at the end of a word root indicates that *gastr-* is not a complete word. Adding a vowel to it, in this case an "o," solves the problem. The result, *gastr/o*, is referred to as a combining form because it is used when combining the root with other roots or suffixes. *Gastr/o* + *megaly* makes *gastromegaly*, or enlargement of the stomach. If the suffix begins with a vowel, a combining vowel is unnecessary. For example, *gastr-* + *-ic* = *gastric*. No additional letters are needed to form the word.

When adding combining vowels to root words, use the following guidelines:

- Use a combining vowel before a suffix that begins with a consonant (eg, *cyt/o* + *logy*).
- Use a combining vowel to join other root words (eg, *gastr/o/enteritis*).

- Do not use a combining vowel before a suffix that begins with a vowel (eg, *gastritis*, not *gastroitis*).

Some other examples of combining forms and vowels are:

- *cardi/o* + *logy* = cardiology (study of the heart)
- *neur/o* + *logy* = neurology (study of the nervous system)

Compound Words

Some medical terms contain more than a one-word root. These words are called **compound words.** In compound words, each word root retains its basic meaning. Simple examples of compound words containing two word roots are *electrocardiogram* and *thermometer*. A more complicated example is *osteoarthritis*. The combining form *oste/o* comes from the word root *ost-*, meaning bone. The word root *arthr-* means joint or joints. The suffix *-itis* means inflammation. Therefore, the combined word *osteoarthritis* means inflammation of the bone joints.

Plural Endings

To change a medical term from singular to plural, certain rules apply. In most cases, as with other words in English, the plural is formed simply by adding an *-s* to the singular word. *Lung* becomes *lungs*, for instance. However, for some medical terms forming the plural is more complicated:

Singular words ending in *-a* change to *-ae* in the plural.

- Example: *vertebra* becomes *vertebrae*

Singular words ending in *-is* change to *-es* in the plural.

- Example: *diagnosis* becomes *diagnoses*

Singular words ending in *-ex* or *-ix* change to *-ices*.

- Example: *apex* becomes *apices*

Singular words ending in *-on* or *-um* change to *-a*.

- Examples: *ganglion* becomes *ganglia; ovum* becomes *ova*

Singular words ending in *-us* change to *-i*.

- Example: *bronchus* becomes *bronchi*

Topographic Anatomy

The surface of the body has many superficial visible features that serve as guides or landmarks indicating the structures that lie beneath them. Taken together, these features make up the body's topography (from the Greek word *topos,* meaning place, and *-graphy,* meaning description). Familiarize yourself with these living landmarks—the body's **topographic anatomy**—to perform a thorough assessment.

To describe topography accurately, you must imagine the body in a fixed position, known as the **anatomic position**: the person is standing, facing you, arms at his or her sides, with the palms of the hands facing forward, so the thumbs point away from the body. This position serves as a shared reference point, so the meaning of

YOU are the Paramedic PART 3

You explain to Tommy that your partner is going to hold his head still and you are going to roll him over onto his back so you can check where it hurts. He presents with a golf ball size hematoma and a small laceration just above his right eye. Bleeding is controlled, and his pupils are equal and reactive. His abdomen is very tender on the right side just below his ribs, and you note bruising in the area. He denies pain in any other area. He tells you he took his insulin this morning and ate breakfast before school.

Recording Time: 8 Minutes	
Respiration	22 breaths/min
Pulse	108 beats/min
Skin	Cool and dry
Oxygen saturation (Spo_2)	99%
Pupils	PERRLA

6. Describe the position of the patient's head injury.
7. What is the abbreviation for the abdominal quadrant that is tender to the touch?

various directional terms stays constant, regardless of body position or movement. For example, let's say a person reports pain in his arm and you need to document it. Whose left or right do you use? To be consistent, the reference point health care providers use is the patient's left and right in the anatomic position.

Words of Wisdom

There is only one anatomic position. Don't confuse this with the patient's position—prone or supine, for instance—or with patient positioning, such as the Fowler or Trendelenburg position.

Anatomic Planes and Axes of the Body

An anatomic plane of the body is an imaginary flat surface—imagine sheets of glass slicing through the body, dividing it horizontally and vertically into sections Figure 7-2. An *axis* is an imaginary line that divides the body equally and creates a point of rotation. Think of a skewer or pole through the middle of an object. The body can be divided along three main axes, to create the following planes:

1. **Coronal plane.** Imagine a sheet of glass (the plane) slicing the body vertically, from ear to ear, dividing it into front (ventral) and back (dorsal) portions. We call this the frontal or **coronal plane**—easy to remember, since "corona" means head.
2. **Transverse plane.** Now imagine a plane passing horizontally through the body at the waist, creating top and bottom portions. This slice is referred to as the **transverse (axial) plane**.
3. **Sagittal (lateral) plane.** Finally, let's divide the body vertically again, but this time slicing it from front to back. This is the **sagittal (lateral) plane**. *Sagitta*, Latin for arrow, describes the way in which the straight line of this plane divides the body into two sides. A sagittal plane might or might not go through the midline of the body. If it does, it's called the **midsagittal plane (midline)**, which divides the body into equal left and right halves. Your nose and navel are found along this imaginary line. Other sagittal planes lie parallel to the midline.

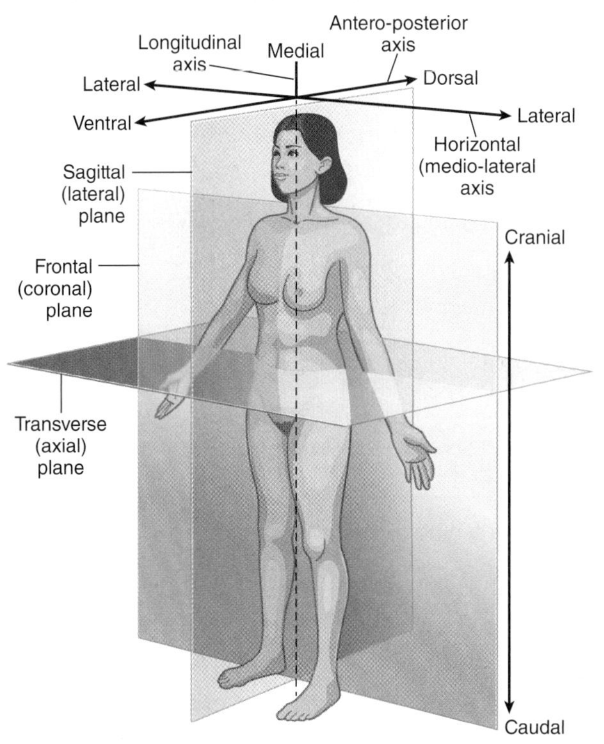

Figure 7-2 Planes and axes of the body.

The three axes along which the body can be divided are as follows:

1. The **anteroposterior axis** runs perpendicular to the coronal plane.
2. The **longitudinal axis** runs perpendicular to the transverse plane.
3. The **horizontal axis**, also called the mediolateral axis, runs perpendicular to the sagittal plane.

These planes and axes help you to identify the location of internal structures and understand the relationships between and among the organs Table 7-7.

A **cross section** is taken by slicing across an object, perpendicular to its long axis, as you would do if you wanted to count the rings in a tree trunk. A **longitudinal section**, in contrast, is a view of an object cut along its long axis. In medicine, this slicing, of course, is often imaginary, or can be accomplished with, say, a camera or a beam of radiation, rather than a scalpel.

Table 7-7 Anatomic Planes of the Body

Plane of the Body	Description
Coronal	Front and back
Transverse	Top and bottom
Sagittal ▪ Midsagittal (midline)	Left and right (divides the body at any point on or parallel to the midline) ▪ Left and right (divides the body into equal left and right halves)

▶ Specific Areas of the Body

In addition to using planes and topographic landmarks, many body areas have specific names. When a person is injured, paramedics rely on anatomic planes, body surfaces, and imaginary lines to describe the location of the injury. Familiarizing yourself with these body regions will not only help you communicate with other professionals, but it will also help you break down other terms, because many of them are used as root words. For example, "sternocleidomastoid" is a combination of *sterno-*, *cleido-*, and *-mastoid*, which refers to the sternum, clavicle, and mastoid process, respectively. If you understand those roots, you will be able to locate the origin and insertion of this large neck muscle. The most common body regions are described in Table 7-8.

▶ Body Cavities

The human body contains several cavities, each containing various organs and other structures. These cavities can be grouped into dorsal cavities, which are more posterior, and ventral cavities, which are anterior. The dorsal cavities include the cranial cavity, which contains the brain, and the spinal cavity, which surrounds the spinal cord. The ventral cavities include the thoracic cavity, which encloses

Table 7-8 Terminology Associated With Specific Body Regions

Term	Word Parts	Definition
Abdominal	abdomin- = abdomen -al = pertaining to	Pertaining to the abdomen
Axillary	axill- = armpit -ary = pertaining to	Pertaining to the armpit
Brachial	brachi/o = arm between the shoulder and elbow -al = pertaining to	Pertaining to the upper arm
Buccal	bucc/o = cheek -al = pertaining to	Pertaining to the cheek
Cardiac	cardi/o = heart -ac = pertaining to	Pertaining to the heart
Cervical	cervic- = neck -al = pertaining to	Pertaining to the neck
Cranial	crani/o = cranium or skull -al = pertaining to	Pertaining to the skull or cranium
Cutaneous	cutane- = skin -ous = pertaining to	Pertaining to the skin
Deltoid	N/A – word root	Pertaining to the shoulder muscle
Femoral	femor/o = femur -al = pertaining to	Pertaining to the thigh
Gastric	gastr/o = stomach -ic = pertaining to	Pertaining to the stomach
Gluteal	glute- = buttocks -al = pertaining to	Pertaining to the buttocks
Hepatic	hepat/ic = liver -ic = pertaining to	Pertaining to the liver
Inguinal	inguin- = groin -al = pertaining to	Pertaining to the groin (depressions in the abdominal wall near the thighs)
Lumbar	lumb- = loin -ar = pertaining to	Pertaining to the loin (the lower back between the ribs and pelvis)

Term	Word Parts	Definition
Mammary	mamm/o = breast -ary = pertaining to	Pertaining to the breast
Nasal	nas/o = nose -al = pertaining to	Pertaining to the nose
Occipital	occiput = the back of the head or skull -al = pertaining to	Pertaining to the inferior posterior region of the head
Orbital	orbit = the bones surrounding the eye -al = pertaining to	Pertaining to the bones surrounding the eye
Pectoral	pector- = breast or chest -al = pertaining to	Pertaining to the chest
Perineal	peri- = around -eal = pertaining to	Pertaining to the perineum, the area between the sacrum and pubis
Plantar	plant/o = sole of the foot -ar = pertaining to	Pertaining to the sole of the foot
Popliteal	poplit- = posterior knee -al = pertaining to	Pertaining to the posterior knee
Pulmonary	pulm/o, pulmon/o = lungs -ary = pertaining to	Pertaining to the lungs
Renal	ren- = kidney -al = pertaining to	Pertaining to the kidneys
Sacral	sacr/o = the lowest portion of the spine -al = pertaining to	Pertaining to the lowest portion of the spine
Temporal	temp/o, tempor/o = temples -al = pertaining to	Pertaining to the temples of the head
Umbilical	umbilic- = navel -al = pertaining to	Pertaining to the navel
Volar	vol- = palm of hand or sole of foot -ar = pertaining to	Pertaining to the sole of the foot or palm of the hand

the heart, lungs and great vessels; the abdominal cavity, which holds several digestive and endocrine organs; and the pelvic cavity, which contains many digestive organs as well as the female reproductive organs. The abdominal and pelvic cavities can be referred to together as the abdominopelvic cavity Figure 7-3. Another cavity is the retroperitoneal cavity, which is separate from and lies posterior (dorsal) to the abdominal cavity and contains different organs, most notably the kidneys.

▶ Directional Terms

Directional terms used in the study of anatomy describe relative positions of body parts as well as imaginary anatomic divisions. When you discuss, describe, or document the location of pain or injury, use the correct directional terms Figure 7-4. Table 7-9 provides the basic terms used in medicine. Since every direction has an opposite—above and below, front and behind, and so on—directional terms in medicine tend to occur in pairs.

Superior and Inferior

The **superior** portion of any body part is the portion above or closest to the head from a specific reference point. The body part closest to the feet is the **inferior** portion. These terms are used to describe the relationship of one structure to another. For example, the knee is superior to the foot and inferior to the pelvis.

Lateral and Medial

Parts of the body that lie farther from the midline are described as **lateral** (outer). The parts that lie closer to the midline are described as **medial** (inner). For example,

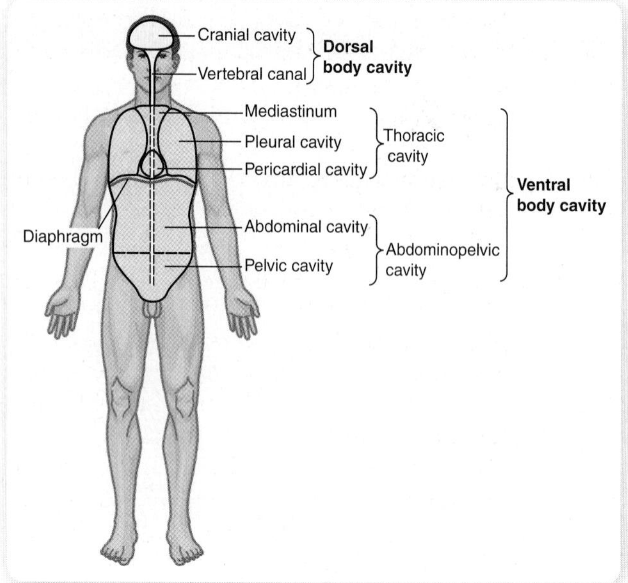

Figure 7-3 Body cavities.

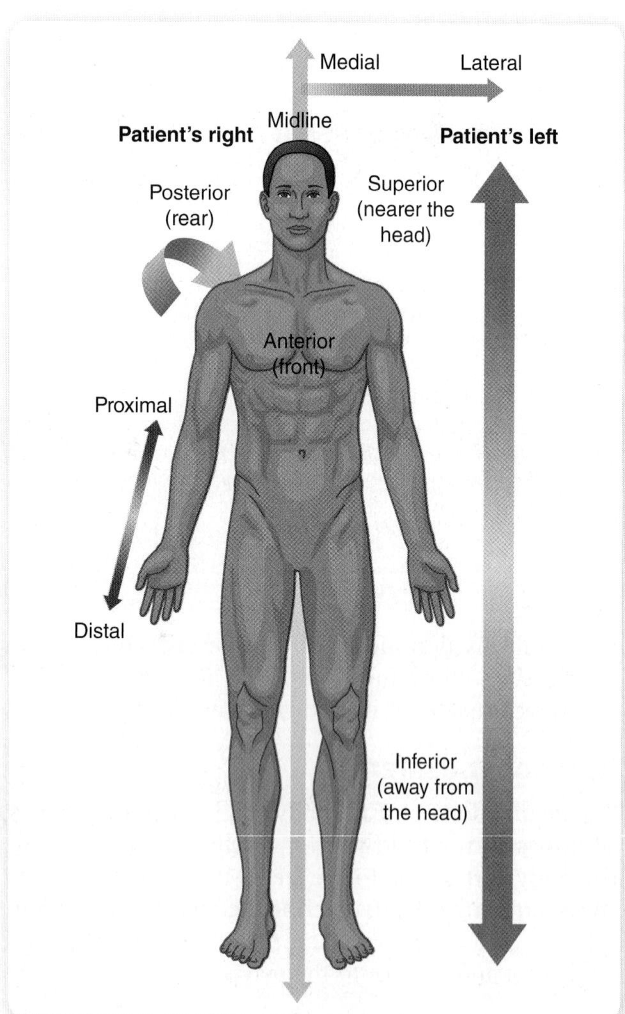

Figure 7-4 Directional terms indicate distance and direction from the midline.

Table 7-9 Common Directional Terms

Common Term	Directional Term	Definition
Right and left	Right Left	The patient's right The patient's left
Top and bottom	Superior Inferior	Closest to the head Closest to the feet
Middle and side	Medial Lateral	Closest to the midline Farthest from the midline
Closest and farthest	Proximal Distal	Closest to the point of attachment Farthest from the point of attachment
In and out	Superficial Deep	Closest to the surface of the skin Farther inside the body
Front and back	Anterior (ventral) Posterior (dorsal)	The front of the body The back of the body

the knee has medial (inner) and lateral (outer) aspects (surfaces).

Proximal and Distal

It is sometimes useful to describe a portion of an extremity relative to its distance from the midline of the body. **Proximal** describes structures that are closer to the body. For example, a fracture of the proximal humerus would involve the end of the bone that's closest to the shoulder. **Distal** indicates structures that are farther from the trunk—that is, nearer to the free end of the extremity. Using our previous example, a fracture of the distal humerus is one that involves the end of the bone farther from the body (adjacent to the elbow). You can use these terms to describe the relationship of one structure to another. For example, the elbow is distal to the shoulder and proximal to the wrist and hand.

Superficial and Deep

Superficial means closer to or on the surface of the skin. **Deep** means farther inside the body and away from the skin.

Anterior and Posterior

Anterior refers to the belly side of the body. Another term for anterior is **ventral**. **Posterior** refers to the spinal side of the body, including the back of the hand (recall, the palms face forward when the body is in the anatomic position). Another term for posterior is **dorsal**. In human medicine, the terms anterior and posterior are used more frequently than the terms ventral and dorsal, which are more common in the veterinary and zoological sciences.

Palmar and Plantar

The front region of the hand is referred to as the palm or **palmar** or volar surface. The bottom of the foot is referred to as the **plantar** or volar surface.

Apex

The **apex** (the plural is *apices* or *apexes*) is the tip of a structure. For example, the apex of the heart is the bottom (inferior portion) of the ventricles in the left side of the chest.

▶ Movement and Positional Terms

All body movement, from the simplest grasp to the most graceful ballet step, can be broken down into a series of simple components and described with specific terms. As with the terms describing anatomic location and direction, an accepted set of terms describes body movement. These are particularly useful in explaining mechanism of injury.

Range of motion is the full distance that a joint can be moved. In the anatomic position, moving the distal point of an extremity toward the trunk is usually called **flexion**. For example, flexion of the elbow brings the hand closer to the shoulder, flexion of the knee brings the foot up to the buttocks, and flexion of the fingers forms the hand into a fist.

In certain cases, specific terms are used to clarify movement, such as in the foot. Dorsiflexion is movement of the foot toward the dorsal aspect, while plantar flexion describes movement toward the sole. **Extension** is the return of a body part from a flexed position to the anatomic position. In the anatomic position, all extremities are in extension. **Abduction** of an extremity moves it away from the midline. **Adduction** moves the extremity toward the midline **Figure 7-5**. A patient's neck can be in one of several positions when the patient is lying supine **Figure 7-6**.

The prefix "hyper-" is often added to the terms *flexion* or *extension* to indicate a mechanism of injury. "Hyper-" indicates that the normal range of motion for the particular

YOU are the Paramedic PART 4

"Well, Tommy, we need to take you to the hospital so they can check that bump on your head and find out why your tummy hurts. Matt and I are going to put you on a board with some seat belts and fix it so your head doesn't move. Don't worry, it won't hurt, and we'll be right here with you. Miss Hawthorne called your mom and dad, and they're going to meet us at the hospital."

After applying a cervical collar and securing the patient on a backboard with straps and a cervical immobilization device, the child is loaded onto the stretcher and into the ambulance. You place him on the cardiac monitor, which shows a sinus rhythm at 98 beats/min. His blood pressure is 96/54 mm Hg and respirations are 18 breaths/min and normal, but his skin is a little cool and clammy to touch. He has good, equal breath sounds. His oxygen saturation (Spo_2) is 96%. You apply a small bandage to his forehead and reassess his abdomen. You note that it is still very tender to the touch and appears a little more discolored than it was initially.

Recording Time: 13 Minutes	
Respiration	18 breaths/min, normal
Pulse	98 beats/min
Skin	Cool, clammy
Blood pressure	96/54 mm Hg
Oxygen saturation (Spo_2)	96%
Pupils	PERRLA

8. Why is knowledge of anatomy pertinent when assessing and treating this patient?
9. What is the medical term for clammy skin?
10. What is the medical term for a phenomenon (such as pain, swelling, or a rash) affecting both sides of the body?

joint was maximized or even exceded, possibly resulting in injury. The term **hyperflexion** refers to a body part that was flexed to the maximum level or even beyond the normal range of motion. **Hyperextension** refers to extension of a body part to the maximum level or even beyond the normal range of motion. An example of a hyperextension injury is one that occurs when a person falls on an outstretched hand, resulting in a distal radius fracture. A hyperflexion injury of the back can occur while bending. Wrist injuries can also be described using the terms **supination** and **pronation**. Turning the palms upward (toward the sky) constitutes supination of the forearm. Turning the palms downward (toward the ground) pronates the forearm.

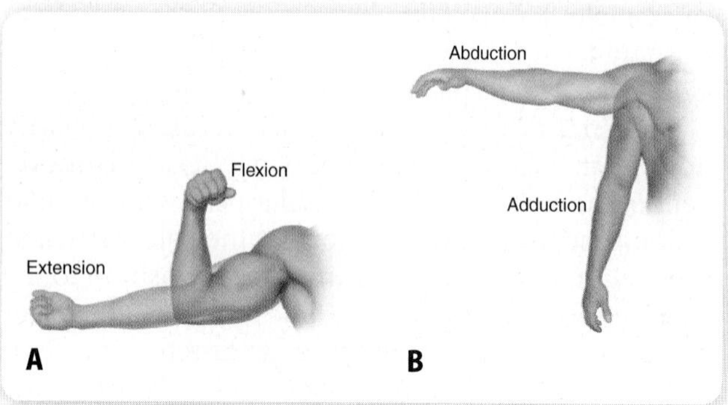

Figure 7-5 A. Flexion and extension. **B.** Abduction and adduction.

Internal rotation means turning the anterior portion of an extremity toward the midline. The lower extremity is internally rotated when the toes are turned inward. **External rotation** means turning an extremity away from the midline. Often, when you are comparing an injured extremity with the uninjured extremity, you will note rotational deformities. A hip can be dislocated anteriorly or posteriorly. In an anterior hip dislocation, the foot is externally rotated and the head of the femur is palpable in the inguinal area (the lower lateral regions of the abdomen and the groin). In the more common posterior hip dislocation, the knee and foot are usually flexed and internally rotated. The term *rotation* also can be applied to the spine. The spine is rotated when it twists on its axis. Placing the chin on the shoulder rotates the cervical spine.

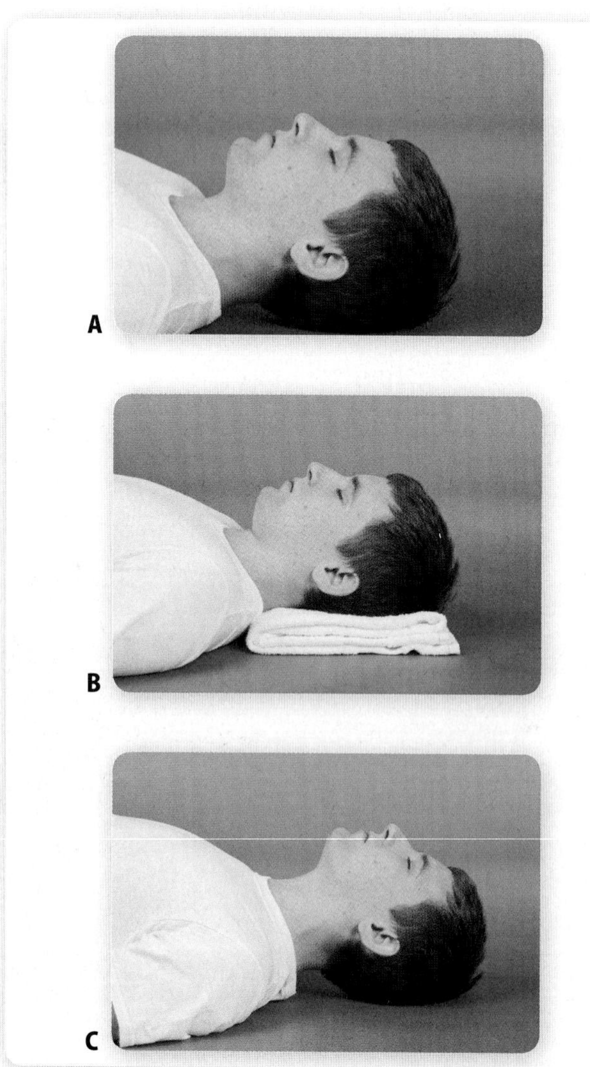

Figure 7-6 Positions of the neck in a patient found in a supine position. **A.** Neutral. **B.** Flexed. **C.** Extended.

Words of Wisdom

Use the correct anatomic terminology in your patient care report (PCR). It makes the report more useful to hospital personnel and enhances your professional image as a paramedic.

Other Directional Terms

A body part or condition that appears on both sides of the midline is said to be **bilateral**. For example, the eyes, ears, hands, and feet are bilateral structures. This is also true of structures inside the body, such as the lungs and kidneys. Structures that appear on only one side of the body are said to be **unilateral**. For example, the spleen is only on the left side of the body, and the liver is predominantly on the right side. The terms *unilateral* and *bilateral* can also describe the location of pain, numbness, itching, or other phenomena; for example, pain on only one side of the body is unilateral pain. You may also use the terms ipsilateral and contralateral. The term **ipsilateral** refers to the same side of the body. A patient having a stroke in the right hemisphere of the brain will usually have facial drooping ipsilaterally, in this case on the right side. **Contralateral** refers to the opposite side of the body. The same patient would have hemiplegia on the contralateral, or the opposite, side from the area of brain injury.

As part of your assessment process, you will palpate the abdomen and report your findings. Therefore, you must be able to describe the exact location of areas of the abdomen. The abdominal cavity is divided into four equal parts called **quadrants**: the right upper quadrant (RUQ), left upper quadrant (LUQ), right lower quadrant (RLQ), and left lower quadrant (LLQ). The quadrants are formed from two lines intersecting at the umbilicus Figure 7-7. Pain or injury in a given quadrant usually arises from or involves the organs that lie in that quadrant. Again, remember right and left refer to the patient's right and left, not yours.

To describe location even more specifically, the abdomen can also be divided into nine regions Figure 7-8.

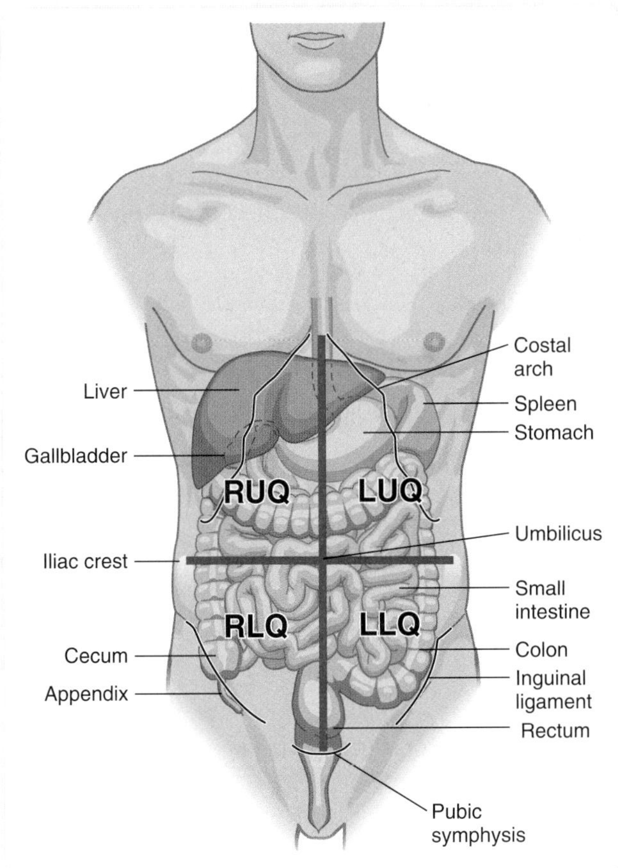

Figure 7-7 The abdomen is divided into four quadrants. RUQ indicates right upper quadrant; LUQ, left upper quadrant; RLQ, right lower quadrant; and LLQ, left lower quadrant.

▶ Prefixes Indicating Position, Direction, and Location

Specialized prefixes are used to specify position, direction, or location. Such terms describe, for instance, movement of the body or something within it, such as a blood clot or tumor metastasis. These prefixes indicate the location of an organ, foreign body, or mass, describe a surgical procedure and the medical instrument used to perform it, or refer to the direction of radiation or ultrasound waves used in diagnosis or treatment. Of course, these are just a few examples of how these versatile prefixes are used in medicine. Which words come to mind as you study Table 7-10?

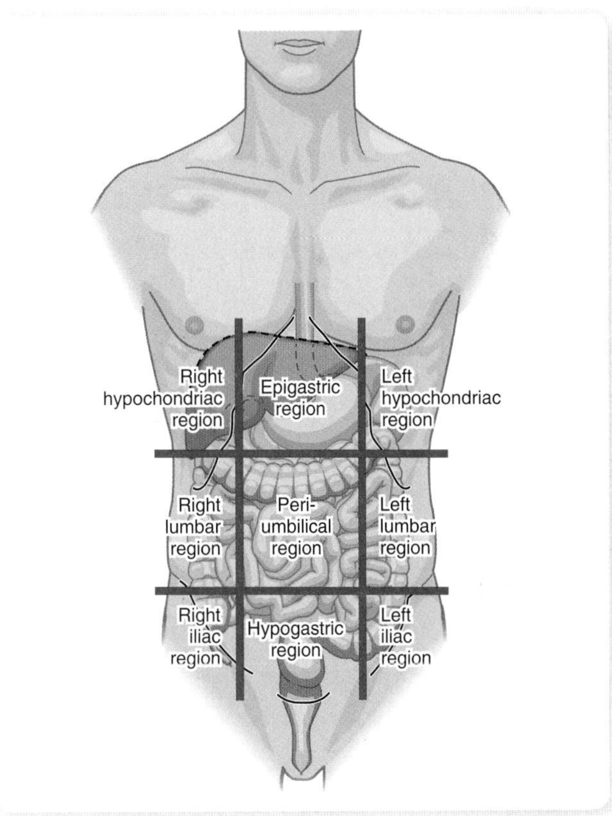

Figure 7-8 Abdominal regions.

Data from Shier, D.N., Butler, J.L., and Lewis, R. Hole's Essentials of Human Anatomy and Physiology, Tenth Edition, McGraw-Hill Higher Education, 2009.

Table 7-10 Prefixes Specifying Position, Direction, or Location

Prefix	Definition	Example	Definition
To/From			
ab-	away from	abduction	Away from the midline of the body, or a specified point of reference
ad-	to, toward	adduction	Toward the midline of the body
Above/Below/Around			
de-	down from, away	decay	To waste away
circum-	around, about	circumferential burn	A burn around an entire area (arm, chest, abdomen, etc)

(continued)

Table 7-10 Prefixes Specifying Position, Direction, or Location *(Continued)*

Prefix	Definition	Example	Definition
Above/Below/Around			
peri-	around	pericardium	Sac around the heart
trans-	across, through, beyond	transvaginal	Across or through the vagina
epi-	above, upon, on	epigastric	Above or over the stomach
supra-	above, upper	suprasternal notch	Top of the sternum
retro-	behind	retroperitoneal	Area behind the peritoneum
sub-	under, below	subcutaneous	Under the skin
infra-	below, under	infrathoracic	Below or at the bottom of the thorax
para-	near, beside, beyond, apart from	parasternal	Near the sternum
contra-	against, opposite	contraindicated	Something that is not indicated
Outside/Inside			
ecto-	out, outside	ectopic pregnancy	Pregnancy where the embryo develops outside of the uterus
endo-	within	endoscopy	View inside the body (with an endoscope)
extra-	outside, in addition	extraneous	Existing or belonging outside the organism
intra-	inside, within	intrauterine	Within the uterus
ipsi-	same	ipsilateral	On or affecting the same side
Within			
inter-	between	intercostal	Between the ribs

▶ Position of the Patient

You will use specific terms to describe the patient's position as you find him or her on the scene or when you are ready to transport the patient to the emergency department Figure 7-9.

Prone and Supine

The body is in the **prone** position when lying face down; it is **supine** when lying face up.

Fowler Position

The **Fowler position** was named after an American surgeon, George R. Fowler, at the end of the nineteenth century. Dr. Fowler placed his patients in a sitting position with their heads elevated to a 90° angle to help them breathe easier and to control their airway. A patient who is sitting straight up, with the knees either bent or straight, is described as being in the Fowler position. A patient in the semi-Fowler position is sitting with his or her back at a 45° angle. This position is generally a position of comfort for those who do not need spinal immobilization.

Recovery Position

The recovery position helps maintain a clear airway in an unresponsive patient. In this position, the patient is lying on his or her left side, with the head resting on the bottom arm. The top knee is bent, angling the front of the patient's body slightly toward the floor or ground. This position, also referred to as the *left lateral recumbent*

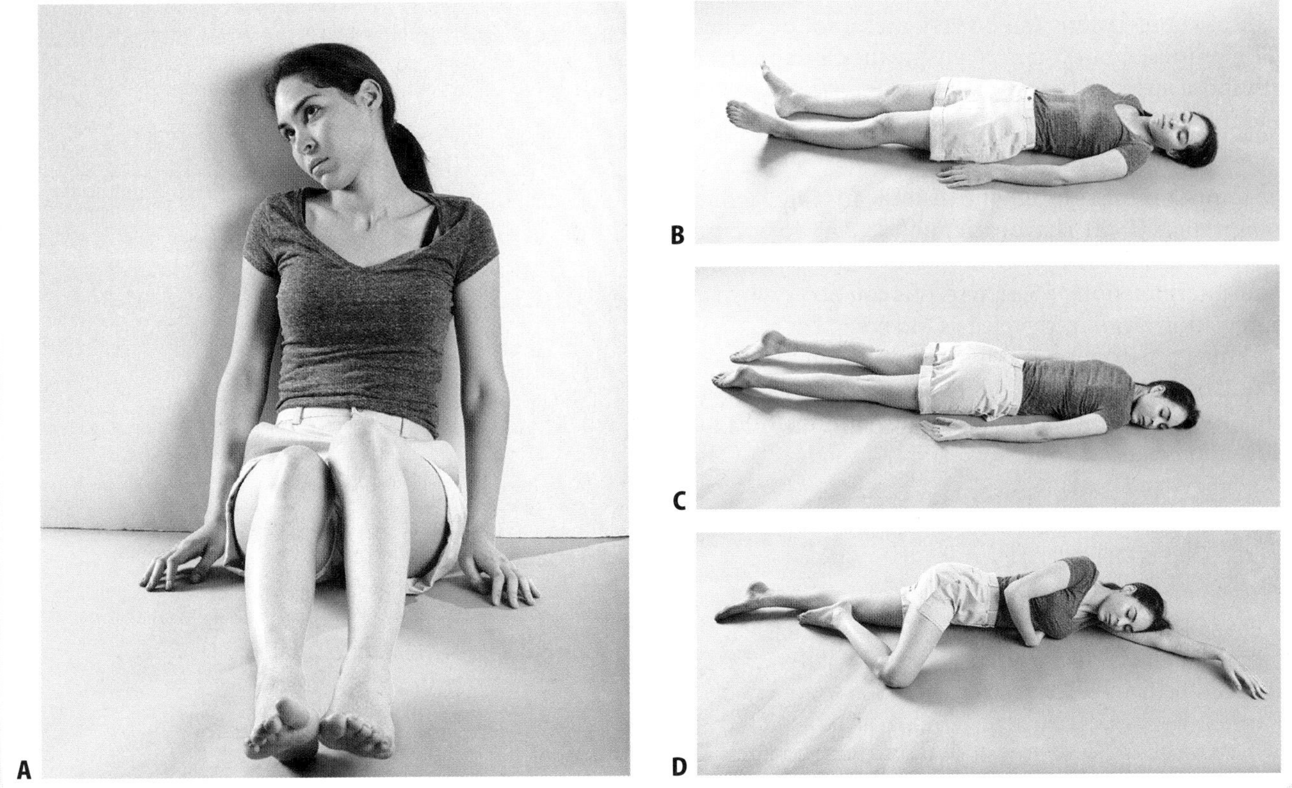

Figure 7-9 Anatomic positions. **A.** Fowler position. **B.** Supine. **C.** Prone. **D.** Recovery (left lateral recumbent) position.

position, helps prevent aspiration of vomitus. It's discussed in greater detail in Chapter 15, *Airway Management*.

Abbreviations, Acronyms, and Symbols

Medical abbreviations, acronyms, and symbols are a type of shorthand used to communicate in the medical world. They evolve for the same reason we abbreviate words in text messages and chats—they allow us to communicate faster. However, in patient care, it's important not to trade speed for accuracy. To minimize misinterpretation and errors, use only commonly understood acronyms and other abbreviations

All acronyms are abbreviations, but not all abbreviations are acronyms. When you shorten a word using an abbreviation, you pronounce each letter of the abbreviation separately. For example, emergency medical technician is abbreviated "EMT," pronounced E–M–T. Acronyms form shortened words from the initials of several words to produce a new word. Acronyms and other abbreviations are sometimes combined to shorten a phrase. For example, the acronym for Urban Search and Rescue, USAR, is pronounced "U-sar."

An abbreviation is still considered an acronym if it's pronounced as a word, even if the word formed isn't part of the English language. An example is HIPAA, short for the Health Insurance Portability and Accountability Act, a law that protects patients' privacy. This abbreviation is classified as an acronym because it's pronounced "hippa," not spelled out letter by letter. DEA, on the other hand, is not considered an acronym because it's spelled out as "D-E-A," rather than pronounced "dia."

Words of Wisdom

In addition to medical terminology, the population of a specific geographic area can have its own slang or regional jargon. Familiarize yourself with this language to improve your communication when responding to calls in these locations. For example, in the south most older adults refer to diabetes as "the sugars" and hypertension as "high blood."

Medical Abbreviations

Abbreviations take the place of the words they represent, to shorten patient care notes or other documentation. Some acronyms have become a common part of the English language. ASAP, for example, stands for "as soon as possible," but is commonly spoken as its own word. Medical abbreviations can be very useful for documentation purposes, but you must ensure they are consistent with those approved for use in your EMS system.

▶ Error-Prone Abbreviations

The Joint Commission and the Institute for Safe Medication Practices (ISMP) have each published a "do not use" list of abbreviations they believe to be especially prone to misinterpretation.[1,2] Serious errors can occur when an abbreviation is not interpreted as intended. For example, "HS" on a prescription can mean either "hour of sleep" (take at bedtime) or "half strength." To avoid such errors, some agencies limit the use of abbreviations or do not allow abbreviations at all.

Patient Safety

Be careful with *look-alike, sound-alike* drug names. Pay close attention to labels to ensure you accurately write down the names. Some common mistakes are listed below. Each drug is different, yet each can be confused because of similar spelling and/or pronunciation:

- Zantac – Xanax
- Toradol – Tegretol
- Clonazepam – Lorazepam
- Alprazolam – Lorazepam
- Amiodarone – Amrinone
- Celebrex – Celexa
- Sinequan – Singulair
- Prozac – Prilosec

Trailing Zeros and Naked Decimals

Another common problem area concerns *trailing zeros* and *"naked" decimals*. Avoid using trailing zeros after a decimal point. For example, 5.0 mg may be read as 50 mg if the decimal is not seen. The same is true if a leading zero is left off before a decimal. If 0.5 mg is written without the leading zero as .5 mg, it may be mistaken for 5 mg if the decimal is not seen. Always leave off trailing zeros after the decimal, but include leading zeros prior to the decimal to avoid errors.

▶ Symbols

Like abbreviations, symbols are sometimes used as a shortcut in documentation and other communication. As with abbreviations, it is important that you use only symbols that are widely understood and accepted (Table 7-11). The symbols > or < may be mistaken for the number "7," the letter "L," or each other. The symbol µ may be mistaken for "mg," resulting in a one thousand times overdose. It is better to spell it out than to use symbols that may be misinterpreted.

To protect patients' safety, The Joint Commission requires every hospital to issue a list of approved abbreviations.

Table 7-11	Common Symbols
°	degrees
1°	first, first degree, primary
2°	secondary, second degree
↑	increase(d)
↓	decrease(d)
Ⓡ	right
Ⓛ	left
α	alpha
β	beta
Ø	null or none
~, ≈	approximately
N	normal
×2	times two
/	per
±	plus or minus
≠	not equal
>	greater than
<	less than
≥	greater than or equal to
≤	less than or equal to
?	questionable, possible
Δ	change
–	negative
♀	female
♂	male

This list cannot include certain abbreviations prohibited by the commission, such as *µm* for micrograms. Each EMS system should also keep a list of approved medical abbreviations available for reporting and documentation purposes. Learn which abbreviations are acceptable in your service area before you use them in a report. For example, some agencies do not use "SOB" as an abbreviation for "shortness of breath." When in doubt, write out the term in full. Accuracy, neatness, and completeness reflect a professional writing style.

Medical Terminology Related to Pharmacology

As a paramedic, you must be familiar with terminology related to medications and medication administration, such as common prefixes Table 7-12, common metric conversions used in drug calculation Table 7-13, and common medical abbreviations related to pharmacology Table 7-14.

Table 7-12 Prefixes Commonly Used in Medication Administration

Prefix Name	Prefix Symbol	Prefix Value
micr/o	mc	1/1,000,000 or 0.000001
milli-	m	1/1,000 or 0.001
centi-	c	10 or 0.01
kil/o	k	1,000
mega-	M	1 million or 1,000,000

Master Tables

Table 7-15 through Table 7-18 provide a reference list of prefixes, suffixes, common word roots, and abbreviations.

Table 7-13 Metric Conversions Used in Drug Calculation

Weight	
1 kilogram (kg)	2.2 pounds (lb) 1,000 grams (g)
1 gram (g)	1,000 milligrams (mg)
1 milligram (mg)	1,000 micrograms (mcg)
Volume	
1 liter (L)	1,000 milliliters (mL)
Temperature	
37° Celsius (°C)	98.6° Fahrenheit (°F)
Length	
1 centimeter (cm)	0.39 inches (in.) 10 millimeters (mm)
100 centimeters (cm)	1 meter (m)

YOU are the Paramedic PART 5

You cover Tommy with a blanket and start an IV line in the back of his left hand, using a 20-gauge catheter to infuse normal saline at a rate of 10 drops per minute. You also assess the patient's blood glucose level, which is now 147 mg/dL.

You and your crew transport the patient to a pediatric trauma center, where the child's parents are waiting, and give a verbal report to the receiving staff. Then you sit down in the EMS office to write your report while Matt cleans and restocks the ambulance.

Recording Time: 18 Minutes	
Respiration	20 breaths/min
Pulse	98 beats/min
Skin	Cool and clammy
Blood pressure	98/60 mm Hg
Oxygen saturation (Spo_2)	99%
Pupils	PERRLA
Blood glucose level	147 mg/dL

Table 7-14 Selected Medical Abbreviations Associated With Pharmacology

Abbreviation	Meaning	Abbreviation	Meaning
amp	ampule	max	maximum
caps	capsules	MDI	metered-dose inhaler
elix	elixir	mEq	milliequivalents
gtt	drop(s)	MS or MSO_4	morphine sulfate
HHN	handheld nebulizer	pr	per rectus (by rectum)
IC	intracardiac	RL	Ringer lactate (solution)
IVP	intravenous push	SVN	small-volume nebulizer
IVPB	intravenous piggyback	tid	ter in die (three times a day)
KO	keep open	TKO	to keep open
KVO	keep vein open	ut dict	ut dictum (as directed)
LR	lactated Ringer (solution)		

Table 7-15 Selected Prefixes Used in Medical Terminology

Prefix	Meaning	Prefix	Meaning	Prefix	Meaning
a-	without, lack of	arteri/o	artery	cephal/o	pertaining to the head
ab-	away from	arthro-	pertaining to a joint	cerebr/o	pertaining to the cerebrum, a part of the brain
abdomin/o	abdomen	auto-	self	cervic/o	pertaining to the neck or the uterine cervix
acr/o	to, toward	bi-	two	chole-	pertaining to bile
aden/o	pertaining to a gland	bio-	pertaining to life	chondr/o	pertaining to cartilage
an-	without, lack of	blast/o	germ or cell	circum-	around, about
ana-	up, back, again	blephar/o	pertaining to an eyelid	contra-	against, opposite
angio-	vessel	brady-	slow	cost/o	pertaining to a rib
ante-	before, forward	calc-	stone; also heel	cyan/o	blue
anti-	against, opposed to	cardi/o	pertaining to the heart	cyst/o	pertaining to the bladder or any fluid–containing sac

Prefix	Meaning	Prefix	Meaning	Prefix	Meaning
cyt/o	pertaining to a cell	glyc/o	sugar	latero-	side
de-	down from	gynec/o	pertaining to females or the female reproductive organs	leuk/o	pertaining to anything white or to leukocytes (white blood cells)
dermat/o	pertaining to the skin	hemat/o	pertaining to blood	lith/o	pertaining to a stone
di-	twice, double	hemi-	half	macro-	large
dia-	through, across	hem/o	pertaining to blood	mal-	bad or abnormal
dys-	difficult, painful, abnormal	hepat/o	pertaining to the liver	medi-	middle
ect/o	out, out from	heter/o	other, different	mega-	large
electro-	pertaining to electricity	hom/o	same or like	melan-	black
end/o	within	hydr/o	water	mening/o	pertaining to a membrane, particularly the meninges
enter/o	pertaining to the intestines or gut	hyper-	over, excessive	micro-	small
epi-	upon, on, above	hypo-	under, deficient	mono-	one
erythr/o	pertaining to anything red or to erythrocytes (red blood cells)	hyster/o	pertaining to the uterus	myel/o	pertaining to the spinal cord, the bone marrow, or myelin
eu-	easy, good, normal	infra-	below	my/o	pertaining to muscle
ex/o	outside	inter-	between	nas/o	pertaining to the nose
extra-	outside, in addition	intra-	within	neo-	new
gastr/o	pertaining to the stomach	iso-	equal	nephr/o	pertaining to the kidney

(continued)

Table 7-15 Selected Prefixes Used in Medical Terminology *(Continued)*

Prefix	Meaning	Prefix	Meaning	Prefix	Meaning
neur/o	pertaining to nerves or the nervous system	pharyng/o	pertaining to the throat, or pharynx	quat-	four
noct-	night	phleb/o	pertaining to a vein	retr/o	backward or behind
olig/o	little, deficient	pneum/o	pertaining to respiration, the lungs, or air	rhin/o	pertaining to the nose
oophor/o	pertaining to the ovary	poly-	many	salping/o	pertaining to a tube
ophthalm/o	pertaining to the eye	post-	after, behind	scler/o	hard; also means pertaining to the sclera of the eye
orchid/o	pertaining to the testicles	pre-	before	semi-	half or partial
orchi/o	pertaining to the testicles	pro-	before, in front of	sub-	under, moderately
oro-	pertaining to the mouth	proct/o	pertaining to the rectum	super-	above, excessive, or more than normal
ortho-	straight or normal	pseud/o	false	supra-	above
oste/o	pertaining to bone	psych/o	pertaining to the mind	tachy-	fast
ot/o	pertaining to the ear	pulm/o	pertaining to the lung	therm-	pertaining to temperature
para-	by the side of	pur-	pertaining to pus	thorac/o	pertaining to the chest
path/o	pertaining to disease	pyel/o	pertaining to the kidney or pelvis	trans-	across
per-	through	py/o	pertaining to pus	tri-	three
peri-	around	quadr/i	four	uni-	one
phag/o	pertaining to eating, ingesting, or engulfing	quart-	fourth, four	vas/o	vessel

Table 7-16 Selected Suffixes Used in Medical Terminology

Suffix	Meaning	Suffix	Meaning	Suffix	Meaning
-algia	pertaining to pain	-lysis	decline, disintegration, or destruction	-ptosis	drooping
-asthen/o	weakness	-megaly	enlargement of	-rrhage or -rrhagia	abnormal or excessive flow or discharge
-blast	immature cell	-ology	science of	-rrhaphy	suture of; repair of
-cele	tumor or swelling	-oma	tumor	-rrhea	flow or discharge
-centesis	procedure in which an organ or body cavity is punctured, often to drain excess fluid or obtain a sample for laboratory analysis	-osis	disease process (see also -sis)	-scope	instrument for examination
-cyte	cell	-ostomy	surgical creation of an opening, or hole	-scopy	examination with an instrument
-ectomy	surgical removal of	-otomy	surgical incision	-sis	process, action, or condition
-emia	pertaining to the presence of a substance in the blood	-pathy	pertaining to disease or a system for treating disease	-taxis	order, arrangement of
-genic	causing	-phobia	an irrational fear	-trophic	nutrition
-gram	record (as in written documentation or results of a study)	-plasty	plastic or reconstructive surgery	-uria	pertaining to a substance in the urine or the condition so indicated
-graph	record or the instrument used to create the record	-plegia	pertaining to paralysis		
-itis	inflammation	-pnea	pertaining to breathing		

Table 7-17 Selected Word Roots and Combining Forms Used in Medical Terminology

Word Root	Meaning	Word Root	Meaning	Word Root	Meaning
acou-	pertaining to hearing	carcin/o	cancer	foramen	opening
adip-	fat	carotid	pertaining to the great arteries of the neck	fract-	break
alb-	white	carp/o	pertaining to the carpus, or wrist	gest-	carry, produce, congestion
alges-	pertaining to pain	cent/i	a fraction in the metric system; one hundredth or 100	gno-	know
andr-	male	cent/e	to puncture (a body cavity)	-gram	something written or recorded
aort/o	pertaining to the aorta, the large artery exiting from the left ventricle of the heart	cili-	eyelid	graph-	write, record
aqua-	water	cleid/o	clavicle	humer/o	pertaining to the humerus, the long bone of the upper arm
asphyxia	lack of oxygen or excess of carbon dioxide in the body that results in unconsciousness	cubitus	elbow	idi-, idi/o	separate, distinct or pertaining to the self
asthen-	weak	cycl-	circle or cycle	iod/o	iodine
audi-	to hear	digit	finger or toe	lact/o	milk
bronch/o	windpipe	edema-	swelling	lingu/o	tongue
bucc-	cheek	esthesi/o	pertaining to sensation or perception	men-	month
bursa	pouch or sac	febr-	fever	ocul/o	eye
callus	hard, thick skin; also a lattice of connective tissue that forms during the healing process after a fracture	flex	bend	ov-	egg

Word Root	Meaning	Word Root	Meaning	Word Root	Meaning
palpate	to examine by touch	retina	inner nerve–containing layer of the eye	stoma	any small opening on the surface of the body, such as a pore; also, the opening created in the abdominal wall for the passage of urine or feces
ped-	child or foot	sangui/n	blood	tact-	touch
percuss	to examine by striking	seb/o	pertaining to sebum, a fatty secretion of the sebaceous glands	tetra-	four
phagia	pertaining to eating or swallowing	sect-	cut	tom/o	cut
phasia	pertaining to speech	seps-	literally means "decay"; refers to the presence of microorganisms or their toxins in the blood, or to the toxic condition that their presence causes in the body	toxic	poisonous
phot/o	light	sept-	wall, divider; also refers to the number seven	trich-	hair
pleur-	rib, side	ser/o	pertaining to serum, the clear portion of body fluids, including blood	ur-	urine
pod-	foot	sin/o	pertaining to a cavity, channel, or hollow space	varic-	varicose vein
pto-	fall	som/a or somat/o	body or soma	vertigo	a disordered sensation in which one's own body or the surroundings are perceived as moving
ptyal-	saliva	spir-	coil	viscer-	internal organs
pyr-	fire	stasis	slowing or stopping of the normal flow of a fluid, such as blood	viscum	sticky
radius	the forearm bone on the thumb side; also a line from the center of a circle or sphere to the edge	stature	height	xen/o	foreign (material)
ren-	kidney	stern/o	sternum (breastbone)	xer-	dry

Table 7-18	Common Abbreviations in Medical Terminology[a]		
Abbreviation	**Meaning**	**Abbreviation**	**Meaning**
A&P	anatomy and physiology	ARDS	adult respiratory distress syndrome
ā	before	ASA	aspirin (acetylsalicylic acid)
AAA	abdominal aortic aneurysm	ASHD	arteriosclerotic or atherosclerotic heart disease
abd	abdomen	AV	atrioventricular
ABCDE	airway, breathing, circulation, disability, and exposure	BBB	bundle branch block
ac	before meals	BGL	blood glucose level
ACLS	advanced cardiac life support	bid/b.i.d./BID	twice daily
ACS	acute coronary syndrome	BKA	below the knee amputation
ADL	activities of daily living	BM	bowel movement
ad lib	as desired	BMD	bag-mask device
AED	automated external defibrillator	BMV	bag-mask ventilation
AF, A-fib, A fib, AFib	atrial fibrillation	BP, B/P	blood pressure
AICD	automatic implantable cardioverter-defibrillator	BPM	beats per minute
AIDS	acquired immunodeficiency syndrome	BS	blood sugar, breath sounds, bowel sounds, bachelor of science (degree)
AK	above the knee	BSA	body surface area
AKA	above the knee amputation	BVM	bag-valve-mask
AMA	against medical advice	bx, Bx	biopsy
amb	ambulatory	c̄	with
AMI	acute myocardial infarction	°C	degrees Celsius (centigrade)
AMS	altered mental status	CA	cancer, carcinoma, cardiac arrest, chronologic age, coronary artery, cold agglutinin
ant	anterior	CABDE	circulation, airway, breathing, disability, and exposure
AO × 4, A/O × 4, A&O × 4	alert and oriented to person, place, time, and event	CABG	coronary artery bypass graft
AP	anteroposterior, front-to-back, action potential, angina pectoris, anterior pituitary, arterial pressure	CAD	coronary artery disease

Abbreviation	Meaning	Abbreviation	Meaning
CBC	complete blood cell count	DON	director of nursing
CC or C/C	chief complaint	DPT	diphtheria and tetanus toxoids and pertussis vaccine, Doctor of Physical Therapy
CCU	coronary care unit or critical care unit	DSD	dry sterile dressing
C diff	*Clostridium difficile*	DtaP	diphtheria and tetanus toxoids and acellular pertussis vaccine
cm	centimeter	DTP	diphtheria and tetanus toxoids and pertussis vaccine
CNS	central nervous system	DTs	delirium tremens
c/o	complaining of	DVT	deep venous thrombosis
CO	cardiac output, carbon monoxide	Dx	diagnosis
CO_2	carbon dioxide	EBL	estimated blood loss
COLD	chronic obstructive lung disease	ECG	electrocardiogram
COPD	chronic obstructive pulmonary disease	ED	emergency department, erectile dysfunction
CP	chest pain, chemically pure, cerebral palsy	EDC	estimated date of confinement
CPAP	continuous positive airway pressure	EDD	expected (estimated) date of delivery
CPR	cardiopulmonary resuscitation	EEG	electroencephalogram
CR	capillary refill	EKG	electrocardiogram (the "k" comes from the German word "Elektrokardiogramm")
CRNA	certified registered nurse anesthetist	ENT	ears, nose, and throat
CRT	capillary refill time, cathode ray tube	EOC	Emergency Operations Center
CSF	cerebrospinal fluid	ER	emergency room
CVA	cerebrovascular accident	ET, ETT	endotracheal tube, endotracheal
DM	diabetes mellitus	ETA	estimated time of arrival
DNR	do not resuscitate	$ETCO_2$	end-tidal carbon dioxide
DOA	dead on arrival	ETOH	ethyl alcohol
DOB	date of birth	°F	degrees Fahrenheit
DOD	date of death	FIO_2	fraction of inspired oxygen
DOE	dyspnea on exertion	FBS	fasting blood sugar

(continued)

Table 7-18 Common Abbreviations in Medical Terminology[a] *(Continued)*

Abbreviation	Meaning	Abbreviation	Meaning
Fe	iron	HPI	history of present illness
FHR	fetal heart rate	HPV	human papilloma virus
FHx	family history	HR	heart rate
fl or fld	fluid	hr	hour
fx	fracture	HTN	hypertension
GB	gallbladder	Hx	history
GCS	Glasgow Coma Scale	I&O	intake and output
GERD	gastroesophageal reflux disease	ICP	intracranial pressure
GI	gastrointestinal	ICS	incident command system, intercostal space
GSW	gunshot wound	ICU	intensive care unit
GTT	glucose tolerance test	IDDM	insulin-dependent diabetes mellitus
GU	genitourinary	IHD	ischemic heart disease
GYN, gyn	gynecology	IM	intramuscular
h	hour	IMS	incident management system
H&P	history and physical	IO	intraosseous
H/A	headache	IPPB, IPPV	intermittent positive pressure breathing, intermittent positive pressure ventilation
Hb, Hgb	hemoglobin	IUD	intrauterine (contraceptive) device
HBV	hepatitis B virus	IV	intravenous
HCV	hepatitis C virus	JVD	jugular venous distention
HCVD	hypertensive cardiovascular disease	kg	kilogram
HF	heart failure	KVO	keep vein open
HH	hiatal hernia	L	liter
HIV	human immunodeficiency virus	lac, LAC	laceration
H_2O	water	lb	pound

Abbreviation	Meaning	Abbreviation	Meaning
LE	lower extremity, left eye, lupus erythematosus	MVP	mitral valve prolapse
LLL	left lower lobe (of the lung)	NA, N/A	not applicable
LLQ	left lower quadrant (of the abdomen)	NAD	no apparent distress, no appreciable disease
L/M, LPM	liters per minute	NARD	No apparent respiratory distress
LMP	last menstrual period	NC	nasal cannula
LOC	level of consciousness, loss of consciousness	NG	nasogastric (tube)
LOM	loss of motion	NICU	neonatal intensive care unit
LUL	left upper lobe (of the lung)	NIDDM	non–insulin-dependent diabetes mellitus
LUQ	left upper quadrant (of the abdomen)	NKA	no known allergies
LVAD	left ventricular assist device	NKDA	no known drug allergies
MAE	moves all extremities	NPA	nasopharyngeal airway
MAEW	moves all extremities well	NPO	nil per os (nothing by mouth)
mcg	microgram	NRB, NRBM	nonrebreathing mask
mg	milligram	NS	normal saline
MI	myocardial infarction	NSR	normal sinus rhythm
MICU	mobile intensive care unit; medical intensive care unit	NTG	nitroglycerin
min	minute	N/V, N&V	nausea and vomiting
mL	milliliter	N/V/D	nausea, vomiting, and diarrhea
mm	millimeter	O_2	oxygen
mm Hg	millimeters of mercury	OB	obstetrics
MOI	mechanism of injury	OBS	organic brain syndrome
MRI	magnetic resonance imaging	OD	overdose, right eye, optical density, outside diameter, doctor of optometry
MRSA	methicillin-resistant *Staphylococcus aureus*	OP	outpatient
MVA	motor vehicle accident	OPA	oropharyngeal airway
MVC	motor vehicle crash	OR	operating room

(continued)

Table 7-18 Common Abbreviations in Medical Terminology[a] *(Continued)*

Abbreviation	Meaning	Abbreviation	Meaning
oz	ounce	pt	patient
p̄	after	PT	physical therapy, prothrombin time
pc	after meals	PTA	prior to admission, plasma thromboplastin antecedent
PCI	percutaneous coronary intervention	PTT	partial thromboplastin time
Pco_2	partial pressure of carbon dioxide	PVC	premature ventricular complex, polyvinyl chloride
PDR	*Physicians' Desk Reference*	PVD	peripheral vascular disease
PE	pulmonary embolism, physical examination	q̄	every
PEARL or PERL	pupils equal and reactive to light	RA	rheumatoid arthritis, right atrium
PEARLA	pupils equal and reactive to light and accommodation	RAD	reactive airway disease, right axis deviation
PEARRL	pupils equal and round, regular in size, react to light	RBC	red blood cell
ped or peds	pediatric	Rh	Rhesus blood factor, rhodium
PEEP	positive end-expiratory pressure	RLL	right lower lobe (of the lung)
PERRL	pupils equal, round, and reactive to light	RLQ	right lower quadrant (of the abdomen)
PERRLA	pupils equal, round, and reactive to light and accommodation	RML	right middle lobe (of the lung)
PID	pelvic inflammatory disease	RN	registered nurse
PMH	past medical history	R/O	rule out
PND	paroxysmal nocturnal dyspnea	ROM	range of motion, rupture of membranes
po	per os (by mouth)	RUL	right upper lobe (of the lung)
PO	postoperative, "post op"	RUQ	right upper quadrant of the abdomen
PRN	pro re nata (as needed)	Rx	prescription
psi	pounds per square inch	s̄	without
PSVT	paroxysmal supraventricular tachycardia	SAH	subarachnoid hemorrhage

Abbreviation	Meaning	Abbreviation	Meaning
Sao_2	oxygen saturation	tech	technician, technologist
SARS	severe acute respiratory syndrome	TIA	transient ischemic attack
SICU	surgical intensive care unit	tid/t.i.d./TID	three times a day
SIDS	sudden infant death syndrome	Tx	treatment
SL	sublingual	UA, U/A	urinalysis
SOB	shortness of breath	UE	upper extremity
Spo_2	saturation of peripheral oxygen	URI	upper respiratory infection
S/S, S&S	signs and symptoms	UTI	urinary tract infection
stat	immediately	VF/V fib/VFib	ventricular fibrillation
STI	sexually transmitted infection	VRE	vancomycin-resistant enterococcus
STEMI	ST-segment elevation myocardial infarction	VS	vital signs
subcut	subcutaneous	VT/V tach	ventricular tachycardia
SUID	sudden unexpected infant death	W/	with
SVN	small-volume nebulizer	WBC	white blood cell
SVT	supraventricular tachycardia	WMD	weapon of mass destruction
sym or Sx	symptoms	WNL	within normal limits
T	temperature	W/O	without
tab	tablet	wt	weight
TB	tuberculosis	yo; y.o.; y/o	year old
TBA	to be admitted, to be announced	$\bar{x}$	except

[a]Sometimes abbreviations are written with periods (for example, abd. and a.c.), and sometimes different capitalization might be used and might convey a different meaning. Not all possible meanings for each abbreviation are given in this table. Unless you are certain about the meaning, ask the person who used the abbreviation and do not use it yourself.

YOU are the Paramedic SUMMARY

1. What is the correct medical term for the position in which the child is lying?

He's lying on his left side, which is the recovery position, also called the *left lateral recumbent* position.

2. How can knowledge of medical terminology assist in your documentation of care for this patient?

Medical terminology is the language of medicine and health care. As a paramedic, you should have a good understanding of medical terminology and be able to identify and use terms correctly. This not only allows you to communicate effectively with other health care providers, but also ensures you use accurate and concise documentation, resulting in better continuity of care.

3. Why would you want to avoid using medical terminology when talking to this patient?

Patients, especially children, are rarely familiar with medical terminology. Therefore, using medical terms during a patient interview will probably lead to misunderstanding and a lack of pertinent information. When you talk with patients, use everyday terms to improve the likelihood of communicating clearly. As a paramedic, you must also be familiar with terms and phrases that are common in the geographic area in which you work.

4. What are the correct medical terms to describe Tommy's mental status and blood glucose level?

His mental status is documented as AOx4 because he is alert to person, place, time, and event. The appropriate term for a high blood glucose level is *hyperglycemia*. It is formed from the prefix *hyper-* (excessive) + the word root *glyc/o* (glucose) + the suffix *-emia* (pertaining to the blood).

5. How would you document that the patient has no medication allergies?

The correct abbreviation for "no known drug allergies" is *NKDA*.

6. Describe *the* position of the patient's head injury.

His injury is on the right side of his forehead, just above his eye. Since *superior* is the term for above and *orbit* is the eye socket, it would be documented as *superior to the right orbit*. You could also use Ⓡ to replace the directional term "right" in your documentation.

7. What is the abbreviation for the abdominal quadrant that is tender to the touch?

The abdomen is divided into quadrants by two imaginary lines intersecting at the umbilicus. The area where Tommy reports having pain is the upper quadrant on the right side. The abbreviation is *RUQ*.

8. Why is knowledge of anatomy pertinent when assessing and treating this patient?

Familiarity with the structures and functions of the body's systems will allow you to better assess a patient as well as predict potential complications resulting from occult injuries (those not visible to the eye). In this instance, if you know what organs are located in the RUQ, you can predict possible injuries, which allows for a greater index of suspicion resulting in more appropriate treatment and transport to the proper facility.

9. What is the medical term for clammy skin?

The term for clammy skin associated with signs of shock is *diaphoresis*.

10. What is the medical term for a phenomenon (such as pain, swelling, or a rash) affecting both sides of the body?

Many body structures are bilateral, and certain medical conditions tend to occur either unilaterally or bilaterally. A phenomenon affecting or appearing on both sides of the midline is said to be *bilateral*.

YOU are the Paramedic SUMMARY *(continued)*

EMS Patient Care Report (PCR)					
Date: 4-20-18	**Incident No.:** 050109		**Nature of Call:** Fall		**Location:** 184 Primary Way
Dispatched: 0935	**En Route:** 0936	**At Scene:** 0942	**Transport:** 0957	**At Hospital:** 1009	**In Service:** 1027

Patient Information	
Age: 8 **Sex:** M **Weight (in kg [lb]):** 25 kg (56 lb)	**Allergies:** NKDA **Medications:** insulin **Past Medical History:** IDDM **Chief Complaint:** Fall

Vital Signs				
Time: 0945	**BP:**	**Pulse:** 104	**Respirations:** 22	**Spo_2:** 98%
Time: 0950	**BP:**	**Pulse:** 108	**Respirations:** 22	**Spo_2:** 99%
Time: 0955	**BP:** 96/54	**Pulse:** 98	**Respirations:** 18	**Spo_2:** 96%
Time: 1000	**BP:** 98/60	**Pulse:** 98	**Respirations:** 20	**Spo_2:** 99%

EMS Treatment (circle all that apply)				
Oxygen @ ______ L/min via (circle one): **NC NRM Bag-mask device**		**Assisted Ventilation**	**Airway Adjunct**	**CPR**
Defibrillation	**Bleeding Control**	**Bandaging:** Hematoma Ⓡ forehead (circled)	**Splinting**	**Other:** Spinal immobilization (circled)

Narrative
9-1-1 dispatch for a male patient who fell. On arrival at the scene, found the patient, an 8-y/o male, lying Ⓛ lateral recumbent in fetal position and holding abdomen; comforted by teacher. Teacher states pt fell approximately 5 feet from top of playground equipment and has not been moved. Patient AOx4, c/o pain in right upper quadrant. Presents with a golf ball–size hematoma superior to the Ⓡ orbit ⓒ small laceration—bleeding controlled. Patient states he has been "dizzy" this morning, causing his fall. PEARL, slightly tachycardic and tachypneic. Hx—IDDM, for which he takes insulin and has NKDA. Teacher states blood glucose level was 183 mg/dL upon arrival this a.m. Pt states he ate and took insulin this a.m. Further assessment of patient's abdomen revealed that it was soft, but very tender to palpation of the RUQ, with discoloration of the area. Patient fully c-spine immobilized on LSB ⓒ c-collar and CID and loaded into ambulance for transport to the pediatric trauma center. En route, vital signs reassessed and noted above, breath sounds clear and equal bilaterally, skin cool and diaphoretic, glucose 147 mg/dL. Pt covered to maintain warmth, head wound bandaged, placed on cardiac monitor showing sinus rhythm ⓢ ectopy, and 20 g IV Ⓛ DH ⓒ NS KVO. Reassessment of abdomen finds increased tenderness and darker discoloration. Met patient's parents and transferred care of patient to receiving hospital without incident. Written report completed and ambulance cleaned and restocked. Departed the hospital and returned to service.**End of report**

Prep Kit

Ready for Review

- Knowledge of medical terminology is essential for health care team members to communicate effectively and document calls.
- You must be able to identify superficial landmarks of the body. These landmarks indicate which structures lie underneath the skin, so you can perform an accurate patient assessment.
- Understanding how terms are formed, and the definitions for the various parts of a medical term, will to help you determine the meaning of an unknown term.
- To strengthen your grasp of medical terminology, become familiar with commonly used medical eponyms, homonyms, and antonyms, as well as symbols and terms used in pharmacology.
- A prefix is the part of a term that appears at the beginning of a word. It generally describes location and intensity of the word root that follows.
- A suffix is placed at the end of a word to change the original meaning. In medical terminology, a suffix usually indicates a procedure, condition, disease, or part of speech.
- The word root is the foundation of the term. It establishes the basic meaning of the word.
- A combining vowel is the part of a term that connects a word root to a suffix or other word root to make it easier to pronounce.
- Prefixes can also indicate numbers or direction. Word roots can also describe color.
- Compound words are words that contain more than one word root.
- To make some terms plural, an s is added to the term. Other terms use other plural forms.
- Anatomic position refers to the position of the body; for example, the position the patient is in when you arrive on scene. Anatomic positions include prone, supine, and Fowler.
- Anatomic planes of the body include coronal, transverse, and sagittal (lateral).
- Directional terms indicate distance and direction from the midline. These include right, left, superior, inferior, lateral, medial, proximal, distal, superficial, deep, ventral, dorsal, anterior, posterior, palmar, plantar, and apex.
- Terms related to movement and position include flexion, extension, adduction, abduction, supination, pronation, and rotation.
- Other directional terms relate to a position on one or both sides of the body. Such terms include bilateral, unilateral, ipsilateral, and contralateral.
- The concept of quadrants is useful in medical terminology. The abdomen is commonly categorized into quadrants to help specify an area of pain or injury.
- Abbreviations, acronyms, and symbols are used as shorthand to communicate and document in a concise manner. To avoid potentially dangerous misinterpretation of your documentation, ensure you use only abbreviations that are commonly understood in your system; avoid using abbreviations that are not recommended.

Vital Vocabulary

abduction Movement of a limb away from the midline.

adduction Movement of a limb toward the midline.

anatomic position The position of reference, in which the patient stands facing you, arms at the side, with the palms of the hands facing forward.

anterior The front surface of the body; the side facing you in the anatomic position.

anteroposterior axis The axis that runs perpendicular to the coronal plane.

antonyms Pairs of word roots, prefixes, or suffixes that have opposite meanings.

apex (plural *apices* or *apexes*) The pointed extremity of a conical structure.

bilateral In anatomy, a body part or condition that appears on both sides of the midline.

combining form A word root followed by a vowel.

combining vowel The vowel used to combine two word roots or a word root and a prefix or suffix.

compound word A word containing more than one word root.

contralateral On the opposite side of the body.

coronal plane An imaginary plane in which the body is cut into front and back portions.

cross section The product of slicing an object crosswise, perpendicular to its long axis.

deep Farther inside the body and away from the skin.

distal Farther from the trunk and nearer to the free end of the extremity.

dorsal The posterior surface of the body, including the back of the hand.

eponym The name of a disease, device, procedure, or drug that is based on the person who invented, discovered, or first described it.

extension The straightening of a joint.

external rotation Rotating an extremity at its joint away from the midline.

flexion The bending of a joint.

Fowler position A sitting position, with the head elevated at a 90° angle (sitting straight upright).

Prep Kit *(continued)*

homonyms Words that sound alike but are spelled differently and have different meanings.

horizontal axis The axis that runs perpendicular to the sagittal plane; also called the mediolateral axis.

hyperextension Maximum extension or extension beyond the normal range of motion.

hyperflexion Maximum flexion or flexion beyond the normal range of motion.

inferior Below or closer to the feet.

internal rotation Rotating the anterior surface of an extremity toward the midline.

ipsilateral On the same side of the body.

lateral In anatomy, parts of the body that lie farther from the midline.

longitudinal axis The axis that runs perpendicular to the transverse plane.

longitudinal section The view of an object cut along its long axis.

medial Closer to the midline.

midsagittal plane (midline) An imaginary vertical line drawn from the middle of the forehead through the nose and the umbilicus (navel) to the floor.

palmar The forward-facing part of the hand in the anatomic position.

plantar The sole or bottom surface of the foot.

posterior In anatomy, the back surface of the body; the side away from you in the standard anatomic position.

prefix Part of a term that appears before a word root, changing the meaning of the term.

pronation Turning the palms downward (toward the ground).

prone Lying flat, face down.

proximal Closer to the trunk.

quadrants The four sections of the abdominal cavity shown by two imaginary lines intersecting at the umbilicus, dividing the abdomen into four equal areas.

range of motion The full distance that a joint can be moved.

sagittal (lateral) plane A plane of the body that passes vertically from front to back, dividing the body into left and right portions.

suffix The part of a term that comes after the word root, at the end of the term.

superficial Closer to or on the surface of the skin.

superior Above or closer to the head.

supination Turning the palms upward (toward the sky).

supine Lying face up.

synonyms Pairs of word roots, prefixes, or suffixes that have the same or almost the same meaning.

topographic anatomy Superficial landmarks of the body that serve as guides to the structures that lie beneath them.

transverse (axial) plane An imaginary plane passing horizontally through the body at the waist, dividing it into top and bottom halves.

unilateral Occurring or appearing on only one side of the body.

ventral The anterior surface of the body.

word root The foundation of a word; establishes the basic meaning of a word.

▶ References

1. ISMP's list of error-prone abbreviations, symbols, and designations. Institute for Safe Medication Practices website. http://www.ismp.org/Tools/errorprone abbreviations.pdf. Accessed February 5, 2016.
2. Facts about the official "do not use" list of abbreviations. The Joint Commission website. http://www.jointcommission.org/facts_about _the_of cial_/default.aspx. Updated June 30, 2016. Accessed February 5, 2016.

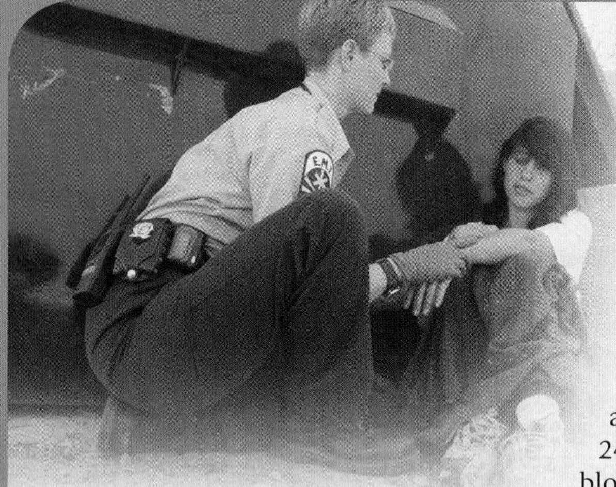

Assessment *in Action*

You respond to a call for a stabbing outside a local bar. Upon arrival, you find a 37-year-old man lying on his back on the sidewalk, bleeding from his abdomen and right upper arm. He is screaming in pain and holding the right side of his abdomen. During your assessment, you note his breathing is 24 times per minute, his pulse rate is 132 beats per minute, his blood pressure is 92/60 mm Hg, he is diaphoretic, his skin is pale, and his pupils are equal and reactive bilaterally. He presents with a 1-inch (3-cm) puncture just above and to the right of his umbilicus and a slashing wound approximately 2 inches (5 cm) in length on his right upper arm, just above the elbow. He tells you he's not allergic to any medications and takes lisinopril for high blood pressure. You place him on oxygen; put him in a position of comfort, with his legs drawn up and the head of the stretcher elevated to a 45° angle; gain intravenous access; and provide rapid transport. Just prior to arrival at the trauma center, you notice that his mental status has deteriorated and he is now responsive only to pain.

1. The term for high blood pressure is *hypertension*. What is the abbreviation?

A. HBP
B. HYP
C. HTN
D. HYN

2. The patient has been stabbed in which abdominal quadrant?

A. RUQ
B. LUQ
C. RLQ
D. LLQ

3. The patient initially was found in what position?

A. Prone
B. Supine
C. Fowler
D. Recovery

4. The wound to his right arm is in what position relative to his right elbow?

A. Medial
B. Lateral
C. Distal
D. Proximal

5. The patient has an elevated respiratory rate and an elevated heart rate. What is the prefix for "fast"?

A. brady-
B. tachy-
C. hyper-
D. supra-

6. The patient's blood pressure is 92/60 mm Hg. What is the appropriate term for this reading?

A. Hypotensive
B. Normotensive
C. Hypertensive
D. Hemotensive

7. What is the appropriate abbreviation for the patient's pupillary response?

A. PEEP
B. PMH
C. PERRLA
D. PRRLL

8. What is the term for the position in which the patient is transported?

A. Recumbent
B. Lateral
C. Fowler
D. Semi-Fowler

9. What are some possible misunderstandings that could occur if a paramedic uses incorrect medical terminology on the job?

10. Rewrite the scenario using medical terminology and abbreviations.

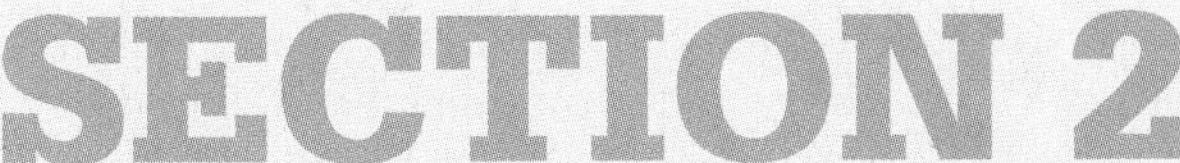

SECTION 2

The Human Body and Human Systems

CHAPTER 8

Anatomy and Physiology

National EMS Education Standard Competencies

Anatomy and Physiology

Integrates a complex depth and comprehensive breadth of knowledge of the anatomy and physiology of all human systems.

Knowledge Objectives

1. Discuss the characteristics shared by all living things. (p 231)
2. Describe the levels of organization in the body, from the least complex to the most complex. (p 231)
3. Discuss the chemical composition of the body, including key substances: carbohydrates, proteins, lipids, nucleic acids, trace elements, and enzymes. (pp 231-238)
4. Discuss the atomic composition of the body, including chemical bonds and chemical reactions. (pp 231-239)
5. Explain the concept of fluid balance, including the purpose and mechanisms for maintaining homeostasis. (pp 237, 387-388)
6. Differentiate between anabolism and catabolism. (p 239)
7. Describe the components of the cell, including the function of cellular structures. (pp 240-245)
8. Discuss the life cycle of a cell, including interphase, mitosis, cytokinesis, and differentiation. (pp 244-246)
9. Discuss aerobic and anaerobic cellular metabolism. (pp 247-248)
10. Identify the major fluid compartments of the body. (p 248)
11. Discuss cell transport mechanisms, including diffusion, facilitated diffusion, osmosis, and active transport. (pp 248-252)
12. Define isotonic, hypotonic, and hypertonic. (p 250)
13. Describe the types of tissues found in the body, including epithelial tissue, connective tissue, muscle tissue, neural tissue, and membranes. (pp 252-260)
14. Discuss how the body maintains homeostasis. (pp 260-262)
15. Describe the anatomy and physiology of the integumentary system, including function, layers of the skin, and other structures present in the skin. (pp 262, 264-266)
16. Discuss the components of the skeletal system, including types of bones. (pp 266-267)
17. Describe the characteristics and composition of bones, including long bone architecture. (pp 267-268)
18. Discuss bone formation, growth, and related hormones. (pp 268-270)
19. Discuss the classifications and types of joints. (pp 270-274)
20. List the sections of the spine. (pp 278-279)
21. Discuss the anatomy and physiology of the muscular system, including gross and microscopic anatomy, actions of muscles, contraction of skeletal muscle fibers, and major muscles of the body. (pp 286-292)
22. List the divisions and subdivisions of the nervous system. (pp 292-293)
23. Describe the structures involved in conduction of electrical impulses between the brain and the rest of the body. (pp 292-295)
24. List the structures of the central nervous system and their functions. (pp 295-306)
25. Define the terms cerebral perfusion pressure and pulse pressure. (p 298)
26. Describe the components of the subdivisions of the peripheral nervous system. (pp 306-316)
27. Describe the sensory function of the nervous system, including types of pain. (pp 316-317)
28. Describe the basic anatomy of the sense organs and explain how they function. (pp 317-323)
29. Discuss the anatomy and physiology of the endocrine system, including endocrine and exocrine glands, chemistry of hormones, regulation of hormone secretion, and the roles of hormones in various processes in the body. (pp 323-332)
30. Discuss the anatomy and physiology of the circulatory system, including the composition and

function of blood, the heart, the blood vessels, and the blood groups. (pp 332-340)

31. Discuss the concepts of cardiac output, stroke volume, preload, afterload, and systemic vascular resistance. (pp 341-342)
32. Discuss the Frank-Starling mechanism. (p 342)
33. Discuss the anatomy and physiology of the lymphatic and immune systems, including their primary structures. (pp 353-355)
34. Discuss the anatomy and physiology of the respiratory system, including the structure and function of the nasal cavities, pharynx, larynx, trachea, bronchial tree, alveoli, lungs, and pulmonary capillaries. (pp 355-364)
35. Discuss the lung volumes and dead space. (pp 364-365)
36. Differentiate between ventilation, oxygenation, and respiration. (p 365)
37. Describe the process of gas exchange in the alveoli. (pp 368-369)
38. Explain how oxygen and carbon dioxide are transported in the blood. (pp 369-370)
39. Discuss the mechanisms that regulate breathing. (pp 369-373)
40. Describe the concept of hypoxic drive. (pp 371-372)
41. Explain how the level of carbon dioxide in the blood and the pH of blood relate to ventilation. (pp 372-373)
42. Explain the anatomy and physiology of the digestive system, including general function, organs and structures involved in digestion, and the process of digestion. (pp 373-382)
43. Describe the anatomy and physiology of the urinary system, including its components, general function, the process of urine formation, and the role of the kidneys in regulating electrolyte balance, acid-base balance, and blood pressure. (pp 382-388)
44. Discuss the anatomy and physiology of the reproductive system, including the hormones and structures involved in reproduction, spermatogenesis and oogenesis, and the menstrual cycle. (pp 388-397)

Skills Objectives

There are no skills objectives for this chapter.

Introduction

Knowledge of anatomy and physiology is fundamental to the education of any health care provider and is paramount for successful practice as a paramedic. In every patient encounter, you will call on your knowledge of anatomy and physiology to help you understand the patient's presentation, anticipate or understand the suspected disease process, and make a decision regarding the care you will provide. A strong foundation of anatomy and physiology is also required to help you fully understand the concepts you will learn in many other chapters of this text, including patient assessment, pharmacology, and the sections describing specific disease processes. **Anatomy** is the study of the structure and makeup of the organism. This knowledge can be divided into gross anatomy, which studies organs and their location in the body, and microscopic anatomy, which studies the tissue and cellular components that cannot be seen with the naked eye. **Physiology** is the study of the processes and functions of the body. These systems, operating simultaneously and relying on a myriad of interactions, all work to maintain a state of balance in which organs and systems can function effectively, known as **homeostasis**. Maintaining homeostasis preserves a range of temperature, acid/base balance, gas and mineral concentrations, and other conditions necessary for normal life processes to function correctly.

YOU are the Paramedic PART 1

You and your crew are dispatched to a "truck versus motorcycle" collision on a two-lane highway. On arrival, you learn that a ¾-ton pickup truck was stationary in the left turn lane waiting for traffic to clear. A motorcycle with a single rider was moving toward the truck at highway speed in the opposite lane of traffic when it drifted across the yellow line and struck the truck in the center of the front bumper. The collision caused the truck to be deformed. The motorcycle rider was ejected from the motorcycle and collided with the truck windshield, after which the rider rolled to the ground.

1. What anatomic areas of the motorcyclist's body may be injured as a result of this collision?
2. Which anatomic areas of the motorcyclist's body may have life-threatening injuries in this scenario?

Adding the prefix *patho-*, meaning "disease," to the word *physiology* forms the term *pathophysiology*, which is the study of how body functions change and react when the body encounters disease or when homeostasis is otherwise disturbed. See Chapter 9, *Pathophysiology*, for more information.

Characteristics of Life

To understand the design and function of the body, it is beneficial to consider the following characteristics shared by all living things:

- **Absorption.** The ability to absorb materials through various membranes, such as the absorption of material through the digestive tract.
- **Circulation.** The ability to move substances in the body by way of body fluids.
- **Digestion.** The ability to convert food sources into simpler compounds.
- **Excretion.** The ability to excrete waste materials.
- **Growth.** The ability to increase in size.
- **Movement.** The ability of the organism to move locations, change position, or move internal structures.
- **Reproduction.** The ability to create new cells, such as in cellular reproduction, or the ability to create new organisms, such as offspring.
- **Respiration.** The ability to use food sources in combination with oxygen to release the energy contained within those sources into the environment
- **Responsiveness.** The ability to respond to internal and external stimuli.

Organizational Structure

To achieve the functions listed previously, the body is organized to ensure the organism works as a whole. This is one of the most important concepts to understand in anatomy and physiology; in fact, the term organism comes from *organize* + *-ism*, which indicates that organization is crucial in the body.[1] The levels of organization progress from the simplest (chemical) to the most complex (body as a whole). The six basic units of organization are presented in Table 8-1.

Chemical Level

Chemical changes within cells influence body functions and the status of the structures of the body. Chemicals of the body include water, **proteins**, **carbohydrates**, **lipids**, **nucleic acids**, and salts, as well as foods, drinks, and medications.

Matter, Elements, Atoms

Mass is a physical property that determines the weight of an object, based on the gravitational pull of the earth. Matter includes liquids, gases, and solids both inside and outside of the human body. All living and nonliving matter is made up of elements, which are the simplest form of matter. Elements cannot be broken down into two or more different substances. Carbon, hydrogen, oxygen, and nitrogen are examples of elements that make up 96% of a human's body weight. Table 8-2 lists the major and trace elements required by the human body.

Table 8-1 Levels of Organization in the Human Body

Level	Description
Chemical	The chemical level consists of atoms and molecules. Atoms are small particles that form the building blocks of matter, which is anything (liquids, gases, and solids) that takes up space and has weight. A molecule is formed when two or more atoms unite through their electron structures.
Cellular	The cellular level is made up of cells, which are the basic living units of structure and function in the human organism. Each of the cells in the body has a specific purpose or function.
Tissue	**Tissues** are created when several cells with common functions join. For example, many muscle cells join to create **muscle tissue**.
Organ	Organs are created when several types of tissue join to perform a function. For example, the heart contains muscle tissue as well as epithelial and nervous tissue.
Organ system	Organ systems are created when several organs combine to perform a common function. For example, the digestive system includes several organs that each have a role in breaking down food into components the body can utilize.
Organism	The organism is the combination of all lower levels of organization working together to ensure survival.

Table 8-2 Elements of the Human Body

Major Elements (totaling 99.9%)	Percentage in the Body
Oxygen (O)	65%
Carbon (C)	18.5%
Hydrogen (H)	9.5%
Nitrogen (N)	3.2%
Calcium (Ca)	1.5%
Phosphorus (P)	1%
Potassium (K)	0.4%
Sulfur (S)	0.3%
Chlorine (Cl)	0.2%
Sodium (Na)	0.2%
Magnesium (Mg)	0.1%
Trace Elements (totaling 0.1%)	
Chromium (Cr)	—
Cobalt (Co)	—
Copper (Cu)	—
Fluorine (F)	—
Iodine (I)	—
Iron (Fe)	—
Manganese (Mn)	—
Zinc (Zn)	—

Atomic Structure

Atoms are small units of an element that vary in size, weight, and how they combine and interact with other atoms. The characteristics of living and nonliving objects result from the atoms they contain. Thus, by forming chemical bonds, atoms can combine and interact with other atoms that are not similar to them.

Atoms are composed of particles that include the proton, which carries a positive charge, the electron, which carries a negative charge, and the neutron, which is neutral. When an atom has the same number of protons and electrons, the atom has no net charge (it is neither positive nor negative). Protons and neutrons are similar in size and mass and are located in the **nucleus**. The mass of an atom is determined mostly by the number of protons and neutrons in its nucleus. The mass of a larger object, such as the human body, is the sum of the masses of all of its atoms.

Electrons orbit the nucleus of an atom at high speed, forming a spherical electron cloud. Atoms normally contain equal numbers of protons and electrons. The number of protons in an atom is known as its atomic number. Thus, hydrogen (H), the simplest atom, has one proton, giving it the atomic number 1, whereas magnesium, with 12 protons, has the atomic number 12.

The atomic weight of an atom of an element equals the number of protons and neutrons in its nucleus. For example, oxygen (O) has eight protons and eight neutrons, so its atomic weight is 16. Atoms that have nuclei containing the same number of protons, but different numbers of neutrons, are isotopes.

▶ Chemical Bonds

Atoms can bond with other atoms by using chemical bonds that result from interactions between their electrons. During this process, the atoms may gain, lose, or share electrons. Chemically inactive atoms are known as *inert* atoms. An example of a chemical that is made up of inert atoms is helium.

An atom that gains or loses electrons carries an electrical charge. Electrically charged atoms or groups of atoms are **ions**. Ions with a positive charge ($^+$) are *cations*, and those with a negative charge ($^-$) are *anions*. When electrons are transferred or shared between atoms, chemical bonds are formed that hold the atoms together, thus forming a molecule. An **ionic bond** is a type of chemical bond formed from the attraction between two oppositely charged ions. For example, when sodium forms an ionic bond with chloride, sodium chloride (table salt) is created.

A covalent bond occurs when atoms are bonded to form molecules by sharing electrons. Some covalent bonds do not share electrons equally, resulting in a *polar molecule*—one that has an uneven distribution of charges. Polar molecules have equal numbers of protons and electrons, but one end of the molecule is slightly negative whereas the other end is slightly positive. An example of a polar molecule is water, created by one hydrogen and two oxygen atoms. A peptide bond, which is another type of covalent bond, is discussed with proteins later in this chapter.

A hydrogen bond is a type of chemical bond formed between a hydrogen atom and a negatively charged atom such as oxygen, nitrogen, or fluorine. Hydrogen bonds are important in protein and nucleic acid structure, and form between polar regions of different parts of a single, large molecule.

The numbers and types of atoms in a molecule are represented by a molecular formula. The molecular formula for water is H_2O, signifying the two atoms of hydrogen and the one atom of oxygen. Structural formulas are used to signify how atoms are joined and arranged inside molecules. Single bonds are represented by single lines, and double bonds are represented by double lines. When structural formulas are represented in three-dimensional models, different colors are used to show different types of atoms.

▶ Compounds

A **compound** is a substance that can be broken down into the two or more elements contained within it. Examples of compounds include water, table sugar, baking soda, alcohol as used in beverages, natural gas, and most medicinal drugs. A molecule of a compound has specific types and amounts of atoms. For example, water consists of two hydrogen atoms and one oxygen atom. When two hydrogen atoms bind with two oxygen atoms, they form hydrogen peroxide instead of water.

A **mineral** is a naturally occurring, inorganic element. Minerals are used in the chemical reactions that occur in the body and are necessary to sustain normal cell function. Humans obtain minerals from plant foods, or from animals that have eaten plants. Minerals are most concentrated in the bones and teeth. Minerals are classified as *macrominerals* (also called macronutrients, trace minerals, or trace elements) when the daily dietary requirement is 100 milligrams (mg) or more and *microminerals* when the body needs less than 100 mg daily. Examples of macrominerals include calcium, magnesium, and phosphorus. Chromium, copper, iodine, iron, selenium, and zinc are examples of microminerals.

Organic Compounds

Organic compounds contain the element carbon. Many organic molecules are made up of long chains of carbon atoms linked by covalent bonds. The carbon atoms usually form additional covalent bonds with hydrogen or oxygen atoms and, less commonly, form covalent bonds with nitrogen, phosphorus, sulfur, or other elements.

Organic compounds that occur in living organisms are *biochemical compounds*. Biochemical compounds are essential for many of the chemical reactions necessary to sustain life and include carbohydrates, proteins, lipids, vitamins, and nucleic acids.

Carbohydrates. Carbohydrates (saccharides) are sugars or starches. They are compounds made up of carbon, hydrogen, and oxygen. Energy from carbohydrates mostly is used to power cellular processes.

Types of carbohydrates include **monosaccharides** (simple sugars), **oligosaccharides** (simple sugars made up of 2 to 10 monosaccharides), disaccharides (double sugars), and **polysaccharides** (complex sugars). Glucose (dextrose), an important simple sugar, is normally found in the blood (the fluid that moves within the cardiovascular system). Fructose, found in fruit juices and honey, and galactose, found in milk and dairy products, are also simple sugars. **Enzymes** in the liver (the largest internal organ in the body) convert fructose and galactose into glucose, which is the form of carbohydrate most commonly oxidized for use as cellular fuel. Ribose and deoxyribose are simple sugars used in the manufacture of ribonucleic acid (RNA) and **deoxyribonucleic acid (DNA)**, which are the so-called blueprint of the cell.

Disaccharides must be broken down into monosaccharides before they can be absorbed and used by the cells of the human body. Examples of disaccharides include sucrose (table sugar), maltose (malt sugar), and lactose (milk sugar).

Plant starch, animal starch, and cellulose are examples of polysaccharides, which are long chains of monosaccharides linked together. Sources of plant starch include potatoes, rice, and peas. **Glycogen**, which is animal starch, is the main polysaccharide in the body and is the form in which glucose (sugar) is stored in the human body, primarily in the liver and skeletal muscle. Cellulose is a complex carbohydrate not digestible by humans. It provides bulk (fiber, or roughage) that helps the muscular digestive system walls to push food through its tubes.

Proteins. Proteins are the most abundant of the body's organic compounds. All proteins contain carbon, oxygen, hydrogen, and nitrogen. Many proteins also contain sulfur, iron, zinc, and magnesium, and some include phosphorus.

Proteins include enzymes, plasma proteins, muscle components (actin and myosin), hormones, and antibodies. **Hormones** are substances formed in tiny amounts by one specialized organ or group of cells and then carried to another organ or group of cells in the same organism to perform regulatory functions (chemical messengers). *Antibodies* (also called immunoglobulins) are proteins that detect and destroy foreign substances. After digestion breaks down proteins into amino acids, they may also supply energy. They are transported to the liver, where deamination occurs, which is the loss of their nitrogen-containing portions. They react to form the waste urea, which is excreted in urine. Other types of proteins include structural proteins such as collagen, a twisted ropelike protein which gives strength to ligaments and **connective tissues**, and keratin, which functions to prevent water loss through the skin. Proteins of the **cell membrane** (cell wall) may serve as receptors and carriers for specific molecules.

Twenty-two different amino acids make up the proteins that exist in humans and most other living organisms. Protein molecules consisting of amino acids held together by peptide bonds are **peptides**. A **polypeptide** is formed from many amino acids bound into a chain. Polypeptides usually have specialized functions. When a polypeptide has more than 100 molecules, it is considered a protein. Certain protein molecules have more than one polypeptide.

All except nine of the required amino acids can be synthesized by an adult's body. Essential amino acids are required for proper growth and tissue repair, but the body cannot produce them on its own; therefore, essential amino acids must be obtained from dietary sources.

Nonessential amino acids are produced by the liver and are therefore not dietary requirements. Complete proteins (found in milk, meats, and eggs) have adequate amounts of the essential amino acids. Incomplete proteins (such as those found in corn) have too little tryptophan and lysine to maintain human tissues or support growth and development. A partially complete protein (such as gliadin, found in wheat) does not have enough lysine to promote growth, but does have enough to maintain life.

Lipids. Lipids are composed of carbon, hydrogen, and oxygen. Many lipids also contain nitrogen and phosphorus. Lipids are not soluble in water. They may dissolve in other lipids, oils, ether, chloroform, or alcohol.

The most common lipids in the body are triglycerides, **phospholipids**, and steroids (which includes cholesterol) Table 8-3. Triglycerides (fats) are made up of glycerol and fatty acids. Triglycerides are the most common lipids found in the diet and they are found in both plant- and animal-based foods. Fats that have a liquid consistency at room temperature are often called oils. **Prostaglandins** are derivatives of an essential fatty acid that are widely distributed in cells throughout the body.

Saturated fats are found mostly in meats, eggs, milk, animal fat (lard), palm oil, and coconut oil. These fats, when consumed excessively, are a risk factor for cardiovascular disease. Unsaturated fats exist in nuts, seeds, and plant oils. Monounsaturated fats are the healthiest type of fats and are found in olive, peanut, and canola oils. Cholesterol is found in animal products, including liver, egg yolk, whole milk, butter, cheese, and meats. It is not present in foods of plant origin.

Lipids have many functions, but mostly they supply energy to the body. Triglyceride molecules must first undergo hydrolysis (breakdown in the presence of water) before they can release energy. When this process occurs, fatty acids and glycerol are released, absorbed, and transported in lymph and blood to the tissues. Some fatty acid portions react to form molecules of acetyl coenzyme A by means of reactions known as *beta oxidation*. Excess amounts of this coenzyme convert into ketone bodies such as acetone, and can be reconverted in reverse.

Table 8-3 Types of Lipids

Type	Examples
Lipids	▪ Phospholipids ▪ Steroids (eg, cholesterol, bile salts, adrenocortical hormones, sex hormones) ▪ Triglycerides
Lipoid substances	▪ Fat-soluble vitamins ▪ Lipoproteins ▪ Prostaglandins

Certain fatty acids cannot be synthesized by the liver. These are known as essential fatty acids. For example, linoleic acid (necessary for phospholipid synthesis, cell membrane formation, and transport of lipids) is an essential fatty acid found in corn, cottonseed, and soy oils. Another essential fatty acid is linolenic acid.

Free fatty acids are used by the liver to synthesize triglycerides, phospholipids, and lipoproteins. Lipids are less dense than proteins; therefore, the proportion of lipids in a lipoprotein increases as the density of the particle decreases. The reverse is also true. Very low-density lipoproteins have a relatively high concentration of triglycerides. Low-density lipoproteins have a relatively high concentration of cholesterol. High-density lipoproteins have a relatively high concentration of proteins.

The liver controls cholesterol in the body. It synthesizes cholesterol and releases it into the bloodstream, or removes it from the bloodstream to be excreted via bile, or to produce bile salts. Cholesterol does not create energy but provides structural materials for cell membranes, and contributes to certain sex hormones and adrenal hormones. Triglycerides are stored in adipose tissue (fat tissue) and may be hydrolyzed (broken down) into free fatty acids and glycerol when blood lipid concentration drops, such as during fasting. Lipid functions are shown in Table 8-4.

Vitamins. Vitamins are organic compounds that are required for normal metabolism. Metabolism may be generally defined as the chemical changes that occur within cells that are necessary to maintain life. Body cells cannot synthesize adequate amounts of vitamins, so they must come from foods. Vitamins are classified by their solubility. Fat-soluble vitamins include A, D, E, and K. Water-soluble vitamins include the B vitamin group and vitamin C.

Bile salts in the small intestine promote absorption of fat-soluble vitamins. Bile salts accumulate in various tissues and their intake must be controlled. For example, when too much vitamin A is consumed, the body receives too much beta-carotene, and the skin may appear orange in color. Table 8-5 explains the fat-soluble vitamins.

The water-soluble vitamins include the B vitamins and vitamin C. The B vitamins consist of compounds essential for normal metabolism, and help to oxidize carbohydrates, lipids, and proteins. The B vitamins are often present together in foods; hence, they are referred to as the vitamin B complex. Cooking and food processing destroy some of these vitamins. Vitamin C (ascorbic acid) is one of the least stable vitamins. It is found in many plant foods, and is necessary for the body to produce collagen, convert folacin to folinic acid, and metabolize certain amino acids. Vitamin C also promotes synthesis of hormones from cholesterol and is vital for iron absorption.

Nucleic Acids. Nucleic acids are large organic molecules (macromolecules) formed by the joining of many smaller molecules (nucleotides). Nucleic acids carry genetic information or form structures within cells. They contain

Table 8-4 Functions of Lipids

Lipid Type	Function
Lipid	
Triglycerides	Long-term energy storage; protection and insulation of body organs
Phospholipids	Essential component of cell membranes
Steroids	
Cholesterol	Helps stabilize cell membranes; necessary for many reactions within the cell
Bile salt	Assists in fat digestion and absorption
Lipid hormones	Sex hormones secreted by **ovaries** and testes; adrenocortical hormones influence blood pressure and fluid volume
Lipoid Substances	
Fat-soluble vitamins	Assist in regulation of biologic processes
Prostaglandins	Help regulate inflammation and tissue repair; regulate effects of several hormones; stimulate smooth muscle; inhibit gastric secretion; influence blood pressure; affect platelet aggregation (clumping)
Lipoproteins	Assist in transportation of fatty acids to and from cells

Table 8-5 Fat-Soluble Vitamins

Vitamin	Sources	Characteristics	Functions
A	Liver, fish, whole milk, butter, eggs, leafy green vegetables, yellow and orange vegetables, and fruits	Several forms; synthesized from carotenes; stored in the liver; stable in heat, acids, and bases; unstable in light	Necessary for synthesis of visual pigments, mucoproteins, and mucopolysaccharides; for normal development of bones and teeth; and for maintenance of epithelial cells
D	Produced when skin is exposed to ultraviolet light; also exists in milk, egg yolk, fish liver oils, and fortified foods	A group of steroids; resistant to heat, oxidation, acids, and bases; stored in the liver, skin, brain, spleen, and bones	Promotes absorption of calcium and phosphorus, as well as development of teeth and bones
E	Oils from cereal seeds, salad oils, margarine, shortenings, fruits, nuts, and vegetables	A group of compounds; resistant to heat and visible light; unstable in the presence of oxygen and ultraviolet light; stored in muscles and adipose tissue	An antioxidant; prevents oxidation of vitamin A and polyunsaturated fatty acids; may help maintain stability of cell membranes
K	Leafy green vegetables, egg yolk, pork liver, soy oil, tomatoes, cauliflower	Occurs in several forms; resistant to heat, but destroyed by acids, bases, and light; stored in the liver	Required for synthesis of prothrombin, which functions in blood clotting

carbon, hydrogen, oxygen, nitrogen, and phosphorus. Nucleic acids are found in all living things, cells, and viruses

Nucleic acid molecules are of two types: DNA and RNA. DNA is the genetic material of the cell and is arranged in hereditary units called genes. This genetic information is stored in the genetic code, which specifies the structure and function of the organism. For example, the DNA in your cells determines your inherited characteristics, including hair color, eye color, and blood type. DNA molecules encode the information needed to build proteins. By directing structural protein synthesis, DNA controls the shape and physical characteristics of the human body.

RNA is important in the process of manufacturing proteins by using the information provided by DNA. Human cells have three types of RNA: (1) messenger RNA, (2) transfer RNA, and (3) ribosomal RNA.

Important structural differences distinguish RNA from DNA. An RNA molecule consists of a single chain of nucleotides. A DNA molecule consists of a pair of nucleotide chains **Figure 8-1**. The two DNA strands

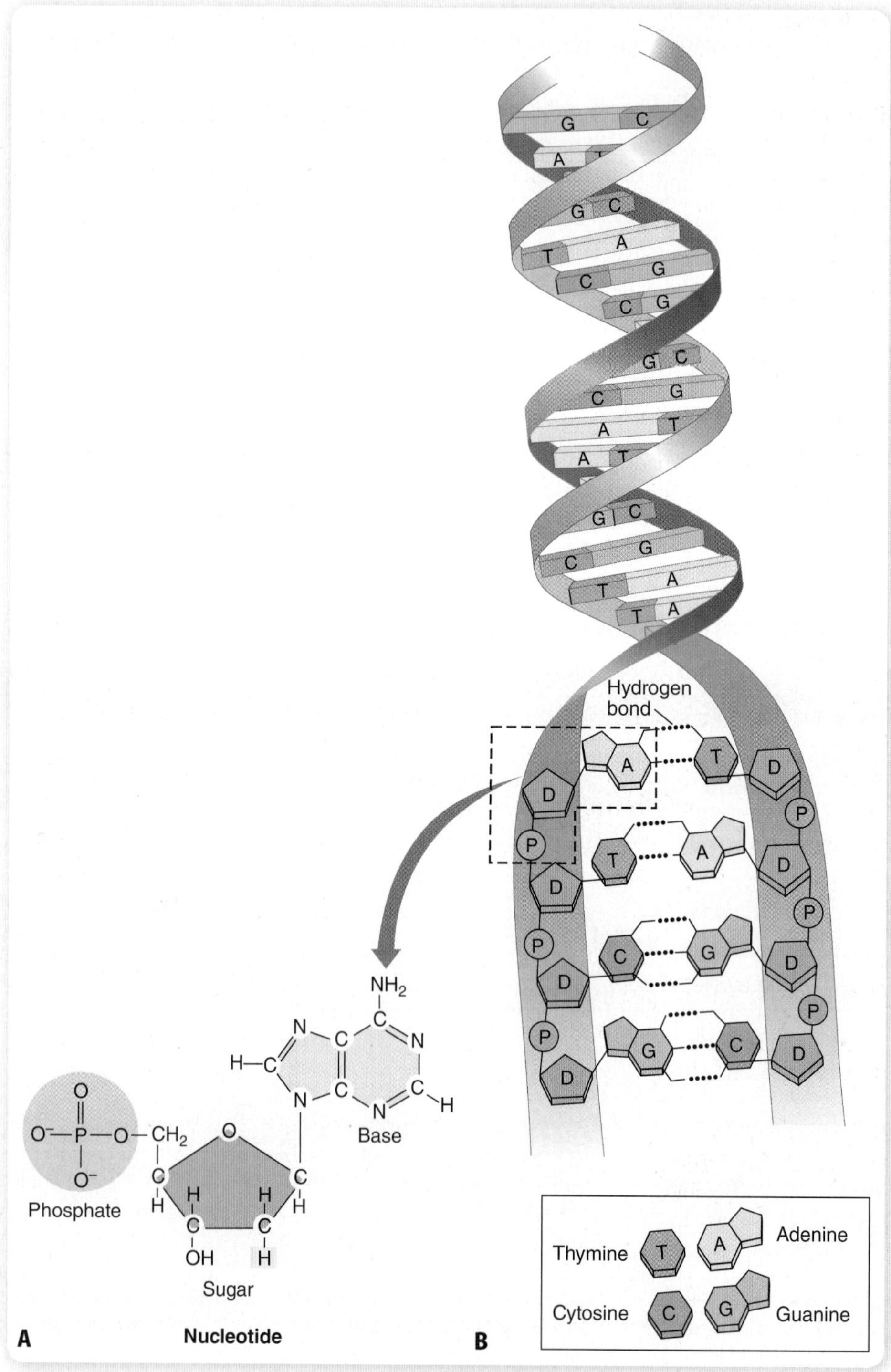

Figure 8-1 DNA. **A.** Nucleotide. **B.** The spiral staircase structure of DNA.

twist around each other in a double helix that resembles a spiral staircase.

Inorganic Compounds

Inorganic compounds are necessary for fluid balance and for transporting materials through cell membranes. **Fluid balance** is the process of maintaining homeostasis through equal intake of fluids (water taken into the body) and output of fluids (water excreted from the body). Inorganic substances in body cells include oxygen, carbon dioxide, compounds that are known as salts, and water. The most abundant compound in the human body is water, accounting for nearly two-thirds of body weight. A **solute** is a dissolved substance. Because solutes dissolved in water are more likely to react with each other as they break down into smaller particles, most metabolic reactions occur in water. In the blood, the watery (aqueous) portion carries vital substances such as oxygen, salts, sugars, and vitamins among the digestive tract, respiratory tract, and the cells.

Oxygen enters the body through the respiratory organs and it is transported in the blood. The red blood cells (RBCs) are also known as erythrocytes and carry the largest amount of oxygen to the tissues. **Organelles** are structures inside the cells, which use oxygen to release energy from **nutrients** such as glucose and drive cellular metabolic activities. Carbon dioxide is an inorganic compound produced as a waste product when some metabolic processes release energy. Carbon dioxide is exhaled via the lungs, the two primary organs of breathing.

Salts are compounds of oppositely charged ions that are abundant in tissues in fluids. Many ions required by the body are supplied in salts. Salt ions are important for transporting substances to and from the cells, as well as for muscle contractions and nerve impulse conduction. Common inorganic substances are summarized in Table 8-6.

▶ Chemical Reactions

Chemical substances can be altered by chemical reactions that form and break chemical bonds. Nerve, muscle, and blood cells are specialized to carry out distinctive chemical reactions; however, every type of cell performs basic chemical reactions. These reactions include the buildup and breakdown of carbohydrates, lipids, nucleic acids, and proteins.

Enzymes are among the most important of all the body's proteins because they catalyze the reactions that sustain life. *Catalysts* are chemical substances that speed up the rate of a chemical reaction without being consumed in the process. A cell makes an enzyme molecule to promote a specific reaction. Enzyme molecules that are not used in the reactions they catalyze are recycled.

Table 8-6 Inorganic Substances in Cells

Molecule or Ion	Function
Carbon dioxide molecule	Metabolic waste product; forms carbonic acid via reaction with water
Oxygen molecule	Used for energy release from glucose molecules
Water molecule	Major component of body fluids, biochemical reactions, chemical transport, and temperature regulation
Bicarbonate ions	Assists in acid-base balance
Calcium ions	Used in bone development, muscle contraction, and blood clotting
Carbonate ions	Used in formation of bone tissue
Chloride ions	Assists in maintaining water balance
Magnesium ions	Used in formation of bone tissue and certain metabolic processes
Phosphate ions	Used in adenosine triphosphate, nucleic acid, and other vital substance synthesis; important for formation of bone tissue and to maintain cell membrane polarization
Potassium ions	Used in cell membrane polarization
Sodium ions	Used in cell membrane polarization and maintenance of water balance
Sulfate ions	Assists in cell membrane polarization

Nearly every chemical reaction that occurs in the human body is facilitated by a specific enzyme. In the body, enzymes assist in the digestion of food, drug metabolism, protein formation, and many other types of reactions. Enzymes make metabolic reactions possible inside cells by controlling temperature conditions that otherwise would be too mild for reactions to occur. Enzymes promote chemical reactions by lowering the amount of activation energy needed for metabolic reactions, which speeds up the rates of the reactions through a process known as catalysis.

Each enzyme acts on a substrate, which is a particular chemical affected by the enzyme. Enzymes are often named after their substrates using the suffix *-ase*. For example, a lipid is broken down to glycerol or other alcohols with the help of an enzyme called a lipase. Another enzyme, called a catalase, facilitates the breakdown of hydrogen peroxide into water and oxygen. Hydrogen peroxide is a toxic substance that results from certain metabolic reactions.

Every cell holds hundreds of various enzymes, each of which recognizes its specific substrates. Enzyme molecules have three-dimensional shapes (conformations) that allow them to identify their substrates. The coiled and twisted polypeptide chain of each enzyme fits the shape of its substrate. The active site of an enzyme molecule combines with portions of its substrate molecules temporarily to form an enzyme-substrate complex. When enzyme-substrate complexes are formed, some chemical bonds within the substrates are distorted or strained. As a result, less energy is required, and the enzyme is then released as it was originally configured. These reactions are often reversible. Sometimes, the same enzyme catalyzes the reaction in both forward and reverse directions. The reactions occur at differing rates, based on the number of molecules of the enzyme and its substrate. Some enzymes process a few substrate molecules every second, whereas others can process thousands in the same length of time.

Enzymes can change because of exposure to heat, electricity, chemicals, radiation, or fluids that have extreme pH levels. Many enzymes are inactive at 45°C (111°F), and most of them are denatured at 55°C (131°F). Denaturation is a process that changes or alters some of the structures of the enzyme. Poisons such as potassium cyanide denature enzymes to achieve their effects. The poison stops the cells from being able to release energy from nutrient molecules.

Some enzymes must combine with a nonprotein component to be active. These nonprotein components are referred to as cofactors, and may be the ion of an element (such as calcium, magnesium, copper, iron, or zinc). Cofactors may also be small, nonprotein, organic molecules called coenzymes. The human body converts many vitamins into essential coenzymes. An example of a coenzyme is coenzyme A, which is involved in **cellular respiration**. Cellular respiration is discussed later in this chapter.

Chemical reactions are represented by chemical equations, which indicate the number and type of molecules involved in the reaction. Four types of chemical reactions are important to the study of physiology: synthesis reactions, decomposition reactions, exchange reactions, and reversible reactions.

Synthesis Reactions

Chemical reactions change the bonds between atoms, molecules, and ions to generate new chemical combinations. Synthesis reaction occurs when two or more reactants (atoms) bond to form a more complex product or structure. The formation of water from hydrogen and oxygen molecules is a synthesis reaction. Synthesis always involves the formation of new chemical bonds, whether the reactants are atoms or molecules. Synthesis requires energy, and it is important for growth and the repair of tissues. Synthesis is symbolized as follows:

$$A + B \rightarrow AB$$

Decomposition Reactions

Decomposition reaction is a reaction that occurs when bonds within a reactant molecule break, forming simpler atoms, molecules, or ions. For example, a typical meal contains molecules of sugars, proteins, and fats that are too large and too complex to be absorbed and used by the body. Decomposition reactions in the digestive tract break down these molecules into smaller fragments before absorption begins. Decomposition is symbolized as follows:

$$AB \rightarrow A + B$$

Exchange Reactions

An exchange reaction occurs when two substances are decomposed and synthesized to produce new compounds. An example of an exchange reaction is the reaction of an acid with a base, which forms water and a salt. An exchange reaction is symbolized as follows:

$$AB + CD \rightarrow AD + CB$$

Reversible Reactions

A reversible reaction is one wherein the products of the reaction can change back into the reactants they originally were. These reactions can proceed in opposite directions, depending on the relative proportions of reactants and products, as well as how much energy is available. So, if $A + B \rightarrow AB$, then $AB \rightarrow A + B$. Many important biologic reactions are freely reversible. Such reactions can be represented as the equation $A + B \rightarrow AB$.

Cellular Metabolism

As evidenced by the structural hierarchy of the human body, the ability of the tissues, organs, and organ systems to function depends on the function of individual cells.

As a result, cells are constantly breaking down substances and building substances necessary for the survival of the organism. Because of metabolism, organisms grow, maintain body functions, release or store energy, produce and eliminate waste, digest nutrients, and destroy toxins. These reactions alter the chemical nature of a substance, and allow the organism to maintain a state of homeostasis.

Metabolic processes include both catabolism and anabolism. With **catabolism**, chemical reactions occur that result in the breakdown of larger molecules into smaller ones that the body can use for its own needs. Energy is released during catabolism that is eventually converted to **adenosine triphosphate (ATP)**, which is the powerful energy source of the body and is used to drive chemical reactions. Catabolism occurs continuously to differing degrees. Excessive catabolism leads to wasting of tissues.

Anabolism is the building of larger substances from smaller substances, such as the building of proteins from amino acids. Anabolic reactions generally require energy in the form of ATP. When a person is healthy and has adequate nutrition, simple nutrients (such as amino acids, fats, and glucose) are used by the body to build the basic chemicals that support cellular functioning and sustain life. Cellular metabolism is discussed in more detail later in this chapter.

▶ Electrolytes

Electrolytes are substances that release ions in water. The ability of the body to perform normal functions, such as nervous impulse transmission, depends on the presence of appropriate amounts of these substances. When electrolytes dissolve in water, the negative and positive ends of water molecules cause ions to separate and interact with water molecules instead of each other. The resulting solution contains electrically charged particles (ions) that will conduct electricity.

A **solution** is a mixture of two substances: (1) a **solvent**, which is the fluid that does the dissolving, or the substance that contains the dissolved components, and (2) a solute, which is the dissolved particles contained in the solvent. Water in the body serves as the universal solvent, dissolving a variety of solutes. These solutes can be classified as electrolytes or nonelectrolytes.

The unit of measurement for electrolytes is the milliequivalent (mEq); it represents the chemical combining power of the ion and is based on the number of available ionic charges in an electrolyte solution. One mEq of any cation reacts completely with 1 mEq of any anion. For example, sodium (Na^+) is a singly charged (monovalent) cation, and chloride (Cl^-) is a singly charged anion. Thus, 1 mEq of Na^+ will react with 1 mEq of Cl^- to form NaCl, which is table salt. Calcium (Ca^{+2}) has two positive charges (bivalent); thus, the Ca^{+2} ion represents 2 mEq and reacts completely with 2 mEq of a singly charged anion.

The primary cations in the body are sodium, potassium, calcium, and magnesium.

- **Sodium.** Sodium (Na^+) is the main extracellular cation and the most significant solute in determining total body water and the distribution of water in the body's intravascular and interstitial fluid compartments. Its role in maintaining adequate cellular perfusion gives rise to the saying, "Where sodium goes, water follows."
- **Potassium.** About 98% of all the body's potassium (K^+) is found inside the cells of the body, making it the principal intracellular cation. Potassium plays a major role in neuromuscular function and in the conversion of glucose into glycogen. Cellular potassium levels are regulated by insulin. The **sodium-potassium pump** (discussed later in this chapter) is helped by the presence of insulin and epinephrine. Hypokalemia, which is a low potassium level in the serum, or blood **plasma**, can lead to decreased skeletal muscle function, gastrointestinal (GI) disturbances, and alterations in cardiac function. High potassium levels in the serum (hyperkalemia) can lead to hyperstimulation of neural cell transmission, resulting in cardiac arrest.
- **Calcium.** Calcium (Ca^{+2}) is the principal cation needed for bone growth. It also plays an important role in the functioning of heart muscle, nerves, and cell membranes and is necessary for proper blood clotting. Low serum calcium levels (hypocalcemia) can lead to overstimulation of nerve cells. High serum calcium levels (hypercalcemia) can lead to decreased stimulation of nerve cells.
- **Magnesium.** Magnesium (Mg^{+2}) has an important role as a coenzyme in the metabolism of proteins and carbohydrates. In addition, it acts in a manner similar to calcium in controlling neuromuscular irritability.

The primary anions in the body are bicarbonate, chloride, and phosphate.

- **Bicarbonate.** Bicarbonate (HCO_3^-) levels are a determining factor between metabolic acidosis and alkalosis in the body (discussed next). Bicarbonate is the primary buffer used in circulating all body fluids.
- **Chloride.** Chloride (Cl^-) primarily regulates the pH level of the stomach. It also regulates extracellular fluid levels.
- **Phosphorus.** Phosphorus (P) is an important component in ATP.

▶ Acids, Bases, and the pH Scale

Acids are electrolytes that release hydrogen ions in water. An example of an acid is hydrochloric acid, made up of hydrogen and chloride ions. A *base*, or alkali, is an electrolyte that release ions that bond with hydrogen ions. An example of a base is sodium hydroxide (NaOH), made up of sodium (Na^+), oxygen, and hydrogen ions. The oxygen and hydrogen atoms, held together by a covalent bond, form hydroxide (OH^-). The acidity or basicity (alkalinity)

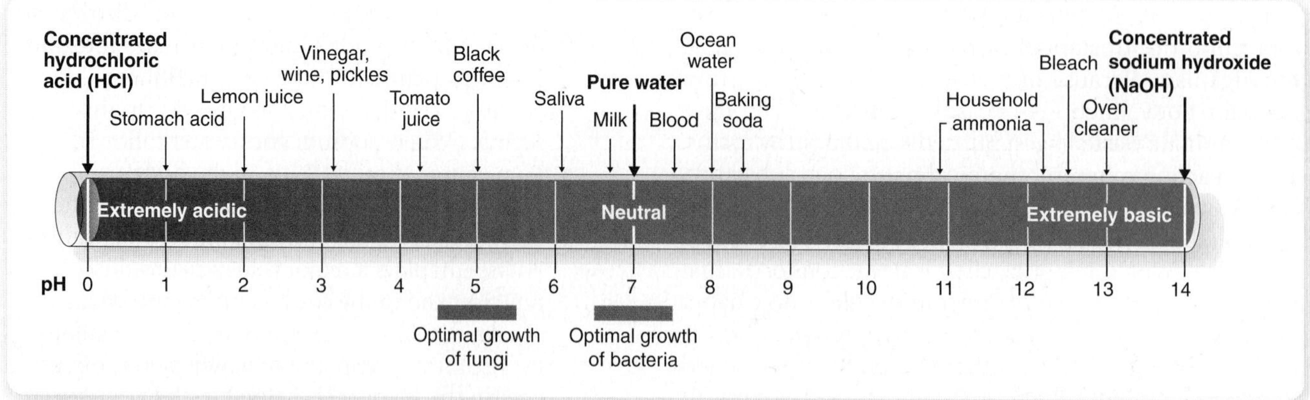

Figure 8-2 The pH scale.

of a solution is determined by the amount of free hydrogen in the solution. In body fluids, the concentrations of hydrogen and hydroxide ions greatly affect chemical reactions. These reactions control certain physiologic functions such as blood pressure (the pressure that the blood exerts against the walls of the arteries as it passes through them) and breathing rates.

Hydrogen ion concentrations can be measured by a value called **pH**. The hydrogen ion concentration in body fluids is vital. It is expressed in a type of mathematical shorthand based on concentrations calculated in moles per liter (with a mole representing an amount of solute in a solution). The pH of a solution is a measurement of its acidity or alkalinity. The pH scale ranges from 0 to 14, with 7 being the midpoint (meaning it has equal numbers of hydrogen and hydroxide ions) **Figure 8-2**. Pure water has a pH of 7, and this midpoint is considered to be neutral (neither acidic nor alkaline). Milk is an example of a slightly acidic solution owing to the lactic acid concentration. A pH of less than 7 is considered acidic, meaning the substance has more hydrogen ions than hydroxide ions. A pH of more than 7 is considered basic, also known as alkaline, meaning the substance has more hydroxide ions than hydrogen ions. Any solution with a very high a pH (such as liquid drain cleaner, which can have a pH approaching 14) is considered a strong base, whereas any solution with a very low pH (such as stomach acid, with a pH ranging from 1.5 to 3.5) is considered a very strong acid.

Normally, the human body is slightly alkaline, with a pH between 7.35 and 7.45. Abnormal fluctuations in pH can damage cells and tissues, change the shapes of proteins, and alter cellular functions. **Acidosis** is an abnormal physiologic state caused by blood pH that is lower than 7.35. If pH falls below 7, then coma may result. **Alkalosis** results from blood pH that is higher than 7.45. If pH rises above 7.8, then it generally causes uncontrollable and sustained skeletal muscle contractions.

To maintain the delicate acid-base balance, the body relies on its buffer systems. *Buffers* are molecules or compounds that limit changes in pH by neutralizing excessive acids or bases. In the absence of buffers, the rapid buildup of acid can cause an abrupt change in pH. Buffers regulate changes in pH to avoid such swift changes. For example, bone acts as a buffer by absorbing excess acids and bases and by releasing calcium into the bloodstream.

The ability of weak acids to bond weakly to H^+ ions makes them ideal buffers because they can accept or donate H^+ ions, depending on the needs of the body. Buffer systems include proteins, phosphate ions, and bicarbonate (HCO_3^-). Because acid production is the major challenge to pH homeostasis, most physiologic buffers combine with H^+. Protein buffering refers to the fact that charged proteins in the cells can accept or donate hydrogen ions, thereby helping to regulate acid-base balance by moving hydrogen into or out of the blood.

Cellular Level

As discussed previously, cells are the basic functional unit of the body. The cells of the body are extremely varied in their shape and function. Over time cells mature, or differentiate. Through this process of **differentiation**, cells become specialized to perform a specific function. For example, some cells make hair, other cells are involved in storing memory, and others help to move your eyes as you read this page. Cells with a common job are grouped closely together and are called tissues. Groups of tissues that all perform interrelated jobs form organs. A series of organs working together make up the body systems that are discussed in this chapter.

Cells perform the following seven general functions:

1. Movement (muscle cells)
2. **Conductivity** (nerve cells)
3. Metabolic absorption (kidney and intestinal cells)
4. Secretion (mucous gland cells)
5. Excretion (all cells)
6. Respiration (all cells)
7. Reproduction (most cells)

Cell Structure

The human body contains two general classes of cells. Sex cells (also called germ cells or reproductive cells) are discussed in more detail later in this chapter. Somatic cells (derived from the term *soma*, meaning "body") include

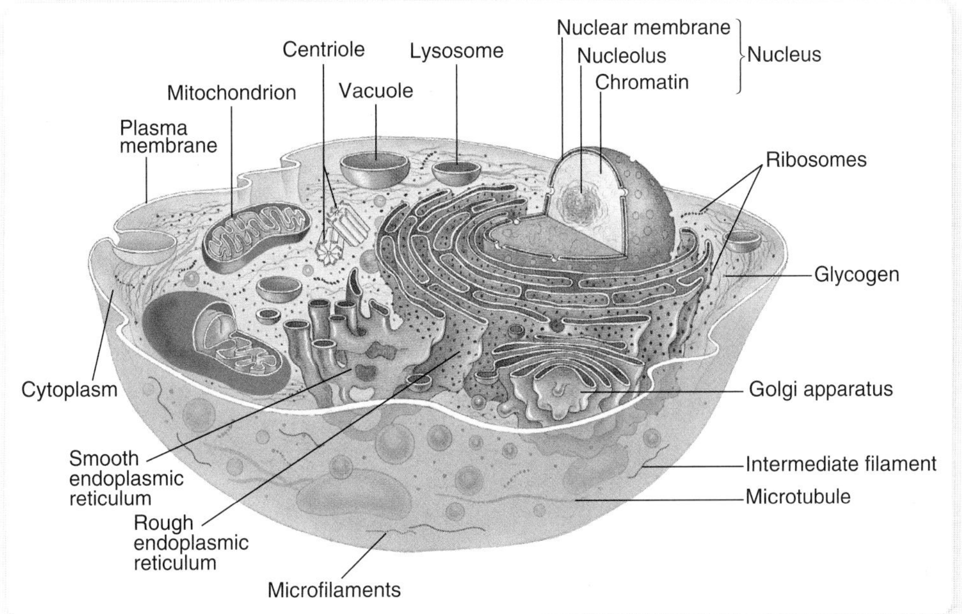

Figure 8-3 Cell structure. The cell is divided into nuclear and cytoplasmic compartments. The cytoplasm is packed with organelles.

all the other cells in the human body. This section focuses on somatic cells.

Cells are highly organized structures surrounded by a cell membrane, also called the cytoplasmic membrane or plasma membrane **Figure 8-3**. Numerous structures with specific functions are contained within the cell. Together these structures are called organelles and are suspended within a substance called the **cytoplasm**. Most of the cells of the body also contain a nucleus. Genetic material is stored in the nucleus, allowing reproduction and new cell growth.

Cell Membrane

The cell membrane encloses the cytoplasm and its organelles. This membrane gives form to the cell and is where most cellular activity takes place. Molecules in the cell membrane form pathways that allow the signals from outside the cell to be detected and transmitted inside. When cells form tissues, the cell membrane assists by adhering the cell to other cells. The membrane of each cell is extremely thin and delicate, able to stretch to differing degrees. Tiny folds on the surface help the cell to increase its surface area.

The cell membrane is composed of a bilayer (two layers). The bilayer is composed of phosphate and fat molecules called phospholipids. This bilayer forms a fluidlike framework for the membrane **Figure 8-4**. The membrane also forms the outer border of the cell and separates the interior of the cell from the fluid surrounding the cell. Any substances within this membrane are *intracellular*, and substances outside this membrane are *extracellular*.

In addition to providing physical isolation between the intracellular and extracellular compartments, one of the major functions of the cell membrane is to regulate the transfer of substances in and out of the cell. This

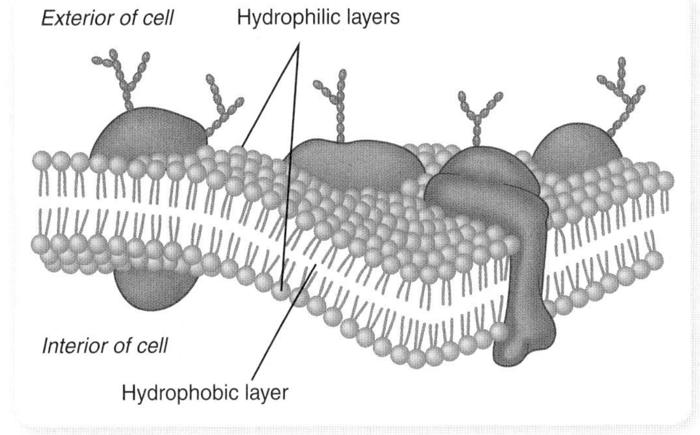

Figure 8-4 The phospholipid bilayer.

function is accomplished by the structure of the membrane. Cell membranes can be either differentially permeable or **semipermeable**. A semipermeable membrane allows certain elements to pass through while not allowing others to do so. In some instances, and often depending on various factors, only certain substances can enter or leave each cell (a condition known as selective permeability). Visualize the design of the cell membrane as a series of balloons with their strings tied together and the balloons facing outward. The balloons represent the phosphate molecules, and the strings represent the lipid molecules. The phosphate molecules attract water and the lipid molecules repel water, which results in a selectively permeable membrane in which oxygen, carbon dioxide, alcohol, and other substances that are soluble in lipids can freely pass through the membrane. However, water and other substances such as amino acids, proteins, nucleic acids, certain ions, and sugars are unable to pass through the membrane itself. The transport of substances in and out of the cell is discussed in more detail later in this chapter.

The cell membrane also has several proteins, known as membrane proteins, embedded and floating within it. These proteins serve the following functions:

- **Channel proteins.** Channel proteins act as a pore through the membrane that allows the passive passage of substances into the intracellular compartment. One example is the manner in which water enters and leaves the cell. As previously mentioned, water is unable to cross through the membrane itself; however, because of the amount of channel proteins that allow the passage of water, it can essentially freely enter and exit the cell. Another category of channel proteins are gated ion channels. These channels open and close at specific times and generally only allow specific substances to pass through. Calcium, for example, passes through calcium channels, and sodium passes through the sodium channels. Both are examples of voltage-gated ion channels. As a paramedic, a variety of medications that you administer (such as calcium channel blockers or sodium channel blockers) cause a dramatic effect on cellular function by altering transport through membrane channel proteins.
- **Enzyme receptors.** Enzyme receptors act as sites where enzymes can bind. Binding occurs inside the cell and the enzyme acts as a catalyst for a reaction to take place in the cell itself.
- **Proteins that act as receptor sites.** These proteins have their binding site on the outside of the cell membrane. The majority of these receptor sites are specific to certain molecules; when the correct molecule binds to the receptor site, a change in cellular function occurs. These changes are crucial to the proper function of the cell; however, as a paramedic, you will also use these sites. For example, the administration of a narcotic or narcotic antagonist results in the medication binding to narcotic receptor sites.
- **Identifier proteins.** These proteins identify the cell as part of a particular organism. This identification is used by the immune system to determine "self" from "nonself" in the defense against outside invaders.
- **Carrier proteins.** These proteins bind to substances and transport them across the cell membrane, which is generally an active process. For example, the sodium-potassium pump moves sodium out of the cell and potassium into the cell.

In addition, some membrane proteins attach to the cytoskeleton of the cell and help determine its shape. Other membrane proteins adhere to membrane proteins of adjacent cells, allowing tissues to form.

Words of Wisdom

Fatty compounds (such as those found in the cell membrane) are chemically neutral (uncharged), whereas electrolytes (such as sodium and potassium) are water based (charged). Thus, for a charged molecule to permeate a cell membrane, it has to travel through a special pathway. These transport channels—the so-called ion channels—consist of protein-lined pores (openings) specifically sized for each substance (for example, calcium and potassium). Local anesthetics (such as lidocaine) and antidysrhythmic drugs (such as amiodarone) exert their effects by blocking ion channels.

Cytoplasm

The cytoplasm is the fluid-like material in which the organelles of the cell are suspended. It lies between the cell membrane and the nucleus. The fluid contained within the nucleus is the *nucleoplasm*. Cytoplasm usually appears clear with scattered specks, though more powerful magnification reveals that it contains membranous networks, protein frameworks, and a cytoskeleton (cell skeleton).

Cytosol, which is the fluid portion of cytoplasm, contains mostly water, as well as glucose, amino acids, fatty acids, ions, lipids, proteins, ATP, and waste products. Many of the chemical reactions necessary for life take place within the cytoplasm. One of the most important of these reactions is glycolysis, the first step in cellular respiration.

Organelles

The organelles within the cytoplasm work like miniature factories within the cell to perform a series of specific functions related to cell structure, growth, maintenance, and metabolism. The following organelles have specific actions that help the cell to carry out its activities:

- **Centrioles.** Cell division requires a pair of centrioles, which are cylindrical structures made up of short microtubules. During cell division, the centrioles form the spindle-shaped structure needed for movement of DNA strands. Cardiac muscle cells, skeletal muscle cells, mature RBCs, and typical **neurons** (nerve cells) have no centrioles; therefore, these cells are incapable of dividing. The centrosome is the cytoplasm surrounding the centrioles. Microtubules of the cytoskeleton usually begin at the centrosome and radiate through the cytoplasm.
- **Cilia and flagella.** These structures extend from certain cell surfaces. Cilia are hair-like, moving in a coordinated sweeping motion to move fluids over the surface of tissues. They are found on cells lining both the respiratory and reproductive tracts. The cells that line the respiratory tract have a large number of cilia to move particles that have

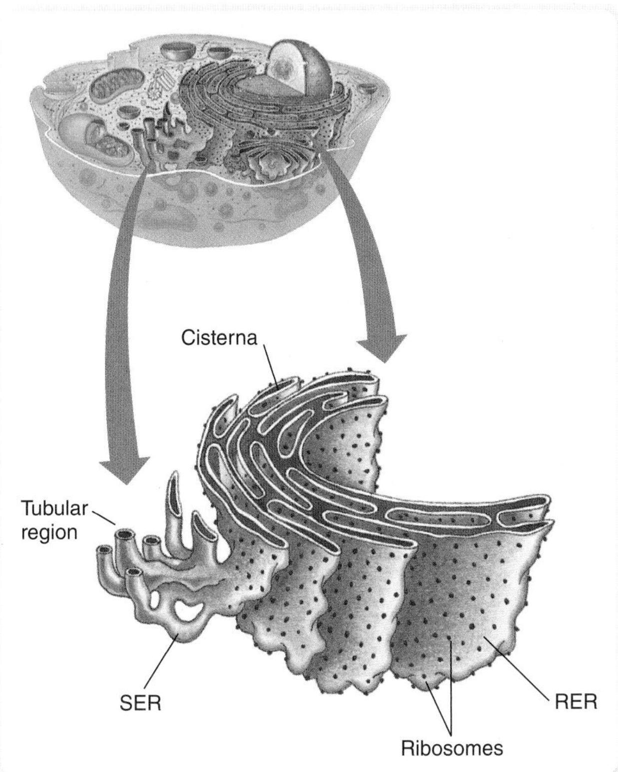

Figure 8-5 Rough endoplasmic reticulum with fixed ribosomes on its outer surface.

been inhaled and trapped in the **mucus** into the **oropharynx** to be swallowed or expelled. Whereas cilia propel other substances, flagella, which are longer than cilia, propel the cells to which they are attached. In humans, a flagellum appears as the tail of a sperm cell).

- **Ribosomes.** Ribosomes are made of complex strands of macromolecules of protein and RNA.[2,3] Ribosome chains form the framework for the genetic blueprint and the synthesis of proteins. Ribosomes may be found either floating freely within the cytoplasm or attached to the endoplasmic reticulum. Because their functions involve the formation of proteins, ribosomes are the so-called protein factories of the cell.
- **Endoplasmic reticulum (ER).** The ER is a chain of canals and sacs that wind through the cytoplasm and connect the nuclear membrane to the cell membrane. The ER moves substances and proteins through the cell. The ER also plays a part in the detoxification process. The ER is either smooth or rough based on the presence or absence of ribosomes on its surface Figure 8-5. The smooth endoplasmic reticulum (SER) lacks ribosomes and it can synthesize phospholipids and cholesterol, which are needed for the growth and maintenance of the cell membrane. The rough endoplasmic reticulum (RER) has ribosomes on its surface and it is found in cells that produce protein to be excreted for use outside the cell. Both free and fixed ribosomes synthesize proteins via instructions from messenger RNA. After creating proteins, the ribosomes transfer the protein into the RER for transport to the Golgi apparatus, where it will be further processed.
- **Golgi apparatus.** This organelle, also called the Golgi complex, consists of a stack of several flattened sacs. These pancake-like structures are hollow, with cavities called cisternae inside them. The Golgi apparatus deals primarily with proteins synthesized on the ribosomes. The end of the Golgi apparatus is specialized to receive glycoproteins, modifying them by removing or adding sugar molecules. The Golgi apparatus has three main functions: (1) concentrating and packaging secretions (such as hormones or enzymes) that are released for secretion out of the cell, (2) packaging special enzymes inside vesicles for use in the cytosol, and (3) renewing or modifying the cell membrane. Mucus is an example of a Golgi apparatus product.
- **Lysosomes.** These tiny sacs perform "housekeeping" tasks within the cell. The enzymes contained within these structures help digest nucleic acids, fats, proteins, polysaccharides, and lipids. Certain white blood cells (WBCs, or leukocytes), have large amounts of lysosomes that contain enzymes designed to digest bacteria. Lysosomes also digest nonfunctional organelles.
- **Microfilaments.** The smallest of the cytoskeletal elements, microfilaments are composed of the proteins actin and myosin. They are typically found in muscle cells. Microfilaments provide cell movement and contraction via interaction with actin and myosin. This process can also change the shape of the entire cell.
- **Mitochondria.** The so-called power plants of the cell and the body, mitochondria are the site of aerobic respiration. Aerobic respiration results in the creation of ATP, which serves as a source of energy throughout the body. The number of mitochondria (singularly called a mitochondrion) in a particular cell varies, based on the energy demands of the cell. The liver, kidneys, and muscles have a large number of mitochondria in their cells because they use ATP at a high rate. A mitochondrion is surrounded by two membranes. The outer membrane gives the organelle its shape, and the inner membrane creates several folds called cristae. These two membranes are important in cellular respiration. Mitochondria contain their own DNA, but in a more primitive form than that found within the nucleus of the cell.

- **Peroxisomes.** These sacs have enzymes that speed up many biochemical reactions. They are abundant in the liver and kidney cells, and their diverse actions include the synthesis of bile acids, detoxification of hydrogen peroxide or alcohol, and breakdown of lipids and biochemicals.
- **Thick filaments.** These organelles are relatively massive bundles of subunits composed of the protein myosin. Thick filaments appear in muscle cells only, where they interact with actin filaments to produce powerful contractions.
- **Vesicles.** Also known as vacuoles, these sacs are formed when a part of a cell membrane folds inward, establishing a bubble-like structure within the cytoplasm. They transport a wide variety of substances inside the cell (endocytotic vesicles) and to the exterior of the cell (exocytotic vesicles).

Nucleus

The nucleus is usually a large structure located near the center of a typical cell. The nucleus is surrounded by the nuclear membrane. This membrane (similar to the cell membrane) encases the nucleoplasm. Within the nucleoplasm are specialized structures that carry the genetic material that the cell uses for reproduction. This material serves as a blueprint for function. DNA resides on threads of chromatin, which are tangles of **chromosomes** that contain thousands of genes. The nucleus also contains a suborganelle called the nucleolus, which is nonmembranous. The nucleolus is densely packed with RNA and surrounded by chromatin. RNA is responsible for ribosome production. Ribosomes are then passed through pores in the nuclear envelope (the outer boundary between the nucleus and the rest of the cell) to the ER for protein synthesis. Recall that RNA and DNA are the so-called blueprint of the cell. Because of this function, the products, appearance, reproduction, and all other aspects of the cell are controlled by the nucleus. Cells without a nucleus, such as RBCs, have a limited lifespan. Table 8-7 summarizes cell structures and function.

▶ Life Cycle of the Cell

The life cycle of the cell is regulated via stimulation from hormones or growth factors. Disruption of the cycle can affect the health of the body. Most human cells divide between 40 to 60 times before they die. The life cycle of a cell includes the following four steps:

1. **Interphase.** The cell obtains nutrients to grow and duplicate.
2. **Cell division (mitosis).** The nucleus divides.
3. **Cytoplasmic division (cytokinesis).** The cytoplasm divides.
4. **Differentiation.** The cell becomes specialized.

Interphase

A cell must grow and duplicate most of its contents before it can actively divide. *Interphase* describes this period of preparation to divide. During interphase, the cell manufactures new living material by duplicating membranes, lysosomes, mitochondria, and ribosomes. The cell also replicates its own genetic material.

Cell Division and Cytoplasmic Division

The two types of cell division are meiosis and mitosis/cytokinesis. **Meiosis** is cell division that occurs in the production of eggs (**oocytes**) and sperm. During meiosis, the number of chromosomes is reduced by half, from 46 to 23. When a sperm joins with an egg and fertilization takes place, the resulting cell will have 46 chromosomes, having received 23 from the sperm and 23 from the egg.

In the rest of the body, cell numbers are increased by **mitosis**, the division of the nucleus of a cell, and cytokinesis, the division of the cytoplasm of a cell. The nucleus must divide precisely so an accurate copy of the DNA can be made by the new cell. Most of the cells of the human body, with the exception of sex cells and RBCs, reproduce by mitosis.

In this continuous process of division and multiplication, one cell divides to become two new cells that are identical to the original cell (the two cells are referred to as daughter cells). Many cells of the body reproduce in this fashion throughout life (eg, skin cells). Other cells divide until near birth (eg, nerve and skeletal cells).

The four stages of mitosis are as follows Figure 8-6:

1. **Prophase.** The two new centriole pairs move to opposite ends of the cell. The chromatin becomes shorter and thicker. Spindle fibers develop, whereas the nucleolus and nuclear membrane disappear.
2. **Metaphase.** The chromosomes line up near the middle portion of the cell, between the centrioles, and spindle fibers attach to them.
3. **Anaphase.** The central areas of each chromosome, called centromeres, are pulled apart to become individual chromosomes, and move toward opposite ends of the cell.
4. **Telophase.** The spindle fibers disappear and the chromosomes lengthen and unwind, with a nuclear envelope forming around them and nucleoli appearing in each newly formed nucleus.

Cytoplasmic division (cytokinesis) begins during anaphase, when the cell membrane constricts down the middle portion of the cell. This process continues through telophase to divide the cytoplasm. The two newly formed nuclei are then separated and nearly half of the organelles are distributed into each new cell.

Differentiation

As discussed previously, differentiation, the process of specialization of a cell, makes each cell unique. New cells must be generated for growth and tissue repair to occur. **Stem cells** can divide repeatedly without specializing. They can either divide into two identical daughter cells or divide so that one daughter cell becomes partially specialized

Table 8-7 Cell Structures and Function

Location	Cell Structure	Function
Nucleus ▪ Control center of the cell ▪ Stores genetic information ▪ Responsible for cell reproduction	Chromatin	Long, slender threads on which DNA is present; during cell division or replication, the chromatin coils to form chromosomes that contain genes
	Nuclear membrane	Composed of two layers and surrounds the nucleus; contains pores (openings) for transport of materials; controls movement of material into and out of the nucleus
	Nucleolus	Small, spherical-shaped structure that has a high concentration of RNA and is the site of ribosome formation
Cytoplasm ▪ Clear, sticky, fluidlike material found outside the nucleus but within the cell membrane that surrounds, supports, and protects organelles ▪ Medium through which nutrients and waste move	Centrioles	Tiny cylinders that help separate the chromosomes during mitosis (cell division)
	Cytoskeleton	Protein rods that provide intracellular shape and support and aid movement of materials into and out of cells
	Endoplasmic reticulum (ER)	Membranous channels that serve as the transport system of the cell through the cytoplasm; rough ER contains ribosomes where protein is synthesized; smooth ER is the site of steroid, phospholipid, and fatty acid synthesis; smooth ER in liver cells break down alcohol and some drugs, such as amphetamines
	Golgi apparatus	Membranous structures that resemble a stack of pancakes; found near the nucleus and serve to package and export proteins
	Lysosomes	Small, round structures that perform "housekeeping" tasks within the cell, digesting cell waste through powerful enzymes
	Mitochondria	Fluid-filled sacs that serve as the so-called power plants of the cell and carry on cellular respiration, converting energy in nutrients to ATP
	Ribosomes	Small granules of RNA that, when fully assembled, function like miniature protein factories
	Vesicles	Tiny membranous sacs used for storage and transport of cellular products and digestion of the metabolic waste of the cell
Surface ▪ Encloses the cytoplasm and forms the outer boundary of the cell	Plasma membrane	Provides support and protection; the plasma membrane is selectively permeable, allowing some substances to enter and leave the cell while not allowing other substances to cross

(progenitor cells). In the human body, all differentiated cell types are created because of the variance of stem and progenitor cells. Researchers are exploring the use of stem cells in treating diseases such as diabetes, heart disease, stroke, macular degeneration, burns, osteoarthritis, and rheumatoid arthritis, as well as spinal injuries.

Cell Division and Cancer

Cell division and growth normally occur at approximately the same rate as cell death. However, when cell division and growth occur at a higher rate than the cell death rate, tissues enlarge. A **neoplasm** (tumor) is a mass of tissue produced by abnormal cell growth and division. A tumor is *benign* when it remains within the epithelium (a capsule made of connective tissue). A benign tumor seldom becomes life threatening and can usually be surgically removed if it affects tissue function.

In contrast, a *malignant* tumor spreads into surrounding tissues in a process called invasion. Malignancy often occurs when a normal gene mutates. These mutated genes are called oncogenes. When cancer develops, the mutations disrupt normal cell growth. The tumor of origin (the primary tumor or primary neoplasm) may result in malignant cells that escape the primary tumor to invade other organs or tissue, resulting in secondary

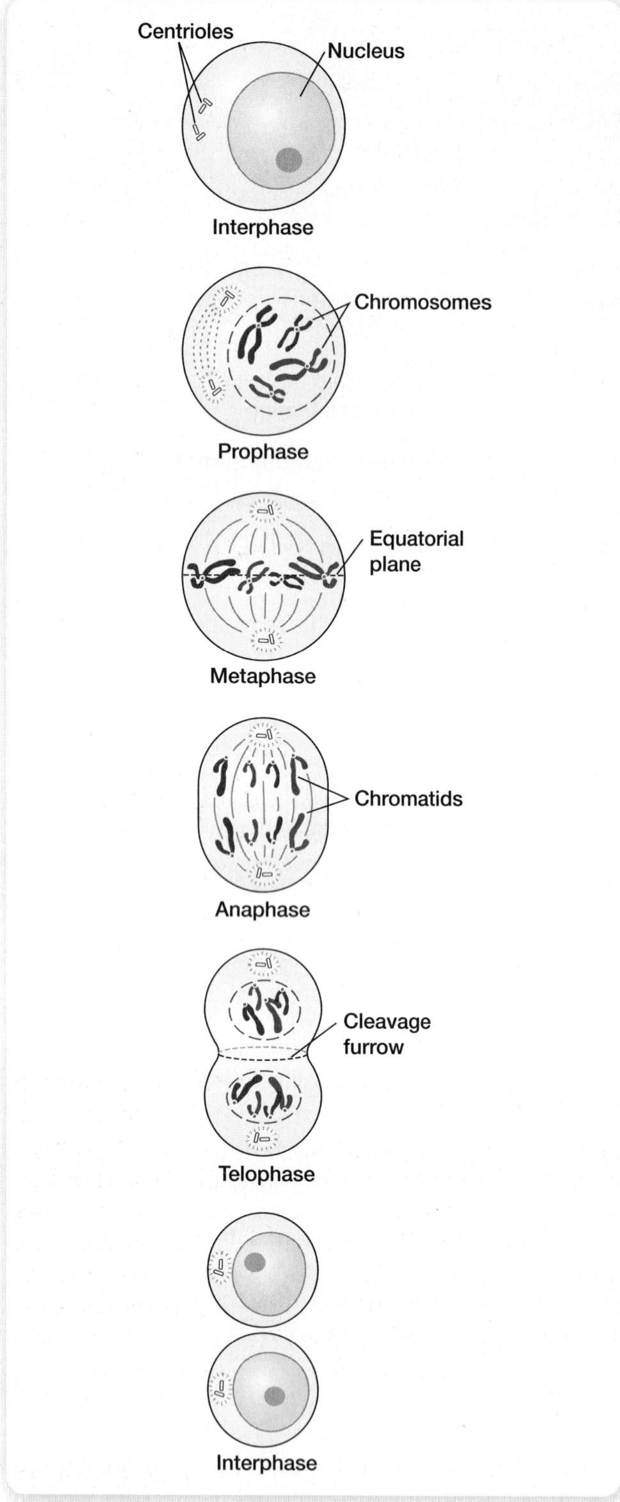

Figure 8-6 Mitosis and cell division.

tumors. This process—metastasis—is not easily controlled. Usually, tumor cells are daughter cells of just one malignant cell. Cancer often begins where stem cells divide because the more frequently that chromosomes are copied for cell division, the greater the chance of errors in the DNA copying process—thereby leading to mutations in the new cells.

Cancer cells change shape as they grow and gradually resemble normal cells less and less. If tumor cells penetrate blood vessels, then they circulate throughout the body. If tumor cells enter the **lymphatic system**, then they build up in **lymph nodes**. The presence of tumor cells stimulates the growth of new blood vessels where the cells situate themselves, which supplies them with more nutrients and accelerates their growth and further metastasis.

As metastasis increases, organ function changes. Cancer cells grow and multiply by taking nutrients and space from normal cells, causing weight loss in most patients with cancer as the normal cells deteriorate. Death may occur when cancer cells compress vital organs or replace healthy cells in vital organs.

▶ Cellular Signaling

To work collectively as a cohesive unit, cells must be able to communicate with other cells and within individual cells. The means by which cells electrochemically communicate is called intercellular communication or cellular signaling. Cellular signaling is used to maintain homeostasis, fight infection, reproduce, and perform other normal functions. Alterations in signals also can lead to dysfunction. Some tumors and cancers are believed to be the result of disruptions in this process. Cellular signaling is discussed in more detail later in this chapter.

▶ Cellular Respiration

Almost all metabolic functions require energy. The major source of energy for the cells is the six-carbon sugar, glucose ($C_6H_{12}O_6$). Use of glucose by the cell is called oxidation, and the result is carbon dioxide (CO_2), water (H_2O), and the high-energy molecule ATP. ATP is the true source of cellular energy because of the high-energy bonds contained between its phosphate molecules. When needed for cellular function, these bonds are broken to release their stored energy. However, despite the large amount of energy contained in these bonds, glucose contains an even higher amount of energy. If glucose molecules were to be broken down in one step, then a considerable loss of energy to heat would occur, with minimal production of ATP. As a result, cellular respiration occurs in three stages to maximize the number of molecules of ATP created for each molecule of glucose.

Glycolysis

As the first step in cellular respiration, **glycolysis** occurs in the cytoplasm and does not require oxygen; it is therefore an *anaerobic* process Figure 8-7. After the glucose molecule moves into the cell, two phosphate molecules, gained from breaking two molecules of ATP, immediately attach to it in separate steps. This process prevents both the glucose from leaving the cells and the concentration of glucose inside the cells from becoming higher than the concentration outside the cells. It also prepares the glucose molecule for further breakdown. Next, a series of complex steps occurs to break down the glucose molecule

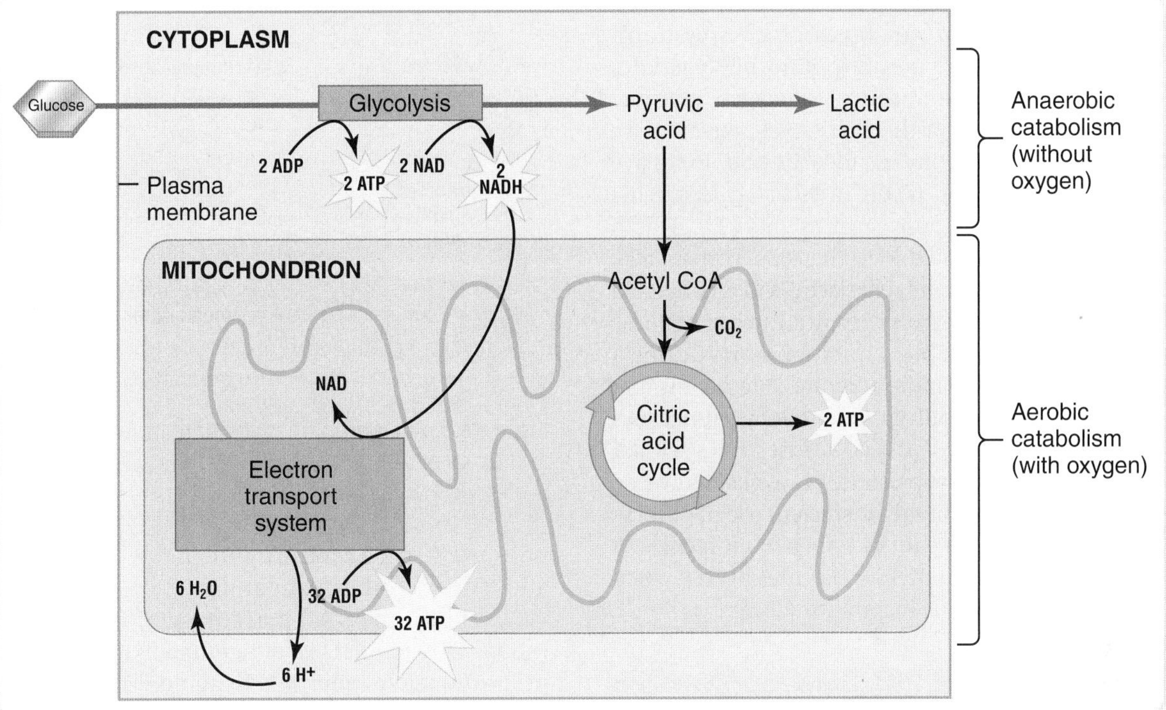

Figure 8-7 During anaerobic metabolism, which occurs in the cytoplasm, the breakdown of glucose results in lactic acid. During aerobic metabolism, which occurs in the mitochondrion, the breakdown of glucose results in carbon dioxide, water, and ATP.

into its final product, two molecules of pyruvic acid. During this phase of cellular respiration, two molecules of pyruvic acid and four molecules of ATP are formed. However, recall the expenditure of two molecules of ATP in the early steps of this process; therefore, the net result of glycolysis is two molecules of pyruvic acid and two molecules of ATP. This process is obviously an inefficient use of glucose, but fortunately it does not end here.

Krebs Cycle

The second step in cellular respiration is the Krebs cycle, also known as the **citric acid cycle** (tricarboxylic acid cycle). The key to this stage in the breakdown of glucose is the presence or absence of oxygen, because the Krebs cycle only occurs in the presence of oxygen (**aerobic metabolism**) (see Figure 8-7). After occurring in the matrix (nonliving material that separates cells in the connective tissue) of the mitochondria, the pyruvic acid formed during glycolysis undergoes a complex series of steps that produces several products, including three molecules of carbon dioxide and one molecule pf ATP. Because two molecules of pyruvic acid are produced during glycolysis, the Krebs cycle occurs twice for each molecule of glucose that is oxidized. Therefore, the result of the Krebs cycle is six molecules of carbon dioxide (this principle is important in the concept of capnography) and two molecules of ATP for every glucose molecule. To summarize ATP production thus far in cellular respiration, four molecules of ATP have been produced—two from glycolysis and two from the Krebs cycle, and only a minimal amount of energy has been gained from the original glucose molecule.

Electron Transport System

The final step in the oxidation of glucose is the electron transport chain, which occurs on the inner cristae of the mitochondria. During this step, the production of ATP takes place. In addition to the production of ATP and carbon dioxide from glycolysis and the Krebs cycle, several other products are created. After moving to the inner cristae, these products transfer their electrons during a series of reactions that ultimately produces 34 molecules of ATP. Because the electron transport system depends on the Krebs cycle, this process is considered a part of aerobic respiration.

Results of Cellular Respiration

At the completion of all steps of cellular respiration, 38 molecules of ATP are produced: two molecules from glycolysis and 36 molecules from aerobic respiration (two from the Krebs cycle and 34 from the electron transport system). Although this result represents an efficient use of the energy contained in one molecule of glucose, it is not 100% efficient because some energy loss occurs in the form of heat.

Aerobic Versus Anaerobic Respiration

As described previously, the presence of oxygen is crucial to the efficient oxidation of glucose by the cells. When oxygen is present, the majority of the respiration that takes place is aerobic (see Figure 8-7). However, respiration can also occur in the absence of oxygen (anaerobic respiration). In this situation, glycolysis occurs as it normally would. However, because of the absence of oxygen, pyruvic acid cannot be oxidized in the Krebs cycle. As a result, the pyruvic acid quickly converts to **lactic acid**. Excessive anaerobic respiration can result in *lactic acidosis*. This condition occurs in situations such as shock, in which sufficient oxygen is unavailable to the cells. Fortunately, when oxygen is restored to the cells, lactic acid is converted back to pyruvic acid and aerobic respiration can resume. It is often said that anaerobic respiration starts during a lack of oxygen; however, a more accurate statement is that aerobic respiration stops during a lack of oxygen because anaerobic respiration (glycolysis) is the first step in cellular respiration, regardless of the presence of oxygen. However, anaerobic respiration is a highly inefficient use of glucose by itself, resulting in a net gain of only two molecules of ATP compared with a gain of 38 molecules of ATP when both anaerobic and aerobic respiration occur.

Words of Wisdom

When cells function with oxygen, they use aerobic and anaerobic components of metabolism. They generate large amounts of ATP (cellular energy) and produce wastes of carbon dioxide and water. When cells function without oxygen, they use purely **anaerobic metabolism**. They generate small amounts of ATP (cellular energy) and produce waste of lactic acid.

Body Fluid Composition

For the cells, tissues, organs, and organ systems to perform their functions efficiently, certain parameters must be maintained. These parameters include the amount, distribution, and movement of body fluids; electrolyte balance; and the amount of hydrogen ions, or acid-base balance.

The most prevalent fluid in the human body is water, which is an essential part of all the chemical reactions that regularly occur in the body. Water also serves as a transport medium for nutrients, hormones, and waste materials. The total amount of fluid in the body at any given time is referred to as **total body water (TBW)**. TBW constitutes about 60% of the weight of a healthy adult male and is made up of **intracellular fluid (ICF)** and **extracellular fluid (ECF)**. Cell membranes separate the intracellular and extracellular fluid compartments. ICF consists of the fluid found within the cells. This intracellular compartment contains about 63% of TBW, and the extracellular compartment contains about 37% of TBW **Figure 8-8**. ICF contains large amounts of potassium, magnesium, and phosphate ions. In contrast, ECF contains large amounts of sodium, chloride, and bicarbonate ions plus nutrients for the cells, such as oxygen, glucose, fatty acids, and amino acids.[4] ECF also contains waste

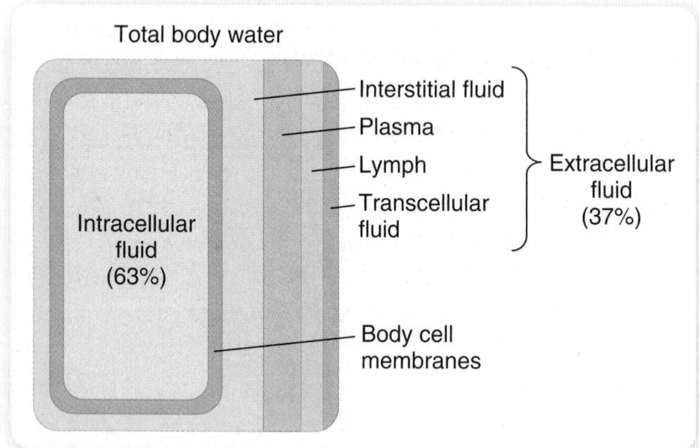

Figure 8-8 Cell membranes separate intracellular and extracellular fluids.

products to be excreted by the lungs (carbon dioxide) and kidneys (other cellular waste).

At birth, the total percentage of fluid in the body (about 75% to 80%) is higher than that of an adult, with proportionately more ECF in adults. This percentage decreases during the first year of life. Infants have a loss of body water for physiologic reasons as they adjust to their new environment outside the womb. This age group is at an increased risk for negative consequences of excessive fluid losses (dehydration) because of their greater metabolic rate and higher body surface area. By the time the child reaches adolescence, the TBW drops to about 60%, or normal adult values. This trend continues throughout a person's life. As the body ages and the amount of muscle mass and adipose tissue changes, the TBW decreases because muscle mass is composed of more water than adipose tissue, which repels water. Infants are also at risk for deadly consequences from fluid and electrolyte imbalances.

The extracellular fluid is composed of **interstitial fluid**, plasma, lymph, and **transcellular fluid**. The intravascular component is the fluid contained within the chambers of the heart and the blood vessels. *Blood volume* refers to the total volume of the intravascular compartment. About 3 L of the total blood volume is blood plasma, referred to as the plasma volume. The remaining 2.5 L consists of RBCs, WBCs, and **platelets** (thrombocytes), which make up the formed elements of the blood. Most of the ECF is composed of interstitial fluid that is outside the intravascular compartment, where it bathes the nonblood cells of the body.[5] The walls of capillaries separate the intravascular and interstitial compartments. Transcellular fluid is found in spaces that are surrounded by epithelial cells, such as the **synovial fluid** within joints (formed where two bones come in contact) and the clear, watery **cerebrospinal fluid (CSF)** that surrounds the brain and spinal cord (discussed later in this chapter).[5]

Cellular Transport Mechanisms

To maintain homeostasis, it is essential to maintain a delicate balance among the fluid compartments of the body.

Under normal conditions, the total volume of water in the body and its distribution in the body compartments remain relatively constant, even though the amount of water that enters and is excreted from the body each day fluctuates.

The fluids in the body exist in a solution of dissolved elements and water. Recall that the cell membrane is semipermeable, allowing lipid-soluble substances to move in and out of the cell freely while not allowing water-soluble substances to cross the membrane. However, to sustain life both types of substances must be allowed to enter and exit the cell.

Water and electrolytes move among the fluid compartments of the body according to some basic chemical and biologic principles. One governing principle is that unequal concentrations on different sides of a cell membrane will move to balance themselves equally on both sides of the membrane. Balance across a cell membrane has two components: (1) the balance of compounds (for example, water and electrolytes) on either side of the cell membrane, and (2) the balance of charges [the positive ($^+$) or negative ($^-$) charges carried on the atoms] on either side of the cell membrane.

When concentrations of charges or compounds are greater on one side of the cell membrane than on the other side, a gradient is created. The natural tendency for materials is to flow from an area of higher concentration to one of lower concentration, establishing a *concentration gradient*. The concentration gradient is the difference in concentrations of a substance on either side of a semipermeable membrane. Gradients are categorized according to the type of material that flows down them: chemical compounds flow down chemical gradients, whereas electrical currents flow down electrical gradients. The process of flowing down a gradient depends on whether the cell membrane will allow the material to pass through it. Certain compounds can travel freely across the cell membrane (a kinetically favorable situation that requires little energy), whereas others require **active transport** across the membrane because of the size of the compound or because of an incompatible charge. Active transport is discussed in more detail later in this chapter.

Each of the compartments of the body is separated by a membrane. **Osmotic pressure** is the pressure exerted by the concentration of the solutes in a given space to stop the flow of solvent across a semipermeable membrane. The osmotic pressure of a solution, or the ability to affect the movement of water, is *osmolality*. It is expressed in osmoles or milliosmoles per kilogram of water. Generally, the amount of water in each compartment is tightly regulated in an effort to maintain the osmolality of TBW in equilibrium. The body uses several mechanisms to accomplish a balanced osmolality in each of the compartments.

Diffusion

Diffusion is the process of particles moving from an area of higher concentration to an area of lower concentration along a concentration gradient until equilibrium is achieved **Figure 8-9**. Because diffusion does not require energy, it is considered a passive transport mechanism. Diffusion applies to both solids and gasses in the human body. By moving some of the solute from one side of the membrane to the other, the body reduces or eliminates the concentration gradient and creates balance as much as possible. As discussed previously, this is the natural tendency of the body and is referred to as moving with the concentration gradient. Complete elimination of concentration gradients is impossible because ions and molecules are always in motion in a random pattern. However, the net change is close to zero. This process is how the body is able to move some nutrients and waste products into and out of the cell. With gases, the molecules are spread farther apart and the diffusion rate depends on the weight of the gas.

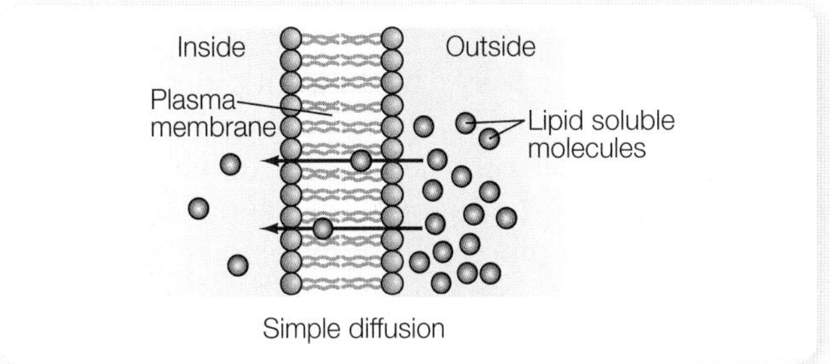

Figure 8-9 Diffusion.

To visualize diffusion, imagine that too many people show up for a theater performance. The theater manager decides to open another seating area to accommodate the crowd. Patrons (charges or compounds) are concentrated in a small area (the cell) outside the door (the cell membrane) leading to the new seating area. When the theater manager opens the door, patrons can move through it (selective cell membrane permeability) from the congested area (down a concentration gradient). The patrons spread themselves out evenly (diffuse) throughout the total area, with some choosing to stay behind in the original seating area as others move into the new area, until all patrons have an equal amount of room.

Substances that can freely cross the cell membrane, such as oxygen and carbon dioxide, move by the process of diffusion in the human body. For example, blood returning to the lungs from the body has a high concentration of carbon dioxide and a low concentration of oxygen. The lungs, however, have a high concentration of oxygen and a low concentration of carbon dioxide. As the blood passes through the pulmonary vasculature, carbon dioxide leaves the blood and enters the lungs until an equal amount of carbon dioxide is present in both. By the same process, oxygen leaves the lungs and enters the blood until an equal amount of oxygen is present in both. By this principle, the amount of expired carbon dioxide is nearly equal to the amount of carbon dioxide contained in the arterial blood.

Filtration

Filtration is commonly used by the kidneys to clean blood. Water carries dissolved compounds across the cell membranes of the tubules of the kidney. The tubule membrane traps these dissolved compounds but allows the water to pass through. This process cleans the blood of wastes and removes the trapped compounds from circulation so they can be flushed out of the body. The antidiuretic hormone (ADH) prevents the loss of water from the kidneys by causing its reabsorption into the tubules.

Facilitated Diffusion

It is sometimes necessary to move molecules across a membrane that either cannot use diffusion or must move against the concentration gradient. In these situations, the movement occurs by either active transport or facilitated diffusion.

Active transport is used to move substances against the concentration gradient or toward the side with a higher concentration. This type of transport, just as it sounds, requires the use of energy by the cell, but it is faster than diffusion. Active transport is similar to operating a motor vehicle in that the vehicle can roll down a hill in neutral gear without the engine being on, but the vehicle has to be running and in gear to go uphill.

Facilitated diffusion is a passive transport mechanism similar to diffusion in that it involves particles moving from an area of higher concentration to an area of lower concentration. However, in this type of diffusion, the molecule entering the cell cannot enter without the assistance of a carrier protein. During facilitated diffusion, the substance needed in the cell binds with the carrier protein, and one of two processes takes place. The combination of the molecule and carrier protein may be lipid soluble and pass through the cytoplasmic membrane, or the two may enter the cell through a membrane protein. This step is possible either because of the new shape of the carrier molecule combination, or the combination of the two can attach to a binding site in the membrane protein Figure 8-10. The membrane protein then changes shape to allow passage of the carrier molecule combination into the cell. After the carrier protein is in the cell, it breaks off from the molecule and returns to the surface of the membrane to transport other molecules into the cell. Glucose enters the cell by this process. Glucose is not lipid soluble and therefore cannot cross the cell membrane; it is also too large a molecule to cross through the membrane proteins. By attaching to a carrier protein, glucose is allowed to enter the cell. Insulin is a hormone that is responsible for regulating the speed with which carrier proteins move glucose into cells.

Osmosis

Osmosis is the movement of a solvent, such as water, from an area of low solute concentration to one of high concentration through a selectively permeable membrane. Osmosis is another passive transport mechanism; however, unlike diffusion, the particles themselves do not move in osmosis.

Recall that solutions contain both a liquid (solvent) and particles suspended in the liquid (solutes). The primary solvent in the body is water, which is considered the universal solvent. Within this solvent are several solutes. In the human body, solutes consist of electrolytes, such as sodium and potassium, and molecules, such as glucose. Water can generally move without much difficulty between the different compartments of the body because the membranes that separate the compartments are permeable to water. The cell membrane is semipermeable because it also is selectively permeable to certain solutes Figure 8-11. Selective permeability is accomplished through pores in the membrane that are selective on the basis of the size, shape, or electrical charge of the molecule. The body tries to maintain an equal solute concentration on each side of the membrane. An **isotonic solution** is one in which an equal concentration of solutes and water is present on either side of a semipermeable membrane.

For example, if a solution on one side of a membrane has 25 sodium ions and 100 water molecules (25% solution), and a solution on the other side of the membrane has 50 sodium ions and 100 water molecules (50% solution), then the water will move from the area of lower solute concentration to higher solute concentration in an effort to reach an equal concentration on both sides of the membrane. In this example, the end result will be 25 sodium molecules and 66 water molecules on one side (37%), and 50 sodium molecules and 134 water molecules on the other (37%).

The concentration of a solution, or ability to draw or give water, is its *tonicity* Figure 8-12, and the difference in concentrations from one side of a selectively permeable membrane to the other is the *osmotic gradient*. The degree of difference between the two concentrations determines how much osmotic pressure is present and how quickly the two concentrations will tend to equalize. A solution with a higher solute concentration compared with another solution is **hypertonic**, and a solution with a lower solute concentration is **hypotonic**. If too much water moves out of a cell, then the cell shrinks abnormally, a process known as crenation. If too much water enters a cell, then it will swell and burst, a process known as lysis.

Active Transport

As discussed previously, in some situations, ions and molecules must be transported from an area of low concentration to an area of high concentration. Active transport, which involves the expenditure of energy, is required because of this "uphill" movement (see Figure 8-10B). For example, most of the sodium in the body is contained in the extracellular fluid, whereas the majority of the potassium in the body is contained in the intracellular

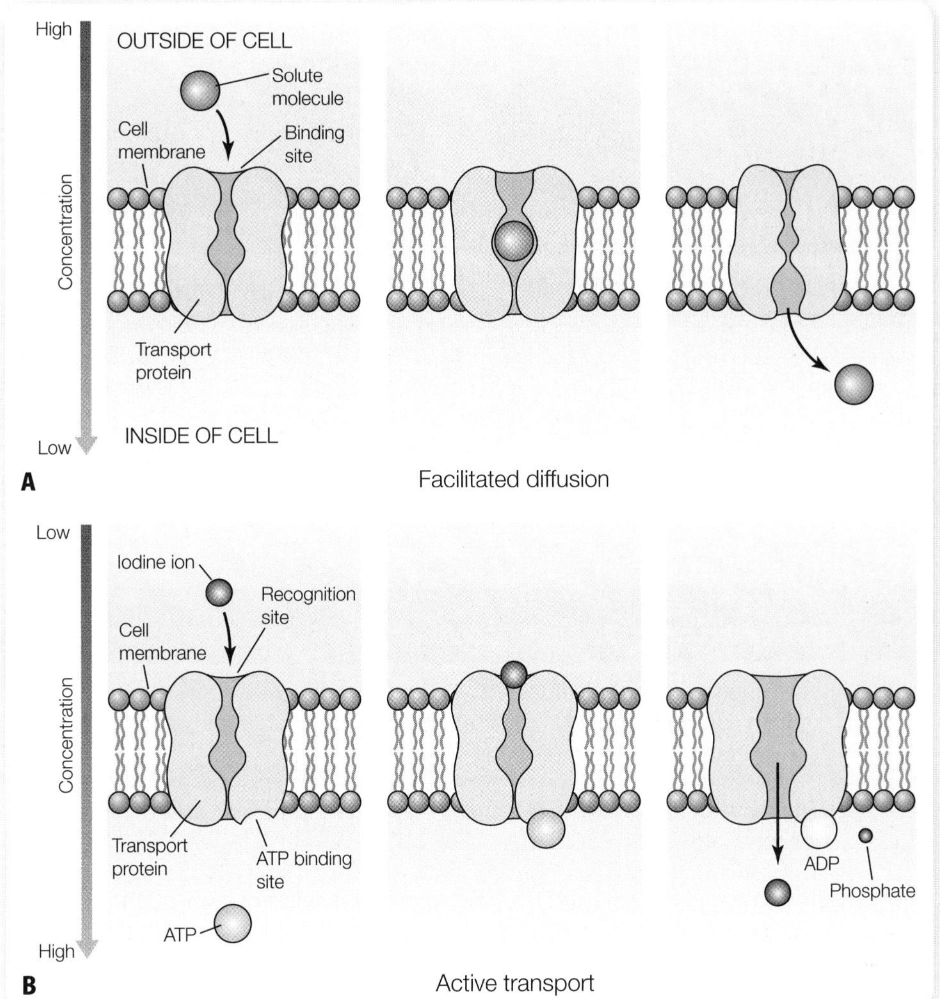

Figure 8-10 A. Facilitated diffusion involves particles moving from an area of higher concentration toward an area of lower concentration with the assistance of a protein. **B.** Active transport uses energy from adenosine triphosphate (ATP) to open a pathway for compounds to move against a concentration gradient.

fluid. Sodium enters the cell through simple diffusion when the sodium channels open, and potassium leaves the cell by the same process when the potassium channels open. To move sodium out of the cell or potassium into the cell, these channels cannot simply be opened again because a higher concentration of sodium on the outside and potassium on the inside is always present. An active transport process—the sodium-potassium pump—must be used to move these ions against their concentration gradient. As with facilitated diffusion, this process uses a system in which the particle being moved binds with a carrier protein. However, unlike facilitated diffusion, this binding requires the use of energy. After the particle is bound, it is transported through the membrane and then released. Although active transport demands a high-energy expenditure, its benefits outweigh the initial use of ATP. Pumping sodium out of the cell and potassium into the cell has the added benefit of moving glucose into the cell at the same time.

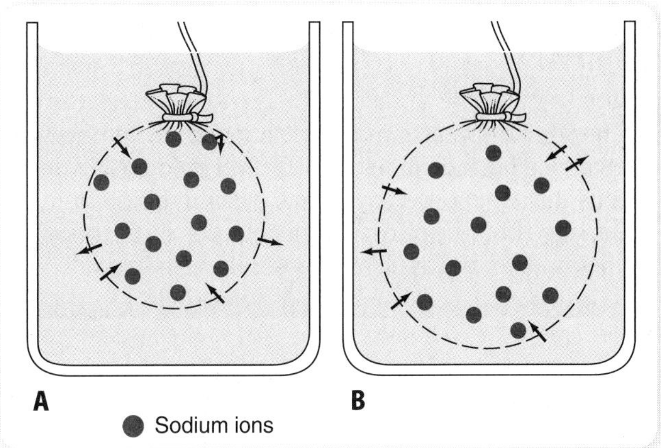

Figure 8-11 A. An example of osmosis occurs when a permeable bag of salt water is immersed in a solution of pure water. **B.** Water moves into the bag (toward the area with lower water concentration) equalizing the concentrations on each side of the membrane.

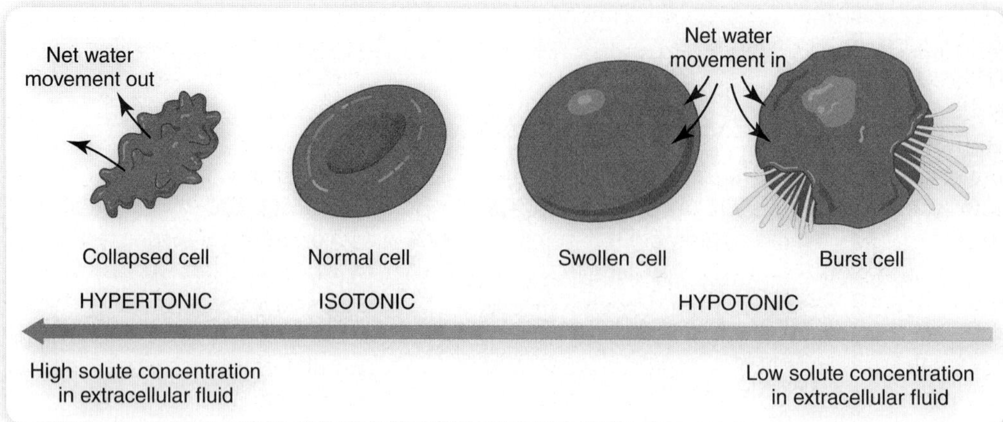

Figure 8-12 Tonicity.

Table 8-8 Cellular Transport Mechanisms

Mechanism	Movement
Diffusion	The movement of a solvent, such as water, from an area of low solute concentration to one of high concentration through a selectively permeable membrane to equalize the solute concentration on both sides of the membrane
Filtration	The movement of water and a dissolved substance from an area of high pressure to an area of low pressure
Facilitated diffusion	The easing of the passage of a substance from an area of higher concentration to an area of lower concentration by a transport (helper) molecule within the membrane
Osmosis	The movement of a solvent, such as water, from an area of low solute concentration to one of high concentration through a selectively permeable membrane to equalize the solute concentration on both sides of the membrane
Active transport	Movement via transport molecules, or pumps, that require energy to move substances from an area of low concentration to an area of high concentration

Words of Wisdom

The sodium-potassium pump continuously removes three sodium ions from the cell for every two potassium ions that are moved back into the cell. If this pump is impaired because of insufficient potassium in the body, then sodium builds up and causes the cells to swell.

Endocytosis and exocytosis are processes that use energy from the cell to move substances into or out of the cell without crossing the cell membrane. In endocytosis, a secretion from the cell membrane moves particles too large to enter the cell by other processes within a vesicle of the cell. The three forms of endocytosis are pinocytosis, phagocytosis, and receptor-mediated endocytosis. **Pinocytosis** ("cell drinking") is the transport of droplets of extracellular fluid into the cell membrane. With **phagocytosis** ("cell eating"), a cell surrounds a foreign particle and engulfs it. Receptor-mediated endocytosis involves the movement of specific kinds of particles into the cell, with protein molecules extending through part of the cell membrane to the outer surface. The opposite process to endocytosis is exocytosis, in which a substance stored in a vesicle is secreted from the cell. Cellular transport mechanisms are summarized in Table 8-8.

Tissue Level

Recall that a tissue is a group of cells that are similar in structure and function. Tissue results from the process of differentiation, which occurs early in the development of a cell and is the process by which the cell becomes specialized for a specific purpose. For example, a cell can become specialized as a cardiac cell or a bone cell. When stem cells undergo mitosis, one daughter cell remains an undifferentiated stem cell whereas the other differentiates and takes on the characteristics of a particular tissue.

The human body is primarily made up of four types of tissue that are classified by their shape, structure, and function. The four types are epithelial, connective, muscle, and nervous tissues. **Epithelial tissues** cover body surfaces, cover and line internal organs, and make up the glands. Connective tissues are widely distributed throughout the body, fill the internal spaces, and function to bind, support, and protect body structures. Muscle tissues are specialized for contraction, and include the skeletal muscles of the body, the heart, and the muscular walls of hollow organs. Skeletal muscles are attached to bones, and are used for movement of the body. **Nervous tissues** carry information from one part of the body to another via electrical impulses. They are found in the brain, spinal cord, and nerves.

Epithelial Tissues

Epithelial tissue covers most of the surfaces of the body (both external and internal surfaces) and the interior of hollow organs. This type of tissue is composed of many cells that fit tightly together, forming a continuous layer of cells with little or no intercellular material (material between the cells). Epithelial tissue has two surfaces. Because epithelial tissue forms coverings and linings, one surface of the tissue is typically unattached and is exposed to the outside (eg, outer surface of the skin, inner lining of the mouth) or internally to an open space (eg, intestinal lining). On the side opposite the free surface (ie, the undersurface), the cells are attached to a basement membrane, which is very thin layer of tissue that anchors the epithelium to the underling structure, such as connective tissue. Because epithelial tissue is generally avascular, which means it has no blood supply of its own, it receives oxygen and nutrients by diffusion from the blood vessels that supply the underlying connective tissues. Glands are secretory structures derived from epithelia.

Words of Wisdom

Epithelial tissue is able to repair itself (regenerate) quickly if injured.

Epithelia perform four essential functions:

1. **Physical protection.** Epithelia protect exposed and internal surfaces from abrasion, dehydration, and destruction from biologic or chemical agents.
2. **Permeability.** Any substance entering or leaving the body must cross an epithelium, so the epithelia control permeability. Some epithelia are relatively impermeable, whereas others are crossed easily by compounds of various sizes. In response to stimuli, the epithelial barrier may be modified and regulated. Hormones can affect ion and nutrient transport through epithelial cells. Physical stress can also alter the structure and properties of epithelia. An example is the formation of calluses on the hands after repeated manual labor.
3. **Sensation.** Most epithelia are sensitive to stimulation because they have a large supply of sensory nerves.
4. **Specialized secretions.** Epithelial cells that produce secretions are called gland cells, and individual cells of this type are scattered among other types of cells in an epithelium. Most or all of the epithelial cells in a glandular epithelium produce secretions, which are either discharged onto the surface of the epithelium or released into the surrounding interstitial fluid and blood.

Epithelial tissue can be divided into groups according to its microscopic shape and the number of layers in the tissue Table 8-9. It is classified by shape as squamous (flat, thin, and scalelike), cuboidal (cubed), columnar (taller than wide), or transitional Figure 8-13. Transitional cells, typically found in the **urinary system**, have the ability to stretch and change their appearance to look like any of the other three types. Epithelial tissue can also be classified according to the number of layers. *Simple epithelium* is composed of a single layer of cells. *Stratified epithelium* is composed of two or more layers. *Pseudostratified epithelium* is made up of epithelium that appears to have multiple layers but does not. The pseudostratified impression, which means falsely stratified, occurs because the cells are irregularly shaped and their nuclei appear at different levels in the tissue, giving the impression of multiple layers.

Epithelial tissue is sometimes subdivided into membranous epithelium and glandular epithelium. Membranous epithelium covers the body; lines the pleural, pericardial, and peritoneal cavities; lines the respiratory, digestive, and genitourinary tracts; and lines the blood and lymphatic vessels. Glandular epithelium consists of specialized cells that produce and secrete substances into ducts or body fluids. It is usually found in **exocrine glands** (which have ducts that open onto surfaces or into the digestive tract) or in **endocrine glands** (which have no ducts and secrete into tissue fluid or blood). The three types of exocrine glands are merocrine, apocrine, and holocrine Figure 8-14. Merocrine glands release fluid by exocytosis. Apocrine glands lose parts of their cell bodies during secretion. Holocrine glands release entire cells that disintegrate to release secretions.

Connective Tissues

Connective tissue is the most abundant type of body tissue and also is the most widely distributed. These

Table 8-9 Types of Epithelial Tissue

Type	Description	Function	Location
Simple squamous	Single layer of thin, flat cells	Permit diffusion of oxygen and carbon dioxide between alveolar air and blood	Alveoli of lungs
		Absorption by diffusion, filtration, and osmosis	Lines walls of capillaries and lymphatic vessels
		Filtration of water and electrolytes	Kidneys
Simple cuboidal	Single layer of cells that are as wide as they are tall (cube-shaped)	Absorption of water and electrolytes	Lines kidney tubules
		Secretion of enzymes and hormones	Lines the ovary surface, ducts of some glands (salivary glands, thyroid gland, pancreas)
Simple columnar	Single layer of cells that are taller than they are wide; some cells are equipped with cilia	Protection; secretion of digestive enzymes; absorption of nutrients	Lines stomach and intestines
		Moves particles of dust and other foreign material away from lungs by means of cilia	Lines parts of respiratory tract
Pseudostratified columnar	Single layer of cells of differing heights, some of which do not reach the unattached surface	Protection; secretion of mucus	Lines trachea and most of upper respiratory passages; lines male urethra
		Moves egg toward uterus	Lining of fallopian tubes
Stratified squamous	Multiple cell layers	Protection	Outer layer of the skin; surface lining of mouth, esophagus, vagina, and anus
Stratified cuboidal	Typically two layers of cubelike cells	Protection	Linings of larger mammary gland ducts, sweat gland ducts, salivary glands
Stratified columnar	Multiple cell layers	Protection; secretion	Part of male urethra, parts of the pharynx, and large ducts of some glands
Transitional	Cells appear simple when stretched and appear stratified when unstretched	Protection; stretch and change appearance	Inner urinary bladder lining, linings of ureters, and part of urethra

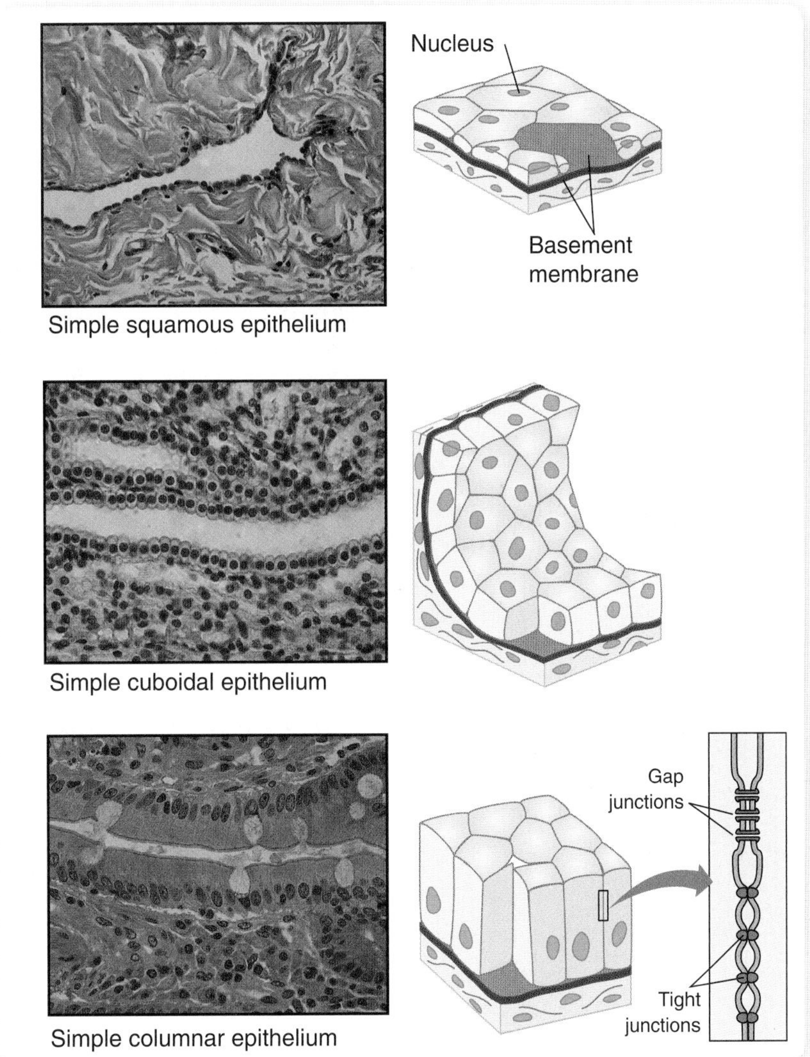

Figure 8-13 Shapes of epithelial cells.

A, C and E: © Donna Beer Stolz, PhD, Center for Biologic Imaging, University of Pittsburgh Medical School; **B, D and F:** © Jones & Bartlett Learning.

tissues bind body structures, provide support and protection, create frameworks, fill body spaces, store fat, produce blood cells, transport fluids and dissolved materials, repair damaged tissues, and protect the body from infection.

Unlike the tightly fitting cells of epithelial tissue, connective tissue is composed of cells that are separated from each other by the matrix. This intercellular substance serves as the cement that gives the connective tissue its basic characteristics (connection of tissue). Although cells make up the majority of epithelial tissue, the matrix usually accounts for the majority of connective tissue.

Most connective tissue cells divide, have good blood supply, and require large amounts of nourishment. Connective tissues include those of bone, cartilage, and fat. Connective tissues contain different types of cells, including those that are fixed or wandering. The most common type of fixed cell is the star-shaped fibroblast, which produces fibers via protein secretion into the extracellular matrix. Table 8-10 summarizes the major cells and tissue fibers of connective tissue.

Fibroblasts produce three connective tissue fibers:

1. **Collagenous fibers**. Important for body parts that hold structures together (ie, ligaments, which connect bone to bone and tendons, which connect muscle to bone); collagenous fibers are also called dense connective tissue or white fibers.
2. **Elastic fibers.** Common in body parts that are often stretched, such as the vocal cords; they are composed of a protein called elastin, and are also called yellow fibers.
3. **Reticular fibers.** Form delicate supporting networks in the spleen and other tissues.

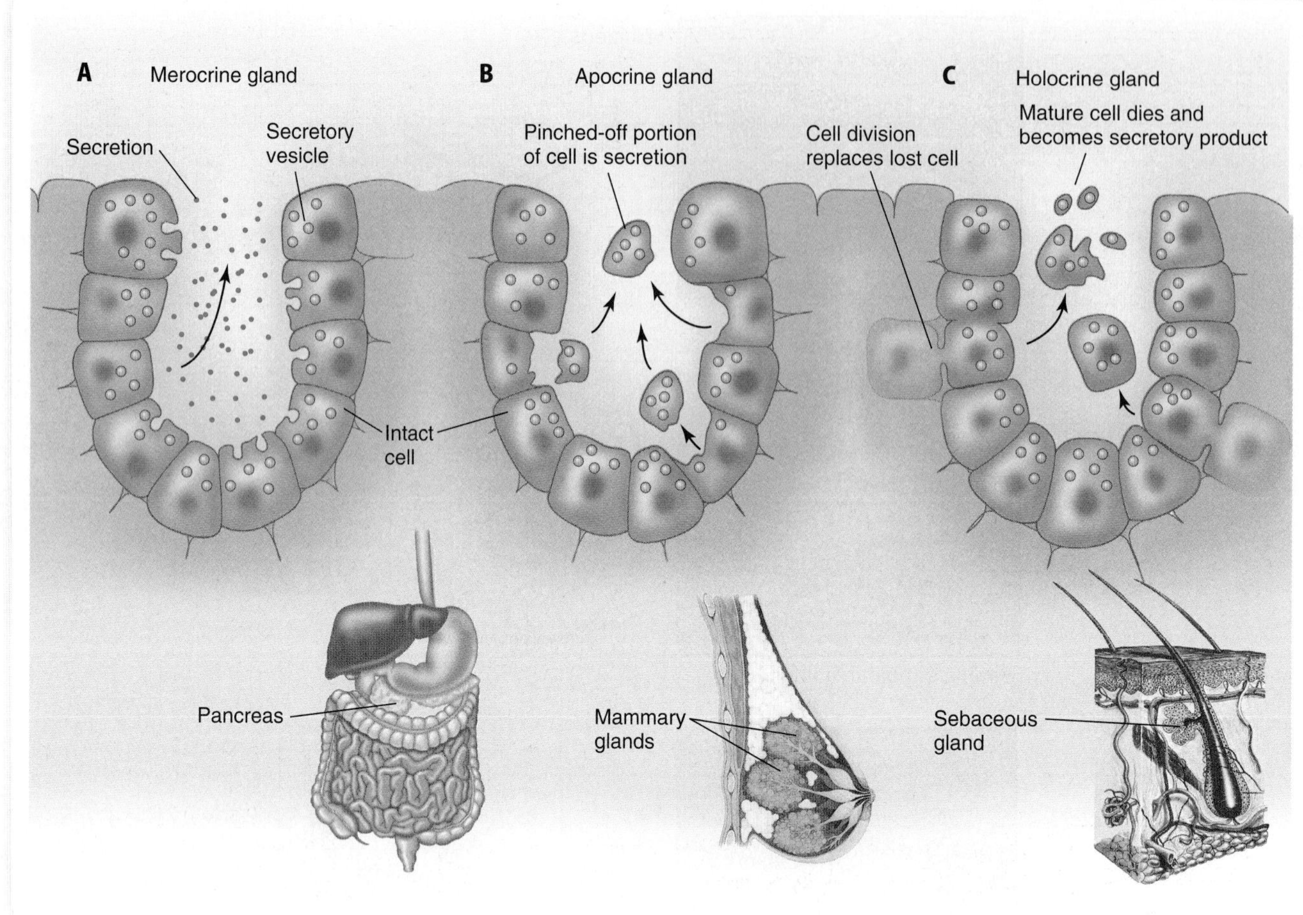

Figure 8-14 Exocrine glands. **A.** Merocrine. **B.** Apocrine. **C.** Holocrine.

Table 8-10 Connective Tissue Cells and Tissue Fibers

Tissue Cell Type	Action
Fibroblasts	Produce fibers
Macrophages	Engulf and devour unwanted microorganisms
Mast cells	Secrete histamine and heparin
Tissue Fiber Type	**Action**
Collagenous	Bind structures together with high tensile strength
Elastic	Ease of stretching
Reticular	Form delicate support networks

The other types of cells found in connective tissue include mast cells, macrophages, adipocytes, and melanocytes. **Mast cells** are distributed throughout connective tissues, usually near blood vessels, and release both heparin (to prevent blood clotting) and histamine (for the inflammatory and allergic response). **Macrophages** are responsible for phagocytosis. Adipocytes (fat cells) store body fat. Melanocytes are specialized cells in the deeper epithelium and are responsible for the production of the pigment **melanin,** which gives skin its color.

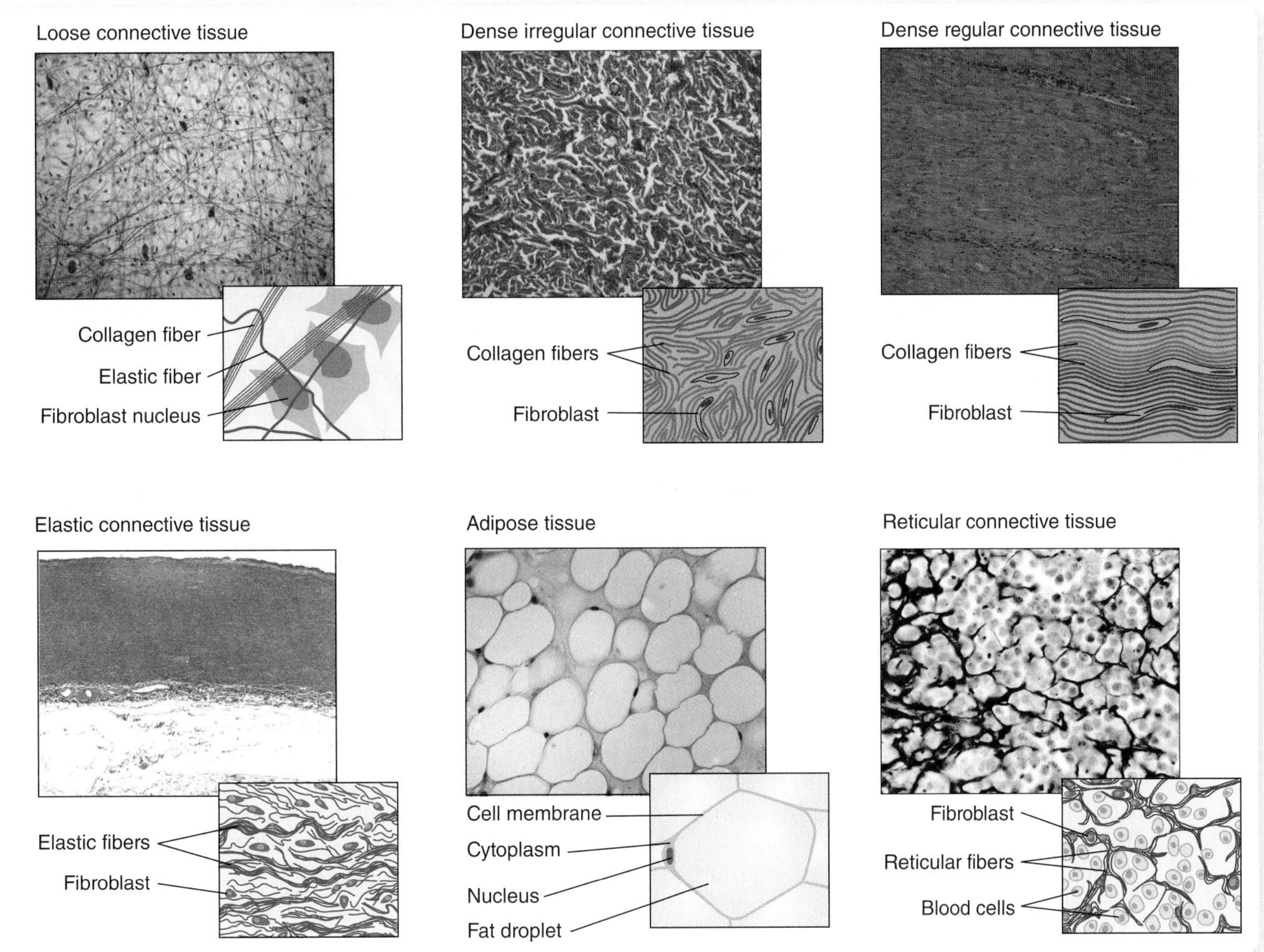

Figure 8-15 Types of typical connective tissues.

Classifications of Connective Tissues

Connective tissues are classified based on their physical properties **Figure 8-15**. The three general categories of connective tissue are connective tissue proper, supporting connective tissues, and fluid connective tissues:

1. Connective tissue proper includes those connective tissues with many types of cells and extracellular fibers in a syrupy ground substance. Ground substance gives the skin resistance to compression. They are divided into dense connective tissue and loose connective tissue.
   - Dense connective tissue is composed of bundles of strong, white, collagenous fibers in parallel rows. Tendons are composed of this type of tissue; they are relatively strong and inelastic. Dense connective tissue also exists in the eyeballs and deep skin layers. This type of tissue is repaired very slowly because it has a poor blood supply.
   - Loose connective tissue includes adipose tissue, areolar tissue, and reticular connective tissue. Adipose tissue lies beneath the skin, between muscles, around the kidneys, behind the eyes, in certain membranes of the abdomen, on the surface of the heart, and around some of the joints. It functions as a cushion for these body parts. Adipose tissue is also important for storing energy in fat molecules (triglycerides). **Areolar tissue** binds skin to underlying organs, fills in spaces between muscles, supports other tissues, holds body fluids, defends against infection, and stores nutrients as fat. It is found beneath most layers of the epithelium. Reticular connective tissue helps to create a framework inside internal organs such as the spleen and liver.
2. Supporting connective tissue differs from connective tissue proper because it has a less diverse cell population and a matrix that contains many more densely packaged fibers. Supporting connective tissue protects soft tissues and some or all of the weight of the

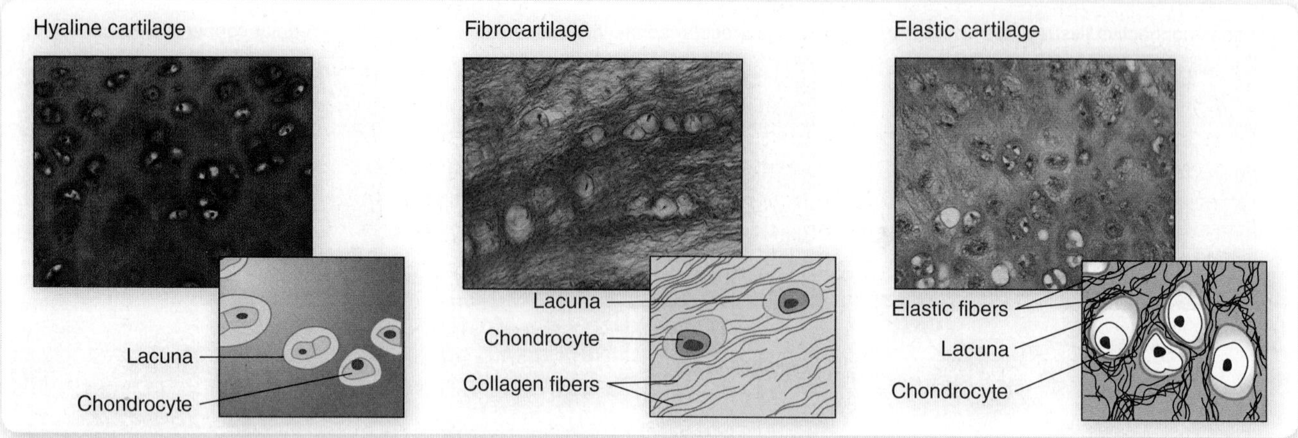

Figure 8-16 Types of cartilage.

body. The two types of supporting connective tissue are cartilage and bone.

- Cartilage is a tough but flexible connective tissue that protects the body from excessive tension and compression. It is composed of cells called chondrocytes. These cells are distributed in a somewhat rigid matrix. The exact makeup of cartilage varies depending on its location and function in the body. Cartilage is harder than dense connective tissue but softer than bone. It also lacks nerve fibers. A covering called the perichondrium provides needs nutrients to cartilage via diffusion. Because it has a limited supply of blood vessels, cartilage heals very slowly. The three major types of cartilage are as follows Figure 8-16:
  - **Hyaline cartilage.** This type of cartilage is smooth and firm and is found on the ends of bones in many joints, the soft portion of the nose, and in the supporting rings of the respiratory passages. It is important for bone growth. Hyaline cartilage is the most common type of cartilage.
  - **Elastic cartilage.** This flexible cartilage provides a framework for the **epiglottis** (a thin, flap-like structure at the roof of the tongue) and the pinna (external part of the ear).
  - **Fibrocartilage.** This tough form of cartilage absorbs shock in the intervertebral disks of the spinal column, in the spongy cartilages of the knees, and in the pelvic girdle (bony pelvis).
- Bone is the most rigid type of connective tissue and establishes the framework of the body. It consists of a matrix of connective tissue, blood vessels, and minerals (particularly calcium and phosphorus). Bones are classified according to their shape. Bone tissue is also classified as either cancellous (spongy) or compact (solid). **Bone marrow** is the soft tissue that fills the inside of bones, and is a site of production of RBCs, platelets, and most WBCs.

3. Blood is classified as connective tissue because the matrix (the RBCs, WBCs, and platelets between the cells) is liquid (mainly water). This matrix allows the transportation of nutrients, oxygen, and waste products. Lymph forms as interstitial fluid enters the lymphatic vessels, which return the lymph to the cardiovascular system. Unlike other connective tissues, blood and lymph do not connect structures or provide any mechanical support.

Muscle Tissues

Muscle tissue is contractile tissue. It is the basis of movement of the body. Muscle tissue is specialized to contract forcefully (shorten). Muscle tissue is classified by its anatomic location (skeletal, smooth, and cardiac) and function.

1. **Skeletal muscle tissue.** Also called voluntary muscle tissue because its use is usually under conscious control. It is connected to the skeletal framework of the body by tendons. Skeletal muscle is sometimes referred to as striated muscle because of the long, threadlike cells that have light and dark markings called striations that are visible under a microscope Figure 8-17. This appearance is the result of alternating dark, thick bands of myosin and light, thin bands of actin. Skeletal muscle also contains several nuclei per cell. Skeletal muscle tissue moves the head, trunk, and limbs, allowing all voluntary movements in these

body areas. Injury to skeletal muscle can result in considerable bleeding because of its rich blood supply.

2. **Smooth muscle tissue.** Also called nonstriated involuntary muscles or unstriated muscles. Smooth muscle tissue is composed of elongated, spindle- shaped cells in hollow internal organ walls (such as the intestines, stomach, blood vessels, and **uterus**). Smooth muscle cannot, in most cases, be controlled by conscious effort. Its main functions include constricting the lumen of blood vessels in response to the needs of the body, aiding in the breakdown and digestion of food, moving fluid through the body, and assisting in the elimination of waste products. Smooth muscle fibers are shorter than striated fibers, having only one nucleus per spindle-shaped fiber. Smooth muscle cells can divide; therefore, they regenerate after being injured.
3. **Cardiac muscle tissue.** Also called **myocardium**; it is a thick, contractile middle layer of the heart wall. Cardiac muscle is similar to skeletal muscle in that it is striated, yet it differs in its structure. Cardiac cells generally have one nucleus and occasionally have two nuclei. In addition, the connection between cells is different. These cells form tight connections called intercalated disks. Cardiac muscle also differs in that it is not under conscious control, but is rather completely involuntary. Cardiac muscle relies on pacemaker cells or nodes of tissue in the conduction system of the heart to stimulate contraction Table 8-11.

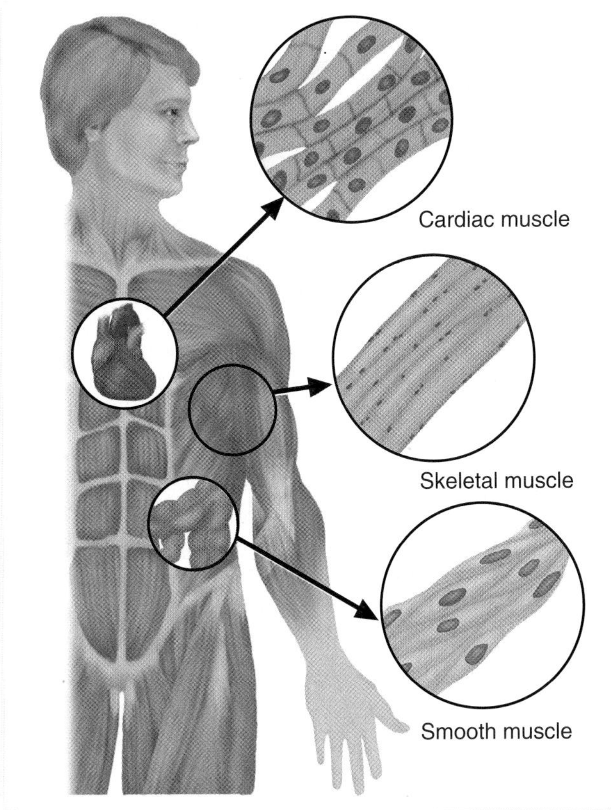

Figure 8-17 The three types of muscle are cardiac, skeletal, and smooth.

Words of Wisdom

Muscles are supplied by a rich collection of blood vessels and nerves. Loss of proper blood supply or the loss of innervation, which refers to the nerve supply of an organ or body part, results in muscle wasting, or atrophy. In patients with permanent nerve injuries or poor distal circulation, muscle atrophy is often observed and may be a clue regarding an underlying disease process.

Table 8-11 Types of Muscle

Type	Control	Striations	Location	Purpose
Skeletal muscle (voluntary muscle)	Voluntary	Yes	Attached to bone	To produce movement
Smooth muscle (nonstriated involuntary muscles or unstriated muscle)	Involuntary	No	In the walls of hollow internal structures and blood vessels	Various: some organ functions, pupil contraction, changes in blood vessel diameter, gland duct operation, hair movement
Cardiac muscle (myocardium)	Involuntary	Yes	Heart	To pump blood

▶ Nervous Tissues

The nervous tissue of the body has the ability to conduct electrical impulses that allow communication between body structures and control body functions. Nervous tissues contain two basic types of cells: (1) neurons and (2) several kinds of supporting cells, collectively called neuroglia, or glial cells. Nervous tissues are found in the brain, peripheral nerves, and spinal cord; the basic cells of these tissues are the neurons. Neurons are the basic structure of neural tissue. When connected to one another, neurons act as conduits that send signals to and from other neurons, muscles, and glands and receive sensory information from the outside world.

Neuroglia are the supporting cells of nervous tissue that are crucial to neuronal functioning. The functions of neuroglia include nourishment, protection, and insulation. They also phagocytize other cells and help in communications between cells.

Types of Membranes

Membranes form a barrier or an interface. Epithelial membranes are thin structures made up of epithelium and underlying connective tissue. They cover body surfaces and line body cavities. The four types of membranes are as follows Table 8-12:

1. **Serous membrane.** Lines body cavities that lack openings to the outside of the body, such as the thoracic, abdominal, and pelvic cavities. Serous membranes are made up of two layers. The parietal membrane adheres to the cavity wall and the visceral membrane adheres to the organ. Serous membranes secrete serous fluid, which lubricates membrane surfaces.
2. **Mucous membrane.** Lines body cavities that open to the outside of the body, including the nose and mouth as well as digestive, respiratory, urinary, and reproductive tubes. Mucous membranes contain goblet cells that secrete mucus.
3. **Cutaneous membrane.** The skin, which covers the body surface.
4. **Synovial membrane.** Forms an incomplete lining within the cavities of the **synovial joints.** It is entirely made up of connective tissues.

Homeostasis

As discussed previously, adaptive responses to various stimuli allow the cells and tissues to respond and function within their respective environments, in a constant effort to preserve a degree of stability or equilibrium. This process is known as homeostasis (from the Greek words for "same" and "steady"); it is also called the dynamic steady state. Physiologic cell turnover refers to the process in which older cells are eliminated and replaced by newer cells. This process occurs via apoptosis, which is normal cell death. Apoptosis is genetically programmed into the cell as a part of normal development, organogenesis (the formation of organs and organ systems), immune function, and tissue growth. It has a normal role in aging, early development, menses, lactating breast tissue, thymus involution, and RBC turnover. Appropriate cell turnover is one component of homeostasis; for example, it allows damaged cells to be replaced so that proper tissue function can continue.

Table 8-12 Membranes of the Body

Membrane Type	Name	Location
Cutaneous	Skin	All exterior surfaces of the body
	Periosteum	Surrounds mature bone
	Perichondrium	Surrounds developing bone
Mucous	Oral mucosa	Soft, mucus-producing membranes lining the nose and mouth
Serous	Visceral pleura	Inner lining covering the lungs
	Parietal pleura	Outer lining separating the visceral pleura and the interior of the chest wall
	Pericardium	Surrounds the heart
	Peritoneum	Surrounds the abdominal organs
	Meninges	Coverings between the brain and skull
Synovial	Knee capsule	Surrounds the synovial fluid contained in the knee joint

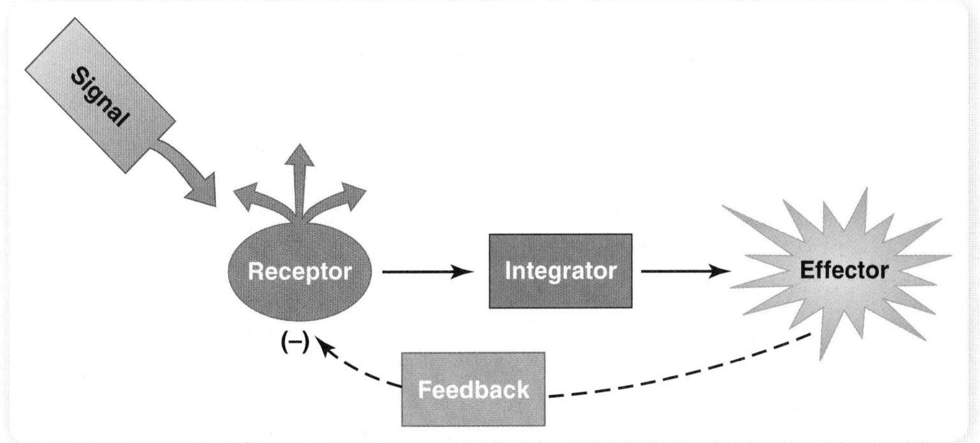

Figure 8-18 Most cellular communication (cellular signaling) includes a component of negative feedback in which the product of a reaction returns information about its own manufacture, thereby stopping its own production.

Homeostasis is maintained in the body because normal regulatory systems are counterbalanced by counterregulatory systems. Thus, for every cell, tissue, or organ that performs one function, at least one component exists that performs the opposing function. Other homeostatic mechanisms include the control of internal body temperature despite fluctuations in the external temperature, the regulation of pH and acid-base balance in the body, and the balance of water or hydration in the cells and body of the organism.

Regulatory systems communicate within the body mainly at the cellular level. Recall that cells communicate electrochemically through cellular signaling, in which they release molecules (such as hormones) that bind to protein receptors on the cell surface. This signaling triggers chemical reactions in the receptor cells that initiate a biologic action. When the action has been completed, the opposing system is alerted to discontinue the action through a process called feedback inhibition or **negative feedback** Figure 8-18.

The thermostat mechanism in a home is a good example of a feedback mechanism. In the middle of the winter, heat loss continually occurs through drafty windows, doors, and poorly insulated areas such as the roof or walls. The thermostat detects decreases in temperature and signals the furnace to produce heat to rewarm the house. After the temperature has risen to a certain point, the thermostat gives negative feedback to the furnace, causing it to shut down to prevent overheating. This feedback process keeps the temperature of the house within a selected range Figure 8-19. Similarly, the body constantly generates heat through cellular processes. Five primary mechanisms help the body reduce excess temperature or eliminate heat: (1) convection, (2) conduction, (3) radiation, (4) evaporation, and (5) respiration. In short, the thermostat of the body balances the generation of heat with the elimination of heat.

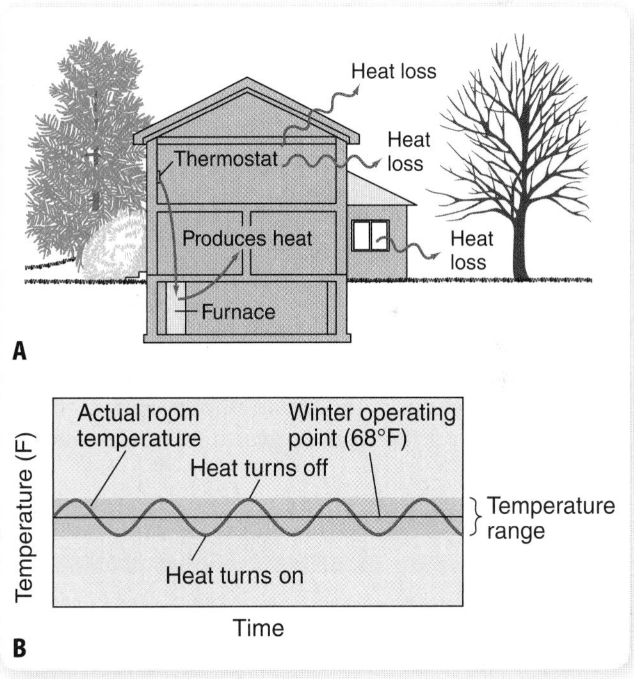

Figure 8-19 Homeostasis and the house. **A.** Heat is maintained in a house by a furnace, which compensates for heat loss. The thermostat monitors the internal temperature and switches the furnace on and off in response to temperature changes. **B.** A hypothetical temperature graph showing temperature fluctuation around the set point.

The human body maintains homeostasis by balancing what it takes in with what it puts out. For example, the body takes in chemicals and electrolytes, food, and water. It uses the nutrients, proteins, sugars, and oxygen and then eliminates the unnecessary chemicals and by-products through respiration (carbon dioxide), sweating (excess liquids), urination, and defecation (feces). Figure 8-20 illustrates this normal balance.

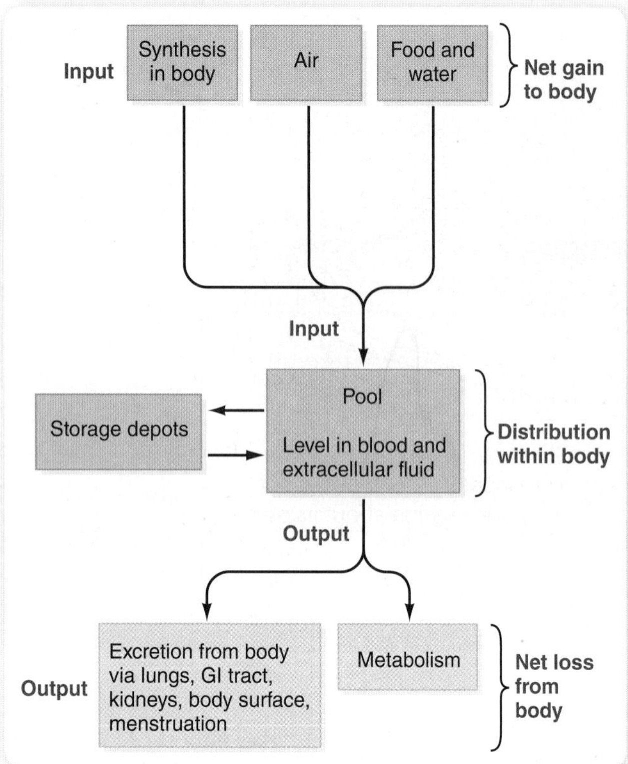

Figure 8-20 Generalized view of the homeostatic system. Inputs and outputs are balanced to maintain more-or-less constant chemical and physical parameters.

When normal cellular signaling is interrupted, disease occurs. The counterregulatory mechanisms of the body are rendered ineffective, and its regulatory systems begin to operate autonomously. The system stops providing critical negative feedback; instead, it gives unopposed positive feedback.

Organ Systems

Recall that an organ is composed of at least two kinds of tissue that are organized to perform a more complex task than a single tissue can. An organ system is composed of at least two kinds of organs that, again, are organized to perform a more complex task than a single organ can. The twelve major organ systems of the body include the integumentary, skeletal, muscular, nervous, endocrine, circulatory, lymphatic, immune, respiratory, digestive, urinary, and reproductive systems **Figure 8-21**.

The Integumentary System

The **integumentary system** is the largest system in the human body and serves as the interface between the body and the outside world. It consists of the skin (integument) and accessory structures, such as hair, nails, **sebaceous glands** (oil glands), and **sweat glands** (sudoriferous, or odor forming, glands). The integumentary system has a crucial role in maintaining the constancy of the internal environment (homeostasis) and does so by performing the following functions:

- **Protection.** The skin protects the underlying tissue from injury, including injury caused by extremes of temperature, ultraviolet radiation, mechanical forces, toxic chemicals, and invading microorganisms. These organisms are everywhere and are routinely found lying on the skin surface. However, they never penetrate the skin unless it is broken by injury; thus, the skin provides a constant protection against outside invaders.
- **Temperature regulation.** Blood vessels in the skin constrict when the body is in a cold environment and dilate when the body is in a warm environment. In a cold environment, constriction of the blood vessels shunts the blood away from the skin to decrease the amount of heat radiated from the body surface. When the outside environment is hot, the vessels in the skin dilate, the skin becomes flushed or red, and heat radiates from the body surface. Also, in a hot environment, sweat is secreted to the skin surface from the sweat glands. Evaporation of the sweat requires energy. This energy, as body heat, is taken from the body during the evaporation process, which causes the body temperature to fall. Sweating alone will not reduce body temperature; evaporation of the sweat must also occur.
- **Fluid regulation.** As a watertight seal, the skin prevents excessive loss of water from the body and drying of tissues, thereby helping maintain the chemical stability of the internal environment.
- **Sensation.** The skin serves as a sense organ, keeping the brain informed about the external environment. Information from the environment is carried to the brain through a rich supply of **sensory nerves** that originate in the skin. Nerve endings that lie in the skin are adapted to perceive and transmit information about heat, cold, external pressure, pain, and the position of the body in space. The skin thus recognizes any changes in the environment. The skin also reacts to pressure, pain, and pleasurable stimuli.
- **Inflammatory response.** The integument responds to injuries and wounds with inflammation, which causes redness, increased warmth, and painful swelling. The blood vessels of the wounded area dilate and allow fluids to leak into the damaged tissues. This provides more nutrients and oxygen to the tissues, aiding in healing.

The skin covers the entire external surface of the body. The various orifices—including the mouth, nose, anus, and vagina—are not covered by skin. Orifices are

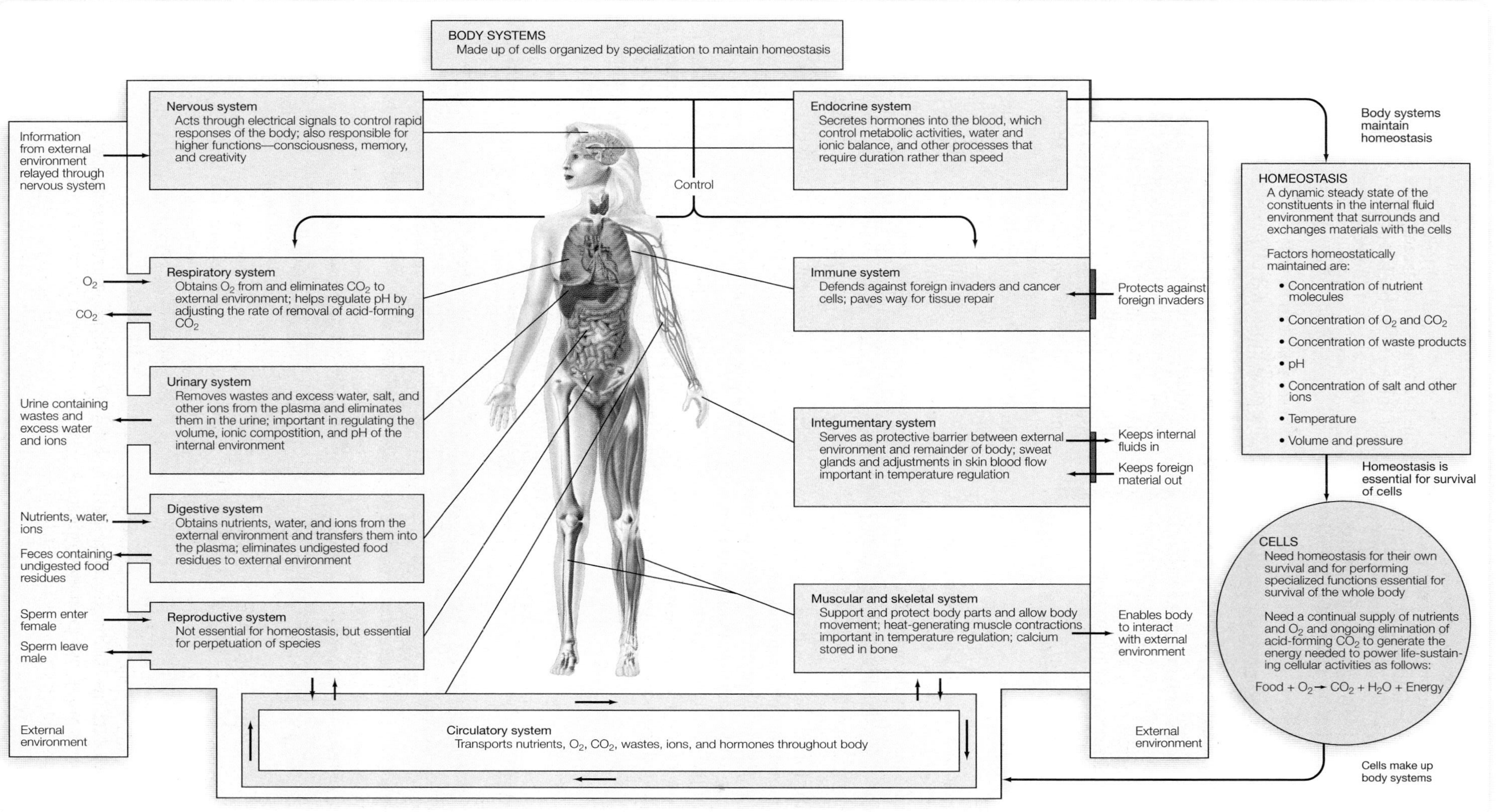

Figure 8-21 Systems of the body.

lined with mucous membranes. Mucous membranes are similar to skin in that they provide a protective barrier against bacterial invasion. Mucous membranes differ from skin in that they secrete mucus, a sticky substance that lubricates the openings. Thus, mucous membranes are moist, whereas the skin is dry. For example, a mucous membrane lines the entire digestive tract from the mouth to the anus.

Words of Wisdom

Considerable damage to the skin may make the body vulnerable to bacterial invasion, temperature instability, and major disturbances of fluid balance, which is precisely what happens when an injury results in an opening in the skin.

▶ Skin

The skin is the largest organ of the integumentary system. It is composed of two layers, the epidermis and dermis. Below the skin lies the subcutaneous tissue layer Figure 8-22. The cells of the epidermis are sealed to form a watertight protective covering for the body. The subcutaneous tissue is composed largely of fat. The fat serves as an insulator for the body and as a reservoir to store energy. The amount of subcutaneous tissue varies greatly from person to person. Beneath the subcutaneous tissue lie the muscles and the skeleton. The subcutaneous layer helps to anchor the skin to the structures below. As a person ages, the loss of the subcutaneous layer causes the skin to have limited support. This process is why wrinkles form in the skin.

Epidermis

The epidermis is the outermost layer of the skin and varies in thickness in different areas of the body. On the soles of the feet, the back, and the scalp, it is quite thick, but in some areas of the body, the epidermis is only two or three cell layers thick.

The epidermis is composed of several layers of cells. These layers can be separated into two regions. The cells of the outermost layer of the epidermis, the **stratum corneum**, are dead cells that have had their cytoplasm replaced with keratin, which is a tough, waterproof substance that provides further protection to the underlying tissues from light, heat, microorganisms, some chemicals, and minor trauma. Because cells of the stratum corneum are dead, they are constantly shed and replaced by new cells that move up through the layers of the epidermis. The innermost epidermal layer, known as the germinal layer, the stratum germinativum, or the stratum basale, is the only location in the epidermis in which the cells are able to undergo mitosis. New cells that are being produced work their way through the layers of the epidermis until they are eventually keratinized, become part of the stratum corneum, and are shed. The ability to reproduce allows the epidermis to repair itself if injured, providing further protection against injury and infection. The germinal layer also contains melanocytes, which produce melanin. The darkness of a person's skin is directly proportional to the amount of melanin present.

Dermis

The dermis lies below the epidermis. These two layers are joined together by the dermal-epidermal junction. One cause of blisters is injury to this junction. The dermal layer is much thicker than the epidermis. It

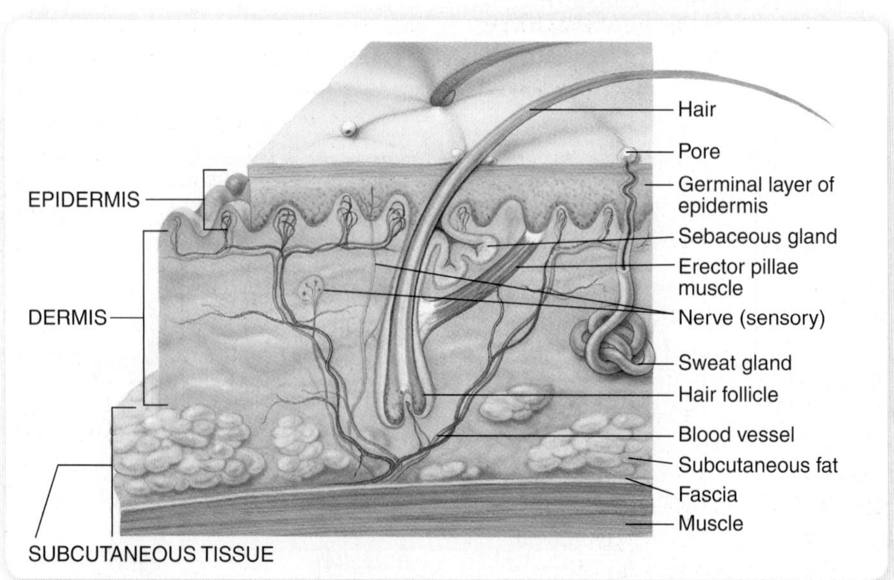

Figure 8-22 The skin has two principal layers: the epidermis and the dermis. Below the skin is a layer of subcutaneous tissue.

mainly consists of connective tissue containing both collagen and elastin fibers, which connect the cells together. The collagenous fibers are tough fibers that give the skin its resiliency, and the elastin fibers give the skin its ability to stretch and (usually) spring back to its normal contour.

The dermis is subdivided into two layers: the papillary layer and the reticular layer. The vasculature inside the papillary dermis serves two functions: It provides nutrients to the epidermis, which does not have its own blood supply, and it aids in **thermoregulation** (the process of maintaining homeostasis). Dilation of these vessels increases blood flow to the skin, allowing heat to dissipate. Conversely, blood vessel constriction results in retention of heat. The size and presence (or absence) of oxygen in these blood vessels cause color variations such as redness or cyanosis. The reticular layer is made of dense, irregular connective tissue, which provides strength and elasticity.

Macrophages and **lymphocytes** are also found within the dermal layer. Both are part of the inflammatory process and are responsible for combating microorganisms that breach the epidermal layer. After a pathogen enters the dermis, macrophages and lymphocytes destroy the invading microorganism and signal other cells to migrate into the area. Physical injury will trigger mast cells to release granules into the surrounding tissue (degranulate) and produce special chemical mediators. The result is increased blood flow to the affected area, manifested as redness and warmth.

The dermis contains the following specialized structures:

- **Nerve endings**. These structures mediate the senses of touch, temperature, pressure, and pain.
- **Blood vessels**. These structures carry oxygen and nutrients to the skin and remove carbon dioxide and metabolic waste products. Cutaneous blood vessels also have a crucial role in regulating body temperature by regulating the volume of blood that flows from the warm core of the body to its cooler surface.
- **Sweat glands**. These glands produce sweat and discharge it through ducts passing to the surface of the skin.
- **Hair follicles.** These small, tubelike structures produce hair and enclose the hair roots. Each follicle contains a single hair. Attached to the hair follicle is a small muscle that, on contraction, causes the follicle to assume a more vertical position. Hairs in each part of the body have definite periods of growth, after which they are shed and replaced.
- **Sebaceous glands.** These glands, located at the neck of each hair follicle, are a specialized secretory mechanism that produce an oily substance (sebum). The secretions of the sebaceous glands empty into the hair follicles and from there, reach the surface of the skin.

Fascia

Between the dermis and the underlying muscle and bone is a thick layer of connective tissue known as subcutaneous tissue, or the superficial **fascia**. This subcutaneous tissue is composed of adipose tissue and areolar tissue. Blood vessels, **lymph vessels**, and hair follicle roots are also found in this layer. The subcutaneous tissue insulates, protects, and stores energy in the form of fat. Subcutaneous injections are given in this layer.

Below the subcutaneous tissue is a thick, dense layer of fibrous tissue known as the **deep fascia**. The deep fascia is composed of tough bands of tissue that surround muscles and other internal structures. It supports and protects underlying structures from injury. Muscles and bones are found below this layer.

▶ Accessory Structures

The accessory structures of the integumentary system include hair, nails, and sebaceous and sweat glands.

Hair

The main function of hair is protection from physical injury, the sun, or the entry of dust and other particles into the eyes and nose. Hair goes through stages of growth and rest. Blood vessels provide nutrients and oxygen to the skin.

Hair growth begins in a hair follicle. Within each follicle is a small cluster of cells known as the hair papilla. The growth of hair begins in this cluster of cells, which is hidden in the follicle, and the cells move upward to become keratinized and to form the shaft of the hair. Each follicle is surrounded by arrector pili, a smooth muscle responsible for goose bumps (the pulling upward of the hair and downward of the skin in response to cold, fear, or excitement).

Nails

Nails protect the ends of the fingers and toes, and consist of a nail plate above a skin surface called the nail bed. The part of the nail plate that grows most actively is covered by a white, crescent-moon-shaped lunula, where epithelial cells divide and become keratinized. The nail cells push forward over the nail bed, causing the nail to continually grow outward. The nail of the middle finger grows fastest, whereas the nail of the thumb grows slowest.

Words of Wisdom

Evaluate the nails of a patient for color, shape, attachment, and presence of indentations to obtain valuable information during the physical exam.

Glands

Two types of glands are located under the skin: sebaceous and sweat glands. As discussed previously, sebaceous glands are found in the dermis and secrete oil (sebum) in the shaft of the hair follicle and the skin. Sebum prevents excessive drying of the skin and hair, prevents water loss, and keeps the skin pliable. Sebum also protects the skin from some forms of bacteria.

The two types of sweat glands are merocrine and apocrine glands. Merocrine (eccrine) glands are the predominant type of sweat glands and are present at birth. These glands open directly to the surface of the body and are found on the forehead, neck, back, and upper lip, though the palms and soles have the highest numbers. When the body temperature rises, these glands respond by producing sweat, which consists of water and salts. This evaporation of water from the skin surface is one of the major mechanisms of the body for shedding excess heat. Apocrine glands open into hair follicles, including in and around the genitalia, axillae, and anus. These glands secrete an organic substance (which is odorless until acted upon by surface bacteria) into the hair follicles.

Mammary glands and ceruminous glands are modified sweat glands. Mammary glands, found in the breasts, secrete milk. Ceruminous glands, located in the external auditory canal of the ear, secrete cerumen (earwax). Cerumen is an oily, sticky substance that traps foreign material.

Words of Wisdom

The skin is affected by the process of aging and environmental exposure. With age, a loss of skin elasticity occurs. In addition, sebaceous glands produce less oil, the epidermis and subcutaneous layers become thinner, and skin cells are replaced at a slower rate. Exposure to ultraviolet light can cause pigment changes, loss of skin elasticity, thickening of the skin, and skin cancer.

The Skeletal System

The integrated structure formed by the 206 bones of the body is the skeleton. The functions of the skeletal system include the following:

1. **Support.** The skeletal system provides a rigid framework and bears the weight of the body.
2. **Leverage.** Many muscles of the body attach to various locations on the skeletal system, which provides movement through leverage of the attachment sites.
3. **Protection.** The internal structures of the body are protected by the skeletal system.
4. **Storage.** The matrix that gives the bone its strength is composed of calcium phosphate material. This combination of minerals is stored in a usable form of bone. In addition, bone serves as a storage location for yellow bone marrow, which is an inactive, fatty bone marrow that stores lipids.
5. **Maintenance of calcium levels.** Calcium is the main element the various bones cells use to create a structure that is hard and resilient. Bones act as a reservoir from which calcium can be withdrawn and deposited. When the concentration of calcium in the blood and tissue fluid is too low, **parathyroid hormone (PTH)** stimulates the release of calcium from bones. When the concentration of calcium is too high, the hormone calcitonin is secreted by the thyroid gland, acting to inhibit the removal of calcium from bone.
6. **Blood cell production.** The bones have cavities within them that contain red marrow. This red marrow is responsible for making RBCs, WBCs, and platelets. The location of the red marrow, or site of blood cell production, varies with age. However, after the age of 4 years, blood cell production is limited to the ribs, sternum (breastbone), **pelvis**, skull, spinal column, and the proximal ends of the humerus and femur (thighbone). The production of blood cells in the bone marrow is referred to as *hematopoiesis* (discussed later in this chapter).

The skeleton may be divided into two distinct portions: the **axial skeleton** and the **appendicular skeleton**. The axial skeleton is composed of the bones of the central part, or axis, of the body; its divisions include the skull, thoracic cage, and vertebral column (spine). The skull is composed of the **cranium** (the vaultlike portion of the skull behind and above the face), basilar skull, face, and inner ear. The spine is composed of 33 irregular bones known as the spinal vertebrae. Moving anteriorly, the thorax (thoracic cavity) is formed by the sternum and 12 pairs of ribs. The appendicular skeleton is made up of the shoulder girdle, the pelvic girdle, and the bones of the upper and lower extremities.

Bones constitute the major structure of the skeletal system. Cartilage, tendons, and ligaments are important connective tissues that work with bones to provide the support framework of the skeleton.

Cartilage covers the ends of the bones where they form joints and is known as articular cartilage. These pieces of connective tissue provide cushioning and allow the bones to move smoothly against each other. Tendons are specialized tough cords or bands of dense, white connective tissue that connect muscles to bones. Ligaments are tough white bands of tissue that connect bones to each other. Tendons and ligaments are composed of densely packed fibers of collagen. A sprain occurs when the bone ends partially or temporarily dislocate and the supporting ligaments are partially stretched or torn.

When a muscle contracts, tendon pulls on bone, resulting in motion at the joint, the point where two or more bones come together, allowing movement to occur. A strain, or muscle pull, occurs when a muscle is stretched or torn. A strain results in pain, swelling, and bruising of surrounding soft tissues. No ligament or joint damage occurs with a strain. Sprains and strains are graded based on their severity and findings during the physical exam.

Words of Wisdom

The collagenous fibers in bone act much like reinforcing rods in a concrete structure, lending flexible strength to the bone. The mineral components of the bone supply strength for bearing weight, much like concrete does in a structure. Bone without the necessary amount of mineral is flexible; bone without enough collagen is extremely brittle.

Characteristics and Composition of Bones

Bones are classified because of their shape. *Long bones* are found in limbs and they are longer than they are wide. They have a body (called a shaft) and two ends that permit movement at joints. These bones have attachment points for muscles, which allow the mechanical basis of movement. The humerus, ulna, radius, femur, tibia (shinbone), and fibula are good examples of long bones. *Short bones* are nearly as wide as they are long and are found only in the wrists and feet. They include the phalanges (which make up the fingers and toes), **metacarpals** (which form the bony portion of the hand), and metatarsals (which form the arches of the feet). Short bones assist with fine movements in several anatomic planes and are compact and strong. *Flat bones* are thin, broad bones that usually protect and encase vital organs and often are curved to help form walls of cavities. The sternum, ribs, scapulae, and certain skull bones are examples of flat bones. *Irregular bones* have unique shapes and functions that are designed to perform a specific function. These bones include the mandible (lower jaw), many facial bones, and those that make up the vertebrae in the spine and the pelvis. Sesamoid bones, which are generally considered a type of irregular bone, are sometimes grouped into a separate category of their own. Sesamoid bones, such as the patella (kneecap), develop in certain tendons to protect the tendons from excessive wear where they cross major joints. Sesamoid bones are so named because they resemble the size and shape of a sesame seed.

Typical Long Bone Architecture

Each type of bone shares common characteristics despite the difference in shape. The long bones are used as an example for this description. Bones are composed of two layers, compact (solid or cortical) bone and spongy bone (also called cancellous bone or trabecular bone) **Figure 8-23**.

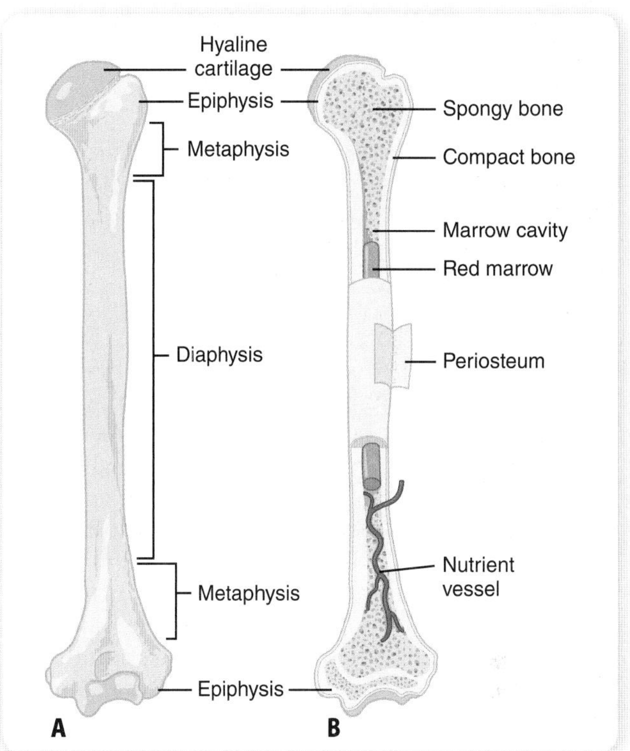

Figure 8-23 The components of the long bone. **A.** Illustration of the humerus. Notice the long shaft and dilated ends. **B.** Longitudinal section of the humerus showing compact bone, spongy bone, and marrow.

Compact bone is mostly solid, with few spaces and contains a central space called the marrow cavity or marrow canal. Cancellous bone consists of a lacy network of bony rods called trabeculae. The trabeculae are oriented along the lines of stress to increase the weight-bearing capacity of the long bones.

Special Populations

Fractures are more common in older people because of a decrease in bone mineral density. The result is weaker bones.

The long bone is divided into three regions: the diaphysis, the epiphysis, and the metaphysis. The **diaphysis** is the shaft of a long bone and is composed of compact bone tissue. Although long bones look solid, the diaphysis is a hollow tube that serves to lighten the bone while maintaining strength. The hollow area within the diaphysis is the medullary canal. It is lined with a thin membrane called the endosteum, which contains specialized cells that are important in forming and repairing bone. The medullary canal contains blood vessels and yellow bone marrow.

Words of Wisdom

In adults, most bone marrow in the long bones in the extremities contains adipose tissue and it is called yellow marrow. The bones of the axial skeleton and girdles contain red marrow, where most RBCs are manufactured.

At each end of the diaphysis is the epiphysis. This area is made of spongy bone, which is composed of several thin plates of bone with spaces between them that contain the red marrow and also serve to lighten the bone. Between and joining the diaphysis and epiphysis is the metaphysis. During childhood and adolescence, when bones are lengthening, this region also contains the physis, also called the **epiphyseal plate** or growth plate. The physis is made up of cartilage that is replaced by bone as it lengthens. After a person reaches adulthood, the growth plate closes and the mature adult bone is complete. Covering the end of the epiphysis is a thin, slick layer of cartilage called the articular cartilage. The term articulate, or articulation, is used where structures come together. Articular cartilage absorbs shock and reduces friction between bones, allowing them to move smoothly and efficiently.

The periosteum is a double layer of connective tissue that lines the outer surface of the entire bone with the exception of areas covered by the articular cartilage. The periosteum contains a rich supply of blood vessels, lymphatic vessels, nerves, bone cells, and elastic fibers. Pain results when the periosteum is disrupted (such as with a fracture). An extensive network of Haversian canals and Volkmann canals supply nutrients and remove waste products from the bone. Blood vessels, lymphatic vessels, and nerves originating in the periosteum enter the compact bone through the horizontal Volkmann canals. After entering the bone they join with the Haversian canals, which run along the length of the bone, and provide blood and nerve supply to the entire bone. A bone stripped of its periosteum will ultimately die, just as the heart muscle dies when the arteries supplying the muscle become blocked.

Bone Formation and Growth

Bone (osseous tissue) is a type of connective tissue that is composed of bone cells and matrix. Three main types of cells found in bone. **Osteoblasts** form bone and maintain the strength of existing bone. **Osteoclasts** break down and reabsorb bone. **Osteocytes** are mature osteoblasts found in lacunae (small cavities or chambers) within the bony matrix. Osteocytes, connected by long, threadlike extensions of the osteocyte cytoplasm, move nutrients and waste through the matrix of the bone. Osteoclasts produce enzymes that cause bone minerals to dissolve, releasing calcium and phosphate into the bloodstream.

Bones begin to form in utero during the first 6 weeks after fertilization. Intramembranous bones originate between layers of connective tissues that are sheetlike in appearance. Examples of intramembranous bones are the flat, broad bones of the skull. These bones begin development when unspecialized connective tissues form at the sites where future bones will be developed. Osteoblasts develop, depositing bony matrix around them. When extracellular matrix has surrounded the osteoblasts, they are termed osteocytes. The surrounding membranous tissues begin to form the periosteum, or membrane that lines the surface of all bones. Inside the periosteum, the osteoblasts form a compact bone layer over the new spongy bone.

Endochondral bones begin as cartilaginous masses that are eventually replaced by bone tissue. These bones develop from hyaline cartilage that is shaped similarly to the bones they will become. They grow rapidly at first, and then begin to change in appearance. When spongy bone begins to replace the original cartilage, a primary ossification center is created, with bone tissue developing outward toward the ends of the structure. Eventually, secondary ossification centers will appear in the epiphyses, forming more spongy bone.

During the first 6 weeks of fetal development, the skeleton is cartilaginous. The bones increase greatly in size as the fetus develops, and throughout childhood **Figure 8-24**. Bone growth continues through adolescence. The process of replacing other tissues with bone is called **ossification**, which involves the deposition of calcium salts.

Osteogenesis is the formation of bone. Long bones are first formed of hyaline cartilage, and later replaced by bony tissue that becomes compact bone. This process begins with the diaphysis and ends with the epiphyses of each long bone. This process of bone formation is called endochondral ossification, and it is the manner in which most bones of the body develop.

Flat bones are not formed in this manner. These bones develop from connective tissue membranes that are replaced by spongy bone, and then compact bone. This process is called intramembranous ossification. In infants, **fontanelles** (so-called soft spots) are sheets of tough connective tissue between the flat bones of the skull; they soften and expand during childbirth and are gradually replaced as the bones of the skull fuse together **Figure 8-25**.

When the bones are growing, the diaphyses meet the epiphyses at the epiphyseal plate. Growth of long bones depends on good nutrition and several hormones, including human growth hormone. Other hormones involved in long bone growth include thyroid hormone, **estrogen**, and **testosterone** **Table 8-13**. After the epiphyseal plate experiences closure, the long bones can no longer grow **Figure 8-26**. Length of bone is balanced by increased bone width. Osteoblast and osteoclast activity is balanced in the body so that the bones grow with uniformity.

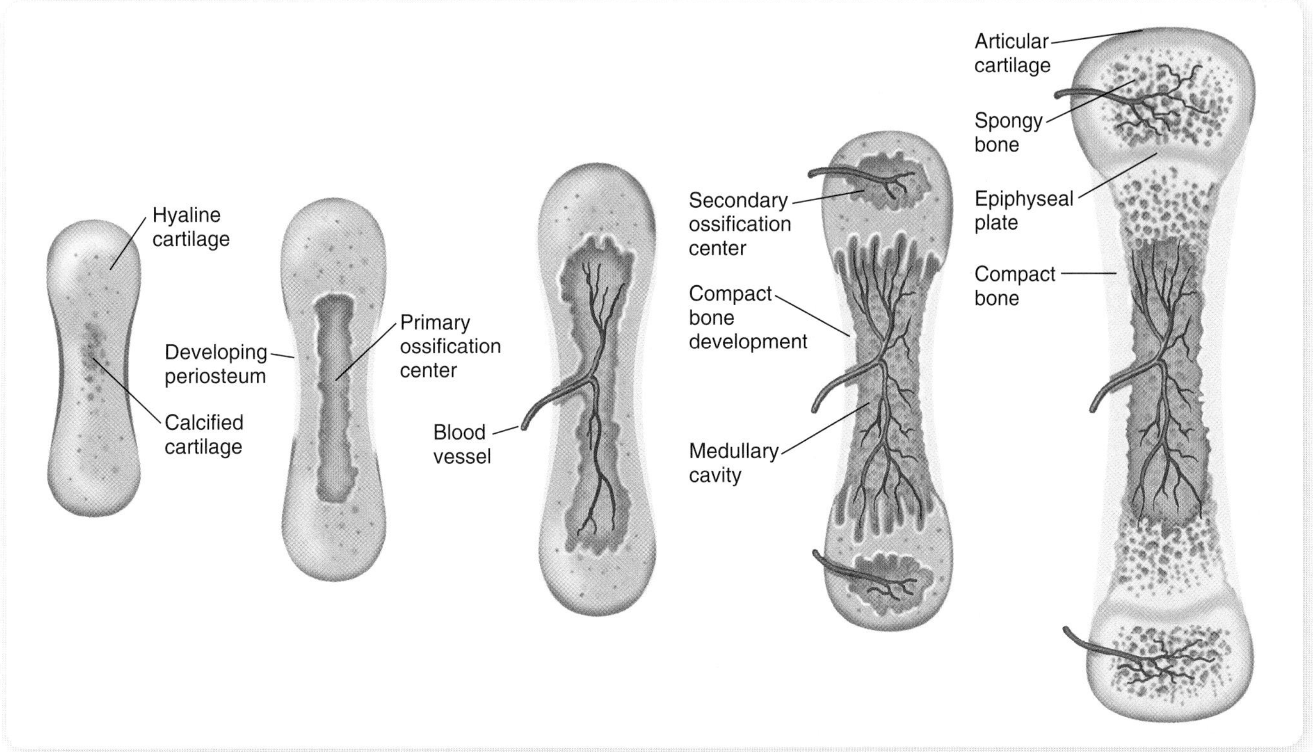

Figure 8-24 The major stages in the development of an endochondral bone.

Data from: Shier, D. N., Butler, J. L., and Lewis, R. Hole's Essentials of Human Anatomy & Physiology, Tenth edition. McGraw-Hill Higher Education, 2009.

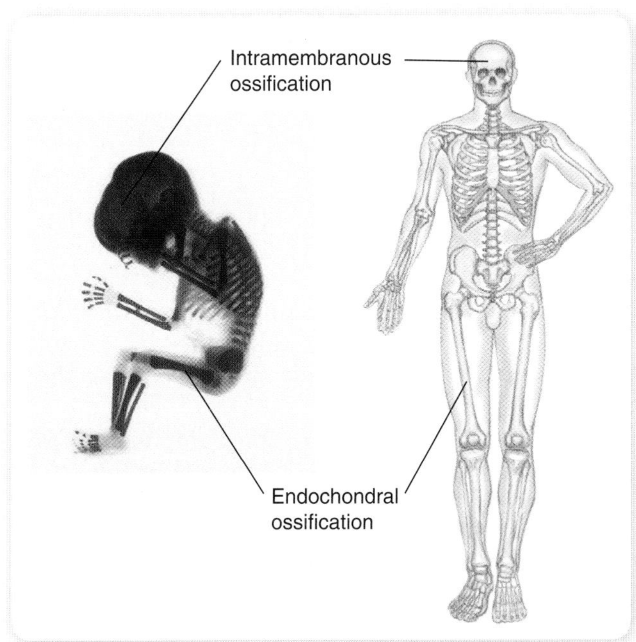

Figure 8-25 Intramembranous ossification results in the development of flat bones. Endochondral ossification results in the production of long bones.

Bone development, growth, and repair are influenced by heredity, nutrition, hormones, and exercise. Vitamin D is required for the absorption of calcium in the small intestine. Without it, calcium is not absorbed well, softening bones and potentially causing deformity. Growth hormone from the **pituitary gland** (an endocrine gland responsible for directly or indirectly affecting all body functions) stimulates cell division in the epiphyseal plates, and sex hormones stimulate ossification of these plates. Exercise stresses the bones, stimulating them to become thickened and strong.

Table 8-13 Hormones Involved in Bone Growth and Maintenance

- Human growth hormone
- Thyroxine
- Insulin
- Parathyroid hormone
- Calcitonin
- Estrogen
- Testosterone

▶ Joints

Recall that wherever two long bones come in contact, a joint (articulation) is formed. A joint consists of the ends of the bones that make up the joint and the surrounding connecting and supporting tissue. Joints allow movement of the extremities that rigid bone would not allow. Another important function of joints is to allow **proprioception**, the awareness of motion and position of a body part. Most joints in the body are named by combining the

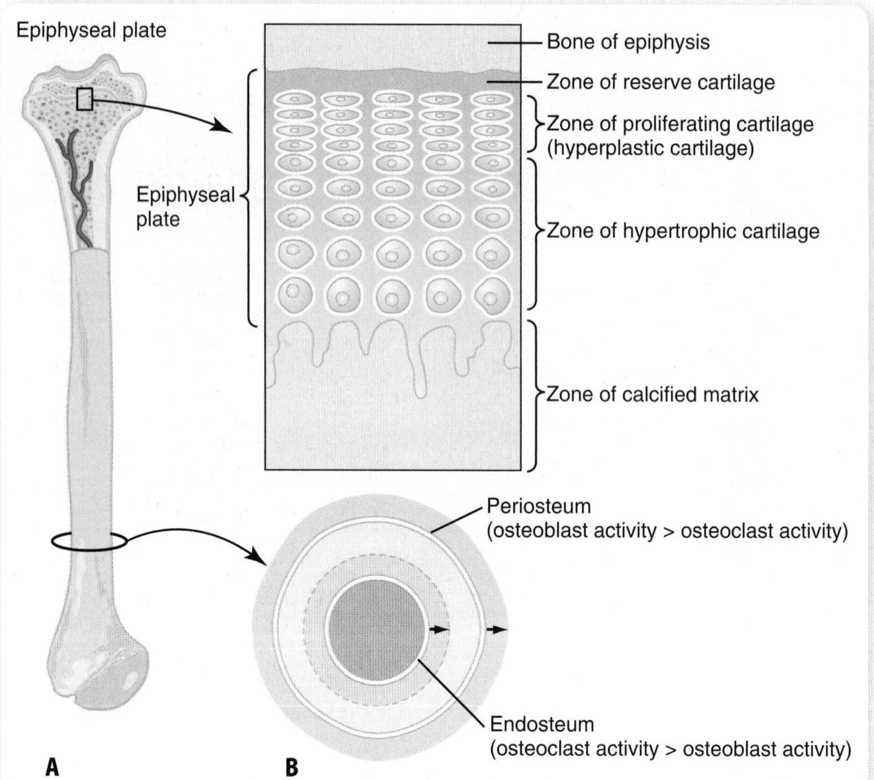

Figure 8-26 A. Lengthwise growth occurs at the epiphyseal plate until people reach the age of skeletal maturity (typically around age 14 years in girls and age 17 years in boys) when the epiphyseal plate closes, becoming the epiphyseal line. **B.** Growth in diameter involves altered rates of osteoclast and osteoblast activity at the periosteum and endosteum.

names of the two bones that form that joint. For example, the sternoclavicular joint is the articulation between the sternum and the clavicle (collarbone).

Types of Joints

Anatomists classify joints according to structure. The structural classification of a joint is determined by the type of soft tissue that connects the bones of a joint to each other (eg, fibrous, cartilaginous, synovial) Table 8-14 Figure 8-27. Physiologists classify joints according to function (the type and degree of movement it allows). Functionally, joints fall into three categories. Synarthroses are separated by a thin layer of fibrous connective tissue and are immovable. Synarthroses include joints such as the gomphosis, suture, and syndesmosis. The temporary joints formed in the growth plates in the long bones of children are examples of synchondroses. Amphiarthroses are connected by a cartilaginous disk, hyaline cartilage, or a fibrocartilage pad and are slightly movable. Amphiarthroses include joints such as the symphysis and synchondrosis. Diarthroses are freely movable and include the synovial joints.

The 230 joints in the human body are summarized as follows:

- **Fibrous joints**. Lying between bones that closely contact each other, fibrous joints are joined by thin, dense connective tissue. An example of a fibrous joint is a suture between flat bones of the skull. No real movement takes place in most fibrous joints, making them synarthrotic in classification. Those with limited movement (amphiarthrotic) include the joint between the distal tibia and fibula.
- **Cartilaginous joints**. Also called amphiarthroses, these joints allow for minimal movement between the bones. The soft tissue that unites the bones of a cartilaginous joint consists of either hyaline cartilage (synchondroses) or fibrocartilage (symphyses). The pubic symphysis and the joints connecting the ribs to the sternum are examples of this type of joint.
- **Synovial joints**. These diarthrotic joints are the most mobile and complex joints of the body. Articular cartilage covers each end of the opposing bones, which reduces the friction of movement of the bone ends and absorbs vibrations and shocks. The bones of a synovial joint are connected by a **joint capsule**, which encloses a joint cavity. The joint capsule is an extension of the periosteum and insulates the joint from surrounding tissues Figure 8-28

Table 8-14 Structural and Functional Classifications of Joints

Structural Name	Functional Name	Type	Description	Example
Fibrous joints	Synarthroses (no movement)	Gomphosis	Fibrous connection with peg-in-hole–shaped bones	Between teeth and mandible; between teeth and maxilla
		Suture	Fibrous connections and interlocking projections	Between skull bones
		Syndesmosis	Bones united by a strong membrane or by interosseous ligaments	Between distal tibia and fibula; between radius and ulna
Cartilaginous joints	Amphiarthroses (little movement)	Symphysis	Connections via a fibrocartilage pad	Symphysis pubis of pelvis; joints formed by intervertebral disks
		Synchondrosis	Bones united by hyaline cartilage	Between the ribs and costal cartilages of rib cage
Synovial joints	Diarthroses (free movement)	(no subcategories)	Complex joint in a joint cavity with synovial fluid	Numerous (wrist, elbow, shoulder, hip, ankle); subdivided according to range of movement

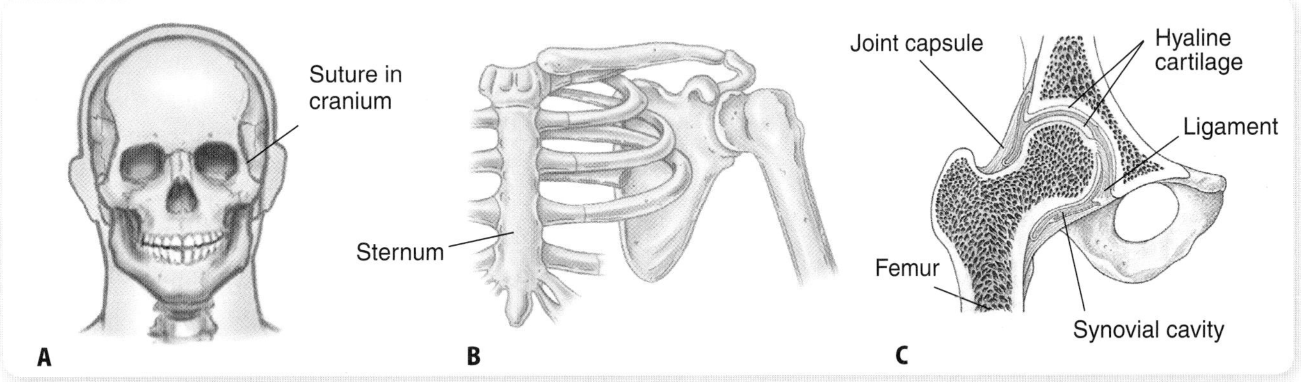

Figure 8-27 Types of joints. **A.** Fibrous. **B.** Cartilaginous. **C.** Synovial.

Figure 8-29. The joint capsule is made up of an outer layer of fibrous connective tissue and an inner synovial membrane layer. The synovial membrane secretes synovial fluid into the joint cavity, which lubricates and nourishes the inner surfaces of the joint. Because cartilage is avascular, the synovial membrane also removes waste products, microorganisms, and debris. The articulating bones of the joint are held in place by strong ligaments, which add support. Because the ligaments are flexible, they allow movement; however, they are strong enough to resist dislocation. Although synovial joint ligaments are usually located outside of the joint capsule, they are sometimes found inside it. The cruciate ligaments of the knee joint are examples of ligaments that are found within the joint capsule. Ligaments found outside the joint capsule may be completely independent of the capsule or they may be attached to the outer layer of the capsule. Examples of synovial joints include the ball-and-socket, hinge, pivot, condyloid, saddle, and gliding

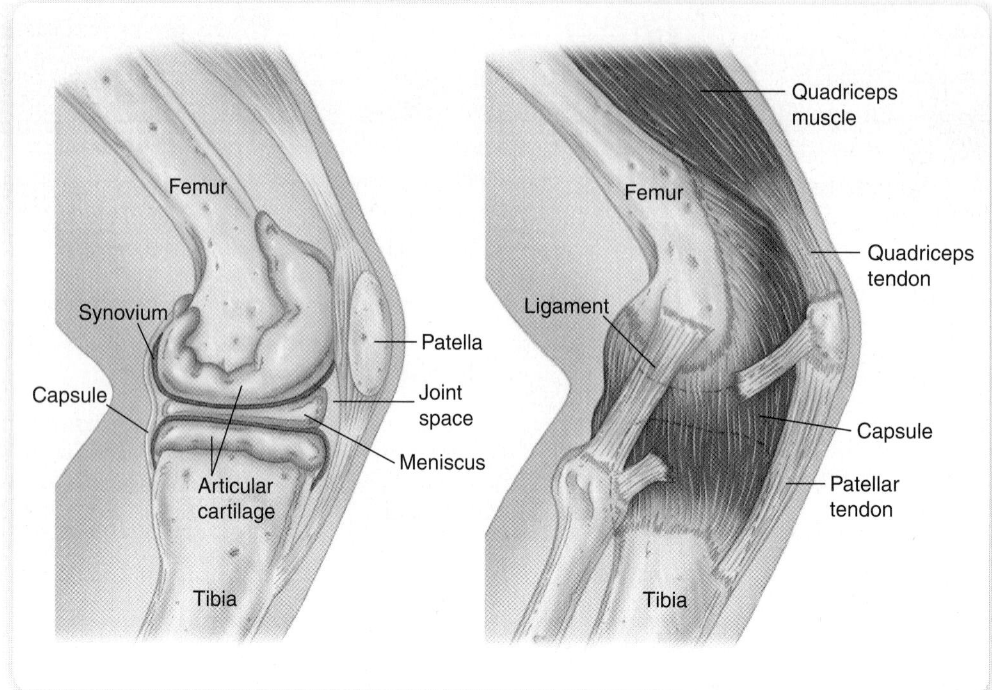

Figure 8-28 A synovial joint consists of bone ends, the fibrous joint capsule, the synovial membrane, and ligaments. The degree to which a synovial joint can move is determined by how the ligaments hold the bone ends and by the configuration of the bones themselves.

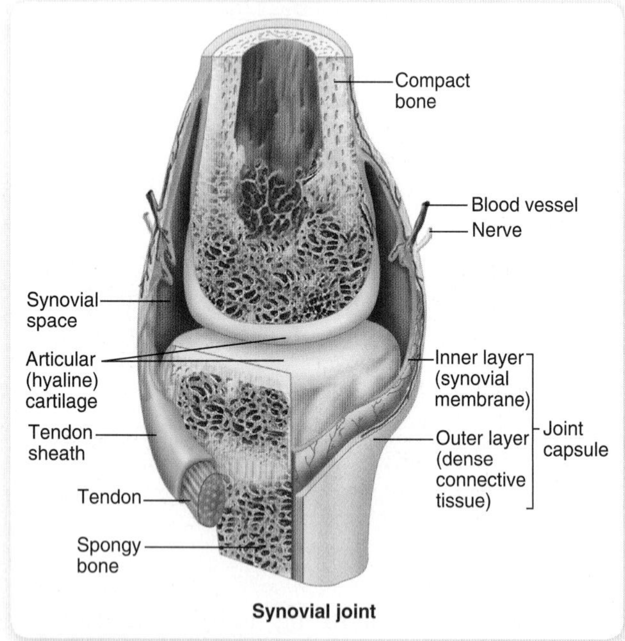

Figure 8-29 A synovial joint.

joints Figure 8-30 Table 8-15. Some synovial joints have shock-absorbing fibrocartilage pads called menisci. They may also have fluid-filled sacs called bursae, commonly located between tendons and underlying bony prominences, such as in the knee or elbow.

Words of Wisdom

A joint that is virtually surrounded by tough, thick ligaments has little motion, whereas a joint such as the shoulder, with few ligaments, is free to move in almost any direction (and will, as a result, be more prone to dislocation).

Bursa

A **bursa** is a small, padlike sac or cavity filled with a small amount of fluid that helps reduce the amount of friction between a tendon and a bone or between a tendon and a ligament. A bursa is usually located near a joint. Examples include the olecranon bursa of the elbow and the prepatellar bursa of the knee. Bursitis is inflammation of a bursa.

▶ Axial Skeleton

The axial skeleton is composed of the skull, thoracic cage, and vertebral column. The brain lies within the skull. The heart, lungs, and great vessels are enclosed in the thorax (thoracic cavity), which is part of the torso. Much of the liver and spleen are protected by the lower ribs. The spinal cord is contained within and protected by a bony spinal canal formed by the vertebrae. It connects the brain to skeletal muscle, skin, and other structures by means of the spinal nerves. Thirty-one pairs of **spinal nerves** attach to the spinal cord and communicate with structures primarily located in the neck, trunk, and extremities.[6]

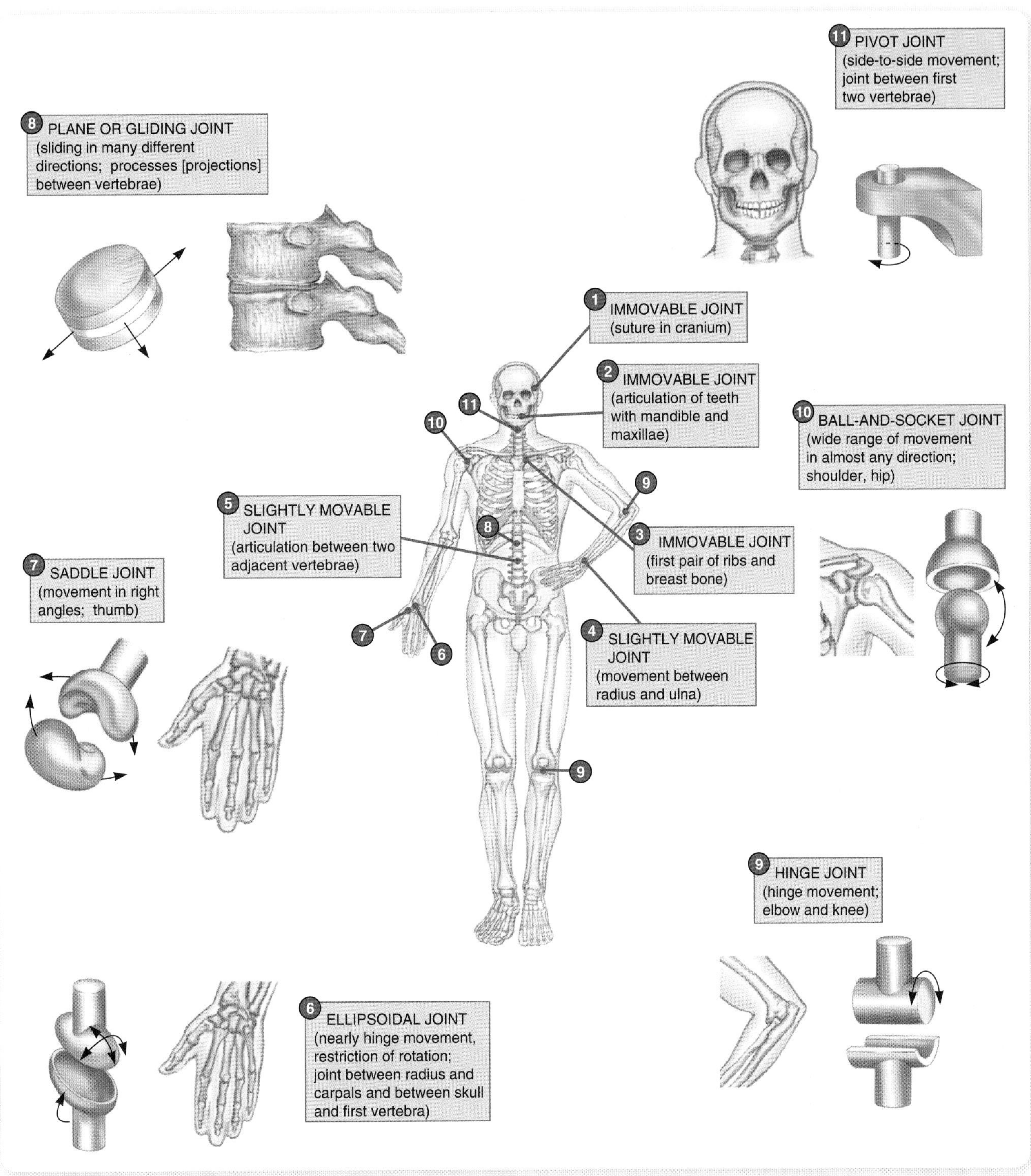

Figure 8-30 Joints in the body.

Skull

At the top of the axial skeleton is the skull, which consists of 28 bones in three anatomic groups: the auditory ossicles, the cranium, and the face **Figure 8-31**. The six auditory ossicles function in hearing and are located deep within cavities of the temporal bone, with three on each side of the head. The remaining 22 bones comprise the cranium and the face.

Auditory Ossicles. Contained within the middle ear are the ossicles, three tiny auditory bones responsible for converting sound waves collected by the eardrum into pressure waves transmitted to the **cochlea**, which is a bony structure resembling a tiny snail shell. These bones are known as the hammer (malleus), anvil (incus), and stirrup (stapes) for their shapes.

Table 8-15 Types of Synovial Joints

Type	Movement	Example
Ball-and-socket	Flexion, extension, abduction, adduction, and rotation	Shoulder and hip joints
Hinge	Flexion, extension, pronation, supination	Elbow and knee joints
Pivot	Rotation	Atlas-axis joint; proximal ends of radius and ulna (elbow joint)
Condyloid (ellipsoidal)	Flexion, extension, abduction, adduction; no rotation	Metacarpophalangeal joints (knuckles); temporomandibular joint (jaw)
Saddle	Flexion, extension, abduction, adduction; limited rotation	Carpometacarpal joint (thumb)
Gliding (plane)	Sliding motion without rotation	Intercarpal joints (wrist); intertarsal joints (ankle)

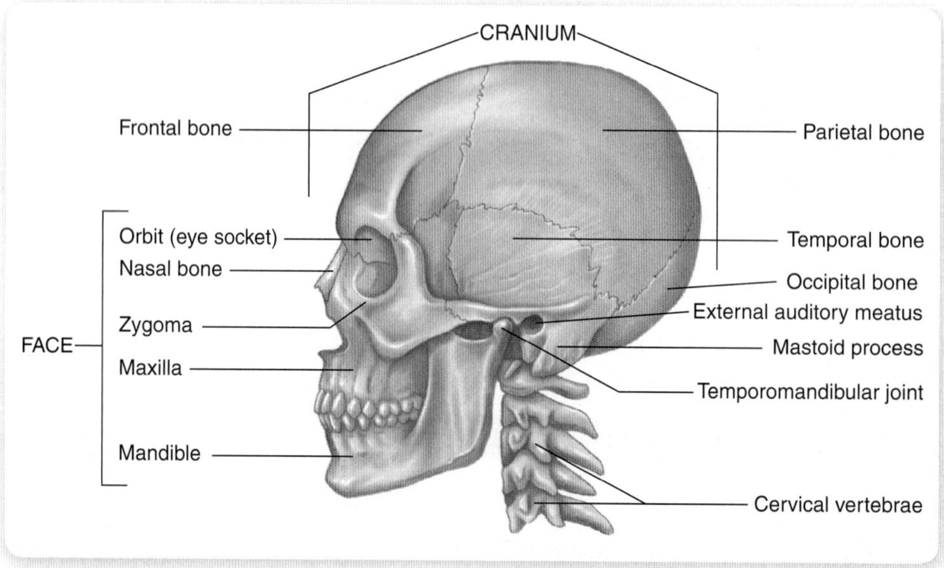

Figure 8-31 The skull consists of 28 bones in three anatomic groups: the auditory ossicles, the cranium, and the face.

Cranial Bones. The dome-shaped roof of the skull, the **cranial vault**, surrounds and protects the upper portion of the brain. Together, eight bones form the cranial vault: two each of the parietal and temporal bones, and the frontal, occipital, sphenoid, and ethmoid bones Figure 8-32. The frontal bone forms the forehead and the roof of the bony sockets that contain the eyeballs. The parietal and temporal bones are considered paired bones because one is on each side of the skull. The parietal bones form the roof and upper part of the sides of the cranium. The temporal bones form the lower sides and base of the cranium. At the base of the temporal bone is a cone-shaped section of bone known as the mastoid process. This area is an important site for attachment of various muscles. The occipital bone forms the back and base of the skull and joins the parietal and temporal bones. The *foramen magnum* is an opening in the occipital bone at the base of the skull through which the spinal cord passes. The sphenoid bone is a bat-shaped bone that joins with the frontal, occipital, and ethmoid bones and forms part of the base of the skull. The thin ethmoid bone contains many small holes. It forms part of the **orbits** (cone-shaped depressions that enclose and protect the eyes) and supports the nasal cavity (the chamber inside the nose that lies between the floor of the cranium and the roof of the mouth).

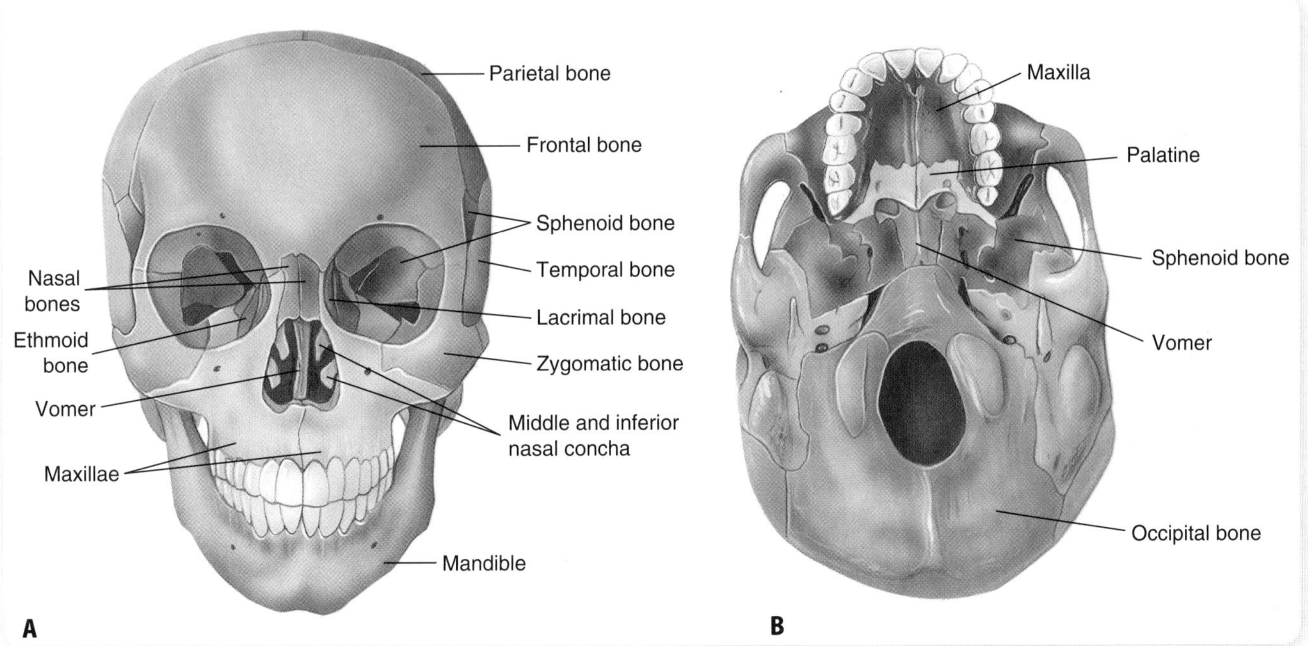

Figure 8-32 The skull and its components. **A.** Front view. **B.** Bottom view.

The bones of the skull are connected together at special joints known as **sutures** Figure 8-33. The paired parietal bones join together at the sagittal suture. The parietal bones abut the frontal bone at the coronal suture. The occipital bone attaches to the parietal bones at the lambdoid suture. As discussed previously, fibrous tissues called fontanelles link the sutures. The tissue felt through the fontanelles are layers of the scalp and thick membranes overlying the brain. Under normal conditions, the brain may not be felt through the fontanelles. By the time a child reaches age 2 years, the sutures should have solidified and the fontanelles closed.

Viewed from above, the floor of the interior of the skull is divided into three compartments: the anterior fossa, middle fossa, and posterior fossa Figure 8-34. The crista galli forms a prominent bony ridge in the center of the anterior fossa and is the point of attachment of the meninges, the membranes that surround the brain. On either side of the crista galli is the **cribriform plate** of the ethmoid bone, the horizontal bone that is perforated with numerous openings (foramina) for the passage of the olfactory nerves from the nasal cavity.

When the mandible is removed, the base of the skull appears amazingly complex, with numerous foramina visible (see Figure 8-34B). The occipital condyles on the occipital bone, which are the points of articulation (connection) between the skull and the vertebral column, lie on either side of the foramen magnum. Portions of the maxilla and the palatine bone, the irregularly shaped bone in the posterior nasal cavity, form the **hard palate**, which is the bony, anterior part of the **palate** (roof of the mouth). The zygomatic arch is the bone that extends along the front of the skull below the orbit.

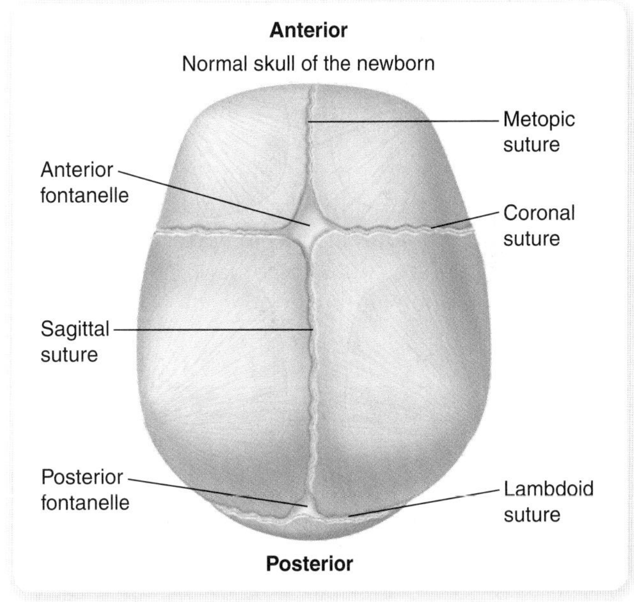

Figure 8-33 The sutures of the skull.

Facial Bones. The facial bones consist of 14 separate bones that form the structure of the face. These bones protect the eyes, nose, and tongue and provide attachment points for the muscles that allow chewing. They are relatively thin but protect the entrances to the digestive system and the **respiratory system**. The 14 facial bones are the paired maxillae, the single mandible (the only freely moving bone in the skull), the paired zygomatic

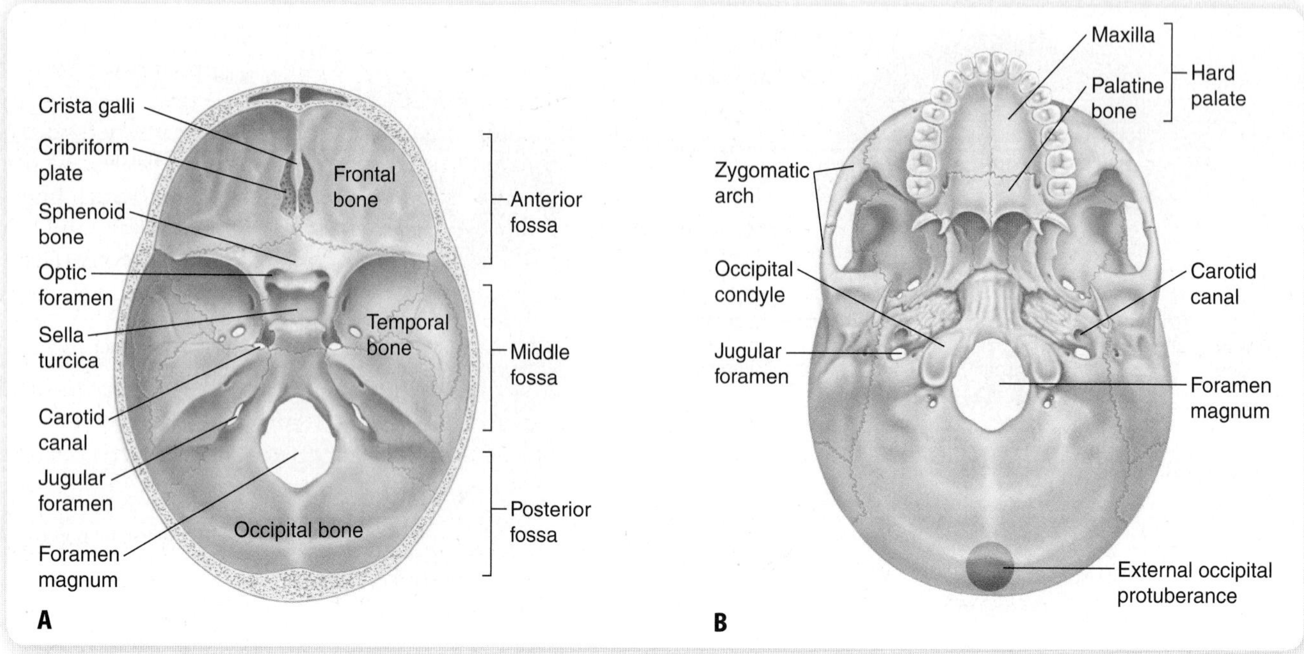

Figure 8-34 A. The floor of the cranial vault and its anatomy. **B.** The base of the skull from below.

bones, the paired palatine bones, the paired nasal bones, the paired lacrimal bones, the single vomer bone, and the paired inferior nasal conchae bones. Both the frontal and ethmoid bones contribute to the cranial vault and the face.

The facial portion of the cranium contains two orbits. In addition to the eyeball and muscles that move it, the orbit contains blood vessels, nerves, and fat. The frontal, sphenoid, zygomatic, maxilla, lacrimal, ethmoid, and palatine bones each form portions of the orbits.

Words of Wisdom

A blow to the eye may result in fracture of the floor of the orbit. This bone is extremely thin and breaks easily. The result is transmission of forces away from the eyeball itself to the bone. Blood and fat then leak into the maxillary sinus below. (The **sinuses** are cavities formed by the cranial bones.) This type of fracture is called a blowout fracture.

The right and left upper jawbones (maxillae) are located between the orbits and the upper teeth and help form the upper face, the infratemporal region, the orbital floor, the lateral wall of the nasal cavity, the floor of the nasal cavity, and the roof of the oral cavity. A condition known as cleft palate results if the right and left maxilla do not join before birth. The lower jaw consists of the body of the mandible anteriorly and the ramus of the mandible posteriorly. The body and ramus meet posteriorly to form the angle of the mandible. The mandible is the only facial bone that is capable of movement. The mandible joins the skull in the area of the temporal bone, forming the temporomandibular joint on each side of the skull. The zygoma (cheekbone) forms the anterior wall of the infratemporal area and the lateral wall of the orbit. The zygoma meets the lateral skull to form the zygomatic arch, which lends shape to the cheeks.

The palatine bones help form the lateral wall and floor of the nasal cavity, the oral cavity (posterior third of the hard palate), and a small portion of the posterior wall of the orbit. The nasal bones help form part of the bony bridge of the external nose, the lateral wall of the nasal cavity, and a small part of the bony nasal septum. The lacrimal bones form the medial wall of the orbits and the lateral wall of the nasal cavity. The vomer is a thin, flat bone that forms a large part of the bony nasal septum. The inferior conchae help form the lateral wall of the nasal cavity and part of the maxillary sinus. The external portion of the nose is formed mostly of cartilage.

The **paranasal sinuses**, are hollow air-filled spaces that help to reduce the weight of the skull as well as provide resonance for the voice. They are located around the nasal cavity and drain into it Figure 8-35. The paranasal sinuses are a group of four pairs, as follows: the ethmoid sinuses within the ethmoid bone, the frontal sinuses within the frontal bone, the maxillary sinuses within the right and left maxillae (the largest of the paranasal sinuses), and the sphenoid sinuses within the body of the sphenoid bone. The paranasal sinuses are lined with epithelium. The cilia of the epithelium move in a

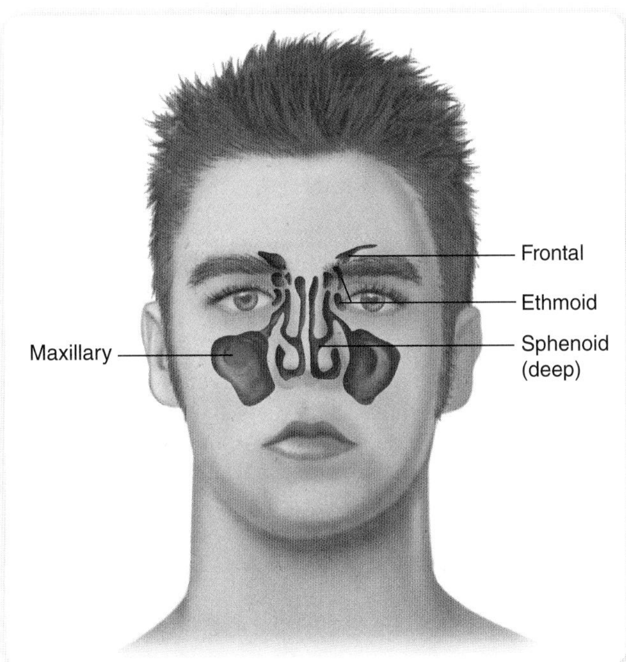

Figure 8-35 The paranasal sinuses.

synchronized beating pattern toward the anterior portion of the nasal cavity. Tiny goblet cells in the epithelium secrete a sticky mucus substance onto the cilia, trapping contaminants as they enter the nasal cavity and moving them toward the front where the mucus is either removed by blowing the nose, or moved down to the throat where it can enter into the digestive system. During sleep, this mucus may flow backward (postnasal drip).

Words of Wisdom

Sinusitis is a relatively common inflammation of the paranasal sinuses. Sinusitis may range in severity from a simple upper respiratory tract infection consisting of headache and nasal drainage to a potentially life-threatening brain infection, depending on the extent of the infection and which sinuses are affected.

The **hyoid bone** is a horseshoe-shaped bone that "floats" beneath the mandible with the open end of the horseshoe pointed posteriorly. Every bone in the body connects (articulates) with at least one other bone, except for the hyoid bone. Although the hyoid is not part of the skull, it is attached to the skull by muscles and ligaments. It serves to anchor the tongue and is a point of attachment for many important neck and tongue muscles. If the hyoid bone is damaged by a blow to the anterior neck, then the patient may have a hoarse and low-volume voice because of airway swelling.

The nerves that provide sensory and motor control to the face are discussed in detail later in this chapter.

Neck

The neck contains many important structures. It is supported by the cervical spine, or the first seven vertebrae in the spinal column. The spinal cord exits from the foramen magnum and lies within the spinal canal formed by the vertebrae. The upper part of the esophagus (which helps transport food from the mouth to the stomach) and the trachea (windpipe) lie in the midline of the neck. The carotid arteries are found on either side of the trachea, along with jugular veins and several nerves.

Several useful landmarks can be palpated and seen in the neck **Figure 8-36**. The most obvious is the firm prominence in the center of the anterior surface commonly known as the Adam's apple. Specifically, this shield-shaped prominence is the upper part of the **thyroid cartilage**. It is more prominent in men than in women. The lower portion is the **cricoid cartilage**, a firm ridge of cartilage inferior to the thyroid cartilage, which is somewhat more difficult to palpate. The **cricothyroid membrane** is a soft depression made up of a thin sheet of connective tissue (fascia) that joins the thyroid cartilage and the cricoid cartilage in the midline of the neck. The cricothyroid membrane is covered at this point only by skin.

Inferior to the **larynx** (voice box), several additional firm ridges are palpable in the anterior midline. These ridges are the cartilage rings of the trachea. The trachea connects the larynx with the main air passages of the lungs (the bronchi). On either side of the lower larynx and the upper trachea lies the thyroid gland. Unless this gland is enlarged, it is usually not palpable.

Pulsations of the carotid arteries are easily palpable in a groove about half an inch (1 cm) lateral to the larynx. Lying immediately adjacent to these arteries, but not palpable, are the internal jugular veins and several

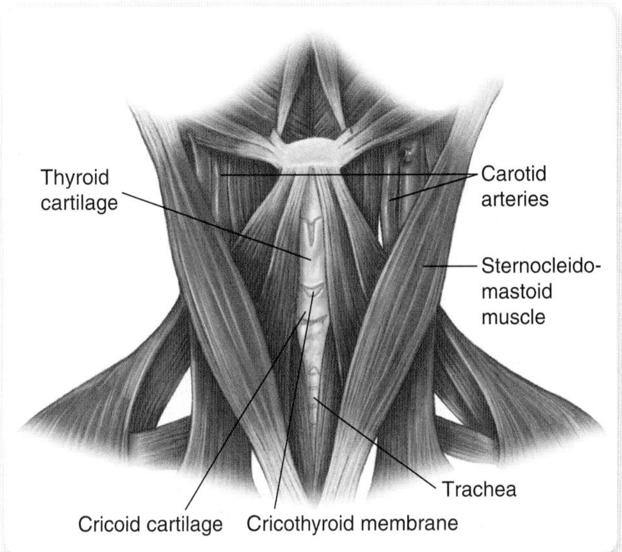

Figure 8-36 The principal structures of the neck include the trachea, along with many blood vessels, muscles, and nerves.

important nerves. Lateral to these vessels and nerves lie the sternocleidomastoid muscles, which allow movement of the head. These muscles originate from the mastoid process of the cranium and insert into the medial border of each clavicle and the sternum at the base of the neck.

Vertebral Column

The spinal cord is encased by the vertebral column (spine), which consists of the 33 bones of the vertebrae. The vertebrae articulate to form the vertebral column, which is the major structural component of the axial skeleton. These skeletal components are stabilized by both ligaments and muscle. Together, these components support and protect neural elements while allowing for fluid movement and an erect stature.

The vertebrae are divided into the following five regions:

- 7 cervical vertebrae
- 12 thoracic vertebrae
- 5 lumbar vertebrae
- 5 sacral vertebrae (fused together in adults to form the sacrum)
- 4 coccygeal vertebrae (fused together in adults to form the coccyx, or tailbone) Figure 8-37.

Each vertebra is identified by its region (eg, cervical, thoracic) and then given a number. Thus the first vertebra is cervical 1, or C1. Starting at C1 and following the spinal column inferiorly, each vertebra gets progressively larger than the previous one because each vertebra must support more weight than the bone above it. The fifth lumbar vertebra is the largest, after which the sacral and coccygeal vertebrae get progressively smaller until the most distal coccygeal vertebrae, the tailbone. To add strength, assist in balance, and prevent injury, the spinal column has four curves: two that curve posteriorly (the cervical and lumbar curvatures) and two that curve anteriorly (the thoracic and sacral curvatures).

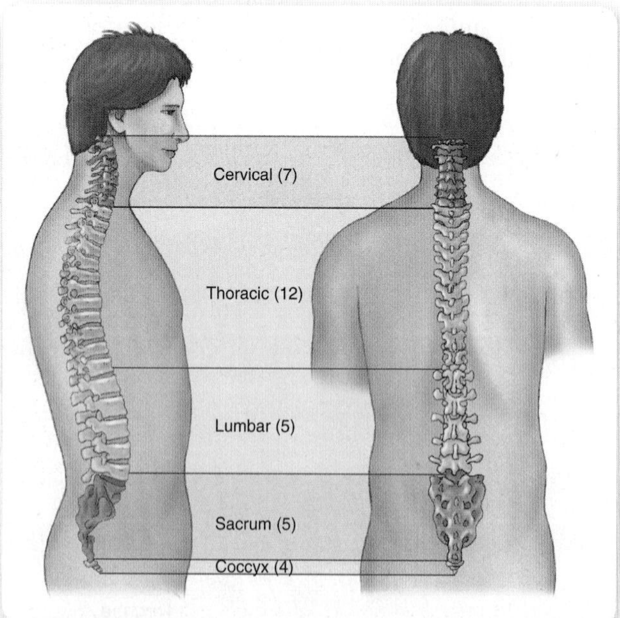

Figure 8-37 The spinal column consists of 33 bones divided into five sections. Each vertebra is numbered and referred to by a letter corresponding to the section of the spine where it is located. For example, the fifth thoracic vertebra is referred to as T5.

Words of Wisdom

Variations of the spinal curvatures exist. Lordosis is an exaggeration of the lumbar curvature, creating a swayback appearance; kyphosis is an exaggeration of the thoracic curvature, causing a humpback appearance; and scoliosis is an abnormal lateral curvature of the spine. As a paramedic, you must be familiar with these conditions because they can affect breathing, immobilization, and other aspects of the patient's condition or care.

The five sections of the spine, from the top down, include the following:

- **Cervical spine**. The first seven vertebrae (C1 through C7) in the neck form the cervical spine. The skull rests on the first cervical vertebra and articulates with it. The first and second cervical vertebrae—named the **atlas** and the **axis**, respectively—are highly specialized, providing support for the head and permitting it to articulate with the spinal column Figure 8-38. The atlas articulates with the occipital condyles at the base of the skull at the atlanto-occipital joint, permitting the head to nod and rotate left to right. The axis has an upward projection

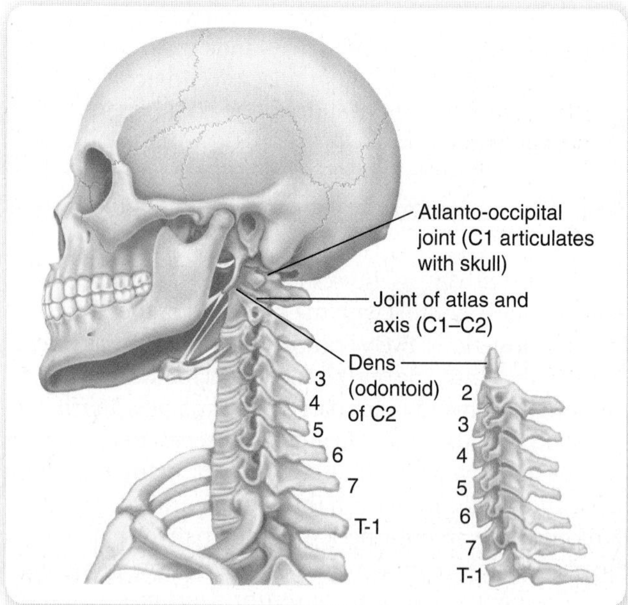

Figure 8-38 The cervical vertebrae.

called the odontoid process. The atlas sits on this process, which acts as a pivot point and allows rotation of the head.

- **Thoracic spine**. The next 12 vertebrae make up the thoracic spine. One pair of ribs is attached to each of the thoracic vertebrae. In addition to the supporting muscles and ligaments found in the vertebral column, the thoracic spine is further stabilized by the rib attachments. The spinous processes are slightly larger; these bony projections serve as attachment points for muscles that hold the upper body erect and assist with the movement of the thoracic cavity during breathing.
- **Lumbar spine**. The lumbar spine includes the five largest bones in the vertebral column, and is integral in carrying a large portion of the upper body weight. This area of the spine is especially susceptible to injury because of its weight-bearing capacity.
- **Sacrum**. The five sacral vertebrae are fused together to form one bone. The sacrum is joined to the iliac bones of the pelvis with strong ligaments at the **sacroiliac joints** to form the pelvis.
- **Coccyx**. The last four vertebrae, also fused together, form the coccyx.

With the exception of C1, each vertebra consists of an inner, thick, round anterior portion, called the vertebral body, which is the weight-bearing component of the spine that provides support and stability **Figure 8-39**. The posterior, or rear-facing, side of a vertebra is the vertebral arch (also called the bony arch, posterior arch, or dorsal arch). The vertebral arch is made up of a spinous process and a thin plate of bone called the lamina between each transverse process and the spinous process. When you feel the midline of the spine, you are feeling the spinous process (thus the reason the vertebral column is also called the spine). The vertebral arch serves as a connection point for muscles and ligaments, allows movement by acting as a lever for muscles, and is the site of interlocking articulation between multiple vertebrae. Thoracic vertebrae also articulate with ribs at the vertebral arch. The vertebral body and vertebral arch form a space called the vertebral foramen. When all vertebrae are aligned, this space forms a large canal running the length of the spinal column. The spinal cord, spinal nerve roots, meninges, and many vessels are housed within this canal, protected by the vertebrae and intervertebral disks.

The pedicle is a short, thick bony projection that connects the vertebral body to the transverse process of the vertebra. Each pedicle joins with a lamina. The articular process is a bony structure that projects outward from the vertebra. The transverse spinous processes comprise the junction of each pedicle and lamina on each side of a vertebra. They project laterally and posteriorly and form points of attachments for muscles and ligaments. The posterior spinous process is formed by the fusion of the posterior lamina and serves as an attachment site for muscles and ligaments.

A cartilaginous cushion called the intervertebral disk rests between most vertebrae to provide padding and space for flexibility. No disk is located between the occiput and C1, or between C1 and C2.[7] The space created by the intervertebral disks allows the spinal nerves to exit the spinal cord. These spinal nerves allow control over the periphery of the body.

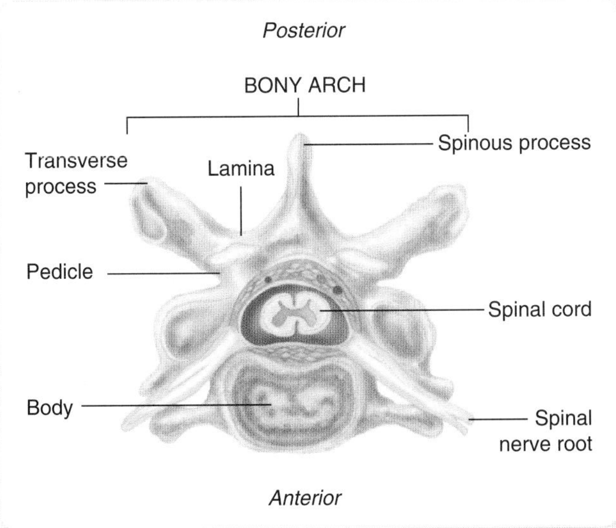

Figure 8-39 A general representation of the human vertebra. Vertebrae in different sections of the spinal column vary in shape. The space through which the spinal cord passes is the canal, and the space through which a nerve root passes is a foramen.

Words of Wisdom

As the body ages, loss of water content occurs in the intervertebral disks and they become thinner as a result. This process causes the height loss associated with aging. Stress on the vertebral column may cause a disk to herniate into the spinal canal, resulting in an injury to the spinal cord or a nerve root injury. Nerves can also be injured at the peripheral level (anywhere in the body outside of the spinal cord), which is called peripheral nerve injury.

The ligaments and intervertebral disks allow some motion so the trunk can bend forward (flex) and back (extend), and they allow for rotation and lateral movement. However, they also limit motion of the vertebrae so the spinal cord will not be injured. An injury to the spine may damage part of the spinal cord and its nerves that may not be protected by the vertebrae. As a paramedic, you must therefore use extreme caution in caring for the patient with a suspected spinal injury to prevent secondary damage to these structures.

Thorax

The thorax (chest) consists of a bony cage overlying some of the most vital organs in the human body. The dimensions of the thorax are defined posteriorly by the thoracic vertebrae and ribs, inferiorly by the **diaphragm** (a specialized skeletal muscle) anteriorly and laterally by the ribs, and superiorly by the thoracic inlet **Figure 8-40**.

The bony structures of the thorax include the sternum, clavicle, scapula, thoracic vertebrae, and 12 pairs of ribs. The sternum is a dagger-shaped bone located in the midline of the chest. It consists of the superior manubrium (the handle), the central sternal body (the blade), and the inferior xiphoid process (the blunt tip) **Figure 8-41**. The space superior to the manubrium is the **suprasternal notch** (also known as the jugular notch) the junction of the manubrium and sternal body is the **angle of Louis** (also called the sternal angle or manubriosternal junction).

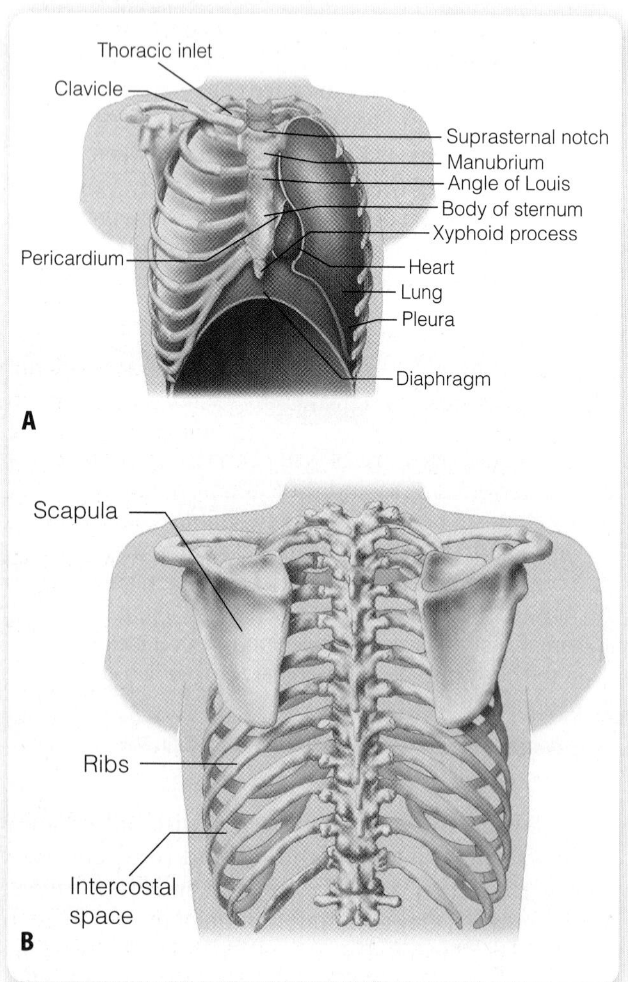

Figure 8-40 The thorax. **A.** Anterior view. **B.** Posterior view.

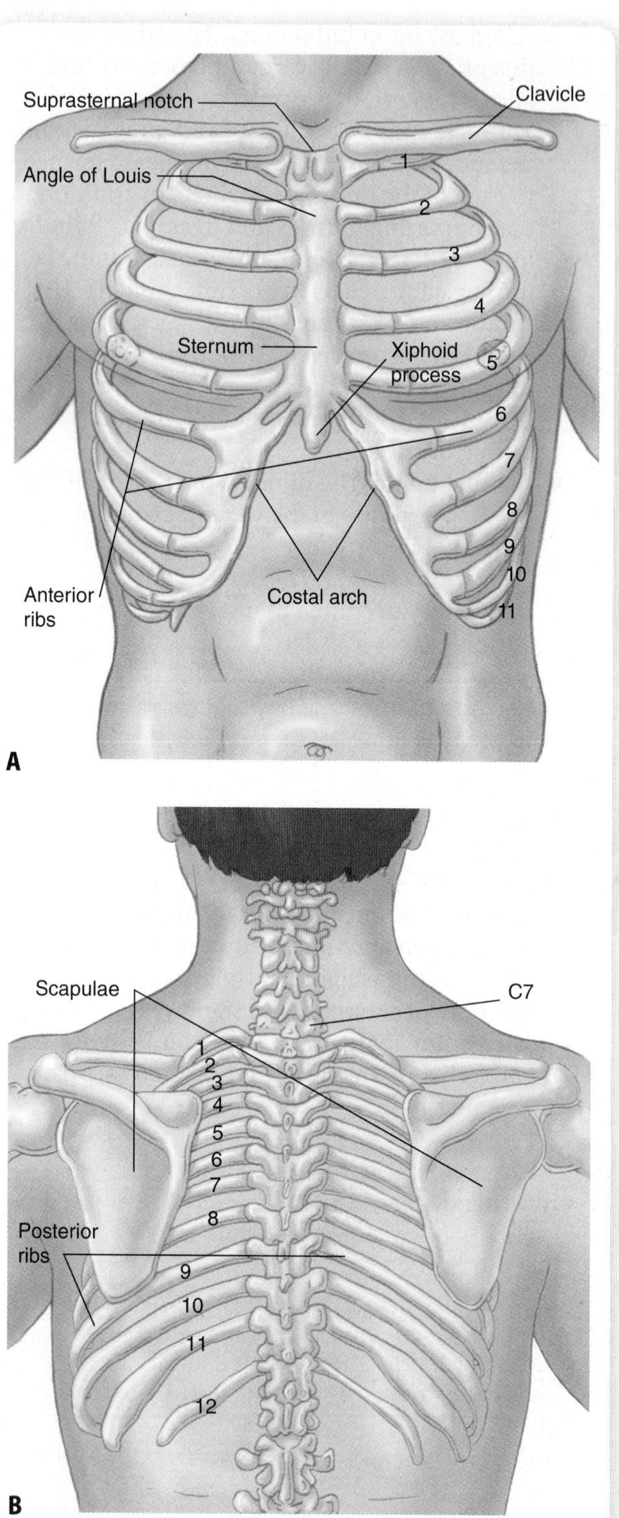

Figure 8-41 The rib cage. **A.** Anterior view. **B.** Posterior view.

The central region of the thorax is the **mediastinum**, which contains the heart, great vessels, part of the esophagus, lymphatic channels, trachea, primary bronchi, and paired vagus and phrenic nerves. Anteriorly, the lungs extend down to the surface of the diaphragm at the level of the xiphoid process. Posteriorly, the lungs extend farther inferiorly to the surface of the diaphragm at the level of the 12th thoracic vertebra.

Words of Wisdom

The dimensions of the thorax are of great importance in the physical assessment of the patient. Although the thoracic cavity extends to the 12th rib posteriorly, the diaphragm inserts into the anterior thoracic cage just below the fourth or fifth rib. With the movement of the diaphragm during breathing, the size and dimensions of the thoracic cavity will vary, which could in tum affect the organs or cavities (thoracic versus abdominal) in patients with a blunt or penetrating injury.

The heart lies immediately behind the sternum (retrosternal). It extends from the second to the sixth ribs anteriorly and from the fifth to the eighth thoracic vertebrae posteriorly. The inferior border of the heart extends into the left side of the chest. Diseased hearts may be larger or smaller than normal. The major blood vessels that travel to and from the heart also lie in the chest cavity. On the right side of the spinal column, the superior and inferior venae cavae carry blood to the heart.

Just beneath the manubrium of the sternum, the arch of the **aorta** (the body's largest artery) and the **pulmonary artery** exit the heart. The arch of the aorta passes to the left and lies along the left side of the spinal column as it descends into the abdomen. The esophagus lies behind the great vessels and directly on the anterior aspect of the spinal column as it passes through the chest into the abdominal cavity.

Each of the 12 matched pairs of ribs attaches posteriorly to the 12 thoracic vertebrae. Anteriorly, the first seven pairs of ribs (true ribs) attach directly to the sternum via the costal cartilage. The costal cartilage then continues inferiorly from the 7th rib and provides an indirect connection between the anterior portions of the 8th, 9th, and 10th ribs (false ribs) and the sternum. The 11th and 12th ribs (floating ribs) are held in place by cartilage and have no anterior connection to the sternum.

Between each rib lies an intercostal space. These spaces are numbered according to the rib superior to the space (that is, the space between the second and third ribs is the second intercostal space). The intercostal spaces house the intercostal muscles and the neurovascular bundle, which consists of an artery, vein, and nerve that run on the bottom aspect of each rib.

Words of Wisdom

The intercostal spaces become important landmarks when you report the anatomic location of injuries or when you perform procedures.

▶ Appendicular Skeleton

The appendicular skeleton includes the bones of the shoulder and pelvic girdles, the upper extremities (arms [more commonly thought of as the upper arms], forearms, wrist, hands, and fingers), and lower extremities (thighs, legs, ankles, instep, and toes).

Shoulder and Upper Extremities

The scapula (shoulder blade) is a flat, triangular bone held to the rib cage posteriorly by powerful muscles that buffer it against injury. The scapulae are attached to the posterior thorax by muscles. The scapula is divided into two posterior components by a sharp diagonal ridge (or spine), at the end of which forms the **acromion process.** The acromion process protects the shoulder joint and provides a site of attachment for the clavicle and various shoulder muscles. Important muscles of the shoulder, including those of the rotator cuff, originate here.

The clavicle is a slender, S-shaped bone attached by ligaments at the medial end to the manubrium of the sternum. The clavicle acts as a strut to keep the shoulder propped up; however, because it is slender and exposed, this bone is vulnerable to injury. The lateral portion of the clavicle articulates with the acromion of the scapula, forming the acromioclavicular joint. Anterior to the acromion process is a fingerlike projection called the coracoid process, which also provides an area for muscle attachment. Between these two processes is a saucer-shaped portion of the scapula known as the glenoid fossa, where the head of the humerus articulates.

Words of Wisdom

The clavicle is one of the most commonly fractured bones in the body whereas the scapula is extremely difficult to fracture.

The scapula and clavicle form the pectoral girdle, also called the shoulder girdle, which serves as an attachment for the upper extremities to the axial skeleton **Figure 8-42**. The upper extremity joins the shoulder girdle at the glenohumeral (shoulder) joint, which is a ball-and-socket joint.

The proximal portion of the humerus, which is the second largest bone in the human body, has a head that articulates with the scapula **Figure 8-43**. On this proximal portion of the humerus are two small extensions off either side of the bone (tubercles). These tubercles serve as muscular attachments for the shoulder joint. The distal end of the humerus articulates with the proximal ends of the forearm bones—the radius and ulna—to form the hinged elbow joint. Several ligaments connect the humerus, radius, and ulna at the elbow joint, and a fluid-filled bursa cushions and protects the joint posteriorly.

The forearm extends from the elbow to the wrist. The radius lies on the lateral or thumb side of the forearm. The proximal portion of the radius is the radial head. The distal portion contains a small bony protrusion, the styloid process, to which some of the ligaments of the wrist are attached. Distally, the ulna is narrow and is on the medial or little-finger side of the forearm. It serves as the pivot around which the radius turns at the wrist to rotate the palm upward (supination) or downward (pronation). The proximal end of the

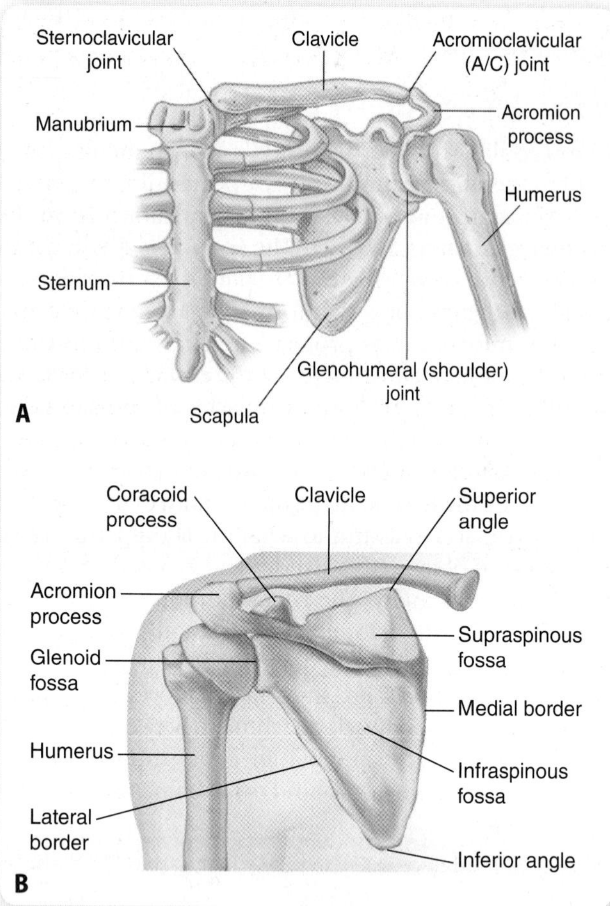

Figure 8-42 The pectoral (shoulder) girdle. **A.** Anterior view, including the clavicle. **B.** Posterior view, including the scapula.

ulna has a large, blunt bony process (olecranon process). This bony process forms the tip of the elbow. Lateral to this process, the proximal end of the radius articulates with the humerus. The distal end of the radius articulates with the irregularly shaped **carpal bones** of the wrist. The distal end of the ulna articulates directly to the radius.

The carpal bones of the wrist are arranged in two rows of four bones each (Figure 8-44). The carpals include the triquetrum, pisiform, capitate, lunate, hamate, trapezoid, trapezium, and scaphoid (carpal navicular) bones. The carpal tunnel is formed by the space bounded by the trapezium and hamate dorsally and the flexor retinaculum, a sheath of tough connective tissue that forms the roof of the carpal tunnel, on the palmar side. Tendons, nerves, and blood vessels lie within the carpal tunnel. Structures within the carpal tunnel include the long flexor tendon to the fingers and the median nerve, which supplies sensory and motor function to the radial half of the palm of the hand. Carpal bones, especially the scaphoid, are vulnerable to fracture when a person falls on an outstretched hand.

Five metacarpals form the bony portion of the hand. The phalanges in the fingers form hinge joints. Each finger has three phalanges, except the thumb, which has only two phalanges. The carpometacarpal joint of the thumb is a **saddle joint**, consisting of two saddle-shaped articulating surfaces that are oriented at right angles to one another so that the complementary surfaces articulate with each other. Movement in these joints can occur in two planes. Arthritis commonly affects the carpometacarpal joint, resulting in stiffness and deformity.

Innervation of the upper extremities arises from the brachial plexus. **Plexuses** are areas where spinal nerves

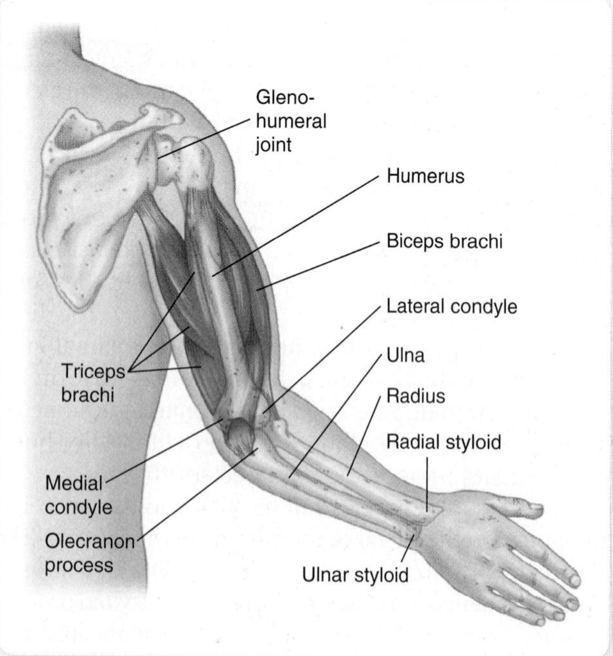

Figure 8-43 The upper arm contains the humerus; the forearm contains the radius and ulna.

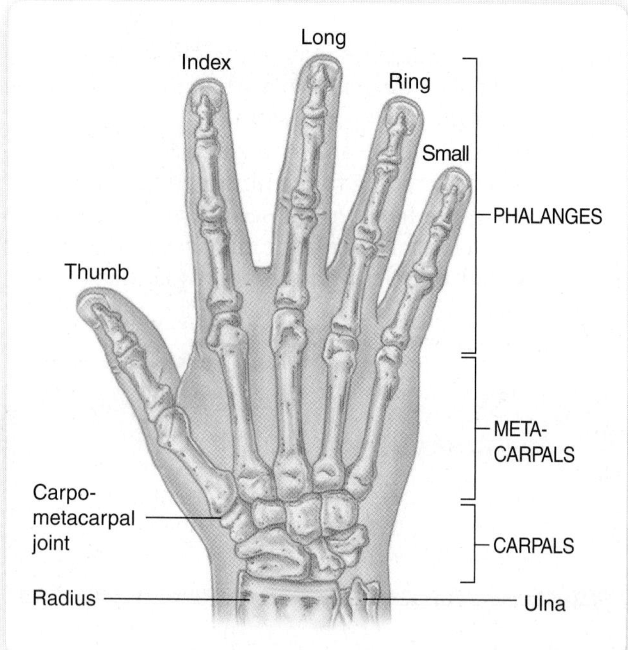

Figure 8-44 The principal bones in the wrist and hand include the carpals, the metacarpals, and the phalanges.

come together and transmit their impulses to areas of the body through a common nerve. The brachial plexus is formed by a network of nerves that originate from the spinal cord at the C5 to T1 levels. After the fibers of these nerves network with one another, five distinct nerves are formed: the axillary, radial, musculocutaneous, ulnar, and median.

The blood supply to the upper extremity originates from the subclavian artery. When the subclavian artery reaches the axilla, it is referred to as the axillary artery. After giving off several branches that supply the shoulder region with blood, the artery leaves the axilla and becomes the brachial artery. After the brachial artery passes through the elbow, it divides into the radial artery and ulnar artery. In the hand, the radial and ulnar arteries form superficial and deep arcades of blood vessels that branch to form the arteries of each finger, the digital arteries.

Words of Wisdom

Here is a tip to help remember which bones are carpals (hand bones) and which bones are tarsals (foot bones): "I steer my CAR (pal) with hands and walk through TAR (sal) with my feet."

Pelvis and Lower Extremities

The pelvis is a ring formed anteriorly from the fusion of the ilium, ischium, and pubis bones on either side of the body to form the right and left innominate bones during early adulthood. Posteriorly, these two innominate bones articulate with the sacrum to form the pelvic ring. The pelvis supports the weight of the trunk, serves as a place of attachment for the thighs, and protects the organs of the pelvic cavity including the intestines, **urinary bladder** (where urine is stored before its elimination from the body), and internal reproductive organs **Figure 8-45**. During pregnancy, the bones protect the developing fetus and provide a passageway through which the newborn passes during delivery. The two innominate bones articulate anteriorly at the symphysis pubis and posteriorly with the sacrum at the sacroiliac joints. An extensive nerve and vascular supply travels along either side of the pelvis to the lower extremities.

Words of Wisdom

Pay attention to the spelling of medical terminology to prevent misunderstandings. Even though *ilium* and *ileum* are pronounced the same, they refer to two different parts of the body.

- Ilium is the bony prominences of the pelvis.
- Ileum is the lower three-fifths of the small intestine.

The lower extremity is made up of the thigh, knee, leg, ankle, foot, and toes **Figure 8-46**. The femur is the

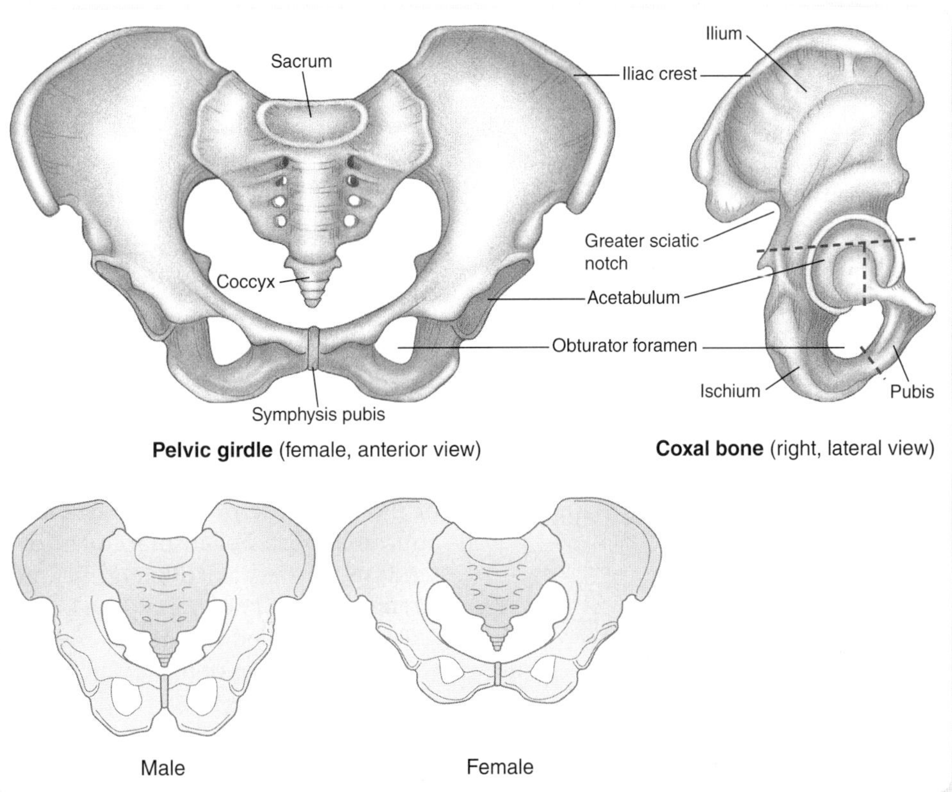

Figure 8-45 The pelvic girdle.

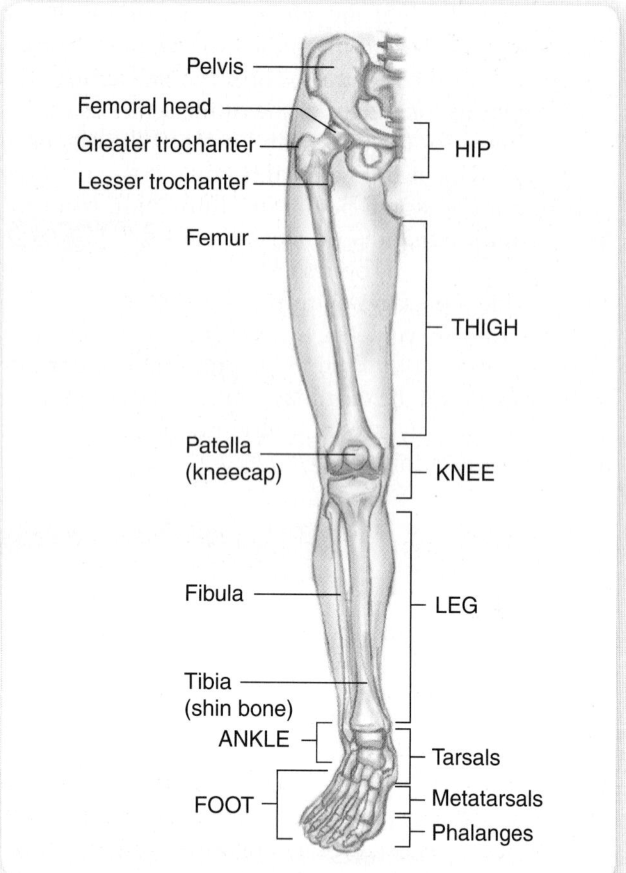

Figure 8-46 The principal parts of the lower extremity, including the femur, femoral head, greater and lesser trochanters, patella, tibia, and fibula.

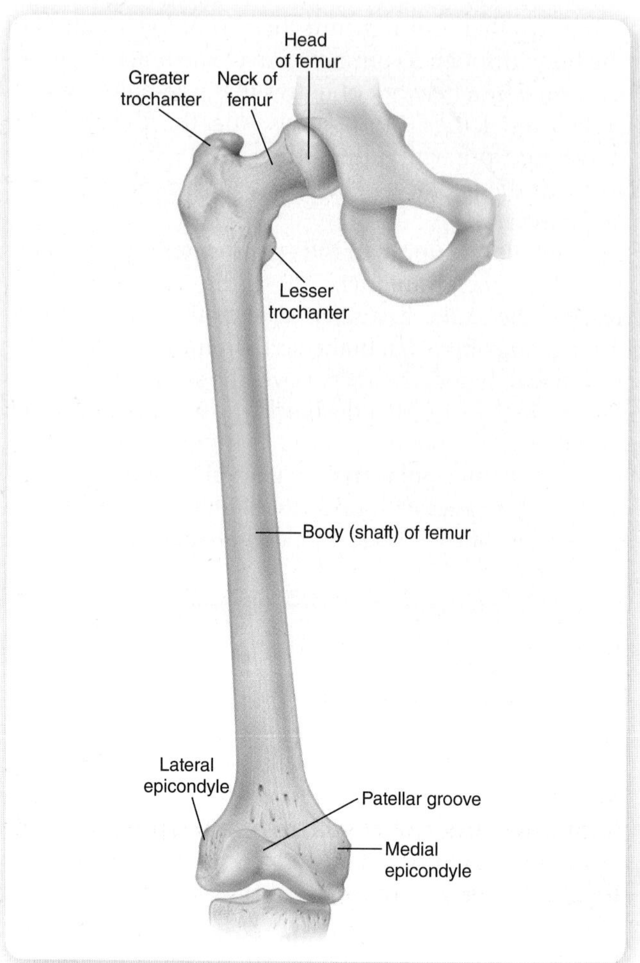

Figure 8-47 The femur.

longest and one of the strongest bones in the body. It articulates proximally in the ball-and-socket joint of the pelvis and distally in the hinge joint of the knee. The femoral head is the ball-shaped part that fits into the **acetabulum**, which is a cup-shaped structure formed by the coxal bones. The femoral head is connected to the shaft, or long tubular portion of the femur, by the femoral neck and intertrochanteric region. The proximal portion of the femur has two separate points of muscular attachment, the greater trochanter, and the lesser trochanter Figure 8-47. The greater trochanter arises lateral to the juncture of the neck and shaft and is clinically considered as part of the hip. Several ligaments and muscle tendons provide integrity to the hip joint. The articular capsule is supported by strong ligaments; they support much of the weight of the body.

Words of Wisdom

The femoral neck is a common site for hip fractures, especially in the older population.

At the distal end of the femur, the lateral and medial condyles articulate with the proximal tibia at the knee Figure 8-48. These are important sites of muscle and ligament attachment. The patella lies within the major anterior tendon of the thigh muscles and articulates with the femur. The knee joint is traditionally classified as a hinge joint and is unusual because it contains ligaments within the joint. Thick, crescent-shaped articular disks (menisci) cover the margins of the tibia to cushion the articular surface. The anterior cruciate ligament, which extends between the tibia and femur, prevents abnormal anterior movement (hyperextension) of the tibia. The posterior cruciate ligament prevents abnormal posterior displacement of the tibia. Several tendons, as well as collateral ligaments, lend further strength to the knee joint. The knee is surrounded by several fluid-filled bursae.

The two bones of the lower leg are the tibia and fibula. The tibia is the longer and thicker of the two bones and is located on the anteromedial side of the leg. It is vulnerable to direct blows and can be felt just beneath the skin. Proximally, the tibia articulates with the distal

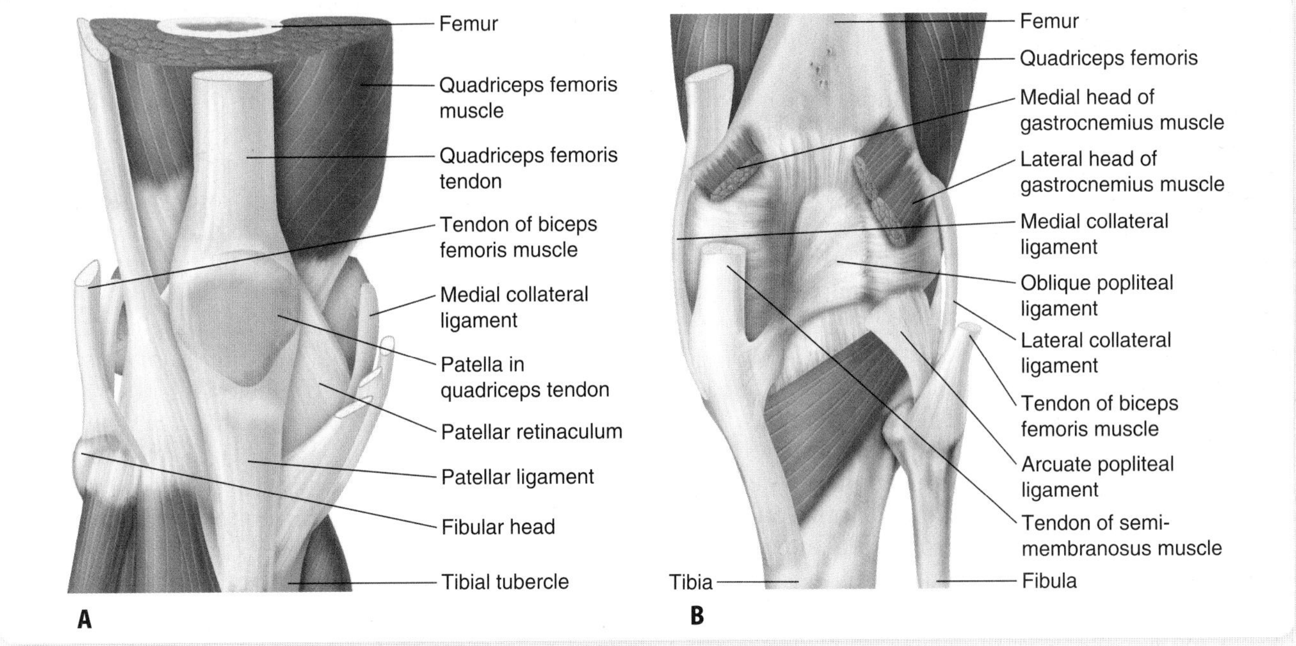

Figure 8-48 The knee. **A.** Anterior view. **B.** Posterior view.

femur and is the weight-bearing bone of the leg. The flat medial and lateral condyles of the proximal tibia articulate with the condyles of the femur at the knee. The tibial tuberosity is a projection on the anterior surface of the proximal tibia and serves as an attachment point for the quadriceps muscle. Distally, the tibia forms the medial malleolus, which is the medial side of the ankle joint. The fibula is a long, slender bone that is much smaller than the tibia. It does not bear any weight, and does not articulate directly with the femur, but rather with the tibia at the head. An enlargement of the distal end of the fibula forms the lateral wall of the ankle joint, the lateral malleolus.

Words of Wisdom

The tibial tuberosity is an important landmark for you to identify before inserting an intraosseous needle into the tibia.

The foot (tarsus) is made up of seven bones called tarsals. The largest of these bones is the **calcaneus** (heel bone). The talus articulates with the tibia and fibula to form the ankle **Figure 8-49**. The bones of the ankle are arranged so that the talus forms a hinge with the lower portion of the tibia and fibula.

The calcaneus lies inferior and lateral to the talus, providing additional support. It is subject to injury when a person falls from a height and lands on the feet. A fibrous capsule surrounds the ankle joint; the medial and lateral portions are thickened to form ligaments. Movements of the ankle and posterior foot include dorsiflexion and plantar flexion, as well as limited inversion and eversion.

The metatarsals and phalanges of the foot are arranged much like the bones of the hand. The toes have

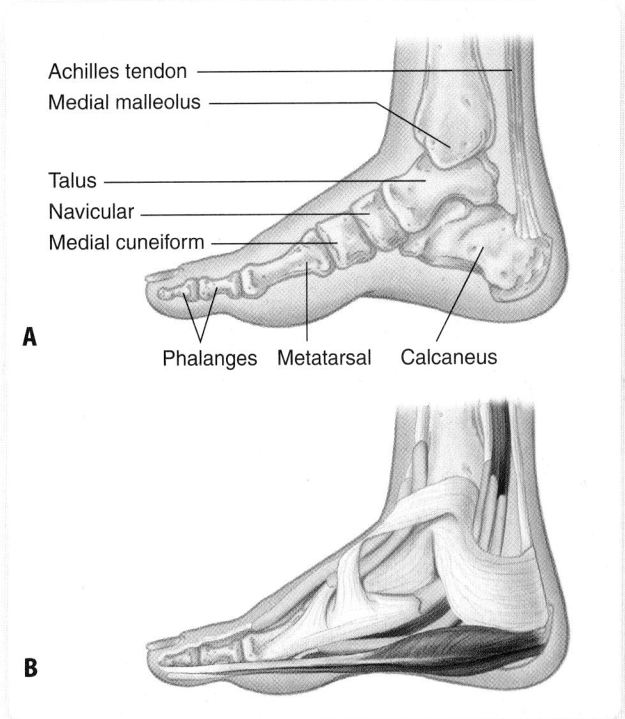

Figure 8-49 A. The surface landmarks of the foot, including the talus, the calcaneus, and the phalanges. **B.** Soft tissues of the ankle.

three phalanges each, except the big toe, which has two phalanges. The ball of the foot is the junction between the metatarsals and the phalanges.

Innervation of the lower extremities is provided by the lumbar and lumbosacral plexuses, which are formed by the spinal nerves that originate from L1 to S4. The networking of nerves within these two plexuses leads to the formation of multiple distinct nerves, including the sciatic nerve—which branches in the popliteal fossa to form the peroneal and tibial nerves—and the femoral nerve.

The blood supply of the lower extremity originates from the external iliac artery. When the external iliac artery reaches the leg, it becomes the femoral artery. When it reaches the knee, the femoral artery turns posteriorly and laterally and it is referred to as the popliteal artery. The popliteal artery divides into the anterior tibial artery and posterior tibial artery. The anterior tibial artery travels along the anterior and lateral surface of the tibia until it reaches the ankle, where it proceeds along the dorsal surface of the foot toward the great toe and becomes the dorsalis pedis artery. The posterior tibial artery travels along the posterior aspect of the tibia until it reaches the ankle, where it follows a path just behind the medial malleolus until it reaches the plantar aspect of the foot. Within the foot, arcades of arteries supply the various structures with blood and give off branches that form the digital arteries of the toes.

The Musculoskeletal System

The term **musculoskeletal** refers to the bones and voluntary muscles of the body. Muscles are a form of tissue that allows body movement. The musculoskeletal system contains more than 600 muscles. Three important functions of the musculoskeletal system are movement and maintenance of posture, joint stability, and production of heat.

Skeletal muscle, so named because it attaches to the bones of the skeleton, forms the major muscle mass of the body. As discussed previously, other types of muscle outside of the musculoskeletal system include smooth muscle and cardiac muscle. Skeletal muscle is also called voluntary muscle because all skeletal muscle is under direct voluntary control of the brain and can be stimulated to contract or relax at will. Movement of the body, like waving or walking, results from skeletal muscle contraction or relaxation. Usually, a specific motion is the result of several muscles contracting and relaxing simultaneously.

Skeletal muscle includes all of the muscles attached to the skeleton and forms the bulk of the tissue of the arms and legs. It is also found along the spine and buttocks. By maintaining a state of partial contraction, this type of muscle allows the body to maintain its posture and to sit or stand. Skeletal muscle varies greatly in size and shape,

YOU are the Paramedic PART 2

The motorcycle rider is lying facedown on the pavement next to the front driver's door of the pickup truck. He is unresponsive. You apply manual cervical spine stabilization and, with assistance, log roll the patient onto his back. You immediately note the patient is pale and sweaty. His upper front teeth have been knocked out and his eyes are swollen shut. You find the patient has a rapid pulse and his breathing is rapid and shallow. He has a large abrasion in the middle of his left chest just below the clavicle. He has deformity and a large laceration on the lower right leg immediately above the inner ankle bone.

Recording Time: 3 Minutes	
Appearance	Found prone on pavement; minimal bleeding from right leg laceration
Level of consciousness	Unresponsive
Airway	Open; fresh blood in mouth
Breathing	24 breaths/min, shallow
Circulation	118 beats/min

3. Given the broken upper teeth and facial swelling, what body structures may have been injured?
4. What is the best way to describe the location of the injury on the left chest?
5. What is the best way to describe the location of the deformity and injury on the right leg?

from thin strands to the large muscles of the thigh and back. It also constitutes the muscles of the tongue, **soft palate**, scalp, pharynx, upper esophagus, and eye.

Skeletal muscle cells possess the following properties that relate to their functions:

- **Excitability.** The ability to receive and respond to a stimulus
- **Contractility.** The ability to shorten (contract)
- **Extensibility.** The ability to stretch (extend)
- **Elasticity.** The ability to rebound toward their original shape and length after contraction

Words of Wisdom

About 40% to 50% of normal body weight is skeletal muscle, because it has a high water content. In addition, because skeletal muscle has a high metabolic rate and demand for energy and oxygen, it has a very rich blood supply, which causes it to bleed extensively when injured.

Components of Connective Tissue

A skeletal muscle is considered an organ of the muscular system, whose function is to contract and create a pulling force. Skeletal muscles are made up of hundreds of skeletal muscle cells bundled together to form muscle fibers, which are surrounded by a delicate sheath of connective tissue called the endomysium. The endomysium is the location of the metabolic exchange between muscle fibers and capillaries.[8] Muscle fibers are arranged in bundles called fascicles that provide a conduit for blood vessels and nerves. Each fascicle is covered with a layer of connective tissue called the perimysium, which holds the fascicles together. The entire skeletal muscle is sheathed in a tough covering of connective tissue called the epimysium. The epimysium, perimysium, and endomysium are continuous with one another. Recall that muscles are separated by muscular fascia or deep fascia, located outside the epimysium, which merges with the tissue of the tendon. The many layers of connective tissue that enclose and separate skeletal muscles allow a great deal of independent movement.

Muscle Attachments

Skeletal muscles form attachments to other structures either directly or indirectly. For example, a direct attachment is formed when extensions of the epimysium merge with the periosteum of a bone. When extensions of epimysium form tendons, an indirect attachment is made. Tendons cross joints to create a pulling force between two bones when a muscle contracts.

One end of a skeletal muscle—the origin—usually is fastened to a relatively immovable part (**origin**) at a moveable joint Figure 8-50. The other end—referred to as the **insertion**—connects to a movable part on the other side of the joint. As contraction occurs, the insertion is pulled toward the origin. More than one origin or insertion may be present, such as in the biceps brachii muscle of the arm. When this muscle contracts, the insertion is pulled toward its origin, which causes the forearm to flex at the elbow. The head of a muscle is the part closest to its origin.

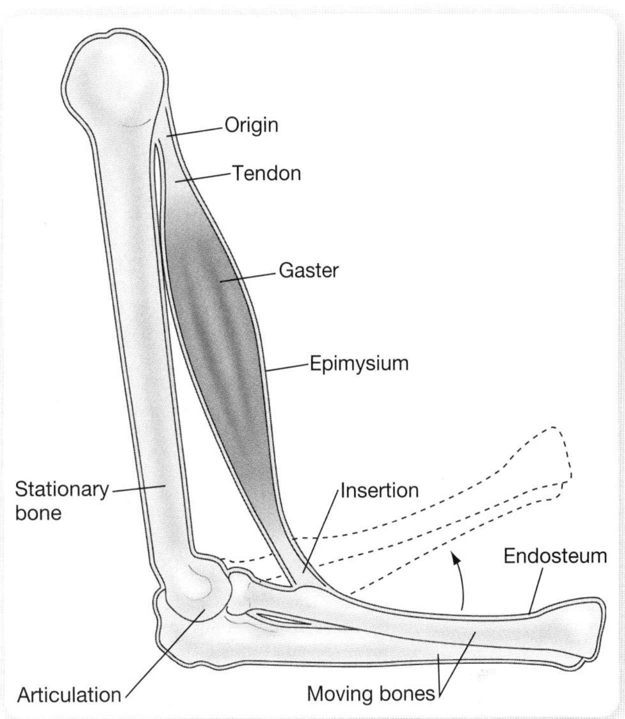

Figure 8-50 The parts of a muscle. The actual origin of the muscle shown is in the scapula. Origin on humerus is shown for clarity.

Muscle Function

Skeletal muscles usually function in groups, with the **nervous system** stimulating the desired muscles to perform the intended function. A muscle that contracts to provide most of the desired movement is called a prime mover or agonist. Other muscles, known as synergists, work with a prime mover to make its action more effective. For example, when you bend your elbow, the agonist muscles are the biceps, whereas the brachialis functions as a synergist.

Other muscles act as antagonists to prime movers. They cause movement in the opposite direction. In the above example, the triceps would be an antagonist to the biceps. Smooth body movement depends on antagonists relaxing while prime movers contract. Muscles may work together or opposite each other to control various movements. Figure 8-51 and Table 8-16 show the major muscles, their locations, and their functions.

Muscle Fibers

A single cell that contracts in response to stimulation and relaxes when the stimulation ceases is known as a skeletal muscle fiber. These fibers are thin, elongated cylinders with rounded ends. The cell membrane of a muscle cell

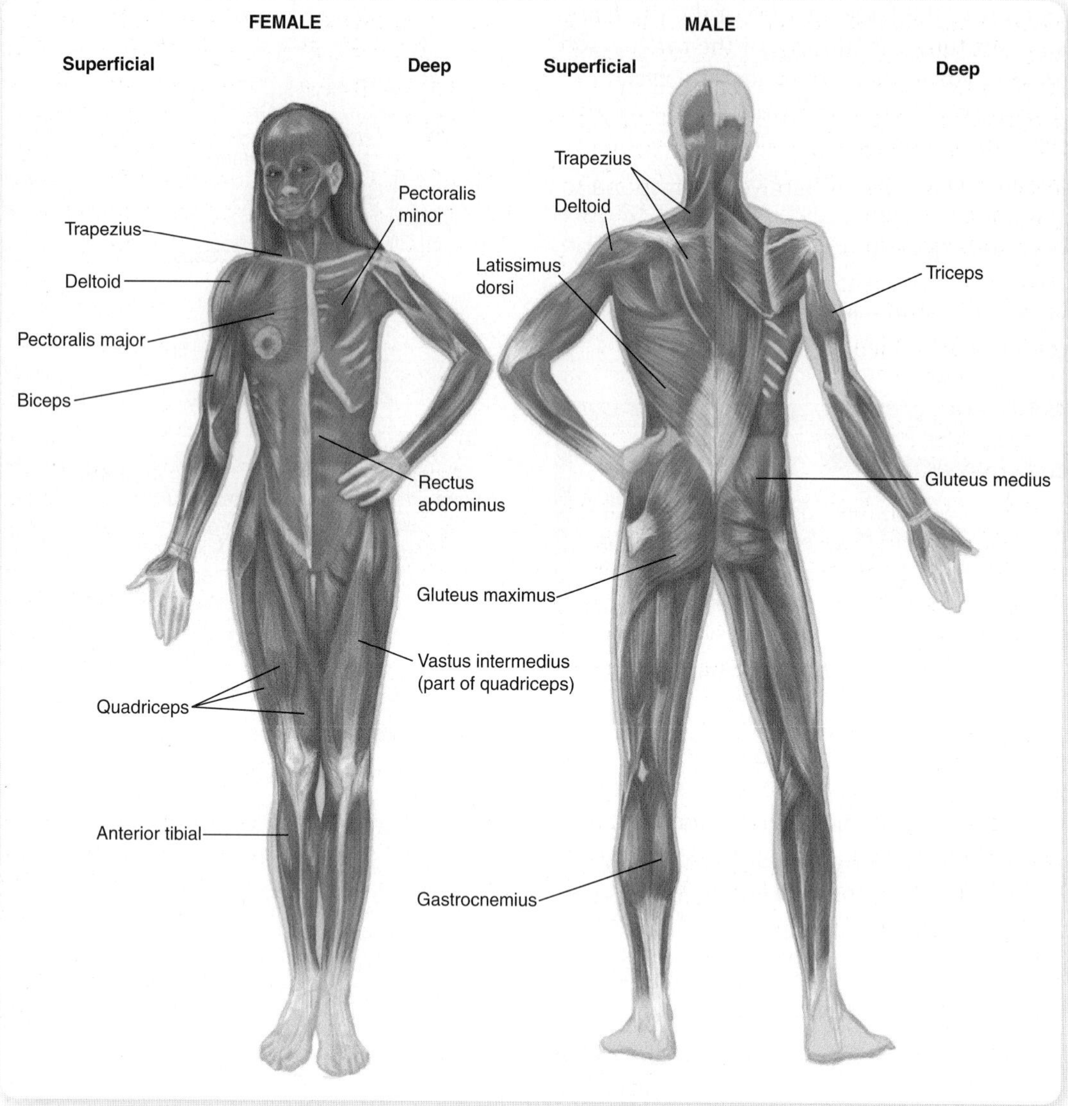

Figure 8-51 The major muscle groups.

Table 8-16 Location and Function of Major Muscles

Name of Muscle	Origin	Function
Biceps	Anterior, humerus	Flexes elbow
Triceps	Posterior, humerus	Extends elbow
Pectoralis	Anterior, thorax	Flexes and rotates arm
Latissimus dorsi	Posterior, thorax	Extends and rotates arm
Rectus abdominis	Anterior, abdomen	Flexes and rotates spine
Tibialis anterior	Anterior, tibia	Points toes toward head
Gastrocnemius	Posterior, tibia	Points toes away from head
Quadriceps (four separate muscles)	Anterior, femur	Extends knee
Biceps femoris	Posterior, femur	Flexes knee
Gluteus (three separate muscles)	Posterior, pelvis	Extends and rotates leg

is the sarcolemma and the cytoplasm of a muscle cell is the sarcoplasm. Sarcoplasmic reticulum, a special type of smooth endoplasmic reticulum that is found in smooth and striated muscle fibers, stores and releases calcium ions. Each muscle fiber is made up of long, cylindrical, threadlike myofibrils that are arranged parallel to each other. Myofibrils are made up of contractile units called sarcomeres. Muscles are basically considered to be collections of sarcomeres.

Sarcomeres are made up of myofilaments that are formed by threads of contractile proteins. Four types of proteins make up myofilaments: **actin**, **myosin**, **troponin**, and **tropomyosin**. Myosin molecules are made up of two protein strands with globe-shaped cross-bridges that project outward. Groups of many myosin molecules make up a myosin filament.

Actin molecules are globe-shaped with a binding site that attaches to myosin cross-bridges. Groups of many actin molecules twist in double strands (helixes) to form an actin filament, which includes troponin and tropomyosin. When at rest, the binding sites on actin molecules are covered by tropomyosin molecules, which are held in place by troponin molecules. A noncontractile protein called **titin** (connectin) is found in sarcomeres of cardiac and skeletal muscle. Titin is important for alignment of the thick myosin filaments in the sarcomere. *Dystrophin*, another noncontractile protein, holds the thin actin filaments to the sarcolemma and contributes to muscle fiber strength. Dystrophin deficiency has been established as one of the causes of muscular dystrophy, a group of genetically transmitted conditions that cause progressive weakness and loss of muscle mass.

The overlap of thick and thin filaments creates striations that can be seen in skeletal and cardiac muscle, which leads to the name striated muscle. The striation pattern of skeletal muscle fibers contain two main parts. The light bands (I bands) are made up of thin filaments of actin attached to Z lines. The dark bands (A bands) are made up of thick filaments of myosin that overlap thin filaments of actin. is A central region (H zone) is composed of thick filaments, with a thickened area (the M line) that consists of proteins holding them in place. Sarcomeres extend from one Z line to another Z line, as shown in **Figure 8-52**.

Inside the sarcoplasm of a muscle fiber, a network of channels surrounds each myofibril. These membranous channels form the sarcoplasmic reticulum. Transverse tubules (T-tubules) are other membranous channels extending inward and passing through the fiber. These tubules open to the outside of the muscle fiber, and contain extracellular fluid. Each tubule lies between enlarged structures called cisternae, near the point where actin and myosin filaments overlap. Together, the sarcoplasmic reticulum and T-tubules activate muscle contraction when stimulated.

To understand how muscles move, you must understand how they are stimulated, which is discussed in detail later in this chapter.

▶ Muscle Contraction

A **motor nerve** is made up of many nerve cells called **motor neurons**. A motor unit is a group of muscle fibers innervated by one motor neuron. When stimulated, the motor unit contracts as a whole. This contraction is a steady contraction throughout the muscle because motor neuron axons are present throughout the fleshy part of the muscle (the muscle belly). The impulse that stimulates muscle

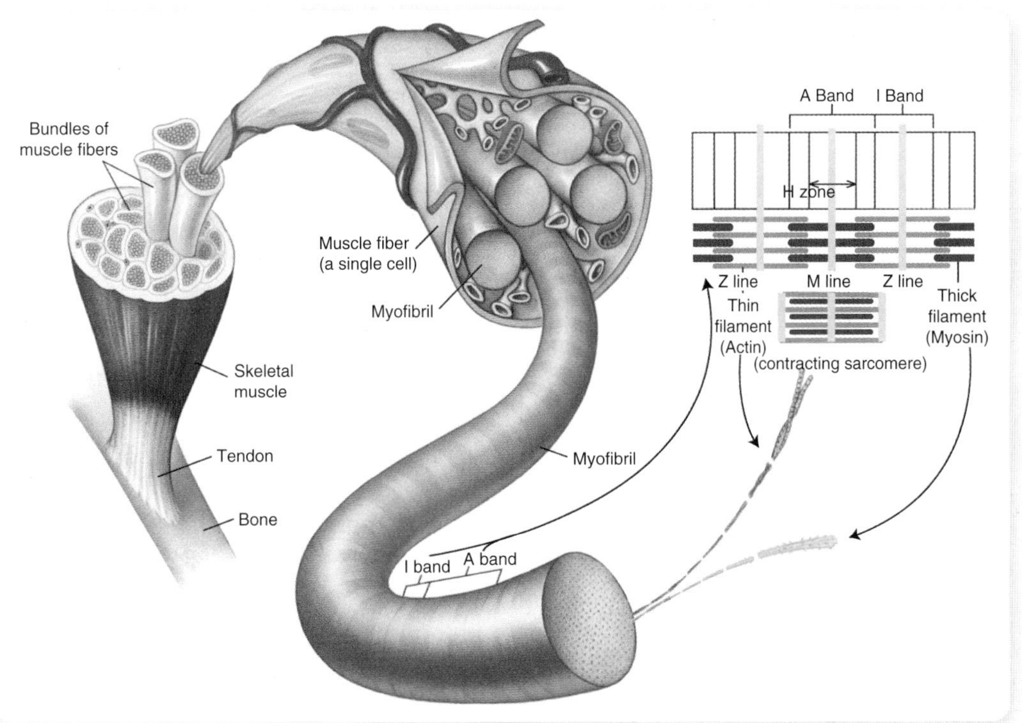

Figure 8-52 Details of the contractile machinery of the muscle cell.

contraction enters the muscle fibers at the **neuromuscular junction**. At this junction, the muscle fibers of the motor unit create the motor end plate, which has receptors for the neurotransmitter **acetylcholine (ACh)**. ACh stimulates skeletal muscle to contract.

Words of Wisdom

Myasthenia gravis is an autoimmune disorder in which the immune system attacks the ACh receptors on the motor end plate, resulting in muscular weakness or failure. A myasthenic crisis is a life-threatening presentation of this disorder in which weakness of the respiratory muscles can lead to respiratory failure or arrest.

The impulse that causes contraction of skeletal muscle is transmitted through motor neurons as a nerve impulse. These impulses are also known as **action potentials**, and are transmitted from one cell to another in the nervous system, causing each successive cell in the chain to fire. The process by which cells activate in response to the action potential is **depolarization**.

When the cell is at rest, ions are actively transported into and out of the cell to create an electrochemical gradient across the cell membrane, resulting in a **polarized** state. When the cell is activated by the release of a neurotransmitter, proteins in the cell wall open rapidly, allowing a rapid influx of ions that equalizes the charges on either side of the cell wall. When the charges are equal, the cell has depolarized, and the protein channels close. Then begins the process of **repolarization**, which again creates the electrochemical gradient so the cell can fire again.

ACh is synthesized in the cytoplasm of motor neurons and released into the synaptic clefts between motor neuron axons and motor end plates. It rapidly diffuses, binding to certain protein receptors in the muscle fiber membrane, and increasing permeability to sodium. These charged particles stimulate a muscle impulse that passes in many directions over the muscle fiber membrane. This impulse eventually reaches the sarcoplasmic reticulum.

The sarcoplasmic reticulum has a high calcium ion concentration, and it responds by making the cisternae membranes more permeable, diffusing calcium into the sarcoplasm. Calcium binds to troponin in the thin filaments, causing tropomyosin molecules to shift, thereby exposing the binding sites on the actin molecules. Because actin and myosin are chemically attracted to each other, the heads of the myosin molecules bind to the exposed actin molecules, creating cross-bridges. The actin and myosin filaments pull themselves toward each other, thereby shortening their length and causing contraction. Because the actin "slides" over the myosin during this process, this is known as the **sliding filament theory** of muscle contraction **Figure 8-53**. The cycle repeats as long as there is enough ATP for energy, and muscular stimulation occurs.

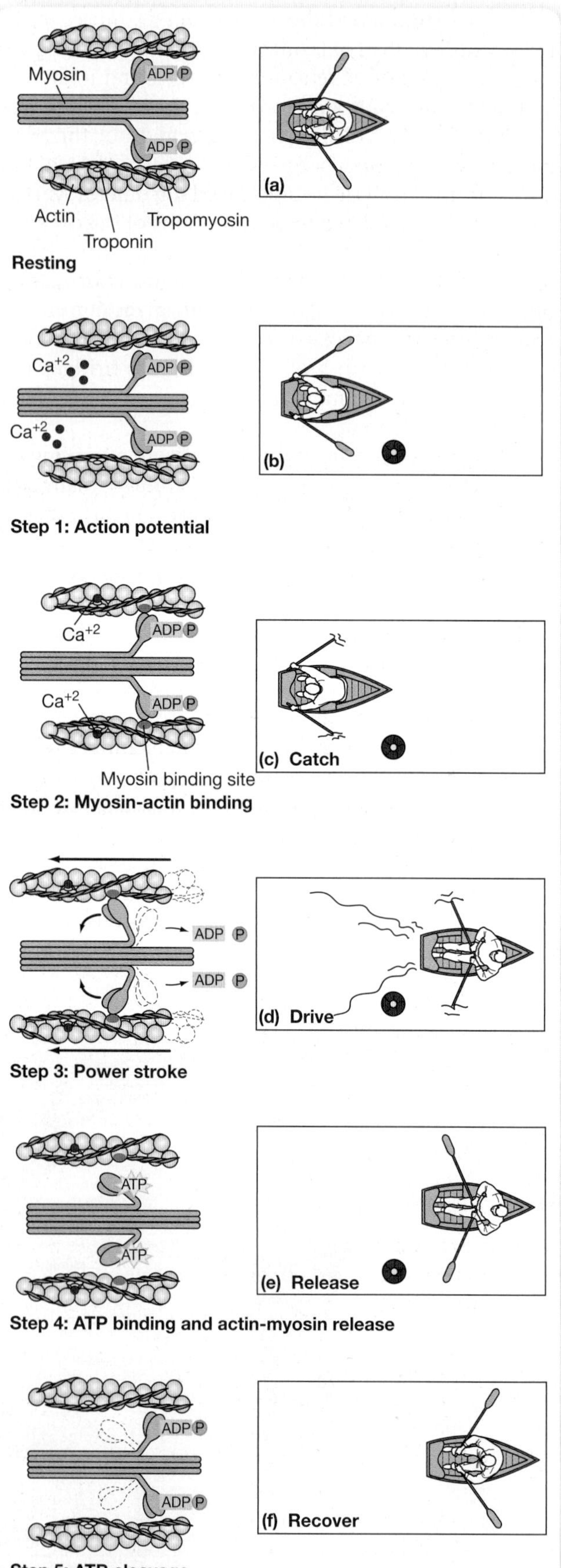

Figure 8-53 The sliding filament theory describes how muscle fibers contract.

Words of Wisdom

Muscle contraction requires energy. This energy is derived from the metabolism of glucose and results in the production of lactic acid (lactate). Lactic acid, in turn, is converted into carbon dioxide and water, a process that requires oxygen. For that reason, vigorous muscular activity is often followed by an increased ventilatory rate, which increases both the delivery of oxygen to, and removal of carbon dioxide from, the tissues.

Muscle Tone

Skeletal muscles cause unique movements based on the type of joint they attach to and where the attachment points are located. Muscle tone is the amount of tension that is in a muscle at any one point in time. It is the result of a constant state of partial contractions in the body. While some motor units contract, others relax. Muscle tone in the skeletal muscles helps maintain balance and body position. In the maintenance of posture, muscle tone allows the head to stay upright and the back to remain straight.

Words of Wisdom

In smooth muscle, tone maintains the size of the blood vessels and aids in digestion.

Muscle Relaxation

Muscle relaxation is caused by the decomposition of ACh via the enzyme **acetylcholinesterase**. This process prevents a single nerve impulse from stimulating the muscle fiber continuously. When the stimulus ceases, calcium ions are transported back to the sarcoplasmic reticulum. Without calcium, the actin and myosin linkages break, and the muscle relaxes.

Energy Sources

Muscular contraction requires ATP and continues as long as ACh is released. Muscle fibers have just enough ATP for short-term contraction. ATP must be regenerated when fibers are active, using existing ATP molecules in the cells. ATP is regenerated from adenosine diphosphate (ADP) and phosphate. Creatine phosphate is an organic compound in muscle tissue that can store and provide energy for muscle contraction with high-energy phosphate bonds. Creatine phosphate is between four and six times more abundant in muscle fibers than ATP; however, it does not directly supply energy. Rather, it stores excess energy from the mitochondria in the phosphate bonds.

When ATP breaks down, energy from creatine phosphate is transferred to ADP molecules to convert them back into ATP. Creatine phosphate stores are exhausted rapidly when muscles are active; therefore, the muscles use cellular respiration of glucose as energy to synthesize ATP.

Oxygen Use and Debt

Oxygen is required for the breakdown of glucose in the mitochondria. RBCs carry oxygen, bound to hemoglobin molecules. **Hemoglobin** is the pigment that makes blood appear red. One hemoglobin molecule reversibly binds with four oxygen molecules. The pigment **myoglobin** is synthesized in the muscles to give skeletal muscles their red-brown color. Myoglobin can also combine with oxygen and temporarily store it to reduce muscular requirements for continuous blood supply during contraction.

When skeletal muscles are used for a minute or more, anaerobic respiration is required for energy. In one type of anaerobic respiration, glucose is broken down via glycolysis to yield pyruvic acid, which reacts by producing lactic acid. Recall that lactic acid can accumulate in muscles, but diffuses in the bloodstream, reaching the liver, where it is synthesized into glucose.

When a person exercises strenuously, oxygen is used mostly to synthesize ATP. As lactic acid increases, an oxygen debt develops. Oxygen debt is equivalent to the amount of oxygen that liver cells require to convert the lactic acid into glucose, as well as the amount needed by muscle cells to restore ATP and creatine phosphate levels.

It may take several hours for the body to convert lactic acid back into glucose. Muscles may experience a change in their metabolic activity as exercise levels change. Increased exercise raises the capacity of the muscles for glycolysis. Aerobic exercise increases the capacity of the muscles for aerobic respiration. This process is summarized in Table 8-17.

Table 8-17 Changes in Muscular Metabolism

Type of Exercise	Pathway Needed	Production of ATP	Result
Low to moderate intensity: blood flow provides enough oxygen for the needs of the cell	Glycolysis, which leads to formation of pyruvic acid and aerobic respiration	For skeletal muscle, 36 molecules of ATP per glucose	Exhalation of carbon dioxide
High intensity: oxygen supply is not enough for the needs of the cell	Glycolysis, which leads to formation of lactic acid	2 molecules of ATP per glucose	Buildup of lactic acid

Words of Wisdom

Skeletal muscles are profoundly affected by the amount of training and work to which they are subjected. Unused muscles tend to atrophy (shrink or waste away), whereas physical training promotes hypertrophy (increase in size).

Muscle Fatigue

Prolonged exercise may cause a muscle to become unable to contract. This condition is called fatigue, and it may also occur because of interruption of muscular blood supply, or occasionally a lack of ACh in the motor neuron axons. The accumulation of lactic acid is the usual cause of muscular fatigue. As lactic acid lowers pH levels, muscle fibers cannot respond to stimulation. When a muscle becomes fatigued and cramps, it experiences a sustained, involuntary contraction. Though not fully understood, muscle cramps appear to be caused by changes in the extracellular fluid surrounding muscle fibers and motor neurons.

Heat Production

Muscles need a great deal of energy to contract. This energy is delivered in the form of ATP. The energy required by muscular contraction is developed during the breakdown of ATP (breaking of bonds). One of the by-products of this breakdown is heat, which is used to maintain a normal body temperature. If the body temperature drops below a set point, then the nervous system stimulates the muscles to start shivering (a form of rapid contractions). Shivering, in turn, generates heat used to elevate the body temperature.

The Nervous System

The nervous system is perhaps the most complex organ system within the human body. It is composed of two major structures, the brain and the spinal cord, and thousands of nerves that allow every part of the body to communicate. This system is responsible for fundamental functions such as controlling breathing, pulse rate, and blood pressure. However, the true complexity of the nervous system is evident in its ability to allow higher-level functions such as reading a book, enjoying music, having a discussion with a friend, and watching television. All of these activities require the brain to engage memory, thought, intelligence, and understanding.

The main functions of the nervous system include the following:

- Monitoring of internal and external environments
- Integration of sensory information
- Coordination of voluntary and involuntary responses

The major structures of the nervous system are divided into two main categories: the **central nervous system (CNS)**, which is responsible for thought, perception, feeling, and autonomic body functions, and the **peripheral nervous system (PNS)**. The PNS consists of the somatic nervous system and the autonomic nervous system. The **somatic nervous system** is the part of the PNS that regulates activities over which there is voluntary control, such as walking, talking, and writing. The **autonomic nervous system (ANS)** controls the many body functions that occur without voluntary control. These activities include body functions such as digestion, dilation and constriction of blood vessels, sweating, fight-or-flight response, and all other involuntary actions that are necessary for basic body functions. Thus, the nervous system as a whole can be divided anatomically into the CNS and PNS and functionally into somatic (voluntary) and autonomic (involuntary) components Figure 8-54.

▶ Neurons and Impulse Transmission

The nervous system is composed of specialized tissue that conducts electrical impulses between the brain and the rest of the body. Recall that neural tissue contains two basic types of cells: neuroglia and neurons.

Neuroglia

Neuroglia are supporting cells that form about half the mass of the brain.[9] They perform the following basic functions: (1) provide a supporting skeleton for neural tissue, (2) isolate and protect the cell membranes of neurons, (3) regulate the composition of interstitial fluid, (4) defend neural tissue from pathogens, and (5) aid in the repair of injury. Neuroglia can divide, whereas most neurons cannot. Types of neuroglia include the following Figure 8-55:

- **Astrocytes.** Found in the CNS, these are the most numerous type of neuroglia. They attach to neurons and blood capillaries of the brain and provide nourishment to neurons by picking up glucose from the blood, converting it to lactic acid, and passing it to the neurons to which they are connected.[10] Astrocytes form tight sheaths around the brain capillaries and participate in recycling some neurotransmitter substances after their release.
- **Ependymal cells.** Found in the CNS, these line fluid-filled cavities, such as the ventricular system of the brain. Some ependymal cells secrete CSF; others have cilia that serve to circulate fluid within the cavities they line.
- **Microglial cells.** Found throughout the CNS, these phagocytize bacterial cells and cellular debris.
- **Oligodendrocytes.** Found in the CNS, these help hold nerve fibers together and form insulating myelin sheaths around axons within the brain and spinal cord.
- **Schwann cells.** Found in the PNS, these manufacture myelin.
- Satellite cells. Found in the PNS, these have similar functions to the astrocytes of the CNS.[9]

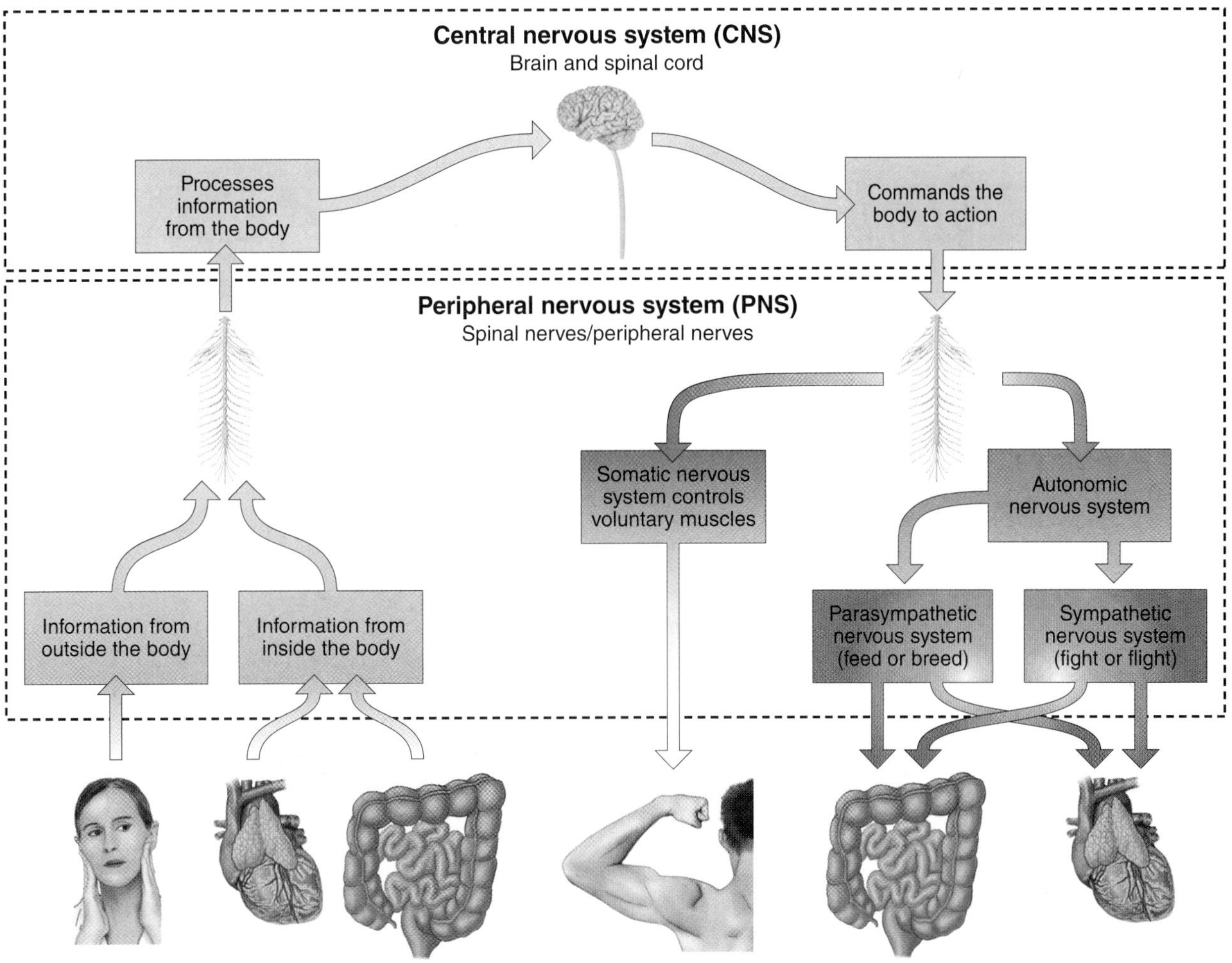

Central nervous system (CNS)
Brain and spinal cord
Processes information from the body
Commands the body to action
Peripheral nervous system (PNS)
Spinal nerves/peripheral nerves
Somatic nervous system controls voluntary muscles
Autonomic nervous system
Information from outside the body
Information from inside the body
Parasympathetic nervous system (feed or breed)
Sympathetic nervous system (fight or flight)

Figure 8-54 Organization of the nervous system. The brain and spinal cord work together to process information in the form of signals generated in response to stimuli from both inside and outside the body. The peripheral nervous system commands the body to act, and the autonomic nervous system oversees involuntary responses.

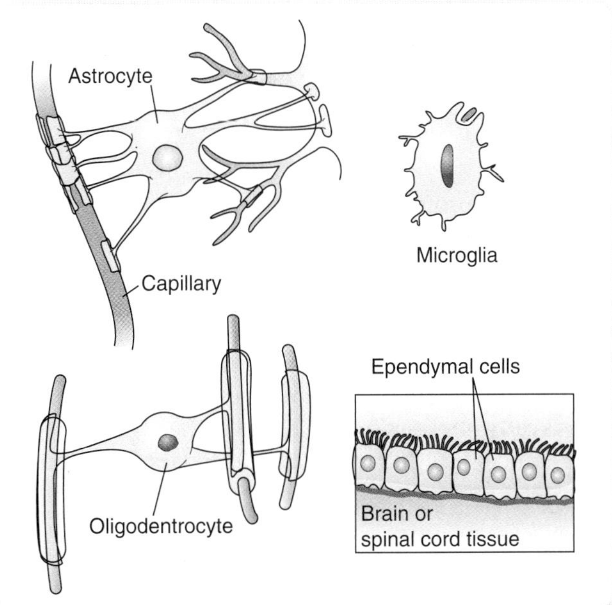

Figure 8-55 Examples of neuroglia that are found in the central nervous system.

Neurons

To understand how muscles move, you must first understand how they are stimulated. Neurons are nerve cells and are the fundamental element of the nervous system. They are present throughout the body. Groups of nerve cells are bundled together to form nerve fibers. Groups of nerve fibers are bundled together to form a nerve, which is tissue that connects the nervous system with body parts or organs.

The neurons that compose a nerve are supplied with oxygen and nutrients from the bloodstream by blood vessels also contained in the nerve. Nerves are information highways. Impulses travel to and from the brain and spinal cord along these highways.

Neurons are composed of three basic parts: dendrites, the cell body, and the axon. **Dendrites** are short, branchlike projections that conduct impulses from nearby cells toward the cell body. Essential cell functions, such as energy production and waste removal, are performed within the nucleus of the cell body. After being conducted through the cell body, the impulse exits the neuron through the

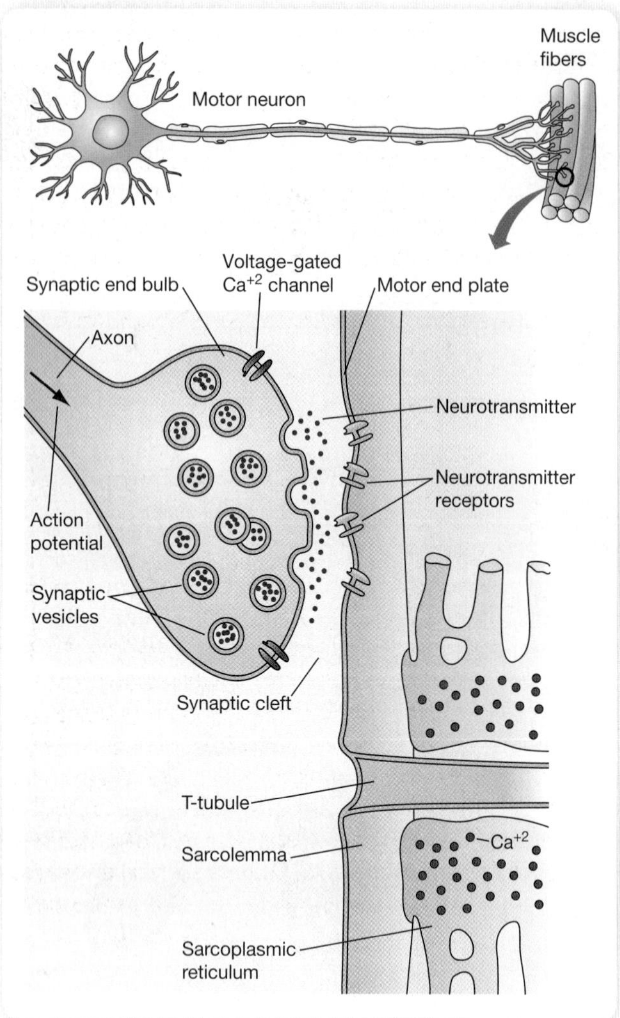

Figure 8-56 A synapse or neuroeffector junction.

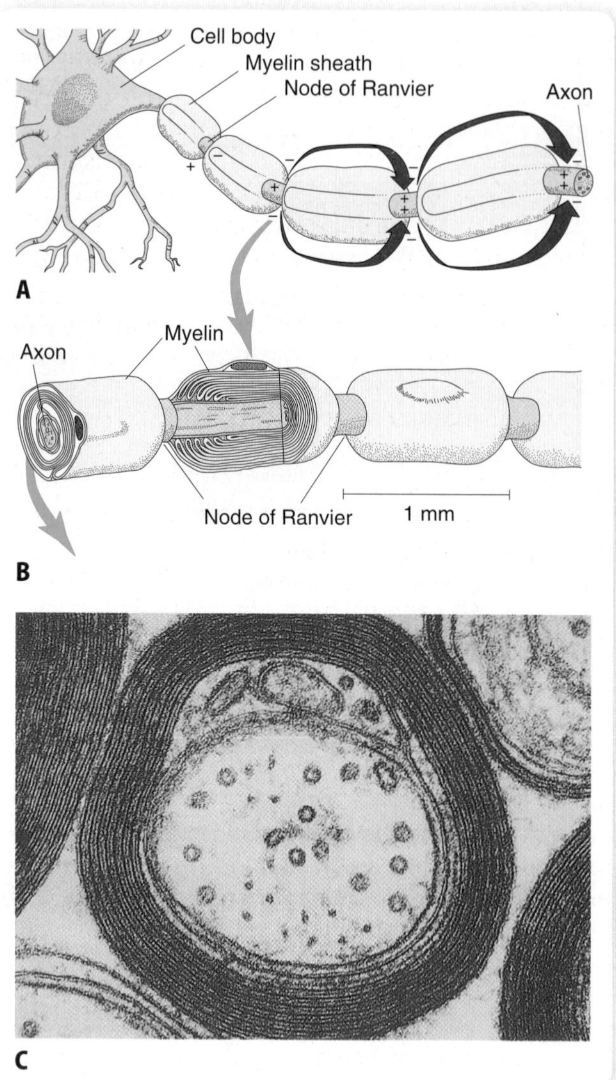

Figure 8-57 A myelinated nerve. **A.** The myelin sheath allows impulses to jump from node to node, greatly accelerating the rate of transmission. **B.** The node of Ranvier. **C.** A transmission electron micrograph shows a cross section of an axon with a myelin sheath.

axon. An **axon** is another projection that sends the signal from the cell body to target tissues or other neurons **Figure 8-56**. Neurons may have dozens of dendrites but usually only one axon. An axon is long and highly branched, allowing it to link with many other cells.

The axon may or may not be wrapped in myelin. Myelin is manufactured by oligodendrocytes in the CNS and by Schwann cells in the PNS. Because myelin is white, this appearance leads to the term **white matter**. Myelinated axons form the white matter in the brain, **brainstem** (which connects the brain to the spinal cord), and spinal cord. Myelin allows the cell to transmit its signal consistently, without "shorting out" or losing electricity to surrounding fluids and tissues. Myelin also increases the speed of conduction. Gaps between the myelinated regions are called nodes of Ranvier **Figure 8-57**. These nodes speed impulse transmission through the axon because the impulses cannot travel through the insulating myelin, but rather jump from node to node as they travel along the axon (saltatory conduction). Axons without myelin sheaths are termed gray matter. Because these axons lack the myelin sheath, impulses travel slower than they do in white matter. An axon terminal is the portion of the axon where the neurotransmitters are manufactured. Dendrites project off the nucleus, but they carry signals from other cells toward the nucleus.

Nerve cells are classified by the direction in which they transmit impulses. Afferent (sensory) nerves carry impulses from sensory receptors in the internal organs and skin to the brain and spinal cord. Efferent (motor) nerves carry impulses from the CNS to the organs, muscles, and glands. Interneurons carry impulses from sensory neurons to motor neurons.

Synapses and Synaptic Transmission

Dendrites and axons of adjacent nerve cells are not in physical contact with each other. Rather, they are separated by a small gap called a **synapse**. This slight gap between each cell allows for a far greater level of fine control than if each cell were in direct contact with the next. A synapse is made up of three main parts. The first is the presynaptic plasma membrane (or terminal), which is the membrane on the signal-passing side of the synapse. The second part is the **synaptic cleft** (synaptic gap), which is a small, fluid-filled space (see Figure 8-56). The third part of the synapse is the postsynaptic plasma membrane, which is the membrane on the signal-receiving side of the synapse.

The two types of synapses are chemical and electrical. Most neurons use **neurotransmitters** to transmit their signal across the synapse to other neurons. Because a synapse may exist between a neuron and a muscle or between a neuron and a gland, neurotransmitters also may be used to transmit a nerve signal across the synapse to muscle cells or to gland cells. Electrical synapses occur between cardiac muscle cells and between some smooth muscle cells where the presynaptic and postsynaptic cell membranes are joined by channels called gap junctions. Because gap junctions are capable of passing electric current, the nerve impulse is able to spread rapidly to neighboring cells.

At the end of the axon of the presynaptic (signal-passing) neuron are tiny bulges called synaptic knobs or synaptic terminals. Within each synaptic knob are many small sacs called **synaptic vesicles** that contain neurotransmitter molecules. When the presynaptic neuron releases its neurotransmitters, they diffuse across the synaptic cleft to receptor sites on the postsynaptic (signal-receiving) plasma membrane, to which the released neurotransmitters bind. The released neurotransmitter may be either excitatory (initiating an impulse on the postsynaptic side) or inhibitory (stopping the impulse at that point). As a paramedic, you may administer a variety of medications to enhance, slow, or even stop these neurotransmissions.

The following process details how transmission of nervous impulses occurs. When the cell is at its resting potential, greater concentrations of extracellular sodium and intracellular potassium are available. Also in the cell is the negatively charged ion chloride. This ion results in a relative negative charge inside the cell compared with the outside. As with the muscle cell, depolarization of the nerve cell results from the opening of the sodium channels and the influx of sodium into the cell. This influx creates a positive charge, causing an action potential inside the cell. This process creates a wave of depolarization along the nerve fiber as each cell depolarizes when stimulated by the previous neuron. Repolarization occurs as potassium leaves the cell in an attempt to restore the negative charge inside the cell. Repolarization is complete when the sodium-potassium pump restores sodium and potassium to their original positions. As the wave of depolarization continues, it eventually reaches the end of the nerve fiber at the synaptic cleft. The end may be the junction of an axon and the dendrite of another neuron, or the neuromuscular junction where the nerve impulse stimulates muscular contraction.

Neurotransmitters

Many neurotransmitters are present within the brain and throughout the body. These substances are grouped by categories: ACh, biogenic amines, amino acids, and neuropeptides (Table 8-18).

Neurotransmitters of the somatic nervous system include ACh; neurotransmitters of the ANS include ACh and **norepinephrine**; and neurotransmitters of the CNS include dopamine, serotonin, and gammaaminobutyric acid, among others. After the neurotransmitter is released from the presynaptic (signal-passing) terminal, it binds with receptor sites on the postsynaptic (signal-receiving) membrane, triggering an impulse that is propagated in the manner previously described. The neurotransmitters are quickly deactivated by substances such as acetylcholinesterase (which breaks down ACh) and monoamine oxidase (which breaks down monoamines such as norepinephrine). After being broken down, these substances are reabsorbed by vesicles in the presynaptic terminal, where the neurotransmitters are recreated.

▶ Central Nervous System

As discussed previously, the CNS consists of the brain and the spinal cord. The CNS is responsible for the integration and coordination of sensory information and motor responses.

Protection

Because the structures of the CNS can be easily damaged with potentially devastating results, the body has four

Table 8-18 Examples of Neurotransmitters

Category	Examples
Amino acids	Gammaaminobutyric acid (GABA), glutamate, glycine
Biogenic amines	Dopamine, epinephrine, histamine, norepinephrine, serotonin
Choline esters	Acetylcholine (ACh)
Neuropeptides	Adrenocorticotropin, cholecystokinin, dynorphins, endorphins, enkephalins, glucose-dependent insulinotropic peptide, glucagon, neurotensin, oxytocin, secretin, substance P, thyrotropin-releasing hormone, vasopressin, vasoactive intestinal peptide

protective mechanisms in place to protect it—bone, meninges, CSF, and the blood-brain barrier. The brain has an additional protective layer, called the scalp.

Scalp. The scalp consists of the following layers, given in descending order:

- Skin, with hair
- Subcutaneous tissue that contains major scalp veins that bleed profusely when lacerated
- Galea aponeurotica, a tendon expansion that connects the frontal and occipital muscles of the cranium
- Loose connective tissue (alveolar tissue) that is easily stripped from the layer beneath in so-called scalping injuries. The looseness of the alveolar layer also provides room for blood to build up between the scalp and skull bone after blunt trauma.
- Periosteum, the dense fibrous membrane covering the surface of bones.

Bone. Bone provides physical protection for the CNS. The brain is protected from mechanical injury by the cranium, and the spinal cord is protected by the vertebral column.

Meninges. The **meninges** form a covering over the brain and spinal cord. Three distinct connective tissue layers compose the meninges: the **dura mater**, the arachnoid, and the **pia mater** Figure 8-58. In common usage the mater is often dropped, and the three layers are referred to simply as the dura, arachnoid, and pia.

The dura is the outermost, thickest, and toughest of the three layers (*dura mater* means "tough mother" in Latin). The dura has two layers: a parietal (outer) layer and a visceral (inner; from the Greek *viscera,* meaning "guts") layer. The parietal layer is tightly adhered to the cranial vault and serves as the periosteum of the inner surface of the skull, and the visceral layer lies over the CNS. In some areas of the CNS, the parietal and visceral layers of the dura are fused. The dura has two projections. The falx cerebri is a vertical projection that separates the two hemispheres of the brain. The tentorium cerebelli, or **tentorium**, is a horizontal projection of the dura that separates the cerebellum from the cerebrum. The temporal lobes are positioned on an opening in the tentorium (tentorial notch, or tentorial incisura). This opening allows passage of the midbrain and oculomotor nerves. These structures play an important role in increased intracranial pressure (ICP) and herniation of the brain. Above the dura is a potential space referred to as the epidural space. The meningeal arteries run in the periosteal layer of the dura. If one of these vessels is injured, such as with an injury to the skull, then bleeding can occur between the dura and the skull, opening up the potential epidural space and causing an epidural hematoma.

The arachnoid, the second meningeal layer, is semitransparent, thin, delicate, and weblike (the Greek word *arachne* means "spider's web"). The dura and arachnoid layers end at the level of the second sacral vertebra.[11] The subdural space, located between the dura and the arachnoid, contains a small amount of serous fluid. Collection of blood in the subdural space, usually resulting from tearing of a cerebral vein, causes a subdural hematoma.

The innermost meningeal layer, the pia mater ("tender mother" in Latin), is delicate and tightly adheres to the CNS. The pia that adheres to the brain contains a network of small blood vessels. The pia that surrounds the spinal cord is less vascular. The **subarachnoid space**, located between the arachnoid and pia, has a vast network of cerebral arteries and veins running through it that are held against the pia by sheets and strands of connective tissue before penetrating the brain.[12] The meninges float in CSF.

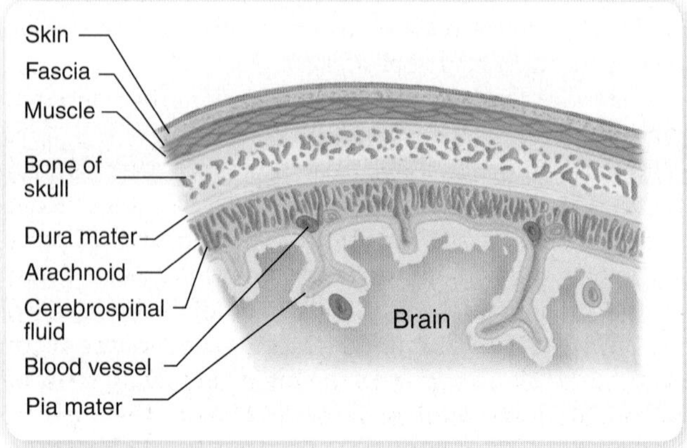

Figure 8-58 The meninges.

> **Words of Wisdom**
>
> A tip to help you remember the names of the meningeal layers is to think of them as a PAD from the inside out, as follows:
>
> **P** Pia mater (innermost layer)
> **A** Arachnoid (middle layer)
> **D** Dura mater (outermost layer)

Cerebrospinal Fluid. The brain contains four hollow, fluid-filled cavities called ventricles. Each cerebral hemisphere contains a lateral ventricle, which communicates with the third ventricle located in the diencephalon, which in turn communicates with the fourth ventricle of the pons and medulla oblongata in the brainstem.

Each ventricle houses a specialized spongelike structure called the **choroid plexus.** CSF is secreted within by the brain by the choroid plexuses. The choroid plexus is the so-called kidney of the brain because it stabilizes the composition of CSF, just as the kidney stabilizes the composition of blood plasma.[13] The cerebral ventricles are linked by small openings that allow CSF to flow easily among them. CSF circulates through the ventricles and then leaves the fourth ventricle through three openings to flow through the subarachnoid spaces of the brain and spinal cord where it eventually enters the venous blood system.

The total volume of CSF in adults is about 155 mL; 30 mL is found within the cerebral ventricles and about 125 mL in the subarachnoid space.[14] CSF is constantly produced and reabsorbed with the total amount of CSF being replaced every 6 to 8 hours.[15] It is important that CSF be produced and reabsorbed at the same rate to maintain a relatively constant pressure within the skull. Excess CSF is eliminated through the venous sinuses located in the folds of the dura in the cranium.

Because the brain and spinal cord essentially float in the CSF, one of its main functions is to absorb outside forces that might otherwise be transmitted to the CNS, causing damage. The CSF also plays a role in the delivery of nutrients and elimination of waste products, and it helps to maintain a constant ionic environment.

Blood-Brain Barrier. The brain must have a stable chemical environment for optimum functioning. Endothelial cells that line capillaries in many parts of the body have openings between them that enable the passage of substances by diffusion. In contrast, endothelial cells in the walls of the capillaries leading to the brain form tight junctions. Extensions of astrocytes, which are one type of neuroglia, wrap around these capillaries to provide additional protection. The combination of the two forms a barrier (the **blood-brain barrier**) between the blood within brain capillaries and the extracellular fluid in brain tissue. This barrier requires substances to pass through it by diffusion or active transport, rather than between the cells. Water-soluble substances such as water, glucose, and essential amino acids pass easily. Most lipid-soluble molecules such as alcohol and gases such as oxygen, carbon dioxide, and volatile anesthetics can also diffuse easily across the barrier. Substances that may be damaging to CNS function such as bacteria, viruses, and many pharmaceuticals are normally not permitted to cross the blood-brain barrier; however, the barrier may be compromised by diseases such as encephalitis, multiple sclerosis, stroke, or tumors.

Words of Wisdom

Whereas the protective qualities of the blood-brain barrier are generally beneficial, they can present a problem when the delivery of therapeutic medications is needed to treat conditions such as Alzheimer disease, multiple sclerosis, and infections and cancers of the CNS. To bypass the blood-brain barrier, medications are sometimes administered directly into the subarachnoid space (intrathecal injection) to enhance delivery of the drug into the brain. The development of techniques to open the blood-brain barrier and the development of therapeutic agents with improved barrier penetrability are areas of ongoing research.

Brain

The **brain** is the primary organ of the nervous system. At birth, the typical brain contains about 100 billion nerve cells. This number declines with age. Each neuron may have thousands or tens of thousands of synapses. The brain occupies 80% of the cranial vault and is the control center for nearly all the functions of the body. The remaining intracranial contents include cerebral blood (12%) and CSF (8%).

Words of Wisdom

Because the brain, CSF, and blood are enclosed within the bony cranium and the relatively inelastic dura, an increase in the size (volume) of the brain, any increase in the amount of CSF, or blood can lead to a marked increase in pressure within the system (that is, intracranial pressure or ICP) unless there is a corresponding decrease in the volume of one of the other components. Increased ICP can disrupt brain **perfusion** (circulation of blood within an organ or tissue) and function. The many possible causes of increased ICP include bleeding into the brain, fluid around the brain, swelling within the brain secondary to injury, increased pressure within the brain because of a mass (eg, tumor), increased CSF production, or an obstruction to the flow or absorption of CSF.

The brain accounts for only 2% of the total body weight, yet it is the most metabolically active and perfusion-sensitive organ in the body. To function properly, the brain must receive a constant supply of oxygen and nutrients, such as glucose. The brain receives about 15% of the *cardiac output* (CO), or the amount of blood that is pumped by the ventricles in 1 minute. The brain also metabolizes 25% of the body's glucose (approximately 60 mg/min) and consumes 20% of the total body oxygen (45 to 50 L/min). Because the brain has no effective means of storing oxygen or glucose, it is sensitive to decreases in glucose, oxygen, and blood flow through it. As a result, the brain continually manipulates the physiology as needed to guarantee that a ready supply of oxygen and glucose are available. If blood supply to the brain is disrupted, then the patient may undergo changes in mental status and vital signs.

The brain consists of four primary areas: the cerebrum, diencephalon, brainstem, and cerebellum **Figure 8-59**. The brain and much of the spinal cord receives their arterial blood supply by means of the internal carotid arteries and the vertebral arteries. The vertebral arteries form the basilar artery. Branches of the internal carotid arteries and the basilar artery form a circle of arteries at the base of the brain called the circle of Willis. The internal carotid arteries provide about 80% of the blood supply to the brain, supplying most of the cerebrum and much of the diencephalon. The vertebral system provides the remaining 20%, supplying the brainstem and cerebellum, as well as parts of the diencephalon, spinal cord, and occipital and temporal lobes.

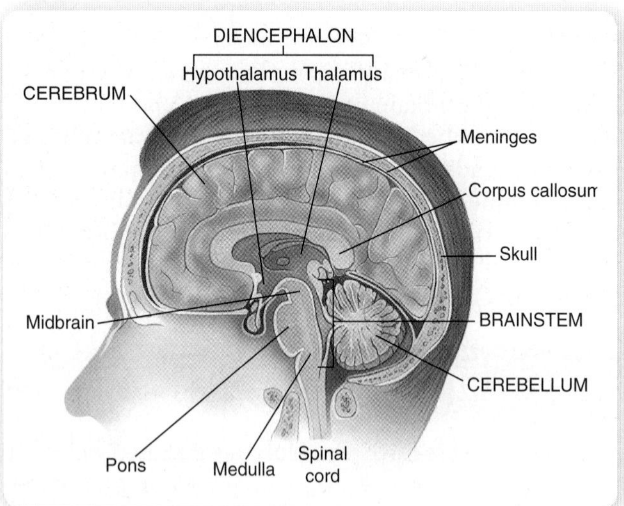

Figure 8-59 The major structures and landmarks of the brain.

Venous drainage of the brain occurs by means of a series of superficial and deep veins that contain no valves. These vessels empty into venous sinuses located in the folds of the dura and into a network of veins around the base of the brain. These veins empty into the internal jugular veins at the base of the skull and ultimately join the general circulation.

Cerebral Blood Flow. Blood flow through the brain (cerebral blood flow) depends on cerebral perfusion pressure. **Cerebral perfusion pressure (CPP)** is the pressure of the blood filling the arteries of the brain. CPP is determined by the difference between mean arterial blood pressure (MAP) and ICP.

$$\text{CPP} = \text{MAP} - \text{ICP}$$

Pulse pressure is the difference between the systolic blood pressure and diastolic blood pressure (DBP). MAP can be closely approximated by adding the DBP plus one-third of the pulse pressure. The MAP is an indicator of how well the brain is being supplied with nutrients, such as oxygen and glucose.

$$\text{MAP} = \text{DBP} + 1/3\ \text{PP}$$

The normal ICP is between 5 mm Hg and 15 mm Hg, and the normal MAP is between 85 mm Hg and 95 mm Hg. This results in a normal CPP of 70 mm Hg to 90 mm Hg. At these pressures, the brain receives sufficient blood flow, with associated oxygen and glucose, to meet its metabolic needs. Cerebral blood flow (CBF) and therefore CPP is affected by the diameter of the vessels in the brain.

A mechanism called autoregulation refers to the ability of the brain to regulate the diameter of the vessels within the brain (and therefore CBF) in response to a wide range of mean arterial pressures. The brain is able to autoregulate and ensures adequate CBF when the CPP is between 60 mm Hg and 160 mm Hg. CPP of less than 60 mm Hg results in inadequate perfusion of the brain, whereas pressures greater than 160 mm Hg result in hypertensive encephalopathy. Increased ICP disrupts autoregulation by decreasing CPP based on the mathematical formula above. As CPP decreases, blood vessels within the brain dilate. This increases the volume of blood in the brain. As a result, ICP increases. This further decreases CPP, which leads to further cerebral vasodilation, and so on.

In an effort to combat increasing ICP, the body invokes the Monro-Kellie doctrine. As stated previously, the cranial vault is a rigid, nondistensible box that is filled by the brain, CSF, and cerebral blood. In response to an expanding intracranial mass, the body attempts to regulate ICP by expelling CSF and venous blood out of the cranial vault. This creates more space for the mass and keeps ICP within normal limits during the early stages of the expanding mass, which can result in subtle signs and symptoms that are easily missed without a high index of suspicion. As with all compensatory mechanisms, there is a limit to the effectiveness of this process. At the point where no additional CSF or venous blood can be expelled, ICP will increase exponentially.

After the ICP begins to rise, the body attempts to maintain CPP by increasing the MAP. This process is evidenced by not only an increased blood pressure (both systolic and diastolic), but also by a widening pulse pressure.

Other factors also interfere with CPP. For example, too much carbon dioxide in the blood causes cerebral vasodilation. This results in increased cerebral blood volume, which leads to increased ICP, and so on. Hypotension results in a decreased MAP, which causes a decrease in the CPP. As stated previously, when the MAP drops to 60 mm Hg or less, CBF begins to decrease. This decrease leads to cerebral vasodilation, and the cycle repeats itself.

When swelling or bleeding occurs in the brain, the brain sends out signals requesting more oxygen. This process triggers a vicious cycle. The more blood that enters the brain, the more oxygen it requires, which in turn results in increased swelling. If the ICP gets too high, then the brain tissue has nowhere to go except through the tentorium incisura, foramen magnum, or both.

Cerebrum. The **cerebrum** is the largest part of the brain, making up about three-fourths of the volume of the brain. The surface of the cerebrum is composed of a thin layer of folded gray matter known as the **cerebral cortex**. White matter lies just beneath the gray matter and makes up the bulk of the cerebrum. Additional areas of gray matter called the **basal ganglia** or basal nuclei are scattered throughout the white matter with connections to other areas of the CNS including the cerebral cortex, cerebellum, and thalamus. The basal ganglia are involved with control of the body's motor tone, and automatic movements (eg, swallowing saliva, blinking), specific body movement sequences associated with skeletal muscle activity (eg, the arms swinging alternating with the legs during walking). The basal ganglia may play a role in thinking and learning.

The cerebral cortex folds onto itself forming ridges called gyri to maximize surface area. Gyri are separated by grooves that are called sulci if they are shallow or fissures if they are deep. Although the cerebrum is partially divided into right and left hemispheres by the longitudinal fissure, a large band of white matter called the **corpus callosum** provides a communication pathway between them.

Each cerebral hemisphere can be subdivided into five lobes—insula, frontal, temporal, parietal, and occipital. Four of the lobes have the same name as the skull bone that lies over it (eg, frontal, parietal, occipital, and temporal) **Figure 8-60**. The insula, also called the central lobe or the Island of Reil, is covered by parts of the frontal, parietal, and temporal lobes in the lateral fissure. The primary functions of each lobe are summarized in **Table 8-19**.

The frontal lobe extends from the anterior cerebrum and continues roughly halfway to the rear of the brain. This area regulates many important functions, including speech, abstract thinking, and personality. Behind and inferior to the frontal lobe lies the temporal lobe. Here impulses from the ears are received and then processed into sounds. One portion of the temporal lobe, the Wernicke area, is the center of the brain that is responsible for understanding speech. Directly above the temporal lobe lies the parietal lobe. This area also contains functions related to speech. In addition, the sense of body positioning (proprioception) is regulated within the parietal lobe. When you raise your arm above your head, you know the location of your arm because of activity in the parietal lobe. The most posterior portion of the cerebrum is the occipital lobe. The primary function of this lobe is to process information from the optic nerve and form the sense of sight (discussed later in this chapter).

The three distinct areas of the cerebral cortex are the motor area, sensory area, and association area. The motor area of the cerebral cortex is located in the frontal lobes (except for the anterior portion) and can be divided into two portions. Just in front of the division of the frontal

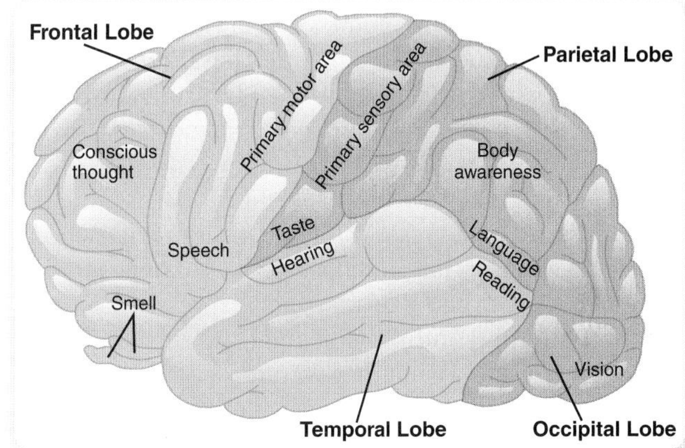

Figure 8-60 The cerebral cortex. Four of the lobes of the brain and the primary functions of those lobes are shown. The fifth lobe, the insula, is hidden.

Table 8-19 Functions of the Cerebral Lobe

Cerebral Lobe	Function
Frontal	Higher cognitive functions (eg, ability to form concepts, plan, problem-solve, reason, judge); voluntary motor function; expressive language (verbal and written); long-term memory storage; sexual behavior; and emotions (eg, aggression, motivation, impulse control, and mood)
Insula	Processes information from receptors in the skin and internal organs including perception of temperature, itch, pain, taste, hunger, thirst, and sense of body position in space; assists in motor function, regulation of homeostasis, and social emotions (eg, lust and disgust, pride and humiliation, gratitude and resentment, self-confidence and embarrassment, trust and distrust, truthfulness and deception, guilt and atonement)
Occipital	Processes and perceives visual information; responsible for color vision, spatial perception, recognition of movement, and linking images from the eyes with experiences, images, and knowledge stored in memory
Parietal	Processes information from sensory receptors in the skin and joints including perception of pain, temperature, and vibration; processes and integrates information related to sight, sound, and taste; determines shapes, sizes, distances; determines right from left; responsible for ability to perform mathematical calculations and recognize and manipulate numbers as well as ability to process language and understand speech
Temporal	Processes higher-order visual information (eg, facial recognition); speech comprehension; memory formation and retrieval; processes, perceives, and integrates memories and sensations of taste, smell, sound, sight, and touch

lobe and parietal lobe is a small strip known as the primary motor center, or the motor strip. This area provides the impulses for precise muscular control of the voluntary muscles. Impulses from the motor strip are conducted down the spinal cord to the muscles of the body. Specific portions of the motor strip are responsible for certain areas of the body. Just anterior to the motor strip is the premotor area. The premotor area is responsible for muscular coordination after the decision to perform a certain movement has been made. As an example of how the motor and premotor areas work together, imagine the decision to turn to the next page of this text. After you make the decision, the premotor area determines what muscles must be used and transmits that information to the motor strip. The motor strip then transmits impulses by way of the spinal cord to the specific muscles of your arm and hand, allowing you to turn the page. The Broca region, located in the inferior left frontal lobe just anterior to the motor cortex, is responsible for the muscular actions associated with speech. Patients who have damage to this area, such as from a stroke, may have expressive aphasia. Patients with this condition are able to understand what they hear and know what they want to say, but they have difficulty producing language. They may speak slowly with long pauses between words, use incorrect or imprecise words, or say something that does not resemble a sentence.

The primary sensory area is a strip that lies just posterior to the motor strip. However, sensory areas are distributed across the cerebral cortex. These areas receive sensory stimuli from the body and interpret what they mean or what actions are needed. For example, the primary sensory area receives sensations from the skin. Other sensory areas contained in the visual cortex of the occipital lobe interpret visual stimulus. The Wernicke area is located at the junction of the temporal and parietal lobes. This is the sensory area for speech recognition and allows comprehension and understanding of speech. The Broca region and Wernicke area are physically connected and work together to allow verbal communication.

Words of Wisdom

Damage to the Wernicke area can result in receptive aphasia. Patients with this condition can usually speak normally, but have difficulty understanding written and spoken words. As a result, they often use nonsense words when speaking and they may not recognize the words they are saying are not appropriate to the situation.

The association areas of the cerebral cortex are located in the anterior frontal lobe as well as the lateral portions of the temporal, occipital, and parietal lobes. These areas are responsible for the analysis and interpretation of sensory information the brain receives and allow effective interaction with the environment. The association areas of the frontal lobes deal with judgment, concentration, abstract thought, and problem solving. Areas within the parietal lobes are used in the understanding of speech and the choosing of words to express emotions. The temporal lobe association areas interpret complex sensory information such as reading, visual memory, and the understanding of speech. The visual association area is located in the occipital lobe near the visual cortex. This area provides the ability to analyze visual patterns and combine visual information with other sensory information.

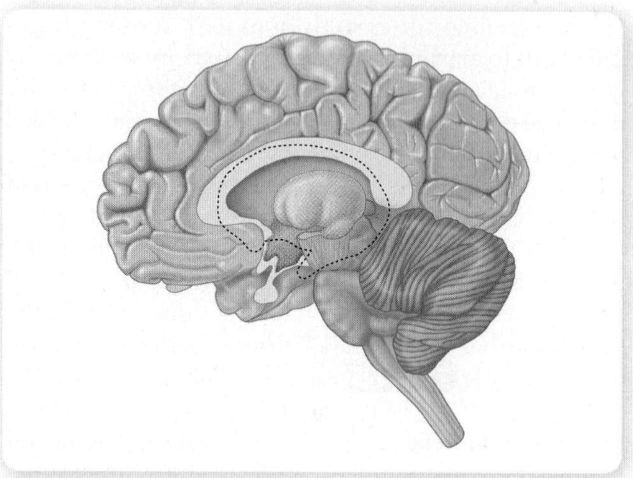

Figure 8-61 The diencephalon.

Diencephalon. The **diencephalon** is located above the brainstem and between the cerebral hemispheres **Figure 8-61**. The diencephalon is composed of several structures including the epithalamus, the thalamus, the hypothalamus, and the subthalamus.

The epithalamus is the uppermost portion of the diencephalon. It contains the **pineal gland**, which synthesizes melatonin, a hormone associated with the body's sleep-wake cycle. The **thalamus** is the sensory switchboard, receiving and relaying sensory information (except the sense of smell) to the sensory cortex for processing. The thalamus is located deep inside the brain and makes up 80% of the diencephalon.[9] The **hypothalamus** is inferior to the thalamus and plays a key role in the emotions and sexuality of the body through the limbic system. The hypothalamus also contains the temperature regulatory

Words of Wisdom

One of the major roles of the diencephalon is to filter out unnecessary information before it reaches the cerebral cortex. For example, the diencephalon keeps you from having to think about shifting your weight on a chair when it becomes uncomfortable. Instead, signals of pressure or pain sent through the peripheral nerves initially stop in the diencephalon, which dispatches the command for you to switch positions slightly without being conscious of doing so.

Table 8-20 Functions of the Hypothalamus

Function/Regulation	Description
Autonomic	Regulates involuntary body functions, including the activity of cardiac muscle, smooth muscles, and glands
Eating and drinking	Promotes and inhibits eating through the hunger and satiety centers; promotes drinking through thirst
Emotional	Regulates psychosomatic illness, stress-related conditions, fear, and rage; exerts emotional influence over body functions
Endocrine	Regulates pituitary gland secretions and affects metabolism and sexual development and functions
Muscular	Stimulates shivering in some muscles; controls muscles responsible for swallowing
Sleep	Regulates responses to the sleep-wake cycle in coordination with other areas of the brain
Temperature	Regulates temperature through sweat to promote heat loss and through shivering to promote heat generation

centers of the body, controls the pituitary gland, and is the site of integration of the nervous system and the endocrine system Table 8-20. The subthalamus controls motor functions. A lesion in the area of the subthalamus is characterized by involuntary but violent flinging movements of the limbs on one side of the body.

Body Temperature. Temperature is one of the oldest and most common factors measured when assessing the body. Heat is a by-product of many cellular and chemical processes, so it follows that the presence of body heat is one of the most basic signs of life. In fact, the **calorie** is a measure of heat that may be produced from a given amount of food, not nutritional value. (The technical term is a **kilocalorie**.) However, many cells and enzymes require that the body temperature be strictly regulated to allow certain processes to function. As discussed previously, this process of maintaining homeostasis of temperature is known as thermoregulation.

The body's average temperature is maintained through a balance of gains and losses. Skeletal muscle generates heat with each contraction. The process of digesting food, with its innumerable decomposition reactions, also generates heat. These processes are controlled in part by secretion of thyroxine, which has many functions, one of which being regulation of body temperature. These processes can also be influenced by activation of the sympathetic nervous system. The body also has means for releasing heat. The simplest of these mechanisms can be seen when a person exercises in warm atmospheres: The pulse quickens, circulating more blood to the periphery, where it can give off heat through the skin; the skin itself begins to perspire, which amplifies heat loss through evaporation; and the respirations accelerate, which exchanges warmed air for cooler air with each breath. Inhibition of digestion and other mechanisms of heat generation also contribute to net heat loss.

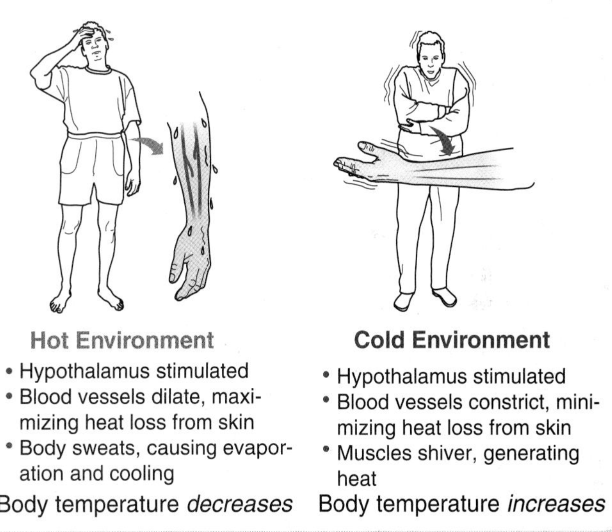

Figure 8-62 The hypothalamus notes a rise or fall in core body temperature and elicits responses to regulate it.

The commonly accepted average body temperature is 98.6°F (37°C). However, body temperature can vary slightly from person to person and also vary based on conditions without causing any adverse effect on the body; therefore, these variances are not necessarily considered abnormal or pathologic. Body temperature regulation begins in the hypothalamus, which acts similar to a thermostat in activating the mechanisms for increasing or decreasing body temperature Figure 8-62.

In many disease processes, the hypothalamus is influenced to raise the body temperature. When the target body temperature is more than 1° above the patient's "normal" temperature, a fever is present. Although the usefulness of fever is a matter of debate, it is known that a fever increases metabolism and activity of phagocytes, which may aid in the destruction and removal of infectious organisms. In most patients, a fever of only a few degrees above normal is generally not harmful other than creating the characteristic body aches and fatigue that make it so uncomfortable. This fact, combined with the theory that fever may actually be beneficial in the healing process, makes treatment of mild fevers controversial. However, moderate fevers that persist for significant periods can cause or exacerbate other symptoms and effects of illness, such as dehydration. High fevers can cause febrile seizures in children and, if they persist, have the potential to cause long-term CNS damage in children and adults. For this reason, moderate to high fevers are usually treated with antipyretics such as acetaminophen or ibuprofen, and dangerously high fevers are sometimes treated with active cooling measures.

Limbic System. The limbic system is the so-called emotional brain, or the feeling and reacting brain. It is composed of several structures beneath the cerebral cortex with connections to other parts of the brain, including the thalamus, hypothalamus, and the frontal and temporal lobes of the cerebrum Figure 8-63.

The limbic system is involved in the generation, integration, and control of emotions and connects them with behavioral responses (eg, anger, rage, fear, surprise, sadness, anxiety, tension).[16] This system is important in motivation, learning, and the transition of information from short- to long-term memory. The limbic system is also closely linked to functions necessary for self-preservation, particularly in response to emotional stimuli.

Words of Wisdom

The limbic system constantly generates emotional impulses (referred to as raw emotions), filtered by the anterior portions of the frontal lobe (referred to as the conscience, or judgment). Inhibition of the frontal lobe can stop this filtering process and allow these raw emotions to be displayed. These emotional outbursts may present in many ways, including verbal or physical aggression, choice of language, or behavior the individual would not normally display.

Brainstem. Recall that the brainstem connects the brain to the spinal cord. It is so called because the brain appears to be sitting on this portion of the CNS as a plant sits on its stem. The brainstem lies deep within the cranium and is the best-protected part of the CNS. It is responsible for many of the essential functions the body requires to survive (vegetative functions).

The brainstem is permeated by a group of specialized neurons that are collectively called the **reticular activating system (RAS)** or reticular formation. More of a network than a structure, the RAS is a mixture of gray and white matter and extends from the spinal cord into the diencephalon. Sensory axons from many different sources,

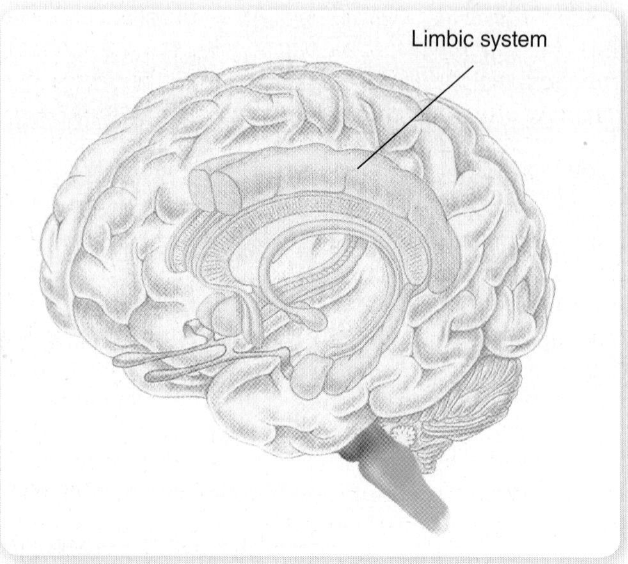

Figure 8-63 The limbic system.

particularly the cranial nerves, send impulses into the RAS. The **cranial nerves** are twelve pairs of peripheral nerves that are associated with the brain and innervate structures primarily in the head.

The RAS filters and then sends impulses that excite the cerebrum and keep the body awake. Consciousness is maintained by the interaction of the RAS and the cerebral cortex. Disruption to this interaction, or a loss of connection between the RAS and the cerebral cortex, results in an altered level of consciousness.

The divisions of the brainstem are the midbrain, pons, and medulla (see Figure 8-59). The **midbrain** (mesencephalon) is the most superior portion of the brainstem. It contains reflex centers for pupillary reflexes and eye movements. The midbrain is also involved in the coordination of motor activity and muscular tone, and serves as a relay for impulses from the cerebral cortex to the pons and spinal cord.

The **pons** is the middle portion of the brainstem and serves as a relay of both afferent (ascending) nerve fibers and efferent (descending) nerve fibers. The pons plays a role in the arousal and sleep cycles of the body and contains respiratory centers that, along with the medulla, control movements associated with breathing.

The **medulla oblongata** is the inferior part of the brainstem. It is continuous with the spinal cord at the foramen magnum. The medulla contains three vital centers that are crucial for survival: the cardiac center, the vasomotor center, and the respiratory center. The cardiac center is responsible for altering heart rate (HR; the number of cardiac contractions per minute—in other words, the pulse rate) and the strength of cardiac contraction to meet the body's demands. The vasomotor (vessel muscle) center affects changes in the diameter of blood vessels, thereby regulating blood pressure. The respiratory center works with the pons to regulate the rhythm of breathing. The medulla also contains centers responsible for coughing, sneezing, vomiting, swallowing, and hiccupping.

Ascending and descending nerve fibers that connect the brain and spinal cord pass through the medulla. About three-fourths of the descending (motor) fibers leave the cerebral cortex, descend through the pons, cross sides in the medulla (right fibers move to the left side and vice versa), and extend down the spinal cord. As a result, the motor area of the left cerebral hemisphere controls motor movement on the right side of the body, and vice versa. About one-fourth of the descending motor fibers leave the cerebral cortex, descend through the pons, but do not cross over or decussate in the medulla, continuing down the same side of the spinal cord from which they came and connecting with motor neurons in the spinal cord.

Cerebellum. The **cerebellum** is the second largest part of the human brain and is similar in size and shape to two large walnuts (see Figure 8-59). It is located inferior to the occipital lobes of the cerebrum and is involved in both fine (small muscle groups) and gross (major muscle groups) muscle coordination. The cerebellum is responsible for interpreting movement and correcting any movements that interfere with coordination and body position. To accomplish this, the cerebellum receives information from the sensory and motor cortexes. The cerebellum determines the direction, force, and duration of the movement and sends this information back to the motor cortex. The jerky tremors of patients with Parkinson disease are an example of cerebellar dysfunction.

Words of Wisdom

In the brainstem, most nerves cross from one side to the other. Motor and sensory nerves on the left side of the brain, for example, serve the right side of the body. This is why a person who has had a stroke or trauma in one hemisphere has nerve deficits on the opposite side of the body. Because the cranial nerves do not cross over, their function will be affected on the same side of the face as the injury or stroke.

Spinal Cord

Recall that the spinal cord is the part of the CNS that connects the brain to skeletal muscle, skin, and other structures by means of the spinal nerves. The spinal cord leaves the skull through the foramen magnum and extends through the spinal column **Figure 8-64**. It is encased within the vertebral canal, which also contains blood vessels, a cushion of adipose tissue, the meninges, and CSF. The vertebrae and their associated ligaments provide additional protection for the cord. In most adults, the spinal cord ends at the level of L2; however, in some patients, the spinal cord may end as high as the disk between the T11 and T12 vertebrae or as low as the L3 vertebra. The end of the spinal cord is known as the conus medullaris. A group of spinal nerves (the cauda equina) continue to travel through the remainder of the spinal column. The cauda equina, which is the collection of nerve roots just below the level of the conus medullaris, is not part of the spinal cord or even the central nervous system.

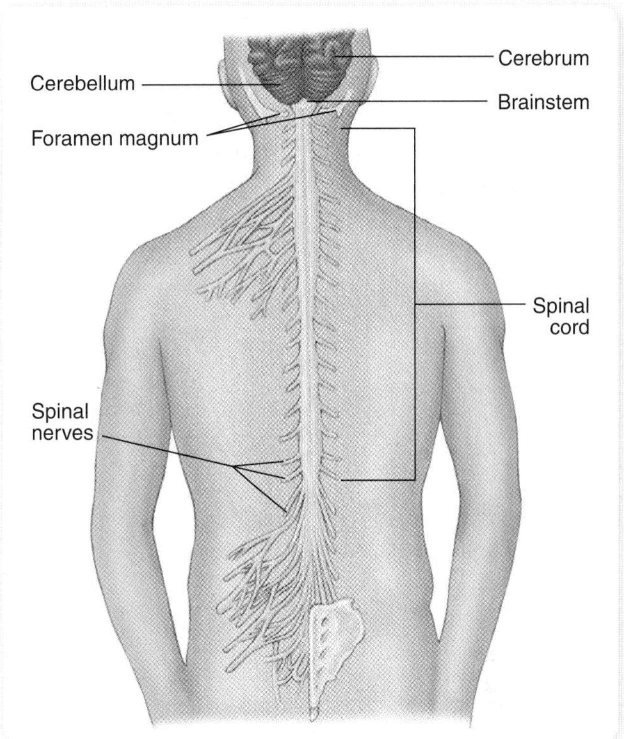

Figure 8-64 The spinal cord exits the skull at the foramen magnum and extends down to the level of the second lumbar vertebra in most adults.

Physically, the spinal cord has a texture similar to a carrot, with many long, stringlike strands running through it. Two grooves, the anterior median fissure and the posterior median sulcus, incompletely divide the spinal cord into symmetrical halves. Each half is further divided into three longitudinal columns (anterior, lateral, and posterior) that run the length of the cord. Within each column are bundles of nerve fibers (tracts) that share the same function. The tracts may be ascending or descending, with each tract carrying specific signals. Ascending tracts transmit impulses and sensations from the body to the brain. Descending tracts transmit motor impulses from the brain to the body.

The spinal cord has a central canal through which CSF flows that extends the entire length of the spinal cord **Figure 8-65**. The central canal is surrounded by gray and white matter. The gray matter of the cord, which is primarily responsible for motor function, is rich in nerve cell bodies that form longitudinal columns (horns) along the cord. When cut transversely, these columns form a characteristic butterfly or H shape in the central regions of the cord. The anterior portions of the letter H are the *anterior horns,* the posterior areas are the *posterior horns,* and the *lateral horns* (found only in the thoracic region and upper two or three lumbar nerve roots) are located between the anterior and posterior horns.

The white matter of the spinal cord is rich in axons. The white matter is divided by the gray matter into three longitudinal columns on each side, known as the anterior,

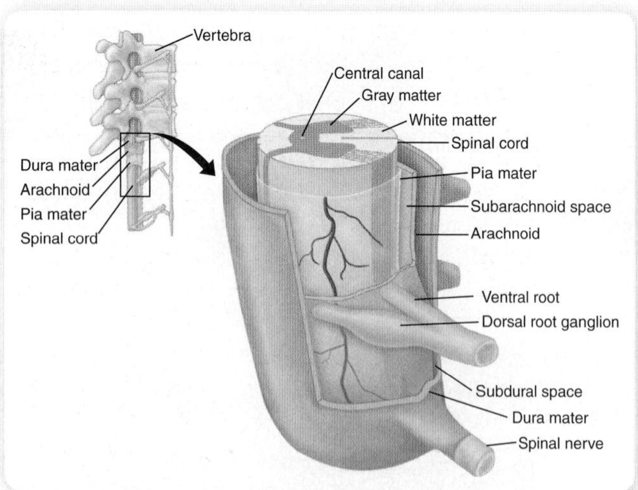

Figure 8-65 Components of the spinal cord. The meninges enclose the brain and spinal cord.

lateral, and posterior funiculi (from the Latin *funiculus*, meaning "string") or white columns. Lateral and posterior white matter both return sensory signals from the body to the brain, whereas the anterior white matter, like the gray matter, carries motor signals to the body. The funiculi contain both ascending and descending tracts that are often named according to their points of origin and termination. The ascending spinal cord tracts and their functions are described as follows:

- **Fasciculus gracilis and fasciculus cuneatus.** The posterior funiculi, which may also be referred to as the *posterior column–medial lemniscus system*, contains the fasciculus gracilis and fasciculus cuneatus tracts. These tracts conduct sensations of discrimination such as light touch, deep pressure, vibration, proprioception, and recognition of objects by touch (stereognosis). These tracts travel the same side of the spinal cord as the impulses they receive and do not cross to the opposite side of the body until they reach the medulla. Although this process does result in the right brain sensing impulses from the left body and the left brain sensing impulses from the right body, in the setting of injury to these tracts, the physical deficits will be ipsilateral (on the same side as the injury).
- **Spinothalamic tracts.** The anterior spinothalamic tract and lateral spinothalamic tract lie within the anterior and lateral funiculi, respectively. Although these two tracts represent a cruder system than the posterior funiculi, they transmit certain sensations. The anterior spinothalamic tract transmits crude touch and pressure, whereas the lateral spinothalamic tract transmits pain and temperature sensations. These tracts travel on the opposite side of the body compared with the impulses they receive. This process not only results in the right brain sensing impulses from the left body and vice versa, but also in the setting of injury, physical deficits will be contralateral (on the opposite side of the injury).
- **Spinocerebellar tracts.** The spinocerebellar tracts are found near the lateral funiculi and have both posterior and anterior tracts. The fibers of the posterior spinocerebellar tract are uncrossed and are more numerous than the anterior spinocerebellar tract fibers. The posterior spinocerebellar tract transmits sensations associated with motor function, equilibrium, proprioception, muscle tone, and movement of the limbs. The fibers of the anterior spinocerebellar tract are mostly crossed (although some fibers do remain uncrossed) and receive less information than the posterior tract. The anterior tract is stimulated by motor signals arriving from the brain through the corticospinal tracts and from internal motor pattern generators in the cord itself. The main function of the anterior tract is to provide feedback to the brain that motor signals have arrived to the anterior horns of the gray matter. In the setting of a lesion or injury, physical deficits will be ipsilateral.

The descending spinal cord tracts originate in the brain and convey impulses to various muscle groups by inhibiting or exciting spinal activity.[17] A motor neuron that originates in the motor cortex of the cerebrum and travels down in a descending white matter tract is called an upper motor neuron. Upper motor neurons can impact movement only through the lower motor neurons. Lower motor neurons originate in the spinal cord, extend into the PNS, and transmit impulses directly to muscles to affect movement. Upper motor neurons begin and end within the CNS; in contrast, lower motor neurons are found in both the CNS and the PNS. Because the lower motor neurons and their fibers (axons) constitute the only connection between the spinal cord and skeletal muscles, they are considered the final common pathway to the muscle. This principle of the final common pathway is important to understand the differences between upper and lower motor neuron diseases and injuries, and the differences between their physical findings and prognoses. For example, when upper motor neurons are injured, the injury results in initial flaccid (floppy) paralysis with a loss of tendon reflexes that is followed by partial recovery (typically including spasticity with abnormally brisk reflexes [hyperreflexia]) over an extended period.[17] When lower motor neurons supplying a muscle are destroyed or interruption of their axons occurs, the injury results in paralysis or weakness of that muscle.

Functions of the descending spinal cord tracts are described as follows:

- **Corticospinal tracts.** The corticospinal tracts (pyramidal tracts) originate in the cerebral cortex (with most arising from the frontal lobe area of the cerebrum) and descend through the anterior and lateral funiculi toward the spinal cord. Most of the fibers of the corticospinal tract cross to the side of the body to which they transmit impulses at the level of the medulla, becoming the lateral corticospinal tract. Those fibers that do not cross at the level of the medulla continue down the same side of the cord as the side of the brain they originated in, becoming the anterior corticospinal tract. However, the fibers of the anterior corticospinal tract also cross to the side of the body contralateral to their origination in the brain. This process generally occurs in the neck or upper thoracic region. Both tracts transmit motor impulses from the cortex to the spinal nerves, where they are distributed to the voluntary muscles. The majority of the fibers of the corticospinal tract terminate at interneurons near the gray matter of the spinal cord. However, those fibers that are responsible for the fine motor function of the fingers and hands terminate directly on the anterior horn(s) of the gray matter, allowing fine motor control. When these tracts are injured, physical findings such as loss of motor control occur on the ipsilateral side as the injury.

- **Extrapyramidal tracts.** Although the corticospinal tracts are primarily responsible for voluntary movement, additional tracts play a role in motor activity. Often called the *extrapyramidal system*, the extrapyramidal tracts are not well defined and lie outside the pyramidal system. They are responsible for some degree of movement and posture that are not under the control of the pyramidal system, as well as control of the sweat glands.
- **Reticulospinal tracts.** The lateral reticulospinal tract is located in the lateral funiculi. The majority of these fibers cross at the level of the medulla, but a few do not. The medial reticulospinal tract is contained in the anterior funiculi, and these fibers do not cross to the opposite side of the body after they leave the brain. These tracts transmit impulses to the body that control muscular tone and the activity of the sweat glands.
- **Rubrospinal tracts.** Upon leaving the brain, these tracts immediately cross to the opposite side of the body and travel down the lateral funiculi. Their primary function is to transmit impulses from the brain that control muscle coordination and posture. Important spinal tracts are summarized in Table 8-21.

Table 8-21 Major Spinal Tracts

Name	Function	Comments
Ascending Tracts (transmit impulses and sensations from the body to the brain)		
Anterior spinothalamic	Conveys light touch and pressure, tickle, and itch sensations on opposite side	In the setting of a lesion or injury, physical deficits will be contralateral.
Fasciculi gracilis and cuneatus	Proprioception, vibration, light touch, deep pressure, two-point discrimination, and stereognosis	In the setting of a lesion or injury, physical deficits will be ipsilateral; fasciculus cuneatus carries impulses from upper body; fasciculus gracilis carries impulses from lower body.
Lateral spinothalamic	Conveys pain and temperature sensations on opposite side	In the setting of a lesion or injury, physical deficits will be contralateral.
Spinocerebellar	Transmit sensations to the cerebellum associated with motor function, equilibrium, proprioception, muscle tone, and limb movement	In the setting of a lesion or injury, physical deficits will be ipsilateral.
Descending Tracts (transmit motor impulses from the brain to the body)		
Anterior corticospinal (pyramidal)	Voluntary motor commands on same side of the body	In the setting of a lesion or injury, physical deficits will be ipsilateral.
Lateral corticospinal (crossed pyramidal)	Voluntary motor commands on the opposite side of the body	In the setting of a lesion or injury, physical deficits will be contralateral.
Reticulospinal (extrapyramidal)	Maintain posture during movement	In the setting of a lesion or injury, physical deficits will be ipsilateral.
Rubrospinal (extrapyramidal)	Muscle coordination and posture	In the setting of a lesion or injury, physical deficits will be contralateral.

▶ Peripheral Nervous System

To respond effectively to its surrounding environment, the CNS needs both input from structures outside it and a means to send output to the body's smooth muscle, cardiac muscle, skeletal muscle, and glands. This process is accomplished by means of the PNS, which is responsible for communication between the CNS and the rest of the body.

As discussed previously, the PNS is functionally divided into two divisions: the somatic division and the visceral division. The somatic division is mainly involved with sensing and responding to information from the external environment. The skin, joints, tendons, and skeletal muscle are innervated by somatic nerve fibers (both sensory and motor). The body's internal environment is monitored and controlled by the visceral (autonomic) division of the PNS. Visceral fibers carry afferent information from body organs to the CNS and provide efferent control of smooth muscle, cardiac muscle, and glands.[6]

Spinal Nerves

A spinal nerve attaches to the lateral surface of the spinal cord by two roots: a posterior (dorsal) root and an anterior (ventral) root. The nerve root is either sensory or motor. The posterior root contains afferent nerve fibers that conduct sensory information to the spinal cord. The cell bodies vvof peripheral neurons are often grouped into clusters called *ganglia* (singular, *ganglion*). The anterior root contains efferent nerves that conduct motor impulses to the body.

The spinal nerves are named for the vertebra at which they exit the spinal column: cervical (8), thoracic (12), lumbar (5), sacral (5), and coccygeal spinal nerve (1). The first seven cervical spine nerves exit above their respective cervical vertebrae. The eighth cervical nerve exits between C7 and T1 (ie, inferior to C7). All spinal nerves below the eighth cervical nerve exit below their respective vertebrae.

The eight cervical roots perform different functions in the scalp, neck, shoulders, and arms. The 12 thoracic nerve roots have varying functions; the upper thoracic nerves supply muscles of the chest that help in breathing and coughing, whereas the lower thoracic nerves provide abdominal muscle control and contain nerves of the sympathetic nervous system. The five lumbar nerve roots supply hip flexors and leg muscles, as well as provide sensation to the legs. The five sacral nerves provide for bowel and bladder control, sexual function, and sensation in the posterior legs and rectum (the lowermost end of the colon). The coccyx has a single nerve root.

> **Words of Wisdom**
>
> Compression of a spinal nerve as it passes through the intervertebral foramen can result in symptoms such as tingling, numbness, muscle weakness, reduced reflexes, and radiating pain. It is often called radiculopathy or, generically, sciatica.

Plexuses. Recall that the spinal nerves combine in five areas of the body to form networks (plexuses) where spinal nerve roots come together and transmit their impulses to areas of the body through a common nerve. This principle allows several spinal nerves to control one area of the body. A plexus in the body acts similar to an electrical junction box that distributes wires to different parts of a house.

The five main plexuses in the body are the cervical plexus, the brachial plexus, the lumbar plexus, the sacral plexus, and the coccygeal plexus **Figure 8-66**. The cervical plexus innervates the neck, the back of the head, the upper shoulders, and the diaphragm. The brachial plexus supplies the lower shoulders, the arm, and the hand. The lumbar plexus innervates muscle and skin in the lower trunk and lower extremities. The sacral plexus supplies the buttocks, the posterior thigh muscles, and the leg and foot muscles. The coccygeal plexus supplies the perineum. Damage to these areas can result in widespread neurologic deficits such as pain, weakness, and loss of sensation because a large number of nerves will be affected.

> **Words of Wisdom**
>
> The lumbar and sacral plexuses are often considered together as the lumbosacral plexus because of overlap between their nerve fibers.

Dermatomes. A myotome is a region of skeletal muscle innervated by a single spinal nerve. Sensory spinal nerves carry sensory information from a specific area of skin on the surface of the body. These areas, known as **dermatomes,** correspond to specific spinal nerves at various levels **Figure 8-67**. It is important that you become familiar with the dermatomes throughout the body. Keep in mind the anatomic variations between people, be aware that dermatomal areas overlap, and recognize that the relationship between dermatomes and vertebral levels is an approximation because spinal cord length may vary among patients.[18] Familiarize yourself with the dermatomes to better understand the presentation of a patient's symptoms if the spinal cord is injured. Spinal cord injuries generally do not result in a lack of function to a specific part of the body (eg, numbness and tingling from the knee down); rather, some impairment of motor and sensory skills is found along the path of specific dermatomes. An injury may be isolated to one dermatome, or the injury may begin along that dermatome and continue distally. Injured nerves manifest with motor impairment, sensory impairment, or both. Musculoskeletal injuries

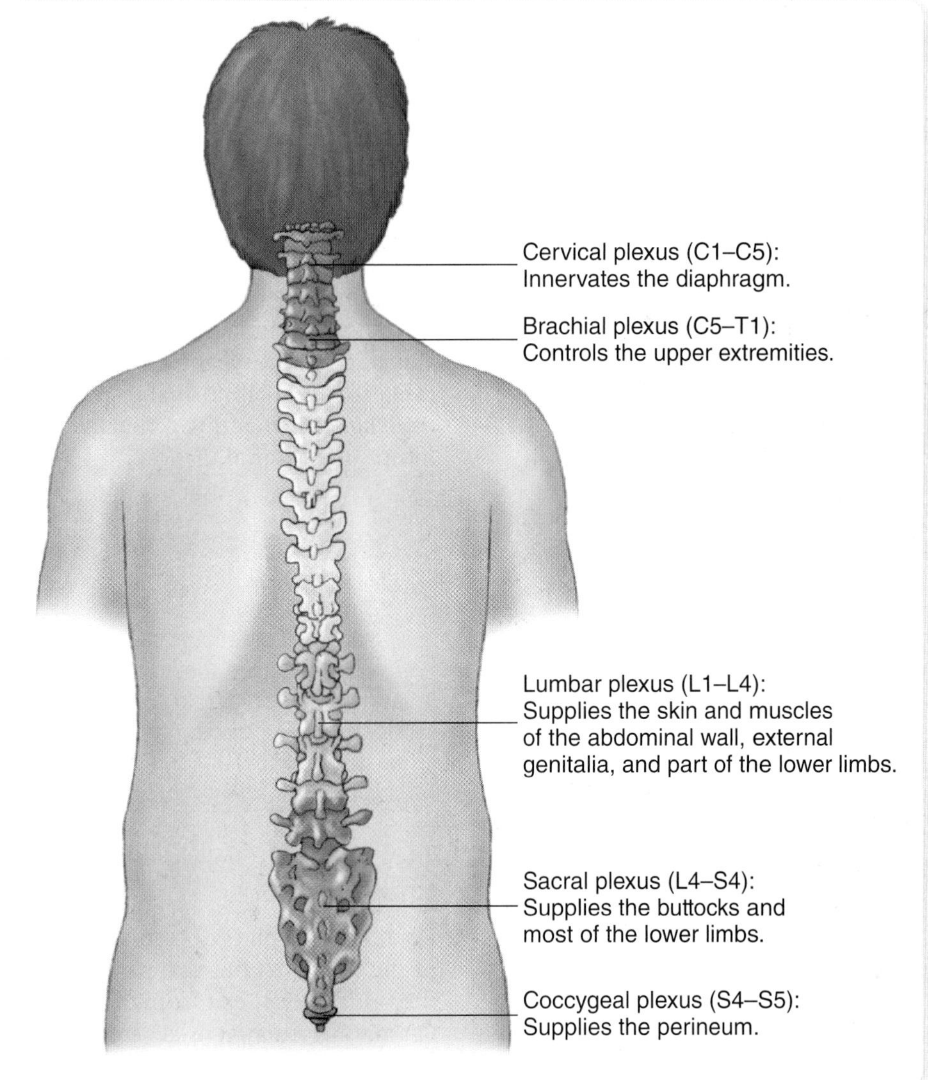

Figure 8-66 Nerve roots originating from groups of vertebrae along the spine converge in plexuses, allowing them to function as a group.

often lead to neurovascular bundle impairment, which is seen with a loss of circulation as well as motor and sensory function distal to the injury site.

Reflexes. The spinal cord contains the main reflex centers of the body. A **reflex arc** is a sensory message that reaches the spinal cord and meets with a motor nerve to cause an action; the reflex action occurs without the message first having to reach the brain to voluntarily cause the action.[19] Components of a reflex arc generally include a sensory receptor, an afferent neuron, one or more interneurons, an efferent neuron, and an effector organ (eg, skeletal muscle, gland).

An example of a simple reflex arc is the patellar reflex (knee-jerk reflex). When the tendon is stretched, such as a collapsing knee when walking, the reflex is to straighten the knee to avoid a fall. If this process required the involvement of the brain, then the fall would likely occur before the conscious thought of straightening the knee could occur. In this example, while the tendon is stretched, sensory impulses travel along afferent axons to the posterior root ganglia. This impulse is then transmitted through an interneuron that determines the motor response to the sensory impulse. From that point, the impulse travels by efferent axons to the skeletal muscles.

A flexor reflex (flexor-withdrawal reflex) involves many interneurons. It is initiated by receptors in the skin, occurring in response to a tactile, painful, or noxious stimulus. For example, after accidentally touching a hand to something hot or sharp, you automatically flex the muscles of the affected limb, thereby withdrawing the hand from the area. (The term withdrawal reflex may be more appropriate because extensor muscles are sometimes used.) For example, because flexion would drive the thigh into a painful stimulus applied to its anterior surface,

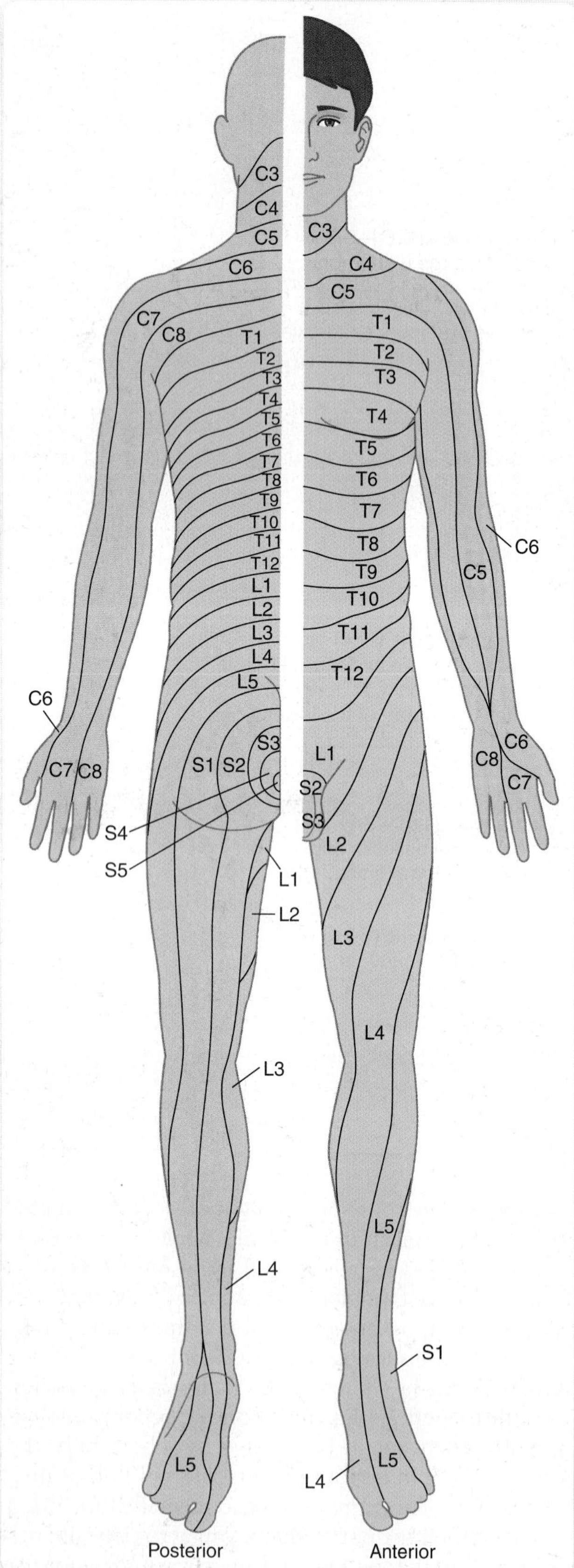

Figure 8-67 Dermatome map showing the association of the spinal nerves and the cutaneous areas of the body.

the appropriate withdrawal response uses the extensor muscles of the affected limb.

Stroking the skin with a firm object elicits a superficial reflex (cutaneous reflex), causing the muscles to contract. The plantar reflex is an example of a superficial reflex that is used to detect corticospinal tract dysfunction. It is assessed by stroking the lateral aspect of the sole of the foot from the heel forward with a firm object, such as the examiner's gloved thumb or the end of a reflex hammer. In patients older than 2 years, the normal response to this stimulus is curling under of all the toes (plantar flexion). Extension of the great toe with or without fanning of the other toes is an abnormal response called *Babinski reflex* or *Babinski sign* and is generally an indication of upper motor neuron dysfunction.

Words of Wisdom

Assessment of reflexes can provide the examiner with useful information about the integrity of peripheral nerves and specific areas of the spinal cord and the presence or absence of upper motor neuron dysfunction such as spinal cord injury or brain injury.

Cranial Nerves

Recall that 12 pairs of cranial nerves arise from the base of the brain. All but two pairs, the olfactory nerves and the optic nerves, exit from the brainstem **Figure 8-68**. Cranial nerves are either referred to by name or abbreviated as CN I, II, and so forth. The number reflects the order in which they connect to the brain from anterior to posterior. Some pairs of cranial nerves transmit motor information, some transmit sensory information, and others are mixed nerves.

Two major nerves provide sensory and motor control to the face: the trigeminal nerve (fifth cranial nerve) and the facial nerve (seventh cranial nerve). The trigeminal nerve branches into the ophthalmic nerve, maxillary nerve, and mandibular nerve. The ophthalmic nerve (a sensory nerve) supplies the skin of the forehead, upper eyelid, and conjunctiva. The maxillary nerve (another sensory nerve) supplies the skin on the posterior part of the side of the nose, lower eyelid, cheek, and upper lip. The mandibular nerve (a sensory and motor nerve) supplies the muscles of chewing (mastication) and skin of the lower lip, chin, temporal region, and part of the external ear. The facial nerve supplies the muscles of facial expression.

Blood supply to the face is provided primarily through the external carotid artery, which branches into the temporal, mandibular, and maxillary arteries. Because the face is highly vascular, it tends to bleed heavily when injured.

A summary of the cranial nerves is shown in **Table 8-22**.

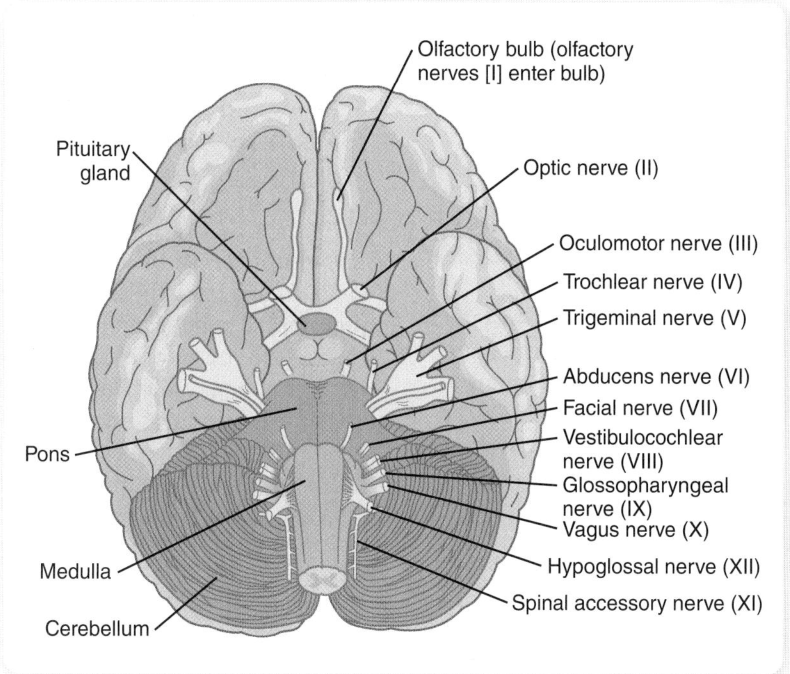

Figure 8-68 The 12 cranial nerves.

Table 8-22 Cranial Nerves

Number	Name	Type	Function
I	Olfactory	Sensory	Reception and interpretation of smell
II	Optic	Sensory	Sense of sight
III	Oculomotor	Motor	Eye movement; elevation of upper eyelids; regulation of pupil size
IV	Trochlear	Motor	Movement of eyeball in a downward, inward direction
V	Trigeminal	Mixed	Jaw clenching and chewing movements; corneal reflex; sensations (touch, pain) in face, cornea, scalp, and teeth
VI	Abducens	Motor	Movement of eyeball in a lateral direction
VII	Facial	Mixed	Facial expressions; secretion of saliva and tears; blinking; sensation of taste on anterior two-thirds of tongue (sweet, salty)
VIII	Vestibulocochlear	Sensory	Sense of hearing and balance
IX	Glossopharyngeal	Mixed	Swallowing movements; secretion of saliva; sensation of taste on posterior one-third of tongue (bitter, sour); prevents aspiration as part of the gag reflex
X	Vagus	Mixed	Swallowing; part of the gag reflex; sensation behind ear; innervation of pharynx and epiglottis; parasympathetic innervation of organs of thorax and abdomen
XI	Accessory	Motor	Movement of shoulders; turning of head
XII	Hypoglossal	Motor	Movement of tongue muscles for speech and swallowing

Autonomic Nervous System

The ANS is the part of the PNS that is not under voluntary control. The two main branches of the ANS are the sympathetic and the parasympathetic divisions. Most structures innervated by the ANS are innervated by both sympathetic and parasympathetic fibers. However, most blood vessels, the spleen, and the piloerector muscles are examples of structures that are solely innervated by the sympathetic division.[20]

Recall that with a neuromuscular junction, the target tissue (the effector), a skeletal muscle fiber, is innervated by a single motor neuron Figure 8-69. Axons of motor neurons course directly to skeletal muscles. ACh receptors are localized on the motor end plate. In contrast, autonomic pathways, which are used to innervate organs, vessels, or glands, require two neurons: preganglionic neurons (synonymous with presynaptic) and postganglionic (synonymous with postsynaptic) neurons Figure 8-70. The somatic nervous system and the ANS are compared in Table 8-23.

The cell body of the preganglionic (signal-passing) neuron is located within a root of the spinal cord or within some cranial nerves exiting the brainstem. Axons of the preganglionic neurons exit the CNS and pass out to the periphery to synapse with autonomic ganglia, which function as relay centers; thus, the CNS and the PNS connect at the autonomic ganglia. The axons of the postganglionic (signal-receiving) neurons travel from the autonomic ganglia to the desired structure to which it provides innervation. Typically, the sympathetic division has a larger number of postganglionic neurons associated with each preganglionic fiber than does the parasympathetic division.

For a physiologic action at the target organ to occur, the preganglionic neuron must first send an impulse to the ganglia and then from the ganglia to the postganglionic neuron. Remember, these neurons are not physically connected; they meet at the synaptic cleft, which is the space between them. Each nerve impulse that is conducted along the nerve generates an action potential and the chemical discharge of a neurotransmitter. When the preganglionic neuron releases its neurotransmitters, they diffuse across the synaptic cleft and interact with specific receptor sites on the dendrites and cell body of the postganglionic neuron or on the cells of the target (effector) organ. This process causes either another nerve impulse or a physiologic action at the effector organ.

Nerves are traditionally classified by the chemical transmitters that they contain; those containing norepinephrine are **adrenergic** and those containing ACh are **cholinergic**. The term cholinergic also refers to other structures or functions that are related to ACh. For instance, cholinergic receptors are proteins in cell membranes that react with ACh and cause the cell to respond in a characteristic way (eg, muscles contract, glands secrete).[20] Similarly, adrenergic refers to structures or functions that are related to norepinephrine and epinephrine (adrenaline). A summary of the characteristics of the sympathetic and parasympathetic divisions of the ANS is shown in Table 8-24.

Sympathetic Division. The sympathetic division of the ANS mobilizes the body for activity Figure 8-71. When exposed to a stressful situation, the sympathetic division prepares the body's fight-or-flight response. These responses include diversion of blood from the skin and GI tract to the brain, heart, and skeletal muscles; increased mental activity and alertness, increased blood glucose concentration, increased HR and arterial pressure, dilation of the bronchial tree, sweating of the skin, pupil dilation, and slowing of digestion and urination.

Sympathetic Nerve Fibers. Preganglionic neuron cell bodies of the sympathetic division are located in the thoracic and upper lumbar segments of the spinal cord (T1 to L2 or L3). Thus, the sympathetic division is sometimes called the thoracolumbar division of the ANS. Sympathetic preganglionic axons—which are usually myelinated—are relatively short because the ganglia are located near the spinal cord, but their postganglionic axons are long because they must travel to the periphery and innervate the effector organs. Sympathetic preganglionic fibers release ACh at the synapse, which then acts on nicotinic receptors in the postganglionic neuron, discussed later in conjunction with cholinergic receptors (see Figure 8-70).

Most of the sympathetic preganglionic axons extend to paravertebral ganglia. The paravertebral ganglia form two sets of autonomic ganglia, one lateral to each side of the vertebral column. Each set of ganglia is linked by axons that run longitudinally to form a structure resembling a ladder or a chain of beads called the sympathetic trunk, sympathetic chain, or paravertebral chain (see Figure 8-71). The sympathetic trunk extends from the second cervical vertebrae to the level of the coccyx. The long postganglionic fibers leave the sympathetic trunk and innervate their effector organs (heart, blood vessels, visceral organs, and glands), where they relay information at synapses. Most sympathetic postganglionic axons are unmyelinated.

Adrenergic Receptors. Most sympathetic postganglionic fibers release norepinephrine as their neurotransmitter, which acts on adrenergic receptors. Sympathetic postganglionic fibers that supply sweat glands and some blood vessels in the skin and skeletal muscles use ACh as their neurotransmitter.

Adrenergic receptors are categorized into the following main types: alpha$_1$, alpha$_2$, beta$_1$, beta$_2$, and beta$_3$. Alpha$_1$ and alpha$_2$ receptors are each known to contain three

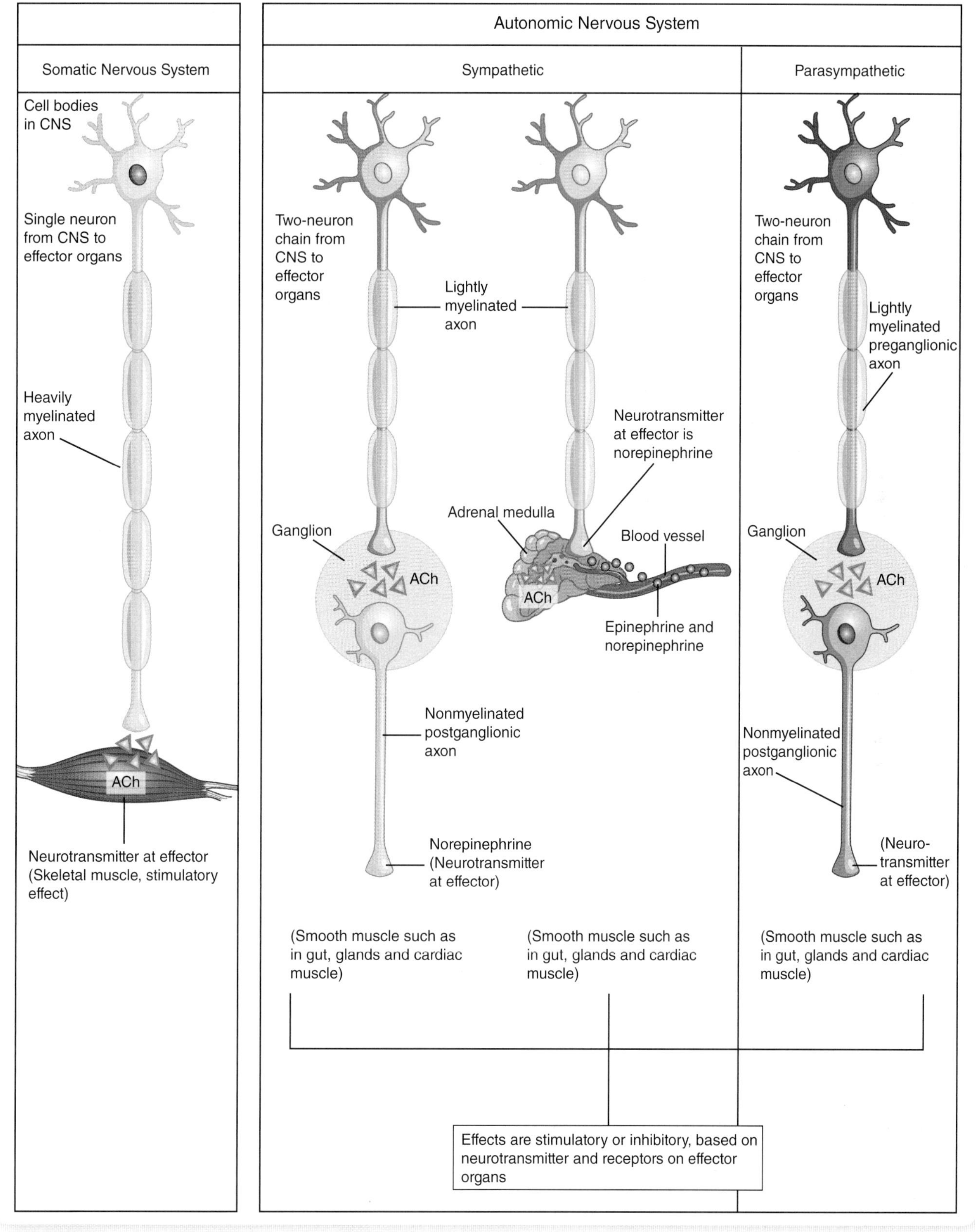

Figure 8-69 Neurons and neurotransmitters of the somatic nervous system and the autonomic nervous system.

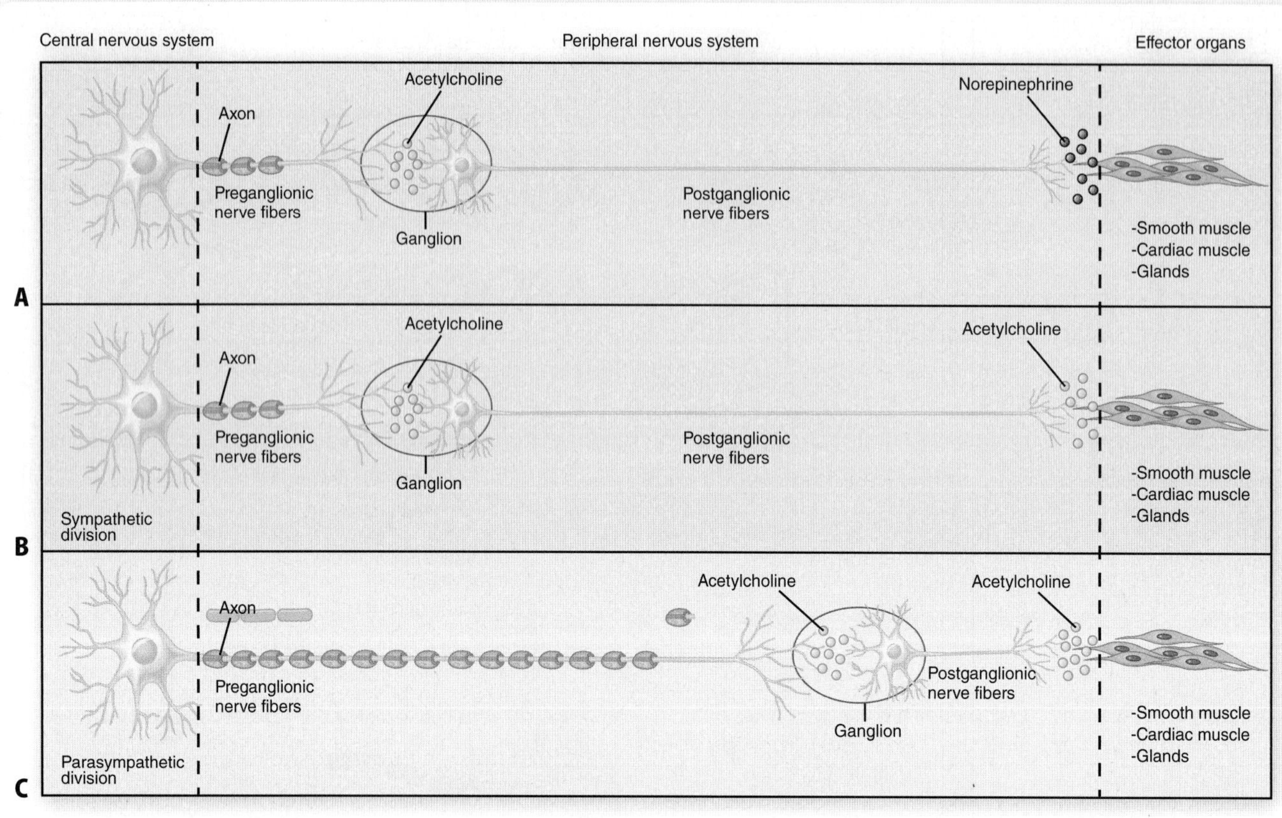

Figure 8-70 All preganglionic fibers secrete ACh. **A.** Sympathetic preganglionic fibers are short. Sympathetic postganglionic fibers are relatively long; most are adrenergic because they secrete norepinephrine and stimulate alpha or beta receptors in effector cells. **B.** Sympathetic postganglionic fibers that innervate sweat glands are cholinergic because they secrete ACh and stimulate muscarinic receptors in effector cells. **C.** Parasympathetic preganglionic fibers are relatively long and their postganglionic fibers are short. All parasympathetic fibers are cholinergic. Postganglionic fibers stimulate muscarinic receptors in effector cells.

Table 8-23 Somatic Nervous System Versus Autonomic Nervous System

Characteristic	Somatic Nervous System	Autonomic Nervous System
Control	Usually voluntary	Usually involuntary
Target (effector) organ	Skeletal muscle	Smooth muscle, cardiac muscle, glands
Pathway	Single motor neuron and skeletal muscle fiber	Two neurons: a preganglionic neuron and postganglionic neuron
Location of cell bodies	Cell body of motor neuron located in the CNS	Cell body of preganglionic neuron located in the CNS
Synaptic location	Axon synapses with skeletal muscle	Preganglionic axons synapse with postganglionic neurons at autonomic ganglia; postganglionic neurons synapse with effector organ
Neurotransmitter	ACh	Preganglionic: ACh; postganglionic: ACh or norepinephrine
Effect on target cells	Excitatory	Excitatory or inhibitory

Table 8-24 Autonomic Nervous System: Sympathetic Versus Parasympathetic Divisions

Characteristic	Sympathetic Division	Parasympathetic Division
General functions	Mobilizes the body for activity and, when exposed to a stressful situation, prepares the body's fight-or-flight response	Conserves energy and maintains organ function
Origin of preganglionic nerve cell bodies	Thoracic and upper lumbar segments of spinal cord (T1 to L2 or L3); thoracolumbar	Cranial nerves III, VII, IX, and X and sacral segments S2 to S4 of the spinal cord; craniosacral
Effector (target) organs	Cardiac muscle, smooth muscle, glands	Cardiac muscle, smooth muscle, glands
Preganglionic fibers	Short, located near the CNS	Relatively long, located near the structures they innervate
Preganglionic neurotransmitter	ACh	ACh
Postganglionic fibers	Long	Relatively short
Postganglionic neurotransmitter	Primarily norepinephrine; postganglionic neurons to sweat glands release ACh	ACh
Effects of stimulation	Effects often widespread; affecting many organs	Localized effects; may be limited to one organ

additional subtypes.[21] Stimulation of these receptors has the following effects:

- **Alpha$_1$ receptors** primarily cause vasoconstriction (narrowing of the blood vessel).
- **Alpha$_2$ receptors** generally cause smooth muscle contraction, inhibition of insulin release, induction of glucagon release, and suppression of further norepinephrine release.
- **Beta$_1$ receptors** are found in the heart and kidneys. Stimulation of these sites in the heart results in an increase in HR (positive chronotropy), an increase in the strength of cardiac contraction (positive inotropy) and, ultimately, irritability of cardiac cells. Stimulation of beta$_1$ receptor sites in the kidneys results in the release of **renin** into the blood. Renin is a hormone that promotes the production of angiotensin, which is a powerful vasoconstrictor.
- **Beta$_2$ receptors** are found in several locations in the body. In the lungs, stimulation causes bronchodilation. These receptors also cause mild vasodilation; **glycogenolysis** (breakdown of glycogen to glucose); and relaxation of the intestines, bladder, and uterus. Beta$_2$ receptors have also been found in the heart and account for about 20% of beta-receptors in the left ventricle and about 40% of beta-receptors in the atria.[22]
- **Beta$_3$ receptors** are localized in fat cells. When activated, they are thought to promote lipolysis and heat production in fat.

The inner portion of the adrenal gland, the *adrenal medulla,* is also a part of the sympathetic division of the ANS. The adrenal medulla is supplied by sympathetic preganglionic axons, which release ACh as their neurotransmitter. Sympathetic preganglionic axons directly innervate chromaffin cells found within the adrenal medulla. Chromaffin cells synthesize and secrete norepinephrine (20%) and epinephrine (80%) into the circulation. Norepinephrine and **epinephrine** are examples of **catecholamines**, which are substances that function as neurotransmitters, hormones, or both. Epinephrine and norepinephrine are broken down into inactive compounds by the actions of enzymes catechol-O-methyltransferase and monoamine oxidase. The by-products are reused to make new molecules of norepinephrine.

Sympathetic neurotransmitters do not interact with adrenergic receptors in the same way. Norepinephrine stimulates alpha$_1$, alpha$_2$, beta$_1$, and beta$_3$ receptors[21] and

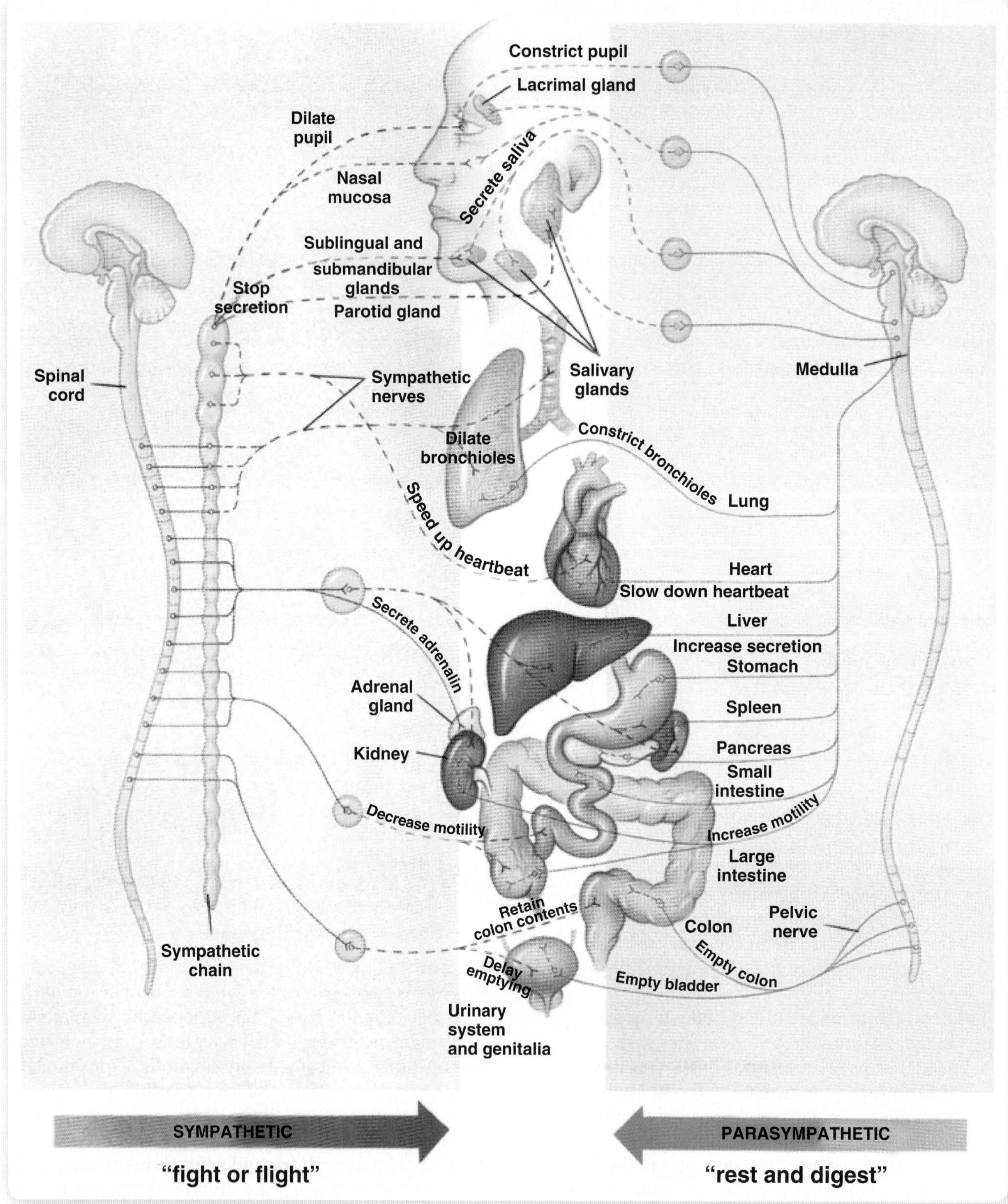

Figure 8-71 Comparison of the divisions of the autonomic nervous system.

has minimal $beta_2$ receptor activity.[20] Epinephrine stimulates all types of alpha and beta receptors about equally.[21] Adrenergic receptors are summarized in Table 8-25.

Parasympathetic Division. The parasympathetic division of the ANS is responsible for conserving energy and maintaining organ function, counterbalancing the sympathetic division (see Figure 8-71). The parasympathetic division is the so-called resting and digesting response of the ANS. The body is taking care of functions such as digestion, growth, healing, and the removal of toxins.

Parasympathetic Nerve Fibers. Preganglionic neuron cell bodies of the parasympathetic division are located in the nuclei of cranial nerves III, VII, IX, and X and in sacral segments S2 to S4 of the spinal cord; hence, the parasympathetic division is also called the craniosacral division of the ANS. Cranial nerves III (oculomotor),

Table 8-25 Adrenergic Receptors

Receptor Type	Location	Effects of Stimulation
$Alpha_1$	Bladder sphincters	Constriction
	Eye	Contraction of radial muscle of iris causes increased pupil size
	GI sphincters	Constriction
	Male reproductive organs	Ejaculation
	Peripheral small arteries and arterioles	Constriction
	Smooth muscle of GI system	Inhibits movement
	Urethral sphincter	Contraction
	Vascular smooth muscle	Constriction
$Alpha_2$	Pancreatic enzymes and insulin	Inhibits release
	Presynaptic nerve terminals in PNS	Inhibits norepinephrine release
	Smooth muscle of GI system	Inhibits motility
$Beta_1$	Adipose tissue	Lipolysis
	Heart	Increased rate and force of contraction
	Kidneys	Release of renin
$Beta_2$	Arterioles of heart, lungs, skeletal muscle	Dilation
	Bronchi	Dilation
	Ciliary muscle of eye	Relaxation
	Liver	Increased glycogenolysis and gluconeogenesis
	Pancreas	Increased release of glucagon
	Uterus	Relaxation
$Beta_3$	Adipose tissue; brown adipose tissue	Promote lipolysis (adipose tissue) and heat production (brown adipose tissue)

VII (facial), IX (glossopharyngeal), and X (vagus) innervate structures in the head and neck, and in the thoracic and abdominal cavities. Think of the two vagus nerves as the superhighways of parasympathetic function because they make up 90% of all preganglionic parasympathetic fibers in the body.[9] The vagus nerves supply the heart, tracheobronchial tree, liver, spleen, kidney, and entire GI tract except for the distal part of the colon.[20] The sacral division of the parasympathetic system forms the pelvic nerve, which innervates a portion of the GI tract and the pelvic organs, including the bladder and reproductive organs. A small number of blood vessels receive parasympathetic innervation.

Parasympathetic preganglionic fibers join with autonomic ganglia near the organ that will be innervated. Short postganglionic fibers leave the autonomic ganglion and innervate the target organ. Parasympathetic preganglionic fibers release ACh, which then stimulates nicotinic receptors in the postganglionic neuron (see Figure 8-70). Parasympathetic postganglionic fibers release ACh that then acts on muscarinic receptors.

Cholinergic Receptors. Two main types of cholinergic receptors are found in the parasympathetic division of the ANS: nicotinic and muscarinic receptors. These receptors received their names by their responsiveness to nicotine (commonly found in cigarettes) and muscarine (found in mushrooms). Nicotinic receptors are found on skeletal muscle, on cells of the adrenal medulla, and on the cell bodies of all postganglionic neurons of the parasympathetic and sympathetic divisions of the ANS.

Five subtypes of muscarinic receptors have been identified (M_1 to M_5). M_1 receptors are generally located in autonomic ganglia, M_2 receptors are located in the heart, M_3 receptors are located in many glands and smooth muscles, and although the locations of M_4 and M_5 receptors are less certain, all five types of muscarinic receptors are found in the CNS.[21] Some muscarinic receptors are located on sympathetic preganglionic neurons and these receptors inhibit the release of norepinephrine. Others are located on parasympathetic preganglionic neurons and, when stimulated, they inhibit the further release of ACh.

Some of the effects of muscarinic receptors are facilitated by specific second messenger systems. A second messenger (biochemical messenger) is a molecule that relays signals from a receptor on the surface of a cell to target molecules in the nucleus of the cell or internal fluid where a physiologic action is to take place. Second messengers can greatly amplify the strength of the signal received.

When ACh binds to nicotinic receptors, an excitatory response occurs. When ACh binds with muscarinic receptors, the result may be excitation or inhibition, depending on the target tissues in which the receptors are found. ACh interacts with these receptors and causes a physiologic response. After ACh has bound with its receptor, it must be broken down to make way for a new molecule of ACh. Acetylcholinesterase is the enzyme that breaks down ACh into smaller molecules. The by-products are recycled and reused to make new molecules of ACh.

Enteric Division. A third division of the ANS, the **enteric nervous system (ENS)**, is embedded in the lining of the digestive system. The ENS contains millions of neurons, distributed in many thousands of small ganglia. Most of these ganglia are found in the myenteric and submucosal plexuses, which are interconnected networks of ganglia. Connections between the ENS and CNS are carried by the vagus and pelvic nerves and sympathetic pathways.[23] Because the ENS includes efferent neurons, afferent neurons, and interneurons, coordinated and purposeful GI function can continue independently even after its connections with the CNS are severed. The ENS releases many different neurotransmitters including nitric oxide, ACh, norepinephrine, serotonin, ATP, and a variety of peptides.

The myenteric plexus receives its messages from the vagus nerve. This plexus extends from the upper esophagus to the internal anal sphincter.[23] The myenteric plexus controls the tone and the intensity of muscle contractions of the intestinal wall. The submucosal plexus is primarily responsible for absorption, secretion, and mucosal blood flow.

Sensory Function

Sensation is an awareness of a body state or condition that results from stimulation of sensory receptors that respond to specific internal or external stimuli. Through the process of sensation, the PNS is able to collect and relay information about the body and the external environment. These messages are generated and transmitted by thousands of **sensory receptors** that monitor conditions within or external to the body. Receptors are capable of sensing monitoring for more than one type of sensation but often become specialized for one specific or a few related sensations.

Sensory receptors convert the energy of a stimulus into action potentials, which are then transmitted along an afferent nerve fiber to the CNS. After these action potentials reach the CNS, they are routed to the specific center with responsibility for interpreting that stimulus, where the message is processed and is brought to conscious thought through **perception**. Perception is an automatic response that is generated through reflexes or other mechanisms, or the message is discarded as unimportant. The intensity of the stimulus is determined by how many nerve endings are activated, how frequently the action potentials are created and propagated, and how many messages are received by the CNS. However, through **adaptation**, the CNS may temporarily or permanently reduce sensitivity to a particular stimulus. For example, when you walk into a crowded restaurant, the noise of a bustling wait staff and dozens of conversations being held over background music may initially strike you as loud and may rise to your consciousness so that you might even mention it to the rest of your party. However, over the next several minutes, the cerebral cortex adjusts to that level of noise and after that, the noise level may not enter your thoughts again until you walk out of the restaurant into the much quieter environment. The perception that a stimulus is still present after the stimulus has been removed is called an **afterimage**. The spots of light you see after glancing at the sun or after a camera flash are examples of afterimages.

General Senses

The **general senses** of pain, temperature, touch, pressure, and position are the means by which the body gathers information from its environment. Sensory receptors for the general senses are widely distributed throughout many tissues of the head and body. Somatic general senses are those that provide sensory information about the body and the environment. Visceral general senses supply information about the body's internal organs.

Pain and Temperature. Pain receptors, or nociceptors, have nerve endings that are sensitive to mechanical, thermal, electrical, or chemical stimuli that could damage the body. Temperature receptors, or thermoreceptors, are nerve endings that respond to heat. The sensations of pain and temperature are related because their receptors overlap, they are conveyed by the same types of fibers in the PNS, and they use the same pathways in the CNS.[14]

Visceral pain is deep pain caused by activation of pain receptors in internal areas of the body that are enclosed within a cavity, such as the chest, abdomen, or pelvis. Visceral sensory nerve fibers travel with autonomic nerves to communicate with the CNS. Visceral pain is poorly localized and generally described as cramping, burning, or gnawing. It often is accompanied by sweating, restlessness, nausea, vomiting, perspiration, and pallor. The patient may move about in an effort to relieve the discomfort.

Somatic pain is caused by the activation of pain receptors in the body's superficial tissues, such as the skin, bones, muscles, and joints. In contrast to visceral pain, somatic pain is generally more intense and more precisely localized. The discomfort that accompanies acute appendicitis is an example of both visceral and somatic pain associated with the GI system. In early acute appendicitis, the patient typically reports vague abdominal pain in the area around the umbilicus (visceral pain). As the inflammation spreads, the patient is able to localize the pain in the right lower quadrant of the abdomen (somatic pain).

Referred pain is pain perceived as occurring in one part of the body other than its true source. This occurs frequently with GI disorders. For example, pain from gallbladder disease often is described as, or accompanied by, pain in the right shoulder. Similarly, when the heart muscle lacks sufficient oxygen to meet the body's demand, pain is often felt in the chest wall, left arm, and left jaw.

Phantom pain may occur secondary to damage to a peripheral nerve. This type of pain may be present after a limb amputation in some patients. For example, the patient may report a cramping, squeezing, shooting, or burning pain in the foot of a limb that no longer exists.

Peripheral and central thermoreceptors are integrated with the CNS, enabling a balance of heat loss and heat production while maintaining the core body temperature within relatively normal limits.[24] Peripheral thermoreceptors that are present on the surface of the body relay information to the hypothalamus about ambient temperature. These receptors are most numerous on the face, lips, and fingers and least numerous on the surface of the trunk. Temperature extremes stimulate pain receptors. Information from thermoreceptors on the skin also travels to the cerebral cortex, enabling conscious awareness of the environmental temperature. Core thermoreceptors that are present in the brain and spinal cord are monitored by the hypothalamus, which adjusts the body's rate of heat production and dissipation as needed, such as during exercise.[24]

Touch and Pressure. Mechanoreceptors (stretch sensors) monitor for changes in physical properties. Among them are tactile receptors that sense touch, proprioceptors responsible for tracking position in space, and **baroreceptors** that measure changes in pressure. Tactile receptors are mechanoreceptors that are located in the skin. Some mechanoreceptors are sensitive to light touch whereas others are stimulated by heavy pressure.

Baroreceptors play an especially important role in many autonomic functions. The most important of these may be measuring the so-called stretch produced in the great vessels. The ANS uses this information to regulate various cardiovascular functions to maintain sufficient CO. Similarly, **chemoreceptors** measure the content of various chemicals in the body and/or bloodstream. By sending messages regarding the amount of carbon dioxide, for example, the ANS can regulate the rate and depth of breathing to ensure proper levels.

Proprioception. Proprioceptors are found in joint capsules, skeletal muscles, and tendons.[14] They provide information about body limb position, muscle stretch, and movement. This information is used by the cerebellum to coordinate motor functions and by the cerebral cortex for conscious awareness of the position of body parts.

Special Senses

The special senses, which serve as the body's first line of protection against environmental hazards, are integrated with the CNS by means of the cranial nerves. Sensory receptors for the special senses of smell, taste, sight, hearing, and balance are localized in a particular area.

Olfaction. The sense of smell, olfaction, is controlled by the first cranial nerve (CN I) with nerve fibers that lie in the upper part of the nasal cavity. Olfactory chemoreceptor

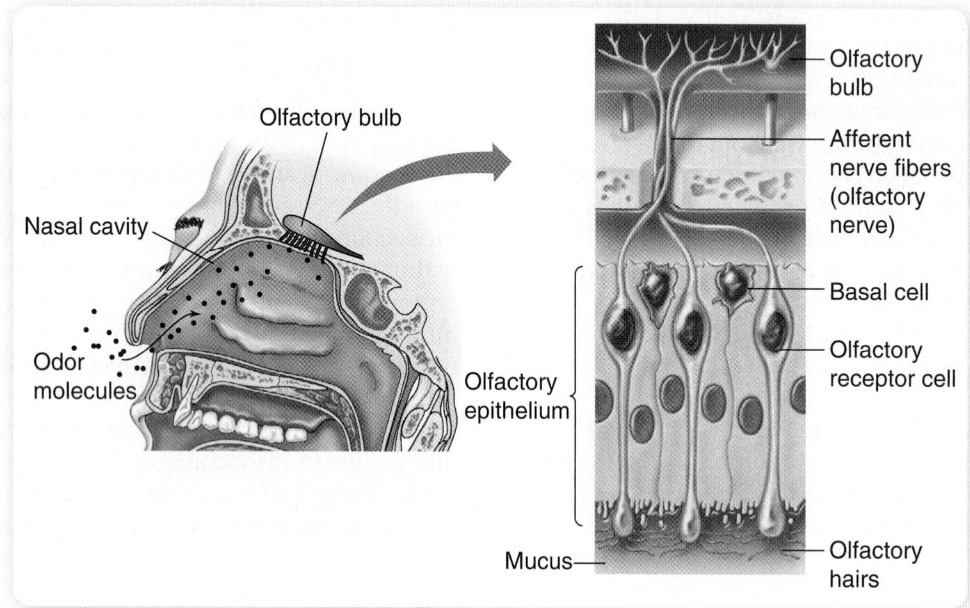

Figure 8-72 Location and structure of olfactory cells.

cells are nerve cells that allow people to perceive smells. One end of the olfactory cell has dendrites that identify chemical stimuli and the other end has an axon that projects directly into the brain. The dendrites of the olfactory neurons extend from the olfactory bulb (in the brain) to the upper part of the nasal cavity **Figure 8-72**. Olfactory cells respond to chemicals dissolved in the mucus covering these cells. After those chemicals reach a threshold level, which may be attained by sniffing to introduce more airflow and therefore more of the substance to be smelled, the chemicals bind with proteins in the olfactory receptors and cause a change in membrane permeability, which in turn creates an action potential. The resulting impulses travel through the olfactory nerves to the olfactory centers in the brain, which interpret these impulses as odors.

Words of Wisdom

Unlike other senses, olfactory signals are transmitted directly to the cerebral cortex without first being filtered by the thalamus. This process creates a close connection to the emotional centers in the brain, and is why you can often recall a feeling or mood associated with a smell even before you remember from where you recognize it. The sense of smell is also important in helping you decipher the taste signals sent by the taste buds. You have probably noticed that when your sense of smell is hampered, such as when you have a cold, foods that normally have mild flavors may have none at all, and others require a much stronger taste stimulus to trigger a response.

Gustation. The senses of smell and taste (gustation) work together to enable you to distinguish among foods. Taste receptor cells are not neurons; they are modified epithelial cells that synapse onto the axons of sensory neurons that communicate with the CNS.[25] Taste receptors respond to four primary taste sensations: sweet, salty, sour, and bitter. Taste is sensed by taste buds, which are located in small elevations called papillae **Figure 8-73**. One taste bud contains 50 to 150 chemoreceptors.[25] Most people have 2,000 to 5,000 taste buds, although the taste buds of some people range from 500 to 20,000.[25]

The facial nerve (CN VII) supplies taste buds on the anterior two-thirds of the tongue, the glossopharyngeal nerve (CN IX) supplies taste buds on the posterior one-third of the tongue, and the vagus nerve (CN X) supplies a few taste buds in the larynx and upper esophagus.[14] Dissolved chemicals from the substance introduced into the mouth combine with specific receptors and cause an action potential that is transmitted to the thalamus for further processing.

Sight. The sense of sight is conducted by the second cranial nerve (CN II). It is facilitated by the eyes, accessory structures, the optic nerve, and the tracts that conduct the impulses to the brain. Recall that each eyeball is recessed into a small frontal skull cavity called the orbit. The eye has two major components: an optical part to gather and focus light and to form an image and a neural part (the retina) to convert the optical image into a neural code.[25] The eye distinguishes two aspects of light: brightness (luminance) and wavelength (color).

The Eye. The eyeball, or globe, is the source of the information the brain processes into pictures **Figure 8-74**. It is imperfectly round and fills the space of the orbit along

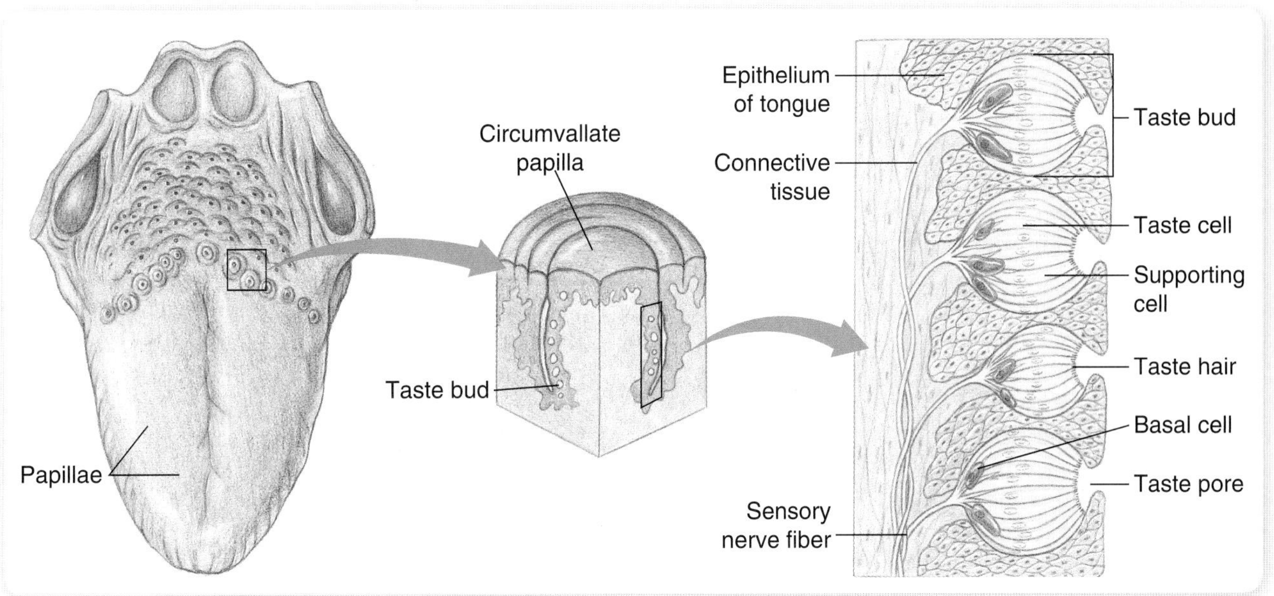

Figure 8-73 The taste buds of the tongue.

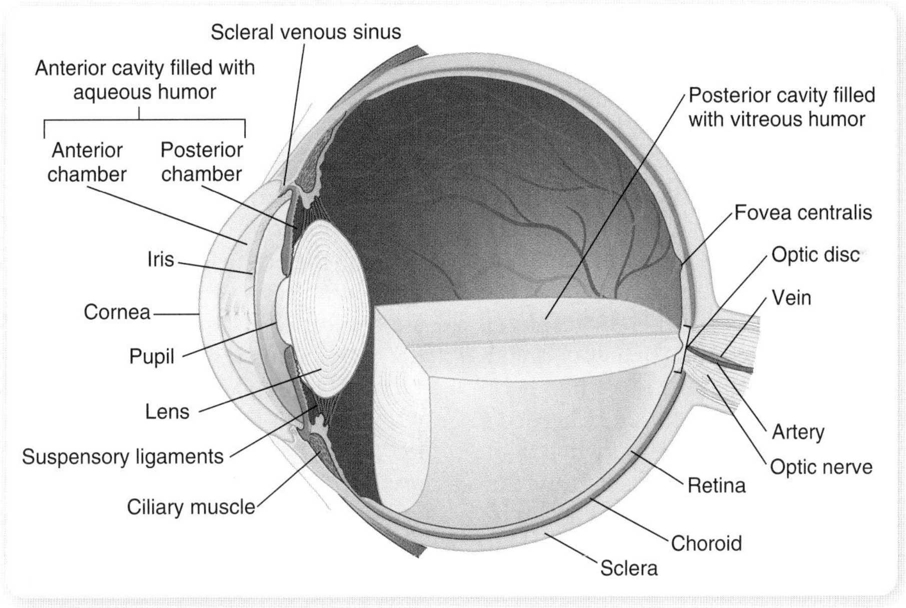

Figure 8-74 The eye.

with the external muscles and a layer of orbital fat that provides cushioning and support. The lens, suspensory ligaments, and ciliary body form a partition that divides the interior of the eyeball into an anterior cavity and a posterior cavity. The posterior cavity, which is between the lens and retina, is filled with **vitreous humor**, a jellylike fluid that helps the globe maintain its shape without distorting light. It also helps hold the retina in place against the wall of the eye.

The iris divides the anterior cavity into anterior and posterior chambers. The anterior chamber is the portion of the globe between the iris and the cornea; the posterior chamber is the portion of the globe between the iris and the lens.[9] Both chambers of the anterior cavity are filled with **aqueous humor**, a clear, watery fluid that maintains intraocular pressure, provides nutrients to the inner surface of the eye, and helps to bend light.[26] Aqueous humor is continuously being formed and reabsorbed. Therefore, if loss of aqueous humor occurs through a penetrating injury to the eye, it will gradually be replenished. The aqueous humor circulates through the pupil and drains into the venous system by the canal of Schlemm, which is a thin-walled vein that extends around the eye. **Glaucoma** is a common cause of blindness that is caused by blockage of the outflow of aqueous humor, which results in an increase in intraocular pressure. A persistent increase in intraocular pressure can permanently destroy optic nerve fibers.

The globe is controlled and directed within the orbit by six **extrinsic muscles**, that attach to the exterior of the globe. The oculomotor (CN III), trochlear (CN IV), and abducens (CN VI) nerves provide the motor nerve supply to these six muscles. CN III also supplies the muscles of the upper eyelid and the sphincter of the pupil and ciliary muscle.

As light passes into the globe, it enters a series of transparent structures that create a **refracting system** responsible for miniaturizing and focusing the image onto the specialized nerve endings of the eye. This process is accomplished through redirecting, or refracting, light as it passes through mediums of different densities. A classic demonstration of this concept occurs when you attempt to retrieve an object from shallow water—for example, retrieving an item at the beach. Because the light is refracted, putting your hand exactly where you see the object will result in a failed attempt to grab the object because the direction of the light is changed as it goes from water to air, leading to a misperception of the actual position of the object in space. The **lens** is a transparent, biconvex elastic disc suspended by ligaments that are attached to ciliary muscles. Contraction and relaxation of the ciliary muscles causes changes in the shape of the lens (making it more rounded or flatter), which affects how light rays entering the eye are refracted, or bent. By altering the shape and thickness of the lens, it is possible for the eye to bring an image into focus. **Accommodation** refers to the ability of the lens to change its shape to focus on a close object. When light rays entering the eye are not refracted at the correct angle, they do not focus on the retina, thereby resulting in visual defects such as farsightedness (hyperopia) and nearsightedness (myopia). **Hyperopia** results when light rays focus behind the retina because the distance between the lens and retina is too short. **Myopia** results when light rays converge and focus in front of the retina because the eyeball is too elongated. In **astigmatism**, irregularities in the shape of the lens create visual defects because parts of the image are out of focus when other parts are in focus. Prescription eyeglasses or contact lenses are used to treat errors of refraction. The increased difficulty in focusing that occurs with aging is **presbyopia**, although debate exists as to the actual mechanism. Although the lens is normally transparent, it can develop **cataracts**, which can cause varying levels of obstruction ranging from a light film to complete obstruction.

The walls of the globe are composed of three layers of connective tissue with the lens suspended inside them. These layers include the fibrous tunic, the vascular tunic, and the nervous tunic. The outermost layer, or fibrous tunic, is continuous with the dura mater. It consists of the sclera and cornea. The **sclera** is a firm, opaque, white outer layer of the eye. It is nonvascular and helps maintain the shape of the eye. The sclera continues posteriorly as the sheath of the optic nerve. It also serves as an attachment for the extrinsic muscles that move the eye. The **cornea** is an avascular, transparent structure that permits light through to the interior of the eye. The cornea is sensitive to pain and is nourished by the aqueous humor.

The middle layer, the vascular tunic, is aptly named because it contains the blood vessels that supply the eye tissues, as well as the lymph vessels and intrinsic eye muscles. It is composed of the iris, the ciliary body, and the choroid. This vascular layer is the primary route through which blood vessels and nerves (other than the optic nerve) travel within the wall of the eye. The iris is the colored (pigmented) part of the eye. It consists of a ring of smooth muscle that surrounds the pupil, which regulates the amount of light entering the eye. The pupil is not actually a structure itself; its boundaries are simply the empty space left by changing the size of the iris. Light enters through the pupil, and the iris controls the size (diameter) of the pupil. The **ciliary body** supports the ciliary muscles that control the curvature of the lens by means of a ring of fibers called the suspensory ligament. The ciliary muscles are supplied by parasympathetic fibers of CN III. The **choroid** is a thin, vascular membrane of venous and arterial capillaries that covers the posterior two-thirds of the eyeball. It supports the outer layers of the retina and contains pigment that absorbs stray light.

The innermost layer, the nervous tunic, contains the **retina**, which consists of an outer pigmented area and an inner sensory layer that responds to light. Light passes through the structures of the eye in this order: cornea, aqueous humor, lens, vitreous humor, and then through the entire layer of the retina.[9] The retina receives light impulses and converts them to nerve signals that are conducted to the brain by the optic nerve. The optic nerve transmits the image to the brain, where it is converted into conscious images in the visual cortex. The retina is part of the CNS, receiving oxygen and nutrients from the choroid plexus and retinal blood vessels. As a result, the retina is the only place where the circulatory system of the brain can actually be viewed directly with an ophthalmoscope.[27]

The sensory part of the retina contains photoreceptor cells (rods and cones), which convert light energy into electrical signals. Photoreceptor cells, which are supplied by capillaries from the choroid, relay impulses to the optic nerve. **Cones** are used for day and color vision, and **rods** are used for night vision. Each of the three kinds of cones are sensitive to a different color: red, green, or blue. Rods and cones transmit information through intermediary cells that synapse with ganglia cells whose axons form the optic nerve. The point where these nerves penetrate the posterior globe to form the base of the optic nerve is a structure known as the optic disk. The optic disk contains no rods or cones and therefore creates a blind spot in the visual field of each eye. As these signals follow the optic nerve toward the CNS, they pass through the **optic chiasm**, where about half of the nerve fibers from each eye cross over to the opposite side of the brain.

> **Words of Wisdom**
>
> An absence of one or more of the color-sensitive pigments in the cone cells of the retina results in color blindness. For example, an individual whose cones lack red pigment is unable to distinguish between red and green (the most common form of color blindness). Sometimes all cone cell pigments are present, but one cell type functions abnormally, detecting a different color than normal.

The vision centers on each side of the brain interpret information separately but then combine those signals to create one image that the brain "sees." This merging of two images into one is known as **binocular vision**. Binocular vision creates the perception of depth when both eyes are able to focus on the same target. In **strabismus**, however, there is a loss of perception of depth and overlapping or doubled images because the eyes fail to coordinate their movement and may become crossed or separated. The opposite condition is also possible. In *amblyopia* (so-called lazy eye), the eyes may be oriented correctly but one fails to send adequate signals to the vision centers, also causing a loss of depth perception and poor-quality images.

The fovea centralis is located in the center of the retina. It lies in the visual axis, which is a line passing from the center of the visual field of the eye, through the center of the lens. The fovea has a higher concentration of cones than any area of the retina and it is the point of the most acute vision (eg, sharpest visual acuity and acute color vision). The **macula** is an area that surrounds the fovea. It is relatively free of blood vessels and has a high concentration of cones. Many of the photoreceptor cells in the macula contain yellow pigment.

Two types of vision exist: central and peripheral. Central vision aids in the visualization of objects directly in front of you, and is processed by the macula. The remainder of the retina processes peripheral vision, which allows the visualization of lateral objects while you are looking forward.

Accessory Structures. The accessory structures of the eye protect, lubricate, move, and aid in the function of the eye. These structures include the eyebrows, eyelids, **conjunctivae**, and **lacrimal glands** (tear glands) **Figure 8-75**.

Eyebrows protect the eyes by providing shade and preventing perspiration and foreign material (eg, sweat, dust) from entering the eye from above. The eyelids protect the eyes from foreign objects. Blinking lubricates the eyes by spreading tears over the surface of the eye. The medial canthus is the site of union of the upper and lower eyelids near the nose. The lateral canthus is the site of union of the upper and lower eyelids away from the nose. The eyelashes help prevent small particles from falling into the eye when it is open.

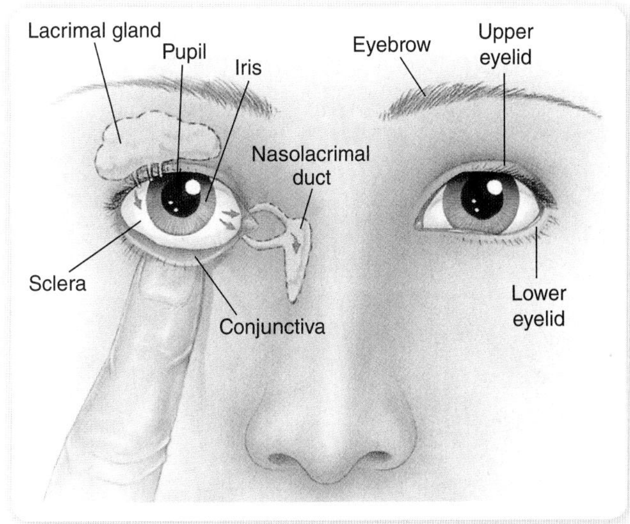

Figure 8-75 The accessory structures of the eye include the eyebrows, eyelids, conjunctiva, and lacrimal glands.

The conjunctivae are a layer of soft mucous membranes lining the inside of the eyelid that cushion and allow smooth movement. **Conjunctivitis** is an inflammation of the conjunctiva. Bacterial conjunctivitis (pink eye) is a common eye infection that results in inflammation and pain.

The lacrimal gland is one of a pair of glands situated superior and lateral to the eye bulb. It makes lacrimal fluid (tears). This fluid is a watery, slightly alkaline secretion that consists of tears and saline that moistens the conjunctiva. Lacrimal fluid also contains enzymes that help protect the eye from protein material (eg, bacteria). The act of blinking, whether voluntary or involuntary, uses tears to sweep debris, bacteria, or other material from the surface of the eye. Excess fluid is collected at the medial corner of the eye and drains into the nasal cavity through the nasolacrimal duct. The nasolacrimal duct is a superficial structure on the outer lateral aspects of the nose. Superficial lacerations to this area can disrupt these ducts, which can lead to life-long complications with the drainage of tears.

Hearing and Balance. The organs of hearing are divided into three portions: external, middle, and inner ear **Figure 8-76**. The external and middle ear are involved in hearing only. The inner ear functions in both hearing and balance, which occur by way of the vestibulocochlear cranial nerve (CN VIII). CN VIII arises from the brainstem and supplies the inner ear, which lies within the temporal bone. It divides within the temporal bone into a cochlear portion to the cochlea, where it carries information about sound, and a vestibular portion to the semicircular canals, where it conveys impulses concerned with balance, position, and movement of the head.

The external ear includes the auricle (**pinna**), and the external auditory canal (external auditory meatus).

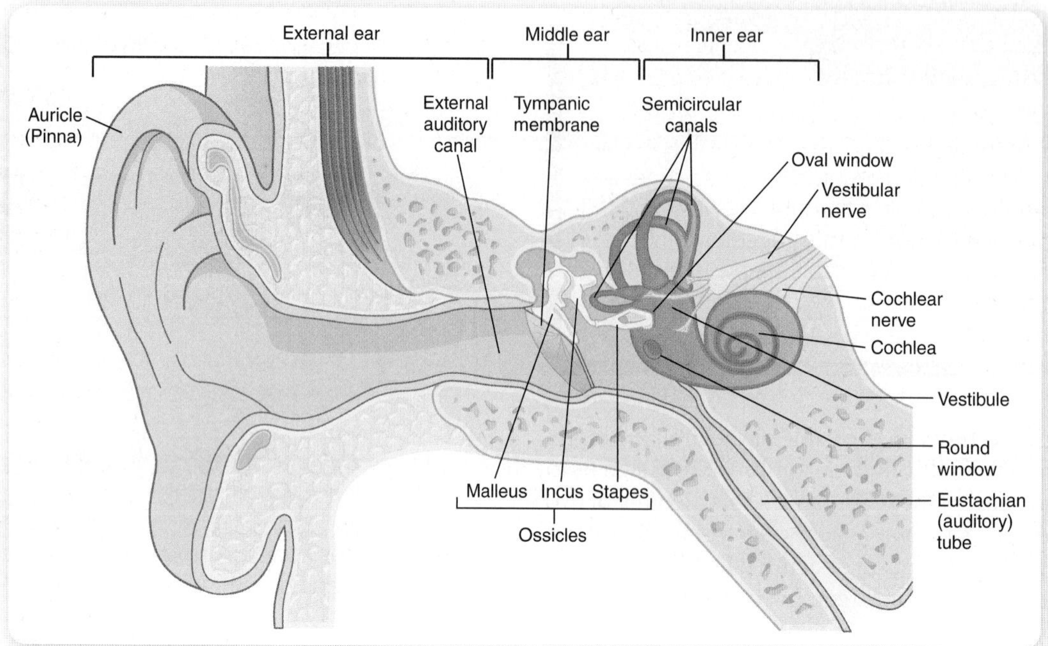

Figure 8-76 The ear.

Recall that the pinna is a formation of cartilage that is covered with skin and protects the ear. The external canal is lined by hair and ceruminous glands, which produce cerumen (earwax). The external ear conducts sound to the tympanic membrane, or eardrum. This thin membrane separates the ear canal from the middle ear. Vibration of the tympanic membrane ultimately results in movement of the fluids of the inner ear.

The middle ear is an air-filled chamber within the temporal bone. As discussed previously, the middle ear contains the auditory ossicles. The malleus, incus, and stapes articulate with each other to transmit sound waves to the cochlea. The **eustachian tube** joins the middle ear cavity to the nasopharynx. The eustachian tube is normally closed, but it opens during swallowing or yawning allowing air to enter the middle ear. This process allows pressure to equalize on both sides of the tympanic membrane. The medial end of the stapes is attached to another membrane, the **oval window**, which separates the middle ear from the entrance to the cochlea. Sound is amplified by the middle ear and transmitted through this membrane to the delicate structures of the inner ear, which are filled with fluid. This movement of fluid within an enclosed space is made possible by the round window, which allows fluid to move in minute amounts as it flexes out of the canal.

The fluid-filled inner ear holds the sensory organs for hearing and balance. The inner ear is composed of a series of canals called the labyrinth. A series of sacs and tubes make up the membranous labyrinth, which contains a thick fluid called **endolymph** that is similar to intracellular fluid. Auditory and vestibular receptor cells (hair cells) are located in the walls of this labyrinth. Some of these hair cells respond to sound, others to head movement, and still others to head position. The membranous labyrinth is suspended within the **bony labyrinth**, which is a cavity in the temporal bone. Between the bony and membranous labyrinths is a fluid called **perilymph**, which is similar to CSF.

Sound waves are conducted through the inner ear by endolymph and perilymph. The bony labyrinth is separated into three areas, the vestibule, the cochlea, and the semicircular canals. The vestibule, which is the space or cavity that serves as the entrance to the inner ear, leads directly to the cochlea. The semicircular canals, which are three bony fluid-filled loops, are involved in balance. The utricle and the saccule are two membranous expansions located within the vestibule. The cochlea contains the organ of hearing, the **organ of Corti**, which contains many hair cells. Permanent damage to the cochlea can result from exposure to high-intensity sounds, such as those produced by subway trains, jet engines, and chain saws.

The auricle of the external ear is designed to collect sound waves directed toward the tympanic membrane. Sound waves cause this membrane to vibrate. This vibration is transmitted to the middle ear, causing the ossicles to vibrate. This vibration results in movement of the fluids of the inner ear. Motion of theses fluids stimulates the hair cells, which stimulates the nerve endings of CN VIII, resulting in the relay of information to the brain for interpretation.

Any condition that results in the partial or complete loss of hearing is known as deafness. Deafness can result from many causes. If any of the structures that normally transmit, or conduct, the vibration of sound from the outer ear to the inner ear fail to do so, then this is termed a conductive deafness. If, instead, the sound is transmitted correctly by the physical structures but some dysfunction or malformation of the organ of Corti or the receptor cells is present, then this is known as a nerve deafness. In the least common case, the nerve impulses may reach the auditory centers of the brain appropriately, but the brain may have a damaged ability to interpret those signals. This is termed central deafness.

Also contained within the inner ear is the vestibular system, composed of a pair of fluid-filled sacs known as **otoliths** and three more fluid-filled, looping passageways known as semicircular canals. These formations have no effect on hearing, but instead are used by the CNS to collect information about movement and orientation in space. The semicircular canals use the movement of fluid to sense rotational movement in each of three planes. The saccule gathers information from its mass of fluid to capture linear movements, while the utricle monitors the degree of head tilt. By processing all of these sensations simultaneously, the vestibular system keeps you upright and aware of your position in space (proprioception).

The Endocrine System

The **endocrine system** consists of the following structures: the hypothalamus, the pituitary gland, the thyroid gland, the parathyroid glands, the thymus gland, the pancreas, the adrenal glands, the pineal gland, and the gonads **Figure 8-77**. Although the hypothalamus is not a gland, its endocrine functions include the production and release of hormones; therefore, it is considered a neuroendocrine organ.[9]

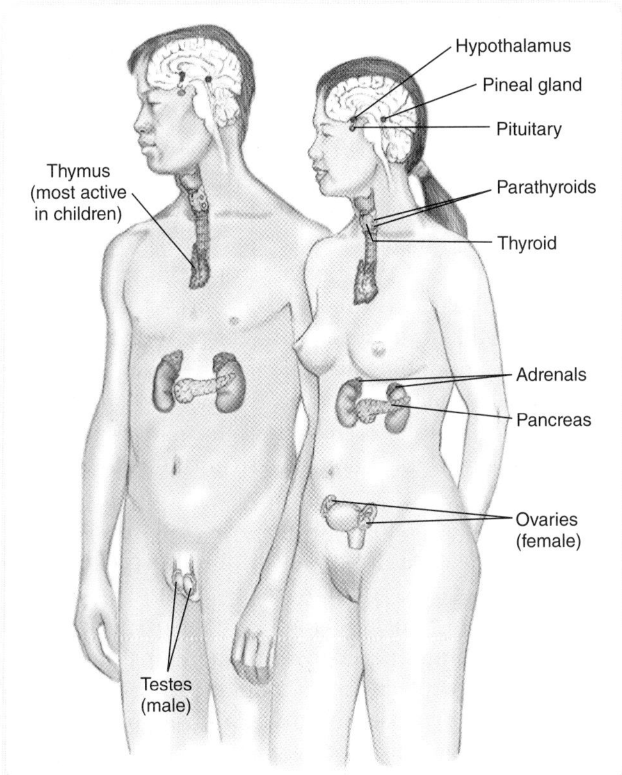

Figure 8-77 The endocrine system uses various glands to deliver chemical messages to organ systems throughout the body.

The endocrine glands send hormones throughout the body to maintain homeostasis. Through its hormones, the endocrine system regulates many of the metabolic functions of the body. Some hormones may only affect tissues in one body system; other hormones may have target tissues in many body systems.

The endocrine glands secrete hormones directly into the interstitial fluid and then into the circulatory system without the use of ducts. These hormones are then distributed to the entire body to affect the activity of other cells. Exocrine glands contain ducts and release their chemical products through those ducts directly to the site where they are to be used. For example, the lacrimal glands produce lacrimal secretions and are exocrine glands. These secretions are deposited directly onto the eye by the lacrimal ducts to bathe the eye with nutrients and protect it. Some cells and tissues outside the endocrine system also produce hormones, which will be discussed later in this chapter.

Words of Wisdom

The nervous system is like a telephone system. It communicates through a complex system of hard wires. This system works well for crisis management and in situations requiring quick fixes or corrections. However, when long-term management is required, the endocrine system starts to work. The so-called hard wiring of the nervous system reaches only a percentage of the body. In contrast, the endocrine system and its hormones reach every cell of the body, enabling a level of cellular control that is not possible with the nervous system. This hormonal control is relatively slow compared with the control exerted by the nervous system. The nervous and endocrine systems of the body operate in parallel toward a common goal: homeostasis.

Intercellular Communication

The human body is a complex organism composed of multiple interconnected systems. To function effectively, these body systems must be regulated and coordinated down to the cellular level. To achieve this level of coordination, cells from within a body system and between body systems must be able to interact. Recall that the means by which cells communicate is called intercellular communication or cellular signaling.

To maintain homeostasis, the body uses many different types of chemical messengers (signaling molecules) to relay information to neighboring or distant cells. Examples of chemical messengers include neurotransmitters, hormones, ions, growth factors, and products of cellular metabolism. Most chemical messengers act on specific receptors on target cells that, once activated, trigger a series of secondary events that mediate the response of the target cell to that stimulus.[28]

In a few special situations, cells with the same function may communicate with each other through direct communication or contact-dependent communication. For direct communication to occur, the cells must share extensive physical contact. A number of cells possess gap junctions that enable adjacent cells to connect. Recall that gap junctions function as electrical connections and permit the exchange of nutrients, metabolites, ions, and small molecules.

You have learned that the nervous system relies on neurotransmitters for nerve cells to communicate. This form of intercellular communication is called synaptic communication or synaptic transmission. After their release into the synapse between nerve cells, neurotransmitters rapidly trigger receptors on the next neuron. Neurotransmitters are rapidly broken down and reabsorbed for future use. Because the nervous system is located throughout the entire body, this form of intercellular communication is capable of rapidly transmitting messages over long distances.

With endocrine communication, glands or specialized cells secrete an endocrine hormone into blood that then circulates throughout the body, thereby influencing tissues distant from the site of manufacture. Different body systems have target cells containing receptors that are activated by specific hormones floating in the bloodstream. After these cells have been activated, they have preprogrammed responses that regulate important body functions. Most hormones have antagonizing hormones that act to balance, or buffer, each other. For example, consider the two competing hormones, insulin and glucagon. Through complex mechanisms, insulin acts to lower blood glucose levels, whereas glucagon acts to raise blood glucose levels. In this manner, the body is better able to achieve homeostasis.

Another form of intercellular communication is known as paracrine communication. Paracrine hormones are chemical messengers that are released into the circulation by one type of cell and act on a neighboring cell of a different type. They are usually taken up by target cells or rapidly broken down by enzymes. The release of ACh at the neuromuscular junction is an example of paracrine signaling.[28] Chemical messengers that are released into the circulation and that affect the function of the same cells that produced them or cells of the same type are autocrine hormones. Cytokines are peptides that are released into the extracellular fluid and that can function as autocrine, paracrine, or endocrine hormones.

▶ Hormones

Hormones are manufactured in endocrine glands within the body and are released directly, without ducts, into the circulatory system. Next, they travel to specific target cells, which have receptors that carry out a complex set of instructions and actions when exposed to the specific hormone for which they are designed. These target cells can exist anywhere in the body. Effects to an individual cell are more gradual and have a longer effect (duration) than the effects of the nervous system. Each target cell has specific receptor sites on the cell membrane, or inside the cell, to which the specific hormone can attach or bind. These receptors have two main functions: (1) to recognize and bind to their particular hormones and (2) to initiate an appropriate signal. After the hormone has attached to the receptor site of the cell, the message to alter the cellular function is delivered.

Many cells contain multiple receptors and act as targets for several hormones—or for molecules introduced into the body as therapy. *Agonists* are molecules that bind to a cell's receptor and trigger a response by that cell; they produce some kind of action or biologic effect. **Antagonists** are molecules that bind to the receptor of a cell and block the action of agonists, thereby preventing a biologic response. Hormone antagonists are widely used as drugs.

Chemistry of Hormones

The endocrine system is composed of several glands spread throughout the body that are not physically connected. Each gland is responsible for creating specific hormones that create specific responses in specific target cells. The three general classes of hormones are as follows: proteins and polypeptides, amine hormones, and steroid hormones.

Proteins and Polypeptides. Proteins and peptides are the most abundant of the body hormones. They are secreted by the anterior and posterior pituitary gland, the hypothalamus, the pancreas, the parathyroid gland, and many other tissues. Proteins are polypeptides with 100 or more amino acids; peptides are polypeptides with fewer than 100 amino acids. Because peptide hormones are water soluble, they are able to enter the circulatory system easily. Protein hormones are not lipid soluble and therefore are unable to cross the cell membrane. These hormones attach to receptor sites on the surface of the cell membrane. This process, in turn, creates a reaction in the cell. This reaction activates a second messenger in the cell, such as cyclic adenosine monophosphate (cyclic AMP), which starts a chain of events resulting in cellular change. These may include changes in the permeability of the cellular membrane, changes in the shape of the cell, or an increase or decrease in cellular production. Insulin and epinephrine are examples of protein hormones that also may be administered as medications. Insulin binds with the cell membrane and causes an increase in the absorption of glucose, whereas epinephrine binds with alpha and beta receptors, causing vasoconstriction, bronchodilation, increased HR, and other effects specific to these receptors.

Amine Hormones. Amine hormones that are derivatives of the amino acid tyrosine are secreted by the adrenal medullae and the thyroid gland. Examples of amine hormones include dopamine, epinephrine, and norepinephrine. Serotonin is an amine hormone made from tryptophan by endocrine cells located within the mucosa of the gut.

Steroid Hormones. Steroid hormones, which are derivatives of cholesterol, are secreted by the adrenal cortex, the ovaries, and the testes (also called the testicles or gonads). Examples of steroid hormones include aldosterone, cortisol, progesterone, and testosterone. Steroid hormones are lipid soluble and can readily cross the cell membrane and act on receptors within the cell. Once inside the cell, they combine with a protein receptor to form a steroid-protein complex. This complex enters the nucleus, causing the cell to create proteins used as enzymes.

Regulation of Hormones

Hormones operate within feedback systems (either positive or negative) to maintain an optimal internal operating environment in the body. Release of hormones is regulated by chemical factors, other hormonal factors, and neural control. Endocrine regulation, through negative feedback, is the most important method by which hormonal secretion is maintained within a physiologic range.

One example of this negative feedback mechanism is the release of epinephrine from the adrenal medulla in response to stress. When stress stimulates the body's neural regulation by means of the sympathetic nervous system, it releases epinephrine into the bloodstream from the adrenal medulla to help the body respond. When the stressor is removed, nervous system stimulation decreases and less epinephrine is released.

Positive feedback mechanisms are those in which an effect leads to or causes another effect. Normal positive feedback mechanisms in the body include the clotting cascade and childbirth. Positive feedback mechanisms also can occur in harmful situations. In decompensated shock, the lack of perfusion to the tissues leads to failure of the cardiac and vasomotor centers, which leads to decreased HR and decreased vasoconstriction. This leads to further decreases in perfusion, which further depress the body's ability to combat the shock, thereby creating a vicious circle.

Prostaglandins (PGs)

Recall that PGs are derivatives of an essential fatty acid. Although PGs are not hormones, they are mentioned here because their effects are similar to those of hormones. PGs are sometimes called tissue hormones because their effects are usually localized on or near the cell in which it is made. At least 16 different PGs exist, and their effects are of short duration.

Examples of changes caused by PGs are changes in capillary permeability, smooth muscle tone, platelet aggregation (clumping), endocrine and exocrine functions, and the inflammatory process (including the development of fever and pain). Several PGs produced in the kidneys cause vasodilation of arterioles. In uterine smooth muscle, PGs increase the intracellular concentration of calcium, thereby increasing uterine contractility. Although some PGs functions are beneficial to the body, PG synthesis has also been implicated in the mechanisms of cardiovascular disease, cancer, and inflammatory diseases.[28] Nonsteroidal antiinflammatory drugs (eg, aspirin, ibuprofen) inhibit the synthesis of PGs.

Leukotrienes and thromboxanes are examples of fatty acid compounds that are tissue hormones similar to PGs. Their effects are localized but potent. Leukotrienes play an important role in the body's inflammatory response. Thromboxane A_2 is a short-lived compound that can cause platelet clumping and constrict small blood vessels.[28]

▶ Hypothalamus

The human body regulates itself by communicating at the cellular level through the nervous and endocrine systems. The hypothalamus is the link between the two systems. Recall that the hypothalamus is located deep in the cerebrum of the brain. It contains cells that function both as nerve cells and as glandular cells. The neuron functions of these cells receive input from the ANS. This input includes feedback from the body's self-monitoring system.

Information processed by the hypothalamus includes, among other things, reports on blood pressure, HR, body temperature, and blood glucose levels. Some hypothalamic neural cells pass this information on to the CNS, some neural cells conduct impulses to the posterior pituitary gland, and some glandular cells produce and release hormones that trigger target tissue in the anterior and posterior lobes of the pituitary gland. These hormones, sometimes called regulatory hormones, regulate the release of hormones by the pituitary gland Table 8-26. The primary effect of these regulatory hormones is to direct the pituitary gland to increase or decrease production of hormones that coordinate body systems.

Hormones that are secreted by neurons into the circulating blood and that influence the function of target cells in another location in the body are called neuroendocrine hormones. The hypothalamus contains neuroendocrine cells whose axons terminate in the posterior pituitary gland.

▶ Pituitary Gland

The pituitary gland (hypophysis) is often referred to as the master gland because its secretions control the secretions of other endocrine glands. It is a small gland, about the size of a grape, found just inferior to the hypothalamus inside a depression in the sphenoid bone. It rests just above the roof of the mouth and is connected to the hypothalamus by a thin piece of tissue called the pituitary

Table 8-26 Hormones of the Hypothalamus

Hormone	Target Site	Effect
Corticotropin-releasing hormone (CRH)	Anterior pituitary	Stimulates release of adrenocorticotropic hormone
Growth hormone–releasing hormone (GHRH)	Anterior pituitary	Stimulates release of growth hormone
Growth hormone–inhibiting hormone (GHIH)	Anterior pituitary	Inhibits release of growth hormone
Gonadotropin-releasing hormone (GnRH)	Anterior pituitary	Stimulates release of luteinizing hormone and follicle-stimulating hormone
Prolactin-inhibiting hormone (PIH)	Anterior pituitary	Inhibits release of prolactin
Prolactin-releasing hormone (PRH)	Anterior pituitary	Stimulates release of prolactin
Thyroid-releasing hormone (TRH)	Anterior pituitary	Stimulates release of thyroid-stimulating hormone

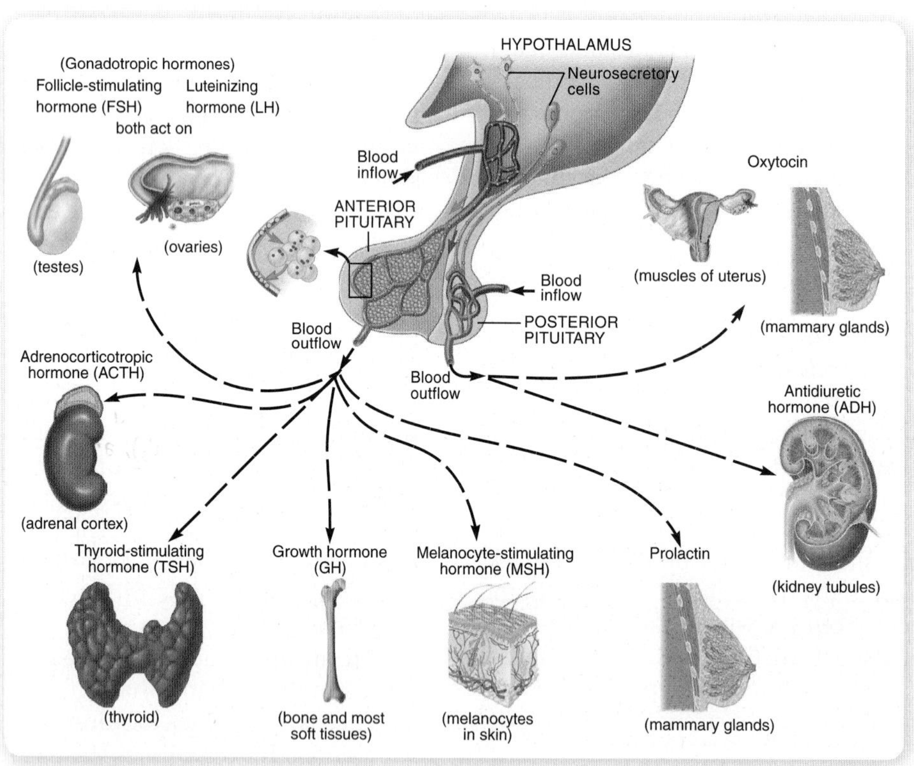

Figure 8-78 The pituitary gland secretes hormones from its two regions: the anterior pituitary lobe and the posterior pituitary lobe.

stalk. The pituitary is divided into the anterior lobe and the posterior lobe Figure 8-78.

The anterior lobe is controlled by hormones released from the hypothalamus. Because the anterior lobe is not physically connected to the hypothalamus, these hormones are released into circulation and absorbed in the anterior lobe by small blood vessels called the hypothalamic-hypophysial portal veins. The anterior lobe contains endocrine cells that produce several hormones when stimulated by the hypothalamus. Some of the hormones released by the anterior lobe of the pituitary gland do not directly affect body systems. Instead, they stimulate other glands to release hormones that regulate body functions. The hormones released by the anterior

Table 8-27 Hormones of the Pituitary Gland

Hormone	Target Site	Effect
Pituitary Gland, Anterior		
Adrenocorticotropic hormone (ACTH)	Adrenal cortex	Stimulates release of steroidal hormones by the adrenal cortex
Follicle-stimulating hormone (FSH)	Ovaries or testes	Stimulates development of ovum or sperm
Growth hormone (GH)	All cells, especially growth cells	Stimulates cell growth and replication, especially in skeletal muscles and cartilage
Luteinizing hormone (LH)	Ovaries or testes	Stimulates release of hormones by the ovaries or testes
Prolactin	Mammary glands	Stimulates production and release of milk
Thyroid-stimulating hormone (TSH)	Thyroid	Stimulates release of thyroid hormones
Pituitary Gland, Posterior		
Antidiuretic hormone (ADH)	Kidneys	Stimulates increased reabsorption of water into bloodstream
Oxytocin	Uterus and breasts of women	Stimulates uterine contractions and milk release

lobe of the pituitary gland are shown in Table 8-27. These hormones are inhibited when the hypothalamus releases the appropriate inhibitory hormone.

The posterior lobe of the pituitary gland contains the distal ends of some hypothalamic neurons. These hypothalamic neurons produce hormones, but do not release them directly into the bloodstream. Instead, the axons that originated in the hypothalamus extend directly into the posterior lobe of the pituitary gland, where they are stored in secretory vesicles. These hormones are then secreted into the bloodstream when stimulated by nerve impulses from the hypothalamus. The hormones released in the posterior lobe of the pituitary gland include ADH and oxytocin. ADH, also called arginine vasopressin, increases the reabsorption of water into the bloodstream. In the absence of ADH, an individual may develop diabetes insipidus, in which the kidneys pass copious amounts of water because they are not told to retain it. Arginine vasopressin also acts as a peripheral vasoconstrictor. Oxytocin stimulates milk release and smooth muscle contractions in the uterine wall, prompting fetal delivery.

▶ Thyroid Gland

The large gland at the base of the neck is the **thyroid gland**. The thyroid affects almost every organ in the body, including the nervous, cardiovascular, and GI systems; reproductive organs; and the skin, hair, and nails. The thyroid gland is critical for normal metabolism.

The thyroid gland consists of two lobes that are connected by a narrow band of tissue, and is covered by a capsule of connective tissue with secretory parts called follicles. The thyroid is filled with a clear substance called colloid, which stores hormones produced by the follicles. The two main hormones of the thyroid gland, triiodothyronine (T_3) and thyroxine (also known as tetraiodothyronine or T_4), are produced in the thyroid follicles Table 8-28. Of the two thyroid hormones, T_3 is the more potent, but it is present in the circulation in much smaller quantities than T_4.

Thyroid-stimulating hormone, which is released by the pituitary gland, causes the thyroid gland to release T_3 and T_4. The thyroid hormones regulate metabolism of carbohydrates, lipids, and proteins, determining the body's **basal metabolic rate** (the rate at which nutrients are consumed in the body). Increasing the body's metabolic rate increases oxygen consumption and heat production. Thyroid hormones are required for growth, development, and maturation of the nervous system.

Because iodine is essential to form normal quantities of thyroid hormones, the thyroid follicles use iodine absorbed through the digestive tract. Without the proper level of dietary iodine intake, thyroxine cannot be produced, and the person's physical and mental growth is diminished.

The thyroid gland also secretes calcitonin, though it is produced by its extrafollicular cells rather than the follicular cells. Calcitonin, in conjunction with PTH, regulates concentrations of calcium in body fluids. This hormone

Table 8-28 Hormones of the Thyroid Gland

Hormone	Target Site	Effect
Calcitonin	Bone	Works in conjunction with PTH to maintain homeostasis of calcium; increases storage of calcium in bone, thereby lowering blood calcium levels
Triiodothyronine (T_3)	All cells	Stimulates cellular metabolism
Thyroxine (T_4)	All cells	Stimulates cellular metabolism

Table 8-29 Hormones of the Parathyroid Gland

Hormone	Target Site	Effect
PTH	Bones, intestines, kidneys	Stimulates calcium release from bones, calcium uptake from intestinal tract, and calcium reabsorption in kidneys, with a net increase in blood calcium levels

Table 8-30 Hormones of the Thymus Gland

Hormone	Target Site	Effect
Thymosin	WBCs	Promotes the development and maturation of lymphocytes (WBCs involved in immunity)

Abbreviation: WBC, white blood cell

is secreted directly into the bloodstream when the thyroid detects high levels of calcium in the extracellular fluid. Calcitonin travels to the bones, where it stimulates the bone-building cells to absorb the excess calcium. It also stimulates the kidneys to absorb and excrete excess calcium.

Parathyroid Glands

The **parathyroid glands** are embedded in the posterior portion of each lobe of the thyroid. They produce and secrete PTH, which maintains normal levels of calcium in the blood and normal neuromuscular function Table 8-29. The effects of PTH are opposite to those of calcitonin. Parathyroid hormone is secreted when calcium blood levels are low. It stimulates the bone-dissolving cells to break down bone and release calcium into the bloodstream. In the kidneys, PTH decreases the amount of calcium released in the urine.

Thymus Gland

The **thymus** is located in the mediastinum, just behind the sternum. It is soft, and consists of two lobes that are enclosed in a connective tissue capsule. The function of the thymus is to help the immune system identify and destroy foreign intruders. During infancy and early childhood, an individual's thymus is large. It diminishes in size as the person reaches adulthood. The thymus, which is often associated with the lymphatic system, releases several hormones that are together called thymosin Table 8-30.

Thymosin promotes the maturation of **T lymphocytes** (T cells), the WBCs primarily responsible for immunity. **Immunity** refers to the body's ability to protect itself from acquiring a disease.

Pancreas

The **pancreas** is located partially in the retroperitoneal space behind the stomach (see Figure 8-77). It is a slender organ with both endocrine and exocrine functions Table 8-31. About 99% of the pancreatic volume consists of exocrine gland cells called pancreatic acini. These cells connect to ducts that deposit an alkaline, enzyme-rich fluid that is involved in the digestion of lipids, carbohydrates, and proteins directly into the digestive tract. The remainder of the pancreas is composed of clustered endocrine cells forming islets. These pancreatic islets are also known as the **islets of Langerhans**. These cell groups within the pancreas act like an organ within an organ. Four types of cells are found in the islets of Langerhans: (1) alpha cells, which produce glucagon; (2) beta cells, which produce insulin; (3) delta cells, which produce somatostatin; and (4) F cells, which produce pancreatic polypeptide. Somatostatin is identical to growth hormone-inhibiting hormone released by the hypothalamus. Somatostatin also decreases the motility of the digestive system and decreases absorption and secretion in the digestive system.

Insulin and glucagon work in opposition to each other and play an important role in maintaining a proper blood glucose balance. Recall that these two hormones

Table 8-31 Hormones of the Pancreas

Hormone	Target Site	Effect
Glucagon	All cells, primarily in liver, muscle, and fat	Excreted when blood glucose level is low (hypoglycemia); increases conversion of glycogen to glucose (glycogenolysis)
Insulin	All cells, primarily in liver, muscle, and fat	Excreted when blood glucose is high (hyperglycemia); increases conversion of glucose to glycogen; assists glucose across cell membrane
Pancreatic polypeptide	Gallbladder; pancreatic exocrine glands	Inhibits gallbladder contraction; regulates some pancreatic enzymes
Somatostatin (identical to growth hormone-inhibiting hormone)	Alpha and beta cells in the pancreas	Excreted with increased levels of insulin and glucagon; decreases secretion of insulin and glycogen; slows the absorption of nutrients

compose a negative feedback system; when the level of one rises, the level of the other lowers. As blood glucose levels in the body rise, parasympathetic stimulation causes the release of insulin into the bloodstream. This promotes the movement of glucose from the bloodstream into the cells. (Note that brain cells do not depend on insulin to help move glucose from the bloodstream into the cells.) Insulin also prompts the liver to convert circulating glucose into glycogen. All of these actions work to reduce the blood glucose level.

Conversely, when the blood glucose levels begin to drop, sympathetic stimulation causes the release of glucagon into the bloodstream, which inhibits the release of insulin. Glucagon causes the liver and skeletal muscles to convert glycogen back into glucose. This process is known as glycogenolysis. In addition, glucagon causes an increase in the breakdown of fats into fatty acids and body proteins into amino acids for conversion by the liver into glucose. This formation of glucose in the liver is called **gluconeogenesis**. Depending on the metabolic needs of the body, the free fatty acids and glycerol may be metabolized directly or converted to ketones. In small amounts, ketone production is normal. In disease states, such as diabetic ketoacidosis, increased plasma glucagon concentrations and unopposed glucagon activity lead to excessive production, resulting in possible harm to the patient.

Glycogen is used by the body when blood glucose levels may not be high. Glycogen is also stored in skeletal muscle cells in a lesser amount that is not readily available for systemic use. Insulin also increases amino acid absorption, protein synthesis, and triglyceride synthesis and inhibits the release of glucagon.

Somatostatin inhibits both insulin and glucagon production. By inhibiting the release of both of these hormones, the body is able to avert wide swings in blood glucose levels as insulin and glucagon compete.

Adrenal Glands

The **adrenal glands** are located on each side of the body on the superior aspect of each kidney. Each adrenal gland is a yellow, pyramid-shaped gland composed of two distinct layers. The outer cortex surrounds the inner medulla Figure 8-79. The **adrenal cortex** is made up of endocrine tissue but, like the hypothalamus, the adrenal medulla contains cells that function both as neural cells and as endocrine cells. The cortex and the medulla manufacture and secrete different hormones.

The adrenal medulla interacts closely with the sympathetic division of the ANS. When stimulated by sympathetic

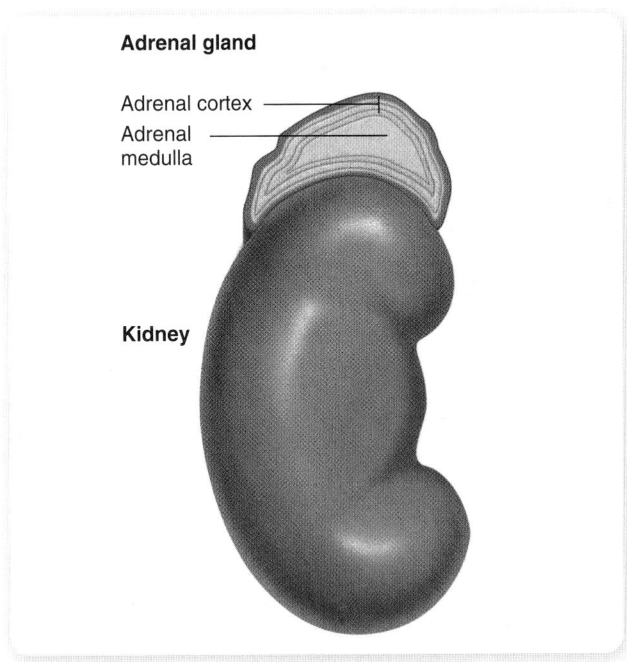

Figure 8-79 The adrenal glands sit on top of the kidney and consist of the adrenal medulla and adrenal cortex.

neurons, the medullar cells release epinephrine and norepinephrine. Instead of being secreted near an organ and acting as neurotransmitters, these catecholamines are released into the bloodstream and act as hormones that cause an increase in cardiac activity, vasoconstriction, and glycogenolysis, which are all key components in the body's fight-or-flight response.

The adrenal cortex is composed of three zones (layers) of secreting cells, each of which releases different steroidal hormones known as **corticosteroids** (adrenocortical steroids). Corticosteroids, which are synthesized from cholesterol, are essential to life. Cells of the innermost zone secrete small amounts of glucocorticoids and gonadocorticoids (sex hormones). The middle zone makes up most of the adrenal cortex and secretes glucocorticoids. Cells of the outer zone secrete mineralocorticoids. Mineralocorticoids are important in regulating the mineral salts (the electrolytes) of the extracellular fluid, particularly sodium and potassium. Between them, these corticosteroids assist in the regulation of blood glucose levels, promote the peripheral use of lipids, stimulate the kidneys to reabsorb sodium, and exert antiinflammatory effects.

During times of stress, the hypothalamus secretes a hormone that stimulates the anterior pituitary to release **adrenocorticotropic hormone (ACTH)**. ACTH targets the adrenal cortex and causes it to secrete cortisol (a glucocorticoid). **Cortisol** influences protein and fat metabolism, inhibits protein synthesis, promotes fatty acid release, and stimulates the liver to synthesize glucose from noncarbohydrates. Cortisol helps balance blood glucose and is controlled by negative feedback; stress plays an important part in triggering cortisol release. Cortisol also helps regulate the immune response by decreasing histamine response, which results in lessened swelling, as well as protecting healthy tissues from unnecessary lysosome activation.

If the body experiences a drop in blood pressure or volume, a decrease in sodium level, or an increase in the potassium level, then the adrenal cortex is stimulated to secrete **aldosterone** (a mineralocorticoid). Aldosterone helps the kidneys to balance sodium and potassium, and stimulates water retention via the process of osmosis. This mechanism is an excellent example of the complex interplay of multiple hormones found in many areas of the body. In this instance, if blood sodium decreases or blood potassium increases, then the adrenal cortex secretes renin. Recall that renin stimulates an increase in angiotensin I, which is then converted into angiotensin II. The presence of increased levels of angiotensin II stimulates the production of aldosterone, as well as several other endocrine functions that help preserve water balance and improve perfusion. Conversely, many stimuli from many systems can also produce this reaction. Because of the multitude of interactions, the endocrine system is constantly adjusting to maintain homeostasis and is considerably complex. The hormones of the adrenal gland are summarized in Table 8-32.

▶ Gonads

In both males and females, the primary functions of the gonads are to promote sexual maturation to puberty and

Table 8-32 Hormones of the Adrenal Gland

Hormone	Target Site	Effect
Adrenal Gland, Cortex		
Cortisol (glucocorticoid)	Most cells	Stimulates release of amino acids from skeletal muscles, lipids from adipose tissue, and glucose and glycogen from liver (mimics effects of glucagon); antiinflammatory effects
Aldosterone (mineralocorticoid)	Kidneys, blood	Increases renal reabsorption of sodium and water (more so in the presence of antidiuretic hormone) and increases urinary loss of potassium; net increase in blood volume
Estrogen	Most cells	Stimulates development of secondary sexual characteristics
Progesterone	Uterus	Stimulates uterine changes in preparation for gestation
Testosterone	Most cells	Stimulates development of secondary sexual characteristics
Adrenal Gland, Medulla		
Epinephrine	Muscle, liver, cardiovascular system	Stimulates cardiac activity; increases vasoconstriction; stimulates glycogenolysis; raises blood glucose levels
Norepinephrine	Muscle, liver, cardiovascular system	Stimulates vasoconstriction

Table 8-33 Hormones of the Gonads

Hormone	Target Site	Effect
Estrogen	Most cells, primarily those in the female reproductive system	Stimulates development of secondary sexual characteristics; involved in pregnancy; regulation of menstrual cycle
Progesterone	Uterus	Stimulates uterine changes in preparation for gestation; regulation of menstrual cycle; prevents maturation of additional egg during ovulation
Testosterone	Most cells, primarily those in the male reproductive system	Stimulates development of secondary sexual characteristics

fulfill any subsequent reproductive needs. In males, the gonads, or testes, are located in the scrotum. Cells of the testes produce male hormones known as *androgens*. The most prominent of these hormones is testosterone. Testosterone promotes healthy sperm production, determines secondary male sex characteristics (eg, deepening of the voice, growth of facial and pubic hair), and stimulates growth. Testosterone has also been shown to affect muscle production and aggressive behavioral responses.

In females, the gonads are the ovaries, which are located inside the pelvic cavity on either side of the uterus. The anterior pituitary gland directs the actions of the ovaries through follicle stimulating hormone (FSH) and luteinizing hormone (LH). The ovaries produce estrogen, progesterone, and a small amount of testosterone. Estrogen promotes follicular maturation (egg development) before ovulation, secondary sex characteristics (eg, enlargement of the breasts, uterine enlargement, fat deposits in the hips and thighs, development of hair under the arms and in the pubic area), and associated behaviors. **Progesterone** prepares the uterus for implantation of the fertilized egg. During pregnancy, progesterone ensures that the uterine wall maintains functionality and prepares the mammary glands for activity. The hormones of the gonads are summarized in Table 8-33.

Pineal Gland

The pineal gland is located in the posterior end of the third ventricle of the brain. It synthesizes and secretes melatonin Table 8-34, which is a hormone that has an effect on sleep-wake patterns and seasonal functions (behavior patterns that occur in mammals, such as the mating season).

YOU are the Paramedic — PART 3

While in transit to the hospital, you begin your rapid exam. When you assess the chest, you feel instability and a grating sensation upon palpation of the anterior chest. You observe that the chest does not rise and fall equally. It is extremely difficult to obtain breath sounds because of noise from traffic and running diesel engines.

Recording Time: 5 Minutes	
Respirations	24 breaths/min, shallow
Pulse	120 beats/min
Skin	Pale, moist, and warm
Blood pressure	106/70 mm Hg
Oxygen saturation (Spo_2)	90% on room air; ventilations assisted with a bag-mask device
Pupils	PERRLA

6. What is the obvious injury you find to the patient's chest?
7. What are the potential hidden injuries you should consider?

Table 8-34	Hormones of the Pineal Gland	
Hormone	**Target Site**	**Effect**
Melatonin	Specific nervous system tissues	Regulates sleep-wake cycle

The Circulatory System

The **circulatory system** includes the heart and a complex arrangement of connected tubes, including the arteries, arterioles, capillaries, venules, and veins (Figure 8-80). Another name for this system is the cardiovascular system.

The circulatory system is entirely closed. The two circuits in the body are as follows: the systemic circulation, which travels throughout the body, and the **pulmonary circulation**, which travels only between the heart and lungs. The systemic circulation carries oxygen-rich blood from the left ventricle through the body and back to the right atrium. In the systemic circulation, as blood passes through the tissues and organs, it gives up oxygen and nutrients and absorbs cellular wastes and carbon dioxide. The cellular wastes are eliminated as blood passes through the liver and kidneys. The pulmonary circulation carries oxygen-poor blood from the right ventricle through the lungs and back to the left atrium. In the pulmonary circulation, as blood passes through the lungs, it is refreshed with oxygen and gives up carbon dioxide.

The vasculature, which is a system of blood vessels, provides the internal piping of the body. It is responsible for bringing nutrients (eg, oxygen, carbohydrates, proteins,

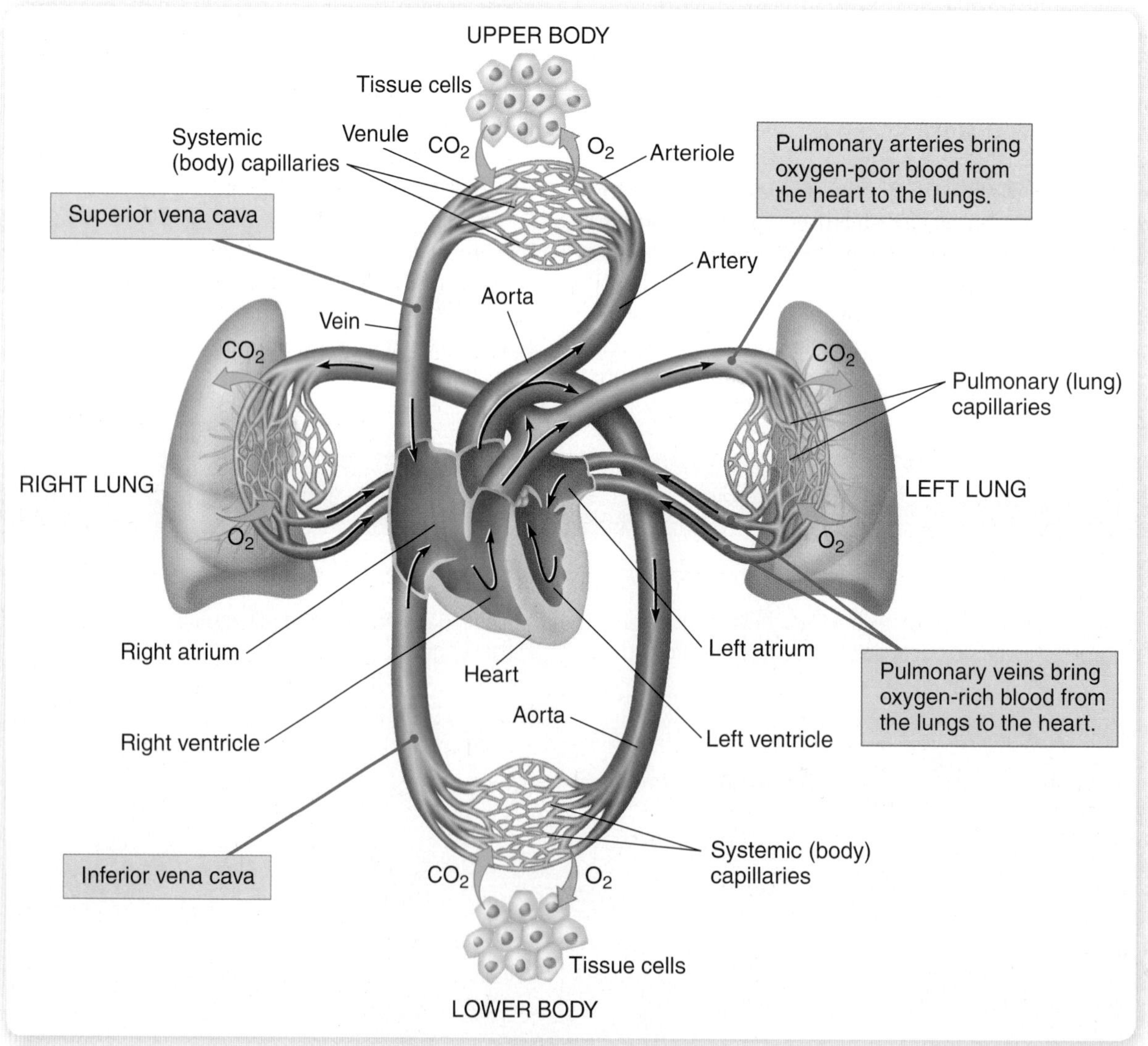

Figure 8-80 The circulatory system includes the heart, arteries, veins, and interconnecting capillaries. The capillaries are the smallest vessels and connect venules and arterioles. At the center of the system, and providing its driving force, is the heart. Blood circulates through the body under pressure generated by the two sides of the heart.

and fats) to cells and transporting waste products away for elimination (eg, carbon dioxide, nitrogen waste products). Blood also plays a key role in the regulation of temperature and fluid balance in the body and helps protect the body from pathogens. The heart works as a pump that provides the force needed to move the blood around the body.

▶ Blood

As mentioned previously, hematopoiesis is the process of blood cell formation. The **hematopoietic system** is the blood components and the organs involved in their development and production. The primary site of hematopoietic cell production is the bone marrow. Secondary hematopoietic organs that participate in this process include the lymphoid tissues, consisting of the thymus, lymph nodes, and spleen. The spleen is involved with the filtering and breakdown of RBCs, assists with the production of lymphocytes (one type of white blood cell), and has an important role in providing homeostasis and infection control.

Two types of hematopoietic tissue are found in the body: myeloid and lymphoid. Myeloid tissue is mainly found in the bone marrow. This type of tissue produces RBCs, WBCs, and blood platelets. Lymphoid tissue is found in the lymph nodes, spleen, and thymus. This type of tissue is the home to lymphocytes and other cells derived from them, such as **plasma cells**. Plasma cells produce antibodies (immunoglobulins) to destroy **antigens** (proteins recognized by the immune system) or antigen-containing particles.

Functions of Blood

Blood is the so-called fluid of life, and performs the following five functions:

1. **Respiratory.** Transports oxygen from the lungs to the tissues and carbon dioxide from the tissues to the lungs.
2. **Nutritional.** Carries nutrients (glucose, proteins, and fats) from the digestive tract to cells throughout the body.
3. **Excretory.** Ferries the waste products of metabolism from the cells where they are produced to the excretory organs.
4. **Regulatory.** Transports hormones to their target organs and transmits excess internal heat to the surface of the body to be dissipated.
5. **Defensive.** Carries defensive cells and antibodies, which protect the body against foreign organisms.

Blood Composition

Blood is primarily composed of plasma (55%) and formed cellular fragments (45%). Plasma is the liquid portion of the blood in which the formed elements of blood are suspended. It comprises the major portion of whole blood. The formed elements are a mixture of RBCs, WBCs, and platelets. Human adult male bodies contain about 70 mL/kg, or about 5 L, of blood, whereas female bodies contain about 65 mL/kg. Table 8-35 outlines the major functions of blood components.

Plasma

Plasma is made up of the following substances Figure 8-81:

- **Water.** Constitutes 92% of plasma. Water enters the plasma from the digestive tract, from fluids between cells, and as a by-product of metabolism.

Table 8-35 Major Functions of Blood Components

Component	Function
Basophils	Inflammatory response; release histamine and heparin
Chemicals within the plasma	Control (buffer) pH
Eosinophils	Help control allergic reactions and inflammation; release enzymes that weaken or destroy parasites
RBCs (erythrocytes)	Oxygen transport (hemoglobin)
Lymphocytes	Immune response
Monocytes	Phagocytize pathogens and cellular debris
Neutrophils	Immune defenses; find and phagocytize bacteria
Plasma	Transport of carbon dioxide, waste, and nutrients
Platelets (thrombocytes)	Control blood loss from disrupted vessels; begin clotting (coagulation) process

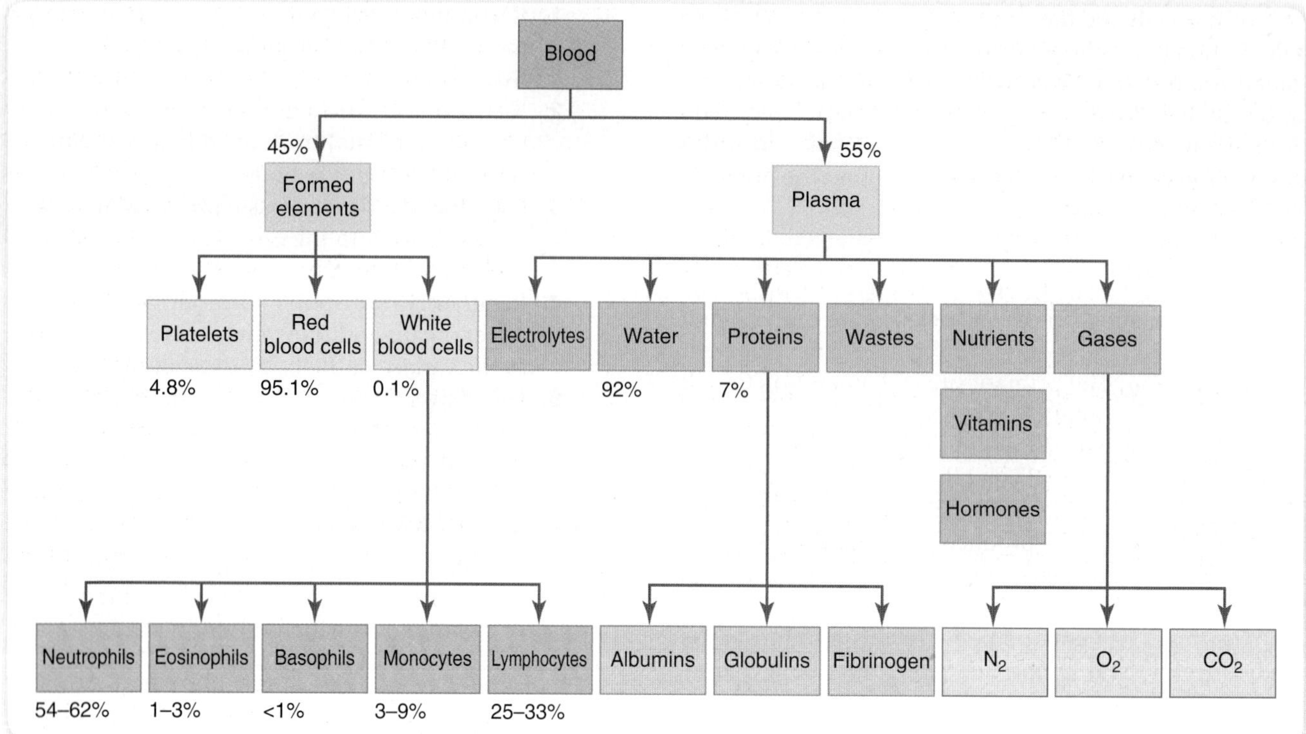

Figure 8-81 Composition of blood.

- **Proteins.** Constitute 7% of the plasma.
  - **Albumins.** Make up the majority of the plasma proteins. Albumins function mainly to regulate oncotic pressure, and thereby control the movement of water into and out of the circulation.
  - **Globulins.** Antibodies made by the liver that make up around 36% of the plasma proteins. As a paramedic, the most important globulins for you to be aware of are the gamma globulins. These are produced in the lymphatic tissue and they include proteins that act as antibodies in the immune system.
  - **Fibrinogen.** Important for blood clotting, makes up about 4% of the plasma proteins.
- **Gases**
  - **Oxygen.** Little oxygen is dissolved in the plasma; almost all oxygen is bound to hemoglobin.
  - **Carbon dioxide.** Transported as bicarbonate in the plasma.
  - **Nitrogen.** The air that you breathe is mostly nitrogen; therefore, this gas is dissolved within the plasma.
- **Electrolytes.** Calcium, sodium, potassium, and chloride are examples of electrolytes in plasma.
- **Nutrients, vitamins, and hormones.** Glucose, amino acids, fatty acids, and glycerol together with mineral salts and vitamins are used by body cells for energy, heat, and for the production of other blood components and body secretions.
- **Wastes.** Carbon dioxide from tissue metabolism is carried to the lungs for elimination. Waste products of protein metabolism such as urea, uric acid, and creatinine are formed in the liver and transported by the blood to the kidneys for elimination.

Hematopoietic Stem Cells

Hematopoiesis starts with a common stem cell that has the ability to change into multiple different types of cells. Through a series of transformations, most of which begin in the bone marrow in mature humans, a type of stem cell specific to the circulatory system, known as a hematocytoblast, forms and begins the process of maturation. Through multiple changes and stages, the hematocytoblasts gradually differentiate into one of the blood components discussed further in this chapter. Some will become normoblasts and eventually mature into reticulocytes, the precursors to RBCs. Other hematocytoblasts will randomly follow a different path to become other formed elements.

Red Blood Cells

Recall that RBCs carry oxygen to the tissues. They are disc-shaped, and are the most numerous of the formed elements. An average human has between 4.2 and

5.8 million RBCs per cubic millimeter of blood. RBCs are unable to move on their own; the flowing plasma passively propels them. RBCs contain hemoglobin, which gives them their red color. Each hemoglobin molecule is capable of binding up to four gaseous molecules, most often oxygen. Oxygen is then carried to end organs, where it diffuses into tissues.

Erythropoiesis is the ongoing process by which RBCs are made. Erythropoietin, a hormone produced mainly by the kidneys, stimulates the production of RBCs by stem cells within the bone marrow. The RBCs may take as long as 5 days to mature and have an average life span of 120 days. Those cells that are destined for destruction decompose in the spleen and other tissues that are rich in macrophages. (Recall that macrophages protect the body against infection.) The body "recycles" some components of hemoglobin, such as the protein, globin, and iron. The part of hemoglobin that is not recycled is converted to **bilirubin**, which is a waste product that undergoes further metabolism in the liver. Normally, a chemical derivative of bilirubin, urobilinogen, is excreted in the stool and in the urine.

The following laboratory tests are commonly performed on blood:

- **RBC count.** Measures the number of RBCs in a sample of blood.
- **Hemoglobin level.** Identifies the amount of hemoglobin found within the RBCs.
- **Measurement of hematocrit.** Gives the overall proportion of RBCs in the blood. The patient's blood is considered balanced (even if the numbers are too high or low) if the hemoglobin level is one-third of the hematocrit value and the RBC count is one-third of the hemoglobin level.

White Blood Cells

The structure of the WBC allows movement through the capillary walls and into the tissues. The total WBC count averages between 4,500 and 10,000 cells/mm^3 in a healthy person and is elevated during an inflammatory response, immune response, or both.

WBCs are derived from stem cells. Many different types of WBCs have varying functions. These jobs include phagocytosis, production of antibodies, secretion of heparin and histamine, and secretion of other chemokines. The lifespan of WBCs generally ranges from 13 to 20 days. After this time, they are destroyed in the lymphatic system. Most WBCs are motile and leave the blood vessels by a process known as **diapedesis** to move toward the tissue where they are needed most.

WBCs are named according to their appearance in a stained preparation of blood. In general, granulocytes have large cytoplasmic granules that are easily seen with a simple light microscope; *agranulocytes* are WBCs that lack these granules. The three types of granulocytes are neutrophils, eosinophils, and basophils. The two types of agranulocytes are monocytes and lymphocytes.

Neutrophils are normally the most common type of granulocyte in the blood. Neutrophils spend their short lives, usually a day or less, circulating in blood and tissues. Because neutrophils are widely dispersed in the body and are highly specialized for finding and destroying bacteria, they are a primary defense against bacterial infection. These cells are also a major component of the inflammatory response. **Eosinophils** release substances that damage or kill parasitic invaders. They also have a major role in mediating the allergic response. Eosinophils release chemotactic factors, which are substances that cause cells to migrate into an area. These can trigger severe bronchospasm. **Basophils** are the least common of all granulocytes and play a role in both allergic and inflammatory reactions. When activated, these cells release histamine and heparin. **Histamine** dilates blood vessels, speeds blood flow to injured tissue, and makes blood vessels more permeable so that neutrophils, clotting proteins, and other blood components can enter connective tissues more quickly.[29] The release of *heparin*, a substance that inhibits blood clotting, enhances the mobility of other WBCs in the area.[29]

Lymphocytes are the smallest of the granulocytes. Although most lymphocytes are found in the lymphoid tissues, many are found in circulating lymph and blood as well. Two major types exist: T lymphocytes and **B lymphocytes** (B cells). T lymphocytes, which are formed in the thymus, mainly work to rid the body of bacteria and viruses through direct invasion. B lymphocytes, which are formed in the bone marrow, mainly work to rid the body of bacterial and viral organisms through the production of antibodies.

Monocytes are one of the first lines of defense in the inflammatory process. In response to infection, monocytes migrate out of the blood vessels and into the tissues where they differentiate into macrophages. Macrophages function primarily as scavengers, engulfing microbes and digesting them during phagocytosis.

Platelets

As you have learned, platelets (thrombocytes) are a key component in the formation of clots, or coagulation. Platelet production is mainly controlled by thrombopoietin, a protein hormone that is related to erythropoietin. Cells in the liver and kidneys secrete thrombopoietin at a constant rate. About two-thirds of the total platelets circulate in the blood, whereas one-third of the platelets are stored in the blood vessels of the spleen. Platelets circulate in the blood for about 7 to 10 days.

Normal Hemostasis. Following injury to a blood vessel wall, a predictable series of events takes place, resulting in **hemostasis** (cessation of bleeding) and formation of the final blood clot. The coagulation process is a complex set of events involving platelets, clotting proteins in the plasma (clotting factors), other proteins, and calcium. Most of the clotting factors are produced in the liver, and they require vitamin K for their production.

The immediate physiologic response to bleeding is vasoconstriction, to clamp down and cut off blood flow at the affected site. Locally, vasoconstrictors such as thromboxane are released. Should the bleeding prove a significant threat to homeostasis, the adrenal glands release epinephrine (a potent vasoconstrictor), leading to systemic vasoconstriction. The secondary response to hemorrhage is platelet plugging. Recall that platelets are cellular fragments that stick to collagen and become activated. Collagen exists within the deep membranes of blood vessels, and a cut or rupture exposes it to the platelets within the circulation. The first platelets to be activated release chemicals that cause the aggregation (clumping) of additional platelets at the site of injury. This process of coagulation involves about a dozen clotting factors that are activated when the body is injured. These factors each require the presence and activation of the preceding factor to work.

Activated platelets express a surface protein that stimulates the **clotting cascade** (coagulation cascade), which is a set of interactions that lead to the formation of a clot **Figure 8-82**. These steps are typically organized into extrinsic and intrinsic pathways that converge into a common pathway. The extrinsic pathway (tissue factor pathway) is the result of damage to the tissues, which then release clotting factors. These factors react with other clotting factors and calcium. The final product is tissue **thromboplastin**. The intrinsic pathway (contact activation pathway) is the result of damaged platelets releasing clotting factors. These factors also react with other clotting factors and calcium. The final product is platelet thromboplastin. These two pathways occur at the same time. Both tissue thromboplastin and platelet thromboplastin join at the common pathway, ultimately converting **prothrombin** (produced by the liver) to its active form, **thrombin**. Thrombin, in turn, acts on another blood protein fibrinogen, also produced by the liver. When activated, fibrinogen is converted into fibrin. **Fibrin** are long, branching fibers that produce a weblike network in the wall of the damaged blood vessel. Fibrin binds to the platelet plug, forming a plug that stops the flow of blood to the tissue. Calcium acts as a binding agent, holding fibrin fibers close together to form the meshwork of the clot.

After the bleeding has stopped and the injured vessel is healed, plasma proteins break down the fibrin fibers of the clot into fragments. During the clot-dissolving portion of coagulation, which is called fibrinolysis, the enzyme plasminogen is converted to **plasmin**, which dissolves the fibrin fibers of the clot.

Words of Wisdom

Any process that interferes with the activation or continuation of the clotting cascade or hemostasis is known as a coagulopathy. Coagulopathies are bleeding disorders that can lead to heavy or prolonged bleeding.

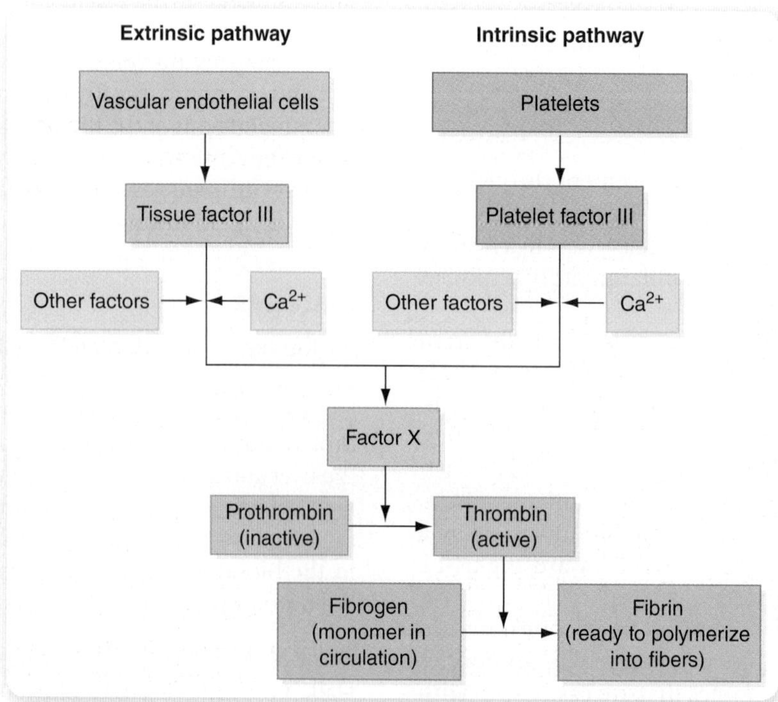

Figure 8-82 The clotting cascade. The extrinsic and intrinsic pathways merge into the final common pathway, forming fibrin.

Table 8-36 ABO Blood Groups

Blood Type	Antigen	Antibody	Potential Donor
A	A	Anti-B	A, O
B	B	Anti-A	B, O
AB	A and B	Neither antibody	AB, A, B, O
O	Neither antigen	Anti-A and Anti-B	O

ABO and Rh Blood Groups

RBCs contain antigens on their surface. Within the plasma are antibodies, which react with antigens. To ensure compatibility and prevent medical complications during blood component replacement, people are classified as having one of four blood types based on the presence or absence of these specific antigens. This process of classification is referred to as blood typing, or determining the ABO blood group. In the **ABO system**, the RBC classification types are O, A, B, and AB, which indicate the antigens found in the plasma membrane Table 8-36.

Type A blood contains RBCs with type A surface antigens and plasma containing type B antibodies; type B blood contains type B surface antigens and plasma containing type A antibodies. Type AB blood contains both types of antigens but the plasma contains no ABO antibodies. Type O contains neither A nor B antigens but contains both A and B plasma antibodies. A person's blood type determines which type of blood he or she may receive in a blood transfusion.

Type O blood, because it has no ABO antigens, can be given to anyone; a person with type O blood is known as a universal donor. A person with type AB blood can receive blood from any donor without having an ABO reaction because type AB blood has no ABO antibodies; therefore, the person is known as a universal recipient.

Blood contains a secondary antigen, known as the Rh antigen (the name signifies that the antigen was first discovered in rhesus monkeys). The Rh blood group consists of several antigens, with D being the most prevalent. The Rh antigen D (**Rh factor**), determines an immune response. A person with the Rh factor present in the blood is Rh-positive; Rh-negative means that the antigen is not present. Unlike the ABO antigens, human plasma does not normally contain Rh antibodies. A person with Rh-negative blood must first be exposed to Rh-positive blood before developing antibodies. The same applies to a person with Rh-positive blood. Rh antibodies are produced within about 2 weeks of the exposure and the antibodies remain in the blood. The second time the person is exposed, a severe reaction may occur.

Another situation in which the Rh blood group may present a problem is in pregnancy. For example, if an Rh-negative mother is exposed to the Rh-positive blood of her unborn child during pregnancy, birth, miscarriage, or abortion, then her immune system will develop antibodies to the Rh antigens. This exposure is generally not an issue with the first pregnancy. However, in subsequent pregnancies, if the unborn child has Rh-positive blood, then the mother's immune system will launch an attack against the RBCs of the fetus. This incompatibility can be addressed through treatment provided at the time of delivery. In order for this to be possible, prenatal testing of the mother's blood is necessary.

Heart

The driving force behind the cardiovascular system is the heart Figure 8-83. This remarkable pump sits in the chest, above the diaphragm, behind and slightly to the left of the lower sternum. The tip of the heart is the apex, and the top of the heart is its base. The base lies at about the area of the second intercostal space, and the apex (bottom) lies at about the fifth intercostal space near or a little medial to the midclavicular line. The heart is not much larger than a person's fist and weighs about 9 ounces (between 250 g and 300 g). Despite its relatively small size, the heart is strong enough to circulate 7,000 L to 9,000 L of blood around the body every day!

The large vessels that carry blood to the heart include the superior and inferior venae cavae (vessels that return venous blood from the upper and lower parts of the body to the right atrium), and the pulmonary veins (vessels that return oxygenated blood from the lungs to the left atrium). The large vessels that carry blood away from the heart include the aorta (which delivers blood from the left ventricle to the body) and the pulmonary arteries (which deliver unoxygenated blood from the right ventricle to the lungs).

Heart Wall

The **pericardium** (pericardial sac) is a thick, fibrous membrane that surrounds the heart. The pericardium anchors the heart within the mediastinum and prevents overdistention of the heart. It has an outer, fibrous membrane (parietal), and an inner membrane (visceral). The fibrous pericardium is made of dense connective tissue. This tissue is attached to the central diaphragm, posterior sternum, vertebral column, and large blood vessels connected to the heart. An inner, double-layered visceral pericardium covers the heart as well. At the base of the heart, the visceral pericardium folds back to become the parietal pericardium. Between the parietal and visceral layers is the pericardial cavity, containing a small volume of serous fluid (about 5 mL) that reduces friction between the pericardial membranes as the heart moves within them.

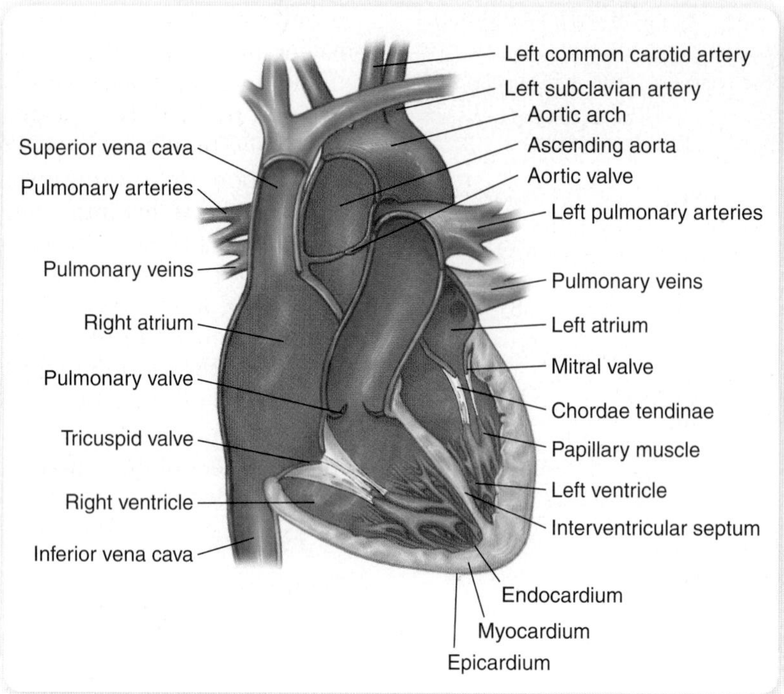

Figure 8-83 Anatomy of the heart.

The wall of the heart consists of three layers Figure 8-84:

- The **epicardium** protects the heart by reducing friction, and is the visceral portion of the pericardium on the surface of the heart. It consists of connective tissue and some deep adipose tissue.
- The myocardium is the middle layer of the heart wall found between the epicardium and endocardium. Recall that the thick myocardium is made mostly of cardiac muscle tissue and is responsible for cardiac contraction and efficient ejection of blood from the heart. The myocardium has a large capillary supply to meet the oxygen demands of the heart; most areas of the myocardium have a 1:1 ratio of capillaries to muscle cells.
- The **endocardium** is made up of epithelium and connective tissue with many elastic and collagenous fibers. This surface is smooth so as not to disrupt blood flow or platelets as they pass through the heart. This lining is continuous with the innermost lining of the blood vessels of the body.

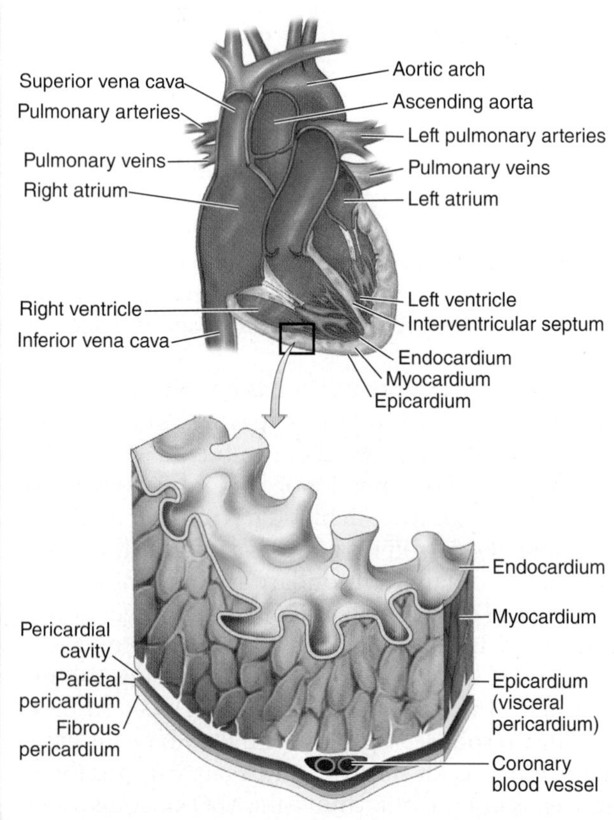

Figure 8-84 The three layers of the heart include the epicardium, the myocardium, and the endocardium.

Heart Chambers

The normal human heart consists of four chambers: two receiving chambers called **atria** and two pumping chambers called ventricles (see Figure 8-83). The heart is divided into right and left halves by a tough piece of tissue called the septum. The interatrial septum separates the two atria; a thicker wall, the interventricular septum, separates the right and left ventricles.

Cardiac Muscle

Cardiac muscle is unique to the heart. However, like other muscles, contraction occurs when calcium interferes with troponin and tropomyosin, allowing the actin and myosin fibers to create cross links that pull against each other to contract (shorten).

Recall that cardiac muscle fibers are long, branching cells that fit together tightly at intercalated disks. The arrangement of these tight-fitting junctions gives an appearance of a syncytium; that is, resembling a network of cells with no separation between the individual cells. The intercalated disks fit together and form gap junctions. As a result, an electrical impulse can be quickly conducted throughout the wall of a heart chamber. This characteristic allows the walls of both atria (likewise, the walls of both ventricles) to contract almost at the same time. The heart consists of two sets of chambers: atrial and ventricular.

Heart Valves

The heart has four valves: two **atrioventricular (AV) valves** and two **semilunar (SL) valves** Figure 8-85. AV valves separate the atria from the ventricles. The right AV valve is the **tricuspid valve**, and the left AV valve is the **mitral valve** (bicuspid valve). These valves direct the flow of blood between the chambers. They also prevent backward flow during ventricular contraction (regurgitation). The valves have fibrous bands of tissue called **chordae tendineae** attached to each part, or cusp, of the valve. Attached to the chordae tendineae and the endocardium of the ventricles are **papillary muscles**. During ventricular contraction (ventricular systole) the AV valves are closed because of the increase in pressure in the chamber. The papillary muscles also contract during ventricular systole, providing counterpressure to the cusps of the AV valves. This pressure prevents the AV valves from "blowing out" or being forced open into the atria. During ventricular relaxation (ventricular diastole), the papillary muscles relax and the AV valves open by the force of blood flowing downward from the atria to the ventricles.

The SL valves separate the ventricles and their associated great vessel. These valves each have three cusps. The right SL valve is the **pulmonic valve**. It separates the right ventricle and the pulmonary trunk. The SL valve on the left is the **aortic valve**. This valve separates the left ventricle from the aorta. These valves have no tendon or muscular support. Moreover, they function only by the relative pressure differences between the ventricles and great vessels they separate. When the ventricle contracts, the pressure in the ventricle exceeds the pressure in the

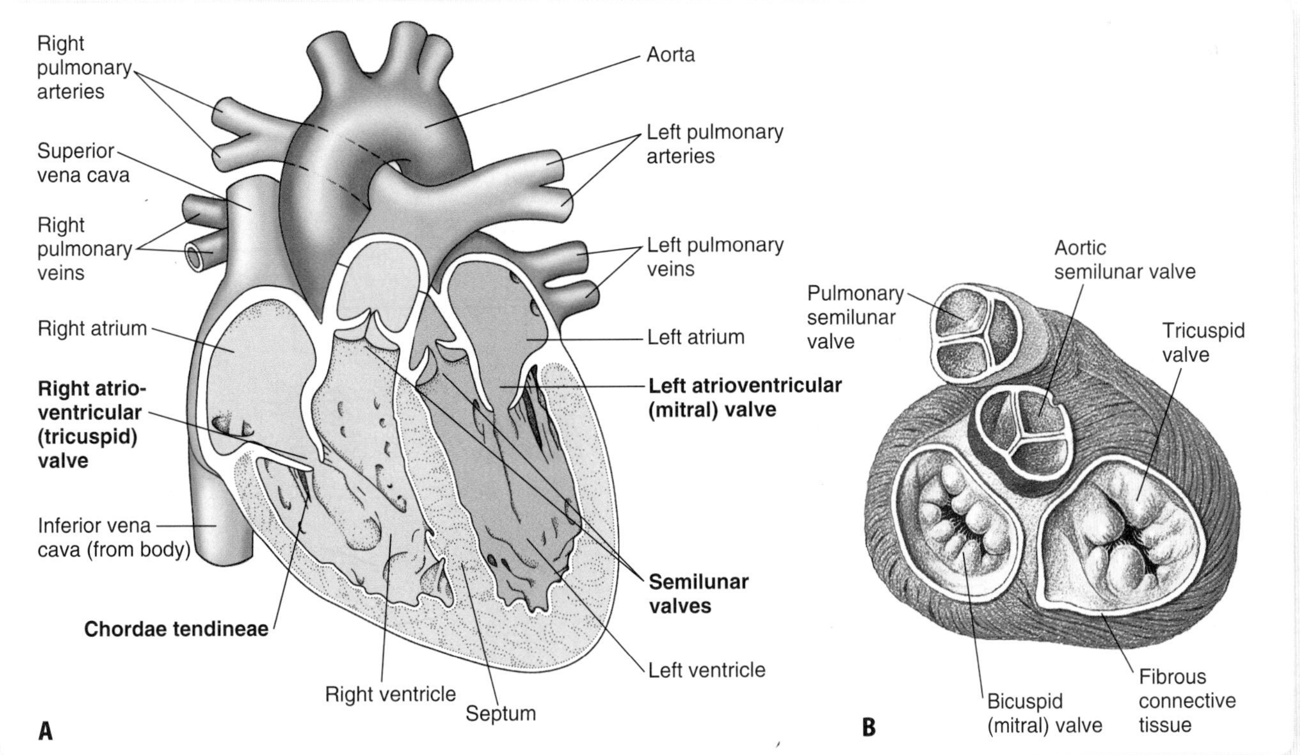

Figure 8-85 A. Heart valves. **B.** Cross section of heart valves.

pulmonary trunk; therefore, the valve opens, allowing blood to enter the great vessel. When the pressure in the great vessel exceeds the pressure of the ventricle, the valve closes.

Blood Flow Through the Cardiovascular System

The body's total blood volume can be divided into the following: the systemic circulation (85%), the pulmonary circulation (about 10%), and the heart chambers (about 5%).[30] Blood enters the right atrium by way of the superior and inferior venae cavae and the coronary sinus (the venous drain for the coronary circulation). About 70% to 80% of this blood flows passively from the right atrium through the tricuspid valve and into the right ventricle. The remaining 20% to 30% is forced into the right ventricle during atrial contraction (atrial kick). The right ventricle expels the blood through the pulmonic valve into the pulmonary trunk. The pulmonary trunk divides into a right and left pulmonary artery, each of which carries blood to one lung (pulmonary circulation; see Figure 8-80).

Blood flows through the pulmonary arteries to the lungs. Blood that is low in oxygen passes through the pulmonary capillaries. There it comes in direct contact with the alveolar-capillary membrane, where oxygen and carbon dioxide are exchanged. Blood then flows into the **pulmonary veins**. The left atrium receives oxygenated blood from the lungs by the four pulmonary veins (two from the right lung and two from the left lung). Again, about 70% to 80% of the blood moves passively from the left atrium into the left ventricle through the mitral valve. The remaining 20% to 30% of the blood is forced into the ventricle through the atrial kick. With contraction of the left ventricle, blood is ejected through the aortic valve to the aorta. Blood is distributed throughout the body (systemic circulation) through the aorta and its branches.

Cardiac Cycle

The **cardiac cycle** refers to a repetitive pumping process that includes all the events associated with blood flow through the heart. The cycle has two phases for each heart chamber: systole and diastole. *Systole* is the period during which the chamber is contracting and blood is being ejected. The atria and ventricles each have a distinct systolic phase. **Diastole** is the period of relaxation during which the chambers are allowed to fill. The atria and ventricles each have a distinct diastolic phase. The myocardium receives its fresh supply of oxygenated blood from the coronary arteries during ventricular diastole. The cardiac cycle depends on the ability of the cardiac muscle to contract and on the condition of the conduction system of the heart. The efficiency of the heart as a pump may be affected by abnormalities of the cardiac muscle, the valves, or the conduction system.

During the cardiac cycle, the pressure within each chamber of the heart rises in systole and falls in diastole. The valves of the heart make sure that blood flows in the proper direction. Blood flows from one heart chamber to another if the pressure in the chamber is more than the pressure in the next. This pressure relationship depends on the careful timing of contractions. The conduction system of the heart provides the necessary timing of events between atrial and ventricular systole.

Think of the heart as a two-sided pump, with the low-pressure right side being responsible for pulmonic circulation and the high-pressure left side being responsible for systemic circulation. However, it is important to realize that the atria and the ventricles function together. As both atria undergo systole, the ventricles are in diastole; conversely, as both ventricles undergo systole, the atria are in diastole.

Heart Sounds. Heart sounds are created by the contraction and relaxation of the heart and flow of blood. These sounds can be heard during auscultation with a stethoscope. Normal heart sounds are often described as sounding like "lub-DUB, lub-DUB, lub-DUB. . . ." The "lub" is called the first heart sound or S_1, and the "DUB" is called the second heart sound or S_2 (Figure 8-86). S_2 ("DUB") is often louder than S_1 ("lub").

S_1 occurs near the beginning of ventricular contraction (systole), when the tricuspid and mitral valves close.

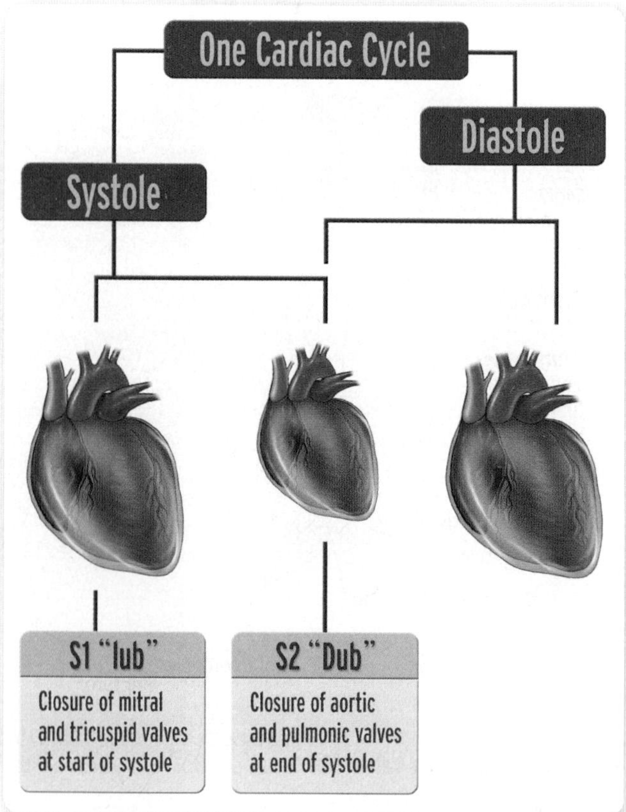

Figure 8-86 The normal S_1 and S_2 heart sounds.

Normally, the closing of these two valves occurs simultaneously as the pressure within the ventricles increases. Any delay in the closing of these two valves, heard as a split sound, is considered abnormal. S_2 occurs near the end of ventricular contraction (systole), when the pulmonary and aortic valves close. The two valves can close simultaneously or with a slight delay between them under normal physiologic circumstances.

Two other heart sounds, S_3 and S_4, are not usually heard in people with normal heart sounds **Figure 8-87**. S_3 is a soft, low-pitched heart sound that occurs about one-third of the way through ventricular diastole. It is caused by vibrations of the ventricular walls, resulting from the rapid filling period of the ventricle during the beginning of diastole. When an S_3 sound is present, the heart beat cycle is described as sounding like "lub- DUB-da." S_3 is sometimes present in healthy children and in young adults. When S_3 is heard in older adults, it is often associated with abnormally increased filling pressures in the atria secondary to moderate to severe heart failure.

S_4 is a medium-pitched heart sound that occurs immediately before the normal S_1 sound. When an S_4 sound is present, the heart contraction cycle sounds like "bla-lub-DUB." The S_4 sound represents either decreased stretching (compliance) of the left ventricle or increased pressure in the atria. An S_4 heart is almost always abnormal.

Other sounds, all abnormal, may be heard when you auscultate the heart and great vessels. Some of these sounds are easy to auscultate; others may require years of experience to identify. These sounds include murmurs, bruits, ejection clicks, and opening snaps. A **murmur** is an abnormal whooshing sound heard over the heart that indicates turbulent blood flow through the heart valves. Although many murmurs are functional (benign) and often go away, several are characteristic of heart disease. A **bruit** is an abnormal whooshing sound heard over a main blood vessel that indicates turbulent blood flow within the blood vessel. A bruit often indicates localized atherosclerotic disease (plaque formation in the arteries). Both ejection clicks and opening snaps indicate abnormal cardiac valve function. They occur at different times in the cardiac cycle, depending on which valve is diseased. Although these sounds are clinically significant, most of these sounds are fleeting and difficult to hear.

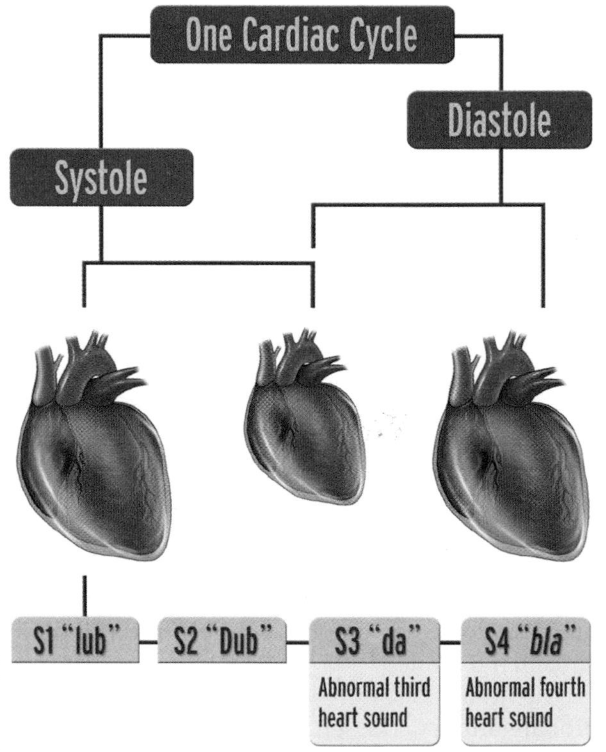

Figure 8-87 The abnormal S_3 and S_4 heart sounds.

Cardiac Output. To understand how the heart functions as a pump, it is necessary to learn the following technical terms:

- **Cardiac output (CO).** Recall that CO is the amount of blood that is pumped by the ventricles in 1 minute. The left and right ventricles are approximately equal in interior size, so the two ventricles have relatively equivalent outputs. Normal CO for an average adult is 5 to 6 L/min.
- **Stroke volume (SV).** The amount of blood pumped out by either ventricle in a single cardiac contraction (heartbeat). Normally, the SV is between 60 and 100 mL for a healthy adult, but the heart has considerable capacity and can easily increase SV by at least 50%.
- **Heart rate (HR).** Recall that HR is the number of cardiac contractions per minute (the pulse rate) The normal HR for an adult at rest is 60 to 100 beats/min.
- **Ejection fraction (EF).** The percentage of blood that leaves the heart each time it contracts. This measurement is usually taken from only the left ventricle because it is the primary pump for the heart. The left ventricular ejection fraction has a normal range of 55% to 70% in an adult, but may be lower if the heart sustains some type of damage (eg, myocardial infarction, heart valve disease, cardiomyopathy, or chronic hypertension).

To meet changing demands, the heart must be able to increase its output several times over in response to the body's increased demand for oxygen—for example, during exercise. CO is a function of both the SV and the HR, which is mathematically expressed as follows:

$$CO = SV \times HR$$

For example, assuming SV is 70 mL and the HR is 80 beats/min, CO would be 70 mL × 80 beats/min, or 5600 mL/min (5.6 L/min). This equation indicates that the heart can increase its output by increasing its SV, increasing its rate, or both. Factors that influence the SV, the HR, or both will affect CO and, thus, oxygen delivery (perfusion) to tissue.

SV is influenced by preload, afterload, and the contractile state (contraction or relaxation) of the myocardium. **Preload** (end-diastolic volume) is the volume of blood in the ventricle at the end of diastole and is primarily a reflection of venous return (the amount of blood returned to the heart).[31] **Afterload** is the force against which the ventricles must contract to eject blood. Afterload is influenced by arterial blood pressure, the ability of the arteries to become stretched (arterial distensibility), and arterial resistance. The greater the afterload, the harder the ventricle must work to pump the blood.

The heart has several ways of increasing SV. One characteristic of cardiac muscle is that, when it is stretched, it contracts with greater force to a limit-a property called the *Frank-Starling mechanism*, or Starling's law. If an increased volume of blood is returned from the systemic veins to the right side of the heart or from the pulmonary veins to the left side of the heart, then the muscle surrounding the cardiac chambers must stretch to accommodate the larger volume. The more the cardiac muscle stretches, the greater the force of its contraction, the more completely it empties, and, therefore, the greater the SV. From the CO equation, it is clear that any increase in SV, with the HR held constant, will cause an increase in the overall CO. Think of a latex balloon. If you blow up the balloon a bit and then let the air escape, then it does so slowly and with little force. This is because the elastic walls of the balloon were not stretched very much. However, if you blow up the balloon as much as possible without popping it, and then let the air out, then it does so very quickly and much more forcefully. The heart works the same way. If the walls are stretched a bit, then a small amount of blood is released. If the walls are stretched a great deal, then a large amount of blood is released.

As mentioned earlier, the pressure under which a ventricle fills (the preload) is influenced by the volume of blood returned by the veins to the heart. In situations of increased oxygen demand, the body returns more blood to the heart (preload increases), and CO consequently increases through the Frank-Starling mechanism. In a diseased heart, the same mechanism is used to achieve a normal resting CO (which explains why some diseased hearts become enlarged).

The heart can also vary the degree of contraction of muscle without changing the stretch on the muscle—a perty called contractility. Changes in contractility may duced by medications that have a positive or negative **pic effect** (inotropic refers to affecting the contractil- nuscle tissue). The ventricles are never completely emptied of blood with any single heartbeat. However, if the heart squeezes into a tighter ball when it contracts, then a larger percentage of the ventricular blood will be ejected, thereby increasing SV and overall CO. Nervous controls regulate the contractility of the heart from heartbeat to heartbeat. When the body requires increased CO, nervous signals increase myocardial contractility, thereby augmenting SV.

The heart can also increase its CO, given a constant SV, by increasing the number of contractions per minute—that is, by increasing the HR. Increasing the rate of contraction is known as a positive **chronotropic effect**. The Frank-Starling mechanism is an intrinsic property of heart muscle, meaning that it is not under nervous system control. By contrast, contractility and changes in the HR are regulated by the nervous system.

Blood Pressure. As mentioned earlier, blood pressure is the pressure that the blood exerts against the walls of the arteries as it passes through them. Systole and diastole are the phases that occur when the left ventricle contracts and when the ventricle relaxes, respectively. The pulsed forceful ejection of blood from the left ventricle of the heart into the aorta is transmitted through the arteries as a pulsatile pressure wave. This pressure wave keeps the blood moving through the body.

The measure of blood pressure is one method of evaluating the effectiveness of CO. Blood pressure is a function of both CO and **systemic vascular resistance** (the resistance to blood flow within all of the blood vessels except the pulmonary vessels). The resistance to the flow of blood is determined by the diameter of the blood vessel and the tone (the normal state of balanced tension in body tissues) of the vascular musculature. A dilated (widened) vessel offers less resistance to blood flow. A constricted (narrowed) vessel offers more resistance to blood flow.

Coronary Circulation

Like all cells in the body, myocardial cells require an uninterrupted supply of oxygen and nutrients. However, the cardiac demand for oxygen is particularly unrelenting because the heart never stops to rest (not without catastrophic consequences), so it is essential for the heart to have a reliable blood supply. Oxygenated blood reaches the heart through the coronary arteries **Figure 8-88**, which branch off the aorta at the coronary ostia, located just above the leaflets of the aortic valve. The coronary arteries are the first vessels that receive blood after left ventricular contraction. Because the coronary arteries are compressed during ventricular systole, they fill during ventricular diastole.

The two main coronary arteries are the left and right coronary arteries. The left main coronary artery is the largest and shortest of the myocardial blood vessels. It rapidly divides into the **left anterior descending artery**

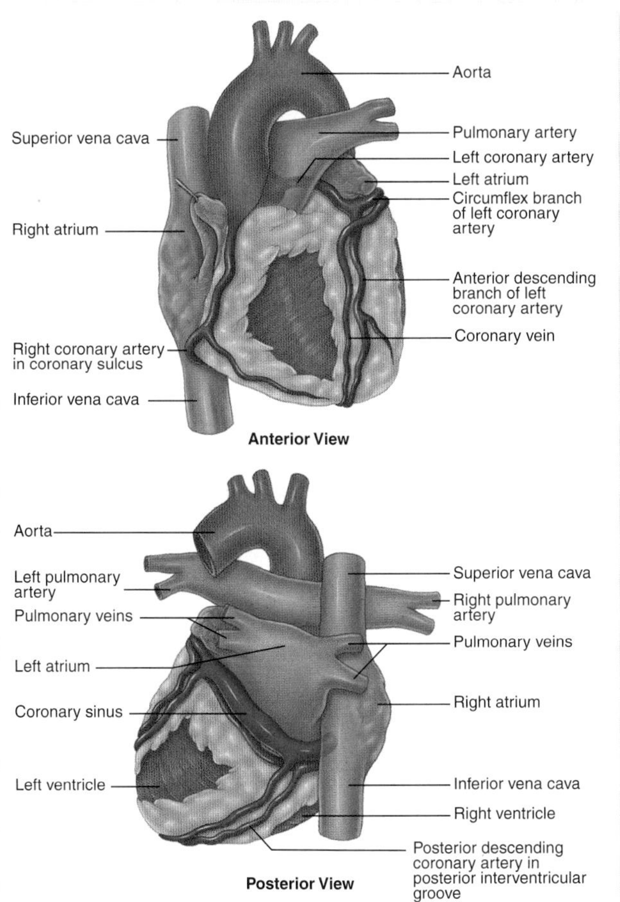

Figure 8-88 The two main coronary arteries and their branches supply the heart with blood.

and the **circumflex coronary artery**, both of which branch widely to supply the more muscular left ventricle of the heart along with the interventricular septum and part of the right ventricle. The **right coronary artery** travels between the right atrium and right ventricle by way of the atrioventricular groove. Branches of this artery supply blood to the walls of the right atrium and ventricle, a portion of the inferior part of the left ventricle, and portions of the conduction system.

The numerous connections (anastomoses) between the arterioles of the various coronary arteries allow for the development of alternative routes of blood flow. In the early stages of coronary heart disease, the inside diameter of the coronary arteries begins to narrow as plaque deposits on the vessel walls. In response to the decreased ability to perfuse the myocardium, *collateral circulation* develops to overcome the imbalance. Collateral circulation is the formation of additional blood vessels connecting arterioles originating from other blood vessels. The result is an increase in oxygenated blood delivery to the myocardium.

The arteries and the main coronary vein cross the heart in a groove (coronary sulcus) that separates the atria from the ventricles. Venous blood empties into the **coronary sinus**, a large vessel in the posterior part of the coronary sulcus, which in turn ends in the right atrium of the heart.

Conduction System

The mechanical pumping action of the heart can only occur in response to an electrical stimulus. This impulse causes the heart to beat via a set of complex chemical changes within the myocardial cells. The CNS and the endocrine system can influence the rate, strength, and speed of contraction.

In general, cardiac cells have either a mechanical (contractile) or an electrical (pacemaker) function. Myocardial cells (working cells) contain contractile filaments. When these cells are electrically stimulated, the contractile filaments slide together, and the myocardial cell contracts. These myocardial cells form the thin, muscular layer of the atrial walls and the thicker muscular layer of the ventricular walls (the myocardium). These cells do not normally generate electrical impulses on their own. Pacemaker cells (conducting cells) are specialized cells of the electrical system of the heart. They are responsible for spontaneously generating and conducting electrical impulses. Myocardial cells respond to impulses from the pacemaker cells by contracting.

Cardiac cells demonstrate four important properties that help the heart to function as an efficient machine: (1) automaticity, (2) excitability, (3) conductivity, and (4) contractility. **Automaticity** is the ability of cardiac pacemaker cells to create an electrical impulse without being stimulated from another source. As discussed previously, excitability refers to the ability of cardiac muscle cells to respond to a stimulus. Conductivity enables a cardiac cell to receive an electrical impulse and pass it on to an adjoining cardiac cell. Contractility refers to the ability of myocardial cells to shorten in response to an impulse, which results in contraction.

Pacemakers of the Heart. The cardiac conduction system consists of six parts: the sinoatrial (SA) node, the atrioventricular (AV) node, the bundle of His, the right and left bundle branches, and the Purkinje fibers **Figure 8-89**.

The **sinoatrial (SA) node** is a mass of specialized tissue located high in the right atrium and is the normal site of origin of the electrical impulse. Cells of the SA node can reach threshold on their own, initiating impulses through the myocardium, stimulating contraction of cardiac muscle fibers. Because it creates these impulses more frequently than other sites in the heart, the SA node is the most common natural pacemaker. The impulse then travels to the **atrioventricular (AV) node.** The AV node is a group of cells composed of thin fibers located in the floor of the right atrium immediately behind the tricuspid valve and near the opening of the coronary sinus. The function of the AV node is to delay the impulse, allowing atrial systole to occur before ventricular systole starts.

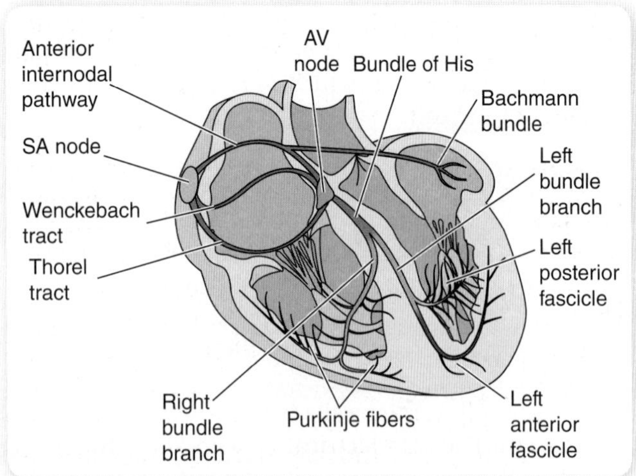

Figure 8-89 The electrical conduction system of the heart. Impulses that originate in the sinoatrial node spread through the atria and along the internodal pathways to the atrioventricular (AV) node. From the AV node, they travel down the bundle of His and right and left bundle branches and into the Purkinje network of the ventricles. Note that the Bachmann bundle is an interatrial pathway that initiates depolarization of the left atrium.

After passing through the AV node, the impulse enters the **bundle of His**, which is located in the upper portion of the interventricular septum. From here, it proceeds rapidly to the right and left bundle branches. The right bundle branch innervates the right ventricle. The left bundle branch spreads the electrical impulse to the interventricular septum and left ventricle, which is thicker and more muscular than the right ventricle. The right and left bundle branches divide into smaller and smaller branches and then into a special network of fibers called the **Purkinje fibers**. The impulse then spreads out, via the Purkinje fibers, to the left, then the right ventricular myocardium, resulting in ventricular contraction or systole.

Regulation of Heart Function

The sympathetic division of the ANS innervates the heart by means of cardiac nerves. Branches of the vagus nerves provide parasympathetic innervation. Networks of these sympathetic and parasympathetic fibers form cardiac plexuses, which are located close to the arch of the aorta. From the cardiac plexuses, fibers course along the base of the heart on the surface of the great vessels and are distributed to the various heart chambers.[32] The fibers then penetrate the myocardium, usually accompanying the right and left coronary arteries. Although most of the fibers terminate in the SA node, some of the fibers end in the AV node and in the atrial myocardium. A few parasympathetic fibers extend to the ventricles.

Stimulation of sympathetic (accelerator) nerves results in an increased force of contraction and increased HR. Increases in HR shorten all phases of the cardiac cycle. When the length of time for ventricular relaxation is shortened, less time is available for the ventricles to fill adequately with blood. Stimulation of parasympathetic (inhibitory) nerve fibers slows the rate of discharge of the SA node, slows conduction through the AV node, decreases the strength of atrial contraction, and can cause a small decrease in the force of ventricular contraction.

Other factors that influence HR include electrolyte and hormone levels, metabolic rate, medications, stress, anxiety, fear, and body temperature.

▶ Blood Vessels and Circulation

The vasculature is a closed system of vessels that distributes blood from the heart to the tissues of the body and returns blood from the tissues to the heart (see Figure 8-80). It can be divided into the following components: (1) the arterial system, which takes blood from the heart and distributes it to the tissues; (2) the venous system, which returns blood from the tissues to the heart; and (3) the microcirculation, where nutrients and cellular waste products are exchanged between the blood and tissues.

Blood vessels are composed of different layers of an elastic tissue and smooth muscle called tunics. The innermost layer is the **tunica intima**, or endothelium **Figure 8-90**. It is composed of a single layer of epithelial cells and provides almost no resistance to blood flow. The middle layer, the **tunica media**, is composed of elastic connective tissue and smooth muscle cells that provide support for the vessel walls. The smooth muscle tissue of this layer is innervated by nerve fibers of the ANS, which can alter the diameter of the lumen of the vessel. The outermost layer of the vessels is the **tunica adventitia**. This layer is composed of nerves and connective tissue that contains elastic and collagenous fibers. The collagenous fibers of the tunica adventitia help hold the vessel open and are the means by which the vessel attaches to nearby body tissues. Tiny blood vessels called the vasa vasorum extend from the tunica adventitia to the tunica media, providing the blood supply for the tissues of the vessel wall. The opening within the blood vessel is the lumen.

Although each blood vessel may hold only a small amount of blood, the total volume of all vessels in the body forms a large container when considered together. It is important to understand that the size of this container is dynamic—that is, it changes in response to conditions present within and outside of the body. For example, if the body is moderately or severely dehydrated, then the amount of circulating blood volume falls. If the total volume of the circulatory system (the container) were to remain constant, then the patient's SV, blood pressure, and CO may drop significantly. To prevent this, the blood vessels receive constant feedback from the ANS. If baroreceptors in the central circulation detect a drop in pressure, then the blood vessels constrict to shrink the

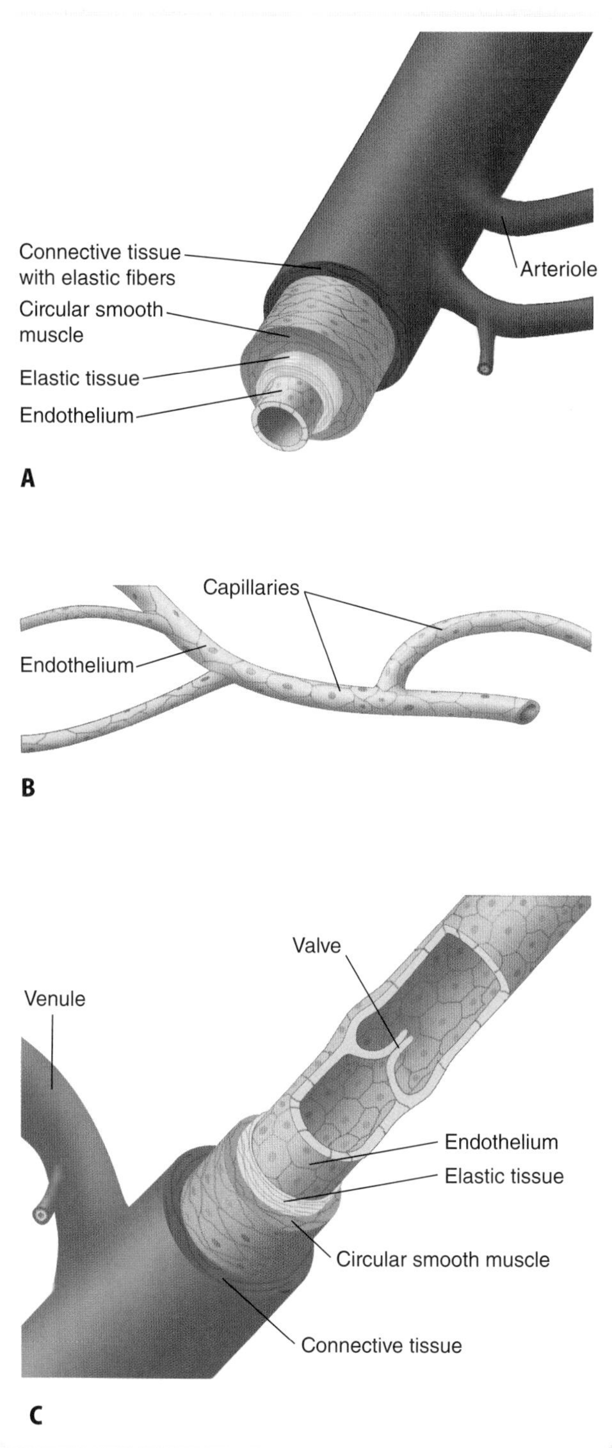

Figure 8-90 The walls of the blood vessels are composed of three layers of tissue: the endothelium (tunica intima), elastic tissue (tunica media), and connective tissue (tunica adventitia). **A.** Artery. **B.** Capillary. **C.** Vein.

size of the container proportionally. These adjustments are coordinated by a wide array of feedback mechanisms to maintain homeostasis. In some cases, the ANS also changes the distribution of blood by constricting peripheral blood vessels to a greater degree than those supplying the vital organs. This process is known as shunting and is a sign of shock.

Arterial System

The arteries make up the body's distribution system **Figure 8-91**. The aorta is the largest artery of the body and its branches deliver blood to all body organs and tissues. The aorta has three main regions: (1) the ascending aorta, (2) the aortic arch, and the (3) descending aorta. The *ascending aorta* originates from the base of the heart and terminates by becoming the arch of the aorta. The aorta curves posteriorly and to the left at the level of the second costal cartilage and forms the segment called the *aortic arch*. The aortic arch descends to vertebral level T4 and continues inferiorly as the **descending aorta**. The descending aorta is named according to its location within the body cavities. The thoracic aorta is the portion of the descending aorta that extends from the aortic arch to the diaphragm. The thoracic aorta ends by passing through the diaphragm to become the abdominal aorta at about vertebral level T12. The main divisions of the aorta and its principal branches are shown in **Table 8-37**.

Conducting arteries are the large arteries that arise from the aorta and its main branches. Because their function is to transport blood under high pressure to the tissues, these vessels are equipped with more elastic tissue and less smooth muscle, allowing them to stretch under great pressures and quickly return to their original shape. Examples of large arteries include the aorta and the brachiocephalic, common carotid, common iliac, and subclavian arteries. The elasticity of the large arteries helps to reduce the workload of the heart. If these arteries were rigid rather than elastic, then the pressure would rise dramatically during systole. This increased pressure would require the ventricles to pump against increased afterload, thereby increasing the work of the heart. Instead, as blood is ejected into these vessels, they distend, and the resultant increase in systolic pressure, and thus the work of the heart, is reduced.[32]

Medium and small arteries are called distributing arteries or muscular arteries. These arteries supply individual organs and larger amounts of smooth muscle, which gives the body the ability to adjust blood flow. Examples include the brachial, gastric, and superior mesenteric arteries.

The smallest of the arteries are arterioles (resistance vessels). The strong muscular walls of these vessels act as stopcocks through which blood is released into the capillaries.

The Head and Neck. The brachiocephalic artery is the first vessel to branch from the aortic arch. It is relatively short and rapidly divides into the right common carotid artery and the right subclavian artery. The carotid arteries transport blood to the head and neck, whereas the subclavian arteries transport blood to the upper extremities.

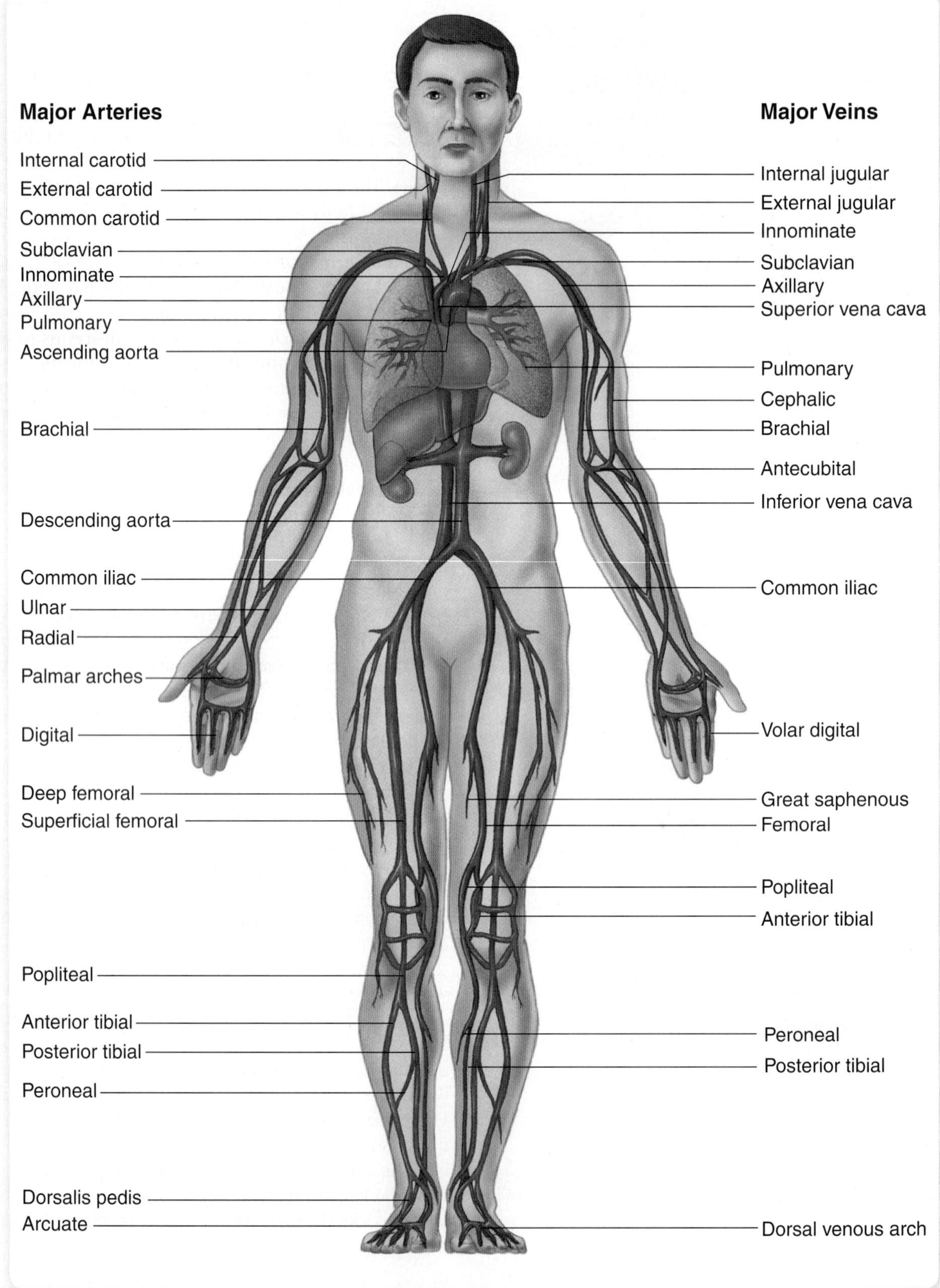

Figure 8-91 The major arteries and veins.

Table 8-37 Major Arteries

Branch of the Aorta	Artery	Area Supplied
Ascending	Right and left coronary arteries	Myocardium
Aortic arch	Brachiocephalic (innominate)	Head and neck, shoulder, upper extremity
	Common carotid	Head and neck
	Subclavian	Head and upper extremity
Descending (thoracic)		
Visceral branches	Supply the organs contained within the thorax	
	Bronchial	Bronchi of lungs
	Esophageal	Esophagus
Parietal branches	Supply the wall of the thoracic cavity	
	Posterior intercostal	Intercostal muscles, lateral rib cage
	Subcostal	Chest wall
	Superior phrenic	Superior surface of diaphragm
Descending (abdominal)		
Visceral branches	Supply the organs contained within the abdomen	
	Celiac trunk	Esophagus, liver, pancreas, spleen, stomach
	Inferior mesenteric	Descending colon, rectum
	Middle suprarenal arteries	Adrenal gland
	Ovarian	Ovary, fallopian tube, ureter
	Renal	Kidney
	Superior mesenteric	Colon, pancreas, small intestine
	Testicular	Testis, ureter
Parietal branches	Supply the walls of the abdomen	
	Common iliac	Pelvis, lower extremity
	Inferior phrenic	Inferior surface of diaphragm, adrenal gland
	Lumbar	Back muscles, lumbar vertebrae
	Median sacral	Sacrum

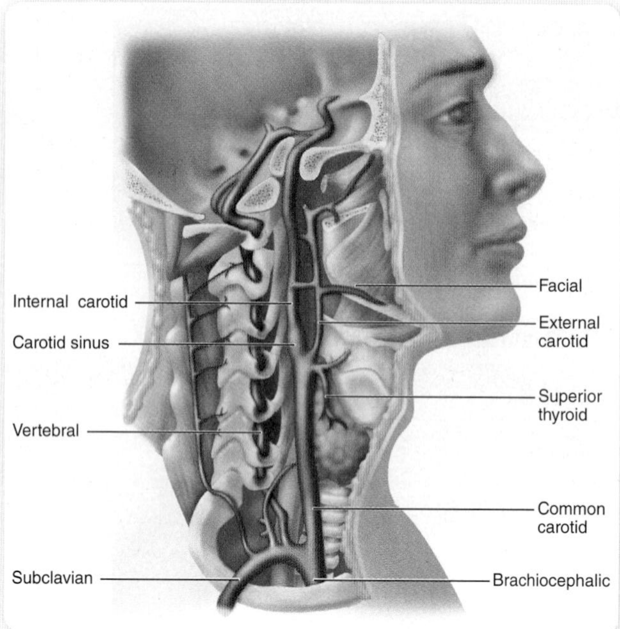

Figure 8-92 The arteries of the head and neck.

Each common carotid artery branches at the angle of the mandible into the internal and external carotid arteries. This point of division is called the carotid bifurcation. Here, a slight dilation, the carotid sinus, contains structures that are important in regulating blood pressure. Branches of the external carotid artery supply blood to the face, nose, and mouth. The internal carotid arteries, together with the vertebral arteries (branches of the subclavian arteries), supply blood to the brain **Figure 8-92**.

The Upper Extremity. The subclavian artery supplies blood to the brain, neck, anterior chest wall, and shoulder. Shortly after its point of origin, the subclavian artery gives rise to the vertebral arteries. The subclavian system then continues from the thorax into the upper extremity. At the shoulder joint, it becomes the axillary artery, then the brachial artery below the head of the humerus. The brachial artery divides into the ulnar and radial arteries **Figure 8-93**.

The Thoracic Aorta. Two types of branches of arteries make up the thoracic aorta: the visceral arteries and the parietal arteries. Visceral arteries supply blood to the thoracic organs, and parietal arteries supply blood to the thoracic wall.

Intercostal arteries run along the ribs and provide circulation to the chest wall. Intercostal arteries branch into anterior and posterior intercostal arteries. The anterior intercostal arteries originate as branches of the subclavian system. The posterior intercostal arteries arise directly from the aorta. Visceral branches of the thoracic aorta supply the bronchial arteries in the lungs and the esophageal arteries.

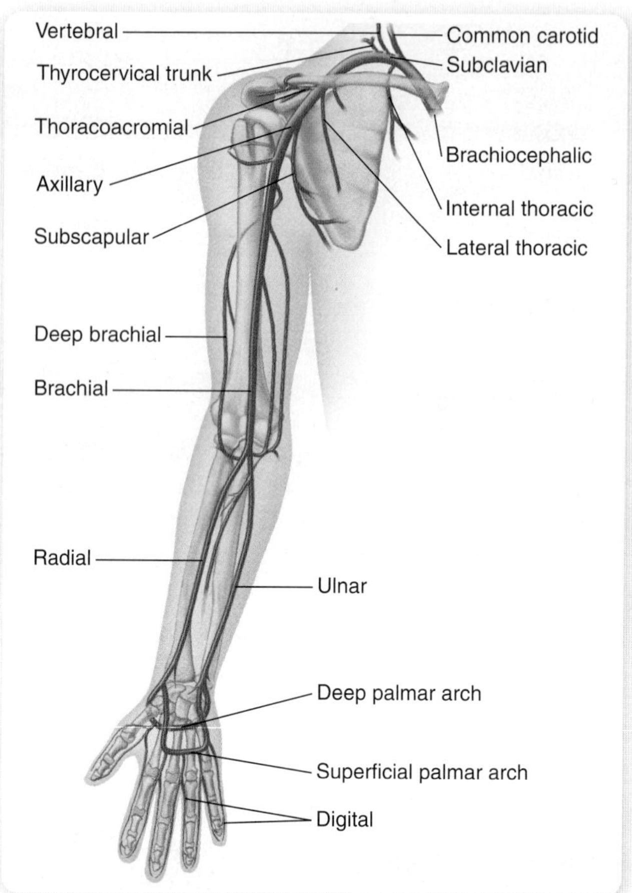

Figure 8-93 The arteries of the upper extremity.

The Abdominal Aorta. Like their thoracic counterpart, branches of the abdominal aorta are divided into visceral and parietal portions. The visceral arteries are subdivided into paired and nonpaired arteries. The three major unpaired branches of the visceral arteries of the abdominal aorta include the celiac trunk, the superior mesenteric, and the inferior mesenteric arteries **Figure 8-94**. The celiac trunk supplies blood to the esophagus, stomach, duodenum, spleen, liver, and pancreas **Figure 8-95**. The superior mesenteric artery and its branches supply blood to the pancreas, small intestine, and colon. The inferior mesenteric artery and its branches supply blood to the descending colon and rectum. Paired branches of the visceral abdominal aorta supply blood to the kidneys, adrenal gland, and gonads. The parietal branches supply blood to the diaphragm and abdominal wall.

The Pelvis and Lower Extremity. At the level of the fifth lumbar vertebra, the aorta divides into the two common iliac arteries. These arteries further divide into the internal iliac arteries, which supply blood to the pelvis, and the external iliac arteries, which enter the lower extremity **Figure 8-96**. The internal iliac artery sends out visceral branches to the rectum, vagina, uterus, and ovary. Parietal branches supply blood to the sacrum, gluteal muscles of

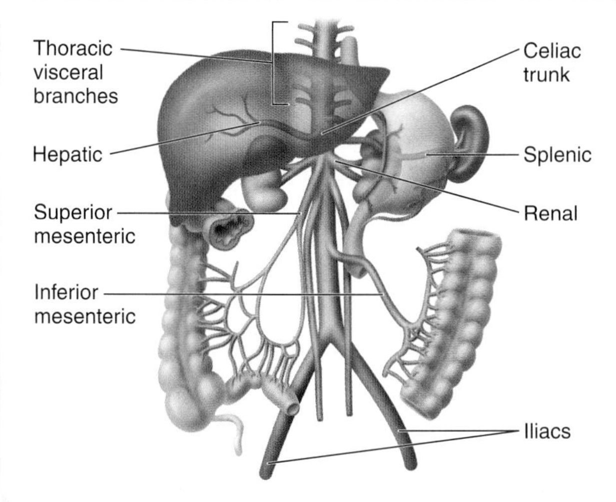

Figure 8-94 The branches of the abdominal aorta.

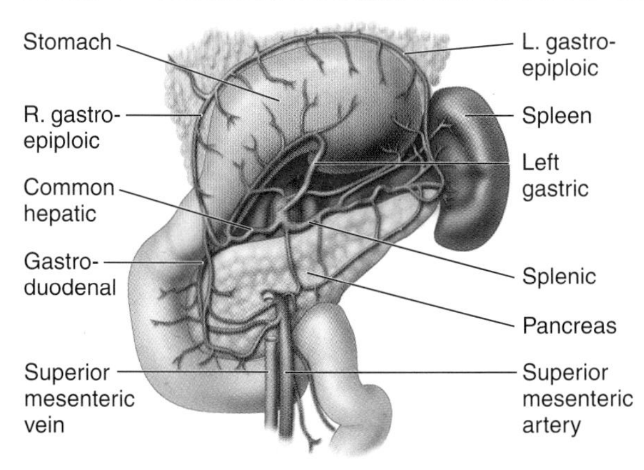

Figure 8-95 The celiac trunk and superior mesenteric vessels.

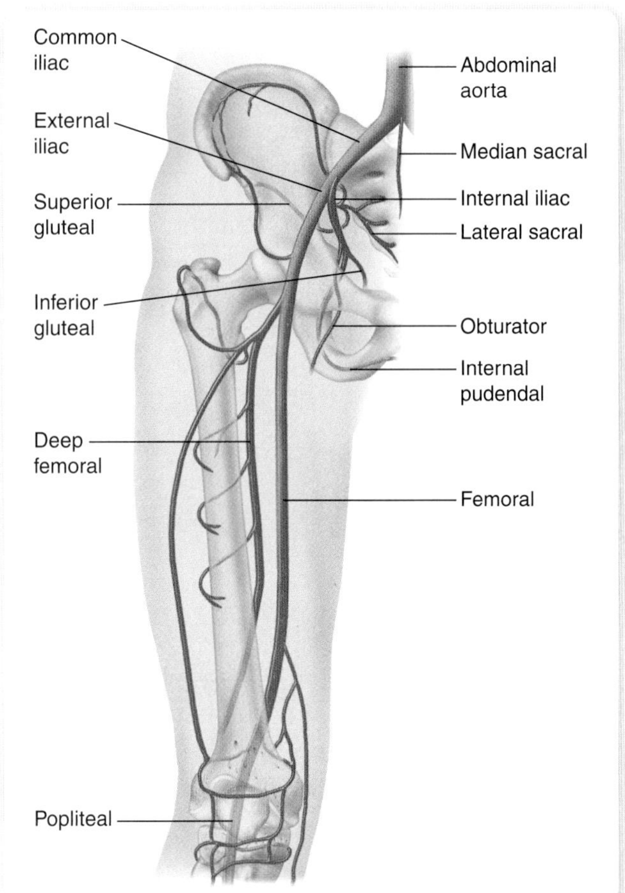

Figure 8-96 The arteries of the pelvis and thigh.

the buttocks region, the pubic region, rectum, external genitalia, and proximal thigh.

Like the upper extremity, the vessels of the lower extremity form a continuum. The external iliac arteries become the femoral arteries. Each femoral artery supplies blood to the thigh, external genitalia, anterior abdominal wall, and knee. The femoral artery becomes the popliteal artery in the lower thigh. Each popliteal artery then branches into the anterior tibial, posterior tibial, and peroneal arteries. At the foot, the anterior tibial artery becomes the dorsalis pedis artery. Plantar arteries arise from the posterior tibial artery and subdivide into digital branches that supply blood to the toes **Figure 8-97**.

Venous System

Think of the venous system as a collection system (see Figure 8-91). Venules are the smallest of the venous vessels, with very little smooth muscle in their middle layer. Venules are called capacitance (storage) vessels because they are capable of holding large amounts of volume. Because 70% of the body's blood is contained in the venous system, the veins are able to adjust blood volume returning to the heart (preload) so the needs of the body can be met when cardiac output is altered, such as shock.[32]

The venules gradually increase in thickness and become medium-sized vessels. Venous blood flow depends on skeletal muscle action, respiratory movements, and gravity. Medium and large veins have valves within them that prevent a backward flow of blood. Veins of the arms and legs have more valves than other veins of the body, where they prevent the backflow of blood in response to gravity. Veins become progressively larger as they approach the heart. The two largest veins of the body are the superior vena cava and inferior vena cava, which empty into the right atrium. In the pulmonary circulation, the pulmonary veins transport oxygenated blood from the lungs to the left atrium of the heart. From the systemic circulation, veins transport blood with a reduced oxygen content from the body tissues to the right atrium of the heart. The major veins of the body and the areas they drain of blood are shown in **Table 8-38**.

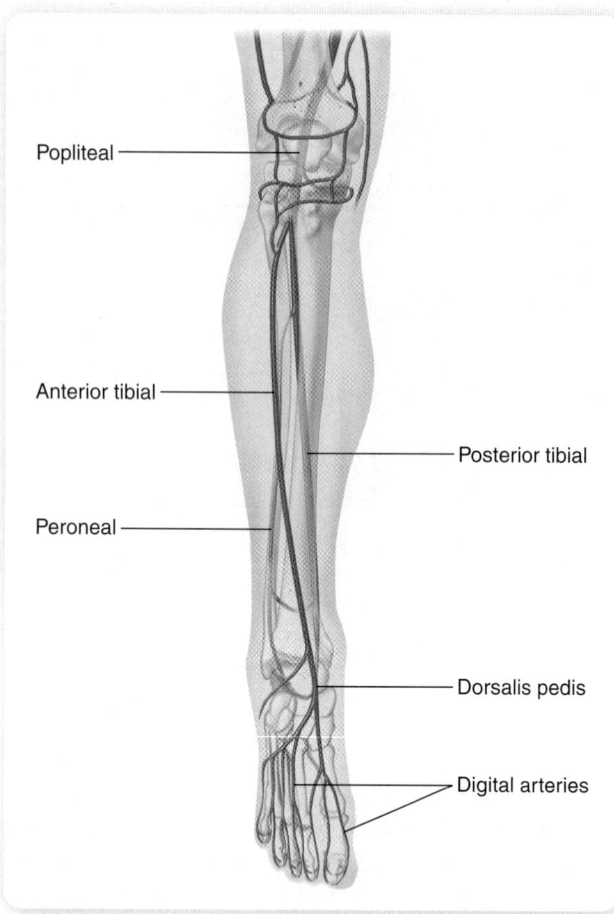

Figure 8-97 The arteries of the lower extremity.

The Head and Neck. The two major veins that drain the head and neck of blood are the external and internal jugular veins. The external jugular vein is more superficial and often is visible immediately beneath the skin. The external jugular vein primarily drains the posterior head and neck. The internal jugular vein drains the cranial vault as well as the anterior portion of the head, face, and neck. Spaces between membranes surrounding the brain form venous sinuses. These sinuses are the primary means of venous drainage from the brain and feed into the internal jugular vein.

The external and internal jugular veins join the subclavian veins (the proximal part of the main vein of the arm) to form the brachiocephalic veins, which drain into the superior vena cava Figure 8-98.

The Upper Extremity. The veins of the upper extremity vary somewhat from person to person Figure 8-99. The names of the veins of the hands, wrists, and forearm follow the arteries of the same name. In the upper forearm, these veins combine to form the basilic vein and the cephalic vein, the major veins of the arm. The basilic and cephalic veins combine to form the axillary vein, which drains into the subclavian vein.

The Thorax. In the thorax, venous drainage begins at the anterior and posterior intercostal veins. The intercostal veins empty into the azygos vein on the right side of the thorax and the hemiazygos vein on the left side. These veins, along with the right and left brachiocephalic veins, provide the major source of flow into the superior vena cava.

Table 8-38 Major Veins

Vein	Areas Drained
Veins That Empty Into the Superior Vena Cava	
Azygos	Bronchi, esophagus, mediastinum, pericardium, posterior wall of thorax and abdomen
Brachiocephalic (innominate)	Head, neck, upper extremity
External jugular	Muscles and skin of face, neck, and scalp
Internal jugular	Brain, skull
Subclavian	Mammary glands, upper extremity
Veins That Empty Into the Inferior Vena Cava	
Common iliac	Lower extremities
Hepatic	Liver
Ovarian	Ovaries
Renal	Kidneys
Testicular	Testes

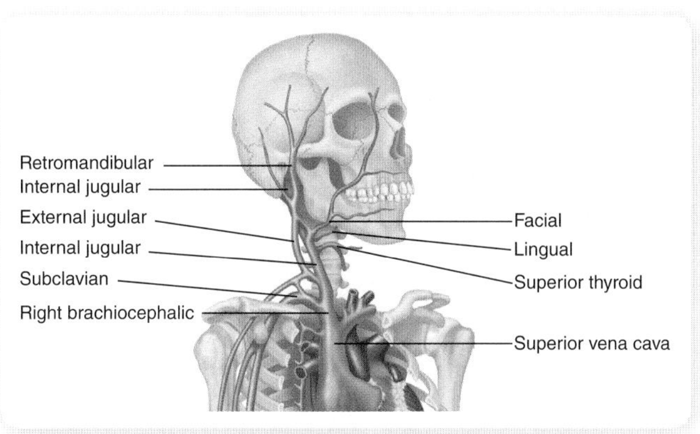

Figure 8-98 The veins of the head and neck.

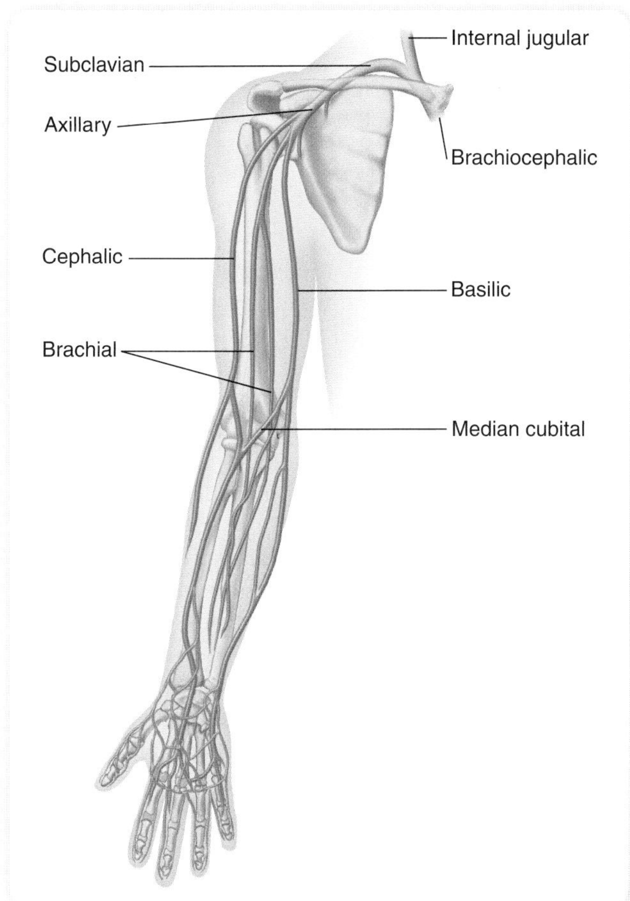

Figure 8-99 The veins of the upper extremity.

The Abdomen and Pelvis. Ultimately, all venous drainage from the lower part of the body passes through the inferior vena cava. The inferior vena cava returns deoxygenated blood from the lower parts of the body to the right atrium for **oxygenation**, the process of loading oxygen molecules onto hemoglobin molecules in the bloodstream. Within the abdominal and pelvic cavities, veins of the same name accompany the major arteries, providing venous drainage from structures including the kidney, adrenal glands, gonads, and diaphragm. The internal iliac veins drain the pelvis, and the external iliac veins drain the lower limbs. The internal and external iliac veins combine in the pelvis, forming the common iliac veins, which combine to form the inferior vena cava.

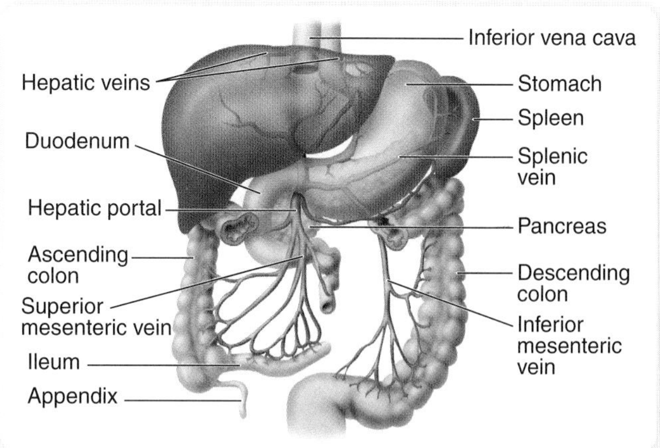

Figure 8-100 The hepatic portal system.

Hepatic Portal Circulation. The **hepatic portal system** is a specialized part of the venous system that carries capillary blood that is rich in digestive nutrients from the digestive organs to the liver. Venous blood from most abdominal organs is returned directly to the inferior vena cava. However, venous blood from the gallbladder, intestines, pancreas, spleen, and stomach first enters the hepatic portal system before being transported to the liver and then to the inferior vena cava **Figure 8-100**. The portal system refers to the passage of blood returning from the digestive tract through two sets of capillaries before it returns to the heart: the first in the capillaries of the abdominal organs, and the second in the liver capillaries. The hepatic portal vein collects blood from capillaries in the abdominal organs, enters the liver, and ultimately ends as a capillary bed, where the liver extracts needed nutrients and stores others. The capillary beds of the hepatic portal vein are drained by hepatic veins. The hepatic veins return blood to the inferior vena cava, which empties into the right atrium of the heart

The Lower Extremity. The longest vein in the body is the great saphenous vein. It drains the foot, leg, and thigh. The saphenous vein originates over the dorsal and medial side of the foot, ascends along the medial side of the leg and thigh, and empties into the femoral vein, which then drains into the external iliac vein. Laterally, the small saphenous vein helps drain the leg and lateral side of the foot. The veins of the feet also drain into the anterior and posterior tibial veins, which accompany their respective arteries, uniting at the knee to form the popliteal vein. The popliteal vein ascends through the thigh, becoming the femoral vein **Figure 8-101**.

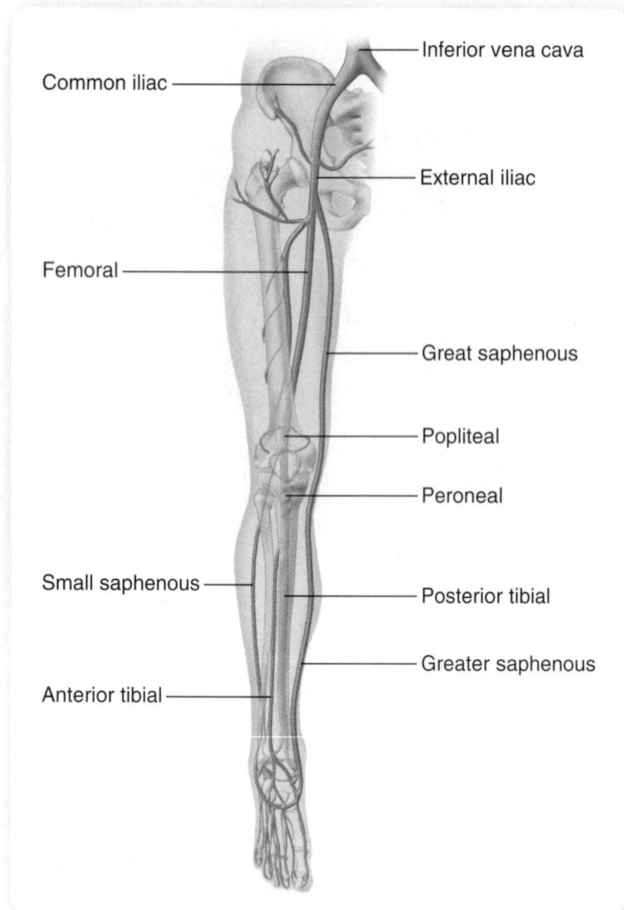

Figure 8-101 The veins of the lower extremity.

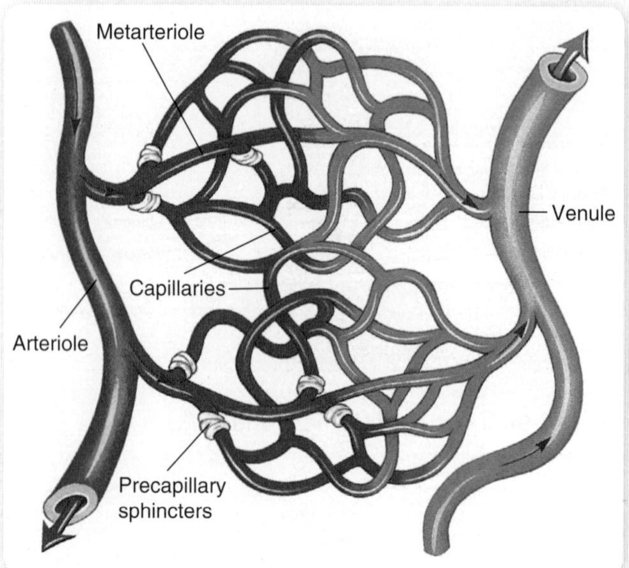

Figure 8-102 The microcirculation is the portion of the vasculature consisting of the arterioles, capillaries, and venules.

Microcirculation

The microcirculation is the portion of the vasculature consisting of the arterioles, capillaries, and venules Figure 8-102. Think of it as a diffusion and filtration system. The most important functions of the microcirculation are the transport of nutrients to the tissues and the removal of cellular waste.[33]

As you have learned, the arterioles are the major resistance vessels. Their lining of smooth muscle allows them to alter their diameter, thereby directing and regulating blood flow into the capillaries. Thus, the arterioles can alter blood flow in each tissue in response to its needs.

Capillaries form the connection between arterioles and venules in most body tissues. The capillary walls are very thin and contain pores, enabling the exchange of gases, water, nutrients, electrolytes, hormones, and waste products between the blood and the interstitial fluid that bathes the tissue cells. Pores are absent in cerebral capillaries, where the blood-brain barrier blocks the entry of many small molecules.[32]

In some tissues, arterioles branch directly into capillaries and control the flow of blood through the capillary bed (network of capillaries) by constricting or dilating. In other tissues, arterioles branch into smaller arterioles (metarterioles). Metarterioles are short, connecting vessels that can either directly link to capillaries or bypass the capillary bed and connect to venules. The proximal ends of metarterioles are encircled by a small cuff of smooth muscle called a **precapillary sphincter**. These sphincters function as regulatory valves, controlling blood flow into the capillary bed. Metarterioles are partially lined with smooth muscle, enabling them to adjust their diameter.

Metarterioles and precapillary sphincters are not found in all tissues. Where metarterioles and precapillary sphincters are present, they are in close contact with the tissues they serve and are responsive to its needs. For example, the precapillary sphincters will constrict and reduce blood flow or relax and increase blood flow in each area depending on local tissue oxygen requirements and the concentrations of nutrients, end products of metabolism, and hydrogen ions. The intermittent contraction and relaxation of the arterioles, metarterioles, precapillary sphincters, and some small arteries is called vasomotion.[32]

In some tissues of the body, a direct connection exists between arteries and veins. These connections, called arteriovenous anastomoses, serve to shunt blood away from the capillary bed and route it from small arterioles directly into small venules of the tissue in need of oxygen and nutrients. Examples of sites where arteriovenous anastomoses can be found include the skin (eg, hands, feet, nose, ear, lips) and the mucosa of the nose and gut.

Capillary Filtration. The exchange of nutrients and waste products between the intravascular space and the intracellular space is crucial to survival. The majority

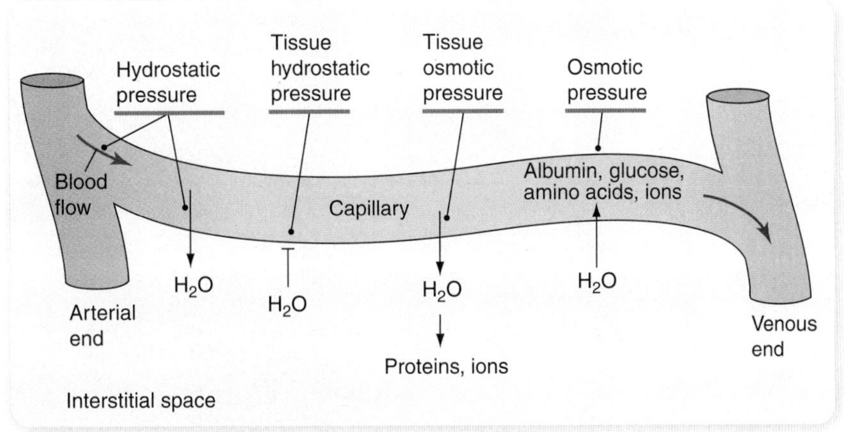

Figure 8-103 Movement of water into and out of capillaries is a result of four separate forces.

of substances, such as oxygen and carbon dioxide, pass between these spaces by way of diffusion, facilitated diffusion, and osmosis. However, many substances depend on the process of capillary filtration for this exchange to take place. Capillary filtration depends on three factors: (1) capillary membrane permeability, (2) arterial hydrostatic pressure, and (3) venous oncotic pressure.

Capillaries do not share the same membrane permeability. For example, the liver capillaries are permeable, enabling plasma proteins (such as albumin) to pass easily. In contrast, the capillaries of skeletal muscle contain few pores. Permeability is not uniform along the length of a capillary. The precapillary side is arterial and the postcapillary side is venous **Figure 8-103**. The venous ends of the capillary are more permeable than the arterial ends and permeability is greatest in the venules, probably because of the greater number of pores in these areas.[32]

The movement of water between the plasma in the intravascular compartment and the **interstitial space** (the space between the cells) is a result of pressure. This pressure occurs at the capillary level by filtration. Recall that filtration is the movement of fluid from **intravascular fluid** under high pressure to interstitial fluid, which generally is under lower pressure.

The two main forces at work inside the capillary are hydrostatic pressure and oncotic pressure. **Hydrostatic pressure** is pressure exerted by a liquid and occurs when blood is moved through the artery at relatively high pressures. In the vascular system, hydrostatic pressure is the pressure generated in vessels by the contraction of the heart (ie, blood pressure), gravity, and other forces. When blood meets the capillary walls, the pressure of the fluid pushes against the walls to force fluid out of the capillary. The opposing force is oncotic pressure. **Oncotic pressure** is a form of osmotic pressure exerted by proteins in the blood plasma that usually tends to pull water into the circulatory system. These proteins tend to make the blood thicker. This thickness means that relative to the interstitial space, more water is present outside the capillary than inside. Diffusion occurs, and water seeks to move into the capillary.

The precapillary and postcapillary sphincters help maintain the delicate balance of pressure gradients. This process is called net filtration and is described by Starling's hypothesis, which states that the net filtration is equal to the combined forces favoring filtration (ie, capillary hydrostatic pressure and interstitial oncotic pressure) minus the combined forces opposing filtration (ie, plasma oncotic pressure and interstitial hydrostatic pressure).

Figure 8-104 shows the entire process. Blood flows into the arterial side of the capillary. Plasma is trying to enter the capillary from the interstitial space, but hydrostatic pressure on the arterial side of the capillary is higher, so plasma, carrying nutrients, leaves the capillary and enters the interstitial space. The hydrostatic pressure is greatly diminished by the time the fluid reaches the venous side of the capillary because the effort of pushing the fluid out of the capillary decreased its force. This decrease in pressure is beneficial because now oncotic pressure can push fluid into the capillary; plasma, with all of the wastes from the cells, enters the venous side of the capillary. These wastes are then carried away.

▶ The Lymphatic System

The lymphatic system is considered part of the circulatory system. The lymphatic system has the following three primary functions:

1. **Removal of excess fluid from tissues of the body and the recovery of fluid needed to maintain the proper balance of water.** Lymph is drained from the tissues and returned to the venous side of the vascular system.
2. **Production and circulation of lymphocytes.** These lymphocytes are produced within lymphoid organs, which provide a significant portion of the body's immune function.

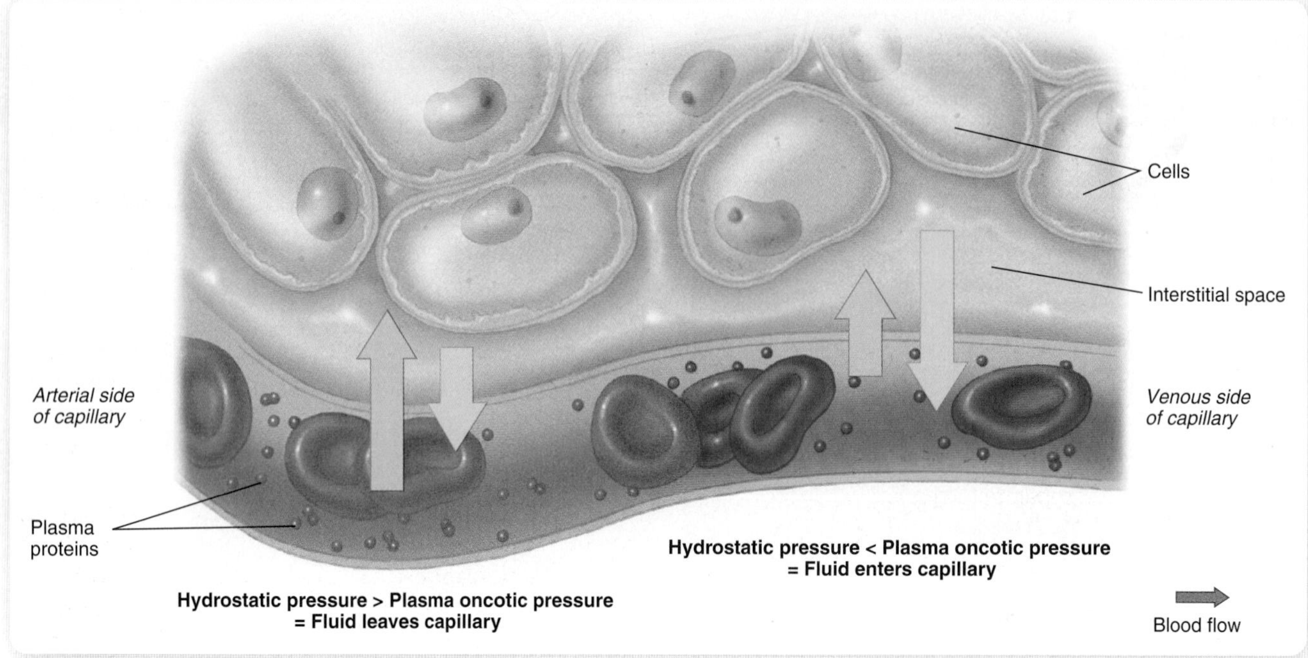

Figure 8-104 Fluid movement from capillaries to interstitial space and back.

3. **Distribution of various products unable to enter the bloodstream directly.** These products include nutrients and some hormones.

The lymphatic system transports lymph by passive circulation. Recall that **lymph** is a thin, plasma-like fluid formed from interstitial or extracellular fluid that bathes the tissues of the body. Lymphatic capillaries pick up the lymph and drain it into larger vessels. Lymph circulates through the body in thin-walled lymph vessels that travel close to the major arteries and veins Figure 8-105. Like veins, lymphatic vessels contain valves that limit backflow. Foreign material such as debris or bacteria is filtered from the lymph in the lymph nodes, round or bean-shaped structures that are interspersed along the course of the lymph vessels, and returns to the main circulatory system via the **thoracic duct**, one of two great lymph vessels. The thoracic duct collects lymph from the lower body, the left side of the head and neck, and the left arm. This duct returns lymph to the central circulation by a connection with the left subclavian vein. The right lymphatic duct collects lymph from the right arm, the right side of the thorax, and the right side of the head and neck. This duct returns lymph to the central circulation by a connection with the right subclavian vein. Various body dynamics, such as changes in respiratory pressure, muscular contractions, and movement of organs surrounding lymphatic vessels, combine to move lymph through the lymphatic system.

Lymphatic Vessels

Lymphatic vessels only carry fluid away from the tissues. In the lymphatic capillaries, the epithelial cells contain one-way valves that allow fluid to enter the vessel but prevent it from flowing back into the tissues. Lymphatic capillaries are present in all tissues except the CNS, bone marrow, cartilage, epidermis, and cornea. Generally, fluid flows from the blood capillaries to the tissues, then out of the tissue spaces into lymph capillaries. In the major blood capillary beds of the body, the internal hydrostatic pressure allows a normal and continuous leak of a total of 3 mL/min to 4 mL/min of fluid into the interstitial spaces. To prevent the tissues from becoming edematous (swollen), the lymphatic vessel must absorb this excess fluid and return it to the central venous circulation.

Thymus

The thymus is located in the thorax, anterior to the aorta and posterior to the upper sternum. It is divided into lobules by inward-extending connective tissues. The lobules contain large amounts of lymphocytes, including primarily inactive thymocytes, which formed from stem cells in the bone marrow and settled in the thymus. Some thymocytes mature into T lymphocytes, which leave the thymus after 3 weeks and provide immunity in the body. Thymosin is secreted by the epithelial cells of the thymus. This hormone causes T lymphocytes to mature.

Spleen

The spleen is located in the upper left abdominal cavity, inferior to the diaphragm and posterior and lateral to the stomach. It is the body's largest lymphatic organ, resembling a large, subdivided lymph node. The spleen contains the largest amount of lymphatic tissue in an adult's body. It differs from lymph nodes in that its venous sinuses are filled with blood, not lymph. Two types of tissues exist inside the splenic lobules. White pulp is located throughout the spleen in small

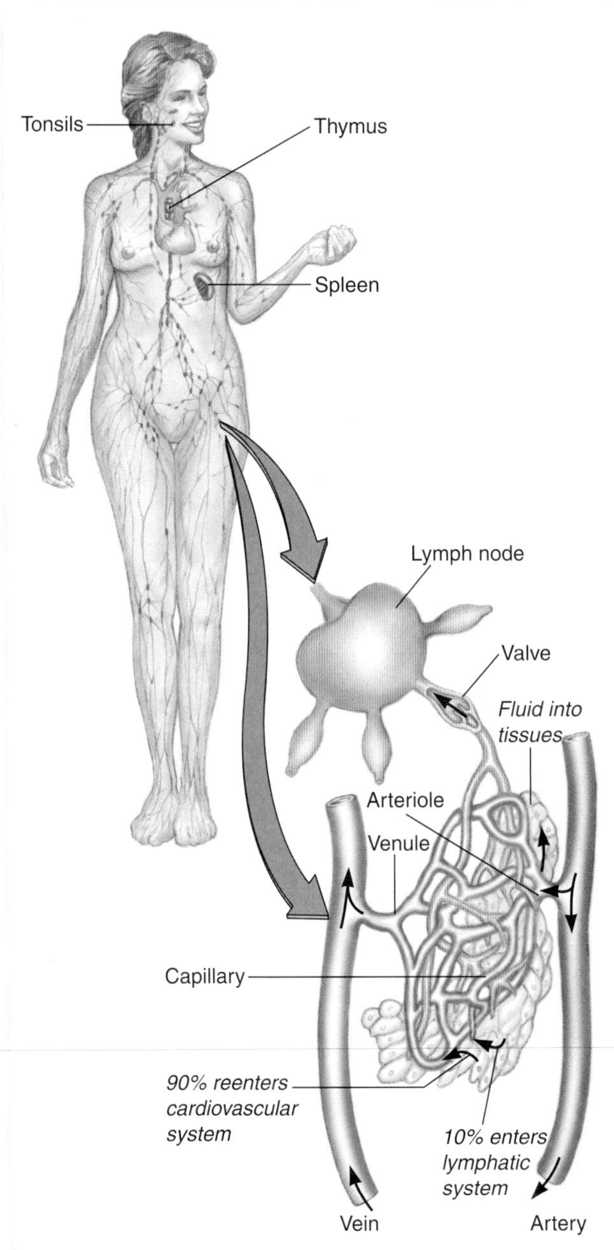

Figure 8-105 The lymphatic system consists of vessels that transport lymph and excess tissue fluid back to the circulatory system. Lymph is picked up by lymphatic capillaries that drain into larger vessels. Like the veins, the lymphatic vessels contain valves that prohibit backflow. Lymph nodes are interspersed along the vessels and filter the lymph.

"islands," made up of splenic nodules containing many lymphocytes. The remainder of the lobules are filled by red pulp, which contains many RBCs, lymphocytes, and macrophages.

The blood capillaries of the red pulp are extremely permeable, and RBCs easily squeeze through the capillary walls to enter the venous sinuses. Older RBCs may be damaged during this process, so they are engulfed by macrophages inside the splenic sinuses. Via the action of macrophages and lymphocytes, the spleen filters blood similarly to the way that lymph nodes filter lymph.

Words of Wisdom

The spleen is prone to injury during rapid deceleration or compression and may be punctured if the overlying left lower ribs are fractured.

Immune System

The human body has multiple defense mechanisms that work together to provide immunity, which is the ability to fight disease, illness, and infection. An infection may be caused by the presence and multiplication of a disease-causing agent (pathogen), which can be a virus, bacterium, fungus, or protozoan.

The immune system has two anatomic components: the lymphoid tissues and the cells that are responsible for the immune response. Lymphoid tissues are distributed throughout the body. The two primary lymphoid tissues are bone marrow and the thymus gland. Bone marrow is specialized soft tissue found within bone. Red bone marrow, which is widespread in the bones of children and is found in some adult bones (in the sternum and ribs), is essential for formation of mature blood cells; it produces B lymphocytes. T lymphocytes originate from precursor cells in the bone marrow, leave the bone marrow, and mature in the thymus gland.

Clusters of lymphoid tissue, which are collectively called mucosa-associated lymphoid tissue, are associated with the skin and the respiratory, urinary, GI, and reproductive tracts. Lymphoid tissues contain immune cells that are in a position to intercept pathogens before they reach the general circulation. The tonsils are perhaps the best known type of mucosa-associated lymphoid tissue. Unencapsulated lymphoid tissue is particularly prominent in the GI tract. Called the gut-associated lymphoid tissue, this tissue lies just under the inner lining of the esophagus and intestines.

The salivary glands (accessory organs of the digestive system) and the lacrimal glands play a role in the immune system as well; the salivary and lacrimal glands produce an antibody, secretory immunoglobulin A, which bathes mucous membranes. As a result, saliva contains antibodies that fight pathogens that enter the mouth, and tears contain antibodies that fight pathogens that enter the eye. Secretory immunoglobulin A is also found in the mammary glands. Though secretory immunoglobulins play an important role in immunity, the primary cells of the immune system are the WBCs, which were discussed earlier in this chapter. Immunity and the immune response is discussed in detail in Chapter 9, *Pathophysiology*.

The Respiratory System

The cells of the body must have energy to function. This energy is produced through a series of complicated steps that require oxygen. The primary function of the respiratory system is to bring oxygen into the body and eliminate carbon dioxide. This system also provides nonspecific defenses against disease, helps control pH, and permits vocalization. The respiratory system is composed of the following parts:

1. The respiratory tract, which consists of passages to move air to and from the exchange surfaces
2. The **respiratory membrane**, where gas exchange takes place (oxygen is picked up in the bloodstream and carbon dioxide is eliminated through the lungs)
3. The lungs, which allow the mechanical movement of air to and from the respiratory membrane
4. The diaphragm, the muscles of the chest wall, and the **accessory muscles** of breathing, which permit normal respiratory movement, and the nerves from the brain and spinal cord to those muscles

The airway is separated into upper and lower structures. The upper and lower structures can be distinguished on the basis of their location above or below the **glottis** or glottic opening (the vocal cords and the opening between them) **Figure 8-106**.[34] Stated another way, the upper airway includes respiratory structures in the head and neck; the lower airway includes respiratory structures in the chest.

▶ Upper Airway

Structures of the upper airway include the nose, mouth, tongue, jaw, oral cavity, larynx, and **pharynx**. The major functions of the upper airway are to warm, filter, and humidify air as it enters the body through the nose and mouth so that by the time it reaches the trachea, it is at body temperature and fully humidified. Humidification is accomplished as the air picks up moisture from the soft tissues of the airway.

The entrance to the respiratory tract begins at the nasal and oral cavities. The area between the nasal cavity and the larynx and posterior to the oral cavity is referred to as the pharynx. The pharynx (throat), which extends from the base of the skull to the level of the sixth cervical vertebrae, allows passage of air to the lower airway and food to the esophagus. For anatomic purposes, the pharynx is divided into three regions, although no physical structures separate these areas.

Nasopharynx

On **inhalation** (the active, muscular part of breathing), air normally enters the body through the nose and passes into the **nasopharynx**, which extends from the back of the nasal cavity to the level of the soft palate. Recall that the palate is the roof of the oral cavity and separates

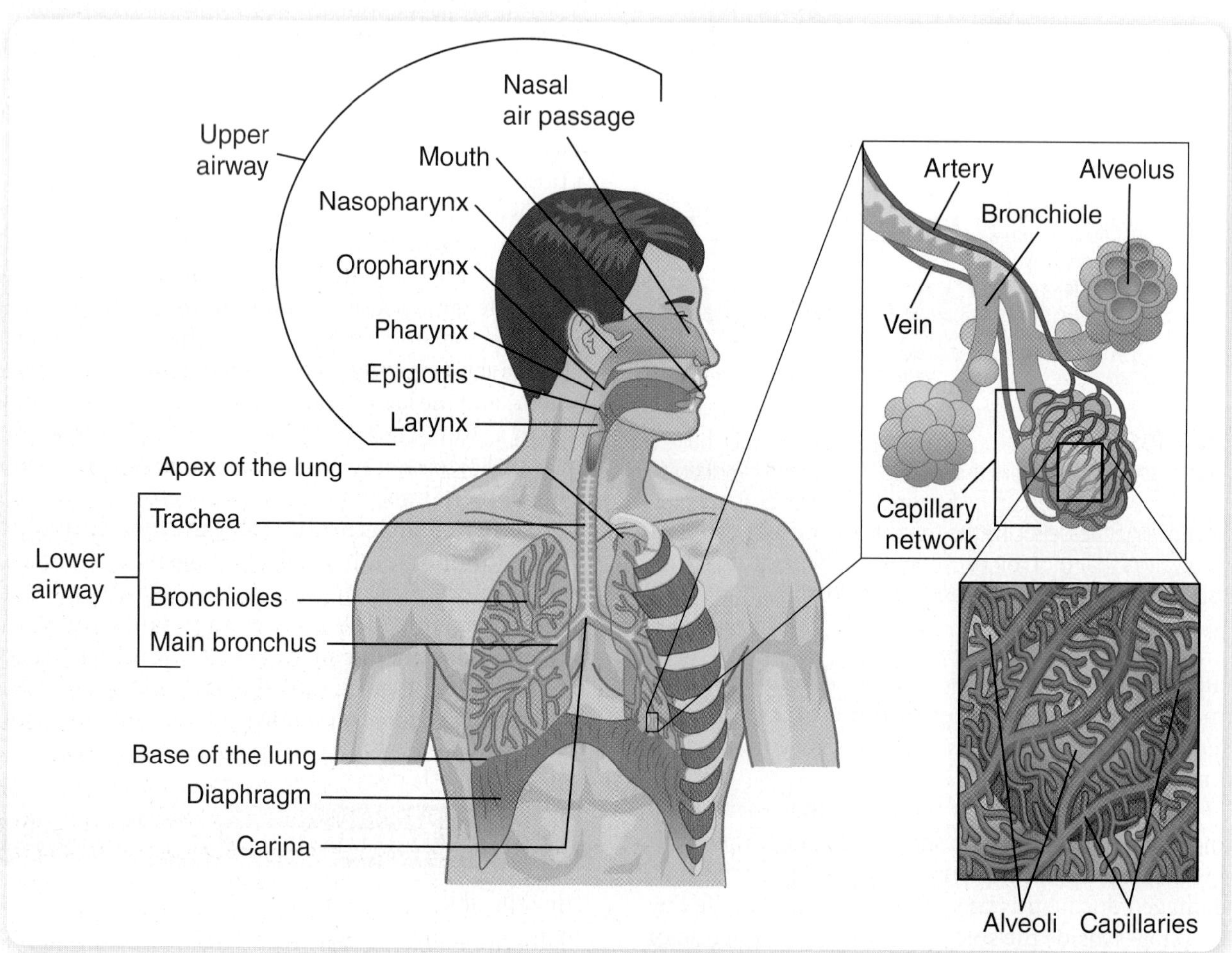

Figure 8-106 The respiratory system consists of all structures of the body that contribute to the process of breathing.

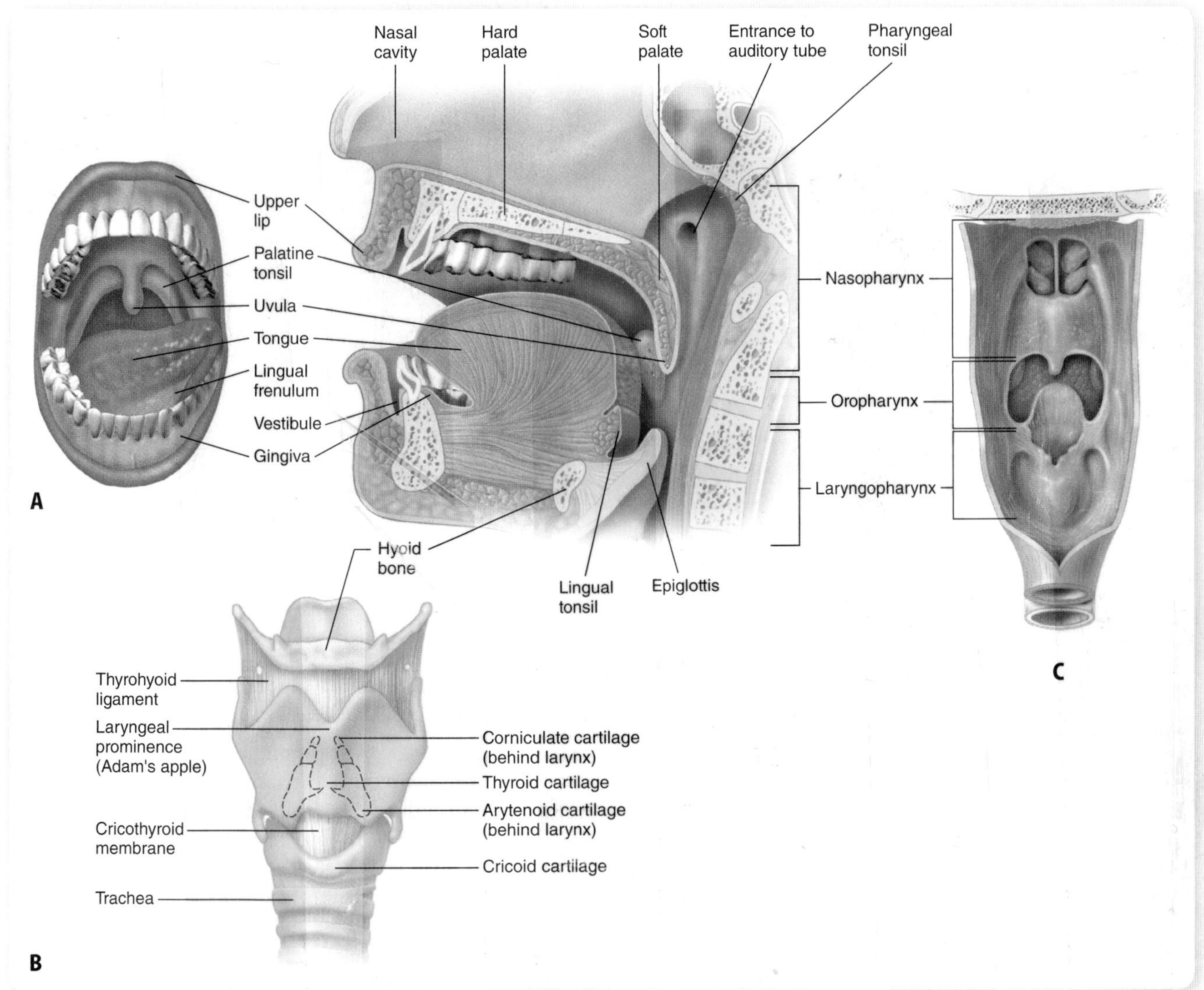

Figure 8-107 A. The oral cavity. **B.** The larynx. **C.** The pharynx.

the nasal cavity from the oral cavity. The hard palate, which is the anterior portion of the palate, is supported by bone (primarily the maxillary bone) Figure 8-107. The posterior portion is the soft palate because it is made up of mucous membrane, muscular fibers, and mucous glands and has no bony support. The palatoglossal arch, the posterior border of the oral cavity, is an extension of the soft palate. The uvula, a small, fleshy tissue structure that resembles a punching bag, projects downward from the posterior part of the soft palate and extends into the palatoglossal arch. When swallowing, muscles elevate the soft palate so that it touches the posterior wall of the pharynx, sealing off the nasopharynx from the oropharynx.

The entire nasal cavity is lined with a ciliated mucous membrane that keeps contaminants such as dust and other small particles out of the respiratory tract. In illness, the body produces additional mucus to trap potentially infectious agents. This mucous membrane is extremely delicate and has a rich blood supply. Olfactory receptors located in the epithelium in the nasal cavity are responsible for recognizing odors.

The nasopharynx is divided into two passages by the nasal septum, a rigid partition that has a rich blood supply. It is composed of the ethmoid and vomer bones and cartilage. Normally, the nasal septum is in the midline of the nose. In some people, the septum may be deviated to one side or the other—a condition that becomes important when contemplating insertion of a nasal airway device. Three bony shelves (turbinates) protrude from the lateral walls of the nasal cavity and extend into the nasal passageway, parallel to the nasal floor. The turbinates increase the surface area of the nasal mucosa and cause turbulence in airflow, making inhaled particles stick to the mucus-coated walls of the nostrils. This combination of vascular supply and turbulence warms, filters, and humidifies the air as it is inhaled.

Along the lateral walls of the nasal passageway are numerous openings that extend into the frontal and maxillary sinuses. Sinuses lessen the weight of the skull,

Words of Wisdom

Any trauma to the nasal passages, such as improper or overly aggressive placement of airway devices, may result in profuse bleeding from the posterior nasal cavity. Bleeding from this area cannot be controlled by direct pressure. Extrinsic factors (such as cocaine use) can also damage the delicate nasal passages or the nasal septum. See Chapter 15, *Airway Management*, for more information.

give resonance to a person's voice, and prevent contaminants from entering the respiratory tract. They also act as tributaries for fluid to and from the eustachian tubes and tear ducts. Because the sinuses help trap particles, they are a common source of infection.

Words of Wisdom

Because of their closeness to underlying brain structures and the thin nature of the bones forming the sinuses, fractures of the bones that comprise the sinuses may cause CSF to leak from the nose (cerebrospinal rhinorrhea) or the ears (cerebrospinal otorrhea). In some patients, CSF may drain from the posterior nasopharynx down the throat, causing a salty taste in the mouth.

Eustachian tubes (auditory tubes) are passages from the inner ear that allow drainage of fluid as well as equalization of pressure that may occur behind the tympanic membrane. Because these tubes are connected to nasal passages, which may contain bacteria, infections can migrate to the middle ear by way of these tubes, especially in toddlers. The back of the nasal cavity opens into the oropharynx.

Oropharynx

The oropharynx is the portion of the pharynx visible within the mouth (see Figure 8-107). Whereas the nasopharynx is a passageway for air only, the oropharynx functions as a passageway for both air and food. The oropharynx begins superiorly at the level of the soft palate and extends to the epiglottis inferiorly.[34] The posterior pharynx has a rich supply of sensitive nerves. Stimulation of this area triggers the gag reflex. Recall that as a protective mechanism, the **gag reflex** initiates coughing or retching to prevent aspiration.

The palatopharyngeal arch is the entrance to the throat, or pharynx **Figure 8-108**. Associated structures in the back of the throat include the tonsils. Tonsils are lymphatic tissue responsible for filtering bacteria and other foreign materials, especially from the mouth and nose.

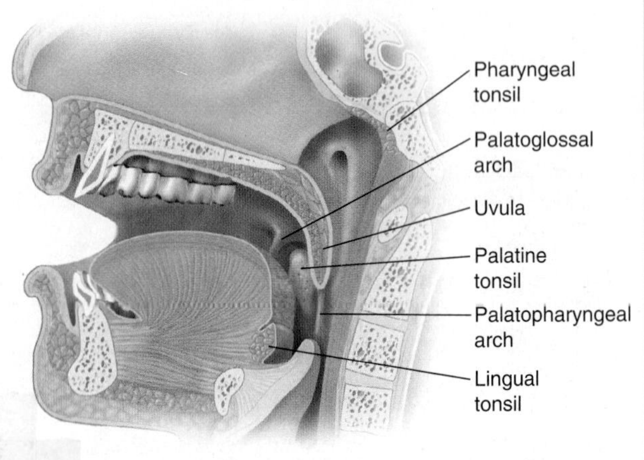

Figure 8-108 The tonsils.

When inflamed and swollen, tonsils become sore and may make swallowing difficult. Two sets of tonsils are located on each side of the throat. The palatine tonsils are located just behind the walls of the palatoglossal arch, anterior to the palatopharyngeal arch. The *adenoids*, also called the pharyngeal tonsils, are located on the upper rear wall of the oral cavity near the opening of the eustachian tubes. The adenoids, when inflamed, can pose an increased risk of ear infection during childhood because they may block drainage exiting the tube. The lingual tonsils are at the base of the tongue.

Within the mouth are several structures that have relevance to the airway, namely the teeth and the tongue. Adults who have retained all their teeth normally have 32 teeth. Teeth provide a supporting structure for the oral cavity and aid in digestion with the chewing of food.

Words of Wisdom

The 32 adult teeth are embedded in the gums in such a manner that significant force is required to dislodge them. However, trauma of lesser severity may result in fracture or avulsion of the teeth, potentially obstructing the upper airway or causing aspiration of tooth fragments into the lungs.

The tongue, a muscular structure in the floor of the mouth, is the primary organ of taste; it is also important in the formation of speech and in the chewing and swallowing of food. The tongue is attached at the mandible and hyoid bone. The hyoid bone is buried in the soft tissues behind the chin. Recall that it is unique in that it does not articulate with any other bones. Serving as a primary anchor of the tongue, the hyoid bone also allows support of the trachea and larynx by means of several ligaments.

Words of Wisdom

Keep in mind that the tongue has a tendency to fall back and block the posterior pharynx when the mandible relaxes. In fact, the tongue is the most common cause of anatomic upper airway obstruction in an unresponsive patient.

Laryngopharynx

The laryngopharynx (hypopharynx) functions in respiration and digestion and extends from the epiglottis to the top of the esophagus. It is the shortest of the three divisions of the pharynx. The laryngopharynx opens into the larynx anteriorly and the esophagus posteriorly.

Two passageways are located at the bottom of the pharynx: the esophagus behind and the trachea (windpipe) in front. Food and liquids enter the pharynx and pass into the esophagus, which carries them to the stomach. Air and other gases enter the trachea and go to the lungs. The epiglottis protects the opening of the trachea. The epiglottis is attached inferiorly to the thyroid cartilage. The superior portion of the epiglottis is movable, flexing up and down when swallowing. The epiglottis serves as a gatekeeper, covering the opening into the larynx during swallowing so that ingested materials enter the esophagus, thereby preventing the passage of foreign matter into the trachea. Recall that the vocal cords, which are white bands of tough tissue, and the opening between them are collectively called the glottis or the glottic opening.[34] At rest, the vocal cords are partially separated (that is, the glottis is partially open). During forceful inhalation, the vocal cords open widely to provide minimum resistance to air flow.

Words of Wisdom

The epiglottis is an important landmark when you perform orotracheal intubation with a straight laryngoscope blade. The epiglottis must be lifted out of the way so you are able to visualize and pass an endotracheal tube between the vocal cords. More of an anatomic landmark than an actual structure, the vallecula (which means "little valley") is the depression (or pocket) between the base of the tongue and the epiglottis. The vallecula is an important landmark when you intubate with a curved laryngoscope blade.

Larynx. Serving as a bridge extending from approximately the fourth through the sixth cervical levels, the larynx joins the pharynx to the trachea. It marks where the upper airway ends and the lower airway begins. The larynx has three purposes: (1) to facilitate the passage of air; (2) as a sphincter, to prevent foreign solids and liquids from entering the lungs; (3) and to produce speech.

The larynx is composed of an outer cage of nine cartilages that protect and support the vocal cords (see Figure 8-107). These cartilages are connected by muscles and ligaments. The thyroid cartilage is the anterior part of the larynx and is the largest of these cartilages. It is usually identifiable externally as the Adam's apple. The glottic opening is located directly behind the thyroid cartilage.

The superior border of the glottis is the epiglottis **Figure 8-109**. At the inferior border of the glottic opening are the corniculate and cuneiform cartilages, which appear as bumps just below the glottis. The pyramid-shaped **arytenoid cartilages** form the posterior attachment of the vocal cords; they are valuable guides for endotracheal intubation. The vestibular folds (false vocal cords) and the true vocal cords are found within the larynx. The vocal folds move to the sides of the larynx during inhalation, allowing air to pass freely. A person is able to produce sound during **exhalation** (the passive part of the breathing process) by controlling the distance between these folds, which vibrate when air is forced through them.

The piriform fossae are two pockets of tissue on the lateral borders of the larynx. Airway devices are occasionally inadvertently inserted into these pockets, resulting in a tenting of the skin under the jaw.

Words of Wisdom

When the airway is stimulated (such as during aspiration of foreign material or submersion incident), defensive reflexes cause spasmodic closure of the vocal cords (laryngospasm), which seals off the airway This reflex normally lasts a few seconds. Persistent laryngospasm, however, can threaten airway patency by preventing **ventilation** (the mechanical process of moving air into and out of the lungs) altogether.

As discussed previously, directly inferior to the thyroid cartilage is the cricoid cartilage; it forms the lowest portion of the larynx (see Figure 8-107). Considered the first cartilage to begin the trachea, it is unique as a complete ring of cartilage, whereas the others are C-shaped rings on the posterior surface. The C-shaped rings are open to permit the esophagus, which lies behind the trachea, to bulge forward as food moves to the stomach.

Located between the thyroid and cricoid cartilage is the cricothyroid membrane (see Figure 8-107). The membrane does not contain many blood vessels and it is covered only by skin and minimal subcutaneous tissue. It is a potential site for performing a cricothyrotomy (an incision through the skin and cricothyroid membrane to relieve difficulty breathing caused by an airway obstruction) if the airway cannot be secured with an advanced airway device.

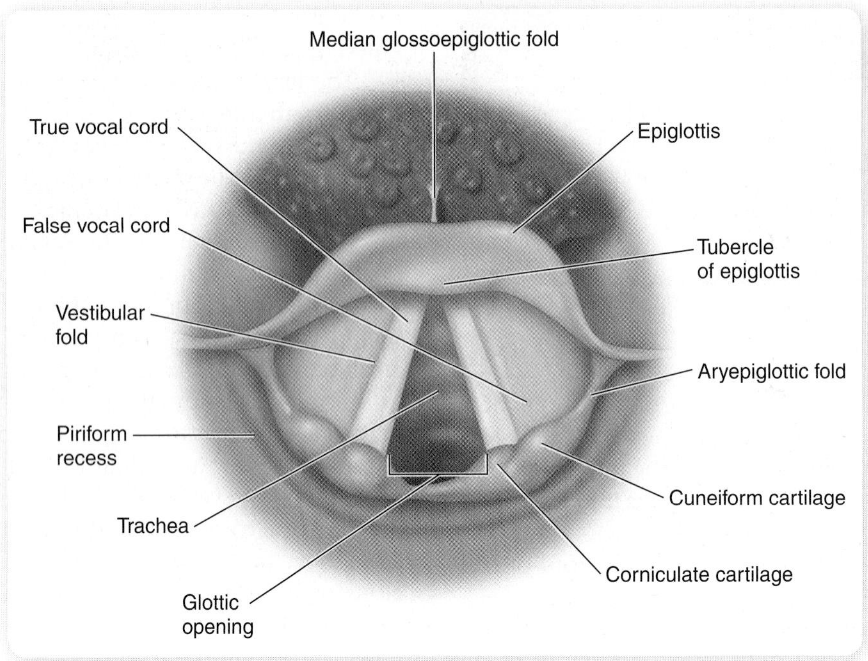

Figure 8-109 The glottis and surrounding structures.

> **Words of Wisdom**
>
> Be aware of other associated structures in proximity to the larynx. Specifically, the thyroid gland is a bow tie–shaped gland that lies across the trachea just inferior to the cricoid cartilage. Several blood vessels, including the carotid arteries, jugular veins, and several vessels branching off these arteries, run alongside the trachea as well as across it.

▶ Lower Airway

Below the glottis is the lower airway. The structures of the lower airway include the trachea, bronchial tree, **alveoli** (tiny sacs of tissue where gas exchange takes place), and lungs. The connective tissue, small airways, and alveoli are collectively referred to as the lung parenchyma. The lower airway is where gas exchange occurs. Functionally, oxygen diffuses from the alveoli into the pulmonary capillaries while carbon dioxide diffuses in the opposite direction.

Trachea

Recall that the trachea (windpipe) is the air passage that connects the larynx to the lungs. Structurally, the trachea is composed of C-shaped cartilaginous rings that support its anterior and lateral walls. The area between the tracheal cartilages is composed of connective tissue and smooth muscle that allow changes in diameter of the trachea. These rings protect the trachea and prevent it from collapsing.

The trachea lies anterior to the esophagus and bifurcates (branches) into two primary bronchi, also called mainstem bronchi (right and left). The point at which this bifurcation occurs is called the **carina** Figure 8-110. An external landmark for the carina is the junction of the body and manubrium of the sternum, referred to as the angle of Louis.

> **Words of Wisdom**
>
> The carina is an important anatomic landmark because the tip of an endotracheal tube is often documented on radiographic study in relation to the carina.

The trachea is lined with columnar epithelial tissue and goblet cells. Goblet cells also line the airways. These cells produce mucus that blankets the entire lining of the conducting airways. The mucus covers the cilia, forming a two-layered blanket that is thick on the surface (gel layer) and thin and watery next to the cilia (sol layer). The gel layer is thick and floats over the sol layer. In a healthy person, cilia constantly push the gel layer up and out of the airway Figure 8-111. As the cilia beat, they reach out into the gel layer, pushing it up and toward the glottis. On the return stroke, the cilia collapse into the sol layer, so that they do not pull the gel layer back down. In this manner, the cilia slowly move the entire gel layer up and out of the tracheobronchial tree, where it is swallowed or expectorated.

Bronchial Tree

The right and left primary bronchi divide into secondary (lobar) bronchi (one for each lobe of the lung). In turn,

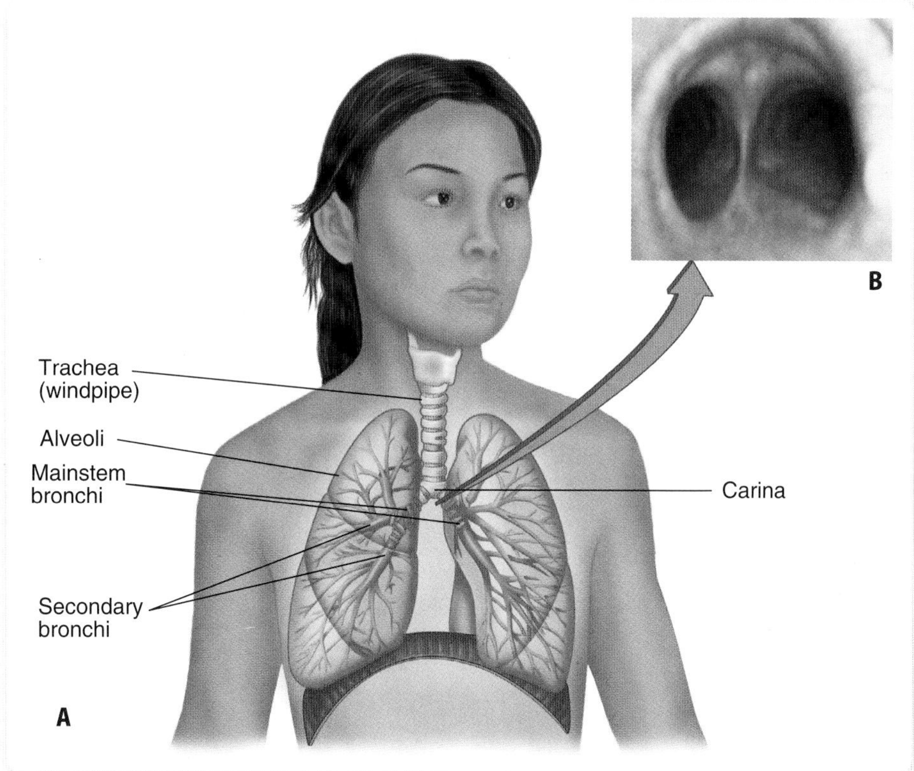

Figure 8-110 The point of bifurcation of the right and left primary (mainstem) bronchi is at the carina. In an adult, this location is at roughly the fifth intercostal space.

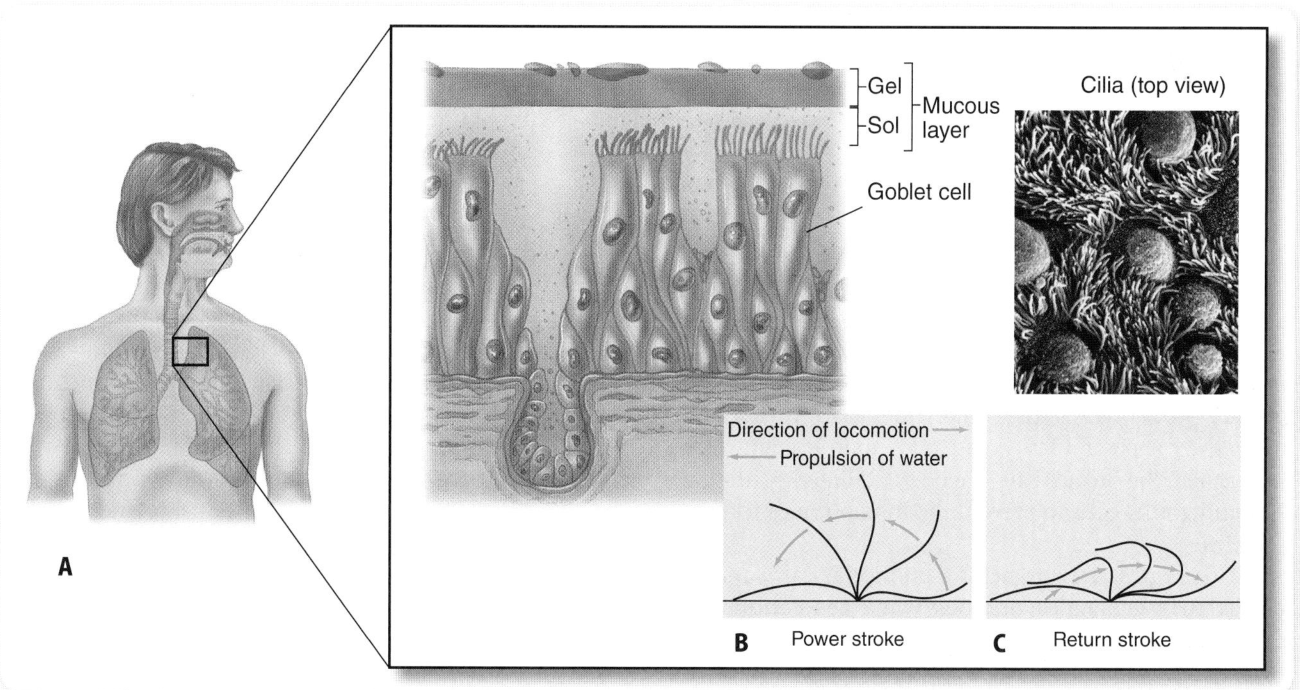

Figure 8-111 Cilia line the larger airways of the respiratory tract **(A)**. Their regular pattern of movement between the gel and sol layers of mucus helps move foreign material out of the tracheobronchial tree **(B** and **C)**.

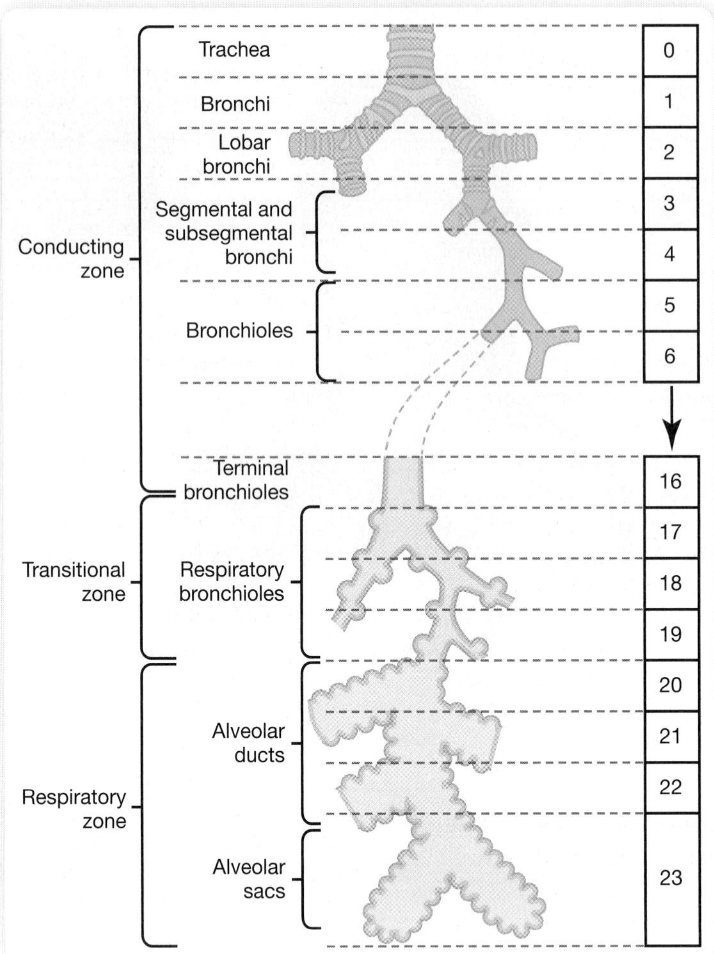

Figure 8-112 The first 16 generations of the lower airway are conducting airways. Transitional airways (generations 17 through 19) consist of respiratory bronchioles that lead into the airways that make up the respiratory zone (generations 20 through 23), where gas exchange occurs.

the secondary bronchi divide into tertiary (segmental) bronchi and continue to subdivide into smaller and smaller bronchi, finally becoming bronchioles. Each bronchus directs air into its respective lung. The right primary bronchus is shorter and wider than the left and leaves the carina at a less-acute angle than the left. Like the trachea, the bronchi are lined with ciliated epithelial cells and goblet cells to prevent the inhalation of foreign particles.

The progressively branching pulmonary airways are referred to by generation numbers where generation zero is the trachea, the first-generation airways are the right and left primary bronchi, and so on **Figure 8-112**. About 23 generations of airways are present in the human body.[35] As the airway passages become smaller, their generation number increases and the amount of cilia, the number of mucus-secreting cells, the presence of submucosal glands, and the amount of cartilage in the airway walls all gradually decrease and smooth muscle and elastic fibers become prominent.[35] Bronchi possess cartilage (up to about the 10th generation) whereas bronchioles (beginning about the 11th generation) lack cartilage. Because bronchioles lack cartilaginous support, they are especially susceptible to collapse during expiration. They can maintain an open lumen only because the pressure surrounding them may be more negative than the pressure inside and because of the outward pull of surrounding tissues.[35] Terminal bronchioles are present at about the 16th generation and are distinguished by being the smallest airways without alveoli.[36] The conducting airways, whose function is to move air to those areas of the lung that participate in gas exchange, begin at the nose and lips and end at the terminal bronchioles.[35]

Respiratory bronchioles (generations 17 to 19) make up the transitional airways (also called the transitional zone). The respiratory bronchioles participate in gas exchange over at least part of their surface and contain an increasing number of alveolar ducts (generations 20 to 22) that direct air into the alveoli (generation 23).[35] Generations 20 through 23 are referred to as the respiratory zone of the lung. The respiratory bronchioles, the alveolar ducts, and the alveoli are considered the respiratory, or gas-exchanging, units of the lungs.[36]

Alveoli

Each alveolar duct ends in alveoli. Think of alveoli as small balloons at the end of a straw. Each alveolus is composed of multiple alveoli that have very thin walls consisting of a single layer of epithelial tissue and elastic fibers. These walls become thinner as they expand, making diffusion of oxygen and carbon dioxide possible. The elastic fibers allow the alveolus to expand and recoil during breathing. Each alveolus is surrounded by a network of capillaries. The thin alveolocapillary membrane lies between the alveolus and the capillary and consists of only one cell layer. Respiratory exchange between the lung and blood vessels occurs in the alveoli at the alveolocapillary membrane.

Alveoli are made up of two types of cells:

1. Type I alveolar cells (pneumocytes) are almost empty, allowing for better gas exchange. They lack cellular components that would permit them to reproduce.
2. Each alveolus has several type II pneumocytes, which can make new type I cells and also produce a substance known as **surfactant**, which reduces surface tension and helps keep the alveoli expanded. When alveoli are damaged by infection, cigarette smoking, or other trauma, their ability to repair themselves correlates directly to the number of type II cells that remain. After all of the type II cells in an alveolus have been destroyed, the alveolus cannot make new cells or surfactant and is essentially dead.

Alveoli function best when they are kept partially inflated. Blowing up a balloon takes a lot of pressure. Once the balloon is partially inflated, however, it is much easier to inflate it the rest of the way. The same is true of alveoli. By reducing the surface tension of the alveoli, surfactant makes it easier for them to expand. When surfactant is washed out of the alveoli, as may occur in pulmonary edema, submersion incidents, or severe shock, they are much more likely to collapse.

Collapsed, fluid-filled, or pus-filled alveoli do not participate in gas exchange. Instead, these alveoli contribute to a shunt, in which blood from the right side of the heart bypasses the alveoli and returns to the left side of the heart in an unoxygenated state, perhaps resulting in hypoxemia. Conditions related to ventilation, perfusion, or both can prevent oxygen from reaching the bloodstream.

Lungs

The lungs are two large, paired structures located within the pleural cavities. The lungs are attached to the heart by the pulmonary trunk (arterial) and the pulmonary veins. The point of entry for bronchial vessels, bronchi, and nerves in each lung is the hilum. The base of each lung rests on the diaphragm, and its apex extends about 1 inch (2.5 cm) above each clavicle. The apex of the left lung is slightly more superior than that of the right. Significantly more blood is circulated to the lung bases compared with the lung apices. Because humans are upright, gravity-dependent creatures, most infections and pathologic conditions occur at the base of the lung.

The right lung is divided into three lobes: the upper, middle, and lower. The left lung has only two lobes, one upper and one lower. The left lung has a notch where the heart lies (cardiac notch). Each lobe is composed of separated lobules; these lobules can be surgically removed, leaving the rest of the lung intact.

The right and left pleural cavities are separate compartments on either side of the mediastinum.[37] Each pleural cavity encloses a lung and its associated bronchial tree and vessels, nerves, and lymphatics.[37] Each lung is contained within a double-layered serous membrane called the **pleura**. The **visceral pleura** is tightly attached to the lung surface. At the hilum, the visceral pleura is continuous with the **parietal pleura**, which lines the wall of the thorax. The parietal pleura is attached to the interior of the mediastinum, the superior surface of the diaphragm, and the inner surface of the rib cage. This design is important in the physiology of breathing.

The parietal pleura contains blood vessels that are believed to produce a filtrate of the plasma called pleural fluid.[35] The visceral pleura contains lymphatic vessels that drain the pleural fluid from the pleural space.[35] The **pleural space** is a potential space between the visceral and parietal pleura **Figure 8-113**. Normally, this space contains nothing but a small amount (about 2 teaspoons [10 mL]) of pleural fluid that separates the parietal and visceral pleurae.[35] The surface tension caused by the fluid between the two pleural layers causes the layers to stick together. As a result, when the parietal pleura moves with the chest wall, it takes the visceral pleura with it, expanding the lungs. The pleural fluid also allows the movement of each lung with little friction. Think of the pleural layers and the fluid between them as two pieces of glass separated by a thin film of water. Because of the surface tension between the membranes and the fluid, the layers glide easily over each other but can be pulled apart with difficulty.[38]

Pleural fluid occasionally can become infected, causing an irritation of the surface of the lung with respiratory movement (pleuritis or pleurisy). Under certain disease conditions or following trauma, the pleural space can fill with fluid, air (pneumothorax), or blood (hemothorax).

As you have learned, the lungs receive blood in two ways. Deoxygenated blood flows from the right ventricle

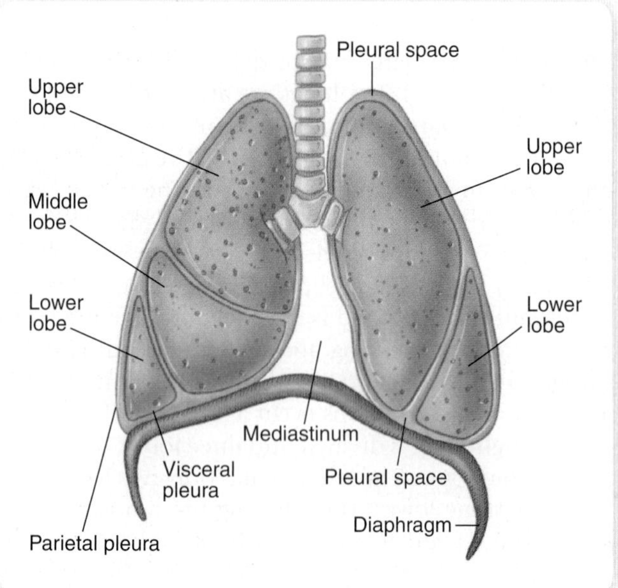

Figure 8-113 The pleura lining the chest wall and covering the lungs is an essential part of the breathing mechanism. The pleural space is not an actual space until blood or air leaks into it, causing the pleural surfaces to separate.

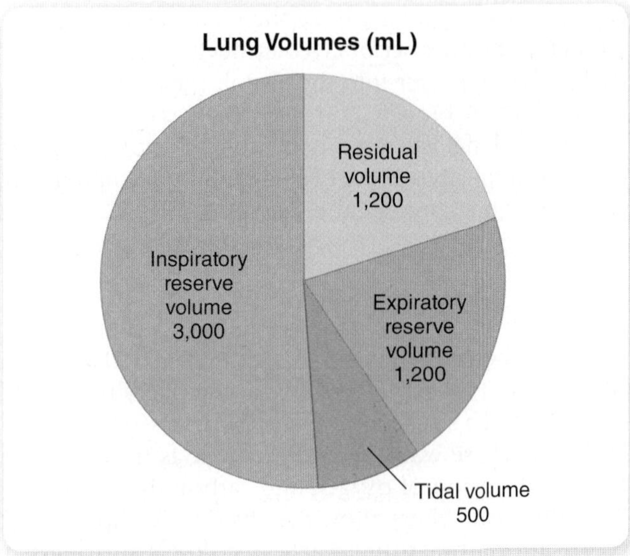

Figure 8-114 Lung volumes.

via the pulmonary arteries. This blood flows through pulmonary capillaries, is reoxygenated at the alveoli, and then returns to the heart via the pulmonary veins. In addition, bronchial arteries branch off of the thoracic aorta and supply the lung tissues themselves with blood. Deoxygenated blood returns to the heart via the bronchial veins. Peripherally in the lungs, venous blood from the bronchi enters the pulmonary veins, returning with oxygenated blood from the alveoli.

▶ Lung Volumes

A substantial amount of air can be moved within the respiratory system. Figure 8-114 shows the typical lung volumes. An adult man has a total lung capacity of 6,000 mL (equivalent to three 2-liter bottles of soda). An adult woman has about one-third less total capacity because the lung size is smaller.

As you are reading this book, the amount of your air movement is about 500 mL (unless you just finished exercising). This measurement is called **tidal volume**. Tidal volume is the amount of air that is moved into or out of the lungs during a single breath. **Inspiratory reserve volume** is the additional amount of air that can be inhaled after the normal tidal volume has been reached. The average person can inhale an additional 3,000 mL of air when needed in times of physiologic stress. Conversely, **expiratory reserve volume** is the additional amount of air that can be exhaled after the normal tidal volume is expelled. The average person can exhale an additional 1,200 mL of air when needed in times of physiologic stress. The **residual volume** is the amount of air that remains in the lungs after maximal exhalation, which serves to prevent alveolar collapse (atelectasis) by keeping the alveoli slightly inflated. The residual volume is 1,200 mL in the average person. Some loss of residual volume occurs when a person is hit in the chest and has the "wind knocked out" of him or her. **Vital capacity** is the amount of air moved in and out of the lungs with maximum inspiration (inhalation) and expiration (exhalation).

When you assist a patient's breathing, you move air in and out of the lungs. You will use a bag-mask device—a large bag filled with air that, when squeezed, pushes air out one end. The typical device holds approximately 1,000 to 1,200 mL of air. Note that although a person's resting tidal volume is 500 mL, you need to use a bag mask device that provides more than twice that volume because of dead space. *Anatomic dead space* is the portion of the respiratory system that has no alveoli, and, therefore, little or no exchange of gas between air and blood occurs. The mouth, trachea, bronchi, and bronchioles are all considered anatomic dead space. When you ventilate a patient with any device, you create more dead space. Gas must first fill the device before it can be moved into the patient.

Typically, anatomic dead space is about 1 mL per pound of ideal body weight (a 150-pound [68-kg] person has about 150 mL of anatomic dead space). If a 150-pound (68-kg) patient took an average breath (tidal volume) of 700 mL, then about 550 mL would participate in ventilation at the alveolar level; the other 150 mL would fill the conducting airways and it would never be exposed to blood flow. If the same patient were to have a tidal volume of 500 mL, then only 350 mL would participate in ventilation, because 150 mL would be stuck in the tubes.

Physiologic dead space is a function of the amount of damaged alveoli that cannot participate in gas exchange. Unlike anatomic dead space, which is fairly constant among patients, the physiologic dead space varies widely based on medical history and exposure to toxins that damage the alveoli, among other factors. Physiologic dead space is the anatomic dead space plus the amount of space occupied by damaged alveoli and can be as much as 1 to 2 L of volume.

Words of Wisdom

Although physiologic dead space cannot be measured in the prehospital setting, you must keep this principle in mind and apply it to an individual's history and presentation when determining the effectiveness of ventilation.

One of the critical determinants in the effectiveness of ventilation is the amount of air moved in and out of the respiratory system in 1 minute, known as **minute volume**. Calculating the minute volume helps you to determine how deeply a patient is breathing.

$$\text{Minute volume} = \text{Respiratory Rate} \times \text{Tidal Volume}$$

▶ Ventilation

The respiratory and cardiovascular systems work together to ensure that a constant supply of oxygen and nutrients is delivered to every cell in the body and that carbon dioxide and other waste products are removed from every cell. If one of these systems is compromised, then oxygen delivery is ineffective and cellular death may occur.

Recall that ventilation is the mechanical process of moving air into and out of the lungs. The two separate phases of ventilation are inhalation (inspiration) and exhalation (expiration) Table 8-39. Each combination of inhalation and exhalation is a *respiratory cycle*. Essential to this process is a change in pressures within the thoracic cavity that allow the passive flow of air into and out of the lungs.

Table 8-39 Ventilation, Oxygenation, and Respiration

Function	Definition
Oxygenation	The process of loading oxygen molecules onto hemoglobin molecules in the bloodstream
Respiration	The actual exchange of oxygen and carbon dioxide in the alveoli and the tissues of the body
Ventilation	The physical act of moving air into and out of the lungs

The lungs have no muscle tissue; therefore, they cannot move on their own. They need the help of other structures to be able to expand and contract during inhalation. Therefore, the ability of the lungs to function properly is dependent on the movement of the chest and supporting structures. These structures include the thorax, the thoracic cage (chest cage), the diaphragm, the intercostal muscles, and the accessory muscles. Muscles of the chest wall are innervated by the intercostal nerves.

Recall that the diaphragm is connected to the sternum anteriorly, the ribs laterally, and the vertebrae posteriorly. The diaphragm is innervated by the phrenic nerves, which arise from the third through fifth cervical nerve roots (hence the phrase, "C3 to C5 keep the diaphragm alive"). The diaphragm functions as a voluntary (skeletal) and an involuntary (smooth) muscle. It acts as a voluntary muscle when you take a deep breath, cough, or hold your breath. However, unlike other skeletal or voluntary muscles, the diaphragm performs an automatic function. Breathing continues during sleep and at all other times. Even though you can hold your breath or temporarily breathe faster or slower, you cannot continue these variations in breathing pattern indefinitely. When the concentration of carbon dioxide rises in the blood, the autonomic regulation of breathing resumes under control of the brainstem. Therefore, although the diaphragm looks like voluntary skeletal muscle and is attached to the skeleton, it behaves, for the most part, like an involuntary muscle.

Inhalation is governed by **Boyle's law**, which states that the pressure of a gas is inversely proportional to its volume. The air pressure outside the body—atmospheric pressure—is normally higher than the air pressure within the thorax. During inhalation, the diaphragm and external intercostal muscles between the ribs contract. When the diaphragm contracts, it moves down slightly, enlarging the thoracic cage from top to bottom. When the external intercostal muscles contract, they move the ribs up and out. These actions combine to enlarge the chest cavity in all dimensions. Pressure in the thorax then falls, making it lower than atmospheric pressure, creating a slight vacuum. This vacuum pulls air in through the trachea, causing the lungs to fill—a process called **negative pressure ventilation**. The alveoli inflate, allowing gases such as oxygen and carbon dioxide to move from an area of higher pressure to an area of lower pressure (diffusion) until the pressures are equal. Thus, oxygen moves from the alveoli into the pulmonary capillaries while carbon dioxide moves into the alveoli for removal from the body. The combined actions of these muscles enlarge the thorax in all dimensions. Maximum inhalation occurs when the diaphragm and intercostal muscles are contracted and the lungs fill with air. When the air pressure inside the thorax equals the air pressure outside the body, air stops moving and inhalation stops. The diaphragm and inspiratory muscles relax allowing the chest to recoil. As these muscles relax, all dimensions of the thorax decrease, and the ribs and muscles assume a normal resting position. When the volume of the chest cavity decreases, air in the lungs is compressed into a smaller space and pressure is greater than atmospheric pressure. *Intrapulmonic pressure* (the pressure within the lungs and airways) is increased, and air is pushed out through the trachea.

Exhalation is normally a passive process, which means that it does not typically require muscular effort. If more forceful exhalation is required, then the posterior internal intercostals muscles contract, pulling the ribs and sternum downward and inward to further increase the pressure in the lungs. Exhalation ends when the *intrapleural pressure* (the pressure between the pleura of the lungs) is equal to the atmospheric pressure, at which point air stops flowing from the lungs to the outside. At the point of equilibration, all pressures in the respiratory system are exactly equal to atmospheric pressure except the intrapleural pressure. Intrapleural pressure stays just slightly negative as the visceral pleura is pulled inward by the tendency of the lungs to collapse and the parietal pleura is pulled outward by its adhesion to the chest wall.

It may help you to understand the ventilation process if you think of the thoracic cage as a bell jar in which balloons are suspended **Figure 8-115**. In this example, the balloons are the lungs. The base of the jar is the diaphragm, which moves up and down slightly with each breath. The ribs, which are the sides of the jar, maintain the shape of the chest. The only opening into the jar is a small tube at the top, similar to the trachea. During inhalation, the bottom of the jar moves down slightly, causing a decrease in pressure in the jar and creating a slight vacuum. As a result, the balloons fill with air.

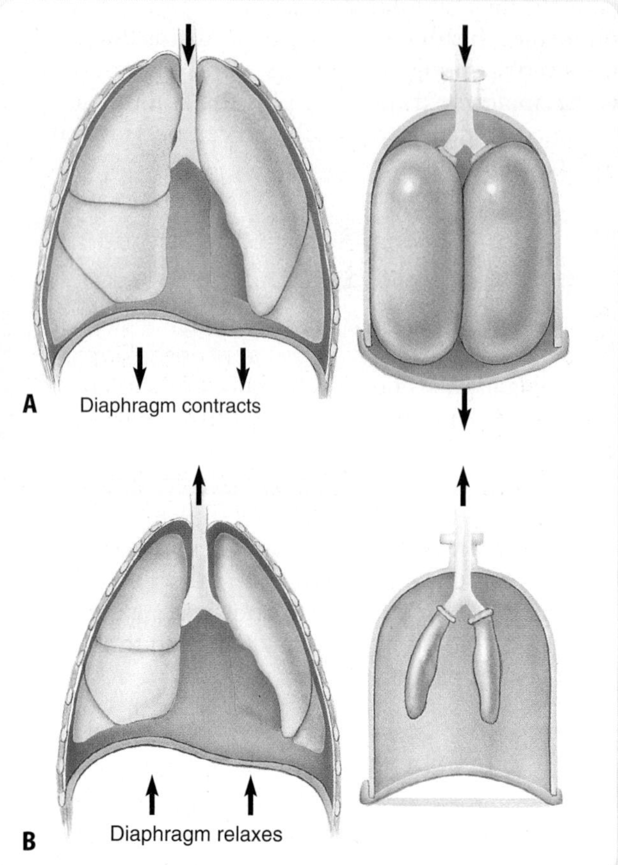

Figure 8-115 The mechanism of ventilation can be illustrated by a bell jar. **A.** Inhalation and chest expansion, anatomic (left) and bell jar (right). **B.** Exhalation and chest contraction, anatomic (left) and bell jar (right).

Words of Wisdom

The process of breathing is typically easy and requires little muscular effort. Now imagine breathing through a straw, and suddenly the diameter of the straw decreases. The smaller the diameter of the straw, the more effort you will have to exert to move air. As the resistance in the airway increases, you begin to use more muscle groups, namely your abdominal and pectoral muscles, to assist the diaphragm in moving air.

Accessory muscles are not generally active during quiet breathing **Table 8-40**. When greater amounts of air must be moved, such as during exercise or illness, accessory muscles (some of which are innervated by cranial nerves) can be recruited to cause more dramatic pressure changes. The intercostal muscles attach each rib to the ribs above it. These muscles allow the ribs to be pulled up and out, expanding the thoracic cavity and allowing more air to be taken in. Accessory muscles of the neck and back and elsewhere, such as the shoulder girdle, can also help open up the thorax.

Words of Wisdom

Normal breathing involves negative intrathoracic pressure and the pulling of air into the lungs (negative pressure ventilation). With ineffective chest movement (such as with reduced tidal volume) or no chest movement (as in apnea), negative intrathoracic pressure cannot be created. When this occurs, the only way to move air into the lungs is by *positive pressure ventilation*, the forcing of air into the lungs. Positive pressure can be created with a bag-mask device, pocket face mask, or mechanical ventilation device.

▶ Oxygenation

Recall that oxygenation is the process of loading oxygen molecules onto hemoglobin molecules in the bloodstream.

Table 8-40 Accessory Muscles of Breathing

Ventilatory Phase	Role	Muscles
Inhalation	Primary	Diaphragm External intercostals
	Accessory	Latissimus dorsi (lower back) Pectoralis major (anterior chest) Scalene muscles (neck) Serratus anterior (anterior chest) Sternocleidomastoid (neck) Trapezius (upper back)
Exhalation	Primary	External oblique muscles (abdomen) Internal intercostal muscles (chest) Internal oblique muscles (abdomen) Rectus abdominis (abdomen)
	Accessory	Latissimus dorsi (lower back)

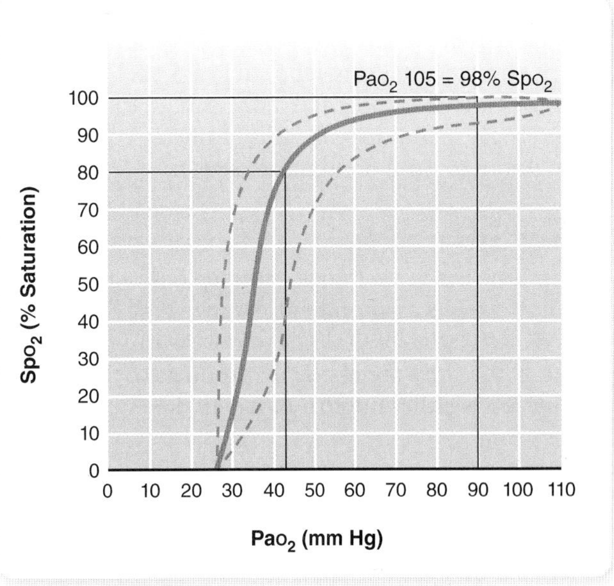

Figure 8-116 The oxyhemoglobin dissociation curve. Shifts are represented by the dotted lines.

Adequate oxygenation is required for internal respiration; however, it does not guarantee that internal respiration is taking place. Oxygenation requires that the air used for ventilation contain an adequate percentage of oxygen. Whereas oxygenation cannot occur without ventilation, ventilation is possible without oxygenation. Ventilation without oxygenation may occur in places where the oxygen level in the air has been depleted, such as in mines and confined spaces. Oxygenation can also be impeded when other gases—for example, carbon monoxide—prevent oxygen from binding to hemoglobin.

Ventilation without adequate oxygenation also occurs in climbers who ascend too quickly to an altitude with inadequate atmospheric pressure. At high altitudes, the percentage of oxygen remains the same (20.8%), but the atmospheric pressure makes it difficult to bring sufficient amounts of oxygen into the body.

The **fraction of inspired oxygen (Fio_2)** is the percentage of oxygen in inhaled air. The Fio_2 increases when supplemental oxygen is given to a patient and is commonly documented as a decimal number. A person breathing room air, which contains about 21% oxygen, would be documented as having an Fio_2 of 0.21.

Oxyhemoglobin Dissociation Curve

Hemoglobin is an iron-containing molecule that has a great affinity for oxygen molecules. **Oxyhemoglobin** is hemoglobin that has oxygen molecules bound to it. About 95% of the protein in an RBC is hemoglobin. Recall that one hemoglobin molecule reversibly binds with four oxygen molecules. Oxygen saturation (expressed as Spo_2 if measured by pulse oximetry and as Sao_2 if measured in the arterial blood gases) is proportional to the amount of oxygen dissolved in the plasma component of the blood (Pao_2). The relationship between the Pao_2 and Sao_2/Spo_2 is represented by the oxyhemoglobin dissociation curve **Figure 8-116**. Under normal conditions (Pao_2 = 105 mm Hg), the Spo_2/Sao_2 level is about 98%.

Whereas *deoxygenated* is the term often used to describe the venous blood returning to the heart during circulation, the blood is not completely devoid of oxygen. Some oxygen is still bound to the hemoglobin because the ability of the respiratory system to supply oxygen to the rest of the body exceeds the demand in normal resting conditions. When metabolism increases, however, the demand for oxygen increases and venous blood contains less oxygen. As blood is circulated to the tissue level, the Pao_2 begins to drop. At this point, the hemoglobin releases its oxygen molecules to make them available for cellular respiration.

In response to changes in metabolism, hemoglobin changes how tightly it holds onto oxygen. More oxygen molecules are released as the acidity of the blood increases (when the pH decreases). This change results in a shift in position of the oxyhemoglobin dissociation curve. Various other conditions can also shift the entire curve to the left or right. A shift to the right causes the hemoglobin to give up its oxygen faster and earlier. A shift to the left has the opposite effect. Acidosis (decreased pH) and increased carbon dioxide levels cause the curve to shift to the right. Alkalosis (increased pH) and a decrease in carbon dioxide levels cause the curve to shift to the left, causing the hemoglobin to hold on to more oxygen.

▶ Respiration

Respiration is the exchange of gases between a living organism and its environment. Human respiration provides oxygen to the body while removing carbon dioxide as one of the chief metabolic by-products of the system. Respiration is either internal or external.

Words of Wisdom

It is important to recognize the differences between ventilation and respiration, although these terms are often used interchangeably. For example, *ventilation*, the mechanical movement of air into and out of the lungs, is often misnamed *respiration*, which is the exchange of gases during cellular metabolism. Similarly, assessment of a patient's respiratory rate is an assessment of his or her ventilatory rate, or the number of times air is inhaled and exhaled per minute.[39]

External Respiration

External (pulmonary) respiration is the exchange of gases between the alveoli of the lungs and the RBCs traveling through the pulmonary capillaries **Figure 8-117**. Fresh air that is inspired into the lungs contains about 21% oxygen, 78% nitrogen, and 0.3% carbon dioxide. As this air reaches the alveoli, it comes into contact with surfactant, which reduces surface tension within the alveoli and keeps them expanded; this expansion facilitates the exchange of oxygen and carbon dioxide. Remember that although adequate ventilation is necessary for external respiration to take place, it does not guarantee that external respiration is being achieved.

After the oxygen crosses the alveolar membrane, it is bound to hemoglobin. Hemoglobin molecules that are low in oxygen concentration are pumped from the right side of the heart into the capillaries of the pulmonary circulation. The capillaries surround the alveoli containing high concentrations of oxygen (from inspired air). The hemoglobin molecules pick up fresh oxygen as it crosses the alveolar membrane and transport it back to the left side of the heart, where it is pumped out to the rest of the body. Under normal conditions, 96% to 100% of the hemoglobin receptors contain oxygen.

Internal Respiration

Once in the bloodstream, gases exchanged between blood cells and tissues constitute internal (cellular) respiration **Figure 8-118**. Without an intact cardiovascular system, internal respiration cannot occur.

Recall that in the presence of oxygen, the mitochondria of the cells convert glucose into energy through aerobic metabolism (aerobic respiration). Energy in the form of ATP is produced through the Krebs cycle and oxidative phosphorylation, which is the process by which the liberated energy (via oxidation of metabolites) is used to synthesize ATP. Together, these chemical processes yield nearly 40 molecules of energy-rich ATP for each molecule of glucose metabolized. Without adequate oxygen, the cells do not completely convert glucose into energy, and lactic acid and other toxins build up in the cell. This process, anaerobic metabolism (anaerobic

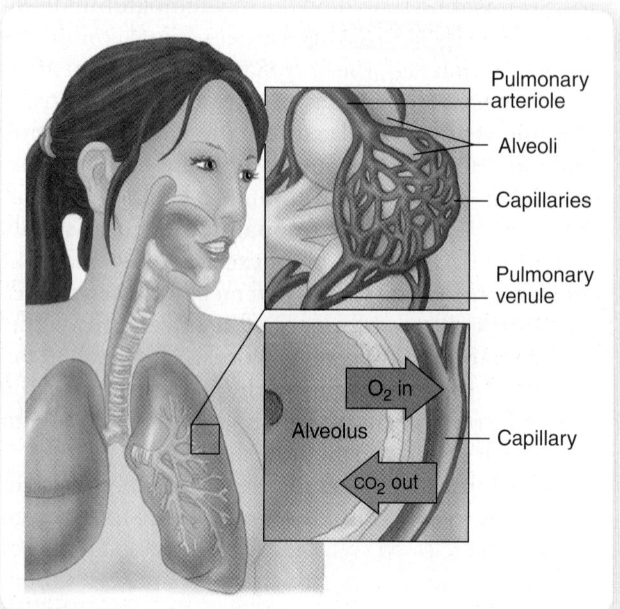

Figure 8-117 External (pulmonary) respiration.

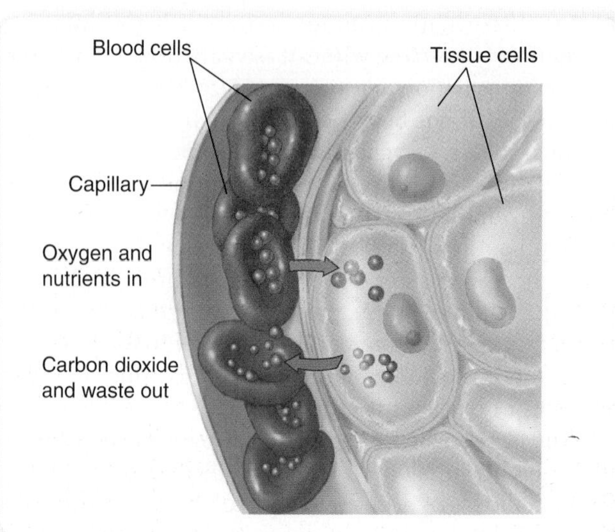

Figure 8-118 Internal (cellular) respiration.

respiration), cannot meet the metabolic demands of the cell. Although another intracellular process, glycolysis, also contributes to production of ATP and does not require oxygen. Glycolysis results in less production of ATP, and lactic acid waste products and toxins are produced. If anaerobic metabolism is not corrected, then the cells will eventually die. To support sufficient production of ATP and, therefore, aerobic internal respiration, adequate perfusion and ventilation must be present. Although perfusion and ventilation are necessary for internal respiration, they do not guarantee that aerobic internal respiration will occur.

When the mitochondria within each cell use oxygen to convert glucose to energy, carbon dioxide—the main waste product—builds up in the cell. Carbon dioxide is then transported through the circulatory system and back to the lungs for exhalation.

Without oxygen, anaerobic metabolism creates a series of events that will eventually lead to cellular death. Initially, cells become hypoxic, and as stores of glucose are depleted, lactic acid, which is the by-product of glycolysis, remains. The increased acidic environment destroys the cellular proteins, in turn leading to cellular death.

Words of Wisdom

Physiologic dead space is an example of a *ventilation/perfusion mismatch*. This situation occurs when an area of the lung is either ventilated but not perfused or perfused but not ventilated. Respectively, these are situations in which oxygen is in the alveoli but no blood flow can pick up the oxygen, or blood flow to the alveoli is present but no oxygen is available at that location to be absorbed. Regardless of the cause of the ventilation-perfusion mismatch (lack of oxygen or lack of blood flow), the condition that occurs is called a *right-to-left shunt*. In essence, the unoxygenated blood from the right atrium is returning to the left atrium in an unoxygenated state.

Role of Diffusion

The process of oxygen transfer from air into the capillaries in the alveoli involves diffusion. Several concepts are useful in understanding this process.

Partial pressure is a term used to describe the amount of gas in air or dissolved in liquid, such as the blood, and is governed by **Henry's law**, which states that the amount of a gas in a solution varies directly with the partial pressure of a gas over a solution. In other words, as the pressure of a gas over a liquid decreases, the amount of gas dissolved in the liquid will also decrease. As more pressure is applied over the liquid, more gas can be dissolved in the liquid. In practical terms, this law states that molecules of a gas can be dissolved in a liquid and remain in the liquid as long as the liquid is in a pressurized, closed container (eg, the cardiovascular system). The partial pressure of a gas is not the same as its concentration. Partial pressure is measured in millimeters of mercury (mm Hg). One mm Hg is equivalent to one torr (symbol: Torr).

When multiple gases are present, each gas exerts a pressure. When several gases are contained within the same space, their partial pressures can be measured. Four main gases are found in the atmosphere of the earth: nitrogen, oxygen, water vapor, and carbon dioxide. The average total pressure exerted by the gases composing the atmosphere is sufficient to elevate a column of mercury (Hg) 760 mm. Therefore, at sea level the total atmospheric pressure is 760 Torr.

Inspired air is a mixture of 78% nitrogen, 21% oxygen, 0.04% carbon dioxide, and a nominal amount of other gases exerting a pressure of 760 mm Hg at sea level. Each gas represents a portion of the air mixture and therefore exerts a partial pressure. The sum of the partial pressures is equal to the total pressure of the mixture. Because gases are lipid soluble, they freely cross the cell membrane and move by diffusion. Partial pressures of the air mixture are responsible for diffusion across cell membranes. When considering the normal lung, normal partial pressure of oxygen in arterial blood is 80 Torr to 100 Torr (commonly abbreviated PaO_2). Normal level of carbon dioxide in arterial blood is 35 Torr to 45 Torr (commonly abbreviated $PaCO_2$).

Of the gases dissolved in the venous blood returning to the lungs, carbon dioxide exerts a high partial pressure and oxygen exerts a low partial pressure, in contrast to the high partial pressure of oxygen and low partial pressure of carbon dioxide in the lungs. As a result, carbon dioxide diffuses out of the venous blood into the lungs **Figure 8-119**. Oxygen diffuses out of the alveoli and into the arterial blood, where about 97% of oxygen combines with the hemoglobin molecule of the RBC for transport.

When arterial blood reaches the tissues, the arterial blood has a high partial pressure of oxygen and a low partial pressure of carbon dioxide. When arterial blood reaches the capillaries, oxygen diffuses out of the arterial blood and into the interstitial fluid (and eventually into the intracellular fluid), whereas carbon dioxide diffuses out of the interstitial fluid and into the venous blood.

Unlike oxygen, which is transported by the hemoglobin, carbon dioxide is transported by one of three methods by the venous blood. Carbon dioxide may be dissolved in the blood, attached to the hemoglobin, or be present in the form of bicarbonate ions, which are created when carbon dioxide combines with water. The carbon dioxide that is attached to the hemoglobin attaches to amino groups, whereas oxygen attaches to iron atoms. Because of this, the two molecules may both be carried at the same time without competing for binding sites on the hemoglobin.

▶ Control of Breathing

The body's need for oxygen is dynamic; it is constantly changing. The respiratory system must be able to accommodate the changes in oxygen demand by altering the

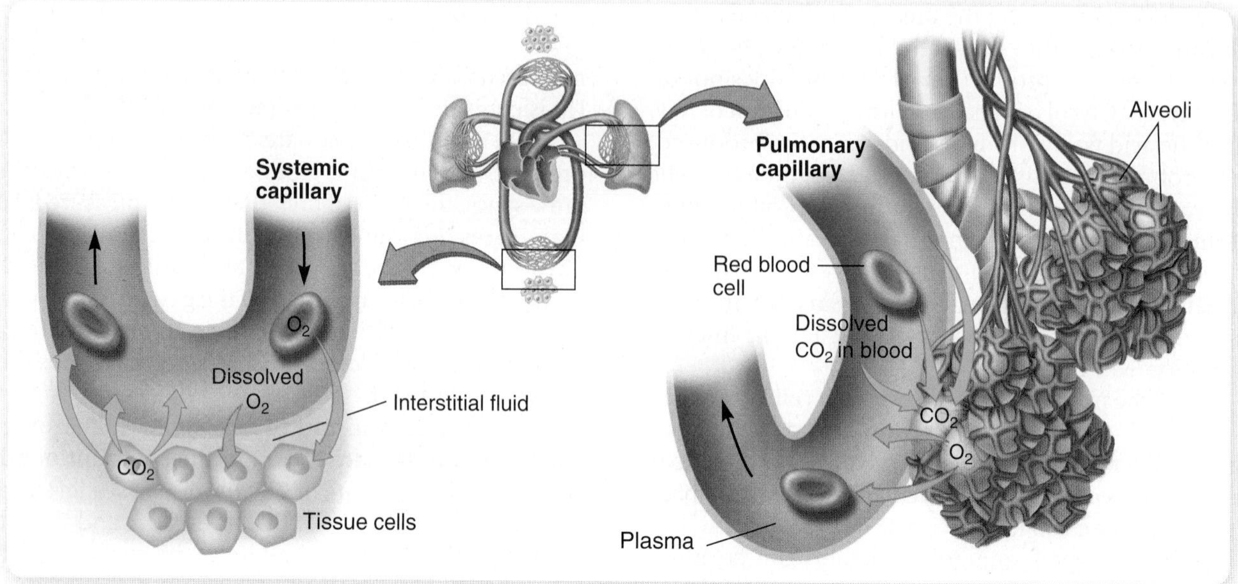

Figure 8-119 In the capillaries of the lungs, oxygen passes from the blood to the tissue cells, and carbon dioxide and waste pass from the tissue cells to the blood. Diffusion occurs when molecules move from an area of higher concentration to an area of lower concentration.

rate and depth of ventilation. These changes are regulated primarily by the pH of the CSF, which is directly related to the amount of carbon dioxide dissolved in the plasma portion of the blood (Pa_{CO_2}). The regulation of ventilation involves a complex series of receptors and feedback loops that sense gas concentrations in the body fluids and send messages to the respiratory centers in the brain to adjust the rate and depth of ventilation accordingly.

Neural Control of Ventilation

Breathing is usually an involuntary mechanism that can be consciously altered for a short period. Involuntary breathing is controlled by the respiratory centers of the brainstem (the medulla and pons), which relay impulses by means of nerves to the inspiratory and expiratory muscles, causing them to contract and relax. Voluntary breathing is necessary for activities such as speaking, singing, holding one's breath, laughing, and blowing up a balloon. With voluntary breathing, control begins in the motor cortex of the cerebrum. Impulses travel down the corticospinal tracts to integrating centers in the spinal cord, thereby bypassing the brainstem.[34]

The control system that regulates involuntary breathing is made up of three components:

1. **Control center.** The control center consists of three pairs of respiratory centers in the reticular formation of the medulla oblongata and pons; there is one of each on the right and left sides of the brainstem.[34] The respiratory centers consist of the **ventral respiratory group (VRG)** and the **dorsal respiratory group (DRG)** of the medulla and the **pontine respiratory group (PRG)** located in the pons (formerly called the pneumotaxic center) **Figure 8-120**.

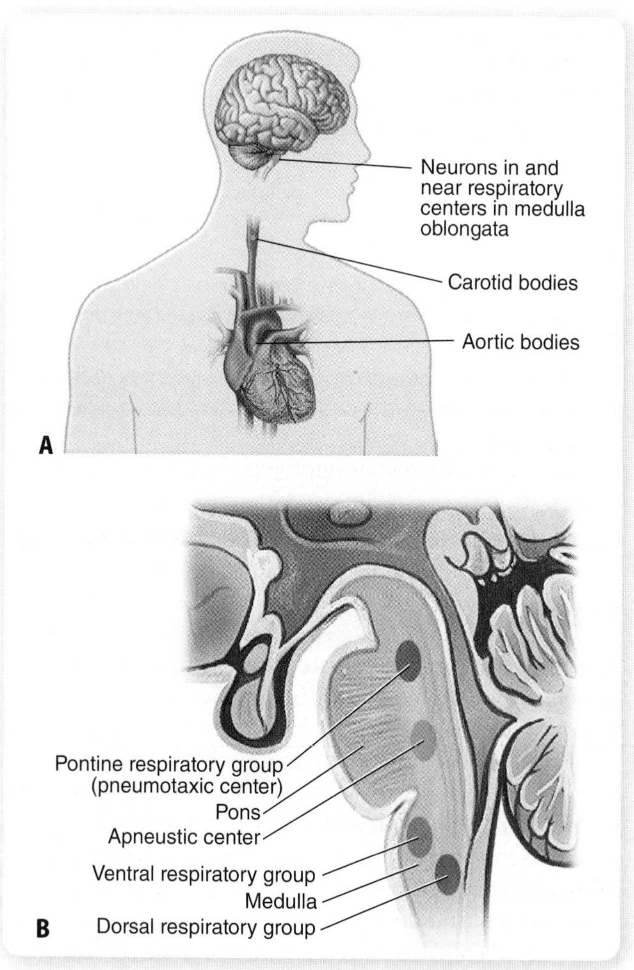

Figure 8-120 Important structures in the regulation of ventilation. **A.** Chemoreceptor locations. **B.** Respiratory centers.

2. **Effectors.** The effectors are the respiratory muscles, whose activity is directed by the respiratory centers, resulting in muscle contraction and relaxation.
3. **Sensors.** Sensors include central chemoreceptors in the medulla (which respond to changes in P_{CO_2} and pH), peripheral chemoreceptors in the carotid and aortic bodies (which respond to changes in P_{O_2}, P_{CO_2} and pH), mechanoreceptors (which are located in the chest wall and lungs, lung stretch receptors, and skin thermoreceptors); proprioceptors in muscles, tendons, and joints;[40] and irritant receptors in the trachea and large airways.

The VRG is a network of inspiratory and expiratory motor neurons with nuclei located in the ventral portion of the medulla. The rhythm of normal, quiet breathing is the result of alternating patterns of stimulation and inhibition of the motor neurons that innervate the diaphragm (the phrenic nerves) and external intercostal muscles (the intercostal nerves). During inhalation, inspiratory neurons of the VRG send impulses by way of these motor nerves, resulting in contraction of the diaphragm and external intercostals, enlargement of the thoracic cage, and the inhalation of air. As the activity of the inspiratory neurons decline, the expiratory neurons fire. Signals are sent to the internal intercostal and abdominal muscles, the inspiratory muscles relax, the lungs recoil, and air is exhaled from the lungs. As the activity of the expiratory neurons decreases, the inspiratory neurons resume firing, and the cycle repeats.

The DRG, also located in the medulla, functions as an integration center. It receives input from several sources, including the PRG, glossopharyngeal (CN IX) and vagus (CN X) nerves,[41] central chemoreceptors in the medulla, and peripheral chemoreceptors.[34] The DRG signals the VRG to alter the rhythm and depth of ventilation to restore homeostasis.

The PRG receives input from the cerebral cortex, the hypothalamus, and the limbic system and communicates information to both the VRG and DRG.[34] Although the respiratory centers of the medulla can generate a basic respiratory rhythm, the PRG influences and modifies the ventilatory rate and depth established by the medullary centers.[40] For example, the PRG is thought to smooth the transition between each phase of the ventilatory cycle and alter breathing by making each breath shorter and shallower or longer and deeper, depending on the body's needs. The **apneustic center** of the pons is thought to work with the PRG to regulate the length and depth of inspiration.[42]

Chemical Control of Ventilation

The goal of the respiratory system is to keep the blood concentrations of oxygen and carbon dioxide and its acid-base balance within narrow ranges. The body has a number of receptors that monitor variables and provide feedback to the respiratory centers to adjust the rate and depth of breathing based on the body's needs. These chemoreceptors have important effects on ventilatory rate and depth.

Chemoreceptors that constantly monitor the chemical composition of body fluids are located throughout the body to provide feedback on many metabolic processes. Central and peripheral chemoreceptors affect respiratory function (see Figure 8-120).

Central chemoreceptors, located in the medulla, respond to changes in carbon dioxide and pH of the CSF. Any changes noted in the P_{CO_2} of arterial blood are quickly reflected in the pH level of the CSF. The acidity of the CSF is an indirect measure of the amount of carbon dioxide in arterial blood because the carbon dioxide in the blood readily diffuses across the blood-brain barrier and combines with water to form carbonic acid. The carbonic acid dissociates, and the pH drops as the hydrogen ion concentration increases. An increase in the acidity of the CSF triggers the central chemoreceptors to increase the rate and depth of breathing to blow off excess carbon dioxide building up in the body. Conversely, when pH levels of the CSF become more alkaline because of low levels of P_{CO_2} in the blood, ventilatory rate decreases.

Peripheral chemoreceptors in the carotid bodies and aortic bodies respond to changes in P_{O_2}, P_{CO_2} and pH. These receptors sense tiny changes in the carbon dioxide level and send signals to the respiratory center via the cranial nerves. The carotid bodies send signals to the brainstem via the glossopharyngeal nerves (CN IX). Chemoreceptors in the aortic arch communicate by way of the vagus nerves (CN X).

When serum carbon dioxide or hydrogen ion levels increase because of a medical condition or traumatic injury involving the respiratory system, chemoreceptors stimulate the respiratory control centers in the medulla to increase the ventilatory rate, thus removing more carbon dioxide or acid from the body.

Hypoxic Drive. Patients with chronic obstructive pulmonary disease (COPD), such as emphysema and chronic bronchitis, have difficulty eliminating carbon dioxide through exhalation; therefore, they always have higher blood levels of carbon dioxide. The high level can potentially alter their primary respiratory drive, which is based on increased arterial carbon dioxide levels and the pH of the CSF. The theory is that the respiratory centers in the brain gradually accommodate elevated carbon dioxide levels. In patients with end-stage COPD, the body uses a backup system to control breathing. This theory of secondary control, called the **hypoxic drive**, stimulates breathing when the arterial oxygen level falls. However, the nerves in the brain, the walls of the aorta, and the carotid arteries that act as oxygen sensors (chemoreceptors) are easily satisfied with a minimal level of oxygen. Therefore, the hypoxic drive is much less sensitive and less powerful than the carbon dioxide sensors in the brainstem. Hypoxic drive is typically found in end-stage COPD and not in patients with a recent diagnosis of COPD.

Lung Receptors

Mechanoreceptors are located in the smooth muscles of the bronchi, bronchioles, and in the visceral pleura.[34] When the lungs inflate, these stretch receptors are stimulated and nerve signals are sent to the respiratory centers by the vagus nerves to inhibit inspiration. This reflex, called the **Hering-Breuer reflex**, is designed to prevent overinflation of the lungs in a conscious, spontaneously breathing person. Because this reflex also increases ventilatory frequency, it maintains a constant alveolar ventilation.[41]

Irritant receptors are located among the epithelial cells in the airway mucous membrane. These receptors are stimulated by smoke, pollen, dust, excess mucus, chemical fumes, and cold air. When irritant receptors are stimulated, the vagus nerves conduct the signals to the brainstem which then signals the respiratory and bronchial muscles, triggering protective reflexes such as coughing, bronchoconstriction, or shallow breathing.[34]

Buffer Systems. Recall that a buffer is a substance that can absorb or donate hydrogen. Buffers absorb hydrogen ions when they are in excess and donate hydrogen ions when they are depleted. Therefore, **buffer systems** act as rapid defenses for acid-base changes, providing almost immediate protection against changes in the hydrogen ion concentration of the extracellular fluid. Problems occur when the amount of acid in circulation is too great for the buffer system to accommodate. To grasp this concept, imagine the buffer system as a bucket that contains the acid in the body **Figure 8-121**. Like a bucket, the buffer system can hold only a certain amount before it overflows.

Three primary buffer systems help the body maintain pH within the optimal range: (1) the circulating bicarbonate buffer component, (2) the respiratory system, and (3) the renal system. The body's fastest means of restoring acid-base balance is the so-called blood buffer—the bicarbonate content of intracellular and extracellular fluid. When an excessive level of acid builds up, it is eliminated through the respiratory system, when carbon dioxide is expelled from the lungs. Conversely, slowing the rate of breathing encourages the retention of carbon dioxide. The renal system regulates pH by filtering out hydrogen and retaining bicarbonate when necessary, or by doing the reverse.

Circulating Bicarbonate Buffer Component. During cellular metabolism, large amounts of carbon dioxide are produced as a waste product. Most of this carbon dioxide is stored in intracellular and extracellular fluid in the form of bicarbonate, the body's most important buffer system. This system is like a bucket that holds and neutralizes excess acid.

In the bicarbonate buffer system, excess acid (H^+) combines with bicarbonate (HCO_3^-) to form carbonic acid ($H_2CO_3^-$). This compound rapidly dissociates into water and carbon dioxide, which is then exhaled. Because the acid is eliminated as water and carbon dioxide, the total pH does not change significantly. A similar process occurs with the production of metabolic base (bicarbonate).

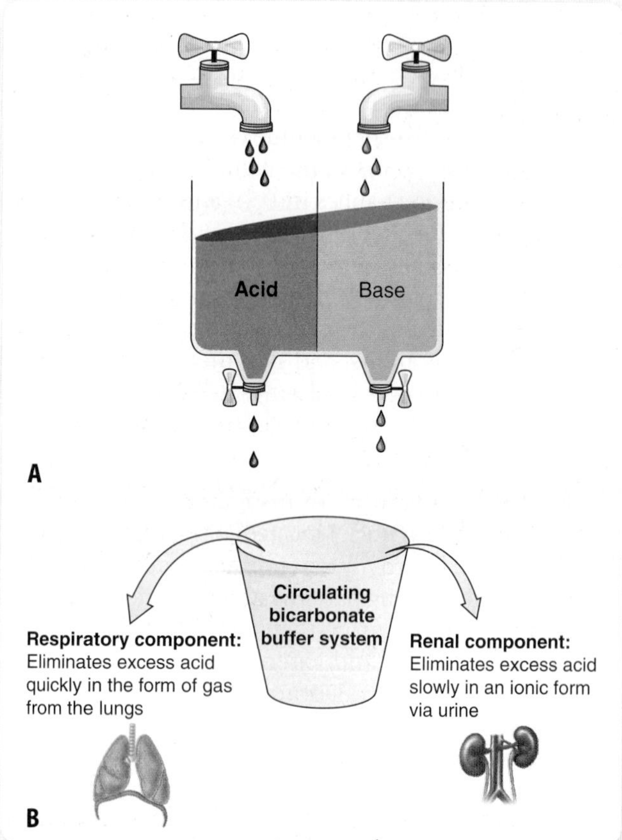

Figure 8-121 Buffer systems. **A.** As the acid or base levels fluctuate, the body must work to ensure that the acid-base balance is maintained. **B.** The respiratory component and the renal component are two systems for eliminating excess acid.

Carbonic acid is a weak acid that can give up an extra hydrogen ion to reform as the bicarbonate ion. The extra hydrogen ion is then converted during metabolism into compounds that are easily expelled from the body, thereby eliminating excess acid.

Respiratory Buffer Component. Aside from the circulating bicarbonate buffer component, the fastest way the body can eliminate excess hydrogen ions is to create water and carbon dioxide, which can be expelled as gases from the lungs.

Carbonic acid is created when carbon dioxide combines with circulating water in the blood. Chemoreceptors in the brain sense the rising level of carbonic acid and signal the respiratory centers to increase the ventilatory rate in an effort to reduce the amount of circulating carbon dioxide. Although the respiratory buffer reacts within minutes, it is much slower to respond than the circulating bicarbonate buffer component.

Acidosis can develop because of abnormal ventilatory function, including a breathing rate that is too fast or too slow, labored breathing, or shallow breathing (reduced tidal volume). At the other end of the acid-base spectrum, alkalosis can develop if the ventilatory rate is too high or the volume too large.

Renal Buffer Component. The kidneys monitor hydrogen and bicarbonate levels in the tubules of nephrons to maintain pH. This system, however, responds more slowly than the bicarbonate and respiratory buffer components to an increasing acid level. It could take hours or even days for the renal buffer system to restore the body's pH to normal.

When the blood contains high levels of carbonic acid, the kidneys respond by excreting more hydrogen ions and breaking down carbonic acid into carbon dioxide and water. In the tubule cell, the carbon dioxide is reabsorbed; a new bicarbonate ion is formed and diffuses through peritubular capillaries into the blood. Reabsorbed bicarbonate is neutralized by reabsorbed sodium ions, which are exchanged for hydrogen ions excreted in the urine. When the blood contains low levels of carbonic acid, the kidneys excrete fewer hydrogen ions and more bicarbonate.

Control of Ventilation by Other Factors

Multiple other factors influence control of ventilatory rates. Factors such as elevated body temperature, CNS stimulants, pain, emotion, hypoxia, and acidosis cause an increased ventilatory rate. Sleep, decreased metabolic states, and CNS depressants, including alcohol, decrease the ventilatory rate.

The Digestive System

The digestive system is composed of two major divisions: (1) the alimentary canal and (2) the accessory digestive organs. The alimentary canal is a series of muscular tubes that is specialized along its length for the sequential processing of food.[43] These tubes are designed to move food and liquid from its entrance into the body (typically the mouth) to its elimination from the body through the anus. The GI tract is the portion of the alimentary canal that consists of the stomach and intestines. The accessory digestive organs produce and secrete enzymes and juices essential in the digestive process.

The digestive system is responsible for the following six processes:

1. **Ingestion**. This process brings material into the digestive tract via the mouth.
2. **Mechanical processing**. Materials are crushed and broken into smaller fragments, making them easier to move through the digestive tract; enzymes begin to attack the particles during chewing, while the teeth and tongue are used to tear and mash food; additional mechanical processing is provided by the mixing motions of the stomach and intestines.
3. **Digestion**. The chemical breakdown of food material into smaller fragments that can be absorbed into the circulatory system; simple molecules such as glucose are absorbed intact whereas others (polysaccharides, proteins, triglycerides) must first be broken down before they can be absorbed.
4. **Secretion**. The release of water, acids, enzymes, and buffers that aid in the breakdown and digestion of food in the digestive tract; this secretion comes from both the digestive tract and the accessory organs.
5. **Absorption.** The movement of organic substrates (molecules acted on by enzymes), electrolytes, vitamins, and water across the epithelium of the digestive tract and into the interstitial fluid.
6. **Excretion.** The removal of waste products from body fluids via secretions from the digestive tract and glandular organs; after mixing with residue that cannot be digested, these waste products become *feces*, the undigested food particles that are eliminated during the process of defecation.

In succession, different secretions, primarily enzymes, are added to the food by the salivary glands, the stomach, the liver, the pancreas, and the small intestine to convert the food into basic sugars, fatty acids, and amino acids. These basic products of digestion are carried across the wall of the intestine and transported through the portal vein to the liver. In the liver, the products are processed further and stored or transported to the heart through veins draining the liver. The heart then pumps the blood with these nutrients throughout the arteries to the capillaries, where the nutrients pass through the capillary walls to nourish the body's individual cells.

The alimentary canal extends from the mouth to the anus. It includes the mouth, pharynx, esophagus, stomach, intestines, rectum, and anus. The walls of the alimentary canal consist of four layers, specialized in certain regions for particular functions, as follows Figure 8-122:

- **Mucosa (mucous membrane).** Surface epithelium, underlying connective tissue, and a small amount of smooth muscle; it is folded in some regions, with projections extending into the lumen that increase its absorptive surface. The mucosa carries out secretion and absorption.
- **Submucosa.** Loose connective tissue with glands, blood vessels, lymphatic vessels, and nerves; it nourishes surrounding tissues and carries away absorbed materials.
- **Muscular layer.** Produces movements of the tube, and is made of two smooth muscle tissue coats: circular fibers of the inner coat encircle the tube, causing contraction, and

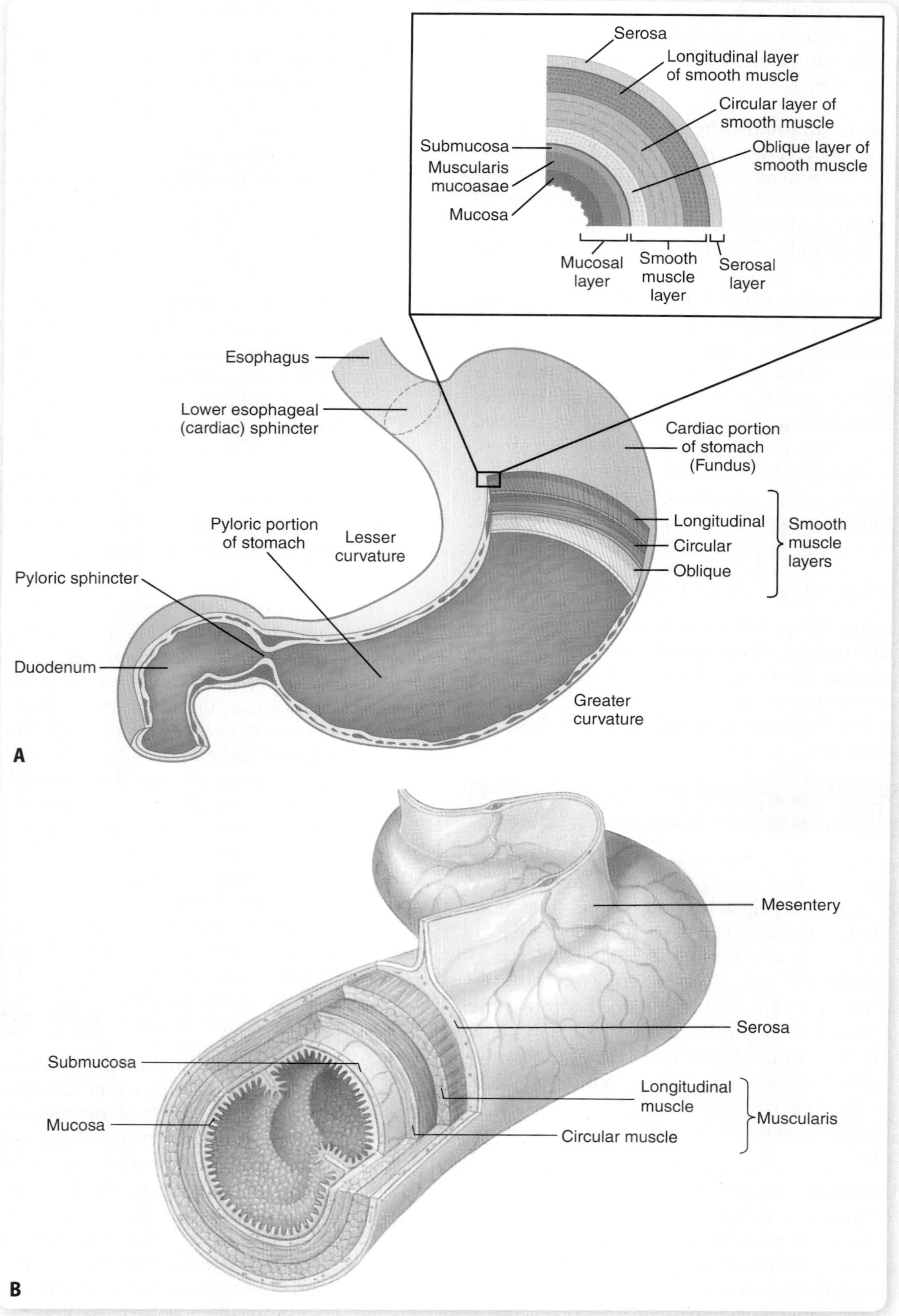

Figure 8-122 The layers of the alimentary canal. **A.** Layers of the stomach. **B.** Layers of the intestines.

longitudinal fibers run lengthwise, causing shortening of the tube.
- **Serosa (serous layer).** Composed of a visceral peritoneum on the outside and connective tissue beneath; it protects underlying tissues and secretes serous fluid so that abdominal organs slide freely against each other.

The accessory organs of the alimentary canal include the teeth, tongue, salivary glands, liver, gallbladder, and pancreas. The secretions from these accessory organs empty via ducts into the digestive tract. The organs of the digestive system are found within the abdomen.

▶ Abdomen

The abdomen contains the major organs of digestion and excretion. The diaphragm separates the thoracic cavity from the abdominal cavity. Thick, muscular abdominal walls create the boundaries of this space anteriorly and posteriorly. Inferiorly, the abdomen is separated from the pelvis by an imaginary plane that extends from the pubic symphysis through the sacrum Figure 8-123. Some organs lie in the abdomen and the pelvis, depending on the posture of the patient.

The simplest and most common method of describing the portions of the abdomen is by quadrants, the four equal areas formed by two imaginary lines that intersect at right angles at the umbilicus. On the anterior abdominal wall, the quadrants thus formed are the right upper quadrant (RUQ), the right lower quadrant (RLQ), the left lower quadrant (LLQ), and the left upper quadrant (LUQ) Figure 8-124. The area around the umbilicus is the periumbilical area.

In the RUQ, the major organs are the liver, the gallbladder, and a portion of the colon and small intestine. Most of the liver lies in this quadrant, almost entirely under the protection of the 8th to 12th ribs. The liver fills the entire anteroposterior depth of the abdomen in this quadrant. Therefore, injuries in this area are frequently associated with injuries of the liver.

In the LUQ, the principal organs are the stomach, the spleen, and a portion of the colon and small intestine. The spleen is almost entirely under the protection of the left rib cage, whereas the stomach may sag well down into the left lower quadrant when full. The spleen lies in the lateral and posterior portion of this quadrant, under the diaphragm and immediately in front of the 9th to 11th ribs. The spleen is frequently injured, especially when these ribs are fractured.

The RLQ contains two portions of the large intestine: the cecum, the first portion into which the small intestine (ileum) opens, and the ascending colon. The *appendix* is a small, tubular structure (about 3 to 4 inches [8 to 10 cm] long) that is effectively a small pouch attached to the lower border of the cecum. This structure contains many bacteria and it may easily become obstructed, resulting in inflammation and infection. The descending and the sigmoid portions of the colon lie in the LLQ.

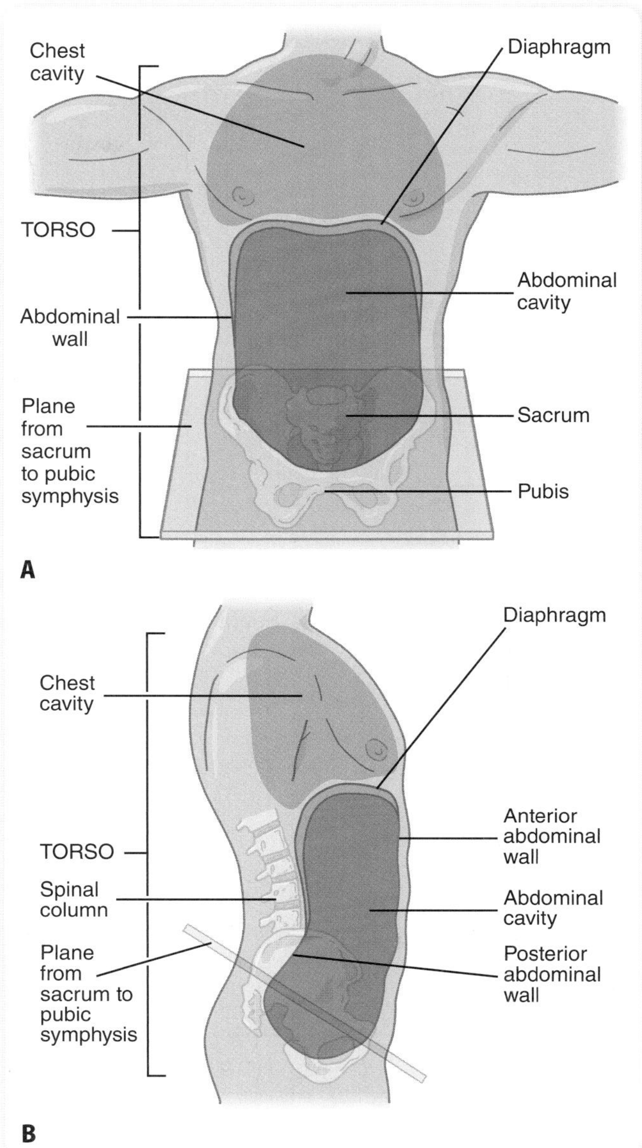

Figure 8-123 The boundaries of the abdomen are the anterior and posterior abdominal cavity walls, the diaphragm, and an imaginary plane from the pubic symphysis to the sacrum. **A.** Anterior view. **B.** Lateral view.

Several organs lie in more than one quadrant. The small intestine, for example, occupies the central part of the abdomen around the umbilicus, and parts of it lie in all four quadrants. The pancreas lies just behind the abdominal cavity on the posterior abdominal wall in both upper quadrants. The large intestine also traverses the abdomen, beginning in the RLQ and ending in the LLQ as it passes through all four quadrants. The urinary bladder lies just behind the pubic symphysis in the middle of the abdomen, and therefore lies in both lower quadrants and also in the pelvis. Less commonly, the abdomen and pelvis can be divided into nine sections to assist in describing the location of abdominal organs, pain, incisions, or scars Figure 8-125.

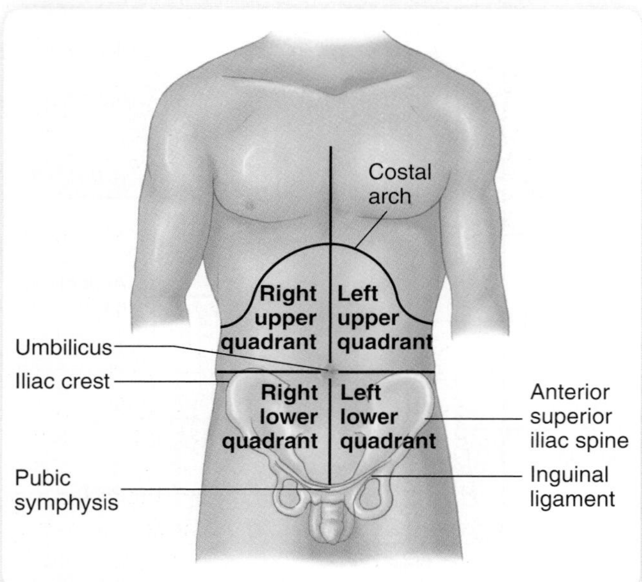

Figure 8-124 The four abdominal quadrants.

Figure 8-125 The nine abdominal regions.

Most of the intraabdominal structures are covered by a large, moist, continuous sheet of serous membrane called the **peritoneum**. The peritoneum is composed of two parts: the parietal peritoneum, which lines the walls of the abdominal cavity, and the visceral peritoneum, which covers the organs within the abdominal cavity. The potential space between these two layers is the peritoneal cavity. Organs in the abdominopelvic cavity are located either inside the peritoneum (intraperitoneal) or behind the peritoneum (retroperitoneal) **Figure 8-126**. The upper peritoneal cavity, also known as the thoracoabdominal component of the abdomen, is covered by the

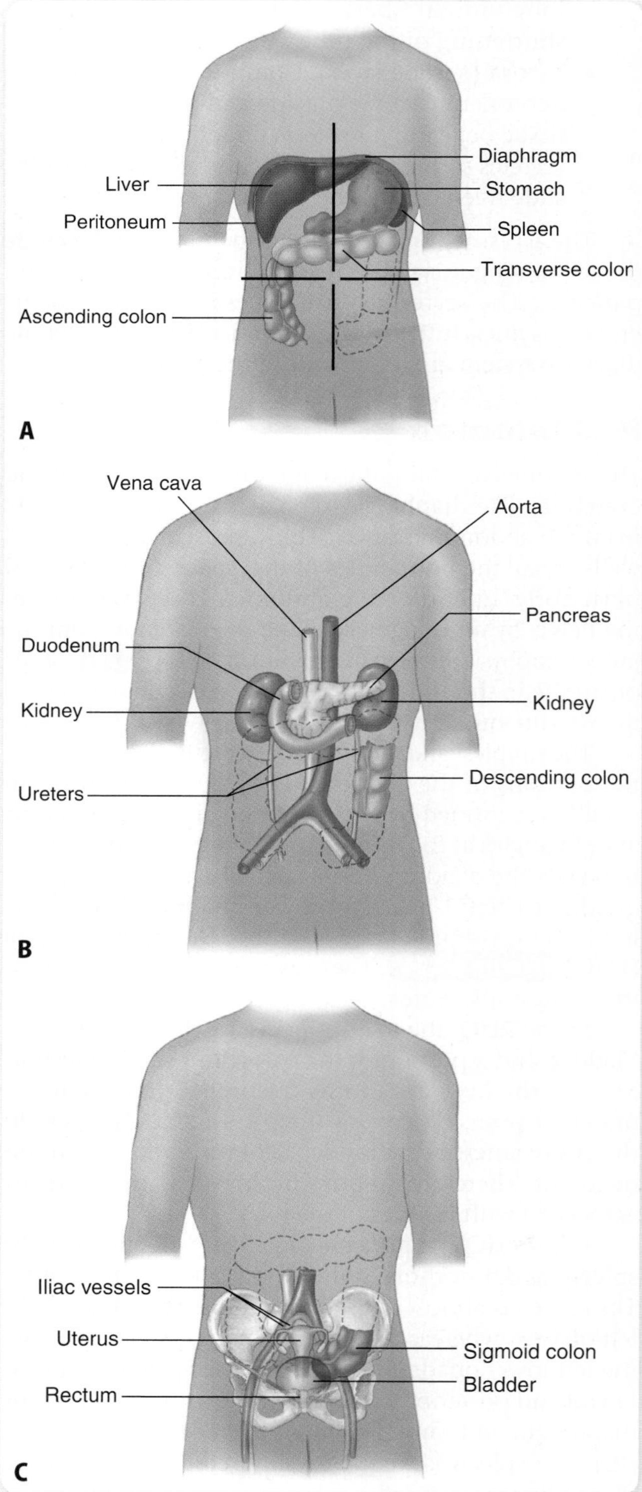

Figure 8-126 Different organs of the abdomen are contained in the peritoneum **(A)**, the retroperitoneal space **(B)**, and the pelvis **(C)**.

lower part of the thorax. The diaphragm, liver, spleen, stomach, gallbladder, and transverse colon are located here. The lower peritoneal cavity contains the small bowel, sigmoid colon, parts of the descending and ascending colon, and, in women, the internal reproductive organs. The retroperitoneal space contains the abdominal aorta, inferior vena cava, pancreas, kidneys, adrenal glands, **ureters** (tubes that carry urine from the kidneys to the bladder) and most of the duodenum and the posterior aspects of the descending and ascending colon, as well as the retroperitoneal components of the pelvic cavity. The rectum, ureters, bladder, iliac vessels, pelvic vascular plexus, major vascular structures, pelvic skeletal structures, and reproductive organs lie in the pelvis.

The abdominal organs are suspended within the abdominal cavity by folds of peritoneum called mesentery. The mesentery contains the nerves, arteries, veins, and lymph vessels that supply the intestines and other intraabdominal structures.

Finally, the abdomen includes many vital vessels, including the abdominal aorta, the superior and inferior mesenteries, the renal artery, the gonadal arteries, the gastric artery, the splenic artery, the hepatic artery, the iliac arteries, the hepatic portal system, and the inferior venae cavae **Figure 8-127**.

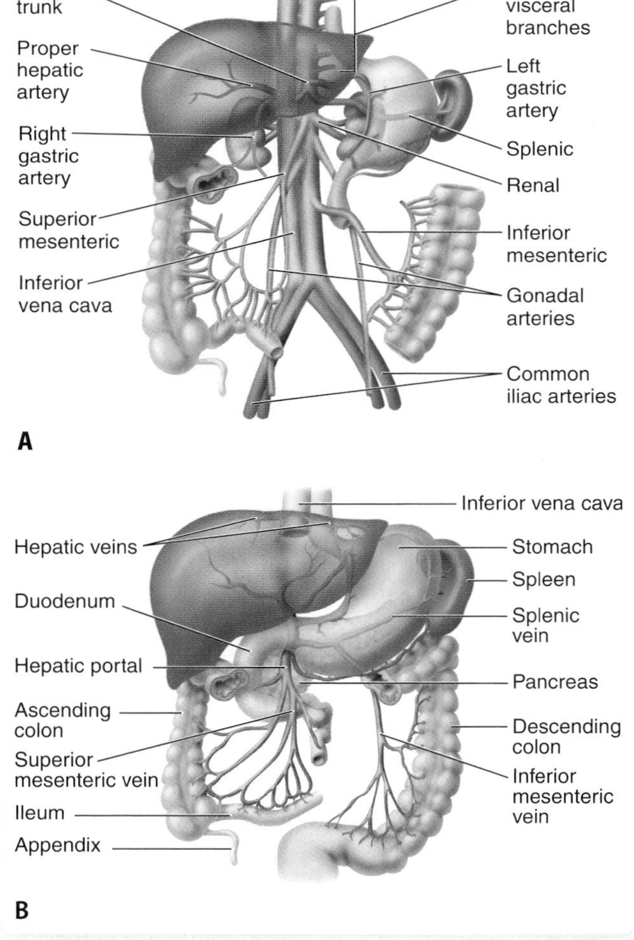

Figure 8-127 A. Arteries of the abdomen. **B.** Veins of the abdomen.

Words of Wisdom

The solid organs of the abdomen include the liver, spleen, pancreas, and kidneys. The hollow organs of the abdomen include the stomach, gallbladder, urinary bladder, and small and large intestines.

Oral Cavity

The first part of the digestive system is the oral cavity (mouth). The mouth consists of the lips, cheeks, gums, teeth, and tongue. A mucous membrane lines the mouth. The roof of the mouth is formed by the hard and soft palates. The hard palate is a bony plate lying anteriorly; the soft palate is a fold of mucous membrane and muscle that extends posteriorly from the hard palate into the throat. The soft palate is designed to hold food that is being chewed within the mouth and to help initiate swallowing. The cheeks make up the lateral walls of the oral cavity. The floor of the oral cavity is formed mainly of soft tissues, such as the tongue.

Digestion begins in the mouth with mastication, or the chewing of food by the teeth. The hypoglossal (CN XII), glossopharyngeal (CN IX), trigeminal (CN V), and facial (CN VII) nerves supply the mouth and its structures. The hypoglossal nerve provides motor function to the muscles of the tongue. The glossopharyngeal nerve provides taste sensation to the posterior portions of the tongue and carries parasympathetic fibers to the salivary glands on each side of the face. The mandibular branch of the trigeminal nerve provides motor innervation to the muscles of mastication. The facial nerve, in addition to supplying motor activity to all muscles of facial expression, provides the sense of taste to the anterior two-thirds of the tongue and cutaneous sensations to the tongue and palate.

Teeth

Recall that the normal adult mouth contains 32 permanent teeth. Loss of the primary or deciduous teeth occurs during childhood. Adult teeth are distributed about the maxillary and mandibular arches. The teeth on each side of the arch are mirror images of each other and form four quadrants: right upper, left upper, right lower, and left lower. Each quadrant contains one central incisor, one lateral incisor, one canine, two premolars, and three molars **Figure 8-128**. The third molars (wisdom teeth) do not appear until late adolescence.

The top portion of the tooth, external to the gum, is the crown, containing one or more cusps. Below the crown lie the neck and the root. The pulp cavity fills the center of the tooth and contains blood vessels, nerves, and specialized connective tissue, called pulp. Dentin and enamel surround the pulp cavity and protect the tooth from damage. Dentin, which forms the principal mass of the tooth, is much denser and stronger than

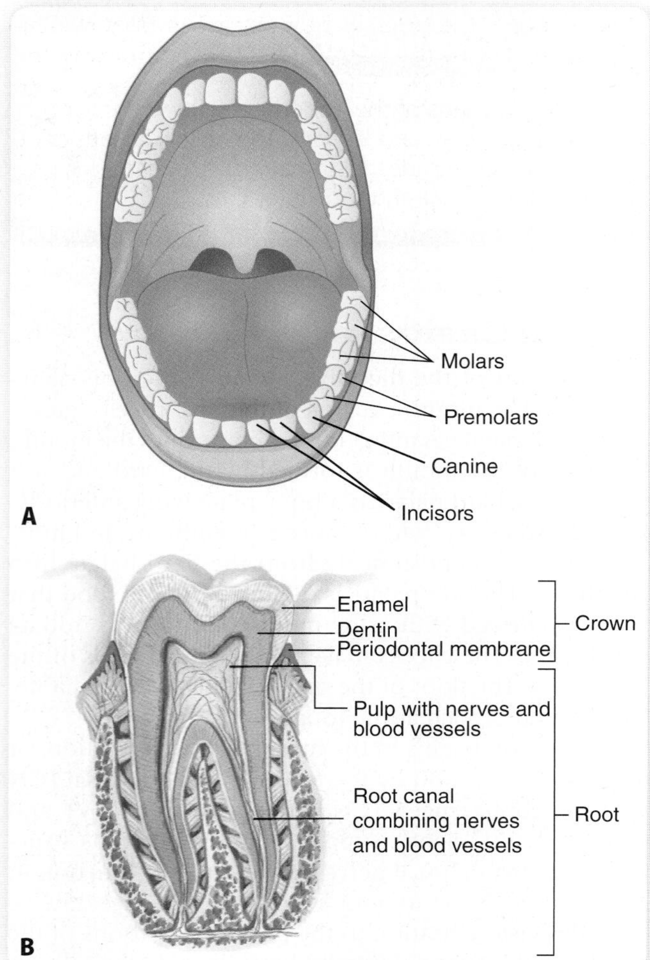

Figure 8-128 The teeth of the adult mouth. **A.** The incisors are used for biting. Canines are used for tearing food. The premolars and molars are used for grinding and crushing. **B.** Each tooth contains nerves and blood vessels.

bone. The bony sockets for the teeth that reside in the mandible and maxilla are alveoli. The ridges between the teeth, the alveolar ridges, are covered by the gingiva, or gums, which are thickened connective tissue and epithelium. Teeth are attached to the alveolar bone by a periodontal membrane.

Your front teeth are mainly used to tear or cut the food. While chewing, the food is worked toward the back of the mouth, where the flat surfaces of the molars crush and grind the food into a more easily swallowed consistency. This mechanical activity eases food down the esophagus during swallowing and helps to prevent aspiration of food into the lungs.

Salivary Glands

As mentioned previously, the salivary glands are accessory organs of digestion. During mastication, food is mixed with secretions from the salivary glands. The location of

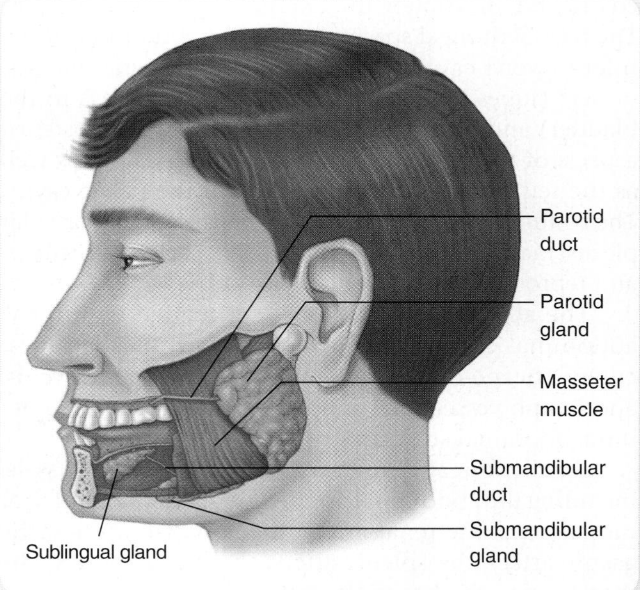

Figure 8-129 The glands and muscles of the mouth.

the salivary glands are as follows: two under the tongue, one on each side of the lower jaw, and one inside each cheek Figure 8-129. The salivary glands are composed of two types of cells. The serous cells produce amylase, a salivary enzyme that begins the digestive process of starchy food material. The mucous cells produce mucus that binds and lubricates material placed in the mouth, such as food.

The oral cavity opens posteriorly into the pharynx. The oropharynx extends vertically from the back of the mouth to the esophagus and trachea. An automatic movement of the pharynx during swallowing lifts the larynx to permit the epiglottis to close over it so that liquids and solids are moved into the esophagus and away from the trachea.

Esophagus

Starting from the pharynx, the esophagus proceeds distally through the chest cavity, passes through the diaphragm, and terminates at the stomach. The esophagus is a hollow tube about 10 inches (25 cm) long that is surrounded by smooth muscle. It helps transport food from the mouth to the stomach, but is unable to absorb nutrients. The esophagus typically lies collapsed in on itself, like a dry fire hose. This deflated position allows air to flow easily into the lungs, and not into the stomach. The esophagus dilates, however, when food or liquid travels through it. The esophagus lies posterior to the trachea. It begins to the right of the aorta and then passes anterior to the aorta as it traverses inferiorly. At the inferior end of the esophagus is the stomach.

Intertwined around the esophagus are veins that drain into another, more complex series of veins that ultimately converge to form the portal vein. The portal vein transports venous blood from the GI tract directly to the liver for processing of the nutrients that have been absorbed.

The esophagus propels material into the stomach by a series of wavelike contractions called **peristalsis**. Peristalsis is not limited to the esophagus; it is responsible for movement throughout the GI tract.

▶ Stomach

The stomach is an intraperitoneal hollow organ that lies just inferior to the diaphragm in the LUQ of the abdomen. It is partially covered by the left lobe of the liver and largely protected by the lower left ribs. The stomach is concave (the lesser curvature) on its right side, and convex (the greater curvature) on its left side. The entrance into the stomach is surrounded by the cardiac sphincter, which controls the movement of material into the stomach. When empty, the stomach is rather small, but it has the capacity to stretch to many times its normal size to accommodate meals. The principal function of the stomach is to receive food in large quantities intermittently, store it, and provide for its movement into the small intestine in small amounts.

The fundus of the stomach (its uppermost part), and it is able to adapt to varying amounts of food. This part is also where gas bubbles rise to, particularly after a meal. The largest part of the stomach is known as the body. It serves primarily as the storage area for ingested food and liquid. The lower part of the stomach is known as the antrum, and is somewhat funnel-shaped, with its narrow end connecting to the pyloric canal, which empties into the duodenum.

The stomach wall is composed of three layers (see Figure 8-122). The external layer, the longitudinal muscle, is continuous with the longitudinal muscle of the esophagus. The middle, or circular layer, the strongest of the three layers, completely covers the stomach. This circular muscle becomes significantly thicker to form the pyloric sphincter. The inner layer, or oblique layer, is the strongest in the fundus region and becomes progressively weaker toward the pylorus (a circumferential muscle at the end of the stomach that acts as a valve).

Blood is supplied to the stomach via the celiac trunk that branches from the abdominal portion of the aorta. Blood from the stomach is returned to the venous system via the portal vein, which carries blood to the liver. The nerve supply is provided by the sympathetic (celiac or solar plexus) and parasympathetic (vagus nerve or CNX) divisions of the ANS.

The stomach contains acid that assists in the digestive process. The gastric juice that is secreted is a mixture of water, hydrochloric acid (strong enough to dissolve metal with a pH of 1.5 to 3), organic substances (mucus, pepsin, and protein), and electrolytes (potassium, sodium, bicarbonate, sulfate, and phosphate). As food enters the stomach, hydrochloric acid is secreted, which helps to break down the food. The stomach contracts to help mix the acid with the food more evenly; churning the acid and food mixture together until a relatively smooth consistency is achieved. The resulting substance is called chyme. Chyme is expelled by the stomach through the pyloric sphincter and into the duodenum, the first part of the small intestine.

▶ Small Intestine

The small intestine is the major hollow organ of the abdomen. The cells lining the small intestine produce enzymes and mucus to aid in digestion. Enzymes from the pancreas and the small intestine carry out the final processes of digestion. More than 90% of the products of digestion (amino acids, fatty acids, and simple sugars), together with water, ingested vitamins, and minerals are absorbed across the wall of the lower end of the small intestine into veins to be transported to the liver.

The small intestine is composed of the duodenum, the jejunum, and the ileum. The duodenum, which is 9 to 11 inches (23 to 28 cm) long, is the part of the small intestine that receives food from the stomach. It forms a C-shaped curve around the head of the pancreas. The duodenal bulb is the widest part of the small intestine. As contents pass through the stomach, they move through the pylorus, which acts as a valve between the stomach and the duodenum. The duodenum connects the pancreas, liver, and gallbladder to the digestive system **Figure 8-130**.

The jejunum, a major site of nutrient absorption, and ileum together measure more than 20 feet (6 m) on average to make up the rest of the small intestine. The ileum, an area of decreased nutrient absorption, is where the chyme is prepared for entry into the large intestine.

In the small intestine, water-soluble and fat-soluble vitamins are absorbed by diffusion into the bloodstream. The small intestine also produces enzymes that work with the pancreatic enzymes to turn chyme into substances that can be directly absorbed into the bloodstream through the capillaries on its surface. Blood enriched with these energy molecules exits the intestinal circulation and flows to the liver, where fat and protein metabolism takes place. The blood then leaves the liver and enters the subclavian vessels.

Words of Wisdom

The duodenum is the last section of what is called the upper GI system. The jejunum is the first part of the lower GI system.

▶ Large Intestine

The large intestine is about 5 feet (2 m) long and encircles the outer border of the abdomen around the small intestine. The main role of the large intestine is to complete

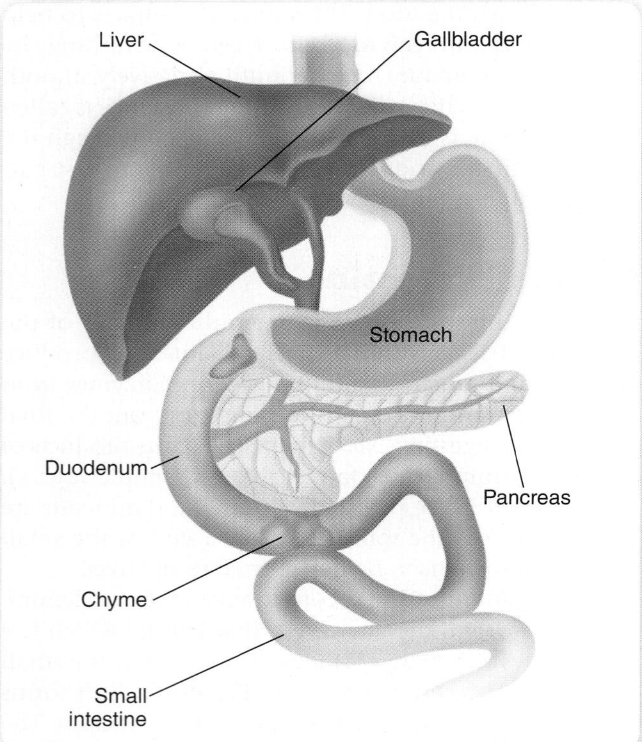

Figure 8-130 The duodenum connects the pancreas, liver, and gallbladder to the digestive system.

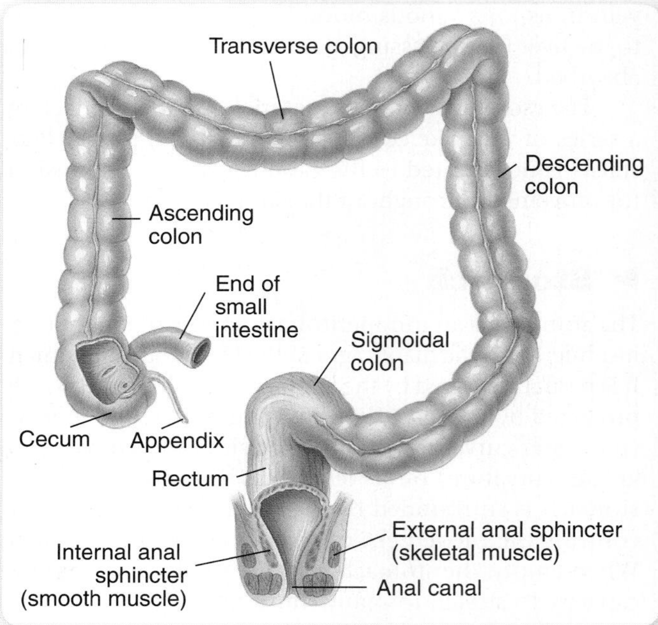

Figure 8-131 The large intestine.

the reabsorption of water. Most water is reabsorbed in the small intestine. This osmotic function of the colon helps to solidify the stool. Intestinal flora (normal bacteria) synthesize some vitamins such as folic acid, vitamin K, riboflavin, and nicotinic acid. Cellulose, which is indigestible by humans, moves through the small intestine with little change and provides bulk to the contents of the large intestine.

The first segment of the large intestine is the cecum and its accessory structure, the appendix Figure 8-131. The ileocecal valve joins the ileum to the cecum. The appendix opens into the cecum in the RLQ of the abdomen. Rising up from the cecum is the ascending colon. It attaches to the transverse colon, which runs from right to left. A 90-degree turn occurs, and the descending colon begins. The sigmoid colon then takes an S-shaped turn. Feces travel through the descending colon, then progress to the sigmoid colon and then through the rectum, which joins the anal canal, to exit the body by the anus. The anus has two **sphincters** (internal and external). The internal anal sphincter (under autonomic control) has stretch receptors that give the sensation of the need to defecate. The external anal sphincter (under voluntary control) allows a controlled bowel movement.

The peristaltic waves of the large intestine happen only between twice and three times per day. The intestinal walls constrict vigorously (mass movements) to force contents toward the rectum. These movements usually follow a meal, but they may also be caused by irritations of the intestinal mucosa. Table 8-41 provides a summary of the organs and functions of the digestive system.

Accessory Organs

The liver, gallbladder, and pancreas are considered part of the digestive system because they are involved in the digestion of food and elimination of waste.

Liver

The liver takes up most of the area immediately beneath the diaphragm in the RUQ and extends into the LUQ of the abdomen. The liver is a complex organ with many functions. It is responsible for the maintenance of blood glucose. It detoxifies the blood by removing drugs and other poisonous substances such as ammonia, which it converts into urea, which is then excreted in urine. The liver is also responsible for the manufacturing of plasma proteins (albumin, fibrinogen, and globulins) and clotting factors, which allow the body to seal off damaged vessels to prevent blood loss. Finally, it plays a role in regulating fats. As old RBCs enter the liver, they are broken down into bile, which is necessary to break down ingested fats. The liver also produces cholesterol and proteins that carry fats through the body to ultimately drain into the small intestine.

The liver is a highly vascular organ through which 100% of the body's blood circulates. This vascular supply has two sources: the hepatic artery and the portal vein. The hepatic artery is how the liver receives its blood and nutrient supply from the circulatory system. The portal vein is composed of a group of vessels that originate from the digestive system. These vessels ensure that all nutrients

Table 8-41 Functions of the Digestive Organs

Organ/Structure	Function
Mouth	Mechanically breaks down food; begins chemical breakdown of food with saliva
Esophagus	Moves food from the mouth to the stomach; provides muscular and vascular structure
Stomach	Performs mechanical and chemical breakdown of food (food in, chyme out)
Small intestine	Major site for chemical breakdown of food; major site of absorption of water, fat, proteins, carbohydrates, and vitamins
Large intestine	Absorption of water; formation of feces; bacterial digestion of food
Rectum/anus	Controls release of feces
Accessory Organs	
Liver	Produces bile; assists with metabolism of carbohydrates, proteins, and fat; stores and manufactures vitamins; responsible for detoxification of blood and elimination of waste
Gallbladder	Stores bile
Pancreas	Exocrine: produces enzymes for protein, carbohydrate, and fat breakdown within the duodenum Endocrine: produces insulin, glucagon, and somatostatin

absorbed from the intestinal tract first are detoxified in the liver before their release into the general venous circulation (first pass).

Gallbladder

The liver is connected to the intestine by the bile ducts. The gallbladder is an outpouching from the bile ducts that serves as a reservoir and concentrating organ for bile produced in the liver. Together, the bile ducts and the gallbladder form the biliary system. The gallbladder is connected to the common bile duct via the cystic duct. Bile is expelled through the common bile duct into the duodenum. The presence of food in the duodenum triggers a contraction of the gallbladder to empty it. The sphincter of Oddi is located at the end of the common bile duct and regulates the movement of bile into the duodenum. The liver connects to the common bile duct via the hepatic duct.

Pancreas

Recall that the pancreas performs both endocrine and exocrine functions. Through its endocrine functions, it is responsible for the synthesis of glucagon, insulin, and somatostatin. Glucagon and insulin are critical in the maintenance of blood glucose. Its exocrine functions include the production of pancreatic digestive juices (pancreatic amylase, trypsin, chymotrypsin, and carboxypeptidase), which aid in the digestion of carbohydrates, fats, proteins, and nucleic acids. The amylase continues the digestion of starchy material begun in the mouth. The pancreatic duct expels these substances at its junction with the duodenum that is next to the opening of the common bile duct.

▶ Digestion and Absorption of Nutrients

Throughout this discussion of human anatomy and physiology, you have learned about numerous chemical and biologic processes that run continuously as long as the organism is alive, and some that continue after the organism has died. *Metabolism* is the sum of all of these reactions. Lay people use this term to describe the rate at which the body processes food. For example, someone with a so-called high metabolism burns more calories at rest than those with a low metabolism. These terms are simplistic but essentially true, because a large part of the body's resting metabolism is devoted to the intake, processing, and use of nutrients, or the substances on which the "engine" of each individual cell runs. Recall that the correct term for the rate at which nutrients are consumed in the body is the basal metabolic rate.

The body obtains nutrients through a variety of processes, but the most common are through inhalation, as is the case with oxygen, and ingestion, as in the food you eat. The various systems of the body break down these substances into usable forms. As discussed previously, nutrients include carbohydrates, lipids, proteins, vitamins, minerals, and water. Macronutrients are those required in large amounts (carbohydrates, lipids, and proteins); they provide energy and have other specific functions. Micronutrients are those required in much smaller amounts (vitamins and minerals); they do not directly provide energy, but allow biochemical reactions that extract energy from macronutrients. Essential nutrients are those that human cells cannot synthesize (such as certain amino acids).

A calorie is the amount of heat needed to raise the temperature of a gram of water by 1°C. The calorie used to measure food energy is greater, by 1,000 times. Cellular oxidation causes the following calorie releases:

- 1 gram of carbohydrate yields about 4 calories.
- 1 gram of protein yields about 4 calories.
- 1 gram of fat yields about 9 calories.

Digestion breaks down nutrients so they can be absorbed and transported via the bloodstream. If the amounts of nutrients are more abundant than the body's needs, then some nutrients can be stored (as in the case of lipids, which are stored as fatty tissue). In this way, the body can be prepared for times when nutrients are not plentiful and draw on those reserves. In other cases, excesses cannot be stored and are simply excreted through elimination of waste. When the amount of nutrients and energy consumed by the body exceeds the amount available in the diet, body structures may be metabolized to sustain life.

Typical meals contain carbohydrates, lipids, proteins, water, electrolytes, and vitamins. The digestive system handles each of these components differently. Digestion involves breaking down large organic molecules before absorption can occur. Water, electrolytes, and vitamins can be absorbed without preliminary breakdown, but may require special transport mechanisms.

Energy from carbohydrates is primarily used to power cellular processes. Digestion breaks carbohydrates down into monosaccharides (which include fructose, galactose, and glucose) for easy absorption. Liver enzymes convert fructose and galactose into glucose, which is the form of carbohydrate most commonly oxidized for use as cellular fuel.

Many cells get their energy by oxidizing fatty acids, though neurons require continuous glucose to survive. The nervous system can be seriously impaired by a lack of glucose. When carbohydrates are not consumed sufficiently, the liver may convert amino acids (from proteins) into glucose.

Some excess glucose is changed to glycogen, which is stored in the liver and muscles. Glucose can be rapidly mobilized from glycogen, but only a certain amount of glycogen can be stored. Excess glucose is usually converted into fat and stored in adipose tissue. For energy, the body first metabolizes glucose, then glycogen into glucose, and lastly, fats and proteins. Proteins supply essential amino acids and provide nitrogen and other elements.

The Urinary System

The urinary system controls the discharge of certain waste materials filtered from the blood by the kidneys. In the urinary system, the kidneys are solid organs; the ureters, bladder, and **urethra** (through which urine is expelled) are hollow organs **Figure 8-132**. The main functions of the urinary system are (1) to control fluid balance in the body, (2) to filter and eliminate wastes, and (3) to control pH balance.

YOU are the Paramedic PART 4

Your physical exam of the patient's abdomen reveals rigidity throughout both lower quadrants. When you press on his pelvis, you feel instability and grinding. The patient remains unresponsive during your assessment.

Recording Time: 10 Minutes	
Respirations	24 breaths/min, shallow
Pulse	118 beats/min
Skin	Pale, moist, and warm
Blood pressure	102/66 mm Hg
Oxygen saturation (Spo_2)	97% (assisted with a bag-mask device)
Pupils	PERRLA

8. What structures are located in the lower abdominal quadrants?
9. What might the instability of the pelvis indicate?

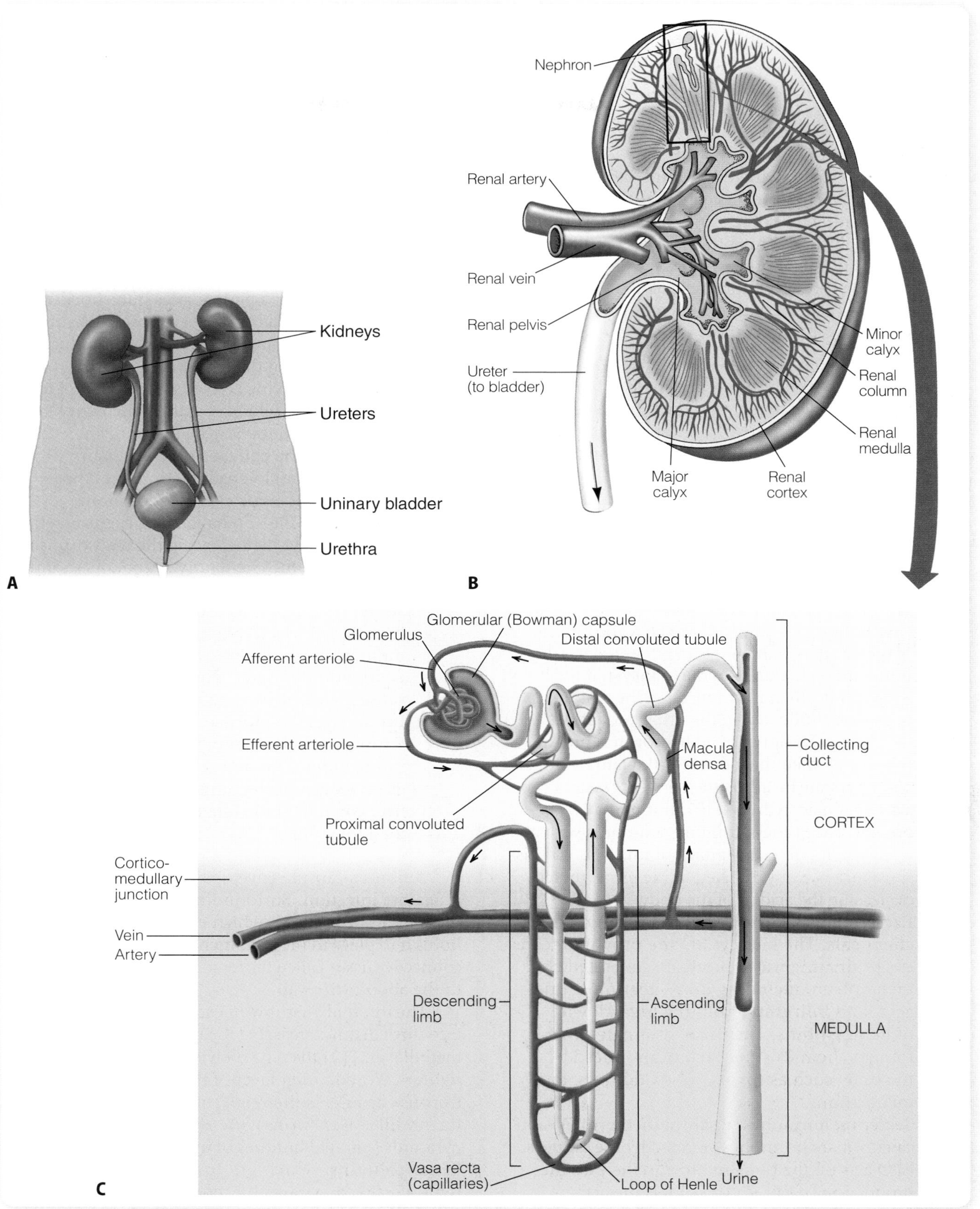

Figure 8-132 The urinary system. **A.** Anterior view showing the relationship of the kidneys, ureters, urinary bladder, and urethra. **B.** Cross-section of the human kidney showing its structures and blood flow through it. **C.** Blood flow through a nephron.

▶ Kidneys

The body has two bean-shaped kidneys that are located on either side of the spine between the 12th thoracic vertebra and the third lumbar vertebra. The right kidney is positioned lower than the left to make room for the liver. Both kidneys are located between the back muscles and the peritoneum. The kidneys are located in the retroperitoneal space, which is behind and outside the peritoneal cavity. These organs help to maintain homeostasis by regulating the composition, pH, and volume of the extracellular fluid. This process is accomplished by their removal of metabolic wastes from the blood and diluting them with water and electrolytes. This process forms urine, which the kidneys excrete. The other important functions of the kidneys include the following:

- **Regulating water and electrolytes.** Water and electrolyte excretion must be matched to water and electrolyte intake to achieve homeostasis. The kidneys alter their filtration and excretion rates to match the body's intake of water and electrolytes.
- **Regulating acid-base balance.** The renal system functions as a compensatory mechanism for maintaining acid-base balance. This is the slowest method for returning the pH to a normal range. It sometimes takes days to accomplish the task. The kidneys regulate the pH by monitoring the elimination of hydrogen and the reabsorption of bicarbonate in the tubules of **nephrons**, (the urine-producing units of the kidneys). If the body is too acidic, then it will increase the amount of hydrogen eliminated in the urine and recover bicarbonate. If not enough hydrogen is present (alkalosis), then the kidneys will retain hydrogen and eliminate bicarbonate. The renal system can also eliminate hydrogen if ammonia (NH_3) is present. The kidneys combine ammonia with a hydrogen ion to create ammonium (NH_4^+). This substance is easily excreted in the urine, thereby decreasing the acidity of the body.
- **Excreting waste products and foreign chemicals.** The kidneys are the primary means of eliminating waste products generated by metabolism, including urea, creatinine, uric acid, and bilirubin (from the breakdown of hemoglobin). They also eliminate other foreign chemicals ingested or produced by the body such as toxins, food additives, and medications.
- **Secreting hormones.** Erythropoietin (EPO) and calcitriol are hormones secreted by the kidneys. EPO acts on the bone marrow to increase the production of RBCs. Calcitriol is the active form of vitamin D. It promotes the absorption of calcium from food and mobilizes calcium from bones to the blood. Renin is a hormone formed in the kidney that initiates the eventual formation of angiotensin II, which is discussed in the next section.
- **Regulating arterial blood pressure.** The kidneys primarily regulate blood pressure by excreting large amounts of sodium and water. However, over a short period the kidneys exert control over arterial blood pressure by the renin-angiotensin-aldosterone mechanism. This mechanism consists of secreting renin, which leads to the formation of angiotensin II, a powerful vasoconstrictor. This is an important concept, especially when you consider a patient in shock. When a patient goes into shock, the kidneys respond by producing renin. Renin combines with angiotensinogen to produce angiotensin I. In the lungs, angiotensin-converting enzyme converts angiotensin I to angiotensin II, which constricts the peripheral arteries as a compensatory mechanism to maintain the patient's blood pressure. In addition, angiotensin II stimulates the production of aldosterone. Aldosterone, produced by the adrenal glands, exerts an effect on the kidneys by increasing the reabsorption of sodium into the circulatory system. As sodium is reabsorbed, so is water and the circulating fluid volume is maintained. ADH is produced by the hypothalamus and released by the posterior pituitary. Increases in ADH cause decreased elimination of water, whereas decreases in ADH cause increased elimination of water.
- **Producing new glucose.** During prolonged fasting, the kidneys produce new glucose from amino acids and other chemicals. This gluconeogenesis is comparable to that of the liver when the individual has gone without food for a long time.

A fibrous capsule envelops the kidney and protects it against infection. Surrounding this capsule is a fatty mass of adipose tissue, which cushions the kidney and holds it in place in the abdomen. A layer of dense fibrous connective tissue called the renal fascia anchors the kidney to the abdominal wall.

The internal anatomy of each kidney can be divided into three distinct areas: (1) the renal cortex, (2) the renal medulla, and (3) the renal pelvis (see Figure 8-132). The lighter-colored, outer layer of the kidney, closest to the fibrous capsule, is the **renal cortex**. The **renal medulla**, the middle layer, forms cone-shaped areas called renal pyramids (parallel bundles of urine-collecting tubules). Renal columns, which are inward extensions of the renal cortex, separate the renal pyramids. The renal pyramids point toward the **renal pelvis**, which collects urine and forms the upper portion of the ureter. The edges of the renal pelvis are called calyces, which collect urine. The major and minor calyces branch off the renal pelvis and connect with the renal pyramids to receive the urine that drains from the collecting tubules. This arrangement has been said to resemble several strands of uncooked spaghetti (the collecting tubules) sitting in a thimble (the papilla, or tip, of the renal pelvis). The collected urine flows through the renal pelvis and into the ureter on its way to the bladder.

About one-fourth of the body's systemic cardiac output flows through the kidney each minute. Blood ejected from the heart flows from the abdominal aorta into the kidney by way of the renal artery. Each kidney has a medial indentation (known as the hilus) through which the renal artery, vein, lymphatic vessels, and nerves enter and leave. After it enters the kidney at the hilus, the renal artery branches several times to become the afferent arteriole. The afferent arteriole quickly branches into a tuft of capillaries called a glomerulus, the main filter of the kidney. From the glomerulus, the blood enters the efferent arteriole, which branches into the peritubular capillaries, where tubular reabsorption occurs. This secondary set of capillaries is unique to the kidney; no other organ in the body has two distinct capillary beds. The capillaries then merge, forming venules and veins, until the renal vein leaves the hilus, carrying the cleansed blood to the inferior vena cava.

Nephrons

Nephrons (found in the cortex) filter the blood, collect excreted water and waste products, and reabsorb water, nutrients, and electrolytes. Each normal adult kidney contains more than 1 million nephrons. Blood flow to the kidneys is supplied by the renal arteries, which divide into arterioles and capillaries.

A nephron contains a glomerulus; a glomerular capsule (Bowman capsule), which surrounds the glomerulus; the proximal convoluted tubule (PCT); the loop of Henle; and the distal convoluted tubule (DCT), which connects with the collecting tubules of the kidney. The glomerulus and glomerular capsule compose the **renal corpuscle**. Blood enters the glomerulus by an afferent arteriole and leaves by an efferent arteriole. Pores in the walls of the capillaries in the glomerulus allow the blood to be filtered. Filtered water and wastes (filtrate) flow from the glomerular capsule through **renal tubules**.

The glomerular capsule is a double-layered cup in which the inner layer infiltrates and surrounds the capillaries of the glomerulus. Special cells in the inner membrane called podocytes wrap around the capillaries in the glomerulus, forming filtration slits. The filtrate passes through these slits, across the filtration membrane, and into the capsule. In this manner, the filtration membrane prevents large molecules, such as proteins, from entering the glomerular capsule **Figure 8-133**.

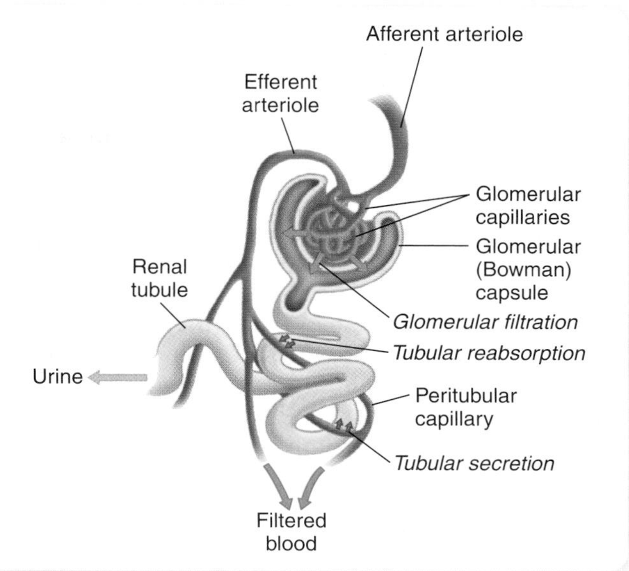

Figure 8-133 The glomerulus of the kidneys. The nephron carries out three blood-filtering processes: glomerular filtration, tubular reabsorption, and tubular secretion.

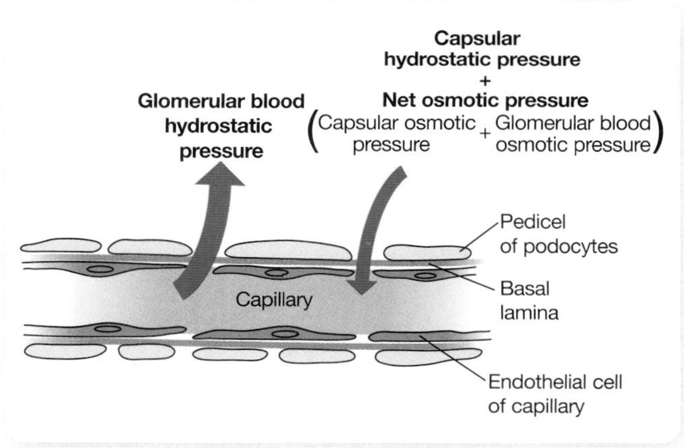

Figure 8-134 The presence of an efferent arteriole results in a high glomerular (blood) hydrostatic pressure. This pressure exceeds the sum of the pressures that oppose the movement of fluid through the glomerular filtration membrane. Filtration is the outcome of this balance of pressures.

Imagine watering your garden with an open-ended hose. If you place your finger over half of the opening of the hose, then the same amount of water must now pass through half the space. As a result, the pressure increases and you can spray the water farther. The same effect occurs at the glomerulus. As blood moves from the relatively large afferent arteriole into the smaller capillaries of the glomerulus, the pressure increases. This effect, along with the smaller diameter of the efferent arteriole, causes the pressure in the glomerulus to rise enough to force the filtrate from the blood into the glomerular capsule **Figure 8-134**.

The amount of filtrate produced, called the glomerular filtration rate, is maintained at a relatively constant rate of 125 mL/min in healthy adults. Initially, the filtrate contains everything that can pass through the filtration membrane: salts, minerals, glucose, water, and metabolic wastes. As the filtrate passes through the rest of the nephron, **tubular reabsorption** and **tubular secretion** convert the filtrate into urine Figure 8-135. As the fluid passes through the PCT, the cells lining the PCT remove all organic nutrients and plasma proteins, as well as some ions, from the filtrate. These compounds are deposited in the interstitial fluid surrounding the PCT. As these solutes accumulate, the concentration of the surrounding fluid becomes higher than that of the filtrate. Water will then move from the filtrate by osmosis. The fluid and nutrients in the interstitial fluid, in turn, move into the peritubular capillaries around the PCT. This process reestablishes the homeostatic balance in the blood and reduces the volume of the tubular filtrate.

Additional reabsorption of water and electrolytes occurs in the loop of Henle. The loop of Henle has two sections: the descending limb, extending toward the medulla, and the ascending limb, moving toward the cortex. The cells in the descending limb are permeable to water, but impermeable to sodium and chloride ions; the cells in the ascending limb are permeable to sodium and chloride ions, but impermeable to water. As a consequence, when the sodium and chloride ions move out of the ascending limb, they increase the solute concentration of the fluid surrounding the descending limb. Water moves by osmosis from the descending limb into the surrounding tissue and eventually into the vasa recta, a series of peritubular capillaries that surround the loop of Henle. This countercurrent multiplier process allows the body to produce either concentrated or diluted urine, depending on the body's needs.

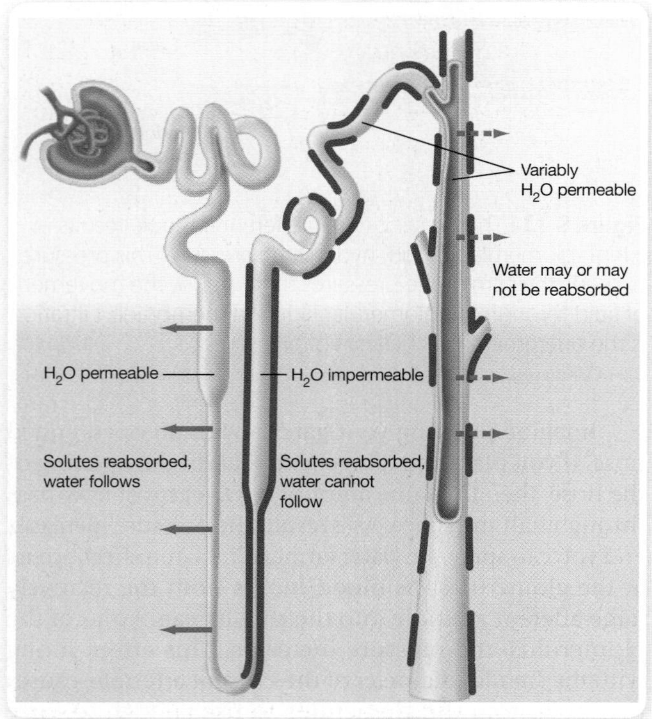

Figure 8-135 A single nephron and the tubular reabsorption of water.

After leaving the loop of Henle, the fluid enters the DCT. At this point, about 80% of the water and 85% of the solutes originally forced out of the glomerulus have been reabsorbed. As the urine passes through the DCT and the collecting ducts to which it is attached (both of which are impermeable to solutes), its composition undergoes its final adjustments. Ions are actively secreted or reabsorbed, and the body alters the permeability of the DCT and collecting ducts to water as necessary, depending on the body's homeostatic needs. These adjustments to the final composition of the urine facilitate the removal of metabolic wastes while maintaining the body's fluid-electrolyte balance.

At the site where the efferent arteriole comes in contact with the DCT, a structure called the juxtaglomerular apparatus is formed. The pressure-sensitive cells in the efferent arteriole (juxtaglomerular cells) monitor the blood pressure. The cells in the DCT (macula densa cells) are sensitive to chemical changes and monitor the concentration of the filtrate in the DCT. When triggered by changes in the blood pressure of the filtrate content, the juxtaglomerular cells release renin. Renin stimulates an increase in angiotensin I, which is then converted into angiotensin II. The presence of increased levels of angiotensin II stimulates the production of aldosterone.

The final adjustments to the composition of the urine at the DCT and collecting duct are controlled primarily by two hormones: ADH and aldosterone. Neurons in the hypothalamus monitor the solute concentration of the blood. When the solute concentration of the blood increases (eg, sweating, decreased fluid intake), ADH is released into the bloodstream. This hormone travels to the DCT and collecting ducts, increasing the permeability of these structures to water. Water therefore leaves the DCT and collecting ducts, and reenters the bloodstream. As the solute concentration returns to normal, secretion of ADH will stop.

Aldosterone increases the rate of active reabsorption of sodium and chloride ions into the blood; a corresponding increase occurs in water reabsorption. This hormone also decreases the reabsorption of potassium ions, resulting in excess potassium being secreted in the urine.

Other hormones also influence the retention or secretion of various substances. For example, PTH causes a decrease in the amount of calcium excreted in the urine. **Atrial natriuretic peptide** is a hormone produced by the atria when they are distended by increased blood volume. This hormone inhibits the absorption of water and sodium in the renal tubules, thereby increasing the elimination of water.

Urea is a result of amino acid catabolism, and its plasma concentration reflects the amount of protein in the diet. Urea filters into the renal tubule. About 80% of urea is reabsorbed, while the remainder is excreted in the urine. Uric acid is a result of metabolism of certain organic bases in nucleic acids. Active transport reabsorbs most of the uric acid present in the glomerular filtrate.

The composition of urine is related to water volume and the amount of solutes that the kidneys must eliminate or retain to maintain homeostasis. Urine is about 95% water, and usually contains urea and uric acid. It is slightly heavier than water, with a specific gravity of 1.003 to 1.035. Its pH is usually close to neutral, but can vary widely depending on many factors, not the least of which being what the patient has eaten. It can be clear to straw-colored, but a darker color usually indicates a concentration of solutes that may indicate dehydration or some other malady. It may have traces of amino acids and electrolytes. Urine production varies between 0.6 and 2.5 L per day. Urine production of 50 to 60 mL per hour is normal, with output of less than 30 mL per hour (or approximately 0.5 mL/kg/hour) suggestive of renal failure.

Ureters

After the urine enters the collecting ducts (the renal pyramids of the medulla), it passes through the minor calyx, into the major calyx, and then into the renal pelvis. From there, the urine is drained from each kidney through thin-walled muscular tubes called ureters. These tubes are about 12 inches (30 cm) in length. Urine is moved out of the kidney by peristaltic contractions that begin inside the kidney and minor and major calyces. These contractions continue in the renal pelvis and move the urine along the ureters toward the urinary bladder.

Urinary Bladder

The urinary bladder is a hollow, muscular sac surrounded by smooth muscle. Recall that it is responsible for storing urine before it is eliminated from the body. Most of the bladder rests in the anterior abdominal cavity, but the dome of the bladder sits in the posterior abdominal cavity, (retroperitoneum), where the ureters and kidneys reside. When empty, the bladder collapses and the muscular walls fold over onto themselves. In contrast, as urine accumulates, the bladder expands and becomes pear-shaped. The stretching of the bladder walls ultimately stimulates nerve impulses to produce the micturition reflex. This spinal reflex causes contraction of the bladders smooth muscle, which in turn produces the urge to void as pressure is exerted on the internal urinary sphincter. Normally, the brain controls this urge, keeping the external urinary sphincter contracted until conditions are favorable for urination. At this point, inhibition of the external urinary sphincter is reduced and the urine passes from the urinary bladder into the urethra.

Urethra

The urinary bladder and the urethra make up the lower urinary tract. The beginning of the urethra, sits at the inferior aspect of the bladder. In males, the urethra passes

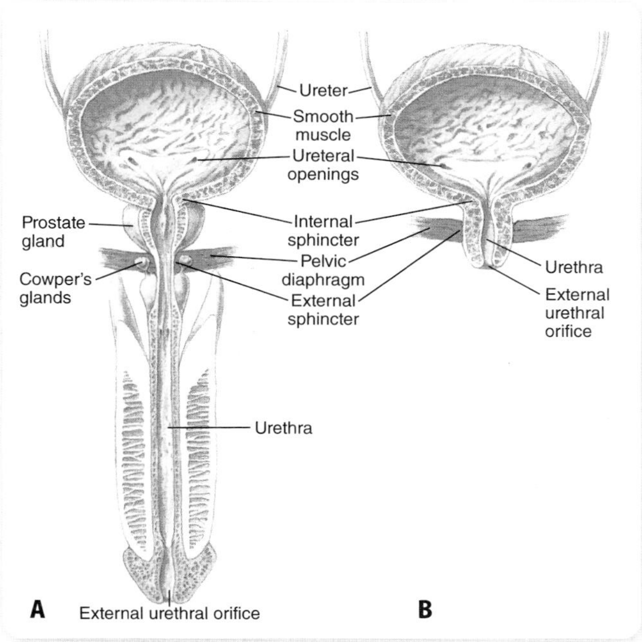

Figure 8-136 Comparison of the urethra in males **(A)** and females **(B)**.

from the anterior base of the bladder through the penis. In females, the urethra opens in front of the vagina. The female urethra is shorter than the male urethra (2 inches [4 cm] versus 8 inches [20 cm]) Figure 8-136.

The male urethra is divided into three regions:

- **Prostatic urethra**. This region begins at the bladder and extends through the prostate gland.
- **Membranous urethra.** This region extends from the prostate gland through the abdominal wall and into the penis.
- **Spongy (penile) urethra.** This region passes through the penis to the external urethral opening.

Fluid Balance

Certain mechanisms in the body maintain the balance between what is taken in and what is excreted. For example, when the fluid volume drops, the pituitary gland secretes ADH Figure 8-137. ADH causes the kidney tubules to reabsorb more water into the blood and excrete less urine, allowing fluid volume in the body to build up. Thirst also regulates fluid intake. The sensation of thirst occurs when body fluids become decreased, stimulating a person to take in more fluids. Conversely, when too many fluids enter the body, thirst decreases, the kidneys are activated, and more urine is excreted, eliminating the excess fluid.

It is important to maintain the proper balance of fluids and electrolytes within the body, because this is necessary for life. A person's body can become depleted of fluids and electrolytes for several reasons, including severe burns or dehydration. The body can maintain fluid balance by

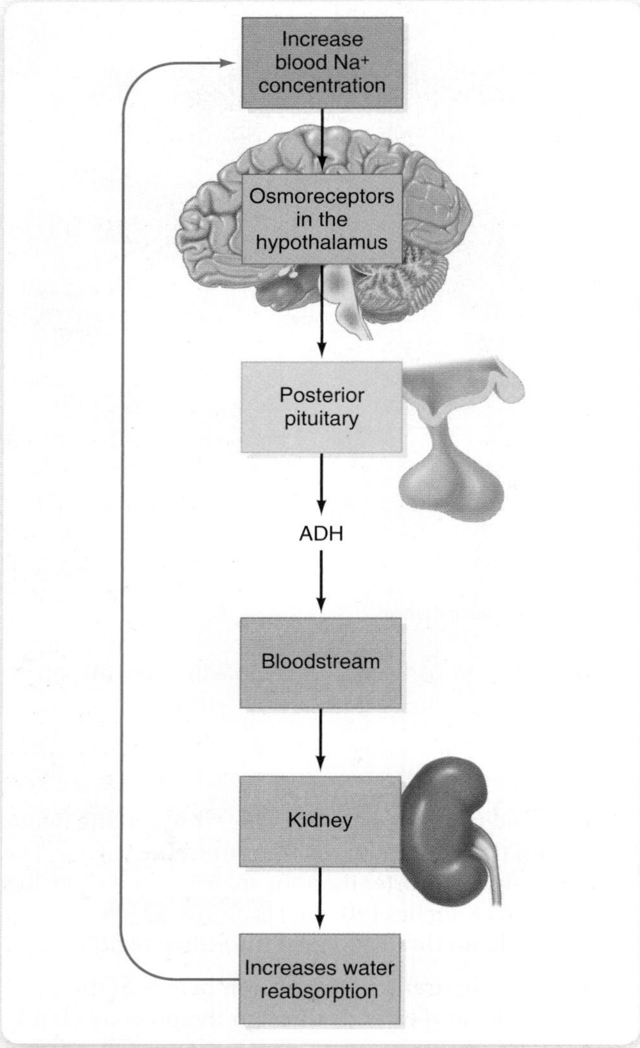

Figure 8-137 The role of ADH in regulating fluid levels.

shifting water from one compartment to another. Water moves in response to osmotic forces as well as hormonal stimuli such as ADH. By moving unequal amounts of electrolytes into and out of the cells, it is also possible for the body to balance other properties of intracellular fluid. For a patient whose fluids or electrolytes are depleted, rapid restoration of fluid balance may mean the difference between life and death **Table 8-42**.

Table 8-42	Major Mechanisms for Fluid Homeostasis
▪ ADH ▪ Thirst ▪ Kidneys ▪ Water shifts	

The Reproductive System

The **reproductive system** controls the reproductive processes by which life is created. The male and female reproductive systems contain organs and glands that create sex cells and transport them to areas where fertilization can occur. The male and female reproductive systems are functionally very different, but the first step in reproduction for each is to produce cells specially created to combine with a partner's to create a new organism. These cells are known as sex cells or gametes. Male gametes are sperm. Female gametes are oocytes or eggs. Gametes are described as **haploid cells** because they carry genetic instructions via 23 individual chromosomes. When sex cells from a man and woman unite during fertilization, the chromosomes from each partner unite with their accompanying chromosome from the opposite gamete, called a **homologous chromosome**, to form 23 pairs of chromosomes, for a total of 46 chromosomes. This first fertilized cell, from which all other body cells are created, is known as the zygote. It, and all other cells besides the gametes, are described as **diploid cells** because they carry two of each of the 23 chromosomes—one from the father and one from the mother. Among these, 22 chromosomes are **autosomes**, which have a corresponding homologous chromosome in both men and women. The 23rd chromosome pair is made up of **sex chromosomes**—one X chromosome, which both men and women have, and the other being either a second copy of the X chromosome or a Y chromosome. If the 23rd pair in the zygote is XX, then the organism will be biologically female; if it is XY, then a male will develop.

It is crucial to understand how critical these chromosomes are and how far-reaching their effects can be on the developing organism. These chromosomes contain the entire sequence of genetic information the organism will have throughout its entire life (unless some artificial change is effected). This genetic information contains the instructions for every structure and process in the body. Chromosomes also contain sequences that will determine or influence various characteristics such as hair color, skin color, body composition, height, and predisposition to certain diseases. These traits are determined through the action of dominant and recessive **alleles** of the same gene. For example, the allele that contains instructions for red hair color is recessive. If it is paired with an allele from the other parent that is dominant, then the cell is said to be heterozygous, and hair color will be dictated by the dominant allele (the allele for red hair will be overridden by the dominant allele). If, however, it is paired with another "redhead" allele, then the cell is said to be homozygous, and the new organism's hair color will be red. The arrangement of genes and their characteristics is known as the person's **genotype**, whereas the set of characteristics that results from expression of those genes is known as a **phenotype**.

▶ Male Reproductive Anatomy

The structures of the male reproductive system include the scrotum, testes, epididymis, ductus deferentia (also called the vas deferentia), ejaculatory ducts, the urethra, and the penis Figure 8-138. The two testes, in which sperm cells and male sex hormones are formed, are the essential organs of the male reproductive system. Accessory glands include seminal vesicles, the prostate gland, and the bulbourethral glands (Cowper glands). The scrotum, penis, and spermatic cords are supporting structures. In males, the urethra is shared by the reproductive and urinary systems.

Scrotum

The **scrotum** consists of a pouch of skin and subcutaneous tissue that extends below the abdomen, posterior to the penis. An internal partition divides the scrotum into two compartments, each enclosing a testis. This partition protects each testis from possible infection from the other. Generally, the left testis is suspended lower than the right so the two are not compressed against each other between the thighs.[44] Each testis is also enclosed in a serous membrane so that it moves smoothly inside the scrotum.

The cremaster and dartos muscles of the scrotum react to temperature changes. When environmental temperatures are cold, the scrotum contracts and wrinkles, moving the testes closer to the pelvic cavity to absorb heat. When it is warmer outside, the scrotum relaxes and hangs loosely to ensure that the testes are about 38°F (3°C) lower than body temperature. This cooler temperature is better for the sperm cells to be produced and to survive.

Testes

The testes, or testicles, are part of the endocrine system because they produce testosterone, and also part of the male reproductive system because they produce sperm. About 2 months before birth or shortly thereafter, the oval-shaped testes typically descend from the pelvis into the scrotum. This descent occurs through the inguinal canal, which is an opening in the abdominal wall.

A testicular artery, which arises from the abdominal aorta just below the renal artery, supplies blood to each testis. The testes are served by the sympathetic and parasympathetic divisions of the ANS. In the testes, the ductus deferens, testicular artery and vein, lymphatic vessels, and nerve fibers compose the spermatic cord, which passes through the inguinal canal.

A tough, fibrous, white capsule surrounds each testis. This tissue extends inward, forming a partition that divides each testis into about 250 to 300 lobules. Each lobule contains up to four highly coiled seminiferous tubules. These tubules merge to form a straight tubule that leads to a tubular network called the rete testis. Efferent ductules connect the rete testis to the epididymis. Sperm cells are produced in the seminiferous tubules.

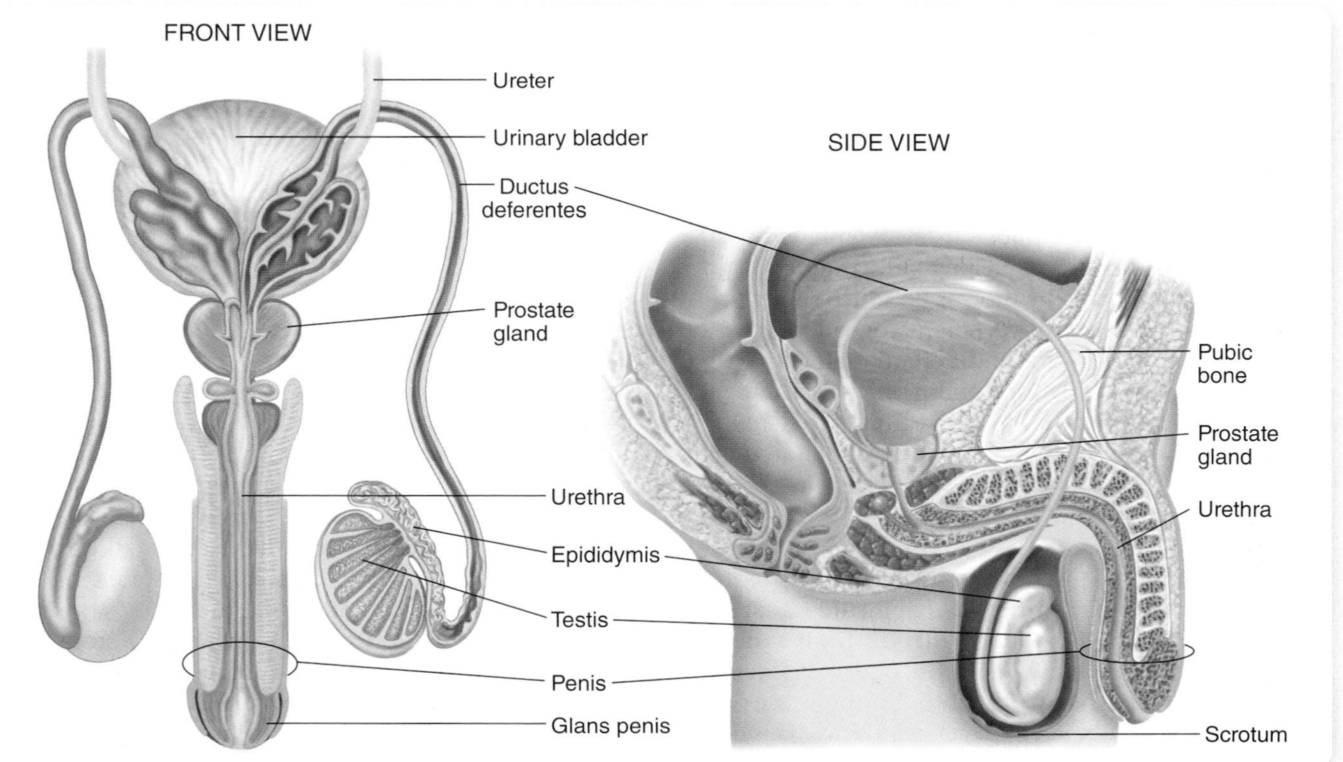

Figure 8-138 The male reproductive system.

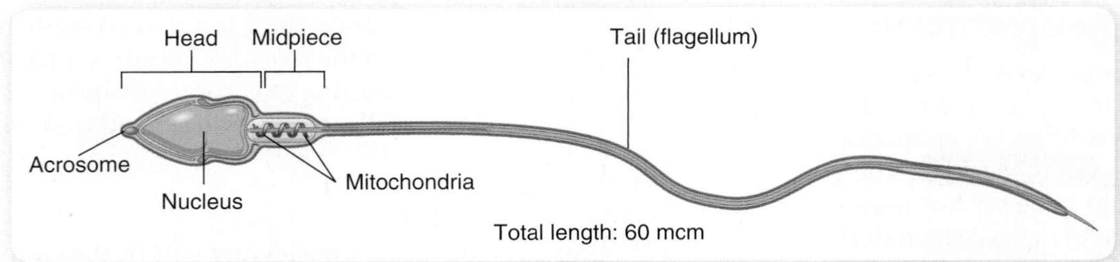

Figure 8-139 The mature sperm cell.

Between the seminiferous tubules are interstitial cells that secrete testosterone. Testosterone enlarges the testes and accessory reproductive organs, and develops the male secondary sex characteristics. These characteristics include the following:

- Increased body hair on the face, chest, armpits, and pubic region
- Decreased hair growth on the scalp (varies by individual)
- Enlargement of the larynx and thickening of the vocal folds, which lower the pitch of the voice
- Thickening of the skin
- Increased muscular growth, broadening of the shoulders, and narrowing of the waist
- Thickening and strengthening of the bones

Testosterone also increases cellular metabolism and the production of RBCs. The more testosterone received by the interstitial cells, the greater the speed at which the male secondary sex characteristics develop. A period in a man's life known as the male climacteric marks a decrease in testosterone level and a decline in sexual function.

Spermatogenesis. At puberty, testosterone levels increase and spermatozoa production begins. Each mature sperm cell appears like a tiny tadpole. It has a flattened head, a cylinder-shaped body, and a long tail Figure 8-139.

Spermatogenesis is the process by which sperm cells are formed. In a male embryo, spermatogenic cells (also called spermatogonia) are undifferentiated. They contain 46 chromosomes. During embryonic development, spermatogonia undergo mitosis, creating two daughter cells. One of these is a new "type A" spermatogonium that maintains supplies of undifferentiated cells; the other is a "type B" spermatogonium that enlarges to become a primary spermatocyte.

During puberty, primary spermatocytes reproduce via meiosis, a type of cell division that includes first and second meiotic divisions. It is different from mitosis, which is the process by which most body cells divide. Meiosis I (the first division) separates chromosome pairs that are homologous, meaning "gene for gene." This does not mean they are identical; genes may vary because of hereditary factors. Each homologous chromosome is replicated before meiosis I occurs, so it consists of two complete DNA strands (chromatids). These attach at areas called centromeres, and carry all the genetic information associated with that specific chromosome. Each of the four daughter cells produced have half as many chromosomes as a typical diploid body cell.

Meiosis II causes one member of each homologous pair to separate its chromatids. This produces other haploid cells (with one set of chromosomes), but with the chromosomes no longer in the replicated form. Meiosis II causes each of the chromatids to become an independent chromosome. Each primary spermatocyte divides into two secondary spermatocytes; these divide again to form two spermatids, which mature. For each primary spermatocyte that undergoes meiosis, four sperm cells, with 23 chromosomes in each of their nuclei, are formed Figure 8-140. The final part of spermatogenesis is called spermiogenesis, in which each spermatid matures into a single sperm or *spermatozoon*.[45]

Spermatic Ducts

To reach the outside of the body, sperm cells must first pass through a series of ducts. Sperm travel from the seminiferous tubules to the rete testes, to the efferent ductules, to the epididymis, to the ductus deferens, to the ejaculatory ducts, to the urethra, and finally to outside the body.[46]

Efferent Ductules. Efferent ductules are small tubes that carry sperm produced in the seminiferous tubules through the rete testis to reach the epididymis. These small ducts have clusters of ciliated cells that help to move the sperm through them.

Epididymis. Sperm cells mature in the epididymis. These epididymides are tightly coiled tubes that are connected to the posterior border of the testes. Each of them lie along the top, descend behind the testis, and then course upward to become the vas deferens. The epididymis can be felt through the skin of the scrotum.

The epididymis stores and protects spermatozoa and aids in their maturation. Immature sperm cells are nonmotile when they reach the epididymis; therefore, rhythmic peristaltic contractions move them through the duct as they mature. It takes about 20 days for sperm to travel from the head and body of the epididymis to the tail. Upon reaching the tail, the sperm are stored and

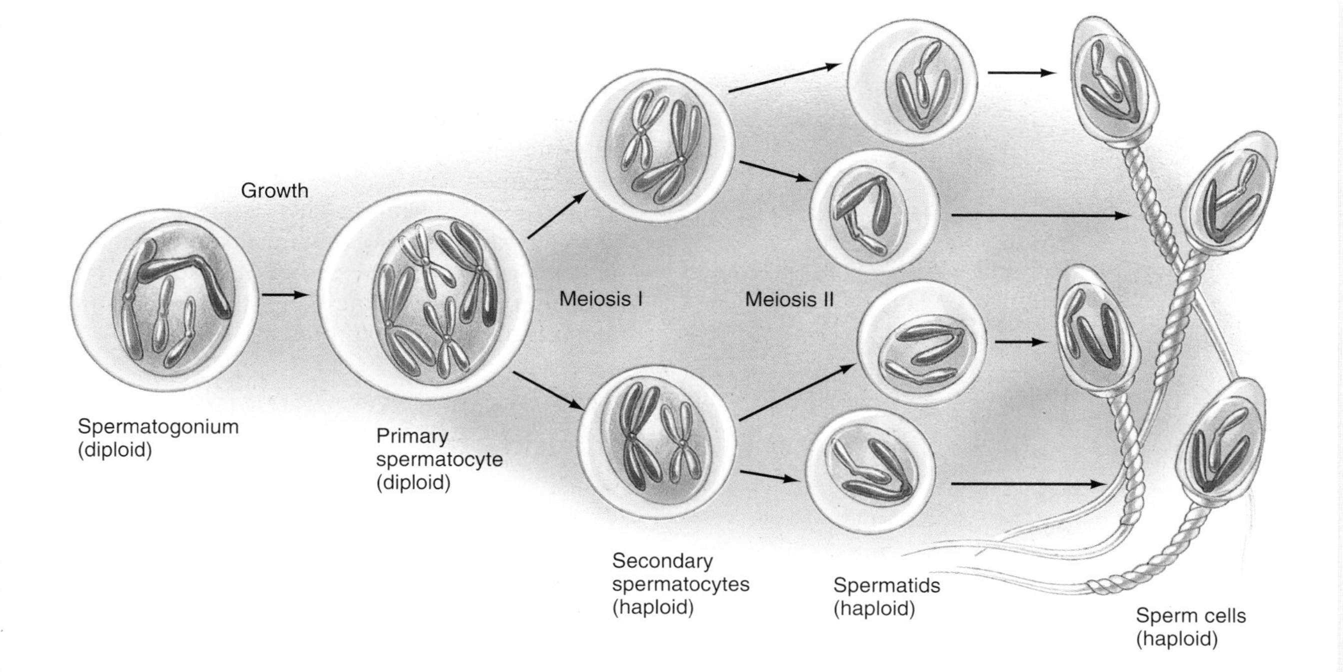

Figure 8-140 Meiosis.

remain viable for 40 to 60 days.[46] Once mature, sperm cells can move independently to fertilize egg cells, but usually do not "swim" until after ejaculation. Sperm that are not ejaculated disintegrate and are picked up by the epididymal blood vessels for reabsorption.

Ductus Deferens and Ejaculatory Duct. At the tail of each of the epididymides, the sperm duct turns 180 degrees and becomes the ductus deferentia. These muscular tubes pass upward along the medial side of the testes, through the spermatic cord and inguinal canal, and into the pelvic cavity. They end behind the urinary bladder, joining just outside the prostate gland with the duct of a seminal vesicle. This forms a short ejaculatory duct, passing through the prostate gland to empty into the urethra.

Male Accessory Glands

The seminal vesicles are a pair of saclike structures that attach to the ductus deferentia near the base of the urinary bladder. They have glandular tissue linings that contribute nearly 60% of semen volume (the fluid that the male urethra conveys to outside of the body during ejaculation). The seminal vesicles secrete a thick, yellow fluid. This fluid contains fructose and other carbohydrates that provide energy for sperm cells, a protein that helps semen stick to the vaginal walls, and PGs that stimulate muscular contractions within the female reproductive organs. These contractions aid the movement of sperm cells toward the egg cell. The secretions of the seminal vesicles are discharged into the ejaculatory duct at emission (when peristaltic contractions are occurring in the vas deferens, seminal vesicles, and prostate gland). These contractions are controlled by the sympathetic division of the ANS.

The prostate gland surrounds the proximal portion of the urethra, slightly inferior to the urinary bladder. It is composed of glandular tissue that produces a thin, white fluid that enhances the motility of sperm and a muscular portion that contracts during ejaculation to prevent urine flow. Prostatic fluid is alkaline, which helps to protect sperm from the acidic environment of the vagina.[46]

The bulbourethral glands lie inferior to the prostate gland surrounded by the fibers of the external urethral sphincter muscle. A short duct connects these glands with the penile portion of the urethra. During sexual arousal, a mucus-like, alkaline fluid is secreted that counteracts the acid present in the male urethra and female vagina. The fluid also lubricates the end of the penis to prepare for sexual intercourse.

Semen is made up of prostatic fluid (about 30%), seminal vesicle fluid (60%), and sperm (10%).[44] Semen has an alkaline pH between 7.2 and 8.0 and includes PGs and nutrients.[45] Between 2 and 5 mL of semen is released at one time, with between 20 and 150 million sperm per milliliter.[45] Sperm cells begin to swim as they mix with accessory gland secretions. They acquire the ability to fertilize a female egg cell once they are inside the female reproductive tract.

Penis

The **penis** is cylindrical in shape, and conveys urine and semen through the urethra. When erect, it stiffens and enlarges, enabling insertion into the vagina during sexual intercourse. The penis is divided into three regions: the

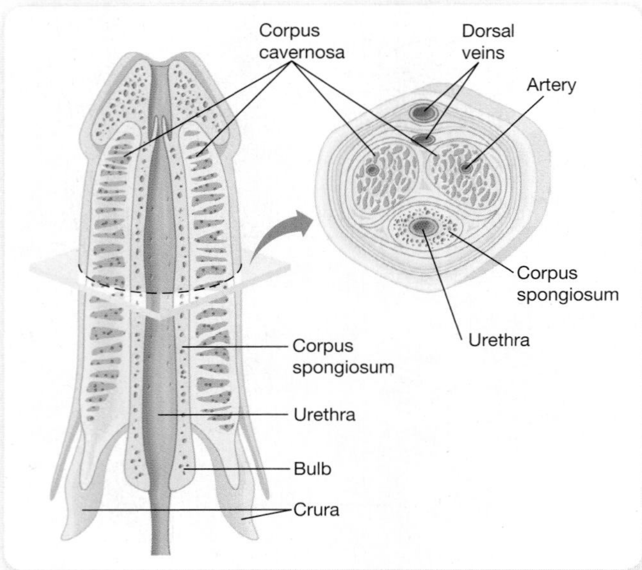

Figure 8-141 The penis.

root, body, and glans. The root of the penis is the fixed portion that attaches the penis to the body wall. The shaft (or body) of the penis is the tubular, movable portion of the organ. It contains three columns of erectile tissue Figure 8-141. Dense connective tissue surrounds each column in a capsule. The penis is enclosed by a layer of connective tissue, a thin layer of subcutaneous tissue, and skin.

The glans penis is the expanded distal end of the penis that surrounds the external urethral orifice. This structure covers the ends of the corpora cavernosa and opens as the external urethral orifice. Skin in this area is thin and hairless, with sensory receptors for sexual stimulation. Boys are born with a loose fold of skin called the foreskin (prepuce) that extends to cover the glans, as a sheath. It is often removed soon after birth by a surgical procedure called circumcision.

When sexual arousal occurs, parasympathetic nerve fibers trigger the local release of nitric oxide. This release results in relaxation of the smooth muscle in the walls of the penile blood vessels and dilation of local arterioles leading into the penis. As the erectile tissue expands with blood, the penis swells and elongates to produce an erection.

Physiologic and emotional release, known as an orgasm, is the culmination of sexual stimulation. Male orgasm is accompanied by emission and ejaculation. During emission, sperm cells from the testes, along with secretions of the prostate gland and seminal vesicles, are moved into the urethra. Emission occurs as a result of sympathetic nerve impulses that stimulate peristaltic contractions in the testicular ducts, epididymides, ductus deferentia, and ejaculatory ducts. Other sympathetic impulses simultaneously cause rhythmic contractions of the seminal vesicles and prostate gland. The urethra fills with semen as sensory impulses pass into the sacral portion of the spinal cord. Somatic motor impulses are then transmitted to certain skeletal muscles, causing rhythmic contractions of the penile erectile columns. This process increases pressure inside the erectile tissues, helping to force semen through the urethra to outside of the body (ejaculation).

Fluid from the bulbourethral glands is expelled first during emission and ejaculation, followed by fluid from the prostate gland, passage of sperm cells, and lastly, fluid from the seminal vesicles. After ejaculation, the arteries of the erectile tissue immediately constrict. Smooth muscles in the vascular spaces contract partially, and veins of the penis carry away excess blood, gradually returning the penis to its flaccid state. Table 8-43 summarizes the functions of the male reproductive structures.

▶ Female Reproductive Anatomy

The female reproductive organs consist of two ovaries, two uterine (fallopian) tubes, the uterus (womb), the **cervix**, the vagina (birth canal), the mammary glands, and the external genitalia Figure 8-142. The ovaries are the essential organs of the female reproductive system because they produce the female gametes. The uterine tubes, uterus, vagina, mammary glands, and external genitalia are considered accessory organs.

Ovaries

The ovaries are solid structures that are about the size and shape of an unshelled almond. They are positioned in the lateral wall of the pelvic cavity in shallow depressions on each side of the uterus. The ovaries perform three main functions: (1) production of immature female gametes (oocytes), (2) secretion of female sex hormones (including estrogens and progestins), and (3) secretion of inhibin.

The ovaries are suspended in the pelvic cavity by ligaments. They receive their blood supply from the ovarian artery, which runs alongside the ovarian ligament, and the ovarian branch of the uterine artery. Each ovary has an outer cortex and an inner portion called the ovarian medulla. Within the cortex are small follicles. Each follicle contains an oocyte, the female germ cell. Each month, during the menstrual cycle, about 20 of these follicles begin the process of maturation, but only a single follicle ultimately matures and releases an ovum. The remaining follicles die off and are reabsorbed by the body.

Oogenesis. During fetal development, diploid (46 chromosomes) germ cells in the ovaries differentiate into oogonia, which are cells that have the potential to develop into ova. Although many oogonia die, those that survive enter a growth phase, enlarge, and become primary oocytes. The primary oocytes begin to undergo meiosis early in development, but then the process stops and does not restart until puberty.

Oogenesis is the process of oocyte formation, which begins at puberty under the influence of FSH. During this time, some primary oocytes continue meiosis, with each primary oocyte producing two daughter cells—a

Table 8-43 Male Reproductive Structures

Structure	Function
Scrotum	Regulates the temperature of the testes by enclosing and protecting them
Testis	Interstitial cells produce and secrete sex hormones; seminiferous tubules produce sperm cells
Epididymis	Stores and protects spermatozoa and aids in their maturation
Ductus deferens	Transfers sperm cells to the ejaculatory duct
Seminal vesicle	Secrete fluid that contains carbohydrates that provide energy for sperm cells, a protein that helps semen stick to the vaginal walls, and PGs that stimulate muscular contractions within the female reproductive organs
Prostate gland	Secretes an alkaline fluid that helps to protect sperm from the acidic environment of the vagina
Bulbourethral gland	Secretes fluid into the penile urethra that counteracts the acid present in the male urethra and female vagina
Penis	Copulatory organ that surrounds the urethra and introduces semen into the female vagina; also part of the urinary system.

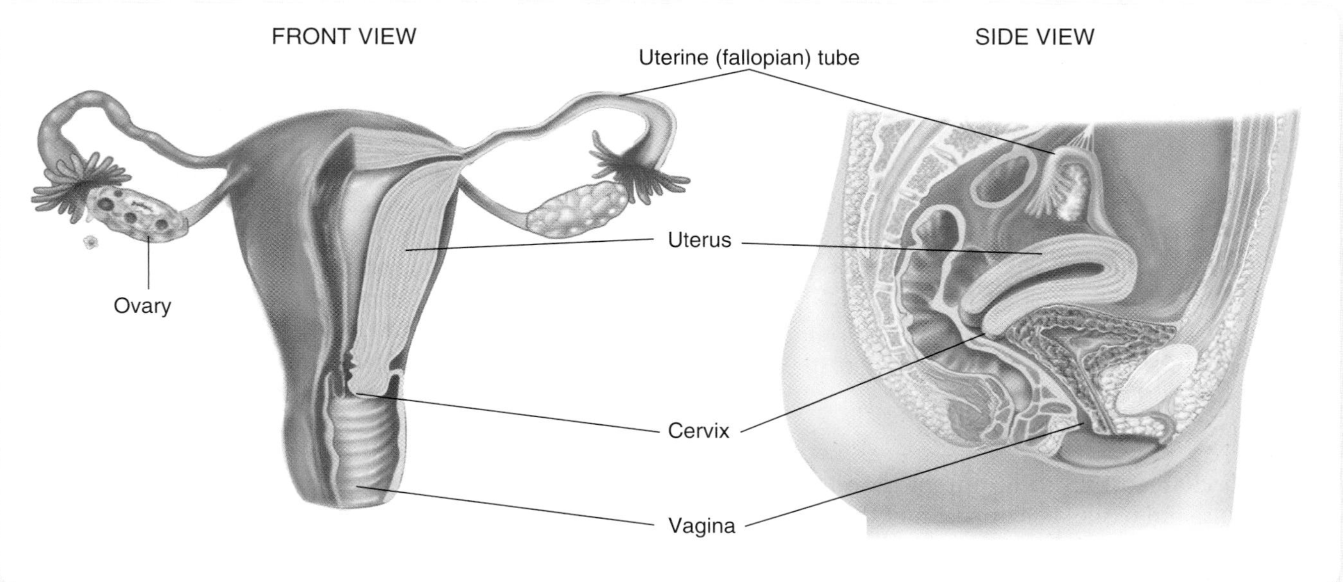

Figure 8-142 The female reproductive system.

secondary oocyte and a first polar body **Figure 8-143**. The secondary oocyte is large and contains 23 chromosomes, cytoplasm, and organelles. The first polar body is small, containing 23 chromosomes but lacking cytoplasm and organelles. The large secondary oocyte can be fertilized by a sperm cell. Because the first polar body is not a functional oocyte, it degenerates and dies. If fertilization of the secondary oocyte occurs, then it divides unequally, producing a tiny second polar body and a large fertilized egg cell (zygote). If fertilization does not occur, then the secondary oocyte deteriorates and is expelled from the uterus, with its second polar body, during menstruation.

The Menstrual Cycle. Also called the menses, period, or menstrual cycle, **menstruation** is the cyclic and periodic

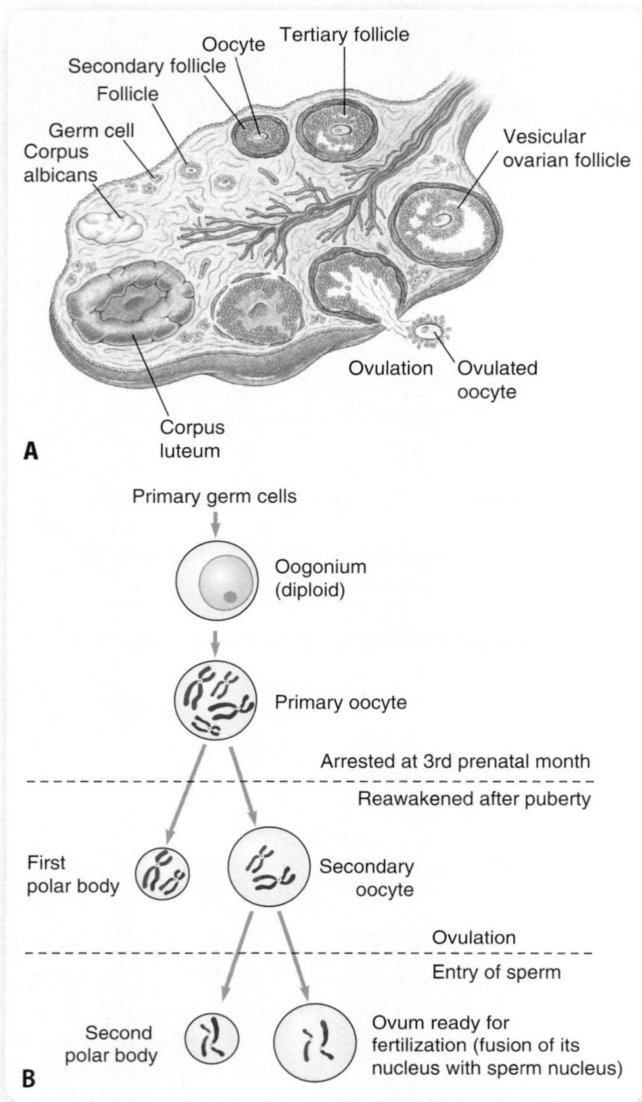

Figure 8-143 Ovarian follicle development and oogenesis. **A.** Secretion from the ovary. **B.** Differentiation of the oocyte.

vaginal discharge of 25 to 65 mL of blood, epithelial cells, mucus, and tissue. The duration of the cycle differs from woman to woman, ranging from an average of 24 days to 35 days. The onset of the first menses, when a girl reaches childbearing age, is called **menarche**. Depending on genetics, socioeconomic factors, and individual health, this event may take place anywhere between the ages of 11 and 14 years. The last menses, when a woman has reached the end of childbearing age, is called **menopause** or the female climacteric. The advent of menopause typically begins between the ages of 40 and 50 years, with menstrual cycles becoming less frequent.

The menstrual cycle is composed of two phases, the ovarian cycle (ovarian changes) and the uterine cycle (changes in the uterus). The ovarian and uterine cycles are linked; that is, events that occur in the ovarian cycle affect those of the uterine cycle.

The ovarian cycle is divided into the follicular phase (days 1 to 13) and the luteal phase (days 14 to 28). Secretion of gonadotropin releasing factor from the hypothalamus stimulates the release of FSH and LH from the anterior pituitary gland. FSH stimulates ovarian follicles to develop and to secrete estrogen and some progesterone. LH stimulates some ovarian cells to secrete hormones such as testosterone, which is used to produce estrogen. As the follicular phase of the menstrual cycle progresses, peak levels of estrogen and LH cause the mature ovarian follicle to rupture and release its oocyte. This process is called **ovulation**. The term ovum (plural: ova) is used after ovulation has occurred.

The luteal phase of the ovarian cycle occurs during days 14 to 28. This is the time from when the oocyte is released from the ovary (ovulation) until the first day of menstruation. LH continues to be excreted throughout the ovarian cycle and subsequent pregnancy, should it occur. What is left of the follicle after the egg has been released becomes the corpus luteum, which in turn secretes estrogen, progesterone, and inhibin. All three hormones inhibit secretion of FSH from the anterior pituitary gland, thereby preventing the further development of follicles. If the egg is fertilized, then the corpus luteum will continue to secrete hormones to support the pregnancy for 90 days. If fertilization does not occur, then the corpus luteum gradually shrinks, turns white, stops secreting hormones, and is gradually absorbed into the tissue of the ovary.

The uterine cycle is divided into the proliferative phase (days 5 to 14) and the secretory phase (days 15 to 28). The proliferative phase is the time after menstruation and before the next ovulation occurs. During this phase, in response to the estrogen released by the follicle, the uterine lining (endometrium) increases in thickness in preparation to receive a fertilized oocyte. The time after ovulation until menstruation is the secretory phase. During this phase, the uterine lining continues to thicken. After ovulation, the corpus luteum mainly secretes progesterone, which stimulates glands in the uterine lining to secrete glycogen, a nutritional source for a fertilized egg. If fertilization does not occur, then estrogen and progesterone levels decrease and the thick lining of the uterus is shed from the woman's body. Based on a 28-day cycle, the menstrual phase (discharge) lasts about 5 days **Figure 8-144**.

The female body undergoes many major changes during pregnancy, including development of the placenta, umbilical cord, and of course, the fetus. These changes, as well as fetal circulation, fetal respiration, stages of labor, and physiologic changes in the infant after birth, are covered in Chapter 41, *Obstetrics*, and in Chapter 42, *Neonatal Care*.

Uterine Tubes

The uterine tubes (fallopian tubes or oviducts) open near the ovaries, and are each about 4 inches (10 cm) long. They pass medially to the uterus, penetrating its wall, and opening into the uterine cavity. Normally, there is one uterine tube associated with each ovary. When the oocyte

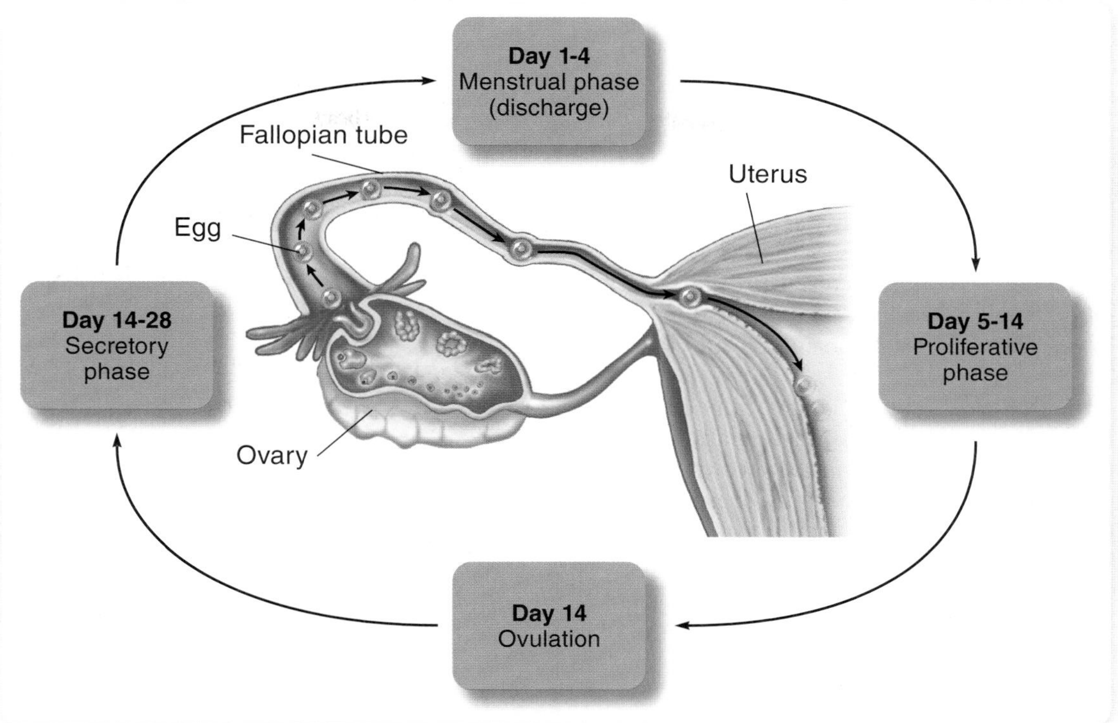

Figure 8-144 The menstrual cycle, based on an average 28-day cycle. The length of the cycle and number of days in each phase vary from woman to woman, but generally fall within a range of 24 to 35 days.

is released, it travels through the fallopian tube to the uterus. The fertilization of the oocyte by a sperm usually occurs when the oocyte is inside the fallopian tube. The fertilized oocyte then continues to the uterus, where it continues to develop into an embryo (early stages of the fetus) and implants into the wall of the uterus.

Each uterine tube extends out laterally from the uterus, terminating just short of an ovary. The proximal end of each fallopian tube is very thick and narrow and connects to the uterus itself. Each uterine tube is composed of three layers of tissue. The outer layer consists of a serous membrane that protects the tubes. The middle layer is made of smooth muscle that contracts to help move the ovum through the tube and into the uterus. The innermost layer contains secretory cells and cilia that also move the ovum along and may also play a part in providing nutrition to the ovum.

In summary, when an ovary releases an egg, the ciliary motion sweeps the egg into the uterine tube. Smooth muscle contractions and the inner mucosa move the ovum through the tube to the uterus. If the egg encounters a sperm cell along the way, then it may become fertilized. Fertilization can occur at any time within about a 24-hour window after ovulation.

Uterus

The uterus (womb) is the organ where the embryo grows. It is responsible for contractions during labor and ultimately helps to push the newborn, placenta, and membranes through the birth canal at delivery. The uterus is hollow and muscular, shaped slightly like an inverted pear. It is located in the anterior pelvic cavity and lies between the urinary bladder and the rectum. The dome-shaped top of the uterus is the fundus. Below the dome, the uterus begins to taper and narrow, forming the body. The narrowest portion of the uterus (the cervix), opens into the vagina. The interior of the body of the uterus is the uterine cavity, and the interior of the cervix is the **cervical canal**.

The uterine wall is thick, with three layers of tissue: the perimetrium (outer protective layer), the myometrium (middle layer), and the endometrium (inner lining). The myometrium is composed of three layers of muscle fibers; the contractions of these muscles help expel the fetus during childbirth. The endometrium is a mucouvs membrane composed of two layers; the layer innermost to the uterine cavity, is shed during menstruation. As the follicle starts developing and pumping out estrogen, the endometrium is stimulated to increase its thickness in preparation for the reception and future growth of a fertilized egg.

Vagina

The vagina is a distensible muscular structure lined with mucous membranes. It extends from the cervix to the outside of the body. The functions of the vagina include the following: (1) serves as a passageway for the elimination of menstrual fluids, (2) receives the penis during sexual intercourse, (3) holds the spermatozoa before their passage into the uterus, and (4) serves as the passageway for childbirth.

The interior of the vagina is acidic owing to the breakdown of glycogen (found in large amounts in the vaginal mucosa), which creates a low-pH environment that inhibits bacterial growth. This acidity, while beneficial, is injurious to sperm cells. Semen is alkaline in nature and likewise has antibacterial properties. The alkalinity of seminal fluid neutralizes the acidity of the vagina, allowing the sperm cells to survive and fertilize the ovum.

Just inside the lower vagina are two tiny openings that lead to the Bartholin glands. These glands secrete mucus that acts as a lubricant during intercourse. Before first sexual intercourse, the vaginal orifice is protected by the hymen. This membrane, made up of connective tissue and epithelium, forms a border around the vaginal orifice, partially enclosing it. It has a central opening that allows uterine and vaginal secretions to pass to the outside of the body.

Breasts and Mammary Glands

The breasts, located above the pectoralis major muscles, extend from the second to the sixth ribs, from the sternum to the axillae. Each breast is mainly composed of adipose tissue and collagen. The main purpose of the mammary glands, which are modified sweat glands housed within the breasts, is lactation (milk secretion) to provide nourishment to the newborn. Milk is carried to the surface of each breast through lactiferous ducts that terminate in a nipple. The nipple of the breast is surrounded by a darker pigmented area called the areola. Prolactin, an anterior pituitary hormone, stimulates milk production. Oxytocin, from the posterior pituitary, stimulates ejection of milk into the ducts of the mammary glands.

External Genitalia

The female external genitalia, collectively called the vulva or pudendum, are the structures seen from the outside of the body **Figure 8-145**. The mons pubis is an anatomic landmark that is a rounded pad of adipose tissue that overlies the symphysis pubis, located anterior to the urethral and vaginal openings. Coarse, dark hair normally appears here in early puberty, becoming sparser later in life with the advent of menopause. The **labia majora** and **labia minora**, described as "lips," surround and protect the vaginal opening together with the more anterior opening of the urethra. The labia majora are covered with pubic hair, but the labia minora are not. The area between the vaginal opening and the anus is called the perineum. The clitoris is located at the anterior junction of the labia minora, just below a layer of skin called the prepuce. The clitoris is a small, cylindrical mass of erectile tissue and nerves that is similar to the glans penis of the male.

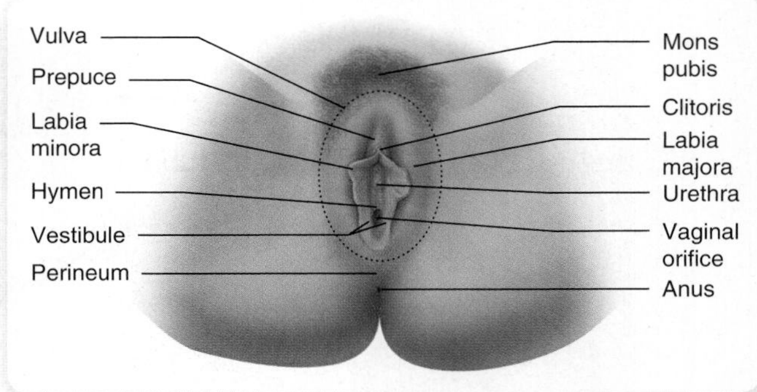

Figure 8-145 The female external genitalia.

Between the labia minora is a cleft referred to as the **vestibule**. Located within the vestibule is the urethral opening (orifice), the vaginal opening, and the hymen. One vestibular gland lies on each side of the vaginal opening. The urethra, which leads to the bladder, allows for passage of urine. The length of the urethra in females averages about 1.6 inches (4 cm). This short length is one reason why women are more prone than men to urinary tract infections and bladder infections.

The erectile tissues of the clitoris and vaginal entrance respond to sexual stimulation. Parasympathetic nerve impulses release nitric oxide to dilate the erectile tissues, increase blood flow, and swell the tissues. The vagina expands and elongates. If sexual stimulation is sufficiently intense, then parasympathetic impulses cause the vestibular glands to secrete mucus into the vestibule, moistening and lubricating the surrounding tissues and lower vagina. This facilitates insertion of the penis. The clitoris responds to local stimulation, culminating in an orgasm if stimulation is sufficient. Just before orgasm, the outer one-third of the vagina is engorged with blood. This increases friction on the penis, with orgasm initiating reflexes directed by the sacral and lumbar spinal cord. The muscles of the perineum and walls of both the uterus and uterine tubes contract rhythmically. This contraction helps transport sperm through the female reproductive tract toward the upper uterine tubes. **Table 8-44** summarizes the functions of the female reproductive structures.

Table 8-44 Female Reproductive Structures

Structure	Function
Ovary (ovaries)	The female reproductive organ that produces oocytes and sex hormones
Uterine (fallopian) tubes	Transports secondary oocytes in the direction of the uterus; fertilization occurs here, with the developing embryo conveyed to the uterus
Uterus	The muscular organ of the female reproductive tract, in which implantation, placenta formation, and fetal development occur
Vagina	Transports uterine secretions to outside of the body, receives the erect penis during intercourse; the fully developed fetus passes through the vagina during normal delivery
Labia majora	Protects and encloses the external reproductive organs
Labia minora	Protects the openings of the vagina and urethra
Clitoris	Gives pleasurable sensations during sexual stimulation
Vestibule	Contains the vaginal and urethral openings
Vestibular glands	Moisten and lubricate the vestibule with a secretion

YOU are the Paramedic SUMMARY

1. What anatomic areas of the motorcyclist's body may be injured as a result of this collision?

Possible areas of injury include the face, skull, brain, thoracic cavity, pelvis, limbs, and spine.

2. Which anatomic areas of the motorcyclist's body may have life-threatening injuries in this scenario?

Possible areas of the body that may have life-threatening injuries include the brain, the airway, the pelvis, the femurs, and the mediastinum.

3. Given the broken upper teeth and facial swelling, what body structures may have been injured?

Structures that may have been injured include the maxilla (upper jaw) and zygomas (cheekbones).

4. What is the best way to describe the location of the injury on the left chest?

The patient has an injury to the superior chest at the left midclavicular line.

5. What is the best way to describe the location of the deformity and injury on the right leg?

The patient has a deformity and a laceration just proximal to the right medial malleolus.

6. What is the obvious injury you find to the patient's chest?

The patient has an injury to the left anterior ribs.

7. What are the potential hidden injuries you should consider?

Because there is obvious injury to the patient's chest, you must also suspect internal injuries to the underlying structures, such as the heart and great vessels, and abdominal organs. Also, the findings of unequal chest rise and fall, as well as a grating sensation, indicate that the patient has a substantial injury, as you will learn in later chapters.

YOU are the Paramedic SUMMARY *(continued)*

8. What structures are located in the lower abdominal quadrants?

The large and small intestine, bladder, and (in women) ovaries and uterus are located in the lower abdominal quadrants.

9. What might the instability of the pelvis indicate?

This finding suggests a pelvic fracture and the potential for significant internal bleeding. Knowledge of anatomy, physiology, and signs/symptoms of internal injury will be the key to treating your patient.

EMS Patient Care Report (PCR)

Date: 04-02-18	**Incident No.:** 245	**Nature of Call:** MVC	**Location:** N/B I-95 @ county line		
Dispatched: 1430	**En Route:** 1430	**At Scene:** 1440	**Transport:** 1450	**At Hospital:** 1507	**In Service:** 1515

Patient Information

Age: 22 **Sex:** M **Weight (in kg [lb]):** 91 kg (200 lb)	**Allergies:** Unknown **Medications:** Unknown **Past Medical History:** Unknown **Chief Complaint:** Unresponsive from MVC

Vital Signs

Time: 1443	**BP:** Not yet obtained	**Pulse:** 118	**Respirations:** 24	**Spo_2:** Not yet obtained
Time: 1445	**BP:** 106/70	**Pulse:** 120	**Respirations:** 24	**Spo_2:** 90% (ambient air)
Time: 1453	**BP:** 102/66	**Pulse:** 118	**Respirations:** 24	**Spo_2:** 97% (assisted with bag-mask device)

EMS Treatment (circle all that apply)

Oxygen @ 15 **L/min via (circle one):** **NC** **NRM** **(Bag-mask device)**		**(Assisted Ventilation)**	**Airway Adjunct**	**CPR**
Defibrillation	**Bleeding Control**	**Bandaging**	**Splinting**	**Other:**

Narrative

Crew dispatched to truck versus motorcycle crash. While traveling at highway speeds, motorcycle struck front bumper of a stationary pickup, pushing truck back 10 feet (3 m). Motorcyclist was ejected from bike, collided with truck windshield, then rolled to the ground. On arrival, found pt unresponsive, lying prone on the pavement. Pt's spine immobilized manually immediately and patient logrolled onto his back. Pt placed in full spinal immobilization per protocol. Physical exam revealed missing upper front teeth with dried blood present, bilateral swelling of the orbital tissue, and an abrasion to superior chest at left midclavicular line. Instability and grating of anterior chest noted on palpation. Unequal chest rise and fall. Bilateral rigidity of lower abdominal quadrants. Palpation of pelvis revealed instability and grinding. Deformity and laceration present just proximal to the right medial malleolus. Pt remains unresponsive. Vital signs as noted above. Ventilations assisted with bag-mask device. Pt condition remained unchanged during transport to Regional Trauma Center. Reported on arrival to Dr. Warren.**End of report**

Prep Kit

▶ Ready for Review

- To care for your patients properly, you must have a thorough understanding of human anatomy and physiology, as well as homeostasis, so you can assess the patient's condition and communicate with hospital personnel and other health care providers.
- To achieve the functions necessary for life, the body is organized by levels. Levels of organization, from least complex to most complex, include chemical, cellular, tissue, organ, organ system, and the organism as a whole.
- If you understand the basics of chemistry, then your understanding of anatomy and physiology will be improved. Chemical changes within cells influence body functions and the status of the body's structures.
- Chemicals can basically be divided into two main groups: organic and inorganic. Organic substances include carbohydrates, lipids, proteins, and nucleic acids. Inorganic substances in body cells include oxygen, carbon dioxide, compounds that are known as salts, and water.
- Chemical reactions occur in the body; an enzyme is often involved. Individual cells are supplied the nutrients and use them in various processes. As a result of cellular metabolism, organisms grow, maintain body functions, release or store energy, produce and eliminate waste, digest nutrients, or destroy toxins. These reactions alter the chemical nature of a chemical substance, maintaining homeostasis.
- Body functions also often require electrolytes. Important ions for bodily functions include sodium, potassium, calcium, magnesium, bicarbonate, chloride, and phosphorus.
- Another important concept is acid-base balance. Abnormal fluctuations in pH level can cause damage to cells, tissues, and proteins. The buffer system of the body helps neutralize excessive acids or bases.
- Cells are the foundation of the human body. Cells with a common job grow close to each other and are called tissues. Groups of tissues that all perform interrelated jobs form organs.
- The life cycle of a cell is regulated via stimulation from hormones or growth factors. The life of a cell includes interphase, cell division or mitosis, cytoplasmic division, and differentiation. Cell division and growth that occur at a rate higher than cell death is cancer. Tumors can be benign or malignant.
- Cellular respiration is a process that releases energy from organic compounds. It occurs in three stages: glycolysis, the Krebs cycle, and the electron transport chain. The result is molecules of adenosine triphosphate, in which energy is stored.
- Cell transport mechanisms, or how materials enter and exit cells, relates to maintenance of fluid quantity and distribution. Several mechanisms, such as diffusion, filtration, osmosis, facilitated diffusion, osmosis, active transport, endocytosis, and exocytosis allow material to pass through the cell wall.
- The human body is primarily made up of four major types of tissue: epithelial, connective, muscle, and nervous tissues. Tissue results from the process of differentiation, the process by which the cell becomes specialized for a specific purpose.
- Membranes form a barrier or an interface. The four types of membranes are serous membranes, mucous membranes, cutaneous membranes, and synovial membranes.
- Homeostasis is the adaptive process by which cells and tissues respond to preserve equilibrium. Cellular signaling—electrochemical communication between cells—triggers chemical reactions needed to maintain homeostasis. Feedback occurs to stop the reaction once it is no longer needed.
- Organ systems include the integumentary, skeletal, muscular, nervous, endocrine, circulatory, lymphatic, immune, respiratory, digestive, urinary, and genital systems.
- The integumentary system is the interface between the body and the outside world and includes the skin, hair, nails, sebaceous glands, and sweat glands. Its functions include protection, temperature regulation, fluid regulation, sensation, and inflammatory response.
- The skin is divided into two parts: the superficial epidermis, which is composed of several layers of cells including the germinal layer and the stratum corneal layer, and the deeper dermis, which contains the specialized skin structures such as sweat glands, sebaceous (oil) glands, nails, hair follicles, blood vessels, and specialized nerve endings.
- Subcutaneous tissue is below the skin and is composed largely of fat, serving as an insulator for the body and as a reservoir to store energy. The subcutaneous layer also helps to anchor the skin to the structures beneath it.
- The skeleton gives the body its recognizable human form through a collection of bones, ligaments,

Prep Kit *(continued)*

tendons, and cartilage. Functions of the skeletal system include support, leverage, protection, storage, maintenance of calcium levels, and blood cell production.

- Bones are classified according to their shape, as long bones, short bones, flat bones, and irregular bones. The bones increase greatly in size as the fetus develops and throughout adolescence.
- A joint is where two bones come into contact. Joints are classified as immovable (synarthrotic), slightly moveable (amphiarthrotic), or freely movable (diarthrotic). Most joints allow motion (knee, hip, elbow), and some bones fuse with one another at joints to form a solid, immobile, bony structure (skull). The 230 joints in the human body are categorized as fibrous, cartilaginous, or synovial.
- The axial skeleton forms the foundation on which the arms and legs are hung. The appendicular skeleton consists of the arms and legs, their connection points, and the pelvis.
- The five sections of the spine are as follows: the cervical spine, thoracic spine, lumbar spine, sacrum, and coccyx.
- The contraction and relaxation of the musculoskeletal system gives the body its ability to move. Skeletal muscle, so named because it attaches to the bones of the skeleton, forms the major muscle mass of the body. It is also called voluntary muscle, because all skeletal muscle is under direct voluntary control.
- The nervous system is perhaps the most complex organ system within the human body. It consists of the brain, spinal cord, and nerves.
- The nervous system is responsible for fundamental functions such as controlling breathing, heart rate, and blood pressure. This system also allows the performance of higher-level activity, such as memory, understanding, and thought.
- The nervous system is divided into the central nervous system (CNS) and the peripheral nervous system (PNS). The CNS includes the brain and the spinal cord. The somatic nervous system is the part of the PNS that regulates activities over which there is voluntary control, such as walking, talking, and writing. The autonomic nervous system (ANS) is the part of the PNS that controls the many body functions that occur without voluntary control such as digestion, dilation and constriction of blood vessels, and sweating.
- The ANS is split into two areas. The sympathetic nervous system is responsible for fight-or-flight response, and the parasympathetic nervous system is responsible for conserving energy and maintaining organ function, including digestion, growth, healing, and the removal of toxins.
- The endocrine system is made up of various glands located throughout the body. Major endocrine glands include the pituitary gland, the thyroid gland, the parathyroid glands, the adrenal glands, the pancreas, the thymus gland, and reproductive glands.
- The hypothalamus serves as the communication center between the nervous and endocrine systems.
- Endocrine glands help regulate metabolism, control chemical reactions, transport substances, regulate water and electrolyte balances, and aid in reproduction, growth, and development.
- The circulatory system is a complex arrangement of connected tubes, including the arteries, arterioles, capillaries, venules, and veins.
- Blood consists of plasma and formed elements or cells that are suspended in the plasma. These cells include red blood cells (erythrocytes), white blood cells (leukocytes), and platelets (thrombocytes).
- Blood has many functions including fighting infection, transporting oxygen and carbon dioxide, controlling pH, transporting wastes and nutrients, and clotting.
- Cardiac muscle has the property of automaticity; it can generate and conduct electricity without influence from the brain.
- The cardiac cycle begins with myocardial contraction and concludes at the beginning of the next contraction. The contraction of the heart results in pressure changes within the cardiac chambers, resulting in the movement of blood from areas of high pressure to areas of low pressure.
- The pressure in the aorta against which the left ventricle must pump blood is called the afterload. The greater the afterload, the harder it is for the ventricle to eject blood into the aorta. This reduces the stroke volume—the amount of blood ejected per contraction.
- Cardiac output is the amount of blood pumped through the circulatory system in 1 minute. Cardiac output is expressed in liters per minute (L/min). The cardiac output equals the heart rate multiplied by the stroke volume.
- Increased venous return to the heart stretches the ventricles, resulting in increased cardiac contractility. This relationship is known as the Frank-Starling mechanism.

Prep Kit *(continued)*

- The lymphatic system helps maintain fluid balance in the body, fight infection by producing and circulating lymphocytes, and distribute various products unable to enter the bloodstream directly (such as nutrients and some hormones). The spleen is the body's largest lymphatic organ.
- The immune system is composed of lymphoid tissues and cells involved in immune response. The body's defense mechanisms work together to resist disease, illness, and infection.
- The respiratory system consists of all the structures of the body that contribute to the process of breathing. It includes the nose, mouth, throat, larynx, trachea, bronchi, and bronchioles. The system also includes the lungs, diaphragm, the muscles of the chest wall, and the accessory muscles of breathing.
- The primary function of the respiratory system is to conduct respiration. Oxygen is essential for the body to function. Gas exchange of oxygen into the blood and carbon dioxide out of the blood occurs at the alveoli of the lungs via diffusion.
- The respiratory center in the brainstem controls breathing. Nerves in this area sense the level of carbon dioxide in the blood and spinal fluid. The brain adjusts breathing as needed if the level of carbon dioxide or oxygen in the arterial blood is too high or too low.
- Increases in the level of carbon dioxide in the blood ($Paco_2$) cause decreased pH levels in the respiratory center, which triggers an increase in ventilation. Decreases in the $Paco_2$ result in increased pH levels in the respiratory center and a decrease in ventilation.
- Hypoxic drive is a backup system the body uses to control respiration. Areas in the brain, walls of the aorta, and carotid arteries act as oxygen sensors and stimulate breathing if the oxygen level falls.
- The functions of the digestive system consist of a series of steps, which include ingestion, mechanical processing, digestion, secretion, absorption, and excretion.
- The alimentary canal extends from the mouth to the anus. It includes the mouth, pharynx, esophagus, stomach, small intestine, large intestine, rectum, and anus. The accessory organs of the alimentary canal include the teeth, tongue, salivary glands, liver, gallbladder, and pancreas.
- The main functions of the urinary system are to control fluid balance in the body, to filter and eliminate wastes, and to control pH balance.
- In the urinary system, the kidneys are solid organs; the ureters, bladder, and urethra are hollow organs.
- The kidneys rid the blood of toxic waste products and control its balance of water and salt.
- The male and female reproductive systems contain organs and glands that create sex cells and transport them to areas where fertilization can occur.
- Chromosomes contain the entire sequence of genetic information the organism will have throughout its entire life. This genetic information contains the instructions for every structure and process in the body. They also contain sequences that will determine or influence various characteristics such as hair color, skin color, body composition, height, and predisposition to certain diseases.
- The primary sex organs (gonads) of the male consist of the two testes, in which sperm cells and male sex hormones are formed. The testes are considered part of both the endocrine system and part of the male reproductive system because they produce testosterone (a hormone) and sperm.
- Testosterone enlarges the testes and accessory reproductive organs, and develops the male secondary sex characteristics. These characteristics include increased amount of body hair; enlargement of the larynx and thickening of vocal folds, which lowers the pitch of the voice; thickening of the skin; increased muscular growth; and thickening and strengthening of bones.
- The female reproductive organs produce and maintain the oocytes (eggs), which are the female sex cells.
- The primary sex organs (gonads) of the female are the two ovaries, which reproduce female sex cells and sex hormones.
- In nonpregnant females, the ovaries are the main source of estrogens, and they secrete increasing amounts of estrogens beginning at puberty. These hormones stimulate enlargement of accessory sex organs and develop and maintain the female secondary sex characteristics including development of breasts and mammary gland systems.
- The female reproductive cycle involves regular, recurring changes in the uterine lining as well as menstrual bleeding (menses).

▶ Vital Vocabulary

ABO system The commonly used blood classification system, based on the antigens present or absent in the blood.

accessory muscles The muscles not normally used during quiet breathing; examples include the

Prep Kit *(continued)*

sternocleidomastoid muscles of the neck, the chest pectoralis major muscles, and the abdominal muscles.

accommodation The ability of the lens of the eye to change its shape to focus on a close object.

acetabulum The socket formed by the coxal (hip) bone into which the ball-shaped femoral head fits snugly.

acetylcholine (ACh) A neurotransmitter released at synapses within the autonomic nervous system and by motor neurons to stimulate skeletal muscle contraction.

acetylcholinesterase An enzyme found in the central nervous system, in red blood cells, and in motor endplates of skeletal muscle that causes the decomposition of acetylcholine.

acid Any molecule that can give up a hydrogen ion, and therefore increases the concentration of hydrogen ions in a water solution.

acidosis A pathologic condition resulting from the accumulation of acids in the body (blood pH less than 7.35).

acromion process The tip of the shoulder and the site of attachment for the clavicle and various shoulder muscles.

action potential Sequence of changes in the membrane potential that occurs when an excitable cell (neuron or muscle) is stimulated.

actin A contractile protein found in the thin filaments of skeletal muscle cells.

active transport A method used to move compounds across a cell membrane to create or maintain an imbalance of charges, usually against a concentration gradient and requiring the expenditure of energy.

adaptation The temporary or permanent reduction of sensitivity to a particular stimulus.

adenosine triphosphate (ATP) The nucleotide formed from the metabolism of nutrients in the cell; involved in energy metabolism; used to store energy.

adrenal cortex The outer layer of the adrenal gland; it produces hormones that are important in regulating the water and salt balance of the body.

adrenal glands Paired endocrine glands located on top of the kidneys that release epinephrine and norepinephrine when stimulated by the sympathetic nervous system; each adrenal gland consists of an inner adrenal medulla and an adrenal cortex.

adrenergic Having the characteristics of the sympathetic division of the autonomic nervous system.

adrenocorticotropic hormone (ACTH) Hormone that targets the adrenal cortex to secrete cortisol (a glucocorticoid).

aerobic metabolism Metabolism that can proceed only in the presence of oxygen.

afterimage The perception that a stimulus is still present after the stimulus has been removed.

afterload The pressure in the aorta against which the left ventricle must pump blood.

albumins The smallest of plasma proteins; they make up around 60% of the plasma proteins and are responsible for the oncotic pressure in the vasculature, thereby controlling the movement of water into and out of the circulation.

aldosterone A hormone responsible for the reabsorption of sodium and water from the kidney tubules.

alkalosis A pathologic condition resulting from the accumulation of bases in the body (blood pH greater than 7.45).

alleles Variant forms of a gene, which can be identical or slightly different in a sequence of deoxyribonucleic acid.

alveoli The air sacs of the lungs in which the exchange of oxygen and carbon dioxide takes place; also, the bony sockets for the teeth that reside in the mandible and maxilla (singular, alveolus).

anabolism The building of larger substances from smaller substances, such as the building of proteins from amino acids.

anaerobic metabolism Metabolism that occurs in the absence of oxygen.

anatomy The study of the structure of an organism and its parts.

angle of Louis A prominence of the sternum that indicates the point where the second rib joins the sternum; also called the sternal angle or manubriosternal junction.

antagonist A molecule that blocks the ability of a given chemical to bind to its receptor, preventing a biologic response.

antigens Proteins, polysaccharides, glycoproteins, or glycolipids commonly found on the surfaces of red blood cells that stimulate an immune system response and cause formation of antibodies; cells learn to recognize antigens as either "self" or "nonself" (foreign).

aorta The principal artery leaving the left side of the heart and carrying freshly oxygenated blood to the body; the largest artery in the body.

Prep Kit *(continued)*

aortic valve The semilunar valve that regulates blood flow from the left ventricle to the aorta.

apneustic center A portion of the pons that is thought to work with the pontine respiratory group to regulate the length and depth of inspiration.

appendicular skeleton The portion of the skeletal system made up of the upper extremities, shoulder girdle, pelvic girdle, and lower extremities.

aqueous humor Watery fluid filling the anterior eye cavity; the quantity determines the intraocular pressure, which is critical to sight.

areolar tissue A type of loose connective tissue that binds skin to underlying organs and fills in spaces between muscles.

arytenoid cartilages Six paired cartilages stacked on top of each other in the larynx.

astigmatism Condition where parts of the image are out of focus and others are in focus; caused by irregularities in the shape of the eye lens.

atlas The first cervical vertebra (C1), which provides support for the head.

atria The two upper chambers of the heart (singular, atrium).

atrial natriuretic peptide A hormone produced by the atria when they are distended by increased blood volume; it inhibits the absorption of water and sodium in the renal tubules, thereby increasing the elimination of water.

atrioventricular (AV) node A group of cells that conduct an electrical impulse through the heart; located in the floor of the right atrium immediately behind the tricuspid valve and near the opening of the coronary sinus.

atrioventricular (AV) valves The mitral and tricuspid valves through which blood flows from the atria to the ventricles.

automaticity Ability of cardiac pacemaker cells to initiate an electrical impulse spontaneously without being stimulated from another source (such as a nerve).

autonomic nervous system (ANS) A subdivision of the nervous system that controls primarily involuntary body functions; comprised of the sympathetic and parasympathetic nervous systems.

autosomes The chromosomes that do not carry genes that determine sex.

axial skeleton The portion of the skeleton made up of the skull, thoracic cage, and vertebral column.

axis Imaginary line joining the positive and negative electrodes of a lead; also the second cervical vertebra.

axon Long, slender extension of a neuron (nerve cell) that conducts electrical impulses away from the nerve cell body to adjacent cells.

B lymphocytes Lymphocytes that exist in the blood, and are abundant in the lymph nodes, bone marrow, intestinal lining, and spleen; also called B cells.

baroreceptors Nerve endings that are stimulated by pressure changes, including increased arterial blood pressure; they are located in the aortic arch and carotid sinuses.

basal ganglia Structures located deep within the cerebrum, diencephalon, and midbrain that have an important role in coordination of motor movements and posture.

basal metabolic rate The rate at which nutrients are consumed in the body.

basophils White blood cells that contain histamine granules and other substances that are released during inflammatory and allergic responses.

bilirubin A waste product of red blood cell destruction that undergoes further metabolism in the liver.

binocular vision The merging of two images into one.

blood-brain barrier A layer of tightly-adhered cells that protects the brain and spinal cord from exposure to medications, toxins, and infectious particles.

bone marrow Soft tissue that fills the inside of bones and is the site of production of red blood cells, platelets, and most white blood cells.

bony labyrinth The collection of hollows in the bone of the inner ear that provide protection to the structures of the inner ear from damage and from extraneous stimulation.

Boyle's law Gas law that demonstrates that as pressure increases, volume decreases; at a constant temperature, the volume of a gas is inversely proportional to its pressure (if the pressure on a gas is doubled, then its volume is halved); written as $PV = K$, where P = pressure, V = volume, and K = a constant.

brain The part of the central nervous system located within the cranium; contains billions of neurons that serve a variety of functions including consciousness, perception, control of reactions to the environment, emotional responses, and judgment.

brainstem The area of the brain between the spinal cord and cerebrum that contains the midbrain, pons,

Prep Kit *(continued)*

and medulla; controls functions that are necessary for life, such as breathing.

bruit Abnormal whooshing sounds indicating turbulent blood flow within a narrowed blood vessel, usually heard in the carotid arteries.

buffer system Fast-acting defenses for acid-base changes, providing almost immediate protection against changes in the hydrogen ion concentration of extracellular fluid.

bundle of His The portion of the conduction system of the heart located in the upper portion of the interventricular septum that conducts an electrical impulse from the atrioventricular junction to the right and left bundle branches.

bursa A small, padlike sac or cavity filled with a small amount of synovial fluid that helps reduce the amount of friction between a tendon and a bone or between a tendon and a ligament, usually located near a joint.

calcaneus The heel bone; the largest of the tarsal bones.

calorie The amount of heat needed to raise the temperature of a gram of water by 33°F (1°C); the amount of energy that can be obtained from the nutrients you eat; also called a kilocalorie.

carbohydrates Substances (including sugars and starches) that provide much of the energy required by the body's cells, as well as helping to build cell structures.

cardiac cycle The repetitive pumping process that begins with the onset of cardiac muscle contraction and ends just before the beginning of the next contraction; each one consists of ventricular contraction (systole) and relaxation (diastole).

carina The point of bifurcation of the right and left primary (mainstem) bronchi.

carpal bones The eight small bones of the wrist.

cartilaginous joints Those connected by hyaline cartilage, or fibrocartilage, such as the joints that separate the vertebrae.

catabolism The breakdown of larger molecules into smaller ones.

cataract Clouding of the lens of the eye or its surrounding transparent membrane.

catecholamines Amine substances such as dopamine, epinephrine, and norepinephrine that function as neurotransmitters, hormones, or both.

cell membrane The cell wall; a selectively permeable layer of cells that surround intracellular contents and control movement of substances into and out of the cell; also called the cytoplasmic membrane or plasma membrane.

cellular respiration A biochemical process resulting in the production of energy in the form of adenosine triphosphate.

central nervous system (CNS) The brain and spinal cord.

cerebellum Area of the brain involved in fine and gross muscle coordination; responsible for interpretation of actual movement and correction of any movements that interfere with coordination and the body's position.

cerebral cortex The outer covering of gray matter that covers the cerebral hemispheres; regulates voluntary skeletal movement and plays an important role in one's level of awareness.

cerebral perfusion pressure (CPP) Pressure inside the cerebral arteries and an indicator of brain perfusion; calculated by subtracting intracranial pressure from mean arterial pressure.

cerebrospinal fluid (CSF) Fluid produced in the ventricles of the brain that flows in the subarachnoid space and bathes the meninges.

cerebrum The largest part of the brain; made up of several lobes that control movement, hearing, balance, speech, visual perception, emotions, and personality; divided into right and left hemispheres; also called gray matter.

cervical canal The interior of the cervix.

cervix The lower one-third or neck of the uterus.

chemoreceptors Sense organs that monitor the levels of oxygen and carbon dioxide and the pH of cerebrospinal fluid and blood and provide feedback to the respiratory centers to modify the rate and depth of breathing based on the body's needs at any given time.

cholinergic Having the characteristics of the parasympathetic division of the autonomic nervous system; also refers to other structures or functions that are related to acetylcholine.

chordae tendineae Thin bands of fibrous tissue that attach to the atrioventricular valves in the heart and prevent them from inverting.

choroid The vascular, pigmented middle layer of the eye wall.

choroid plexus Group of specialized cells in the ventricles of the brain; filters blood through cerebral capillaries to create cerebrospinal fluid.

chromosomes Structures formed from condensed fibers and protein of deoxyribonucleic acid; they are threadlike, and are contained within the nucleus of the cells.

Prep Kit *(continued)*

chronotropic effect Related to the effect of the rate of contraction of the heart.

ciliary body The structure associated with the choroid layer of the eye that secretes aqueous humor and contains the ciliary muscle.

circulatory system The complex arrangement of connected tubes, including the arteries, arterioles, capillaries, venules, and veins, that moves blood, oxygen, nutrients, carbon dioxide, and cellular waste throughout the body.

circumflex coronary artery One of two branches of the left main coronary artery.

citric acid cycle A sequence of enzymatic reactions involving the metabolism of carbon chains of glucose, fatty acids, and amino acids to yield carbon dioxide, water, and high-energy phosphate bonds; also known as the Krebs cycle or tricarboxylic acid cycle.

clotting cascade A set of interactions that lead to the formation of a fibrin clot; also called the coagulation cascade.

cochlea The portion of the inner ear that has hearing receptors.

compound A substance that can be broken down into the two or more elements contained within it.

conductivity The property that allows a cardiac cell to receive an electrical impulse and pass it on to an adjoining cardiac cell.

cones One of two photoreceptors of the retina that can distinguish colors, but requires a greater amount of light to activate and create an image.

conjunctiva The membranous covering on the anterior surface of the eye that also lines the eyelids.

conjunctivitis Inflammation of the conjunctiva.

connective tissues Tissues that bind, support, protect, frame, and fill body structures; they also store fat, produce blood cells, repair tissues, and protect against infection.

contractility The ability of myocardial cells to shorten in response to an impulse, which results in contraction.

cornea The transparent tissue layer in front of the pupil and iris of the eye.

coronary sinus Venous drain for the coronary circulation into the right atrium.

corpus callosum A deep bridge of nerve fibers connecting the brain hemispheres.

corticosteroids Any of several steroids secreted by the adrenal gland.

cortisol A glucocorticoid of the middle adrenal cortex that influences protein and fat metabolism and stimulates glucose to be synthesized from noncarbohydrates.

cranial nerves The 12 pairs of nerves that arise from the base of the brain.

cranial vault The bones that encase and protect the brain, including the parietal, temporal, frontal, occipital, sphenoid, and ethmoid bones; the roof of the skull (cranium).

cranium The area of the head above the ears and eyes; the part of the skull that houses the brain.

cribriform plate A horizontal bone perforated with numerous openings for the passage of the olfactory nerve filaments from the nasal cavity.

cricoid cartilage A firm ridge of cartilage that forms the lower part of the larynx; the first ring of the trachea and the only upper airway structure that forms a complete ring; also called the cricoid ring.

cricothyroid membrane A thin sheet of fascia located between the thyroid and cricoid cartilage that is relatively avascular and contains few nerves; the site for emergency access to the airway.

cytoplasm The gel-like material that fills out a cell; it makes up most of the volume of the cell, and suspends the organelles of the cell.

deep fascia A dense layer of fibrous tissue below the subcutaneous tissue; composed of tough bands of tissue that surround muscles and other internal structures.

dendrites Branchlike projections of nerve cells that receive impulses or sensory information from nearby cells and conduct impulses toward the nerve cell body.

deoxyribonucleic acid (DNA) Specialized structure within the cell that carries genetic material for reproduction.

depolarization In response to an action potential, the rapid movement of electrolytes across a cell membrane that changes overall charge of the cell. This rapid shifting of electrolytes and cellular charges is the main catalyst for muscle contractions and neural transmissions.

dermatome The area of the skin supplied by a specific sensory spinal nerve.

descending aorta The portion of the aorta that extends through the thorax and abdomen into the pelvis.

diapedesis A process whereby leukocytes move through the wall of a capillary and out to the tissues where they are needed most.

Prep Kit *(continued)*

diaphragm Large skeletal muscle that plays a major role in breathing and separates the chest cavity from the abdominal cavity.

diaphysis The shaft of a long bone.

diastole Phase of the cardiac cycle in which the atria and ventricles relax between contractions and blood enters these chambers.

diencephalon Portion of the brain between the brainstem and cerebrum; contains the epithalamus, the thalamus, the hypothalamus, and the subthalamus.

differentiation The process of specialization of a cell.

diffusion The process of particles moving from an area of higher concentration to an area of lower concentration along a concentration gradient until equilibrium is achieved.

digestion The chemical breakdown of food material into smaller fragments that can be absorbed into the circulatory system.

diploid cells Cells that carry two of each of the 23 chromosomes—one from the father and one from the mother.

dorsal respiratory group (DRG) A portion of the medulla oblongata that functions as an respiratory integration center; it receives input from several sources including the pontine respiratory group, sensory input through the glossopharyngeal and vagus nerves, central chemoreceptors in the medulla, and peripheral chemoreceptors.

dura mater The outermost of the three meninges that enclose the brain and spinal cord; it is the toughest meningeal layer.

electrolytes Salt or acid substances that become ionic conductors when dissolved in a solvent (such as water); chemicals dissolved in the blood.

endocardium The thin membrane lining the inside of the heart.

endocrine glands Glands that have no ducts and secrete directly into tissue fluid or blood.

endocrine system The complex message and control system that integrates many body functions, including the release of hormones.

endolymph The fluid containing nerve receptors that resides inside the membranous labyrinth. Sound waves converted into pressure waves are transmitted through this fluid to the auditory nerves.

enteric nervous system (ENS) A subdivision of the autonomic nervous system that controls the digestive system.

enzymes Substances designed to speed up the rate of specific biochemical reactions.

eosinophil A leukocyte that may play a role following infection in various areas in the body.

epicardium The layer of the serous pericardium that lies closely against the heart; also called the visceral pericardium.

epiglottis A thin, flaplike structure that allows air to pass into the trachea but prevents food and liquid from entering.

epinephrine A hormone produced by the adrenal medulla that has a vital role in the function of the sympathetic division of the autonomic nervous system; mediates the fight-or-flight response; also called adrenaline.

epiphyseal plate The growth plate of a long bone; a major site of bone development during childhood; also called the physis.

epithelial tissues Body tissues that cover organs, form the inner lining of cavities, and line hollow organs.

estrogen A hormone released from the ovaries that stimulates the uterine lining during the menstrual cycle.

eustachian tube A branch of the internal auditory canal that connects the middle ear to the oropharynx.

excitability The ability of cardiac muscle cells to respond to an electrical, chemical, or mechanical stimulus.

exhalation The passive part of the breathing process in which the diaphragm and the intercostal muscles relax, forcing air out of the lungs.

exocrine glands Glands that secrete chemicals into ducts that open onto a surface for elimination.

expiratory reserve volume The amount of air that can be exhaled following a normal exhalation; average volume is about 1,200 mL.

extracellular fluid (ECF) Fluid outside of the cell, in which most of the body's supply of sodium is contained; accounts for 15% to 20% of body weight.

extrinsic muscles Referring to the eye; six muscles that attach to the exterior of the globe and are controlled by the cranial nerves.

fascia A sheet or band of tough fibrous connective tissue that covers, supports, and separates muscles, and which also covers arteries, veins, tendons, and ligaments.

fibrin A white, insoluble protein formed by the action of thrombin on fibrinogen during the blood clotting process; forms the matrix of a blood clot.

Prep Kit *(continued)*

fibrinogen A plasma protein that is important for blood clotting.

fibrous joints Joints that lie between bones that closely contact each other, joined by thin, dense connective tissue.

filtration The movement of fluid from intravascular fluid under high pressure to interstitial fluid, which is generally under lower pressure.

fluid balance The process of maintaining homeostasis through equal intake (water taken into the body) and output (water excreted from the body) of fluids.

fontanelles The soft spots in the skull of a newborn and infant where the sutures of the skull have not yet grown together.

fraction of inspired oxygen (FIO_2) The percentage of oxygen in inhaled air.

gag reflex A normal neural reflex elicited by touching the soft palate or posterior pharynx; the responses are symmetric elevation of the palate, retraction of the tongue, and contraction of the pharyngeal muscles.

general senses Sensations monitored throughout the body by receptors scattered throughout many different tissues.

genotype The arrangement of a person's genes and their characteristics is based on the combination of alleles, for one gene or many.

glaucoma A disease of the eye caused by an increase in intraocular pressure; when severe enough, this may damage the optic nerve and potentially cause permanent loss of vision.

globulins Antibodies made by the liver or lymphatic tissues that make up around 36% of the plasma proteins.

glottis The true vocal cords and the opening between them.

gluconeogenesis A process that stimulates both the liver and the kidneys to produce glucose from noncarbohydrate molecules.

glycogen A long polymer from which glucose is converted in the liver (animal starch).

glycogenolysis The breakdown of glycogen to glucose.

glycolysis Process by which glucose and other sugars are broken down to yield lactic acid (anaerobic glycolysis) or pyruvic acid (aerobic glycolysis). The breakdown releases energy in the form of adenosine triphosphate.

haploid cells Cells that carry genetic instructions via 23 individual chromosomes.

hard palate The anterior portion of the palate that is supported by bone (primarily the maxillary bone).

hematocrit A measure of the relative percentage of blood cells (mainly erythrocytes) in a given volume of whole blood.

hematopoietic system The blood components and the organs involved in their development and production.

hemoglobin An iron-containing pigment found in red blood cells that carries oxygen to the cells from the lungs and carbon dioxide away from the cells to the lungs.

hemostasis The stoppage of bleeding; involves the steps of blood vessel spasm, platelet plug formation, and blood clotting.

Henry's law A law of gas that states that the amount of a gas in a solution varies directly with the partial pressure of a gas over a solution.

hepatic portal system A specialized part of the venous system that carries blood from the digestive tract to the liver and then to the inferior vena cava.

Hering-Breuer reflex A protective mechanism that terminates inhalation, thus preventing overexpansion of the lungs.

histamine A substance found in large amounts in basophils that increases tissue inflammation.

homeostasis A tendency to constancy or stability in the body's internal environment; processes that balance the supply and demand of the body's needs.

homologous chromosome A chromosome of the same numbered pair from the opposite parent.

hormone A substance that is produced in one tissue or organ and is released into the blood and carried to other (target) organs, where it acts to produce a specific response.

hydrostatic pressure The pressure of water against the walls of its container.

hyoid bone A small, horseshoe-shaped bone to which the jaw, tongue, epiglottis, and thyroid cartilage attach.

hyperopia Farsighted; the ability to see distant objects with difficulty focusing on objects close.

hypertonic Concentration of solute is higher compared with another solution.

hypothalamus An area of the diencephalon that is the primary link between the endocrine system and the nervous system; responsible for control of many body functions, including heart rate,

Prep Kit *(continued)*

digestion, sexual development, temperature regulation, emotion, hunger, thirst, and regulation of the sleep cycle.

hypotonic Concentration of solute is lower compared with another solution.

hypoxic drive A situation in which a person's stimulus to breathe comes from a decrease in PaO_2 rather than the normal stimulus, an increase in $PaCO_2$.

immunity The body's ability to protect itself from acquiring a disease.

inhalation The active process of moving air into the lungs; also called inspiration; also a route of medication delivery.

inotropic effect The effect on the contractility of muscle tissue, especially cardiac muscle.

insertion A moveable part of the body to which a skeletal muscle is fastened at a moveable joint; its action opposes that of an origin.

inspiratory reserve volume The additional amount of air that can be inhaled after the normal tidal volume has been reached.

integumentary system The largest organ system in the body, consisting of the skin and accessory structures (eg, hair, nails, glands).

interstitial fluid The fluid located outside of the blood vessels in the spaces between the body's cells.

interstitial space The space in between the cells.

intracellular fluid (ICF) Fluid within cells in which most of the body's supply of potassium is contained; accounts for 40% to 45% of body weight.

intravascular fluid Fluid outside cells but inside the circulatory system; the majority of it is plasma, which is the fluid component of blood.

ionic bond A chemical bond where oppositely charged ions attract each other.

ions Atoms that have become positively or negatively charged, either by giving up or acquiring an electron.

islets of Langerhans Groups of cells located in the pancreas that produce insulin, glucagon, somatostatin, and pancreatic polypeptide.

isotonic solution A solution in which there is an equal concentration of solutes and water on either side of a semipermeable membrane. In this case, water does not shift, and no change in cell shape occurs.

joint capsule A saclike envelope that encloses the cavity of a synovial joint.

kilocalorie The amount of heat needed to raise the temperature of a gram of water by 33°F (1°C); the amount of energy that can be obtained from the nutrients you eat; also known as a calorie.

labia majora Two prominent, rounded folds of skin lateral to the labia minora of the female external genitalia.

labia minora A pair of skin folds in the female external genitalia that border the vestibule.

lacrimal glands The glands that produce fluids to keep the eye moist; also called tear glands.

lactic acid A metabolic end product of the breakdown of glucose that accumulates when metabolism proceeds in the absence of oxygen.

larynx A complete structure formed by the epiglottis, thyroid cartilage, cricoid cartilage, arytenoid cartilage, corniculate cartilage, and cuneiform cartilage; also called the voice box.

left anterior descending artery One of the two branches of the left main coronary artery that supplies blood to the left ventricle and other areas of the heart.

lens The transparent disc within the eye that refracts light to focus images on the retina.

lipids Fats, fatlike substances (cholesterol and phospholipids), and oils that supply energy for body processes and building of certain structures.

lymph A thin liquid formed from interstitial fluid that flows through the lymphatic vessels and lymph nodes and aids in immune response and debris removal.

lymph nodes Round or bean-shaped structures interspersed along the course of the lymph vessels, which filter the lymph and serve as a source of lymphocytes.

lymph vessels Unidirectional, thin-walled vessels through which lymph circulates through the body; they travel close to the major veins.

lymphatic system A network of capillaries, vessels, ducts, nodes, and organs that helps to maintain the fluid environment of the body by producing lymph and transporting it through the body.

lymphocytes A type of white blood cell that has an important role in immunity.

macrophages Large cells, usually derived from monocytes, that are specialized for phagocytosis; they kill pathogens, absorb foreign materials, and slow infections and infectious agents.

Prep Kit *(continued)*

macula A yellow depression in the retina where acute vision arises; also known as the macula lutea.

mast cells Cells located in connective tissues to which antibodies, formed in response to allergens, attach, bursting the cells and releasing chemical mediators in response to an antigen-antibody reaction.

mediastinum The space between the lungs, in the center of the chest, that contains the heart, great vessels, part of the esophagus, lymphatic channels, trachea, primary bronchi, and paired vagus and phrenic nerves.

medulla oblongata Inferior part of the brainstem that is continuous inferiorly with the spinal cord; serves as a conduction pathway for ascending and descending nerve tracts; responsible for maintenance of basic life functions, such as heart rate and breathing.

meiosis A type of cell division that occurs in the production of eggs and sperm.

melanin The pigment that gives skin its color.

menarche The first menstrual cycle; the onset of menses.

meninges A set of three tough membranes, the dura mater, arachnoid, and pia mater, that enclose the entire brain and spinal cord.

menopause The period when a woman's reproductive cycle ceases; also called the female climacteric.

menstruation Cyclical shedding of the endometrial lining.

metacarpals The five bones that form the palm and back of the hand.

midbrain The most superior portion of the brainstem; it works with the pons to route information from higher within the brain to the spinal cord and vice versa.

mineral An inorganic element essential for human metabolism.

minute volume The amount of air that moves in and out of the lungs per minute minus the dead space; also called minute ventilation.

mitosis The division of chromosomes in a cell nucleus.

mitral valve The atrioventricular valve in the heart that separates the left atrium from the left ventricle.

monocytes White blood cells that mature in the blood and then travel to the tissues, where they differentiate into macrophages; these function primarily as scavengers for the tissues.

monosaccharides The simplest carbohydrate molecule.

motor nerve Nerve that carries information from the central nervous system to the muscles of the body.

motor neurons Nerve cells that transmit instructions from the central nervous system to the end organs; also known as efferent neurons.

mucous membranes The lining of body cavities and passages that communicate directly or indirectly with the environment outside the body.

mucus The opaque, sticky secretion of the mucous membranes that lubricates the body openings.

murmur An abnormal heart sound, heard as a "whooshing," indicating turbulent blood flow within the heart.

muscle tissue Contractile tissue consisting of filaments of actin and myosin, which slide past each other, shortening cells.

musculoskeletal The bones and voluntary muscles of the body.

myocardium The middle and thickest layer of the heart; it contains the cardiac muscle fibers that cause contraction of the heart, as well as the conduction system and blood supply.

myoglobin A pigment synthesized in the muscles to give skeletal muscles their red-brown color.

myopia Nearsighted; the ability to see objects close with difficulty seeing objects far away.

myosin A contractile protein found in the thick filaments of skeletal muscle cells.

nasopharynx The part of the pharynx that lies above the level of the palate.

negative feedback The concept that once the desired effect of a process has been achieved, further action is inhibited until it is needed again; also called feedback inhibition.

negative pressure ventilation Drawing of air into the lungs; airflow from a region of higher pressure (outside the body) to a region of lower pressure (the lungs); occurs during normal breathing.

neoplasm A mass of tissue produced by abnormal cell growth and division that may be malignant (cancerous) or benign.

nephrons The functional (urine-producing) units of the kidneys.

nervous system The system that controls virtually all activities of the body, both voluntary and involuntary.

nervous tissue Composed of neurons and neuroglia.

Prep Kit *(continued)*

neuroglia Supporting cells that provide a supporting skeleton for neural tissue, isolate and protect the cell membranes of neurons, regulate the composition of interstitial fluid, defend neural tissue from pathogens, and aid in the repair of injury.

neuromuscular junction The connection between a motor neuron and a muscle fiber.

neurons The basic nerve cells of the nervous system, containing a nucleus within a cell body and extending one or more processes; they exist in masses to form nervous tissue.

neurotransmitter A chemical released from one nerve that crosses the synaptic cleft to reach a receptor.

neutrophils One of the three types of granulocytes; they have multi-lobed nuclei that resemble a string of baseballs held together by a thin strand of thread; they destroy bacteria, antigen-antibody complexes, and foreign matter.

norepinephrine A naturally occurring catecholamine that functions as a neurotransmitter and adrenal hormone; it is synthesized by the adrenal medulla, the peripheral sympathetic nerves, and the central nervous system. It is also available as a drug sometimes used in the treatment of severe hypotension; produces vasoconstriction through its alpha-stimulator properties.

nucleic acids Large organic molecules, or macromolecules, that carry genetic information or form structures within cells, and include deoxyribonucleic acid and ribonucleic acid.

nucleus In the context of the cell, a cellular organelle that contains the genetic information; controls the function and structure of a cell. In the context of an atom, the central portion of an atom that contains protons and neutrons.

nutrients Substances that provide nourishment for growth such as carbohydrates, lipids, proteins, vitamins, minerals, and water.

oligosaccharide A simple sugar composed of 2 to 10 monosaccharides.

oncotic pressure The pressure of water to move, typically into the capillary, as the result of the presence of plasma proteins.

oocyte Immature female sex cell produced in the ovary that may develop by meiosis into an ovum (egg).

oogenesis The process of egg cell formation, which begins at puberty.

optic chiasm Location where approximately half of the nerve fibers from each eye cross over to the opposite side of the brain.

orbit An eye socket of the skull.

organ of Corti The organ that is the primary receptor for sound, and is made up of thousands of individual cilia, each with their own associated nerve.

organelles Structures within cells that have specialized functions.

origin A relatively immovable part of the body where a skeletal muscle is fastened at a moveable joint; its action opposes that of an insertion.

oropharynx A tubular structure that extends vertically from the back of the mouth to the esophagus and trachea.

osmosis The movement of a solvent, such as water, from an area of low solute concentration to one of high concentration through a selectively permeable membrane to equalize concentrations of a solute on both sides of the membrane.

osmotic pressure The pressure exerted by the concentration of the solutes in a given space to stop the flow of solvent across a semipermeable membrane.

ossification The formation of bone by osteoblasts.

osteoblasts Cells involved in the formation of bony tissue.

osteoclasts Macrophages of the bone surface that dissolve the matrix and return minerals to the extracellular fluid.

osteocytes Mature bone cells.

otoliths A pair of fluid-filled sacs within the inner ear that are used by the central nervous system to collect information about movement and orientation in space.

oval window The opening between the stapes and inner ear.

ovaries Female glands that produces sex hormones and ova (eggs).

ovulation Midcycle release of an ovum during the menstrual cycle.

oxygenation The process of loading oxygen molecules onto hemoglobin molecules in the bloodstream.

oxyhemoglobin Hemoglobin that has oxygen molecules bound to it.

palate The roof of the nasal cavity; it separates the nasal cavity from the oral cavity.

Prep Kit *(continued)*

pancreas An organ with both endocrine and exocrine functions; it is a major source of digestive enzymes and produces the hormone insulin.

papillary muscles Muscles attached to the chordae tendineae of the atrioventricular heart valves and the ventricular muscle of the heart.

paranasal sinuses The sinuses, or hollowed sections of bone in the front of the head, which are lined with mucous membrane and drain into the nasal cavity; the frontal, ethmoid, sphenoid, and maxillary sinuses.

parathyroid glands Four glands that are embedded in the posterior portion of each lobe of the thyroid; they produce and secrete parathyroid hormone.

parathyroid hormone (PTH) Hormone produced and secreted by the parathyroid glands; it maintains normal levels of calcium in the blood and normal neuromuscular function.

parietal pleura The lining of the pleural cavity attached tightly to the interior of the chest cage.

partial pressure The pressure exerted by an individual gas in a mixture.

pelvis The attachment of the lower extremities to the body, consisting of the sacrum and two pelvic bones.

penis The cylindrical male sex organ; it conveys urine and semen through the urethra.

peptide Protein molecule consisting of amino acids held together by peptide bonds.

perception Becoming aware of or understanding something using the senses.

perfusion The circulation of oxygenated blood within an organ or tissue in adequate amounts to meet the cells' current needs.

pericardium A thin, double-layered membrane made up of the fibrous pericardium and serous pericardium.

perilymph Fluid within the bony labyrinth that surrounds and protects the membranous labyrinth while allowing transmission of pressure waves caused by sound.

peripheral nervous system (PNS) The part of the nervous system that consists of 31 pairs of spinal nerves and 12 pairs of cranial nerves that are responsible for communication between the central nervous system and the rest of the body. These may be sensory nerves, motor nerves, or connecting nerves.

peristalsis The wavelike contraction of smooth muscle by which the ureters or other tubular organs propel their contents.

peritoneum Double-layered serous membrane that lines the abdominal cavity and covers the organs located in the abdominopelvic cavity.

pH The measure of acidity or alkalinity of a solution.

phagocytosis A form of endocytosis in which a cell surrounds a foreign particle and engulfs it.

phantom pain A sensation of pain in a part of the body that is no longer present.

pharynx The area between the nasal cavity and the larynx and posterior to the oral cavity; the throat.

phenotype The appearance, health condition, or other characteristics associated with a particular genotype.

phospholipid A type of lipid molecule that comprises the cell membrane.

physiology The study of the processes and functions of the living organism.

pia mater The innermost of the three meninges that enclose the brain and spinal cord; it rests directly on the brain and spinal cord.

pineal gland A gland in the brain that synthesizes and secretes melatonin, a hormone that affects patterns of sleep and wakefulness.

pinna A formation of cartilage within the inner ear that protects the ear and collects sounds into the ear canal, while allowing some perception of the direction from which the sound comes; also called the auricle.

pinocytosis A form of endocytosis in which the cell membrane sinks inward and ingests droplets of extracellular fluid.

pituitary gland An endocrine gland responsible for directly or indirectly affecting all body functions; also called the hypophysis.

plasma A watery, yellow fluid that carries the blood cells and nutrients and transports cellular waste material to the organs of excretion.

plasma cells Cells that produce antibodies (immunoglobulins) to destroy antigens or antigen-containing particles; formed from divided and differentiated B cells.

plasmin A naturally occurring enzyme that dissolves the fibrin fibers in blood clots; usually present in the body in its inactive form, plasminogen.

platelets Formed elements of the blood that function in blood clotting; also called thrombocytes.

Prep Kit *(continued)*

pleura The serous membranes covering the lungs and lining the thoracic cavity.

pleural space The potential space between the parietal pleura and the visceral pleura.

plexus A cluster of nerve roots that permits peripheral nerve roots to rejoin and function as a group.

polarized When a cell is at rest, ions are actively transported into and out of the cell to create an electrochemical gradient across the cell membrane.

polypeptide Formed from many amino acids bound into a chain. When this has more than 100 molecules, it is considered to be a protein. Certain protein molecules have more than one.

polysaccharides Complex carbohydrates that contain many simple joined sugar units, such as plant starch. Some, such as cellulose, cannot be broken down for nutrition in humans but play important roles in digestion.

pons Area of the brainstem that contains the sleep and respiratory centers for the body, which along with the medulla, control breathing.

pontine respiratory group (PRG) A portion of the pons that communicates information to both the ventral and dorsal respiratory groups; it is thought to smooth the transition between each phase of the ventilatory cycle and alter breathing by making each breath shorter and shallower or longer and deeper, depending on the body's needs.

precapillary sphincters Smooth muscle located at the entrances to the capillaries; responsive to local tissue needs.

preload The volume of blood in the ventricle at the end of diastole; it is primarily a reflection of venous return (the blood that is returned to the heart).

presbyopia The increased difficulty in focusing on objects that occurs with aging.

progesterone A female hormone released from the ovaries that promotes changes in the uterus during the reproductive cycle, affects the mammary glands, and helps regulate gonadotropin secretion.

proprioception The awareness of motion and position of a body part.

prostaglandins Lipids made from arachidonic acid that usually act more locally than hormones, are very potent, stimulate hormone secretions, and help to regulate blood pressure.

proteins Created from amino acids, they include enzymes, plasma proteins, muscle components (actin and myosin), hormones, and antibodies.

prothrombin A protein made in the liver and released into the blood where it is converted into thrombin during the process of blood clotting.

pulmonary artery One of two arteries that carry deoxygenated blood from the right ventricle to the lungs.

pulmonary circulation The flow of blood from the right ventricle through the pulmonary arteries and all of their branches and capillaries in the lungs and back to the left atrium through the venules and pulmonary veins; also called the lesser circulation.

pulmonary veins The four veins that return oxygenated blood from the lungs to the left atrium of the heart.

pulmonic valve The semilunar valve that regulates blood flow between the right ventricle and the pulmonary artery; also called the pulmonary semilunar valve.

pulse pressure The difference between the systolic and diastolic pressures.

Purkinje fibers A system of fibers in the ventricles that conducts the excitation impulse from the bundle branches to the myocardium.

referred pain Pain that feels as if it is originating from a body part other than the site being stimulated.

reflex arc A sensory message that reaches the spinal cord and meets with a motor nerve to cause an action; the reflex action occurs without the message first having to reach the brain to voluntarily cause the action.

refracting system A series of transparent structures within the eye that redirect light as it passes through mediums of different densities.

renal corpuscle The initial blood-filtering component of the nephron.

renal cortex The outer portion of each kidney; it forms renal columns and has tiny tubules associated with the nephrons.

renal medulla The inner portion of each kidney; it is made of conical renal pyramids, and has striations.

renal pelvis A cone-shaped collecting area that connects the ureter and the kidney.

renal tubule The portion of the nephron containing the tubular fluid filtered through the glomerulus.

renin A hormone produced by cells in the juxtaglomerular apparatus when the blood pressure is low.

repolarization The process by which ions are moved across the cell membrane to return to a polarized state.

Prep Kit (continued)

reproductive system The system in males and females that controls the reproductive processes via organs and glands that create sex cells and transport them to areas where fertilization can occur.

residual volume The amount of air remaining in the lungs and airway passages that is unable to be expelled after a maximal forced exhalation.

respiration The exchange of gases between a living organism and its environment.

respiratory membrane Where gas exchange takes place; oxygen is picked up in the bloodstream and carbon dioxide is eliminated through the lungs.

respiratory system All the structures of the body that contribute to the process of breathing, consisting of the upper and lower airways and their component parts.

reticular activating system (RAS) Group of specialized neurons in the brainstem; involved in sleep and wake cycles; maintains consciousness.

retina The inner layer of the eye wall, including the visual receptors.

Rh factor An antigen found on the red blood cells of most people; when a woman without this protein is impregnated by a man with this protein, the woman's body can create antibodies against the protein and attack future pregnancies.

right coronary artery Blood vessel that provides oxygenated blood to the right side of the heart muscle.

rods One of two photoreceptors of the retina sensitive to light, but does not discriminate colors, producing a picture that is somewhat less focused and essentially black and white.

sacroiliac joint The point of attachment of the ilium to the sacrum.

saddle joint Two saddle-shaped articulating surfaces oriented at right angles to each other so that complementary surfaces articulate with each other, such as is the case with the thumb.

Schwann cells Neuroglial cells in the peripheral nervous system that form a myelin sheath around axons.

sclera The white, fibrous outer layer of the eyeball.

scrotum A pouch of skin and subcutaneous tissue hanging from the lower abdominal region, posterior to the penis.

sebaceous glands Glands that produce an oily substance called sebum, which discharges along the shafts of the hairs.

semilunar (SL) valves The two valves, the aortic and pulmonic valves, that are shaped like half-moons and separate the heart from the aorta and pulmonary arteries.

semipermeable Property of the cell membrane that describes the ability to allow certain elements to pass through while not allowing others to do so.

sensory nerves The nerves that carry sensations of touch, taste, heat, cold, pain, and other modalities from the body to the central nervous system.

sensory receptors Structures located in the dermis that initiate nerve impulses that can reach one's conscious awareness.

sex chromosomes The X and Y chromosomes, which determine sex.

sinoatrial (SA) node The normal site of the origin of electrical impulses; located high in the right atrium, it is the natural pacemaker of the heart.

sinuses Cavities formed by the cranial bones that trap contaminants from entering the respiratory tract and act as tributaries for fluid to and from the eustachian tubes and tear ducts.

skeletal muscle tissue Voluntary muscle tissue attached to bones and composed of long, threadlike cells that have light and dark striations.

sliding filament theory A method of action of muscle contraction involving how sarcomeres shorten, with thick and thin filaments sliding past each other toward the center of the sarcomere from both ends.

sodium-potassium pump The mechanism by which the cell brings in two potassium ions and releases three sodium ions.

soft palate The posterior portion of the palate that is made up of mucous membrane, muscular fibers, and mucous glands; it is so named because it has no bony support.

solute The dissolved particles contained in a solvent.

solution A mixture of a solvent and a solute.

solvent The fluid that dissolves a solute, or the substance in which a solute is dissolved or mixed.

somatic nervous system The part of the nervous system that regulates activities over which there is voluntary control.

somatic pain Pain caused by the activation of pain receptors in the body's superficial tissues, such as the skin, bones, muscles, and joints; in contrast to visceral pain, this is generally more intense and more precisely localized.

spermatogenesis The process by which sperm cells are formed.

Prep Kit *(continued)*

sphincters Muscles arranged in circles that are able to decrease the diameter of tubes. Examples are found within the rectum, bladder, and blood vessels.

spinal nerves 31 pairs of nerves that originate from the spinal cord and exit the spine on either side between vertebrae; each has a sensory root and a motor root and is responsible for sending and receiving sensory and motor messages to and from the central nervous system from a portion of the body.

stem cells Cells that retain the ability to divide repeatedly without specializing, and that allow for continual growth and renewal.

strabismus Loss of perception of depth and overlapping or doubled images.

stratum corneum The outermost or dead layer of the skin.

stroke volume (SV) The volume of blood pumped forward with each ventricular contraction.

subarachnoid space The space located between the pia mater and the arachnoid membrane.

suprasternal notch The indentation formed by the superior border of the manubrium and the clavicles, often used as a landmark for procedures such as subclavian vein access; also known as the jugular notch.

surfactant A liquid protein substance that coats the alveoli in the lungs, decreases alveolar surface tension, and keeps the alveoli expanded; a low level in a premature infant contributes to respiratory distress syndrome.

sutures Seams that occur only between the bones of the skull; they are a type of fibrous joint.

sweat glands The glands that secrete sweat, located in the dermal layer of the skin.

synapse A functional connection where neurons communicate with other cells.

synaptic cleft The space between neurons; also called the synaptic gap.

synaptic vesicles Small sacs that contain neurotransmitters.

synovial fluid The fluid secreted by synovial membranes that lubricates synovial joints.

synovial joints Complex joints that allow free movement of the component bones and are lubricated with synovial fluid.

synovial membrane The lining of a joint that secretes synovial fluid into the joint space.

systemic vascular resistance The resistance that blood must overcome to be able to move within the blood vessels; related to the amount of dilation or constriction in the blood vessel.

T lymphocytes Lymphocytes that interact directly with antigens, producing the cellular immune response; they also stimulate the B lymphocytes to produce antibodies; also called T cells.

tentorium A horizontal projection of the dura that separates the cerebellum from the cerebrum.

testosterone The most important male sex hormone (androgen).

thalamus Structure of the diencephalon that is the sensory switchboard of the brain, through which almost all signals travel on their way in or out of the brain.

thermoregulation The process by which the body maintains temperature through a combination of heat gain by metabolic processes and muscular movement and heat loss through breathing, evaporation, conduction, convection, and perspiration.

thoracic duct One of two great lymph vessels; it empties into the superior vena cava.

thrombin An enzyme that causes the conversion of fibrinogen to fibrin, which binds to a platelet plug, forming a final mature clot.

thromboplastin A chemical that stimulates blood clotting.

thymus A lymphatic organ located in the thorax that is important in early immunity; it shrinks with age and is eventually replaced by other types of tissue.

thyroid cartilage A firm prominence of cartilage that forms the upper part of the larynx; the Adam's apple.

thyroid gland A large endocrine gland that is located at the base of the neck and produces and excretes hormones that influence growth, development, and metabolism.

tidal volume The amount of air moved in and out of the lungs in one relaxed breath; about 500 mL for an adult.

tissue A group of cells that are similar in structure and function.

titin A noncontractile protein found in sarcomeres of cardiac and skeletal muscle.

total body water (TBW) Total amount of fluid in the human body; accounts for about 60% of the weight of a healthy adult male; divided into various compartments.

transcellular fluid Fluid classified as extracellular but distinct because it is formed from the transport

Prep Kit *(continued)*

activities of cells. Examples include cerebrospinal fluid, bladder urine, the aqueous humor, and the synovial fluid of the joints.

tricuspid valve The atrioventricular valve that separates the right atrium from the right ventricle.

tropomyosin An actin-binding protein that regulates muscle contraction and other actin-related mechanical functions of the body.

troponin A regulatory protein in the actin filaments of skeletal and cardiac muscle that attaches to tropomyosin.

tubular reabsorption The process that moves substances from the tubular fluid into the blood, within the peritubular capillary.

tubular secretion The process that moves substances from the blood in the peritubular capillary into the renal tubule.

tunica adventitia The outer layer of tissue of a blood vessel wall, composed of elastic and fibrous connective tissue.

tunica intima The smooth, thin, inner lining of a blood vessel.

tunica media The middle and thickest layer of tissue of a blood vessel wall, composed of elastic tissue and smooth muscle cells that allow the vessel to expand or contract in response to changes in blood pressure and tissue demand.

ureter A small, hollow tube that carries urine from the kidneys to the bladder.

urethra The canal that conveys urine from the bladder to outside the body.

urinary bladder A sac behind the pubic symphysis made of smooth muscle that collects and stores urine.

urinary system The organs that control the discharge of certain waste materials filtered from the blood and excreted as urine.

uterus A muscular, inverted pear-shaped organ that lies situated between the urinary bladder and the rectum.

ventilation The mechanical process of moving air into and out of the lungs in two separate phases: inhalation (inspiration) and exhalation (expiration).

ventral respiratory group (VRG) An area of the medulla oblongata that can cause inspiration or expiration depending on which motor neurons are stimulated.

vestibule The structure into which the vagina opens posteriorly, and the female urethra opens into in the midline; also the central part of the labyrinth of the ear, behind the cochlea and in front of the semicircular canals.

visceral pain Deep pain caused by activation of pain receptors in internal areas of the body that are enclosed within a cavity, such as the chest, abdomen, or pelvis.

visceral pleura Lining of the pleural cavity that adheres tightly to the surface of the lung.

vital capacity The amount of air moved in and out of the lungs with maximum inspiration and exhalation.

vitamins Organic compounds required for normal metabolism.

vitreous humor A jellylike fluid filling the posterior eye cavity that helps the globe maintain its shape without distorting light.

white matter Bundles of myelinated nerves.

▶ References

1. Online Entymology Dictionary. © 2001-2006 Douglas Harper. http://www.etymonline.com/index.php?term=organism&allowed_in_frame=0. Accessed June 22, 2016.
2. Moini J. Cells. In: *Anatomy and Physiology for Health Professionals.* 2nd ed. Burlington, MA: Jones & Bartlett Learning; 2016:45-66.
3. Patton KT, Thibodeau GA. Anatomy of cells. In: *Anatomy & Physiology*. 8th ed. St. Louis, MO: Mosby; 2013:66-89.
4. Hall JE. Functional organization of the human body and control of the "Internal Environment". In: Hall JE, ed. *Guyton and Hall Textbook of Medical Physiology*. 13th ed. Philadelphia, PA: Elsevier; 2016:3-10.
5. Aronson PS, Boron WF, Boulpaep, EL. Transport of solutes and water. In: Boron WF, Boulpaep EL, eds. *Medical Physiology: A Cellular and Molecular Approach.* 2nd ed. Philadelphia, PA: Saunders; 2012:106-146.
6. Darby SA. General anatomy of the spinal cord. In: Cramer GD, Darby SA, eds. *Clinical Anatomy of the Spine, Spinal Cord, and ANS.* 3rd ed. St. Louis, MO: Mosby; 2014;65-97.
7. Cramer GD. General characteristics of the spine. In: Cramer GD, Darby SA, eds. *Clinical Anatomy of the Spine, Spinal Cord, and ANS.* 3rd ed. St. Louis, MO: Mosby; 2014;15-64.
8. Neumann DA. Muscle: The primary stabilizer and mover of the skeletal system. In: *Kinesiology of the Musculoskeletal System: Foundations for Rehabilitation.* 2nd ed. St. Louis, MO: Mosby; 2010:47-76.
9. Moini J. Control and coordination. In: *Anatomy and Physiology for Health Professionals.* 2nd ed. Burlington, MA: Jones & Bartlett Learning; 2016:223-346.

Prep Kit *(continued)*

10. Patton KT, Thibodeau GA. Nervous system cells. In: *Anthony's Textbook of Anatomy & Physiology*. 20th ed. St. Louis, MO: Mosby; 2013:380-419.
11. Jenkins DB. The back. In: *Hollinshead's Functional Anatomy of the Limbs and Back,* 9th ed. St. Louis, MO: Saunders; 2009:204-237.
12. Nolte J. Meningeal coverings of the brain and spinal cord. In: *The Human Brain: An Introduction To Its Functional Anatomy,* 6th ed. Philadelphia, PA: Mosby; 2009:80-98.
13. Ransom BR. The neuronal microenvironment. In: Boron WF, Boulpaep EL, eds. *Medical Physiology: A Cellular and Molecular Approach.* 2nd ed. Philadelphia, PA: Saunders; 2012:289-309.
14. Rubinson K, Lang EJ. The nervous system. In: Koeppen BM, Stanton BA, eds. *Berne & Levy Physiology.* 6th ed. Philadelphia, PA: Mosby; 2010:49-229.
15. Privitera MD, Zakaria T, Khatri R. Nervous system. In: Kaplan LA, Pesce AJ, eds. *Clinical Chemistry: Theory, Analysis, Correlation.* 5th ed. New York, NY: Mosby; 2009:904-928.
16. Braun K. The prefrontal-limbic system: development, neuroanatomy, function, and implications for socioemotional development. *Clin Perinatol.* 2011;38(4):685-702.
17. Seidel HM, Ball JW, Dains JE, Flynn JA, Solomon BS, Stewart RW. Neurologic system. In: Seidel HM, Ball JW, Dains JE, Flynn JA, Solomon BS, Stewart RW, eds. *Mosby's Guide to Physical Examination.* 7th ed. St. Louis, MO: Mosby; 2010:702-748.
18. Darby SA, Frysztak RJ. Neuroanatomy of the spinal cord. In: Cramer GD, Darby SA, eds. *Clinical Anatomy of the Spine, Spinal Cord, and ANS.* 3rd ed. St. Louis, MO: Mosby; 2014;341-412.
19. Brand RW, Isselhard DE. Nervous system. In: Brand RW, Isselhard DE, eds. *Anatomy of Orofacial Structures: A Comprehensive Approach.* 7th ed. St. Louis, MO: Mosby; 2014:376-391.
20. Glick DB. The autonomic nervous system. In: Miller RD, *Cohen NH, Eriksson LI, Fleisher LA, Wiener*-Kronish JP, Young WL, eds. *Miller's Anesthesia.* 8th ed. Philadelphia, PA: Saunders; 2015:346-386.
21. Wecker L, Crespo LM, Dunaway G, Faingold C, Watts S. Introduction to the autonomic nervous system. In: *Brody's Human Pharmacology: Molecular to Clinical.* 5th ed. Philadelphia, PA: Mosby; 2010:93-106.
22. Opie LH., Hasenfuss G. Mechanisms of cardiac contraction and relaxation. In: Bonow RO, Mann DL, Zipes DP, Libby P, eds. *Braunwald's Heart Disease: A Textbook of Cardiovascular Medicine.* 9th ed. Philadelphia, PA: Saunders; 2012:459-486.
23. Furness JB, Callaghan BP, Rivera LR, Cho HJ. The enteric nervous system and gastrointestinal innervation: integrated local and central control. *Adv Exp Med Biol.* 2014;817:39-71.
24. Stitt J. Regulation of body temperature. In: Boron WF, Boulpaep EL, eds. *Medical Physiology: A Cellular and Molecular Approach.* 2nd ed. Philadelphia, PA: Saunders; 2012:1237-1248.
25. Connors BW. Sensory transduction. In: Boron WF, Boulpaep EL, eds. *Medical Physiology: A Cellular and Molecular Approach.* 2nd ed. Philadelphia, PA: Saunders; 2012:371-407.
26. Rizzo, DC. The nervous system: The brain, cranial nerves, autonomic nervous system, and the special senses. In: *Fundamentals of Anatomy and Physiology.* 4th ed. Boston, MA: Cengage Learning; 2016:250-277.
27. Page CP, Curtis MJ, Walker, MJ, Hoffman BB. Drugs and the eye. In: *Integrated Pharmacology*. 3rd ed. Philadelphia, PA: Mosby; 2006:545-562.
28. Cantley L. Signal transduction. In: Boron WF, Boulpaep EL, eds. *Medical Physiology: A Cellular and Molecular Approach.* 2nd ed. Philadelphia, PA: Saunders; 2012:48-74.
29. Saladin KS. The circulatory system: blood. In: *Anatomy & Physiology: The Unity of Form and Function.* 7th ed. New York, NY: McGraw-Hill Education; 2015:672-707.
30. Boulpaep EL. Arteries and veins. In: Boron WF, Boulpaep EL, eds. *Medical Physiology: A Cellular and Molecular Approach.* 2nd ed. Philadelphia, PA: Saunders; 2012:467-481.
31. Lohr NL, Benjamin IJ. Structure and function of the normal heart and blood vessels. In: Benjamin IJ, Griggs RC, Wing EJ, Fitz JG, eds. *Andreoli and Carpenter's Cecil Essentials of Medicine.* 9th ed. Philadelphia, PA: Saunders; 2016:16-21.
32. Pappano AJ. The cardiovascular system. In: Koeppen BM, Stanton BA, eds. *Berne & Levy Physiology.* 6th ed. Philadelphia, PA: Mosby; 2010:285-413.
33. Hall JE. The microcirculation and lymphatic system. In: Hall JE, ed. *Guyton and Hall Textbook of Medical Physiology.* 13th ed. Philadelphia, PA: Elsevier; 2016:189-202.
34. Saladin KS. The respiratory system. In: *Anatomy & Physiology: The Unity of Form and Function.* 7th ed. New York, NY: McGraw-Hill Education; 2015:848-888.
35. Boron WF. Organization of the respiratory system. In: Boron WF, Boulpaep EL, eds. *Medical Physiology: A Cellular and Molecular Approach.* 2nd ed. Philadelphia, PA: Saunders; 2012:613-629
36. Cloutier MM, Thrall RS. The respiratory system. In: Koeppen BM, Stanton BA, eds. *Berne & Levy*

Prep Kit *(continued)*

Physiology. 6th ed. Philadelphia, PA: Mosby; 2010:414-483.

37. Drake RL, Vogl AW, Mitchell AW. Thorax. In: *Gray's Basic Anatomy.* Philadelphia, PA: Churchill Livingstone; 2012:57-132.
38. Waugh A, Grant A. The respiratory system. In: *Ross and Wilson Anatomy and Physiology in Health and Illness.* 12th ed. Edinburgh, Scotland: Churchill Livingstone; 2014:242-273.
39. Brashers VL. Structure and function of the pulmonary system. In: McCance KL, Huether SE, Brashers VL, Rote NS, eds. *Pathophysiology: The Biologic Basis for Disease in Adults and Children* 7th ed. St. Louis, MO: Mosby; 2014:1225-1247.
40. Spyer KM, Gourine AV. Chemosensory pathways in the brainstem controlling cardiorespiratory activity. *Philos Trans R Soc Lond B Biol Sci.* 2009;364(1529):2603-2610.
41. Richerson GB, Boron WF. Control of ventilation. In: Boron WF, Boulpaep EL, eds. *Medical Physiology: A Cellular and Molecular Approach.* 2nd ed. Philadelphia, PA: Saunders; 2012:725-745.
42. Corne S, Bshouty Z. Basic principles of control of breathing. *Respir Care Clin N Am.* 2005;11(2):147-172.
43. Binder HJ. Organization of the gastrointestinal system. In: Boron WF, Boulpaep EL, eds. *Medical Physiology: A Cellular and Molecular Approach.* 2nd ed. Philadelphia, PA: Saunders; 2012:883-894.
44. Saladin KS. The male reproductive system. In: *Anatomy & Physiology: The Unity of Form and Function.* 7th ed. New York, NY: McGraw-Hill Education; 2015:1028-1057.
45. Moini J. Reproductive system. In: *Anatomy and Physiology for Health Professionals.* 2nd ed. Burlington, MA: Jones & Bartlett Learning; 2016:553-584.
46. Roiger D, *Bullock* NJ. The male reproductive system. In: *Anatomy, Physiology, & Disease: Foundations for the Health Professions*. New York, NY: McGraw-Hill Education; 2014:592-621.

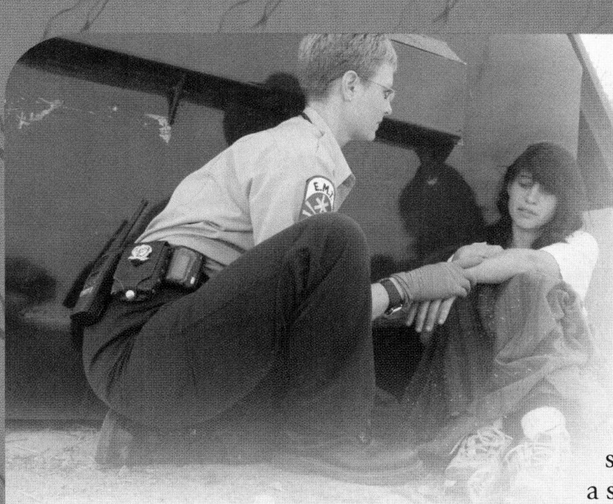

Assessment *in Action*

You are dispatched to a patient who fell from a third floor balcony of a local hotel. When you arrive at the patient's side, you find her to be responsive and breathing. She has no sensation below the level of her umbilicus. She cannot move her legs or flex her hips. You and your partner provide spinal immobilization to this patient because the fall was from a substantial height.

1. Which of the following terms are used to describe the hip bones?

A. Lumbar or coccygeal bones
B. Pelvic or innominate bones
C. Sesamoid, irregular, or long bones
D. Spongy, compact, or cancellous bones

2. What are the two main divisions of the nervous system?

A. Internal and external
B. External and central
C. Central and peripheral
D. Peripheral and cerebral

Assessment in Action (continued)

3. How many pairs of spinal nerves exist in the normal human body?

- **A.** 28
- **B.** 29
- **C.** 30
- **D.** 31

4. What is the function of afferent nerves?

- **A.** Carry information to the central nervous system.
- **B.** Carry information away from the central nervous system.
- **C.** Control breathing.
- **D.** Control thermoregulation.

5. What is the function of the lumbar nerve roots?

- **A.** Supply muscles of the chest that help with breathing.
- **B.** Provide abdominal muscle control.
- **C.** Provide bowel and bladder control.
- **D.** Supply hip flexors and leg muscles.

6. You decide to use a dermatome because of the lack of sensation in the patient's lower body. What is a dermatome designed to do?

- **A.** It determines how the internal organs function.
- **B.** It measures the degree of burn injury on the body.
- **C.** It helps determine a level of spinal injury on the body.
- **D.** It assesses level of consciousness.

7. If this patient were found not breathing, what would you expect the patient's blood pH to be?

- **A.** Higher than 7.35
- **B.** Lower than 7.35
- **C.** At 7.35

8. Explain the differences between ventilation and respiration.

9. Which of the body's buffer systems responds the most rapidly to keep the hydrogen ion concentration within normal limits?

10. Within which vessels is most of the body's blood contained?

CHAPTER 9

Pathophysiology

National EMS Education Standard Competencies

Pathophysiology

Integrates comprehensive knowledge of pathophysiology of major human systems.

Knowledge Objectives

1. Define pathophysiology, including its role in diagnosing and treating disease. (p 420)
2. Compare atrophy, hypertrophy, hyperplasia, dysplasia, and metaplasia as means of cellular adaptation. (p 420)
3. List factors that can affect or upset homeostasis. (p 420)
4. Explain the causes, clinical manifestations, assessment, and management of edema. (pp 421-422)
5. Discuss types of fluid deficits and potential resulting complications. (pp 422-423)
6. Explain the physiologic consequences of electrolyte imbalances in sodium, potassium, calcium, phosphate, and magnesium. (pp 422-425)
7. Compare respiratory acidosis, respiratory alkalosis, metabolic acidosis, and metabolic alkalosis. (pp 426-429)
8. Outline how cellular injury occurs in patients with hypoxia, chemical exposures, infection (sepsis), immunologic exposures (hypersensitivity reactions), inflammatory conditions, genetic disorders, nutritional imbalances, physical damage (mechanical injury), and other harmful exposures, such as extremes of hot and cold. (pp 429-434)
9. Examine the concept of apoptosis. (p 433)
10. Define perfusion, including the physiologic consequences of hypoperfusion. (pp 434-435)
11. Analyze the mechanisms by which the body compensates for hypoperfusion. (pp 434-435)
12. Discuss the causes of central and peripheral shock, including cardiogenic, obstructive, hypovolemic, and distributive shock. (pp 435-437)
13. Explain how to manage a patient in shock. (pp 437-438)
14. Describe multiple organ dysfunction syndrome. (pp 438-439)
15. Examine the body's three defense mechanisms against pathogens: anatomic barriers, the immune response, and the inflammatory response. (pp 439-451)
16. Explain how plasma protein systems—the complement system, the coagulation (clotting) system, and the kinin system—modulate the inflammatory response. (pp 447-448)
17. Compare wound healing by primary intention with wound healing by secondary intention. (p 450)
18. Outline each of the four types of hypersensitivity reactions and mechanisms for immunologic injury. (pp 451-453)
19. List several autoimmune reactions. (pp 453-454)
20. Compare inherited and acquired immunodeficiencies. (pp 454-455)
21. Analyze the controllable and uncontrollable risk factors that intersect in order to cause disease. (pp 455-456)
22. Outline how incidence, prevalence, morbidity, and mortality data are used to analyze disease risk. (pp 456-457)
23. Recognize autosomal dominant and autosomal recessive patterns of inheritance. (pp 456-458)
24. Analyze risk factors for cancer and cardiovascular disease. (pp 458-462)
25. Describe how hematologic disorders occur. (p 460)
26. Name common renal, gastrointestinal, and neuromuscular disorders. (pp 462-464)
27. List the stages of the general adaptation syndrome, and explore the relationship between stress and disease. (pp 465-467)

Skills Objectives

There are no skills objectives for this chapter.

Introduction

The human body is made up of cells, tissues, and organs. These structures function in a constantly changing microenvironment. The study of the origin, growth, structure, behavior, and reproduction of living organisms is known as *biology*. **Pathophysiology** is the study of the physiology of altered functioning in the presence of disease. The word is derived from the Greek words *pathos*, meaning "suffering," and *physis*, meaning "form." When the structure and function in cells, tissues, and organs break down in response to stressors and the body can no longer maintain homeostasis, disease may result. Determining the origin of a disease process often helps paramedics choose the best approach to patient evaluation and initial treatment.

To understand disease processes, you must understand the ways disease alters the structure and function in cells. We begin this chapter by reviewing the changes that affect cells, disrupt the body's ability to maintain homeostasis, and lead to disease. Next, we consider the influence inflammation and shock have on disease development. We also discuss the role of immunity and defense mechanisms in protecting the organism from disease. We conclude with a discussion on the effects genetics and stress have in disease development.

Adaptations in Cells and Tissues

When cells are exposed to adverse conditions, cells undergo a process of adaptation in an attempt to guard against injury. In some situations, the cells change permanently; in others, the structure or function of the cells change only temporarily.

Atrophy is a decrease in cell size due to a loss of subcellular components, which in turn leads to a decrease in the size of the tissue and organ. The actual number of cells remains unchanged. The decreased size represents an attempt to cope with a new steady state in less-than-favorable conditions or a lack of use. For example, a casted, immobilized limb shrinks in muscle mass as a result of disuse atrophy.

Hypertrophy is an increase in the size of the cells due to synthesis of more subcellular components, which in turn leads to an increase in tissue and organ size. For example, the left ventricle in the heart may hypertrophy owing to chronic high resistance pressures from hypertension (elevated blood pressure).

Hyperplasia is an increase in the actual number of cells in an organ or tissue, usually resulting in an increase in the size of the organ or tissue. For example, a callus represents hyperplasia of the keratinized layer of the epidermis of the foot in response to increased friction or trauma.

Dysplasia is an alteration of the size, shape, and organization of cells. It is most often found in epithelial cells that have undergone irregular, atypical changes in response to chronic irritation or inflammation. For example, the development of cervical dysplasia in women is strongly associated with exposure to certain human papillomaviruses.

Metaplasia refers to the reversible cellular adaptation in which one adult cell type is replaced by another adult cell type. For example, in squamous metaplasia, the ciliated epithelium in the airways of smokers may be replaced by metaplastic epithelium.

Disturbances in Fluid Balance

The human body is composed primarily of water. Therefore, all biochemical reactions taking place within the body are occurring in an aqueous environment. As a result, changes in fluid and electrolyte balance that disrupt homeostasis can either cause or exacerbate various disease processes. The result may be an emergent condition.

Homeostasis can be upset in a number of ways such as excessive output or input of fluids. Profuse sweating can cause dehydration, while excessive salt intake can contribute to hypertension.[1] Not drinking enough water can also alter homeostasis. In fact, a person deprived of water for 3 days or more may die.

The degree of fluid imbalance required to compromise homeostasis and cause illness depends on the patient's size, age, and any underlying medical conditions. In healthy adults, loss of more than 30% of total body fluid is required, but in a small child, a loss of only 10% to

YOU are the Paramedic PART 1

You and your partner are dispatched to a single-family residence to assist a 72-year-old man who is having difficulty breathing. On arrival, a neighbor greets you at the door. She tells you the resident of the home—your patient—lives alone, has had numerous heart attacks, and is not doing well. As you approach him, you assess his surroundings. You observe a large number of used facial tissues on the side table, along with an array of prescription medication bottles. The patient is sitting upright in a chair. He is wearing a nasal cannula attached to a home oxygen unit. He is able to speak only a few words at a time. He says he can't breathe, and you note that he looks pale.

1. What is your general impression of the patient?
2. What can you learn about the patient from his surroundings?

15% of total body fluid could easily produce symptoms. Consequently, fluid therapy is a fundamental step in resuscitation.

Special Populations

The total volume of water in the body varies by age and body composition throughout the lifespan. At birth, a healthy full-term neonate has about 80% total body water; however, the percentage of total body water decreases with age Figure 9-1. After several weeks, an infant's total body water drops to about 70%.[2] In childhood, the percentage of total body water falls to around 60%. Adults have 50% to 60% total body water, but water may constitute only 45% of body weight in older adults. Dehydration, then, can be a serious concern in older adults. Dehydration also remains a concern in the pediatric population. Despite infants having higher total body water content than adults, infants are at higher risk of dehydration due to increased rate of fluid loss during disease and pathologic states.

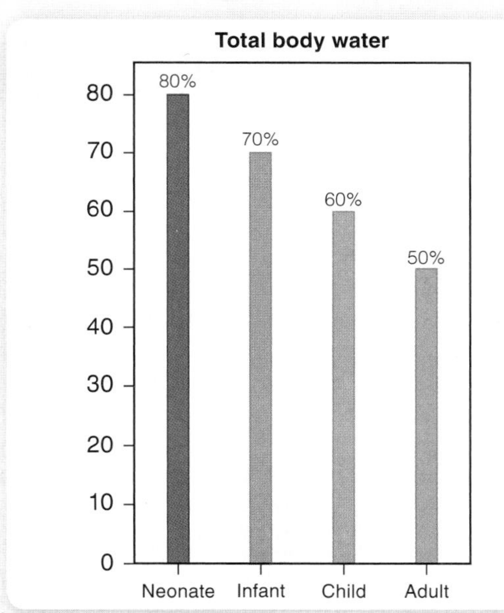

Figure 9-1 Average total water volume in the body by age.

Words of Wisdom

A hypertonic solution has a relatively higher osmotic pressure—that is, it contains more solute—than does the interstitial fluid or the fluid within and surrounding the brain. Administering a hypertonic solution such as mannitol, sodium bicarbonate, or hypertonic saline can cause excess fluid to drain from the tissues and into the blood, and can decrease swelling in the brain.

▶ Edema

Edema is swelling caused by excessive fluid trapped in the body tissues Figure 9-2. Edema may have any of several causes. One possible cause is increased capillary hydrostatic pressure, which may be associated with any of the following:

- Arteriolar dilation (for example, from allergic reactions or inflammation)
- Venous obstruction (for example, hepatic obstruction, heart failure, or thrombophlebitis)
- Increased vascular volume, as occurs in patients with heart failure
- An increased level of adrenocortical hormones
- Premenstrual sodium retention
- Pregnancy
- Environmental heat stress
- The effects of gravity from prolonged standing

Decreased colloidal osmotic pressure in the capillaries, another possible cause of edema, can be associated with various processes:

- Decreased production of plasma proteins, such as occurs in starvation and in patients with liver disease or severe protein deficiency
- Increased loss of plasma proteins attributable to protein-losing kidney diseases, extensive burns, or other causes

Obstruction of lymphatic vessels can also cause edema. Such obstruction can be associated with infection, lymphatic disease, or removal of lymphatic structures (for example, removal of lymph nodes during mastectomy can cause upper-extremity edema). When lymph vessels are blocked, the amount of fluid exiting through the arterial end of the capillaries is not equal to the amount of fluid being returned to the venous side. Consequently, more fluid leaves the arterial side, where the mean forces favoring outward movement are slightly higher. This additional fluid is picked up by the lymphatic system.

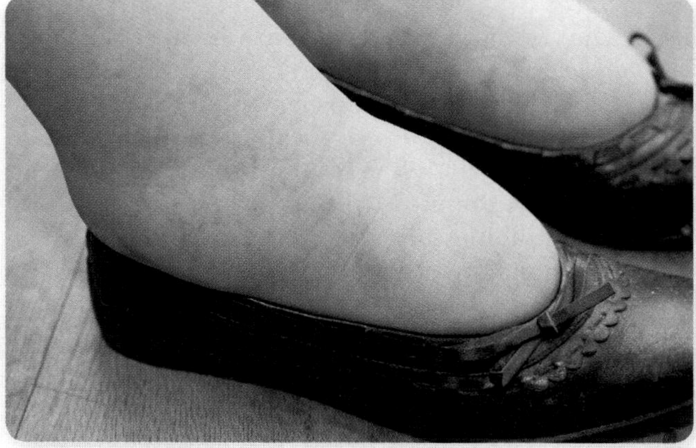

Figure 9-2 Edema is an excessive amount of fluid in the interstitial space.

Severe edema, then, may be caused by long-standing lymphatic obstruction. Peripheral edema (as in the ankles and feet) is the most common form. If a person is unable to get out of bed for an extended period, then edema may occur in the sacral area (sacral edema). *Ascites,* the abnormal accumulation of fluid in the peritoneal cavity, is also a type of edema.

The clinical manifestations of edema may be local or generalized. Patients with cardiac disease may have pulmonary edema, or edema may occur after submersion, narcotic overdose, or high altitude pulmonary edema (HAPE). Patients with acute pulmonary edema have an excessive amount of fluid in their lungs, which impairs the diffusion of oxygen into pulmonary capillaries, making the patient hypoxic and severely short of breath.

Paramedics must perform an in-depth physical assessment that includes auscultation of breath sounds, evaluation for pedal and sacral edema and jugular venous distention, an electrocardiogram (ECG), and vital signs. Along with a thorough exam, it is important to determine a patient's medical history and his or her current and past medications. Often, treatment is dictated by the patient's chief complaint and presenting problem. The definitive treatment of edema depends on the underlying medical condition that caused it. Possible interventions may include the use of continuous positive airway pressure, supplemental oxygen, positional therapy, nitrates, and diuretics.

Words of Wisdom

When you eat a bag of potato chips, you ingest a large quantity of salt. Acutely, the body responds by holding on to water. Hence, urine output temporarily declines. In healthy people, however, the kidneys and other regulatory mechanisms return both sodium and water levels to normal homeostatic balance.

Isotonic Fluid Deficit

Recall the concept of tonicity from Chapter 8, *Anatomy and Physiology*. An isotonic fluid deficit is a decrease in extracellular fluid with proportionate losses of sodium and water Table 9-1. This is the most common form of fluid loss, and is often the result of sweating. Excessive sweating or combining increased physical exertion with other comorbidities may complicate the fluid loss and cause additional problems. An isotonic fluid excess is a proportionate increase of sodium and water in extracellular fluid; common causes include kidney, heart, and liver failure. The manifestations of these conditions depend on the serum sodium level. When the body becomes dehydrated, orthostatic hypotension and decreased urine output (**oliguria**) often occur. When the sodium level is very high (>160 mEq/L), the patient is at risk of delirium and coma.

Table 9-1 Isotonic Fluid Deficit/Excess (Hypovolemia/Hypervolemia)

Imbalance	Common Causes
Fluid deficit (Proportionate loss in both water and sodium; decreased total body sodium)	Vomiting, diarrhea, loss of plasma or whole blood (eg, burns, hemorrhage), loop diuretic use, excessive sweating, fever, decreased oral fluid intake
Fluid excess (Proportionate gain in both water and sodium; increased total body sodium)	Heart failure, cirrhosis, renal failure, steroids, excessive sodium intake

Data from: Monahan FD. *Phipps' Medical-Surgical Nursing: Health and Illness Perspectives.* 8th ed. St. Louis, MO: Mosby; 2007:359; Potter P, Perry A, Stockert P, Hall A. *Basic Nursing.* 7th ed. St. Louis, MO: Mosby; 2011:466.

Electrolyte Imbalances

Sodium

Sodium, an element essential to the human body, is found primarily in the blood and fluid outside the cells. It regulates fluid balance, total fluid volume, and blood pressure by controlling the movement of water across cellular membranes. It also facilitates muscle contraction and nerve impulse transmission. Abnormal sodium levels may result in nausea, seizures, and cardiac dysrhythmias. A blood test can determine the level of serum sodium (Na); the normal range is 136 to 142 mEq/L.[3] A *hypertonic fluid deficit* occurs when there is water loss in the body without a proportionate loss of sodium—in other words, there is a relative water loss Table 9-2. This condition, called **hypernatremia**, is clinically defined as a serum sodium level greater than or equal to 143 mEq/L. A hypotonic fluid deficit occurs when there is sodium loss in the body without a proportionate loss of water (there is a relative water excess). This deficit causes **hyponatremia**, characterized by a serum sodium level of less or equal to 135 mEq/L.

Causes of hypernatremia and hyponatremia include excessive sweating in the heat or during exercise, gastrointestinal losses through vomiting or diarrhea, and inappropriate use of IV fluids or diuretics. Some patients have nausea and headaches. In others, seizures and coma develop. Clinical findings typically depend not only on the absolute sodium level, but also on when the abnormality developed. People who become hyponatremic over a period of days tend to have fewer symptoms than people in whom the abnormality develops acutely.

Table 9-2 Hypotonic and Hypertonic Fluid Deficit	
Imbalance	**Common Causes**
Hypotonic	
Fluid *deficit* with hyponatremia	Vomiting, diarrhea, prolonged sweating, thiazide diuretic use
Fluid *excess* with hyponatremia	Heart failure, cirrhosis, renal failure
Normal fluid volume with hyponatremia	Syndrome of inappropriate antidiuretic hormone (SIADH)
Hypertonic	
Fluid *deficit* with hypernatremia	Diabetic ketoacidosis, diabetes insipidus, high protein intake, severe diarrhea
Fluid *excess* with hypernatremia	Administration of hypertonic sodium solutions

Data from: Monahan FD. *Phipps' Medical-Surgical Nursing: Health and Illness Perspectives.* 8th ed. St. Louis, MO: Mosby; 2007:359; Potter P, Perry A, Stockert P, Hall A. *Basic Nursing.* 7th ed. St. Louis, MO: Mosby; 2011:466.

▶ Potassium

Potassium (K^+), the major intracellular cation, is crucial to many cellular functions, including neuromuscular control, regulating skeletal, smooth, and cardiac muscles, regulating acid-base balance, facilitating intracellular enzyme reactions, and maintaining intracellular osmolarity. The normal serum level of potassium ranges from 3.5 to 5.0 mEq/L.[3]

Hypokalemia is a decreased serum potassium level. Common causes include the following:

- Decreased dietary potassium intake and absorption
- Decreased shift of potassium into the cells as a result of insulin administration, alkalosis, or beta-adrenergic stimulation, such as with epinephrine
- Renal potassium loss, such as with increased aldosterone activity or diuretic use
- Extrarenal potassium loss, such as with vomiting, diarrhea, or laxative use

Muscular weakness, fatigue, and muscle cramps are the most frequent symptoms associated with mild to moderate hypokalemia. If the potassium level dips below 2.5 mEq/L, then flaccid paralysis, hyporeflexia, and sustained muscle contraction (tetany) may occur. Although acute hypokalemia can be treated with IV potassium supplementation, this therapy is rarely undertaken in the prehospital setting.

Hyperkalemia is an elevated serum potassium level. Here are some common causes you may see in the prehospital setting:

- Decreased excretion (from renal failure or from medications that inhibit potassium excretion [spironolactone, angiotensin-converting enzyme inhibitors, nonsteroidal anti-inflammatory drugs])
- Shifts of potassium from within the cell (as with burns, crush injuries, metabolic acidosis, and insulin deficiency)
- Excessive dietary potassium intake

An elevated potassium level interferes with normal neuromuscular function, leading to muscle weakness and, rarely, flaccid paralysis. While changes in the ECG may increase your index of suspicion for a given pathology, it is impossible to diagnose an electrolyte imbalance based entirely on findings from a cardiac monitor.

▶ Calcium

Nearly all (98%) of the body's calcium (Ca^{+2}) is found in the bones and teeth. This element lends strength and stability to the collagen and ground substance that form the matrix of the skeletal system. Calcium enters the body through the gastrointestinal tract. Its absorption from the intestine is aided by vitamin D Figure 9-3, which is manufactured largely by the body in a complex process that begins with exposure of the skin to sunlight. Calcium is then stored in bone tissue and ultimately excreted by the kidney. A normal level of serum calcium ranges from 8.2 to 10.2 mg/dL.[3]

Hypocalcemia, a decreased serum calcium level, can be caused by the following:

- Decreased calcium intake or absorption (as in malabsorption and vitamin D deficit)
- Increased calcium loss (as in alcoholism and diuretic therapy)
- Endocrine disease (such as hypoparathyroidism)
- Sepsis

Signs and symptoms of hypocalcemia stem from the increased excitation of the neuromuscular and cardiovascular systems. Skeletal muscle spasm can cause cramps or sustained muscle contraction (tetany). Laryngospasm with stridor can obstruct the airway. Seizures can occur, as can abnormal sensations (paresthesias) affecting the lips and extremities. Prolongation of the QT interval and the development of cardiac dysrhythmias may be observed on the ECG.

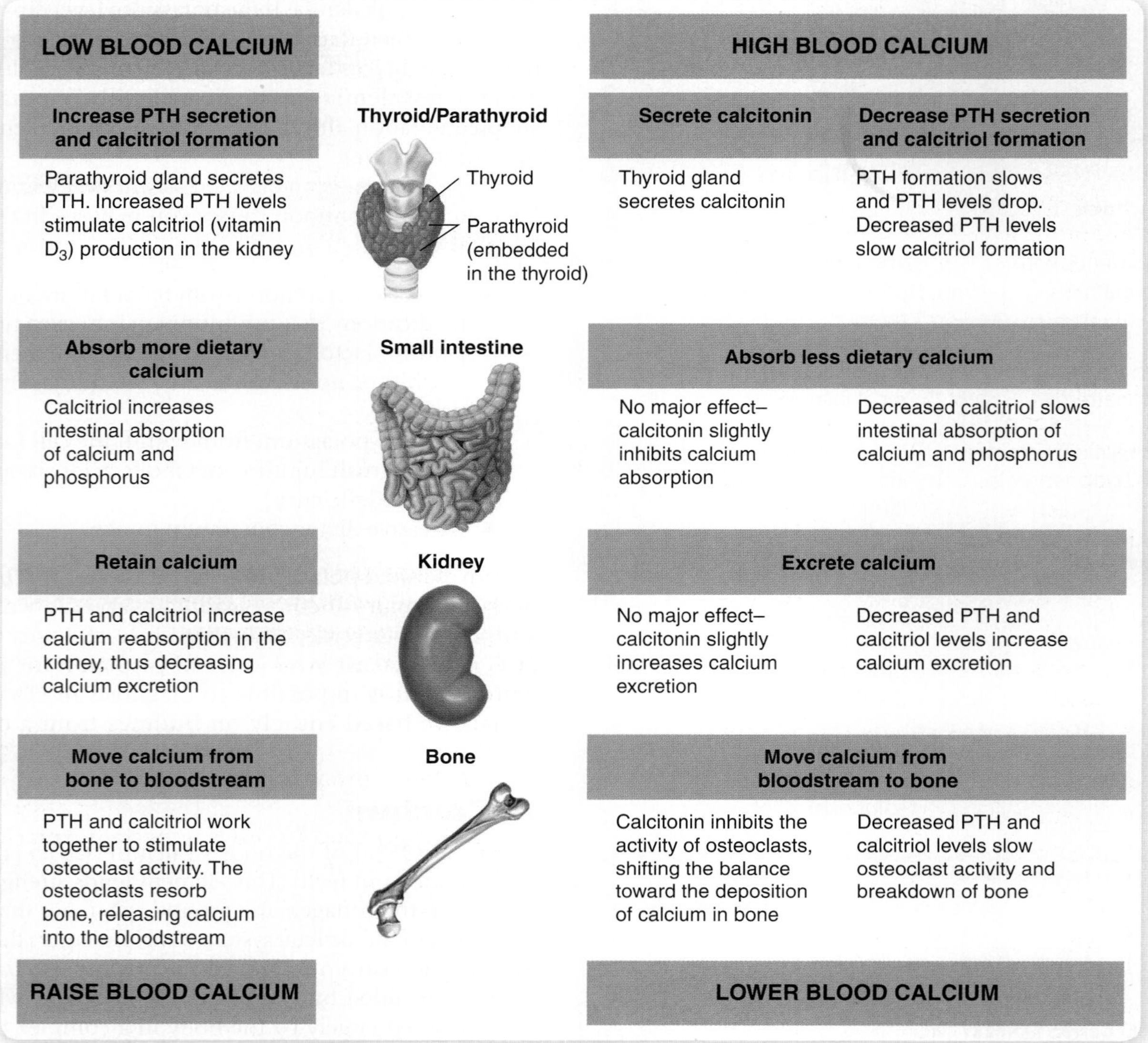

LOW BLOOD CALCIUM		HIGH BLOOD CALCIUM	
Increase PTH secretion and calcitriol formation	**Thyroid/Parathyroid**	**Secrete calcitonin**	**Decrease PTH secretion and calcitriol formation**
Parathyroid gland secretes PTH. Increased PTH levels stimulate calcitriol (vitamin D_3) production in the kidney	Thyroid; Parathyroid (embedded in the thyroid)	Thyroid gland secretes calcitonin	PTH formation slows and PTH levels drop. Decreased PTH levels slow calcitriol formation
Absorb more dietary calcium	**Small intestine**	**Absorb less dietary calcium**	
Calcitriol increases intestinal absorption of calcium and phosphorus		No major effect– calcitonin slightly inhibits calcium absorption	Decreased calcitriol slows intestinal absorption of calcium and phosphorus
Retain calcium	**Kidney**	**Excrete calcium**	
PTH and calcitriol increase calcium reabsorption in the kidney, thus decreasing calcium excretion		No major effect– calcitonin slightly increases calcium excretion	Decreased PTH and calcitriol levels increase calcium excretion
Move calcium from bone to bloodstream	**Bone**	**Move calcium from bloodstream to bone**	
PTH and calcitriol work together to stimulate osteoclast activity. The osteoclasts resorb bone, releasing calcium into the bloodstream		Calcitonin inhibits the activity of osteoclasts, shifting the balance toward the deposition of calcium in bone	Decreased PTH and calcitriol levels slow osteoclast activity and breakdown of bone
RAISE BLOOD CALCIUM		**LOWER BLOOD CALCIUM**	

Figure 9-3 Regulation of the blood calcium level. Calcitonin is a fast-acting hormone, but has only a weak effect, because any decrease in Ca^{+2} ion concentration triggers the release of parathyroid hormone (PTH). PTH almost completely overrides the calcitonin effect. In a patient with a prolonged calcium elevation or deficiency, the action of PTH is the most powerful hormonal mechanism for maintaining a normal blood calcium level.

Hypercalcemia is an increased serum calcium level. Selected causes are listed below:

- Increased calcium intake or absorption (such as with excessive antacid ingestion)
- Endocrine disorders (such as primary hyperparathyroidism and adrenal insufficiency)
- Neoplasms (cancers)
- Miscellaneous causes (such as diuretics and sarcoidosis)

The signs and symptoms associated with hypercalcemia are sometimes vague and can include fatigue, weakness, nausea, constipation, and frequent urination (**polyuria**). In severe cases, stupor, coma, or renal failure may develop. Treatment of hypercalcemia depends on addressing the underlying cause. On an acute basis, volume replacement with boluses of 0.45% or 0.9% sodium chloride solution may be helpful.

▶ Phosphate

Phosphate (PO_4^{-3}), primarily an intracellular anion, is essential to many body functions.

Hypophosphatemia is a decrease in the level of serum phosphate. Causes include the following:

- Decreased supply or absorption, as can occur in starvation, malabsorption, or blocked absorption (such as with aluminum-containing antacids)
- Excessive loss of phosphate associated with use of diuretics, or in patients with

hyperparathyroidism, hyperthyroidism, or alcoholism
- Intracellular shift of phosphorus (for example, after administering glucose, anabolic steroids, or oral contraceptives, or in patients with respiratory alkalosis or salicylate poisoning)
- Electrolyte abnormalities, such as hypercalcemia and hypomagnesemia
- Abnormal loss of nutrients followed by inadequate replenishment, as can occur in patients with diabetic ketoacidosis or chronic alcoholism

Signs and symptoms can include dysrhythmias, hypotension, muscle weakness, and altered mental status. Acute, severe hypophosphatemia can lead to seizures, acute blood disorders, and increased susceptibility to infection. The breakdown of muscle fibers (rhabdomyolysis) may also occur. Treatment involves oral replenishment in mild to moderate cases. Severe cases and symptomatic patients require hospital IV phosphate replacement.

Hyperphosphatemia, an increased serum phosphate level, has many possible causes:

- Massive loading of phosphate into the extracellular fluid
  - Excessive use of vitamin D, laxatives, or enemas containing phosphate
  - IV phosphate supplements
  - Chemotherapy
  - Metabolic acidosis
- Decreased excretion into the urine (such as in renal failure and hypoparathyroidism, and with excessive administration of growth hormone [which results in acromegaly]).

Signs and symptoms vary widely but may include tremor, paresthesia, hyperreflexia (overactive reflexes), confusion, seizures, muscle weakness, decreased mental status, coma, hypotension, heart failure, or a prolonged QT interval.[4-6] The normal range for serum phosphate is 2.3 to 4.7 mg/dL.[3]

▶ Magnesium

Magnesium (Mg^{+2}) is the second most abundant intracellular cation, after potassium. About 50% of the body's magnesium is stored in the bones, 49% in other body cells, and the remaining 1% in the extracellular fluid. The normal range of serum magnesium is 1.3 to 2.1 mEq/L.[3]

Hypomagnesemia, a decreased serum magnesium level, has several possible causes:

- Diminished magnesium absorption or intake (as occurs in malabsorption, chronic diarrhea, laxative abuse, or malnutrition)
- Increased renal loss of magnesium (related to diuretics, hyperaldosteronism, hypercalcemia, or volume expansion)
- Miscellaneous causes, such as diabetes, respiratory alkalosis, and pregnancy

Table 9-3 Major Electrolytes

Electrolyte	Symbol	Normal Serum Level
Sodium	Na	136–142 mEq/L
Chloride	Cl^-	96–106 mEq/L
Potassium	K^+	3.5–5.0 mEq/L
Calcium	Ca^{+2}	8.2–10.2 mg/dL
Phosphate	PO_4^{-3}	2.3–4.7 mg/dL
Magnesium	Mg^{+2}	1.3–2.1 mEq/L

Data from: AMA Manual of Style, 10th edition. Table 2: Selected Laboratory Tests, With Reference Ranges and Conversion Factors.

Weakness and muscle cramps are common symptoms. A person with hypomagnesemia may have marked neuromuscular and CNS hyperirritability, with tremors and jerking. Hypertension, tachycardia, or ventricular dysrhythmias may occur, and confusion and disorientation can be pronounced.

Hypermagnesemia is an increased serum magnesium level. It almost always occurs as a result of kidney insufficiency, in which the body is unable to excrete magnesium taken in from food or drugs, especially antacids and laxatives. Symptoms include muscle weakness, decreased deep tendon reflexes, and altered mental status. Weakness is common, and respiratory muscle paralysis and cardiac arrest are possible.

Table 9-3 summarizes the major electrolytes of the body.

Disturbances of Acid-Base Balance

The concept of pH was discussed in Chapter 8, *Anatomy and Physiology*; recall that pH represents the concentration of hydrogen ions (H^+) in a solution. In other words, it is a measure of the acidity or alkalinity of a solution. There is an inverse relationship between pH and H^+ ion concentration: the lower the pH, the higher the acidity.

In the human body, maintaining pH within a narrow range is vital. Acids and bases neutralize each other; therefore, they must remain in balance for the body to preserve homeostasis. Every patient complaint you encounter as a paramedic will have a component of acid-base balance and imbalance. For example, a patient experiencing an asthma attack may have a resulting alkalosis (pH greater than 7.45), whereas a patient in diabetic ketoacidosis will experience an underlying acidosis (pH less than 7.35).

Acidosis is an increase in extracellular H^+ ions; **alkalosis** is a decrease in extracellular H^+ ions.

$$\downarrow \text{pH means} \uparrow H^+ \text{ concentration} = \text{Acidosis}$$
$$\uparrow \text{pH means} \downarrow H^+ \text{ concentration} = \text{Alkalosis}$$

If intracellular pH is low, then the excessive concentration of H^+ ions in the extracellular fluid (the fluid outside the cell) will signal the cell to accept more H^+ ions, giving it an overall positive charge. To return its charge to neutral, the cell begins to shift potassium and other cations (positively charged ions) into the interstitial fluid.

Disturbances of acid-base balance are associated with disturbances of potassium balance, in part because of the kidney transport system that moves H^+ and K^+ in opposite directions. In acidosis, the kidneys excrete H^+ and resorb K^+. Conversely, in alkalosis, the kidneys resorb H^+ and excrete K^+. A potassium imbalance usually manifests itself as a disturbance in excitable tissues, especially those of the heart.

In addition, Ca^{+2} ions shift out of the cell in response to an influx of hydrogen. Because calcium acts at the neuromuscular junction, a high serum calcium level (hypercalcemia) decreases the rate of neural transmission—the speed at which an impulse is conveyed by a neuron. This slowed signaling will cause some minimal ECG changes but seldom precipitates a dysrhythmia. A low serum calcium level (hypocalcemia), on the other hand, is characterized by hypersensitive neurons and an accelerated rate of neural transmission. Signs of hypocalcemia include wheezing, stridor, bradycardia, crackles, and an S_3 heart sound. Hypocalcemia can be identified on ECG and can cause a dysrhythmia.

Types of Acid-Base Imbalance

Acid-base disorders are associated with four main clinical presentations: respiratory acidosis, respiratory alkalosis, metabolic acidosis, and metabolic alkalosis. Fluctuations in the level of bicarbonate in the body cause metabolic acidosis or alkalosis, whereas respiratory disorders cause respiratory acidosis or alkalosis. When the body's buffering systems, discussed in Chapter 8, *Anatomy and Physiology*, cannot immediately correct an acid-base imbalance, compensatory mechanisms respond to help restore the normal balance. For example, respiratory alkalosis may occur as a compensatory response to metabolic acidosis. Thus, patient management often involves treating more than one acid-base imbalance.

Respiratory Acidosis

The following equation demonstrates how a diminished rate of respiration can precipitate acidosis:

$$\downarrow \text{Respiration} \rightarrow \uparrow CO_2 \rightarrow \uparrow H_2CO_3 \rightarrow \text{Acidosis}$$

Respiratory acidosis is always related to hypoventilation. Decreased lung tidal volume reduces the amount of CO_2 that is exhaled, causing hypercapnia (increased CO_2). Because the acidosis is linked to inadequate breathing, the renal buffer system is initiated as a compensatory mechanism. Some causes of respiratory acidosis include the following:

- Airway obstruction
- Cardiac arrest
- Overdose of a CNS depressant drug, such as heroin
- Submersion
- Respiratory arrest
- Pulmonary edema
- Closed head injury
- Chest trauma
- Carbon monoxide poisoning

Hypoventilation associated with any of these conditions can devolve quickly into an overwhelming, life-threatening acidosis, making it impossible for the renal system to compensate in time to accomplish a pH shift. The decrease in pH increases permeability of cell membranes, causing a leakage of potassium into the blood. The release of potassium ions into the extracellular fluid can cause a potentially fatal cardiac dysrhythmia. The discharge of calcium into extracellular spaces causes hypercalcemia, characterized by lethargy, a diminished level of consciousness, and a generalized slowing of the nervous system. This nervous system inhibition may also be evidenced by a delayed pupillary response or a weakened or delayed response to painful stimuli.

Signs and symptoms of respiratory acidosis include the following:

- Systemic or cerebral vasodilation (or both)
- Headache, light-headedness
- Warm, flushed skin[7]
- CNS depression
- **Bradypnea** (slow respiratory rate)
- Nausea and vomiting

Chronic obstructive pulmonary disease (COPD) gradually destroys lung tissue and inhibits oxygen and carbon dioxide exchange, eventually resulting in respiratory acidosis Figure 9-4. In patients with COPD, the normal stimulus for gas exchange is absent. Carbon dioxide retention leads to an increasing level of carbonic acid. Chemoreceptors eventually become unable to detect the presence of metabolic acids. As a result, the only remaining breathing stimulus is the hypoxic drive, which stimulates breathing by sensing a decreased oxygen level in the blood.

The slow onset of this form of respiratory acidosis in patients with COPD makes it survivable. The renal system slowly moderates the acidosis, preventing the life-threatening cardiac dysrhythmias often associated with acute acidosis.

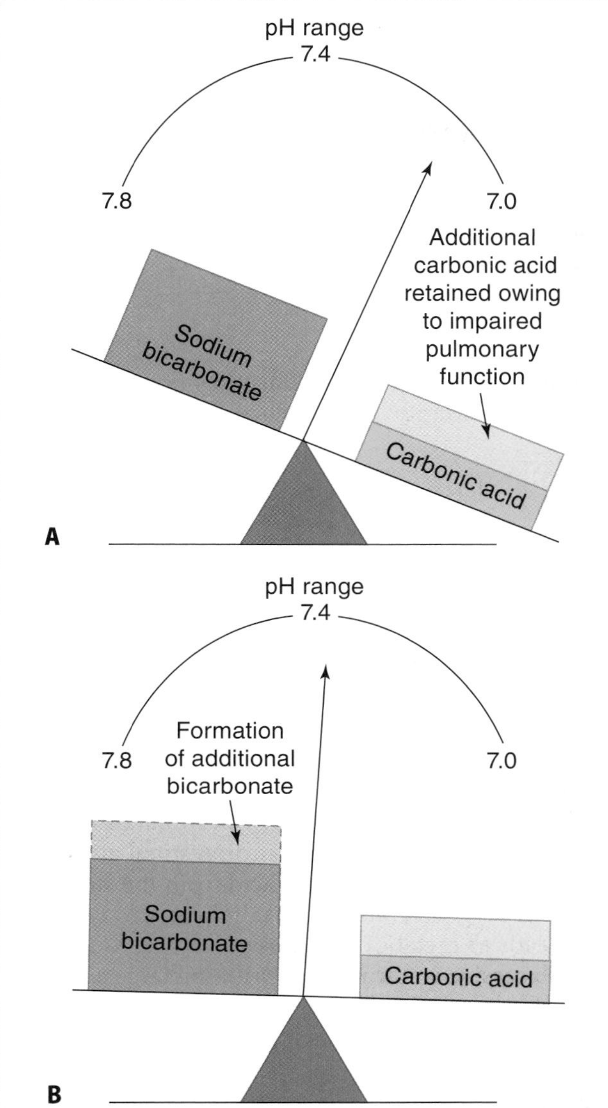

Figure 9-4 A. Derangement of acid-base balance in respiratory acidosis. **B.** Compensation by formation of additional bicarbonate.

Words of Wisdom

Compensatory mechanisms for pH imbalances bring the pH closer to normal. Respiratory compensation (acidosis or alkalosis) occurs rapidly and relatively predictably. Metabolic compensation, if it occurs at all, takes hours or days. Acute compensation is never complete. Chronic compensation, such as that which occurs in patients with COPD, often returns the pH to normal.

Respiratory Alkalosis

The following equation demonstrates how an increased respiratory rate can produce alkalosis:

$$\uparrow \text{Rate of respiration} \rightarrow \downarrow CO_2 \rightarrow \downarrow H_2CO_3 \rightarrow \text{Alkalosis}$$

Respiratory alkalosis is associated with conditions that result in hyperventilation. Over time, an increased respiratory rate decreases the amount of circulating carbon dioxide in the body. In respiratory alkalosis, the carbon dioxide level in the blood drops, which reduces the level of circulating carbonic acid. The renal system then begins to retain H^+ ions to rebalance the depleted acid level. As the same time, H^+ ions begin to shift from the extracellular fluid compartment to the intracellular fluid. Calcium moves into the intracellular fluid to rebalance the depleted hydrogen level. The resulting hypocalcemia causes muscle contractions. In fact, hyperventilation accompanied by **carpopedal spasm** (a contorted position in which the fingers or toes flex in a clawlike manner) is the classic sign of respiratory alkalosis.

Some causes of hyperventilation and respiratory alkalosis include the following:

- Drug overdose, especially an overdose of aspirin
- Fever
- Overzealous bag-mask ventilation

Some signs and symptoms of respiratory alkalosis are listed below:

- Diminished level of consciousness
- Light-headedness
- Carpopedal spasm
- Paresthesias of the lips and face
- Chest tightness
- Confusion
- Vertigo
- Blurred vision
- Nausea and vomiting

Metabolic Acidosis

The following equation demonstrates how an increased carbonic acid level can produce **metabolic acidosis**:

$$\uparrow H_2CO_3 \rightarrow \uparrow H^+ + HCO_3^- \rightarrow \text{Acidosis}$$

Any acidosis unrelated to the respiratory system is considered metabolic. An increased rate of breathing (tachypnea) represents the body's attempt to restore acid-base balance, by eliminating excess carbon dioxide through the respiratory system. For example, patients with diabetic ketoacidosis often experience Kussmaul respirations (deep, closely spaced, sighing breaths), in which the body hyperventilates in an attempt to blow off carbon dioxide and correct the acidosis.

As with any acidosis, the extracellular hydrogen level increases and extracellular buffers attempt to neutralize the excess acid. Ion shifts occur, hydrogen leaks into the cells, and potassium shifts into the extracellular spaces, raising the serum potassium level and putting the patient at risk of a life-threatening dysrhythmia. Calcium also shifts into the extracellular spaces. The resulting hypercalcemia obstructs impulse transmission to neurons in muscle and other tissues. Consequently, the patient becomes lethargic and has a decreased level of consciousness.

Causes of metabolic acidosis include the following:

- **Lactic acidosis.** Lactic acidosis is the product of anaerobic cellular respiration, which occurs when tissues and organs are inadequately perfused, as in shock and cardiac arrest.
- **Ketoacidosis.** Ketoacidosis is associated with insulin deficiency or desensitization of cells to insulin. Unable to use glucose for energy, cells must instead begin metabolizing fatty acids. Extremely acidic compounds called ketones are the byproducts of such metabolism.
- **Aspirin (acetylsalicylic acid) overdose.** A dose of 10 to 30 g aspirin in an adult constitutes an overdose. Aspirin directly stimulates the respiratory centers of the brain, producing tachypnea. Rapid breathing leads to respiratory alkalosis, and initiation of renal compensatory mechanisms leads to metabolic acidosis.
- **Alcohol ingestion.** Ingesting an excessive amount of ethyl alcohol can induce alcoholic ketoacidosis. Ingesting as little as 30 mL of either methanol (wood alcohol) or ethylene glycol (antifreeze) can also induce fatal forms of acidosis.
- **Gastrointestinal losses.** Gastrointestinal losses can precipitate metabolic acidosis. Diarrhea, for example, removes bases from the lower intestinal tract.

The clinical presentation of metabolic acidosis is similar to that of respiratory acidosis:[7,8]

- Vasodilation
- CNS depression
- Headaches
- Warm, flushed skin
- Tachypnea
- Nausea and vomiting
- Cardiac dysrhythmias

Metabolic Alkalosis

The following equation demonstrates how a decreased H^+ ion concentration can produce alkalosis:

$$\downarrow H^+ \rightarrow \downarrow H_2CO_3 \rightarrow \text{Alkalosis}$$

Metabolic alkalosis occurs when increased urine output or a decreased gastric acid level leads to an excessive loss of acid. This is rarely an acute condition, but it is common among chronically ill patients, especially those who require nasogastric suctioning.

Several factors associated with upper gastrointestinal losses can lead to metabolic alkalosis:

- **Excessive vomiting.** Illness or an eating disorder, such as anorexia nervosa or bulimia, can be responsible for upper gastrointestinal acid loss. Expelling a great deal of acid from the stomach can trigger a complex metabolic pathway that leads to metabolic alkalosis.
- **Excessive water intake.** Drinking large amounts of water during vigorous exercise not only dilutes the stomach acid, but also stimulates the

YOU are the Paramedic — PART 2

You ask your partner to obtain a baseline oxygen saturation level and obtain baseline vital signs, including waveform capnography. While she's setting up her equipment, you ask the patient about his past medical history. With great difficulty, he replies, "Heart failure."

Recording Time: 1 Minute	
Appearance	Awake, in distress, anxious
Level of consciousness	Alert (oriented to person, place, and day)
Airway	Open
Breathing	Accelerated rate; accessory muscle use; productive cough
Circulation	Weak radial pulses; moist, pale, cool skin

3. How does the recruitment of accessory muscles facilitate breathing?
4. How might the productive cough help you identify the source of the patient's breathing difficulty?

small intestine to prepare for incoming food from the stomach. An outpouring of strongly alkaline digestive enzymes into the lower gastrointestinal tract exacerbates any existing acid-base imbalance.

- **Nasogastric suctioning.** Removal of contents directly from the gastrointestinal tract eliminates acids from the body, resulting in alkalosis.
- **Excessive intake of alkaline substances.** Metabolic alkalosis can stem from excessive reliance on antacids or similar alkaline substances. This possibility is important to remember when assessing a patient with cardiac disease who reports having self-medicated for hours or days with over-the-counter antacids.

  Another cause of excessive intake of bases is the overzealous administration of sodium bicarbonate during resuscitation. Introducing copious amounts of sodium bicarbonate into the circulatory system can dramatically alter the pH level.

The respiratory system serves as the compensatory mechanism for metabolic alkalosis. Bradypnea develops to correct the diminished H^+ ion level by retaining carbon dioxide, thereby driving up levels of circulating acids.

Signs and symptoms of metabolic alkalosis include the following:

- Confusion
- Muscle tremors and cramps
- Bradypnea
- Hypotension

Cellular Injury

The manifestations of cellular injury or death depend on how many and which types of cells are damaged. Various processes may cause cellular injury:

- Hypoxia (lack of oxygen)
- Ischemia (lack of blood supply)
- Chemical injury
- Infectious injury
- Immunologic (hypersensitivity) injury
- Physical damage (mechanical injury)
- Inflammatory injury

Manifestations of cellular injury occur at the microscopic (structural) and functional levels. Common microscopic abnormalities (such as cardiac cell **necrosis** [a process in which the cell breaks down] as a result of long-standing hypoxemia) include cell swelling, rupture of cell membranes or nuclear membranes, and breakdown of nuclear material such as chromosomes **Figure 9-5**. This kind of damage often distorts the shape of a cell and disrupts its function. Functional disturbances may include inefficient oxygen utilization, intracellular acidosis, toxic waste accumulation, and derangement of nutrient metabolization.

Changes in individual cells often affect the entire organism. In some cases, the changes are associated with only minor systemic abnormalities, such as fever. At other times, such as when renal failure occurs, entire organ systems collapse and the patient's condition becomes critical. Because all body systems are connected, dysfunction in one system inevitably affects the function of other systems, upsetting the homeostatic balance on which the body depends to sustain life.

Words of Wisdom

The fatty compounds of which the cell membrane is composed are chemically neutral (uncharged); however, electrolytes such as sodium and potassium are water based and therefore carry a charge. To permeate a cell membrane, charged molecules must travel along special pathways. Such transport channels—the so-called ion channels—consist of protein-lined pores specifically sized for a given substance (for example, calcium or potassium). Lidocaine and other local anesthetics, as well as antidysrhythmic drugs such as amiodarone, exert nerve-blocking effects on these ion channels.

With proper treatment, cellular injury can be repaired, up to a point; however, when irreversible injury occurs, no treatment will help. Cell death is followed by necrosis. The cell membrane becomes abnormally permeable, allowing an influx of electrolytes and fluids. Then the cell and its organelles swell, and lysosomes release enzymes that destroy intracellular components. These processes occur during and after cell death.

Hypoxic Injury

Hypoxic injury is a common—and often deadly—cause of cellular injury. It may result from decreased amounts of oxygen in the air or loss of hemoglobin function (such as in carbon monoxide poisoning), a decreased number of red blood cells (as from bleeding), disease of the respiratory or cardiovascular system (such as COPD), or loss of cytochromes (mitochondrial proteins that convert oxygen to adenosine triphosphate [ATP], like that seen in cyanide poisoning).

Although hypoxia has deleterious effects on cells, the damage does not stop there. Cells that are hypoxic for more than a few seconds produce mediators (substances) that may damage areas near or far from the initial area of damage in the body. The result is a positive feedback cycle in which mediators lead to more cell damage, which leads to more hypoxia, which leads to further mediator production, and so forth.

The earliest and most dangerous mediators produced by cells in response to hypoxia are **free radicals**. A free radical molecule is missing one electron in its outer shell. The presence of an odd, unpaired electron causes chemical instability as free radicals randomly attack cells

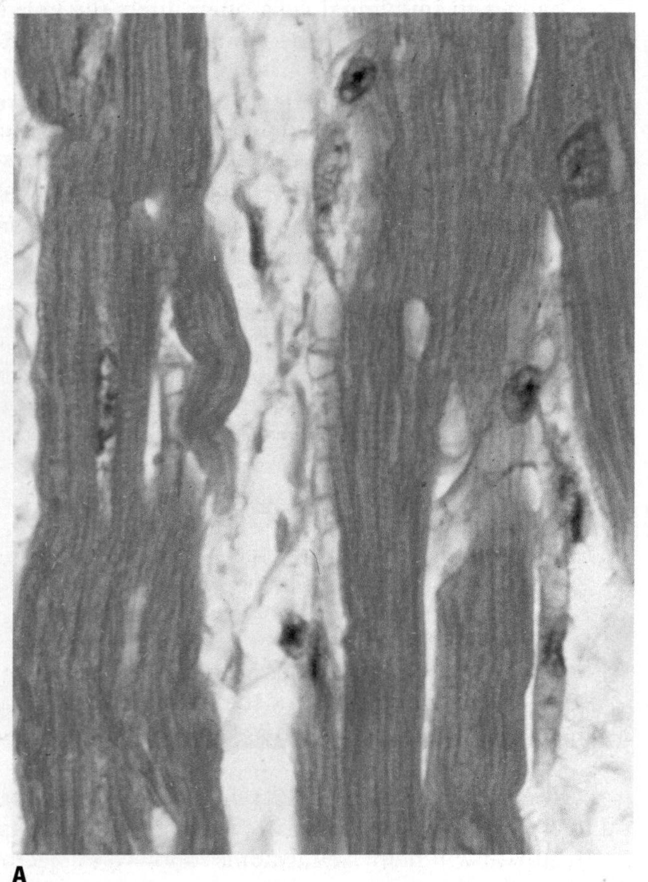

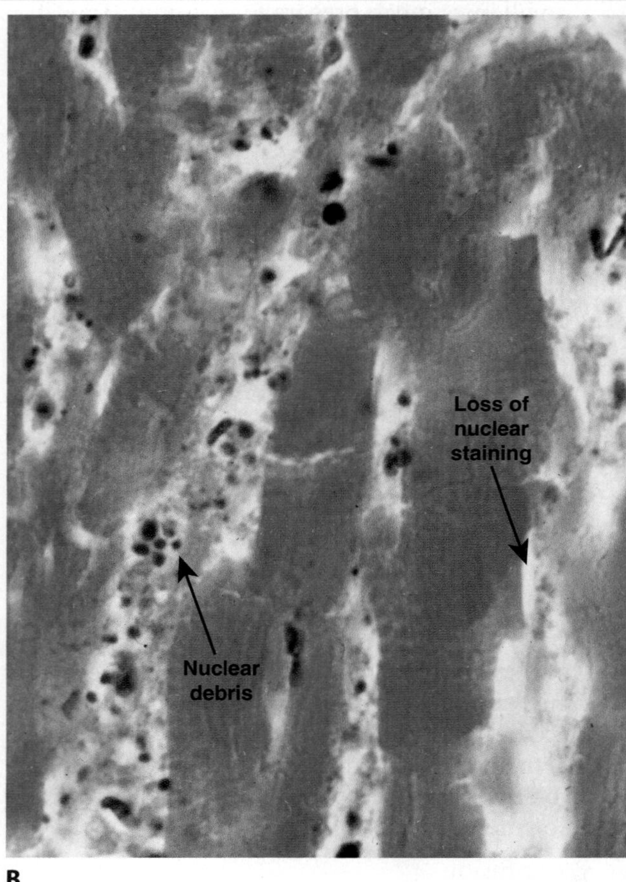

Figure 9-5 Comparison of cardiac muscle fibers **(A)** with necrotic fibers **(B)**. Note fragmentation of fibers, loss of nuclear staining, and fragmented bits of nuclear debris. Cellular injury causes swelling, resulting in nuclear membrane rupture and breakdown of the nuclear material (original magnification ×400).

From: An Introduction to Human Disease, 7th Edition. Photo courtesy of Leonard V. Crowley, MD, Century College.

and membranes in an attempt to steal back the missing electron. The result is widespread and potentially deadly tissue damage.

▶ Chemical Injury

A variety of chemicals, including poisons, lead, carbon monoxide, ethanol, and pharmacologic agents, may injure and ultimately destroy cells. Common poisons include cyanide and pesticides. Cyanide induces cell hypoxia by blocking oxidative phosphorylation in the mitochondria and preventing the metabolism of oxygen. Pesticides block an enzyme, acetylcholinesterase, thereby preventing proper transmission of nerve impulses.

Long-term ingestion of lead, such as that caused by chewing on windowsills painted with lead-based paint, leads to brain injury and neurologic dysfunction. The ability of lead to substitute for calcium (molecules of lead and calcium are a similar size) is a common factor in many of its toxic actions. Mostly likely, lead occupies the space normally held for calcium in vital biochemical reactions, leading to abnormal results and dysfunction.

Carbon monoxide binds to hemoglobin more easily than does oxygen, preventing adequate oxygenation of the tissues. A low-level exposure of carbon monoxide causes nausea, vomiting, and headache. A higher level can be fatal in less than 2 hours.[9]

At lower doses, ethanol, as found in drinking alcohol, causes the well-known effects of inebriation. Higher doses produce severe CNS depression and hypoventilation, sometimes precipitating cardiovascular collapse.

Some pharmacologic agents produce toxic products when the agents are metabolized in the body, especially in overdose conditions. For example, acute overdose occurs when an excessive dose of acetaminophen (Tylenol) is ingested. If an adult takes a dose of more than 140 mg/kg, or 4 g, then the toxins that accumulate can poison the liver and can sometimes be fatal.

▶ Infectious Injury

Infectious injury to cells occurs as a result of an invasion of bacteria, fungi, or viruses. Bacteria may cause injury by direct action on cells or by the production of toxins. Viruses often initiate an inflammatory response that leads to cell damage and patient symptoms.

Virulence measures the disease-causing ability of a microorganism. The pathogenicity of any particular microorganism is a function of its ability to reproduce and cause disease within the human body. In particular, the growth and survival of bacteria in the body depend on the effectiveness of the body's own defense mechanisms and on the bacteria's ability to resist the mechanisms. A depressed immune system is less capable of fighting off microorganisms that the body perceives as harmful; populations with weaker immune systems include newborn infants, older adults, people with diabetes, and people with cancer or other chronic diseases.

Bacteria

Many bacteria have a capsule that protects them from ingestion and destruction by **phagocytes**—cells (that is, white blood cells) that engulf and consume foreign material such as microorganisms and cellular debris **Figure 9-6**.

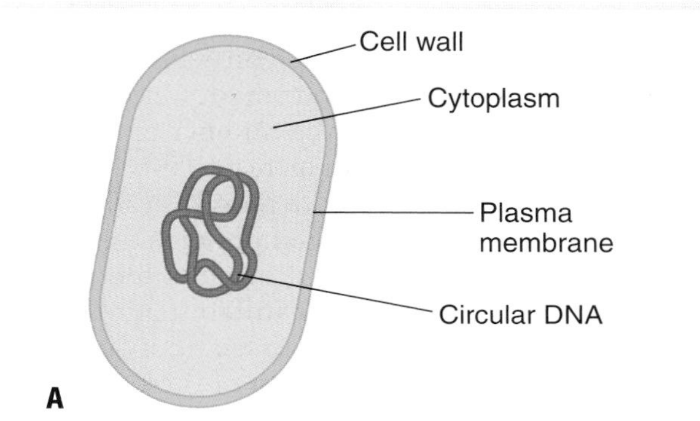

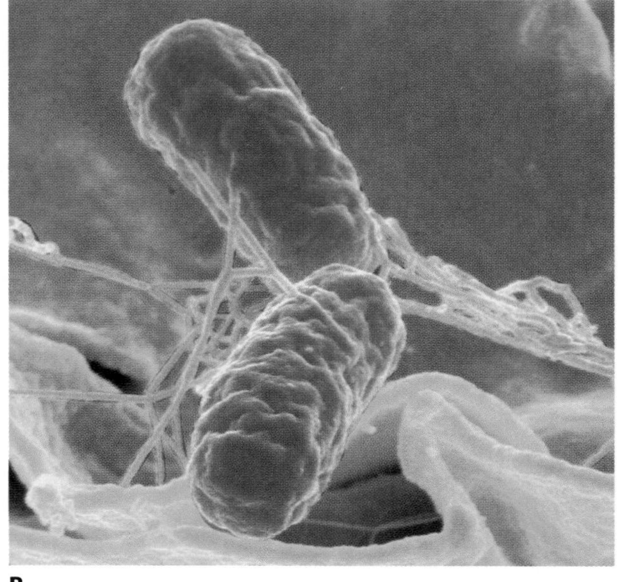

Figure 9-6 General structure of a bacterium. **A.** Bacteria come in many shapes and sizes, but all have a circular strand of deoxyribonucleic acid (DNA), cytoplasm, and a plasma membrane. A cell wall surrounds the membrane in many bacteria. **B.** An electron micrograph of *Salmonella* bacteria. Many bacteria have a capsule that protects them from ingestion and destruction by phagocytes.

A: © Jones & Bartlett Learning; B: Courtesy of Rocky Mountain Laboratory, NIAID, NIH.

However, not all bacteria are encapsulated. *Mycobacterium tuberculosis*, for example, lacks a capsule, yet stubbornly resists destruction; it can be transported by phagocytes throughout the body.

Bacteria can be categorized depending on the results of Gram staining. In Gram staining, a dried, fixed suspension of bacteria, prepared on a microscopic slide, is stained first with a purple dye and then with an iodine solution. Next, the slide is decolorized with alcohol or another solvent; it is then stained with a red dye. Bacteria that resist decolorization and retain the purple stain are called **gram-positive** bacteria, whereas those that have been decolorized and accept the red counterstain are termed **gram-negative** bacteria. Gram-positive bacteria are distinguished by thick cell walls composed of many layers of peptidoglycan (amino acids and glucose); conversely, the cell walls of gram-negative bacteria consist largely of lipids. The pathogenic qualities of gram-negative bacteria, which include the microorganism that causes bubonic plague, make them especially problematic for humans.

Bacteria also produce exotoxins or endotoxins—substances such as enzymes or toxins—that can injure or destroy cells. Staphylococci, streptococci, and *Clostridium tetani*, for example, secrete exotoxins into the medium surrounding the cell. Exotoxins are produced within the cell and are released into surrounding tissues or fluids (blood or lymph). They are poisonous and their actions vary depending on the organism; for example, neurotoxins damage nervous tissue, enterotoxins affect the tissues of the gastrointestinal tract, and cytotoxins damage a variety of host tissues. Inactive exotoxins are sometimes used as the basis for vaccines.

Endotoxins are lipopolysaccharides that are part of the cell walls of gram-negative bacteria. Endotoxins cause inflammation, fever, chills, and malaise, as well as effecting vascular tone. When large amounts of endotoxins are present in the body, septic shock may develop. Endotoxins remain active even after the bacteria are destroyed, which may be one reason why there is a delay in seeing the effects of antibiotics.

When cells are injured, circulating white blood cells are attracted to the site of injury. White blood cells release endogenous **pyrogens**, which then cause a fever to develop. Indeed, the body's most common reaction to the presence of bacteria is inflammation. Some bacteria have the ability to produce hypersensitivity reactions. The presence of bacteria in the blood is called bacteremia; septicemia (sepsis) is systemic disease, which may be life threatening, caused by the proliferation of microorganisms (or related toxins) in the blood.

Viruses

Viruses are among the most common causes of afflictions. Viruses are intracellular parasites that take over the metabolic processes of the host cell and use the cell to help them replicate. A virus consists of a nucleic acid core of RNA or DNA. Surrounding the viral core is a protein coat known as the capsid, which protects the virus from phagocytosis. Some viruses have an additional protective coat known as the envelope.

The replication of a virus occurs inside the host cell because viruses do not have their own organelles. Viral infection of a host cell leads to a decreased synthesis of macromolecules that are vital to the host cell. Unlike bacteria, however, viruses do not produce exotoxins or endotoxins. Viruses induce pathology by disrupting the normal metabolic processes, but are protected from antibiotics by living and replicating inside the host cell and effectively hiding from the medication.

A symbiotic relationship may exist between a virus and normal cells that allows the virus to persist without causing an active infection. Viruses such as the human immunodeficiency virus (HIV) can elicit a strong immune response, rapidly producing an irreversible, lethal injury in susceptible cells.

▶ Immunologic and Inflammatory Injury

Inflammation is a protective response occurring in the presence of cellular injury, including trauma, infection, and hypoxia. Infection is characterized by an invasion of microorganisms that causes cell or tissue injury, which leads to the **inflammatory response**. The inflammatory response can be triggered by an agent that is physical (heat or cold), chemical (such as concentrated acid or alkali or another caustic chemical), or microbiologic (such as a bacterium or virus). The inflammatory response is characterized by both local and systemic effects, as shown in **Figure 9-7**, and discussed in detail later in this chapter.

Local effects consist of dilation (expansion) of blood vessels and increased vascular permeability. Leukocytes (white blood cells) are attracted to the site of injury. The leukocytes adhere to the endothelium of the small blood vessels, exert force to break through the cell walls, and migrate to the area of tissue damage. The characteristic signs of inflammation are heat, redness, tenderness, swelling, and pain. The increased warmth and redness of the inflamed tissues are caused by dilation of capillaries and slowing of blood flow through the vessels. Swelling occurs because the extravasation (leakage) of plasma from the dilated and more permeable vessels causes the volume of fluid in the inflamed tissue to increase. The tenderness and pain are secondary to irritation of sensory nerve endings at the site of the inflammatory process.

If the inflammatory process is severe, then systemic effects become evident. The person feels ill, and the temperature is elevated. The bone marrow accelerates its production of leukocytes so the number of leukocytes circulating in the bloodstream increases; this increase in the number of leukocytes in the blood is called **leukocytosis**. The liver produces several proteins called acute phase proteins that are released into the bloodstream in response to tissue injury or inflammation, which help protect the body from the tissue injury caused by the inflammation. The best known of these proteins is called C-reactive protein, which is often measured to

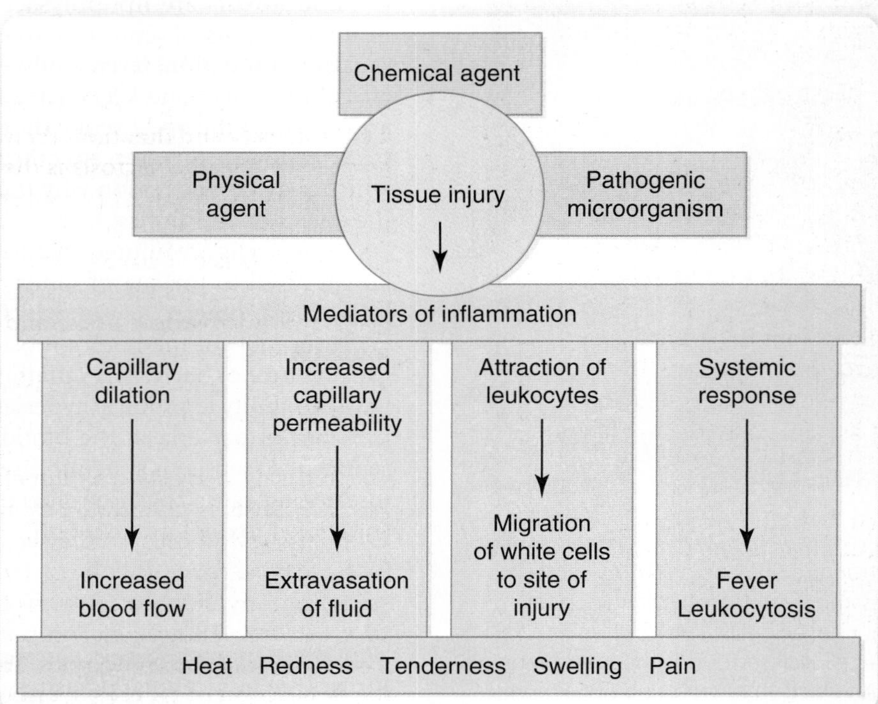

Figure 9-7 Local and systemic effects of tissue injury caused by various agents.

monitor the activity of diseases characterized by tissue inflammation.

The outcome of an inflammation depends on the amount of tissue damage. If the inflammation is mild, then it soon subsides, and the tissues return to normal. If the inflammatory process is more severe, then tissue is destroyed to some extent and must be repaired. During healing, damaged cells are replaced, and the framework of the injured tissue is repaired as an ingrowth of cells produces connective-tissue fibers and new blood vessels. Scar tissue replaces large areas of tissue destruction. Sometimes, the scarring subsequent to a severe inflammation is so severe that function is seriously disturbed.

Cellular membranes may be injured when they come in direct contact with the cellular and chemical components of the immune or inflammatory process, such as phagocytes (neutrophils and macrophages), histamine, antibodies, and lymphokines. In such a case, potassium leaks out of the damaged cell and water flows inward, causing the cell to swell. The nuclear envelope, organelle membranes, and cell membrane may rupture, leading to cell death. The degree of swelling and chance of membrane rupture depend on the severity of the immune and inflammatory responses.

▶ Injurious Genetic Factors

Genetic factors that may damage cells include chromosomal disorders, premature development of atherosclerosis, and, sometimes, obesity. An abnormal gene may develop in a person in one of three ways: by mutation of the gene during meiosis, which affects the newly formed fetus; by heredity; or due to other causes later in life. In trisomy 21 (Down syndrome), the child is born with an extra chromosome 21. Rheumatoid arthritis has a genetic link as well.

▶ Injurious Nutritional Imbalances

Good nutrition is required to maintain good health and assist the cells in fighting disease. Injurious nutritional imbalances that can injure cells and the organism as a whole include obesity, malnutrition, vitamin excess or deficiency, and mineral excess or deficiency. These conditions can lead to alterations in physical growth, mental and intellectual retardation, and even death.

▶ Injurious Physical Agents or Conditions

Physical agents, such as heat, cold, and radiation, may also cause cell injury—for example, burns, frostbite, radiation sickness, and tumors. The degree of cell injury that results is determined by the strength of the agent and the length of exposure.

▶ Apoptosis

Apoptosis is normal cell death. It is unique in that it is genetically programmed into the cell as a part of normal development, organogenesis, immune function, and tissue growth. It has a normal role in aging, early development, menses, lactating breast tissue, thymus involution, and red blood cell turnover.

During apoptosis, cells exhibit characteristic nuclear changes, and they typically die in well-defined clusters rather than in a random manner. The molecular mechanism underlying apoptosis involves the activation of genes that encode for proteins known as caspases (*c*ysteine-*asp*artic prote*ases*). The production of these proteins essentially leads to cell suicide. Unlike in the case of cell death from disease processes, proteins and DNA undergo controlled degradation that allows their remnants to be taken up and reused by neighboring cells. In this way, apoptosis allows the body to eliminate a cell but recycle many of its components. Pathologically, areas that have undergone apoptotic death do not show any evidence of inflammation. In contrast, an inflammatory response is typically observed when cells undergo necrosis from hypoxia or cellular toxins.

Apoptosis can be activated prematurely by pathologic factors such as cell injury. This sort of premature stimulation, which occurs in some forms of heart failure, causes early cell death. Another example of pathologic apoptosis is the death of hepatocytes (liver cells) in patients with viral hepatitis. The dying cells form lumps of chromatin known as Councilman bodies. Inhibition of the normal course of apoptosis allows destructive cellular proliferation, such as in cancer and rheumatoid arthritis (uncontrolled synovial tissue proliferation). **Figure 9-8** illustrates the process by which cancerous cells develop from normal cells.

▶ Abnormal Cell Death

If the injury leading to cellular degeneration is of sufficient intensity and duration, then irreversible cell injury leads to cell death. Necrosis is the term for tissue death. Necrosis is the result of the morphologic changes that occur following cell death in living tissues. It may be simple necrosis or derived necrosis.

Simple necrosis refers to areas of necrosis where the gross and microscopic tissue and some of the cells are recognizable. It may be caused by acute ischemia, acute toxicity (such as from heavy metals), or direct physical injury (such as from caustic chemicals and burns).

Derived necrosis includes caseation necrosis, dry gangrene, fat necrosis, and liquefaction necrosis. Caseation necrosis is manifested by the loss of all features of the tissue and cells, so they come to resemble cheese when viewed through a microscope. Dry gangrene results from invasion and putrefaction of necrotic tissue, after the blood supply is compromised and the tissue undergoes coagulation necrosis. Fat necrosis results from the destruction of fat cells, usually by enzymes (such as pancreatic proteases and lipases). Liquefaction necrosis results from coagulation necrosis followed by conversion of tissues into a liquid form and invasion by putrefying

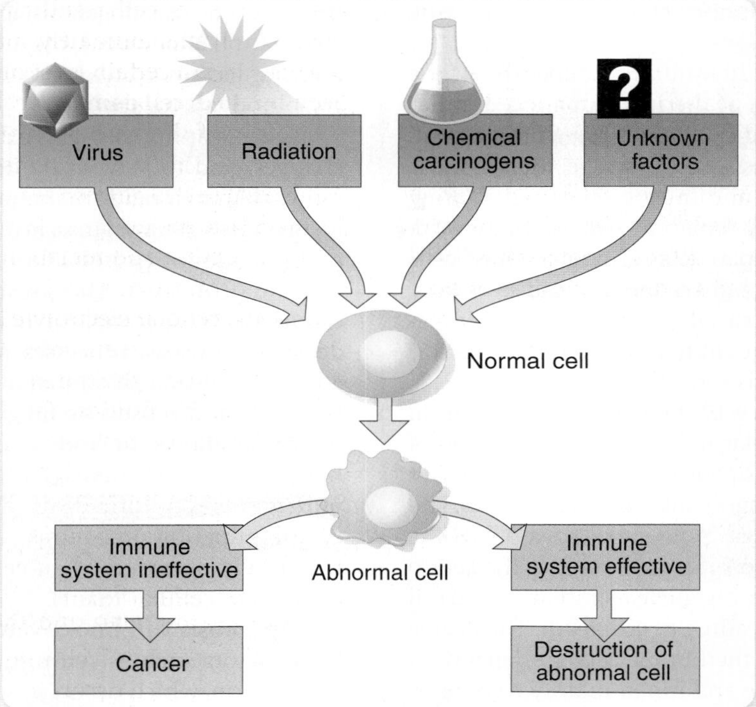

Figure 9-8 The onset of cancer. Viruses and other factors induce a normal cell to become abnormal. When the immune system is working effectively, it destroys the abnormal cells, so no cancer develops. When abnormal cells evade the immune system, they form a tumor and may become a spreading cancer.

bacteria that grow rapidly in a warm moist environment; the bacteria produce lytic enzymes and gas.

Hypoperfusion

Perfusion is defined as the delivery of oxygen and nutrients and removal of wastes from the cells, organs, and tissues by the circulatory system. Adequate circulation is dependent upon a pumping heart, intact vascular system, and an appropriate amount of oxygen-carrying blood. A deficiency in any of these areas will cause problems with perfusion. **Hypoperfusion** occurs when the level of tissue perfusion decreases below normal. It is important to evaluate a patient's level of organ perfusion during emergency medical care, especially in diagnosing shock.

When the body senses tissue hypoperfusion, it sets compensatory mechanisms into motion. In some cases, this action is sufficient to stabilize the patient's condition. At this point, the shock is called compensated shock. In other cases, the hypoperfusion overwhelms the normal compensatory mechanisms and the patient's condition progressively deteriorates; this is called decompensated (hypotensive) shock Table 9-4.

Documentation & Communication

The terms shock and hypoperfusion are often used interchangeably; however, the terms are not synonymous. Localized hypoperfusion, such as from arterial occlusion, is not shock.

In response to hypoperfusion, the body releases catecholamines (epinephrine and norepinephrine), which produce increased strength of cardiac contraction (positive inotropy), increased pulse rate, vasoconstriction and, consequently, increased systemic vascular resistance. In addition, the renin-angiotensin-aldosterone system (RAAS) is activated and antidiuretic hormone is released from the pituitary gland. Together, these actions trigger salt and water retention and peripheral vasoconstriction, thereby increasing the amount of fluid in the vascular space and improving blood pressure and cardiac output. Depending on the severity of the insult, variable amounts of fluid will shift from the interstitial tissues into the vascular compartment. The spleen also releases some red blood cells that are normally sequestered there, to augment

Table 9-4 Signs and Symptoms of Compensated and Decompensated Hypoperfusion (Shock)

Compensated	Decompensated
Agitation, anxiety, restlessness	Altered mental status (verbal to unresponsive)
Sense of impending doom	Hypotension
Weak, rapid (thready) pulse	Labored or irregular breathing
Clammy (cool, moist) skin	Thready or absent peripheral pulses
Pallor with cyanotic lips	Ashen, mottled, or cyanotic skin
Shortness of breath	Dilated pupils
Nausea, vomiting	Diminished urine output (oliguria)
Delayed capillary refill time in infants and children	Impending cardiac arrest
Thirst	
Normal blood pressure	

the oxygen-carrying capacity of the blood. The overall response of the initial compensatory mechanisms is to increase the preload (venous return), stroke volume, and heart rate to ensure adequate cardiac output. The result is usually an increase in cardiac output and myocardial oxygen demand.

As hypoperfusion persists, myocardial stress increases. Eventually, the above-normal compensatory mechanisms can no longer keep up with the increased oxygen demand. Myocardial function worsens, with decreased cardiac output and ejection fraction. Tissue perfusion decreases, leading to impaired cell metabolism. Often, the blood pressure decreases, especially in progressive hypoperfusion. Fluid may leak from the blood vessels, causing systemic and pulmonary edema. At this point, other signs of hypoperfusion may be present, such as dyspnea, dusky skin, low blood pressure, oliguria, and impaired mentation.

Shock is an abnormal state associated with inadequate oxygen and nutrient delivery to the metabolic apparatus of the cell, resulting in impairment of cellular metabolism and, ultimately, inadequate perfusion of vital organs. Once a certain level of tissue hypoperfusion has been reached, cell damage proceeds in a similar manner regardless of the type of initial insult. Impairment of cellular metabolism prevents the body from properly using oxygen and glucose at the cellular level. Cells revert to anaerobic metabolism, which causes increased lactic acid production and metabolic acidosis, decreased oxygen affinity for hemoglobin, decreased ATP production, changes in cellular electrolyte levels, cellular edema, and release of lysosomal enzymes. Glucose impairment raises the level of blood glucose as catecholamines and cortisol are released. In addition, fat breakdown (lipolysis) with ketone formation may occur.

Types of Shock

Shock can occur due to inadequacy of the central circulation (the heart and the great vessels) or of the peripheral circulation (the remaining vessels, including the microscopic circulation—that is, arterioles, venules, and capillaries, as illustrated in Chapter 8, *Anatomy and Physiology*.) From a mechanistic approach, two types of shock are distinguished: central and peripheral. **Central shock** consists of cardiogenic shock and obstructive shock. **Peripheral shock** includes hypovolemic shock and distributive shock.

The following sections provide an overview of types of shock. These topics are also discussed in later chapters.

Central Shock

Cardiogenic Shock

Cardiogenic shock occurs when the heart cannot circulate enough blood to maintain adequate peripheral oxygen delivery. In the case of ischemic heart disease, this condition occurs when there is a loss of 40% or more of functioning myocardium. The most common cause of cardiogenic shock is myocardial infarction, as a single event or by cumulative damage. Other forms of cardiac dysfunction may also precipitate cardiogenic shock (such as a large ventricular septal defect or hemodynamic significant dysrhythmias; see Chapter 17, *Cardiovascular Emergencies*).

Obstructive Shock

Obstructive shock occurs when blood flow becomes blocked in the heart or great vessels. In **pericardial tamponade** Figure 9-9, diastolic filling of the right and left ventricles of the heart is impaired due to significant amounts of fluid in the pericardial sac surrounding the heart. Decreased ventricular filling associated with pericardial tamponade leads to a decrease in the cardiac output. Aortic dissection leads to a false lumen

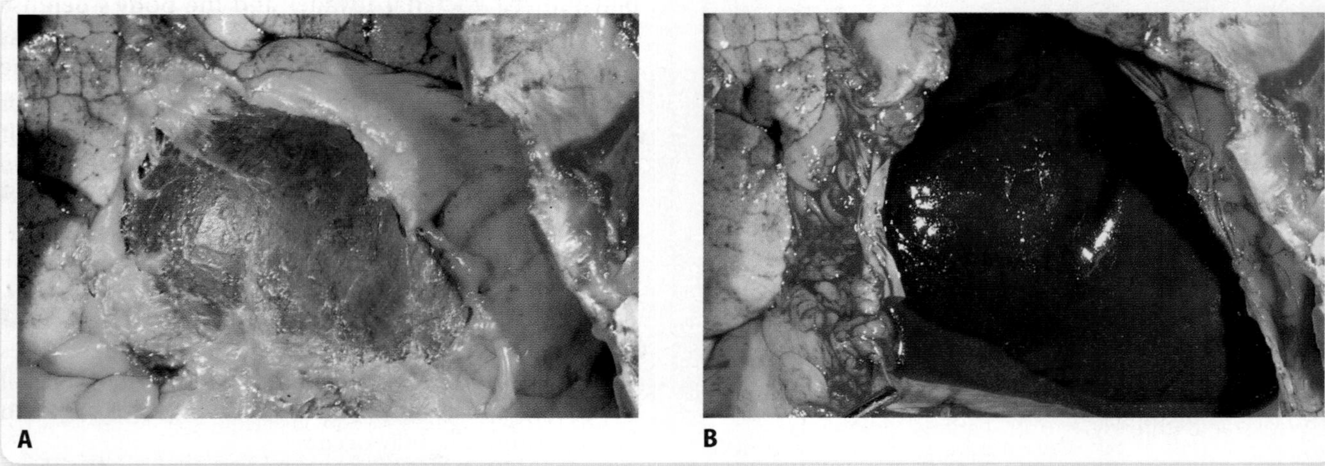

Figure 9-9 Cardiac tamponade following myocardial rupture. **A.** Distended pericardial sac. **B.** Pericardial sac opened, showing clotted blood surrounding the heart, which compressed the heart and prevented filling of the right ventricle in diastole.

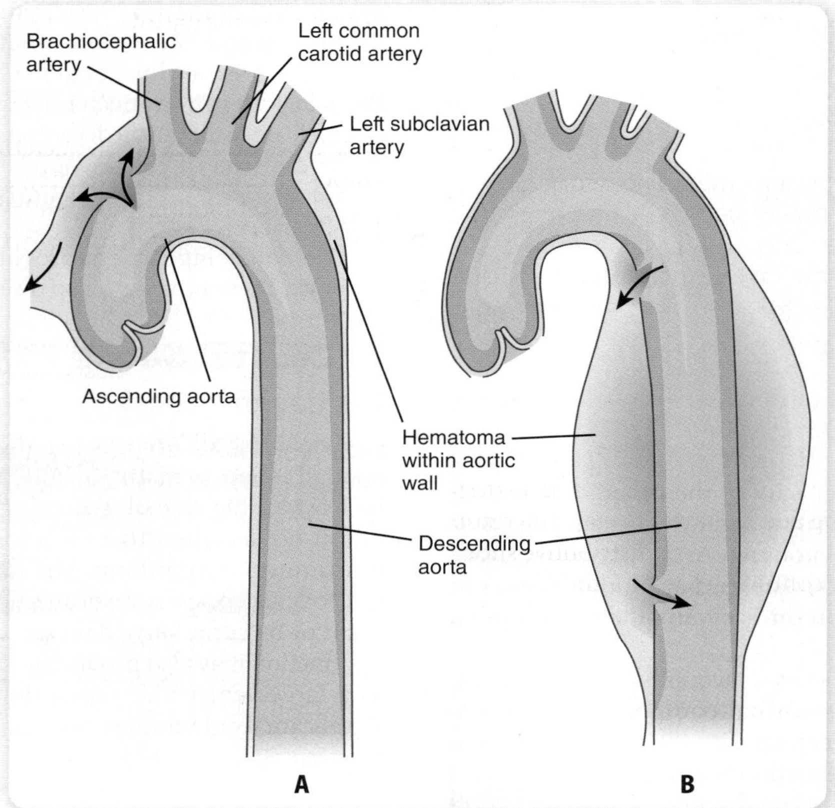

Figure 9-10 Sites of thoracic aortic dissection. **A.** A tear in the ascending aorta causes proximal and distal dissection. **B.** A tear in the descending aorta may cause extensive distal dissection.

(aortic opening), with loss of normal blood flow Figure 9-10. A left atrial tumor may obstruct flow between the atrium and ventricle and decrease cardiac output. Obstruction of the superior or inferior vena cava (vena cava syndrome) decreases cardiac output by decreasing venous return. A large pulmonary embolus (blood clot in the lung) or a tension pneumothorax (lung collapse) may prevent adequate blood flow to the lungs, resulting in inadequate venous return to the left side of the heart.

Words of Wisdom

Neurogenic shock can involve bradycardia if the injury is in the high thoracic region because of disruption in the sympathetic autonomic pathway. Cardiogenic shock can involve bradycardia when myocardial infarction is the cause and there is a disruption in the electrophysiologic pathway.

▶ Peripheral Shock

Hypovolemic Shock

In **hypovolemic shock**, the circulating blood volume is insufficient to deliver adequate oxygen and nutrients to the body. Two types of hypovolemic shock—exogenous and endogenous—are possible, depending on where the fluid loss occurs. The most common type of exogenous hypovolemic shock is external bleeding (such as from an open wound); it may also result from loss of plasma volume caused by diarrhea or vomiting. Endogenous hypovolemic shock occurs when the fluid loss is contained within the body.

Distributive Shock

Distributive shock occurs when there is widespread dilation of the resistance vessels (small arterioles), the capacitance vessels (small venules), or both. The circulating blood volume then pools in the expanded vascular beds, and tissue perfusion decreases. The three most common types of distributive shock are anaphylactic shock, septic shock, and neurogenic shock.

Anaphylactic shock (also called anaphylaxis) occurs when histamine and other vasodilator proteins are released on exposure to an **allergen** (any substance that causes a hypersensitivity reaction). Anaphylactic shock is also accompanied by wheezing and **urticaria** (hives). The result is widespread vasodilation that causes distributive shock and blood vessels that continue to leak. Fluid leaks out of the blood vessels into the interstitial spaces, resulting in intravascular hypovolemia.

Septic shock occurs as a result of widespread infection, usually bacterial. Complex interactions occur between the bacterial invader and the body's defense systems. Initially, the body's own defense mechanisms may keep the infection at bay. If the normal immune mechanisms become overwhelmed, then the body produces a multitude of substances that cause vasodilation and decreased cardiac output. If left untreated, then the result is multiple organ dysfunction syndrome (discussed later) and often death.

Words of Wisdom

In anaphylaxis, interstitial fluid may cause significant swelling. In some cases, this swelling may occlude the upper airway, resulting in a life-threatening condition manifesting as the adventitious sound of stridor. Recurrent large areas of subcutaneous edema of sudden onset, usually disappearing within 24 hours, are called angioedema. This condition is seen frequently as a result of allergy to food or drugs, such as ACE inhibitors.

Words of Wisdom

Typically, the earliest signs of shock are restlessness and anxiety. The patient looks scared!

Neurogenic shock usually results from spinal cord injury. The effect is loss of normal sympathetic nervous system tone and vasodilation **Figure 9-11**. Patients often have fluid-refractory hypotension due to the degree of vasodilation.

▶ Management of Shock

Most types of shock are characterized by reduced cardiac output, circulatory insufficiency, and rapid heartbeat. Although low blood pressure is classically associated with shock, it is a late sign, especially in children.

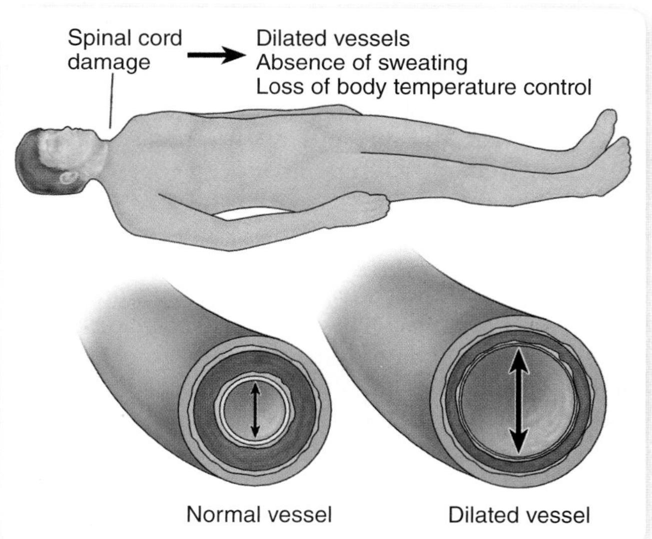

Figure 9-11 Damage to the spinal cord can cause significant injury to the part of the nervous system that controls the size and muscle tone of blood vessels. If the smooth muscle in the blood vessels is cut off from its impulses to contract, then the vessels dilate widely, increasing the size and capacity of the vascular system. The blood in the body can no longer fill the enlarged vessels, which results in inadequate perfusion and neurogenic shock.

Words of Wisdom

A possible exception to the standard use of IV fluid therapy to treat shock is hypovolemic shock caused by ongoing bleeding. Permissive hypotension, in which the provider attempts to achieve an appropriate mental status and the presence of peripheral pulses, may be safer than attempting restoration of normotension, which may aggravate ongoing bleeding. As always, follow your local protocols. $ETCO_2$ is also beneficial in developing target outcomes for patients in shock.

Clinically, determining the presence or absence of shock requires you to evaluate the presence and volume of the peripheral pulses and assess end-organ perfusion and function. Strength of the peripheral pulses is related to stroke volume of the heart and pulse pressures. Peripheral pulses should be readily palpable if the person is not in shock, although cold environments or obesity may compromise the presence or strength of these pulses. Normal skin perfusion is indicated by warm, dry, pink extremities, fingers, and toes, whereas a slow, delayed, or prolonged **capillary refill time** indicates shock (although this technique is more reliable in children). To test the capillary refill time, briefly squeeze the toenail or fingernail, and then observe the time it takes for color to return. A normal capillary refill time is less than 2 seconds after blanching of the toe or finger, whereas a person in shock may have a capillary refill time of more than 2 seconds. Mottling, pallor, peripheral or central cyanosis, and delayed capillary refill may signal the presence of shock, whereas altered mental status indicates inadequate brain tissue perfusion. The accuracy of a capillary refill measurement decreases after age 6 years; it is most useful in young children but not as useful in the adult population.

Measuring end-tidal carbon dioxide ($ETCO_2$) may also be useful to the astute clinician. While $ETCO_2$ provides valuable information regarding the respiratory and ventilatory status of the patient, you can also interpret the effectiveness of perfusion in your patient based on changes in capnography and capnometry. Carbon dioxide is one of the byproducts of cellular metabolism, so decreasing levels of $ETCO_2$ are an early indicator of shock. Low levels of $ETCO_2$ combined with other signs and symptoms of shock such as hypotension and altered mental status are ominous clinical findings.

Treatment primarily addresses the underlying condition (see Chapter 30, *Bleeding*).

Multiple Organ Dysfunction Syndrome

Multiple organ dysfunction syndrome (MODS), first described in 1975, is a progressive condition that occurs in some critically ill patients. It is characterized by the concurrent failure of two or more organs or organ systems that were initially unharmed by the acute disorder or injury that caused the patient's current illness. Six organ systems are surveyed in diagnosing MODS: respiratory, hepatic, renal, hematologic, neurologic, and cardiovascular. Each system is assigned a score to determine the patient's overall risk. For example, the Glasgow Coma Scale score is used to score the patient's neurologic system function. While MODS may begin in one physiologic system, the disease process often progresses in a cyclical method, including multiple organ systems and complicating factors throughout its course.

In MODS, the overall mortality rate varies widely depending on the underlying etiology and ensuing diagnosis and treatment. Despite the inevitability its name suggests, the condition is often reversible, particularly in patients who were healthy before the physiologic insult occurred.[10] Multiple organ dysfunction syndrome is the major cause of death following sepsis, trauma, and burn injuries, with mortality rates of up to 70%.[10]

Primary MODS is a direct result of an insult, such as a pulmonary contusion from striking the chest on the steering wheel during a motor vehicle crash. Secondary MODS is a slower, more progressive organ dysfunction.

MODS occurs when injury or infection (septic shock) triggers a massive systemic immune, inflammatory, and coagulation response accompanied by endotoxin release. Overactivating the complement system further increases inflammation and cellular damage. Vascular endothelial damage triggers overactivation of the coagulation system, which leads to uncontrolled coagulation in the venules and arterioles. This coagulation, in turn, causes microvascular thrombus formation and tissue ischemia. In addition, MODS activates the kallikrein-kinin system, stimulating the release of bradykinin, a potent vasodilator. Kallikrein is an inactive enzyme of the pancreas. When it becomes activated, it can dilate blood vessels, influence blood pressure, modulate salt and water excretion by the kidneys, and influence cardiac remodeling after AMI. Bradykinin increases vascular permeability, dilates blood vessels, contracts smooth muscle, and causes pain when injected into the skin. Vasodilation leads to tissue hypoperfusion and may also contribute to hypotension.

The net outcome of the activation of these systems is maldistribution of systemic and organ blood flow. Often the body attempts to compensate for this problem by accelerating tissue metabolism. The result is an imbalance in oxygen supply and demand that causes tissue hypoxia, initiating a cascade of ill effects including tissue hypoperfusion, exhaustion of the cells' fuel supply (ATP), metabolic failure, lysosome breakdown, anaerobic metabolism, and acidosis and impaired cellular function.

Typically, MODS develops hours or days following resuscitation. The signs and symptoms include hypotension, insufficient tissue perfusion, uncontrollable bleeding (coagulopathy), and multisystem organ failure. A low-grade fever may develop from the inflammatory response, tachycardia, and dyspnea. Patients may also be difficult to oxygenate because of acute lung injury and acute respiratory distress syndrome.

During a 14- to 21-day period, renal and liver failure can develop in patients with MODS, along with collapse of the gastrointestinal and immune systems. The kidneys are dependent on adequate perfusion pressure. Once the mean arterial pressure drops, the kidneys stop functioning. Oliguria occurs early in shock. Renal studies show elevated serum urea nitrogen and creatinine levels. Many patients require continuous bedside dialysis.

The liver is a complex organ with a key role in excreting wastes and toxins. Adequate liver function is also essential for the synthesis of blood proteins and coagulation proteins, as well as the storage of glycogen, iron, and vitamins. Patients with MODS have elevated levels of total bilirubin and of the liver enzymes aspartate aminotransferase and alanine aminotransferase. Unfortunately, there are no definitive treatments for liver failure. Treatment focuses on minimizing the effects of liver damage.

The brain, adrenal glands, and heart are also affected early in MODS. The level of consciousness deteriorates quickly in hypoxic states, but it declines precipitously in patients with MODS. Cerebral hypoxia and subsequent ischemia can cause permanent deficits as a result of anoxic brain injury.

Perhaps the heart suffers more than any other organ in a patient with MODS. As the heart struggles to maintain arterial perfusion pressure, it too becomes hypoxic. Hypotension cannot be controlled despite the administration of fluids and vasopressors. Compensatory tachycardia consumes even more oxygen, and dysrhythmias such as bradycardia, ventricular tachycardia, and ventricular fibrillation develop. Cardiovascular collapse and death typically occur within days to weeks of the initial insult.

The Body's Self-Defense Mechanisms

The **immune system** includes all structures and processes associated with the body's defense against foreign substances and disease-causing agents. The body has three lines of defense: anatomic barriers, the inflammatory response, and the immune response.

Anatomic Barriers

Several anatomic barriers decrease the chances of foreign substances invading the body. The skin serves as a major deterrent. Hairs in the upper respiratory tract (the nose) and the lining of the lower respiratory tract (cilia-covered epithelial cells) help repel foreign matter, especially small particles and some bacteria. Acid in the stomach prevents many infectious agents from entering the body via the gastrointestinal tract.

Immune Response

The **immune response** is the body's defense reaction to any substance it recognizes as foreign. This response is often directed toward invading microbes, such as bacteria or viruses. It is also triggered by foreign bodies, such as a splinter, and even abnormal cell growths, such as tumors. The immune response involves only one type of white blood cells, namely lymphocytes.

YOU are the Paramedic — PART 3

Your partner is administering high-flow oxygen, attaching the $ETCO_2$, assessing vital signs, placing the cardiac monitor, and setting up an IV line. You auscultate lung sounds and hear little air movement. You hear coarse crackles (rales) bilaterally in all fields. The patient coughs, and you notice pink, foamy sputum. You ask your partner to assess the medications on the side table while you establish the IV line.

Recording Time: 2 Minutes	
Respirations	22 breaths/min; shallow
Pulse	110 beats/min
Skin	Cool, moist, and pale
Blood pressure	140/90 mm Hg
Oxygen saturation (Spo_2)	89% before high-flow oxygen administration
Pupils	PERRLA

5. On the basis of what you know about physiology, what is causing the pink, foamy sputum?
6. How do you account for the decreased Spo_2 level?

Not all invaders can be destroyed by the body's immune system. In some cases, the best compromise the body can reach is to control the damage and keep the invader from spreading. Often, the immune system succeeds in preventing severe disease following infection. When the normal systems become overwhelmed or fail, serious disease occurs.

The body responds to different kinds of immune challenges in remarkably similar ways. Although the details depend on the particular challenge, the basic pattern is the same—the innate response starts first and is then reinforced by the more specific acquired response. These two pathways are interconnected.

Consider what happens when bacteria enter the body. If the bacteria are not encapsulated, then macrophages begin immediately to ingest the bacteria. If the bacteria are encapsulated, then antibodies (opsonins) must coat the capsule before it can be ingested by phagocytes.

Components of the cell wall then activate the complement system. Some components of the activated complement system, termed **chemotaxins**, attract leukocytes from the circulation to help fight the infection. The complement cascade ends with the formation of a set of proteins called the **membrane attack complex**. These molecules insert themselves into the bacterial membrane, weakening those areas in the membrane. Ions and water enter the cell through the weakened areas, leading to lysis of the bacterium (a chemical process that does not involve immune cells).

If antibodies to the bacteria are already present in the body, then these antibodies will assist the innate response by acting as opsonins and neutralizing bacterial toxins. Although it often takes several days, memory B cells attracted to the infection site will be activated if a recognized antigen is encountered. If the infection is new to the body—that is, preexisting antibodies are not present—then B cells will be activated. Combined with helper T cells and cytokine release, antibodies are produced and memory B and T cells are formed.

Table 9-5 describes the types of immune system cells.

Table 9-5 Immune System Cells

Type of Cell	Description
Basophil	A type of white blood cell that releases histamine during inflammation.
Eosinophils	A type of white blood cell that phagocytizes the antigen-antibody complex; attacks parasites.
Neutrophils	A type of white blood cell that phagocytizes bacteria.
Monocytes	A type of white blood cell that phagocytizes bacteria, dead cells, and cellular debris.
Lymphocyte	A type of white blood cell involved in immune protection; attacks cells directly or produces antibodies.
Macrophage	White blood cells within tissues; produced by differentiation of monocytes. Functions include phagocytosis and stimulating lymphocytes and other immune cells to respond to pathogens; one of the first lines of defense in the inflammatory process.
Mast cells	Cells that are found in the connective tissues, beneath the skin, in the gastrointestinal mucosa and in the mucosal membranes of the respiratory system. Functions relate to allergic reactions, immunity, and wound healing.
Plasma cells	White blood cells that develop from B cells and produce large volumes of specific antibodies.
B cells (B lymphocytes)	Cells that mature in the bone marrow where they differentiate into memory cells or immunoglobulin-secreting (antibody) cells. Functions include eliminating bacteria, neutralizing bacterial toxins, preventing viral reinfection, and producing immediate inflammatory response.
Helper B cells	A type of regulator cell that activates B cells to produce antibodies.
Memory B cells	A type of B cell that aids in the quick response to subsequent exposures to an antigen because memory cells recall the antigen as foreign. These cells rapidly produce antibodies.
T cells (T lymphocytes)	Cells that are produced in the bone marrow and mature in the thymus. Two major types work to destroy antigens—regulator cells and effector cells.
Killer T cells	A type of T cell that destroys cells infected with viruses by releasing lymphokines that destroy cell walls; also called cytotoxic or effector cells.

Characteristics of the Immune Response

The native and acquired immune responses protect the body from infectious agents such as viruses and bacteria and from foreign substances that have gained access to the body through the skin or the lining of internal organs.

Natural immunity, also called native immunity, is a nonspecific cellular and humoral (antibody) response that operates as the first line of defense against pathogens. Most natural immunity is associated with the initial inflammatory response.

Acquired immunity (also called adaptive immunity) is a highly specific, inducible, discriminatory method by which armies of cells respond to an immune stimulant, such that the immune system will never fail to recognize the same stimulant when it is subsequently encountered, even years later. It arises when the body is exposed to a foreign substance or disease and produces antibodies to the invader. Passively acquired immunity is the receipt of preformed antibodies to fight or prevent infection. Examples of passively acquired immunity include the transplacental passage of antibodies and the passage of antibodies in colostrum (the mother's initial breast milk to her infant), which protects the infant until his or her immune system matures sufficiently to take over. The injection of immunoglobulin (a concentrated form of antibodies obtained from donors) is also a form of passively acquired immunity.

The primary (initial) immune response takes place during the first exposure to an **antigen** (a foreign substance; a neoantigen is an antigen associated with cancerous cells). Clinical symptoms may not be apparent. Sometimes, the body's initial response is to produce an antibody that triggers symptoms on subsequent exposures. The secondary (amnestic) immune response occurs with reexposure to a foreign substance. The body has already developed a memory, of sorts, for that substance, so a reaction occurs on reexposure to it.

An **antibody** binds a specific antigen so the complex can attach itself to specialized immune cells that ingest the complex to destroy it or release biologic mediators such as histamine to induce an allergic or inflammatory response. The specific features of the antigen-antibody interaction depend on the foreign substance involved **Figure 9-12**.

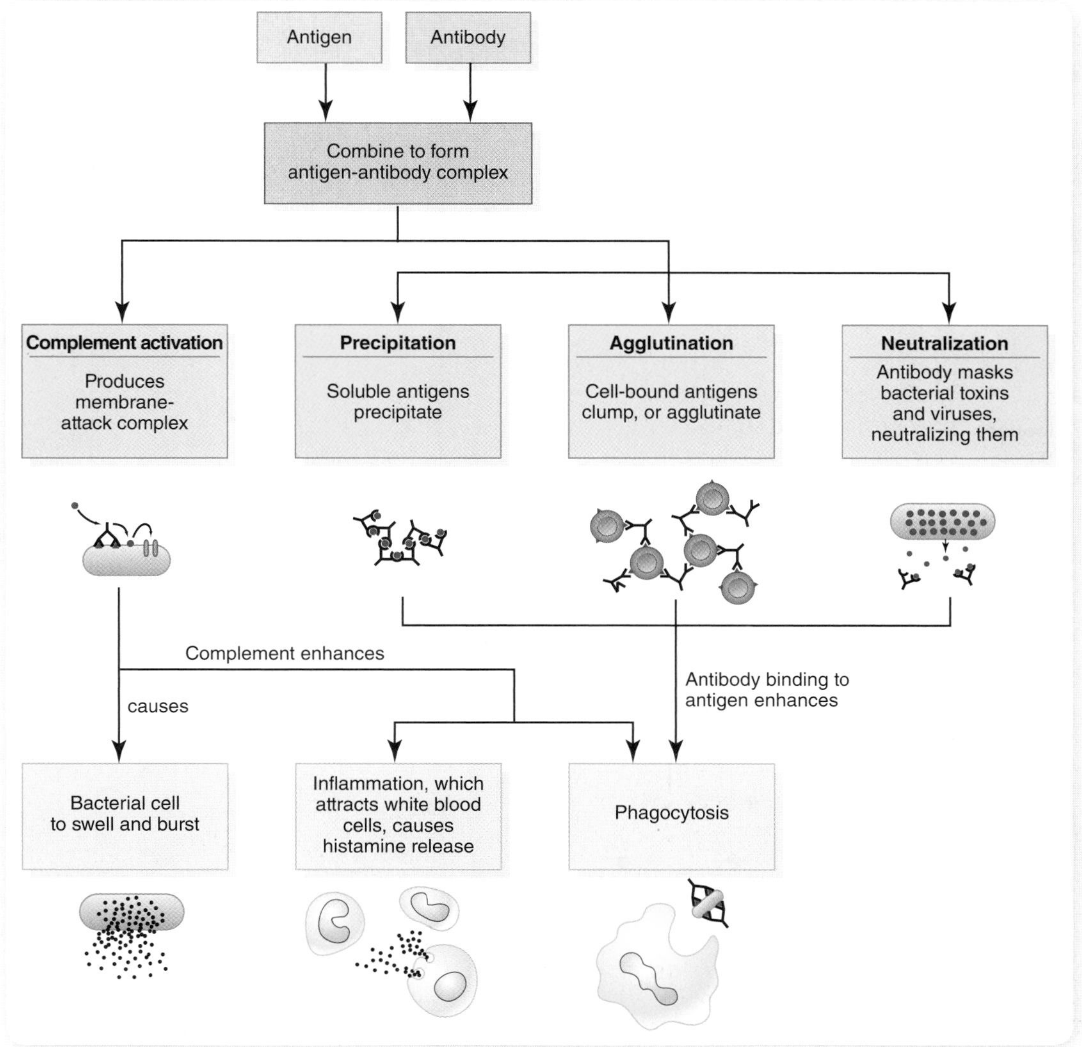

Figure 9-12 How antibodies work.

An **immunogen** is an antigen capable of generating an immune response. Thus, an immunogen is an antigen, but an antigen is not necessarily an immunogen. Antigens and immunogens can be categorized by size. Proteins, polysaccharides, and nucleic acids are larger, whereas amino acids, monosaccharides, and fatty acids are smaller. A **hapten** is a substance that normally does not stimulate an immune response but that can be combined with an

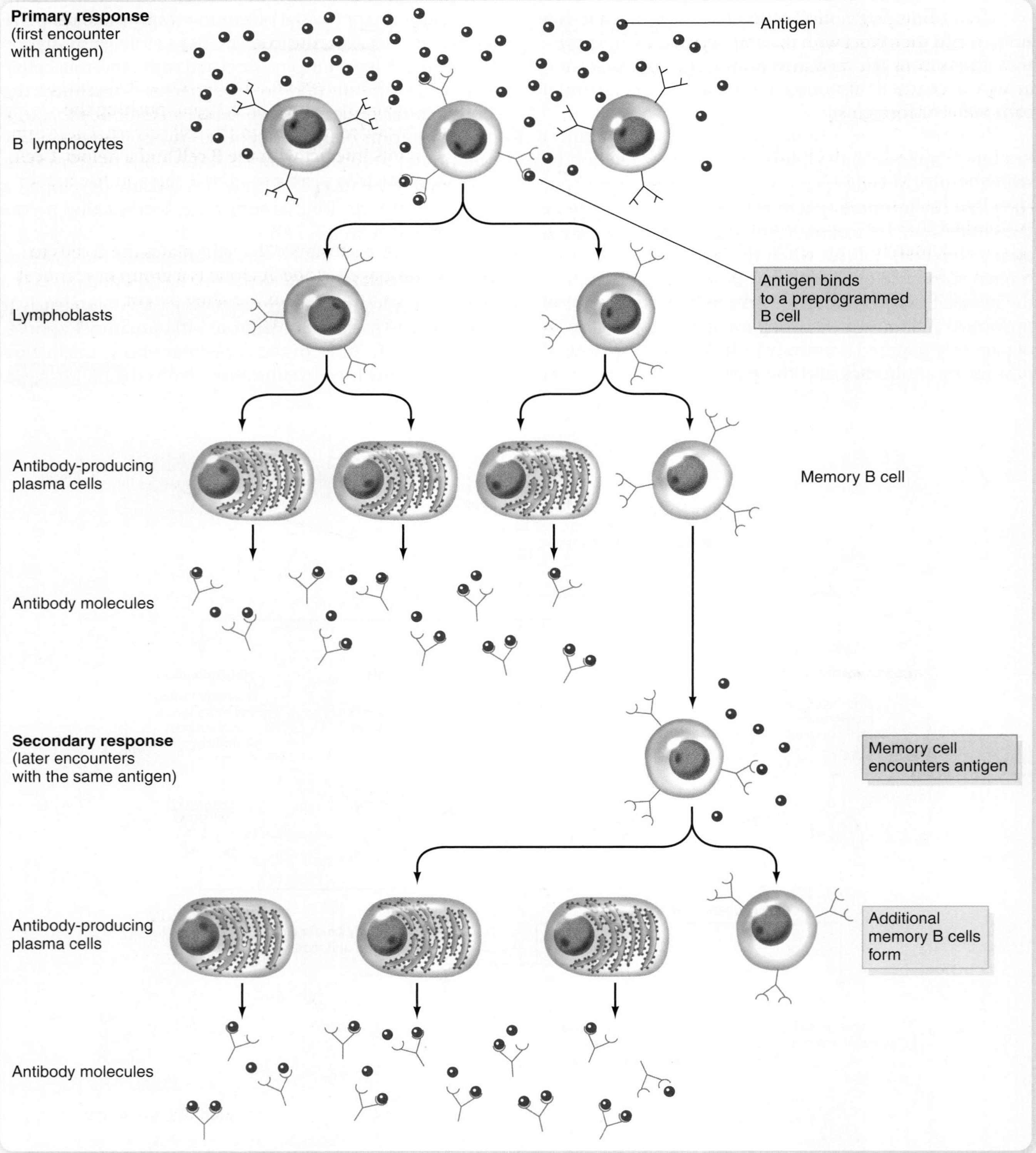

Figure 9-13 B-cell activation. Immunocompetent B cells are stimulated by the presence of an antigen, producing an intermediate cell, the lymphoblast. The lymphoblasts divide, producing plasma cells and some memory B cells. Memory B cells respond to subsequent antigen encroachment, yielding a rapid secondary response.

antigen and, at a later time, initiate a specific antibody response on its own.

Humoral Immune Response

In **humoral immunity**, B-cell lymphocytes produce antibodies called immunoglobulins, which recognize a specific antigen and then react with it, as shown in Figure 9-13. This differs from cell-mediated immunity, discussed later, in which macrophages and T cells attack and destroy pathogens or foreign substances.

B Lymphocytes. Like all blood cells, B cells are born in the bone marrow, where they are descended from stem cells. The clonal selection theory holds that each B cell makes antibodies that have only one type of antigen-binding region and, therefore, are specific for a particular antigen, known as the cognate antigen. Antibodies are found on the surface of B cells, where they are able to recognize the presence of their cognate antigens. When a B cell recognizes the cognate antigen, it proliferates to make more identical B cells in an exponential manner, each of which can make antibodies that recognize the same antigen.

For B cells to produce antibodies, B cells must first be activated. The most common way this occurs is via **helper T cells** Figure 9-14:

1. A macrophage engulfs the antigen via phagocytosis. It digests the antigen, pushing the discarded particles to the cell surface. These remnants interact with the B cell and a helper T cell.
2. The antigen binds to the B cell and the helper T cell, activating both.
3. The activated helper T cell secretes a lymphokine, a substance that stimulates the B cells to produce a clone. A clone is a group of identical cells formed from the same parent cell. The

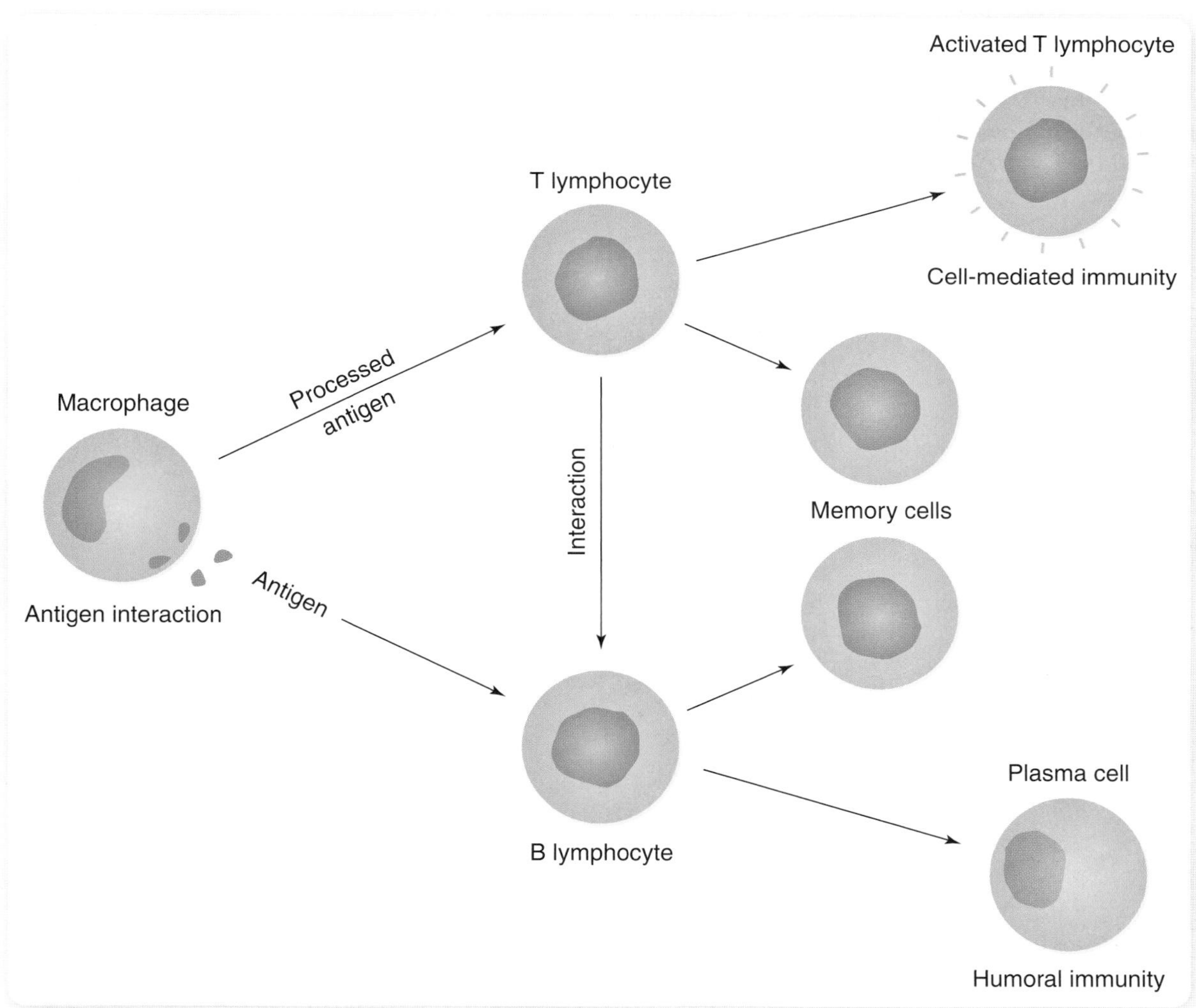

Figure 9-14 Interaction of cell-mediated and humoral immunity. A macrophage presents processed antigen fragments to the T lymphocyte. The B lymphocyte processes the intact antigen and displays fragments of the same antigen on its cell membrane. The T lymphocyte, which has responded to the same antigen, stimulates the B lymphocyte to proliferate, mature into plasma cells, and make antibodies.

clone comprises two types of identical cells that have different functions: plasma cells, which make the antibodies, and memory cells, which "remember" the initial encounter with the antigen. B cells produce many such clones, called polyclonal antibodies. It is also possible for monoclonal antibodies to be created. These are very specific antibodies used in laboratory research and in some cancer therapies, but are not particularly relevant to paramedic field practice.

The human body distinguishes between foreign substances and its own cells and tissues by means of the major histocompatibility complex, a group of genes located on a single chromosome that permits a person who is capable of generating an immune response to distinguish *self* from *nonself* (namely, what is foreign). The human leukocyte antigen gene complex is the human major histocompatibility complex and is present in all nucleated human cells. It encodes for numerous antigens that are unique to a person. When the immune system encounters these particular antigens, it recognizes them as self, and no immune response occurs.

Immunoglobulins. The antibodies secreted by B cells are called **immunoglobulins** (this text uses the terms *immunoglobulins* and *antibodies* interchangeably, unless otherwise stated). These Y-shaped proteins consist of a crystallizable fragment (Fc) portion and two antigen-binding fragment (Fab) regions that bind only a specific antigen. The basic antibody molecule has four chains linked into a Y shape. Each side of the Y is identical, with one light chain attached to one heavy chain Figure 9-15. The two arms, or Fab regions, contain antigen-binding sites. The stem, or Fc region, determines to which of the five immunoglobulin classes an antibody belongs Figure 9-16.

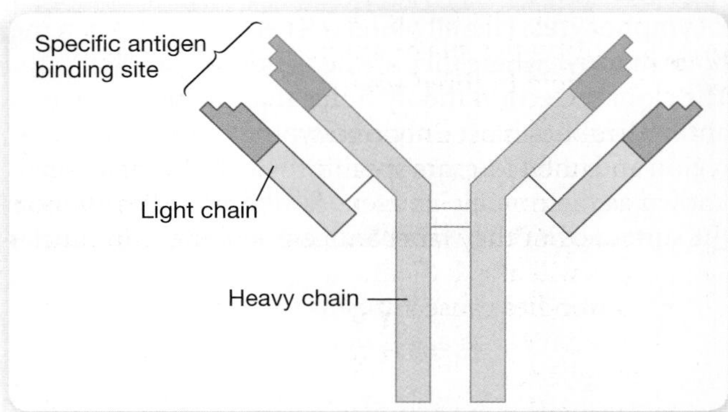

Figure 9-15 Structure of an immunoglobulin molecule.

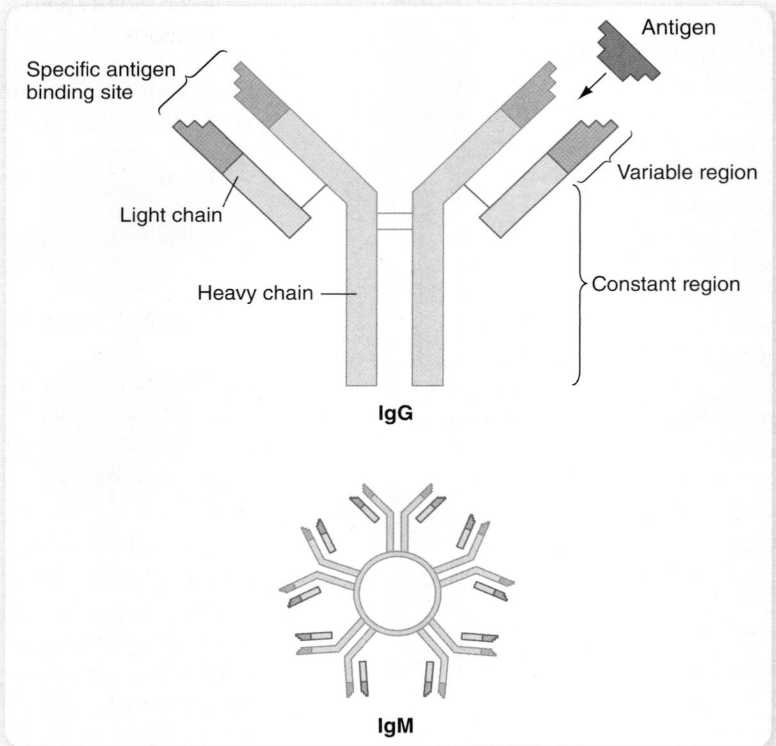

Figure 9-16 General structure of an antibody. Note that IgG is a monomer; it is one molecule. IgM is a pentamer; it is a cluster of five antibodies and is effective in combining with foreign antigens. Also note that the antigen fits exactly into the antigen–binding site (if it did not, it would not be able to bind). Antigen binding sites therefore have different structures depending on the antigen to which they are designed to bind.

There are three main categories of antigens on antibodies: isotypic, allotypic, and idiotypic. An isotypic antigenic marker occurs in all members of a subclass of an immunoglobulin class. An allotypic antigenic marker is found on some members of a subclass of an immunoglobulin class, but not on all of them. An idiotypic antigenic determinant is a unique structure that is created on the light and heavy chains of an immunoglobulin molecule. Some of these structures are involved in immune regulation.

Most antibodies are found in the plasma. Antibodies make up about 20% of the plasma proteins in a healthy person. Antibodies make antigens more visible to the immune system in three ways:

- Antibodies act as opsonins. In **opsonization**, an antibody coats an antigen to facilitate its recognition by immune cells. Antibodies are not toxic, but they label antigens so other immune cells will attack them.
- Antibodies cause antigens to clump (precipitate, also known as agglutinate) for easier phagocytosis.
- Antibodies bind to and inactivate some toxins produced by bacteria. Macrophages can then ingest and destroy the inactivated toxins.

Antibodies are divided into five general classes of immunoglobulins Table 9-6. Fetal immunity is a passively acquired immunity that is derived primarily from maternal IgG and IgM antibodies. As a fertilized ovum grows, its peripheral cells differentiate into a group of cells called the trophoblast. The trophoblast forms the placenta and other structures that will support and nourish the embryo. The pregnant woman's immunity passes through the trophoblast. In fact, the umbilical cord's blood cells contain immunologic properties and have been used in medical treatment, which is a reason why some people decide to store their children's umbilical cord blood. The fact that the umbilical cord contains immunologic properties relates to paramedicine in that, when cutting the umbilical cord, the position of the newborn is important; ensure the newborn is not held too high or too low relative to the mother; otherwise, the newborn could have a loss or gain of excess blood and, therefore, immunity. Following delivery, the antibodies that were passed to the fetus persist until the neonate's own B cells take over. A substantial number of antibodies are also transferred through breast milk, which is one of many reasons that many experts favor breastfeeding.

Cell-Mediated Immune Response

Cell-mediated immunity is characterized by the formation of a population of lymphocytes that can attack and destroy foreign material. It is the main defense against viruses, fungi, parasites, and some bacteria. Cell-mediated immunity is the mechanism by which the body rejects transplanted organs and eliminates the abnormal cells that sometimes arise spontaneously in cell division.

Table 9-6 General Classes of Immunoglobulins

Class	Description
IgG	The most common immunoglobulin. Accounts for 75% of the antibodies in the blood. Found in lymph, synovial fluid, peritoneal fluid, cerebrospinal fluid, and breast milk. IgG is the only immunoglobulin that crosses the placenta, giving infants immunity during the first few months of life.
IgA	Accounts for 15% of the antibodies in the blood. Also found in tears, saliva, respiratory tract secretions, and the stomach. IgA combines with a protein in the mucosa and defends body surfaces against invading microorganisms.
IgM	Accounts for 5% to 10% of the antibodies in the blood and is the dominant antibody in ABO (blood type) incompatibilities. IgM is the initial antibody formed in most infections.
IgE	Accounts for less than 1% of the antibodies in the blood and is associated with allergic reactions. When mast cell receptors combine with IgE and antigen, the mast cells degranulate and release chemical mediators such as histamine.
IgD	Accounts for less than 1% of the antibodies in the blood. The physiologic role of IgD is unclear.

In cell-mediated immunity, T-cell lymphocytes recognize antigens and contribute to the immune response in two major ways: (1) by secreting cytokines that attract other cells or (2) by becoming cytotoxic and killing infected or abnormal cells. There are five subgroups of T cells:

1. **Killer T cells.** Killer T cells (also called cytotoxic T cells) destroy the antigen. Killer T cells help rid the body of cells that have been infected by viruses and cells that have been transformed into cancer cells. Killer T cells are also responsible for the rejection of tissue and organ grafts.
2. **Helper T cells.** Helper T cells activate many immune cells, including B cells and other T cells (also called T4 or $CD4^+$ cells).
3. **Suppressor T cells.** Suppressor T cells (also called T8 or $CD8^+$ cells) suppress the activity of other lymphocytes so they do not destroy normal tissue.

4. **Memory T cells.** Memory T cells remember the reaction for the next time it is needed.
5. **Lymphokine-producing cells.** Secreted by lymphocytes, these cells work to damage cells; for example, lymphokines destroy cells that have been infected with a virus.

During the cell-mediated response, macrophages ingest pathogens. When a macrophage digests a pathogen, it releases small particles of antigen. This antigen pushes its way to the macrophage surface, where it is recognized by specific T cells. Other T cells, such as helper T cells and killer T cells, bind to the antigen and macrophage, destroying the invader.

Special Populations

T-cell and B-cell function is deficient in older adults. Depressed lymphocyte function is accompanied by a decrease in macrophage activity. Therefore, older adults are more prone to experience infections and recover slowly. In addition, older adults have an increased level of **autoantibodies** (antibodies directed against the self), which partly explains why older adults are prone to autoimmune disease.

▶ Inflammatory Response

The inflammatory response is a response of the tissues of the body to irritation or injury. It is characterized by pain, swelling, redness, and heat. White blood cells of various types are a major component of this response.

The inflammatory reaction and the immune response are independent processes, although the processes often occur simultaneously. Inflammation can be present without activation of the immune response, and vice versa. Inflammation is a dynamic process that, once initiated, triggers a complex cascade involving local and systemic events. The two most common causes of inflammation are infection (such as bacterial or viral) and injury.

Acute Inflammation

The acute inflammatory response involves vascular and cellular components. Initially, the arterioles constrict in an attempt to limit blood loss, but then dilate, allowing an influx of blood under increased pressure. This leads to increased intravascular pressure and causes the blood vessel to expand; as in a balloon that is being inflated, the vessel walls become thinner. The higher pressure combined with increased vessel wall permeability causes fluid to leak into the interstitial spaces (edema). When enough fluid has escaped into the surrounding area and the intravascular pressure has been released, the vessel wall contracts and the flow slows, leading to pooling of blood in the capillaries.

A variety of blood cells participate in tissue inflammatory reactions: white blood cells (leukocytes), platelets, mast cells, and plasma cells (B lymphocytes that create antibodies). Specific cell types include neutrophils, monocytes, lymphocytes, eosinophils, basophils, and activated platelets. Chemical mediators, primarily produced by the mast cells, account for the vascular and cellular events that occur during the acute inflammatory response. Cell-derived mediators include histamine, arachidonic acid derivatives, and cytokines such as interleukins and tumor necrosis factor.

Words of Wisdom

Corticosteroids can decrease the initial inflammatory response, which is a necessary part of wound healing. However, as immunosuppressants, corticosteroids also increase the risk of wound infection. This consideration is important in patients with diabetes because of their propensity to develop such infections.

Mast Cells. Mast cells have a major role in inflammation. During inflammation, mast cells degranulate and release a variety of substances. The primary stimuli for the degranulation of mast cells during the inflammatory response are physical injury (trauma), chemical agents (for example, bacterial toxins), and immunologic substances (for example, interaction of an antigen and an IgE antibody).

After degranulation, mast cells release **vasoactive amines**. The most important of these substances, **histamine** and **serotonin**, increase vascular permeability, cause vasodilation, and can cause bronchoconstriction, nausea, and vomiting. Because histamine is a preformed vasodepressor amine stored in mast cells, it can be released quickly, so its actions are seen early in the inflammatory response. Mast cells also synthesize chemotactic factors that attract neutrophils (neutrophil chemotactic factor) and eosinophils (eosinophilic chemotactic factor).

Mast cells also synthesize leukotrienes. **Leukotrienes**—also known as slow-reacting substances of anaphylaxis—are a family of biologically active compounds derived from arachidonic acid. The clinically important leukotrienes participate in host defense reactions and pathophysiologic conditions that paramedics commonly see in the field, such as immediate hypersensitivity and inflammation. Leukotrienes have potent actions on many parts of the body, including the cardiovascular, pulmonary, immune, and central nervous systems and the gastrointestinal tract.

Leukotrienes are primarily endogenous mediators of inflammation. They contribute to the signs and symptoms seen in acute inflammatory responses, including responses resulting from the interaction of allergens with IgE antibodies on mast cells. Certain leukotrienes are bronchoconstrictors, stimulate airway mucus secretion, and are very effective at increasing the permeability of postcapillary venules (including those in the bronchial circulation), thereby causing plasma protein exudation (oozing out of the tissue) and edema. Certain leukotrienes may also promote eosinophil migration into the airways of animals and people with asthma, and they may also increase bronchial hyperresponsiveness through an action on sensory nerves.

Finally, mast cells synthesize **prostaglandins**. These substances, which are derived from arachidonic acid, comprise a group of about 20 lipids that are composed of modified fatty acids attached to a five-member ring. Prostaglandins are found in many vertebrate tissues, where they act as messengers in reproduction, the inflammatory response to infection, and pain perception. Aspirin and nonsteroidal anti-inflammatory drugs inhibit prostaglandin synthesis, leading to reduced inflammation and pain.

Plasma Protein Systems. There are plasma-derived mediators that modulate the inflammatory process; these are called plasma protein systems. They include the complement system, the coagulation (clotting) system, and the kinin system. The interaction of these systems is vital to a normal inflammatory response. Each system consists of a cascade of biochemical reactions such that as one compound is produced, it catalyzes the formation of the next compound—much like knocking over a line of dominoes.

- **Complement system.** The **complement system** is a group of plasma proteins that attract white blood cells to sites of inflammation, activate white blood cells, and directly destroy cells. The central compound in this complement cascade is called C3. C3 is produced by one of the two complement pathways: the classic pathway or the alternative pathway. The classic pathway starts when an antigen-antibody complex binds to a complement component (C1); activation of this pathway is dependent on the presence of antibodies. The alternative pathway can be triggered by bacterial toxins and does not need antibodies to be activated.

  Regardless of which pathway is taken, the main products are the same: C3b, anaphylatoxins, and the membrane attack complex. C3b coats bacteria, making it easier for macrophages to engulf them. Anaphylatoxins (C3a, C4a, and C5a) stimulate smooth-muscle contraction and increase vascular permeability by stimulating the release of histamine from mast cells and platelets. The membrane attack complex is a set of complement proteins (C5b, C6, C7, C8, and C9) that bind to form a hollow tube, much like a short straw, that can puncture into the plasma membrane of a cell. In this way, transmembrane channels are formed that allow ions, water, and other small molecules to pass through, resulting in loss of cellular osmolarity and death of the cell.
- **Coagulation system.** The **coagulation system** serves a vital role in the formation of blood clots in blood vessels. Inflammation triggers the coagulation cascade, initiating a complex series of reactions that encourage fibrin formation. **Fibrin** is the protein that polymerizes (bonds) to form the fibrous component of a blood clot. The various coagulation factors are counterbalanced by a variety of inhibitors, so the coagulation is restricted to one area. Simultaneously, the **fibrinolysis cascade** is activated to dissolve the fibrin and create fibrin split products (namely, fragments of the dissolving clot).
- **Kinin system.** The **kinin system** leads to the formation of the vasoactive protein bradykinin from kallikrein. Kallikrein is an enzyme that is normally found in blood plasma, urine, and body tissue in an inactive state. When it becomes activated, it can dilate blood vessels, influence blood pressure, modulate salt and water excretion by the kidneys, and influence cardiac remodeling after AMI. Bradykinin increases vascular permeability, dilates blood vessels, contracts smooth muscle, and causes pain when injected into the skin.

  The kinin system is spurred into action by the activation of Hageman factor (coagulation factor XII). (Table 9-7 lists the various coagulation factors.) In addition to its role in the kinin system, Hageman factor participates in the clotting, fibrinolytic, and complement cascades. Its activators include bacterial lipopolysaccharides and endotoxin. Activated factor XII triggers the intrinsic clotting cascade, which occurs when blood is exposed to collagen or other substances. For example, when a blood vessel is cut, the skin cells are damaged and the blood comes in contact with collagen. The extrinsic clotting cascade is activated by substances released from injured cells when tissue damage occurs.

Cellular Components of Inflammation. The goal of the cellular components of the acute inflammatory response is for inflammatory cells—namely, **polymorphonuclear neutrophils (PMNs)**—to arrive at the sites in the tissue where they are needed. This process involves two major stages: an intravascular phase and an extravascular phase. During the intravascular phase, leukocytes move to the sides of blood vessels and attach to the endothelial cells. During the extravascular phase, leukocytes travel to the site of inflammation and kill organisms. The cellular event sequence is as follows:

1. **Margination.** Loss of fluid from the blood vessels into the inflamed or infected tissue gives the blood that remains in the vessels increased viscosity, which slows the flow of

Table 9-7 Coagulation Factors

Factor Number	Name	Description
I	Fibrinogen	Protein synthesized in liver; converted into fibrin in stage 3
II	Prothrombin	Protein synthesized in liver (requires vitamin K); converted into thrombin in stage 2
III	Tissue thromboplastin	Released from damaged tissue; required in extrinsic stage 1
IV	Calcium ions	Required throughout entire clotting sequence
V	Proaccelerin (labile factor)	Protein synthesized in liver; required to form prothrombin activator in intrinsic and extrinsic stage 1
VII	Serum prothrombin conversion accelerator (stable factor, proconvertin)	Protein synthesized in liver (requires vitamin K); functions in extrinsic stage 1
VIII	Antihemophilic factor (antihemophilic globulin)	Protein synthesized in liver; required for intrinsic stage 1
IX	Plasma thromboplastin component	Protein synthesized in liver (requires vitamin K); required for intrinsic stage 1
X	Stuart factor (Stuart-Prower factor)	Protein synthesized in liver (requires vitamin K); required to form prothrombin activator in intrinsic and extrinsic stage 1
XI	Plasma thromboplastin antecedent	Protein synthesized in liver; required for intrinsic stage 1
XII	Hageman factor	Protein required for intrinsic stage 1
XIII	Fibrin-stabilizing factor	Protein required to stabilize the fibrin strands in stage 3

blood and produces stasis. PMNs, which usually travel toward the center of the vessel, settle toward the sides as the blood flow slows. As stasis develops, leukocytes also move (marginate) toward the sides of the vessels, where they bump into the endothelial cells and bind to them. Stress can lead to demargination of some white blood cells, which stimulates the bone marrow to produce more, in turn increasing the white blood cell count.

2. **Activation.** Mediators of inflammation trigger the appearance of selectins and integrins on the surfaces of endothelial cells and PMNs, respectively.
3. **Adhesion.** PMNs attach to endothelial cells, as mediated by selectins and integrins.
4. **Transmigration (diapedesis).** The PMNs permeate the vessel wall, passing into the interstitial space.
5. **Chemotaxis.** The PMNs move toward the site of inflammation in response to chemotactic factors released by bacteria or formed from activated complement, chemokines, or arachidonic acid derivatives (such as leukotrienes) in response to cell injury. Figure 9-17 illustrates the inflammatory response.

Cellular Products of Inflammation. **Cytokines** are products of cells that affect the function of other cells. Monocytes release monokines, and lymphocytes release lymphokines.

Interleukins include IL-1 (interleukin-1) and IL-2 (interleukin-2), which attract white blood cells to the sites

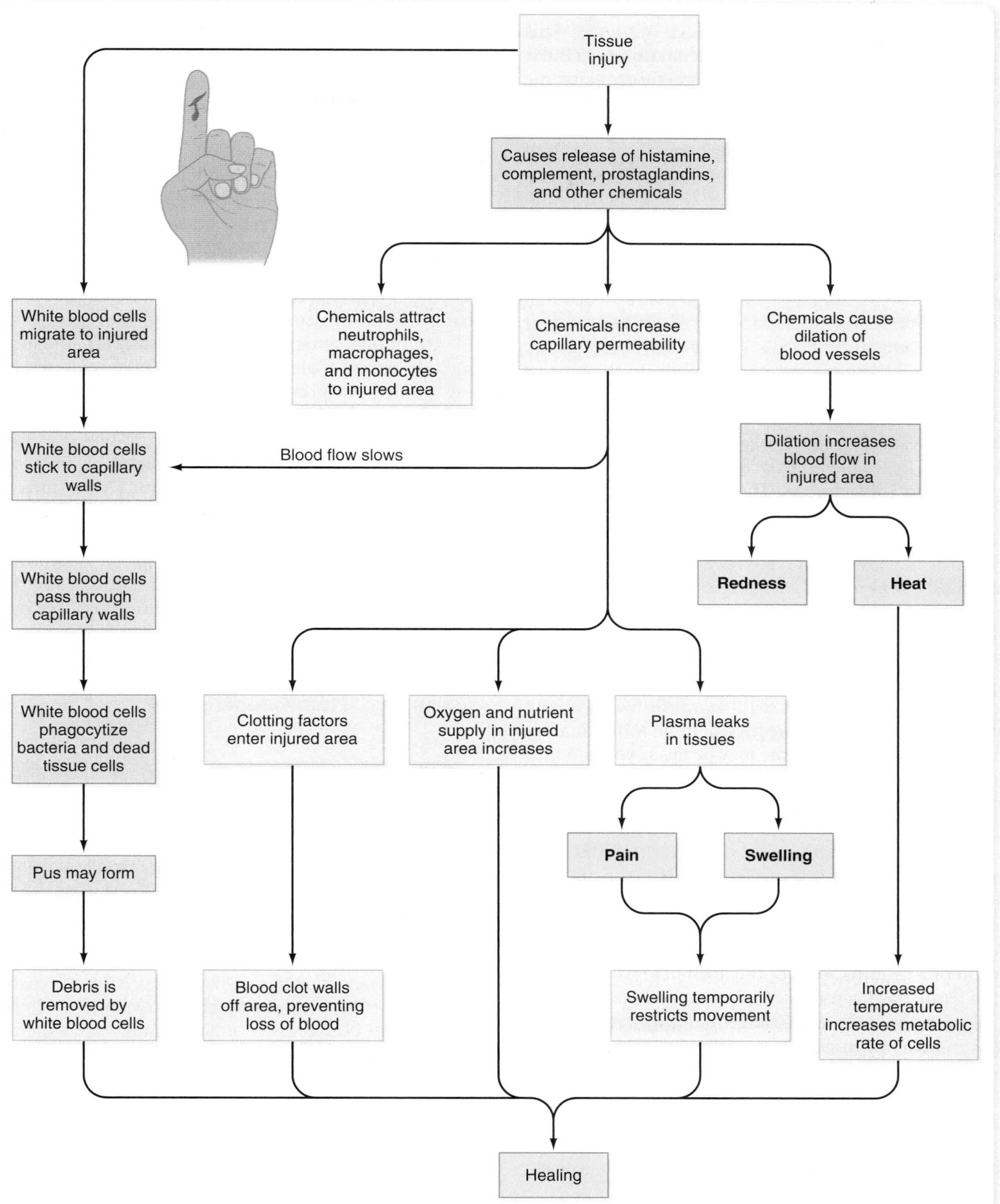

Figure 9-17 The inflammatory response.

of injury and bacterial invasion. **Interferon** is a protein produced by cells when they are invaded by viruses. This cytokine is released into the bloodstream or intercellular fluid to induce healthy cells to manufacture an enzyme that counters the infection.

Lymphokines stimulate leukocytes. Macrophage-activating factor stimulates macrophages to help engulf and destroy foreign substances. Migration inhibitory factor keeps white blood cells at the site of infection or injury until they can perform their designated task.

Injury Resolution and Repair. Normal wound healing involves four steps—repair of damaged tissue, removal of inflammatory debris, restoration of tissues to a normal state, and regeneration of cells. Healing after tissue injury or loss caused by inflammation depends on the type of cells that make up the affected organ. Labile cells divide continuously, so organs derived from these cells (such as skin and intestinal mucosa) heal completely. Stable cells are replaced by regeneration of remaining cells, which are stimulated to enter mitosis. These cells are found in the liver and kidney. Permanent cells, such as nerve cells and cardiac myocytes, cannot be replaced; scar tissue is laid down instead. However, research is being done on the use of stem cells to replace damaged nerve cells.

Wounds may heal by primary or secondary intention. Healing by primary intention occurs in clean wounds with opposed margins (such as clean surgical wounds or surgically débrided wounds). First, blood fills the defect and coagulates, forming a scab—a mesh-like structure composed of fibrin and fibronectin. If the inflammatory process was severe, then tissue may be destroyed and may require repair. Next, macrophages remove cellular debris and secrete growth factors. These growth factors stimulate angiogenesis and growth of fibroblasts, encouraging the formation of granulation tissue. The epithelium then regenerates, covering the surface defect. Deposition of collagen produces fibrous union. By the end of the first week, 10% of the preinjury strength is regained. Scar maturation occurs as collagen cross-linking takes place. By the end of 3 months, 80% of the normal tensile strength of the tissue has been restored.

Healing by secondary intention occurs in large, gaping or infected wounds. Wounds that heal by secondary intention have a more pronounced and prolonged inflammatory phase, causing the neutrophils to persist for days. They also have more abundant granulation tissue. Wound contraction is mediated by myofibroblasts, which help to draw the margins of the wound closer to each other as time passes.

Dysfunctional Wound Healing. Factors that can lead to dysfunctional wound healing may be local or systemic. Local factors include infection (when the body's healing efforts are diverted to fight off the cause of the infection); an inadequate blood supply (as in diabetes) that produces tissue hypoxia, which slows wound healing and may promote infection; and foreign bodies (when present in a wound, they stimulate acute and chronic inflammation, both of which interfere with wound healing).

There are several systemic factors that influence wound healing. Collagen is necessary for wound healing, but inadequate nutritional intake can lead to insufficient levels of collagen, which in turn can lead to inadequate scar formation and suppression of the immune system. Anything that interferes with epithelialization (the process during which epithelial cells begin to form a scab that protects the wound from the outside world) will prevent proper wound healing. *Wound contraction* is the process during which the size of the wound becomes smaller, as part of healing. Anything that interferes with wound contraction can also prevent healing.

Additional systemic factors that disrupt wound healing include hematologic abnormalities (proper wound healing requires the presence of adequate numbers of white blood cells). Patients who have impaired bone marrow stores of white blood cells are susceptible to infection and their wounds often heal more slowly. Diabetes and acquired immunodeficiency syndrome (AIDS) affect the cells of the immune system, which has a direct role in wound healing, and increase the likelihood of wound infection. Corticosteroids suppress the initial inflammatory response required for the proper formation of scar tissue and increase the risk of wound infection by slowing the immune system response.

Finally, if a wound separates, for example from stress, this will slow down the healing process as healing needs to start over, at least to some extent.

Special Populations

Neonates and older adults often have relative impairment of their immune systems, potentially slowing their inflammatory responses. As a consequence, signs of inflammation may be more subtle in these populations. In addition, wound healing often takes longer, especially in older patients. The immune system is not fully developed until a child is between 2 and 3 years old; therefore, when you treat fever in younger children, you must be aggressive and thorough. Many experts recommend hospital admission for a temperature greater than 100.4°F (38°C) in a child younger than 3 months.

Chronic Inflammatory Responses

Chronic inflammatory responses are usually caused by an unsuccessful acute inflammatory response to a foreign body, a persistent infection, or the presence of an antigen. They are associated with an infiltrate (pus) containing monocytes and lymphocytes and usually involve tissue destruction and repair (or scar formation). The vascular events are similar to those that take place in acute inflammation but also include the growth of new blood vessels (a process known as **angiogenesis**).

Variances in Immunity and Inflammation

Hypersensitivity

Hypersensitivity is any response of the body to any substance to which a patient has increased sensitivity. It is a generic term for a variety of reactions. **Allergy** is a hypersensitivity reaction to the presence of an agent (allergen). **Autoimmunity** is the production of antibodies or T cells that work against the tissues of one's own body, producing hypersensitivity reactions or autoimmune disease (as in systemic lupus erythematosus [SLE]). **Isoimmunity** is the formation of T cells or antibodies directed against the antigens on another person's cells (typically after the transplantation of an organ or tissues). A blood transfusion reaction is an example of an isoimmune reaction to another person's red blood cells. The destruction of cells by antibodies or T cells may be an autoimmune or an isoimmune reaction.

Transient neonatal diseases are those that are present at birth, but which eventually resolve. There are many examples; some include transient neonatal hyperglycemia, transient neonatal myasthenia gravis, and transient neonatal neutropenia. Transient neonatal diseases occur due to pathogenic immunoglobulins passing from the pregnant woman to the fetus during pregnancy. In some cases the disease can become permanent, for example if pathogenic immunoglobulins develop in the infant.

Types of Hypersensitivity Reactions

A hypersensitivity reaction may be immediate, occurring within seconds to minutes, or delayed, occurring hours to days after exposure to an antigen. The speed of symptom evolution depends on the antigen and the type of response the body mounts against it. Hypersensitivity reactions are typically classified based on how the immune system caused the injury. **Table 9-8** describes the four types of injuries.

Type I: Immediate Hypersensitivity Reactions. A type I hypersensitivity reaction is an acute reaction that occurs in response to a stimulus (such as a bee sting, penicillin, or shellfish). The mechanism involves interaction between the stimulus (antigen) and a preformed antibody of the IgE type. At first exposure to a specific antigen, specific IgE antibodies bind to mast cells via the nonspecific region (Fc) portion. On secondary exposure to the same antigen, these bound antibodies are cross-linked by the antigen, resulting in degranulation of the mast cell and release of histamine and other mediators **Figure 9-18**. The released histamine feeds back on mast cells and eosinophils, leading to the release of additional histamine and other mediators. The severity of the symptoms that develop in a particular patient depends on the extent of mediator release.

The degree of severity of hypersensitivity reactions varies from severe, life-threatening reactions, such as anaphylaxis, to milder reactions, such as allergic rhinitis (edema and irritation of the nasal mucosa), bronchial asthma (bronchial constriction, mucus production, and airway inflammation), wheal and flare (such as an insect

Table 9-8 Mechanisms of Immunologic Injury

Type	Mechanism	Examples
I: Immediate hypersensitivity	IgE antibodies fix to mast cells and basophils. Later contact with a sensitizing antigen triggers mediator release and clinical manifestations.	Localized response: hay fever, food allergy Systemic response: bee sting, penicillin, anaphylaxis
II: Cytotoxic hypersensitivity reactions	Antibody binds to cell or tissue antigen, and complement is activated, which damages cell, causes inflammation, and promotes destruction of antibody-coated cell by phagocytosis.	Autoimmune hemolytic anemia Blood transfusion reactions Rh hemolytic disease Some types of glomerulonephritis
III: Immune complex disease	Circulating antigen-antibody complexes form, which activate complement and cause inflammatory reaction	Some types of glomerulonephritis Lupus erythematosus Rheumatoid arthritis
IV: Delayed (cell-mediated) hypersensitivity	Sensitized (delayed hypersensitivity) T cells release lymphokines that attract macrophages and other inflammatory cells.	Tuberculosis Fungus and parasitic infections Contact dermatitis

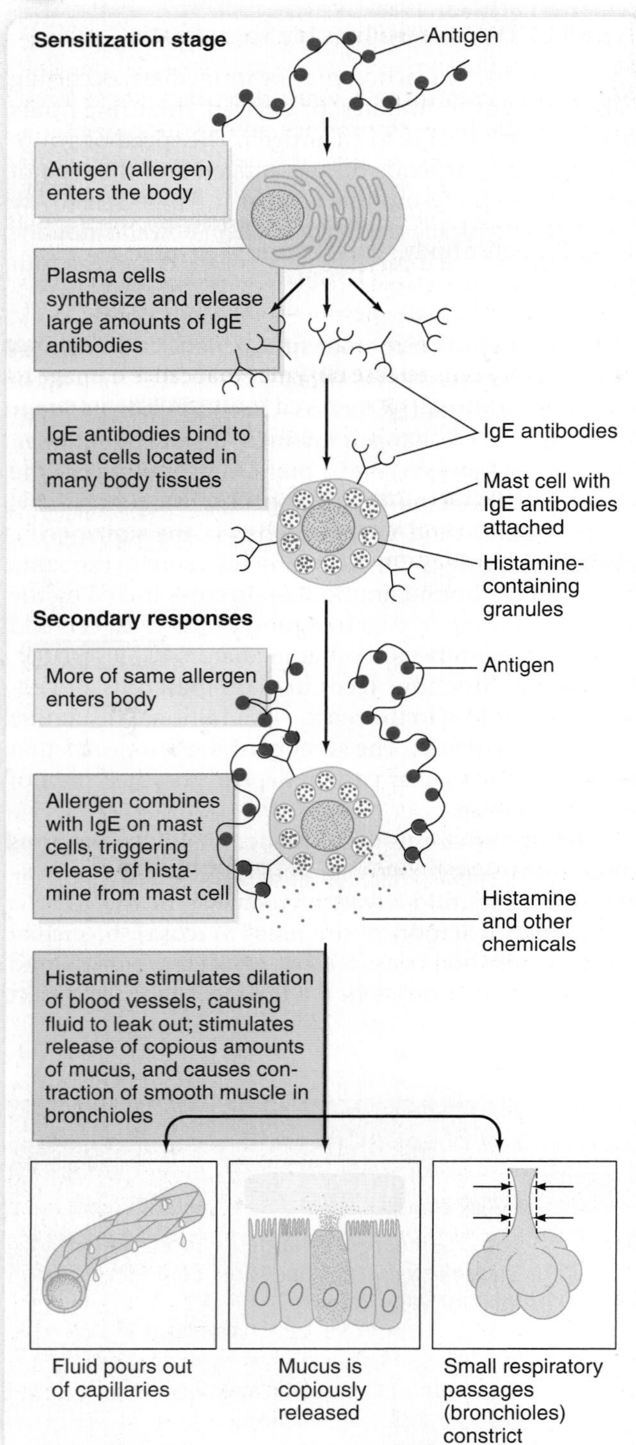

Figure 9-18 Type I allergic reaction. The antigen stimulates the production of massive amounts of IgE, a type of antibody produced by plasma cells; the IgE, in turn, attaches to mast cells. This is a sensitization stage. When the antigen enters again, it binds to the IgE antibodies on the mast cells, triggering a massive release of histamine and other chemicals. Histamine causes blood vessels to dilate and become leaky, and it promotes increased production of mucus in the respiratory tract. Mast cell degranulation may also cause bronchospasm in some people.

bite leading to vasodilation and swelling), and mild food allergy (leading to diarrhea, gastrointestinal distress, and vomiting). A propensity to type I reactions may be diagnosed through skin tests (such as the patch test and scratch test) and other laboratory procedures (measurement of specific IgE antibody levels). Treatment is avoidance of the antigen, but desensitizing injections may be helpful in severe cases.

It is impossible to predict the severity of any given reaction. If a person has had a severe reaction in the past, then he or she is at an increased risk for another one with subsequent antigen exposures. Always assume an IgE-mediated reaction could rapidly become a life-threatening event. These reactions need to be treated quickly in the field, and most prehospital providers are trained to administer epinephrine by using an EpiPen auto-injector or by giving a subcutaneous injection.

Type II: Cytotoxic Hypersensitivity. Type II hypersensitivity reactions are cytotoxic (cell destructive) and classically involve the combination of IgG or IgM antibodies with antigens on the cell membrane. Cells are lysed (destroyed) by complement fixation or by other antibodies. This process also destroys many of the body's healthy cells. Histamine release from mast cells is not involved, and IgG-mediated allergic responses occur within a few hours of antigen exposure. Examples of IgG-mediated responses include transfusion reactions and newborn hemolytic disease.

Type III: Tissue Injury Caused by Immune Complexes. Type III hypersensitivity responses involve primarily IgG antibodies that form immune complexes with antigen to recruit phagocytic cells, such as neutrophils, to a site where they can release inflammatory cytokines. Because histamine release from mast cells is not involved, IgG-mediated allergic responses occur within a few hours of antigen exposure. Reactions may be systemic or localized.

The systemic form is called **serum sickness** and results from a large, single exposure to an antigen, such as horse antibody serum. Antigen-antibody complexes formed in the bloodstream are then deposited in sites around the body, most notably in the kidney, with resultant inflammatory reactions (such as serum sickness from penicillin). Signs and symptoms of serum sickness may include fever, malaise, rashes, joint aches, lymphadenopathy, and splenomegaly.

The localized form of a type III response is called an Arthus reaction. Arthus reactions consist of a circumscribed area of vascular inflammation (**vasculitis**). An example of an Arthus reaction is farmer's lung (a type of hypersensitivity pneumonitis reaction in the lung caused by inhalation of moldy hay dust).

Type IV: Delayed (Cell-Mediated) Hypersensitivity. Type IV allergic responses, also known as cell-mediated hypersensitivity, are primarily mediated by soluble molecules that are released by specifically activated T cells. These reactions are classified into two subtypes: delayed hypersensitivity and cell-mediated cytotoxicity.

Delayed hypersensitivity involves lymphocytes and macrophages. T cells respond to an antigen and activate CD4 (a helper T cell) lymphocytes. These lymphocytes release mediators that are designed to destroy the foreign substance. An example is contact hypersensitivity to poison ivy.

Cell-mediated cytotoxicity involves only sensitized T cells (CD8 lymphocytes or **killer T cells**). These cells kill the antigen-bearing target cells rather than activating the CD4 lymphocyte to do so. Examples include the body's response to viral infections, tumor immune surveillance, and the mechanism by which transplant rejection occurs.

Targets of Hypersensitivity Reactions

The immune system targets different molecules, depending on the type of hypersensitivity reaction. In allergic reactions, the target is an antigen or allergen. Allergens are substances that cause a hypersensitivity reaction, such as those listed in Table 9-9.

Autoimmune Reactions. In autoimmune reactions, the target is a person's own tissues. For reasons that are unclear, normal tolerance of "self" tissues breaks down and the immune system treats the body's own tissues as foreign.

Graves disease is an autoimmune disease caused by thyroid-stimulating or thyroid-growth immunoglobulins. These antibodies activate receptors for thyroid-stimulating hormone, causing increased activity by the thyroid gland. In addition to hyperthyroidism, Graves disease is associated with characteristic eye changes—lid retraction, stare, and exophthalmos (protrusion of the eyes)—and skin changes (pretibial myxedema—localized edematous skin in the pretibial area).

Table 9-9 Allergens That Can Cause Hypersensitivity Reactions

Type	Examples
Inhalants	Pollen, dust, smoke, fungi, plastic, odors
Food	Eggs, dairy, wheat, chocolate, strawberries
Drugs	Aspirin, antibiotics, serums, codeine
Infectious agents	Bacteria, viruses, fungi, animal parasites
Contactants	Animals, plants, metals, chemicals
Physical agents	Light, pressure, radiation, heat and cold

Type 1 diabetes mellitus is also considered an autoimmune disease. Although the exact insult is unknown (but is suspected to be a viral infection), some agent stimulates the body to produce autoantibodies against beta cells in the pancreas that produce insulin. The results are a deficiency of insulin and, therefore, diabetes.

Rheumatoid arthritis is a chronic systemic disease that affects the entire body. One of the most common forms of arthritis, it is characterized by inflammation of the synovium (the connective tissue membrane lining the joint) with resulting pain, stiffness, warmth, redness, and swelling. Inflammatory cells release enzymes that cause damage to bone and cartilage. The involved joint can lose its shape and alignment, resulting in pain and loss of movement. Rheumatoid arthritis is associated with the formation of rheumatoid factor—that is, IgM antibodies to tissue IgG. In the joints, the synovial membrane is thickened due to infiltration of inflammatory cells (lymphocytes).

Myasthenia gravis is an acquired autoimmune disease that is characterized by autoimmune attack on the nerve-muscle junction. The circulating autoantibodies cause abnormal muscle fatigability and typically involve the smallest motor units first, such as the extraocular muscles. This produces ptosis (droopy eyelid) and diplopia (double vision). Other muscles may be involved, causing problems with swallowing (dysphagia). Characteristically, repeated contraction of the affected muscles makes the symptoms worse. Two thirds of people with myasthenia gravis have thymic abnormalities, with the most common being thymic hyperplasia. A minority of people have a tumor of the thymus, called a thymoma.

Neutropenia refers to a decrease in circulating neutrophils. Neutrophils are usually the first to arrive at the scene of an infection and serve to scavenge pathogenic microorganisms so infection cannot spread. Once the neutrophils are fully used, they die and become part of the yellow wound drainage (pus). When a patient has neutropenia, an insufficient level of neutrophils decreases the body's ability to fight infection. Isoimmune neutropenia refers to this condition in a neonate. It develops when a pregnant woman produces antibodies against neutrophils, which then cross the placenta and cause neutropenia in the fetus.

Idiopathic thrombocytopenic purpura (ITP), also known as immune thrombocytopenic purpura, is a blood disorder in which antibodies form to blood platelets that cause their destruction. Thrombocytopenia describes a decrease in blood platelets; purpura is purple areas of the skin and mucous membranes (such as the lining of the mouth) where bleeding has occurred as a result of decreased numbers of or ineffective platelets. Some cases of ITP are caused by certain types of medications, whereas others are associated with infection, pregnancy, or immune disorders such as lupus (SLE, systemic lupus erythematosus).[11] About half of all cases are classified as idiopathic (the cause is unknown).

Bleeding is the main symptom of ITP and can include bruising and tiny red dots on the skin or mucous membranes. In some cases, bleeding from the nose, gums, and digestive or urinary tracts may occur. Rarely, the patient has bleeding within the brain.

Treatment of idiopathic ITP is based on the severity of the symptoms and the patient's platelet count. In some cases, no therapy is needed. In most cases, drugs that alter the immune system's attack on the platelets are prescribed, such as corticosteroids (prednisone, for example) and IV infusions of immunoglobulin. Another treatment that usually increases the number of platelets is removal of the spleen, the organ that destroys antibody-coated platelets.

SLE is a chronic autoimmune disease with many manifestations. In SLE, the body's immune system is directed against the body's tissues. The cause of SLE is not known. Although SLE is more common in young women, it can occur in either sex at any age. The production of autoantibodies leads to immune complex formation. These immune complexes can then be deposited in glomeruli, skin, lungs, synovium, and mesothelium, among other places. Symptoms include arthritis, a red rash over the nose and cheeks, fatigue, weakness, fever, and photosensitivity. Glomerulonephritis (kidney disease), pericarditis, anemia, and neuritis may develop. In addition, many people with SLE have renal complications.

▶ Immune Deficiencies

Immunodeficiency is an abnormal condition in which some part of the body's immune system is inadequate, and, consequently, resistance to infectious diseases is decreased. It may be congenital or acquired.

Congenital Immunodeficiencies

Patients with severe combined immunodeficiency disease have defects that involve lymphoid stem cells. As a consequence, T cells (cellular immunity) and B cells (humoral immunity) are affected. Patients are at risk for infection with all types of organisms (bacteria, mycobacteria, fungi, viruses, parasites, and prions). There are two forms of this disease, both of which are inherited.

X-linked agammaglobulinemia (XLA) is one of the most common forms of inherited primary immunodeficiency, and occurs predominantly in males. XLA results in a decrease in the level of mature B cells.[12] The result is a decreased ability to produce antibodies, and therefore decreased ability to effectively protect against bacteria and viruses.[12,13]

The result is a markedly decreased level of all immunoglobulins and of mature B lymphocytes; however, T lymphocytes function normally. Recurrent pyrogenic infections develop, but patients have no problems with fungal and viral infections because their cell-mediated immunity is unaffected. These infections first emerge in affected infants at about 6 months of age, when the level of maternal immunoglobulin has decreased.

Isolated deficiency of IgA is probably the most common form of immunodeficiency. This disease results from a block in the terminal differentiation of B lymphocytes. Most patients are asymptomatic, but in some, chronic sinus infections may develop. Patients also have an increased incidence of autoimmune disease.

YOU are the Paramedic PART 4

Your partner reports all of the medication bottles are out of date and empty. You ask the patient about this and he states he does not have the means necessary to buy the medications. When you look at the list of medications, you find one for a diuretic. Your cardiac monitor indicates a sinus tachycardia matching the pulse rate. No ectopy is noted. $ETCO_2$ waveform appears appropriate in shape and reads 36 mm Hg.

Recording Time: 7 Minutes	
Respirations	24 breaths/min; shallow
Pulse	114 beats/min
Skin	Cool, pale, and moist
Blood pressure	138/88 mm Hg
Oxygen saturation (SpO_2)	92% with high-flow oxygen administration
Pupils	PERRLA

7. Why would a diuretic be prescribed for a patient with congestive heart failure?
8. Why would this patient have a normal or slightly high blood pressure?

Acquired Immunodeficiencies

Any nutritional deficiency can hamper normal immune function and the inflammatory response. Nutritional deficiencies may depress bone marrow function and diminish white blood cell development. A lack of protein in the diet, for example, decreases the liver's ability to manufacture inflammatory mediators and plasma proteins.

The stress of trauma can also cause immunodeficiency. Other contributors to this condition may include hypoperfusion or shock, mediator production, damage to vital organs, and the decreased nutrition occurring during trauma states.

Iatrogenic (treatment-induced) immunodeficiency is most often caused by medications. For example, corticosteroids, whether taken orally or inhaled, suppress the immune system. This immune system suppression is often of therapeutic benefit. However, in a small number of patients the immunosuppression leads to other diseases, such as tuberculosis. Because of its potential for adverse effects, physicians are usually cautious about prescribing this therapy for a prolonged period. In addition, idiosyncratic reactions to antibiotics may cause bone marrow suppression. Bone marrow suppression in cancer is often a direct side effect of chemotherapy and not a true idiosyncratic reaction.

Physical or mental stress has been shown to decrease white blood cell and lymphocyte function. It may also lead to decreased production of various antibodies.

AIDS is an immunodeficiency disease that is caused by the RNA retrovirus HIV. HIV binds to the CD4 surface protein of helper T cells, infects these cells, and kills them. The destruction of the cells causes decreased humoral and cell-mediated reactions.

Treatment of Immunodeficiencies

Replacement therapy is available for immunodeficiencies such as common variable immunodeficiency. Intravenous gamma globulin has been used in the therapy for a number of immunologic disorders of the nervous system, especially myasthenia gravis and inflammatory neuropathies, with considerable success. Bone marrow transplantation may restore immune competence in patients with acquired causes of immunodeficiency, such as following chemotherapy to treat cancer. Transfusion is another form of replacement therapy for immunodeficiencies. In the future, gene therapy may be useful to treat congenital and acquired causes of immunodeficiency.

Factors That Cause Disease

Genetic, environmental, age-related, and sex-associated factors can cause or contribute to disease. Genetic factors are present at birth and are passed on through a person's genes to future generations. Environmental factors include microorganisms, immunologic vulnerabilities, personal habits and lifestyle, exposure to chemicals and other toxins, the physical environment, and the psychosocial environment. Family violence, for example, might be a key factor in causing depression or substance abuse, perhaps even years later. A sedentary lifestyle and a high-fat diet can cause or contribute to obesity, diabetes, heart disease, stroke, and other diseases.

Disease can also have anatomic causes. For example, malrotation of the colon is a disease in which the colon does not form properly, resulting in partial blockage. Another example is degenerative diseases of the spine; as intervertebral disks age, they may degenerate to the extent that the patient experiences pain due to nerve compression. *Aortic stenosis* is a condition in which the aortic valve becomes very tight and narrowed, resulting in chest pain from decreased perfusion of the coronary arteries or congestive heart failure.

Finally, an immunologic reaction may result in disease. An example is exposure to an agent that triggers an abnormal immune response against myelin, leading to the development of multiple sclerosis.

Controllable Versus Uncontrollable Risk Factors

Some uncontrollable factors, such as genetics and race, influence the development of disease, but many other factors can be controlled. For example, behaviors such as smoking, drinking alcohol, inadequate nutrition (excessive fat, salt, and sugar intake or insufficient intake of protein, fruits, vegetables, and fiber), lack of physical activity, and stress can be modified.

Age-Related Risk

The risk of a particular disease often depends on a person's age. For example, newborns are at greater risk of certain diseases because their immune systems are not fully developed (see Chapter 42, *Neonatal Care*). Teenagers are at high risk of injury due to trauma and illicit drug and alcohol use. As people get older, the risk of having cancer, heart disease, stroke, and Alzheimer disease increases (see Chapter 44, *Geriatric Emergencies*).

Sex-Associated Factors

In some cases, sex is related to the risk of having a certain disease. Note: A person's physical sex and gender are not necessarily the same. In this discussion, we are referring to a person's genetic sex; for example, a person born with an XY sex chromosome is genetically and physically male, even if the person's gender is female.

Some diseases present differently in women compared with men (eg, presentation of AMI). For example, the hormones found in a premenopausal woman have been shown to have protective benefits in major head trauma and certain cardiac conditions.

Finally, genetic disorders are related to a person's sex when a defective gene is located on a sex chromosome.

Most sex-linked disorders are X linked. X-linked disorders may be either recessive or dominant. Because females have two X chromosomes, those with a defective X gene may not have the disorder; if the disorder is recessive, the X chromosome without the defect will mask the defective X chromosome. Men with a defective X gene will always be affected because they only have one X chromosome; the defect cannot be masked.

▶ Analysis of Disease Risk

Analyzing disease risk involves consideration of disease rates and disease risk factors (causal and noncausal). Risk factors that can directly cause a disease to develop are called causal risk factors. For example, *Mycobacterium tuberculosis* is a causal risk factor for a person becoming infected with tuberculosis. Risk factors that are associated with risk for a disease but not a direct cause are called *noncausal risk factors*. For example, poverty is a noncausal risk factor for tuberculosis.

All studies of a disease should consider the incidence, prevalence, and mortality of the disease. The **incidence** is the number of new cases of a disease in a population (for example, six cases of West Nile virus infection were identified in the county). **Prevalence** refers to the number of cases of a disease or condition in a particular population within a particular period (for example, last year, more than 100,000 patients had this disease). **Morbidity** refers to the presence of disease or to the incidence or prevalence of a disease. **Mortality** is most often discussed as the mortality rate, which is the number of deaths from a disease in a given population, expressed as a proportion (for example, 1 in 50 affected people in the United States). Table 9-10 illustrates how the concepts of incidence, prevalence, morbidity, and mortality might be expressed, using statistics on diabetes as an example.

Interaction of Risk Factors

Risk factors, age, and sex differences often interact. For example, suppose a person has a genetic tendency toward coronary artery disease; the risk of myocardial infarction or sudden death is higher in this person even if he or she exercises regularly and has no other risk factors. A person who smokes heavily but has no other risk factors may have a similarly elevated risk. Table 9-11 shows the interplay of various risk factors in causing respiratory disease.

▶ Common Familial Diseases and Associated Risk Factors

The terms *genetic risk* and *familial tendency* are often used interchangeably. A true genetic risk is one that is passed through generations by inheritance of a gene. In contrast, with a familial tendency, diseases seem to cluster in family groups despite lack of evidence for heritable gene-associated abnormalities.

Table 9-12 lists some of the traits and diseases carried on human chromosomes. **Autosomal recessive** is a pattern of inheritance that involves genes located on autosomes (any chromosome other than sex chromosomes). A person needs to inherit two copies of a particular form of a gene to show that trait. A parent who carries the gene for an autosomal recessive trait but does not display the trait has a 25% chance of passing the inherited condition to his or her child if the other parent is also a carrier for the trait. If both parents have the inherited condition, then all of their children will have the condition. Hemochromatosis, which causes the accumulation of too much iron in the body, has an autosomal recessive pattern of inheritance—a person must inherit a copy of the hemochromatosis gene from each parent for the disease to develop.

Table 9-10 Incidence, Prevalence, Morbidity, and Mortality Rate of Diabetes in the United States

Term	Example
Incidence	In 2012, 1.7 million people 20 years or older were newly diagnosed with type 1 or type 2 diabetes. An additional 86 million people aged 20 years and older are categorized as prediabetic.
Prevalence	A total of 9.3% of the total US population (adults and children) had diabetes in 2012.
Morbidity	In 2012, 29.1 million adults and children in the United States had diabetes (21.0 million diagnosed and an estimated 8.1 million undiagnosed).
Mortality rate	In 2010, diabetes was responsible for or a key contributor to the deaths of 234,051 people.

Data from: Centers for Disease Control and Prevention. *National Diabetes Statistics Report: Estimates of Diabetes and Its Burden in the United States, 2014.* Atlanta, GA: U.S. Department of Health and Human Services; 2014.http://www.cdc.gov/diabetes/pubs/statsreport14/national-diabetes-report-web.pdf. Accessed January 6, 2017. American Diabetes Association. Statistics About Diabetes. http://www.diabetes.org/diabetes-basics/statistics/. Accessed January 6, 2017.

Table 9-11 Common Respiratory Diseases

Disease	Pathology and/or Symptoms	Causes and Possible Contributing Causes
Emphysema	Breakdown of alveoli, shortness of breath	Smoking Air pollution Possible genetic susceptibility Exacerbated by obesity
Chronic bronchitis	Cough, shortness of breath	Smoking Air pollution Possible genetic susceptibility Exacerbated by obesity
Acute bronchitis	Inflammation of the bronchi; coughing up yellow mucus; shortness of breath	Many viruses and bacteria Possible genetic susceptibility Smoking Exacerbated by obesity
Sinusitis	Inflammation of the sinuses; characterized by mucus discharge, blocked nasal passages, and headache	Many viruses and bacteria Poor general health
Laryngitis	Inflammation of larynx and vocal cords, sore throat, hoarseness, mucus buildup, and cough	Many viruses and bacteria Poor general health
Pneumonia	Inflammation of the lungs, ranging from mild to severe; cough and fever, shortness of breath at rest, chills, sweating, chest pain, blood-tinged mucus	Bacteria, viruses, fungi, or inhalation of irritating gases Lack of physical activity
Asthma	Constriction of bronchioles, mucus buildup in bronchioles, periodic wheezing, difficulty breathing	Allergy to pollen, certain foods, food additives; dander (dead skin cells and other debris shed by dogs, cats, or birds) Physical activity (exercise-induced asthma) Probable genetic link

In **autosomal dominant** inheritance, a person needs to inherit only one copy of a particular form of a gene to show that trait; it does not matter which form of the gene is inherited from the other parent. A parent has at least a 50% chance of passing on an autosomal dominant inherited condition to his or her child. Familial adenomatous polyposis, which places people at extremely high risk for the development of colorectal (colon) cancer, has an autosomal dominant pattern of inheritance.

Immunologic Disorders

Immunologic diseases are caused by hyperactivity or hypoactivity of the immune system. Most immunologic diseases that exhibit familial tendencies involve an overactive immune system—for example, allergies, asthma, and rheumatic fever. Significant overlap exists often among causative factors, including the person's environment.

Allergies are acquired following initial exposure to an allergen. Repeated exposures cause the immune system to react to the allergen Figure 9-19. Although the clinical presentation varies, it usually includes swelling and itching, runny nose, coughing, sneezing, wheezing, and nasal congestion. A person who has an allergic tendency is said to be **atopic**. Environmental conditions may also increase a person's susceptibility to an allergic reaction.

Asthma is a chronic inflammatory condition of the lower airway resulting in intermittent wheezing and excess mucus production. Nearly 60% of attacks are precipitated by viral infections. Allergies account for another 20% of asthma attacks, with stress and emotions causing the remainder. In addition to the familial component, chromosomal differences in certain patients may enhance their susceptibility to asthma.

Table 9-12 Traits and Diseases Carried on Human Chromosomes

Trait or Disease	Result
Autosomal Recessive	
Albinism	Lack of pigment in eyes, skin, and hair
Cystic fibrosis	Pancreatic failure, mucus buildup in lungs
Sickle cell anemia	Abnormal hemoglobin characterized by sickle-shaped red blood cells that obstruct vital capillaries
Tay-Sachs disease	Improper metabolism of gangliosides in nerve cells
Phenylketonuria	Accumulation of phenylalanine in blood; causes mental retardation
Attached earlobe	Earlobe attached to skin of the neck
Hyperextensible thumb	Thumb bends past a 45° angle
Autosomal Dominant	
Achondroplasia	Dwarfism resulting from a defect in the epiphyseal plates that interferes with the formation of long bones
Marfan syndrome	Defect of connective tissue resulting in excessive growth and a high risk of aortic rupture
Widow's peak	Hairline coming to a point on forehead
Huntington disease	Progressive deterioration of the nervous system beginning in a person's late 20s or early 30s; causes mental deterioration and early death
Brachydactyly	Disfiguration of hands, shortened fingers
Freckles	Permanent aggregations of melanin in the skin

Special Populations

Rheumatic fever is an inflammatory disease that occurs primarily in children. This disease results from a delayed reaction to an untreated streptococcal infection of the upper respiratory tract (such as strep throat). Symptoms, which appear several weeks after the acute infection, may include fever, abdominal pain, vomiting, arthritis, palpitations, and chest pain. Recurrent episodes of rheumatic fever may cause permanent myocardial damage, especially to the cardiac valves. A family history of acute rheumatic fever may predispose a person to the disease.

Cancer

Cancer describes the pathology associated with malignant growths (neoplasms) in various anatomic areas of the human body. The prognosis often depends on the extent of its spread (metastasis) and the effectiveness of treatment.

A major risk factor associated with lung cancer is cigarette smoking. Research has identified eight alterations in the genetic material of lung cancers that suggest a genetic tendency to develop the disease. Other predisposing factors include exposure to asbestos, coal products, and other industrial and chemical products. Symptoms include cough, difficulty breathing, blood-tinged sputum, and repeated infections. Treatment depends on the type,

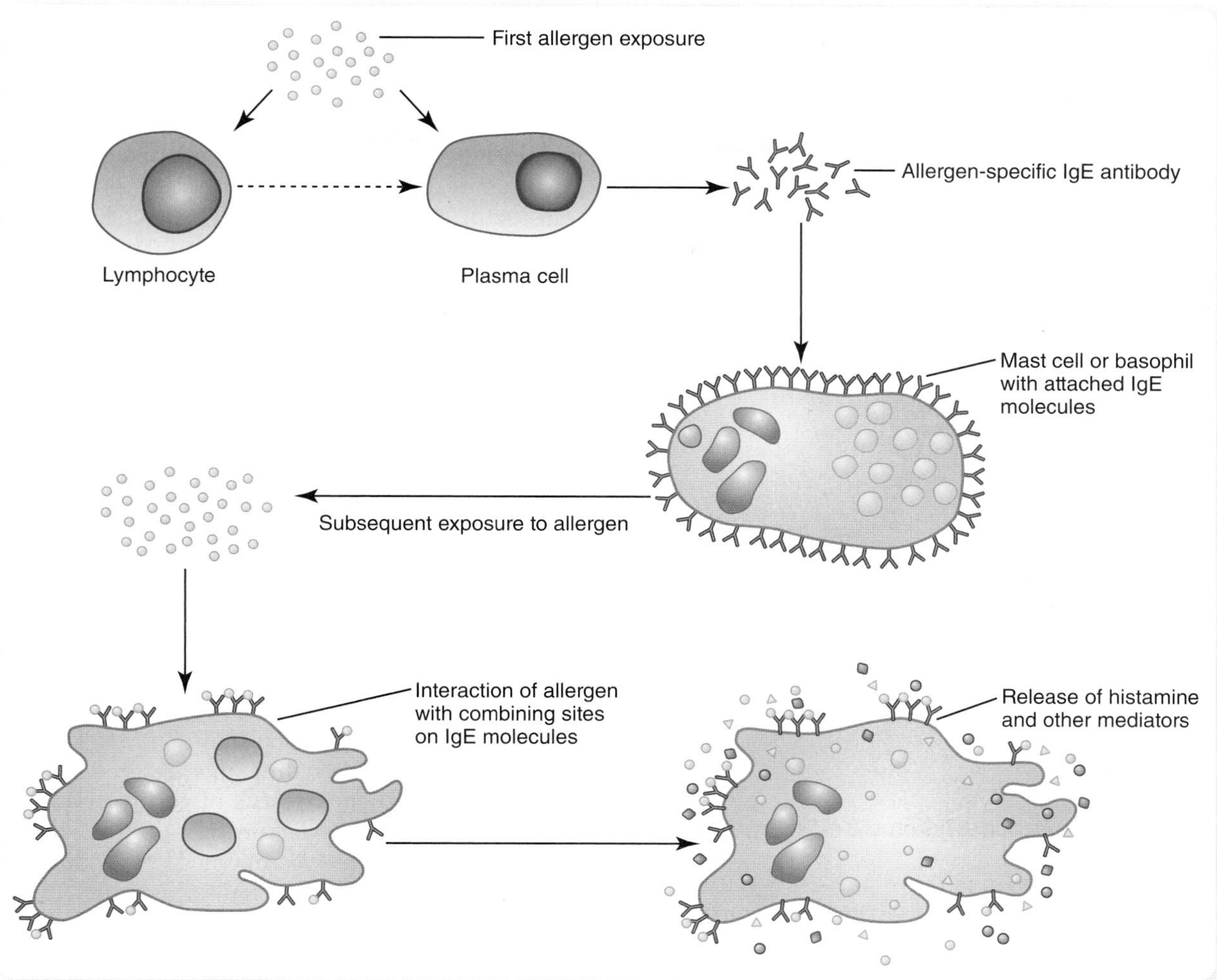

Figure 9-19 Pathogenesis of allergy. First, exposure to an allergen induces formation of specific IgE antibodies in susceptible patients, which then bind to mast cells and basophils. Subsequent exposure to the same allergen leads to antigen-antibody interaction through activation of memory cells, liberating histamine and other mediators from mast cells and basophils. These mediators induce allergic manifestations.

site, and extent of the cancer and may include surgery, chemotherapy, and/or radiotherapy.

Breast cancer is the most common type of cancer occurring among women and accounts for as many as 231,840 newly diagnosed cases and 40,290 deaths each year in the United States.[14] Women whose first-degree relatives (ie, parent, sister, or daughter) have breast cancer are 2.1 times more likely to have the disease. Risk varies with the age at which the affected relative was diagnosed; the younger the age at occurrence, the greater the risk posed to relatives. Approximately 5% to 10% of patients with breast cancer have a pattern of autosomal dominant inheritance, in which cancer predisposition is transmitted from generation to generation.[15] The susceptibility may be inherited through the mother's or the father's side of the family.

Early symptoms of breast cancer are usually detected by the woman during breast self-examination and include a small, painless lump, thick or dimpled skin, or a change in the nipple **Figure 9-20**. Later symptoms include nipple discharge, pain, and swollen lymph glands in the axilla. Treatment depends on the location, size, and metastasis of the tumor.

Colorectal cancer is the third most common type of cancer in men and women. In 2016, the American Cancer Society expected 95,270 new cases and an estimated 49,190 deaths from colorectal cancer in the United States.[14] Relatives of people diagnosed with colorectal cancer are more likely to have the disease themselves, and parents can pass on to their children changes in certain genes that can lead to colorectal cancer. Symptoms may be minimal, consisting only of small amounts of blood in the stool. Treatment involves surgery and sometimes chemotherapy. Periodic rectal examinations and colonoscopy are recommended for adults age 50 years and older to detect the disease at an early stage.

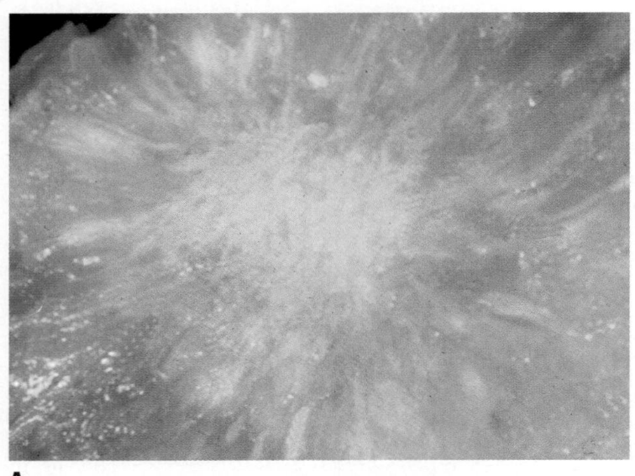

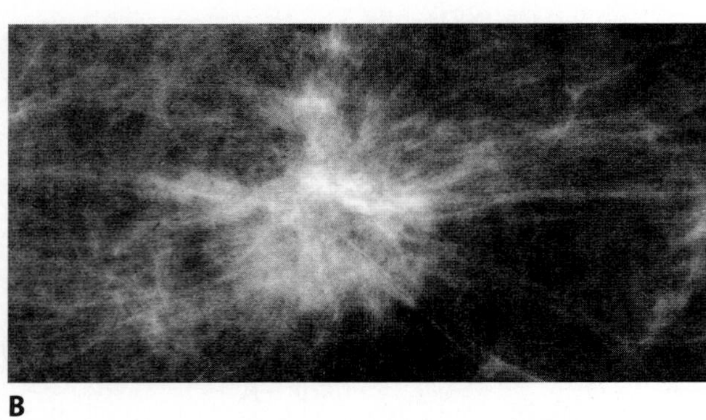

Figure 9-20 Breast carcinoma. **A.** Cross-section of breast biopsy specimen. The tumor appears as a firm mass with poorly defined edges that infiltrate the surrounding fatty breast tissue. **B.** Appearance of breast carcinoma in a mammogram. The tumor appears as a white area with infiltrating margins.

Endocrine Disorders

Diabetes mellitus is one of the most significant endocrine diseases. This chronic disorder of metabolism is associated with partial insulin secretion or total lack of insulin secretion by the pancreas, which in turn affects the body's ability to use glucose. Symptoms include excessive thirst and urination, weight abnormalities, and the presence of excessive glucose in the urine and the blood.

Ketoacidosis-prone (type 1) diabetes is also known as insulin-dependent diabetes mellitus because patients need exogenous insulin to survive. Non–ketoacidosis-prone (type 2) diabetes is called non–insulin-dependent diabetes, even though many people with type 2 diabetes require exogenous insulin injections. Both forms have a hereditary predisposition. Type 1 diabetes has no known cure (other than pancreas transplantation) at the present time; type 2 diabetes can occasionally be brought under control with weight loss, regular physical activity, and medications.

Hematologic Disorders

Hemolytic anemia is characterized by increased destruction of red blood cells. This disorder has a number of causes, such as an Rh factor blood transfusion reaction (which would most likely occur in the neonate population), a disorder of the immune system, and exposure to bacterial toxins or chemicals such as benzene. **Figure 9-21** depicts how the body handles iron. Hemolytic anemia following an aspirin overdose or penicillin administration is rare; it is much more common, albeit still rare, with sulfa drugs used to treat urinary tract infections, such as the trimethoprim-sulfamethoxazole combination (known as Septra and Bactrim). An inherited enzyme deficiency (glucose-6-phosphatase dehydrogenase deficiency) markedly increases a person's susceptibility to sulfa drug–induced hemolytic anemia.

Hemophilia is an inherited disorder characterized by excessive bleeding. It is a sex-linked condition, occurring predominantly in males, and is passed from asymptomatic mothers to sons.[16] In this disorder, one of the blood-clotting proteins (usually factor VIII) necessary for normal blood coagulation is missing or is present in abnormally low amounts. Patients experience greater than usual blood loss in dental extractions and following simple injuries. They may also have bleeding into joints and, rarely, into the brain. Treatment consists of administration of the missing blood-clotting factors.

Hemochromatosis is an inherited (autosomal recessive) disease in which the body absorbs more iron than it needs. The excess iron is stored in various organs, including the liver, kidneys, and pancreas. Hemochromatosis can lead to diabetes, heart disease, liver disease, arthritis, impotence, and a bronzed skin color. These symptoms can be avoided by regularly drawing blood (phlebotomy).

Cardiovascular Disorders

Several cardiovascular disorders are known to follow specific patterns of inheritance. Still others have strong familial tendencies (such as coronary heart disease).

Long QT Syndrome. Long QT syndrome is a cardiac conduction system abnormality characterized by prolongation of the QT interval on the ECG. Because most cases of long QT syndrome are inherited in an autosomal dominant manner, all first-degree relatives of affected people must be screened. Sometimes these syndromes are associated with congenital hearing loss, hypertrophic cardiomyopathy, or mitral valve prolapse (MVP). Patients are at risk for palpitations and ventricular dysrhythmias, especially torsades de pointes. Many patients are asymptomatic until they have a dysrhythmia, causing syncope or sudden death. Always consider syncope under the following conditions to be due to a life-threatening dysrhythmia until proven otherwise:

- Exercise-induced syncope
- Syncope associated with chest pain

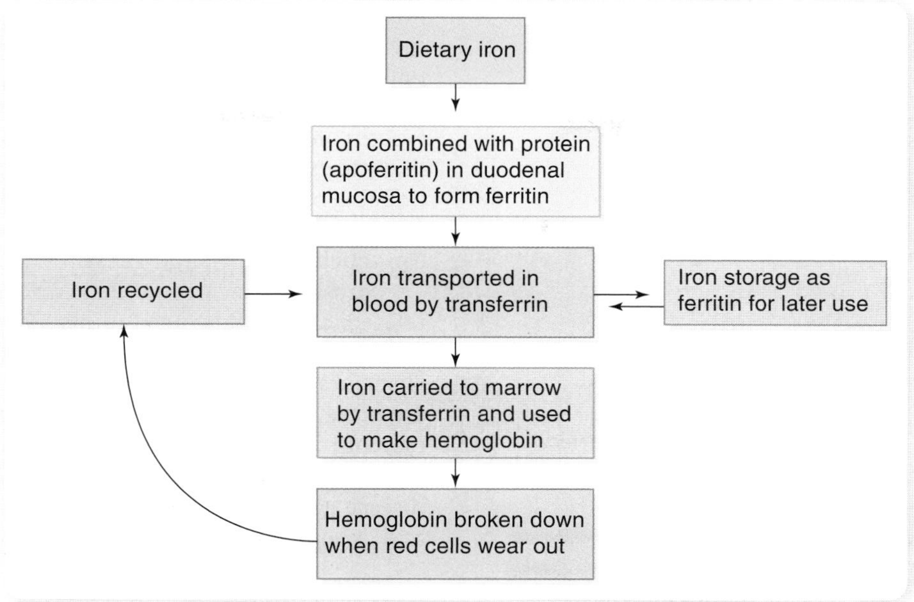

Figure 9-21 Iron uptake, transport, storage, and utilization for hemoglobin synthesis. Most of the iron used for hemoglobin synthesis is recycled from worn-out red blood cells. Chronic blood loss removes iron-containing cells from the circulation, and the iron contained in the red blood cells can no longer be recycled to make hemoglobin, leading to iron deficiency anemia.

- A history of syncope in a close family member (ie, parent, sibling, or child)
- Syncope associated with startle (for example, loud noises such as phones or alarm clocks)

Cardiomyopathy. *Cardiomyopathy* is a general term for diseases of the myocardium (heart muscle) that ultimately progress to heart failure, AMI, or death. These diseases cause the heart muscle to become thin, flabby, dilated, or enlarged. One variant, hypertrophic cardiomyopathy, is genetically autosomal dominant. The main feature of hypertrophic cardiomyopathy is an excessive thickening of the heart muscle (hypertrophy means to thicken or grow excessively) **Figure 9-22**. In addition, microscopic examination of the heart muscle shows that it is abnormal. Patients may have shortness of breath, chest pains, palpitations, or syncope; sudden cardiac death is also possible. Beta-blockers are effective treatment in some patients. Others require surgery or an automatic implantable cardiac defibrillator designed to deliver a shock to the heart.

Mitral Valve Prolapse. Also referred to as a floppy mitral valve, mitral valve prolapse (MVP) is relatively common, affecting 2.5% of males and 7.6% of females. A familial tendency toward MVP exists, but the condition is usually associated with other cardiovascular conditions. The mitral valve leaflets balloon into the left atrium during systole. Although MVP is often benign and asymptomatic, some patients have chest pain, fatigue, dizziness, dyspnea, or palpitations. Generally, the only physical finding is a clicking sound heard during cardiac auscultation. Cardiac dysrhythmias develop in a small number of patients.

Sometimes MVP leads to mitral regurgitation (also called mitral insufficiency), in which a large amount of blood leaks backward through the defective valve. Mitral regurgitation can lead to thickening or enlargement of the heart wall, caused by the extra pumping of the heart to make up for the backflow of blood. It sometimes causes people to feel tired or short of breath. Mitral regurgitation usually can be treated with medication, but some people need surgery to repair or replace the defective valve.

Coronary Heart Disease. *Coronary heart disease*, often called coronary artery disease, is caused by impaired circulation to the heart. Typically, patients have occluded coronary arteries from atherosclerotic plaque buildup. The effects can range from ischemia to infarction and necrosis (death) of the myocardium. Almost half of all cardiovascular deaths are caused by coronary heart disease.[17] This condition has a familial tendency; significant risk factors for coronary artery disease development include having a father who had an AMI or died suddenly before 55 years of age or having a mother who had an AMI or died suddenly before 65 years of age. Other risk factors include hypercholesterolemia, cigarette smoking, hypertension (high blood pressure), age (as age increases, the risk for coronary heart disease increases), and diabetes.

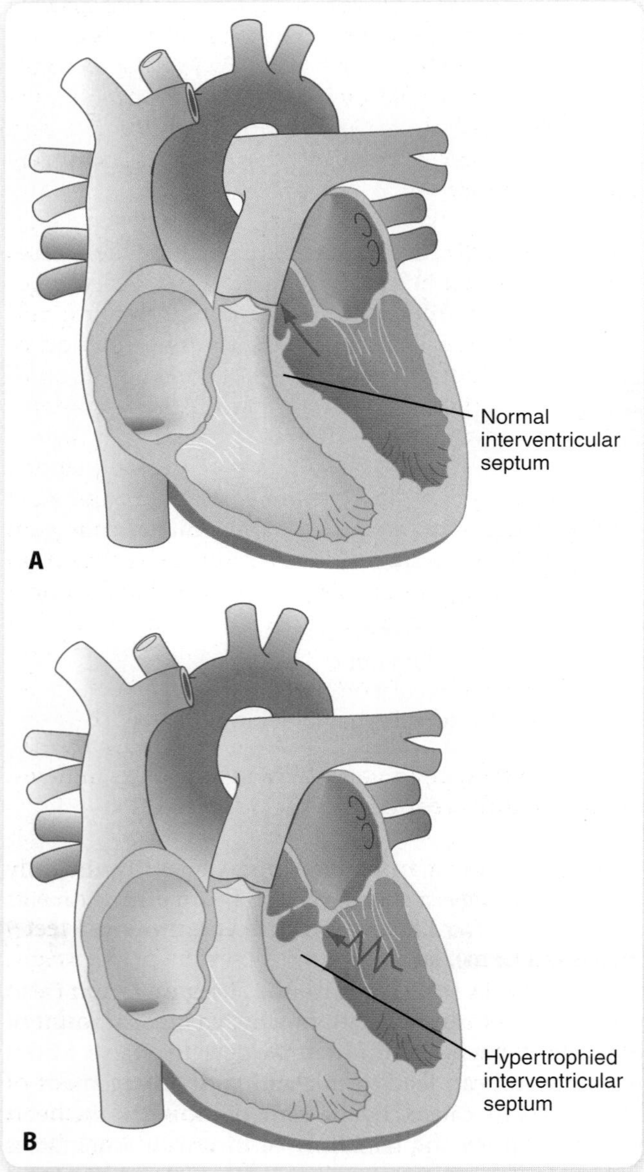

Figure 9-22 Comparison of normal cardiac function with malfunction characteristic of hypertrophic cardiomyopathy. **A.** Normal heart, illustrating unobstructed flow of blood from left ventricle into aorta during ventricular systole. **B.** Hypertrophic cardiomyopathy, illustrating obstruction to outflow of blood from left ventricle by hypertrophied septum, which impinges on the anterior leaflet of mitral valve.

Hypercholesterolemia is an elevation of the blood cholesterol level. The blood cholesterol level is divided into high-density lipoprotein ("good cholesterol") and low-density lipoprotein ("bad cholesterol"). Despite having a normal total cholesterol level, having an abnormally low level of high-density lipoprotein and/or an elevation of low-density lipoprotein increases the risk of coronary heart disease.

Hypertension and Stroke. Hypertension (high blood pressure) is associated with an increased risk of coronary artery disease and is also strongly associated with an increased risk of stroke. Risk factors for developing hypertension can be categorized as genetic or lifestyle-related and include age (as age increases, the risk increases), race (more common in African Americans), sex (men are more likely to experience hypertension), family history, obesity or being overweight, sedentary lifestyle, tobacco use, diet (too much salt, too little potassium, too little vitamin D, too much alcohol), and stress.

Stroke risk factors are also either genetic or lifestyle-related, and include age (adults 55 years or older are at increased risk), race (more common in African Americans, Hispanics, and American Indian/Alaska Natives), sex (men are more likely to have a stroke), family history, obesity or being overweight, sedentary lifestyle, hypertension, hypercholesterolemia, tobacco use, diabetes, cardiovascular disease, using birth control pills or hormone therapies, and excessive alcohol consumption.

Renal Disorders

Gout. *Gout* is an abnormal accumulation of uric acid due to a defect in metabolism. As a result of this defect, uric acid accumulates in the blood and joints, causing pain and swelling of the joints, especially the big toe. Often, the patient has fever and chills. Gout is more common among men than women and usually has a genetic basis. If left untreated, gout causes destructive tissue changes in the joints and kidneys. Treatment includes diet and medications to reduce inflammation and to increase the excretion of uric acid or decrease its formation.

Kidney Stones. *Kidney stones* are small masses of uric acid or calcium salts that form in any part of the urinary system (kidney, ureter, or urinary bladder). Kidney stones may cause severe pain, nausea, and vomiting when the body attempts to pass them. Although most stones are small, occasionally they become large enough to adopt the internal contours of the kidney Figure 9-23. Researchers have found a gene that causes the intestines to absorb too much calcium, which can lead to the formation of kidney stones. Uric acid stones also often have a genetic basis. Some are small enough to pass in the urine, with or without pain; others must be removed surgically.

Gastrointestinal Disorders

Malabsorption Disorders. *Malabsorption disorders* are caused by defects in the function of the bowel wall that prevent adequate nutrient absorption. The result is a complex of symptoms, including loss of appetite, bloating, weight loss, muscle pain, and stools with high fat content. Diarrhea, which may be bloody, may also be a prominent symptom.

Lactose intolerance is caused by a defect or deficiency of the enzyme lactase, resulting in an inability to digest lactose (milk sugar). Symptoms include bloating, flatulence, abdominal discomfort, nausea, and diarrhea after ingesting dairy or dairy products.

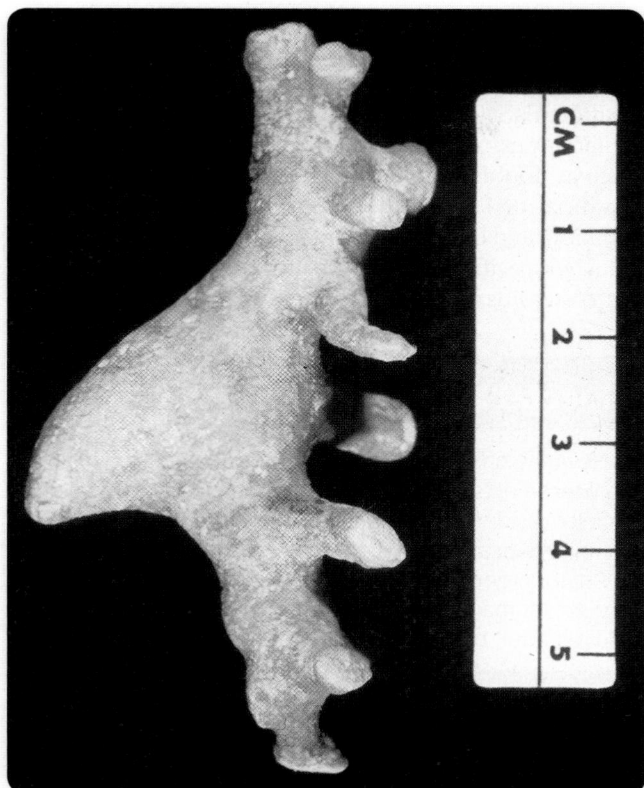

Figure 9-23 Large staghorn-shaped kidney stone.

Courtesy of Leonard V. Crowley, MD, Century College.

Ulcerative colitis is a serious chronic inflammatory disease of the large intestine and rectum. This disease, which shows a familial tendency, is characterized by recurrent episodes of abdominal pain, fever, chills, and profuse diarrhea, with stools containing pus, blood, and mucus. Treatment consists of anti-inflammatory agents, including corticosteroids. Patients with severe cases may require surgery to remove parts of the intestinal tract. Patients are at increased risk for the development of colorectal cancer.

Crohn disease is a serious chronic inflammatory condition affecting the colon and/or the terminal portion of the small intestine. It is believed to be associated with as-yet-undetermined gene abnormalities. Symptoms include frequent episodes of diarrhea, melena, abdominal pain, nausea, fever, weakness, and weight loss. Management is by anti-inflammatory agents, antibiotics, proper nutrition, and sometimes surgery to remove the damaged portion of the bowel, fistulas, or scar tissue.

Peptic Ulcer Disease. *Peptic ulcer disease* is characterized by circumscribed erosions (ulcerations) of the mucous membrane lining of the gastrointestinal tract—specifically, in the esophagus, stomach, duodenum, or jejunum. Peptic ulcers may be associated with excess acid production or from a breakdown in the normal mechanisms protecting the mucous membranes. Although this disease seems to have a genetic component, a major contributor to its development is infection with the bacterium *Helicobacter pylori*—the observed familial patterns seem to be due to shared infections with *H pylori*. Symptoms include gnawing pain, which is often worse when the stomach is empty, after the person eats certain foods, or when the person is under stress. Treatment includes avoiding irritants such as tobacco, alcohol, and certain foods, antibiotics, and medications to decrease acidity. In refractory cases, surgery may be necessary.

Gallstones. *Gallstones* (choleliths) are stonelike masses in the gallbladder or its ducts caused by precipitation of substances contained in bile (such as cholesterol and bilirubin). Factors that contribute to the formation of gallstones include abnormalities in the composition of bile, or stasis of bile. Gallstones may be asymptomatic, but they cause symptoms when they obstruct the flow of bile. They may cause inflammation of the gallbladder. Small stones that are able to pass into the common duct produce indigestion and biliary colic. Biliary colic pain has a sudden onset and increases steadily to its maximum in approximately 1 hour. The pain is located in the upper right quadrant or the epigastric area and may be referred to the back. Larger stones may cause jaundice (yellow skin and sclerae). Although genetic factors are responsible for at least 30% of symptomatic gallstone disease, heredity probably has an even larger role in gallstone pathogenesis. Data based on symptomatic gallbladder disease underestimate the true prevalence in the population.

Obesity. **Obesity** is an unhealthy accumulation of body fat, and is defined as a body mass index of greater than or equal to 30 kg/m^2. For example, an adult who is 5 feet 9 inches tall (2 m), is considered obese if he or she weighs more than 203 pounds (92 kg). Body mass index, and therefore definitions of obesity, is different for children and adolescents.

Morbid obesity is defined as a body mass index of greater than or equal to 40 kg/m^2. Using the example again of an adult who is 5 feet 9 inches tall (2 m), he or she is considered morbidly obese if he or she weighs more than 270 pounds (122 kg). Morbid obesity includes all of the health risks associated with obesity, but it also makes basic functions such as walking or breathing difficult.

People who are overweight are also at increased risk for disease, although the risk is not as high as for those who are obese. Being **overweight** is defined as a body mass index of 25 to 29.9 kg/m^2. Using the previous example of an adult who is 5 feet 9 inches tall (2 m), he or she would be overweight if he or she weighed between 169 and 202 pounds (77 and 92 kg).

Obesity has a significant negative impact on a person's health and life span; simply put, it has been statistically proven that the life span of a person with obesity is decreased by an average of 8 to 13 years.[18,19] Obesity has become an epidemic among adults and children in the United States. Approximately two thirds of adults in the United States have obesity or are overweight. Approximately 30% of children and adolescents in the United States are obese.[18,19]

Obesity has many deleterious effects, both medical and social. Health risks associated with obesity include hypertension, hyperlipidemia, cardiovascular disease, glucose intolerance, insulin resistance, diabetes, gallbladder disease, infertility, and cancer of the endometrium, breast, prostate, and colon. Social and psychological effects of obesity include depression, anxiety, shame, rejection, and discrimination in various environments including school and the workplace.

Although some people likely have a genetic predisposition to obesity, the roles of specific genes in its development have yet to be determined. Behavioral and environmental factors are better known. Behavioral factors that contribute to obesity include choosing a sedentary lifestyle, overeating, or eating foods high in calories and low in nutritional value, such as fast food and soda. A person's community or work environment may make it difficult to choose to be physically active or to eat properly. For example, a lack of sidewalks in a community would contribute to the risk of members of that community becoming obese. Large portion sizes offered by restaurants contribute to a lack of understanding of what is a proper portion size. Finally, interest in television and technological media may take time away from physical activity and encourage unhealthy product consumption. Because people tend to snack while watching TV or using a computer, they consume unnecessary additional calories.

Neuromuscular Disorders

Although environmental contributions are highly likely, certain neuromuscular disorders have a familial and genetic basis. The next few sections present several of the better known and more worrisome disorders in this category.

Huntington Disease. *Huntington disease* (also called Huntington chorea), for example, is a hereditary condition (autosomal dominant) characterized by progressive chorea (involuntary rapid, jerky motions) and mental deterioration, leading to dementia. Symptoms usually first appear in the third or fourth decade of life and progress to death, often within 15 years.

Muscular Dystrophy. Muscular dystrophy is a generic term for a group of hereditary diseases of the muscular system characterized by weakness and wasting of groups of skeletal muscles, leading to increasing disability. The various forms differ in age of onset, rate of progression, and mode of genetic transmission. Duchenne muscular dystrophy is a sex-linked recessive disease (affecting only males); symptoms first appear around the age of 4 years. Progressive wasting of leg and pelvic muscles produces a waddling gait and abnormal curvature of the spine. Usually by age 12, the person becomes unable to walk and begins to use a wheelchair. No known treatment exists, and the person often dies, most often of a heart disorder, by age 20.

Multiple Sclerosis. *Multiple sclerosis* is a progressive disease in which the myelin sheath surrounding the nerve fibers of the brain and spinal cord become damaged.[20] Although the disease is not directly inherited, some patients have a familial predisposition, suggesting a genetic influence on susceptibility. The disease usually begins in early adulthood and progresses slowly, with periods of remission and exacerbation. Early symptoms include abnormal sensations in the face or extremities, weakness, and visual disturbances (such as double vision), which progress to ataxia (lack of coordination), abnormal reflexes, tremors, difficulty in urination, and difficulty in walking. Depression is also common. No specific treatment or cure has been developed, but corticosteroids and other drugs are used to treat symptoms.

Special Populations

Never assume that new or worsening confusion in an older adult is due solely to Alzheimer disease, without first considering potentially correctable causes such as new medications, infections, or myocardial infarction. An apparent emotional, psychological, or behavioral disorder may have an organic cause, especially in the older adult population.

Alzheimer Disease. *Alzheimer disease* is characterized by cortical atrophy and loss of neurons in the frontal and temporal lobes of the brain; in addition, as the brain ventricles become enlarged a loss of brain tissue occurs. Alzheimer disease affects over 5 million Americans.[21] Histologic changes in the brain of a person with Alzheimer disease include neurofibrillary tangles and senile plaques Figure 9-24. Studies of the genetics of inherited early-onset Alzheimer disease have been linked to mutations on three genes.

Alzheimer disease is progressive. Early in its progression, it is characterized by memory loss, lack of spontaneity, subtle personality changes, and disorientation to time and date. It may then progress to including impaired cognition and abstract thinking, restlessness and agitation, wandering, inability to carry out activities of daily living, impaired judgment, and inappropriate social behavior. Advanced Alzheimer disease involves indifference to food, inability to communicate, urinary and fecal incontinence, and seizures.

Psychiatric Disorders

Some common psychiatric disorders seem to have a familial and perhaps even genetic component. Two of the most important are schizophrenia and bipolar disorder.

Schizophrenia. *Schizophrenia* comprises a group of mental disorders characterized by gross distortions of reality (psychoses), withdrawal from social contacts, and disturbances of thought, language, perception, and emotional response. Its symptoms are highly varied but may include apathy, catatonia or excessive activity, bizarre actions, hallucinations, delusions, and rambling speech. Although the cause of schizophrenia has not been identified, a combination of hereditary or genetic predisposing factors is likely in most cases.

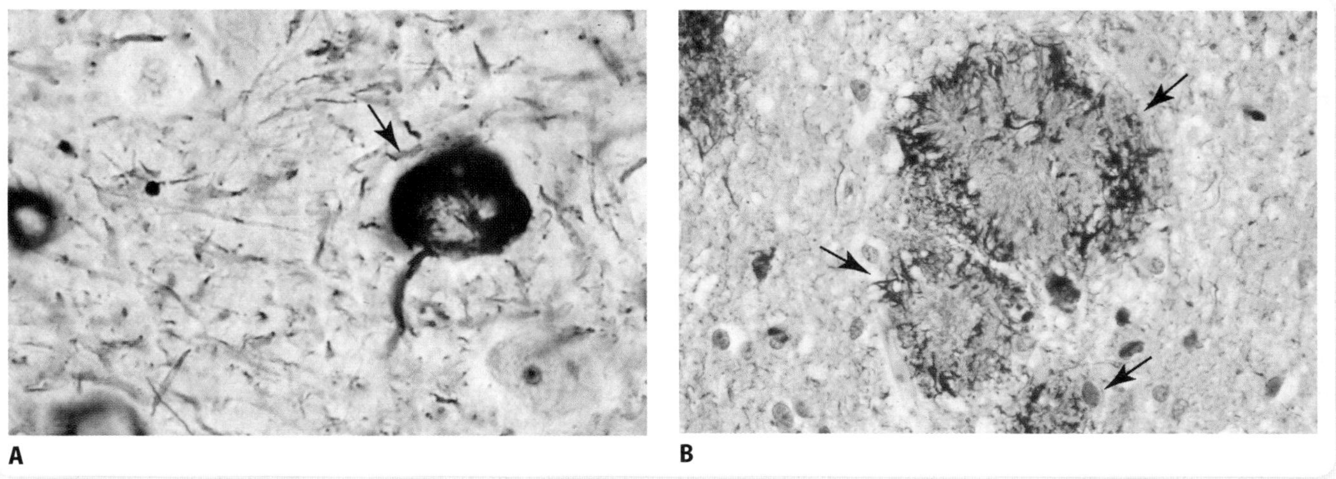

Figure 9-24 Alzheimer disease. **A.** Thickened neurofilaments encircle and obscure the nuclei of nerve cells (arrow), forming a neurofibrillary tangle (original magnification, ×400). **B.** Three senile plaques (arrows) composed of broken masses of thickened neurofilaments (original magnification, ×100).

Courtesy of Leonard V. Crowley, MD, Century College.

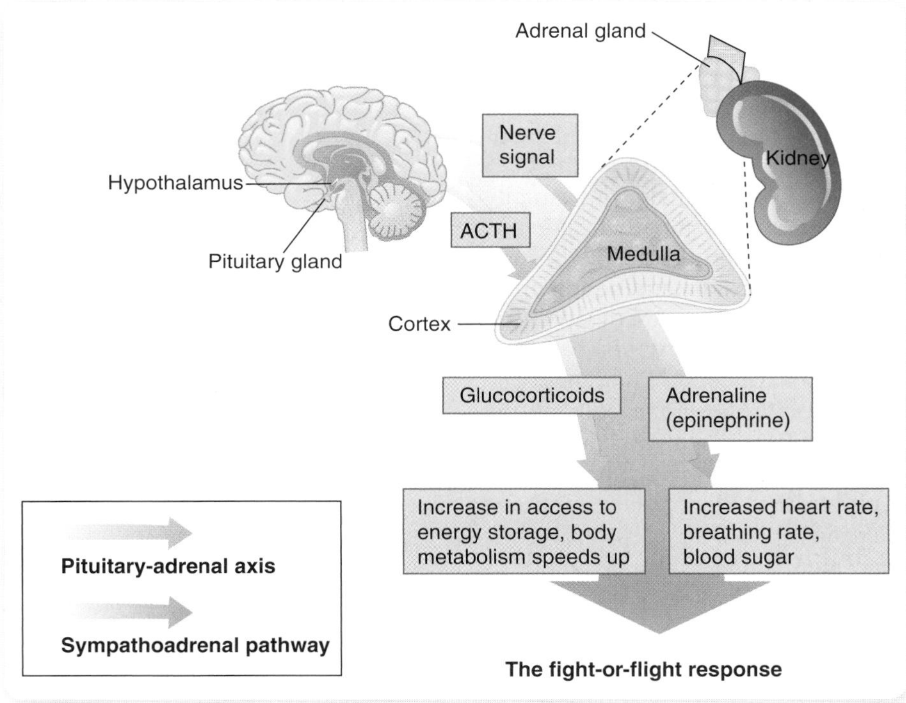

Figure 9-25 Physiologic response to stress.

Bipolar Disorder. *Bipolar disorder* (formerly known as manic-depressive disorder or manic-depressive psychosis) is a mental disorder characterized by episodes of mania and depression. One or the other phase may be dominant at any given time, the phases may alternate, or aspects of both phases may be present at once. The higher rates of bipolar disorder among relatives, identical twins, and biologic parents versus adoptive parents have been cited as evidence of the role of genetics in this disorder; the risk within the general population as a whole is approximately 2.6%.[22] Treatment consists of psychotherapy plus antidepressants and tranquilizers.

Stress and Disease

Stress is the medical term for a wide range of strong external stimuli, physiologic and psychological, that can cause a physiologic response. Physiologic stress is defined as a change that makes it necessary for the cells of the body to adapt. Figure 9-25 shows the series of events that occur when the body responds to a stimulus or stressor. Three concepts related to physiologic stress include the stressor itself, its effect in the body, and the body's response to the stress.

The brain and central nervous system (CNS) constantly interact with a person's consciousness. Research has shown a strong connection between the human psyche and brain physiology. When a person experiences stress, the body's defense mechanisms are activated. Usually, the response to stress is appropriate and beneficial. However, an unchecked stress response can have deleterious outcomes, including chemical dependency, heart attack, stroke, depression, headache, and abdominal pain.

▶ General Adaptation Syndrome

The **general adaptation syndrome**, a term introduced by Hans Selye, an Austrian endocrinologist, in the 1920s, characterizes a three-stage reaction to stressors, physical (such as injury) and emotional (such as loss of a loved one).

Stage 1: Alarm

The body reacts to stress first by releasing catecholamines, chemical compounds derived from the amino acid tyrosine that act as hormones or neurotransmitters. They are produced mainly from the adrenal medulla and the postganglionic fibers of the sympathetic nervous system. Catecholamines are soluble, so they circulate dissolved in blood. The most abundant catecholamines are epinephrine (adrenaline), norepinephrine (noradrenaline), and dopamine. Adrenaline acts as a neurotransmitter in the CNS and as a hormone in the blood. Noradrenaline is primarily a neurotransmitter of the peripheral sympathetic nervous system but is also present in the blood (mostly through spillover from the synapses of the sympathetic system).

As shown in Figure 9-25, stress causes the sympathetic nervous system to be stimulated. When the body senses stress, the brain causes the adrenal medulla of the endocrine system to send catecholamines (the hormones epinephrine and norepinephrine) that activate the sympathetic nervous system by binding to **receptor** sites. In the sympathetic nervous system, the receptors that allow certain responses to be activated are called alpha and beta receptors. Whenever one of these is activated, a predictable sequence of responses occur. Activation of alpha receptors results in vasoconstriction, while activation of beta receptors results in increased heart rate, increased force of contraction, and increased conduction velocity. Beyond those cardiac effects of catecholamines, other physiologic effects include an increase in respiratory rate, decreased blood flow to the skin, smooth-muscle constriction, and various effects on the liver that increase the body's use of glucose.

Normally, the fight-or-flight response that occurs in the alarm reaction prepares the body to deal with stress, but it can also weaken the immune system, leading to infection.

Stage 2: Resistance or Adaptation

During stage 2, the resistance or adaptation stage, the body adapts to stressors. It does so primarily by stimulating the adrenal gland to secrete two types of corticosteroid hormones that increase the blood glucose level and maintain blood pressure: glucocorticoids and mineralocorticoids. The most significant glucocorticoid in the body is cortisol, which controls carbohydrate, fat, and protein metabolism. Cortisol also has potent anti-inflammatory actions. Mineralocorticoids (predominantly aldosterone) control electrolyte and water levels in the body, mainly by promoting sodium retention by the kidneys.

During times of stress, the hypothalamus secretes a hormone that stimulates the anterior pituitary to release adrenocorticotropic hormone (ACTH) **Figure 9-26**. ACTH targets the adrenal cortex, resulting in cortisol secretion. Cortisol stimulates body cells to increase their energy production in response to increased stressors;

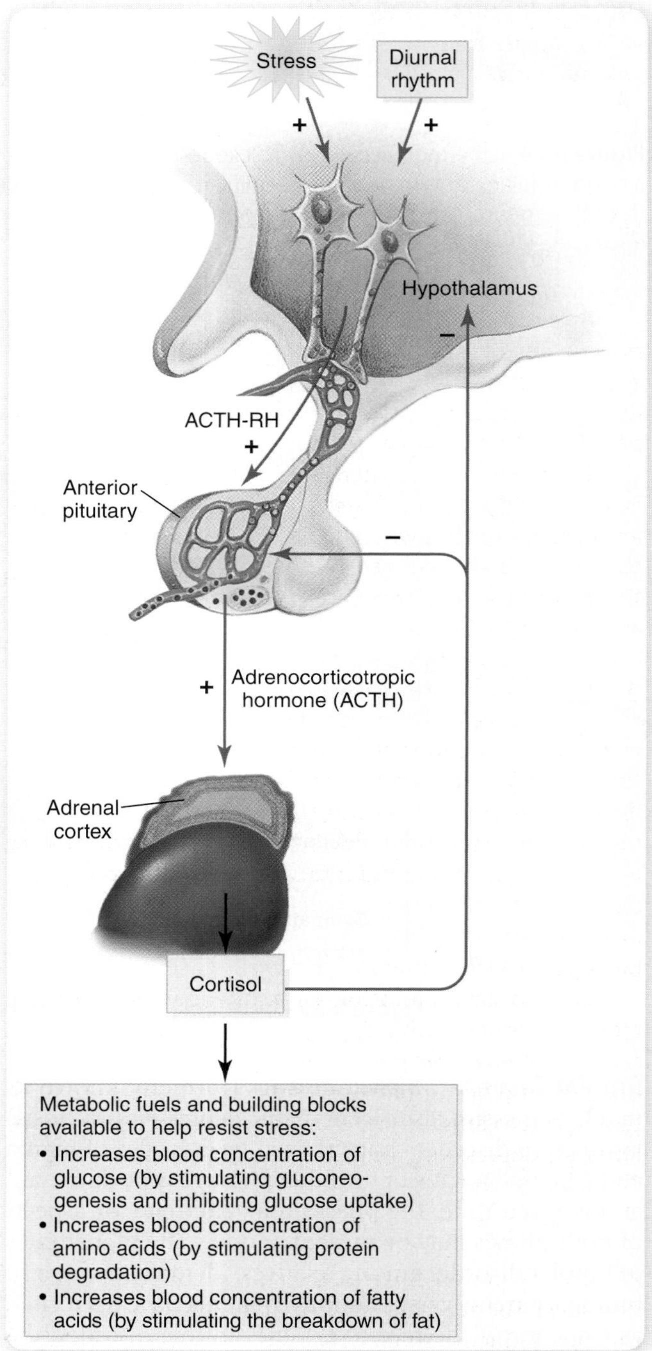

Figure 9-26 Stress triggers secretion of adrenocorticotropic hormone, which results in cortisol secretion.

cortisol increases serum glucose levels and impairs the use of glucose by peripheral tissues. It also decreases protein reserves and permits mobilization of fatty acids by epinephrine and growth hormone. It reduces inflammation when inflammation has served its purpose; therefore, it has a role in wound healing. Cortisol also increases red blood cell production and affects electrolyte levels. However, it also decreases the size of lymphoid tissue. Since the lymphatic system has an important role in immunity, this may explain why stress and disease are linked.

Other hormones related to stress include endorphins, which are neurotransmitters released during times of stress. Endorphins help reduce pain and stress by activating opiate receptor sites. They essentially produce a type of analgesia.

Additional hormones include growth hormone, prolactin, and testosterone. Growth factor is a hormone that promotes cell and tissue growth and repair. In the context of stress, growth factor is reduced. Since growth factor correlates to the body's ability to heal, this means that there is a reduced ability to heal when the body is under chronic stress.

Prolactin is a hormone that stimulates breast milk production. It is also believed to play a role in the immune system. In times of stress, prolactin levels increase. Research suggests that prolactin levels increase more in people with ineffective coping mechanisms.

The hormone testosterone is affected by stress. There is a direct link between cortisol levels and testosterone levels; namely, that when cortisol levels are high, testosterone levels are reduced. When the body is not under stress, testosterone levels are protected from cortisol by an enzyme. In the presence of stress, cortisol levels are too high for the enzyme to sufficiently handle them. As a result the excess cortisol causes testosterone levels to decrease.

It was once believed that elevated testosterone levels were linked to a suppressed immune system. Now, research suggests that testosterone may be related to the distribution of white blood cells in the body. It is thought that in times of stress, white blood cells are sent to the skin to protect against wound infection. But in the context of chronic stress, this would mean fewer white blood cells in other parts of the body on a regular basis, making those parts more susceptible to infection.

Cortisol levels and the sympathetic nervous system return to normal during this resistance or adaptation stage, causing fight-or-flight symptoms to disappear. Continuation of stress and accompanying corticosteroid release eventually lead to fatigue, lapses in concentration, irritability, lethargy, depression, and a depressed immune system.

Stage 3: Exhaustion

After a long period of stress, the person enters the exhaustion stage. The adrenal glands become depleted, decreasing the blood glucose level, which results in decreased stress tolerance, progressive mental and physical exhaustion, illness, and collapse. At this point, the body's immune system is compromised, significantly reducing a person's ability to resist disease. Heart attack, high blood pressure, or severe infection may result.

▶ Effects of Chronic Stress

The **hypothalamic-pituitary-adrenal axis** is a major part of the neuroendocrine system that controls reactions to stress. The hypothalamic-pituitary-adrenal axis triggers a set of interactions among the glands, hormones, and parts of the midbrain that mediate the general adaptation syndrome. Continued stress, however, leads to loss of these normal control mechanisms. As a result, the adrenals continue to produce cortisol, which exhausts the stress mechanism and leads to fatigue and depression. Cortisol also interferes with serotonin activity, furthering the depressive effect.

A consistently high cortisol level suppresses the immune system by increasing production of interleukin-6, an immune system messenger. Not surprisingly, then, research indicates that stress and depression have a negative effect on the immune system. Reduced immunity makes the body more susceptible to everything from colds and flu to cancer. For example, the incidence of serious illness, including cancer, is significantly higher among people whose spouse has died during the past year.

Although severe, prolonged stress does not cause death directly, it does cause the body to lose its ability to fight disease in its effort to manage the stress. Stress also encourages the body to release fat and cholesterol into the bloodstream, which in turn block the arteries and can eventually cause a heart attack or stroke. Many people start drinking alcohol to excess to combat their stress. Other diseases and conditions related to chronic stress include depression, headaches, insomnia, ulcers, diuresis, acne, diabetes mellitus, rheumatoid arthritis, and asthma. The variety in this list shows that stress affects most every organ system in the body.

However, it is important to note that a person's reaction to stressful events correlates to elevation or reduction in hormone levels. Therefore, coping mechanisms play a role in the physiologic response to stress. When a healthy person experiences stress, he or she may be able to manage the stress with minimal negative effects to the immune system if he or she has effective coping mechanisms. But in any patient, ineffective coping mechanisms will have deleterious effects on immune status. Effects will be worst in those whose immune systems are already compromised and who do not have effective coping mechanisms to combat the stress. Conversely, effective coping mechanisms can go a long way in helping a patient improve his or her immune system's response. Finally, a person's outlook has been shown to relate to the effectiveness of his or her medical treatment; much like a placebo effect, if a patient believes that the treatment will be effective, it is more likely to be effective.

Fortunately, this immune suppression process can be corrected with psychotherapy, medication, or any number of other positive influences that restore hope and a feeling of self-esteem. The ability of human beings to recover from adversity is remarkable.

YOU are the Paramedic SUMMARY

1. What is your general impression of the patient?

The patient is in obvious respiratory distress because he is not able to speak complete sentences without taking a breath. This finding is very important in the assessment of your patient because it indicates there is not enough oxygen available to the patient to speak effectively.

2. What can you learn about the patient from his surroundings?

The scene assessment gives numerous indications that the patient has a significant medical history. The first significant finding is you were met at the door by a neighbor. The neighbor tells you the patient has had medical issues and lives alone. Once you enter the residence, you observe multiple medication containers and an abundance of used facial tissues adjacent to the patient. These items need to be investigated further. The patient is also wearing a nasal cannula attached to a home oxygen unit, which indicates a preexisting respiratory condition.

3. How does the recruitment of accessory muscles facilitate breathing?

As you have learned, the act of breathing relies on positive and negative pressures. The chest and other related muscles expand and contract to create the pressure. When the act of breathing becomes difficult, accessory muscles assist with the mechanical aspect of breathing. The nasal passages will flare in an attempt to gain as much space as possible to increase airflow into the airways. Musculature in the chest will work visibly harder to move the chest wall and diaphragm to assist in creating the pressure gradient necessary for breathing. Sitting upright aligns the airway to decrease the amount of pressure needed within the chest.

4. How might the productive cough help you identify the source of the patient's breathing difficulty?

The productive cough could indicate many disease processes. The color of the sputum is of particular interest in your assessment. Thick green, brown, or yellow sputum may indicate infection. Pink, frothy sputum indicates pulmonary edema. Hemoptysis may indicate trauma or carcinoma. After you assess the color, determine how much of it is present. In this case, the numerous used facial tissues can help indicate an amount.

5. On the basis of what you know about physiology, what is causing the pink, foamy sputum?

Pink, foamy sputum is an indication of pulmonary edema that, in this case, may be a sign of exacerbation of congestive heart failure. If the left ventricle of the heart is not pumping effectively, then blood backs up in the system. The result of the backup causes an increase in pressure within the pulmonary vasculature. The increased pressure forces fluid through the alveolar membrane and into the alveoli. Blood will enter the alveoli through the alveolar membrane in small amounts, producing a pink rather than red appearance. The froth comes from the additional fluid being exposed to the air in the patient's lungs and airways.

6. How do you account for the decreased Spo_2 level?

In this case, the patient would have a decreased amount of surface area for oxygen exchange due to pulmonary edema. Less surface area means less oxygen will "saturate" the cells, which in turn will be read by the pulse oximeter as a decrease in saturation. It is important to note that the saturation amount shown on the electronic device represents any gas that is saturating the cells. Oxygen is one of many gases that can affect the reading. In addition, saturation levels may be compromised by the patient's own lack of circulation.

7. Why would a diuretic be prescribed for a patient with congestive heart failure?

If a patient has congestive heart failure, then the heart is not pumping blood effectively. This causes a backup within the circulatory system, which in turn causes fluid to back up into the pulmonary vasculature. A diuretic helps to eliminate some of the fluid from the system to lessen the workload on the heart. Most diuretics work on the kidneys to eliminate water and electrolytes. The elimination moves fluid from the extracellular to the intravascular space, which will transport it out of the body. The goal is to reduce the cardiac preload, which will reduce the amount of work the cardiac system has to do and reduce the fluid backup.

8. Why would this patient have a normal or slightly high blood pressure?

In patients with heart failure, the heart is working harder to pump fluid volume. According to the Starling law, increased venous return to the heart increases cardiac preload. The heart muscle stretches in response to the increased amount of fluid. The heart muscle will then contract with greater force—up to a point—to expel the fluid. This accounts for a normal or higher blood pressure because the body is trying to compensate for a lack of the heart's muscular ability.

YOU are the Paramedic SUMMARY (continued)

EMS Patient Care Report (PCR)					
Date: 08-01-18	**Incident No.:** 1234		**Nature of Call:** Difficulty breathing	**Location:** 420 Beach Street	
Dispatched: 2041	**En Route:** 2041	**At Scene:** 2045	**Transport:** 2052	**At Hospital:** 2107	**In Service:** 2122
Patient Information					
Age: 72 **Sex:** M **Weight (in kg [lb]):** 80.2 kg (177 lb)			**Allergies:** No known drug allergies **Medications:** Numerous **Past Medical History:** Congestive heart failure **Chief Complaint:** Difficulty breathing		
Vital Signs					
Time: 2047	**BP:** 140/90	**Pulse:** 110	**Respirations:** 22	$\mathbf{Spo_2}$: 89%	
Time: 2052	**BP:** 138/88	**Pulse:** 114	**Respirations:** 24	$\mathbf{Spo_2}$: 92%	
Time:	**BP:**	**Pulse:**	**Respirations:**	$\mathbf{Spo_2}$:	
EMS Treatment (circle all that apply)					
Oxygen @ 15 **L/min via (circle one):** **NC** **(NRM)** **Bag-mask device**		**Assisted Ventilation**	**Airway Adjunct**	**CPR**	
Defibrillation	**Bleeding Control**	**Bandaging**	**Splinting**	**Other:**	
Narrative					
Arrived to find this 72-year-old man being attended by his neighbor. Pt lives alone in this residence. Pt alert (oriented to person, place, and day). Pt unable to speak in completed sentences due to respiratory effort. Pt states he has not been compliant with his medications for a time. Pt states he has a history of "heart failure" and is using 2 L/min O_2 via cannula. Assessment shows vital signs as above; lung sound assessment shows coarse crackles in all fields. Pt has productive cough with pink foamy sputum. O_2 via NRM applied at 15 L/min on scene and throughout transport. IV line of NS established TKO, ECG shows sinus tach @114, no ectopy noted. $ETCO_2$ waveform appears appropriate in shape and reads 36 mm Hg. Treatment per local protocol, radio report during transport, and verbal report to Halifax Health on arrival. Pt transferred to room A-20.**End of report**					

Prep Kit

▶ Ready for Review

- Pathophysiology is the study of the physiology of altered functioning in the presence of disease.
- Pathophysiology in the cellular environment includes disturbances in fluid balance and electrolyte imbalances. These various imbalances can upset homeostasis and may result in or contribute to emergency conditions.
- Cellular injury is caused by factors such as hypoxia, chemical exposure, infectious agents, inappropriate immunologic responses, inflammatory responses, genetic factors, nutritional imbalances, physical agents such as radiation, and adverse conditions such as extreme cold.

Prep Kit *(continued)*

- When cells are exposed to adverse conditions, cells undergo a process of temporary or permanent adaptation to protect themselves from injury. Examples of adaptation include atrophy, hypertrophy, hyperplasia, dysplasia, and metaplasia.
- Inflammatory response is characterized by both local and systemic effects. Local effects consist of dilation (expansion) of blood vessels and increased vascular permeability. If the inflammatory process is severe, then systemic effects such as fever become evident. The outcome of an inflammation depends on how much tissue damage has resulted from the inflammation.
- Immunologic diseases occur because of hyperactivity or hypoactivity of the immune system. Allergies are acquired following initial exposure to a stimulant known as an allergen. Repeated exposures generate an immune system reaction to the allergen.
- Perfusion is the delivery of oxygen and nutrients to cells, organs, and tissues through the circulatory system. Hypoperfusion occurs when the level of tissue perfusion falls below normal.
- Shock is an abnormal state associated with inadequate oxygen and nutrient delivery to the metabolic apparatus of the cell, resulting in an impairment of cellular metabolism.
- Central shock consists of cardiogenic shock and obstructive shock. Cardiogenic shock occurs when the heart cannot circulate enough blood to maintain adequate peripheral oxygen delivery. Obstructive shock occurs when blood flow within the heart or great vessels (aorta and pulmonary vein) becomes blocked.
- Peripheral shock includes hypovolemic shock and distributive shock. In hypovolemic shock, the circulating blood volume is insufficient to deliver adequate oxygen and nutrients to the body. Distributive shock occurs when there is widespread dilation of the resistance vessels (small arterioles), the capacitance vessels (small venules), or both.
- Multiple organ dysfunction syndrome (MODS) occurs in acutely ill patients and is characterized by the dysfunction of two or more organs that were not affected by the physiologic insult for which the patient was initially being treated. Six organ systems are surveyed to determine whether a patient has MODS and, if so, how high is the risk of mortality: respiratory, hepatic, renal, hematologic, neurologic, and cardiovascular.
- The immune system includes all of the structures and processes that mount a defense against foreign substances and disease-causing agents.
- The body has three lines of defense: anatomic barriers, the inflammatory response, and the immune response.
- There are two general types of immune response: native and acquired.
- Immunity may be humoral or cell-mediated.
- Important white blood cells in the immune system include neutrophils, eosinophils, basophils, monocytes, and lymphocytes. Other important cells of the immune system include macrophages, mast cells, plasma cells, B cells, and T cells.
- The antibodies secreted by B cells are called immunoglobulins. Antibodies make antigens more visible to the immune system in three ways: by acting as opsonins, by making antigens clump, and by inactivating bacterial toxins.
- The inflammatory response is the reaction of the body's tissues to cellular injury. It is characterized by pain, swelling, redness, and heat.
- The two most common causes of inflammation are infection and injury.
- The plasma protein systems that modulate the inflammatory process include the complement system, the coagulation (clotting) system, and the kinin system.
- Cytokines are products of cells that affect the functioning of other cells; they include interleukins, lymphokines, and interferon.
- Chronic inflammatory responses are usually caused by an unsuccessful acute inflammatory response after the invasion of a foreign body, a persistent infection, or an antigen.
- Normal wound healing involves four steps: repairing damaged tissue, removing inflammatory debris, restoring tissues to a normal state, and regenerating cells.
- Wounds may heal by primary or secondary intention. Healing by primary intention occurs in clean wounds with opposed margins. Wounds that heal by secondary intention have a prolonged inflammatory phase and more abundant granulation tissue.
- Hypersensitivity is an increased response of the body to any substance to which the person is abnormally sensitive. A hypersensitivity reaction may be immediate, occurring within seconds to minutes, or delayed, occurring hours to days after exposure to the antigen.
- Hypersensitivity reactions may be classified as autoimmune, idiopathic, or blood incompatibility reactions.
- Immunodeficiency may be congenital or acquired.

Prep Kit *(continued)*

- Age- and sex-associated factors interact with a combination of genetic and environmental factors, lifestyle, and anatomic or hormonal differences to cause disease.
- Analyzing disease risk involves consideration of disease rates (incidence, prevalence, morbidity, and mortality) and controllable and uncontrollable disease risk factors (causal and noncausal). These risk factors, age, and sex differences interact to influence a person's level of risk.
- A true genetic risk is passed through generations on a gene. In contrast, a familial tendency may cluster in family groups despite lack of evidence for heritable gene-associated abnormalities. In autosomal dominant inheritance, a person needs to inherit only one copy of a particular form of a gene to show the trait. In autosomal recessive inheritance, the person must inherit two copies of a particular form of a gene to show the trait.
- Stress does not cause death directly, but it can permit diseases to flourish, ultimately leading to death.
- The general adaptation syndrome describes the body's short- and long-term reactions to stress.
- Stress causes the sympathetic nervous system to be stimulated. This occurs through the release of catecholamines that activate the sympathetic nervous system by binding to alpha and beta receptor sites, resulting in effects categorized as fight-or-flight response.
- Stress also causes secretion of cortisol, which has many useful effects such as increasing serum glucose levels, decreasing protein reserves, and permitting mobilization of fatty acids. However, continuous secretion of cortisol has deleterious effects.

▶ Vital Vocabulary

acidosis An increase in extracellular H^+ ions; a blood pH of less than 7.35.

acquired immunity The immunity that occurs when the body is exposed to a foreign substance or disease and produces antibodies to the invader.

activation Mediators of inflammation trigger the appearance of molecules known as selectins and integrins on the surfaces of endothelial cells and polymorphonuclear neutrophils, respectively.

adhesion The attachment of polymorphonuclear neutrophils to endothelial cells, mediated by selectins and integrins.

alcoholic ketoacidosis The metabolic acidotic state that manifests because of the inadequate nutritional habits associated with chronic alcohol abuse. The liver and body experience inadequate fuel reserves of glycogen and, thus, have to switch to fatty acid metabolism.

alkalosis A decrease in extracellular H^+ ions; a blood pH greater than 7.45.

allergen Any substance that causes a hypersensitivity reaction.

allergy A hypersensitivity reaction to the presence of an agent (allergen) that is intrinsically harmless.

anaphylactic shock A severe hypersensitivity reaction that involves bronchoconstriction and cardiovascular collapse.

angiogenesis The growth of new blood vessels.

antibody A protein secreted by certain immune cells that bind antigens to make them more visible to the immune system.

antigen A foreign substance recognized by the immune system.

apoptosis Normal, genetically programmed cell death.

asthma A chronic inflammatory lower airway condition resulting in intermittent wheezing and excess mucus production.

atopic An allergic tendency.

atrophy A decrease in cell size due to a loss of subcellular components.

autoantibodies Antibodies directed against the person's own proteins.

autoimmunity The production of antibodies or T cells that work against the tissues of a person's body, producing autoimmune disease or a hypersensitivity reaction.

autosomal dominant A pattern of inheritance that involves genes that are located on autosomes or the nonsex chromosomes. Inheritance of only one copy of a particular form of a gene is needed to show the trait.

autosomal recessive A pattern of inheritance that involves genes located on autosomes or the nonsex chromosomes. Inheritance of two copies of a particular form of a gene is needed to show the trait.

bradypnea A slow respiratory rate.

capillary refill time A test performed on the fingernails or toenails that involves briefly squeezing the toenail or fingernail and evaluating the time it takes for the color to return.

cardiogenic shock A condition caused by loss of 40% or more of the functioning myocardium; the heart is no longer able to circulate sufficient blood to maintain adequate oxygen delivery.

Prep Kit *(continued)*

carpopedal spasm A contorted position of the hand or foot in which the fingers or toes flex in a claw-like manner; may result from hyperventilation or hypocalcemia.

cell-mediated immunity The immune process by which T-cell lymphocytes recognize antigens and then secrete cytokines (specifically lymphokines) that attract other cells or stimulate the production of cytotoxic cells that kill the infected cells.

central shock A type of shock caused by central pump failure, including cardiogenic shock and obstructive shock.

chemotaxins Components of the activated complement system that attract leukocytes from the circulation to help fight infections.

chemotaxis The movement of additional white blood cells to an area of inflammation in response to the release of chemical mediators, such as neutrophils, injured tissue, and monocytes.

coagulation system The system that forms blood clots in the body and facilitates repairs to the vascular tree.

complement system A group of plasma proteins whose function is to do one of three things: attract leukocytes to sites of inflammation, activate leukocytes, and directly destroy cells.

cytokines The products of cells that affect the function of other cells.

distributive shock The type of shock caused by widespread dilation of the resistance vessels (small arterioles), the capacitance vessels (small venules), or both.

dysplasia An alteration in the size, shape, and organization of cells.

edema Swelling caused by excessive fluid trapped in the body tissues

fibrin A whitish, filamentous protein formed by the action of thrombin on fibrinogen; the protein that polymerizes (bonds) to form the fibrous component of a blood clot.

fibrinolysis cascade The breakdown of fibrin in blood clots and the prevention of the polymerization of fibrin into new clots.

free radicals A molecule that is missing one electron in its outer shell.

general adaptation syndrome A three-stage description of the body's short- and long-term reactions to stress.

gram-negative A reaction of bacteria to a Gram stain in which the bacteria do not retain the dark purple stain; this type of bacteria has cell walls that consist largely of lipids, and have pathogenic qualities that make them especially problematic for humans.

gram-positive A reaction of bacteria to a Gram stain in which the bacteria retain the dark purple stain; this type of bacteria has thick cell walls composed of many layers.

hapten A substance that normally does not stimulate an immune response but can be combined with an antigen and at a later point initiate an antibody response.

helper T cells A type of T lymphocyte that is involved in cell-mediated and antibody-mediated immune responses. It secretes cytokines that stimulate the B cells and other T cells.

hemochromatosis An inherited disease in which the body absorbs more iron than it needs and stores it in the liver, kidneys, and pancreas.

hemolytic anemia A disease characterized by increased destruction of the red blood cells. It can occur from an Rh factor reaction (primarily in Rh-positive neonates born to sensitized Rh-negative mothers), exposure to chemicals, or a disorder of the immune system.

hemophilia An inherited sex-linked disorder characterized by excessive bleeding.

histamine A vasoactive amine that increases vascular permeability and causes vasodilation.

humoral immunity A type of immunity in which B-cell lymphocytes produce antibodies called immunoglobulins which recognize a specific antigen and then react with it.

hypercalcemia An elevated blood calcium level.

hypercholesterolemia An elevated blood cholesterol level.

hyperkalemia An elevated serum potassium level.

hypermagnesemia An increased serum magnesium level.

hypernatremia A serum sodium level greater than or equal to 143 mEq/L.

hyperphosphatemia An elevated serum phosphate level.

hyperplasia An increase in the actual number of cells in an organ or tissue, usually resulting in an increase in the size of the organ or tissue.

hypersensitivity A generic term for responses of the body to a substance to which a patient has increased sensitivity.

hypertrophy An increase in the size of the cells due to synthesis of more subcellular components, leading to an increase in tissue and organ size.

hypocalcemia A decreased serum calcium level.

hypokalemia A decreased serum potassium level.

hypomagnesemia A decreased serum magnesium level.

Prep Kit *(continued)*

hyponatremia A serum sodium level that is less than or equal to 135 mEq/L.

hypoperfusion A condition that occurs when the level of tissue perfusion decreases below that needed to maintain normal cellular functions.

hypophosphatemia A decreased serum phosphate level.

hypothalamic-pituitary-adrenal axis A major part of the neuroendocrine system that controls reactions to stress. It is the mechanism for a set of interactions among glands, hormones, and parts of the midbrain that mediate the general adaptation syndrome.

hypovolemic shock A condition that occurs when the circulating blood volume is inadequate to deliver adequate oxygen and nutrients to the body.

immune response The body's defense reaction to any substance that is recognized as foreign.

immune system The body system that includes all of the structures and processes designed to mount a defense against foreign substances and disease-causing agents.

immunodeficiency An abnormal condition in which some part of the body's immune system is inadequate, and, consequently, resistance to infectious disease is decreased.

immunogen An antigen that is capable of generating an immune response.

immunoglobulins Antibodies secreted by the B cells.

incidence The number of new cases of a disease in a population.

inflammatory response A reaction by tissues of the body to irritation or injury, characterized by pain, swelling, redness, and heat.

interferon A protein produced by cells in response to viral invasion that is released into the bloodstream or intercellular fluid to induce healthy cells to manufacture an enzyme that counters the infection.

interleukins Chemical substances that attract white blood cells to the sites of injury and bacterial invasions.

isoimmunity The formation of antibodies or T cells that are directed against antigens or another person's cells.

ketoacidosis An acidotic state created by the production of ketones via fat metabolism.

ketones Acidic by-products of fat metabolism.

killer T cells The cells released during a type IV allergic reaction that kill antigen-bearing target cells.

kinin system A group of polypeptides that mediate inflammatory responses by stimulating visceral smooth muscle and relaxing vascular smooth muscle to produce vasodilation.

lactic acidosis Anaerobic cellular respiration due to hypoperfusion of tissues and organs.

leukocytosis An elevated white blood cell count, often due to inflammation.

leukotrienes Arachidonic acid metabolites that function as chemical mediators of inflammation; also known as slow-reacting substances of anaphylaxis.

lymphokines Cytokines released by lymphocytes, including many of the interleukins, gamma interferon, tumor necrosis factor beta, and chemokines.

margination The loss of fluid from the blood vessels into the tissue, causing the blood left in the vessels to have increased viscosity, which in turn slows the flow of blood and produces stasis.

membrane attack complex Molecules that insert themselves into the bacterial membrane, leading to weakened areas in the membrane.

metabolic acidosis A pathologic condition characterized by a blood pH of less than 7.35 and caused by an accumulation of acids in the body from a metabolic cause.

metabolic alkalosis A pathologic condition characterized by a blood pH of greater than 7.45 and caused by an accumulation of bases in the body from a metabolic cause.

metaplasia A reversible, cellular adaptation in which one adult cell type is replaced by another adult cell type.

morbidity Number of nonfatally injured or disabled people; usually expressed as a rate, meaning the number of nonfatal injuries in a certain population in a given time period divided by the size of the population.

morbid obesity An excessively unhealthy accumulation of body fat, defined as a body mass index of greater than or equal to 40 kg/m^2.

mortality The quality of being mortal; number of deaths from a disease in a given population.

multiple organ dysfunction syndrome (MODS) A grave but sometimes reversible condition in an acutely ill patient characterized by the progressive dysfunction of two or more organs or organ systems not affected by the patient's initial illness or injury.

natural immunity A nonspecific cellular and humoral response that operates as the body's first line of defense against pathogens; also called native immunity.

Prep Kit *(continued)*

necrosis The death of tissue, usually caused by a cessation of the blood supply.

neurogenic shock A type of shock that usually results from spinal cord injury; loss of normal sympathetic nervous system tone and vasodilation occur.

obesity An unhealthy accumulation of body fat, defined as a body mass index of greater than or equal to 30 kg/m^2.

obstructive shock The type of shock that occurs when blood flow to the heart or great vessels is obstructed.

oliguria Decreased urine output.

opsonization The process by which an antibody coats an antigen to facilitate its recognition by immune cells.

overweight An unhealthy accumulation of body fat, defined as a body mass index of 25 to 29.9 kg/m^2.

pathophysiology The study of the physiology of altered functioning in the presence of disease.

perfusion The delivery of oxygen and nutrients to the cells, organs, and tissues of the body; also involves the removal of wastes.

pericardial tamponade The impairment of diastolic filling of the right ventricle due to significant amounts of fluid in the pericardial sac surrounding the heart, leading to a decrease in the cardiac output.

peripheral shock Shock caused by peripheral circulatory abnormalities; includes hypovolemic shock and distributive shock.

phagocytes The cells that engulf and consume foreign material such as microorganisms and debris.

polymorphonuclear neutrophils (PMNs) The type of white blood cells formed by bone marrow tissue that have a nucleus consisting of several parts or lobes connected by fine strands.

polyuria Frequent and plentiful urination.

prevalence The number of cases of a disease in a specific population within a given period.

prostaglandins A group of lipids that act as chemical messengers.

pyrogens Chemicals or proteins that travel to the brain and affect the hypothalamus and stimulate a rise in the body's core temperature.

receptor A specialized area in tissue that initiates certain actions after specific stimulation.

respiratory acidosis A pathologic condition characterized by a blood pH of less than 7.35 and caused by an accumulation of acids in the body from a respiratory cause.

respiratory alkalosis A pathologic condition characterized by a blood pH of less than 7.45 and caused by an accumulation of bases in the body from a respiratory cause.

septic shock The type of shock that occurs as a result of widespread infection, usually bacterial; untreated, the result is multiple organ dysfunction syndrome and often death.

serotonin A vasoactive amine that increases vascular permeability to cause vasodilation.

serum sickness A condition in which antigen-antibody complexes formed in the bloodstream deposit in sites around the body, most notably the kidneys, with resultant inflammatory reactions.

transmigration (diapedesis) The polymorphonuclear neutrophils permeate through the vessel wall, moving into the interstitial space.

urticaria Multiple small, raised areas on the skin that may be one of the warning signs of impending anaphylaxis; also known as hives.

vasculitis An inflammation of the blood vessels.

vasoactive amines Substances such as histamine and serotonin that increase vascular permeability.

virulence A measure of the disease-causing ability of a microorganism.

▶ References

1. He F, Li J, MacGregor GA. Effect of longer term modest salt reduction on blood pressure: Cochrane systematic review and meta-analysis of randomised trials. *BMJ.* 2013; 346:f1325.
2. Friis-Hansen BJ, Holiday M, Stapleton T, Wallace WM. Total body water in children. *Pediatrics.* 1951; 7(3):321-327.
3. Fontanarosa PB, Christiansen S. Units of measure. Table 2: selected laboratory tests, with reference ranges and conversion factors. In: American Medical Association, ed. *AMA Manual of Style: A Guide for Authors and Editors.* 10th ed. New York, NY: Oxford University Press; 2007:798-815.
4. Paz J, West M. *Acute Care Handbook for Physical Therapists.* 4th ed. St. Louis, MO: Elsevier/Saunders; 2014.
5. Speakman E. *Body Fluids & Electrolytes: A Programmed Presentation.* 8th ed. St. Louis, MO: Elsevier/Mosby; 2002.
6. Stipanuk MH, Caudill M. *Biochemical, Physiological, and Molecular Aspects of Human Nutrition.* 3rd ed. St. Louis, MO: Elsevier/Saunders; 2013.
7. Brown AFT, Cadogan M. *Emergency Medicine: Diagnosis and Management.* 6th ed. Boca Raton, FL: CRC Press; 2011.
8. Goldman L, Schaffer A. *Goldman-Cecil Medicine,* 25th ed. St. Louis, MO: Elsevier/Saunders; 2016.

Prep Kit *(continued)*

9. Rose JJ, Wang L, Xu Q, et al. Carbon monoxide poisoning: pathogenesis, management and future directions of therapy. *Am J Resp Crit Care.* 2016, Oct 18. [Epub ahead of print] DOI:10.1164/rccm.201606-1275CI.
10. Schmidt H, Müller-Werdan U, Hoffmann T, et al. Autonomic dysfunction predicts mortality in patients with multiple organ dysfunction syndrome of different age groups. *Crit Care Med.* 2005;33(9), 1994-2002.
11. Mayo Clinic Staff. *Diseases and conditions: Lupus: Causes.* Mayo Clinic.© 1998-2016 Mayo Foundation for Medical Education and Research. All rights reserved. http://www.mayoclinic.org/diseases-conditions/lupus/basics/causes/con-20019676. Accessed November 8, 2016.
12. Genetics Home Reference. X-linked agammaglobulinemia (XLA). https://ghr.nlm.nih.gov/condition/x-linked-agammaglobulinemia. Accessed October 31, 2016.
13. American Academy of Allergy, Asthma & Immunology. X-linked agammaglobulinemia (XLA). https://www.aaaai.org/conditions-and-treatments/primary-immunodeficiency-disease/x-linked-agammaglobulinemia. Accessed October 31, 2016.
14. American Cancer Society. *Cancer Facts & Figures 2015*. Atlanta: American Cancer Society; 2015. http://www.cancer.org/acs/groups/content/@editorial/documents/document/acspc-044552.pdf. Accessed October 31, 2016.
15. Howlader N, Noone AM, Krapcho M, et al. (eds). SEER Cancer Statistics Review, 1975-2013, National Cancer Institute. Bethesda, MD, http://seer.cancer.gov/csr/1975_2013/, based on November 2015 SEER data submission, posted to the SEER web site, April 2016. Accessed May 6, 2016.
16. National Hemophilia Foundation. Hemophilia A. https://www.hemophilia.org/Bleeding-Disorders/Types-of-Bleeding-Disorders/Hemophilia-A. Accessed October 31, 2016.
17. CDC, NCHS. Underlying Cause of Death 1999-2013 on CDC WONDER Online Database, released 2015. Data are from the Multiple Cause of Death Files, 1999-2013, as compiled from data provided by the 57 vital statistics jurisdictions through the Vital Statistics Cooperative Program. Accessed January 3, 2017.
18. Flegal KM, Carroll MD, Kit BK, Ogden CL. Prevalence of obesity and trends in the distribution of body mass index among US adults, 1999–2010. http://jama.jamanetwork.com/article.aspx?articleid=1104933External Link Disclaimer. *JAMA.* 2012;307(5):491–97.
19. Ogden CL, Carroll MD, Kit BK, Flegal KM. Prevalence of obesity and trends in body mass index among US children and adolescents, 1999–2010. http://jama.jamanetwork.com/Mobile/article.aspx?articleid=1104932External Link Disclaimer. *JAMA.* 2012;307(5):483–90.
20. National Multiple Sclerosis Society. What Is MS? http://www.nationalmssociety.org/What-is-MS/What-Causes-MS. Accessed October 31, 2016.
21. Alzheimer's Foundation of America. About Alzheimer's Disease. https://www.alzfdn.org/AboutAlzheimers/statistics.html. Published January 28, 2016. Retrieved January 3, 2017.
22. Depression and Bipolar Support Alliance. Bipolar Disorder Statistics. http://www.dbsalliance.org/site/PageServer?pagename=education_statistics_bipolar_disorder. Retrieved January 3, 2017.

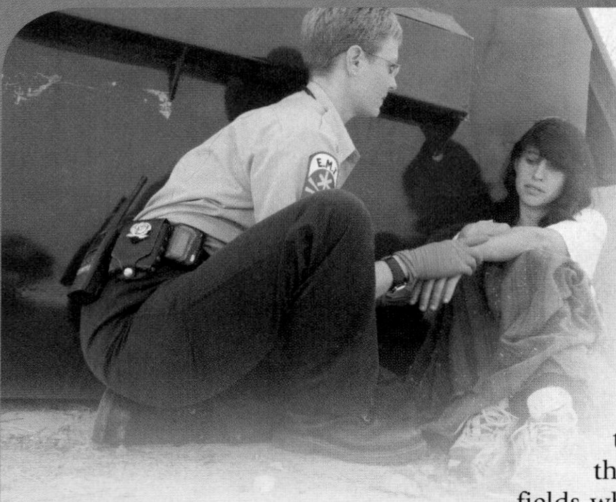

Assessment *in Action*

You are dispatched to a local park for a 20-year-old woman who was stung by a bee. On arrival, you are met by a law enforcement officer who directs you to the patient. The patient is sitting upright on a park bench in obvious distress. You can see urticaria covering her arms, legs, and face. Her tongue is swollen, and she points to a medical alert bracelet that says, "Allergic to bee stings." You can hear wheezing in all fields when assessing lung sounds. When you assess her pulse, you find it weak at the radial site.

1. The strength of a person's peripheral pulses is related to:

A. heart rate and preload.
B. stroke volume.
C. physical size.
D. mast cells.

2. Anaphylactic shock is characterized by:

A. hypertension and vasoconstriction.
B. wheezing and widespread vasodilation.
C. hypotension and hives.
D. crackles (rales) and stridor.

3. When oxygen does not reach the cell, the cell reverts to:

A. anaerobic metabolism.
B. aerobic metabolism.
C. production of ketones.
D. production of bicarbonate.

4. Distributive shock occurs when:

A. blood moves from the core of the body.
B. blood pools in expanded vascular structures.
C. microorganisms attack the body.
D. a significant decrease in stroke volume occurs.

5. How does the body respond to hypoperfusion?

A. Decreased preload and heart rate
B. Increased systemic vascular resistance
C. Systemic hypoxia increases vascular resistance
D. Decreased cardiac oxygen demand

6. The worst respiratory sign in a patient with anaphylactic shock is:

A. diminished lung sounds.
B. loud expiratory wheezing.
C. diffuse coarse crackles.
D. labored breathing.

7. Based on your knowledge of the pathophysiology of anaphylaxis, what do you anticipate the patient's vital signs to be?

A. Bradycardic and hypertensive with elevated $ETCO_2$
B. Tachycardic and hypotensive with elevated $ETCO_2$
C. Tachycardic and hypotensive with decreased $ETCO_2$
D. Tachycardic and normotensive with $ETCO_2$ of 40 mm Hg

8. In arterial blood gas analysis, a patient has a low pH and a high $Paco_2$. What type of acidosis or alkalosis does the patient have?

9. Will a patient who has been hyperventilating have signs and symptoms of respiratory acidosis or respiratory alkalosis?

10. Stridor is an ominous finding in anaphylaxis as it indicates swelling of the ________ ________, and impending respiratory distress.

CHAPTER 10

Life Span Development

National EMS Education Standard Competencies

Life Span Development

Integrates comprehensive knowledge of life span development.

Knowledge Objectives

1. Know the terms used to designate the following developmental stages of life: infants, toddlers and preschoolers, school-age children, adolescents (teenagers), early adults, middle adults, and late adults. (pp 477, 482, 484, 485, 487, 488)
2. Describe the major physiologic and psychosocial characteristics of an infant's life. (pp 478-482)
3. Describe the major physiologic and psychosocial characteristics of a toddler and preschooler's life. (pp 482-484)
4. Describe the major physiologic and psychosocial characteristics of a school-age child's life. (pp 484-485)
5. Describe the major physiologic and psychosocial characteristics of an adolescent's life. (pp 485-487)
6. Describe the major physiologic and psychosocial characteristics of an early adult's life. (p 487)
7. Describe the major physiologic and psychosocial characteristics of a middle adult's life. (pp 487-488)
8. Describe the major physiologic and psychosocial characteristics of a late adult's life. (pp 488-492)

Skills Objectives

There are no skills objectives for this chapter.

Introduction

One of the most interesting things about humans is that people evolve over the life span. As a paramedic, you must be aware of the obvious and subtle changes that humans undergo physically and mentally at various stages of life, and understand how these changes may affect your approach to patient care.

Infants

As any parent or caregiver can attest, **infants** develop at a startling rate Figure 10-1. In medicine, an infant is defined as a baby who is age 1 month to 1 year. Babies younger than age 1 month are categorized as either newborns or neonates depending on their age, and are covered in detail in Chapter 42, *Neonatal Care*.

YOU are the Paramedic — PART 1

Your unit is dispatched to a private residence for a 3-year-old girl who has fallen in the backyard. The dispatcher advises that the child was running and fell, striking her head on a wooden deck. The dispatcher states that the child is crying audibly over the phone. As you arrive in front of the residence, the father comes toward your vehicle to meet you, carrying the child in his arms. The child appears to be vigorously struggling to be set down and is crying loudly.

1. What is your first concern at this scene?
2. Which stage of development describes a 3-year-old child, and how will this information affect your assessment?

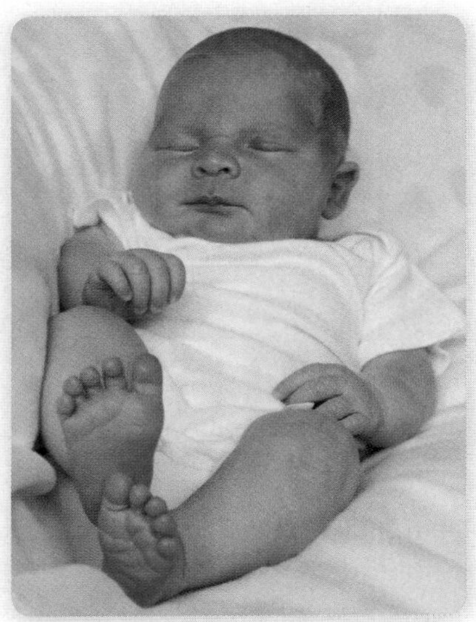

Figure 10-1 An infant.

Infants both grow and develop. Growth is defined as an increase in size, while development represents increased function or mastery of skills.[1]

▶ Physical Changes

Vital Signs

Normal ranges of vital signs for various age groups are outlined in Chapter 11, *Patient Assessment*, and Chapter 43, *Pediatric Emergencies*. The younger the person, the faster the pulse rate and respirations. At birth, an average pulse rate of 140 beats/min and a respiratory rate of 30 to 60 breaths/min are considered normal.[2] Tidal volume in infants starts at 6 to 8 mL/kg. By age 1 year, the tidal volume increases to 10 to 15 mL/kg. Normal oxygen saturation level is 94% or greater.[2] Blood glucose level is normally 45 mg/dL or greater at birth, then increases to 60 mg/dL or greater from age 1 month on.[2]

In children, blood pressure often directly corresponds to the patient's weight, so it typically increases with age. At birth, systolic blood pressure of an infant is usually in the range of 67 to 84 mm Hg. By age 1 year, systolic blood pressure is in the range of 85 to 104 mm Hg.[2]

Weight

A full-term newborn usually weighs around 7.5 pounds (3.4 kg) at birth.[3,4] In the first week after birth, infants usually have a loss of 5% to 10% of their birth weight due to the loss of fluid. By the second week of life, infants normally gain weight. From here on, infants grow at a rate of about 1 ounce (30 g) per day, doubling their weight by age 6 months and tripling it by age 1 year.[3]

Cardiovascular System

Prior to birth, fetal circulation occurs through the placenta. Just after birth, physiologic changes take place in the cardiovascular system that allow independent circulation via the newborn's own vasculature. This process will be covered in detail in Chapter 42, *Neonatal Care*.

Pulmonary System

Prior to an infant's first breath, the lungs have never been inflated. An infant's first breath is therefore forceful—it has to be! An infant's first breath results from chemical, mechanical, thermal, and sensory triggers.[5]

Young infants are primarily "nose breathers" for the first several months of their lives.[6-10] Infants younger than 6 months are particularly prone to nasal congestion, which can cause viral upper respiratory infections. If you respond to a call for an infant who is choking, then always make sure the infant's nasal passages are clear and unobstructed by mucus.

The rib cages of infants are less rigid than those of older people. The diaphragm is the newborn's major respiratory muscle. Intercostal muscles are not well developed. Thus you observe the abdomen bulge with each inspiration, but see little thoracic expansion.[8,11] Because of the immaturity of the accessory muscles, the infant can quickly become fatigued.

An infant's airway is different from an adult's airway. The infant's tongue is larger in proportion to the oral cavity, and the airway is proportionally shorter and narrower. As a result of these two factors, the airway in an infant can be occluded more easily than the airway in older children or adults. An infant also has fewer alveoli in the lungs, which decreases the surface area for gas exchange.

Words of Wisdom

Infants often land headfirst when they fall because an infant's head accounts for a much larger percentage of the body weight than the head of an adult. Also, most infants cannot stretch out their arms in time to cushion or slow their fall. Keep this point in mind when you assess an infant for potential head, neck, and spine injuries.

Words of Wisdom

When you count respirations in an infant, you may choose to count the number of times the abdomen rises instead of concentrating solely on chest rise.

Fluid and heat loss occur through exhalation. The rapid respiratory rate of infants can lead to significant heat and fluid loss. Keep infants warm, and monitor for signs of dehydration.

When you provide bag-mask ventilations to an infant, be aware that an infant's lungs are fragile. Ventilations that are delivered with excessive force or excessive volume can result in trauma from pressure, or **barotrauma** Figure 10-2. It is imperative to use a bag-mask device that is the correct size for the patient Figure 10-3.

Renal System

Newborns and infants can become easily dehydrated. Newborn kidneys are less able than adult kidneys to concentrate urine and excrete water. Therefore when dehydration occurs, newborns and infants cannot compensate to the same extent adults can.[12]

Also, an infant's urine consists mainly of water, which can cause the child to develop electrolyte imbalances.

Immune System

While in the womb, infants collect antibodies from the maternal blood. For the first year of life, the infant maintains some of the mother's immunities, so he or she has naturally acquired passive immunities. Infants can also receive antibodies via breastfeeding, further bolstering their immune systems.

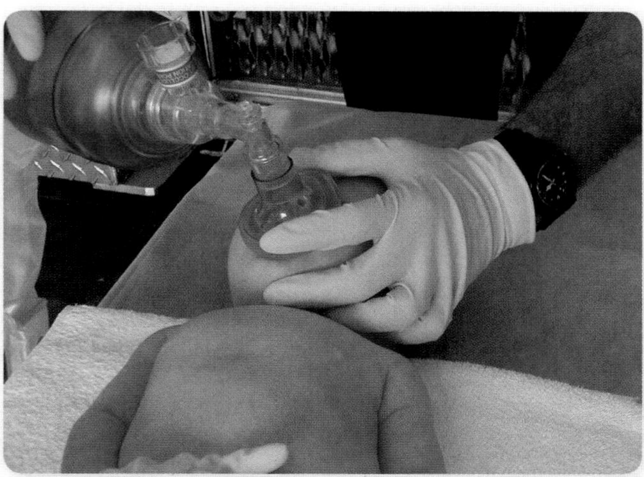

Figure 10-2 An infant's lungs are fragile. Use caution when providing bag-mask ventilations to avoid barotrauma.

Courtesy of Marianne Gausche-Hill, MC, FACEP, FAAP.

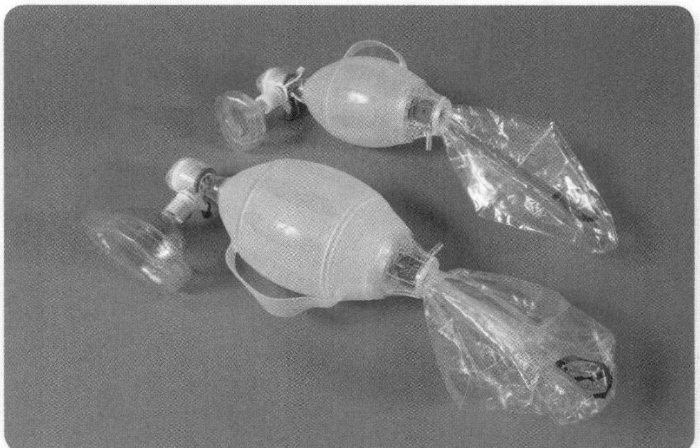

Figure 10-3 Different sizes of bag-mask devices.

Nervous System

Although an infant's nervous system is developed at birth, its evolution continues after birth. For example, a newborn lacks the ability to localize and isolate a particular response to sensation. An infant's brainstem and spinal are present and functioning, but memory and fine motor coordination are not yet fully developed. Also, ability to control body temperature is limited.[13]

An infant is born with certain reflexes. The cranial nerves control important infant reflexes, such as blinking, sucking, and gag reflexes. The **Moro reflex** (startle reflex) occurs when an infant is caught off guard by something or someone; the infant opens his or her arms wide, spreads the fingers, and seems to grab at things. A **palmar grasp** occurs when an object is placed into the infant's palm; the infant will close the fingers around the object. The **rooting reflex** occurs when something touches an infant's cheek; the infant will instinctively turn his or her head toward the touch. In conjunction with the **sucking reflex**, which occurs when an infant's lips are stroked, these reflexes are often tested during feeding.

An infant's **fontanelles** (soft spots) allow the head to be molded Figure 10-4—for example, when the newborn passes through the birth canal. These three or four bones of the skull eventually bind together and form suture joints by age 2 years. The fontanelles play a key role in your assessment of an infant. An anterior fontanelle that is sunken may be a sign of dehydration.

Perhaps the neurologic development that is of most interest to parents and/or caregivers is the development of a sleep pattern. Sleep pattern is developed through a combination of central nervous system development and parental efforts. Most infants develop the ability to sleep for five hours by age 3 months, but some do not develop this until age 1 year.[14] A concern related to infant sleep is sudden infant death syndrome (SIDS); this is discussed in Chapter 43, *Pediatric Emergencies*.

Musculoskeletal System

Growth plates (often called epiphyseal plates) are located on either end of an infant's long bones, and are the centers where longitudinal bone growth occurs. Growth charts are used to track the growth of an infant or child and provide percentiles comparing the child's growth with the growth that is expected for an average infant or child of that age.

Teeth

Teething (ie, when teeth erupt or break through the gums) often starts between the ages of 4 and 7 months and can be a challenge to both parents and infants. As with many of the changes in life, this time frame is an estimate, and some infants will have teeth erupt as early as 1 month, and some may have to wait as long as 1 year. Teeth usually

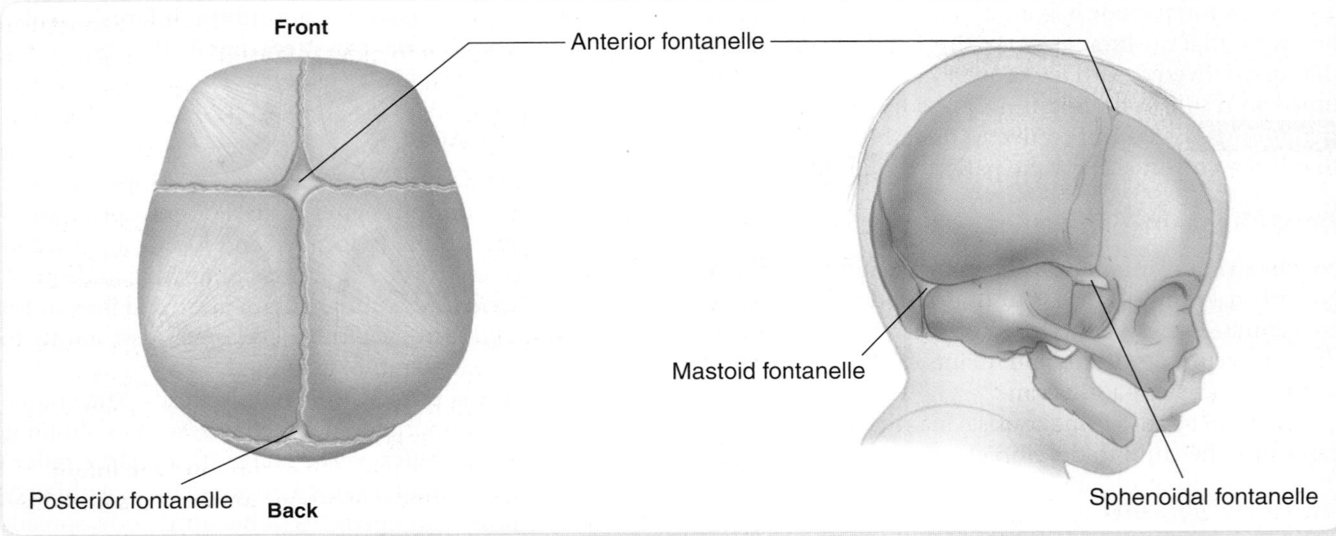

Figure 10-4 The fontanelles.

erupt in a predetermined order, and a child should have a full set by the age of 3 years. The child will usually keep this set of "baby teeth" until around the age of 6 years, when permanent teeth start to come in.

▶ Psychosocial Changes

An infant's psychosocial development begins at birth and continues to evolve as the infant interacts with and reacts to the environment. Parents and/or caregivers are often concerned about whether their child is developing within the socially accepted norms. Table 10-1 outlines typical ages at which major psychosocial changes are noticed.

One key to having a happy, healthy infant is spending quality time with the child. Nevertheless, infants often have their own timetables as to when they will become attached to their parents and other family members. **Bonding**, or the formation of a close, personal relationship, is usually based on a **secure attachment**. A secure attachment occurs when an infant understands that parents and/or caregivers will be responsive to his or her needs. This realization encourages an infant to reach out and explore, knowing that his or her parents will provide a so-called safety net.

Another type of attachment, referred to as **anxious avoidant attachment**, is observed in infants who are

YOU are the Paramedic PART 2

You and your partner convince the mother and father to sit down on the front steps of the residence rather than immediately climb up into your vehicle. You ask the child her name and she buries her face in her father's chest. The mother tells you her name is Juliet. The father tries to forcefully turn Juliet so she will face you, and the child clings to him even harder and cries louder.

Recording Time: 2 Minutes	
Appearance	Actively moving and crying
Level of consciousness	Conscious and agitated
Airway	Open
Breathing	Loud crying
Circulation	Adequate

3. Why is Juliet clinging to her father and turning away from you?
4. What are some of the measures you can take to alleviate the child's distress?

Table 10-1 Psychosocial Characteristics at Various Ages

Age (in months)	Noticeable Characteristics
2	Recognizes familiar faces; tracks objects with the eyes
3	Brings objects to the mouth; smiles and frowns
4	Reaches out to people; drools
5	Sleeps through the night; recognizes family from strangers
6	Teething begins; sits upright in a chair; speaks one-syllable words
7	Afraid of strangers; has mood swings
8	Responds to "no"; sits upright alone; plays peek-a-boo
9	Pulls himself or herself up; places objects in mouth to explore them
10	Responds to his or her name; crawls efficiently
11	Starts to walk without help; frustrated with restrictions
12	Knows his or her name; can walk

repeatedly rejected by their parents and/or caregivers. These children develop an isolated lifestyle in which they do not have to depend on the support and care of others. Child neglect will be covered in more detail in Chapter 43, *Pediatric Emergencies*.

In most infants, the primary method of communicating distress is through crying. Parents and/or caregivers can often tell what is upsetting their child simply by listening to the tone of the child's crying—that is, they know the difference between a basic cry (which conveys hunger, discomfort, frustration, or sleepiness) and one that conveys anger or pain. Infants occasionally make another distinct cry—an alarming, distressed cry. This cry may be heard when an unexpected event occurs, causing a **situational crisis** (crisis caused by a specific set of circumstances) for the infant.

Infants who have bonded well with their parents and/or caregivers and have good relationships will usually respond predictably when a situational crisis occurs. The most prevalent example of a situational crisis is being separated from a parent and/or caregiver. Separation anxiety is common in older infants. The normal reaction peaks between the ages of 10 and 18 months, and involves clingy behavior and fear of unfamiliar places and people. An infant's reaction to a situational crisis is classified into the following three phases:

- The **protest phase** can start immediately and usually lasts about a week. It is easily recognized by loud crying, irritability, restlessness, and rejection of other caregivers' efforts.
- The **despair phase** follows, which is characterized by the monotonous wailing indicating that the infant begins to believe the situation is not going to change.
- **Withdrawal** eventually occurs, and the infant becomes almost apathetic and appears bored by his or her surroundings.

As infants become accustomed to their homes and families, they begin to need the security of a predictable environment. If an infant's environment is too unpredictable, then the infant may despair and become withdrawn, which may lead to problems in the development of trust. **Trust and mistrust** refers to a stage of development from birth to about 18 months of age. Most infants desire that their worlds be planned, organized, and routine. If the infant perceives that his or her parents and/or caregivers will provide this predictable environment for him or her, then the infant gains trust in them. The opposite also holds true; if an infant perceives that his or her parents and/or caregivers will not provide an organized and routine environment, then the infant may develop behavioral problems.

Infants respond well to an instructional technique called **scaffolding**. Scaffolding is a technique in which a person builds on what has already been learned. As a student, you can also benefit from this technique! For example, the basic assessment skills that you learned in your emergency medical technician course will now be used as building blocks for the advanced assessments taught in this paramedic course.

Temperament

With regard to temperament (behavioral style), children are classified as being easy, difficult, or slow to warm up to their surroundings and lifestyles. Easy children are characterized by the relative ease by which they adapt. Their body functions work properly, they have low-intensity reactions, and they accept new surroundings well. Difficult children usually have intense reactions, and do not acclimate to new surroundings well. Children who are slow to warm up usually have low-intensity reactions, but generally exhibit negative moods.

As a paramedic, you can adjust your approach according to the developmental stage of your patient. Effective techniques include having the parent or caregiver hold the infant and allowing the infant to hold a toy **Figure 10-5**. In fact, you may complete your physical assessment of an

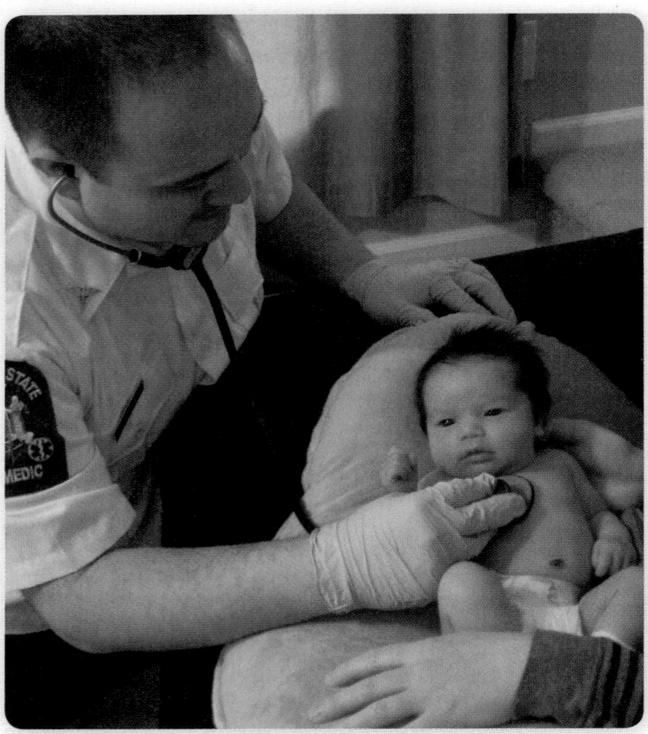

Figure 10-5 Have the parent or caregiver hold the infant while you perform your assessment and treatment, if possible.

infant with the infant in the parent or caregiver's arms—unless the child is in respiratory failure, in need of spinal immobilization, or has a reduced level of consciousness. You may also distract the child and save the most difficult part of the assessment and treatment for last.

Toddlers and Preschoolers

Physical Changes

In **toddlers** (children ages 1 to 2 years Figure 10-6) and **preschoolers** (children ages 3 to 5 years Figure 10-7), the pulse rates and respiratory rates are slower than in infants, whereas the systolic blood pressure is higher (approximately 100 mm Hg). At the same time, weight gain should level off.

A toddler's cardiovascular system is not dramatically different from that of an adult. A toddler's lungs continue to develop more bronchioles and alveoli. Although toddlers and preschoolers have more lung tissue, they do not have well-developed lung musculature, which prevents them from sustaining deep or rapid respirations for an extended time.

The loss of passive immunity in the immune system is possibly the most obvious development at this stage of human life. Common colds often develop that may manifest as gastrointestinal distress or upper respiratory tract infections. As toddlers spend more time around playmates and classmates, they acquire their own immunity as the body is exposed to various pathogens.

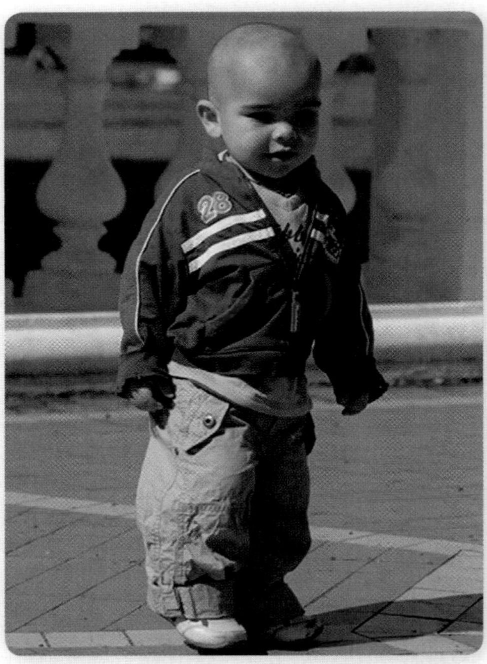

Figure 10-6 A toddler.

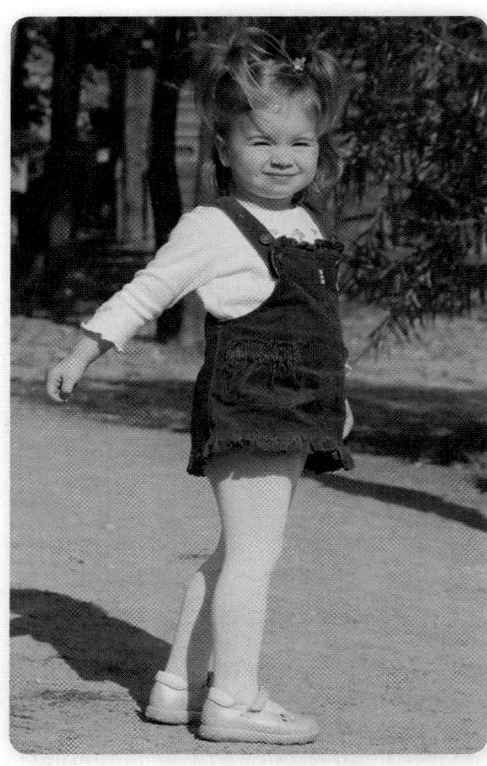

Figure 10-7 A preschooler.

Neuromuscular growth also makes considerable progress at this age. Toddlers and preschoolers spend a great deal of time finding out exactly how to use their expansive

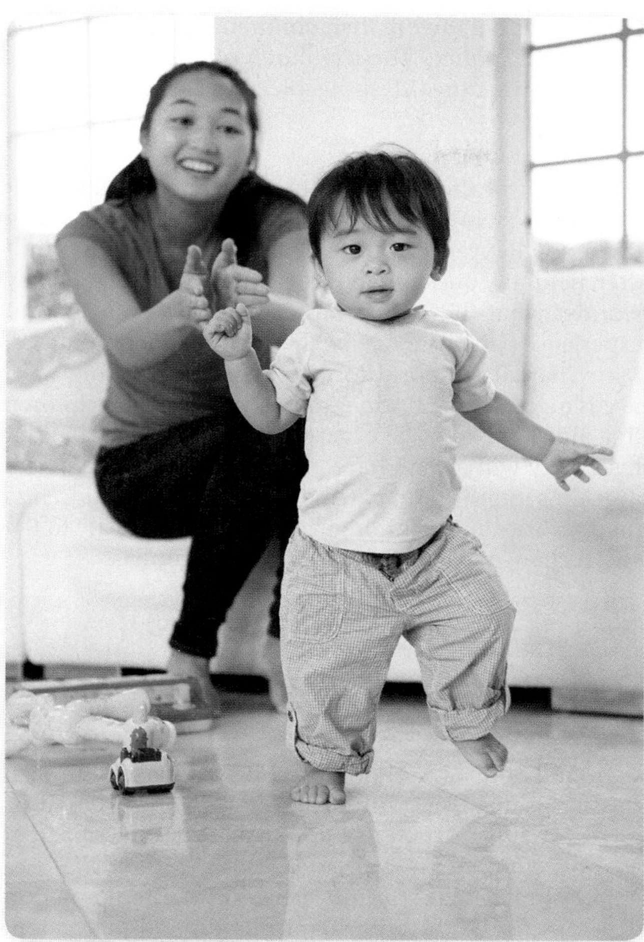

Figure 10-8 Toddlers learn to walk, one of the major milestones in life.

nervous system and the muscles it controls by walking, running, jumping, and playing catch (Figure 10-8). By age 3 years, bone density and muscle mass increase to become more like those of an adult. Watching children play as they age from 1 to 5 years demonstrates how they move from gross motor activities (grabbing an object with the full palm) to fine motor activities (picking up a crayon). By the end of this stage, a preschooler will have a brain that weighs 90% of its final adult weight. In addition, all of this playing places stress on the muscles and bones. Consequently, muscle mass increases, as does bone density.

This stage also includes the continued development of the renal system and perhaps the most anticipated event of this stage of life: toilet training! Physiologically, toddlers develop bowel control prior to bladder control.[15] Toddlers have the neuromuscular control needed for bladder control and can feel when the bladder is full by 12 to 15 months of age. On average, the 18-month-old child has the ability to control his or her muscles to delay excretion for a short time. However, the child may not be psychologically ready until 18 to 30 months of age. There might not be any greater satisfaction for a child of this age than to run up to his or her parents and tell them, "I'm a big kid now—I used the potty!"

Other developments that continue during this time frame include the emergence of baby teeth. Teething can be painful and accompanied by fever. In addition, parents and/or caregivers and toddlers are enthralled with sensory development—for example, tickling.

Psychosocial Changes

This period of development is often exciting for parents and/or caregivers. Toddlers are learning to speak and express themselves, thereby taking a major step toward independence. At the same time, toddlers are very attached to their parents and feel safe with them. As mentioned previously, separation anxiety peaks between 10 and 18 months of age. It is fascinating to watch a child struggle through the conflict of wanting to play, yet also wanting to be protected.

Children understand language long before they begin to speak, and language acquisition occurs in phases, beginning with the ability to speak one or two words at age 1 year, to basic language mastery at 36 months of age.[16] From ages 2 to 5, the number of words in a spoken sentence typically equals the child's age; in other words, at age 3, a toddler speaks three-word sentences.[17] Refinement of language skills continues throughout childhood. By the age of 3 or 4 years, most children can use and understand full sentences. As they progress through this stage of their life, they will go from using language to communicate what they want to using language creatively and playfully.

This period is also the time when toddlers begin to interact with other children and start to play games. Playing games teaches control, obedience, and even competitiveness. A lot of learning and development take place when children watch their peers during group outings, such as playdates. Of course, behavior observed on television and the Internet can also be learned, which is why some parents and/or caregivers limit their children's viewing choices or the amount of time they devote to these activities. During this phase of development, children also learn to recognize sexual differences by observing their role models and siblings.

Words of Wisdom

When you interact with patients who are very young, try to keep their routines the same by keeping family and familiar items nearby.

With toddlers and preschoolers, you might try to "break the ice" by giving them a teddy bear and explaining what you are going to do by showing them on the teddy bear. Such children may be able to understand by show-and-tell more clearly than by listening to a verbal description. Be sure that the toy has no removable parts, and store it in a clean plastic bag between calls.

As with infants, it is important to include the parent or caregiver when working with a toddler or preschooler. Also, position yourself at the child's level so that you are making eye contact. Explain to the child what you are going to do before you do it, and allow the child to make choices when possible. As with infants, save the most difficult part of the assessment and treatment for last.

Another tip—do not try to reason with a child as to why a procedure (such as establishing an intravenous line) has to be done. Explain it briefly at a level they can understand, then do it! Often the psychological experience can be worse than the physical one if you give a child too much time to worry about a minor procedure.

Documentation & Communication

When you document your assessment of an infant or young child, it is often best to avoid struggling with a stable patient to obtain a blood pressure. Simply documenting breath sounds, an apical pulse, work of breathing, and the child's interactions with his or her surroundings can more than adequately describe your patient's condition.

Parenting Styles

A child's development is affected by the parenting style employed by his or her parents. Although the process of parenting is a complex behavior, rarely well defined in any one individual, three idealized approaches may be examined. An **authoritarian** parenting style demands absolute obedience from a child no matter what the situation. This style of parenting shows no regard for the child's personal freedoms; for example, a child is punished for simply questioning a parent. Children who are raised in this manner often develop self-esteem problems; girls are more likely to become shy and boys are more likely to become argumentative or hostile.

Authoritative parenting is based on respect for parental authority and balance with individual freedom of the child. These parents regularly respond to the personal needs of the child. They set rules and enforce them fairly; however, they believe that children need certain freedoms and attempt to maintain a balance between the two. This style can allow children to develop into adults who are independent, well socialized, and easygoing.

Permissive parenting does not impose many rules, if any, on the child. The child is in control and the parent takes a tolerant approach to the child's behavior, including socially unacceptable behaviors. Permissive parenting is broken into two subcategories—indifferent and indulgent. The former style describes parents who just do not care; the latter style describes parents who are excessively lenient. Permissive parents rarely, if ever, punish their children, and therefore their children may grow up to be considered spoiled. These children often become adults who are immature, irresponsible, and lack self-control.

Divorce

About half of the marriages in the United States result in divorce.[18] No matter what stage of life a child is in, a divorce will have a profound effect on him or her. Children naturally question if the divorce was their fault, may wonder what they could have done to prevent it, and experience pain from having their environment changed. Many parents respond to their children's feelings and needs together, and by doing so, they assure their children that although they will experience some changes in their lives, they will always have parents who love them very much. As long as both parents maintain their children as their priority, most children adapt relatively easily to the social changes a divorce brings upon a family.

School-Age Children

▶ Physical Changes

School-age children are those age 6 to 12 years. The vital signs and body of a school-age child gradually approach those observed in adulthood **Figure 10-9**. Obvious physical traits and body function changes become apparent as most children grow about 5.5 to 7.7 pounds (2.5 to 3.5 kg) and 2 inches (5 cm) each year.[19,20] Brain function develops further in both hemispheres, and permanent teeth also come in during this period. Also, the onset of puberty may begin in elementary school-age children and has been documented at age 10 years or younger.

▶ Psychosocial Changes

Children are engaged in a great deal of psychosocial growing up during the school years, though the pace

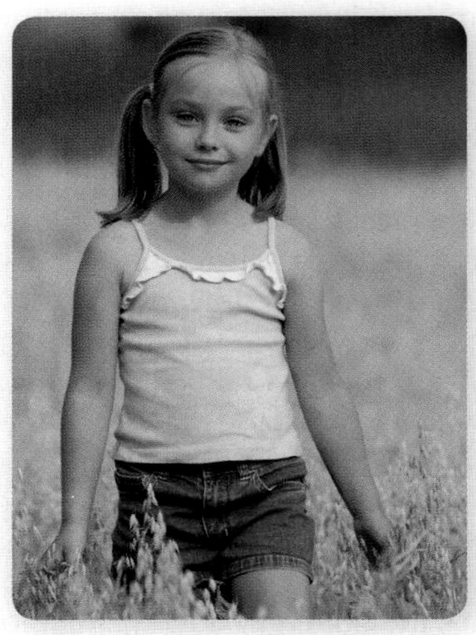

Figure 10-9 A school-age child.

of development varies from child to child. Parents as a whole do not devote as much time to their children during this phase. Nevertheless, it is at this critical time in human development that children learn various types of reasoning. In **preconventional reasoning**, children act almost purely to avoid punishment and to get what they want. In **conventional reasoning**, they look for approval from their peers and society. In **postconventional reasoning**, children make decisions guided by their conscience.

During this stage, children begin to develop their **self-concept** and **self-esteem**. Self-concept is a person's perception of himself or herself; self-esteem is how a person feels about himself or herself, and how a person feels about how he or she fits in with peers.

When you are working with a school-age child, use the same techniques you would use with a preschooler (that is, position yourself at the child's level, explain what you are going to do, and give choices when possible). Always be honest about what you are doing. For example, if a procedure might hurt, then say that to your patient. The biggest issue with school-aged children is trust. You have to earn it quickly through open and honest communication and you must never lose it through lies or sneaky maneuvers. If you are direct with them and remain assertive, then school-aged children will respond well most of the time.

Adolescents (Teenagers)

Physical Changes

The vital signs of **adolescents** (children ages 13 through 18 years) begin to level off within the adult ranges, with a systolic blood pressure between 110 and 131 mm Hg, a pulse rate between 60 and 100 beats/min, and respirations in the range of 12 to 20 breaths/min Figure 10-10.

Adolescence is also the phase of life when humans experience a rapid, 2- to 3-year growth spurt (that is, an increase in muscle and bone growth) as well as changes in blood chemistry. Growth begins with the hands and feet, then moves to the long bones of the extremities, and finishes with growth of the torso. As a whole, boys experience this stage of development later in life than girls do. When this period of growth has finished, however, boys are generally taller and physically stronger than girls. Muscle mass and bone density are nearly at adult levels.

One of the more subtle changes during this phase of life is the maturation of the human reproductive system. Secondary sexual development begins, along with enlargement of the external sex organs. Pubic hair and axillary hair begin to appear. Voices start to change in range and depth. In girls, the breasts and thighs increase in size as adipose tissue is deposited there. Menstruation

YOU are the Paramedic PART 3

Your partner asks the mother what Juliet's favorite item is and she answers, "Her pink blanket." Your partner asks the mother to retrieve the blanket and to show her where the fall occurred. The mother agrees and both enter the residence. The father is still struggling with the child and you ask him to loosen his embrace and allow the child to pick her position of comfort. Your partner and the mother return with the child's blanket. Your partner sits down on the ground, slightly lower than the child, and offers her the blanket. Juliet takes the blanket from her and appears to calm down considerably. You carefully begin your assessment.

Recording Time: 7 Minutes	
Respirations	Crying
Pulse	130 beats/min
Skin	Hot, dry, red
Blood pressure	Unable to obtain
Oxygen saturation (Spo_2)	Unable to obtain
Pupils	PERRLA

5. Measurement of Spo_2 level and blood pressure requires equipment. How can you gain the child's trust to use your equipment?

6. What is the expected normal range for a 3-year-old child's pulse rate and respiratory rate?

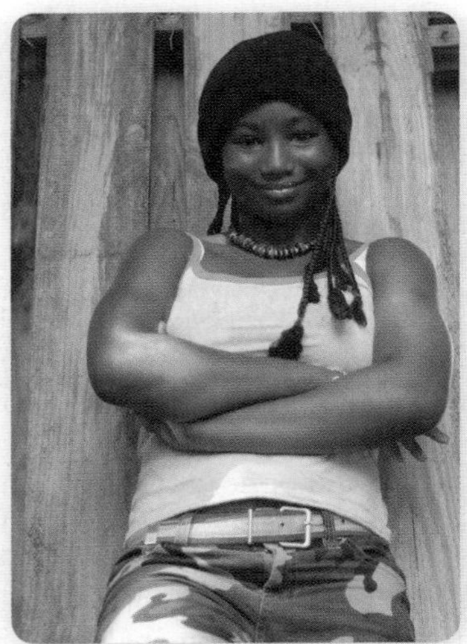

Figure 10-10 An adolescent.

begins during this time; however, **menarche** (the first menstrual bleeding) is starting to occur at increasingly younger ages, so it is common to begin menstruation prior to becoming a teenager.

Another key development in girls is the release of follicle-stimulating hormone and luteinizing hormone, both of which increase estrogen and progesterone production. In contrast, the hormone gonadotropin is secreted in boys and results in the production of testosterone. Acne can occur due to hormonal changes.

These changes in the endocrine and reproductive systems provide the platform for reproduction. By the middle of adolescence, boys are able to produce sufficient sperm and girls are able to develop eggs for reproduction to take place.

▶ Psychosocial Changes

Adolescents and their families often deal with conflict as teenagers try to gain control of their lives from their parents. Privacy becomes an issue among adolescents, their siblings, and their parents. Self-consciousness also increases. Adolescents may struggle to create their own identities—to define who they are, for example, by dressing in a certain style of clothing to fit their personalities **Figure 10-11**. Adolescents use the feedback from their family and peers to help create their adult images. Adolescents are often caught between two worlds. They want to be treated like adults, yet want to be cared for like younger children.

Rebellious behavior can be part of an adolescent trying to find his or her own identity. Adolescents continually compare themselves with their peers, which makes peer pressure a major factor in the psychological growth of an adolescent. Antisocial behavior peaks during the eighth or ninth grade. Adolescence is also a time when eating disorders may develop as teenagers become obsessed with body image. Self-destructive behaviors such as smoking, drinking alcohol, and experimenting with drugs may begin. Although these behaviors can be troubling to parents, the adolescent is trying to determine if he or she is ready to take control of his or her own life. An adolescent's struggle toward independence may include setbacks that can be devastating. Patience and support from family and friends are essential in assisting an adolescent's transition into adulthood.

Adolescents may also show greater interest in sexual relations. Many adolescents are fixated on their public images and are terrified of being embarrassed. At this age, the adolescent develops a code of personal ethics, based partly on the ethics and values of the parents and partly on the influence of his or her own environment. At this tumultuous time, adolescents are at a higher risk than other populations for suicide and depression.

When you work with adolescents, be respectful and discreet. Remember, privacy is important to adolescents. If possible, have your partner speak with the parent in a separate area while you talk with the patient **Figure 10-12**. This may make the adolescent more comfortable and provide you more accurate answers than you would receive in the presence of a parent.

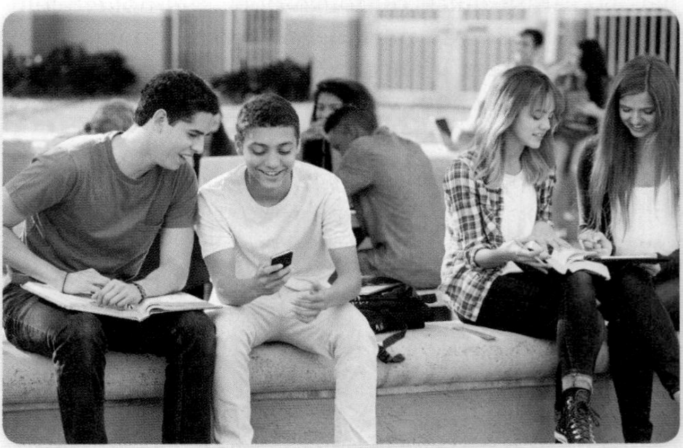

Figure 10-11 Adolescents want to fit in and may struggle to create their identities.

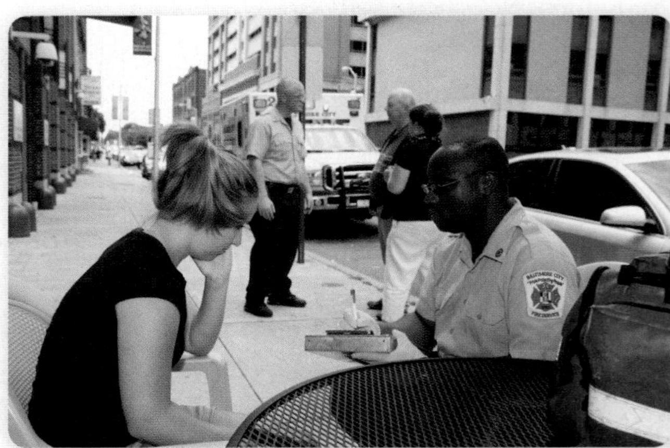

Figure 10-12 Try to interview adolescent patients in private, if possible.

> **Words of Wisdom**
>
> It is best to ask adolescents certain questions in total privacy, where they feel they can answer without constraint.

Early Adults

Physical Changes

Early adults range in age from 19 to 40 years Figure 10-13. Their vital signs do not vary greatly from those seen throughout adulthood. Ideally, the pulse rate is around 70 beats/min, the respiratory rate is in the range of 12 to 20 breaths/min, and the systolic blood pressure is approximately 120/80 mm Hg.

From age 19 years to just a little after age 25 years, the human body should be functioning at its optimal level. After this point, the discs in the spine begin to settle, and height can sometimes be affected, causing a "shrinking." Fatty tissue increases, which leads to weight gain. Muscle strength decreases, and the reflexes slow.

Psychosocial Changes

During this period, humans strive to create a place for themselves in the world, and many do everything they can to "settle down." As early adults struggle to find stability in their careers, stress on the job increases. Along with this natural tendency to settle come the experiences of romantic and affectionate love. Childbirth is most common in this age group. Despite all of this stress and change, this age group enjoys one of the more stable periods of life. People in early adulthood generally experience fewer psychological conditions related to well-being.

Middle Adults

Physical Changes

Middle adults range in age from 41 to 60 years Figure 10-14. Even though the body is still functioning at a high level, this age group is vulnerable to vision and hearing loss along with other varying degrees of degradation. Cardiovascular health also becomes an issue for many people in this age group. Cardiac output (the amount of blood circulated each minute) decreases, while cholesterol levels increase, leading to higher incidences of cardiovascular disease. Owing to the decrease in metabolism, it becomes more difficult for middle adults to control weight. Middle adults also experience a greater incidence of cancer. In women, **menopause**—the cessation of menstruation—begins in the late 40s or early 50s. This change can result in both the loss of bone density and the development of cardiovascular disease. Subsequently, these women are at a higher risk for fractures and cardiac conditions.

Psychosocial Changes

Middle adults tend to focus on achieving their life's goals, as they realize that they are past the halfway point

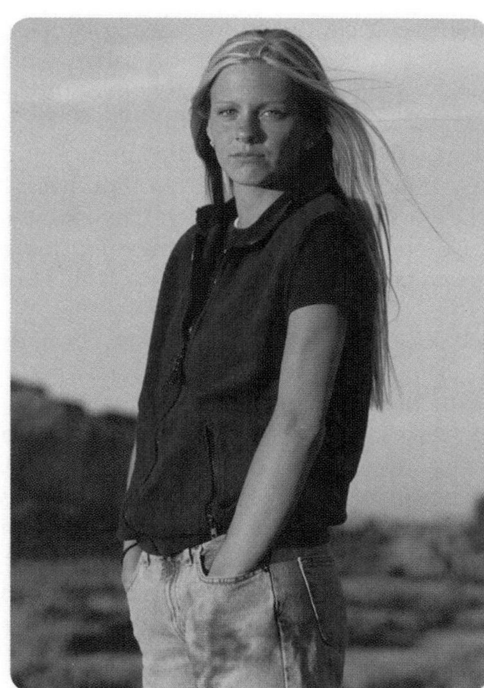

Figure 10-13 An early adult.

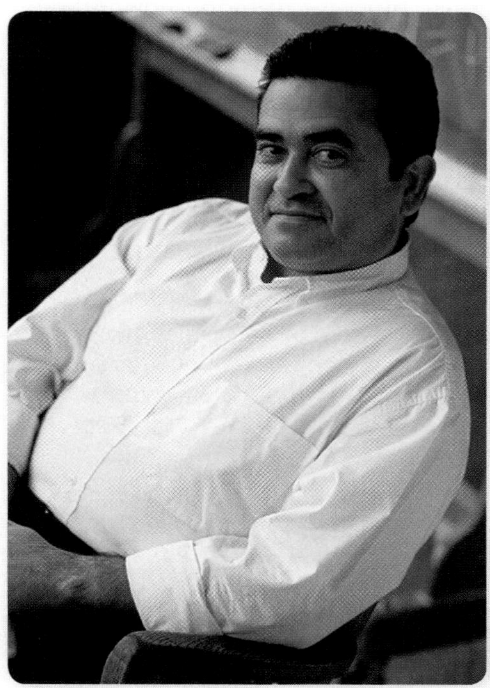

Figure 10-14 A middle adult.

in human life expectancy (discussed next). After years of nurturing and living with children, parents must readjust their lifestyle as their children leave the home, commonly called the empty nest syndrome. Finances may become a worrisome issue, as people plan for retirement while still managing everyday financial demands. During this time, people often view crisis as a challenge to be overcome rather than a threat to be avoided.

Late Adults

Physical Changes

Late adults include those ages 61 and older Figure 10-15. **Life expectancy** is constantly changing. When the first edition of this text was printed in 1979, human life expectancy was about 73 years. It is now approximately 78 years, with maximum life expectancy generally estimated at 115 years.[21]

Later in life, the vital signs depend on the patient's overall health, medical conditions, and medications taken. Today's late adults are staying active longer than their ancestors did. Thanks to medical advances, they are often able to overcome numerous medical conditions, but may need multiple medications to do so Figure 10-16.

Cardiovascular System

Cardiac function declines with age consequent to anatomic and physiologic changes that are largely related to **atherosclerosis**. In this disorder, which most commonly affects coronary vessels, cholesterol and calcium build up inside the walls of blood vessels and form plaque. The accumulation of plaque eventually leads to partial or complete blockage of blood flow. Atherosclerosis can also contribute to development of an **aneurysm**, or weakening and bulging of the blood vessel wall; an aneurysm may potentially rupture if it is subjected to high stretching forces. Many people older than age 65 have atherosclerotic disease.

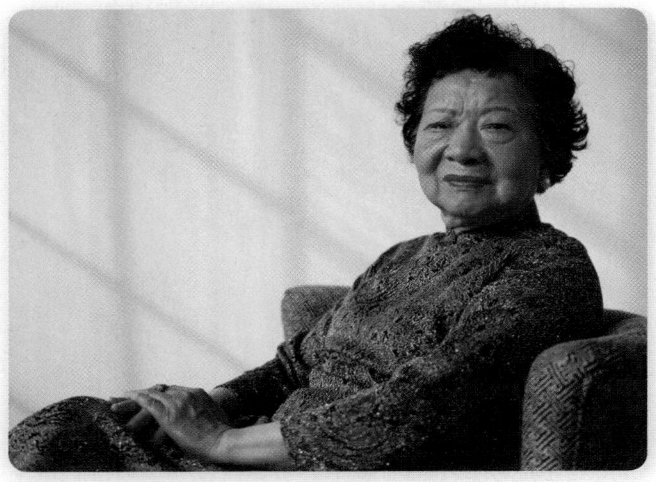

Figure 10-15 A late adult.

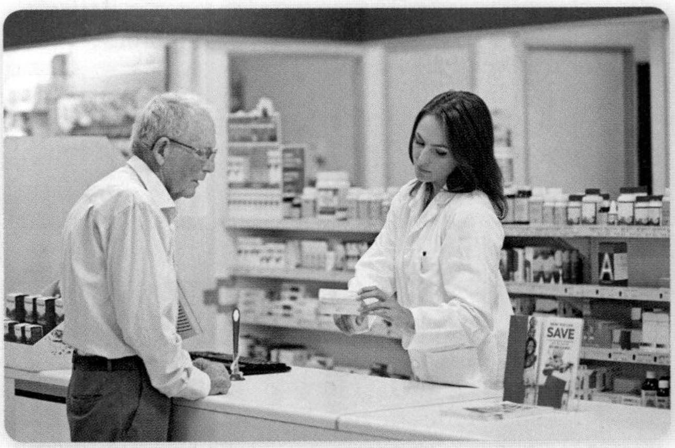

Figure 10-16 Older people are often prescribed multiple medications to help them stay active.

Other age-related changes typically include a decrease in pulse rate, a decline in cardiac output, and an inability to elevate cardiac output to match the demands of the body. These changes translate into a heart that is less able to respond to exercise or disease (for example, by an increased pulse rate). In the event of a life-threatening illness, the body typically needs to increase the pulse rate to ensure adequate blood pressure. Because heart muscle may be weakened with age, the increase in pulse rate can cause damage to the heart itself.

The vascular system also becomes stiff. Because of this change, the diastolic blood pressure increases with age. The left ventricle must then work harder to move blood effectively, so it becomes thicker. A loss of elasticity occurs. The thickening and stiffening of the left ventricle hinders filling in the ventricle, thereby decreasing cardiac output. Similar stiffening occurs in the heart valves, which may impede normal blood flow into and out of the heart. As the blood passes through these stiffened valves, a heart murmur may be heard, even in the absence of disease. Decreases in elastin and collagen in blood vessel walls reduce the elasticity of the peripheral vessels by as much as 70%. Compensation for blood pressure changes will be hampered because these vessels are less able to distend and contract.

Blood cells are also affected by aging. The body's cells originate from within the bone marrow. As a person ages, more of the bone marrow is replaced with fatty tissue. This replacement decreases the ability of the bones to manufacture more blood cells when needed. Although typically the fatty tissue does not pose a problem by itself, if an older person sustains trauma, then the ability of the body to produce blood cells to replace those lost is diminished. Finally, functional blood volume gradually declines over time.

Respiratory System

In late adults, the size of the airway increases and the surface area of the alveoli decreases. Metabolic changes cause the natural elasticity of the lungs to decrease, forcing people to increasingly rely on their intercostal muscles to breathe. In addition, the chest becomes more rigid because of calcification of the ribs to the sternum, which adds to the difficulty of breathing. As the elasticity of the lungs decreases, the overall strength of the intercostal muscles and diaphragm also decreases. These factors together make breathing more labor-intensive for older people. You might think that a rigid chest would be more protective, but this rigidity makes the chest more fragile. Overall, the bone structure of late adults is weakened. Instead of the chest being able to bend and give if struck, the calcified bony structure of the chest can fracture. As with all of the physical changes related to aging, however, the changes in the respiratory system are often gradual and go unnoticed until a severe, life-threatening condition occurs. An older person will then have less respiratory reserve to maintain adequate breathing.

Within the mouth and nose, there is a gradual loss of the mechanisms that protect the upper airway. This loss leads to decreased ability to clear secretions and decreased cough and gag reflexes. The number of cilia that line the airways diminishes with age, which results in decreased sensation to foreign objects such as dust or smoke, and less responsiveness when structures of the airway are innervated. With a lessened ability to maintain upper airway function, aspiration and obstruction become more likely.

When a younger patient inhales, the airway maintains its shape, allowing air to enter. As the smooth muscles of the lower airway weaken with age, strong inhalation can make the walls of the airway collapse inward and cause inspiratory wheezing **Figure 10-17**. The collapsing airways result in low flow rates, because less air can move through the smaller airways, and air trapping, because air does not completely exit the alveoli (incomplete expiration).

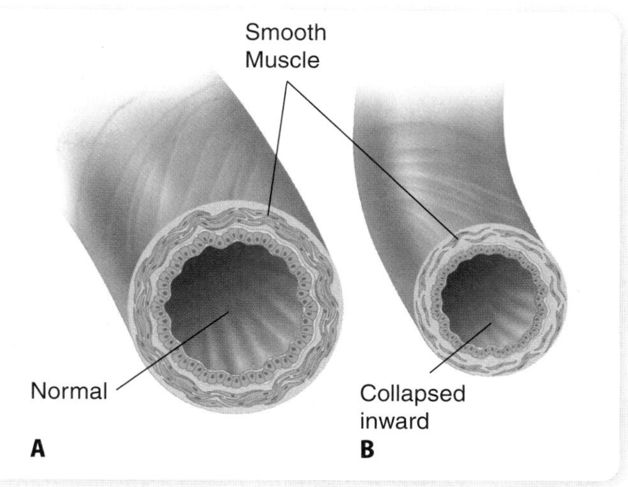

Figure 10-17 A. Healthy muscle in a younger patient's airway helps maintain the open airway during the pressures of inhalation. **B.** Muscle weakening with age can lead to airway collapse that may produce wheezing.

In older adults, the vital capacity (the volume of air moved during the deepest inspiration and expiration) is significantly decreased as compared with the vital capacity noted in young adulthood. Factors contributing to this decline include loss of respiratory muscle mass, increased stiffness of the thoracic cage, and decreased surface area available for the exchange of air.

Physiologically, vital capacity decreases and residual volume (the amount of air left in the lungs after expiration

YOU are the Paramedic PART 4

You and your partner are slowly gaining the trust of your patient. You are able to see a 0.5-inch (1-cm) laceration on the child's forehead with a corresponding abrasion and hematoma. The wound is not actively bleeding.

Recording Time: 17 Minutes	
Respirations	20 breaths/min
Pulse	118 beats/min
Skin	Hot, dry, pink
Blood pressure	Unable to obtain
Oxygen saturation (Spo_2)	99% on room air
Pupils	PERRLA

7. You need to bandage your patient's laceration. Offer some ideas to make this process more acceptable to the patient.
8. How should you transport this patient?

of the maximum possible amount of air) increases with age. As a consequence, stagnant air remains in the alveoli and hampers gas exchange. This effect can produce **hypercapnia** (increased carbon dioxide in the bloodstream) and acidosis, even when the person is at rest.

Endocrine System

As with other systems of the body, the function of the endocrine system gradually declines. As people get older, they tend to slow their physical activity. Unfortunately, many people do not decrease their food intake. When a person gains weight, more insulin is needed to control the body's metabolism and blood glucose (sugar) level. However, insulin production and glucose metabolism gradually decrease, so late adults are more prone to the development of diabetes mellitus. Changes in a late adult's mental status may also be the result of changes in his or her blood glucose level. The reproductive systems of both men and women change with age. Men are able to produce sperm long into their 80s, but the rigidity of the penis tends to decrease over time. It is unclear whether this decrease is due to aging itself or other conditions such as cardiovascular disease. During menopause, decreased production of regulating hormones results in atrophy of the woman's reproductive organs. The uterus and vagina both decrease in size. Hormone production for both sexes gradually decreases as people age. Sexual desire may diminish with age but does not cease.

Renal and Gastrointestinal Systems

In the kidneys, both structural and functional changes occur in the late adult. The filtration function of these organs, for example, declines significantly between the ages of 20 and 90 years. Kidney mass also decreases over the same span of time.[21] The number of **nephrons**—the sophisticated capillaries that are basic filtering units in the kidneys—also declines between the ages of 30 and 80 years. One portion of the nephron is the glomeruli. The decreased blood supply causes more abnormal glomeruli to be present as a person ages. Aging kidneys respond less efficiently to hemodynamic stress (ie, stress relating to the circulation of blood) and to fluid and electrolyte imbalances. Therefore, a decrease occurs in the body's ability to eliminate wastes, as well as a decreased ability to conserve fluids when needed.

Changes in gastrointestinal function may inhibit nutritional intake and utilization in older adults, resulting in vitamin and mineral deficiencies. In the mouth, for example, taste bud sensitivity to salty and sweet sensations decreases. Teeth become weaker during this phase of life, making it more difficult for late adults to chew certain foods. The secretion of saliva decreases, which reduces the body's ability to process complex carbohydrates. Gastric motility (movement of the gastrointestinal system and the contents within it) slows with age because of the loss of intestinal tract neurons, which can lead older adults to feel constipated or not hungry. Likewise, gastric acid secretion diminishes. Blood flow in the vessels supplying the mesentery (membranes that connect organs to the abdominal wall) may drop by as much as 50%, decreasing the ability of the intestines to extract nutrients from digested food. Gallstones become increasingly common with age, and anal sphincter changes reduce elasticity and can produce fecal incontinence. Bowel movements are often a great concern to patients in this age group. Many patients keep meticulous track of their bowel movements and can become concerned if they do not have a bowel movement for a day or two. Although this situation does not necessarily constitute a medical emergency, it can still be a valid fear that the patient has. Ask about bowel habits during the interview, and remember that the patient has the right to define his or her own emergency.

Nervous System

Nervous system changes can result in the most debilitating of age-related ailments. In the central nervous system, the brain weight may shrink 10% to 20% by age 80 years.[23] A selective loss of 5% to 50% of neurons occurs, and the surviving neurons shrink in size. The frontal lobe may have a loss of as much as 20% of its synapses (the junctions between neurons) during the course of a person's life. Motor and sensory neural networks become slower and less responsive. The metabolic rate in the older adult's brain does not change, however, and oxygen consumption remains constant throughout life.

One natural consequence of aging is a change in sleep patterns. For example, instead of sleeping through the night, older people may take a nap during the day and be up late at night. The sleep cycle may move into a biphasic (two-phased) sleep cycle—for example, sleep from 0100 hours to 0600 hours and nap from 1200 hours to 1500 hours.

The brain, which is surrounded by the meninges, takes up almost all of the space in the skull. Cerebrospinal fluid protects the brain inside these membranes. Unfortunately, age-related shrinkage creates a void between the brain and the outermost layer of the meninges, which provides room for the brain to move when stressed. This shrinkage also stretches the bridging veins that return blood from inside the brain to the dura mater. If trauma moves the brain forcibly, then the bridging veins can tear and bleed **Figure 10-18**. Bleeding can empty into this void, resulting in a subdural hematoma, which may go unnoticed for some time in this age group. Increased intracranial pressure is required for signs of head trauma to be present; the intracranial pressure will not rise—and, therefore, its signs will not be present—until the void has been filled and pressurized. (For more information, see Chapter 34, *Head and Spine Trauma*.)

Functioning of the peripheral nervous system also slows with age. Sensation becomes diminished and misinterpreted. The ability to know where the body is in space (proprioception) can be diminished. Increased reaction times cause longer delays between stimulation and motion. The resulting slowdown in reflexes and decreased kinesthetic sense may contribute to the incidence of falls

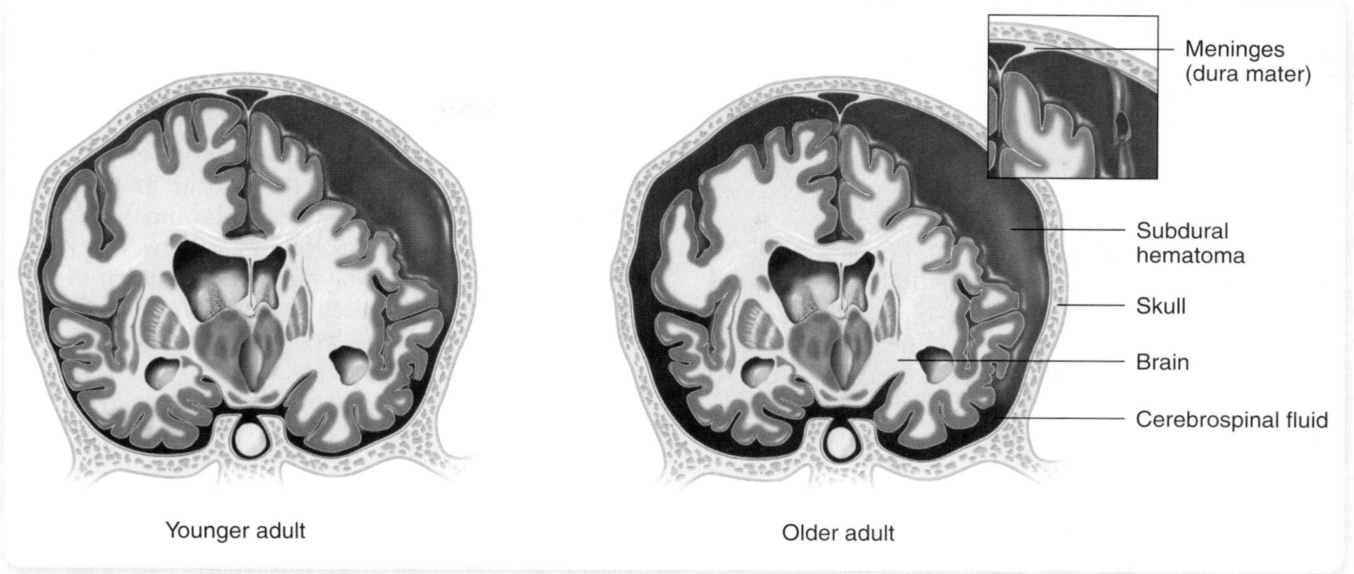

Figure 10-18 Age-related atrophy or shrinkage of the brain results in a space between the brain and its cover, the dura mater. Bleeding into this area can occur more easily from trauma because veins are stretched. Because of the additional space, bleeding in an older adult's brain does not always produce immediate signs of increased intracranial pressure.

and trauma. Nerve endings deteriorate, and the ability of the skin to sense the surroundings becomes hindered. Hot, cold, sharp, and wet items can all create dangerous situations for late adults because reaction time and pain perception are both diminished in this population.

Sensory Changes

In addition to a diminished sensation of touch, the other senses are also affected by aging. Often it is assumed that older people are hard of hearing and have difficulty seeing. It is true that in all late adults, changes occur that diminish the effectiveness of the eyes and ears; however, most older people can still hear well and are able to see clearly. They may need eyeglasses or hearing aids, but it is wrong to assume that your older patient is deaf and nearly blind. Pupillary reaction and ocular movements become more restricted with age. The pupils are generally smaller in older patients, and the opacity of the lens of the eye diminishes visual acuity and makes the pupils sluggish when responding to light. Visual distortions are also common in older people. Thickening of the lens makes it harder for the eye to focus, especially at close range. Peripheral fields of vision become narrower, and a greater sensitivity to glare constricts the visual field.

Hearing loss is about four times more common than loss of vision in late adults. Changes in several hearing-related structures may lead to a loss of high-frequency hearing, or even deafness.

Finally, loss of taste bud sensation and a decline in olfactory (sense of smell) perception are normal occurrences. Unfortunately, these changes make eating less pleasurable, which can contribute to an older person's lack of adequate nutrition.

▶ Psychosocial Changes

As a paramedic, you should treasure your opportunities to spend time with and communicate with late adults. Many of them have amazing stories and experiences to share, yet younger people often take them for granted. Older people have a great amount of wisdom to share, and they may need to be reminded of their worth. Indeed, until about 5 years before death, most late-stage adults retain high brain function. In the 5 years preceding death, however, mental function is presumed to decline, a theory referred to as the **terminal drop hypothesis**.

As the geriatric population continues to grow, we as a society have the responsibility to seek out unique ways to accommodate their needs during their last 20 to 40 years of life. Many older people live at home. They certainly may have the assistance of family, friends, or home health care providers, but they are relatively healthy, active, and independent. Although most older adults live at home, the number of assisted-living communities is growing across the nation. These facilities allow older adults to live in campus-based communities with people in their own age group, while enjoying the privacy of their own apartment and the security of nursing care, maintenance, and food preparation, if desired **Figure 10-19**. Unfortunately, these facilities can be expensive.

Most people need to deal with financial issues throughout their lives. Few things in life produce more worry and stress than money problems. Late adults, in particular, may constantly worry about rising costs of health care and are often forced to make decisions such as whether to pay for groceries or their medications. Modern families often take less responsibility for their older family members than earlier generations did. Today, many single women

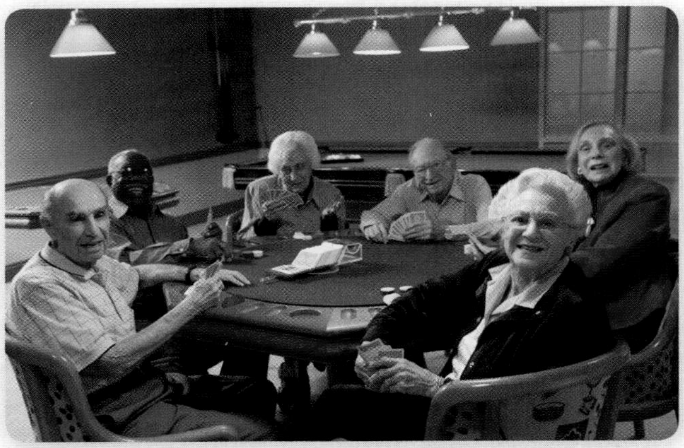

Figure 10-19 Many older adults live in assisted-living facilities.

in the United States who are 60 years of age or older are living at or below the poverty level.[24,25] This problem remains to be resolved.

One of the important issues that older people need to face is their own mortality. The fact is, everyone dies. Yet for most of us, this concept is an intellectual exercise with a distant connection to reality. It is difficult for late adults to watch as their friends, relatives, and companions grow older and die, leaving them seemingly alone. Late adults may feel useless or worry about being a burden to their families as their health declines and they are no longer able to take care of themselves. Isolation and depression are challenges for older people.

Many older people are happy and actively participating in life. With good financial resources and a good support system of family and friends, older people in their 80s and beyond can enjoy life and continue to feel productive.

YOU are the Paramedic SUMMARY

1. What is your first concern at this scene?

Because the family is actively moving toward your vehicle, scene safety is the primary concern. The mother and father may try to open the vehicle doors to get their daughter inside for your emergency medical care. A fall or other unintended injury could occur as a result. Remember, in this case you actually have three patients to care for until you can gain control of the situation.

2. Which stage of development describes a 3-year-old child, and how will this information affect your assessment?

In this patient you should suspect bone injuries. By age 3 years, bone density and muscle mass increase to become more like those of an adult. On impact, they are less flexible because they have less cartilage and fat storage.

3. Why is Juliet clinging to her father and turning away from you?

Fear of strangers is pronounced in toddlers and preschoolers. Juliet has also had an interruption in her normal routine and a loss of control over her environment. She may also be sensing her parents' sense of urgency, reinforcing the thought, "Something is really wrong here." These are all issues that will need to be overcome in the successful treatment of this child.

4. What are some of the measures you can take to alleviate the child's distress?

Gaining the trust of the father and mother is paramount to gain the trust of the toddler. After you gain their support, approach the toddler in a calm, friendly manner. If you can find a favorite toy or object that will normally comfort the child, then use it. In this case, Juliet prefers her pink blanket. The father is actively forcing his daughter to turn around and face you. Toddlers look for their parents and/or caregivers to protect them from harm, not to hurt them. Allowing the toddler to move as she wishes (condition permitting), rather than being physically forced, is always preferred.

5. Measurement of Spo_2 level and blood pressure requires equipment. How can you gain the child's trust to use your equipment?

Unfamiliar equipment can be especially frightening for a child. Any item that attaches to the child may present a problem. One of the best methods to overcome the child's fear is to show the equipment to the child. Show Juliet what it is and, how it is used, and let her touch it prior to using it (condition permitting). If any part of your exam or treatment is going to hurt, then never lie and say it will not. It will completely eliminate any trust that you have built.

6. What is the expected normal range for a 3-year-old child's pulse rate and respiratory rate?

A normal pulse rate for a toddler ranges from 80 to 140 beats/min, depending on whether the child is awake or sleeping, and on his or her level of physical development. A normal respiratory rate ranges from 22 to 37 breaths/min.

7. You need to bandage your patient's laceration. Offer some ideas to make this process more acceptable to the patient.

As mentioned earlier, it is important to explain what you are going to do before you do it. In this case, you

YOU are the Paramedic SUMMARY *(continued)*

need to bandage a laceration on the toddler's forehead. Ask the parents to assist you with the bandaging (condition permitting). Allow the child to hold a toy or other special item during bandaging so the situation will be less scary.

8. How should you transport this patient?

Most EMS providers have a policy on family members accompanying patients to the hospital. Please make sure you are familiar with this policy. Younger children have a strong fear of being left alone or of being taken away from their family. It is preferable to have one of the parents ride in the patient compartment with the child for his or her comfort. This practice is only advisable if the family member can be properly seated with an acceptable automotive restraint firmly fastened.

EMS Patient Care Report (PCR)					
Date: 05-01-18	**Incident No.:** 0909		**Nature of Call:** Fall	**Location:** 215 Shady Glen Way	
Dispatched: 1400	**En Route:** 1400	**At Scene:** 1407	**Transport:** 1429	**At Hospital:** 1449	**In Service:** 1459
Patient Information					
Age: 3 years **Sex:** F **Weight (in kg [lb]):** 13.6 kg (30 lb)			**Allergies:** Family denies **Medications:** Family denies **Past Medical History:** Family denies **Chief Complaint:** Laceration & abrasion to forehead		

Vital Signs				
Time: 1414	**BP:** Unable to obtain	**Pulse:** 130	**Respirations:** Crying	**Spo_2:** Unable to obtain
Time: 1424	**BP:** Unable to obtain	**Pulse:** 118	**Respirations:** 20	**Spo_2:** 99% room air
EMS Treatment (circle all that apply)				
Oxygen @ _______ L/min via (circle one): **NC NRM Bag-mask device**		**Assisted Ventilation**	**Airway Adjunct**	**CPR**
Defibrillation	**Bleeding Control**	**Bandaging** (circled)	**Splinting**	**Other:**

Narrative

Arrived in front of this residence to find the father carrying the 3-year-old girl to this unit. Mother is also present. The child appears to be actively resisting the father who is trying to hold her. Family asked to move from the roadway to the front steps of the residence. Father allowed to hold the child who is actively crying. The mother states the child was running in the backyard of this residence when she fell forward, striking her head on the deck. Assessment of the injured area shows a 0.5-inch (1-cm) laceration approx 1 inch (2.5 cm) superior to the right eye, with a corresponding hematoma and area of abrasion around the laceration. Pt initially resisted attempts at assessment but was able to be calmed sufficiently. Area of injury successfully bandaged with assistance from family. Pt transported to Children's Hospital with further calming noted during transport. Father allowed per policy in the patient compartment with seat belts in place. Report to Jim RN on arrival at Children's Hospital.**End of report**

Prep Kit

▶ Ready for Review

- The developmental stages of life include the following: infants, toddlers and preschoolers, school-age children, adolescents (teenagers), early adults, middle adults, and late adults.
- Each developmental stage is marked by different physical and psychosocial changes and characteristics.
- Infants (ages 1 month to 1 year) develop at a startling rate, experiencing specific developmental milestones during every month of the first year of life.
- Two important points regarding an infant's airway are that an infant's tongue can more easily occlude the airway, and the infant's lungs are fragile.
- An infant's primary means of communication is crying. With regard to temperament, children are classified as being easy, difficult, or slow to warm up to their surroundings and lifestyles.
- The vital signs of toddlers (ages 1 to 2 years) and preschoolers (ages 3 to 5 years) differ somewhat from those of infants.
- Toddlers and preschoolers learn to speak and express themselves. Toilet training is usually accomplished around age 28 months.
- A child's development is affected by the parenting style employed by his or her parents. Types of parenting styles include authoritarian, authoritative, and permissive. Divorce may begin to affect children when they are toddlers.
- From ages 6 to 12 years, the school-age child's vital signs and body gradually approach those observed in adulthood.
- School-age children develop self-esteem and reasoning abilities and receive their permanent teeth.
- The vital signs of adolescents (ages 13 to 18 years) begin to level off within the adult ranges.
- Adolescents (teenagers) undergo significant reproductive development. They also focus on creating their self-images and are self-conscious. They also may engage in self-destructive behavior.
- Vital signs do not vary greatly through adulthood; however, the vital signs of late adults do vary depending on each person's health.
- Early adults (ages 19 to 40 years) focus on work and family. The body should function at an optimal level, and lifelong habits are developed.
- Middle adults (ages 41 to 60 years) focus on achieving life goals. During this stage, medical conditions such as diabetes, hypertension, and cancer become more common.
- Late adults (ages 61 years and older) undergo significant physical changes. They also focus on their mortality. Suicide and depression are concerns in this age group.

▶ Vital Vocabulary

adolescents People who are 13 to 18 years of age.

aneurysm A swelling or enlargement of part of a blood vessel, resulting from weakening of the vessel wall.

anxious avoidant attachment A bond between an infant and his or her parent or caregiver in which the infant is repeatedly rejected and develops an isolated lifestyle that does not depend on the support and care of others.

atherosclerosis A disorder in which cholesterol and calcium build up inside the walls of the blood vessels, forming plaque, which eventually leads to partial or complete blockage of blood flow.

authoritarian A parenting style that demands absolute obedience.

authoritative A parenting style that balances parental authority with the child's freedom by setting and enforcing rules, but also allowing the child to have some freedom.

barotrauma Trauma resulting from increased pressure; for example from too much pressure in the lungs.

bonding The formation of a close, personal relationship.

conventional reasoning A type of reasoning in which a child looks for approval from peers and society.

despair phase The second phase of an infant's response to a situational crisis; characterized by monotonous wailing.

early adults People who are 18 to 40 years of age.

fontanelles Areas where the infant's skull has not fused together; usually disappear at approximately 18 months of age; also called soft spots.

growth plates Structures located on either end of an infant's bone that aid in lengthening bones as the child grows.

hypercapnia Increased carbon dioxide levels in the bloodstream.

infants People who are 1 month to 1 year of age.

late adults People who are 61 years of age or older.

life expectancy The average amount of years a person can be expected to live.

menarche A female's first menstrual period.

menopause The cessation of menstruation, which begins in a woman's late 40s or early 50s, and which marks the end of the reproductive years.

middle adults People who are 41 to 60 years of age.

Moro reflex An infant reflex in which, when caught off guard, the infant opens his or her arms wide, spreads the fingers, and seems to grab at things.

nephrons The basic filtering units in the kidneys.

palmar grasp An infant reflex that occurs when something is placed in the infant's palm; the infant grasps the object.

permissive A parenting style in which the parent does not impose many rules, if any, on the child; two subcategories include indifferent and indulgent.

Prep Kit (continued)

postconventional reasoning A type of reasoning in which a child bases decisions on his or her conscience.

preconventional reasoning A type of reasoning in which a child acts almost purely to avoid punishment and to get what he or she wants.

preschoolers People who are 3 to 5 years of age.

protest phase An infant's initial response to a situational crisis; characterized by loud crying.

rooting reflex An infant reflex that occurs when something touches an infant's cheek, and the infant instinctively turns his or her head toward the touch.

scaffolding An instructional technique that builds on what has already been learned.

school-age children People who are 6 to 12 years of age.

secure attachment A bond between an infant and his or her parent or caregiver, in which the infant understands that parents and/or caregivers will be responsive to his or her needs and provide care when help is needed.

self-concept A person's perception of himself or herself.

self-esteem How a person feels about himself or herself, and how a person feels about how he or she fits in with peers.

situational crisis A crisis caused by a specific set of circumstances.

sucking reflex An infant reflex in which the infant starts sucking when his or her lips are stroked.

terminal drop hypothesis The theory that a person's mental function declines in the last 5 years of life.

toddlers People who are 1 to 3 years of age.

trust and mistrust A phrase that refers to a stage of development from birth to approximately 18 months of age, during which infants gain trust of their parents and/or caregivers if their world is planned, organized, and routine.

withdrawal In the context of infant behavior, the final phase of an infant's response to a situational crisis; characterized by apathy and boredom.

▶ References

1. Leifer G, Fleck E. *Growth and Development Across the Lifespan.* 2nd ed. St. Louis, MO: Saunders; 2012:94.
2. Chameides L, Ashcraft J, Berg M. *Pediatric advanced life support.* Dallas, TX: American Heart Association; 2011.
3. Leifer G, Fleck E. *Growth and Development Across the Lifespan.* 2nd ed. St. Louis, MO: Saunders; 2012:95.
4. Kliegman RM, Stanton B, Geme J, Schor N. *Nelson Textbook of Pediatrics.* 20th ed. Philadelphia, PA: Elsevier; 2016:63.
5. Lowdermilk D, Perry S, Cashion MC, Alden KR. *Maternity and Women's Health Care.* 11th ed. St. Louis, MO: Mosby; 2015:524.
6. Duderstadt K. *Pediatric Physical Examination: An Illustrated Handbook.* 2nd ed. St. Louis, MO: Mosby; 2013:106.
7. McCance K, Huether S. *Pathophysiology: The Biologic Basis for Disease in Adults and Children.* 6th ed. St. Louis, MO: Mosby; 2009:1310.
8. Jarvis C. *Physical Examination and Health Assessment.* 6th ed. St. Louis, MO: Saunders; 2011:436.
9. Stillwell SB. *Mosby's Critical Care Nursing Reference.* 4th ed. St. Louis, MO: Mosby; 2006:647.
10. Mahadevan SV, Garmel G. *An Introduction to Clinical Emergency Medicine.* 2nd ed. New York, NY: Cambridge University Press; 2012:539.
11. Hazinski MF. *Nursing Care of the Critically Ill Child.* 3rd ed. St. Louis, MO: Mosby; 2012:14.
12. Hazinski MF. *Nursing Care of the Critically Ill Child.* 3rd ed. St. Louis, MO: Mosby; 2012:8-9.
13. Hazinski MF. *Nursing Care of the Critically Ill Child.* 3rd ed. St. Louis, MO: Mosby; 2012:15-16.
14. Leifer G, Fleck E. *Growth and Development Across the Lifespan.* 2nd ed. St. Louis, MO: Saunders; 2012:105-106.
15. Leifer G, Fleck E. *Growth and Development Across the Lifespan.* 2nd ed. St. Louis, MO: Saunders; 2012:113.
16. Leifer G, Fleck E. *Growth and Development Across the Lifespan.* 2nd ed. St. Louis, MO: Saunders; 2012:114-115.
17. Kliegman RM, Stanton B, Geme J, Schor N. *Nelson Textbook of Pediatrics.* 20th ed. Philadelphia, PA: Elsevier; 2016:77.
18. Marriage and Divorce. Centers for Disease Control and Prevention website. https://www.cdc.gov/nchs/fastats/marriage-divorce.htm. Updated June 13, 2016. Accessed March 14, 2017.
19. Leifer G, Fleck E. *Growth and Development Across the Lifespan.* 2nd ed. St. Louis, MO: Saunders; 2012:132.
20. Kliegman RM, Stanton B, Geme J, Schor N. *Nelson Textbook of Pediatrics.* 20th ed. Philadelphia, PA: Elsevier; 2016:79.
21. Dong X, Milholland B, Vijg J. Evidence for a limit to human lifespan. *Nature.* 2016;538(7624): 257-259. https://www.ncbi.nlm.nih.gov/pubmed/27706136. Accessed November 13, 2016.
22. Meiner S. *Gerontologic Nursing.* 5th ed. Maryland Heights, MO: Mosby; 2014:549-550.
23. Balter M. The incredible shrinking human brain. Science website. http://www.sciencemag.org/news/2011/07/incredible-shrinking-human-brain. Published July 25, 2011. Accessed November 13, 2016.
24. Munnell AH. *Why are so many older women poor?* Just the Facts on Retirement Issues. April 2004, Just the Facts 10. Center for Retirement Research at Boston College. http://crr.bc.edu/wp-content/uploads/2004/04/jtf_10.pdf. Accessed September 26, 2016.
25. Weiss L. *Unmarried Women Hit Hard by Poverty.* Center for American Progress. https://www.americanprogress.org/issues/women/news/2009/09/10/6683/unmarried-women-hit-hard-by-poverty/. Accessed September 26, 2016.

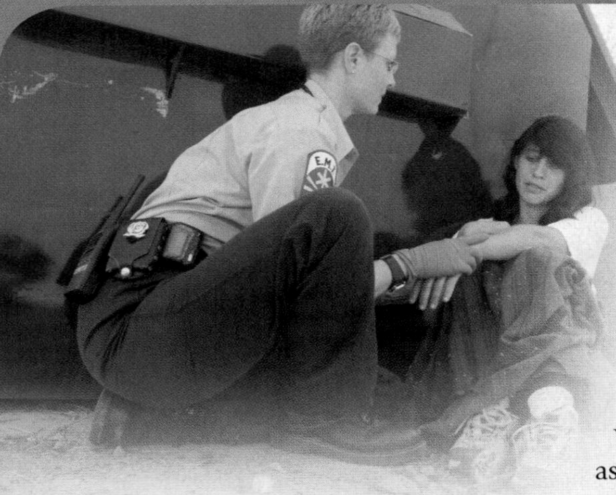

Assessment in Action

Your unit arrives at an apartment complex for a call involving a 16-year-old girl with severe abdominal pain. After entering the apartment, you find the patient curled in a fetal position and reporting intense pain and moderate nausea. Her mother is with her, attempting to console her. You and your partner quickly survey the scene and begin your assessment of the patient.

1. An adolescent is classified as:

A. age 12 to 18 years.
B. age 10 to 19 years.
C. age 13 to 21 years.
D. age 8 to 18 years.

2. Which of the following characteristics describe the development of an adolescent?

A. Permanent teeth come in and remain.
B. Privacy issues arise, especially regarding parents and siblings.
C. The human body is functioning at its peak performance.
D. A decreased interest in sexual relations occurs.

3. Using your knowledge of human anatomy, what possible organ systems could be involved in this patient's illness?

A. Reproductive
B. Respiratory
C. Cardiac
D. Neurologic

4. Adolescents typically struggle with creating their own identities, and which of the following psychosocial concerns?

A. Public image
B. Career success
C. Education
D. Family

5. Hormonal changes in adolescent girls cause which of the following developments?

A. Beginning of menopause
B. Production of testosterone
C. Menarche
D. Release of gonadotropin

6. Adolescents are at a higher risk than other population groups for:

A. pneumonia and bronchitis.
B. cardiovascular disease.
C. prostate and breast cancer.
D. suicide and depression.

7. Personal ethics are usually developed during the adolescent phase, and are often primarily influenced by:

A. childhood friends.
B. clergy.
C. teachers.
D. parents.

8. What are some of your differential diagnoses for this patient?

9. Using your knowledge of adolescent psychosocial concerns, how would you choose to interview and assess this patient to ensure that you are receiving honest and complete information?

10. *Terminal drop hypothesis* refers to the period of decline prior to death. When should you expect this finding, and how can you alter your patient rapport to engage older patients?

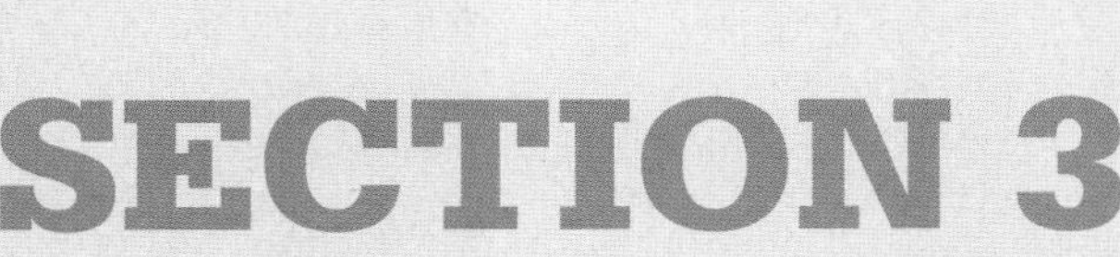

Patient Assessment

CHAPTER 11

Patient Assessment

National EMS Education Standard Competencies

Assessment

Integrate scene and patient assessment findings with your knowledge of epidemiology and pathophysiology to form a field impression. Use clinical reasoning to develop a list of differential diagnoses, modify the assessment, and formulate a treatment plan.

Scene Size-up

- Scene safety (pp 505-508)
- Scene management (pp 505-508)
  - Impact of the environment on patient care (pp 505-507)
  - Addressing hazards (pp 505-508)
  - Violence (pp 506-507)
  - Need for additional or specialized resources (pp 505-506, 508)
  - Standard precautions (p 509)
  - Multiple patient situations (pp 506, 508)

Primary Survey

- Primary survey for all patient situations
  - Initial general impression (p 510)
  - Level of consciousness (pp 511-512)
  - ABCs (pp 511-515)
  - Identifying life threats (pp 510-515)
  - Assessment of vital functions (pp 512-516)
- Begin interventions needed to preserve life (pp 511-515)
- Integration of treatment/procedures needed to preserve life (pp 511-515)

History Taking

- Determining the chief complaint (pp 503-504, 519-520)
- Investigation of the chief complaint (pp 531-532)
- Mechanism of injury/nature of illness (pp 508, 535-537)
- Past medical history (pp 534-535)
- Associated signs and symptoms (pp 532-533, 537-539)
- Pertinent negatives (p 537)
- Components of the patient history (pp 532-535)
- Interviewing techniques (pp 519-525)
- How to integrate therapeutic communication techniques and adapt the line of inquiry based on findings and presentation (pp 520-523, 527-529)

Secondary Assessment

- Performing a rapid full-body scan (pp 516, 540-542)
- Focused assessment of pain (pp 540-541, 549, 552)
- Assessment of vital signs (pp 543-548)
- Techniques of physical examination (pp 510, 541, 543)
- Respiratory system (pp 563-567)
  - Presence of breath sounds (pp 563-567)
- Cardiovascular system (pp 568-570)
- Neurologic system (pp 583-588)
- Musculoskeletal system (pp 575-579)

Techniques of physical examination for all major

- Body systems (pp 568-570, 575-581, 583-588)
- Anatomic regions (pp 554-567, 570-575, 581-583)

Assessment of

- Lung sounds (pp 563-567)

Monitoring Devices

- Obtaining and using information from patient monitoring devices including (but not limited to)
  - Pulse oximetry (p 547)
  - Noninvasive blood pressure (pp 546-548)
  - Blood glucose determination (pp 552-553)
  - Continuous ECG monitoring (p 590)
  - 12-lead ECG interpretation (p 591)
  - Carbon dioxide monitoring (pp 591-592)
  - Basic blood chemistry (p 592)

Reassessment

- How and when to reassess patients (pp 593-594)
- How and when to perform a reassessment for all patient situations (pp 593-594)

Medicine

Integrates assessment findings with principles of epidemiology and pathophysiology to formulate a field impression and implement a comprehensive treatment/disposition plan for a patient with a medical complaint.

Medical Overview

Assessment and management of a

- Medical complaint (pp 504, 510-516, 531-535)

Pathophysiology, assessment, and management of medical complaints to include
- Transport mode (pp 504, 510-518, 531-535)
- Destination decisions (pp 504, 510-518, 531-535)

Knowledge Objectives

1. Name the components of the patient assessment process; include the most important determination made by paramedics. (pp 501-504)
2. Explain how to determine the mechanism of injury (MOI) or nature of illness (NOI) at an emergency medical scene; include why it is important to differentiate trauma patients from medical patients. (pp 504, 508)
3. Discuss possible hazards that may be present at an emergency medical scene, ways to recognize them, and precautions to protect personal safety. (pp 505-508)
4. List the minimum standard precautions EMS personnel should follow and the personal protective equipment that should be worn at an emergency medical scene; include examples of when additional precautions would be appropriate. (p 509)
5. Describe the principal goals of the primary survey process. (pp 510-512)
6. Describe how a general impression of a patient is formed as part of the primary survey; include why this step is critical to patient management. (pp 510-512)
7. Recall how to identify life threats by inspecting and palpating for open and closed findings during the primary survey. (pp 510, 541-543)
8. Explain how to assess the airway status in responsive and unresponsive patients; include examples of possible signs and causes of airway obstruction in each case, and the appropriate response by paramedics. (p 512)
9. Explain how to assess a patient's breathing status; include the key information paramedics must obtain during this process and the care required for patients with adequate and inadequate breathing. (pp 512-513)
10. Explain how to assess a patient's circulatory status; include the different methods to obtain a pulse and appropriate management depending on the patient's status. (pp 513-515)
11. Explain how to assess a patient's skin using color, temperature, and condition (CTC); include examples of normal and abnormal findings, and how this information relates to the patient's status. (p 514)
12. Determine the priority of patient care and transport at an emergency scene, include examples of conditions that necessitate immediate transport. (pp 516-518)
13. Identify the MOIs most likely to produce life-threatening injuries. (pp 517-518)
14. Discuss the process of obtaining a patient history; include the purpose and the initial approach to a patient. (pp 519-520)
15. Give examples of different techniques paramedics may use to obtain full and accurate information from patients during the history-taking process. (pp 520-523)
16. Discuss challenges paramedics may face when obtaining a patient history in which sensitive information must be collected; include strategies to facilitate such situations. (pp 522-525)
17. Understand the unique challenges that arise during history taking involving pediatric and geriatric patients. (pp 529-531)
18. Identify the elements of the history to be obtained from responsive medical patients, from family or bystanders in the case of unresponsive medical patients, and from trauma patients. (pp 531-537)
19. Recognize which aspects of the body systems should be covered during the history-taking process. (pp 537-539)
20. Apply clinical reasoning, based on the results of the primary survey and patient history, to form a differential diagnosis. (p 539)
21. Explain the purpose of performing a secondary assessment; include physical exam techniques, and equipment used in the secondary assessment. (pp 540-543, 547-548)
22. Name the devices used to monitor a patient's medical condition during the secondary assessment and reassessment. (pp 546-548, 590-592)
23. Explain the importance of assessing a patient's mental status; include examples of different methods used to assess alertness, responsiveness, and orientation. (pp 552-554)
24. Explain general (systemic) conditions considered during the secondary assessment; include examples of what the secondary assessment should include based on a patient's chief complaint. (pp 554-588)
25. Describe normal and abnormal lung sounds heard during auscultation. (pp 563-567)
26. Explain the importance of performing patient reassessment; include reassessing mental status and ABCDE as well as reassessing transport priority and any interventions applied. (pp 593-594)

Skills Objectives

1. Demonstrate how to evaluate and document a patient's orientation and status. (pp 512, 515-516, 552-554)
2. Demonstrate how to assess a patient's airway and breathing, and correctly obtain information on respiratory rate, rhythm, quality/character, and depth. (pp 512-513, 544-546)

3. Demonstrate how to assess a patient's circulation by evaluating pulses and assessing the skin CTC. (pp 513-514)
4. Demonstrate how to perform a rapid full-body scan. (pp 541-542, Skill Drill 11-1)
5. Demonstrate how to perform percussion as an assessment technique. (pp 543-544, Skill Drill 11-2)
6. Demonstrate how to compare the patient's serial vital signs with baseline measurements to identify trends in the patient's status. (pp 543-547)
7. Demonstrate how to perform a full-body exam for patients with potentially serious—and potentially hidden—injuries. (pp 549-551, Skill Drill 11-3)
8. Demonstrate how to assess a patient's blood glucose level using a glucometer. (pp 552-553, Skill Drill 11-4)
9. Demonstrate how to examine a patient's head, assessing for open and closed findings. (pp 556-557, Skill Drill 11-5)
10. Demonstrate how to perform a general eye exam. (pp 558-560, Skill Drill 11-6)
11. Demonstrate how to examine a patient's neck for injury. (pp 560-563, Skill Drill 11-7)
12. Demonstrate how to examine a patient's chest and auscultate the lung fields. (pp 563-565, Skill Drill 11-8)
13. Demonstrate how to auscultate heart sounds. (p 568)
14. Demonstrate how to obtain a patient's orthostatic vital signs to assess the extent of any internal bleeding. (p 571)
15. Demonstrate how to examine a patient's abdomen, including inspection, auscultation, percussion, and palpation techniques. (pp 571-574, Skill Drill 11-9)
16. Demonstrate how to examine a patient's musculoskeletal system. (pp 575-579, Skill Drill 11-10)
17. Demonstrate how to examine a patient's peripheral vascular system, including the upper and lower extremities. (pp 579-581, Skill Drill 11-11)
18. Demonstrate how to examine and palpate a patient's spine for abnormalities, and evaluate range of motion. (pp 581-583, Skill Drill 11-12)
19. Demonstrate how to perform a neurologic exam, including using the COASTMAP mnemonic and AVPU scale to test for patient responsiveness. (pp 583-587, Skill Drill 11-13)
20. Demonstrate how to evaluate deep tendon reflexes and score the patient's responses. (pp 587-588, Skill Drill 11-14)

Introduction

As a paramedic, one of the most important skills you will develop is the ability to assess a patient. Assessment combines a number of steps—assessing the scene, obtaining the patient's **chief complaint** (the reason the patient called for help) and medical history, and performing a secondary assessment (physical exam). One of the most encouraging things about your patient assessment skills is *there is no limit to how good they can be.* In the hospital setting, physicians and nurses are able to use additional tools (eg, x-rays, ultrasound, and lab work) to help them develop a diagnosis. However, most paramedics do not have these resources available and must rely on their ability to obtain an accurate patient history, perform a systematic physical exam, and use available diagnostic tools (eg, cardiac monitor, capnography, and glucometry) wisely.

To the patient, the entire assessment process should appear seamless. To the provider, the process usually unfolds by integrating questions and answers into the physical exam. What varies from patient to patient is the number and types of questions that must be asked and the extent to which the patient should be examined before a working diagnosis is reached. Your **differential diagnosis** is the list of possible diagnoses based on the patient's assessment findings. The **working diagnosis** is the one diagnosis from the differential list on which you are basing your treatment plan. It is important for you to develop experience in prioritizing patients,

YOU are the Paramedic — PART 1

You are working the night shift, and your unit is dispatched for a "man down" in a questionable part of town. The dispatcher says he has no further information because the call was relayed from a third party. Your unit is the first on the scene. You see a man lying on his left side on the sidewalk in front of an abandoned strip mall. There appears to be no one else around. Your partner turns on the scene lights, and you see what appears to be blood near the man on the sidewalk.

1. What is your first concern at this scene?
2. How will you address this concern?

Patient Assessment

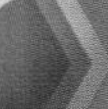

Scene Size-up

Ensure scene safety
Determine mechanism of injury/nature of illness
Take standard precautions
Determine number of patients
Consider additional/specialized resources

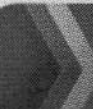

Primary Survey*

Form a general impression

Assess
- Responsiveness/level of consciousness

Assess and Treat
- Airway
- Breathing
- Circulation

Also Assess
- Disability
- Exposure

Identify
- Chief complaint/life threats (treat)
- Priority of patient care
- Transport decision

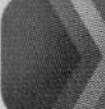

History Taking

History of present illness (OPQRST)
Past medical history (SAMPLE)

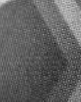

Secondary Assessment

Is the patient medical or trauma?

Assess
- Baseline vital signs
- Monitoring devices (as appropriate)

Systematic physical exam
- Full-body exam or rapid full-body scan
- Focused on injury
- Based on body system (respiratory, cardiovascular, neurologic, reproductive, etc)

Reassessment

- Repeat the primary survey
- Obtain vital signs
- Reassess the chief complaint
- Recheck interventions
- Identify and treat changes in the patient's condition

Reassess patient
- Unstable patients: every 5 minutes
- Stable patients: every 15 minutes

***Note:** The primary survey usually follows an ABCDE sequence (Airway, Breathing, Circulation, Disability, Exposure) but if the patient appears lifeless or has severe external bleeding, use a CABDE sequence (Circulation, Airway, Breathing, Disability, Exposure).

since some patients must be evaluated quickly and transported immediately to the facility best equipped to handle their suspected condition (ie, life-threatening trauma, a stroke, a heart attack, etc). The entire patient assessment process should be organized and thorough, yet be flexible because of the varied environments where patients are found.

Aside from the **primary survey**, which focuses on the identifying and correcting life threats, the sequence of the remaining components of the patient history and secondary assessment is flexible. In other words, you can perform most of your assessment and physical exam in the order that is in the patient's best interest *once the primary survey has been completed and life threats addressed.*

A key to making your prehospital practice successful is developing and cultivating your own assessment style and overall strategy for evaluating and providing patient care in unique and varied circumstances in the field. Within the parameters of applicable standards of care, you can add personal touches—for example, deciding which gear to take with you on a given call or choosing to kneel, sit, or stand while you interview a particular patient.

Remember, your overall job as a paramedic is to quickly identify your patient's problem(s), set care priorities, develop a patient care plan, and quickly and efficiently execute it.

Words of Wisdom

The acronym SOAP sums up the general approach to assessment. That is, we acquire ***s***ubjective information from an interview (the symptoms), as well as observe and measure ***o***bjective information (the signs), and compare the data with our previous experiences to arrive at an ***a***ssessment of what we believe is wrong (the differential diagnosis), so we can ***p***lan the most appropriate treatment for our working diagnosis.

Sick Versus Not Sick

The most important assessment skill for you to acquire, and one that comes only from much experience, is being able to quickly determine whether the patient is *sick* or *not sick*. This quick, early assessment is based on the chief complaint (the reason the patient called for help), respiration, pulse, mental status, and skin color, temperature, and condition (CTC). Together, these items reflect the overall performance of the patient's respiratory, cardiovascular, and neurologic systems. These three critical systems balance the body like a three-legged stool. Together they support the body. However, if you kick out one leg such as the respiratory system, then the other two systems will only momentarily support the body before all systems collapse. For trauma patients, the mechanism of injury (MOI) and obvious signs of trauma should be factored in as well.

If the patient is sick, the next step is to determine how sick. On one end of the sickness scale is a patient with a miserable sinus infection. Is the patient sick? Yes. Is this a life-threatening event? Probably not. On the other end of the scale is a patient with blue lips and drenched in sweat who is struggling to answer your questions but is so short of breath that only one- or two-word bursts are possible. Is the patient sick? Yes. Is this a life-threatening event? Based on these signs and symptoms, the answer is yes.

Every time you assess a patient, you must *qualify* whether your patient is sick or not sick, and then you must *quantify* how sick is the patient (ie, a patient in respiratory distress is considered to be "sick" and the use of accessory muscles and retractions indicate the sickness is "severe"). Once you've done so, you're in a position to decide what, if any, care must be provided at the scene, versus in the ambulance en route to the hospital.

Establishing a Field Impression

More often than not, you'll form your **field impression** based on the patient's history and chief complaint. A field impression is an initial summary of the patient's conditions based on the clinical presentation and the exclusion of other possible causes based on the differential diagnoses. You must be able to obtain quality information from patients with differing cognitive abilities and educational, cultural, and ethnic backgrounds, some of whom may be impaired by alcohol or drugs.

Being good at patient assessment is like being a good detective. As you interview your patient, sift through the information you obtain to glean clues throughout the process. On that basis, ask more questions relevant to the patient's chief complaint. Your questions about current medications may yield nothing important, for example, yet, your next line of questioning may yield a wealth of pertinent information about medical history. Just as a veteran detective methodically collects and analyzes clues to crack a case, you must also follow a similar process to deliver the best care to your patient.

In time, every paramedic develops his or her own patient assessment style. As you work at developing this most important job skill, it's critical to think of patient assessment as a fluid process. As the patient interview unfolds, be able to change the sequence of your questioning as the situation or the patient's condition dictates. Develop a feel for when to expand your questioning to focus on important information. Of course, your style must be based upon sound medical practice as taught in your paramedic program keeping in mind: (1) how you learn and how you practice technical skills as a student will carry over to how you deliver care and perform technical skills in the field, and (2) there is a psychomotor examination for assessment that students must pass, which follows a relatively prescriptive format.

▶ Is This Medical or Trauma?

Just as hospitals are organized into medical and surgical units, in prehospital care there are two basic patient classifications: medical and trauma. For patients with medical conditions, your priorities are to identify the chief complaint and sift carefully through the medical history for clues to the patient's current condition. In contrast, trauma calls are generally the result of unexpected events. When trauma is the primary culprit, the patient's medical history is often less relevant to your care plan, and the specific destination may be very important. Some trauma patients can be stabilized only under the "bright lights and cold steel" of a surgical suite. Other patients may require specific destinations for treatment such as the STEMI (ST-segment elevation myocardial infarction) patient, a burn patient, a cardiac arrest patient with return of spontaneous circulation (ROSC), or a stroke patient, each needing specialty care centers. Prioritizing and determining the appropriate destination for critical trauma patients is discussed in detail in Chapter 29, *Trauma Systems and Mechanism of Injury*.

That said, never forget that medical events can cause trauma. For example, a patient with diabetes who takes insulin may crash her vehicle if she misses breakfast, causing a subsequent drop in her blood glucose level. By the same token, traumatic events can produce medical conditions. For example, the stress of an assault might trigger breathing difficulties in a patient with asthma. In other words, sometimes what seems obvious turns out not to be the whole story. For example, you may be called to a nursing home, where an elderly man is on the floor with an obvious fracture of the right hip. It is important to look beyond this obvious deformity and find out how he ended up on the floor. A twist, snap, and fall to the floor is different from passing out and waking up on the floor, which could indicate that a dysrhythmia caused the syncopal episode. Keep your mind open to the varied patient care scenarios you may encounter in your practice so you are mentally ready to respond to your patient's needs. Remember, any given call may be 100% trauma, 100% medical, or any combination of the two. As a medical professional, you must look beyond the obvious and consider the list of conditions that could account for the patient's illness—that is, the differential diagnosis.

Patient Assessment

Scene Size-up

- Ensure scene safety
- Determine the mechanism of injury/nature of illness
- Take standard precautions
- Determine the number of patients
- Consider requesting additional/specialized resources

Primary Survey

History Taking

Secondary Assessment

Reassessment

Scene Size-up

Dynamic scene management begins by assessing the scene itself, a process known as **scene size-up**. Regardless of when or where you respond to an emergency call, the first step—before initiating any patient care—is to evaluate the overall safety and stability of the scene. Look for any threats to you or any member of the rescue team, the patient, and any friends, family, or bystanders. Additionally, ensure you have safe and secure access into the scene for your team and its equipment, and ready egress from the scene as well. Lastly, consider any special resources you may need, such as a hazmat team or police support, and get them headed in your direction. Remember, the sooner you call for help, the sooner help arrives.

If you don't take a few moments to evaluate the scene and address safety issues, you may find that you and/or your partner have joined the list of casualties. An injured paramedic simply adds to the rescue team's burden and subtracts from available resources.

The success of the overall coordination of any incident can be greatly affected by your ability to perform an adequate scene size-up. This step sets the tone for the remainder of the incident. Without this early assessment, the scene is likely to be chaotic and patient care will suffer.

Scene Safety

The main focus of your size-up is the safety and well-being of your emergency medical services (EMS) team and any other emergency responders. Ask yourself, "Is it safe for me and my team to enter this scene and approach the patient?" To answer that question, use a wide-angle lens to evaluate the scene. If you determine it's safe, establish patient contact and proceed with your assessment. However, if the scene does not appear to be safe (ie, there is an obvious danger present), or if it's not clear whether it is safe (ie, danger may be present), then either secure the scene or call in additional resources before you begin patient care. Remember, it may become necessary to exit an unsafe or uncertain scene until law enforcement have arrived. Doing so is not abandonment—it's self-preservation!

Ensuring scene safety is a dynamic process requiring constant reassessment. Scene and environmental conditions can change rapidly, so maintaining vigilance is an important concept to understand for all EMS personnel. The EMS occupation is dangerous, and every effort should be made to reduce the potential for injuries or fatalities. The National Institute for Occupational Safety and Health (NIOSH) reports in 2013, on-the-job injuries were linked to 65 EMS fatalities. The leading cause of these fatalities was motor vehicle crashes (23 fatalities), followed by aircraft crashes (20 fatalities). EMS personnel struck by vehicles made up half of the remaining deaths, and homicide and other causes were responsible for the rest.[1]

Crash and rescue scenes often include multiple threats and extrication hazards, such as unstable vehicles, leaking fuel, jagged metal and broken glass, fire or explosion hazards, downed power lines, and hazardous materials **Figure 11-1**. In addition, just conducting EMS and rescue operations on an active roadway poses a hazard. Many motorists are distracted by trying to view the incident scene as they pass, commonly referred to as "rubbernecking." These drivers may not be alert for EMS personnel in the roadway. Therefore, even at incidents in which there appears to be limited danger involved in the extrication process, the threat of another motorist disrupting your scene is always a possibility. When working next to a public roadway, wear, at a minimum, an American National Standards Institute (ANSI/ISEA) 107 or 207 certified high-visibility public safety vest **Figure 11-2**.

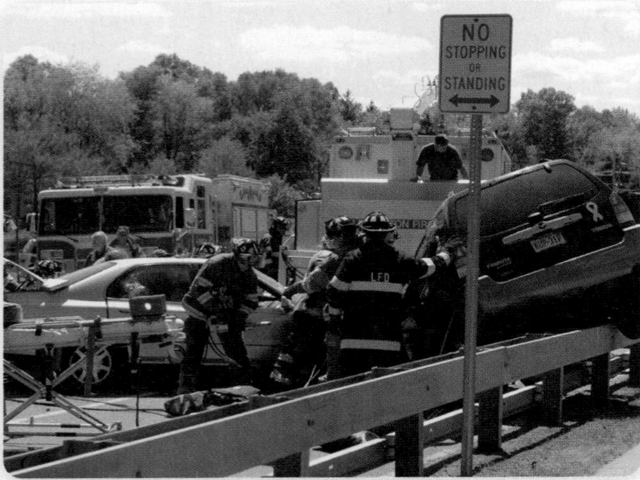

Figure 11-1 Crash scenes pose many threats to you, your partners, and the patient.

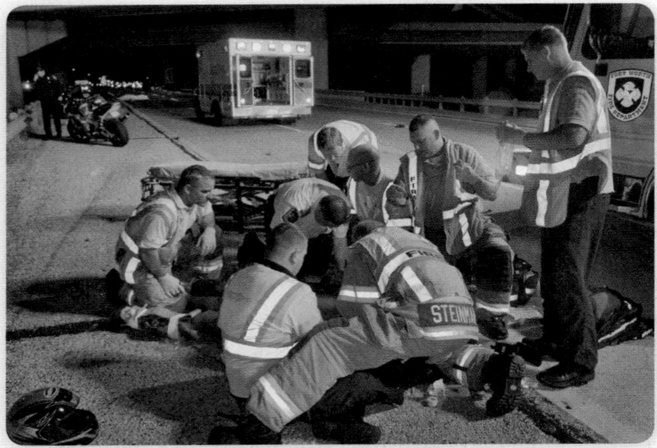

Figure 11-2 Wear a certified high-visibility public safety vest when working on any roadway.

NFPA 1901, 2009 edition, requires one traffic vest for each seating position. The vest must have a five-point breakaway feature. Wearing a vest gives you adequate visibility while minimizing interference with your other clothing and equipment. In addition, several manufacturers offer specialty gloves, coats, and boots with reflective properties. It is always better to be overly safe rather than not safe enough.

Another major consideration is access and egress. You and your team must be able to safely gain access to the scene and the patient, and then safely exit with the patient. If the scene cannot be secured to your standards, consider making a snatch and grab—that is, a quick entry to find the patient, do the *absolute least* care that will allow him or her to be moved safely, and make a quick exit with your patient to a more secure, stable location. In many cases, that will be within the confines of your ambulance.

In all cases, establish a safe perimeter to keep bystanders out of harm's way. At some point, scene tape or barricades may be required. Initially, though, scene security is usually established simply with personnel assigned that task. Without that perimeter, allowing bystanders uncontrolled entry into the emergency scene can quickly cause chaos, greatly complicating the call, hindering patient care, and increasing the likelihood of injury to patients, bystanders, and EMS personnel.

Arriving at a scene with hazards and multiple patients can become overwhelming to you and your EMS team. Formulate a basic plan with your team and visually scan the scene before exiting your vehicle. This promotes better coordination of patient care and early identification of the need for additional resources. For example, when you arrive at the scene of a motor vehicle crash (MVC), you may notice multiple patients in potentially unstable vehicles. In addition, the incident may have occurred at a busy intersection, with multiple motor vehicles driving past the scene. It's apparent that the fire department and perhaps specialized rescue resources and police are needed at the scene. Fire department and rescue personnel can help stabilize vehicles and extricate patients, and police officers can control traffic. In addition, since multiple patients are involved, this would be a good time to request additional ambulances if necessary.

Toxic substances are found at many scenes. From the cleaning products found in almost every home to the countless chemicals used in industry and manufacturing facilities, always be alert for the presence of toxic substances. Be wary of working in environments in which the atmosphere itself is toxic. Smoke is the by-product of incomplete combustion. It can contain many toxins, pathogens, and carcinogens. Having proper body and respiratory protection is a must before entering such a scene and initiating patient care **Figure 11-3**.

All too often, EMS personnel are the first to arrive—sometimes unknowingly—at a crime scene. Don't think of crime scenes in the past tense, because there is always a possibility that more violence may occur. Under ideal circumstances, when EMS personnel are dispatched

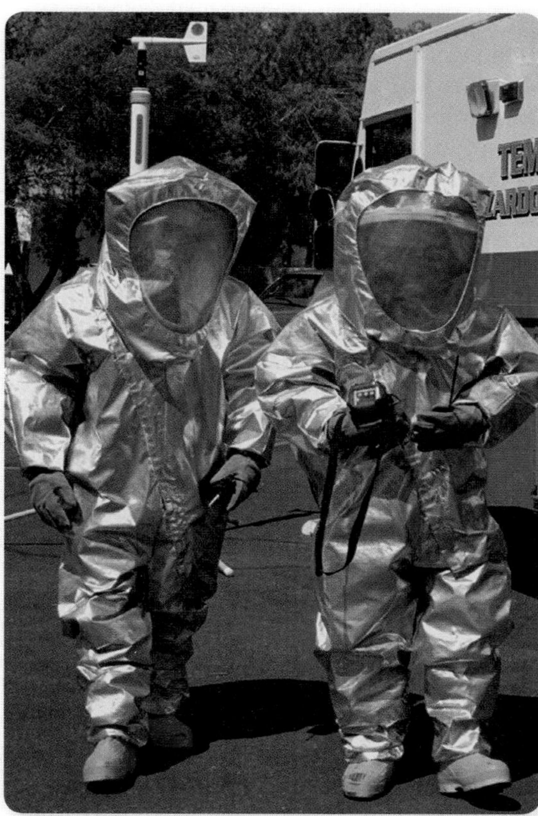

Figure 11-3 Scenes involving toxic substances may require specially trained rescuers with extra protective equipment.

Courtesy of Tempe Fire Department.

to a possible crime scene, law enforcement personnel should enter and secure the scene first. For example, dispatch might receive a call for an injured person; on arrival, EMS might discover that the patient has a gunshot wound. Request law enforcement immediately because it is nearly impossible for you and your partner to control such a scene and care for the patient at the same time Figure 11-4. The scene must be considered insecure because the perpetrator could return.

When faced with an unstable scene or one that is beginning to deteriorate (for instance, people are becoming progressively louder or more unruly, or making aggressive gestures or threats), consider retreating to your rig until the scene has been secured and deemed safe. If you believe you can maneuver safely and remove the patient from the scene with you, then do so—but remember making such an attempt is a judgment call. When dispatched to a scene in which the potential for violence is high, you and your partner must formulate a plan of escape should the scene become unsafe. When you arrive, park your vehicle away from the scene, lock it, and refrain from entering the scene until law enforcement personnel have secured the area.[2]

Carefully and thoroughly survey the scene to look for clues that indicate a potential for violence. In addition to the threat from bystanders, the risk of a patient becoming aggressive is always present, particularly when cocaine or methamphetamines are involved. With the increase

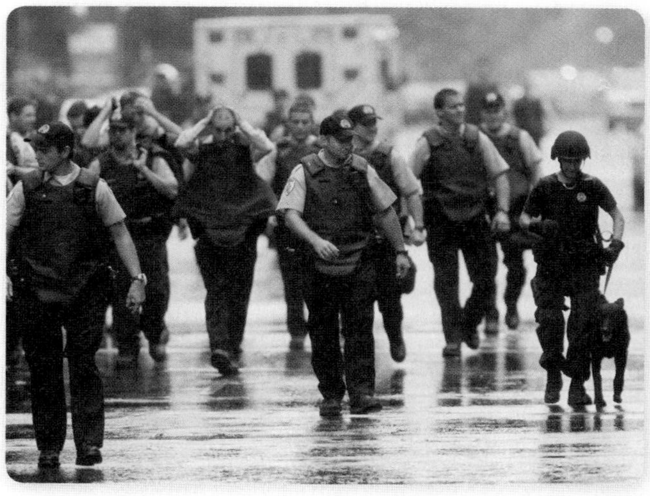

Figure 11-4 After you request law enforcement support, wait in your vehicle at a safe distance.

© Paul Chiasson, CP/AP Photo.

in manufacture and abuse of methamphetamines, EMS personnel are seeing a growing number of patients who are at the tail end of multiple sleepless days fueled by methamphetamine. Such people are often paranoid, emotionally unstable, and almost always armed, making them a far more serious threat than an average patient with a non–drug-induced behavioral emergency. In addition, methamphetamine and crack users are at high risk of experiencing excited or agitated delirium. **Delirium** is characterized by an acute sudden change in mental status, secondary to some significant underlying factor/incident. They may present in a blind rage and be almost uncontrollable. Never hesitate to call for law enforcement assistance in managing any patient who may become violent. Further information about violent patients is provided in Chapter 28, *Psychiatric Emergencies*.

Other risks at the scene relate to the physical environment at the scene. Unstable surfaces are everyday occurrences in the field. In some parts of the United States, snow- or ice-covered surfaces can persist for 3 or 4 months out of the year. Rain occurs most everywhere. The longer a patient is exposed to wind and rain, the more likely it is that hypothermia will become a factor. Conversely, a hot asphalt highway is not a good place for a patient either. When the environment is unfriendly, perform the primary survey, address life threats, and move the patient into the controlled environment of the ambulance as quickly as possible.

In addition, most of the country has terrain issues ranging from hills to mountains to sandy beaches. Thus, working on unstable surfaces is an inevitable part of prehospital medicine Figure 11-5. Take the time to make all of your patient lifts and moves as safe and controlled as possible. Focusing on this aspect of your practice will go a long way toward preventing falls and injuries.

Also, consider the stability of the structures around you and the threat of a secondary collapse. If you have any doubt about the structural integrity of any scene, leave

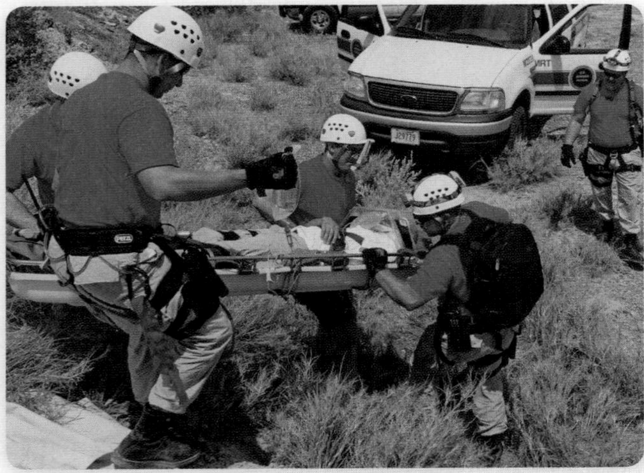

Figure 11-5 At times, you may need a team to carry patients out of areas with unstable terrain.

Courtesy of James Tourtellotte/U.S. Customs & Border Control.

the area, establish a safe perimeter, and request additional resources to secure the scene.

Once the safety of EMS personnel has been established, the safety of the patient and any bystanders is the next priority. If at any time the scene becomes unsafe for EMS personnel, it also becomes unsafe for the patient. The first step, then, is to minimize the likelihood that any such hazard could injure EMS personnel or the patient. If you cannot do so, move the patient to a safe area, as long as taking this action does not place you, your partner, or other responders at unreasonable risk. Next, consider bystanders' safety. Many bystanders attempt to help during an emergency; always remember they are probably not trained to handle EMS equipment, or to treat or manage illnesses or injuries. If a bystander happens to be a health care provider by profession, it's best to contact medical control to ask whether this person should play a role, and, if so, to determine what that role should be.

Establish a perimeter or barrier around the emergency scene to prevent bystanders and the media from entering. It may be best to isolate the patient or bystanders to facilitate appropriate patient care or to establish a safer environment. If the scene becomes unsafe for bystanders, have them removed from the scene immediately with the help of law enforcement.

Mechanism of Injury or Nature of Illness

Most calls to 9-1-1 will be for a medical emergency or some form of trauma. Remember, a call for an injured man could prove to be for a man who fell and injured himself as a result of a low blood glucose level. Similarly, a trauma victim may have crashed her vehicle when she passed out because of an abnormal heart rhythm. Prudent paramedics keep their minds open to multiple possibilities when trying to figure out what is going on with patients. Failure to do so leads to tunnel vision and results in poor patient care.

The **mechanism of injury (MOI)** is the way in which a traumatic injury occurs—the forces that act on the body to cause injury. Assess and evaluate the MOI to help you predict the likelihood that certain injuries have occurred and estimate their severity. The patterns of injury sustained in traumatic events are discussed in detail in Chapter 29, *Trauma Systems and Mechanism of Injury*.

On medical calls, quickly determine from the patient (or family, friends, or bystanders) why EMS personnel were requested. The **nature of illness (NOI)** is the general type of illness a patient is apparently experiencing.

At this point of the call, if there is more than one patient or if the patient is morbidly obese (so that multiple responders or a specialty unit is needed to remove the person from the scene), then you may need to request additional resources. On a medical call, if multiple patients have similar symptoms or complaints, consider carbon monoxide poisoning (or contact with some other noxious agent) or food poisoning as prime candidates. Irrespective of the cause of the problem, the presence of multiple patients means that they must be triaged to determine which additional resources you need and how you'll allocate them.

Likewise, when multiple patients require care at a trauma scene, you must triage them. Identify the number of patients and estimate the severity of their injuries. Then request enough additional resources to support the emergency medical responders already on the scene—for example, additional EMS, fire, police, specialty rescue, public utilities, or hazardous materials personnel. Listen for clues in the dispatch information, such as the number of patients and bystanders, and any hazards identified; this information might lead you to request additional resources sooner or activate the incident command system (ICS) if necessary. Consider calling in law enforcement early if protecting the patient or securing the scene from bystanders is necessary. Don't underestimate the value of overkill. Remember, you can always cancel the extra help if it's not needed!

Be familiar with the various specialized resources available to you. To ensure their safety, these specialized agencies use specific equipment when carrying out their operations. Chemical and biological suits, specialized extrication equipment, and ascent or descent gear may be needed at a given scene. Only specially trained responders may participate in these rescue operations.

The process of scene size-up must be completed quickly. Once you've analyzed the dispatch information, evaluated overall scene safety, determined the MOI or NOI, and summoned additional help, you're ready to manage patient care. If the responding crew can manage the situation without further assistance, assess the need for spinal immobilization and proceed with patient care. Based on the scene size-up and MOI, EMS must ensure manual stabilization takes place on reaching the patient.

Throughout this textbook, the terms *manual stabilization* and *spinal immobilization* are used. Some literature use the term *spinal motion restriction* because traditionally applying a cervical collar and backboarding do not completely immobilize the spine. The same is likely true with all forms of splinting. This textbook uses the terms *manual stabilization* and *spinal immobilization* which represent the *intended consequence* of these actions.

Indications for manual stabilization and spinal immobilization are covered in Chapter 34, *Head and Spine Trauma*.

Standard Precautions

To reemphasize the point made earlier, your first and foremost concern on any call is to ensure your own safety and that of the other EMS personnel. After all, you cannot help the patient if you become injured. Suppose you contract an infectious disease because you neglected to follow standard precautions? You would then miss time from work. Worst-case scenario, you might contract a career-ending or life-threatening disease.

Any patient with whom you come into contact should be considered potentially infectious. Diseases do not discriminate; they can be found in suburban children and urban children, older adults in residential homes or nursing homes, and prosperous business professionals and homeless people. Standard precautions were developed to ensure health care workers would treat all patients the same way—that is, as potentially infectious.

Wear properly fitting gloves on every call. If blood or other fluids could splash or spray, wear eye protection. When inhaled particles are a risk, wear a properly sized and fitted mask (HEPA or N95). In rare cases, a gown may also be indicated. Always take the steps necessary to protect yourself on calls. When in doubt, it is always better to err on the side of caution. Infection control is covered in depth in Chapter 2, *Workforce Safety and Wellness*.

Words of Wisdom

Remember to change your gloves between patients to prevent any possible contamination. Immediately wash your hands or use an alcohol-based hand sanitizer/rub every time you remove or change your gloves.[3] Handwashing is the number one way to prevent the transmission of disease.

Also, consider other hazards involved in patient care and take the necessary precautions to protect yourself. Personal protective equipment includes clothing or specialized equipment that provides some protection from substances that may pose a health or safety risk. It includes items like steel-toe boots to protect your feet and toes, leather gloves, a helmet, heat-resistant outerwear, and a self-contained breathing apparatus.

Patient Safety

In addition to scene safety, the topic of patient safety has become a central topic in EMS. The Health and Medicine Division (HMD [formerly known as the Institute of Medicine]) of the National Academies of Sciences, Engineering, and Medicine defines patient safety as "freedom from accidental injury," while the National Patient Safety Foundation defines its goal as the "avoidance, prevention, and amelioration of adverse outcomes or injuries stemming from the process of care." Patient safety is defined as the reduction of risk of unnecessary harm associated with EMS care to an acceptable minimum which is defined by the limits of the best available medical evidence, equipment, technology, and human skill.

Patient Assessment

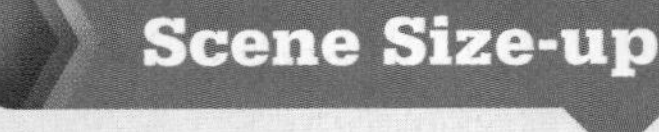

Primary Survey*

Form a general impression

Assess
- Responsiveness/level of consciousness

Assess and Treat
- Airway
- Breathing
- Circulation

Also Assess
- Disability
- Exposure

Identify
- Chief complaint/life threats (treat)
- Priority of patient care
- Transport decision

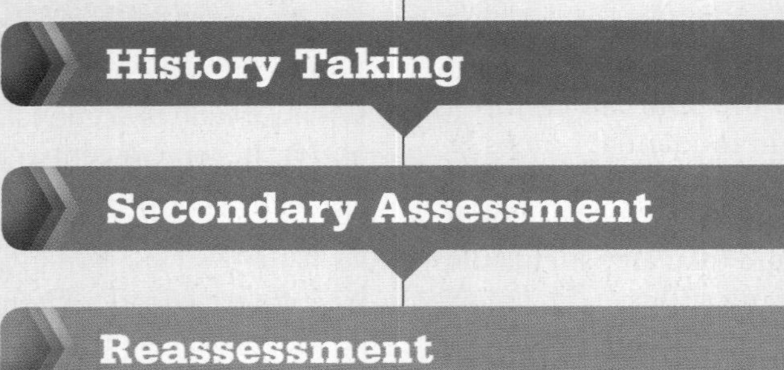

***Note:** The primary survey usually follows an ABCDE sequence (Airway, Breathing, Circulation, Disability, Exposure) but if the patient appears lifeless or has severe external bleeding, use a CABDE sequence (Circulation, Airway, Breathing, Disability, Exposure).

Primary Survey

Examination Techniques

Before we discuss the primary survey, there are three important examination techniques to use during your assessment that are worth mentioning at the outset. You may use these during the primary survey or the secondary assessment, depending on the urgency of the patient's condition.

- **Inspection.** Inspection is simply looking over your patient and noting any abnormalities or asymmetry (for example, swelling, deformity, or discoloration) that may indicate soft-tissue injuries.
- **Palpation.** Palpation is the process of touching to feel for abnormalities (swelling or deformities, for instance). At times, palpation is gentle, but a firm touch will help you to identify areas in which the patient has pain or tenderness. Your fingertips are well suited for detecting texture and consistency, while the back of your hand is better at noting skin temperature.
- **Auscultation.** Auscultation is the act of listening to sounds within the body (eg, bowel, lung, and blood pressure sounds) using a stethoscope.

Form a General Impression

The primary survey can be the most intense portion of the assessment process because it focuses on identifying and managing life-threatening problems. In the first 60 to 90 seconds, as you look at, talk with, and touch your patient, you will form a **general impression**, which is your overall initial impression that determines the priority for patient care; based on the patient's surroundings, the mechanism of injury, signs and symptoms, and the chief complaint. Forming a general impression enables you to identify threats to the ABCDE (Airway, Breathing, Circulation, Disability, and Exposure). As additional information becomes available, remain objective and avoid tunnel vision—that is, making a field diagnosis with limited clinical information.

Each of us, without even trying or being conscious of doing so, makes dozens of observations about the appearance of another person during the first few seconds of an encounter—for example, whether the other person is sitting or standing, overweight or thin, smiling or frowning, dressed neatly or unkempt. When assessing a patient, you must make similar observations, but in a much more conscious, objective, and systematic manner. Look for specific clues to give you an immediate sense of the seriousness of the situation. A patient who gasps "I just. . .can't. . .catch. . . my breath" is clearly very sick. An even more obvious example of a priority is a patient who reports thoracic pain after having been stabbed in the chest.

An important note regarding the National Registry Paramedic Portfolio follows. You will be tested on this should you choose to pursue National Registration. The assessment format described in this section is designed for sick or injured patients. In some situations, patients may have no complaints and may not be in any distress. Those patients may be given a *well-patient exam*, which is more comprehensive than the medical or trauma exams, and takes more time. In the National Registry Paramedic Portfolio, there is a form for a lab session involving the comprehensive normal adult physical assessment. The well-patient exam includes more detail than needs to be practiced in the streets. For example, the general impression for the well-patient exam includes: the patient's appearance, whether the patient speaks when approached, facial expression, skin color, eye contact, weight estimated in kilograms, work of breathing, posture, ease of movement, odors of body or breath, dress, hygiene, and grooming. Performing these assessments during an emergency call could take time that would be better spent providing lifesaving care and transportation.

In the field, when time is of the essence and patients are often in distress, use the assessment format presented in this chapter, which follows the National Registry Paramedic Portfolio for medical and trauma assessment. The National Registry Paramedic Portfolio is available at nremt.org.

The goal here is to answer two questions: First, is my patient stable or unstable? If my patient is stable, might he or she become unstable? These questions can be simplified by rephrasing them as a single question. Second, is my patient sick or not sick? In the case of trauma, the question takes a slightly different form: Is my patient hurt? If so, how seriously?

Whether the call is for a medical or trauma patient the first question is a qualification and the second is a quantification: "Is my patient sick?" requires a yes or no answer, whereas "How sick is my patient?" attempts to rate the severity of the situation. With time and experience, you will answer both questions and form your general impression within that 60- to 90-second window.

The patient's mental status is often one of the primary indicators of how sick he or she really is. Changes in the level of consciousness (LOC) may provide the first clue to an alteration in the patient's condition. Thus, establish a baseline as soon as you encounter the patient. As you assess mental status in a trauma patient, decide whether to implement spinal immobilization procedures. Other considerations for mental status include observing the patient's speech (quality, rate, volume, articulation of words, fluency), mood, orientation (to person, place, and time), memory (short term, long term). These are discussed further in the secondary assessment.

Once you've established the severity of the patient's complaint, determine your care priorities, develop a care plan, and put it into action. If the primary problem seems to be a traumatic injury, identify and evaluate the MOI. If the primary problem seems to be medical, identify the NOI. Identify the age and sex of your patient, because this information may change how your patient presents. For example, an older woman having a heart attack might have no chest pain, whereas an older man with the same condition may have severe chest pain. Likewise, a school-age girl will often be more emotionally mature than a boy of the same age, changing how each child answers your questions and reacts to the emergency itself.

The information gleaned from the primary survey is crucial to your patient's overall outcome. Treat life threats as you find them, but also decide what additional care

Words of Wisdom

The primary survey consists of: GI, MS, ABCDE (or CABDE), and priority decision.

To be specific, first form a general impression (GI) of the patient, then quickly determine the mental status (MS) using the AVPU scale (discussed next). Then, assess and manage life threats found in the ABC order. The exception to this is when the patient looks lifeless or has life-threatening external bleeding, in which case follow the CAB order. If the patient has no pulse, begin chest compressions. If the patient has life-threatening bleeding, apply a tourniquet immediately.

The DE portion of the acronym is to remind you that disability and exposure are important because they help identify all potentially life-threatening injuries. It is important to assess disability, and to expose the patient, then cover up the patient. The treatment of airway, breathing, and circulation threats to life are emphasized because they must be managed within seconds. Remember the saying "When seconds count, your treatment can't be minutes away." This sums up the importance of assessing and managing life threats identified during the primary survey.

is needed, what must be done on scene versus en route, when to initiate transport, and which facility is most appropriate given your patient's unique needs.

A patient's mental status is initially assessed using the **AVPU** scale:

A *Alert* (responds appropriately; further define mental status as follows)
Alert and Oriented × *4* = Person, place, time, and event
Alert and Oriented × *3* = Person, place, and time
Alert and Oriented × *2* = Person and place
Alert and Oriented × *1* = Person only
V Responsive to *verbal* stimuli
P Responsive to *pain*
U *Unresponsive*

As shown above, mental status can be assessed by determining whether the patient is **alert and oriented (A × O)** in four areas: person, place, time, and event. Regarding orientation to time, if the patient knows the correct day but he or she is unsure about the time, then this could indicate disorientation. Similarly, if the patient knows the time but he or she is unsure of the day, month, or year, then this also indicates disorientation. Ask the day, month, and year if you suspect disorientation, and document the patient's responses in your patient care report.

When patients exhibit mental status changes, they remain awake but become disoriented. Generally, patients first become disoriented to events. Then they forget the time and then they forget where they are. Forgetting who they are is the last orientation lost.

Describing how a patient is acting is more helpful than simply documenting the patient's level of responsiveness. For example, you may describe a patient as "alert and cooperative," or "awake and combative," or even "awake but slow to respond to questions."

As you classify the response to stimuli, grade the patient according to the best response you can elicit. For example, a patient passed out on the street who moans in response to a loud shout from you would score a "V" on the AVPU scale. Response to tactile stimuli (for instance, pinching the nail bed, twisting the skin of the forearm, pinching the muscle mass above the clavicle) would earn a "P." Is it an appropriate response (that is, withdrawal from the pain source) or does it merely represent neurologic posturing (ie, decorticate posturing [flexing the arms and extending the legs] or decerebrate posturing [extension of both arms and legs])? No response to verbal or tactile stimuli would be classified as "U." A mental status of "U," means you applied painful stimuli and received no response.

Assess the Airway

Assess the patient's airway status by focusing on two questions: Is the airway open and patent? If it is open, is it likely to remain so? Immediate life threats may be caused by the tongue, foreign body airway obstruction, liquids, and anatomic (crush/swelling) obstruction. For air to be drawn into the lungs, the airway must be properly positioned and unobstructed (anatomically open). Responsive patients who are talking or crying will give the paramedic a clue about the adequacy of the airway. If you hear sonorous breath sounds (snoring respirations), think "position problem"—the sounds are most likely caused by partial obstruction of the airway by the tongue. If you hear gurgling or bubbling sounds, think "suction"—there are most likely fluids, such as blood, mucus, or vomit, in the mouth or posterior pharynx.

As you consider airway management options, move from simple to complex. The easiest problem to solve is the position of the head. No equipment is required and it can be improved quickly. In the case of obstruction, such as by food, use basic life support (BLS) procedures (eg, chest compressions/Heimlich maneuver) to clear the obstruction. Suctioning takes longer, because of the need to set up and use the equipment, and is more complicated than repositioning the patient. In addition, suctioning for too long may create new problems, such as hypoxia and bradycardia secondary to vagal stimulation.

The possibility of a spine injury (or lack thereof) drives the decision of which technique to use to open the airway (head tilt–chin lift maneuver in medical patients or the jaw-thrust maneuver in trauma patients).

Special Populations

If you perform the head tilt–chin lift maneuver, remember the anatomic differences among the various age groups. Ensure you don't create an airway obstruction by improperly positioning the head. Infants and young children do not have well-developed cartilaginous rings to provide tracheal support, as adults do. Thus, a child's trachea is easily collapsed or occluded as the head position changes.

If a mechanical means is required to keep the airway open, you must choose an airway adjunct. If you opt to place an oropharyngeal airway (OPA) or nasopharyngeal airway (NPA), you must retrieve the equipment, choose the right size for the specific patient, and then place the airway. This procedure takes time, so always bring all the equipment needed for a primary survey.

If you determine the patient cannot maintain his or her airway and you cannot maintain it by any other means, use a more invasive technique, such as endotracheal intubation or a rescue airway (eg, a multilumen airway (Combitube), King LT airway, laryngeal mask airway, or surgical airway), as discussed in Chapter 15, *Airway Management*.

Assess Breathing

Assess a patient's breathing in the same way regardless of his or her age. Focus on two key questions: First, is the patient breathing? If no, then you have to breathe for the patient. Second, if the patient is breathing, is the breathing adequate? Examples of life threats to breathing include open pneumothorax, tension pneumothorax, flail chest, and inadequate minute volume.

Expose the chest and inspect for injuries. If you locate a flail segment, then ensure adequate ventilations and support them as needed. If you locate a sucking chest wound, then seal it with a three-sided occlusive dressing and oxygenate, and ventilate the patient as needed. If a patient shows signs of respiratory failure or shock and has diminished or absent breath sounds on one side of the chest, then consider the possibility of a tension pneumothorax. Needle decompression of the chest should be performed, if indicated.

The amount of air moved in and out of the lungs each minute is the best measure of breathing adequacy. This is called the *minute volume*. As discussed in detail in Chapter 15, *Airway Management*, minute volume is calculated by multiplying the respiratory rate by the tidal volume, that is, the volume of air inspired with each inhaled breath. For example, an adult patient breathing slowly and deeply, at 12 breaths/min and 500 mL/breath, has a minute volume of 6,000 mL. By comparison, a patient breathing faster and shallower, at a rate of 24 breaths/min and 250 mL/breath, would have a minute volume of 6,000 mL. On a per-minute basis, the volumes of the two patients are identical, even though the second patient is breathing twice as fast as the first patient. As a general rule, a breathing rate of *greater* than 24 breaths/min is considered too fast for the adult patient. Likewise, a breathing rate of 8 breaths/min is considered too slow. In both cases prompt treatment needs to be initiated; although more so with the patient breathing at 8 breaths/min versus 24 breaths/min.

Besides assessing tidal volume, note the patient's breathing rate, and the work of breathing (ie, respiratory effort). Signs of increased work of breathing may include the use of accessory muscles, chest retractions, restlessness, and leaning forward to inhale. Assess for chest rise and fall, note the symmetry of the chest wall, and the depth and rhythm of respirations (eg, regular, irregular, periodic). Auscultate lung sounds, note the presence, clarity, and any abnormal sounds. Alternate from side to side and compare your findings. During the primary survey, the type of lung sounds a patient has is as important as noting whether they are present and equal. If the breathing assessment reveals hypoxia or inadequate ventilations, then it is important to begin correcting these problems by utilizing supplemental oxygen and/or positive pressure ventilation as needed.

Assess Circulation

Assess circulation by performing a full-body scan. Look for major hemorrhage or other life-threatening injuries, check for a pulse, and evaluate the skin. In some cases, blood loss can be very rapid, quickly leading to shock, exsanguination, or even death. Signs of blood loss include active bleeding from wounds and/or other evidence of bleeding, such as blood on the patient's clothing or pooled nearby. Profuse bleeding from a large vein is characterized by steady blood flow. Bleeding from an artery is characterized by spurting blood. Of course, if the patient already has significant blood loss, then his or her systolic blood pressure (BP) will have dropped, and blood will be ejected less forcefully. If a major artery has been severed, then the patient can exsanguinate in a couple of minutes.

When you evaluate an unresponsive patient, scan for blood quickly and lightly by running your gloved hands from head to toe, pausing periodically to see if your gloves are bloody. Immediately control all life-threatening external bleeding. If an extremity is hemorrhaging, then it is appropriate to immediately apply a tourniquet. Apply the tourniquet in less than 30 seconds to address arterial bleeding.[4] In a responsive patient, this step should come before you assess the patient's pulse, airway or breathing. More information about applying tourniquets and controlling blood loss is discussed in Chapter 30, *Bleeding*.

Assessing the pulse allows a rapid check of the rate, quality, and rhythm of the heartbeat. To palpate the pulse, gently compress an artery against a bony prominence, which allows you to feel the pressure wave generated by the heart's contraction. In responsive adults and children, the pulse is best palpated over the radial artery, and in unresponsive patients, it's most readily assessed at the carotid artery. Use the tips of your index and middle fingers to palpate the pulse. In responsive or unresponsive infants, palpate the pulse over the brachial artery. In any patient, if you can't find a pulse, begin chest compressions.

For most patients, it is best to count the pulses felt in a 30-second period and then multiply by 2 to obtain the rate per minute. A pulse that is weak and difficult to palpate, irregular, or extremely slow should be palpated and counted for a full minute. The normal pulse rate in resting adults is between 60 and 100 beats/min. People who are physically fit may have a resting rate in the high 40s, whereas people who are out of shape might have a resting pulse rate of perhaps 112 beats/min. In general, a rate of less than 60 beats/min is considered slow and is referred to as *bradycardia*. A rate higher than 100 beats/min is considered fast and is referred to as *tachycardia*.

Compare the strength and quality of central and peripheral pulses. Assess the quality or strength of the pulse to evaluate cardiac output. A normal pulse is easily felt, as if a strong wave were passing beneath your fingertips. A weak pulse is difficult to feel and a thready pulse is one that is weak and fast. In contrast, a patient who has hypertension will produce a pulse that is more forceful than usual—a so-called bounding pulse. A weak central pulse may indicate hypotensive shock (discussed in Chapter 40, *Management and Resuscitation of the Critical Patient*). A peripheral pulse that is difficult to find, weak, or irregular suggests poor peripheral perfusion and may be a sign of shock, hemorrhage, or a cardiac dysrhythmia.

Note the rhythm of the pulse. A normal rhythm is regular, like the ticking of a clock. If some beats come early or late or are skipped, the pulse is considered irregular. Although many cardiac dysrhythmias are not life threatening, an irregular pulse can indicate a serious condition. As such, consider all patients with an irregular pulse to be at risk of deterioration until proven otherwise. Report your findings by describing the rate, quality, and rhythm of the pulse. For example, you might say, "the patient's pulse is 72, strong, and regular," or "the pulse is 138, thready, and regular."

As part of this phase of the primary survey, assess the patient's skin for color, temperature, and condition (CTC). Collectively, these criteria provide insight into the patient's overall **perfusion**. To assess the warmth and moisture of the patient's skin, use the back of your hand. It tends be more sensitive than your palm **Figure 11-6**.

The color of the skin **Table 11-1**, especially in light-skinned patients, reflects the status of the circulation immediately beneath the skin, including the oxygen saturation of the blood. In people of color, changes may not be readily evident in the skin but may be assessed by examining the mucous membranes (such as the lips or conjunctivae). When the blood vessels supplying the skin are fully dilated in a light-skinned person, the skin becomes warm and pink. When the blood vessels supplying the skin constrict or cardiac output drops, the skin becomes pale or mottled and cool. If the patient does not get enough oxygen (for example, a narcotic overdose may cause respiration as slow as 4 breaths/min) the blood will desaturate as the oxygen level drops. The skin will then turn a dusky gray or blue—a condition described as **cyanosis**). **Pallor**, or paleness, occurs if arterial blood flow ceases to part of the body, as in the case of a blood clot or massive bleeding. Hypothermia will also result in pallor as the body shunts blood to the core and away from the extremities.

Skin temperature rises as peripheral blood vessels dilate; it falls as vessels constrict. Fever and a high environmental temperature usually stimulate vasodilation, whereas shock elicits vasoconstriction. Normal skin is moderately warm and dry and does not feel "oily." The dryness or moisture of the skin is largely determined by the sympathetic nervous system. Stimulation of the sympathetic nervous system, as in shock or any other severe stress or pain, causes intense or excessive sweating (**diaphoresis**). Depression of the sympathetic nervous system, as occurs when the thoracic or lumbar spine is injured, can cause the affected skin to become abnormally dry and cool **Table 11-2**.

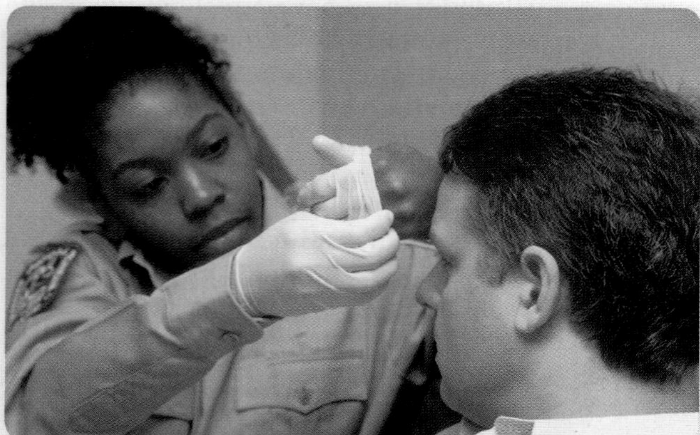

Figure 11-6 Assessing the skin CTC: color, temperature and condition. Use the back of the hand to assess the temperature and moisture of the skin.

Table 11-1 Inspection of the Skin

Skin Color	Possible Cause
Red (flushed)	Fever Hypertension Superficial burns Allergic reaction Alcohol intake Carbon monoxide poisoning (late sign)
White (pallor)	Excessive blood loss Anaphylaxis Hypoglycemia Anxiety
Blue (cyanosis)	Hypoxemia, oxygen desaturation
Mottled	Cardiovascular embarrassment (as in shock), disseminated intravascular coagulopathy (DIC)
Jaundice	Liver dysfunction

Table 11-2 Skin Palpation

Skin Condition	Possible Cause
Hot, dry	Excessive body heat (heatstroke)
Hot, wet	Reaction to increased internal or external temperature
Warm, dry	Fever
Cool, dry	Exposure to cold
Cool, wet	Shock

Special Populations

Capillary refill time (CRT) is included as part of the assessment of children in many pediatric training programs as a tool to evaluate the child's cardiovascular status. Because of variability in peripheral perfusion, the use of nail polish, and hand hygiene, many physicians and nurses view capillary refill in adults as a less reliable proxy for peripheral perfusion than it is in children. Delayed capillary refill can actually be normal in some adults. Capillary refill is discussed in Chapter 43, *Pediatric Emergencies*.

Evidence-Based Medicine

A 2015 study found that CRT was 2 seconds or less when measured on the finger in healthy children and older infants, but may extend to 4 seconds when measured on the chest or foot. Study results revealed that CRT is an important "red flag" for identifying children with serious illness; that is, finding an abnormal CRT increases the likelihood of a serious outcome including death and dehydration. However, a normal CRT does not make a serious outcome less likely. Therefore, a normal CRT should not be used to rule out serious illness in children.[5]

Restoring Circulation

If a patient has inadequate circulation, take immediate action to restore or improve circulation, control severe bleeding, and improve oxygen delivery to the tissues. Remember to follow standard precautions, which may specify gloves, protective eyewear, and use of a barrier device for ventilation. Prolonged impaired circulation is devastating because it deprives the body's cells of oxygen, which is necessary for normal cell functioning.

The apparent absence of a palpable pulse in a responsive patient indicates low cardiac output, not cardiac arrest. However, if you cannot detect a pulse in an unresponsive adult, then begin chest compressions and, as soon as the defibrillator (AED or manual) is available, turn it on and follow the steps of applying the pads and assessing the need for defibrillation. Although patients with traumatic cardiac arrest will probably require intravenous fluid therapy for blood loss, certain medications will be needed to treat the cardiac arrest itself. Identify the patient's cardiac rhythm with a cardiac monitor/defibrillator to enable you to administer the most appropriate medication. CPR and control of bleeding are intended to maintain circulation. Oxygen delivery is improved by administering supplemental oxygen. Patients with impaired circulation should receive high-flow oxygen via a nonrebreathing mask or assisted ventilation to improve oxygen delivery at the cellular level. CPR and defibrillation procedures are discussed in Chapter 17, *Cardiovascular Emergencies*.

Remember, there are only a few medical conditions through which sudden death occurs: airway obstruction, respiratory arrest, cardiac arrest, and severe bleeding. Often (but certainly not always) these conditions are reversible, but to reverse them, you must be able to recognize them quickly and take immediate steps to correct them. This is the purpose of the primary survey.

Evidence-Based Medicine

Research from military operations has shown the majority of combat wounds occur in the extremities, and 7% of battlefield deaths could be prevented with properly applied tourniquets.[6,7]

Assess the Patient for Disability

Once you've examined the patient's airway, breathing, and circulation and addressed any life-threatening conditions, perform a brief neurologic evaluation of the patient. A mini-neurologic exam includes the AVPU scale and pupils (eg, size, equality, reactivity to light), a quick assessment for neurologic deficits, and the **Glasgow Coma Scale (GCS)**. The GCS is the most commonly employed, reliable, and consistent method of assessing mental status and neurologic function. It assigns a point value (score) for eye opening, verbal response, and motor response; these values are added for a total score Table 11-3. While it may take slightly longer to perform than the AVPU scale, calculating a GCS score provides much greater insight into the patient's overall neurologic function. When you report and record your findings, be sure to include the score for each GCS category, not just a cumulative score.

To illustrate how the GCS works, let's walk through a sample scenario. You encounter an older man who tracks you with his eyes as you enter his room. As you speak with the man, you note that his verbal response is disoriented, even though he follows your commands. His GCS values would be 4, 4, and 6, for a total score of 14. By comparison, if the patient opened his eyes only to pain, moaned as the only verbal response, and withdrew to pain, then he would be assigned GCS values of 2, 2, and 4, for a total score of 8.

Finally, as part of your brief neurologic evaluation, assess for any gross neurologic deficits by having the patient carefully move all extremities to pinpoint any motor deficits. Assess bilaterally for motor strength or weakness by asking the patient to move each extremity against the resistance of your hands. Assess grip strength by having the patient squeeze two of your fingers bilaterally and simultaneously, so that any unilateral neurologic deficits will be obvious. Quickly assess for any loss of sensation

Table 11-3 Glasgow Coma Scale

Eye Opening		Best Verbal Response		Best Motor Response	
Spontaneous	4	Oriented conversation	5	Follows commands	6
To verbal command	3	Disoriented conversation	4	Localizes pain	5
To pain	2	Nonsensical speech	3	Withdraws to pain	4
No response	1	Unintelligible sounds	2	Abnormal flexion	3
		No response	1	Abnormal extension	2
				No response	1
Scores: 15: Indicates no neurologic disabilities 13–14: Mild dysfunction 9–12: Moderate to severe dysfunction 8 or less: Severe dysfunction (The lowest possible score is 3.)					

by touching the distal portions of the extremities with a blunt or sharp object to assess for any gross sensory defects.

Expose Then Cover

As you physically examine the patient, visually inspect each area to ensure an accurate and thorough assessment. Although not every patient needs to be completely exposed for appropriate assessment to occur, it is important to keep in mind that you can't assess what you can't see. Therefore, adequate exposure of each area being examined is essential to the physical exam process. When you are finished, cover up the patient to respect his or her privacy and to maintain body heat.

Words of Wisdom

When a patient is a high priority and there is no time for a complete secondary assessment on scene, perform a rapid full-body scan (sometimes called a rapid full-body sweep) before you apply a cervical collar on the patient. The rapid full-body scan is discussed in the Secondary Assessment section later in this chapter.

Make a Transport Decision

As noted previously, early in the assessment process, identify priority patients who will benefit from limited time at the scene and rapid transport. Priority patients are typically deemed to be in either an unstable or potentially unstable condition and need definitive care that cannot be accomplished in the field setting.

Patients in stable condition are generally deemed not to be high-priority cases. These patients, while injured or ill, are not necessarily in critical (unstable) condition and therefore do not require expedient transport.

In transporting patients to the hospital, safety should always be of the utmost importance. With a priority patient, expedite transport, doing only what is absolutely necessary at the scene and handling everything else en route, including the appropriate patient history taking,

Patient Safety

The National Academy of Science's 2001 report, *Crossing the Quality Chasm: A New Health System for the 21st Century* identified six quality aims that health care should embrace:[8,9]

- **Safety.** Avoid injuries to patients from the care that is intended to help them.
- **Timeliness.** Reduce waits and sometimes harmful delays for both those who receive and those who give care.
- **Effectiveness.** Provide services based on scientific knowledge to all who could benefit, and refrain from providing services to those not likely to benefit.
- **Efficiency.** Avoid waste, including waste of equipment, supplies, ideas, and energy.
- **Equity.** Provide care that does not vary in quality because of personal characteristics such as gender, ethnicity, geographic location, and socioeconomic status.
- **Patient centeredness.** Provide care that is respectful of and responsive to individual patient preferences, needs, and values, and ensure that patient values guide all clinical decisions.

secondary assessment, and reassessment. The following is a list of priority patients:

- **Patients receiving CPR, in respiratory arrest, or being given life-sustaining ventilatory/circulatory support.**
- **Poor general impression.** The patient is in obvious distress and does not look well.
- **Unresponsive.** Unresponsiveness is never a good sign and typically points to a patient in serious or critical condition who may not be able to protect his or her airway.
- **Responsive but does not or cannot follow commands.** Altered mentation is another bad sign; the question you must answer is exactly how bad, especially if there is a possible traumatic brain injury.
- **Difficulty breathing.** Breathing difficulties are one of the most common chief complaints in prehospital care. Patients having difficulty breathing are in trouble; those who are working to breathe are in much bigger trouble.
- **Hypoxia that fails to correct rapidly** (within 1 to 2 minutes of field intervention).
- **Hypoperfusion or shock.** Without question, hypoperfusion or shock is an obvious sign of a high-risk patient. A weak or absent peripheral pulse, sustained tachycardia, and pale, cool, wet skin all point to a very ill patient.
- **Complicated childbirth.** Any part of the neonate that presents from the birth canal other than the newborn's head—a shoulder or foot, for example—represents a situation unlikely to be managed successfully in the field setting.
- **Chest pain with a systolic blood pressure of less than 100 mm Hg.** Especially in the context of tachycardia, this sign may indicate shock or cardiac compromise and a high-risk patient in unstable condition.
- **Suspected acute myocardial infarction (AMI) with electrocardiogram (ECG) showing STEMI.** This patient must be managed quickly and taken to the most appropriate cardiac facility in your region, since "time is muscle."
- **Suspected stroke.** When the signs and symptoms of a stroke are identified, it's important to establish the last time the patient was seen normal and begin transport to a hospital with a stroke unit.
- **Uncontrolled bleeding.** Whether internal or external, such bleeding is a serious life threat.
- **Severe pain anywhere.** Any person with severe pain, especially enough to wake the person up

YOU are the Paramedic PART 2

You immediately request law enforcement personnel to respond to the scene and advise the dispatcher of what you see. You use the public address (PA) system to say to the patient, "If you can hear me, wave at me." The patient gestures in your direction. Law enforcement personnel arrive with two patrol cars. The officers approach the patient, and then motion for you to come to them. The first officer informs you the patient has been stabbed in the chest. The patient's shirt is bloody, but you can't see a knife or other implement that may have been used as a weapon. The patient looks up at you but says nothing when you ask him what happened.

Recording Time: 3 Minutes	
Appearance	Awake
Level of consciousness	Not following simple commands
Airway	Open and clear
Breathing	Adequate
Circulation	Adequate
Disability	"V" verbal; equal strength in four extremities
Exposure	A single injury to chest; blanket applied

3. What is your general impression of this patient?
4. What is your next step in assessing this patient?

in the middle of the night, should be considered a priority patient.

- **Multiple injuries (including severe burns).** Whereas a patient may have multiple minor injuries that by themselves are not serious, several small problems can add up to one large problem.
- **Abdominal injuries.** Consider any signs or symptoms of abdominal injury as serious and indicative of a high-priority patient in unstable condition.
- **Severe hypertension.** Patients can be in a hypertensive crisis or having a stroke.
- **Inability to move** any part of the body.
- **Apparent life-threatening event (ALTE).** An episode characterized by a combination of apnea (central or obstructive), color change (cyanotic, pallid, erythematous, or plethoric), change in muscle tone (usually diminished), and choking or gagging.

When time is of the essence, the transport decision for a patient should follow regional protocols to ensure the patient is taken to the most appropriate hospital destination for his or her condition. This includes those who should be taken to a Level I trauma center (see the CDC 2011 decision scheme for field triage of injured patients discussed in Chapter 29, *Trauma Systems and Mechanism of Injury*), and STEMI patients, or stroke patients who should be taken to the appropriate level cardiac care center or stroke center, respectively.

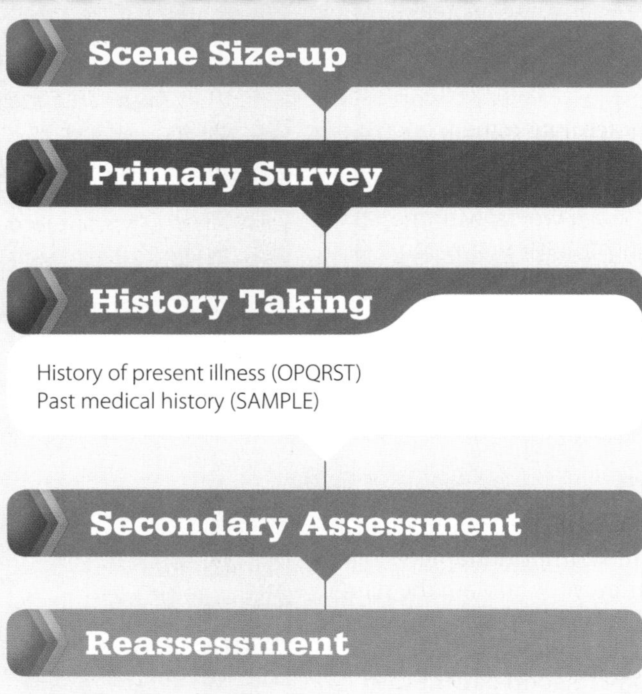

History Taking

Purpose

The purpose of obtaining a **patient history** (the patient's chief complaint, present symptoms, and previous illnesses) is to gain information about the patient and learn about the events surrounding the incident. Your goal is to obtain a clear and accurate patient history of the immediate event and pertinent past medical history (discussed in detail later in the chapter), noting details to help you distinguish life threats from nonemergency complaints. When pertinent, expanded details about the patient history help narrow down your differential diagnosis.

As a general rule, open-ended questions typically yield more information, as they allow patients to respond in their own words with a variety of answers. Closed-ended questions, answered yes or no, yield valuable information but with limited detail. Avoid asking leading questions, because they may take the patient down an irrelevant information pathway. At times you must ask very direct questions, such as with a depressed patient: "Have you had thoughts about hurting yourself or committing suicide?"

Ensure your questions are age appropriate and education appropriate. Also, be patient. Ask a question and then wait for the answer. Rushing your patient along almost guarantees you won't capture the information you want and need. During the assessment process, you may even find time to do some patient teaching, for example, "You may want to consider using a week-at-a-time pill box to help you keep up with your medications."

Words of Wisdom

A good provider is able to gather data about the patient's current medical conditions as well as the patient's medical history. Gathering data is not always as easy as it sounds. You must determine how reliable the patient is in his or her ability to provide an accurate medical history. If for some reason the patient is unable to provide a reliable history, then you must find a caregiver or bystander who can speak to the patient's medical issues. For example, a patient who was involved in a high-speed MVC may not be able to provide an accurate history because of alterations in mental status from a head injury. Similarly, a patient who is under the influence of alcohol or other drugs may not be in a state of mind to provide a reliable history.

Words of Wisdom

How you approach the interview can make or break a therapeutic relationship. Patients must know you are interested in their well-being as a whole and not simply their condition or injury. Learn to listen carefully to what patients have to say without interrupting them and before initiating a physical examination. More often than not, the cause of the patient's symptoms can be determined from the patient's own words, with the physical examination and diagnostic tests simply confirming the suspected cause or differential diagnosis. It has often been said, "patients don't care how much you know until they know how much you care."

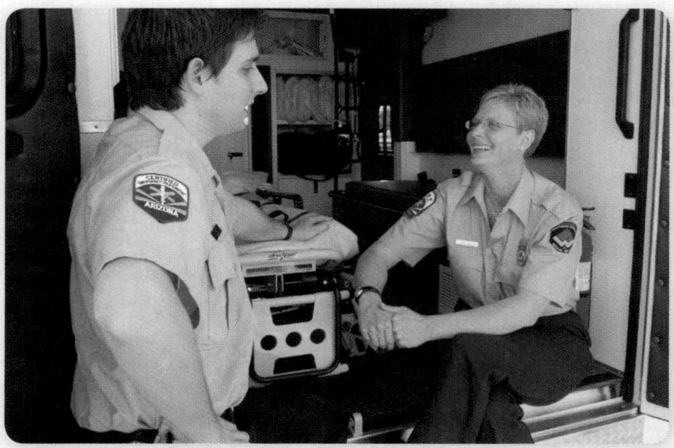

Figure 11-7 Your appearance should be professional and your demeanor positive and friendly.

© Jones & Bartlett Learning.

Patient Information

A number of components collectively make up the patient history. On most runs, the two most important pieces of patient history information you must obtain are the patient's name and the chief complaint. After that, you can obtain the rest of the patient history in whatever order is most convenient and conducive to good patient care.

Techniques for History Taking

Your Appearance and Demeanor

Every time you care for a patient, you must first establish a professional relationship. In most cases, this is a short-term relationship, often less than 2 hours, lasting only until you provide your handoff report and turn over the patient to the emergency department staff.

Although time is short, you will want to leave a positive impression in the communication you establish with all involved. When you first meet your patients, they should be looking at a clean, neat, health care provider. Maintain good personal hygiene and grooming, and wear attire that is professional, clean, and pressed **Figure 11-7**. If you look professional, your patients will likely form a good first impression of you. By comparison, if you look unprofessional, then it may be difficult for your patients to trust that they will indeed receive competent care. Remember, this perception is in the eyes of the patient, not the eyes of the provider, and in many communities *most* patients are older adults, who may have traditional views. Gaining the trust of your patients is an important aspect of care.

Along with your appearance, be aware of your demeanor. On every call, your attitude is on display. If you are unhappy, you may look sad or gloomy. Remember, your facial expressions and body language send powerful messages. If you have come to believe that calls to 9-1-1 must meet *your* expectations, *you are wrong*. If patients think a problem is serious enough to merit a call to 9-1-1, you have an obligation to treat those patients and their complaints accordingly—professionally and to the best of your ability.

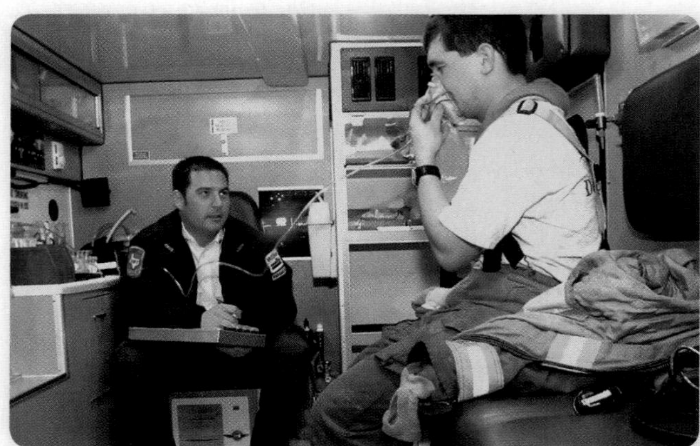

Figure 11-8 You may want to take notes on an assessment card during the patient history.

© Glen E. Ellman.

Note Taking

As you begin to gather information, let the patient know you will be asking a number of questions and while he or she is answering, you or your partner will be taking notes. This lets patients know they are not being ignored and that the information being provided is important enough to write down **Figure 11-8**.

With this approach, remember to make eye contact with the patient. Too often, EMS personnel reel off a list of questions to patients to fill in all the blanks on the patient care report. Do not bury your nose in the tablet computer or clipboard! If possible, position yourself at the patient's eye level. Maintain good eye contact and pay attention.

Communication Techniques

Introducing Yourself and Addressing the Patient. Introduce yourself to your patient, tell him or her you are a paramedic, and give the name of your service. Introduce your partner as well. Then ask the patient his or her name and how he or she would like to be addressed. Err on the side of formality, using Mr, Miss, Mrs, or Ms. There is a world of difference between Mr. John Markham (formal), John (more casual), or Johnnie (really casual). Your patient will say, "Call me Johnnie" if that's what he prefers. Addressing patients by the name they prefer is professional, but until then, assuming formality is respectful and will help establish better rapport than being too familiar.

Avoid catch-all nicknames like "pal," "buddy," "sport," "chief," "dude," "friend," "honey," "sweetie, "cutie," and "darling." You can bog down the process of obtaining a patient history by demeaning the patient and treating the patient unprofessionally. Using casual nicknames can also be problematic when there are cultural differences. Certain terms have negative connotations in some cultures. Become familiar with the cultural groups in your area and with issues that could lead to misunderstanding. It's helpful for paramedics to develop this sort of cultural intelligence—the ability to function effectively across various cultural contexts, interacting with people of all nationalities and getting along with those of all ethical, political, and even generational stripes.

Asking About Feelings. Asking about a patient's feelings is one of the most difficult conversations you may have as a paramedic. But as part of obtaining a good health history, ask if a patient is tired, depressed, or having any number of feelings that are most easily dealt with by denial. (Even ask these questions of a colleague if you see the signs in him or her.)

Keep any unpleasant sights, sounds, and smells from disturbing a patient who is feeling bad. You can also validate your patient's feelings: "This is a tough situation." That's empathy in action. Do your best to attend to the patient's psychological needs continuously throughout the call. It is a challenging part of your job, but such needs can profoundly affect a person's physical health.

Communicating Empathy. Empathy is often described as one step further than sympathy; empathy is a psychological gift that allows you to feel what your patient is feeling—the ability to put yourself in his or her shoes. At times as you gather the patient history, you'll hear sad or even tragic information from your patients. Don't hesitate to communicate your feelings and address the emotional impact of what you've heard **Figure 11-9**. Empathy can help you set your patient on the path to healing—no matter what the diagnosis.

While being empathetic with your questioning, it is important to remain effective. Don't ask, "Are you okay?" This is the most tempting of all yes or no questions! Instead, ask for facts first, and then follow up. When asked, for example, most people would deny they feel exhausted, frazzled, scared, or depressed. After all, your patient met you only a few minutes ago. Establish that you are a caring health professional by asking a series of "safe" questions about physical health before you ask about mental health conditions.

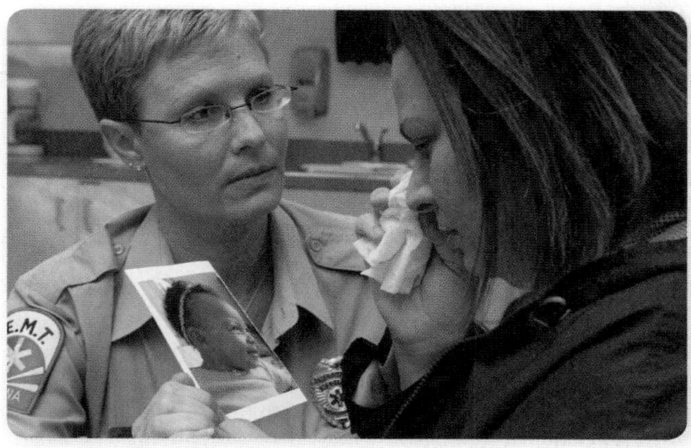

Figure 11-9 Be as empathetic as possible if a patient conveys sad or tragic information.

Words of Wisdom

An empathic statement such as, "I could see how this chest pain would make you worried about having a heart attack" shows the patient that you can identify with him or her as another human being. Such mutual understanding allows the patient to feel comfortable revealing information to you and often helps improve patient satisfaction with the encounter. On the other hand, sympathetic statements, can sometimes be misconstrued by patients as insincere gestures of comfort. True sympathy is difficult to express unless you have personally experienced what the patient is encountering. Providing empathic responses to patient concerns is an art that can only be learned with time, observation, and practice.

Offering Reassurance. With that positive demeanor also comes the temptation to reassure your patients, sometimes inappropriately. Be cautious about what you tell your patients so you do not make promises you cannot deliver.

For example, you may be tempted to reassure a metal worker who caught his wedding ring on a piece of metal that a few stitches are all that is needed in terms of treatment. In reality, many circumferential finger cuts can result in an amputation. Imagine how much distress you will cause your patient when he arrives at the hospital and receives news that is not so positive.

In addition, if your reassurance is inappropriate, then your patient could choose not to share quite as much information as he or she might have under other circumstances, leaving you with less information rather than more.

Sometimes, however, it's appropriate to offer some reassurance. When an unexpected event occurs, it can overwhelm people emotionally. Patients and their family members, along with their friends and neighbors, can suddenly find themselves under extreme levels of stress as a result of the emergency situation. Just as some people react with anger and hostility to a stressful situation, others cry when they're overcome by sadness, happiness, fear, or anxiety. Patience and some soothing words, such as "We're here to take care of you now," go a long way.

Fortunately, the presence of EMS arriving on the scene often exerts a calming effect. During the course of your career, you will be surprised at how often you hear someone say—usually the moment you walk in the door—"Thank goodness, the paramedics are here!" Collectively, your calm demeanor and patient approach; appropriate touch, such as a hand on the shoulder; and a quiet, "I'm in control now" tone of voice will help a person stop crying and allow you to begin your assessment and care.

Reading Nonverbal Cues. Remain alert for nonverbal signs of distress. Pain, psychological distress, or fear often registers in body movements and facial expressions. As you work in the field as a student, you will learn how to read patients' many nonverbal cues. The paramedics you work with will help you decipher them, as will experienced caregivers in the emergency department and at the hospital.

One of the most important elements of the interview process is for you to be a *great listener,* and a big part of being a great listener is being a *patient listener.* For a number of reasons, a patient can be slow to respond. Don't let a period of silence make you uneasy. Maybe the person didn't hear your question, didn't understand you, is afraid to answer, is trying to recall distant details related to the question you just asked, or is trying to decide if he or she trusts you enough to reply truthfully or at all. Ask and then wait, give patients time to think before they answer; otherwise a patient may become silent if you display a lack of sensitivity. If you cannot seem to determine the cause of your patient's silence, consider whether your manner could be responsible, and adjust your approach.

Throughout the assessment process, look for nonverbal communication, such as changes in facial expression, heavy sighs, or aggressive gestures (such as finger pointing), any of which can affect your information processing.

When you communicate with patients, be poised and confident, with a positive demeanor. Always keep in mind that any information you fail to obtain could be the information you need to treat your patient.

Encouraging Dialogue. You'll make patient care decisions on the basis of the answers to your questions, combined with data from your diagnostics. Certain approaches and conversation techniques can improve the volume and quality of information you obtain during the patient interview. These techniques are discussed in Chapter 5, *Communications* and are summarized in Table 11-4.

Documentation & Communication

As you move through your assessment, use open-ended questions whenever you can. If possible, avoid asking questions that can be answered only with a yes or no—but ask your patient a closed-ended question if that's what the situation requires. Avoid leading questions, which are phrased in a way that suggests your opinion, rather than encouraging the patient to give an answer based on his or her own observations. Examples of leading questions are "Do you think this is a cardiac emergency?" or "Is the pain in your chest a dull ache? Does it radiate behind your sternum and into your jaw?" You don't want to put words into patients' mouths or ideas into their heads. Either give them a choice of answers to choose from, or simply ask them to describe in their own words how they feel. Many patients, particularly older adults, are eager to please and will give the answer they think the interviewer wants to hear. Asking leading questions may lead to the wrong diagnosis and hinder patient care.

Avoiding Medical Jargon. Remember to speak in layperson's terms, not in the language of medicine. Patients with no background in medicine will generally use nonmedical terms to answer your assessment questions. Do not try to impress patients with medical terminology. Simple phrases will be much more readily understood by patients, especially those with developmental challenges and those whose primary language is different from yours. On the one hand, asking someone, "Do you think you're having an attack of unstable angina?" may get you little more than a blank stare in return. On the other hand, asking, "Are you having chest pain?" may get you just the information you need to proceed with patient care.

Match your terminology to the patient's level of knowledge and understanding. While a patient who is an emergency department nurse or a retired surgeon will understand medical terminology, a patient who speaks little English may need simple and focused communication.

Dealing With Sensitive Topics

The **social history** is not typically gathered in the prehospital arena. However, it provides valuable information regarding the patient's overall health status and helps to identify risk factors for various disease processes. Examples of components of the social history include tobacco use, alcohol and drug use, sexual behavior, diet, travel history, housing environment, and occupation.

Obtaining a History of Alcohol and Drug Abuse. According to the National Highway and Traffic Safety Administration (NHTSA), in 2014 there were 9,967 fatalities in motor vehicle traffic crashes involving a driver with a known blood alcohol content (BAC) of 0.08 g/dL or higher.[10]

Table 11-4 Communication Techniques

Technique	Meaning	Examples
Facilitation	Encourage your patient to feel open to give you any information you need.	Pay attention. Make eye contact. Repeat key information from the patient's answers. Nod your head. Use phrases such as: ▪ "That's helpful." ▪ "Anything else you can think of?" ▪ "Please go on."
Reflection	Pause to consider something significant your patient has told you.	Patient: "I couldn't catch my breath." You: "That's very helpful. Hold on a second, and let me think about that for a moment."
Clarification	Ask for more information when some aspect of the patient history is vague or unclear to you.	You: "What's going on today, Mrs. Hendrickson?" Patient: "Oh, I don't know. I'm just . . . well, I'm just not feeling like myself." You: "I'm sorry. Could you try to be a little more specific? If you could give me some details, it'll help me figure out what's going on with you today." Patient: "I'm always full of energy first thing in the morning, but I'm so weak right now that I couldn't even take Princess outside."
Confrontation	Make your patient aware that you perceive an inconsistency between her behavior (or the information she's giving you) and the actual scene or your exam/diagnostic findings.	Use a direct approach; for example, with a chronically depressed patient, ask whether he or she is contemplating suicide and, if so, if he or she has a plan. Remain professional and nonjudgmental, but direct.
Interpretation	Infer the cause of the patient's distress, then asking the patient if you're right.	Maintain a diplomatic approach. Use the phrase: "So, if I understand you correctly . . ."

That number represents 31% of the total traffic fatalities for that year in the United States **Figure 11-10**.

Keep in mind that alcohol can mask any number of signs and symptoms, including pain. When a patient who experienced a significant traumatic event denies neck or back pain, and you smell what you believe to be alcohol on the patient's breath, or if the patient's behavior raises your suspicion of alcohol or drug use, perform manual stabilization of the neck.

The patient may offer an unreliable history of pain, alcohol consumption, or drug use. If asked how much they've consumed, people who abuse drugs or alcohol routinely understate the amount. Experienced paramedics say the typical answer to the question of how many drinks a person has had is "a couple" even when the person's behavior and the physical signs indicate the person has had many more. People who regularly abuse drugs or alcohol become adept at hiding the signs and symptoms from their friends, family, and workplace associates, and at denying there is a problem. Such denial can go on for years.

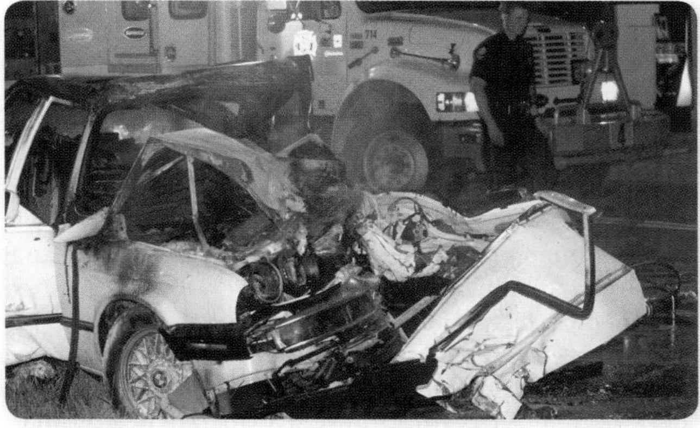

Figure 11-10 Many crashes involve alcohol. In these cases, the patient history may not be reliable.

With intoxication also comes a decrease in patience; as the patient tries to explain things to you, his or her hostility or anger can escalate faster than if he or she were not intoxicated. A common scenario for this type of situation occurs at minor MVCs, when an intoxicated driver wants to get back into his or her vehicle and continue driving. The patient's behavior can become explosive. In such cases, do not aggravate the patient. Your ability to be patient and diplomatic is paramount in such dangerous situations. Dealing with intoxicated people can be frustrating for you and can stand in the way of your best efforts to care for the health of your patients; however, remain objective and nonjudgmental. Remember, you're there to help.

Alcohol is a legal drug. Marijuana is now also legal in some states. If your patient is using other substances to "get high," either the substances themselves or the manner in which they're used (for example, huffing paint fumes) is most likely illegal. The fear of punishment might lead patients to deny use. Let your patient know you are a medical provider and anything he or she tells you will be kept in confidence to the extent the law allows. Do your best to win your patient's trust, because you need accurate information to provide proper treatment.

Keep your best professional attitude as you work with patients whom you suspect of having used drugs or alcohol. Never judge your patients by their appearance or behavior. An unkempt homeless person might be in desperate need of assessment and immediate care for head trauma, not alcoholism. Remember, no one calls EMS to be judged!

Words of Wisdom

The patient may be unable to provide an accurate history for a variety of reasons (eg, altered mental status, intoxication). A patient's information may also not be reliable because the patient cannot remember, does not trust the provider, or is not motivated to assist the provider. Remember to judge the reliability of your source of information at the end of your evaluation, not at the beginning. If you determine the reliability of the information at the beginning, then you may not accurately listen to the history and may miss vital information.

Taking a Sexual History. The social history may include information regarding sexual behavior. Discussing sexual activity is an uncomfortable topic, even for seasoned paramedics. Use caution and tact as you ascertain this information; few patient encounters require a detailed sexual history. However, for some patients, obtaining a sexual history is important. For instance, a woman in her 20s with left lower quadrant pain and a missed menstrual cycle could have an ectopic pregnancy, a potentially life-threatening emergency. A sexual history of this patient will be an important aspect of the overall patient assessment. Interview the patient in a setting that is as private as possible. Remember, patients of all ages are hesitant to share private or embarrassing information. Ensure your patients feel so secure with you they'll give you the information you need.

A number of factors may influence patients to be less than forthcoming about their sexual history. Having had a religious upbringing, wanting to conform with cultural or societal mores, and having engaged in sexual practices that are outside the perceived mainstream may inhibit a patient from giving an accurate sexual history. You may need to ask patients if they have ever been tested for HIV, AIDS, or hepatitis, or in some cases, if the patient has male or female genitalia. Do not interject any opinions or biases about sexual choices or behavior. Their choices are not your choices, just as your choices are not theirs. Today, there are more patients who are open about being transgender. Be sure to use the name or pronoun (Mr, Ms, Sir, Madam) they prefer or, better yet, simply use their name as they introduce themselves. Every patient you care for deserves to be treated with compassion and respect.

Special Populations

Some preteens may be confused when asked about their sexual activities. Be direct and avoid using questions like "Are you sexually active?" Some young people may think "active" means "often."

Domestic Violence and Sexual Assault or Rape

As a paramedic, you're required to report a case if you have reason to suspect physical abuse or domestic violence. Although it would be inappropriate for you to accuse someone of abuse at the scene, never hesitate to call for law enforcement personnel if you have reason to believe abuse has occurred. Police can help stabilize the scene, provide another set of professional eyes, and, if necessary, take someone into custody.

A number of clues may lead you to suspect domestic violence. Injuries inconsistent with the information you are being given are common in such cases, as are multiple injuries in various stages of healing. Unspoken messages may be given by the family's behavior. You may notice the fearful posture of the woman at the kitchen table as her husband or significant other stands over her and answers your questions for her. If the injured family member does not give you the information but waits for someone else to speak up, that may be a clue that the injured family member is being repressed. You can suggest the significant other who is doing all the talking go to the ambulance to help with the stretcher. The moment the door shuts, you may receive valuable information, such as "My husband is beating me and I'm scared to death. You have got to get me out of here before he kills me or one of the kids." *Immediately* request law enforcement personnel if this or if anything resembling this situation occurs.

Words of Wisdom

If you find yourself suddenly in a dangerous position and your partners are not aware of it, use a predetermined code word to alert them. One inconspicuous code is to use the trade name of something in your ambulance—"Could you get the ambulance cot?" Your partners should know that it means there is danger and that they should summon law enforcement personnel.

Emergency scenes involving domestic violence are some of the most dangerous for EMS and law enforcement personnel alike **Figure 11-11**. Do not even think of handling them without law enforcement personnel on hand.

In cases of sexual assault or rape, handle all clothing per local protocol, and bag it with any other evidence (use paper bags rather than plastic). Sexual assault and rape have a devastating psychological impact. Be supportive, caring, and nonjudgmental during your care. Ideally, have an EMS provider of the same sex care for the person who has been assaulted.

Handling Physical Attraction to Patients

It is not abnormal for clinicians and patients to be attracted to each other. Although these feelings are normal, it is *never* appropriate for a clinician to act on them. If a patient becomes seductive or makes sexual advances, politely, but firmly, make clear that your relationship is professional, rather than personal. Should this occur, try to keep your partner, a member of law enforcement, or a family member in the room with you at all times to witness any events that occur, and as a support person to help the patient recognize that his or her behavior is inappropriate. Make absolutely certain that you do not cross the line that separates personal from professional behavior, and do not allow the patient to cross that line either.

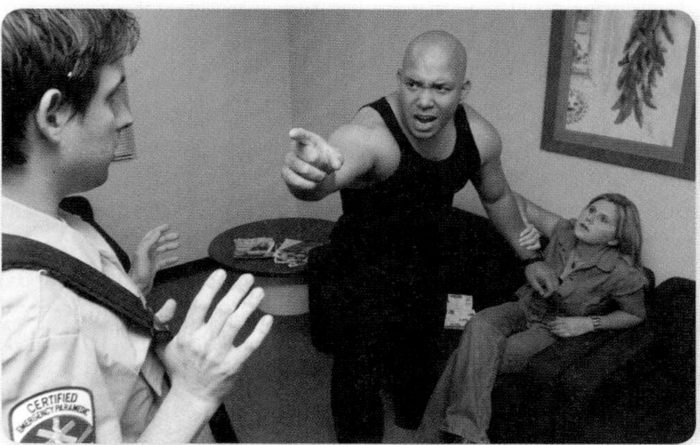

Figure 11-11 Do not handle potentially violent calls alone. Summon law enforcement personnel.

Ensuring Confidentiality

As discussed in Chapter 4, *Medical, Legal, and Ethical Issues*, it is your duty to maintain confidentiality of the patient's information. HIPAA and state laws govern the disclosure of patient information. Be familiar with the relevant laws. Also, show the patient that you respect the confidentiality of his or her medical information to help build rapport and contribute to a favorable overall patient care experience.

Protecting the Patient's Privacy

Interview patients in a private setting. Most people do not want to admit to having some bad habits, such as smoking, or drug or alcohol abuse. If the patient seems reluctant to divulge such information, perhaps out of fear of prosecution, you must be persistent enough to obtain it. Do not hesitate to ask nonessential personnel to leave the room or at least to step back, because you'll frequently find yourself asking your patient personal or intimate questions to elicit necessary information. If the setting makes the patient feel threatened or uncomfortable, he or she may choose to not answer your questions, or to answer inaccurately. Privacy is usually readily available in your office—that is, the ambulance—should you need to move the patient to get a clearer medical history. Ensuring the patient's privacy, confidentiality, and comfort level goes a long way toward establishing positive patient rapport and encouraging more honest, open communication.

Gathering Information From Third Parties

Some patients might not be able to give you any or much information, and you'll have to turn to their family and friends for assistance. It is important to document the sources of such information in your record. Although you need the information to help your patient, be aware the further you go from the primary source, the greater the chance the information will contain inaccuracies. Like working with interpreters, family and friends often function as filters for information. They may be able to describe the patient's chief complaint, history of the present illness, past medical history, and possibly current health status.

Remember, you cannot reveal medical information about your patients to their family, so forming your questions will be difficult. However, obtaining information about your patient is critical, so work with people who can help your patients.

Law enforcement personnel and bystanders can also be valuable sources of information. Never forget that the best source of information is your patient. Answers provided by others may be less accurate, and therefore less helpful.

If emergency medical responders are already on the scene, find out what information they've already obtained and the results of any care they provided, such as whether any bleeding has been controlled or oxygen administered. Ask if the patient's medications have been obtained (prescriptions, over-the-counter (OTC) medications, recreational drugs, and supplements). Gather this information to save time and avoid having to ask the same question again.

Words of Wisdom

Patients' medications, their living conditions, and the name of their physicians can often give clues about their medical history. For example, insulin means the patient has diabetes, and an oxygen tank and nebulizer in the home probably denotes chronic lung disease. The name of a specialist physician, such as an oncologist or psychiatrist, may indicate the patient is being treated for cancer or mental illness, respectively.

Many day-to-day patient contacts in EMS are routine transfers from assisted living or extended care facilities to the hospital and back. Take a few moments to review the transfer paperwork. Know the patient's medical history so you'll be prepared to provide care should your planned routine transfer take an unexpected turn.

Keep in mind the importance of evaluating your sources of information for reliability. Although the medical records in the transfer packet from an extended care or other health care facility should be assumed to be reasonably accurate, the reliability of individual caregivers' documentation inevitably varies. When all is said and done, you are ultimately responsible for patient care decisions, so ensure you work with information that is as accurate as possible.

Cultural Competence

To communicate effectively, you must strive to understand the differences inherent in all people. Only then can you adjust your efforts to accommodate and overcome cultural barriers. The most common barriers to communication are those related to race, ethnicity, age, gender, language, education, religion, geography, and economic status. The collection of all these characteristics can be termed "culture." Culture and ethnicity are *not* the same thing, though a person's culture may be affected by his or her ethnicity.

You cannot treat your patients effectively if you use your own culture as your only reference—EMS personnel cannot impose their morality on patients. Take time to understand other cultures, especially the cultures in your region. This knowledge is important and help you communicate effectively when you care for patients who have different cultural backgrounds than yours. Culture has an impact on our modern society in a number of ways. Cultural beliefs can affect many medical decisions and treatment plans. For example, some cultures believe illness may be caused by evil spirits. When you're treating a patient who believes an evil spirit is the cause of an illness, do not dismiss the belief and fear. Be compassionate. Your approach will ensure the communication is kept open to maintain continuity of care.

Dietary practices and family relationships must be considered during patient care. In some cultures, people may eat certain foods that may not be healthy, and may make them more prone to diabetes and heart disease. When you have the opportunity, making recommendations about healthy eating choices can improve the health of the entire family.

In cultures that have an identified leader in the household who makes most of the decisions regarding diet and medical care, it's important to establish a good relationship with that person to help facilitate patient care.

With regard to health care, certain cultures and religions don't believe in administering vaccinations and medications for disease prevention and treatment. Some of these groups object to the transfusion of blood products, no matter how serious the illness. For this reason, always gain consent before administering any medication to a patient. However, remember, as long as the patient is a mentally competent adult, he or she has the right to refuse treatment of any kind.

A person's economic status may relate to the person's overall physical health. People of low income have fewer financial resources to maintain good health. You must provide the best possible care for all patients regardless of income.

Classes and seminars are available that focus on handling cultural differences. What do all of these classes and seminars actually teach? In a word, respect. You may not get everything right when you encounter a person from another culture, but your efforts to communicate will reflect your respect, which makes a positive impression. Remember the importance of manners. Use phrases such as "Yes, sir," "No, ma'am," "Thank you," "Please," "Would you," "Could you," and "May I." If at any time you notice that the patient seems to have become embarrassed or uncomfortable, adjust your approach, if possible, to help maintain the patient's dignity.

Facilitating Cross-Cultural Communication

The world has many groups of people who do not speak the primary language of the countries in which they live. But when they are sick, you want to give them the best possible care Figure 11-12.

The first person to look to for help is someone who speaks your language and your patient's language—an interpreter. (If there are large groups of people who speak one language in your service area, it would be wise to learn how to ask for an interpreter in that other language.) However, using an interpreter comes with inherent risks, because, ultimately, the interpreter acts as a filter. How a question is phrased can make a world of difference; therefore, it is best to ask closed-ended questions that

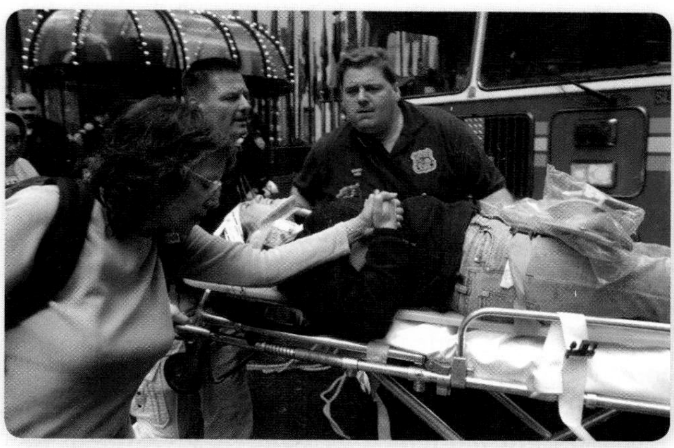

Figure 11-12 You will work with people of other cultures, which may require using an interpreter.

yield short answers. For example, "Are you having trouble breathing?" The tradeoff is these types of questions do not yield a large amount of information; however, if you ask thoughtful questions and wait for the patient's reply, you will be able to extract the information you need to provide care. Lastly, take a moment and remind the interpreter that he or she should not share this private information about the patient with anyone else.

Often, the only person available to interpret will be your patient's child—children absorb a new language quickly in their schools. However, if you can find someone older and not so intimately attached to your patient, then it would be better for getting a good patient history. Keep your questions as straightforward as possible, and do your best not to scare a child.

Documentation & Communication

Be aware, medical terms and jargon often do not translate well, such as "ECG leads," "CAT scan," "JAWS," and "stool."

Maintaining patient confidentiality should be considered when selecting an appropriate interpreter. For this reason, using a certified medical interpreter is the preferred choice. Not only are certified interpreters trained to understand medical terminology, they are also aware of patient confidentiality laws. Confidentiality may become a potential problem when choosing a family member or a bystander to interpret. The patient may not want certain medical information divulged through an interpreter. Therefore, every attempt should be made to find a qualified medical interpreter to ensure the patient's rights are not violated. Realistically, finding a medical interpreter in the EMS environment may not be practical, but it should be considered.

However, do not let a few broken words of yours be a substitute for an interpreter. Also, simply speaking louder during your questioning will not overcome a language barrier.

Finally, remember, manners, hand gestures, and body language have different meanings in different cultures. Develop a communication style that is free of mannerisms or gestures that could be misinterpreted or that could have culture-specific meanings.

Special Challenges in History Taking

Dealing With Talkative or Reserved Patients

Another challenge you're likely to face is patients who talk too much or not enough. You'll need to help some patients filter the information they offer. They may want to tell you about every cold and splinter they've ever had. Some people learn to talk endlessly as a way of socializing, but you must consider possible clinical reasons for the chattiness. Recovering from a fight-or-flight situation, consuming a triple espresso 15 minutes ago, or taking an illegal drug—cocaine, crack, or methamphetamine—might be the reason.

Whatever the cause, the first requirement in caring for a talkative patient is, once again, to remain patient. Give the patient free reign for several minutes. When patients are given free reign, the majority of them will talk for less than 2 minutes. During the first couple of minutes, you will typically gain the most valuable information you need. Try not to interrupt them unless it is necessary to clarify something that was said. If the patient continues to talk for longer, or if what he or she is saying is simply incomprehensible, then try interrupting to ask for clarification of a piece of information. This gives you an opportunity to quickly summarize what you've just heard.

Other patients will offer very little information or take you so literally that it may obscure your assessment. For example, if you ask a patient, "Do you have any heart problems," such a patient might say, "No." When you open the patient's shirt, however, you find a scar running down the middle of the chest from open-heart surgery. You reply, "I thought you said you didn't have any heart problems." The patient replies: "I don't have any heart problems. I did a few years ago, but they fixed it." With reserved patients, it's especially important to ask open-ended questions, since they're unlikely to volunteer additional information.

Handling Patients With Anxiety

Although you may not want to believe it, you may be a cause for many of your patients being overly anxious. No matter how much the public loves to watch emergencies on television, it is frightening to see an ambulance, fire engine, or squad car pull up and stop in front of your house. Expect your patient to initially be somewhat anxious, but he or she should start to calm down shortly after your arrival. If not, consider other possibilities. High anxiety is an early sign of physiologic shock, which must be treated immediately. Alternatively, your patient could be hiding something, such as physical abuse or illegal drug use.

> **Words of Wisdom**
>
> A common cause of anxiety is hypoxia, or low levels of oxygen in the blood. The patient may be sweaty and restless and become agitated easily. Hypoxia is often misinterpreted as panic.

Talking to Patients With Depression. Paramedics, unlike most other health care providers, see people when an illness or traumatic event just occurred. Your patients are uniquely vulnerable and uniquely demanding. Try your best to develop empathy for them.

If a patient doesn't have an obvious medical condition, consider the possibility that he or she might be depressed and that a mental health condition referral might be needed. Depression is a common reason for seeking medical attention. If a patient seems sad, hopeless, restless, and irritable; has sleep or eating disruptions; says he or she has low energy; or has pain for which you cannot find a source, consider that your patient might be depressed.

There are two basic types of depression: situational and chronic. Situational depression describes a normal reaction to a stressful event, such as a job loss, divorce, or the death of a loved one. Chronic depression is ongoing and has no apparent cause.

Most people with situational depression are eventually able to accept what has happened and begin to get on with their lives. Others develop chronic depression. Either form of depression can lead to harmful behavior, including suicide. Ask about your patient's feelings to assess the risk of suicide. If the patient admits to having had thoughts about taking his or her own life, follow your protocol to ensure this patient is connected to a mental health professional.

Earlier chapters discussed ways of being knowledgeable of the various resources that may be of help for your patients.

Dealing Safely With Anger and Hostility

Frequently, you will find yourself the target of patients' and family members' frustrations, which may manifest as anger or hostility. Such reactions to unfairness and harsh realities are normal. Remember, do not take these situations personally—take them professionally.

A valuable coping skill is not to get angry yourself. When you're in control of your own anger, you can work to calm the situation. Be attentive to changes in body language, such as threatening gestures or an escalating volume of the conversation or, worse yet, having a heated dialog melt down into an outright yelling match. When people are angry or hostile, the worst thing you can do is get angry yourself.

On any call, establishing a safe and secure scene is your first order of business. If you cannot calm the patient or family members, it is time to call for law enforcement personnel. If the patient or a family member is hostile, you might need to tell the person directly that if he or she continues to shout, you won't feel safe enough to provide care and, you will have to seek the assistance of law enforcement personnel before you can resume. However, if the patient and/or the family members are already angry, then telling them the police are on the way will not suddenly make them happy. In worst case scenarios, you may have to withdraw to the safety of your ambulance and wait for the police to arrive.

> **Special Populations**
>
> Most patients are older than the paramedics taking care of them. They can feel threatened by strange "youngsters" telling them what is best for them. Listen and be respectful to your older patients. Without talking down to them or becoming impatient, explain what you are doing and why. They may not know what is in their best interest, and a calm, courteous explanation may put them at ease.

If the hostile person suddenly leaves the room, especially in the middle of the conversation, then you or your partner should consider that a threat as he or she may be going to obtain a weapon and potentially come back and shoot you, your partner, and maybe even the patient. If law enforcement has not yet arrived, then it may be best to retreat to a safe location until they arrive.

Clarifying a Confusing History or Unusual Behavior

Paramedics sometimes find that the patient's history given at the scene is different from the history the patient gives to the physician in the hospital emergency department. Sometimes, the information is so different that it seems as if this is an entirely different patient. Patients may be too frightened or embarrassed to give particular information to a paramedic, but they will give a physician the vital information by telephone.

The human brain is an impressive organ, but it may malfunction for any number of reasons. More often than not, confusing behavior is related to a lack of glucose or oxygen, two fuels that are essential to the brain, although it cannot store either of them. There are many other possibilities that could account for confusing behavior on the part of your patients, such as a toxic environment, a cerebrovascular accident (stroke), or a transient ischemic attack. Also, consider the possibility of mental illness or drug-induced delirium. In addition, organic causes such as Alzheimer disease, other forms of dementia, or a brain tumor can contribute to discrepancies.

Managing Patients With Sensory or Developmental Challenges

Limited Education or Intellectual Challenges. *Never, ever* presume you will not be able to obtain a history directly from the patient—any patient. Some patients will not have much knowledge of the health care system or its specialized vocabulary. Other patients will be developmentally challenged. Assume you can get at least some worthwhile history from all patients. Assume it is your job to keep asking questions in different ways until you get the answers you need.

Words of Wisdom

Never, never, never assume it is impossible to talk to a patient until you have tried.

With a skillful question-answer approach (and patience), you can frequently obtain adequate information from patients who have limited education or intellectual capabilities. Be alert for omissions or partial answers to your questions. These patients may not know or be able to recall the information you're requesting. For patients who are severely mentally challenged, you may need to get information from family members, friends, or another caregiver.

Hearing Loss, Low Vision, or Blindness. Another interesting challenge relates to working with patients with hearing or vision loss. Hearing loss can range from a slight loss to total deafness. For patients with only minimal loss, such as older people, speaking slowly and slightly louder may be all that is necessary. For people with more severe hearing loss, you may want to let them wear your stethoscope as you hold the bell and speak to them. If you do this, clean the earpieces before you offer them to the patient and before you put them back on.

Words of Wisdom

After successful completion of a paramedic program, two of the best investments in continuing education you can make for your future are learning conversational Spanish and learning sign language.

Many patients with varying degrees of low vision are self-sufficient and live independently. People who are blind have the greatest challenge. When interacting with a patient who is blind or has low vision, first and foremost, announce yourself, giving the patient your identity and your reason for being there. If you pull up a chair to sit next to a patient with low vision or blindness, remember to put it back exactly where you found it; the same is true if furniture has to be moved to provide access or egress. People who are blind have arranged their living environments situated in the way they want it, so they can get around with remarkable ease. Ensure you leave things the way you found them.

Once you move the patient to the ambulance, he or she is in a foreign environment and requires assistance from EMS personnel for transport and an orderly transition into the emergency department. Inform the person what you are doing and the location of the transport vehicle at all times (for example, "We'll be at the hospital in about 10 minutes" or "We're at the hospital, and we will be wheeling you off the ambulance and into the emergency department in just a minute").

Managing Age-Related Considerations

Pediatric Patients

Most of the problems encountered in the field for pediatric patients are respiratory related or fluid related. Just a day or two of vomiting or diarrhea can put a small child at high risk. With trauma, pediatric patients are top-heavy, more likely to fall and strike their heads, especially in vehicle-versus-pedestrian incidents). A full discussion of pediatric assessment appears in Chapter 43, *Pediatric Emergencies*. The initial approach to any pediatric patient should be similar to an adult—with a few exceptions. Always begin with a scene size-up; assessment and treatment of life-threatening conditions affecting airway, breathing, or circulation; and forming a general impression and treatment strategy. There are differences, however, in the overall interaction you have with the patient and the parents.

Obtaining an accurate **history of the present illness**, which is a narrative detail of the symptoms that the patient is experiencing, can be difficult in the pediatric population. Whereas every effort should be made to include the child in the history-taking process, the most accurate and complete history will come from the parents or a responsible caregiver. Typically, the parents are familiar with their children's habits and demeanor and know when something is wrong. Therefore, listen when a parent shows concern and tells you the child is not acting appropriately.

Many times parents call for EMS out of fear for the welfare of their child. It is important for you as the health care provider not only to understand the fears the parents might have, but also to continue to ascertain and investigate those concerns in more detail. For instance, a febrile seizure in a pediatric patient is a fairly common entity encountered by EMS personnel and a relatively benign condition; however, for a new parent, it can be a frightening, emotionally traumatic event. Parents want to know what is wrong with their child and will typically go to sources like the internet for answers. The problem with this approach is that it leaves a great deal to the imagination, and online sources are not always credible. Therefore, a parent of a child experiencing a febrile seizure is probably not just thinking about the immediate event, but is also worried about all of the possible causes of a seizure (for example, bleeding into the brain, a brain tumor, cancer), when in reality it may be a benign condition. Be aware of these fears and take them into consideration when caring for parents or other legal guardians.

As you obtain information from the parent or caregiver, pay attention to the relationship between this person and the child. Typically, sick children cling to the parent or caregiver and are reluctant to allow a paramedic to examine them or remove them from the arms of the parent or caregiver. A child who readily allows you to remove him or her from the parent for examination should raise your concern that the child may be seriously ill and should also bring into consideration the possibility of neglect and/or abuse.

In neonates and infants, a maternal health history is important. Ask about the mother's health status during pregnancy, the type of prenatal care provided, use of medications, hormones, and vitamins, and alcohol or drug use during pregnancy. A birth history should also be obtained: find out the duration of pregnancy, the location of the birth, labor conditions, any delivery complications, whether it was a vaginal or cesarean delivery, the condition of the infant at birth, and the birth weight. Ask about maternal gestational history and any other pregnancies or children, including stillbirths and any deceased children.

The first month following birth, otherwise known as the neonatal period, is an important part of the pediatric history. Questions should be asked about congenital anomalies, feeding problems, the presence of jaundice, evidence of any illness, and developmental landmarks.

Around the age of 3 to 5 years, children become very capable of providing history of the current problem. Once in school, the focus of questioning should change based on the child's age. Asking about the child's school performance helps to determine whether there are any developmental challenges or intellectual disabilities. Questioning should also focus on the child's dentition, growth, sexual development, illnesses, and immunizations.

If the child is an adolescent, focus more on him or her than on the parent in the history taking. Adolescents struggle for independence and want to be in charge of their bodies. Gather your history from the adolescent to help establish trust and a good rapport. As the line of questioning for an adolescent becomes more private, consider interviewing the patient in a more private location, in the presence of your partner. Focus your questioning on risk-taking behaviors, self-esteem issues, rebelliousness, drug and alcohol use, and sexual activity. Some patients may be reluctant to discuss these issues with you, which is why establishing trust and rapport is so important.

YOU are the Paramedic PART 3

You immediately determine that the patient has the potential to deteriorate quickly. Your partner pulls the stretcher out of the ambulance with the help of a police officer. Meanwhile, you determine that the patient is responsive and disoriented. You cut off the patient's shirt and find an approximate 1-inch (2.5 cm) penetration on the left side of the chest, just inferior to the center of the clavicle. The wound has stopped bleeding. You apply a three-sided occlusive dressing. The patient is breathing rapidly and appears to be very restless.

Recording Time: 5 Minutes	
Respiration	28 breaths/min, shallow
Pulse	122 beats/min, weak
Skin	Cool, pale, clammy
Blood pressure	90/64 mm Hg
Oxygen saturation (Spo_2)	93% on room air
Pupils	PERRLA

5. On the basis of your assessment of ABCDE, what is your first priority in the care of this patient?
6. Can you determine the transport priority of this patient at this point?

In addition to gathering information about the child, ensure you gather an accurate family medical and recent travel history. More information on the relevance of recent travel history is found in Chapter 26, *Infectious Diseases*.

A review of body systems should also be included in the pediatric history. While every system should be covered, pay special attention to any skin **lesions** (localized areas of the skin that do not resemble the area surrounding it); any history of otitis media (inner ear infections); any snoring, mouth breathing, and environmental allergies; and any dental problems.

Geriatric Patients

Geriatric patients can pose a rather different challenge for paramedics. This patient population is growing and frequently represents the primary customer for EMS. This population has a variety of medical and traumatic conditions not seen in other patients.

With aging often comes decreased sensorium, so complaints of pain are less frequent. Diabetes will add the problems of peripheral neuropathy, further diminishing pain sensitivity, as well as eyesight and kidney diseases. Balance and equilibrium problems increase the likelihood of falls. Many older patients are on blood thinners as part of an atrial fibrillation treatment regimen. Even a minor fall may be deadly if blood cannot clot in a timely fashion. Even if it does, a fall can be lethal for an older adult, as evidenced by the data (see Chapter 44, *Geriatric Emergencies*).

An older adult may have difficulty seeing you or hearing your questions during the patient assessment. If the patient wears eyeglasses or a hearing aid, ensure these aids are available during the interview. You may need to speak more slowly and louder when treating older patients; however, do not assume all older adults have difficulty hearing. In addition, it may be helpful to face your patient when asking questions, in case the patient is adept at speech reading (lip reading) to help with communication. Accommodating these sensory losses can improve the amount and the quality of information gathered during the patient assessment.

Medication compliance is a challenge for any patient, but much more so for older adults. They tend to have multiple chronic medical conditions that can complicate the history-taking process. Multiple chief complaints can make it difficult for you to distinguish between acute and chronic complaints. Suppose a 64-year-old man tells you, "I'm really weak, and it feels like there are butterflies in my chest." Determine whether these symptoms are related. If you believe they're related, to provide appropriate care you must identify the *origin of the problem*. In this case, you may want to ask, "Have you had this problem before?" to see if the patient has had problems in the past with tachycardia and weakness.

You also need to prioritize multiple complaints. Suppose the patient complains of being dizzy and having pain in her left ankle. You might then ask questions and further determine the two complaints are unrelated. Decide which condition is your priority.

In addition, patients often take a multitude of prescription and OTC medications that may contribute to their various complaints, a phenomenon called *polypharmacy*, or cause **iatrogenic** illnesses. An iatrogenic condition—that is, one caused by medications or other medical treatment—can mask other illnesses that may need immediate medical attention.

Words of Wisdom

It is known that any patient taking five or more drugs likely has some form of drug interaction.

Accidental overdoses and adverse drug reactions are a common issue with older adults. Gather an accurate medication history, along with current dosages, to assist other health care providers with continued care of the patient.

Disease symptoms may become less dramatic in the older patient. As the body ages, responses to things like shock and pain are often dulled. This can complicate the assessment process because these patients do not always exhibit the "textbook" response to an illness. Their symptoms may be vague and nonspecific, especially in postmenopausal women with AMI. Maintain a high clinical index of suspicion when treating older adults, and always consider the worst-case scenario.

Consider including a functional assessment during the body systems review in the older adult with an apparent disability. This typically includes assessment of mobility at home and in the community, upper extremity function and limitations, and activities of daily living (ADLs). Physicians will typically assess instrumental ADLs (IADLs) when examining older patients. This includes assessing tasks like getting dressed, bathing, and cooking, and may even extend to areas like financial management and shopping. Assist in this process by assessing some of these functions in the field; this evaluation should be part of your assessment of patients in both stable and unstable conditions, as time allows.

Responsive Medical Patients

For a responsive patient with a medical condition, you will usually form a working field impression based on information gathered during the history-taking process. The secondary assessment and any diagnostic tests you perform after obtaining the history will help you further pinpoint the problem.

Chief Complaint

Ensure the patient is as comfortable as possible before you start—warm or cool enough, privacy ensured—and that you have gained the patient's confidence and trust. Then ask your patient why he or she called for your help (the chief complaint). The patient's chief complaint is the most serious thing that concerns the patient. Ideally, the chief complaint should be recorded in the patient's own words. For example, if the patient says, "My ribs hurt," then you write "My ribs hurt" in quotation marks as the chief complaint in your documentation. For patients who are unresponsive or otherwise unable to speak, writing their primary medical condition or simply "unresponsive" is generally considered acceptable.

In addition to the patient's name and chief complaint, ask about the *day of the week and location,* to determine if the patient is alert. Next, ask about *events* surrounding the current situation, to begin to elaborate on the chief complaint. Your EMS system may require you to collect some additional identifying data, such as age, sex, address, and occupation. You'll also want to know who called 9-1-1: Did the patient place the call for help, or did a friend, family member, or bystander make the call?

Look for items on the scene or in the home that may help you learn more about the patient's condition. Items such as pill containers and medical jewelry can provide invaluable insight into a patient's underlying conditions. Medical identification devices may take the form of a bracelet, necklace, or wallet card. Such an item is used to identify patients with a history of allergies, certain medical conditions (such as, diabetes, cardiac conditions, pacemaker placement, hypertension, and renal disease), and other conditions that may need to be addressed, such as the existence of an automated implantable cardioverter defibrillator (AICD).

With a responsive medical patient, some type of pain, discomfort, or body dysfunction ("I haven't had a bowel movement in 4 days") prompts the call for help. In some cases, the complaint may be vague ("I just don't feel right today"). Vague complaints are common among older people, especially among postmenopausal women. Such complaints challenge you to ask the right questions and be a patient listener as you work to obtain the information you need to make good care decisions **Figure 11-13**.

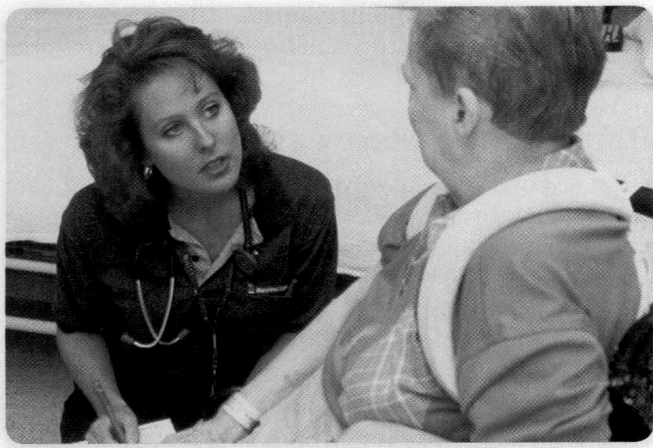

Figure 11-13 Be especially patient when obtaining information about a vague complaint.

History of the Present Illness

After determining the chief complaint, obtain the history of the present illness. This information should provide you with a clear sequence and chronologic account of the patient's **signs** and **symptoms**—specifically, *what happened* and *when.* Signs are objective observations or measurements that you make, and symptoms are subjective information that the patient tells you.

Be sure to ask about the *region* or location of the pain, including the following:

- Where exactly does it hurt?
- Can you point to where it hurts with one finger; is it in a specific area?
- Does the pain stay right there, or does it move or radiate anywhere else?
- If your pain does move or radiate, where does it go?

To obtain a full, clear, chronologic account of the symptoms the patient is experiencing, the OPQRST mnemonic offers a useful approach to analyzing a patient's chief complaint. For example, when exploring a complaint of pain:

- **Onset.** What were you doing when the pain started?
- **Provocation/Palliation.**
  - Did the pain start all of a sudden or come on over a period of time?
  - Does anything make the pain go away or feel better or worse?
- **Quality.** If you were trying to make me feel the way you do, what would you do to me to give me that same feeling?
- **Region/Radiation/Referral.**
  - Can you point to the place where it hurts?
  - Does the pain stay there, or does it go somewhere else?
- **Severity.** On a scale of 0 to 10, with 0 being no pain and 10 the worst pain you have ever felt, how would you rank this pain?[11,12]
- **Time.** How long have you felt this way?

Documentation & Communication

Documenting the pain severity rating is important. Also, note how distressed the patient appears: mildly, moderately, or severely distressed.

The SAMPLE mnemonic may also be useful in the interview process: Signs and symptoms of current complaint; Allergies; Medications; Pertinent past medical history; Last oral intake; and Events leading up to current injury or illness.

The history of the present illness starts with one of the most open-ended of all medical questions: "What is going on today that made you call 9-1-1?" This or a similar question will get the conversation moving. If your patient's behavior is inappropriate, consider the possibility that it might be due to hypoxia, to a medical cause such as sepsis or stroke, low blood glucose level or hypothermia, or to a behavioral emergency, or the patient may have altered mentation secondary to drug or alcohol ingestion.

One of the more challenging aspects of the history-taking process is pulling together the patient's **current health status**, because it is made up of many unrelated pieces of information. However, it often ties together some of the past medical history with the history of the present illness or current event, so it is unquestionably of value to the assessment process. The patient's current health status focuses on environmental and personal habits of the patient that may influence his or her general state of health.

Questions that are most helpful to obtain a useful history of the patient's current health status include:

- What prescription medicines are you taking? How much and how often? Patients can, and often do, confuse when and how to take their medications—and, if so, you could be witnessing a drug reaction. As you gain experience as a paramedic, your familiarity with drugs and drugs' effects will give you an idea of the patient's illness. Medications will also give you a clue about mental health conditions or dementia without you needing to antagonize a reluctant patient.
- Do you take any OTC medications, such as aspirin, or supplements, such as herbs or vitamins?
- Are you allergic to anything? Can you describe the reaction you experienced?
- Do you drink beer, wine, or cocktails? How much? How often? If necessary, remind the patient that certain information is necessary to know for you to treat him or her appropriately.
- Do you smoke? Gather information about the quantity of smoking, along with the length of time. (This history is typically recorded in "pack years." A patient who smokes one pack of cigarettes per day for 15 years is charted as having a 15 pack-year history. A patient who smokes half a pack of cigarettes per day for 15 years is charted as having a 7½ pack-year history.)
- Do you take any illicit drugs? (Assure your patient of confidentiality as you make such inquiries, to the extent that the law allows.)
- What did you have to eat yesterday and today?
- Ask about screening tests that are relevant. For example, for difficulty breathing, ask, "Have you had a chest x-ray lately?"
- Are your immunizations up to date? Have you had a flu shot or pneumococcal vaccine? Ask about childhood immunizations, too.
- Have you been getting a good night's sleep? Look for maladaptive sleep patterns.
- Do you exercise? How much? How often?
- Ask about specific hazards (ie, cleaners, chemicals, or environmental hazards) that may be present at home or at a worksite that would make the patient more vulnerable to injury or illness.
- With regard to safety measures, ask about use of safety belts, protective eyewear, bicycle helmets, gun locks, medication lockboxes, and outlet covers (if small children are present in the home).
- Do you have a family history of any specific diseases? Conditions that should be evaluated in family members include alcoholism, anemia, arthritis, cancer, diabetes, drug addiction, epilepsy, headaches, heart disease, hypertension, kidney disease, mental illness, stroke, and tuberculosis.
- Where do you live? What do you like to do at home? Is there anyone in your life whom you might be afraid of? (You might need to assess a difficult home situation, such as failure to thrive.)
- How do you spend your time during the day? The response to this question may help assess the patient's ability to function independently in society.
- Have you had any important experiences recently? Ask about any recent significant life events such as divorce, job changes or a move to a new home. Even some of the positive experiences in life such as weddings can be some of the most stressful to patients.
- Do you have any religious beliefs that would prevent me from administering treatment? Ask about religious preference to ensure you are respectful of the patient's personal belief systems.
- Are you an optimistic person? (It is important to get your patient's overall outlook on life to assess for depression or other psychiatric conditions.)
- Have you traveled recently to any countries with infectious diseases?

Of course, you do not have to obtain every piece of information on this list for every patient. It takes time, practice, and a certain amount of common sense to know the right questions to ask each patient. Decide which of the listed items you want to explore and which you do not. For a sick patient with immediate life threats, you may not have time to explore any of them. For a patient in stable condition who does not appear to be in apparent distress, you may have time and decide to explore all relevant topics.

A brief family medical history helps to establish patterns and risk factors for diseases. If a 35-year-old man with chest pain tells you his father died of a heart attack at age 39, for instance, be concerned this patient could be experiencing a massive heart attack as well. Remember, not every aspect of the family history is necessarily important in the immediate emergent setting. Your goal is to collect information pertinent to the patient's current medical condition.

Special Populations

In some cases, a patient's religious beliefs may be relevant—for example, if the beliefs pertain directly to medical care. If your patient indicates such beliefs are important, this information should be passed along to ED staff.

A patient's occupation, living environment, and travel history may need to be questioned to complete the social history. Occupation identification provides information about possible exposure to toxic substances and gives details regarding physical health. The environment in which the patient resides provides details regarding lifestyle and chronic exposures. A travel history may point to the possibility of certain illnesses that are uncommon in the United States. In that case, consider whether any of those illnesses put you at risk of contracting a communicable disease. A travel history is also useful when pulmonary embolism (PE) is suspected. People who have been on long flights are prone to developing blood clots from not having moved their lower extremities for extended periods of time. Anytime a patient presents with an unusual or puzzling illness, obtain a travel history.

Words of Wisdom

When a patient has a fever of unknown origin, you may want to inquire about recent travel, as certain infectious diseases are associated with specific areas of the world.

Questions about the patient's diet are also part of the patient's social history. It's appropriate to ask about your patient's typical daily food intake, as well as the timing and quantity of food consumption. This information may help you narrow down the list of possible differential diagnoses. For example, patients who do not eat certain foods because of personal, cultural, or religious reasons may experience nutritional deficiencies that are reflected in their symptoms.

Past Medical History

The **past medical history** gives you an opportunity to learn about any pertinent or chronic underlying medical conditions the patient may have. Some aspects of the past medical history may not seem important now, but taking a careful and thorough history will help paint a clear picture of the patient's overall health status. Not only might this help in your assessment, but it will also help maintain the overall continuity of care with the health care providers who assume responsibility for the patient at the hospital.

The past medical history is frequently linked to the patient's current condition. For example, people with diabetes who don't manage their blood glucose levels may have progressively worsening problems with peripheral circulation, eyesight, wound healing, or kidney function. Likewise, most patients with stable angina will eventually develop unstable angina; at some point, the patient may have a heart attack.

The past medical history should include current medications and dosages. Once again, while this information may not seem important at the time, it may be quite helpful later. Not only should information about prescription medications be obtained, but any OTC medications, recreational drugs, and herbal/alternative medication therapies or dietary supplements should be identified as well. In addition, any allergies the patient has should be documented. This includes allergies to medications, as well as allergies to other substances (food, detergents, pet dander). As you record this information, ask the patient what his or her reaction is to each specific allergen. This information will be valuable later in the patient care process.

Childhood illnesses and immunizations should be assessed briefly if time allows. This will help you rule in or out various disease processes as you take the history and perform a secondary assessment.

Ask the patient to tell you about any illnesses or any conditions for which he or she is currently being treated by a physician. This information will provide insight and details that may pertain to the current emergent medical condition. For example, if the patient reports chest pain, a past medical history of hypertension, hyperlipidemia, and diabetes is pertinent because each of those conditions is considered an independent risk factor for AMI. Ask the patient about past surgeries. A great way to approach this is if you notice a surgical scar in your primary survey, ask the patient how he or she got it. However, not all surgical scars are noticeable, and some procedures leave no scar at all. Therefore, ask each patient about past surgeries, including when they occurred.

A history describing past hospitalizations and any disabilities from previous illnesses will help you fine-tune your assessment. A history of hospitalization for chronic obstructive pulmonary disease (COPD), for example, gives you clues as to how advanced or severe the disease might be. A neurologic deficit from a previous traumatic event might obscure the physical exam findings in a suspected stroke patient; therefore, it is important to ask about previous disabilities.

The patient's emotional affect—that is, his or her expression of emotion or lack thereof—provides insight into the patient's overall mental health and helps you assess his or her mental status. A patient who has just been involved in a MVC is likely to be upset. However, when a patient appears to have an emotional response that is not typical or appropriate for the current circumstances, consider the possibility of altered mental status. Ask about any mental health conditions the patient might be having and whether he or she has ever been hospitalized for a mental health condition. Although it's often difficult for patients and families to admit to mental health conditions, if you are matter-of-fact and dignified in asking the question, you can get an honest answer.

As you inquire about the patient's past medical history, take the time to explore how some of his or her problems were solved ("It took a couple of breathing treatments before I felt better" or "After my last asthma attack, I had to be intubated and was in the hospital on a ventilator for a week").

Equally important is the situation in which the patient presents with an illness he or she has never experienced. An acute presentation of a new illness or condition is best considered serious until proven otherwise.

Unresponsive Patients

You start at a disadvantage when you assess an unresponsive patient because your most reliable source of information—the patient—cannot answer your questions. Owing to this serious limitation, history taking and secondary assessment of an unresponsive patient is much like a trauma assessment. You must rely on a thorough head-to-toe physical exam, plus the normal diagnostic tools (pulse oximetry, capnography, cardiac monitor, and glucometer) to acquire the information necessary for patient care (discussed later in the section Secondary Assessment of Unresponsive Patients).

Trauma Patients

As you move into the history taking for a trauma patient, quickly revisit all of the information from the primary survey, including reconsidering the MOI. Collectively, these data may help you identify patients who must be transported quickly to the trauma center. Unresponsiveness can indicate serious injury, usually a traumatic brain injury, even if the MOI does not seem significant.

A number of mechanisms of injury and evidence of high-energy impact may produce life-threatening injuries Figure 11-14.[13]

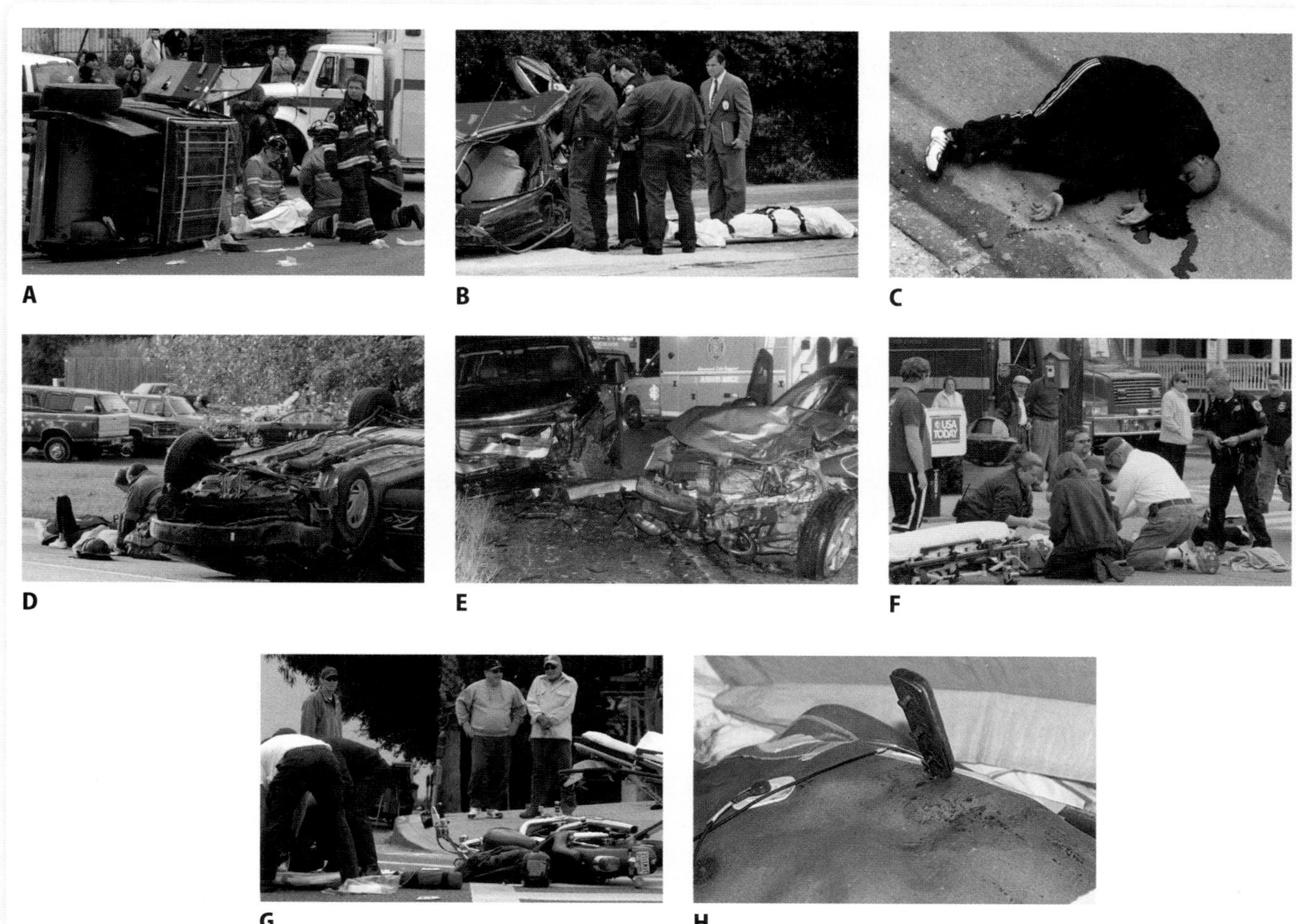

Figure 11-14 Significant mechanisms of injury. **A.** Ejection (partial or complete) from *any* motor vehicle (car, motorcycle, all-terrain vehicle). **B.** Death of another patient in the same passenger compartment. **C.** Adult fall from more than 20 feet. **D.** Vehicle telemetry data consistent with high-risk injury. **E.** High-speed MVC. **F.** Vehicle-pedestrian collision. **G.** Motorcycle crash greater than 20 mph. **H.** Penetrating injuries to the head, neck, torso, or extremities.

- Falls
  - Adults: greater than 20 feet (6 m; one story is equal to 10 feet, or 3 m)
  - Children: greater than 10 feet (3 m) or two or three times the height of the child
- High-risk motor vehicle crash
  - Intrusion, including roof: greater than 12 inches (30 cm) occupant site; greater than 18 inches (46 cm) any site
  - Ejection (partial or complete) from a motor vehicle
  - Death in same passenger compartment
  - Vehicle telemetry data, available in many new vehicles, consistent with a high risk of injury
  - Vehicle versus pedestrian/bicyclist: thrown, run over, or with significant (greater than 20 mph) impact
- Motorcycle or ATV crash greater than 20 mph

If the patient is an infant or a child, MOIs that would indicate a high-priority patient include the following Figure 11-15:

- Fall from more than 10 feet (3 m), or two to three times the child's height
- Fall of less than 10 feet with loss of consciousness
- Bicycle collision
- Medium- to high-speed motor vehicle crash (25 miles per hour or greater)

In many cases, multiple MOIs come into play during a traumatic event—for example, a lateral collision may leave the patient with a crushed upper arm and pelvic girdle as well as penetrating trauma from a piece of door trim impaled in the chest. A patient with any of the previously mentioned mechanisms should immediately raise your index of suspicion.

Words of Wisdom

Two or more serious MOIs markedly increase the likelihood that a patient will sustain a serious or fatal injury.

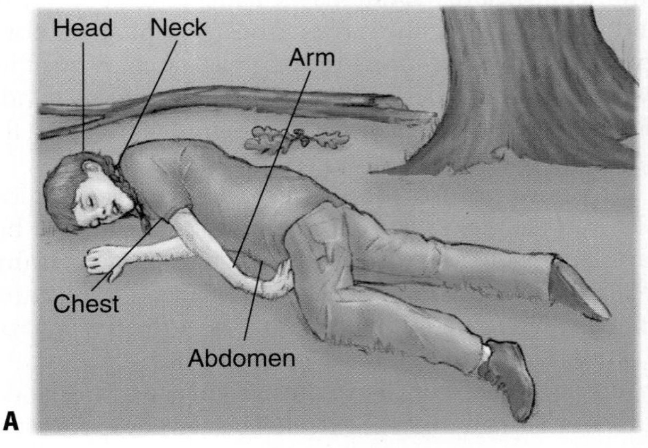

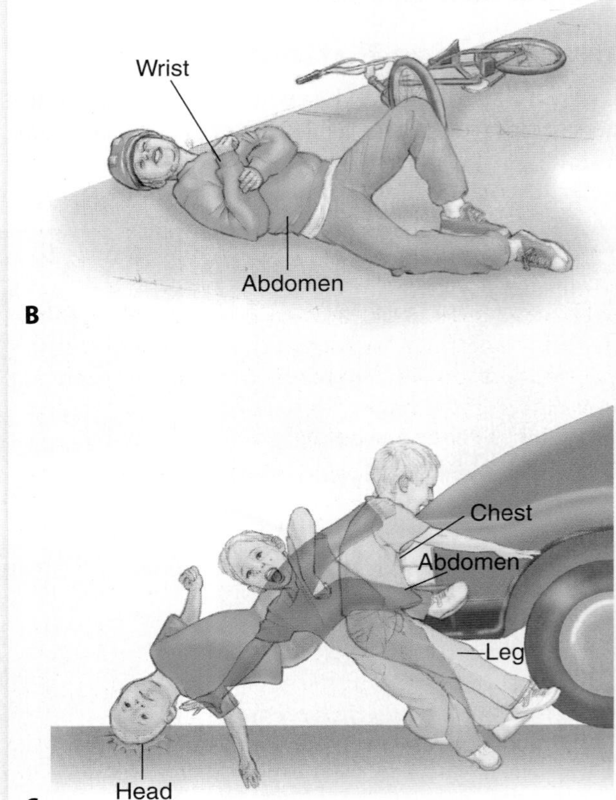

Figure 11-15 Significant MOIs for an infant or child. **A.** Falls from more than 10 feet. **B.** Bicycle collision. **C.** Vehicle–pedestrian collision.

Seat belts and air bags have significantly reduced the prevalence of death and disability associated with MVCs. However, be aware seat belts and air bags can also cause injury. As you evaluate a patient who was involved in a MVC, look for signs and ask questions to determine whether seat belts and/or air bags were involved. Check the clavicle where the shoulder strap crosses. The clavicle is a small bone, and the subclavian vein and artery run directly beneath it. In shorter patients, the shoulder strap mounted on the B column in a car can ride up across the neck, increasing the risk of soft-tissue and cervical spine injury. Examine the area where the lap belt crosses the pelvic girdle. If the belt is not across the iliac spine but has ridden up over the lower abdomen, a person has an increased risk of organ damage and thoracic or lumbar spine injury. Passengers who tuck the shoulder harness under their arms for comfort and are then involved in rollover crashes are at high risk of death from liver injury caused by the improperly positioned belt.

Air bags have saved countless lives, but many people do not realize that an air bag is a secondary restraint system, designed to work with seat belts to reduce injuries.

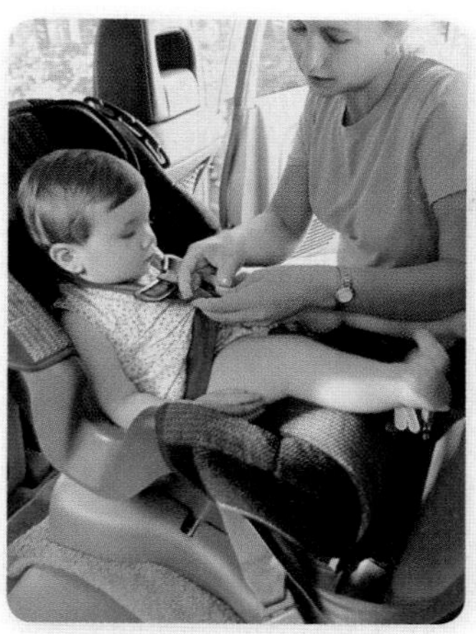

Figure 11-16 A child should be correctly positioned in a properly sized and fitted child safety seat in the rear seat of the vehicle.

When the seat belt is not used and a crash occurs, the air bag deploys, momentarily catching the patient. As the air bag deflates, it releases the driver or passenger, who continues moving forward and may go down-and-under (into the dashboard) or up-and-over (into the steering wheel and/or windshield) if he or she is not restrained by a seat belt. At the scene of any crash with air bag deployment, lift the bag and look beneath it for a bent steering wheel—another possible source of life-threatening internal injuries. During your handoff report at the hospital, inform the hospital personnel whether seat belts were used and properly positioned, and whether the air bag deployed.

Child safety seats have also saved countless lives **Figure 11-16**. If they are improperly installed or positioned in the vehicle, however, they can be rendered useless as a safety device. If the child safety seat comes loose during a crash, the risk of face, head, neck, and spine trauma to the child increases markedly. Similarly, if the child is too large or too small for the seat, it won't provide the intended level of protection.

Most trauma calls involve patients with a single, isolated injury or, on occasion, several minor injuries. In nearly all of these cases, the lack of serious or critical injuries is consistent with the absence of a significant MOI: A collision on the basketball court results in a sprained ankle; a skater crashes and ends up with a Colles fracture; a loose piece of metal spins off a lathe in the machine shop, lacerating the machinist's forearm. Patients should not show any sign of systemic involvement (hypotension). If they do, there is more going on than an isolated injury. Continue your assessment with the goal of finding and correcting the more serious injury.

Review of Body Systems

The review of body systems during history taking provides additional information that could help you form an accurate field impression. To collect even more information, many prehospital providers include **pertinent negatives**—that is, an absence or lack of certain signs and symptoms characteristic of particular illnesses. For instance, people experiencing an AMI typically have chest pain. In addition, such patients often report shortness of breath, nausea and/or vomiting, sweating, and syncope. The absence of these additional symptoms tells you just as much as their presence does, helping you form a more accurate field impression. Another example would be a patient who struck his head but denies any loss of consciousness.

General Symptoms

Many patients present with vague, nonspecific signs and symptoms that tend to be classified as "generalized weakness" and "flulike symptoms." In these patients, it's often difficult to differentiate among various field diagnoses; asking questions about fever, chills, malaise, fatigue, night sweats, and weight variations can be helpful in focusing on a likely diagnosis.

Skin, Hair, and Nails

Questions about the integumentary system should focus on items like rashes (particularly in the pediatric population), itching or hives, and sweating. This system tends to be one of the most forgotten systems when performing the physical exam, and yet it is one of the most important. Symptoms vary because they are subjective, but the significance of signs such as sweating and pallor should not be downplayed. Look for and ask about these conditions, because many patients will dismiss such subtle complaints or neglect to communicate them to you.

Musculoskeletal

Issues with the musculoskeletal system tend to be attributed to trauma, but many medical conditions affect this system as well. For patients reporting signs and symptoms that could be associated with the musculoskeletal system, ask about joint pain, loss of range of motion, and any swelling, redness, erythema, and localized heat or deformity.

Head and Neck

There are multiple structures within the head and neck that could affect the overall health status of a patient. Pay particular attention to patients experiencing a severe headache or loss of consciousness, because these could be the result of a life-threatening condition.

Eyes and Ears. Ask questions regarding the eyes and vision, including visual acuity, blurred vision, **diplopia** (double vision), photophobia (sensitivity to light), pain, changes in vision, and flashes of light seen in the field of vision. Questions about the ears should focus on hearing loss, pain, discharge, tinnitus (ringing in the ears), and vertigo (sensation of the room spinning).

Nose, Throat, and Mouth. Ask patients about their sense of smell, rhinorrhea (runny nose), obstruction, epistaxis, postnasal discharge, and sinus pain. Questions about the throat and mouth should focus on complaints such as sore throat, bleeding, pain, dental problems, ulcers, and changes in the sense of taste.

Endocrine System

The endocrine system is a complicated network of hormone-secreting glands that help regulate various functions in the human body. Many diseases of the endocrine system are seen in the EMS environment and should be included in your review of systems. Because multiple glands and organs are part of the endocrine system, there is a broad range of questions pertaining to this system. Ask if your patient has ever been told he or she has an enlarged thyroid gland. While subtle enlargement is typically noticed only with palpation, excessive enlargement is generally noticed by the patient.

Additional questions about the endocrine system pertain to temperature intolerance, skin changes, swelling of hands and feet, weight changes, polyuria (increased frequency of urination), polydipsia (increased thirst), polyphagia (increased appetite), and any changes in body or facial hair.

Chest and Lungs

Complaints regarding the heart and lungs are common reasons for requesting EMS. A review of systems would not be complete without screening for possible cardiac and respiratory conditions. Always screen patients for dyspnea and chest pain. Other respiratory questions should focus on coughing, wheezing, hemoptysis (coughing up blood), and the presence of active tuberculosis. With regard to coughing, obtain a description of the cough, including production of mucus or phlegm. When you question a patient about cardiac complaints, focus initially on whether this is a first-time or recurring event. The next priority will be questions about pain or discomfort. As described earlier, elaborate on the chief complaint using the OPQRST questions. Other questions related to the heart and blood vessels pertain to orthopnea, edema, and past cardiac evaluation and tests.

Hematology and Lymph Nodes

Ask patients about any history of anemia, bruising, or fatigue. Anemia may exacerbate multiple medical conditions that could be seen during an EMS call. Note any bruising, especially when it is atraumatic. This could suggest a clotting disorder that may affect traumatic injuries as well as other medical conditions. Note any bruising that may point toward physical abuse; keep in mind, paramedics are mandatory reporters.

Tender and enlarged lymph nodes can be seen with conditions ranging from infection to cancer. Many patients encountered by EMS personnel have an infection. Questioning about tender or enlarged lymph nodes can point toward a possible field impression.

Gastrointestinal

Gastrointestinal (GI) complaints are common among calls for EMS. Paramedics must understand GI ailments and ask appropriate questions in the review of systems to help distinguish among various illnesses. Ask patients about appetite, general digestion, food allergies and intolerances, heartburn, any nausea or vomiting, diarrhea, hematemesis (blood in vomit), bowel irregularity, changes in stool (size, shape, smell, or color), flatulence, jaundice, and any past GI evaluations. Pay particular attention to signs and symptoms that point toward active GI bleeding, a life-threatening condition.

Many patients hesitate to offer information about urination. Some people attribute changes in urinary habits to aging, but often such changes are a new finding that could indicate an underlying infection or other problem that should be addressed. Ask about urinary habits or changes in urinary habits, including dysuria (painful urination), increased frequency of urination, urgency (sudden need to urinate), nocturia (waking up in the middle of the night to urinate), hematuria (blood in urine), or polyuria (excessive urination). Ask about flank pain and pain in the suprapubic region if you suspect that the chief complaint could represent an underlying urinary problem.

Genitourinary

The genitourinary system also includes the genitals. As mentioned earlier, patients may not find it easy to discuss their genitals with a complete stranger. However, medical conditions such as sexually transmitted diseases can be serious. Even though this may be an embarrassing topic for both patients and paramedics, ask about any current or history of sexually transmitted diseases. Some questions are specific to the male and female sexes. Recall, both the male and the female sex organs secrete hormones belonging to the endocrine system.

Keep your questions focused. For a woman reporting acute abdominal pain, foul-smelling vaginal discharge, pain on urination, or genital lesions, ask if her menstrual cycle is regular, when she last had her period, and if she has dysmenorrhea (menstrual pain). Ask when she last had sexual intercourse, whether she has had multiple sex partners, what kind of contraception she uses (if any), and whether she has ever been pregnant. Female gynecologic and obstetric conditions are discussed further in Chapter 22, *Gynecologic Emergencies*, and Chapter 41, *Obstetrics*.

When you question male patients, ask about erectile dysfunction, any fluid discharge, and testicular pain. It may seem trivial to the patient, but problems with erectile dysfunction are frequently related to systemic diseases like hypertension or diabetes. In addition, the medications used to treat many of these conditions can affect the care provided by paramedics, such as not giving nitroglycerin to a patient taking erectile dysfunction drugs like Viagra or Cialis.

For men who report pain on urination, discharge from the penis, or genital lesions, ask when their most recent sexual encounter was and if they use condoms. Ask them to describe the characteristics of any discharge or lesions.

Neurologic

The nervous system is intricate and often difficult to understand. When a patient summons EMS for a neurologic complaint, you must understand the importance of assessing for neurologic pathology. That means asking certain questions during the review of systems that cover or involve the nervous system. Ask about a history of seizures or syncope, loss of sensation, weakness in the extremities, paralysis, loss of coordination or memory, and muscle twitches or tremors. Be alert for signs of facial asymmetry, especially when the chief complaint is headache. If you suspect stroke or a transient event, then perform the Cincinnati Prehospital Stroke Scale, the Los Angeles Prehospital Stroke Screen, or another stroke assessment tool used in your region. Stroke scales are discussed in detail in Chapter 18, *Neurologic Emergencies*.

Psychiatric

Paramedics are often called to the scene of a behavioral health emergency. Considering the wide array of behavioral health conditions, question patients appropriately to differentiate among the various mental illnesses. This step is important not only to deliver appropriate patient care, but also to ensure the safety of yourself, the crew, and the patient. Ask the patient about a history of or any current depression, mood changes, difficulty concentrating, anxiety, irritability, sleep disturbances, daytime fatigue, and suicidal or homicidal ideation.

Critical Thinking

When all is said and done, the aim of your assessment should be to figure out the most likely reason for your patient's chief complaint and how best to address it. In Chapter 12, *Critical Thinking and Clinical Decision Making*, you'll learn the details of critical thinking. For now, recognize that there are five aspects of critical thinking: (1) concept formation, (2) data interpretation, (3) application of principles (guidelines or algorithms), (4) reflection in action (being willing to change course as you interpret your patient's condition), and (5) reflection on action (doing honest and thorough postrun critiques to benefit learning).

Being able to think and perform well under pressure is a big part of becoming a good paramedic. In many ways, critical thinking and decision making are just two more skills you'll need to work on, not just while you are a student, but for the rest of your career.

Clinical Reasoning

Clinical reasoning combines your knowledge of anatomy, physiology, and pathophysiology with information about the patient's complaints in order to direct questioning as you take a history. Note any abnormal symptoms or physical findings, as well as their anatomic location. Pay careful attention to any signs or symptoms inconsistent with your working diagnosis, because they may point you in a different direction. As the patient answers your interview questions, you'll begin to analyze the information based on your medical knowledge. Once the history of the chief complaint, history of the present illness, past medical history, and review of systems have been completed, you can begin to develop the differential diagnosis—a working hypothesis of the nature of the problem. Your differential is the list of possible causes of the patient's complaint. Take, for instance, a patient with a sudden onset of shortness of breath in the absence of trauma. You could begin to refine your differential by ruling out myocardial infarction, pulmonary edema, pneumonia, allergy, reactive airway disease, and so on. Part of your history and physical exam is to rule in or rule out possible diagnoses in your differential. Using the above example, since the shortness of breath began suddenly, the dyspnea is probably not due to pneumonia if the patient has no fever. There is no trauma, so it is unlikely to be the result of a fractured rib.

Like a detective, you can then begin to test this hypothesis to determine whether it holds true. You can accomplish this through further assessment and testing (for example, a 12-lead ECG or a glucose check). The process evolves as you ask different questions based on the patient's answers. This exploration, in turn, helps you focus your physical assessment and narrow down your possible field diagnoses even further.

As you develop your differential diagnosis, begin with broad possibilities—that is, decide which body systems might be contributing to the patient's complaint. For instance, chest pain could involve the cardiac, respiratory, or gastrointestinal systems. This approach helps you avoid tunnel vision, which means locking into a diagnosis too early, before considering all the possibilities and systematically ruling out each one to determine a diagnosis.

The physical exam (discussed later in this chapter) is another important aspect of clinical reasoning. Tenderness or other specific exam findings help point you toward specific anatomic locations that can tighten up your diagnostic possibilities. Once you identify the possible organ systems involved, use your knowledge of pathophysiology to determine the most likely diagnosis. Once you determine your working diagnosis, continue your questioning of the patient to help confirm your diagnosis. In addition, reevaluate the overall situation and complaint to ensure you address all of the patient's complaints.

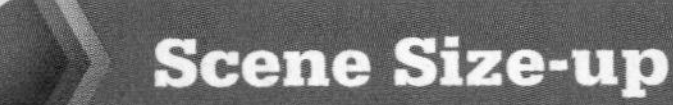

Patient Assessment

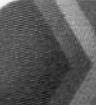

Scene Size-up
Primary Survey
History Taking
Secondary Assessment
Is this patient medical or trauma?
Assess
■ Baseline vital signs
■ Monitoring devices (as appropriate)
Systematic physical exam
■ Full-body exam or rapid full-body scan
■ Focused on injury
■ Based on body system (respiratory, cardio-vascular, neurologic, reproductive, etc)
Reassessment

Secondary Assessment

Secondary assessment is the process by which quantifiable, objective (based on fact or observable) information is obtained from a patient about his or her overall state of health. This information is compared with subjective (observed or perceived by the patient), historic information obtained from the patient. Armed with these two types of information, you can obtain a field impression and develop a differential diagnosis for the patient. While performing an assessment, you may see the patient's condition as a clinical phenomenon; however, a caring and empathetic approach will yield better results and a more accurate evaluation. Likewise, putting forth a professional appearance and demeanor will instill trust and confidence in your abilities as a care provider.

The secondary assessment consists of two elements:

1. Obtaining baseline vital signs that measure overall body function
2. Performing a systematic physical exam such as the full-body exam (also called the head-to-toe survey), a focused exam on a specific injury, or the exam which is based on the body system of the chief complaint (ie, respiratory, cardiovascular, neurologic, reproductive, etc.)

Of course, the conditions in the prehospital setting may determine precisely how the secondary assessment is performed. Sometimes it may be condensed. For example, for an unresponsive medical patient or a trauma patient with a significant MOI, there may only be time to perform a rapid full-body scan, discussed later in this section.

The overall patient assessment helps you determine whether a medical condition exists, so actions can be taken to manage it. Before you can appreciate abnormalities on examination, you must understand the wide variety of normal presentations. This is something that can be learned only through direct, hands-on experience and patient interaction. Thus, every patient encounter represents an opportunity for you to gain experience about the normal human condition.

As you approach your patient, keep in mind the major body systems and their anatomic locations. An understanding of anatomy and physiology helps you tremendously during the assessment and in determining your field impression. For example, as you palpate the chest, it is important to remember the heart, lungs, great vessels, and esophagus are located in that anatomic region and should be considered when a patient reports pain in that area. In addition, understanding the gastrointestinal system and the location of specific organs in the abdominal cavity can help narrow down a differential diagnosis.

As stated earlier, the general approach to examining a patient should be systematic. However, the actual start of your exam is determined by several factors, such as the patient's stability of the patient, the chief complaint, the history, the patient's ability to communicate, and the potential for unrecognized illness or injury. A patient who reports isolated ankle pain does not necessarily warrant an exam that begins with assessment of the head. With that said, a multisystem trauma patient may require a rapid assessment of the patient from head to toe at the beginning of the assessment. Some patients, depending on their level of stability, may never get a complete assessment because you will be too busy managing the life-threatening injuries identified in the primary survey. Therefore, not every aspect of the secondary assessment will be completed in every patient. In addition, the additional challenge of underlying comorbidities (the simultaneous existence of two or more chronic conditions found in a patient) exists when examining a patient. For example, a patient involved in a MVC who is unresponsive may have an underlying diabetic emergency that contributed to the crash.

Other factors to consider when beginning an exam include location of the exam, the patient's position and point of view, and maintaining professionalism. Always consider your environment when examining a patient, and ask yourself if this is the most appropriate environment in which to conduct the exam. Factors such as noise, lighting, and the patient's position might hinder your assessment. In addition, the patient's privacy should always be considered, not only because of the need to expose your patient, but also to discourage bystanders from watching and listening during the exam process. If necessary and feasible, move the patient to a more private location, such as the ambulance, before conducting an in-depth secondary assessment. Remember, the patient is probably going through an emotional and traumatic event.

Your touch during the exam will contribute to the patient's stress level. Explain everything to the patient before you actually perform the exam to help alleviate the patient's stress. This helps you establish a high level of professionalism and show that you are attentive to the patient's needs. Keep in mind, most people do not care for physical exams, so being kind, professional, and compassionate will go a long way toward calming their anxiety and fears.

Physical Exam of Priority Patients

The physical exam you perform is based on the needs of your patient. If the patient is an unresponsive medical patient or a trauma patient with significant MOI, then you may not have the time to perform the physical exam traditionally done in the secondary assessment. It may be necessary to do a **rapid full-body scan** (sometimes called the rapid full-body sweep) and get moving to the hospital. The rapid full-body scan is a 60- to 90-second nonsystematic review and palpation of the patient's body to identify injuries that must be managed or protected immediately. If there is time to do the traditional head-to-toe physical exam, then that should be performed as discussed in the next section.

During the rapid full-body scan, *inspect* the soft tissue, look for open or closed wounds and *palpate* for pain or tenderness. Evaluate each area of the body for the following:

- **Open:**
  - Abrasions/amputations/avulsions
  - Punctures/penetrations
  - Lacerations
- **Closed:**
  - Deformities or swelling
  - Burns
  - Contusions/crush injuries

To perform a rapid full-body scan of the patient, follow the steps in Skill Drill 11-1. Remember, this should take no longer than 60 to 90 seconds!

Assessment Techniques

The techniques of inspection, palpation, auscultation, and percussion allow you to use your physical senses to obtain information and learn about the normal (versus abnormal) functions of a patient's body. Recall inspection involves looking at the patient, either in general or at a specific area. For example, you might take in a patient's overall appearance from the doorway and then look specifically at the chest wall for abnormalities or deformities Figure 11-17.

Recall palpation is touching for the purpose of obtaining information, such as detecting tenderness (eliciting pain), feeling for any deformity, **crepitus** (a grating or grinding sensation or sound made when two pieces of broken bone rub together), mass, or abnormal organ enlargement, and judging pulse quality Figure 11-18. You will typically use your fingertips to check pulses, but you'll use your palms to sweep across and around the skull, for example, to assess structural integrity as well as to assess for defects (ie, knots or dents). Use the back of your hand to touch a patient's skin for fever assessment, because it's more sensitive than your palm.

Various palpation techniques are used to examine specific areas. Palpation with the hands and fingertips is typically performed on the chest, abdomen, and extremities. Accomplish this by keeping your hand and forearm on a horizontal plane, with fingers together and flat on the

Skill Drill 11-1 Performing a Rapid Full-Body Scan

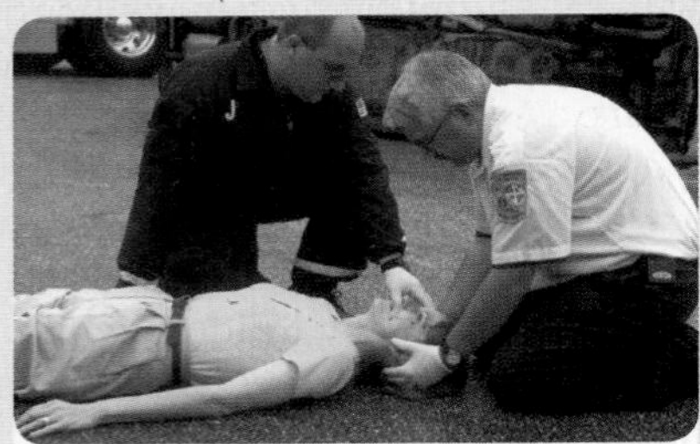

Step 1 Inspect and palpate the head for open/closed findings and crepitus.

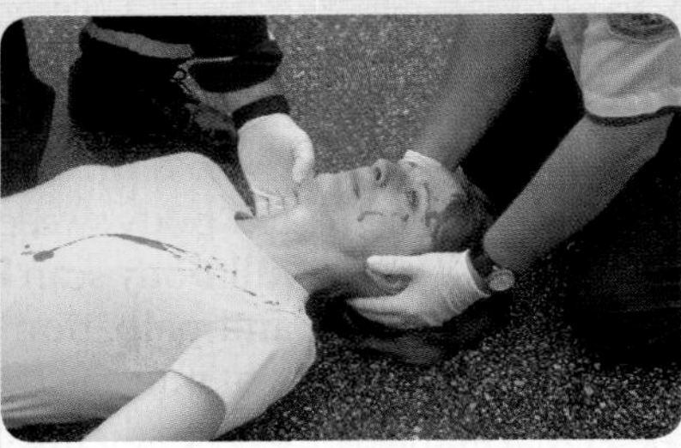

Step 2 Inspect and palpate the neck for open/closed findings, **jugular venous distention (JVD)** (the visible bulging of the jugular veins when a patient is in semi-Fowler or full Fowler position), tracheal deviation, and crepitus. In trauma patients, consider applying a cervical spinal immobilization device. It is particularly important to assess the neck before covering it with a cervical collar.

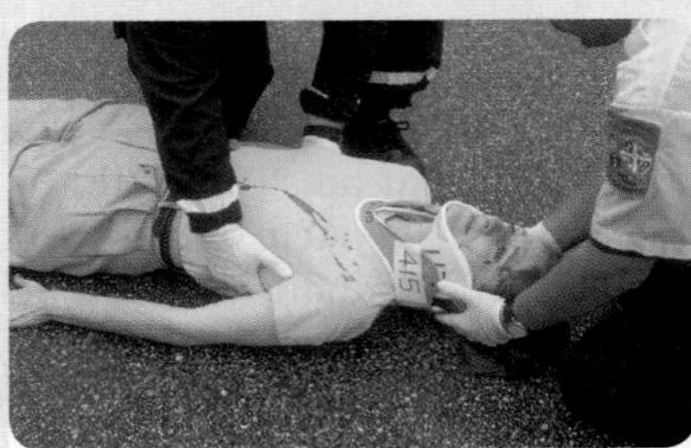

Step 3 Inspect and palpate the chest for open/closed findings, paradoxical motion, and crepitus. Listen to breath sounds on both sides of the patient's chest.

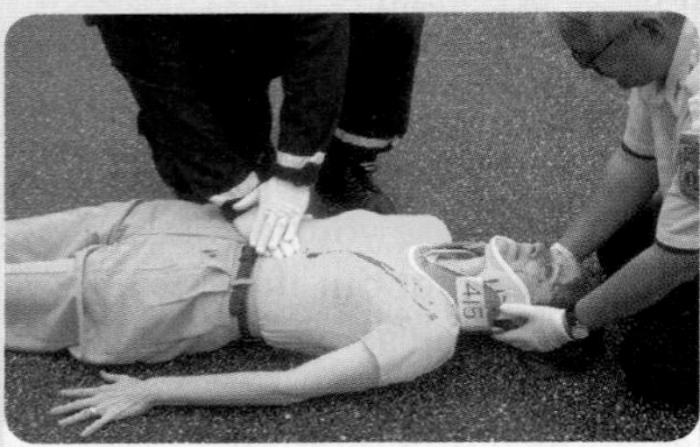

Step 4 Inspect and palpate the abdomen for open/closed findings, rigidity (firm or soft), and distention.

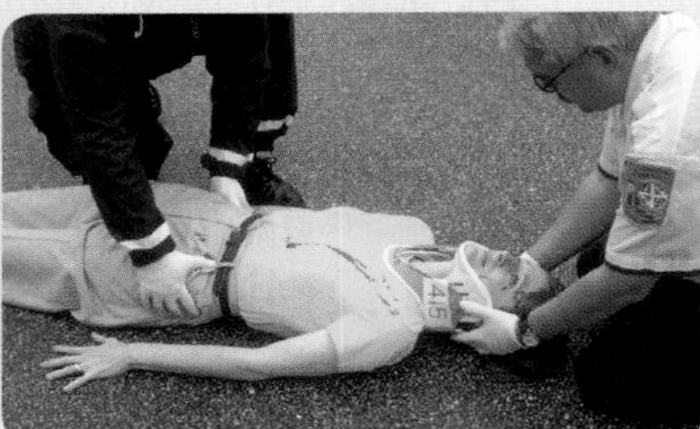

Step 5 Inspect and palpate the pelvis for open/closed findings. If there is no pain, gently compress the pelvis downward and inward to look for tenderness and instability.

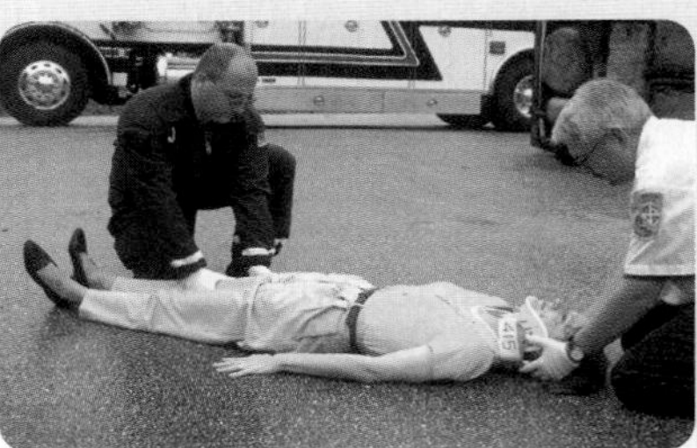

Step 6 Inspect and palpate all four extremities for open/closed findings. Assess bilaterally for distal pulses and motor and sensory functions.

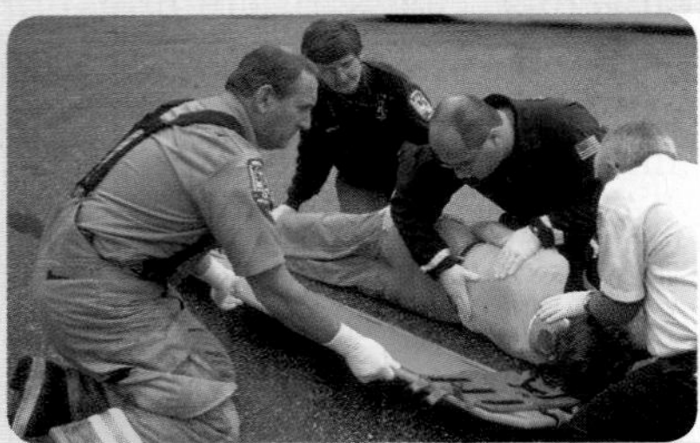

Step 7 Inspect and palpate the back and buttocks for open/closed findings. In all trauma patients, maintain in-line stabilization of the spine while rolling the patient on his or her uninjured side in one smooth motion. If you place the patient on a backboard, check the back before you finish log rolling the patient onto the board. If you use a scoop stretcher, you won't be able to inspect or palpate the lower thoracic and lumbar spine.

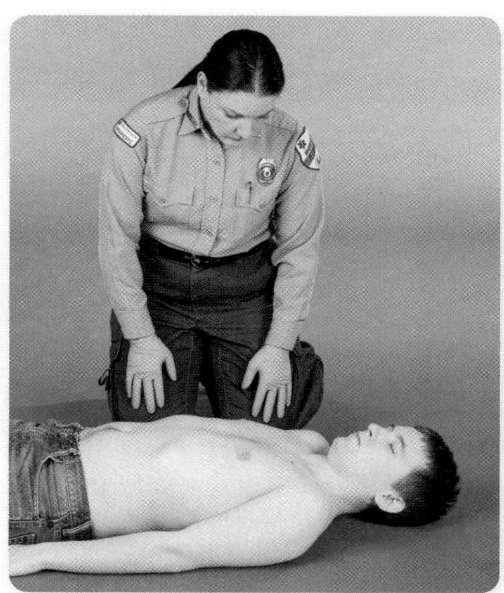

Figure 11-17 Physical exam: inspection.

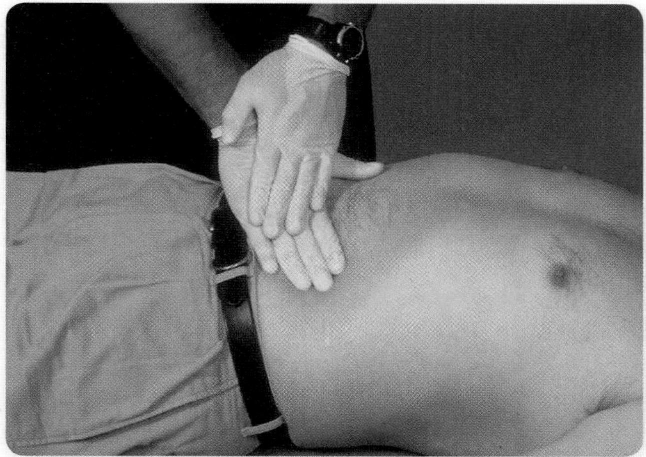

Figure 11-18 Physical exam: palpation.

patient, and palpating with a sliding or dipping motion, depending on the area being examined. Palpation with the fingertips may be reserved for examining the distal extremities, the head, and the neck. Use the ulnar surface of the hand when examining the abdomen. Some patients will immediately tense their abdominal muscles during the exam, regardless of whether there is pain. When you use only the ulnar surface of one hand, the exam seems less intrusive to the patient, and the results are more likely to be accurate. Use the dorsal aspect of the hand in the same manner as the ulnar surface. This technique is also used when assessing skin temperature.

Words of Wisdom

When done properly, palpation should not cause harm. Deep palpation is rarely done in EMS, and requires practice and an understanding of when to stop.

Percussion entails gently striking the surface of the body, typically where it overlies various body cavities. This technique allows you to detect changes in the densities of the underlying structures. For example, percussion of a normal lung will yield medium to loud, low-pitched, resonant sounds. Percussion sounds over muscle and bone should be soft, high-pitched, and flat. Percussion sounds over hollow organs such as the intestines are often described as loud, high-pitched, and tympanic (like a drum).

Percussion is a skill that requires a lot of practice to perfect. An internist who performs this skill a dozen times a day becomes competent quickly. By comparison, percussion is rarely done in the field and, as such, is a minimally developed skill for most providers. Follow the steps in Skill Drill 11-2 to perform percussion.

Recall auscultation is listening to sounds within the body with a stethoscope. The body generates a variety of high- and low-frequency sounds—both normal and abnormal—that can be detected via auscultation. You can assess bowel sounds via auscultation, as you can lung and heart sounds. Appreciating the presence of and differences in auscultated sounds requires keen attention, a thorough understanding of what "normal" sounds like, and lots of practice.

Vital Signs

Vital signs consist of a measurement of pulse rate, rhythm, and quality; respiratory rate, rhythm, and quality; blood pressure; temperature; and pulse oximetry. Other than overall patient appearance, vital signs provide the most objective data for determining patient status. Measuring vital signs requires you to use the techniques of auscultation, palpation, and inspection. The first set of vital signs, commonly taken in the secondary assessment, is called the *baseline*. The additional sets of readings, commonly taken during reassessment, are called *serial vital signs*. Reviewing the serial vital signs and comparing the measurements against the baseline readings helps you establish trends showing patient improvement or deterioration. This is called *vital sign trending*. Because vital signs can change dramatically over relatively short time periods, failing to check them frequently and observe trends, especially in the context of a significantly ill or injured patient, can lead to poor patient care.

Pay strict attention vital signs, as they measure critically important parameters. Normal limits, as shown in Table 11-5, can vary, depending on factors such as age and medication use. Interpret the readings with those factors in mind.

Pulse

Pulse measurements should assess the rate, presence, location, quality, and regularity of the heartbeat. Pulses can be obtained at several points in the body,

Secondary Assessment

Skill Drill 11-2 Performing Percussion

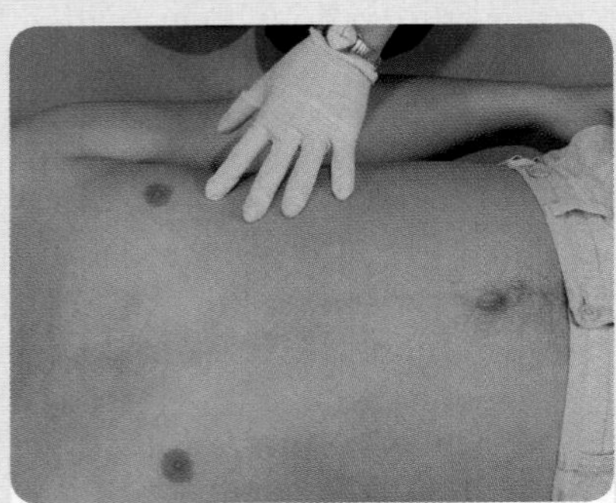

Step 1 Place your hand lightly against the surface to be examined.

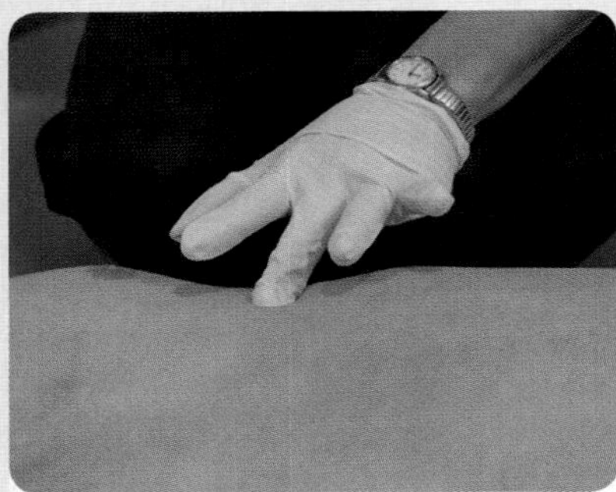

Step 2 Hyperextend your middle finger, and apply firm pressure to the surface to be percussed.

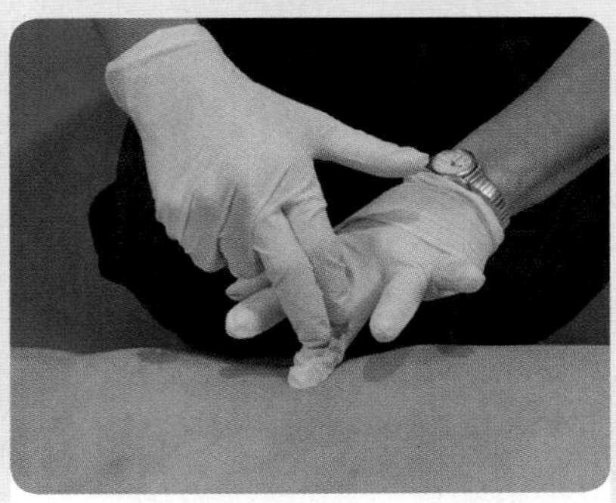

Step 3 Directly strike the middle phalanx of your middle finger with one or two fingertips of your other hand. Apply the same force over each area of the body to accurately compare the sounds produced by percussion.

Table 11-5 Normal Vital Signs at Various Ages

Age	Pulse Rate (beats/min)	Respirations (breaths/min)	Blood Pressure (mm Hg)	Temperature (°F)
Neonate (0 to 1 month)	Awake: 100 to 205 Asleep: 90 to 160	30 to 60	Systolic: 67 to 84 Diastolic: 35 to 53 Mean arterial pressure: 45 to 60	98 to 100 (37 to 38°C)
Infant (1 month to 1 year)	Awake: 100 to 180 Asleep: 90 to 160	30 to 53	Systolic: 72 to 104 Diastolic: 37 to 56 Mean arterial pressure: 50 to 62	96.8 to 99.6 (36 to 37.5°C)
Toddler (1 to 2 years)	Awake: 98 to 140 Asleep: 80 to 120	22 to 37	Systolic: 86 to 106 Diastolic: 42 to 63 Mean arterial pressure: 49 to 62	96.8 to 99.6 (36 to 37.5°C)
Preschool age (3 to 5 years)	Awake: 80 to 120 Asleep: 65 to 100	20 to 28	Systolic: 89 to 112 Diastolic: 46 to 72 Mean arterial pressure: 58 to 69	98.6 (37°C)
School age (6 to 12 years)	Awake: 75 to 118 Asleep: 58 to 90	18 to 25	Systolic: 97 to 120 Diastolic: 57 to 80 Mean arterial pressure: 66 to 79	98.6 (37°C)
Adolescent (12 to 15 years)	Awake: 60 to 100 Asleep: 50 to 90	12 to 20	Systolic: 110 to 131 Diastolic: 64 to 83 Mean arterial pressure: 73 to 84	98.6 (37°C)
Early adult (18 to 40 years)	60 to 100	12 to 20	Systolic: 90 to 140	98.6 (37°C)
Middle adult (41 to 60 years)	60 to 100	12 to 20	Systolic: 90 to 140	98.6 (37°C)
Older adult (61 years and older)	60 to 100	12 to 20	Systolic: 90 to 140	98.6 (37°C)

Pediatric data from: American Heart Association (AHA). Vital signs in children. In: AHA. *Pediatric Advanced Life Support.* Dallas, TX: AHA; 2015.

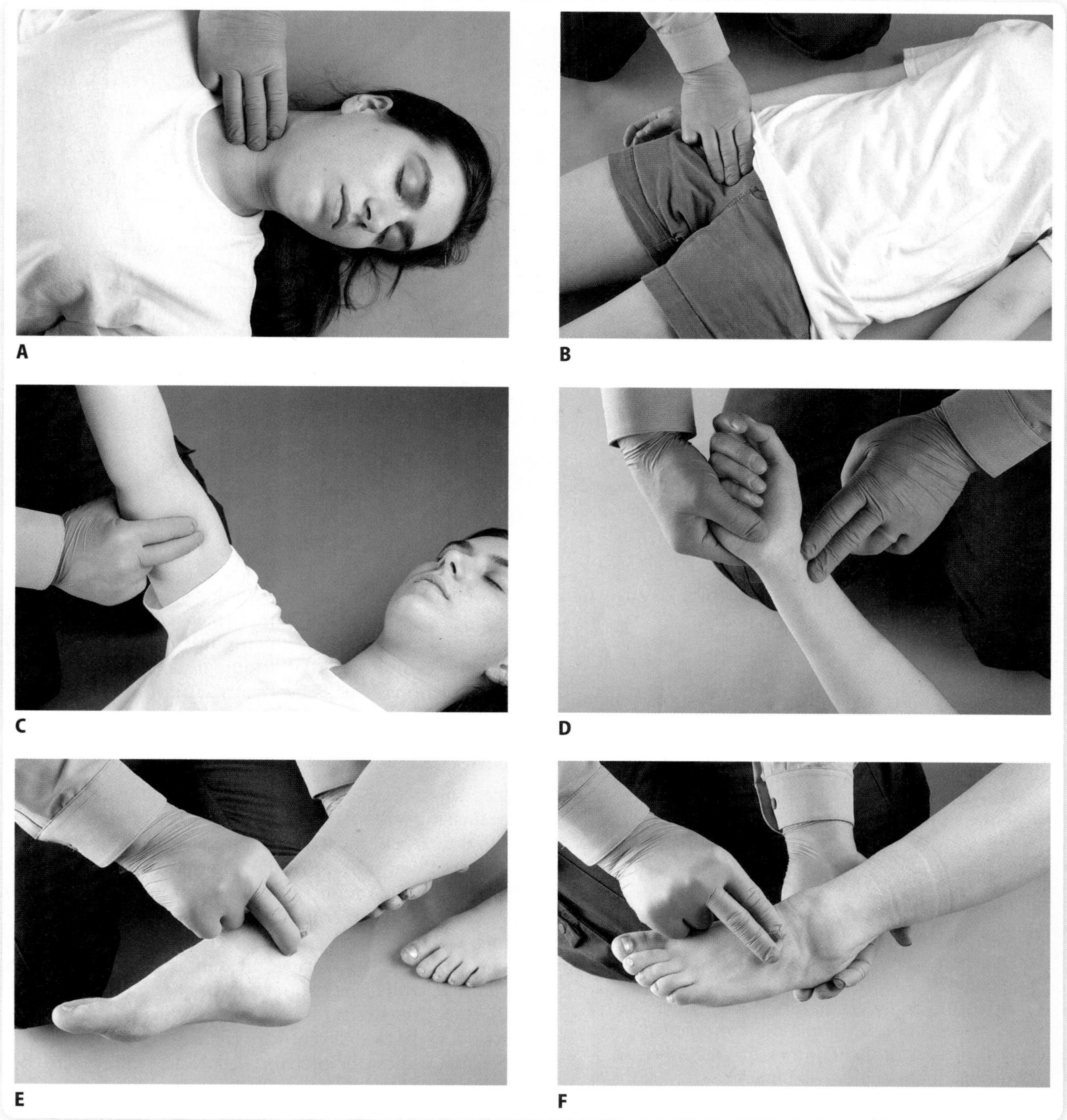

Figure 11-19 Common pulse points. **A.** Carotid pulse. **B.** Femoral pulse. **C.** Brachial pulse. **D.** Radial pulse. **E.** Posterior tibial pulse. **F.** Dorsalis pedis pulse.

including the radial, brachial, femoral, and carotid arteries **Figure 11-19**. As mentioned in the Primary Survey section, when you are formally counting the pulse rate, time the pulses for a minimum of 30 seconds and then multiply by 2 to obtain the rate per minute.

EMS personnel should compare proximal and distal pulses during patient evaluation. If the pulse is irregular or slow, it's best to count for a full minute. If for some reason you're unable to palpate a radial pulse, reassess for a pulse using the carotid artery.

Although it is appropriate to check for the presence of a central pulse in an unresponsive patient, the actual pulse rate should be counted in the most peripheral location that can be palpated. In the responsive patient, determine the respiratory rate while you appear to be checking the pulse; this may decrease patients' tendency

Table 11-6 Pathologic Respiratory Patterns

Pattern Name	Description and Indication
Apnea, bradypnea, or dyspnea	Breathing that stops from any cause is called *apnea*. Slowed breathing is called *bradypnea*. Labored or difficult breathing is known as *dyspnea*. Common causes of breathing trouble (dyspnea) in adults include allergic reactions, asthma or other lung diseases, cardiac arrest, choking, drug overdose (especially an overdose of alcohol, narcotic painkillers, barbiturates, anesthetics, or other depressants), fluid in the lungs, and obstructive sleep apnea. Other causes of apnea include head injury, heart attack, irregular heartbeat, metabolic disorders (ie, a body's chemical, mineral, or acid-base imbalance), submersion, and stroke.
Biot (ataxic) respiration	An irregular breathing pattern, rate, and depth of respiration with intermittent periods of apnea; caused by increased intracranial pressure.
Cheyne-Stokes respiration	A gradual increase in respiratory rate and depth, followed by a gradual decrease with intermittent periods of apnea; associated with brainstem injury
Kussmaul respiration	A pattern of deep, gasping respiration; common in diabetic ketoacidosis.
Tachypnea	Excessively rapid and shallow breathing; common with lung disease or other medical cause (such as anxiety, asthma, choking, chronic obstructive pulmonary disease, heart failure, or pulmonary embolus).

to inadvertently alter their breathing pattern or rate when they become aware of being evaluated.

Respiration

The respiratory rate is typically measured by observing the rise and fall of the patient's chest. Overall respiratory effort can be assessed by visualizing portions of the abdominal wall, neck, and face, and by assessing accessory muscle use. Although the absolute respiratory rate is important, the quality of the respiratory effort should be evaluated as well. Learn to recognize pathologic respiratory patterns Table 11-6. Refer to Chapter 16, *Respiratory Emergencies* for depictions of these. Similarly, learn to recognize when patients exhibit tripod positioning, accessory muscle use, or retractions. This is especially critical information in assessing pediatric patients.

Special Populations

The respiratory rate should be measured for a minimum of 30 seconds, and then multiplied by 2 to obtain the rate per minute for pediatric patients.

Assessing the work of breathing in a pediatric patient is one of the single most predictive signs available; therefore, when you see a child with excessive work of breathing who begins to show signs of ventilatory fatigue, a physiologic collapse is usually moments away.

Special Populations

Palpating the pulse in an infant often presents a real challenge. Because an infant's neck is often short and fat, and the pulse rate is quite fast, you may have a hard time finding the carotid pulse. Therefore, in infants younger than 1 year, palpate the brachial artery to assess the pulse.

Blood Pressure

Blood pressure (BP) is the measurement of the force exerted against the walls of the blood vessels. It is commonly measured in a peripheral artery, although it can be obtained essentially anywhere in the circulatory system. Blood pressure is the product of cardiac output and peripheral vascular resistance, so it includes two components: systolic pressure and diastolic pressure, reported in millimeters of mercury (mm Hg). **Systolic pressure** is created by the left ventricle while it is contracting (that is, during systole). **Diastolic pressure** is the result of residual pressure in the system while the left ventricle is relaxing (during diastole). Normally, diastolic pressure should not fall to zero, because peripheral vascular resistance in the arteriolar side of the circulatory system should continually provide for a diastolic pressure. The coronary arteries receive blood flow by this mechanism, so a drop in diastolic pressure means less myocardial perfusion.

Words of Wisdom

Many patients exhibit an increase in blood pressure (BP) because of anxiety and the stress of an acute injury or illness. Look at your patient as well as trends in vital signs before concluding the BP is truly abnormal.

Blood pressure must be measured using a cuff appropriate to the patient's size and habitus (physique or body build). The cuff should be one half to two thirds the size of the upper arm. Cuffs that are too small or tight yield an artificially high pressure; cuffs too large or loose give inaccurately low results. Although BP should ideally be auscultated, it can be palpated to estimate the systolic pressure; however, this method introduces the potential for error. Periodic inspection of the BP cuff's gauge is important because it can lose accuracy and require recalibration.

> **Words of Wisdom**
>
> Whenever possible, avoid taking blood pressure on a painful/injured extremity, on an arm with an arteriovenous shunt or fistula, or on a post-mastectomy side. Doing so can cause pain and/or result in inaccurate readings.

Temperature

Many methods can be used to evaluate body temperature. If you use a device to measure the tympanic membrane temperature to obtain a patient's body temperature, be aware that extrinsic factors may increase or decrease the temperature reading. Ensure the external auditory canal is free of **cerumen** (ear wax), which can lower the temperature reading. Position the probe in the canal so the infrared beam is aimed at the tympanic membrane; otherwise the measurement will be invalid. Wait 2 to 3 seconds until the digital temperature reading appears. This method measures core body temperature, which is usually higher, and more accurate, than the oral temperature. The oral temperature is considered a proxy of the actual temperature, which is the core body temperature.

Pulse Oximetry

Arterial oxygen saturation is determined via **pulse oximetry**, which has earned a place in health care as part of regular vital signs monitoring Figure 11-20. Typically, oxygen is a consideration for symptomatic patients (those with signs of hypoxia) who have an Spo_2 of less than 94%. Although pulse oximetry is a valuable tool, it shouldn't be used as an absolute indicator of the need for oxygen therapy. Pulse oximetry measures the percentage of hemoglobin saturation and can be inaccurate in certain situations. Know the limitations of pulse oximetry to appropriately process the information it provides. Inaccurate readings may be obtained for a variety of reasons, including hypotension, hypothermia, carbon monoxide poisoning, sickle cell disease, anemia, vascular dyes, patient motion, incorrect placement, and even certain types of nail polish.

Equipment Used in the Secondary Assessment

Equipment used to perform the secondary assessment includes a stethoscope, **sphygmomanometer**, or blood pressure cuff, pulse oximeter, capnography and glucometry equipment, reflex hammer, scissors, a reliable light source, gloves, and a sheet or blanket.

> **Words of Wisdom**
>
> Remember to look at your patient, not the number. If the patient looks sick but the pulse oximetry reading is normal, then the patient is still sick.

Stethoscopes are available in two forms: acoustic and electronic Figure 11-21. The acoustic stethoscope does not amplify sounds; rather, it simply blocks out ambient noises, allowing you to hear and appreciate the sounds of the body. An electronic stethoscope, on the other hand, converts the acoustic sound waves into an electronic signal that is then amplified.

Today's acoustic stethoscope, which is the most commonly seen in the prehospital setting, consists of two earpieces attached to an air-filled tube connected to a chest piece. The chest piece has two sides—a diaphragm (plastic

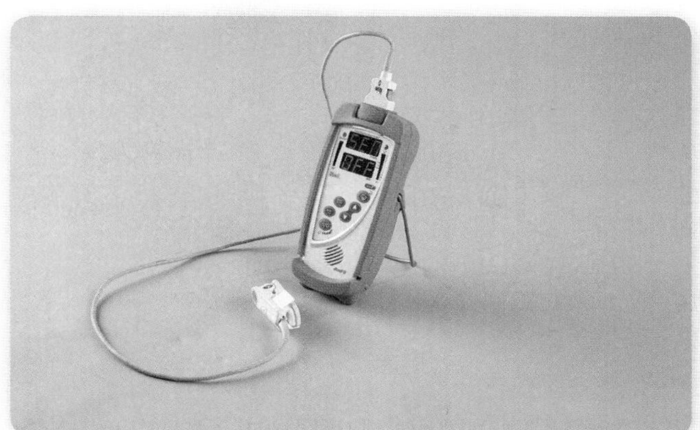

Figure 11-20 A pulse oximeter.

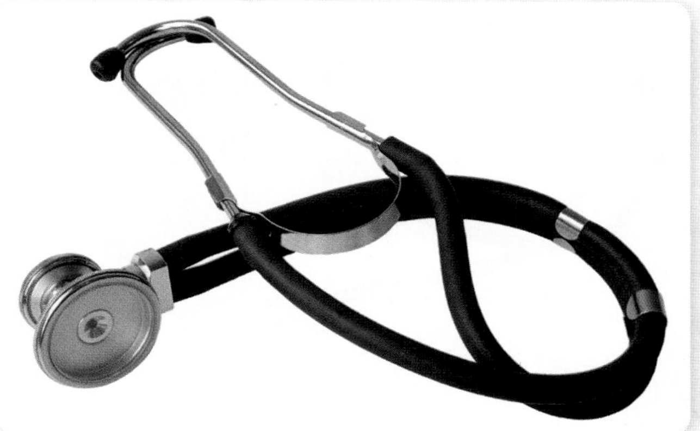

Figure 11-21 A stethoscope.

disk) and a bell (hollow cup)—that can be placed against the patient to sense sounds. The diaphragm is vibrated by the sounds of the body, which are then transmitted up to the stethoscope's earpieces; thus, the diaphragm side is used to pick up higher-frequency sounds. The bell, which usually transmits lower-frequency sounds, senses the sounds directly off the skin of the patient. Some stethoscopes have attenuated diaphragms, meaning they have an outer metal ring and another ring closer to the center of the head. Pushing lightly on the head allows you to listen to one set of sounds while pressing firmly seats the diaphragm against the inner ring, allowing you to hear a different set of sounds.

Words of Wisdom

There are important differences between the bell and the diaphragm of the stethoscope. The cup-shaped bell is used to listen for deep and low-pitched sounds (heart sounds). It is placed lightly on the skin, just enough to form a seal. The flat diaphragm is used to listen for high-pitched sounds (breath, bowel, and normal heart sounds); it is placed firmly on the skin.

A sphygmomanometer, or blood pressure cuff, measures blood pressure Figure 11-22. The traditional device consists of an inflatable cuff, which occludes blood flow, and a manometer (pressure meter), which is used to determine the pressure in the artery. These two components are connected by tubing. In manual cuffs, a separate tube is attached to an inflation bulb. Bladderless blood pressure cuffs are also available, but they can be uncomfortable against bare skin.

The **ophthalmoscope** allows you to examine a patient's eyes and view the retina and aqueous fluid. An **otoscope** is used to evaluate a patient's ears. However, these two devices are rarely used in paramedicine. Chapter 19, *Diseases of the Eyes, Ears, Nose, and Throat* discusses assessment of these structures in detail.

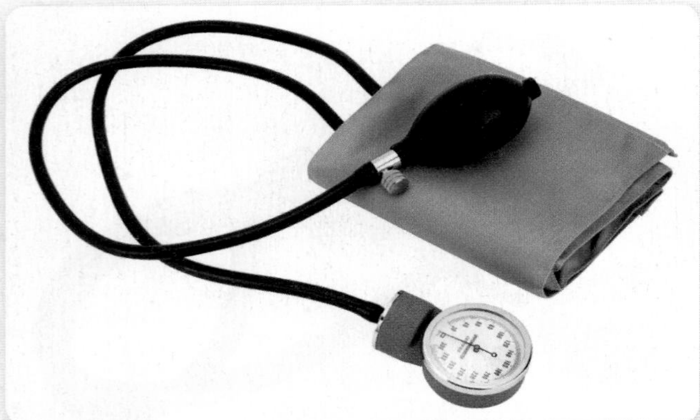

Figure 11-22 A sphygmomanometer.

The Physical Exam

The physical exam of a patient in the prehospital setting is the most important skill a health care provider can master. Establishing vascular access, administering medications, and performing endotracheal intubation are mechanical skills that require extensive practice to achieve proficiency. By comparison, the skills of assessing a patient and interpreting the findings of a physical exam truly separate the accomplished paramedic from the novice. The physical exam consists of a review of systems to determine the nature and extent of the patient's illness or injury.

Remember, as soon as you approach the scene, you will have already begun to gather information about the patient's overall presentation Figure 11-23. A patient lying on the ground on a rainy, cool evening, for instance, should be considered hypothermic until proven otherwise. A quick look at the environment in which you find the patient and his or her general appearance provides a substantial amount of information before you even begin to ask questions.

Look for signs of significant distress, such as mental status changes, anxiousness, labored breathing, difficulty speaking, diaphoresis, obvious pain, obvious deformity, and guarding or splinting of a painful area. It is not uncommon for people experiencing substantial and incapacitating pain to present with a quiet and still affect.

Other aspects that may be readily apparent and worth noting include dress, hygiene, expression, overall size, posture, foul or unusual odors, and overall state of health. As you characterize the patient's overall state, use the appropriate terms to describe the degree of distress: no apparent distress, mild (slight or not harsh), moderate (small or average), acute (very great or bad), and severe (dangerous or difficult to endure). Other acceptable terms to describe the general state of a patient's health include chronically ill, frail, feeble, robust, and vigorous.

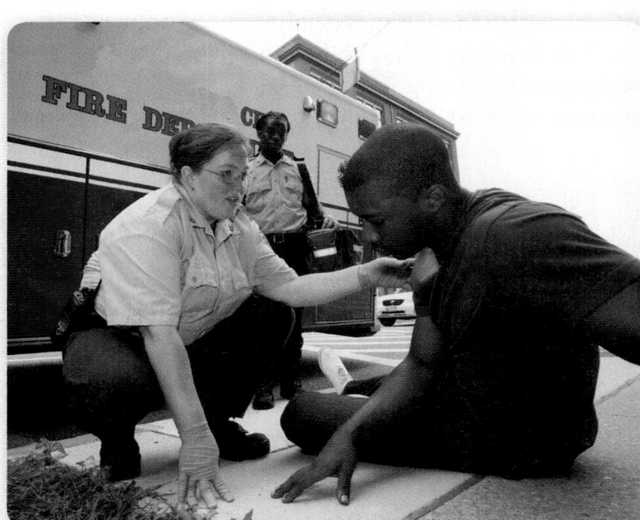

Figure 11-23 Get a general impression of the overall situation as you approach the patient.

The secondary assessment should be driven by the information you gathered during the primary survey and the history-taking phase. For a patient who tells you, "I just can't catch my breath," early assessment of breath sounds is a must. If the patient tells you, "My leg feels numb," assessment of pulse, motor function, and sensation in the affected and unaffected extremities is indicated. Exercise good judgment to make the best use of your time. Don't waste time palpating a patient's abdomen or auscultating heart sounds if the person reports knee pain. In general, the care you provide for a responsive medical patient will be driven by your local protocols in conjunction with your consultation with the base station physician.

The Full-Body Exam

The **full-body exam** is a systematic head-to-toe exam. Like the rapid full-body scan, the full-body exam includes inspection, palpation, and auscultation. It also includes percussion and clearly takes more time to complete. The goal of this process is to identify hidden injuries or other problems you may not have found during the primary survey. Any patient who has sustained a significant MOI, is unresponsive, or is in critical condition should receive this type of exam. An unresponsive patient is unable to tell you what's wrong; therefore, this type of exam may give you clues to identify the problem. Based on the severity of the patient this exam is often done en route to the ED.

To perform a full-body exam of a patient with no suspected spinal injuries, follow the steps in Skill Drill 11-3. To perform a full-body exam in which the patient has sustained significant trauma, ensure manual stabilization is still in place and follow the steps in Skill Drill 11-3.

A **focused exam**, sometimes called a focused assessment, is generally performed on patients who have sustained insignificant MOIs and on responsive medical patients. This type of exam is based on the chief complaint. The most common complaints from a responsive medical patient involve the head, heart, lungs, or abdomen, individually or in combination.

For example, if a patient reports a headache, then carefully and systematically assess the head and/or the

Skill Drill 11-3 Performing the Full-Body Exam

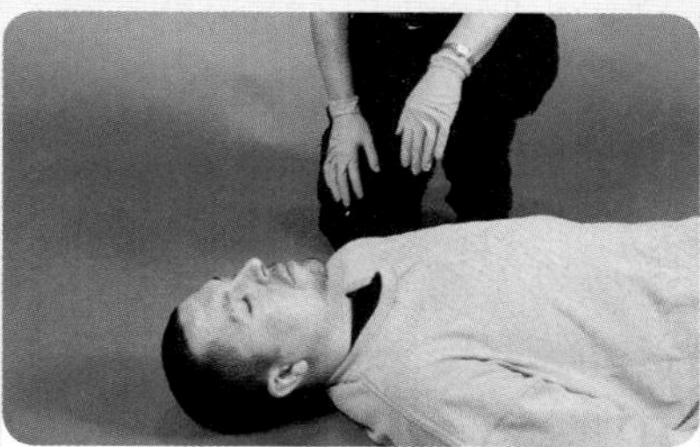

Step 1 Examine the face for obvious lacerations, bruises, fluids, and deformities.

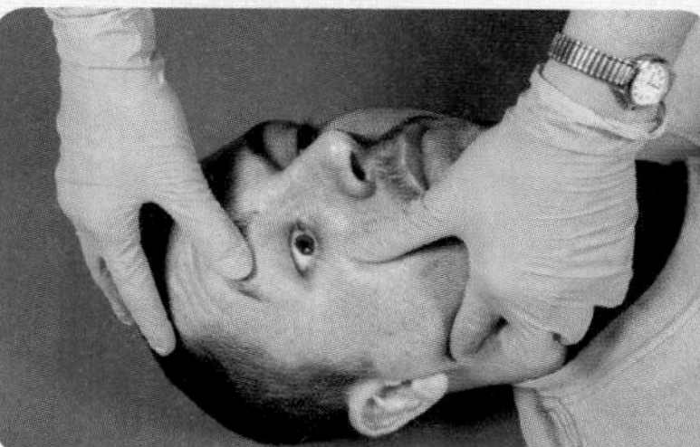

Step 2 Inspect the area around the eyes and eyelids.

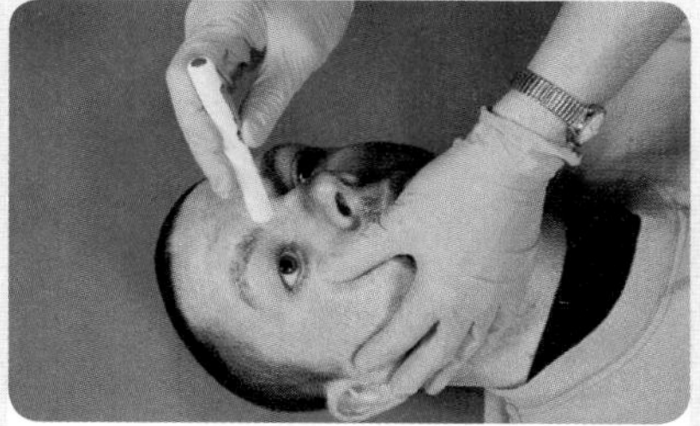

Step 3 Examine the eyes for redness and for contact lenses. Use a penlight to assess the pupils.

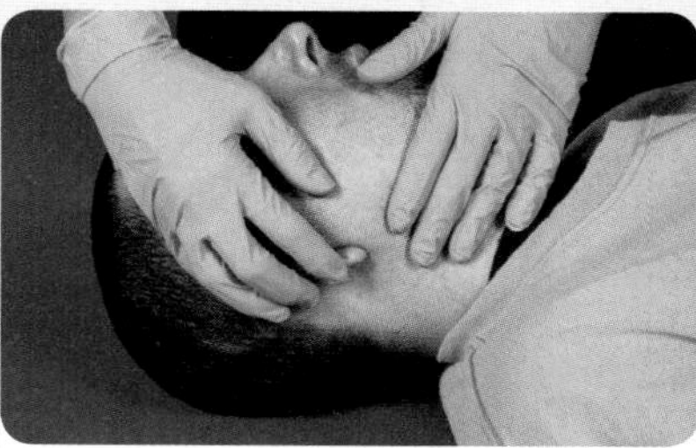

Step 4 Look behind the ears for bruising (Battle sign).

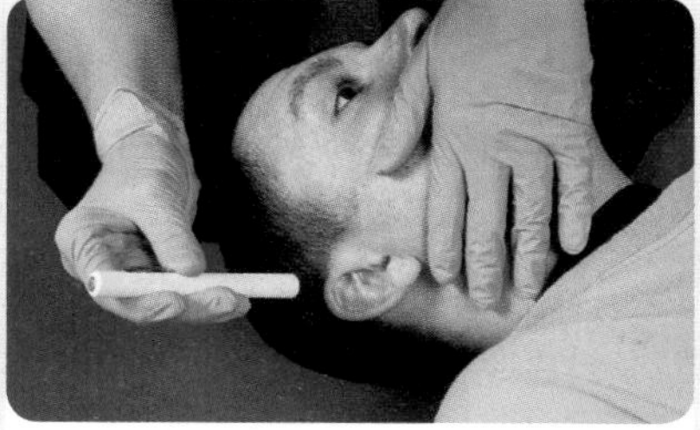

Step 5 Use the penlight to look for drainage of spinal fluid or blood in the ears.

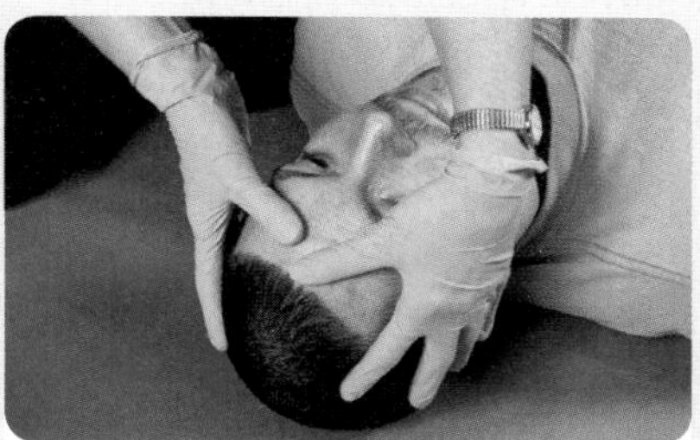

Step 6 Examine the head for bruising and lacerations. Palpate for tenderness, skull depressions, and deformities.

Skill Drill 11-3 Performing the Full-Body Exam *(continued)*

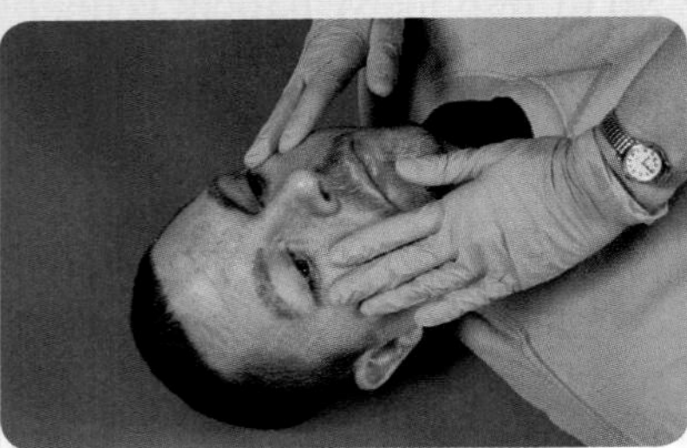

Step 7 Palpate the zygomas for tenderness, symmetry, and instability.

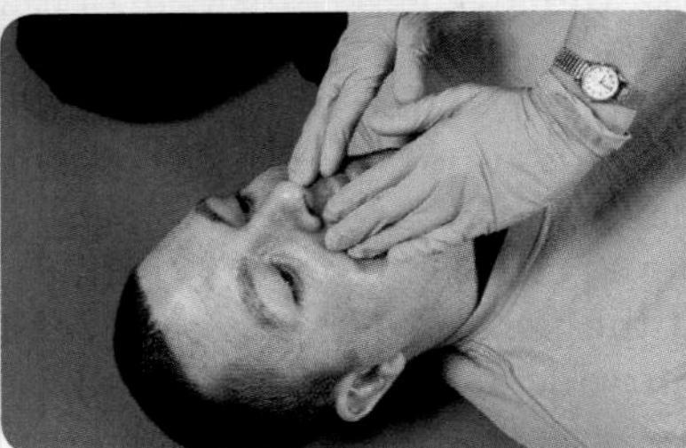

Step 8 Palpate the maxillae.

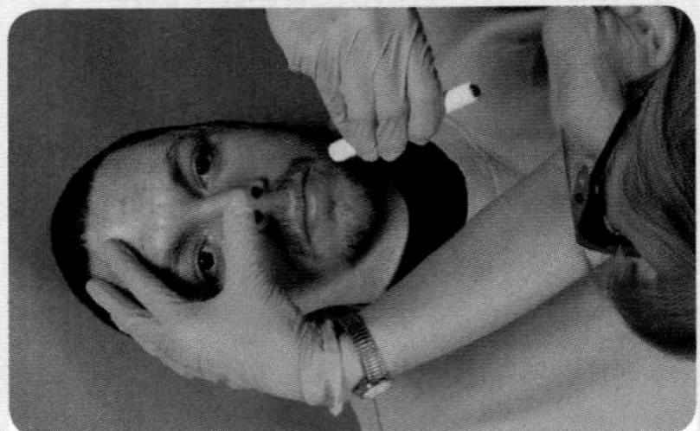

Step 9 Check the nose for blood and drainage.

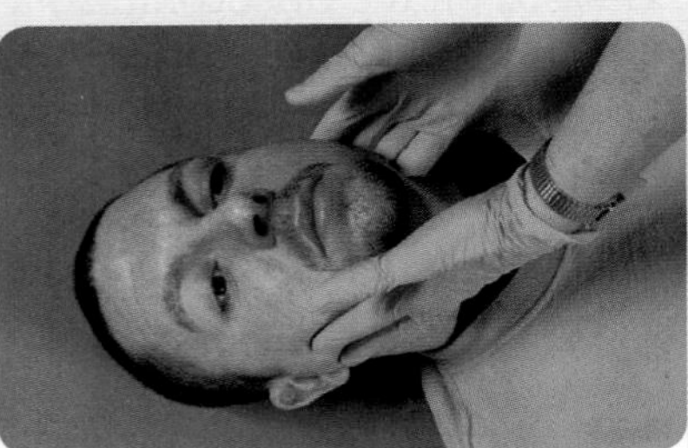

Step 10 Palpate the mandible.

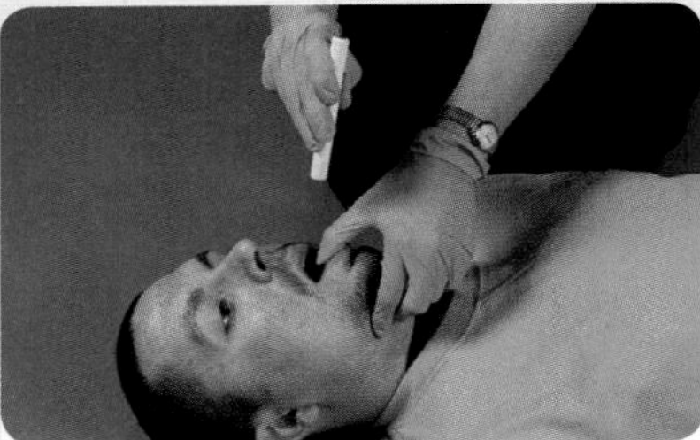

Step 11 Assess the mouth and nose for cyanosis, foreign bodies (including loose or broken teeth or dentures), bleeding, lacerations, and deformities.

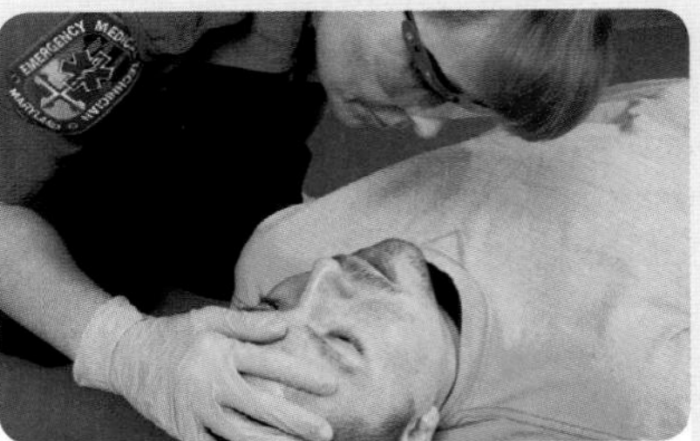

Step 12 Check for unusual odors on the patient's breath.

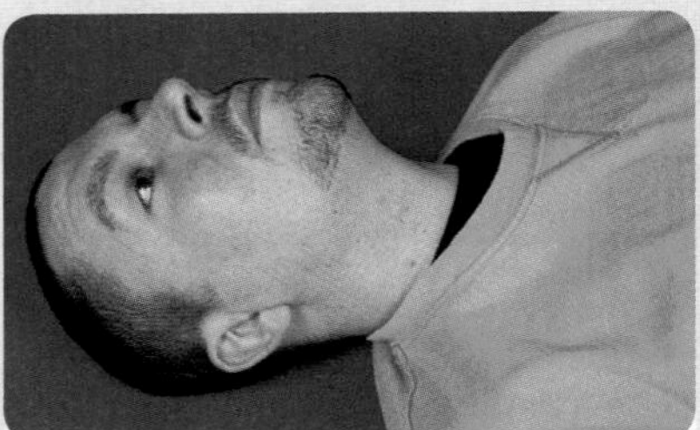

Step 13 Inspect the neck for obvious lacerations, bruises, and deformities. Observe for jugular venous distention and/or tracheal deviation.

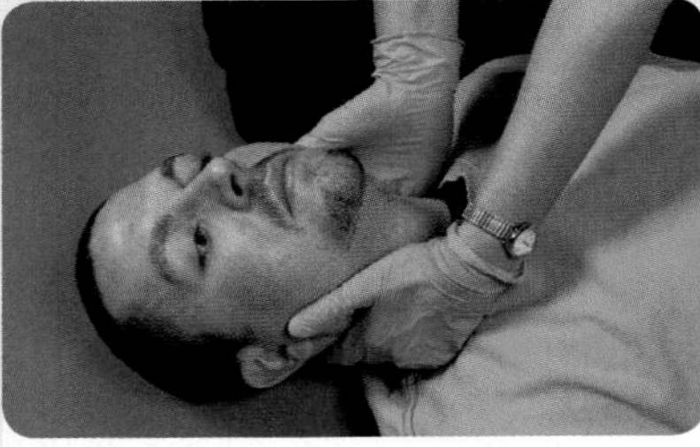

Step 14 Palpate the front and the back of the neck for tenderness and deformity.

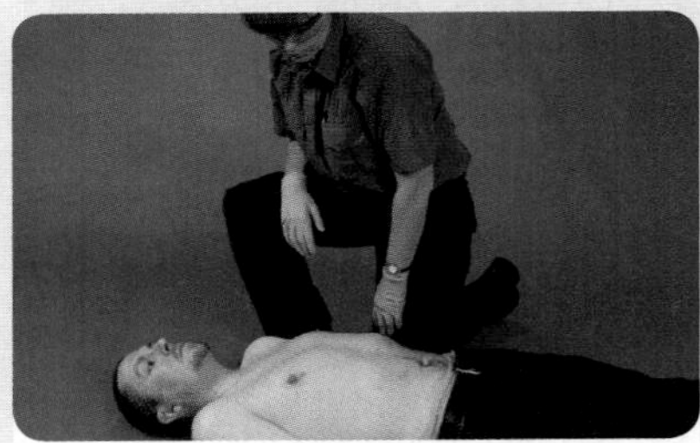

Step 15 Inspect the chest for obvious signs of injury before you begin palpation. Watch for movement of the chest with respiration. Assess the work of breathing.

Skill Drill 11-3 Performing the Full-Body Exam *(continued)*

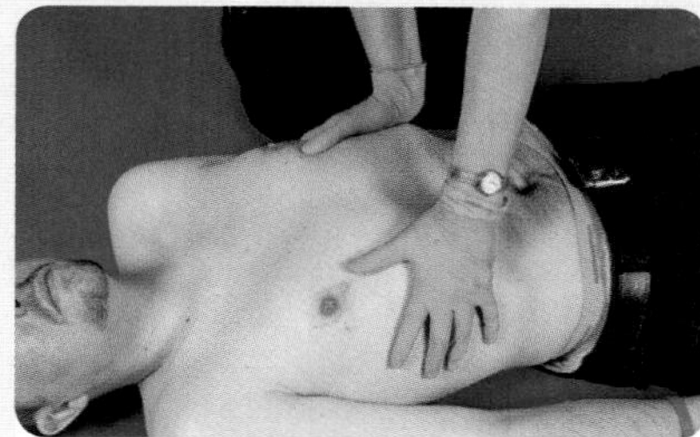

Step 16 Gently palpate over the ribs to assess structural integrity and elicit tenderness. Avoid pressing over obvious bruises and fractures.

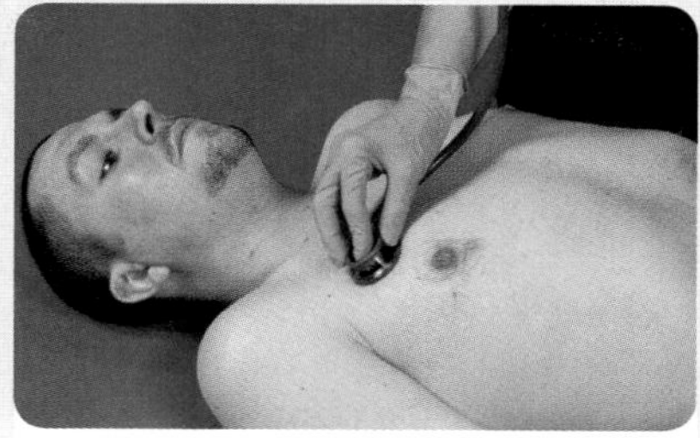

Step 17 Listen for breath sounds over the midaxillary and midclavicular lines—a minimum of four fields if you check the anterior chest, and six fields if you are assessing the posterior chest.

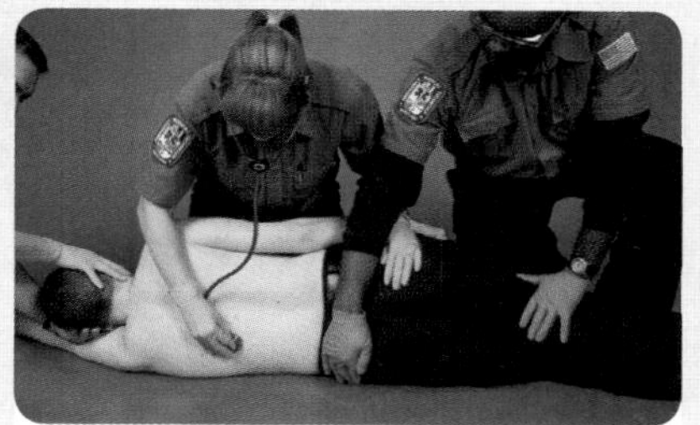

Step 18 Assess the lungs including the bases and apexes of the lungs. At this point, also assess the back for tenderness and deformities, so you log roll the patient only once. Remember, if you suspect a spinal cord injury, then use spinal precautions as you log roll the patient.

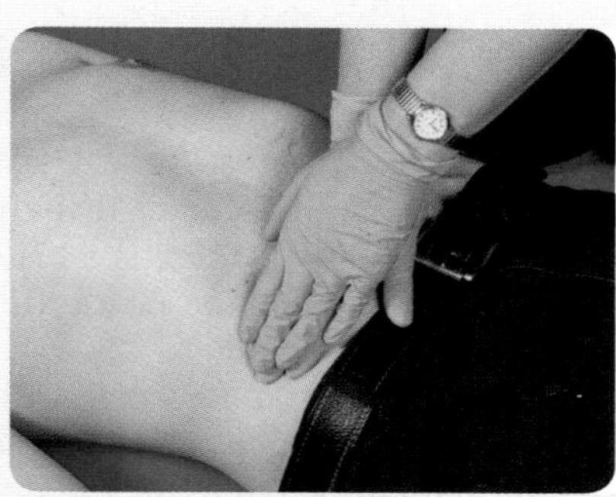

Step 19 Look for obvious laceration, bruising, and deformity of the abdomen and pelvis. Gently palpate the abdomen for tenderness. Palpate the quadrant diagonal from where any pain is located. If the patient indicates his or her pain is localized to one quadrant, then palpate that area last. The contraction of abdominal muscles in response to palpation is seen with underlying conditions such as appendicitis and is described as "guarding." When the contraction persists throughout the abdominal musculature, the abdomen is described as "rigid," a condition seen with severe abdominal inflammation such as peritonitis.

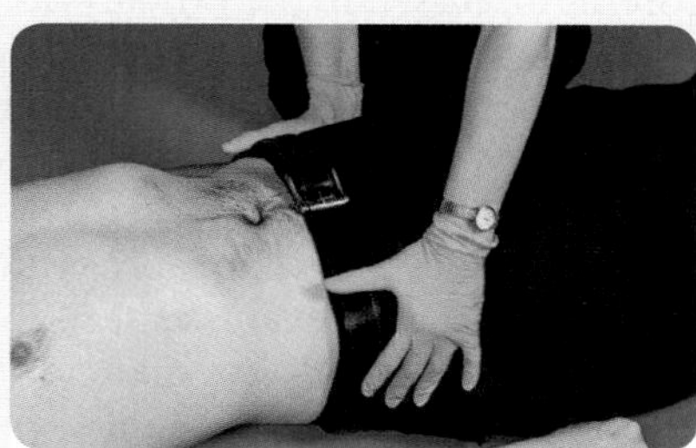

Step 20 Gently compress the pelvis from the sides to assess for tenderness.

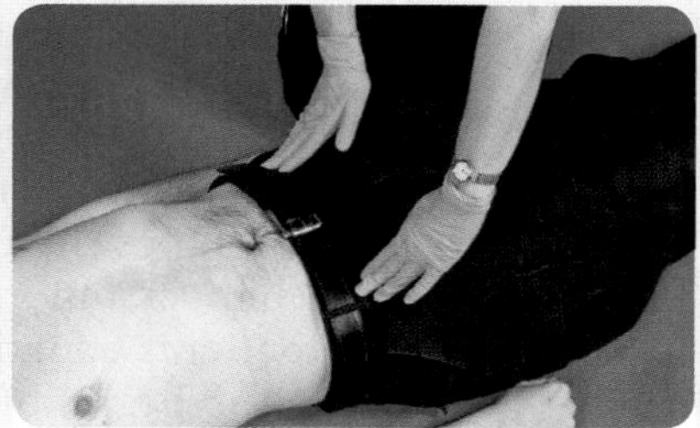

Step 21 Gently press the iliac crests to elicit instability, tenderness, and/or crepitus.

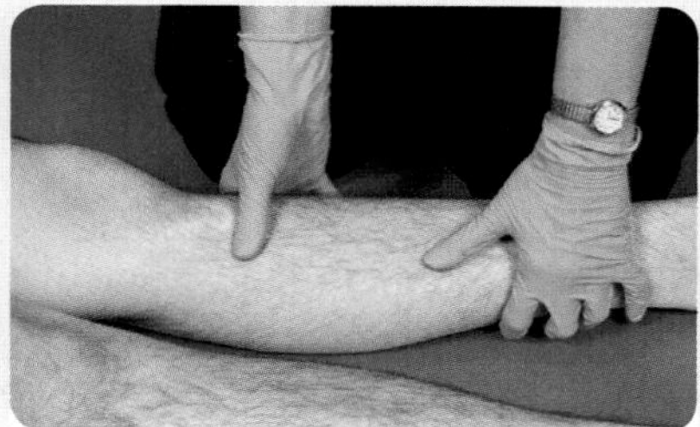

Step 22 Inspect all four extremities for any lacerations, bruises, swelling, deformities, or medical alert jewelry. Also, assess distal pulses and motor and sensory functions in all extremities. Compare right and left sides whenever possible.

Table 11-7 Common Chief Complaints and Focused Exams

Chief Complaint	Focused Exam
Chest pain	Evaluate skin, pulse, and blood pressure. Look for trauma to the chest, assess the external jugular veins, and listen to breath sounds. Assess for pedal/dependent edema. Obtain a 12-lead ECG.
Abdominal pain	Evaluate skin, pulse, and blood pressure. Look for trauma to the abdomen, and palpate the abdomen for tenderness or **rigidity**.
Shortness of breath	Evaluate skin, pulse, blood pressure, and rate and depth of respiration. Assess for airway obstruction. Listen carefully to breath sounds, and assess for hypoxemia (ie, use pulse oximetry). Assess for pedal/dependent edema. Obtain a 12-lead ECG.
Dizziness	Evaluate skin, pulse, blood pressure, and adequacy of respiration. Monitor the level of consciousness and orientation carefully. Check the head for signs of trauma. Evaluate for signs of stroke, including facial droop, slurred speech, and one-sided weakness. Check for a history of inner ear problems. Assess blood glucose level. Obtain an ECG.
Any pain associated with bones or joints	Evaluate skin, pulse, movement, and sensation adjacent and distal to the affected area.

neurologic system. A patient with an arm laceration may need only to have that arm evaluated. The goal of a focused exam is to focus your attention on the immediate complaint. Table 11-7 gives examples of common chief complaints and the appropriate corresponding focused exams.

Words of Wisdom

Many technologic devices are available to EMS personnel to aid in patient assessment. Although this equipment is considered excellent, always remember you are assessing a patient—not a machine. Take the time to explain what your tools are and why you are using them. This simple action may help lessen a patient's anxiety.

Mental Status

For patients with head-related symptoms (confusion, headache, altered mentation), assess and palpate the head to look for signs of trauma. Check for facial asymmetry, such as facial droop or other signs of a suspected stroke. Dilated or constricted pupils may indicate recreational drug use, whereas red conjunctiva may suggest drug or alcohol use. Elevated blood pressure often accompanies a headache, possibly secondary to hypertension.

Evaluate a patient's mental status by assessing cognitive function (the ability to use reasoning). At a minimum, evaluate the patient's degree of alertness. Use the AVPU scale, as described in the Primary Survey section, to help identify the patient's LOC. Test the patient's blood glucose using a glucometer if there is an altered mental status, especially if there is a history of diabetes. The steps for using a glucometer are shown in Skill Drill 11-4.

You can further assess mental status by considering whether the patient is alert and oriented (A × O) in four areas: person, place, time, and the event itself, and determining the GCS score, as discussed in the Primary Survey section of this chapter. Assessing whether the patient can recall his or her name tests long-term memory, whereas assessing whether the patient knows where he or she is and what happened tests short-term memory.

Once the basic mental status has been assessed, conduct a thorough mental status exam, especially in patients experiencing a behavioral emergency. This exam begins by assessing the patient's general appearance, including posture, facial expression, and ability to relax. Does the posture change with topics of discussion, with activities, or as certain people draw near the patient? A tense posture, restlessness, and fidgeting suggest the patient may be anxious, while a slumped posture and slow movements might indicate underlying depression. Observe the patient's face, both at rest and as he or she interacts with others. Watch for variations in expression with topics of discussion. Are the facial expressions appropriate? A relatively immobile face (ie, a patient who does not blink, or whose face appears to be frozen in a stare) throughout the exam may indicate Parkinson disease.

Skill Drill 11-4 Using a Glucometer to Assess Blood Glucose Level

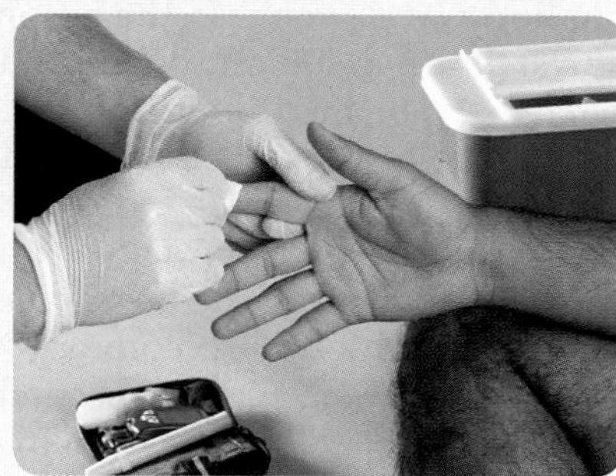

Step 1 Identify the need to obtain a blood glucose level, normal parameters for blood glucose level, contraindications, and possible complications. Take standard precautions. Clearly explain the procedure to the patient. Select, check, and assemble the equipment (glucometer, test strip, needle or spring-loaded puncture device, alcohol prep pads). Turn on the glucometer and insert a test strip. Cleanse the fingertip with an alcohol prep pad.

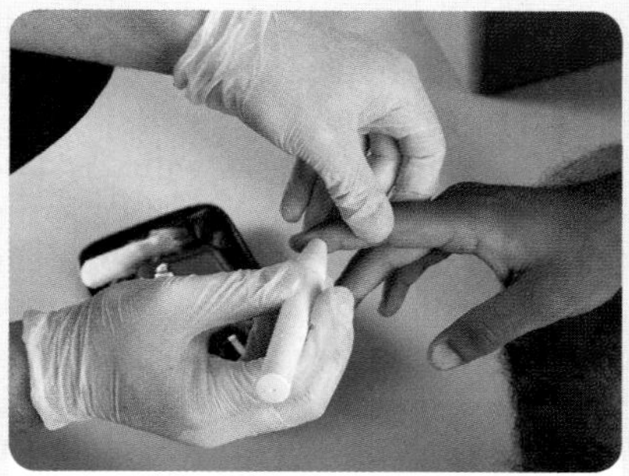

Step 2 Puncture the prepped site with lancet needle or puncture device, drawing capillary blood.

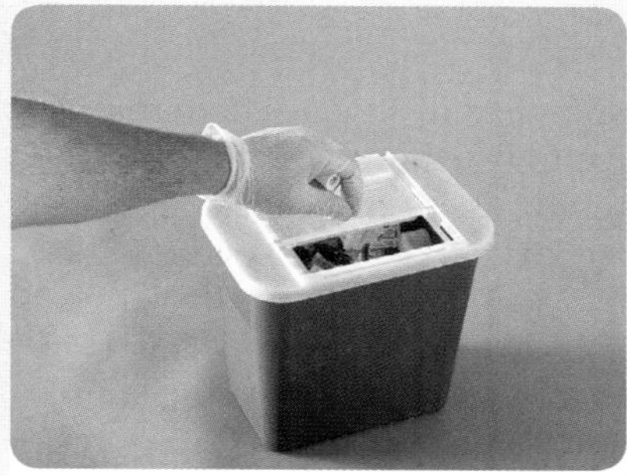

Step 3 Dispose of the lancet needle in a sharps container.

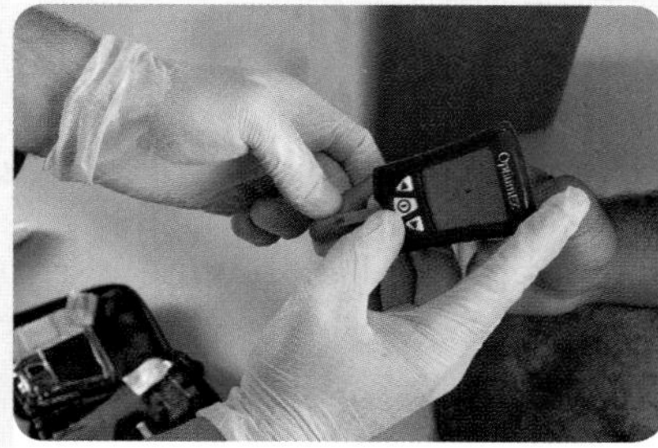

Step 4 Express a blood sample and transfer it to the test strip. Insert the test strip into the glucometer and activate the device per the manufacturer's instructions.

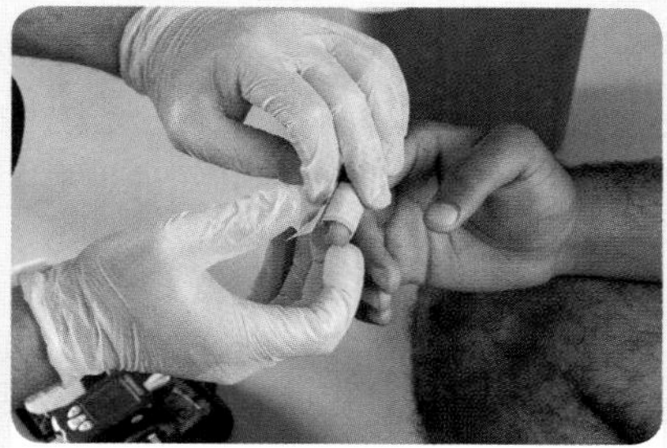

Step 5 Dress the fingertip wound with pressure and an alcohol prep pad, then place a bandage over the puncture site. Record the reading from the glucometer and document appropriately.

Special Populations

Clearly, a child or infant will respond differently than an adult, and mental status may be difficult to evaluate. A modified assessment should be used for these patients. First, determine whether the child is alert. Even infants should be alert to your presence and should follow you with their eyes (a process called "tracking"). Ask the parent whether the child is behaving normally, particularly with regard to alertness. Most children older than 2 years know their names and the names of their parents and siblings. Evaluate mental status in school-age children by asking about holidays, recent school activities, or teachers' names. This issue is addressed in Chapter 43, *Pediatric Emergencies.*

Note the patient's speech and language patterns. Pay attention to the quantity, rate, volume, articulation, and fluency of speech. Alterations in language suggest an underlying psychiatric or central nervous system (CNS) disease.

Ask the patient about his or her mood. This is an objective statement similar to the chief complaint. Simply asking, "how do you feel" may give you an appropriate response; however, more direct questioning regarding mood might be needed. All patients should be asked about suicidal ideation. Any patient who expresses thoughts of suicide should be evaluated at an appropriate facility.

Assessing the patient's thoughts and perceptions is an important part of the complete mental status exam. Assess the logic, relevance, organization, and coherence of the patient's thoughts simply by listening to his or her conversation. Listen for irregularities such as abrupt shifting of the conversation from one subject to another, invented or distorted words, and largely incomprehensible speech, which may indicate an underlying disorder such as schizophrenia. The patient's perceptions deal with senses. Ask your patient if he or she sometimes hears, sees, or feels things that others do not, even when no one else is there. Patients who answer "yes" to any of these questions may be experiencing hallucinations related to an underlying psychiatric illness or CNS disorder.

Listen for thought content that suggests phobias, obsessions, anxieties, or delusions. Delusions are false, fixed, personal beliefs not shared by most other members of the patient's culture. It is important that any observations made regarding the patient's thought content be relayed to the hospital.

Assess the patient's insight and judgment. Insight shows the patient's awareness of his or her illness and need for treatment. You can simply ask, "What do you think is wrong?" Some patients may respond by saying, "I'm depressed, and I know I need to get help." This demonstrates that the patient has positive insight into his or her illness. However, some patients may believe it's normal to hear voices and to feel they do not need treatment. These patients are considered to be lacking insight.

You can usually assess judgment by noting the patient's response to family and interpersonal conflict, jobs, and use of money. You can ask, "Who's going to look after your home while you're in the hospital?" Any inappropriate response may indicate delirium, dementia, a developmental delay, or a psychotic state.

Finally, the complete mental status exam includes a further assessment of the patient's cognitive function. This can be accomplished by assessing the patient's attention, memory, and ability to learn. There are several ways to assess the patient's attention. Two common ways are *serial 7s* and *spelling backward*: Serial 7s is conducted by having the patient start at 100, subtract 7, and continue subtracting 7. Note the patient's effort, speed, and accuracy. Spelling backward is another way to assess attention. Ask the patient to spell a five-letter word, such as W-O-R-L-D, forward and then backward. Once again, note the patient's effort, speed, and accuracy.

To assess memory, begin by assessing remote memory, such as birthdays, anniversaries, schools attended, and jobs held. It can be difficult to assess accuracy of remote memory if there is no one available to confirm the patient's answers, and, thus, it is not always the most accurate assessment tool. Next, inquire about the patient's recent memory. This could involve the events of the day. Ask the patient which medications he or she took today. Ask what the patient ate for breakfast, but like remote memory, someone must be available to confirm the answer. Finally, assess the patient's memory recall by giving him or her three or four words to remember, such as ball, key, and lawnmower. Ask the patient to recite the words 3 to 5 minutes later.

Skin, Hair, and Nails

Skin. Perhaps the quickest and most reliable initial way to evaluate a patient's overall degree of distress is to look at the skin. Relatively subtle but serious changes in overall circulation are usually manifested early on in the skin's appearance.

The skin, which is the largest organ system in the body, serves three major functions:

1. Transmit information from the environment to the brain
2. Protect the body from the environment
3. Regulate body temperature (thermoregulation)

In a cold environment, blood vessel constriction shunts blood away from the skin to decrease the amount of heat loss through radiation from the body surface (observed as pale skin). When the environment is hot, the blood vessels dilate, the skin becomes flushed or red, and heat loss occurs as it radiates from the body surface. Also, in a hot environment, sweat is secreted by sweat glands and carried to the skin surface by tiny ducts. A loss of energy, in the form of body heat, occurs during the evaporation process, which causes body temperature to fall. It is worth noting that at a humidity level of more than 85%, evaporation does not work.

Examine the skin by both inspection and palpation. Pay careful attention to the skin's CTC: color, temperature, and condition (moisture or texture), as well as **turgor** and any significant lesions or obvious deformities. Look for evidence of diminished perfusion, evaluate for pallor and cyanosis, and be wary of diaphoresis. Reddened or pink skin can be seen in a variety of normal states, but it is also evident in states of relative **vasodilation** (flushing). Flushed skin is usually apparent in patients with fever, and it may be seen in patients experiencing an allergic process. Reddened skin should also be considered in the context of superficial burns.

Examining the skin for changes in perfusion is usually best accomplished in areas in which the epidermis is thinnest, such as the fingernails, lips, and conjunctivae. It is sometimes useful to examine the palms and soles as well. Recall, pallor or paleness, occurs when red blood cell perfusion to the capillary beds of the skin is poor. You may also be able to detect pallor by looking at the patient's lips or the conjunctivae of the eyes. Pale skin is a relatively common finding in the seriously ill patient and may indicate severe **vasoconstriction**, as seen in profound anemia, acute cardiovascular events, other shock-like states, and hypothermia. Local areas of blanched, cool, white skin are typical of frostbite.

Cyanosis indicates a relative lack of oxygen perfusion, although the number of red blood cells may be adequate to carry any available oxygen. Cyanosis correlates extremely closely with low arterial oxygen saturation. Generally, it can be visualized in the skin, but more specifically in the fingernail beds, face, and lips. Although cyanotic skin is commonly seen in states of oxygen desaturation, it can also be a function of hypothermia, especially in young patients. **Mottling** is a typical finding in states of severe, protracted hypoperfusion and shock and is easily recognized in seriously ill or injured pediatric patients. However, when mottling is seen in a pediatric patient, do not immediately consider the finding "normal." It is important to consider all aspects of the history and physical to ensure there is no evidence of hypoperfusion.

Ecchymosis is localized bruising or blood collection within or under the skin. Evaluate large ecchymoses for the possibility of serious underlying soft-tissue, bony, or organ injury. Serious wounds to the head, neck, and torso should also be noted, as well as any evidence of a hemorrhage.

It takes practice to accurately gauge patients' relative perfusion and hydration status. Becoming familiar with the abnormal findings of the skin and mucous membranes is an excellent aid in judging both. Turgor relates directly to hydration. Poor skin turgor is an expression of poorly hydrated skin, with associated **tenting** evident in extreme cases, particularly in young children. Tenting is when skin slowly retracts—rather than quickly springing back into place—when it is pinched and pulled away slightly from the body. Just a few hours of profuse vomiting and diarrhea can leave an infant seriously dehydrated. Because of normal changes in elastin and connective tissues with advanced age, skin turgor is an insignificant indicator in older adult (geriatric) patients, as is skin that is abnormally dry to the touch.

Special Populations

When assessing skin turgor in an older patient, use the skin of the upper chest. This is a much more reliable indicator than the extremities.

Pay attention to skin temperature, as it can sometimes prove useful in determining the etiologies of different medical conditions (eg, respiratory distress). Sometimes it can help you make a clinical distinction between pneumonia and congestive heart failure with pulmonary edema.

Words of Wisdom

As you inspect the skin, always be alert for signs of possible abuse or maltreatment. Multiple bruises at different stages of healing or even pressure sores should raise concerns about possible physical abuse or neglect, and should be reported. Fingerprint bruises, that is, bruises caused by being grabbed, lifted, or dragged, should always make you suspicious.

Be aware that some medical conditions and folk medicine practices may be mistaken for abuse. For example, Mongolian spots are benign and not associated with any conditions or illnesses. Ehlers-Danlos syndrome is a condition associated with cuts, bruises, and scars attributable to the fragility of the patient's skin. Blood disorders such as hemophilia, von Willebrand disease, and leukemia can also cause skin changes such as those seen in abuse situations.

Examine the skin for lesions. Lesions result from many causes that are often difficult to determine. An accurate description of skin lesions is essential. They may be elevated, flat, or depressed. Lesions may also be categorized as vascular (associated with a blood vessel), infectious, traumatic, or inflammatory. They may be the result of a localized skin process or a manifestation of systemic disease. Examples of common lesions include birthmarks, moles, blisters, ulcers, scars, and warts. Skin lesions may sometimes be the only external evidence of a serious internal injury. Take note of any large areas of ecchymosis, palpable crepitus (palpable fractures), and open wounds. Devastating internal injuries can produce external signs that look relatively benign. Be aware of any body areas hidden by clothing or by devices such as a backboard and head immobilizer. Always visually inspect and

Table 11-8 **Abnormal Findings in the Nails**

Condition	Findings	Possible Cause
Beau lines	Transverse depressions in the nails indicating a period of growth inhibition	Systemic illness, severe infection, or nail injury
Clubbing	The angle between the nail and the nail base approaches or exceeds 180°	Flattening and enlargement of the fingertips is associated with chronic respiratory disease
Psoriasis	Pitting, discoloration, and subungual thickening of the nail	Autoimmune disease
Splinter hemorrhages	Red or brown linear streaks in the nail bed	Bacterial endocarditis or trichinosis
Terry nails	Transverse white bands covering the nail except for the distal tip	Cirrhosis

manually palpate the patient's back and expose the entire body. Likewise, evaluate the skin for rashes by discreetly examining areas of skin otherwise hidden by clothing.

Hair and Nails. Examine the hair by inspection and palpation. In this survey, note the quantity, distribution, and texture of the hair. Recent changes in the growth or loss of hair can indicate an endocrine disorder, such as diabetes, or may be the result of treatment modalities for disease processes such as chemotherapy or radiation treatment of cancer. Although recent hair loss may be related to a disease process, it can also be a normal finding in the older patient. Hair that has been forcibly ripped out often points to an abuse scenario.

Examine the fingernails and toenails to reveal many subtle findings Table 11-8 Figure 11-24. The color, shape, texture, and presence or absence of lesions should all be assessed. The normal nail should be firm and smooth on palpation. Normal changes to the nails with aging include the development of striations and a color change (yellow tint) related to the reduction in body calcium. Overly thick nails or nails that have lines running parallel to the finger often suggests a fungal infection.

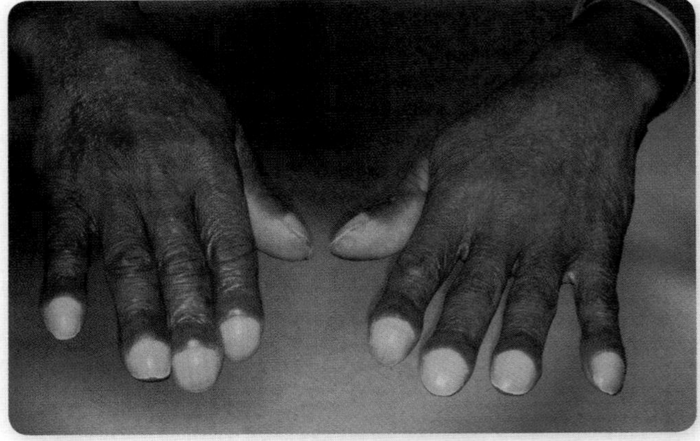

Figure 11-24 Clubbing is associated with chronic respiratory disease.

Head, Eyes, Ears, Nose, and Throat

The head, eyes, ears, nose, and throat (HEENT) exam consists of an evaluation of the head and related structures. It is crucial because the head contains the brain, numerous important sensory organs, and all of the upper airway anatomy. The eyes are a nervous system structure that involves both motor pathways (lids, extraocular muscles, pupillary constrictors, corneal blink reflex) and sensory pathways. The ears provide for both hearing and balance control. The nose is a sensory organ involved with the senses of smell and taste; it also plays an important role in assisting with breathing. The throat consists of the mouth, posterior pharynx, and all the structures intrinsic to them. This complicated organ simultaneously coordinates many motor and sensory functions, while also coordinating the initial activities of the respiratory and digestive systems.

Head. Examine the head by feeling it and inspecting it visually. This step is important in managing possible trauma patients, those with altered mental status, and those who are unresponsive. Inspect and feel the entire cranium for signs of deformity or asymmetry. Do not palpate any depressions so you do not push bone fragments into the cranial vault or the brain Figure 11-25. Note any warm, wet areas; they usually represent blood, cerebrospinal fluid (CSF), or a combination of the two. If you find evidence of external bleeding, attempt to separate the hair manually and irrigate the clot; this should allow you to identify the source of bleeding. Evaluate the skull for any deformity, or tenderness. Observe the general shape and contour of the skull. Look for scars or shunts that suggest a history of trauma or problems with the CNS. If you suspect the presence of a cerebral shunt, ask the patient where the shunt was placed and where it drains in the body.

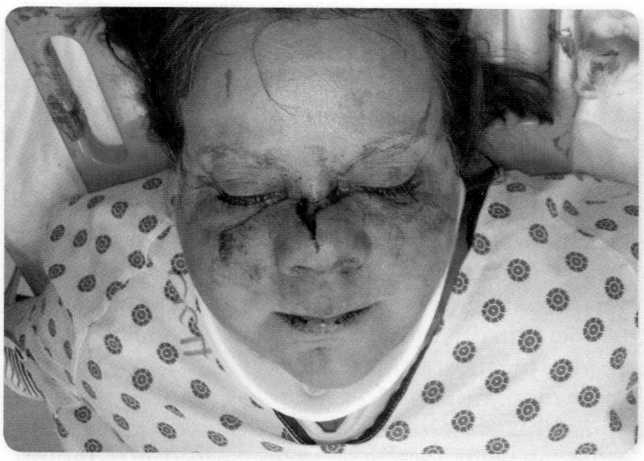

Figure 11-25 When examining the head and face, do not palpate any depression in the skin; you could push bone fragments into the cranial vault or brain.

Words of Wisdom

Protecting fragile CNS structures from further damage is vital to the patient's prospect of living a normal life. Lean toward caution and overprotection in assessing and treating possible brain and spinal cord injuries.

As you evaluate the face, assess the color and moisture of the skin, as well as expression, symmetry, and contour of the face itself. Asymmetry of the face could suggest an underlying nervous system problem, such as a stroke or facial nerve palsy. Also, pay attention to any swelling or apparent areas of injury, and note any signs of respiratory distress. Follow the steps in Skill Drill 11-5 to assess the head.

Skill Drill 11-5 Assessing the Head

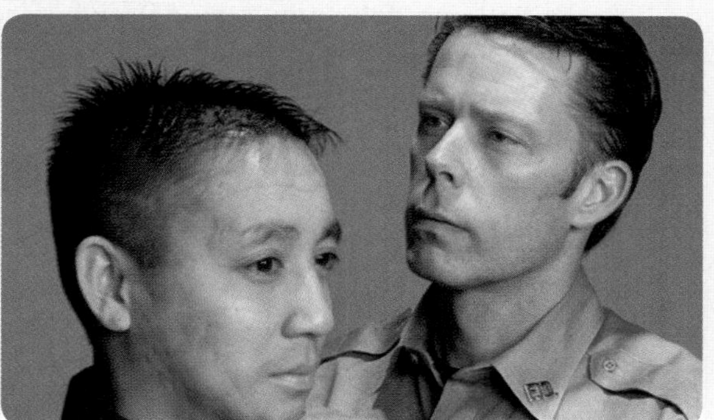

Step 1 Inspect and palpate the head for open/closed findings and crepitus.

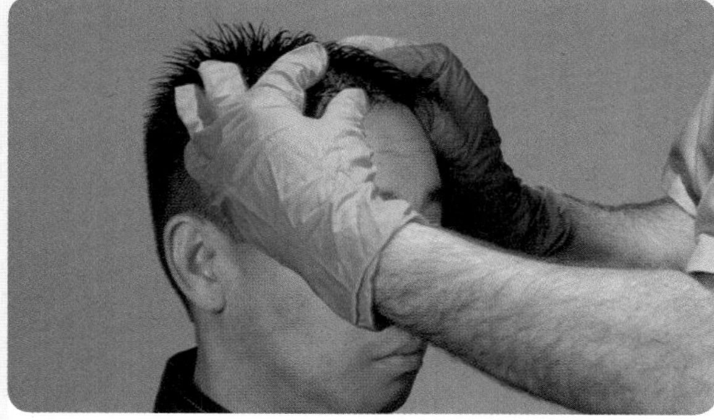

Step 2 Palpate the top and back of the head to locate any subtle abnormalities. Use a systematic approach, going from front to back, to ensure nothing is missed.

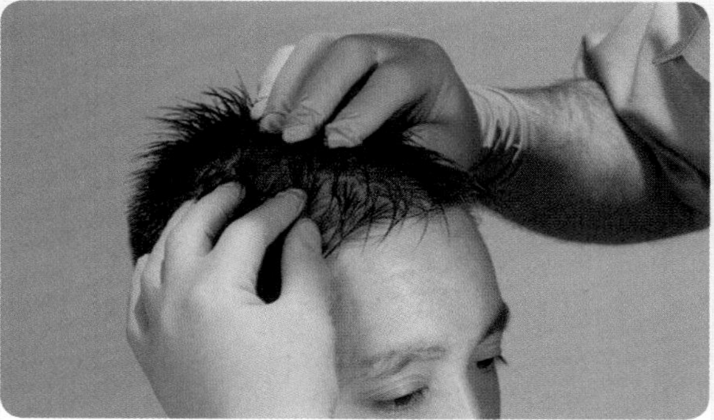

Step 3 Part the hair in several places to examine the condition of the scalp. Identify any lesions beneath the hair.

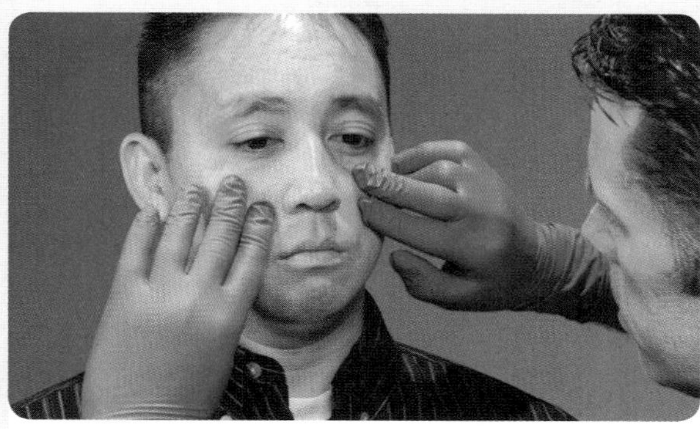

Step 4 Palpate the structure of the face. Note any open/closed findings and crepitus. Pay attention to the condition of the skin, hair distribution, and the shape of the face.

Eyes. The eyes are a tremendously complex sensory organ. They process light stimuli for the brain, so the brain can translate light impulses into visual images. The eyes are a critical link to the CNS, and as such they allow the examiner to more precisely assess the functions of the CNS.

Each eye consists of an anterior chamber and a posterior chamber, which are always assessed in a standardized fashion, from front to back. The outer aspects of the eye are checked first, with deeper structures subsequently evaluated. After you assess the outer eye, assess the patient's **visual acuity**—that is, how well the patient can see—by examining each eye in isolation. The standard tool for checking visual acuity is the Snellen (E chart) chart **Figure 11-26**, although it's not appropriate in the prehospital setting. More appropriate tools in this environment are simple tests, such as light/dark discrimination and finger counting. Reporting on visual acuity must include the distance from which finger counting was measured.

The pupil is a circular opening in the center of the pigmented iris of the eye. The diameter and reactivity of the patient's pupil to light reflect the status of the brain's perfusion. The pupils are normally round and of approximately equal size; they serve as optical diaphragms, adjusting their size to accommodate the available light. In the absence of light, the pupils will become fully relaxed and dilated. In normal room light, the pupils appear to be midsized. With high light levels or when a bright light is suddenly introduced, the pupils instantly constrict, allowing less light to enter, thereby protecting the sensitive receptor cells at the back of the eye.

Pupil size is regulated by a series of continuous motor commands that the brain automatically sends through the oculomotor nerves (third cranial nerve) to each eye. When a bright light is introduced into one eye (or higher levels of light enter one eye only), both pupils should constrict equally to the appropriate size for the pupil receiving the most light.

Asymmetric pupils (**anisocoria**, specifically, unequal pupils with greater than 1-mm difference, and which can be found in 19% of the population) may indicate significant ocular or neurologic pathology, but the condition must be correlated with the patient's overall presentation[14] **Figure 11-27**. Topical application of certain medications and substances can also provoke pupillary changes.

Also test muscle movement. Muscles are responsible for physically moving the eyes from side to side and up and down, which allows for seamless binocular vision.

To examine the eye, follow the steps in **Skill Drill 11-6**.

After the general eye exam, a more precise penlight exam is typically undertaken **Figure 11-28**.

Words of Wisdom

Failure of the eyes to track in a certain direction indicates weakness of an extraocular muscle or dysfunction of the cranial nerve that innervates it.

Words of Wisdom

Cataracts appear as opaque black areas against the red reflex.

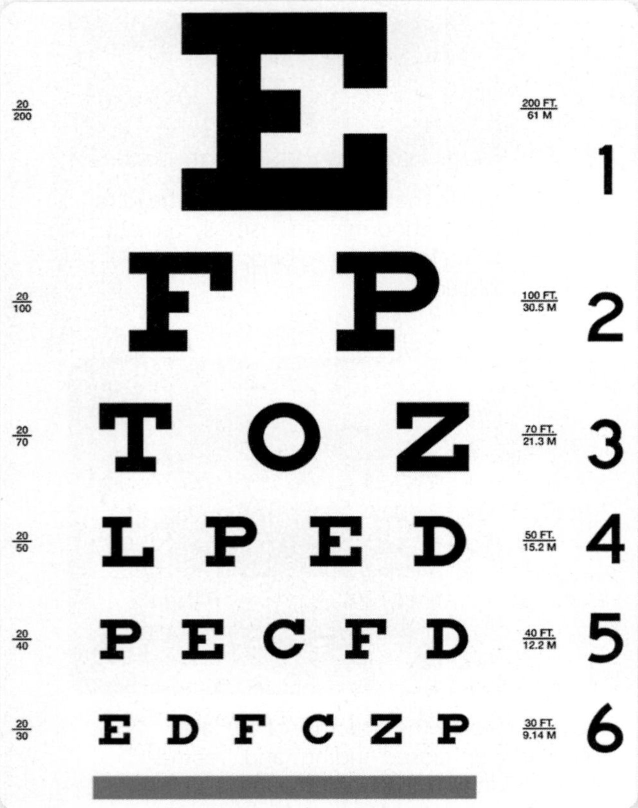

Figure 11-26 Because of its size and complexity, the Snellen chart is not a good prehospital tool.

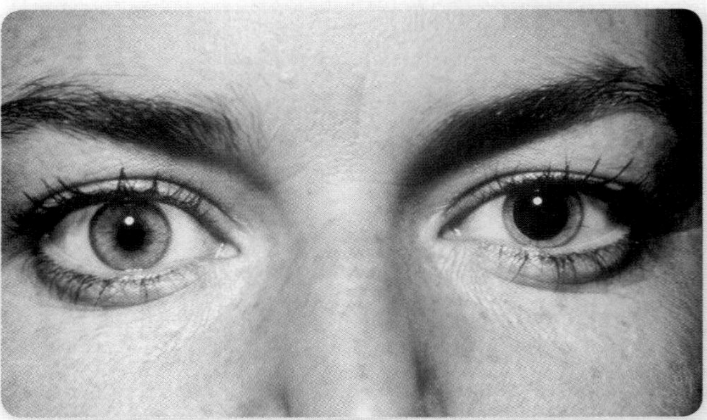

Figure 11-27 Asymmetric pupils may be normal or could signify a severe brain injury.

Skill Drill 11-6 Examining the Eye

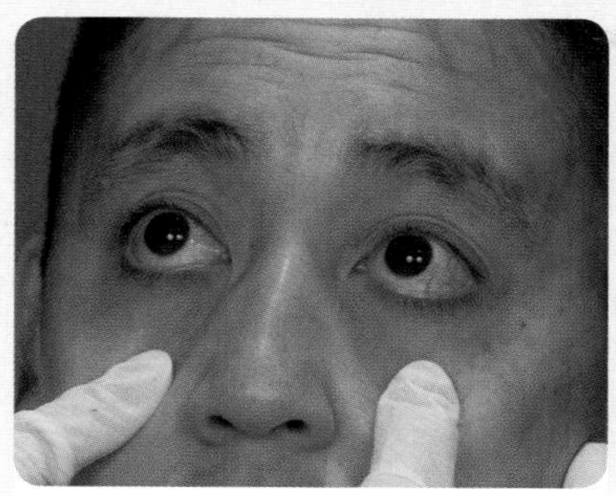

Step 1 Examine the exterior portion of the eye. Carefully inspect and palpate the upper and lower orbits, starting at the nose and working toward the lateral edge. Look for any obvious trauma or deformity. Ask about general problems, including any pain or redness, altered vision, vision loss, diplopia (double vision), photophobia, blurring, discharge, sensitivity to light, and corrective lens use. Note periorbital ecchymosis (raccoon eyes).

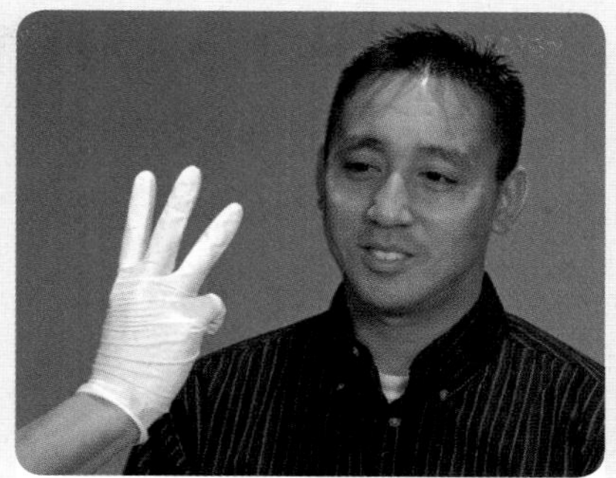

Step 2 Measure visual acuity by having the patient count the number of fingers you are holding up at varying distances (usually 6 feet (2 m), 3 feet (1 m), and 1 foot (0.3 m) away from the patient). Perform this exam on each eye independently. If corrective lenses are normally worn, check visual acuity with the correction in place.

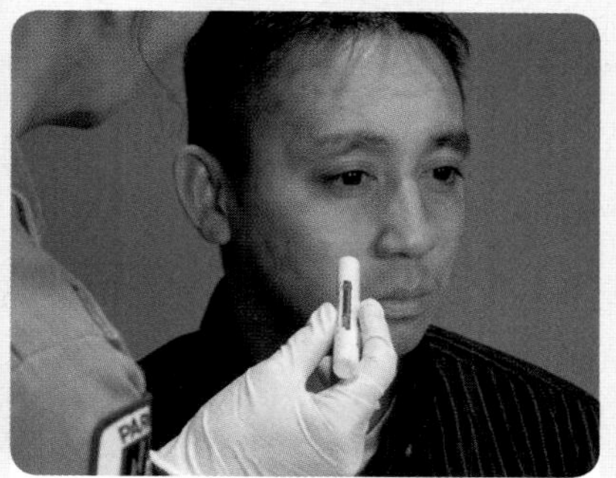

Step 3 Examine the pupils for size (in millimeters), shape, and symmetry. They should be equal. Test the pupils for their reactivity to light in as dark an environment as possible. Both pupils should constrict when exposed to light, and they should be equal in their response.

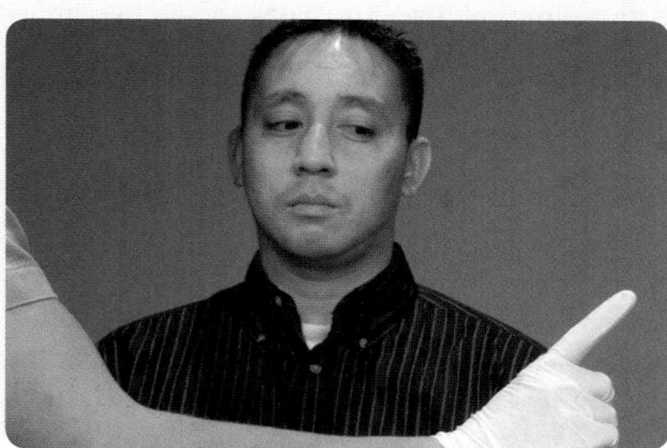

Step 4 Test for cranial nerve function by asking the patient to follow your fingers in a Z or H pattern. The eyes should move smoothly and symmetrically, tracking your finger movement. Evaluate whether the eyes move in sync (conjugate gaze) and whether they can track in all fields (up, down, left, right). Note any abnormal movement of the eyes. A visual field exam assesses the retina's (and therefore the optic nerve's) ability to perceive light. This is done by checking the patient's peripheral vision, examining each eye separately.

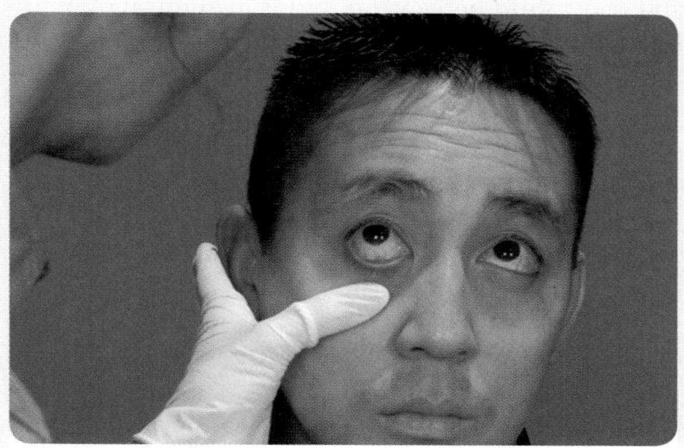

Step 5 Inspect the eyelids, lashes, and tear ducts for evidence of trauma or discharge. Turn up the lids to look for foreign bodies, and inspect the conjunctivae and sclera. The sclera ought to be white, not jaundiced or injected (red). Painless subconjunctival hemorrhage is a common but benign presentation. The conjunctivae should be pink—not cyanotic, pale, or overly reddened. The cornea and lens will be difficult to examine without additional assessment tools, although in a trauma situation, you should note whether the globe is patent. Next, examine the anterior chamber and iris for clarity, noting any cloudiness or bleeding.

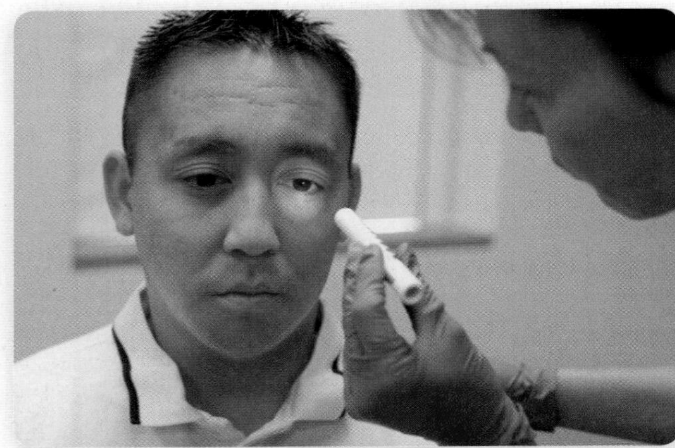

Figure 11-28 Penlight exam of the eye.

Words of Wisdom

Use of the ophthalmoscope requires *frequent practice*. It is not used in the traditional prehospital care setting, but may be used in situations where paramedics have received significant additional training and are working in an expanded scope setting.

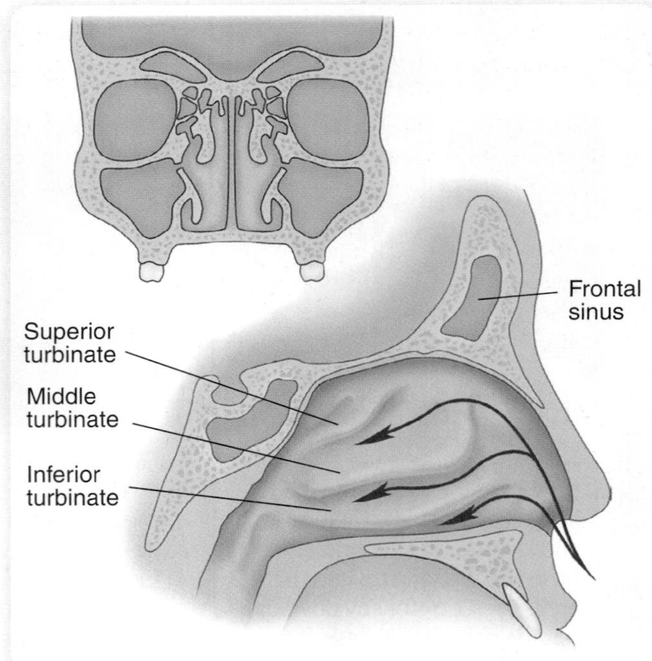

Figure 11-29 The nose has two chambers, divided by a septum. Each chamber is composed of layers of bone called *turbinates*. Above the nose are the frontal sinuses. On either side of the nose are the orbits of the eyes.

Ears. The ear is a sensory organ chiefly involved with hearing and sound perception, but is also intimately involved with balance control. The ear consists of an outer portion, a middle portion, and an inner portion.

Assessing the ears essentially involves checking for new aberrations in hearing perception and inspecting and palpating for wounds, swelling, or drainage (pus, blood, CSF). Often the mastoid process of the skull, which is palpated immediately posterior to the auricle, is assessed for discoloration and tenderness (**Battle sign**).

Nose. The nose is a sensory organ involved with smell and taste; it is also part of the respiratory system. As you assess injuries of the nose, it helps to picture the inside of the nose itself **Figure 11-29**. The nasal cavity is divided into two sections, or chambers, by the nasal septum, which is made of cartilage. Each nasal chamber contains three layers of bone (the turbinates) covered with a moist lining. Both chambers have superior, middle, and inferior turbinates. During nasal breathing, the air moves through the nasal chambers and is filtered and humidified as it passes over the turbinates.

As you check the nose, assess it both anteriorly and inferiorly. Look for evidence of asymmetry, deformity, wounds, foreign bodies, discharge or bleeding, and tenderness. Note any evidence of respiratory distress, such as flaring of the nostrils. Inspect the exterior of the nose, looking for color changes, symmetry, and structural abnormalities. The nose should be firm and the nares clear of obstruction. Examine the column of the nose; it should be midline with the face. Inspect the septum for any deviation from midline. The nares should be symmetric. Slight deviation or asymmetry of the nares, septum, and column are normal findings; however, gross abnormalities should be noted. Note any drainage or discharge.

Words of Wisdom

Frank blood or clear, watery drainage (CSF) from the ears or nose following trauma suggests a basilar skull fracture.

Throat. Assess the throat by evaluating the mouth, the pharynx, and sometimes the neck. The throat is a conduit for both respiration and digestion, and it is close to numerous vital neurovascular structures.

As part of assessing overall hydration status, pay close attention to the lips, teeth, oral mucosa, and tongue. In patients who present with markedly altered mental status, rapidly determine upper airway status; prompt assessment of the throat and upper airway structures is mandatory. Depending on the situation, assess for the presence of a foreign body or **aspiration** in either the throat or lower airway structures. Situations requiring removal of foreign bodies, secretions, or blood can manifest in many types of emergency cases. Always be prepared to assist with clearing the pharynx using manual techniques and suction.

Examine the mouth beginning with the lips, which should be pink and free of edema or surface irregularities.

Confirm the mouth is symmetric. The gums should be pink, with no lesions or edema. Cyanosis often presents early around the lips. Be alert for this sign! Listen for hoarseness and note any unusual odors.

Inspect the airway for obstructions. Visually inspect the tongue, noting its color, size, and moisture. The tongue should be located at midline, without swelling, and it should be moist.

Inspect and palpate the maxilla and the mandible, assessing the integrity and symmetry of both structures. Open the mouth, and look for signs of trauma (such as cracked or missing teeth, or missing crowns or onlays). Check the bite for fit.

Examine the oropharynx, identifying any discoloration or pustules that might indicate an infection. Be alert for any unusual odors on the patient's breath (such as alcohol or ketones). Check the posterior pharynx for fluids that may need to be suctioned. Inspect the uvula for edema and redness.

The neck is an extraordinarily muscular region, through which many vital structures pass. External anatomy includes the jaw, cricothyroid membrane, external jugular veins, thyroid cartilage, suprasternal notch, and cervical spinous processes. As you assess the neck, look for any abnormalities, including those related to symmetry, masses, and venous distention. When a patient is lying supine and sitting up at as much as a 45° angle, the jugular veins are naturally distended in a patient with an adequate blood volume. If JVD is present when the patient is sitting up at more than a 45° angle, then it is a sign of venous system overload or hypertension. JVD can be most readily observed by evaluating the anterolateral aspects of the neck; it can be provoked in a normal person by having the person lie supine and elevate the legs. Note how much distention is present, measured in centimeters from the origin of the jugular vein at the base of the neck to the angle of the jaw. Note the angle of the patient's position relative to 0° angle (flat) when you take the measurement. Palpate the carotid pulses and note the relative strength of the impulse. Look for any pulsating or expanding mass near the carotid pulse point. Palpate the suprasternal notch to identify any tracheal deviation. Look for a tracheal stoma. These are present in patients who have had a laryngectomy, and the stoma serves as their only means of a patent airway. If one is present, assess to ensure it is free of any obstruction. In these patients, all airway management should focus around the stoma. Have the patient open and close the jaws as you palpate over the temporomandibular joint during your examination of the jaw. Palpate for swollen lymph nodes, which are a sign of infection. Normally, lymph nodes are about the size of peas. When full of infectious material, they can increase to the size of grapes. To examine the neck, follow the steps in Skill Drill 11-7.

Cervical Spine

The cervical spine is the pathway by which the spinal cord makes its way out of the brain and into the torso, enabling the spinal nerves to reach and innervate the rest of the body Figure 11-30. It is also the point at which the head connects to the body. The spine is supported by a large muscle mass, as well as multiple tendinous and ligamentous supports. Cervical injury can present in a variety of ways, and the assessment for such injury must be conducted carefully.

Evaluate the patient first for the MOI and then for the presence of pain. Does the patient have an altered mental

Skill Drill 11-7 Examining the Neck

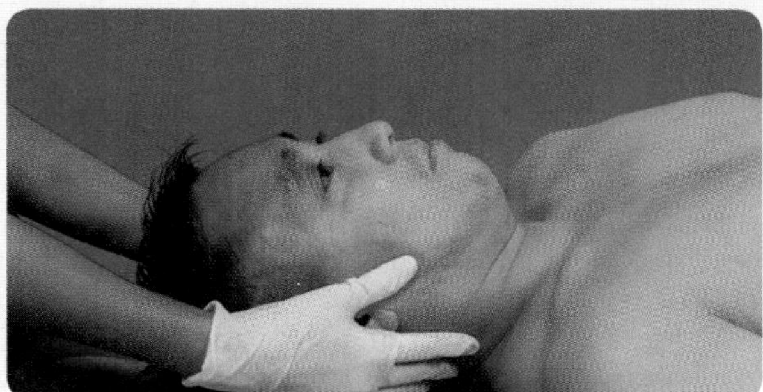

Step 1 If spinal trauma is suspected, take precautions to protect the cervical spine in accordance with your protocol. Assess for the usage of accessory muscles during respiration.

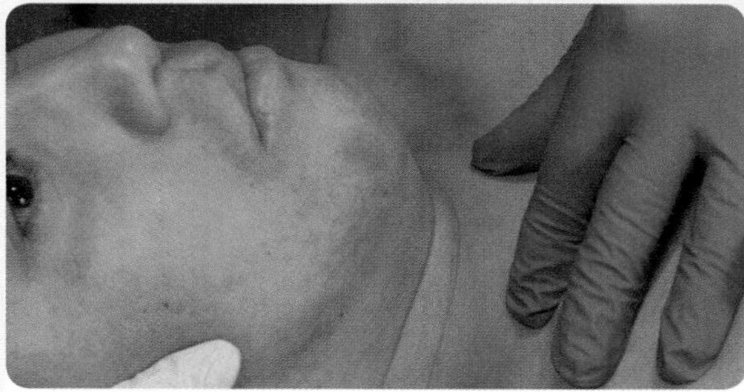

Step 2 Palpate the neck to find any structural abnormalities or subcutaneous air, and to ensure the trachea is midline. Begin at the suprasternal notch and work your way toward the head. Be careful when applying pressure to the area of the carotid arteries, because doing so may stimulate a vagal response.

(continued)

Skill Drill 11-7 Examining the Neck *(continued)*

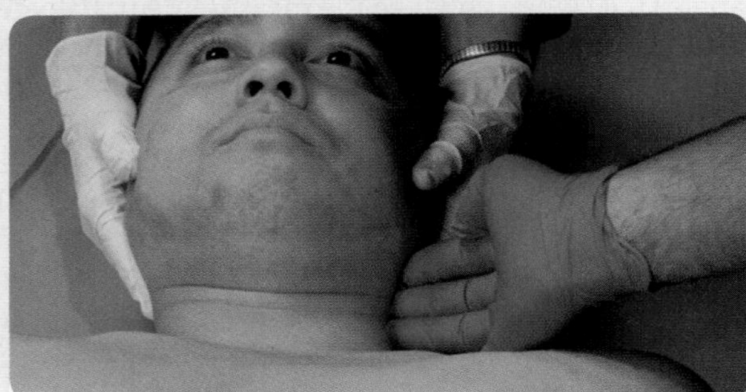

Step 3 Assess the lymph nodes and note any swelling, which may indicate infection.

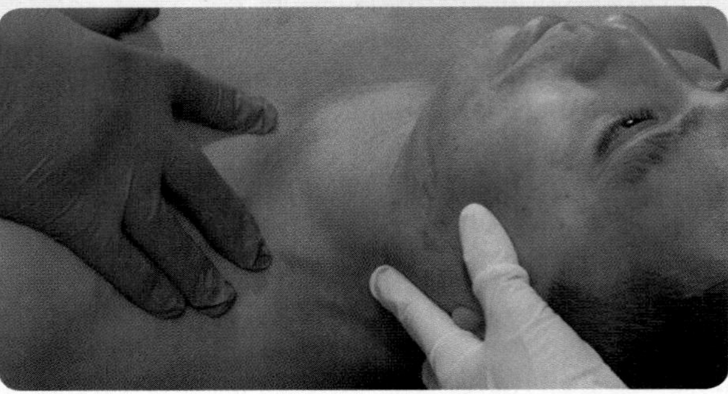

Step 4 Assess the jugular veins for distention, which may indicate a problem with venous return to the heart.

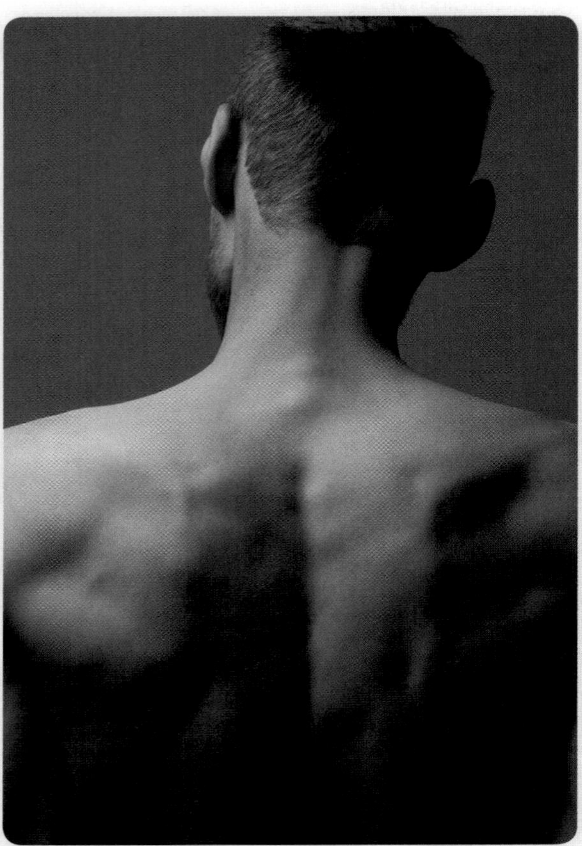

Figure 11-30 The cervical spine, as seen from the back of the neck.

status, or did a loss of consciousness occur at the time of the event? According to the 8th edition of *Prehospital Trauma Life Support,* indications for spinal immobilization include:

- Tenderness on palpation of the spinal column
- Complaint of pain in the spine
- Altered mental status (eg, traumatic brain injury, under the influence of ethyl alcohol or intoxicating substances)
- Inability to communicate effectively (eg, extremely young age, language barrier)
- GCS of less than 15
- Evidence of a distracting injury
- Paralysis or other neurologic deficit or complaint

As you examine the cervical spine, inspect and palpate it, look for evidence of tenderness and deformity. Pain is the single most reliable indicator of a spine injury or spinal cord injury. Midline posterior tenderness involving the bony spinous processes should always arouse concern. Palpable discomfort over the lateral aspects of the neck usually signals a muscular or ligamentous problem, not an injury to the bony spinal column itself. Any manipulation that results in pain, tenderness, or tingling should prompt you to stop the exam *immediately* and place the patient into a properly sized cervical collar. Any complaint of neck pain in patients who have sustained a significant MOI warrants careful evaluation and, depending on the findings, may warrant stabilization with a cervical collar and backboard depending on your local protocol. Continued assessment of a patient's range of motion should take place only when there is no potential for serious injury.

As you evaluate the neck, if there is no complaint of pain, no neurologic abnormalities such as weakness or numbness in the arms or legs, and no midline tenderness, then ask the patient to actively move his or her neck through a range of motion. Instruct the patient to stop if he or she encounters discomfort or any neurologic symptoms. Never move the patient's neck yourself (referred to as *passive motion* because the patient's participation is passive). This could result in spinal cord injury. To check range of motion, first have the patient slowly rotate his

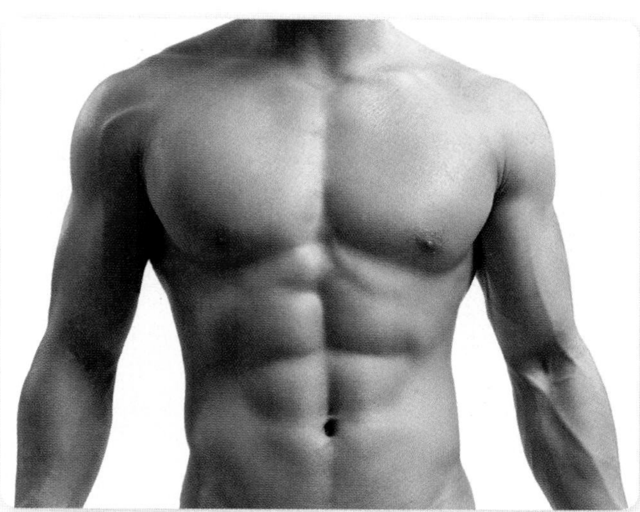

Figure 11-31 The chest (thorax) consists of the superior aspect of the torso, from the base of the neck to the diaphragm, as delineated by the costal arch.

or her head from shoulder to shoulder. Then, if there is no pain or discomfort, then have the patient extend the head back and flex the head and neck, touching chin to chest. Any discomfort elicited by these maneuvers should prompt you to terminate the exam immediately and protect the patient's spine.

Chest

The chest (or thorax) consists of the superior aspect of the torso, from the base of the neck to the diaphragm, as delineated by the costal arch Figure 11-31. The chest wall is divided into anterior and posterior portions—literally, the patient's front and back. The back of the chest extends down the patient's back, to the level of the diaphragm posteriorly, which moves up and down with breathing. The chest contains many vital structures, including the lungs and mediastinal elements (heart, great vessels). The chest wall serves as a protective covering for the internal components. It consists of numerous musculoskeletal, vascular, nervous, connective, and lining structures.

Typically, the chest exam proceeds in three phases: The chest wall is checked, a pulmonary evaluation is conducted, and the cardiovascular assessment is performed. The chest must be inspected to assess for deformities in wall patency and to look for external clues of respiratory distress. Expose the chest and begin your assessment, using the techniques of inspection, palpation, percussion, and auscultation. The examination of the posterior chest is the same as the examination of the anterior chest. Follow the steps in Skill Drill 11-8 to examine the chest.

Pay close attention to any signs of abnormal breathing movements (paradoxical or accessory muscle use, impaired or diminished breathing movement) and retractions (suprasternal, sternal, intercostal, or subcostal). Look for the signs of ventilatory fatigue, such as decreased mentation or a tired, worn-out appearance that often precedes ventilatory failure and, frequently, respiratory or cardiac arrest. Watch for the appearance of JVD with respiratory patients. It may point to pneumothorax or heart failure.

Look for signs of accessory muscle use or retractions, which suggest respiratory distress. Note any chest deformities, such as barrel chest (COPD), flail segments/subcutaneous air (trauma), kyphoscoliosis of the spine (compression fractures), significant bruising, and any suspicious wounds. Remember, flail segments may not be accompanied by paradoxical movement early on, because of the splinting effect of muscle spasms.

Palpate areas of the chest wall that were initially noted to be abnormal on inspection. Palpation will also enable you to better appreciate respiratory symmetry and expansion, and the overall work of breathing. Although often impractical in the prehospital environment, chest wall percussion can allow enhanced evaluation of the underlying chest cavity by distinguishing either dullness or hyperresonance.

The lungs have five discrete lobes: The right side contains upper, middle, and lower lobes; the left side contains upper and lower lobes. During your exam, listen over each lobe comparing from side to side, both anteriorly and posteriorly. To facilitate your auscultatory assessment, have the patient take as deep a breath as he or she can through an open mouth. Listen to as many portions of the lungs as possible, avoiding, of course, any bony prominences, attached medical equipment, and clothing. You can often hear a patient's breath sounds better from the patient's back; therefore, if the patient's back is accessible, listen there and assess six fields Figure 11-32. If you have stabilized the patient or if the patient is in a supine position, listen from the front and sides and assess four fields. Always use the best stethoscope available.

Normal breath sounds are clear and quiet during inspiration and expiration and are heard in three areas. **Bronchial sounds**, heard over the trachea, are hollow, tubular sounds that are lower pitched. The inspiration/expiration ratio is 1:3. The normal sounds found in the mid-chest or in the posterior chest between the scapula reflect a mix of pitch between the vesicular and bronchial sounds. The inspiration/expiration ratio is 1:1 and they are called **bronchovesicular sounds**. The soft and low-pitched sounds, normally heard over most of the lung surface, with a rustling quality during inspiration and softer sound during expiration are known as **vesicular sounds**.

Words of Wisdom

The lungs are hyperinflated in patients with chronic emphysema, resulting in hyperresonance where you would expect to hear cardiac dullness.

Secondary Assessment

Skill Drill 11-8 Examining the Chest

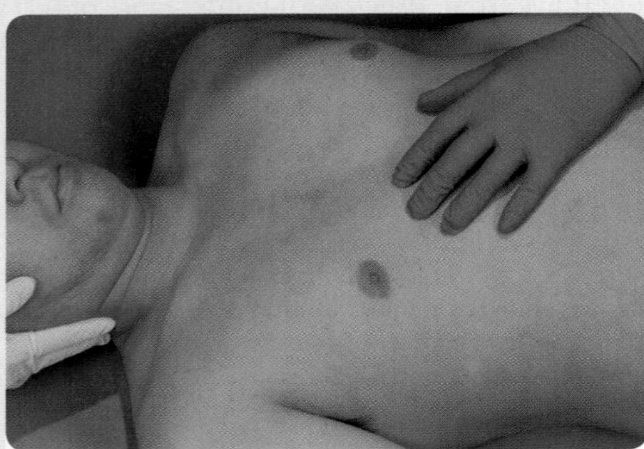

Step 1 Ensure the patient's privacy as best you can. Inspect and palpate the chest for open/closed findings, paradoxical motion, and crepitus. Observe the chest wall for respiratory effort, and document the respiratory rate, depth, and rhythm. If you find any open wounds, dress them appropriately.

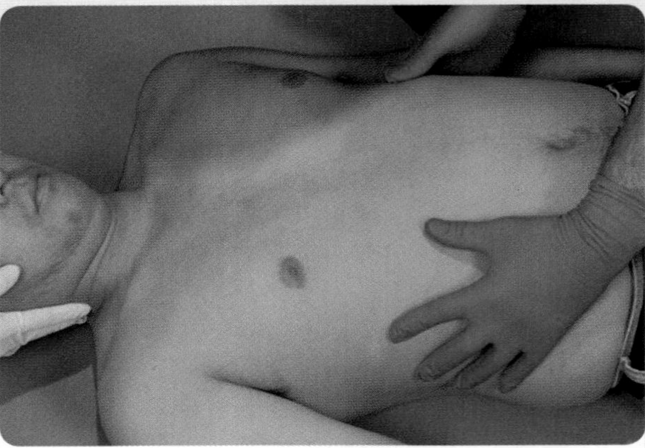

Step 2 Compare the two sides of the chest for symmetry. Note the shape of the patient's chest—it can give you clues to many underlying medical conditions, such as emphysema. Look for any surgical scars, such as a midline "zipper" scar, which may be the result of a previous cardiac surgery. Palpate the chest to reveal any air under the skin (as occurs in subcutaneous emphysema).

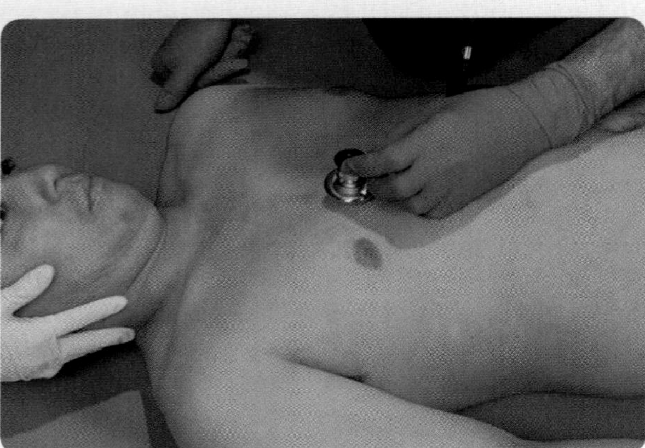

Step 3 Auscultate the lung fields. Note any abnormal lung sounds. Auscultate for heart tones. Always auscultate directly to the patient's skin, not through his or her clothing. Listening over the fabric will result in breath sounds being muted by the clothing. With each stethoscope placement, listen to at least one full inhalation and exhalation. If the patient is able to cooperate, then have him or her breathe through an open mouth to help emphasize the lung sounds.

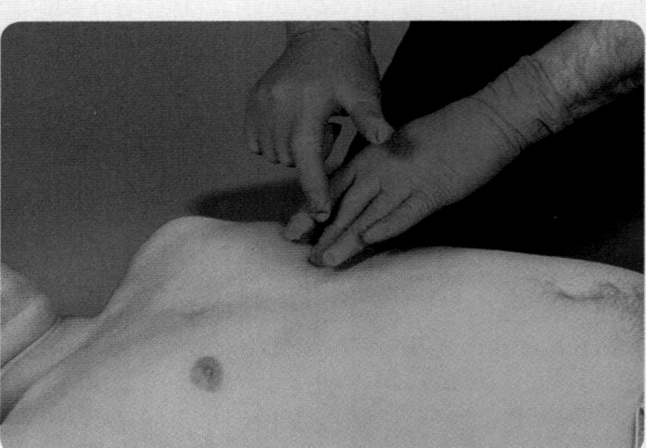

Step 4 Percuss the chest to detect any abnormalities. Repeat the appropriate portions of the exam for the posterior aspect of the thorax.

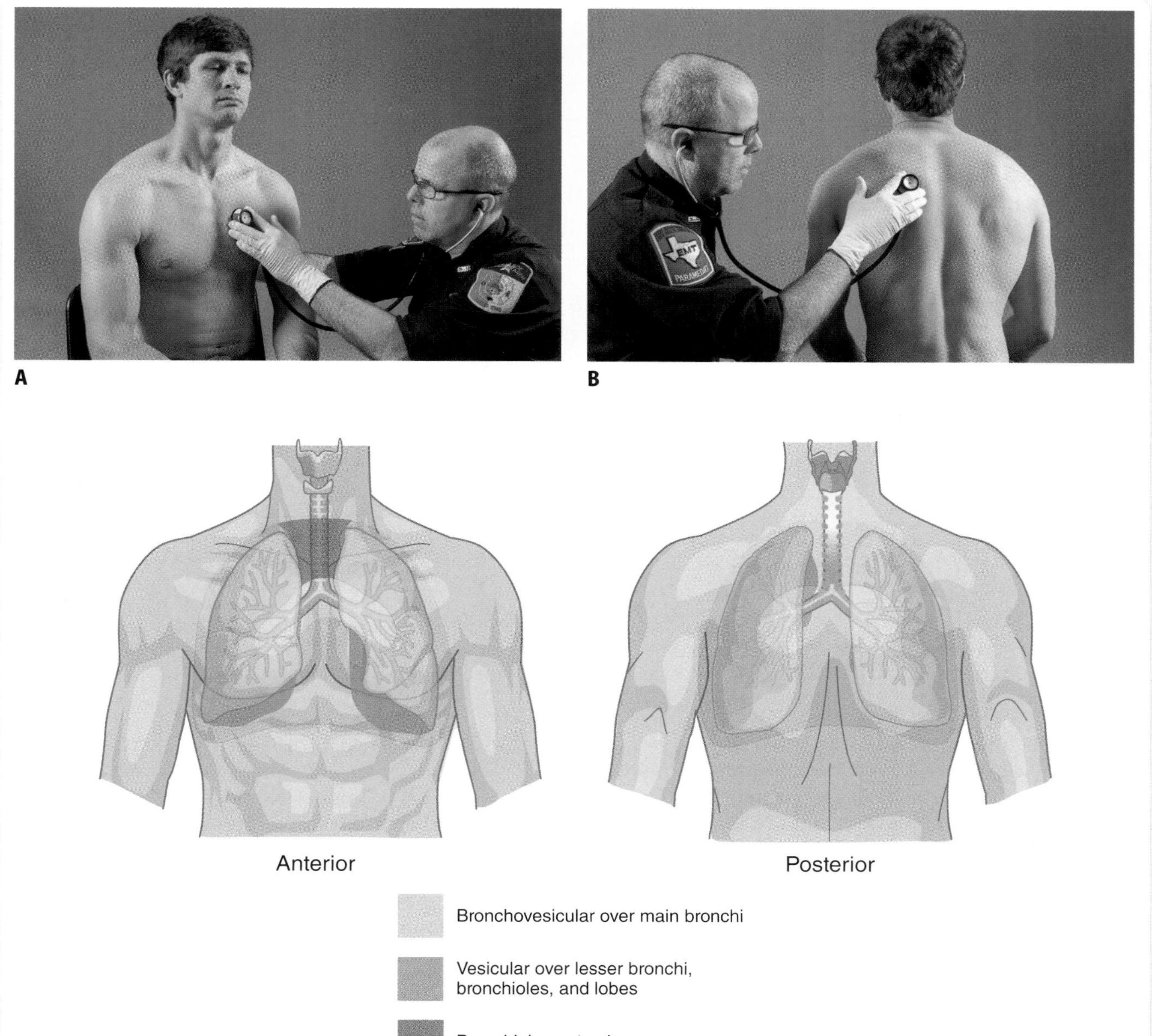

Figure 11-32 Locations for auscultating breath sounds: both sides of the chest in multiple lung fields, as shown. **A.** Stethoscope position for auscultating the front of the chest. **B.** Stethoscope position for auscultating the back. **C.** Colors in illustration correspond to areas where sounds are heard.

For patients with respiratory complaints, assess breath sounds early and often. Pathologic or **adventitious breath sounds** include the following **Figure 11-33**:

- **Wheezing breath sounds.** These sounds suggest lower airway obstruction. **Wheezing** is a high-pitched whistling sound that is most prominent on expiration but can be heard on inspiration in sicker patients. If wheezing is unilateral, an aspirated foreign body or infection should be suspected. If wheezing is bilateral, suspect asthma. Other causes include an inhaled irritant, such as chlorine, or other, less common lung diseases, such as asbestosis, may be the problem.
- **Crackles** (also called *rales*). Wet breath sounds may indicate cardiac failure or infection, especially in a young child. Such sounds are often difficult to hear, especially in the back of a moving ambulance. A moist crackling, usually on inspiration and expiration, is called *crackles.* Crackles are produced by oxygen passing

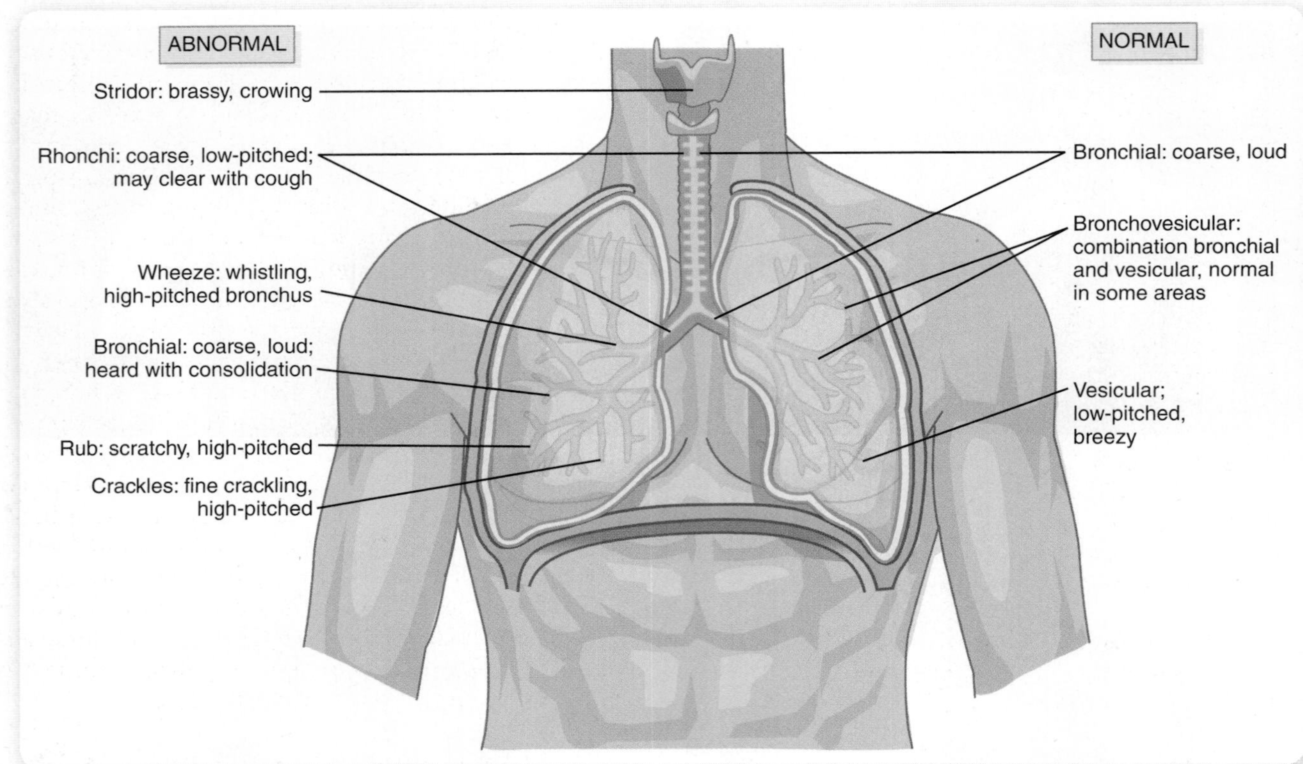

Figure 11-33 Locations and descriptions of abnormal (adventitious) breath sounds versus normal breath sounds.

through moisture in the bronchoalveolar system, or by closed alveoli opening abruptly. Examples of conditions in which crackles may be heard include pneumonia, heart failure, asthma, and restrictive pulmonary diseases.

- **Rhonchi.** Rhonchi, or congested breath sounds, are continuous sounds with a lower pitch and a rattling quality. They indicate fluid in the larger airways. They may indicate the presence of mucus in the lungs, for example, as a result of infection (such as pneumonia) or inflammation (such as bronchitis). Expect to hear low-pitched, noisy sounds that are most prominent on expiration. The patient often reports a productive cough associated with these sounds. Aspiration of fluid may also produce rhonchi.
- **Stridor.** Stridor is a brassy crowing sound often heard without a stethoscope. It is caused by the narrowing, swelling, or obstruction of the upper airway and may indicate the patient has an airway obstruction in the neck or upper part of the chest. It is most prominent on inspiration. Stridor may be caused by bacterial epiglottitis, viral croup, swelling from upper airway burns, or a partial foreign body airway obstruction. Stridor often indicates a life-threatening condition, because it equates to an 85% reduction in airway size. The onset of crowing or stridor in the presence of fever or upper respiratory infection should be recognized as a threat to life.
- **Pleural friction rubs.** These squeaking or grating sounds occur when the pleural linings rub together. If this occurs, the pleural layers have lost their lubrication, most commonly because of pleural inflammation. This condition is usually associated with pain on inspiration. The sounds may be heard anytime the chest wall moves; therefore, they can be heard on inspiration, expiration, or both.

Words of Wisdom

Percussion of the chest produces hyperresonance when the thorax is full of air and hyporesonance, or dullness, when it is full of blood.

At times even the most experienced provider has difficulty deciphering the various pathologic lung sounds. In these instances, it might be helpful to describe the sounds rather than attempt to classify them immediately. Ask yourself if the sounds appear to be dry or moist. Moist sounds might suggest pneumonia or pulmonary edema. Are the sounds continuous or intermittent? Continuous sounds suggest a pathologic process, whereas intermittent sounds could be from a partial foreign body obstruction or a reversible process, such as bronchospasm. Define the sounds as coarse or fine. Coarse sounds are louder and harsher and suggest a possible problem in the bronchial tree, whereas fine sounds are quieter and sometimes associated with a lower airway problem.

Words of Wisdom

One of the most important—and perhaps most often overlooked—aspects of pulmonary assessment is appreciating when breath sounds are diminished or absent. Numerous medical conditions can cause decreased breath sounds, including pneumothorax, hemothorax, pleural effusion, pulmonary edema, atelectasis/consolidation, exacerbated COPD, status asthmaticus, opiate intoxication, pneumonia, bronchitis, and altered mental status. You cannot be aware of diminished or absent breath sounds without first developing an appreciation of the wide spectrum of normal presentations that exist. Before going out into the field, spend many hours listening to normal breath sounds so you develop an understanding of what constitutes the many variations of normal breathing. After that, spend time listening to patients with respiratory difficulty, preferably alongside an experienced provider who can point out the significant variations in the presenting abnormalities.

Decreased breath sounds can be localized to a portion of one lung, or they can encompass the entire chest. When hypoventilation is suspected, take immediate action. Decreased breath sounds typically signal a lack of respiratory excursion or decreased tidal volume. If decreased breath sounds are localized to a specific area, assess transmitted voice sounds to see if there is any increased vocal resonance, which is a sign of consolidation in the lung, suggesting possible pneumonia. Further assessment of increased vocal resonance can be made by testing for **bronchophony**. Place the diaphragm of the stethoscope over the suspected area of consolidation and ask the patient to say, "ninety-nine." In healthy lung tissue, the term should sound muffled and indistinct; however, if the sound is loud and clear, this is considered bronchophony and suggests an area of consolidation. A similar test, called **whispered pectoriloquy**, is performed in the same manner, but with the patient whispering "ninety-nine." Once again, a normal response should be muffled and indistinct. A louder and clearer whisper is considered a positive test. Another test for consolidation is **egophony**. Here you place the diaphragm over the area of decreased breath sounds and ask the patient to say a drawn-out *"eeee."* A normal response will elicit a muffled long vowel sound. However, if there is any consolidation in the area, the sound will sound like an "A." Keep in mind, these tests require an optimal listening environment—something that's hard to find at an emergency scene.

Words of Wisdom

Normal breathing should be quiet and not grossly evident to you. If you can see or hear the patient working hard to breathe, there's a problem.

YOU are the Paramedic PART 4

Your crew has finished moving the patient onto your stretcher, and you're moving the patient to the ambulance for transport to the trauma center. En route you plan to start an IV line for fluid administration, oxygenate the patient, and closely monitor his ventilation.

Recording Time: 10 Minutes	
Respirations	28 breaths/min, shallow
Pulse	120 beats/min, weak
Skin	Cool, pale, clammy
Blood pressure	92/62 mm Hg
Oxygen saturation (Spo_2)	99% on 15 L/min O_2 via nonrebreathing mask
Pupils	PERRLA

7. How can you determine the level of internal damage if you do not have the implement that was used to stab the patient?

8. What is the relevance of past medical history in this case?

Secondary Assessment

Cardiovascular System

The cardiovascular system circulates blood throughout the body, an activity that maintains perfusion of the body's tissues. Blood flows through two circuits: the systemic circulation in the body and the pulmonary circulation in the lungs. The systemic circulation carries oxygen-rich blood from the left ventricle through the body and back to the right atrium. As this blood passes through the tissues and organs, it gives up oxygen and nutrients and absorbs cellular wastes and carbon dioxide. The cellular wastes are, in turn, eliminated as the blood is filtered by the liver and kidneys. The pulmonary circulation carries oxygen-poor blood from the right ventricle through the lungs and back into the left atrium.

The cardiac cycle consists of the events of cardiac relaxation (diastole), filling, and contraction (systole). These mechanical events are coordinated electrically with the heart's pacing and conduction system.

The contraction and relaxation of the heart, combined with the flow of blood, generates characteristic heart sounds during auscultation with a stethoscope. The normal pattern sounds much like this: "lub-DUB, lub-DUB, lub-DUB . . ." The "lub" is referred to as the first heart sound or S_1, and the "DUB" (emphasized because it is often louder) is the second heart sound, or S_2. S_1 represents the closure of the atrioventricular valves, marking the onset of ventricular contraction, or systole. S_2 represents the closure of the semilunar valves, marking the onset of ventricular relaxation, or diastole.

Pathologic heart sounds include S_3 and S_4. The S_3, or third heart sound, is a soft, low-pitched rare sound occurring early in ventricular diastole as the mitral valve opens allowing passive filling of the left ventricle. Although S_3 is sometimes present in healthy young people, it is most commonly associated with abnormally increased filling pressures in the atria secondary to moderate to severe heart failure. S_4, which is considered a "gallop" rhythm, is a low-pitched sound occurring with late diastolic filling of the ventricle due to atrial contraction. S_4 occurs immediately before the normal S_1 sound; it is always abnormal. The S_4 sound represents either decreased stretching (compliance) of the left ventricle or increased pressure in the atria. Events on the right side of the heart usually occur slightly later than those on the left side, creating two discernible sounds, rather than one heart sound. This is known as **splitting**. This most often occurs with S_2 and is a finding upon auscultation of the S_2 heart sound. It is caused when the closure of the aortic valve and the closure of the pulmonary valve are not synchronized normally. A split S_2 that does not change with respiration may indicate a serious heart problem and warrants further evaluation.

> **Words of Wisdom**
>
> The S_3 sound is associated with heart failure and should be considered abnormal in patients older than age 35.

You can appreciate heart sounds by listening to the chest wall in the parasternal areas superiorly and inferiorly, as well as in the region superior to the left nipple. To auscultate heart sounds, place the patient in a position that will bring the heart closer to the left anterior chest wall, such as sitting up and leaning slightly forward. Place your stethoscope at the fifth intercostal space over the apex of the heart; this should correspond approximately to the mitral valve. **Figure 11-34** shows where to place the stethoscope to hear various heart sounds.

Korotkoff sounds are related to a patient's blood pressure. There are five Korotkoff sounds, but only the first and fifth are clinically significant. The sounds are as follows, and occur in this order:

1. Phase I—Clear, faint, tapping sounds that gradually increase in intensity; correlates to systolic contraction.

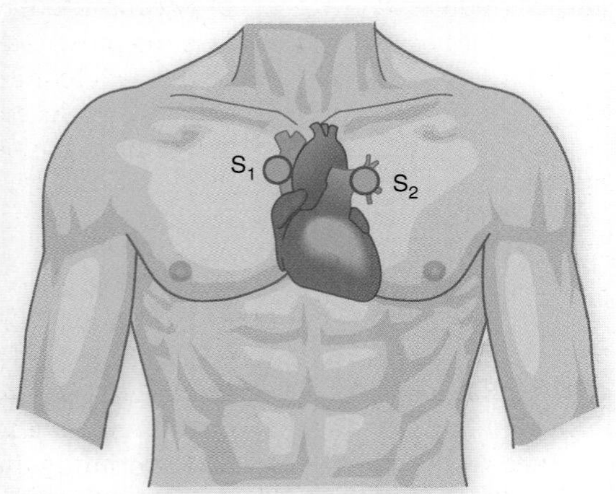

Heart Sound	Represents	Where Heard
S_1	Aortic region—closure of atrioventricular valve	2nd to 3rd intercostal space at right sternal border
S_2	Pulmonic region—closure of semilunar valve	2nd to 3rd intercostal space at left sternal border
S_3	Tricuspid region	4th, 5th, 6th intercostal space at left sternal border
S_4	Mitral region—closure of the mitral valve	Apex of the heart—5th to 6th intercostal space at left midclavicular line

Figure 11-34 Locations for stethoscope placement when auscultating heart sounds. To appreciate the S_2 sound, ask the patient to breathe normally and hold his or her breath on inhalation. Auscultate the area above the left nipple to listen for S_3 and S_4 heart sounds.

2. Phase II—Sounds change to a soft *swishing* sound.
3. Phase III—Sounds become crisper again and increase in intensity; softer than tapping sounds in Phase I
4. Phase IV—Sounds become muffled.
5. Phase V—All sounds disappear; correlates to diastolic pressure.

The second and third Korotkoff sounds have no known clinical significance.

In some patients, between Phases II and III, sounds may disappear briefly. This is referred to as auscultatory gap.

While inspecting and palpating the chest, listen for heart sounds. Feel the chest wall to locate the point of maximum impulse (PMI) and appreciate the apical pulse. Palpate for any **lifts** (also called **heaves**—the perception of the heart beating very strongly) in the chest wall, suggesting hypertrophy. Be aware of any **thrills** (humming vibrations). A palpable thrill suggests an underlying bruit or murmur and warrants further investigation. Listen over the areas in which the cardiac valves are located: The aortic valve is near the second intercostal space, to the right of the sternum. The pulmonic valve lies near the second intercostal space, to the left of the sternum. The tricuspid valve is auscultated over the lower left sternal border. The mitral valve can be assessed over the cardiac apex, lateral to the lower left sternal border near the midclavicular line. Note the intensity of the heart sounds, and listen for S_1, S_2, and any extra sounds and murmurs.

A **bruit** is an abnormal *whooshing* sound that indicates turbulent blood flow moving through a narrowed artery (most significant in the carotid arteries). A **murmur** is an abnormal *whooshing* sound heard over the heart that indicates turbulent blood flow around a cardiac valve. Murmurs are graded according to intensity, from 1 (softest) to 6 (loudest). Many people have normal physiologic murmurs. In some patients, they can represent a degree of pathology, depending on the nature of the underlying condition and the specific anatomy of the valve involved. To fully appreciate the nature and quality of normal heart sounds and murmurs, you must thoroughly practice your listening skills using excellent equipment.

Arterial pulses represent systolic blood pressure. They occur when contraction of the left ventricle and subsequent ejection of blood into the systemic circulation generate a pressure wave, which then travels throughout the arterial system. Arterial pulses are palpable wherever an artery crosses a bony prominence.

Venous pressure tends to be low. In fact, in the normal setting, the pressure in the venae cavae just before blood is received into the right atrium is close to zero. Veins are relatively nonmuscular, thin-walled vessels do not affect systemic vascular resistance or support systemic blood pressure. Blood flows through the venous system and returns to the heart in part because it is propelled continuously from behind, draining the capillary network. Most venous blood return is a function of the respiratory cycle, propelled by negative intrathoracic pressure generated at inspiration during normal breathing.

Assess the extremities, particularly the lower extremities, for any sign of venous obstruction or insufficiency. Signs include venous engorgement, palpable edema, swelling, hyperpigmentation, and mild erythema. Patients may report swelling, painful superficial veins, heaviness in the extremities, or changes in skin color.

Occasionally, jugular venous pressure helps you estimate the capacity of the venous system. Anytime you see JVD, determine the location of the venous obstruction that's impeding blood return to the heart. If the patient has penetrating left chest trauma, JVD may indicate cardiac tamponade. If the patient has pedal edema, consider heart failure. Specifically, in right-sided heart failure, blood flow into the right atrium tends to be sluggish. Venous capacitance increases in an effort to compensate, which in turn elevates pressure and results in JVD. If you palpate the liver and see significant JVD, this suggests liver disease or inflammation secondary to hepatitis.

In situations involving hypotension, evidence of JVD may be absent, even while the patient is supine. However, hypotensive patients with JVD must be carefully assessed as to the nature of their condition. Depending on the clinical situation, patients with JVD may be experiencing cardiogenic shock or have a ruptured cardiac valve. In the setting of chest trauma, neck vein distention and hypotension may point to a tension pneumothorax or pericardial tamponade.

The ability of the circulatory system to constrict and dilate can diminish markedly as a person ages. Although this limitation varies considerably from patient to patient, an older patient's ability to compensate for a cardiovascular insult may be profoundly curtailed by age-related changes, especially arterial atherosclerosis and diabetes. In addition, many medications that older people routinely take to manage medical conditions such as high blood pressure can impair the body's ability to handle sudden changes in the demand for blood supply (for instance, the body wants to increase the pulse rate, but a beta-blocker medication won't let it accelerate). By contrast, the vessels of children and young adults are better able to vasoconstrict and increase the pulse rate to compensate for a vascular insult; this compensation mechanism can fool you into believing young patients are less sick than they actually are.

As you examine a patient's cardiovascular system, pay attention to arterial pulses, noting their location, rate, rhythm, and quality. In addition, note the amplitude of the pulses (for example, weak and thready versus strong and bounding). Obtain an accurate blood pressure, and repeat this measurement periodically to monitor the patient's hemodynamic stability. Note if the patient has a history of hypertension, and if so, note which class of hypertension the patient falls into Table 11-9. Palpate the carotid arteries and listen to them with the bell of the stethoscope to assess for any bruits (discussed later).

Table 11-9 Hypertension Classification

Hypertension Classification	Systolic Blood Pressure (mm Hg)	Diastolic Blood Pressure (mm Hg)
Normal	< 120	and < 80
Prehypertension	120–139	or 80–89
Stage 1 hypertension	140–159	or 90–99
Stage 2 hypertension	≥ 160	or ≥ 100

For a suspected heart problem, assess the pulse for regularity and strength, and examine the skin for signs of hypoperfusion (pallor and cool, moist skin) or oxygen desaturation (cyanosis). If the pulse feels irregular, assess it over 1 minute, rather than for only 30 seconds, to obtain a more accurate measurement of the rate. Listen to breath sounds, since many cardiac conditions are associated with respiratory problems—crackles secondary to pulmonary edema, for instance. Obtain baseline vital signs. Serious hypotension with sustained or progressive tachycardia is common in cardiogenic shock; stay alert for this condition, because it has a mortality rate of more than 80%. Check for JVD, too. It can indicate heart failure, cardiac tamponade, or pneumothorax. Examine the extremities for signs of peripheral edema, which may indicate right-sided heart failure.

Abdomen

Because of the large number of organs within the abdomen, the location of those structures, and the complexity of associated medical complaints, the abdomen is easily described by mentally dividing it into four quadrants. The diaphragm—the large, dome-shaped muscle used for respiration—is at the top of the abdominal cavity, and the pelvis is at the bottom. The quadrants—left upper quadrant (LUQ), right upper quadrant (RUQ), left lower quadrant (LLQ), right lower quadrant (RLQ)—are marked by a set of imaginary perpendicular lines intersecting at the umbilicus, which serves as the central reference point Figure 11-35.

Alternatively, assess the abdominal organs by dividing the abdomen into nine regions: right hypochondrial, RH; epigastric, E; left hypochondrial, LH; right lumbar, RL; umbilical, U; left lumbar, LL; right iliac, RI; hypogastric, H; left iliac, LI Figure 11-36.

The abdomen contains almost all of the organs of digestion, the organs of the genitourinary system, and significant neurovascular structures. The abdominal wall is a relatively thick muscular organ overlying the peritoneum. The peritoneum is a well-defined layer of fascia made up of the parietal peritoneum and visceral peritoneum. Abdominal organs are often characterized as being intraperitoneal or extraperitoneal, depending on their location relative to this layer. Intraperitoneal organs include the stomach, proximal duodenum of the small

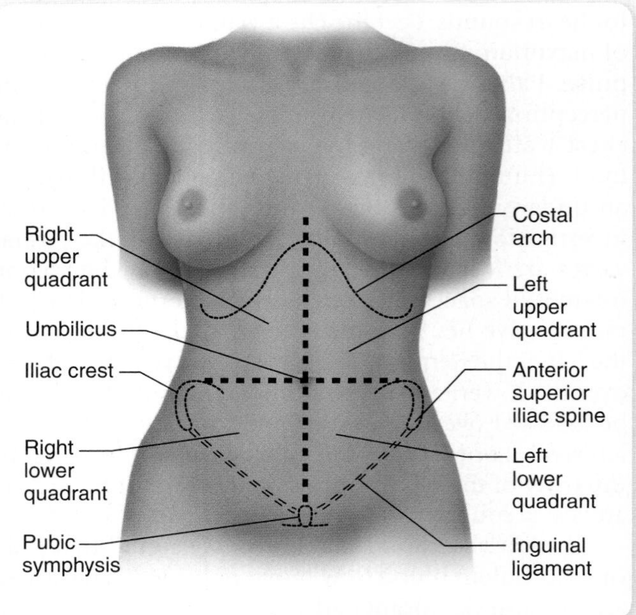

Figure 11-35 The abdomen is divided into quadrants by imaginary vertical and horizontal lines that intersect at the umbilicus.

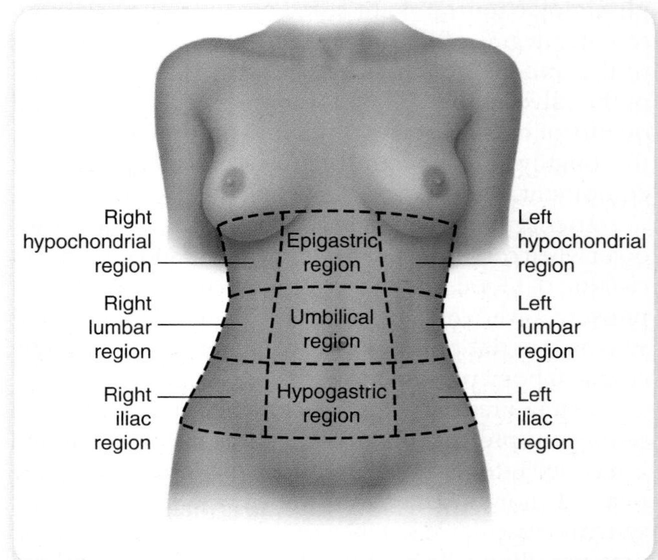

Figure 11-36 The abdomen can be divided into nine regions.

intestine, pancreas, jejunum, ileum, appendix, cecum, transverse colon, sigmoid colon, proximal rectum, liver, gallbladder, spleen, omentum, and female internal genitalia. Extraperitoneal organs include the mid- and distal duodenum, abdominal aorta, mid- and lower rectum, kidneys, pancreatic tail, adrenal glands, ureters, renal blood vessels, male gonadal blood vessels, ascending colon, descending colon, and urinary bladder.

One of the most challenging complaints for you to assess in the field setting is abdominal pain because it can have multiple causes and often presents with little or no external signs. Three basic mechanisms produce abdominal pain:

- *Visceral pain* occurs when hollow organs are obstructed, thereby stretching the smooth muscle wall, which in turn produces cramping and more diffuse, widespread pain.
- *Inflammation* or irritation of the somatic pain fibers located in the skin, the abdominal wall, and the musculature may produce sharp, localized pain, as in the case of pelvic inflammatory disease or appendicitis. If gastric contents, blood, or urine enters the peritoneum, it will also produce somatic pain, albeit usually much less localized and more diffuse.
- *Referred pain* occurs when pain originates in a particular organ, but the patient perceives it in a different location. Examples include flank pain associated with kidney stones, inner thigh pain from appendicitis or pelvic inflammatory disease, capsular pain from cholecystitis, and groin pain (waves of pain) from renal colic.

Obtaining baseline vital signs is an integral part of any secondary assessment. Clues provided help you determine the seriousness of the patient's condition and the function of internal organs. Remember, shock, whether medical or trauma related, is seen in different stages. Changes in a patient's blood pressure may be the last piece of evidence you see when shock changes from one level to the next. Keep in mind, blood pressure must be sufficient to maintain adequate end-organ perfusion.

Normally, baroreceptors in the body sense dropping blood pressure and volume and stimulate a catecholamine and renin-aldosterone response. This, in turn, causes peripheral vasoconstriction, increased pulse rate, and fluid retention, which puts more blood into the core circulation and increases volume and blood pressure. In patients with volume depletion, there is not enough circulating blood to push into the core circulation, especially as they move from a supine position to sitting or standing. **Orthostatic vital signs**, also called the "tilt test," are measurements of a patient's blood pressure and pulse taken in the supine and sitting or standing positions. The results of the test can help you determine the extent of volume depletion and indicate whether the patient needs fluid replacement. The tilt test is generally used for patients with complaints of nausea, vomiting, diarrhea, syncope, and gastrointestinal problems.

Words of Wisdom

If a patient becomes dizzy when moving from a supine position to a sitting position, *do not* have him or her stand up, because he or she will probably pass out.

In some studies, a tilt test or orthostatic change is considered positive when the patient's systolic blood pressure decreases up to 20 mm Hg, diastolic pressure increases more than 10 mm Hg (a narrowing pulse pressure), and the pulse rate increases by 20 beats/min. Take vital signs at 1-minute intervals between moving a patient to a new position, and the place the cuff on the same arm in the same location. Document whether the pulse was regular, if the patient is being monitored and there is an attached ECG strip, and whether the patient is experiencing other symptoms. If a fluid bolus for volume replacement is given, repeat the orthostatic assessment after assessing lung sounds.

Words of Wisdom

Assess all four quadrants of the abdomen for pain/tenderness, rigidity, swelling, guarding, and distention. Begin in an area where the patient has no pain.

As you examine a patient's abdomen, make the patient as comfortable as possible. Sometimes this requires administering pain medication first, which usually helps the patient to be more cooperative and better able to focus with less discomfort. Assess the abdomen with the patient in a supine position. To examine and palpate/percuss over the posterior aspects of the abdomen, however, ask the patient to sit up or log roll him or her into position. Always proceed with abdominal assessment systematically, routinely performing inspection, auscultation, and palpation, as shown in Skill Drill 11-9.

The abdomen can be described as flat, rounded, protuberant (bulging), scaphoid (hollow or boat [skiff] shaped), or pulsatile (pulsing or throbbing). In a normal abdomen, the cavity should appear soft with no tenderness or masses. Any abdominal distention must be distinguished from obesity. An obese patient's abdomen tends to be more protuberant than distended (tense and bloated), and is typically exceptionally pliable.

Some patients may have **ascites**, a collection of fluid within the peritoneal cavity. Ascites is similar to edema, but instead of affecting the interstitial tissues of the legs, it involves the abdomen. The patient's abdomen may appear markedly distended, and a visible or palpable fluid wave may be evident during examination, with shifting dullness noted on percussion. Ascites typically

Skill Drill 11-9 Examining the Abdomen

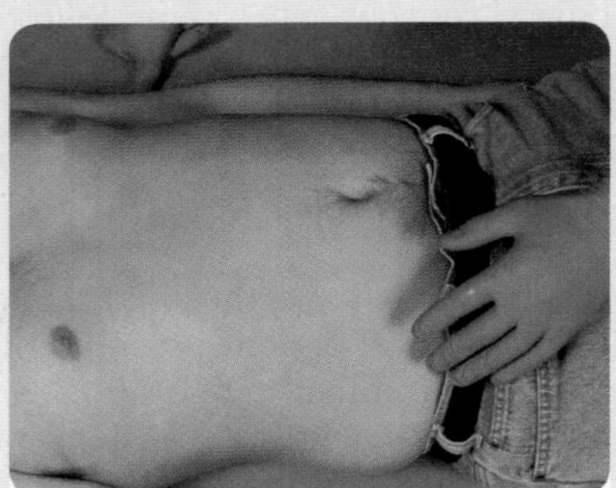

Step 1 Inspect and palpate the abdomen for open/closed findings, rigidity (firmness), tenderness, distention, swelling, or bruising. Look at the skin as well as the contour and overall appearance of the abdominal wall. Note any surgical scars, because they may be clues to an underlying illness, previous trauma, or surgeries. Look for symmetry and distention. Look for a rash or other signs of an allergic reaction. Finally, note any wounds, striae, dilated veins, or generalized distention or localized masses.

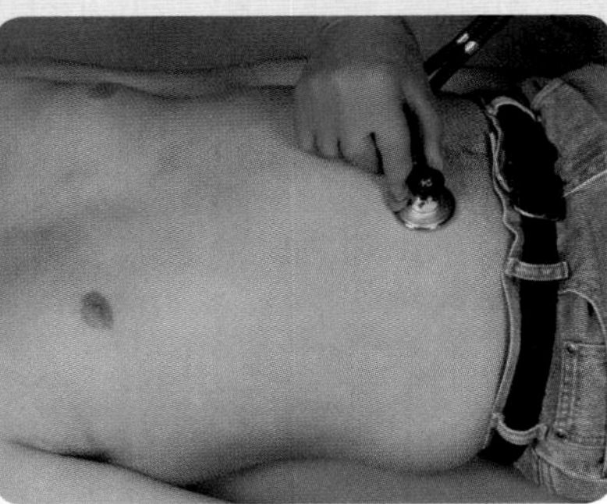

Step 2 Auscultate the abdomen for bowel sounds (if time and noise level permit). Note the presence or absence of bowel sounds. Note the frequency and character of any hyperactive sounds.

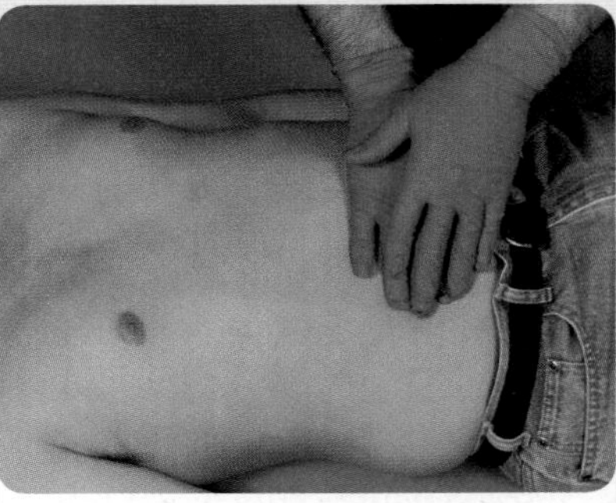

Step 3 Before palpating the abdomen, ask the patient to point to the area of greatest discomfort. Avoid touching that area until last. Systematically palpate the four quadrants of the abdomen, beginning with the quadrant farthest from the patient's complaint. Work slowly, and avoid quick movements. Perform percussion as appropriate. Pay special attention to the patient's expressions because they may yield valuable information.

occurs in patients with liver disease, but it can also be associated with a malignancy or even renal or cardiac insufficiency.

Blue discoloration in the periumbilical area (Cullen sign) or along the flanks (Grey Turner sign) is indicative of intraperitoneal hemorrhage, with two of the more common causes being ruptured ectopic pregnancy and acute pancreatitis.

Abdominal auscultation is part of a routine abdominal exam, although it may have limited utility in the prehospital setting. To hear bowel sounds, the environment must be fairly quiet and the patient must remain still. Take time to ensure an adequate assessment. Sometimes an abnormality is characterized by hyperactivity (increased) or hypoactivity (decreased), rather than a total absence of bowel sounds. Obstruction typically produces a high-pitched or tinkling sound. Differentiating normal from abnormal findings can sometimes be challenging, so practice this skill on many healthy people to develop a full appreciation for the abnormal situations you're likely to encounter.

Words of Wisdom

The increased intestinal motility that occurs in bowel hyperactivity produces loud, high-pitched, rushing, or tinkling sounds. Hypoactive or absent sounds may follow recent abdominal surgery or in response to peritoneal inflammation.

In addition to auscultating for bowel sounds, use the bell of the stethoscope to listen for any bruits in the abdomen. Recall, bruits are sounds made from turbulent blood flow through the arteries. In the abdominal cavity, listen for bruits over the aorta, right and left renal arteries, and common iliac arteries. Bruits in these areas suggest arterial stenosis or blockage.

Palpation yields the most significant diagnostic information during the abdominal exam—that is, tenderness (elicited pain). A moan, facial grimace, or sudden withdrawal all send the same message. You have touched something or somewhere that causes pain or discomfort. A patient who contracts his or her abdominal muscles shows guarding. **Guarding** can be either voluntary or involuntary and typically indicates underlying conditions such as appendicitis. Marked persistent contraction throughout the abdominal musculature is described as rigid and often indicates peritonitis. This is clinically important and often results in urgent surgical evaluation and intervention.

You may then be able to correlate these findings with historical information related to the patient's current illness or situation to determine what's wrong. Tightness or guarding can result from internal bleeding, an inflamed organ, and many other causes. Possible sources of LUQ pain include a ruptured spleen or mononucleosis. Unless it can be ruled out, LUQ pain should always be assumed to be the spleen, since misdiagnosing a ruptured spleen could be fatal. Patients with LLQ abdominal pain, especially if they have a history of constipation, nausea, vomiting, and fever, should be suspected of having diverticulitis. With RLQ abdominal pain, appendicitis is a likely culprit. Generalized abdominal pain in women of childbearing age can be caused by an ectopic pregnancy, a ruptured ovarian cyst, or some other obstetric or gynecologic condition, which can be life threatening.

Words of Wisdom

Restlessness and constant changes of position occur with the colicky pain of gastroenteritis or bowel obstruction. Absolute stillness, resisting any movement, is demonstrated with the pain of peritonitis (inflammation of the peritoneum). Knee flexion, facial grimacing, and rapid/uneven respiration are also signs of pain.

When appropriate, speak with the patient about the NOI while palpating the abdomen. Palpate each quadrant gently but firmly, and recognize that the patient may respond in many ways. Once an area of tenderness has been localized, attempt to visualize which structures may underlie it, and think about what might be causing the problem. If the patient has penetrating trauma, this step is less of a priority; it's difficult to localize areas damaged with a high-velocity MOI by visualizing and palpating the abdominal wall. Consider any signs or symptoms of abdominal injury as serious and indicative of a high-priority patient in unstable condition. That key information is worth pursuing in your assessment.

Rebound tenderness is rarely checked in the field, primarily because doing so can be painful. It requires slowly pushing down and then rapidly releasing sections of the abdomen. A positive sign (the patient cries out or withdraws) indicates peritoneal irritation. Such irritation may arise when a peritoneal organ becomes inflamed, or when a hollow organ ruptures, emptying its contents into the peritoneal cavity. Large-volume bleeding with peritoneal distention may also produce this phenomenon. However, be aware, in trauma cases, solid-organ bleeding does not always cause peritoneal irritation, guarding, and rigidity.

Words of Wisdom

Pain on release of pressure is described as *rebound tenderness*, a reliable sign of peritoneal inflammation, such as that seen in appendicitis. Do not repeatedly check for rebound tenderness since it hurts the patient.

Patients with less discrete (localized), guarded tenderness to palpation may have a more visceral problem. Although this may represent an early manifestation of a serious condition, it can also be associated with various degrees of bowel obstruction, renal colic, biliary colic, or urinary tract infection. The pain is often deep-seated and poorly described by the patient. Cases of colic typically involve a problem with peristalsis, the wave-like contraction motion of a hollow tubular structure such as the small or large intestine, common bile duct, or ureter. A stone may obstruct the tube, for example, or an adhesion or hernia may prevent proper intestinal peristalsis. Some patients will describe the pain as wavelike or waxing and waning. Other lower-abdominal sources of pain and tenderness include genitourinary processes.

As you palpate the abdominal cavity, attempt to palpate the liver, gallbladder, and spleen. To palpate the liver, place your left hand behind the patient, parallel to and supporting the right 11th and 12th ribs and adjacent soft tissues below. Place your right hand on the patient's right abdomen just below the rib cage. Ask the patient to take a deep breath. Try to feel the liver edge as it comes down to meet your fingertips. If you feel it, slightly lighten the pressure of your palpating hand so the liver can slip under your finger pads and you can feel its anterior surface.

Use the same technique to assess the gallbladder. While the gallbladder is typically not palpable, eliciting pain or a sudden gasp indicates possible inflammation. The difference in the technique is when the patient takes a deep breath, attempt to move your fingertips under the edge of the liver, rather than palpating its anterior surface. This will bring your fingertips closer to the gallbladder.

The spleen is a very difficult organ to palpate, and it is likely you will be able to palpate the spleen only if it is inflamed. With your left hand, reach over and around the patient to support and press forward the lower left rib cage and adjacent soft tissue. With your right hand below the left costal margin, press in toward the spleen. Begin palpation low enough so you are below a possible enlarged spleen. Ask the patient to take a deep breath, and try to feel the tip or edge of the spleen as it comes down to meet your fingertips.

Vascular sources can cause significant abdominal pain, most notably aortic aneurysm. Occasionally, a markedly dilated aorta can be seen pulsating in the midline of the upper abdomen. If the patient has an obvious pulsatile mass, do not palpate it. However, if no pulsatile mass is seen, then proceed with abdominal palpation. A ruptured aortic aneurysm also tends to be tender to palpation. Once you suspect an aortic aneurysm, take extreme care to minimize manipulation. The aorta is a retroperitoneal structure, so a lack of obvious findings while assessing the anterior abdomen does not rule out this diagnosis.

Another notable palpable abdominal wall mass is a *hernia*, a localized weakening of the abdominal wall musculature. Occasionally, you might find a hernia in the ventral wall of the abdomen. This is different from a hernia that might be found in the groin. Many of these types of hernias, such as umbilical hernias, are congenital, whereas others are the result of a previous abdominal surgery (incisional hernia). Hernias in the ventral wall are not always visible. If you suspect a hernia but do not see an umbilical or incisional hernia, place the patient in the supine position and ask him or her to raise his or her head and shoulders off the table. This maneuver will usually produce the bulge of a hernia. Most of the time, such findings are considered benign in the EMS environment. However, it is a true medical emergency if a section of bowel becomes entrapped and strangled in the hernia. In such cases, the patient's symptoms will include pain, fever, and possibly shock.

Female Genitalia

The female genitalia consist of the ovaries, fallopian tubes, uterus, vagina, and external genitalia. The ovaries lie in the lowermost portion of the abdomen, in the inguinal region, just superior to the inguinal crease. In the nonpregnant state, the uterus is a small structure not palpable on external examination.

In general, assessment of female genitalia is performed in a limited and discreet manner. Always keep the patient appropriately draped during the course of the exam. Male paramedics should be assisted by a woman. Reasons to examine the genitalia include concern over life-threatening hemorrhage or when you suspect delivery is imminent in a pregnant patient.

As you assess the abdomen, palpate both the bilateral inguinal region and the hypogastric region. If the decision is made to examine the genitalia specifically, limit the exam to inspection only. Pain and tenderness in the fallopian tubes and ovaries can be elicited during patient assessment. Clinically significant causes of this pain include an ectopic pregnancy, complications of third-trimester pregnancy, and ovarian disorders or pelvic infections in nonpregnant patients. In the trauma patient where pelvic fracture is a concern, genital bleeding is a possibility, albeit an unlikely one. In the case of injury involving intentional trauma, significant bleeding is possible; if you must intervene in this kind of situation, then preserve any garments and give them to law enforcement personnel as soon as possible. Note the amount and quality of any bleeding, as well as any inflammation, discharge, swelling, or genital lesions.

Male Genitalia

The male reproductive system consists of the testes, reproductive ducts, seminal vesicles, prostate, penis, and urethra Figure 11-37. The testes are analogous to the ovaries, in that they are the principal organs of reproduction. The testes, which lie outside the torso in a sac called the *scrotum*, produce hormones), and reproductive cells

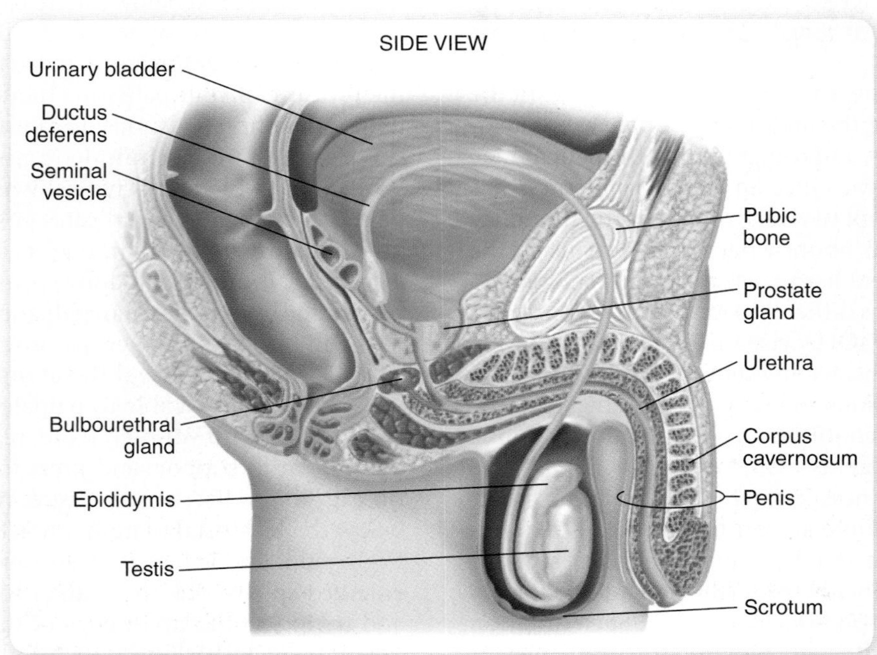

Figure 11-37 The male genitalia.

(sperm). The sperm is then transported from the testes to the pelvis, where it mixes with semen from the seminal vesicles and fluid from the prostate and is then released during the process of ejaculation.

As you examine the male genitalia, ensure your partner is present, and perform the exam in a limited and discreet manner. In the prehospital setting, situations requiring assessment of the male genitalia are limited. Always assess the entire abdomen and note any pertinent findings, because lower abdominal problems are occasionally referred from the genitalia. Patients with testicular torsion or an inguinal hernia sometimes present with complaints of lower abdominal pain but minimal abdominal tenderness. In the case of a trauma patient, assess for the possibility of significant genital bleeding and injury or underlying fracture. Note any inflammation, discharge, swelling, or lesions. Also, note priapism, a prolonged erection of the penis, usually the result of a spinal cord injury. In addition, look for evidence of urinary incontinence, especially in an unresponsive patient. Incontinence in an unresponsive patient may be associated with spinal cord injury or seizure.

Anus

The anus—the distal orifice of the alimentary canal—is often evaluated at the same time as the genitalia. It is examined in only a limited number of circumstances, and is always done with the patient appropriately draped and your partner present. With a positive history (eg, rectal bleeding, severe anal pain) or signs or symptoms of trauma, examine the area to assess the need to control bleeding or initiate another intervention (such as treatment for shock or care of eviscerated parts). The exam usually involves inspection only and occurs with the patient in a laterally recumbent position. Examine the back, posterior buttocks, and perineum, noting obvious bleeding, trauma, lumps, ulcers, inflammation, rash, abrasions, or evidence of fecal incontinence.

Musculoskeletal System

The extremities consist of both soft tissue and bones. Joints are areas where the ends of bones abut each other to form a kind of hinge. This hinge is held together by ligaments, creating a jointed appendage. Each joint has a shock-absorbing lining (the cartilage) and is filled with fluid (synovial fluid). Joints allow the body to perform mechanical work. Indeed, the mechanical process of motion becomes possible when the joints are alternately flexed and extended by skeletal (striated) muscles that traverse the joints. These skeletal muscles are anchored to bone by tendons. Each muscle is named according to its location and function.

The principal joints of the upper extremities are the shoulder (acromioclavicular and glenohumeral joints), elbow (olecranon), and wrist (radiocarpal). The principal joints of the lower extremities are the hip (acetabulum), knee (patellar), and ankle (tibiotalar).

In older patients, musculoskeletal complaints are common. As joints age, they become more vulnerable to repetitive-motion stress and trauma, and the loss of articular cartilage due to inflammatory or mechanical breakdown leads to osteoarthritis in older adults. These patients are likely to have decreased mobility and range of motion secondary to joint and muscle changes. Disruption of the bones, joints, and soft tissues can take a variety of forms, and discomfort or disability may be a manifestation of an acute problem, a chronic problem, or both. In addition to joint changes, muscle mass begins to decrease with age and from a lack of use. Older adults tend to live a more sedentary lifestyle, which contributes to these conditions. A common finding when assessing joints is crepitus with movement. Whereas this would be considered an abnormal finding in the younger population, it is a normal variant of aging, typically associated with advanced arthritis.

Common types of musculoskeletal and soft-tissue injuries include fractures, sprains, strains, dislocations, contusions, hematomas, and open wounds. Fractures may be characterized in a number of ways. For example, an open fracture is essentially a fracture with direct communication to the exterior surface of the body, whereas a closed fracture is associated with intact surrounding skin. While there are occasions when what looks like an open fracture is simply an open wound in close proximity to the site of fracture but not actually in contact with the fracture, any fracture with a nearby wound is considered an open fracture until the actual communication between the fracture and the wound is proven to be absent, typically based on results of a surgical exploration.

While fractures always involve a pathologic process, it is important to distinguish a **pathologic fracture** from a **traumatic fracture**. A pathologic fracture occurs when normal forces are applied to abnormal bone structures, producing a fracture. A traumatic fracture occurs when abnormal forces are applied to normal bone structures, producing a fracture. Traumatic fractures usually occur in high-intensity blunt trauma. Pathologic fractures often occur as a result of decreased bone density, such as osteopenia or occult malignancy, and can occur with relatively little application of force.

Examine the skeleton and joints, paying attention to their structure and function. Consider how the joint and associated extremity look and how well they function. Does the extremity look normal and move easily? In particular, note any limitation in range of motion, as well as any bony crepitus or pain with motion. Look for evidence of inflammation or injury, such as swelling, tenderness, increased heat, redness, ecchymosis, and decreased function. Also evaluate the joint or extremity for obvious deformity, diminished strength, atrophy, or asymmetry. The musculoskeletal exam shouldn't cause the patient any pain; if pain occurs, it should be considered an abnormal finding. Follow the steps in **Skill Drill 11-10** to examine the musculoskeletal system.

Skill Drill 11-10 Examining the Musculoskeletal System

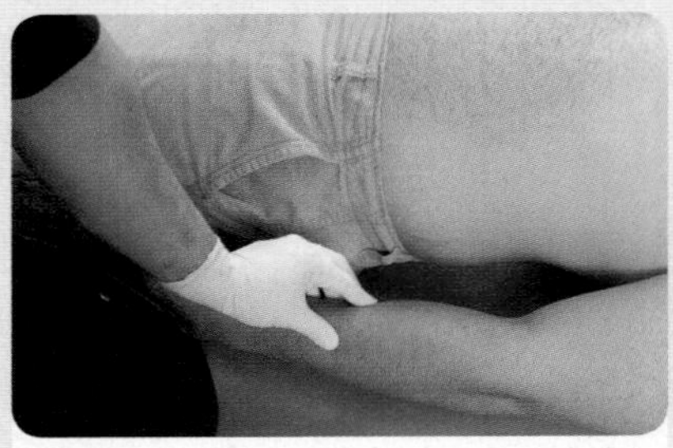

Step 1 Beginning with the upper extremities, inspect the skin overlying the muscles, bones, and joints for soft-tissue damage. Note any deformities or abnormal structures.

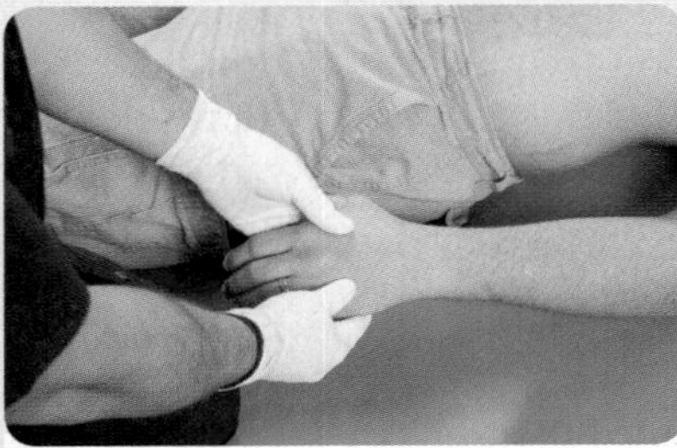

Step 2 Inspect and palpate the hands and the wrists. Note any open/closed findings and crepitus.

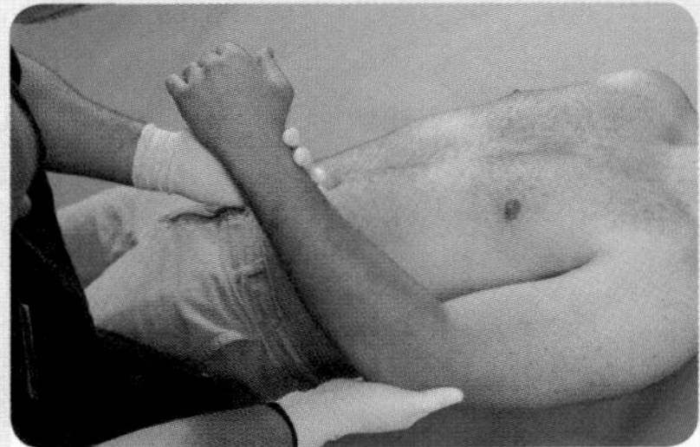

Step 3 Inspect and palpate the elbows. Ask the patient to flex and extend the elbow to establish the range of motion. Note any abnormalities.

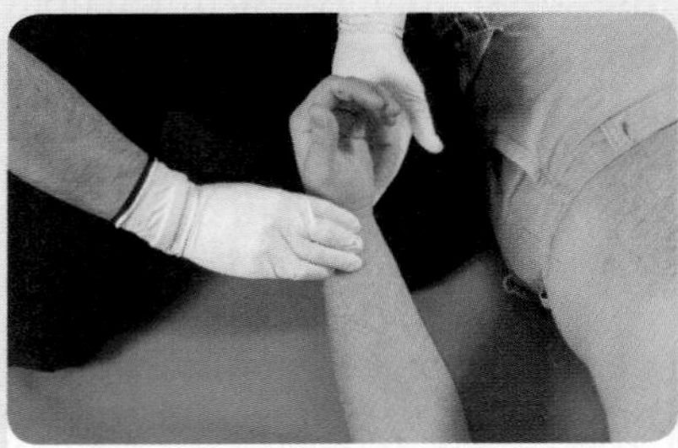

Step 4 Check for adequate distal pulse, motor function, and sensation in each extremity.

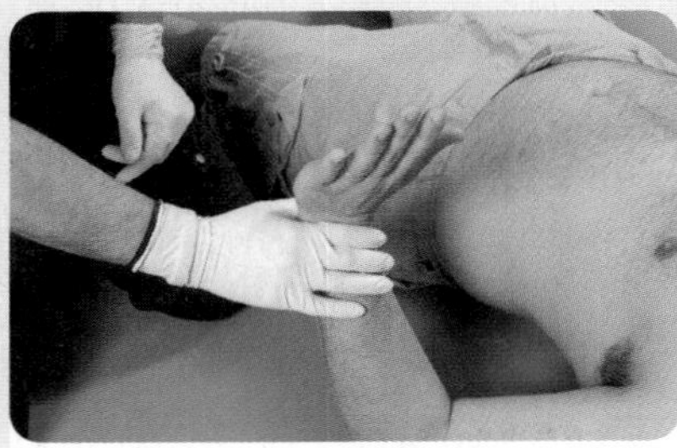

Step 5 Ask the patient to flex and extend the joints of the fingers, hands, and wrist to establish range of motion. If the patient experiences any discomfort, immediately stop that portion of the exam.

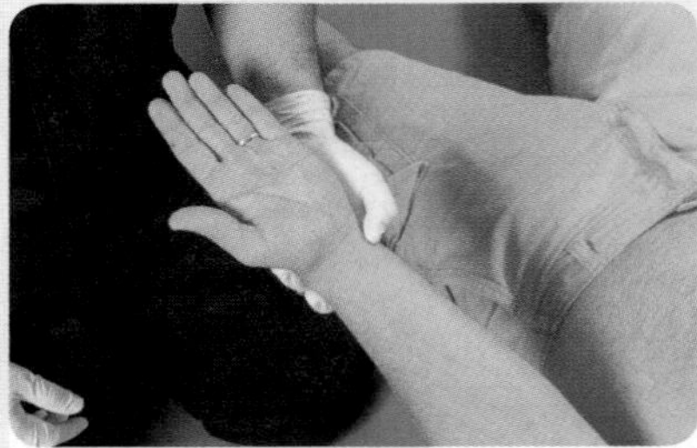

Step 6 Ask the patient to turn his or her hand from the palm-down position to the palm-up position and back again.

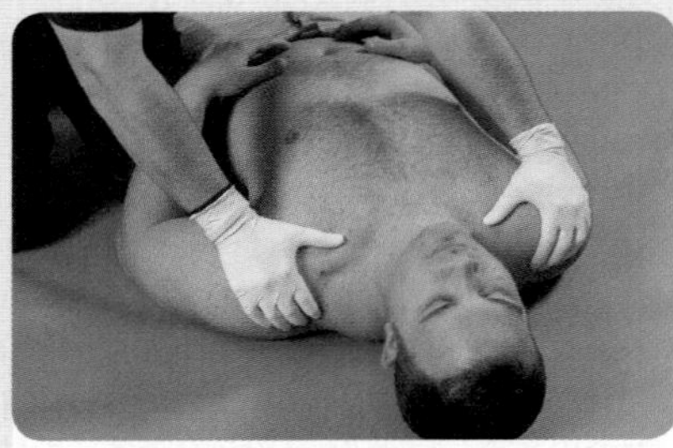

Step 7 Inspect and palpate the shoulders. Ask the patient to shrug the shoulders and raise and extend both arms.

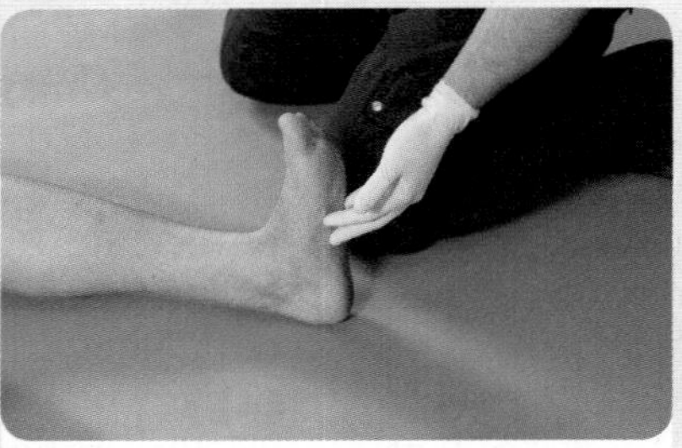

Step 8 Inspect and palpate the bony structures to establish range of motion. Ask the patient to point and bend his or her toes.

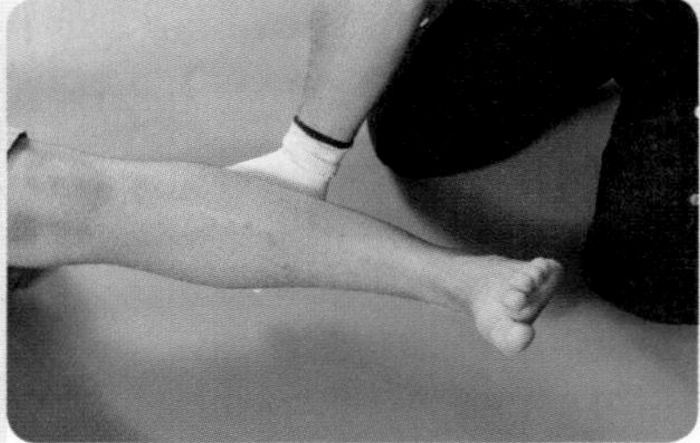

Step 9 Ask the patient to rotate the ankle to check for pain or restricted range of motion.

Skill Drill 11-10 Examining the Musculoskeletal System *(continued)*

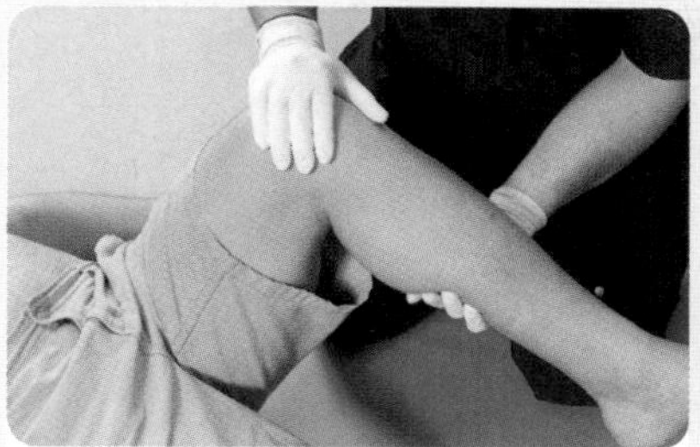

Step 10 Inspect and palpate the knee joints and patella to establish range of motion. Ask the patient to bend and straighten both knees.

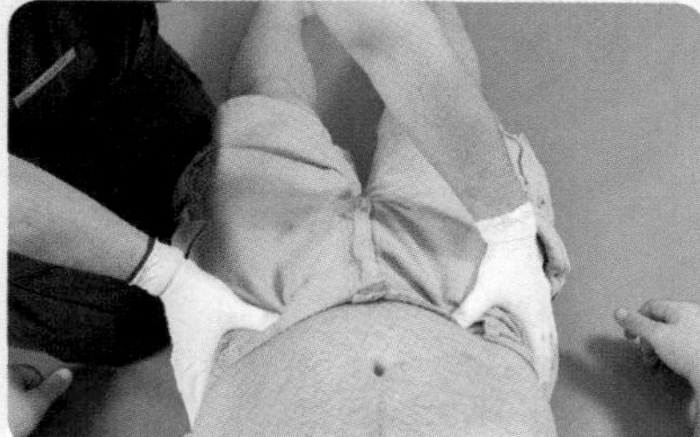

Step 11 Check for structural integrity of the pelvis by applying gentle pressure to the iliac crests, pushing in and then down.

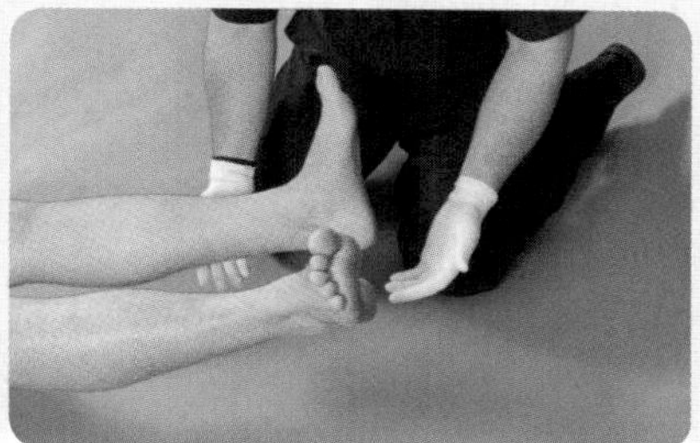

Step 12 Ask the patient to lift both legs, bend at the hip and turn the legs inward and outward. Note any abnormalities.

Words of Wisdom

Point tenderness is the most reliable indicator of an underlying fracture.

Often the diagnosis of a problem involving the shoulders and related structures can be made simply by noting the patient's posture at the time of your first contact. For example, a glenohumeral joint dislocation may be manifested as the loss of normal contour of the shoulder, with abnormal squaring of the lateral aspect of the shoulder, and the humeral head visible and/or palpable in the soft tissues of the chest wall, in the subacromial region Figure 11-38.

Palpate the proximal upper extremity and shoulder. Assess the sternoclavicular joint, acromioclavicular joint, subacromial area, and bicipital groove (origin of the biceps, just distal to the anterior aspect of the humeral head). Note any tenderness, swelling, crepitus, deformity, rotation, or ecchymosis in these areas.

Words of Wisdom

To assess a patient with a possible shoulder dislocation, position yourself behind the patient and compare the shoulders. The dislocated side is usually lower than the uninjured side.

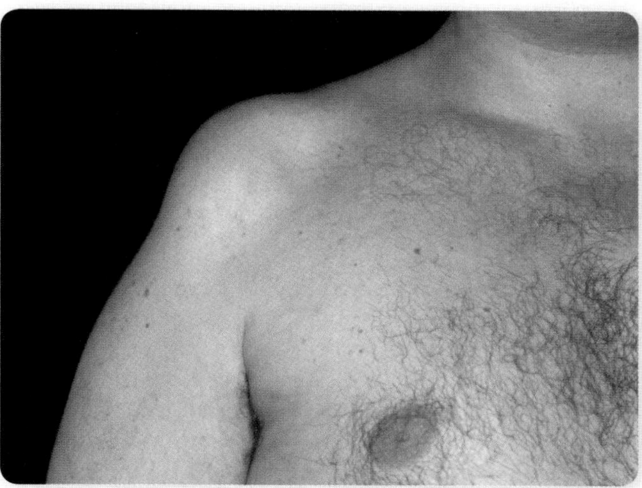

Figure 11-38 Abnormal squaring of the shoulder.

When possible, check range of motion by asking the patient to raise his or her arms to the vertical position, above the head. Next, ask the patient to demonstrate external rotation and abduction by placing both hands behind the neck, with the elbows out to the sides. Finally, perform internal rotation by asking the patient to place both hands behind the lower back.

Evaluate the elbows by performing an overall inspection for gross deformity or abnormal rotation. Palpate the elbow between the epicondyles and olecranon, and also palpate each epicondyle and the olecranon Figure 11-39. Note any tenderness, crepitus, swelling, or thickening.

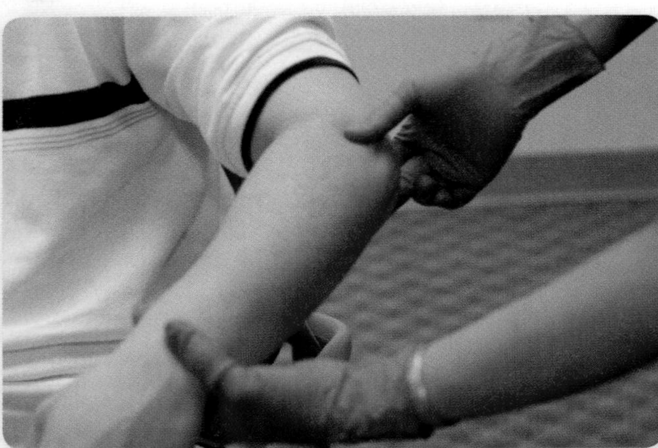

Figure 11-39 Palpate the elbow.

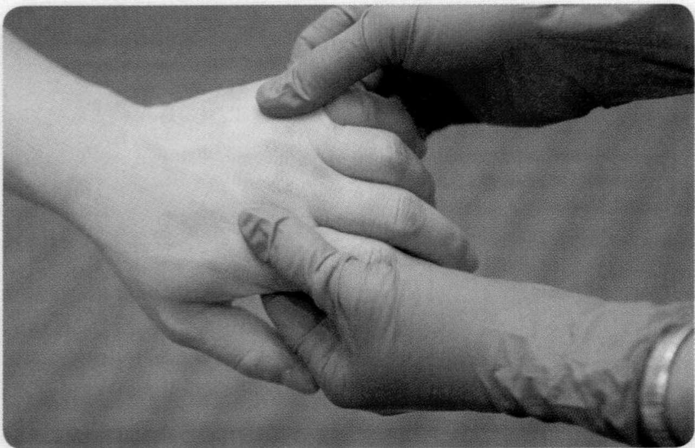

Figure 11-40 Palpate the hand and fingers.

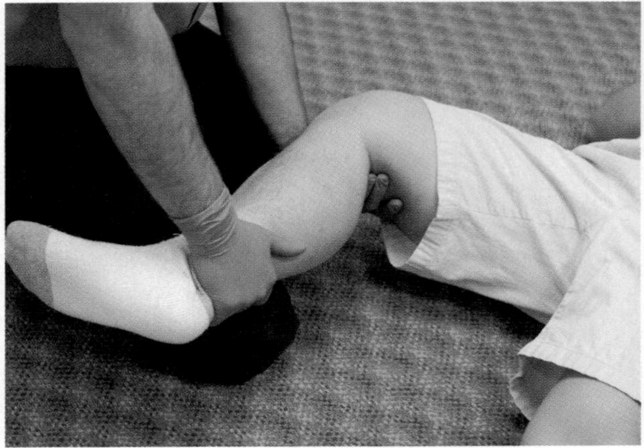

A

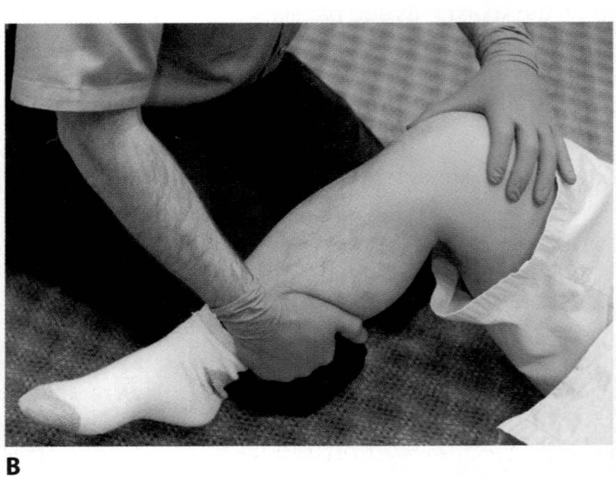

B

Figure 11-41 Examination of the lower extremities. **A.** Hip. **B.** Knee.

Perform range-of-motion testing last because suspicion of significant pathology or fracture of the elbow mandates appropriate immobilization as soon as possible. When testing the elbows, flex and extend them both passively and actively. Then have the patient supinate and pronate the forearms while the elbows are flexed at the patient's sides.

Inspect the hands and wrists for any abnormalities, including swelling, redness, contusions, wounds, nodules, deformities, or atrophy. Palpate the hands, feeling the medial and lateral aspects of each interphalangeal joint on each finger Figure 11-40. Squeeze the hands, compressing the metacarpophalangeal joints. Palpate the carpal bones of the wrists, noting any areas of swelling, tenderness, or bogginess. Perform range-of-motion evaluations by asking the patient to make fists with both hands, then extend and spread the fingers, then flex and extend the wrists, and, finally, move the hands laterally and medially, with the palms facing down. At this point, check capillary refill (in pediatric patients), symmetry of radial pulses, and overall limb temperature.

A rapid appreciation of injury or disability involving the lower extremities can be gained by evaluating the patient's ability to walk. Of course, this may not be a practical first approach to assessment in many prehospital cases.

Examine the knees and hips by inspecting the overall alignment and symmetry of the lower extremities Figure 11-41. Identify any lower extremity deformity, especially shortening and/or rotation, either internal or external; these findings are often evident with an injury to the proximal aspect of the lower extremity or hip joint. In particular, an open-book pelvic fracture, which presents with both feet rotated outward, is a life-threatening injury. Look for evidence of thickening, swelling, or bruising of the thigh. Note any crepitus or palpable tenderness. If possible, test the range of the knees and hips in an effort to determine the presence of underlying injury to those structures. Ask the patient to bend each knee and raise the bent knee toward the chest. Assess for rotation and abduction of the hips, both passively and actively. Palpate each hip individually—specifically, distal to the inguinal crease and over the anterior, lateral, and posterior aspects. Finally, palpate and gently compress the pelvis downward and then inward.

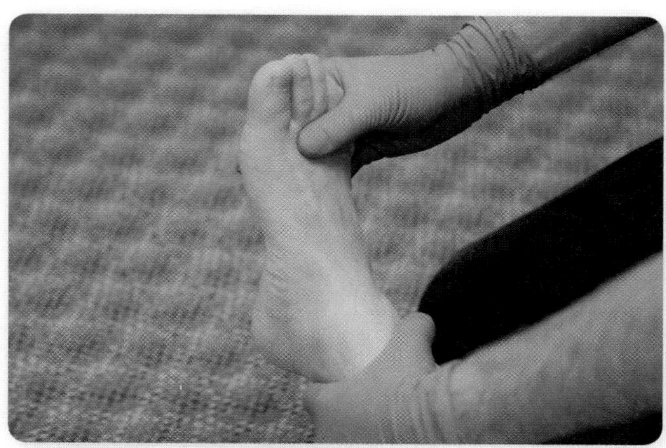

Figure 11-42 Inspect the feet.

Examine the ankles and feet, observing all surfaces. Note any wounds, deformities, discolorations, nodules, or swelling. Palpate all aspects of the feet and ankles, noting tenderness, bogginess, swelling, or crepitus. Measure distal pulses over the dorsalis pedis and posterior tibialis, and assess the overall limb temperature. Pulse strength may decrease in older patients, especially those with a history of moderate edema and peripheral vascular disease. Because of the small anatomic size of young pediatric patients, pulses may be difficult to palpate. In this situation, capillary refill, discussed in Chapter 43, *Pediatric Emergencies*, will be a more reliable indicator of perfusion. Assess range of motion by having the patient plantar flex, dorsiflex, and invert and evert the ankles and feet. Check the forefoot and toes by inspection, palpation, and range-of-motion testing **Figure 11-42**.

Peripheral Vascular System

The peripheral vascular system comprises all aspects of the circulatory system except the heart, the great vessels immediately involved with the mediastinum, and the coronary circulation. Thus, it includes all of the body's arteries, veins, arterioles, venules, capillaries, lymphatics, and the respective fluids these structures carry.

The lymphatic system is an intricate network of nodes and ducts of various sizes dispersed throughout the body **Figure 11-43**. Lymph nodes are larger accumulations of lymphatic tissue, and smaller amounts of lymph are distributed in tissue throughout the body. All lymphatic tissue contains large numbers of immunologically active cells; thus, the lymphatics manage a key function in the body's immune system. The ducts contain a fat-rich fluid known as lymph, which transports materials from the lymph tissue into the central venous circulation via the thoracic ducts.

Perfusion occurs in the peripheral circulation via a network of capillary beds. Blood cells and plasma in close proximity to tissue offload substances required by the cells for proper metabolic functioning and simultaneously transport metabolic wastes out of the tissues for eventual elimination from the body. Impaired functioning of the peripheral vascular system means the capillary beds cannot adequately perfuse tissues and organs, causing significant morbidity and mortality.

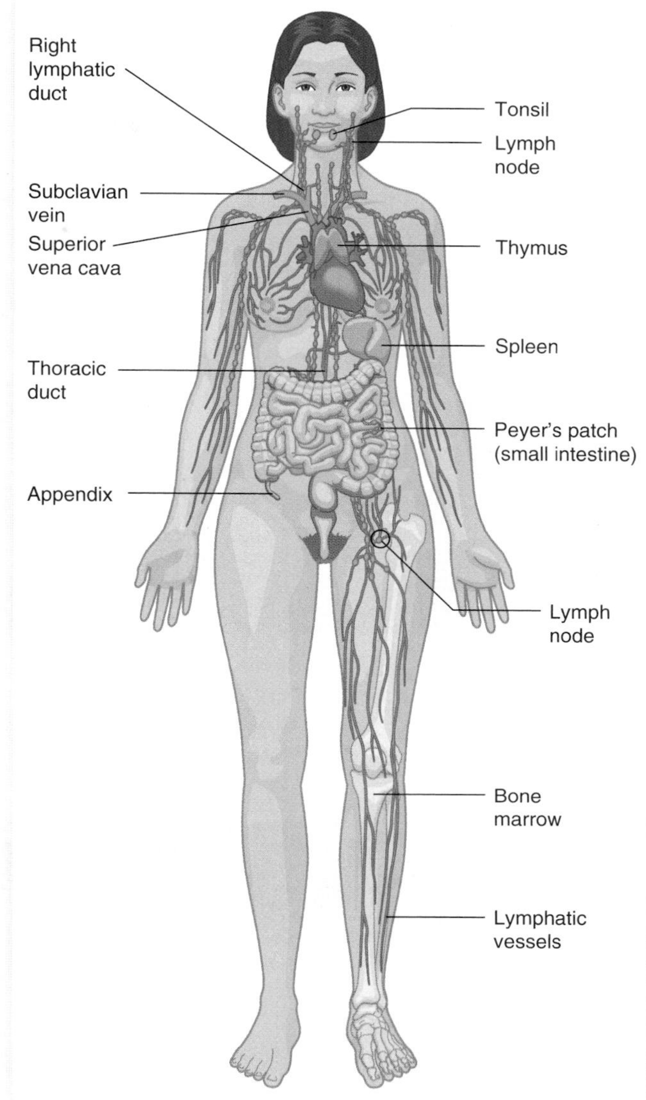

Figure 11-43 Lymphatic system.

Diseases of the peripheral vascular system are often seen in patients with other underlying medical conditions, such as diabetes, hypertension, dyslipidemia, obesity, and those caused by tobacco use. These disease processes typically damage the smaller-diameter vessels of the peripheral vascular system, resulting in disease of the tissues and organs that depend on those vessels for proper functioning. With age and the advance of these various disease processes, the vasculature can no longer manage rapid changes in perfusion requirements, thereby becoming a source of illness.

As you assess the peripheral vascular system, pay attention to both the upper and lower extremities. Look for signs that indicate either acute or chronic vascular problems. A wide range of disorders—from chronic venous stasis and lymphedema to intermittent claudication (cramp-like pain in the lower legs because of poor circulation or low potassium levels) and acute arterial occlusion—can affect the peripheral vascular system. Peripheral vascular disease can manifest in many forms, depending on the point in the vasculature where the abnormality is located. Carotid artery disease can manifest as a stroke, for example, while arterial embolization involving the mesenteric vessels can cause bowel ischemia and necrosis. In the extremities, involvement of the peripheral vasculature can lead to limb ischemia. Follow the steps in Skill Drill 11-11 to examine the peripheral vascular system.

Skill Drill 11-11 Examining the Peripheral Vascular System

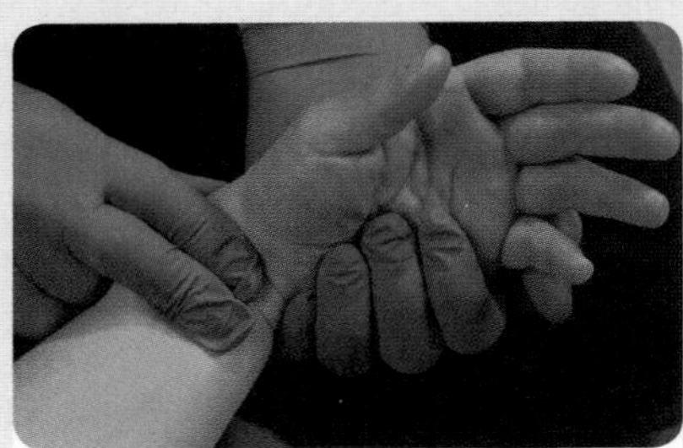

Step 1 As you examine the upper extremities, note any abnormalities in the radial pulse, skin color, temperature, or condition.

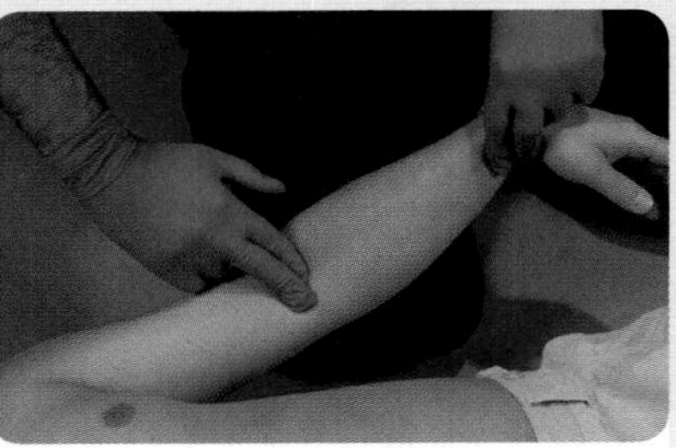

Step 2 If you note abnormalities in the distal pulse, work your way proximally, check those pulse points, and note your findings.

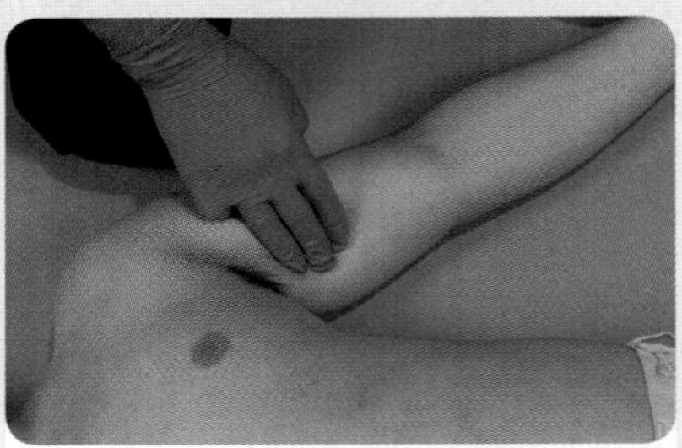

Step 3 Palpate the epitrochlear and brachial nodes of the lymphatic system. Note any swelling or tenderness.

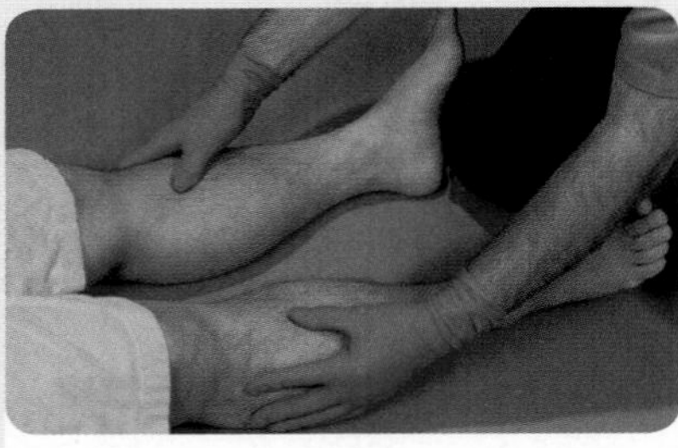

Step 4 Examine the lower extremities, noting any abnormalities in the size and symmetry of the legs. Evaluate the temperature of each leg relative to the rest of the body and to each other.

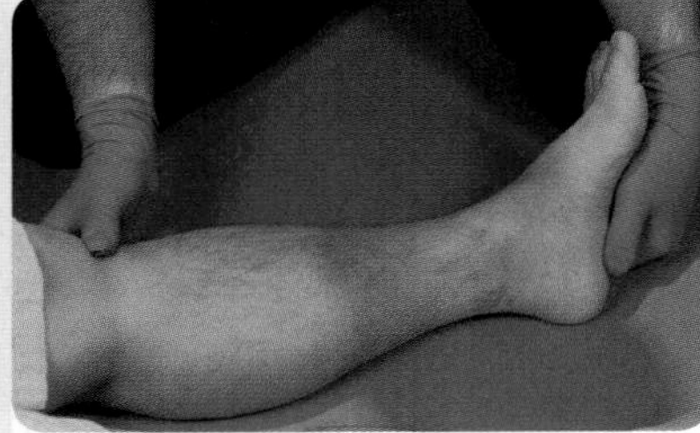

Step 5 Inspect the skin color and condition. Note any abnormal venous patterns or enlargement.

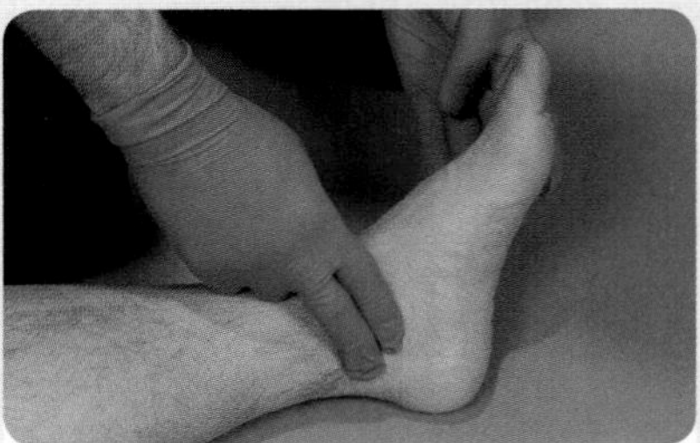

Step 6 Check distal pulses, noting any abnormalities.

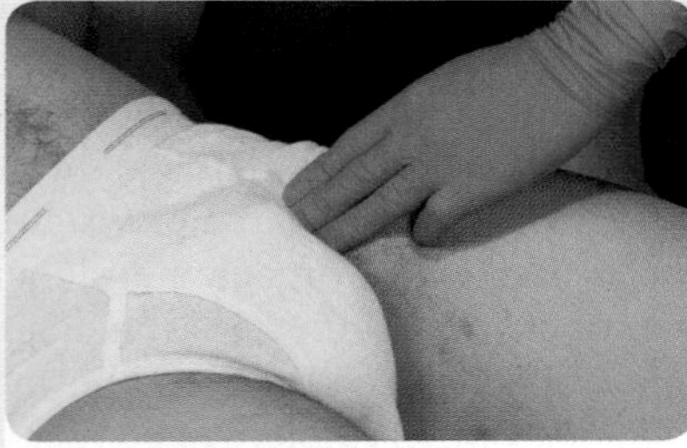

Step 7 Palpate the inguinal nodes for swelling or tenderness.

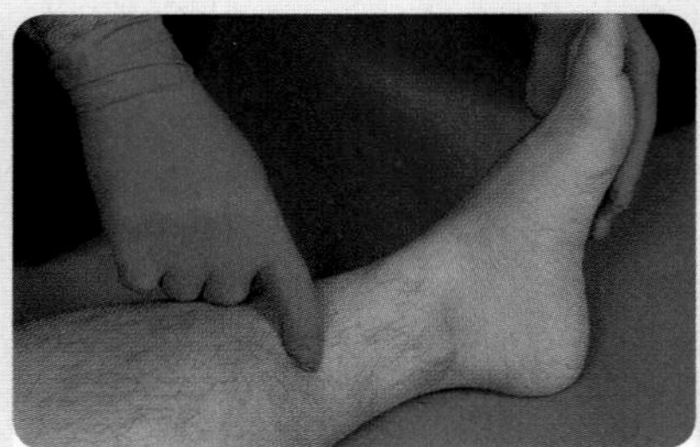

Step 8 Evaluate for pitting edema in the legs and feet.

Inspect the upper extremities from fingertips to shoulders. Note each extremity's relative size, and evaluate it for symmetry by comparing one side with the other. Pay attention to any obvious swelling, unusual venous patterns, the color, temperature, and condition of the skin, and the color of the nail beds. If indicated, palpate the epitrochlear and axillary lymph nodes, noting their size, tenderness, mobility, and overlying redness. Palpate the radial pulses simultaneously, and compare them. In situations of unilaterally absent pulses, check proximally over the brachial pulse sites. As you evaluate a limb for ischemia, consider the five Ps of acute arterial insufficiency that you learned in EMT training: Pain, Pallor, Paresthesia, Paresis, and Pulselessness. The loss of a palpable pulse is probably the worst indicator of such a problem because it is considered a late finding.

Proper evaluation of the vascular status of the lower extremities requires the patient to be lying down and draped appropriately. Remove the patient's socks, stockings, and shoes before proceeding with the exam. Inspect the lower extremities from the groin and buttocks to the feet. Always compare the right side with the left side. Look at the size and symmetry of the legs, noting any localized versus generalized swelling. Pay attention to any remarkable superficial venous patterns or venous enlargement. Observe the skin pigmentation, as well as the skin color and texture. **Rubor**, ecchymosis, or pallor may all be encountered in patients with significant vascular insufficiency. Also note the presence of any rashes, scars, or ulcers, and determine whether they are shallow or deep.

Words of Wisdom

Bilateral, dependent, pitting edema occurs with systemic conditions such as heart failure and hepatic cirrhosis. Unilateral edema occurs with local conditions such as deep vein occlusion.

Palpate pulses in the lower extremities to assess the arterial circulation. In particular, palpate pulses over the dorsalis pedis and posterior tibialis, and in the femoral regions. The popliteal pulse can also occasionally be appreciated. Note the temperature of the feet and legs, and attempt to palpate any edema in the legs. To do so, press your thumb over the dorsum of the foot and anteriorly over the tibias, and hold the thumb with firm, gentle pressure for at least 5 seconds. If indicated, palpate the superficial inguinal lymph nodes, noting their mobility, size, tenderness, any overlying redness.

Words of Wisdom

Pitting edema 4-point scale:
+1 = 0 inch – 1/4 inch (0 cm – 0.635 cm)
+2 = 1/4 inch – 1/2 inch (0.635 cm – 1.27 cm)
+3 = 1/2 inch – 1 inch (1.27 cm – 2.54 cm)
+4 = > 1 inch (> 2.54 cm)

Spine

Assessment of the cervical spine was introduced earlier. This section covers the complete assessment of the spine. The spine represents the core of the axillary skeleton. It consists of 33 individual vertebrae, the lower nine of which are fused.

Assess the spine, begin by inspecting the back from both the posterior and lateral aspects. The spine features several curves, representing the cervical, thoracic, and lumbar regions. Some amount of curvature in the spine is normal, however, lordosis and kyphosis are abnormal amounts of spine curvature. **Lordosis** refers to the inward curve of the lumbar spine just above the buttocks. *Exaggerated* lordosis results in swayback **Figure 11-44**. **Kyphosis** refers to the outward curve of the thoracic spine **Figure 11-45**. It is frequently exaggerated in older adults because of degenerative joint disease, osteoporosis, and vertebral compression fractures. At its worst, kyphosis can become a source of restrictive lung disease, a form of COPD. **Scoliosis**, a sideways curvature of the spine, is also abnormal **Figure 11-46**. As you examine the spine, look for differences in the height of the shoulders as well as differences in the height of the iliac crests of the pelvis. Look at the entire back, noting any wounds or ecchymosis.

Palpation of the spine is typically done while the patient is supine, often after he or she has been log rolled onto one side to facilitate access to the back and placement of a spinal immobilization device. As you palpate the spine, use your thumb to touch each spinous process. This allows you to identify any tenderness, step-off, or crepitus.

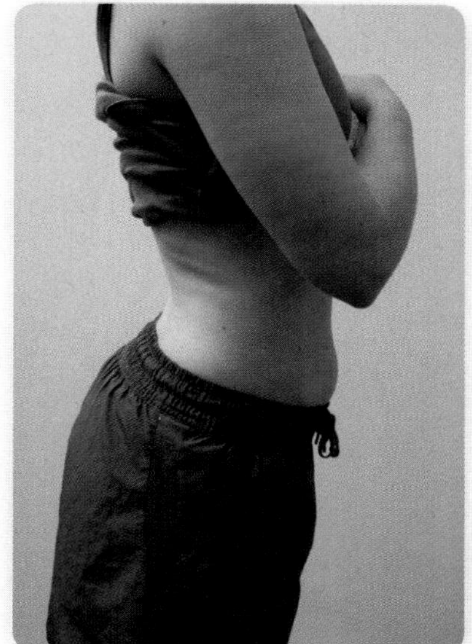

Figure 11-44 Lordosis is inward curvature of the lumbar spine just above the buttocks.

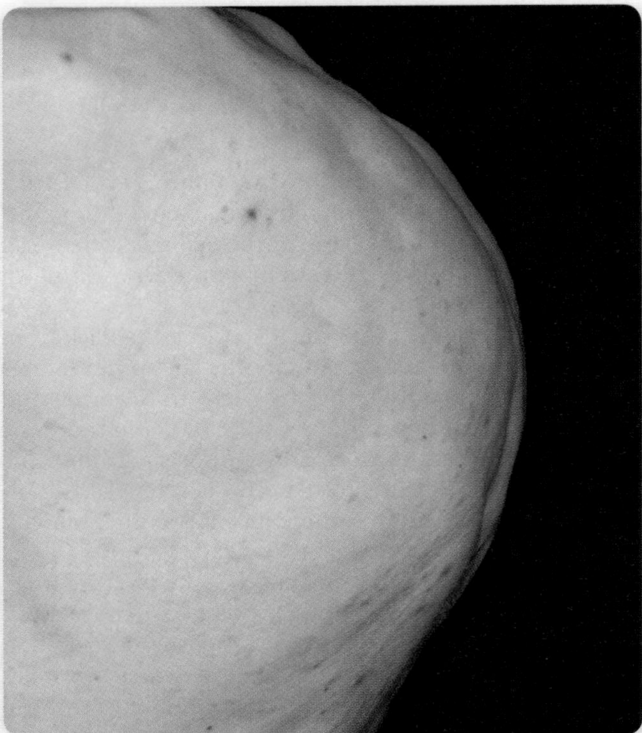

Figure 11-45 Kyphosis is outward curvature of the spine; it can be exaggerated in older adults.

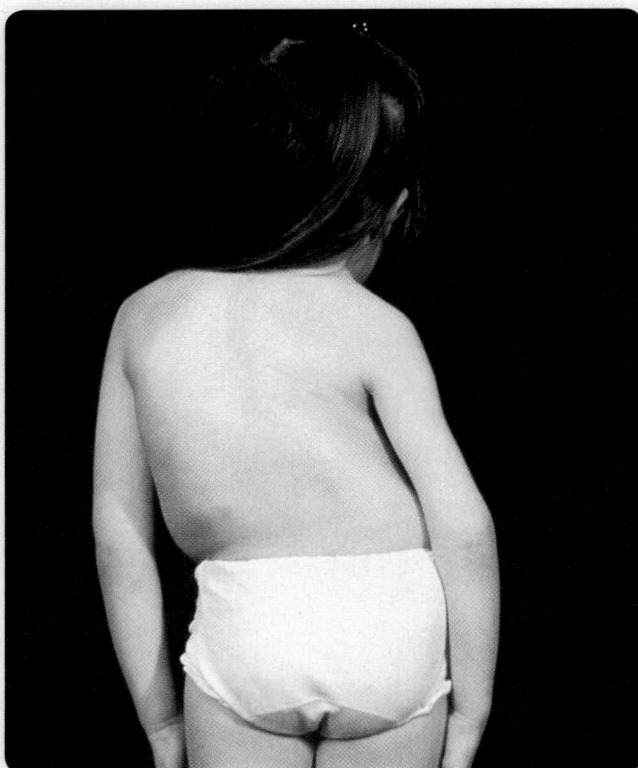

Figure 11-46 Scoliosis is the sideways curvature of the spine.

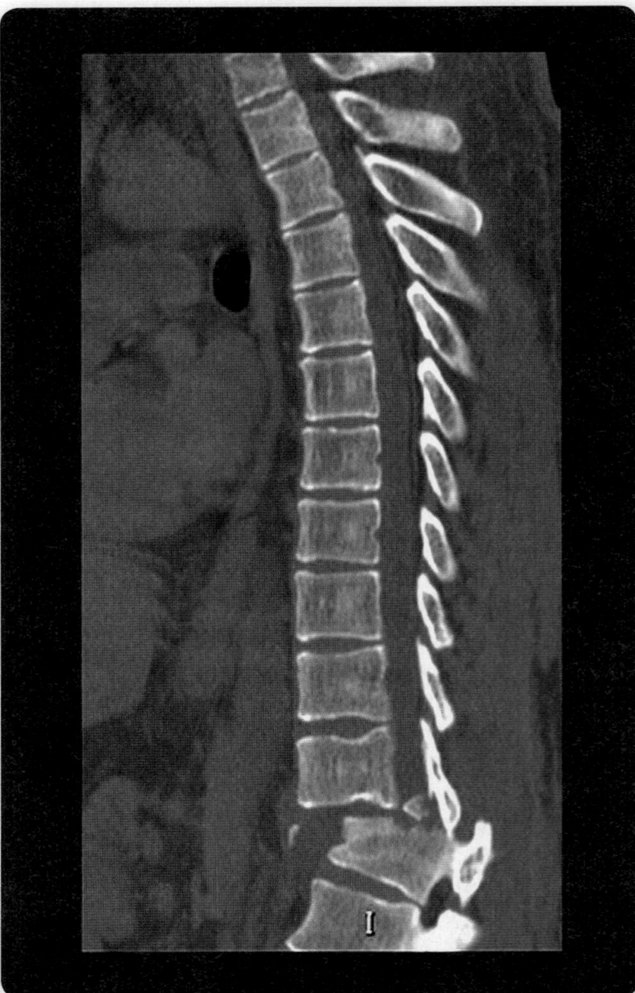

Figure 11-47 In the context of a displaced fracture or a dislocation, there may be a step-off when palpating from one vertebra to the next, as shown here.

Step-off occurs in the context of a displaced fracture or a dislocation and is shown in Figure 11-47. If you identify any abnormality, promptly institute proper splinting and protective measures per your regional protocols.

> **Words of Wisdom**
>
> Log rolling the patient onto a backboard always gives you a valuable opportunity to inspect and palpate the back quickly for signs of injury. Instruct and position your assistants to facilitate this brief exam.

Check the rest of the back for any other significant findings on palpation. Tap over the costovertebral angles, and palpate the scapulae, paraspinal areas, and base of the neck. Also, check the buttocks. Finally, perform a range-of-motion evaluation. Although this evaluation may be of limited utility in the prehospital setting, in areas that practice selective spinal immobilization, it may prove quite helpful. Range of motion should *never* be done passively. The awake and alert patient will protect himself and will not transect his own spinal cord by actively moving his neck. Conversely, you can do just that. Always ask the patient to move his or her neck through a comfortable range of motion. If at any time during ranging the patient experiences pain in the spine or tingling in the extremities, immediately stop that phase of assessment and immobilize the spine per your regional protocols.

During your assessment of the patient's active range of motion, pay attention to the smoothness and symmetry of the patient's movement, along with the actual degree of motion elicited or accomplished. Follow the steps in Skill Drill 11-12 to examine the spine.

Nervous System

As you learned in Chapter 8, *Anatomy and Physiology*, the brain is an extraordinarily complex structure, with an enormous perfusion requirement. With the exception of the cranial nerves, all nerves are ultimately channeled to the brain via the spinal cord. The spinal cord plays the role of a large conduit, passing information back and forth along its sensory pathways. Recall that the nervous system is divided into involuntary (autonomic) and voluntary portions, with the autonomic nervous system being further subdivided into the sympathetic and parasympathetic systems.

Skill Drill 11-12 Examining the Spine

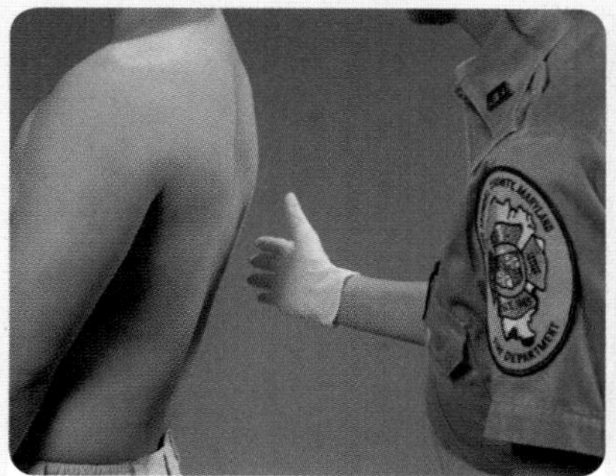

Step 1 Inspect the cervical, thoracic, and lumbar curves for any abnormalities.

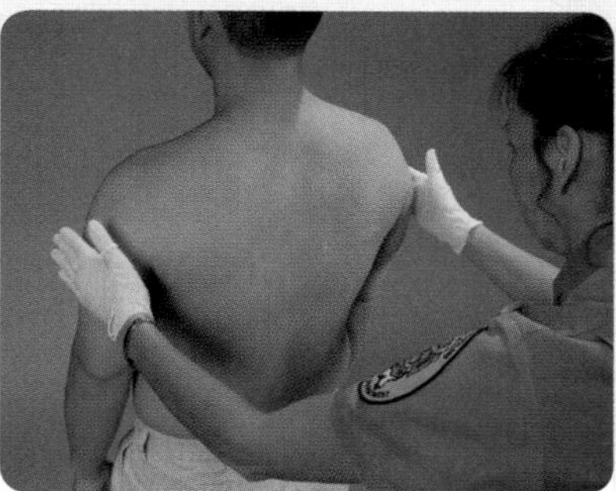

Step 2 Evaluate the height of the shoulders and iliac crests. Differences between one side and the other may indicate abnormal spinal curvature.

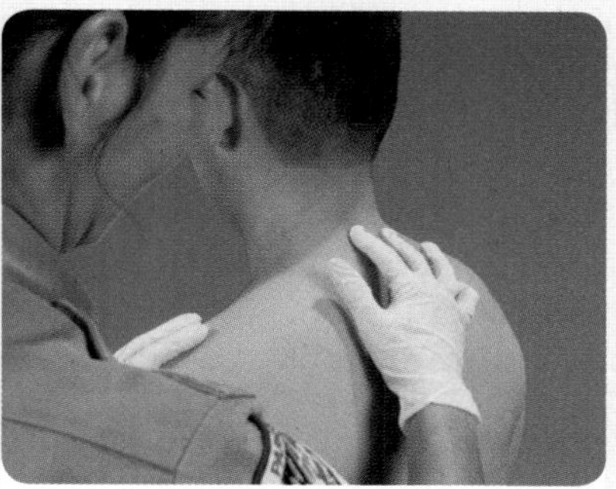

Step 3 Palpate the posterior portion of the cervical spine, noting any point tenderness or structural abnormalities.

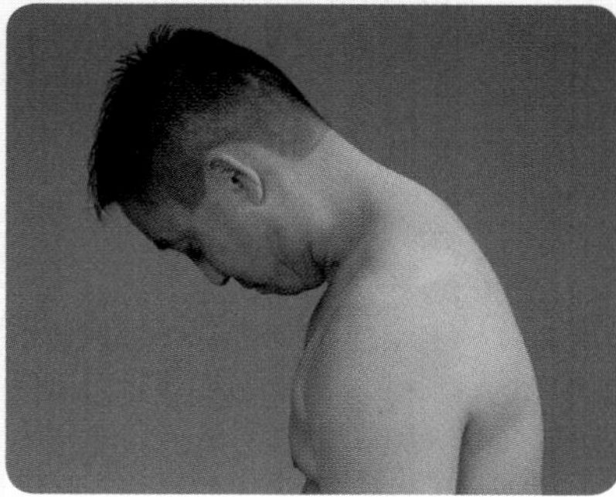

Step 4 In the nontrauma patient, and in the absence of reported pain, ask the patient to move his or her head forward, backward, and from side to side.

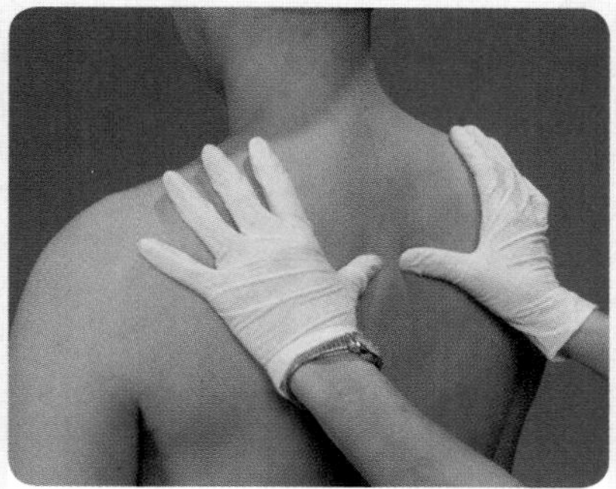

Step 5 Palpate each vertebra with the thumbs.

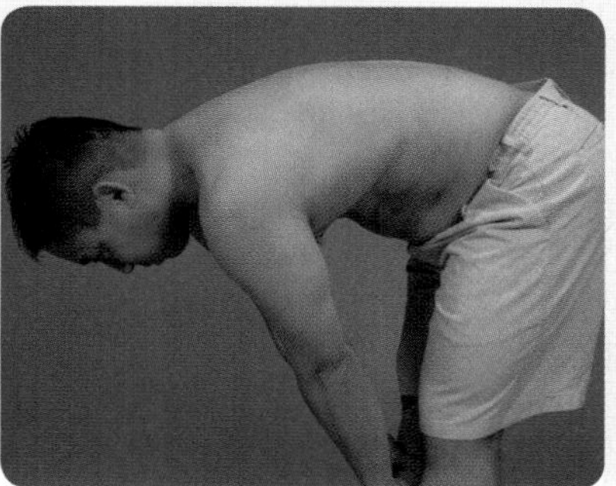

Step 6 In the absence of pain or trauma, ask the patient to bend at the waist in each direction to establish the range of motion.

Reflexes are involuntary motor responses to specific sensory stimuli, such as giving a tap on the knee or stroking the eyelash. The location of what is stimulated determines which muscle will contract reflexively. Spinal reflexes occur when sensory input comes from receptors in the muscles, joints, and skin. The motor response to this stimulation occurs entirely within the spinal cord; no brain processing is required. Other reflexes include the deep tendon reflexes and the superficial and brainstem reflexes. **Primitive reflexes**—including the Babinski, grasping, and sucking signs—are normal findings in infants. In older people, once the long motor pathways of the peripheral nervous system (PNS) have become fully myelinated, these primitive reflexes represent abnormal findings, typical of injury or disconnection between the cerebral cortex and the brainstem.

A Babinski reflex test may be used to check neurologic function. It is accomplished by stimulating the sole of the foot by rubbing it with your thumb or by running a pen or other pointed object along the length of it. In a normal reaction, the great toe will flex. However, *do not* perform a Babinski reflex test on a patient who has lower-extremity injuries. Doing so could prompt the patient to pull the leg back, causing pain.

The Neurologic Exam. The check of the nervous system is one of the most time-consuming elements of the physical exam. Most of the time a complete and thorough neurologic exam will be impossible in the field and would be inappropriate; however, if the patient displays signs and symptoms of a neurologic condition, every attempt should be made to perform relevant portions of the neurologic exam. At a minimum, the neurologic exam should determine the patient's baseline mental status (AVPU), cranial nerve function (pupils, eyes, smile, speech, swallow, shoulder shrug), distal motor function (ability to move), and distal sensory function (ability to feel). It may also test deep tendon reflexes if necessary.

First, assess the patient's overall mental status. Is the patient awake? If so, is the patient alert, and to what degree? If a change in LOC has occurred, what kind of stimulus does it take to get a response, and to what degree does the patient's mental status improve? In the case of altered mental status, do you observe any unusual postures? Is there any alteration in physical status (for example, can the patient move successfully and symmetrically)? A detailed explanation of the mental status exam was covered earlier in the chapter. Here is a quick review using the COASTMAP mnemonic:

- **C - Consciousness.** Along with level of consciousness, note the patient's ability to pay attention and concentrate. Is he or she easily distracted?
- **O - Orientation.** Ask about the year, season, month, day, and date. Have the patient identify the present location—that is, state, city or town, and specific location. Can the patient recall and describe current event?
- **A - Activity.** Does the patient appear anxious or restless? Is he or she sitting still, scarcely moving at all? Is he or she making any strange or repetitive motions (possibly because of methamphetamine use)?
- **S - Speech.** Note the rate, volume, articulation, and intonation of the patient's speech. Does it sound pressured (forced)? Does the speech have a flat, monotonous delivery consistent with depression? Is the speech garbled or slurred (dysarthria)? Garbled or slurred speech has many possible causes, including alcohol or drug impairment, stroke, and traumatic brain injury.
- **T - Thought.** Listen to the patient's story. What's on his or her mind? Is the patient making sense? Is there anything unusual about his or her reasoning? Is the patient expressing apparently false ideas (delusions)? Are voices telling the patient what to do or think (psychosis)? Does the patient report thoughts that people are "out to get me" (paranoia)?
- **M - Memory.** You can form an impression of the patient's memory by listening to him or her reconstruct past events. A more precise assessment requires asking a few questions. Explain to the patient that you'd like him or her to try to remember three words. Then slowly say the names of three unrelated words (such as apple, bicycle, sewing machine). Ask the patient to repeat those words to ensure he or she has heard and understood them. A few minutes later, ask the patient if he or she can remember the three words you named before; this tests retention and memory.
- **A - Affect.** The patient's affect (mood) may be most apparent in his or her body language. A posture of shoulders drooping and head bent, for example, conveys depression. Note whether the affect seems appropriate to the situation.
- **P - Perception.** Detecting disorders of perception may be difficult, because patients are often hesitant to answer questions about hallucinations. Sometimes it's helpful to ask the patient, "Do you ever hear things that other people can't hear?"

Words of Wisdom

Restlessness is a danger signal!

After assessing the patient's overall mental status, begin the comprehensive neurologic exam. Of course, this exam is not needed in every case. Its details may vary greatly, depending on the nature of the patient's problem. Also, many portions of the neurologic exam may have been completed earlier, during other aspects of the patient assessment. Keep track of your initial findings so you can report them, so they are not needlessly repeated, and so any subsequent changes in mental status can be noted. Are left- and right-sided motor and sensory findings symmetric? If not, how do they differ? Does the presenting problem appear to be more of a CNS or a PNS malfunction, or is it secondary to swelling or bone displacement from trauma?

When testing the cranial nerves, a number of simple maneuvers can be employed to determine the presence and degree of disability Table 11-10. With practice, the entire cranial nerve examination can be performed in less than 3 minutes. That said, don't waste time performing this exam if the patient has more pressing needs.

Adequate evaluation of the motor system involves assessing several distinct areas. Although motor activity may represent the localized workings of the musculoskeletal system, the nervous system has an overriding influence on motor activity. Observe the patient's initial posture and body position Figure 11-48 as well as his or her body position both at rest and with movement, if appropriate. Observe any apparent involuntary movements,

Table 11-10 Tests for Cranial Nerve Dysfunction

Cranial Nerve	Function	Assessment Technique
I. Olfactory	Smell	Not usually assessed. Use ammonia or another known scent as an inhalant.
II. Optic	Vision	Place finger in front of patient's face. Ask if he or she can see your finger.
III. Oculomotor	Movement of the eye, pupil, and eyelid	Have the patient follow your finger as you move it in an "H" shape. Ask the patient to blink.
IV. Trochlear	Movement of the eye	(Tested in the same way as the oculomotor nerve.)
V. Trigeminal	Chewing Pain Temperature Touch of the mouth and face	Ask the patient to smile.
VI. Abducens	Movement of the eye	(Tested in the same way as the oculomotor nerve.)
VII. Facial	Movement of the face Tears Salivation and taste	(Tested in the same way as the trigeminal nerve.)
VIII. Auditory	Hearing and balance	Ask the patient to follow your spoken commands.
IX. Glossopharyngeal and X. Vagus	Glossopharyngeal: Swallowing, taste, and sensations in the mouth and pharynx Vagus: Sensation and movement of the pharynx, larynx, thorax, and GI system	Ask the patient to smile and then swallow.
XI. Accessory	Movement of the head and shoulders	Ask the patient to shrug his or her shoulders; hold both of the patient's shoulders at the same time to assess symmetry.
XII. Hypoglossal	Movement of the tongue	Ask the patient to stick out his or her tongue.

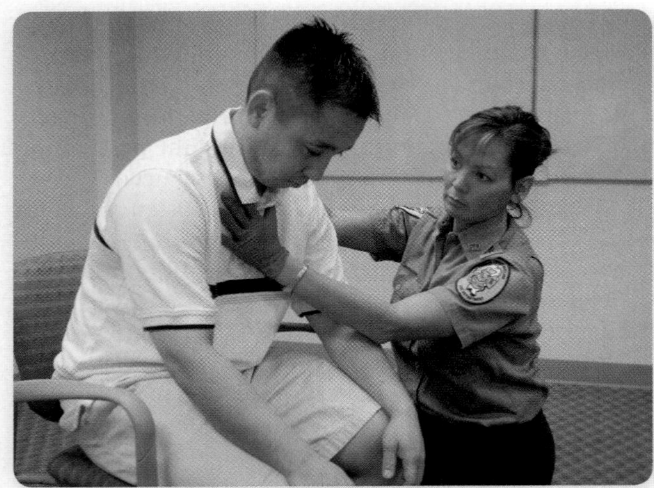

Figure 11-48 Note the patient's posture and body position.

and document the quality, rate, rhythm, and amplitude. Determine whether these involuntary movements are related to the patient's posture or activity, and consider whether their presentation includes a component of fatigue or emotion. Make a general assessment of the bulk of the patient's major muscle groups. Compare the size of these muscles and the symmetry of their contours. Document associated muscle tone by checking for resistance to passive motion.

An important part of the motor exam is the evaluation of overall muscle strength. To perform this assessment, ask the patient actively move against your resistance. Grade strength on a scale of 1 to 5:

1. No muscle contraction or only a twitch detectable
2. Only active movement with gravity eliminated (side to side)
3. Active movement against gravity obtained (leg lift)
4. Active movement against some resistance or with fatigue evident
5. Active movement against full resistance without evident fatigue

Strength is expressed as a ratio, with 5/5 representing normal muscle tone—for example, "strength is 4 over 5 (4/5) in the bilateral upper and lower extremities." When checking strength, be prepared to test for flexion, extension, grip, abduction, adduction, and opposition, depending on the location of the muscle groups involved.

Check coordination as part of the neurologic exam because it tests a variety of nervous system functions, especially those involving cerebellar function. Assess coordination by evaluating a patient's ability to perform rapid alternating movements, point-to-point movements (including finger-to-nose and heel-to-shin testing), stance, and gait. Evaluate gait and stance but only in those patients whose status allows them to be placed safely in a standing position. Note any upper extremity tremors or **pronator drift**. Pronator drift is seen when the patient is asked to hold his or her arms straight out with palms up and with his or her eyes shut. When the eyes are shut, you can observe one arm drifting downward towards their feet. This could be a sign of a stroke.

In addition to coordination, test **proprioception**— the patient's awareness of motion and position of a body part. Proprioception is a function of the cerebellum. Loss of proprioception can be seen in medical conditions such as trauma, multiple sclerosis, vitamin B_{12} deficiency, and peripheral neuropathy. Test for proprioception by grasping the patient's great toe, holding it by its sides between your thumb and index finger, and then pulling it away from the other toes. Demonstrate for the patient "up" and "down" as you move the patient's toe clearly upward and downward. Then, with the patient's eyes closed, ask for a response of "up" or "down" as you move the large toe.

Of course, it is also helpful to assess the GCS as discussed in the Primary Survey section. The steps in Skill Drill 11-13 summarize examination of the nervous system.

Just as you use the motor function to test nervous system function from the brain to the body, use the sensory function to test the nervous system's communication between the body and the brain. Test sensory processes bilaterally, looking for asymmetry and comparing proximal to distal processes. When performing the primary survey of a patient who appears to be gravely ill, a sensory exam is typically the first evaluation performed. In this exam, assess both primary and cortical sensory functions. Attempt initial "shake and shout" maneuvers to check for any evidence of higher cerebral functioning and determine whether the patient's primary sensory functioning is intact. Typically, these tests look for any response to gross stimuli (such as a loud shout in the face) or more noxious forms (for example, squeezing the nail bed, twisting the skin of the forearm).

To appropriately assess cortical functioning, the patient's primary functioning must be intact. The brain's primary sensory cortex gathers sensory information and uses it to perform higher-level cortical functions. Therefore, if the primary function is disrupted, any examination of cortical function will be unreliable. However, if primary sensory functioning seems to be intact, proceed with testing the patient's perception of gross versus light touch (the fingers are used; no equipment is required). This test evaluates areas of cortical sensory function. More involved sensory evaluation requires checking sharp versus dull perception and two-point discrimination. Sensation is commonly reported relative to dermatomal location on the body's surface. Dermatomes are areas of the skin that are supplied by a specific sensory nerve.

Skill Drill 11-13 Examining the Nervous System

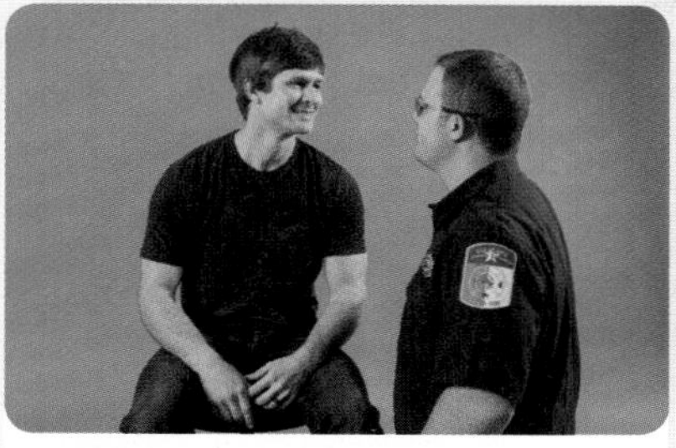

Step 1 Use the AVPU scale to assess the patient's mental status. Note the patient's posture. Evaluate cranial nerve function (see Table 11-10).

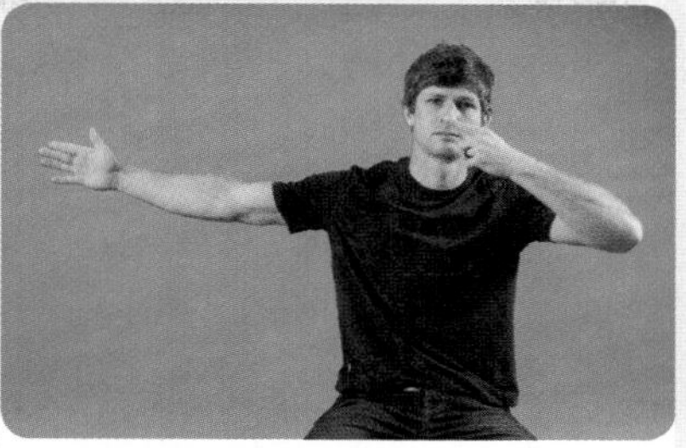

Step 2 Evaluate the patient's coordination by performing the finger-to-nose test using alternating hands.

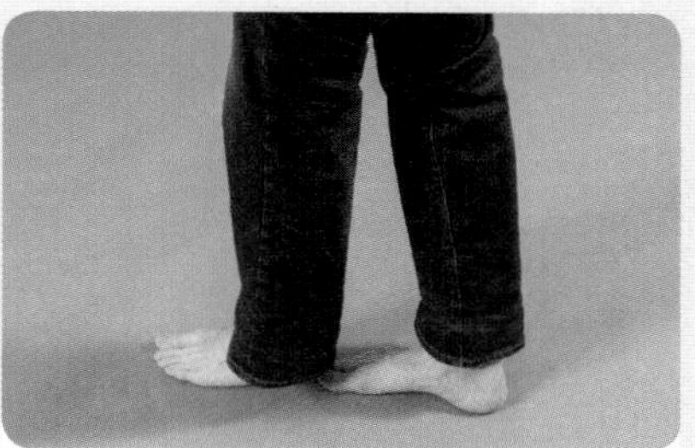

Step 3 If appropriate, test the patient's gait and balance by having him or her walk heel-to-toe or take a heel-to-shin stance.

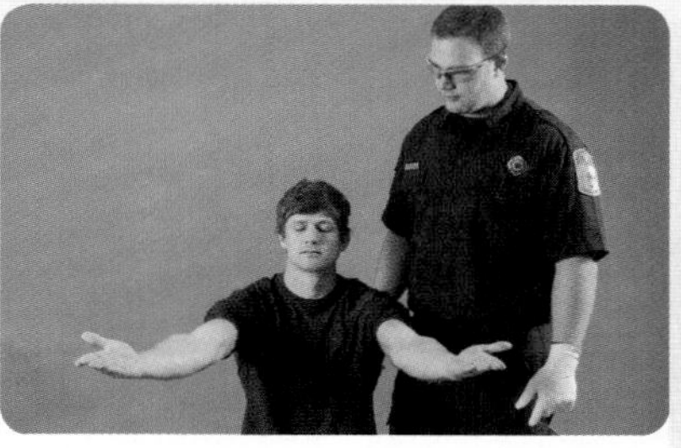

Step 4 Perform the pronator drift test by asking the patient to close his or her eyes and hold both arms out in front of the body. There should not be a difference in movement on either side.

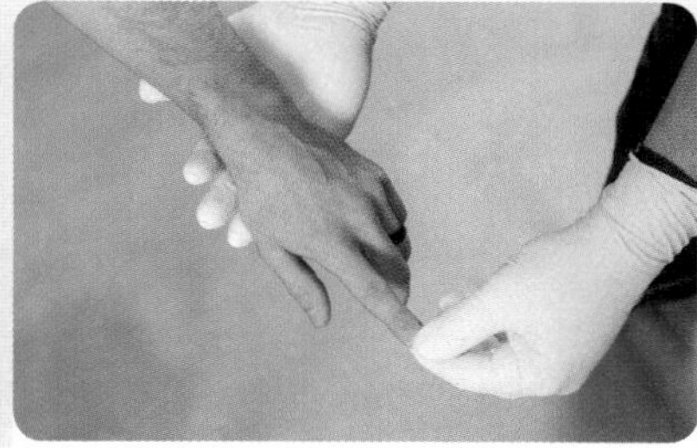

Step 5 Evaluate the patient's sensory function by checking his or her responses to both gross and light touch. If appropriate, check for deep tendon reflexes.

Follow the steps in Skill Drill 11-14 to evaluate deep tendon reflexes. A method of scoring deep tendon reflexes is covered in Table 11-11.

Results of the Neurologic Exam. Abnormal findings on the neurologic exam can take a wide variety of forms. Most common are mental status changes that can represent any number of acute or chronic processes, many of which have a non-neurologic origin. Mental status changes are often associated with inadequate perfusion or are encountered as a subtle indicator of early sepsis (which is common among older adults).

When caring for a patient with abnormal mental status, distinguishing between delirium and dementia is important. Recall, delirium is an acute sudden change in mental status, secondary to some significant underlying factor/incident.

Table 11-11 Scoring Deep Tendon Reflexes

Grade	Deep Tendon Reflex Response
0	No response
1+	Sluggish
2+	Active (expected response)
3+	Slightly hyperactive
4+	Hyperactive

Skill Drill 11-14 Evaluating Deep Tendon Reflexes

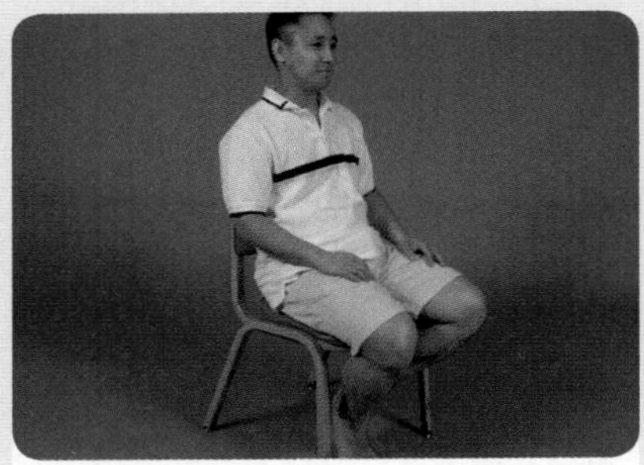

Step 1 Place the patient in a sitting position.

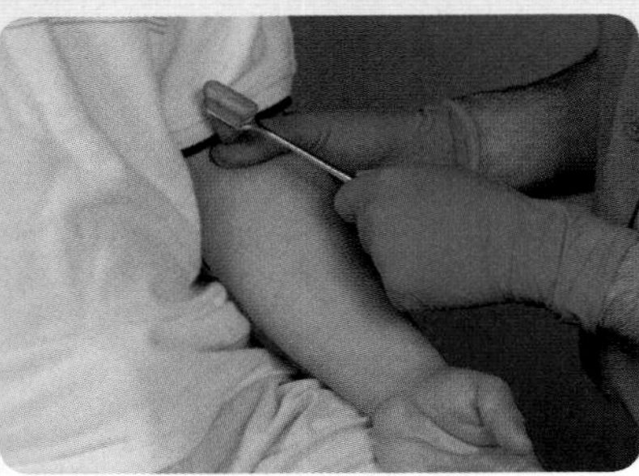

Step 2 Flex the patient's arm at the elbow to a 45° angle. Locate the biceps tendon in the antecubital fossa. Place your thumb over the tendon, with your fingers behind the elbow. Strike your thumb with the reflex hammer, note the flexion of the elbow.

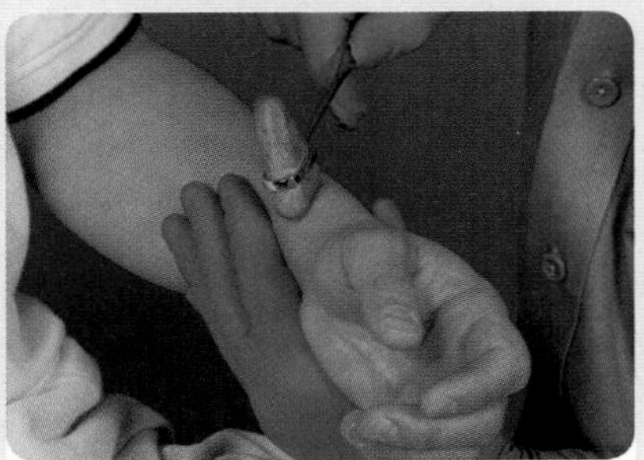

Step 3 With the patient's arm remaining at a 45° angle, rest the patient's forearm on your arm, with the hand slightly pronated. Strike the patient's brachioradialis tendon proximal to the wrist, note the flexion of the elbow.

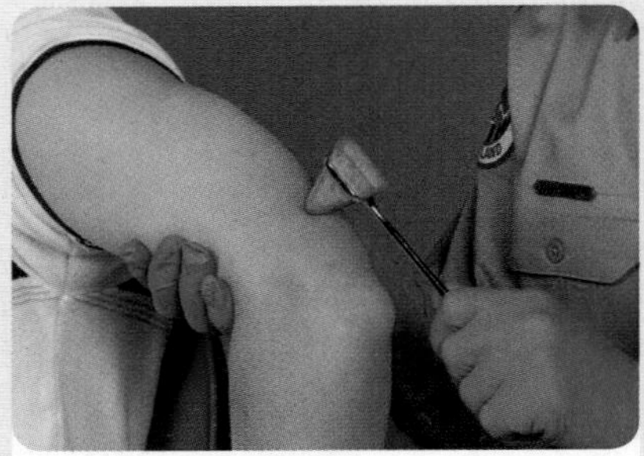

Step 4 Flex the patient's arm at the elbow to a 90° angle, and rest his or her hand against the body. Locate and strike the triceps tendon, noting contraction of the triceps or extension of the elbow.

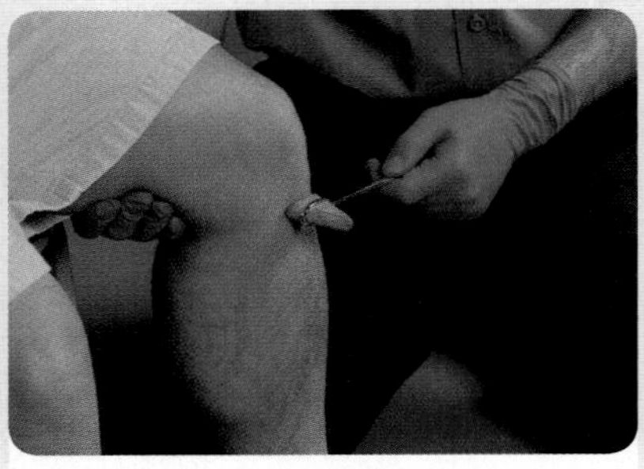

Step 5 Flex the patient's knee to a 90° angle, allowing the leg to dangle. Support the upper leg with your hand, and strike the patellar tendon just below the patella. Note the contraction of the quadriceps and the extension of the lower leg.

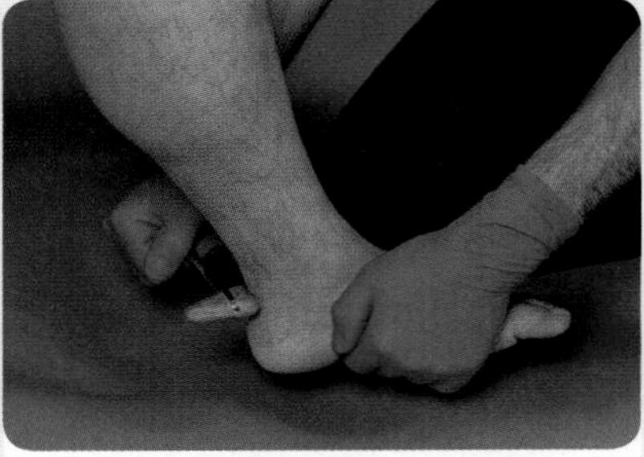

Step 6 With the patient's leg in the same position, hold the heel of the patient's foot in your hand. Strike the Achilles tendon, noting the plantar flexion of the foot.

Dementia is a gradual and pervasive deterioration of cognitive cortical functions, typically secondary to the slow progression of a disease such as Alzheimer disease.

Commonly encountered motor abnormalities include facial and extremity strength asymmetry along with difficulty in speaking (expressive **aphasia**). These signs are typical of cerebrovascular disease. Other commonly encountered abnormalities include ataxia, dystonia, seizures, vertigo, visual changes, tinnitus, and tremor. In the setting of trauma, global changes in mental status are more indicative of intracranial mass lesions, whereas decreased extremity motor function may present with proximal versus distal asymmetry and objective **paresthesias** (tingling or sensory changes), which is more consistent with a spinal lesion.

Secondary Assessment of Unresponsive Patients

After completing the primary survey—and assuming you've ruled out trauma—position an unresponsive patient in the recovery position (left lateral recumbent position) to facilitate drainage of vomit, blood, or other fluids and to help prevent aspiration. If spinal trauma is suspected, position the patient in neutral alignment, fitted with a properly sized rigid cervical collar, and implement spinal immobilization procedures as per your regional protocol.

Perform a thorough assessment of the head, neck, chest, abdomen, pelvis, posterior body, and extremities, looking for signs of illness, such as rash or urticaria (hives), fever, unusual or excessive bruising, pulmonary or peripheral edema, and irregular pulse. Follow up your exam with at least two sets of vital signs—one taken now and another obtained a few minutes after you begin your initial interventions (for example, supplemental oxygen and IV therapy). The first set of readings establishes a baseline (baseline vital signs); the second and additional sets (serial vital signs) provide comparative data to help you evaluate whether the patient's condition is improving, staying status quo, or worsening. If time allows, take additional sets of vital signs to obtain further data, and allow you to map trends such as a steadily accelerating pulse rate. Ensure the vital signs include an auscultated blood pressure, accurate pulse and respiratory rates, and temperature. Recheck breath sounds as well. All unresponsive patients should have their posture assessed. If there is no spontaneous movement, you may need to apply a painful stimulus. If the patient responds normally, he or she will push the stimulus away or withdraw from it. Abnormal postural responses include decorticate and decerebrate posturing of the trunk and extremities. More information on postural presentations can be found in Chapter 18, *Neurologic Emergencies*.

Words of Wisdom

Unresponsive patients should always be considered in unstable condition and at high risk, so rapid transport to the appropriate facility is indicated. Throughout transport, perform reassessment, which includes rechecking ABCDE and reassessing any sign or symptom associated with the patient's chief complaint.

Secondary Assessment of Trauma Patients

Trauma patients can be classified into two broad groups: patients with an isolated injury and patients with multisystem trauma. From a secondary assessment perspective, the difference is an isolated injury allows you to focus immediately on the main injury. In contrast, with multisystem trauma, first, find all of the various injuries, or as many of them as you reasonably can. Then, prioritize the injuries by severity and plan the order in which you will address them. During the assessment, continually think about how each injury or condition relates to the others. For example, the mortality rate doubles for a patient with a serious traumatic brain injury who has just a single episode of hypotension. In such a case, if you do not recognize and address the hypotension, and the consequent lack of adequate perfusion pressure, this can have a huge impact on the patient—in some cases, a fatal impact.

Another important consideration is the high "visibility factor" of many injuries, which sometimes creates a distraction. A compound fracture of the lower leg and ankle, with the foot twisted sideways and jammed under the brake pedal of a vehicle, is not a pretty sight—but it's not life threatening. Because the grossly deformed ankle draws your attention, though, you may miss the early signs and symptoms of shock associated with the more serious—but probably invisible—internal injuries and bleeding that you can't see.

Words of Wisdom

The salvage of lives takes precedence over the salvage of limbs.

Any unresponsive trauma patient with altered mentation should be considered a high-risk, priority patient requiring immediate transport to a trauma center. This patient may have a traumatic brain injury, stroke, hypoglycemia, or alcohol or drug intoxication. All are serious—possibly lethal—circumstances or devastating injuries.

Recall, you will perform the primary survey and, if indicated, a rapid full-body scan on trauma patients. Though there may not always be time for further physical examination of a trauma patient, take advantage of the opportunity to continue the exam if time and the patient's condition do allow for it. Remember, examining a trauma patient *takes lots and lots of practice*.

Before you physically examine a trauma patient, if you suspect a spine injury, ensure the cervical spine is manually immobilized in the neutral position. Quickly reassess the patient's current mental status, comparing it with baseline readings. Last, revisit your transport decision. If you decide the patient needs immediate transport, perform the rapid full-body scan and do not delay transport to pursue a more thorough examination.

Also, mentally piece together all that you now know about your patient, including the chief complaint, the history of the present event, the medical history, and any information about the patient's current health status. Combine that knowledge with the other information and insights you gained from your various assessments, along with the data from your diagnostics, and you should have more than enough information to make good clinical choices for your patient.

Recording Secondary Assessment Findings

Medical information may be presented in both verbal and written forms. Documentation should always be recorded in an orderly, concise way, without omitting important facts. The information you obtain may then be practically and accurately relayed to the receiving medical staff. In addition, thorough documentation ensures an accurate accounting of the patient's history prior to entering the hospital will be legally entered into the formal medical record. A number of acceptable formats are currently in use, including electronic records. Use the documentation method that is required by your local protocols.

Secondary assessment requires physical interaction between you and the patient and can be performed successfully on a patient who cannot communicate. As you record your exam findings, note objective signs, pertinent negatives, and similar relevant information. Objective information is usually recorded in a standard format, in the same order used for the written patient care report (PCR).

Words of Wisdom

Remember the legal and ethical components of assessment:

1. Respect the patient's decision-making autonomy.
2. Be accountable to the patient.
3. Respect the patient's confidentiality and privacy.
4. Obtain consent.
5. Understand and respect advance directives.
6. Document facts accurately and nonjudgmentally.

Limits of the Secondary Assessment

The ability to perform a secondary assessment competently is one of the most valuable skills you can possess. This assessment can, for example, uncover information that the patient is unable or unwilling to share. An accomplished clinician will use this skill in conjunction with the history taking and other diagnostic tools to form an impression and formulate a treatment plan.

Nevertheless, despite the emphasis placed on a comprehensive physical exam, the secondary assessment has some limitations. Even the most experienced provider understands not everything can be discovered in such an assessment. Learn to keep the total time in the field to a minimum. There is no reason to proceed with a thorough secondary assessment in the field, including an assessment of deep tendon reflexes, when the result is going to be transportation to the ED regardless. The ED physician will need to repeat the exam. A secondary assessment should rarely take more than a few minutes. Move things along expeditiously, especially if the patient has a priority condition where time is crucial In the prehospital setting, it is important to remember the evaluation by a trained physician coupled with laboratory and radiographic studies is needed for a definitive diagnosis.

Monitoring Devices

Whereas the history-taking and secondary assessment process is the best method for determining a differential diagnosis of your patient, certain diagnostic and monitoring devices and laboratory tests are typically used to aid in the assessment process. Keep in mind, although these devices are helpful, they cannot replace a good past medical history and secondary assessment. Avoid the pitfall of relying on monitoring devices and not on the physical exam and patient presentation. Always remember to treat your patient—not the monitor.

Continuous ECG Monitoring

The purpose of continuous ECG monitoring in the prehospital environment is to establish a baseline ECG rhythm and monitor the patient for dynamic changes in cardiac electrical activity.

Patients should be on continuous cardiac monitoring if they present with cardiac signs and symptoms or with signs and symptoms of illnesses that could affect the heart. Many patients' illnesses meet this threshold, which is why paramedics frequently place patients on cardiac monitors as part of their routine advanced life support (ALS) care.

Most ECG monitors designed for the prehospital environment work in the same fashion. To monitor the cardiac rhythm accurately, the electrodes must be placed correctly Figure 11-49. Cardiac rhythm monitoring devices typically use three to five leads. The leads are usually colored and labeled to help with placement. The lead wires are attached to electrodes, which are adhesive disks with a gel center to aid in skin contact. Some manufacturers offer a "diaphoretic" electrode that sticks more effectively to a sweating patient.

Whereas continuous ECG monitoring provides real-time visibility of cardiac electrical activity, it shows you only one aspect of the heart's electrical activity. An ECG tracing gives you limited information about the muscular function of the heart, nor will it always accurately assess the adequacy of the blood supply to the cardiac muscle via the coronary vessels. The heart is like a light bulb in a socket—the bulb contains everything it needs in order to function; however, it requires a supply of electricity. When a light bulb burns out and stops working, electricity is still flowing to the socket. As long as the switch remains on, the electricity is there whether the bulb works or not. The same principle is true here. There are times when the ECG looks normal, but the heart is nevertheless not functioning properly. More information on ECG interpretation can be found in Chapter 17, *Cardiovascular Emergencies*.

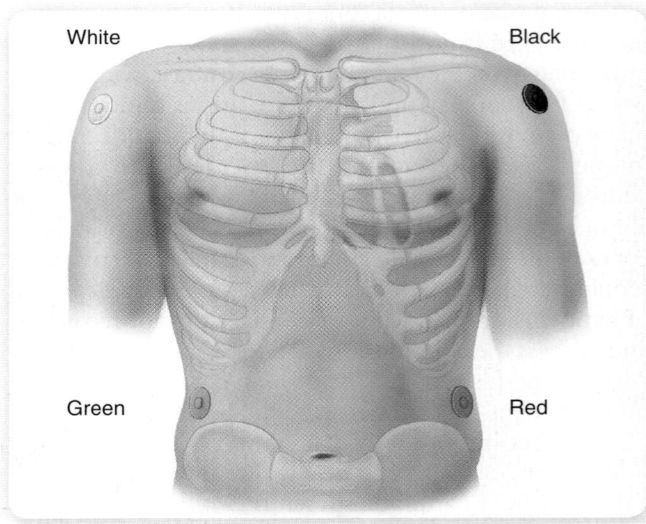

Figure 11-49 4-lead electrode placement.

12-Lead ECG Monitoring

For the purposes of rhythm interpretation, a single lead (usually lead II) is often sufficient. However, to localize the site of injury to the heart muscle, you must be able to look at the heart from several angles. That's precisely the purpose of a 12-lead ECG.

The addition of the 12-lead ECG to the paramedic's toolbox has opened the door for more advanced patient care in the field. Paramedics are now able to diagnose AMI in the patient's home. This early recognition of allows hospitals to prepare before patients arrive, thus, decreasing the amount of time it takes to receive definitive care. In addition, paramedics in some areas of the United States are performing early intervention in the field by administering fibrinolytics to STEMI patients or by diverting them to cardiac centers with catheterization labs.

The only way to learn how to take a 12-lead ECG is to practice with the equipment itself. Here are some guidelines to ensure the ECGs you obtain are of the highest quality possible.

- The patient should be supine. If the patient feels shortness of breath in that position, you may elevate the back of the stretcher to about a 30° angle.
- Ensure the patient does not become chilled, because shivering will produce artifact in the ECG tracing. Note that 12-lead ECGs are more sensitive to artifact than 3-lead monitoring ECGs.
- Prepare the patient's skin as you would for placement of monitoring electrodes.
- Connect the four limb electrodes. Double-check that the correct electrode is on each limb (the "LA" electrode is on the left arm, the "RA" electrode is on the right arm, and so on).
- Connect and apply the precordial leads as indicated in Figure 11-50.
- Record the ECG.

Interpretation of 12-lead ECGs is discussed in detail in Chapter 17, *Cardiovascular Emergencies*.

Carbon Dioxide Monitoring

As you learned in Chapter 8, *Anatomy and Physiology*, carbon dioxide is a naturally occurring by-product of cellular metabolism in the human body. As the metabolism reacts in response to stressors, change in the output of carbon dioxide can be seen and measured. Recognize carbon dioxide output in a patient and use that information to determine treatment strategies.

There are two ways in which carbon dioxide is monitored in the field: capnometry and capnography. **Capnometry** typically consists of a disposable or electronic device that provides you with a means of measuring carbon dioxide output. **Capnography** includes not only a measurement of carbon dioxide output, but also provides a waveform based on serial measurements. It's the ECG of ventilation, so to speak. A capnograph is a practical device that's simple to use in the prehospital environment. Whereas the older models were heavy and sometimes difficult to operate,

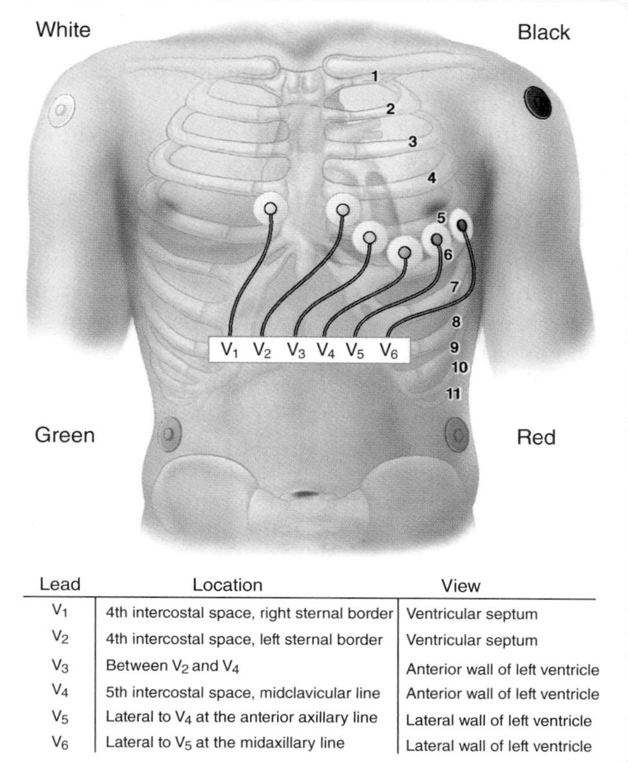

Lead	Location	View
V_1	4th intercostal space, right sternal border	Ventricular septum
V_2	4th intercostal space, left sternal border	Ventricular septum
V_3	Between V_2 and V_4	Anterior wall of left ventricle
V_4	5th intercostal space, midclavicular line	Anterior wall of left ventricle
V_5	Lateral to V_4 at the anterior axillary line	Lateral wall of left ventricle
V_6	Lateral to V_5 at the midaxillary line	Lateral wall of left ventricle

Figure 11-50 12-lead electrode placement.

newer devices are user friendly and easy to interpret. These devices can be used to confirm endotracheal tube placement, or they can also be used in conscious and breathing patients to produce a continuous picture of ventilatory status and alert you to bronchospasm, shock, or acidosis.

Evidence-Based Medicine

The correlation between $ETCO_2$ and cardiac output has two important implications during CPR. First, the effectiveness of CPR in producing adequate cardiac output can be monitored based on the $ETCO_2$ values. Second, abrupt increases in $ETCO_2$ values suggest concomitant increases in cardiac output and are indicative of ROSC.

In intubated patients, the device is placed on the proximal end of the endotracheal tube and then connected to your portable ECG monitor or a separate monitoring device. For breathing patients, a special nasal cannula adapted for collecting carbon dioxide while administering oxygen is used. Although the capnograph is superior in monitoring quality to the capnometer, it too has limitations. Such devices typically require a minimum airflow to calculate a reading and are sometimes affected by secretions in the tubing. They also require periodic calibration.

The purpose of capnometry is to verify correct endotracheal tube placement. The idea is that the capnometer is placed on the proximal end of an endotracheal tube. If the tube is in the trachea, exhaled CO_2 should pass by the sensor and provide information about tube placement. This sounds easy enough; however, it is not without limitations.

Capnometry and capnography are discussed in more detail in Chapter 15, *Airway Management*.

Basic Blood Chemistry

A variety of elements found in blood can aid you in differentiating between possibilities within the differential diagnosis. Although results from the history taking and secondary assessment are paramount in initially determining the differential diagnosis, sometimes a laboratory result helps to narrow the scope of possibilities.

Glucometer. Measuring the blood glucose level of every patient with altered mentation is a must. It's a relatively easy test to perform and provides you with rapid information about the patient's available level of available glucose. A low glucose level helps you in forming the differential diagnosis for an unresponsive patient. Likewise, a high glucose level in a patient with nausea, vomiting, and abdominal pain may indicate diabetic ketoacidosis.

Blood glucose should be assessed in all known diabetic patients, all patients who are unresponsive for unknown reasons, and for patients with generalized malaise/weakness. In addition, a blood glucose level can be assessed on any patient whom you feel has a poor general impression.

There are generally two ways to obtain a rapid blood glucose reading in the field: from the hub of an IV catheter or from a finger stick. When obtaining a blood sample from an IV catheter, establish IV access as usual, place the test strip against the hub of the catheter before you connect the IV tubing, and allow a drop of blood to touch the test strip. For patients with an IV line already placed, use a lancet needle to obtain a drop of blood. Cleanse the site (finger) with antiseptic, and puncture the site with the lancet. Immediately dispose of the needle in a sharps container, and collect a drop of blood on the test strip. When you're finished, place a bandage over the puncture site.

Most glucometers take only a few seconds to give you a reading. Keep in mind, while this is convenient for you, rapid does not always equal accurate. Glucometers must be calibrated on a regular basis to maintain accuracy. In addition, verify the test strips are correct for the glucometer you are using and haven't expired. Ensure you've prepped the site adequately, and that the finger is clean.

Cardiac Biomarkers. Cardiac biomarkers are used to assess for cardiac muscle damage. Typically, such blood tests are performed to determine whether the patient has had an AMI. Earlier in this chapter, we covered the use of 12-lead ECGs in the field to help determine whether a STEMI has occurred; however, most heart attacks are known as non-ST elevation MIs (NSTEMIs). These events are typically diagnosed by means of lab results, using cardiac biomarkers; however, several devices are now available to measure these cardiac markers quickly in the field.

In the EMS environment, cardiac biomarkers should be assessed in all cardiac patients, provided doing so is consistent with local protocol. They should also be assessed in any patient with signs and symptoms of a stroke. The procedure is similar to obtaining a blood glucose level. The accuracy of the test depends on proper calibration of the equipment and use of an appropriate unexpired testing medium (that is, test strips). In addition, understand that it can take several hours for cardiac biomarkers to appear in a patient's blood after an AMI. Therefore, if elevated levels are not seen in the field, you cannot necessarily rule out the possibility that an AMI is taking place. AMI is discussed in greater detail in Chapter 17, *Cardiovascular Emergencies*.

Other Blood Tests. With the invention of rapid laboratory testing devices, more EMS systems—particularly those that handle specialty care transports—are beginning to perform basic laboratory tests in the field.

The i-STAT handheld operates with single-use, disposable i-STAT test cartridges Figure 11-51. Test cartridges for the i-STAT cover a broad menu of the most commonly performed diagnostic tests, such as those for cardiac markers, lactate, coagulation, blood gases, chemistries and electrolytes, and other hematology studies.

Tests such as a basic and complete metabolic profile (CHEM 7 and CHEM 12) reveal the patient's electrolyte status, along with his or her renal and, sometimes, liver function. The brain natriuretic peptide (BNP) level is typically elevated in a patient experiencing an exacerbation of chronic heart failure. A BNP test helps you to differentiate cardiac versus pulmonary causes of respiratory distress. These tests are not generally used in the field unless you are working in a specialty clinic setting.

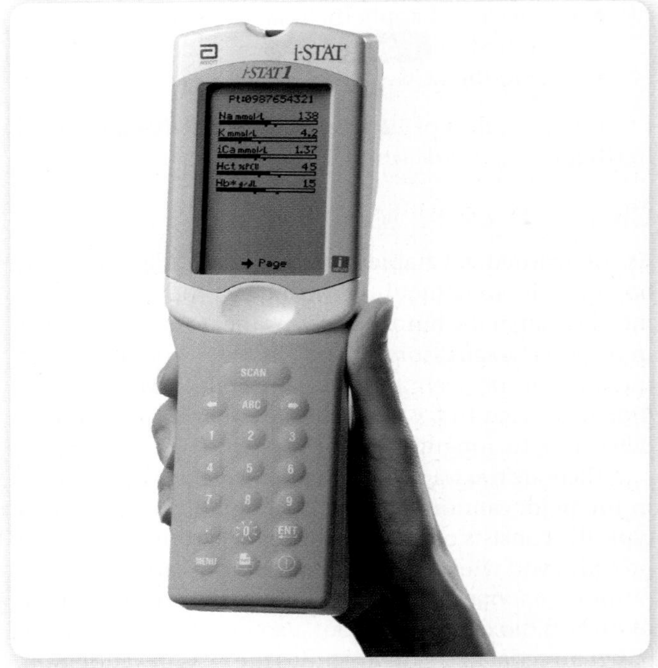

Figure 11-51 The i-STAT portable testing device.

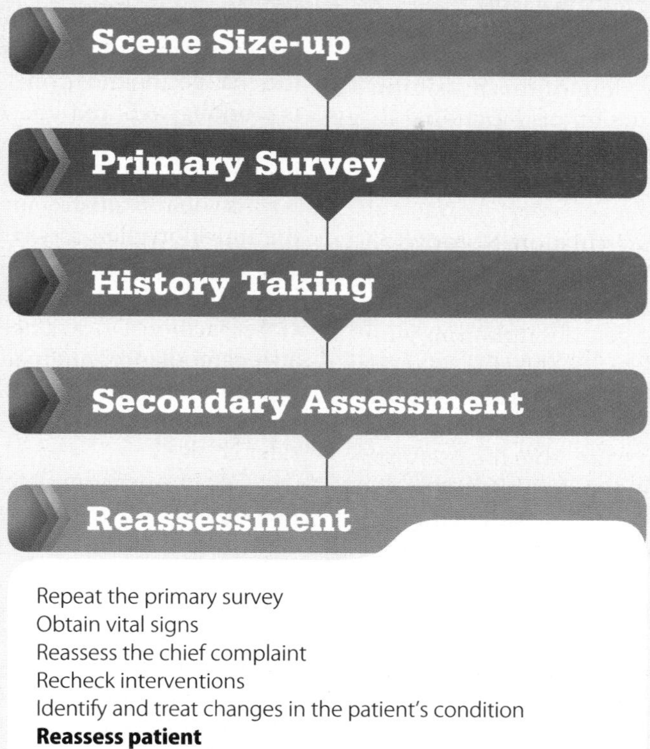

Reassessment

After the primary survey, **reassessment** is the single most important assessment process you will perform. When performing reassessment, reassess ABCDE, to ensure you adequately address the chief complaint, obtained another set of vital signs, and closed any other patient care loops, such as dressing small wounds and placing ice packs. Reassessment represents a continuous, yet cyclical, process you perform throughout transport, right up to the time you turn over patient care to the emergency department staff. For patients in stable condition, do a reassessment every 15 minutes or so. For patients in unstable condition, make a concerted effort to repeat the reassessment every 5 minutes.

Reassessment of the Primary Survey

Reassessment combines repetition of the primary survey, reassessment of vital signs and breath sounds, and repetition of the secondary assessment. During the reassessment, continue to evaluate and reevaluate the patient's status and the efficacy of any treatments already administered by comparing serial vital signs. This information indicates which changes have occurred and which critical conditions have been addressed and corrected.

First, compare the patient's LOC with your baseline assessment. Is the LOC changing? If so, how? If mentation is decreasing, can the patient still protect the airway? If you have doubts, consider inserting an advanced airway.

Second, review the patient's airway. Is it patent? Swelling, bleeding, or just a change of position can quickly obstruct the airway, so ensure the airway is properly positioned and dry. Always be prepared to suction, and don't delay if you hear gurgling in the upper airway. It's far better to prevent aspiration than to treat it later. If the airway needs to be secured, *prepare the patient for intubation and perform the procedure immediately*. Then recheck lung sounds and perform oximetry and capnography periodically to confirm correct tube placement.

Third, reassess breathing. Is the patient breathing adequately? If not, figure out why and correct the problem. For hypoventilation, assist breathing with oxygen and a bag-mask device. Correct hypoxia with high-concentration oxygen therapy. For patients with diminished or absent breath sounds, JVD, and progressive dyspnea (signs of pneumothorax), decompress the chest.

Stay alert for signs of ventilatory fatigue, such as a decreasing pulse oximetry reading or a patient who looks increasingly tired. Be especially alert for this possibility in children, because it's a classic sign of impending disaster. Patients of any age who show signs of ventilatory fatigue need to have their airway aggressively managed for them.

Finally, reassess the patient's circulation. Note overall skin color as an initial gauge of cardiovascular function and hemodynamic status. With pale, cool, wet skin, think shock; with cyanosis, think oxygen desaturation; with mottling, think end-stage shock.

Ensure all bleeding is controlled. If you find blood-soaked dressings, add fresh dressings to the stack and rebandage in place. Reassess the blood pressure, watch closely for signs that the patient is beginning to decompensate.

Reassess the pulse, including its rate, strength, and regularity. Progressive tachycardia may indicate that the patient's problem has not been corrected (he or she is still bleeding, is hypoxic, or is developing cardiogenic shock). In contrast, sustained or progressively worsening bradycardia may reflect rising intracranial pressure (from trauma or a stroke) or end-stage shock.

Special Populations

During a crisis, the responses of children and older adult patients may differ. Therefore you may have to take a different approach to reassessment. Adult patients have a tendency to show signs of deterioration as their condition becomes unstable. Children, however, will decompensate much faster; therefore, frequent reassessment is imperative. Any indication of deteriorating mental status or changes to airway, breathing, or circulation should prompt immediate intervention.

Geriatric patients differ from other adult and pediatric patients in that they may lack appropriate compensatory mechanisms and therefore may not show signs of deterioration as their medical condition becomes unstable. In addition, many of these patients have underlying diseases or take medications that mask the relevant assessment findings. For example, a patient who is going into shock would typically demonstrate an increased pulse rate. However, many older adult patients either lack the ability to increase their pulse rate or take medications that regulate the pulse rate. Reassessment of mental status may also prove challenging in this population. For some patients, a seemingly altered mental status is their baseline behavior; therefore, it becomes difficult to assess whether the patient is improving. Frequent reassessment is necessary to determine and monitor a patient's overall progress and stability.

Reassessment of Patient Care and Transport Priorities

After reassessing the patient, think about your care plan. Have you addressed all life threats? Based on what you know, do you need to revise your priority list? If so, make the change and move on. On the other hand, if your plan is working well and you have addressed most or all of the patient's chief complaints, there's no need to revise the care plan.

As you reevaluate your patient care priorities, reassess the transport plan as well. Should routine transport be stepped up to priority? Is the patient's condition worsening to the point that you should consider diverting to a closer facility? Do you need to set up a rendezvous with an air ambulance? Alternatively, if your patient's condition has improved and stabilized, step down from priority and transport the patient as a routine case—clearly the safer choice.

Get another complete set of vital signs, and compare them with the expected outcomes from your therapies. For example, if you administered a 500-mL bolus of normal saline to a patient with gastrointestinal bleeding, you would expect blood pressure to rise and pulse rate to drop. With any priority patient, even with a short transport, you should have, at a minimum, obtain three sets of vital signs. With most priority patients, you'll have four or five sets of vital signs. Thus, you can look for trends or patterns, such as the slowing pulse, rising blood pressure, and erratic respiratory patterns that represent the **Cushing reflex**, a grave sign for patients with head trauma. Alternatively, narrowed pulse pressure, muffled heart tones, and JVD are associated with cardiac tamponade (**Beck triad**), usually secondary to penetrating chest trauma.

Words of Wisdom

You cannot recognize narrowing pulse pressures until you've taken two or three sets of blood pressure readings. Multiple checks provide the comparative data you need.

The last element of the reassessment is to revisit the patient's chief complaint(s) (from the history taking), along with your interventions. Have any complaints improved or resolved? For instance, has the 9 over 10 chest pain improved with the nitroglycerin you administered? Did the second albuterol treatment ease the patient's breathing? Which situations remain unresolved? Worsening situations are especially worrisome because they could indicate an unseen problem or ineffective interventions. With each reassessment, document your findings so the medical record is accurate and complete. Finally, if you haven't reached the receiving facility, begin the process again—that's why it's called *reassessment*.

YOU are the Paramedic SUMMARY

1. What is your first concern at this scene?

You don't know at this point what happened to the patient. This may or may not be a crime scene. Either way, the main priority is to ensure the safety and well-being of you and your partner. Consider whether it's safe to enter this scene and approach the patient. Assess and evaluate the scene through a wide-angle lens. If you're in doubt as to whether the scene is safe, then request the appropriate additional resources before you proceed. In this case, the scene safety issue is related to the potential for violence. You are not trained to make this scene safe; therefore, it is mandatory that you request law enforcement prior to exposing yourself to the danger.

2. How will you address this concern?

Request law enforcement personnel immediately in cases that could involve a crime, because it's nearly impossible for you and your partner to control the scene and care for the patient at the same time, and because the perpetrator could return with additional weapons. If you are unsure what to do, protect yourself and your crew before anything else. This may mean staying in the ambulance until law enforcement personnel arrive to secure the scene.

3. What is your general impression of this patient?

You know the patient is responsive and bleeding from a chest wound, but he is not responsive to simple commands. Even with this limited information, you know this patient could deteriorate rapidly into shock and could require rapid transport.

4. What is your next step in assessing this patient?

Changes in the level of consciousness (LOC) may provide the first clue to an alteration in the patient's condition, so establish a baseline as soon as you encounter the patient. As you assess mental status, if trauma is involved, decide whether you suspect spinal trauma and implement spinal immobilization procedures. The quickest and simplest way to assess the patient's mental status or LOC is to use the AVPU scale.

5. On the basis of your assessment of ABCDE, what is your first priority in the care of this patient?

Airway assessment focuses on two questions: Is the airway open and patent? Is it likely to remain so? If you determine the patient cannot maintain his or her airway, an oropharyngeal or nasopharyngeal airway may resolve the problem. However, if you cannot maintain it by any other means, use a more invasive technique, such as endotracheal intubation. Breathing is proportional and related to airway adequacy. Assessing breathing likewise focuses on two questions: Is the patient breathing? If not, then you have to breathe for the patient. If the patient is breathing, is breathing adequate? Again, if breathing is not adequate, do what is necessary to support the patient's breathing or consider performing rapid-sequence intubation.

6. Can you determine the transport priority of this patient at this point?

Yes. When you have a priority (unstable) patient, expedite transport, doing only what is absolutely necessary at the scene and handling everything else en route, including the appropriate history taking and physical exam. This patient presents with a poor general impression, is responsive but does not or cannot follow commands, and has difficulty breathing because of a penetrating injury to his chest. Based solely on these three criteria, rapid transport of this patient is a priority.

7. How can you determine the level of internal damage if you do not have the implement that was used to stab the patient?

Any chest injury, regardless of the object used, can cause significant internal damage. The chest contains many structures that are vital to life, including the lungs and mediastinal elements (heart, great vessels). The chest (or thorax) consists of the superior aspect of the torso, from the base of the neck to the diaphragm, as delineated by the costal arch. The chest wall is divided into anterior and posterior portions—literally, the patient's front and back. The back of the chest extends down the patient's back, to the level of the diaphragm posteriorly, which tends to move up and down with breathing. The chest wall serves as a protective covering for the internal components. It consists of numerous musculoskeletal, vascular, nervous, connective, and lining structures.

8. What is the relevance of past medical history in this case?

The past medical history gives you an opportunity to learn about any pertinent or chronic underlying medical conditions the patient may have. Although some aspects of the past medical history may not seem important with this patient, a careful and thorough history will help paint a clear picture of his overall health status. However, he may not be willing or able to give you this information. Rely on what you learned during your patient assessment and inspection as much as possible. Always look for any medical alert jewelry or devices and note of any scars that may indicate prior open heart or chest wall surgery, such as placement of a pacemaker or an automated implantable cardioverter defibrillator.

YOU are the Paramedic SUMMARY *(continued)*

EMS Patient Care Report (PCR)

Date: 04-28-18	**Incident No.:** 902	**Nature of Call:** Stabbing		**Location:** 4th Ave/Main St	
Dispatched: 0200	**En Route:** 0201	**At Scene:** 0205	**Transport:** 0215	**At Hospital:** 0225	**In Service:** 0240

Patient Information

Age: Approx 30 **Sex:** M **Weight (in kg [lb]):** 75 kg (165 lb)	**Allergies:** Unknown **Medications:** Unknown **Past Medical History:** Unknown **Chief Complaint:** 1-inch (2.5 cm) penetrating wound to upper left chest

Vital Signs

Time: 0210	**BP:** 90/64	**Pulse:** 122	**Respirations:** 28	**Spo_2:** 93% on room air
Time: 0215	**BP:** 92/62	**Pulse:** 120	**Respirations:** 28	**Spo_2:** 99% on 15 L/min
Time: 0220	**BP:** 92/60	**Pulse:** 118	**Respirations:** 26	**Spo_2:** 99% on 15 L/min

EMS Treatment (circle all that apply)

Oxygen @ 15 **L/min via (circle one):** **NC** (**NRM** circled) **Bag-mask device**		**Assisted Ventilation**	**Airway Adjunct**	**CPR**
Defibrillation	**Bleeding Control**	**Bandaging**	**Splinting**	(circled) **Other:** Occlusive dressing

Narrative

Unit 84 dispatched for a man down in front of the strip mall at 4th Avenue & Main Street. This unit arrived on scene prior to all other responders to find this pt lying left lateral recumbent on the sidewalk. There appears to be no one else present on the scene. Prior to exiting the vehicle, scene lights reveal what appears to be blood on the sidewalk near the pt's chest. Because of safety concerns, level of consciousness was assessed via the PA system. Pt demonstrated following commands at that time. PD on scene approximately 1 minute after our arrival. Scene secured for pt assessment and treatment. pt is an approx. 30-year-old man with a penetrating wound, approx. 1 inch in length just inferior to the center of the left clavicle. Bleeding has stopped. Three-sided occlusive dressing applied. Pt is responsive, responds to commands, but is not verbal. Sensation and motion is normal in all four extremities so based on the clinical evaluation no spinal immobilization was applied. VS as noted and 15 L/min O_2 via NRM applied. IV NS established with 16ga, right AC. Pt able to maintain own airway but having increased difficulty breathing upon lying supine on the stretcher. Pt transport to the regional trauma center with early notification. Head of the backboard raised 15%, which provided some relief to breathing effort. Pt report given to Dr. Solomon upon arrival.**End of report**

Prep Kit

▶ Ready for Review

- Patient assessment is the foundation on which quality prehospital care is built and the single most important skill you bring to bear on patient care.
- There are five components in the patient assessment process: scene size-up, primary survey, history taking, secondary assessment, and reassessment.
- The first step of the patient assessment process is the scene size-up, because your first and foremost concern on any call is to ensure your safety and the safety of other EMS personnel.
- During the scene size-up, you also determine the mechanism of injury or nature of the patient's illness.
- Another important step in protecting yourself is to take standard precautions. Don all the necessary personal protective equipment before approaching the patient.
- The first step in the primary survey is to form a general impression of the patient's condition. As you approach the patient, note whether he or she appears to be in stable or unstable condition, and observe the environment for clues.
- During the primary survey, identify threats to ABCDE and address them immediately.
- Assess the patient for disability, then make a transport decision. If the patient has sustained trauma, perform a rapid full-body scan (from the secondary assessment portion of the assessment process) to identify injuries that require care before you immobilize the patient.
- Once the primary survey is completed and all life threats are addressed, move into the history-taking component of patient assessment.
- Patient history is a primary means of diagnosing the chief complaint in the field; its value depends on your ability to skillfully elicit complete and accurate information.
- Use constructive communications skills as you talk with patients: facilitation, reflection, clarification, empathy, confrontation, interpretation, and direct questions about feelings.
- At times you must ask patients about sensitive topics, such as alcohol or drug abuse, physical abuse or other violence, or sexual history. Be familiar with techniques for successfully interviewing patients about these topics.
- Within your service and with your partner, work on strategies for communicating positively with patients who are silent, overly talkative, anxious, angry or hostile, intoxicated, crying, depressed, or seeking reassurance. Discuss how to determine the chief complaint in a patient with multiple symptoms. Discuss how to remain professional when treating a patient to whom you are physically attracted.
- For responsive medical patients, obtain the past medical history directly from the patient, although certain patients, such as children, may need assistance. For responsive medical patients, ask questions about each body system to obtain a thorough picture of the patient's health.
- For unresponsive medical patients and trauma patients, it may be necessary to obtain the medical history from family members or bystanders.
- The first part of a patient's medical history also serves as a good mental status examination: ask for the patient's name; the date, time, and location; the chief complaint; and the events leading up to the call for EMS.
- After clarifying the history of the present illness, ask the patient about his or her past medical history, the general state of his or her health, and any pertinent family history. Ask for a list of the patient's medications and allergies, as part of this questioning.
- Obtaining a medical history from an older adult patient may be challenging. Older patients may have multiple medical conditions, take numerous medications, and have a different patient presentation than other adults, which can make their emergencies more complex. They may also have sensory losses that require you to adjust your approach to collect the necessary information.
- Secondary assessment (also known as the head-to-toe physical exam) is the process by which you obtain quantifiable, objective information from a patient about his or her overall state of health.
- The two types of physical examinations performed during the secondary assessment are the full-body exam and the focused assessment. If the patient has serious life threats, you may not have time to perform a secondary assessment at all. Or, you may focus on the area of the chief complaint first, and then move on to other body systems if time permits.
- The secondary assessment includes obtaining vital signs that measure overall body function, and performing a head-to-toe physical exam that evaluates the function of specific body systems. This exam is done in a sequential manner to ensure every aspect of the body's function is evaluated.
- The techniques of inspection, palpation, percussion, and auscultation allow you to use your physical senses to obtain physical information and understand the normal (versus abnormal) functions of a patient's body.

Prep Kit (continued)

- Vital signs consist of a measurement of blood pressure; pulse rate, rhythm, and quality; respiratory rate, rhythm, and quality; body temperature; and, if indicated, pulse oximetry. Other than overall patient appearance, vital signs are some of the most valuable objective data for determining patient status.
- Monitoring devices used by the paramedic include continuous ECG monitoring, 12-lead ECG, carbon dioxide monitoring (capnography and capnometry), blood chemistry analyses, blood glucose monitoring, and cardiac biomarkers, among others.
- Alter your approach to patient assessment when caring for infants and children. If a young child cannot speak, assess his or her condition based largely on what you can see and hear. Family members or caregivers may also be able to provide useful information.
- After the primary survey, the reassessment is the single most important assessment process you will perform.
- The reassessment is performed on all patients. It gives you an opportunity to reevaluate the chief complaint and to reassess your interventions to ensure they are still effective. Information from the reassessment may be used to identify and treat changes in the patient's condition.
- A patient in stable condition should be reassessed every 15 minutes, whereas a patient in unstable condition should be reassessed every 5 minutes. A critical patient must be evaluated continuously.

▶ Vital Vocabulary

adventitious breath sounds Abnormal breath sounds, such as wheezing, rhonchi, crackles, stridor, and pleural friction rubs.

alert and oriented (A × O) A determination made when assessing mental status by looking at whether the patient is oriented in four areas: person, place, time, and the event itself. Each element provides information about different aspects of the patient's memory.

anisocoria Unequal pupils with a greater than 1-mm difference.

aphasia The language impairment that affects the production or understanding of speech and the ability to read or write.

apparent life-threatening event (ALTE) An episode characterized by some combination of apnea (central or obstructive), color change (cyanotic, pallid, erythematous, or plethoric) change in muscle tone (usually diminished), and choking or gagging.

ascites Abnormal accumulation of fluid in the peritoneal cavity; typically signals liver failure.

aspiration The entry of fluids or solids into the trachea, bronchi, and lungs; the act of drawing material in or out by suction.

auscultation The act of using a stethoscope to listen to sounds within the body.

AVPU A method of assessing mental status by determining whether a patient is Awake and alert, responsive to Verbal stimuli or Pain, or Unresponsive; used principally in the primary survey.

Battle sign Bruising over the mastoid process, which may indicate a basilar skull fracture; also known as retroauricular ecchymosis or raccoon eyes.

Beck triad The combination of a narrowed pulse pressure, muffled heart tones, and jugular venous distention associated with cardiac tamponade; usually caused by penetrating chest trauma.

blood pressure (BP) The measurement of the force exerted against the walls of the blood vessels as the heart contracts and relaxes; it is calculated as the product of cardiac output and peripheral vascular resistance.

bronchial sounds Hollow, tubular, lower-pitched sounds heard over the trachea.

bronchophony A test of decreased breath sounds performed by placing the diaphragm of the stethoscope over the area in question while the patient says "ninety-nine;" a loud, clear sound indicates lung consolidation.

bronchovesicular sounds A combination of the tracheal and vesicular breath sounds; heard where airways and alveoli are found, in the upper part of the sternum and between the scapulae.

bruit An abnormal whooshing sound of turbulent blood flow moving through a narrowed artery; usually heard in the carotid arteries.

capnography The use of a noninvasive diagnostic tool that can quickly and efficiently provide information on a patient's ventilatory and circulatory status with a graphic and digital depiction similar to an electrocardiogram.

capnometry The use of a capnometer, which is a monitoring device used to measure the amount of expired carbon dioxide. The reading is usually given as a digital reading.

cerumen Ear wax.

chief complaint The reason the patient is seeking help.

crackles Wet rattling, bubbling, or crackling lung sounds indicative of fluid in the small airways; also known as *rales*.

Prep Kit *(continued)*

crepitus A crackling, grating, or grinding sound often heard when fragments of broken bones rub together.

current health status A composite picture of a number of factors in a patient's life, such as dietary habits, current medications, allergies, exercise, alcohol or tobacco use, recreational drug use, sleep patterns and disorders, and immunizations.

Cushing reflex The combination of a slowing pulse, rising blood pressure, and an erratic respiratory pattern; a grave sign for patients with head trauma or cerebrovascular accident.

cyanosis A blue-gray skin color that is caused by inadequate levels of oxygen in the blood.

delirium An acute confusional state characterized by global impairment of thinking, perception, judgment, and memory.

dementia The gradual and pervasive deterioration or loss of cognitive cortical functions.

diaphoresis Excessive sweating; it is often associated with shock.

diastolic pressure The result of residual pressure in the circulatory system while the left ventricle is relaxing (ie, in diastole).

differential diagnosis The process of weighing the probability of one disease versus other diseases by comparing clinical findings that could account for a patient's illness; also refers to the list of possible conditions considered based on the patient's signs and symptoms.

diplopia Double vision.

ecchymosis Localized bruising or collection of blood within or under the skin.

egophony A test of decreased breath sounds performed by placing the diaphragm of the stethoscope over the area in question while the patient saying a drawn-out "ee;" an "A" sound indicates lung consolidation.

field impression A field conclusion of the patient's problem based on the clinical presentation and the exclusion of other possible causes through considering the differential diagnoses.

focused exam A type of physical exam that is typically performed on responsive patients who have sustained an isolated injury. This type of exam is based on the chief complaint and focuses on one body system or part.

full-body exam A systematic head-to-toe exam performed during the secondary assessment of a patient who has sustained a significant mechanism of injury, is unresponsive, or is in critical condition.

general impression The overall initial impression that determines the priority of patient care; based on the patient's surroundings, the mechanism of injury, signs and symptoms, and the chief complaint.

Glasgow Coma Scale (GCS) An evaluation tool used to determine level of consciousness by evaluating and assigning point values (scores) for eye opening, verbal response, and motor response, which are then totaled; effective in helping predict patient outcomes.

guarding Contraction of the abdominal muscles indicating peritoneal irritation.

heave The perception that the heart is beating very strongly; felt upon palpation of the chest wall, this finding suggests hypertrophy; also called a lift.

history of the present illness A narrative detail of the symptoms that a patient is experiencing, usually obtained using the OPQRST mnemonic.

iatrogenic Related to a side effect or complication of medications or other medical treatment.

inspection Looking at the patient, either in general or at a specific area (ie, a patient's overall appearance from the doorway, versus looking specifically at the chest wall for abnormalities/deformities).

jugular venous distention (JVD) The visible bulging of the jugular veins when a patient is in semi-Fowler or full Fowler position; indicates inadequate blood movement through the heart and/or lungs.

Korotkoff sounds Sounds related to blood pressure measurement that are heard by stethoscope.

kyphosis Outward curve of the thoracic spine.

lesions Localized areas of the skin that do not resemble the area surrounding it.

lift A sensation felt upon palpation of the chest wall, in which the heart beats extremely strongly; suggests hypertrophy; also called a heave.

lordosis Inward curve of the lumbar spine just above the buttocks. An exaggerated form results in the condition known as swayback.

mechanism of injury (MOI) The series of events that result in traumatic injuries; the forces that act on the body to cause injury.

mottling A blotchy pattern on the skin; a typical finding in states of severe protracted hypoperfusion and shock.

murmur An abnormal *whooshing* sound heard over the heart that indicates turbulent blood flow around a cardiac valve.

nature of illness (NOI) The general type of illness a patient is apparently experiencing.

Prep Kit *(continued)*

ophthalmoscope An instrument used to examine a patient's eyes and view the retina and aqueous fluid; consists of a concave mirror and a battery-powered light that is usually contained in the handle.

orthostatic vital signs Multiple sets of vital signs taken from the patient in different positions. (for example, in the supine and sitting or standing positions) to determine the degree of hypovolemia; also called a tilt test.

otoscope An instrument used to examine the ears of a patient; consists of a head and a handle. The head contains an electric light source and a low-power magnifying lens.

pallor Paleness.

palpation Physical touching for the purpose of obtaining information (for example, to detect tenderness).

paresthesias Tingling feeling or sensory change.

past medical history Information obtained during the history-taking process, such as the patient's general state of health, childhood and adult diseases, surgeries and hospitalizations, psychiatric and mental illnesses, or traumatic injuries, which may relate to the patient's current condition.

pathologic fracture A fracture that occurs when normal forces are applied to abnormal bone structures.

patient history Information about the patient's chief complaint, present symptoms, and previous illnesses.

percussion Gently striking the surface of the body, typically overlying various body cavities, to detect changes in the densities of the underlying structures.

perfusion The circulation of oxygenated blood through the body tissues and vessels.

pertinent negatives The absence of certain signs and symptoms normally expected of specific illnesses or conditions; these findings warrant no medical care or intervention, but demonstrate the thoroughness of the patient exam and history.

pleural friction rubs Squeaking or grating sounds that occur when the pleural linings rub together, which may be heard on inspiration, expiration, or both; commonly caused by inflammation of the pleura.

primary survey The part of the assessment process that focuses on identifying immediate or potential life-threatening conditions so you can initiate lifesaving care.

primitive reflexes Reflex reactions such as Babinski, grasping, and sucking signs normally found in infants.

pronator drift The drifting of one arm downward toward a patient's feet while he or she holds out his or her arms, palm side up, with his or her eyes shut; can be a sign of a stroke.

proprioception The perception of the position and movement of the body or limbs.

pulse The wave of pressure created as the heart contracts and forces blood out the left ventricle and into the major arteries; palpated at a point where an artery passes close to a bone.

pulse oximetry An assessment tool used to measure oxygen saturation of hemoglobin in the capillary beds.

rapid full-body scan A 60- to 90-second nonsystematic review and palpation of the patient's body to identify injuries that must be managed or protected immediately; also called the rapid full-body sweep.

reassessment The portion of the assessment process in which a patient's condition is reevaluated and responses to treatment is assessed.

reflexes Involuntary motor responses to specific sensory stimuli, such as a tap on the knee or stroking the eyelash.

rhonchi Coarse, low-pitched breath sounds heard in patients with chronic mucus in the upper airways.

rigidity A clinically important sign characterized by marked peritoneal irritation and guarding, indicating an injury or illness for which urgent surgical intervention may be required.

rubor Redness; one of the classic signs of inflammation.

scene size-up A step in the patient assessment process involving a quick assessment of the scene and its surroundings to gather information about the overall safety and stability of the scene and the mechanism of injury or nature of illness. This process is carried out before you enter and begin patient care.

scoliosis Sideways curvature of the spine.

secondary assessment The process by which more detailed, quantifiable, objective information is obtained from the patient about his or her overall state of health.

signs Objective observations that can be seen, heard, felt, smelled, or measured.

social history A subsection of the patient history that provides valuable information regarding the patient's overall health status and helps to identify risk factors for various disease processes; includes items such as tobacco use, alcohol and drug use, sexual behavior, diet, travel history, living environment, and occupation.

sphygmomanometer A blood pressure cuff.

splitting In the context of heart sounds, a situation in which events on the right side of heart occur slightly later than those on the left side, and create two discernible sounds rather than one heart sound.

Prep Kit *(continued)*

stridor A harsh, high-pitched respiratory sound produced as air moves past an obstruction within or immediately above the glottic opening; associated with severe upper airway obstruction.

symptoms Subjective information the patient feels, such as pain, discomfort, or other abnormality.

systolic pressure Blood pressure created by the left ventricle as it contracts (that is, in systole).

tenting A condition in which the skin slowly retracts after being pinched and pulled away slightly from the body; a sign of dehydration.

thrill A humming vibration that can be palpated through the chest wall, suggesting an underlying bruit or murmur.

traumatic fracture A fracture that occurs when abnormal forces are applied to normal bone structures.

turgor Loss of skin elasticity.

vasoconstriction Narrowing of the diameter of a blood vessel.

vasodilation Widening of the diameter of a blood vessel.

vesicular sounds Normal breath sounds made by air moving in and out of the alveoli.

visual acuity Determined by the ability or inability to see, and by how far.

wheezing A high-pitched whistling sound that may be heard on inspiration, expiration, or both, indicating air movement through a constricted lower airway, as in asthma.

whispered pectoriloquy A test of decreased breath sounds performed by placing the diaphragm of the stethoscope over the area in question as the patient whispers "ninety-nine;" a loud, clear sound indicates lung consolidation.

working diagnosis The one diagnosis from a differential list used to base the patient's treatment plan.

▶ References

1. Emergency Medical Services Workers Injury and Illness Data. Centers for Disease Control and Prevention. The National Institute for Occupational Safety and Health (NIOSH). http://www.cdc.gov/niosh/topics/ems/data2013.html. Accessed June 14, 2016.
2. Reichard AA, Marsh SM, Moore PH: Fatal and nonfatal injuries among emergency medical technicians and paramedics. *Prehosp Emerg Care*. 2011 Oct-Dec;15(4):511-7.
3. Centers for Disease Control and Prevention. Guideline for Hand Hygiene in Health-Care Settings: Recommendations of the Healthcare Infection Control Practices Advisory Committee and the HICPAC/SHEA/APIC/IDSA Hand Hygiene Task Force. *MMWR*. 2002;51(No. RR-16).
4. Terrorism Response Tactics: Active Shooter Level II: Participant Guide. Texas State University. Advanced Law Enforcement Rapid Response Training. www.ALERRT.com. Accessed December 6, 2016.
5. Fleming S, Gill P, Jones C, et al. The diagnostic value of capillary refill time for detecting serious illness in children: a systematic review and meta-analysis. Huy NT, ed. *PLoS OneE*. 2015;10(9):e0138155.
6. Kragh JK, Littrel ML, Jones JA, et al. Battle casualty survival with emergency tourniquet use to stop limb bleeding. *J Emerg Med*. 2011 Dec; 41(6):590-597.
7. Beekley AC, Sebesta JA, Blackbourne LH, et al.: Prehospital tourniquet use in operation iraqi freedom: effect on hemorrhage control and outcomes. *J Trauma*. 2008 Feb;64(2 Suppl):S28-37.
8. The National Academies of Sciences, Engineering, and Medicine. https://www.nationalacademies.org/hmd/About-HMD.aspx. Accessed August 23, 2016.
9. Institute of Medicine Committee on Quality of Health Care in America. Crossing the Quality Chasm: A New Health System for the 21st Century. March 2001. Copyright © 2000 by the National Academy of Sciences. http://www.nationalacademies.org/hmd/~/media/Files/Report%20Files/2001/Crossing-the-Quality-Chasm/Quality%20Chasm%202001%20%20report%20brief.pdf. Accessed August 31, 2016.
10. Traffic Safety Facts, 2014. US Department of Transportation, National Highway Traffic Safety Administration, Washington, DC. http://www-nrd.nhtsa.dot.gov/Pubs/812231.pdf. Accessed June 22, 2016.
11. Krebs EE, Carey TS, Weinberger M. Accuracy of the pain numeric rating scale as a screening test in primary Care. *J Gen Intern Med*. 2007 Oct;22(10):1453-1458. Published online 2007 Aug. 1. http://www.ncbi.nlm.nih.gov/pmc/articles/PMC2305860/. Accessed August 18, 2016.
12. Lord B. The Assessment of Pain in Paramedic Practice. May 1, 2016. http://www.emsworld.com/article/12187476/the-assessment-of-pain-in-paramedic-practice. Accessed August 18, 2016.
13. Guidelines for Field Triage of Injured Patients: Recommendations of the National Expert Panel on Field Triage, 2011, Centers for Disease Control and Prevention. www.cdc.gov/mmwr/preview/mmwrhtml/rr6101a1.htm.
14. Lam BL, Thompson HS, Corbett JJ. The prevalence of simple anisocoria. *American Journal of Opthalmology*. Elsevier, Inc. July 1987;104(1):69-73. http://www.ajo.com/article/0002-9394(87)90296-0/fulltext. Accessed July 31, 2016.

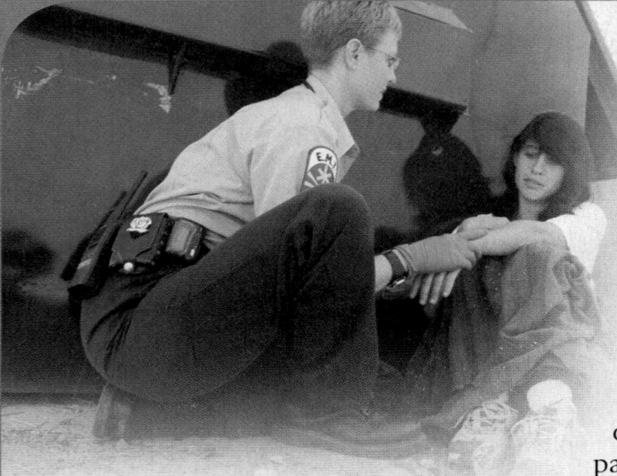

Assessment in Action

You and your partner are on scene with a patient who is having chest pain. You've already completed your primary survey and have administered high-flow oxygen to the patient, delivered by a nonrebreathing mask. You introduce yourself and ask the patient to rate his pain. He says it's a 10 on a scale of 0 to 10, and he describes it as a squeezing sensation. The patient has no prior history of cardiac problems.

1. Which will yield the most helpful information for developing a differential diagnosis?

A. Capnography reading
B. Vital signs
C. Cardiac monitor
D. History and physical exam

2. As part of your secondary assessment of this patient, you should obtain:

A. a blood glucose test.
B. a 12-lead ECG.
C. the Cincinnati Prehospital Stroke Scale.
D. a complete assessment of bowel sounds.

3. Given the patient's history, which finding on his 12-lead ECG would be unexpected?

A. A pacemaker rhythm
B. Sinus bradycardia
C. Sinus tachycardia
D. ST segment elevation

4. When listening to this patient's lung sounds, which finding would be the most likely if he is having an AMI?

A. Clear in all lung fields
B. Rales or crackles at the bases
C. A pleural rub
D. Rhonchi in all lung fields

5. Arriving at the presumptive field diagnosis of a "rule out AMI" will help you determine:

A. transport to the closest hospital.
B. transport to a hospital with percutaneous coronary intervention (PCI) capability.
C. administer a liter of normal saline.
D. discontinue oxygen administration.

6. This patient is likely to be transported to a cardiac hospital. The diagnosis of MI can involve blood tests to identify elevation of cardiac biomarker readings. How long can it take for this elevation to develop after an AMI?

A. Seconds
B. Minutes
C. Hours
D. Days

7. When taking this patient's history, what is the best way to phrase questions about pain?

A. Use open-ended questions.
B. Begin with yes or no questions.
C. Pose indirect questions.
D. Focus on location, not severity or quality.

8. How should you address this patient, and why?

9. What is a differential diagnosis?

10. Which of the five elements of critical thinking have you and your partner demonstrated so far in this situation?

CHAPTER 12

Critical Thinking and Clinical Decision Making

National EMS Education Standard Competencies

Assessment

Integrate scene and patient assessment findings with knowledge of epidemiology and pathophysiology to form a field impression. This includes developing a list of differential diagnoses through clinical reasoning to modify the assessment and formulate a treatment plan.

Knowledge Objectives

1. Describe the four cornerstones of effective paramedic practice. (pp 603-606)
2. Explain the benefits and drawbacks of patient protocols or standing orders and patient care algorithms in the emergency medical services (EMS) system. (p 605)
3. Explain how to distinguish patients with critical life threats from those in serious condition and those with minimal, non–life-threatening injuries. (pp 606-607)
4. Describe the five stages of critical thinking and thought processing in the prehospital setting. (pp 607-611)
5. Describe the *Six Rs of clinical decision making.* (pp 611-614)

Skills Objectives

There are no skills objectives for this chapter.

Introduction

The most fundamental description of what a paramedic does on a day-to-day basis is as follows: identify problems, set patient care priorities, develop a treatment plan, and, finally, execute that plan. While these steps are crucial, **cookbook medicine**—the practice of blindly following steps without thinking about what you are doing or whether it is working—is not an effective way to practice paramedicine. Effective paramedicine requires you to be a "thinking cook" because many patients present atypically when compared with classic textbook descriptions. To further complicate matters, the prehospital environment is dynamic; you must always maintain situational awareness because the stability of the scene can deteriorate without warning **Figure 12-1**. Some paramedics who have worked in hospital emergency departments (EDs) say that working in the ED is less chaotic than working in the streets. Most EDs are generally well lit, located in well-known areas, and are generally safe places for health care professionals to work. That is not always the case when working in the field or in patients' homes! Still, as a paramedic working in the prehospital setting, you are expected to provide quality patient care.

This chapter is divided into two parts: first, an explanation of critical thinking, followed by a practical discussion about how you can apply critical thinking skills in the streets. To become a master at critical thinking and clinical decision making, you need to know the cornerstones of the thinking processes and the terms that describe them.

Cornerstones of Effective Paramedic Practice

Gathering, Evaluating, and Synthesizing Information

The first cornerstone of your paramedic practice involves gathering, evaluating, and synthesizing (processing) information. Every day, call by call, you will find yourself challenged as you try to obtain information from patients of different age groups and educational backgrounds, with varying abilities to communicate. At times, alcohol, drugs, language barriers, or hearing impairments will impair a patient's ability to respond to your questions, further complicating the patient assessment process.

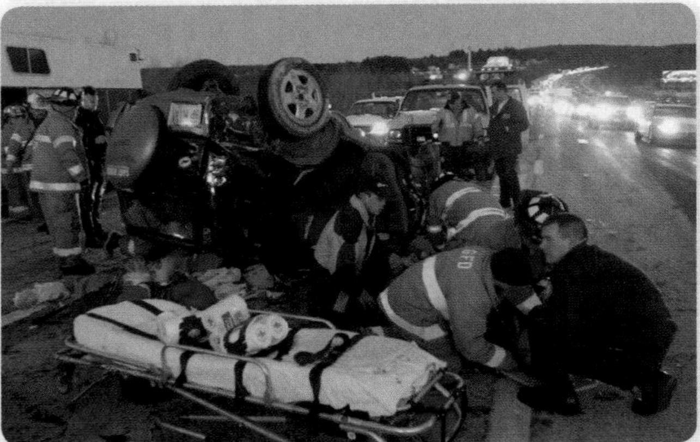

Figure 12-1 Your work as a paramedic is rarely done in a quiet, stress-free setting. Learn the skill of making decisions in a chaotic environment.

After you have gathered the information, you must assess and evaluate it to formulate a treatment plan. You must check the validity of the information—often relying on your own judgment and communication skills. For example, you may encounter a patient with a minor sprained ankle who asks you for morphine for pain. You may initially think this person is seeking an illicit drug. Another consideration, however, is that your patient may be a health care professional or is knowledgeable about medications and has a low tolerance for pain. Because morphine is not typically a first-line drug for a sprained ankle, you may need to explain to your patient why the drug cannot be administered. As a thinking paramedic, you must be as objective as possible in the decision-making process.

After you have evaluated the information you obtained from the scene, the patient, or a bystander, and determined which information is valid or invalid, you need to synthesize this information.

Words of Wisdom

Your professional ethics demand that you consider all the possibilities when communicating with a patient. No one calls emergency medical services (EMS) to be judged! Focus on how you can best meet your patient's needs.

For example, consider the following patient, a 64-year-old man having chest pain. He has had type 1 diabetes mellitus since childhood, started smoking in high school, and has had chronic obstructive pulmonary disease (COPD) since his 50s. Synthesis requires that you consider how each element interacts with the others, and ultimately how they impact your patient's current condition Figure 12-2.

Words of Wisdom

After you have established a differential diagnosis, your treatment plan will be determined by the patient care protocols or standing orders in the EMS system where you work.

In this scenario, the patient has diabetes. A comorbidity like diabetes is directly related to circulatory complications. A **comorbidity** is when the patient has two or more chronic diseases or conditions. Diabetes often leads to the development of vascular disease. In addition, in the context of shock, a high blood glucose level can make progressively thickening blood stickier, further worsening the situation. Also, whereas an extremely low blood glucose level may kill someone or result in brain damage quickly, a chronic, higher-than-normal blood glucose level takes its toll on every organ and body system. Think about how many people with long-term diabetes you encounter with vision impairment or amputated fingers or toes. The patient's other comorbidity, COPD, is a disease of poor gas exchange that frequently results in a combination of hypoxia and hypercapnia. You must consider the patient's comorbidities while you assess his new symptom, the onset of chest pain. It is likely that coronary artery disease has caused one or more of the vessels of the heart muscle to become blocked, in turn causing this part of the heart to begin to necrose, or die. If you take all the information you have gathered and synthesize it, then your conclusion would sound something like this: "I have a patient with diseases of both circulation and gas exchange. There is a possibility that part of the patient's heart is dying because blood vessels are unable to deliver oxygenated blood to a portion of the heart muscle."

You must treat the combined effect of your patient's disease processes to prevent the unperfused section of the

YOU are the Paramedic PART 1

At 1102 hours, you and your partner are dispatched to Winner's Cheerleading Gym for a 15-year-old girl who injured her shoulder during cheerleading practice. On arrival, you ascend to the third floor and see a girl surrounded by people. A coaching staff member is holding the girl's left arm. A second staff member tells you the patient was practicing a pyramid maneuver and was not caught upon dismount. The patient fell approximately 8 feet (2 m) onto a spring floor with her arms outstretched.

1. Summarize your general impression of this emergency call and what factors may be involved.
2. What is included in your primary survey and initial management steps for this patient?

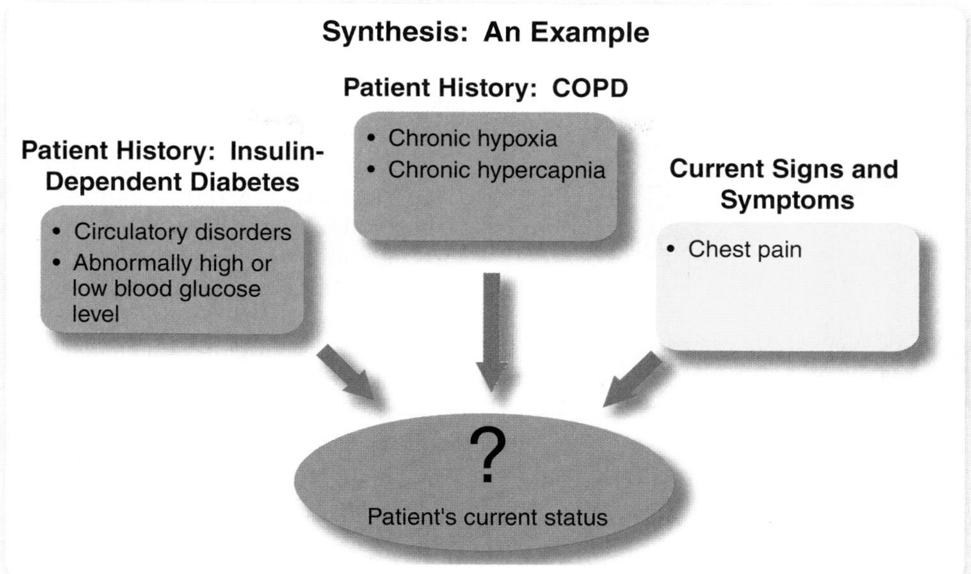

Figure 12-2 When you synthesize the patient information you have gathered, assess the relative importance of the patient's medical history (blue boxes) and his or her current signs and symptoms (yellow box). These factors usually affect each other.

heart from dying, which may cause the death of your patient. This is the synthesis part—taking individual conditions and mentally gluing them together to determine their potential for having a life-threatening impact. In the scenario described above, you should consider the working diagnosis of acute coronary syndrome, a potentially life-threatening condition.

▶ Developing and Implementing a Treatment Plan

The second cornerstone of your paramedic practice is your ability to develop and implement a treatment plan. This step is much simpler than analyzing the validity of the information you have gathered. After you have determined the patient's primary problem by identifying the chief complaint and establishing your working diagnosis, your treatment plan is defined and guided by the patient care protocols or standing orders in the EMS system where you work. Remember that your differential diagnosis is the list of possible diagnoses based on the patient's assessment findings. The working diagnosis is the one diagnosis from that differential list on which you are basing your treatment plan. As discussed in Chapter 1, *EMS Systems*, protocols or standing orders define the essential clinical standard of care for patients with certain injuries, illnesses, or behavioral conditions. They further specify performance parameters (ie, what therapies or interventions you can or cannot do without contacting medical control) as well as when you need to contact medical control before providing additional care. Collectively, protocols promote both a standard approach and a standard of quality care as defined by regional, state, or national standards. Protocols also provide parameters for medical control so they do not order treatment with medications beyond your level of training or what is usually carried on your unit.

Unfortunately, protocols, standing orders, and patient care algorithms only address the classic textbook list of patient care presentations. As a rule, they do not address vague patient complaints that do not fit into a neat clinical description—nor do they address patients with multiple disease etiologies (remember synthesis?). Those patients will require multiple treatment modalities as part of the treatment plan.

Therefore, your next step is to decide what to do to best meet your patient's needs.

Patient Safety

Several studies have examined clinical decision making by EMS personnel and have looked at how paramedics determine medical necessity for transport, appropriate cancellation of ALS calls, effectiveness of paramedic scope of practice, and other clinical issues. Collectively, the results of such studies suggest that perhaps EMS providers are being asked to make decisions that they are not trained to make. Furthermore, as procedures and tasks have been added to the paramedic scope of practice, a sort of "scope creep" (uncontrolled change) may result in decisions that could harm the patient. Although this observation points to an increased potential for error due to increasing demands on EMS providers' skills and decision making, no concrete recommendations have been proposed. Nevertheless, it would seem likely that additional training in complex decision making; low-frequency, high-risk skills; and advanced equipment will be needed, as well as additional real-time support from medical control physicians.

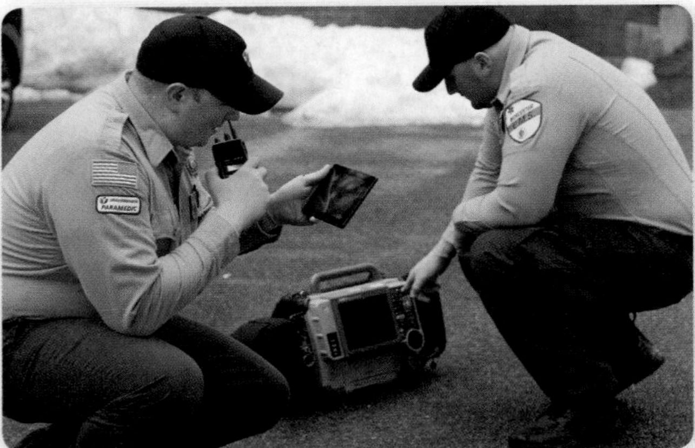

Figure 12-3 Every call has its own unique circumstances and challenges. Much of your patient care relies on the use of careful, open-minded decision making.

▶ Using Judgment and Independent Decision Making

The third cornerstone of your paramedic practice is the use of judgment and independent decision making **Figure 12-3**. For example, you have been called to a factory where a machinist has been injured on the job and has a serious gash to the upper part of his leg. You see a substantial amount of blood gushing from the area of his femoral artery with every contraction of his heart. In such a situation, it is in the patient's best interest to delay any contact with medical control until the bleeding is controlled and you are en route. You must take lifesaving action or this patient may die. Even under the best circumstances, your patient may have died well before you completed a call with medical control. To save the patient, you immediately recognize the severed artery as an immediate life threat and apply continuous direct pressure, and, ideally, a tourniquet or hemostatic dressing to ensure bleeding control.

Consider another scenario in which you have a patient who is in cardiac arrest on her front porch. In such a situation, you would immediately perform high-quality cardiopulmonary resuscitation on scene, including defibrillation if indicated. Then, once en route, you would provide advanced life support (ALS) care (ie, obtaining intravenous or intraosseous access, administering vasopressors, and inserting an advanced airway). Imagine that same patient were instead located in a third-story attic apartment with a small, treacherous exterior stairway as your only access point. Because of the physical environment, you realize it is impossible to quickly and efficiently remove the patient from the apartment for transport to the receiving facility. As such, you have a decision to make. Either you terminate resuscitation at the scene, or you resuscitate and stabilize the patient before transport. As circumstances change, so may your treatment plan. However, necessary treatment changes will only happen if you are using your critical thinking and decision-making skills to the best of your abilities.

▶ Thinking and Working Under Pressure

The fourth and final cornerstone of your paramedic practice is your ability to think and work under pressure. Imagine ringing the doorbell at the address to which you have been dispatched and a hysterical mother opens the door. She hands you a cyanotic, apneic 14-month-old child who has been submerged in the bathtub. Critical thinking tells you the child must start breathing within the next few seconds or cardiac arrest will occur, further decreasing the likelihood of saving the child's life. Only a combination of knowledge coupled with excellent clinical skills will allow you to avert a patient care disaster: the death of the child. You must be able to work under extreme pressure and be able to think, analyze the situation, and perform quickly and effectively.

The Range of Patient Conditions

One of the key elements of your paramedic practice is to be able to quickly determine if your patient is sick or not sick. For patients who are sick, you must be able to quantify how sick they are, which in turn allows you to make the best choices as to the care you provide at the scene and the care you provide in the ambulance while en route. This process becomes more complicated when you have multiple sick or injured patients.

Special Populations

It can be difficult to recognize whether an infant or child is sick or not sick because these patients tend to be "low frequency yet high acuity." That is to say, paramedics do not go on many calls for children, but when they do, these tend to be serious calls. To improve your ability, consider taking continuing education courses and reading research articles on the topic of pediatrics.

Clear thinking in a chaotic emergency starts with triage, a process of sorting your patients into four categories based on the severity of their injuries **Figure 12-4**. Patients in critical condition need immediate care and transport to survive (red tags). Patients in unstable condition are a second priority; their care and transport can be temporarily delayed by a few minutes to possibly the next half hour, or else they become critical patients (yellow tags). The two groups of patients who are left are those with nonsurvivable injuries or the obviously dead (black tags, also called Priority Zero), and those often termed the walking wounded or minimally injured (green tags). For the sake of discussion, the walking wounded will be referred to as non-life threats. The triage process

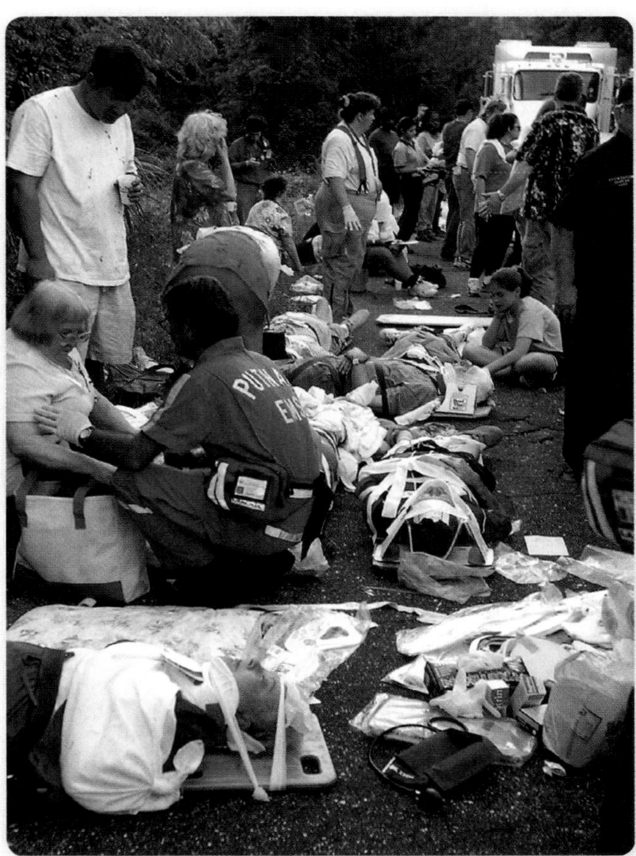

Figure 12-4 With multiple patients, you must quickly assess and prioritize the urgency of each patient's condition.

is discussed further in Chapter 47, *Incident Management and Mass-Casualty Incidents*.

Examples of patients with life *threats* would include those with the following injuries or illnesses:

- Major multisystem trauma
- Devastating single-system trauma
- End-stage disease presentations
- Acute presentations of chronic conditions

Examples of patients in unstable condition would include those with the following injuries or illnesses:

- Serious multisystem trauma
- Acute presentations of "first-time" medical events
- Multiple disease etiologies

Examples of patients who have minimal, non–life-threatening injuries would include those with the following injuries or illnesses:

- Simple abrasions
- Partial-thickness burns of an extremity of less than 5% body surface area
- Small lacerations with only capillary bleeding

Critical Thinking and Clinical Decision Making

It is important for you to understand the processes of thinking and decision making. By having a better understanding of how your thoughts are formed and processed, you can learn to think more effectively.

YOU are the Paramedic PART 2

As you talk with the staff member, he tells you he saw the patient fall, and reports that only her arm seems injured. He did not witness any trauma to the head or neck. You examine the patient and find that her left arm has an angular deformity in the region of the humerus. You observe abnormal motion every time she tries to move the arm, and she is unable to move it without "really bad" pain. The patient rates her level of pain as 9 on the 1 to 10 scale, but denies having any head, neck, or back pain. You obtain her vital signs while a staff member continues holding her arm. The patient's parents are not on scene, but the staff member tells you they are being contacted. Although the patient is visibly shaken, she is not crying and is answering questions appropriately.

Recording Time: 0 Minutes	
Appearance	Visibly upset, obvious deformity to the arm
Level of consciousness	Alert and oriented
Airway	Open and patent
Breathing	Normal, 22 breaths/min
Circulation	Radial pulse, tachycardic

3. Have you gathered enough data to turn your field impression into a treatment plan?
4. Should you administer pain medication?

▶ Concept Formation

The first stage of the thought process in prehospital care is that of gathering information—things you see, hear, smell, or feel and that which you gather from your diagnostic tools. This process is called **concept formation**.

Concept formation starts as you arrive at the scene, become situationally aware, and evaluate the scene to ensure the safety of yourself, your crew, and your patient. In the patient assessment process, this step is known as the scene size-up. Determine the mechanism of injury (MOI) for trauma, or in the case of medical calls, the nature of the present illness (NOI). How does your patient present? Does the patient appear uncomfortable, frightened, or deathly ill? Assess the patient's level of consciousness (LOC), in part to determine whether the patient can provide you with reliable information to act on. This initial evaluation of his or her LOC will also establish a baseline to refer to later as the call progresses and the patient's condition changes.

You move further into the information-gathering process as you perform your primary survey, focusing on the identification and correction of any immediate threats to your patient's life relative to the ABCDEs (Airway, Breathing, Circulation, Disability, and Exposure). You continue on as you perform the secondary assessment and physical exam and identify the patient's chief complaint. By obtaining a SAMPLE (Signs and symptoms; Allergies; Medications; Pertinent past medical history; Last oral intake; Events leading up to the illness or injury) history, you will be able to gather important information from the patient, including any medications the patient is taking (prescription, over-the-counter, illicit, or possibly herbal).

Words of Wisdom

As part of your situational awareness, observe family members for clues. Do they seem worried or nervous? Does calling 9-1-1 seem routine for them? Are they huddled in a corner crying or are they trying to watch television during your assessment? Be alert for situations that are not what they seem to be.

One of the most important observations you need to judge is your patient's **affect**, or emotional state reflected in physical behavior **Figure 12-5**. The affect might not tally with what the patient tells you. For example, you may treat a patient who presents with manic behavior that can be associated with amphetamine abuse, yet the patient denies any drug use. You might even see drug paraphernalia. You must assess the accuracy of the information you are receiving if it does not match what you are seeing and hearing.

Last, you need to obtain the patient's vital signs and relevant clinical test results by using your primary diagnostic tools (for example, a glucometer, pulse oximeter, capnometer, electrocardiogram (ECG) monitor, blood pressure cuff, and stethoscope).

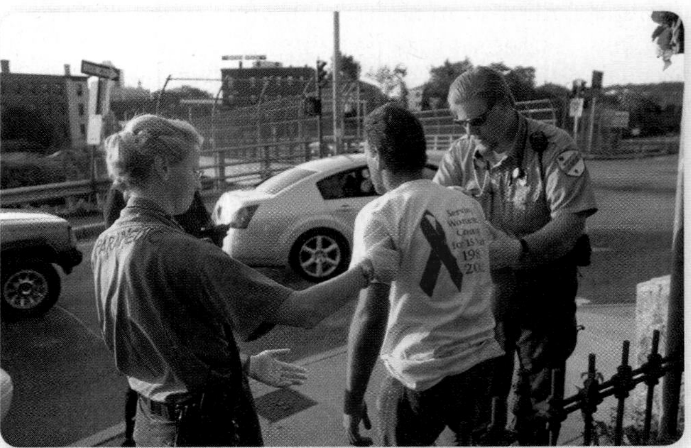

Figure 12-5 Take in clues not only from your patient's affect, but also from his or her surroundings. Assess the entire environment to make sure you fully understand its impact on your patient's condition.

▶ Data Interpretation

During the second stage of the critical thinking process, you must evaluate all the information you have gathered and form a conclusion, which is called **data interpretation**. You need a solid background in anatomy, physiology, and pathophysiology to understand how the body works and how it responds when complications arise. Another key element is your level of education and experience. If you have come to the paramedic program with considerable experience as an emergency medical technician (EMT), then you will have an excellent platform to build on. However, even without that background, applying yourself in your studies will help you to meet the challenges of working in EMS.

How you think and form conclusions is affected not only by the attitudes of your patients, but also by your attitude as a health care provider. This means, for example, you should never consider a call a waste of your time or talent. Furthermore, unprofessional comments such as, "I can't believe you called us for *this*!" show a lack of compassion and interest in providing quality patient care. Having a negative attitude about any patient or patient care situation will almost guarantee that the care you provide will be suboptimal. To maintain the standards of care set by your profession, you must provide the best care you can for every patient you encounter.

▶ Application of Principle

The third stage of the critical thinking process comes when your field impression becomes your working diagnosis. The key word here is *working*. The working diagnosis is what you tentatively believe to be the problem and the focus of your treatment. It is important to note that your working diagnosis may not simply be narrowed down to just one problem. It could be a number of conditions from your differential diagnosis and the conditions for which you are treating the patient.

From this point on, your treatment plan is driven by the patient care protocols, or standing orders, in the system where you work.

▶ Reflection in Action

In the fourth stage of the critical thinking process, you are actively treating your patient while monitoring the effects of your interventions. Think of *reflection in action* as simply *thinking while doing*.

For example, if your patient is having considerable difficulty breathing (Spo_2 level less than 94% combined with obvious signs of hypoxia), then you would apply a nonrebreathing mask with oxygen flowing at 15 L/min. After a few minutes you would ask the patient, "Is it getting any easier for you to breathe?" If the situation does not improve, then additional interventions (ie, a drug or more aggressive ventilation) may be appropriate. It is important to periodically check your interventions to see whether they are making the patient feel better. If you ask your patient how your treatment is working, then you will also be reassuring your patient that you are concerned and on top of the situation **Figure 12-6**. Reassessment is an important part of your patient care.

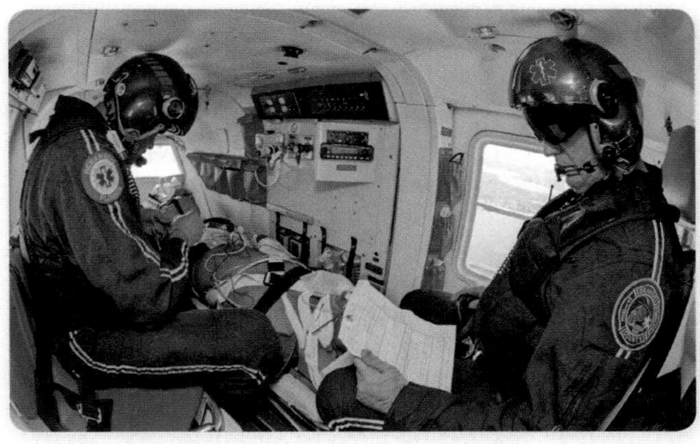

Figure 12-6 A patient's condition can change rapidly—especially when he or she is critically ill or injured. Continually monitor any changes to a patient's condition.

Documentation & Communication

It is important to document not only what procedures are done and what medications are given, but also what effect the procedure or medication had, if any.

Consider a scenario in which a 58-year-old man has experienced chest pain while moving rocks to landscape his yard. Although he has no history of cardiac disease, he is in the right age group for you to suspect a heart condition. When you ask him if he can pinpoint where the pain seems to be, his index finger curls into a fist as he points to the location on his chest directly over his heart. His heart could still be the issue, so you continue with the same treatment plan.

Then you ask if anything makes the pain better or worse and the patient explains that if he holds his left arm still, then the pain goes away. However, with arm movement the pain is severe. This is key information, because you know that the pain associated with a heart attack is not relieved by simply sitting still and not moving. You now revise your general impression and focus your assessment on the possibility of a musculoskeletal injury, and your treatment plan and interventions change accordingly. Prior to this information, you would have immediately given the patient aspirin, nitroglycerin, and oxygen therapy to improve delivery of oxygen to a potentially infarcting heart. Instead, you might now consider providing an analgesic for pain relief for an isolated musculoskeletal injury.

One of the key elements of this stage of the critical thinking process is to avoid **tunnel vision**. Tunnel vision occurs when you focus on or consider only one aspect of a situation without first taking into account all possibilities. Keep your mind open to all the possible causes of your patient's current condition. Keep in mind that your patient might be having a heart attack that presents in a way that differs from the typical signs and symptoms, so perform an ECG and reassess constantly.

Words of Wisdom

To provide optimal patient care, avoid tunnel vision when it comes to determining the cause of a patient's condition. Do not focus only on your general impression. As you gather information, modify your treatment plan according to the patient's needs.

▶ Reflection on Action

The last stage in the critical thinking process occurs after the call is over and is commonly associated with run review, run critiques, or debriefings. This is the time when you look back at the call and reflect on how you gathered and processed information and reached the decisions that you did. One of the most difficult aspects of this stage is learning to accept that something went wrong or that better treatment choices could have been made. It is important to establish an attitude that there is always room for personal and professional improvement. A review of the run is an excellent opportunity to evaluate what might have gone wrong and how to improve your skills as a paramedic.

Patient Safety

Medical error can be defined as the failure of a planned action to be completed as intended or the use of a wrong plan to achieve an aim. Rather than deeming every medical error to be the result of a single human error, it is necessary to look deeper and see other factors that may have set the stage for failure. Medical errors can be categorized as adverse drug events, wrong-site surgeries, falls, burns, pressure ulcers, and mistaken patient identities. High error rates with serious consequences are most likely to occur in the intensive care unit, operating room, ED, and with paramedics in the field or during critical care transports.

A just culture (the beliefs, customs, and acceptable behaviors within an organization) focuses on identifying issues that lead to errors or unsafe behaviors, while still maintaining individual accountability for reckless behavior. It helps distinguish various types of errors, including human error (ie, slips), at-risk behavior (ie, taking shortcuts), and reckless behavior (ie, ignoring required safety steps). Humans are not perfect, so any human-made system should anticipate some level of error. A mistake or lapse can happen to even the best paramedics. Human error is typically a product of the system design and behavioral choices, and therefore should not be viewed as a punishable action, but rather an opportunity to think critically about, and ultimately improve, the system.

You will periodically encounter patients with atypical presentations, meaning they do not follow classic signs and symptoms. For example, you may see a patient with a neck fracture who has no pain. Even though pain is the single best predictor of a possible spine injury, it is not an absolute predictor. To make an accurate diagnosis, you must also use all that you have learned about communication with patients. For instance, your patient might come from a culture that minimizes the presence of pain.

Reflection gives you the chance to continuously improve your thinking and decision making skills. In turn, your patient care improves as you become more experienced. Be open to learning and remember that every run you go on, every class you take, and every run review you attend is another opportunity to improve your skills Figure 12-7. Personal and professional growth will not happen if you cannot admit mistakes or if you are unwilling to continue to learn. The successful completion of the paramedic course is only the starting point in your career as an ALS provider. To provide the best possible care, you must commit to a lifetime of learning. The most important trait for a successful lifetime career in EMS is a true desire to continuously improve as a paramedic.

A list of the fundamental elements that contribute to the critical thinking and clinical decision-making process follows. As you look over each item on the list, ask yourself, "Do I have this quality already, or do I need to develop it?"

YOU are the Paramedic PART 3

The staff member tells you she has tried calling the parents twice but has not reached them yet. She says she will continue to try. Because of the patient's extreme pain, you decide to call medical control regarding pain medication. You give the physician a report, including her height (5 feet [2 m]) and weight (100 lb [45 kg]), and he advises you to administer 2 mg of morphine followed by another 2-mg dose of morphine 10 minutes later. The patient agrees and you start an intravenous line and administer 2 mg of morphine.

Recording Time: 5 Minutes	
Respirations	26 breaths/min
Pulse	110 beats/min
Skin	Warm and dry
Blood pressure	110/80 mm Hg before pain medication (morphine) 2 min after morphine administration: 100/50 mm Hg
Oxygen saturation (Spo_2)	100%
Pupils	PERRLA

5. What is your working diagnosis?
6. What effects can be expected from the administration of morphine?

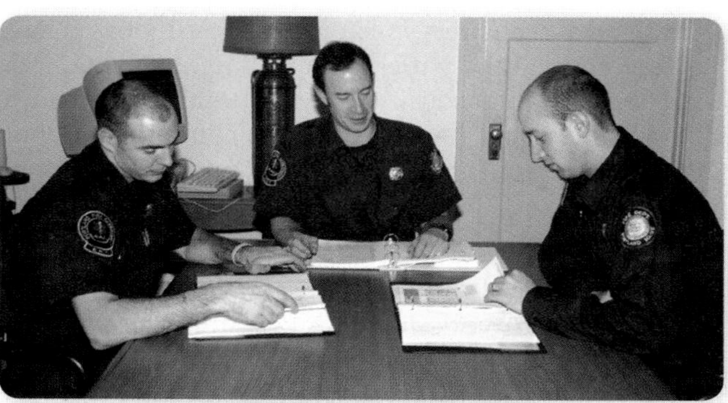

Figure 12-7 A formal review, or audit, of your performance can seem intimidating. However, it is also an opportunity for you to gain important feedback and improve as a paramedic.

- Adequate knowledge of anatomy, physiology, and pathophysiology
- Ability to gather and organize data and form concepts
- Ability to focus on specific and multiple elements of data
- Ability to identify and deal with **medical ambiguity**—the uncertainty regarding the specific cause of the patient's condition; few calls follow the scripts in your protocols to the letter.
- Skill in differentiating between relevant and irrelevant data
- Capability to analyze and compare similar situations
- Capability to analyze and compare contrary situations
- Ability to articulate your reasoning and construct arguments

From Theory to Practical Application

A number of unique factors come into play with every call. Consider the following scenario:

You are dispatched to a "car off the road" involving a single vehicle with four passengers that has spun off the slippery road into a ditch at an estimated speed of 35 miles per hour (mph). Think about how each of the following variables might change how you respond to and manage this call.

- The passengers were not wearing seat belts.
- The vehicle was traveling at 65 mph and not 35 mph.
- The vehicle flipped over and is on its roof.
- It is 20°F (–7°C) outside and the crash was not discovered for at least an hour.

As you can see from the list, changes in variables create many possible new outcomes for patients, and therefore your ability to manage the call and patient care properly also becomes more challenging.

Even if only a few of the calls you respond to on a day-to-day basis represent life-threatening emergencies, you must handle every call in the same professional manner and provide the best possible care.

Words of Wisdom

Never be fooled by patients who initially appear uninjured or healthy. Never hesitate to take a thorough history and perform a complete physical exam.

As discussed in Chapter 2, *Workforce Safety and Wellness*, you have to learn to cope with your own reactions, such as the impact of the fight-or-flight response, when you are confronted with extreme medical emergencies. This response can impair your critical thinking skills and diminish your concentration and assessment abilities. One way to counter these negative effects is to improve your mental conditioning and your skill performance. Practice your skills until you can do them instinctively (known as muscle memory) and can perform them on command in the skills lab setting. Once you reach that level of skill performance, you can quickly draw on them in a real-life setting, allowing you to better focus on patient assessment or other decision-making areas.

Facilitate better thinking under pressure by memorizing the following mental checklist for all calls:

1. Take a moment to scan the scene.
2. Take another moment to stop and think.
3. Move forward and make decisions and act on behalf of your patient.
4. Stay calm and in control, and maintain situational awareness.
5. Regularly and continually reevaluate your patient.

Taking It to the Streets

When you are out on a call, critical thinking can be summed up with the *Six Rs of clinical decision making* **Figure 12-8**.

▶ 1. Read the Scene

An emergency scene is filled with information readily available to you. This information tells a story that is only available at the scene; it becomes unavailable the moment you initiate transport to the hospital. To effectively read the scene, you must evaluate the following items: (1) the overall safety of the situation, (2) the environmental conditions, (3) the immediate surroundings, (4) any access and egress issues, and (5) the MOI or NOI **Figure 12-9**. In particular, when you are considering the MOI, take time to evaluate all aspects of the incident. For example, with a motor vehicle crash, note the length of the skid marks or whether there are none; what object the vehicle struck; how

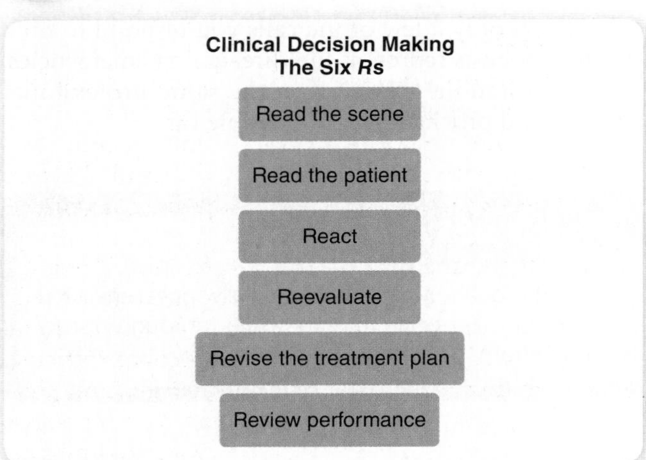

Figure 12-8 The *Six Rs of clinical decision making.*

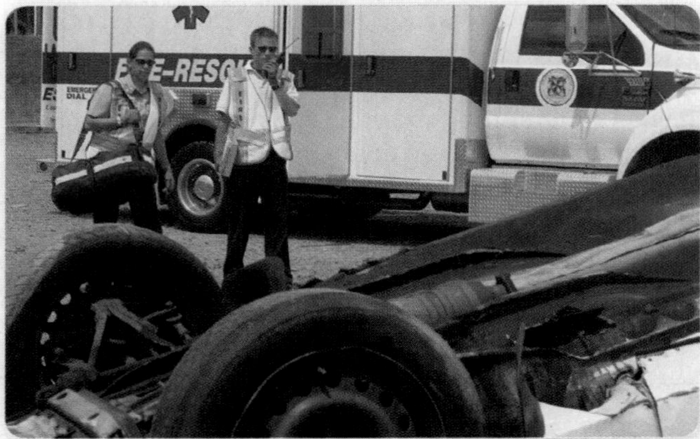

Figure 12-9 Although you need to focus on treating patients as soon as possible, always take a moment to register important information about the scene. As you learned in Chapter 11, *Patient Assessment*, an effective scene size-up will help you remain safe and provide quality patient care.

much intrusion into the passenger compartment occurred; whether seat belts were worn; and whether the headrests were properly positioned. In another example, involving a patient who fell, you would look for the height of the fall, how the patient landed, and the surface or object on which the patient landed.

Other issues to consider when you size up the scene include assessing the environment. Was it hot, cold, or wet? Also, are eyewitnesses, friends, or family members available to provide additional information?

▶ 2. Read the Patient

One of the greatest skills you can develop is learning to read a patient quickly. As you approach the patient, does the patient see you and track you with his or her eyes? Offer the patient your hand to shake (or an appropriate gesture based on his or her culture and customs), introduce yourself, and ask why 9-1-1 was called. If the patient takes your hand and answers you appropriately, then you have just determined the patient has a Glasgow Coma Scale score of 15 (spontaneous eye opening, follows commands, appropriate verbal response). Other components of an effective primary survey and history taking include the following:

- **Observe the patient.** What is the patient's LOC and level of comfort or discomfort? Skin color? Position? Work of breathing? Any obvious deformity or asymmetry?
- **Talk to the patient.** Determine the chief complaint. Is this a new condition or the worsening of a preexisting condition? Obtain the medical history and the events leading up to the illness or injury.
- **Touch the patient.** Assess the skin for color, temperature, and condition. Assess the rate, regularity, and strength of the pulse.
- **Auscultate breath sounds.** Confirm the adequacy or inadequacy of breathing and assess the patency of the airway.
- **Identify and correct any life threats** relative to the ABCDEs in the order you find them.
- **Obtain complete and accurate vital signs** Figure 12-10. For every patient, even for routine transfer patients, you must obtain a baseline set of vital signs. For patients with serious conditions, two sets of serial vital signs provide comparative data to begin to establish trends. For patients in critical condition, three or more sets of vital signs allow you to assess trends and to reassess whether the patient's condition is stabilizing, improving, or getting worse. If your patient's condition is deteriorating, then multiple sets of vital signs will track the progression.

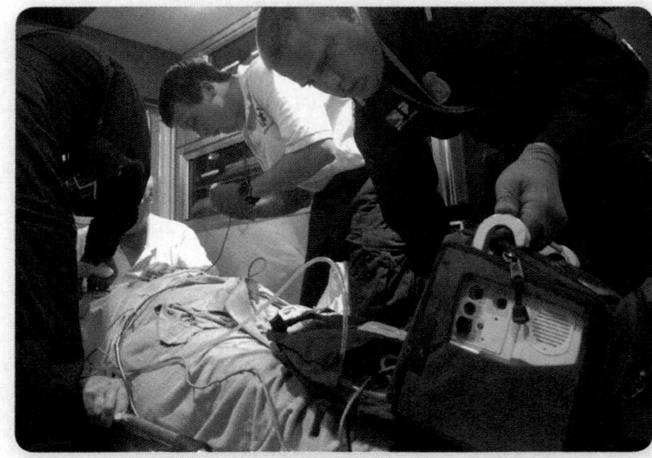

Figure 12-10 The more accurate your patient information, the more reliable your diagnosis. Take the time to obtain a set of baseline vital signs for every patient.

Patient Safety

Effective communication is vital to those participating in the aftermath of an adverse patient safety event, such as serious physical or psychological injury. Communicating effectively helps a patient care team navigate competing priorities, overcome issues related to human factors, and reduce error. A *huddle* is a communication technique and event that often takes the form of a structured, short meeting in which a patient care team comes together to talk about a patient, procedure, or situation. A huddle can also be called whenever a team needs to regroup and share concerns, discuss resource allocation, anticipate outcomes, and create contingency plans. After a serious adverse event, the team is advised to huddle and discuss the event that occurred, including the stabilization of the patient and situation; determine the facts of what happened; mitigate any ongoing harm; address staff safety concerns; secure equipment or materials; and alert others as deemed necessary by the senior staff member leading the huddle. The huddle is critical to ensure that actual events, sequences, and timing are accurately recorded to aid in further analysis and corrective actions related to the situation. It is also the only opportunity to preserve equipment in the actual state when the incident occurred—for example, a problem caused by a faulty ventilator or intravenous pump cannot be properly analyzed if the settings are changed or the equipment is returned to use.

▶ 3. React

Your first priority in patient care is to treat any life threats. Next, consider possible causes of your patient's symptoms and rule in certain conditions or rule them out as you gather more information and develop your differential diagnosis, and ultimately, a working diagnosis.

If you are unable to narrow down the differential diagnosis to a working diagnosis by the end of your assessment, then provide care based on the presenting signs and symptoms. If your patient has difficulty breathing, then administer high-flow oxygen and place the patient in a position of comfort. For signs and symptoms of shock, keep the patient warm, administer high-flow oxygen, and establish one or two large-bore IV lines en route while you continue to try to search for the cause of the condition. You will often care for patients whose conditions cannot be diagnosed until they reach the ED. In fact, some patients are admitted to a critical care unit for further tests and monitoring (for example, to R/O MI or "rule out myocardial infarction"). Many conditions cannot be treated in the field; in some cases, transport to an appropriate facility may be one of the most important aspects of the care you provide. Therefore, it is just as important to determine a treatment plan as it is to treat life threats. This plan must include rapid transport if your analysis of the patient's condition warrants it.

YOU are the Paramedic — PART 4

On reassessment, the patient feels less pain and rates it as 5 on the 1 to 10 scale. You proceed to immobilize the arm with a sling. After you and your partner place the patient onto a stretcher and move her to the ambulance, the patient's aunt arrives on the scene. You give the aunt a complete report and tell her you will be transporting her niece to the local ED for treatment. You advise the aunt that you are administering a second dose of morphine. The aunt tells you "No!" and says you should not have given pain medication to her niece.

Recording Time: 10 Minutes	
Respirations	18 breaths/min
Pulse	70 beats/min
Skin	Warm and dry
Blood pressure	100/60 mm Hg
Oxygen saturation (Spo_2)	100%
Pupils	PERRLA
ECG	Sinus without ectopy

7. How should you respond to the aunt's statement that pain medication should not have been administered?
8. Did you have the right to give the patient pain medication without a parent present?

Controversies

For many years EMS personnel have provided patients with effective prophylactic treatments even though the need for treatment has not been supported by evidence-based research. Should every trauma patient be immobilized on a backboard? Probably not. Should every unresponsive person be given naloxone? Probably not. Should EMS personnel be aggressive with fluids or limit them? Paramedicine is always evolving, so expect lifelong learning and learn to embrace change!

▶ 4. Reevaluate

As you continue to provide patient care, make certain you follow up on your interventions. Check whether the splint you applied has eased the pain in your patient's injured leg. If you are treating a patient with pain medication, then reevaluate his or her pain level to see if the medication is effective. On challenging calls, it is easy to get into "treatment mode" and focus on doing things while forgetting to follow up on whether what you are doing is actually improving the patient's condition.

As you reassess your patient, take the time to add any information you may have gathered from the secondary assessment to the primary survey. For example, you find that your patient has no breath sounds in the upper right lobe secondary to a fractured rib that caused a small pneumothorax. By itself, the small pneumothorax is not an immediate life threat to a relatively healthy person. The patient, however, also has bilateral fractured femurs, substantial blood loss, and a minor head injury. Under those circumstances, a small pneumothorax may complicate matters far more than if it were a single, isolated condition. When you care for patients, especially trauma patients with multiple injuries, it is up to you to assess the cumulative impact of all factors as you develop your treatment plan. Your goal is to ensure nothing that should be addressed in the field is overlooked.

▶ 5. Revise the Treatment Plan

As you continue to care for your patient, you may get indications that what you previously thought was a head injury is an issue secondary to glue sniffing—two very different causes. As a thinking paramedic—no matter how sure you are of the working diagnosis—you must always keep your mind open to other possibilities. As the call unfolds and additional information becomes available, be prepared to revise your treatment plan as necessary. By remaining mentally "light on your feet," you position yourself to be receptive to changing presentations or circumstances, which, in turn, helps you avoid tunnel vision.

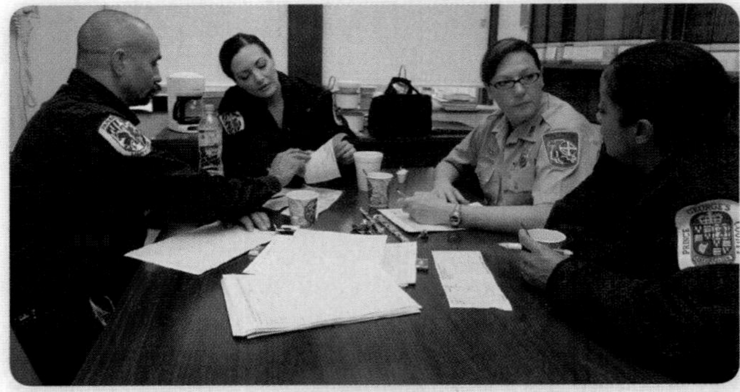

Figure 12-11 You can learn something new with every call you run. One of the best ways to review your performance—and to continually learn and improve—is to talk it over with peers.

▶ 6. Review Performance

Again, after a call is over, you have the opportunity to look back and reexamine your work Figure 12-11. Whether this review is in the formal setting of a continuous quality improvement meeting, a simple debriefing after a field code, or a conversation with your partner back at the station, taking the time to critically look at your work allows for real growth opportunities. This is particularly true when you have made a mistake. Whereas success is satisfying and certainly feels good, there is little growth opportunity to be achieved. However, when you make a mistake, you can learn how to avoid repeating the mistake and how to do better the next time. Excellence in prehospital care is the gradual result of you constantly striving to improve your performance, which requires that you *always* have an attitude that is open to learning.

Being a thinking paramedic will only happen if you choose to work on your critical thinking skills day by day, call by call, throughout your career. If you continue to improve the way you think and make decisions, then your patient care will improve as well. Your reward will be excellence in your practice—the ultimate job satisfaction.

YOU are the Paramedic SUMMARY

1. Summarize your general impression of this emergency call and what factors may be involved.

The call was for a child who injured her shoulder during cheerleading practice. On scene, you are told by a staff member that the patient fell 8 feet (2 m) onto a spring floor with her arms outstretched. You realize that you will be caring for a pediatric patient with injuries that may be severe. The process of gathering your general impression based on everything you see, hear, smell, and feel is called concept formation.

2. What is included in your primary survey and initial management steps for this patient?

You need to immediately rule out any injury to the patient's cervical spine, back, or head. Assess the patient's vital signs, including her level of consciousness and the ABCDEs (Airway, Breathing, Circulation, Disability, and Exposure). Monitor the patient's respiratory status and place the patient on oxygen if there are any signs of difficulty breathing. Also, ask the patient whether pain medication would be helpful to her prior to immobilizing her arm in a sling. Remember that parental consent must be obtained, if possible, before providing emergency treatment to a minor.

3. Have you gathered enough data to turn your field impression into a treatment plan?

You have enough information to make a treatment plan. The patient has sustained an isolated trauma to her arm. You must complete the following critical actions: immobilize the arm, make the patient comfortable, and transport the patient to a hospital for further treatment.

4. Should you administer pain medication?

You are ethically responsible for making your patient as comfortable as possible. In the absence of parental consent, you may administer medication to pediatric patients to help relieve pain, but this varies from jurisdiction to jurisdiction. Recent studies have shown, however, that prehospital providers are less likely to give pain medication to pediatric patients than to adults. If a parent or guardian is unavailable to give consent to emergency treatment, then you may undertake emergency treatment to sustain life without consent under the doctrine of implied consent. When in doubt, obtain online guidance from medical control. Know your state laws and local protocols concerning the treatment of minors.

5. What is your working diagnosis?

You have ruled out multisystem trauma and determined that the patient has an isolated extremity trauma. There is no medical condition associated with the emergency, and the patient denies having any significant medical history or medication allergies. Your treatment includes immobilization of the injury and providing the patient comfort while en route to the hospital.

6. What effects can be expected from the administration of morphine?

Morphine is a common narcotic analgesic that is carried by many emergency medical services (EMS) agencies. The effect of morphine is different for each patient. Although pain medication may not eliminate the patient's pain, it will reduce the level of pain. Some benefits to giving pain medication are a more relaxed patient, which will result in positive changes in vital signs and a decreased level of anxiety. Some patients may be allergic to pain medications; any allergies should be established prior to medication administration. Pain medications sometimes cause adverse effects, such as nausea and/or vomiting. Those effects should be anticipated and can be treated with an antiemetic medication.

7. How should you respond to the aunt's statement that pain medication should not have been administered?

Minors present special issues for the paramedic. Usually a parent is the legal decision maker for a child; a relative is not a legal decision maker unless there is documentation signed by the mother or father stating otherwise. Recognizing that the relative may have a valid concern, explain that your treatment was authorized by a physician and is standard care. Advise the aunt to contact the patient's parents to discuss her concerns. Remember to stay friendly and do not argue with the family member as that tends to unnecessarily escalate the situation.

8. Did you have the right to give the patient pain medication without a parent present?

Under certain circumstances you do have the right to treat a minor without a parent present. In this situation, you have been given the authority by medical control to treat the patient. Often, obtaining consent to treat a child may be difficult. At times, a parent or guardian of a child may not want you to treat the child for a variety of reasons. In such cases, you must respect the parent's (or guardian's) wishes and discuss the medical consequences of that decision with him or her. However, you may not withhold care from the patient when the person requesting this is not the parent or guardian. As a patient advocate, you need to be aware of the challenges associated with obtaining permission and be prepared to discuss the need for care.

YOU are the Paramedic SUMMARY *(continued)*

EMS Patient Care Report (PCR)					
Date: 04-24-18	**Incident No.:** 110435		**Nature of Call:** Child injured	**Location:** Winner's Cheerleading Gym	
Dispatched: 1102	**En Route:** 1103	**At Scene:** 1105	**Transport:** 1130	**At Hospital:** 1145	**In Service:** 1200
Patient Information					
Age: 15 **Sex:** F **Weight (in kg [lb]):** 45 kg (100 lb)			**Allergies:** None **Medications:** None **Past Medical History:** None **Chief Complaint:** Upper arm pain		
Vital Signs					
Time: 1110	**BP:** 110/80; 2 min after morphine admin, 100/50	**Pulse:** 110	**Respirations:** 26	**Spo$_2$:** 100%	
Time: 1115	**BP:** 100/60	**Pulse:** 70	**Respirations:** 18	**Spo$_2$:** 100%	
Time:	**BP:**	**Pulse:**	**Respirations:**	**Spo$_2$:**	
EMS Treatment (circle all that apply)					
Oxygen @ _______ L/min via (circle one): **NC NRM Bag-mask device**		**Assisted Ventilation**	**Airway Adjunct**	**CPR**	
Defibrillation	**Bleeding Control**	**Bandaging**	**Splinting** (circled)	**Other:**	
Narrative					

Arrived on scene to find 15-year-old girl in care of coaching staff. Staff states pt was on top of a pyramid performing a cheerleading maneuver and was not caught upon dismount. Pt states she fell about 8 feet (2 m) onto her left arm and right arm, with most of the force absorbed by the left arm. The floor at gym was on springs and was able to absorb most of the energy of the fall. Pt states she has "really bad" pain in her left upper arm. Pt denies any head, neck, or back pain. Pt denies any other injury, problem, or pain other than in her left arm. Assessment of the pt's arm reveals extreme pain with arm movement. Pt agreed to receive medication treatment for pain. Medical control at Midtown Hospital authorized 2 mg of morphine initially and another 2 mg after 10 minutes if pain is still severe. Hospital staff will be awaiting our arrival. IV line established in right AC vein with 20-gauge needle, saline well attached, and saline drip started at KVO rate. 2 mg of morphine administered at 1115 followed by 10-mL flush. Minutes later the pt stated the pain level changed from 9/10 to 5/10, and pt's arm was immobilized with a sling. Pt moved to ambulance and reassessed; vital signs taken and noted above. Pt stated pain level was still at 5 after 10 minutes. Pt was given second dose of 2 mg of morphine. Pt's aunt met us prior to leaving for hospital and expressed displeasure with EMS giving her niece morphine. EMS reassured aunt that pt treatment was authorized by medical control physician and stated that pt was feeling much better and in less pain. Pt transported without further incident. Vital signs monitored and pt's pain decreased from 5 to 4. Pt released to nurse in ED room 4 with report. IV patent and less than 200-mL infused. RN witnessed waste of 6 mg of morphine. Waste form attached to PCR.**End of report**

Prep Kit

▶ Ready for Review

- The first cornerstone of your paramedic practice is having the ability to gather, evaluate, and synthesize (process) information.
  - After you have gathered information, assess and evaluate its validity and the impact it may have on the treatment plan you are developing.
  - After you have evaluated the information you obtained from the scene, the patient, or any bystanders and determined what information is valid, then you need to synthesize that information.
- The second cornerstone of your paramedic practice is developing and implementing a treatment plan.
  - Your treatment plan is almost always defined by the patient care protocols or standing orders in the emergency medical services (EMS) system where you work.
- The third cornerstone of your paramedic practice is judgment and making independent decisions.
- The fourth and final cornerstone of your paramedic practice is your ability to think and work under pressure.
- The first stage of the thought process in prehospital care is gathering information—things you see, hear, smell, or feel or obtain with your diagnostics. This is concept formation.
  - As part of your primary survey, focus on the identification and correction of any immediate life threats relative to the ABCDEs (Airway, Breathing, Circulation, Disability, and Exposure).
- The second stage of the critical thinking process is data interpretation—evaluating the information you have gathered and forming a conclusion.
- The third stage of the critical thinking process is the application of principle—when your field impression becomes your working diagnosis.
- The fourth stage of the critical thinking process is reflection in action—actively treating your patient while monitoring the effects of your interventions.
- The last stage in the critical thinking process is reflection on action. It occurs after the call is over and is commonly associated with run reviews, run critiques, or debriefings. Look back at the total call and reflect on how you processed all the information you gathered and reached the decisions that you did.
- Use the *Six Rs of clinical decision making* to summarize what must be done on a call:
  - Read the scene.
  - Read the patient.
  - React.
  - Reevaluate.
  - Revise the treatment plan.
  - Review performance.
- Excellence in prehospital care results from a constant effort to improve your practice, which requires that you always have an attitude that is open to learning.

▶ Vital Vocabulary

affect The patient's emotional state as reflected in the patient's physical behavior.

comorbidity The existence of two or more chronic diseases or conditions in a patient.

concept formation Pattern of understanding based on initially obtained information; the first stage of the critical thinking process in prehospital care.

cookbook medicine Blindly following a protocol or algorithm without thinking about what is being done and whether or not it is working.

data interpretation The process of reaching conclusions based on comparing the patient's presentation with information from your training, education, and past experiences; the second stage of the critical thinking process in prehospital care.

medical ambiguity Vague or unclear aspects of medicine.

tunnel vision Focusing on or considering only one aspect of a situation without first taking into account all possibilities.

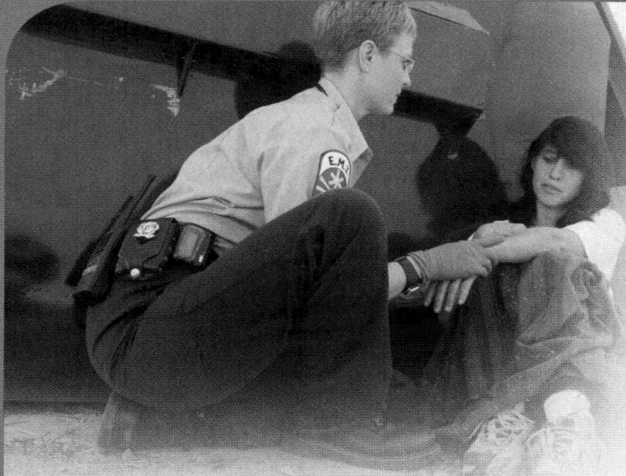

Assessment in Action

You are dispatched to a domestic dispute between brothers. The police are on the scene and state that two patients were involved in a street brawl. You arrive on the scene and find a 16-year-old boy with a swollen, bruised eye with a laceration (bleeding is controlled) and a 7-year-old boy with a bruise to his right arm. The mother is on the scene.

1. Which of the following elements is not involved in reading the scene?

- **A.** Evaluating the scene safety
- **B.** Evaluating environmental conditions
- **C.** Evaluating the location of the ambulance
- **D.** Evaluating access and egress issues

2. After reading the scene, the next step in the *Six Rs of clinical decision making* is:

- **A.** relieving the patient of worry.
- **B.** readying the ambulance for transport.
- **C.** requesting advanced life support.
- **D.** reading the patient.

3. The third step of critical thinking, called *React*, involves which of the following steps as your first priority in patient care?

- **A.** Correct life threats.
- **B.** Consider the worst-case scenario.
- **C.** Complete a full-body exam.
- **D.** Establish command of the scene.

4. The patients are both alert and have calmed down. You and your partner apply ice packs to each patient while you continue your assessments and begin treatment, including splinting the injured arm and providing pressure to maintain bleeding control for the laceration. You each inquire as to how your patient is feeling. Which step of the *Six Rs of clinical decision making* does this describe?

- **A.** Request
- **B.** Reevaluate
- **C.** React
- **D.** Review

5. You and your partner decide that both patients should be transported to the hospital for evaluation. With the process of concept formation, including the primary survey of each patient, you determine that the 7-year-old requires a radiograph to ascertain whether there is a broken bone, and the 16-year-old needs stitches for the laceration. Evaluating all the information you have gathered is called:

- **A.** data interpretation.
- **B.** working diagnosis.
- **C.** reflection in action.
- **D.** reading the scene.

6. A few days after the call, you receive a message from your quality improvement supervisor saying that your documentation and care were exceptional. This feedback helps you:

- **A.** realize you are an exceptional health care provider.
- **B.** review your performance.
- **C.** understand that you cannot make mistakes.
- **D.** revise your patient treatment plan for future runs.

7. If you arrived on the scene and found the fight still occurring and no police presence, using your best judgment and independent decision making, then what would you do?

- **A.** Stop your vehicle and remain inside.
- **B.** Get out of your vehicle and stop the fight.
- **C.** Stop your vehicle and yell for them to stop.
- **D.** Leave the scene until police arrive and secure the scene.

8. You are in your station doing chores and a 16-year-old walks in reporting chest pain. How do you treat the patient?

9. From your experience, give an example of the issues that can result by not gathering, evaluating, and synthesizing information about the patient.

10. If a paramedic does not make a practice of following the *Six Rs of clinical decision making* as discussed in this chapter, then what potential challenges could result in scene management and patient care?

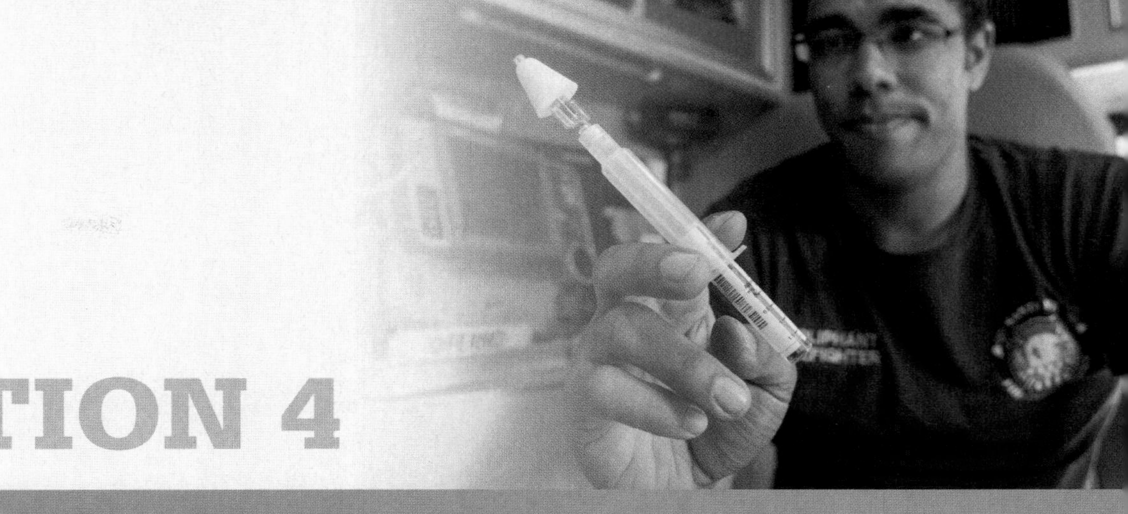

SECTION 4

Pharmacology

CHAPTER 13

Principles of Pharmacology

National EMS Education Standard Competencies

Pharmacology

Integrates comprehensive knowledge of pharmacology to formulate a treatment plan intended to mitigate emergencies and improve the overall health of the patient.

Principles of Pharmacology

- Medication safety (pp 628, 647-650)
- Medication legislation (pp 622-623)
- Naming (p 625)
- Classifications (pp 623, 627)
- Schedules (p 623)
- Pharmacokinetics (p 641)
- Storage and security (pp 627-628)
- Autonomic pharmacology (pp 649-653)
- Metabolism and excretion (pp 646-647)
- Mechanism of action (pp 626-631)
- Phases of medication activity (pp 646-647)
- Medication response relationships (pp 630-631, 635-639)
- Medication interactions (pp 639-640)
- Toxicity (pp 628, 636-638)

Medication Administration

- Routes of administration (pp 641-644)
- Self-administer medication (see Chapter 14, *Medication Administration*)
- Peer-administer medication (see Chapter 14, *Medication Administration*)
- Assist/administer medications to a patient (see Chapter 14, *Medication Administration*)
- Within the scope of practice of the paramedic, administer medications to a patient (pp 648-649, and see Chapter 14, *Medication Administration*)

Knowledge Objectives

1. Explain how pharmacology relates to paramedic clinical practice. (p 622)
2. Describe the regulatory measures affecting medications administered in the prehospital setting. (pp 622-623)
3. Describe how drugs are classified. (pp 623, 627)
4. Outline reliable sources of medication information available to paramedics. (pp 625-627)
5. List the components of a medication profile. (p 626)
6. Discuss requirements for medication storage, security, and accountability. (pp 627-628)
7. Describe the pharmacokinetic and pharmacodynamic properties of medications in general. (pp 628-630, 641)
8. Identify situations in which medication effects will be altered by the age, sex, weight, and other characteristics of a particular patient. (pp 631-635)
9. Present steps to reduce the incidence of medication errors and limit the severity of harmful effects associated with medication administration. (pp 635-636, 647-650)
10. Discuss the prevention, recognition, and management of adverse medication reactions. (pp 636-637)
11. Select the optimal medication and method of medication administration for patients with a particular clinical condition or situation. (pp 641-645)
12. Identify the various classes of medications that influence the sympathetic nervous system. (pp 649-653)
13. Describe specific medications used by paramedics in the prehospital setting. (pp 653-657)
14. List notable classes of medications that may be taken by patients in the prehospital setting. (pp 654-657)
15. Explain the medications likely to be used by patients with respiratory conditions, including what each medication is used for. (pp 659-660)
16. Recognize the medications commonly prescribed to patients with cardiovascular diseases. (pp 660-669)

Skills Objectives

There are no skills objectives for this chapter.

Introduction

Medication administration is a defining element of paramedic clinical practice. When given appropriately, medications have the unique ability to correct or decrease the severity of an illness or injury, manage many life-threatening conditions, and substantially reduce patient discomfort. If you administer the incorrect medication, use the incorrect route, select an inappropriate dose, or fail to follow the correct technique for administration, severe and often life-threatening consequences are possible in many situations. This chapter will assist you in minimizing the risks associated with medication administration while providing patients with a large variety of benefits available from pharmacologic interventions. Throughout this chapter, the terms *medications* and *drugs* are used interchangeably. As commercial medications, illicit drugs, and other chemicals enter the human body, many share common characteristics and produce similar clinical effects, despite entering the body under vastly different circumstances.

Words of Wisdom

The terms *medication* and *drug* are often used interchangeably but have differing meanings. A **medication** refers to a substance used to treat an illness or condition. A **drug**, generally speaking, is any substance that produces a physiologic effect, whether therapeutic or not; when used in a clinical sense, it is understood to refer to a substance that produces a therapeutic effect when given in the appropriate circumstances and in the appropriate dose. Therefore, every medication is a drug, but not every drug is a medication.

Pharmacology is the scientific study of how various substances interact with or alter the function of living organisms. You will use the science of pharmacology in a variety of ways, such as when treating patients who already receive medications on an intermittent or long-term basis. You will also encounter patients who are experiencing adverse effects of medications taken at home, so it is crucial to obtain a medication history during patient assessment. It is also important to understand pharmacology when administering medications to treat patient symptoms during an emergency medical services (EMS) response or while treating a patient who has been exposed to a potentially toxic chemical, drug, or medication.

Historical Perspective on Medication Administration

Chemicals, primarily derived from plants or animals, have been used for many centuries to cure disease or relieve symptoms. Early Chinese, Mesopotamian, and Egyptian societies used chemical remedies to treat everything from pain to baldness. Diseases were poorly understood, and natural remedies were directed toward various symptoms rather than the disease process itself. Formal scientific study of the effects of medication on the body began to emerge during the late 17th century and into the 18th century. Today, the science of pharmacology has evolved into a highly profitable and highly regulated industry. Many unique subspecialties such as genetic manipulation and toxicology continue to blur the line between pharmacology, medicine, and a variety of other scientific fields. Although the science of pharmacology has evolved into a sophisticated area of health care, certain medications discovered in ancient times are still in use.

The process of medication selection and administration is no longer random or anecdotal as it was in previous centuries. Evidence-based guidelines assist clinicians using pharmacologic interventions across the spectrum of medical specialties. Medications now undergo extensive testing and numerous clinical trials before widespread use is permitted. Despite the advanced science of pharmacology, adverse reactions are commonplace.

Medication and Drug Regulation

The United States has implemented a comprehensive system of medication and drug regulation. The first significant regulation was enacted in 1906 with the passage of the Pure Food and Drug Act. As its name implies, this act prohibited altering or mislabeling medications. In 1909, opium was prohibited from being imported under the Opium Exclusion Act. The Harrison Narcotics Act became law in 1914, restricting the use of various opiates and cocaine.

YOU are the Paramedic PART 1

The communications center dispatches you and your partner to a skilled nursing facility for an 88-year-old woman reported to have altered mental status. Additional dispatch information advises that the patient has a pulse and is breathing, but she has a decreased level of consciousness.

1. What medical conditions would you expect to encounter in a skilled nursing facility or long-term care facility?

Under the Food, Drug, and Cosmetic Act (1938), the US Food and Drug Administration (FDA) was given enforcement authority for rules requiring that new drugs were safe and pure. The FDA remains the federal agency responsible for approving new medications and removing unsafe medications from use. Approval of a new medication typically takes several years. Occasionally, breakthrough medications for life-threatening conditions may receive preferential expedited consideration. Only a small fraction of medications submitted to the FDA are approved, and many medications, once approved, are used "off-label"—that is, for a purpose not approved by the FDA, at doses different from the recommended doses, or by a route of administration not approved by the FDA. Off-label use is extremely common in health care, but a physician medical director or paramedic may have an increased risk of liability for ill-advised off-label use of a medication that results in a bad outcome for a patient. Medications should be administered off-label only when they are specifically approved for this use by the service's medical director or by agency/regional protocol. Intranasal use of naloxone and the use of intravenous tranexamic acid for trauma, both discussed later in this chapter, are frequently cited examples of off-label medication use in EMS.

It is essential that you be familiar with the rules and regulations implemented under the Controlled Substances Act (also known as the Comprehensive Drug Abuse Prevention and Control Act) of 1970. This act classifies certain medications with the potential of abuse into five categories (schedules) with corresponding security, dispensing, and record-keeping requirements Table 13-1. The US Drug Enforcement Agency is responsible for enforcing this act.

Schedule I medications may not be prescribed, dispensed, used, or administered for medical use. Marijuana, prescribed for medical purposes, remains a controversial Schedule I controlled substance. Various states permit prescription marijuana for certain medical conditions, and some allow both medical and recreational use. All marijuana use remains in conflict with federal controlled substances regulation.

Paramedics are likely to carry and administer Schedule II medications such as fentanyl (Sublimaze) and morphine sulfate, and Schedule IV medications such as midazolam (Versed), diazepam (Valium), and lorazepam (Ativan). All Schedule II through V medications require locked storage, significant record keeping, and controlled wasting procedures. State EMS, pharmacy, or law enforcement agencies may impose additional requirements for the security and accountability of these controlled substances.

Words of Wisdom

Careful accountability of controlled substances protects the paramedic and the EMS organization. Failure to adequately control and waste controlled substances may jeopardize your job, your reputation, and your professional certification or licensure.

Table 13-1 Classification of Medications Considered Controlled Substances

Schedule	Description	Examples
I	High abuse potential; no recognized medical purpose	Heroin, marijuana, LSD
II	High abuse potential; legitimate medical purpose	Fentanyl (Sublimaze), methylphenidate (Ritalin), cocaine
III	Lower potential for abuse than Schedule II medications	Hydrocodone (Vicodin), acetaminophen with codeine (Tylenol with codeine #3), ketamine
IV	Lower potential for abuse than Schedule III drugs	Diazepam (Valium), lorazepam (Ativan)
V	Lower potential for abuse than Schedule IV drugs	Narcotic cough medicines

Abbreviation: LSD, lysergic acid diethylamide

Sources of Medication

Medications can be derived or manufactured from a wide variety of possible sources. Ancient societies used medications isolated from the roots, leaves, or bark of certain plants. Animals, particularly animal endocrine systems, are used as the source of other medications. Minerals provide yet another source of many medications used for a wide variety of clinical conditions. Microorganisms such as bacteria, fungi, and mold also are used for the manufacture of medication. Table 13-2 lists sources of many common medications.

Many other medications are either synthetic (made completely in a laboratory setting) or semisynthetic (made from chemicals derived from plant, animal, or mineral sources that have been chemically modified in a laboratory setting). Genetic engineering is also used to manufacture certain medications that cannot otherwise be obtained from natural sources.

During the manufacturing process, pharmaceutical companies tightly control the concentration, purity, preservatives, and other ingredients present in medications. The

Table 13-2 Sources of Medications

Source	Examples
Plant	Atropine, aspirin, digoxin, morphine
Animal	Heparin, antivenom, thyroid preparations, insulin
Microorganism	Streptokinase, numerous antibiotics
Mineral	Iron, magnesium sulfate, lithium, phosphorus, calcium

United States Pharmacopeia–National Formulary ([USP-NF] discussed later) is a great source of information regarding the manufacturing details of a particular medication. On the packaging of the medication, you will notice a manufacturing lot number and expiration date.

▶ Forms of Medication

You will manage and administer medication in various forms. The vast majority of medications are administered as sterile injectable solutions. These solutions require careful handling and aseptic technique during administration to avoid contamination with microorganisms or other harmful substances. These solutions are supplied in larger intravenous (IV) bags, vials, and ampules and occasionally in glass bottles for medications such as nitroglycerin or ethanol. Other forms of medication are outlined in Table 13-3.

Table 13-3 Forms of Medication

Form	Description	Examples
Capsule	Powdered or solid medication enclosed in a dissolvable cylindrical gelatin shell	Acetaminophen (Tylenol), ibuprofen (Motrin), diphenhydramine (Benadryl)
Tablet	Solid medication particles bound into a shape designed to dissolve or be swallowed	Aspirin (ASA), nitroglycerin SL
Powder	Small particles of medication designed to be dissolved or mixed into a solution or liquid	Glucagon, vecuronium (Norcuron)
Droplet	Sterile solution or nonsterile liquid intended for direct administration into the nose or ear	Phenylephrine (Neo-Synephrine, Afrin), tetracaine (Paramedics may use the parenteral form of certain medications to administer through an alternate route, such as when administering intranasal naloxone [Narcan])
Parenteral solution	Sterile solution for direct injection into a body cavity, tissue, or organ	Fentanyl (Sublimaze), epinephrine
Skin preparation	Gel, ointment, or paste substance designed to permit transdermal (through the skin) absorption	Nitroglycerin paste, fentanyl (Sublimaze) patch
Suppository	Medication in a wax-like material that dissolves in the rectum or other body cavity	Promethazine (Phenergan), acetaminophen (Tylenol)
Liquid	Medication dissolved or suspended in liquid intended for oral consumption	Infant acetaminophen (Tylenol), cough syrup
Inhaler/spray	Medication in gas or fine mist form intended for inhalation and absorption through the lung, airway, or oral tissues	Albuterol (Ventolin), nitroglycerin spray

Abbreviation: ASA, acetylsalicylic acid; SL, sublingual

Patient Safety

If glass bottles are being used during interfacility transport, carefully secure them to prevent injury to the patient or yourself in the event of a crash.

Medication Management for Paramedics

Medication Names

Every medication in the United States is given three distinct names: a chemical name, a generic or nonproprietary name, and a brand or proprietary name. During initial development, medications are given a chemical name, which is often long and difficult to pronounce and may contain specific letters or numbers according to the medication's chemical composition. The chemical name is rarely used in clinical practice. Sodium bicarbonate, potassium chloride, and certain other medications are the few exceptions in which the chemical name is used in clinical practice. The majority of medication reference sources used by paramedics do not publish the chemical name or structure of a medication.

Every medication also receives a nonproprietary, or generic, name. The generic name is proposed by the manufacturer and must be approved by the United States Adopted Names Council and the World Health Organization. The generic name is regulated internationally to promote consistency and avoid duplication in drug names. Generic names typically include a "stem" that links them to other medications in the same **class** (the grouping to which a medication belongs). Often the stem is at the end of the name, but it may also appear at the beginning or within the drug name. Many benzodiazepine medications, such as midazolam, diazepam, and lorazepam have the stem "am." Angiotensin-converting enzyme (ACE) inhibitor medications, such as enalapril (Vasotec), captopril (Capoten), and lisinopril (Prinivil, Zestril), have the stem "pril" that signifies that each medication is a member of the ACE inhibitor class. Numerous other examples of stems exist.

Be careful not to rely entirely on a stem when attempting to determine the class of a medication because different classes might have the same stem. Tricyclic antidepressants, such as amitriptyline (Elavil) and desipramine (Norpramin), have the same stem as certain selective serotonin reuptake inhibitors (SSRIs) such as fluoxetine (Prozac) and paroxetine (Paxil). An overdose of a tricyclic antidepressant is often life threatening, whereas an overdose of an SSRI medication does not typically pose the same risk. Besides knowing that stems provide information about the class of drugs, paramedics need to know the specific names of and indications for the drugs they administer.

The final type of medication name is the brand name, which is chosen by the manufacturer and approved by the FDA. The brand name does not have the same functional requirements as the generic name, but it must meet certain minimum criteria set by the FDA. Brand names are often selected for marketing purposes. Creative examples are sometimes linked to a particular condition. Metoprolol, a beta-adrenergic blocking agent, has the brand name Lopressor, which may be a subtle reference to lowering pressure (of the blood). Oseltamivir has the brand name Tami*flu* and is used to treat in*flu*enza. The three distinct medication names are illustrated with the following example of a medication commonly administered by paramedics:

Chemical name: 4-chloro-*N*-furfuryl-5-sulfamoylanthranilic acid
Generic name: furosemide
Brand name: Lasix

You will observe that many reference sources now use "tall man" lettering to print the names of certain medications. This approach is intended to avoid confusion among medications with similarly spelled names. The capitalized letters highlight a portion of the name in medications with similar names. One example is DOBUTamine and DOPamine, and another is diphenhydrAMINE and dimenhyDRINATE.

Patient Safety

Many medication names look and sound the same. Minimize the risk of medication errors by double-checking the medication container label every time you are preparing to administer a medication. Concentrations and packaging may change unexpectedly.

Medication Reference Sources

There is a vast array of medication reference sources available to assist you in clinical practice. When selecting a reference source to use or purchase, consider a variety of factors, including the reliability of the reference source; whether the source is printed, electronic, or both; the depth of information needed or provided; accessibility; cost; availability of updates; and size of materials used (if a printed product).

Medication information is typically compiled in a format called a **medication monograph** or medication profile. The detail may vary dramatically between reference sources, but the basic structure remains consistent. Table 13-4 highlights common components of medication profiles.

Table 13-4 Components of Medication Profiles

Component	Description
Medication names	Sources typically include both the brand and the generic names. Print sources often alphabetize by generic name. Electronic sources can typically be searched by either brand or generic name.
Category or class of medication	The grouping to which a medication belongs. Medications are grouped according to their characteristics, traits, or primary components.
Use/**indication**	A sign, symptom, or condition that would potentially benefit from a particular medication; the reason for giving a medication.
Mechanism of action (pharmacodynamics)	The way in which a medication produces the intended response.
Pregnancy risk factor	A scale indicating the likelihood of potential harm to the fetus if the medication is administered to a pregnant patient.
Contraindications	Any condition, especially a disease, that is known to render some particular line of treatment improper or undesirable.
Available forms (how supplied)	The manner in which the manufacturer packages the medication for distribution and sale. Typical methods of packaging are prefilled syringes, vials, or ampules.
Dosage (often differentiated based on age or indication)	The typical or average volume or dose of the medication that is to be administered to the patient and the route of introduction of the medication to the patient.
Administration and monitoring considerations	Any additional information needed to safely administer the medication and any important parameters that should be observed following administration.
Potential incompatibilities	Problems that may occur when two or more medications are administered together, which could be at the same time, in the same solution, or through the same IV tubing or delivery device (nebulizer, syringe, etc).
Adverse effects	Any abnormal or harmful effects caused by exposure to a chemical. Adverse effects are indicated by such results as death, a change in food or water consumption, altered body and organ weights, altered enzyme levels, or visible illness. An effect may be classified as adverse if it causes functional or anatomic damage, causes irreversible change in the person's homeostasis, or increases the person's susceptibility to other chemical or biologic stress.
Pharmacokinetics	The medication's effects on the body, as described by the following terms: ▪ **Onset.** The estimated amount of time it will take for the medication to enter the body/system and begin to take effect. ▪ **Peak.** The estimated amount of time it will take for the medication to have its greatest effect on the patient/system. ▪ **Duration (of action).** The estimated amount of time that the medication will have any effect on the patient/system.

Special Populations

Pediatric and older patients often have slower medication absorption and elimination times, necessitating modification of the doses of many drugs administered to these patients. Pregnant patients are limited in the medications they can take because of risk to the fetus.

The *USP-NF* and the *Physicians' Desk Reference* (*PDR*) provide a wealth of reliable, detailed information about thousands of medications. The information includes graphic diagrams of the chemical structure and other specific chemical properties. The printed forms of these sources are impractical in prehospital settings because of their size and amount of information. Much of the information in these sources is not needed in prehospital settings, and it may be difficult for paramedics to locate needed information rapidly. The electronic versions of the *USP-NF* and *PDR* may be helpful to EMS educators and administrators developing agency-specific medication protocols or creating training materials.

Manufacturers provide written materials with every package of medication distributed. These "package inserts" are written by manufacturers and approved by the FDA. The package inserts include information on **dosing**, route of administration, contraindications, adverse effects, and a variety of other characteristics of a particular medication.

Hospital pharmacies often compile medication information into formularies that are specific to the information needs of specific hospitals. The hospital formulary typically includes much of the same information as that included in the medication package insert, *USP-NF*, or *PDR*, but it is tailored to the needs of prescribers in the hospital. Paramedics in hospital-based or hospital-affiliated EMS systems may have access to the hospital formulary.

The American Medical Association (AMA) publishes another reliable source of medication information. *AMA Drug Evaluations* provides great detail about medication selection and administration. It contains much of the same information included in the *USP-NF* and *PDR*, with additional discussion of investigational medications. Paramedics must use caution when referencing the AMA publication because not every medication in the compendium has received FDA approval.

You have many other choices for commercially published medication information references. Some resources are specifically for prehospital or critical care transport providers, with an emphasis on medication selection, dosing, and administration for patient conditions encountered in these settings. Other references focus exclusively on IV medications or emphasize only information needed during hands-on patient care. With the advancements in portable electronic devices and "smart" cell phones, many medication references can be accessed electronically, making vast amounts of information available without requiring additional space or weight in an ambulance. State EMS agencies and individual fire and EMS organizations frequently compile information on approved medications given by paramedics in a particular setting through specific protocols or a medication formulary.

Words of Wisdom

Find a pocket-sized medication reference source (print or electronic) that works well for you, and always keep it with you while on duty.

AHA Classification of Recommendations and Level of Evidence

In most EMS settings you will follow guidelines established and distributed by the American Heart Association (AHA). These guidelines may be referenced directly or may be incorporated into more extensive department or agency policies or protocols. The medications and interventions listed within the AHA guidelines have varying degrees of support through reliable scientific evidence. Chapter 1, *EMS Systems*, discusses the distinction and relationship between *class* and *level of evidence*. You can generally infer the level of evidence by the assigned class of a proposed intervention. To provide greater clarity to health care providers regarding the level of evidence, the AHA uses the following system to describe the relative importance of certain medications or interventions:

- *Class I* indicates there is strong evidence supporting the use of the medication for the condition.
- *Class IIa* indicates moderate evidence.
- *Class IIb* indicates weak evidence.
- *Class III* indicates the evidence does not support that there is a benefit and may support that there is a harmful consequence; the treatment is not helpful and may be harmful.
- *Class indeterminate* indicates either that research is beginning on a treatment or that research is continuing on a treatment. There are no recommendations until further research is performed (ie, cannot recommend for or against).

Medication Storage

Medication storage is an important consideration for paramedics. The uncontrolled prehospital environment is a difficult place to maintain the safety and integrity of medication packages. It is important to keep medication in a location that provides adequate protection for medication supplies yet is convenient enough to allow quick access in emergency situations. Devices such as medication refrigerators and secure cabinets may be impractical in some prehospital settings or response vehicles.

The most basic concern regarding medication storage is the integrity of the medication container. Medication should be stored in a manner that prevents physical damage to the medication vial, ampule, solution, or tablets. It is often necessary to remove most of the packaging provided by the manufacturer, leaving only the bare medication container in the vehicle or response bag. Because drug boxes or bags may be dropped accidentally during a call, medication containers should be placed in protective bins or surrounded by enough padding to avoid damage during response or patient care at the scene. Paramedics should organize medication containers in a manner that facilitates quick, accurate identification of the medication during emergency situations. Needs of individual EMS organizations dictate the type and quantity of medications that are available on a particular response vehicle or in a provider's bag. Excessive quantities of medication may make storage difficult or cause unnecessary waste due to expiration. Insufficient quantities may undermine patient care or necessitate frequent restocking.

Direct sunlight, extremes of heat and cold, and physical damage to medication containers can make medications ineffective or unsafe for use. Temperature extremes hasten the expiration of many medications. Medications in general require secure storage in a climate-controlled environment. Special medication warmers or refrigerators may be necessary if safe temperatures cannot be maintained in an ambulance or EMS response vehicle. A recent multicenter study demonstrated that ambulance interiors in a variety of geographic regions had temperature extremes outside the *USP-NF*-recommended range of 15°C to 30°C (59°F to 86°F) for the storage of most medications used in the prehospital setting.[1] You may need to discard medication that has been exposed to extremes of temperature. EMS agencies in environments where temperature extremes are common need to invest in equipment such as heaters, coolers, and refrigerators for transport vehicles to ensure the safety and integrity of the medications they carry.

▶ Medication Security

Controlled substances (as described in Table 13-1) require additional security, record keeping, and disposal precautions. These medications must be kept in locked storage or continuously held by an on-duty EMS provider responsible for administration. Disposal of partially used or damaged medication containers requires verification by a witness or return of the damaged or unused portion to the department responsible for dispensing the medication. EMS agencies and individual paramedics are jointly responsible for adhering to all federal, state, and local regulations regarding the security and accountability of controlled substances. These regulations vary slightly from region to region. In general, every last milliliter or milligram of a controlled substance needs to be documented from ordering, to receipt by the EMS agency, to administration by the EMS provider (or discard as waste). The particular forms and procedures may vary from place to place, but the standard for accountability remains constant.

Controlled substances are often the target of tampering or diversion. Inspect medication vials, ampules, and the like for subtle signs of tampering that may be as small as a pinhole. Suspect tampering in situations in which appropriate doses of analgesic or sedative medications seem ineffective, especially when patient tolerance is unlikely.

The Physiology of Pharmacology

The purpose of medications is to produce a desired effect in the body, usually in response to a particular illness, injury, or medical condition, but occasionally to prevent a specific harmful situation. As a medication is administered, it begins to alter a function or process within the body. This action is known as **pharmacodynamics**.

Any medication capable of beneficial clinical effects can cause toxic effects when given at an excessive dose. Toxic effects may also occur if a medication is given by an incorrect route or when a delivery device, such as an IV catheter or intraosseous (IO) needle, malfunctions. In other cases, medications may become ineffective when given at an inadequate dose or through the incorrect route. Even in the absence of error, many factors related to the patient, the patient's condition, and the particular medication may cause toxicity or adverse effects.

The human body simultaneously begins the process of **absorption**, **distribution**, possibly **biotransformation**, and, ultimately, **elimination** of a medication or chemical following administration. The action of the body on a medication is known as **pharmacokinetics**. You must always consider the principles of pharmacodynamics and pharmacokinetics when deciding whether to administer a particular medication.

▶ Principles of Pharmacodynamics

Scientific research has demonstrated the presence of **receptor** sites in proteins connected to cells throughout the body. Various receptors are activated by **endogenous** chemicals, those occurring naturally within the body, and by the presence of medications and chemicals absorbed into the body. Activation of these receptors produces a specific response by individual cells, tissues, organs, and, ultimately, body systems. When a medication binds with a receptor site, one of four possible actions will occur:

1. Channels permitting the passage of ions (charged particles) in cell walls are opened or closed.
2. A biochemical messenger becomes activated, initiating other chemical reactions within the cell.

3. A normal cell function is prevented.
4. A normal or abnormal function of the cell begins.

For purposes of this chapter, **exogenous** (from outside the body) chemicals will be referred to as medications, even though exposure to chemicals in the environment can cause effects similar to those of medications, including adverse effects. Clandestine methamphetamine laboratories are a great example of environmental exposure to a chemical. Law enforcement officers and other emergency responders may experience accidental inhalation or dermal exposure to methamphetamines during an emergency response and demonstrate clinical effects identical to those of people who intentionally abuse these substances. In another example, toddlers who accidentally ingest certain mouse poisons have clinical effects identical to those experienced following the therapeutic administration of warfarin (Coumadin). In each instance, the exposure is different from normal therapeutic administration, yet the clinical effects are identical.

Later sections of this chapter will discuss specific medications and chemicals used by paramedics and introduce the properties of various classes of medications pertinent to prehospital care. Chapter 27, *Toxicology*, discusses the adverse properties of commonly abused drugs. Functionally, the distinction between the terms *therapeutic medications*, *exogenous chemicals*, and *illicit drugs* is largely irrelevant. These terms reflect substances that follow similar (and often predictable) patterns when interacting with the body.

Medications are developed to reach and bind with particular receptor sites of target cells. Newer medications are designed to target only specific receptor sites on certain cells in an attempt to minimize the adverse effects. Many older medications, including those used by paramedics, affect cells and tissues totally unrelated to the condition being treated, causing adverse effects throughout the body.

Two types of medications or chemicals directly affect cellular activity by binding with receptor sites on individual cells. **Agonist medications** initiate or alter a cellular activity by attaching to receptor sites, prompting a cell response. **Antagonist medications** prevent endogenous or exogenous agonist chemicals from reaching cell receptor sites and initiating or altering a particular cellular activity **Figure 13-1**. Certain notable agonist-antagonist pairs are discussed at various points later in this chapter. Opiate medications such as morphine sulfate and fentanyl are agonist chemicals that cause **analgesia** and respiratory depression. The effects of these chemicals can be reversed by the opiate antagonist naloxone (Narcan). In certain circumstances, the clinical effects from benzodiazepine

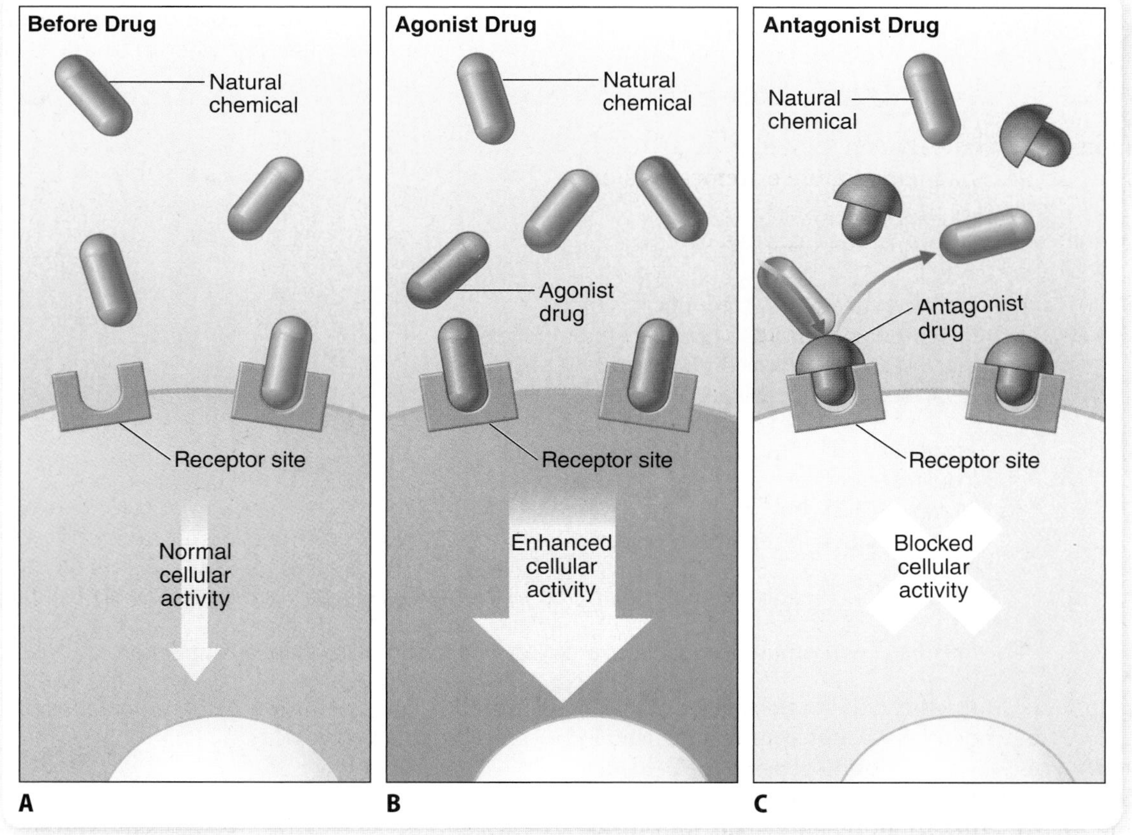

Figure 13-1 A. Normally, natural chemicals bind to receptor sites to cause actions. **B.** When an agonist drug is present, it binds to the receptor site and enhances cellular activity. **C.** When an antagonist drug is present, it binds to the receptor site and blocks cellular activity.

agonist medications can be reversed by the benzodiazepine antagonist medication flumazenil (Romazicon).

Agonist Medications

The dose of a particular medication, the route of administration, and a large number of other factors determine the concentration of a medication present at target cell receptor sites. **Affinity** is the ability of a medication to bind with a particular receptor site. Medication concentration and affinity determine the number of receptor sites bound by that medication. Agonist medications bind with receptor sites, initiating or altering an action by the cell Table 13-5.

A certain minimum concentration of agonist medication must be present for cellular activity to be initiated or altered. As the concentration of the medication increases and crosses the **threshold level**, initiation or alteration of cellular activity begins. Increasing concentrations of medication cause increased effects until all receptor sites become occupied or the maximum capability of the cell is reached. The concentration of the medication required to initiate a cellular response is known as the medication's **potency**. As the potency of a medication increases, the concentration or dose required for a particular cellular response decreases. Conversely, a higher concentration is required when the potency of a medication is low. The ability to initiate or alter cell activity in a therapeutic or desired manner is referred to as **efficacy**. Once all the cellular receptor sites become bound with agonist medications, cellular activity plateaus and no increase or further change in activity is possible. At this point, the effect of the medication has peaked and additional doses or higher concentrations of the medication will not cause additional cellular action. The **dose-response curve** illustrates the relationship of medication dose (or concentration) and efficacy. Relative potency is demonstrated when the dose-response curves of two different medications causing the same effect are compared. The threshold dose is lower for medications with a higher potency Figure 13-2.

Antagonist Medications

Antagonist medications bind with receptor sites to prevent a cellular response to agonist chemicals. Antagonists may be used to inhibit normal cellular activation by naturally occurring agonist chemicals within the body. Antagonist medications may also be used to treat the harmful agonist effects of exogenous medications or chemicals, possibly following an overdose or a toxic exposure.

Table 13-5 Important Receptor Sites Within the Body

Receptor	Agonist Effect
Alpha (α)-1	Vasoconstriction of arteries and veins
Alpha (α)-2	Insulin restriction Glucagon secretion Inhibition of norepinephrine release
Beta (β)-1	Increased heart rate (chronotropic effect) Increased myocardial contractility (inotropic effect) Increased myocardial conduction (dromotropic effect) Renin secretion for urinary retention
Beta (β)-2	Bronchus and bronchiole relaxation Insulin secretion Uterine relaxation Arterial dilation in certain key organs
Dopaminergic	Vasodilation of renal and mesenteric arteries (Numerous receptor subtypes exist.)
Nicotinic	Present at neuromuscular junction, allowing ACh to stimulate muscle contraction
Muscarinic-2	Present in the heart; activated by ACh to offset stimulation of the sympathetic nervous system, decreasing heart rate, contractility, and electrical conduction velocity
Opioid	Present in central and peripheral nervous system, bowels, and various tissues; activated by opioid substances to produce analgesia, euphoria, respiratory depression, and numerous other clinical effects. There are three types of opioid receptors (mu, kappa, and delta). The mu (μ) opioid receptors are most prominent, with the greatest affinity for both morphine and naloxone (opioid antagonist).

Abbreviation: ACh, acetylcholine

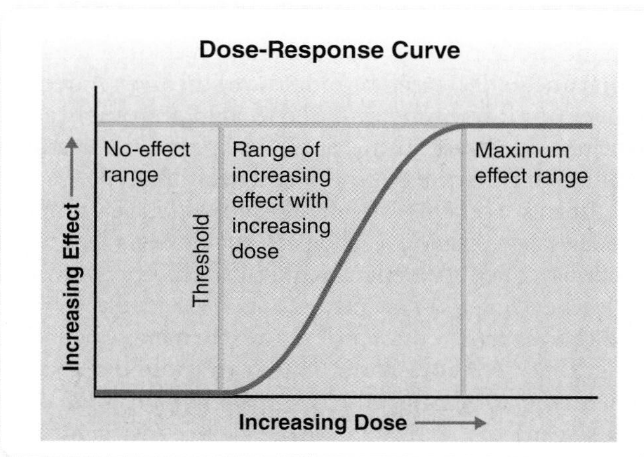

Figure 13-2 Dose-response curve.

Antagonists may be competitive or noncompetitive. **Competitive antagonists** temporarily bind with cellular receptor sites, displacing agonist chemicals. The efficacy of a competitive antagonist medication is directly related to its concentration near the receptor sites. As the concentration of a competitive antagonist increases near the receptor sites, it is able to prevent a greater number of agonist chemicals from reaching the receptor, thus decreasing cellular action. This effect can apply to a large quantity of one particular agonist chemical or the presence of multiple chemicals with similar agonist effects. As the competitive antagonist concentration falls (due to elimination of the drug or substance, such as through the kidneys) or when the concentration of agonist chemicals increases, a greater number of agonist chemicals bind with receptor sites and continue or resume cellular activation.

The efficacy of a competitive antagonist medication is also related to its affinity (ability to bind at a receptor site) compared with the affinity of the agonist chemicals present. Competitive antagonist medications with a lower affinity require a higher concentration to be effective.

Noncompetitive antagonists permanently bind with receptor sites and prevent activation by agonist chemicals. Effects of noncompetitive antagonist medications continue until new receptor sites or new cells are created, which may be a long time after the last dose of antagonist medication was given. Ketamine (discussed later) is a noncompetitive antagonist of the agonist glutamate on *N*-methyl-D-aspartate receptors in the central nervous system (CNS). Effects of ketamine last for only approximately 25 minutes. Aspirin (also discussed later) is a noncompetitive antagonist that binds to the enzyme cyclooxygenase, causing antiplatelet effects that last up to 10 days when platelets are regenerated. Even increased doses of agonist chemicals will not overcome the presence of noncompetitive antagonist chemicals on cellular receptor sites.

Partial Agonist Chemicals

It is also possible to have a **partial agonist** chemical attach to cellular receptor sites. Partial agonists bind to the receptor site but do not initiate as much cellular activity or change as do other agonists. Partial agonists effectively lower the efficacy of other agonist chemicals that may be present at the cells. Buprenorphine (Buprenex, Subutex) is a partial agonist medication used for both analgesia and the management of opioid addiction. Buprenorphine has a high affinity for binding to the mu opioid receptors (described in Table 13-5), preventing agonism by other opioid chemicals. Buprenorphine provides some degree of agonism, causing analgesia and euphoria, but has a "ceiling effect" that allows only partial activation of the opioid receptors, minimizing the risk of toxicity and physical dependence. The maximum effects possible from buprenorphine are much less than the effects from other opioid chemicals.

Alternative Mechanisms of Drug Action

It is possible for medications to alter cell, tissue, organ, and system function in the body without directly interacting with receptors on individual cells. Medications are engineered to target other sites throughout the body, including microorganisms, lipids, water, and exogenous toxic substances. **Antimicrobials**, such as **antibiotics** and **antifungals**, may be designed to target specific substances present in the cell walls of a particular bacterium or fungus. Other medications, known as **chelating agents**, bind with heavy metals such as lead, mercury, and arsenic in the body and create a compound that can be eliminated. Sodium bicarbonate (discussed in detail later in this chapter), a medication used for a wide variety of medical conditions, breaks down after administration, producing bicarbonate ions. Bicarbonate ions are able to bind with excess hydrogen (H^+) ions, raising the pH and decreasing the acidity of various body fluids.

Mannitol (Osmitrol) is a **diuretic** medication, designed to distribute into water in the body, creating **osmotic** changes that alter the distribution of fluids and electrolytes. The resulting diuretic effect draws excess water from certain body tissues, including the brain and eyes, while enhancing excretion of urine by the kidneys. Plasma expanders and bulk laxatives target water in the body and alter the distribution of various body fluids.

Electrolyte-based medications such as magnesium, potassium, and calcium change the concentration and distribution of ions in cells and fluids throughout the body, affecting a wide variety of cell activities. An alteration in the concentration of certain electrolytes at the cellular level affects the ability of various cells to function. Alterations of cell function occur without chemicals directly binding to cell receptor sites.

Factors Affecting Response to Medications

A wide variety of factors determine how a particular medication will affect a patient. These factors may influence the choice of medication, dose, route, timing, manner of administration, and monitoring necessary after a patient receives a medication. Even weight-based medication dosing, which is common in the prehospital setting, produces profound differences in how a medication affects an individual patient because of the factors described in the following sections.

Age. The distribution, metabolism, and elimination of medication continue to change throughout the human life span. Older adult and pediatric patients can have a response to a variety of medications that is much different from responses in adolescents and adults. You may encounter unusual situations that require you to consult with online medical control to adjust the dose of medication for infants, children, and older patients to obtain the desired response.

Medications distribute into three primary types of body substances (water, lipids or fat, and protein) following administration. The percentage of body fat is lowest in preterm infants, increases significantly in toddlers, decreases through adolescence, and increases in adults, including older adults. The percentage of body water is highest in newborns and steadily decreases throughout the life span. The percentage of body protein varies throughout the life span, generally peaking in preteens, adolescents, and adults. Infants and older adults have the lowest percentage of body protein. If a medication is **water-soluble**, higher weight-based doses must be administered to infants (with a higher percentage of body water) than to adults and older adults. Fat- and lipid-soluble medications require higher weight-based doses in older adults because of their higher body fat percentage and increased fat distribution.

When you are treating pediatric or older patients with altered percentages of body water, fat or lipid, and protein, consider careful titration of medication rather than simply administering a weight-based bolus. Water-soluble and lipid-soluble medications may require increased initial doses to overcome widespread distribution. Older adult patients, for example, generally have a lower percentage of body water. Therefore, water-soluble medications, such as digoxin, cause higher serum levels in older patients compared with other patients who weigh the same and are given the same dose. There is less body water for the digoxin to spread into, causing a greater concentration in the body water present, particularly in the blood (serum). Older adult patients also generally have a higher percentage of body fat. Lipid-soluble medications such as diazepam initially produce much lower serum levels for a given dose, but they take much longer for the body to eliminate, dramatically prolonging the effects of the medications. Without careful monitoring, it is easy to exceed therapeutic serum levels when administering repeated doses, causing adverse or toxic effects that may persist for hours to days. Solubility is typically included with other information in medication reference materials.

Alteration of metabolism and elimination in pediatric and older patients may prolong the effects of medications or result in higher medication concentrations in various tissues. Medication metabolism in the liver is affected by the **cytochrome P-450 system** (discussed later in this chapter). This system works differently on different types of medications, is extremely variable in infants and children, and has a functional decline in older adults. Hepatic metabolism is also generally impaired in older adults due to decreased blood flow to the liver. A decline in liver or kidney function, due to aging or other cause, requires a decrease in the dosage of many medications because elimination from the body is impaired.

Patients at extremes of age are disproportionately prone to **paradoxical** medication reactions. In paradoxical medication reactions, patients experience clinical effects opposite from the intended effects of the medication. For example, sedative medications can produce profound excitement or agitation rather than sedation. Barbiturates can cause unexpected excitement or agitation in older patients. Promethazine (Phenergan), diphenhydramine (Benadryl), chloral hydrate, and various benzodiazepines, such as midazolam, can cause paradoxical excitement or agitation in children. Paradoxical reactions frequently complicate an already delicate clinical situation in which patients who need sedation become even more excited, agitated, or combative.

Weight. Many medications used in prehospital care and critical care transport are administered using weight-based dosing. A quantity of medication (usually grams, milligrams, micrograms, or milliliters) is multiplied by the patient's weight in kilograms to obtain the recommended dose for the individual patient. This method of medication dosing has advantages and limitations. The major advantage of this method is that the amount of medication administered is proportional to the size of the patient. Medication manufacturers and clinicians have already calculated factors affecting absorption, distribution, metabolism, rates of elimination, and desired quantity present at target cells or tissues when giving a particular medication at a weight-based dose. You can use the weight-based formula to calculate the appropriate medication dose for patients ranging from preterm neonates through large adults.

Special Populations

When you are caring for a pediatric patient, before administering any medication, ask the parents whether the child has had a previous reaction, such as a paradoxical reaction.

There are several limitations associated with this method as well. To calculate a weight-based medication dose, the patient's weight in kilograms is needed. In emergency situations, a patient's weight must be estimated and, often, converted from pounds to kilograms. Even in controlled settings, health care providers might have difficulty accurately estimating patient weights. A study revealed that a significant portion of health care providers' estimates of patient weight were off by more than 10% to 15%.[2] Patients are generally more accurate at estimating their own weight than are health care providers. An inaccurate estimate of a patient's weight, depending on the degree of inaccuracy, could result in administration of an incorrect dose of medication. Multiplication of numbers in the formula during a stressful situation or at an uncontrolled scene may also lead to dosing errors. Using a calculator or a preprinted medication dose chart when administering weight-based medications can help reduce errors.

The weight-based method of dose calculation does not consider the various alterations in distribution, metabolism, and elimination discussed earlier. Data regarding the percentages of body water, fat, and protein at various ages become less reliable as obesity and malnutrition affect society. Weight-based medication doses can be calculated by using the patient's actual body weight or ideal body weight. For example, lidocaine, an antidysrhythmic medication, is administered based on a patient's actual body weight. The cardiac medication digoxin is given based on a patient's ideal body weight. Unfortunately, many reference sources do not provide guidance about whether the patient's actual or ideal body weight should be used for medication dose calculations. The formulas for ideal body weight in adults are as follows:

For men: Ideal Weight (kg) = 50 + (2.3 times patient's height in inches over 5 feet)
For women: Ideal Weight (kg) = 45.5 + (2.3 times patient's height in inches over 5 feet)

For example, the ideal weight for a 6-foot-tall man is 77.6 kg [$50 + (2.3 \times 12)$], and the ideal weight for a 5-foot 5-inch woman is 57 kg [$45.5 + (2.3 \times 5)$].

Environment. Hyperthermia and hypothermia can affect medication absorption, metabolism, and efficacy. Fever causes tachycardia that may increase hepatic blood flow, theoretically increasing the initial metabolism of drugs in the liver and reducing the amount of drug returned to circulation by the liver. Fever also suppresses the function of the cytochrome P-450 system in the liver, which ultimately decreases the rate of metabolism of certain classes of medications. Individual patient responses may vary from the expected response.

Hypothermia is known to impair the effectiveness of medications used in traditional advanced cardiac life support (ACLS). Atropine sulfate and lidocaine are generally viewed as ineffective and are not indicated for hypothermic cardiac arrest. Epinephrine has demonstrated the ability to maintain coronary perfusion pressure during hypothermic cardiac arrest but remains controversial in patients with cardiac arrest resulting from hypothermia.[3-5]

Genetic Factors. Paramedics should be extremely careful when deciding whether to administer medications to patients with specific genetic disorders. Primary pulmonary hypertension, sickle cell disease, and glucose-6-phosphate dehydrogenase deficiency require special consideration and may exclude certain medications frequently used by paramedics. Patients with primary pulmonary hypertension may have acute decompensation when vasopressor medications are used. Salicylate medications such as aspirin (acetylsalicylic acid) may precipitate **hemolysis** (destruction of red blood cells [RBCs] by disruption of the cell membrane) in patients with glucose-6-phosphate dehydrogenase deficiency. Patients with sickle cell disease require adequate hydration and intravascular fluid volume. Medications that cause diuresis, such as furosemide (Lasix), or vasoconstriction, such as epinephrine or dopamine, may cause or worsen potentially fatal complications of sickle cell disease. Many other genetically linked conditions require careful consideration when administering medications in the prehospital setting.

Subtle genetic variations among individuals may cause significantly different responses to the same medication. ACE inhibitors, beta-2 agonists, antipsychotic medications, warfarin, aspirin, and glycoprotein IIb/IIIa inhibitors are all linked to the actions of particular genes. Variations in the expression of these linked genes will cause differing responses to each of these medications or medication groups (along with many others). The profound impact of genetic variations on medication response has prompted a vast array of genetic screening tests specific to certain disease states or medications.

Patients with genetic disorders and their family members are often excellent sources of information specific to the disorder. You should use the knowledge of patients and family members about genetic conditions; admitting a lack of knowledge about an unusual genetic condition and treating patients and families as experts on the genetic condition can help build their confidence in you.

Pregnancy. Pregnancy causes an array of physiologic changes in the body, which can affect medication decisions significantly. Cardiac output and intravascular volume increase dramatically, each by about 40% above baseline. The **hematocrit**, or the percentage of RBCs in the intravascular space, decreases in response to an increase in overall blood plasma volume. Respiratory tidal volume and minute volumes increase, while the inspiratory and expiratory reserve volumes decrease. Gastrointestinal (GI) motility decreases as pregnancy progresses. Renal blood flow and urinary elimination increase, roughly in proportion to cardiac output and intravascular volume. Pregnant patients have better renal function in a supine position than when upright. The majority of endocrine glands undergo some degree of change during pregnancy, causing emotional instability, altered glucose metabolism, thyroid-generated tachycardia, and other problems.

Each of these changes can affect the absorption, distribution, or elimination of medications during pregnancy. The stress imposed on the body during pregnancy from these changes can also exacerbate an underlying disease process, potentially threatening the life or health of the patient and fetus. In addition to considering maternal alterations during pregnancy, you must consider potential harmful effects on the developing fetus when administering medication to a pregnant patient. During the research, approval, and marketing process, medications are assigned into one of five possible FDA pregnancy risk categories based on potential harm to the fetus. This five-category system is being replaced by a more detailed system that uses narrative summaries to convey prescribing information related to pregnancy (including labor and delivery), lactation, and the risks of a medication to male and female users with reproductive potential. Medications approved after June 2015 have only the narrative summary. Medications approved before June 2015 have a 3-year period to transition to this new format.[6,7] This change was driven by concerns that the five-category system oversimplified risks related to pregnancy and lactation, leading to poor prescribing decisions.[6] Table 13-6 outlines the pregnancy categories for both classification systems.

Table 13-6 FDA Pregnancy Category Classification

Pregnancy Categories by Letter	Implications
A	Controlled studies in women fail to demonstrate a risk to the fetus in the first trimester (and there is no evidence of a risk in later trimesters), and the possibility of fetal harm appears remote.
B	Either animal-reproduction studies have not demonstrated a fetal risk but there are no controlled studies in pregnant women, or animal-reproduction studies have shown an adverse effect (other than a decrease in fertility) that was not confirmed in controlled studies in women in the first trimester (and there is no evidence of a risk in later trimesters).
C	Either studies in animals have revealed adverse effects on the fetus (teratogenic or embryocidal or other) and there are no controlled studies in women, or studies in women and animals are not available. Drugs should be given only if the potential benefit justifies the potential risk to the fetus.
D	There is positive evidence of human fetal risk, but the benefits from use in pregnant women may be acceptable despite the risk (eg, if the drug is needed in a life-threatening situation or for a serious disease for which safer drugs cannot be used or are ineffective).
X	Studies in animals or humans have demonstrated fetal abnormalities, there is evidence of fetal risk based on human experience, or both, and the risk of the use of the drug in pregnant women clearly outweighs any possible benefit. The drug is contraindicated in women who are or may become pregnant.
Drug Categories (Pregnancy, Lactation, and Reproductive Potential)[a]	**Type of Information in Narrative Summary[b]**
Pregnancy (includes labor and delivery)	Pregnancy exposure registry Risk summary Clinical considerations Data
Lactation (includes nursing mothers)	Risk summary Clinical considerations Data
Female and male users with reproductive potential	Pregnancy testing Contraception Infertility

[a] Effective June 30, 2015.

[b] Medications approved after June 2015 will have only the narrative summary. Medications approved before June 2015 have a 3-year period to transition to this new format.

Data from: US National Archives and Records Administration. *Code of Federal Regulations*. Title 21, Volume 4, Parts 200 to 299. Revised as of April 1, 1997; FDA pregnancy categories. Drugs.com website. https://www.drugs.com/pregnancy-categories.html. Accessed March 9, 2017; and Pregnancy and lactation labeling (drugs) final rule. US Food and Drug Administration website. http://www.fda.gov/Drugs/DevelopmentApprovalProcess/DevelopmentResources/Labeling/ucm093307.htm. Updated November 18, 2016. Accessed March 9, 2017.

In general, medications and interventions that protect the life and health of the mother are usually in the best interest of the dependent fetus. The majority of medications given by paramedics do not pose an unacceptable risk to a fetus. However, you must consider pregnancy risk implications whenever considering administration of medication to a potentially pregnant patient. Avoid medications known to cause harm to the fetus in all but the most extreme, life-threatening situations for the mother. In situations where there is a direct threat to the life of the patient, it is often necessary to administer a higher-risk medication to preserve the life of the mother, regardless of risk to the unborn child. Online medical control physicians can often provide guidance in these difficult situations. Most commercial reference sources provide the FDA pregnancy risk category for each medication. A medication's pregnancy risk category is listed within its medication monograph. Aspirin and certain benzodiazepines such as diazepam and midazolam are common prehospital medications known to cause fetal harm.

Special Populations

Treat every female of childbearing age as though she could be pregnant.

Psychosocial Factors. You should be aware of the role of psychosocial factors in the effectiveness of medications when they select and administer medications. Pain, anxiety, and overall discomfort can vary dramatically among individual patients with the same illness or injury. Unlike measurable vital signs and readily observable clinical findings, patient perceptions and responses to discomfort remain largely subjective. Psychological, cultural, emotional, and situational factors may influence the amount of discomfort reported by patients in relation to the underlying medical condition, patient positioning, environmental stressors, and the interventions you may perform during treatment. You should be alert to verbal and nonverbal cues when assessing for discomfort and administering medications for anxiety, pain, and sedation. Nonverbal cues may be indicated by vital sign changes, facial expression, posture and movement changes, altered respiratory patterns, tears or crying, and other behaviors. The cues provide potentially useful information about patient pain, anxiety, or discomfort but can have different meanings to different people, so interpretations of the cues should be confirmed with patients.

Medication administration is further complicated by the **placebo effect**. Numerous studies have demonstrated that patients experience measurable clinical improvement or have unexplained adverse effects after receiving a medication with no pharmacologic properties. Placebos were used commonly in 17th- and 18th-century medical practice, and use continued until the early 1900s. Pharmacologically inactive medications continue to be used by health care researchers to validate the efficacy or adverse effects of investigational medications by quantifying the placebo effect present in the particular study. The physiologic mechanism of the placebo effect remains under speculation. Pain relief from a placebo may be from endorphins released by the brain in anticipation of pain relief from the placebo. Adverse effects following placebo administration may somehow be linked to negative expectations or anxiety, but this mechanism remains uncertain. The efficacy of a placebo may be related to the timing of administration in relation to medications that are pharmacologically active.

It may be tempting to exploit the placebo effect by administering inactive substances to a patient as an alternative to pharmacologic treatment. This practice is demeaning to patients and may lead to discipline or criminal prosecution if the act involves the diversion of controlled substances. Placebo use by paramedics violates ethical principles, deceives patients, and undermines the credibility of the EMS profession.

▶ Types of Medication Responses

Every medication capable of a therapeutic benefit also has the potential for adverse or toxic effects at excessive doses. Even at appropriate doses, many medications produce harmful or undesired effects in susceptible people. You may prevent or minimize adverse effects by properly selecting the correct medication, route, dose, method of administration, and supportive treatment necessary for each patient.

Patient Safety

Many types of errors can occur in health care. Perhaps most notable are medication and prescription errors, but other, less common errors include wrong patient identification, transfusion errors, preventable suicides, falls, burns, wrong-sided procedures, and errors in transition of care or handoffs. Types of medical errors are listed in Table 13-7.

Therapeutic (Desired) Response

Pharmacologic interventions are based on a patient's actual or anticipated illness, injury, presenting complaint, sign, or symptom. This condition should match the use or indication listed on the profile for the specific medication. EMS agencies and organizations often formulate protocols that specify which medications should or can be administered in certain situations. Medical directors may authorize off-label uses (discussed earlier) for approved medications when this use reflects accepted medical practice. When protocols or guidelines do not seem appropriate for the needs of a patient, in many EMS systems you may

Table 13-7 Types of Medical Errors

Error Category	Specific Errors
Diagnostic	Error or delay in diagnosis Failure to employ indicated tests Use of outmoded tests or therapy Failure to act on results of monitoring or testing
Treatment	Error in the performance of an operation, procedure, or test Error in administering the treatment Error in the dose or method of using a drug Avoidable delay in treatment or in responding to an abnormal test Inappropriate care
Preventive	Failure to provide prophylactic treatment Inadequate monitoring or follow-up of treatment
Other	Failure of communication Equipment failure Other system failure

Data from: Kohn LT, Corrigan JM, Donaldson MS, eds. *To Err Is Human: Building a Safer Health System.* Washington, DC: National Academy Press; 2000.

be able to contact online medical control for advice or authorization for medication administration.

Medication is administered in a dose intended to produce a desired clinical response for the patient. This response may be complete resolution of the problem following a single dose of medication. In other cases, you may need to administer multiple doses of the same medication to obtain a desired response. Certain medications require frequent repeated dosing, careful titration, or continuous administration to obtain or maintain the desired response. These medications are capable of demonstrating **cumulative action**. Several smaller doses of a medication produce the same desired clinical effect as a larger, single dose of that same medication. This approach allows the same therapeutic benefit while decreasing any risks associated with administering too much of a medication by a single, larger dose. Not every medication or situation allows cumulative action. Many medications require a minimum threshold concentration to cause a clinical effect. Metabolism and elimination (discussed later) may remove medication molecules before the threshold concentration is reached if the doses are too small or infrequent. The clinical situation and medication choice determine which manner of medication administration is necessary or optimal.

Adverse Medication Effects

Adverse and toxic effects are important considerations during medication selection and administration. Pharmaceutical researchers and manufacturers attempt to

YOU are the Paramedic PART 2

Upon arrival, you are directed to the patient's room. The nursing staff report that she is normally awake, alert, and oriented; however, she was noted to be "not herself" over the past several hours and now looks much worse. The staff also report that the patient was admitted to the skilled nursing facility for complications of diabetes mellitus and was slowly improving until she developed nausea, vomiting, and diarrhea over the past 36 to 48 hours. The patient's temperature was 99.7°F (37.6°C) just prior to your arrival.

Recording Time: 0 Minutes	
Appearance	Pale skin
Level of consciousness	Decreased responsiveness, moaning and incoherent speech, eyes open to deep tactile stimuli
Airway	Patent
Breathing	Clear breath sounds, slightly diminished at bases bilaterally
Circulation	Normal pulse strength, slightly increased heart rate

2. Based on this brief history and physical examination, what problems do you suspect?
3. What additional information would assist you with identifying possible causes of her condition?

develop medications that target only specific receptor sites on particular types of cells. Unfortunately, the vast number of possible receptor sites within the body makes medications selective (rather than specific) at best. Even medications that bind with a limited group of receptor sites cause undesired responses in a variety of cells.

The term *side effect* is often used to mean *adverse effect*. Although both terms are usually used to mean harmful or potentially harmful effects, the term *adverse effect* more clearly indicates the possibility of serious consequences. Some side effects can be beneficial; for example, a physician may prescribe a specific antidepressant to treat postmenopausal symptoms, such as "hot flashes," because a positive side effect of the drug was identified. Also, a side effect of a medication can be desirable in certain situations and harmful in others. For example, benzodiazepines are used to treat seizure activity and are known to cause sedation. Sedation may be desirable for a combative patient with a head injury but could also jeopardize the life of the same patient if he or she is vomiting.

Various sources may also refer to adverse effects as **untoward effects**. Both adverse and untoward effects are clinical changes, caused by medication, that are not desired and that cause some degree of harm or discomfort to the patient.

Patient Safety

The process of a patient receiving a medication is complex and fraught with opportunities for error, including prescribing, dispensing, administering, and monitoring errors. The uncontrolled prehospital environment creates additional challenges for paramedics administering medications. In a recent study, approximately 9% of paramedics reported making a medication error within the previous 12 months.[8] The authors of the study noted that approximately 4% of these errors were not reported.[8]

Undesired or harmful responses to a medication may be directly related to the intended cellular response or to random activation of unrelated cells throughout the body. Examples of undesired or harmful responses include hypoglycemia after the administration of insulin (exaggerated "therapeutic" effect); profound bradycardia after taking metoprolol, a beta-adrenergic antagonist medication (exaggerated therapeutic effect); and an allergic reaction to a medication (not a therapeutic effect). Common adverse effects include nausea, vomiting, sedation, palpitations, hypotension, hypertension, bradycardia, tachycardia, respiratory depression, endocrine abnormalities, dizziness, and a variety of others. Medication reference sources often categorize adverse effects by body system, frequency of occurrence, or severity.

When selecting medications, consider possible adverse effects in relation to the patient's condition. For example, the respiratory depressant properties of opioid analgesics, such as morphine sulfate, are unlikely to adversely affect a patient with burns who is intubated and being mechanically ventilated; however, an immediate threat to life might result if morphine is given to a patient becoming fatigued during an asthma attack. Another example involves the choice between two or more medications that can be given for the same condition, such as ondansetron (Zofran) and promethazine (Phenergan), antiemetic medications. Promethazine causes significant hemodynamic and electrocardiographic changes that are not known to occur with ondansetron. Ondansetron may prove to be a safer antiemetic medication for patients who are particularly susceptible to adverse effects known to be associated with promethazine. In general, a medication should be avoided or used with caution in patients who are particularly susceptible to adverse effects associated with that medication.

Patients with certain chronic medical conditions are generally more susceptible to the adverse effects of medications than are patients without such conditions. Significant cardiovascular disease, diabetes, impaired immune function, and renal failure are more often associated with greater severity or frequency of adverse effects. Many adverse effects of medications directly relate to these conditions; for example, renal failure hinders the ability of the kidneys to eliminate medications properly. In addition, patients with respiratory distress, shock, multiple trauma, or other life-threatening conditions may be unable to tolerate even mild adverse effects. You must use caution when selecting medications for patients with these conditions. You also need to be alert for adverse effects once medications have been given.

Adverse effects may range in severity from barely perceptible by patients and paramedics to an immediately life-threatening condition, requiring aggressive intervention. Cardiomyopathy, a disease of the heart muscle, can be caused by certain antidepressant medications. Certain antibiotics and antiseizure medications are known to cause **Stevens-Johnson syndrome**, a severe, possibly fatal medication reaction that mimics a burn. A wide variety of medications are known to cause anemia (low RBC count) through bone marrow suppression or direct hemolysis.

Adverse effects occasionally occur that are completely unexpected and not previously known to occur with a particular medication. These effects are **idiosyncratic** medication reactions. Idiosyncratic medication reactions involve abnormal susceptibility to a medication, possibly due to genetic traits or dysfunction of a metabolic enzyme that is peculiar to an individual patient.

Therapeutic Index

Pharmaceutical companies and scientists evaluate the safety and effectiveness of a potential medication before it is made available to the public. Animal testing establishes the **median lethal dose (LD_{50})**, which is the weight-based dose of a medication that causes death in 50% of the animals tested. Manufacturers determine the **median toxic dose (TD_{50})** for a particular adverse effect of the medication, which means that 50% of the animals tested had toxic effects at or above this weight-based dose. Human or animal testing also reveals the **median effective dose (ED_{50})** for a particular use or indication of the medication. The relationship between the median effective dose and the median lethal dose or median toxic dose is known as the **therapeutic index**, or therapeutic ratio. If there is a large difference between the median effective dose and the median toxic dose or median lethal dose, the medication is considered safe or possibly even nontoxic. If the ratio is relatively small, careful patient selection, medication use, and monitoring of the medication are essential. A relatively unsafe medication may be used in clinical practice if it is the only choice available for an otherwise fatal medical condition.

Immune-Mediated Medication Response

Medications and substances present in the environment have the potential to trigger an exaggerated response from the body's immune system. This response is described generally as an allergic reaction. It can range from mild skin changes to a multisystem, life-threatening reaction. You may encounter patients with this condition who request EMS assistance or may encounter it immediately after medication administration to a patient being treated for an unrelated condition.

Patients who are genetically predisposed have an initial exposure and sensitization to a particular allergen. Various components of the body's immune system evolve into antibodies that specifically target this type of allergen. When the patient is reexposed to this type of allergen, a potentially massive cascade of immune system activity, known as **anaphylaxis**, begins. In severe cases, this reaction dramatically alters the function of the skin, GI, respiratory, and cardiovascular systems, ultimately manifesting as shock and respiratory failure. Chapter 25, *Immunologic Emergencies*, includes additional discussion of the pathophysiology and management of an immune-mediated medication response.

Patients predisposed to an allergic reaction, anaphylaxis, or other immune-mediated medication response may report previous reactions to medications, latex, foods, or other substances in the environment. Aspirin and antibiotics, most commonly penicillin and sulfa-based antibiotics, are the major culprits in immune-mediated medication responses. It is possible for a very small amount of any medication to cause this reaction. An immune-mediated reaction can occur days or weeks after initiating a medication.

Patients may also have **medication sensitivity** that is not related to an exaggerated immune system response. A mild to severe reaction may occur after the first exposure to a medication or other substance, often with many of the same signs and symptoms as an immune-mediated reaction. The treatment for medication sensitivity is similar to the treatment for an immune-mediated response. You should avoid administering medications to patients who have had a serious reaction to the specific medication (or a medication in the same class), unless the adverse effect was clearly dose-related and can be mitigated by judicious administration and careful monitoring.

Words of Wisdom

Do not be afraid to ask the same patient about allergies more than once if multiple medications are being administered.

Medication Tolerance

Certain medications are known to have decreased efficacy or potency when taken repeatedly by a patient, a state known as **tolerance**. Theories suggest that tolerance results from a mechanism reducing available cell receptors for a particular medication, a process known as **down-regulation**. The body also compensates for the effects associated with a medication by increasing the metabolism and/or elimination of the medication, resulting in a decreased concentration of the medication present near receptor sites. In certain cases, the desirable effects continue while other unintended or adverse effects decrease. In other situations, adverse effects persist or increase while additional medication is required to achieve the same therapeutic goal.

Repeated exposure to a medication within a particular class, such as opioids or benzodiazepines, can cause a tolerance to other medications in the same class. This phenomenon is known as **cross-tolerance**. Cross-tolerance becomes problematic when patients use or abuse medications, drugs, or chemicals on a regular basis and then require medications from that class for a legitimate medical purpose. It becomes extremely difficult to determine the appropriate dose for the patient, often resulting in inadequate or excessive doses of therapeutic medications.

A similar condition, known as **tachyphylaxis**, occurs with certain medications. Repeated doses of medication within a short time rapidly cause tolerance, making the medication virtually ineffective. Tachyphylaxis is prone to occur with certain sympathomimetic medications (discussed later) and may occur with other medications that you may administer, such as nitroglycerin and dobutamine.

Words of Wisdom

Consider patient tolerance, IV infiltration or disconnect, or possible medication tampering every time a controlled substance does not demonstrate the expected clinical effect.

Medication Abuse and Dependence

Certain classes of medications, along with similar groups of illicit chemicals, have serious potential for misuse and abuse. People may choose to experience many of the desirable clinical effects from medications or chemicals without the presence of an underlying medical condition or symptom. Patients who receive certain medications for legitimate medical conditions may continue to use these medications long after the legitimate medical condition has resolved. It is often difficult to determine whether an appropriate medical indication for certain medications continues to exist. You are almost certain to encounter patients who misuse or abuse medications, illicit drugs, and other chemicals.

Two distinct groups of medications and chemicals are prone to misuse and abuse: stimulants and depressants. **Stimulant** chemicals cause a transient increase in physical, mental, or emotional performance. Caffeine, cocaine, and amphetamines are stimulants that have serious potential for misuse or abuse. In general, these medications increase a person's level of alertness, increase the heart rate, increase blood pressure, and otherwise activate the sympathetic nervous system. The immediate or long-term effects of stimulant medications have the potential to become life threatening.

Depressant medications and chemicals, in contrast to stimulants, reduce CNS and sympathetic nervous system functioning, causing sedation, anxiolysis, respiratory depression, bradycardia, hypotension, and a variety of similar clinical symptoms. Benzodiazepines, alcohol, and opioid chemicals are common depressant substances. Toxicity from depressant substances is also potentially life threatening following acute or long-term exposure.

Repeated exposure to certain medications or chemicals causes a patient to experience **habituation**, the abnormal tolerance to adverse or therapeutic effects associated with a substance. In essence, the body adapts to accommodate the exposure and protect itself from the severity of clinical changes associated with a substance. Prolonged or significant exposure to depressants, stimulants, and other medications and chemicals can cause some degree of **dependence**. Dependence is the physical, emotional, or behavioral need for these substances to maintain a level of "normal" function. The person has adapted to the frequent presence of the substance. In absence of the substance, adverse clinical effects occur. In severe cases, abrupt withdrawal from a substance can precipitate life-threatening clinical changes.

Medication Interactions

Patients receiving multiple medications, drugs, or other chemicals are at risk of an unintended interaction between the various substances, possibly with unexpected results. Undesirable medication interactions are referred to as medication **interference**. You should consider the possibility of illicit drugs, over-the-counter and prescribed medications, and herbal remedies interacting with any medication that might be given to a patient. As patients are prescribed a greater number of medications to treat chronic medical conditions, the risk of a medication interaction increases dramatically.

The most obvious concern with medication interactions is incompatibility during administration. When given simultaneously through the same IV tubing, certain medications will change chemical composition, possibly creating solid particles in the tubing, which then travel into the patient. Other medication combinations will deactivate one or more of the medications, making them ineffective. Medications require the proper IV solution. Various medications can be mixed only in normal saline or dextrose-containing solutions. You should consult a reliable medication reference source before administering multiple medications, especially continuous medication infusions, through the same IV tubing. Sodium bicarbonate and furosemide are two medications used frequently in the prehospital setting that are incompatible with several other common prehospital medications.

It is possible for a medication to increase the effect, decrease the effect, or alter the effect of another medication within the body. Table 13-8 describes various types of medication interactions.

Table 13-8 Medication Interactions

Type of Interaction	Description	Example
Addition or summation	Two medications with a similar effect combine to produce an effect equal to the sum of the individual effect of each medication (eg, 1 + 1 = 2).	The antipyretic properties of acetaminophen (Tylenol) and the antipyretic properties of ibuprofen (Motrin, Advil) combine to reduce a fever in patients with fevers that could not be controlled by either medication alone.
Synergism	Two medications with a similar effect combine to produce an effect greater than the sum of the medications' effects.	Patients experience profound sedation when IV opioid medications such as fentanyl (Sublimaze) are given with IV benzodiazepines such as midazolam (Versed), greater than the expected sum of these two medications.

(continued)

Table 13-8 Medication Interactions *(Continued)*

Type of Interaction	Description	Example
Potentiation	The effect of one medication is greatly enhanced by the presence of another medication, which does not have the ability to produce the same effect.	Promethazine (Phenergan) is given to increase the effects of codeine or other antitussives (cough suppressants) for more improved relief of cough than is achieved with the antitussive alone.
Altered absorption	The action of one medication increases or decreases the ability of another medication to be absorbed by the body. For example, medications that increase or decrease the gastrointestinal pH or motility may increase or decrease the absorption of other medications that are taken orally.	Ranitidine (Zantac), an H_2 blocker, can reduce absorption of ketoconazole (an antifungal) or certain cephalosporin antibiotics.
Altered metabolism	The action of one medication increases or decreases the metabolism of another medication within the body. For example, many medications (and certain foods) alter the performance of the cytochrome P-450 system in the liver, which is responsible for the metabolism of a variety of other medications.	Fluconazole (Diflucan), an antifungal medication, inhibits the function of cytochrome P-450 enzyme CYP3A4, significantly increasing bleeding risks associated with warfarin (Coumadin), an anticoagulant medication.
Altered distribution	The presence of one medication alters the area available for the distribution of another medication in the body, which becomes important when both medications are bound to the same site, such as plasma proteins. If proteins are already occupied by one medication, toxic levels of the other medication may develop.	The anticonvulsant medication valproic acid (Depakote, Depakene) competes with another anticonvulsant medication, phenytoin (Dilantin), causing potentially increased or decreased serum levels and possibly unpredictable clinical effects.
Altered elimination	Medications may increase or decrease the functioning of the kidneys or other route of elimination, influencing the amount of or duration of effect of another medication in the body.	Ethanol decreases the metabolism of warfarin (Coumadin), which may predispose the patient to bleeding risk.
Physiologic (drug) antagonism	Two medications, each producing opposite effects, are present simultaneously, resulting in minimal or no clinical changes.	Sodium nitroprusside (Nipride) and dobutamine (Dobutrex) are often given simultaneously for cardiogenic shock. By itself, dobutamine increases cardiac output, possibly causing an elevated blood pressure. Sodium nitroprusside causes vasodilation and possibly hypotension. When given together, these medications can be titrated to maintain a normal patient blood pressure.
Neutralization	Two medications bind together in the body, creating an inactive substance.	Digoxin-specific antibodies (Digibind, Digifab) are administered to patients with toxicity to the medication digoxin. These medications combine, rendering digoxin molecules inactive.

Abbreviations: H_2, histamine-2 receptor antagonist; IV, intravenous

Data from: Schelleman H, Bilker WB, Brensinger CM, Han X, Kimmel SE, Hennessy S. Warfarin with fluoroquinolones, sulfonamides, or azole antifungals: interactions and the risk of hospitalization for gastrointestinal bleeding. *Clin Pharmacol Ther*. 2008 (Nov);84(5):581-588.

▶ Principles of Pharmacokinetics

You must carefully consider the pharmacokinetic properties of any medication you are considering administering to a patient. As a medication is administered, the body begins a complex process of moving the medication, possibly altering the structure of the medication and ultimately removing the medication from the body. The medication dose, route of administration, and clinical status of a patient will largely determine the duration and effectiveness of the medication (see the section *Principles of Pharmacodynamics*, earlier in this chapter). Actions of absorption, distribution, metabolism, and elimination are discussed in detail in the following text.

The pharmacokinetics section of medication profiles typically states the *onset*, *peak*, and *duration of effect* for most medications. These values vary by route of administration and may have a broad range, depending on characteristics of individual patients. The onset and peak of a medication are generally related to absorption and distribution. A minimum dose or concentration of medication must be present at certain sites in the body for clinical effects to occur (see the earlier section, *Principles of Pharmacodynamics*).

The duration of effect is generally related to medication metabolism and elimination. As the amount of a medication near cell receptors (or other site of action) decreases, the clinical effects caused by the medication begin to decrease and normal function resumes.

If a medication permanently binds with a receptor site or irreversibly alters the function of a cell, the duration of the medication is determined by the body's ability to regenerate cells. In these cases, the duration of effect of a medication may be almost entirely unrelated to the dose or concentration present in the body. A single dose of aspirin, for example, is rapidly eliminated by the body, usually within several hours, but can cause an inhibition of platelet activity lasting for 3 to 10 days.

Documentation & Communication

Communicating the time of onset and peak of a medication to the patient will build trust and credibility.

▶ Routes of Medication Administration

Absorption

Medication must enter the body to provide a clinical benefit. As such, it is essential for you to select a route of administration capable of delivering an appropriate amount of medication to the correct location within a patient's body. The route of administration is determined by the physical and chemical properties of the medication, the routes of administration available for a specific patient, and how quickly the effects of the medication are needed.

The chosen route of administration determines the percentage of the unchanged medication that reaches systemic circulation. This percentage, known as **bioavailability**, varies significantly from one medication to another, except when administered by the IV route. Medications administered by the IV route, by definition, have 100% bioavailability. Bioavailability is irrelevant for medications that are sequestered in the GI tract, such as activated charcoal and certain cathartic medications. Bioavailability is a critical consideration for other medications that are poorly absorbed by certain routes or subject to immediate metabolism by the liver before reaching systemic circulation. A number of important medication groups, such as beta-blockers and calcium channel blockers, have a relatively low bioavailability when taken orally. The IV doses of these medications are many times lower than the oral doses when given for the same indication. Lidocaine and fentanyl are generally not given orally because of their low bioavailability with this route. Various routes of administration available to paramedics are discussed in the following sections.

Oral, Orogastric Tube, and Nasogastric Tube

A large number of medications prescribed for chronic medical conditions and several important prehospital medications are administered into the GI system. Use of this route requires that a patient be responsive and able to swallow or have a nasogastric tube or an orogastric tube in place. Aspirin, antipyretic medications, activated charcoal, diphenhydramine, and oral glucose are prehospital medications that may be administered into the GI system. Once administered, medication absorption varies depending on several factors, as described in Table 13-9.

Table 13-9 GI Medication Absorption

Factor	Medication Absorption
GI motility	Ability of medication to pass through the GI tract into the bloodstream
GI pH	Perfusion of the GI system (may be decreased during systemic trauma or shock)
Presence of food, liquids, or chemicals in the stomach	Injury or bleeding in the GI system (both can alter GI motility, decreasing the time that oral medications can be absorbed)

Abbreviation: GI, gastrointestinal

In addition to these factors, GI medications may be subject to first-pass metabolism. Medication passes from the GI tract into the portal vein and travels directly into the liver. Once in the liver, metabolism occurs, altering and potentially inactivating the medication before it ever reaches systemic circulation. First-pass metabolism can be exploited if metabolism changes a previously inactive medication into an active medication. Codeine, for example, undergoes a significant **first-pass effect** and a portion of the medication can be converted to morphine, a more potent analgesic, by the liver. Metabolism of a medication may also occur within the GI tract and as the medication enters the bloodstream. Bioavailability of medications given orally or through a nasogastric or an orogastric tube can range from 5% to 100%, depending on the particular medication and the effect of first-pass metabolism. Several important cardiac medications such as metoprolol and verapamil are subject to significant first-pass metabolism when taken orally. The reduction in bioavailability due to first-pass hepatic metabolism is already calculated into oral dosing, explaining why the oral dose of these medications is significantly higher than the IV doses of these medications for the same purpose. Patients with hepatic (liver) dysfunction are at risk of toxicity of these medications when given orally, even at conventional doses, because first-pass effect is impaired and a greater quantity of this medication reaches systemic circulation.

Endotracheal

The endotracheal route is no longer considered a reliable method of medication administration. The ACLS protocols deemphasize the usefulness of medication administration via the endotracheal tube. If endotracheal medications must be given, sources recommend administering at least 2 to 2.5 times the IV dose for medications approved for this route, followed by a 5- to 10-mL flush with sterile water or normal saline.[9] With improved IO techniques and devices, it is likely that use of the endotracheal route of medication administration will become increasingly limited. You may still administer bronchodilators or mucolytic medications in certain critical care settings via the endotracheal route.

Intranasal

The intranasal route of medication administration seems to be gaining popularity in the prehospital setting. Liquid medications are converted into a fine mist that is sprayed into one or both nostrils. Fentanyl, midazolam, and naloxone can be administered using this route, often with effectiveness equal to or better than conventional methods. Medication absorption is rapid, and the bioavailability of intranasal medications appears close to 100% in certain studies. Other studies suggest that this method is superior to the IV and rectal routes of administration for a variety of reasons. Nasal medication administration can occur almost immediately, without delay for initiating an IV line, especially in situations where IV access is difficult or impossible to obtain. Additionally, nasal administration does not place you at risk for a needlestick injury when treating uncooperative patients.

Intravenous

The IV route remains the preferred method for the administration of the majority of medications used in the prehospital setting. A small-diameter catheter is inserted into a peripheral or external jugular vein, allowing medications to be administered directly into systemic circulation. In special situations, you may be permitted to use permanent indwelling venous catheters or large-bore catheters that have already been inserted into central veins by other health care professionals. The bioavailability of IV medication is 100% by definition. Medications administered by the IV route have an onset of action that is significantly quicker than the onset of medications given orally or through an orogastric or nasogastric tube, often allowing an immediate response or creating the ability to titrate a medication carefully in a rapidly evolving clinical situation.

There are several important limitations regarding the IV route of medication administration. Access is difficult in several noteworthy groups of patients: patients who have abused IV drugs, patients in profound shock or having cardiovascular collapse, and patients with certain chronic medical conditions such as diabetes and renal failure. The IV access procedure has the potential to cause pain or infection and is somewhat time consuming. Uncontrolled scenes, environmental extremes, and movement of the transport vehicle make IV access challenging in the prehospital setting. Establishing IV access is discussed further in Chapter 14, *Medication Administration*.

> **Words of Wisdom**
>
> Frequently reassess the IV site for infiltration or tubing disconnect during transport. Confirm that the IV is still working properly during patient turnover, especially if the medication being administered has a high potential to cause an adverse effect.

The infiltration of IV medication into tissues around the blood vessel is a significant concern for paramedics. Certain classes of medications such as **sympathomimetics** and electrolyte solutions can cause significant pain and tissue damage when they accumulate in surrounding tissues. In extreme cases, tissue death will occur in affected areas, leaving a large area of necrotic tissue or skin.

Intraosseous

The IO route of medication administration provides a viable alternative when IV access cannot be obtained in the prehospital setting. A needle is inserted through the

Table 13-10 Veins Used During IO Infusion

Intraosseous Site	Vein
Proximal tibia	Popliteal vein
Femur	Femoral vein
Distal tibia (medial malleolus)	Great saphenous vein
Proximal humerus	Axillary vein
Manubrium (sternum)	Internal mammary and azygos veins

Abbreviation: IO, intraosseous

patient's skin and into the bone. The tip of the needle pierces the hard, outer layer of bone and enters the softer bone marrow. Vascular uptake from the bone marrow provides a reliable route for medications and IV fluids Table 13-10. Chapter 14, *Medication Administration,* describes the technique for IO access in greater detail.

Any medication that can be administered by the IV route can also be administered by the IO route. Infusion rates for IO fluids are comparable to IV rates when a pressure bag or mechanical infusion device is used. The IO devices can generally be left in place for up to 24 hours, allowing a route of medication or fluid administration until IV access can be obtained.

Administration by the IO route is contraindicated in bones that are fractured. It is also discouraged when patients have various bone diseases or a skin infection over a possible insertion site. Newer devices allow IO insertion in a variety of anatomic locations and across the spectrum of patient age and weight.

Intramuscular

Various medications used in the prehospital setting can be administered by the intramuscular (IM) route. Sterile medication is drawn into a syringe attached to a needle and injected into one of the larger muscles of the patient. This route is used when IV access cannot be established or when the clinical situation requires immediate medication administration that cannot wait for IV access. Medications have a bioavailability from 75% to 100% following IM administration. The absorption rate is determined by the accuracy of the injection landmark and the perfusion to the chosen muscle.

You should use caution when performing an IM injection. Uncooperative patients may move suddenly, placing you or other responders at risk for a contaminated needlestick. Auto-injection devices, such as the EpiPen® and DuoDote Auto-Injector®, are commercially available, are spring-loaded, and deliver a predetermined quantity of medication. These devices usually do not retract the needle following administration, which means they do present the risk of a contaminated needlestick.

You should confirm that a medication is appropriate for IM use before administering it. Even if a medication is safe for IM use, medication reference sources may indicate that a particular muscle should be used or may recommend a particular technique for the injection. Many medications are safe for IV use but cause significant injury if given by the IM route. Certain medications are indicated only for IM use and cause a variety of complications if given by the IV route.

Subcutaneous

Subcutaneous medication administration is similar to IM administration. A sterile medication solution is drawn into a syringe attached to a needle. The medication is then injected into various subcutaneous tissue sites throughout the body. The anterior part of the abdomen, just outside the umbilicus, and the skin overlying the triceps muscle are common sites for subcutaneous injection. Compared to IM needles, the needles for subcutaneous administration are shorter and have a smaller diameter. Certain medications may be indicated for subcutaneous use only and should not be given by the IV route, even if a patent IV line is already in place. Slower absorption through the subcutaneous tissue may prevent adverse cardiovascular effects compared with IV administration of the medication. Consult advanced life support (ALS) protocols or a reliable medication reference for specific information about the subcutaneous administration of a medication. The techniques for subcutaneous and IM medication administration are discussed in greater detail in Chapter 14, *Medication Administration*.

Dermal and Transdermal

You may encounter patients in the prehospital setting who are receiving medication via the transdermal route. Patches commonly containing nicotine, antiemetics, analgesics, nitroglycerin, or other medications are placed in various locations on the body. Transdermal medications may alter a patient's clinical presentation or interfere with medications administered by a paramedic. It is often helpful to ask a patient or family member if a transdermal medication patch is in place while obtaining a medication history for the patient. Transdermal patches deliver a relatively constant dose of medication during a long period. Changes in patient temperature or perfusion may alter the delivery of medication to the patient, potentially causing significant clinical changes. Transdermal patches often contain a large quantity of medication. If these patches are chewed or ingested, particularly by children, life-threatening toxic effects are possible.

Sublingual

Nitroglycerin is frequently given to patients using the sublingual (SL) route of administration. Nitroglycerin tablets are placed under a patient's tongue or nitroglycerin is sprayed under the patient's tongue, where it is absorbed rapidly by the mucous membranes, resulting in a relatively quick onset. Bioavailability of nitroglycerin administered sublingually is quite low. Relatively large doses of SL nitroglycerin are required compared with an IV infusion, close to 100 times larger for initial dosing. Patients must be responsive and alert to receive SL medications. In addition, a lack of moisture or saliva in a patient's mouth may significantly delay the absorption of SL medications. In this case, the spray formulation is preferable over SL tablets. You may also encounter patients receiving certain analgesic medications by lozenges and other medications administered sublingually using lollipops, gums, and orally dissolving tablets.

Inhaled or Nebulized

The respiratory system is an extremely important route of medication administration for paramedics. In the prehospital setting, medications may be inhaled or nebulized into the respiratory tract. Inhaled prehospital medications are limited to oxygen and, possibly, the antidote, amyl nitrate, which is given in laboratory and industrial settings for cyanide exposure. You may also administer or assist patients administering respiratory medication using a metered-dose inhaler (MDI), typically for asthma or chronic obstructive pulmonary disease (COPD). Activation of the MDI converts liquid medicine into a gas, allowing the medication to pass into the patient's lungs. When used with a spacer, MDIs are at least as effective as nebulizers for the administration of bronchodilator medications.

Medication in liquid form may also be nebulized (converted into a fine spray) for administration directly into the respiratory system. Tubing with oxygen or compressed air is attached to a small chamber, creating a mist as the gas passes through the liquid medication. The chamber is attached to a mouthpiece or a mask, allowing patients to receive droplets of medication with each inspired breath. Unfortunately, a portion of the medication is lost during exhalation and during any pauses in patient respiration. Nebulized medications are typically administered for the treatment of bronchospasm or airway edema. Racemic epinephrine, albuterol, levalbuterol (Xopenex), and ipratropium bromide (Atrovent) are nebulized medications available in the prehospital setting. In some instances, you may be instructed to administer other medications by nebulizer. Calcium gluconate may be nebulized following inhalation exposure to hydrofluoric acid. Be aware that nebulized medications have the potential to cause bronchospasm. You should not routinely administer calcium, lidocaine, or other nontraditional medications by nebulizer without approval from medical control.

Rectal

Certain medications used in the prehospital setting may be administered via the rectal route. The rectal route is preferred over the oral route in several situations. The rectal route can be used when the patient is unresponsive, having seizures, vomiting, or unable to swallow oral medications. In addition, rectal medications are usually not subject to first-pass metabolism, which decreases the bioavailability of many oral medications. Certain medications administered rectally may have greater than 90% bioavailability. If a medication is administered into the proximal rectum, some first-pass effect is still possible. Medications administered into the lower rectum are less likely to have any dose reduction due to first-pass effect. Whenever possible, medications should be administered into the lower, rather than proximal, rectum.

Rectal medications are manufactured in suppository form, which is a waxlike substance molded into a shape similar to a bullet. The suppository is lubricated and inserted into the patient's rectal cavity. Antiemetics and antipyretic medications are often available in suppository form. Absorption of rectal medications can be unpredictable, often related to the specific site of absorption within the rectum. The rectal dose of a medication is often higher than is the oral or IV dose.

You may administer or assist with the administration of rectal diazepam for the emergency control of seizures, particularly in children. This method has been proven effective, with minimal risk of subsequent respiratory depression. You may administer the IV solution rectally, using a commercial device for this purpose, a lubricated feeding tube attached to a syringe, or a lubricated small-diameter syringe, such as a tuberculin syringe with the needle removed. (Never insert a needle into a patient's rectum; doing so may cause trauma, bleeding, or perforation into the abdominal cavity.)

Ophthalmic

EMS systems may approve the administration of medications by the ophthalmic route. In the prehospital setting, the ophthalmic route is generally limited to ocular **anesthetic** agents given to facilitate the irrigation of eyes following a chemical exposure. Although the role of ophthalmic medications in the prehospital setting is generally limited, you should be aware that it is possible for medications to cause systemic toxic effects following ophthalmic administration.

Other Methods of Medication Administration

Hemodialysis is one of the rare exceptions in which medications produce their beneficial effects outside the patient's body. Blood from a patient is pumped through a dialysis machine, exposing the blood to dialysate solution that removes toxins, excess electrolytes, and other chemicals from the blood before returning it to the patient. Paramedics working in the prehospital setting are unlikely to use this method.

You may encounter patients receiving medication through a variety of other routes. These methods are not generally used in the prehospital setting and may cause serious or life-threatening complications if used by untrained personnel. You should not use any unfamiliar catheters, lines, tubes, or other devices for medication or fluid administration unless you have received appropriate training and authorization.

Distribution of Medication

Chemical and physical properties of a medication determine how the medication moves through the body. Many medication factors such as the size of medication molecules, the ability to bind with other substances within the body, and the ability to dissolve in certain body fluids determine which cells, tissues, and organs a particular medication will reach. Individual patient factors such as fat, water, and protein content will also determine how much of a medication is available to cause physiologic changes at a given dose.

The human body has an elaborate system of barriers designed to prevent the introduction of foreign substances into the body and into specific cells, tissues, and organs. Medication molecules need to pass through various barriers to reach target sites within the body. To cross these barriers, medication molecules must move through spaces between individual cells or pass directly through the center of individual cells.

The process of **osmosis** is used to enhance the distribution of certain medications, electrolytes, and IV fluids. During osmosis, free water along with certain particles such as sodium and potassium can pass through a semipermeable membrane to equalize the concentration of the water and other particles on each side of the membrane. This process allows IV fluids to leave the intravascular space and enter various tissues and cells. Osmosis is also one of the mechanisms that the kidneys use to regulate the fluid balance within the body.

Filtration is a process within the body, similar to osmosis, that is used to redistribute water and other particles. Most discussion of filtration within the body focuses on renal sodium and water filtration in the glomerular capillaries. Hydrostatic pressure forces various body fluids against semipermeable membranes, causing the passage of certain substances into an adjacent compartment.

The skin, GI tract, eyes, and urinary tract contain epithelial cells that create a continuous barrier. This barrier prevents the movement of medication molecules between the epithelial cells. For medications to cross the epithelial barrier, the medication molecules must pass directly through cells to enter the body. Small medication molecules that are **nonionic** (uncharged) and **lipophilic** (attracted to fats and lipids) pass easily through cell membranes. All but the largest lipid-soluble medications can pass easily through cell membranes.

Larger, **hydrophilic** (attracted to water molecules) and ionic (charged) medication molecules must find another route of entry into cells. For larger medication molecules, cells use a process called **pinocytosis** to ingest extracellular fluids and their contents. Medication molecules may also bind with carrier proteins for transport into cells. This process of binding with carrier proteins is called **facilitated diffusion** when no energy is expended and is called **active transport** when energy is used to move the molecules against a concentration gradient.

In addition to the epithelial barrier, the human body has capillary barriers near specific tissues. Once inside blood vessels, medication molecules must pass through capillary walls to reach target cells or other sites. The blood-brain barrier, the blood-placenta barrier, and the blood-testes barrier are areas where capillary cells form a continuous barrier, preventing the passage of medication molecules through openings in capillary walls. These three anatomic barriers prevent various medication molecules from reaching underlying tissues. Only certain medications are able to pass through cell membranes in these areas and enter adjacent tissues.

Capillaries in the kidney, thyroid, pancreas, and other areas allow medication molecules to pass freely through the capillary walls into surrounding tissues. Only protein-bound medications have difficulty passing through the capillaries in these areas. The lungs and peritoneum also permit medication molecules to enter and exit easily through capillary walls.

Plasma protein binding significantly alters the distribution of certain medications within the body. Medication molecules temporarily attach to proteins in the blood plasma. Albumin and other plasma proteins effectively store a quantity of medication largely independent of the concentration of the medication present in the blood or other body tissues. Patient age, nutritional status, and medical condition influence the amount of plasma protein present in the body. As plasma protein levels change or when another medication that binds with plasma proteins is introduced, the concentration of the original medication in blood and body tissues may change significantly.

Protein binding increases the amount of medication necessary for a desired clinical effect. This reversible process also releases medication as circulating levels of a particular medication begin to fall, leading to a longer duration of action for the medication. It is possible for a patient to have a therapeutic (safe) level of a protein-bound medication until a second protein-bound medication with greater affinity is administered. The second medication displaces the original medication attached to plasma proteins, causing a dramatic increase in the amount of the original medication present in circulation and subsequent toxic effects.

Fat tissue is another site of medication distribution that alters the amount of medication available for action within the body. Large quantities of lipophilic medications can be sequestered in the fat tissues of people with obesity. The medication is released slowly, causing prolonged effects compared with the same dose in people with a lean body composition. As the percentage of body fat increases, the same weight-based dose of a hydrophilic medication results in a higher concentration in the plasma and water throughout the body.

▶ Volume of Distribution

The **volume of distribution** for a medication describes the extent to which a medication will spread within the body. Certain medications do not readily leave the plasma. Other medications spread into water throughout the body. Still other medications readily bind with bone, teeth, or other tissues, resulting in a relatively low concentration in the blood. The volume of distribution relates medication dose to the anticipated plasma level of a given medication in an "average" patient. Medications with a lower volume of distribution have higher levels present in the plasma at a given dose than do medications with a higher volume of distribution. In the alternative, if a medication has a high volume of distribution, a larger total dose is needed to obtain a certain level in the plasma than with a medication with a lower volume of distribution. It is also possible to estimate the amount of a medication or chemical present in the body by knowing the level of the medication present in the plasma and the known volume of distribution for a particular medication. This value may help explain why a large dose of additional medication may cause only a modest increase of available medication.

▶ Medication Metabolism

Many medications undergo some degree of chemical change by the body, known as biotransformation. As a medication undergoes biotransformation, it becomes known as a metabolite. Metabolites can be either active or inactive. **Active metabolites** remain capable of some pharmacologic activity, such as altering a cell process or body function. It is possible for active metabolites to go from helpful or therapeutic to harmful. **Inactive metabolites**, however, no longer possess the ability to alter a cell process or body function. Biotransformation has four possible effects on a medication absorbed into the body:

1. An inactive substance can become active, capable of producing desired or unwanted clinical effects (active metabolite).
2. An active medication can be changed into another active medication (active metabolite).
3. An active medication can be completely or partially inactivated (inactive metabolite).
4. A medication can be transformed into a substance (active or inactive metabolite) that is easier for the body to eliminate.

Most biotransformation occurs in the liver. The cytochrome P-450 system in the liver uses a complex, enzyme-based process to alter the chemical structure of a medication or other chemical. Separate pathways within the cytochrome P-450 system are responsible for the metabolism of different medication groups. These pathways can be selectively influenced by other medications, chemicals, and diet choices, altering the metabolism of certain groups of medications. Ethanol, oral contraceptives, and grapefruit juice are known to cause potentially

YOU are the Paramedic — PART 3

You give the patient oxygen via a nonrebreathing mask; however, the patient resists keeping the mask in place. One of the staff nurses assists with providing oxygen to the patient while you establish IV access by placing an 18-gauge catheter into the patient's right antecubital space and obtain a blood glucose level. Your partner obtains vital signs and places the patient on the cardiac monitor.

Recording Time: 10 Minutes	
Respirations	22 breaths/min
Pulse	108 beats/min, regular
Skin	Pale, warm, dry
Blood pressure	96/64 mm Hg
Oxygen saturation (Spo_2)	98% on 10 L/min oxygen via nonrebreathing mask
Blood glucose level	132 mg/dL
ECG	Sinus tachycardia with motion artifact

4. Would intravenous dextrose solution be indicated for this patient?
5. Do the electrocardiogram (ECG) findings assist in identifying the cause of this patient's condition?

life-threatening alterations in the cytochrome P-450 metabolism of certain medications.

The kidneys, skin, lungs, GI tract, and many other body tissues have some ability to cause biotransformation as well. Microorganisms present in the GI tract begin biotransformation of certain medications taken orally. In general, biotransformation makes medications and chemicals more water-soluble and easier for the kidneys and other organs to eliminate from the body. You should suspect altered metabolism of medications in patients with chronic alcoholism, liver disease, or any condition known to affect the liver.

Medication Elimination

Medications and other chemicals are primarily removed from the body by the kidneys. The original medication or its metabolite (the chemical produced following biotransformation) is filtered by the kidneys and excreted into the urine. A variety of factors influences how quickly medication is eliminated from the body. Kidney dysfunction or disease impairs elimination of many substances. Patients with acute or chronic renal failure are at significant risk for toxic effects of medications or metabolic waste products in the body. Renal blood flow, urinary tract obstruction, and alterations in the pH of urine affect the ability of the kidneys to remove medication and toxins from the body.

Medications and chemicals in the body follow two distinct patterns of metabolism and elimination: zero-order elimination and first-order elimination. Under **zero-order elimination**, a fixed amount of a substance is removed during a certain period, regardless of the total amount in the body. Ethanol is a classic example of zero-order elimination. Chronic consumption of ethanol increases the liver's ability to metabolize ethanol because of enhanced activation of the cytochrome P-450 system. Despite the increased rate of elimination, only a fixed amount of ethanol will be eliminated each hour, regardless of initial plasma levels. The duration of intoxication is directly related to the initial plasma level.

The majority of medications and chemicals undergo **first-order elimination**. The rate of elimination is directly influenced by the plasma levels of the substance. In essence, the more substance in the plasma, the more the body works to eliminate the substance. First-order elimination is quantified as a medication **half-life** on the medication profile. The half-life of a medication is the time needed in an average person for metabolism or elimination of 50% of the substance in the plasma. It takes much longer than two half-lives to eliminate a medication completely, despite the literal connotation of the term. A medication half-life is altered by factors such as disease states, changes in perfusion, and medication interactions. Consider the following example of half-life calculations:

Patient A has taken an overdose of medication X, which has a half-life of 2 hours. The plasma level of the medication on arrival to the emergency department was 100 mcg/mL. After 2 hours, the plasma level will be 50 mcg/mL. Four hours after arrival, the plasma level will be 25 mcg/mL. After another 2 hours, the plasma level will be 12.5 mcg/mL.

A medication half-life pertains only to the quantity of medication within the body, not necessarily to the clinical effects of the medication. Aspirin, as discussed earlier, has a half-life of only 15 to 20 minutes, but it causes antiplatelet effects that last for 3 to 10 days. Adenosine, a medication given in the prehospital setting for dysrhythmias, has a half-life of less than 10 seconds, but it may permanently resolve supraventricular tachycardia. The benzodiazepine clonazepam (Klonopin) has a long half-life—19 to 50 hours in adults. Patients often remain sedated for several days following an intentional overdose.

Physicians and other health care providers attempt to create a steady state of certain medications. Medications are administered at a dose and frequency that equals the body's rate of elimination, resulting in a constant level of medication within the body. A medication steady state is desirable for anticoagulants, antibiotics, antiseizure medications, and certain antidysrhythmic medications. You should suspect alterations in the steady state of a medication when patients manifest symptoms of an underlying disease (such as seizures or a dysrhythmia) that is usually well controlled by long-term medications.

Smaller amounts of medication can be eliminated through other body systems. Medication, medication metabolites, and other chemicals can be eliminated in expired air from the lungs, stool, saliva, breast milk, and perspiration. When given orally, activated charcoal is capable of binding with certain oral toxins (and several chemicals present in the bloodstream) and eliminating them through the GI tract. (Activated charcoal is discussed further in Chapter 27, *Toxicology*.)

Reducing Medication Errors

As a paramedic, you will have the difficult tasks of assessing patients, performing invasive procedures, and administering medications in the uncontrolled prehospital setting. In this environment, patient history is often limited, inaccurate, or nonexistent. You will not always have the time or resources for a careful evaluation of the risks and benefits associated with medications that you are considering administering to a patient. Medication decisions are often based on memory and frequently occur in the context of a stressful, life-threatening patient situation. You and other paramedics are constantly at risk for a cognitive error, such as choosing the wrong medication or dose, or a technical error, such as administering a greater volume of medication than was intended. Table 13-11 lists the 10 rights of medication administration.

Patient safety experts strongly recommend using specific practices to decrease the likelihood of medication

Table 13-11 The 10 Rights of Medication Administration
1. Right Patient
Although you will typically treat one patient at a time, sometimes you may have to manage multiple patients. It is essential to confirm the identity of a patient before administering any medication—especially when patients are unresponsive or are unable to communicate (because of extremes of age, altered level of consciousness, or other factors). Always make an attempt to have the patient confirm his or her identity verbally, or confirm the identity of the patient yourself through identification devices (such as bracelets or ID cards), to the extent possible. A critical issue, as identified in the SAMPLE (Signs/symptoms, Allergies, Medications, Pertinent past history, Last oral intake, Events leading to injury or illness) history, is to ensure that the patient does not have allergies to the medication(s) you intend to give Figure 13-3 .
2. Right Medication
Administration of the wrong medication is the most common pharmacology-related error. Several factors may lead to "wrong medication" errors, including similar packaging and labeling, similar names and storage practices, and ineffective communication. Always repeat (echo) the medication order, and confirm that the packaging matches the intended order. Avoid using abbreviations, and always recheck the order before administration.
3. Right Dose
Doses of nearly every medication depend on patient-specific factors (such as condition, weight, and age). The actual dose needed is often not equal to the amount supplied in an ampule or a prefilled syringe in the prehospital setting. Therefore, you will have to calculate the patient-specific dose. When calculating the correct dose, always recheck your math, and, if possible, have your partner recheck and verify the final dose.
4. Right Route
Many medications can be administered by a variety of routes; the optimal route depends on the patient's condition and the speed with which the medication needs to take effect. Errors can occur when medication doses and routes are confused. For example, IV drip doses can be different from doses for the same medication injected into an IV as a bolus. Another important route-related issue is the patient's condition. If a patient is in profound shock, you must consider how well the medication will be absorbed and distributed to target tissues. Choosing the right route helps enable the medication to have the correct effect. Always verify the route of administration.
5. Right Time
Because all medications take a certain amount of time to take effect and may have the potential to interfere with other medications, you must always follow the recommended guidelines for the proper frequency of medication administration. Evaluate the patient's condition before and after you administer any medication, and document any noted response or change in the patient's condition. Also remember that some medications require a specific administration frequency to maintain a therapeutic level.
6. Right Documentation and Reporting
Because paramedics almost always transfer care of a patient to other health care providers, it is critical to document in writing the medications administered, the dose, when they were administered, and the effects the patient experienced. Whenever possible, communicate this information in writing (on the patient care report) and in a verbal report to the next level of care.
7. Right Assessment
Confirm indications and contraindications. Ensure that the medication is appropriate for the patient's medical condition and medical history.
8. Right to Refuse
Respect patient autonomy. Patients with decision-making capacity or a surrogate decision maker may refuse medications and other interventions, even if refusing a medication may result in harm. Consult online medical control in any high-risk situation. Make sure the patient is aware of the potential consequences of refusing a medication or treatment.

9. Right Evaluation
Continually monitor your patient. Observe for desired effects and any possible adverse reactions for any medication administered. Certain medications may require careful monitoring; other medications may require multiple doses to achieve the desired effect.
10. Right Patient Education
Patient education should begin as soon as possible. Responsive patients should be informed of any pertinent risks and benefits prior to medication administration. Involve responsive patients in ongoing evaluation and monitoring by informing them of any important symptoms they may experience or that should be reported.

Abbreviation: IV, intravenous

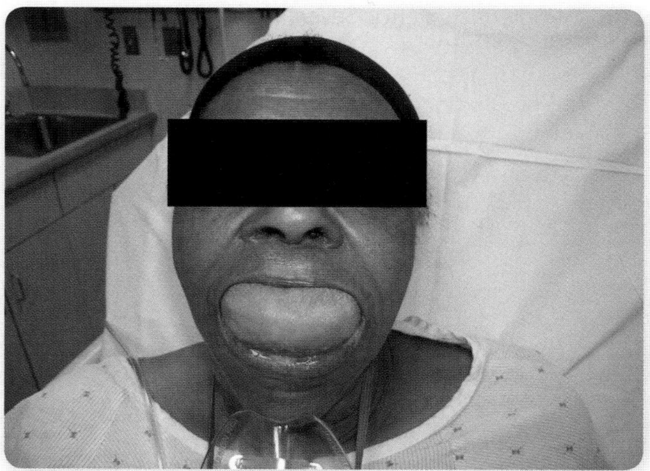

Figure 13-3 Angioedema is acute swelling, sometimes of the lips and tongue, that may be caused by an allergic reaction. Some medications cause angioedema after the first or second dose.

errors. Perform a verbal read-back of any orders received from online medical control. The read-back should include the medication, dose, and route. When multiple providers are present, call out the medication name and dose prior to administration. Both of these practices allow your colleagues the opportunity to catch potential medication errors before they reach the patient.

Unlabeled syringes pose a significant hazard in health care. Many medications are supplied in vials, requiring that providers draw the medication into a syringe. Because most injectable medications are supplied as a clear liquid, and because even the same medication may be supplied in different concentrations, a medication drawn into a syringe may present no identifying characteristics. Whenever possible, paramedics should use premade stickers or hand-written labels that indicate at least the medication's name and concentration, even if the medication is intended to be administered immediately. In EMS, workflow is frequently disrupted, which may result in the presence of several syringes on the scene. In addition, there may be delays between when a medication is drawn into a syringe and when it is administered to the patient.

Patient safety experts recommend building an environment in which EMS providers feel comfortable reporting errors (and near misses). In these environments, errors are identified/disclosed and evaluated, and system changes are implemented to prevent future occurrences. In this type of environment, often referred to as a "just culture," the focus is on improving systems rather than seeking to punish individuals.

Paramedics are encouraged to bring a patient's home medications when transporting the patient to a health care facility. Having the medications on hand allows the receiving health care providers to accurately transcribe the various medications, doses, frequency, and other pertinent information, rather than rely on the patient's memory or notes from EMS personnel.

You should use a current, reliable medication reference source whenever administering potentially unfamiliar medications or whenever considering an unusual dose or route of administration. Technical errors can be avoided by having a partner confirm the volume in a syringe or a weight-based medication calculation. Many health care settings require that two providers check pediatric and high-risk medication calculations. You should also evaluate for a patient medication allergy or hypersensitivity before each medication administration.

The Institute for Safe Medication Practices has developed a list of medication abbreviations prone to causing errors. When physicians, paramedics, and other health care providers use these symbols and abbreviations, there is an increased likelihood of a medication error due to miscommunication. The full list is exhaustive. Table 13-12 lists several important sources of error relevant to the prehospital setting.

Drugs That Act on the Sympathetic Nervous System

As discussed earlier, receptor sites exist in proteins connected to cells throughout the body. Receptors are activated by chemicals, whether naturally occurring or in the form

Table 13-12 Examples of Errors and Misinterpretations in Reporting

Error Source	Intended Meaning	Possible Misinterpretation	Correction
Trailing zero after the decimal point (eg, 4.0 mg)	4 mg	40 mg	Avoid trailing zeros when the decimal place is not needed.
No leading zero before decimal point (eg, .8 mg)	0.8 mg	8 mg	Use a zero before the decimal point when the dose is less than 1 unit.
MSO_4	Morphine sulfate	Magnesium sulfate	Write out "morphine sulfate."
$MgSO_4$	Magnesium sulfate	Morphine sulfate	Write out "magnesium sulfate."
SC	Subcutaneous	SL (sublingual)	Write out "subcutaneous."
IN	Intranasal	IV (intravenous) or IM (intramuscular)	Write out "intranasal."

Table 13-13 Responses to Stimulation of the Sympathetic Nervous System

Organ	Sympathetic Stimulation	Receptor Type
Heart	Increased heart rate (positive chronotropic effect) Increased force of contraction (positive inotropic effect) Increased conduction velocity (positive dromotropic effect)	Beta-1 (mnemonic: one heart = beta-1)
Arteries	Constriction	Alpha
Lungs	Bronchial muscle relaxation	Beta-2 (mnemonic: two lungs = beta-2)

of a medication. Drugs that influence the sympathetic nervous system are classified according to the receptors with which they interact.

A drug receptor is analogous to the ignition switch in a car. When the proper key is inserted into the car's ignition and turned, a predictable sequence of events follows: the battery sends a current to the starter and the spark plugs, which fire; combustion of gasoline and air occurs; and the engine starts. Although many keys may fit into a specific car's ignition, not every key that fits will turn and start the car—but all that do turn cause the same reaction. Likewise, the organs of the body have a number of "ignition switches." In the sympathetic nervous system, those switches (receptors), are labeled alpha and beta. Whenever one of those switches is activated by a "key" (a drug or hormone), a predictable sequence of responses occurs Table 13-13.

The heart has only one ignition switch for a beta agent. Any beta agent will have the same effect on the heart: it will increase the heart's rate, force, and **automaticity** (generation of a spontaneous impulse from within). The arteries, by contrast, have receptors for alpha and beta agents. An alpha drug will turn on the switch that causes **vasoconstriction**; a beta agent will activate the switch that causes **vasodilation**. Similarly, the lungs have alpha and beta receptors. Alpha agents do not have much effect on the lungs; at most, they cause minor **bronchoconstriction**. By contrast, beta adrenergic agonists (such as drugs used to treat asthma) trigger significant **bronchodilation**. Figure 13-4 represents these concepts schematically.

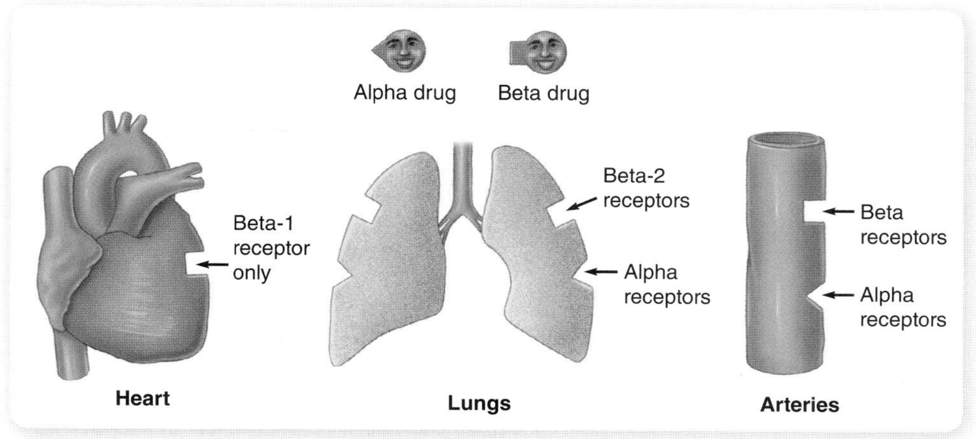

Figure 13-4 Receptor sites of the sympathetic nervous system in the heart, lungs, and arteries.

Drugs that have alpha or beta sympathetic properties are called sympathomimetic drugs because they imitate (mimic) the actions of naturally occurring sympathetic chemicals. If you know whether a sympathomimetic drug is an alpha or a beta agent, you can predict the response by the heart, lungs, and arteries. Consider, for example, isoproterenol (Isuprel). It is a pure beta agent. Armed with this knowledge, you can immediately recognize that isoproterenol acts in the manner shown in Figure 13-5; it stimulates the heart, dilates the bronchi, and dilates the arteries. Phenylephrine (Neo-Synephrine), by contrast, is a pure alpha agent. It has no direct effect on the heart but causes slight bronchoconstriction and marked vasoconstriction Figure 13-6.

Unfortunately, predicting the effects of a drug is not always so simple. Although isoproterenol and phenylephrine are pure beta and alpha agents, respectively, most other sympathomimetic drugs have varying degrees of alpha and beta activity Figure 13-7. Norepinephrine (Levophed) is chiefly an alpha agent, and its alpha effects predominate; because it also has some beta activity, however, it will have effects on the heart. Conversely, epinephrine (Adrenalin) is chiefly a beta agent, and its beta effects predominate; nevertheless, when administered in high doses, epinephrine will produce some alpha effects, especially on the arteries.

Table 13-14 lists several sympathomimetic agents that are commonly encountered in the field. Two of the drugs, norepinephrine and epinephrine, are also naturally occurring chemicals of the sympathetic nervous system. Their actions are the same whether they are produced in the body and released from the nervous system or manufactured in a factory and injected.

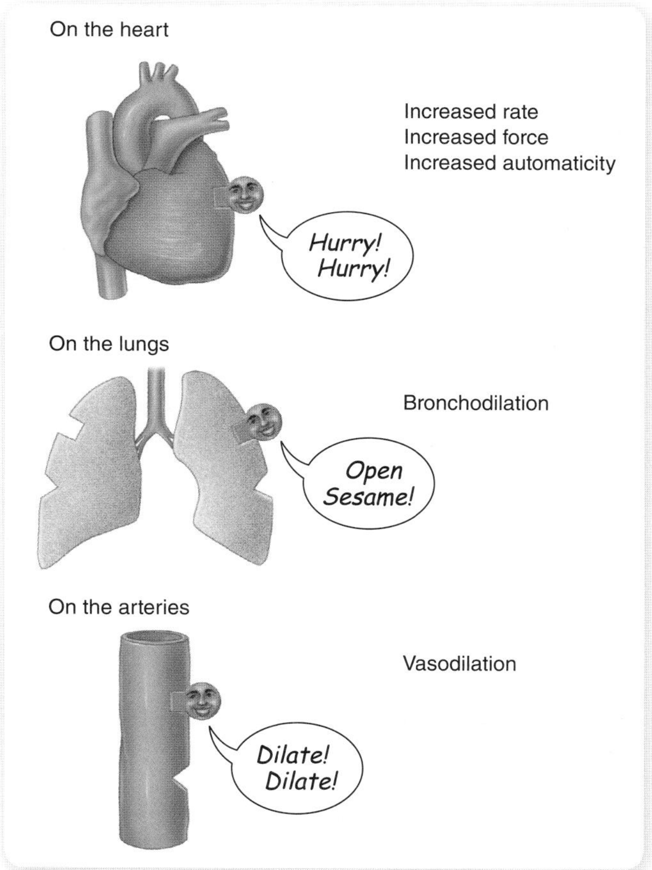

Figure 13-5 Beta sympathetic agents increase the rate, force, and automaticity of the heart; dilate the bronchi; and dilate peripheral arteries.

Beta sympathetic agents can be classified into two groups based on the subtle differences between the beta receptors in the heart and the lungs. Drugs that act primarily on cardiac beta receptors are called beta-1 adrenergic agonists; those that act chiefly on pulmonary beta receptors are called beta-2 adrenergic agonists. Commonly prescribed bronchodilators (beta-2 adrenergic agonists) include albuterol, formoterol, salbuterol, levalbuterol, and salmeterol.

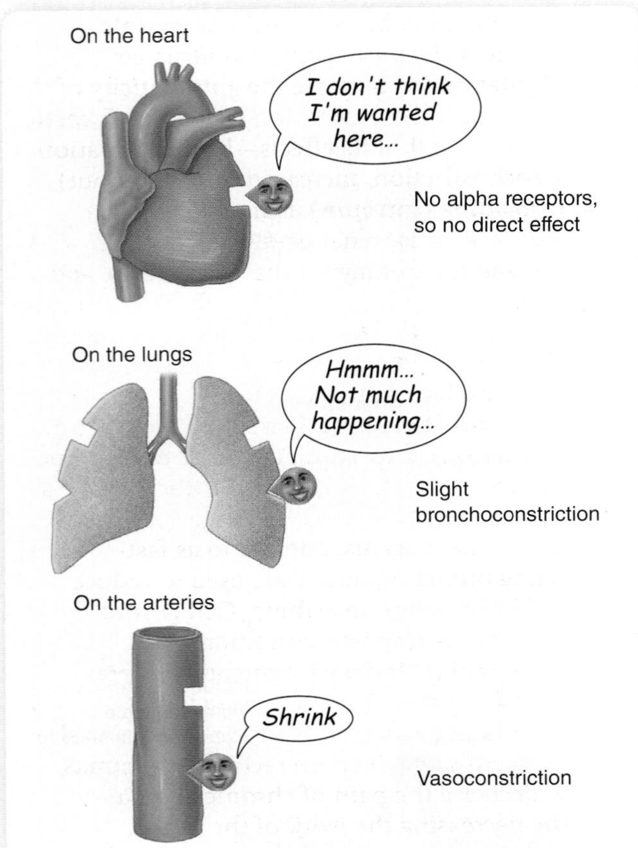

Figure 13-6 Alpha agents have no direct effect on the heart; they cause slight bronchoconstriction and marked vasoconstriction.

Alpha — Beta

Phenylephrine Norepinephrine Epinephrine Isoproterenol

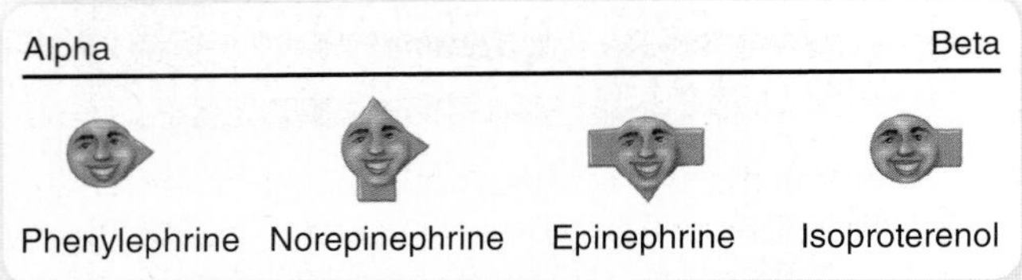

Figure 13-7 Many sympathomimetic agents have both alpha and beta properties.

Words of Wisdom

To remember which type of adrenergic agonist (beta-1 or beta-2) acts on which type of beta receptor, ask yourself, "How many hearts do I have?" One heart—beta-1. "How many lungs do I have?" Two lungs—beta-2.

Another class of drugs that acts on the sympathetic nervous system comprises the sympatholytic or sympathetic blockers. As their name implies, they block the action of sympathetic agents by beating them to the receptor sites and preventing these agents from turning on the ignition. The receptor sites cannot distinguish a blocker from a stimulator until it is too late. With the blocker occupying the receptor site, the stimulating agent cannot get in to turn on the switch **Figure 13-8**.

Beta adrenergic blockers occupy beta receptors in the heart, lungs, and arteries, and elsewhere in the body. Thus beta agents, whether released from sympathetic nerve endings or given intravenously, cannot exert their full effects when a beta-blocker such as propranolol (Inderal) or metoprolol has been administered previously **Figure 13-9**.

The indications for the major autonomic stimulating and blocking agents can be deduced once you know the

Table 13-14 Common Sympathomimetic Agents

Receptor	Agent
Alpha	Phenylephrine (Neo-Synephrine) Norepinephrine bitartrate (Levophed)
Alpha or beta, depending on dose	Dopamine
Beta	Epinephrine Albuterol (Proventil; beta-2–specific) Isoproterenol (Isuprel; pure beta-specific)

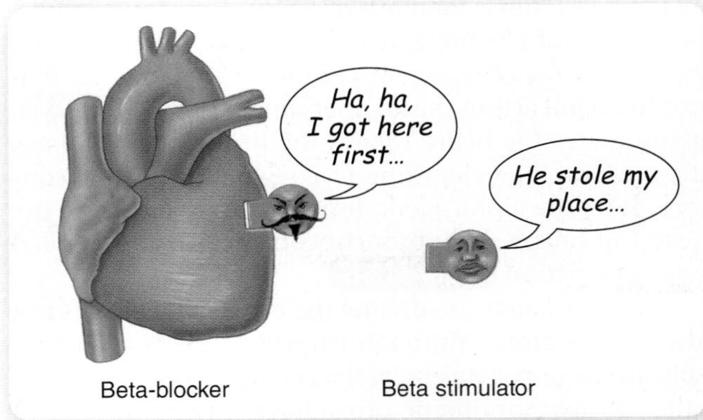

Figure 13-8 A sympathetic blocker occupies the receptor site for the stimulating drug, thereby preventing the stimulating drug from exerting its usual effect.

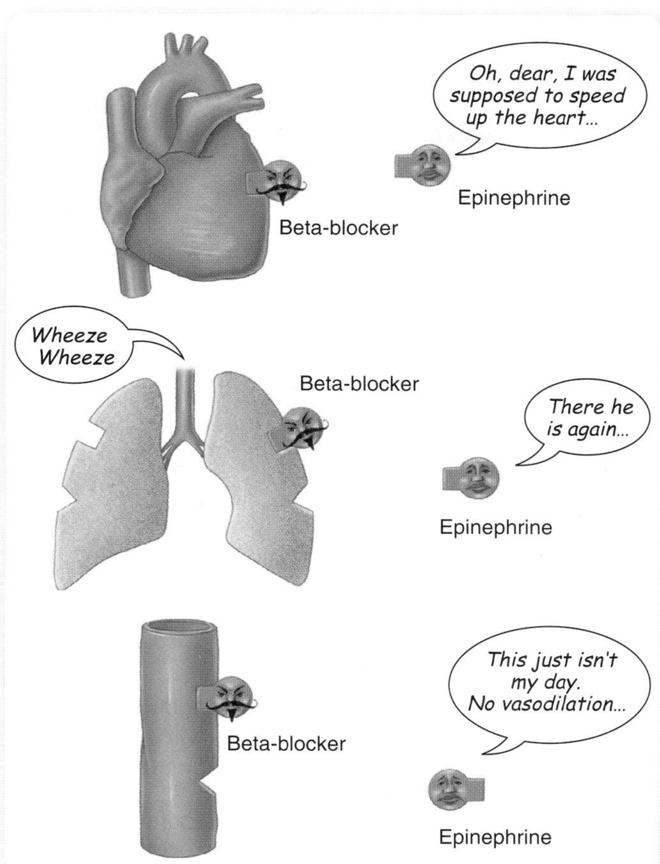

Figure 13-9 By occupying beta receptor sites, the beta-blocker prevents epinephrine from exerting its usual effects on the heart, lungs, and blood vessels.

properties of the drugs and the manner in which they interact with the autonomic nervous system:

- **Atropine.** Parasympathetic blocker, opposing the vagus nerve. It is used to speed the heart when excessive vagal firing has caused bradycardia.
- **Norepinephrine (Levophed).** Sympathetic agent (primarily alpha), causing vasoconstriction. It is used to increase the blood pressure when hypotension is caused by vasodilation (as in neurogenic shock).
- **Isoproterenol (Isuprel, Medihaler-Iso).** Sympathetic agent (almost pure beta), causing a strong increase in the heart rate and dilation of the bronchi. It is used in extreme cases to increase cardiac output and to dilate bronchi in asthma.
- **Epinephrine (Adrenalin).** Sympathetic agent (predominantly beta), with actions similar to those of isoproterenol, but having an additional, primarily peripheral vasoconstrictor effect. Indications for epinephrine are similar to those for isoproterenol, but also include asystole, pulseless electrical activity, ventricular fibrillation (to increase the automaticity of the heart and vasoconstriction), and anaphylactic shock (for all of its effects—bronchodilation, vasoconstriction, increased cardiac output).
- **Dopamine (Intropin).** Sympathetic agent, used to increase renal perfusion, increase rate and force of myocardial contraction, and constrict peripheral blood vessels. Dopamine is a unique medication because it causes different physiologic effects at different dosages, as discussed later in this chapter.
- **Albuterol (Proventil, Ventolin), isoetharine (Bronkosol, Bronkometer), and terbutaline (Brethine, Bricanyl, Brethaire, Terbulin).** Sympathetic beta-2 agents that act on the lungs. These agents, referred to as fast-acting bronchodilators, are used to induce bronchodilation in asthma, COPD, and other bronchospastic conditions.
- **Propranolol (Inderal).** Sympathetic beta-blocker, opposing the actions of beta-stimulating agents. It is used clinically to slow the heart rate in certain tachydysrhythmias, to decrease the pain of chronic angina (by decreasing the work of the heart), and to depress irritability in the heart (by decreasing the tendency of the heart to fire automatically). Its use is contraindicated in asthma.

Important Medications in the Prehospital Setting

It is essential that you understand the indications and limitations of several important groups of medications. The following sections contain an overview of medications and medication groups used to treat medical conditions primarily affecting certain body systems. Many medication groups have indications for a wide range of medical conditions, including outside the context of a particular body system Table 13-15.

▶ Medications Used in Airway Management

In certain EMS systems you may be permitted to use a variety of medications for airway management. Rapid-sequence intubation and medication-facilitated airway placement are controversial procedures in the prehospital setting and are not permitted in all locations. When these procedures are performed, various sedative medications with or without chemical paralytic medications are used to secure an artificial airway in patients with an intact gag reflex and some degree of responsiveness. Patients become adequately

Table 13-15 Notable Medication Groups Affecting Prehospital Patient Care

Medication Class	Common Indications or Purposes	Primary Body System Affected	Examples
Alkalinizing agents	Increase serum or urine pH	Renal	Sodium bicarbonate
Alkylating agents	Group of cancer medications that attack the DNA of cancer cells, causing cell death	Varied	Cisplatin, cyclophosphamide (Cytoxan), ifosfamide (Ifex)
Antacids	Neutralize excess acids present in the stomach	GI	Sucralfate (Carafate), aluminum salts, calcium carbonate
Anthelmintics	Treat intestinal parasites	GI	Mebendazole (Vermox)
Antibiotics	Treat bacterial infection	Varied	Penicillin, ciprofloxacin (Cipro)
Anticoagulants	Reduce efficacy of clotting factors present in the blood	Hematologic	Heparin, warfarin (Coumadin)
Antidiarrheals	Decrease GI motility, alter GI secretion activity	GI	Loperamide (Imodium), diphenoxylate-atropine combination (Lomotil)
Antidysrhythmics	Prevent or control various cardiac dysrhythmias	Cardiovascular	Lidocaine, amiodarone (Cordarone)
Antiemetics	Treat or prevent nausea and vomiting	GI, CNS	Promethazine (Phenergan), ondansetron (Zofran)
Antiflatulents	Prevent or treat excess intestinal gas	GI	Simethicone, lactase
Antifungals	Treat fungal infections	Varied	Fluconazole (Diflucan), ketoconazole (Nizoral)
Antiglaucoma agents (usually eyedrops)	Treat glaucoma	Varied	Brinzolamide (Azopt), bimatoprost (Lumigan)
Antihistamines	Block histamine receptors, dry mucous membranes, inhibit immune response in allergic reactions	Varied	Diphenhydramine (Benadryl), loratadine (Claritin)
Antihyperlipidemics	Decrease blood cholesterol, sequester cholesterol chemicals in bile	Hematologic, cardiovascular	Cholestyramine (Questran), colesevelam (Welchol)
Antimetabolites	Cancer medications that mimic normal substances within a cell, disrupt cell metabolism, and kill cancer cells	Varied	Methotrexate (Rheumatrex, Trexall) 5-fluorouracil (5-FU, Adrucil)
Antiparasitic agents	Treat parasitic infections	Varied	Nitazoxanide (Alinia)
Antipsychotics	Treat psychoses, including schizophrenia	Sympathetic nervous system	Haloperidol (Haldol), olanzapine (Zyprexa)

Medication Class	Common Indications or Purposes	Primary Body System Affected	Examples
Antitumor antibiotics	Antibiotic medications (as above) that have the additional ability to target and kill certain cancer cells	Varied	Doxorubicin (Adriamycin), mitomycin (Mutamycin)
Antivirals	Treat viral infections	Varied	Acyclovir (Zovirax), famciclovir (Famvir)
Barbiturates	Reduce or prevent seizures, provide sedation	CNS	Phenobarbital
Benzodiazepines	Treat anxiety and seizures, provide sedation	CNS	Lorazepam (Ativan), diazepam (Valium), oxazepam (Serax)
Beta-agonists	Bronchodilation	Respiratory	Albuterol, levalbuterol (Xopenex)
Beta-blocking agents	Reduce heart rate and blood pressure	Cardiovascular	Metoprolol (Lopressor), atenolol (Tenormin)
Calcium channel blockers	Reduce heart rate and blood pressure	Cardiovascular	Diltiazem (Cardizem), verapamil (Calan), nicardipine (Cardene)
Cardiac glycosides	Decrease heart rate and improve contractility	Cardiovascular	Digoxin (Lanoxin)
Chemotherapeutic agents	Treat cancer or malignancy	Varied	Vincristine (Oncovin, Vincasar), cisplatin (Platinol)
Cholesterol synthesis inhibitors	Prevent cholesterol conversion in the liver	GI	Atorvastatin (Lipitor), simvastatin (Zocor)
Cholinergics	Activate secretory glands in eyes and GI tract; improve muscle weakness in myasthenia gravis	Parasympathetic nervous system	Pilocarpine (Isopto); pyridostigmine (Mestinon)
Corticosteroids	Decrease inflammation; immunosuppressant; replace or augment function of the adrenal cortex (see glucocorticoids and mineralocorticoids below)	Endocrine and immune	Prednisone, dexamethasone (Decadron)
Cough suppressants	Decrease bronchial irritation causing cough	CNS	Codeine, dextromethorphan
Digestants	Enhance digestion of food; may include supplemental pancreatic enzymes	GI	Glutamine
Diuretics	Promote excretion of urine; manage fluid overload	Renal	Mannitol (Osmitrol), furosemide (Lasix)

(continued)

Table 13-15 Notable Medication Groups Affecting Prehospital Patient Care *(Continued)*

Medication Class	Common Indications or Purposes	Primary Body System Affected	Examples
Fibrinolytics	Dissolve clots present in blood vessels or vascular access devices	Hematologic	Tissue plasminogen activator (tPA), tenecteplase (TNKase)
Glucocorticoids	Replacement or maintenance therapy, treat systemic inflammation, numerous other uses	Endocrine and immune	Hydrocortisone, beclomethasone (Beconase)
Glycoprotein IIb/IIIa inhibitors	Deactivate proteins involved in platelet aggregation	Hematologic	Tirofiban (Aggrastat), eptifibatide (Integrilin)
Histamine-2 receptor antagonists	Block histamine receptors, including those responsible for gastric acid secretion	GI and immune	Ranitidine (Zantac), famotidine (Pepcid)
Hormone replacement drugs	Replace hormones, improve bone density that has decreased due to aging and hormone loss; replace or augment function of impaired pituitary or thyroid glands	Endocrine	Estrogen, progesterone, levothyroxine (Synthroid), testosterone, recombinant human growth hormone
Immunomodulators	Inhibit or enhance functioning of the immune system	Immune	Interferon, levamisole (Ergamisol)
Immunosuppressants	Prevent rejection of transplanted organs and tissues; treat rheumatoid arthritis	Immune	Cyclosporine (Gengraf), tacrolimus (Prograf)
Insulin	Positive inotropic effects, allows cellular glucose uptake, treat hyperkalemia	Endocrine	Insulin (Humalog, Humulin)
Laxatives	Increase GI motility	GI	Bisacodyl (Dulcolax), docusate (Colace)
Mineralocorticoids	Promote sodium and water retention	Endocrine and immune	Fludrocortisone (Florinef)
Mucolytics	Assist with elimination of mucus in the respiratory tract	Pulmonary	Acetylcysteine (Mucomyst)
Mydriatics	Dilate pupils for ocular diagnostic and treatment procedures	Ocular and parasympathetic nervous system	Cyclopentolate (Cyclogyl)
Narcotic analgesics	Relieve pain and relieve or suppress cough	CNS	Morphine, oxycodone
Nasal decongestants	Decrease upper airway mucus secretion	Sympathetic nervous system	Pseudoephedrine (Sudafed), phenylephrine (Neo-Synephrine)

Medication Class	Common Indications or Purposes	Primary Body System Affected	Examples
Neuromuscular blocking agents	Provide chemical paralysis in intubated and ventilated patients	Peripheral nervous system and musculoskeletal	Succinylcholine (Anectine), rocuronium (Zemuron)
Nonsteroidal anti-inflammatory drugs	Treat pain and inflammation	Endocrine	Ibuprofen (Motrin, Advil), ketorolac (Toradol), indomethacin (Indocin)
Oral contraceptives	Prevent conception (pregnancy)	Endocrine and genitourinary	Estrogen, progesterone
Oral hypoglycemic agents	Manage type 2 diabetes mellitus	Endocrine	Glyburide (Diabeta), metformin (Glucophage), glipizide (Glucotrol)
Phosphodiesterase inhibitors	Treat erectile dysfunction	Cardiovascular	Sildenafil (Viagra), tadalafil (Cialis)
Plant alkaloids	Cancer medications derived from plants	Varied	Vincristine (Vincasar), etoposide (Toposar)
Platelet inhibitors	Decrease platelet aggregation in patients at risk of thrombus formation	Hematologic	Aspirin, clopidogrel (Plavix)
Protein pump inhibitors	Suppress activity of parietal cell acid secretion	GI	Omeprazole (Prilosec), esomeprazole (Nexium)
Selective serotonin reuptake inhibitors	Treat depression, anxiety, and related conditions	CNS	Paroxetine (Paxil), sertraline (Zoloft)
Sympathomimetics	Increase blood pressure, heart rate, and cardiac output; constrict blood vessels	Cardiovascular	Epinephrine (Adrenalin), phenylephrine (Neo-Synephrine)
Tocolytics	Decrease or eliminate uterine contractions during preterm labor	Endocrine and genitourinary	Magnesium sulfate
Tricyclic antidepressants	Treat depression, neuropathy, and chronic pain syndromes	CNS	Amitriptyline (Elavil), doxepin, desipramine (Norpramin)
Xanthines	Bronchodilation	Respiratory	Theophylline (Uniphyl)

Abbreviations: CNS, central nervous system; GI, gastrointestinal

sedated, the gag reflex disappears, and trismus or other facial muscle tension ceases following the correct use and sequence of airway medication. If performed correctly, patients have no awareness or memory of the procedure.

Sedative-Hypnotic Agents Used in Airway Management

Etomidate (Amidate) and ketamine (Ketalar) are two ultra-short-acting sedative medications used to facilitate airway placement. Etomidate is an imidazole derivative that works as a single-dose profound sedative. It is preferred for its minimal effect on blood pressure and other hemodynamic parameters. Etomidate begins working in 30 to 60 seconds, peaks in approximately 60 seconds, and lasts approximately 5 minutes. The short duration is usually desirable for airway procedures, but you need to resedate patients promptly with an alternative sedative medication during or immediately after inserting an airway device. Etomidate causes adrenal suppression (if multiple doses are given) that has the potential to further compromise the condition of an already critically ill patient. No more than one dose of etomidate should be given.

Ketamine is another possible adjunct to airway placement. It has a chemical composition similar to that of phencyclidine (PCP) and causes profound dissociation and general anesthesia. Ketamine can maintain the blood pressure and heart rate, but it also raises intracranial pressure, making it less than optimal for patients with head injury who require airway placement. Ketamine causes some degree of bronchodilation, which is potentially helpful in patients with asthma or another COPD who require airway placement for respiratory failure. An emergence reaction with brief psychosis, disorientation, hallucinations, and other effects is possible following ketamine administration. Certain providers and settings are using ketamine for control of refractory pain or delirium that is unresponsive to other medications. Check with your medical director on his or her thoughts on this medication. Emergence reactions may be eliminated or reduced by administering benzodiazepine medications with ketamine during airway procedures.

Benzodiazepines

Benzodiazepine medications are widely used in the prehospital setting. This group of medications includes diazepam, lorazepam, and midazolam. Patients may be prescribed other benzodiazepines such as clonazepam and temazepam (Restoril) for use on a long-term basis. Benzodiazepines have potent antiseizure, anxiolytic, and sedative properties, making them desirable in many situations. It is possible for benzodiazepines to be used as the primary sedative for airway placement procedures, but high doses of these medications are required to achieve adequate sedation. At high doses, benzodiazepines cause hypotension, further complicating the conditions of patients with shock or multiple trauma. Benzodiazepines are best used for maintenance sedation following airway placement. Benzodiazepines provide some degree of seizure protection in patients with head injuries. Active seizures can be treated initially with IV, IM, intranasal, and rectal administration of benzodiazepines. Lower doses of benzodiazepines may also be helpful to reduce anxiety, although this use is not approved in all EMS systems. You should be aware that the three prehospital benzodiazepine medications are pregnancy class D, which means they have demonstrated potential harm to the fetus. These medications should be administered to pregnant patients only during life-threatening situations when no safer alternative medications are available.

Flumazenil is a competitive benzodiazepine antagonist available in certain health care settings. Using flumazenil to reverse a benzodiazepine overdose has the serious potential of exposing patients to numerous life-threatening conditions. There are several important contraindications to flumazenil that require careful consideration before it can be administered. Death from isolated benzodiazepine toxicity is rare. The risks associated with flumazenil outweigh its potential benefits in most clinical situations. Flumazenil can precipitate benzodiazepine withdrawal symptoms in patients who receive benzodiazepines on a long-term basis. Reversal of benzodiazepine sedation may cause combative behavior, anxiety, and possibly elevated intracranial pressure in susceptible patients. Additionally, if seizures occur following flumazenil administration, benzodiazepine anticonvulsant medications will be minimally effective or ineffective in controlling seizure activity and other effective anticonvulsant medications may not be immediately available.

Chemical Paralytic Agents

Two classes of chemical paralytic agents may be used in the prehospital setting. These medications provide muscle relaxation that facilitates airway device placement and prevents patient-ventilator asynchrony during mechanical ventilation. Paralytic agents allow better visualization of airway structures than when only sedative medications are used. The class of chemical paralytic agent used largely influences the onset and duration of muscle relaxation.

Under normal circumstances, nerve cells release acetylcholine (ACh), which binds to nicotinic receptor sites on muscle cells, causing muscle contraction. Chemical paralytic (neuromuscular blocking) medications bind with nicotinic receptor sites on muscle cells, antagonizing (preventing activation by) ACh **Figure 13-10**.

Succinylcholine (Anectine) is a **competitive depolarizing** paralytic agent. It reaches the neuromuscular junction, binds with nicotinic receptors on muscles, causes a brief activation known as **fasciculation**, and prevents additional activation by ACh. Many health care providers prefer succinylcholine because of its rapid onset (30 to 60 seconds) and relatively brief duration (3 to 8 minutes). Succinylcholine has several important adverse effects. It may cause or worsen hyperkalemia (elevated potassium level), cause bradycardia (especially in children), and elevate intraocular pressure in susceptible patients. Malignant hyperthermia is a rare, but immediately life-threatening, adverse reaction to succinylcholine. This disorder is characterized by severe hyperthermia (elevated temperature), muscle rigidity, and metabolic acidosis. Other anesthetic agents also can cause this disorder. Patients able to communicate should be screened for personal or family reactions to anesthesia before administering succinylcholine. The serious adverse reactions associated with succinylcholine cause many clinicians to prefer other neuromuscular blocking agents, even if the other agents have a significantly longer duration of action.

Several **nondepolarizing** paralytic agents are used in the prehospital or critical care transport setting. Nondepolarizing agents compete with ACh at nicotinic receptor sites. They occupy but do not activate receptor sites, preventing activation by ACh. These medications generally have a longer duration than succinylcholine and fewer adverse effects. Rocuronium (Zemuron) has the most

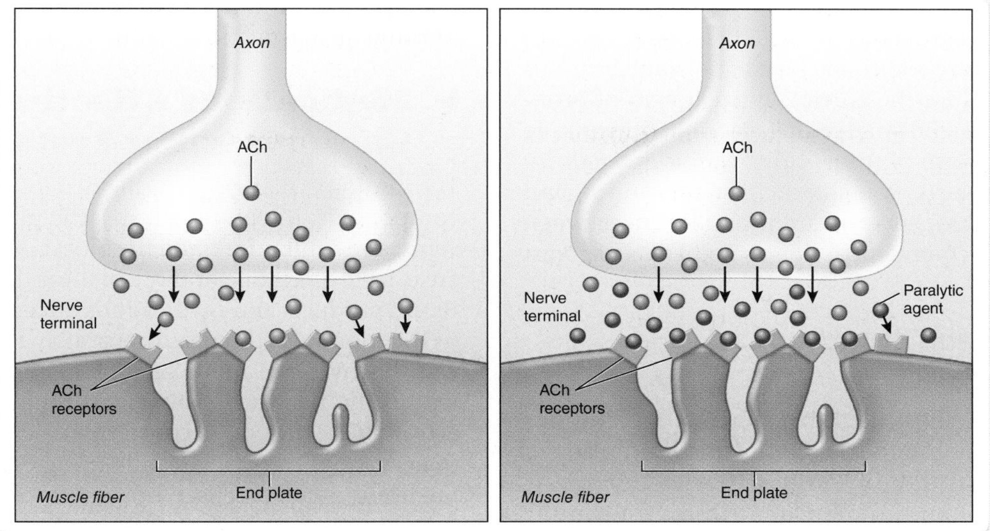

Figure 13-10 Chemical paralytic medications bind with nicotinic receptor sites on muscle cells, antagonizing acetylcholine (ACh).

rapid onset (1 to 3 minutes) combined with a shorter duration (15 to 60 minutes), making it an appropriate nondepolarizing agent for placement of airway devices in emergency situations. Vecuronium (Norcuron) may also be administered either as an adjunct or as a sole chemical paralytic agent for emergency airway procedures. The onset of vecuronium is slightly longer than that for rocuronium, but it is available as a powder for reconstitution, giving it a longer room-temperature shelf life than rocuronium has.

Depolarizing and nondepolarizing chemical paralytic agents create an immediate threat to life if they are administered by paramedics who are not able to secure an artificial airway. Paramedics who are authorized to administer these medications must be proficient with bag-mask ventilation and skilled with the placement of backup "rescue" airway devices, as discussed in Chapter 15, *Airway Management*. If you are not able to oxygenate and ventilate a patient adequately following administration of a chemical paralytic agent, potentially fatal complications are likely.

Other Airway Medications

Paramedics in certain EMS systems use medication to treat upper airway edema in patients who are responsive and spontaneously breathing. Corticosteroid, vasoconstrictor, and bronchodilator medications may be used when upper airway edema is present. These medications are discussed later in this chapter.

▶ Medications Used in Respiratory Management

Effective respiration requires adequate oxygenation and ventilation. Respiratory emergencies can be a primary complaint or the manifestation of a disease process in another body system. Medication groups discussed in this section relate to primary respiratory conditions such as asthma and COPD.

Beta-Agonist Medications

Beta-adrenergic agonist medications remain the primary treatment for acute bronchospasm associated with asthma, COPD, and a variety of other conditions. The walls of lower airways contain smooth muscles that contract (causing a smaller airway lumen) or relax (increasing the airway lumen) in response to biochemical changes and external irritants. Beta-2 receptor sites on bronchial smooth muscle cause muscle relaxation and bronchodilation when activated by beta-2 agonist chemicals. Norepinephrine and epinephrine are naturally occurring beta-2 agonists in the body. Paramedics are able to administer a variety of beta-2 agonist medications for patients experiencing bronchospasm.

Beta-agonist medications can be selective, targeting only beta-2 receptor sites, or nonselective, affecting beta-1 and beta-2 receptor sites. Despite advertised selectivity, many beta-2 agonist medications demonstrate some degree of beta-1 activation. Albuterol (Ventolin, Proventil) is a selective beta-2 agonist medication used in the prehospital setting and throughout health care. This medication is typically nebulized or administered using an MDI for the emergency treatment of bronchospasm. Albuterol may cause varying degrees of tachycardia, especially during prolonged administration. Metabolic acidosis may also develop if patients receive prolonged, continuous administration of nebulized albuterol. Albuterol can promote cellular uptake of potassium, making it a potential temporary treatment for hyperkalemia until definitive potassium removal occurs.

Levalbuterol is structurally similar to albuterol, without many of the reported beta-1 effects. Terbutaline (Brethaire) and epinephrine are additional beta-agonist medications that may be used for the emergency treatment of bronchospasm in the prehospital setting. Racemic epinephrine is the nebulized form of epinephrine engineered to limit cardiovascular effects. You should exercise caution and carefully monitor for adverse cardiovascular effects when administering racemic epinephrine and other beta-agonist medications.

Mucokinetic and Bronchodilator Medications

Paramedics may supplement beta-agonist medications with ipratropium bromide or a similar medication when treating patients with bronchospasm or reactive airway disease. Ipratropium bromide antagonizes muscarinic receptors, causing bronchodilation and decreased mucus in the upper and lower airways. Ipratropium is administered only every 6 to 8 hours, so you should administer only a single dose to patients in the prehospital setting. Cardiovascular effects from ipratropium are usually limited because of its poor systemic absorption.

Corticosteroids

Many respiratory emergencies involve some degree of airway inflammation. In the prehospital setting, corticosteroid medications are administered to reduce airway inflammation and, ultimately, improve oxygenation and ventilation. These medications significantly reduce the severity of respiratory compromise from asthma, COPD, allergic reactions, and other causes of airway inflammation. Methylprednisolone (Solu-Medrol), dexamethasone (Decadron), and prednisone are administered in certain prehospital systems. Corticosteroid medications have immunosuppressant properties and can alter a vast array of endocrine functions. These medications have a wide variety of contraindications and adverse effects, so EMS systems may limit or restrict their use by paramedics. If you are permitted to administer these medications, you must take care to evaluate the potential risks and benefits for each patient.

Leukotriene Receptor Antagonists

Patients with asthma have an overproduction of chemicals called leukotrienes, which bind to receptor sites within the lungs causing powerful bronchoconstriction as well as inflammatory, mucus-promoting, and vascular permeability effects. Leukotrienes are reported to be exponentially more potent at causing bronchoconstriction than histamines. Levels of leukotrienes are significantly elevated in patients with asthma. Leukotriene receptor antagonist medications, such as Montelukast (Singulair) and Zafirlukast (Accolate) are taken by patients with asthma and certain allergies on a long-term basis. These medications are taken for long-term symptom management, and not used to treat emergent episodes of bronchospasm and inflammation.

▶ Medications Affecting the Cardiovascular System

The cardiovascular system is divided into three functional components: the pump (heart), the plumbing (arteries, veins, and capillaries), and the blood. Many medications are used to affect one or more of these three components. Blood products and medications affecting the functions of the blood are discussed separately in other chapters. Antidysrhythmic medications specifically target cells within the heart to resolve a dysrhythmia or suppress **ectopic foci** (sites of electrical impulse generation other than normal pacemaker cells). Many antidysrhythmic medications affect cells in other parts of the cardiovascular system or throughout the body. Other cardiovascular medications alter the activity of the heart or change the tone of blood vessels.

Several of the medications discussed in this section are not generally used in the prehospital setting. However, you may encounter these medications during interfacility transport or while responding to an emergency in a health care setting outside of a hospital.

Antidysrhythmic Medications

A variety of medications have the ability to improve or correct abnormalities in a patient's cardiac rhythm. Many of the medications used to treat cardiac dysrhythmias have a similar ability to cause cardiac dysrhythmias and a large number of adverse effects in patients receiving these medications. You must carefully consider the risks and benefits of a particular medication in the context of an individual patient. In many cases, you will benefit from the expert guidance of a physician through online medical control when treating patients in hemodynamically stable condition with a cardiac dysrhythmia. Medications used to treat cardiac dysrhythmias are grouped into four classes according to mechanism using the **Vaughan-Williams classification** scheme. Adenosine (Adenocard) is a medication used to treat certain cardiac dysrhythmias but is not included in the Vaughan-Williams classification. The Vaughan-Williams classification scheme is based on mechanism of action rather than on specific medication groups. Certain medications have a mechanism of action in more than one class.

A brief overview of cardiac cellular activity is essential to understanding the action of antidysrhythmic medications. There are five phases of cardiac cell activity, 0 through 4. The cardiac cycle begins at phase 4. During phase 4, cardiac cells are at rest, waiting for the generation of a spontaneous impulse from within (automaticity) or transfer of an impulse from an adjacent cardiac cell. This period coincides with diastole of the heart.

Phase 0 begins when the cardiac muscle cells receives an impulse. Sodium ions rapidly enter the cell through

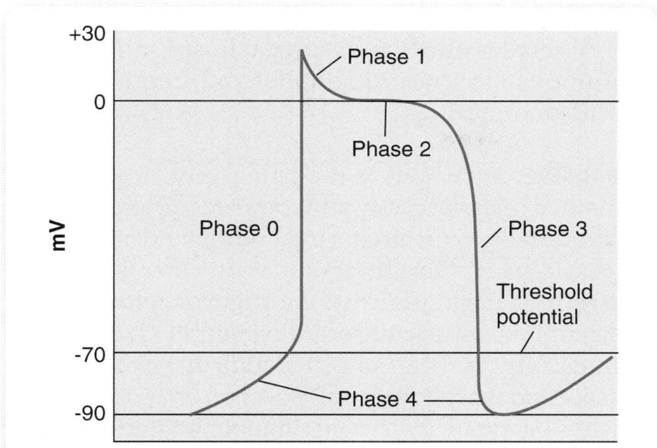

Figure 13-11 Action potential in a cardiac muscle cell.

Reproduced from *12-Lead ECG: The Art of Interpretation*, courtesy of Tomas B. Garcia, MD.

sodium channels in the cardiac cell. Calcium, entering more slowly through calcium channels, causes the release of calcium for muscle contraction. **Depolarization** occurs, altering the electrical charge present in the cell, and contraction begins **Figure 13-11**. During phase 1, sodium channels close while potassium exits the cell. During phase 2, sodium and calcium slowly enter the cell, while potassium continues to leave the cell. During phase 3, calcium channels slowly close and calcium leaves the cell while potassium channels open, enabling the rapid movement of potassium out of the cell. Repolarization, which began during phase 2, is complete at the end of phase 3.

Throughout phases 0, 1, and 2 and up to the middle of phase 3, no additional depolarization may occur because of external stimuli. This protection limits the potential maximum heart rate by ensuring that a certain amount of time elapses between myocardial contractions. This period is known as the **absolute refractory period** or effective refractory period. Immediately following the absolute (effective) refractory period, there is a brief window for an unusually powerful stimulus to initiate depolarization, known as the **relative refractory period**.

It is possible for nonpacemaker cells to initiate electrical activity spontaneously. During periods of cellular hypoxia, certain ion channels become altered. These changes permit calcium (instead of sodium) to initiate depolarization, resulting in ectopic beats that frequently accompany myocardial ischemia.

Class I Antidysrhythmic Medications. Class I antidysrhythmic medications slow the movement of sodium through channels in certain cardiac cells. Procainamide (Pronestyl) is a class IA medication that can suppress activity of ectopic foci and slow conduction velocity. This action has the potential to prolong the QRS and QT intervals. This medication is effective for a variety of atrial and ventricular dysrhythmias but requires careful administration and monitoring.

Lidocaine is a class IB antidysrhythmic medication that has been used in the prehospital setting for many years. It blocks sodium channels in the Purkinje fibers and ventricle, effectively resolving various ventricular dysrhythmias and suppressing ectopic foci. Lidocaine is poorly absorbed orally and quickly metabolized by the liver. Administration typically involves a larger bolus dose, followed by a continuous infusion. You may also see lidocaine used as a local anesthetic during soft-tissue repair and as an adjunct to sedation in patients who are at risk of increases in intracranial pressure during intubation attempts. Lidocaine has numerous significant medication interactions and should be used with caution in patients with liver or kidney disease.

Class II Antidysrhythmic Medications/Beta-Adrenergic Blocking Agents. Beta-adrenergic blocking agents (beta-blockers) constitute the second major class of antidysrhythmic agents. Beta-blockers competitively inhibit catecholamine (epinephrine and norepinephrine) activation of beta receptor sites. At therapeutic doses, certain beta-blockers are capable of some beta-1 selectivity, affecting heart rate, contractility, or cardiac conduction velocity, without substantial impact on beta-2 receptors in the lungs. Selectivity is lost when higher doses or nonselective beta-blockers are administered. Toxic effects from beta-blockers typically include bradycardia, hypotension, conduction delays, and a variety of other cardiovascular effects. Beta-blockers should be used with extreme caution in patients with reactive airway disease because of the potential beta-2 antagonism causing bronchospasm. Beta-blockers may also cause massive conduction abnormalities when given simultaneously with calcium channel blockers or other medications that slow atrioventricular node conduction.

Metoprolol is a beta-blocking agent used to reduce the heart rate during myocardial ischemia and in certain atrial tachycardias. This medication decreases the heart rate with a modest reduction in blood pressure. In the setting of myocardial ischemia, metoprolol is used to decrease the heart rate, resulting in lower myocardial oxygen consumption. In certain EMS systems, you may carry and administer metoprolol. It is essential to monitor patient heart rate and blood pressure carefully while slowly administering metoprolol in select situations.

Class III Antidysrhythmic Medications. Class III antidysrhythmic medications increase the duration of phases 1, 2, and 3 of the cardiac cycle. By extending the cellular action potential, these medications prolong the absolute refractory period, treating atrial or ventricular tachycardias. In certain class III medications, the degree of prolongation of action potential is inversely proportional to the baseline heart rate, essentially making the medications less effective for treating extremely rapid heart rates while dramatically decreasing relatively slower baseline heart rates.

Amiodarone (Cordarone) is a class III antidysrhythmic medication that has gained popularity in recent years. Amiodarone is useful for treating atrial and ventricular tachycardia. The role of amiodarone in the treatment of Wolff-Parkinson-White syndrome remains controversial. It is recommended in the ACLS algorithm, but several studies suggest that the risks of amiodarone for the treatment of Wolff-Parkinson-White syndrome outweigh potential benefits. Amiodarone is administered by the IV route in the prehospital or critical care setting and can be continued orally for long-term maintenance. Amiodarone is widely distributed throughout the body, potentially causing a wide range of adverse effects. In addition to severe adverse cardiovascular effects, amiodarone causes various life-threatening pulmonary conditions in up to 10.7% of patients.[10] Patients typically develop pulmonary complications after several months on oral amiodarone; however, these complications can occur at any point during treatment.

Sotalol (Betapace) is another class III medication that you may encounter. This medication is often taken orally by patients for either ventricular or atrial dysrhythmias. It can be used intravenously for termination of ventricular tachycardia.

Class IV Antidysrhythmic Medications/Calcium Channel Blockers. Calcium channel blockers have a variety of potential uses in the prehospital setting. These medications can be used for reducing blood pressure and controlling the heart rate and may increase myocardial oxygen delivery during periods of ischemia. In addition, these medications may be used to inhibit uterine contractions during preterm labor, for long-term management of migraines, and for the treatment of cardiomyopathy.

Calcium channel blockers displace calcium at certain receptor sites or enter smooth muscle cells in place of calcium. This action relaxes smooth muscle present in the heart, blood vessels, GI tract, and uterus. Calcium channel blockers slow conduction through the atrioventricular node, decrease the automaticity of ectopic foci within the heart, and decrease the velocity of cardiac contraction. Cardiac workload and oxygen consumption are decreased by lowering peripheral vascular resistance (afterload) while simultaneously reducing cardiac output.

Verapamil (Calan) and diltiazem (Cardizem) are two calcium channel blockers commonly used in prehospital and critical care transport settings. In most cases, these medications are used for the control of the heart rate in patients with atrial fibrillation or atrial flutter. Diltiazem appears to have less effect on blood pressure, making it more desirable for patients at risk for hypotension. Many EMS agencies stock verapamil rather than diltiazem because it has a longer room-temperature shelf life and lower cost. IV calcium preparations such as calcium chloride and calcium gluconate may mitigate hypotension or bradycardia following an overdose of or toxicity from a calcium channel blocker. Both medications are administered by the IV route over at least 2 minutes with continuous electrocardiographic and frequent blood pressure monitoring.

Adenosine. Adenosine is the only member of the fifth (unnamed) class of antidysrhythmic medications that is used routinely in the prehospital setting. Adenosine can be used to treat paroxysmal supraventricular tachycardia or to assist in diagnosis when the origin or pattern cannot be determined on an electrocardiogram (ECG) because of an unusually fast heart rate. It is difficult to identify the presence and morphology of P waves on an ECG when the patient's heart rate is elevated. Immediately after administration, adenosine decreases cardiac conduction velocity and prolongs the effective refractory period, producing a several-second pause in cardiac activity. One or two doses of adenosine are often successful in resolving an episode of paroxysmal supraventricular tachycardia. For diagnosis, paramedics and other health care providers use adenosine to evaluate the ECG tracing as cardiac electrical activity terminates and resumes to determine the presence of P waves, flutter waves, or other evidence of supraventricular activity, especially when a wide (0.12 seconds or greater) QRS complex is present. This technique may distinguish between ventricular tachycardia and atrial tachycardia with aberrancy. Adenosine is occasionally used in cardiac and neurologic surgical settings to produce a brief, predictable cessation of cardiac activity during blood vessel repair.

Patients and health care providers often experience similar levels of anxiety during the 5- to 15-second pause in electrical and mechanical cardiac activity caused by adenosine. Adenosine has a rapid onset, a brief duration, and a half-life of less than 10 seconds. You should administer adenosine through a large-bore proximal IV site, immediately followed by a 10-mL normal saline flush. This technique often requires planning and coordination, possibly with two providers, to maximize adenosine's clinical effects. Run a continuous paper ECG recording whenever administering adenosine. Doing so will assist you and other health care providers with dysrhythmia identification if conversion with adenosine is unsuccessful.

▶ Additional Cardiovascular Medications

Alpha-Adrenergic Receptor Antagonists

Alpha-adrenergic receptor antagonists (alpha blockers) prevent endogenous catecholamines from reaching alpha receptors, primarily in the smooth muscle of blood vessels. In general, these medications lower blood pressure (particularly diastolic) and decrease systemic vascular resistance. Nonselective blockade of alpha-2 receptors causes a "reflex" tachycardia by allowing an increase of norepinephrine secretion from the sympathetic nervous system.

Patients taking alpha-blocking medications at home are frequently prone to orthostatic hypotension (hypotension related to sudden position changes) and tachycardia. Alpha-adrenergic receptor antagonists are prescribed for patients with hypertension, an enlarged prostate gland, and glaucoma. Alpha receptor antagonism occurs frequently as a seemingly unrelated adverse effect of other medications.

It is conceivable that you may administer one of three alpha-adrenergic medications in the prehospital or critical care transport settings. Clonidine (Catapres) is a primarily alpha-2 receptor agonist, often given orally for emergency treatment of hypertension. By activating alpha-2 receptors, clonidine suppresses the release of norepinephrine, a potent vasoconstrictor, causing vasodilation. You may also administer phentolamine (Regitine). Catecholamines and sympathomimetics (discussed later) can cause profound tissue necrosis if **extravasation** (seepage of blood and medication into the tissue surrounding the blood vessel) occurs during administration through a peripheral IV line. As extravasation occurs, blood vessels in the skin and soft tissue constrict, cutting off blood flow to cells in the affected area. Phentolamine can be delivered by subcutaneous injection to reverse vasoconstriction in affected soft tissue, preventing tissue death.

You may also administer labetalol (Trandate), an unusual medication with a combination of alpha-1, beta-1, and beta-2 antagonism properties. It is administered in emergency settings for hypertension. The IV form has a far greater effect on beta-1 and beta-2 receptors than it has on alpha-1 receptors. Patients at risk for unopposed alpha stimulation, such as patients with a pheochromocytoma or cocaine overdose, should receive another alpha-adrenergic antagonist before receiving labetalol for a hypertensive emergency. In this case, a declining cardiac output from the beta-1 antagonism prompts the secretion of endogenous catecholamines, causing potentially uncontrolled hypertension.

Angiotensin-Converting Enzyme Inhibitors

The medications known as ACE inhibitors alter the function of the renin-angiotensin system in the body. This system causes vasoconstriction and fluid retention in response to hypotension or hypoperfusion. When the conversion of angiotensin I to angiotensin II is altered by the use of ACE inhibitor medications, a variety of clinically beneficial effects occur. Blood pressure is reduced and cardiac afterload is decreased without significantly altering cardiac output or causing an increased heart rate. These medications are useful for treating hypertension, cardiomyopathy, and heart failure. In addition, they protect kidney function in certain groups of susceptible people.

Patients taking ACE inhibitors are known to have a chronic, dry cough that is thought to be linked to an accumulation of chemicals from the now-altered renin-angiotensin system. Patients taking ACE inhibitors may experience sudden, life-threatening angioedema. This swelling of the mouth, face, and airway is a result of a rapid increase in subdermal and submucosal vascular permeability. When angioedema occurs, normal treatments such as epinephrine and antihistamines are not as effective. You should expect to provide close monitoring and supportive treatment or, in severe situations, prepare for an extremely difficult endotracheal intubation. Select EMS systems may utilize ACE inhibitors, particularly enalapril (Vasotec). You should follow local protocols regarding indications and administration, and be aware of important contraindications if enalapril or another ACE inhibitor is used in your EMS system.

Anticholinergic Medications

Anticholinergic medications are used in prehospital and other health care settings for several important clinical purposes. The parasympathetic and sympathetic nervous systems continually respond to internal and external stimuli by releasing various biochemicals. These chemicals enhance or suppress the function of many tissues, organs, and body systems. Throughout the day, activity of either the sympathetic or the parasympathetic nervous system will predominate, depending on perceived needs of the body. The sympathetic nervous system predominates in response to stress, releasing catecholamines to improve cardiovascular performance, enhance respiration, and retain body water. As the stressful stimulus disappears, the parasympathetic nervous system predominates, allowing vital functions such as rest, digestion, and urination to resume.

The vagus nerve (cranial nerve X) is a major component of the parasympathetic nervous system. This nerve controls parasympathetic stimulation of receptor sites in the heart, lungs, and digestive system and throughout the chest and abdomen. The vagus nerve releases ACh that acts on muscarinic-2 receptors in the heart to decrease heart rate and contractility and cardiac conduction velocity. Excessive activation of muscarinic-2 receptors in the heart by ACh causes bradycardia and conduction delays. Excessive activation of other muscarinic receptors causes increased salivation, bronchoconstriction, pulmonary secretions, vomiting, emesis, diarrhea, tearing, and a vast array of unwanted clinical effects. Many of these symptoms are present when patients are exposed to acetylcholinesterase inhibitors in pesticides and nerve agents, which permits excessive release of ACh and leads to elevated ACh levels in the body. Atropine sulfate is used in the prehospital and other health care settings to treat many **cholinergic** symptoms associated with excessive release of ACh.

Atropine is considered a competitive muscarinic receptor antagonist. The effectiveness of atropine is largely related to its concentration at receptor sites compared with ACh. When ACh increases dramatically due to inhibition of **acetylcholinesterase** (the enzyme that breaks down ACh), massive doses of atropine may be required.

Atropine is used for the treatment of bradycardia when vagal (vagus nerve) stimulation of muscarinic-2 receptors is suspected. This condition may occur when a patient strains to defecate or has mechanical pressure applied to his or her neck or when another event causes the vagus nerve to release excessive ACh. In many cases, atropine is administered empirically to exclude the possibility of vagal stimulation during episodes of bradycardia with an unidentified cause. As atropine is administered for bradycardia, ACh activation of muscarinic-2 receptors is prevented, allowing underlying sympathetic stimulation to predominate. Atropine is unlikely to be effective for the treatment of bradycardia caused by blocked cardiac conduction such as in second- and third-degree atrioventricular blocks.

Atropine is used before airway manipulation, especially in children. Laryngoscopy can stimulate the vagus nerve, causing ACh-induced bradycardia. In addition to preventing bradycardia, atropine can suppress the release of saliva and other secretions in the patient's airway. Low doses (<0.1–0.2 mg) of atropine can cause CNS stimulation and paradoxical bradycardia.

Atropine is the lifesaving antidote for acetylcholinesterase inhibitor toxicity. When patients are exposed to pesticides and nerve agents, atropine is continuously administered until respiratory and hemodynamic status improves, regardless of the total dose required. Ambulance and hospital atropine supplies can be quickly exhausted following severe exposures, especially when multiple patients are involved. Atropine does not bind with nicotinic receptors; consequently it will not improve muscle weakness, fasciculations, or paralysis from cholinergic poisoning.

Catecholamines and Sympathomimetics

Catecholamines are naturally occurring chemicals in the body that stimulate receptor sites in the sympathetic nervous system. These chemicals contain two structures: the catechol group and the monoamine group. Endogenous catecholamines include epinephrine, norepinephrine, and dopamine. These chemicals stimulate alpha, beta, and dopaminergic receptor sites, causing the "fight-or-flight" response to stressful stimuli. These three chemicals are manufactured commercially for administration to patients with certain medical conditions. Catecholamines are rapidly metabolized by monoamine oxidase and catechol O-methyltransferase (an enzyme), resulting in a brief duration of action after administration. You may encounter certain catecholamine and sympathomimetic medications in the prehospital setting. Other medications in this category may be encountered during critical care transport.

Sympathomimetic chemicals are not found naturally within the body. These synthetic chemicals mimic naturally occurring catecholamines, activating receptor sites in the sympathetic nervous system. Various amphetamines, albuterol, phenylephrine, and cocaine have sympathomimetic properties. Sympathomimetic medications do not undergo the same metabolism as catecholamines, thus allowing for a longer duration of action following administration.

Epinephrine (Adrenalin), also known as adrenaline (note the similarity with the brand name), is a catecholamine used in the prehospital setting. Epinephrine stimulates alpha, beta-1, and beta-2 receptor sites, causing potent vasoconstriction; a marked increase in heart rate, contractility, and cardiac output; and powerful bronchodilation. Epinephrine can be administered via the IV, IO, IM, subcutaneous, endotracheal, and nebulized routes, depending on the clinical situation and type of medication access available. Nebulized epinephrine is used for airway edema and bronchospasm from various causes. Epinephrine may be given by the IM and subcutaneous routes for anaphylaxis and by the IV route in severe cases of anaphylactic shock. Epinephrine is administered by the IV and IO routes and through the endotracheal tube for cardiac arrest. Epinephrine infusions are used for profound hypotension, shock, and refractory bradycardia.

Epinephrine, like many catecholamines and sympathomimetic chemicals, can dramatically increase the cardiac workload and myocardial oxygen demand. These medications should be used with extreme caution in patients with myocardial ischemia, cardiomyopathy, or cardiogenic shock.

Norepinephrine is another naturally occurring catecholamine that has been manufactured commercially for use in health care. This medication stimulates beta-1 and alpha receptor sites, causing an increase in blood pressure, cardiac contractility, and heart rate. Vasoconstrictor (alpha) effects are usually greater than cardiac (beta-1) effects. Conditions that involve loss of vasomotor tone, such as sepsis, neurogenic shock, and anaphylactic shock, are the primary indications for norepinephrine as intravascular volume is being restored.

Norepinephrine is administered by continuous IV infusion and titrated according to patient response. Paramedics may administer norepinephrine in the critical care transport setting using an infusion pump. Norepinephrine is not typically used as an initial vasopressor in the prehospital setting, although EMS treatment guidelines may continue to evolve with advances in the management of sepsis. Norepinephrine and other vasopressor medications have the potential to cause tissue necrosis if extravasation occurs during IV administration. Alpha receptor activation causes constriction of blood vessels in the affected area, cutting off the blood supply and leading to tissue death if not treated promptly. Frequent assessment of the IV site is imperative if norepinephrine is being administered through a peripheral IV site. Paramedics who have been appropriately trained should ideally administer norepinephrine and other vasoconstrictor medications through a central venous catheter when available.

Table 13-16 Physiologic Effects of Dopamine Categorized by Dose

Dose (mcg/kg per minute)	Receptor	Effect
5–10	Beta-1	Increased rate/force
10–20	Alpha	Vasoconstriction

Data from: Dopamine: drug information. UpToDate website. http://cursoenarm.net/UPTODATE/contents/mobipreview.htm?29/10/29870?source=see_link. Accessed March 9, 2017.

Dopamine (Intropin) is frequently used in the prehospital setting as the primary medication for hypotension refractory to volume resuscitation, although you may begin to see greater emphasis on other vasopressor medications for particular medical conditions. Dopamine is administered using a weight-based infusion calculation, typically micrograms per kilogram per minute. The clinical effects of dopamine vary dramatically depending on the dose range being administered **Table 13-16**. There is some overlap among the various receptors being activated. At 5 to 10 mcg/kg per minute, dopamine activates beta-1 receptor sites, causing an increased heart rate and increased contractility. From 10 to 20 mcg/kg per minute, alpha effects predominate, causing profound vasoconstriction.

Dobutamine is a synthetically manufactured catecholamine that is similar to dopamine. It activates beta-1 and, to a lesser degree, beta-2 and alpha receptor sites. Dopaminergic receptors. Dobutamine may slightly increase heart rate, while providing a significant improvement in inotropic effects (force of cardiac contraction). When used for the treatment of cardiogenic shock, dobutamine is frequently combined with an IV vasodilator medication to increase inotropic effects and decrease afterload, resulting in improved cardiac output. A dobutamine infusion is not routinely initiated in the prehospital setting. During use in a hospital or critical care transport, dobutamine is administered with an infusion pump with careful cardiac and hemodynamic monitoring. Hypotension is possible, especially when initiating a dobutamine infusion. Some clinicians recommend briefly using another beta-1 agonist medication while initiating a dobutamine infusion or temporarily delaying administration of a vasodilator medication if patient condition permits.

Milrinone (Primacor) is an agent that is functionally similar to dobutamine. This medication can be given either orally or intravenously for the treatment of heart failure. It has the ability to increase cardiac contractility while simultaneously causing dilation of systemic arteries and veins. This combination improves cardiac output but increases patient mortality when used long term.

Phenylephrine is a synthetic, almost pure, alpha agonist medication. Minimal beta effects may be possible at high doses, but for all purposes, it is a pure alpha agonist medication. It is a potent vasoconstrictor with a longer duration of action than is offered by catecholamine medications. Clinically, phenylephrine is used for the treatment of hypotension resulting from a loss of vascular tone. You may also use phenylephrine as a mucosal vasoconstrictor during artificial airway placement. Phenylephrine may cause reflex tachycardia, and tachyphylaxis (discussed in the earlier section, *Principles of Pharmacodynamics*) is relatively likely. Extravasation is a major concern with phenylephrine because of powerful alpha receptor activation. If you are administering phenylephrine during a critical care transport, careful monitoring of the IV site is essential, and phentolamine (discussed earlier) should be available.

Digitalis Preparations

Digitalis preparations are prescribed for treatment of chronic heart failure or certain rapid atrial dysrhythmias (such as rapid atrial flutter, atrial fibrillation, and supraventricular dysrhythmias). Digitalis acts by increasing the strength of cardiac contractions, thereby improving cardiac output and slowing conduction through the atrioventricular junction (such as in atrial fibrillation or flutter), allowing fewer impulses to be conducted to the ventricles and thereby slowing the overall heart rate. Patients may experience a wide variety of signs and symptoms as an adverse reaction to digitalis preparations, including loss of appetite, nausea, vomiting, headache, blurred vision, yellow vision, or various cardiac dysrhythmias. *Virtually any cardiac dysrhythmia may be caused by the toxic effects of digitalis*, so it is important to ask all patients with disturbances in cardiac rhythm whether they are taking digitalis.

Patients taking digitalis are sensitive to calcium preparations. They are also highly sensitive to a decline in serum potassium levels. Therefore, you must exercise caution when giving agents that might reduce the body's potassium stores (such as diuretics or large quantities of sodium bicarbonate). Commonly used digitalis preparations include digoxin (Lanoxin) and digitoxin (Crystodigin).

Direct Vasodilator Medications

Various direct vasodilator medications are used for the management of uncontrolled hypertension, heart failure, myocardial infarction, cardiac ischemia, and cardiogenic shock. These medications act on arteries, veins, or both, causing vascular smooth muscle relaxation and vasodilation. These medications have the potential to reduce cardiac preload and afterload and pulmonary vascular resistance.

Nitroglycerin (Nitro-Bid, Nitrostat) is a direct vasodilator that is administered for a variety of cardiovascular conditions. Nitroglycerin primarily dilates veins and coronary arteries, decreasing cardiac preload, reducing myocardial oxygen demand, and improving coronary circulation. When administered sublingually by tablet or spray, effects begin in 1 to 3 minutes and peak in 4 to 10 minutes. Effects begin almost immediately following IV administration but persist only a few minutes after the IV infusion is discontinued. The rapid physiologic responses associated with the administration of IV nitroglycerin (relief of chest pain, decreased blood pressure) make it a relatively safe medication to titrate to desired clinical effect. The IV doses begin at 5 mcg/min in adults and can be increased to 400 mcg/min if symptoms persist and an acceptable blood pressure is maintained.[11] As mentioned earlier in this chapter, the SL dose of nitroglycerin is substantially higher than the IV dose. Nitroglycerin is prone to causing tolerance after 24 to 48 hours of continuous IV infusion. Some clinicians recommend obtaining a 15-lead ECG (12-lead ECG with additional evaluation for ischemia of the right side of the heart) prior to initiating treatment with nitroglycerin. Right-sided myocardial infarction requires an adequate preload to maintain adequate cardiac output, which may be compromised by the administration of nitroglycerin.

SL nitroglycerin tablets are prone to degradation. Tablets must be stored in a closed, light-protected container. Nitroglycerin binds with the plastic of containers and IV fluids or tubing. Glass bottles should be used for IV administration as safety and availability permit. The use of nitroglycerin should be avoided in patients taking phosphodiesterase-5 inhibitors used for erectile dysfunction, such as sildenafil (Viagra) and tadalafil (Cialis) Figure 13-12. When combined, nitroglycerin and phosphodiesterase-5 inhibitors may cause severe, refractory hypotension. (Note: Nitroglycerin is a component of dynamite, but medical preparations of nitroglycerin have no explosive hazards.)

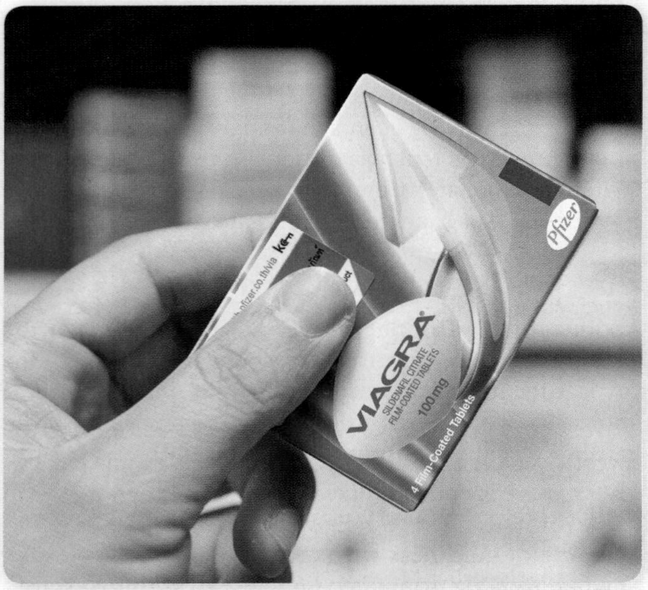

Figure 13-12 Administration of nitroglycerin in patients who have taken erectile dysfunction medication within certain timeframes is contraindicated.

Sodium nitroprusside (Nipride) is a potent IV vasodilator, affecting the smooth muscle of veins and arteries. Frequently, it is used in conjunction with inotropic medications for the management of cardiogenic shock. Sodium nitroprusside is used for malignant hypertension and in situations where intentional hypotension is desired, such as with an unstable vascular aneurysm. The IV infusion rates can be adjusted to maintain optimal blood pressure and cardiac output.

Sodium nitroprusside is administered by continuous IV infusion with frequent or constant blood pressure monitoring. Effects from sodium nitroprusside decrease rapidly once the infusion is discontinued. Sodium nitroprusside is metabolized into cyanide and thiocyanate, which can cause toxicity during a prolonged infusion. When it is administered in the critical care transport setting, you should ask the sending facility staff or provider about obtaining plasma cyanide and thiocyanate levels before departure with the patient.

Words of Wisdom

Antianginal Agents

Three major classes of drugs are used to relieve the pain of angina: nitrates, beta-blockers, and calcium channel blockers. All of them work exclusively or primarily on the demand side of the oxygen supply-demand equation; that is, all of them diminish, in one way or another, myocardial oxygen demand.

Hydralazine (Apresoline) is a direct vasodilator that paramedics may administer for hypertensive emergencies, for pulmonary hypertension, or, in pregnant patients, for eclampsia or preeclampsia. This medication dilates arterioles, lowering pulmonary and systemic vascular resistance. In emergency situations, an IV bolus dose is administered over at least 1 minute and repeated (or increased) up to every 20 to 30 minutes as clinically indicated.

A subgroup of patients with idiopathic pulmonary artery hypertension may be dependent on life-sustaining, continuous infusions of epoprostenol (Flolan). This medication is a potent vasodilator, impacting both pulmonary and systemic blood vessels. Additionally, epoprostenol inhibits platelet aggregation, which likely decreases the prevalence or severity of pulmonary thrombus (blood clot) formation.

You may encounter patients who are on continuous epoprostenol infusions. These patients often have compact infusion pumps and long-term IV access in place, typically a peripherally inserted central catheter or similar device. EMS assistance may be requested if there is an unexpected failure of either the infusion device or IV access. EMS systems may provide protocols for paramedics to assist with administration of a patient's own epoprostenol; however, it is not typically administered to patients for the first time in the prehospital setting. Adverse effects include tachycardia, palpitations, dysrhythmia, bleeding, and flushing. You should consult with online medical control if considering adjustments to the continuous infusion rate. In most cases, paramedic involvement will be limited to reestablishing IV access and troubleshooting the infusion pump, unless a concurrent medical condition is present.

Words of Wisdom

Contact online medical control if you encounter a patient in the community who is receiving an infusion of a medication you are not accustomed to administering.

Diuretic Medications

Paramedics administer diuretic medications to correct volume overload, manage heart failure, and improve respiration in patients experiencing pulmonary edema. Diuretic medications also have the potential to preserve kidney function when large quantities of by-products from cellular destruction, such as from muscle breakdown or blood cell hemolysis, are released. Diuretic medications are used to eliminate certain toxins from the body and to promote the excretion of excess electrolytes. Table 13-17 lists commonly prescribed diuretic medications.

Furosemide is a diuretic medication used in the prehospital setting. People may also take furosemide on a long-term basis for the management of hypertension, heart failure, liver disease, or kidney dysfunction. Furosemide is generally administered for treatment of pulmonary edema, often related to cardiac dysfunction. Careful consideration is necessary before administering furosemide to patients with hemodynamic instability and known electrolyte disturbances. Furosemide is administered by the IV route over 1 to 2 minutes per 40-mg dose. In emergency situations, furosemide can be administered by the IM route, although effects are significantly delayed compared with the IV route. Some research studies suggest that furosemide causes renal artery vasodilation in addition to promoting urinary excretion from the kidneys.

Mannitol is an osmotic diuretic that may or may not be available to paramedics. In critical care settings, mannitol is used to decrease intracranial pressure associated with cerebral edema. Osmotic diuretics can target specific body tissues, removing excess water from the brain and eyes. Osmotic pressure gradients also draw water out of selected body tissues and through the kidneys to maintain urine flow when the kidneys risk becoming clogged with cellular by-products. Many electrolyte disturbances are possible following mannitol administration. Prolonged mannitol infusions have been known to cause a paradoxical increase in intracranial pressure.

Table 13-17 Commonly Prescribed Diuretics

Category	Generic Name (Trade Name)
Loop diuretics: disrupt sodium reabsorption in the thick ascending limb in the loop of Henle within the kidneys	Furosemide (Lasix) Bumetanide (Bumex) Torsemide (Demadex)
Potassium-sparing diuretics: impair sodium reabsorption in the cortical collecting tubule of the kidney	Spironolactone (Aldactone) Triamterene (Dyrenium)
Thiazide diuretics: inhibit sodium transport within the distal tubule of the kidney	Chlorothiazide (Diuril) Hydrochlorothiazide Metolazone (Diulo, Zaroxolyn)
Vasodilator/nitrate	Hydralazine (Apresoline)
Combination drugs	Hydrochlorothiazide and spironolactone (Aldactazide) Triamterene and hydrochlorothiazide (Dyazide, Maxzide)

Antihypertensive Agents

As the name implies, antihypertensive agents are used to treat hypertension (high blood pressure). Many of the diuretic agents already mentioned are also used as antihypertensives or in combination with antihypertensives for a synergistic effect. Similarly, beta-blockers are used in the treatment of hypertension.

It is often difficult to regulate the dosage of antihypertensives so that the patient's blood pressure is lowered enough but not too much. As a consequence, some patients taking these agents may have symptoms of hypotension, including weakness and dizziness. Many will experience a feeling of giddiness with a change in position (such as when moving from a recumbent to a sitting or standing position); this phenomenon is termed **orthostatic hypotension**. Every patient taking antihypertensive drugs, therefore, should have his or her blood pressure checked in the recumbent and sitting positions to detect orthostatic

Table 13-18 Commonly Prescribed Antihypertensive Agents

Category	Generic Name (Trade Name)
Nonselective beta-blockers (have both beta-1 and beta-2 effects)	Labetalol (Normodyne, Trandate) Propranolol (Inderal)
Angiotensin-converting enzyme (ACE) inhibitors (The generic drug names in this class of medications end in *-pril*)	Benazepril (Lotensin) Captopril (Capoten) Enalapril (Vasotec) Fosinopril (Monopril) Lisinopril (Prinivil, Zestril) Quinapril (Accupril) Ramipril (Altace)
Alpha agonist	Clonidine (Catapres) Methyldopa (Aldomet)
Alpha blocker	Prazosin (Aldomet)
Other antihypertensive	Reserpine (Sandril, Ser-Ap-Es, Serpasil)

hypotension. Table 13-18 lists commonly prescribed antihypertensive agents.

Other Cardiac Medications

In addition to those discussed thus far, Table 13-19 lists medications that may be prescribed for patients with cardiac conditions.

▶ Blood Products and Medications Affecting the Blood

In the body, blood acts as the primary transport mechanism for oxygen, carbon dioxide, nutrients, waste products, biochemicals, and medications. Health care providers have the ability to manipulate or enhance many characteristics of the blood for a therapeutic clinical purpose. In certain situations, they will want to suppress the clotting ability of the blood to enhance circulation or mitigate the effects of hypoperfusion. In other cases, they will need to augment the oxygen-carrying or clotting ability of the blood when these functions become impaired. A variety of medications affecting the blood are used in the prehospital and critical care transport settings. In addition, many EMS systems allow paramedics to initiate or monitor the administration of various blood products in appropriate clinical situations.

Blood Product Administration

The average adult has about 5 L of blood, constituting approximately 7% to 8% of body weight. Blood is roughly 55% plasma. Water makes up approximately 50% of the total intravascular volume. RBCs account for approximately 45% of the blood volume. Many chemicals, cells, proteins, and hormones make up the remainder of blood composition. Trauma and a vast array of medical conditions alter the total amount, composition, or performance of the blood. Health care providers, including paramedics, may administer several different blood products to correct these abnormalities. Patients receive transfusions of specific components of the blood that are diminished or have impaired function. Whole blood transfusions are no longer used clinically in the United States.

Blood components are unmatched, type-specific to a particular patient, or cross-matched to a particular recipient.

YOU are the Paramedic PART 4

As you prepare to transport, a 250-mL normal saline fluid bolus is infusing from a 1-L bag through 10-gtt tubing. The patient remains on oxygen, and her cardiac rhythm remains unchanged. The nursing staff provide the following additional information on this patient:

- Allergies:
  - Penicillin
  - "Sulfa" medications
- Scheduled/daily medications:
  - Metformin
  - Aspirin, once daily
  - Lisinopril
  - Atorvastatin
  - Vitamin C
  - Folate
- As-needed medications:
  - Acetaminophen
  - Diphenhydramine
  - Metoclopramide
  - Ondansetron
  - Promethazine
  - Docusate

6. Does the patient's allergy and medication list add any possible causes of her current condition?
7. Which medications on this list, if any, should be used with particular caution in older patients?

Table 13-19	Other Medications Prescribed to Treat or Prevent Heart Disease
Category	**Generic Name (Trade Name)g**
Angiotensin II receptor blockers (ARBs) (The generic drug names in this class of medications end in *-sartan*)	Losartan (Cozaar); valsartan (Diovan); irbesartan (Avapro); candesartan (Atacand)
Cholesterol-lowering drugs	Statins: lovastatin (Altacor, Mevacor); fluvastatin (Lescol); pravastatin (Pravachol); atorvastatin (Lipitor); simvastatin (Zocor) Niacins: nicotinic acid (Niacor); extended-release niacin (Niaspan) Bile acid resins: colestipol (Colestid); cholestyramine (Questran); colesevelam (Welchol) Fibrates: clofibrate (Atromid); gemfibrozil (Lopid); fenofibrate (Tricor)
Vasodilators	Isosorbide dinitrate[a] (Dilatrate-SR, Iso-Bid, Isonate, Isorbid, Isordil, Isotrate, Sorbitrate); isosorbide mononitrate (Imdur); hydralazine[a] (Apresoline)

[a]Isosorbide dinitrate and hydralazine are given together.

Type-specific blood products can be used as soon as the decision has been made and the recipient patient's blood type is known, but there is a somewhat greater risk of an adverse, potentially life-threatening transfusion reaction. Cross-matched blood has a decreased risk of transfusion reaction but requires a blood sample from the patient, followed by careful analysis in the blood bank before the blood product can be released for administration to the patient.

In the prehospital setting, you will most likely use unmatched blood, possibly carried by air-medical crews or sent to the scene of a prolonged extrication where a patient has a profound hemorrhage and will remain entrapped for a long period. Unmatched blood is almost always type O, Rh-negative (O negative). (Rh is the antigen responsible for hemolytic disease of the newborn.) Type O-negative blood products can theoretically be administered to patients with any blood type, although other proteins and chemicals in the blood product may cause a transfusion reaction.

During interfacility patient transports, you may face the dilemma of deciding whether to administer unmatched, type O-negative blood products or delay transport to obtain type-specific or cross-matched blood products. The stability of the patient's clinical condition and the duration of anticipated delays for blood typing or cross-matching often make the decision obvious. In the absence of a clear choice, online medical control and the sending physician are valuable resources for guidance.

Blood products require careful patient monitoring during administration. Many types of transfusion-related reactions are possible. Any paramedic who is expected to initiate or monitor blood product transfusion should become very familiar with the recognition and management of potential transfusion reactions during transport. In addition to pulse rate and blood pressure monitoring, temperature should be reassessed frequently during transport. If an indwelling urinary catheter is present, you should monitor for changes in urine color that may indicate a life-threatening hemolytic transfusion reaction.

Most blood products require special filtered IV tubing. This tubing may become clogged during massive blood product transfusions. Certain IV fluids are incompatible with blood products in the same IV tubing. Normal saline is the preferred IV fluid for Y-site tubing administration during blood product transfusions.

Packed Red Blood Cells

Packed RBCs (PRBCs) can be administered by paramedics to correct anemia resulting from blood loss, inadequate RBC production, or the massive destruction of circulating RBCs, known as hemolysis. Patients without a concurrent serious medical condition may compensate well for profound anemia that has developed during weeks to months. When blood cell loss occurs suddenly from trauma, hemorrhage, or hemolysis, patients are far less able to compensate. In general, the rate of administration of PRBCs should be proportional to the rate of blood cell loss.

A unit of PRBCs contains approximately 225 to 250 mL of concentrated RBCs, along with a preservative. Administration of 1 U of PRBCs will increase the hematocrit value, the percentage of RBCs in the blood, by roughly 3% (less with continued RBC loss). In children and infants, a patient-specific volume of PRBCs is administered. Patients at risk for volume overload, such as patients with renal failure or heart failure, require slow PRBC administration and careful monitoring of fluid volume and respiratory status.

Typically, PRBCs are administered over no longer than 4 hours per unit. In patients in critical condition, PRBCs can be administered rapidly through a commercial pressure infuser-warmer or by using pressure bags. You should use the largest IV catheter possible. In adults, at least a 20-gauge IV catheter should be used, preferably an 18-gauge or larger. Patients with trauma and hemorrhage should have adequate IV fluid resuscitation before or concurrently with PRBC administration. For blood cells, AB is the universal recipient and O the universal donor.

Units of PRBCs usually contain a citrate-based preservative. Hypocalcemia may develop as the citrate binds with calcium in the body. During massive PRBC transfusions, you should monitor for signs of hypocalcemia, such as tetany and a prolonged QT interval on the ECG tracing.

Patients receiving PRBCs are also at risk for hyperkalemia. If PRBCs are stored for a long period or if hemolysis occurs during PRBC administration, large amounts of intracellular potassium are released. In severe situations, hyperkalemia can be life threatening. Peaked T waves on the ECG tracing are highly suggestive of hyperkalemia.

Fresh Frozen Plasma

Impaired blood clotting can be treated by the administration of fresh frozen plasma (FFP). Because FFP contains many clotting factors, it is often given following trauma, hemorrhage, warfarin toxicity, disseminated intravascular coagulation, and other conditions. Whenever large volumes of other blood components (such as PRBCs) are administered, FFP should also be used. The FFP must be compatible with a patient's blood type but does not need to be Rh compatible.

In general, units of FFP hold the same volume as units of PRBCs (225–250 mL). These units require adequate defrosting before administration. FFP is used for replacement of clotting factors, not volume expansion. Volume expansion is usually best accomplished with IV fluids and PRBC transfusion. Some medical centers and EMS agencies have started using liquid plasma, also known as never-frozen plasma, which has superior stability and efficacy to FFP.[12]

Cryoprecipitate is a blood product that contains a concentrated assortment of blood clotting factors, without the additional volume present in FFP. It is unlikely that you will administer cryoprecipitate in the prehospital setting. Type AB plasma and cryoprecipitate can be given to patients with any blood type.

Platelets

Paramedics and other health care providers administer platelets to correct thrombocytopenia, a low platelet level in the blood. Thrombocytopenia can be caused by trauma, hemorrhage, various and chronic medical conditions and by certain anticoagulant medications. Patients may also have a normal level of platelets that are dysfunctional because of a clotting disorder or antiplatelet medication. Platelets must be blood type and Rh compatible.

Medications That Alter Blood Performance

Blood platelets combine with clotting or coagulation chemicals in the bloodstream to terminate bleeding when a blood vessel ruptures. This complicated process is essential for human survival. Without this process, spontaneous bleeding would readily occur and otherwise minor trauma would cause death from exsanguination. When blood clotting occurs in a blood vessel, a thrombus (blood clot) is created. This thrombus can occlude the blood vessel, jeopardizing dependent cells, tissues, and organs. During prehospital care and interfacility transport, you may administer or monitor several important medications that alter the blood's ability to form a thrombus, preventing or limiting the injury to vital organs such as the heart and lungs.

Tranexamic Acid

Tranexamic acid (Lysteda) has emerged as a powerful medication intervention to promote blood clotting and reduce mortality in trauma patients with severe bleeding. This medication is being used by many trauma centers, by the military, and in an increasing number of EMS settings.

Trauma patients begin the process of blood clot formation in response to an injury and bleeding. This clot formation is often coupled with *hyperfibrinolysis*, resulting in the rapid dissolving of new blood clots. Left unchecked, hyperfibrinolysis leads to dramatically increased mortality of trauma patients. Tranexamic acid is a commercial preparation of lysine, an amino acid in the body responsible for preventing breakdown of fibrin clots. When administered within 3 hours of the traumatic event, tranexamic acid significantly decreases patient mortality. Currently, the recommended dose is 1 g in an IV infusion administered over 10 minutes. This protocol may change as clinical practice evolves.[13]

Anticoagulant Medications

Anticoagulant medications impair the function of clotting or coagulation chemicals in the bloodstream. Human blood contains a balance of substances that promote the formation of blood clots or are capable of dissolving blood clots. This balance permits the termination of bleeding while simultaneously allowing blood clots to dissolve once blood vessel integrity is restored. Anticoagulant medications enhance the function of substances in the blood that inhibit clot formation. These medications prevent the formation of new blood clots and the growth of existing clots, but they do not dissolve existing blood clots.

Heparin and enoxaparin (Lovenox) are frequently used anticoagulant medications that enhance antithrombin

III to inhibit blood coagulation. Both medications are used to treat or prevent acute coronary syndrome, deep vein thrombosis, and pulmonary embolus. These medications are not generally initiated in the prehospital setting, although it is conceivable that paramedics in remote locations or ambitious EMS systems may administer these medications in specific clinical situations. Enoxaparin is administered as a single IV or subcutaneous dose, usually every 12 hours. In addition to the possibility of prehospital administration, paramedics may continue an IV heparin infusion during interfacility transport. If only one IV site is available, heparin infusions are compatible with nitroglycerin and several other prehospital medication infusions through Y-site IV tubing. Both heparin and enoxaparin have the potential to cause bleeding, thrombocytopenia, and a variety of other adverse effects.

You may also encounter patients receiving fondaparinux (Arixtra), another anticoagulant medication. Fondaparinux is typically administered to prevent deep vein thrombosis, to treat thrombosis, or during the period immediately following an ST-elevation myocardial infarction to prevent reinfarction.

Warfarin (Coumadin) is a common anticoagulant medication that patients take orally on a short- or long-term basis for treatment or prevention of blood clots. Warfarin works by preventing the production of four different blood clotting factors that use vitamin K. Patients are at risk of life-threatening bleeding when warfarin levels are not adequately controlled, following trauma, or when any other hemorrhage occurs. Certain foods, alcohol, and a variety of medications can increase effects from warfarin. A wide variety of physiologic conditions can predispose patients taking warfarin to severe bleeding. Warfarin levels are inferred by blood prothrombin time (PT) and international normalized ratio (INR) levels. During interfacility and critical care transports, the patient's PT and/or INR values are essential to understanding the severity of the patient's situation and should be included in the handoff report to the receiving facility's personnel.

Several treatment options are available if patients taking warfarin develop severe bleeding or require emergent surgery. It is important to carefully weigh the risk of hemorrhage against the risks associated with reversing the protective effects from warfarin. In many instances, providers will attempt to control bleeding without completely reversing the warfarin. This decision usually requires specialty consultation and thoughtful deliberation among providers. Warfarin can be reversed through administration of vitamin K, also known as phytonadione, given as intermittent IV infusions. Patients anticoagulated by warfarin may receive a clotting factor concentrate in response to severe bleeding or prior to surgery. Four-factor prothrombin complex concentrate is available in the United States under the brand name Kcentra. This medication is given by IV infusion at a rate based on the patient's weight and INR value. FFP is an additional option for individuals with hemorrhage or impaired blood clotting ability due to warfarin. FFP may take longer to administer and can cause fluid volume overload in susceptible individuals. You are unlikely to be involved in the decision to reverse warfarin-related coagulopathy; however, understanding this complication is important and enables efficient communication during interfacility and critical care transports.

Antiplatelet Medications

Platelets perform an essential role in blood clotting and thrombus formation. Medications can be used to reduce platelet aggregation (clumping), preventing new thrombus formation or the extension of an existing thrombus. You may encounter several oral and IV antiplatelet medications. **Table 13-20** lists commonly prescribed anticoagulant and antiplatelet agents.

Aspirin is an oral antiplatelet medication used extensively for the treatment and prevention of thrombus formation. Aspirin is administered in the prehospital setting for treatment of acute coronary syndrome, often suspected in patients reporting chest pain. Aspirin is also indicated for the treatment of a stroke once the presence of hemorrhage has been reliably excluded. You should carefully assess for the possibility of an occult aneurysm when considering aspirin for a patient with chest pain. Platelet inactivation from aspirin has the potential to seriously complicate any condition associated with bleeding.

When indicated, aspirin is crushed or chewed before swallowing, promoting rapid GI absorption. Aspirin is rapidly eliminated by the body, but the antiplatelet effects persist until all affected platelets are replaced, which may take up to 10 days. Patients may claim an aspirin allergy based on GI upset. You should ask about

Table 13-20 Commonly Prescribed Anticoagulant and Antiplatelet Agents

Category	Generic Name (Trade Name)
Antiplatelet agents	Clopidogrel (Plavix); ticlopidine (Ticlid); aspirin; prasugrel (Effient)
Coumarin anticoagulant	Warfarin (Coumadin)
Direct thrombin inhibitor	Dabigatran (Pradaxa)

the specific circumstances when a patient reports an aspirin allergy or sensitivity and aspirin is otherwise clinically indicated.

Clopidogrel (Plavix) and ticlopidine (Ticlid) are two additional oral antiplatelet medications that paramedics may administer as an aspirin alternative. These medications inhibit platelet aggregation by a mechanism different from that of aspirin. Clopidogrel has been shown to be superior to aspirin in certain clinical situations. Ticlopidine has several serious adverse effects that limit its role in prehospital and long-term treatment. Aspirin, clopidogrel, and ticlopidine may cause various types of bleeding in patients, depending on the medication, dose, or combination.[14,15]

You may encounter various glycoprotein IIb/IIIa inhibitor medications during interfacility transport. Abciximab (ReoPro), tirofiban (Aggrastat), and eptifibatide (Integrilin) provide potent platelet inhibition in a manner more effective than that of the aforementioned oral antiplatelet medications. These medications are administered by an IV infusion, which is often continued during interfacility transport to a tertiary cardiac care center. Bleeding and thrombocytopenia are adverse effects observed in roughly 5% to 7% of patients receiving these medications.[16]

Fibrinolytics

Fibrinolytics (eg, Activase) dissolve blood clots in arteries and veins. These medications are administered for the emergency treatment of acute myocardial infarction and stroke. In addition, fibrinolytics are administered in lower doses to open certain vascular catheters that have become occluded by a presumed blood clot.

Fibrinolytics have the serious potential to cause life-threatening hemorrhage. Careful patient selection and exclusion are essential before these medications are administered. Any condition suggestive of blood clot formation elsewhere in the body, such as recent trauma or surgery, is likely to prevent a patient from receiving fibrinolytics. There are numerous other absolute and relative contraindications to fibrinolytic therapy.

Fibrinolytics remain valuable in remote locations and smaller community hospitals but have a limited role in the treatment of acute myocardial infarction when interventional cardiology services are readily available. Many hospitals have developed rapid diagnostic and treatment procedures to optimize the effectiveness of fibrinolytics for acute ischemic strokes.

Avoid multiple IV attempts and unnecessary trauma in any patient who is a likely candidate for fibrinolytics. A careful determination of the time of onset of symptoms will influence the decision about whether fibrinolytics will be administered. You should not unnecessarily delay patient transport; these medications are indicated only within a short period after the onset of symptoms. Prolonged prehospital time may preclude the administration of fibrinolytics.

Patient Safety

The potential for medication errors in the EMS environment is enhanced by issues such as packaging and labeling changes. Unfortunately, in recent years, EMS agencies have been dramatically affected by medication manufacturing shortages (eg, shortages in $D_{50}W$, sodium bicarbonate, dopamine, morphine sulfate, and glucagon). As substitutes for the unavailable medications, agencies may use medications with which paramedics are less familiar, medications from different manufacturers that use different labeling or packaging, and medications that have different dosing regimens. In a high-pressure, uncontrolled environment, such as the back of a moving ambulance with a patient who is decompensating or going into cardiac arrest, errors can easily occur.

Words of Wisdom

Consider carrying a magnifying glass to read small print on labels (eg, concentration, expiration date). The zoom function of a cell phone's camera can also be used for this purpose.

▶ Medications Used for Neurologic Conditions

As a paramedic, you may encounter and treat a large number of patients with neurologic complaints and conditions. Pain accompanies the vast majority of traumatic injuries and is a common symptom associated with many medical conditions. Seizure activity is another event that frequently triggers EMS activation. Many patients encountered by EMS would benefit clinically from the treatment of anxiety or the administration of sedative medications.

Paramedics rely heavily on opioid (narcotic) medications for analgesia (treatment of pain) in the prehospital setting. These medications are effective at eliminating or reducing pain caused by a variety of conditions. You will likely also need to administer naloxone, a powerful reversal agent for patients who have received dangerous amounts of opioid chemicals.

Benzodiazepine medications (discussed earlier in the *Medications Used in Airway Management* section) are the primary treatment modality for persistent seizure activity. These medications also work well for sedation and the treatment of anxiety. Benzodiazepines are arguably underused in the prehospital setting.

Opioid Analgesic Medications

Paramedics administer medications that stimulate opioid receptors in the body to relieve or prevent pain associated with an injury, medical condition, or medically related procedure or movement. The human body contains at least seven types of opioid receptors in the CNS, peripheral nervous system, and GI tract. Medications used by paramedics act on mu (μ) opioid receptor sites. Natural endorphins also stimulate (activate) mu receptor sites, causing analgesia, euphoria, constricted pupils, respiratory depression, and decreased GI motility. Opioid medications are also known to suppress the cough reflex, which can be a desirable or an adverse clinical effect.

Opioid chemicals, medications, and illicit drugs are known for causing tolerance, cross-tolerance, and addiction. Patients who receive opioid substances on a long-term basis often require unusually high doses of opioid medications for relief of pain from an acute illness or injury. They may also experience severe withdrawal symptoms if opioid reversal is required following an error during treatment.

Opioid medications can cause profound sedation, respiratory depression, and apnea when excessive doses are administered. Other adverse effects include hypotension, bradycardia, palpitations, dysrhythmias, and noncardiogenic pulmonary edema. The severity or likelihood of adverse effects may vary significantly among different opioid medications.

Of the opioid medications, paramedics administer morphine sulfate or fentanyl most commonly in the prehospital setting. Meperidine (Demerol), hydromorphone (Dilaudid), and newer synthetic opioid medications may be used in select EMS or critical care transport settings. Depending on the medication chosen, paramedics may use the IV, IM, or intranasal route of administration.

Morphine sulfate is used frequently in EMS. In addition to the aforementioned adverse effects, morphine sulfate is known to cause nausea or vomiting in up to 60% of patients.[17] Always use extreme caution when administering morphine to patients who are unable to protect their airway. Patients with an altered level of consciousness and patients secured to a backboard may experience a life-threatening airway obstruction if vomiting occurs after morphine administration. Morphine may also prompt a histamine release that causes pruritus (itching), flushing, and diaphoresis. These symptoms are often inaccurately described as an allergic reaction.

Fentanyl is gaining popularity as an opioid analgesic in the prehospital setting. It is generally not as prone to causing hypotension, making it the preferred analgesic for patients in critical or unstable condition. Fentanyl also does not have the same risk of nausea and histamine release that morphine has, and it can be administered intranasally.

Opiate Antagonist Medication

Naloxone is a powerful opioid receptor antagonist that is used by paramedics and other health care providers to reverse the effects of excessive opioid chemicals in the body. Naloxone competes with opioid chemicals at opioid receptor sites, causing a complete or partial reversal of the clinical effects of opioids. Efficacy is dose-dependent. Large doses of naloxone are often required to reverse the effects of potent opioid chemicals. In addition, the duration of naloxone in the body is less than that of many opioid chemicals. Recurrent toxic effects are a risk when naloxone is eliminated more rapidly than the opioid chemicals in the body. Severe opioid overdose situations require repeated naloxone administration or continuous IV infusion.

When administering naloxone to patients who receive opioids on a long-term basis, administer only enough naloxone to correct life-threatening conditions such as respiratory depression and airway compromise. Complete opioid reversal is likely to cause severe withdrawal symptoms, endangering the patient and health care providers.

Phenytoin and Fosphenytoin

Phenytoin (Dilantin) and fosphenytoin (Cerebyx) are administered to prevent seizure activity. Patients may receive either of these medications on a long-term basis for control of a seizure disorder. You may also encounter these medications while performing an interfacility transport of patients with a head injury, intracranial hemorrhage, or status epilepticus. Both medications are administered by IV infusion, usually during 10 to 30 minutes, depending on medication and dose. Phenytoin and fosphenytoin decrease the potential for seizure activity by altering sodium channels, limiting cellular sodium in portions of the CNS. In general, fosphenytoin has fewer adverse effects than phenytoin has, but both medications can cause a wide variety of adverse effects throughout the body.

▶ Medications Affecting the Gastrointestinal System

Paramedics administer two major groups of medications that affect the GI system. Histamine-2 receptor antagonists are administered to reduce the acid in the stomach and GI tract and also augment other medications used in the treatment of allergic reactions. Antiemetic agents are administered to prevent and treat nausea and vomiting.

Histamine-2 Receptor Antagonists

Histamine-2 receptor antagonist medications (H_2 blockers) decrease acid secretion in the stomach. You may encounter patients who receive H_2 blockers for short-term and episodic treatment of acid-related GI conditions. These medications are also administered in emergency settings to offset histamine release during an immune-mediated medication reaction or other type of allergic reaction. H_2 blockers prevent histamine from stimulating receptor sites on parietal cells in the stomach. Acid secretion is reduced, protecting against ulcers, GI bleeding, acid-aspiration pneumonitis, and a variety of other related conditions. Ranitidine (Zantac), cimetidine (Tagamet), and famotidine (Pepcid) are available for oral and IV administration.

Antiemetic Medications

Several types of antiemetic medications are available for use in the prehospital setting. Patients may activate EMS with a primary complaint of nausea or vomiting. Nausea and vomiting occur as symptoms associated with events such as head injury, pregnancy, overdose, and myocardial ischemia. Beyond the obvious discomfort associated with nausea and vomiting, vomiting may dramatically worsen many serious medical conditions. Protracted vomiting may cause a Mallory-Weiss tear (a tear in the mucous membrane of the lower part of the esophagus or the upper part of the stomach), leading to GI bleeding. Vomiting can raise intracranial and intraocular pressure, adversely affecting patients with head or eye injuries. Vomiting can also cause pulmonary aspiration in patients with an inadequately protected airway because of a decreased level of consciousness or positioning (such as being secured to a backboard or lying supine). Vomiting with aspiration of activated charcoal, administered following a toxic exposure, is often lethal. Patients with epiglottitis, peritonsillar abscess, or other airway disease may have increased edema due to vomiting. You are strongly encouraged to use antiemetic medications to prevent nausea and vomiting in at-risk patients.

Promethazine and prochlorperazine (Compazine) are phenothiazine antiemetic medications used in various health care settings. Phenothiazine medications have antiemetic and antipsychotic properties. These medications activate dopaminergic receptors in the brain, releasing hormones that depress the reticular activating system of the brain, and, ultimately, inhibit emesis.

Both promethazine and prochlorperazine are available in oral and IV preparations. IV administration of these medications is associated with a number of serious adverse effects. Depending on the setting, you may administer these medications, diluted in a large syringe, by the IV route over 1 to 2 minutes. In ideal situations, you should dilute either medication in 50 mL of normal saline and administer over approximately 10 minutes. Promethazine is notorious for tissue injury during IV administration. Prochlorperazine is known for causing hypotension if administered rapidly through an IV line. **Dystonic** reactions are possible with promethazine and prochlorperazine, causing unusual muscle activity and significant patient discomfort. Dystonic reactions can be treated with IV diphenhydramine. Many other adverse effects are possible.

Metoclopramide (Reglan) is a novel antiemetic medication that may be available in the prehospital setting. Metoclopramide increases GI motility by enhancing the effects of ACh at receptor sites in the upper GI tract. Increased GI motility promotes gastric emptying that is useful in a variety of clinical situations. Metoclopramide can be administered orally, by slow IV injection, and by IV infusion. Dystonic reactions are also a possible adverse effect of metoclopramide and are again treated with IV diphenhydramine.

Antiemetic medications that antagonize the 5-hydroxytryptamine$_3$ (5-HT$_3$) receptor sites have experienced a recent surge in popularity. The 5-HT$_3$ receptors are present in the brain and GI tract. These receptors have a prominent role in activation of the vomiting center of the brain. Medications with the ability to occupy these receptor sites prevent certain (but not all) mechanisms that induce vomiting. For example, 5-HT$_3$ antagonists do not prevent vomiting related to motion sickness.

Ondansetron, granisetron (Kytril), and dolasetron (Anzemet) are 5-HT$_3$ receptor antagonists available for clinical use. These medications are available in oral and IV preparations. Certain 5-HT$_3$ medications are now available in orally dissolving tablets. This preparation may eliminate the need for starting an IV in patients who are actively vomiting but not showing signs of dehydration. Adverse effects are minimal but include the potential for QT prolongation shown on an ECG tracing. You should expect to encounter these medications more frequently as costs decrease and use becomes more widespread.

Octreotide

You may encounter octreotide (Sandostatin) during interfacility transport of certain patients. Octreotide is not routinely administered in the prehospital setting. This medication is a synthetic version of somatostatin, a hormone that inhibits serotonin release, causing decreased secretion of insulin, glucagon, growth hormones, and various other chemicals. Octreotide has many potential uses. You may be requested to monitor an IV octreotide infusion during interfacility transport of patients with bleeding esophageal varices. Octreotide decreases blood flow through esophageal blood vessels, reducing bleeding until definitive treatment can be provided. You should carefully monitor patients for a wide assortment of adverse effects, including bradycardia and chest pain related to octreotide.

▶ Miscellaneous Medications Used in the Prehospital Setting

Certain medications are used widely in the prehospital setting but do not belong to one of the medication classes discussed. You should expect to use these medications for a variety of clinical situations. Additional dosing and administration information is available in the Appendix, *Emergency Medications*.

Acetaminophen

Acetaminophen (Tylenol, APAP) is a medication with antipyretic (fever reduction) and mild analgesic properties. Paramedics and other EMS providers may administer acetaminophen as an adjunct to other analgesic medications, to reduce discomfort by treating fever symptoms, or to prevent febrile seizures in pediatric patients. Acetaminophen is not indicated for hyperthermia related to the toxic effects of medications or environmental exposure.

Acetaminophen is available as a tablet and capsule, liquid, and rectal suppository. At least two liquid concentrations are available, which may lead to dose calculation errors if you do not confirm the concentration before administration. Oral administration should be avoided in patients who are at high risk for seizures or airway compromise.

Adverse effects are rare when acetaminophen is given at therapeutic doses. Toxicity from acetaminophen overdose is insidious and often mismanaged by health care providers. Elevated acetaminophen levels can cause severe, potentially fatal liver damage. Toxicity is determined by patient history and evaluation of a serum acetaminophen level, calculated according to the likely time of overdose. Once toxicity has been determined, many providers continue to mistakenly associate toxicity with serum acetaminophen levels. Liver damage will continue to occur from the presence of a harmful metabolite, rather than from the acetaminophen itself.

Calcium Preparations

In the prehospital setting, IV calcium has many potentially lifesaving uses. Calcium can be used for all of the following purposes:

- As an antidote to calcium channel blocker overdose
- To treat magnesium (sulfate) toxicity
- To prevent dysrhythmia during severe hyperkalemia
- For calcium repletion in patients with hypocalcemia
- For calcium restoration after hydrofluoric acid exposure
- As a pretreatment to prevent hypotension associated with IV verapamil administration

Calcium is not indicated for routine use during cardiac arrest resuscitation.

Typically, IV calcium is available as calcium chloride or calcium gluconate. Calcium chloride contains approximately three times the amount of elemental calcium per gram as calcium gluconate contains. Both medications are known to be extremely irritating to blood vessels and should be diluted for slow IV infusion whenever possible. Carefully monitor IV catheter sites to avoid extravasation. Avoid subcutaneous or IM administration and assess for incompatibility when administering simultaneously with other medications. Precipitation in IV tubing has been known to occur.

Dextrose

Intravenous dextrose solution is administered to patients with known or presumptive hypoglycemia. In most cases, hypoglycemia is diagnosed with a handheld glucometer, now available on most ALS ambulances. When a glucometer is not immediately available, various clinical clues, such as a known history of diabetes, concurrent ethanol intoxication, and altered mental status, will prompt an astute paramedic to suspect hypoglycemia.

Once hypoglycemia is diagnosed, dextrose solution is administered through a large-bore IV catheter while the IV site is continually observed for signs of infiltration. Extravasation of IV dextrose can cause tissue destruction and edema. You should confirm IV placement with an adequate flush or free-flowing IV fluid before administering dextrose.

The initial adult dose for moderate to severe hypoglycemia is 25 g of a 50% dextrose solution for a total volume of 50 mL. Patients with mild hypoglycemia receive a reduced dose. Issues with availability and concerns regarding administration may prompt EMS agencies to consider lower dextrose concentrations for treatment of hypoglycemia in adults. Children receive weight-based doses of a 25% dextrose solution. Infants and smaller children receive weight-based doses of a 10% dextrose solution. Any of these patients may receive dextrose as a continuous infusion, rather than intermittent bolus, depending on the clinical situation. Rebound hypoglycemia is possible following dextrose administration. You should continue to monitor a patient's clinical status and blood glucose level following dextrose administration.

Diphenhydramine

EMS providers frequently use diphenhydramine for a variety of clinical situations. Diphenhydramine is a competitive histamine-1 receptor antagonist, preventing receptor activation by histamine released during various medical conditions. Diphenhydramine has a wide range of potential uses in the prehospital setting:

- Treatment of anaphylaxis in conjunction with other medications and interventions
- Sole treatment of mild allergic or immune-mediated medication reactions
- Mild sedative
- Mild antitussive (cough suppressant)
- Treatment of dystonic reaction or extrapyramidal symptoms
- Treatment of pruritus from an unknown cause
- Drying of the mucous membranes in patients with symptomatic rhinorrhea

Paramedics will administer diphenhydramine by the IV or IM route most commonly. Oral capsule, tablet, and liquid preparations are also available commercially and are routinely taken by many people to treat minor conditions, such as seasonal allergies. Adverse effects from therapeutic doses of diphenhydramine are usually limited to mild sedation, palpitations, and anxiety. These symptoms become more significant if excessive amounts of diphenhydramine are administered in error. Profound toxicity and death are possible following large overdoses.

Glucagon

Glucagon (GlucaGen) is another medication with a variety of potential uses in the prehospital setting. Glucagon is a naturally occurring peptide hormone, secreted by the pancreas, that is also manufactured commercially for the treatment of certain medical conditions.

You may use glucagon for the treatment of hypoglycemia. Glucagon converts glycogen stores in the liver to circulating blood glucose, which can be used by various cells. This medication is useful if you are unable to initiate IV access in diabetic patients who would otherwise be given IV glucose (dextrose). Patients who are combative because of moderate hypoglycemia and unresponsive patients without IV access are likely recipients of glucagon by the IM route. Glucose production takes 5 to 20 minutes following IV administration of glucagon and 30 minutes following IM administration. Blood glucose levels remain increased for only a limited time after glucagon is administered. Be sure to continually monitor for a return of hypoglycemia. An IV dextrose solution remains the preferred treatment for patients with hypoglycemia.

Glucagon is also used to provide increased heart rate and contractility following a beta-adrenergic antagonist (beta-blocker) overdose. It produces positive chronotropic and inotropic effects without directly activating beta-1 receptors. Glucagon is used in the treatment of severe calcium channel blocker overdoses to reverse myocardial depression. These two clinical situations require large amounts of glucagon, often more than 10 mg, which is rarely carried by EMS. In addition, glucagon is supplied as a dry powder in a vial with a separate phenol vial for reconstitution. Large doses of phenol during treatment of beta-blocker or calcium channel blocker overdoses will cause phenol toxicity. In these cases, you should reconstitute glucagon with sterile water if more than one vial (1 mg) of glucagon will be administered.

You may also administer glucagon to patients who present with a foreign body or large food particle lodged in the esophagus. Glucagon relaxes the smooth muscle in the GI tract, possibly allowing the object to pass into the stomach for digestion. Glucagon for this purpose should typically be administered only after consultation with online medical control.

Ketorolac

Certain EMS systems use ketorolac (Toradol) as an alternative or adjunct to opioid analgesic medications. Ketorolac is a nonsteroidal anti-inflammatory drug (NSAID) that inhibits prostaglandin synthesis, treating both pain and inflammation. It is typically administered via IV or IM route, although oral forms are available. GI irritation and headache are the most common adverse effects. Ketorolac is also known to cause pain at the injection site. Avoid or use with caution in any patient known to be susceptible to GI bleeding or a similar disorder.

Magnesium Sulfate

Magnesium sulfate is an IV electrolyte medication with several important clinical indications. Magnesium sulfate is used for the following:

- Emergency treatment of torsades de pointes or similar ventricular dysrhythmia
- Correction of known or presumptive hypomagnesemia, common in patients who are malnourished or consume ethanol on a long-term basis
- Prevention or treatment of seizures in pregnant patients with preeclampsia or eclampsia
- Adjunctive treatment with bronchodilators and other treatments for severe, refractory asthma

In cardiac arrest situations, 1 to 2 g of magnesium sulfate can be given by slow IV push during 1 to 2 minutes. In other emergency situations, magnesium sulfate is administered as an IV infusion during at least 5 minutes, although slower infusion rates are preferred for patients in less critical condition.

Magnesium sulfate replaces magnesium deficiencies in the body. Magnesium is essential for the movement of other electrolytes such as sodium, calcium, and potassium through channels of cell membranes. Hypomagnesemia causes seizure activity and cardiac dysrhythmias. As magnesium sulfate is administered, it decreases the excitability of cell membranes and slows conduction through the atrioventricular node, prolonging conduction time.

Magnesium sulfate acts to relax various smooth muscle tissues. Clinical effects on smooth muscle are most notable in the lower airways, causing bronchodilation, and in the uterus, causing tocolysis. Respiratory depression, decreased muscle tone, and loss of deep tendon reflexes are possible from excessive doses of magnesium sulfate. Toxic effects from magnesium sulfate are treated by discontinuing the infusion and administering an IV calcium preparation.

Sodium Bicarbonate

Sodium bicarbonate is an alkalinizing agent used in the prehospital and other health care settings. It is administered to do the following:

- Raise the blood pH in patients with a severe metabolic acidosis.
- Stabilize profound hyperkalemia in an emergency situation.
- Provide cardiac cell membrane stabilization following tricyclic antidepressant overdose.
- Promote urinary excretion of salicylate chemicals and certain tissue waste products.
- Replace bicarbonate lost due to various medical conditions.

Sodium bicarbonate can be administered by rapid IV push or added to IV fluids for intermittent or continuous infusion. You should evaluate potential incompatibility when sodium bicarbonate is administered in the same IV tubing as other prehospital medications, especially calcium preparations and catecholamines. Patients receiving sodium bicarbonate should be monitored for changes in electrolyte and blood pH levels. Excessive bicarbonate administration can cause fluid volume overload, alkalosis, numerous electrolyte abnormalities, and cerebral and pulmonary edema. In many cases, sodium bicarbonate is titrated to maintain a desired arterial or urinary pH value.

Tetracaine

Tetracaine, a mild opthalmic anesthetic, is used when inserting the Morgan Lens into an eye, to facilitate flushing the eyes. This procedure is discussed in Chapter 19, *Diseases of the Eyes, Ears, Nose, and Throat.*

Thiamine

Thiamine is a commercial medication preparation of vitamin B_1. Paramedics administer thiamine to correct a presumptive thiamine deficiency before dextrose administration in patients who are malnourished or who consume alcohol on a long-term basis. Thiamine deficiency can cause Wernicke encephalopathy, a neurologic disorder, which may be exacerbated by the sudden administration of IV dextrose. Thiamine is usually administered by the IV route in the prehospital setting, either by IV push or added to IV fluids. Toxic and adverse effects are unlikely when therapeutic doses are administered.

YOU are the Paramedic SUMMARY

1. What medical conditions would you expect to encounter in a skilled nursing facility or long-term care facility?

A vast array of medical conditions may be present in patients living in a skilled nursing facility or long-term care facility. Many medical interventions that previously have been used only in hospitals and rehabilitation facilities are now commonplace in skilled nursing facilities and long-term care facilities. These interventions include IV therapy, dialysis, complex wound care, and orthopaedic treatment. Dementia is the most common reason for skilled nursing facility placement. Other conditions such as stroke (cerebrovascular accident), heart failure, Parkinson disease, osteoarthritis, and complications from diabetes mellitus are common.

2. Based on this brief history and physical examination, what problems do you suspect?

This brief history and physical examination cannot exclude any of the possible causes or conditions that the patient may have.

3. What additional information would assist you with identifying possible causes of her condition?

Vital signs, blood glucose level, physical examination, thorough history of the present illness, and medication list would be helpful in identifying possible causes of the altered mental status in this patient.

4. Would intravenous dextrose solution be indicated for this patient?

Intravenous dextrose solution is not indicated for this patient. Normal blood glucose levels range from 70 to 99 mg/dL. This patient has a blood glucose level of 132 mg/dL and would be considered hyperglycemic. It is unlikely that this patient would benefit from IV dextrose solutions. Additionally, administration of dextrose solution could worsen other possible causes of altered mental status in older patients.

5. Do the electrocardiogram (ECG) findings assist in identifying the cause of this patient's condition?

The ECG tracing reveals sinus tachycardia. This finding indicates a state of physiologic stress on the body, but it is not specific enough to identify the cause of this patient's condition. Sinus tachycardia typically represents an increased catecholamine release from a wide variety of causes, such as exercise or physical exertion, fever, hypovolemia, shock, sepsis, pain, anxiety, hypoxia, or anemia, among numerous other possible causes. Many potential causes of altered mental status in older patients cause sinus tachycardia. It is not diagnostic in this scenario.

6. Does the patient's allergy and medication list add any possible causes of her current condition?

This patient is currently receiving 12 different medications on either a regularly scheduled or an as-needed basis. While certain medications on this patient's profile are relatively benign, other medications on her profile are extremely likely to alter many body organs, systems, and function. Medication interactions and medication side effects are frequently implicated as the cause of altered mental status in older patients. Medication toxicity, medication side effects, and medication interactions should be evaluated whenever searching for causes of altered mental status, particularly in older patients.

7. Which medications on this list, if any, should be used with particular caution in older patients?

Both promethazine (Phenergan) and metoclopramide (Reglan) require caution when used in older patients. Each of these medications can cause a number of serious cardiovascular and neurologic symptoms. Neurologic symptoms range from mild drowsiness to serious reactions, such as seizures and hallucinations. Promethazine is notorious for causing bizarre and unpredictable responses in older patients, including paradoxical excitation rather than sedation.

YOU are the Paramedic SUMMARY *(continued)*

EMS Patient Care Report (PCR)

Date: 7-23-18	**Incident No.:** 2056	**Nature of Call:** Altered mental status	**Location:** 1 Goldenbridge Lane

Dispatched: 1510	**En Route:** 1511	**At Scene:** 1516	**Transport:** 1545	**At Hospital:** 1600	**In Service:** 1620

Patient Information

Age: 88 **Sex:** F **Weight (in kg [lb]):** 60 kg (133 lb)	**Allergies:** Penicillin, sulfa medications **Medications:** Metformin, aspirin QD, lisinopril, atorvastatin, vitamin C, folate **Past Medical History:** Diabetes mellitus, nausea and vomiting **Chief Complaint:** Altered mental status

Vital Signs

Time: 1521	**BP:** 96/64	**Pulse:** 108	**Respirations:** 22	**Spo_2:** 98% on O_2
Time: 1531	**BP:** 104/68	**Pulse:** 106	**Respirations:** 22	**Spo_2:** 99% on O_2
Time: 1541	**BP:** 112/72	**Pulse:** 104	**Respirations:** 20	**Spo_2:** 99% on O_2
Time: 1551	**BP:** 114/76	**Pulse:** 98	**Respirations:** 20	**Spo_2:** 98% on O_2

EMS Treatment (circle all that apply)

Oxygen @ 10 **L/min via (circle one):** **NC** **(NRM)** **Bag-mask device**	**Assisted Ventilation**	**Airway Adjunct**	**CPR**	
Defibrillation	**Bleeding Control**	**Bandaging**	**Splinting**	(**Other:** Cardiac monitoring)

Narrative

On arrival, found 88-year-old woman in bed with decreased responsiveness, moaning and incoherent speech, eyes open to deep tactile stimuli. Pt admitted for complications of diabetes mellitus. Pt developed nausea, vomiting, and diarrhea over past 36 to 48 hours. Pt noted to be "not herself." Pt temp. 99.7°F (37.6°C) just prior to arrival. Pt given 100% O_2 via nonrebreathing mask. Blood glucose checked with a result of 132 mg/dL. Pt vitals taken and noted above. Slightly elevated pulse noted, and cardiac monitor applied. ECG tracing shows sinus tachycardia. Started IV in the right antecubital space with an 18-gauge catheter. Normal saline bag hung with 10-drop set at KVO rate. Pt placed on stretcher and vitals taken. Pt transported to Memorial Hospital without further changes. Report given to RN in room 4; IV patent and rhythm shown on the monitor.**End of report**

Prep Kit

▶ Ready for Review

- Although the science of pharmacology has evolved into a sophisticated area of health care, certain medications discovered in ancient times are still in use.
- Paramedics need to be familiar with the rules and regulations implemented under the Controlled Substances Act (also known as the Comprehensive Drug Abuse Prevention and Control Act) of 1970.
- Schedule I medications may not be prescribed, dispensed, used, or administered for medical use.
- All Schedule II through V medications require locked storage, significant record keeping, and controlled wasting procedures.
- Every medication in the United States is given three distinct names:
  - Chemical name
  - Generic name
  - Brand name
- Reference sources, such as the *United States Pharmacopeia–National Formulary* and the *Physicians' Desk Reference*, provide details about thousands of medications.
- Direct sunlight, extremes of heat and cold, and physical damage to medication containers can make medications ineffective or unsafe for use.
- Controlled medications require additional security, record keeping, and disposal precautions. They must be kept in locked storage or continuously held by an on-duty EMS provider responsible for administration.
- As a medication is administered, it begins to alter a function or process in the body. This action is known as pharmacodynamics.
- Medications are developed to reach and bind with particular receptor sites of target cells. Alpha and beta receptors include alpha-1 (vasoconstriction), alpha-2 (insulin restriction, glucagon secretion, inhibition of norepinephrine release), beta-1 (cardiac effects), and beta-2 (smooth muscle relaxation and bronchodilation).
- Newer medications are designed to target only very specific receptor sites on certain cells in an attempt to minimize side effects.
- A wide variety of factors, including the patient's genetic makeup, determine how a particular medication will affect a patient and may influence the choice of medication, dose, route, timing, manner of administration, and monitoring necessary after a patient receives a medication.
- The terms *side effect* and *adverse effect* are often used interchangeably, but adverse effect is usually meant in prehospital settings. Adverse effects are undesired or harmful responses to a medication.
- The relationship between the median effective dose and the median lethal dose or median toxic dose is known as the therapeutic index or therapeutic ratio.
- Repeated exposure to a medication within a particular class has the potential to cause a tolerance affecting other medications in the same class.
- Patients receiving multiple medications, drugs, or other chemicals are at risk of an unintended interaction between the various substances, possibly with unexpected results.
- As a medication is administered, the body begins a complex process of moving the medication, possibly altering the structure of the medication and ultimately removing the medication from the body. The medication dose, route of administration, and clinical status of a patient will largely determine the duration of action and effectiveness of the medication.
- Many medication factors such as the size of medication molecules, the ability to bind with other substances in the body, and the ability to dissolve in certain body fluids determine which cells, tissues, and organs a particular medication will reach.
- Biotransformation is a process that has four possible effects on a medication absorbed into the body:
  - Can become active, producing wanted or unwanted clinical effects
  - Can be changed into another active medication
  - Can become completely or partially inactivated
  - Can be transformed into a substance that is easier for the body to eliminate
- Paramedics are constantly at risk for a cognitive error (such as choosing the wrong medication or dose) or a technical error (such as administering more volume of medication than intended).
- There are 10 rights of medication administration:
  - Right patient
  - Right medication
  - Right dose
  - Right route
  - Right time
  - Right documentation and reporting
  - Right assessment
  - Right to refuse
  - Right evaluation
  - Right patient education
- Medications that influence the sympathetic nervous system are classified according to the receptors with which they interact—alpha or beta.

Prep Kit *(continued)*

- Medications and medication groups often used in the prehospital setting include medications used for airway and respiratory management; medications used to manage conditions affecting the cardiovascular, gastrointestinal, and neurologic systems; and blood products and medications used to manage conditions affecting the blood.

▶ Vital Vocabulary

absolute refractory period The early phase of cardiac repolarization, wherein the heart muscle cannot be stimulated to depolarize; also known as the effective refractory period.

absorption The process by which the molecules of a substance are moved from the site of entry or administration into systemic circulation.

acetylcholinesterase An enzyme that breaks down acetylcholine.

active metabolite A medication that has undergone biotransformation and is able to alter a cellular process or body function.

active transport The process of molecules binding with carrier proteins when energy is used to move the molecules against a concentration gradient.

adverse effect Abnormal or harmful effect to an organism caused by exposure to a chemical. It is indicated by some result such as death, a change in food or water consumption, altered body and organ weights, altered enzyme levels, or visible illness.

affinity The ability of a medication to bind with a particular receptor site.

agonist medications The group of medications that initiates or alters a cellular activity by attaching to receptor sites, prompting a cellular response.

analgesia The state of being insensible to pain while still conscious.

anaphylaxis An extreme systemic form of an allergic reaction involving two or more body systems.

anesthetic A medication that causes the inability to feel sensation.

antagonist medications The group of medications that prevent endogenous or exogenous agonist chemicals from reaching cell receptor sites and initiating or altering a particular cellular activity.

antibiotics The medications used to fight infection by killing the microorganisms or preventing their multiplication to allow the body's immune system to overcome them.

antifungals The medications used to treat fungal infections.

antimicrobials The medications used to kill or suppress the growth of microorganisms.

automaticity A state in which cardiac cells are at rest, waiting for the generation of a spontaneous impulse from within.

bioavailability The percentage of the unchanged medication that reaches systemic circulation.

biotransformation A process with four possible effects on a medication absorbed into the body: (1) An inactive substance can become active, capable of producing desired or unwanted clinical effects. (2) An active medication can be changed into another active medication. (3) An active medication may be completely or partially inactivated. (4) A medication is transformed into a substance (active or inactive) that is easier for the body to eliminate.

bronchoconstriction Narrowing of the bronchial tubes.

bronchodilation Widening of the bronchial tubes.

chelating agents Medications that bind with heavy metals in the body and create a compound that can be eliminated; used in cases of ingestion or poisoning.

cholinergic A term used to describe the fibers in the parasympathetic nervous system that release a chemical called acetylcholine.

class The grouping to which a medication belongs. Medications are grouped according to their characteristics, traits, or primary components.

competitive antagonists Medications that temporarily bind with cellular receptor sites, displacing agonist chemicals.

competitive depolarizing A term used to describe paralytic agents that act at the neuromuscular junction by binding with nicotinic receptors on muscles, causing fasciculations and preventing additional activation by acetylcholine.

contraindication Any condition, especially any condition of disease, that renders some particular line of treatment improper or undesirable.

cross-tolerance A process in which repeated exposure to a medication within a particular class causes a tolerance that may be "transferred" to other medications in the same class.

cumulative action Several smaller doses of a particular medication capable of producing the same clinical effects as a single larger dose of that same medication.

cytochrome P-450 system A hemoprotein involved in the detoxification of many drugs.

Prep Kit *(continued)*

dependence The physical, behavioral, or emotional need for a medication or chemical to maintain "normal" physiologic function.

depolarization The process of discharging resting cardiac muscle fibers by an electric impulse that causes them to contract.

depressant A chemical or medication that decreases the performance of the central nervous system or sympathetic nervous system.

digitalis preparation A drug used in the treatment of heart failure and certain atrial dysrhythmias.

distribution The movement and transportation of a medication throughout the bloodstream to tissues and cells and, ultimately, to its target receptor.

diuretic A chemical that increases urinary output.

dose-response curve A graphic illustration of the response of a drug according to the dose administered.

dosing The specified amount of a medication to be given at specific intervals.

down-regulation The process in which a mechanism reducing available cell receptors for a particular medication results in tolerance.

drug A substance that has some therapeutic effect (such as reducing inflammation, fighting bacteria, or producing euphoria) when given in the appropriate circumstances and in the appropriate dose.

duration (of action) In a pharmacologic context, the time a medication concentration can be expected to remain above the minimum level needed to provide the intended action.

dystonic Pertaining to voluntary muscle movements that are distorted or impaired because of abnormal muscle tone.

ectopic foci Sites of generation of electrical impulses other than normal pacemaker cells.

efficacy In a pharmacologic context, the ability of a medication to produce the desired effect.

elimination In a pharmacologic context, the removal of a medication or its by-products from the body.

endogenous Originating from within the organism (body).

exogenous Originating outside the organism (body).

extravasation Seepage of blood and medication into the tissue surrounding the blood vessel.

facilitated diffusion The process of medication molecules binding with carrier proteins when no energy is expended.

fasciculation Brief, uncoordinated, visible twitching of small muscle groups; may be caused by the administration of a depolarizing neuromuscular blocking agent (namely, succinylcholine).

filtration Use of hydrostatic pressure to force water or dissolved particles through a semipermeable membrane.

first-order elimination The process in which the rate of elimination is directly influenced by plasma levels of a substance.

first-pass effect The alteration of a medication via metabolism within the gastrointestinal tract before it reaches systemic circulation.

habituation The unusual tolerance to the therapeutic and adverse clinical effects of a medication or chemical.

half-life The time needed in an average person for metabolism or elimination of 50% of a substance in the plasma.

hematocrit The percentage of red blood cells in a blood sample.

hemolysis The destruction of red blood cells by disruption of the cell membrane.

hydrophilic Attracted to water molecules.

idiosyncratic In a pharmacologic context, abnormal susceptibility to a medication, possibly due to genetic traits or dysfunction of a metabolic enzyme, that is peculiar to an individual patient (and usually unexplained).

inactive metabolite A medication that has undergone biotransformation and is no longer able to alter a cell process or body function; not pharmacologically active.

indication A circumstance that points to or shows the cause, pathology, treatment, or issue of an attack of disease; that which points out; that which serves as a guide or warning.

interference One medication or chemical taken by a patient that undermines the effectiveness of another medication taken by or administered to a patient.

lipophilic Attracted to fats and lipids.

mechanism of action The way in which a medication produces the intended response.

median effective dose (ED_{50}) The weight-based dose of a medication that was effective in 50% of the humans and animals tested.

median lethal dose (LD_{50}) The weight-based dose of a medication that caused death in 50% of the animals tested.

median toxic dose (TD_{50}) The weight-based dose of a medication that demonstrated toxicity in 50% of the animals tested.

Prep Kit *(continued)*

medication A substance used to treat an illness or condition.

medication monograph A document that gives detailed information about drugs, such as the indications and uses, dosing information, precautions, contraindications, and adverse effects.

medication sensitivity A mild to severe reaction after the first exposure to a medication or other substance, often with many of the same signs and symptoms as an immune-mediated reaction.

noncompetitive antagonists Medications that permanently bind with receptor sites and prevent activation by agonist chemicals.

nondepolarizing A term used to describe drugs that produce muscle relaxation by interfering with impulses between the nerve ending and muscle receptor.

nonionic Uncharged.

onset The time needed for the concentration of the medication at the target tissue to reach the minimum effective level.

orthostatic hypotension A fall in blood pressure when changing to a standing position.

osmosis The movement of a solvent, such as water, from an area of low solute concentration to one of high concentration through a selectively permeable membrane to equalize concentrations of a solute on both sides of the membrane.

osmotic Characterized by the movement of a solvent, such as water, across a semipermeable membrane (eg, the cell wall) from an area of lower solute concentration to one of higher concentration.

paradoxical Opposite from expected.

partial agonist A chemical that binds to the receptor site but does not initiate as much cellular activity or change as other agonists do; lowers the efficacy of other agonist chemicals present at the cells.

peak In a pharmacologic context, the point of maximum effect of a drug.

pharmacodynamics The biochemical and physiologic effects and mechanism of action of a medication in the body.

pharmacokinetics The activity of medications in the body over time, such as absorption, distribution, and elimination.

pharmacology The scientific study of how various substances interact with or alter the function of living organisms.

pinocytosis A process by which cells ingest the extracellular fluid and its contents.

placebo effect In a pharmacologic context, the positive and negative effects of an inactive medication on a person that are related to the person's expectations and other factors.

plasma protein binding A process in which medication molecules temporarily attach to proteins in the blood plasma, significantly altering medication distribution in the body.

potency The relationship between the desired response of a medication and the dose required to achieve the response.

receptor A specialized area in tissues that initiates certain actions after specific stimulation.

relative refractory period The period in the cell-firing cycle at which it is possible but difficult to restimulate the cell to fire another impulse.

Stevens-Johnson syndrome A severe, possibly fatal reaction that mimics a burn; may be due to a medication.

stimulant A medication or chemical that temporarily enhances central nervous system and sympathetic nervous system functioning.

sympathomimetics Medications administered to stimulate the sympathetic nervous system.

tachyphylaxis A condition in which repeated doses of medication within a short period rapidly cause tolerance, making the medication virtually ineffective.

therapeutic index The relationship between the median effective dose and the median lethal dose or median toxic dose; also known as the therapeutic ratio.

threshold level In a pharmacologic context, the concentration of medication at which initiation or alteration of cellular activity begins.

tolerance A condition that develops following repeated use by a patient of a medication that results in decreased efficacy or potency.

untoward effect A clinical change caused by a medication that causes harm or discomfort to a patient; also known as adverse effect.

vasoconstriction Narrowing of the diameter of a blood vessel.

vasodilation Widening of the diameter of a blood vessel.

Vaughan-Williams classification A classification scheme based on the mechanism of action rather than on specific medication groups.

volume of distribution The extent to which a medication will spread within the body.

water-soluble A property that indicates a material can be dissolved in water.

Prep Kit *(continued)*

zero-order elimination A process in which a fixed amount of a substance is removed during a certain period, regardless of the total amount in the body.

► References

1. Brown LH, Bailey LC, Medwick T, Okeke CC, Krumperman K, Tran CD. Medication storage on US ambulances: a prospective multi-center observational study. *Pharm Forum*. 2003;29:540-547.
2. Lin BW, Yoshida D, Quin J, Strehlow M. A better way to estimate adult patients' weights. *Am J Emerg Med*. 2009;27(9):1060-1064.
3. American Heart Association. Highlights of the 2015 American Heart Association Guidelines Update for CPR and ECC. American Heart Association website. http://eccguidelines.heart.org/wp-content/uploads/2015/10/2015-AHA-Guidelines-Highlights-English.pdf. Accessed March 3, 2017.
4. Zafren K, Mechem CC. Accidental hypothermia in adults. UpToDate website. http://www.uptodate.com/contents/accidental-hypothermia-in-adults. Updated February 6, 2017. Accessed March 3, 2017.
5. Tveita T. Pharmacodynamics in hypothermia. *Critical Care*. 2012;16(2):A6. https://ccforum.biomedcentral.com/articles/10.1186/cc11264. Accessed March 3, 2017.
6. FDA pregnancy categories. Drugs.com website. https://www.drugs.com/pregnancy-categories.html. Accessed March 9, 2017.
7. Pregnancy and lactation labeling (drugs) final rule. U.S. Food and Drug Administration website. http://www.fda.gov/Drugs/DevelopmentApprovalProcess/DevelopmentResources/Labeling/ucm093307.htm. Page last updated November 18, 2016. Accessed March 9, 2017.
8. Vilke GM, Tornabene SV, Stepanski B, et al. Paramedic self-reported medication errors. *Prehosp Emerg Care*. 2006 (Oct-Dec);10(4):457-462.
9. Pozner CN. Advanced cardiac life support (ACLS) in adults. UpToDate website. https://www.uptodate.com/contents/advanced-cardiac-life-support-acls-in-adults?topicKey=EM%2F278&elapsedTimeMs=6&view=print&displayedView=full#. Updated March 6, 2017. Accessed March 8, 2017.
10. Patterson SJ, Oliphant CS, Self TH. Amiodarone-induced lung disease *Consultant*. 2014;54(3):207-208.
11. Reeder GS. Nitrates in the management of acute coronary syndrome. UpToDate website. http://www.uptodate.com/contents/nitrates-in-the-management-of-acute-coronary-syndrome?source=search_result&search=Intravenous+nitroglycerin&selectedTitle=1%7E51. Updated December 27, 2016. Accessed March 8, 2017.
12. Matijevic N, Wang YW, Cotton BA, et al. Better hemostatic profiles of never-frozen liquid plasma compared with thawed fresh frozen plasma. *J Trauma Acute Care Surg*. 2013;74(1):84-91.
13. Napolitano LM, Cohen MJ, Cotton BA, et al. Tranexamic acid in trauma: how should we use it. *J Trauma Acute Care Surg*. 2013;74(6):1575-1586.
14. Katzan IL. Antiplatelet agents in secondary stroke prevention. Cleveland Clinic Center for Continuing Education website. http://www.clevelandclinicmeded.com/medicalpubs/diseasemanagement/neurology/antiplatelet-agents/. Published January 2009. Accessed January 8, 2017.
15. Bhatt DL, Fox KAA, Hacke W, et al. Clopidogrel and aspirin versus aspirin alone for the prevention of atherothrombotic events. *N Engl J Med*. 2006;354(16):1706-1717.
16. Anondo Stangi P, Lewis S. Review of currently available GP IIb/IIIa inhibitors and their role in peripheral vascular interventions. *Semin Intervent Radiol*. 2010;27(4):412-421.
17. Smith HS, Smith JM, Seidner P. Opioid-induced nausea and vomiting. *Ann Palliat Med*. 2012;1(2):121-129.

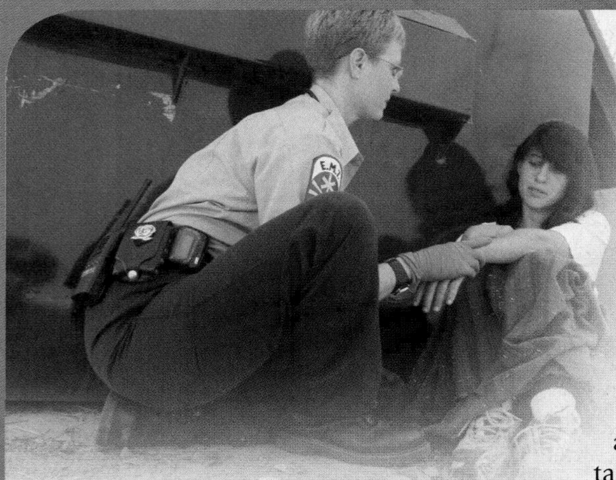

Assessment *in Action*

You arrive at a moderately well-kept apartment of a 76-year-old man who called EMS because of heart palpitations and dizziness. The patient states that his physician recently prescribed some new medications for an irregular heartbeat and high blood pressure. The new medications are an "ACE inhibitor" and a "calcium channel blocker." He started taking the medication 2 days ago, and the symptoms began this morning. He also takes a low-dose aspirin each day.

The patient says he does not want to go to the hospital; he just wants you to check him out because he is worried. His family members do not visit him often, and he lives alone.

1. The primary action of an ACE inhibitor is to:

A. suppress the conversion of angiotensin I to angiotensin II.
B. promote the conversion of angiotensin I to angiotensin II.
C. block the alpha receptor.
D. block the beta-1 receptor.

2. On which system does an ACE inhibitor focus?

A. Sympathetic nervous system
B. Renin-angiotensin system
C. Parasympathetic nervous system
D. Sodium potassium pump

3. Calcium channel blockers have which type(s) of properties?

A. Antihypertensive
B. Anticonvulsant
C. Antiplatelet
D. Anticoagulant

4. Taking a low-dose aspirin helps the patient by:

A. keeping pain under control.
B. keeping the blood pressure low.
C. keeping platelets from coagulating.
D. altering the patient's mood.

5. Based on the characteristics of the patient's medications, which portion of his assessment would you expect to be abnormal?

A. Blood glucose level
B. Pupils
C. Blood pressure
D. Lung sounds

6. A direct biochemical interaction between two drugs is referred to as:

A. synergism.
B. interference.
C. potentiation.
D. summation effect.

7. During your conversation with the patient, he mentions that he is having ringing in his ears (tinnitus). Which medication do you suspect might be causing this symptom?

A. Beta-blocker medication
B. Calcium channel blocker
C. ACE inhibitor
D. Aspirin

8. You have a patient who intentionally overdosed on acetaminophen (Tylenol) and states the pills were ingested 20 minutes ago. Is there an effective antidote for acetaminophen toxicity if administered promptly?

9. You are transporting a patient with respiratory distress, who has a history of reactive airway disease. The total transport time is 15 minutes. First responders have already administered the following medications to the patient: albuterol, ipratropium bromide, and methylprednisolone. Which medication should you repeat if the patient's symptoms are not improving?

10. Give an example of a medication that would be contraindicated in a patient with a suspected cerebrovascular accident with profoundly altered mental status before the patient reaches the hospital.

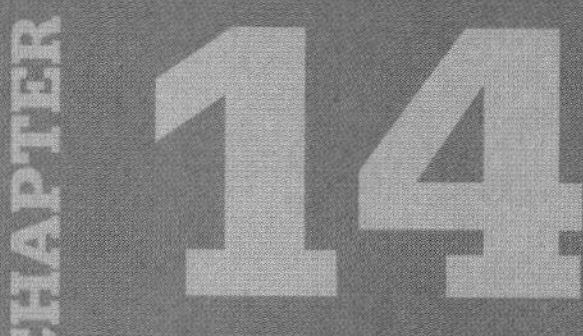

Medication Administration

National EMS Education Standard Competencies

Pharmacology

Integrates comprehensive knowledge of pharmacology to formulate a treatment plan intended to mitigate emergencies and improve the overall health of the patient.

Medication Administration

- Routes of administration (see Chapter 13, *Principles of Pharmacology*)
- Self-administer medication (p 729)
- Peer-administer medication (p 761)
- Assist/administer medications to a patient (pp 694-705, 717-719, 729-746, 749-758)
- Within the scope of practice of the paramedic, administer medications to a patient (pp 687-688, and see Chapter 13, *Principles of Pharmacology*)

Knowledge Objectives

1. Describe the role of medical direction in medication administration. (p 687)
2. Discuss the benefits of performing a *Medication Administration Cross-Check© (MACC)* before administering a medication. (p 688)
3. Explain the importance of properly documenting medication administration. (p 688)
4. Discuss paramedics' responsibilities related to security of medications stocked on the ambulance. (p 689)
5. Explain the difference between aseptic, clean, and sterile techniques. (p 689)
6. Describe the use of standard precautions related to medication administration. (p 690)
7. Discuss the signs and symptoms that can occur when there are changes in fluid status in the body. (pp 690-691)
8. List commonly used intravenous (IV) fluid compositions and types of IV solutions. (pp 692-694)
9. Discuss the techniques for performing IV therapy. (pp 694-707)
10. Discuss the factors to consider when choosing an IV solution. (p 695)
11. Discuss the factors to consider when choosing an administration set. (pp 695-698)
12. Discuss the factors to consider when choosing an IV site. (pp 698-699)
13. List the types of IV catheters. (pp 699-700)
14. Describe special considerations when performing IV therapy on a pediatric or older adult patient. (pp 707-708)
15. List the factors to check if the IV flow rate is incorrect. (pp 708-709)
16. Describe complications that can occur as a result of IV therapy. (pp 709-712)
17. Discuss transport considerations for a patient undergoing a blood transfusion. (p 713)
18. Discuss the advantages, disadvantages, and techniques for establishing an intraosseous (IO) IV line. (pp 714-720)
19. List the types of IO devices available. (pp 715-717)
20. Discuss the potential complications of IO infusion. (pp 719-720)
21. Discuss the systems of weights and measures used when administering medication. (pp 721-723)
22. Explain the principles of drug dose calculations, including desired dose, concentration on hand, volume on hand, volume to administer, and IV drip rate. (pp 725-729)
23. Discuss the advantages, disadvantages, and techniques of oral medication administration. (pp 729-730)
24. Discuss the advantages, disadvantages, and techniques of rectal medication administration. (pp 730, 732)
25. Discuss the advantages, disadvantages, and techniques of intradermal medication administration. (p 737)
26. Discuss the advantages, disadvantages, and techniques of subcutaneous medication administration. (pp 737-739)
27. Discuss the advantages, disadvantages, and techniques of intramuscular medication administration. (pp 738-742)
28. Discuss the advantages, disadvantages, and techniques of intravenous medication administration. (pp 740, 742-746)
29. Discuss the advantages, disadvantages, and techniques of IO medication administration. (pp 749-750)

30. Discuss the advantages, disadvantages, and techniques of transdermal medication administration. (pp 749-751)
31. Discuss the advantages, disadvantages, and techniques of sublingual medication administration. (pp 751-752)
32. Discuss other methods of medication administration, including the buccal, ocular, and aural routes. (pp 751-753)
33. Discuss the advantages, disadvantages, and techniques of intranasal medication administration. (pp 753-754)
34. Discuss the advantages, disadvantages, and techniques of inhaled medication administration. (pp 753, 755-758)
35. Discuss the rates at which medication is absorbed through various routes. (pp 761-762)

Skills Objectives

1. Demonstrate how to spike an IV bag. (pp 696-697, Skill Drill 14-1)
2. Demonstrate how to obtain vascular access. (pp 700-705, Skill Drill 14-2)
3. Demonstrate how to obtain a blood sample. (p 712)
4. Demonstrate how to gain IO access. (pp 717-719, Skill Drill 14-3)
5. Demonstrate how to administer oral medication to a patient. (pp 729-730)
6. Demonstrate how to administer medication via a gastric tube. (pp 730-731, Skill Drill 14-4)
7. Demonstrate how to draw medication from an ampule. (pp 733-734, Skill Drill 14-5)
8. Demonstrate how to draw medication from a vial. (pp 734-736, Skill Drill 14-6)
9. Demonstrate how to administer a subcutaneous medication to a patient. (pp 737-739, Skill Drill 14-7)
10. Demonstrate how to administer an intramuscular medication to a patient. (pp 738-742, Skill Drill 14-8)
11. Demonstrate how to administer a medication via the IV bolus route. (pp 740, 742-744, Skill Drill 14-9)
12. Demonstrate how to administer a medication via IV piggyback. (pp 744-746, Skill Drill 14-10)
13. Demonstrate how to perform an IO infusion. (pp 749-750, Skill Drill 14-11)
14. Demonstrate how to administer a sublingual medication to a patient. (pp 751-752, Skill Drill 14-12)
15. Demonstrate how to administer an intranasal medication to a patient. (pp 753-754, Skill Drill 14-13)
16. Demonstrate how to assist a patient with a metered-dose inhaler. (p 756, Skill Drill 14-14)
17. Demonstrate how to assist a patient with a small-volume nebulizer. (p 758, Skill Drill 14-15)
18. Demonstrate how to access a tunneling device. (pp 759-760, Skill Drill 14-16)

YOU are the Paramedic PART 1

You respond to a private residence for a call concerning a 26-year-old man who experienced a syncopal episode. Upon arrival, the patient states that while in the bathroom he had a sudden onset of palpitations and felt dizzy. He lowered himself to the ground before briefly losing consciousness. The patient reports that palpitations are still present, but he denies chest discomfort or dyspnea. Your primary survey reveals no immediate life threats. As your partner applies the cardiac monitor and obtains a baseline set of vital signs, you note a rapid, irregular pulse.

Recording Time: 1 Minute	
Appearance	Warm and dry skin
Level of consciousness	Alert (oriented to person, place, time, and event)
Airway	Spontaneously patent
Breathing	20 breaths/min, nonlabored
Circulation	Strong, rapid, irregular radial pulse

1. Given this scenario, what route of delivery do you anticipate using to administer medications? What are the advantages of this route?
2. What aspects of the patient history are important to consider prior to administering any medication to this patient?

Introduction

Your paramedic education will furnish you with knowledge of anatomy and physiology, pathophysiology, and how pharmacologic treatments will affect your patients. It is your responsibility to administer the appropriate medications and the appropriate dosage when needed, and to determine the most effective route by which to administer them. It is also important to remember that any procedure, including medication administration, that you perform must be approved by a medical director either by established protocols or online medical direction.

Vascular access is often needed in emergency medicine for patients who are hemodynamically unstable and in need of intravenous (IV) fluids, various medications, or both. A number of techniques are used to gain vascular access in the prehospital setting, including cannulation of a peripheral extremity vein, external jugular (EJ) vein cannulation, intraosseous (IO) access, and long-term vascular access devices (VADs). **Cannulation** is the insertion of a catheter, such as into a vein to allow for fluid flow. In critically ill or injured patients, survival often depends on your ability to obtain vascular access quickly and effectively. Because these procedures are invasive, you must be proficient, yet cautious. Significant harm to the patient can result from improper technique, insufficient knowledge of the medications being administered, or both.

This chapter discusses the various types of IV solutions used in the prehospital setting and the techniques of IV/IO therapy. It describes the mathematical principles used in pharmacology, and for calculating medication doses (**bolus** [a single dose, usually administered by the IV route], as well as maintenance infusion). Paramedics administer medications in different forms. The chapter concludes with a discussion of routes for administering medications.

Patient Safety

A concept that contributes to an effective safety culture is the *high-reliability organization* (HRO).[1,2] The airline and nuclear power industries that are populated with HROs share some common traits. For example, all HROs are preoccupied with failure, and there is an understanding in each organization's culture that failures will inevitably occur. However, HROs focus on managing these failures, so a failure does not reach the public (the patient, in the health care industry). This drive has led to the redundancy in training, equipment, and maintenance seen in the airline industry. The airlines and nuclear power plants recognize that an individual person or piece of equipment may fail, so they have put considerable effort into ensuring a single failure does not cause a catastrophic event (plane crash, nuclear meltdown). In health care, an HRO would focus on double checks (for example, cross-checking a medication being administered) and other systems to ensure a single failure, which is inevitable, does not lead to patient harm.

Medical Direction

Medical direction is discussed in Chapter 1, *EMS Systems*, but some points specific to medication administration are also important to highlight here. For example, your medical director may not allow you to perform certain procedures (for example, administering certain narcotics) before making contact with him or her. When requesting orders from online medical control, be confident and detailed. Gather all patient information prior to contacting medical control. You should be able to paint a picture of the patient to the physician and demonstrate the need for the medication you are requesting.

Local policies and procedures are designed to guide you in specific situations. The principles of crew resource management, discussed in Chapter 5, *Communications*, and Chapter 39, *Responding to the Field Code*, suggest you should use any resources available to help reduce cognitive load. This means that if you are not confident with a drug dose, indication, contraindication, or any other aspect of medication administration, then you should use your protocols, a drug formulary, a flip guide, a smartphone or tablet application, or any other available resource. Beyond the resources available on your response unit, consider medical control. Online medical control is not just for approval of medications that are outside of your protocols. You can also use medical control for general consultation of treatment modalities with which you are not confident. *If you have any doubt regarding the correct action, then consult medical control!*

Ensuring Correct and Safe Medication Administration

It is your responsibility to ensure the medications you deliver are administered accurately and safely. Medication errors are an issue throughout health care. Paramedics administer medications based on standing orders or online medical direction. However, actual oversight in the moment of administration is minimal. This is why the emergency medical services (EMS) system must develop tools to mitigate errors arising from human factors, and why paramedics must make a conscious effort to use these tools.

The 10 rights of medication administration are discussed in Chapter 13, *Principles of Pharmacology*, and should always be followed. The danger of something going wrong when you are administering a drug—for example, administering the incorrect drug or the incorrect dose of a drug—can also be minimized by utilizing a tool to verify the drug dose, name, route, rate of administration, indication for

Words of Wisdom

Wichita-Sedgwick County EMS System in Kansas developed a tool known as *Medication Administration Cross-Check*© (MACC) Figure 14-1.[4] This tool uses principles of crew resource management by requiring a process for verification for every medication, every time. The tool employs job aids to help reduce cognitive load and ensure the process is completed each time a medication is administered.

Because EMS systems vary in configuration—for example, a paramedic working with a basic life support (BLS) provider—the tool is designed to work with all provider levels. Although BLS providers may lack familiarity with all medications, they can verify quantities, medication names, expiration dates, etc.

More important, the second provider, regardless of certification level, acts as a sounding board for the first provider. This forces the first provider to validate the medication administration. Some providers may catch the error as they read it back to themselves. Others may catch it when the second provider asks them to repeat something that did not sound right. Sometimes the second provider can catch the error and bring it to the first provider's attention. The tool will not eliminate all medication errors. However, with proper use of this tool, medication errors can be significantly reduced.

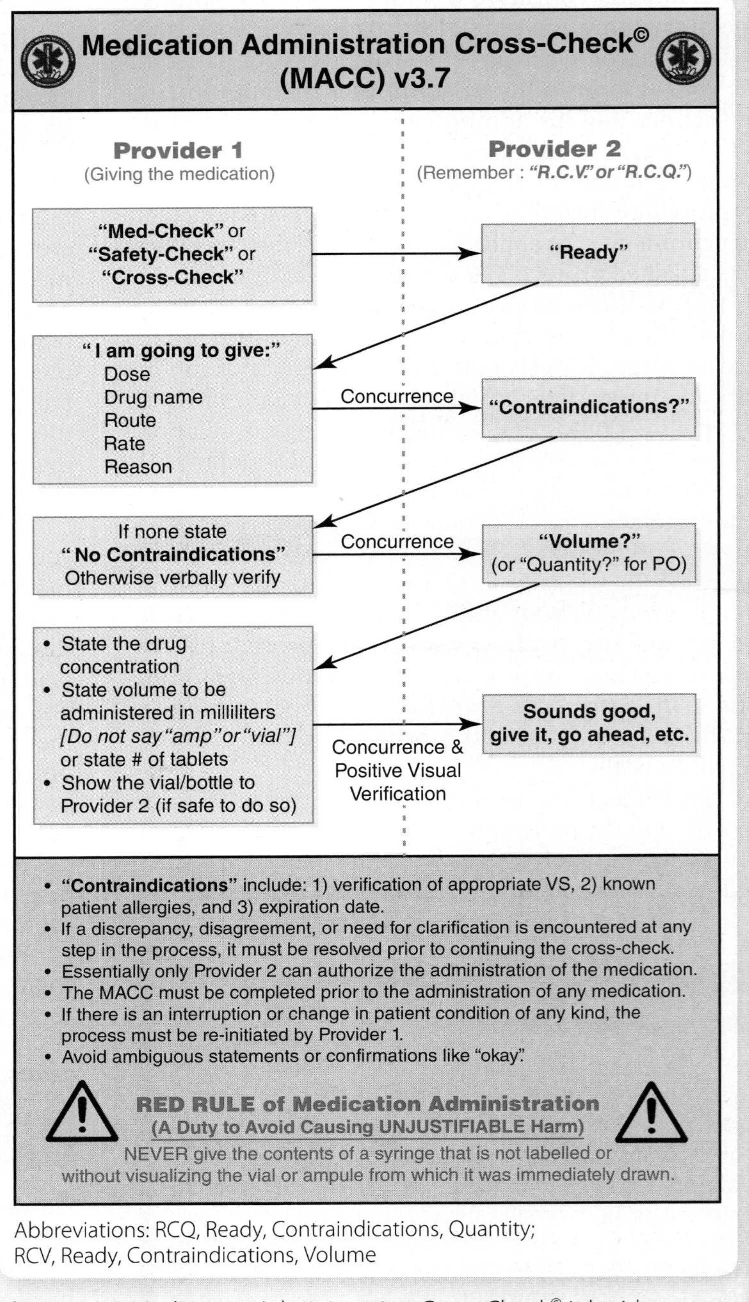

Abbreviations: RCQ, Ready, Contraindications, Quantity; RCV, Ready, Contraindications, Volume

Figure 14-1 Medication Administration Cross-Check© job aid.

Reproduced from: Misasi P, Braithwaite S. The Medication Administration Cross-Check© (MACC) User's Manual. Wichita-Sedgwick County EMS System. March 2012. https://kansasemstransition.files.wordpress.com/2012/08/macc-user-manual-v2-0.pdf. Accessed May 26, 2016.

administration, contraindications, drug **concentration**, and volume to be administered.[3] Never guess what the physician has ordered. Ask, when in doubt.

Documenting medication administration is extremely important. You must list the dose administered, name of the medication, route, rate, time of administration, who administered the drug, who helped perform the medication check, and the patient's response. The dose should be listed by the total quantity administered during that administration, the units of measure for that drug, and the volume administered to the patient. Verify the spelling of the drug name; this is where medication errors commonly occur. The rate should be documented in reference to a bolus, infusion, or other administration method.

Local Drug Distribution System

Before responding to an EMS call, you must ensure all equipment on the ambulance is fully functional; this verification is made during your check of the ambulance at the beginning of your shift. All medications must be checked to ensure they are not expired or damaged and they are readily available in the right quantity. You must be thoroughly familiar with the system used to exchange and replace outdated or damaged drugs in your EMS system.

You are also responsible for the documentation and security of all controlled substances carried on your ambulance, including accounting for all controlled substances that were wasted (ie, residual medication that was not administered to the patient). Follow the specific policies and procedures of your local drug distribution, security, and accountability system.

Documentation & Communication

If you administer a controlled substance to your patient (eg, morphine, midazolam [Versed], fentanyl [Sublimaze, Duragesic]), then document the amount of medication that you gave to the patient and the amount of medication that you wasted (did not give to the patient). Have your partner, nurse or physician from the receiving facility, or supervisor witness (actually see) you wasting the medication. Both of you should sign the form—you as the paramedic who administered and wasted the medication—and the witness who observed you waste the medication.

Medical Asepsis

Medical asepsis is the practice of preventing contamination of the patient by using **aseptic technique**. This method of cleansing is intended to prevent contamination of a site when you are performing an invasive procedure such as starting an IV line or administering a medication. Medical asepsis may be accomplished through the use of sterilization of equipment, antiseptics, or disinfectants.

Clean Technique Versus Sterile Technique

Some of the equipment you will use in the field has been sterilized for patient safety. For example, some medications have been packaged using **sterile** technique. Sterile technique refers to the destruction of all living organisms and is achieved by using heat, gas, or chemicals.

For a sterile field to exist, multiple pieces of sterile equipment must be used and rules must be followed. You will need to wear sterile sleeves or a gown that covers you from the wrist to 2 inches (5 cm) proximal to the elbow. Then, appropriate-size sterile gloves, using numeric sizes rather than small to extra large sizing, will need to be used. Sterile drapes need to be placed around the procedural area. Anything below the drapes should be considered nonsterile. In order for the area to remain sterile, only sterile items and personnel may enter the sterile field.

Because it may not be feasible to maintain a sterile environment in the field, you must practice medical asepsis to reduce the risk of contamination and infection. Examples of medical asepsis include handwashing, wearing gloves, and keeping equipment as clean as possible. For example, the site on a patient's hand that has been cleaned with iodine and alcohol before starting an IV line is said to be "medically clean."

If you open an IV catheter package and the IV catheter inadvertently falls to the ground or otherwise comes in contact with a contaminated surface, discard it and use a new IV catheter. If you have already cleaned the injection port on the IV tubing where you intend to inject a medication and you inadvertently touch the cleaned injection port, then recleanse the port before injecting the medication. You must always make a conscious effort to prevent contamination—whether handling equipment, supplies, or the patient. This is the cornerstone of maintaining a medically clean environment.

Words of Wisdom

In addition to ensuring medications have not expired or become contaminated, you must ensure the medications are kept at the recommended temperatures while stored in your ambulance. Some medications become inactive in extreme heat or cold conditions. Refer to the package insert for the medication for this information.

Antiseptics and Disinfectants

Antiseptics are used to cleanse an area before performing an invasive procedure such as IV therapy or medication administration. Even though antiseptics are capable of destroying pathogens, they are not toxic to living tissues. Isopropyl alcohol (rubbing alcohol), iodine, and 2% chlorhexidine gluconate (ChloraPrep) are the three most common antiseptics you will use in the field.

Disinfectants, by contrast, are toxic to living tissues; therefore, you should never use them on a patient. Use disinfectants only on nonliving objects such as the inside of the ambulance, laryngoscope blades, and other nondisposable equipment.

Standard Precautions and Contaminated Equipment Disposal

The first rule of standard precautions is to treat any body fluid as being potentially infectious. Chapter 2, *Workforce Safety and Wellness*, discusses these principles in detail.

▶ Disposal of Contaminated Equipment

After an IV catheter or needle has penetrated a patient's skin, it is contaminated. Considering the fact that accidental needlesticks are the most common route for disease transmission in the health care setting, you must always handle contaminated equipment carefully and dispose of it immediately and properly. **Sharps** include IV/intramuscular (IM) and subcutaneous needles and catheters, scalpels, broken ampules or vials, and anything else that can penetrate or lacerate the skin.

Immediately dispose of all sharps in a puncture-proof sharps container that bears a biohazard logo Figure 14-2. Sharps containers should be readily accessible; place at least two in the back of the ambulance so your handling of needles, catheters, and other sharps is kept to a minimum amount of time. In addition, you should have a smaller sharps container in your jump kit for immediate disposal of sharps while not in the ambulance. Table 14-1 lists some safe practices that will minimize your risk of an inadvertent needlestick. Many EMS systems have transitioned to Luer-lock IV tubing to help minimize risks during medication administration. Some systems have begun using blunt-tip needles to draw up medications. While retractable needles are commonplace in EMS for IV catheters, they are not commonly used for **subcutaneous** (injections administered into the loose connective tissue between the dermis and the muscle layer) or IM injections. Retractable needle systems for subcutaneous and IM injections is a concept that is popular in hospitals and beginning to gain traction in EMS Figure 14-3. As always, follow your agency's exposure control plan.

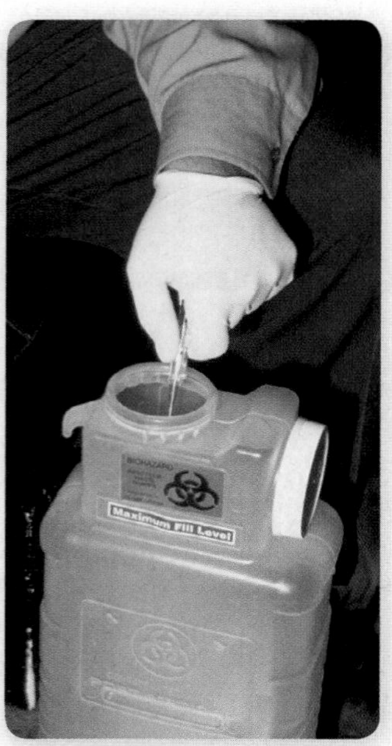

Figure 14-2 Always dispose of sharp objects or blood-filled items in a puncture-proof sharps container.

Cellular Fluid Composition and Status

▶ Body Fluid Composition

The human body is composed mostly of water, which provides the environment where the chemical reactions necessary for life take place. The healthy body maintains a delicate balance between intake and output of fluids and electrolytes, ensuring the internal environment remains fairly constant. The ill or injured body, however, may be

Table 14-1 Minimizing Your Risk of a Needlestick
Use blunt-tip needles when drawing medication from vials or infusing medications directly into an IV solution.
Use a needleless delivery system. Needleless delivery systems "recap" themselves, which greatly reduces the risk of a needlestick.
Immediately dispose of all sharps in a puncture-proof sharps container. *Do not* drop the sharps on the floor for later disposal, and *do not* attempt to recap a needle and syringe before placing it in the sharps container. Even if you use a needle or IV line that automatically retracts, you still must discard it in a sharps container.
When possible, perform all invasive procedures at the scene. If your patient's condition warrants starting an IV line or administering a medication en route to the hospital, then *use extreme caution.* Although most paramedics become proficient at starting IV lines in the back of a moving ambulance, it may be necessary to have your partner briefly stop the ambulance, especially if you are traveling over rough terrain.
Recap needles *only* as an absolute last resort. If you must recap a needle, then use the one-handed technique: Place the needle cover on a stationary surface, then slide the needle—with one hand—into the needle cap.

Abbreviation: IV, intravenous

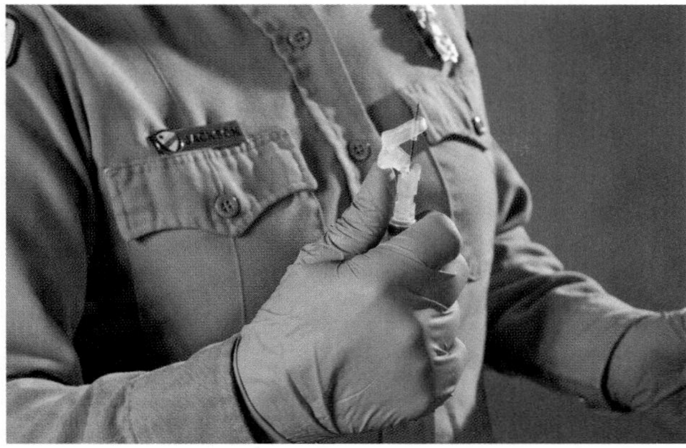
A

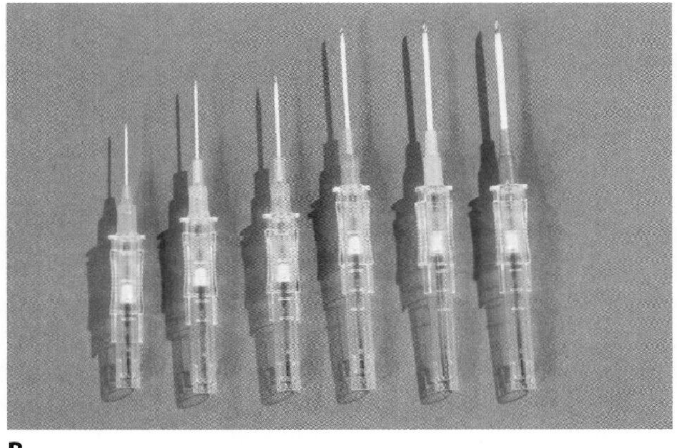
B

Figure 14-3 Safety hypodermic needle **(A)** and safety catheters **(B)**.

unable to maintain homeostasis, and excesses or deficits of fluids and electrolytes may occur. You need to know when IV fluids are indicated, what kinds of fluids are required in different situations, and when IV fluids can be dangerous.

A healthy person loses approximately 2 to 2.5 L of fluid daily through urine output, through the lungs (exhalation), and through the skin. These losses are replaced by intake of fluids and by nutrients that are partially converted to water in their metabolism. In illness, abnormal states of hydration may occur where intake and output are no longer in balance.

Dehydration

Dehydration is defined as inadequate total systemic fluid volume. It is usually a chronic condition of young and older patients and may take days to manifest. As fluid loss occurs from the vascular compartment, the body reacts by shifting interstitial fluid into the vascular area; fluid also shifts from the intracellular to the extracellular compartments. As a consequence, a total systemic fluid deficit occurs.

Signs and symptoms of dehydration include decreased level of consciousness, orthostatic hypotension, tachypnea, dry mucous membranes, decreased urine output, tachycardia, poor skin turgor, and flushed, dry skin. Causes of dehydration include diarrhea, vomiting, gastrointestinal drainage, infections, metabolic disorders such as diabetic ketoacidosis, hemorrhage, environmental emergencies, high-caffeine diet, and insufficient fluid intake.

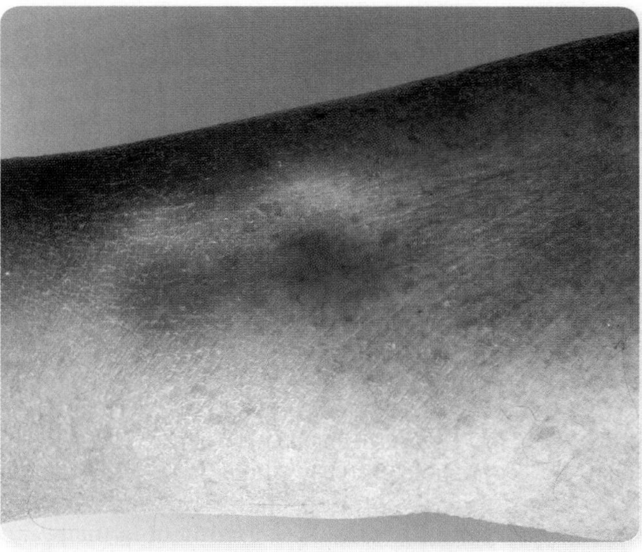

Figure 14-4 One sign of fluid backup is pitting edema, shown in this patient. Pitting edema occurs when the skin is pressed with a finger and an indentation remains after removal of the finger, as seen here.

Words of Wisdom

The cardinal sign of overhydration is edema.

Overhydration

When the body's total systemic fluid volume increases, **overhydration** occurs. Fluid fills the vascular compartment, filters into the interstitial compartment, and is forced from the engorged interstitial compartment into the intracellular compartment. This fluid backup can lead to death **Figure 14-4**. Overhydration may occur in patients with impaired kidney function, and also when health care professionals administer an amount of fluid that is beyond what the body can excrete. Neonates (children younger than 1 month) are also more likely to experience overhydration because their kidneys are not yet fully developed.

Signs and symptoms of overhydration include shortness of breath, puffy eyelids, edema, polyuria, moist crackles (rales), and acute weight gain. Causes of overhydration include unmonitored IV lines (in pediatric patients), kidney failure, water intoxication in endurance sports, and prolonged hypoventilation.

IV Fluid Composition

The use of IV fluids can significantly alter the patient's condition and facilitate patient treatment. Each bag of IV solution must be sterile and safe; therefore, each bag of IV solution is individually sterilized Figure 14-5.

Human plasma contains a variety of electrolytes, as discussed in Chapter 9, *Pathophysiology*. The compounds and ions dissolved in IV solutions are identical to the ones found in the body, although the concentrations may vary. Table 14-2 lists the electrolyte composition of various IV fluids.

Sodium is used as the benchmark to calculate a solution's tonicity. The concentration of sodium in the cells of the body is approximately 0.9%. Altering the concentration of sodium in the IV solution, therefore, can move the water into or out of any fluid compartment in the body.

When selecting the appropriate IV solution for your patient, it is important to understand how electrolytes operate. A patient's electrolytes can become altered from excessive vomiting, diarrhea, dietary issues, medications (taken regularly or administered by the EMS crew), blood loss, or a variety of other injuries. Understanding the role of each electrolyte, along with the clinical presentation you may encounter if the patient has too much or not enough of an electrolyte, is beneficial in selecting the appropriate IV solution.

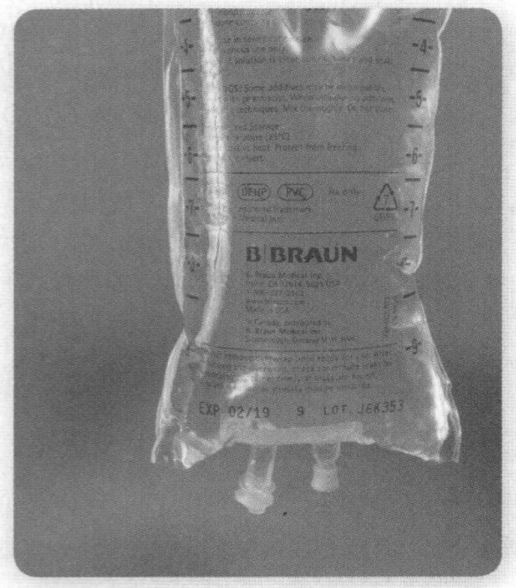

Figure 14-5 Each bag of intravenous solution must be sterile, leak-free, clear, and not expired.

Types of IV Solutions

Based on their dissolved components, or makeup, IV solutions are categorized as either crystalloid or colloid. Based on their tonicity, they are also categorized as isotonic, hypotonic, or hypertonic. IV fluids use combinations of these solutions to create the desired effects inside the body.

Crystalloid Solutions

Crystalloid solutions are dissolved crystals (eg, salts or sugars) in water. The ability of these fluids to cross membranes and alter fluid levels makes them the best choice for prehospital care of injured patients who need body fluid replacement. When you use an **isotonic crystalloid solution** for fluid replacement to support blood pressure after blood loss, remember the 3-to-1 replacement rule: 3 mL of isotonic crystalloid solution is needed to replace 1 mL of patient blood. This amount is needed because approximately two thirds of the infused isotonic crystalloid solution will leave the vascular spaces in about 1 hour. The two-thirds of infused crystalloids is either absorbed into the interstitial space or excreted. You should closely monitor urine output when heavy fluid resuscitation occurs. This may alert you to potential kidney abnormalities.

When you replace volume loss in a patient, it is imperative to remember crystalloid solutions cannot carry oxygen. Fluid boluses should be administered as appropriate based on the working diagnosis to maintain perfusion (ie, radial pulses, adequate mental status) but not to restore blood pressure to the patient's normal level. Increasing blood pressure too much with IV solutions not only dilutes remaining blood volume, thereby decreasing the proportion of hemoglobin, but in the case

Table 14-2 Electrolyte Composition of Intravenous Fluids

Fluid	Sodium (Na)	Chloride (Cl)	Potassium (K)	Calcium (Ca)	Magnesium (Mg)
Human plasma	135–145	95–105	3.5–5	8–10.5	1.5–2.5
0.45% sodium chloride	77	77	0	0	0
0.9% sodium chloride	154	154	0	0	0
3.0% sodium chloride	513	513	0	0	0
Lactated Ringer	130	109	4	3	0

All values are represented as milliequivalents per liter.

of hemorrhagic shock, may also increase internal bleeding by interfering with **hemostasis**—the body's internal blood-clotting mechanism. Blood pressure should be titrated to 90 mm Hg systolic in adults, unless otherwise noted by local protocol.[5]

Words of Wisdom

In trauma, isotonic crystalloid solutions—normal saline and lactated Ringer solution (LR)—replace volume loss but do not carry oxygen. Replace volume loss to maintain perfusion, but recognize the need for blood product administration and surgery. Fluid resuscitation should not take precedence over rapid transport.

Colloid Solutions

Colloid solutions contain molecules (usually proteins) that are too large to pass through the capillary membranes and, therefore, remain in the vascular system. These large protein molecules give colloid solutions a high osmolarity. As a result, they draw fluid from the interstitial and intracellular compartments into the vascular compartments. Colloid solutions work well in reducing edema (eg, in pulmonary or cerebral edema) while expanding the vascular compartment. They could cause dramatic fluid shifts and place the patient in considerable danger if they are not administered in a controlled setting. For this reason, along with a short duration of action and low cost-to-benefit ratio in the prehospital setting, colloids are rarely used in prehospital medicine but may be seen in interfacility transports. Examples of colloid solutions include albumin, dextran, Plasmanate, and hetastarch (Hespan).

Isotonic Solutions

As mentioned, IV solutions are also categorized by their tonicity. The three categories related to tonicity are:

- *Isotonic:* 0.9% sodium chloride (normal saline), LR
- *Hypotonic:* 5% dextrose in water (D_5W)
- *Hypertonic:* 3% saline, blood products, albumin

The effects of osmotic pressure on a cell are referred to as the tonicity of the solution. Tonicity is the concentration of sodium in a solution and the movement of water in relation to the sodium levels inside and outside the cell:

- An **isotonic solution** has the same concentration of sodium as does the cell. In this case, water does not shift and no change in cell shape occurs.
- A **hypertonic solution** has a greater concentration of sodium than does the cell. Water is drawn out of the cell, and the cell may collapse from the increased extracellular osmotic pressure.
- A **hypotonic solution** has a lower concentration of sodium than does the cell. Water flows into the cell, causing it to swell and possibly burst from the increased intracellular osmotic pressure.

Fluid movement across a cell membrane resulting from hypertonic, isotonic, and hypotonic solutions is illustrated in **Figure 14-6**. IV fluids introduced into the circulatory system can affect the tonicity of the extracellular fluid, resulting in serious consequences unless care is used.

Isotonic solutions such as **normal saline** (0.9% sodium chloride) have almost the same **osmolarity** (concentration of sodium) as serum and other body fluids. As a consequence, isotonic solutions expand the contents of the intravascular compartment without shifting fluid to or from other compartments, or changing cell shape—an important consideration when you are caring for hypotensive or hypovolemic patients. When you are administering isotonic solutions, you must be careful to avoid fluid overloading. Patients with hypertension and congestive heart failure are at greatest risk of this problem.

Lactated Ringer (LR) solution is generally used in the field for patients who have significant blood loss. It contains lactate, which is metabolized in the liver to form bicarbonate—the key buffer that combats the intracellular acidosis associated with severe blood loss. LR solution should not be given to patients with liver problems because they cannot metabolize the lactate.

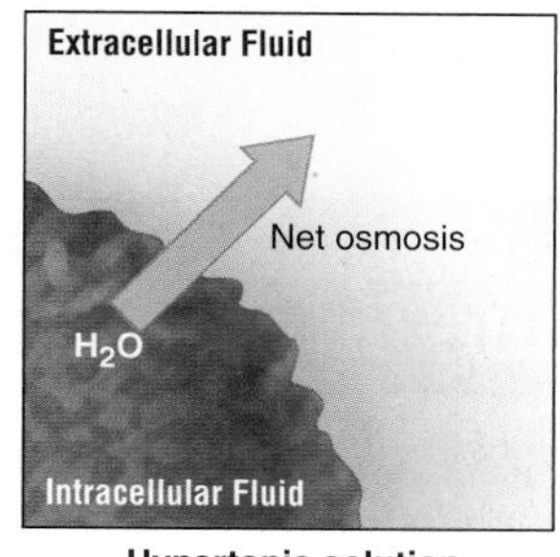

Hypertonic solution

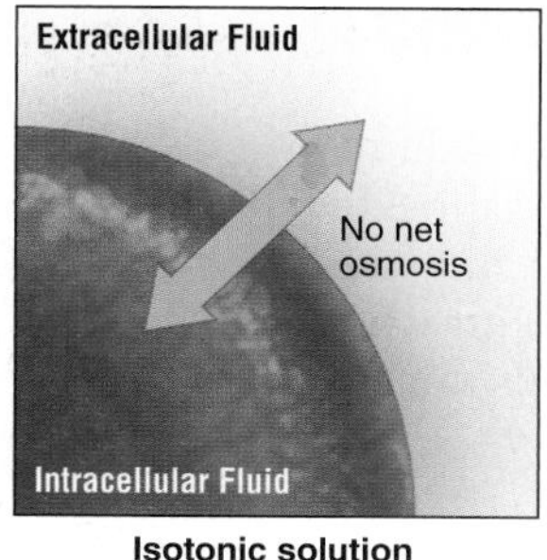

Isotonic solution

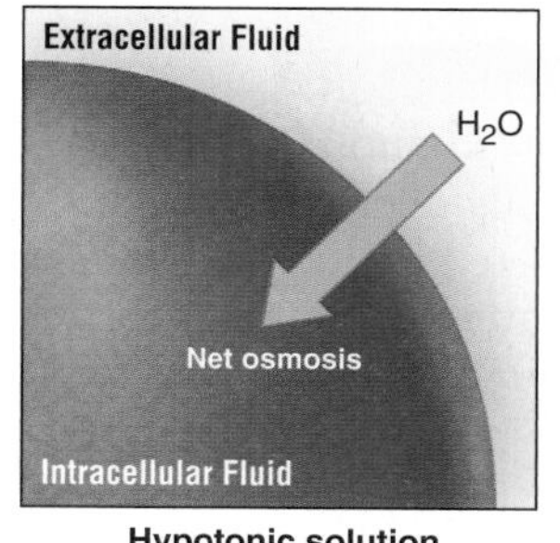

Hypotonic solution

Figure 14-6 Fluid movement with hypertonic, isotonic, and hypotonic solutions.

LR has not shown an overwhelming benefit over normal saline for fluid resuscitation. LR is contraindicated during blood product transfusions because the calcium binds to the **anticoagulants** added to transfused blood, creating a possible blood clot. LR is also contraindicated for mannitol, methylprednisolone, nitroglycerin, nitroprusside, norepinephrine, procainamide, and propranolol infusions.

D_5W, 5% dextrose in water, is a unique type of isotonic solution. As long as it remains in the bag, it is considered an isotonic solution. Once it is administered, however, the dextrose is quickly metabolized, and the solution becomes hypotonic. D_5W is rarely administered by itself. It is usually administered when you are preparing medication infusions such as dopamine (Intropin) or amiodarone (Cordarone).

Hypotonic Solutions

A hypotonic solution has a lower concentration of sodium (osmolarity) than the cell's serum. When this fluid is placed in the vascular compartment, it begins diluting the serum. Soon the serum osmolarity is less than that of the interstitial fluid; water is pulled from the vascular compartment into the interstitial fluid compartment and eventually the same process is repeated, pulling water from the interstitial compartment into the cells. Eventually cells swell and possibly burst from the increased intracellular osmotic pressure.

Hypotonic solutions hydrate the cells while depleting the vascular compartment. They may be needed for a patient who is receiving dialysis when diuretic therapy dehydrates the cells. Solutions such as hypotonic saline may be used for hyperglycemic conditions such as diabetic ketoacidosis, where high serum glucose levels draw fluid out of the cells and into the vascular and interstitial compartments.

Hypotonic solutions can cause a sudden fluid shift from the intravascular space to the cells, leading to cardiovascular collapse and increased intracranial pressure from shifting fluid into the brain cells. For example, giving D_5W for an extended period can increase intracranial pressure. This makes hypotonic solutions dangerous for patients with stroke or any head trauma. Administering these solutions to patients with burns, trauma, malnutrition, or liver disease is also hazardous because these patients are at risk for developing **third spacing**, an abnormal fluid shift into the serous linings.

One hypotonic solution you may see is 0.45% sodium chloride, commonly referred to as half-normal saline. It is rarely administered in the prehospital setting, but you may see it during interfacility transports for patients who have normal sodium levels but need fluid replenishment.

Hypertonic Solutions

A hypertonic solution has an osmolarity higher than that of serum, meaning that the solution has a higher **ionic concentration** than serum and pulls fluid and electrolytes from the intracellular and interstitial compartments into the intravascular compartment. The danger is that the cells may collapse from the increased extracellular osmotic pressure. Hypertonic solutions shift body fluids into the vascular spaces and help stabilize blood pressure, increase urine output, and reduce edema. These fluids are rarely used in the prehospital setting but may be commonly found during interfacility transports. The high electrolyte concentration of hypertonic solutions may be used for a variety of problems.

Often the term "hypertonic" is used to refer to solutions that contain high concentrations of proteins. These proteins have the same effect on fluid as sodium. Careful monitoring is needed to guard against fluid overloading when you are using hypertonic fluids, especially with patients with impaired heart or kidney function. Also, hypertonic solutions should not be given to patients with diabetic ketoacidosis or others at risk of cellular dehydration.

You may encounter the hypertonic solution 3% sodium chloride in your EMS protocols or during interfacility transport. Due to the fluid shifts that occur with sodium, 3% sodium chloride is administered to patients with severe traumatic brain injuries. It is used as a temporizing measure to draw out fluid in an effort to reduce intracranial pressure until the patient can be taken into neurosurgery.

Oxygen-Carrying Solutions

The best fluid to replace blood loss is whole blood. Unlike the crystalloid and colloid solutions, whole blood contains hemoglobin, which carries oxygen to the body's cells. On occasion (eg, aeromedical transports, multiple-casualty incidents), O-negative blood—a universally compatible blood type—may be used outside a hospital setting. However, because of the refrigeration requirements and other storage issues, general use of whole blood is impractical in the prehospital setting.

Synthetic blood substitutes, which do have the ability to carry oxygen, are being researched and, in some places, field-tested. They show great potential for improving treatment of patients who have significant blood loss. Not only would these synthetic blood substitutes expand circulating volume, but they would also carry and deliver oxygen to the part of the body that needs it the most—the cells.

IV Techniques and Administration

Intravenous means "within a vein." **Intravenous therapy** involves cannulation of a vein with a catheter to access the patient's vascular system. It is one of many invasive techniques you will perform as a paramedic.

Peripheral vein cannulation involves cannulating veins of the periphery—that is, veins that can be seen and/or palpated (eg, veins of the hand, arm, or lower extremity and the EJ vein).

The most important point to remember about IV therapy is to keep the IV equipment sterile. Forethought and attention to detail will help prevent mental and procedural errors while starting the IV line. One way to ensure proper technique is to develop a routine to follow as you assemble the appropriate equipment.

Assembling Your Equipment

To avoid delays and IV site contamination, gather and prepare all your equipment before you attempt to start an IV line. In some cases, the patient's condition may make full preparation difficult, so working as a team becomes critical. The members of your own crew, by anticipating your needs, often can assemble the needed IV equipment. Whereas procedures may vary from service to service, some variation of the following equipment will be available. Equipment includes Figure 14-7:

- Elastic tourniquet (preferably non-latex)
- Antiseptic wipe or solution
- Gauze
- Tape or adhesive bandage
- Appropriate-size IV catheter
- IV extension set
- A saline flush
- IV administration set

Choosing an IV Solution

When you are choosing the most appropriate IV solution, you must identify the needs of your patient. Ask yourself the following questions:

- Is the patient's condition critical?
- Is the patient's condition stable?
- Does the patient need fluid replacement?
- Will the patient need medications?

In the prehospital setting, the choice of IV solution is usually limited to two isotonic crystalloids, normal saline and LR solution. D_5W is often reserved for administering medication because the presence of dextrose has the potential to alter fluid and electrolyte levels in the body.

Each IV solution bag is wrapped in a protective sterile plastic bag and is guaranteed to remain sterile until the posted expiration date. Once the protective wrap is torn and removed, however, the IV solution must be used within 24 hours. Each IV bag has two ports: an injection port for medication and an **access port** for connecting the administration set. A removable pigtail protects the sterile access port. Once this pigtail is removed, the bag must be used immediately or discarded.

IV solution bags come in different fluid volumes Figure 14-8. Volumes commonly used in hospitals are 1,000 mL, 500 mL, 250 mL, 100 mL, and 50 mL; the more common prehospital volumes are 1,000 mL and 500 mL. The smaller volumes (250 mL and 100 mL) typically contain D_5W or saline and are used for mixing and administering maintenance medication infusions.

Choosing an Administration Set

An **administration set** moves fluid from the IV bag into the patient's vascular system. IV administration sets are sterile as long as they remain in their protective packaging. Each set has a **piercing spike** protected by a plastic cover. Once this spike is exposed and the seal surrounding the cap is broken, the set must be used immediately or discarded.

On most drip sets, a number on the package indicates the number of drops it takes for a milliliter of fluid

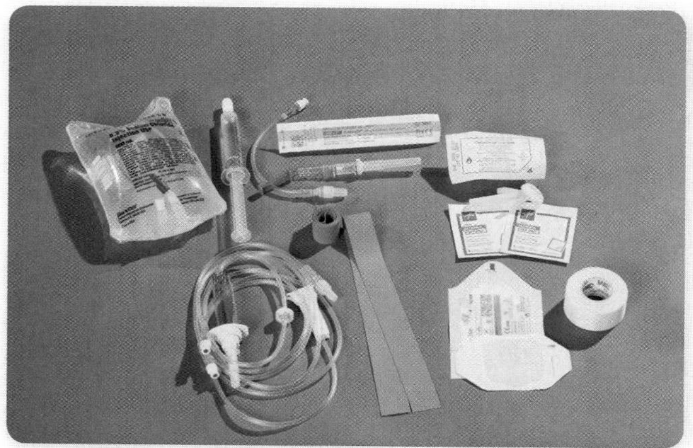

Figure 14-7 Intravenous equipment.

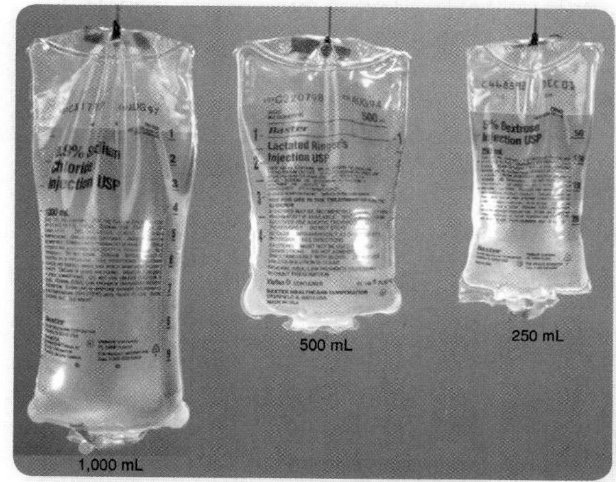

Figure 14-8 Intravenous solution bags come in different fluid volumes.

to pass through the orifice and into the **drip chamber** Figure 14-9. Administration sets come in two primary sizes: microdrip and macrodrip. **Microdrip sets** allow 60 gtt (drops) per milliliter (mL) through the needlelike orifice inside the drip chamber. They are ideal for medication administration or pediatric fluid delivery because it is easy to control their fluid flow. **Macrodrip sets** allow 10 or 15 gtt/mL through a large opening between the piercing spike and the drip chamber. They are best used for rapid fluid replacement. Some drip sets allow the provider to dial the desired drip set in; those allow the provider to adjust the drip set to 10, 15, or 60 drops.

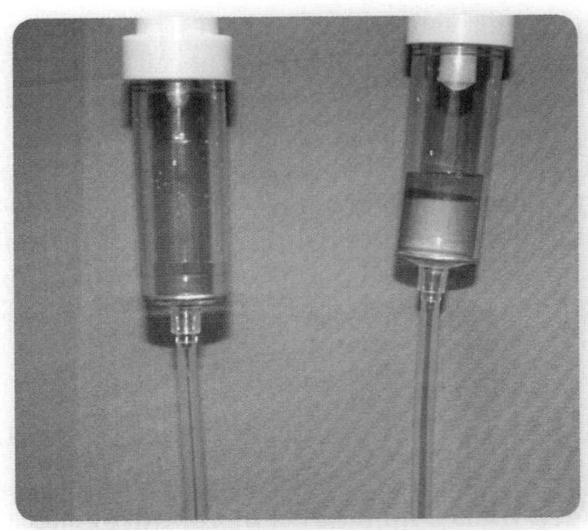

Figure 14-9 A drip set's packaging contains a number referring to the number of drops it takes for 1 milliliter of fluid to pass through the orifice into the drip chamber. Two different-size drip sets are shown here.

Preparing an Administration Set

After choosing the IV administration set and the IV solution bag, verify the expiration date of the solution and check for solution clarity. Prepare to spike the bag with the administration set. The steps for this procedure are shown in Skill Drill 14-1.

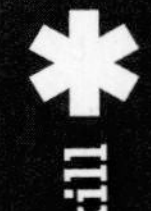

NR Skill

Skill Drill 14-1 Spiking the Bag

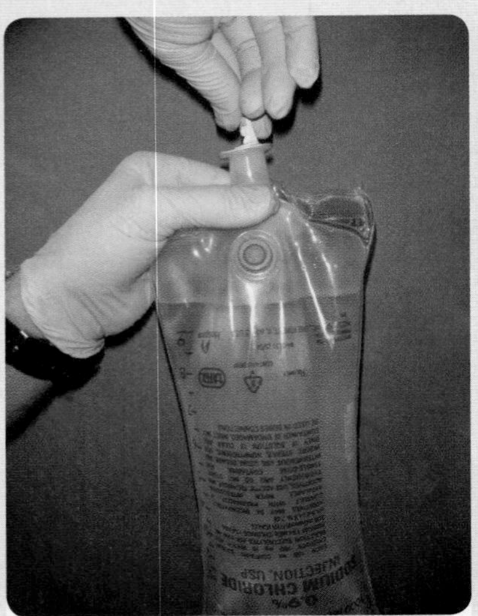

Step 1 Take standard precautions. Ensure you've chosen the correct administration set (primary or piggyback), tubing is not tangled, and protective covers are in place. Ensure you have the proper solution, that it is clear and has not expired, and that the protective tail port covers are in place. Move the roller clamp to the off position.

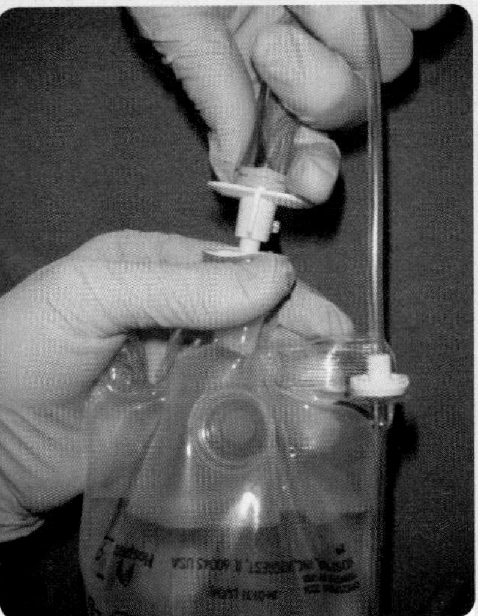

Step 2 Remove the protective covering found on the end of the IV bag. The bag is still sealed and will not leak until the piercing spike punctures this port. Remove the protective cover from the piercing spike (remember, this spike is sterile and sharp!) and slide the spike into the IV bag port until it is seated against the bag.

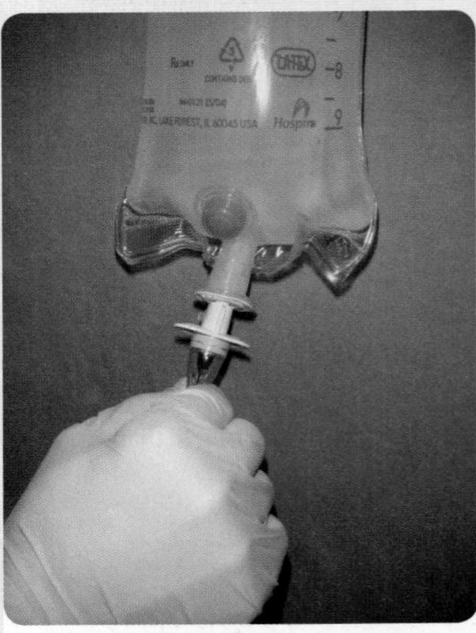

Step 3 Squeeze the drip chamber to fill to the line marking the chamber, then run fluid into the line to flush the air out of the tubing.

Skill Drill 14-1 Spiking the Bag *(continued)*

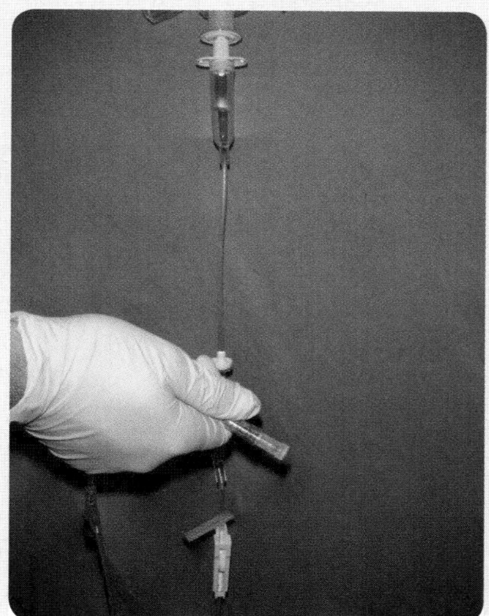

Step 4 Twist the protective cover of the opposite end of the IV tubing to allow air to escape. Do not remove this cover yet because the cover keeps the tubing end sterile until it is needed. Let the fluid flow until air bubbles are removed from the line before turning the roller clamp wheel to stop the flow, or setting the drip rate per the required dose.

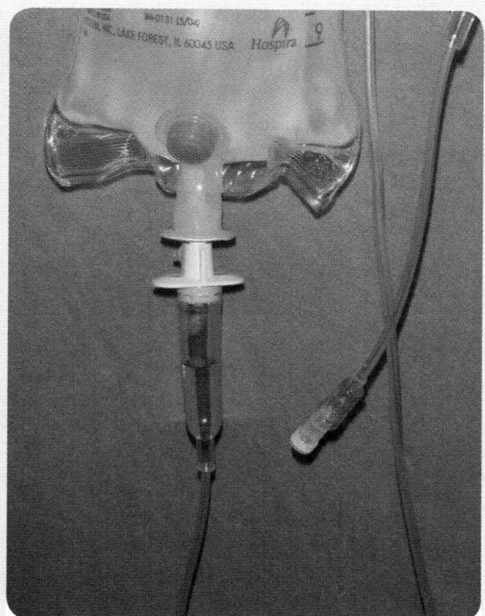

Step 5 Next, go back and check the drip chamber; it should be only half-filled. The fluid level must be visible to calculate drip rates. If the fluid level is too low, then squeeze the chamber until it fills; if the chamber is too full, with the roller clamp in the off position, invert the bag and the chamber and squeeze the chamber to empty the fluid back into the bag. Hang the bag in an appropriate location with the end of the IV tubing easily accessible.

Other Administration Sets

Blood tubing is a macrodrip administration set that is designed to facilitate rapid fluid replacement by manual infusion of multiple IV bags or IV and blood replacement combinations. Most blood tubing administration sets have dual piercing spikes that allow two bags of fluid to be used simultaneously for the same patient **Figure 14-10**. The central drip chamber has a special filter designed to filter the blood during transfusions.

Fluid control for pediatric patients and certain older adult patients is important. A microdrip set called a **Volutrol** (also called Buretrol or burette) allows you to fill a 100- or 200-mL calibrated drip chamber with a specific amount of fluid and administer only that amount to avoid inadvertent fluid overload. This type of set is commonly used in pediatric patients. A proximal roller

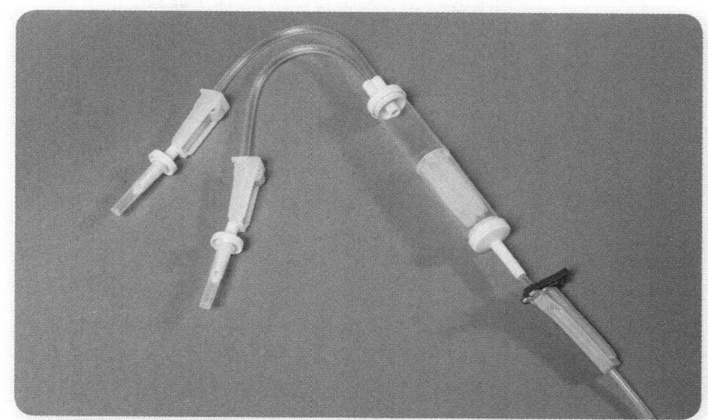

Figure 14-10 Most blood sets have dual piercing spikes that allow two bags of fluid to be used at once for the same patient.

clamp enables you to shut off the Volutrol drip chamber from the IV bag. If the patient needs additional fluids, then simply open the proximal roller clamp and fill the Volutrol with more fluid.

▶ Choosing an IV Site

It is important for you to select the most appropriate vein for IV catheter insertion. Common sites for IV catheter insertion are shown in Figure 14-11. Avoid areas of the vein that contain valves and bifurcations because a catheter will not pass through these areas easily and the needle may cause damage. Valves can be recognized as small bumps located in the vein. Bifurcations are points where one vein may split into two. Use the following criteria to select a vein:

- Locate the vein section with the straightest appearance Figure 14-12.
- Choose a vein that has a firm, round appearance or is springy when palpated.
- Avoid areas where the vein crosses over joints.
- Avoid edematous extremities and any extremity with a dialysis fistula or on the side a mastectomy was done.

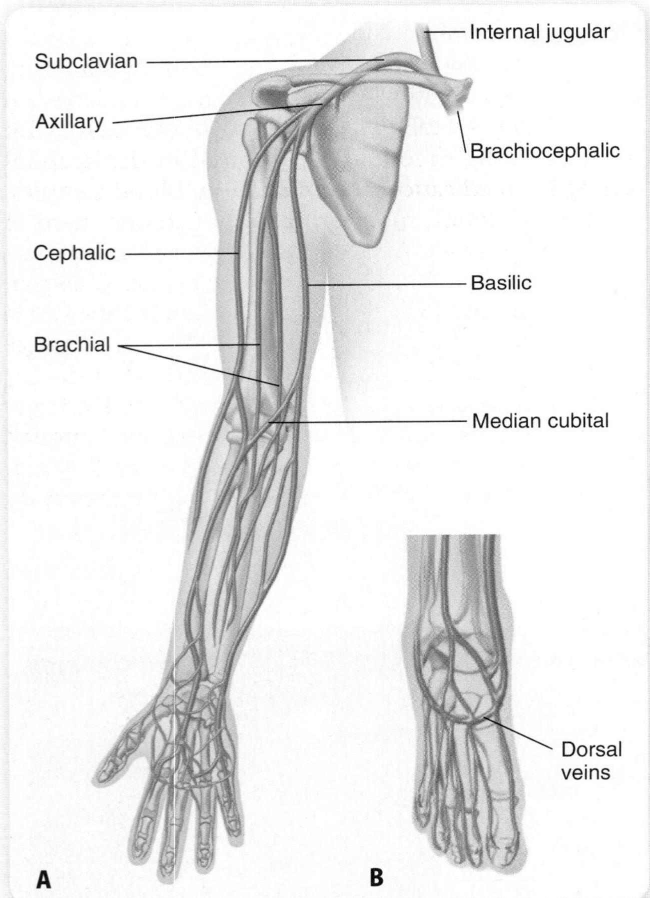

Figure 14-11 A. Common intravenous (IV) sites in the upper extremity include the brachial and cephalic veins in the proximal arm, the radial and ulnar veins in the distal arm, the antecubital veins that lie anterior to the elbow, and the dorsal veins of the hands. **B.** Common IV sites in the lower extremity include the dorsal veins of the feet.

Words of Wisdom

As a general rule, you should start distally and work your way up the patient's extremity when starting an IV line. For patients who need rapid fluid replacement, are in cardiac arrest, or are otherwise in hemodynamically unstable condition, however, you should use a vein that is readily available without a great deal of searching such as the antecubital vein. Unlike other extremity veins (eg, hand, forearm), this vein is usually visible and easier to palpate. Cannulating an EJ vein or obtaining IO access in the leg or humerus can also be considered.

If you think you may be able to establish a larger IV catheter, but are certain you can establish a smaller IV catheter, then choose the smaller IV catheter. Whereas fluid resuscitation may be important, establishing IV access is the priority.

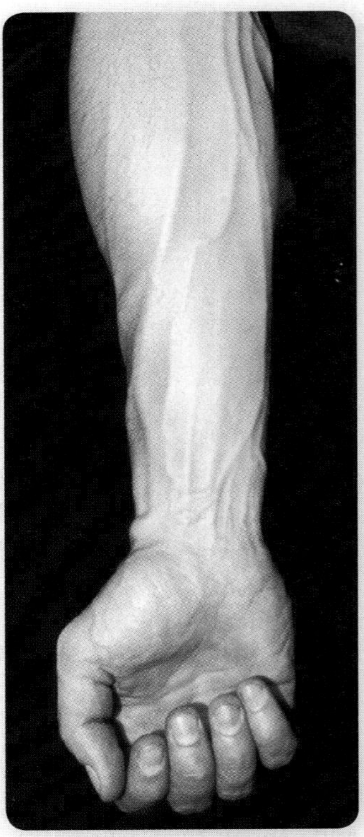

Figure 14-12 Look for veins that are relatively straight and spring back when palpated.

If IV therapy is being given for a life-threatening illness or injury, then this choice is often limited to the areas that remain open during hypoperfusion. Otherwise, limit IV access to the more distal areas of the extremities: *Start distally; work proximally*. If the most distal site ruptures or infiltrates, then you can move up the extremity to the next appropriate site. Because failed cannulation brings the possibility of leakage into the surrounding tissues, any fluid introduced immediately below an open wound has the potential to enter the tissue and cause damage.

Large protruding arm veins can be deceiving in terms of their ease of cannulation. Often these bulging veins can roll from side to side during a cannulation attempt, causing you to miss the vein. A remedy is to apply manual traction to the vein to lock it into position. Traction techniques differ depending on the location chosen for cannulation. Hold hand veins in place by pulling the skin over the vein taut with the thumb of your free hand as you flex the patient's hand **Figure 14-13**. Stabilize wrist veins by flexing the wrist and pulling the skin taut over the vein. Applying lateral traction to the vein with your free hand can stabilize veins in the forearm and **antecubital** areas. Stabilizing and cannulating the EJ vein requires a different approach (discussed later in this chapter).

The patient's opinion should also be considered when you are selecting an IV site because he or she may know an IV location that has worked in the past. Avoid attempts to insert an IV in an extremity if it shows signs of trauma, injury, or infection. Also, pay careful attention to areas of the vein that have **track marks**; they are usually a sign of sclerosis caused by frequent cannulation or puncture of the vein, for example from IV drug abuse.

Hospitals prefer that IV lines be located in nonarticulating areas such as the top of the hand or forearm. This may be taken into consideration if you anticipate long emergency department (ED), intensive care unit (ICU), or medical/surgical unit stays. Otherwise, the hospital may reestablish your IV line in a more desirable position. However, in critical situations, you may be unable to take this into consideration.

Some protocols allow IV cannulation of leg veins. Use caution when you are cannulating veins in these areas because they can place the patient at greater risk of **venous thrombosis** and subsequent **pulmonary embolism**.

▶ Choosing an IV Catheter

Catheter selection should reflect the purpose of the IV line, the age of the patient, and the location for the IV line. The most common types used in the prehospital setting are over-the-needle catheters and butterfly catheters. An **over-the-needle catheter** **Figure 14-14** is a Teflon catheter inserted *over* a hollow needle (eg, Angiocath, Terumo, Jelco). A **butterfly catheter** is a hollow, stainless steel needle with two plastic wings to facilitate its handling **Figure 14-15**. These catheters are most common in phlebotomy, but are sometimes used for IV placement in scalp veins for pediatric patients. An intracatheter is a tube that enters the bloodstream with the puncturing needle. It can be used in the hospital setting for medication administration, blood samples, and hemodynamic monitoring. Although once used in the prehospital setting, they are rarely used today.

Over-the-needle catheters are sized by their diameter, which is referred to as the **gauge**. The smaller the gauge of the catheter, the larger the diameter. Thus, a 14-gauge catheter is of larger diameter than a 22-gauge catheter; 14-gauge is the largest, 27-gauge is the smallest. The larger the diameter, the more fluid that can be delivered through it. The most common lengths are $1\frac{1}{4}$ inch and $2\frac{1}{4}$ inch (3 cm and 6 cm). While 10- and 12-gauge catheters do

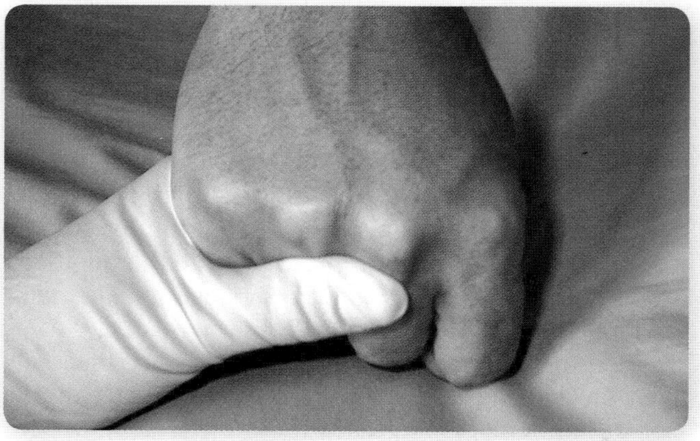

Figure 14-13 Hold hand veins in place by pulling the skin over the vein taut with the thumb of your free hand as you flex the patient's hand.

Courtesy of Rhonda Hunt.

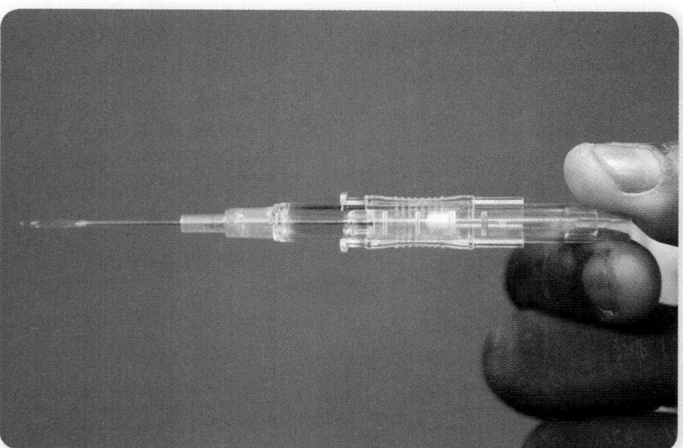

Figure 14-14 A catheter is a hollow tube that is inserted into a vein to keep the vein open, allowing a passageway into the vein. This photo shows an over-the-needle catheter (needle plus catheter).

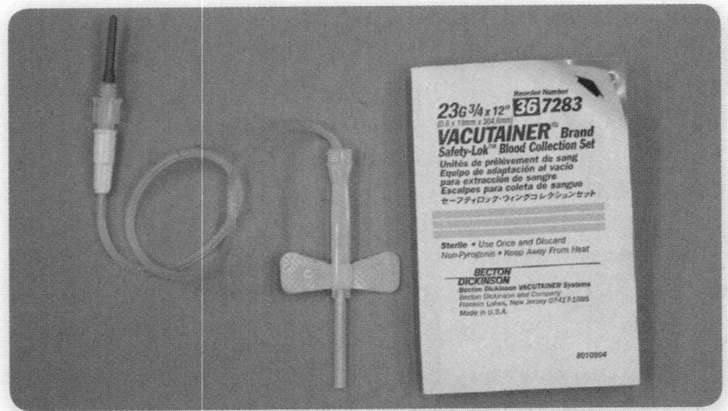

Figure 14-15 Butterfly catheters allow providers to see a flash of blood, similar to over-the-needle catheters. The wings facilitate handling.

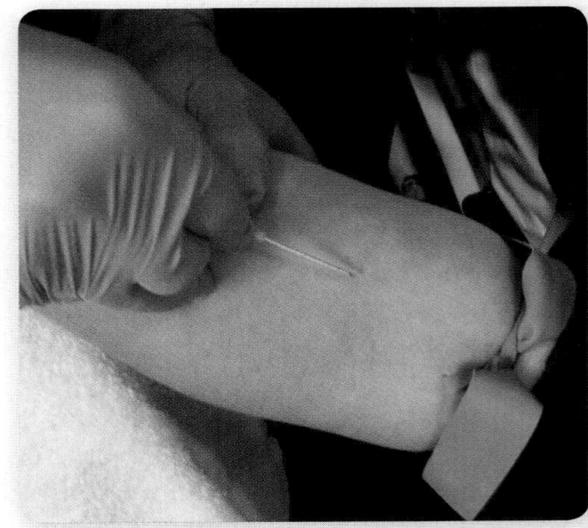

Figure 14-16 Keep the beveled side of the catheter up when inserting the needle in a vein.

exist, they are not typically used by EMS providers for vascular access. Their presence in the prehospital realm is reserved for needle decompression.

Select the largest-diameter catheter that will fit the vein you have chosen or that will be the most appropriate and comfortable for the patient. An 18- or 20-gauge catheter is usually a good size for adults. Metacarpal veins of the hand can usually accommodate 18- or 20-gauge catheters. An 18-gauge catheter should be used when the patient requires fluid replacement (eg, for hypovolemic shock); larger catheters do not help enough to make a difference, and with them, the miss rate is higher and the pain factor significant. You should be able to insert an 18-gauge catheter into an antecubital vein or EJ vein in the average adult.

Words of Wisdom

Typically, hospitals prefer to have an 18-gauge catheter or larger if they need to administer blood products or IV contrast agents (a dye administered to improve the view during radiologic studies). However, do not waste time trying to establish an IV line of that size if you do not see a vein that will accommodate it. It is possible that if you establish vascular access using a 22-gauge catheter, this may be sufficient until the hospital can insert a larger gauge catheter. If the hospital is unable to obtain a larger gauge vascular access, then they can still utilize the smaller gauge peripheral IV line (that was established prior to arrival at the hospital) for blood transfusions or other management needs. Smaller gauge peripheral IV lines may not be able to infuse as quickly as hospital staff would like, but the patient can still receive the necessary treatment. Ultimately, you should obtain the best vascular access you are capable of in your current situation without prolonging scene time.

In recent years, an attempt has been made to create over-the-needle catheters that minimize the risk of a **contaminated stick**—when a paramedic punctures his or her skin with the same catheter that was used to cannulate the vein of a patient. Newer over-the-needle catheters use automatic needle retraction after insertion, usually accomplished with a locking slide mechanism or a spring-loaded slide mechanism.

▶ Inserting the IV Catheter

Each paramedic has a unique technique to insert an IV line, and you should observe many different techniques to determine what works best for you. Two considerations, however, apply to *any* technique:

1. Keep the beveled side of the catheter up when you are inserting the needle in a vein (Figure 14-16).
2. Maintain adequate traction on the vein during cannulation.

Apply a constricting band above the site you have chosen for the insertion to allow blood to fill the veins. This creates additional vascular pressure to engorge the veins with blood below the band. It should be snug enough to significantly diminish venous flow but should not hamper arterial flow. The constricting band should be left in place only long enough to complete the IV insertion, obtain blood samples (if needed), and attach the line. *Do not leave the constricting band in place while you assemble the IV equipment.*

Constricting bands can be difficult to manage, especially if you are wearing gloves. You should develop a technique that will allow you to release the constricting band with a small tug on one end. The most common constricting band is a latex-free IV tourniquet. Unlike tourniquets used for bleeding control, these constricting bands only stop venous flow. It looks like a long, flat, 1-inch-wide (3 cm) rubber band. It is often packaged in IV start kits.

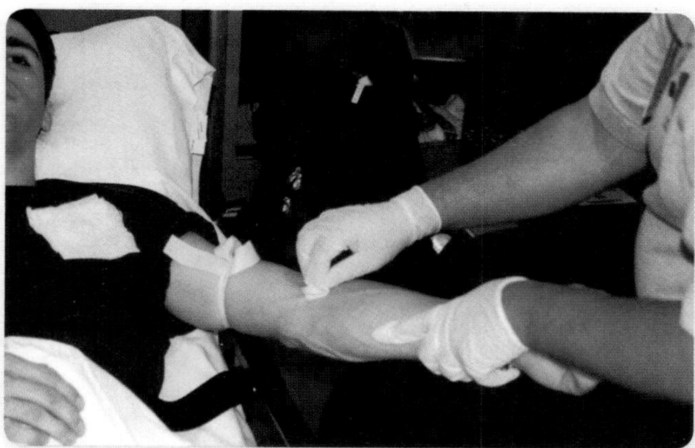

Figure 14-17 Always use aseptic technique when cleansing the site for intravenous cannulation. Use the first alcohol pad to clean in a circular motion from the inside out, then use the second to wipe straight down the center.

Courtesy of Rhonda Hunt.

At times, visualizing or palpating IV sites may be difficult. Providers may choose to replace the constricting bands with another device that may apply more pressure, such as a larger diameter and denser band known as a **Penrose drain**, a blood pressure cuff, or in a pinch, surgical hose. Some services may have an infrared light that is designed to visualize a patient's vasculature. Since there are numerous devices available, ensure you follow the manufacturer's recommendations.

Once you have selected an insertion site, prep it with an alcohol swab, iodine swab, or chlorhexidine (ChloraPrep). Do not touch the site after it has been prepped. If you contaminate the site, then you will need to clean it again **Figure 14-17**. Apply gentle downward or lateral traction on the skin over the vein, **distal traction** with your free hand while holding the catheter, bevel side up, in your dominant hand. Use caution as you apply traction to avoid collapsing the vein. Distal traction will stabilize the vein and keep it from "rolling" as you stick. Begin by establishing an insertion angle of about 45°. Advance the catheter through the skin until the vein is pierced (you should see a flash of blood in the catheter **flash chamber**); then immediately drop the angle down to about 15° and advance the catheter a few more centimeters to ensure the catheter sheath is in the vein. Slide the sheath off the needle and into the vein; do not advance the needle too far because it can puncture the other side of the vein. After the catheter is fully advanced, apply pressure to the vein just proximal to the end of the indwelling catheter, remove the band, remove the needle, and dispose of it in a sharps container, or in the case of other style catheters, trigger the shielding device.

Words of Wisdom

Iodine helps to make veins more visible by changing ambient light reflection. This technique is particularly beneficial in dark-skinned people.[6,7] As with any patient, ensure the patient is not allergic to iodine.

Ultrasonographically Guided Peripheral IV

As ultrasonography becomes more prevalent in the EMS community, it may become an available technique for difficult peripheral IV placement. Ultrasonography is used in many EDs with patients for whom IV insertion with traditional techniques is predicted to be a difficult. Ultrasonography allows providers to see deeper veins, often in the upper arm, that are not visible to the naked eye and may not be palpable.

The process begins similarly to traditional IV insertion. After placing a constricting band on the upper arm near the humeral neck, apply sterile gel to the transducer and the arm. Place the transducer in your nondominant hand, and place the probe at the antecubital fossa. Run the probe up the humerus looking for the basilic vain, brachial vein, and the cephalic vein. After identifying a vessel that is 1/6 inch (0.4 cm) or larger in diameter and 1/2 inch (1.5 cm) or less in depth, begin to apply pressure on the vessel. To differentiate veins from arteries, remember veins are easily compressed when pressure is applied. Arteries may deform mildly when pressure is applied but are not likely to completely compress. Furthermore, you may be able to notice pulsation from an artery.

After it is determined that the vessel is a vein, hold the needle in your dominant hand and align the transducer so the needle shadow is visible on the screen. Insert the needle through the skin at a 45° angle and visualize the needle tip on the screen. Advance the needle while watching the screen. As you visualize the needle penetrating the vein, verify IV success with the presence of blood in the flash chamber. Advance the catheter and withdraw the needle. Then connect the device as you would a normal peripheral IV.

Securing the Line

Once the catheter is in position and the contents of the IV bag are flowing properly, you must secure the IV line. Tape the area so the catheter and tubing are securely anchored in case of a sudden pull on the line **Figure 14-18**. Tear the tape before you start the IV line, because you will need one hand to stabilize the site while you apply the tape. Double back the tubing to create a loop that will act as a shock absorber if the line is pulled accidentally. Cover the insertion site with sterile gauze, and secure it with tape or use a commercially manufactured device (eg, Veniguard, Opsite). Avoid circumferential taping around any extremity because it may impair circulation. If the tubing needs to be secured circumferentially because the patient is attempting to

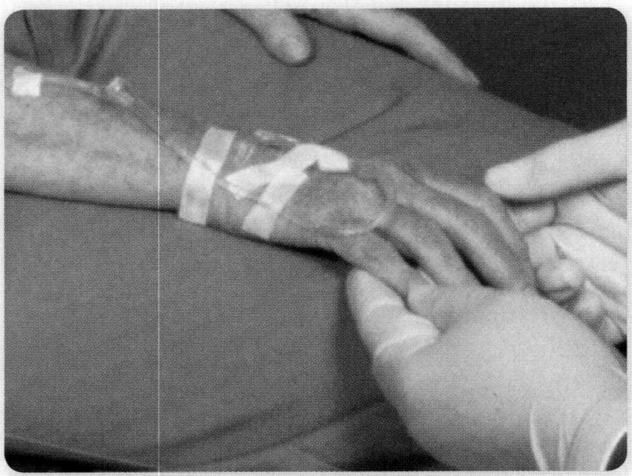

Figure 14-18 Tape the area so the catheter and tubing are securely anchored.

Documentation & Communication

To document the establishment of an IV line, you need to include the following:

1. The gauge of the needle
2. The IV attempts versus successes
3. The site (for example, left forearm, left EJ)
4. The type of fluid you are administering
5. The rate at which the fluid is running

For example, if you initiated an IV line in the left antecubital fossa with an 18-gauge catheter and are infusing normal saline at a rate of 120 mL per hour, the documentation should appear as follows:

18g IV × 1 in left AC with NS @ 120 mL/h by Medic 785

Words of Wisdom

Helpful IV hints:

- Allow the patient's arm to hang off the stretcher.
- Pat or rub the area, without being too firm. If this is done too vigorously, then it can initiate a vasoconstriction reflex.[6]
- Apply wrapped chemical heat packs for about 60 seconds.
- If you meet resistance from a valve, then elevate the extremity.
- After two misses, let your partner try.
- Try sticking without a constricting band if the IV line keeps infiltrating.
- Never pull the catheter back over the needle.
- The more IV insertions you perform, the more proficient you will become.

pull the line, then consider wrapping the extremity and tubing with roller gauze.

To establish vascular access, follow the steps in Skill Drill 14-2.

▶ Changing an IV Bag

You may have to change the IV bag for some patients, particularly those who require larger volumes of IV fluid (ie, for hypovolemic shock). Do not allow an IV fluid bag to become *completely* depleted of fluid. Change the bag when about 25 mL of fluid is left.

Like the initial setup of the IV bag and administration set (Skill Drill 14-1), replacing the IV bag is a sterile process. If the equipment becomes contaminated, then replace it and use new equipment. Always ensure some fluid remains in the drip chamber and tubing of the set. This simple action will prevent air from entering the patient's vein.

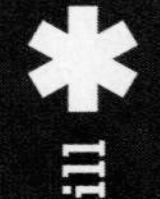

NR Skill

Skill Drill 14-2 Obtaining Vascular Access

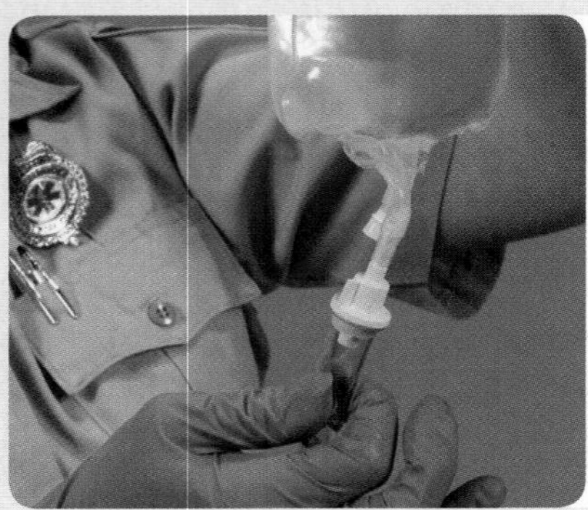

Step 1 Choose the appropriate fluid, and examine the bag for clarity and expiration date. Ensure no particles are floating in the fluid and that the fluid is appropriate for the patient's condition and not expired.

Choose the appropriate drip set, and attach it to the fluid. A macrodrip set (eg, 10 gtt/mL) should be used for a patient who needs volume replacement; a microdrip set (eg, 60 gtt/mL) should be used for a patient who needs a medication infusion. If an IV extension set is available, then attach it to the end of the tubing to assist the hospital staff in manipulating the IV tubing at the hospital.

Fill the drip chamber by squeezing it.

Skill Drill 14-2 Obtaining Vascular Access *(continued)*

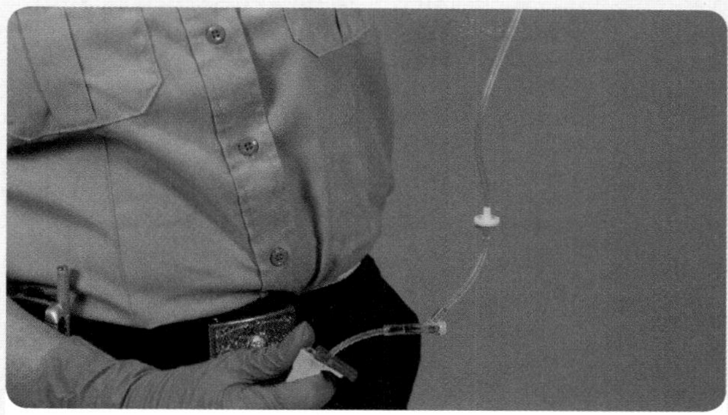

Step 2 Flush or "bleed" the tubing to remove any air bubbles by opening the roller clamp. Ensure no errant bubbles are floating in the tubing.

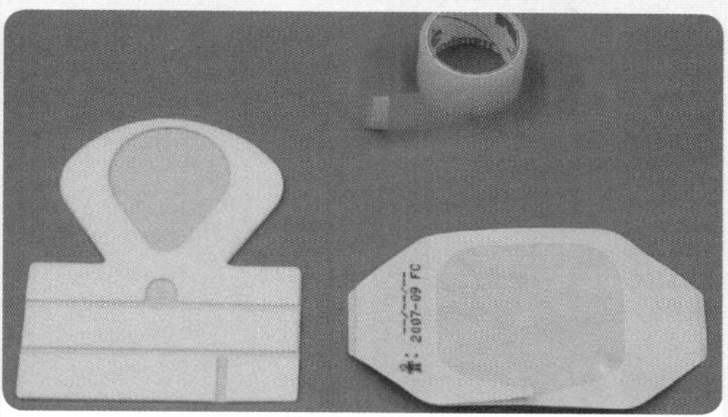

Step 3 Before the venipuncture; tear tape needed to secure the site, collect and open antiseptic swabs, gauze pads, and anything else needed for vascular access per local practice.

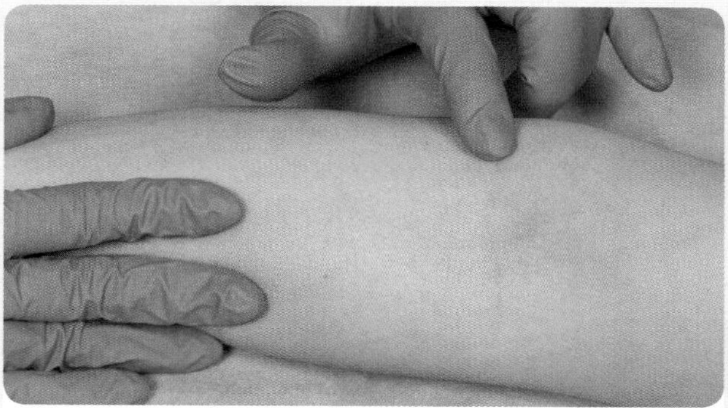

Step 4 Take standard precautions before making contact with the patient. Palpate a suitable vein. Veins should be "springy" when palpated. Avoid areas that are hard when palpated.

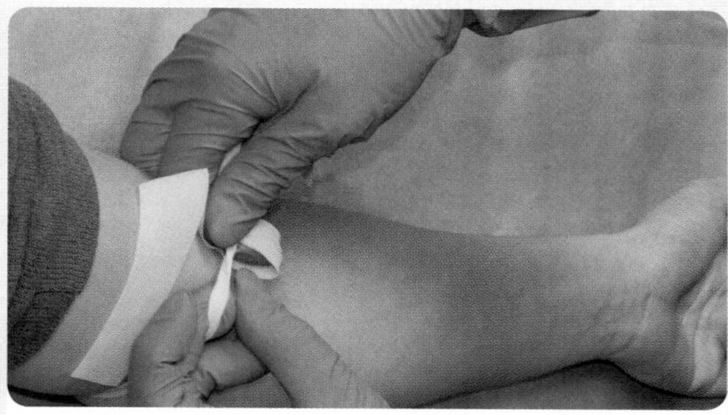

Step 5 Apply the constricting band above the intended IV site. It should be placed approximately 4 to 8 inches (10 to 20 cm) above the intended site.

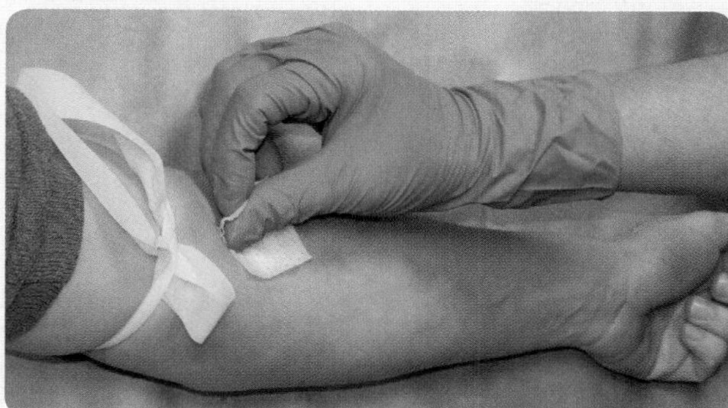

Step 6 Clean the area using aseptic technique. Use an alcohol pad to cleanse in a circular motion from the inside out. Use a second alcohol pad to wipe straight down the center.

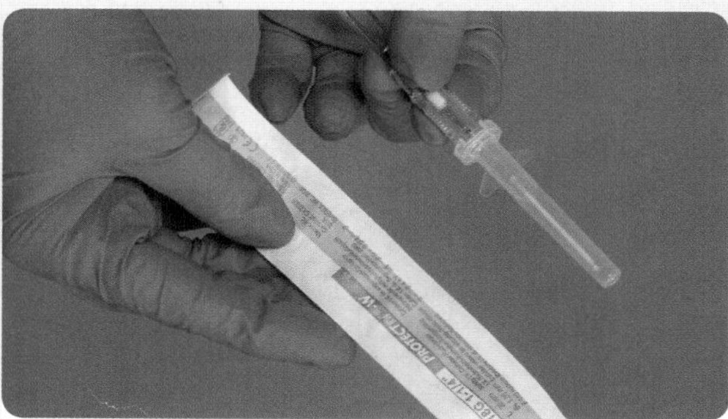

Step 7 Choose the appropriate-size catheter and twist the catheter to break the seal. Do not advance the catheter upward because this may cause the needle to shear the catheter. Examine the catheter and discard it if you discover any imperfections. Loosen the catheter hub.

(continued)

Skill Drill 14-2 Obtaining Vascular Access *(continued)*

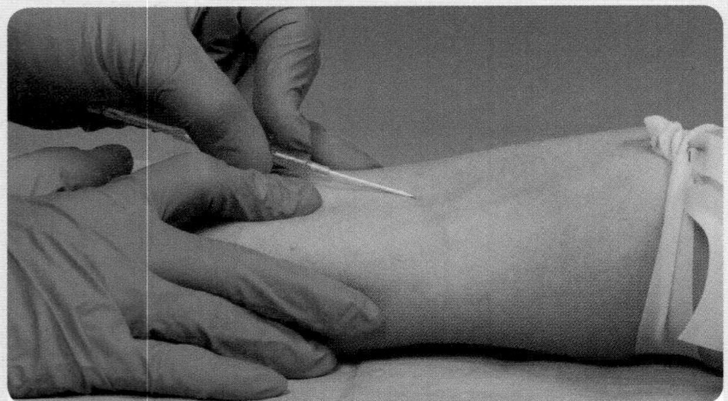

Step 8 Advise the patient to expect a needlestick. While applying distal traction at the site with one hand, insert the catheter at an angle of approximately 45° with the bevel up.

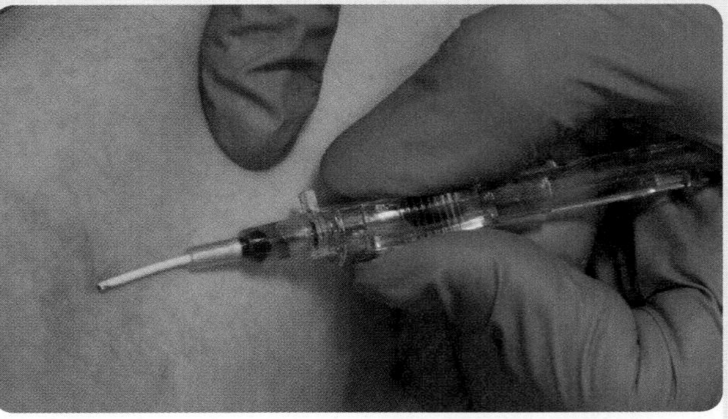

Step 9 Feel for a "pop" as the stylet enters vein and observe for "flashback" as blood enters the catheter. The clear chamber at the top of the catheter should fill with blood when the catheter enters the vein. If you note only a drop or two, then you should gently advance the catheter farther into the vein, approximately ⅛ to ¼ inch (0.3 to 0.6 cm).

Apply pressure to the site to occlude the catheter and prevent blood from leaking while removing the stylet. Hold the hub while withdrawing the needle so as not to pull the catheter out of the vein.

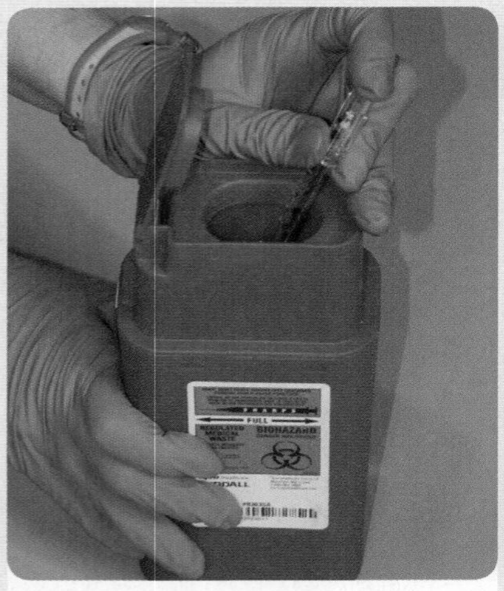

Step 10 Immediately dispose of all sharps in the proper container.

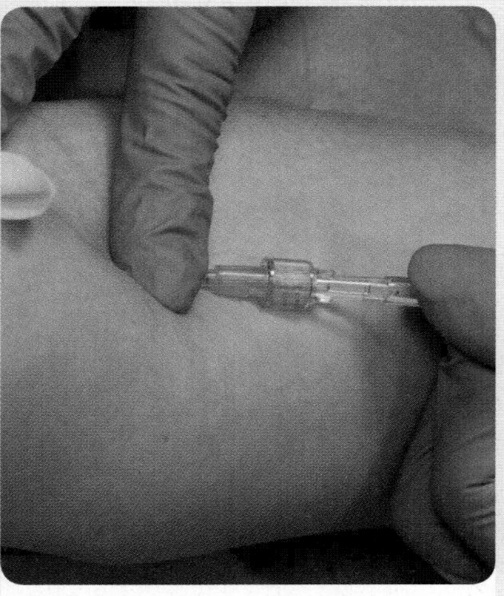

Step 11 Attach the prepared IV line. Hold the hub of the catheter while connecting the IV line.

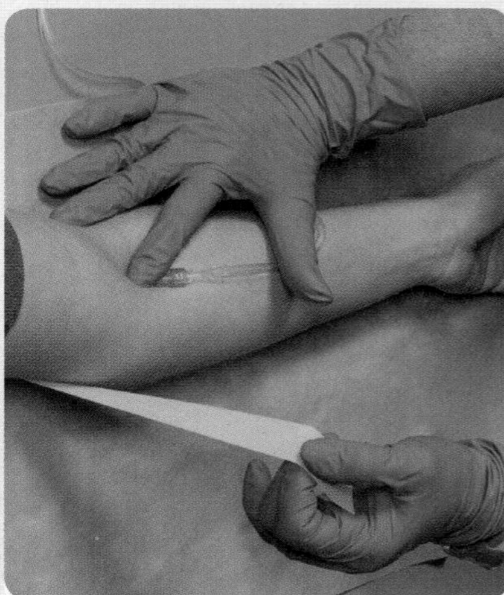

Step 12 Remove the constricting band.

Skill Drill 14-2 Obtaining Vascular Access *(continued)*

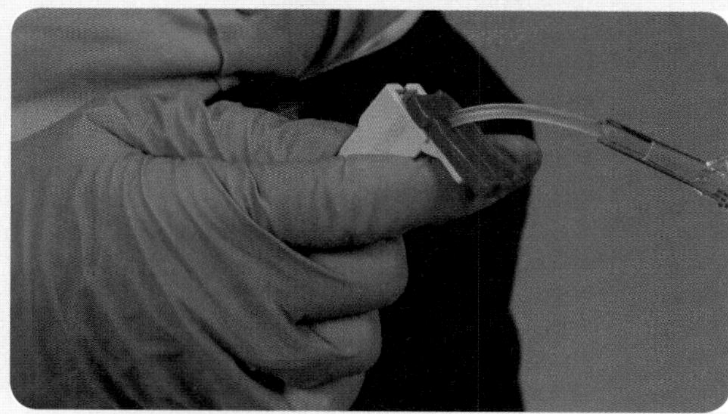

Step 13 Open the IV line to ensure fluid is flowing and the IV is patent. Observe for any swelling or **infiltration** (the escape of fluid into the surrounding tissue, causing a localized area of edema) around the IV site. If the fluid does not flow, then check whether the constriction band has been released. If infiltration is noted, then immediately stop the infusion and remove the catheter while holding pressure over the site with a piece of gauze to prevent bleeding.

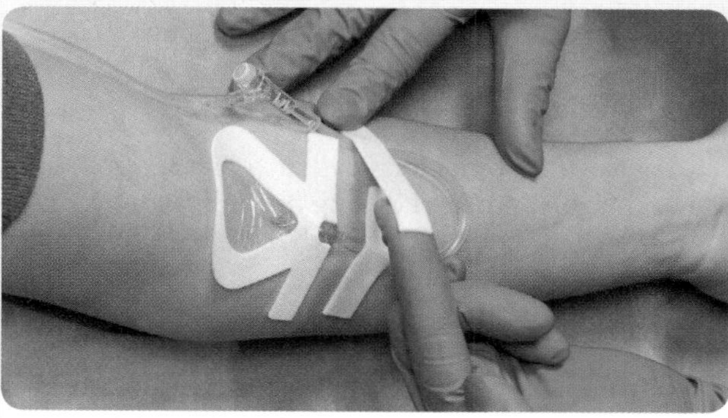

Step 14 Secure the catheter with tape or a commercial device.

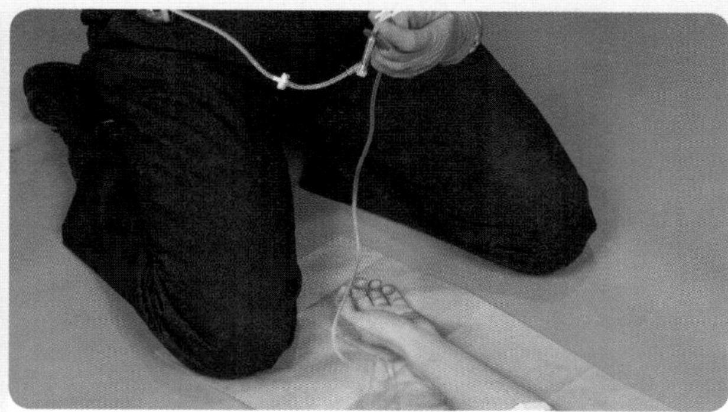

Step 15 Secure IV tubing and adjust the flow rate while monitoring the patient.

The steps for changing an IV fluid bag are as follows:

1. Stop the flow of fluid from the depleted bag by closing the roller clamp.
2. Prepare the new IV bag by removing the pigtail from the piercing spike port. Inspect the new bag of IV fluid for clarity and discoloration; also ensure it has not expired.
3. Remove the piercing spike from the depleted bag and insert it into the port on the new bag. *Do not touch the piercing spike of the administration set.*
4. Ensure the drip chamber is appropriately filled, and then open the roller clamp and adjust the fluid rate accordingly.

► Discontinuing the IV Line

To discontinue the IV line, shut off the flow from the IV with the roller clamp. Gently peel the tape back toward the IV site. As you get closer to the site and the catheter, stabilize the catheter while you loosen the remaining tape holding the catheter in place. Do not remove the IV tubing from the hub of the catheter. Fold a 4-inch × 4-inch (10-cm × 10-cm) piece of gauze and place it over the site, holding it down while you pull back on the hub of the catheter. Gently pull the catheter and the IV line from the patient's vein while applying pressure to control bleeding **Figure 14-19**.

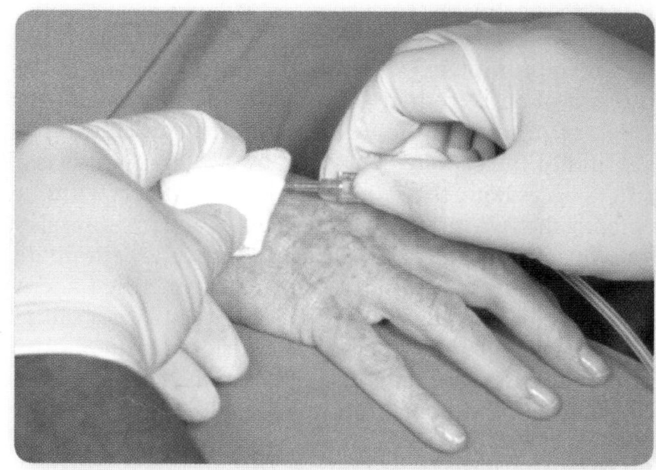

Figure 14-19 When removing a catheter and IV line, pull gently and apply pressure to control bleeding.

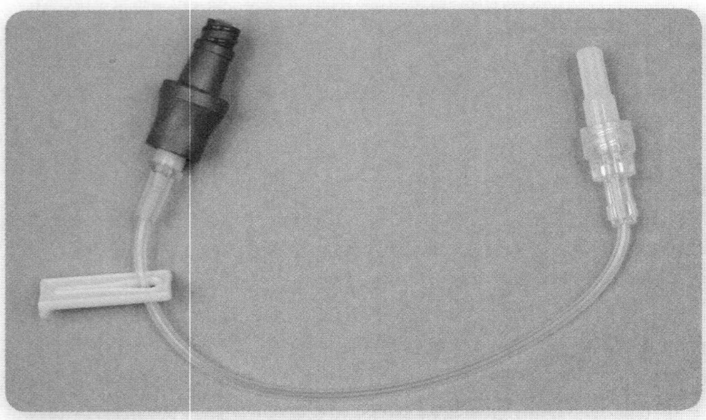

Figure 14-20 A saline lock is attached to the end of an intravenous catheter and filled with approximately 2 mL of normal saline to keep blood from clotting at the end of the catheter.

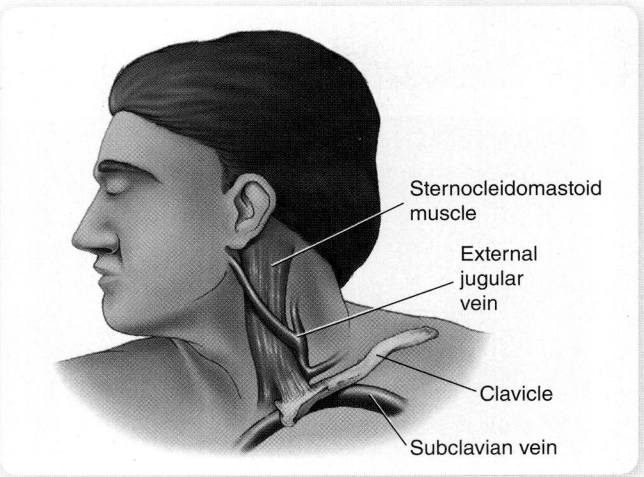

Figure 14-21 Anatomy of the external jugular vein.

▶ Alternative IV Sites and Techniques

Saline Locks

Saline locks (buff caps) are a way to maintain an active IV site without running fluids through the vein. A saline lock is comprised of a male Luer lock connector, from the standardized Luer taper system created by Hermann Luer, that attaches to the hub of an IV catheter and a female Luer lock connector that can connect to syringes for medication administration or to an IV administration set. Saline locks may have tubing ranging from 1 to 5 inches (3 to 13 cm) between the male and female Luer lock connectors. These access ports are used primarily for patients who do not need additional fluids but who may need rapid medication delivery (eg, in case of heart failure or pulmonary edema). A saline lock is attached to the end of an IV catheter and filled with approximately 2 mL of normal saline to keep blood from clotting at the end of the catheter **Figure 14-20**. Because this is a sealed-access site, the saline remains in the port without entering the vein, preventing clotting. These devices are also known as intermittent (INT) sites because they eliminate the need to reestablish an IV line each time the patient needs medication or fluid. Some services place a saline lock on every patient to ease the transfer of patient care. This allows the hospital to temporarily disconnect the IV administration without having to reestablish the IV catheter.

External Jugular Vein Cannulation

The **external jugular (EJ) vein** **Figure 14-21** runs downward and obliquely backward behind the angle of the jaw until it pierces the deep fascia of the neck just above the middle of the clavicle. It ends in the subclavian vein, where valves retard the backflow of blood. The EJ vein is fairly large and usually easy to cannulate; however, because the vein lies so near the surface of the skin, it rolls if the vein is not appropriately anchored during cannulation. It is also near other vessels (such as the carotid artery) that may be damaged during cannulation.

You should exhaust all other means of cannulating a peripheral vein (ie, in the arm or hand) before attempting cannulation of the EJ vein. Although it is a "peripheral" vein, more risks are associated with cannulation of this vein—namely, inadvertent puncture of the carotid artery, a *rapidly* expanding **hematoma** (an accumulation of blood in the tissues surrounding an IV site) if infiltration occurs, and air embolism.

Follow these steps to cannulate the EJ vein:

1. Place the patient in a supine, head-down position to fill the jugular vein. Turn the patient's head to the side opposite the intended venipuncture site. ***Always** feel carefully for a pulse before cannulating an EJ vein. It is imperative not to pierce the carotid artery.*
2. Appropriately cleanse the venipuncture site.
3. Occlude the jugular vein with your finger, distal to the catheter insertion site, to facilitate backflow of blood; this will allow the vein to become more visible.
4. Align the catheter in the direction of the vein, with the point aimed toward the shoulder on the side of the venipuncture **Figure 14-22**.
5. Make the puncture midway between the angle of the jaw and the midclavicular line. Stabilize the vein by placing a finger lightly on top of it just above the clavicle.
6. Proceed as described for cannulation of a peripheral vein. *Do not let air enter the catheter once it is in the vein.* Patients can draw in as much as 10% of their tidal volume through an open EJ vein, causing a large air embolism.
7. Tape the line securely but do *not* put circumferential dressings around the neck.

Special Populations

IV Therapy Considerations for Special Populations

Pediatric IV Therapy Highlights

- Use smaller gauge catheters or butterfly needles for peripheral IV access due to smaller vasculature.
- IV catheters and tubing may need additional gauze to secure them from being pulled out.
- Arm boards or splints may be needed to assist in securing the lines
- Access may be obtained in other locations such as scalp veins or umbilical veins

Geriatric IV Therapy Highlights

- Use smaller gauge catheters to increase comfort and prevent extravasation.
- Distal traction is needed due to increased skin elasticity, but caution should be taken. Aggressive traction can cause skin tears.
- Slower flow rates should be considered to reduce the possibility of rupturing a vein or causing complications from fluid overload.
- Avoid smaller, spider, veins which are not likely to tolerate a catheter.

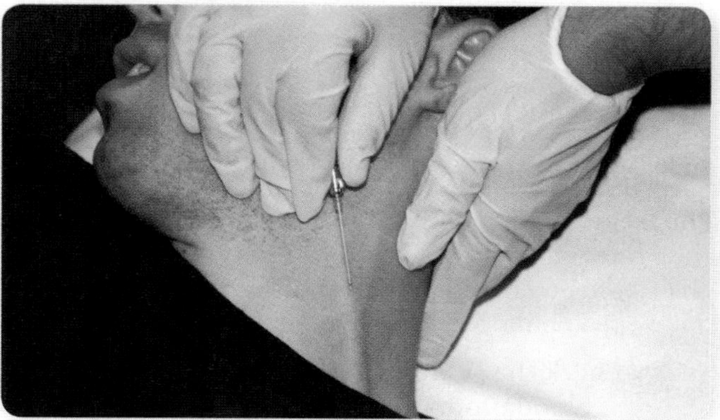

Figure 14-22 The external jugular vein requires a specific insertion site midway between the angle of the jaw and the midclavicular line with the catheter pointed toward the shoulder on the same side as the venipuncture.

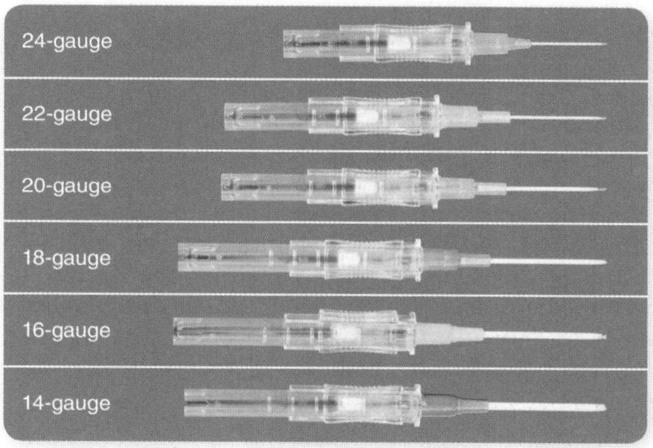

Figure 14-23 Note the difference in sizes of the catheters.

► Pediatric IV Therapy Considerations

The same IV solutions and equipment can be used on pediatric patients as on adults, with a few exceptions.

Catheters

If you are using over-the-needle catheters to start a pediatric IV line, then the 20-, 22-, 24-, or 26-gauge catheters are best for insertions Figure 14-23 . Butterfly catheters can be used in pediatric patients and can be placed in the same locations as over-the-needle catheters and in visible scalp veins. Scalp veins are best used in young infants.

IV Locations

When you are starting an IV line, explain what you are doing to both the child and the parent. A parent can become as stressed as a child, so take time to thoroughly explain the procedure.

The younger the pediatric patient, the fewer choices you have for IV sites. Hand veins are painful and difficult to manage in younger pediatric patients but remain the location of choice for starting peripheral IV lines. Sometimes the best choice is an antecubital vein line with full arm immobilization to avoid dislodging the IV line. Protecting the IV site after it has been established is crucial and is sometimes best accomplished by immobilizing the site before cannulation with an arm board. While securing the site, ensure the catheter hub and tubing connection are covered with a clear dressing so they can be continually assessed. If there is a fear of the child pulling the catheter out, then consider wrapping the tubing and catheter with roller gauze. Do not wrap so tightly that it impedes circulation or tubing flow. It must be able to be displaced quickly and easily near the IV hub and all ports so that you can inspect them regularly.

One of the better techniques for starting pediatric IV lines is to use a penlight to illuminate the veins on the back of the hand. Shine the light through the palm side of the hand to illuminate the veins on the backside of the hand. Be sure not to burn the patient with the penlight, even though this is unlikely. Once a suitable site is located, slightly graze the surface of the hand with your fingernail so you can find the location after you turn off the penlight. Proceed with the IV insertion, using the mark you created as a guide.

Scalp vein cannulation is often aesthetically unpleasant for both the child and the parents and can produce apprehension in both simply because of the location. In addition, scalp veins can be difficult to cannulate and do not allow for rapid fluid resuscitation. When you are securing a scalp vein, tape a paper cup over the site to avoid applying any direct pressure to the butterfly catheter. Pressure may cause the needle to puncture the other side of the vein and let fluids escape into the tissues (extravasation).

Older Adult IV Therapy Considerations

Smaller catheters may be preferable with older patients unless rapid fluid replacement is needed. Some medications commonly used by older patients have the tendency to increase the fragility of already frail skin and veins. Often, simply puncturing the vein will cause a massive hematoma. The use of tape can lead to skin damage, so be careful when establishing IV lines in older patients. Consider using alternative options such as paper tape or commercial devices that reduce the risk of skin damage.

Catheters

Try using the smaller catheters (such as 20, 22, or 24 gauge), because they may be more comfortable for the patient and can reduce the risk of extravasation.

IV Sets

Be careful when you are using macrodrips because they can allow rapid infusion of fluids, which may lead to edema if they are not monitored closely. With both older and pediatric patients, fluid overloading is potentially serious. Always monitor fluid administration carefully.

Locations

In choosing an IV site, you should consider the possibility of poor vein elasticity. One of the consequences of aging is the loss of elasticity in the body tissues. Veins become sclerosed, making them brittle. Certain medications, such as prednisone, can also affect the structure of the vein, making the veins of older patients even more fragile and easily ruptured. Avoid small spidery veins that weave back and forth Figure 14-24 because they may rupture easily. Do not use **varicose veins**; although they often appear to be ideal choices for IV starts, they are almost completely closed off and allow very little circulation.

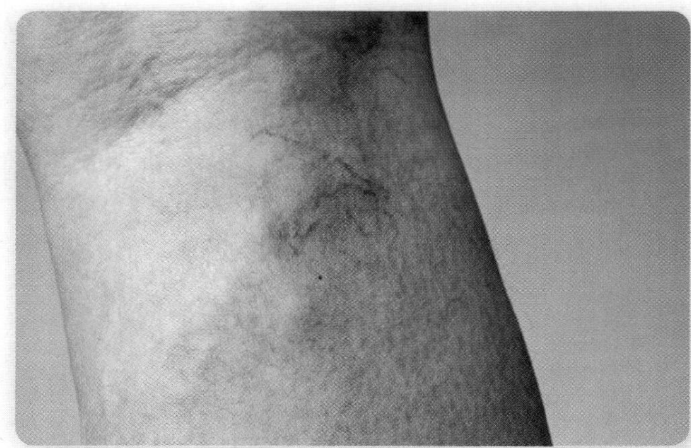

Figure 14-24 When you are looking for an intravenous site, avoid small spidery veins and varicose veins.

Factors Affecting IV Flow Rates

Several factors can influence the flow rate of an IV line. For example, if the IV bag is not hung high enough, the flow rate will not be sufficient. Perform the following checks after completing IV administration and whenever a flow problem occurs:

- **Check the IV fluid.** Thick, viscous fluids such as blood products and colloid solutions infuse slowly and may be diluted to help speed delivery. Cold fluids run more slowly than warm fluids. If possible, warm IV fluids before administering them in a cold environment.
- **Check the administration set.** Macrodrips are used for rapid fluid delivery; microdrips deliver a more controlled flow.
- **Check the height of the IV bag.** The IV bag must be hung high enough to overcome gravity. Hang it as high as possible. The closer it is to the patient, the slower it will be. If it falls below the level of the patient, then it will begin to draw blood out of the vein.
- **Check the type of catheter used.** The larger the diameter of the catheter (the smaller the number—for example a 14 gauge is of larger diameter than a 20 gauge), the faster fluid can be delivered.
- **Check the constricting band.** Do not leave the constricting band on the patient's arm after establishing the IV line.
- **Check the entire line to ensure it is not clamped at any point.** Occasionally, the roller clamp or the clamp from an extension set is left closed.

- **Check the positioning of the IV line.** The problem with the IV line may be positional, requiring you to ask the patient to keep his or her arm straight, place gauze underneath the catheter hub, or manipulate the line into position in another fashion.

Potential Complications of IV Therapy

Problems associated with IV therapy can be categorized as local or systemic reactions. **Local reactions** include problems such as infiltration and thrombophlebitis. **Systemic complications** include allergic reactions, circulatory overload, air embolus, vasovagal reactions, and catheter shear.

Local IV Site Reactions and Local Complications

Most local reactions require you to discontinue the IV and reestablish the IV line in the opposite extremity or in a proximal location. Examples of local reactions include infiltration; thrombophlebitis; occlusion; vein irritation; hematoma; nerve, tendon, or ligament damage; and arterial puncture.

Infiltration

Infiltration is the escape of fluid into the surrounding tissue, which causes a localized area of edema. Causes of infiltration include the following problems:

- The IV catheter passes completely through the vein and out the other side.
- The patient moves excessively.
- The tape used to secure the IV line becomes loose or dislodged.
- The catheter is inserted at too shallow an angle and enters only the fascia surrounding the vein (this problem is more common with IV lines in larger veins, such as those in the upper arm and neck).

Signs and symptoms of infiltration include edema at the catheter site, continued IV flow after occlusion of the vein above the insertion site, and the patient reporting tightness, burning, and pain around the IV site.

If infiltration occurs, then discontinue the IV line and reestablish it in the opposite extremity or in a more proximal location on the same extremity. Apply direct pressure over the swollen area to reduce further swelling or bleeding into the tissue. Avoid wrapping tape around the extremity because it could create a constricting band.

Occlusion

Occlusion is the physical blockage of a vein or catheter. If the flow rate is not sufficient to keep fluid moving out of the catheter tip such that blood enters the catheter, then a clot may form and occlude the flow. The first sign of an occlusion is a decreasing drip rate or the presence of blood in the IV tubing. With a positional IV site, fluid flows at different rates depending on the position of the catheter within the vein; these differences can produce occlusions. Positional IVs may be necessary because of proximity to a valve or because of patient movement that allows the line to become physically blocked, such as the patient resting on the line or crossing his or her arms. Occlusion may also develop if the IV bag nears empty and the patient's blood pressure overcomes the flow, causing fluid backup in the line.

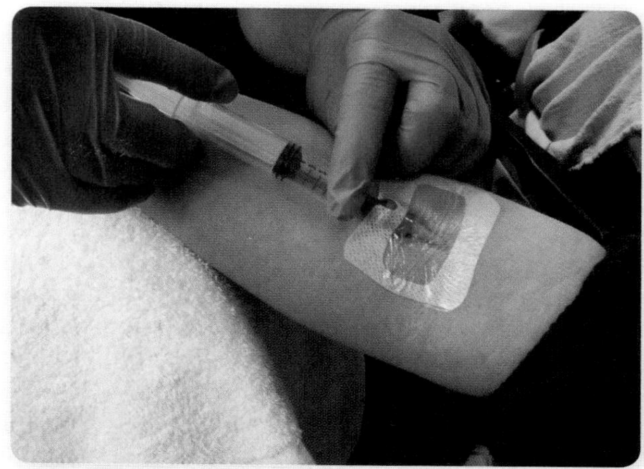

Figure 14-25 To check if an intravenous line is viable, gently flush the catheter to disrupt the occlusion and reestablish flow. This photo shows a syringe prefilled with saline.
Courtesy of Rhonda Hunt.

To determine whether an IV line should be reestablished, you may use a syringe prefilled with saline, or you may draw the saline from an IV bag. Once you have the full syringe of clean IV fluid, you will use it to add pressure to the line. Gently apply pressure to the plunger to disrupt the occlusion and reestablish flow **Figure 14-25**. If flow is reestablished, then ensure the line is free and the rate is sufficient. If the occlusion does not dislodge, then discontinue the administration and reestablish the IV line in the opposite extremity or at a proximal location on the same extremity.

Vein Irritation

Occasionally, a patient will experience vein irritation from the IV fluid or medication administration. Patients who have this problem often immediately report that the solution is bothering them (ie, tingling, stinging, itching, and burning). In such cases, observe the patient closely in case an allergic reaction to the fluid develops.

Vein irritation is usually caused by a too-rapid infusion rate. If redness develops at the IV site—a sign suggesting thrombophlebitis—discontinue the IV line and save the equipment for later analysis. Reestablish the IV line in the other extremity with new equipment in case the old equipment contained unseen contaminants.

Thrombophlebitis

Infection and **thrombophlebitis** (inflammation of the vein) may occur in association with venous cannulation; both conditions are most frequently caused by lapses in aseptic technique. Thrombophlebitis is commonly encountered in patients who abuse drugs as well as in patients who are receiving long-term IV therapy in a hospital or hospice setting or with vein-irritating solutions (eg, dextrose solutions, which have a low pH, or hypertonic solutions of any sort). It can also be produced by mechanical factors, such as excessive motion of the IV needle or catheter after it has been placed.

Thrombophlebitis is usually manifested by pain and tenderness along the vein and redness and edema at the venipuncture site. These signs generally do not appear until after several hours of IV therapy, so you are unlikely to see a case of thrombophlebitis in the field setting unless you are conducting an interhospital transport of a patient with an established IV line. In such a case, stop the infusion and discontinue the IV at that site. Warm compresses applied to the site may provide some relief.

It is far better to prevent thrombophlebitis or infection than to treat it afterward. To prevent thrombophlebitis, take the following measures:

- Use a povidone-iodine preparation to scrub and disinfect the skin over the venipuncture site; then do a final wipe with an alcohol swab. Make certain the site has had time to dry before initiating the venipuncture.
- Always wear gloves when you are performing a venipuncture.
- Never touch or otherwise contaminate the site after it has been prepped.
- After inserting the catheter, cover the puncture site with a sterile dressing.
- Anchor the catheter and tubing securely to prevent motion of the catheter within the vein.

Hematoma

A hematoma is an accumulation of blood in the tissues surrounding an IV site, often resulting from vein perforation or improper catheter removal. Blood can be seen rapidly pooling around the IV site, leading to tenderness and pain (Figure 14-26). Patients with a history of vascular diseases (including diabetes) and patients taking certain medications (eg, corticosteroids or a blood thinner such as warfarin [Coumadin]) or drinking alcohol can have a predisposition to vein rupture or to hematoma development with IV insertion.

If a hematoma develops while you are attempting to insert a catheter, then stop and apply direct pressure to help minimize bleeding. If a hematoma develops after a successful catheter insertion, then evaluate the IV flow and the hematoma. If the hematoma appears to be controlled and the flow is not affected, then monitor the IV site and leave the line in place. If the hematoma develops as a result of discontinuing the IV line, then apply direct pressure with a 4-inch × 4-inch (10-cm × 10-cm) gauze pad to the site.

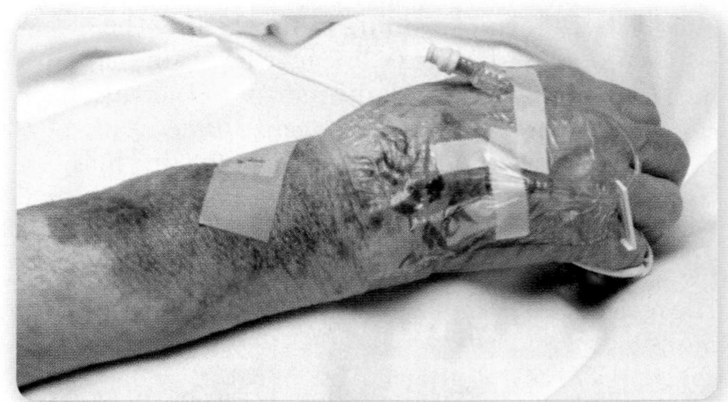

Figure 14-26 Hematomas can be caused by the improper removal of a catheter, resulting in pooling of blood around the intravenous site, leading to tenderness and pain.

Courtesy of Rhonda Hunt.

Nerve, Tendon, or Ligament Damage

Improper identification of anatomic structures around the IV site can lead to perforation of tendons, ligaments, and nerves. Selecting an IV site located near joints increases the risk for perforation of these structures. When this type of injury occurs, patients will experience sudden and severe shooting pain. Numbness or tingling in the extremity after the incident is common. Immediately remove the catheter and select another IV site.

Arterial Puncture

You may accidentally puncture the wrong blood vessel if the vein selected for cannulation lies near an artery. The risk of arterial puncture is especially high when cannulating an EJ vein; therefore, use extreme care. If you insert a catheter into an artery by mistake, then bright red blood will spurt back through the catheter. The blood's color and its flow characteristics will alert you to your error. Be aware that patients with extremely high blood pressures may have a rapid backflow into the bag. Carefully evaluate the incident, the landmarks, and the patient. Immediately withdraw the catheter, and apply direct pressure over the puncture site for at least 5 minutes or until bleeding stops.

To avoid cannulating an artery, always check for a pulse in any vessel you intend to cannulate. Under normal circumstances, veins are near the skin surface and arteries lie much deeper. On occasion, an anatomic anomaly occurs and the vessels become transpositioned, resulting in an artery being superficial.

▶ Systemic Complications

Systemic complications can evolve from reactions or complications associated with IV line insertion. They usually involve other body systems and can be life-threatening. If the IV line is established and patent in a patient experiencing a systemic complication, then do not remove it because it may be needed for treatment. Potential systemic complications include allergic reactions, pyrogenic reactions, circulatory overload, air embolus, vasovagal reactions, and catheter shear.

Pyrogenic Reactions

Pyrogens are foreign proteins capable of producing fever. The presence of pyrogens in the infusion solution or administration set may induce a **pyrogenic reaction**, which is characterized by an abrupt temperature elevation (as high as 106°F [41.1°C]) with severe chills, backache, headache, weakness, nausea, and vomiting. Occasionally, vascular collapse occurs, with all the signs and symptoms of shock. The reaction usually begins within 30 minutes after the IV infusion has been started.

If you observe *any* signs of such a reaction—for example, if the patient reports a headache or backache after you have started running fluids—*stop the infusion immediately!* Start a new IV line in the other arm with a *fresh infusion solution,* and remove the first IV line. If the patient is showing signs of shock, then treat as any other case of shock.

Pyrogenic reactions can be largely avoided by carefully inspecting the IV bag before use. If the bag has any leaks or if the fluid looks cloudy or discolored, then select another bag.

Circulatory Overload

Healthy adults can handle as much as 2 to 3 extra liters of fluid without compromise. Problems occur, however, when the patient has cardiac, pulmonary, or renal dysfunction; these types of dysfunction do not tolerate any additional demands from increased circulatory volume. The most common cause of circulatory overload in the prehospital setting is failure to readjust the drip rate after flushing an IV line immediately after insertion. Always monitor the IV line to ensure the proper drip rate. If an IV delivery device (eg, Volutrol, Buretrol, infusion pump) is available, consider using it for patients who are at risk for circulatory overload.

> **Special Populations**
>
> It is easy to overload older adult patients who need large amounts of IV fluids. Administer small boluses of fluid (200 to 300 mL), and check breath sounds before and after each bolus to ensure the lungs remain "dry."

Signs and symptoms of circulatory overload include dyspnea, jugular vein distention, and hypertension. Crackles are often heard when you are evaluating breath sounds. Acute peripheral edema can also be an indication of circulatory overload.

To treat a patient with circulatory overload, slow the IV rate to keep the vein open and raise the patient's head to ease respiratory distress. Administer high-flow oxygen, and monitor vital signs and breathing adequacy. Consider the use of continuous positive airway pressure (CPAP) to push fluid out of the lungs (alveoli).

Air Embolus

Healthy adults can tolerate as much as 200 mL of air introduced into the circulatory system. For patients who are already ill or injured, however, any air introduced into the IV line can present a problem. Properly flushing an IV line will help eliminate the likelihood of an air embolus. Although IV bags are designed to collapse as they empty to help prevent this problem, this collapse does not always occur. Be sure to replace empty IV bags with full ones.

If your patient begins developing respiratory distress with unequal breath sounds, then consider the possibility of an air embolus. Other associated signs and symptoms include cyanosis (even in the presence of high-flow oxygen), signs and symptoms of shock, loss of consciousness, and respiratory arrest.

Treat a patient with a suspected air embolus by placing the patient on his or her left side with the head down to trap any air inside the right atrium or right ventricle, administering 100% oxygen, and rapidly transporting to the closest appropriate facility. Be prepared to assist ventilations if the patient experiences inadequate breathing.

Vasovagal Reactions

Some patients have anxiety concerning needles or the sight of blood. Such anxiety may cause vasculature dilation, leading to a drop in blood pressure and patient collapse. Patients can present with anxiety, diaphoresis, nausea, and **syncopal episodes**.

> **Words of Wisdom**
>
> Once a catheter has been advanced over a needle, never, never, never pull it back!

Treatment for patients with vasovagal reactions (also known as "vagaling down") centers on treating them for shock:

1. Place patient in the position dictated by protocol for shock management.
2. Administer high-flow oxygen.
3. Monitor vital signs.
4. Establish an IV line in case fluid resuscitation is needed.

Catheter Shear

Catheter shear occurs when part of the catheter is pinched against the needle, and the needle slices through the catheter, creating a free-floating segment. The catheter segment can then travel through the circulatory system and possibly end up in the pulmonary circulation, causing a pulmonary embolus. Treatment involves surgical removal of the sheared tip. If you suspect a catheter shear, then place the patient in a left lateral recumbent position with the legs down and the head elevated to try to keep the catheter remnant out of the pulmonary circulation.

Catheter hubs are **radiopaque** (ie, they appear white on a radiograph) to aid in diagnosing this type of problem. Never rethread a catheter. Dispose of the used one and select a new catheter.

Patients who have experienced catheter shear with pulmonary artery occlusion present with sudden dyspnea, shortness of breath, and possibly diminished breath sounds. The symptoms mimic the presentation of an air embolus and can be treated the same way. Such patients need continued IV access, and you must try to obtain an IV site in the other extremity.

Obtaining Blood Samples

If blood samples are needed—usually at the request of the hospital for laboratory analysis—you should obtain them at the same time you start the IV line. If you have difficulty drawing blood, however, then stop and finish establishing the IV line. While some critical care transport settings may obtain arterial blood samples as well, the paramedic scope of practice is generally limited to obtaining venous blood samples.

To obtain blood samples when you are starting an IV line, you will need the following equipment:

- 15- or 20-mL syringe
- 18- or 20-gauge needle
- Self-sealing blood tubes

The blood-tube tops usually come in red, blue, green, and lavender, and should be filled in that order. Use the following mnemonic to help you remember the order for filling the tubes: Red Blood Gives Life. The *red*-topped tube contains clot activator in plastic tubes (not glass tubes) and is used for serum-based tests. The *blue*-topped tube contains citrate, a reversible anticoagulant; citrate binds calcium, which is required for blood clotting, and is used for coagulation assays such as prothrombin time, partial thromboplastin time, and international normalized ratio. The *green*-topped tube (plasma separator tube) contains heparin and is used for some plasma-based determinations. The *lavender*-topped tube contains the anticoagulant EDTA and is used for blood counts (eg, RBC, hematocrit, WBC, platelet counts).

After the IV catheter is in place, occlude the catheter and remove the constricting band. Attach a 15- or 20-mL syringe to the hub of the IV catheter and draw the necessary amount of blood. Do not pull back on the plunger of the syringe aggressively. Too much pressure can cause hemolysis, which will make the sample useless. *Do not leave the constricting band on while drawing blood with the syringe; doing so may cause waste products to build up in the blood and could skew laboratory test results.* Detach the syringe after the required amount of blood has been obtained, attach the IV tubing, and begin the infusion. Attach an 18- or 20-gauge needle to the syringe, fill the blood tubes with the necessary amount of blood, and immediately dispose of the syringe and needle in a puncture-proof sharps container. *Exercise extreme caution when you are filling blood tubes with this technique; you are handling a "live" needle!*

If IV therapy is not indicated but blood samples are required, then obtain them by using a cylindrical device that attaches to an 18- or 20-gauge sampling needle (a **Vacutainer**). The blood tubes are inserted into the Vacutainer after the needle it is attached to has entered the vein. To obtain blood using a Vacutainer, follow these steps:

1. Apply a constricting band, and locate a suitable vein—typically, the antecubital vein. Take standard precautions.
2. Prep the vein as you would when starting an IV line—use an alcohol prep or iodine swab, and cleanse the area in a circular motion, starting from the inside and working your way out.
3. Insert the needle (already attached to the Vacutainer) into the vein.
4. Remove the constricting band, and insert blood tubes into the Vacutainer to obtain the necessary amount of blood Figure 14-27.
5. Remove the needle from the vein, and apply direct pressure.
6. Dispose of the needle in a puncture-proof sharps container.
7. Label all the tubes with the patient's name, the date, the time, and your name with your credentials as soon as possible to avoid mixing tubes with those of another patient.

Once the blood tubes are filled, gently turn them back and forth several times to mix the anticoagulant and blood evenly. The exception is the red-topped tube, which is intended to separate the serum from the other blood components. Avoid shaking this tube after the blood has clotted, because the motion may destroy the sample.

For blood tubes to be viable for testing, they must be at least three fourths full. Follow local protocols for the types of blood tubes to fill.

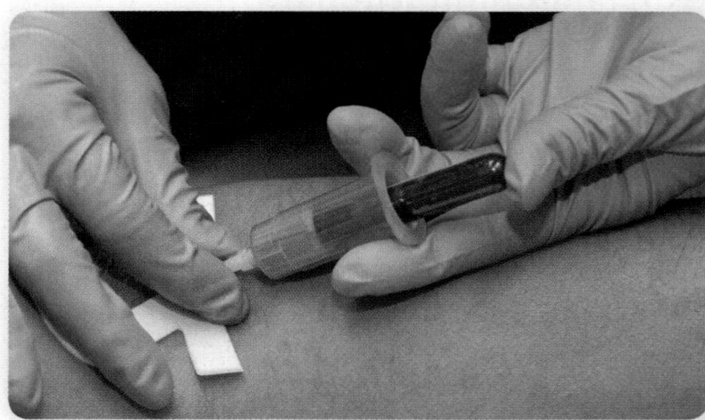

Figure 14-27 Obtaining blood samples with a Vacutainer.

Blood Transfusions

Some states allow paramedics to transport blood and blood products in the interfacility setting. This generally implies that blood infusion was initiated at a transferring facility prior to arrival and that EMS will continue the infusion. Preparation for transports involving blood transfusion can be time consuming because of the amount of data that must be gathered, checked, and rechecked prior to transport.

> **Patient Safety**
>
> Incorrect patient identification is a potentially serious problem in health care that can lead to a medication administration error. Practice recommendations to help avoid this error include always using multiple patient identifiers. Providers administering medications should always use two patient identifiers (ie, name and date of birth). This is particularly important for EMS crews picking up a patient for an interfacility transport. While the 9-1-1 EMS call for a single patient yields one obvious patient in most cases, it is entirely possible for a crew to pick up the wrong patient at a hospital or health care facility and transport him or her.

Blood type is identified by obtaining a type and crossmatch from the patient's bloodwork. After obtaining the patient's blood type, the facility will place a bracelet on the patient that will identify his or her blood type. Any time the bag of blood is changed or care is transferred, the blood being transfused or about to be transfused must be checked against the patient's bracelet and verified by two advanced life support (ALS) providers. This can be a paramedic and a nurse, or two paramedics, depending on local, regional, or state regulations. This verification includes:

- The patient's complete name
- The patient's medical record number
- The product that is being transfused
- The unit number of the product being transfused
- ABO and Rh type of the product
- The expiration date of the unit

In emergency medical settings, the patient's ABO blood type and Rh factor may not be known. In these cases, the hospital will have type O blood available for transfusion. If your crew is expected to switch out units during the transport, then verify the ABO type and Rh factor before leaving the transferring hospital even if you have two ALS providers on the transporting crew. This ensures you do not accidentally accept a unit that will not be usable. Any blood accepted must be used within 4 hours or returned to the blood bank.

Any time you accept a transport involving a blood transfusion, ensure the patient has at least one available vascular site that does not have blood running. If a transfusion reaction occurs, then any IV lines that have blood transfusing should be discontinued.

When blood is being transfused, it is administered through specific blood tubing that has a filter and then mixed with normal saline. Vital signs should be obtained prior to transport and compared with previous vital signs to identify trends of patient improvement or decline. Vital signs must be assessed every 5 minutes after any additional units of blood are exchanged. When new units are added, you should closely monitor the patient for signs of hemolytic reactions such as tachycardia, hives, airway compromise, wheezing, chest pain, or signs of impending doom. Transfusion reactions are discussed in Chapter 24, *Hematologic Emergencies*.

Intraosseous Infusion

Intraosseous means "within the bone." **Intraosseous infusion** is a technique of administering fluids, blood and blood products, and medications into the **intraosseous space** of the proximal tibia, humeral head, or sternum.

Long bones, such as the tibia, consist of a shaft (**diaphysis**), the ends (**epiphyses**), and the growth plate (**epiphyseal plate**) Figure 14-28.

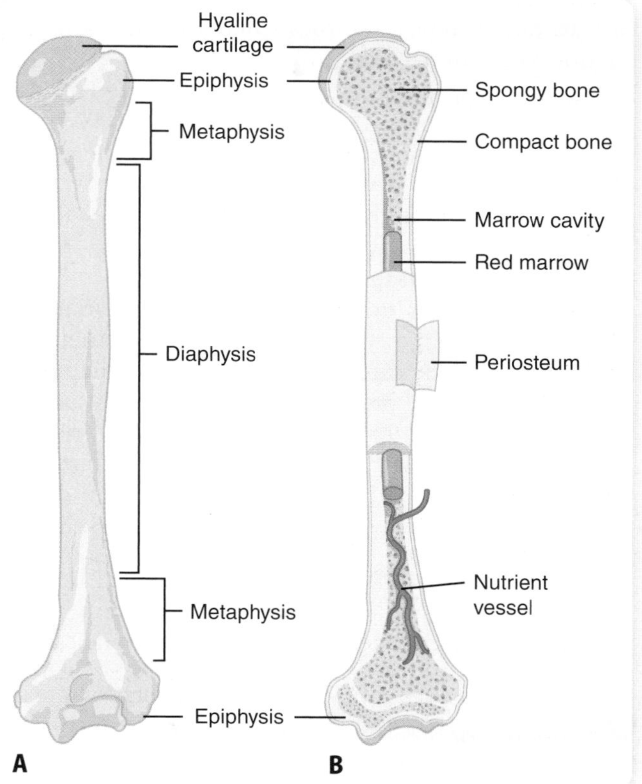

Figure 14-28 The components of a long bone.
A. The humerus. Note the long shaft and dilated ends.
B. Longitudinal section of the humerus showing compact bone, cancellous (spongy) bone, and marrow.

Table 14-3 Vascular Access Time and Flow Rate for Various IO Sites

IO Site	Reported Flow Rate (mL/min)
Sternal	469
Humeral	148.1–286
Proximal tibial	154–204.6

Abbreviation: IO, intraosseous

Data from: Pasley J, Miller CHT, DuBose JJ, et al. Intraosseous infusion rates under high pressure: a cadaveric comparison of anatomic sites. *J Trauma Acute Care Surg*. 2015;78(2):295-299; Ngo ASY, Oh JJ, Chen Y, et al. Intraosseous vascular access in adults using the EZ-IO in an emergency department. *Int J Emerg Med*. 2009;2(3):155-160; and Ong MEH, Chan YH, Oh JJ, Ngo AS-Y. An observational, prospective study comparing tibial and humeral intraosseous access using the EZ-IO. *Amer J Emerg Med.* 2009;27:8-15.

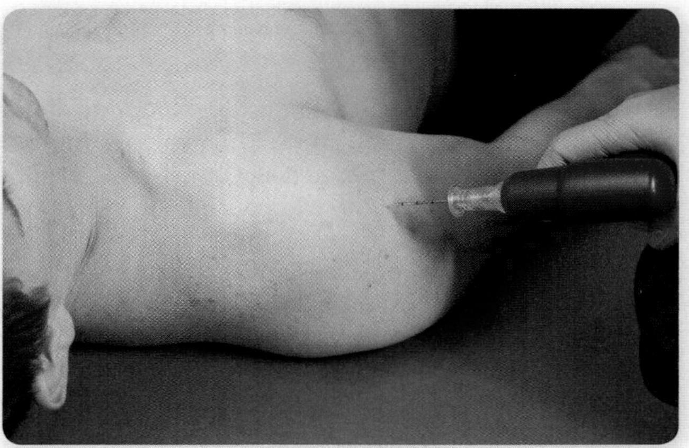

Figure 14-29 The humeral site for intraosseous insertion.

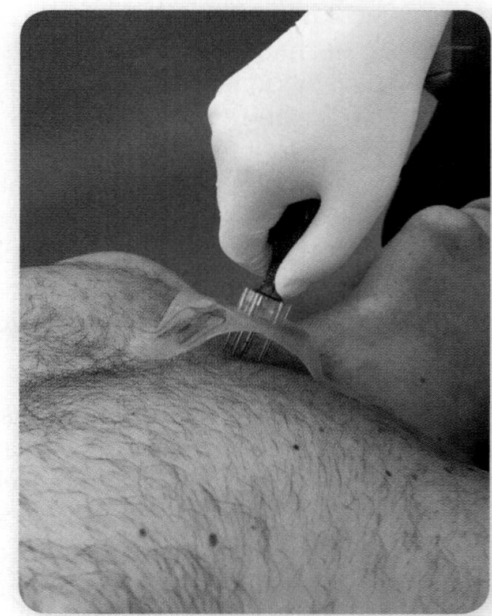

Figure 14-30 The sternal site for intraosseous insertion.

Courtesy of Stephen J. Rahm, NRP.

The **intraosseous (IO) space** collectively comprises the spongy cancellous bone of the epiphyses and the medullary cavity of the diaphysis. Its vasculature drains into the central circulation by a network of venous sinuses and canals.

When a patient is in shock, cardiac arrest, or an otherwise hemodynamically compromised condition, peripheral veins often collapse, making IV access extremely difficult, if not impossible. However, the IO space remains patent, unless the patient has sustained trauma to its bony structure (eg, a fracture). For this reason, the IO space is commonly referred to as a "noncollapsible vein." It quickly absorbs IV fluids and medications and rapidly gets them to the central circulation—as rapidly as is possible with the IV route. Anything that can be given via the IV route—crystalloids, medications, and blood and blood products—can be given via the IO route.

IO infusion is indicated when you are unable to obtain IV access in a critically ill or injured patient (eg, in profound shock, cardiac arrest, or status epilepticus). Depending on local protocol, you will typically attempt two IV lines within 90 seconds prior to an IO infusion attempt. Some situations, such as cardiac arrest, may warrant going immediately to an IO infusion due to the time savings, likelihood of success, and ease of use. Vascular access times and flow rates for various IO sites are presented in Table 14-3.

► IO Sites

Three common sites you will use for IO insertion are the sternum, humerus, and proximal tibia. The technique for performing IO infusion requires proper anatomic landmark identification.

To locate the humeral IO site, you will need to manipulate the patient's arm and palpate the humeral head Figure 14-29. Begin by placing the patient's hand over his or her abdomen, which causes an external rotation of the humeral head. Place the ulnar aspect of one of your hands vertically over the axilla near the humeral head that will be used for insertion. Place the ulnar aspect of your other hand laterally along the midline of the upper portion of the patient's humerus. Place your thumbs together, palpating up the surgical neck to the humeral head. When this site is used, medications can reach the right atrium within 3 seconds of rapid IV push. Appropriate needle selection and stabilization are crucial to use this site successfully.

Identify the sternal IO site by palpating the sternal notch and using the IO device's adhesive target Figure 14-30. The sternal site has an extremely rapid flow rate. The device location is near the chest compression landmarks; however, the device does not impede chest compressions.

The flat bone of the proximal tibia is located medial to the tibial tuberosity, the bony protuberance just below the knee. It is necessary to feel the leg to know

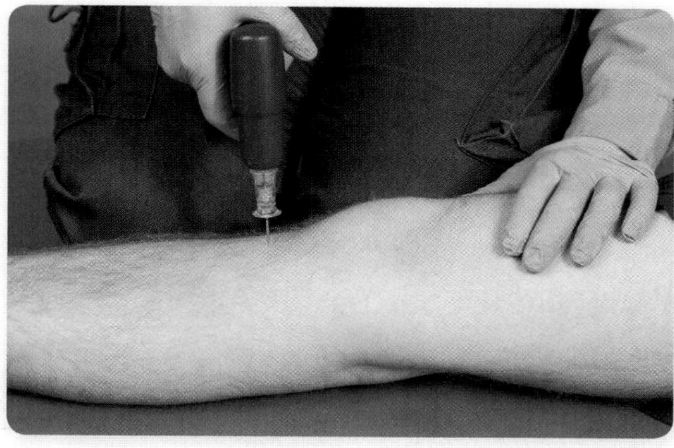

Figure 14-31 The proximal tibia site for intraosseous insertion in adults.

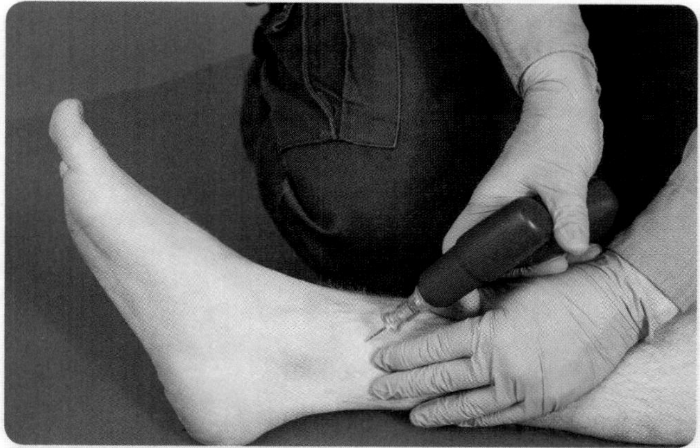

Figure 14-32 The distal tibia site for intraosseous insertion in adults.

the difference between the first and second landmarks (these cannot be seen; they must be felt). To locate the proximal tibia IO site, palpate the tibial tuberosity, then palpate 2 cm medially. This is the site for adult patients Figure 14-31. For pediatric patients, palpate 1 to 2 cm distally to avoid the epiphyseal plate.

For the distal tibia IO site, use palpation as well. First, identify the medial malleolus. Then palpate 2 to 3 cm above that site Figure 14-32. For pediatric patients, you should palpate 1 to 2 cm above the medial malleolus.

▶ Equipment for IO Infusion

Several products are used for placing an IO needle into the IO space: manually inserted IO needles, the FAST1, the EZ-IO, the Bone Injection Gun (BIG), and the New Intraosseous (NIO) device. Use of these devices requires specialized training and thorough familiarity with each device's features, functionality, and clinical application.

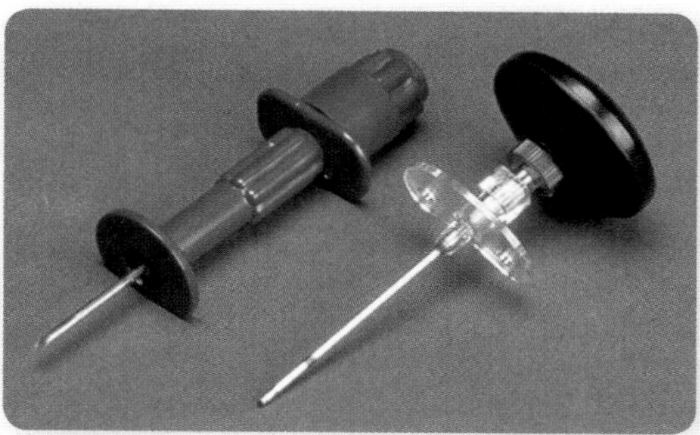

Figure 14-33 Manually inserted intraosseous needles.

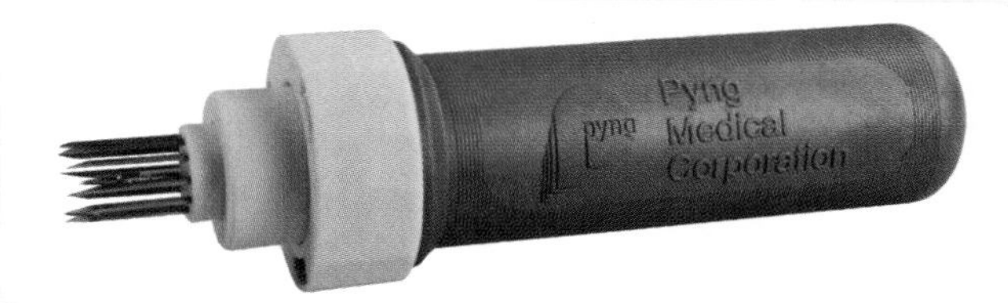

Figure 14-34 The FAST1 intraosseous insertion device.

If your EMS system uses any of these devices, then follow local protocols regarding their application.

Manually inserted IO needles (ie, Jamshedi needle, Cook catheter) were the original devices used for establishing IO access in children and are still widely used in the prehospital setting. They consist of a solid boring needle (**trocar**) inserted through a sharpened hollow needle Figure 14-33. The IO needle is pushed into the bone with a screwing, twisting action. Once the needle pops through the bone, the solid needle is removed, leaving the hollow steel needle in place. The IV tubing is attached to this catheter.

Because manually inserted IO needles are long, rest at a 90° angle to the bone, and are easily dislodged, they require full and careful immobilization. Stabilization is critical for these lines to maintain adequate flow. Stabilize the IO needle in the same manner that you would any impaled object.

FAST Devices

The **FAST devices** (First Access for Shock and Trauma) were the first IO devices approved for use in patients age 12 years and older. Four design elements allow for IO placement in the sternum using FAST devices: an infusion tube and subcutaneous portal, an introducer, a target/strain relief patch, and a protective dome Figure 14-34. FAST devices can be used during cardiac arrest. While chest compressions can coincide with FAST IO use, mechanical CPR devices must be paused during the insertion phase. Mechanical CPR can continue once the FAST device is stabilized.

The company that developed the FAST devices chose sternum placement based on the ease of locating the manubrium and because it is easier to penetrate than other bones. The landmarks can be felt on the vast majority of adults even in low-light situations. The target device is shaped so that it lines up with the sternal notch, minimizing the margin for error.

The FAST1 is the original sternal IO device. It consists of a 14-gauge infusion tube and 10 stabilization needles. It has been field tested in the military and used in civilian EMS for over a decade. The device is completely manual (no batteries required).

The FAST Responder (FASTR) is an updated device that has some advantages. Many of the components are already assembled, expediting the insertion process. For example, the adhesive target comes attached to the device. The device also has a safety lock that must be removed before insertion. The FASTR only requires 32 pounds (15 kg) of pressure for insertion. If sternal IOs are the preference for your EMS system, then familiarize yourself with both devices.

Both devices are designed to remain in place for a maximum of 24 hours. To remove either FAST device, firmly grasp the insertion tube and pull steadily until the device is dislodged. Use one continuous motion for removal; avoid starting and stopping.

EZ-IO Device

The **EZ-IO** features a handheld battery-powered driver, to which a special IO needle is attached Figure 14-35. This device is used to insert an IO needle into the proximal or distal tibia of adults and children and the humeral head in adults when IV access is difficult or impossible to obtain. The battery-powered driver of the EZ-IO is universal, but different sizes of needles are available depending on the patient. The needle size is estimated based on the insertion site and patient's weight; however, the ultimate determining factor in needle size selection is the amount of subcutaneous tissue present over the insertion site Table 14-4. When sizing the needle, you should ensure at least one hash mark (5 mm) can be seen after insertion.

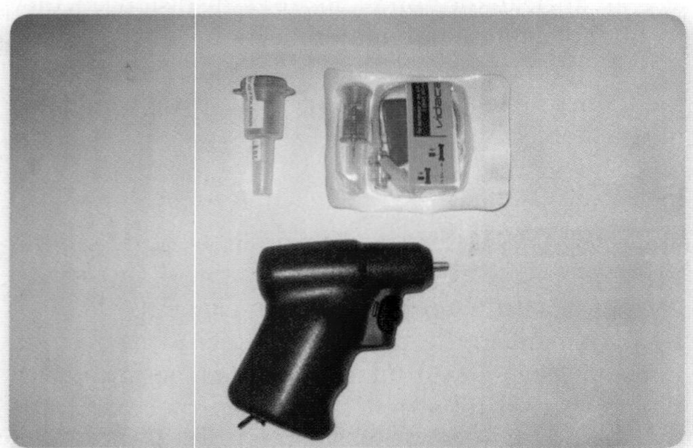

Figure 14-35 The EZ-IO insertion device features a handheld battery-powered driver, to which a special intraosseous needle is attached. The battery-powered driver of the EZ-IO is universal, but different sizes of needles are available.

Courtesy of VidaCare Corporation.

Use a 10-mL syringe to remove an EZ-IO. Attach the syringe to the IO's Luer lock, twist the syringe clockwise, and pull the device out in one swift motion.

Bone Injection Gun Device

The **Bone Injection Gun (BIG)** is a spring-loaded device that is used to insert an IO needle into the proximal tibia of adult and pediatric patients and the humeral head in adults Figure 14-36. It comes in an adult size and a pediatric size. Although both versions offer the same operational features, the depth of insertion is different for the adult and pediatric devices.

The BIG uses the safety lock as the stabilization device once the device has been inserted. When you are ready to remove the device, use the stabilization device as the removal tool. Place the wider side of the removal tool over the connection port. Pull the device out in one swift motion while grasping onto the removal tool.

New Intraosseous Device

The **New Intraosseous (NIO) device** is a device that is placed in the proximal tibia of an adult patient

Table 14-4 EZ-IO Needle Sizes and Determination Criteria

EZ-IO Needle[a]	EZ-IO Needle Size (mm)	Needle Determination Criteria[b]
	15	3–39 kg
	25	> 40 kg
	45	Excessive subcutaneous tissue and humeral IO insertion

[a]All needles are 15 gauge.

[b]Determination criteria may vary based on the amount of subcutaneous tissue present.

Abbreviation: IO, intraosseous

Data from: Arrow EZ-IO Intraosseous Vascular Access. EZ-IO Intraosseous Vascular Access Needles: Instructions for Use. 8082 Rev A. July 2014. http://www.teleflex.com/en/usa/ezioeducation/documents/8082_Rev_A_US_FDA_Intraosseous_Infusion_System_IFU.PDF. Accessed February 15, 2017.

Figure 14-37. The humeral head is an alternative site for this device. The spring-loaded device contains neither drill nor battery. It is inserted by unlocking a safety cap. Then, while applying downward pressure with the dominant hand, the fingers of the other hand are used to pull trigger wings up to deploy the device. The device is then pulled up in a rotating motion while the needle stabilizer is held against the skin. Once the introducing trocar is removed, any Luer-lock tubing can be attached.

A pediatric version, NIO Pediatric (NIO-P), is also available. This device has an adjustable dial, allowing the provider to adjust by age or depth (if excessive girth for the age is anticipated). At the time of this writing, the NIO-P is approved for placement in the proximal tibia only.

▶ Performing IO Infusion

Follow these steps to perform IO infusion using an EZ-IO device Skill Drill 14-3.

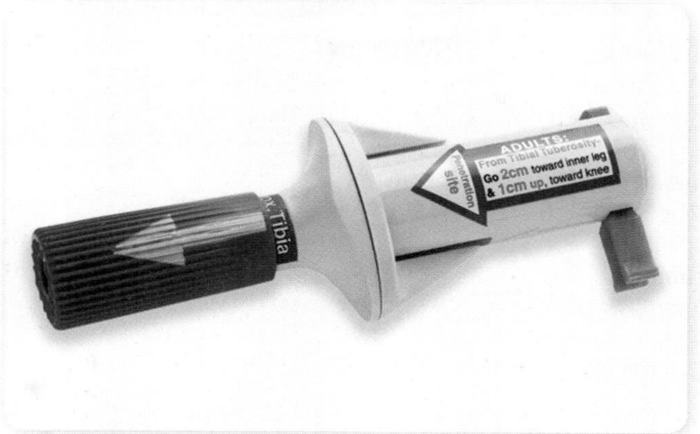

Figure 14-36 The Bone Injection Gun (BIG).

Courtesy of PerSys Medical.

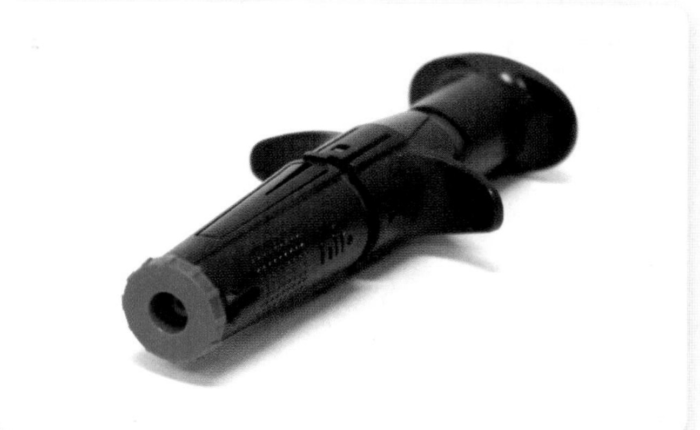

Figure 14-37 The New Intraosseous (NIO) device.

Courtesy of PerSys Medical.

Skill Drill 14-3 Gaining Intraosseous Access With an EZ-IO Device

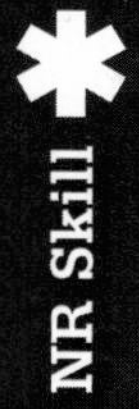

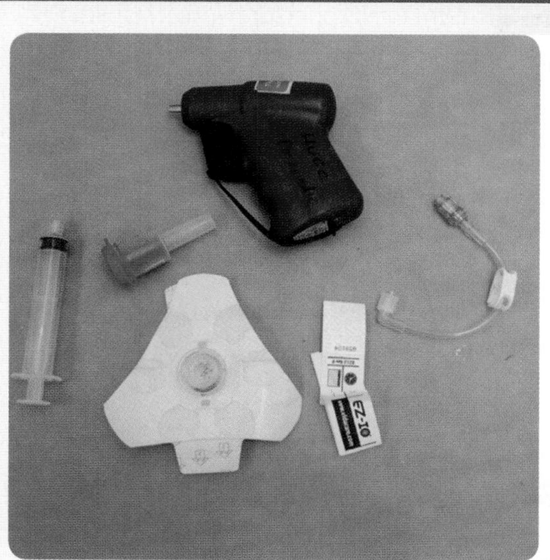

Step 1 Check the selected IV fluid for proper fluid, clarity, and expiration date. Look for discoloration and for particles floating in the fluid. If particles are found in the fluid, then discard the bag and choose another bag of fluid.

Select the appropriate equipment, including an IO needle, syringe, saline, extension set, antiseptic swabs, and gauze pads.

A three-way stopcock may also be used to facilitate easier fluid administration.

Select the proper administration set. Connect the administration set to the bag. Prepare the administration set. Fill the drip chamber and flush the tubing. Ensure all air bubbles are removed from the tubing.

Prepare the syringe and extension tubing. Ensure the tubing is not tangled.

Cut or tear the tape and prepare bulky dressings. This can be done at any time before IO puncture.

(continued)

Skill Drill 14-3 Gaining Intraosseous Access With an EZ-IO Device *(continued)*

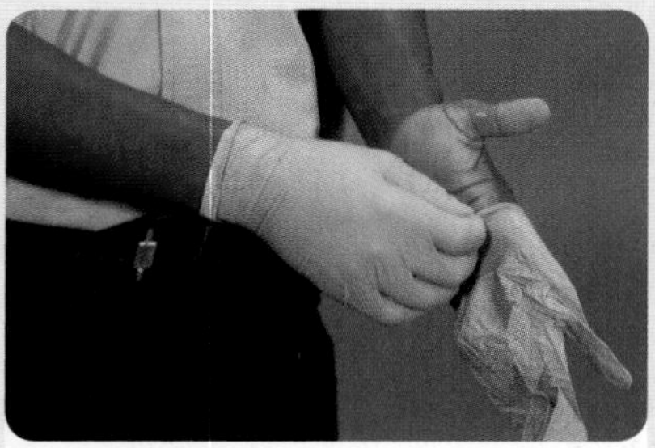

Step 2 Take standard precautions.

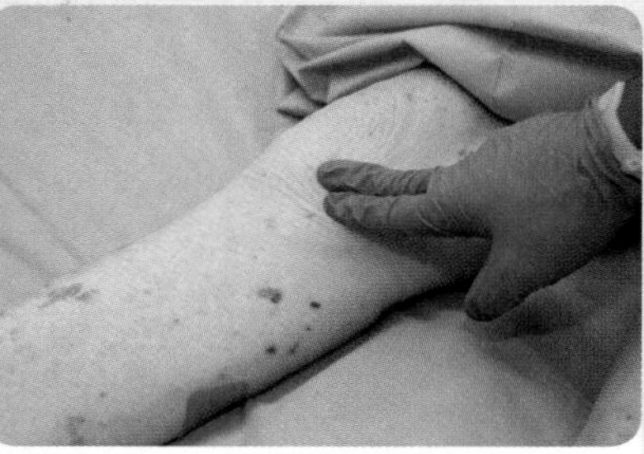

Step 3 Identify the proper anatomic site for IO puncture. Palpate the landmarks and then prepare the site.

- **Tibia placement.** This site is reserved for the EZ-IO and the BIG.
- **Humerus placement.** Humeral placement is typically reserved for adults when using the EZ-IO or the BIG.

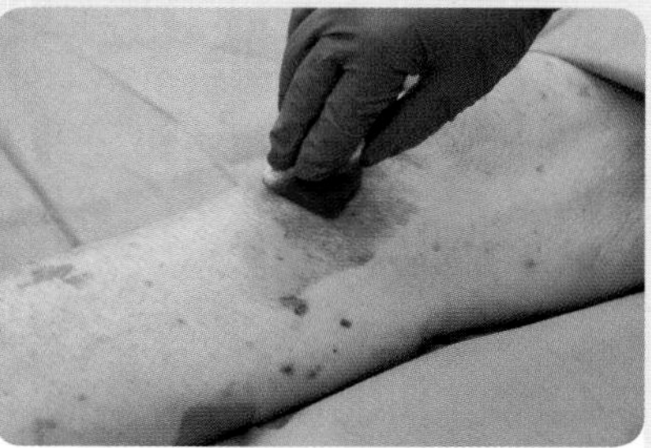

Step 4 Cleanse the site appropriately. Follow aseptic technique by cleansing in a circular manner from the inside out.

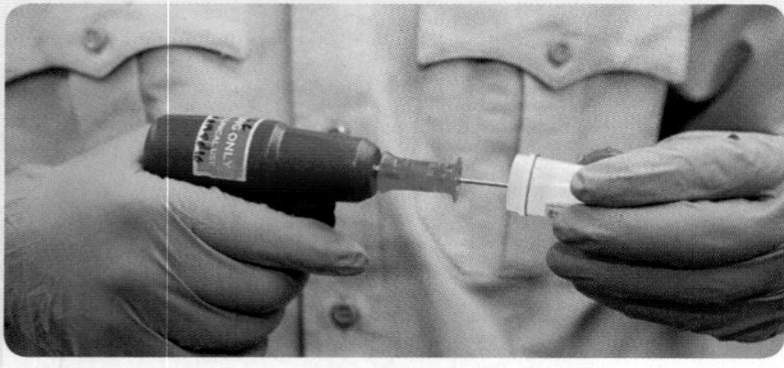

Step 5 Attach the needle to the EZ-IO gun and remove the protective cover. Examine the needle. If you find any imperfections, then discard the needle and select another one.

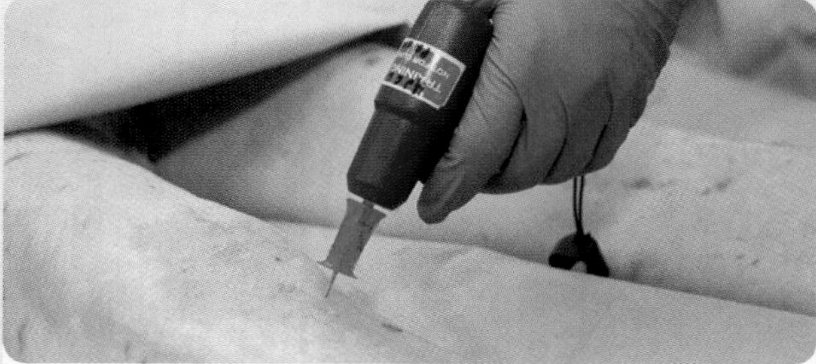

Step 6 Perform the IO puncture by first stabilizing the tibia, then placing a folded towel under the knee, and finally holding the extremity in a manner to keep your fingers away from the site of puncture. For humeral placement, continue to apply pressure on the anterior and inferior aspects of the humerus. Insert the needle at a 90° angle to the insertion site. Advance the needle with a twisting motion until a "pop" is felt. Unscrew the cap, and remove the stylet from the needle.

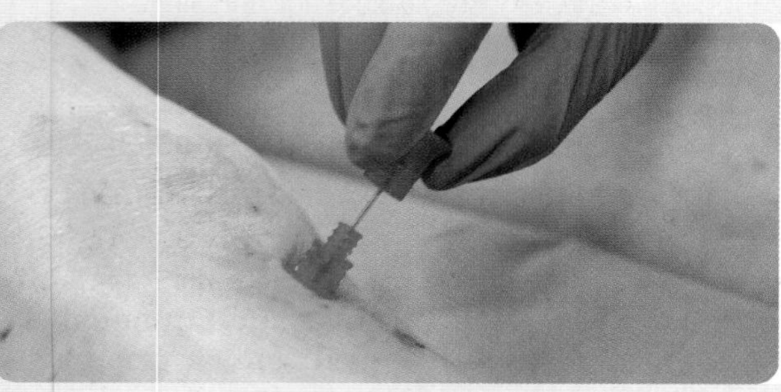

Step 7 Remove the stylet from the catheter.

Skill Drill 14-3 Gaining Intraosseous Access With an EZ-IO Device *(continued)*

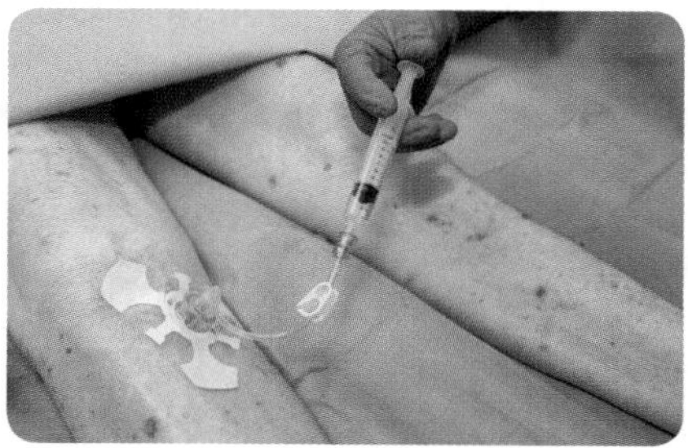

Step 8 Attach the syringe and extension set to the IO needle. Pull back on the syringe to aspirate blood and particles of bone marrow to ensure proper placement. The absence of marrow does not mean the access failed. Check the site for other signs of extravasation.

Slowly inject saline to ensure proper placement of the needle. Responsive patients should receive 1% lidocaine prior to infusion of fluids. Watch for extravasation, and stop the infusion immediately if it is noted. It is possible to fracture the bone during insertion of the IO needle. If this happens, then remove the IO needle and switch to the other insertion site.

Connect the administration set and adjust the flow rate as appropriate. Fluid does not flow as rapidly through an IO catheter as through an IV line; therefore, crystalloid boluses should be given with a syringe in children and a **pressure infuser device** (a sleeve placed around the IV bag and inflated to force fluid from the IV bag) in adults.

Secure the needle with tape, and support it with a bulky dressing. Stabilize in place in the same manner that an impaled object is stabilized. Use bulky dressings around the catheter, and tape securely in place. Be careful not to tape around the entire circumference of the leg because this could impair circulation and potentially result in compartment syndrome.

Dispose of the needle in the proper container.

To attach the FAST1 device, follow these steps:

1. Align the adhesive target on the patient and prepare to insert the device into the manubrium. The manubrium is approximately 15 mm below the sternal notch, and at 13.3 mm, it is the thickest part of the sternum. The stabilization needles prevent you from pushing the insertion tube to an inappropriate depth.
2. Prepare the insertion site on the patient's manubrium.
3. Position yourself behind the patient's head, place two hands on the FAST1 device, align the stabilization needles with the target, and apply approximately 45 pounds (20 kg) of pressure until you feel the infusion tube separate from the FAST1 introducer **Figure 14-38**.
4. Discard the stabilization needle in a sharps container and attach the IV tubing to the insertion tube's Luer-lock. Aspirate blood and particles of bone marrow to ensure proper placement. Slowly inject the IV solution to ensure proper placement of the needle. Adjust the flow rate as appropriate. Place the protective dome, and begin using the device.

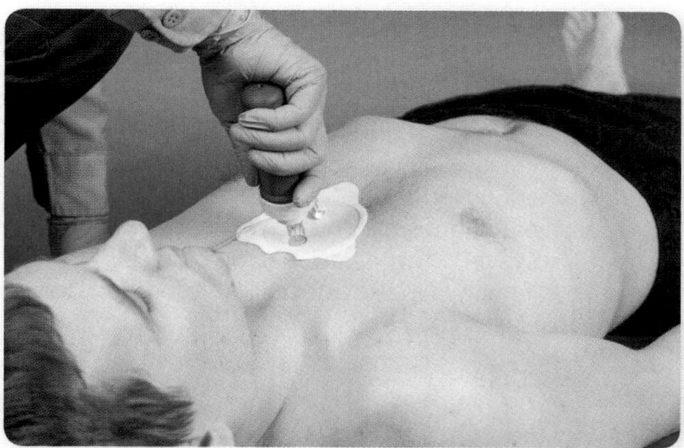

Figure 14-38 To use the FAST1 device, first align the adhesive target along the patient's sternal notch, and match the insertion site with the patient's manubrium. Position yourself behind the patient's head, place two hands on the FAST1 device, align the stabilization needles with the target, and apply pressure until you feel the infusion tube separate from the FAST1 introducer.

▶ Potential Complications of IO Infusion

If the proper technique is used (ie, proper anatomic landmark identification, aseptic technique), then IO infusion is associated with a relatively low complication rate. The same potential complications associated with IV therapy—thrombophlebitis, local irritation, allergic reaction, circulatory overload, and air embolism—can occur with IO infusion, as well as several others unique to this method of infusion.

Extravasation occurs when the IO needle does not rest in the IO space, but rather rests outside the bone (because the bone was missed completely or is fractured). In such a case, IV fluid will collect in the soft tissues. The risk of extravasation can be reduced significantly by using the proper insertion technique: *Insert the IO needle at a 90° angle to the bone*. Extravasation should be suspected if the infusion does not run freely or if the site—especially the posterior aspect of the leg—rapidly becomes edematous. If this occurs, then discontinue the infusion immediately and reattempt insertion in the opposite leg. Undetected extravasation could result in compartment syndrome.

Osteomyelitis is inflammation of the bone and muscle caused by an infection. Osteomyelitis can occur from IO insertion, but is rare.

Failure to identify the proper anatomic landmark can damage the growth plate, potentially resulting in long-term bone growth abnormalities in children.

If your insertion technique is too forceful, or if you use an IO needle that is too large for the patient's age or size, then fractures can occur. Through-and-through insertion occurs when the IO needle passes through *both* sides of the bone. To avoid this, stop inserting the needle when you feel a pop. If you feel a "pop, pop," then you have likely passed the needle through both sides of the bone. If either occurs, then remove the needle and attempt insertion on the opposite extremity.

> **Words of Wisdom**
>
> With the exception of the FAST1 sternal IO device, all IO devices—manual, spring-loaded, and battery-powered—are primarily used to insert an IO needle into the IO space of the proximal tibia, distal tibia, or humeral head. However, other anatomic locations, such as the distal femur, may also be acceptable locations for IO needle insertion.

A pulmonary embolism can occur if particles of bone, fat, or marrow enter into the systemic circulation and lodge in a pulmonary artery. You should suspect a pulmonary embolism if the patient experiences acute shortness of breath, pleuritic chest pain, and cyanosis.

> **Documentation & Communication**
>
> When you start an IV line for the purpose of administering a medication, you should set the flow rate just slow enough to keep the vein patent. This slow flow rate can be documented using the acronym KVO, which stands for Keep Vein Open, or TKO, which stands for To Keep Open.

Contraindications to IO Infusion

Cannulation of a peripheral vein remains the preferred route for administering IV fluids and medications. If a functional IV line is available—in a pediatric patient or an adult—IO cannulation is *not* indicated. Other contraindications to IO cannulation and infusion include fracture of the bone intended for IO cannulation, osteoporosis, **osteogenesis imperfecta** (a congenital disease resulting in fragile bones), bilateral knee replacements, and a prosthetic limb at the IO site.

Medication Administration

Before administering any medication to a patient, you must have a thorough understanding of how the medication will affect the human body—negatively and positively. This includes familiarity with the medication's mechanism of action, indications, contraindications, side effects, routes of administration, pediatric and adult doses, and antidotes (if available) for adverse reactions.

The first rule of medicine is *primum non nocere*, "The first thing (is) to do no harm." For example, administering the drug atropine to a patient with asymptomatic bradycardia could result in undesirable tachycardia and potential hemodynamic compromise. As a result, you have caused harm to the patient who otherwise did not need the drug. Therefore, it is paramount for you to ensure a particular drug is clearly indicated to treat the patient's condition.

You must also have an understanding of basic math for pharmacology to calculate the appropriate medication dose. This section begins with a review of basic mathematical principles as they apply to pharmacology and concludes with the various methods of medication administration.

Drug doses and flow rate calculations are often sources of confusion for many prehospital personnel, yet they are skills you will need to use frequently in the field and during your initial training while practicing at skill stations. As a paramedic, you must learn to quickly and accurately calculate medication doses to maximize the chance for a positive patient outcome. Disastrous results, including death, may be the outcome if you administer an inappropriate medication or dose, administer it by the incorrect route, or give the medication too rapidly or too slowly.

Mathematical Principles Used in Pharmacology

Mathematics Review

This section will discuss the use of fractions, percentages, and decimals. Having basic math skills is imperative for paramedics to appropriately administer medications.

Understanding fractions is important in formula calculation. Fractions represent a portion of a whole number expressed. Fractions are expressed as a numerator (the top number representing the portion available) over the denominator (representing the total quantity). For example, if you have four EMS units available and one of them is dispatched to an emergency, then one-fourth (1/4) of your units are occupied. Think of fractions as the numerator divided by the denominator. For example, 1/4 is the same as 1 ÷ 4.

Decimals distinguish numbers that are greater than zero from numbers that are smaller than zero. Whole numbers appear to the left side of the decimal point, and fractions of numbers on the right. Fractions can be easily converted to decimals by dividing the numerator by the denominator. For example, when you are administering atropine to bradycardic adult patients, you administer 1/2 of a milligram. By dividing 1 by 2, you get 0.5 (1 ÷ 2 = 0.5).

Dividing or multiplying by 10 is simple when you remember the following method. If you are dividing a number by 10, then simply move the decimal point to the left. If you are multiplying a number by 10, then simply move the decimal point to the right. In other words, if you are dividing the number 20 by 10, moving the decimal point one space to the left results in 2, which is the correct answer. The following examples show this method.

Multiplication problem: 20 × 10

Step 1: Place the decimal point:

20.0

Step 2: To multiply by 10, move the decimal point one space to the right:

200.0
→

The answer is 200.

Division problem: 20 ÷ 10

Step 1: Place the decimal point:

20.0

Step 2: To divide by 10, move the decimal point one space to the left:

2.00
←

The answer is 2.

Percentages are a part of 100 and are denoted by the % symbol. Percentages can be represented as a fraction with the denominator being 100; for example, 21% = 21/100. Decimals can also be turned into percentages easily by moving the decimal point over two places (0.21 is equal to 21%).

The Metric System

The **metric system** is a decimal system based on multiples of ten Figure 14-39. It is used to measure length, volume, and weight, which are represented as follows:

- Meter (m): The basic unit of length
- Liter (L): The basic unit of volume
- Gram (g): The basic unit of weight

In the metric system, prefixes demonstrate the fraction of the base being used. Commonly used prefixes, from smallest to largest, include the following:

- micro- = 0.000001
- milli- = 0.001
- centi- = 0.01
- kilo- = 1,000.0

Table 14-5 lists examples of units and abbreviations.

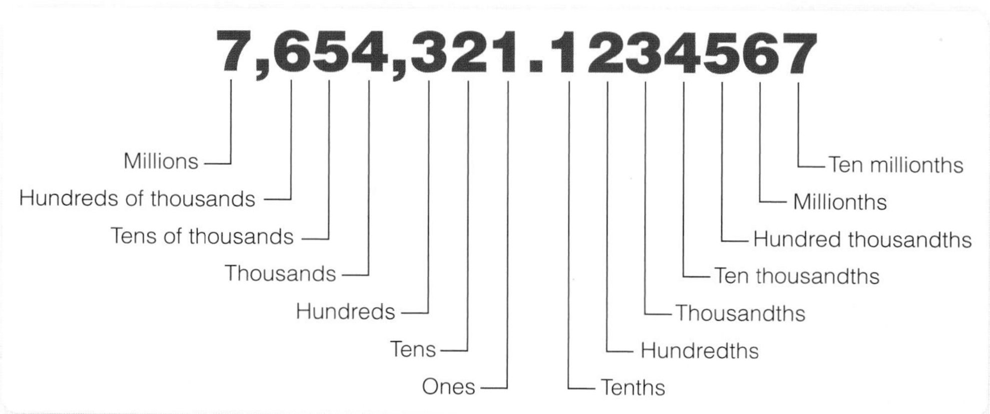

Figure 14-39 Decimal scale.

Table 14-5 Units of Measurement

Volume		Numeric Value	Concentration	
Abbreviation	**Unit**		**Abbreviation**	**Unit**
kL	Kiloliter	1,000	kg	Kilogram
L	Liter	1	g	Gram
mL	Milliliter	0.001	mg	Milligram
mcL	Microliter	0.000001	mcg	Microgram

Table 14-6 Symbols Used in the Metric System

Unit	Symbol
Weight (smallest to largest)	
Microgram	mcg
Milligram	mg
Gram	g (or gm)
Kilogram	kg
Volume (smallest to largest)	
Milliliter	mL
Deciliter	dL
Liter	L

Table 14-7 Metric Units

Unit	Equivalent
Weight (smallest to largest)	
1 mcg	0.001 mg
1 mg	1,000 mcg
1 g	1,000 mg
1 kg	1,000 g
Volume (smallest to largest)	
1 mL	1 cc*
100 mL	1 dL
1,000 mL	1 L

*Cubic centimeters (cc) is a unit also used to represent milliliters (mL); therefore, 1 cc is the same as 1 mL (1 cc = 1 mL).

Words of Wisdom

A cubic centimeter (cc) is equal to a milliliter (mL), and these units may be used interchangeably.

Medications are supplied in a variety of weights and volumes, and you will be required to convert those weights to volume to administer the appropriate dose of a medication to your patient. Table 14-6 lists the symbols of weight and volume, with their respective abbreviations, that are used in the metric system. Table 14-7 lists the metric units of weight and volume.

To administer the appropriate dose of a medication to a patient, you must be able to convert larger units of weight to smaller ones (for example, g to mg) and larger units of volume to smaller ones (for example, L to mL). Conversely, you must be able to convert smaller units of weight to larger ones (for example, mg to g) and smaller units of volume to larger ones (for example, mL to L).

Drugs are packaged in different units of weight and volume. However, the weight (for example, mcg, mg, g) and volume (for example, mL) of the drug to be administered usually comprise only a fraction of the total amount of its packaged form. For example, a physician may order 50 mg of a drug for a patient, but the drug is packaged in grams. Therefore, you must be able to convert grams to milligrams and then determine how much volume is required to achieve the desired dose. (**Desired dose** refers to the amount of a drug that the physician orders, or protocol dictates, you to give to a patient).

Volume Conversion. In the prehospital setting, you will usually be dealing with only two measurements of volume: milliliters and liters. Because 1 L equals 1,000 mL, simply divide or multiply by 1,000 or move the decimal point three places to the left or right.

When you are converting mL to L, divide the smaller unit of volume by 1,000 *or* simply move the decimal point three places to the left, as demonstrated in the following example:

Example 1:
Converting 500 mL of normal saline to L
(500 mL = *x* L)

500 mL ÷ 1,000 = 0.5 L *or* 500. = 0.5 L normal saline
←

Conversely, when you are converting L to mL, multiply L by 1,000 *or* simply move the decimal point three places to the right, as demonstrated in the following example:

Example 1:
Converting 1.5 L of lactated Ringer solution to mL
(1.5 L = *x* mL)

1.5 L × 1,000 = 1,500 mL *or* 1.500 = 1,500 mL
→

Example 2:
Converting 25 L of lactated Ringer solution to mL
(25 L = *x* mL)

25 L × 1,000 = 25,000 mL *or* 25.000 = 25,000 mL
→

Words of Wisdom

Carry a calculator, EMS field guide, pocket infusion charts, or use a smartphone app to assist you in converting pounds to kilograms or when calculating a drug dosage.

YOU are the Paramedic PART 2

You have completed a secondary assessment and obtained vital signs. The patient denies any chronic medical conditions and says he has never experienced anything like this before. He takes no medications and has no known drug allergies. The cardiac monitor has been applied, and you note that the patient is currently in atrial fibrillation with a rapid ventricular response. You contact medical control and provide a brief report. The physician asks you to administer diltiazem 0.25 mg/kg IV push over 2 minutes; he would like a target heart rate of less than 110 beats/min. The patient weighs 231 pounds (105 kg). Your diltiazem comes prepackaged in a syringe with 30 mg/5 mL.

Recording Time: 5 Minutes	
Respirations	20 breaths/min
Pulse	180 beats/min, irregular
Skin	Warm and dry
Blood pressure	134/90 mm Hg
Oxygen saturation (Spo_2)	99%
Pupils	PERRLA
ECG	Atrial fibrillation with a rapid ventricular response

3. What information must you and your partner be sure to communicate to one another as you are preparing to administer this medication?
4. Why is it prudent to contact medical control in this scenario to discuss management options?
5. What dose will you administer to the patient? Given the supplied medication, what volume will you administer?

Weight Conversion

Converting weight is simply a matter of multiplying or dividing by 1,000 *or* moving the decimal point three places to the right or left.

To convert a larger unit of weight to a smaller one, *multiply* the larger unit of weight by 1,000 *or* move the decimal point three places to the *right*, as demonstrated in the following examples:

Example 1:
Converting 25 g of dextrose to mg (25 g = *x* mg)

25 g × 1,000 = 25,000 mg *or* 25.000 = 25,000 mg (→)

Example 2:
Converting 0.15 mg of fentanyl to **mcg** (0.15 mg = *x* **mcg**)

0.15 mg × 1,000 = 150 mcg *or* 0.150 = 150 mcg (→)

Conversely, to convert a smaller unit of weight to a larger unit when the difference is 1,000 (such as mg to g or mcg to mg), divide the mg by 1,000 *or* simply move the decimal point three places to the left, as demonstrated in the following examples. Remember, 1 g equals 1,000 mg and 1 mg equals 1,000 mcg.

Example 1:
Converting 200 mcg of fentanyl to mg (200 mcg = *x* mg)

200 mcg ÷ 1,000 = 0.2 mg *or* 200. = 0.2 mg (←)

Example 2:
Converting 250 mg of dextrose to g (250 mg = *x* g)

250 mg ÷ 1,000 = 0.25 g *or* 250. = 0.25 g (←)

Converting Pounds to Kilograms

Most likely your patients will not be able to tell you how much they weigh in kilograms (kg). However, if your patient is able to tell you his or her weight in pounds, you can easily convert that number to kilograms. This information will frequently be available during interfacility transports. For patients who do not know their weight in pounds or who are unresponsive and unable to provide you with this information, you must perform the following steps:

1. Estimate the patient's weight in pounds (lb).
2. Convert pounds to kilograms (kg).

Although many of the drugs given in emergency medicine are administered in a standard dose (eg, 1 mg of epinephrine), others are administered based on the patient's weight in kilograms (eg, 1 to 1.5 mg/kg of lidocaine). In addition, most drugs administered to pediatric patients are based on their weight in kilograms.

Two formulas can be used to convert pounds to kilograms. Use whichever one is easiest for you to remember.

For example, when converting a 170-pound man's weight to kilograms, the formula would be as follows:

Formula 1:
Divide the patient's weight in pounds by 2.2 (1 kg = 2.2 lb)

170 lb ÷ 2.2 = 77.27 kg
250 lb ÷ 2.2 = 113.64 kg
479.6 lb ÷ 2.2 = 218 kg
6.6 lb ÷ 2.2 = 3 kg
30 lb ÷ 2.2 = 14.09 kg
68 lb ÷ 2.2 = 30.91 kg

Because the value following the decimal point in this example is less than 0.5, you may round the patient's weight in kilograms to 77. If the value after the decimal point in the first example had been greater than 0.5, then you would round up the weight in kilograms to 78. Although this may seem negligible, it is good practice to administer the *most* appropriate amount of the drug to the patient.

Formula 2:
Divide the patient's weight in pounds by 2 and subtract 10% of that number

For example, when converting a 120-pound woman's weight to kilograms, the formula would be as follows:

Example 1:
Converting a 120-pound woman's weight to kilograms

Step 1: 120 lb ÷ 2 = 60
Step 2: 60 lb × 10% = 6
Step 3: 60 − 6 = 54 kg

NOTE: This formula provides an approximate weight and is not exact.

Words of Wisdom

A teaspoon is approximately 5 mL, and a tablespoon is approximately 15 mL. A cup is approximately 240 mL. Drops vary based on the diameter of the dropper. These measurements may be useful to remember if you need to calculate exact amounts of a patient's medication.

Temperature Conversion

The Fahrenheit and Celsius (or centigrade) temperature scales are commonly used to measure temperature. On the **Celsius scale**, water freezes at 0° and boils at 100°. On the **Fahrenheit scale**, water freezes at 32° and boils at 212°. Normal body temperature is 98.6° Fahrenheit (37° Celsius). Values on each of these scales can easily be interconverted by using the following equations:

- To convert Fahrenheit to Celsius: Subtract 32, then multiply by 0.555 (5/9)

Fahrenheit → Celsius
98.6°F − 32 × 0.555 = 36.9 (37°C)

- To convert Celsius to Fahrenheit: Multiply by 1.8 (9/5), then add 32

Celsius → Fahrenheit
37°C × 1.8 + 32 = 98.6°F

Examples:

Fahrenheit → Celsius
104.2°F − 32 × 0.555 = 40.1°C
100.9°F − 32 × 0.555 = 38.2°C
92.4°F − 32 × 0.555 = 33.5°C

Celsius → Fahrenheit
37.9°C × 1.8 + 32 = 100.2°F
38.6°C × 1.8 + 32 = 101.4°F
32.2°C × 1.8 + 32 = 90°F

► Calculating Medication Doses

There are multiple formulas for calculating medication doses. This chapter focuses on those formulas that most students find easy to understand. For other calculation formulas, you should consult with your instructor. The method of drug dose calculation demonstrated in this chapter is based on the following three factors:

- Desired dose
- Concentration of the drug available (dose on hand)
- Volume to be administered

Desired Dose

The desired dose (ie, the drug order) is the amount of a drug that the physician orders, or protocol dictates, you to give to a patient. It may be expressed as a standard dose (eg, 5 mg of diazepam [Valium], 25 g of 50% dextrose) or as a specific number of micrograms, milligrams, or grams per kilogram of body weight (eg, 1 to 1.5 mg/kg of lidocaine [Xylocaine]).

Drug Concentrations

After you have received a drug order (desired dose), you must determine how much of the drug you have available. In other words, you must know its concentration—the total weight (mcg, mg, or g) of the drug contained in a specific amount of volume (mL or L). Sometimes this information is printed on the label of the drug container (eg, Drug X at a concentration of 5 mg/mL); other containers may list the total weight and total volume of the drug separately (eg, 8 mg of morphine sulfate in 2 mL). The following are examples of common prepackaged drug concentrations:

- Lidocaine, 100 mg/10 mL
- Epinephrine, 1 mg/10 mL (1:10,000)
- Furosemide, 40 mg/4 mL
- Adenosine, 6 mg/2 mL
- 50% dextrose, 25 g/50 mL
- Fentanyl, 100 mcg/1 mL
- Naloxone, 2 mg/2 mL

In the preceding examples, notice that the drugs are contained in different volumes of solution. This is your **volume on hand**. *To administer a drug, you must know the weight of the drug that is present in* ***1 mL***. This information will tell you the concentration of the drug that you have on hand. The formula for calculating this is as follows:

Total Weight of the Drug ÷ Total Volume in Milliliters = Weight per Milliliter

By using this formula, you can easily calculate how much of the drug is contained in each milliliter.

Example:
Amiodarone, 150 mg/3 mL

150 mg (total weight) ÷ 3 mL (total volume) = 50 mg/mL

Ondansetron, 4 mg/2 mL

4 mg ÷ 2 mL = 2 mg/mL

Epinephrine, 1 mg/10 mL

1 mg ÷ 10 mL = 0.1 mg/mL

Thiamine, 100 mg/2 mL

100 mg ÷ 2 mL = 50 mg/mL

Things become slightly more complex when the label of the drug lists the drug concentration as a percentage—for example, "1% lidocaine (Xylocaine)." What *percentage* means in terms of drug concentration is the number of *grams present in 100 mL*. Thus, 1% lidocaine (Xylocaine) contains 1 g of drug in every 100 mL (1 dL). By dividing the numerator and denominator by 100, you will arrive at a concentration of 10 mg/mL:

$$\frac{1\text{ g}}{100\text{ mL}} = \frac{1{,}000\text{ mg}}{100\text{ mL}} = 10\text{ mg/mL}$$

Documentation & Communication

To prevent errors when you are documenting decimals, write 0.2 mg or 2 mg instead of .2 mg or 2.0 mg, which could easily be mistaken for 2 mg or 20 mg, respectively.

Volume to Be Administered

After you have determined the concentration of the drug present in each milliliter, you must calculate how much volume is needed to give the amount of the drug ordered (desired dose). Use the following formula to calculate the volume to be administered:

Desired dose (mg) ÷ concentration of drug on hand (mg/mL) = volume to be administered

Example 1:
According to your protocols, you should administer 5 mg of midazolam (Versed) for your patient who is having a seizure. You have a vial of midazolam, which contains 10 mg in 5 mL. How many milliliters of midazolam must you give to achieve the ordered dose of 5 mg?

Step 1: Determine the concentration (in mg/mL).

10 mg ÷ 5 mL = 2 mg/mL (concentration)

Step 2: Determine how much volume to administer.

5 mg (desired dose) ÷ 2 mg/mL (concentration) = 2.5 mL

Example 2:
Your protocols dictate that you administer 12.5 g of dextrose to a hypoglycemic patient. You have a prefilled syringe of 50% dextrose containing 25 g in 50 mL. How many milliliters of dextrose will you give?

Step 1: Determine the concentration (in g/mL).

25 g ÷ 50 mL = 0.5 g/mL (concentration)

Step 2: Determine how much volume to administer.

12.5 g (desired dose) ÷ 0.5 g/mL (concentration) = 25 mL

Example 3:
You are treating a patient who has nausea and feels like she is going to vomit. Your protocol says you can administer 4 mg of ondansetron (Zofran). Ondansetron is packaged in a vial of 4 mg in 2 mL.

Step 1: Determine the concentration (in g/mL).

4 mg ÷ 2 mL = 2 mg/mL (concentration)

Step 2: Determine how much volume to administer.

4 mg (desired dose) ÷ 2 mg/mL (concentration) = 2 mL

Example 4:
During a cardiac arrest your protocols allow you to administer 300 mg of amiodarone (Cordarone) as an antidysrhythmic after epinephrine or vasopressin when ventricular fibrillation or ventricular tachycardia is present. Amiodarone is packaged as 150 mg in 3 mL.

Step 1: Determine the concentration (in g/mL).

150 mg ÷ 3 mL = 50 mg/mL (concentration)

Step 2: Determine how much volume to administer.

300 mg (desired dose) ÷ 50 mg/mL (concentration) = 6 mL

▶ Weight-Based Drug Doses

As mentioned earlier, some medication doses are based on the patient's weight in kilograms. Determining the appropriate dose for the patient requires simply adding one step to the formula that was previously discussed—conversion of the patient's weight in pounds to kilograms. Remember, 1 kg = 2.2 pounds.

Example 1:
A 7-year-old girl requires 0.02 mg/kg of atropine to treat symptomatic bradycardia. You have a prefilled syringe of atropine containing 1 mg in 10 mL. The child's mother tells you the child weighs 60 pounds. How many milligrams will you give to this child (that is, what is the desired dose)? How much volume will you give to achieve the required dose?

Step 1: Convert the child's weight in pounds to kilograms.

Formula 1: 60 lb ÷ 2.2 = 27.2 kg (round to 27 kg)

Formula 2: 60 lb ÷ 2 − 10% = 27 kg

Step 2: Determine the desired dose.

$$0.02 \text{ mg/kg} \times 27 \text{ kg} = 0.54 \text{ mg}$$
(round to 0.5 mg [desired dose])

Step 3: Determine the concentration.

$$1 \text{ mg} \div 10 \text{ mL} = 0.1 \text{ mg/mL (concentration)}$$

Step 4: Determine how much volume to administer.

$$0.5 \text{ mg (desired dose)} \div 0.1 \text{ mg/mL (concentration)} = 5 \text{ mL}$$

Example 2:
You are managing a patient with excited delirium. Your protocol suggests you can administer 1 to 2 mg IV or 3 to 4 mg/kg IM of ketamine. The patient weighs 110 pounds and you are unable to get vascular access. The ketamine is packaged in a vial of 500 mg in 10 mL.

Step 1: Convert the patient's weight in pounds to kilograms.

Formula 1: $110 \text{ lb} \div 2.2 = 50 \text{ kg}$

Step 2: Determine the desired dose.

$$3 \text{ mg/kg} \times 50 \text{ kg} = 150 \text{ mg}$$

Step 3: Determine the concentration.

$$500 \text{ mg} \div 10 \text{ mL} = 50 \text{ mg/mL (concentration)}$$

Step 4: Determine how much volume to administer.

$$150 \text{ mg (desired dose)} \div 50 \text{ mg/mL (concentration)} = 3 \text{ mL}$$

Calculating Fluid Infusion Rates

Once the IV or IO catheter is in place, you need to adjust the flow rate according to the patient's clinical condition or as dictated by medical control. To do so, you must know the following information:

- The volume to be infused
- The period over which it is to be infused
- The properties of the administration set you are using—that is, how many drops per milliliter (gtt/mL) it delivers

By knowing in advance the volume to be infused, the period over which it will be infused, and the properties of the administration set, you can calculate the flow rate.

For example, suppose the physician orders an infusion of 1 L (1,000 mL) of normal saline to be infused in 4 hours, and the macrodrip administration set provides 10 gtt/mL:

$$\frac{\text{Volume to be infused} \times \text{gtt/mL of administration set}}{\text{total time of inusion } \textit{in minutes}} = \text{gtt/min}$$

Information:

Total volume to be infused	=	1,000 mL
gtt/mL of the administration set	=	10
Time of infusion (in minutes)	=	4 h × 60 min/h = 240 min

Calculation:

$$\frac{1{,}000 \text{ mL} \times 10 \text{ gtt/mL}}{240 \text{ minutes}} = \text{approximately } 42 \text{ gtt/min}$$

Words of Wisdom

If the physician orders a specific number of milliliters to be administered per hour (mL/h), then a quick and easy way to calculate the number of drops per minute (gtt/min) with a 60-gtt set is to divide the number of milliliters per hour:

- By 6, if using a macrodrip that provides 10 gtt/mL
- By 4, if using a macrodrip that provides 15 gtt/mL
- By 1, if using a microdrip set that provides 60 gtt/mL

Calculating the Dose and Rate for a Medication Infusion

Non–Weight-Based Medication Infusions

Following the administration of certain drugs, you may need to begin a continuous infusion to maintain a therapeutic blood level of the drug to prevent a recurrence of the condition. Medication infusions are usually ordered to be administered over a specified period, usually per minute.

To calculate a continuous medication infusion that is not weight-based, you must know the following information in advance:

- The desired dose (mcg/min or mg/min)
- The properties of the administration set you are using (eg, microdrip [60 gtt/mL])

Will you be using an infusion pump? (Mechanical infusion pumps are discussed later in this chapter.)

You will use the same formula to calculate a drug dose as previously discussed. Then, however, you will calculate the desired dose to be administered continuously—usually a certain number of micrograms (mcg) or milligrams (mg) per minute.

For example, suppose you have just administered 75 mg of lidocaine to your patient in cardiac arrest, after which time the cardiac rhythm converts to a perfusing rhythm. Medical control then orders you to begin a continuous lidocaine infusion at 2 mg/min. You must determine at how many drops per minute (gtt/min) to set the IV drip rate to deliver the 2 mg/min desired dose. To do so, you will add a certain amount of lidocaine into a bag of IV fluid. In this example, 2 g (2,000 mg) of lidocaine will be added to a 500-mL bag of normal saline, a common combination. The formula to calculate the continuous infusion rate is as follows:

Step 1: Determine the concentration.

2 g (2,000 mg) of lidocaine ÷ 500 mL of normal saline = 4 mg/mL (concentration)

Step 2: Determine the amount of volume to infuse per minute (mL/min).

For this calculation, you must recall the desired dose—in this case, 2 mg/min.

To determine the number of mL/min, you perform the following calculation:

$$\frac{2\text{ mg(desired dose)}}{\text{min}} \times \frac{1\text{ mL}}{4\text{ mg}} = \begin{matrix}0.5\text{ mL/min}\\ \text{(concentration)}\end{matrix}$$

Step 3: Determine how many drops per minute (gtt/min) at which to set the IV flow rate.

For this calculation, you must know the number of drops per milliliter (gtt/mL) that your IV administration set delivers—a microdrip (60 gtt/mL) or a macrodrip (10 or 15 gtt/mL). For a microdrip administration set (typically used when administering a continuous medication infusion), the number of drops per minute for the IV flow rate would be calculated as follows:

0.5 mL/min × 60 gtt/mL = 30 gtt/min

▶ Weight-Based Medication Infusions

Some continuous medication infusions are based on the patient's weight in kilograms. Dopamine (Intropin), for example, is typically administered in a range of 5 to 20 mcg/kg/min. By using the previously discussed formula and factoring in the patient's weight in kilograms to determine the desired dose, you will calculate the IV drip rate for a 70-kg patient who requires a continuous dopamine infusion at 5 mcg/kg/min. In this example, 800 mg of dopamine will be added to a 500-mL bag of normal saline, a common combination.

Example 1:

Step 1: Determine the desired dose.

5 mcg/kg/min × 70 kg = 350 mcg/min (desired dose)

Step 2: Determine the concentration.

800 mg (800,000 mcg) of dopamine ÷ 500 mL of normal saline = 1.6 mg/mL (concentration)

The caveat here is that dopamine is administered in *micrograms*, not milligrams. Therefore, you must convert the 1.6 mg/mL concentration to mcg/mL. Recall, to convert a larger unit of weight to a smaller one, you must multiply by 1,000 *or* move the decimal point three places to the *right;* in other words, 1.6 mg is equal to *1,600 mcg*.

Step 3: Determine the amount of volume to infuse per minute (mL/min).

Again, you must recall the desired dose—in this case, 350 mcg/min. To determine the number of mL/min, the calculation continues as follows:

350 mcg/min (desired dose) ÷ 1,600 mcg/mL (concentration) = 0.22 mL/min

Step 4: Determine how many drops per minute (gtt/min) at which to set the IV flow rate.

Again, you must know the properties of the administration set you are using. In this example, you will use the microdrip (60 gtt/mL). The number of drops per minute for the IV flow rate would be calculated as follows:

$$\frac{0.22\text{ mL}}{\text{min}} \times \frac{60\text{ gtt}}{\text{mL}} = \begin{matrix}13.2\text{ gtt/min}\\ \text{(round to 13 gtt/min)}\end{matrix}$$

Dobutamine (Dobutrex) is usually transferred with an IV pump so calculating gtt is rarely needed for this medication. However, paramedics will see this medication in use during interfacility transports, so the following calculation uses dobutamine as an example.

Example 2:
Dobutamine is a common interfacility medication for cardiogenic shock. The dose is generally 2 to 20 mcg/kg/min. For this example, you are transferring a 60-kg patient who is on a drip of 10 mcg/kg/min. The dobutamine is packaged as 250 mg in a 500-mL bag.

Step 1: Calculate the desired dose.

$$10 \text{ mcg/kg/min} \times 60 \text{ kg} = 600 \text{ mcg/min}$$
(desired dose)

Step 2: Calculate the concentration. The first step in calculating the concentration is to convert the units from mg to mcg.

$$250 \text{ mg} \times \frac{1{,}000 \text{ mcg}}{\text{mg}} = 250{,}000 \text{ mcg}$$

$$250{,}000 \text{ mcg} \div 500 \text{ mL} = 500 \text{ mcg/mL}$$
(concentration)

Step 3: Calculate the amount of volume to infuse per minute (mL/min).

$$600 \text{ mcg/min (desired dose)} \div 500 \text{ mcg/mL (concentration)} = 1.2 \text{ mL/min}$$

Step 4: Calculate how many drops per minute (gtt/min) at which to set the IV flow rate.

$$1.2 \text{ mL/min} \times 60 \text{ gtt/mL} = 72 \text{ gtt/min}$$

Pediatric Drug Doses

There are numerous methods for determining the appropriate dose of medication for a pediatric patient. Many paramedics use length-based resuscitation tape measures or pediatric wheel charts Figure 14-40; others carry an EMS field guide with tables or charts specific to pediatric patients. Most drugs used in pediatric emergency medicine are based on the child's weight in kilograms. With the exception of the obviously smaller doses and volumes, the calculations for pediatric drug dosing and medication infusions are the same as they are for adults.

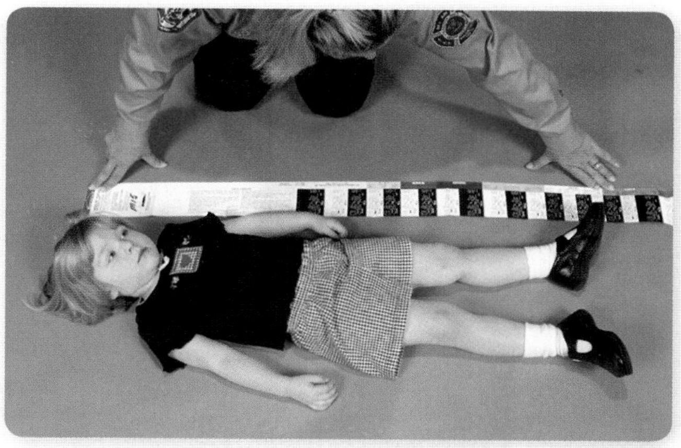

Figure 14-40 Use of a length-based resuscitation tape measure is one method of calculating pediatric drug doses. The tape measure estimates the child's weight (up to 34 kg) based on his or her length.

Enteral Medication Administration

Enteral medications are those that are given through some portion of the digestive or intestinal tract. These are also referred to as alimentary medications. This includes medications that are administered orally, through a feeding tube, or rectally.

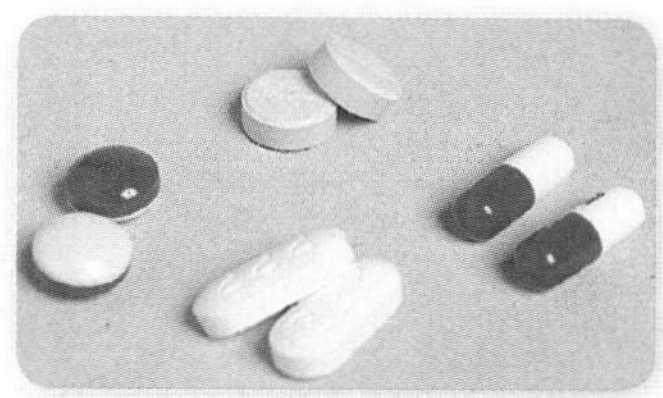

Figure 14-41 Tablets and capsules, oral medications typically taken by mouth, enter the bloodstream through the digestive system.

Oral Medication Administration

Most patients take their daily medications at home by the oral route (PO [per os]). Forms of solid and liquid oral medications include capsules, timed-release capsules, lozenges, pills, tablets, elixirs, emulsions, suspensions, and syrups Figure 14-41.

Drugs taken by mouth are absorbed at a slow rate from the stomach and intestines—usually somewhere between 30 and 90 minutes. Because absorption is slower, it may be necessary for prehospital providers to initiate PO medications early.

To administer oral medications, you may use a small medicine cup, a medicine dropper, a teaspoon, an oral syringe, or a nipple. Gather the appropriate equipment for the form of medication you are administering. Check for indications, contraindications, and precautions, and review the 10 rights before administering any medication.

Follow these steps when administering an oral medication Figure 14-42.

1. Take standard precautions.
2. Determine the need for the medication based on patient presentation.
3. Obtain a history, including any drug allergies.
4. Follow standing orders, or contact medical control for permission.

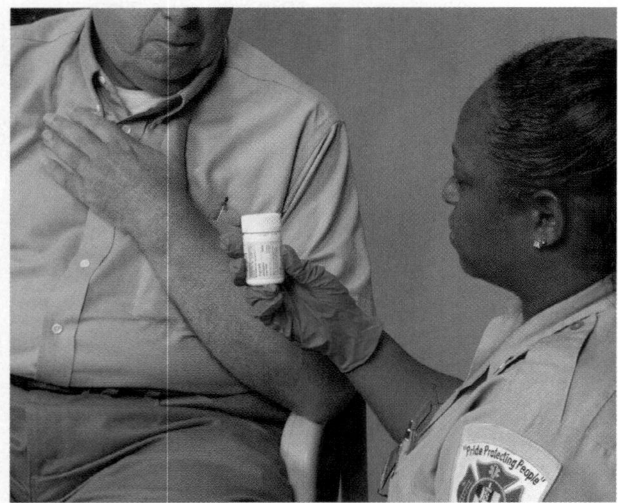
A

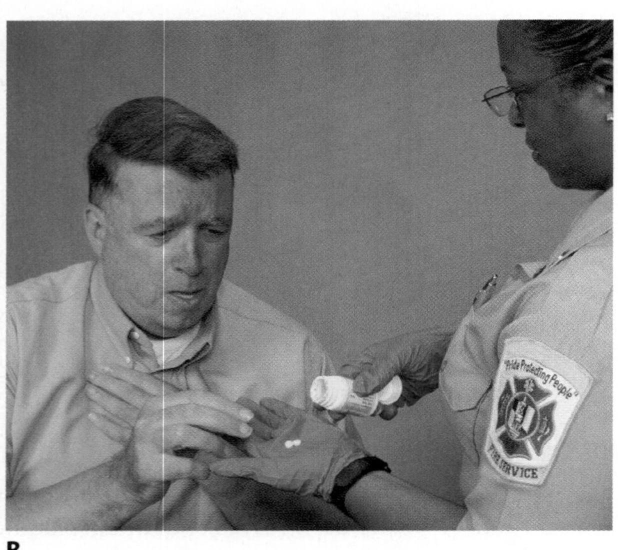
B

Figure 14-42 Administering an oral medication. **A.** Check the medication and its expiration date. **B.** Have the patient take the medication. Provide a glass or cup of water if necessary.

5. Check the medication to be sure it is the right medication, it is not cloudy or discolored, and its expiration date has not passed.
6. Determine the appropriate dose. If using a liquid medication, then pour the desired amount into a calibrated cup or withdraw the appropriate amount into a syringe or dropper. If administering solid medications, then pour the appropriate amount into the lid of the bottle and then place them in the patient's hand.
7. Instruct the patient to swallow the medication with water, if administering a pill or tablet.
8. Monitor the patient's condition, and document the medication given, route, time of administration, and response of the patient.

You may need to calculate the number of pills, capsules, or tablets to give. For PO medications, the concentration is already available on the bottle. For example, during exacerbation of chronic obstructive pulmonary disease, your protocols may call for 60 mg of PO prednisone. The concentration is labeled as 20 mg/tablet.

Calculation:

60 mg (desired dose) ÷ 20-mg tablets (concentration) = 3 tablets

Orogastric and Nasogastric Tube Medication Administration

Gastric tubes (orogastric or nasogastric) are occasionally inserted in the prehospital setting to decompress the stomach, perform gastric lavage, or establish a route for enteral medication administration, though use of this route for medication administration in the field is rare. Some services may allow activated charcoal to be administered by gastric tube for toxic ingestion when PO activated charcoal is contraindicated. Gastric tubes are also commonly present during interfacility transports. The most common solution to be administered through gastric tubes during interfacility transports is liquid nutrition for tube feeding. Chapter 15, *Airway Management*, describes insertion of orogastric and nasogastric tubes. Follow the steps in Skill Drill 14-4 to administer medications via the gastric tube after the tube has been inserted.

Use warm saline for injections. Because the solution will be going directly into the digestive tract with a temperature of approximately 98.6°F, a solution at room temperature has the possibility of placing the patient in hypothermia.

Rectal Medication Administration

Certain drugs may be administered rectally if you are unable to establish IV or IO access. In the field, diazepam (Valium) can be administered rectally (PR) in patients because IV access can be challenging when the patient is having a seizure. Because the rectal mucosa is highly vascular, medication absorption is rapid and predictable Figure 14-43. Because rectal medications are not digested prior to being absorbed by the body's vasculature, they also bypass the first pass metabolism; this is why they have such a rapid onset. Certain antiemetic medications are available in **suppository** form (eg, promethazine [Phenergan]), and under certain circumstances, you might be asked to administer them. A suppository is a drug mixed in a firm base that melts at body temperature and is shaped to fit the rectum. In the clinical setting, medications are sometimes administered via an **enema**, a fluid solution that is administered into the rectum, such as for imaging studies of the gastrointestinal tract.

Skill Drill 14-4 Administering Medication via a Nasogastric Tube

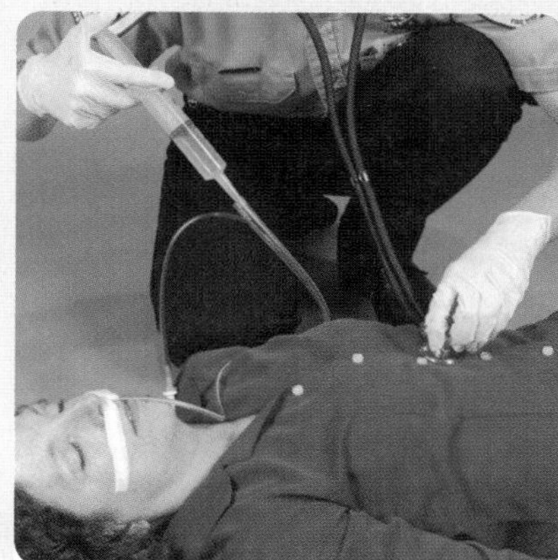

Step 1 Take standard precautions. Confirm proper gastric tube placement. Attach a 60-mL cone-tipped syringe to the gastric tube and slowly inject air as you or your partner auscultates over the epigastrium. To further confirm proper placement, withdraw on the plunger of the syringe and observe for the return of gastric contents in the tube. Leave the gastric tube open to air.

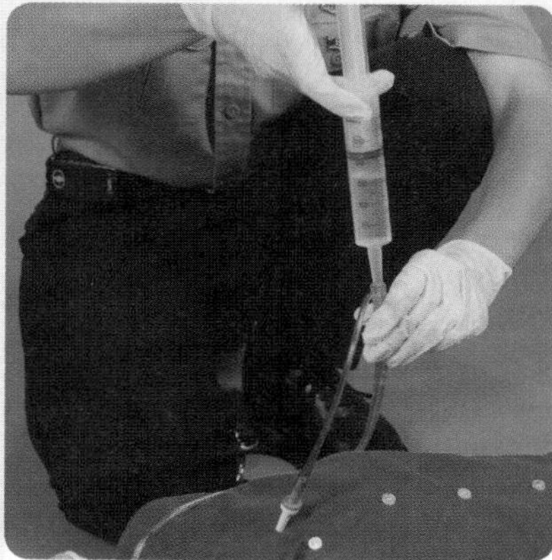

Step 2 Draw up 30 to 60 mL of normal saline into the syringe, and irrigate the gastric tube. If you meet resistance, ensure the tube is not kinked.

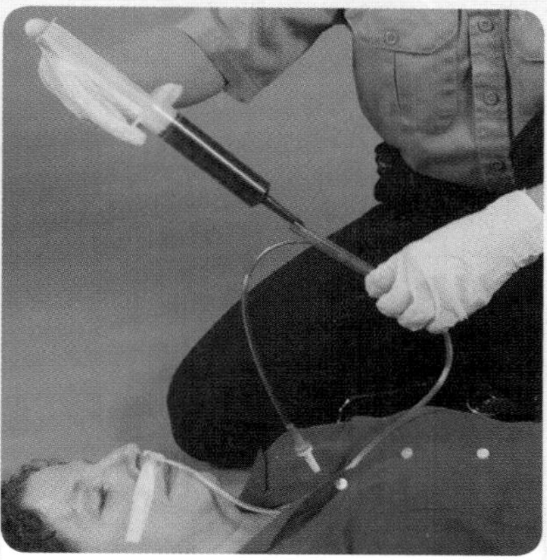

Step 3 Draw up the appropriate amount of medication, ensure it is the correct medication and amount, and slowly inject the medication into the gastric tube.

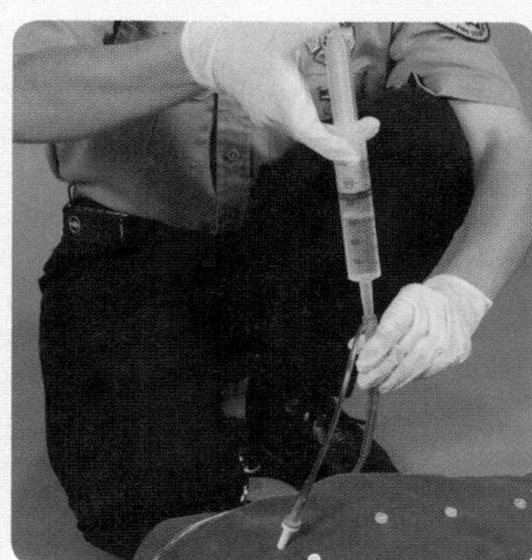

Step 4 Inject 30 to 60 mL of normal saline into the gastric tube following administration of the medication. This will ensure the tube is flushed and the patient has received the entire dose of the medication.

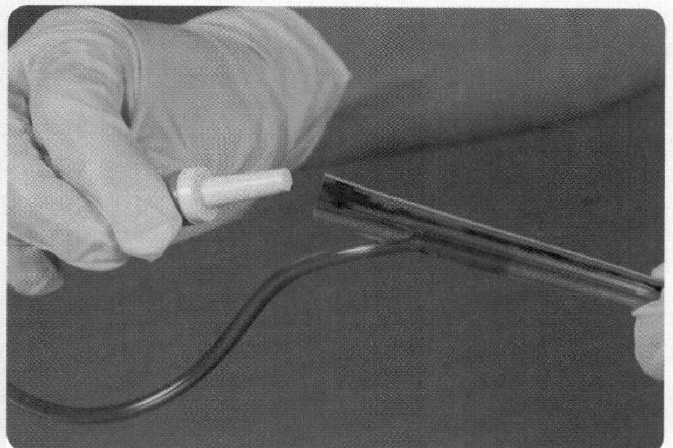

Step 5 Clamp off the proximal end of the gastric tube. Do not attach the gastric tube to suction because this will result in removal of the medication from the stomach. Monitor the patient for adverse reactions. Document the medication given, route, dose, administration time, and condition and response of the patient. Repeat the medication dose if indicated.

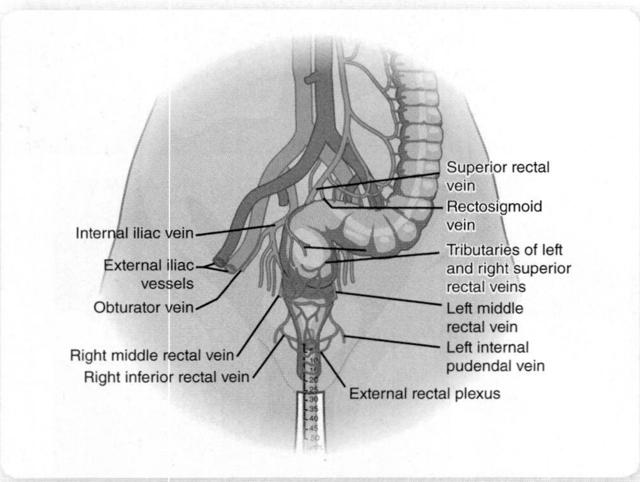

Figure 14-43 The rectal mucosa is highly vascular. It rapidly and predictably absorbs medications.

Follow these steps to administer a drug via the rectal route:

1. Take standard precautions.
2. Determine the need for the medication based on patient presentation.
3. Obtain a history, including any drug allergies.
4. Follow standing orders, or contact medical control for permission.
5. Determine the appropriate dose, and check that the medication is the right medication, there is no cloudiness or discoloration, and the expiration date has not passed.
6. Use a water-soluble gel for lubrication when you insert a suppository. Insert the suppository into the rectum approximately 1 to 1½ inches (3 to 4 cm) while instructing the patient to relax and not to bear down.
7. For medications in liquid form, some modifications are needed. You may use a nasopharyngeal airway, a small endotracheal (ET) tube Figure 14-44, an 18-gauge IV catheter without a needle, or a commercial device as your delivery device.
   - Lubricate the end of the delivery device with a water-soluble gel, and gently insert it approximately 1 to 1½ inches (3 to 4 cm) into the rectum.
   - Instruct the patient to relax and not to bear down, if possible.
   - With a *needleless* syringe, gently push the medication through the tube.
   - Once the medication has been delivered, remove and dispose of the tube or syringe in an appropriate container.
8. Monitor the patient's condition, and document the medication given, route, time of administration, and response of the patient.

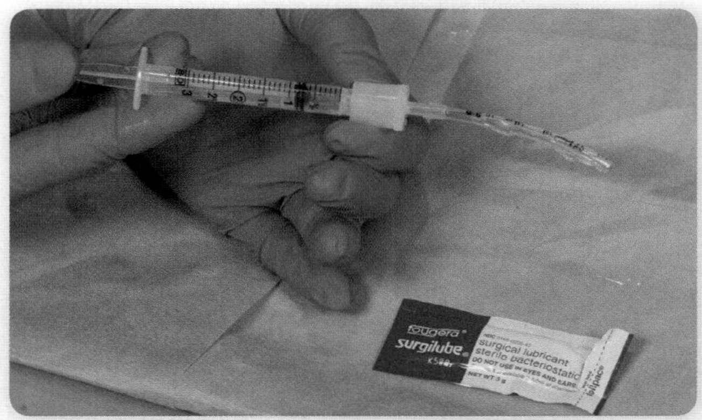

Figure 14-44 Syringe attached to a pediatric endotracheal tube.

> **Words of Wisdom**
>
> Diazepam (Valium) is available in a specially designed container, which is marketed under the name Diastat. The distal end of the container is tapered, which facilitates insertion into the rectum. This feature eliminates the need for syringes or other methods of injecting the medication into the rectum. This is a commonly prescribed medication for children with seizures.

Parenteral Medication Administration

The **parenteral route** refers to any route other than the gastrointestinal tract. Parenteral routes for medication administration include the intradermal, subcutaneous, IM, IV, IO, and percutaneous routes. Compared with enterally administered medications (eg, oral, gastric tube), parenterally administered medications are absorbed into the central circulation more quickly and at a more predictable rate, thus, achieving their therapeutic effects faster. Of the parenteral drug routes, IV administration is the route most commonly used in the prehospital setting and generally is the quickest route for getting medication into the central circulation.

Syringes and Needles

A variety of needles and syringes are used for administering parenteral medications. Many syringes come prepackaged with a needle already attached. The needles and syringes may also be packaged separately. Syringes consist of a plunger, body or barrel, flange, and tip Figure 14-45. Most syringes are marked with 10 calibrations per milliliter on one side of the barrel, where each small line represents 0.1 mL; the other side of the barrel is marked in minims. Syringes vary from 1 mL to 60 mL; the 3-mL syringe is the one most commonly used for injections.

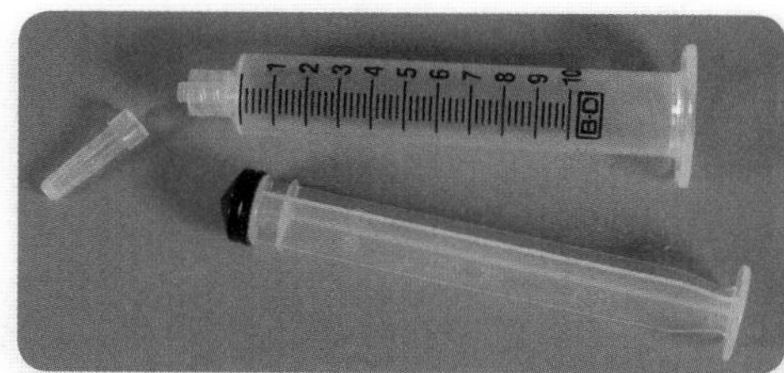

Figure 14-45 A syringe consists of a plunger, body or barrel, flange, and tip.

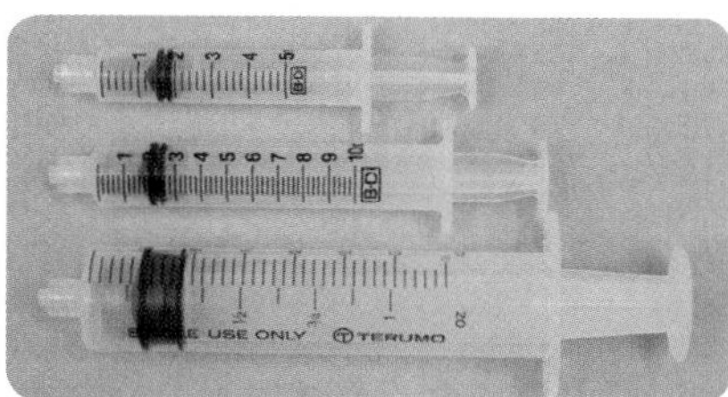

Figure 14-46 Syringes come in a variety of sizes. Some come with needles already attached, others without needles attached.

Syringe selection is based on the volume of medication that you will administer Figure 14-46.

Hypodermic needle lengths vary from 3/8 inch to 2 inches (0.9 cm to 5 cm) for standard injections. As with IV catheters, the gauge of the needle refers to the diameter: The smaller the number, the larger the diameter. Common needle gauges range from 18 to 26. The needle gauge used depends on the route of parenteral medication administration. Smaller-gauge needles, for example, are used for subcutaneous injections, whereas larger-gauge needles are used for IM and IV injections.

The proximal end of the needle, or hub, attaches to the standard fitting on the syringe. The distal end of the needle is beveled.

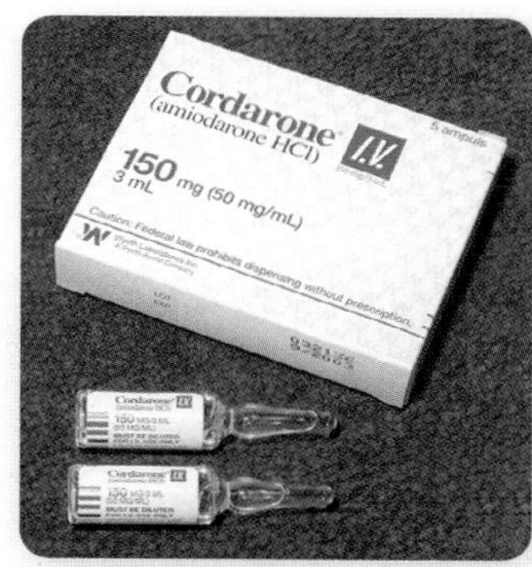

Figure 14-47 Medication stored in ampules.

Packaging of Parenteral Medications

Ampules

Ampules are breakable sterile glass containers that are designed to carry a single dose of medication Figure 14-47. They may contain as little as 1 mL or as much as 10 mL, depending on the medication.

When you are drawing a medication from an ampule, follow the steps in Skill Drill 14-5.

Skill Drill 14-5 Drawing Medication From an Ampule

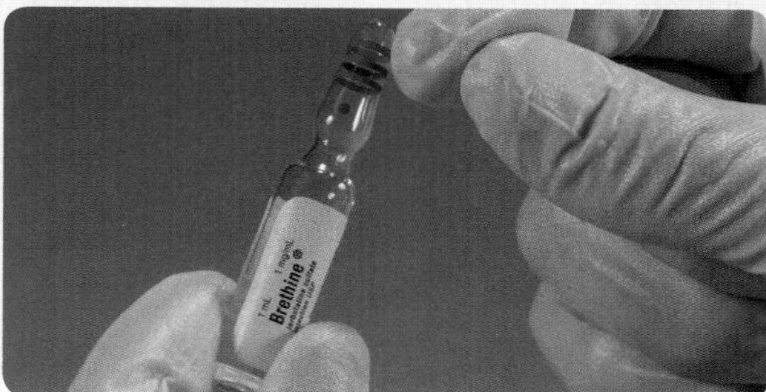

Step 1 Check the medication and ensure the expiration date has not passed and that it is the correct drug and concentration.

Shake the medication into the base of the ampule. If some of the drug is stuck in the neck, then gently thump or tap the stem.

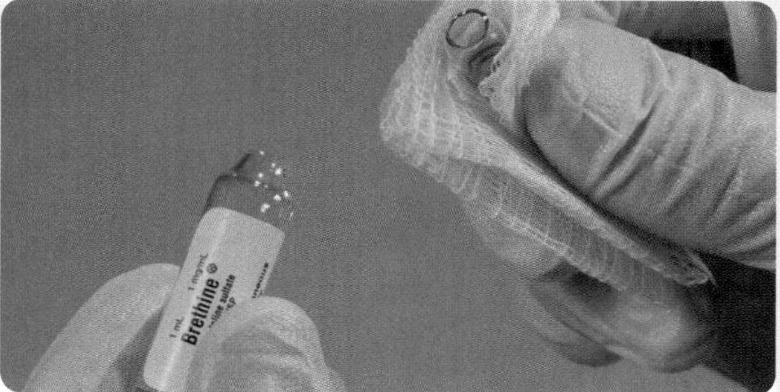

Step 2 Using a 4-inch × 4-inch (10-cm × 10-cm) gauze pad, an alcohol prep, or an ampule breaker, grip the neck of the ampule and snap it off where the ampule is scored. If the ampule is not scored and an attempt is made to break it, some sharp edges may be present. Drop the stem in the sharps container.

(continued)

Skill Drill 14-5 Drawing Medication From an Ampule *(continued)*

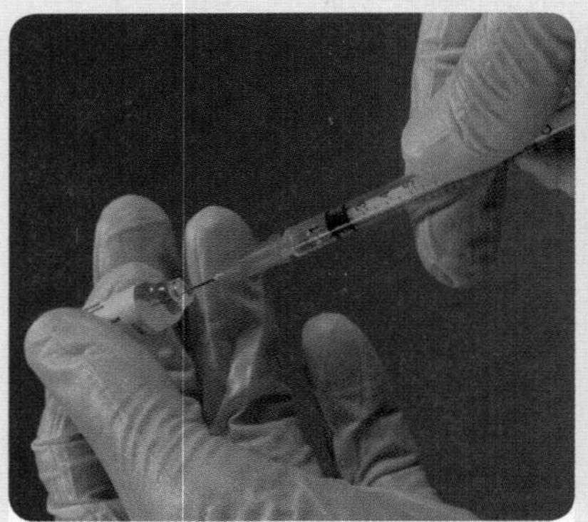

Step 3 Insert a filtered needle into the ampule without touching the outer sides of the ampule. Draw the solution into the syringe, and dispose of the ampule in the sharps container.

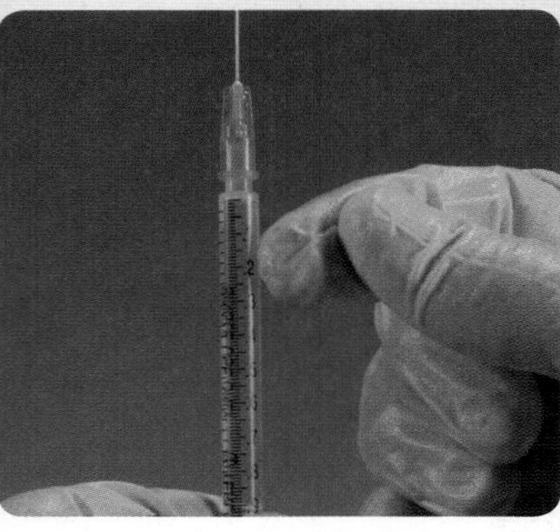

Step 4 Hold the syringe with the needle pointing up, and gently tap the barrel to loosen air trapped inside and cause it to rise.

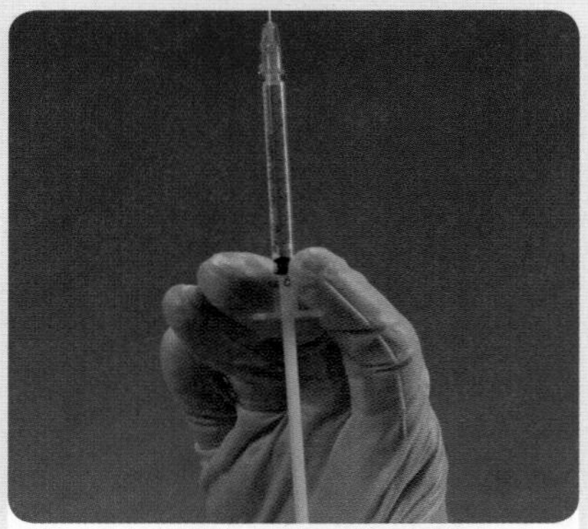

Step 5 Press gently on the plunger to dispel any air bubbles. Recap the needle using the one-handed method. Dispose of the needle in the sharps container and attach a standard hypodermic needle to the syringe if necessary to administer the medication.

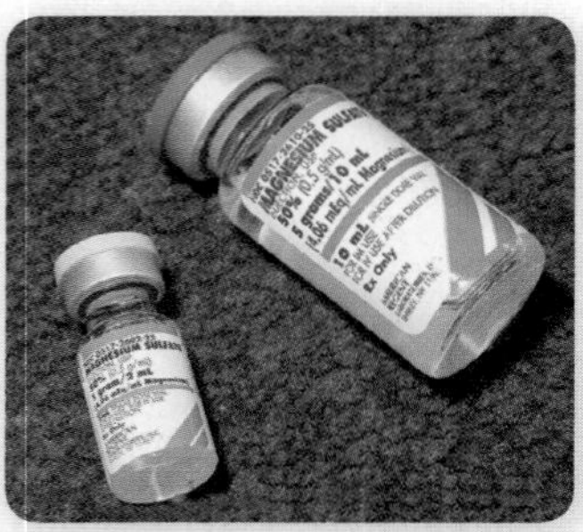

Figure 14-48 Vials (single-dose and multiple dose).

Vials

Vials are small glass or plastic bottles with a rubber-stopper top; they may contain single or multiple doses of a medication **Figure 14-48**. When you are using a vial of medication, you must first determine how much of the drug you will need and how many doses are in the vial.

For a single-dose vial, you may draw up the entire amount in the vial. For multiple-dose vials, you should draw up only the amount needed. Remember, once you remove the cover from a vial, it is no longer sterile. If you need a second dose, then clean the top of the vial with alcohol before withdrawing the medication.

Some medications that are stored in vials may need to be reconstituted, such as methylprednisolone sodium succinate (Solu-Medrol) and glucagon. Glucagon is stored in two vials, one with the powdered form of the drug and the other with sterile water. **Drug reconstitution** involves injecting the sterile water (or provided **diluent**) from one vial into the vial that contains the powder, thereby making a solution for injection. To reconstitute the contents from two vials, draw the fluid out of the first vial and inject it into the vial that contains the powder. Shake the vial vigorously, unless contraindicated, to mix the medication before drawing out the contents for administration.

Methylprednisolone sodium succinate is stored in a **Mix-o-Vial**, a single vial divided into two compartments

Words of Wisdom

Whenever you use a needle to draw up medication from an ampule or vial, to avoid sticking yourself, hold the syringe against your palm with the needle pointing up and draw the ampule or vial down onto the needle using the thumb and forefinger of the palm the syringe is braced against. This especially applies if you are in a moving ambulance.

by a rubber stopper Figure 14-49. To reconstitute a drug that is contained in a Mix-o-Vial, squeeze the two vials together, which releases the center stopper and allows the contents to mix. Shake vigorously to mix the contents before drawing out the medication.

When you are drawing medication from a vial, follow the steps in Skill Drill 14-6.

Prefilled Syringes

Prefilled syringes are packaged in tamper-proof boxes. Two types of prefilled syringes exist: those that are separated into a glass drug cartridge and a syringe Figure 14-50, and preassembled prefilled syringes Figure 14-51. These syringes are designed for ease of use. After all, it is much easier and quicker to use a prefilled syringe when you are treating a patient in cardiac arrest than it is to draw up each individual dose. It is important to remember that with many drug cartridge and syringe systems, both pieces of the assembly may contain sharps and should be disposed of properly. In cases where the medication is too large to fit into a standard sharps container, the medication should be handled with care and disposed of either at the receiving facility's larger sharps container, or at the station in a larger sharps container.

To assemble the two-part prefilled syringe, pop the yellow caps off of the syringe and the drug cartridge,

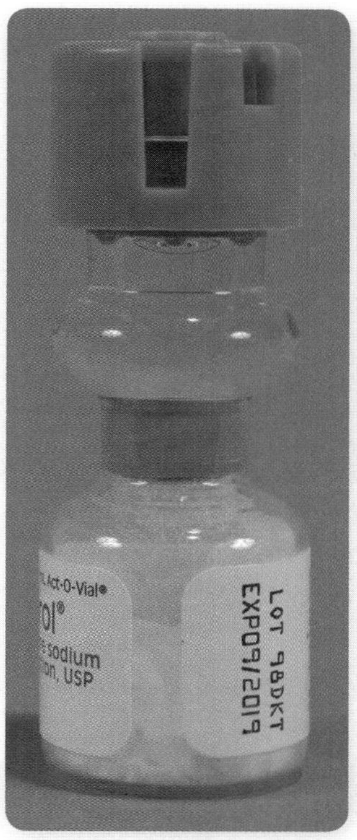

Figure 14-49 A Mix-o-Vial.

Skill Drill 14-6 Drawing Medication From a Vial

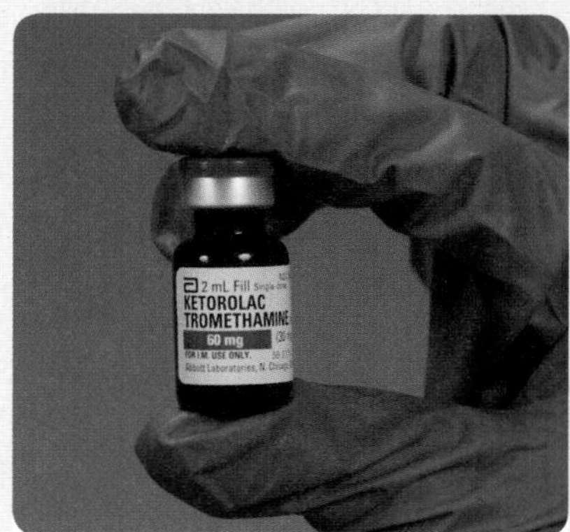

Step 1 Check the medication and ensure the expiration date has not passed and that it is the correct drug and concentration. Remove the sterile cover, or clean the top with alcohol if the vial was previously opened.

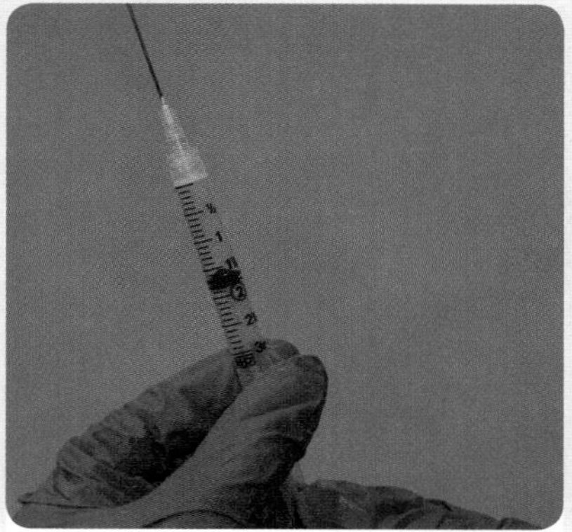

Step 2 Determine the amount of medication that you will need, and draw that amount of air into the syringe. Allow a little extra room to expel some air while removing air bubbles.

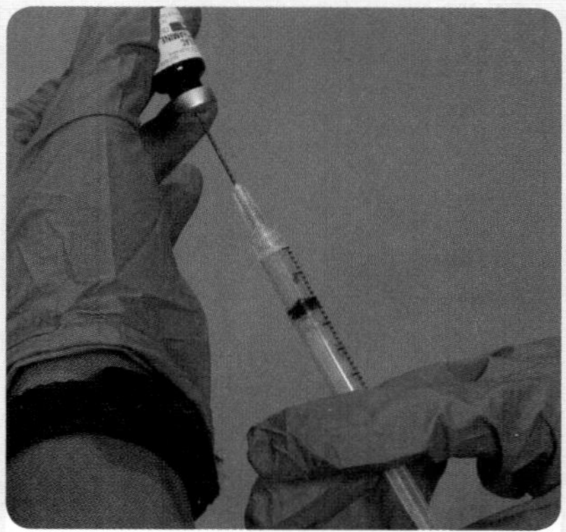

Step 3 Invert the vial, clean the rubber stopper with an alcohol prep, and insert the needle through the rubber stopper into the medication. Expel the air in the syringe into the vial and then withdraw the amount of medication needed.

(continued)

Skill Drill 14-6 Drawing Medication From a Vial *(continued)*

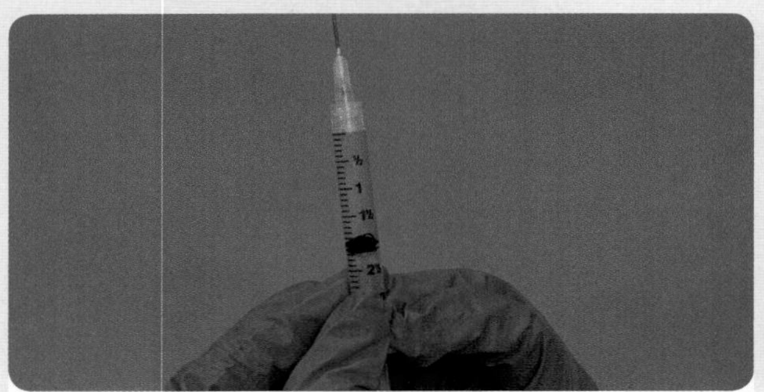

Step 4 Once you have the correct amount of medication in the syringe, withdraw the needle from the vial and expel any air in the syringe.

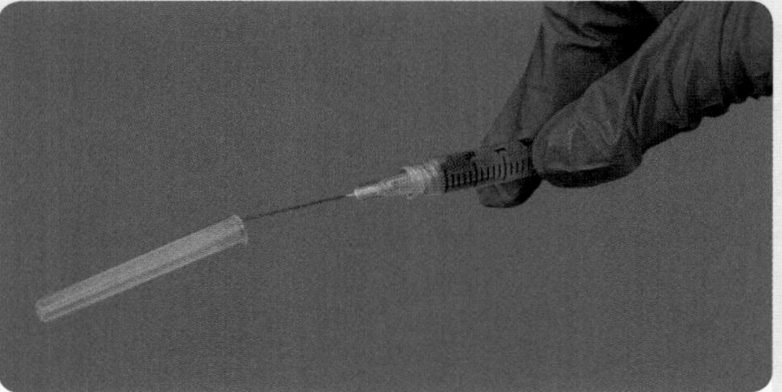

Step 5 Recap the needle using the one-handed method. Label the syringe if it is not immediately given to the patient.

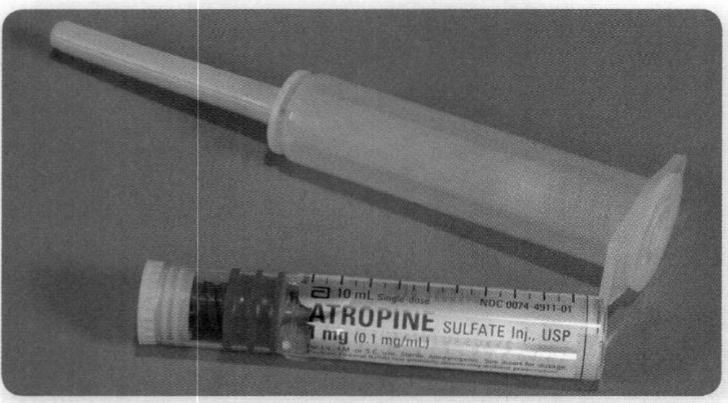

Figure 14-50 Two-part prefilled syringes are separated into a glass drug cartridge and a syringe (for example, Bristojet).

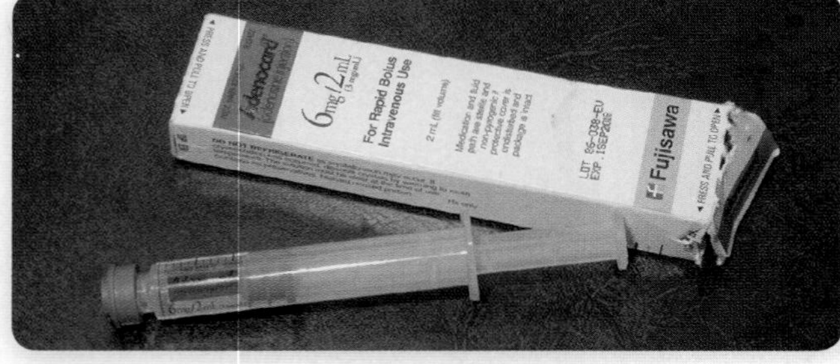

Figure 14-51 Preassembled prefilled syringe.

insert the drug cartridge into the barrel of the syringe, and screw them together. Remove the needle cover, and expel air in the manner previously described. Follow the steps for the route by which the medication is to be given.

Single-dose disposable medication cartridges that are inserted into a reusable syringe are also available. These syringes are commonly referred to by their brand names of Tubex, Aboject, and Carpuject syringes Figure 14-52.

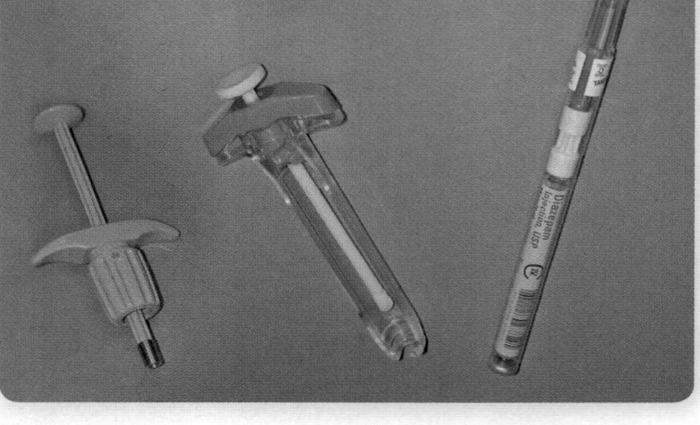

Figure 14-52 Reusable syringes (left). Disposable medication cartridge (right).

Push-Dose Pressors

Some vasopressors are available for administration in a small bolus format. This is generally reserved for patients with transient hypotension or for EMS systems with short transport times. Epinephrine and phenylephrine (Neosynephrine) are currently available in push-dose format. While push-dose phenylephrine is generally seen in ICUs, EDs, and critical care transport, push-dose epinephrine is becoming a popular substitute for dopamine in many EMS systems.

Generally speaking, to use push-dose epinephrine, you have to mix the appropriate concentration yourself. Begin by taking a 10-mL saline flush and wasting 1 mL. Use a blunt-tip needle and draw out 0.1 mg (1 mL) of an epinephrine 1:10,000 (0.1 mg/mL) prefilled syringe.

This gives you a concentration of 0.1 mg or 100 mcg in 10 mL. The typical dosing is 10 to 20 mcg every 2 to 5 minutes as needed or until an infusion is initiated.

▶ Intradermal Medication Administration

Intradermal injections involve administering a small amount of medication—typically less than 1 mL—into the dermal layer, just beneath the epidermis. The technique involves the use of a 1-mL syringe (for example, a tuberculin syringe) and a 25- to 27-gauge, 3/8-inch to 1-inch (0.9-cm to 3-cm) needle.

When you are selecting a site for an intradermal injection, you should avoid areas that contain superficial blood vessels to minimize the risk of systemic medication absorption. Because of their high visibility and relative lack of hair, the most common anatomic locations for intradermal injections are the anterior forearm and upper back.

Medications administered intradermally have a slow rate of absorption; there is minimal to no systemic distribution. The medication remains locally collected at the site of the injection. Unless you are anesthetizing the skin before establishing an IV line, you will rarely use the intradermal route to administer medications in the prehospital setting. Instead, these injections are typically given in a physician's office or in the hospital to test a patient for allergies or to perform a PPD (purified protein derivative)—a skin test for tuberculosis.

Follow these steps to administer a medication via the intradermal route:

1. Take standard precautions.
2. Determine the need for the medication based on patient presentation.
3. Obtain a history, including any drug allergies and vital signs.
4. Follow standing orders, or contact medical control for permission.
5. Check the medication to ensure that it is the correct one, that it is not cloudy or discolored, and that the expiration date has not passed, and determine the appropriate amount to give for the correct dose.
6. Advise the patient of potential discomfort while explaining the procedure.
7. Assemble and check equipment needed: alcohol preps and a 1-mL syringe with a 25- to 27-gauge, 3/8-inch or 1-inch (0.9-cm to 3-cm) needle. Draw up the correct dose of medication.
8. Cleanse the area for administration using aseptic technique.
9. Pull the skin taut with your nondominant hand.
10. Insert the needle at a 10° to 15° angle with the bevel up.
11. Slowly inject the medication while observing for the formation of a wheal, or small bump, which indicates the medication is collecting in the intradermal tissue.
12. Remove the needle. Immediately dispose of the needle and syringe in the sharps container.
13. Monitor the patient's condition, and document the medication given, route, administration time, and response of the patient.

▶ Subcutaneous Medication Administration

Subcutaneous injections are given into the loose connective tissue between the dermis and the muscle layer **Figure 14-53**. Volumes of a drug administered subcutaneously are usually 1 mL or less. The injection is performed using a 24- to 26-gauge ½-inch to 1-inch (1-cm to 3-cm) needle. Common sites for subcutaneous injections—in both adults and children—include the upper arms, anterior thighs, and the abdomen **Figure 14-54**.

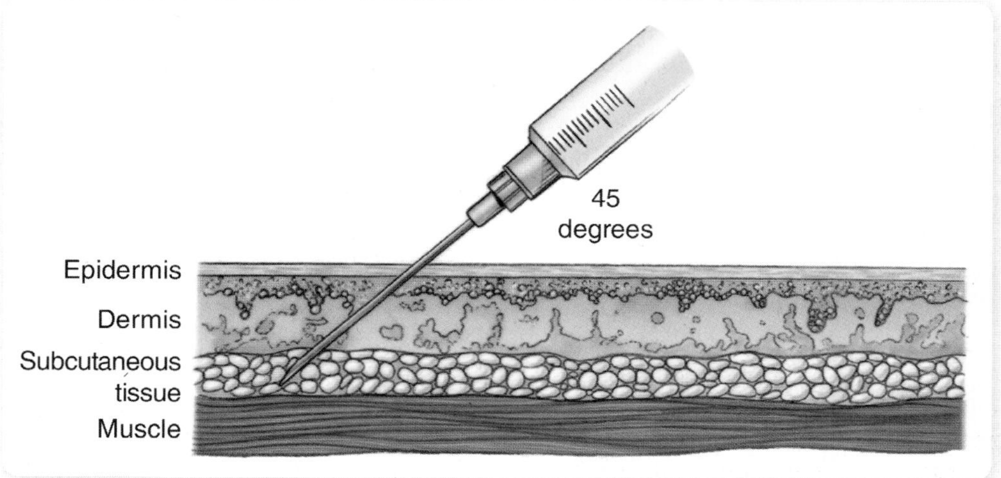

Figure 14-53 A subcutaneous injection is below the dermis and above the muscle.

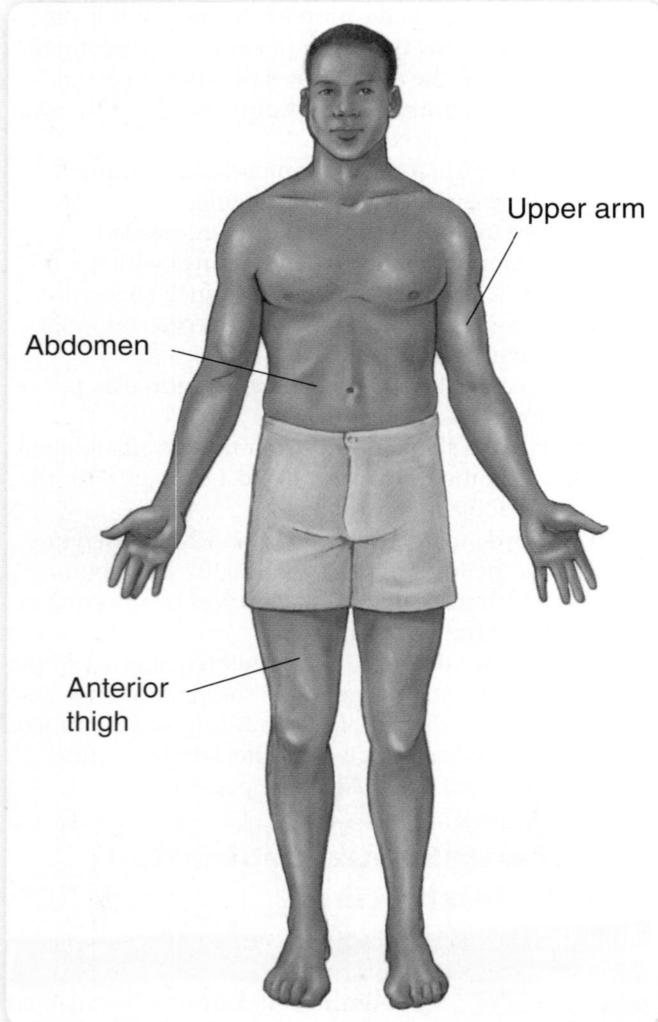

Figure 14-54 Common sites for subcutaneous injections.

Patients who take insulin injections usually vary the sites owing to the multiple (usually daily) injections they require.

Follow the steps in Skill Drill 14-7 to administer a medication via the subcutaneous route.

Intramuscular Medication Administration

Intramuscular (IM) injections are given by penetrating a needle through the dermis and subcutaneous tissue and into the muscle layer Figure 14-55. This technique allows administration of a larger volume of medication (up to 5 mL) than the subcutaneous route. Because there is also the potential for damage to nerves due to the depth of the injection, it is important to choose the appropriate

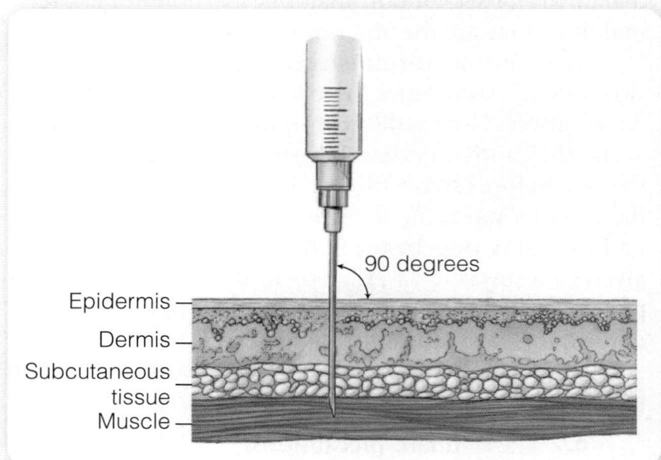

Figure 14-55 An intramuscular injection is below the dermis and subcutaneous layer and into the muscle.

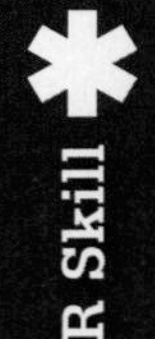

Skill Drill 14-7 Administering Medication via the Subcutaneous Route

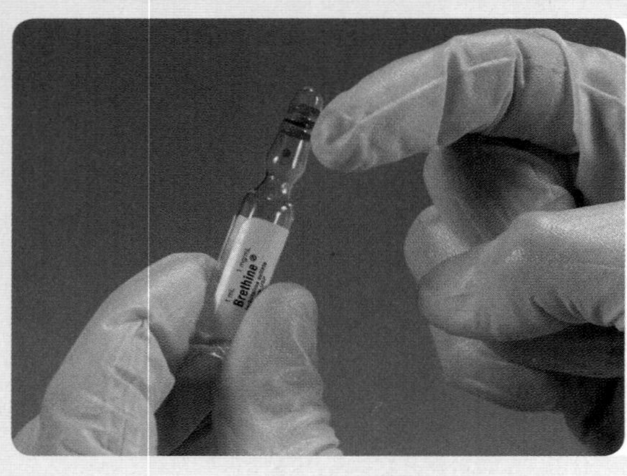

Step 1 Take standard precautions. Determine the need for the medication based on patient presentation. Obtain a history, including any drug allergies and vital signs. Follow standing orders, or contact medical control for permission. Check the medication to ensure that it is the correct one, that it is not cloudy or discolored, and that the expiration date has not passed, and determine the appropriate amount and concentration for the correct dose.

Skill Drill 14-7 Administering Medication via the Subcutaneous Route *(continued)*

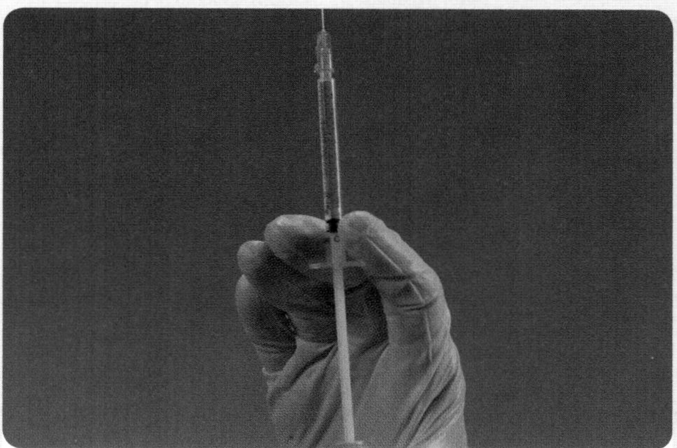

Step 2 Advise the patient of potential discomfort while explaining the procedure.

Assemble and check equipment needed: alcohol preps and a 3-mL syringe with a 24- to 26-gauge needle. Draw up the correct dose of medication and dispel air while maintaining sterility.

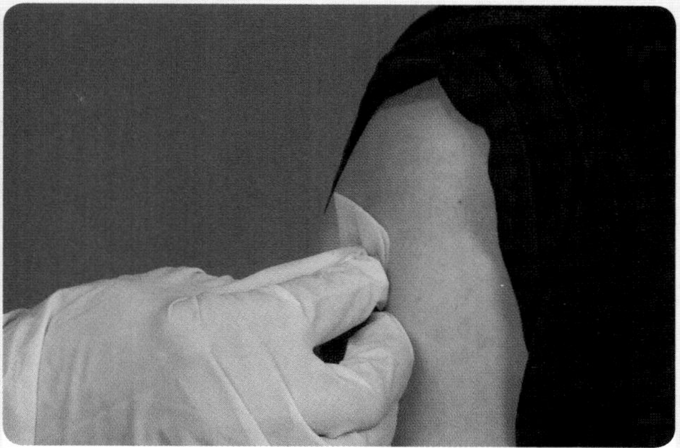

Step 3 Cleanse the area for the administration (usually the upper arm or thigh) using aseptic technique.

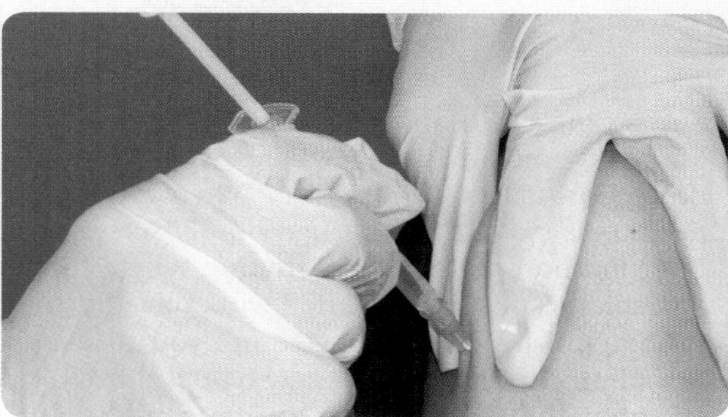

Step 4 Pinch the skin surrounding the area, advise the patient of a stick, and insert the needle at a 45° angle. Inject the medication and remove the needle. Immediately dispose of the needle and syringe in the sharps container.

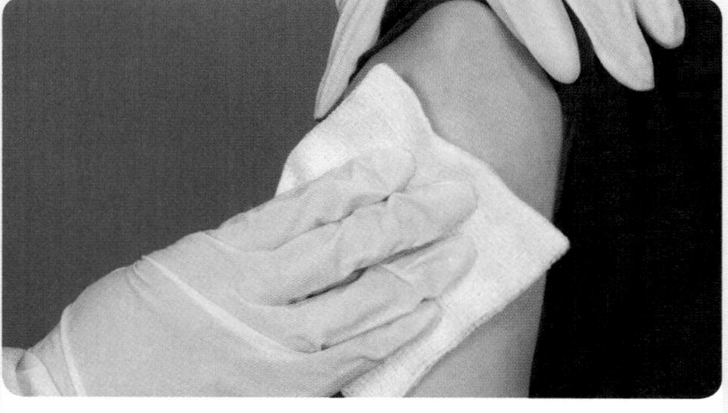

Step 5 To disperse the medication through the tissue, rub the area in a circular motion with your gloved hand (unless contraindicated for the medication). Properly store any unused medication. Monitor the patient's condition, and document the medication given, route, administration time, and response of the patient.

site. Common anatomic sites for IM injections for adults and children include the following:

- **Vastus lateralis muscle**—the large muscle on the lateral side of the thigh.
- **Rectus femoris muscle**—the large muscle on the anterior side of the thigh.
- **Gluteal area**—the buttocks, specifically the upper lateral aspect of either side. When injecting into the gluteal area, you should use the upper, outer quadrant to avoid the sciatic nerve.
- **Deltoid muscle**—the muscle of the upper arm that covers the prominence of the shoulder. The site for injection is approximately 1½ to 2 inches (4 cm to 5 cm) below the acromion process on the lateral side Figure 14-56.

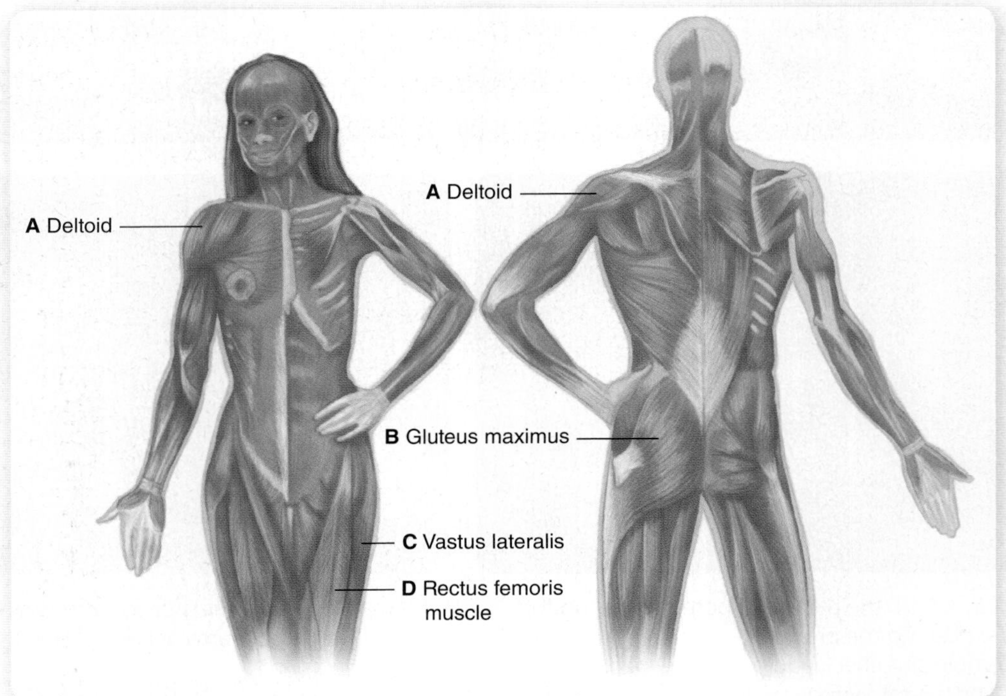

Figure 14-56 Common sites for intramuscular injections. **A.** Deltoid muscle. **B.** Gluteal area. **C.** Vastus lateralis muscle. **D.** Rectus femoris muscle.

Words of Wisdom

Effective absorption of medications administered by the subcutaneous and IM routes requires adequate peripheral perfusion. This is clearly not the case in patients in profound shock or cardiac arrest. Therefore, *subcutaneous and IM injections should not be given to patients with inadequate perfusion* unless no other options exist.

Subcutaneous and IM injections should not be given into skin that is hardened, bruised, red, or otherwise discolored, or stained.

Follow the steps in Skill Drill 14-8 to administer a medication via the IM route.

▶ IV Bolus Medication Administration

The IV route places the drug directly into the circulatory system. It is the fastest route of medication administration because it bypasses most barriers to drug absorption. As a result, *there is no room for error with IV administration*. (See "Potential Complications of IV Therapy" earlier in this chapter for details on what can go wrong.) Drugs are administered by direct injection with a needle and syringe into an established peripheral IV line. Many services now use needleless systems to provide protection against needlesticks. When you are using a needleless system, the syringe simply screws into the injection port of the administration set (IV tubing). If a needleless port is punctured with a needle, then the system will leak. This will require you to switch out the administration set to a new one. If this is a critical situation and time does not warrant you the ability to switch out the drip set, you can provide a "temporary patch" on the system by placing a syringe filled with saline on the needleless port.

Recall, a bolus is a single dose, usually given by the IV route. When given in one mass, it may consist of a small or large quantity of a drug and can be given rapidly or slowly, depending on the drug. Some medications, such as lidocaine and amiodarone, require an initial bolus and then may require a continuous IV infusion to maintain a therapeutic level of the drug. Some medications can have devastating effects if administered too fast. For example, promethazine can cause an extreme burning sensation if administered too fast. Furosemide may cause tinnitus if administered rapidly. Other medications may be ineffective if they are administered too slowly. For example, adenosine has a half-life of 10 seconds and will be ineffective if it does not reach the heart in that time frame.

Follow the steps in Skill Drill 14-9 when you are administering a medication via the IV bolus route.

Skill Drill 14-8 Administering Medication via the Intramuscular Route

NR Skill

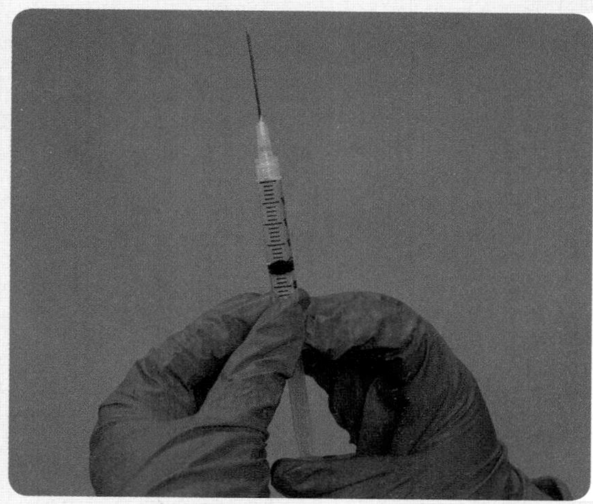

Step 1 Take standard precautions. Determine the need for the medication based on patient presentation. Obtain a history, including any drug allergies and vital signs. Follow standing orders, or contact medical control for permission.

Check the medication to ensure that it is the correct one, that it is not cloudy or discolored, and that the expiration date has not passed, and determine the appropriate amount and concentration for the correct dose.

Advise the patient of potential discomfort while explaining the procedure.

Assemble and check equipment needed: alcohol preps and a 3- to 5-mL syringe with a 21-gauge, 1-inch or 2-inch (4-cm or 5-cm) needle. Draw up the correct dose of medication and dispel air while maintaining sterility.

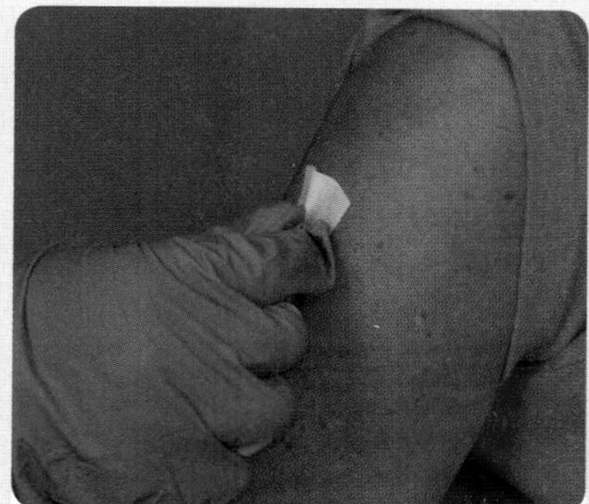

Step 2 Cleanse the area for administration (usually the upper arm or the hip) using aseptic technique.

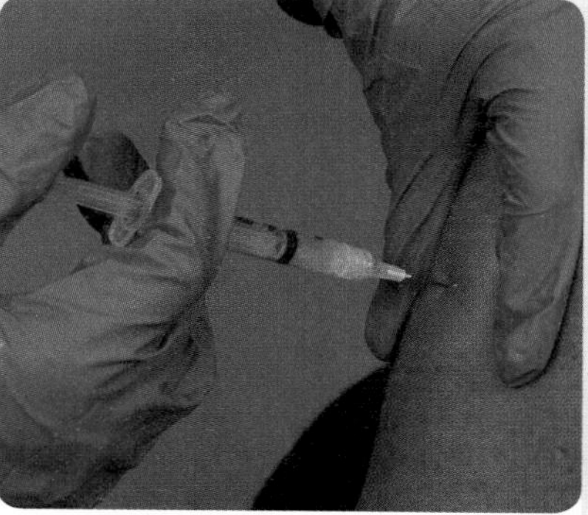

Step 3 Stretch the skin over the cleansed area, advise the patient of a stick, and insert the needle at a 90° angle.

Pull back on the plunger to aspirate for blood. The presence of blood in the syringe indicates you may have entered a blood vessel. In such a case, remove the needle, and hold pressure over the site. Discard the syringe and needle in the sharps container. Prepare a new syringe and needle, and select another site.

If there is no blood in the syringe, then inject the medication and remove the needle.

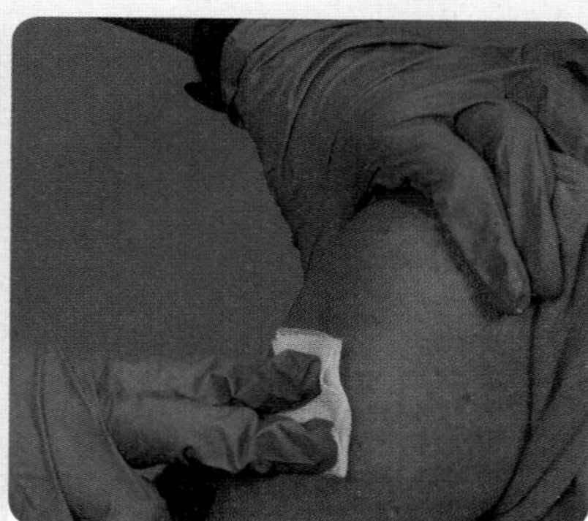

Step 4 Immediately dispose of the needle and syringe in the sharps container. Store any unused medication properly. Monitor the patient's condition, and document the medication given, route, administration time, and response of the patient.

NR Skill

Skill Drill 14-9 Administering Medication via the Intravenous Bolus Route

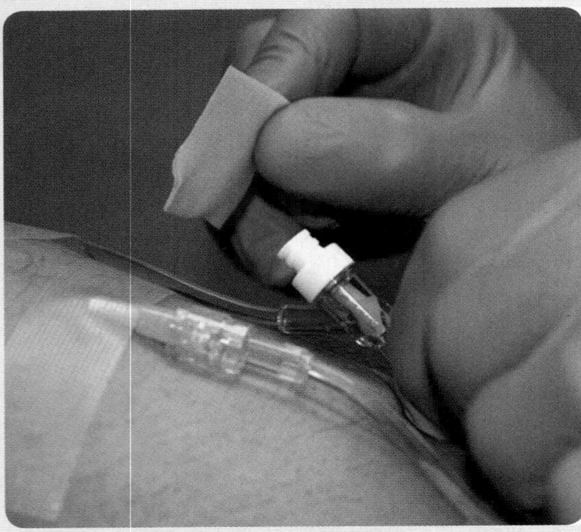

Step 1 Take standard precautions. Determine the need for the medication based on patient presentation. Obtain a history, including any drug allergies and vital signs.

Follow standing orders, or contact medical control for permission.

Check the medication to ensure that it is the correct one, that it is not cloudy or discolored, and that the expiration date has not passed, and determine the appropriate amount and concentration for the correct dose.

Explain the procedure to the patient and the need for the medication. Assemble needed equipment, and draw up the medication. Expel any air in the syringe. Draw up 20 mL of normal saline to use as a flush for the medication.

Cleanse the injection port with alcohol, or remove the protective cap if using the needleless system.

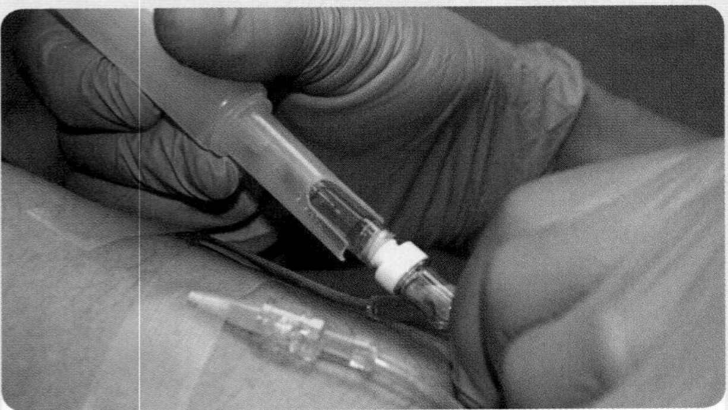

Step 2 Insert the needle into the port, and pinch off the IV tubing proximal to the administration port. Failure to shut off the line will result in the medication taking the pathway of least resistance and flowing into the bag instead of into the patient. Administer the correct dose of the medication at the appropriate rate. Some medications must be administered quickly, whereas others must be pushed slowly to prevent adverse effects.

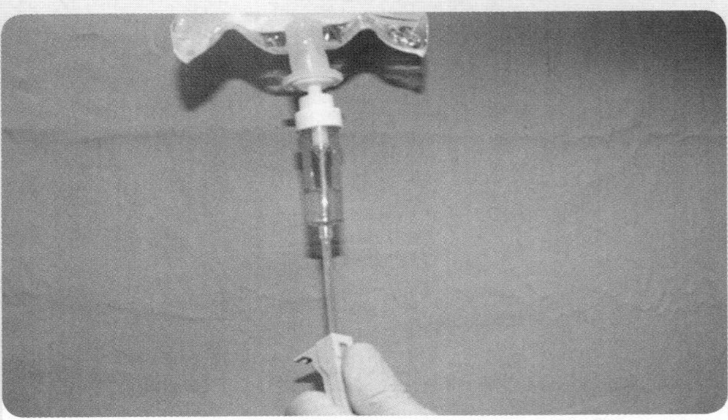

Step 3 Place the needle and syringe into the sharps container.

Unclamp the IV line to flush the medication into the vein. Allow it to run briefly wide open, or flush with a 20-mL bolus of normal saline.

Readjust the IV flow rate to the original setting.

Properly store and label any unused medication.

Monitor the patient's condition, and document the medication given, route, time of administration, and response of the patient.

As discussed earlier in this chapter, saline locks are used for patients who are not in need of IV fluid boluses but may need medication therapy. Follow these steps to administer a medication through a saline lock:

1. Take standard precautions.
2. Determine the need for the medication based on patient presentation.
3. Obtain a history, including any drug allergies and vital signs.
4. Follow standing orders, or contact medical control for permission.
5. Check the medication to ensure that it is the correct one, that it is not cloudy or discolored, and that the expiration date has not passed, and determine the appropriate amount and concentration for the correct dose.
6. Explain the procedure to the patient and the need for the medication.

7. Assemble needed equipment, and draw up the medication. Draw up 20 mL of normal saline to use as a flush for the medication.
8. Cleanse the injection port with alcohol, or remove the protective cap if using the needleless system.
9. Insert the needle into the port while holding it carefully, or screw the syringe onto the port. Clamp off the IV tubing proximally to prevent backflow into the IV solution.
10. Pull back slightly on the syringe plunger, and observe for blood return. If blood appears, then slowly inject the medication, watching for infiltration. If resistance is felt, or if the patient reports any discomfort, then discontinue administration immediately. A new site will need to be established.
11. Place the needle and syringe into the sharps container.
12. Clean the port, and insert the needle with the syringe containing the flush.
13. Flush the saline lock, and place the needle in the sharps container.
14. Store any unused medication properly.
15. Monitor the patient's condition, and document the medication given, route, time of administration, and response of the patient.

Adding Medication to an IV Bag

Certain medications are added to the IV solution itself to be administered as a maintenance infusion—for example, dopamine, lidocaine, and epinephrine. All of these medications require careful titration to achieve the desired effect.

The steps for adding medication to an IV bag are as follows:

1. Check the fluid in the IV bag for clarity or discoloration, and ensure the expiration date has not passed.
2. Check the medication name on the ampule, vial, or prefilled syringe. Check the concentration of the drug it contains (for example, mcg/mL or mg/mL).
3. Compute the volume of the drug to be added to the IV bag. Draw up that amount in a syringe (if a prefilled syringe is used, note the proportion of the volume of the syringe required).
4. Cleanse the medication injection port on the IV bag with an alcohol swab.
5. Inject the desired volume of medication into the IV bag by puncturing the rubber stopper on the medication injection port **Figure 14-57**.
6. Withdraw the needle, and dispose of the needle and syringe in the sharps container. Agitate the

YOU are the Paramedic PART 3

Vascular access has been obtained with an 18-gauge IV needle in the patient's right forearm. The IV line is patent and flushes easily. Your partner connects a 1-L bag of normal saline to the IV line, and the flow rate is set to KVO. Shortly after administering the dosage of diltiazem as ordered, the rhythm on the cardiac monitor changes to a sinus rhythm. You contact medical control to provide an update of the patient's condition. The physician asks that you begin a maintenance infusion of diltiazem at 5 mg/h. You have a premixed bag of diltiazem with 30 mg/100 mL and a microdrip administration set.

Recording Time: 10 Minutes	
Respirations	18 breaths/min
Pulse	90 beats/min
Skin	Warm and dry
Blood pressure	126/78 mm Hg
Oxygen saturation (Spo_2)	100%
Pupils	PERRLA
ECG	Sinus rhythm

6. Why would it be preferable to use an IV pump for a maintenance infusion of a medication?
7. What is the appropriate flow rate to administer the maintenance infusion of diltiazem?

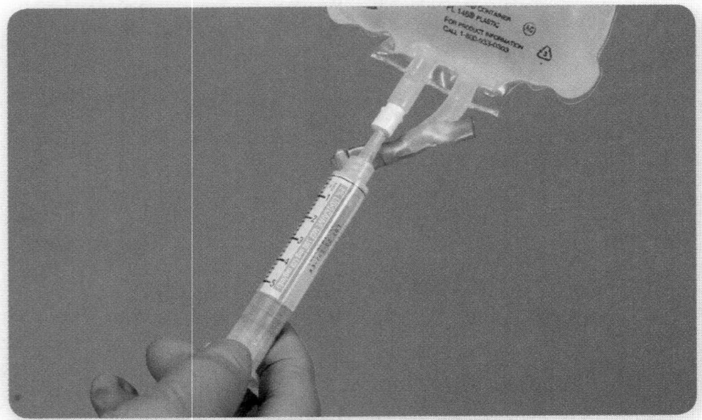

Figure 14-57 Adding medication to an intravenous bag.

IV bag gently to ensure the medication added is well mixed in the solution.

7. Label the IV bag; on a piece of tape, write the name of the medication added, the amount added, the concentration of medication in the IV bag (for example, mcg/mL or mg/mL), the date and time, and your name.
8. Attach the IV administration set, and prepare the IV bag as discussed earlier in this chapter.

IV Piggyback

The IV administration set that is connected directly to the hub of the IV catheter is referred to as the primary line. This line is generally used to administer an isotonic solution. Saline is the preferred isotonic solution because it mixes with all medications in the prehospital and interfacility setting. When you are performing a continuous infusion, take the distal end of the drip set that is attached to the mixed medication and connect it to a port on the primary line. The line that is connected to the continuous infusion is referred to as a "piggyback" or secondary line. Multiple lines can be piggybacked onto a primary IV line. When multiple lines are present on a patient, it is important to label the lines. This will ensure that when medications are administered en route, there are no medication interactions.

Follow the steps in Skill Drill 14-10 to perform IV piggyback infusion.

Words of Wisdom

Medications that are used for maintenance infusions (for example, lidocaine and dopamine) are commonly premixed and prepackaged, which eliminates the need to calculate and draw up the appropriate amount of medication to add to the bag. However, you must still be aware of the concentration (for example, mcg/mL or mg/mL) of the drug in the premixed solution and the appropriate maintenance infusion rate.

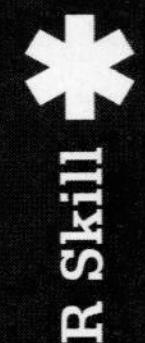

Skill Drill 14-10 Administering a Medication via Intravenous Piggyback Infusion

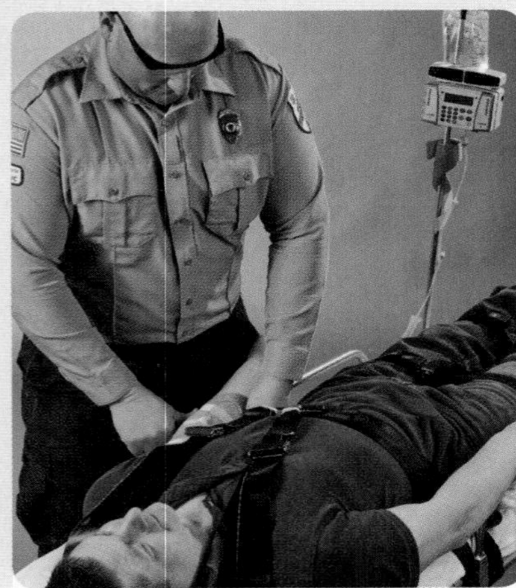

Step 1 Take standard precautions. Ensure the established IV line is patent.

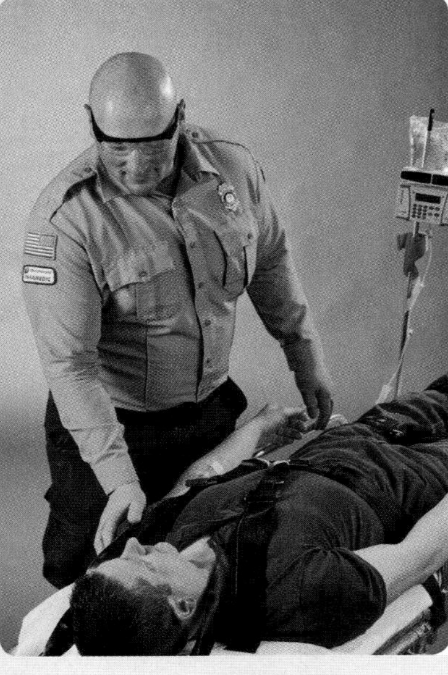

Step 2 Determine the need for the medication based on patient presentation. Obtain a history, including any drug allergies and vital signs. Follow standing orders, or contact medical control for permission. Identify the concentration, then determine the appropriate dose and rate of the infusion. Check the medication to ensure that it is the correct one, that it is not cloudy or discolored, and that the expiration date has not passed, and determine the appropriate amount and concentration for the correct dose. Explain the procedure to the patient and/or parent and the need for the medication.

Skill Drill 14-10 Administering a Medication via Intravenous Piggyback Infusion *(continued)*

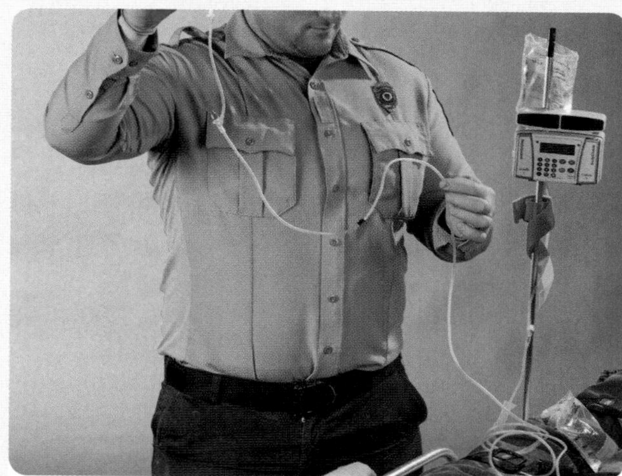

Step 3 Assemble needed equipment. Check medication clarity and expiration date. Ensure you have the proper IV solution, and that it is clear, sterile, and not expired. Ensure you have the correct administration set and correct drip rating. Check for tangling and that the protective covers are on the ends. The flow clamp should be closed.

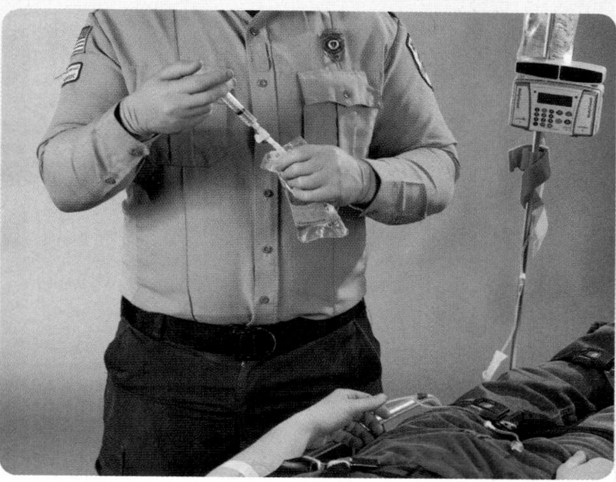

Step 4 Cleanse the injection port of the secondary IV bag (into which the medication will be infused) with alcohol. Inject the medication into the second IV bag and then place the syringe into the sharps container. Gently swirl the IV bag to mix the injected medication into the solution.

Note: Drawing up medications may not be necessary if the manufacturer attaches the medication to the second IV bag (IV antibiotics, some antidysrhythmics, etc).

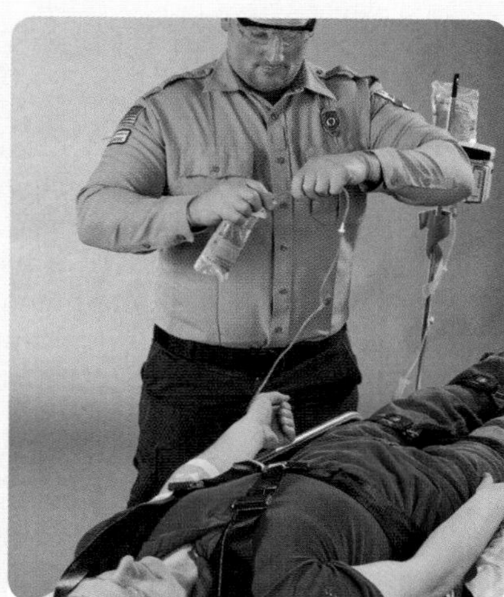

Step 5 Remove the protective cover on the secondary IV bag. Insert the tubing spike into the second IV bag tail port. Turn the bag with the medication upright. Squeeze the drip chamber until it is half full. Maintain sterility.

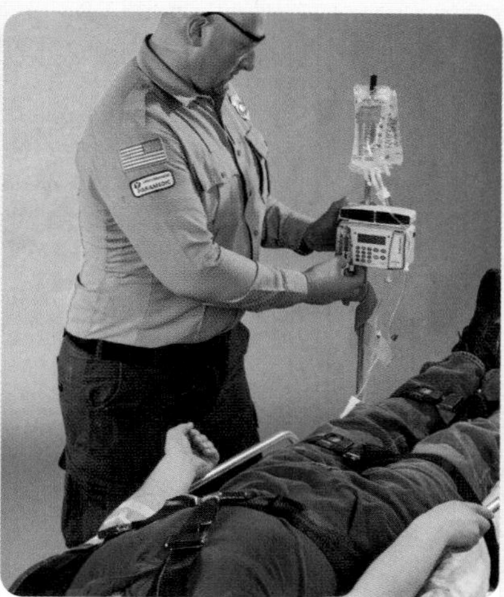

Step 6 Unclamp the line from the secondary IV bag to dispel air from it, or utilize the infusion pump to accomplish this step. Maintain sterility. While removing the air, try to minimize the loss of fluid. Clamp the line after all air bubbles have been removed.

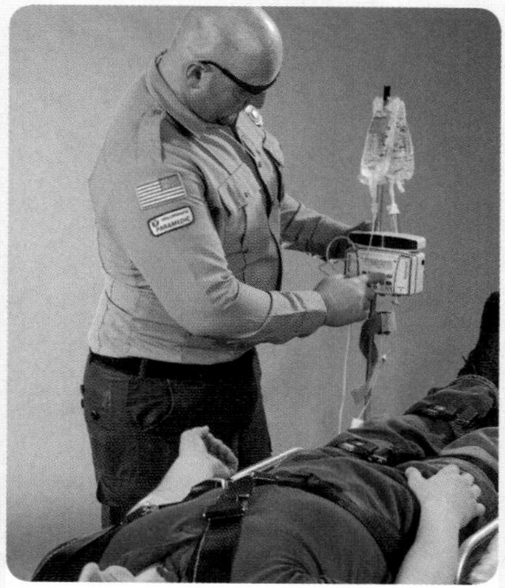

Step 7 If applicable, program the IV infusion pump with the appropriate dose and rate. Place the cartridge from the secondary IV bag in the pump.

(continued)

Skill Drill 14-10 Administering a Medication Via Intravenous Piggyback Infusion *(continued)*

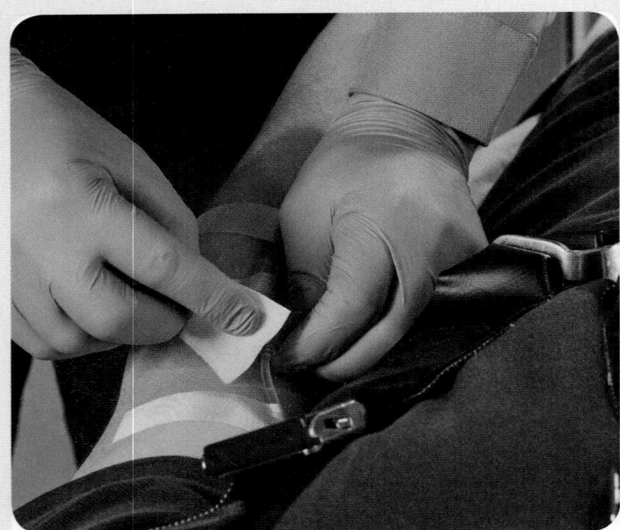

Step 8 Cleanse a port on the primary IV line. Attach the distal end of the secondary IV line to a port on the primary IV line. Begin the flow and ensure that the rate is appropriate. Maintain sterility.

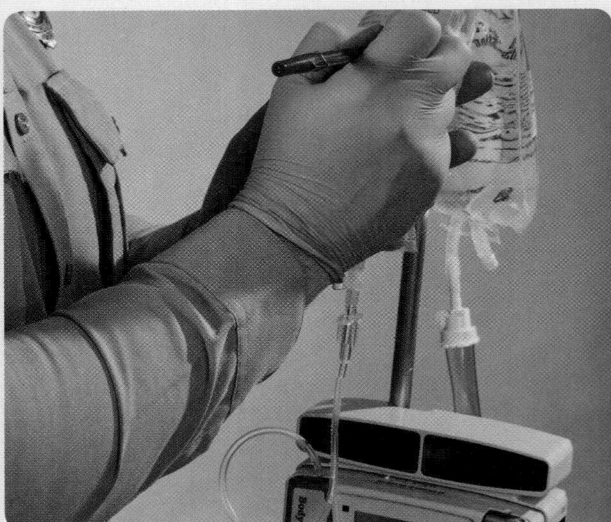

Step 9 Label the secondary IV bag. Monitor the patient's condition, and document the medication given, route, concentration, dose, date time, and your initials. Document the patient's response to the medication.

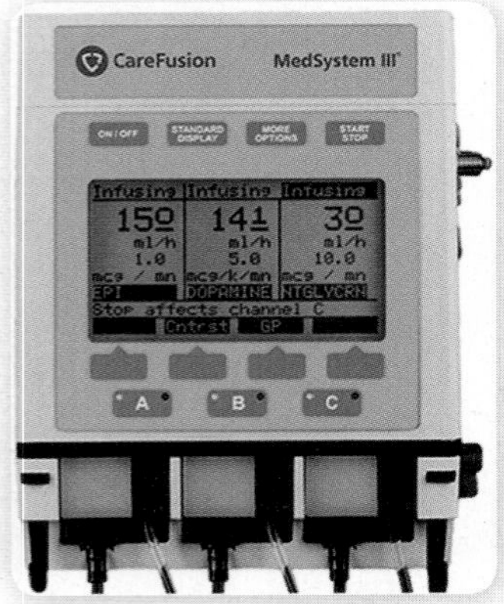

Figure 14-58 Syringe-type infusion pump.

IV Infusion Pumps

When you are administering a medication maintenance infusion where the rate of the medication administration over time is critical, the standard of care within the medical community is to use an IV **infusion pump**, a mechanical device that infuses a precise volume that is programmed by the clinician Figure 14-58. The use of microdrip sets to time infusions is not used in any other area of medicine due to the propensity for medication errors and the variability in drip rate depending on bag height, movement, etc. The infusion pump can also be used to deliver IV fluid maintenance infusions in children and older patients to minimize the risk of a "runaway IV" and subsequent circulatory overload.

IV infusion pumps are used heavily in the hospital and during interfacility transports. They are sometimes used in the prehospital setting as well. IV infusion pumps have many advantages as well as several disadvantages. They are beneficial in that they deliver the rate that is set by the pump without deviating, and they calculate the amount of fluid that has been infused and the amount of fluid remaining. Some problems that can arise include a lack of uniformity among manufacturers. This makes it imperative for you to become familiar with the pumps used by your service.

Pumps can also pose problems during transport because of air trapping in the lines that is detected by the pumps. When air is detected, the pump stops the infusion and an alarm sounds. This becomes problematic during transport when the ambulance travels over

Patient Safety

A tool that is helpful in analyzing potential sources of error or patient harm is *failure mode and effect analysis (FMEA)*. This process was developed by military engineers in the 1940s and further refined and used by NASA (National Aeronautics and Space Administration) engineers working on the Mercury, Gemini, and Apollo space programs. More recently, this process has been used to analyze the potential for health care failures.[8,9] To use FMEA, one constructs a risk matrix for each potential failure that incorporates the likelihood of that failure, the ability to detect the failure, and the potential harm and assigns a risk score to the event Table 14-8. This process can help identify priorities in risk mitigation and process redesign.[10]

potholes, makes hard turns, and is exposed to other applied forces.

IV infusion pumps deliver fluids or medications via positive pressure. Although medications delivered in this manner can result in infiltration of a vein, most infusion pumps are equipped with an alarm that indicates a change in the flow pressure. Other common safety features include alarms that alert you to the presence of occlusion (eg, air in the tubing) or depletion of the medication. IV infusion

Words of Wisdom

Infusion pumps are the standard of care for any medication infusion. As patient clinicians and advocates, you must advocate for their use within the prehospital realm.

Table 14-8 Sample Case Study Using Failure Mode and Effect Analysis

Institute for Safe Medication Practices
Analysis for IV Patient-Controlled Analgesia

Processes and Subprocesses	Failure Modes	Causes	Effects	Severity	Probability	Hazard Score	Actions to Reduce Failure Mode
Prescribing							
Assess patient	Inaccurate pain assessment	Cultural influences; patient unable to articulate	Poor pain control	2	4	8	Standard scale to help assess pain; training on cultural influences
Choose analgesic/ mode of delivery	Incorrect analgesic selected	Clinical situation not considered (age, renal function, allergies, etc); tolerance to opiates not considered; standard PCA protocols not followed (or not available); concomitant use of other analgesics not considered; drug storage; knowledge deficit; improper selection of patients appropriate for PCA	Improper dosing; improper drug; allergic response; improper use of substitute drug	4	3	12	CPOE with decision support, clinical pharmacy program; standard PCA protocol with education on use; point-of-use access to drug information; feedback mechanism on drug shortages with information on substitute drugs available; selection criteria for PCA patients

(continued)

Table 14-8 Sample Case Study Using Failure Mode and Effect Analysis *(Continued)*

Processes and Subprocesses	Failure Modes	Causes	Effects	Severity	Probability	Hazard Score	Actions to Reduce Failure Mode
Prescribe analgesic	Incorrect dose (loading, PCA, constant, lock-out), route, frequency	Knowledge deficit; mental slip; incorrect selection from list; information about drug not available	Overdose; under dose; ADR	4	3	12	CPOE with decision support; clinical pharmacy program; standard PCA protocols
	Proper patient monitoring not ordered	Knowledge deficit; mental slip	Failure to detect problems early to prevent harm	4	3	12	Standard PCA order sets with monitoring guidelines
	Prescribed on wrong patient	Similar patient names; patient identifier not clear; name does not appear on screen when ordering drugs	Incorrect patient receives inappropriate drug and dose; ADR; allergic response	3	3	9	Match therapy to patient's condition; alerts for look-alike patient names; visible demographic information on order form or screen
	No order received	Unable to reach covering physician	Poor pain control	2	2	4	Proper physician coverage and communication channels

Abbreviations: ADR, adverse drug reaction; CPOE, computerized physician order entry; PCA, patient-controlled analgesia.

Modified from: Woodhouse S, Burney B, Coste K. To err is human: improving patient safety through failure mode and effect analysis. *Clin Leadersh Manag Rev.* 2004;18(1):32-36. http://europepmc.org/abstract/med/14968751. Accessed February 3, 2017.

pump tubing is specific to the manufacturer and model and is usually incompatible with other infusion pumps **Figure 14-59**.

You should become familiar with some of the terminology related to infusion pumps. Pumps may have multiple chambers for multiple medications. Each chamber can calculate one medication. If the number of medication lines outweighs the available chambers, then it may be necessary to transport an isotonic fluid on gravity only. This means that your isotonic line will have the gtt/min set manually as opposed to being set by the pump. The rate is always established in mL/hour. Some IV pumps may have medication databases that will calculate the medication rate by the desired dose and the patient's weight as necessary. The volume to be infused is the amount of solution remaining to be infused. For example, if you were infusing 100 mL of amiodarone and 25 mL has already been infused, then 75 mL is your

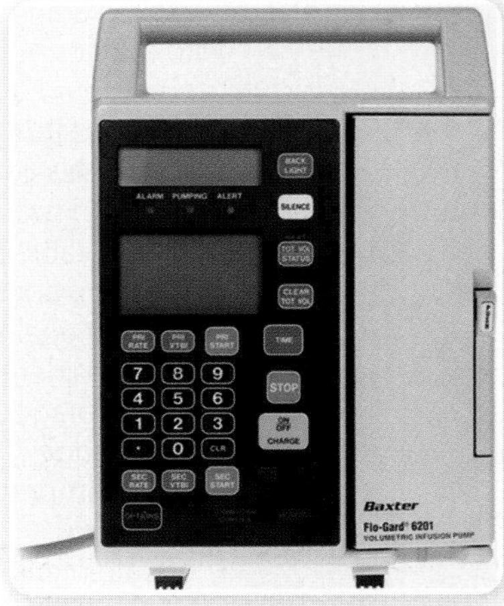

Figure 14-59 Infusion pump that accommodates intravenous tubing.

Courtesy of Baxter International Inc.

volume to be infused. The volume infused is the amount of solution that has already been administered, 25 mL as stated above. If your infusion pump does not perform medication calculations, then this formula will help you determine the rate at which to set the pump:

Example:
Nitroglycerin drips are common interfacility medications for acute coronary syndrome and are being established in the prehospital setting in some areas. The doses range from 5 to 50 mcg/min. This calculation will start at 5 mcg/min. You have 25 mg in 250 mL.

Step 1: Determine the concentration.

$$25 \text{ mg} \times \frac{1{,}000 \text{ mcg}}{\text{mg}} = 25{,}000 \text{ mcg}$$

$$25{,}000 \text{ mcg} \div 250 \text{ mL} = 100 \text{ mcg/mL}$$
(concentration)

Step 2: Determine the amount of volume to infuse per minute (mL/min).

For this calculation, you must recall the desired dose—in this case, 5 mcg/min. To determine the number of mL/min, you perform the following calculation:

$$5 \text{ mcg/min (desired dose)} \div 100 \text{ mcg/mL (concentration)} = 0.05 \text{ mL/min}$$

Step 3: Determine the rate and volume to be infused.

The rate can be established by multiplying the mL/min by 60.

$$\frac{0.05 \text{ mL}}{\text{min}} \times \frac{60 \text{ min}}{\text{h}} = 3 \text{ mL/h}$$

The volume to be infused for nitroglycerin as packaged above is 250 mL unless otherwise requested by medical control. Therefore, infuse this volume at 3 mL/h until it is administered, or until you arrive at the receiving facility.

IV infusion pumps come in a wide variety of configurations. You should be familiar with the basic concepts discussed in this section but seek individual training on the specific infusion pump you will use in practice. Become familiar with the tubing, cartridges, and basic way to navigate the pump and ensure your comfort with the device prior to utilizing it with a patient.

IO Medication Administration

The IO route is used for critically ill or injured children and adults when IV access is difficult or impossible to obtain. Any fluid or medication that may be given through an IV line—bolus or maintenance infusion—can be given by the IO route. Shock, status epilepticus, and cardiac arrest are but a few of the reasons for establishing IO access. Unlike with an IV line, fluid does not flow well into the bone because of resistance; therefore, it is necessary to use a large syringe to infuse the fluid. A pressure infuser device—a sleeve placed around the IV bag and inflated to force fluid from the IV bag—should be used when infusing fluids in adults.

Complications of using the IO route are similar to those of the IV route. Along with the complications discussed earlier in this chapter, there is also the potential for compartment syndrome if fluid leaks outside the bone and into the osteofascial compartment.

Follow the steps in Skill Drill 14-11 to administer a medication via the IO route.

Percutaneous Medication Administration

With **percutaneous** routes of administration, medications are applied to and absorbed through the skin and mucous membranes. Because percutaneously administered medications bypass the gastrointestinal tract, their absorption is more predictable. Percutaneous routes of medication administration include the transdermal, sublingual, buccal, ocular, aural, and nasal routes.

Transdermal Medication Administration

Transdermal medications are applied topically—that is, on the surface of the body. Ordinarily, intact skin is an effective barrier to medication absorption. However, some medications have been specially prepared to cross that barrier at a slow steady rate, so the transdermal route is useful for the sustained release of certain medications.

Nitroglycerin, estrogen, nicotine, and analgesic patches, for example, are applied to the skin and release medications over a specified period. Creams, lotions, and pastes (eg, nitroglycerin paste, corticosteroid cream) are also transdermally administered medications.

Factors that can increase the speed of transdermal absorption include administration of too much of the medication (ie, inadvertent or intentional overdose) and thin or nonintact skin. Decreased speed of transdermal absorption can be caused by factors such as thick skin, scar tissue in the area to which the medication is applied, and peripheral vascular disease.

Some medications, such as nitroglycerin paste, may be applied in the prehospital setting. Usually though, providers will be assisting patients with their own transdermal patches. If your service uses nitroglycerin, or another transdermal medication, then you will perform the following steps:

1. Take standard precautions.
2. Determine the need for the medication based on patient presentation.
3. Obtain a history, including any drug allergies and vital signs.
4. Follow standing orders, or contact medical control for permission.

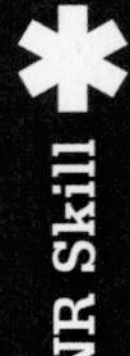

Skill Drill 14-11 Administering Medication via the Intraosseous Route

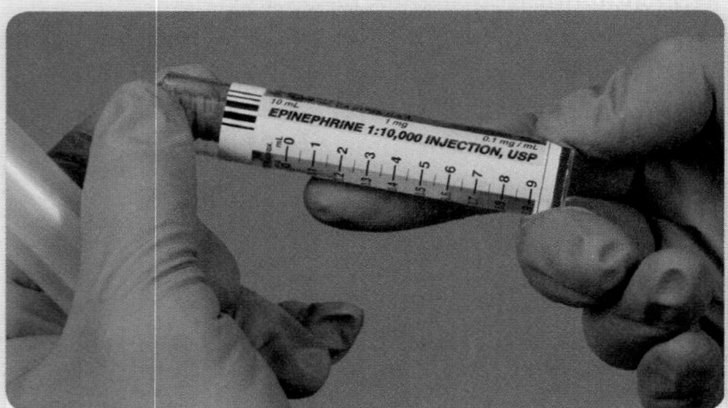

Step 1 Take standard precautions. Determine the need for the medication based on patient presentation. Obtain a history, including any drug allergies and vital signs. Follow standing orders, or contact medical control for permission. Check the medication to ensure that it is the correct one, that it is not cloudy or discolored, and that the expiration date has not passed, and determine the appropriate amount and concentration for the correct dose.

Explain the procedure to the patient and/or parent and the need for the medication.

Assemble needed equipment and draw up the medication. Also draw up 20 mL of normal saline for a flush.

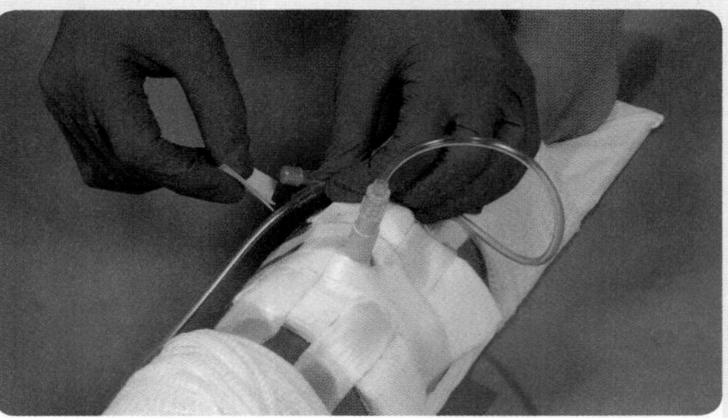

Step 2 Cleanse the injection port of the extension tubing with alcohol, or remove the protective cap if using the needleless system.

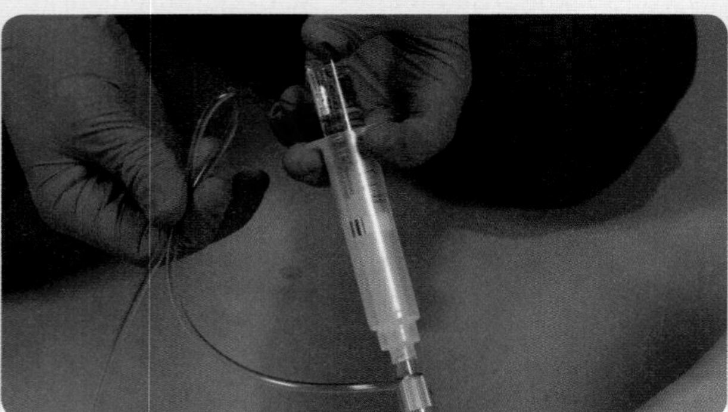

Step 3 Insert the needle into the port, and clamp off the IV tubing proximal to the administration port. This is usually managed with a three-way stopcock. Failure to shut off the line will result in the medication taking the pathway of least resistance and flowing into the bag instead of into the patient.

Administer the correct dose of the medication at the proper push rate. Some medications must be administered quickly, whereas others must be pushed slowly to prevent adverse effects.

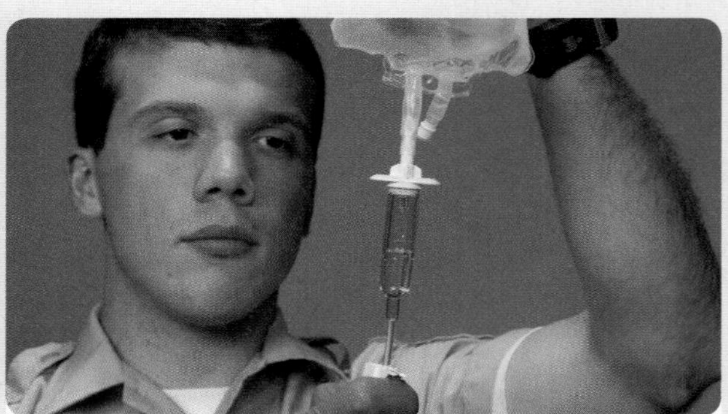

Step 4 Place the needle and syringe into the sharps container. Unclamp the IV line to flush the medication into the site. Flush with at least a 20-mL bolus of normal saline. Readjust the IV flow rate to the original setting. Store any unused medication properly.

Monitor the patient's condition, and document the medication given, route, time of administration, and response of the patient.

5. Check the medication patch or cream to ensure that it is the correct one and that the expiration date has not passed, and determine the appropriate amount for the correct dose.
6. Explain the procedure to the patient and the need for the medication.
7. Clean and dry the area of the skin where the medication will be applied.
8. Apply the medication to the area in accordance with the manufacturer's specifications.
9. Monitor the patient's condition, and document the medication given, route, time of administration, and response of the patient.

Words of Wisdom

During assessment of your patient, look for transdermal medication patches, especially narcotic and nitroglycerin patches, which can result in hypotension. If the patient is already in a hemodynamically unstable condition, then narcotics and nitroglycerin may complicate the clinical picture.

Do not, under any circumstances, administer, assist, or in any other manner come in contact with transdermal medications without taking the proper standard precautions. These medications are designed to go through skin and can easily be absorbed through ungloved hands.

Sublingual Medication Administration

The **sublingual** (under the tongue) region is highly vascular, so medications given via the sublingual route are rapidly absorbed. Sublingually administered medications, relative to enterally administered medications, get into the circulation much faster. Nitroglycerin—spray or tablet—is a medication that is most commonly administered via the sublingual route **Figure 14-60**.

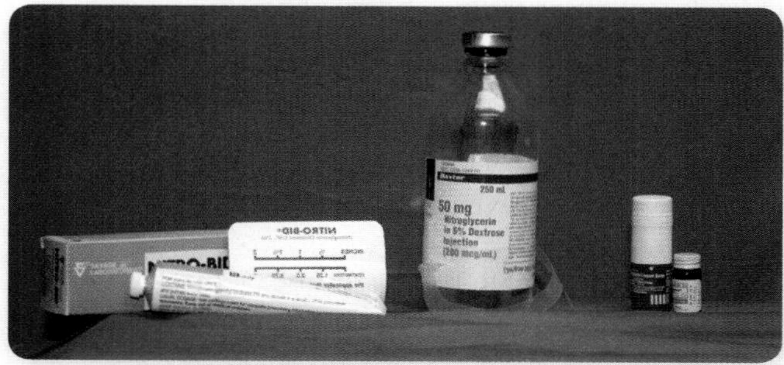

Figure 14-60 Nitroglycerin is often given sublingually as a spray or a tablet. It is also available as a transdermal patch or paste and can be administered as an intravenous drip.

Medications may also be *injected* into the network of veins (venous plexus) under the tongue (basically this is another form of IV injection). This technique is especially useful for giving narcotic antagonists to patients who have overdosed on heroin because finding a suitable vein in such patients may be nearly impossible.

To administer a sublingual medication, follow the steps in **Skill Drill 14-12**.

Words of Wisdom

If using a spray medication dispenser, then spray it once or twice away from the patient and the crew prior to administration. Doing this will ensure the dispenser is primed and that the patient will receive the full dose of the medication. Also, as with transdermal medications, use proper standard precautions because nitroglycerin can be absorbed through your hands.

Buccal Medication Administration

The **buccal** region, which is also highly vascular, lies in between the cheek and gums. Most medications administered via the buccal route are in the form of tablets or gels. Glucose is one of the few medications that may be administered buccally in the prehospital setting.

To administer a medication via the buccal route, follow these steps:

1. Take standard precautions.
2. Determine the need for the medication based on patient presentation.
3. Obtain a history, including any drug allergies and vital signs.
4. Follow standing orders, or contact medical control for permission.
5. Check the medication to ensure that it is the correct one and that its expiration date has not passed. Determine the appropriate amount for the correct dose.
6. Explain the procedure to the patient and the need for the medication.
7. Place the medication in between the patient's cheek and gum, or ask the patient to do so.
8. Advise the patient not to chew or swallow the tablet, but to let it dissolve slowly.
9. Monitor the patient's condition, and document the medication given, route, administration time, and response of the patient.

Ocular Medication Administration

Drops or ointments are commonly administered via the **ocular** route **Figure 14-61**. Ocular medications are typically administered for pain relief, allergies, drying of the eyes, or infections. Other than assisting a patient with

Skill Drill 14-12 Administering Medication via the Sublingual Route

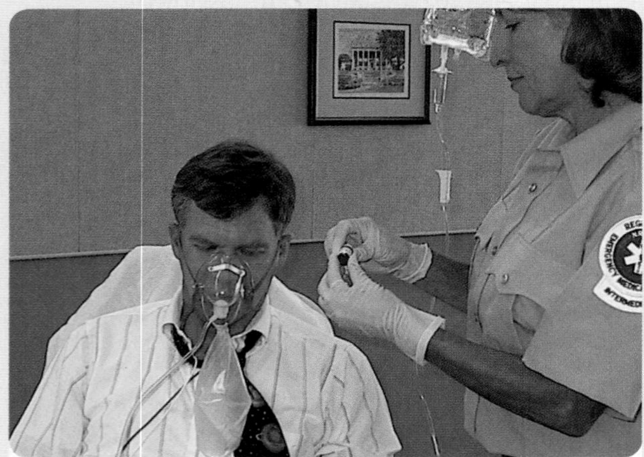

Step 1 Take standard precautions. Determine the need for the medication based on patient presentation. Obtain a history, including any drug allergies and vital signs. Follow standing orders, or contact medical control for permission. Check the medication to ensure that it is the correct one and that its expiration date has not passed, and determine the appropriate amount for the correct dose.

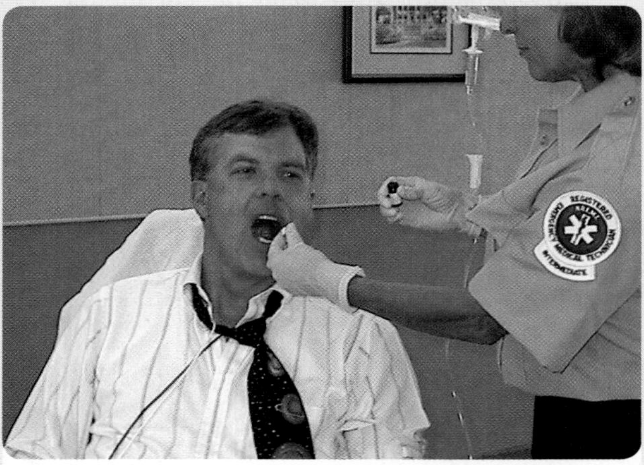

Step 2 Ask the patient to rinse his or her mouth with a little water if the mucous membranes are dry. Explain the procedure, and ask the patient to lift his or her tongue.

Place the tablet or spray the dose under the tongue, or ask the patient to do so. Advise the patient not to chew or swallow the tablet, but to let it dissolve slowly.

Monitor the patient's condition, and document the medication given, route, administration time, and patient's response.

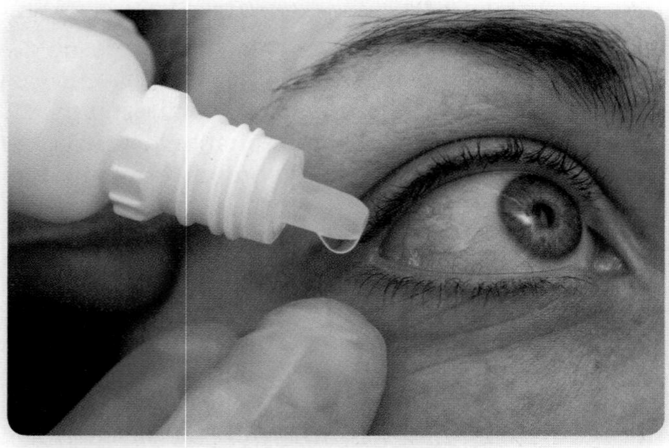

Figure 14-61 The ocular route.

his or her ocular medication or irrigating a patient's eyes following a toxic exposure, medication administration in the prehospital setting via the ocular route is rare. In the hospital and in some prehospital systems, providers utilize bottles to squeeze out the prescribed amount of drops into the eye. A commercial device known as the Morgan lens can be used to administer some ophthalmic medications, particularly local anesthetics. The device uses a proprietary lens that connects to an IV drop set and IV fluids. While it's used predominantly for irrigation, some medications may be used in or with the Morgan lens. The Morgan lens is discussed in Chapter 19, *Diseases of the Eyes, Ears, Nose, and Throat*.

If a patient asks you to assist him or her with ocular medication administration, follow these steps:

1. Take standard precautions.
2. If administering a prescribed medication, then confirm the medication is prescribed to the patient.
3. Place the patient in a supine position, or have the patient place his or her head back and look up.
4. *Without touching the eyeball,* expose the conjunctiva by gently pulling down on the lower eyelid.

5. Administer the required amount of medication on the conjunctival sac by using an eye dropper. Do not apply the medication directly on the eyeball.
6. Advise the patient to close his or her eyes for 1 to 2 minutes.
7. Document the medication name, route, dose, and administration time. Monitor the patient's condition and response.

Aural Medication Administration

Certain medications—mainly antibiotics, analgesics, and earwax removal preparations—are administered via the mucous membranes of the **aural** (ear) canal. As with ocular medications, the aural route is rarely, if ever, used in the prehospital setting.

If you are asked by the patient to assist in administering his or her aural medication, then follow these steps:

1. Take standard precautions.
2. Confirm the medication is prescribed to the patient.
3. Place the patient on his or her side with the affected ear facing up.
4. Expose the ear canal by pulling the ear up and back (adults) or down and back (infants and children).
5. Administer the medication in the appropriate dose with a medicine dropper.
6. Document the medication name, route, dose, and administration time. Monitor the patient's condition and response.

Intranasal Medication Administration

Intranasal (within the nose) medications include nasal spray for congestion or solutions to moisten the nasal mucosa. In recent years, this route of medication administration has become more popular in the prehospital setting. Intranasally administered medications are rapidly absorbed, providing a more rapid onset of action than IM injections. For example, some studies suggest that intranasal fentanyl has an equal onset and duration to IV morphine. Administration of emergency medications via the intranasal route is performed with a **mucosal atomizer device (MAD)** Figure 14-62. The MAD attaches to a syringe and allows you to spray (atomize) select medications into the nasal mucosa.

Owing to the molecular structure of drugs, only a few emergency medications can be given intranasally, including naloxone (Narcan), midazolam (Versed), glucagon (GlucaGen), ketorolac (Toradol), flumazenil (Romazicon), and fentanyl citrate. Typically, intranasal medications require 2 to 2.5 times the dose of IV medications. Follow local protocol, or consult with medical control about the appropriate doses of these medications and any other medications that may be administered intranasally.

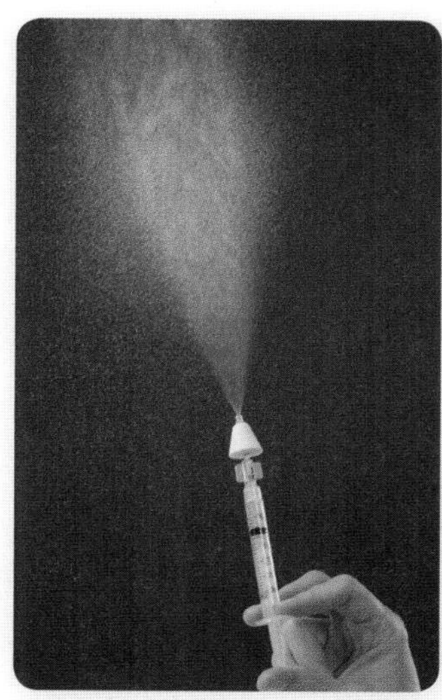

Figure 14-62 Mucosal atomizer device.

To administer a medication via the intranasal route, follow the steps in Skill Drill 14-13.

Medications Administered by the Inhalation Route

Nebulizer and Metered-Dose Inhaler

Many medications used in the treatment of respiratory emergencies are administered via the **inhalation** route. The most common inhaled medication is oxygen. Beta$_2$ agonist bronchodilators (eg, albuterol [Ventolin, Proventil], isoetharine [Bronkosol], metaproterenol [Alupent]) are often administered in the prehospital setting for patients experiencing respiratory distress caused by certain obstructive airway diseases, such as asthma, bronchitis, and emphysema. Other medications, such as ipratropium bromide (Atrovent)—an anticholinergic bronchodilator—are also administered via the inhalation route. Check your drug reference guide or the package insert for the indications, contraindications, and precautions before giving any of these medications.

A patient with a history of respiratory problems will usually have a **metered-dose inhaler (MDI)** to use on a regular basis or as needed Figure 14-63. MDIs are usually administered by the patient using the patient's own prescribed medications, but paramedics must know how to administer via this route because they may assist the patient with administration. Medications administered by the MDI can be delivered through a mouthpiece held by the patient or by a mask—with or without a spacer device—for young children and patients who are unable to hold the mouthpiece Figure 14-64.

Skill Drill 14-13 Administering Medication via the Intranasal Route

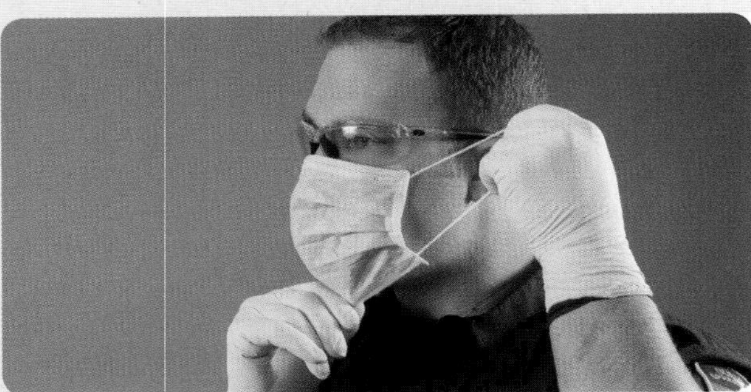

Step 1 Take standard precautions. Determine the need for the medication based on patient presentation. Obtain a history, including any drug allergies and vital signs. Assemble and collect the needed equipment, including the MAD. Follow standing orders, or contact medical control for permission. Check the medication to ensure that it is the correct one, that it is not cloudy or discolored, and that the expiration date has not passed.

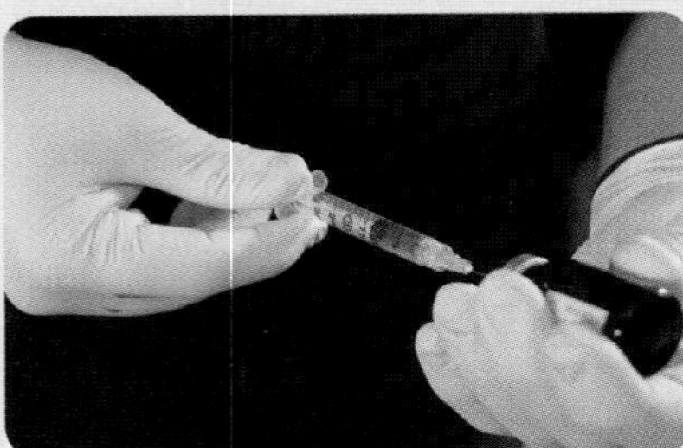

Step 2 Draw up the appropriate dose of medication in the syringe, dispel air, and reconfirm medication. Dispose of needle properly.

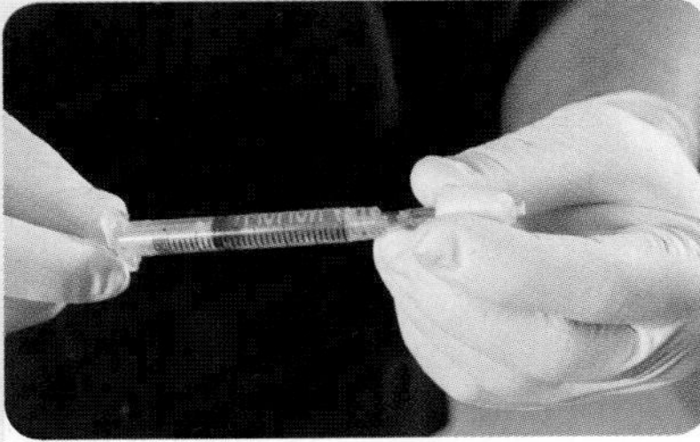

Step 3 Attach the MAD to the syringe, maintaining sterility.

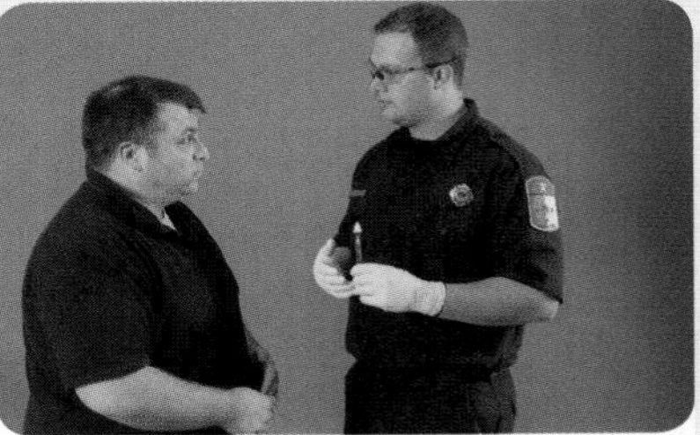

Step 4 Explain the procedure to the patient (or to a relative if the patient is unresponsive) and the need for the medication. Stop ventilation of the patient if necessary; remove any masks. Insert the MAD into the larger and less deviated or less obstructed nostril.

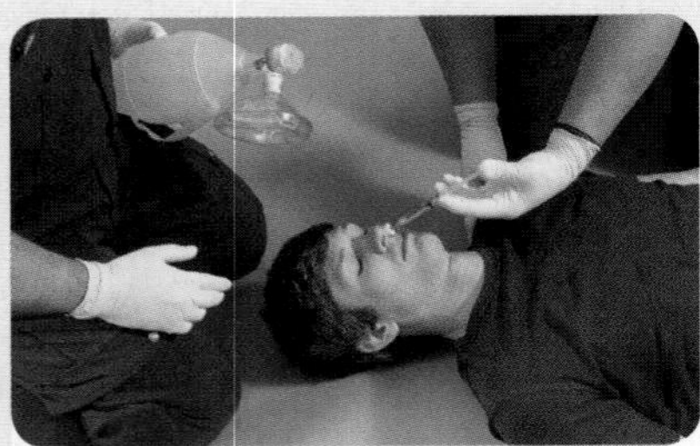

Step 5 Quickly spray the medication dose into a nostril.

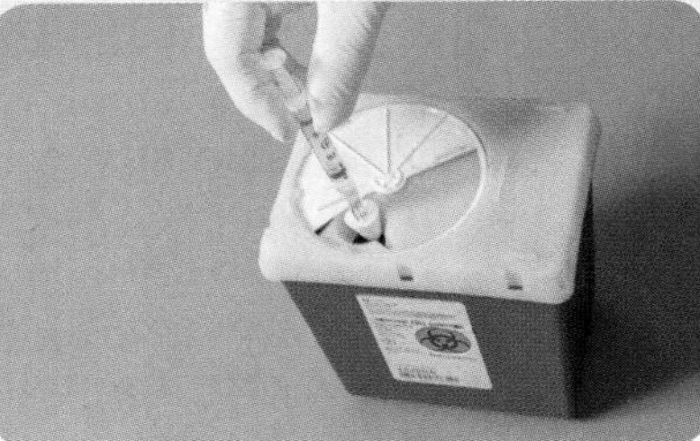

Step 6 Dispose of the MAD and syringe in the appropriate container.

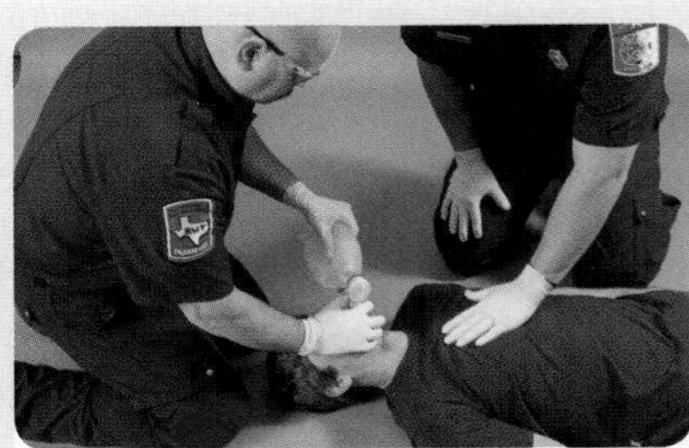

Step 7 Monitor the patient's condition. Document the medication given, route, time of administration, and response of the patient.

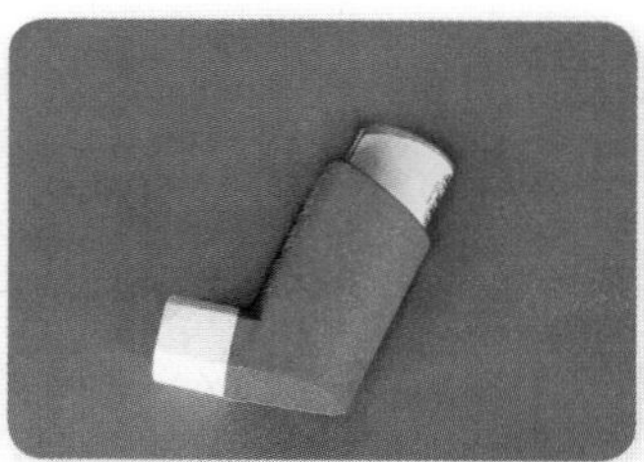

Figure 14-63 Some medications are inhaled into the lungs with a metered-dose inhaler so that they can be absorbed quickly into the bloodstream.

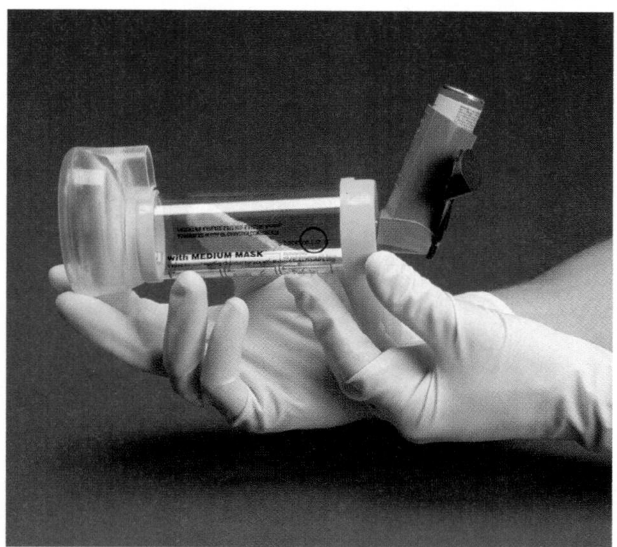

A

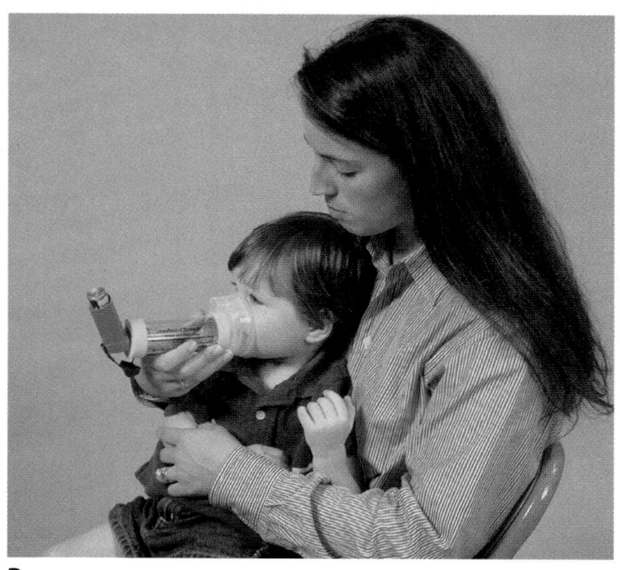

B

Figure 14-64 A. In children, a metered-dose inhaler and spacer can be used with or without a mask. **B.** Children as young as 6 months can use a mask and spacer device.

Follow the steps in Skill Drill 14-14 to help a patient self-administer medication from an inhaler.

Words of Wisdom

MDIs are also called HFAs, after the propellant hydrofluoroalkane that is now used instead of chlorofluorocarbons.

For more severe problems, liquid bronchodilators may be aerosolized in a **nebulizer** for inhalation. Small-volume nebulizers (also called updraft or handheld nebulizers) are the most commonly used method of administration of inhaled medications in the prehospital setting Figure 14-65. Oxygen or a compressed air source is connected to the nebulizer to produce the aerosolized mist.

Some nebulizers have been adapted with child-friendly shapes and images to ease the use with pediatric patients. They may allow for blow-by administration to help the patient tolerate the medication. Other methods used on patients include a nebulized mask that does not require the patient to hold the device. Some adapters have been designed to allow providers to administer nebulized medications to intubated patients with each ventilation Figure 14-66. These devices may also be adapted for use with CPAP masks Figure 14-67.

Follow the steps in Skill Drill 14-15 to administer a medication via a small-volume nebulizer.

Some patients with respiratory emergencies may be breathing inadequately (ie, inadequate tidal volume, fast or slow respiratory rate) and will not be able to effectively inhale beta-agonist medications into the lungs via a nebulizer or an MDI. In this case, utilize a small-volume nebulizer in-line with the assistive device. If the patient is intubated, then assist with bag-mask ventilation or a ventilator by placing a short piece of corrugated tubing, separated by a T-piece, to connect the nebulizer. When utilizing CPAP, most manufacturers have a nebulizer that is designed to work with their device. The nebulizer should be placed between the assistive device and mask, or ET tube if the patient is intubated, with a separate oxygen line connected to the nebulizer.

▶ Endotracheal Medication Administration

If IV or IO access is unavailable, then certain resuscitative medications can be administered down the ET tube. As a paramedic, you should remember absorption rates with this route are poor and other, more effective routes should be utilized prior to attempting medication administration

Skill Drill 14-14 Assisting a Patient With a Metered-Dose Inhaler

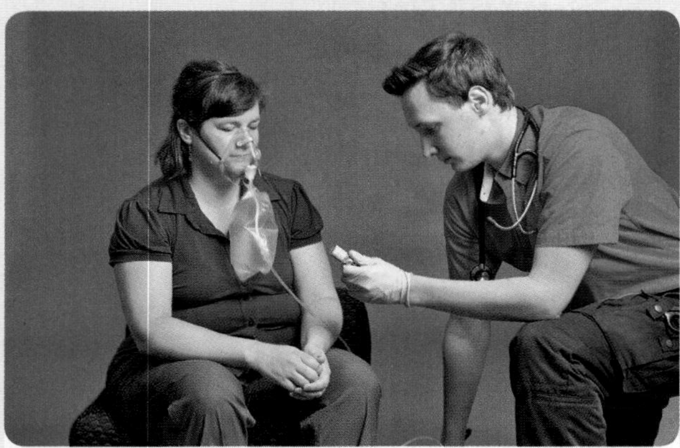

Step 1 Take standard precautions. Obtain an order from medical control or follow local protocol. Assemble the needed equipment.

Ensure you have the right medication, right patient, right dose, right route, and that the medication is not expired.

Ensure the patient is alert enough to use the inhaler. Check to see whether the patient has already taken any doses. Obtain baseline breath sounds for comparison after a few minutes of inhaler use. Ensure the inhaler is at room temperature or warmer.

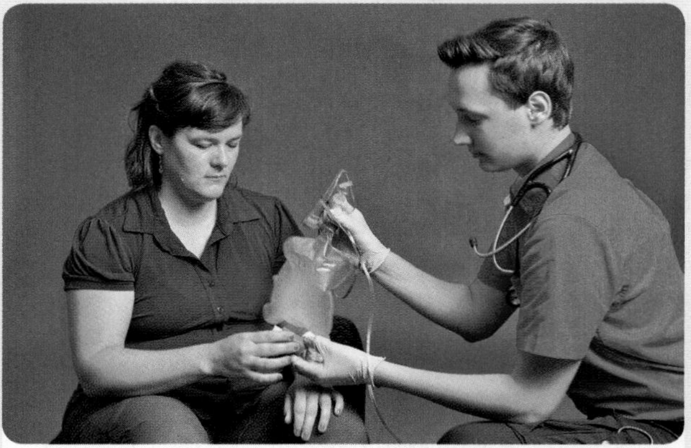

Step 2 Shake the inhaler vigorously several times. Stop administering supplemental oxygen and remove any mask from the patient's face. Ask the patient to exhale deeply and, before inhaling, to put his or her lips around the opening of the inhaler.

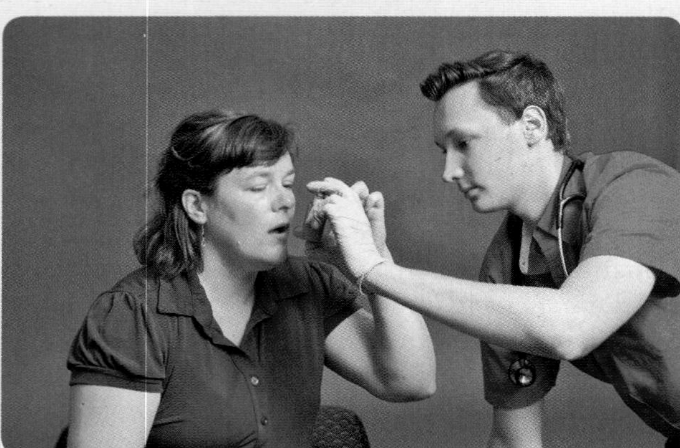

Step 3 If the patient has a spacer, then attach it to allow more effective use of the medication. Have the patient depress the handheld inhaler as he or she begins to inhale deeply.

Instruct the patient to hold his or her breath for as long as he or she comfortably can to help the lungs absorb the medication.

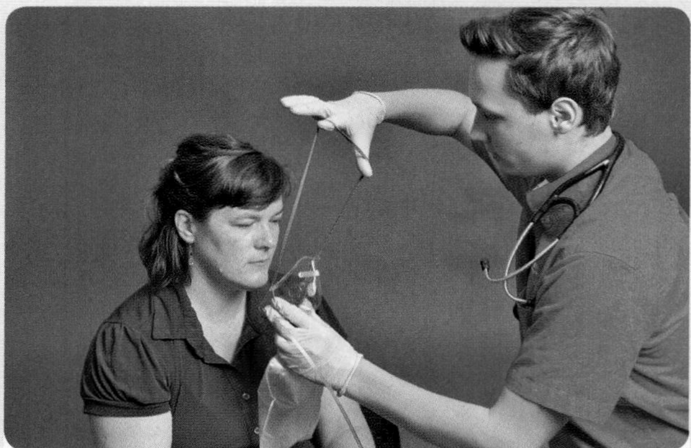

Step 4 Continue administering supplemental oxygen.

Allow the patient to breathe a few times, then give the second dose per direction from medical control or according to local protocol. Monitor the patient's condition, and document the medication given, route, administration time, and response of the patient.

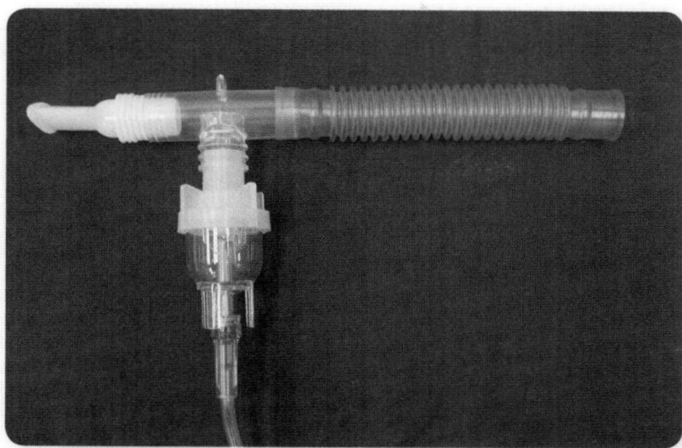

Figure 14-65 A small-volume nebulizer is used to deliver medications via aerosolized mist.

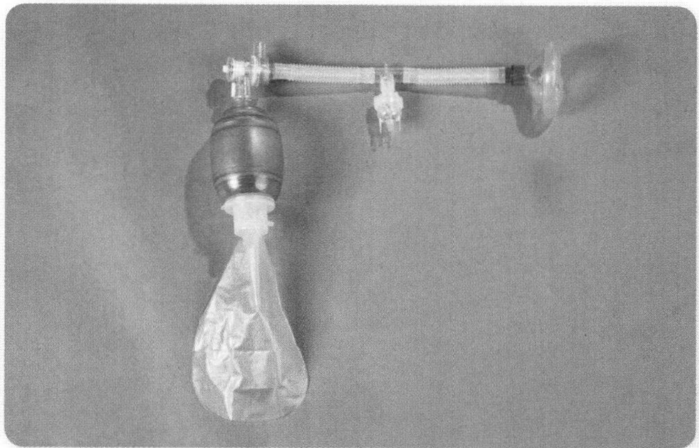

Figure 14-66 A nebulizer can be attached to a bag-mask device and administered through the mask.

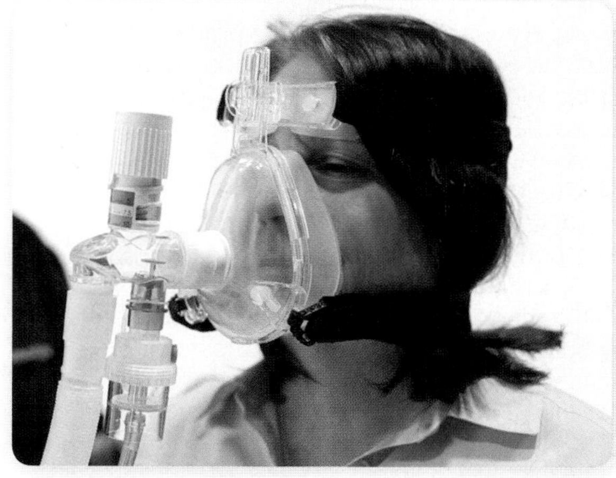

Figure 14-67 A nebulized medication being administered through a continuous positive airway pressure mask.

Controversies

In the past, nebulizers were considered the preferred method of administering beta-agonist medications for the treatment of asthma attacks. Recent studies, however, have shown that MDIs—especially when used with spacing devices—are at least as effective as nebulizers and have several distinct advantages[11,12]:

- MDIs are *more convenient* than nebulizers. They do not require any setup time or a source of compressed gas.
- MDIs are *more reliable* than nebulizers. With a nebulizer, one cannot be certain that the patient is getting the full dose of the drug. MDIs deliver a more consistent amount of drug aerosol.
- Because most people with asthma use MDIs at home, using the MDI in an emergency provides an excellent opportunity to *educate the patient* in proper use of the device. Studies have shown that more than half of patients using MDIs at home employ an incorrect and ineffective technique. Showing a patient the correct technique and demonstrating its effectiveness can improve the outcome of subsequent asthma attacks.

through an ET tube. The optimal ET dose of most medications is unknown, but the usual dose given by the ET route is 2 to 2.5 times the recommended IV dose for the medication to be adequately dispersed throughout the tracheobronchial tree.[13] When necessary, medications that can be administered via the ET route can be remembered with the mnemonic LEAN (or LANE): Lidocaine, Epinephrine, Atropine, and Naloxone (Narcan).[13] While naloxone is accepted to be administered via the ET tube, it is contraindicated for neonates. As always, check your local protocols prior to administration.

Long-Term Vascular Access Devices

There may be some situations where IV access is imperative but difficult to obtain. Some of these patients may have a long-term VAD inserted. These patients may be receiving an antibiotic regimen, chemotherapy, regular blood draws for chronic disorders, hemodialysis, or other acute or chronic illnesses. These patients will be upfront about their medical device and will generally request that you not insert a peripheral line.

If you encounter a patient with a long-term VAD, you will generally see there are two types: non-tunneling and implanted. Most protocols only allow the use of these VADs during critical events. These devices are usually preserved with heparin to prevent clotting. Because these devices are

NR Skill

Skill Drill 14-15 Administering a Medication via a Small-Volume Nebulizer

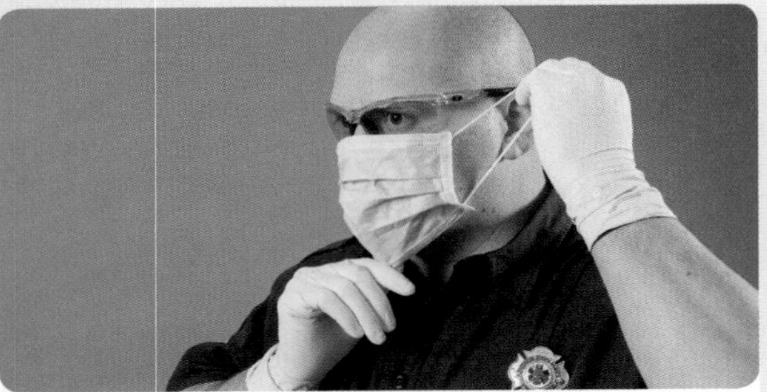

Step 1 Take standard precautions. Determine the need for an inhaled bronchodilator based on patient presentation. Obtain a history, including any drug allergies and vital signs.

Follow standing orders, or contact medical control for permission. Check the medication and its expiration date. Make sure that you have the right medication and that it is not cloudy or discolored. Assemble and check needed equipment.

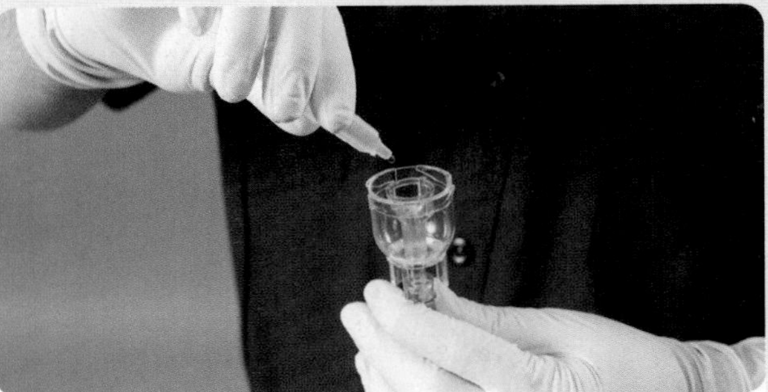

Step 2 If the medication is in a premixed package, then add it to the bowl of the nebulizer. If it is not premixed, then add the medication to the bowl and mix it with the specified amount of normal saline, usually 2.5 to 3 mL.

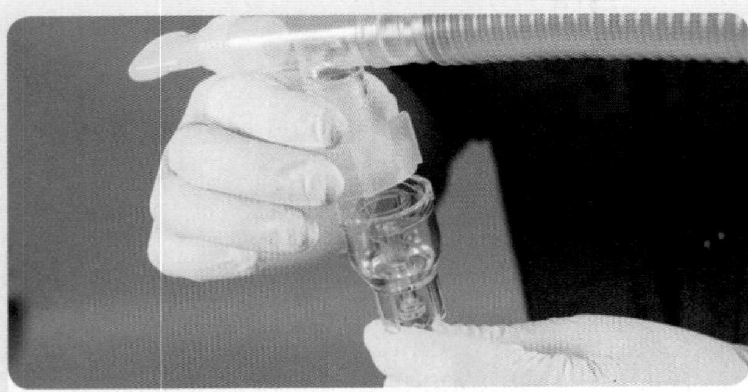

Step 3 Connect the T piece with the mouthpiece to the top of the bowl, or the mask to the bowl, and connect it to the oxygen tubing.

Set the flowmeter at 6 L/min to produce a steady mist. Remove the oxygen mask from the patient if oxygen is being administered.

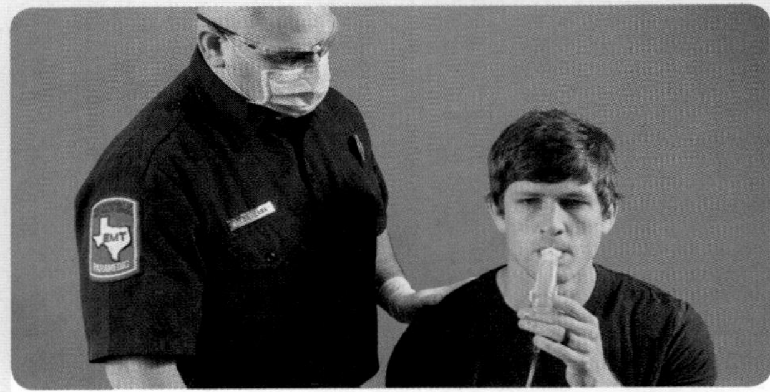

Step 4 With the MDI or handheld nebulizer in position, instruct the patient on the proper way to breathe. Have the patient breathe as deeply as possible and hold his or her breath for 3 to 5 seconds before exhaling. Continue to coach the patient as needed.

Monitor the patient's condition, and document the medication given, route, time of administration, and response of the patient to the medication.

Cardiac monitoring is essential when administering a beta agonist. If cardiac dysrhythmias are noted, then stop administering the medication, manage in accordance with current resuscitation guidelines, and contact medical control.

not accessed frequently in the prehospital or interfacility setting, it is imperative that you seek out regular training on how to access and use these devices.

Non-tunneling. Non-tunneling devices are devices that have been inserted by direct venipuncture through the skin directly into a selected vein. The most common devices that will be encountered in the prehospital and interfacility setting are peripheral inserted central catheters (PICCs), midline, and central venous catheters (CVCs).

PICCs are frequently used for long-term medication administration, chemotherapy, frequent venous sampling, and total parenteral nutrition. PICCs are generally inserted by designated PICC nurses who receive specific training on PICC insertion. The insertion point is usually at the antecubital vein, while the distal end of the PICC usually sits at the superior vena cava and is verified by a radiograph. PICCs may be left in place for 6 to 8 weeks. Some patients may have their PICC accessed by family or home health regularly. The PICC may have a single, double, or triple lumen.

Midlines are also inserted at the antecubital vein. However, unlike a PICC, the distal end of the midline rests at the proximal end of the extremity. Midlines can generally be used for approximately 4 weeks. They can also be used for shorter medication therapies and venous therapies. CVCs are generally inserted in emergent situations by physicians into the subclavian, femoral, or internal jugular vein, and are used for emergent medication administration, fluid resuscitation, blood administration, or blood sampling. These catheters are generally large-bore and may sit near the vena cava.

Follow the steps in Skill Drill 14-16 for how to access a tunneling device.

Implanted. Implanted vascular access devices are implanted in surgery, sutured under the skin. These devices are palpable outside the skin but are not exposed to the outside environment. The device consists of a self-sealing core inserted in a stainless steel, titanium, or plastic shell connected to a catheter that runs into the superior vena

> **Words of Wisdom**
>
> When you are accessing multilumen devices, you should always attempt to access the largest lumen first. If the lumens are the same diameter, then you should access the distal lumen. The lumen that should be used will generally be marked by the number 1.

Skill Drill 14-16 Accessing a Tunneling Device

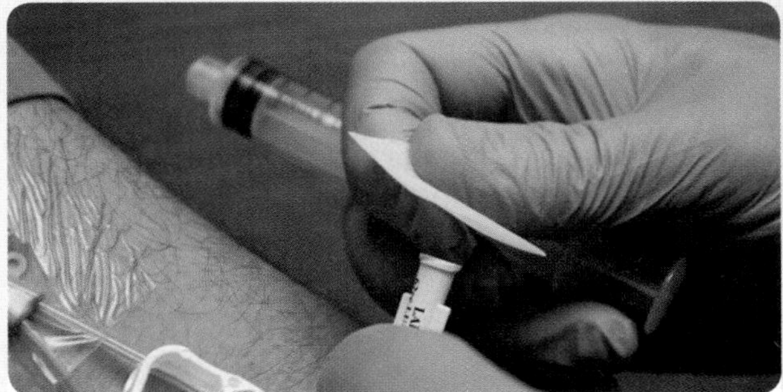

Step 1 Use aseptic technique. Prepare all of the appropriate equipment: Empty 10- to 20-mL syringe (nothing less than a 10-mL syringe should be used), 10-mL normal saline flush, sterile gloves, alcohol prep, 10-gtt administration set, 500 mL normal saline.

Ensure all lumens are clamped. Air embolism is a serious risk with these patients because many of these devices go directly into the vena cava. That is why central lines must be clamped whenever they are not in use.

Use an alcohol prep to prepare the lumen that will be used.

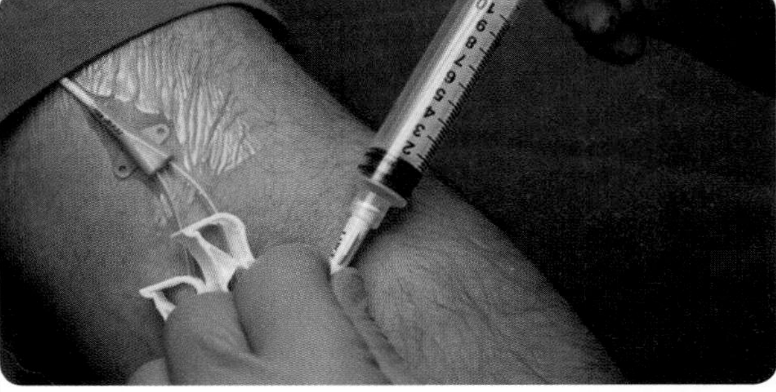

Step 2 Attach the empty syringe and withdraw a minimum of 10 mL of blood from the lumen. Discard this immediately into the sharps container. Do not withdraw too forcefully. If you meet some resistance, then gently flush and withdraw. Ask the patient to turn his or her head in the opposite direction of the central line.

(continued)

Skill Drill 14-16 Accessing a Tunneling Device *(continued)*

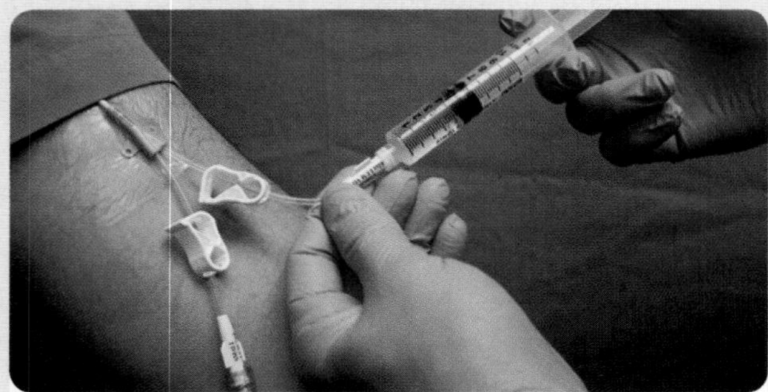

Step 3 After you have withdrawn the 10 mL of blood, attach the 10-mL syringe filled with normal saline and slowly administer it.

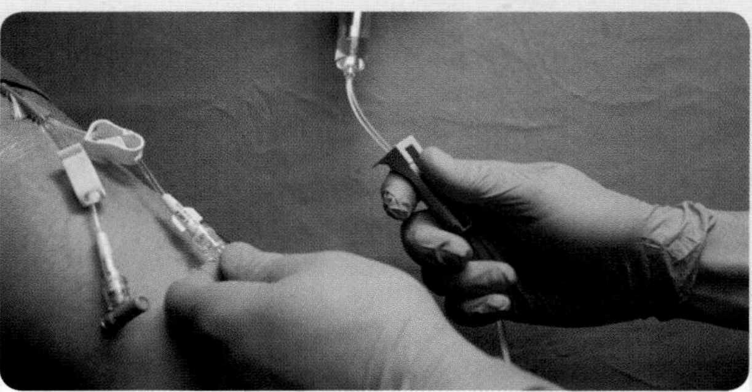

Step 4 Attach the prepared IV drip set and set it up for at least 10 mL/h. Depending on the size of the catheter, you can infuse at a rate of 125 to 250 mL/h. The line must be running continuously because heparin is not available.

Administer IV medications through the attached IV drip set.

Monitor the patient's condition, and document the medication given, route, administration time, and response of the patient.

cava. These devices can only be accessed with a Huber needle that is non coring and has a mild angle. These devices can be used for long-term medication administration, total parenteral nutrition, chemotherapy, blood products, or venous blood sampling.

Arteriovenous (AV) fistulas are used for a variety of disorders. They are created by connecting a vein and an artery. For kidney failure, hemodialysis uses AV fistulas to dialize the blood. AV fistulas are also used for plasmapheresis in various disorders such as myasthenia gravis and Guillain-Barré syndrome. AV fistulas require a unique skill set to access and generally should not be accessed by paramedics.

Accessing an implanted vascular access device is not in the scope of paramedic practice in most places; special training and medical authorization are required to perform this skill. The steps for accessing such as device are summarized as follows:

1. Use aseptic technique. Prepare all necessary equipment: Huber needle, empty 10- to 20-mL syringe (nothing less than a 10-mL syringe should be used), 10-mL normal saline flush, sterile gloves, chlorhexidine gluconate (ChloraPrep) or betadine, 10-gtt administration set, 500 mL normal saline.
2. Identify the site in the upper part of the chest. Stabilize it between the thumb and index finger of your nondominant hand.
3. Clean the site with chlorhexidine. If an allergy is present, then clean the site with betadine Figure 14-68A.
4. Apply pressure around the edges of the port to stretch the skin over the injection site Figure 14-68B.
5. While stabilizing the device, insert the Huber needle at a 90° angle Figure 14-68C.
6. Withdraw at least 10 mL of blood from the needleless extension set Figure 14-68D. Discard it immediately.
7. Flush the set with the 10-mL normal saline flush. Attach the 10-gtt IV administration set.
8. Administer medications directly into the drop set medication port.
9. Monitor the patient's condition, and document the medication given, route, administration time, and response of the patient.

Central lines imply that a patient has a significant medical history that should be investigated and that standard IV access may be difficult to obtain. Accessing these devices is risky and requires proper training. Aseptic technique is imperative considering that many of these devices sit inside the superior vena cava. These devices are all preserved with heparin, which is why providers must withdraw at least 10 mL of blood from

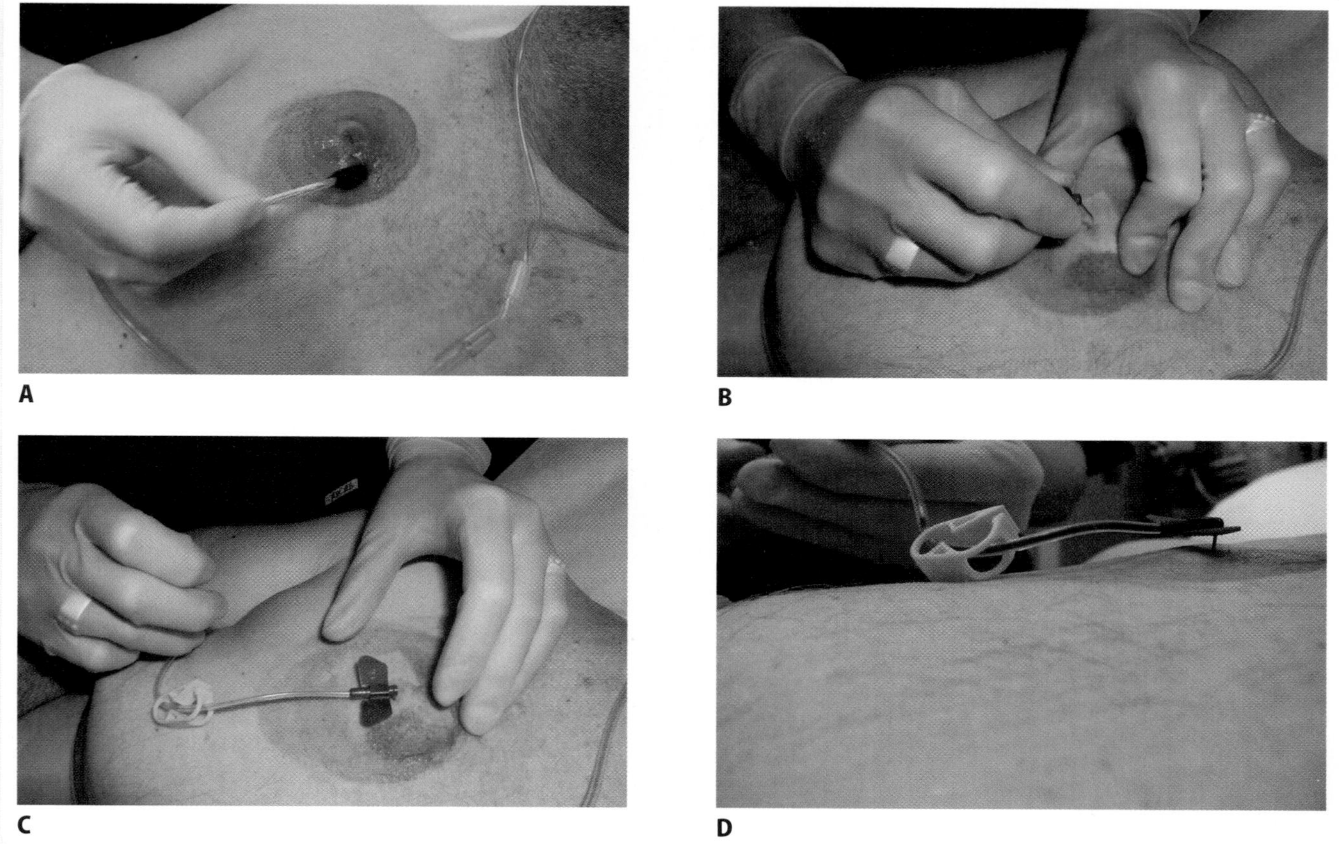

Figure 14-68 Accessing an implanted vascular access device. Using aseptic technique, the general steps include: identifying and cleaning the site **(A)**, stretching the skin over the site **(B)**, inserting the Huber needle at a 90° angle **(C)**, and then withdrawing at least 10 mL of blood **(D)**, discarding it, flushing with 10 mL normal saline, attaching the administration set, and administering medications directly into the medication port.

the device. Because EMS providers do not routinely carry heparin, EMS providers must keep the IV administration set minimally at KVO/TKO to prevent clots from forming.

Words of Wisdom

In rare instances, paramedics may perform peer-assisted medication administration (administering medication to oneself or to one's partner). It may be necessary for the EMS crew to receive medications because they were exposed to a toxic agent. In this case, you would first treat yourself and then your partner.

Rates of Medication Absorption

The speed at which a drug is absorbed is directly related to the route by which it is given. Obviously, drugs injected directly into the bloodstream (ie, as IV or IO injections) gain access to the central circulation the fastest. Oral medications take longer to achieve their therapeutic effects because they must be absorbed through the gastrointestinal tract first. Table 14-9 summarizes the various medication routes and their rates of absorption. Table 14-10 provides examples of medications and their route, onset, peak, and duration. Specific medications are covered in detail in the Appendix to Volume 1, *Emergency Medications*.

Table 14-9 Medication Routes and Rates of Absorption

Route of Administration	Onset of Action[a]
Intraosseous	30–60 s
Intravenous	30–60 s
Endotracheal	2–3 min
Inhalation	2–3 min
Nasal mucosal atomization	3–5 min
Sublingual	3–5 min
Intramuscular injection	10–20 min
Subcutaneous injection	15–30 min
Rectal	5–30 min
Oral	30–90 min
Topical	Minutes to hours

[a]In a healthy person with adequate perfusion

Data from: Verma P, Thakur AS, Deshmukh K, Jha AK, Verma S. Routes of drug administration. *Int J Pharm Sci Res.* 2010 Jul-Sep;1(1):54-59. http://www.technicaljournalsonline.com/ijpsr/VOL%20I/IJPSR%20VOL%20I%20ISSUE%20I%20JULY%20SEPTEMBER%202010/IJPSR%20VOL%20I%20ISSUE%20I%20Article%208.pdf. Accessed February 16, 2017.

Table 14-10 Examples of Specific Medications

Drug	Route	Onset	Peak	Duration
Metoprolol tartrate (Lopressor)	PO	15 min	1 h	6–12 h
	IV	Immediate	20 min	5–8 h
Fentanyl citrate (Sublimaze)	Transdermal	6–8 h	12–24 h	72 h
	IV	Immediate	3–5 min	20–40 min
	IM	7–8 min	20–30 min	1–2 hours
	Intranasal	1–2 min	9–15 min	20–40 min
Naloxone	IV	0–2 min	0–2 min	20–120 min
	IM	2–10 min	2–10 min	20–120 min
	ET	2–10 min	2–10 min	20–120 min
	Intranasal	2–10 min	2–10 min	20–120 min

Abbreviations: ET, endotracheal; IM, intramuscular; IV, intravenous; PO, per os (oral route/by mouth)

YOU are the Paramedic SUMMARY

1. Given this scenario, what route of delivery do you anticipate using to administer medications? What are the advantages of this route?

Given this patient's presentation, you should anticipate giving medications through the IV route. The sudden onset of symptoms suggests some sort of acute cardiac event, possibly involving a dysrhythmia. IV administration will allow for reliable and quick absorption in the body. Subcutaneous or IM administration of medications to a patient experiencing a cardiac event may be unreliable due to perfusion status.

2. What aspects of the patient history are important to consider prior to administering any medication to this patient?

Remember the 10 rights of medication administration that are discussed in Chapter 13, *Principles of Pharmacology*. Verify the drug dose, name, route, rate of administration, indication, contraindications, drug concentration, and volume to be administered. While interviewing the patient, determine what medications (or home remedies) the patient is taking and whether the patient has any known drug allergies.

3. What information must you and your partner be sure to communicate to one another as you are preparing to administer this medication?

The MACC method of confirming specific details regarding medication administration is a useful way to minimize the risk of a medication error. During this preadministration check, communication with your partner should involve, at a minimum, details regarding the dose, volume to be administered, indication, and contraindications.

4. Why is it prudent to contact medical control in this scenario to discuss management options?

Medical control can serve as an invaluable resource while you are in the field. Establishing a line of communication with online medical control early may assist you in reducing the cognitive load and reducing the potential of making a dosing or judgment error. When discussing patient management with the physician, make sure you are confident and detailed in the information that you provide.

5. What dose will you administer to the patient? Given the supplied medication, what volume will you administer?

The desired dose in this case is 26.25 mg, which is calculated as follows:

$$\frac{0.25\text{ mg}}{\text{kg}} \times 105\text{ kg} = 26.25\text{ mg}$$

The drug concentration is 30 mg in 5 mL of fluid. Therefore, the volume to be administered is calculated as follows:

$$26.25\text{ mg} \div \frac{30\text{ mg}}{5\text{ mL}} = 26.25\,\cancel{\text{mg}} \times \frac{\overset{1}{\cancel{5}}\text{ mL}}{\underset{6}{\cancel{30}}\,\cancel{\text{mg}}} = 4.375\text{ mL}$$

Because the order is 26.25 mg and the concentration is 30 mg in 5 mL, there are 6 mg per mL. Therefore, the initial administration of medication is 4.375 mL of diltiazem.

6. Why would it be preferable to use an IV pump for a maintenance infusion of a medication?

IV infusion pumps are the standard of care within the medical community. While they are not available on every ambulance, you should still recognize that their use would be appropriate if they are available. A mechanical device that infuses a precise volume programmed by the paramedic is preferred over the use of a microdrip set. There is a high propensity for errors in IV flow rates and, thus, medication dosing when using microdrip sets. IV infusion pumps do not have variability in drip rate based on bag height, movement, etc.

7. What is the appropriate flow rate to administer the maintenance infusion of diltiazem?

You have a premixed bag with 30 mg/100 mL. The infusion is calculated to provide 5 mg/h.

First, calculate the concentration:

$$30\text{ mg} \div 100\text{ mL} = 0.3\text{ mg/mL (concentration)}$$

Second, determine the amount of volume to infuse per hour (mL/h):

$$\frac{5\text{ mg}}{\text{h}}\text{ (desired dose)} \div \frac{0.3\text{ mg}}{\text{mL}}\text{(concentration)} = 16.67\text{ mL/h}$$

Last, determine the amount of volume to infuse per minute. The rate can be established by dividing the mL/h by 60:

$$\frac{16.67\text{ mL}}{\text{h}} \times \frac{1\text{ h}}{60\text{ min}} = 0.28\text{ mL/min}$$

YOU are the Paramedic SUMMARY *(continued)*

Using a microdrip set (60 gtt/mL), you would administer 16.67 gtt/min to achieve a rate of 0.28 mL/min:

$$\frac{0.28 \text{ mL}}{\text{min}} \times \frac{60 \text{ gtt}}{1 \text{ min}} = 16.67 \text{ gtt/min}$$

Medication calculations like this one help illustrate the importance of understanding the math behind drug administration. As a tip, you should remember that when using a microdrip set (60 gtt/mL), gtt/min is equal to mL/h. Infusing your diltiazem at a rate of 16.67 gtt/min using a microdrip set will give you the 16.67 mL/h and achieve the goal of 5 mg/h. However, as illustrated in the previous question, it would be preferred to have this infusion on a pump to ensure that the proper amount of medication and proper volume are administered.

EMS Patient Care Report (PCR)

Date: 08-01-18	**Incident No.:** 1232	**Nature of Call:** Cardiac	**Location:** 247 Pine Street		
Dispatched: 1115	**En Route:** 1116	**At Scene:** 1119	**Transport:** 1137	**At Hospital:** 1207	**In Service:** 1237

Patient Information

Age: 26 **Sex:** M **Weight (in kg [lb]):** 105 kg (231 lb)	**Allergies:** None **Medications:** None **Past Medical History:** None **Chief Complaint:** Palpitations; syncopal episode

Vital Signs

Time: 1120	**BP:** N/A	**Pulse:** N/A	**Respirations:** 20	**Spo_2:** N/A
Time: 1124	**BP:** 134/90	**Pulse:** 180	**Respirations:** 20	**Spo_2:** 99%
Time: 1129	**BP:** 126/78	**Pulse:** 90	**Respirations:** 18	**Spo_2:** 100%
Time:	**BP:**	**Pulse:**	**Respirations:**	**Spo_2:**

EMS Treatment (circle all that apply)

Oxygen @ ______ L/min via (circle one): **NC NRM Bag-mask device**		**Assisted Ventilation**	**Airway Adjunct**	**CPR**
Defibrillation	**Bleeding Control**	**Bandaging**	**Splinting**	**Other:**

Narrative

EMS arrived on scene to find 26-year-old male complaining of the sudden onset of palpitations. Pt called 9-1-1 before sitting down on the ground because he felt weak. Pt suffered a syncopal episode and had regained consciousness upon EMS arrival. Pt was found awake, alert, and oriented to person, place, time, and event. Pt complained of palpitations. Pt denied having any chest pain or dyspnea. Pt also reported that he no longer feels dizzy or weak but could still feel the palpitations. Pt has no medical history and takes no medications. Pt was found to be in atrial fibrillation with a rapid ventricular response. Online medical direction was obtained with Dr. Adams at Beauregard Hospital. Per Dr. Adams, 0.25 mg/kg of diltiazem (26.25 mg) given IV bolus over 2 minutes. Pt converted to sinus rhythm. Pt reported no complaints. Per Dr. Adams, maintenance infusion of diltiazem initiated at 5 mg/h. Pt transported to Beauregard Hospital without any acute changes. Pt turned over to Dr. Adams in Room 5 in the ED with report to RN.**End of report**

Prep Kit

▶ Ready for Review

- Vascular access is often needed in emergency medicine for patients in hemodynamically unstable condition and in need of intravenous (IV) fluids, various medications, or both.
- It is your responsibility to ensure the medications you deliver are administered correctly and safely. Medication errors are an issue throughout health care. To minimize the danger of incorrect medication administration, you should use a tool to verify the drug dose, name, route, rate of administration, indication for administration, contraindications, drug concentration, and volume to be administered.
- Documenting medication administration is extremely important. You must list the dose administered, name of the drug, route, rate, time of administration, who administered the drug, who helped perform the medication check, and the patient's response.
- Maintaining and securing medication supplies on the ambulance are part of a paramedic's role. Follow the specific policies and procedures of your local drug distribution, security, and accountability system.
- Use the aseptic technique when you are performing any invasive procedure to minimize the risk of patient contamination. Always take standard precautions when performing an invasive procedure to maximize your own safety, and dispose of equipment properly.
- An ill or injured body may be unable to maintain homeostasis, resulting in an excess or deficit of fluids or electrolytes. Understanding the workings of the intracellular and extracellular chemicals and charges will provide you with a better foundation for understanding why different types of IV solutions are administered for different conditions.
- Crystalloid IV solutions are the best choice for injured patients who need fluid replacement. Colloid solutions work well to reduce edema while expanding the vascular compartment.
- A solution can be isotonic, hypotonic, or hypertonic. Isotonic solutions, for example normal saline, have almost the same osmolarity as serum and other body fluids. Lactated Ringer is an isotonic solution often used prehospitally for patients who have significant blood loss.
- Hypotonic solutions may be needed for a patient receiving dialysis, or for patients in diabetic ketoacidosis. Hypertonic solutions may be administered to patients with severe traumatic brain injuries.
- Techniques for gaining vascular access include cannulation of a peripheral extremity vein, cannulation of the external jugular vein, and cannulation of the intraosseous (IO) space. Although the ultimate goal of vascular access is to be able to administer fluids and medications, each of these techniques requires a different approach and must be practiced frequently for initial and ongoing proficiency.
- Several different IV administration sets exist, and you must know which one is most appropriate for a given patient's condition. Microdrip sets (60 gtt/mL) are commonly used for medication infusions. Macrodrip sets (10 or 15 gtt/mL) are used when the patient requires IV fluid boluses to treat dehydration, hypovolemic shock, and other states of hemodynamic instability.
- You must consider two factors when choosing an IV catheter: gauge and length. The larger the gauge (the smaller the number), and the shorter the length, the more fluid that can be infused through it. Over-the-needle catheters are the most commonly used IV catheters in the prehospital setting.
- Cannulation of a peripheral extremity vein is the preferred initial means of establishing vascular access. If it is unsuccessful and the patient is critically ill or injured, proceed with IO cannulation without delay. External jugular vein cannulation is usually attempted only after all other techniques of gaining vascular access have failed.
- The IO space, which acts like a sponge, quickly absorbs fluids and medications and rapidly transports them to the central circulation. Although peripheral veins often collapse when a patient is in shock or cardiac arrest, the IO space tends to remain patent. Thus IO cannulation and infusion may be life-saving measures if peripheral venous access is not possible. Any fluid or medication that can be administered via the IV route can be administered via the IO route and can travel to the central circulation just as rapidly.
- You must be thoroughly familiar with the equipment you are using when performing IO cannulation. Follow local protocols and attend in-service training regarding the specific equipment used for IO cannulation in your EMS system.
- Potential complications of IV therapy include local and systemic reactions. After administering any medication, always monitor the patient for any reaction or improvement.
- You may need to obtain a blood sample, for example for analysis at the receiving facility. Obtain blood samples at the same time you start an IV line.
- At times you may transport a patient who is undergoing a blood transfusion. When receiving

Prep Kit *(continued)*

such a patient, ensure there is at least one available vascular site that is not transfusing blood.

- Good math skills and a thorough understanding of the metric system are imperative to providing the right dose of a drug to your patient. Administering the incorrect drug, using the incorrect route, or giving the incorrect dose can have disastrous effects.
- As a paramedic, you must be familiar with the various routes of medication administration, including the proper use of equipment and proper anatomic locations for administration via each route.
- Parenteral routes are those that do not pass through the gastrointestinal tract, and include the intradermal, subcutaneous, intramuscular, IV, IO, and percutaneous routes. Enteral routes are those that pass through any portion of the gastrointestinal tract (oral, sublingual, gastric tube).
- The IV and IO routes are the fastest routes of medication administration.
- IV medication can be administered as a bolus (single dose), or piggyback (a secondary IV line connected to a port on the primary infusion line).
- The standard of care to administer a medication maintenance infusion is to use an electromechanical infusion pump. An infusion pump delivers fluid at a set rate, and calculates the amount of fluid infused, as well as the remaining amount. You may encounter these most often during interfacility transports.
- When in doubt, always follow local protocols or contact medical control as needed for direction when you are administering a medication. *Never make a hasty critical decision before consulting with a physician.*

▶ Vital Vocabulary

access port A sealed hub on an administration set designed for sterile access to the IV fluid.

administration set Tubing that connects to the IV bag access port and the catheter to deliver IV fluid.

ampules Small glass containers that are sealed and the contents sterilized.

antecubital The anterior aspect of the elbow.

anticoagulant A substance that prevents blood from clotting.

antiseptics Chemicals used to cleanse an area before performing an invasive procedure, such as starting an IV line; not toxic to living tissues; examples include isopropyl alcohol and iodine.

aseptic technique A method of cleansing used to prevent contamination of a site when you are performing an invasive procedure, such as starting an IV line.

aural Pertaining to the ear.

blood tubing A special type of macrodrip administration set designed to facilitate rapid fluid replacement by manual infusion of multiple IV bags or IV–blood replacement combinations.

bolus A term used to describe "in one mass"; in medication administration, a single dose given by the intravenous or intraosseous route; may be a small or large quantity of the drug.

Bone Injection Gun (BIG) A spring-loaded device that is used for inserting an intraosseous needle into the proximal tibia in adult and pediatric patients.

buccal Between the cheek and gums.

butterfly catheter A rigid, hollow, venous cannulation device identified by its plastic "wings" that act as anchoring points for securing the catheter.

cannulation The insertion of a catheter, such as into a vein to allow for fluid flow.

catheter shear Occurs when a needle is reinserted into the catheter, and it slices through the catheter, creating a free-floating segment.

Celsius scale A scale for measuring temperature where water freezes at 0° and boils at 100°.

colloid solutions Solutions that contain molecules (usually proteins) that are too large to pass out of the capillary membranes and, therefore, remain in the vascular compartment.

concentration The total weight of a drug contained in a specific volume of liquid.

contaminated stick The puncturing of an emergency care provider's skin with a needle or catheter that was used on a patient.

crystalloid solutions Solutions of dissolved crystals (for example, salts or sugars) in water; contain compounds that quickly dissociate in solution.

D_5W An intravenous solution made up of 5% dextrose in water.

dehydration Depletion of the body's systemic fluid volume.

desired dose The amount of a drug that the physician orders for a patient; the drug order.

diaphysis The shaft of a long bone.

diluent A solution (usually water or normal saline) used for diluting a medication.

disinfectants Chemicals used on nonliving objects to kill organisms; toxic to living tissues.

Prep Kit *(continued)*

distal traction Gentle downward or lateral traction on the skin.

drip chamber The area of the administration set where fluid accumulates so that the tubing remains filled with fluid.

drug reconstitution Injecting sterile water or saline from one vial into another vial containing a powdered form of the drug.

enema A fluid solution, possibly containing supplemental medications, that can be administered rectally to aid in a variety of gastrointestinal complications.

enteral medications Medication administration that involves the medication passing through a portion of the gastrointestinal tract.

epiphyseal plate The growth plate of a bone; a major site of bone development during childhood.

epiphyses The ends of a long bone.

external jugular (EJ) vein Large neck vein that is lateral to the carotid artery.

EZ-IO A handheld, battery-powered driver to which a special intraosseous needle is attached; used for insertion of the intraosseous needle into the proximal tibia of children and adults.

Fahrenheit scale A scale for measuring temperature where water freezes at 32° and boils at 212°.

First Access for Shock Trauma (FAST) devices Manual sternal intraosseous devices used in patients age 12 and older; include an infusion tube, subcutaneous portal, an introducer, a target/strain relief patch, and a protective dome.

flash chamber The area of an IV catheter that fills with blood to help indicate when a vein is cannulated.

gastric tubes Tubes that are commonly inserted in patients in the prehospital setting to decompress the stomach; can also be used to administer certain enteral medications.

gauge The internal diameter of an IV catheter or needle.

gtt A unit of measure that indicates drops.

hematoma An accumulation of blood in the tissues beneath the skin; a potential complication of IV therapy.

hemostasis The body's natural blood-clotting mechanism.

hypertonic solution A solution that has a greater concentration of sodium than does the cell; the increased osmotic pressure can draw out water from the cell and cause it to collapse.

hypotonic solution A solution that has a lower concentration of sodium than does the cell; the increased osmotic pressure lets water flow into the cell, causing it to swell and possibly burst.

implanted vascular access devices Devices that are implanted in surgery, sutured under the skin, for the purpose of long-term medication administration, total parenteral nutrition, chemotherapy, blood product administration, and venous blood sampling; an arteriovenous fistula is an example.

infiltration The escape of fluid into the surrounding tissue; the result of vein perforation during intravenous cannulation.

infusion pump A mechanical device that infuses a precise intravenous volume programmed by the clinician.

inhalation Breathing into the lungs; a medication delivery route.

intradermal The layer of the dermis, just beneath the epidermis; a medication delivery route.

intramuscular (IM) Into a muscle; a medication delivery route.

intranasal Within the nose.

intraosseous (IO) Within the bone.

intraosseous infusion A technique of administering fluids, blood and blood products, and medications into the intraosseous space of a long bone, usually the proximal tibia.

intraosseous space The spongy cancellous bone of the epiphyses and the medullary cavity of the diaphysis, collectively.

intravenous (IV) Within a vein.

intravenous therapy Cannulation of a vein with an IV catheter to access the patient's vascular system.

ionic concentration The amount of charged particles found in a particular area.

isotonic crystalloid solutions Intravenous solution that does not cause a fluid shift into or out of the cell; examples include normal saline and lactated Ringer solutions.

isotonic solution A solution that has the same concentration of sodium as does the cell. In this case, water does not shift, and no change in cell shape occurs.

lactated Ringer (LR) solution A sterile isotonic crystalloid IV solution of specified amounts of calcium chloride, potassium chloride, sodium chloride, and sodium lactate in water.

local reactions Reactions that occur in a localized area; a potential complication of intravenous therapy.

macrodrip sets Administration sets named for the large orifice between the piercing spike and the drip chamber; allow for rapid fluid flow into the vascular system; allow 10 or 15 gtt/mL, depending on the manufacturer.

Prep Kit *(continued)*

medical asepsis A term applied to the practice of preventing contamination of the patient by using aseptic technique.

metered-dose inhaler (MDI) A pressurized canister that delivers a specific dose of a medication; commonly used for beta-agonist bronchodilators.

metric system A decimal system based on tens for the measurement of length, weight, and volume.

microdrip sets Administration sets named for the small needlelike orifice between the piercing spike and the drip chamber; allow for carefully controlled fluid flow and are ideally suited for medication administration; allow for 60 gtt/mL.

Mix-o-Vial A single vial divided into two compartments by a rubber stopper; methylprednisolone sodium succinate (Solu-Medrol) is stored this way.

mucosal atomizer device (MAD) A device that attaches to the end of a syringe that is used to spray (atomize) certain medications via the intranasal route.

nebulizer A device for producing a fine spray or mist that is used to deliver inhaled medications.

New Intraosseous (NIO) device A spring-loaded device that contains neither drill nor battery, used for inserting an intraosseous needle into the proximal tibia of an adult patient.

non-tunneling devices Devices that have been inserted by direct venipuncture through the skin directly into a selected vein, for the purpose of long-term medication administration, total parenteral nutrition, chemotherapy, and venous blood sampling; peripheral inserted central catheters and central venous catheters are examples.

normal saline A solution of 0.9% sodium chloride; an isotonic crystalloid.

occlusion Blockage, usually of a tubular structure such as a blood vessel or IV catheter.

ocular Pertaining to the eye.

osmolarity The ability to influence the movement of water across a semipermeable membrane.

osteogenesis imperfecta A congenital bone disease that results in fragile bones.

osteomyelitis Inflammation of the bone and muscle caused by infection.

overhydration An increase in the body's systemic fluid volume.

over-the-needle catheter A Teflon (plastic) catheter inserted over a hollow needle.

parenteral route A route of medication administration that involves any route other than the gastrointestinal tract.

Penrose drain A type of surgical drain often used as a constricting band.

percutaneous Through the skin or mucous membrane.

peripheral vein cannulation A technique in which a cannula (tube) is inserted into veins of the peripheral areas, that is, veins that can be seen and/or palpated. Examples of peripheral veins include those of the hand, arm, and lower extremity and the external jugular vein.

piercing spike The hard, sharpened plastic spike on the end of the administration set designed to pierce the sterile membrane of the IV bag.

prefilled syringes Medication syringes that are prepackaged and prepared with a specific concentration.

pressure infuser device A sleeve that is placed around the IV bag and inflated to force fluid to flow from the IV bag and into the tubing.

pulmonary embolism A blood clot or foreign matter trapped within the pulmonary circulation.

pyrogenic reaction A reaction characterized by an abrupt temperature elevation (as high as 106°F [41°C]) with severe chills, backache, headache, weakness, nausea, and vomiting; a potential complication of intravenous or intraosseous therapy.

radiopaque Feature of an IV catheter (or any other object) that allows it to appear on a radiograph.

saline locks Special types of IV devices that eliminate the need to hang a bag of IV fluid; also called a buff cap or INT (intermittent); commonly used for patients who do not require fluid boluses but may require medication therapy.

sharps Any contaminated item that can cause injury; includes IV needles and catheters, broken ampules or vials, or anything else that can penetrate or lacerate the skin.

sterile The destruction of all living organisms; achieved by using heat, gas, or chemicals.

subcutaneous Into the tissue between the skin and muscle; a medication delivery route.

sublingual Under the tongue; a medication delivery route.

suppository A drug mixed in a firm base that melts at body temperature and is shaped to fit the rectum.

syncopal episodes Fainting; brief losses of consciousness caused by transiently inadequate blood flow to the brain.

systemic complications Reactions that affect systems of the body.

third spacing The shifting of fluid into the tissues, creating edema.

Prep Kit (continued)

thrombophlebitis Inflammation of a vein.

track marks The visible scars from repeated cannulation of a vein; commonly associated with illicit drug use.

transdermal Across the skin; a medication delivery route.

trocar A solid boring needle.

Vacutainer A cylindrical device that attaches to an 18- or 20-gauge sampling needle; accommodates self-sealing blood tubes when blood samples are being obtained.

varicose veins Veins on the leg that are large, twisted, and ropelike and can cause pain, swelling, or itching.

venous thrombosis The development of a stationary blood clot in the venous circulation.

vials Small glass or plastic bottles that contain medication; may contain single or multiple doses.

volume on hand The amount of fluid you have on hand, such as the amount of fluid in an IV bag or the amount of fluid in a vial of medication.

Volutrol A special type of microdrip set that features a 100- or 200-mL calibrated drip chamber; used for fluid regulation in patients prone to circulatory overload, such as pediatric and older patients; also called a Buretrol.

▶ References

1. Hines S, Luna, K, Lofthus J, et al. Becoming a High Reliability Organization: Operational Advice for Hospital Leaders. (Prepared by the Lewin Group under Contract No. 290-04-0011.) AHRQ Publication No. 08-0022. Rockville, MD: Agency for Healthcare Research and Quality. April 2008.
2. Chassin MR, Loeb JM. High-reliability health care: getting there from here. The Joint Commission. *Milbank Q.* 2013;91(3):459-490.
3. National Highway Traffic Safety Administration (NHTSA). Patient Safety in Emergency Medical Services: Roundtable Report and Recommendations. www.nhtsa.gov/people/injury/ems/archive/patient_safetyems/patientsafety02.doc. Published 2002. Accessed May 26, 2016.
4. Misasi P, Braithwaite S. The Medication Administration Cross-Check© (MACC) User's Manual. Wichita-Sedgwick County EMS System. https://kansasemstransition.files.wordpress.com/2012/08/macc-user-manual-v2-0.pdf. Published 2012. Accessed May 26, 2016.
5. National Association of Emergency Medical Technicians (NAEMT). *Advanced Medical Life Support.* 2nd ed. Burlington, MA: Jones & Bartlett Learning; 2017:159.
6. Cantor-Peled G, Halak M, Ovadia-Blechman Z. Peripheral vein locating techniques. Open Access Journals. http://www.openaccessjournals.com/articles/peripheral-vein-locating-techniques.html. Accessed February 25, 2017.
7. Mbamalu D, Banerjee A. Methods of obtaining peripheral venous access in difficult situations. *Postgrad Med J.* 1999;75(886):459-462.
8. Lago P, Bizzarri G, Scalzotto F, et al. Use of FMEA analysis to reduce risk of errors in prescribing and administering drugs in paediatric wards: a quality improvement report. *BMJ Open.* 2012; 2(6):e001249.
9. Reiley TT. FMEA in preventing medical accidents. Quality Congress. ASQ's Annual Quality Congress Proceedings; Milwaukee, WI: 2002: 657-664. http://search.proquest.com/openview/57b910167d3a560a21560ab41b48587a/1?pq-origsite=gscholar&cbl=39817. Accessed February 3, 2017.
10. Senders JW. FMEA and RCA: the mantras* of modern risk management. *Qual Saf Health Care.* 2004;13(4):249–250.
11. Hess D. Delivery of inhaled medication in adults. UpToDate. https://www.uptodate.com/contents/delivery-of-inhaled-medication-in-adults. Updated June 27, 2016. Accessed March 23, 2017.
12. Smith C, Goldman RD. Nebulizers versus pressurized metered-dose inhalers in preschool children with wheezing. *Can Fam Physician.* 2012;58(5):528–530.
13. Link MS, Berkow LC, Kudenchuk PJ, et al. Part 7: adult advanced cardiovascular life support: 2015 American Heart Association Guidelines Update for Cardiopulmonary Resuscitation and Emergency Cardiovascular Care. *Circulation.* 2015;132(18 suppl 2):S444–S464.

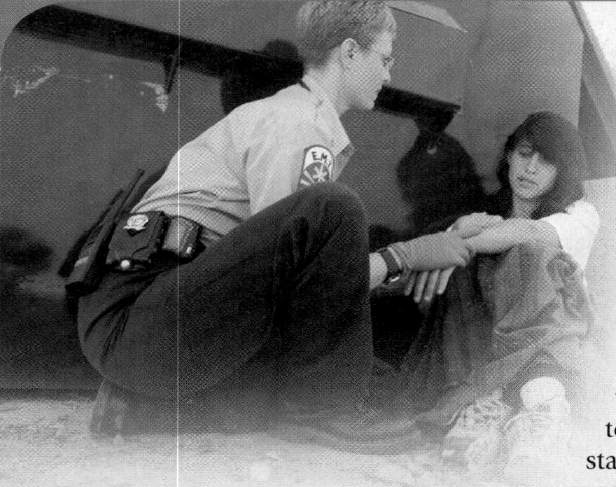

Assessment *in Action*

You and your partner are dispatched to a local diner for a patient with chest pain. You are brought to the patient by staff, where you find a 66-year-old man seated at a table clutching his chest. The patient states he has not been feeling well for the past few days and while he was eating, he began to have some chest pain and trouble breathing. The patient states he recently went to his doctor, who diagnosed him with pneumonia. The patient states he finished his antibiotics several days ago. You obtain his blood pressure and vital signs and find them all to be within normal limits.

1. What should be your first action with this patient?

- **A.** Start an IV line.
- **B.** Administer a nitroglycerin spray.
- **C.** Attach the patient to the cardiac monitor.
- **D.** Place the patient on oxygen.

2. You want to administer a nitroglycerin spray to the patient because all his vital signs are normal. How is nitroglycerin spray administered?

- **A.** Intravenously
- **B.** Sublingually
- **C.** Transdermally
- **D.** Intramuscularly

3. Concerning absorption of the medication in the body for the desired effect, the sublingual administration is absorbed:

- **A.** very slowly.
- **B.** slowly.
- **C.** normally.
- **D.** rapidly.

4. Another name for a sublingual or transdermal administration of medication is:

- **A.** inhalation.
- **B.** parenteral.
- **C.** enteral.
- **D.** percutaneous.

5. Aspirin is indicated in this patient. How is aspirin administered and how fast is it absorbed?

- **A.** Intranasally and quickly, within 5 minutes
- **B.** Intranasally and slowly, within 1 hour
- **C.** Orally chewed and quickly, within 15 minutes
- **D.** Orally swallowed whole and slowly, within 3 hours

6. You have inserted an IV line. All of the following are potential complications EXCEPT:

- **A.** infiltration.
- **B.** flash in the flash chamber.
- **C.** occlusion.
- **D.** hematoma.

7. You want to administer a 250-mL fluid bolus over the next 20 minutes using a 10-drop set. At how many drops per minute would you set the rate?

- **A.** 50 gtt/min
- **B.** 125 gtt/min
- **C.** 150 gtt/min
- **D.** 200 gtt/min

8. You and your partner are treating an older adult patient who reports shortness of breath. The patient is in rapid atrial fibrillation and the physician orders 10 mg of diltiazem. The medication comes in a vial of 25 mg in 5 mL. How much would you administer?

9. You have just resuscitated a patient who was in cardiac arrest and are initiating the return of spontaneous circulation protocol, which calls for you to administer 2 L of saline. You have established an IO line to administer medication and you have attached the first liter of chilled saline but cannot get the fluid to flow rapidly. What is the problem?

10. Calculate the flow rate for the following: Medical control has ordered you to administer 2 mg/min of lidocaine. You have 2 g of lidocaine, a 500-mL bag of normal saline, and a 60-gtt administration set.

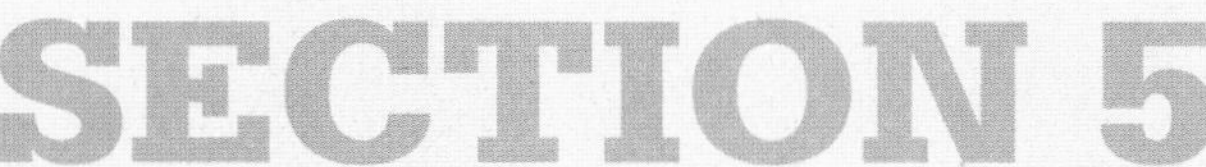

SECTION 5

Airway Management

CHAPTER 15

Airway Management

National EMS Education Standard Competencies

Airway Management, Respiration, and Artificial Ventilation

Integrates complex knowledge of anatomy, physiology, and pathophysiology into the assessment to develop and implement a treatment plan with the goal of ensuring a patent airway, adequate mechanical ventilation, and respiration for patients of all ages.

Airway Management

- Airway anatomy (pp 776-778)
- Airway assessment (pp 782-787)
- Techniques of ensuring a patent airway (pp 782-783)

Respiration

- Anatomy of the respiratory system (pp 776-778)
- Physiology and pathophysiology of respiration (pp 777-782)
  - Pulmonary ventilation (pp 777-780)
  - Oxygenation (pp 777-778, 780-782)
  - Respiration (pp 777-778, 780-782)
    - External (p 778)
    - Internal (p 778)
    - Cellular (p 778)
- Assessment and management of adequate and inadequate respiration (pp 782-787, 794-885)
- Supplemental oxygen therapy (pp 806-808)

Artificial Ventilation

Assessment and management of adequate and inadequate ventilation

- Artificial ventilation (pp 813-814)
- Minute ventilation (p 779)
- Alveolar ventilation (pp 782-787)
- Effect of artificial ventilation on cardiac output (p 781)

Knowledge Objectives

1. Review the anatomy of the respiratory system, including the major structures of the upper and lower airway. (pp 776-778)
2. Discuss the physiology of breathing, including ventilation, oxygenation, and respiration. (pp 777-778)
3. Describe factors related to the pathophysiology of respiration, including ventilation-perfusion ratio mismatch, hypoventilation, hyperventilation, and circulatory compromise. (pp 778-782)
4. Describe factors related to ventilation, including partial pressure and volumes. (pp 779-780)
5. Explain positive pressure ventilation versus negative pressure ventilation. (p 781)
6. Discuss acid/base imbalance, specifically respiratory acidosis and respiratory alkalosis. (pp 781-782)
7. Explain how to assess for a patent airway. (pp 782-783)
8. List the signs of adequate breathing. (p 783)
9. List the signs of inadequate breathing. (pp 783-785)
10. Describe the five abnormal breathing patterns to recognize when assessing a patient's breathing. (p 785)
11. Explain how to assess a patient's breath sounds. (pp 785-787)
12. Explain how to assess for adequate and inadequate respiration, including the use of pulse oximetry. (pp 787-794)
13. Discuss the methods for end-tidal carbon dioxide assessment, including its importance. (pp 790-794)
14. Explain the use of the recovery position to maintain a clear airway. (p 795)
15. Describe how to perform the head tilt–chin lift maneuver. (pp 795-796)
16. Describe how to perform the jaw-thrust maneuver. (pp 795-796)
17. Describe how to perform the tongue-jaw lift maneuver. (p 796)
18. Describe the importance and techniques of suctioning. (pp 797-799)
19. Explain how to measure and insert an oropharyngeal (oral) airway. (pp 800-801)
20. Explain how to measure and insert a nasopharyngeal (nasal) airway. (pp 801-802)
21. Describe the causes of foreign body airway obstruction. (pp 802-803)

22. Describe the management of mild and severe foreign body airway obstruction in an adult, a child, and an infant. (pp 804-806)
23. Describe the importance of giving supplemental oxygen to patients who are hypoxic. (p 806)
24. Describe the basics of how oxygen is stored and the various hazards associated with its use. (pp 806-807)
25. Explain how to use a nonrebreathing mask, including the oxygen flow requirements for its use. (pp 808-809)
26. Describe the indications for using a nasal cannula rather than a nonrebreathing mask. (p 809)
27. Describe the indications for using a humidifier during supplemental oxygen therapy. (pp 810-811)
28. Explain how to perform mouth-to-mask ventilation. (pp 813-814)
29. Describe the assessment and care of a patient with apnea. (pp 813-814)
30. Describe the use of a one- and two-person bag-mask device. (pp 815-816)
31. Describe the signs associated with adequate and inadequate artificial ventilation. (p 816)
32. Discuss automatic transport ventilators and how to use them. (pp 816-817)
33. Describe the indications, contraindications, and complications of using continuous positive airway pressure (CPAP). (pp 817-820)
34. Explain the considerations surrounding gastric distention, including how to perform nasogastric and orogastric decompression. (pp 820-823)
35. Discuss airway management considerations for patients with a laryngectomy, tracheostomy, or stoma. (pp 823-828)
36. List the advanced airway devices and techniques available to you as a paramedic. (p 829)
37. Discuss methods used to predict the difficult airway. (pp 829-831)
38. Describe the advantages, disadvantages, and equipment used when performing endotracheal (ET) intubation. (pp 831-833)
39. Explain how to determine correct ET tube size. (p 832)
40. List factors to consider when determining correct laryngoscope blade size. (p 833)
41. Discuss the indications and contraindications of orotracheal intubation. (p 833)
42. List the methods available for confirming correct ET tube placement and the advantages and disadvantages of each method. (pp 839-840)
43. Describe how to secure an ET tube. (pp 840-841)
44. Discuss the indications, contraindications, advantages, disadvantages, and complications of nasotracheal intubation. (p 847)
45. Discuss the indications, contraindications, advantages, disadvantages, and complications of digital intubation. (pp 849, 851)
46. Discuss the indications, contraindications, advantages, disadvantages, and complications of transillumination intubation. (p 852)
47. Discuss the indications, contraindications, advantages, disadvantages, and complications of retrograde intubation. (p 853)
48. Explain what to do when intubation fails. (p 858)
49. Explain how to perform tracheobronchial suctioning. (pp 858-860)
50. Discuss considerations related to field extubation. (pp 859, 861)
51. List possible pharmacologic adjuncts to airway management and ventilation, including both sedatives and neuromuscular blocking agents used for emergency intubation. (pp 861-864)
52. Discuss the procedure for performing rapid sequence intubation. (pp 864-866)
53. Discuss King LT airway devices, including how they work, the indications, contraindications, and complications, and the procedure for inserting them. (pp 866-869)
54. Discuss the laryngeal mask airway, including how it works, its indications, contraindications, and complications, and the procedure for inserting it. (pp 868-872)
55. Discuss the i-gel supraglottic airway device, including how it works, and the procedure for inserting it. (pp 871-874)
56. Discuss the Cobra perilaryngeal airway, including how it works, its indications, contraindications, and complications, and the procedure for inserting it. (pp 872-875)
57. Discuss the esophageal tracheal Combitube, including how it works, its indications, contraindications, and complications, and the procedure for inserting it. (pp 875-877)
58. Discuss the indications, contraindications, advantages, disadvantages, and complications of performing open cricothyrotomy. (pp 878-879)
59. Discuss the indications, contraindications, advantages, disadvantages, and complications of performing needle cricothyrotomy. (pp 882-883)

Skills Objectives

1. Demonstrate how to use pulse oximetry. (pp 787-789)
2. Demonstrate how to position the unresponsive patient. (pp 794-795)
3. Demonstrate how to place a patient in the recovery position. (p 795)
4. Demonstrate how to perform the head tilt–chin lift maneuver. (pp 795-796)
5. Demonstrate how to perform the jaw-thrust maneuver. (pp 795-796)

6. Demonstrate how to perform the tongue-jaw lift maneuver. (p 796)
7. Demonstrate how to operate a suction unit. (pp 797-798)
8. Demonstrate how to suction a patient's airway. (pp 798-799)
9. Demonstrate how to insert an oropharyngeal (oral) airway. (p 800)
10. Demonstrate how to insert an oropharyngeal airway using a tongue depressor. (pp 800-801)
11. Demonstrate how to insert a nasopharyngeal (nasal) airway. (pp 801-802)
12. Demonstrate how to use Magill forceps to remove an object that is in the airway. (p 805, Skill Drill 15-1)
13. Demonstrate how to place an oxygen cylinder into service. (pp 807-808)
14. Demonstrate how to use partial and nonrebreathing masks in providing supplemental oxygen therapy to patients. (pp 808-810)
15. Demonstrate how to use a Venturi mask in providing supplemental oxygen therapy to patients. (p 810)
16. Demonstrate how to use a humidifier in providing supplemental oxygen therapy to patients. (pp 810-811)
17. Demonstrate mouth-to-mask ventilation. (pp 813-814)
18. Demonstrate how to assist a patient with ventilations using the bag-mask device for one and two rescuers. (pp 815-816)
19. Demonstrate how to use an automatic transport ventilator to assist in delivering artificial ventilation to the patient. (pp 816-817)
20. Demonstrate how to use CPAP. (pp 818-819, Skill Drill 15-2)
21. Demonstrate how to insert a nasogastric tube. (pp 821-822, Skill Drill 15-3)
22. Demonstrate how to insert an orogastric tube. (pp 822-823, Skill Drill 15-4)
23. Demonstrate how to suction a stoma. (pp 824-825, Skill Drill 15-5)
24. Demonstrate ventilation through a stoma using a resuscitation mask. (pp 824-826, Skill Drill 15-6)
25. Demonstrate bag-mask device-to-stoma ventilation. (pp 824-825, 827, Skill Drill 15-7)
26. Demonstrate how to replace a dislodged tracheostomy tube. (pp 825, 827-828, Skill Drill 15-8)
27. Demonstrate the entire procedure for orotracheal intubation using direct laryngoscopy. (pp 833-843, Skill Drill 15-9)
28. Demonstrate how to secure an ET tube. (pp 840-841)
29. Demonstrate the entire procedure for orotracheal intubation using video laryngoscopy. (pp 844-846, Skill Drill 15-10)
30. Demonstrate how to perform blind nasotracheal intubation. (pp 848-850, Skill Drill 15-11)
31. Discuss how to perform digital intubation. (pp 851-852)
32. Demonstrate how to perform transillumination intubation. (pp 852-855, Skill Drill 15-12)
33. Demonstrate how to perform retrograde intubation. (pp 855-857, Skill Drill 15-13)
34. Discuss how to perform face-to-face intubation. (pp 855, 858)
35. Demonstrate how to perform tracheobronchial suctioning. (pp 859-860, Skill Drill 15-14)
36. Demonstrate how to perform rapid sequence intubation. (pp 864-866)
37. Demonstrate insertion of the King LT airway. (pp 868-869, Skill Drill 15-15)
38. Demonstrate insertion of the laryngeal mask airway. (pp 870-872, Skill Drill 15-16)
39. Demonstrate insertion of the i-gel airway. (pp 873-874, Skill Drill 15-17)
40. Demonstrate insertion of the Combitube. (pp 876-877)
41. Demonstrate how to perform open cricothyrotomy. (pp 880-882, Skill Drill 15-18)
42. Demonstrate how to perform needle cricothyrotomy and translaryngeal catheter ventilation. (pp 883-885, Skill Drill 15-19)

YOU are the Paramedic — PART 1

At 1830 hours, your alert tones sound: "Medic 73, respond to 145 Circle Oak Drive for a 39-year-old man who is unresponsive and not breathing." You and your partner proceed to the scene with a response time of approximately 4 minutes. You recognize the address as that of a known heroin user. Law enforcement personnel and a fire engine company are dispatched to provide assistance.

1. What is the difference between ventilation and oxygenation?
2. Would a heroin overdose cause primary ventilation failure or oxygenation failure? Why or why not?

Introduction

Establishing and maintaining a **patent** (open) airway and ensuring effective oxygenation and ventilation are vital aspects of effective patient care. Attempting to stabilize the condition of a patient whose airway is compromised is futile. The human body needs a constant supply of oxygen to carry out the physiologic processes necessary to sustain life; the airway is where it all begins. Few situations will cause such acute deterioration and death more rapidly than airway or ventilation compromise. To preserve life, the airway must remain patent at all times—regardless of the situation.

The function of the respiratory system is simple: It brings in oxygen and eliminates carbon dioxide (the primary waste product of oxygen **metabolism**, the chemical processes that provide the cells with energy from nutrients). If this process is interrupted, then vital organs of the body will not function properly. For example, brain cells can survive for only 6 minutes or so without oxygen before permanent damage occurs.

Failure to manage the airway or inappropriate management of the airway is a major cause of preventable death in the prehospital setting. The basic airway management techniques learned in initial emergency medical technician (EMT) education are among the most crucial skills for you as a paramedic. The failure to use basic airway techniques, improper performance of the techniques (such as improper bag-mask seal or improper airway positioning), a rush to use advanced interventions, and failure to reassess the patient's condition increase mortality and morbidity. Therefore, a large portion of this chapter is dedicated to reinforcement of basic airway management skills.

You must understand the importance of early detection of airway conditions, rapid and effective intervention, and continual reassessment of a patient with airway or breathing compromise.

This chapter begins with a review of anatomy as it relates to the procedures of airway management, followed by the processes of ventilation, oxygenation, and respiration. A basic-to-advanced approach—just as airway management is typically performed in the field—is followed to emphasize the importance of securing a patent airway and ensuring adequate ventilation, oxygenation, and respiration. The chapter then describes the techniques of opening and maintaining a patent airway, recognizing and treating airway obstructions, assessing a patient's ventilation and oxygenation status, administering supplemental oxygen, and providing ventilatory assistance. Although a responsive patient may not need to have you open his or her airway manually and may need only supplemental oxygen, you must remember the order in which steps should be performed, bypassing steps that do not apply to the particular situation. Finally, advanced techniques, including advanced airway devices and procedures, are discussed in detail.

Review of Airway Anatomy

To effectively manage a patient's airway, you must identify key anatomic structures and understand how those structures may need to be manipulated when inserting various airway devices. The following section provides a brief review of airway anatomy. A detailed discussion of airway and respiratory anatomy and physiology is found in Chapter 8, *Anatomy and Physiology*.

Upper Airway

Anatomically, the upper airway includes all structures above the glottic opening (glottis), or the space between the vocal cords. When you perform skills such as endotracheal (ET) intubation, you must identify the upper airway anatomy while you advance the **laryngoscope** blade in the patient's mouth Figure 15-1A. ET intubation is discussed in detail later in this chapter.

Because of its tendency to fall back into the posterior pharynx of an unresponsive patient, the tongue is the first—and largest—anatomic structure that must be manipulated when managing a patient's airway. At the base of the tongue, the uvula extends from the soft palate in the posterior oral cavity; manipulation of the uvula is usually unnecessary, although the uvula is an important anatomic landmark to identify as you proceed to the posterior pharynx.

The pharynx is a muscular tube that extends from the nose and mouth to the level of the esophagus and trachea; it is composed of the nasopharynx, oropharynx, and the laryngopharynx (also called the hypopharynx). The laryngopharynx is the lowest portion of the pharynx; it opens into the larynx anteriorly and the esophagus posteriorly Figure 15-1B.

Lower Airway

The lower airway extends from the glottis to the pulmonary capillary membrane. The larynx is a complex structure formed by many independent cartilaginous structures. It marks where the upper airway ends and the lower airway begins Figure 15-2.

The thyroid cartilage is a shield-shaped structure palpable on the anterior neck. The superior part of the thyroid cartilage forms a V shape called the thyroid notch. The laryngeal prominence, known as the Adam's apple, is immediately inferior to the thyroid notch. The Adam's apple is more prominent in men than in women, and it can also be difficult to palpate in patients with obesity or patients with short necks. The thyroid cartilage is suspended from the hyoid bone by the thyrohyoid ligament and is directly anterior to the glottic opening and vocal cords.

The cricoid cartilage, or cricoid ring, lies inferior to the thyroid cartilage; it forms the lowest portion of the larynx and is the only circumferential ring of the trachea (the other tracheal rings are semicircular). The cricoid ring is more prominent in females than it is in males.

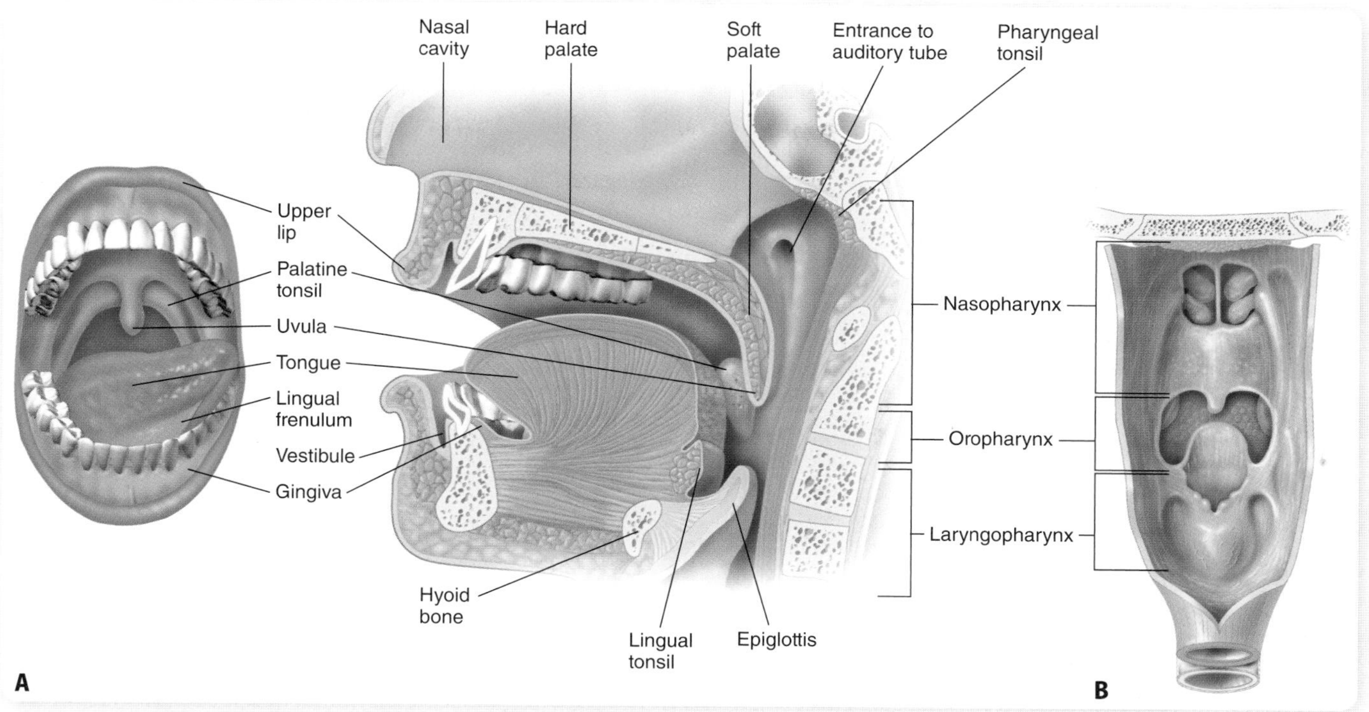

Figure 15-1 A. The oral cavity. **B.** The pharynx.

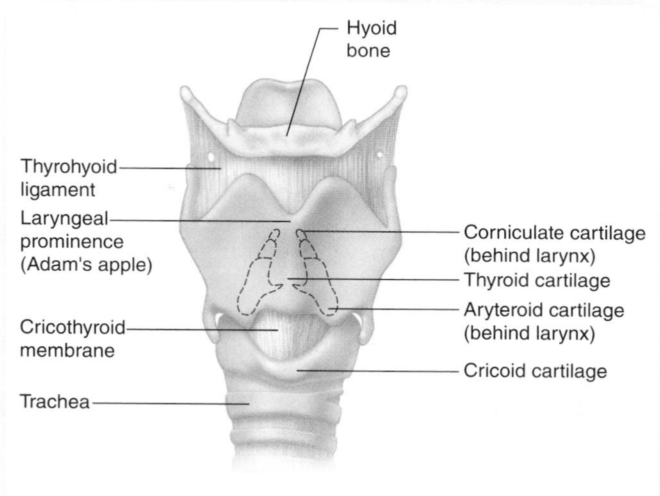

Figure 15-2 The larynx.

The cricothyroid membrane is located between the thyroid and cricoid cartilages; it is a site for emergency surgical and nonsurgical access to the airway (cricothyrotomy). Because it is bordered laterally and inferiorly by the highly vascular thyroid gland, you must locate the anatomic landmarks carefully when accessing the airway via the cricothyroid membrane.

The glottis is the narrowest portion of the adult airway **Figure 15-3**. The vocal cords are located at the lateral borders of the glottis. The **epiglottis** (a leaf-shaped cartilaginous structure that closes over the trachea during swallowing) is located at the superior border of the glottis. When you perform ET intubation, you must visualize the epiglottis, glottis, and vocal cords before inserting the ET tube.

Just beyond the vocal cords, the trachea immediately descends into the thoracic cavity; it is not a straight tube. This information is critical when you prepare an ET tube and place it into the trachea.

Ventilation, Oxygenation, and Respiration

The respiratory and cardiovascular systems work together to ensure that a constant supply of oxygen and nutrients is delivered to every cell in the body and that carbon dioxide and other waste products are removed from every cell **Table 15-1**.

Ventilation is the physical act of moving air in and out of the lungs. The active, muscular part of ventilation is called inhalation. Exhalation, unlike inhalation, is a passive process and does not normally require muscular effort.

Oxygenation is the process of loading oxygen molecules onto **hemoglobin** molecules in the bloodstream. For oxygenation to occur, the percentage of oxygen inhaled during ventilation—that is, the fraction of inspired oxygen (FIO_2)—must be adequate. Although oxygenation cannot occur without ventilation, ventilation is possible without oxygenation.

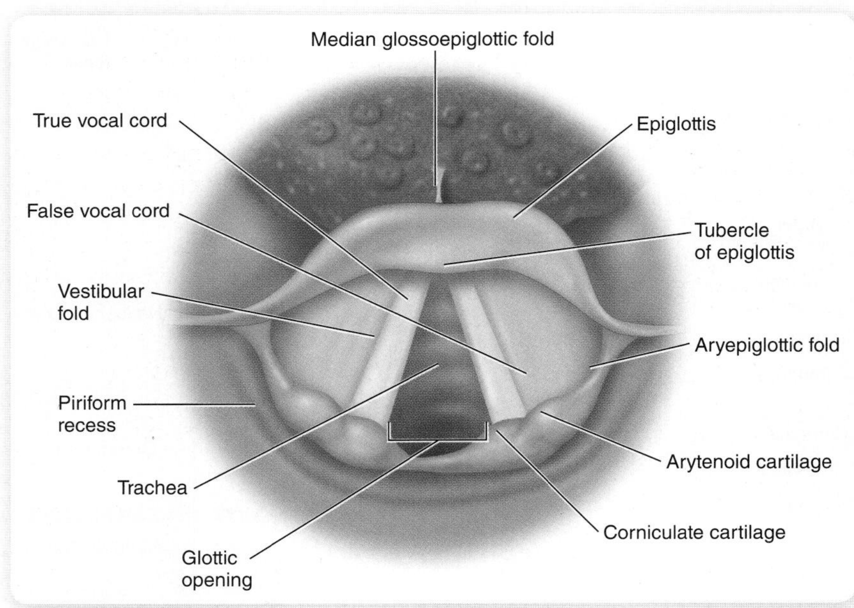

Figure 15-3 The glottis and its surrounding structures.

Table 15-1 Ventilation, Oxygenation, and Respiration

Function	Definition
Ventilation	The physical act of moving air into and out of the lungs
Oxygenation	The process of loading oxygen molecules onto hemoglobin molecules in the bloodstream
Respiration	The exchange of oxygen and carbon dioxide in the alveoli and the tissues of the body

Respiration is the process of exchanging oxygen and carbon dioxide. External respiration (pulmonary respiration) is the process of exchanging oxygen and carbon dioxide between the alveoli and the blood in the pulmonary capillaries. Internal respiration (cellular respiration) is the exchange of oxygen and carbon dioxide between the systemic circulation and the cells of the body. Adequate oxygenation is required for respiration; however, it does not guarantee that respiration is taking place.

Pathophysiology of Respiration

Multiple conditions can inhibit the body's ability to effectively provide oxygen to the cells. Disruption of pulmonary ventilation, oxygenation, and respiration will cause immediate effects on the body. You must recognize these conditions and correct them immediately. It is important to be able to distinguish a primary ventilation problem from a primary oxygenation or respiration problem. For example, overdose of a central nervous system (CNS) depressant drug (ie, narcotic/opiate, barbiturate) suppresses the rate and depth (tidal volume) of breathing, and causes, at least initially, a ventilation problem. If ventilation is impaired, then adequate oxygen will not be taken into the lungs and distributed to the cells and tissues of the body. By contrast, a person trapped in a place that is devoid of oxygen may develop an oxygenation problem first; he or she is ventilating, but is not breathing in adequate amounts of oxygen. As a result, oxygen delivery to the cells and tissues will be compromised, resulting in a respiration problem.

Every cell in the body needs a constant supply of oxygen to survive. Whereas some tissues are more resilient than others, eventually all cells will die if deprived of oxygen Figure 15-4. To provide adequate amounts of oxygen to the tissues of the body, external respiration and perfusion—circulation of blood within an organ or tissue in adequate amounts to meet the current needs of the cells—must take place.

▶ Hypoxia

Failure to meet the body's needs for oxygen may result in hypoxia. **Hypoxia** is a dangerous condition in which the tissues and cells do not receive enough oxygen. If hypoxia is uncorrected, then death may occur quickly.

Patients who are breathing inadequately will show varying signs and symptoms of hypoxia. The onset and degree of tissue damage caused by hypoxia often depend on

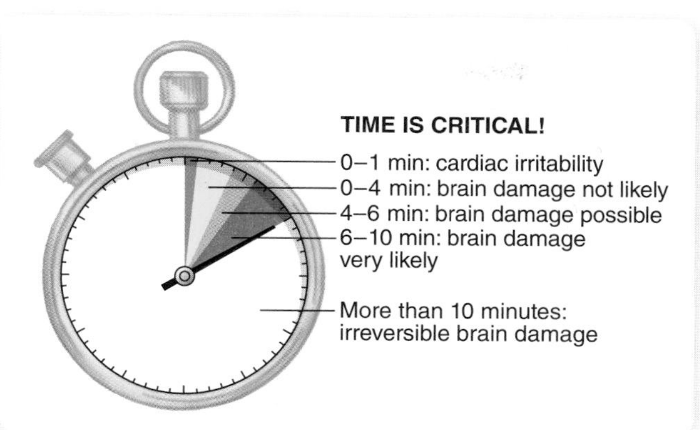

Figure 15-4 Cells need a constant supply of oxygen to survive. Some cells may be severely or permanently damaged after 4 to 6 minutes without oxygen.

the quality of ventilations. Early signs of hypoxia include restlessness, irritability, apprehension, tachycardia, and anxiety. Late signs of hypoxia include changes in mental status, a weak (thready) pulse, and **cyanosis**—a blue or purple skin color. Responsive patients often report a feeling of shortness of breath (**dyspnea**) and may be unable to speak in complete sentences. You should administer supplemental oxygen to a patient with respiratory distress before signs and symptoms of hypoxia appear.

Ventilation-Perfusion Ratio and Mismatch

The lungs have a functional role in placing ambient (room) air in proximity to circulating blood to permit gas exchange by simple diffusion. To accomplish this task, air and blood flow must be directed to the same place at the same time. In other words, ventilation and perfusion must be matched. A failure to match ventilation and perfusion, or **$\dot{V}/\dot{Q}$ mismatch**, contributes to most abnormalities in oxygen and carbon dioxide exchange.

In most people, the normal resting minute ventilation is approximately 6 L/min. About one-third of this volume fills dead space; therefore, resting alveolar volume is approximately 4 L/min. However, pulmonary artery blood flow is approximately 5 L/min, yielding an overall ratio of ventilation to perfusion of 4:5 L/min, or 0.8 L/min. Because neither ventilation nor perfusion is distributed equally, both are distributed to dependent regions of the lungs at rest. However, an increase in gravity-dependent flow is more marked with perfusion (blood) than with ventilation (air). Hence, the ratio of ventilation to perfusion is highest at the apex (top) of the lung and lowest at the base (bottom).

When ventilation is compromised but perfusion continues, blood passes over some alveolar membranes without gas exchange taking place; therefore, not all alveoli are enriched with oxygen. The result is a lack of oxygen diffusing across the membrane and into the circulatory system. Along the same lines, carbon dioxide is also unable to diffuse across the membrane and is recirculated into the bloodstream. This condition results in a $\dot{V}/\dot{Q}$ mismatch and could lead to severe hypoxia if the $\dot{V}/\dot{Q}$ mismatch is not recognized and treated.

Similar problems can occur when perfusion across the alveolar membrane is disrupted. Even though the alveoli are filled with fresh oxygen, disruption in blood flow does not allow for optimal exchange of gases across the membrane. The result of inadequate perfusion is less oxygen absorption in the bloodstream and less carbon dioxide removal. This $\dot{V}/\dot{Q}$ mismatch can also lead to hypoxia, and the patient needs immediate intervention to prevent further damage or death.

Factors Affecting Ventilation

Maintaining a patent airway is critical for the provision of oxygen to the tissues of the body. Many intrinsic (internal) and extrinsic (external) factors can cause airway obstruction. Intrinsic conditions such as infection, allergic reactions, and unresponsiveness (possibly leading to airway obstruction by the tongue) can significantly restrict the ability to maintain a patent airway. Swelling from infections and allergic reactions can be fatal if not aggressively managed with medications and, possibly, advanced airway management techniques. The tongue is the most common airway obstruction in an unresponsive patient. This airway obstruction, while easily corrected, can result in hypoxia and hinder adequate tissue perfusion. Snoring respirations and an improper position of the head and/or neck are good indicators that the tongue may be obstructing the airway. Prompt correction of this obstruction is necessary for adequate ventilation and oxygenation.

Some factors affecting pulmonary ventilation are not necessarily directly part of the respiratory system. The central and peripheral nervous systems have key roles in the regulation of breathing. Interruptions in these systems can have a drastic effect on the ability to breathe effectively. Medications that depress the CNS (such as opiates or opioids and benzodiazepines), if taken in excess, lower the respiratory rate and reduce the tidal volume. This lower rate and tidal volume will decrease alveolar volume and overall minute volume. As a result, the amount of carbon dioxide in the respiratory and circulatory systems is increased, resulting in an overall increase of the carbon dioxide content of the blood. Trauma to the head and spinal cord can also interrupt nervous system control of ventilation, resulting in decreased respiratory function and even failure. Neuromuscular disorders, such as muscular dystrophy and poliomyelitis, can also affect the ability of the nervous system to control breathing. Muscular dystrophy causes degeneration of muscle fibers, slowing motor development, and loss of muscle contractility. Curvature of the spine is also likely in patients with muscular dystrophy and can impair pulmonary function. Polio is a viral neuromuscular disorder that can affect the nerves, including those that regulate ventilation, and result in paralysis. Neuromuscular blocking agents (paralytics), such as those used to facilitate intubation, effectively paralyze a patient and induce apnea (discussed later in this chapter).

Patients with allergic reactions might have not only a potential airway obstruction due to swelling (angioedema), but also a decrease in pulmonary ventilation from bronchoconstriction. As the bronchioles constrict, air is forced through smaller lumens, resulting in decreased ventilation. Bronchoconstriction is also associated with conditions such as chronic obstructive pulmonary disease (COPD) and asthma.

Extrinsic factors affecting pulmonary ventilation can include trauma and foreign body airway obstruction. Trauma to the airway or chest requires immediate evaluation and intervention. Blunt or penetrating trauma and burns can disrupt airflow through the trachea and into the lungs, quickly resulting in oxygenation deficiencies. In addition, trauma to the chest wall can result in structural damage to the thorax, leading to inadequate pulmonary ventilation. For example, a patient with numerous rib fractures or a flail chest may purposely breathe shallowly in an attempt to alleviate the pain caused by the injury. This practice is called respiratory splinting and can result in decreased pulmonary ventilation. Proper ventilatory support is crucial to the outcome of patients with such injuries or conditions.

If carbon dioxide production exceeds the body's ability to eliminate it by ventilation, then the partial pressure of carbon dioxide ($Paco_2$) rises, resulting in **hypoventilation** (slow and/or shallow breathing). Theoretically, hypoventilation can occur in two ways: either carbon dioxide production can exceed the body's ability to eliminate it, or carbon dioxide elimination can be depressed to the extent that it no longer keeps up with normal metabolism.

At the other extreme is **hyperventilation** (rapid and/or deep breathing), which occurs when carbon dioxide elimination exceeds carbon dioxide production. For example, a patient experiencing an anxiety attack tends to breathe very deeply and rapidly, so he or she eliminates carbon dioxide at a rate faster than the body produces it. The level of carbon dioxide in his or her blood then falls below normal, and the patient experiences symptoms such as dizziness and numbness or tingling in the face and extremities.

Hypoventilation and hyperventilation could represent the body's attempt to compensate for various abnormal conditions. For example, if the pH of the blood is too high (alkalosis), the patient's breathing may become slow and/or shallow in an attempt to retain carbon dioxide (and therefore, hydrogen ions [H^+]) in an attempt to decrease the pH. Conversely, hyperventilation could be a compensatory response of the body to a decrease in the pH of the blood (acidosis), such as what occurs with hyperglycemic ketoacidosis or aspirin overdose.

In addition to factors discussed thus far, decreases or increases in minute volume can lead to problems with carbon dioxide levels in the blood Table 15-2.

Table 15-2 Carbon Dioxide Balance

	Hypoventilation	Hyperventilation
Minute volume	↓	↑
CO_2 elimination	↓	↑
$Paco_2$	↑ (hypercapnia)	↓ (hypocapnia)

Abbreviations: CO_2, carbon dioxide; $Paco_2$, partial pressure of carbon dioxide

A decrease in the minute volume decreases carbon dioxide elimination, resulting in a buildup of carbon dioxide in the blood (**hypercapnia**). An increase in the minute volume increases carbon dioxide elimination, which lowers the carbon dioxide content of the blood (**hypocapnia**).

▶ Factors Affecting Oxygenation and Respiration

External elements in the environment can affect the overall process of respiration. For proper respiration to occur at the cellular level, oxygenation and perfusion must function efficiently.

External Factors

Adequate respiration requires proper ventilation and oxygenation. External factors such as atmospheric pressure and the partial pressure of oxygen (Pao_2) in the ambient air have a key role in the overall process of respiration. At high altitudes, the percentage of oxygen remains the same, but the partial pressure decreases because the total atmospheric pressure decreases. The low Pao_2 can make it difficult—or impossible—to adequately oxygenate the tissues, thus interrupting internal respiration. In addition, closed environments, such as mines and trenches, may also have decreases in ambient oxygen, resulting in poor oxygenation and respiration.

Carbon monoxide (CO), along with other toxic gases, displaces oxygen in the environment and makes proper oxygenation and respiration difficult. In particular, CO has a much greater affinity for hemoglobin than does oxygen (250 times more). The attachment of CO molecules to the hemoglobin molecules, which forms carboxyhemoglobin (COHb), inhibits the proper transport of oxygen to the tissues and can cause false pulse oximetry readings. Pulse oximetry is discussed in detail later in this chapter.

Internal Factors

Conditions that reduce the surface area for gas exchange also decrease the body's oxygen supply, leading to inadequate tissue perfusion. Medical conditions such as pneumonia, pulmonary edema, and COPD may also result in a disturbance of cellular metabolism. These conditions decrease the surface area of the alveoli by damaging the alveoli or by leading to an accumulation of fluid in the lungs.

Nonfunctional alveoli create a barrier to the diffusion of oxygen and carbon dioxide. As a result, blood entering the lungs from the right side of the heart bypasses the alveoli and returns to the left side of the heart in an unoxygenated state—a condition called **intrapulmonary shunting**.

Patients who are submerged in water and patients with pulmonary edema have fluid in the alveoli. This accumulation of fluid inhibits adequate gas exchange at the alveolar membrane and results in decreased oxygenation and respiration. In addition, exposure to certain environmental conditions (such as high altitudes) or occupational hazards (such as epoxy resins) can result in fluid accumulation in the alveoli over time, resulting in an overall decrease in respiration. These conditions can result in anaerobic respiration and an increase in lactic acid accumulation. Excess lactic acid in the blood lowers the pH and can result in numerous life-threatening conditions, such as cardiac dysrhythmias, coma, and shock.

Other conditions that affect the cells of the body include hypoglycemia, hormonal imbalances, and infection. As oxygen and glucose levels decrease, the body is unable to maintain a homeostatic balance with regard to energy production. If the metabolic needs of the body cannot be met, then cellular death is likely. Infection also increases the metabolic needs of the body and disrupts homeostasis (the tendency toward stability in the body's internal environment). If the disruption in homeostasis is not corrected, then the cells will die as well. If the levels of the hormone insulin decrease in the body, then the cellular uptake of glucose will decrease. Without sufficient glucose, the cells will metabolize fatty acids, resulting in ketoacidosis—a form of metabolic acidosis.

Circulatory Compromise

The circulatory system must function efficiently for respiration to occur. When the circulatory system is compromised, perfusion becomes inadequate and the body's oxygen demands will not be met.

Obstruction of blood flow to individual cells and tissues is typically related to trauma emergencies. Conditions that you may encounter include simple or tension pneumothorax, open pneumothorax (sucking chest wound), hemothorax, hemopneumothorax, and pulmonary embolism. All of these conditions inhibit gas exchange at the tissue level as a result of their effects on the respiratory and circulatory systems. In addition, conditions such as heart failure and cardiac tamponade inhibit the ability of the heart to effectively pump oxygenated blood to the tissues.

Blood loss and anemia—a deficiency of red blood cells—reduce the oxygen-carrying ability of the blood. Without sufficient circulating red blood cells, not enough hemoglobin molecules are available to bind with oxygen.

When the body is in a state of shock, oxygen is not delivered to the cells efficiently. Hemorrhagic shock (a form of hypovolemic shock) is a decrease in blood volume, because of internal or external bleeding, that causes inadequate oxygen delivery to the body. In contrast, vasodilatory shock is not caused by a decrease in blood volume, but by an increase in the size of the blood vessels. As the diameter of the blood vessels increases, the blood pressure decreases and blood flow diminishes; oxygen is not delivered to the tissues in an effective manner. Both forms of shock result in poor tissue perfusion that leads to anaerobic metabolism. You should aggressively treat any patient suspected of being in shock to prevent further interruptions in tissue perfusion.

Words of Wisdom

The Effects of Ventilation on Cardiac Output

During normal breathing, the negative pressure created by each breath increases venous return of blood to the heart. Just as negative intrathoracic pressure draws air into the chest cavity through the airway (**negative pressure ventilation**), the same pressure also draws venous blood back to the heart from the head (via the superior vena cava) and abdomen (via the inferior vena cava).

When patients transition from negative pressure ventilation to **positive pressure ventilation** (the forcing of air into the lungs [ie, bag-mask ventilation]), they lose this stimulus for venous return, and some patients may experience decreased cardiac output and hypotension as a result. The increased intrathoracic pressure caused by positive pressure ventilation creates a pressure gradient against which the heart must pump. This process increases the **afterload** (the amount of resistance against which the ventricle must contract), which can further decrease cardiac output. The greater the pressure used to ventilate an apneic or a hypoventilating patient, the greater the decrease in **preload** (the volume of blood that returns to the heart), which occurs when the heart is literally squeezed by increased intrathoracic pressure.

Patients who are hypotensive, in shock, or are otherwise hemodynamically unstable may experience profound changes in blood pressure as a result of the hemodynamic effects of positive pressure ventilation. The best way to minimize this complication is to ventilate the patient for a period of 1 second—just enough to cause visible chest rise—and avoid ventilating the patient too fast. Positive and negative pressure ventilation are discussed in more detail later in this chapter.

▶ Acid-Base Balance

Hypoventilation and hyperventilation, along with hypoxia, can cause disruptions in the acid-base balance in the body that may lead to rapid clinical deterioration and death.

The respiratory system and the renal system have roles in maintaining homeostasis. Homeostasis requires a balance between the acids and bases, among other body systems. When an excess of acid is present in the body, the fastest way to eliminate it is through the respiratory system. Excess acid can be expelled as carbon dioxide from the lungs. Conversely, slowing respirations will increase the level of carbon dioxide. The renal system regulates pH by filtering out more (or retaining) hydrogen ions and retaining (or filtering out) bicarbonate when needed. The fastest way the body can eliminate excess H^+ ions is to create water and carbon dioxide, which can be expelled as gases from the lungs.

Anything that inhibits respiratory function can lead to acid retention and acidosis. Any time a patient is in respiratory distress or is unable to breathe, acidosis quickly develops. Acidosis can develop as a result of abnormal respiratory function (such as with bradypnea, labored breathing, or shallow breathing [reduced tidal volume]). Alkalosis can develop if the respiratory rate is too high (or the volume too much).

The four main clinical presentations of acid-base disorders are:

- Respiratory acidosis
- Respiratory alkalosis
- Metabolic acidosis
- Metabolic alkalosis

Fluctuations in pH due to the available bicarbonate in the body result in metabolic acidosis or alkalosis. Fluctuations in pH due to respiratory disorders that result in excess carbon dioxide retention or elimination result in respiratory acidosis or alkalosis. The focus here is on respiratory acidosis and respiratory alkalosis.

Acid-base disorders that are not immediately correctable by the body's buffering systems cause the body to initiate compensatory responses to help return levels to normal. For example, metabolic acidosis may create respiratory alkalosis as a compensatory response. Patient management often involves treating more than one form of acid-base imbalance.

Patient Assessment: Airway Evaluation

The importance of carefully assessing a patient's airway and ventilatory status cannot be overemphasized. In the field, you will encounter patients with a variety of airway conditions—some of these conditions are easily corrected; others require aggressive management. The emergency medical care you provide to a patient with an airway or ventilation problem is only as good as the assessment you perform.

▶ Assessing Airway Patency

When presented with a patient who is experiencing a respiratory problem, first determine if his or her airway is patent. An adult who is responsive, alert, and able to speak in complete sentences with a normal voice has no

YOU are the Paramedic PART 2

You arrive at the scene and find the man lying supine on his porch. The patient's neighbor, who called 9-1-1, advises that he saw the patient suddenly collapse after stumbling out of his house. The neighbor further states that she had talked to the patient 5 minutes prior to his collapse and that he was "fine." While your partner prepares the cardiac monitor/defibrillator, you confirm the patient has a carotid pulse, but is not breathing. His skin is cyanotic, and fluids that smell like beer are draining from his mouth.

Recording Time: 1 Minute	
Appearance	Motionless, cyanotic
Level of consciousness	Unresponsive
Airway	Secretions draining from the mouth
Breathing	Absent
Circulation	Carotid pulse, rapid and weak; skin, cyanotic

3. What should be your most immediate treatment priority?
4. What negative effects can occur if you hyperventilate a patient?

immediate airway problem. However, because his or her status can rapidly change, remain vigilant.

An unresponsive patient has a compromised airway until that is ruled out by a careful assessment. Signs of airway compromise in an unresponsive patient include snoring (caused by partial airway obstruction by the tongue), vomitus (stomach contents) draining from the mouth, and a gurgling sound heard during breathing (which indicates secretions in the airway). Secretions pooling in the patient's mouth is a clear indicator of a markedly depressed or absent gag reflex. The **gag reflex** is a spastic pharyngeal and esophageal reflex caused by stimulating the posterior pharynx to prevent foreign bodies from entering the trachea. The absence of a gag reflex significantly increases the risk of aspiration.

Recognizing Adequate Breathing

Normal breathing in an adult at rest is characterized by a rate between 12 and 20 breaths/min Table 15-3 with adequate depth (tidal volume), a regular pattern of inhalation and exhalation, and clear and equal breath sounds bilaterally. Breathing at rest should appear effortless, and changes in rate and regularity should be subtle (not obvious).

Words of Wisdom

Hypoxemia is defined as a low level of oxygen in arterial blood. Hypoxia, as discussed earlier, is a deficiency of oxygen at the tissue and cellular levels. Although these terms are often used interchangeably, they are different processes. Hypoxemia can often be reversed by administering supplemental oxygen, whereas hypoxia requires more aggressive oxygenation and, in some cases, ventilatory support. Left untreated, hypoxia will lead to **anoxia**—a lack of oxygen that results in tissue and cellular death.

Table 15-3 Normal Respiratory Rate Ranges

Age	Range (breaths/min)
Adults	12 to 20
Children (ages 1 to 18 years)	12 to 37
Infants (ages 1 month to 1 year)	30 to 53

Pediatric data from: American Heart Association (AHA). Vital signs in children. In: *Pediatric Advanced Life Support.* Dallas, TX: AHA; 2015.

Recognizing Inadequate Breathing

Any patient you encounter—especially one with a respiratory complaint—should be assessed for breathing adequacy. Just because a patient is breathing does not indicate that he or she is breathing adequately. Generally speaking, if you can see or hear a patient breathe, then a problem exists.

An adult patient who presents with respiratory distress and is breathing at a rate of less than 12 breaths/min or more than 20 breaths/min must be evaluated for other signs of inadequate ventilation, such as shallow breathing (reduced tidal volume), an irregular pattern of breathing, altered mentation, and **adventitious** (abnormal) breath sounds. Cyanosis is a clear indicator of a low blood oxygen content; however, you may not encounter it as an early sign.

Patients with respiratory distress often compensate with preferential positioning, such as an upright sniffing position (in which the patient is sitting up, with the head moved forward until the earlobes are on the same vertical plane as the manubrium of the sternum), or a tripod position (in which the patient is sitting up and leaning forward with elbows bent). Patients experiencing respiratory distress will avoid a supine position because it will worsen their breathing difficulties.

The potential causes of respiratory distress and inadequate ventilation are numerous and include severe infection (sepsis), trauma, brainstem injury a noxious (poisonous) or oxygen-poor environment, and renal failure. Respiratory distress may be the result of an upper and/or lower airway obstruction, respiratory muscle impairment (such as in spinal cord injury), or CNS impairment (such as in head injury and drug overdose).

If a patient's airway is not patent, or if breathing is absent or inadequate, then all therapies that you may attempt will prove futile. Proper airway management involves opening the airway, clearing the airway, assessing breathing, and providing the appropriate intervention or interventions—in that order.

Evaluation of a patient with a respiratory complaint includes visual observations, auscultation, and palpation. Use visual techniques at first sight of the patient—literally from the door as you enter the room. Determine answers to the following questions when you assess a patient with respiratory distress:

- How is the patient positioned? Is he or she in a tripod position (elbows out)?
- Is the patient experiencing **orthopnea** (positional dyspnea)?
- Is rise and fall of the chest adequate (adequate tidal volume)?
- Is the patient gasping for air (air hunger)?
- What is the skin color? Is the skin moist or clammy (diaphoretic)?
- Is flaring of the nostrils present?
- Is the patient breathing through pursed lips?

- Do you note any **retractions** (skin pulling between and around the ribs during inhalation):
  - Intercostal?
  - At the suprasternal notch?
  - At the supraclavicular fossa?
  - Subcostal?
- Is the patient using accessory muscles to breathe?
- Is the patient's chest wall moving symmetrically? (**Asymmetric chest wall movement**, when one side of the chest moves less than the other, indicates that airflow into one lung is decreased.)
- Is the patient taking a series of quick breaths, followed by a prolonged exhalation phase?

A patient with inadequate ventilation may appear to be working hard to breathe (labored breathing). Labored breathing requires effort and may involve the use of accessory muscles. **Accessory muscles** include the sternocleidomastoid muscles (neck muscles), the pectoralis major muscles, and the abdominal muscles.

Accessory muscles are not used during normal breathing. Signs of inadequate ventilation in adults include the following:

- Respiratory rate of fewer than 12 breaths/min or more than 20 breaths/min in the presence of dyspnea
- Irregular respiratory rhythm, such as taking a series of deep breaths followed by periods of apnea
- Diminished, absent, or noisy auscultated breath sounds
- Abdominal breathing
- Reduced flow of exhaled air at the nose and mouth
- Unequal or inadequate chest expansion, resulting in reduced tidal volume
- Increased effort of breathing (use of accessory muscles)
- Shallow depth of breathing (reduced tidal volume)
- Skin that is pale, cyanotic, cool, moist (clammy), or mottled
- Retractions
- Staccato speech patterns (one- or two-word dyspnea)

When you assess a patient with respiratory distress, consider the external environment, such as high altitude and enclosed spaces, which can be associated with impaired oxygenation. Remember personal safety if the environment is unsafe.

Feel for air movement at the nose and mouth. Observe the chest for symmetry, and note any **paradoxical motion**—the inward movement of a segment of the chest during inhalation and outward movement of the chest during exhalation, opposite normal chest movement and an indication of a flail chest. Assess for **pulsus paradoxus**. Pulsus paradoxus is a clinical finding in which the systolic blood pressure drops more than 10 mm Hg during inhalation. A change in pulse quality, or even the disappearance of a pulse during inhalation, may also be detected. Pulsus paradoxus is generally seen in patients with decompensating COPD, severe pericardial tamponade, or other conditions that cause an increase in intrathoracic pressure (such as tension pneumothorax or a severe asthma attack).

A history of the present illness is a vital part of your assessment of a patient with respiratory distress. Ask the following questions to determine the evolution of the current problem:

- Was the onset of the problem sudden or gradual?
  - Some people may perceive respiratory distress that occurred 2 days earlier as arising gradually, when, in fact, the onset was sudden; the patient may have waited 2 days before calling for help.
- Is any cause or "trigger" of the event known?
  - Asthma is commonly exacerbated by stress, cold weather, or environmental allergens.
  - A foreign body airway obstruction is commonly preceded by a sudden onset of difficulty in breathing during a meal or, in children, while playing with small toys or other objects.
- What is the duration (is the problem constant or recurrent)?
- Does anything alleviate or exacerbate the problem?
- Are any other associated symptoms present, such as a productive cough (if yes, then what color is the sputum?), chest pain or pressure, or fever?
- Were any interventions attempted before the arrival of emergency medical services (EMS)?
- Has the patient been evaluated by a physician or admitted to the hospital for this condition in the past? If so, then what was the diagnosis?
  - Determine specifically whether the patient was hospitalized or seen in the emergency department and then released. If the patient was hospitalized, then ask whether he or she was admitted to an intensive care unit (ICU) or a regular, unmonitored floor. A condition that warranted admission to an ICU is clinically significant.
- Is the patient currently taking any medications?
  - Do not simply ask which medications were taken today. Instead, determine the overall compliance by asking whether the patient has been taking the medications as prescribed. Ask, "Have you been able to take all of your

pills as directed?" "Has anything stopped you from taking your pills as directed, such as running out of some of the pills?" "Is something bothering you about taking a certain pill?" Verify this information by looking at the prescription dates on the medication bottles and by reading the prescription directions.
- Ask whether the patient has had any changes in his or her current prescription, such as a new medication or changes in the prescribing directions of an existing medication.

- Does the patient have any risk factors that could cause or exacerbate his or her condition, such as alcohol or illicit drug use, cigarette smoking, or an inadequate diet?

Evaluate the patient for protective reflexes of the airway. These reflexes include coughing, sneezing, and gagging. A patient whose cough mechanism is suppressed—whether by drugs, by pain, by trauma, or by any other cause—is at serious risk of aspirating foreign material. Sneezing is usually elicited by irritation of the nose.

Sighing is a slow, deep inhalation followed by a prolonged and sometimes audible exhalation. Sighing periodically hyperinflates the lungs, thereby reexpanding atelectatic (collapsed) alveoli. The average person sighs about once per minute. Hiccuping is a sudden inhalation, caused by spasmodic contraction of the diaphragm, cut short by closure of the glottis. Hiccuping serves no physiologic purpose, although persistent hiccups may be clinically significant.

Patients with serious injuries or illnesses may present with changes in their respiratory patterns. Table 15-4 shows various abnormal respiratory patterns and their causes.

▶ Assessment of Breath Sounds

While you are assessing breathing, auscultate breath sounds with a stethoscope. Breath sounds should be clear and equal on both sides of the chest (bilaterally), anteriorly, and posteriorly. Compare each apex (top) of the lung with the opposite apex and each base (bottom) of the lung with the opposite base.

Breath sounds are created as air moves through the tracheobronchial tree. The size of the airway determines the type of sound that will be produced. Significant differences in adult, child, and infant airways exist, resulting in differences in breath sounds. The trachea and bronchi have large diameters; therefore, the sound produced is higher pitched and is heard during inspiration and expiration. Breath sounds are heard over the majority of the chest, representing airflow into the alveoli. **Tracheal breath sounds**, also called bronchial breath sounds, are heard by placing the stethoscope diaphragm over the trachea or over the sternum. Assess breath sounds for duration, pitch, and intensity. **Vesicular breath sounds** are softer, muffled sounds and have been described like wind blowing through the trees. The expiratory phase is barely audible. **Bronchovesicular sounds** are a combination of the two and are heard in locations where airways and alveoli are found—the upper part of the sternum and between the scapulae. Locations for these sounds are shown in Figure 15-6. Figure 15-7 describes the normal breath sounds. Assess bronchovesicular sounds for duration, pitch, and intensity.

Table 15-4	Abnormal Respiratory Patterns
Cheyne-Stokes respirations	Gradually increasing rate and depth of respirations followed by a gradual decrease of respirations with intermittent periods of apnea; associated with brainstem insult Figure 15-5.
Kussmaul respirations	Deep, rapid respirations; seen in patients with diabetic ketoacidosis.
Biot (ataxic) respirations	Irregular pattern, rate, and depth of breathing with intermittent periods of apnea; results from increased ICP.
Apneustic respirations	Prolonged, gasping inhalation followed by extremely short, ineffective exhalation; associated with brainstem insult.
Agonal gasps	Slow, shallow, irregular, or occasional gasping breaths; results from cerebral anoxia. Agonal gasps may be seen when the heart has stopped but the brain continues to send signals to the muscles of respiration.

Abbreviation: ICP, intracranial pressure

Data from: Fontanarosa PB, Christiansen S. Units of measure. Table 2: Selected laboratory tests, with reference ranges and conversion factors. In: American Medical Association, ed. *AMA Manual of Style: A Guide for Authors and Editors.* 10th ed. New York, NY: Oxford University Press; 2007:798-815.

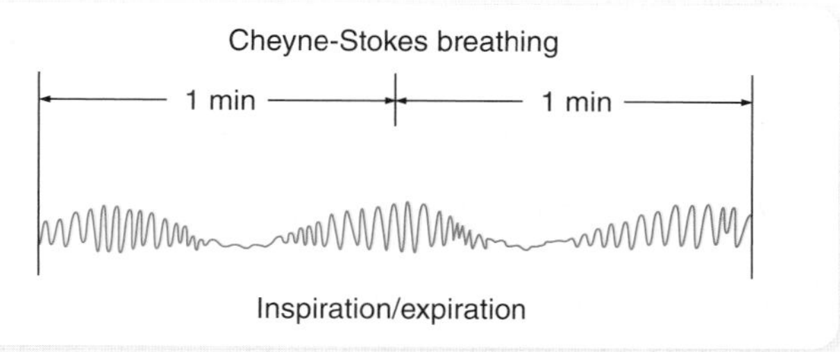

Figure 15-5 Cheyne-Stokes breathing shows a crescendo-decrescendo pattern of respirations followed by periods of apnea.

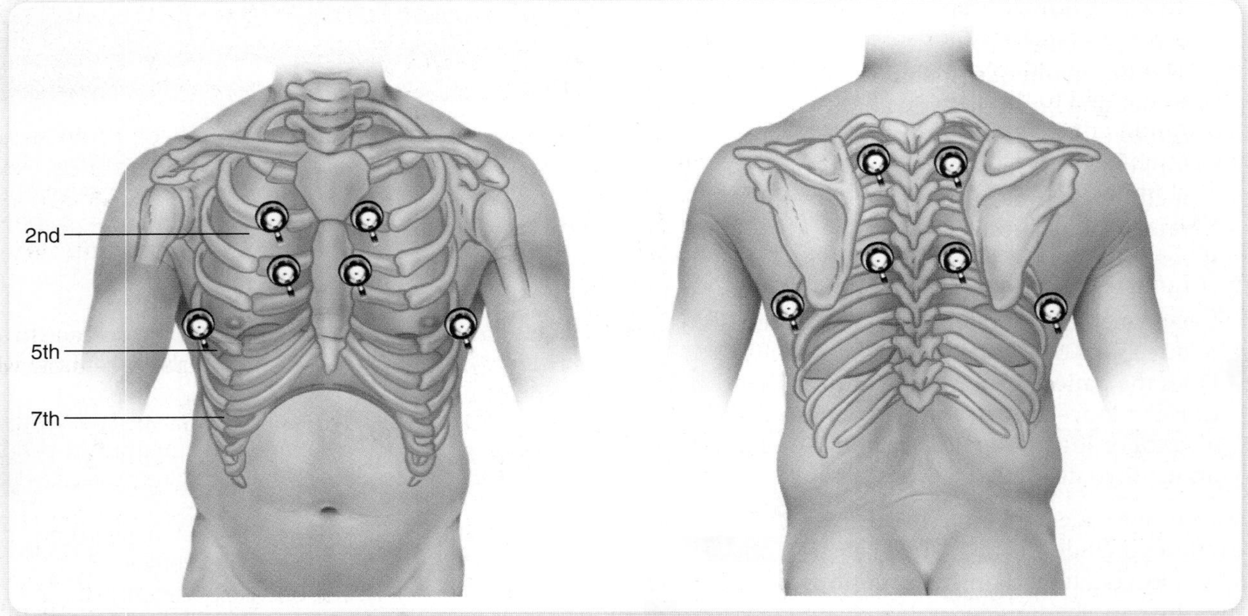

Figure 15-6 Common sites of auscultation include the 2nd, 5th, and 7th intercostal spaces as shown.

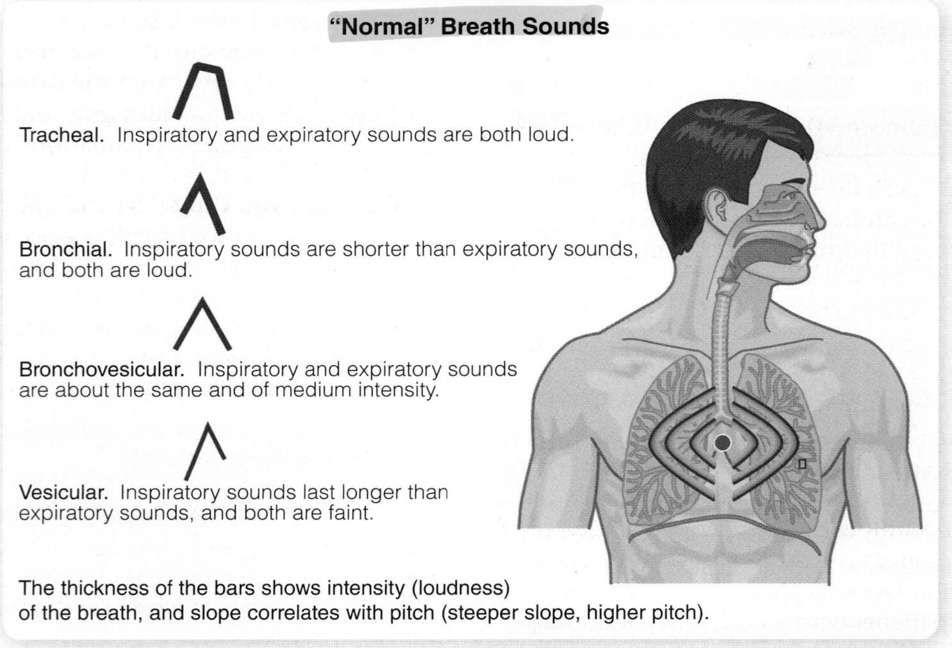

Figure 15-7 Normal breath sounds are heard over different parts of the chest. Breath sounds become softer away from the largest airways. The character during inspiration versus expiration also changes.

Duration refers to the length of time for the inspiratory and expiratory phase of the breath. Normally, expiration is twice as long as inspiration. This relationship is expressed by the **inspiratory/expiratory (I/E) ratio**; a normal I/E ratio is 1:2. When a patient's lower airway is obstructed and he or she has difficulty getting air out (such as in asthma, for example), the expiratory phase is prolonged and may be four to five times as long as inspiration. In the case of a patient with asthma, the I/E ratio would be 1:4 or 1:5. In a patient with tachypnea, the expiratory phase is short and approaches that of inspiration; the I/E ratio may be 1:1.

Pitch is described as intensity of sound that is higher or lower than normal, such as in stridor or wheezing (discussed next). The intensity of sound depends on airflow rate, constancy of flow throughout inspiration, patient position, and the site selected for auscultation. Thickness of the chest wall may affect the intensity. Sounds that are less intense are said to be diminished.

A common error in assessing the intensity of breath sounds occurs when auscultation is performed over the patient's clothing. Always auscultate directly on the patient's skin.

Sounds that might be classified as normal—but are present in an unexpected area—can indicate an abnormal condition. For example, tracheal sounds in areas that should produce vesicular sounds may indicate pneumonia.

Words of Wisdom

When you auscultate breath sounds emergently—for example, when confirming proper ET tube placement, ruling in (or ruling out) a pneumothorax, or confirming adequate bag-mask ventilation—auscultate bilaterally at the third or fourth intercostal space in the midaxillary line. Immediate corrective action is needed if breath sounds are absent altogether or if they are unilaterally diminished or absent.

Adventitious (abnormal) breath sounds are usually classified as either continuous or discontinuous. **Wheezing** is a continuous sound as air flows through a constricted lower airway, such as with asthma or bronchiolitis. Wheezing is a high-pitched sound that may be heard on inspiration, expiration, or both. **Rhonchi** are also continuous sounds, although they are low-pitched; they indicate mucus or fluid in the larger lower airways (such as in pulmonary edema and bronchitis). **Crackles** (formerly known as rales) occur when airflow causes mucus or fluid in the airways to move in the smaller lower airways. The crackles tend to clear with coughing. Crackles may also be heard when collapsed airways or alveoli pop open. Crackles are classified as discontinuous sounds and may occur early or late in the inspiratory cycle. Early inspiratory crackles usually occur when larger, proximal bronchi open and are common in patients with COPD; they tend not to clear with coughing. Late inspiratory crackles occur when peripheral alveoli and airways pop open and are more common in dependent lung regions. These sounds are common in patients with reduced lung volumes.

Stridor results from foreign body aspiration, infection, swelling, disease, or trauma within or immediately above the glottic opening. Stridor produces a loud, high-pitched sound that is typically heard during the inspiration phase. A **pleural friction rub** results from inflammation that causes the pleura to thicken. The pleural space can decrease as a result, allowing the surfaces of the visceral and parietal pleurae to rub together. This decrease often creates stabbing pain with breathing or any movement of the thorax.

Quantifying Ventilation and Oxygenation

In addition to your visual and hands-on assessments of the patient with an airway or breathing problem, several methods and devices are used to quantify—that is, assign a numeric value to—ventilation and oxygenation.

Pulse Oximetry

Pulse oximetry is a simple, rapid, safe, and noninvasive method of measuring—minute by minute—how well a person's hemoglobin is saturated.

A **pulse oximeter** measures the percentage of hemoglobin in the arterial blood that is saturated with oxygen **Figure 15-8**. Under normal circumstances, hemoglobin is saturated with oxygen (Spo_2). A sensor probe, clipped to the patient's finger or earlobe, uses a light-emitting diode to transmit light through the vascular bed to a light-sensing detector. The amount of light transmitted across the vascular bed depends on the proportion of hemoglobin that is saturated with oxygen. To ensure that the instrument is measuring arterial and not venous oxygen saturation, pulse oximeters are designed to assess only pulsating blood vessels. As a consequence, pulse oximeters also measure the patient's pulse. One way to check the functioning of a pulse oximeter is to compare the pulse reading it provides with your own measurement of the patient's pulse by palpation. When you use the pulse oximeter that is attached to the cardiac monitor/defibrillator, you can select the option of viewing the Spo_2 waveform to confirm the device is properly sensing **Figure 15-9**. Refer to the manufacturer's instructions.

A normally oxygenated, normally perfused person should have an Spo_2 level of greater than 95% while breathing room air. A reading of less than 95% in a

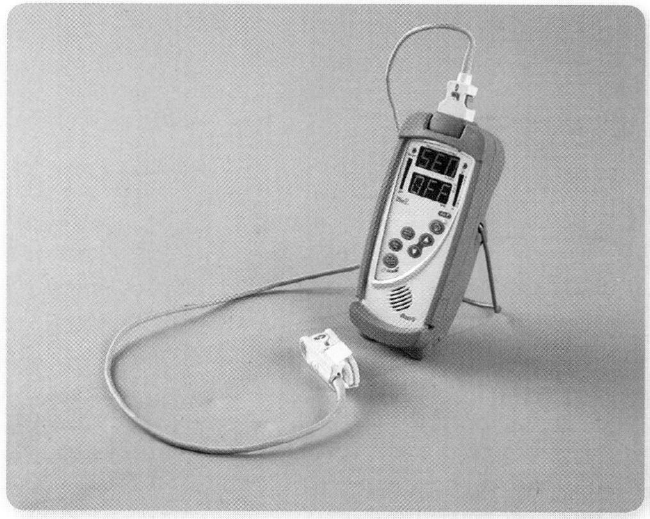

Figure 15-8 Pulse oximetry is a noninvasive method of assessing arterial oxygen saturation.

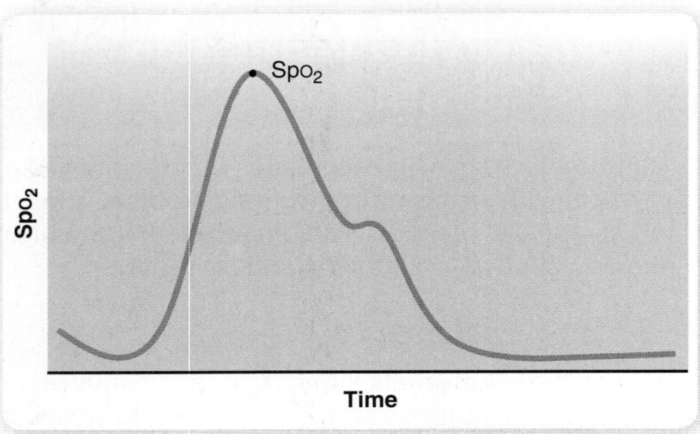

Figure 15-9 The characteristic shape of the pulse oximeter waveform confirms that the device is properly sensing.

nonsmoker suggests hypoxemia; a reading of less than 90% accompanied by respiratory distress signals a need for aggressive oxygen therapy.

Situations in which pulse oximeters may be useful in prehospital emergency medical care include the following:

- **Monitoring the oxygenation status of a patient during an intubation attempt or during suctioning.** The low-saturation alarm on the pulse oximeter can signal that you should abort the intubation attempt and ventilate the patient.
- **Identifying deterioration in the condition of a trauma patient.** In a patient with multiple trauma, the signs of a developing tension pneumothorax may not be evident until the condition is advanced. A declining Spo_2 level can alert you to a problem and prompt a search for the cause of the problem.
- **Identifying deterioration in the condition of a patient with cardiac disease.** Pulse oximetry may enable early identification of patients who are experiencing heart failure in the wake of acute myocardial infarction.
- **Identifying high-risk patients with respiratory conditions.** For example, pulse oximetry may identify patients with asthma who are having serious attacks or patients with emphysema who are in severe decompensation.
- **Assessing vascular status in orthopaedic trauma.** Pulse oximetry is routine practice in assessing a fractured extremity to evaluate circulation distal to the fracture. Loss of a pulse means that the limb is in jeopardy and may require urgent action in the field if transport time is long. A pulse oximeter clipped to a finger or toe on a broken limb might provide critical information about the ongoing circulation to the limb.

The usefulness of a pulse oximeter depends on its ability to provide accurate information. A pulse oximeter that

YOU are the Paramedic PART 3

The patient's oropharynx is now clear of secretions. You insert an oral and a nasal airway and attempt to ventilate the patient with a bag-mask device. You meet resistance during your first ventilation attempt and the patient's chest does not rise, so you reposition the patient's airway and reattempt to ventilate. After failing to produce chest rise after two ventilation attempts, you suspect a severe foreign body upper airway obstruction and instruct your partner to begin chest compressions.

Recording Time: 3 Minutes	
Respirations	Absent
Pulse	130 beats/min; weak and regular
Skin	Cyanotic
Blood pressure	Not available yet
Oxygen saturation (Spo_2)	68%
$ETCO_2$	Not available yet
ECG	Not available yet

5. In addition to your inability to ventilate the patient, do any other indicators suggest that the patient's airway is obstructed?
6. What equipment should you prepare while your partner is performing chest compressions?

gives a reading of 99% when the patient is actually severely hypoxemic will not provide helpful information and could lead to inadequate or erroneous interventions. Be aware of circumstances that might produce erroneous readings:

- **Bright ambient light** may enter the spectrophotometer of the pulse oximeter and create an incorrect reading. Protect the sensor clip by covering it with a towel or aluminum foil.
- **Patient motion** can confuse the pulse oximeter because it may mistake motion for arterial pulsation and read the oxygen saturation level from a vein rather than an artery.
- **Poor perfusion** makes it difficult for the pulse oximeter to sense a pulse and therefore to generate a reading. Poor perfusion occurs in states such as shock, cardiac arrest, and cold exposure. If the vessels in a patient's limbs are constricted and the limbs are cold, then it may be necessary to place the pulse oximeter clip on the earlobe or nose.
- **Nail polish** will prevent the sensor from working properly. Carry disposable acetone (nail polish remover) swabs to quickly remove nail polish.
- **Venous pulsations** may occur in some patients with right-sided heart failure due to the systemic backup of blood. If a vein is pulsating, then the pulse oximeter may regard it as an artery and measure venous oxygen saturation.
- **Abnormal hemoglobin** may produce a falsely normal Spo_2 level.

The two types of hemoglobin normally found are **oxyhemoglobin (Hbo_2)**, hemoglobin that is occupied by oxygen, and **reduced hemoglobin**, the hemoglobin after the oxygen has been released to the cells. However, in the presence of **methemoglobin (metHb)** (a compound formed by oxidation of the iron on the hemoglobin), and **carboxyhemoglobin (COHb)** (hemoglobin loaded with CO), normal Spo_2 values may be observed, even though the body is not receiving sufficient oxygen. As mentioned previously, CO binds to hemoglobin 250 times more readily than oxygen. A **carbon monoxide oximeter**, also called a CO-oximeter or CO monitor, is a device that measures absorption at several wavelengths to distinguish Hbo_2 from COHb and determines the level of Hbo_2 saturation—the percentage of oxygenated Hb compared with the total amount of hemoglobin—including COHb, metHb, Hbo_2, and reduced Hb **Figure 15-10**. When a patient presents with CO poisoning, the CO-oximeter will detect this Hb—expressed as SpCO—and will report a markedly reduced Hbo_2 saturation. Remember, do not make treatment decisions based solely on pulse oximetry, and be aware of its limitations.

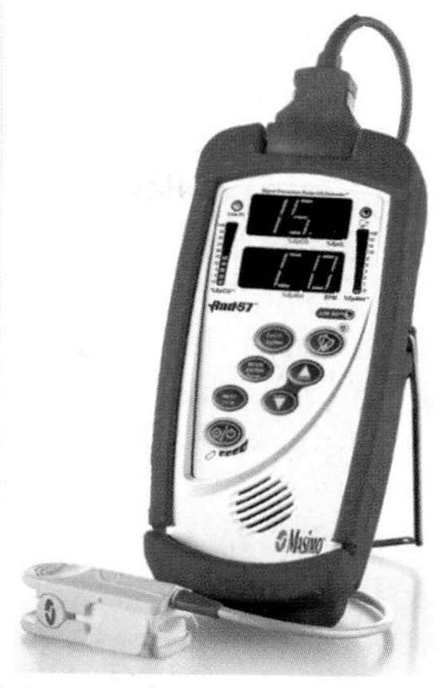

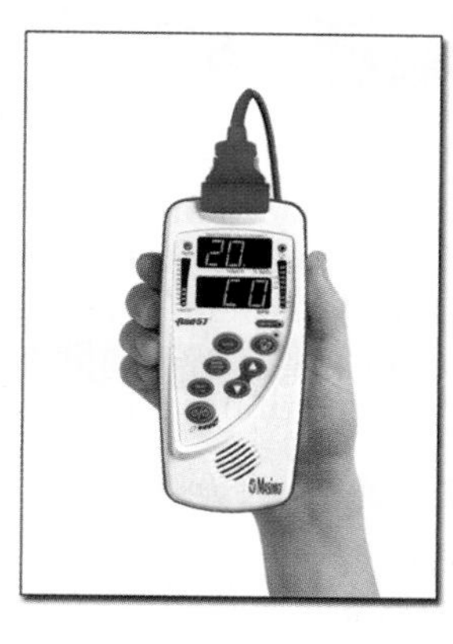

Figure 15-10 A carbon monoxide oximeter has the ability to distinguish oxyhemoglobin from carboxyhemoglobin.

The Masimo® Rad-ST™ Pulse CO-Oximeter™ courtesy of Masimo Corporation (www.masimo.com).

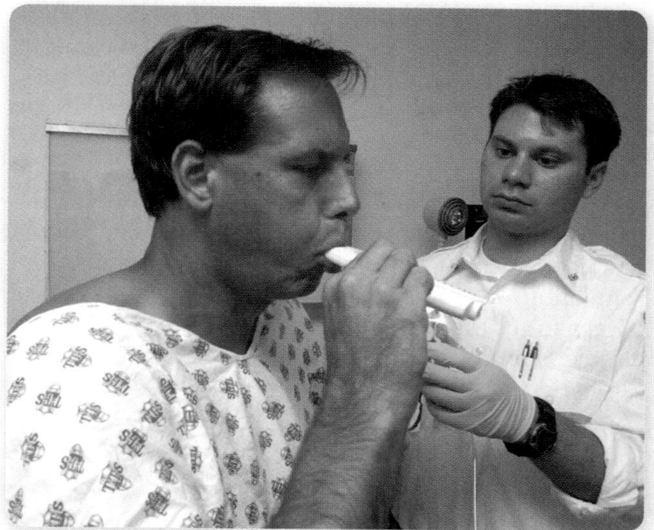

Figure 15-11 Peak expiratory flowmeters are used to quantify the degree of bronchoconstriction.

▶ Peak Expiratory Flow Measurement

In patients with certain reactive airway diseases (such as asthma), you can evaluate bronchoconstriction by measuring the peak rate of a forceful exhalation with a peak expiratory flowmeter **Figure 15-11**. An increasing **peak expiratory flow** suggests that the patient is responding to treatment (such as inhaled bronchodilators). A decreasing peak expiratory flow may be an early indication that the patient's condition is deteriorating.

> **Words of Wisdom**
>
> **When in doubt, look at the patient!**
>
> Always weigh the information provided by the pulse oximeter (or any other device) against clinical observations. If the patient is turning blue and struggling to breathe, then you should ignore the pulse oximeter reading that suggests the patient is adequately oxygenated.

Peak expiratory flow varies based on sex, height, and age. Healthy adults have a peak expiratory flow rate of 350 to 750 mL. To assess peak expiratory flow, place the patient in a seated position with legs dangling. Assemble the flowmeter, and ensure that it reads zero. Ask the patient to take a deep breath, place the mouthpiece in his or her mouth, and exhale as forcefully as possible (ensure no air leaks around the device or comes from the patient's nose). Perform the test three times, and take the best peak flow rate of the three readings.

▶ Arterial Blood Gas Analysis

Paramedics are not typically trained to obtain arterial blood specimens and do not carry the equipment needed to analyze the patient's blood. As a result, you will rely on noninvasive methods of assessing ventilation and oxygenation (such as pulse oximetry and capnography/capnometry).

Analysis of arterial blood gases (ABGs) provides the most comprehensive quantitative information about the respiratory system. In this procedure, blood is obtained from a superficial artery, such as the radial or femoral artery. The blood is then analyzed for pH, $Paco_2$, Pao_2, Hco_3^- (concentration of bicarbonate ions), base excess (indicating acidosis or alkalosis), and Sao_2 levels. Normal ABG values are summarized in Table 15-5.

With ABG measurements, the values of pH and Hco_3^- are used to evaluate the acid-base status of the patient. The $Paco_2$ value is an indicator of the effectiveness of ventilation. The values of Pao_2 and Sao_2 are indicators of oxygenation. To maintain normal ABG values, a balance between alveolar volume and perfusion of the alveolar capillaries must be maintained.

▶ End-tidal Carbon Dioxide Assessment

Carbon dioxide can be described as the "smoke of metabolism." The body uses oxygen as its fuel and makes carbon dioxide as its byproduct. As long as oxygen is delivered to the cells and tissues, the production of carbon dioxide continues. A helpful analogy is a motor vehicle engine. As long as gasoline continues to burn, exhaust is produced. In the human body, carbon dioxide is the exhaust.

End-tidal carbon dioxide ($ETCO_2$) monitors detect the presence of carbon dioxide in exhaled air. These monitoring tools are important adjuncts for determining the adequacy of ventilations and proper placement of advanced airways. The types of $ETCO_2$ monitors include colorimetric, digital, and digital/waveform.

A **colorimetric carbon dioxide detector** provides qualitative information regarding the presence of carbon dioxide in the patient's exhaled breath; that is, it does not assign a numeric value. The colorimetric CO_2 detector is attached between the ET tube and ventilation device. After six to eight positive-pressure breaths—the amount of time it takes for carbon dioxide to accumulate in the device—the specially-treated paper inside the detector should turn from purple to yellow during exhalation Figure 15-12. Air exhaled through an ET tube that has been properly placed in the trachea of a patient with adequate perfusion should contain 4% to 5% carbon dioxide, which will cause the paper to turn yellow during exhalation. If inadvertent esophageal intubation occurs, then a negligible amount (less than 0.5%) of carbon dioxide will be present in the exhaled gas; this amount will cause the paper to remain purple during exhalation.

Several limitations exist with the colorimetric CO_2 detector. The device might give a false-positive reading if the patient has carbon dioxide trapped in the stomach from the ingestion of carbonated beverages. Furthermore, the device is sensitive to extremes of temperature and humidity; it may be less reliable if vomitus or other secretions get inside it; and the paper inside the device degrades over time, resulting in a less reliable reading.

Table 15-5 Normal Arterial Blood Gas Values

pH	7.35 to 7.45
Pao_2	80 to 100 mm Hg
$Paco_2$	35 to 45 mm Hg
Hco_3–	21 to 28 mEq/L
Base (excess or deficit)	−2 to 3 mEq/L
Sao_2	>95%

Abbreviations: Hco_3^-, concentration of bicarbonate ions; $Paco_2$, partial pressure of carbon dioxide; Pao_2, partial pressure of oxygen; Sao_2, oxygen saturation

Data from: Fontanarosa PB, Christiansen S. Units of measure. Table 2: selected laboratory tests, with reference ranges and conversion factors. In: American Medical Association, ed. *AMA Manual of Style: A Guide for Authors and Editors*. 10th ed. New York, NY: Oxford University Press; 2007:798-815.

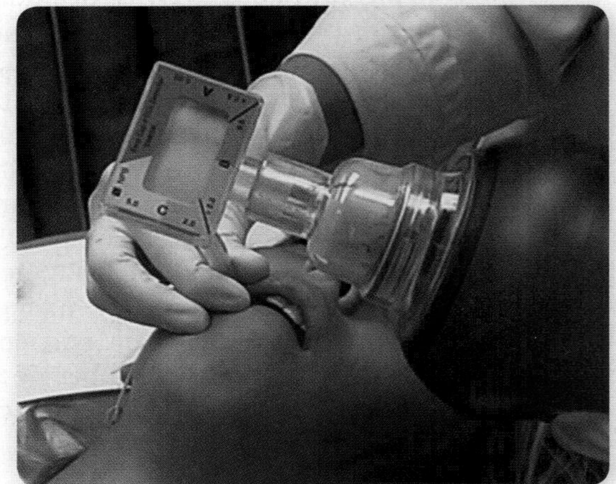

Figure 15-12 The paper inside the colorimetric carbon dioxide detector should turn from purple to yellow during exhalation, indicating the presence of exhaled carbon dioxide.

Courtesy of Marianne Gausche-Hill, MD, FACEP, FAAP.

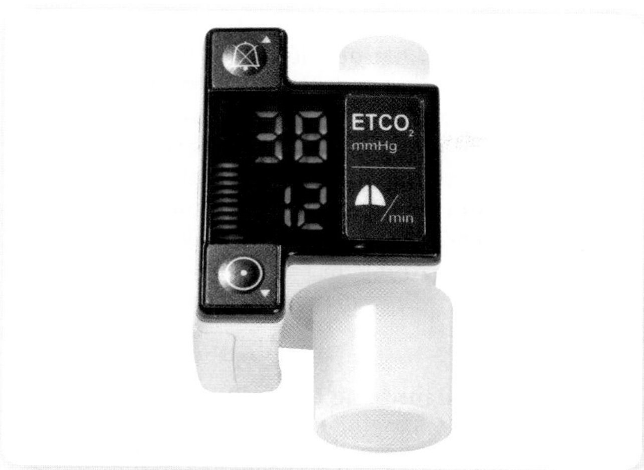

Figure 15-13 A capnometer.

The colorimetric CO_2 detector is a "spot-check" device; you may use it during initial confirmation of ET tube placement, but you should replace it as soon as possible with a more accurate and reliable quantitative device.

A **capnometer** provides quantitative information, in real time, by displaying a numeric reading of exhaled carbon dioxide levels. It uses a special adapter, which attaches between the advanced airway device and ventilation device **Figure 15-13**. Because it provides quantitative data, the capnometer is more reliable than the colorimetric CO_2 detector.

A **capnographer** is a device that provides a graphic representation of exhaled carbon dioxide levels. It performs the same function and attaches in the same way as the capnometer. The two types of capnographers are waveform and digital/waveform.

Waveform capnography provides quantitative, real-time information regarding the patient's exhaled carbon dioxide level. Unlike capnometry, however, waveform capnography displays a graphic waveform. In most cases, portable cardiac monitors/defibrillators provide a numeric reading and a waveform (also called digital/waveform capnography and quantitative waveform capnography).

Quantitative waveform capnography has many applications in emergency medicine, including the detection of bronchospasm, hypoventilation, and hyperventilation. Quantitative waveform capnography is the recommended method of monitoring initial and ongoing placement of an advanced airway device. Capnography can also serve as an indicator of the effectiveness of chest compressions and to detect return of spontaneous circulation (ROSC). The provision of this information is possible because blood must circulate through the lungs for carbon dioxide to be exhaled and measured. When ROSC occurs, you would expect a large amount of carbon dioxide to be returned to the lungs.

Waveform capnography can be monitored in spontaneously breathing patients with an adequate airway by applying a special nasal cannula device to the patient

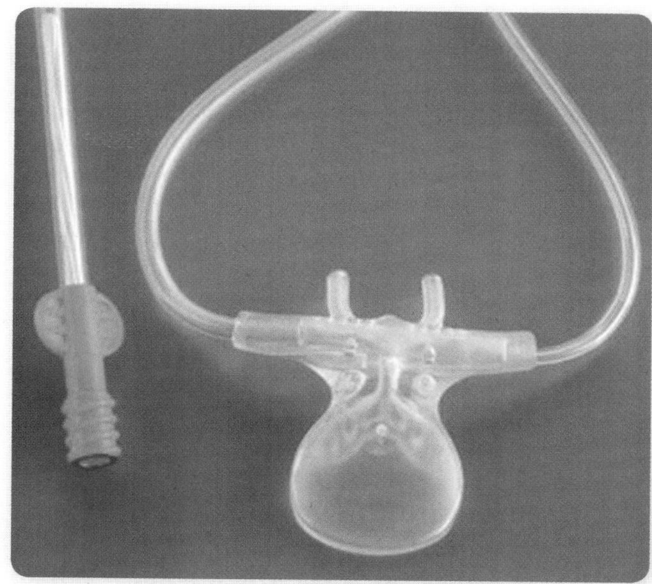

Figure 15-14 FilterLine® nasal cannula device for monitoring end-tidal carbon dioxide in a spontaneously breathing patient.

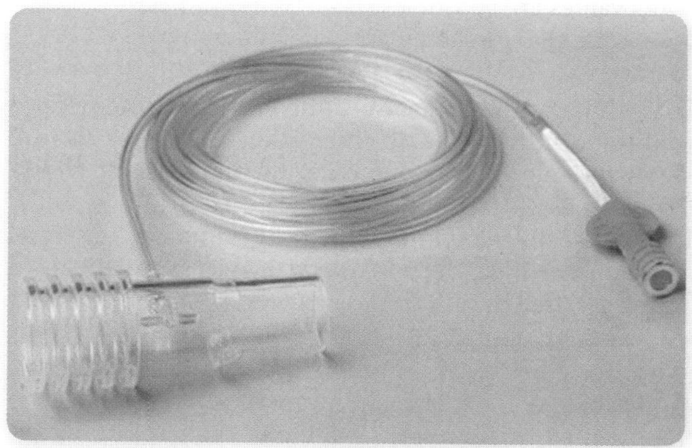

Figure 15-15 FilterLine® inline end-tidal carbon dioxide device for use in the intubated patient.

and connecting the sampling line to the cardiac monitor/defibrillator **Figure 15-14**. If the patient is intubated, then place an in-line adaptor between the ET tube (or other advanced airway) and ventilation device and connect the sampling line to the cardiac monitor/defibrillator **Figure 15-15**.

Because carbon dioxide rapidly equilibrates in the alveolar gases, the carbon dioxide concentration in exhaled gases—particularly the gases present near the end of exhalation—closely approximate arterial $PaCO_2$ levels, which normally range between 35 and 45 mm Hg. Typically, $ETCO_2$ level is approximately 2 to 5 mm Hg lower than the arterial $PaCO_2$ level. Because carbon dioxide is present only in negligible (0.5% or less) concentrations in the esophagus, use of an $ETCO_2$ detector—specifically, quantitative waveform capnography—is a reliable (and essential) method for confirming and monitoring advanced airway placement.

Use of $ETCO_2$ monitoring is limited with patients in cardiac arrest. In a patient with a short arrest interval, exhaled carbon dioxide may be detected despite a lack of perfusion. Patients with prolonged cardiac arrest, however, will have minimal levels of exhaled carbon dioxide because of severe acidosis and minimal carbon dioxide return to the lungs.

Evidence-Based Medicine

Studies of quantitative waveform capnography to verify advanced airway position in patients in cardiac arrest have demonstrated 100% accuracy in identifying correct and incorrect airway placement. In addition to clinical assessment, you should regard continuous quantitative waveform capnography as the most reliable method of confirming initial and ongoing advanced airway placement.

Normal Capnographic Waveform

It is important to understand the features of the normal capnographic waveform, including contour, baseline level, and rate and rise of the carbon dioxide level. A normal waveform has four distinct phases Figure 15-16. Phase I (A-B), also known as the respiratory baseline, is the initial stage of exhalation; the gas sample is dead space gas, free of carbon dioxide. Phase II (B-C) is called the expiratory upslope. At point B, alveolar gas mixes with dead space gas, resulting in an abrupt rise in carbon dioxide levels. The expiratory or alveolar plateau is represented by phase III (C-D), and the gas sampled is essentially alveolar. Point D is the maximal $ETCO_2$ level—the best reflection of the alveolar carbon dioxide level. The height of the waveform at point D correlates with the numeric value of exhaled carbon dioxide that is also displayed on the cardiac monitor/defibrillator. Fresh gas is introduced during phase IV, the inspiratory downstroke (D-E); this downstroke displaces carbon dioxide, causing the waveform to return to the baseline level of carbon dioxide—approximately 0 mm Hg. The duration (width) of each waveform corresponds to the duration of ventilation, and the space between waveforms corresponds with the patient's respiratory rate.

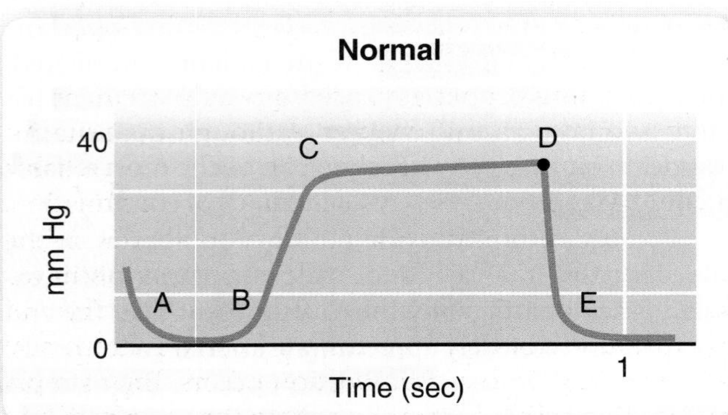

Figure 15-16 Normal capnographic waveform with points A through E shown.

Abnormal Capnographic Waveforms

In addition to quantifying the amount of exhaled carbon dioxide, the shape of the capnographic waveform can provide information regarding abnormal breathing processes, such as hypoventilation, hyperventilation, bronchospasm, and rebreathing. You can also recognize inadvertent **extubation** (the process of removing the tube from an intubated patient) by using waveform capnography.

Hypoventilation is a condition in which the production of carbon dioxide exceeds elimination. Because of increased carbon dioxide levels (hypercapnia), the capnographic waveforms are tall and the $ETCO_2$ value is correspondingly high (greater than 45 mm Hg). Bradypnea, a common feature of hypoventilation, produces a prolonged alveolar plateau (phase III [C-D]) and longer-than-normal intervals between waveforms Figure 15-17. Causes of hypoventilation include respiratory depression (ie, narcotic/opiate overdose) and a ventilatory rate that is too slow in an intubated patient.

Hyperventilation is a condition in which the elimination of carbon dioxide exceeds production. Because of decreased carbon dioxide levels (hypocapnia), the capnographic waveforms are small and the $ETCO_2$ value is correspondingly low (less than 35 mm Hg). Tachypnea, a clinical sign of hyperventilation, produces a short alveolar plateau (phase III [C-D]) and shorter-than-normal intervals between waveforms Figure 15-18. The numerous causes of hyperventilation include anxiety/panic attacks, metabolic acidosis, head injury, and pulmonary embolism.

Waveform capnography in the nonintubated patient is an excellent way to assess the severity of asthma, COPD, or any pathologic process that causes pulmonary air trapping; it can also be used to gauge the effectiveness of treatment. The characteristic "shark fin" of bronchospasm appears as an upsloping phase II (B-C); this shape signifies difficulty during the exhalation phase with incomplete alveolar emptying Figure 15-19.

If the patient is rebreathing previously exhaled carbon dioxide, then $ETCO_2$ values increase and the waveforms elevate and never return to the baseline (0 mm Hg) at the end of the inspiratory downstroke (phase IV [D-E]). Causes of rebreathing include inadequate expiratory time, a malfunctioning inspiratory valve on the mechanical ventilator, or an insufficient inspiratory flow rate Figure 15-20.

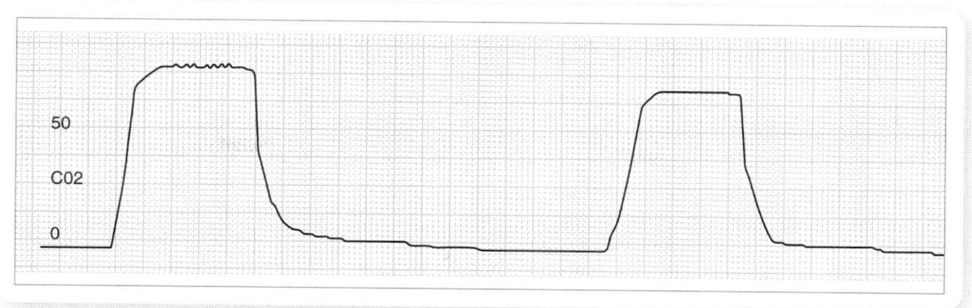

Figure 15-17 Capnographic waveforms caused by hypoventilation.

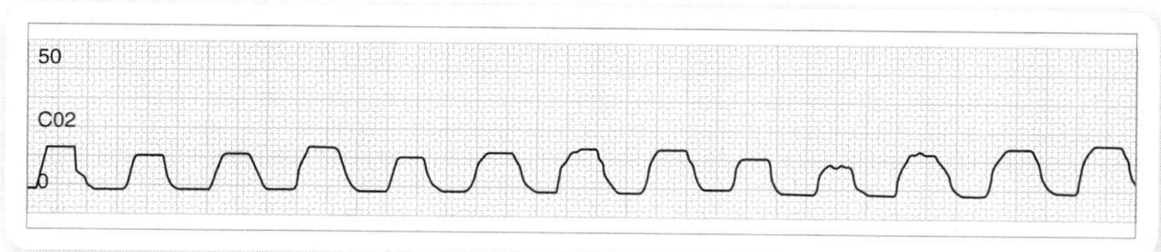

Figure 15-18 Capnographic waveforms caused by hyperventilation.

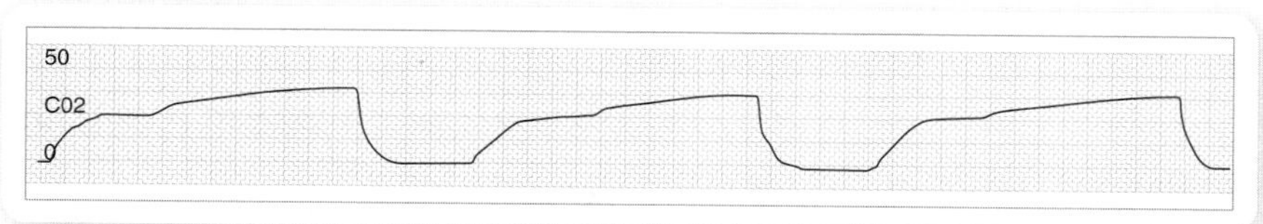

Figure 15-19 A shark fin capnographic waveform indicates bronchospasm and incomplete alveolar emptying.

Patient Safety

A consideration related to patient safety is the availability of appropriate equipment that has been properly maintained and checked. For example, intravenous (IV) pumps and ventilators have backup power supplies, and it is critical to ensure that all devices are in good working order with fully charged batteries prior to initiation of patient care. Waveform capnography is critical for monitoring intubated patients during transport and must be considered a minimum standard of care. Likewise, monitor alarms are critical for monitoring for unexpected changes in the patient's condition. You must correctly set alarm limits and volumes prior to transport to ensure you are alerted immediately to any parameters that move out of range.

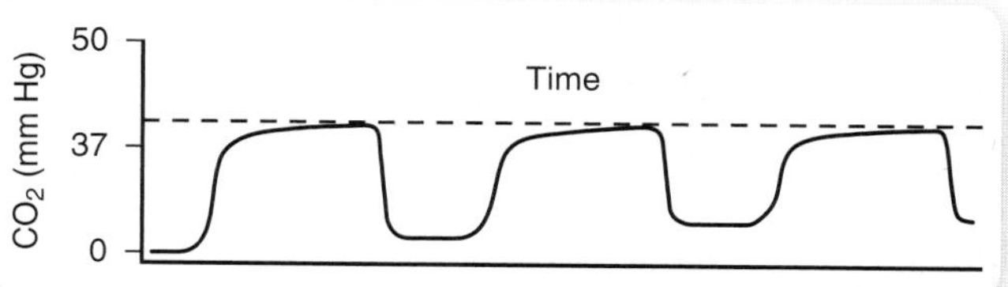

Figure 15-20 Capnographic waveforms caused by rebreathing.

If inadvertent extubation occurs, then you would expect to see a complete loss of a capnographic waveform and ETCO_2 reading **Figure 15-21**. Clearly, this finding requires immediate attention. The numerous methods for confirming proper advanced airway placement are discussed later in this chapter. Although quantitative waveform capnography has shown to be the most reliable method, you should employ all methods of confirmation.

On occasion, the sampling tubing from the in-line adaptor to the cardiac monitor/defibrillator gets obstructed with blood or other debris, thus blocking the flow of gas to the sensor and "zeroing out" the waveform and ETCO_2 reading. If this complication occurs, then simply replace the in-line adaptor to restore the waveform and ETCO_2 reading.

When you assess the ventilation status of any patient, whether he or she is spontaneously breathing, apneic with

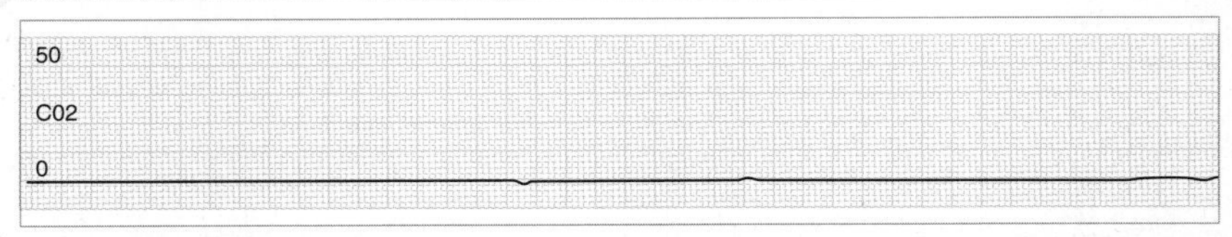

Figure 15-21 The complete loss of a capnographic waveform and end-tidal carbon dioxide reading in the intubated patient requires immediate attention.

Table 15-6 Causes of Increased and Decreased $ETCO_2$ Levels

	↑ $ETCO_2$	↓ $ETCO_2$
Spontaneously breathing	Hypoventilation	Hyperventilation
Apneic with a pulse	Positive pressure ventilation is too slow.	Positive pressure ventilation is too fast.
Apneic and pulseless	Positive pressure ventilation is too slow. Could indicate ROSC[b]	Misplaced ET tube[a] Decreased CO_2 return to the lungs (prolonged arrest) Chest compressions are of inadequate rate and/or depth. Positive pressure ventilation is too fast.[c]

Abbreviations: CO_2, carbon dioxide; ET, endotracheal; ROSC, return of spontaneous circulation

[a] No $ETCO_2$ light-emitting diode reading is displayed, and capnographic waveform is flat.
[b] With ROSC, an abrupt and sustained increase in $ETCO_2$ occurs (typically >40 mm Hg).
[c] In cardiac arrest of short duration.

a pulse, or pulseless and apneic, it is critical to understand and recognize the causes of increased and decreased $ETCO_2$ levels to make necessary adjustments to your treatment Table 15-6.

Airway Management

Air will reach the lungs only if it travels through the trachea. Therefore, a patent airway is essential. Patency is obvious in a responsive patient who is able to talk. In a patient with an altered level of consciousness (LOC), however, the airway is often not patent and you will need to use manual maneuvers to open it. In addition, you may need to use artificial airway adjuncts to assist in maintaining the airway. In a patient with a compromised airway, clearing the airway and maintaining patency are vital. Clearing the airway means removing obstructing material, tissue, or fluids from the nose, mouth, and throat. Maintaining the airway means keeping the airway patent so that air can enter and leave the lungs freely Figure 15-22.

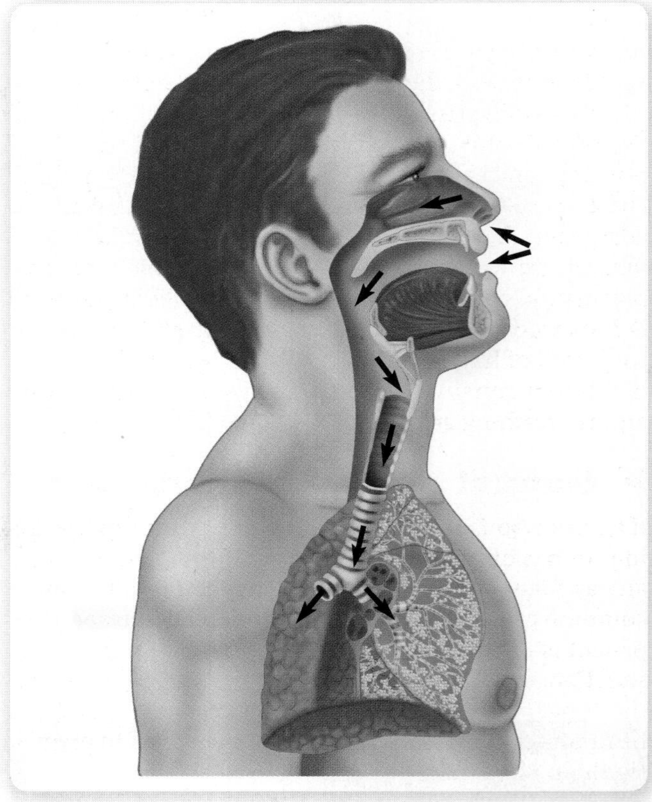

Figure 15-22 Air reaches the lungs only if it travels through the trachea. Maintaining the airway means keeping the airway patent so that air can enter and exit the lungs freely.

Positioning the Patient

In a perfect world, all patients would present in a supine position, so that you could quickly assess them and intervene without moving them. If an unresponsive patient is found in a prone position, however, then reposition

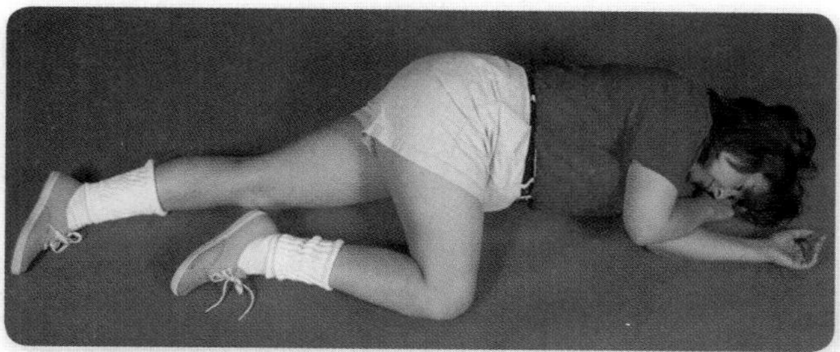

Figure 15-23 The recovery position.

him or her properly so that you can assess the need for ventilations or cardiopulmonary resuscitation (CPR).

To move a patient to a supine position, log roll the person as a unit. After the patient is placed in a supine position, quickly assess for breathing by visualizing the chest for visible movement. If the patient is breathing adequately and is not injured, position him or her in the recovery position. The **recovery position**, which involves placing the patient in a left lateral recumbent position, is indicated if the patient has a decreased LOC; is not suspected of having trauma to the spine, hips, or pelvis; is able to maintain his or her own airway spontaneously; and is breathing adequately **Figure 15-23**.

Manual Airway Maneuvers

If an unresponsive patient has a pulse, but is not breathing (or has only agonal gasps), then you must open the airway manually to provide rescue breathing. The most common cause of airway obstruction in an unresponsive patient is the tongue **Figure 15-24**. To correct this obstruction, manually maneuver the patient's head to propel the tongue forward and open the airway by using the head tilt–chin lift maneuver or the jaw-thrust maneuver (without head tilt).

Evidence-Based Medicine

According to the *2015 Guidelines for CPR and Emergency Cardiovascular Care*,[1] the airway is opened after one of the following circumstances has occurred: the patient is found to be pulseless and 30 chest compressions have been provided, or the patient is found to have a pulse, but is not breathing. To assess for breathing in an unresponsive patient, visualize the chest for obvious movement while simultaneously checking for a pulse; this assessment should take no more than 10 seconds. Chapter 39, *Responding to the Field Code*, covers these topics in detail.

Head Tilt–Chin Lift Maneuver

Opening the airway can often be done quickly and easily by simply tilting the patient's head back and lifting the chin. This **head tilt–chin lift maneuver** is the preferred technique

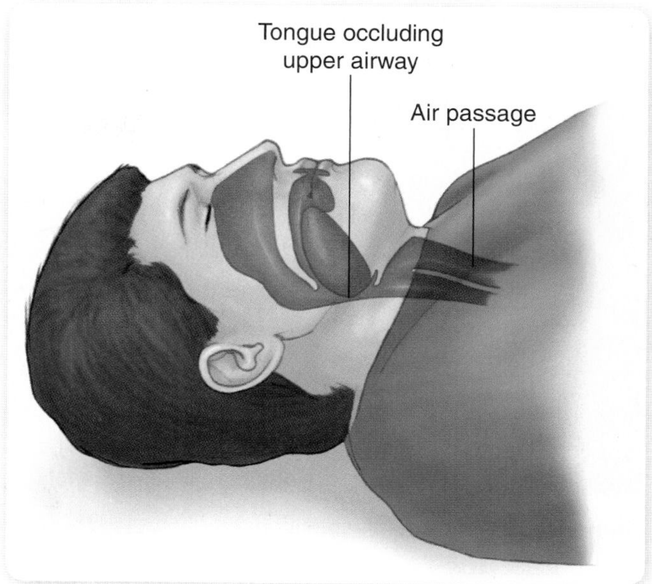

Figure 15-24 When the tongue falls back and occludes the posterior pharynx, it may obstruct the airway.

for opening the airway of a patient who has not sustained trauma. Occasionally, this simple maneuver is all that is required for the patient to resume breathing. Consider the following points when using the head tilt–chin lift maneuver:

- **Indications.** An unresponsive patient; a patient with no mechanism for cervical spine injury; or a patient who is unable to protect his or her own airway
- **Contraindications.** A responsive patient or a patient with a possible cervical spine injury
- **Advantages.** No equipment required and is simple, safe, and noninvasive
- **Disadvantages.** May be hazardous to patients with spinal injury and does not protect against aspiration

To perform the head tilt–chin lift maneuver, position yourself at the patient's side. Place one hand on the patient's forehead and apply backward pressure with your palm to tilt back the patient's head. This extension of the neck will propel the tongue forward, away from the posterior pharynx, and clear the airway. Place the tips of your fingers of your other hand under the lower jaw near the bony part of the chin. Do not compress the soft tissue under the chin, because this may block the airway. Lift the chin upward, bringing the entire jaw with it. Do not use your thumb to lift the chin. Lift so that the teeth are nearly brought together, but avoid closing the mouth completely. Continue to hold the forehead to maintain a backward tilt of the head **Figure 15-25**.

Jaw-Thrust Maneuver

If you suspect that the patient has experienced a cervical spine injury, then open his or her airway with the

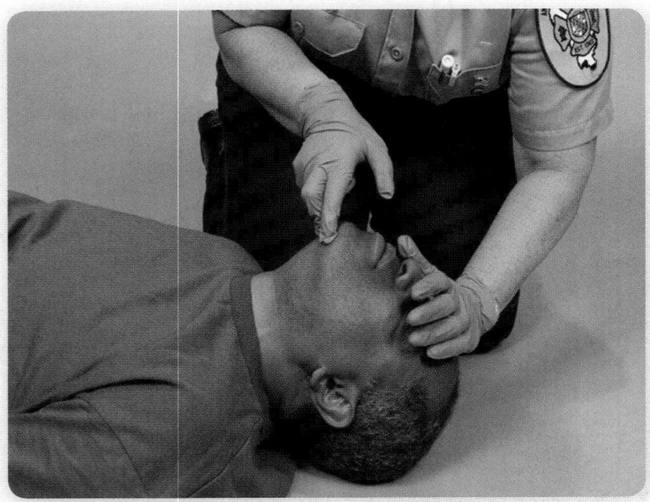

Figure 15-25 The head tilt–chin lift maneuver.

jaw-thrust maneuver. In this technique, you open the airway by placing your fingers behind the angle of the jaw and lifting the jaw forward. The jaw is displaced forward at the mandibular angle. Consider the following points when using the jaw-thrust maneuver:

- **Indications.** An unresponsive patient; a patient with a possible cervical spine injury; or a patient who is unable to protect his or her own airway
- **Contraindications.** A responsive patient with resistance to opening the mouth. The jaw-thrust maneuver may be needed in a responsive patient who has sustained a jaw fracture to keep the tongue away from the back of the throat.
- **Advantages.** May be used in patients with cervical spine injury; may be used with a cervical collar in place; no special equipment is required
- **Disadvantages.** Cannot maintain the jaw-thrust maneuver if the patient becomes responsive or combative; difficult to maintain for an extended time; very difficult to use in conjunction with bag-mask ventilation; thumb must remain in place to maintain jaw displacement; requires a second rescuer for bag-mask ventilation; does not protect against aspiration

To perform the jaw-thrust maneuver, position yourself at the patient's head. Place the meaty portion of your thumbs on the zygomatic arches, and hook the tip of your index fingers under the angle of the mandible, in the indentation below each ear. While holding the patient's head in a neutral, in-line position, displace the jaw upward and open the patient's mouth with the tips of your thumbs Figure 15-26. Because opening and maintaining a patent airway is so critical, you should carefully perform the head tilt-chin lift maneuver if the jaw-thrust maneuver fails to adequately open the airway.

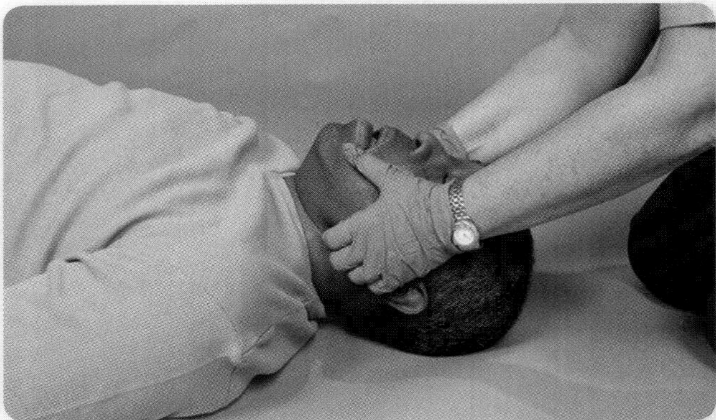

Figure 15-26 The jaw-thrust maneuver.

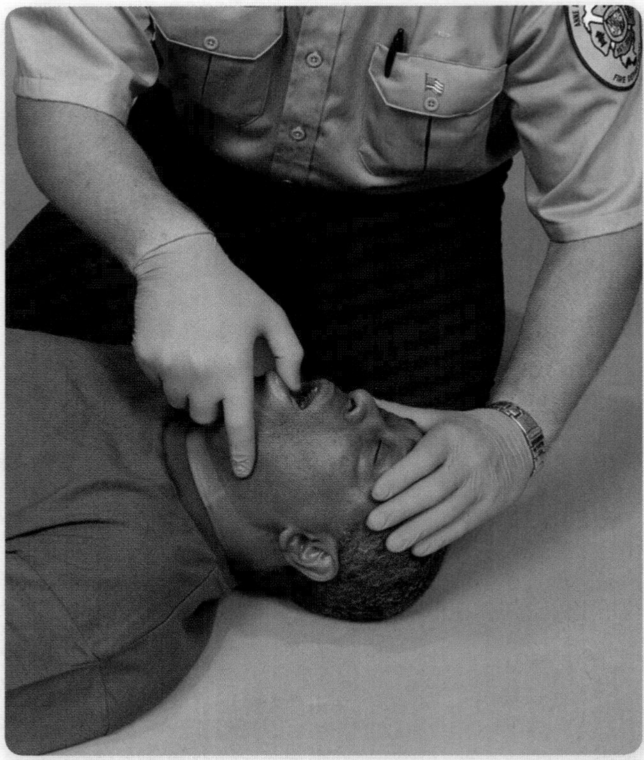

Figure 15-27 The tongue-jaw lift maneuver.

Tongue-Jaw Lift Maneuver

The **tongue-jaw lift maneuver** is used more commonly to open a patient's airway for the purpose of suctioning or inserting an oropharyngeal or supraglottic airway. It cannot be used to ventilate a patient because it will not allow for an adequate mask seal on the patient's face.

To perform the tongue-jaw lift maneuver, position yourself at the side of the patient. Place the hand closest to the patient's head on the forehead. With the other hand, reach into the patient's mouth and hook your first knuckle under the incisors (front teeth) or gumline. While holding the patient's head and maintaining the hand on the forehead, lift the jaw straight up Figure 15-27.

Suctioning

When the patient's mouth or throat becomes filled with vomitus, blood, or secretions, a suction apparatus enables you to remove material quickly and efficiently, thereby allowing you to ventilate the patient. Ventilating a patient with secretions in his or her mouth will force material into the lungs, resulting in an upper airway obstruction or aspiration. Therefore, clearing the patient's airway with suction, if needed, is your next priority after opening the patient's airway with the manual maneuvers previously discussed. Remember: If you hear gurgling, then the patient needs suctioning.

Suctioning Equipment

Ambulances should carry a fixed suction unit (which operates off a vacuum from the engine) and a portable suction unit (battery-operated or hand-powered) **Figure 15-28**. Regardless of your location—in the patient's residence, the middle of a field, or the back of the ambulance—you must have quick access to suctioning equipment. It is essential for effective airway management.

Hand-operated suctioning units with disposable canisters are reliable, effective, and relatively inexpensive; they can easily fit into the bag that you carry to the patient's side. Mechanical or vacuum-powered suction units should be capable of generating a vacuum of 300 mm Hg within 4 seconds of clamping off the tubing. The amount of suction should be adjustable for use in children and intubated patients. Check the vacuum on the mechanical suction unit at the beginning of every shift by turning on the device, clamping the tubing, and making sure the pressure gauge registers 300 mm Hg. Ensure that all battery-charged units have fully charged batteries. **Table 15-7** lists the advantages and disadvantages of the most common types of suction devices.

Regardless of which type of suction unit you are using, the device must generate enough vacuum pressure to adequately suction the patient's mouth and oropharynx. In addition to the suctioning unit, you should have the following supplies readily accessible at the patient's head:

- Wide-bore, thick-walled, nonkinking tubing
- Soft and rigid suction catheters
- A nonbreakable, disposable collection bottle
- A supply of water for rinsing the catheters

A suction catheter is a hollow, cylindrical device that is used to remove fluids and secretions from the patient's airway. A Yankauer catheter (**tonsil-tip catheter**) is a good option for suctioning the oropharynx in adults; it may also be used for infants and children. These plastic-tip catheters have a large diameter and are rigid, so they do not collapse. Rigid catheters are capable of suctioning large volumes of fluid rapidly. Tips with a curved contour allow for easy, rapid placement in the oropharynx **Figure 15-29**.

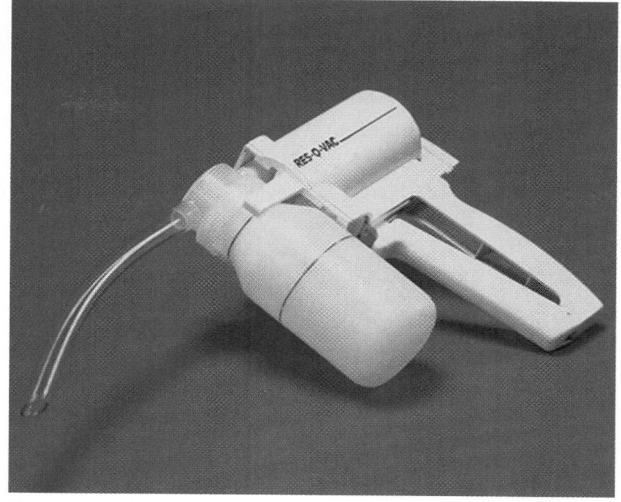

A

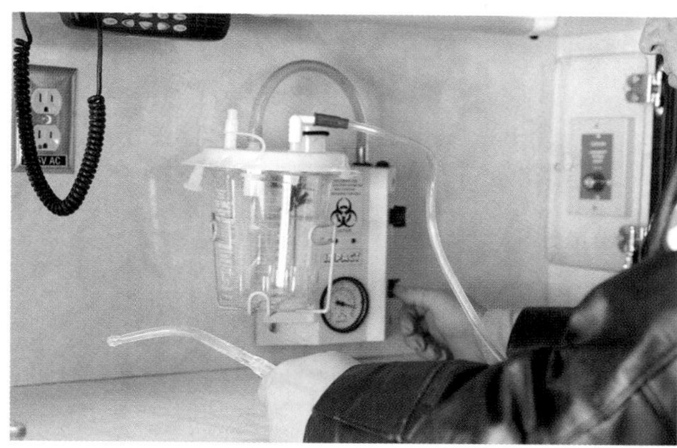

B

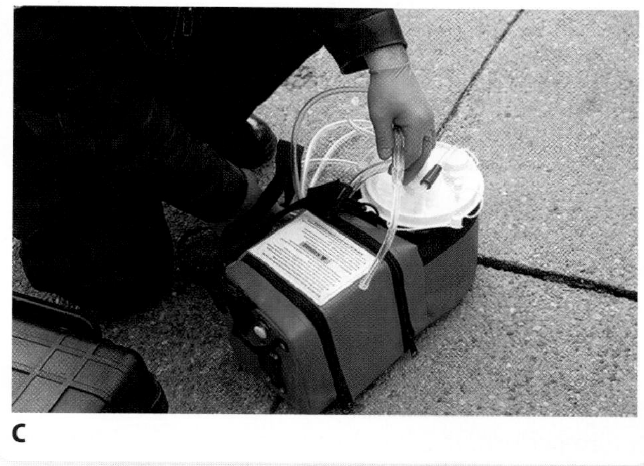

C

Figure 15-28 Effective suctioning equipment is essential for good airway management. **A.** Hand-operated device. **B.** Fixed unit. **C.** Portable unit.

Soft plastic, nonrigid catheters, sometimes called French or **whistle-tip catheters**, can be placed in the oropharynx or nasopharynx or down an ET tube. They come in various sizes and have a smaller diameter than

Table 15-7 Comparison of Common Suction Devices

Device Type	Advantages	Disadvantages
Hand-powered portable	▪ Lightweight ▪ Portable ▪ Mechanically simple ▪ Inexpensive	▪ Limited volume ▪ Manually powered ▪ Body fluid contact ▪ Components not disposable
Oxygen-powered portable	▪ Lightweight ▪ Small	▪ Limited suction power ▪ Uses a lot of oxygen for limited suctioning power
Battery-operated portable	▪ Lightweight ▪ Portable ▪ Excellent suction power ▪ Most problems can be identified and fixed in the field	▪ More complicated mechanics ▪ May lose battery integrity over time ▪ Some body fluid contact ▪ Components not disposable
Mounted vacuum-powered	▪ Extremely strong vacuum ▪ Adjustable vacuum power ▪ Components are disposable	▪ Not portable ▪ Body fluid contact ▪ Cannot be fixed in the field ▪ Cannot substitute power source

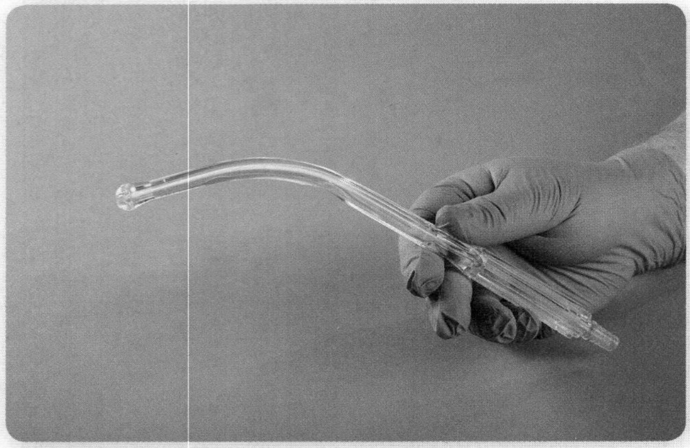

Figure 15-29 Tonsil-tip (Yankauer) catheters are a good choice for suctioning the oropharynx because they have wide-diameter tips and are rigid.

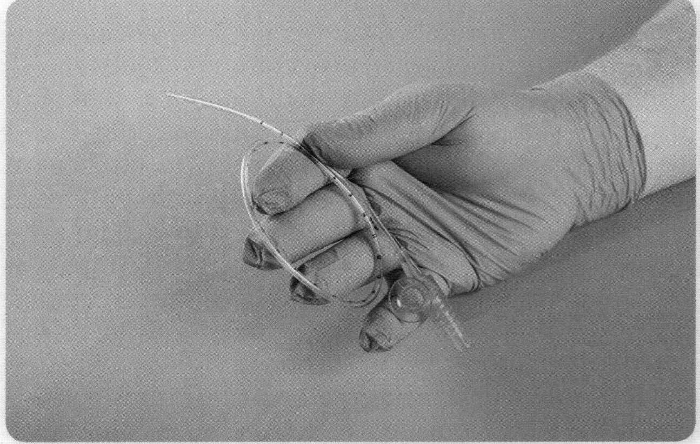

Figure 15-30 Whistle-tip (French) catheters are used in situations in which rigid catheters cannot be used, such as when a patient has a stoma or if the patient's teeth are clenched. Flexible catheters can also be passed down an endotracheal tube.

rigid catheters. Soft catheters are used to suction the nose and liquid secretions in the back of the mouth and in situations in which a rigid catheter cannot be used, such as for a patient with a stoma **Figure 15-30**. (Airway management considerations for such patients are covered later in this chapter.) For example, a rigid catheter could break a tooth in a patient with clenched teeth, whereas a flexible catheter may be worked along the cheeks without causing injury. Suction tubing without the attached catheter facilitates suctioning of large debris in the oropharynx and allows access to the back of the pharynx in a patient with clenched teeth.

▶ Suctioning Techniques

Mortality increases significantly if a patient aspirates; therefore, suctioning the upper airway is critical to avoid this potentially fatal outcome. Suction the patient's airway until it is clear of liquids or other debris. Remember, ventilating a patient whose airway is full of blood, vomit, or other secretions virtually assures aspiration.

Be careful not to stimulate the back of the throat, especially in a young child or an infant, because this can induce a vagal response and cause bradycardia. After the patient has been suctioned, continue ventilation and oxygenation.

Soft-tip catheters are best used when passed through an ET tube. Lubricate the catheter with a water-soluble gel when suctioning the nasopharynx. Insert the catheter, and apply suction during extraction of the catheter to clear the airway. After the patient has been suctioned, reevaluate the patency of his or her airway, and continue to ventilate and oxygenate as needed.

Before inserting any suction catheter into a patient, ensure you measure for the proper size, from the corner of the mouth to the earlobe or the angle of the jaw **Figure 15-31A**. Never insert a catheter past the base of the tongue because it may cause the patient to gag or vomit. Turn the patient's head to the side, or log roll him or her to the side, and insert the suction catheter to the predetermined depth. Apply suction in a circular motion while you withdraw the catheter **Figure 15-31B**. Repeat as needed until the airway is clear of secretions.

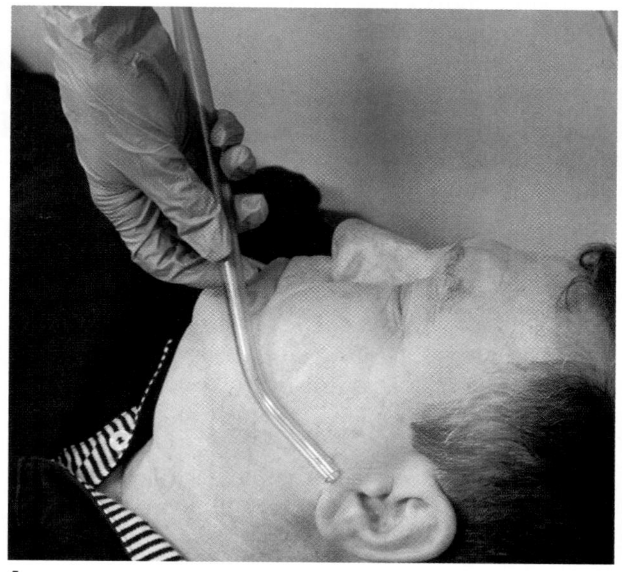

A

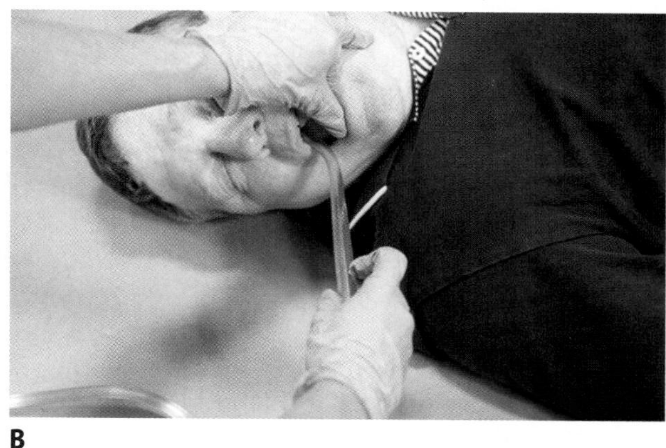

B

Figure 15-31 A. Measure for the proper size suction catheter from the corner of the mouth to the earlobe or angle of the jaw. **B.** Apply suction while you are withdrawing the catheter. Repeat as needed until the airway is clear of secretions.

Airway Adjuncts

After manually opening the airway of an unresponsive patient and using suction as needed to clear away any blood or other secretions, you may need to insert an artificial airway adjunct to help maintain airway patency. An artificial airway is not a substitute for proper head positioning. Even after you insert an airway adjunct, you must manually maintain the appropriate position of the patient's head.

▶ Oropharyngeal Airway

The **oropharyngeal (oral) airway** is a curved, hard plastic device that fits over the back of the tongue with the tip in the posterior pharynx **Figure 15-32**. It is designed to hold the tongue away from the posterior pharyngeal wall, and its use makes it much easier to ventilate patients with a **bag-mask device** (discussed later in this chapter). The oral airway can also serve as an effective bite block, preventing an intubated patient from biting down on the ET tube.

> **Words of Wisdom**
>
> Wear a face mask and protective eyewear whenever you are managing a patient's airway. Body fluids can become aerosolized, and the mucous membranes of your mouth, nose, and eyes can easily come in contact with these contaminants.

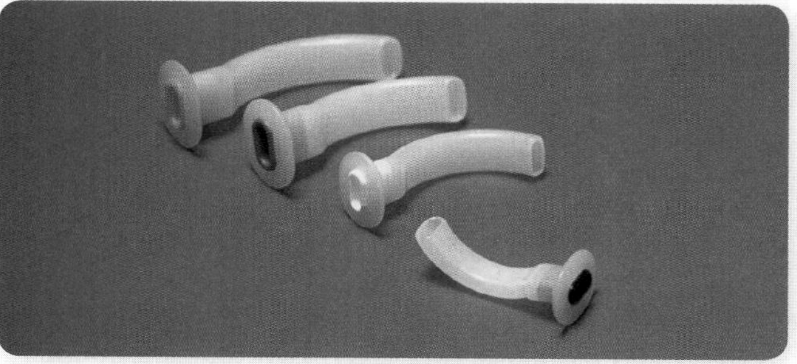

Figure 15-32 An oral airway is used for unresponsive patients who have no gag reflex. It helps to keep the tongue from blocking the airway.

Promptly insert an oral airway in unresponsive patients—breathing or not—who have no gag reflex. Because its distal end sits in the back of the throat, this device will stimulate gagging and retching in a responsive patient. For that reason, you should use the oral airway only in unresponsive patients without a gag reflex. If the patient gags during insertion of the oral airway, then remove the device immediately and be prepared to suction the oropharynx. Consider the following points when using an oral airway:

- **Indications.** Unresponsive patients and patients with an absent gag reflex
- **Contraindications.** Responsive patients and patients with a gag reflex
- **Advantages.** Noninvasive; easily placed; prevents blockage of the glottis by the tongue
- **Disadvantages.** Does not protect against aspiration
- **Complications.** Unexpected gag may cause vomiting, or improper technique may cause pharyngeal or dental trauma

If the oral airway is improperly sized or is inserted incorrectly, then it could push back the tongue into the pharynx, creating an airway obstruction. Rough insertion of the airway can injure the hard palate, resulting in oral bleeding and creating a risk of vomiting and aspiration. Before inserting an oral airway, suction the oropharynx as needed to ensure that the mouth is clear of blood or other fluids.

To select an oral airway that is the correct size for the patient, measure the distance from the corner of the patient's mouth to the earlobe or the angle of the jaw Figure 15-33. You can insert the oral airway in one of two ways, as follows:

- Open the patient's mouth with the cross-finger technique or tongue-jaw lift, hold the airway upside down with your other hand, and insert the airway in the mouth with the tip facing the hard palate Figure 15-34A. Advance the oral airway until it reaches the soft palate and then rotate it 180°, allowing it to follow the curvature of the tongue, until the flange rests on the patient's lips Figure 15-34B.
- Use a tongue blade to depress the tongue, ensuring that the tongue remains forward Figure 15-35A. Insert the oral airway, with the tip pointing down, and follow the curvature of the tongue until the flanges rests on the patient's lips Figure 15-35B.

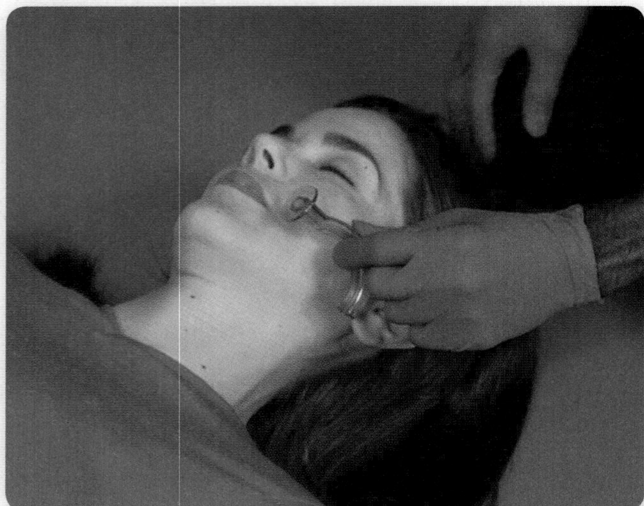

Figure 15-33 Size the oral airway by measuring from the corner of the mouth to the earlobe or the angle of the jaw.

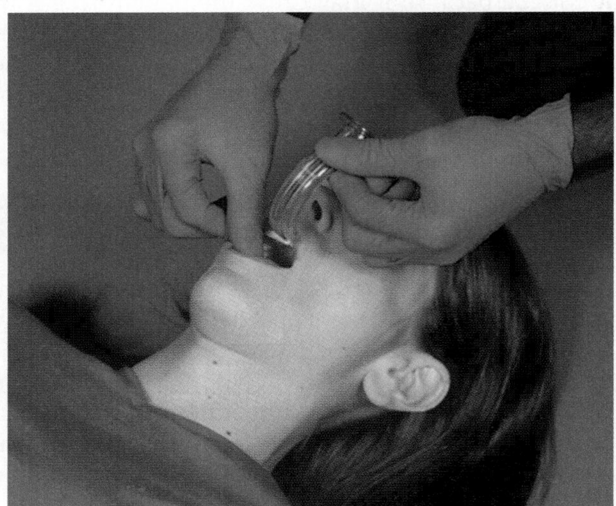

A

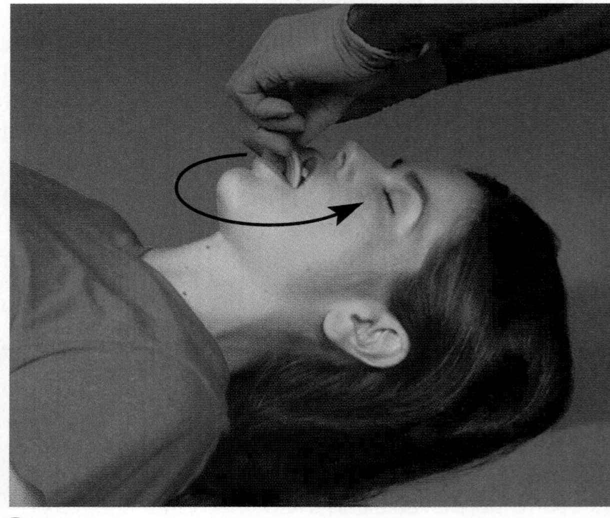

B

Figure 15-34 A. Open the patient's airway and insert the airway with the tip facing the hard palate. **B.** Rotate the oral airway 180° after it reaches the soft palate, allowing it to follow the curvature of the tongue, until the flange rests on the patient's lips.

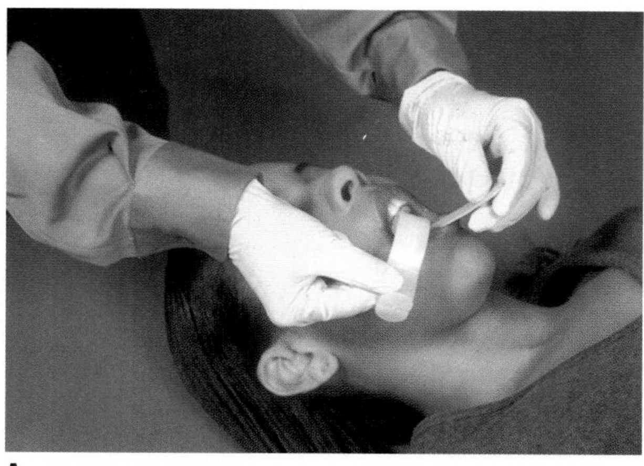

A

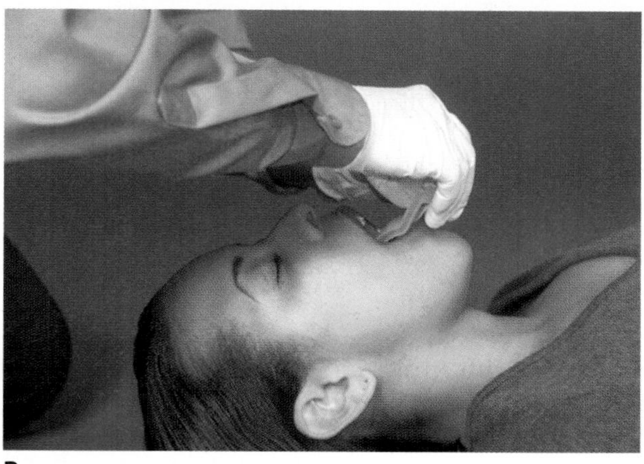

B

Figure 15-35 A. Use a tongue blade to depress the tongue, ensuring that the tongue stays forward. **B.** Insert the oral airway, with the tip pointing down, and allow it to follow the curvature of the tongue until the flange rests on the patient's lips.

▶ Nasopharyngeal Airway

The **nasopharyngeal (nasal) airway** is a soft, rubber tube that is inserted through the nose into the posterior pharynx behind the tongue, thereby allowing passage of air from the nose to the lower airway. Nasal airways are commonly measured using the French (Fr) catheter scale, and range in size from 12 Fr to 36 Fr; the length of the nasal airway depends on its size. A nasal airway is much better tolerated than an oral airway in patients who have an intact gag reflex but an altered LOC **Figure 15-36**. Do not use this device if the patient has experienced trauma to the nose or you have reason to suspect a skull fracture (for example, cerebrospinal fluid [CSF] leakage from the nose). Although rare, inserting the airway in such cases may cause it to enter the cranial vault through the hole caused by the fracture.

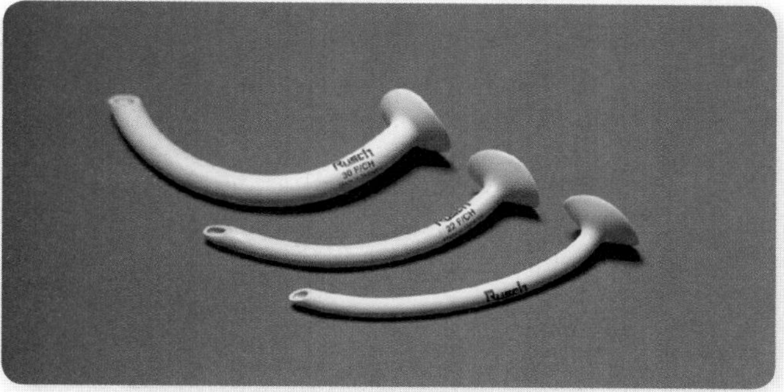

Figure 15-36 A nasal airway is better tolerated by patients who have an intact gag reflex.

Special Populations

In children, using a tongue blade to hold the tongue down while inserting an oral airway is the preferred method. Because the child's hard palate is more fragile than an adult's, rotating the oral airway can lacerate or even fracture the hard palate.

Insert the nasal airway gently to avoid causing epistaxis (nosebleed). Lubricate the airway with a water-soluble gel, preferably one that contains a local anesthetic, and slide it gently, tip downward, into one nostril. Do not force it. If you meet resistance, then try to pass the airway down the other nostril.

If the nasal airway is too long, then it may obstruct the patient's airway. If the patient becomes intolerant of the nasal airway, then gently remove it from the nasal passage. Although a nasal airway is not as likely to cause vomiting as an oral airway, you should still have suction readily available. Consider the following points when using a nasal airway:

- **Indications.** Unresponsive patients and patients with an altered mental status who have an intact gag reflex
- **Contraindications.** Patient intolerance; presence of facial (specifically, the nose) fracture or skull fracture
- **Advantages.** Can be suctioned through; provides a patent airway; can be tolerated by responsive patients; can be safely placed "blindly" (that is, without direct visualization of the vocal cords); no requirement for the mouth to be open
- **Disadvantages.** Improper technique may result in severe bleeding (resulting epistaxis may be extremely difficult to control); does not protect against aspiration.

To select a nasal airway that is the correct size for the patient, measure the distance from the tip of the nostril

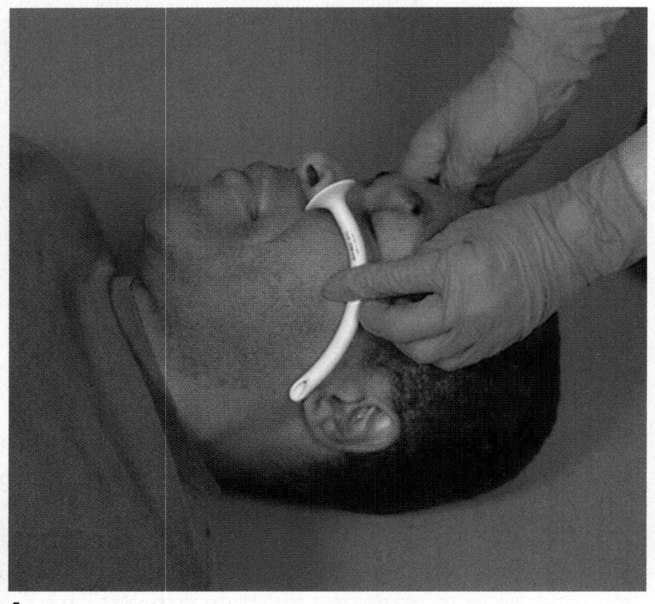
A

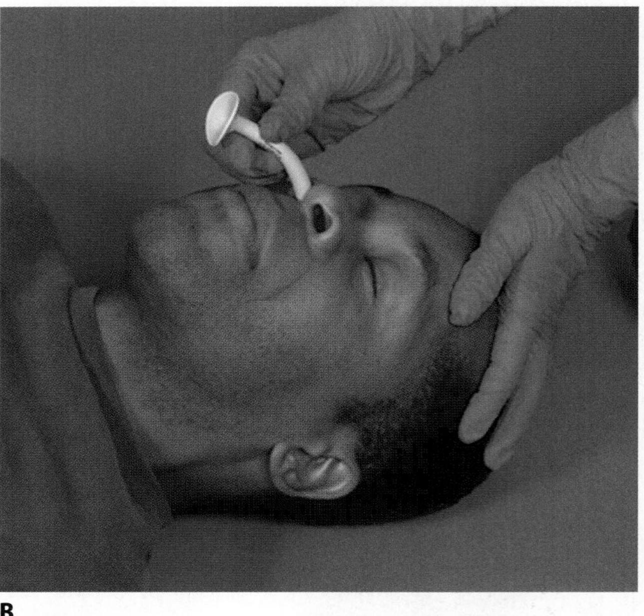
B

Figure 15-37 A. Size the nasal airway by measuring from the tip of the nostril to the angle of the jaw or the earlobe. **B.** Insert the nasal airway into the larger nostril, with the bevel facing the septum, until the flange rests on the patient's nostril.

to the earlobe or the angle of the jaw **Figure 15-37A**. Insert the prelubricated airway into the larger nostril, with the bevel facing the septum, until the flange rests on the patient's nostril **Figure 15-37B**.

Airway Obstructions

The airway connects the body to the life-giving oxygen in the atmosphere. If the airway becomes obstructed, then this lifeline is cut and the patient dies—often within minutes. As a paramedic, you must recognize the signs of an obstructed airway and immediately take corrective action.

Causes of Airway Obstruction

In an adult, sudden foreign body airway obstruction usually occurs during a meal. In children, it typically occurs while eating or playing with small toys. An otherwise healthy child who presents with a sudden onset of difficulty breathing—especially in the absence of fever—should be suspected of having a foreign body airway obstruction. Airway obstruction, however, has many other causes, including the tongue, laryngeal edema, laryngeal spasm (laryngospasm), trauma, and aspiration.

When the airway is obstructed because of an infectious process or a severe allergic reaction, repeated attempts to clear the airway as if it were obstructed by a foreign body will be unsuccessful and potentially harmful. These conditions require specific management and prompt transport to an appropriate medical facility. Airway infection is covered in Chapter 16, *Respiratory Emergencies*; allergic reactions are covered in Chapter 25, *Immunologic Emergencies*.

Tongue

In a patient with an altered LOC, the jaw relaxes and the tongue tends to fall back against the posterior wall of the pharynx, closing off the airway. A patient with partial obstruction caused by the tongue will make a snoring sound when breathing (sonorous breathing); a patient whose airway is completely obstructed cannot breathe at all. Fortunately, obstruction of the airway by the tongue is simple to correct using a manual maneuver (such as head tilt–chin lift or jaw-thrust maneuver).

Foreign Body

A significant number of people die of foreign body airway obstructions each year, often as the result of choking on a piece of food. The typical patient is middle-aged or older and wears dentures. The person has usually consumed alcohol, which depresses protective reflexes and adversely affects judgment about how large a piece of food can be prudently placed in the mouth. In addition, people with conditions that decrease their airway reflexes (such as stroke) are at an increased risk for foreign body airway obstructions.

Signs may include choking, gagging, stridor, dyspnea, **aphonia** (inability to speak), and **dysphonia** (difficulty speaking). Treatment depends on whether the patient is effectively moving air. Techniques for the removal of foreign body airway obstruction are discussed later in this chapter.

Laryngeal Spasm and Edema

A laryngeal spasm (laryngospasm) results in spasmodic closure of the vocal cords, completely occluding the airway.

It is often caused by trauma during an overly aggressive intubation attempt or occurs immediately on extubation, especially when the patient has an altered LOC.

Laryngeal edema causes the glottic opening to become extremely narrow or totally closed. Conditions that commonly cause this problem include epiglottitis, anaphylaxis, or inhalation injury (such as burns to the upper airway).

Airway obstructions caused by laryngeal spasm or edema may be relieved by aggressive ventilation to force air past the narrowed airway or a forceful upward pull of the jaw in an attempt to reposition the airway. In certain patients, muscle relaxant medications may be effective in relieving laryngeal spasm. Do not let your guard down after the laryngospasm has appeared to have resolved; resolution of the crisis does not mean that laryngospasm will not recur. Transport the patient to the hospital for evaluation.

Laryngeal Injury

Airway patency depends on good muscle tone to keep the trachea open. Fracture of the larynx increases airway resistance by decreasing airway size due to decreased muscle tone, laryngeal edema, and ventilatory effort. An advanced airway may be required to maintain a patent airway. Penetrating and crush injuries to the larynx can compromise the airway secondary to swelling and bleeding. As with laryngeal fractures, advanced airway management may be required.

Aspiration

Aspiration of blood or other fluid significantly increases mortality. In addition to potentially obstructing the airway, aspiration destroys delicate bronchiolar tissue, introduces pathogens into the lungs, and decreases the patient's ability to ventilate (or be ventilated).

Suction should be readily available for any patient who is unable to maintain his or her own airway. Always assume that patients who require emergency medical care have a full stomach.

▶ Recognition of an Airway Obstruction

A foreign body lodged in the upper airway can cause a mild (partial) or severe (complete) airway obstruction, depending on the size of the object and its location in the airway. A rapid but careful assessment is required to determine the seriousness of the obstruction because the differences in managing mild versus severe cases are significant.

A patient with a mild airway obstruction is responsive and able to exchange air but may show varying degrees of respiratory distress. The patient will usually have noisy respirations and may be coughing. He or she may wheeze between coughs but does not become cyanotic. Patients with a mild airway obstruction should be left alone. A forceful cough is the most effective means of dislodging

YOU are the Paramedic PART 4

Despite basic life support (BLS) and advanced life support (ALS) procedures to remove the obstruction, you are unsuccessful. The patient remains apneic and positive pressure ventilation is still impossible. The engine company arrives with two EMTs along with law enforcement personnel. Your partner states, "We need to do a needle cricothyrotomy." The patient's pulse is weaker and is now only palpable at the carotid artery. The ECG leads are attached to the patient.

Recording Time: 5 Minutes	
Level of consciousness	Unresponsive
Respirations	Absent
Pulse	140 beats/min; weak and regular
Skin	Cyanotic
Blood pressure	Not available yet
Oxygen saturation (Spo_2)	60%
$ETCO_2$	Not available yet
ECG	Sinus tachycardia

7. Is your partner's suggestion to perform a needle cricothyrotomy the best option? Why or why not?

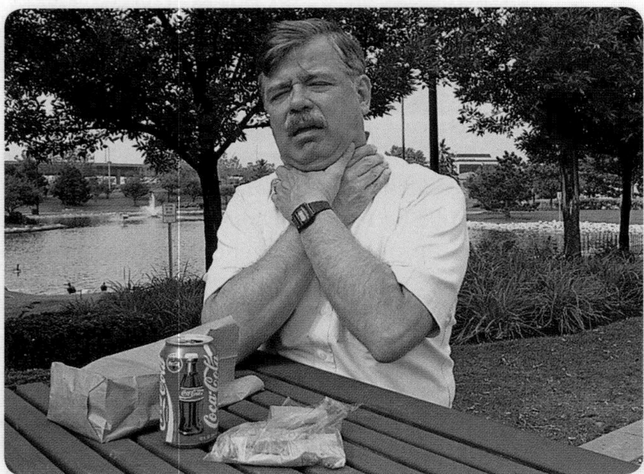

Figure 15-38 The universal sign of choking.

the mild airway obstruction. Attempts to manually remove the object could force it farther down into the airway and cause a severe obstruction. Closely monitor the patient's condition, and be prepared to intervene if you see signs of severe airway obstruction.

A patient with a severe airway obstruction typically experiences a sudden inability to breathe or talk. The patient may grasp at his or her throat (the universal sign of choking) and make frantic, exaggerated attempts to move air **Figure 15-38**. A patient with a severe airway obstruction has a weak, ineffective, or absent cough and is in marked respiratory distress; weak inspiratory stridor and cyanosis are often present.

▶ Emergency Medical Care for Foreign Body Airway Obstruction

If a patient with a suspected airway obstruction is responsive, then ask, "Are you choking?" If the patient nods "yes" and cannot speak, then begin treatment immediately. If the obstruction is not promptly cleared, then the amount of oxygen in the blood will decrease dramatically, resulting in severe hypoxia and death.

Words of Wisdom

Causes of Airway Obstruction

- Relaxation of the tongue in an unresponsive patient
- Foreign objects (food, small toys, balloons, dentures)
- Blood clots, broken teeth, or damaged oral tissue following trauma
- Airway tissue swelling (infection, allergic reaction)
- Aspirated vomitus

If, after opening the airway, you are unable to ventilate the patient (no visible chest rise) or you feel resistance when ventilating (poor lung compliance), then reposition the airway and again attempt to ventilate the patient. **Lung compliance** is the ability of the alveoli to expand when air is drawn into the lungs during negative pressure ventilation or pushed into the lungs during positive pressure ventilation. Poor lung compliance is characterized by increased resistance during ventilation attempts.

If you find large pieces of vomitus, mucus, loose dentures, or blood clots in the airway, then sweep them forward and out of the mouth with your gloved index finger. Blind finger sweeps of the mouth—regardless of the patient's age—are not recommended and may cause further harm; attempt to remove only foreign bodies that you can see and easily retrieve. After the patient's airway is open, insert your index finger down along the inside of the patient's cheek and into his or her throat at the base of the tongue, then try to hook the foreign body to dislodge it and maneuver it into the mouth. Take care not to force the foreign body deeper into the airway. Do not blindly insert any object other than your finger into the patient's mouth to remove a foreign body, because an instrument jammed into the throat can damage the delicate structures of the pharynx and compound the obstruction with hemorrhage. Use suctioning to clear the airway of secretions as needed.

Words of Wisdom

Do not blindly insert any instrument, whether improvised or specially designed, into a patient's pharynx—this practice is extremely dangerous!

The **abdominal thrust maneuver** (also called the Heimlich maneuver) is the most effective method of dislodging and forcing a foreign object out of the airway of a responsive adult or child. It aims to create an artificial cough by forcing residual air out of the person's lungs, thereby expelling the object. You should perform the Heimlich maneuver on any responsive child or adult with a severe airway obstruction until the obstructing object is expelled or until the patient becomes unresponsive. If a responsive patient with a severe airway obstruction is in the advanced stages of pregnancy or has morbid obesity, then perform chest thrusts instead of abdominal thrusts.

If the responsive patient with a severe airway obstruction becomes unresponsive, then carefully position him or her supine on the ground and begin chest compressions. Perform 30 chest compressions (15 compressions if two rescuers are present and the patient is an infant or a child), and then open the airway and look in the mouth. Attempt to remove the foreign body only if you can see it. If you are able to retrieve the object, then attempt to ventilate. If you cannot see the object, then resume chest compressions.

If you are unable to relieve a severe airway obstruction in an unresponsive patient with the basic techniques previously discussed, then proceed with **direct laryngoscopy** (visualization of the airway with a laryngoscope) for the removal of the foreign body. Insert the laryngoscope blade into the patient's mouth. If you see the foreign body, then carefully remove it from the upper airway with **Magill forceps**, a special type of curved forcep **Figure 15-39**. Laryngoscopes and blades are discussed later in this chapter.

To remove an upper airway obstruction with Magill forceps, follow the steps shown in **Skill Drill 15-1**.

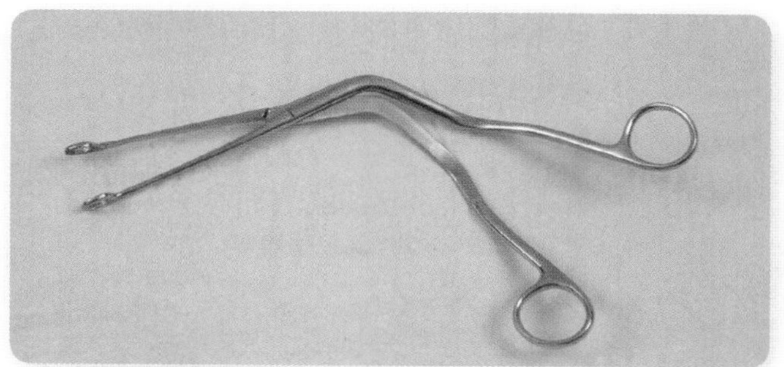

Figure 15-39 Magill forceps.

Skill Drill 15-1 Removing an Upper Airway Obstruction With Magill Forceps

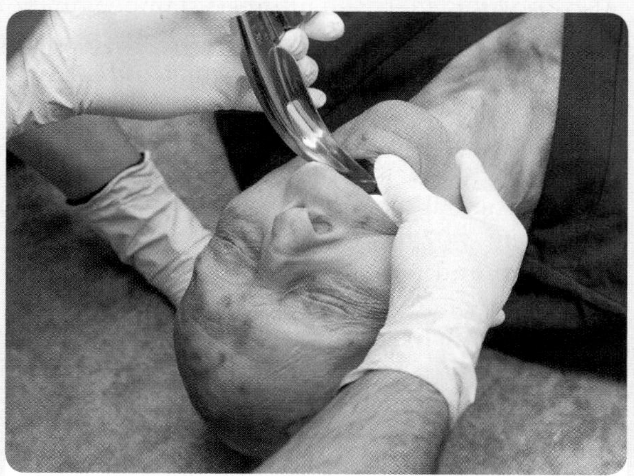

Step 1 With the patient's head in the sniffing position, open the patient's mouth and insert the laryngoscope blade.

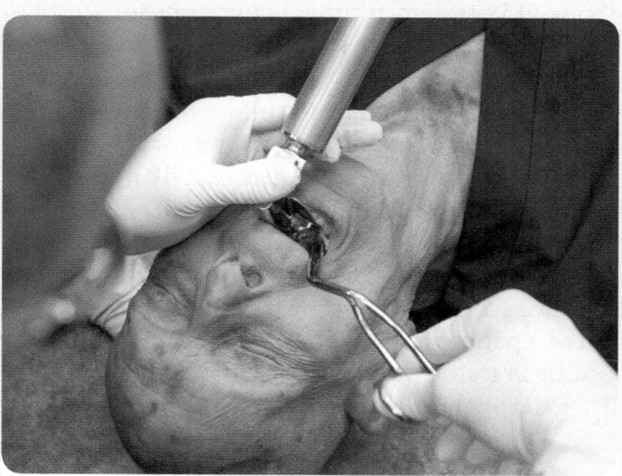

Step 2 Visualize the obstruction, and retrieve the object with the Magill forceps.

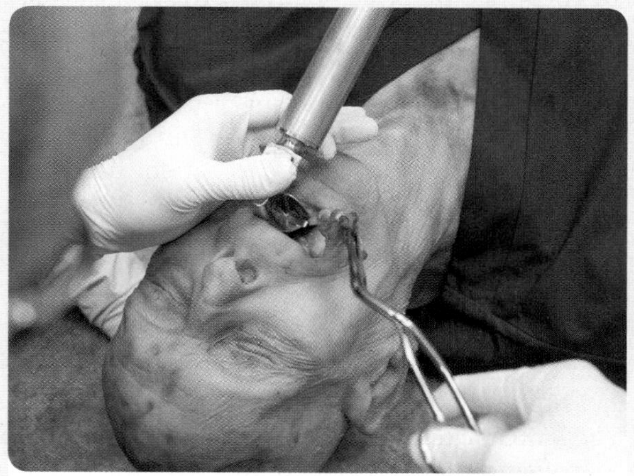

Step 3 Remove the object with the Magill forceps.

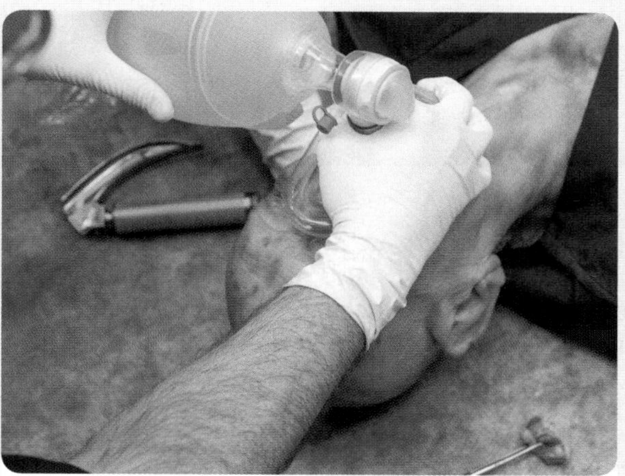

Step 4 Attempt to ventilate the patient.

Words of Wisdom

A patient with a severe upper airway obstruction has very little time before severe hypoxia develops. If several attempts to relieve the obstruction with BLS methods fail, then proceed with direct laryngoscopy without delay. While you are performing BLS maneuvers, your partner should prepare the laryngoscope, a properly sized laryngoscope blade, and Magill forceps.

Supplemental Oxygen Therapy

Supplemental oxygen is indicated for patients with respiratory distress and those with suspected or documented hypoxemia (that is, an oxygen saturation level of less than 94%). Your EMS system protocols may call for supplemental oxygen in other select cases.

Historically, oxygen was administered to patients whose clinical condition did not otherwise indicate its use (that is, no evidence of respiratory compromise, with an oxygen saturation level greater than 94%). Limited evidence suggests that supplemental oxygen in a well-oxygenated patient may not be in his or her best interest, because issues such as oxidative stress and hyperoxic injury are of concern. However, the evidence that oxygen is helpful to a patient with hypoxia is profound, so if you are in doubt as to the patient's oxygenation status, then administer supplemental oxygen.[2,3]

Evidence-Based Medicine

Current guidelines from the American Heart Association state that if the patient is not experiencing respiratory distress *and* has an oxygen saturation level that is greater than or equal to 94%, then supplemental oxygen is not indicated.[4] Follow your local protocols regarding supplemental oxygen administration.

The oxygen-delivery method must be appropriate for the patient's ventilatory status. Reassess frequently and adjust accordingly based on the patient's clinical condition and adequacy of breathing.

▶ Oxygen Sources

Oxygen Cylinders

Pure (100%) oxygen is stored in seamless steel or aluminum cylinders. The colors of the cylinders may vary from silver, to chrome, to green, or some combination thereof. Ensure that the cylinder is labeled "medical oxygen."

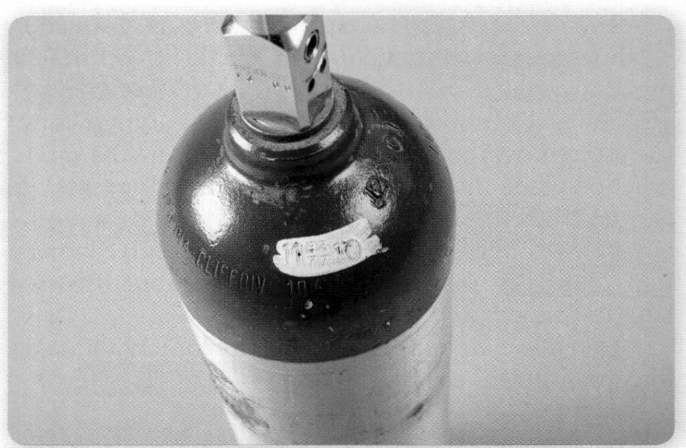

Figure 15-40 Oxygen cylinders for medical use have a series of letters and numbers stamped into the metal on the collar of the cylinder.

Also, look for letters and numbers stamped on the collar of the cylinder Figure 15-40. Of particular importance are the month and year stamps, which indicate when the cylinder was last hydrostatically tested.

Oxygen cylinders are available in various sizes. You will most often use the D cylinder, which contains 350 L of oxygen and is typically carried from the ambulance to the patient, and the M cylinder, which contains 3,000 L of oxygen and remains on board the ambulance as a main supply tank.

Oxygen delivery is measured in terms of liters per minute (L/min). To prevent running out of oxygen at an inconvenient moment, you should replace an oxygen cylinder with a full one when the pressure falls to 200 pounds per square inch (psi) or lower. That level is called the **safe residual pressure**, indicating that it is *unsafe* to continue using the oxygen cylinder. In some EMS systems, the safe residual pressure for an oxygen cylinder is 500 psi. On the basis of the pressure in the oxygen cylinder and the flow rate of oxygen delivery, you can calculate how long the supply of oxygen in the cylinder will last—that is, the tank life Table 15-8.

▶ Safety Reminders

Any cylinder containing compressed gas under high pressure has the potential, under specific conditions, to assume the properties of a rocket. Furthermore, oxygen presents the additional hazard of fire because it supports the combustion process. For these reasons, the following safety precautions are necessary when you are handling oxygen cylinders:

- Keep combustible materials, such as oil and grease, away from contact with the cylinder itself, the regulators, fittings, valves, and tubing.
- Do not permit smoking in any area where oxygen cylinders are in use or on standby.

Table 15-8 Oxygen Cylinders: Duration of Flow

Formula
(Tank Pressure in psi − 200 psi [the safe residual pressure]) × Cylinder Constant/Flow Rate in L/min = Duration of Flow in min
Cylinder Constant
D = 0.16 G = 2.41 E = 0.28 H = 3.14 M = 1.56 K = 3.14
Steps
Determine the life of an M cylinder that has a pressure of 2,000 psi and a flow rate of 10 L/min.

$$\frac{(2{,}000 - 200) \times 1.56}{10} = \frac{2{,}808}{10} = 281 \text{ min, or 4 h 41 min}$$

Abbreviation: psi, pounds per square inch

- Store oxygen cylinders in a cool, well-ventilated area. Do not subject the cylinders to temperatures above 125°F (approximately 50°C).
- Use an oxygen cylinder only with a safe, properly fitting regulator valve. Regulator valves for one gas should never be modified for use with another gas.
- Close all valves when the cylinder is not in use, even if the tank is empty.
- Secure cylinders so that they will not topple over. In transit, keep them in a proper carrier or rack, or strap them onto the stretcher with the patient.
- When working with an oxygen cylinder, always position yourself to its side. Never place any part of your body over the cylinder valve. A loosely fitting regulator can be blown off the cylinder with sufficient force to cause serious injury.
- Have the cylinder hydrostat tested every 10 years to ensure it can still sustain the high pressures required. The original test date is stamped onto the cylinder together with its serial number.

Oxygen Regulators and Flowmeters

High-pressure regulators are attached to the cylinder stem to deliver cylinder gas under high pressure. These regulators are used to transfer cylinder gas from tank to tank, such as when you are refilling a portable oxygen cylinder.

The pressure of gas in a full oxygen cylinder is approximately 2,000 psi. Clearly, this is far too much pressure to deliver directly into a patient's airway. Instead, gas flow from an oxygen cylinder to the patient is controlled by a **therapy regulator**, which attaches to the stem of the oxygen cylinder and reduces the high pressure of gas to a safe range (about 50 psi).

Flowmeters, which are usually permanently attached to the therapy regulator, allow the oxygen delivered to the patient to be adjusted within a range of 1 to 25 L/min. The two types of flowmeters most commonly used are the pressure-compensated flowmeter and the Bourdon-gauge flowmeter.

A **pressure-compensated flowmeter** incorporates a float ball within a tapered calibrated tube; this float ball rises or falls based on the gas flow in the tube. The gas flow is controlled by a needle valve located downstream from the float ball. Because this type of flowmeter is affected by gravity, it must remain in an upright position to obtain an accurate flow reading Figure 15-41. The pressure-compensated flowmeter is most often used with the main oxygen source on the ambulance.

By contrast, the **Bourdon-gauge flowmeter** is not affected by gravity and can be placed in any position. This pressure gauge is calibrated to record the flow rate Figure 15-42. The major disadvantage of this type of flowmeter is that it does not compensate for backpressure. As a result, it will usually record a higher flow rate when there is any obstruction to gas flow downstream.

Preparing an Oxygen Cylinder for Use

Before you administer supplemental oxygen, you must prepare the oxygen cylinder and therapy regulator. Inspect

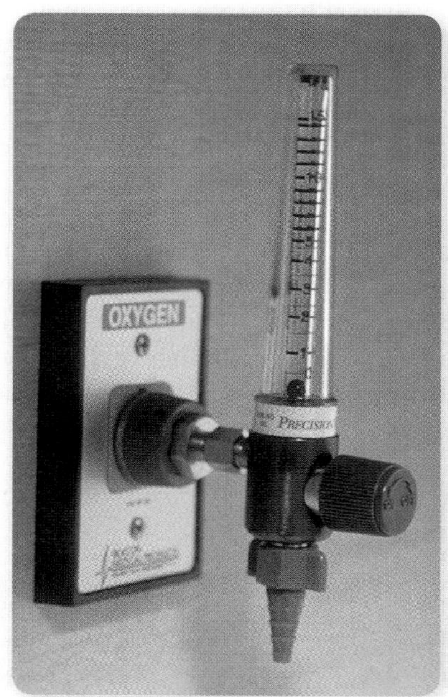

Figure 15-41 Pressure-compensated flowmeters contain a float ball that rises or falls based on the gas flow in the tube. It must remain in an upright position for an accurate flow reading.

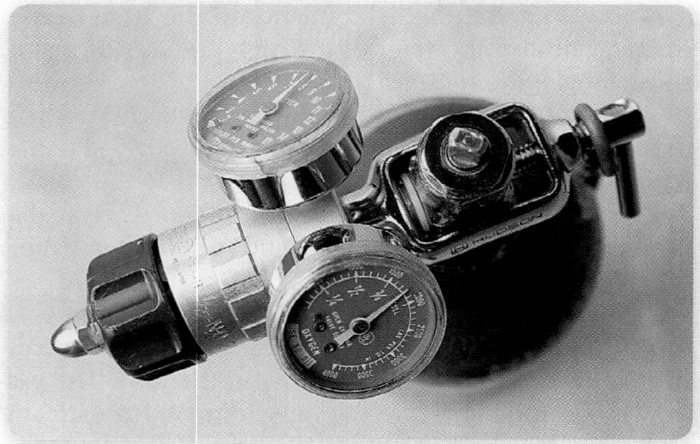

Figure 15-42 The Bourdon-gauge flowmeter is not affected by gravity and can be placed in any position.

the cylinder and its markings and then remove the plastic seal covering the valve stem opening (if commercially filled). Inspect the opening to ensure that it is free of dirt and other debris. With the tank facing away from yourself and others, use an oxygen wrench to "crack" the cylinder—that is, quickly open and close the valve to ensure that dirt particles and other contaminants do not enter the oxygen cylinder.

Attach the regulator/flowmeter to the valve stem, ensuring that the pin-index system is correctly aligned. A metal or plastic O-ring is placed around the oxygen port to optimize an airtight seal between the collar of the regulator and the valve stem. Place the regulator collar over the cylinder valve, with the oxygen port and indexing pins on the side of the valve stem that has three holes. Align the regulator so that the oxygen port and the pins fit into the correct holes on the valve stem; align the screw bolt on the opposite side with the dimpled depression. Tighten the screw bolt until the regulator is firmly attached to the cylinder. At this point, you should not see any space between the sides of the valve stem and the interior walls of the collar **Figure 15-43A**.

With the regulator firmly attached, open the cylinder and read the pressure level on the regulator gauge. A second gauge or selector dial on the flowmeter indicates the oxygen flow rate. Attach the oxygen connective tubing to the "Christmas tree" nipple on the flowmeter and select the oxygen flow rate that is appropriate for the patient's clinical status **Figure 15-43B**.

Supplemental Oxygen-Delivery Devices

In general, the oxygen-delivery equipment that is used in the prehospital setting is limited to nonrebreathing masks, bag-mask devices, and nasal cannulas, depending on local protocol. However, you may encounter other devices during transports between medical facilities.

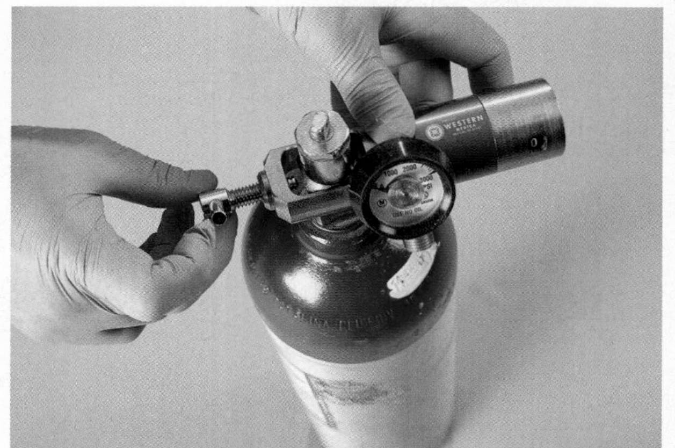

A

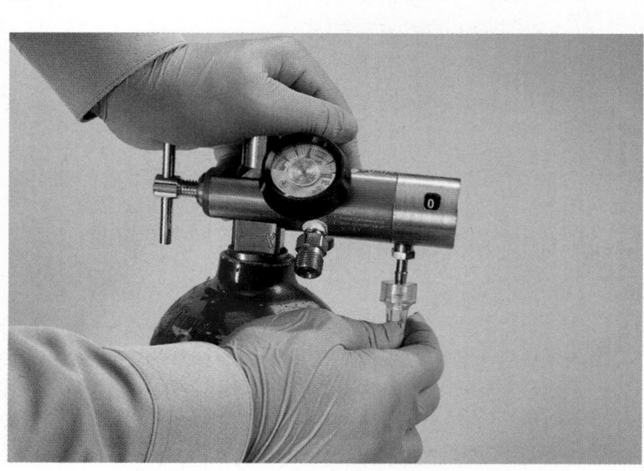

B

Figure 15-43 A. Attach the oxygen regulator, ensuring that the pin-indexing system is properly aligned, and tighten the screw bolt until it is secure. **B.** Attach the oxygen delivery device and select the flow rate that is appropriate for the patient's clinical status.

Nonrebreathing Mask

The **nonrebreathing mask** is used to administer high-flow oxygen to significantly hypoxemic patients who are otherwise breathing adequately. With a good mask-to-face seal and a flow rate of 15 L/min, it is capable of providing up to 90% inspired oxygen (F_{IO_2}).

The nonrebreathing mask is a combination mask and reservoir bag system. Oxygen fills a reservoir bag that is attached to the mask by a one-way valve, permitting the patient to inhale from the reservoir bag but not to exhale back into it. The only gas that can enter the reservoir, therefore, is 100% oxygen piped in from the oxygen cylinder. Exhaled gas escapes through one-way flapper valves located on the side of the mask **Figure 15-44**.

Before you administer oxygen to a patient with a nonrebreathing mask, you must ensure that the reservoir bag is completely filled. The oxygen flow rate is adjusted from 12 to 15 L/min to prevent collapse of the bag during inhalation. Use a pediatric nonrebreathing mask, which

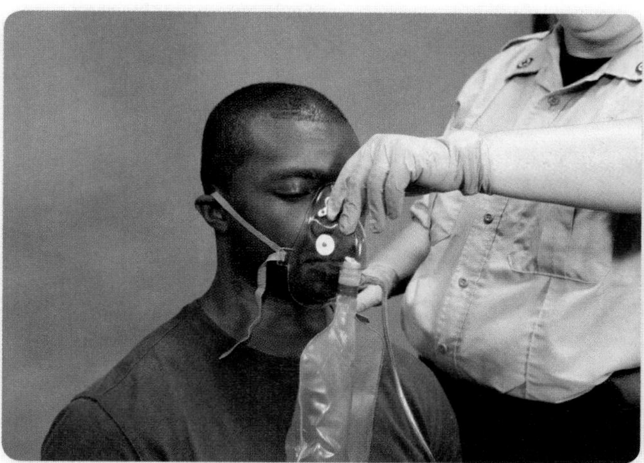

Figure 15-44 Nonrebreathing mask.

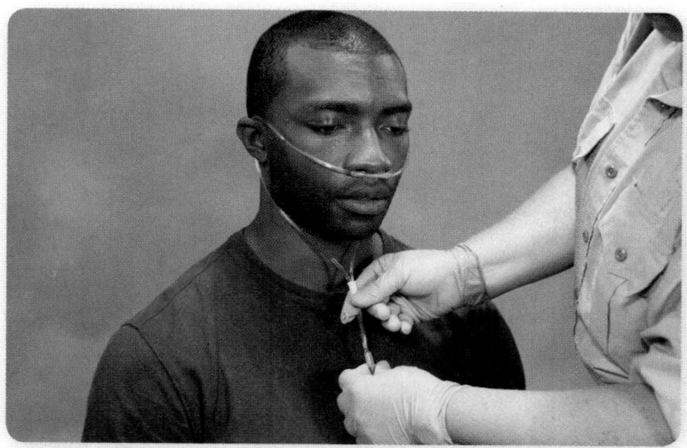

Figure 15-45 Nasal cannula.

has a smaller reservoir bag, for infants and small children; they inhale smaller volumes of air.

The nonrebreathing mask is indicated for spontaneously breathing patients who require high-flow oxygen concentrations (ie, shock, significant hypoxemia) and are breathing adequately (that is, adequate tidal volume, normal rate and regularity). Contraindications include apnea and poor respiratory effort. Because the nonrebreathing mask delivers oxygen passively, the patient's respirations must be of adequate depth to open the one-way valve, thus slightly collapsing the reservoir bag, and drawing air into the lungs. A patient with a marked reduction in tidal volume (shallow breathing) will benefit little, if at all, from a nonrebreathing mask.

▶ Nasal Cannula

The **nasal cannula** delivers oxygen via two small prongs that fit into the patient's nostrils **Figure 15-45**. With an oxygen flow rate of 1 to 6 L/min, the nasal cannula can provide an oxygen concentration of 24% to 44%. Use an oxygen humidifier (discussed next) when giving oxygen via nasal cannula for a prolonged period because it will help prevent mucosal drying and irritation.

The nasal cannula provides low to moderate oxygen enrichment and is most beneficial for patients with mild hypoxemia (oxygen saturation level between 90% and 93%) and in patients who require long-term oxygen therapy (such as for COPD). It is less effective if the patient is apneic, has poor respiratory effort, is severely hypoxic, or is a mouth breather. In the prehospital setting, the nasal cannula is primarily used when patients who need oxygen cannot tolerate a nonrebreathing mask or if they require only low concentrations of oxygen to maintain an oxygen saturation level greater than 94%.

The nasal cannula is generally well tolerated, especially by patients who are claustrophobic and intolerant of an oxygen mask over the face. However, it does not provide high volumes or concentrations of oxygen.

Table 15-9 compares oxygen delivery devices.

Table 15-9 Oxygen-Delivery Devices

Device	Flow Rate	Oxygen Delivered
Nasal cannula	1–6 L/min	24%–44%
Partial rebreathing mask	6–10 L/min	35%–60%
Nonrebreathing mask	15 L/min	Up to 90%
Bag-mask device with oxygen reservoir	15 L/min	Nearly 100%
Mouth-to-mask device	15 L/min	Nearly 55%

▶ Partial Rebreathing Mask

A **partial rebreathing mask** is similar to the nonrebreathing mask except that it lacks a one-way valve between the mask and the reservoir **Figure 15-46**. Room air is not drawn in with inhalation, but residual exhaled air is mixed in the mask and rebreathed.

Contraindications are the same as for the nonrebreathing mask—any patient with apnea or inadequate tidal volume. At flow rates of 6 to 10 L/min, an oxygen concentration of 35% to 60% is possible. Increasing the oxygen flow rate beyond 10 L/min will not enhance the oxygen concentration, and leakage from the mask around the face decreases the amount of oxygen inhaled by the patient.

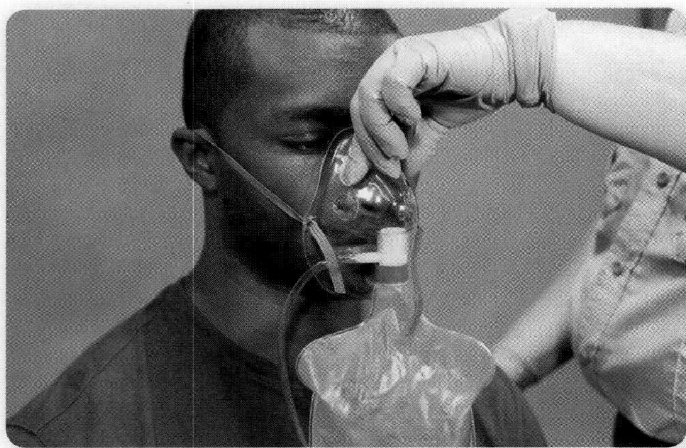

Figure 15-46 Partial rebreathing mask.

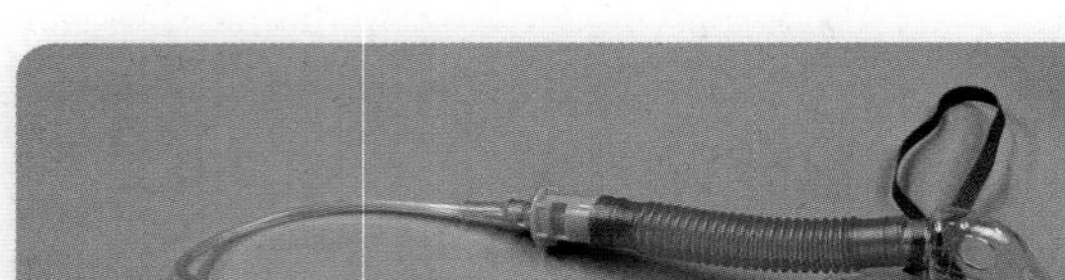

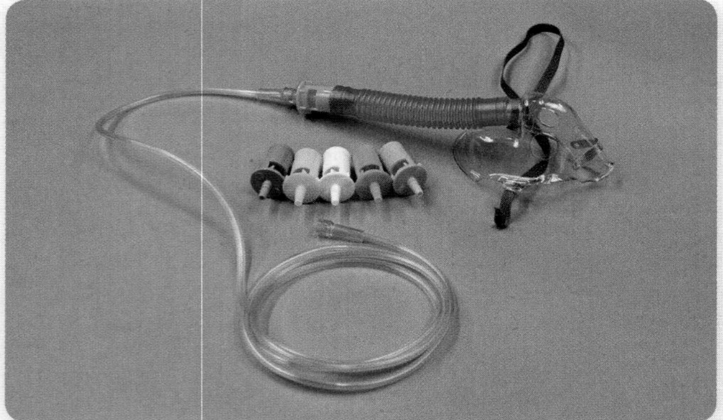

Figure 15-47 Venturi mask.

▶ Venturi Mask

The **Venturi mask** draws room air into the mask along with the oxygen flow, allowing for the administration of highly specific oxygen concentrations **Figure 15-47**. Depending on the adapter used, the Venturi mask can deliver 24%, 28%, 35%, or 40% oxygen. Venturi masks are especially useful in the hospital management of patients with COPD and other chronic respiratory diseases. They can also benefit patients who require precise oxygen concentrations during long-distance interfacility transports.

▶ Tracheostomy Masks

Patients with tracheostomies do not breathe through the nose and mouth; therefore, a face mask or nasal cannula would be ineffective for providing oxygen. Masks designed specifically for patients with tracheostomies cover the tracheostomy hole (stoma) and have a strap that goes around the neck. These masks are usually available in ICUs, where many patients have tracheostomies, and may be unavailable in the emergency setting. If you do not have a tracheostomy mask, then you can improvise by placing a face mask over the stoma. Even though the mask is shaped to fit the face, you can usually get an adequate fit over the patient's neck by adjusting the strap **Figure 15-48**.

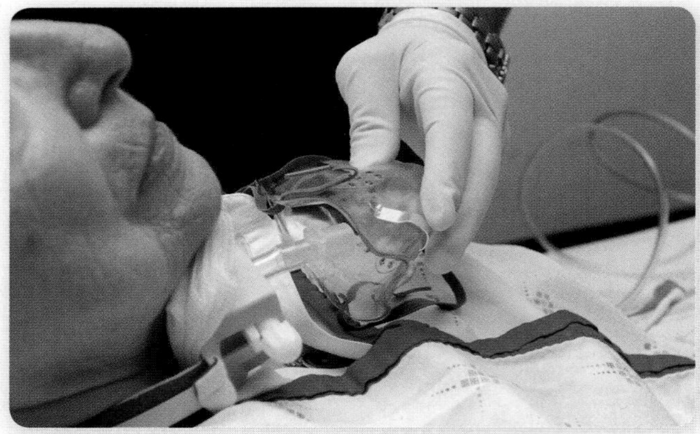

Figure 15-48 If a tracheostomy mask is unavailable, then use a face mask instead.

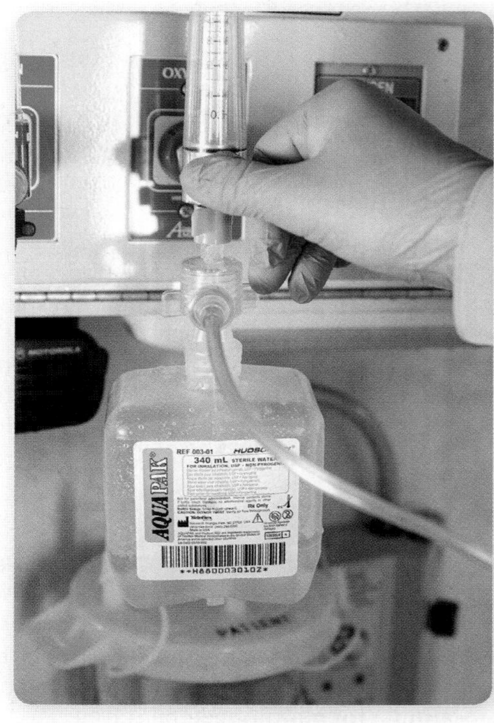

Figure 15-49 Administering humidified oxygen is preferred for long-distance transports to avoid drying the patient's mucous membranes.

▶ Oxygen Humidifier

Oxygen stored in cylinders has zero humidity, and it is not a good idea to deliver dry gases to a patient's airway for long periods. In fact, oxygen that is entirely devoid of moisture will rapidly dry the patient's mucous membranes. An **oxygen humidifier** consists of small bottle of sterile water through which the oxygen leaving the cylinder becomes moisturized before it reaches the patient **Figure 15-49**. Because the humidifier must be kept in an upright position, however, it is practical only for the fixed oxygen unit in the ambulance. In addition, oxygen humidifiers can be a source of infection for the patient. For this reason, use a disposable bottle.

Ventilatory Support

Obviously, a patient who is not breathing needs artificial ventilation and high-flow supplemental oxygen. Artificial ventilation is among the most important skills in EMS—at any level. Artificial ventilation is the skill of providing assisted ventilation to a patient who is breathing spontaneously, or by ventilating a patient who is not breathing at all. Artificial ventilation techniques are extremely effective when performed properly. Mastery of these techniques is imperative.

Patients who are breathing inadequately, such as too fast or too slowly with reduced tidal volume (shallow breathing), are typically unable to speak in complete sentences. An irregular breathing pattern may also require artificial ventilation to assist in maintaining adequate minute volume. Fast, shallow breathing can be just as dangerous as very slow breathing. Fast, shallow breathing moves air primarily in the larger airway passages (dead space) and does not allow for adequate exchange of oxygen and carbon dioxide in the alveoli. Signs of altered mental status and inadequate minute volume are indications for assisted ventilation. In addition, excessive accessory muscle use and fatigue from labored breathing are signs of potential respiratory failure. Patients with these signs need immediate treatment. Two treatment options are available for patients with severe respiratory distress or respiratory failure: (1) positive pressure ventilation with a bag-mask device or (2) continuous positive airway pressure [CPAP] or bilevel positive airway pressure [BPAP]). The purpose of assisted ventilation is to improve the overall oxygenation and ventilatory status of the patient. CPAP and BPAP are discussed later in this chapter; the focus of this section is assisted ventilation with a bag-mask device.

Normal Ventilation Versus Positive Pressure Ventilation

The act of moving air into and out of the lungs is based on pressure changes within the thoracic cavity. During normal ventilation, the diaphragm contracts and negative pressure is generated in the chest cavity. This negative pressure draws air into the chest through the trachea in an attempt to equalize the pressure in the chest with the pressure of the external atmosphere (negative pressure ventilation). However, positive pressure ventilation generated by a device, such as a bag-mask device, forces air into the chest cavity from the external environment. The difference between normal ventilation and positive pressure ventilation can create challenges for paramedics Table 15-10.

Table 15-10 Normal Ventilation Versus Positive Pressure Ventilation

	Normal Ventilation	Positive Pressure Ventilation
Air movement	Air is sucked into the lungs due to the negative intrathoracic pressure created when the diaphragm contracts.	Air is forced into the lungs by means of mechanical ventilation.
Blood movement	Normal breathing facilitates venous return, thus maintaining preload.	Intrathoracic pressure is increased, which impairs venous return (and preload); as a result, stroke volume and cardiac output are reduced.
Airway wall pressure	Not affected during normal breathing	More volume is required to have the same effects as normal breathing. As a result, the walls are pushed out of their normal anatomic shapes.
Esophageal opening pressure	Not affected during normal breathing	Air is forced into the stomach, causing gastric distention that could result in vomiting and aspiration.
Overventilation	Not typical of normal breathing	Forcing volume and rate results in increased intrathoracic pressure, gastric distention, and decreased cardiac output (hypotension).

The physical act of the chest wall expanding and recoiling during breathing aids the circulatory system in returning blood to the heart. During normal ventilation, the chest wall movement works similar to a pump. The pressure changes in the thoracic cavity help draw venous blood back to the heart, which improves preload. However, when positive pressure ventilation is initiated, more air is needed to achieve the same oxygenation and ventilatory effects of normal breathing. This increase in airway wall pressure causes the walls of the chest cavity to push out of their normal anatomic shape. As a result, an increase occurs in the overall intrathoracic pressure within the chest cavity. Positive pressure affects venous return to the heart (reduced preload). The blood flow is decreased due to the increased pressure in the chest. This decreased blood flow results in insufficient venous return to the heart, and as a result, the amount of blood pumped out of the heart is reduced. Therefore, it is imperative that you regulate the rate and volume of artificial ventilations to help prevent this drop in cardiac output. Cardiac output is a function of stroke volume multiplied by the pulse rate. Stroke volume is the amount of blood ejected by the ventricle in one cardiac cycle. The cardiac output is the amount of blood ejected by the left ventricle in 1 minute.

Another difference between normal ventilation and positive pressure ventilation is the control of airflow. When a person breathes, air enters the trachea and, generally, not the esophagus. However, the force generated from positive pressure ventilation allows air to enter not only the trachea, but also the esophagus. Ventilations that are too forceful can open the esophagus—normally a flat tube—and instill air in the stomach. This potential complication—called **gastric distention**—is discussed later in this chapter.

▶ Assisted Ventilation

Follow these steps to assist a conscious patient's ventilations using a bag-mask device. Remember to first explain the procedure to the patient, and take standard precautions (discussed later in this chapter) as needed when managing the patient's airway.

1. Place the mask over the patient's nose and mouth.
2. Squeeze the bag each time the patient inhales, maintaining the same rate as the patient, coaching the patient as needed.
3. After the initial 5 to 10 breaths, slowly adjust the rate and deliver the appropriate tidal volume.
4. Adjust the rate and tidal volume to maintain adequate minute volume.

YOU are the Paramedic PART 5

You achieve access to the airway via the cricothyroid membrane, and you are now able to ventilate the patient. Waveform capnography, the presence of bilaterally equal breath sounds, and an absence of epigastric sounds further confirm correct placement in the trachea. You and your partner secure the patient to the stretcher and load him the ambulance. After obtaining a complete set of vital signs and establishing IV access, you begin transport.

Recording Time: 20 Minutes	
Level of consciousness	Unresponsive
Respirations	12 breaths/min via positive pressure ventilation
Pulse	118 beats/min; weak and regular
Skin	Diaphoretic; cyanosis is quickly resolving
Blood pressure	94/56 mm Hg
Oxygen saturation (Spo_2)	96% (with positive pressure ventilation and supplemental oxygen)
$ETCO_2$	83 mm Hg
ECG	Sinus tachycardia

8. How can the patient's $ETCO_2$ level be so high when his Spo_2 level is 96%?
9. Is it necessary to adjust your current treatment? If so, then how?

Artificial Ventilation

Without immediate treatment, patients who are in respiratory arrest will die. The act of breathing for a patient, or artificial ventilation, is not a skill you should take lightly. After you determine that a patient is not breathing, begin artificial ventilation immediately. The methods that you may use to provide artificial ventilation include the mouth-to-mask technique and the one-, two-, or three-person bag-mask device technique.

Mouth-to-Mask Ventilation

As you learned in your CPR course, ventilation is routinely performed with a barrier device, such as a mask with a one-way valve or a plastic face shield Figure 15-50. A barrier device is a protective item that features a plastic barrier placed on a patient's face with a one-way valve to prevent the backflow of secretions, vomitus, and gases. Barrier devices provide you with adequate protection.

Mouth-to-mask ventilation (or ventilation using another barrier device) is preferred if a bag-mask device is unavailable. Advantages of using a mask include placing a physical barrier between your mouth and the patient's mouth. Most masks feature a one-way valve to prevent exposure to blood and other body fluids. It is also easier to secure an effective seal with a mask because you can use both hands, which enables the provision of adequate tidal volume to the patient.

A mask with an oxygen inlet provides oxygen during mouth-to-mask ventilation to supplement the air from your own lungs. Remember that the gas you exhale contains 16% oxygen, which is adequate to sustain a patient's life for a limited period. With the mouth-to-mask technique, however, the patient receives the additional benefit of significant oxygen enrichment with inspired air—up to 55%. Consider carrying a face mask device with one-way valve in your personal vehicle, in case you encounter an apneic patient while off duty.

The mask may be shaped like a triangle or a doughnut, with the apex (top) placed across the bridge of the nose. The base (bottom) of the mask is placed in the groove between the lower lip and the chin. In the center of the mask is a chimney with a 15-mm connector.

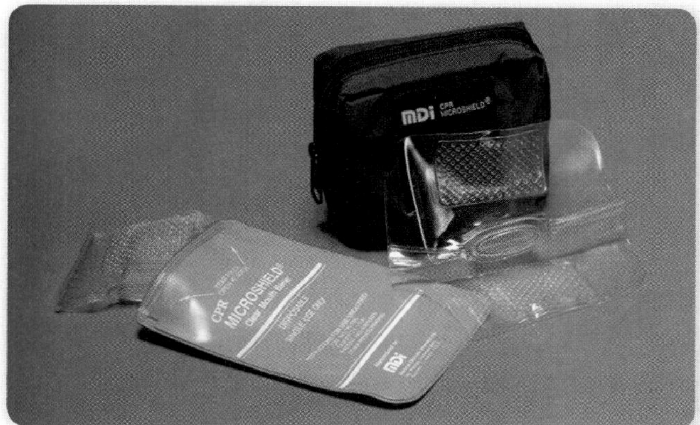

Figure 15-50 Plastic face shield.

Mouth-to-Mask Ventilation Technique

To ventilate a patient using a pocket face mask, open his or her airway with the head tilt-chin lift or jaw-thrust maneuver. Insert an oral or nasal airway to help maintain airway patency. Connect the one-way valve to the face mask and place the mask on the patient's face. Ensure the top of the mask is placed over the bridge of the nose and the bottom is between the lower lip and chin. Hold the mask in position by placing your thumbs over the top part of the mask and your index fingers over the bottom half. Grasp the patient's lower jaw with the next three fingers on each hand. Place your thumbs on the dome of the mask, making an airtight seal by applying firm pressure between the thumbs and fingers. Maintain an upward and forward pull on the lower jaw with your fingers to keep the airway open Figure 15-51A. Exhale slowly over a period of 1 second—just enough to produce visible chest rise—then remove your mouth from the one-way valve and allow the patient to passively exhale Figure 15-51B.

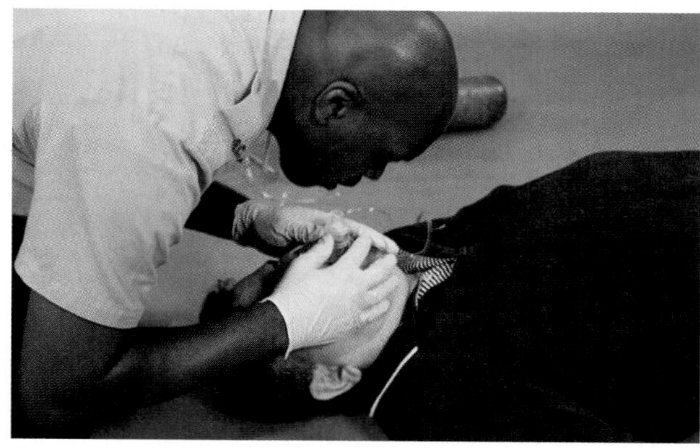

A

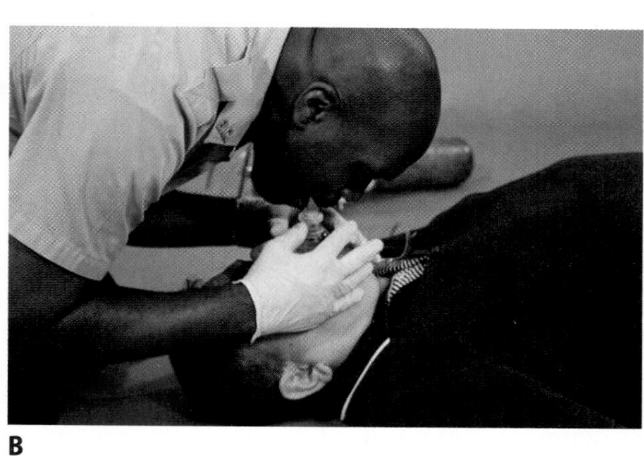

B

Figure 15-51 A. Open the patient's airway and properly position the mask on the face. **B.** Deliver each breath over a period of 1 second, observe for chest rise, and allow the patient to passively exhale.

Table 15-11	Ventilation Rates by Age
Adult	Apneic with a pulse: 10 to 12 breaths/min ▪ With or without an advanced airway in place (eg, ET tube, LMA, i-gel supraglottic airway) Apneic and pulseless: 10 breaths/min ▪ After an advanced airway has been inserted
Infant (ages 1 month to 1 year) and child (ages 1 to 17 years)	Apneic with a pulse: 12 to 20 breaths/min ▪ With or without an advanced airway in place (eg, ET tube, LMA, i-gel supraglottic airway) Apneic and pulseless: 10 breaths/min ▪ After an advanced airway has been inserted

Abbreviations: ET, endotracheal; LMA, laryngeal mask airway
Avoid hyperventilating any patient; hyperventilated lungs may "squeeze" the heart, thus impeding venous return and subsequent cardiac output. Hyperventilation also increases the risks of regurgitation and aspiration.

Data from: Kleinman ME, Brennan EE, Goldberger ZD, Swor RA, Terry M, Bobrow BJ, Gazmuri RJ, Travers AH, Rea T. Part 5: adult basic life support and cardiopulmonary resuscitation quality: 2015 American Heart Association Guidelines Update for Cardiopulmonary Resuscitation and Emergency Cardiovascular Care. *Circulation*. 2015;132(suppl 2):S414-S435; Link MS, Berkow LC, Kudenchuk PJ, Halperin HR, Hess EP, Moitra VK, Neumar RW, O'Neil BJ, Paxton JH, Silvers SM, White RD, Yannopoulos D, Donnino MW. Part 7: adult advanced cardiovascular life support: 2015 American Heart Association Guidelines Update for Cardiopulmonary Resuscitation and Emergency Cardiovascular Care. *Circulation*. 2015;132(suppl 2):S444-S464; Atkins DL, Berger S, Duff JP, Gonzales JC, Hunt EA, Joyner BL, Meaney PA, Niles DE, Samson RA, Schexnayder SM. Part 11: pediatric basic life support and cardiopulmonary resuscitation quality: 2015 American Heart Association Guidelines Update for Cardiopulmonary Resuscitation and Emergency Cardiovascular Care. *Circulation*. 2015;132(suppl 2):S519-S525; and de Caen AR, Berg MD, Chameides L, Gooden CK, Hickey RW, Scott HF, Sutton RM, Tijssen JA, Topjian A, van der Jagt E, Schexnayder SM, Samson RA. Part 12: pediatric advanced life support: 2015 American Heart Association Guidelines Update for Cardiopulmonary Resuscitation and Emergency Cardiovascular Care. *Circulation*. 2015;132(suppl 2):S526-S542.

The effectiveness of ventilation is best determined by watching the patient's chest rise and fall and feeling for resistance of the patient's lungs as they expand. You should also hear and feel air escape as the patient passively exhales. Ensure you provide the correct number of breaths per minute for the patient's age **Table 15-11**.

▶ The Bag-Mask Device

With an oxygen flow rate of 15 L/min and an adequate seal, a bag-mask device with an oxygen reservoir can deliver nearly 100% oxygen **Figure 15-52**. Most bag-mask devices on the market include modifications or accessories (reservoirs) that permit the delivery of oxygen concentration levels approaching 100%. However, the device can deliver only as much volume as can be squeezed out of the bag by hand. The bag-mask device provides less tidal volume than mouth-to-mask ventilation; however, it delivers a much higher level of oxygen concentration.

The bag-mask device is the most common device used to ventilate patients in the prehospital setting. An experienced paramedic will be able to provide adequate tidal volume

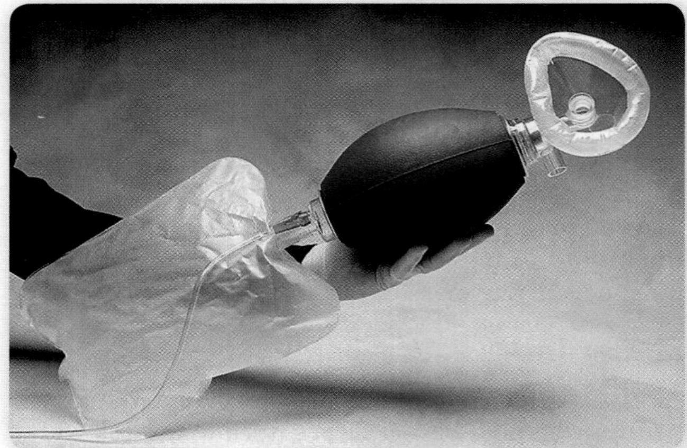

Figure 15-52 A bag-mask device with an oxygen reservoir can deliver nearly 100% oxygen if a good seal between the face and mask is maintained and if supplemental oxygen is attached to the device.

with the bag-mask device. Use of the device is a difficult skill to master, particularly if you do not have many opportunities to practice. Mask seal on a medical patient may be difficult to maintain with only one rescuer. Because it takes two hands to perform a jaw-thrust maneuver, it takes two rescuers to use the bag-mask device on a trauma patient unless an advanced airway has already been inserted. The amount of tidal volume and the concentration of oxygen delivered to the patient are dependent on the integrity of the mask seal. You should practice this skill frequently by ventilating a manikin with the bag-mask device.

Words of Wisdom

Airway management and ventilation procedures often expose you to blood, vomitus, and oral secretions. Although blood is the most potentially infectious body fluid, you should exercise great caution to avoid contact with all body fluids. Wear gloves for all airway and ventilation procedures and when handling airway equipment that might have been contaminated with body fluids. To reduce the risk of splashing or droplets of body fluid coming in contact with your mouth, nose, and eyes, wear a mask and protective eyewear or a face shield, especially when inserting an advanced airway. In cases of significant blood splashing, such as with a trauma, patient you should also wear a protective gown, if possible.

Bag-Mask Device Components

All adult bag-mask devices should have the following components and characteristics:

- A disposable, self-inflating bag
- No pop-off valve or, if one is present, then the capability of disabling the pop-off valve

- An outlet valve that is a true nonrebreathing valve
- An oxygen reservoir that permits delivery of a high concentration of oxygen
- A one-way, no-jam inlet valve system that provides an oxygen inlet flow at a maximum of 15 L/min with a standard 15/22-mm fitting for a face mask and an advanced airway (that is, ET tube, laryngeal mask airway [LMA], King LT, i-gel)
- A transparent face mask
- The ability to perform under extreme environmental conditions, including extreme heat and cold

The total amount of gas in the reservoir bag of an adult bag-mask device is usually 1,200 to 1,600 mL. The pediatric bag contains 500 to 700 mL, and the infant bag holds 150 to 240 mL.

The volume of air (oxygen) to deliver to the patient is based on one key observation—visible chest rise. A delivered tidal volume of 500 to 600 mL (6 to 7 mL/kg) per breath will produce visible chest rise in most adults. When using a bag-mask device, deliver each breath over a period of 1 second—just enough to produce visible chest rise—at the appropriate rate. Breaths that are given too forcefully or too fast can result in two negative effects: gastric distention (and the associated risks of vomiting and aspiration) and decreased venous return to the heart (preload) due to increased intrathoracic pressure.

Improper technique, an ineffective mask-to-face seal, or the presence of gastric distention may cause you to deliver inadequate tidal volume and oxygen. Training and practice are key to the proper use of the bag-mask device.

Bag-Mask Device Technique

Whenever possible, you and your partner should work together to provide ventilation with the bag-mask device. One paramedic can maintain a good mask seal by securing the mask to the patient's face with two hands while the other paramedic squeezes the bag. Ventilation using a bag-mask device is a challenging skill; it may be difficult for you to maintain a proper seal between the mask and the face with one hand while squeezing the bag well enough to deliver an adequate volume of air to the patient. As mentioned previously, effective one-person bag-mask ventilation requires considerable experience. Also, performance of this skill depends on having enough personnel to carry out other actions that need to be done simultaneously, such as chest compressions, putting the stretcher in place, or helping to lift the patient onto the stretcher.

Follow these steps to use the two-person bag-mask device technique:

1. Kneel above the patient's head. If possible, then your partner should be at the side of the head. Select the proper size mask.
2. Maintain the patient's neck in a neutral position. Open the airway and suction the oropharynx as needed. Insert an oral or nasal airway to help maintain airway patency.
3. Connect the bag-mask device to supplemental oxygen.
4. Place the mask on the patient's face. Ensure the top is over the bridge of the nose and the bottom is in the groove between the lower lip and the chin. If the mask has a large, round cuff around the ventilation port, then center the port over the patient's mouth. Inflate (or deflate) the collar to obtain a better fit and seal to the face if necessary.
5. Bring the lower jaw up to the mask with your last three fingers. This step will help to maintain an open airway. Ensure you do not grab the fleshy part of the neck because you may compress structures and create an airway obstruction. If you think the patient may have a spinal injury, then ensure your partner manually stabilizes the cervical spine as you move the lower jaw.
6. Connect the bag to the mask if you have not already done so.
7. Hold the mask in place while your partner squeezes the bag with two hands until the patient's chest visibly rises **Figure 15-53**. If a spinal injury is suspected, then stabilize the patient's head and neck with your forearms while maintaining an adequate mask-to-face seal with your hands. Continue squeezing the bag once every 5 to 6 seconds for adults and once every 3 to 5 seconds for infants and children.
8. If you are alone, then place your thumb and index finger as high up on the mask as you can to form a C. Maintain the airway by lifting the bony prominence of the chin with your remaining fingers to form an E. Do not push the mask to the face; pull the lower jaw into

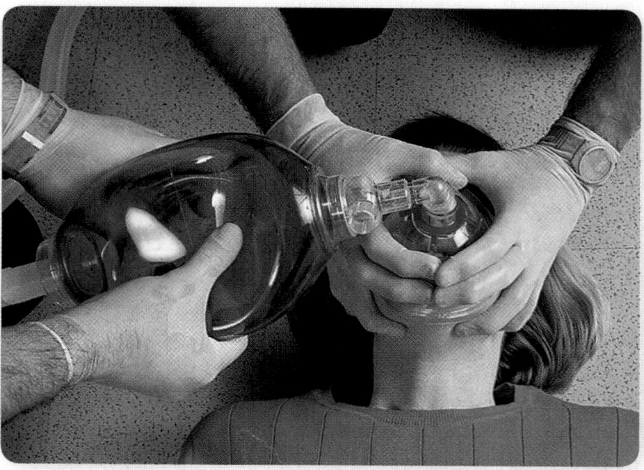

Figure 15-53 With two-person bag-mask ventilation, hold the mask in place while your partner squeezes the bag with two hands until the patient's chest visibly rises.

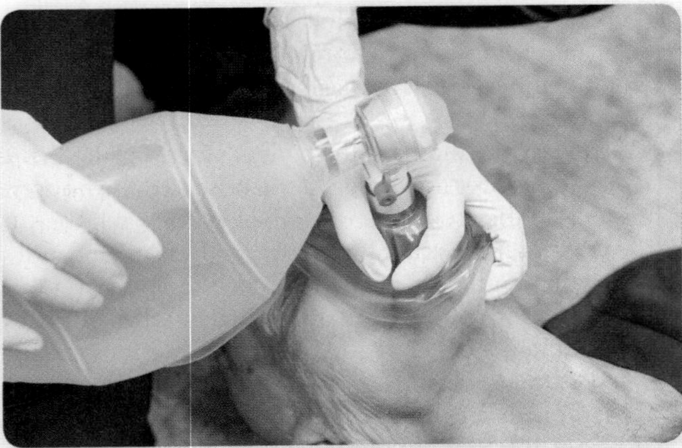

Figure 15-54 Maintain the seal of the mask to the face using the EC clamp technique, if you are ventilating the patient by yourself.

the mask. This practice is called the EC clamp technique, and it will maintain an effective mask-to-face seal Figure 15-54. Use the head tilt–chin lift maneuver to ensure the neck is extended. Squeeze the bag with your other hand in a rhythmic manner once every 5 to 6 seconds for adults and once every 3 to 5 seconds for infants and children.

9. Observe for gastric distention, changes in compliance of the bag with ventilations, and either improvement or deterioration of the patient's clinical status.

When using the bag-mask device to assist ventilation, you should squeeze the bag as the patient inhales. Then, for the next 5 to 10 breaths, slowly adjust the rate and tidal volume until an adequate minute volume is achieved.

To assist ventilations of a conscious patient who is breathing too fast (hyperventilation) with reduced tidal volume, first explain the procedure to the patient if he or she is coherent. Initially assist ventilations at the rate at which the patient has been breathing, squeezing the bag each time the patient inhales. Then, for the next 5 to 10 breaths, slowly adjust the rate and tidal volume until an adequate minute volume is achieved.

As you are ventilating a patient with a bag-mask device, evaluate the effectiveness of your ventilations. Artificial ventilations are inadequate if the patient's chest does not rise and fall with each ventilation, if you are unable to hear breath sounds when auscultating the chest, if the rate of ventilation is too slow or too fast for the patient's age, or if the pulse rate and/or oxygen saturation level do not improve. If the patient's chest does not rise and fall, then you may need to reposition the head or insert an oral and/or nasal airway.

If the patient's stomach, rather than the chest, seems to be rising and falling, then reposition the head. In a patient with a possible spinal injury, you should reposition the jaw rather than the head. If too much air is escaping from under the mask, then reposition the mask for a better seal. If the patient's chest still does not rise and fall after you have made these corrections, then check for an airway obstruction. If an obstruction is not present, then attempt ventilation with another airway device.

Advanced airway techniques are beneficial when ventilation with basic means is ineffective, the patient has a cervical spine injury, or the patient's condition otherwise warrants them.

Words of Wisdom

Indications That Artificial Ventilation Is Adequate[a]

- Adequate and equal chest rise and fall with ventilation
- Breath sounds can be heard during auscultation of the chest
- Ventilations are given at the appropriate rate:
  - 10 to 12 breaths/min for adults
  - 12 to 20 breaths/min for infants and children
- Pulse rate returns to a normal range
- Oxygen saturation level improves

Indications That Artificial Ventilation Is Inadequate

- Minimal or no chest rise and fall
- Breath sounds cannot be heard during auscultation of the chest
- Ventilations given too fast or too slow for patient's age
- Pulse rate does not return to a normal range
- Oxygen saturation level does not improve

[a] In patients who are apneic with a pulse (that is, not in cardiac arrest).

▶ Automatic Transport Ventilators

The **automatic transport ventilator (ATV)** allows the variables of ventilation—ventilatory rate, tidal volume, and peak inspiratory time—to be precisely set; these features allow for consistent ventilation Figure 15-55. Many types of ATVs are available, some with basic settings and others with more advanced settings and features, such as F_{IO_2} titration. The steps for using the ATV are as follows:

1. Attach the ATV to the wall-mounted oxygen source.
2. Set the ventilatory rate, tidal volume, and peak inspiratory time on the ATV as appropriate for the patient's age and condition.
3. Connect the ATV to the 15/22-mm fitting on the ET tube or other advanced airway device.
4. Auscultate the patient's breath sounds, and observe for equal chest rise to ensure adequate ventilation.

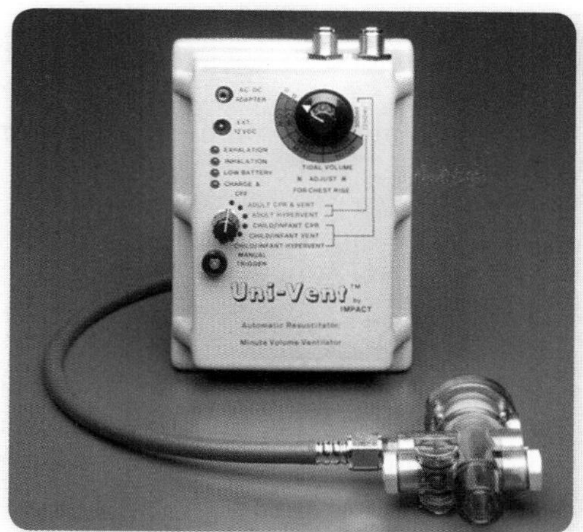

Figure 15-55 Automatic transport ventilator.
Courtesy of Impact Instrumentation, Inc.

Although the ATV lacks the sophisticated controls of a hospital ventilator, it frees your hands to perform other non–airway-related tasks. However, although the ATV is helpful to paramedics, you must always have a bag-mask device readily available should the ATV malfunction.

In most cases, the respiratory rate is set at the midpoint or average for the patient's age. You can estimate tidal volume using a formula based on 6 to 7 mL/kg, which can be adjusted based on chest rise and the patient's physiologic response. ATVs are considered volume-cycled, rate-controlled ventilators, which means that they deliver a preset volume at a preset ventilatory rate, although this does not guarantee that all of the volume is being delivered to the lungs, unless the patient is intubated. When using the ATV in the intubated patient who is in cardiac arrest, it is critical to set the rate and tidal volume accordingly to reduce the risk of hyperventilation.

The ATV is oxygen-powered, although some models may require an external power source. The ATV generally consumes 5 L/min of oxygen, whereas a bag-mask device uses 15 to 25 L/min. In addition, the ATV has a pressure relief valve, which can lead to hypoventilation in patients with inadequate lung compliance, increased airway resistance, or airway obstruction. The possibility of **barotrauma** (trauma resulting from excessive pressure) exists if the pressure relief valve fails or if ventilation is too fast or too forceful.

Continuous Positive Airway Pressure

Continuous positive airway pressure (CPAP) is a noninvasive means of providing ventilatory support for patients experiencing respiratory distress. Many people with obstructive sleep apnea wear a CPAP unit at night to maintain their airways while they sleep. The use of CPAP in the prehospital setting has proven to be an excellent adjunct in the treatment of respiratory distress caused by acute pulmonary edema, obstructive lung disease, and acute bronchospasm (such as in asthma)—especially when used in conjunction with beta-2 agonists. Typically, many patients with these conditions would be managed with advanced airway techniques, such as ET intubation. Early intervention with CPAP is an alternative means of providing ventilatory assistance and can prevent the need for intubation. Because of the simplicity of the device and its great benefit to patients, CPAP is widely used by paramedics.

CPAP increases pressure in the lungs, opens collapsed alveoli and prevents further alveolar collapse (atelectasis), pushes more oxygen across the alveolar membrane, and forces interstitial fluid back into the pulmonary circulation. The desired effect of CPAP is to improve pulmonary compliance and make spontaneous ventilation easier. The therapy is typically delivered through a face mask that is secured to the head with a strapping system.

Special Populations

Artificial Ventilation of Pediatric Patients

The flat nasal bridge of pediatric patients makes it more difficult to achieve an effective mask-to-face seal compared with adult patients. Compressing the mask against the face to improve mask seal may result in obstruction. The best mask seal is achieved by the two-person bag-mask ventilation technique with jaw displacement.

For full-term neonates and infants, use a pediatric bag-mask device with a minimum tidal volume of 450 mL. In children (ages 1 year to the onset of puberty [ages 12 to 14 years]), consider the size of the child when determining bag size. You may use an adult bag-sized mask-device with a volume of 1,500, but a pediatric bag-mask device is preferred. Children older than 12 to 14 years require an adult-sized bag-mask device for adequate ventilation. Choose a size to ensure a proper mask fit. The mask should reach from the bridge of the nose to the cleft of the chin. A length-based resuscitation tape may also be used to estimate the most appropriately sized bag-mask device for pediatric patients who weigh up to 75 pounds (34 kg).

When you are ventilating a pediatric patient, ensure a proper mask seal by using the EC clamp technique (as discussed previously in this chapter). Avoid placing pressure on the soft area under the chin because this pressure may cause an airway obstruction.

Deliver each ventilation over 1 second—just enough to produce visible chest rise. Do not overinflate. Deliver one breath every 3 to 5 seconds (12 to 20 breaths/min), allowing adequate time for exhalation. While ventilating, look for adequate chest rise. Auscultate breath sounds at the third or fourth intercostal space on the midaxillary line bilaterally. Also assess for improvement in skin color and pulse rate.

A good seal with minimal leakage between the face and mask is essential.

The face mask is fitted with a pressure relief valve that determines the amount of pressure delivered to the patient (such as 5 cm of water [cm H_2O]). This pressure results in a high inspiratory flow and the need to push a pressure valve open with exhalation. Although a great deal of effort is often required to achieve this, especially while in respiratory distress, many patients improve dramatically when CPAP is applied.

Indications for CPAP

CPAP is indicated for patients experiencing respiratory distress in which their own compensatory mechanisms cannot keep up with their oxygen demands. Although the condition of most patients improves after the application of CPAP, it is important to remember that CPAP is merely treating the symptoms and not necessarily treating the underlying pathology.

The following are general indications for using CPAP:

- Patient is alert and able to follow commands
- Obvious signs of moderate to severe respiratory distress (such as accessory muscle use, tripod position, retractions) from an underlying disease such as heart failure with pulmonary edema, obstructive lung disease (such as COPD), acute bronchospasm (such as in acute asthma), and suspected pneumonia
- Respiratory distress after a submersion incident
- Breathing that is so rapid that it affects overall minute volume
- Pulse oximetry reading of less than 90%

Consider these guidelines when assessing the need for CPAP, but it is important that you follow your local guidelines and protocols.

Contraindications for CPAP

CPAP has proven to be immensely beneficial to patients experiencing respiratory distress from acute pulmonary edema, acute bronchospasm, and obstructive lung disease; however, at times CPAP is not appropriate.

The following are general contraindications for using CPAP:

- Patient is unresponsive or otherwise unable to follow verbal commands
- Respiratory arrest or agonal respirations
- Patient is unable to speak
- Patient is unable to protect his or her own airway
- Hypoventilation (slow respiratory rate and/or reduced tidal volume)
- Hypotension (systolic blood pressure is less than 90 mm Hg)
- Signs and symptoms of a pneumothorax or chest trauma (either blunt or penetrating)
- Closed head injury
- Facial trauma
- Cardiogenic shock
- Tracheostomy
- Active gastrointestinal bleeding, nausea, or vomiting
- History of recent gastrointestinal surgical procedure
- Patient is unable to sit up
- Inability to properly fit the CPAP system mask and strap
  - Excessive facial hair or dysmorphic facial features can impede your ability to ensure a proper-fitting mask
- Patient cannot tolerate the mask

In addition, always reassess the patient for signs of clinical deterioration and/or respiratory failure. Although CPAP is an excellent tool to assist with ventilation, not all patients will experience improvement in their conditions with this device. After signs of respiratory failure become apparent or the patient is no longer able to follow commands, you should remove the CPAP device and initiate positive pressure ventilation with a bag-mask device attached to high-flow oxygen. In some patients, intubation will be required.

Application of CPAP

Several varieties of CPAP units are available to EMS systems; however, most follow the same general guidelines for use and setup. The CPAP units are generally composed of a generator, a mask, a circuit that contains corrugated tubing, a bacteria filter, and a one-way valve. During the expiratory phase, the patient exhales against a resistance called **positive end-expiratory pressure (PEEP)**. Within the CPAP generator is a valve that determines the amount of PEEP; however, some CPAP models have PEEP valves that connect separately. Depending on the device, the PEEP is controlled by manually adjusting the PEEP using a manometer or predetermined by a fixed setting on the PEEP valve. A PEEP of 5 to 10 cm H_2O is generally an acceptable therapeutic range for a patient using CPAP, although it can be adjusted higher or lower if needed. Always consult the operations manual of a particular CPAP device for proper assembly instructions.

Because most CPAP units are powered by oxygen, it is important to have a full cylinder of oxygen when using CPAP and a backup cylinder. Some CPAP units use a continuous flow of oxygen, whereas others use oxygen on more of a demand basis. Continuously monitor the amount of available oxygen in the cylinder. Some CPAP units will empty a D cylinder in as little as 5 to 10 minutes. Therefore, proper planning for oxygen consumption is necessary when considering applying CPAP. In addition, some of the newer CPAP devices allow you to adjust the FIO_2 level. Most CPAP devices are set to deliver a fixed FIO_2 level of 30% to 35%; however, some can deliver as high as 80%.

Follow the steps shown in Skill Drill 15-2 to use CPAP.

NR Skill

Skill Drill 15-2 Using CPAP

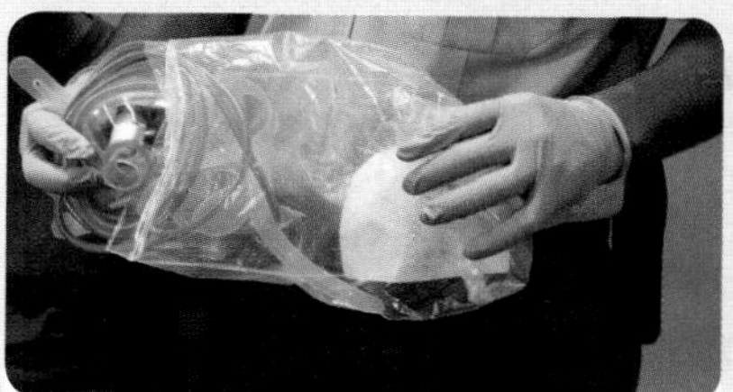

Step 1 Take standard precautions. Assess the patient for indications and contraindications of CPAP. Confirm the patient's blood pressure, and explain the procedure to him or her. Check your equipment, then connect the circuit to the CPAP device.

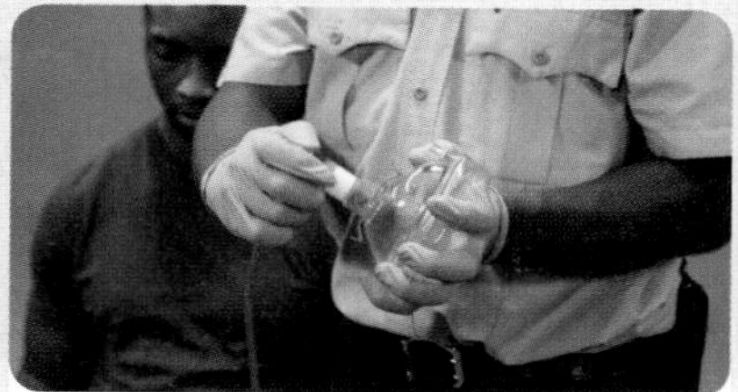

Step 2 Connect the face mask to the circuit tubing. After the system is connected, look for an on/off button or switch. Some models have this feature. Confirm the device is powered on and working before you apply CPAP to the patient.

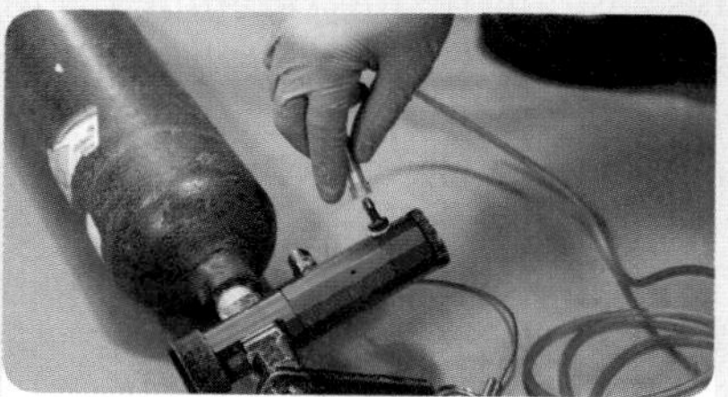

Step 3 Connect the tubing to the oxygen tank.

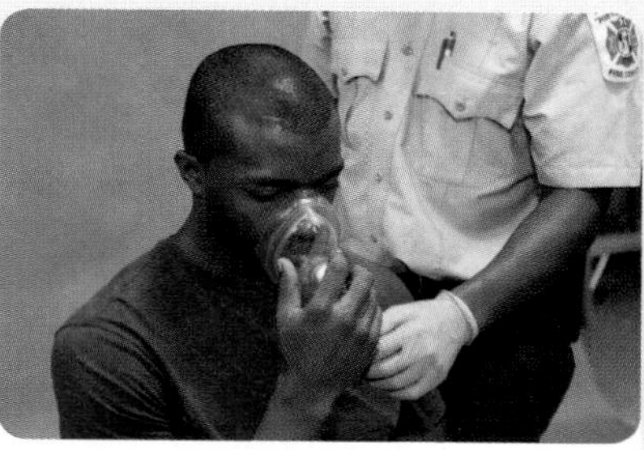

Step 4 Place the mask over the patient's mouth and nose, creating as much of an airtight seal as possible. Place the patient in a high Fowler position to facilitate breathing, and coach him or her through the initial application of the mask. To reduce some of the stress and anxiety associated with the application of CPAP, it may be beneficial to initially allow the patient to hold the mask to his or her face. Allow the patient to get used to the mask.

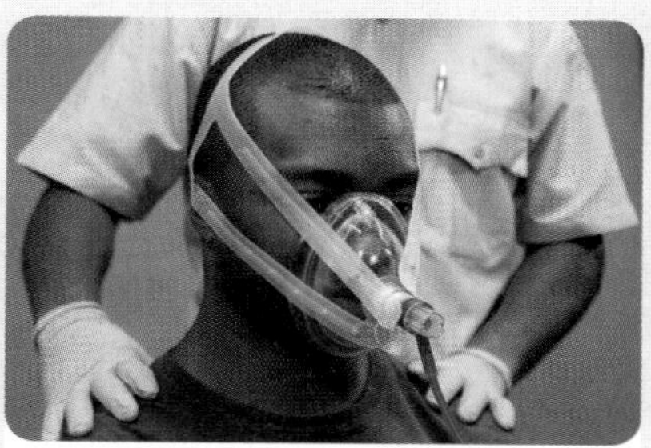

Step 5 After the mask is placed on the face and the patient adjusts to it, use the strapping mechanism to secure it to the patient's head. Ensure the seal between the mask and face remains intact. Consult the manufacturer's guidelines for specific strapping instructions.

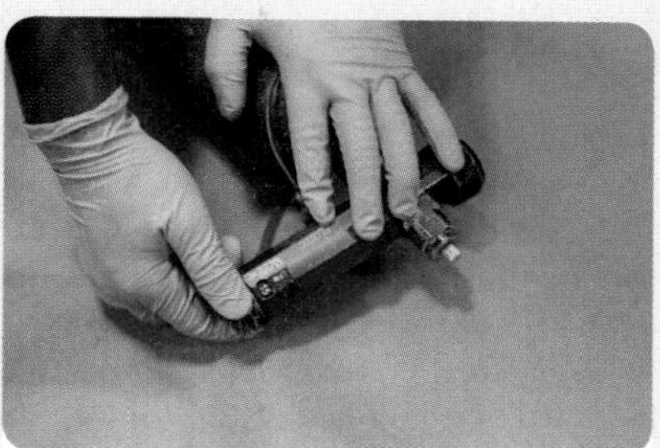

Step 6 Adjust the PEEP valve and the FIO_2 level according to the manufacturer's recommendations to maintain adequate oxygenation and ventilation. With CPAP in place, the patient's oxygenation saturation level should improve, the work of breathing should decrease, the ease of speaking should increase, and breath sounds should improve. Constantly reassess the patient for signs of clinical deterioration and/or complications (ie, pneumothorax).

▶ Complications of CPAP

The application and administration of CPAP is a relatively easy process. However, some patients may find CPAP claustrophobic and will resist the application, and many patients will resist the therapy simply because they are already experiencing respiratory distress. As a patient becomes more hypoxic, the application of the mask to the face is sometimes perceived as suffocation, rather than an attempt to help him or her breathe. In any event, it is important to explain the application to patients and coach them through the process, allowing them to adjust to the situation. Do not force the mask on any patient. Forceful application will create a higher level of anxiety and increase oxygen demand. Coaching patients is not always easy; it takes practice and a willingness to work closely with your patient during a difficult time.

Because of the high volume of pressure generated by CPAP, causing a pneumothorax due to barotrauma is possible. You should be aware of this risk and continually assess your patient for signs and symptoms of a pneumothorax.

In addition to pneumothoraces, increased pressure in the chest cavity can result in hypotension. As the intrathoracic pressure increases, venous blood returning to the heart (preload) meets resistance from the increased pressure in the chest, which can cause hypotension. Although hypotension is uncommon with lower levels of CPAP, it is essential that you continuously monitor the patient's blood pressure.

As with any form of positive pressure ventilation in the unprotected airway, air may enter the stomach, which increases the risk of aspiration if vomiting occurs.

Words of Wisdom

Bilevel positive airway pressure (BPAP), another form of noninvasive positive pressure ventilation, is also used to treat patients with obstructive lung disease, acute bronchospasm, and acute pulmonary edema. Whereas CPAP delivers a single pressure (which is most beneficial to the patient during exhalation), BPAP delivers two pressures—a higher inspiratory positive airway pressure (IPAP), which opens the lower airways, and a lower expiratory positive airway pressure (EPAP), which helps keep the lower airways open. Common BPAP settings deliver 10 cm H_2O during inhalation and 5 cm H_2O during exhalation; the difference between the IPAP and EPAP is called pressure support. The indications, contraindications, and precautions for BPAP are the same as they are for CPAP. Follow your EMS system protocols regarding the use of BPAP and the desired IPAP and EPAP settings.

Gastric Distention

Any form of artificial ventilation that blows air into the patient's mouth—as opposed to blowing air directly into the trachea via an ET tube—may lead to inflation of the patient's stomach with air. Gastric distention—inflation of the patient's stomach with air—is especially likely to occur if excessive pressure is used to inflate the lungs, if ventilations are performed too fast or too forcefully, or if the airway is partially obstructed during ventilation attempts. The pressure in the airway forces open the esophagus, and air flows into the stomach. Gastric distention occurs most often in children but is common in adults as well.

A distended stomach is harmful for at least two reasons. First, it promotes regurgitation of stomach contents, which can lead to aspiration of the stomach contents. Second, a distended stomach pushes the diaphragm upward into the chest, reducing the amount of space in which the lungs can expand.

Signs of gastric distention include an increase in the diameter of the stomach, an increasingly distended abdomen, and increased resistance to bag-mask ventilations. If you observe these signs then reassess and reposition the airway as needed and observe the chest for adequate rise and fall as you continue ventilating. In addition, limit ventilation times to 1 second or the time needed to produce adequate chest rise.

Gastric Decompression

Invasive gastric decompression involves inserting a **gastric tube** into the stomach and removing the contents with suction. The gastric tube is an effective tool for removing air and liquid from the stomach because removal of the stomach contents decreases the pressure on the diaphragm and virtually eliminates the risks of regurgitation and aspiration.

You can insert the gastric tube into the stomach either through the mouth (**orogastric [OG] tube**) or through the nose (**nasogastric [NG] tube**). Consider the use of a gastric tube for any patient who will need positive pressure ventilation for an extended period, especially if the patient is not intubated. You should also insert an NG or OG tube when gastric distention interferes with ventilations—for example, when children are receiving positive pressure ventilation or have swallowed large volumes of air because of increased work of breathing.

Use extreme caution with NG and OG tubes in patients with known esophageal diseases (such as tumors or varices). Never use NG and OG tubes in patients whose esophagi are not patent. After insertion, ensure the tube has been placed into the stomach. Occasionally, the tube may remain in the esophagus without entering the stomach (supragastric placement) or it may have been placed into the trachea.

Nasogastric Tube

An NG tube is inserted through the nose, into the nasopharynx, through the esophagus, and into the stomach **Figure 15-56**. In airway management and ventilation, it decompresses the stomach, thereby decreasing pressure on the diaphragm and limiting the risk of regurgitation.

The NG tube is relatively well tolerated, even by patients who are responsive. Patients can still talk with an NG tube in place, and, after a few hours, most patients get used to it. For these reasons, the NG route of insertion is generally preferred for responsive patients.

During the insertion of an NG tube, most patients who are responsive will gag and may vomit, even if their gag reflexes are suppressed. In a patient with a decreased LOC, vomiting can seriously threaten the airway.

Insertion of an NG tube in patients with severe facial injuries, particularly midface fractures and skull fractures,

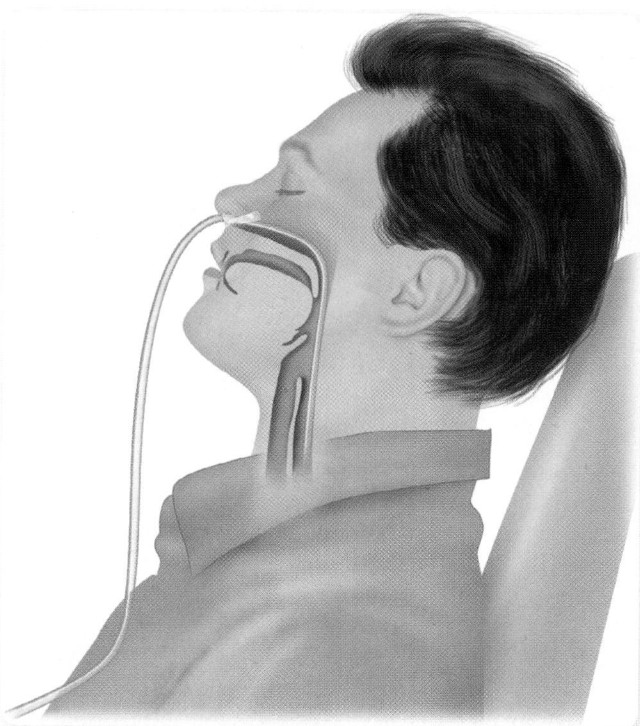

Figure 15-56 Nasogastric tube.

is contraindicated. Although rare, the NG tube may be inadvertently inserted through the fracture and into the cranial vault. For patients with these conditions, use the OG route of insertion.

Improper technique during NG tube insertion can cause trauma to the nasal passageways, esophagus, or gastric lining; therefore, use caution and be gentle when inserting the NG tube.

Use of the NG tube in patients who are not intubated may interfere with the mask seal of the bag-mask device. If you cannot effectively ventilate a patient because of severe gastric distention, however, then you must balance the benefit of gastric decompression against the risk of a poor mask seal and determine which has a higher priority. Of course, if the patient is unresponsive and requires ET intubation, then you can easily pass an ET tube around the NG tube.

The steps of NG tube insertion are shown in Skill Drill 15-3.

Orogastric Tube

An OG tube serves the same purpose as an NG tube, but it is inserted through the mouth instead of the nose Figure 15-57. The advantages and disadvantages of the OG tube are essentially the same as they are for the NG tube. The major differences are that the OG tube carries no risk of nasal bleeding and is safer in patients with severe facial trauma. In addition, you can use larger tubes, which is helpful if the patient requires gastric lavage. Gastric lavage, also called gastric irrigation, is the process of cleaning out the contents of the stomach; it is typically performed in the emergency department for patients with toxic ingestions.

The OG tube, however, is less comfortable for responsive patients, causes gagging much more often, and increases the possibility of vomiting. Responsive patients also

Skill Drill 15-3 Inserting a Nasogastric Tube in a Responsive Patient

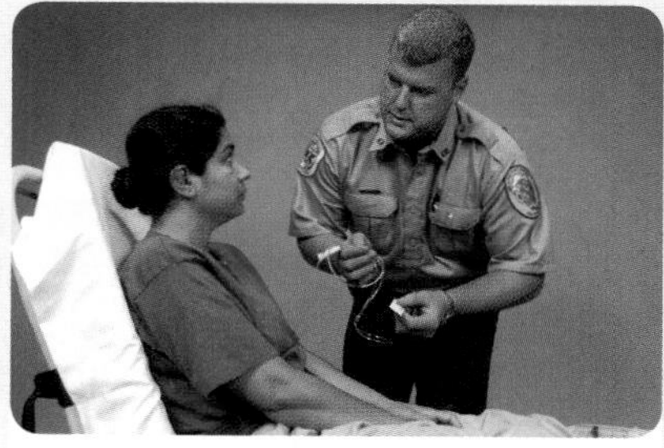

Step 1 Explain the procedure to the patient and oxygenate him or her, if necessary and possible. Ensure the patient's head is in a neutral or slightly flexed position. Suppress the gag reflex with a topical anesthetic spray.

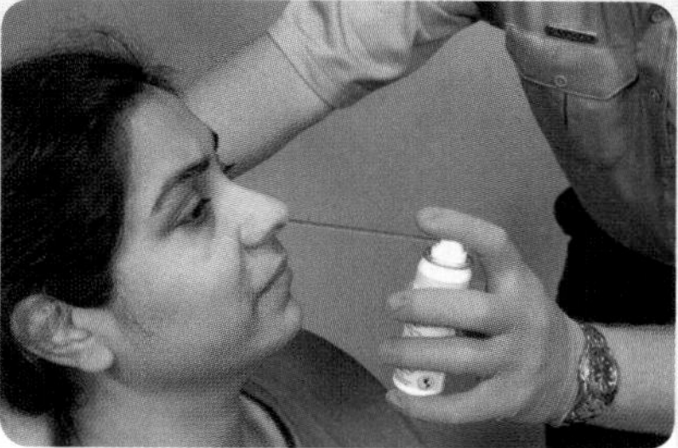

Step 2 Constrict the blood vessels in the nares with a topical alpha-agonist, if available.

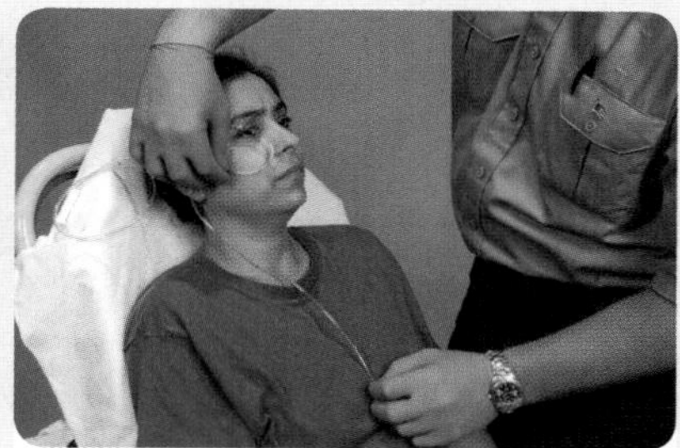

Step 3 Measure the tube for the correct depth of insertion (nose to ear to xiphoid process).

(continued)

Skill Drill 15-3 Inserting a Nasogastric Tube in a Responsive Patient *(continued)*

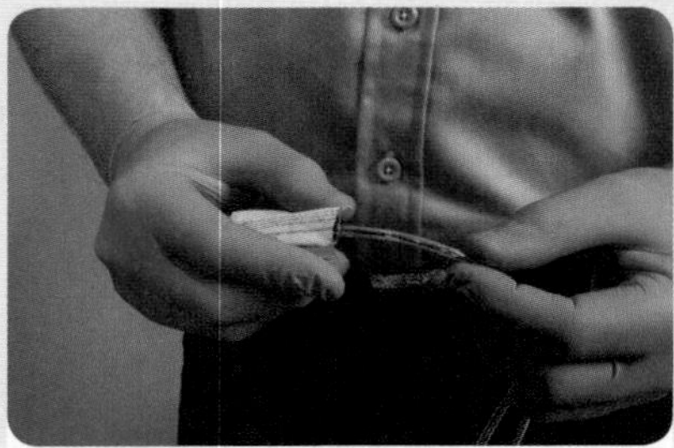

Step 4 Lubricate the tube with a water-soluble gel.

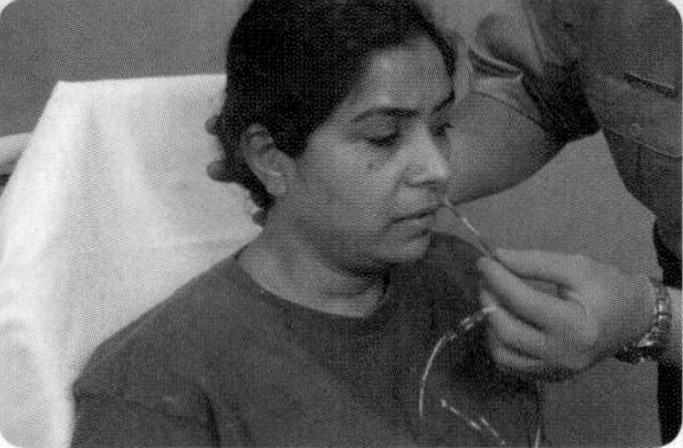

Step 5 Advance the tube gently along the nasal floor.

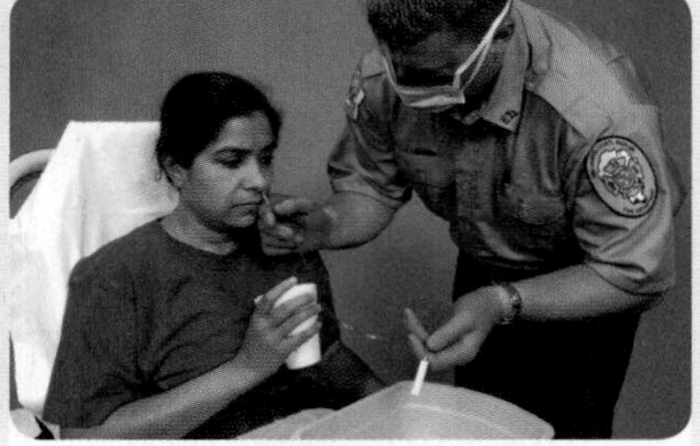

Step 6 Encourage the patient to swallow or drink to facilitate passage of the tube into the esophagus.

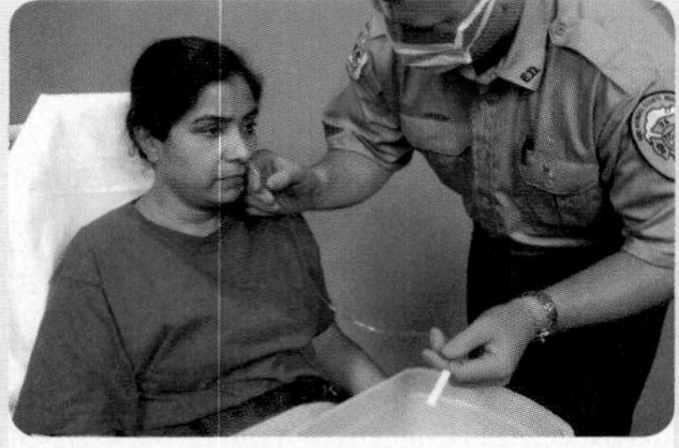

Step 7 Advance the tube into the stomach.

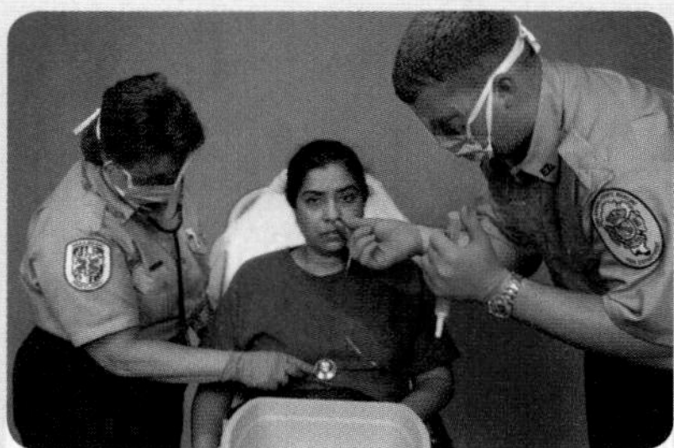

Step 8 Confirm proper placement: Auscultate over the epigastrium while injecting 20 to 30 mL of air into the tube, and/or observe for gastric contents in the tube. There should be no reflux around the tube.

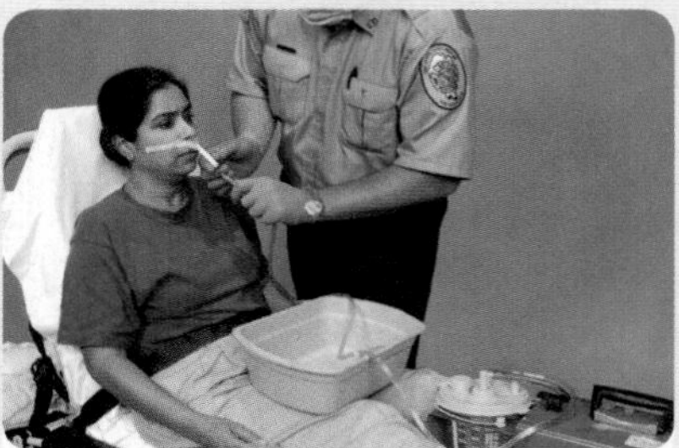

Step 9 Apply suction to the tube to aspirate the stomach contents, and secure the tube in place. The blue extension of the gastric tube should remain open to air.

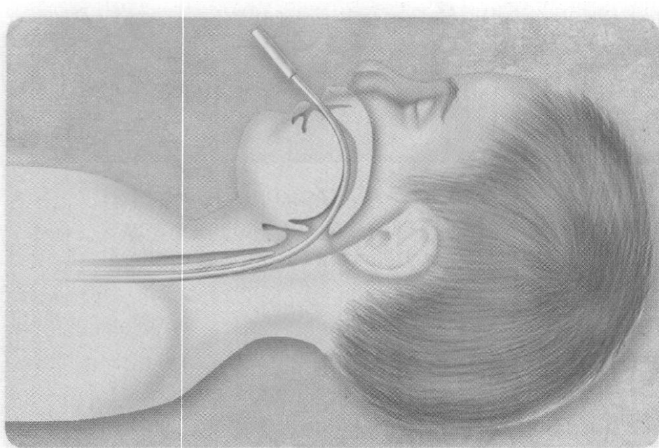

Figure 15-57 Orogastric tube.

tend to bite the tube as it is passed orally. The OG route is generally preferred for patients who are unresponsive without a gag reflex.

The steps of OG tube insertion are shown in Skill Drill 15-4.

Words of Wisdom

After you insert an advanced airway device, consider inserting a gastric tube (orally or nasally) if no contra-indications exist. Doing so will maximize your ability to ventilate the patient by removing air that may have entered the stomach from bag-mask ventilation that occurred before you inserted the advanced airway device.

Skill Drill 15-4 Inserting an Orogastric Tube in an Unresponsive Patient

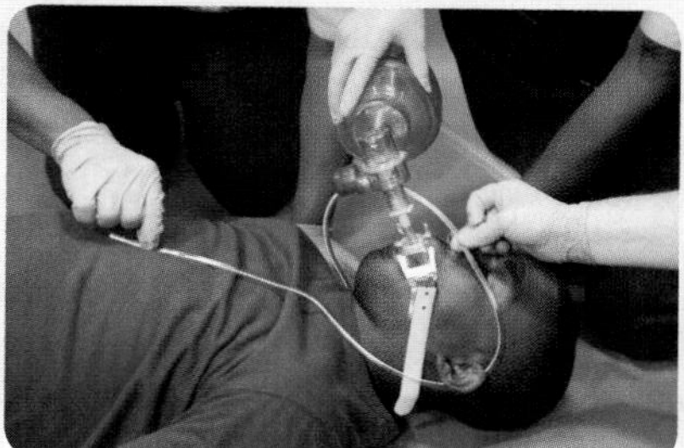

Step 1 Position the patient's head in a neutral or slightly flexed position. Measure the tube for the correct depth of insertion (mouth to ear to xiphoid process).

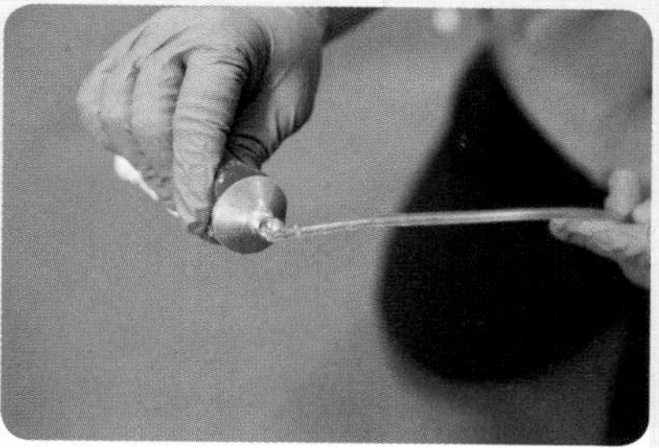

Step 2 Lubricate the tube with a water-soluble gel.

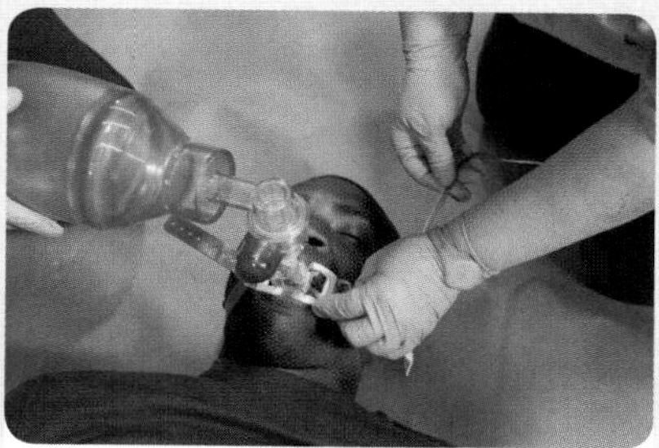

Step 3 Introduce the tube at the midline, and advance it gently into the oropharynx. Advance the tube into the stomach.

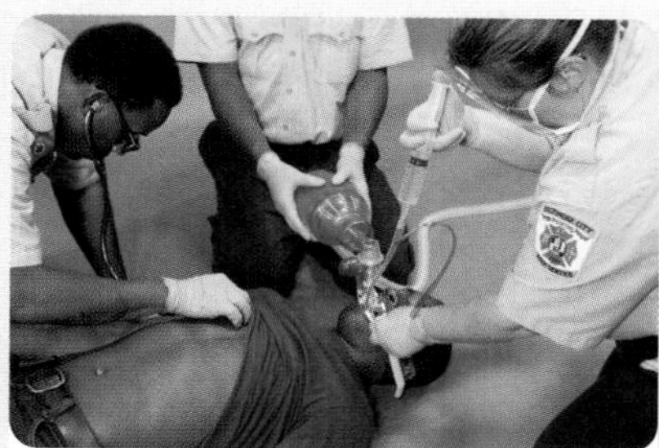

Step 4 Confirm proper placement: Auscultate over the epigastrium while injecting 20 to 30 mL of air and/or observe for gastric contents in the tube. There should be no reflux around the tube. Afterwards, auscultate over the lung fields to confirm the ET tube has not been dislodged.

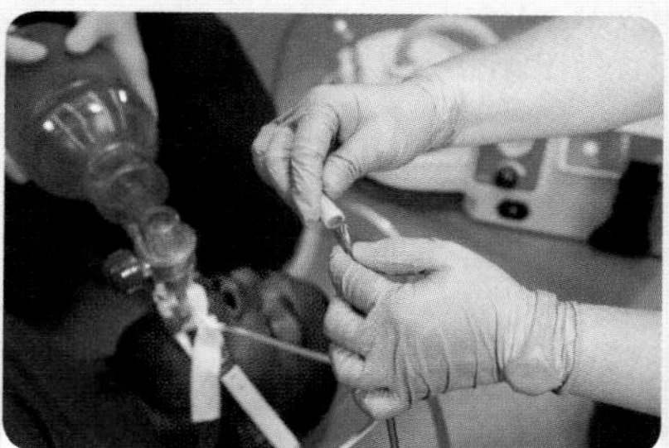

Step 5 Apply suction to the tube to aspirate the stomach contents.

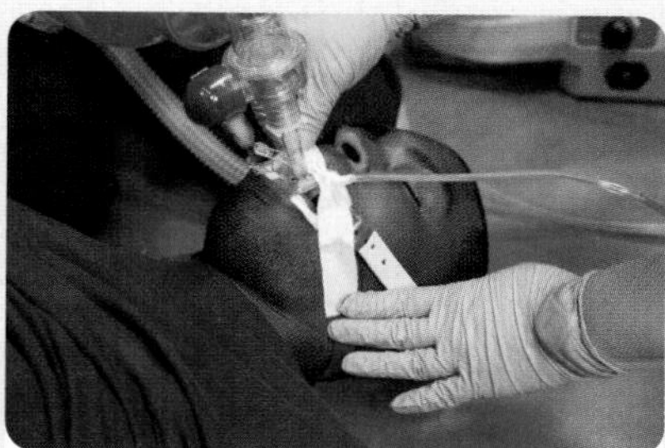

Step 6 Secure the tube in place.

Special Patient Considerations

Laryngectomy, Tracheostomy, Stoma, and Tracheostomy Tubes

A **laryngectomy** is a surgical procedure in which the larynx is removed. This procedure is performed by making a **tracheostomy** (surgical opening into the trachea), thus creating a **stoma**, an orifice that connects the trachea to the outside air. The tracheal stoma is located in the midline of the anterior part of the neck. Surgical removal of the entire larynx is called **total laryngectomy**. A person who has had this procedure is sometimes known as a laryngectomee, or neck breather—he or she breathes through the stoma in his or her neck. Because a connection no longer exists between the patient's pharynx and lower airway, you cannot ventilate the patient through the nose and mouth with a bag-mask device or other face mask. The air blown into the mouth or nose can only go down the esophagus into the stomach; it will not reach the lower airway.

A **partial laryngectomy** entails surgical removal of a portion of the larynx. People who have had this procedure are called partial neck breathers—they breathe through the stoma and the nose or mouth. In practice, you may be unable to tell whether a person has had a total or partial laryngectomy until you attempt artificial ventilation.

Suctioning of a Stoma

You may encounter patients who require suctioning of thick secretions from the stoma. Failure to recognize and identify this need could result in hypoxia. It is not uncommon for a patient's stoma to become occluded with mucous plugs. Patients with a laryngectomy have a less efficient cough and, therefore, have difficulty spontaneously clearing the stoma.

You must perform suctioning of the patient's stoma with extreme care, especially if you suspect laryngeal swelling. Even the slightest irritation of the tracheal wall can result in a violent laryngospasm and complete airway closure. Limit suctioning of the stoma to 10 seconds at a time.

The steps for suctioning a stoma are shown in Skill Drill 15-5.

Ventilation of Stoma Patients

Neither the head tilt–chin lift nor the jaw-thrust maneuver is required for ventilating a patient with a stoma. If the patient has a stoma and no tracheostomy tube (discussed next) in place, then you can perform ventilations using the mouth-to-stoma (with a resuscitation mask) technique or with a bag-mask device. Regardless of the technique used, you should use an infant- or child-sized mask to make an adequate seal over the stoma. Seal the patient's nose and mouth with one hand to prevent the leakage of air up the trachea. Release the seal of the patient's mouth and nose following each ventilation, allowing exhalation to occur through the upper airway. Two rescuers are needed to perform bag-mask device-to-stoma ventilations: one to seal the nose and mouth and the other to squeeze the bag-mask device. If you are unable to ventilate a patient who has a stoma, then try suctioning the stoma and mouth with a soft-tip (French) catheter before providing artificial ventilation through the nose and mouth. Note that this technique would only work if the patient had a partial laryngectomy, not if he or she had a total laryngectomy. If you seal the stoma during ventilation, then the ability to artificially ventilate the patient in this way may be improved, or it may help to clear any obstructions.

YOU are the Paramedic — PART 6

During transport, you observe a marked increase in the patient's heart rate and blood pressure. The patient does not respond to verbal stimuli, but he clenches his fists when you apply a painful stimulus. Normal capnographic waveforms are observed on the cardiac monitor/defibrillator, and no spontaneous respiratory effort is noted. You connect the patient to the ATV and set the rate and tidal volume accordingly.

Recording Time: 25 Minutes	
Level of consciousness	Responsive to painful stimuli
Respirations	20 breaths/min via positive pressure ventilation
Pulse	130 beats/min; strong and regular
Skin	Skin is pink and slightly moist
Blood pressure	164/92 mm Hg
Oxygen saturation (Spo_2)	98% (with positive pressure ventilation and supplemental oxygen)
$ETCO_2$	32 mm Hg
ECG	Sinus tachycardia

10. What is the most likely explanation for the increase in the patient's heart rate and blood pressure? Is additional treatment necessary?

Skill Drill 15-5 Suctioning of a Stoma

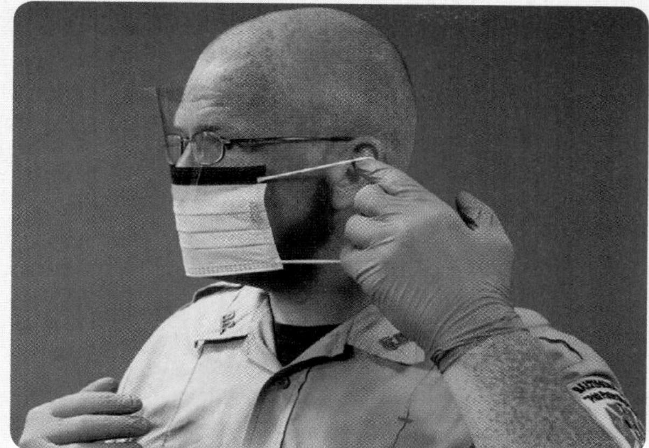

Step 1 Take standard precautions.

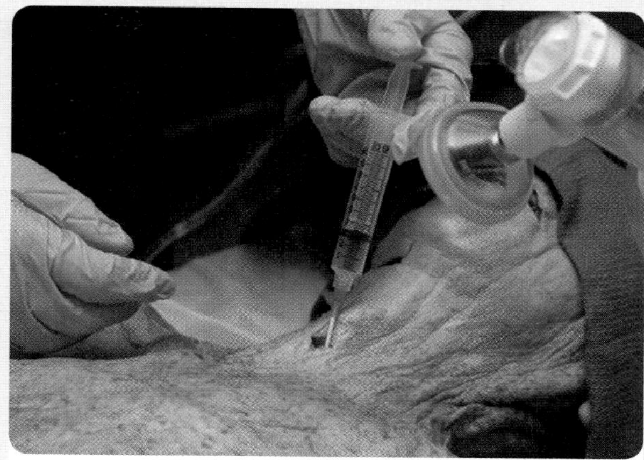

Step 2 Inject 3 mL of sterile saline through the stoma and into the trachea.

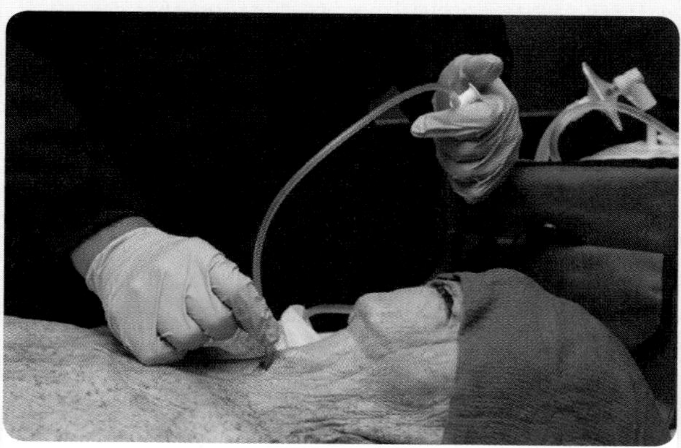

Step 3 Instruct the patient to exhale (if he or she is responsive), and insert the catheter without providing suction until resistance is felt (no more than 12 cm).

Step 4 Suction while withdrawing the catheter.

The steps for performing mouth-to-stoma ventilation with a resuscitation mask are shown in Skill Drill 15-6.

The steps for performing bag-mask device-to-stoma ventilation are shown in Skill Drill 15-7.

Tracheostomy Tubes

A **tracheostomy tube** is a plastic tube placed within the tracheostomy site (stoma) Figure 15-58. It requires a 15/22-mm adapter to be compatible with ventilatory devices, such as a mechanical ventilator or bag-mask device. Patients with a tracheostomy tube may receive supplemental oxygen via tubing designed to fit over the tube or by placing an oxygen mask over the tube. Ventilation is accomplished by simply attaching the bag-mask device to the 15-mm adaptor on the tracheostomy tube.

Patients with a tracheostomy tube who experience sudden dyspnea often have thick secretions in the tube. In this case, perform suctioning through the tracheostomy tube as you would through a stoma.

When a tracheostomy tube becomes dislodged, **stenosis** (narrowing) of the stoma may occur. Stenosis is potentially life-threatening because soft-tissue swelling decreases the diameter of the stoma and impairs the patient's ventilatory ability. In such cases, you may be unable to replace the tracheostomy tube itself and may have to insert an ET tube into the stoma before it becomes totally occluded. Because a patient with a stoma already

Skill Drill 15-6 Ventilating Through a Stoma Using a Resuscitation Mask

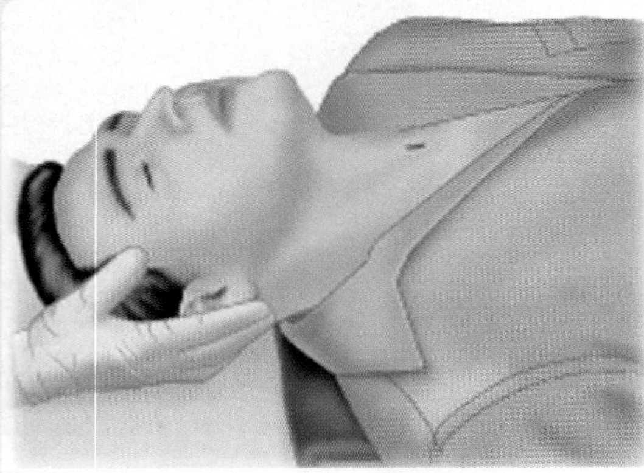

Step 1 Position the patient's head in a neutral position with the shoulders slightly elevated.

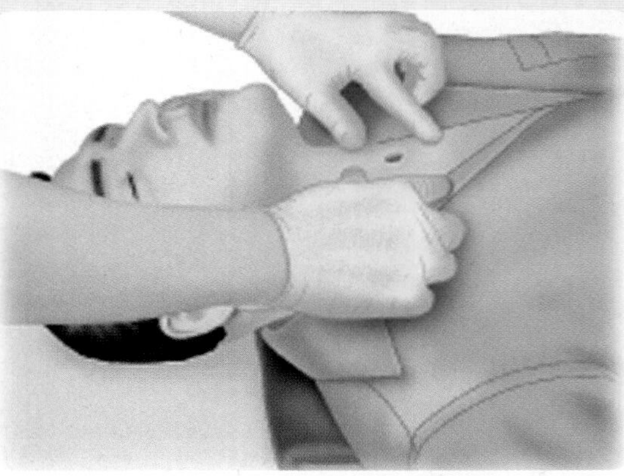

Step 2 Locate and expose the stoma site.

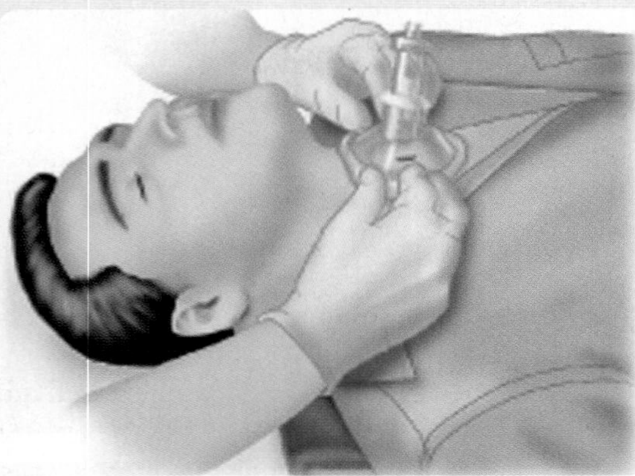

Step 3 Place the resuscitation mask over the stoma, and ensure an adequate seal. For best results, use a pediatric mask.

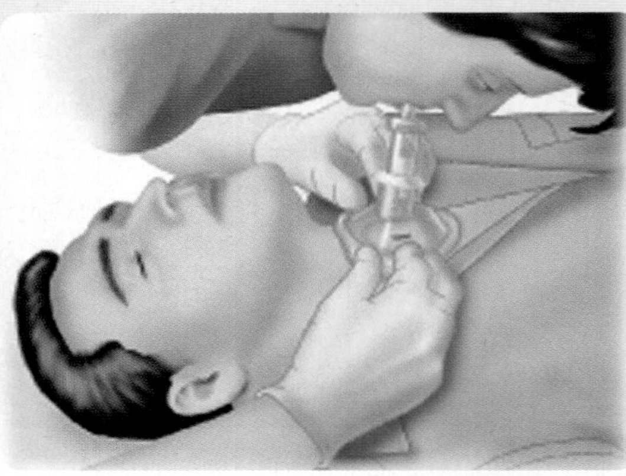

Step 4 Maintain the patient's neutral head position, and ventilate the patient by exhaling directly into the resuscitation mask. Assess the patient for adequate ventilation by observing his or her chest rise and feeling for air leaks around the mask.

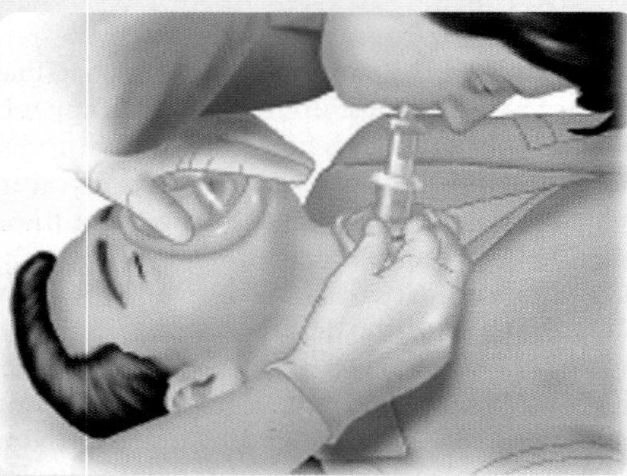

Step 5 If air leakage is evident, then seal the patient's mouth and nose and ventilate.

Skill Drill 15-7 Ventilating a Stoma With a Bag-Mask Device

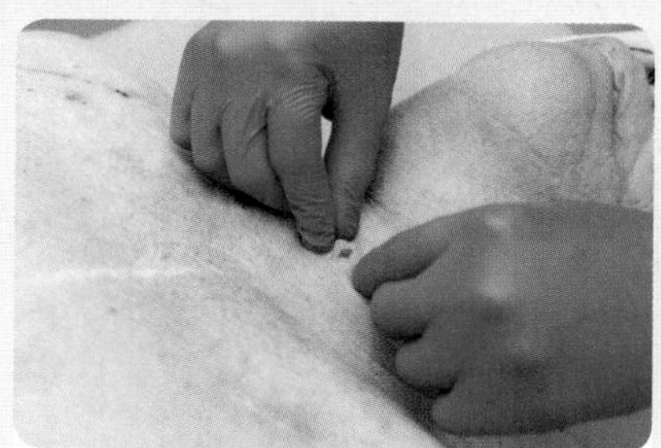

Step 1 With the patient's head in a neutral position, locate and expose the stoma.

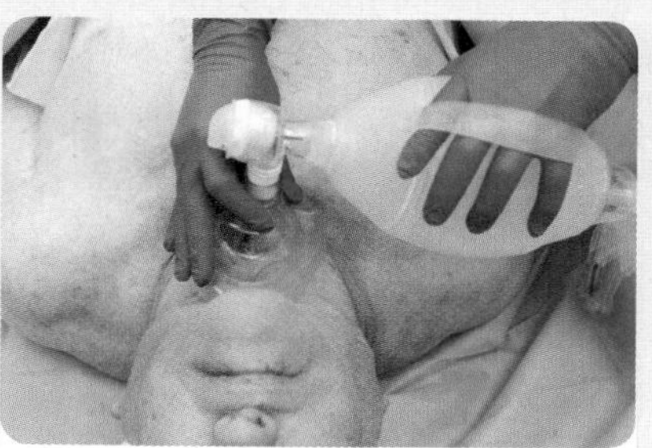

Step 2 Place the bag-mask device (with a pediatric mask) over the stoma, and ensure an adequate seal. Ventilate the patient by squeezing the bag-mask device, and assess for adequate ventilation by observing chest rise and feeling for air leaks when using a mask. Seal the mouth and nose if an air leak is evident from the upper airway.

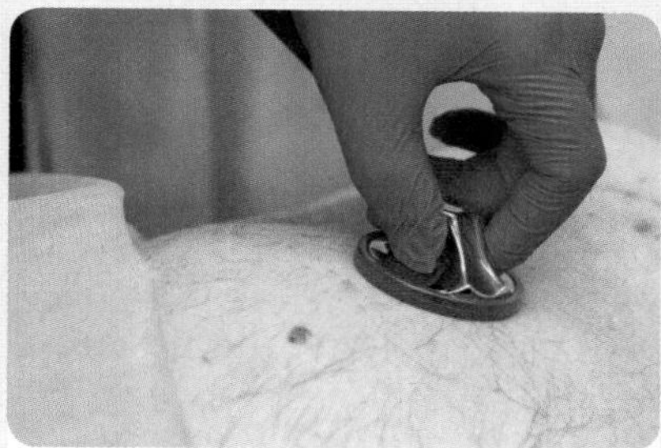

Step 3 Auscultate over the lungs to confirm adequate ventilation.

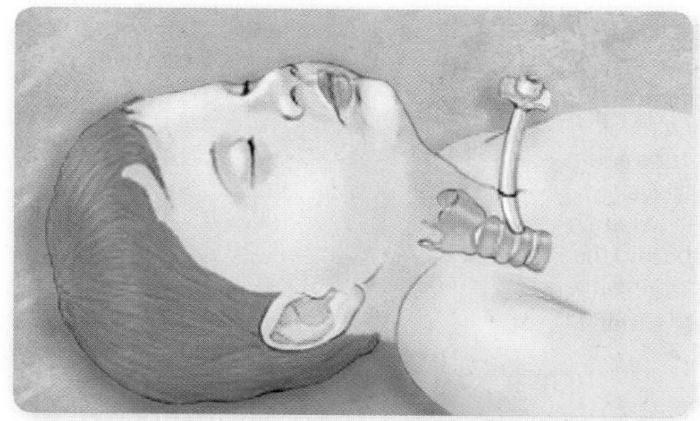

Figure 15-58 A tracheostomy tube.

has a significant medical injury or illness (such as brain injury, chronic respiratory insufficiency), he or she may be less tolerant of even brief periods of hypoxia.

The steps for replacing a dislodged tracheostomy tube are shown in Skill Drill 15-8.

▶ Dental Appliances

Dental appliances, which are frequently encountered in the geriatric population, can take many different forms: dentures (upper, lower, or both), bridges, individual teeth, and braces (in the younger population). When you assess the airway of a patient with a dental appliance, especially one who is unresponsive, you must determine whether the appliance is either loose or fitting well. If the dental appliance fits well, then leave it in place. A well-fitting appliance helps to maintain the structure of the face, facilitating an effective mask-to-face seal if the patient requires mouth-to-mask or bag-mask ventilation. If the appliance is loose, however, then it could easily become an airway obstruction and you should remove it.

If an unresponsive patient has an airway obstruction caused by a dental appliance, then perform the usual steps in clearing an obstruction, such as chest compressions, direct laryngoscopy, and use of the Magill forceps. If the obstruction is caused by a bridge, then you must take great care when clearing the obstruction; these devices often contain sharp metal ends that can easily lacerate the posterior pharynx or larynx.

Often it is not the dental appliance itself that hinders your ability to manage a patient's airway, but rather attempts to identify and remove the device. Do not become overly concerned with the presence of the dental appliance; instead, concentrate on managing the airway. In addition, the oropharyngeal anatomy may be somewhat distorted by the presence of a dental appliance.

Skill Drill 15-8 Replacing a Dislodged Tracheostomy Tube With a Temporary ET Tube

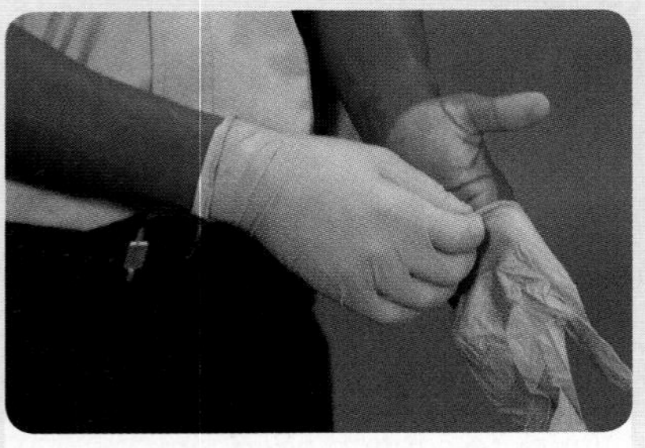

Step 1 Take standard precautions. Assemble the equipment.

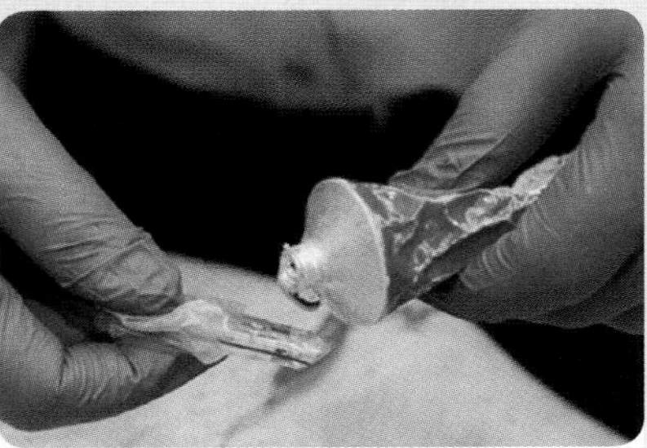

Step 2 Lubricate the same-sized tracheostomy tube or an ET tube (at least 5.0 mm) with a water-soluble gel.

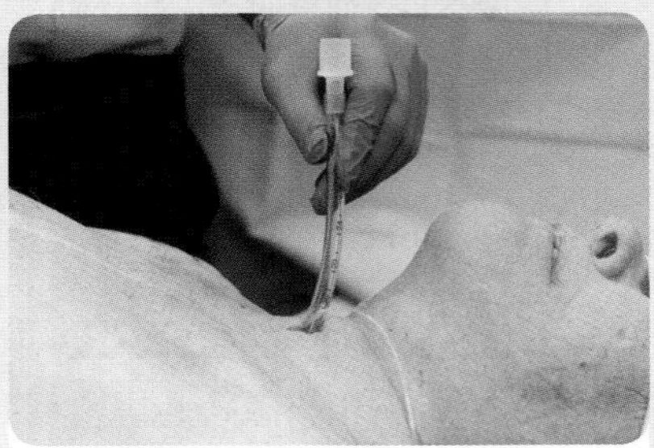

Step 3 Instruct the patient to exhale, and gently insert the tube approximately 0.5 to 0.75 inch (1 to 2 cm) beyond the balloon cuff.

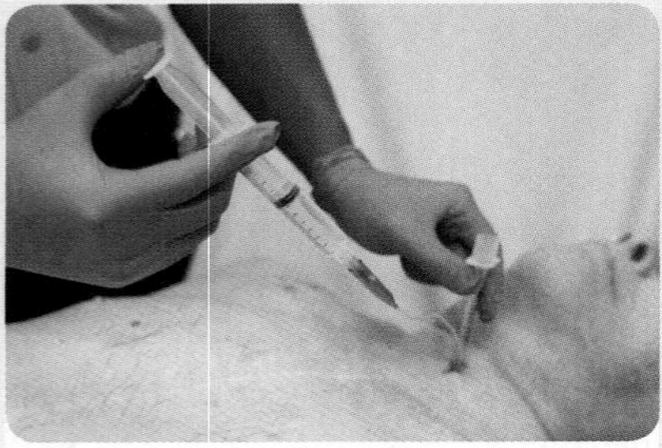

Step 4 Inflate the balloon cuff.

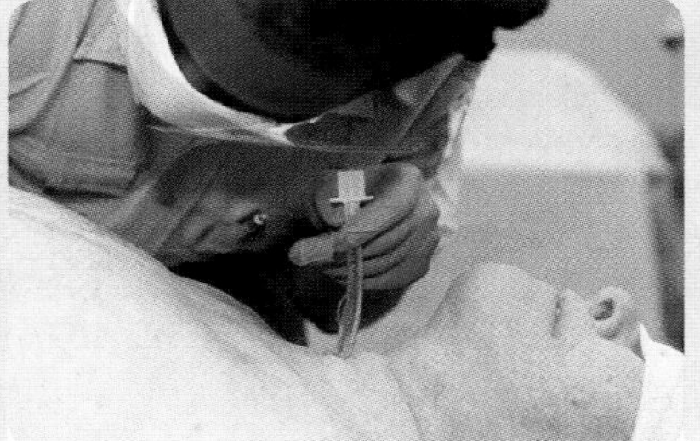

Step 5 Ensure the patient is comfortable, and confirm patency and proper placement of the tube by listening for air movement from the tube and noting the patient's clinical status. Ensure that a false lumen (placement of the tube into the soft tissue of the neck, rather than in the trachea) was not created.

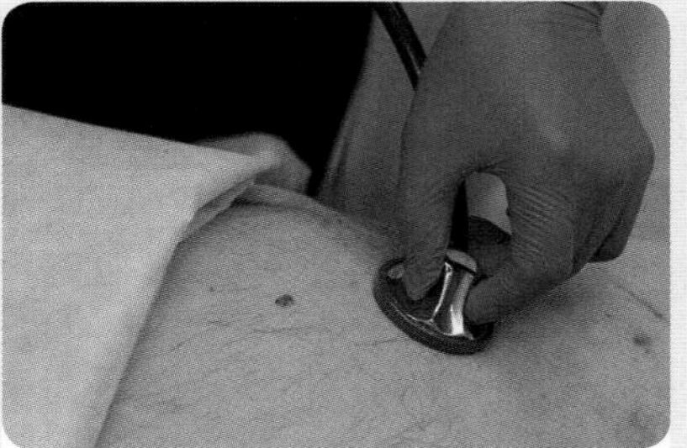

Step 6 Auscultate the lungs to confirm correct tube placement.

In general, it is best to remove dental appliances before intubating a patient. After the ET tube is in place and has been secured, removal of the dental appliance will be extremely difficult and dangerous because it may cause dislodgement of the tube or inflict unnecessary oropharyngeal trauma.

▶ Facial Trauma

It can be especially challenging to effectively manage the airway of a patient with facial injuries Figure 15-59. Because the face is highly vascular, facial trauma can result in severe tissue swelling and bleeding into the airway. Control bleeding with direct pressure, and suction the airway as needed. You may encounter a patient with severe facial trauma who is breathing inadequately and has severe oropharyngeal bleeding—both problems are life-threatening. In this situation, you must suction the airway until it is clear and then ventilate the patient. Remember, ventilating a patient whose airway is full of blood virtually assures aspiration. If you cannot control the source of the oropharyngeal bleeding, then perform continuous suctioning and intubate the trachea.

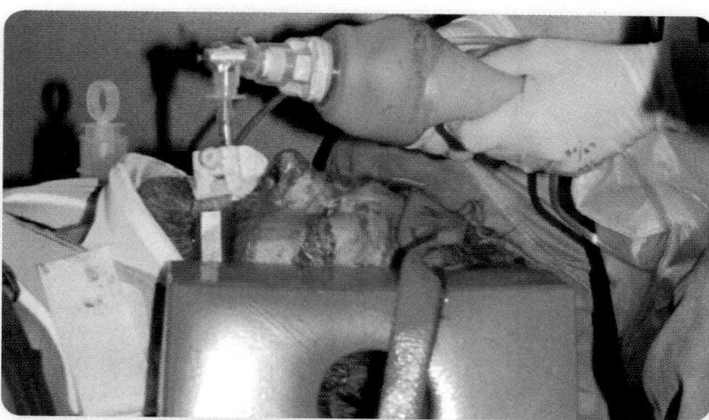

Figure 15-59 Airway management can be especially challenging in patients with facial injuries.

Facial injuries should also increase your index of suspicion for a cervical spine injury. Therefore, when managing the airway, use the jaw-thrust maneuver and keep the patient's head in a neutral, in-line position. ET intubation of a trauma patient is most effectively performed by two paramedics—one who maintains neutral, in-line stabilization of the patient's head and the other who performs the intubation. An alternative technique, especially if you are the only paramedic managing the patient's airway, is to stabilize the patient's head in a neutral, in-line position with your thighs and then perform the intubation.

While you are ventilating a patient with facial injuries, stay alert for changes in ventilation compliance or sounds that may indicate laryngeal edema (such as stridor). If you are unable to effectively ventilate or orally intubate a patient with severe facial injuries, then perform a cricothyrotomy (either surgical or needle). Advanced airway management techniques, including ET intubation, multilumen and supraglottic airway devices, and needle and surgical cricothyrotomy are discussed next.

Advanced Airway Management

One of the most common mistakes in the situation of respiratory or cardiac arrest is to proceed with advanced airway management too early, forsaking the basic techniques of establishing and maintaining a patent airway in a patient who is already hypoxic. Never abandon the basics of airway management—do not immediately proceed with advanced techniques simply because you can.

After establishing and maintaining a patent airway with basic techniques and maneuvers, you should consider advanced airway management. Patients primarily require advanced airway management for two reasons: (1) failure to maintain a patent airway and/or (2) failure to adequately oxygenate and ventilate. Advanced airway management involves the insertion of a number of advanced airway devices that are designed to facilitate adequate oxygenation and ventilation. The remainder of the chapter discusses and illustrates the following advanced airway devices and techniques:

- ET tube
  - Orotracheal intubation
    - Direct laryngoscopy
    - Video laryngoscopy
  - Blind nasotracheal intubation
  - Digital intubation
  - Intubation via transillumination
  - Face-to-face intubation
  - Retrograde intubation
- King LT airway
- Laryngeal mask airway
- i-gel
- Esophageal tracheal Combitube
- Surgical and needle cricothyrotomy

Predicting the Difficult Airway

As a paramedic, you must decide how to accomplish airway management. Ask yourself, "Can I manage this airway with BLS techniques? Can I intubate this patient's trachea?" This section discusses the factors to consider when caring for a patient who has a difficult airway.

History is one factor. Anatomic findings suggestive of a difficult airway may include congenital abnormalities (ie, dysmorphic face), recent operations, trauma, infection, or neoplastic diseases (such as cancer).

A commonly used mnemonic to guide assessment of the difficult airway is LEMON, which stands for:

Look externally
Evaluate 3-3-2
Mallampati classification
Obstruction
Neck mobility

As indicated by the *L* in the mnemonic, simply looking at the patient may indicate the relative difficulty that may be encountered in airway management. Patients with short, thick necks may be difficult to intubate. Morbid obesity significantly complicates intubation. Dental conditions, such as an overbite or "buck" (protruding) teeth, may make intubation difficult.

The *E* stands for Evaluate 3-3-2. Three anatomic measurements are assessed using the **3-3-2 rule** Figure 15-60. The first *3* refers to mouth opening. Ideally, a patient's mouth should open at least three fingerbreadths (approximately 2 inches [5 cm]). A width of less than three fingerbreadths indicates a potentially difficult airway. (Of course, if the patient can open his or her mouth on command, then you should reconsider your decision to intubate.) The second *3* refers to the length of the mandible. At least three fingerbreadths is optimal. This length is measured from the tip of the chin to the hyoid bone. Patients with smaller mandibles have less room for displacement of the tongue and epiglottis and can make airway management more difficult. Finally, the *2* refers to

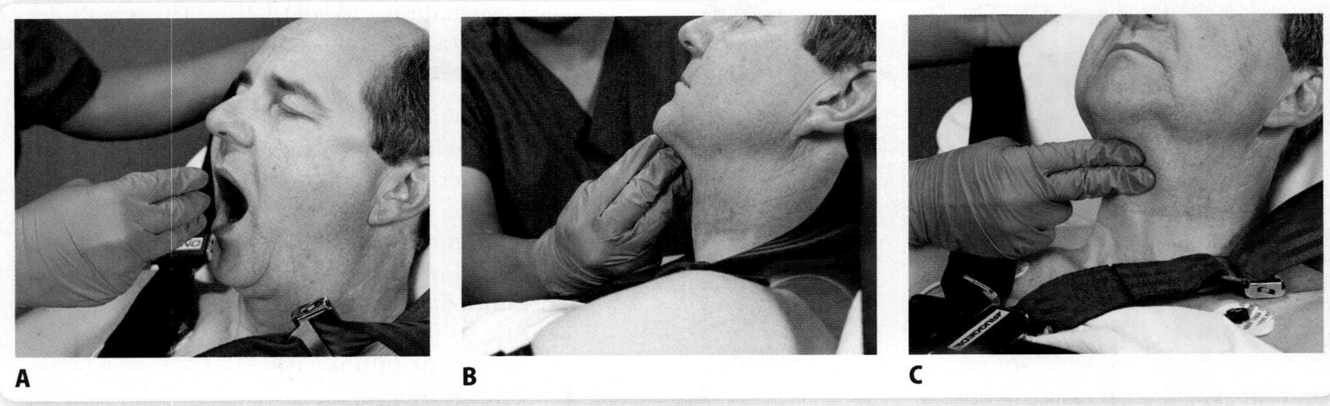

Figure 15-60 The 3-3-2 rule. **A.** The mouth should be at least three fingerbreadths wide when open. **B.** The space from the chin to the hyoid bone should be at least three fingerbreadths wide. **C.** The distance from the hyoid bone to the thyroid notch should be at least two fingerbreadths wide.

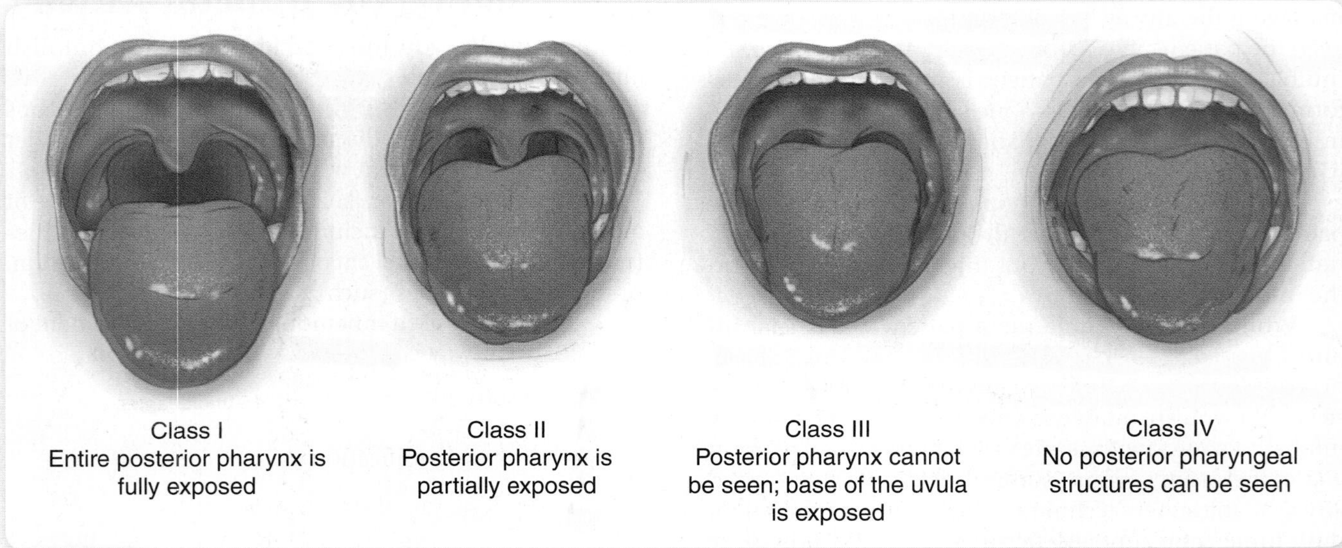

Figure 15-61 Mallampati classification.

the distance from the hyoid bone to the thyroid notch; it should be at least two fingerbreadths wide.

The *M* stands for Mallampati classification. An anesthesiologist, Mallampati, developed the **Mallampati classification** to predict the relative difficulty of intubation **Figure 15-61**. This classification notes the oropharyngeal structures visible in an upright, seated patient who is fully able to open his or her mouth. Although this evaluation is an accurate predictor of intubation difficulty, it is of limited value in unresponsive patients and in patients who cannot follow commands. *If a patient is cooperative and able to comply with this evaluation, then emergency prehospital intubation is probably not indicated.* However, the evaluation is important because it can provide useful information should intubation become necessary.

Compared with the Mallampati classification, the **Cormack-Lehane classification** has more applicability in an emergent setting because it classifies views obtained by direct laryngoscopy based on the structures seen **Figure 15-62**.

The *O* stands for obstruction. Make note of anything that might interfere with visualization or ET tube placement. Foreign body, obesity, hematoma, and masses are all examples of situations that can create a difficult airway.

Finally, the *N* stands for neck mobility. The ideal position for visualization and intubation is the sniffing (tripod) position. Neck mobility problems are most commonly associated with trauma patients (due to cervical collars or injury) and older patients (due to osteoporosis or arthritis). The inability to place the patient in the sniffing position can significantly reduce your ability to visualize the airway.

Cormack-Lehane Class	Class 1: Full view of glottis	Class 2: Partial view of glottis or arytenoids **Modified system:** *Class 2a:* Partial view of the glottis *Class 2b:* Arytenoids or posterior part of the vocal cords only just visible	Class 3: Only epiglottis is visible	Class 4: Neither glottis nor epiglottis is visible
Laryngoscopic view	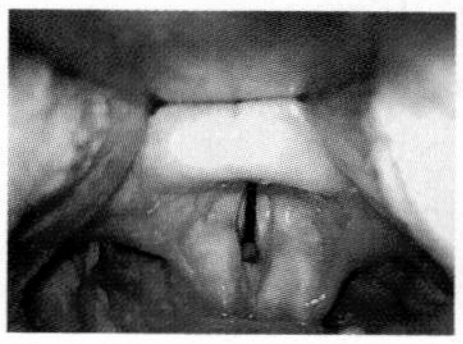 A	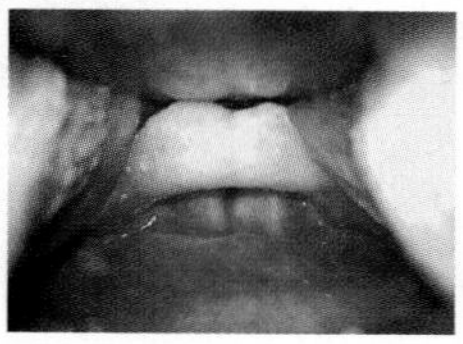 B	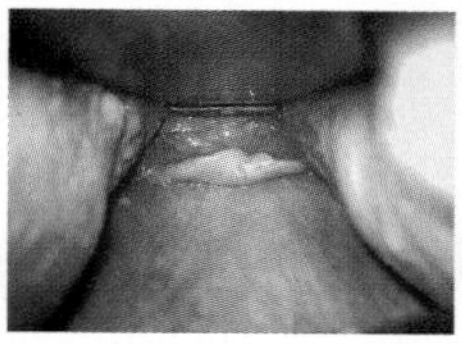 C	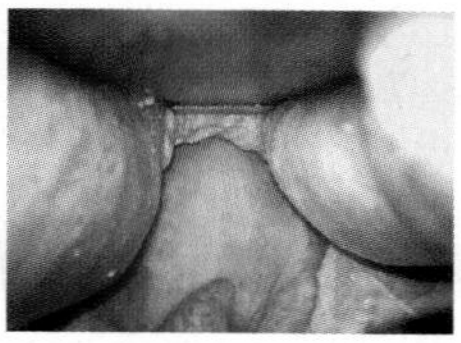 D

Figure 15-62 Cormack-Lehane classification. **A.** Full view of the epiglottis, arytenoid cartilage, and vocal cords (Class 1). **B.** The epiglottis is in full view, but only a portion of the glottis or arytenoid cartilage can be seen (Class 2). **C.** Only the epiglottis can be seen. Neither the glottis nor the arytenoid cartilage is visible (Class 3). **D.** Neither the epiglottis nor the glottis is visible (Class 4).

▶ Endotracheal Intubation

Endotracheal (ET) intubation is defined as passing an ET tube through the glottic opening and sealing the tube with a cuff inflated against the tracheal wall. When the tube is passed into the trachea through the mouth, the procedure is called **orotracheal intubation**. When the tube is passed into the trachea through the nose, the procedure is called **nasotracheal intubation**.

Intubation of the trachea is the most definitive means of achieving complete control of the airway. You need a solid understanding of the basics of this technique when making urgent decisions about when to intubate a patient. Consider the following points when performing ET intubation:

- **Advantages.** Provision of a secure airway and protection against aspiration
- **Disadvantages.** Special equipment required; physiologic functions of the upper airway (warming, filtering, humidifying) bypassed
- **Complications.** Bleeding; hypoxia; laryngeal swelling; laryngospasm; vocal cord damage; mucosal necrosis; and barotrauma

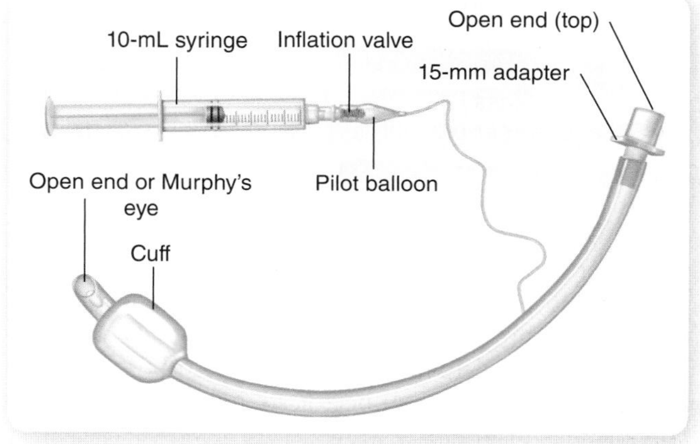

Figure 15-63 Endotracheal tube.

Endotracheal Tubes

The basic structure of an **endotracheal (ET) tube** **Figure 15-63** includes the proximal end, the tube itself, the cuff and pilot balloon, and the distal tip. The proximal end is equipped with a standard 15/22-mm adapter that allows it to be attached to any ventilation device. It also includes an inflation port with a pilot balloon; the distal cuff is inflated with a syringe attached to the inflation port, which has a one-way valve. The pilot balloon indicates whether the distal cuff is inflated or deflated after the tube has been inserted into the mouth.

Centimeter markings along the length of the ET tube provide a measurement of its depth. The distal end of the tube has a beveled tip to facilitate insertion and an

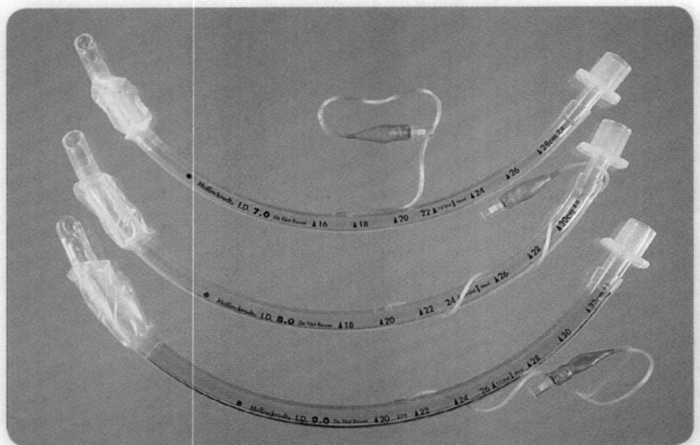

Figure 15-64 Endotracheal tubes are available in a variety of sizes.

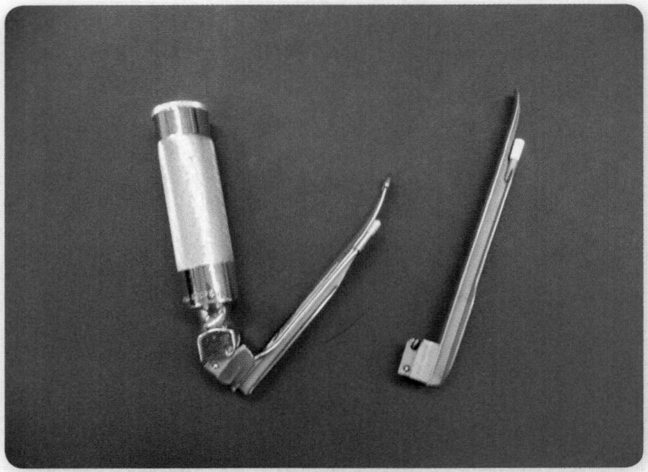

Figure 15-65 A laryngoscope with a straight blade.

opening on the side called the **Murphy eye**, which enables ventilation to occur even if the tip becomes occluded by blood, mucus, or the tracheal wall.

ET tubes range in size from 2.5 to 9.0 mm in inside diameter, and the length ranges from 12 to 32 cm **Figure 15-64**. Sizes ranging from 5.0 to 9.0 mm are equipped with a distal cuff that, when inflated, makes an airtight seal with the tracheal wall. A tube that is too small for the patient will lead to increased resistance to airflow and difficulty in ventilating. A tube that is too large can be difficult to insert and may cause trauma. Usually, a woman will require a 7.0- to 8.0-mm tube, and a man will require a 7.5- to 8.5-mm tube.

The **stylet**, a semirigid wire that is inserted into the ET tube to mold and maintain the shape of the tube, enables you to guide the tip of the tube over the arytenoid cartilage and through the vocal cords. Lubricate this device with a water-soluble gel to facilitate its removal, and bend its end to form a gentle "hockey stick" curve. The end of the stylet should rest at least 0.5 inch (1 cm) back from the end of the ET tube; if the stylet protrudes beyond the end of the tube, then it may damage the vocal cords and surrounding structures. Bend the other end of the stylet over the proximal tube connector, so that the stylet cannot slip farther into the tube.

In pediatric patients, use ET tubes ranging in size from 2.5 to 4.5 mm. In children, the funnel-shaped cricoid ring (the narrowest portion of the pediatric airway) forms an anatomic seal with the ET tube, eliminating the need for a distal cuff in most patients. The proximal end of the tube still has a 15/22-mm adapter for use with standard ventilation devices, and the distal end has a beveled tip with distal end markings. However, because it lacks a balloon cuff, a pilot balloon is not included.

A number of anatomic clues can help determine the proper size of ET tube for adults and children. The internal diameter of the nostril is a good approximation of the diameter of the glottic opening. The diameter of the little finger or the size of the thumbnail is also a good approximation of airway size. Because all attempts to predict the ET tube size required for a given patient are estimates, however, you should always have three ET tubes ready: one tube of the size you think will be appropriate, one a size larger, and one a size smaller.

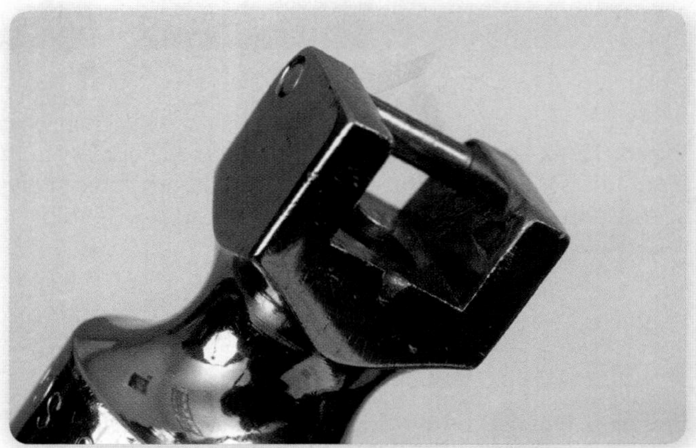

Figure 15-66 The handle of the laryngoscope has a bar designed to connect with a notch on the blade.

Laryngoscopes and Blades

A laryngoscope is required to perform orotracheal intubation by direct laryngoscopy—a procedure in which the vocal cords are directly visualized for placement of the ET tube. The laryngoscope consists of a handle and interchangeable blades **Figure 15-65**. The handle contains the power source for the light on the laryngoscope blade. Most laryngoscopes run on disposable batteries, but some are rechargeable. The handle has a bar designed to connect with a notch on the blade **Figure 15-66**. When the blade is moved into the perpendicular position, the bright light shines near the tip of the blade. Newer laryngoscopes feature a light source within the handle itself, which attaches to a fiberoptic blade.

Laryngoscope blades include the straight (Miller) blade and the curved (Macintosh) blade. The **straight laryngoscope blade** is designed so that its tip will extend beneath the epiglottis and directly lift it up Figure 15-67 —a particularly useful feature in infants and small children, who often have a long, floppy epiglottis that is difficult to elevate out of the way with a curved blade. In an adult, use of a straight blade requires great care; if used improperly and levered across the upper jaw, the straight blade is more likely to damage the patient's teeth. The **curved laryngoscope blade** is less likely to be levered against the teeth by an inexperienced paramedic Figure 15-68 . The direction of the curve conforms to that of the tongue and pharynx, so the blade follows the outline of the pharynx with relative ease. The tip of the curved blade is placed in the vallecula (the space between the epiglottis and the base of the tongue) rather than beneath the epiglottis; it indirectly lifts the epiglottis to expose the vocal cords. Have curved and straight blades readily available during an orotracheal intubation attempt.

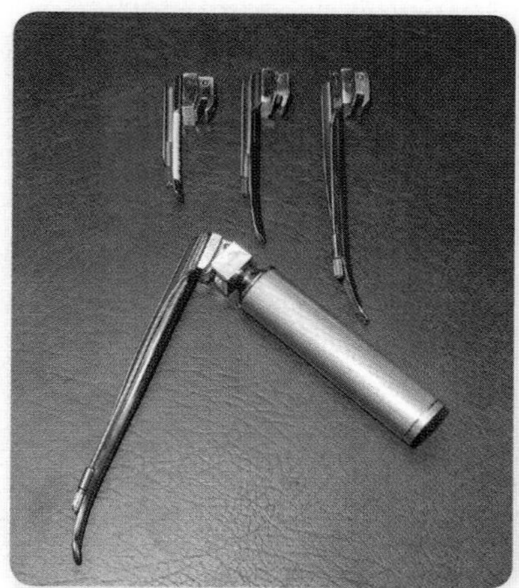

Figure 15-67 A laryngoscope and an assortment of straight (Miller) blades.

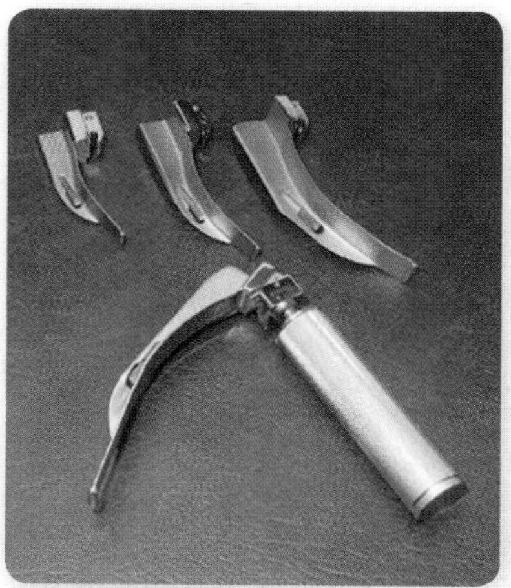

Figure 15-68 A laryngoscope and an assortment of curved (Macintosh) blades.

Blade sizes range from 0 to 4. Sizes 0, 1, and 2 are appropriate for infants and children, whereas 3 and 4 are considered adult sizes. For pediatric patients, blade sizes are often recommended based on the child's age or height. Choose the blade for adults based on your experience and the size of the patient (3 for average-sized adults and 4 for larger people).

▶ Orotracheal Intubation by Direct Laryngoscopy

Orotracheal intubation by direct laryngoscopy involves inserting an ET tube through the mouth and into the trachea while directly visualizing the glottic opening with a laryngoscope. The indications and contraindications for orotracheal intubation include the following:

- Indications
  - Airway control needed as a result of coma, respiratory arrest, and/or cardiac arrest
  - Ventilatory support before impending respiratory failure
  - Prolonged ventilatory support required
  - Absence of a gag reflex
  - Traumatic brain injury
  - Unresponsiveness
  - Impending airway compromise (such as in burns or trauma)
- Contraindications
  - An intact gag reflex
  - Inability to open the patient's mouth because of trauma, dislocation of the jaw, or a pathologic condition
  - Inability to see the glottic opening
  - Copious secretions, vomitus, or blood in the airway

Table 15-12 summarizes the equipment and preparation required before performing orotracheal intubation. Make a copy of this table, and affix it to your intubation kit, so that you can check the kit systematically at the beginning of every shift.

Standard Precautions

Intubation may expose you to blood or other body fluids, so take proper precautions when performing this procedure. In addition to gloves, wear a face shield that covers your entire face, which will be relatively close to the patient's mouth and nose, and that will protect you if the patient vomits or coughs during intubation. If a face shield is unavailable, then wear safety glasses and a mask.

Table 15-12 Preparing Equipment for Intubation

Equipment	What to Check, Prepare, and Assemble
Ventilation equipment	Have your partner ventilate the patient while you are assembling, checking, and preparing your equipment. Ensure the patient is being ventilated with 100% oxygen and the pulse oximeter reading is greater than 95%.
ET tube	Select the proper size tube (7.0–7.5 for women; 7.5–8.5 for men). Inject 10 mL of air into the cuff, and ensure that the cuff holds air. Confirm the 15/22-mm adapter is firmly inserted into the tube. Insert the stylet, and ensure that the tip is proximal to the Murphy eye. Straighten the ET tube completely, and place a slight bend (in the shape of a hockey stick) just proximal to the cuff Figure 15-69. Increase the angle of the bend if the patient's vocal cords are more anterior.
Laryngoscope and blades	Have an assortment of blades (straight and curved) available, because some patients are easier to intubate with one than with the other. Confirm the blade you select is free of nicks, which could easily cause soft-tissue trauma to the upper airway. Check the bulb to ensure that the light is "bright, white, steady, and tight." The light should be bright enough so that it is uncomfortable to look at directly. It should be white, not yellow or dim. The light should not flicker, especially as the blade is moved on the handle. Most important, the bulb must be tightly screwed into the blade to prevent it from being aspirated into the lungs. Newer blades utilize fiberoptics to provide light, in which the light source is located in the laryngoscope handle itself; nonetheless, confirm the batteries have enough power to provide sufficient light.
Towels	You may need towels to properly position the patient's head.
Suction	You may need suction to clear the airway of blood or other secretions to obtain an adequate laryngoscopic view of the glottic opening and vocal cords.
Magill forceps	Have Magill forceps available should you need to guide the ET tube between the vocal cords or if you encounter a foreign body obstruction during laryngoscopy.
Confirmation devices	Stethoscope and an $ETCO_2$ detector (use quantitative capnography to confirm initial and ongoing ET tube placement). Other devices include the colorimetric CO_2 detector and esophageal detector device (bulb or syringe that is attached to the proximal end of the ET tube).
ET tube–securing device	Have the appropriate device readily available to secure the ET tube. A commercial device specifically designed to secure the ET tube is recommended.

Abbreviations: CO_2, carbon dioxide; $ETCO_2$, end-tidal carbon dioxide; ET, endotracheal

Words of Wisdom

Perform ventilations with a bag-mask device and 100% oxygen for at least 2 to 3 minutes before attempting intubation. The patient needs an oxygen reserve to tolerate the period without ventilation that will occur during insertion of an advanced airway. You also need the time to check your equipment properly.

Preoxygenation

Adequate preoxygenation with a bag-mask device and 100% oxygen is a critical step before intubating a patient. You should preoxygenate an apneic or hypoventilating patient for 2 to 3 minutes. During the intubation attempt, the patient will undergo a period of so-called forced apnea, during which time he or she will not be ventilated. The goal of preoxygenation is to prevent hypoxia from occurring during this time. Unfortunately, you will be unable to perform an extensive preintubation evaluation of the patient (such as obtaining hemoglobin and hematocrit values), and patients who are intubated in the prehospital setting are usually in physiologically unstable condition.

Monitor the patient's Spo_2 level and achieve as close to 100% saturation as possible during the 2- to 3-minute period of preoxygenation. During the intubation attempt, you must continually monitor the Spo_2 level and maintain it at greater than 95%.

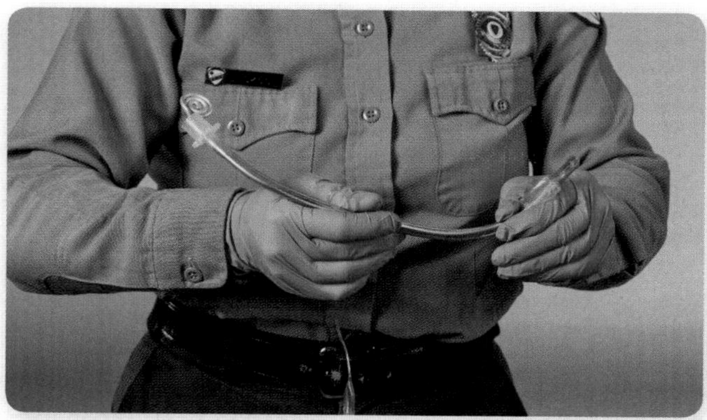

Figure 15-69 Prior to use, straighten the endotracheal tube/stylet combination and place a slight bend just proximal to the cuff.

The consequences of even brief periods of hypoxia can be disastrous. Do not rely solely on pulse oximetry to quantify a patient's oxygenation status; it can produce falsely high readings, even if the patient is severely hypoxic. Although some sequelae of hypoxia are dramatic and occur immediately, most are subtle and occur gradually. Some of the poor neurologic outcomes following aggressive airway management result from intubation-induced hypoxia.

Positioning the Patient

Successful laryngoscopy will be extremely difficult—if not impossible—without proper positioning of the patient's head. The airway has three axes: the mouth, the pharynx, and the larynx. When the head is in a neutral position, these axes are at acute angles, facilitating entry of food into the esophagus rather than into the trachea **Figure 15-70**. Although this positioning is advantageous to a conscious, spontaneously breathing person, the angles of these axes make laryngoscopy difficult.

> **Words of Wisdom**
>
> If the patient has experienced a possible neck injury, then you must place his or her head in a neutral, in-line position. Do not use the sniffing position or extend the patient's head in any way. Intubation of a trauma patient is *most* effectively performed by two paramedics.

To facilitate visualization of the airway, the three axes must be aligned to the greatest extent possible. This alignment is most effectively achieved by placing the patient in the sniffing position. In most supine patients, the sniffing position can be achieved by elevating the occiput about 1 to 2 inches (2.5 to 5 cm). Elevate the head with folded towels, or have your partner elevate the head, until the earlobes are at the level of the sternum **Figure 15-71**.

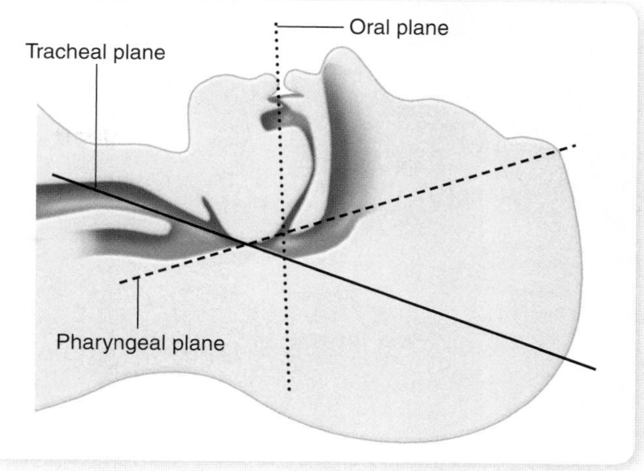

Figure 15-70 In a neutral position, the three axes of the airway—mouth, pharynx, and larynx—are at acute angles and make laryngoscopy difficult.

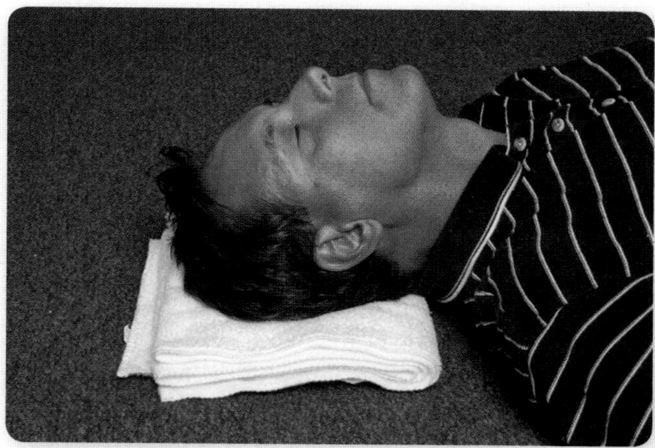

Figure 15-71 The sniffing position is achieved by elevating the head until the earlobes are at the level of the sternum.

When you use towels, the thickness can easily be adjusted by changing the number of folds. For patients with obesity, padding under the head alone may not result in the sniffing position; you may need to add padding under the shoulders and neck as well. To determine whether the patient is in a true sniffing position, view the person from the side to evaluate the adequacy of his or her head position.

Laryngoscope Blade Insertion

After you have properly positioned the patient's head and provided preoxygenation, direct your partner to stop ventilating. Position yourself at the top of the patient's head. If the patient is on a stretcher, then you can squat to put your head at the level of the patient's face. If the patient is on the floor or ground, then you may need to either kneel and lean forward or lie down to get into the proper position **Figure 15-72**.

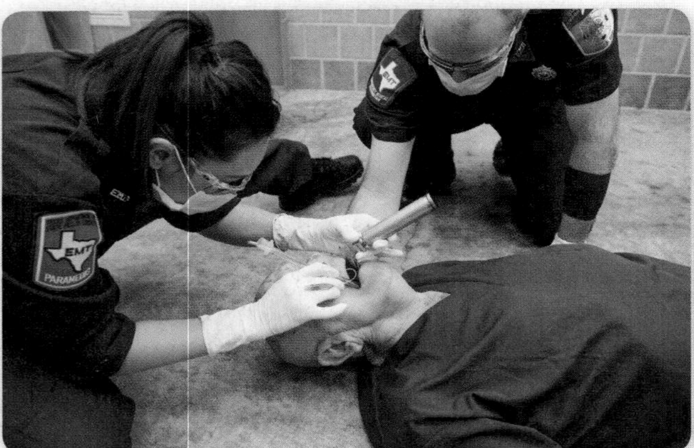

Figure 15-72 If the patient is on the floor or ground, then you may need to kneel and lean forward or lie on the floor to get into the proper position.

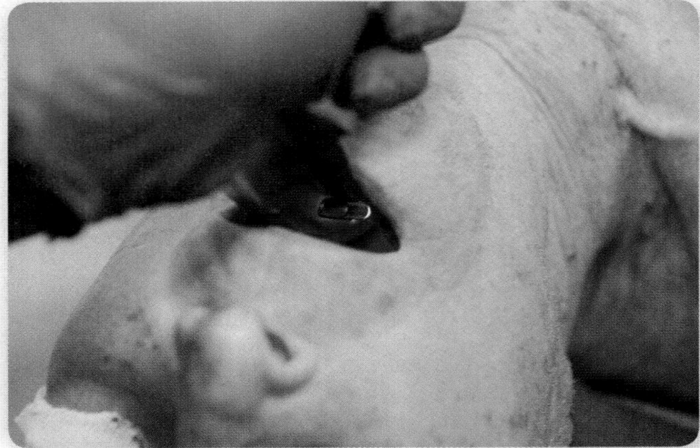

Figure 15-73 The tongue is a sticky, amorphous structure that can hinder visualization of the airway. Proper manipulation of the laryngoscope blade in the mouth is critical to controlling the tongue.

Hold the laryngoscope in your left hand, as far down on the handle as possible. It is not necessary to grasp the laryngoscope in your palm; simply hold it with your fingertips. If the patient's mouth is not open, then place the side of your right-hand thumb just below the bottom lip and push the mouth open, or "scissor" your thumb and index finger between the molars. As an alternative, you can open the mouth with the tongue-jaw lift maneuver.

Insert the blade into the right side of the patient's mouth. Use the flange of the blade to sweep the tongue gently to the left side of the mouth while moving the blade into the midline. Place the little finger of your left hand under the patient's chin; doing so will help you lift the jaw and will help prevent you from levering back against the patient's teeth. Take care not to catch the patient's lips between the laryngoscope blade and the teeth. Moving the tongue from right to left is a critical step. If you simply insert the blade in the midline, then the tongue will hang over both sides of the blade and all you will see is the tongue **Figure 15-73**.

Slowly advance the blade—while continuing to sweep the tongue to the left—until you identify the uvula; you should now be visualizing the posterior pharynx. Continue advancing the blade until the epiglottis comes into view. *The epiglottis is a critical structure to identify during laryngoscopy*. Gently manipulate the blade until you can see the epiglottis. Do not pry back on the laryngoscope; prying will cause you to use the patient's upper teeth as a fulcrum, resulting in breaking and potential aspiration of teeth **Figure 15-74**. Laryngoscopy does not require brute force; it is a technique of finesse. It is critical to relax when using a laryngoscope; a human's jaw is easy to manipulate, unlike that of a manikin. The correct motion is similar to holding a glass and offering a toast **Figure 15-75**.

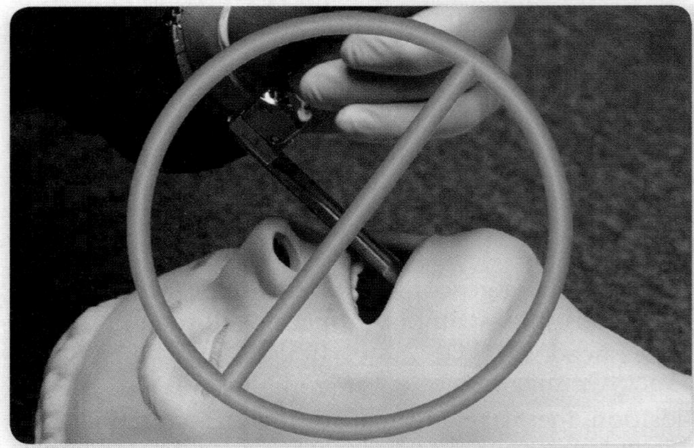

Figure 15-74 Avoid prying against the upper teeth with the laryngoscope, which can result in breaking and potential aspiration of the teeth.

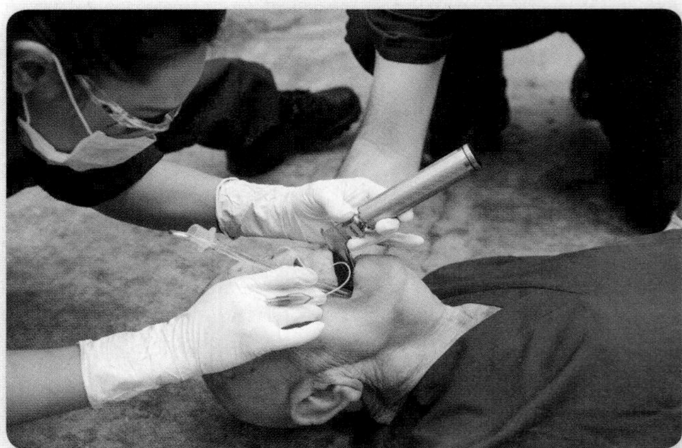

Figure 15-75 Relax your arms and gently advance the laryngoscope blade until the anatomy can be visualized.

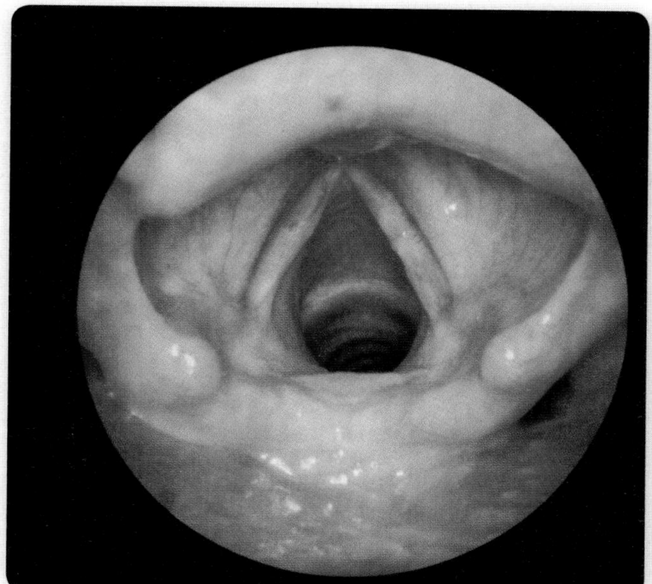

Figure 15-76 Laryngoscopic view of the epiglottis, vocal cords (white fibrous bands), and arytenoid cartilage.

Visualization of the Glottic Opening

After you identify the epiglottis, place the tip of the curved blade in the vallecular space, which is above the epiglottis. The straight blade is positioned directly under the epiglottis. Gently lift until the glottic opening comes into full view. You should see the vocal cords and the arytenoid cartilage. The vocal cords are white fibrous bands that lie vertically within the glottic opening. The arytenoid cartilage is located inferiorly on both sides of the glottic opening Figure 15-76. Identifying these structures enables to you make small adjustments in the position of the blade to ensure maximal visualization of the glottic opening.

The **gum elastic bougie**, also called an ET tube introducer, is a flexible device that is 0.20 inch (5 mm or 15 Fr) in diameter and about 2 feet (70 cm) long. A 30° bend is found at the distal tip Figure 15-77. Reusable and disposable versions are available in both adult and pediatric sizes. The bougie is used in epiglottis-only views to facilitate intubation. It can make intubation possible in some difficult situations, especially when your view of the glottic opening is limited. The bougie is rigid enough that it can be easily directed through the glottic opening, yet flexible enough that it does not cause damage to the tracheal walls.

The bougie is inserted through the glottic opening under direct laryngoscopy. The angle at its distal tip facilitates entry into the glottic opening and enables you to "feel" the ridges of the tracheal wall Figure 15-78. After the bougie is placed deeply into the trachea, it becomes a guide for the ET tube. Simply slide the tube over the bougie and into the trachea. Remove the bougie, ventilate, and confirm proper ET tube placement.

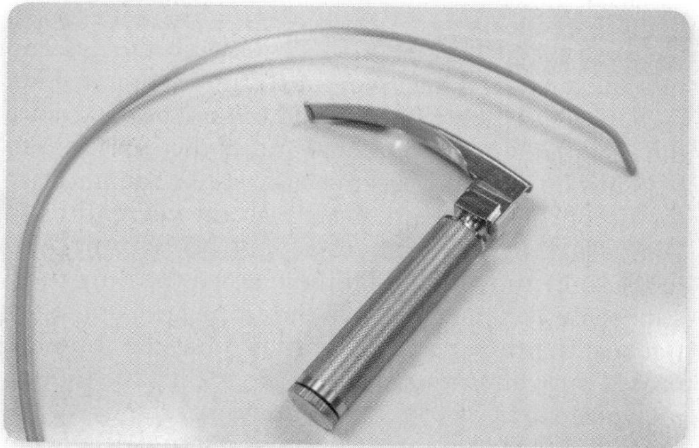

Figure 15-77 A gum elastic bougie is shown next to a laryngoscope.

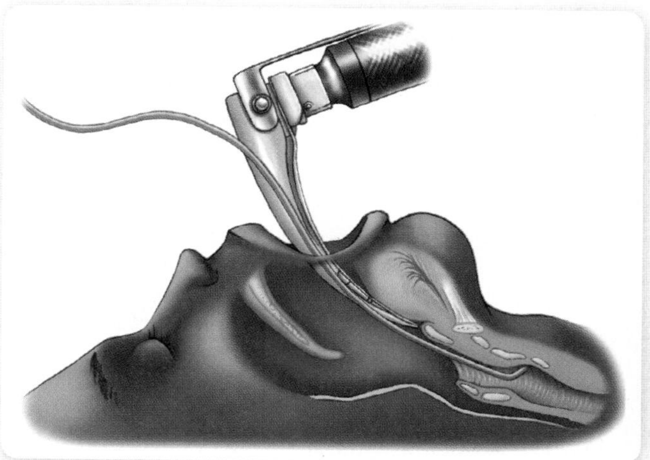

Figure 15-78 The angle at the distal tip of the gum elastic bougie facilitates entry into the glottic opening and enables you to feel the tracheal rings.

Words of Wisdom

When you use the bougie to facilitate intubation, orienting the tip anteriorly will enable you to feel the tracheal rings. Advance it until you meet resistance, which indicates that the bougie is at the level of the carina.

ET Tube Insertion

After you have visualized the glottic opening, pick up the preselected ET tube in your right hand, holding it with two fingers (like a pencil). The lower down you hold the tube, the more control you have over it. Under direct visualization, insert the tube from the right corner of the patient's mouth. As you see the tube pass through the vocal cords, rotate the tube to the right and direct the tip of the ET tube downward, allowing it to descend into the trachea. If the tip of the ET tube is oriented up, then it will hit the cricoid ring and will not pass. Advance the ET tube until the proximal end of the cuff is 0.5 to 0.75 inch (1 to 2 cm) past the vocal cords. You must see the tip of the ET tube pass through the vocal cords. If you cannot see the vocal cords, then do not insert the tube. An ET tube inserted blindly down the throat will almost always come to rest in the esophagus, not in the trachea; the only way to be certain that the tube has passed through the vocal cords is to see it pass through the vocal cords. If you take your eye off the tip of the tube (and the vocal cords), even for a second, then you significantly increase the likelihood of allowing the tube to slip into the esophagus.

Words of Wisdom

Improving Your Laryngoscopic View

During laryngoscopy, you (the intubator) can reach around with your right hand and manipulate the larynx (external laryngeal manipulation) while directly observing the effect on your view of the vocal cords. After the view is optimized, an assistant can maintain the optimum laryngeal position as you insert the ET tube with your right hand. This procedure, called **bimanual laryngoscopy**, is an effective method for improving your laryngoscopic view Figure 15-79.

During external laryngeal manipulation, the intubator (or his or her assistant) can perform the **BURP maneuver**, in which backward, upward, and rightward pressure is applied to the lower one-third of the thyroid cartilage.

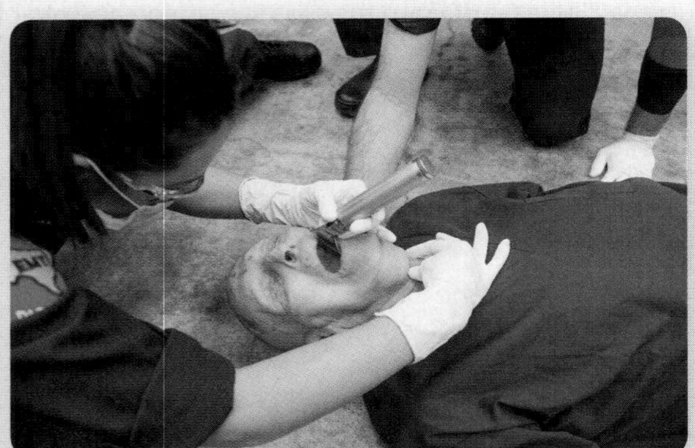

Figure 15-79 Bimanual laryngoscopy using external laryngeal manipulation.

Do not try to pass the ET tube down the barrel of the laryngoscope blade—especially when using a straight blade. The laryngoscope blade is not designed as a guide for the tube; it is a tool used only to visualize the glottic opening. Placing the tube down the barrel of the blade will obscure your view of the glottic opening Figure 15-80.

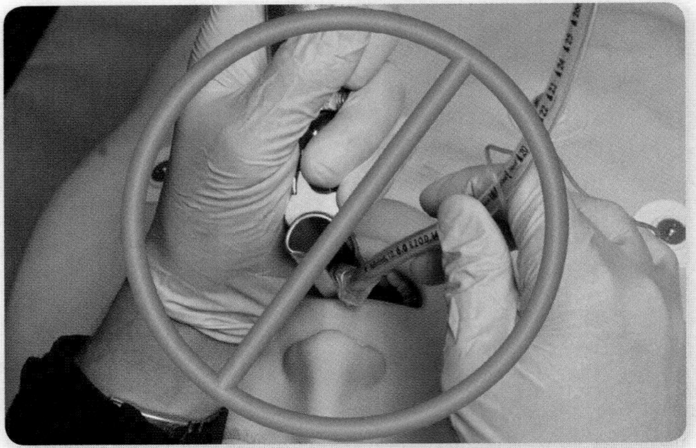

Figure 15-80 Avoid placing an endotracheal tube down the barrel of the blade because it obscures your view of the glottic opening.

Ventilation

After you have seen the cuff of the ET tube pass roughly 0.5 to 0.75 inch (1 to 2 cm) beyond the vocal cords, gently remove the blade, hold the tube securely in place with your right hand, and remove the stylet from the tube. Back out the stylet carefully to avoid extubating the patient.

Inflate the distal cuff with 5 to 10 mL of air, and then detach the syringe from the inflation port. If the syringe is not removed immediately following inflation of the distal cuff, then air from the cuff may leak back into the syringe, resulting in an inadequate seal between the cuff and the tracheal wall. Avoid inflating the distal cuff with excess pressure, which may cause tissue necrosis of the tracheal wall.

Note the depth of the ET tube (in centimeters) at the patient's teeth; this observation will enable you and other health care personnel involved in the medical care of the patient to determine whether the tube has slipped in or out of the trachea. For example, if the depth of the ET tube was initially 20 cm at the teeth, but is now 24 cm, then you know that the tube has advanced into the trachea.

Words of Wisdom

An intubation attempt should not take more than 30 seconds. Thirty seconds begins when you stop ventilating with the bag-mask device and resume ventilations with the ventilation device attached to the ET tube. If you are unable to intubate the patient within 30 seconds, then abort the attempt and reoxygenate the patient with 100% oxygen before attempting intubation again. If the patient is in cardiac arrest, then do not interrupt chest compressions to insert an ET tube.

Have your assistant attach the bag-mask device to the ET tube and continue ventilation. Place an in-line capnography monitor, which is attached to the cardiac monitor/defibrillator, between the bag-mask device and ET tube. While the first ventilations are delivered, look at the patient's chest to ensure that it rises with each ventilation. At the same time, listen with a stethoscope to the stomach over the epigastrium and over both lungs at the third or fourth intercostal space in the midaxillary line. If the ET tube is properly positioned, then you will hear equal breath sounds bilaterally and a quiet epigastrium. However, epigastric sounds may be transmitted to the lungs in patients with obesity or patients with significant gastric distention, leading you to believe that you have inadvertently intubated the esophagus.

Continue ventilation as dictated by the patient's age. Recall from Table 15-11 that you should ventilate an apneic adult with a pulse at a rate of 10 to 12 breaths/min (one breath every 5 to 6 seconds), and an apneic infant or child with a pulse at a rate of 12 to 20 breaths/min (one breath every 3 to 5 seconds). If the patient (adult, child, or infant) is in cardiac arrest, then ventilate him or her at a rate of 10 breaths/min (one breath every 6 seconds).[1,5-7] Do not stop chest compressions to deliver ventilations (asynchronous CPR).

Confirmation of Tube Placement

Visualizing the ET tube passing between the vocal cords is your first—and most reliable—method of confirming that the tube has entered the trachea; however, you must continue gathering information to assess and monitor the location of the tube. A misplaced tube that goes undetected is a fatal error. You must incorporate multiple assessment findings into the determination of where the tube is located.

Auscultation is the next step in confirming proper tube placement. Unequal or absent breath sounds suggest esophageal placement, right mainstem bronchus placement, pneumothorax, or bronchial obstruction.

Bilaterally absent breath sounds or gurgling over the epigastrium when auscultating during ventilation indicates that you have intubated the esophagus rather than the trachea. If copious vomitus is being emitted from the ET tube, then do not remove it! Instead, inflate the distal cuff, turn the tube to the side, and continue ventilation with a bag-mask device. If vomitus is not being emitted from the ET tube, then remove it and resume bag-mask ventilation. Reoxygenate the patient, be prepared to suction the airway as needed, and consider another attempt at intubation.

If breath sounds are heard only on the right side of the chest, then the ET tube has likely been advanced too far and entered the right mainstem bronchus. Follow these steps to reposition the tube:

1. Deflate the distal cuff.
2. Place your stethoscope over the left side of the chest.
3. While ventilation continues, slowly retract the tube while simultaneously listening for breath sounds over the left side of the chest.
4. Stop as soon as bilaterally equal breath sounds are heard.
5. Note the depth of the tube (in centimeters) at the patient's teeth.
6. Reinflate the distal cuff.
7. Secure the tube.
8. Resume ventilations.

If the ET tube has been properly positioned in the trachea, then it should be easy to compress the bag-mask device, and you should see corresponding chest expansion. Increased resistance (decreased ventilation compliance) during ventilations may indicate gastric distention, esophageal intubation, or tension pneumothorax. Each of these conditions warrants immediate reassessment and corrective action.

Continuous waveform capnography (discussed earlier in this chapter), in addition to a clinical assessment (such as auscultation over the epigastrium and over the lung fields bilaterally and assessing for visible chest rise), is regarded as the most reliable method of confirming and monitoring correct placement of the ET tube. The ideal time to attach the in-line capnography monitor is when the bag-mask device is attached to the ET tube. If waveform capnography is unavailable, then you can use a colorimetric $ETCO_2$ detector (also discussed earlier in this chapter) or an esophageal detector device, along with a clinical assessment of the patient.

The **esophageal detector device** is a bulb or syringe with a 15/22-mm adapter. With the syringe model, the syringe is attached to the end of the ET tube and the plunger is withdrawn, creating negative pressure **Figure 15-81**. If the tube is in the trachea (which has rigid, noncollapsible

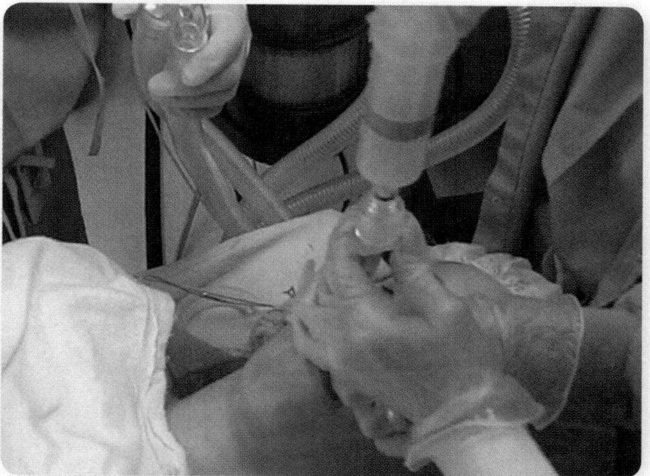

Figure 15-81 With the esophageal detector device syringe, the ability to freely withdraw air indicates placement of the tube in the trachea.

Courtesy of Marianne Gausche-Hill, MD, FACEP, FAAP.

walls), then air is easily drawn into the syringe and the plunger does not move when released. Unlike the trachea, however, the esophagus is a flaccid, easily collapsible tube. Thus, if the tube is in the esophagus, then a vacuum is created as the plunger of the esophageal detector device is withdrawn and the plunger moves back toward the *0 mL* mark when released.

With the bulb model, the bulb is squeezed and then attached to the end of the ET tube. If it remains collapsed or inflates slowly, then the esophageal wall has occluded the distal tip of the tube, indicating that esophageal intubation has likely occurred. If the bulb briskly expands, then the tube is properly positioned in the trachea **Figure 15-82**.

Words of Wisdom

Advance the *straight* end of the gum elastic bougie into the ET tube to help confirm its placement. If the bougie meets resistance and stops advancing—indicating that it has reached the carina—then the ET tube is likely in the trachea. If the bougie does not meet resistance and keeps advancing, then suspect inadvertent esophageal placement.

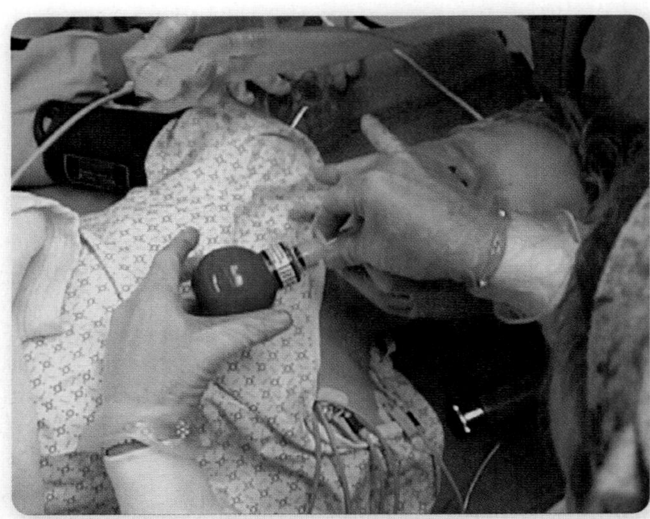

Figure 15-82 If the endotracheal tube is in the trachea, then the bulb of the esophageal detector device should briskly fill with air.

Courtesy of Marianne Gausche-Hill, MD, FACEP, FAAP.

Securing the Tube

The last, and very important step, in orotracheal intubation by direct laryngoscopy is to secure the ET tube. Inadvertent extubation is relatively common and can be

YOU are the Paramedic PART 7

After administering midazolam (Versed) and fentanyl (Sublimaze), you reassess the patient and note his heart rate and blood pressure have improved. However, you note his $ETCO_2$ level has decreased, as has the amplitude of the capnographic waveforms.

Recording Time: 30 Minutes	
Level of consciousness	Sedated with midazolam (Versed)
Respirations	20 breaths/min via positive pressure ventilation
Pulse	110 beats/min; regular and strong
Skin	Pink, cool, and dry
Blood pressure	126/74 mm Hg
Oxygen saturation (Spo_2)	97% (with positive pressure ventilation and supplemental oxygen)
$ETCO_2$	19 mm Hg; decreased waveform height
ECG	Sinus tachycardia

11. What are some possible causes of the patient's decreasing $ETCO_2$ level and waveform height? What should you do to determine the cause?

12. What would you expect the patient's $ETCO_2$ reading and waveform to do if he were not being adequately ventilated?

traumatic to the patient. As a paramedic, it can be discouraging to accomplish a difficult intubation, only to have the ET tube slip out of the trachea. Reintubation will almost certainly be even more difficult. Never take your hand off the ET tube before it has been secured with an appropriate device. Even then, it is a good idea to support the tube manually while you ventilate the patient to avoid a sudden jolt from the ventilation device that pulls the tube from the trachea.

Many commercial tube-securing devices are available. Familiarize yourself with the specific device used by your EMS system. The steps for securing an ET tube are as follows:

1. Note the depth of the ET tube (in centimeters) at the patient's teeth.
2. Remove the ventilation device from the ET tube.
3. Position the ET tube in the center of the patient's mouth.
4. Place the securing device over the ET tube. Tighten the screw to secure it in place. Fasten the strap.
5. Reattach the ventilation device, auscultate again over both lungs and over the epigastrium, and note the capnography reading and waveform.

Many commercially manufactured ET tube–securing devices feature a built-in bite block to prevent the patient from occluding the tube if he or she bites down. If you do not have a commercially manufactured ET tube–securing device, then you can secure the tube in place with tape and insert a bite block or oral airway between the patient's molars to prevent him or her from biting the tube.

It is also important to minimize head movement in an intubated patient. With a firmly secured tube, the tip can move as much as 2 inches (5 cm) during head flexion and extension. If the patient's head is hyperflexed, then the ET tube can be pulled from the trachea completely. If the head is hyperextended, then the ET tube could be pushed further into the trachea, potentially into a mainstem bronchus. Keep the patient's head in a neutral position to reduce the likelihood of tube dislodgement during transport. Consider applying a cervical collar and head blocks to minimize head movement.

The steps for orotracheal intubation by direct laryngoscopy are shown in Skill Drill 15-9.

Documentation & Communication

On the patient care report, document the means of assessing placement of the ET tube, such as breath sounds, visualization, and waveform capnography findings. Also document the depth of the tube, as noted by the centimeter marking at the patient's teeth. In addition, indicate when correct placement was confirmed: at the time the ET tube was placed, any time the patient was moved (ie, from the floor to the stretcher, loaded into the ambulance), and on arrival at the hospital.

Skill Drill 15-9 Performing Orotracheal Intubation Using Direct Laryngoscopy

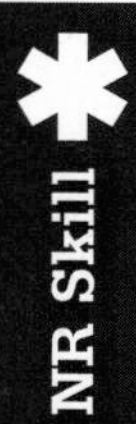

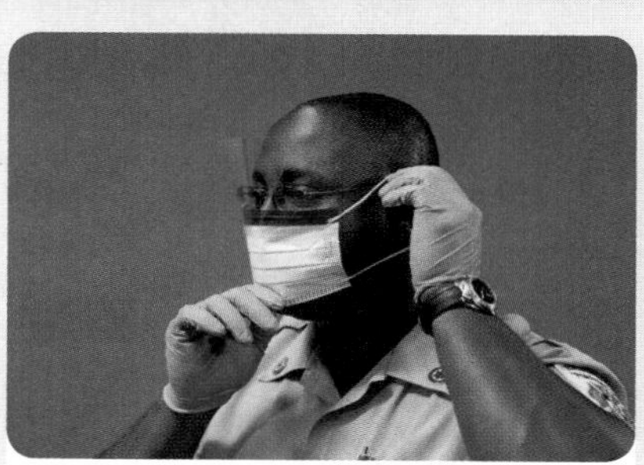

Step 1 Take standard precautions. If you suspect trauma, then maintain manual in-line stabilization of the head.

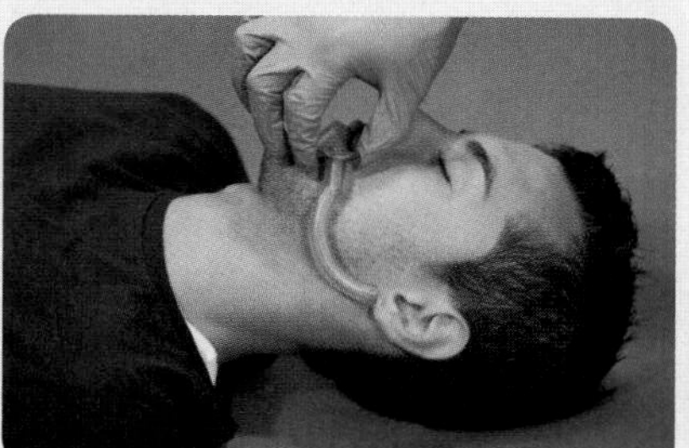

Step 2 Measure for the proper size and insert an oral airway.

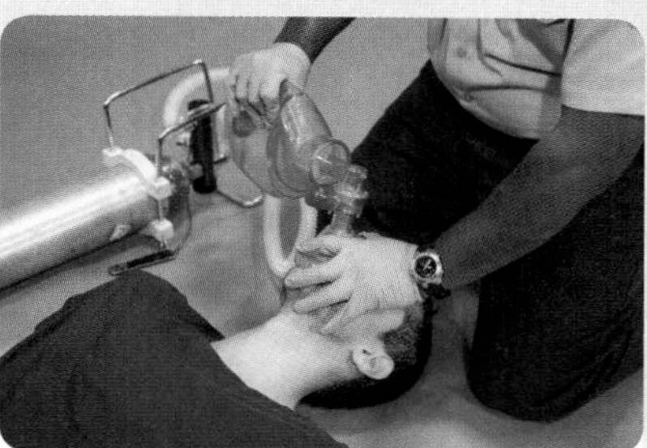

Step 3 Ventilate the patient with a bag-mask device at a rate of 10 to 12 breaths/min with sufficient volume to produce chest rise. Preoxygenate the patient for 2 to 3 minutes with 100% oxygen.

(continued)

Skill Drill 15-9 Performing Orotracheal Intubation Using Direct Laryngoscopy *(continued)*

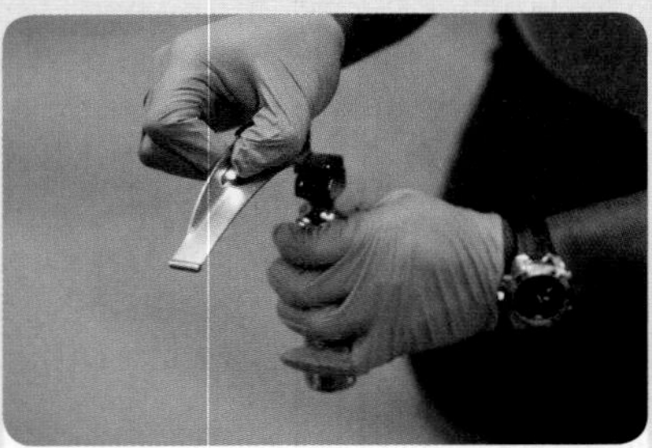

Step 4 Check, prepare, and assemble your equipment.

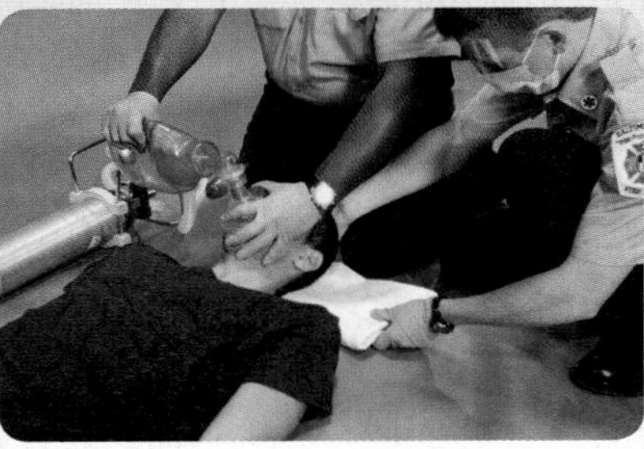

Step 5 Place the patient's head in the sniffing position.

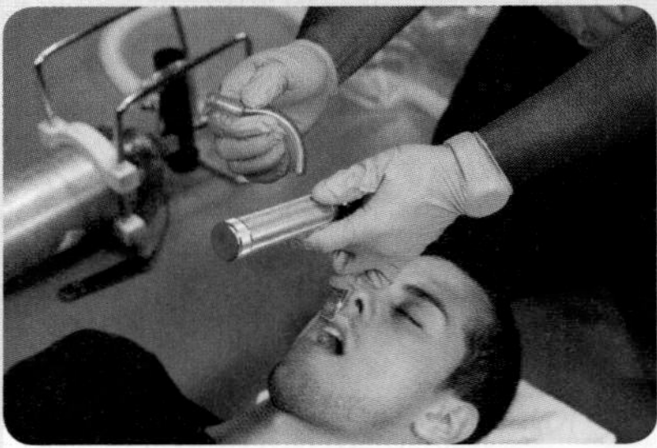

Step 6 Remove the oral airway, then insert the blade into the right side of the patient's mouth, and displace the tongue to the left.

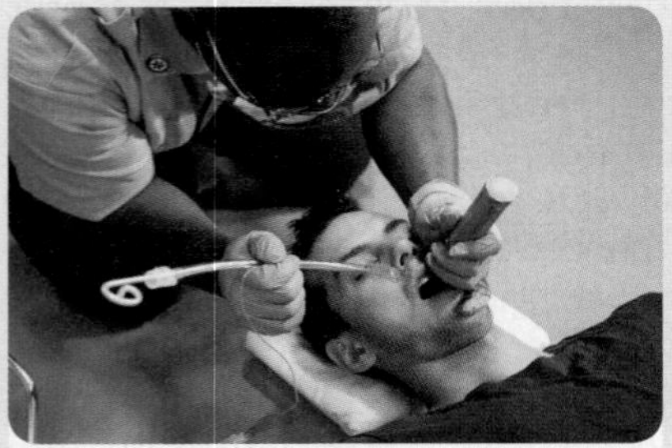

Step 7 Gently lift the long axis of the laryngoscope handle until you can visualize the glottic opening and the vocal cords.

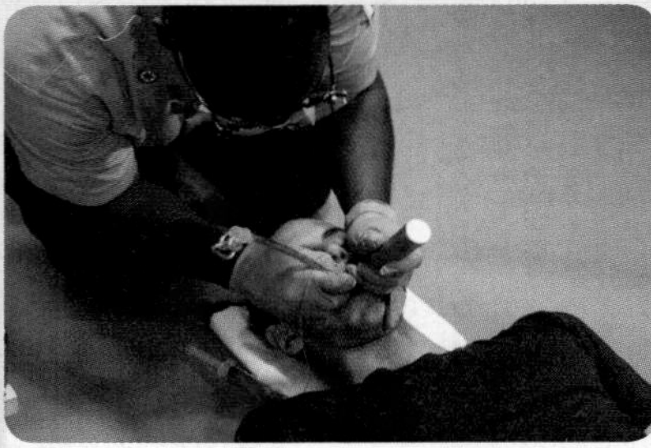

Step 8 Insert the ET tube through the right corner of the mouth.

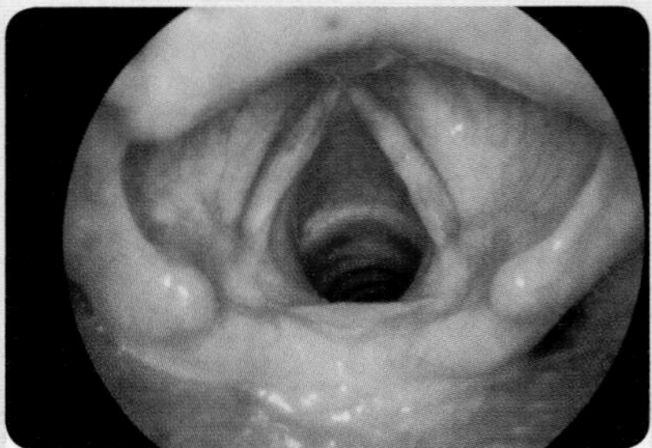

Step 9 Visualize the entry of the ET tube between the vocal cords.

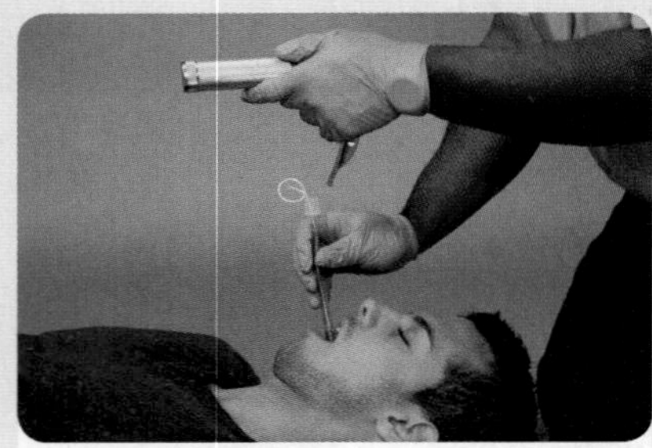

Step 10 Remove the laryngoscope from the patient's mouth.

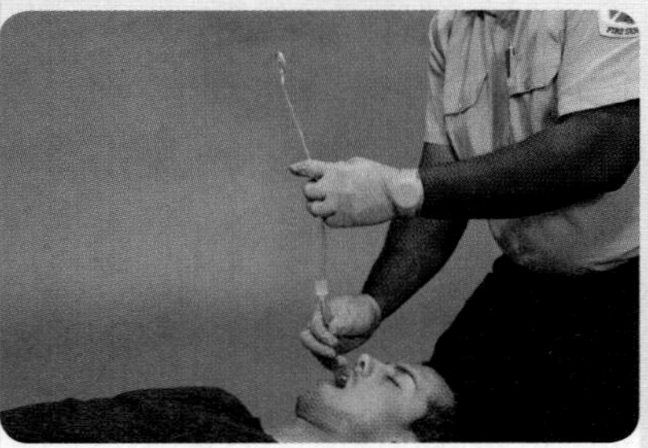

Step 11 Note the depth of the ET tube (in centimeters) at the patient's teeth and remove the stylet from the ET tube.

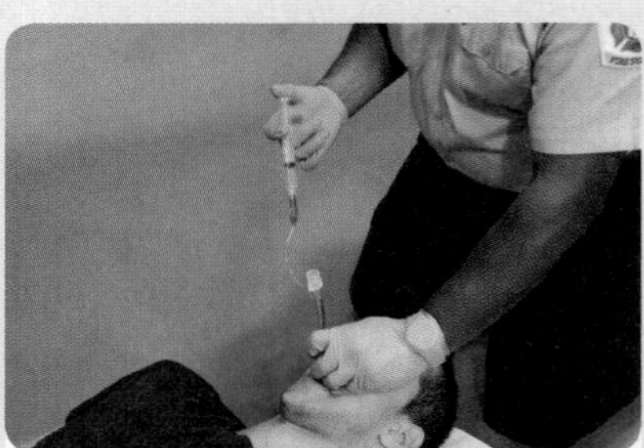

Step 12 Inflate the distal cuff of the ET tube with 5 to 10 mL of air, and immediately detach the syringe from the inflation port.

Skill Drill 15-9 Performing Orotracheal Intubation Using Direct Laryngoscopy *(continued)*

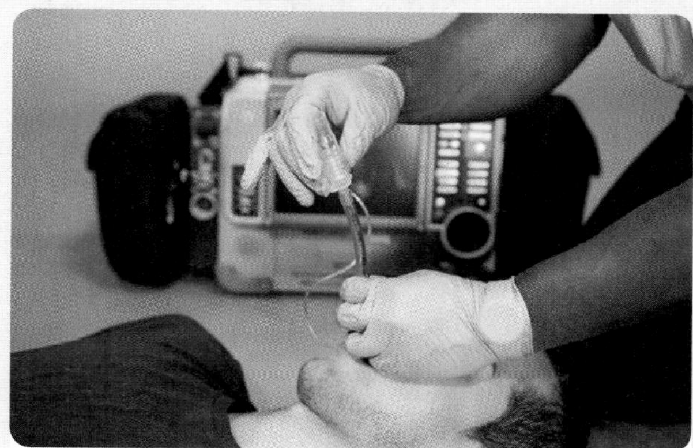

Step 13 Attach the ETCO$_2$ detector (waveform capnography preferred) to the ET tube.

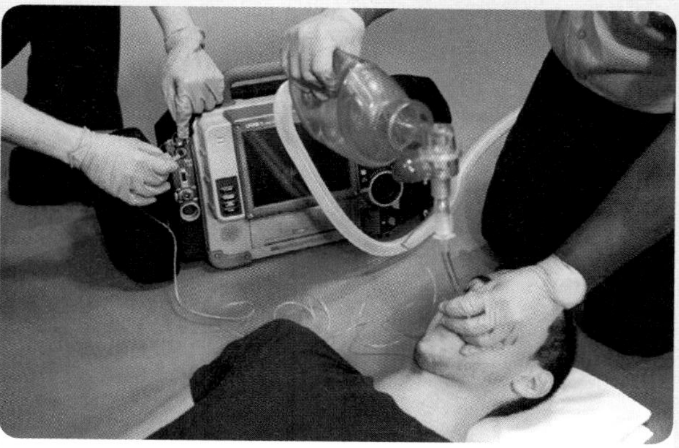

Step 14 Attach the ETCO$_2$ detector to the cardiac monitor/defibrillator and observe for a capnographic waveform and numeric CO$_2$ reading.

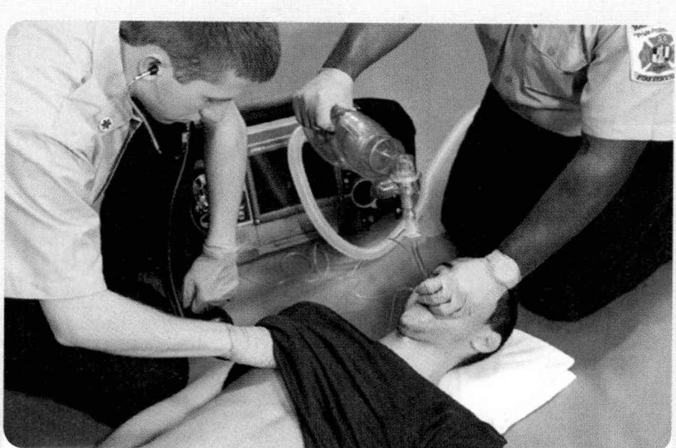

Step 15 Attach the ventilation device and ventilate. Listen over the epigastrium and over both lungs.

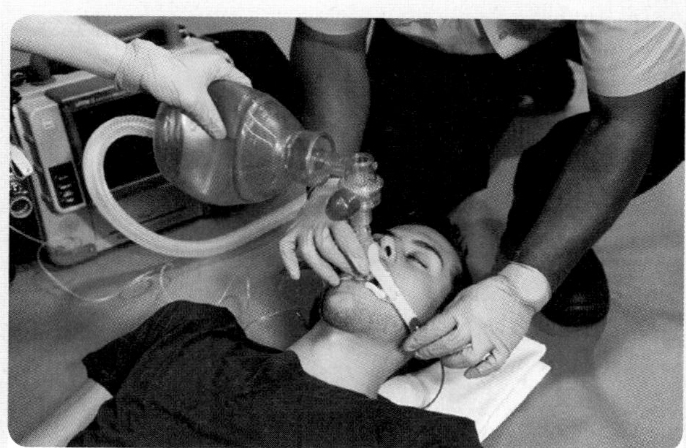

Step 16 Secure the ET tube with a commercial device or tape. Ventilate the patient at the proper rate while monitoring capnography and pulse oximetry.

▶ Orotracheal Intubation by Video Laryngoscopy

Video laryngoscopy is increasingly popular in the prehospital and in-hospital settings because it facilitates visualization of the glottic opening and vocal cords, even in patients with the most difficult airways. Instead of trying to visualize the vocal cords around the laryngoscope, as with direct laryngoscopy, you can guide placement of the ET tube with the use of a video monitor. However, video laryngoscopy requires better hand-to-eye coordination than direct laryngoscopy.

Types of Video Laryngoscopes

A number of video laryngoscopes are commercially available—some with a laryngoscope and separate video monitor **Figure 15-83**, and others with the video monitor attached to the laryngoscope itself **Figure 15-84**. All video laryngoscopes feature single-use blades of various sizes.

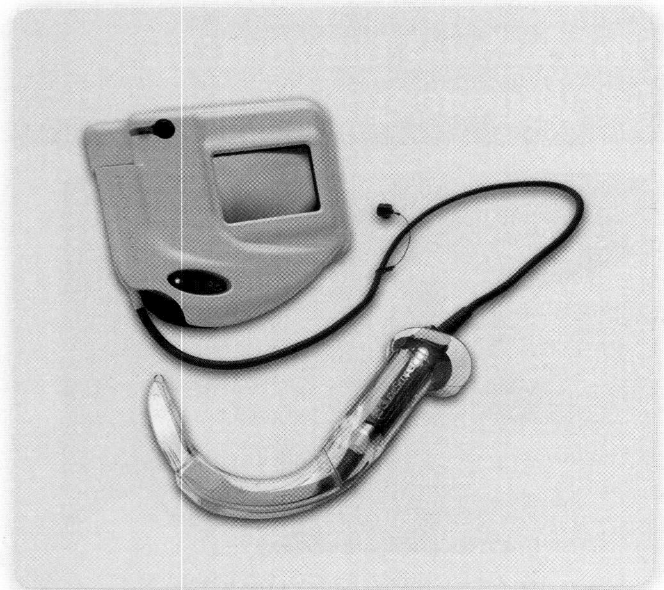

Figure 15-83 The GlideScope® Ranger video laryngoscope.

Courtesy of Verathon®.

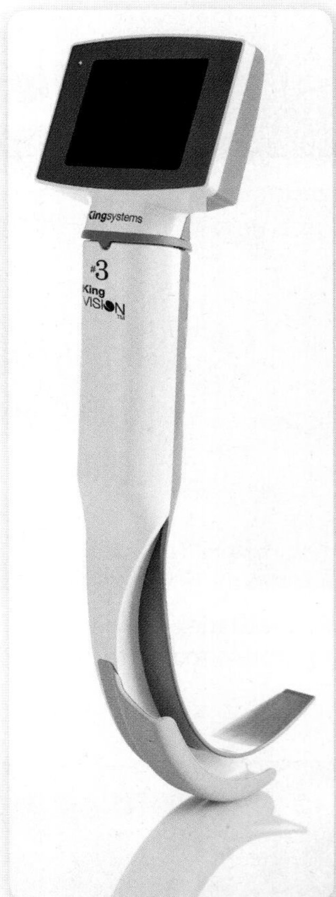

Figure 15-85 The King Vision® video laryngoscope.

© Ambu.

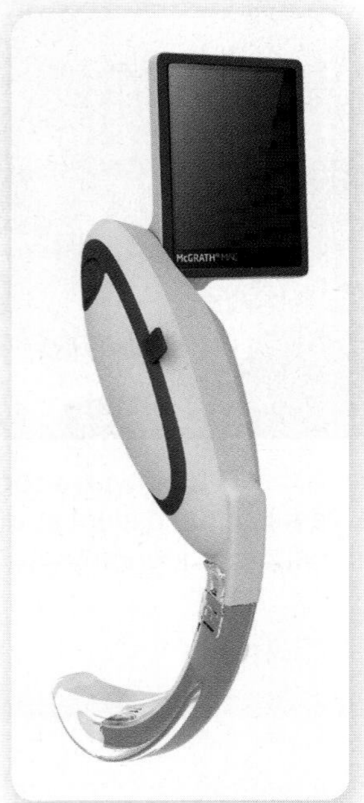

Figure 15-84 The McGrath™ video laryngoscope.

© 2017 Medtronic. All rights reserved. Used with the permission of Medtronic.

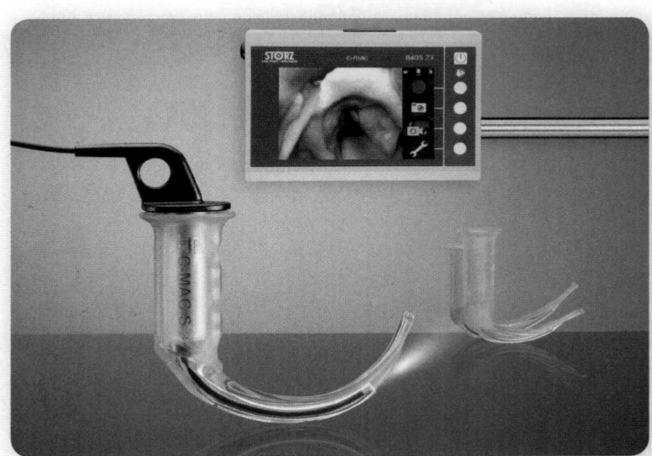

Figure 15-86 The C-MAC® video laryngoscope.

© Photo Courtesy of KARL SOTRZ Endoscopy-America, Inc.

Some video laryngoscopes require displacement of the tongue, such as the McGrath laryngoscope, whereas others are inserted in the midline of the mouth and simply follow the curvature of the tongue, such as the King Vision® Figure 15-85 and Pentax Figure 15-86 laryngoscopes. These nondisplacing devices also feature a channel through which the ET tube is placed, thus avoiding the need for a stylet.

Certain video laryngoscopes, such as the McGrath, can allow you to directly visualize the airway structures if the video monitor suddenly stops working.

Video laryngoscopy can be beneficial in a variety of environments. Consult the manufacturer's guidelines regarding the use of the video laryngoscope used by your service. The steps for orotracheal intubation by video laryngoscopy are shown in Skill Drill 15-10.

Skill Drill 15-10 Performing Orotracheal Intubation Using Video Laryngoscopy

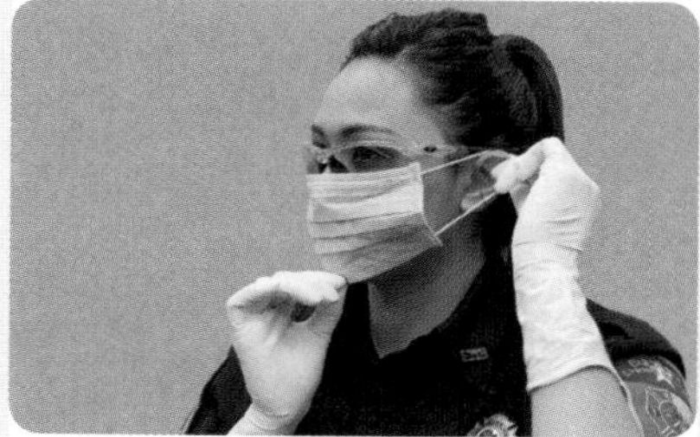

Step 1 Take standard precautions. If you suspect trauma, then maintain manual in-line stabilization of the head.

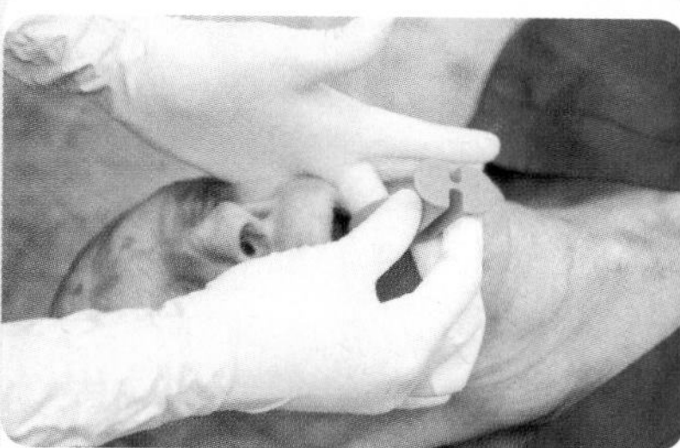

Step 2 Measure for the proper size and insert an oral airway.

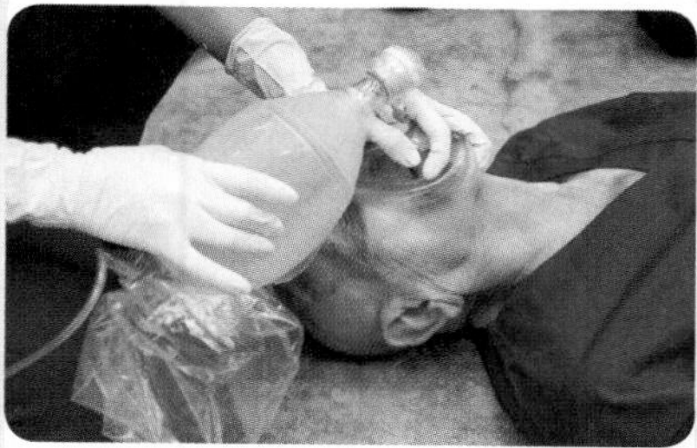

Step 3 Ventilate the patient with a bag-mask device at a rate of 10 to 12 breaths/min with sufficient volume to produce chest rise. Preoxygenate the patient for 2 to 3 minutes with 100% oxygen.

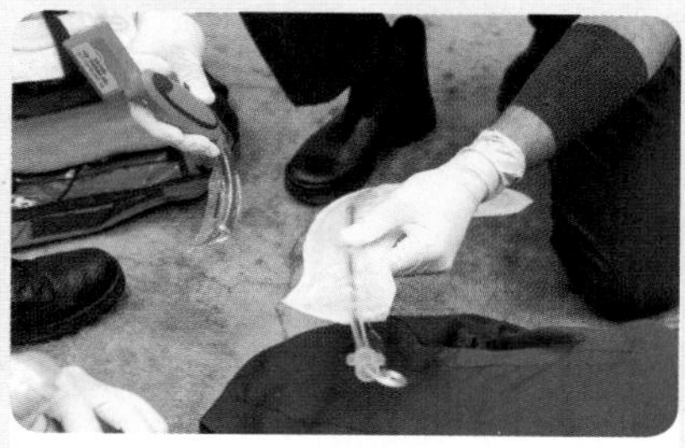

Step 4 Check, prepare, and assemble your equipment. Turn on the video laryngoscope and ensure the light and camera are functioning.

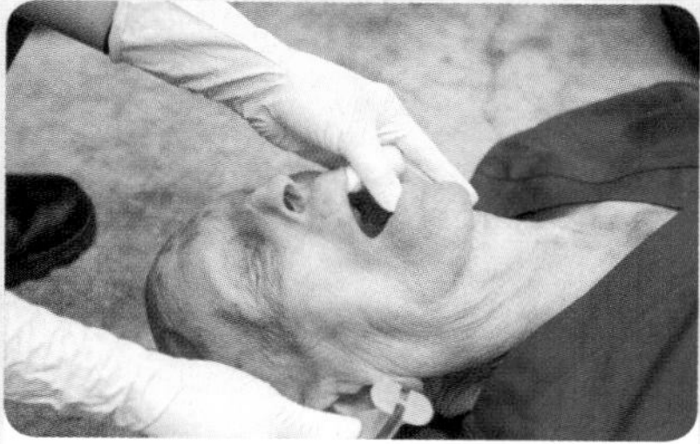

Step 5 Remove the oral airway and place the patient's head in the sniffing position.

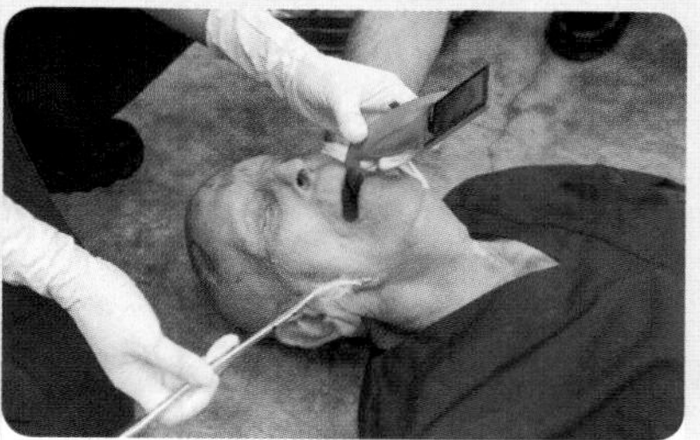

Step 6 Insert the video laryngoscope blade into the right side of the patient's mouth (displacing laryngoscope) or the midline of the mouth (nondisplacing laryngoscope). If using a displacing laryngoscope, sweep the tongue to the left. Visualize the epiglottis, vocal cords, and arytenoid cartilage.

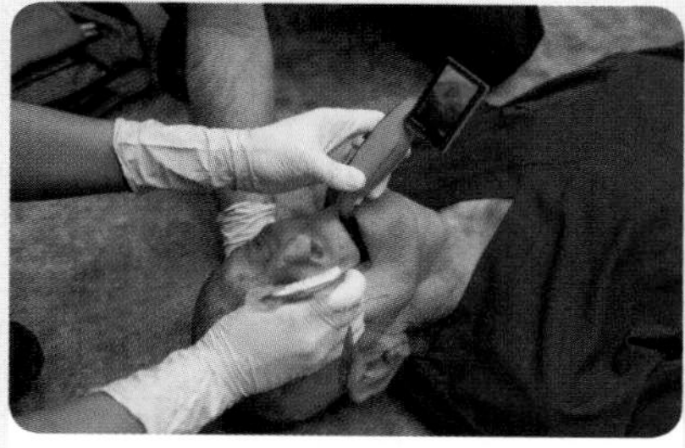

Step 7 Visualize entry of the ET tube between the vocal cords on the video monitor.

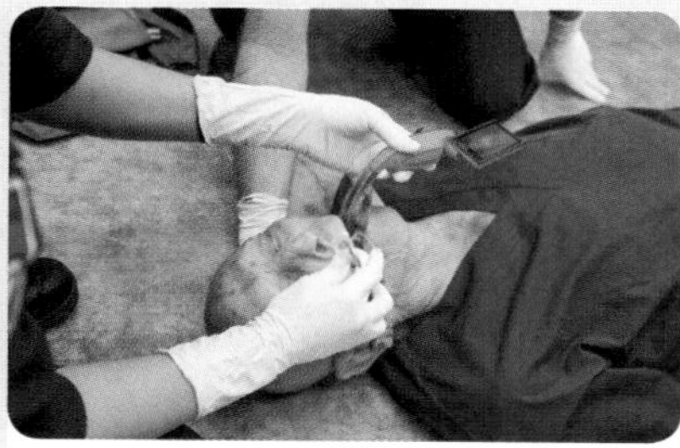

Step 8 Remove the laryngoscope from the patient's mouth.

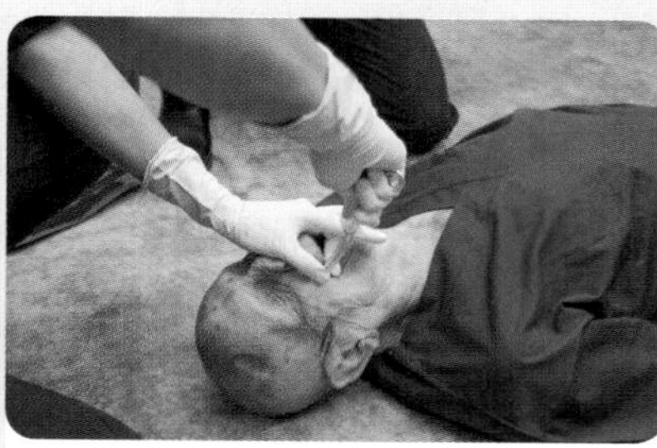

Step 9 Remove the stylet from the ET tube (if used).

(continued)

Skill Drill 15-10 Performing Orotracheal Intubation Using Video Laryngoscopy *(continued)*

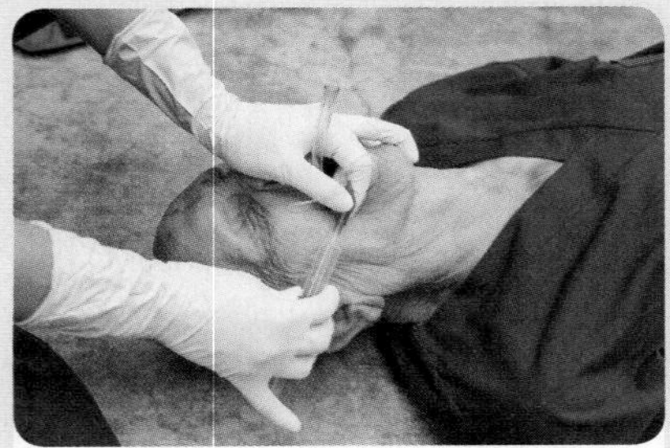

Step 10 Inflate the distal cuff of the ET tube with 5 to 10 mL of air, and immediately detach the syringe from the inflation port.

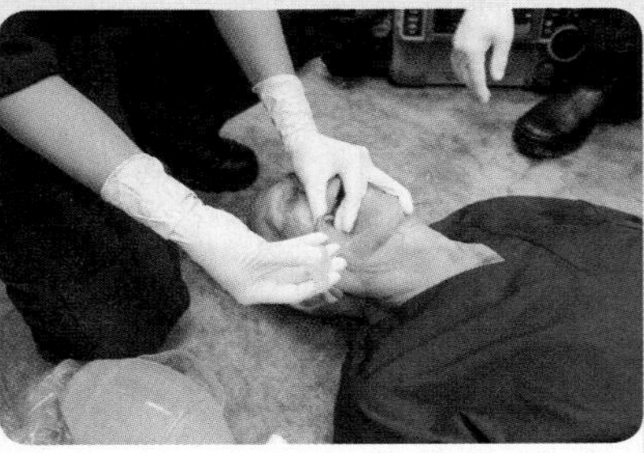

Step 11 Attach the $ETCO_2$ detector (waveform capnography preferred) to the ET tube.

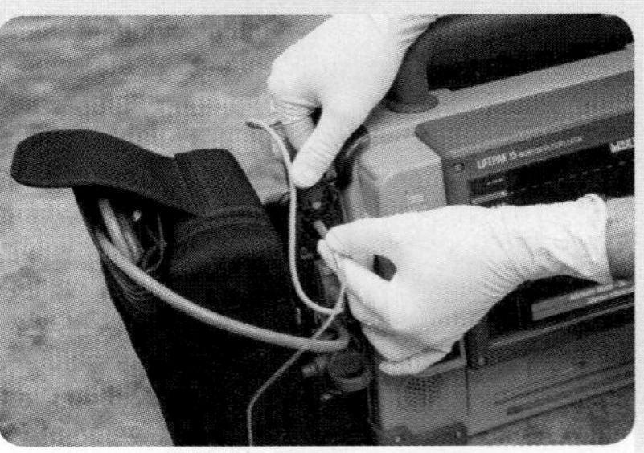

Step 12 Attach the $ETCO_2$ detector to the cardiac monitor/defibrillator and observe for a capnographic waveform and numeric CO_2 reading.

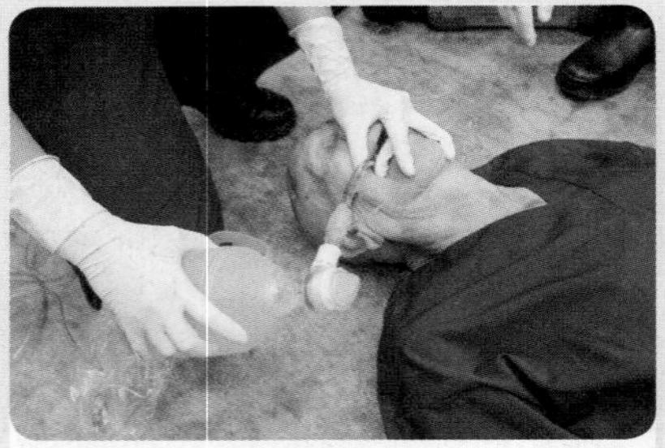

Step 13 Attach the ventilation device and ventilate. Auscultate over the epigastrium and over both lungs.

Step 14 Secure the ET tube with a commercial device or tape.

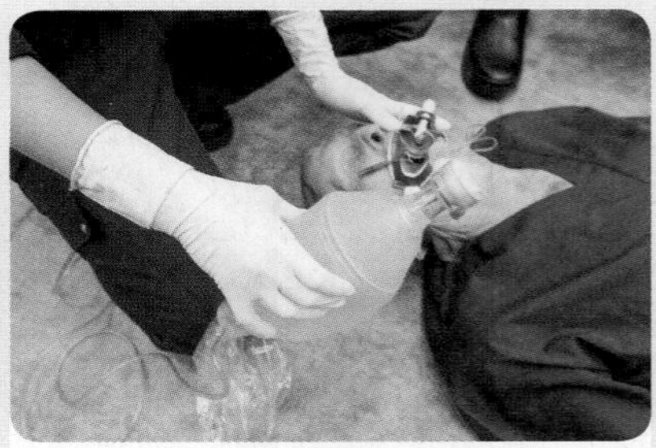

Step 15 Ventilate the patient at the proper rate while monitoring capnography and pulse oximetry.

Evidence-Based Medicine

The results of studies comparing direct laryngoscopy and video laryngoscopy are mixed. However, a systematic review of the literature shows that video laryngoscopy leads to higher rates of first pass success, shorter intubation times, and better overall success when used by less-experienced intubators.[8-10]

Words of Wisdom

The camera on the video laryngoscope is located on the distal end of the device. You will be unable to obtain a view of the airway anatomy if the camera becomes clouded by secretions. Keep the camera ahead of any secretions, and use suction to remove secretions before you advance the blade.

▶ Nasotracheal Intubation

Nasotracheal intubation is the insertion of an ET tube into the trachea through the nose. In the prehospital setting, it is usually performed without directly visualizing the vocal cords—hence the term "blind" nasotracheal intubation.

Blind nasotracheal intubation is an excellent technique for establishing control over the airway in situations when it is difficult or hazardous to perform laryngoscopy, or if it is not in the patient's best interest to administer sedatives and other pharmacologic agents to facilitate orotracheal intubation. Because the procedure must be performed on patients with spontaneous breathing, it is less likely to result in hypoxia.

Indications and Contraindications

Nasotracheal intubation is indicated for patients who are breathing spontaneously but require definitive airway management to prevent further deterioration of their condition. Responsive patients and patients with an altered mental status and an intact gag reflex who are in respiratory failure because of conditions such as COPD, asthma, or pulmonary edema are excellent candidates for nasotracheal intubation.

Nasotracheal intubation is contraindicated in apneic patients (that is, in respiratory or cardiac arrest), who should receive orotracheal intubation. This procedure is also contraindicated in patients with head trauma and possible midface fractures, as evidenced by CSF drainage from the nose following a head injury. In patients with these injuries, a nasally inserted ET tube may enter the cranial vault and penetrate the brain. Other contraindications for nasotracheal intubation include anatomic abnormalities, such as a deviated septum or nasal polyps, and frequent cocaine use. Nasal insertion of an ET tube in patients with these contraindications may result in severe epistaxis.

Avoid nasotracheal intubation, if possible, in patients with blood-clotting abnormalities and in patients who take anticoagulation medications (such as warfarin [Coumadin]). These situations also increase the likelihood and severity of epistaxis following insertion of anything in the nose.

Advantages and Disadvantages

The primary advantage of blind nasotracheal intubation is that you can be perform it on patients who are responsive and breathing. This procedure does not require placement of anything in the mouth (such as a laryngoscope), so the nasotracheal route is associated with much less retching and a lower risk of vomiting in patients with an intact gag reflex.

Another major advantage of nasotracheal intubation is that you do not need laryngoscope, which eliminates the risk of trauma to the teeth or soft tissues of the mouth. Because the patient's mouth does not need to be opened, this technique is better suited to patients with limited temporomandibular joint mobility, such as patients with mandibular wiring, mandibular fractures, seizures, or clenched teeth (**trismus**).

Nasotracheal intubation does not require the patient to be placed in a sniffing position, which makes it an ideal technique for intubating patients with a possible spinal injury, unless you suspect a midface fracture. Finally, because the tube is inserted through the nose, the patient cannot bite the tube. The tube can be secured more easily than a tube that is inserted orally because the nose generally has less secretions than the mouth.

On the downside, because nasotracheal intubation is a blind technique, you cannot use one of the major methods of tube confirmation—visualizing the tube passing through the vocal cords. Confirming proper tube position is critical, regardless of the intubation method used; however, you should be even more diligent when confirming tube placement following nasotracheal intubation.

Complications

Bleeding is the most common complication associated with nasotracheal intubation. If intubation is successful, then the airway is protected and the risk of aspiration is eliminated. However, severe bleeding can occur, especially with rough technique. Severe bleeding poses an additional threat to an already compromised airway because the swallowing of blood greatly increases the likelihood of vomiting and subsequent aspiration.

The incidence of bleeding associated with nasotracheal intubation can be reduced by gentle insertion of the tube into the nostril and lubrication of the tip with a water-soluble gel. If available, then an anesthetic lubricant containing a vasoconstrictive agent (such as phenylephrine hydrochloride [Neo-Synephrine]) will reduce the amount of patient discomfort and the likelihood and severity of nasal bleeding.

Equipment

You can use the same equipment for orotracheal intubation—minus the laryngoscope and stylet—for blind nasotracheal intubation. Standard ET tubes should be 1.0 to 1.5 mm smaller when inserted nasally. When choosing the size of the tube, select one that is slightly smaller than the nostril in which it will be inserted.

Some ET tubes have been designed specifically for blind nasotracheal intubation. For example, the Endotrol tube **Figure 15-87** is slightly more flexible than a standard ET tube and is equipped with a "trigger" that is attached to a piece of line, which is itself attached to the tip of the tube. Pulling the trigger moves the tip of the tube anteriorly and increases the overall curvature of the tube. This feature replaces the function of the stylet.

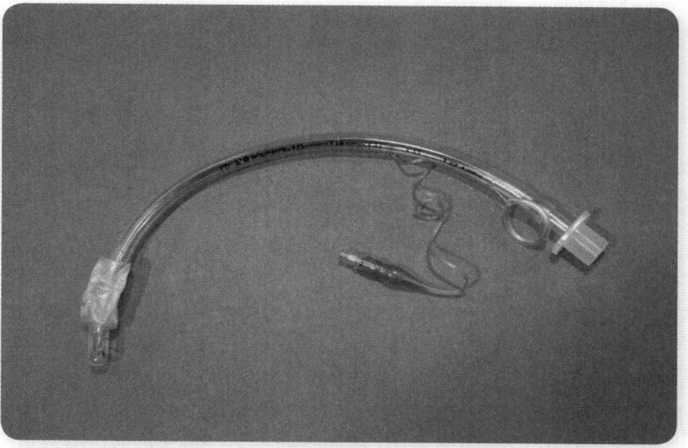

Figure 15-87 The Endotrol tube makes nasotracheal intubation safer, easier, and more efficient.

Table 15-13	Devices Used to Determine Maximum Airflow During Nasotracheal Intubation
Humid-Vent 1	A device that attaches to the 15/22-mm adapter at the end of the ET tube to prevent secretions from being expelled from the tube
Beck Airway Airflow Monitor	A small whistle that attaches to the 15/22-mm adapter and emits a high-pitched sound as air moves in and out of the tube
Stethoscope with head removed	Stethoscope tubing placed in the proximal end (approximately 1 in. [2 to 3 cm]) of the ET tube enables you to hear air movement without placing your face next to the tube

Abbreviation: ET, endotracheal.

The movement of air through the ET tube helps to determine proper tube placement following nasotracheal intubation. A number of devices have been developed to allow you to confirm successful nasotracheal intubation without the need to place your face next to the tube, thus risking contact with contaminants in the patient's exhaled breath Table 15-13.

▶ Technique for Nasotracheal Intubation

When you perform blind nasotracheal intubation, you use the patient's spontaneous respirations to guide a nasotracheal tube into the trachea and confirm proper placement. The tube is advanced as the patient inhales, at which point the vocal cords are open at their widest, which facilitates placement of the tube into the trachea.

After preparing your equipment and preoxygenating the patient, insert the tube into the nostril with the bevel facing toward the nasal septum. The right nostril is typically used because the curvature of the tube is in the correct orientation in relation to the bevel. If the right nostril is obstructed or if significant resistance is met, then insert the tube into the left nostril, but rotate the tube 180° as its tip enters the nasopharynx.

The angle of insertion is critical when performing nasotracheal intubation. Aim the tip of the tube straight back toward the ear Figure 15-88. The goal is to follow the floor of the nasal cavity until the tube enters the nasopharynx. Do not insert the tube with the tip aimed upward

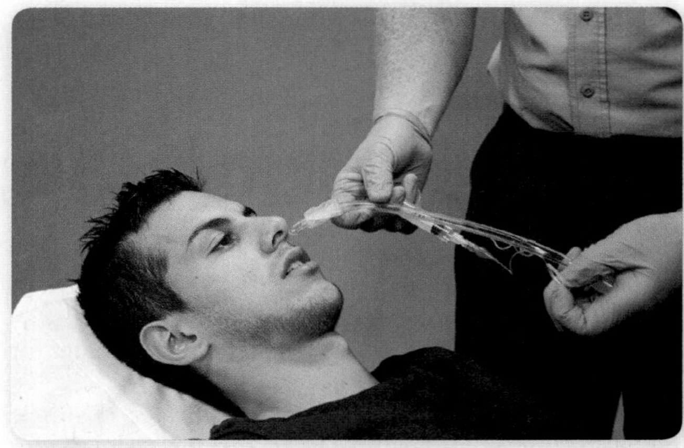

Figure 15-88 Aim the tip of the tube straight back toward the ear.

toward the eye; doing so can damage the turbinates and cause significant bleeding.

As the tube is advanced into the nasopharynx, you will begin to hear air rushing in and out of the tube as the patient breathes. Your goal is to position the tube just above the glottic opening so that the patient will draw the tube into the trachea when he or she inhales deeply. Manipulate the patient's head to control the position of the tip of the tube. Cup your left hand (if the tube is inserted in the right nostril) under the patient's occiput. Move the patient's head until you find the position that offers the maximum amount of air moving through the tube. At this point, the tube should be positioned just above the glottic opening.

As the patient inhales, the negative pressure created by inhalation facilitates movement of the tube through the glottic opening. Instruct the patient to take a deep breath, and gently advance the tube with the inhalation. Placement of the tube in the trachea will be evidenced by an increase in air movement through the tube.

If you see a soft-tissue bulge on either side of the airway, then the tube has probably been inserted into the piriform fossa. Hold the patient's head still and slightly withdraw the tube. After maximum airflow is detected, advance the tube on inhalation. If you do not see a soft-tissue bulge and no air is moving through the tube, then the tube has entered the esophagus. Withdraw the tube until you detect airflow, and then extend the head.

After the tube has been properly positioned, inflate the distal cuff with the minimum amount of air necessary to achieve an airtight seal. Attach a ventilation device to the tube, and ventilate the patient according to his or her clinical condition. Because you do not have the benefit of visualizing the tube passing between the vocal cords, confirmation (by multiple techniques) and continuous monitoring of proper tube position are critical. Although the movement of air in and out of the tube during breathing is a good indicator that the tube is in the trachea, it is not foolproof. In some cases, only the tip of the nasotracheal tube has passed through the glottic opening; even slight patient movement may dislodge the tube into the esophagus, which might not be recognized. Movement of the tube can also result in right mainstem placement.

Clean up any secretions or excess lubricant, and secure the tube with tape. Document the depth of insertion at the nostril, and monitor it frequently to detect movement of the tube. The steps for performing blind nasotracheal intubation are shown in Skill Drill 15-11.

Words of Wisdom

Keep a laryngoscope and Magill forceps within easy reach in case the patient becomes apneic during the procedure or you are unable to thread the tip of the tube through the glottic opening blindly. In these cases, you will need to complete the procedure using direct laryngoscopy.

▶ Digital Intubation

Digital intubation (also referred to as blind or tactile intubation) involves directly palpating the glottic structures and elevating the epiglottis with your middle finger while guiding the ET tube into the trachea by using the sense of touch. This airway management technique does not require a laryngoscope. Because of the variety of alternative airway devices available (such as Combitube, King LT, i-gel, and LMA), digital intubation is rarely performed. Nevertheless, being adept at digital intubation provides you with an option in some extreme circumstances, and you should frequently practice this skill.

Digital intubation is most advantageous in cases of equipment failure. The primary disadvantage of digital intubation is that it requires placing your fingers in the patient's mouth, which places you at risk of being bitten and exposed to an infectious disease. The patient's teeth could easily tear through your gloves, especially if the teeth

Skill Drill 15-11 Performing Nasotracheal Intubation

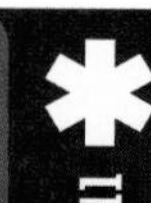
NR Skill

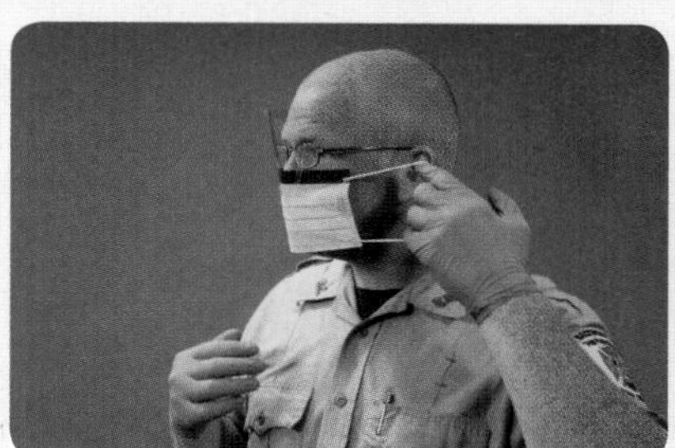

Step 1 Take standard precautions.

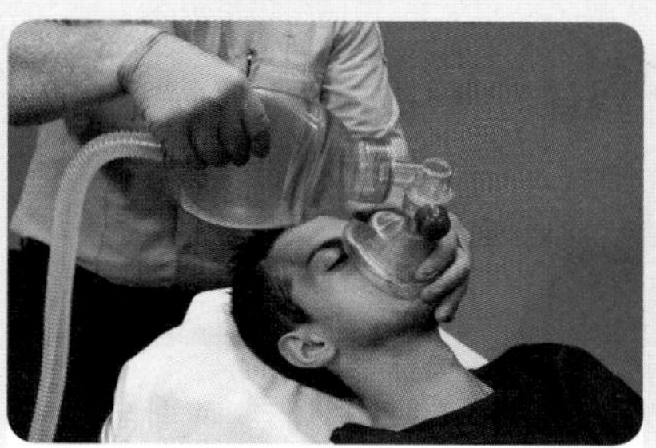

Step 2 Preoxygenate the patient whenever possible with a bag-mask device and 100% oxygen. Auscultate the patient's breath sounds to confirm adequate ventilation.

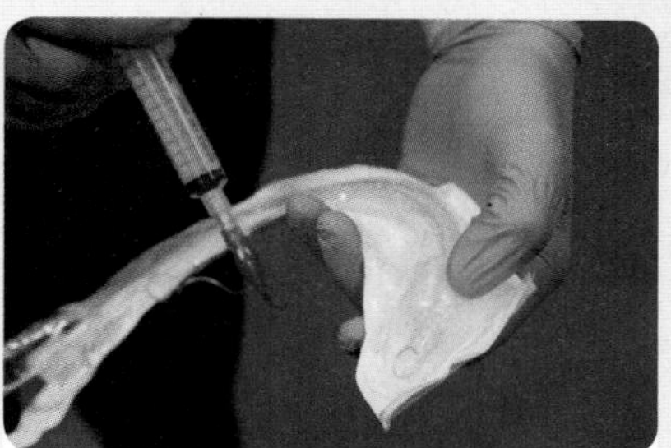

Step 3 Check, prepare, and assemble your equipment.

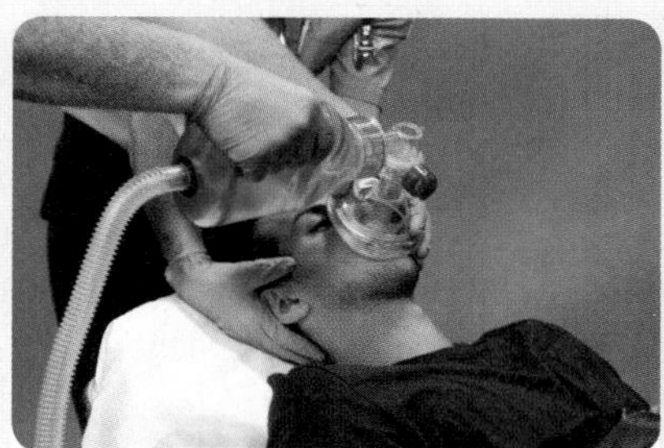

Step 4 Place the patient's head in a neutral position.

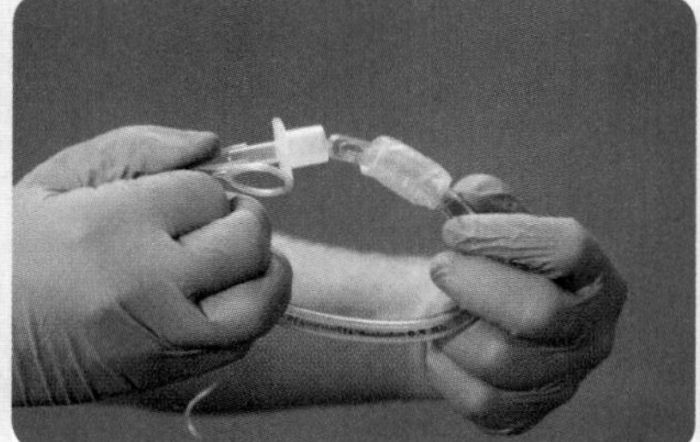

Step 5 Preform the nasotracheal tube by bending it in a circle.

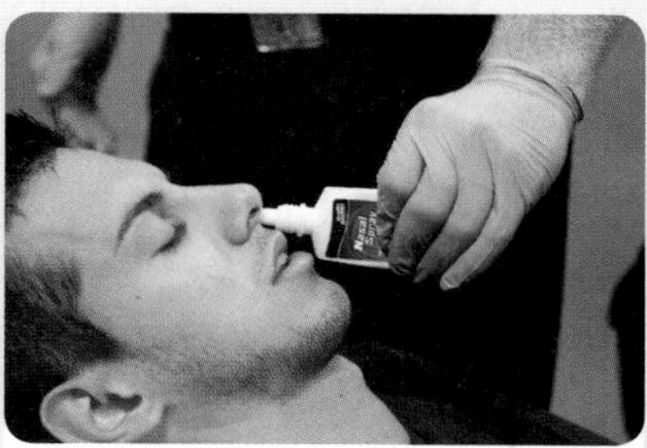

Step 6 Administer nasal spray to cause vasoconstriction of the nasal mucosa

(continued)

Skill Drill 15-11 Performing Nasotracheal Intubation *(continued)*

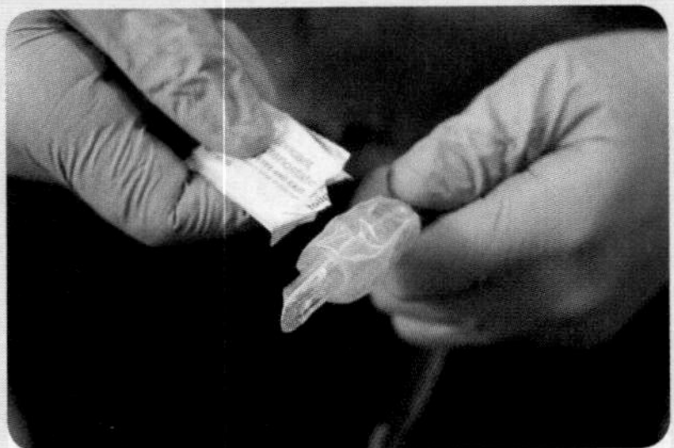

Step 7 Lubricate the tip of the nasotracheal tube with a water-soluble gel.

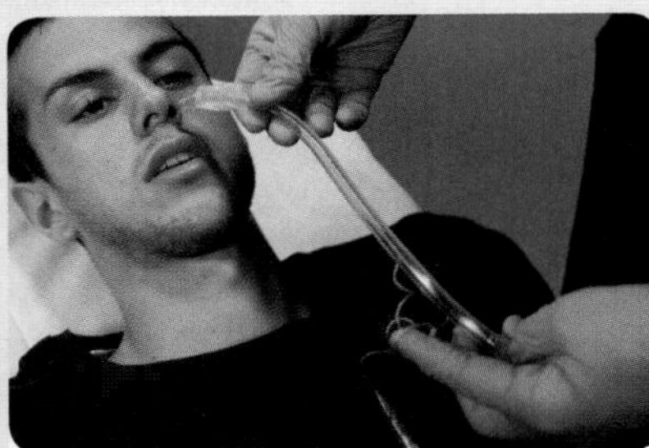

Step 8 Gently insert the nasotracheal tube into the more compliant nostril, with the bevel facing toward the nasal septum, and advance the tube along the nasal floor. Pause to ensure that the tip of the tube is positioned just superior to the vocal cords. Observe for condensation in the tube and note audible breath sounds from the proximal end of the tube.

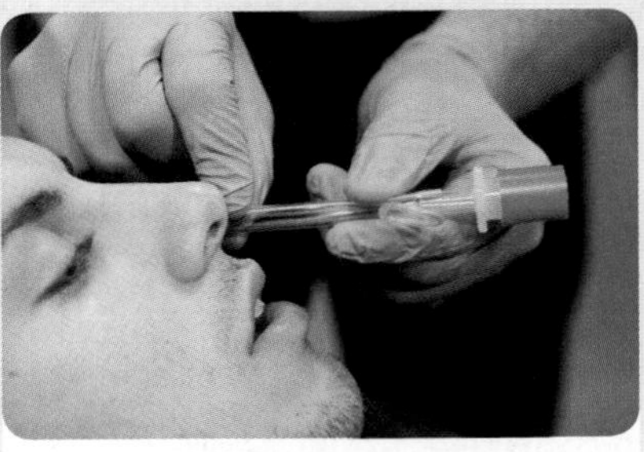

Step 9 Advance the nasotracheal tube through the vocal cords as the patient inhales. The Beck Airway Airflow Monitor device can be helpful in this step. Ensure that the patient is aphonic (unable to speak).

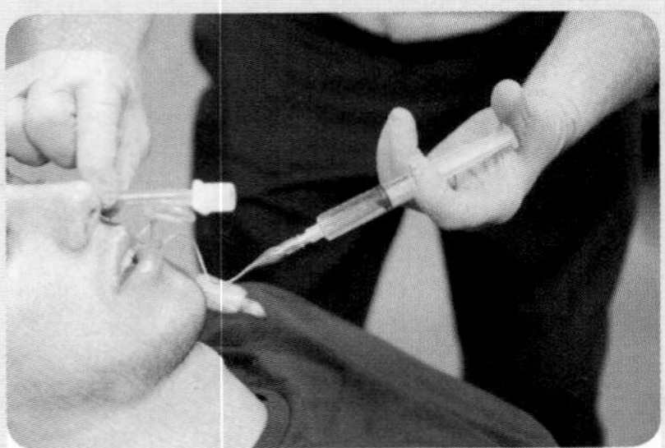

Step 10 Inflate the distal cuff with 5 to 10 mL of air, and immediately detach the syringe.

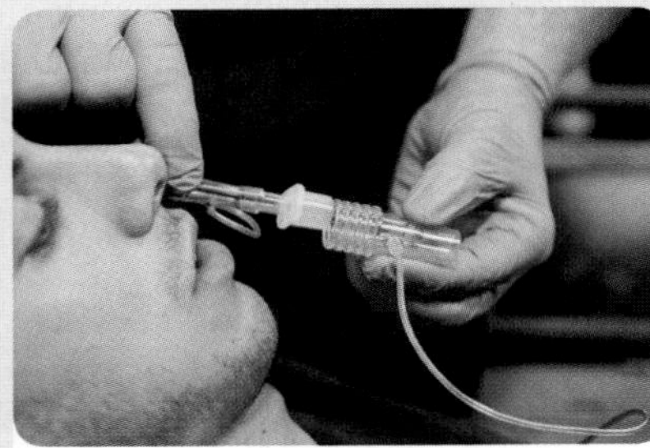

Step 11 Attach the $ETCO_2$ detector (waveform capnography preferred) to the nasotracheal tube.

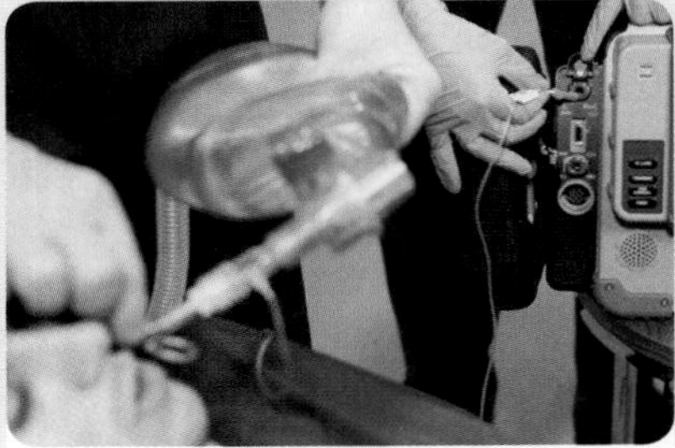

Step 12 Attach the $ETCO_2$ detector to the cardiac monitor/defibrillator.

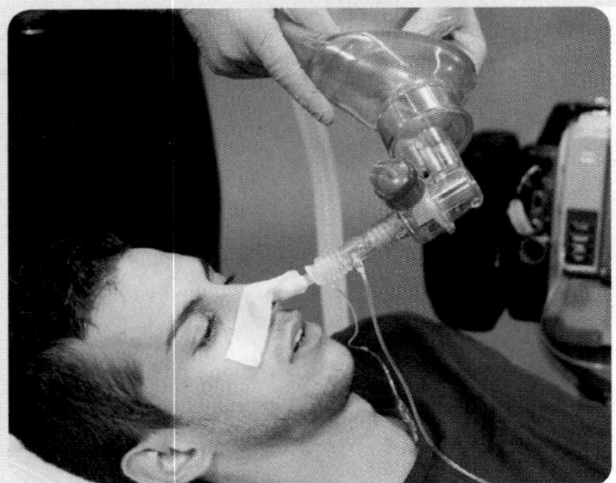

Step 13 Attach the bag-mask device, ventilate, and auscultate over the epigastrium and over both lungs. Ensure proper tube placement with waveform capnography. Secure the nasotracheal tube. Ventilate the patient at the appropriate rate, while monitoring capnography and pulse oximetry.

are sharp or broken. Therefore, perform digital intubation only in patients who are deeply unresponsive and apneic, and who also have a bite block in the mouth to prevent closure. This technique is absolutely contraindicated if the patient is breathing, is not deeply unresponsive, or has an intact gag reflex.

Successful placement of an ET tube via digital intubation depends on frequency of practice, experience, manual dexterity, and the size and length of the fingers. If you have short and/or wide fingers, then you will have greater difficulty performing digital intubation.

Misplacement of the ET tube is the major complication of digital intubation. Although the intubation is guided by the sense of touch, it is easy to misdirect the tip of the tube during insertion. Therefore, diligent attention to tube confirmation is absolutely essential.

To perform digital intubation, select an ET tube that is one-half to a full size smaller than that used for intubation with direct or video laryngoscopy. In this technique, you guide the tip of the tube into the trachea while using your index finger as a leverage point. A stylet provides the tube with the rigidity necessary to make the bend in the tube. Two configurations are recommended; practice with both to determine your preference.

- In an "open J" configuration, the stylet is inserted and a large J shape is made in the distal end of the tube.
- In the "U-handle" configuration, the tube is bent into a U shape and the proximal half of the tube is bent into a 90° handle toward your dominant hand **Figure 15-89**.

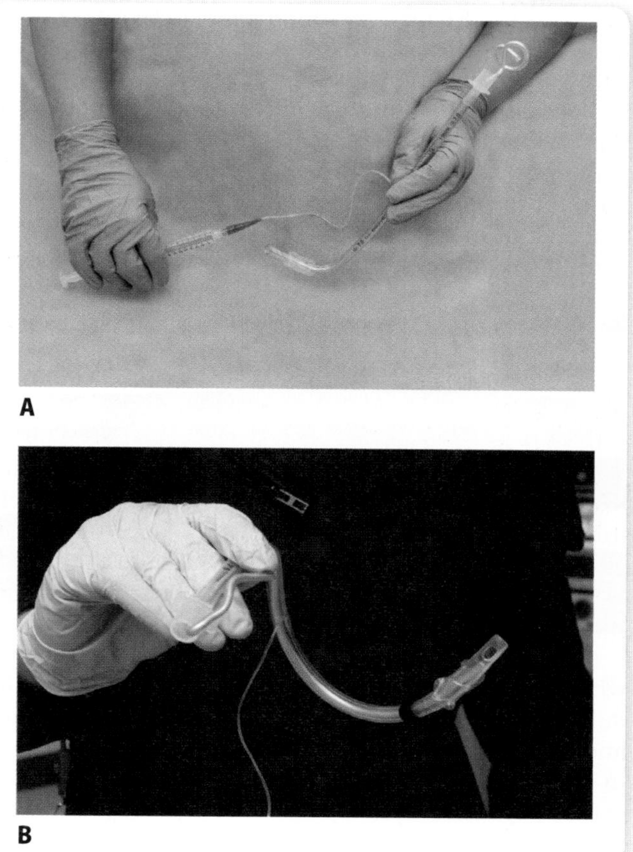

Figure 15-89 Different endotracheal tube configurations. **A.** Open J configuration. **B.** The U-handle configuration.

A: © Jones & Bartlett Learning. Courtesy of MIEMSS; B: © Jones & Bartlett Learning.

Because a sniffing position is not required to perform digital intubation, you can position yourself at the patient's left side facing toward the head. This position facilitates digital intubation if the patient is trapped in a seated or standing position.

Before you consider placing your fingers in the patient's mouth, insert a bite block or the flange of an oral airway, turned sideways, between the patient's molars. This action will prevent complete closure of the patient's mouth, providing protection for your fingers in the event of a sudden change in LOC or seizure.

Insert the index and middle fingers of your left hand into the right side of the patient's mouth. Press down against the tongue as you slide your fingers along the midline of the tongue until you can feel the epiglottis. Then pull the epiglottis forward with your middle finger.

Hold the ET tube in your right hand, like you would hold a pencil, and insert it into the left side of the patient's mouth. Advance the tube along the outer surface of your left index finger or between your middle and index fingers, and guide its tip toward the glottis **Figure 15-90**. After you feel the cuff of the tube pass about 2 inches (5 cm) beyond the tip of your finger, stabilize the tube with your right hand while you gently withdraw your two left fingers from the patient's mouth.

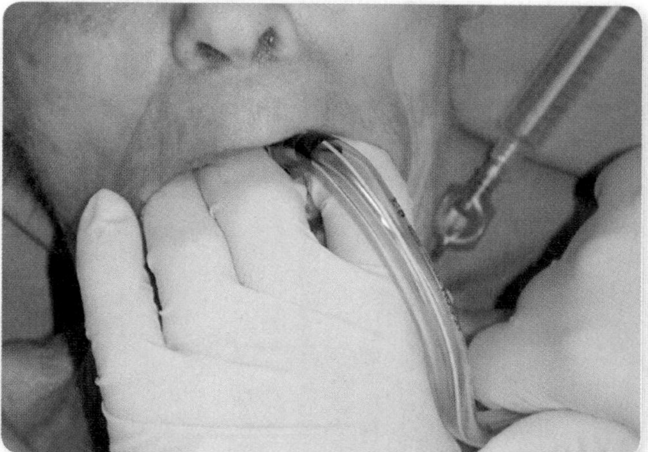

Figure 15-90 Advance the tube with your other hand and guide it between the vocal cords with your index finger.

© American Academy of Orthopaedic Surgeons.

After the tube has been positioned and stabilized manually, carefully remove the stylet and inflate the distal cuff with 5 to 10 mL of air. (Do not forget to detach the syringe from the inflation port.) Attach the ventilation device to the ET tube—with an $ETCO_2$ detector between the ventilation device and tube—and ventilate the patient while observing for visible chest rise.

Because digital intubation is a blind technique, you must follow a rigorous protocol for confirmation of tube placement. Auscultate both lungs and over the epigastrium, monitor the $ETCO_2$ level, and properly secure the tube in place. Continue ventilations according to the patient's clinical condition.

▶ Transillumination Techniques for Intubation

Transillumination intubation, like digital intubation, is rarely considered a first-line technique to definitively secure the airway, but it may prove valuable in some situations. The tissue that overlies the trachea is relatively thin. Therefore, a bright light source placed inside the trachea emits a bright, well-circumscribed light that is visible on the outside of the trachea and the external soft tissue that overlies it.

You can use a number of devices to intubate the trachea with the transillumination technique **Figure 15-91**. Be familiar with the specific equipment used in your service and consult the product documentation for instructions in its use. In this section, the term lighted stylet is used generically to describe any malleable stylet with a bright light source at its distal end that can be used to guide intubation.

Indications and Contraindications

You can use transillumination intubation whenever a patient needs to be intubated, but it is usually performed after other intubation techniques have failed. This technique is absolutely contraindicated in patients with an intact gag reflex and in patients with an airway obstruction. When determining whether to attempt transillumination, consider the amount of soft tissue overlying the trachea. Transillumination may be difficult in patients with obesity and patients with short, muscular necks.

Theoretically, it is possible to perform transillumination in pediatric patients; however, the stylet must fit inside the ET tube. Most lighted stylets will not fit in tubes smaller than 6.0 mm.

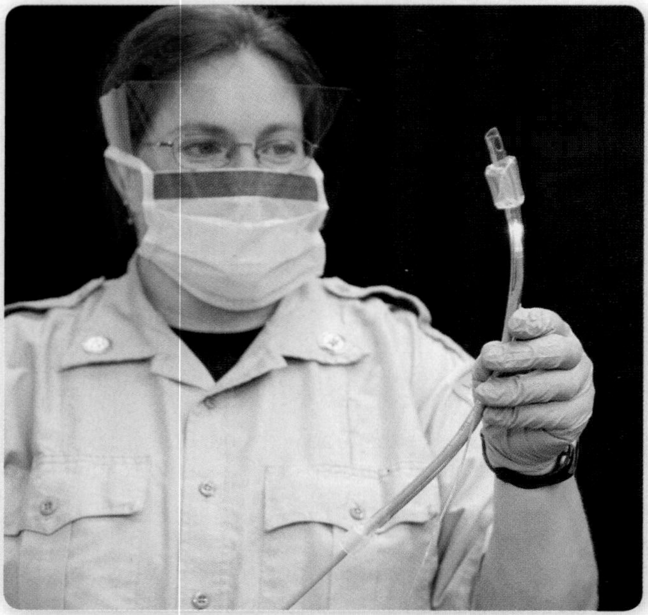

Figure 15-91 In transillumination intubation, a lighted stylet is inserted into the endotracheal tube.

Advantages and Disadvantages

Because transillumination does not involve the use of a laryngoscope, it largely avoids the complications associated with laryngoscopy (such as dental and soft-tissue trauma). In contrast with other blind intubation techniques (such as digital and nasotracheal intubation), transillumination adds a visual parameter—a light at the midline of the neck—that increases the chance for successful tube placement. Furthermore, this technique does not require visualization of the glottic opening, so the tube can be inserted through copious secretions. Finally, because the patient's head does not need to be in a sniffing position, you can safely perform transillumination in patients with a possible spinal injury.

The major disadvantages of transillumination are the requirements for special equipment—namely, a bright light source at the tip of the malleable stylet—and proficiency with its use. As a consequence of the requirement for a bright light source, transillumination can be difficult or impossible in brightly lit areas. If you are inside, you may be able to dim the lights to perform this procedure.

Complications

Although transillumination is not an entirely blind technique, you cannot directly visualize the tube passing between the vocal cords. Therefore, misplacement of the tube in the esophagus is the main complication. Pay strict attention to tube confirmation techniques following transillumination intubation.

Equipment

Whether specifically designed or modified, the single most important piece of equipment required for transillumination-guided intubation is a device with a rigid stylet and a bright light source at the end. Because the light may not always be aimed directly at the skin surface, it should shine laterally and forward. The lighted stylet must be long enough to accommodate a standard-length ET tube, and the stylet must be adequately secured within the tube.

Technique for Transillumination Intubation

As with any intubation technique, the patient must be preoxygenated for at least 2 to 3 minutes with a bag-mask device and 100% oxygen. Your assistant can perform this task while you prepare your equipment.

Select the appropriately sized ET tube, and check the cuff to ensure that it holds air. Lubricate and insert the lighted stylet so that the light is positioned immediately at (but not beyond) the tip of the tube. Ensure the stylet is firmly seated into the tube.

Prepare the tube by bending it into the proper shape to facilitate entry of the tube into the trachea and to ensure the light will be visible at the anterior part of the neck. The stylet should be straight, with a sharp 90° angle in the tube-stylet assembly just proximal to the cuff. This bend in the tube must be sharp because it will act as the pivot point when you direct the stylet into the trachea; it will also place the light in the proper position to illuminate the anterior part of the neck.

Place the patient's head in a neutral or slightly extended position. This position will move the epiglottis off the posterior pharyngeal wall and facilitate entry of the ET tube into the glottic opening. Extension of the patient's head will also provide maximum exposure of the anterior part of the neck, enhancing visualization of the lighted stylet under the soft tissue as it moves down the airway. The intubator is typically positioned at the patient's head.

While holding the lighted stylet in your dominant hand, displace the patient's jaw forwardly by grasping it with your thumb and forefinger. This step will ensure that the epiglottis is not covering the glottic opening. Turn on the lighted stylet, and insert the device in the midline of the patient's mouth, with the tip directed toward the laryngeal prominence. The goal is to lift the epiglottis with the ET tube–stylet combination.

As you continue to insert the tube-stylet assembly, draw your wrist toward you. The light should become visible at the midline of the neck. A tightly circumscribed light slightly below the thyroid cartilage indicates that the tip of the tube has entered the trachea. A faintly glowing light and bulging of the soft tissue above the thyroid cartilage indicates that the tip of the tube is in the vallecular space. If the tip is in this space, then withdraw the tube slightly, displace the jaw forward, and continue to advance the tube-stylet assembly. A dim, diffuse light at the anterior part of the neck typically indicates esophageal placement. In this case, slightly withdraw the tube-stylet assembly and slightly extend the patient's head. You may also consider increasing the angle of the bend in the tube. These actions should reposition the tube-stylet assembly at the glottic opening. If you continue to encounter difficulty, then abort the procedure and ventilate the patient with a bag-mask device and 100% oxygen before reattempting insertion of the tube-stylet assembly.

Once a bright, tightly circumscribed light is visible at the midline and just below the thyroid cartilage, hold the stylet in place and advance the tube approximately 1 to 1.5 inches (2 to 4 cm) into the trachea. When the tube is securely in the trachea, manually stabilize it in place with your nondominant hand and carefully withdraw the lighted stylet.

Inflate the distal cuff of the ET tube with 5 to 10 mL of air, detach the syringe from the inflation port, and attach the bag-mask device to the ET tube. Ventilate the patient while auscultating over the apices and bases of both lungs and over the epigastrium. Following subjective and objective confirmation of proper tube placement, secure the tube in place with the appropriate device and continue ventilations according to the patient's clinical condition.

The steps for performing intubation with the transillumination technique are shown in Skill Drill 15-12.

Retrograde Intubation

When intubation is unsuccessful by standard methods, you may use the technique of **retrograde intubation**. This technique is rarely performed in the prehospital environment and is only relevant in EMS systems where local protocols indicate this method as a paramedic skill. In retrograde intubation, a needle is placed percutaneously within the trachea via the cricothyroid membrane. A wire is placed toward the head through the needle upward through the trachea and into the mouth. The wire is then visualized and secured, and the ET tube is placed over the wire and guided into the trachea. The wire is subsequently removed, and the ET tube is advanced and secured.

Indications for retrograde intubation include the following:

- Copious secretions in the airway that cannot be removed with suction
- Failure to intubate the trachea by less invasive methods (ie, direct or video laryngoscopy)

Contraindications for retrograde intubation include the following:

- Lack of familiarity with the procedure
- Laryngeal trauma
- Unrecognizable or distorted anatomic landmarks
- Coagulopathy (relative contraindication)
- Severe hypoxia (due to inability to ventilate during the procedure and time to perform the procedure)

Complications of retrograde intubation include the following:

- Hypoxia
- Cardiac dysrhythmias
- Mechanical trauma
- Infection
- Increased ICP

The assessment findings and transport complications with retrograde intubation are the same as with standard intubation.

Skill Drill 15-12 Performing Transillumination Intubation

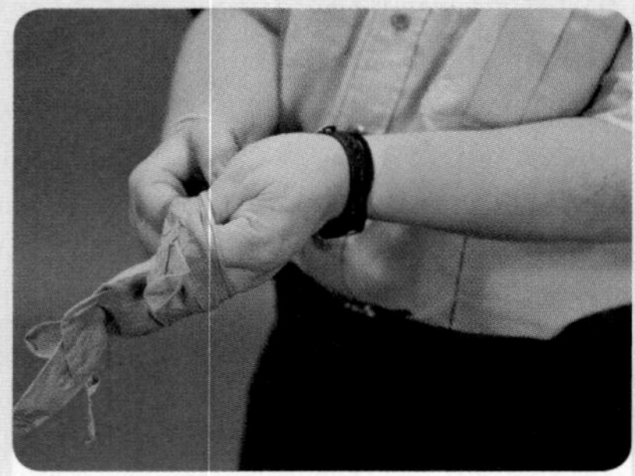

Step 1 Take standard precautions.

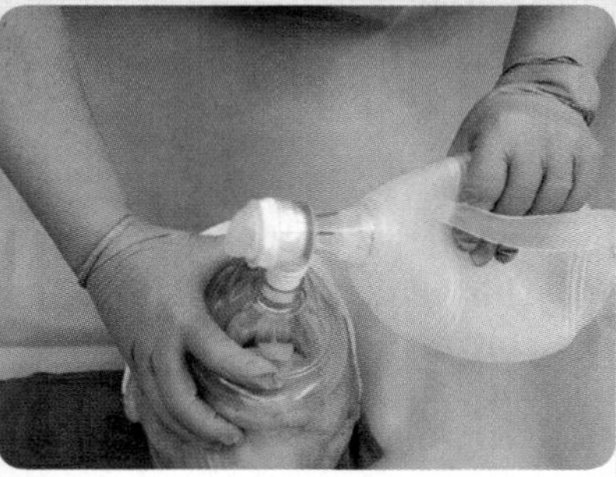

Step 2 Preoxygenate the patient for 2 to 3 minutes with a bag-mask device and 100% oxygen.

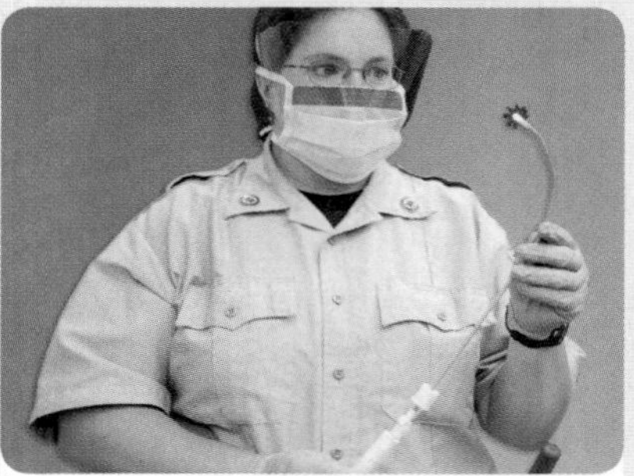

Step 3 Check, prepare, and assemble your equipment.

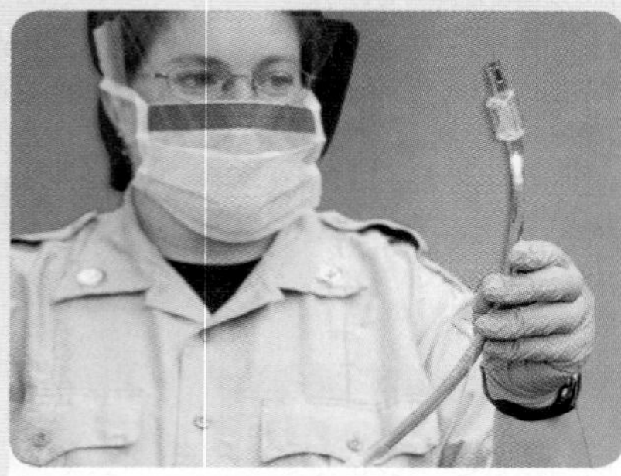

Step 4 Insert the lighted stylet into the ET tube.

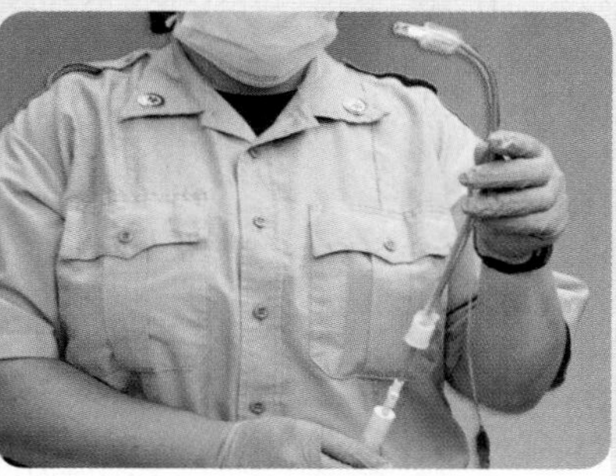

Step 5 Bend the ET tube by placing a slight curve at its distal end (like a hockey stick), and turn on the lighted stylet.

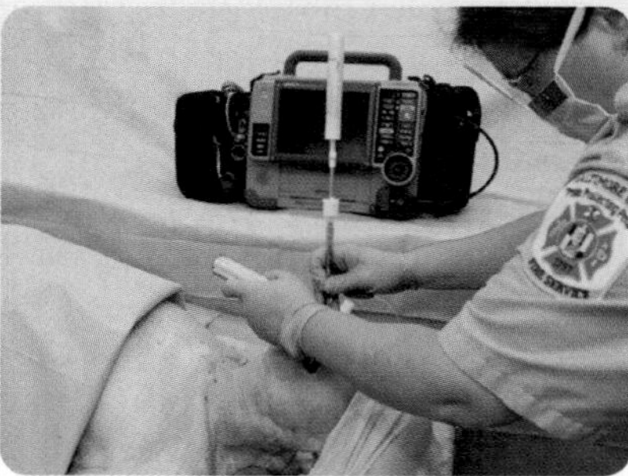

Step 6 Lift the patient's tongue and mandible anteriorly.

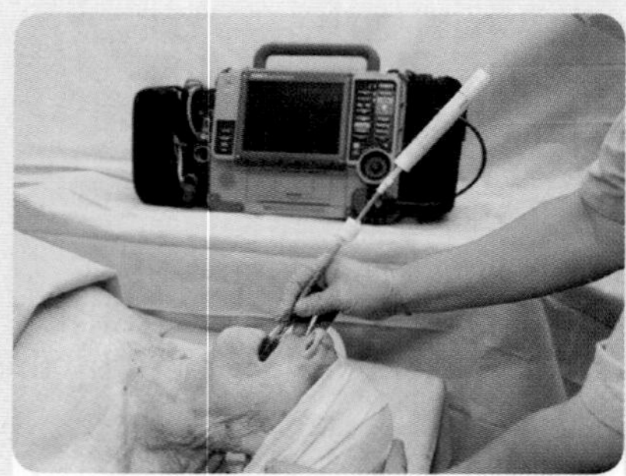

Step 7 Insert the ET tube into the midline of the patient's mouth and slowly advance toward the larynx, but stop before passing through the vocal cords.

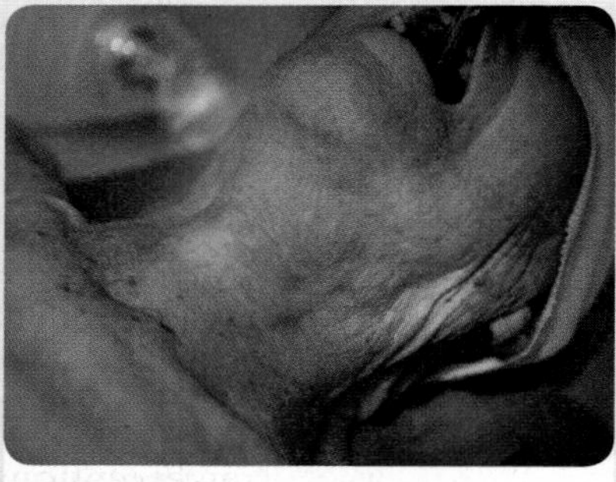

Step 8 Observe for a tightly circumscribed light at the midline of the neck, and advance the ET tube approximately 1 to 1.5 inches (2 to 4 cm) farther.

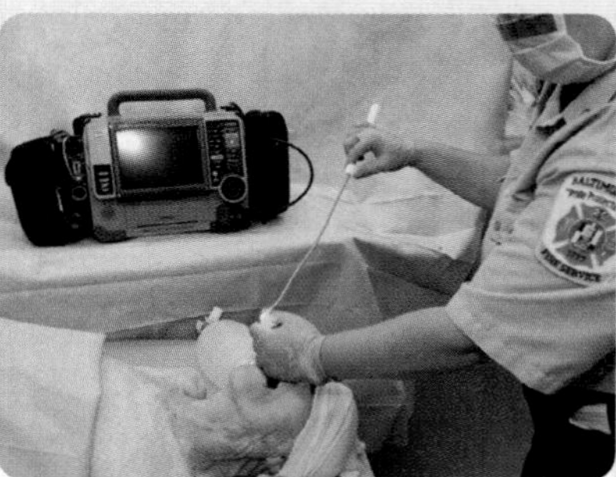

Step 9 Remove the stylet from the ET tube.

Skill Drill 15-12 Performing Transillumination Intubation *(continued)*

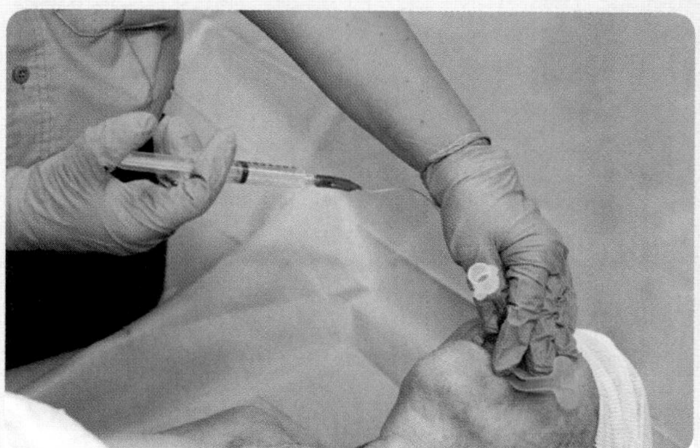

Step 10 Inflate the distal cuff of the ET tube with 5 to 10 mL of air, and immediately detach the syringe.

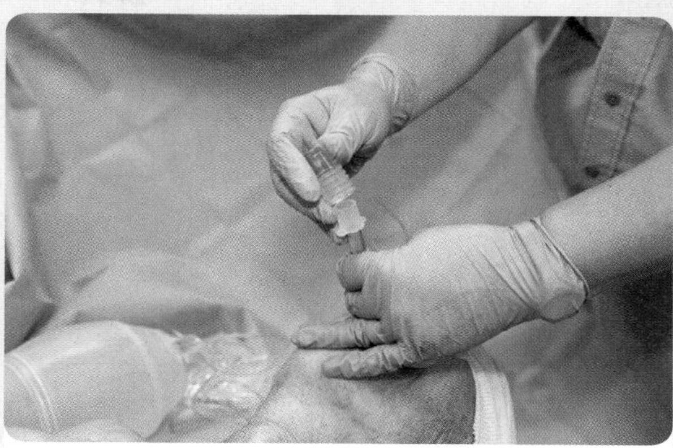

Step 11 Attach the $ETCO_2$ detector (waveform capnography preferred) to the ET tube.

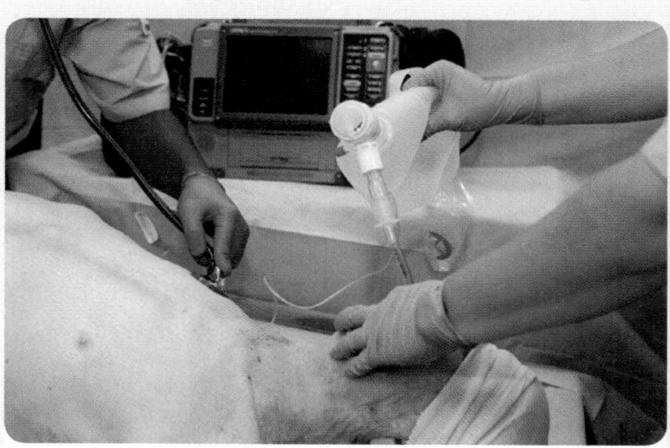

Step 12 Attach the ventilation device, ventilate, and auscultate over the apices and bases of both lungs and over the epigastrium. Ensure proper tube placement with waveform capnography.

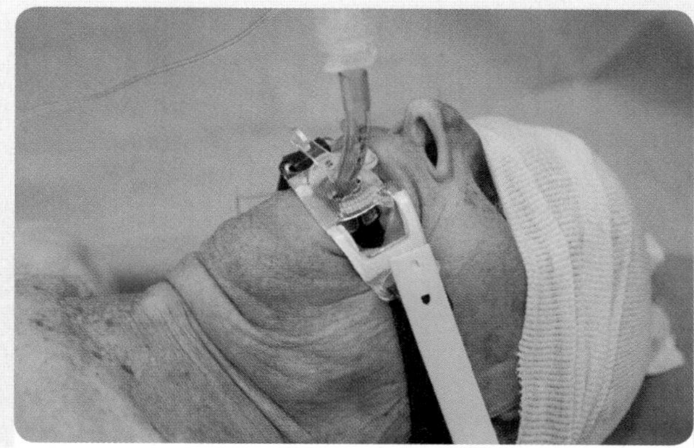

Step 13 Secure the ET tube, and recheck breath sounds.

The steps for performing retrograde intubation are shown in Skill Drill 15-13.

▶ Face-to-Face Intubation

You may perform intubation with the your face at the same level as the patient's face when other positions are not possible—for example, in a motor vehicle crash in which the patient is seated in a tight space and the space above the head cannot be accessed, or when the seated patient suddenly becomes unconscious and apneic. This technique is called **face-to-face intubation**. The procedure is essentially the same as orotracheal intubation using direct laryngoscopy, with the following exceptions:

- The patient's head cannot be placed in the sniffing position. It is manually stabilized by a second paramedic during the entire procedure.
- The laryngoscope (with a curved [Macintosh] blade) is held in the right hand with the blade facing downward like a hatchet, and the ET tube is held in the left hand. The laryngoscope

Skill Drill 15-13 Performing Retrograde Intubation

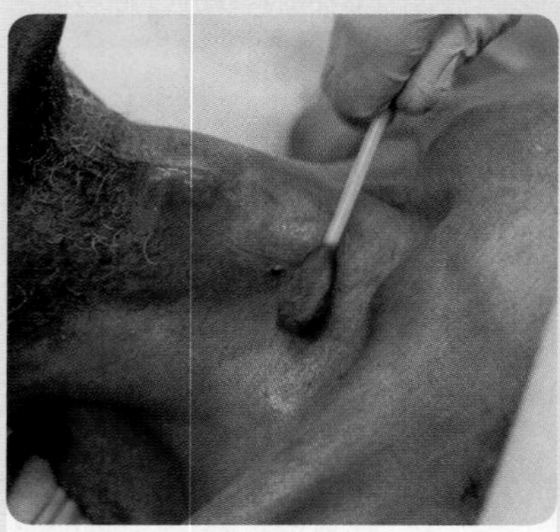

Step 1 Take standard precautions. Place the patient supine. Ventilate the patient with 100% oxygen via the appropriate device while preparing the equipment and the patient. Cleanse the anterior part of the neck from the laryngeal prominence to just below the cricoid ring.

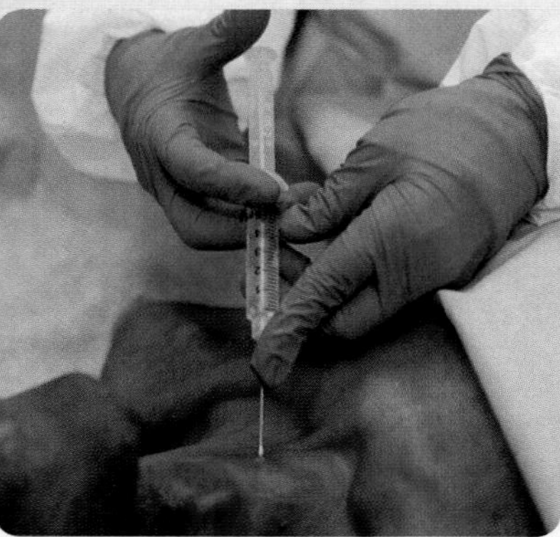

Step 2 If the patient is responsive, then consider numbing the area over the cricothyroid membrane using a local anesthetic.

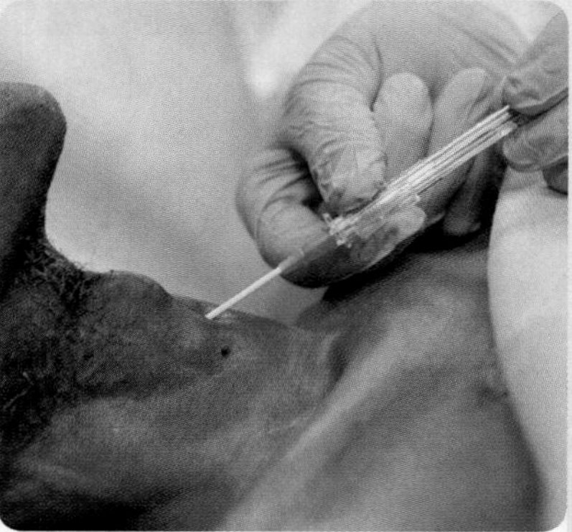

Step 3 Puncture the cricothyroid membrane using a large needle aligned with the airway and pointed approximately 30° cephalad (toward the head), perpendicular at the level of the cricothyroid membrane.

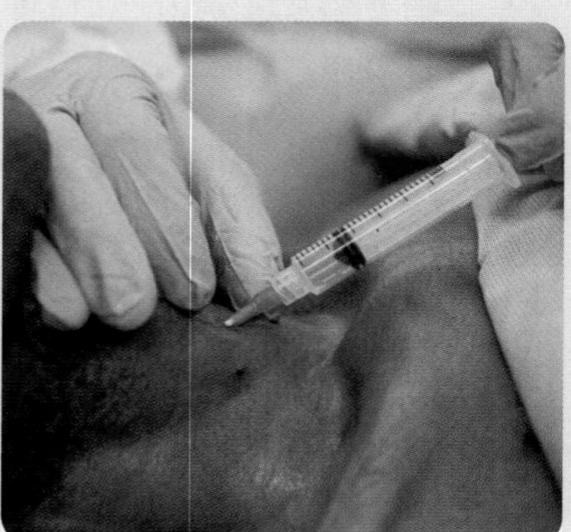

Step 4 Identify the tracheal lumen by aspirating air into the syringe attached to the needle.

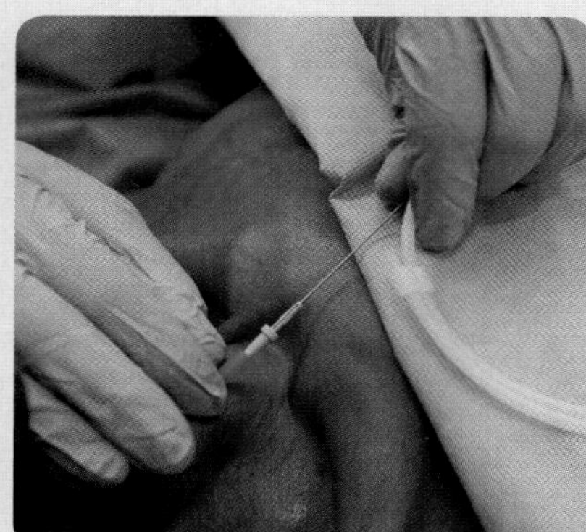

Step 5 Pass the 28-inch (70-cm) guide wire through the catheter until it appears in the oropharynx.

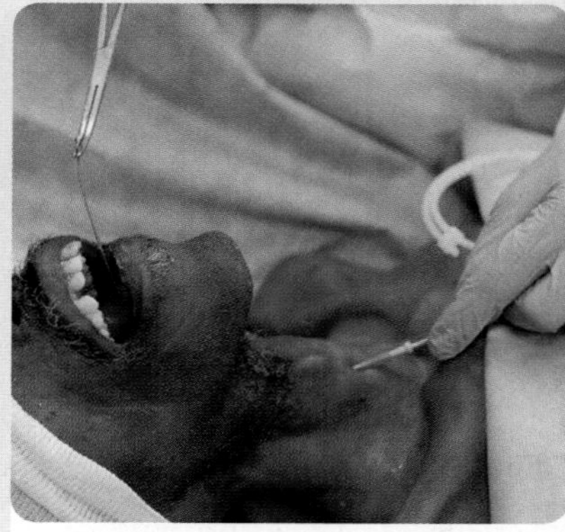

Step 6 Grasp the guide wire with a clamp or Magill forceps, and pull the wire partially out of the mouth, ensuring that the distal end is still emerging from the neck and the wire is pulled taut.

Skill Drill 15-13 Performing Retrograde Intubation *(continued)*

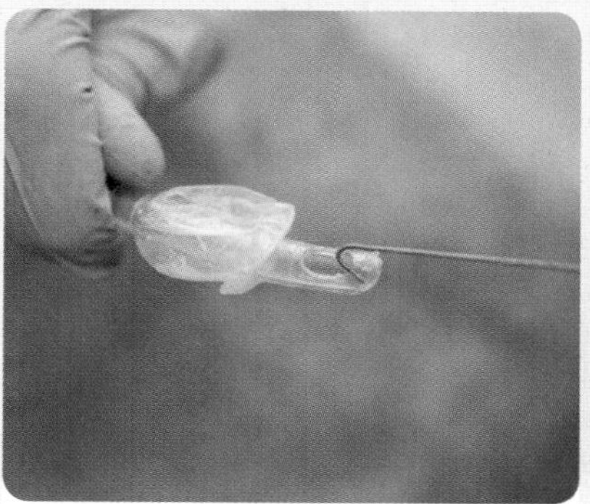

Step 7 Insert the guide wire emerging from the mouth, through the lumen of the ET tube.

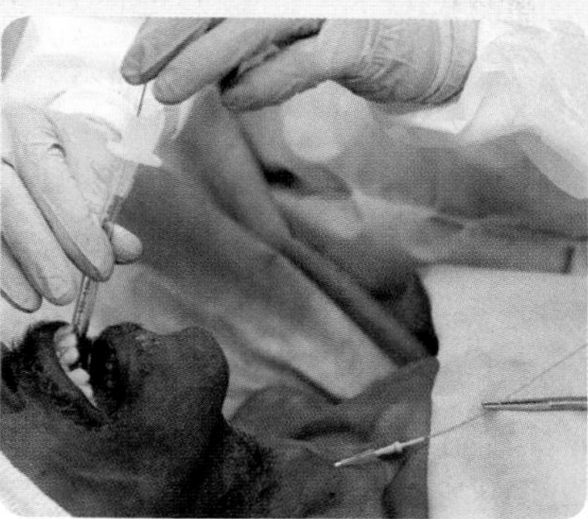

Step 8 Advance the ET tube into the trachea.

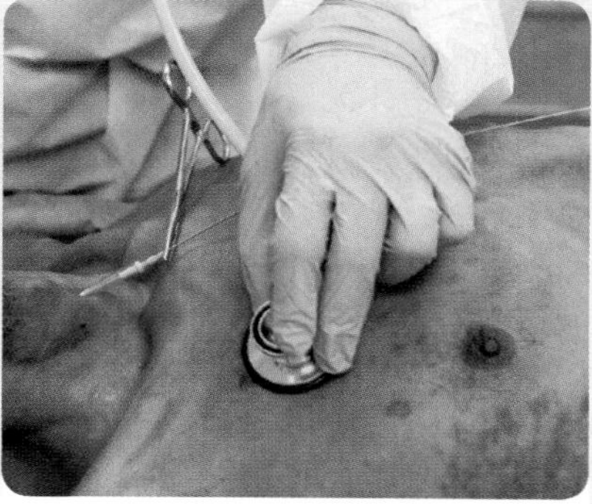

Step 9 Verify tube placement by auscultating the lungs bilaterally and over the epigastrium. Attach an $ETCO_2$ detector (waveform capnography preferred) to ensure proper tube placement.

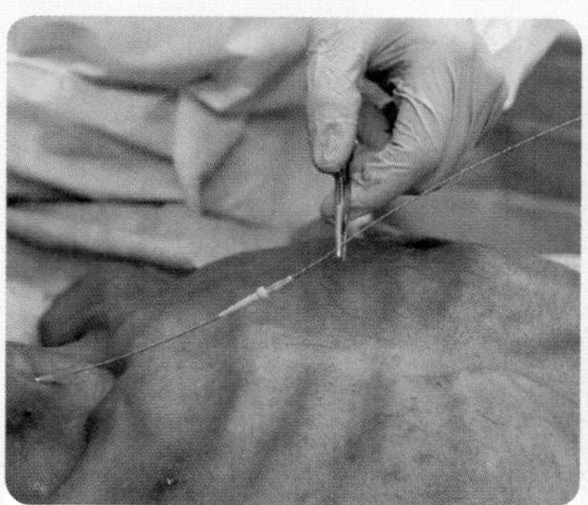

Step 10 After tube placement is confirmed, remove the guide wire by pulling on the distal end emerging from the neck, then advance the tube approximately 1 inch (2 to 3 cm) farther.

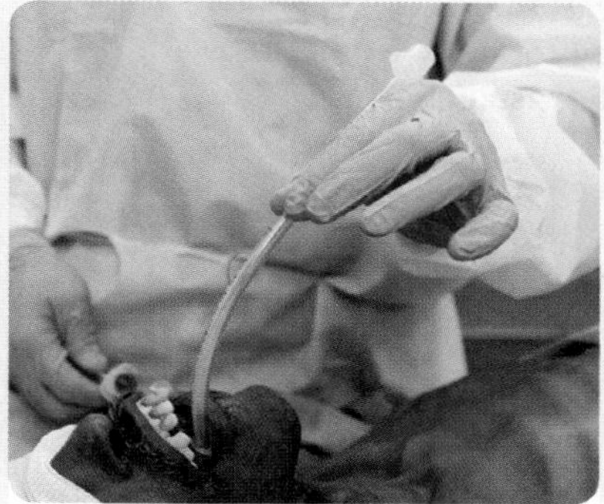

Step 11 If tube placement is incorrect, then remove the tube and attempt to ventilate. If ventilating adequately, then continue to ventilate with high-flow oxygen and reassess. Determine whether additional attempts at retrograde intubation are warranted or whether another means of securing the airway is necessary (such as cricothyrotomy).

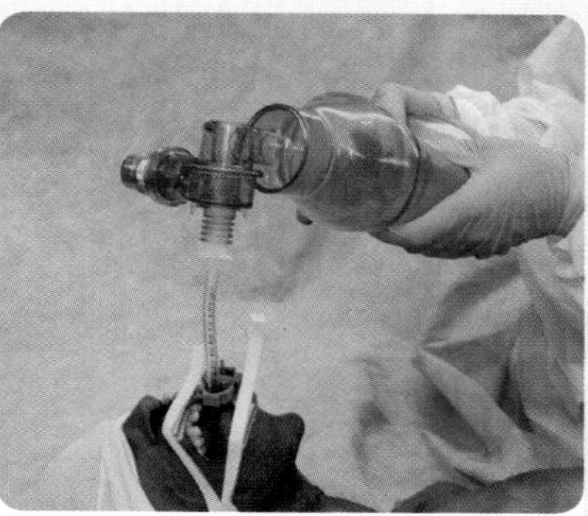

Step 12 Secure the ET tube in place and continue to ventilate.

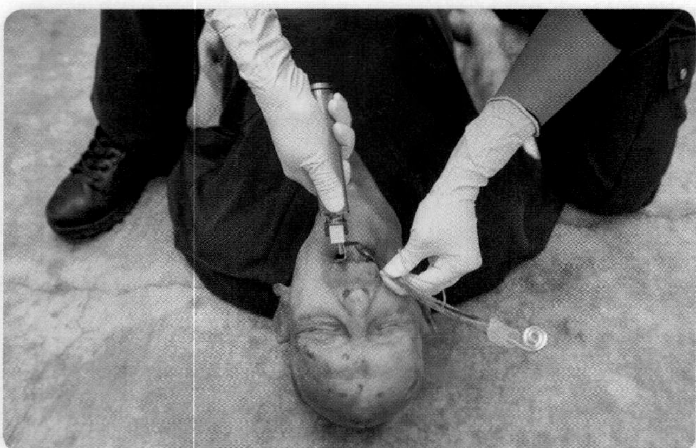

Figure 15-92 To perform face-to-face intubation, hold the laryngoscope in your right hand, with the blade facing downward, and hold the endotracheal (ET) tube in your left hand. Insert the blade in the right side of the patient's mouth and sweep the tongue to the patient's left. Adjust the patient's head, if needed, to improve your view and advance the ET tube until the cuff is 0.5 to 0.75 inches (1 to 2 cm) past the vocal cords.

blade is inserted into the right side of the patient's mouth, the tongue is swept to the patient's left, and the vocal cords are visualized Figure 15-92.

- After the laryngoscope blade has been placed, you may slightly adjust the patient's head for better visualization by pulling the mandible forward while pressing down.

▶ Failed Intubation

A study using data from 40 states demonstrated an overall prehospital ET intubation success rate of 85.3%.[11] At the service and regional level, intubation is an extremely important procedure to be closely monitored by physician-led quality-assurance efforts, because the implications for failed intubation—and, more importantly, an unrecognized misplaced ET tube (in the esophagus)—is significant for the paramedic, the medical director of the EMS agency, and the regional system. In addition, failed intubation can be potentially fatal to the patient.

A failed airway attempt is defined as the failure to maintain an acceptable oxygen saturation level during or after one or more failed intubation attempts, or a total of three failed intubation attempts by an experienced intubator—even when the oxygen saturation level can be maintained. Methods to minimize complications of airway management have been discussed in this chapter. However, you frequently do not have a choice of methods in the prehospital setting. So, what do you do? Many rescue airway techniques are available.

Words of Wisdom

ET Intubation: Points to Remember

- Never attempt ET intubation before the patient has been adequately preoxygenated.
- Assemble and check all equipment before you begin.
- Position is everything! Ensure that the patient's head is in the proper position to align the airway axes.
- Do not rush. Work with deliberate speed.
- Get it right the first time. The second attempt will likely be more difficult. Remember that it is acceptable to manage the airway with BLS techniques until a more experienced provider is available to insert an advanced airway.
- Confirm the ET tube is in the right place. Take nothing for granted.
- Secure the ET tube appropriately. Otherwise, you might soon be trying to reinsert it.
- Even when the ET tube is properly secured, stabilize it with your hand as you ventilate the patient.
- Consider applying head blocks after intubating a patient. Doing so will minimize the amount of head movement and the risk of inadvertent extubation.
- Reconfirm proper ET tube placement after any major patient move (ie, from the ground to the stretcher, after loading into the ambulance, transferring the patient to the hospital stretcher).
- Perform simple BLS airway maneuvers with an oral airway and/or a nasal airway and a bag-mask device. With good technique, you can provide adequate oxygenation and ventilation. The objective is to ventilate and oxygenate—not intubate.
- Consider using a rescue airway device, such as the King LT, LMA, or i-gel (all of which are discussed later in this chapter)

Tracheobronchial Suctioning

Tracheobronchial suctioning involves passing a suction catheter into the ET tube to remove pulmonary secretions. The first rule to remember about performing tracheobronchial suctioning is this: Do not do it if you do not have to! This kind of suctioning requires strict attention to sterile technique, which is nearly impossible to maintain in the prehospital environment. Suctioning the trachea can also cause cardiac dysrhythmias; cardiac arrest has been reported during tracheobronchial suctioning. For these reasons, you should avoid suctioning through an ET tube unless secretions are so massive that they interfere with ventilation. If you must perform tracheobronchial suctioning, then use sterile technique (if possible), and monitor the patient's cardiac rhythm and oxygen saturation during the procedure.

Preoxygenation of the patient is essential before performing tracheobronchial suctioning. Lubricate a soft-tip (whistle-tip) catheter, and ensure maximal preoxygenation. It may be necessary to inject 3 to 5 mL of sterile water down the ET tube to loosen extremely thick pulmonary secretions.

Gently insert the suction catheter down the ET tube until you feel resistance. Apply suction while the catheter is extracted, taking care not to exceed 10 seconds in an adult. After tracheobronchial suctioning is complete, reattach the ventilation device, continue ventilations, and reassess the patient.

The steps for performing tracheobronchial suctioning are shown in Skill Drill 15-14.

▶ Field Extubation

As mentioned previously, extubation is the process of removing the ET tube from an intubated patient. Patients are rarely extubated in the prehospital setting. Generally, the only reason to consider performing extubation in the field is a patient who is unreasonably intolerant of the ET tube (for example, extremely combative, gagging, or retching). In general, it is safer to sedate the patient rather than remove the ET tube, but sedation (discussed next) may not be an option in all EMS systems or for patients in hemodynamically unstable condition. Before performing field extubation, you should contact medical control or follow locally established protocols.

The most obvious risk associated with extubation is overestimation of the patient's ability to protect his or her own airway. In addition, when extubation is performed on responsive patients, a high risk of laryngospasm exists, and most patients experience some degree of upper airway swelling because of the trauma of having the tube in the trachea. These two facts, along with the ever-present potential for vomiting, make successful reintubation challenging, if not impossible. If you are not absolutely sure that you can reintubate the patient, then do not remove the ET tube. Instead, sedate the patient. If you used a paralytic drug to facilitate intubation, then consider administering additional doses, if allowed by local protocol, in conjunction with a sedative. Field extubation is absolutely contraindicated if any risk exists of recurrent respiratory failure or uncertainty about a patient's ability to maintain his or her own airway spontaneously.

If field extubation is necessary, then first ensure that the patient is adequately oxygenated. Discuss the procedure with the patient, and explain what you plan

YOU are the Paramedic — PART 8

After calling in your radio report to the hospital, you note the patient is taking occasional spontaneous breaths, and you can see his eyes moving around beneath his eyelids. You will arrive at the hospital in approximately 8 minutes and the patient's vital signs indicate hemodynamic stability.

Recording Time: 35 Minutes	
Level of consciousness	Spontaneous eye movement noted
Respirations	4 breaths/min (baseline); 12 breaths/min via positive pressure ventilation
Pulse	106 beats/min; regular and strong
Skin	Pink, warm, and dry
Blood pressure	134/78 mm Hg
Oxygen saturation (Spo_2)	98% (with positive pressure ventilation and supplemental oxygen)
$ETCO_2$	41 mm Hg; normal waveform
ECG	Sinus tachycardia

13. Is a neuromuscular blocking agent (paralytic) indicated for this patient? Why or why not?

Skill Drill 15-14 Performing Tracheobronchial Suctioning

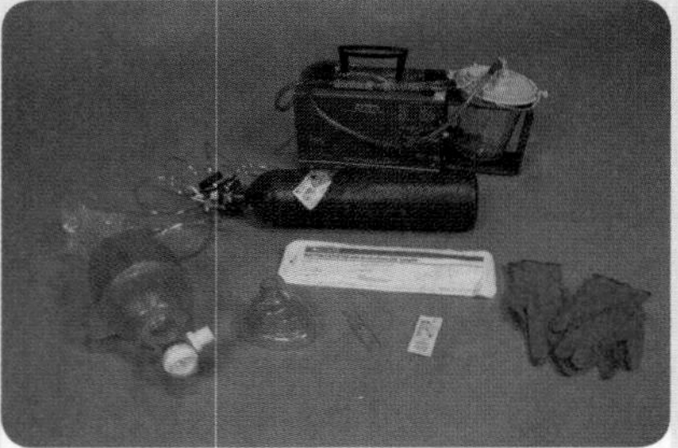

Step 1 Check, prepare, and assemble your equipment.

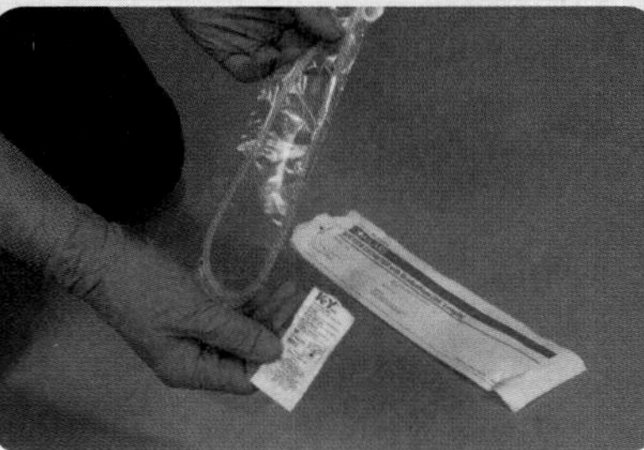

Step 2 Lubricate the suction catheter.

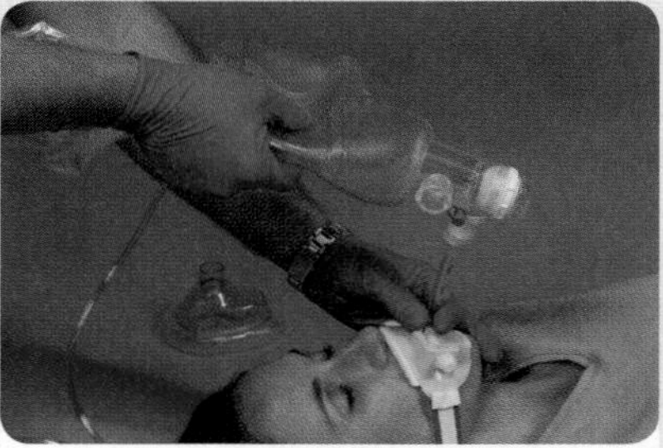

Step 3 Preoxygenate the patient.

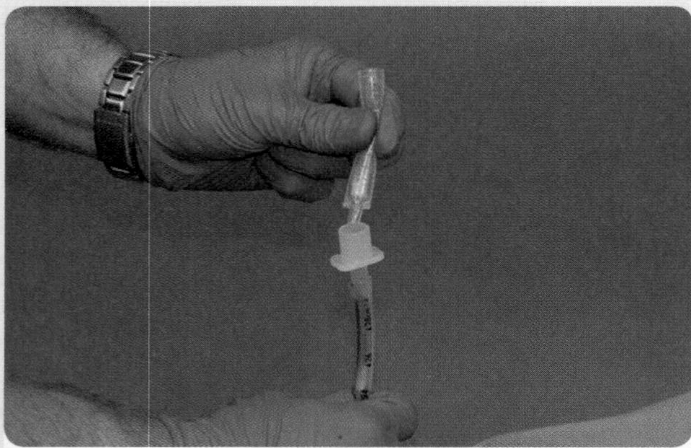

Step 4 Detach the ventilation device. If absolutely necessary to mobilize very thick secretions, consider injecting 3 to 5 mL of sterile water down the ET tube using sterile technique.

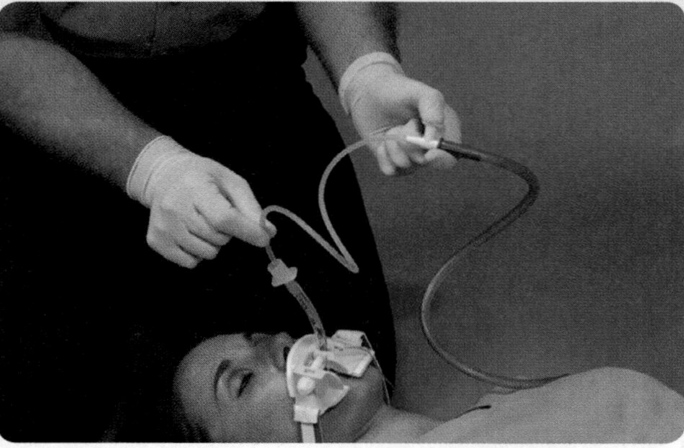

Step 5 Gently insert the catheter into the ET tube until you feel resistance.

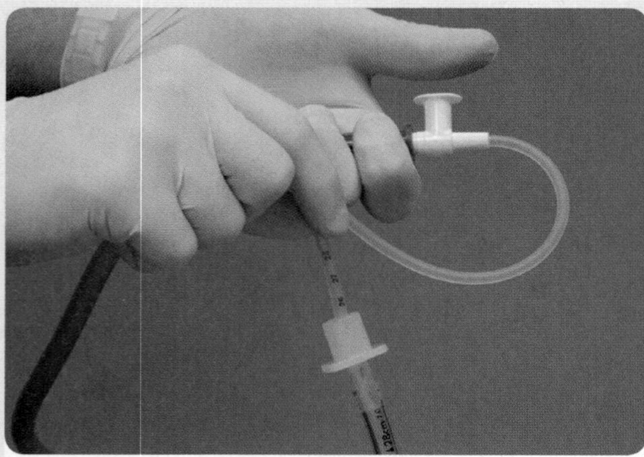

Step 6 Suction in a rotating motion while withdrawing the catheter. Monitor the patient's cardiac rhythm and oxygen saturation level during the procedure.

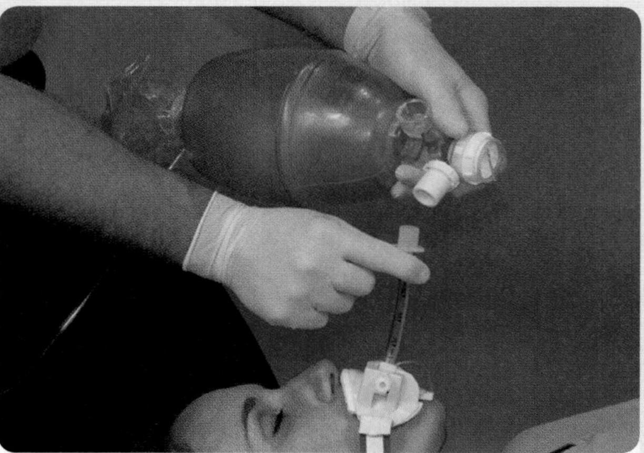

Step 7 Reattach the ventilation device, and resume ventilation and oxygenation.

to do. If possible, then have the patient sit up or lean slightly forward so that he or she is in a safe position should vomiting occur after extubation. Assemble and have available all equipment to suction, ventilate, and reintubate, if necessary. After confirming that the patient remains responsive enough to protect his or her own airway, suction the oropharynx to remove any secretions or debris that may threaten the airway after the tube has been removed. Deflate the distal cuff on the ET tube while the patient begins to exhale so that any accumulated secretions proximal to the cuff are not aspirated into the lungs. On the next exhalation, remove the tube in one steady motion, following the curvature of the airway. Place a towel or emesis basin in front of the patient's mouth in case vomiting occurs.

Pharmacologic Adjuncts to Airway Management and Ventilation

Pharmacologic agents in airway management are used to decrease the discomfort of intubation, decrease the incidence of complications associated with laryngoscopy and intubation, and make aggressive airway management possible for patients who need it but are unable to cooperate.

Sedation in Emergency Intubation

Sedation is used in airway management to reduce a patient's anxiety, induce amnesia, and decrease the gag reflex. It is useful for anxious, combative, or agitated patients and for patients who need aggressive airway management but who are too responsive to tolerate intubation. If used properly and under the correct circumstances, then sedation effectively increases patient compliance and comfort, making definitive airway management easier and safer to perform. If used improperly, however, then it can cause further harm.

The complications associated with sedation in airway management are related primarily to undersedation and oversedation. Undersedation can result in inadequate patient cooperation, the complications of gagging (such as trauma, tachycardia, hypertension, vomiting, and aspiration), and incomplete amnesia of the event. Oversedation can result in uncontrolled general anesthesia,

Words of Wisdom

Hypersensitivity to sedative medications is the primary contraindication to the use of these drugs. Obtain an accurate and thorough medical history, to the extent possible, before giving any drug to any patient.

Table 15-14 Sedatives Used in Airway Management

Drug Type	Examples
Benzodiazepines: sedative-hypnotic	Diazepam (Valium) Midazolam (Versed)
Dissociative anesthetics	Ketamine (Ketalar)
Narcotics (opioids): sedative-analgesic	Fentanyl (Sublimaze) Alfentanil (Alfenta)
Nonnarcotics/ nonbarbiturates: sedative-hypnotic	Etomidate (Amidate)

loss of protective airway reflexes, respiratory depression, complete airway collapse, and hypotension.

The level of sedation desired dictates the amount of medication administered. A patient's response to sedatives is dose-dependent. Follow local protocol or contact medical control regarding the appropriate dose for a given patient.

Two major classes of sedatives are commonly used in airway management: analgesics and sedative-hypnotics Table 15-14. Analgesics decrease the perception of pain. Sedative-hypnotics induce sleep and decrease anxiety; they do not reduce pain.

Benzodiazepines

Benzodiazepines are sedative-hypnotic drugs. Diazepam (Valium) and midazolam (Versed) provide muscle relaxation and mild sedation and are used extensively as anxiolytic and antiseizure medications. They also provide **anterograde amnesia**, which is beneficial for invasive or uncomfortable procedures; the patient likely will not recall the event.

Midazolam is two to four times as potent as diazepam, is faster acting, and has a shorter duration of action. Some clinicians use midazolam to induce general anesthesia before intubation; however, the likelihood of complications increases because of the large dose necessary to induce muscle relaxation. In general, the use of neuromuscular blockers (paralytics) to achieve muscle relaxation is preferred because neuromuscular blockers require smaller doses to achieve the desired effect.

Respiratory depression and hypotension are potential side effects of benzodiazepine administration. Flumazenil (Romazicon) is a benzodiazepine antagonist that can reverse the effects of diazepam and midazolam.

Dissociative Anesthetics

A **dissociative anesthetic** is a medication that produces anesthesia by distorting the patient's perception of sight and sound and inducing a feeling of detachment (dissociation) from environment and self. Unlike benzodiazepines, which primarily produce a sedative state, dissociative anesthetics produce anesthesia through hallucinogenic, amnestic, analgesic, and sedative effects. Ketamine (Ketalar) is a common dissociative anesthetic in emergency medicine; it is rapid-acting and has a relatively short duration of action. At lower (subdissociative) doses (0.2 to 0.3 mg/kg), ketamine is commonly used as an analgesic. Higher doses (2 mg/kg) induce sedation and are commonly given prior to a neuromuscular blocker to facilitate intubation.

Ketamine produces a sympathomimetic effect, which makes it a hemodynamically stable choice among sedative induction agents when performing emergency airway management in patients with hypotension.

In some patients, **reemergence phenomenon** may occur during the end of the half-life of ketamine, when the patient is awakening. Reemergence phenomena may range from pleasant dreams to vivid nightmares and delirium. Benzodiazepines have been shown to reduce the incidence of reemergence phenomenon, as well as to calm the patient if severe reemergence phenomenon occurs.

Opioids/Narcotics

Opioids, a type of narcotic, are potent analgesics with sedative properties. Narcotics are used in emergency airway management as a premedication, during induction, and in maintenance of sedation or amnesia. The two most commonly used narcotics for airway management are fentanyl (Sublimaze) and alfentanil (Alfenta). Fentanyl is 70 to 150 times more potent than morphine. It has a rapid onset of action and a relatively short duration of action. Alfentanil is less potent than fentanyl but has a faster onset of action and a shorter duration of action. It is also eliminated from the body faster.

Opioids can cause profound respiratory and CNS depression and produce severe hypotension and bradycardia, especially in patients who are in hemodynamically unstable condition. These negative effects can be reversed with naloxone (Narcan), a narcotic antagonist.

Nonnarcotics/Nonbarbiturates

Etomidate (Amidate) is a nonnarcotic, nonbarbiturate hypnotic-sedative drug often used in the induction of general anesthesia. It is a fast-acting agent of short duration. This drug has little effect on pulse rate, blood pressure, and ICP and does not cause the histamine release and bronchoconstriction that may occur with other agents. However, a high incidence of uncomfortable myoclonic muscle movement is associated with its use. Etomidate is a useful induction agent in patients with coronary artery disease, increased ICP, or borderline hypotension/hypovolemia.

> **Words of Wisdom**
>
> You should consider combativeness, aggressiveness, and belligerence as signs of cerebral hypoxia until proven otherwise. Be firm and direct, but still treat your patients with respect and empathy. Keep in mind that they are fighting for their lives, not with you.

▶ Neuromuscular Blockade in Emergency Intubation

Cerebral hypoxia can make an ordinarily calm person combative, aggressive, belligerent, and uncooperative, resulting in a difficult and potentially dangerous situation—both for the patient and for you. A patient with cerebral hypoxia must be treated with aggressive oxygenation and ventilation, but combativeness or other resistive behavior often makes this task difficult, if not impossible. Clenching of the patient's teeth due to spasm of the jaw muscles (trismus) and laryngospasm can also hamper your efforts to obtain a definitive airway.

Historically, physical restraint of a combative patient was common to enable obtaining a definitive airway. A safer, more effective approach is chemical paralysis with **paralytics**, collectively known as neuromuscular blocking agents. With the patient chemically sedated and paralyzed, a loss of his or her protective airway reflexes occurs; you can effectively perform oxygenation and ventilation, and the patient will not gag during insertion of an ET tube.

Neuromuscular Blocking Agents

Although sedatives alone can be used to facilitate intubation—especially in patients who already have a markedly depressed gag reflex—it is often necessary to administer a drug specifically designed to induce paralysis. Paralytic drugs affect every skeletal muscle in the body, including the diaphragm and the intercostal muscles. Within approximately 1 to 2 minutes of receiving an IV dose of a paralytic, a patient will become totally paralyzed. That is, the patient will stop breathing; his or her jaw muscles will go slack, and the base of the tongue will fall back against the posterior pharynx and obstruct the airway. Put bluntly, paralytics convert a breathing patient with a marginal airway into an apneic patient with no airway. Before you bring about such a change, you must be absolutely sure that you can protect the patient's airway and ensure adequate oxygenation and ventilation. Although it is optimal to insert an ET tube, you must have other airway devices (such as a King LT or i-gel) readily available if ET intubation is unsuccessful. After a patient is paralyzed, you are completely responsible for the patient's breathing and well-being. Fortunately, paralytic agents do not affect cardiac or smooth muscle.

A paralyzed patient appears to be asleep or unresponsive, but is not! Paralytic agents, unlike sedatives, have no effect on LOC. The patient is fully aware and can hear, feel, and think. Do not administer a paralytic without sedating the patient first!

▶ Pharmacology of Neuromuscular Blocking Agents

To understand how medications induce paralysis, recall how skeletal muscles contract. All skeletal (striated) muscles are voluntary and require input from the somatic nervous system to initiate contraction. As an impulse to contract reaches the terminal end of a motor nerve, **acetylcholine (ACh)** is released into the synaptic cleft (the junction between the nerve cell and the muscle cell). This neurotransmitter diffuses across the short distance of the synaptic cleft and binds to receptor sites on the motor end plate. ACh occupying the receptor sites triggers changes in electrical properties of the muscle fiber, a process called depolarization. When enough motor end plates have been depolarized, a threshold is reached and the muscle fiber contracts. Depolarization lasts for only a few milliseconds because of the presence of acetylcholinesterase, an enzyme that quickly removes ACh from the synaptic cleft and from the receptors on the motor end plate.

Paralytic medications function at the neuromuscular junction and relax the muscle by impeding the action of ACh. They are classified into two categories: depolarizing and nondepolarizing agents. Table 15-15 lists the standard doses for these agents used in the prehospital setting.

Table 15-15 Neuromuscular Blocking Agent Doses

Drug	Standard Dose
Succinylcholine (depolarizing)	1–2 mg/kg via IV push (initial dose); a repeat dose can be given based on the patient's clinical response
Vecuronium bromide[a] (nondepolarizing)	0.1–0.2 mg/kg via IV push (initial adult dose); maintenance dose within 45 to 60 minutes: 0.8 to 1.2 mg/kg. Initial pediatric dose: 0.1 to 0.3 mg/kg IV/IO; maintenance dose within 20 to 40 minutes: 0.01 to 0.015 mg/kg IV push.
Pancuronium bromide[a] (nondepolarizing)	0.06–0.1 mg/kg via slow IV (initial adult dose). Repeat every 30–60 minutes as needed. *Pediatric:* 0.04 to 0.1 mg/kg slow IV/IO.
Rocuronium bromide[a] (nondepolarizing)	0.6–1.2 mg/kg IV/IO. *Pediatric* (older than 3 months): 0.6–1.2 mg/kg IV/IO.

Abbreviation: IV, intravenous

[a] Consider administering 10% of the initial dose (defasciculating dose) before administering succinylcholine.

Words of Wisdom

Paralysis Versus Sedation

Imagine what it must be like to be completely paralyzed. You cannot blink, talk, move, or, most important, breathe! You are completely dependent on others to keep you alive. Paralytic agents do not induce sedation or amnesia. If you administer only a paralytic agent, then the patient will be fully responsive and remember the entire event. Therefore, unless contraindicated, you must sedate a patient before administering a paralytic. Paralysis without sedation is a form of patient abuse!

▶ Depolarizing Neuromuscular Blocking Agent

A **depolarizing neuromuscular blocker** competitively binds with the ACh receptor sites but is not affected as quickly by acetylcholinesterase. Therefore, it causes depolarization of the muscle and prevents future signals for depolarization from having an effect because all of the ACh receptor sites are already occupied.

Succinylcholine chloride (Anectine) is a depolarizing neuromuscular blocking agent. Because succinylcholine causes depolarization, **fasciculations**—characterized by brief, uncoordinated twitching of small muscle groups in the face, neck, trunk, and extremities—can be observed during its administration. These fasciculations tend to cause generalized muscle pain at the termination of paralysis (when the succinylcholine wears off).

Depolarizing neuromuscular blockers are characterized by a very rapid onset (60 to 90 seconds) of total paralysis and a relatively short duration of action (5 to 10 minutes). For this reason, succinylcholine is often used as an initial paralytic. With this drug, if you are unable to secure the patient's airway, then you have to support ventilation for only a short period before the patient can breathe again on his or her own.

Use succinylcholine with caution. The drug may be contraindicated, in patients with burns, crush injuries, and blunt trauma—that is, conditions that can result in hyperkalemia. In addition, because its chemical structure is similar to that of ACh, succinylcholine can cause bradycardia, especially in pediatric patients. Administration of atropine sulfate, which may prevent succinylcholine-induced bradycardia, should be considered prior to administering succinylcholine to pediatric patients.

Words of Wisdom

Not all patients require additional doses of a paralytic medication after intubation. In many cases, additional doses of a sedative medication (ie, midazolam, ketamine) will facilitate patient compliance and allow you to continue to support oxygenation and ventilation. However, if the patient's clinical condition dictates it, then you may need to administer additional doses of a paralytic. Remember to keep the patient adequately sedated.

Nondepolarizing Neuromuscular Blocking Agents

Nondepolarizing neuromuscular blockers also bind to ACh receptor sites; however, unlike depolarizing neuromuscular blockers, they do not cause depolarization of the muscle fiber. When given in sufficient quantity, the amount of nondepolarizing medication exceeds the amount of ACh in the synaptic cleft, and the critical threshold of depolarization cannot be achieved. Thus, when nondepolarizing paralytics are administered in small quantities before administering a depolarizing paralytic, they prevent fasciculations. The defasciculating dose is typically 10% of the normal dose; it does not induce paralysis, but causes weakness.

The most commonly used nondepolarizing neuromuscular blockers are vecuronium bromide (Norcuron), pancuronium bromide (Pavulon), and rocuronium bromide (Zemuron). All three agents have a duration of action longer than that of succinylcholine. **Vecuronium** has a rapid onset of action (2 minutes) and a duration of action of about 45 minutes. **Rocuronium** has a rapid onset of action (less than 2 minutes) and a duration of action of 45 to 60 minutes. **Pancuronium** also has a rapid onset of action (3 to 5 minutes) and a duration of action of approximately 60 minutes.

Nondepolarizing neuromuscular blockers, because of the longer duration of action, are ideal when a patient requires extended periods of paralysis, such as a prolonged transport time or when the patient's airway has been secured and you need to manage other injuries or conditions. However, do not give these agents before you have secured the patient's airway.

▶ Rapid Sequence Intubation

Rapid sequence intubation (RSI), also referred to as rapid sequence induction or drug-assisted intubation, represents a culmination and integration of all of your airway, problem-solving, and decision-making skills into one procedure. RSI includes the safe, smooth, and rapid induction of sedation and paralysis followed immediately by intubation. RSI has been successfully performed in the operating room for years, and its use in the prehospital setting has become increasingly popular. It is generally used for responsive or combative patients who need to be intubated, but are otherwise unable to tolerate laryngoscopy.

Preparation of the Patient and Equipment

The experience of being intubated is frightening for patients, so you must explain what you are going to do and reassure the patient that he or she will be asleep during the procedure and will not feel or remember anything. Apply a cardiac monitor/defibrillator and pulse oximeter. Check, prepare, and assemble your equipment, and ensure that it is in good working order. In particular, have suction immediately available.

Patient Safety

When the decision to perform RSI is made, it is critical for all team members to be aware of exactly what will occur. Side conversations should be avoided so that the entire team can remain focused on performing the procedure safely.

Preoxygenation

All patients undergoing RSI should be adequately preoxygenated before the procedure is begun. If the patient is breathing spontaneously and has adequate tidal volume, then apply high-flow oxygen via nonrebreathing mask. However, if the patient is hypoventilating, then assisted ventilations with a bag-mask device and high-flow oxygen may be necessary. Avoid bag-mask ventilation before RSI whenever possible to avoid gastric distention and the associated risks of regurgitation and aspiration.

Premedication

If your initial paralytic of choice is succinylcholine, then consider administering a defasciculating dose—typically 10% of the normal dose—of a nondepolarizing paralytic, if time permits. You may also consider administering atropine sulfate to decrease the incidence of bradycardia associated with the administration of succinylcholine. The usual dose for an adult is 0.5 mg, and for infants and children it is 0.02 mg/kg.

Sedation and Paralysis

As long as the patient is in hemodynamically stable condition (systolic blood pressure of greater than 90 mm Hg), administer a sedative agent to induce sedation and amnesia. As soon as the patient is adequately sedated, administer the paralytic agent. The onset of paralysis will be quick and should be complete within 2 minutes. Observe for apnea and check for laxity (looseness) of the mandible; these are signs of adequate paralysis.

Intubation

The procedure of intubation is no different for RSI than it is for any other situation. "Rapid sequence" refers to the rapid administration of medications. If you cannot accomplish the intubation within a short period and/or if the patient's oxygen saturation level falls, then stop and ventilate the patient with a bag-mask device and 100% oxygen. When the patient's oxygen saturation level returns to an acceptable level, reattempt intubation. If you must ventilate the patient with a bag-mask device, then do so slowly (1 second per breath—just enough to produce visible chest rise).

After the tube is in the trachea, inflate the cuff, remove the stylet, verify correct position of the ET tube (by auscultation and continuous waveform capnography). Secure the tube in place as usual, and continue ventilations at the appropriate rate.

Maintenance of Paralysis and Sedation

When you are absolutely sure that you have successfully intubated the trachea, depending on your transport time and the patient's clinical status, additional paralytic administration may be necessary. If you administered succinylcholine initially (with a short duration of action), then administer a nondepolarizing agent (such as vecuronium or rocuronium) to maintain long-term paralysis. If you administered a long-acting paralytic initially, then additional dosing is usually not necessary for short transport times. Administer additional sedation as needed if the patient's blood pressure is adequate.

Although the general steps of RSI are the same for all patients, some modification is necessary for patients in unstable condition. If the patient's oxygen saturation level drops, then you have no choice except to ventilate (slowly). If the patient is in hemodynamically unstable condition, then you must judge whether sedation is appropriate or whether the risk of profound hypotension is too great to sedate the patient before inducing paralysis. Table 15-16 lists sample protocols for RSI in patients in hemodynamically stable and unstable condition.

Words of Wisdom

You should attempt RSI only if you are confident that you will be able to intubate and ventilate the patient, or to keep the patient oxygenated and ventilated if intubation is unsuccessful. Otherwise, a patient who has been sedated and paralyzed will die. Above all, do no harm!

Evidence-Based Medicine

Many patients who require ET intubation are hypoxemic, but you cannot preoxygenate them because of their mental status (ie, agitation, delirium, combativeness). In such cases, a procedure called **delayed sequence intubation (DSI)** could offer an alternative to RSI. DSI is intended to facilitate the process of preoxygenation, allowing you to safely secure the airway while avoiding oxygen desaturation. DSI is essentially a procedural sedation, in which case the procedure is preoxygenation.

The procedure for DSI begins by placing the patient in a head-up position of at least 15°, ensuring the earlobes are aligned with the sternum. Continuous monitoring of the patient's ECG and oxygen saturation (Spo_2), $ETCO_2$, and blood pressure values are essential.

After you have prepared the patient and all monitoring parameters are in place, administer a dissociative dose of ketamine (1 to 1.5 mg/kg). Ketamine is the ideal DSI induction agent because it preserves airway reflexes and does not supress the patient's respiratory drive. You may give additional, smaller doses (0.5 mg/kg) of ketamine if needed, until the desired effect is achieved. After 10 to 15 seconds, administer oxygen at 15 L/min via nonrebreathing mask and nasal cannula to the patient, which initiates the process of denitrogenation. **Denitrogenation** attempts to replace alveolar nitrogen with oxygen; the goal is to achieve an intrapulmonary oxygen reserve that will allow apnea to be prolonged as long as possible with the least possible oxygen desaturation. If the patient's Spo_2 level is less than 95%, then use noninvasive positive pressure ventilation with CPAP or a bag-mask device with a PEEP valve.

After ensuring that the patient's Spo_2 can be maintained above 95% for 3 minutes, administer a paralytic (succinylcholine or rocuronium). Leave the nasal cannula in place at 15 L/min. The patient is intubated after approximately 90 seconds.

If the patient's Spo_2 cannot be maintained above 95% during the intubation attempt, then repeat the process of denitrogenation for another 3 minutes. If several intubation attempts prior to desaturation are unsuccessful, the DSI procedure is aborted altogether and the patient is allowed to reassociate (ie, the ketamine is allowed to wear off).

Table 15-16 Sample Protocols for RSI

For patients in hemodynamically stable condition:

1. Prepare the patient and equipment.
2. Preoxygenate with 100% oxygen for at least 2 to 3 min.
3. Consider administering a defasciculating dose of a nondepolarizing paralytic.
4. Sedate.
5. Administer succinylcholine.
6. Intubate and verify correct ET tube placement.
7. Properly secure the ET tube.
8. Administer a nondepolarizing paralytic (standard dose), as needed, and maintain adequate sedation.
9. Clearly document all medications administered, the times administered, and confirmation of tube placement.

For patients in hemodynamically unstable condition:

1. Prepare the patient and equipment.
2. Preoxygenate and ventilate as necessary.
3. Consider sedation.
4. Administer succinylcholine.
5. Intubate and confirm correct ET tube placement.
6. Properly secure the ET tube.
7. Administer a nondepolarizing paralytic. If you are able to achieve hemodynamic stability, then administer sedation as needed.
8. Clearly document all medications administered, the times administered, and confirmation of tube placement.

Abbreviations: ET, endotracheal; RSI, rapid sequence intubation

Evidence-Based Medicine

Oxygen uptake by the alveoli will continue, even when the diaphragm is not moving and the lungs are not expanding. In an apneic patient, approximately 250 mL/min of oxygen will move from the alveoli to the bloodstream. A much smaller amount of carbon dioxide—only 8 to 20 mL/min—moves into the alveoli; the remainder is buffered in the bloodstream. The difference in oxygen and carbon dioxide movement across the alveolar membrane is due to the difference in gas solubility in the blood, as well as the affinity of hemoglobin for oxygen. As a result, the net pressure in the alveoli becomes subatmospheric, which generates a flow of gas from the pharynx to the alveoli. This process is called **apneic oxygenation** and it allows oxygenation to continue, even though the patient is apneic. The administration of supplemental oxygen via nasal cannula at 15 L/min before and after the patient has been chemically sedated and paralyzed has been shown to extend normal oxygen saturations, thereby reducing hypoxic events that can occur during the period of forced apnea that RSI induces.[12]

Alternative Advanced Airway Devices

Supraglottic Airway Devices

King LT Airway

The **King LT airway** is a latex-free, single-use, single-lumen airway that is blindly inserted into the esophagus **Figure 15-93**. You can use the King LT to provide positive pressure ventilation to apneic patients and maintain a patent airway in unresponsive patients who are breathing spontaneously, but who require advanced airway management. The King LT is available in both adult and pediatric sizes.

The device consists of a curved tube with ventilation ports located between two inflatable cuffs. Both cuffs are inflated simultaneously using a single valve. When the airway is properly placed in the esophagus, the distal cuff seals the esophagus, and the proximal cuff seals the oropharynx **Figure 15-94**. Openings located between these two cuffs provide ventilation of the lungs after positioning is confirmed. You can use the King LT as a rescue airway device if intubation is unsuccessful.

Two types of King LT airway are available: the King LT-D and the King LTS-D. The King LTS-D is the more commonly used device; it is available in seven sizes that are based on the patient's height and/or weight. Each size has a different color of proximal connector and requires different cuff inflation pressures. **Table 15-17** lists sizes and patient criteria for the King LTS-D. Each kit contains a single King LT, a syringe for cuff inflation, water-soluble gel, and instructions for use.

The King LT-D (see Figure 15-93) and the King LTS-D share most of the same features. Both have a proximal pharyngeal cuff and a distal cuff and several ventilation outlets at the distal part of the tube. In both, an ET tube introducer (a gum elastic bougie) can be inserted through the tube, where it exits at a "ramp" between the

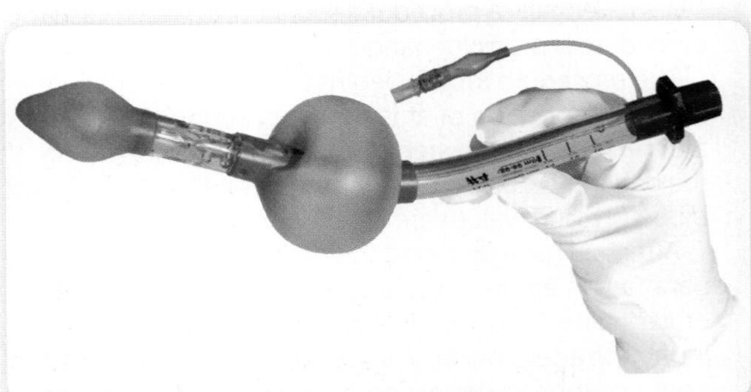

Figure 15-93 The King LT airway is a single-lumen airway that is blindly inserted into the esophagus. The King LT-D model is shown here.

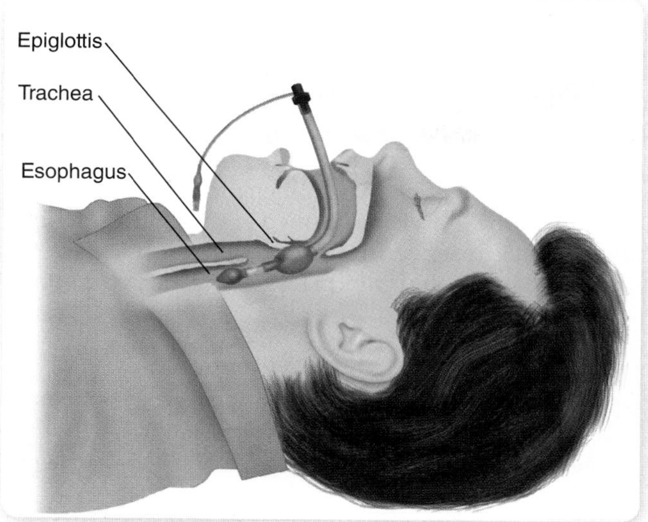

Figure 15-94 Placement of the King LT airway. When properly placed, the distal cuff seals the esophagus, and the proximal cuff seals the oropharynx.

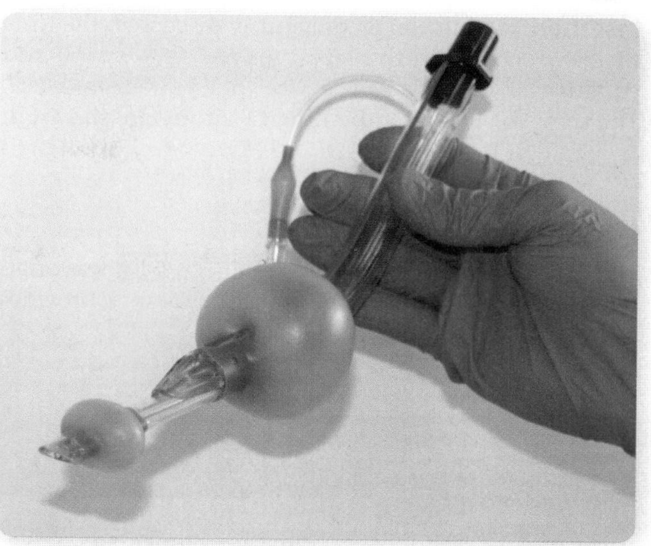

Figure 15-95 The King LTS-D.

Courtesy of Candice M. Thompson, NREMT-P.

Table 15-17 Sizes and Patient Criteria for the King LTS-D

Size	Connector Color	Patient Criteria: Height and Weight[a]	Cuff Volume
0	Transparent	<11 lb (5 kg)	10 mL
1	White	11–26 lb (5–12 kg)	20 mL
2	Green	35–45 in. (90–115 cm) or 26–55 lb (12–25 kg)	35 mL
2.5	Orange	41–51 in. (105–130 cm) or 55–77 lb (25–35 kg)	40–45 mL
3	Yellow	4–5 ft (122–155 cm)	50–60 mL
4	Red	5–6 ft (155–180 cm)	70–80 mL
5	Purple	>6 ft (180 cm)	80–90 mL

[a] Sizes 0 and 1 are weight-based. Sizes 2 and 2.5 are weight- and/or height-based. Adult sizes (sizes 3–5) are height-based.

Data from: Ambu King LTS-D Disposable Laryngeal Tube. Ambu USA website. December 2015 version. http://www.ambuusa.com/usa/products/anesthesia/product/king_lts-d%E2%84%A2_disposable_laryngeal_tube-prod17813.aspx. Accessed February 21, 2017.

pharyngeal and distal cuffs. If you need to insert an ET tube, then simply insert the tube introducer through the King airway and into the trachea. Next, remove the King airway, and direct an ET tube into the trachea by placing it over the tube introducer.

The distal end of the King LT-D is closed, whereas the distal end of the King LTS-D is open. This opening permits insertion of a suction catheter (up to size 18F) through a gastric access lumen on the proximal end of the King LTS-D for gastric decompression **Figure 15-95**.

Indications for the King LT Airway. The King LT airway is an alternative to bag-mask ventilation when a rescue airway device is required for a failed intubation attempt. The King LT airway has the same advantages, disadvantages, complications, and special considerations as the Combitube (discussed later in this chapter).

Contraindications for the King LT Airway. The King LT airway does not eliminate the risk of vomiting and aspiration. High airway pressures can cause air to leak into the stomach or out of the mouth. Do not use the King LT airway in patients with an intact gag reflex, patients with known esophageal disease, or patients who have ingested a caustic substance. As with other advanced airway devices, proper placement is confirmed by observing chest rise, auscultating the lungs and epigastrium, and using waveform capnography.

Complications of the King LT Airway. It is reasonable to assume that laryngospasm, vomiting, and possible hypoventilation may occur. Trauma may also result from improper insertion technique. Ventilation may be difficult if the pharyngeal balloon pushes the epiglottis over the glottic opening. If this complication occurs, then gently withdraw the device—without deflating the cuffs—until ventilation becomes easier.

Insertion Technique. As previously discussed, the King LT airway comes in five sizes; the patient's height and weight will determine the size that you should use. The steps for inserting the King LT airway are shown in Skill Drill 15-15.

Laryngeal Mask Airway

The **laryngeal mask airway (LMA)** Figure 15-96 was originally developed for use in the operating room. It provides a viable option for patients who require more airway and ventilatory support than bag-mask ventilation can provide, but it does not require ET intubation.

The LMA is designed to provide a conduit from the glottic opening to the ventilation device. It surrounds the opening of the larynx with an inflatable silicone cuff positioned in the hypopharynx. When properly inserted, the opening of the LMA is positioned at the glottic opening, and the tip is inserted into the proximal esophagus, the lateral portions in the piriform fossae, and the upper border

NR Skill

Skill Drill 15-15 Inserting a King LT Airway

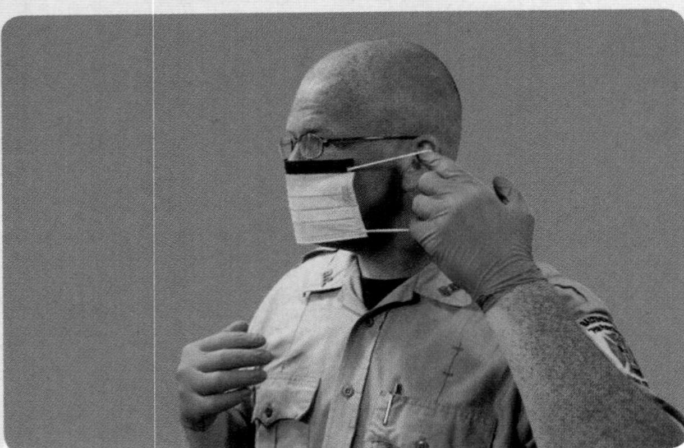

Step 1 Take standard precautions.

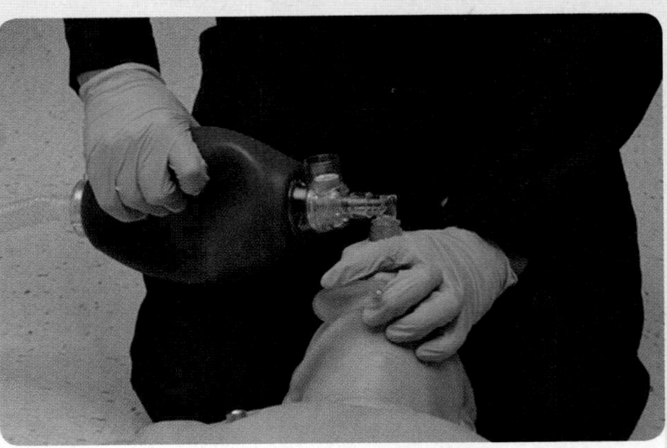

Step 2 Preoxygenate the patient with a bag-mask device and 100% oxygen.

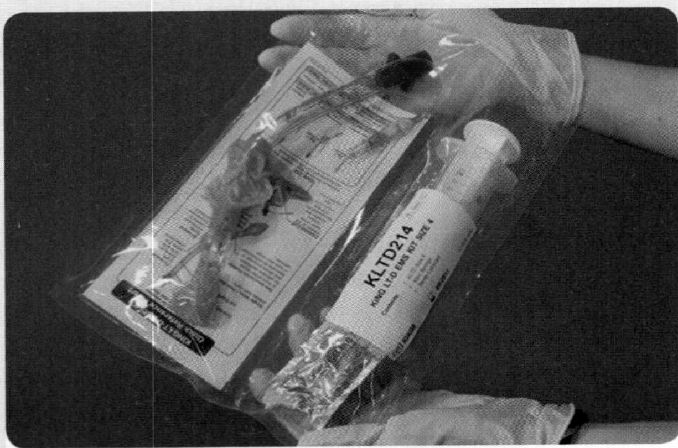

Step 3 Gather your equipment. Choose the proper size of King LT airway for the patient. Test the cuffs for proper inflation. Ensure all air is removed from the cuffs before insertion. Lubricate the tip of the device with a water-soluble gel for easy insertion and minimal airway damage.

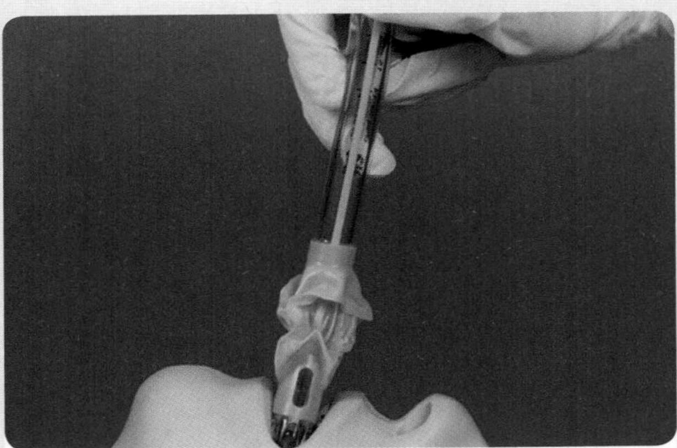

Step 4 Place the patient's head in a neutral position, unless contraindicated (use the jaw-thrust maneuver if you suspect trauma). In your dominant hand, hold the King LT at the connector. With your other hand, hold the patient's mouth open while positioning the head. Insert the tip of the King LT airway into the midline of the mouth.

Skill Drill 15-15 Inserting a King LT Airway *(continued)*

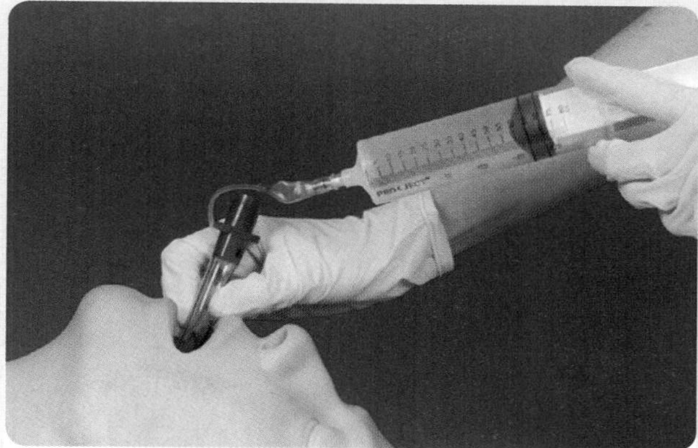

Step 5 Advance the tip beyond the base of the tongue. If you meet resistance, then rotate the device slightly, change your angle, and advance it again. Continue to gently advance the device until the base of the connector is aligned with the patient's teeth or gums. Do not use excessive force. Inflate the cuffs with the recommended amount of air or just enough to seal the device.

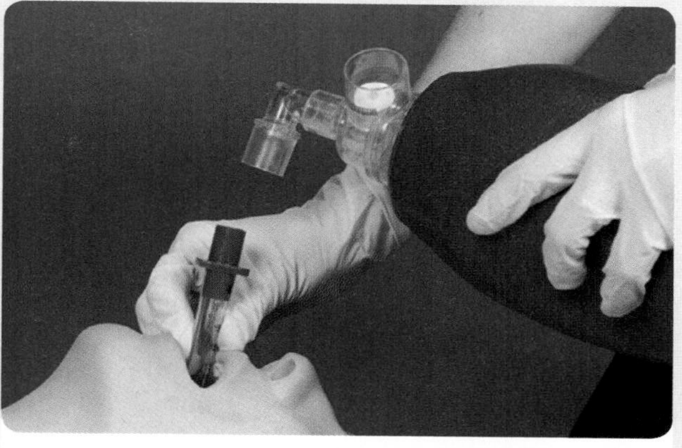

Step 6 Attach the tube to the ventilation device, and confirm tube placement by auscultating the lungs and epigastrium and attaching waveform capnography. Add additional air to the cuffs to maximize airway seal, if needed; however, avoid exceeding the manufacturer's recommended maximum amount of air. After placement is confirmed, continue to ventilate the patient.

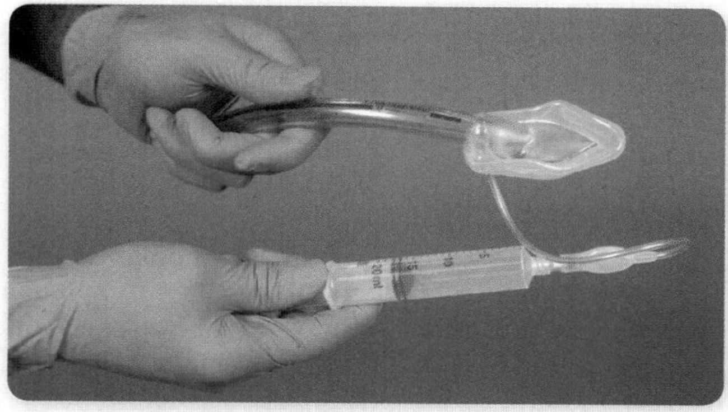

Figure 15-96 The laryngeal mask airway.

at the base of the tongue. The inflatable cuff conforms to the contours of the airway and forms a relatively airtight seal **Figure 15-97**.

Indications and Contraindications for the LMA. Consider the LMA as one possible alternative to bag-mask ventilation when the patient cannot be endotracheally intubated. Do not consider the LMA as a primary airway in emergency situations.

The LMA is less effective in patients with obesity and you should not use it in patients with morbid obesity. Pregnant patients and patients with a hiatal hernia are at an increased risk for regurgitation; evaluate such patients carefully if you are considering use of the LMA. The LMA is ineffective for the ventilation of patients requiring high pulmonary pressures (such as patients with COPD or heart failure).

Advantages and Disadvantages of the LMA. The LMA has many advantages compared with ventilating an unprotected airway with a bag-mask device. The LMA may provide better ventilation than a bag-mask device and an oral and/or nasal airway, and ventilation with an LMA does not require the continual maintenance of a mask seal. Compared with ET intubation, LMA insertion is easier because it does not require laryngoscopy. Significantly less risk exists for soft-tissue, vocal cord, tracheal wall, and dental trauma than with ET intubation and other forms of intubation that rely on blocking the esophagus. The LMA provides protection from upper airway secretions, and the tip of the LMA wedged into the proximal esophagus most likely provides some obturation.

The main disadvantage of the LMA—especially in emergency situations—is that it does not provide protection

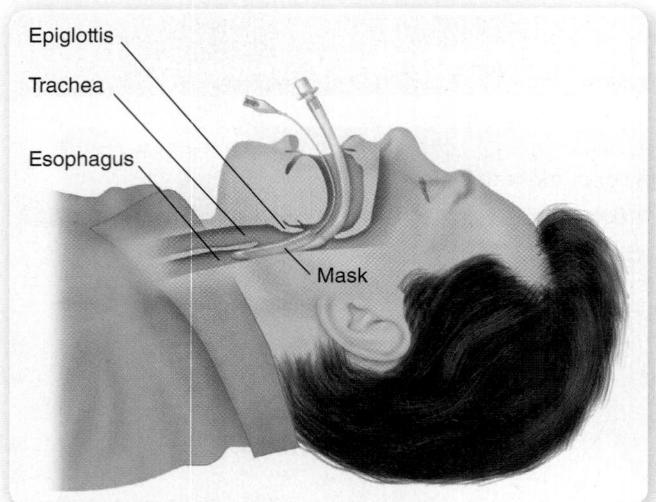

Figure 15-97 When properly positioned, the opening of the laryngeal mask airway is at the glottic opening, the tip is at the entrance of the esophagus, the lateral portions is in the piriform fossae, and the upper border is at the base of the tongue.

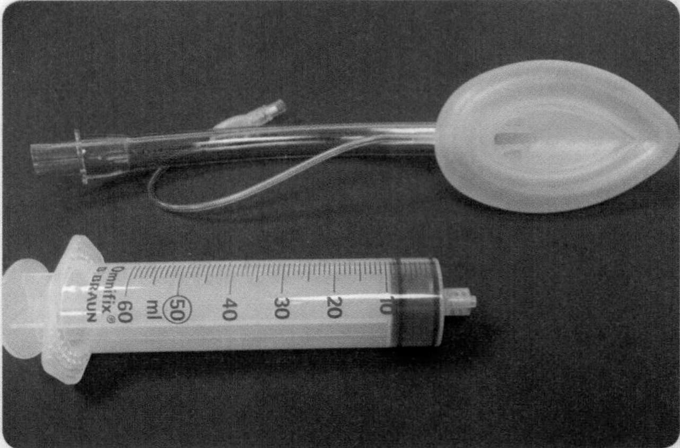

Figure 15-98 The laryngeal mask airway with the cuff inflated.

against aspiration. In fact, the LMA increases the risk of aspiration if the patient regurgitates, because the stomach contents would most likely be directed into the trachea.

During prolonged LMA ventilation, some air may be insufflated into the stomach because the seal made in the airway is not airtight. Because of the risk of aspiration, it is unlikely that the LMA will ever replace ET intubation in prehospital emergency medical care.

Complications of the LMA. The most significant complications associated with use of the LMA involve regurgitation and subsequent aspiration. The product literature states that the LMA should be used only in patients who are fasting. Unfortunately, this limitation would eliminate all patients in emergency situations, who should always be presumed to have full stomachs. You must weigh the risk of aspiration against the risk of hypoventilation with bag-mask ventilation in the context of the clinical scenario.

Observe the patient for clinical indications of adequate ventilation (that is, chest rise and breath sounds) during LMA ventilation. Hypoventilation of patients who require high ventilatory pressures can also occur, and the patient should be monitored for evidence of upper airway swelling.

Equipment for the LMA. Several types of LMA are available, and the sizes are based on the patient's weight. The device consists of a tube and an inflatable mask cuff. The cuff provides a collar that positions the opening of the tube at the glottic opening when inflated. Two vertical bars at the opening of the tube prevent occlusion. The proximal end of the tube is fitted with a standard 15/22-mm adapter that is compatible with any ventilation device. The cuff

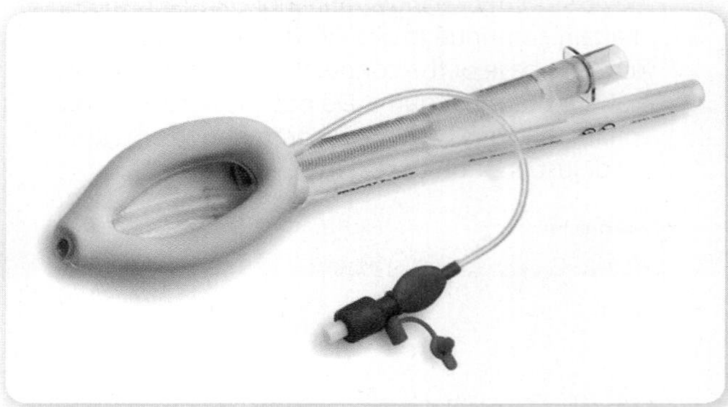

Figure 15-99 The ProSeal laryngeal mask airway.

has a one-way valve assembly and should be inflated with a predetermined volume of air (based on the size of the airway) Figure 15-98.

The LMA ProSeal has a built-in drain tube that allows expelled gastric contents to bypass the pharynx, thus reducing the risk of aspiration Figure 15-99. The LMA Supreme is an anatomically shaped device that features a gastric access port, thus enabling the insertion of a gastric tube without interrupting ventilations Figure 15-100.

A 6.0-mm ET tube can be passed through a size 3 or 4 LMA, allowing for intubation. The vertical bars are designed to allow a well-lubricated tube to pass straight through, and research in the operating room found a high success rate of ET intubation following this technique. The LMA Fastrach is designed to guide an ET tube into the trachea and may prove to be a viable alternative to direct laryngoscopy Figure 15-101.

Insertion Technique. Before insertion, check and prepare all equipment. The steps for inserting an LMA are shown in Skill Drill 15-16.

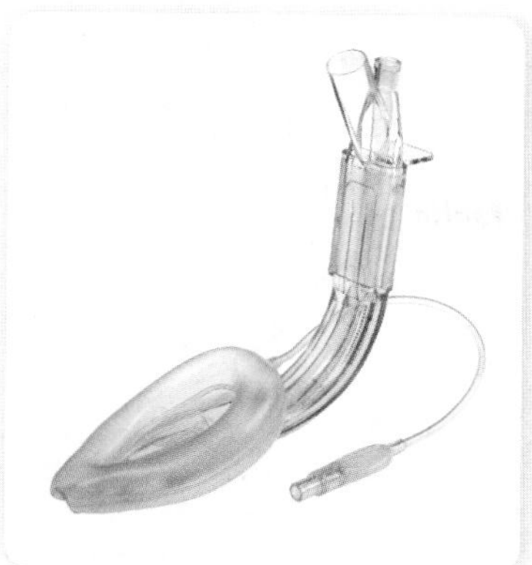

Figure 15-100 The Supreme laryngeal mask airway.

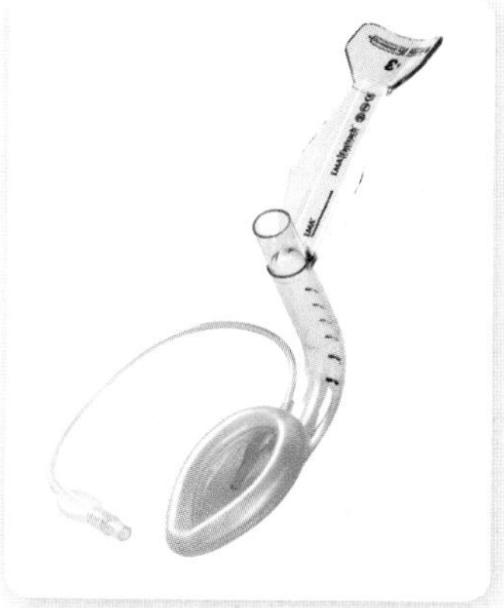

Figure 15-101 The Fastrach laryngeal mask airway with a 6.0-mm endotracheal tube.

Documentation & Communication

If adverse events occur with the use of advanced airway devices, such as bleeding or trauma, then be sure to document these occurrences on the PCR.

i-gel

The **i-gel** supraglottic airway is inserted in a manner similar to the LMA. This particular airway device was designed to create a noninflatable, anatomical seal of the pharyngeal, laryngeal, and perilaryngeal structures, while avoiding compression trauma that may occur from devices with an inflatable cuff Figure 15-102. The i-gel is a common rescue airway device and is a reasonable alternative when intubation is unsuccessful.

The i-gel features an integral bite block, a gastric access channel that allows for passage of a 12-Fr gastric tube, a supplemental oxygen inlet port to facilitate passive oxygenation, and a support strap to secure the i-gel in position. A color-coded, proximal hook ring indicates the size of the i-gel and serves as an anchor for the support strap. Furthermore, the size and weight range for the i-gel is printed on the device.

Like the LMA, the tip of the i-gel is designed to fit into the proximal esophagus, while the sides and proximal parts of the device form a seal around the hypopharynx. This position facilitates air entry into the trachea Figure 15-103. Table 15-18 lists three adult-sized i-gel supraglottic airways and patient weight criteria.

Skill Drill 15-16 Inserting an LMA

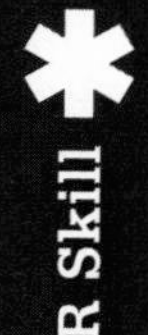

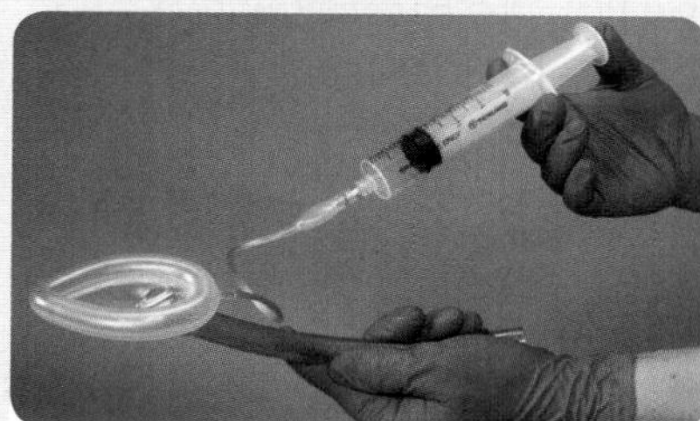

Step 1 Take standard precautions. Check the cuff of the LMA by inflating it with 50% more air than is required for the size of airway to be used.

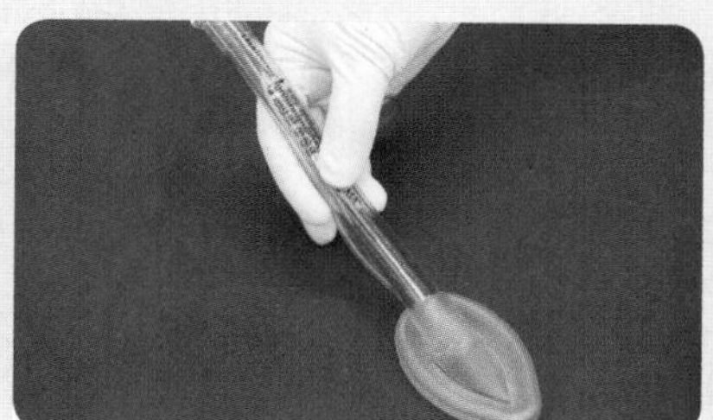

Step 2 Deflate the cuff completely, so that no folds appear near the tip. Deflation is best accomplished by pressing the device, cuff facing down, on a flat surface to remove all wrinkles from the cuff.

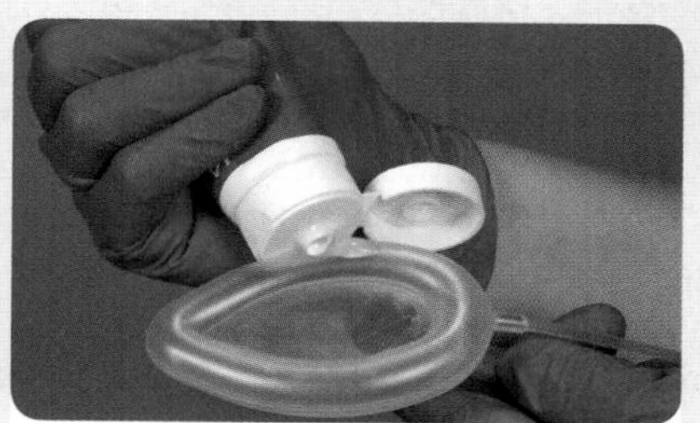

Step 3 Lubricate the outer rim of the device.

(continued)

Skill Drill 15-16 Inserting an LMA *(continued)*

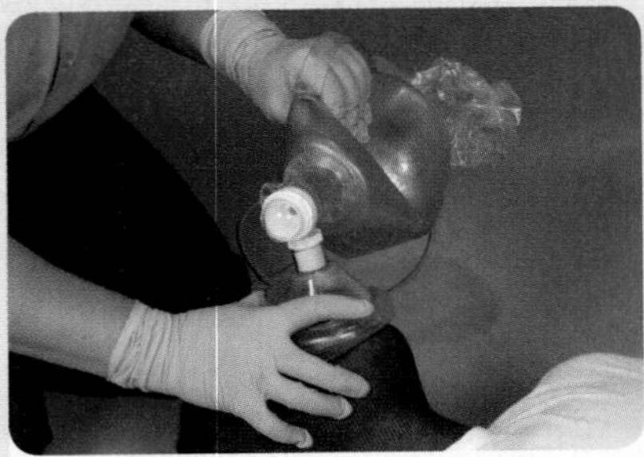

Step 4 Preoxygenate the patient before insertion. Do not interrupt ventilation for more than 30 seconds to accomplish airway placement. Place the patient in the sniffing position.

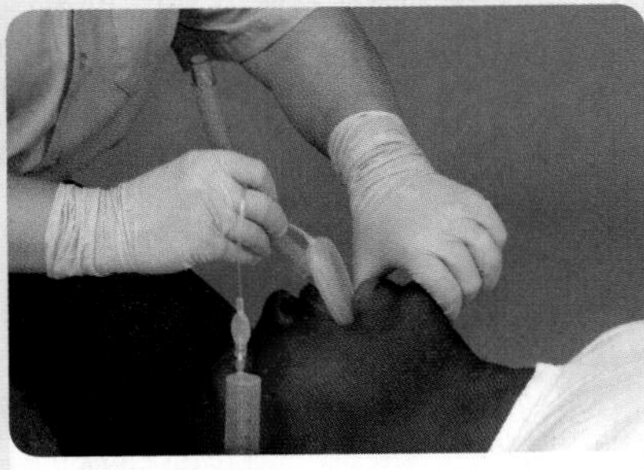

Step 5 Proper insertion of the LMA depends on holding the device properly. Insert your finger between the cuff and the tube. Place the index finger of your dominant hand in the notch between the tube and the cuff. Open the patient's mouth. Lift the jaw with one hand, and begin to insert the device with the other hand.

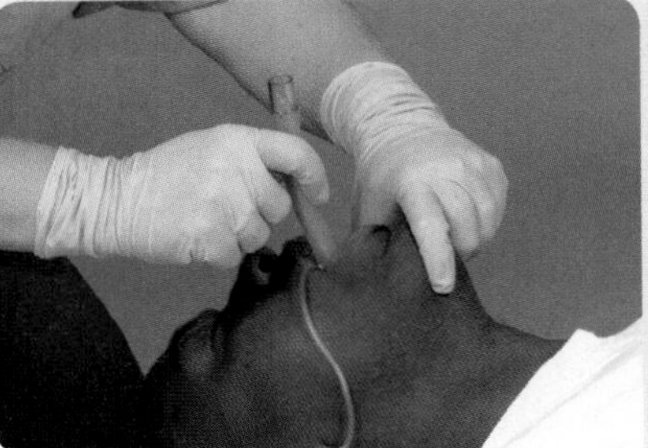

Step 6 Insert the LMA along the roof of the mouth. The key to proper insertion is to slide the convex surface of the airway along the roof of the mouth. Use your finger to push the airway against the hard palate. After it slides past the tongue, the LMA will move easily into position.

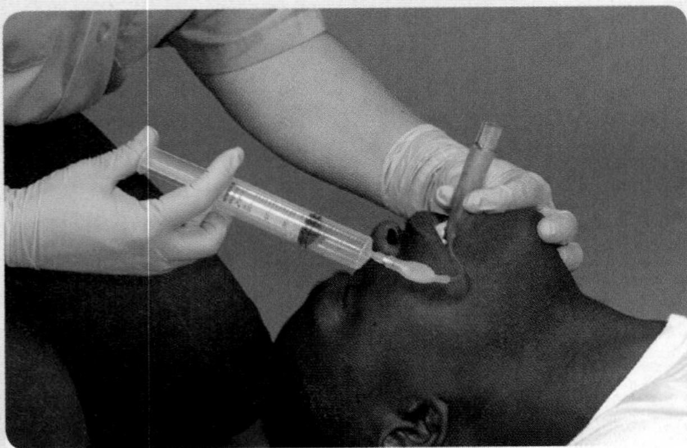

Step 7 Inflate the cuff with the amount of air indicated for the airway being used. If the LMA is properly positioned, then it will move out of the airway slightly 0.5 to 0.75 inch (1 to 2 cm) as it moves into position (a good indication that the LMA is in the correct position).

Step 8 Begin to ventilate the patient. Confirm chest rise and the presence of breath sounds. Ensure proper tube placement with waveform capnography. Continuously and carefully monitor the patient's condition.

The steps for inserting an i-gel supraglottic airway are shown in Skill Drill 15-17.

Cobra Perilaryngeal Airway

The **Cobra perilaryngeal airway (CobraPLA)** was first introduced as a device to ventilate patients with difficult airways. It is so named because of the cobra-like shape of the distal part of the airway Figure 15-104. The shape allows the device to slide easily along the hard palate and to hold the soft tissue of the airway from the laryngeal inlet (hence, *perilaryngeal*) after it is in place. The CobraPLA is a supraglottic device with a tube for ventilation and a circumferential cuff (that sits in the hypopharynx at the

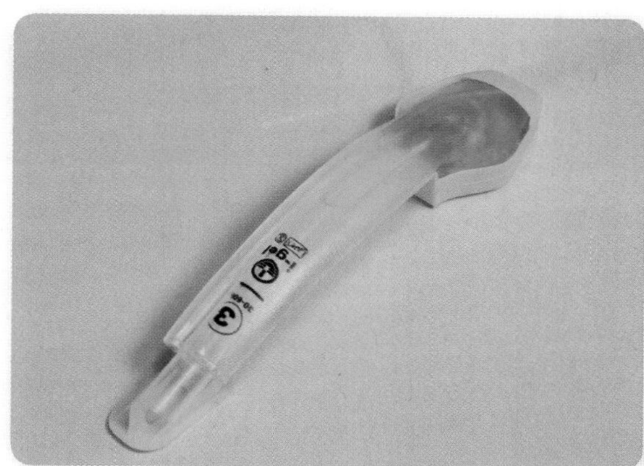

Figure 15-102 The i-gel supraglottic airway.

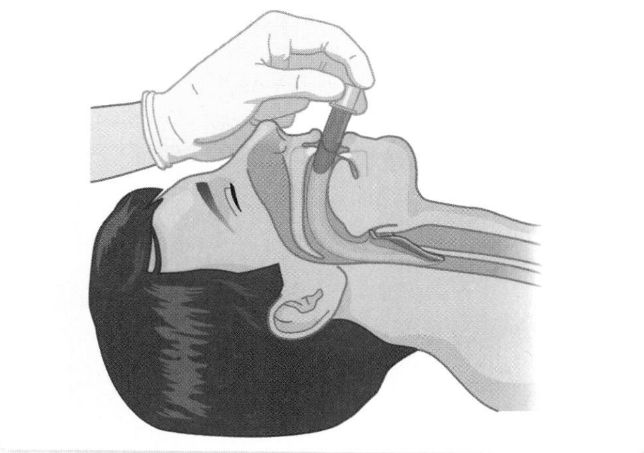

Figure 15-103 Correct position of the i-gel in the airway.

Table 15-18 Sizes and Patient Criteria for Adult i-gel Supraglottic Airway

Size	Connector Color	Weight Criteria
3	Yellow	66–132 lb (30–60 kg)
4	Green	110–198 lb (50–90 kg)
5	Orange	>198 lb (>90 kg)

Data from: i-gel user guide. 9989 issue 1 01.10. Intersurgical Ltd website. http://docsinnovent.com/downloads/i-gel_User_Guide_English.pdf. Accessed February 21, 2017.

base of the tongue) proximal to the distal end, which is the ventilation outlet. The CobraPLA also has a 15/22-mm standard adapter and the distal widened end that holds soft tissue apart and allows for ventilation of the trachea. The distal tip is proximal to the esophagus and seals the hypopharynx. When the cuff is inflated, it raises the tongue and creates an airway seal allowing for ventilation. Because the insertion technique is simple, it is possible to successfully place the device with minimal experience.

The CobraPLA is available in eight sizes. Proper size is determined by the size that comfortably fits through the patient's mouth.

Indications for the CobraPLA. The CobraPLA is used in a manner similar to that for other supraglottic airway

Skill Drill 15-17 Inserting an i-gel Supraglottic Airway

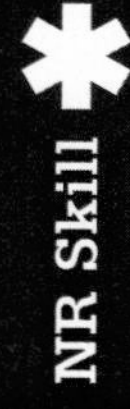

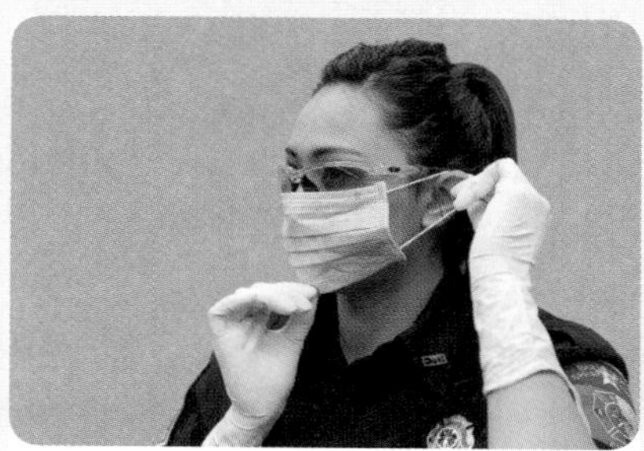

Step 1 Take standard precautions.

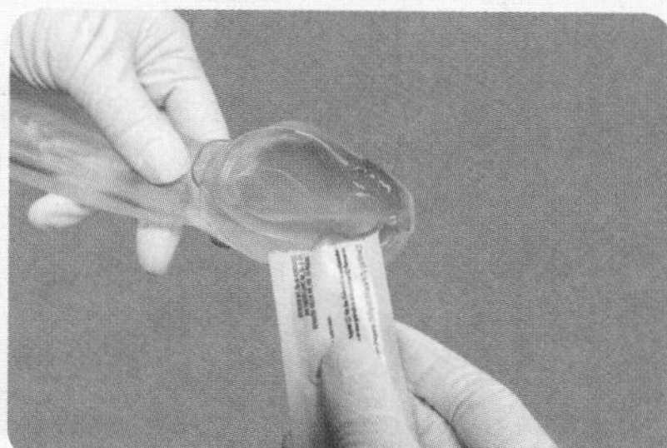

Step 2 Lubricate the back, sides, and front of the cuff with a thin layer of water-soluble gel.

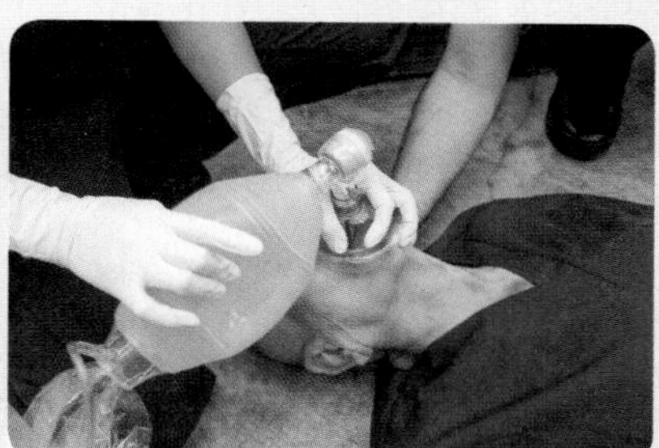

Step 3 Preoxygenate the patient before insertion. Do not interrupt ventilation for more than 30 seconds to accomplish airway placement. Place the patient in the sniffing position.

(continued)

Skill Drill 15-17 Inserting an i-gel Supraglottic Airway *(continued)*

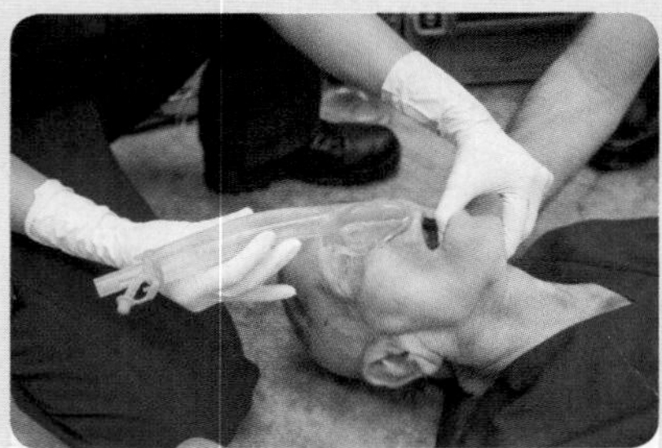

Step 4 Open the airway with the tongue-jaw lift maneuver and position the i-gel so that the cuff outlet is facing towards the patient's chin.

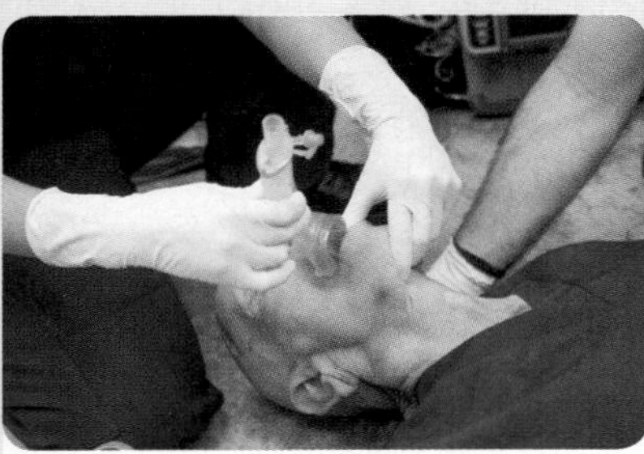

Step 5 Introduce the leading soft tip of the i-gel into the patient's mouth, directing it towards the hard palate.

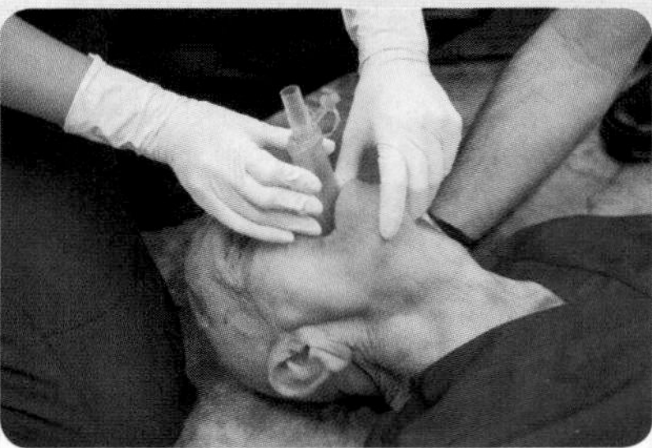

Step 6 Glide the i-gel downwards and backwards along the hard palate with a continuous but gentle push until a definitive resistance is felt.

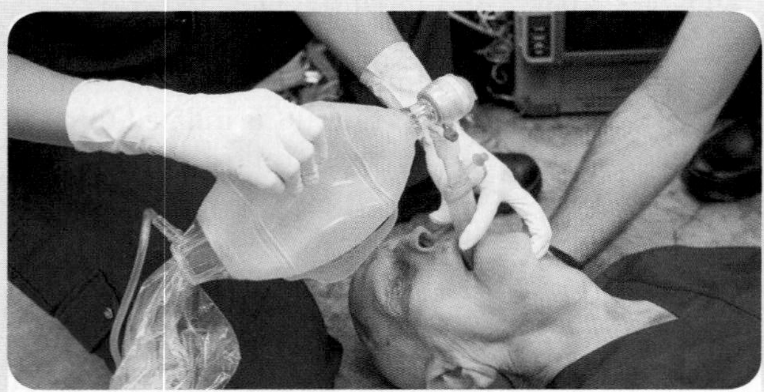

Step 7 Begin to ventilate the patient. Confirm chest rise and the presence of breath sounds. Ensure proper tube placement with waveform capnography. Continuously and carefully monitor the patient's condition.

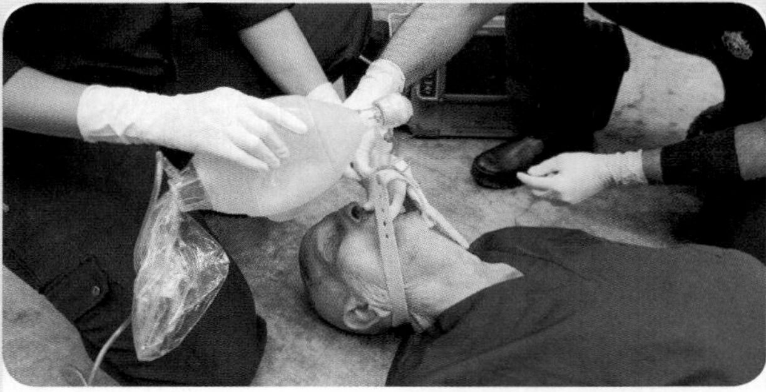

Step 8 Secure the i-gel in place with the provided strap.

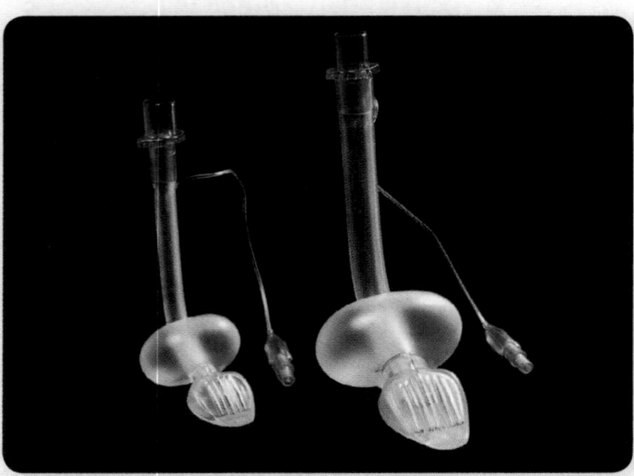

Figure 15-104 The Cobra perilaryngeal airway.

devices and can be used in pediatric patients. Because the device does not provide protection against aspiration, it is recommended for use only in patients who are not at risk for vomiting.

Contraindications for the CobraPLA. Contraindications include the risk for aspiration and massive trauma to the oral cavity.

Complications of the CobraPLA. If the patient has an intact gag reflex, then laryngospasm may occur. If you do not insert the CobraPLA far enough, then inflation of the cuff may cause the patient's tongue to protrude from the mouth, disrupting an adequate seal. Using the proper size is vital because you cannot ventilate the patient if the device is too small and passes into the laryngeal inlet. However, in such cases, you can remove it and insert another size with minimal trauma to the oropharynx.

Insertion Technique. To insert the CobraPLA, fully deflate the cuff and apply a water-soluble gel to the front and back of the device and to the cuff. With the patient's head in the sniffing position, open the airway with the tongue-jaw lift maneuver and direct the distal end of the CobraPLA straight back between the tongue and hard palate. Continue advancing the CobraPLA until modest resistance is felt Figure 15-105A. Inflate the cuff with only enough air to achieve a good seal; do not overinflate the cuff. Ventilate the patient while observing for chest rise and auscultating over the neck, chest, and epigastrium. Use waveform capnography for further confirmation and secure the device in place Figure 15-105B.

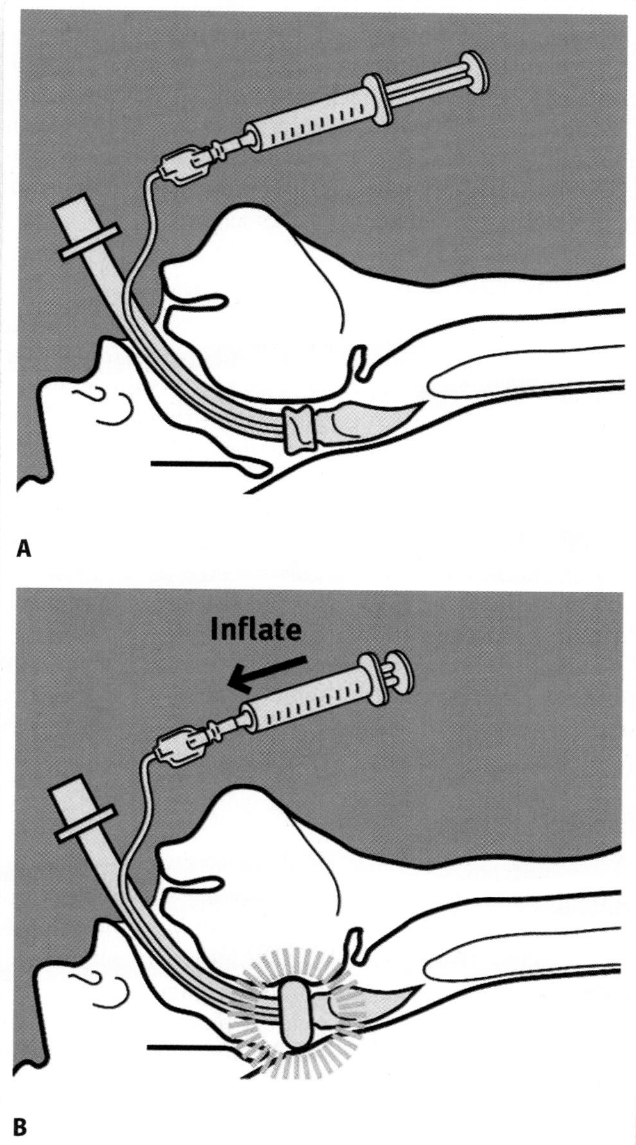

Figure 15-105 A. Open the airway with the tongue-jaw lift maneuver and advance the Cobra perilaryngeal airway until modest resistance is felt. **B.** Inflate the cuff with only enough air to achieve a good seal. Ventilate the patient, confirm proper placement, and secure the device in place.

Multilumen Airways

Combitube

The **Combitube** is a **multilumen airway** device with a long tube that is inserted blindly into the airway Figure 15-106. It is a reasonable alternative to ET intubation and has been clinically proven to secure the airway and allow for better ventilation than a bag-mask device and simple airway adjunct in most cases.

In contrast with single-lumen airways, the tube can be used for ventilation whether it is inserted into the esophagus or trachea. Although this device almost always comes to rest in the esophagus, it can function as an ET tube if inserted into the trachea Figure 15-107. The Combitube contains two lumens, which function appropriately based on tube position and ventilating through the correct lumen. Each lumen has a standard 15/22-mm ventilation adapter, which accommodates any ventilation device (such as a bag-mask device or mechanical ventilator). The proper port for ventilation depends on where the tube is located. It also contains an oropharyngeal balloon, which eliminates the need for a mask seal.

Indications and Contraindications for the Combitube

The Combitube is indicated for airway management of deeply unresponsive, apneic patients with no gag reflex in whom ET intubation is not possible or has failed. If the patient regains consciousness, then you must remove the device.

The Combitube cannot be used in children younger than 16 years, and it should be used only for patients between 5 and 7 feet (1.5 to 2 m) tall. A smaller version of the Combitube—called the Combitube SA (small adult)—can be used for patients between 4 and 5.5 feet (approximately 1 to 2 m) tall. Because the device is inserted into the esophagus most of the time, use is

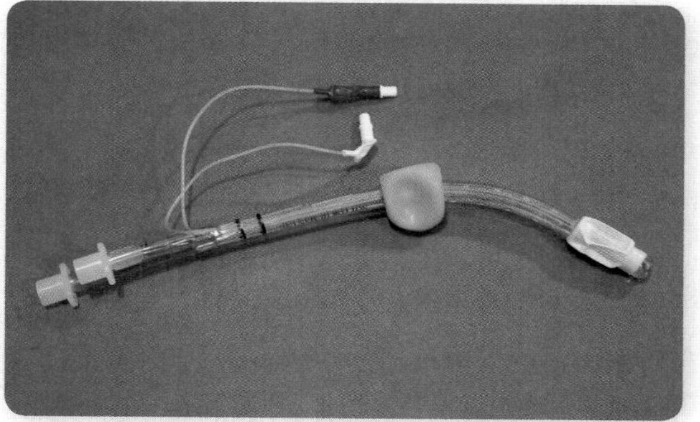

Figure 15-106 Combitube.

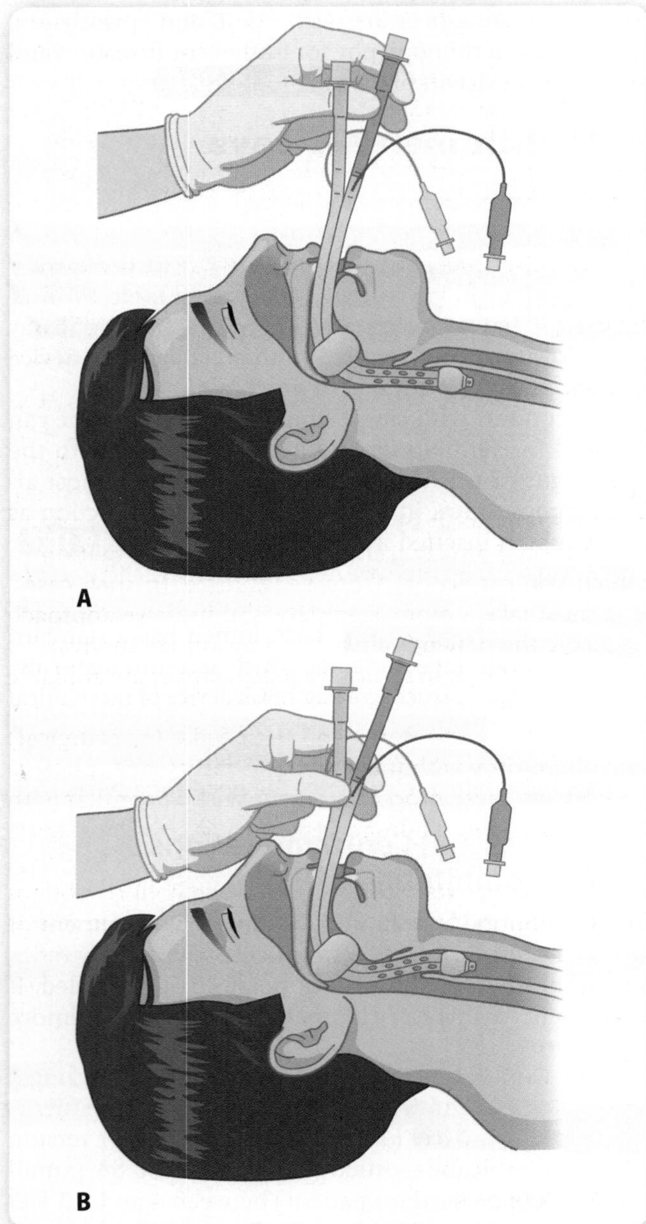

Figure 15-107 A. If the Combitube is inserted into the esophagus, then ventilations can still be provided to the patient. **B.** If the Combitube is inserted into the trachea, then it functions as an endotracheal tube, with ventilations provided directly into the trachea.

contraindicated in patients with esophageal trauma, patients with a known pathologic condition of the esophagus (such as esophageal varices or cancer), patients who have ingested a caustic substance, or patients who have a history of alcoholism.

Advantages and Disadvantages of the Combitube

The major advantage of the multilumen airway is that, in effect, it cannot be improperly placed; effective ventilation is possible whether the tube enters the esophagus or the trachea. Insertion of the Combitube is also technically easier than ET intubation. Furthermore, because insertion of the airway is performed with the patient's head in the neutral position, cervical spine movement is kept to a minimum. In addition, no mask seal is required to ventilate with the Combitube.

The Combitube also provides some patency to the airway. If the tube is placed in the trachea, then it functions exactly like an ET tube, and no upper airway positioning is required. If the tube is placed in the esophagus, then the pharyngeal balloon creates an airtight seal in the oropharynx, making the tongue position less of a factor in the maintenance of a patent airway. A jaw-thrust maneuver should easily alleviate any ventilatory difficulty if the epiglottis partially obstructs the airway.

Use of the Combitube requires strict attention and good assessment skills because ventilation in the wrong port results in no pulmonary ventilation. The device is a temporary airway and you should replace it as soon as possible. The pharyngeal balloon reduces—but does not completely eliminate—the risk of aspiration.

Complications of the Combitube

The most significant complication associated with the use of a Combitube is unrecognized displacement of the tube into the esophagus. (It is acceptable if the tube is placed in the esophagus, but you must realize this to effectively ventilate.) Therefore, good assessment skills are essential to properly confirm tube placement, and use rigorous confirmation protocol following insertion of the device.

Laryngospasm, vomiting, and possible hypoventilation may occur during insertion of a Combitube. In addition, pharyngeal or esophageal trauma may result from improper technique.

Ventilation may be difficult if the pharyngeal balloon pushes the epiglottis over the glottic opening. If this occurs, withdrawing the device approximately 1 to 1.5 inches (2 to 4 cm) should make ventilation easier.

Insertion Technique

The Combitube consists of a single tube with two lumens, two balloons, and two ventilation ports. One of the lumens is open at its distal end, and the other is closed. The closed lumen has side holes to the pharyngeal balloon. The proximal balloon is designed to be inflated with 100 mL of air and provide a pharyngeal seal. The distal balloon is inflated with 15 mL of air and makes an airtight seal with the walls of the trachea (in case of tracheal placement) or provides esophageal obturation (in case of esophageal placement).

Before inserting the Combitube, check and prepare your equipment. Check both cuffs, and ensure that they hold air. Preoxygenate the patient before insertion. Do not interrupt ventilation for longer than 30 seconds to insert the airway. For insertion, place the patient's head in a neutral position.

- **Forwardly displace the jaw.** With the patient's head in a neutral position, insert the thumb of your gloved nondominant hand into the patient's mouth and lift the jaw. This action lifts the hyoid bone and pulls the base of the tongue off the posterior pharyngeal wall.
- **Insert the device.** Following the curvature of the tube, insert the device blindly into the posterior pharynx. Insert the Combitube until the incisors are between the two black lines printed on the tube. Be gentle, and stop advancing the tube if you meet resistance.
- **Inflate the balloons.** The Combitube has two independent inflation valves that must be inflated sequentially. The first inflation valve goes to the balloon on the pharyngeal tube (blue [No. 1] tube) and is inflated with 100 mL of air. The second inflation valve inflates the distal balloon of the tracheal tube (clear [No. 2] tube) and is filled with 15 mL of air.

When inserting a Combitube, confirmation of ventilation is critical. If you ventilate through the wrong tube, then the patient will receive no pulmonary ventilation and you could be instilling air directly into the stomach.

Following inflation of the balloons, begin to ventilate the patient. Ventilate through the longer (blue) tube first. Observe for chest rise and auscultate breath and epigastric sounds. If there are no breath sounds (or epigastric sounds are present) and the chest does not rise and fall with ventilation, then switch immediately to the shorter (clear) tube. Be sure to continuously monitor ventilation. The Combitube is generally secure in the airway owing to the large pharyngeal balloon, although you may consider securing the device in place after ventilations are confirmed. Use continuous waveform capnography to confirm the presence of exhaled carbon dioxide, which further confirms proper ventilation.

Surgical and Nonsurgical Cricothyrotomy

In most cases, you can secure a patent airway with relative ease using basic methods (eg, bag-mask device with oral airway) or advanced methods (eg, ET intubation, supraglottic airway). In some situations, however, the patient's condition or other factors preclude the use of conventional airway techniques, creating a situation in which you cannot intubate or ventilate. In such cases, you must take a more aggressive and invasive approach to secure the patient's airway and maximize survival.

Two methods of securing a patent airway are available when conventional techniques and methods fail: the open (surgical) cricothyrotomy and the needle (nonsurgical) cricothyrotomy with translaryngeal catheter ventilation. To perform these procedures, you must be familiar with the key anatomic landmarks that lie in the anterior aspect of the neck **Figure 15-108**.

In addition, you must be familiar with the important blood vessels in this area. The superior cricothyroid vessels

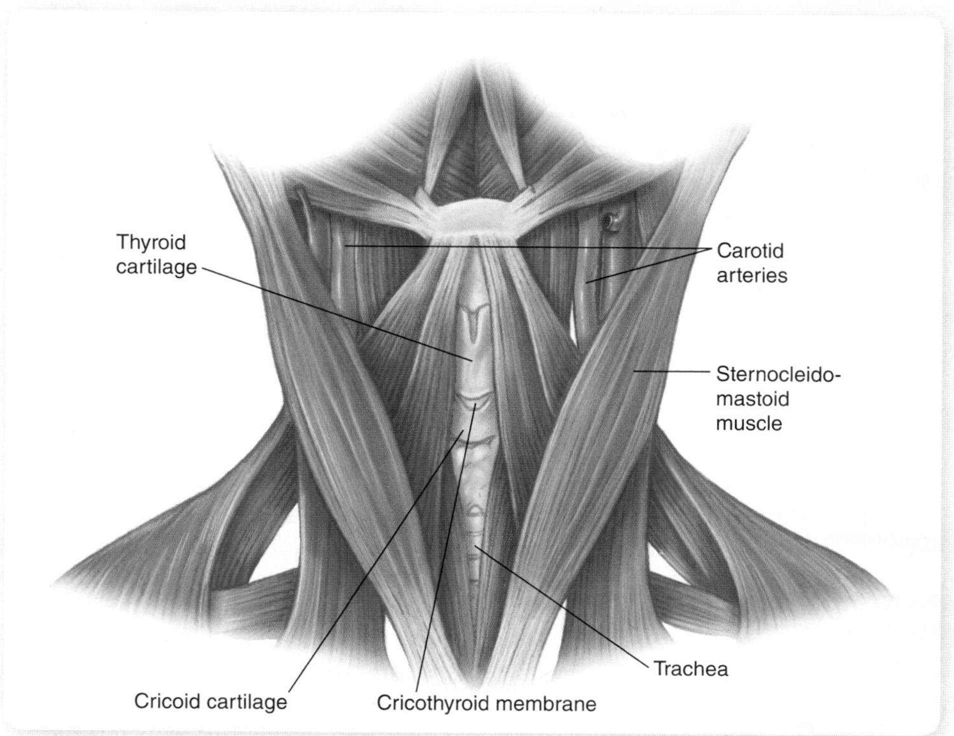

Figure 15-108 Anatomy of the anterior aspect of the neck.

run at a transverse angle across the upper third of the cricothyroid membrane. The carotid arteries run vertically and are located lateral to the cricothyroid membrane. Therefore, use great care when incising the cricothyroid membrane.

When performing a cricothyrotomy, it is important to know that the patient will bleed from the subcutaneous and small skin vessels as you incise down to the cricothyroid membrane. Although this bleeding is usually minor, it will impair your visual reference, making cricothyrotomy a tactile procedure. You should be able to easily control any bleeding with light pressure after you have inserted the tube into the trachea.

▶ Open Cricothyrotomy

Open cricothyrotomy (surgical cricothyrotomy) involves incising the cricothyroid membrane with a scalpel and inserting an ET or tracheostomy tube directly into the subglottic area (below the vocal cords) of the trachea. The cricothyroid membrane is the ideal site for making a surgical opening into the trachea because no important structures lie between the skin and the airway. The airway at this level lies relatively close to the skin (except in patients with obesity) and is easy to enter through the thin cricothyroid membrane. The posterior wall of the airway at this level is formed by the tough cricoid cartilage, which helps prevent accidental perforation through the back of the airway into the esophagus.

Several types of surgical cricothyrotomies exist. As previously discussed, open (surgical) cricothyrotomy involves incising the patient's skin and cricothyroid membrane and inserting an ET tube or tracheostomy tube. A modified cricothyrotomy is another type of cricothyrotomy. Commercial modified cricothyrotomy kits are available, such as the Quicktrach, which may be used in the prehospital setting. The Quicktrach kit features a 4.0-mm cannula over a large-bore needle that punctures through the cricothyroid membrane. A stopper prevents the needle from being inserted too deeply, thus reducing the risk of posterior tracheal wall perforation. The Quicktrach II kit includes all the features of the Quicktrach, but also has an inflatable cuff on the distal end of the cannula that minimizes the risk of aspiration **Figure 15-109**. No scalpel incision is necessary when using the Quicktrach kit.

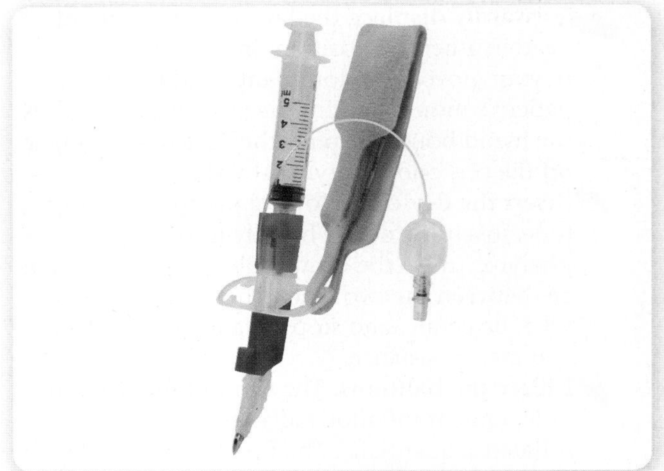

Figure 15-109 The Quicktrach II kit.

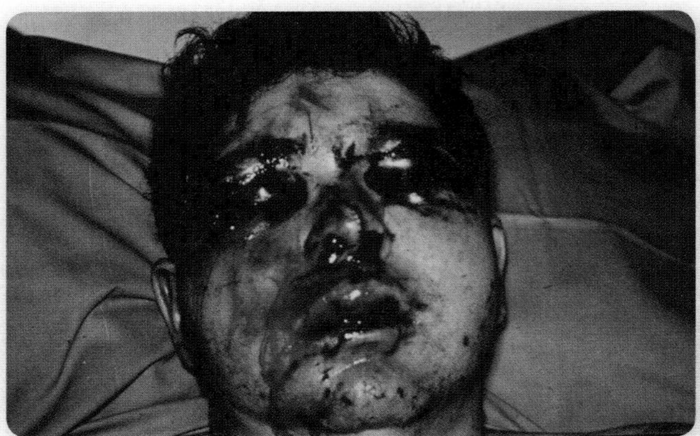

Figure 15-110 Patients with massive maxillofacial trauma often have mandibular fractures or profuse bleeding in the oropharynx, both of which can make bag-mask ventilation and intubation extremely difficult, if not impossible.

Indications and Contraindications

Open cricothyrotomy is indicated when you cannot secure a patent airway with more conventional means. It is not the preferred means of initially securing a patient's airway. For example, if you are unable to intubate a patient but can provide effective bag-mask ventilations, then cricothyrotomy would not be indicated.

Situations that may preclude conventional airway management include severe foreign body obstructions of the upper airway that cannot be extracted with Magill forceps and direct laryngoscopy, airway obstructions from swelling (such as epiglottitis, anaphylaxis, and upper airway burns), massive maxillofacial trauma, and the inability to open the patient's mouth. Patients with massive maxillofacial trauma **Figure 15-110** often have associated mandibular fractures, which makes it extremely difficult to maintain an effective mask-to-face seal with a bag-mask device. Intubation in patients with these injuries would also be extremely difficult because of posterior tongue lacerations with profuse bleeding. In such patients, frequent suctioning to prevent aspiration would delay intubation and increase hypoxia.

Patients with head injuries and trismus (clenched teeth) may require cricothyrotomy, especially if you do not have the resources or protocols to perform RSI. Furthermore, head injury, which is commonly accompanied by facial trauma, is a contraindication for nasotracheal

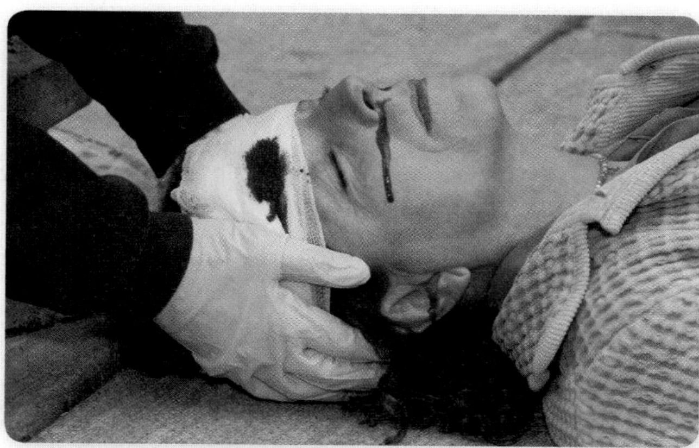

Figure 15-111 Endotracheal intubation may be impossible in patients with a head injury and trismus. Nasotracheal intubation is contraindicated in patients with head injury and fluid drainage from the nose.

intubation and placement of a nasal airway, especially if fluid is draining from the patient's nose Figure 15-111. If this fluid is CSF, then fracture of the cribriform plate likely is present. If you attempt nasotracheal intubation, then the ET tube or nasal airway could inadvertently enter the cranial vault through the fractured plate.

As noted earlier, the main contraindication for open cricothyrotomy is the ability to secure a patent airway by less invasive means. Other contraindications include the inability to identify the correct anatomic landmarks (cricothyroid membrane), crushing injuries to the larynx and tracheal transection, underlying anatomic abnormalities (such as trauma, tumors, or subglottic stenosis), and age younger than 8 years. The larynx of a small child is generally unable to support a tube large enough to produce effective ventilation without causing damage to the larynx; a needle cricothyrotomy (discussed later in this chapter) would be safer for young children.

In situations in which cricothyrotomy is contraindicated, promptly transport the patient to the closest appropriate facility, where an emergency tracheostomy can be performed.

Advantages and Disadvantages

Open cricothyrotomy can be performed quickly, and without manipulating the cervical spine. The latter characteristic is especially advantageous because many cricothyrotomies involve patients with massive facial trauma.

Disadvantages of cricothyrotomy include the difficulty encountered in performing the procedure in children, which is why it is contraindicated in children younger than 8 years. In contrast with needle cricothyrotomy, an open cricothyrotomy is more difficult to perform; however, inserting a large-bore tube (such as an ET tube or a tracheostomy tube) permits achieving greater tidal volume, which facilitates more effective oxygenation and ventilation.

Complications

Expect some minor bleeding when an open cricothyrotomy is performed. More severe bleeding is usually the result of laceration of a larger lateral vein. Incising the cricothyroid membrane vertically, instead of horizontally, will minimize the risk of this potential complication. It will also minimize the risk of damaging the highly vascular thyroid gland. After the incision has been made, gently inserting the tube will minimize the risks of perforating the esophagus and damaging the laryngeal nerves.

You must perform an open cricothyrotomy quickly. Taking too long to complete a cricothyrotomy will result in unnecessary hypoxia, which may result in cardiac dysrhythmias, permanent brain injury, and/or cardiac arrest.

Words of Wisdom

Frequent practice on a cadaver, if available, or a special cricothyrotomy manikin, will maximize your ability to perform cricothyrotomy quickly. In general, skills that are not frequently performed in the field should be routinely practiced to maintain proficiency and competence.

It is possible to create a false passage if the tube undermines the subcutaneous tissue and never enters the trachea through the cricothyroid membrane. Although this complication can occur with any patient, the risk is greater when performing an open cricothyrotomy on a patient with obesity. Suspect tube misplacement when subcutaneous emphysema is encountered after performing a cricothyrotomy. Subcutaneous emphysema occurs when air infiltrates the subcutaneous (fatty) layers of the skin and is characterized by a "crackling" sensation when palpated.

Any invasive procedure performed in the prehospital setting has the risk of infection to patients. Therefore, maintain aseptic technique to the extent possible when performing an open cricothyrotomy.

Equipment

If a commercially manufactured cricothyrotomy kit is unavailable, then you must prepare the following equipment and supplies:

- Scalpel (No. 10 blade)
- ET or tracheostomy tube (6.0 mm minimum)
- Commercial device (or tape) for securing the tube
- Suction apparatus
- Sterile gauze pads for bleeding control
- Bag-mask device attached to 100% oxygen
- $ETCO_2$ detector

Technique for Performing Open Cricothyrotomy

After you determine that an open cricothyrotomy is needed, you must proceed rapidly, yet cautiously. Identify the cricothyroid membrane by palpating for the V notch of the thyroid cartilage, which feels like a high, sharp bump. Stabilize the larynx between your thumb and middle fingers while you palpate with your index finger. When you have located the V notch, slide your index finger down over the thyroid prominence (Adam's apple) and into the depression between the thyroid and cricoid cartilage; that is the cricothyroid membrane.

Males have a prominent thyroid notch and thyroid prominence, whereas females do not. The cricoid ring is more prominent in females than it is in males; therefore, when palpating the anatomy in females, first locate the cricoid ring, then the cricothyroid membrane, and finally, the thyroid cartilage.

While you are locating and preparing the site, your partner should prepare your equipment and ensuring that the cardiac monitor/defibrillator and pulse oximeter are attached to the patient.

Maintain aseptic technique as you cleanse the area with iodine; avoid touching the area once cleansed. While stabilizing the larynx with one hand, make a vertical incision (approximately 0.5 to 0.75 inches [1 to 2 cm]) over the cricothyroid membrane; in patients with obesity, the vertical incision may need to be longer and deeper. A No. 10 scalpel is ideal because it has a pointed tip for puncturing and a beveled edge for incising. After the incision has been made, remove the scalpel and immediately place your index finger on top of the cricothyroid membrane. Remember, the patient will likely bleed after the first incision is made, so your visual reference may be reduced or lost. Therefore, it is critical to maintain stabilization of the larynx and to keep the cricothyroid membrane acquired. Puncture through the cricothyroid membrane and make a horizontal incision (approximately 0.5 inch [1 cm]) in each direction from the midline; do not to incise too far laterally. Remove the scalpel and immediately put your index finger through the cricothyroid membrane. At this point, you can insert the scalpel handle (with the protective sheath over the blade) into the opening and rotate it, or use a tracheal hook or Trousseau tracheal dilator (available in commercial cricothyrotomy kits) Figure 15-112. Your partner should be readily available to control any bleeding that might occur.

With the trachea exposed, gently insert a 6.0-mm cuffed ET tube or a 6.0 cuffed tracheostomy tube Figure 15-113 and direct it into the trachea. After the tube is in place, stabilize it manually and inflate the distal cuff with the appropriate volume of air—typically 5 to 10 mL. Attach the bag-mask device to the standard 15/22-mm adapter on the tube, and ventilate the patient while your partner auscultates to ensure the presence of bilaterally clear breath sounds and the absence of epigastric sounds. If epigastric sounds are heard, then you have likely perforated the trachea and inserted the tube into the esophagus.

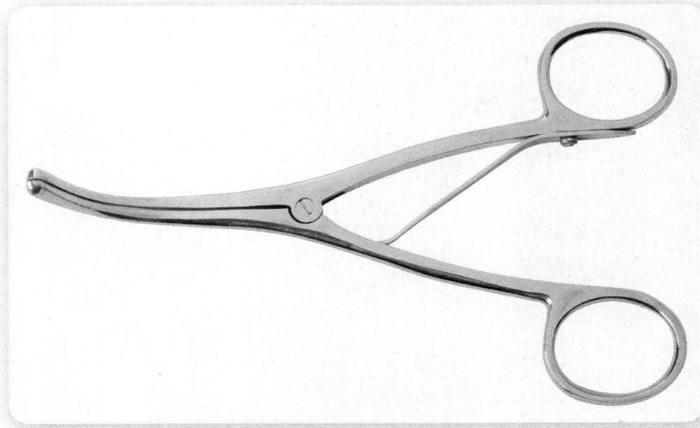

Figure 15-112 Trousseau tracheal dilator.

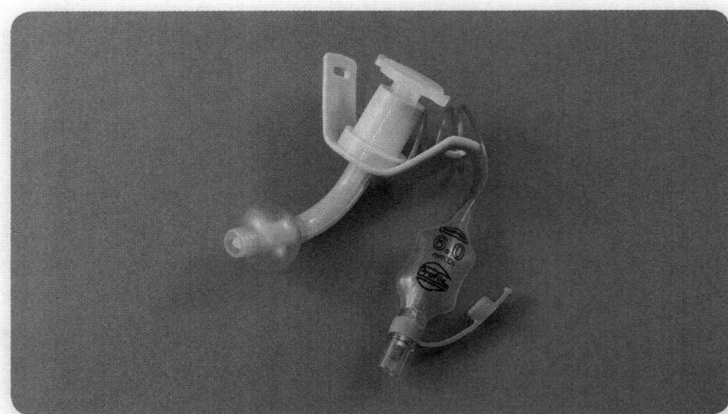

Figure 15-113 Cuffed tracheostomy tube.

Additional confirmation of correct tube placement can be accomplished by attaching an $ETCO_2$ detector between the tube and ventilation device. After confirming proper tube placement, ensure that any minor bleeding has been controlled, properly secure the tube, and continue to ventilate the patient at the appropriate rate.

The steps for performing an open cricothyrotomy are shown in Skill Drill 15-18.

▶ Needle Cricothyrotomy

Needle cricothyrotomy also uses the cricothyroid membrane as an entry point into the airway. In this procedure, a 14- to 16-gauge over-the-needle IV catheter is inserted through the cricothyroid membrane and into the trachea. Adequate oxygenation and ventilation are then achieved by attaching a high-pressure jet ventilator Figure 15-114 to the hub of the catheter. Known as **translaryngeal catheter ventilation**, this procedure is commonly used as a temporary measure until a more definitive airway can be obtained (such as open cricothyrotomy or tracheostomy). When using a high-pressure jet ventilator, watch closely to avoid overinflation of the lungs.

Skill Drill 15-18 Performing an Open Cricothyrotomy

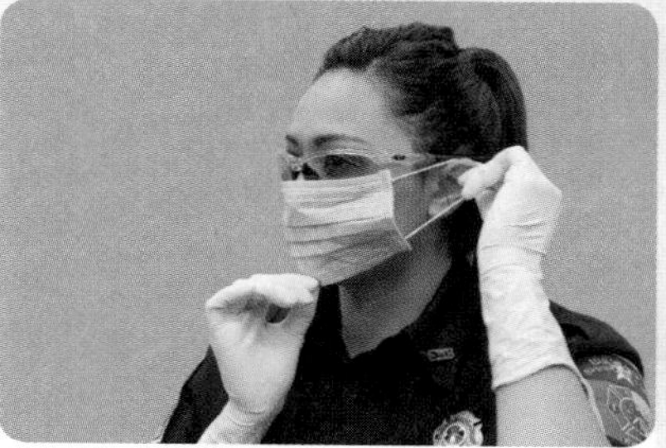

Step 1 Take standard precautions.

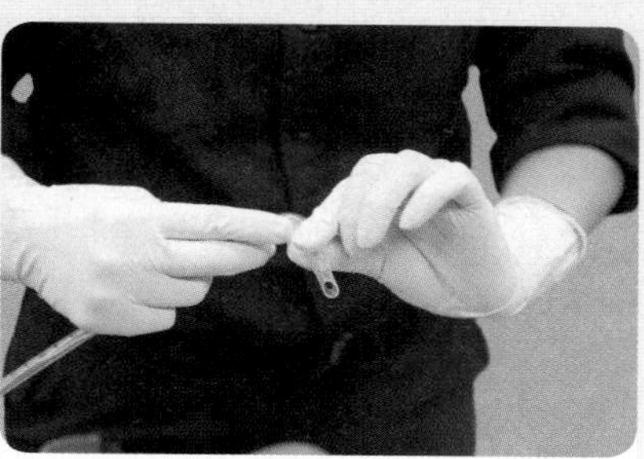

Step 2 Check, assemble, and prepare the equipment. Place a 90° bend in a 6.0-mm ET tube (with a stylet inserted), just proximal to the cuff.

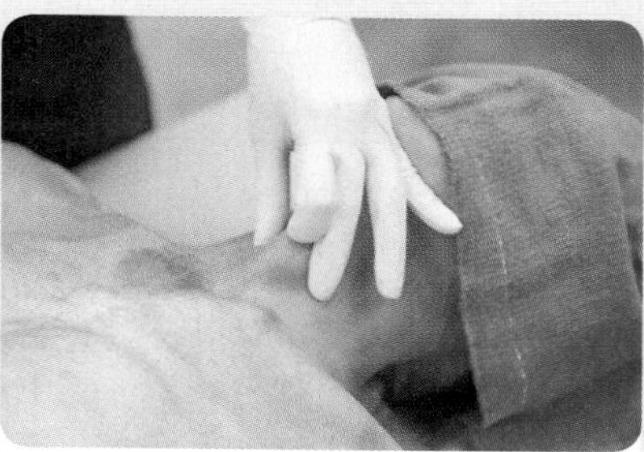

Step 3 With the patient's head in a neutral position, palpate for and locate the cricothyroid membrane.

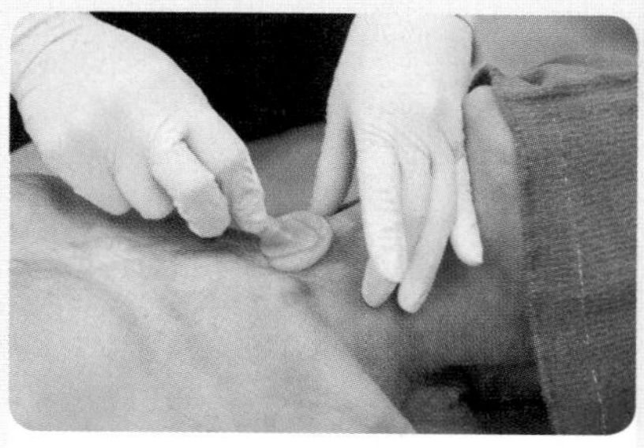

Step 4 Cleanse the area with an iodine- or chlorhexidine-containing solution.

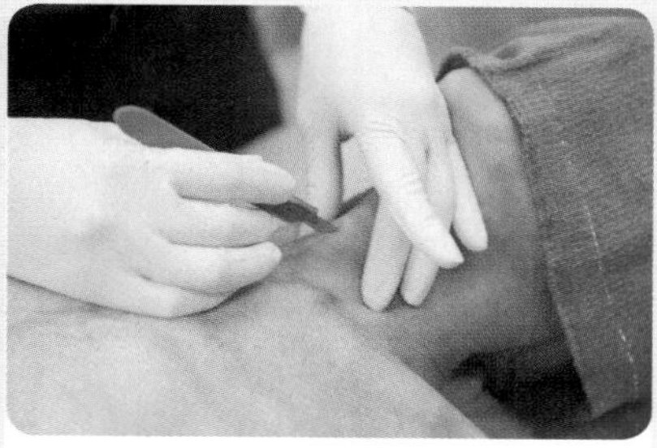

Step 5 Stabilize the larynx, and make a vertical incision (approximately 0.5 to 0.75 inch [1 to 2 cm]) over the cricothyroid membrane.

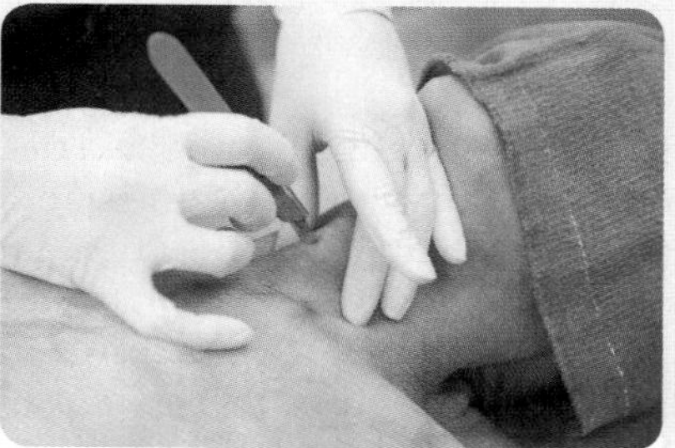

Step 6 Puncture the cricothyroid membrane.

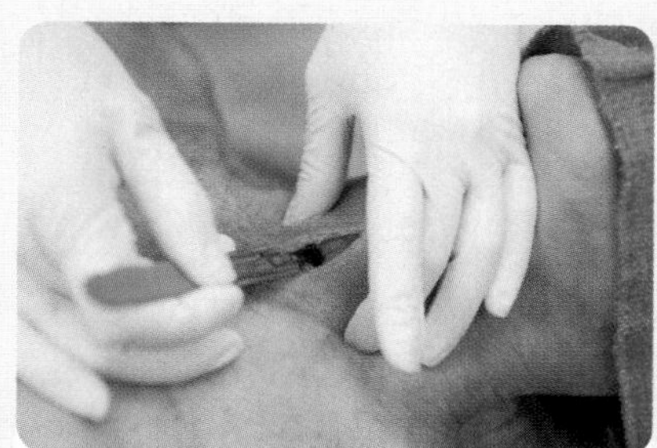

Step 7 Make a horizontal incision (approximately 0.5 inch [1 cm]) in each direction from the midline. Insert the scalpel handle into the opening and rotate it.

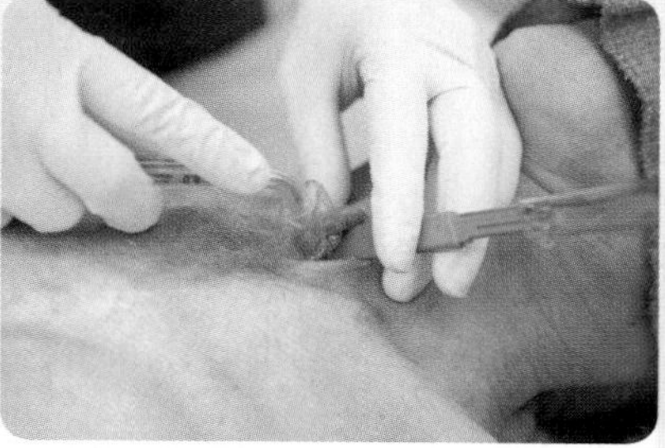

Step 8 Insert the tube into the trachea as you remove the scalpel handle.

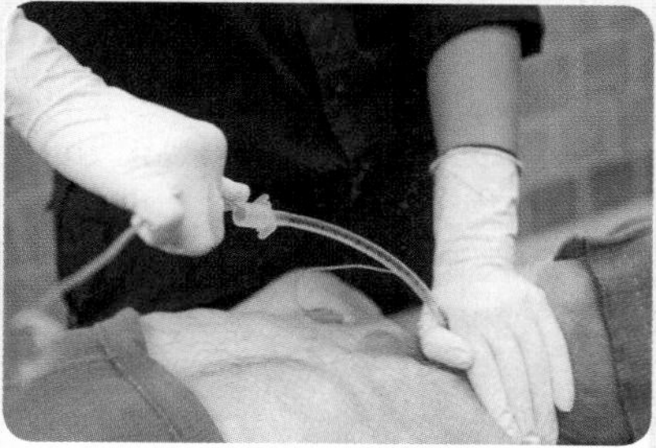

Step 9 Manually stabilize the ET tube between your thumb and index finger, carefully remove the stylet, and inflate the distal cuff.

(continued)

Skill Drill 15-18 Performing an Open Cricothyrotomy *(continued)*

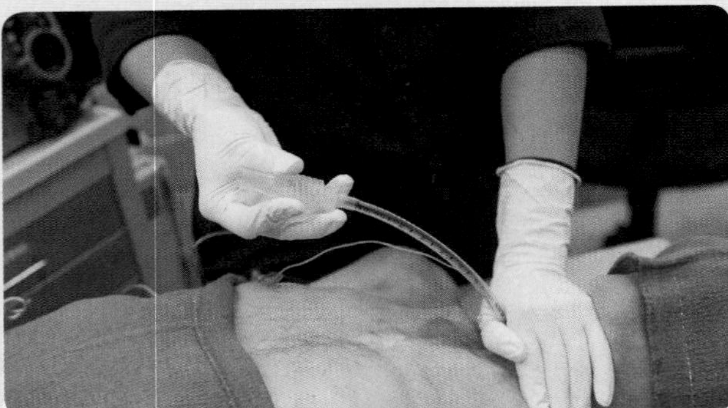

Step 10 Attach an $ETCO_2$ detector between the tube and the ventilation device.

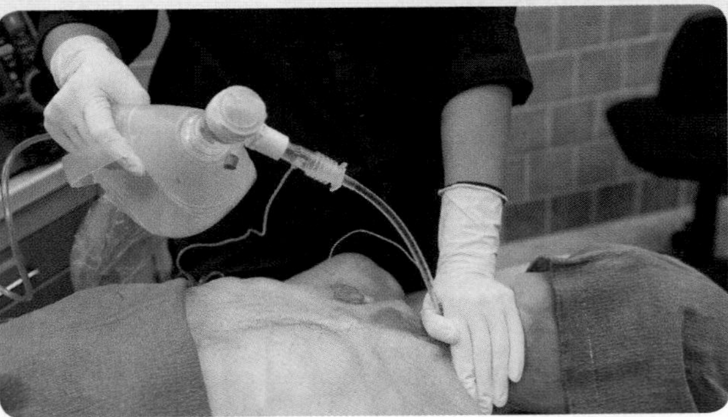

Step 11 Ensure proper tube placement with waveform capnography. Attach the $ETCO_2$ detector to the monitor. Ventilate the patient.

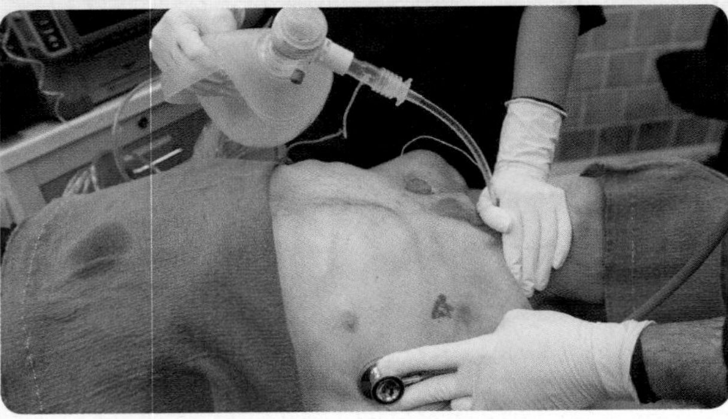

Step 12 Confirm correct tube placement by auscultating the apices and bases of both lungs and over the epigastrium.

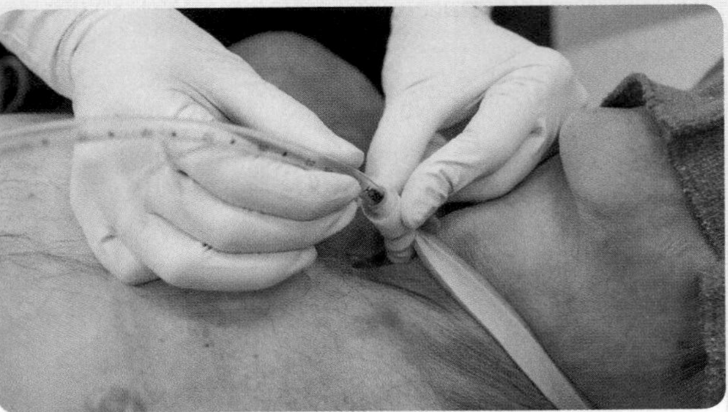

Step 13 Secure the tube with a commercial device or tape. Reconfirm correct tube placement, and resume ventilations at the appropriate rate.

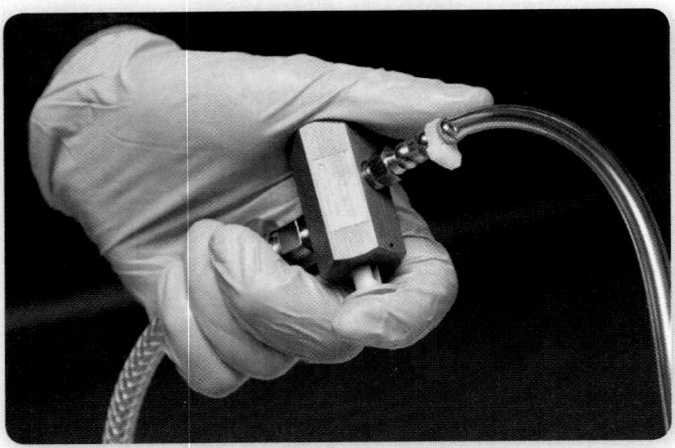

Figure 15-114 High-pressure jet ventilator.

Indications and Contraindications

The indications for needle cricothyrotomy and translaryngeal catheter ventilation are essentially the same as for the open cricothyrotomy—the inability to ventilate the patient by other, less invasive techniques; massive maxillofacial trauma; inability to open the patient's mouth; and uncontrolled oropharyngeal bleeding.

Needle cricothyrotomy is contraindicated in patients who have a severe airway obstruction above the site of catheter insertion. Exhalation cannot occur through the jet ventilation device, so it must occur via the glottic opening. If the airway is completely obstructed above the catheter insertion site, then exhalation will not be possible. As a result, the patient will become hypercapneic. The high-pressure jet ventilator used with needle cricothyrotomy causes an increase in intrathoracic pressure, potentially resulting in barotrauma and risk for a pneumothorax. Barotrauma can also be caused by overinflation of the lungs with the jet ventilator, so take care to open the release valve only until the patient's chest adequately rises.

If the equipment necessary to perform translaryngeal catheter ventilation is not immediately available, then perform an open cricothyrotomy.

Advantages and Disadvantages

Compared with an open cricothyrotomy, needle cricothyrotomy is faster and technically easier to perform. In particular, it is associated with a lower risk of causing damage to adjacent structures because you are puncturing the cricothyroid membrane with an IV catheter—not incising it with a scalpel. Needle cricothyrotomy also allows for subsequent intubation attempts because it uses a small-bore catheter, thus allowing an ET tube to easily pass beside it. This advantage could be particularly beneficial if you do not have the equipment or protocols to perform an open cricothyrotomy. In addition, this procedure does not require manipulation of the patient's cervical spine.

However, disadvantages exist to performing a needle cricothyrotomy. Using a smaller-bore tube (such as an over-the-needle IV catheter) to ventilate the patient does not provide protection from aspiration like a cuffed ET tube or tracheostomy tube would during an open cricothyrotomy (a larger-bore tube, combined with the distal cuff, would fill the diameter of the trachea, protecting it from aspiration). Also, this technique requires a specialized, high-pressure jet ventilator to provide adequate tidal volume. This jet ventilator will expend high volumes of oxygen rapidly.

Complications

Improper catheter placement can result in severe bleeding caused by damage to adjacent structures. Even if the catheter is correctly placed, excessive air leakage around the insertion site can cause subcutaneous emphysema, especially if the patient has undetected laryngeal trauma. If too much air infiltrates into the subcutaneous space, then compression of the trachea and subsequent obstruction may occur.

Exercise extreme care when ventilating a patient by using a jet ventilator. The ventilation valve should be depressed or occluded just long enough for adequate chest rise to occur. Overinflation of the lungs can result in barotrauma, which involves a risk of pneumothorax. Conversely, depressing or occluding the ventilation valve for too short a period could cause hypoventilation, resulting in inadequate oxygenation and ventilation.

Equipment

The following equipment is needed to perform needle cricothyrotomy and translaryngeal catheter ventilation:

- Large-bore IV catheter (14- to 16-gauge)
- 10-mL syringe
- 3 mL of sterile water or saline
- Oxygen source (50 psi)
- High-pressure jet ventilator device and oxygen tubing

Technique for Performing Needle Cricothyrotomy

When preparing your equipment, draw up approximately 3 mL of sterile water or saline into a 10-mL syringe and attach the syringe to the IV catheter. Next, place the patient's head in a neutral position, and locate the cricothyroid membrane. Cleanse the area with an iodine-containing solution.

While you are stabilizing the patient's larynx, carefully insert the needle into the midline of the cricothyroid membrane at a 45° angle toward the feet (caudally). You should feel a pop as the needle penetrates the membrane. After the pop is felt, insert the needle approximately 0.5 inch (1 cm) farther, and then aspirate with the syringe. If the catheter has been correctly placed, then you should be able to easily aspirate air and see the saline or water bubbling within the syringe. If blood is aspirated or if you meet resistance, then reevaluate catheter placement because it is likely outside the trachea.

After confirming correct placement, advance the catheter over the needle until the catheter hub is flush with the skin, then withdraw the needle and place it in a puncture-proof biohazard container. Next, attach one end of the oxygen tubing to the catheter and the other end to the jet ventilator.

Begin ventilations by opening the release valve on the jet ventilator and observing for adequate chest rise. Auscultation of breath and epigastric sounds will further confirm correct catheter placement. To prevent overexpansion of the lungs and subsequent barotrauma, release the ventilation valve as soon as you see the chest rise. Exhalation will occur passively via the glottis. Ventilate the patient as dictated by his or her clinical condition.

Secure the catheter by placing a folded 4 × 4-inch (10 × 10-cm) gauze pad under the catheter and taping it in place. Continue ventilations while frequently reassessing the patient for adequacy of ventilations and for potential complications (such as subcutaneous emphysema from incorrect placement).

The steps for performing needle cricothyrotomy with translaryngeal catheter ventilation are shown in Skill Drill 15-19.

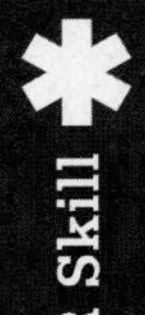

NR Skill

Skill Drill 15-19 Performing Needle Cricothyrotomy and Translaryngeal Catheter Ventilation

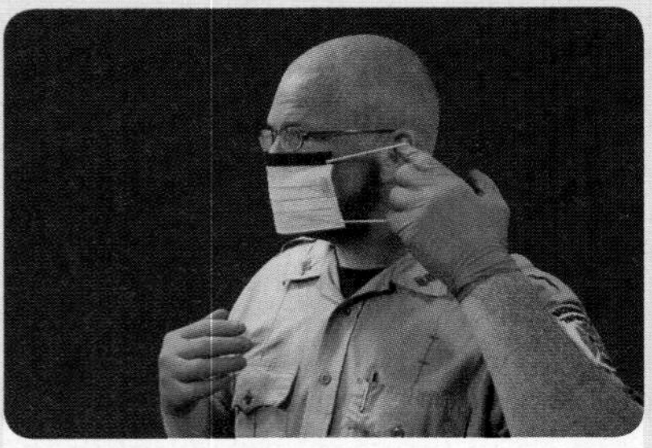

Step 1 Take standard precautions.

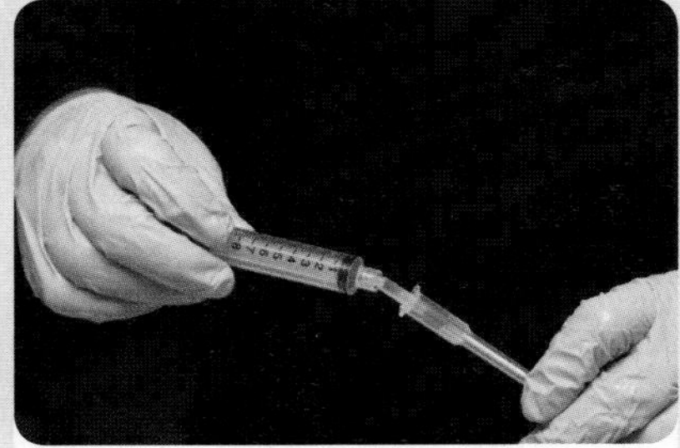

Step 2 Attach a 14- to 16-gauge IV catheter to a 10-mL syringe containing approximately 3 mL of sterile saline or water.

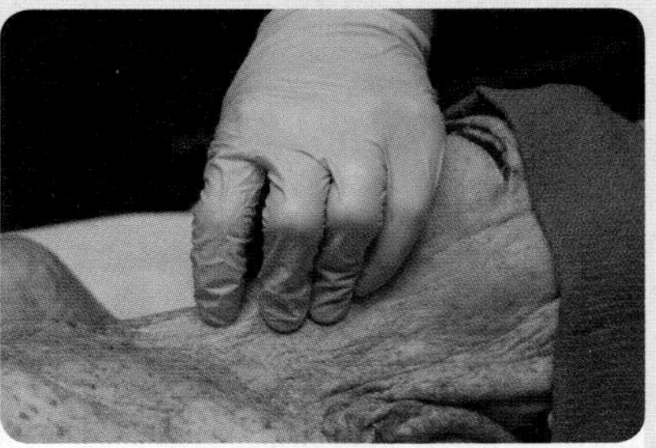

Step 3 With the patient's head in a neutral position, palpate for and locate the cricothyroid membrane.

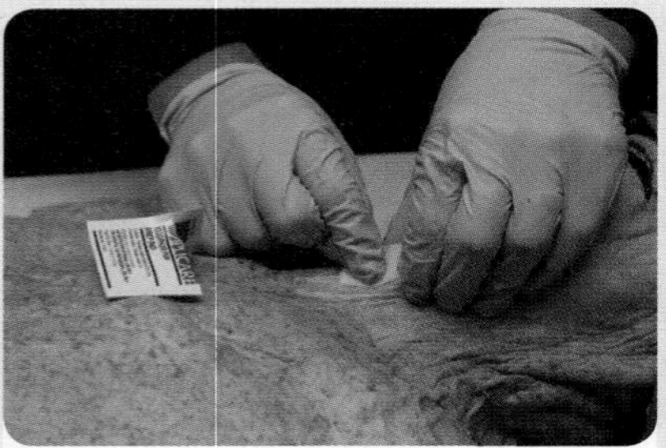

Step 4 Cleanse the area with an iodine-containing solution.

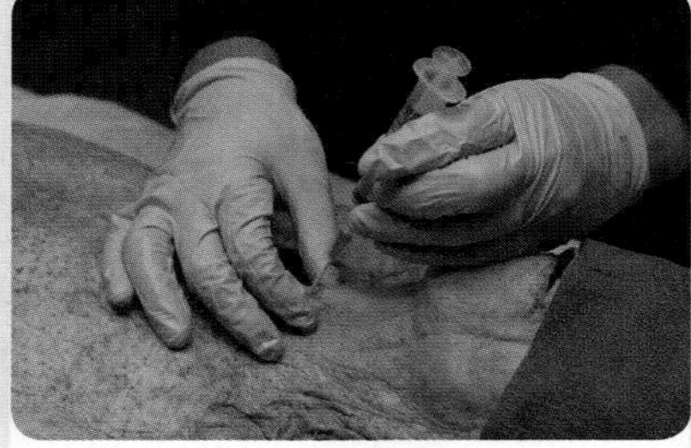

Step 5 Stabilize the larynx, and insert the needle into the cricothyroid membrane at a 45° angle toward the feet.

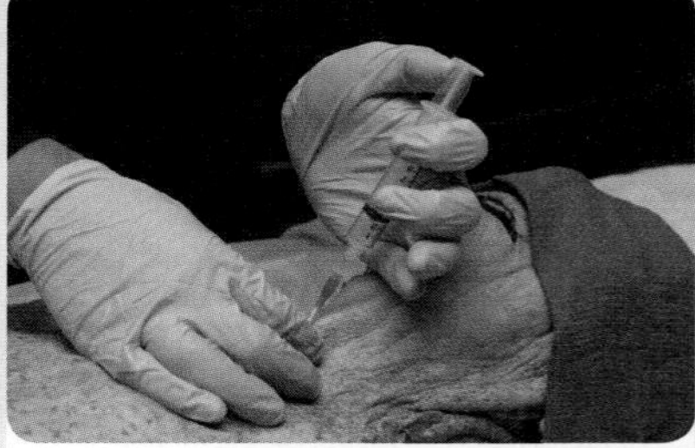

Step 6 Aspirate with the syringe to determine correct catheter placement.

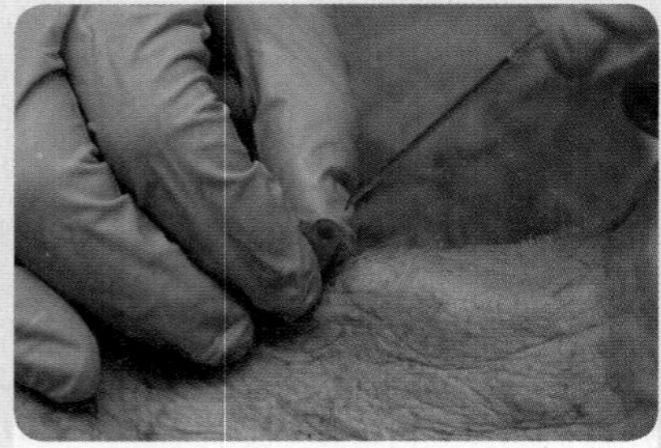

Step 7 Slide the catheter off of the needle until the hub of the catheter is flush with the patient's skin.

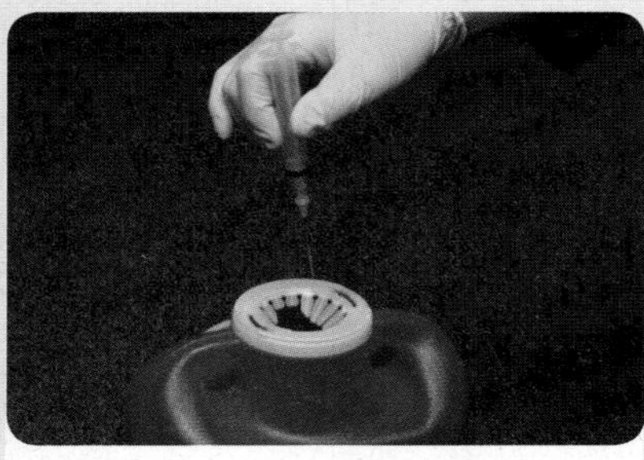

Step 8 Place the syringe and needle in a puncture-proof container.

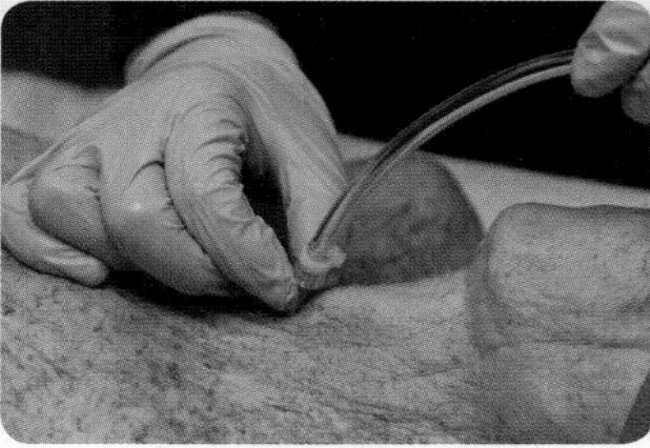

Step 9 Connect one end of the oxygen tubing to the catheter and the other end to the jet ventilator. Maintain manual stabilization of the catheter until it has been secured in place to avoid dislodgment with jet ventilation.

Skill Drill 15-19 Performing Needle Cricothyrotomy and Translaryngeal Catheter Ventilation *(continued)*

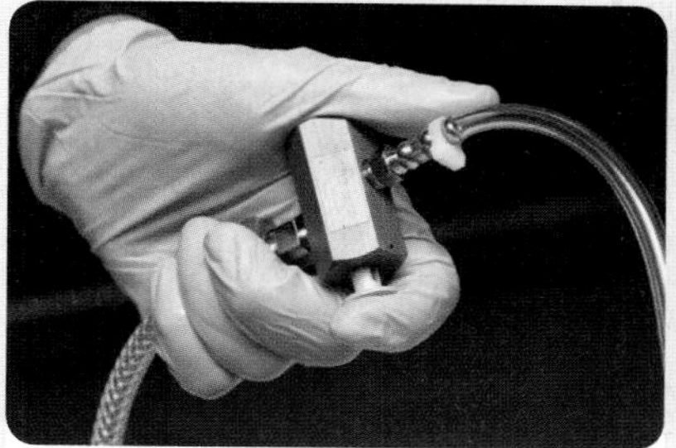

Step 10 Press or occlude the ventilation valve on the jet ventilator for 1 second while observing for chest rise. Release the ventilation valve for 2 to 3 seconds to allow for exhalation.

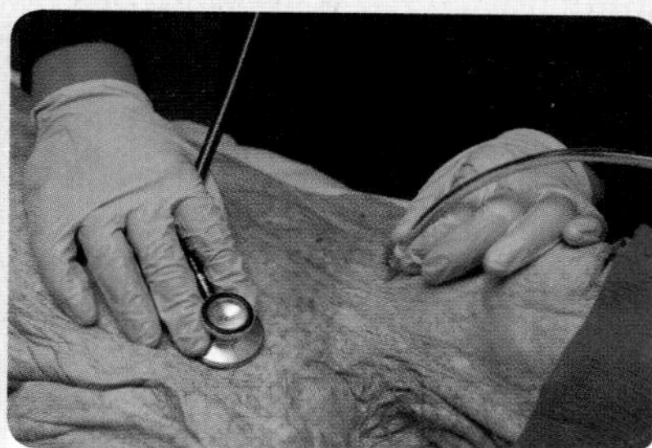

Step 11 Auscultate the apices and bases of both lungs and over the epigastrium to confirm correct catheter placement.

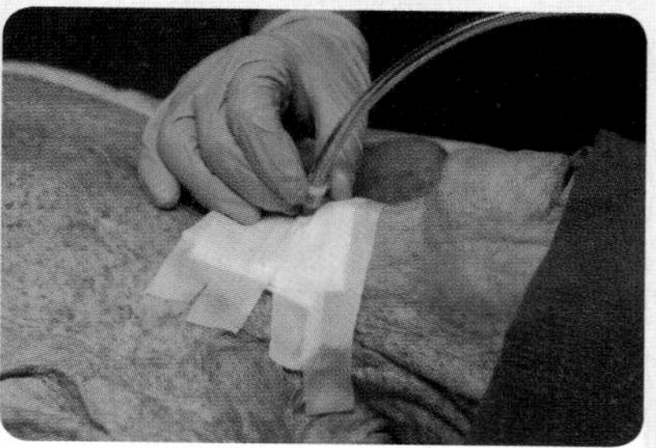

Step 12 Secure the catheter with a 4 × 4-inch (10 × 10-cm) gauze pad and tape. Continue ventilations while frequently reassessing for adequate ventilations and potential complications.

YOU are the Paramedic SUMMARY

1. What is the difference between ventilation and oxygenation?

Ventilation is the act of moving air into and out of the lungs, whereas oxygenation is the process of loading oxygen molecules onto hemoglobin molecules in the bloodstream. The presence of ventilation does not guarantee that oxygenation is taking place; thus, it is possible to ventilate but not oxygenate. An example is a patient who is trapped in a grain silo. The inside of the silo is relatively devoid of oxygen and may contain a number of toxic gases. The patient may continue to ventilate, but is unable to oxygenate because little to no oxygen is available to breathe into the lungs. Conversely, oxygenation is not possible without ventilation; if a patient is not ventilating, then he or she cannot bring any oxygen into the lungs.

2. Would a heroin overdose cause primary ventilation failure or oxygenation failure? Why or why not?

Heroin, an opiate, is a CNS depressant. Along with other vital body functions, such as heart rate and blood pressure, a heroin overdose would depress the patient's respiratory drive and cause primary ventilation failure. If ventilation is absent or inadequate, then the patient cannot intake adequate amounts of oxygen into the lungs. As a result, a subsequent failure of oxygenation would occur.

3. What should be your most immediate treatment priority?

The patient has secretions in his mouth, which is an immediate threat to the airway. Therefore, your most immediate treatment priority should be to turn the patient onto his side—which will allow secretions to drain—and suction his airway until it is clear of secretions. Do not suction a patient's airway while he or she is supine—doing so markedly increases the risk of aspiration. Mortality increases significantly if a patient aspirates, so you must make every effort to prevent this complication.

4. What negative effects can occur if you hyperventilate a patient?

Hyperventilating a patient—that is, ventilating too fast and/or with too much volume—can cause several negative physiologic effects and is associated with poor patient outcomes. It significantly increases intrathoracic pressure and puts pressure on the heart; these effects

YOU are the Paramedic SUMMARY (continued)

can markedly reduce venous return and cardiac output. As the heart is squeezed in the thoracic cavity, coronary filling can also be impaired; therefore, perfusion to the heart can be reduced.

5. In addition to your inability to ventilate the patient, do any other indicators that the patient's airway is obstructed?

The fact that the patient suddenly collapsed is not consistent with a heroin overdose. The patient who overdoses on heroin or other opiates typically experiences a progressive decline in breathing and consciousness. The fact that the patient was seemingly fine 5 minutes before his collapse is also more consistent with a sudden condition (eg, airway obstruction) than what you would expect to encounter with an opiate overdose.

6. What equipment should you prepare while your partner is performing chest compressions?

You should prepare your laryngoscope with the proper size blade and a pair of Magill forceps. If a couple of rounds of chest compressions are ineffective, then you must perform laryngoscopy, attempt to visualize the obstruction, and remove it with the forceps.

Remember, if you can see the obstruction, then you may attempt to remove it with the forceps. However, be sure not to grasp the object tightly or remove it quickly, which may cause it to separate. This separation could cause the remaining material to advance farther into the trachea.

7. Is your partner's suggestion of a needle cricothyrotomy the best option? Why or why not?

If you are unable to remove a foreign body upper airway obstruction and cannot ventilate the patient, then the only viable option is to bypass the obstruction and gain access to the trachea via the cricothyroid membrane.

In this case, a needle cricothyrotomy with transtracheal jet ventilation would not be the best option. Transtracheal jet ventilation requires the ability of the patient to exhale—at least partially—through the upper airway. If the upper airway is completely obstructed, then exhalation will not be possible.

For patients with a severe foreign body upper airway obstruction that cannot be relieved with chest compressions or visualized and removed with Magill forceps, the best option is a surgical cricothyrotomy. If the patient cannot be ventilated by any other means, then access to the trachea via the cricothyroid membrane is his or her only chance for survival.

8. How can the patient's $ETCO_2$ level be so high when his SpO_2 level is 96%?

Because you are now able to ventilate the patient, you would expect his SpO_2 level to increase accordingly, since oxygen can now be delivered to the lungs and bind to hemoglobin in the bloodstream. However, because of the prolonged apnea caused by the airway obstruction, he has retained a lot of carbon dioxide—both in his lungs and at the cellular level. The patient's markedly elevated $ETCO_2$ level reflects this. If the patient remained apneic, then the cells would convert to anaerobic metabolism (metabolism in the absence of oxygen) and begin producing lactic acid. While the patient's $ETCO_2$ level may initially be elevated from residual carbon dioxide retention, it would eventually decrease as cellular anoxia continues. Cellular oxygenation is required for the production of carbon dioxide.

9. Is it necessary to adjust your current treatment? If so, then how?

The patient is markedly hypercapneic, and the only way to correct this condition is to titrate your ventilations. Therefore, increase the rate—and perhaps volume—of positive pressure ventilation until his $ETCO_2$ level returns to its normal range of 35 to 45 mm Hg. However, you must exercise caution and not increase the ventilation rate and volume too much, because this increase can have a negative effect on cardiac output (his blood pressure is marginal at 94/56 mm Hg).

10. What is the likely explanation for the increase in the patient's heart rate and blood pressure? Is additional treatment necessary?

A marked increase in heart rate and blood pressure in an intubated patient—or in this case, the patient who had a cricothyrotomy and was previously unresponsive—should alert you that the patient is likely experiencing pain (a tube in the trachea is painful). Furthermore, the fact that he clenches his fists in response to pain indicates that he is beginning to wake up. This is obviously a positive sign; however, if his mental status continues to improve, then he may become combative, which could result in dislodgement of the tracheotomy tube.

To maintain patient comfort and facilitate his compliance, you should administer a sedative and an analgesic. Midazolam (Versed) and ketamine (Ketalar) are commonly used sedatives. Midazolam is commonly given in a dose of 2 to 5 mg, and ketamine is commonly given in a dose of 1 to 2 mg/kg. Fentanyl (Sublimaze) is a commonly used analgesic; the usual dose is 0.5 to 1 mcg/kg. Administer additional sedation and analgesia as needed, depending on the patient's clinical response and your transport time.

YOU are the Paramedic SUMMARY *(continued)*

11. What are some possible causes of the patient's decreasing $ETCO_2$ level and waveform height? What should you do to determine the cause?

Any change in $ETCO_2$ level should prompt an immediate reassessment of advanced airway placement and ventilation rate and volume. For example, if the ET tube moves out of the trachea and into an area that contains minimal or no carbon dioxide (ie, the esophagus, or in this case, the subcutaneous tissues of the neck), then no numeric $ETCO_2$ value would be displayed and the capnograph would display a flat line. Although the $ETCO_2$ level is decreased in this patient, the cardiac monitor/defibrillator is still displaying a numeric $ETCO_2$ value and capnographic waveform. Therefore, tube displacement is not the likely cause.

The gas sampling tubing that connects the in-line CO_2 detector and cardiac monitor/defibrillator can become partially or completely occluded with secretions. If this occurs, then the patient's $ETCO_2$ level (numeric value and waveform) may markedly decrease. Simply replacing the in-line CO_2 detector should correct this.

Ventilations that are too fast or with too much volume (hyperventilation) will drive the patient's $ETCO_2$ reading down and produce smaller capnographic waveforms because too much carbon dioxide is being eliminated from the lungs. Other causes of decreased $ETCO_2$ level include decreased carbon dioxide production (such as in hypothermia, paralysis, or acidosis) and decreased carbon dioxide delivery to the lungs because of decreased cardiac output (such as with cardiogenic shock).

In the case of this patient, it is likely that the decrease in his $ETCO_2$ level is caused by a ventilatory rate that is too fast.

12. What would you expect the patient's $ETCO_2$ reading and waveform to do if he were not being adequately ventilated?

If an intubated patient with spontaneous perfusion (that is, he or she has a pulse) is not being adequately ventilated, then you would expect to see an increase in his or her $ETCO_2$ value and an increase in the amplitude of the capnographic waveform. This increase would indicate that the patient is not being ventilated fast enough and/or is not receiving adequate tidal volume (hypoventilation), resulting in pulmonary carbon dioxide retention. Increasing the rate, and if necessary, the tidal volume, should restore the $ETCO_2$ value to a therapeutic range.

13. Is a neuromuscular blocking agent (paralytic) indicated for this patient? Why or why not?

A neuromuscular blocking agent, such as rocuronium bromide (Zemuron) or vecuronium bromide (Norcuron) is not the best option for this patient for a number of reasons.

- Although the patient is taking spontaneous occasional breaths and is moving his eyes, he is not combative and appears to be tolerating the tube and your positive pressure ventilation.
- Taking away the patient's respiratory drive through chemical paralysis after he experienced a prolonged period of apnea is not in his best interest.
- The patient's Spo_2 and $ETCO_2$ levels indicate that he is well oxygenated and ventilated.
- Your estimated time of arrival at the hospital is only 8 minutes.

For these reasons, the best option is to administer additional sedation (ie, midazolam, ketamine) and assist his spontaneous respiratory efforts. Depending on the type of transport ventilator you are using, you can either adjust the settings accordingly, or disconnect the mechanical ventilator and manually ventilate him with a bag-mask device.

EMS Patient Care Report (PCR)

Date: 8-01-18	**Incident No.:** 08160005		**Nature of Call:** Unresponsive, not breathing		**Location:** 145 Circle Oak Drive
Dispatched: 1820	**En Route:** 1821	**At Scene:** 1825	**Transport:** 1845	**At Hospital:** 1908	**In Service:** 1929

Patient Information

Age: 39 **Sex:** M **Weight (in kg [lb]):** estimated at 80 kg (176 lb)	**Allergies:** Unknown; information not available **Medications:** Unknown; information not available **Past Medical History:** Heroin abuse; no other medical history available **Chief Complaint:** Unresponsive and apneic

YOU are the Paramedic SUMMARY (continued)

Vital Signs						
Time: 1828	**BP:** N/A	**Pulse:** 130	**Respirations:** 0	**Spo_2:** 68%	**$ETCO_2$:** N/A	**ECG:** N/A
Time: 1830	**BP:** N/A	**Pulse:** 140	**Respirations:** 0	**Spo_2:** 60%	**$ETCO_2$:** N/A	**ECG:** Sinus tachycardia
Time: 1835	**BP:** 94/56	**Pulse:** 118	**Respirations:** 12 (with PPV)	**Spo_2:** 96%	**$ETCO_2$:** 83	**ECG:** Sinus tachycardia
Time: 1840	**BP:** 164/92	**Pulse:** 130	**Respirations:** 20 (with PPV)	**Spo_2:** 98%	**$ETCO_2$:** 32	**ECG:** Sinus tachycardia
Time: 1845	**BP:** 126/74	**Pulse:** 110	**Respirations:** 20 (with PPV)	**Spo_2:** 97%	**$ETCO_2$:** 19	**ECG:** Sinus tachycardia
Time: 1855	**BP:** 134/78	**Pulse:** 106	**Respirations:** 12 (with PPV)	**Spo_2:** 98%	**$ETCO_2$:** 41	**ECG:** Sinus tachycardia

EMS Treatment (circle all that apply)				
Oxygen @ 15 L/min via (circle one): **NC** **NRM** **Bag-mask device** (circled)		**Assisted Ventilation**	**Airway Adjunct:** Oral airway, Nasal airway (circled)	**CPR**
Defibrillation	**Bleeding Control**	**Bandaging/ Splinting**	**IV Therapy** Time: 18:36 Gauge: 18 Site: Left arm Fluid: Normal saline Rate: TKO	(circled) **Other:** Suction, surgical cricothyrotomy (tube size 6.0 mm), cardiac monitoring, $ETCO_2$ monitoring, pulse oximetry **Medication:** Midazolam Time: 1842 Dose: 5 mg Route: IV push **Medication:** Fentanyl Time: 1843 Dose: 100 mcg Route: IV push **Medication:** Midazolam Time: 18:57 Dose: 2.5 mg Route: IV push

YOU are the Paramedic SUMMARY *(continued)*

Narrative
9-1-1 dispatch for a pt who was unresponsive and not breathing. Arrived on scene and found a 39-year-old man, lying supine on his front porch. He was unresponsive and apneic, but had radial and carotid pulses. Secretions that smelled of ETOH were draining from the patient's mouth and he was markedly cyanotic. Suctioned the patient's oropharynx, inserted oral and nasal airways, and began bag-mask ventilation. The patient's neighbor, who was present at the scene, advised that she observed the patient stumble onto his porch and then collapse. She further stated that she had just talked to him 5 minutes prior, and that he was "fine." Chest rise was not noted and resistance was met with initial ventilation, so the patient's head was repositioned. After the second ventilation attempt failed, initiated chest compressions due to suspected foreign body airway obstruction. Direct laryngoscopy was performed, and a large pastry-like substance was impacted in and around the glottic opening. Removal of the object with Magill forceps was unsuccessful, so the decision was made to perform a surgical cricothyrotomy. The patient maintained a spontaneous pulse, although it was notably weaker and only present at the carotid artery. A 6.0-mm ET tube was successfully placed in the trachea via the cricothyroid membrane and ventilation was noted to produce visible chest rise. Successful placement of the ET tube was confirmed with waveform capnography, bilaterally equal breath sounds, and an absence of epigastric sounds. Began ventilation rate of 12 breaths/min. The cardiac monitor revealed sinus tachycardia w/o ectopy, and the patient's cyanosis began resolving. Secured the ET tube in place, secured the patient to the stretcher, and loaded him into the ambulance. Established IV access, assessed vital signs, and began transport. Connected patient to ATV and continued ventilation rate of 12 breaths/min. The patient's $ETCO_2$ level was noted to be 83 mm Hg; bilateral chest rise was noted, and breath sounds were clear to auscultation bilaterally. After adjusting the ventilation rate and tidal volume, the patient's $ETCO_2$ level returned to a range of 40 to 42 mm Hg. The patient's BP and pulse were noted to be markedly elevated, and he clenched his fists in response to a painful stimulus. Administered midazolam and fentanyl for sedation and pain control; these interventions facilitated ventilation and patient compliance. Reassessed the patient's vital signs, which indicated hemodynamic stability, and continued ventilation support. The patient's skin color, condition, and temperature had markedly improved; it was now pink, cool, and dry. The cardiac monitor continued to display sinus tachycardia w/o ectopy, and $ETCO_2$ readings remained within range of 40 and 42 mm Hg. With a short transport time remaining, spontaneous respiratory effort and eye movement was noted, so addition midazolam was administered and ventilatory support was continued for the remainder of the transport. Delivered the patient to the ED w/o incident and gave verbal report to the staff RN. The attending physician reconfirmed correct ET tube placement by noting bilaterally equal breath sounds, no epigastric sounds, and $ETCO_2$ reading of 41 mm Hg. Medic 73 cleared the hospital and returned to service.**End of report**

Prep Kit

▶ Ready for Review

- The upper airway consists of all structures above the vocal cords—the larynx, oropharynx, nasopharynx, and tongue. Its functions include the warming, filtering, and humidification of inhaled air.
- The lower airway consists of all structures below the vocal cords—the trachea, mainstem bronchi, bronchioles, pulmonary capillaries, and alveoli. Pulmonary gas exchange takes place at the alveolar level in the lungs.
- Ventilation, oxygenation, and respiration are crucial for the tissues to receive the needed nutrients.
- Ventilation is the act of moving air into and out of the lungs. For ventilation to occur, the diaphragm and intercostal muscles must function properly.
- Negative pressure ventilation is the drawing of air into the lungs due to changes in intrathoracic pressure. Positive pressure ventilation is the forcing of air into the lungs and is provided via bag-mask device, pocket mask, or mechanical ventilation device to patients who are not breathing (apneic) or are breathing inadequately.
- In contrast to negative pressure ventilation—which favors venous return to the heart—positive pressure ventilation can impair venous return to the heart. Do not hyperventilate any patient; doing so can cause a significant increase in intrathoracic pressure, which can further impair venous return and reduce cardiac output.
- Oxygenation is the process of loading oxygen molecules onto hemoglobin in the bloodstream. Oxygenation may not occur if the environment is depleted of oxygen or if the environment contains carbon monoxide, which prevents oxygen from binding to hemoglobin.
- Respiration is the exchange of oxygen and carbon dioxide in the alveoli and tissues of the body.
- Many conditions exist that can inhibit the body's ability to effectively deliver oxygen to the cells. With $\dot{V}/\dot{Q}$ mismatch, ventilation may be compromised but perfusion continues, leading to a lack of oxygen diffusing into the bloodstream, which can lead to severe hypoxemia.
- Other factors that impede delivery of oxygen to cells include airway swelling, airway obstruction, medications that depress the CNS, neuromuscular disorders, respiratory and cardiac diseases, circulatory compromise, submersion, and trauma to the head, neck, spine, or chest.
- Hypoventilation and hyperventilation, along with hypoxia, can cause disruptions in the acid-base balance in the body that may lead to rapid deterioration in a patient's condition and death. When an excess of acid is present in the body, the fastest way to eliminate it is through the respiratory system. Excess acid can be expelled as carbon dioxide from the lungs. Conversely, slowing respirations will increase the level of carbon dioxide. Respiratory acidosis and respiratory alkalosis can result from a number of conditions and can be life threatening.
- Adequate breathing in the adult features a respiratory rate between 12 and 20 breaths/min, adequate depth (tidal volume), a regular pattern of inhalation and exhalation, symmetric chest rise, and bilaterally clear and equal breath sounds.
- Inadequate breathing in the adult features a rate that is too slow (less than 12 breaths/min) or too fast (greater than 20 breaths/min), a shallow depth of breathing (reduced tidal volume), an irregular pattern of inhalation and exhalation, asymmetric chest movement, adventitious (abnormal) breath sounds, cyanosis, and an altered mental status.
- It is important to be able to recognize abnormal breathing patterns when assessing a patient. These include Cheyne-Stokes respirations, Kussmaul respirations, Biot (ataxic) respirations, apneustic respirations, and agonal gasps.
- While assessing breathing, auscultate breath sounds with a stethoscope. Breath sounds represent airflow into the alveoli. They should be clear and equal on both sides of the chest (bilaterally), anteriorly, and posteriorly. Abnormal breath sounds include wheezing, rhonchi, crackles, stridor, and pleural friction rub.
- The pulse oximeter measures the percentage of hemoglobin that is saturated with oxygen (SpO_2). This type of measurement depends on adequate perfusion to the capillary beds and can be inaccurate when the patient is cold, is in shock, or has been exposed to carbon monoxide.
- Peak expiratory flow is a fairly reliable assessment of the severity of bronchoconstriction. It is also used to gauge the effectiveness of treatment, such as inhaled beta-2 agonists (such as albuterol).
- Carbon dioxide (CO_2) monitors detect the presence of CO_2 in exhaled air and are important adjuncts for determining ventilation adequacy and advanced airway placement. The colorimetric CO_2 detector is a qualitative device that attaches between an advanced airway and ventilation device; specially treated paper inside the detector turns yellow

Prep Kit *(continued)*

during exhalation, indicating the presence of exhaled CO_2. The capnometer is a quantitative device that provides a numeric display of end-tidal CO_2 ($ETCO_2$). The capnographer, also a quantitative device, provides real-time objective data regarding $ETCO_2$ by displaying a waveform (waveform capnography) or a waveform and numeric display (digital/waveform capnography). The capnographer can analyze air samples of a spontaneously breathing patient or can be used when an advanced airway has been inserted and the patient is being manually or mechanically ventilated. Quantitative digital/waveform capnography is the most accurate method for monitoring a patient's $ETCO_2$ level.

- Patients who are apneic or are not breathing adequately require some form of positive pressure ventilation, such as bag-mask ventilation. Patients who are breathing adequately, but have evidence of hypoxemia (SpO_2 level less than 94%) or respiratory distress, should receive an appropriate concentration of oxygen via nasal cannula or nonrebreathing mask. Never withhold oxygen from any patient suspected of being hypoxemic.
- Unrecognized inadequate breathing will lead to hypoxia, a dangerous condition in which the body's cells and tissues do not receive adequate oxygen.
- Regardless of the patient's condition, his or her airway must remain patent at all times. The first step in airway management is to position the patient. The recovery position involves placing the patient in a left lateral recumbent position. It is the preferred position to maintain the airway of unresponsive patients with adequate breathing and no evidence of injury to the spine, pelvis, or hips.
- The patient's head must be properly positioned. Manual airway maneuvers include the head tilt–chin lift, jaw-thrust, and the tongue-jaw lift.
- Clearing the airway means removing obstructing material; maintaining the airway means keeping it open, manually or with adjunctive devices.
- Oropharyngeal suctioning may be required after opening a patient's airway. Rigid (tonsil-tip or Yankauer) catheters are preferred when suctioning the pharynx. Soft plastic (whistle-tip or French) catheters are used to suction secretions from the nose and can be passed down an ET tube to suction pulmonary secretions.
- If a patient has secretions in the airway, then position him or her on his or her side and suction the oropharynx until it is clear of secretions.
- Airway obstruction can be caused by choking on food (or, in children, on toys); epiglottitis; inhalation injuries; airway trauma with swelling; and anaphylaxis. It is critical to differentiate between a mild (partial) airway obstruction and a severe (complete) airway obstruction.
- Chest compressions, finger sweeps (only if the object can be seen and easily retrieved), manual removal of the object, and attempts to ventilate is the recommended sequence of events to attempt to remove a foreign body airway obstruction in an unresponsive adult. Continuously perform abdominal thrusts in a responsive adult or child with an airway obstruction until the obstruction is relieved or he or she becomes unresponsive.
- If BLS maneuvers are not successful in relieving a foreign body airway obstruction in the unresponsive patient, then visualize the airway with a laryngoscope. If you can see the foreign body, then carefully grasp it with Magill forceps and slowly back it out of the airway.
- Basic airway adjuncts include the oropharyngeal (oral) airway and the nasopharyngeal (nasal) airway. The oral airway keeps the tongue off of the posterior pharynx; it is used only in unresponsive patients without a gag reflex. The nasal airway is better tolerated in patients with altered mental status who have an intact gag reflex.
- Administer supplemental oxygen to any patient with respiratory distress or evidence of hypoxemia (SpO_2 level less than 94%). Be familiar with oxygen cylinder sizes and the duration of flow, and always take standard precautions when using oxygen.
- The nonrebreathing mask can deliver up to 90% oxygen when the flow rate is set at 15 L/min. The nasal cannula should be used if the patient cannot tolerate the nonrebreathing mask; it can deliver oxygen concentrations of 24% to 44% when the flowmeter is set at 1 to 6 L/min. Other types of oxygen-delivery devices include the partial rebreathing mask and Venturi mask.
- Methods of providing artificial ventilation include the one- and two-person bag-mask ventilation technique and mouth-to-mask with one-way valve and supplemental oxygen attached. Artificial ventilation is indicated for patients who are apneic or are not breathing adequately.

Prep Kit *(continued)*

- CPAP has been clinically proven to improve a patient's breathing by forcing fluid from the alveoli (in pulmonary edema) or dilating the bronchioles (in obstructive lung diseases and asthma). It involves the patient breathing against a certain amount of positive pressure during exhalation. CPAP has also been shown to reduce the need for intubation.
- Check for loose dental appliances in a patient before providing artificial ventilation. Loose dental appliances should be removed to prevent them from obstructing the airway; tight-fitting dental appliances should be left in place during artificial ventilation.
- If you are going to remove a patient's dental appliance, then do so before intubation. Removing it after the patient has been intubated may result in inadvertent extubation.
- Patients with massive maxillofacial trauma are at high risk for airway compromise due to oral bleeding. Assist ventilations and provide oral suctioning as needed.
- Ventilating too forcefully or too fast can cause gastric distention, which can cause regurgitation and aspiration. Administering ventilations over 1 second—just enough to produce visible chest rise—will reduce the incidence of gastric distention and the associated risks of regurgitation and aspiration.
- Invasive gastric decompression involves the insertion of a gastric tube into the stomach. A nasogastric tube is inserted into the stomach via the nose; an orogastric tube is inserted into the stomach via the mouth.
- Patients with a tracheal stoma or tracheostomy tube may require ventilation, suctioning, or tube replacement. Ventilation through a tracheostomy tube involves attaching the bag-valve device to the 15/22-mm adapter on the tube; ventilation of a patient with a stoma and no tracheostomy tube can be performed with a pocket mask or bag-mask device. Use pediatric-size masks when ventilating a patient through a stoma.
- Unresponsive patients or patients who cannot maintain their own airway should be considered candidates for ET intubation, the insertion of an ET tube into the trachea. In orotracheal intubation, the ET tube is inserted into the trachea via the mouth; in nasotracheal intubation (a blind technique), the ET tube is inserted into the trachea via the nose. Other methods of ET intubation include retrograde intubation, face-to-face intubation, intubation with the use of a lighted stylet (transillumination), and digital (or tactile) intubation.
- Direct laryngoscopy involves directly visualizing the vocal cords with a laryngoscope, and video laryngoscopy involves visualizing the vocal cords on a video screen.
- A critical step in intubation is confirmation of tube placement. Continuous waveform capnography, in addition to a clinical assessment (such as auscultation of breath sounds and over the epigastrium and assessing for visible chest rise), is regarded as the most reliable method of confirming and monitoring correct placement of the ET tube.
- If an attempted intubation does not result in acceptable oxygen saturation levels, then perform BLS maneuvers with an oral airway and/or nasal airway and a bag-mask device, and consider using another airway device.
- Tracheobronchial suctioning is indicated if the condition of an intubated patient deteriorates because of pulmonary secretions in the ET tube.
- Do not perform extubation in the prehospital setting unless the patient is unreasonably intolerant of the tube. It is generally best to sedate an intubated patient who is becoming intolerant of the ET tube.
- RSI involves using pharmacologic agents to sedate and paralyze a patient to facilitate placement of an ET tube. It should be considered when a responsive or combative patient requires intubation but cannot tolerate laryngoscopy.
- Drugs used for RSI include sedatives, such as midazolam (Versed), diazepam (Valium) and ketamine (Ketalar), and neuromuscular blocking agents (paralytics) to induce complete paralysis. The latter agents are classified into depolarizing (such as succinylcholine) and nondepolarizing (such as vecuronium, pancuronium, and rocuronium) paralytics.
- Alternative airway devices, which may be used if ET intubation is either impossible or unsuccessful, include the King LT, laryngeal mask airway, i-gel supraglottic airway, Combitube, and CobraPLA.
- Open (surgical) cricothyrotomy involves incising the cricothyroid membrane, inserting a tracheostomy tube or ET tube into the trachea, and manually or mechanically ventilating the patient. Needle cricothyrotomy involves inserting a 14- to 16-gauge over-the-needle catheter through the cricothyroid membrane and ventilating the patient with a high-pressure jet ventilation device (transtracheal jet ventilation).

Prep Kit (continued)

- Cricothyrotomy is indicated in situations where intubation is not possible and you cannot ventilate the patient by any other means.

▶ Vital Vocabulary

3-3-2 rule A method used to predict difficult intubation. A mouth opening of less than three fingerbreadths, a mandible length of less than three fingerbreadths, and a distance from hyoid bone to thyroid notch of less than two fingerbreadths indicate a possibly difficult airway.

abdominal thrust maneuver Abdominal thrusts performed to relieve a foreign body airway obstruction.

accessory muscles The muscles not normally used during normal breathing; include the sternocleidomastoid muscles of the neck, the pectoralis major muscles of the chest, and the abdominal muscles.

acetylcholine (ACh) A chemical neurotransmitter of the parasympathetic nervous system.

adventitious Abnormal.

afterload The pressure gradient against which the heart must pump; an increase can decrease cardiac output.

agonal gasps Slow, shallow, irregular respirations or occasional gasping breaths that result from cerebral anoxia.

anoxia An absence of oxygen.

anterograde amnesia An inability to remember events after the onset of amnesia.

aphonia The inability to speak.

apneic oxygenation The continued alveolar uptake of oxygen, even when the patient is apneic; can be facilitated by administering oxygen via nasal cannula during intubation.

apneustic respirations Prolonged gasping inspirations followed by extremely short, ineffective expirations; associated with brainstem insult.

asymmetric chest wall movement Unequal movement of the two sides of the chest; indicates decreased airflow into one lung.

automatic transport ventilator (ATV) A portable mechanical ventilator attached to a control box that allows the variables of ventilation (such as rate and tidal volume) to be set.

bag-mask device A manual ventilation device that consists of a bag, mask, reservoir, and oxygen inlet; capable of delivering up to 100% oxygen.

barotrauma Trauma resulting from excessive pressure.

benzodiazepines Sedative-hypnotic drugs that provide muscle relaxation and mild sedation; include drugs such as diazepam (Valium) and midazolam (Versed).

bimanual laryngoscopy An effective technique to improve laryngoscopic view of the vocal cords by external manipulation of the larynx.

bilevel positive airway pressure (BPAP) A form of noninvasive positive pressure ventilation that delivers two pressures (a higher inspiratory positive airway pressure, and a lower expiratory positive airway pressure).

Biot (ataxic) respirations Irregular pattern, rate, and depth of respirations with intermittent periods of apnea; result from increased intracranial pressure.

Bourdon-gauge flowmeter An oxygen flowmeter that is commonly used because it is not affected by gravity and can be placed in any position.

bronchovesicular sounds A combination of the tracheal and vesicular breath sounds; heard where airways and alveoli are found, the upper part of the sternum and between the scapulas.

BURP maneuver The backward, upward, and rightward pressure used during intubation to improve the laryngoscopic view of the glottic opening and vocal cords; also called external laryngeal manipulation.

capnographer A device that attaches between the endotracheal tube and ventilation device; provides graphic information about the presence of exhaled carbon dioxide.

capnometer A device that performs the same function and attaches in the same way as a capnographer but provides a digital reading of the exhaled carbon dioxide.

carbon monoxide oximeter A device that measures absorption at several wavelengths to distinguish oxyhemoglobin from carboxyhemoglobin.

carboxyhemoglobin (COHb) Hemoglobin loaded with carbon monoxide.

Cheyne-Stokes respirations A gradually increasing rate and depth of respirations followed by a gradual decrease with intermittent periods of apnea; associated with brainstem insult.

Cobra perilaryngeal airway (CobraPLA) A supraglottic airway device with a shape that allows the device to slide easily along the hard palate and to hold the soft tissue away from the laryngeal inlet.

colorimetric carbon dioxide detector A device that attaches between the endotracheal tube and ventilation device; uses special paper that should turn

Prep Kit (continued)

from purple to yellow during exhalation, indicating the presence of exhaled carbon dioxide.

Combitube A multilumen airway device that consists of a single tube with two lumens, two balloons, and two ventilation ports; an alternative device if endotracheal intubation is not possible or has failed.

continuous positive airway pressure (CPAP) A method of ventilation that delivers a single pressure, used primarily in the treatment of critically ill patients with respiratory distress; can prevent the need for endotracheal intubation.

Cormack-Lehane classification A system used to predict intubation difficulty based on the airway structures observed during laryngoscopy.

crackles The breath sounds produced as fluid-filled alveoli pop open under increasing inspiratory pressure; can be fine or coarse; formerly called rales.

curved laryngoscope blade A blade designed to fit into the vallecula, indirectly lifting the epiglottis and exposing the vocal cords; also called the Macintosh blade.

cyanosis Blue or purple skin; indicates inadequate oxygen in the blood.

delayed sequence intubation (DSI) A procedure in which a patient is sedated for the purpose of preoxygenation prior to the administration of a paralytic and intubation.

denitrogenation The process of replacing nitrogen in the lungs with oxygen to maintain a normal oxygen saturation level during intubation.

depolarizing neuromuscular blocker A drug that competitively binds with the acetylcholine receptor sites but is not affected as quickly by acetylcholinesterase; an example is succinylcholine chloride.

digital intubation A method of intubation that involves directly palpating the glottic structures and elevating the epiglottis with the middle finger while guiding the endotracheal tube into the trachea by using the sense of touch.

direct laryngoscopy Visualization of the airway with a laryngoscope.

dissociative anesthetic A medication that distorts perception of sight and sound and induces a feeling of detachment from environment and self.

dysphonia Difficulty speaking.

dyspnea Difficult or labored breathing.

endotracheal (ET) tube A tube that is inserted into the trachea for definitive airway maintenance; equipped with a distal cuff, proximal inflation port, a 15/22-mm adapter, and centimeter markings on the side.

endotracheal (ET) intubation Inserting an endotracheal tube through the glottic opening and sealing the tube with a cuff inflated against the tracheal wall.

end-tidal carbon dioxide ($ETCO_2$) monitors Devices that detect the presence of carbon dioxide in exhaled air.

epiglottis A leaf-shaped cartilaginous structure that closes over the trachea during swallowing.

esophageal detector device A bulb or syringe that is attached to the proximal end of the endotracheal tube; a device used to confirm proper endotracheal tube placement.

extubation The process of removing the endotracheal tube from an intubated patient.

face-to-face intubation Performing intubation at the same level as the patient's face; used when the standard position is not possible. In this position, the laryngoscope is held in the provider's right hand and the endotracheal tube in the left.

fasciculations Brief, uncoordinated twitching of small muscle groups in the face, neck, trunk, and extremities; may be seen after the administration of a depolarizing neuromuscular blocking agent (succinylcholine chloride).

gag reflex An automatic reaction when something touches an area deep in the oral cavity that helps protect the lower airway from aspiration.

gastric distention The enlargement or expansion of the stomach, often with air; can be a complication of ventilating the esophagus instead of the trachea.

gastric tube A tube that is inserted into the stomach to remove its contents.

gum elastic bougie A flexible device that is inserted between the glottis under direct laryngoscopy; the endotracheal tube is threaded over the device, facilitating its entry into the trachea. Also called a tracheal tube introducer.

head tilt–chin lift maneuver Manual airway maneuver that involves tilting the head back while lifting up on the chin; used to open the airway of an unresponsive nontrauma patient.

hemoglobin An iron-containing protein within red blood cells that has the ability to combine with oxygen.

Prep Kit *(continued)*

hypercapnia Increased carbon dioxide content in arterial blood.

hyperventilation A condition in which an increased amount of air enters the alveoli; carbon dioxide elimination exceeds carbon dioxide production.

hypocapnia Decreased carbon dioxide content in arterial blood.

hypoventilation A condition in which a decreased amount of air enters the alveoli; carbon dioxide production exceeds the body's ability to eliminate it by ventilation.

hypoxemia A decrease in arterial oxygen level.

hypoxia A lack of oxygen to cells and tissues.

i-gel A supraglottic airway device that uses a non-inflatable, gel-like mask to isolate the larynx and facilitate ventilation.

inspiratory/expiratory (I/E) ratio An expression for comparing the length of inspiration with that of expiration, normally 1:2, meaning that expiration is twice as long as inspiration (not measured in seconds).

intrapulmonary shunting Bypassing of oxygen-poor blood past nonfunctional alveoli.

jaw-thrust maneuver A technique to open the airway by placing the fingers behind the angle of the jaw and bringing the jaw forward; used when a patient may have a cervical spine injury.

King LT airway A single-lumen airway that is blindly inserted into the esophagus; when properly placed in the esophagus, one cuff seals the esophagus, and the other seals the oropharynx.

Kussmaul respirations A respiratory pattern characteristic of diabetic ketoacidosis, with marked hyperpnea and tachypnea; represents the body's attempt to compensate for the acidosis.

laryngeal mask airway (LMA) A device that surrounds the opening of the larynx with an inflatable silicone cuff positioned in the hypopharynx; an alternative to bag-mask ventilation.

laryngectomy A surgical procedure in which the larynx is removed.

laryngoscope A device that is used in conjunction with a laryngoscope blade to perform direct laryngoscopy.

lung compliance The ability of the alveoli to expand when air is drawn into the lungs during negative pressure ventilation or positive pressure ventilation.

Magill forceps A special type of forceps that is curved, thus allowing paramedics to maneuver it in the airway.

Mallampati classification A system for predicting the relative difficulty of intubation based on the amount of oropharyngeal structures visible in an upright, seated patient who is fully able to open his or her mouth.

metabolism The chemical processes that provide the cells with energy from nutrients.

methemoglobin (metHb) A compound formed by oxidation of the iron on hemoglobin.

multilumen airway Airway device with a single long tube that can be used for esophageal obturation or endotracheal tube ventilation, depending on where the device comes to rest following blind positioning.

Murphy eye An opening on the side of an endotracheal tube at its distal tip that permits ventilation to occur even if the tip becomes occluded by blood, mucus, or the tracheal wall.

nasal cannula A device that delivers oxygen via two small prongs that fit into the patient's nostrils; with an oxygen flow rate of 1 to 6 L/min, an oxygen concentration of 24% to 44% can be delivered.

nasogastric (NG) tube A gastric tube is inserted into the stomach through the nose.

nasopharyngeal (nasal) airway A soft rubber tube about 6 inches (15 cm) long that is inserted through the nose into the posterior pharynx behind the tongue, thereby allowing passage of air from the nose to the lower airway.

nasotracheal intubation Insertion of an endotracheal tube into the trachea through the nose.

needle cricothyrotomy Insertion of a 14- to 16-gauge over-the-needle intravenous catheter (such as an Angiocath) through the cricothyroid membrane and into the trachea.

negative pressure ventilation Drawing of air into the lungs; airflow from a region of higher pressure (outside the body) to a region of lower pressure (the lungs); occurs during normal (unassisted) breathing.

nondepolarizing neuromuscular blockers Drugs that bind to acetylcholine receptor sites; they do not cause depolarization of the muscle fiber; examples are vecuronium (Norcuron) and pancuronium (Pavulon); also called paralytics.

Prep Kit *(continued)*

nonrebreathing mask A combination mask and reservoir bag system in which oxygen fills a reservoir bag attached to the mask by a one-way valve permitting a patient to inhale from the reservoir bag but not to exhale into it; at a flow rate of 15 L/min, it can deliver 90% to 100% inspired oxygen.

open cricothyrotomy An emergency incision of the cricothyroid membrane with a scalpel and insertion of an endotracheal or a tracheostomy tube directly into the subglottic area of the trachea; also called surgical cricothyrotomy.

opioids Potent analgesics with sedative properties; examples are fentanyl (Sublimaze) and alfentanil (Alfenta); also called narcotics.

orogastric (OG) tube A gastric tube inserted into the stomach through the mouth.

oropharyngeal (oral) airway A hard plastic device that is curved so that it fits over the back of the tongue with the tip in the posterior pharynx.

orotracheal intubation Insertion of an endotracheal tube into the trachea through the mouth.

orthopnea Positional dyspnea.

oxygen humidifier A small bottle of water through which the oxygen leaving the cylinder is moisturized before it reaches the patient.

oxyhemoglobin (Hbo_2) Hemoglobin that is occupied by oxygen.

pancuronium A nondepolarizing neuromuscular blocking agent; used to maintain paralysis following succinylcholine-facilitated intubation.

paradoxical motion The inward movement of the chest during inhalation and outward movement during exhalation; the opposite of normal chest wall movement during breathing.

paralytics Drugs that paralyze skeletal muscles; used in emergency situations to facilitate intubation; also called neuromuscular blocking agents.

partial laryngectomy Surgical removal of a portion of the larynx.

partial rebreathing mask A mask similar to the nonrebreathing mask but without a one-way valve between the mask and the reservoir; room air is not drawn in with inspiration; residual expired air is mixed in the mask and rebreathed.

patent Open.

peak expiratory flow An approximation of the extent of bronchoconstriction; used to determine whether therapy (such as with inhaled bronchodilators) is effective.

pleural friction rub The result of an inflammation that causes the pleura to thicken, decreasing the pleural space and allowing the pleurae to rub together.

positive end-expiratory pressure (PEEP) Mechanical maintenance of pressure in the airway at the end of expiration to increase the volume of gas remaining in the lungs.

positive pressure ventilation Forcing of air into the lungs.

preload The pressure of blood that is returned to the heart (venous return).

pressure-compensated flowmeter An oxygen flowmeter that incorporates a float ball in a tapered calibrated tube; the float rises or falls according to the gas flow in the tube; is affected by gravity and must remain in an upright position for an accurate reading.

pulse oximeter A device that measures oxygen saturation level (Spo_2).

pulsus paradoxus A drop in the systolic blood pressure of 10 mm Hg or more; commonly seen in patients with pericardial tamponade or severe asthma.

rapid sequence intubation (RSI) A specific set of procedures, combined in rapid succession, to induce sedation and paralysis and intubate a patient quickly.

recovery position Left lateral recumbent position; used in all unresponsive nontrauma patients who are able to maintain their own airway spontaneously and are breathing adequately.

reduced hemoglobin The hemoglobin after the oxygen has been released to the cells.

reemergence phenomenon The occurrence of dreams, nightmares, or delirium that can take place during the end of the half-life of ketamine.

respiratory acidosis A pathologic condition characterized by a blood pH of less than 7.35 and caused by the accumulation of acids in the body from a respiratory cause.

respiratory alkalosis A pathologic condition characterized by a blood pH of greater than 7.45 and resulting from the accumulation of bases in the body from a respiratory cause.

retractions The drawing in of the intercostal muscles and the muscles above the clavicles that can occur in respiratory distress.

Prep Kit *(continued)*

retrograde intubation A technique in which a wire is placed through the trachea and into the mouth with a needle via the cricoid membrane; the endotracheal tube is then placed over the wire and guided into the trachea.

rhonchi A continuous, low-pitched sound; indicates mucus or fluid in the larger lower airways.

rocuronium A nondepolarizing neuromuscular blocking agent; used to maintain paralysis following succinylcholine-facilitated intubation.

safe residual pressure The pressure at which an oxygen cylinder should be replaced with a full one; often is 200 psi.

sedation The reduction of a patient's anxiety, induction of amnesia, and suppression of the gag reflex, usually by pharmacologic means.

stenosis A narrowing, such as of a blood vessel or stoma.

stoma In the context of the airway, the resultant orifice of a tracheostomy that connects the trachea to the outside air; located in the midline of the anterior part of the neck.

straight laryngoscope blade A blade designed to lift the epiglottis and expose the vocal cords; also called the Miller blade.

stridor A high-pitched inspiratory sound representing air moving past an obstruction within or immediately above the glottic opening.

stylet In the context of intubation, a semirigid wire inserted into an endotracheal tube to mold and maintain the shape of the tube.

succinylcholine chloride A depolarizing neuromuscular blocker frequently used as the initial paralytic during rapid sequence intubation; causes muscle fasciculations.

therapy regulator A device that attaches to the stem of the oxygen cylinder and reduces the high pressure of gas to a safe range (about 50 psi).

tongue-jaw lift maneuver A manual maneuver that involves grasping the tongue and jaw and lifting; commonly used to suction the airway and to place certain airway devices.

tonsil-tip catheter A hard or rigid suction catheter; also called a Yankauer catheter.

total laryngectomy Surgical removal of the entire larynx.

tracheal breath sounds Breath sounds heard by placing the stethoscope diaphragm over the trachea or sternum; also called bronchial breath sounds.

tracheobronchial suctioning Inserting a suction catheter into the endotracheal tube to remove pulmonary secretions.

tracheostomy A surgical opening into the trachea.

tracheostomy tube A plastic tube placed within the tracheostomy site (stoma).

transillumination intubation A method of intubation that uses a lighted stylet to guide the endotracheal tube into the trachea.

translaryngeal catheter ventilation A method used in conjunction with needle cricothyrotomy to ventilate a patient; requires a high-pressure jet ventilator.

trismus Clenched teeth caused by spasms of the jaw muscles.

vecuronium A nondepolarizing neuromuscular blocking agent; used to maintain paralysis following succinylcholine-facilitated intubation.

Venturi mask A mask with a number of interchangeable adapters that draws room air into the mask along with the oxygen flow; allows for the administration of highly specific oxygen concentrations.

vesicular breath sounds Soft, muffled breath sounds in which the expiratory phase is barely audible.

video laryngoscopy Visualization of the epiglottis and vocal cords through a video monitor that is attached to a laryngoscope.

$\dot{V}/\dot{Q}$ mismatch An imbalance between the anatomic portions of the lung being ventilated (V) and the anatomic portions being perfused (Q).

waveform capnography A waveform display of exhaled carbon dioxide shown on a portable cardiac monitor/defibrillator.

wheezing A high-pitched whistling sound that may be heard on inspiration, expiration, or both; indicates air movement through a constricted lower airway, such as with asthma.

whistle-tip catheters Soft plastic, nonrigid catheters; also called French catheters.

▶ References

1. Kleinman ME, Brennan EE, Goldberger ZD, et al. Part 5: adult basic life support and cardiopulmonary resuscitation quality: 2015 American Heart Association Guidelines Update for Cardiopulmonary Resuscitation and Emergency

Prep Kit (continued)

Cardiovascular Care. *Circulation*. 2015;132 (suppl 2):S414-S435.

2. O'Connor RE, Al Ali AS, Brady WJ, et al. Part 9: acute coronary syndromes: 2015 American Heart Association Guidelines Update for Cardiopulmonary Resuscitation and Emergency Cardiovascular Care. *Circulation*. 2015;132 (suppl 2):S487.
3. O'Gara PT, Kushner FG, Ascheim DD, et al. 2013 ACCF/AHA guideline for the management of ST-elevation myocardial infarction: executive summary: a report of the American College of Cardiology Foundation/American Heart Association Task Force on Practice Guidelines. *J Am Coll Cardiol*. 2013;61:485-510.
4. O'Connor RE, Al Ali AS, Brady WJ, et al. Part 9: acute coronary syndromes: 2015 American Heart Association Guidelines Update for Cardiopulmonary Resuscitation and Emergency Cardiovascular Care. *Circulation*. 2015;132 (suppl 2):S483-S500.
5. Link MS, Berkow LC, Kudenchuk PJ, et al. Part 7: adult advanced cardiovascular life support: 2015 American Heart Association Guidelines Update for Cardiopulmonary Resuscitation and Emergency Cardiovascular Care. *Circulation*. 2015;132(suppl 2):S444-S464.
6. Atkins DL, Berger S, Duff JP, et al. Part 11: pediatric basic life support and cardiopulmonary resuscitation quality: 2015 American Heart Association Guidelines Update for Cardiopulmonary Resuscitation and Emergency Cardiovascular Care. *Circulation*. 2015;132 (suppl 2):S519-S525.
7. de Caen AR, Berg MD, Chameides L, et al. Part 12: pediatric advanced life support: 2015 American Heart Association Guidelines Update for Cardiopulmonary Resuscitation and Emergency Cardiovascular Care. *Circulation*. 2015;132(suppl 2):S526-S542.
8. Nouruzi-Sedah P, Schumann M, Groeben H. Laryngoscopy via Macintosh blade versus GlideScope: success rate and time for endotracheal intubation in untrained medical personnel. *Anesthesiology*. 2009 Jan;110(1):32-37.
9. Jarvis JL, McClure SF, Johns D. EMS intubation improves with King vision video laryngoscopy. *Prehospital Emergency Care*. 2015;19(4):482-489.
10. Naito H, Guyette FX, Martin-Gill C, Callaway CW. Video laryngoscopic techniques associated with intubation success in a helicopter emergency medical service system. *Prehosp Emerg Care*. 2016;20(3):333-342.
11. Diggs LA, Yusuf JE, De Leo G. An update on out-of-hospital airway management practices in the United States. *Resuscitation*. 2014;85(7):885-92.
12. Weingart SD, Levitan RM. Preoxygenation and prevention of desaturation during emergency airway management. *J Ann Emerg Med*. 2012;59(3):165-175.

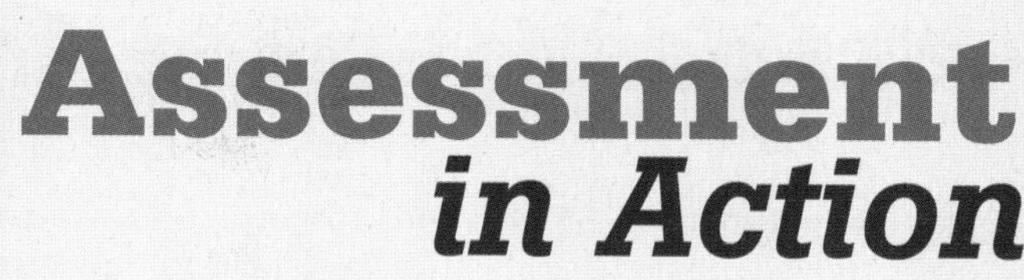

Assessment *in Action*

Your unit is dispatched to a residence for a 68-year-old man with difficulty breathing. The patient was awakened from sleep with the feeling that he was being smothered. You find him sitting on the edge of his bed in obvious respiratory distress.

Your primary survey reveals that the patient is conscious and alert. His airway is patent; however, his breathing is markedly labored and he can speak only in two-word sentences. His pulse is rapid and weak, his skin is pale and diaphoretic, and he has dried blood on his lips. The patient's oxygen saturation level reads 78% and you hear diffuse, coarse crackles when you auscultate his lungs.

1. Immediate treatment of this patient should include:

A. oxygen at 6 L/min via a nasal cannula.
B. CPAP.
C. sedation followed by orotracheal intubation.
D. albuterol via a small-volume nebulizer.

2. In which of the following situations would CPAP be contraindicated for this patient?

A. Oxygen saturation level of less than 80%
B. Inability to follow verbal commands
C. Patient history of sleep apnea
D. Systolic blood pressure of less than 140 mm Hg

3. You hear coarse crackles when auscultating the patient's breath sounds. This finding indicates:

A. widespread collapsing of the alveoli.
B. fluid accumulation in the larger airways.
C. air moving through narrowed air passages.
D. mucus or fluid in the smaller lower airways.

4. If the patient were breathing at a rate of 30 breaths/min, then you would MOST likely encounter:

A. an Spo_2 level of less than 90%.
B. unequal breath sounds.
C. an $ETCO_2$ level of less than 35 mm Hg.
D. tall capnographic waveforms.

5. You anticipate that your patient's condition may deteriorate and that RSI may be required. Which of the following drug-dose combinations would be the MOST appropriate to facilitate intubation?

A. Ketamine, 5 mg/kg; rocuronium, 0.1 mg/kg
B. Etomidate, 0.3 mg/kg; succinylcholine, 1 mg/kg
C. Midazolam, 2 mg; vecuronium, 0.6 to 1.2 mg/kg
D. Diazepam, 5 mg; rocuronium, 0.01 mg/kg

6. In addition to the glottic opening and vocal cords, which of the following anatomic structures is the MOST critical to visualize during laryngoscopy?

A. Epiglottis
B. Vallecula
C. Esophagus
D. Uvula

7. You will know that your patient's condition is improving with CPAP when:

A. his oxygen saturation improves.
B. he appears to be sleepy.
C. he pulls the mask from his face.
D. his respiratory rate increases.

Assessment ***in Action*** *(continued)*

You have intubated a 55-year-old woman who was in respiratory failure; her airway was classified as a 2 on the Cormack-Lehane classification system. You have attached the ATV; the ventilation rate is set at 12 breaths/min and the tidal volume is set at 450 mL. During transport, the capnographic waveform suddenly goes flat, and a numeric value is no longer shown. After correcting the problem, you continue to ventilate the patient. However, despite an $ETCO_2$ level of 39 mm Hg, the patient's SpO_2 level falls below 85% and the monitor alarm begins to sound. You confirm you are delivering an FIO_2 level of 1.0 and continue to search for the cause of her ongoing hypoxemia.

8. How does the Cormack-Lehane airway classification differ from the Mallampati classification?

9. Under which circumstances might you encounter a complete loss of a capnographic waveform in the intubated patient?

10. What are some conditions or situations that would cause persistent hypoxemia, despite ventilation?

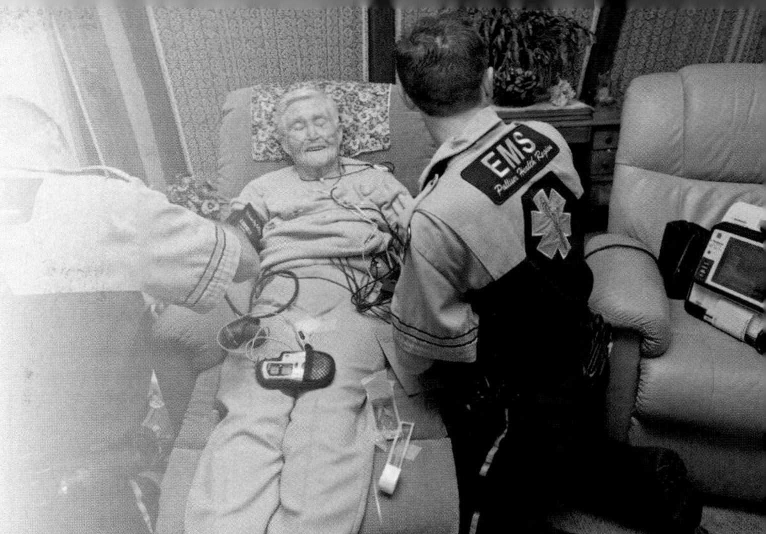

SECTION 6

Medical

CHAPTER 16

Respiratory Emergencies

National EMS Education Standard Competencies

Medicine

Integrates assessment findings with principles of epidemiology and pathophysiology to formulate a field impression and implement a comprehensive treatment/disposition plan for a patient with a medical complaint.

Respiratory

Anatomy, signs, symptoms, and management of respiratory emergencies, including those that affect the

- Upper airway (pp 905-907, 912-921, 936-939)
- Lower airway (pp 905-907, 912-921, 939-944)

Anatomy, physiology, pathophysiology, assessment, and management of

- Epiglottitis (see Chapter 43, *Pediatric Emergencies*)
- Spontaneous pneumothorax (pp 924-925, 945)
- Pulmonary edema (p 947)
- Asthma (pp 939-941)
- Chronic obstructive pulmonary disease (pp 941-944)
- Environmental/industrial exposure (p 947)
- Toxic gas (pp 946-947)
- Pertussis (see Chapter 43, *Pediatric Emergencies*)
- Cystic fibrosis (see Chapter 45, *Patients With Special Challenges*)
- Pulmonary embolism (p 949)
- Pneumonia (pp 944-945)
- Viral respiratory infections (pp 936-938, 944-945)
- Obstructive/restrictive disease (pp 941-942)

Anatomy, physiology, epidemiology, pathophysiology, psychosocial impact, presentations, prognosis, and management of

- Acute upper airway infections (pp 936-938)
- Spontaneous pneumothorax (pp 924-925, 945)
- Obstructive/restrictive lung diseases (pp 941-942)
- Pulmonary infections (pp 944-945)
- Neoplasm (pp 945-946)
- Pertussis (see Chapter 43, *Pediatric Emergencies*)
- Cystic fibrosis (see Chapter 45, *Patients With Special Challenges*)

Shock and Resuscitation

Integrates comprehensive knowledge of causes and pathophysiology into the management of cardiac arrest and pre-arrest states.

Integrates a comprehensive knowledge of the causes and pathophysiology into the management of shock, respiratory failure, or arrest, with an emphasis on early intervention to prevent arrest.

Knowledge Objectives

1. Discuss the morbidity and mortality of respiratory illness in the United States. (p 904)
2. Recall the primary structures of the respiratory system and the role of the respiratory system in breathing, cardiovascular regulation, and renal function. (pp 905-909)
3. Define hypoventilation and hyperventilation, including examples of conditions associated with each. (pp 909-911)
4. Describe the proper measures to ensure scene safety when called to care for a patient with dyspnea. (p 911)
5. Describe factors that contribute to a general impression of the patient's condition and an accurate estimation of his or her degree of respiratory distress. (pp 912-919)
6. Explain the typical presentation of a patient with dyspnea and the signs and symptoms that indicate a high level of respiratory distress. (pp 912-914)
7. Identify breathing alterations that may indicate respiratory distress, and the signs of increased work of breathing. (pp 913-914)
8. Identify the signs of lung consolidation, including abnormal breath sounds associated with excessive fluid in the lungs. (pp 915-917)
9. Explain how to assess the adequacy of the circulation of a patient with dyspnea. (pp 918, 920-921)
10. Describe the abnormal breathing patterns associated with neurologic insults that depress the respiratory center in the brain. (pp 918-920)
11. Discuss how transport decisions are made for patients with respiratory distress. (p 921)

12. Describe how to investigate the chief complaint of a patient who is having trouble breathing. (pp 921-922)
13. Identify each component of the SAMPLE history as it applies to patients with dyspnea. (pp 922-923)
14. Describe the components of the physical examination of a patient with dyspnea. (pp 923-925)
15. Describe the devices used to monitor patients with respiratory complaints. (pp 925-927)
16. Describe interventions available for treating patients with dyspnea. (pp 927-936)
17. Explain the pathophysiology, assessment, and management of a patient with upper airway inflammation caused by infection. (pp 936-938)
18. Explain the pathophysiology, assessment, and management of a patient with an obstructive lower airway disease. (pp 939-944)
19. Explain the three features that characterize asthma and how each is treated. (pp 939-941)
20. Compare the signs and symptoms of asthma, emphysema, chronic bronchitis, and restrictive lung diseases. (pp 939-944)
21. Discuss complications that can cause a patient with chronic obstructive pulmonary disease (COPD) to decompensate. (pp 942-943)
22. Explain the concepts of hypoxic drive and auto-PEEP as they relate to COPD. (pp 943-944)
23. Explain the pathophysiology, assessment, and management of patients with pulmonary infections, atelectasis, cancer, toxic inhalations, pulmonary edema, and acute respiratory distress syndrome. (pp 944-948)
24. Explain the pathophysiology, assessment, and management of patients with pneumothorax, pleural effusion, and pulmonary embolism. (pp 948-949)

Skills Objectives

1. Demonstrate the process of history taking for a patient with dyspnea. (pp 921-923)
2. Demonstrate the application of a CPAP/BPAP unit. (pp 933-935)

Introduction

Few reasons for dialing 9-1-1 are more compelling than the feeling of being unable to breathe (dyspnea). In most cases, respiratory distress originates in the respiratory system itself.

Respiratory disease is one of the most common pathologic conditions, making respiratory distress one of the most common emergency medical services (EMS) dispatches. Asthma and chronic obstructive pulmonary disease (COPD) are among the top 10 chronic conditions that cause restricted activity.[1] Approximately 15 million Americans have COPD.[2] Of all Americans, 25 million have asthma,[3] resulting in half a million hospitalizations and 3,500 deaths annually.[4] **Pneumonia**, first described by Hippocrates in 400 BC, remains one of the most common fatal illnesses in developing countries and accounts for 6% of in-patient deaths—50,000 per year—in the United States.[5] More than 30 types of pneumonia have been identified.[6]

Some respiratory diseases, such as cystic fibrosis, have a genetic (or intrinsic) cause. Others, such as occupational lung diseases, are caused by external (or extrinsic) factors. In approximately 80% of cases, COPD is related to cigarette smoking,[2] for example, but 3% of cases can be attributed to the genetic absence of a critical enzyme (alpha-1 antitrypsin).[7]

YOU are the Paramedic PART 1

You are dispatched to a medical alarm at a large apartment complex. When you arrive, you and your partner find the right building, grab your gear, and head to the closest entrance. You proceed to the fifth-floor apartment from which the call originated. There you find a 74-year-old man with ashen-gray skin who is diaphoretic and struggling to breathe. The patient lives alone and is speaking in one- to two-word sentences.

1. What initial, "from the door" findings make you concerned for this patient?
2. What are your priorities for this patient?

Researchers have yet to fully decipher the multifactorial mechanism by which many respiratory diseases develop. Intrinsic factors, such as genetics, cardiac disease, and even stress, are thought to combine with extrinsic factors, such as smoking and environmental pollutants. Asthma, for example, may be affected by genetics, race, geographic location, diet, allergies, childhood illnesses, or some combination of these factors.

In this chapter, we will examine these complex and sometimes puzzling respiratory conditions. We will start by discussing how to assess a patient whose chief complaint is dyspnea, focusing on aspects to emphasize in obtaining the history and carrying out the physical examination. The chapter will conclude with an in-depth look at some of the disorders that may affect each component of the respiratory system—from the respiratory control centers in the brain to the alveolus, the smallest functional unit of respiration in the lung.

Anatomy and Physiology Review

The primary structures of the respiratory system are often compared with an inverted tree, with the trachea representing the trunk and the **alveoli**—the tiny saclike units in which gas exchange occurs—resembling the leaves. That is a useful analogy, but in reality, a tree would have to branch 24 times and have nearly a billion leaves to rival the intricacy of the respiratory system **Figure 16-1**. Imagine attempting to pull fluid from the ground into the leaves by exerting negative pressure at the leaf ends and the complexities of breathing become apparent.

Tracheobronchial Tree

The trunk of the tracheobronchial tree is the trachea, or windpipe, which carries air to the lungs. The trachea extends about 4 to 5 inches (10 to 13 cm), from the larynx to the left and right mainstem bronchi. The ridgelike point at which the tracheal cartilage bifurcates is called the **carina**. The carina is at roughly the level of the fifth intercostal space **Figure 16-2**. In adults, the right mainstem bronchus typically branches at a less acute angle than the left. This anatomic peculiarity explains why an endotracheal (ET) tube that is advanced too far almost always goes into the right mainstem bronchus in an adult. Similarly, aspirated foreign bodies often end up in the right mainstem bronchus.

Bronchi

The right and left mainstem bronchi continue to branch into the lobes of the lungs. The right lung has three lobes, and the left has two. These secondary or lobar bronchi then divide into tertiary, or segmental, bronchi and then into subsegmental bronchi before ultimately becoming bronchioles. These conducting airways serve as pathways to the parts of the lung in which gas exchange occurs. Collectively, all airways that do not participate in gas exchange represent dead space. Patients with chronic respiratory disease may have increased dead space (physiologic dead space), indicating that an even larger proportion of each breath makes no contribution to respiration.

Bronchioles

Gas transfer is most efficient in the alveoli, but a significant amount of gas is also exchanged across the respiratory bronchioles **Figure 16-3**. The terminal bronchioles are thin and have little cellular structure. This anatomic design is helpful for gas exchange, but it also means the bronchioles lack cilia, have no protective blanket of mucus, and are not shielded by smooth muscle or more rigid structures. With laminar airflow, particles about 5 micrometers in diameter are often carried this deep into the lungs (smaller particles are often exhaled without sticking). Once foreign material reaches the terminal

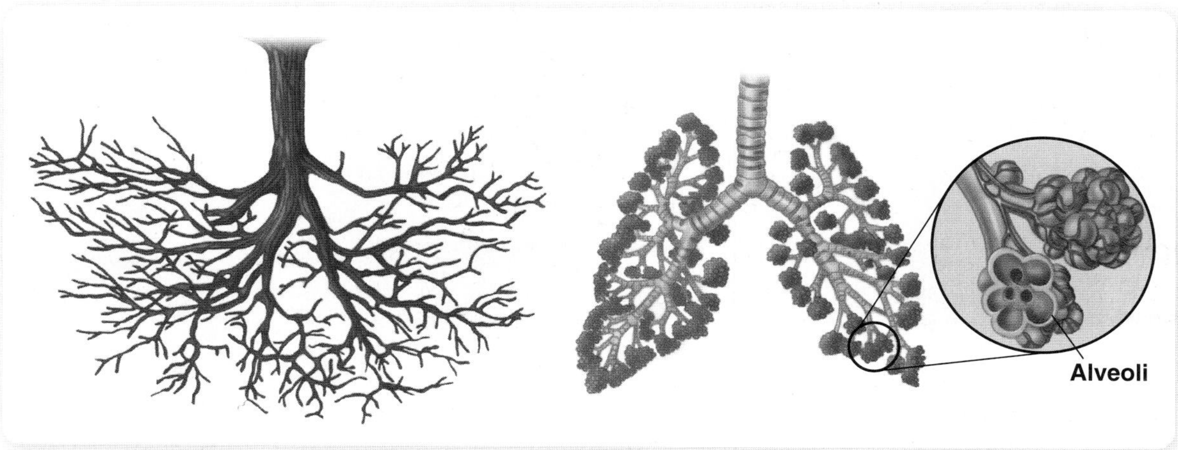

Figure 16-1 The tracheobronchial tree branches in much the same way as a real tree, except that even the most magnificent tree has only a small fraction of the number of branches in a single human lung.

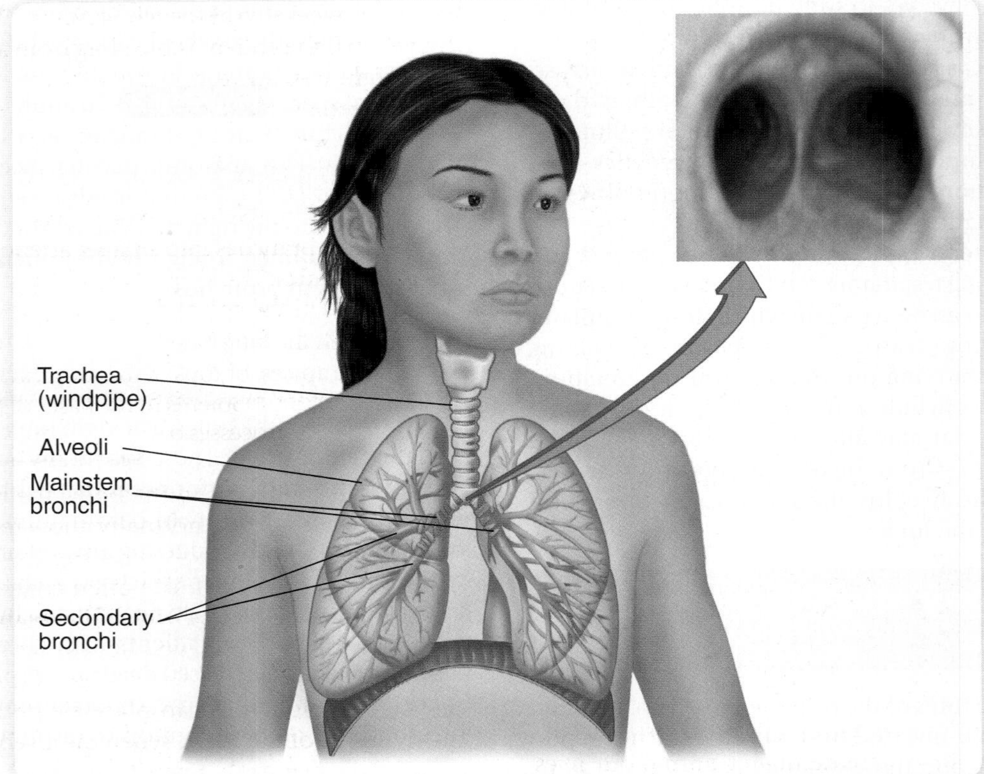

Figure 16-2 The right and left mainstem bronchi bifurcate, or split, at the carina. In an adult, this point is at roughly the fifth intercostal space.

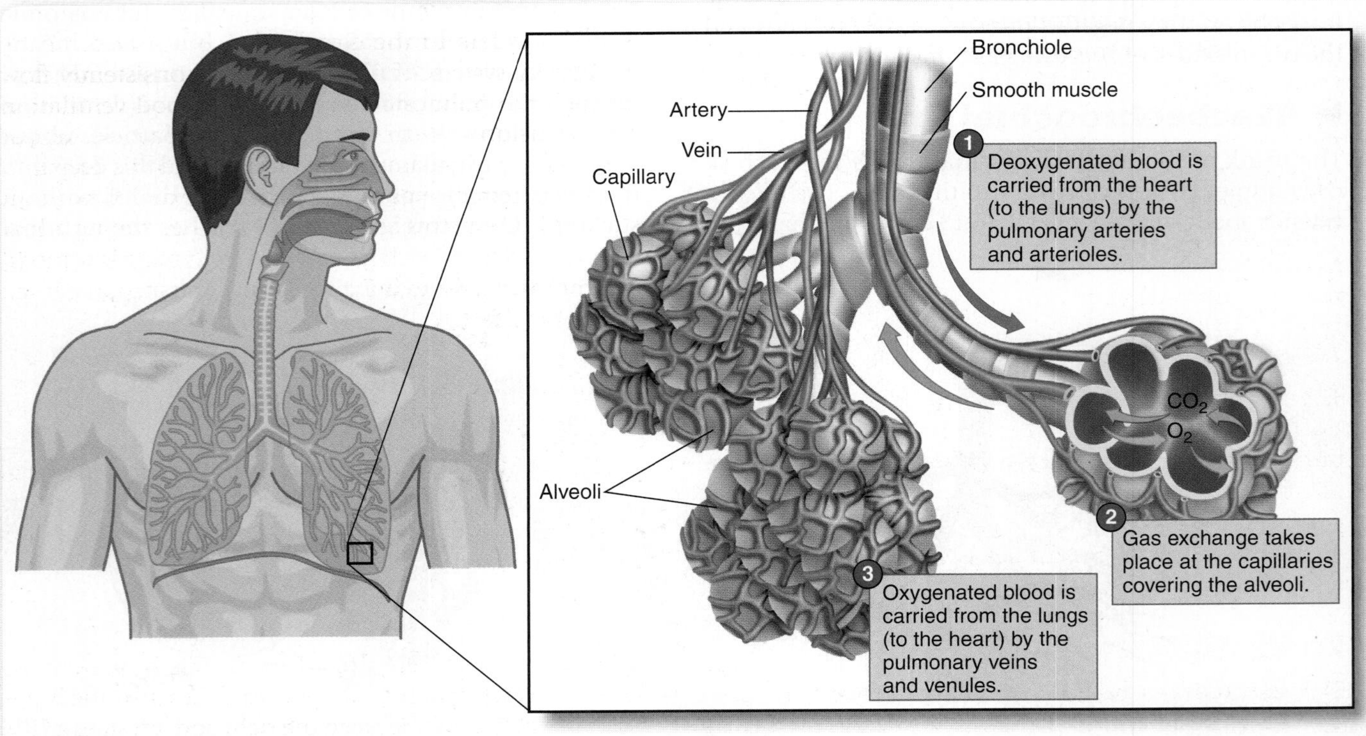

Figure 16-3 The respiratory bronchioles, sometimes called the *terminal bronchioles*, include the alveoli and the last several branches of the tracheobronchial tree. Gas exchange occurs over this entire area.

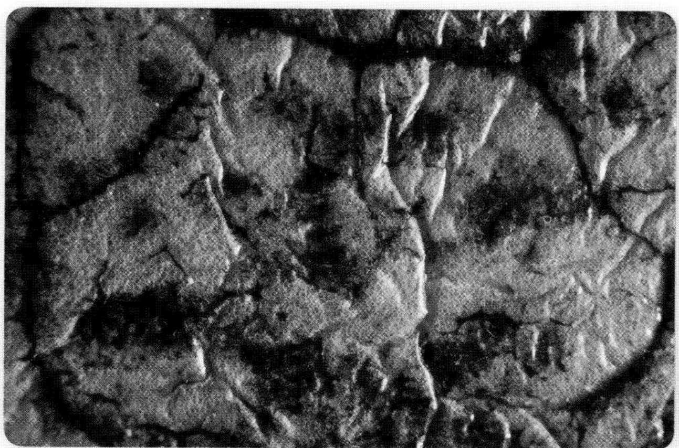

Figure 16-4 Smokers and people who work around coal dust or other particulates may have large areas of discoloration in their lungs.

bronchioles and alveoli, parts of the lung collectively known as the lung **parenchyma**, it may never come out. Common substances that break down to this size include coal dust, asbestos fibers, and the contaminants in cigarette smoke. We all inhale small particulate matter during our lives. At autopsy, most people have many small black spots on their lungs from simply living in an industrialized society. Smokers and people who work around coal dust or other particulates may have significant areas of discoloration, or even completely blackened lungs **Figure 16-4**.

Smooth muscle surrounds the conducting airways down to the subsegmental level. Bronchoconstriction occurs when the smooth muscle narrows these larger airways. Below the subsegmental level, bronchodilator medications have little effect. Wheezing that resolves with administration of bronchodilator medication was probably caused by constriction of the smooth muscle. Wheezing that is not resolved by these medications may have been caused by a pathologic condition deeper in the tracheobronchial tree.

Alveoli

The terminal airways and alveoli include branches 16 through 24 of the tracheobronchial tree, the so-called terminal bronchioles. The typical description of alveoli as a bunch of grapes clustered around a bronchiole isn't completely accurate; rather, the entire surface of the alveoli and terminal bronchioles is covered in capillaries and participates in gas exchange.

▶ Mediastinum

The heart and large blood vessels take up space in the middle of the chest between the lungs. The large conducting airways (trachea and mainstem bronchi) and some other organs, such as the thymus in children, also reside in this space. Collectively, they appear on a chest radiograph as the large white area in the middle of the film. This middle ground is referred to as the *mediastinum*. The mediastinum can widen if the patient is bleeding from a ruptured aorta, or it might trap air from a traumatic injury, a condition called *pneumomediastinum*.

▶ Pulmonary Blood Flow

Blood flows from the heart to the lungs via the pulmonary artery, which branches into smaller arteries, arterioles, and finally capillaries. The lung bases have a greater number of capillaries than the apices do, so more gas exchange takes place between the lung bases and the circulatory system than between the apices, or tops of the lungs, and the circulatory system. Therefore, problems in the bases of the lungs (where most infectious processes occur and fluid builds up) impair **ventilation** more than do problems affecting the apices.

Like all capillaries in the body, the pulmonary capillaries are narrow and normally allow red blood cells to pass through only in single file. People with chronic lung disease and chronic **hypoxia** often generate a surplus of red blood cells over time, which makes their blood thick. Patients with **polycythemia**, for example, have viscous blood. The effort to push this blood through the tiny pulmonary capillaries can place a significant strain on the right side of the heart. When the alveoli are distended by COPD, they push against the capillary bed, further narrowing the capillaries and straining the right side of the heart. Right-sided heart failure that occurs because of chronic lung disease is known as **cor pulmonale**.

▶ Perfusion

Perfusion refers to the circulatory component of the respiratory system. If blood does not consistently flow through the pulmonary vessels, then good ventilation and diffusion are wasted, because an adequate supply of oxygen cannot come into contact with the blood. A large pulmonary embolus can block blood flow to an entire lung. Patients who are anemic (ie, having a low **hemoglobin** level) or hypovolemic (ie, having low blood volume) also have an impaired ability to transport oxygen and carbon dioxide.

▶ Mechanisms of Respiratory Control

Recall from Chapter 8, *Anatomy and Physiology*, that the medulla and portions of the brainstem are involved in neurologic control of respiration. Additional mechanisms of respiratory control are reviewed here.

Cardiovascular Regulation

The lungs are closely linked to cardiac function—so closely, in fact, that some whimsically describe the lungs as an organ that lies between the right and left sides of the heart. While this description is not anatomically correct, it *is* true that changes in the right or left side of the heart can have dramatic pulmonary consequences. When you consider the prevalence of acute cardiac disorders and the total number of patients with respiratory disorders, it's easy to see why dispatches for shortness of breath are common and diagnostically challenging.

Left-sided heart failure typically progresses much faster than does right-sided heart failure. Right-sided heart failure may slowly worsen over many days, whereas left-sided heart failure resulting from a massive acute myocardial infarction can kill a person in a matter of minutes. Thinking of the lungs as lying between the right and left sides of the heart (in terms of function) helps understand why: The right side of the heart pumps blood to the lungs, whereas the left side of the heart receives blood from the lungs and then pumps it through the body to perfuse organs and tissues.

The body's immediate response to mild hypoxemia is to increase the heart rate, sometimes to more than 130 beats/min, a rate that constitutes tachycardia. Severe hypoxia often causes bradycardia. Any uncorrected hypoxic insult may trigger a fatal cardiac dysrhythmia, such as ventricular fibrillation or ventricular tachycardia. Changes in fluid balance, right-sided heart pumping pressure, or left-sided heart pumping pressure can cause various forms of heart failure. Thorough evaluation of the cardiovascular system is essential to proper evaluation of a patient with a respiratory condition.

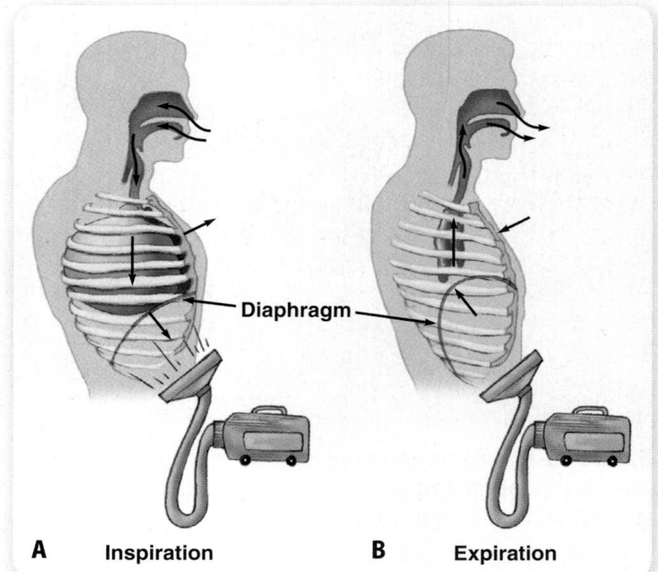

Figure 16-5 Normal ventilation is negative pressure ventilation, meaning that air is sucked into the lungs, much as a vacuum cleaner sucks in air. When the diaphragm contracts, it pulls down into the abdomen, expanding the chest cavity and sucking in air **(A)**. When the pressure is released, the diaphragm relaxes and the lungs empty **(B)**. Compare with positive pressure ventilation, shown in Figure 16-23.

Muscular Control

The body is designed to take in air by means of negative pressure. Picture a vacuum cleaner at the base of the lungs that sucks in air during inhalation. This air is pulled in through the mouth and nose, over the turbinates, and around the complex terrain of the epiglottis and glottis. Air typically does not enter the esophagus and stomach because it is preferentially sucked into the trachea **Figure 16-5**.

This negative pressure vacuum effect occurs because the thorax is essentially an airtight box, with the flexible diaphragm at the bottom and an open tube—the trachea—at the top. During quiet breathing, as the diaphragm flattens, the overall size of the container increases, and air is sucked in through the tube at the top, filling the increasing space within the thorax. The amount of air moved each minute is called *minute ventilation*. Minute ventilation can be increased by breathing deeply, which drops the diaphragm more aggressively, or by breathing more rapidly. Rapid breathing is called *tachypnea*.

Any traumatic opening of the thorax provides an alternative route for air to be sucked in. This air ends up in the pleural space, resulting in a sucking chest wound **Figure 16-6**. When multiple ribs are broken in more than one place (flail chest), free-floating sections of the thorax are pulled in as the patient breathes, limiting the amount of air that can be sucked in through the trachea.

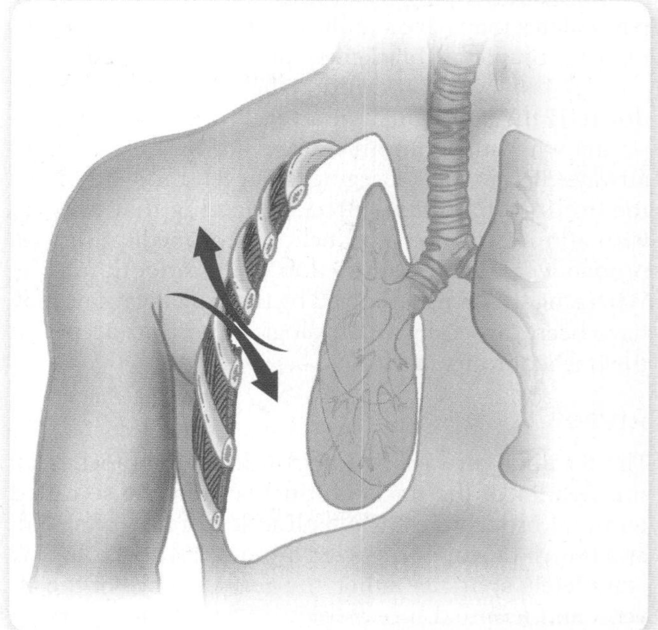

Figure 16-6 A sucking chest wound can compromise ventilation by allowing air to enter the thorax during the inspiratory or negative pressure phase of ventilation.

Renal Status

Fluid balance, acid-base balance, and blood pressure are controlled, in part, by the kidneys. Each of these factors also affects the pulmonary mechanics and, hence, the delivery of oxygen to the tissues. Patients with severe renal disease often present with respiratory signs and symptoms, so paramedics should always note signs of severe renal disease when evaluating a patient's condition. The condition of patients whose heart failure is associated with renal disease can be difficult to manage because **diuresis**—the production of large amounts of urine by the kidney—may be difficult or impossible. Patients with renal disease may also have acid-base disturbances that cause them to hyperventilate, and they are sometimes mistaken for respiratory disorders. Often, a patient's need for emergency dialysis may influence transport decisions and options.

▶ Hypoventilation

When the lungs fail to work properly, the body cannot efficiently dispose of carbon dioxide, and it accumulates in the blood. This excess carbon dioxide combines with water to form bicarbonate ions and hydrogen (H^+) ions, also known as *carbonic acid*. The result is acidosis.

Acidosis can occur if hypoventilation is not recognized. Impaired ventilation can be attributed to a variety of factors, as shown in Table 16-1. We will examine each of these factors in detail later in the chapter.

Recall that pH is an expression of how many free hydrogen ions (H^+) are in a solution. Thus, the carbon dioxide level of the blood is directly related to pH (acid-base balance). Patients who are hypoventilating usually have respiratory acidosis. As their carbon dioxide level goes up, their pH level drops.

Many underlying conditions can cause patients to **hypoventilate**:

- **Conditions that impair lung function.** When a patient is breathing but gas exchange is impaired, the carbon dioxide level in the blood rises. This situation can occur in patients with severe atelectasis, pneumonia, pulmonary edema, asthma, or COPD.
- **Conditions that impair the mechanics of breathing.** Gas flow can be suppressed by a flail chest, diaphragmatic rupture, severe **retractions**, an abdomen full of air or blood, abdominal or chest binding (as may occur during spinal motion restriction), or anything else that restricts the pressure changes that facilitate respiration.

  Obesity hypoventilation syndrome (also known as Pickwickian syndrome) is respiratory compromise caused by morbid obesity. One of the earliest descriptions of this combination of obesity, respiratory compromise, and sleep apnea is found in the character of "Joe the fat boy" in Charles Dickens's *Pickwick Papers*. Joe would fall asleep in midsentence, snore loudly, and generally display signs of hypercapnia. This syndrome is becoming more common, given the nationwide increase in the prevalence of obesity.
- **Conditions that impair the neuromuscular apparatus.** A patient who has had head trauma, an intracranial infection, or a brain tumor may have sustained damage to the respiratory centers of the brain, which may in turn compromise ventilation. Other conditions also may impair the neuromuscular apparatus:
  - Serious injury to the spinal cord above the level of the fifth cervical vertebra (C5) may block the nerve impulses that stimulate breathing.
  - **Guillain-Barré syndrome**, characterized by progressive muscle weakness and paralysis advancing up the body from the feet, can result in ineffective breathing if the paralysis reaches the diaphragm.
  - Amyotrophic lateral sclerosis (ALS; also known as Lou Gehrig disease) also causes progressive muscle weakness. This disease is fatal, with death usually attributable to respiratory failure as the muscles of respiration become unable to maintain adequate ventilation.
  - **Botulism** is caused by the bacterium *Clostridium botulinum*. This somewhat rare disease is usually caused by food poisoning or by giving infants raw (unpasteurized) honey, which may be contaminated with spores of the bacterium. Botulism can cause muscle paralysis and is usually fatal when it reaches the muscles of respiration.
- **Conditions that reduce respiratory drive.** The stimulus to breathe is often referred to as *respiratory drive*. Anything that interrupts or decreases the involuntary stimulus to breathe

Table 16-1 Selected Causes of Impaired Ventilation

Category	Conditions
Upper airway obstruction	Foreign body obstruction Infection Trauma
Lower airway obstruction	Trauma Obstructive disease Increased mucus production Airway swelling (edema)
Chest wall impairment	Pneumothorax Flail chest Pleural effusion Restrictive disease (scoliosis, kyphosis)
Neuromuscular impairment	Overdose Lou Gehrig disease (amyotrophic lateral sclerosis) Carbon dioxide narcosis

can result in hypoventilation or even apnea. Perhaps the most common hypoventilation crisis paramedics see is acute heroin overdose. Intoxication with alcohol, narcotics, or any of a host of other drugs and toxins can reduce the respiratory drive. Head injury, hypoxic drive, and asphyxia are all associated with grossly low respiratory rate and volume. The ultimate expression of hypoventilation is respiratory arrest followed by cardiac arrest.

In these circumstances, aggressive treatment must be initiated to assist the patient's respiratory efforts.

▶ Hyperventilation

Hyperventilation occurs when people breathe in excess of metabolic need by increasing the rate or depth of respiration, or both, expelling more carbon dioxide than normal. The result is alkalosis. As the patient's carbon dioxide level dips, his or her pH level rises. When this cycle is triggered by emotional distress or a panic attack, it may be called *hysterical hyperventilation* or *hyperventilation syndrome*. The falling carbon dioxide level may make the person feel short of breath, so he or she tends to become even more anxious and breathe even more rapidly and deeply. In acute hyperventilation syndrome, patients usually feel as if they cannot breathe at all. Hyperventilation that is not caused by some metabolic crisis is usually self-limiting.

Respiratory alkalosis causes numbness or tingling in the hands and feet and around the mouth. If it persists, then patients may complain of chest pain and will ultimately experience **carpopedal spasm**, in which the hands and feet become clenched into a clawlike position. These symptoms frighten the patient even further and usually make him or her hyperventilate even more. A hysterical patient may eventually lose consciousness, but not before experiencing extreme distress. If the patient begins hyperventilating on awakening, then the process could repeat itself.

The traditional therapy for hyperventilation called for patients to rebreathe their own carbon dioxide from a paper bag or from a partial rebreathing mask set at 21% oxygen (in other words, not attached to supplemental oxygen). This practice can be dangerous for two important reasons:

1. Patients quickly exhaust the oxygen in the gas they are breathing (and rebreathing). Hyperventilation does not mean that the patient has too much oxygen, but rather that he or she is exhaling too much carbon dioxide. Rebreathing carbon dioxide can cause hypoxia, which is counterproductive when trying to terminate a relatively benign hyperventilation episode.
2. Hyperventilation in a patient with acidosis might represent the body's attempt to drive the pH level back up to normal. In a patient with diabetic ketoacidosis, for example, the body produces too much acid because of inadequate glucose metabolism. The body attempts to compensate for the acidosis through hyperventilation or **Kussmaul respirations**. A variety of overdoses, toxic exposures, and metabolic abnormalities, including shock and sepsis, can also produce

YOU are the Paramedic — PART 2

It's evident to you that this patient is struggling to breathe. He tells you that he woke up suddenly with difficulty breathing and weakness. Your partner prepares to obtain vital signs and administer 100% oxygen via nonrebreathing mask. When you initially listen to the patient's lungs, you hear crackles in the apices and diminished lung sounds in the bases. No medication bottles are in obvious view.

Recording Time: 1 Minute	
Appearance	Ashen gray, poor
Level of consciousness	Alert (oriented to person, place, and time)
Airway	Patent
Breathing	Rapid and shallow with crackles (rales)
Circulation	Weak and rapid radial pulse

3. What is your working diagnosis at this time?
4. What assessment and treatment steps will you want to accomplish on scene?

acidosis and compensatory hyperventilation, and *none should be treated by rebreathing carbon dioxide*. Never conclude that a patient is "just hyperventilating" until all possible causes of the presentation have been ruled out, which is difficult or perhaps impossible in the field. Hyperventilation is a diagnosis of exclusion; you cannot presume hyperventilation syndrome until all other medical causes have been ruled out.

Ultimately, treatment may include sedating a person who is truly hysterical and is hyperventilating, but such an extreme measure is rarely taken in the field. Hyperventilation is often triggered by an emotional stressor, such as having a family argument, being involved in a motor vehicle crash, or receiving bad news. More often than not, psychological support is helpful. An important part of care is to help the patient understand that if the behavior that precipitated the hyperventilation is repeated, the hyperventilation will probably recur.

Other useful psychological support techniques include breathing with the patient, having him or her count to two between breaths (gradually increasing to higher numbers), and distracting the person in various ways, such as asking to hear his or her life story. Singing a song with the patient may require him or her to use enough breath control to terminate the episode.

Patient Assessment

Evaluation of the respiratory organs is clearly an important component of assessment during a respiratory emergency. However, the job performed by the respiratory system so dramatically affects other body systems that a thorough respiratory assessment includes much more than simply listening to the patient's lungs.

As always, remember that recognizing and treating life threats, including life-threatening hemorrhage, is the priority during the primary survey and throughout the assessment. Because many respiratory ailments are life threatening, respiratory assessment is always an early step in patient assessment.

Scene Size-up

Paramedics should always think first about safety, including taking standard precautions. Using proper personal protective equipment (PPE) is vital whenever exposure to blood, bodily fluids, or respiratory secretions is possible. In addition, the patient may have a respiratory infection that could be communicable by sputum, respiratory droplets, or airborne particles (see Chapter 26, *Infectious Diseases*). When treating a patient with respiratory distress, the minimum PPE consists of disposable examination gloves and eye protection. A face shield and gown may also be used if the patient is suspected of having or is known to have a communicable respiratory infection, such as methicillin-resistant *Staphylococcus aureus* (MRSA), which could be transmitted in their sputum.

Pulmonary complaints are associated with a broad range of dangerous situations and toxins. The paramedic may be called to a scene where the atmosphere has a diminished oxygen concentration, such as a methamphetamine laboratory, a silo, or another enclosed, improperly ventilated space. The atmosphere on scene may contain carbon monoxide or irritant gases, or the patient may have a highly contagious respiratory illness. It is therefore essential to evaluate scene safety on every call, even on one that appears to be a routine dispatch for shortness of breath.

Words of Wisdom

Respiratory illnesses are common community-acquired "minor" illnesses to which we are all subject. Paramedics are not immune to viruses and the common cold. Unfortunately, a minor illness in a young, healthy EMS provider might represent a deadly disease in very young, very old, or immunocompromised patients. For example, immunity conferred by the pertussis vaccination lasts for 5 to 10 years, so an adult who was vaccinated as a child can contract the disease. An infected adult can transmit the infection to an unvaccinated child. As a paramedic, it's important for you to pay attention to your own health, including your vaccination history and immunity status. You will probably be exposed to tuberculosis, pertussis, hepatitis B, and a variety of other pathogens and contagious diseases during your career (see Chapter 26, *Infectious Diseases*).

Respiratory disease can impair ventilation, diffusion, perfusion, or a combination of the three. The most common complaint of patients with a respiratory disease is dyspnea. The most common cause of dyspnea is hypercapnia, or too much carbon dioxide in the blood. This condition is caused by inadequate ventilation. Although dyspnea is often associated with hypoxia, some patients may be hypoxic without any associated dyspnea. Always evaluate the patient's oxygen saturation, even in the absence of a complaint of dyspnea.

Rapid-onset dyspnea may be caused by acute **bronchospasm**, anaphylaxis, pulmonary embolism, or pneumothorax. **Paroxysmal nocturnal dyspnea** is dyspnea that comes on suddenly in the middle of the night and may be an ominous sign of left-sided heart failure.

Factors that limit the ability of the diaphragm to move (such as advanced pregnancy, obesity, and air or blood in the abdomen), conditions that restrict chest wall movement (such as crush injuries, tightly applied immobilization devices, and an abnormal spinal curvature, as associated with scoliosis or kyphosis), and injuries that disrupt the integrity of the thoracic cage (such as flail chest) hinder a patient's ability to move an adequate supply of air for ventilation.

Primary Survey

The first priority in assessing and managing any respiratory condition is to establish and maintain an open airway. Food, gum, chewing tobacco, and the like should be removed from the patient's mouth. Suction should be applied if necessary and the airway kept in the optimal position, which is typically that in which the patient is most comfortable. See Chapter 15, *Airway Management*, for a more in-depth discussion of airway management techniques.

The following pages discuss signs associated with life-threatening respiratory distress. You may notice a multitude of other signs, both obvious and subtle, during the first few moments of every patient encounter.

One glance at a patient may suggest a body type associated with a particular pathologic condition. The classic presentation of a patient with **emphysema** includes a barrel chest (a chest that is larger in diameter from front to back than from side to side as a result of years of having air trapped in the thorax), muscle wasting (as a result of cannibalizing muscle mass for energy), and pursed-lip breathing (as a result of the obstructive disease). Patients with emphysema are often tachypneic and do not typically present with profound hypoxia and cyanosis.

Severely ill patients with immune system disorders and those with cancer or other end-stage diseases are often easy to identify by their sickly appearance. They may have rigors and pneumonia with accompanying chills. Tall, thin young adults are predisposed to spontaneous pneumothorax, and women who smoke and take oral contraceptives are predisposed to pulmonary embolus.

Patients with **chronic bronchitis** tend to be more sedentary and may be obese as a result. You are likely to encounter such a patient in a chair or recliner, in which he or she sleeps in an upright position. A wastebasket nearby may overflow with tissues, and you may see an ashtray filled with cigarette butts or a cup into which the patient spits his or her copious secretions. A male patient might keep a urinal near the chair to avoid frequent trips to the bathroom. On a table next to the chair, you may see several medication bottles, inhalers, or an aerosol nebulizer. Such a scene can disclose volumes of information about the patient and his or her history long before you place a stethoscope on the patient's chest.

Clues to a variety of pathologic conditions may be evident immediately, but keep in mind that they are only clues. Avoid constructing a hasty field impression based on minimal information. Patients with COPD often get pneumonia, an asthma attack can be triggered by an ongoing infection, and heart failure can develop in a cancer patient. In other words, the patient's presentation may suggest a particular condition, but this suspicion must be confirmed by a thorough assessment.

Words of Wisdom

In the 1950s, John Hickam, MD, Duke University, coined the phrase that became known as Hickam's dictum. He found it necessary to remind medical students that patients often present with multiple pathologies, all of which must be taken into account during assessment. When evaluating respiratory distress, remember Hickam's advice: "Patients can have as many diseases as they damn well please."

Assess Oxygen Demand and Work of Breathing

Oxygen demand increases with exertion of any kind. If a patient's condition is stable at rest, then observe his or her condition during typical exertion. Ask if the patient becomes dyspneic when moving from the chair to the stretcher, when going to the bathroom, or while eating. Note the patient's oxygen saturation while at rest and during any simple exertion.

Increased work of breathing, anxiety, hypoxia, or fever can trigger a sympathetic nervous system response characterized by tachycardia, diaphoresis, and pallor. This effect can be so pronounced that the heart rate often decreases as patients respond to treatment even if they are treated with sympathetic stimulators that normally increase the heart rate.

Note Position and Determine Degree of Distress

Patients in respiratory distress tend to avoid the supine position and seek a sitting position. A person in the tripod position, for example, leans forward and rotates the scapulae outward by placing the arms on a table, elbows out, or by placing the hands on the knees **Figure 16-7**. This position opens up a little more space for airflow in the lung apices and draws the abdominal structures away from the diaphragm. Because considerably less perfusion occurs at the apex of the lung than at the base, the effort required for a person to assume the tripod position may offset the modest gain in oxygenation. Be wary if a patient in respiratory distress wants to lie flat; this could be a sign of sudden deterioration in his or her condition.

A patient may try to maximize airflow through the upper airway by purposeful hyperextension, accomplished by holding his or her head in the head tilt–chin lift position, or so-called sniffing position. This position may also indicate upper airway swelling. Maintaining this position uses up valuable energy. A patient with severe respiratory disease who begins to feel fatigued may hold his or her head up in this position only during inhalation, letting the head and neck fall into flexion during exhalation. This "head bobbing" is an ominous sign of imminent decompensation and may be a clue to the severity of the situation.

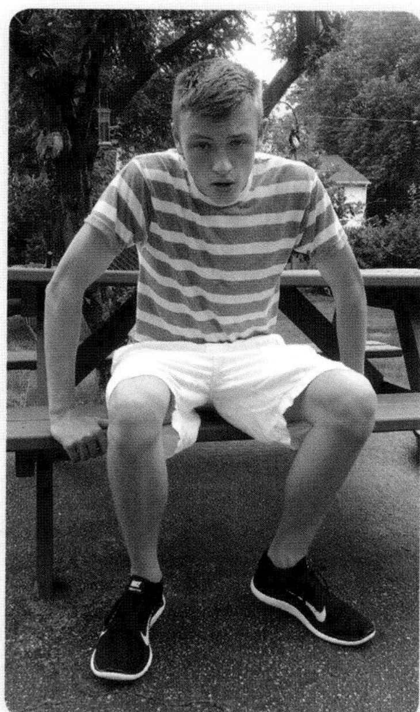

Figure 16-7 The tripod position (elbows out) improves diaphragmatic movement by getting the abdomen out of the way and rotating the scapulae laterally, allowing somewhat more air to flow to the apices. Unfortunately, this position takes work, which requires more oxygen, and may or may not ultimately benefit the patient.

Breathing Alterations

Breathing alterations can involve any of the following:

- The conducting airways (trachea, bronchi, and bronchioles), such as occurs in asthma or bronchitis
- The alveoli, as in pneumonia or emphysema
- The muscles and nerves that control breathing, as in Guillain-Barré syndrome or spinal cord injury
- The rigid structure of the thorax, thereby hampering the pressure changes that facilitate the breathing process, as occurs in flail chest

Increased Work of Breathing

Patients who are relying on accessory muscles to breathe are in danger of tiring out, so noticing such muscle use is important. Is the patient using the muscles of the abdomen to push out air (as in asthma or COPD), or using the muscles of the chest and neck to pull air in Figure 16-8? Infants and small children have substantial chest wall elasticity; when they use accessory muscles to breathe, the flexible cartilage of the sternum or ribs often collapses, causing bony retractions.

By the same mechanism, a patient of any age may pull the soft tissues in between the ribs, above or below

Words of Wisdom

Maintaining the airway and breathing for a patient are not the same thing. Many patients need assistance to establish a patent airway. Having an open airway, however, does not ensure an adequate volume of gas is moving into and out of the lungs. Proper ventilation is necessary to remove carbon dioxide and maintain acid-base balance. Increasing the amount of available oxygen ensures that even a patient who is not moving an adequate volume of gas (that is, a patient who is hypoventilating) can maintain adequate oxygen saturation. If ventilation remains inadequate in a hypoventilating patient, then the patient will become hypercapnic (the blood contains too much carbon dioxide) and acidotic (the pH of arterial blood is too low). These conditions disrupt the balance of important body systems and are fatal if uncorrected. While it is important to maintain an adequate oxygen saturation, adequate oxygenation does not always mean there is adequate ventilation. While closely related, maintaining an airway, maintaining adequate ventilation, and maintaining adequate oxygenation are three different things, and the paramedic must attend to each!

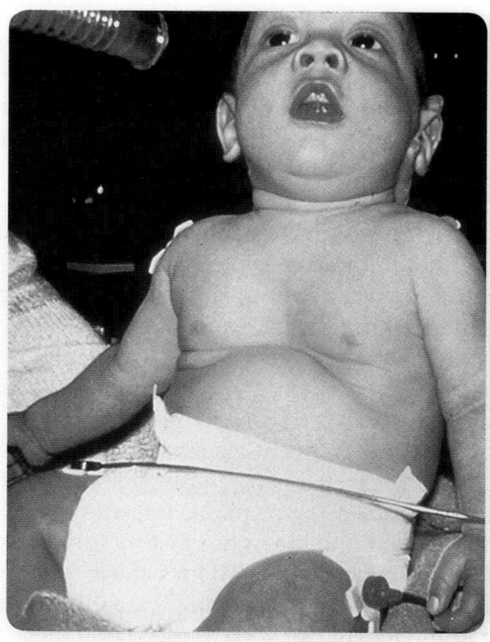

Figure 16-8 Bony retraction not only indicates severe distress and increased work of breathing, but also contributes to respiratory failure. With inhalation, the lower sternum is pulled into the lungs. Every cubic centimeter of space displaced by the retraction represents a cubic centimeter of air that cannot reach the airways.

Courtesy of Health Resources and Services Administration, Maternal and Child Health Bureau, Emergency Medical Services for Children Program.

Table 16-2 Signs of Increased Work of Breathing

Sign	Description
Bony retractions	During inhalation, the sternum or ribs pull back or recede (retract) into the chest, creating a visible deformity with each breath.
Soft-tissue retractions	Soft tissue is drawn in around the bones during inhalation. Dramatic retractions can be seen in the supraclavicular, intercostal, and subxiphoid areas.
Nasal flaring	The nostrils fan wide open during inhalation.
Tracheal tugging	During inhalation, the thyroid cartilage is drawn upward and the area just above the sternal notch is pulled in.
Paradoxical respiratory movement	During inhalation, the epigastrium is pulled in as the abdomen is pushed out, creating a seesaw effect as the two move in opposite directions.
Pulsus paradoxus	Peripheral pulses are weak or absent on inhalation, caused by extreme pressure changes in the thorax.
Pursed-lip breathing	Patients with obstructive diseases (such as COPD and acute asthma) have trouble pushing air out. It is more effective to exhale slowly over a longer period than to try to expel the air forcefully. Many patients learn to purse their lips (like a kiss) and exhale slowly through this restricted orifice. This technique allows more efficient exhalation and provides a diagnostic clue to the disease.
Grunting	In infants and young children with lower airway illness, the glottis closes at the end of exhalation and a grunt is emitted at the end of each breath. The grunting exerts a small amount of pressure that helps keep the alveoli open (as with positive end-expiratory pressure). The grunts may be audible, or a stethoscope may be required to hear them. Grunting is a classic sign of respiratory distress in infants.

Abbreviation: COPD, chronic obstructive pulmonary disease

the sternum or clavicles, causing soft-tissue retractions. In adults and children, profound intrathoracic pressure changes can make the peripheral pulse weak or imperceptible during inspiration and can make it easier to palpate during exhalation, a state known as **pulsus paradoxus**. Patients who are using accessory muscles to breathe may have dramatic pressure changes within the thorax and exhibit these and other signs of increased work of breathing, summarized in Table 16-2. Such signs may indicate life-threatening respiratory distress.

Altered Rate and Depth of Respiration

Assessing the rate and depth of breathing is an obvious component of respiratory assessment. Unfortunately, rate and depth are sometimes inaccurately determined. The conscientious paramedic will observe the patient's respiratory rate and depth without being obvious (patients may breathe faster or deeper if they are aware that you are counting). Count the respiratory rate while you appear to be doing something else, like checking the pulse or taking the blood pressure. The rate may be a commonly "guessed" vital sign, but respiratory depth is even more commonly misjudged. The use of continuous end-tidal carbon dioxide monitoring provides documentation of the patient's respirations and makes it much easier to accurately determine rate and depth. A patient with an adequate rate but a low volume will still have an inadequate minute volume, which is calculated as follows:

$$\text{Respiratory rate} \times \text{Tidal volume} = \text{Minute volume}$$

The respiratory rate can vary significantly from minute to minute. Be sure to monitor trends in respiratory rate—whether it is increasing or decreasing—rather than concentrating on a specific rate from the beginning of the assessment. While assessing the patient's respiration, note the pattern (see Table 16-5) and the inspiratory-to-expiratory (I:E) ratio. Is the patient working hard to inhale, exhale, or both? Does his or her breath have a peculiar odor (such as the acetone odor associated with diabetic ketoacidosis)? Are there any abnormal respiratory noises?

As a general rule, *any* respiratory noises that are audible without a stethoscope are abnormal.

Abnormal Breath Sounds

Whenever possible, auscultate the lungs systematically. Although examiners tend to compare the left and right sides, recall that the lungs are not symmetric. Thus, it's important to understand where to listen in order to hear each lobe Figure 16-9.

Many pathologic conditions are gravity dependent, meaning that most types of pneumonia and heart failure are found in the lung bases. Wheezing is typically diffuse and spread throughout the lung fields. Wheezing confined to only one spot may indicate a foreign body or tumor. The bases are heard almost exclusively by listening with the stethoscope on the patient's back.

The upper lobes, which are less likely to have abnormalities, are heard by listening on the anterior part of the chest. The right middle lobe can best be heard by listening just beneath or lateral to the right breast. The best left-right differentiation can be noted at the midaxillary line; this is the best place to listen to confirm ET tube placement.

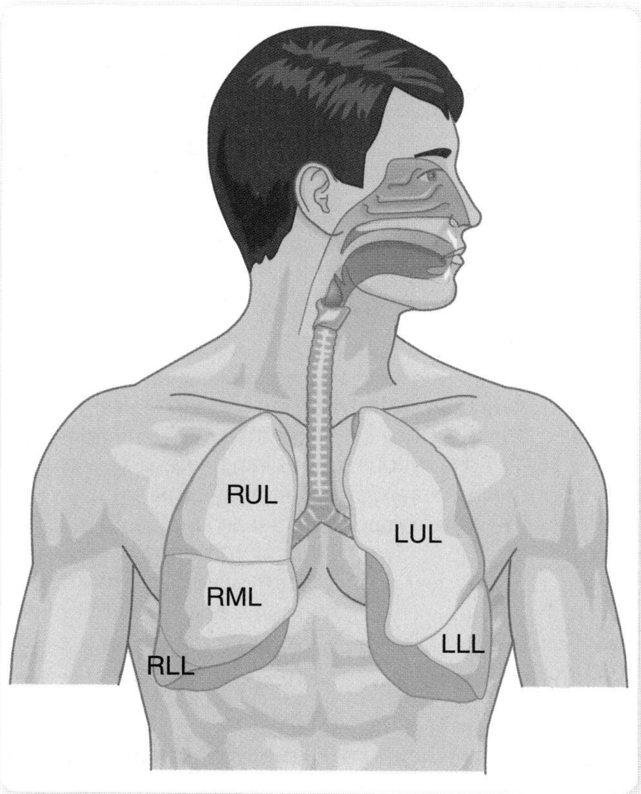

Figure 16-9 The lungs are not symmetric. Most acute pathologic conditions are best heard in the lung bases, requiring that the stethoscope be placed on the patient's back. The right middle lobe is best heard beneath the right breast or just lateral to it. Abbreviations: LUL, left upper lobe; LLL, left lower lobe; RUL, right upper lobe; RML, right middle lobe; RLL, right lower lobe.

Listening to the anterior part of the chest allows the examiner to hear the noisemaker (the ET tube), whether it is in the trachea or the esophagus.

Breath sounds are made by turbulent airflow in the large airways. Using a stethoscope, you will hear these sounds as they are transmitted through the lung tissue. Tracheal breath sounds are not commonly auscultated, but note how harsh and tubular they sound. Bronchial breath sounds are also quite loud, but note that exhalation predominates. Farther toward the periphery, bronchovesicular sounds are softer and stay constant with inspiration and expiration. The most common breath sounds are the soft, breezy vesicular sounds heard in the periphery. They have a much more obvious inspiratory component. Listen to a large number of healthy lungs to become familiar with these four different types of breath sounds Figure 16-10. Some pathologic conditions cause normal breath sounds to be heard in abnormal places.

Sound moves better through fluid than it does through air. The more air in a patient's chest, then, the more distant or diminished the breath sounds are at the periphery, if they are audible at all. Patients with COPD and asthma, for example, may have diminished breath sounds. Conversely, the wetter the patient's lungs are, so to speak, the louder the sounds are at the periphery. Patients with wet lungs include those with pneumonia, heart failure, and **lung consolidation**, which occurs when fluid accumulation makes the lungs firm. Pneumonia in the right middle lobe produces bronchovesicular sounds (equal during inspiration and expiration), and in the periphery you may even hear bronchial sounds (louder during expiration than inspiration) instead of the expected vesicular sounds (louder during inspiration than expiration).

The quality of the breath sounds also depends on how much extra tissue comes between the stethoscope and the patient's respiratory structures. For this reason, it's often helpful to compare breath sounds on the right with those on the left (keeping in mind that the lungs are not symmetrical). In a patient with a one-sided pathologic condition such as pneumonia, the breath sounds may be *louder* over the side with the abnormality than over the healthy side.

Breath sounds and vocalizations travel more efficiently through a firm, fluid-filled lung than through a healthy lung, but they travel poorly through a hyperinflated lung. If a patient speaks during chest auscultation, then the examiner cannot usually understand what he or she is saying through the stethoscope. If the patient's words are audible, then it may mean the patient has consolidation from pneumonia or atelectasis. These sounds are most clearly audible directly over the consolidated lobe. Table 16-3 lists signs of consolidation.

Adventitious (abnormal) breath sounds are the extra noises that can be heard on top of the breath sounds described previously. Continuous sounds (for example, a wheeze) can be heard across some portion of each breath.

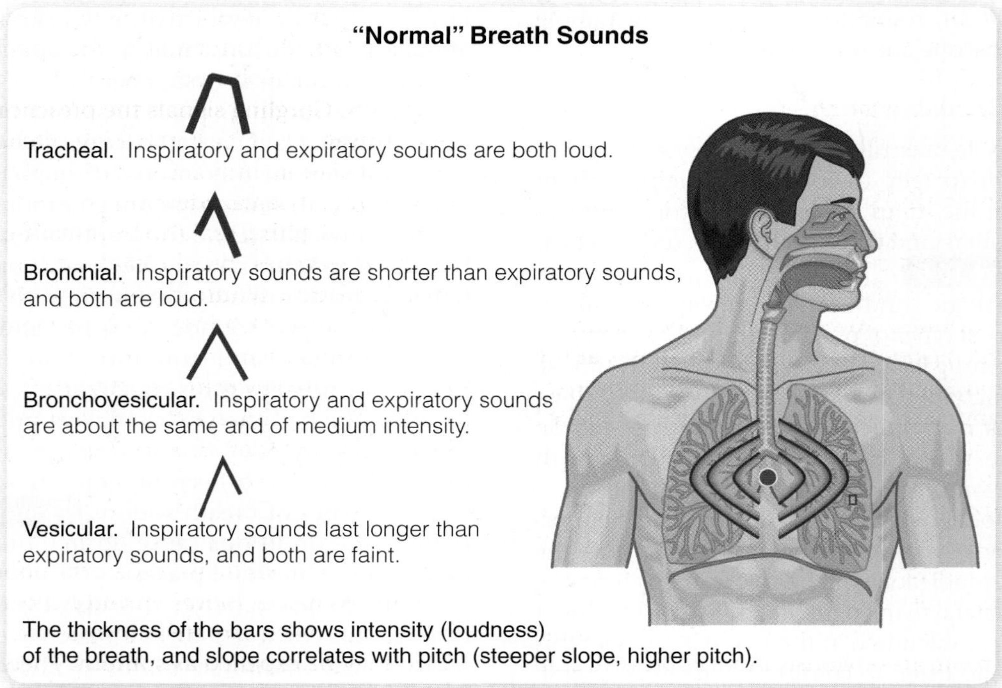

Figure 16-10 Normal breath sounds are heard over different parts of the chest. As the stethoscope moves away from the largest airways, breath sounds become softer. The character of sounds during inspiration versus exhalation also changes.

Table 16-3 Signs of Lung Consolidation

Sign	Test
Bronchophony	When a patient says "99" repeatedly through a normal lung, it sounds like a hum. Through a consolidated lung, you can understand the word "99."
Egophony	The patient says "Eeeeee" while you are auscultating, and you hear "Aaaaaay" (as in "state"). The sound may be heard particularly well over a pleural effusion.
Whispered pectoriloquy	The patient whispers while you are auscultating, and you can understand what is said.

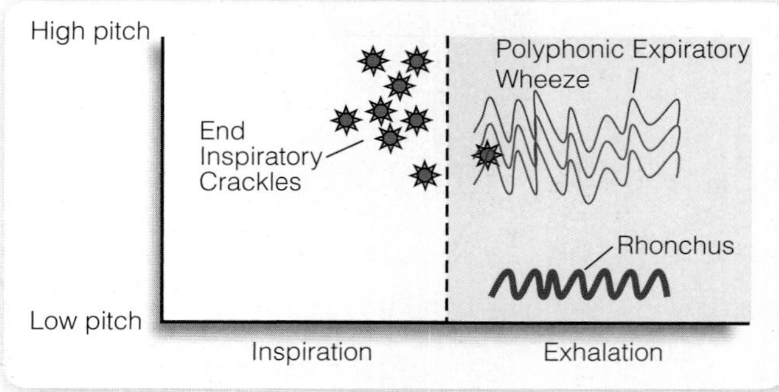

Figure 16-11 Adventitious sounds can be described as continuous (wheezes and rhonchi) or discontinuous (crackles). They can also be characterized by their pitch (such as high or low), by the point at which they occur in the respiratory cycle (end inspiration or forced exhalation), and by their complexity (monophonic versus polyphonic).

Discontinuous sounds are the instantaneous pops, snaps, and clicks known as **crackles** Figure 16-11.

Wheezes are high-pitched whistling sounds made as air is forced through narrowed airways, which makes them vibrate, much like the reed in a musical instrument. Wheezing may be diffuse, as in asthma and heart failure, or localized, as when a foreign body partially obstructs a bronchus. Pathologic conditions such as asthma rarely cause one-sided wheezing. Have the patient cough, and listen again. If the sound seems to originate on only one side, then it could be caused by the movement of secretions. If a single bronchus is vibrating, then the wheeze produces a single note, known as a **monophonic** sound. If many bronchi are vibrating, then the wheeze may have many notes, like a bagpipe. This is called a **polyphonic** sound. Note when the sound is heard in the respiratory cycle. For example, does the wheeze occur during inspiration and exhalation? Just during exhalation? Or just at the end of exhalation?

During auscultation of the lungs, you may hear crackles. Crackles are discontinuous noises caused by the popping open of air spaces (fine crackles) or by the movement of fluid or secretions in the larger airways (coarse crackles). These sounds are usually associated with increased fluid in the lungs. In some parts of the country, the terms *rales* and *rhonchi* continue to be used interchangeably with crackles. The term rales, however, refers specifically to the high-pitched crackles heard in the lung bases at the end of inspiration. Rales are consistent with pulmonary edema. *Rhonchi* are also a type of crackles—the low-pitched sounds caused by secretions trapped in the larger airways.

Certain sounds—stridor from upper airway obstruction and grunting from lower airway obstruction—are audible without a stethoscope. A low-pitched gurgling sound (sometimes called a "death rattle") is sometimes heard as the patient becomes unable to clear his or her own secretions. Wheezes and crackles that are audible when entering a room are obviously more impressive than sounds that require a stethoscope to hear. As a patient becomes sicker, the various emissions become louder and take on a musical character. As respiratory distress worsens, the noises may again diminish. The most ominous breath sounds are no breath sounds at all. An absence of breath sounds indicates that the patient is not moving enough air to ventilate the lungs. *Silence means danger*.

Noisy breathing is obstructed breathing. **Snoring** indicates partial obstruction of the upper airway by the tongue—a form of obstruction easily corrected by head-tilt maneuvers. Gurgling signals the presence of fluid in the upper airway. **Stridor**, a harsh, high-pitched sound heard during inhalation, indicates narrowing, usually as a result of swelling (laryngeal edema).

Quiet breathing can also be revealing. A patient with tachypnea who has crystal-clear breath sounds may have hyperventilation syndrome but may also be breathing rapidly because of acidosis. Quiet tachypnea suggests possible shock. Paramedics occasionally assume that tachypnea caused by pain, anxiety, or a metabolic disorder is the patient's primary condition, when in fact the real cause is diabetic crisis or sepsis.

Sputum

Normally, a mucous blanket coats the upper tracheobronchial tree. As mucus moves up and out of the trachea, it is usually swallowed. Irritated airways secrete more mucus, which may be expelled as sputum. There is a difference between saliva from the mouth (oral secretions) and the thicker, sometimes color-tinged sputum from the lungs. This mucus may be mixed with blood, pulmonary edema fluid, aspirated food particles, or the decaying debris from dead infectious organisms. The sputum may be a variety of colors, which sometimes gives us clues about infection. The patient's level of hydration may affect the thickness

YOU are the Paramedic PART 3

You've administered oxygen to the patient via a nonrebreathing mask, but this intervention doesn't seem to be improving his condition. His oxygen saturation level is still in the low 80s, so you decide to apply continuous positive airway pressure (CPAP). He is visibly anxious and is asking you to help him. Your partner helps assemble the CPAP equipment while you begin continuous electrocardiogram (ECG) monitoring. The 12-lead shows ST elevation in leads 2 and 3. You inquire again if the patient has any chest pain or discomfort, which he denies.

Recording Time: 5 Minutes	
Respirations	34 breaths/min; shallow and rapid
Pulse	110 beats/min; weak
Skin	Gray and clammy
Blood pressure	140/100 mm Hg
Oxygen saturation (Spo_2)	80% with oxygen by nonrebreathing mask
Pupils	PERRLA

5. Does this patient have an airway condition or a breathing disorder?
6. Does the absence of chest pain or discomfort indicate the patient is not having a heart attack?

Table 16-4 Classic Sputum Types

Type	Causes
Frothy, sometimes with a pink tinge	Heart failure
Thick	Dehydration or antihistamine use
Purulent	Infectious process (because the pus contains dead white blood cells)
Yellow, green, brown	Older secretions in various stages of decomposition
Clear or white	Bronchitis
Blood-streaked	Tumor, tuberculosis, pulmonary edema, or trauma from coughing

of the sputum, with very thick secretions clogging the airways of dehydrated patients. It is appropriate to note whether the patient is coughing up discolored sputum Table 16-4. Many smokers and people with chronic respiratory diseases cough up sputum every day (especially first thing in the morning). In such cases, try to determine if the color or amount of the sputum has changed. Some people keep a cup or emesis basin nearby to spit in.

Increased sputum production coupled with fever and chills is a classic presentation of an infection such as pneumonia. Blood-tinged sputum may be a warning sign of **tuberculosis**, or it may mean the patient has been coughing forcefully enough to break small blood vessels in the airway. When air is forced through fluid-filled airways, the pink foam or froth often associated with heart failure is created. It is important to note whether the mucus is **purulent**, or pus-like. Ask the patient if he or she has coughed up any mucus and, if so, whether its color or any other characteristics seem different from normal.

Abnormal Breathing Patterns

Major neurologic insults may also manifest themselves with certain altered respiratory patterns. Brain trauma or any event that disturbs brain function may depress the respiratory control centers in the medulla. For example, the increasing intracranial pressure that occurs in closed head trauma may literally put the squeeze on the medulla, producing a variety of respiratory abnormalities, including apnea. A stroke may have a similar effect by depriving portions of the brain of circulation, and therefore oxygenated blood (see Chapter 17, *Cardiovascular Emergencies*). Overdose with a central nervous system depressant, such as an opiate or barbiturate, may also severely depress respiratory center activity.

Severe traumatic brain injuries result in bizarre respiratory patterns when one or more of the brain's respiratory centers are damaged or deprived of adequate blood flow. Table 16-5 summarizes various breathing patterns.

Most of the brain's respiratory centers are located in and around the brainstem Figure 16-12. Patients with serious trauma to the upper cerebral hemispheres, such as penetrating trauma from a gunshot wound, are often still breathing despite having mortal wounds. Apneustic breathing is caused by damage to the pneumotaxic center in the brain, which regulates the inspiratory pause. In a patient with apneustic respiration, each short, brisk inhalation is followed by a long pause before exhalation. This pattern indicates severe pressure within the cranium or direct trauma to the brain. Similarly, Biot respirations are seen when the center that controls breathing rhythm is damaged. This respiratory pattern is grossly irregular, sometimes with lengthy apneic periods.

Cheyne-Stokes respirations are more of a higher brain function. Many deep sleepers or intoxicated people have this respiratory pattern. The depth of breathing (or volume of snoring) gradually increases and then decreases (crescendo-decrescendo), followed by an apneic period. The apneic period is usually brief in a relatively healthy person. Exaggerated Cheyne-Stokes respirations, in which the crescendo-decrescendo is much more pronounced, may be seen in patients with severe brain injury. In these patients, the apneic period may last 30 to 60 seconds.

Injury high in the spinal cord may paralyze the intercostal muscles and even the diaphragm. Polio attacks the nerves that supply the respiratory muscles, but certain chronic illnesses, such as myasthenia gravis, weaken the respiratory muscles themselves. The net effect of these conditions is the inability of the respiratory muscles to function normally in response to the respiratory drive. As a consequence, tidal volume is shallow and there is a corresponding decrease in minute volume. Patients with such conditions often need assisted ventilation to boost tidal volume, thereby increasing minute volume.

Circulation Assessment in the Context of Respiratory Emergencies

Assessing skin color is a fast way to begin determining the adequacy of the patient's circulation Figure 16-13. Although it is important to note the generalized cyanosis of oxygen desaturation or the profound pallor of shock, more subtle information can be gained by assessing the mucous membranes. The tissue inside the mouth, under the eyelids, and even in the nail beds is usually the same pink color in all healthy patients. A few notable variations are as follows:

- **Cyanosis.** Healthy adults have a hemoglobin level of 12 to 14 g/dL. With a hemoglobin

Table 16-5 Breathing Patterns

Pattern	Description
Agonal	Irregular, widely spaced gasps usually representing stray neurologic impulses in a dying patient; an occasional agonal gasp is not unusual in a patient with no pulse; not actually considered a form of breathing
Apneustic	A prolonged inspiratory hold (sometimes called "fish breathing") that can occur following damage to the pneumotaxic center in the brain; an ominous sign of severe brain injury
Ataxic	Chaotically irregular respirations that indicate severe brain injury or brainstem herniation
Biot respirations	Irregular pattern, rate, and depth of respirations, characterized by intermittent patterns of apnea; indicates severe brain injury or brainstem herniation
Bradypnea	Unusually slow respiration
Central neurogenic hyperventilation	Tachypneic hyperpnea; rapid, deep respirations caused by increased intracranial pressure or direct brain injury; drives carbon dioxide level down and pH up, resulting in respiratory alkalosis
Cheyne-Stokes respirations	Crescendo-decrescendo breathing with a period of apnea between cycles; not considered ominous unless it is grossly exaggerated or occurs in a patient with brain trauma
Cough	Forced exhalation against a closed glottis; an airway-clearing maneuver; also occurs when foreign substances irritate the airways; controlled by the cough center in the brain (antitussive medications work on the cough center to reduce this sometimes annoying physiologic response)
Eupnea	Normal breathing
Hiccup	Spasmodic contraction of the diaphragm, causing short exhalations with a characteristic sound; sometimes seen in cases of diaphragmatic (or phrenic) nerve irritation from acute myocardial infarction, ulcerating disease, or endotracheal intubation
Hyperpnea	Abnormally increased rate and depth of breathing; seen in various neurologic and chemical disorders, including overdose with certain drugs
Hypopnea	Abnormally decreased rate and depth of breathing
Kussmaul respirations	The same pattern as in central neurogenic hyperventilation, but caused by the body's attempt in metabolic acidosis to rid itself of blood acetone via the lungs; seen in diabetic ketoacidosis; accompanied by a fruity (acetone) breath odor and, usually, cracked and dry mouth and lips
Sighing	Periodically taking a deep breath of about twice the normal volume; forces open alveoli that routinely close from time to time
Tachypnea	Unusually rapid breathing; does not reflect depth of respiration and does not mean a patient is hyperventilating (breathing too rapidly and deeply, resulting in a reduced carbon dioxide level); often involves moving only small volumes of air, or *hypo*ventilation (much like a panting dog)
Yawning	Seems beneficial in the same manner as sighing

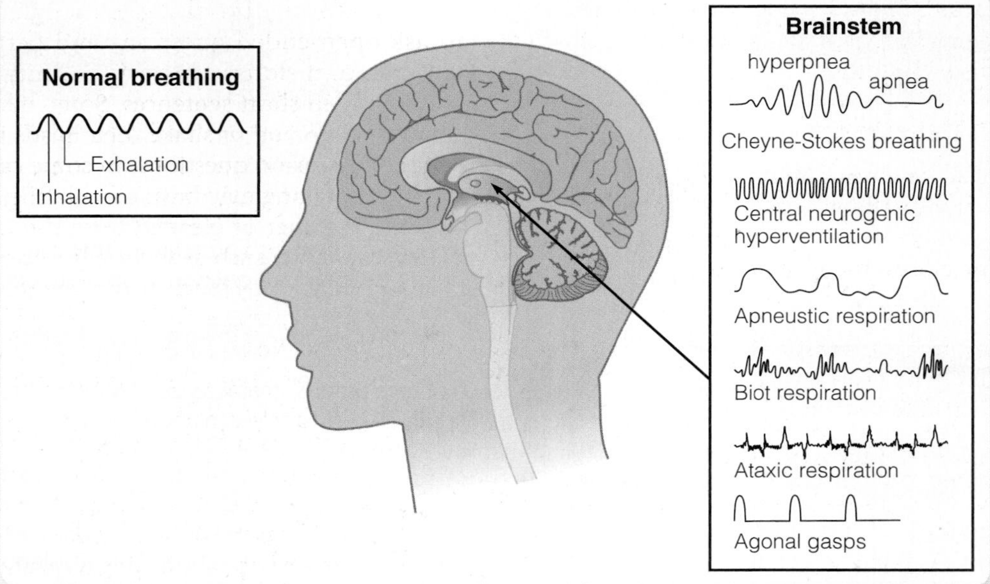

Figure 16-12 The neurologic control of respiration is complex, and many variations in the respiratory pattern may occur in a patient with brain injury. The respiratory patterns shown—each recorded for 1 minute—have been documented using an end-tidal carbon dioxide detector. Note that most irregular breathing patterns are controlled by the brainstem.

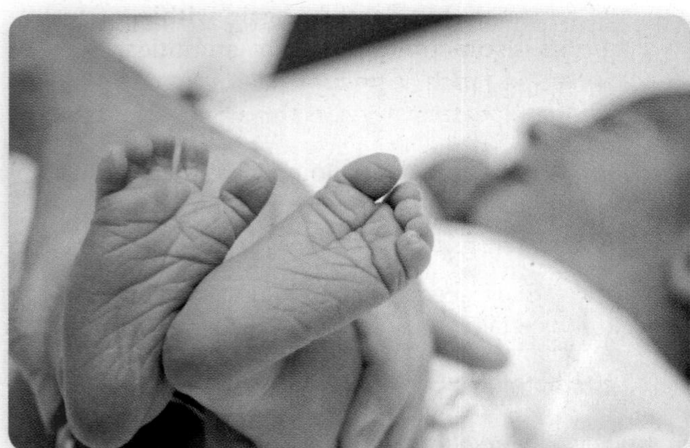

Figure 16-13 Skin color can be an early, fast indicator of several disease processes. Cyanosis (shown here) presents as blue skin and indicates at least 5 g/dL of unoxygenated hemoglobin. Carbon monoxide intoxication can present as cherry-red skin, although this is a late sign. When making any preliminary diagnosis, allow for wide variation in patients' skin color and tone.

level in this range, the blue discoloration of cyanosis becomes apparent when about 5 g/dL becomes desaturated (has no oxygen molecules attached). The person's oxygen saturation would be roughly 65%! If a person's hemoglobin level were only 10 g/dL, then 50% of the hemoglobin molecules (5 of the 10 g/dL) would have to become desaturated before the patient would look cyanotic. Some patients in cardiac arrest have deep blue skin, whereas others are pale. Similarly, in patients with high hemoglobin levels, such as those with chronic respiratory disease, cyanosis may develop earlier than in patients with normal hemoglobin levels. Of course, there are slight variations in what is considered normal. In addition, some patients with chronic respiratory conditions who have an artificially low oxygen saturation may also have a low level of chronic cyanosis. Patients with chronic bronchitis, for example, often have chronically low oxygen levels and relatively high hemoglobin levels, resulting in chronic peripheral cyanosis.

- **Chocolate-brown skin.** High levels of methemoglobin derived from nitrates and certain toxic exposures may turn the mucous membranes brown. This transformation is typically more evident in the patient's venous blood than in the skin and mucous membranes.
- **Pale skin.** Pale skin and mucous membranes are caused by reduced blood flow to the small vessels near the surface of the skin. The source of this condition could be hypoxia, shock, a cold environment, or release of catecholamines, such as epinephrine or norepinephrine.

Note whether the patient's mucous membranes are moist or dry. Dehydration can be seen in the mucous membranes of the mouth and eyes. Dry, cracked lips; a dry, furrowed tongue; and dry, sunken eyes point to obvious dehydration. The skin of an older patient may always look dry because of poor turgor, so skin assessment is of less value in certain older people.

Transport Decision

The treatment of acute cardiac and respiratory disorders is fundamental in virtually all emergency departments (EDs). Patients with respiratory conditions are usually transported to the closest medical facility.

Special Populations

In some settings, specialty pediatric centers are an option for children, particularly children with tracheostomies, home ventilators, or other sophisticated ventilatory support.

Patients whose respiratory distress is related to renal failure would benefit from being taken to a facility that can provide emergency dialysis. (Not all centers that provide routine dialysis offer it on weekends or at night.)

Sometimes multiple EDs are available, separated by only a few minutes of additional travel time. In such cases, you must weigh the benefits of taking a patient to his or her preferred facility, where previous laboratory and radiograph results and the patient's own physician may be available, against the advantages of going to the closest facility. Patients with acute decompensation should usually be taken to the closest facility, but most patients with respiratory conditions can tolerate a few extra minutes if the delay facilitates their care after arrival.

History Taking

Ask patients to explain in their own words what they are feeling. Many patients can identify their conditions and explain the best way to treat it without your having to dig for the information. In fact, a patient with a chronic respiratory condition is often knowledgeable about his or her disease or disorder and may have tried several treatment options already. The patient might relate having been intubated and treated with a ventilator for a previous attack. Many patients with chronic respiratory disease have some symptoms all of the time. The pertinent question, then, is this: "What changed that made you call 9-1-1 today?" Increased cough, a change in the amount or color of sputum, fever, or wheezing may be some of the chief complaints, in addition to the usual dyspnea. Chest pain is also a common chief complaint. Its origin may range from myocardial ischemia leading to acute left-sided heart failure, to pneumonia and pleural infection.

One challenge in assessing patients with respiratory conditions is that they may not be able to talk because of their difficulty breathing. Although it's usually best to ask open-ended questions and permit patients to tell their own stories, dyspneic patients may be able to speak only in short sentences. Some may be able to do no more than nod or shake their heads in response to a series of yes-or-no questions. In some cases, the bulk of the history taking may have to be hastily obtained from a family member or gleaned from the few clues immediately available, such as the medications present in the home. Basic therapy (such as oxygen or aerosol therapy) often must be instituted before getting the complete story from a patient. Sometimes, a patient must immediately be intubated, which precludes the possibility of obtaining a direct history from that point on.

When patients are able to discuss their chief complaints with you, they are often able to tell you exactly what condition they have. If they have one of the common respiratory illnesses (such as asthma, COPD, or heart failure), then they may be having an acute flare-up (called an exacerbation), or they might have one of the following common disorders:

- **Asthma with fever.** When a patient with reactive airways begins wheezing, an inhaler usually helps for only a little while before symptoms return. The typical asthma attack that responds to treatment but flares up again within a few hours is sometimes caused by an underlying infection (such as pneumonia or bronchitis), which repeatedly triggers the asthmalike symptoms. The asthma attack subsides only when the trigger is treated. Be sure to note signs of respiratory infection. Does the patient have a fever or chills? Is he or she coughing up sputum? What color is the sputum?
- **Non-delivery of medication.** Some inhalers indicate how many actuations (puffs) they are designed to deliver and how many doses remain in the canister. Without an automatic counter, most patients do not keep close track of their use. Often the medication has been exhausted even though some propellant remains in the canister. A patient may have been inhaling nothing but propellant for days, which explains why the wheezing is not getting better. Similar difficulties can occur when patients use outdated medications or medications that have overheated or otherwise been improperly stored (for example, left in a hot automobile or similar environment). In such cases, the bronchodilator from your ambulance may be effective, even though the patient's has failed. Another possible scenario is that a patient doesn't fully understand how to use the device and doesn't inhale at an appropriate point, instead spraying the medicine on the inside of the mouth. This potential error is one reason that physicians often prescribe a spacer device to be used with an inhaler.

- **Travel-related conditions.** Advances in technology have given patients with chronic respiratory disease much more freedom to leave the house and to travel. Some patients present with significant pulmonary edema after a lengthy journey. The culprit: not wanting to take diuretics while traveling. Remember to ask the obvious ("What medications do you use?"), always followed by "Did you take them during your trip?"

  In addition, paramedics may be called to assist someone whose oxygen tank has run dry, whose portable ventilator has suddenly malfunctioned, or whose medications were left behind or lost with the luggage.
- **Dyspnea triggers.** Just because a person knows the triggers for his or her reactive airways, such as pet dander, perfume, cigarette smoke or smog, pollen, or excessive heat, humidity, or cold, does not mean the triggers can always be avoided. A social or family situation may be important enough to risk having an episode of dyspnea, and no one can prevent all contact with all triggers, many of which are present in public places.
- **Seasonal conditions.** Bacteria, mold, and fungi can grow in heating ducts or in air conditioning units during their respective off-seasons. When the weather suddenly changes and use of heating or air conditioning systems begins, you can expect an increase in calls from people with chronic respiratory diseases.
- **Noncompliance with therapy.** Some people with chronic respiratory disease rebel against therapy in an attempt to regain control over their lives. Other patients don't understand the long-term nature of the therapy, and they attempt to wean themselves off their medications, oxygen, or respiratory support devices. Unfortunately, a crisis may result. Still other patients have been prescribed home oxygen, aerosol therapy, continuous positive airway pressure (CPAP), bilevel positive airway pressure (BPAP), or a variety of medications that they do not use or that they take only sporadically. Dangerous complications can occur if certain medications, such as oral corticosteroids, are stopped abruptly.

The mnemonic SAMPLE (Signs and symptoms, Allergies, Medications, Pertinent past medical history, Last oral intake, Events preceding the onset of the complaint) helps paramedics systematically obtain information about the history of the present illness and the patient's medical history.

- **Signs and symptoms.** Respiratory difficulty must always be evaluated in light of the patient's cardiovascular and renal status. Many acute myocardial infarctions present as heart failure, as do renal crises. Tachypnea can signal anxiety, diabetes, or shock. In addition, the vast majority of chronically ill patients have a respiratory component to their diseases. A whole host of pathologic conditions can masquerade as respiratory distress, especially in patients with underlying respiratory disease. Don't be too quick to conclude that the patient's *only* condition is a relatively straightforward respiratory disorder. Always dig deeper to determine what else may be triggering or worsening the patient's respiratory distress.
- **Allergies.** A person may know the triggers for his or her respiratory difficulties but be unable to avoid them. In your assessment, ask whether the person has been exposed to a known trigger.
- **Medications.** Part of a thorough history includes reviewing the patient's prescribed and over-the-counter medications. Many patients take multiple medications. A common combination might include a rapid-acting **beta-2 agonist** (rescue inhaler), a corticosteroid, and a slow-acting bronchodilator.

  Dyspneic patients might resort to using—and sometimes misusing—over-the-counter medications in addition to their prescribed medications. The following is a list of over-the-counter medications that a patient may use in conjunction with his or her prescriptions:
  - Antihistamines dry out secretions and should not be taken by people with asthma. Antihistamines are a common ingredient in many over-the-counter cough and cold medications.
  - Antitussives are used to suppress cough. Because coughing helps clear secretions from the airways, suppressing a cough might not be helpful. Coughing can be annoying, particularly if it interrupts sleep. However, the need for comfort must be weighed against the need to rid the airway of excess secretions. Overuse of antitussives can cause sedation, reduce respiratory drive, and partially obstruct the airway with secretions. Many over-the-counter cough syrups also contain antihistamines that can cause respiratory symptoms if not used appropriately.
  - Bronchodilators are available in some over-the-counter preparations. They often produce a nonspecific response, meaning the medication may also have a significant effect on the heart and blood vessels, particularly when used in addition to a prescription bronchodilator. The most common over-the-counter bronchodilators are simply attenuated (diluted) forms of epinephrine.
  - Diuretics can be found in diet pills and in caffeine-containing products, including

  many beverages. People are often told to drink plenty of fluids to maintain hydration, but overindulging in beverages that contain alcohol or caffeine has the opposite effect.
  - Expectorants thin out the pulmonary secretions so that they can be coughed up. Most common expectorants can be purchased over the counter. Many products combine expectorants with antitussives or antihistamines. These combinations are often at odds with each other. People with increased mucus production should avoid antihistamine products, taking only products that contain the expectorant guaifenesin.

  By following a simple interviewing pattern, it's possible to determine which medications the patient is supposed to take (which often yields valuable clues to other conditions), whether the patient is taking the medications correctly, and whether the patient has any medication allergies.

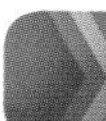

- **Pertinent past medical history.** An asthma attack, heart failure, pneumonia in an immunocompromised patient, and even spontaneous pneumothorax are pathologic conditions that often occur repeatedly. A patient's experience with these types of events can serve as a baseline to assess the current condition. Ask these questions: Do you feel better or worse than last time? How often does this happen to you? What did the doctor tell you it was? What helped you or what happened last time?

  In addition, ask patients about tobacco use, secondhand smoke exposure, and other possible toxic exposures.
- **Last oral intake.** The typical reason for ascertaining the patient's last oral intake is concern about a full stomach should ET intubation be required. Patients with chronic respiratory disease also tend to eat and drink less when they become acutely ill, which can add dehydration, hypoglycemia, or malnutrition to the already complex picture of their illness.
- **Events preceding the onset of the complaint.** It is important to determine what was happening just before or when the patient began having symptoms. In addition, the speed with which the patient's distress has worsened is an important consideration in determining the underlying cause. Did the symptoms arise suddenly, or did they get worse over time? How long have the symptoms been this bad? The position of comfort and difficulty speaking may also indicate the degree of distress. A patient who is comfortable lying flat and who is speaking in full sentences can be assumed to be in little distress. A patient who is sitting in a **Fowler position** (sitting upright) and speaking only in two- or three-word statements is probably in considerable distress, possibly even life-threatening distress. The patient might be described as having "three-word dyspnea."

Documentation & Communication

Remember to consult medical control. Report all pulmonary medications the patient is taking, and note whether they are oral, inhaled, or parenteral. If the patient uses an inhaler, then report when he or she last used it, note how many puffs were used at that time, and record what the label says about dosage and administration.

When respiratory disorders are chronic or recurring, patients may have already developed crisis management strategies. Determine what the patient may have already tried and whether it had any effect (positive or negative). Ask what the patient was doing when the dyspnea began. Patients often know exactly what set off the episode.

Secondary Assessment

By the time you have elicited a patient's history, you should already have gathered some important information about his or her physical signs, such as level of consciousness, position, and degree of distress. This section presents the components of the physical exam in sequence, noting at each step the points of particular relevance to a patient with dyspnea.

Assessing the level of consciousness is imperative in patients with dyspnea. Although the patient's arterial blood gases cannot be measured in the field, the patient's brain is constantly doing precisely that. Any decline in the partial pressure of oxygen (Pa_{O_2}) constitutes hypoxemia and initially manifests as restlessness and confusion. In worst-case scenarios, it may progress to combative behavior. An increase in the partial pressure of carbon dioxide (Pa_{CO_2}), by contrast, usually has sedative effects, making the patient sleepy and difficult to rouse.

If the lungs are not functioning properly, then delivery of oxygen and removal of carbon dioxide may be impaired. Failure to deliver oxygen efficiently results in cellular hypoxia. Hypoxia kills cells by making it impossible for them to make enough energy to do their work; it also causes acidosis. The brain is sensitive to reduced levels of oxygen. For this reason, any alteration in level of consciousness could represent a degree of respiratory compromise. Anxiety can be an early sign of hypoxia, while confusion, lethargy, and coma are typically later signs. A brief seizure often accompanies a hypoxic event or cardiac arrest. Dizziness and tingling extremities could signify hyperventilation.

In the neck, look for **jugular venous distention** when a patient is in a semisitting position. Jugular venous distention is a condition in which the jugular veins are engorged with blood. It is common in patients who have an obstructive lung disease such as asthma or COPD. Healthy young adults often have jugular venous distention when they are supine, and it is common to see gross jugular venous distention when people are laughing or singing Figure 16-14.

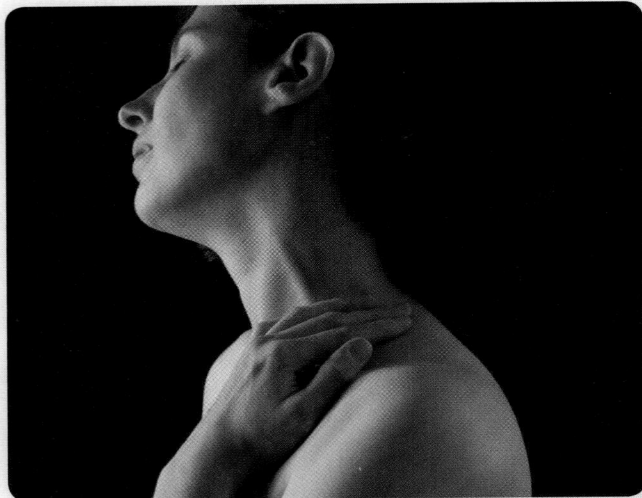

Figure 16-14 Jugular venous distention may be a normal finding in a healthy young adult who is supine or laughing. In an adult who is sitting upright, however, distention may indicate that blood is backing up as it tries to enter the thorax or the right atrium.

Cardiac tamponade, pneumothorax, heart failure, and COPD can all cause jugular venous distention. Distended neck veins may implicate cardiac failure as the source of dyspnea. Jugular venous distention may also indicate that high pressure in the thorax is keeping the blood from draining out of the head and neck.

Jugular venous distention must be interpreted in the light of the patient's position and other vital signs. The presence of jugular venous distention in a patient who is sitting upright provides a rough measure of the pressure in the right atrium of the heart. Grossly distended jugular veins despite a blood pressure of 80/40 mm Hg in a trauma patient should cause considerable concern; however, jugular venous distention in a healthy 20-year-old person who is lying flat (but not while sitting) is of little concern.

While you are examining the neck, note the position of the trachea. Tracheal deviation is a classic—albeit late—sign of a tension pneumothorax Figure 16-15. The deviation occurs behind the sternum, so this sign is difficult to feel except in extreme cases. Consider palpating the trachea at the suprasternal notch. On a radiograph, tracheal deviation caused by tension pneumothorax can be clearly identified.

Next, examine the chest and abdomen. When the right ventricle is not pumping effectively, blood backs up, making it difficult for the jugular veins and the large reservoir of blood in the liver to drain into the thorax. As a result, the combination of jugular venous distention and hepatomegaly (distended liver) may occur in right-sided heart failure. **Hepatojugular reflux** is distention the jugular veins when the liver is gently pressed. It is specific to

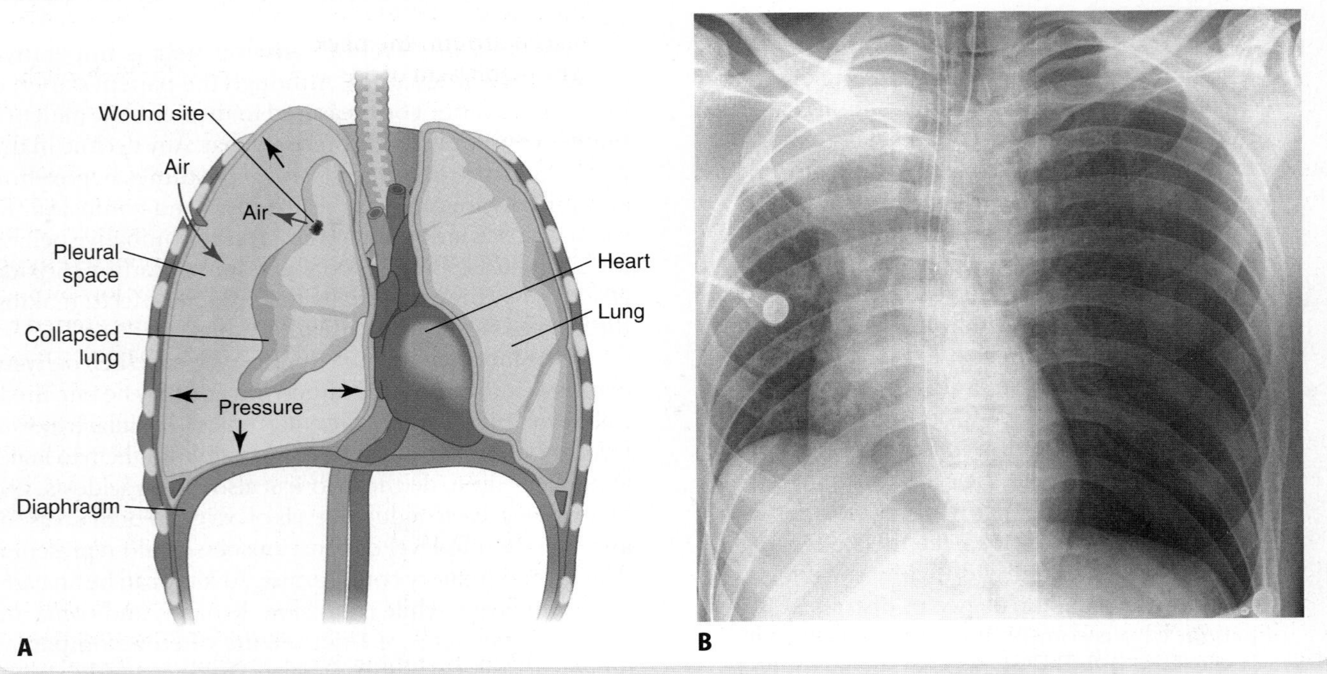

Figure 16-15 Pneumothorax occurs when air leaks into the pleural space between the lung and the chest wall **(A)**. The radiograph **(B)** shows a collapsed right lung, which appears darker.

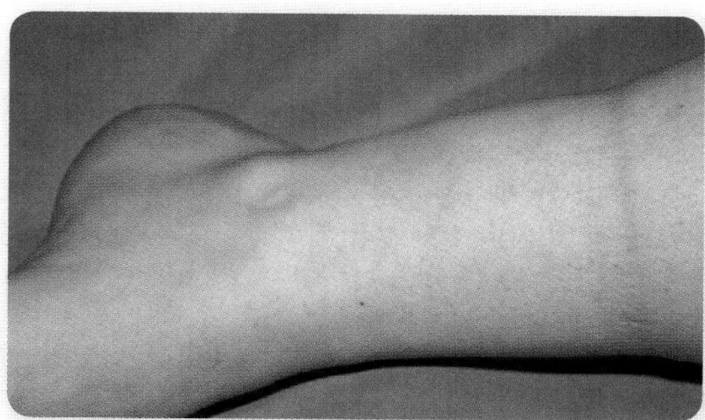

Figure 16-16 Pitting edema is present when the fingers leave a temporary depression in the tissue.

right-sided heart failure. Assess for hepatojugular reflux by pressing gently on the liver while the patient is in a semi-Fowler (45° angle) position.

Feel the chest for vibrations as the patient breathes. Large-airway secretions are usually easy to feel and to hear. These vibrations are called **tactile fremitus**. Some recommend chest percussion. With experience, it's possible to distinguish between the sound of a normal chest and the sound of a chest full of either blood (hemothorax) or air (pneumothorax), which will be hypertympanic to percussion. A chest tumor will be dull to percussion. Percussion remains a difficult procedure to use in the field, however, because of ambient noise.

Chest or abdominal trauma can cause respiratory distress by a variety of mechanisms (see Chapter 35, *Chest Trauma*, and Chapter 36, *Abdominal and Genitourinary Trauma*).

As you examine the patient's extremities, take note of anything unusual. Does the patient have edema of the ankles or lower back? If so, does it pit when a finger is pushed into the edematous tissue **Figure 16-16**? Is there peripheral cyanosis? Check the pulse. Does the patient have profound tachycardia as a result of exertion or hypoxia? Is there a weak or imperceptible peripheral pulse on inspiration (known as pulsus paradoxus)? Note the patient's skin temperature and check for any obvious fever. Is the patient's skin cool and clammy from shock? Is there distal clubbing as a result of chronic hypoxia **Figure 16-17**?

Vital Signs and Monitoring Devices

In addition to respiratory rate and quality of respirations, vital signs provide obvious clues to the respiratory workload. Patients under stress can be expected to have tachycardia because of hypoxemia, the use of sympathomimetic drugs, and the stress of dyspnea. They often also have hypertension for the same reasons. Bradycardia, hypotension, and a falling respiratory rate are ominous signs of impending arrest in patients with respiratory diseases.

As appropriate to the patient care plan, apply any monitors that are immediately available. Repeated vital signs, electrocardiogram (ECG), and pulse oximetry readings are the data most commonly collected. In some situations, depending on available equipment, peak expiratory flow, $ETCO_2$, and transcutaneous carbon monoxide levels might also be recorded.

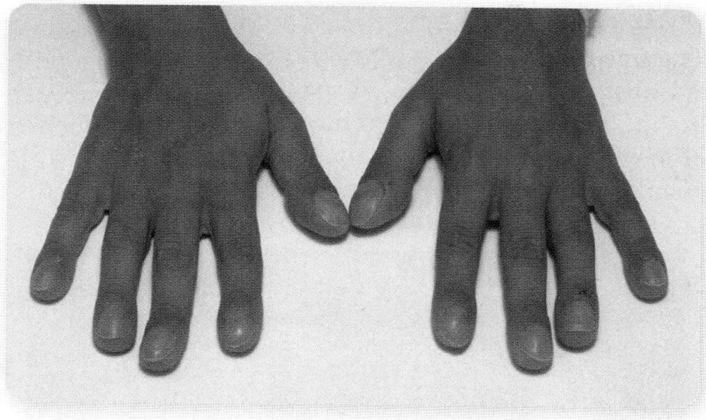

Figure 16-17 Digital clubbing is a sign of chronic hypoxia. It is seen in young people with congenital heart disease and in older people with severe chronic lung disease.

Stethoscope

Your stethoscope is one of the most important and frequently used tools at your command. You should choose one that meets your needs and, of course, your budget. Keep in mind that high-end cardiology stethoscopes are not well suited for taking blood pressures, while low-end models may deliver poor sound quality. Periodically check to ensure the earpieces are clean and clear of earwax. Regularly wipe the length of the main tubing with an all-purpose cleaner to slow the breakdown of the tube from the oils picked up when it's placed around the neck.

The diaphragm of the stethoscope is for high-pitched sounds (breath sounds); the bell (if present) is for low-pitched sounds (some heart tones). Applying firm pressure to the bell stretches the skin beneath it and makes it act like a diaphragm. Therefore, the bell should be placed lightly against the skin to pick up the lower-pitched sounds. Some newer stethoscopes take advantage of this principle by allowing a single head to transmit either high- or low-pitched sounds, depending on the amount of pressure exerted by the operator. In older-style stethoscopes, the bell rotates to allow the examiner to hear the different sounds better.

The ear canals tend to point anteriorly in your skull—that is, toward your eyes. The earpieces on the scope can be tilted farther forward for a better fit. But be careful: accidentally putting the stethoscope in backward causes the earpieces to hit the sides of the ear canal, obscuring nearly all sound.

The longer a stethoscope's tubing, the more extraneous noise you will hear. Higher-quality stethoscopes have a tubing-within-the-tubing design that limits external noise interference. Although the Sprague-Rappaport design is popular, its two parallel tubes often bang against each other while moving, which can create extra noise.

Pulse Oximeter

Under normal circumstances, a pulse oximeter is a noninvasive device that measures the percentage of a patient's hemoglobin to which oxygen molecules are attached Figure 16-18. For example, an oxygen saturation of 97% indicates that 97% of the patient's hemoglobin has oxygen attached to it. Oxygen saturation greater than 94% is considered normal. Medicare will not approve home oxygen use unless a patient's saturation falls below 88%.

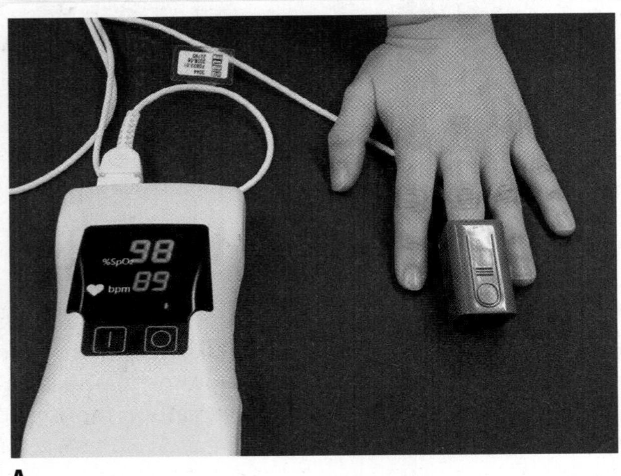

A

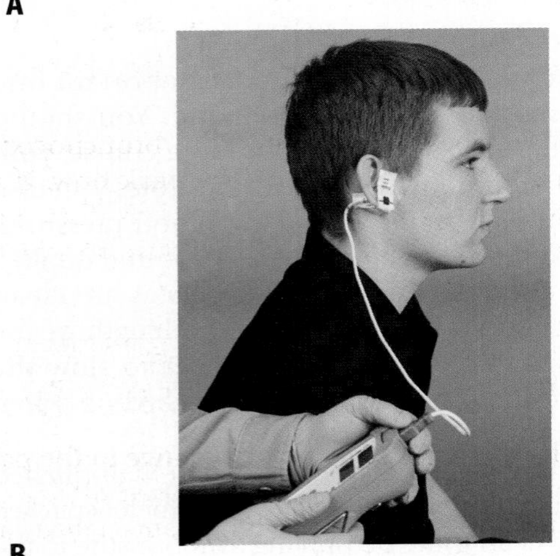

B

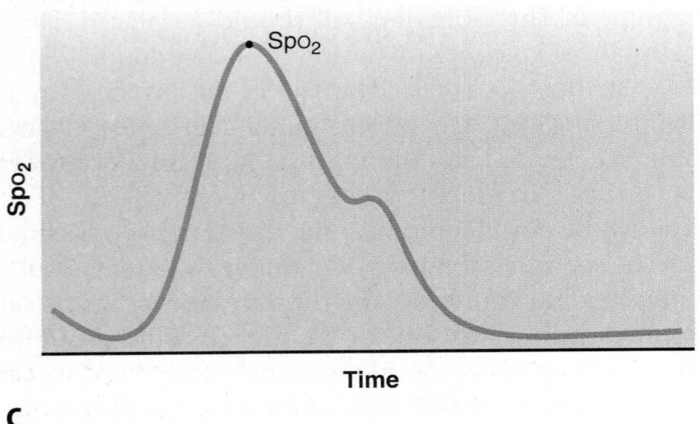

C

Figure 16-18 Pulse oximeters come in many sizes and, increasingly, are built into cardiac monitors **(A** and **B)**. Some oximeters provide a waveform **(C)**, which should demonstrate this characteristic shape when the oximeter is sensing properly.

A pulse oximeter must "see" a pulsatile capillary bed to return an accurate reading. Nail polish may need to be removed with nail polish remover before a reading can be obtained (although some research indicates that if a consistent reading is being taken through nail polish, the reading is probably accurate). Another strategy is to turn the probe so that it reads through the sides of a patient's finger instead of through the nail bed.[8] Inadequate peripheral perfusion, cold extremities, or the patient's movement (tremors or shivering) can make the reading inaccurate. A variety of pulse oximeter probes are available that may allow readings to be taken from the earlobe, forehead, or other areas of the body. Most pulse oximeters also display the patient's pulse rate; this reading should match the palpated heart rate.

If the patient's hemoglobin level is low—as a consequence of trauma or hemorrhage, for example—then the pulse oximetry result will be correspondingly high. If a patient's hemoglobin is only 6 g/dL (normal is 12 to 14 g/dL), then his or her oxygen saturation will probably be 100%. Such a patient needs more hemoglobin in the form of whole blood or packed red cells. Providing additional oxygen would be of little value. Some people, such as those who live at high altitudes or have chronic hypoxia (for example, patients with COPD), have abnormally high hemoglobin levels. Such people have a correspondingly low oxygen saturation. For example, a patient with a combination of moderate hypoxia and polycythemia (excess red blood cell production) may have an oxygen saturation level that normally hovers around 90%.

While it is relatively easy to measure oxygenation, a favorable oxygen saturation result does not necessarily mean all is well. A pulse oximeter cannot differentiate between an oxygen molecule attached to hemoglobin and a carbon monoxide molecule attached to hemoglobin. Most people who live in an industrialized society have a 1% to 2% carbon monoxide level all the time. Smokers may have a level as high as 3% to 4%. Thus, a 97% pulse oximetry reading may actually represent 95% oxygen saturation and 2% carbon monoxide saturation. A patient whose hemoglobin has a toxic or even fatal level of carbon monoxide attachment may nevertheless show a normal or high pulse oximetry value. Portable devices that specifically measure carbon monoxide levels enable paramedics to readily assess for carbon monoxide poisoning in the field Figure 16-19. These devices are available in some systems.

The oxyhemoglobin dissociation curve illustrates the relationship between oxygen saturation and the amount of oxygen dissolved in the plasma (Pao_2) Figure 16-20. It demonstrates that when oxygen molecules are scarce, they bind easily to hemoglobin, so that small changes in Pao_2 bring about relatively large changes in oxygen

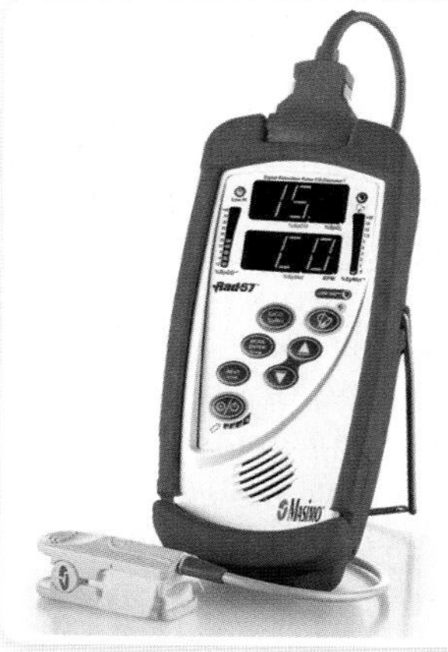

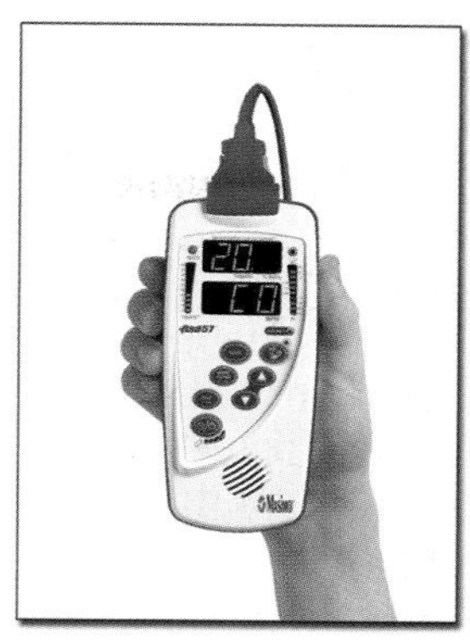

Figure 16-19 Devices are available that can measure oxygen saturation and carbon monoxide levels.

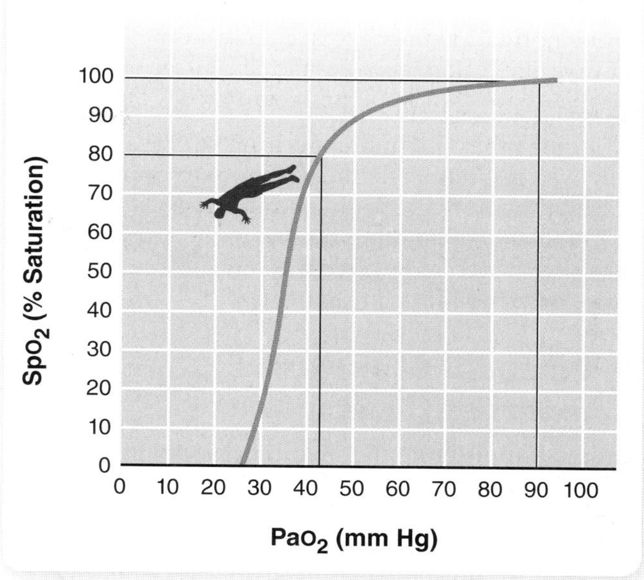

Figure 16-20 The oxyhemoglobin dissociation curve. As a patient becomes increasingly hypoxemic (lower PaO_2), he or she may fall off the curve as saturation drops rapidly.

saturation. As the hemoglobin receptors begin to fill up with oxygen molecules, larger changes in PaO_2 (shown on the horizontal axis of the curve) are required to produce changes in oxygen saturation.

Using a nonrebreathing mask for a healthy patient may increase the saturation level from 96% to 99%, whereas giving oxygen by a nasal cannula at 2 L/min to a hypoxic patient may increase the oxygen saturation from 80% to 92%—a more significant change. Conversely, the more hypoxic a patient becomes, the faster desaturation will occur after the patient falls off the steep part of the oxyhemoglobin dissociation curve. Other factors, such as acid-base balance and body temperature can also affect the entire system, shifting the curve to the left or right.

End-Tidal Carbon Dioxide Monitor

$ETCO_2$ detection, or waveform capnography, is discussed in detail in Chapter 15, *Airway Management*. The absolute value and the shape of the waveform are both important assessment parameters. Waveform capnography can also be used to document unusual respiratory patterns and evaluate the effectiveness of treatment.

Peak Expiratory Flowmeter

Peak flow is the maximum rate at which a patient can expel air from the lungs. (Chapter 15, *Airway Management,* describes the use of a peak expiratory flowmeter.) A lower value indicates that the patient's larger airways are narrowed by bronchial constriction or bronchial edema. Many patients with pulmonary disease check their peak flow twice a day and chart the results. They may present this chart when EMS personnel arrive. Normal peak flow values vary by age, sex, and height, but generally run from about 350 to 700 L/min. A peak flow less than 150 L/min is considered inadequate and signals significant distress, although some people with chronic asthma have a peak flow that never exceeds 100 L/min. Both bronchoconstriction and airway edema can reduce peak flow. If a bronchodilator is administered but peak flow does not improve, then airway edema may be the cause, in which case steroids may be indicated.

Reassessment

Contact medical control to report any change in the patient's level of consciousness or any increased difficulty breathing. Consistent with local protocol, contact medical control before assisting with administration of any prescribed medications. Document any changes, noting the time at which they occurred, and document any orders given by medical control.

Emergency Medical Care

In this section, we will discuss how to manage a patient with dyspnea. Later in the chapter, we will discuss how to manage specific diseases and conditions.

Paramedics have a relatively short list of tools to treat respiratory compromise. At the most basic level, your goal is to provide supportive care, administer supplemental oxygen therapy, and provide monitoring and transport. In actuality, you can do little in the field to alter the course of a pathologic condition such as COPD, pneumonia, or pulmonary contusion.

The primary exception is the treatment of bronchoconstriction. A host of bronchodilators are available to help relax bronchial smooth muscle. Such therapy can be extremely helpful if the patient's primary condition is bronchial muscle spasm caused by anaphylaxis or asthma. Bronchodilator therapy may be somewhat helpful to many other patients as well.

At the other end of the spectrum of care are patients with overt respiratory failure. The primary approach is to take over the work of breathing completely by intubating and manually ventilating the patient. CPAP and BPAP have also proved to be effective strategies and may help avoid intubation in many patients.

▶ Perform Standard Interventions

Before administering the medications discussed in the following sections, a variety of standard interventions should have already been implemented. Administering oxygen to keep the saturation greater than or equal to 94%[9] and establishing an intravenous (IV) line are typical interventions for any patient who needs advanced life support. Psychological support is also an important consideration for a patient with dyspnea. Your efforts to reduce the patient's anxiety with a calm, professional, caring demeanor can help reduce the patient's heart rate and blood pressure and allow maximum breathing effectiveness. Allow the patient to assume the position of greatest comfort. Most patients prefer to sit upright or lean forward, which can also help alleviate some of their distress.

▶ Decrease the Work of Breathing

Even under normal circumstances, muscles must work to allow breathing, and they must work much harder during respiratory distress. This extra work comes at a cost. People with asthma, for example, can often compensate for respiratory distress by devoting substantial energy to breathing. They can maintain their oxygen and carbon dioxide levels in an acceptable range as long as they continue to recruit their muscles for this effort. The tremendous workload consumes large amounts of energy, which must be fueled by even more oxygen and ventilation. A patient in such a condition typically is not in a position to eat and drink normally, thus, becoming progressively more dehydrated, malnourished, and fatigued. At some point, the patient will tire and be unable to continue the necessary work of breathing; he or she will look sleepy, the rate and depth of respiration will slowly drop, and decompensation (respiratory failure) will occur. Some patients with asthma may compensate for days, hoping that their steroids and bronchodilators will resolve an attack. By the time they realize that those approaches aren't working, they may be in too much distress to seek care except by calling 9-1-1.

The Trendelenburg and supine positions, especially in an overweight patient, cause the abdominal organs to compress the diaphragm. With each breath, the patient must move the abdominal contents out of the way to expand the thorax and breathe. Abdominal distention with air or blood compounds the situation. Shortness of breath induced by lying flat is called **orthopnea**. It explains why most people maintain a sitting position when they are short of breath. To decrease the work of breathing, help the patient sit up if he or she is more comfortable in that position. Remove constricting clothing, such as belts and tight collars. *Do not make the person walk*. Relieve gastric distention, perhaps with a nasogastric tube. Do not bind the chest or make the patient lie on the side of the unaffected lung.

▶ Provide Supplemental Oxygen

It is essential to provide supplemental oxygen to any patient who needs it. As with any other medication, you must administer oxygen in the concentrations necessary to be effective. Patients who are not breathing adequately should receive bag-mask ventilation with supplemental oxygen, or more advanced airway management techniques. Closely reassess the patient's breathing status, and adjust treatment accordingly. Pulse oximetry is a useful guide to oxygenation if it is accurate (the pulse rate on the oximeter matches the palpated pulse) and if the patient's hemoglobin level is relatively normal.

It is safe to administer oxygen in concentrations less than 50% to almost anyone, and it is appropriate to do so when there is a reasonable chance the patient would benefit from it. Oxygen concentrations higher than 50% should be reserved for patients with hypoxia that does not respond to lower concentrations. The use of 100% oxygen should be limited to the shortest period necessary.

Of the oxygen in the body, 97% is bound to hemoglobin. The other 3% is dissolved in the plasma. Once all of the hemoglobin in the blood has been saturated with oxygen, further exposure to high concentrations of oxygen begins to damage the lung tissue.

As a paramedic, you will treat many patients who require high-concentration oxygen to maintain acceptable oxygen saturation. You should never hesitate to administer oxygen aggressively to those patients who need it. At the same time, however, most patients with good oxygen saturation (at least 94%) do not benefit from supplemental oxygen.[10-12] Even patients with trauma, stroke, and acute coronary syndrome derive no benefit from supplemental oxygen therapy if oxygen saturation is already at or above 94%.[9] It remains common practice to administer low-flow oxygen to such patients, but **hyperoxia** (an excess of oxygen) should be avoided. In general, the American Heart Association (AHA) recommends maintaining oxygen saturation between 94% and 99%.[9] Oxygen saturation of 100% should be avoided, because it's impossible to predict how high the blood oxygen level may rise once the hemoglobin is completely saturated.

There are a few situations in which the pulse oximeter may not provide an accurate picture of oxygenation, such as in cases of carbon monoxide intoxication. In a pregnant patient, you might hyperoxygenate the pregnant woman in an attempt to deliver oxygen to a potentially compromised fetus. Be sure to follow local protocol and consult medical control in such emergencies.

Words of Wisdom

The Renaissance physician Paracelsus observed that it is the dose of a substance, not its composition, that makes it poisonous. Even water, the most innocuous of all substances, can become toxic if a person ingests too much of it.

Just as any medication administered in high doses can kill a person, so too can the overzealous use of oxygen. It is not necessary and could be dangerous to administer 100% oxygen to a patient whose true oxygen saturation is already above 94%. Conversely, there may be occasions, such as when treating patients with carbon monoxide exposure, in which high-flow oxygen is indicated despite an apparently high oxygen saturation. Use moderation and common sense in deciding whether to administer or continue supplemental oxygen.

Special Populations

In the 1950s, scientists began to understand that administering high concentrations of oxygen could cause blindness in premature neonates. Thus, the medical community began to recognize that oxygen can have toxic effects. Current protocols now discourage administering 100% oxygen in neonatal care, even during initial resuscitation (100% oxygen is still given, however, in neonatal cardiac arrest). Further research is being done on the effects of free radicals and the impact of high-concentration oxygen on all patients.

▶ Administer a Bronchodilator

Many patients with respiratory distress receive some benefit from bronchodilation, and some patients benefit substantially. Today's aerosol bronchodilators rarely harm patients, so paramedics tend to use them aggressively in the field. Patients who do not have bronchospasm usually benefit only slightly from aerosol bronchodilators, however, and the oxygen concentration delivered is often reduced during a typical aerosol treatment. Under these circumstances, application of a nonrebreathing mask is a better choice than the aerosol treatment. Follow local

YOU are the Paramedic — PART 4

While your partner prepares the patient for transport, you transmit the 12-lead ECG to the medical center and administer a dose of nitroglycerin paste. The patient's condition is still deteriorating. You have your partner begin positive pressure ventilation with a bag-mask device, and you establish an IV line. The patient initially resists but eventually becomes more comfortable and tolerates the treatment. As soon as the patient is in the ambulance, you begin priority 1 transport to the medical facility. You contact medical control and request the use of additional nitroglycerin paste. The physician grants the requests and also gives an order to administer 162 to 325 mg of aspirin to the patient. During transport, the patient's oxygen saturation progressively increases with treatment.

Recording Time: 10 Minutes	
Respirations	28 breaths/min; assisted
Pulse	100 beats/min
Skin	Pale and diaphoretic
Blood pressure	130/100 mm Hg
Oxygen saturation (Spo_2)	85% with oxygen by mask at 15 L/min and increasing
Pupils	PERRLA

7. What is the rationale for administering nitroglycerin if the patient has no chest pain or discomfort?

protocol, but remember bronchodilators are of little value in treating conditions such as pneumonia, pulmonary edema, and heart disease.

Bronchodilators relax the smooth muscle around the larger bronchi and are a significant therapy for bronchoconstriction. Administered via so-called rescue inhalers, fast-acting bronchodilators provide almost instant relief, a property that sometimes leads to their misuse. Strictly speaking, bronchodilators do not reduce swelling, kill bacteria, push fluid out of the lungs, or open closed alveoli. However, patients with pneumonia, heart failure, or atelectasis may have a small amount of secondary bronchoconstriction that could be reversed with a bronchodilator.

In the past, the strategy was to give aerosol atropine (the most common parasympathetic blocker). Today, a medication specifically designed for aerosol use, ipratropium, is available. It is also available in an inhaler. The combination of albuterol (a beta-2 agonist) and ipratropium (an anticholinergic) is also available as a premixed cocktail, so to speak, or as an aerosol spray or metered-dose inhaler. Popular long-acting bronchodilators include salmeterol (Serevent) and cromolyn (Intal, NasalCrom). Such agents have dramatically improved the quality of life for many patients with respiratory illness who use the medications correctly.

Aerosol Therapy

An aerosol treatment is a simple method of delivering medications, such as bronchodilators. Aerosol nebulizers deliver liquid medications in the form of a fine mist Figure 16-21. Particles of approximately 5 micrometers ride laminar airflow into the lower respiratory tract. Larger particles rain out in the mouth and pharynx and are swallowed, so they have little ultimate effect. Particles significantly smaller than 5 micrometers may be exhaled with the next breath. To generate the optimal particle size, most nebulizers need to have gas flow of at least 6 L/min. Running the gas slower than that generates particles that are too large; running it significantly faster makes the particles smaller and makes the treatment go faster, with the potential for less medication delivery. While aerosol delivery is fast and convenient, only a small amount of the medication ultimately reaches the intended receptors. You should strive to maximize medication delivery by coaching the patient on proper technique.

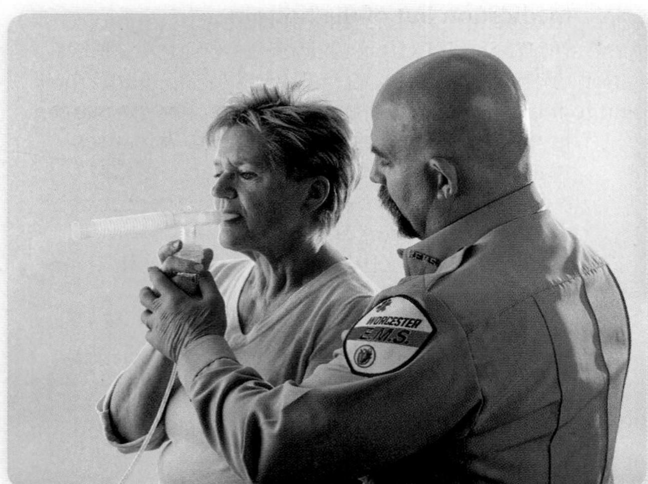

Figure 16-21 Aerosol nebulizers are often used to deliver medication directly to the respiratory tract. Unfortunately, they may supply only 30% to 40% oxygen during a treatment. Flow rate is an important factor in how much medication reaches the lungs.

In the home, most people run their aerosol treatments off of a small air compressor; in the ambulance, this therapy usually runs off of tanked oxygen or a wall unit attached to the main oxygen supply. As a result, the patient might receive only 30% to 40% oxygen via an aerosol treatment; while this amount is still more than the 21% oxygen contained in room air, it may be less than the amount of supplemental oxygen required by a patient with significant hypoxia. The relative drop in the fraction of inspired oxygen that occurs when a patient's nonrebreathing mask is removed to administer an aerosol treatment may be a contraindication to the procedure, particularly if the aerosol therapy is relatively unlikely to improve the patient's condition.

A nebulizer can be attached to a mouthpiece (pipe), face mask, or **tracheostomy** collar, or it can simply be held in front of the patient's face—the so-called blow-by technique. The smaller the amount of mist the patient inhales, however, the less medication he or she receives. Blow-by and mouthpiece treatments are ineffective if patients continually turn their heads or remove the mouthpiece to answer questions. As such, once the decision has been made to deliver a breathing treatment, try to stop the conversation and let the patient focus on inhaling the medication.

Controversies

In some systems, aerosol treatments are given to anyone who is dyspneic in the belief that they might help and are usually harmless; in other systems, use of aerosol bronchodilators is restricted to situations in which they are clearly indicated. Be sure to consult medical direction and your local protocols to keep abreast of how this class of medications is used in your region.

Although bronchodilators are the medications most commonly delivered by this method, corticosteroids, anesthetic agents, antitussives, and mucolytics can be dispersed in an aerosol. Aerosol lidocaine is extremely effective for numbing the upper airway before procedures, and aerosol fentanyl is used to reduce chronic coughing in patients who are terminally ill with lung cancer.

The newer aerosol bronchodilators cause far less tachycardia than is caused by the older, less beta-2–specific ones. As a result, it has become possible to give repeated treatments to patients with bronchospasm. Albuterol (Proventil, Ventolin), which is currently the most common beta-2 agonist, is routinely given every 4 hours, but more frequent treatments and even continuous therapy for hours at a time are often used without the occurrence of tachycardia. Continuous nebulizers that hold up to 10 times the usual medication dosages and run for an hour or more are available. However, they carry the potential for some beta-1 stimulation, causing tachycardia, and some physicians are therefore concerned that aerosol bronchodilators could worsen tachycardia in a patient with underlying cardiac disease. Tachycardia is almost always already present in patients with dyspnea, so consult medical control or local protocols for guidance. The steps for administering medications via small-volume nebulizer are shown in Chapter 14, *Medication Administration*.

Metered-Dose Inhalers

When used correctly, a metered-dose inhaler delivers the same amount of medication as an aerosol treatment. Because it does not require additional equipment (such as a nebulizer or air compressor), it's usually the delivery method of choice for bronchodilators and corticosteroids in the home setting **Figure 16-22**. Because patients use (and may misuse) their own inhalers in the home, be sure to document how often the patient has been taking an extra puff. Do not forget to consult medical control before administering additional doses if this is required in your system.

The metered-dose inhalers on the ambulance should ideally be equipped with **spacers**. A spacer is a device that collects the medication as it is released from the canister, allowing more to be delivered to the lungs and less to be lost to the environment. Remember, the mist coming out of the inhaler is not what reaches the patient's alveoli; rather, the 5-micrometer particles, which remain suspended in the spacer for several minutes, are pulled deep into the lungs by smooth laminar flow. When a spacer is used, the patient doesn't have to time the inhalation to coincide with the discharge of the inhaler. Spacers also reduce deposition of the medication into the mouth and oropharynx, which can occur among inexperienced users.

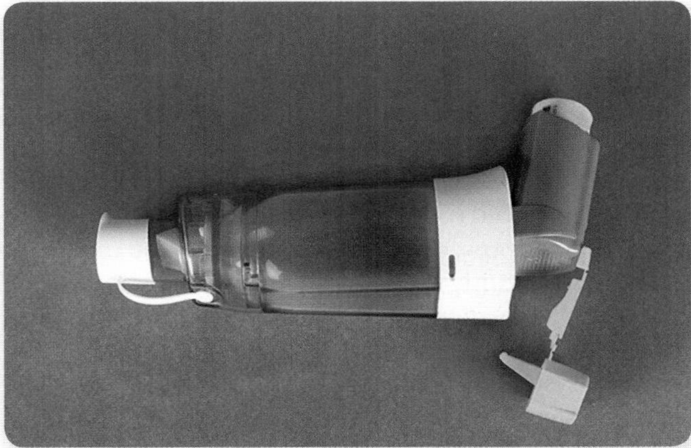

Figure 16-22 Metered-dose inhalers are a common delivery system for respiratory medications. Their effectiveness is greatly increased by the use of a spacer device (shown here), which regulates the release of medication into the inhaler.

In addition to improving medication delivery, the spacer allows paramedics to use the same expensive inhaler for multiple patients. Each patient gets a new spacer, but the inhaler itself is used over and over. Be sure to establish a system to keep track of how many times an inhaler has been used so that patients receive the proper amount of medication, and not just propellant.

Following the correct technique when using a metered-dose inhaler isn't difficult, but it requires constant reinforcement. The steps for administering medication with a metered-dose inhaler are shown in Chapter 14, *Medication Administration*.

The following are some tips on avoiding common errors when using or administering a metered-dose inhaler:

- **The mist from a metered-dose inhaler must enter the lungs.** Patients must inhale deeply as they discharge the inhaler to draw the medication deep into their lungs. Placing the inhaler directly into the mouth (without a spacer) often causes much of the medication to fall on the posterior pharynx, where it is swallowed and subsequently digested, thereby negating its intended effect.
- **Some patients mistakenly blow into the spacer.** Tell them to think of the spacer as a big straw, from which they should try to suck the medication out of the bottom.
- **Many spacers make a harmonica-like sound if the patient sucks too hard.** The best particle deposition comes from smooth, low-pressure laminar flow. Inhaling too forcefully causes turbulent flow, which makes many of the particles stick to the trachea and large bronchi, where they are not as effective.
- **Patients should try to inhale the medication deeply and then hold their breath for a few seconds.** This is a lot to ask of someone who is dyspneic, and it's not always possible. Sometimes the inhalation causes the patient to cough immediately after inhaling the medication, which precludes delivery of a full dose but may be unavoidable.
- **Make sure the inhaler contains medication.** The labels of most inhalers list the number of puffs of medication in the canister. Patients should be encouraged to keep track of how many times they have used the inhaler and to discard it when they reach the recommended

number of uses. The sound of fluid sloshing around when the canister is shaken doesn't indicate that there is medication left in it.

- **Keep the spacer and canister holder clean.** The spacer and canister holder should be rinsed off occasionally to avoid inhaling dust and other particles. In addition, respiratory devices should be dried after they are cleaned to discourage the growth of microorganisms.
- **After using a corticosteroid inhaler, patients should rinse out the mouth with water or mouthwash.** Residual corticosteroid in the pharynx can predispose patients to thrush, an annoying fungal infection of the pharynx or mouth.

Special Populations

In asthma education programs children learn to take a puff from a bronchodilator inhaler, turn over an hourglass egg timer, and wait 1 or 2 minutes before releasing their breath and taking the next puff. This strategy lets the medication delivered in the first puff open up the airways a little so that the medication in the second puff can go deeper into the airways.

Failure of a Metered-Dose Inhaler. Metered-dose inhalers have some drawbacks. Using such a device requires a cooperative patient who is willing and able to perform the maneuver correctly. Because the entire dose is delivered in one or two breaths, little or no medication will reach the lungs if incorrect technique is used to administer the dose. An inhaler may be contraindicated for a patient who is not moving enough air to effectively draw the medication into the lungs. In addition, the patient must be able to recognize when the inhaler is empty; in other words, the canister contains some propellant, but no medication.

A patient who doesn't fully understand how to use the device may inhale at an inappropriate point and end up spraying medication on the inside of the mouth. This potential error is one reason that physicians often prescribe a spacer device to be used with a metered-dose inhaler.

Dry-Powder Inhalers

Some respiratory medications are most stable in the form of a fine powder. Several common corticosteroids and slow-acting bronchodilators are often dispensed by this means. For example, tiotropium (Spiriva), a once-a-day anticholinergic for the management of COPD, is delivered via dry-powder inhaler.

A dry-powder inhaler is a plastic disk that holds about 1 month's worth of medication. Each time the device is opened, the small plastic blister that holds each dose is rotated into position. The patient then pushes a small lever to puncture the blister, presses the disk to his or her lips over the opening, and inhales deeply to suck the powder out of the device. Other dry-powder devices require the patient to insert a capsule of powdered medication, which is then pierced when the patient compresses a button or lever on the device. The patient sucks the powder out using a technique similar to that previously described.

Documentation & Communication

Teach patients to use their rescue inhalers before taking corticosteroids, slow-acting bronchodilators, or other medications. A rescue inhaler dilates the bronchi so that subsequent medications are delivered more effectively.

These devices are reasonably convenient and easy to use, but they are rarely used during emergency care. They deliver relatively expensive medications, so don't open and close a dry-powder inhaler repeatedly; it's possible to waste several days' worth of medication as the blisters rotate into and then past the position in which they can be punctured.

Leukotriene Modifiers

In some patients, bronchoconstricting chemicals called leukotrienes are released, particularly during an allergic response. A leukotriene blocker, such as montelukast (Singulair), which is usually taken orally, may be effective.

Electrolytes

In severe asthma attacks, magnesium sulfate 40 mg/kg (maximum dose 2 g) over 15 to 30 minutes may be ordered or included in standard protocols. IV magnesium can cause hypotension if given too quickly, but it can encourage smooth muscle relaxation in severe asthma and is particularly useful in efforts to avoid intubation in acute asthma patients.

Corticosteroids

Corticosteroids are used to reduce bronchial swelling (edema). These corticosteroids are different from the anabolic corticosteroids that are abused by some athletes. The corticosteroids used in respiratory medications have a variety of adverse effects, and long-term use can cause Cushing syndrome, which is characterized by the classic moon face and generalized edema. Corticosteroids cause rapidly changing blood glucose levels and can blunt the immune system, allowing infection to flourish. The use of corticosteroids such as prednisone must be discontinued gradually. Because of the long-term adverse effects, a course of corticosteroid therapy lasting only 1 or 2 weeks is usually prescribed.

Inhaled Corticosteroids. Inhaled corticosteroids do not seem to have the same adverse effects as their oral counterparts. For that reason, inhaled corticosteroids are becoming standard adjuncts to treat asthma and COPD. Two of the components in the asthma triad can be addressed by administering a slow-acting bronchodilator to reduce bronchospasm and an inhaled corticosteroid to reduce airway edema. (The third component of the triad is increased mucus production. Asthma is discussed in more detail later in the chapter.)

Intravenous Corticosteroids. In a medical emergency, it is common to give corticosteroids intravenously. A single bolus of IV corticosteroids does not seem to cause negative long-term consequences and is reasonably safe. Methylprednisolone and hydrocortisone are IV corticosteroid preparations given as an IV bolus, usually for acute exacerbations of COPD or acute asthma attacks. Their onset of action is measured in hours, so no results will be seen in the field. As always, consult local protocols and medical control before administering these agents.

▶ Administer a Vasodilator

Treatment options for pulmonary edema include a variety of strategies for causing vasodilation, thereby sequestering more fluid in the venous circulation and decreasing preload. Nitrates, from sublingual nitroglycerin tablets or nitroglycerin drips, can be used as long as the patient has adequate blood pressure and does not take a phosphodiesterase inhibitor such as sildenafil (Viagra) or tadalafil (Cialis). Morphine sulfate decreases anxiety but probably does not increase venous capacitance as much as once thought. It is not used as often as it once was in treating pulmonary edema.

▶ Restore Fluid Balance

Rehydration is supplemental therapy for patients with respiratory conditions who are dehydrated (for example, some patients with pneumonia or asthma). It is common to give a fluid bolus to younger patients who are dehydrated. In any older adult or other patient with cardiac dysfunction, administering too much fluid could cause pulmonary edema. Always assess breath sounds before and after giving a fluid bolus to be certain that the patient does not become overhydrated. Hydrating patients with pneumonia may cause the pneumonia to blossom or expand. This is an anticipated complication, but probably not one that must be addressed in the field. Let the medical facility rehydrate the patient after they have more information, labs, and radiographs. Because the condition of a patient with a respiratory condition can deteriorate precipitously, having an IV line in place is a wise precaution.

▶ Administer a Diuretic

Not every patient with crackles has pulmonary edema. Giving diuretics to patients with pneumonia or asthma may worsen their overall condition by dehydrating them and causing secretions to further obstruct smaller airways.

Diuretics are used to help reduce blood pressure and maintain fluid balance in patients with heart failure. Patients with pulmonary edema may benefit from a diuretic to remove excess fluid from the circulation, which ultimately keeps it out of the lungs. Loop diuretics (bumetanide [Bumex] and furosemide) are the most commonly used agents in emergency situations. Thiazide diuretics are often taken orally to treat high blood pressure and heart failure.

Many diuretics cause the loss of not only fluid, but also potassium. Patients who do not take potassium supplements may have low potassium levels and a resulting predisposition to cardiac dysrhythmias and chronic muscle cramping.

Do not give diuretics to patients with pneumonia or to those who are already dehydrated; reserve them for patients who clearly have pulmonary edema. Some EMS systems reserve furosemide only in standing orders for patients with wet lungs and peripheral edema, and others have removed it from their prehospital formulary altogether.

Patients with some degree of renal failure may require sizable doses of diuretics or may not respond to them. If a patient requires dialysis for renal failure, then trying to induce diuresis is unlikely to be effective. Although the management of respiratory distress is routine in virtually all EDs, a dialysis patient in pulmonary edema may be best served in a medical facility with the ability to provide emergency dialysis. This is one of the few circumstances in which a paramedic may decide to transport a patient with respiratory difficulty to a specialty center instead of the local ED.

▶ Support or Assist Ventilation

If the patient becomes fatigued, then breathing might need to be supported more aggressively. Therapy with CPAP and BPAP is becoming increasingly common and can preclude the need for intubation in many patients. Some patients may simply require bag-mask ventilation for a short period to reoxygenate, improve hemoglobin saturation, and reduce the $Paco_2$ level.

Trying to assist breathing for a patient who is *already breathing on his or her own* is one of the most difficult interventions. To avoid worsening a patient's condition, though, it's important to be confident in your bag-mask ventilation technique. Gastric distention and vomiting from overaggressive ventilation can complicate an already worsening situation. As always, *do no harm*. The same is true when providing sedation to anxious and possibly combative patients. The need to control a patient's behavior must be balanced against the possibility of further depressing respiration. It's almost always counterproductive to sedate a patient in the field to treat erratic behavior associated with dyspnea.

Continuous Positive Airway Pressure

CPAP is used in two distinctly different ways: to treat obstructive sleep apnea and to treat respiratory failure. Many people with obstructive sleep apnea wear a CPAP unit at night to maintain the airway during sleep. This type of CPAP may be applied via nasal pillows, a nasal mask, a face mask that resembles a typical mask used for bag-mask ventilation, or a mask that covers the entire face. This is *not* the type of CPAP used to assist breathing in critically ill patients. In people who are not critically ill, the positive pressure delivered maintains the stability of the posterior pharynx, thereby preventing obstruction of the upper airway as the person sleeps. This pressure limits hypoxic episodes and snoring.

The CPAP used as therapy for respiratory failure is almost always delivered through a mask secured to the face by some type of strap. When positive pressure ventilation (that is, with a pocket mask or bag-mask ventilation) is given, air is forced into the upper airway and flows into the trachea and esophagus unless steps are taken to help direct it into the trachea Figure 16-23. Indeed, positive pressure ventilation with bag-mask ventilation or a pocket mask is physiologically the opposite of normal (negative pressure) ventilation.

Using a bag-mask device for ventilation produces positive pressure in the chest. The more forcefully the bag is squeezed, the higher the pressure. Pressure that is too high can be detrimental: simple pneumothorax can evolve into tension pneumothorax, air leaks can produce huge amounts of subcutaneous air, and venous return can be impeded or even completely blocked. In recent years, prehospital providers have begun to understand the ramifications of using positive pressure ventilation during low-flow states such as shock and cardiac arrest. This understanding has led to CPR guidelines that stress lower ventilation rates, smaller volumes, and lower pressures. CPR is based on hemodynamic principles, and the rate, volume, and pressure of delivered breaths can quickly do more harm than good during resuscitation.

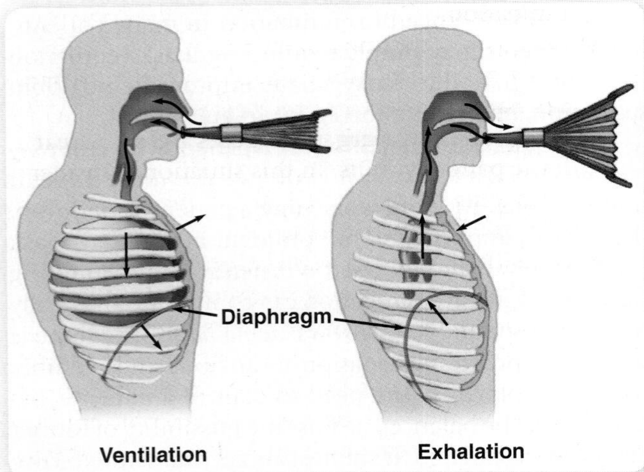

Figure 16-23 Positive pressure ventilation is physiologically the opposite of normal ventilation. Air is pushed into the respiratory tract with bag-mask ventilation and can enter the esophagus, opening the normally flat tube and allowing air to enter the stomach, unless careful technique is used. Compare with negative pressure ventilation, shown in Figure 16-5.

Similarly, administering CPAP increases pressure in the chest. If the patient's blood pressure is already low, then too much CPAP can reduce venous return to the heart, causing a sudden drop in blood pressure. This circumstance is uncommon with lower levels of CPAP, but blood pressure must be carefully monitored whenever CPAP is used (especially at levels more than 10 cm H_2O). CPAP can turn a simple pneumothorax into a tension pneumothorax in only a few breaths.

Remember to ensure a good seal with minimal leakage Figure 16-24. In the field, 100% supplemental oxygen is the most common gas driving the positive pressure. Be vigilant about monitoring the gas supply; depending on the flow rate and the patient's respiratory rate, some CPAP units may empty a D cylinder in as little as 5 or 10 minutes. The mask is fitted with a pressure-relief valve that determines the amount of pressure delivered (such as 5 cm H_2O). The effect is similar to being in a gale-force wind (high inspiratory flow) and having to push a pressure valve open by exhaling. This would seem to require a great deal of effort and tire out a patient in decompensating respiratory failure, but many patients in critical condition make a dramatic turnaround when CPAP is applied.

Sometimes patients find the CPAP mask claustrophobic and fight its application. Some patients can be talked through the mask application with good results, but other patients simply cannot tolerate the process. Don't struggle with a patient who is unwilling to use the mask; doing so will increase the patient's anxiety, cardiac workload, and cardiac oxygen consumption.

When CPAP works as intended, it can provide dramatic relief and avoid intubation. When it fails, it is critical for you to recognize the patient's deteriorating condition and be prepared to move to the next step (usually intubation).

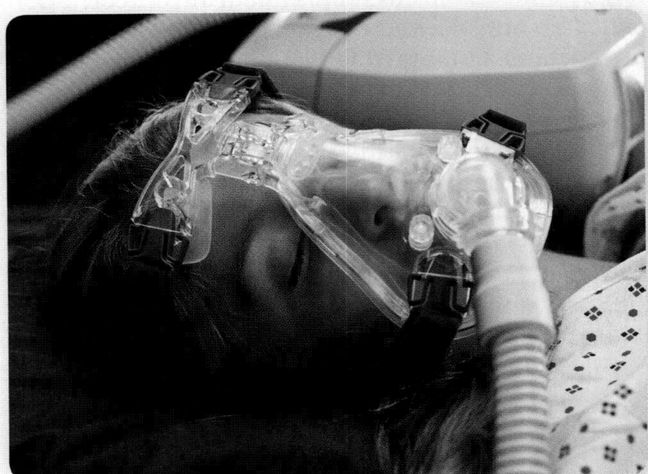

Figure 16-24 The continuous positive airway pressure used in the acute setting is usually administered via face mask, which must achieve a tight seal to function properly.

Within several minutes of application, the patient's oxygen saturation should increase and the respiratory rate should decline. The outcome of CPAP is inversely related to the patient's respiratory rate soon after its application: if this rate *increases*, the therapy is likely to fail; if this rate *decreases*, the therapy is likely to succeed.

Indications, contraindications, application, and complications of CPAP administration are discussed in Chapter 15, *Airway Management*.

Bilevel Positive Airway Pressure

In BPAP, one level of pressure can be delivered during inspiration (inspiratory positive airway pressure) and a different level of pressure can be delivered during exhalation (expiratory positive airway pressure). Instead of delivering 20 cm H_2O as in CPAP, BPAP set at 20/8 delivers 20 cm H_2O pressure during inhalation and 8 cm H_2O pressure during exhalation. Because this type of positive airway pressure is more like normal breathing, it is often more comfortable for patients. It causes a pressure variation in the chest, which allows for more normal blood flow. The BPAP device is also more complex and expensive, and it is not commonly used in the field.

Automated Transport Ventilators

Automated transport ventilators are essentially flow-restricted oxygen-powered ventilation devices with built-in timers. They can be set to deliver a particular volume of oxygen at a particular rate, which can be helpful when an extra pair of hands is needed **Figure 16-25**. They are a particularly good substitute for bag-mask ventilation for patients in cardiac or respiratory arrest. Basic automated transport ventilators may not offer advanced features, such as alarms, flow rate controls, and a selection of ventilatory modes. They are *not* little ventilators and are *not* intended to ventilate patients without direct observation and attention by a skilled paramedic.

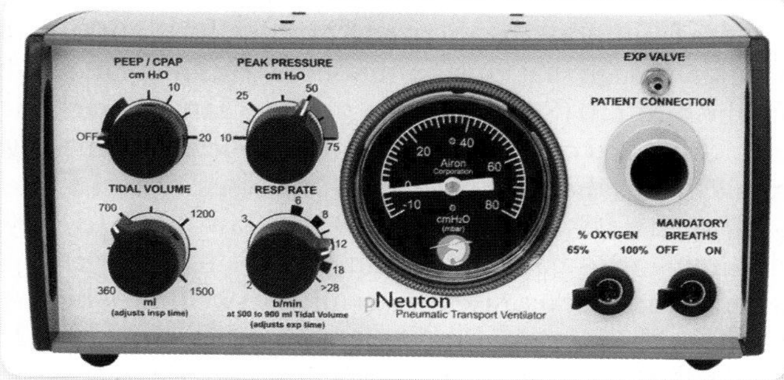

Figure 16-25 Portable versions of this automatic transport ventilator can be used in the field to dial in specific ventilation rates and volumes. This functionality can be useful in ensuring proper ventilation in a patient with cardiac arrest once an advanced airway has been inserted.

Courtesy of Airon Corporation (www.AironUSA.com).

Conscious patients require up to 150 L/min of flow to breathe comfortably. Some automated transport ventilators are permanently set to deliver 40 L/min, which would be extremely inadequate for a spontaneously breathing patient. Flow-restricted oxygen-powered ventilation devices and automated transport ventilators are preset to 40 L/min, which is the optimal flow for ventilating a patient in cardiac arrest—via face mask and without causing gastric distention. A more detailed discussion of ventilators can be found in Chapter 45, *Patients With Special Challenges*.

▶ Intubate the Patient

Ultimately, patients who are in respiratory failure may need to be intubated and ventilated. Intubation can be lifesaving, and many patients can be extubated within a day or two and have an excellent outcome. However, there are some factors to consider when intubating a patient. Paramedics must weigh these matters along with established protocol, medical direction, and any expression of the patient's wishes. Keep these guidelines in mind:

- **Patients with asthma are extremely difficult to ventilate and are prone to pneumothoraces.** Given these risks, intubation should be the last option for such patients.
- **Be proactive; ventilate patients *before* cardiac arrest occurs.** When in doubt, attempt to ventilate. A patient who is combative may not be ready for intubation. If a patient allows intubation, it was probably necessary. For patients who are conscious but in respiratory distress, sedation and neuromuscular blocking medications (through pharmacologically assisted intubation) are necessary to facilitate intubation.
- **Consider intubating a patient who has little or no gag reflex—for example, a patient who has had a stroke or is severely intoxicated.** The absence of a gag reflex poses a grave threat if the patient vomits. In this situation, consider intubating the patient to protect the airway even if ventilation is adequate.
- **Consider bag-mask ventilation.** Some patients who have diabetes or have overdosed are in obvious need of intubation. However, if an ampule of 50% dextrose or naloxone (Narcan) is likely to completely change that picture, it might be better to use bag-mask ventilation for a few minutes to monitor the effect of the initial medication therapy, assuming the patient can be ventilated without causing gastric distention and vomiting. Ventilate slowly (over 1 second), and use only enough ventilation to produce a visible chest rise.

Intubation is discussed in Chapter 15, *Airway Management*.

Words of Wisdom

In addition to the risk of further sedation and incorrect tube placement, the condition of any patient with a spinal cord injury may be worsened during the intubation process. Oral injury or aspiration is possible as well. Intubate the patient only after other, less invasive methods of ventilation have failed.

▶ Inject a Beta-Agonist Subcutaneously

Administration methods that require the patient to inhale medication may be unreliable or ineffective when the patient's breathing effort is inadequate, as evidenced by diminished tidal volume. In some circumstances, it may be beneficial to attempt beta-agonist (beta-2) stimulation the old way—that is, by administering subcutaneous or intramuscular terbutaline or epinephrine. These medications are not as specific to beta-2 as their aerosol cousins, so they will also cause more tachycardia (beta-1 stimulation) and hypertension (alpha stimulation), but when a patient's airways are severely constricted, these agents are sometimes the more effective approach. Be particularly careful using beta-agonists in older adult patients who may not easily tolerate the additional cardiac stimulation.

▶ Instill Medication Directly Through an Endotracheal Tube

It is possible to administer some resuscitation medications through an ET tube; however, AHA guidelines discourage this practice.[13] IV or intraosseous medication administration is preferred due to better predictability of delivery and pharmacologic effect.

Pathophysiology, Assessment, and Management of Obstructive Upper Airway Diseases

▶ Anatomic Obstruction

Pathophysiology

The most common source of upper airway obstruction in an unresponsive patient is the tongue. Every year, obstruction caused by the tongue results in the death of some trauma patients, patients in insulin shock, patients who have had a seizure, or patients who are intoxicated.

Assessment

Assessment of the airway is among the most foundational skills of paramedics. Anyone with a decreased level of consciousness, particularly a person in a supine position, is at risk of some upper airway obstruction. Sonorous (snoring) respiration is an obvious sign that breathing is at least partially obstructed. Other signs include gurgling, squeaking, or bubbling sounds during breathing. Stridor may be associated with accessory muscle use or retractions if the patient is attempting to breathe through an obstructed airway.

Management

Bystanders often place a pillow beneath the head of an unresponsive person, which exacerbates airway obstruction. If the patient is snoring, then remove the pillow and reposition the patient's airway.

Excessive soft tissue in the airway is one cause of obstructive sleep apnea, and some people go so far as to have such tissue surgically removed from the pharynx to limit anatomic obstruction. Fortunately, the soft tissue of the upper airway can be manually displaced with a variety of basic maneuvers, as discussed in Chapter 15, *Airway Management*. If restriction of spinal motion is unnecessary, then place an unconscious patient in the recovery position to avoid blocking the airway. The recovery position is the safest position for many patients who have had a seizure or are hypoglycemic or intoxicated. It also reduces the risk of aspiration if the patient vomits.

▶ Inflammation Caused by Infection

Pathophysiology

A variety of infections can cause swelling in the upper airway. Infection can lead to **laryngotracheobronchitis**, or inflammation of the larynx, trachea, and bronchi. An acute form of laryngotracheobronchitis is a common cause of **croup**, a condition characterized by stridor, hoarseness, and a barking cough that most commonly occurs in infants and small children. (Some authors consider laryngotracheobronchitis and croup to be the same.) The Poiseuille law holds that as the diameter of a tube decreases, resistance to flow increases exponentially. This law explains why children—who have narrow airways—often have croup when an infection causes upper airway swelling, whereas adults with the same infection do not **Figure 16-26**. Viral infection is a more common underlying cause of croup than bacterial infection is. Croup may also be caused by allergies that result in airway swelling and obstruction, or by obstruction with a foreign body.

The **palatine tonsils** can also become impressively inflamed in children, but this condition is rarely life threatening. When a child is properly positioned for intubation, inflamed tonsils do not typically obstruct a

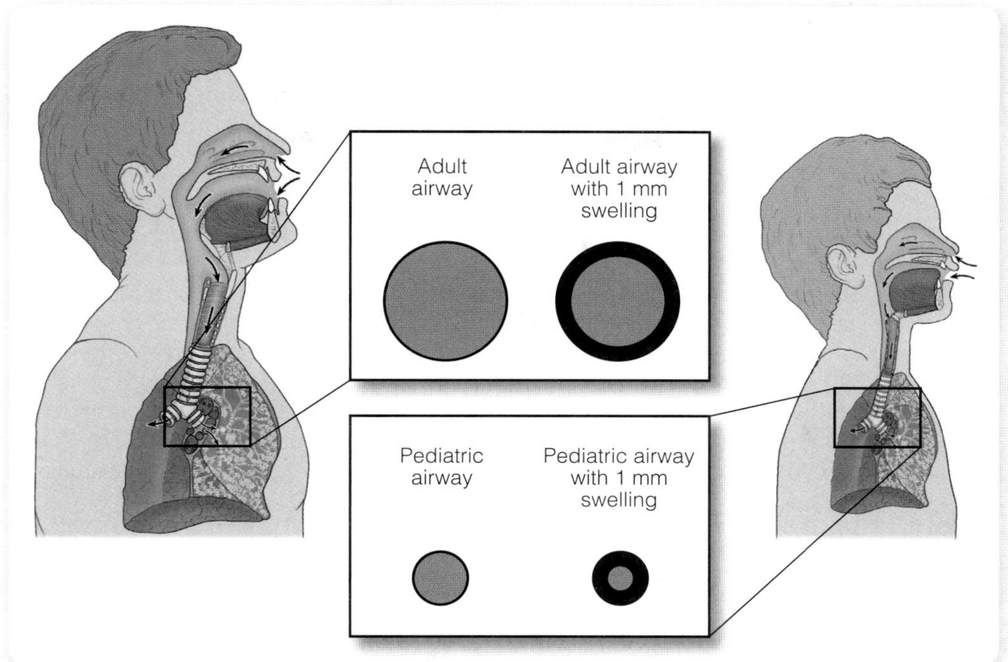

Figure 16-26 Any airway constriction (for example, in a condition such as asthma) can severely reduce the volume of airflow, especially in children. The Poiseuille law states that as the diameter of a tube decreases, resistance to flow increases exponentially.

clear view of the glottis. Take care to avoid injuring the tonsils with the laryngoscope, however, because they can swell and bleed if traumatized.

Assessment

In recent decades, many deadly upper airway conditions, such as epiglottitis, have become rare as a result of widespread immunization efforts. Unfortunately, the rate of childhood immunization has begun to decline as the general public becomes complacent about such diseases. Paramedics must, therefore, remain vigilant for these pathologic conditions. Table 16-6 lists the signs and symptoms of selected inflammatory conditions that can impair the upper airway.

Words of Wisdom

Immunization has significantly reduced the incidence of many infectious diseases, such as diphtheria; however, an increasing number of people in the United States are unable to obtain vaccinations (because of poverty, lack of access to health care, or geographic isolation, for example) or refuse to be vaccinated (because they fear that vaccines cause other diseases or believe that vaccinations are unnecessary). Lack of immunity among unvaccinated adults and children has led to the reemergence of certain diseases. In addition, because immunization does not last forever, conditions such as epiglottitis may be seen (albeit rarely) among adults in their 20s and 30s.

Croup and tonsillitis are common, especially among children, but the other conditions mentioned are rare. When these pathologic conditions occur, they are critical emergencies, because swelling can rapidly obstruct the airway, making orotracheal intubation extremely difficult or impossible. *Avoid manipulating the airway* unless absolutely necessary. Ventilation can usually be accomplished with careful bag-mask technique.

Management

If intubation is essential because the patient cannot be effectively ventilated with bag-mask technique, then the airway may be entirely obscured by the swelling. Attempts at laryngoscopy may worsen the swelling. Ask a partner to press on the patient's chest while you look for a stream of bubbles coming from the airway. Use an ET tube at least two full sizes smaller than would typically be appropriate for that patient. If this effort fails after a single attempt, then a needle or surgical cricothyrotomy is necessary. It is preferable to defer surgical attempts to the staff at the closest medical facility, but time may force you to use an invasive airway approach if permitted in your system.

▶ Aspiration

The inhalation of anything other than breathable gases is called **aspiration**. Patients can aspirate fresh or salt water, blood, vomitus, or food. Aspiration of foreign bodies, such as nuts or broken teeth, may also occur.

In older patients, chronic aspiration of food is a common cause of pneumonia from the bacteria in the

Table 16-6 Inflammatory Conditions That Can Impair the Upper Airway

Condition	Comments
Croup	A condition most often found in children between 6 months and 6 years, but can occur at any age; in northern areas, most common between October and March; characterized by stridor, hoarseness, and a barking cough; distressing but not typically fatal; a viral infection is usually the underlying cause. Do not manipulate the airway.
Epiglottitis	Severe, rapidly progressive inflammation of the epiglottis and surrounding tissues, usually caused by infection (most commonly with *Haemophilus influenzae* type B); may be fatal because of sudden respiratory obstruction; a life-threatening emergency; signs and symptoms include sore throat, fever, drooling, hoarseness, and purposeful hyperextension of the neck; was once more common in children, but is now rare because of widespread immunization against *H influenzae*, leaving unvaccinated adults as the most common susceptible group. Fortunately, the pathology is less life threatening in adults.
Peritonsillar abscess	Uncommon in children, more common in young adults; abscess forms near one pharyngeal tonsil; symptoms include fever and sore throat; may be mistaken for epiglottitis until a lateral abscess (instead of enlarged epiglottis) is seen in the throat. Do not manipulate the airway.
Retropharyngeal abscess	Most common in children; caused by infection in retropharyngeal lymph nodes and by direct pharyngeal trauma; signs and symptoms include fever and sudden stridor; may be mistaken for epiglottitis until laryngoscopic examination reveals retropharyngeal abscess (instead of cherry-red epiglottis). Do not manipulate the airway.
Diphtheria	Causative bacterium attacks and kills a layer of epithelial tissue, creating a **pseudomembrane**, often in the tonsillar area; membrane (and swelling of upper airway associated with the disease) can obstruct the upper airway; no longer common because of diphtheria, tetanus, and pertussis (DTP) vaccination. Do not manipulate the airway.
Enlarged tonsils	The palatine tonsils can swell excessively, sometimes to the size of a golf ball; associated with fever, difficulty swallowing, and throat pain; enlarged tonsils rarely obstruct the airway but can cause snoring and stridor. Do not manipulate the airway.

aspirated material. The aspiration of stomach contents carries the additional risk of aspiration **pneumonitis**, in which gastric acid irritates lung tissue.

Pathophysiology

Most adults choke only when they are intoxicated or traumatized, or when the gag reflex has diminished after a stroke, as a result of other neurologic dysfunction, or as a consequence of aging. Many older adult patients have impaired swallowing. Patients who receive tube feedings are at risk of aspiration, particularly if they are placed supine immediately after receiving a large feeding.

Aspiration is associated with a high mortality rate. It is a common but profoundly dangerous complication in patients who have had a cardiac arrest and in patients who are unresponsive as a result of trauma or overdose. Such patients are at risk of aspirating vomitus.

Assessment

To assess a patient with a sudden onset of dyspnea, consider the circumstances. Did the breathing difficulty occur immediately after eating? Does the patient have a gastric feeding tube, and if so, when was the last feeding and how large was it? Is the material suctioned from the patient's airway the same color as the tube feeding? Is there particulate matter in the suctioned material? A fever and cough may present several hours after an aspiration-prone event, such as a seizure or an episode of unresponsiveness. Some patients aspirate chronically and may have a history of aspiration pneumonia.

Management

Follow these guidelines when treating patients who are at risk of aspiration or who have aspirated:

1. Aggressively reduce the risk of aspiration by avoiding gastric distention when ventilating and by decompressing the stomach with a nasogastric tube whenever appropriate.
2. Aggressively monitor the patient's ability to protect his or her own airway, and protect the patient's airway with an advanced airway when needed.

3. Aggressively treat aspiration with suctioning and airway control if steps 1 and 2 fail.

Patients at risk of aspiration should not eat when they are having difficulty breathing. If basic life support maneuvers fail to clear an obstructed airway, then use laryngoscopy and Magill forceps, and, if necessary, perform a needle or surgical cricothyrotomy if allowed by local protocol.

Pathophysiology, Assessment, and Management of Obstructive Lower Airway Diseases

Obstructive lower airway diseases are characterized by diffuse obstruction of airflow within the lungs. The most common obstructive airway diseases are emphysema, chronic bronchitis, and asthma, an acutely episodic syndrome; these three conditions collectively account for a large portion of the typical provider's calls for dyspnea. Emphysema and chronic bronchitis are collectively classified as COPD because the changes in pulmonary structure and function are chronic, progressive, and irreversible. Asthma is considered a separate entity because—at least in its early stages—the airway narrowing is reversible.

Obstructive disease occurs when the positive pressure of exhalation causes the small airways to pinch shut, trapping gas in the alveoli. The harder the patient tries to push air out, the more air becomes trapped in the alveoli Figure 16-27. Patients with obstructive disease learn that exhaling slowly at a low pressure is more effective than exhaling rapidly at high pressure.

Patients with obstructive airway disease may have a variety of physical findings that suggest the nature of their disease:

- **Pursed-lip breathing.** Breathing in this way allows patients to exhale slowly under controlled pressure.
- **Increased I/E ratio.** The I/E (inspiratory-to-expiratory) ratio is typically 1:2 in healthy people breathing quietly. In other words, it takes about twice as long to exhale as it does to inhale. Patients who are gravely ill with obstructive disease may have an I/E ratio as high as 1:6 or 1:8.
- **Abdominal muscle use.** Abdominal muscles help to push out air (during exhalation). Patients with obstructive disease must work to push out air with every breath. People with asthma, for example, may complain of abdominal pain after an attack because they do the equivalent of hundreds of sit-ups as they struggle to breathe.
- **Jugular venous distention.** The trapped air in the lungs increases pressure in the thorax. Blood draining into the superior vena cava from the head and neck can back up in the jugular veins, causing jugular venous distention.

Asthma

Pathophysiology

The name *asthma* (from a Greek word meaning "panting") was first given to the disease by the second-century Greek physician Areatus "because in the paroxysms [of an asthma attack], the patients also pant for breath." Bronchial asthma is characterized by an increased reactivity of the trachea and bronchi to a variety of stimuli. This hyperreactivity results in widespread, reversible narrowing of the airways, or bronchospasm Figure 16-28. Asthma makes it difficult to exhale. Air becomes trapped in the distal portions of the lung, so that air from the next inhalation cannot enter the alveoli.

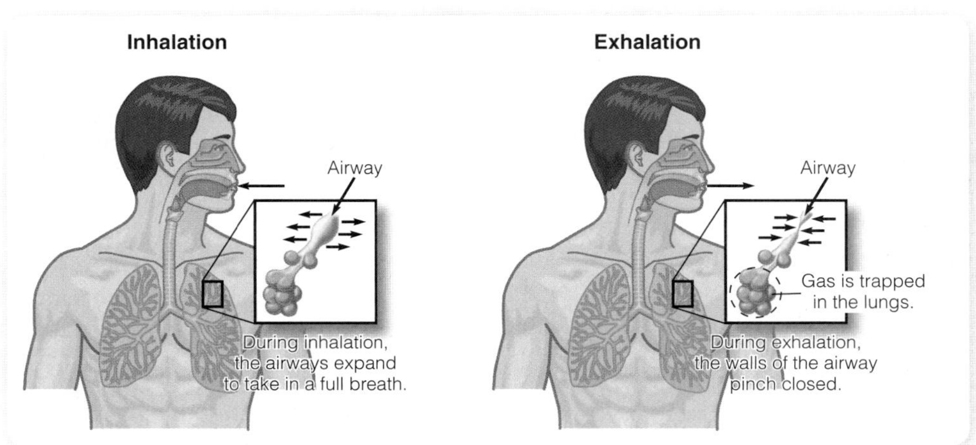

Figure 16-27 Obstructive disease is characterized by changes in the smaller airways that cause them to pinch closed during exhalation, trapping air inside the lungs. Healthy airways narrow during exhalation, but not enough to trap air or obstruct airflow.

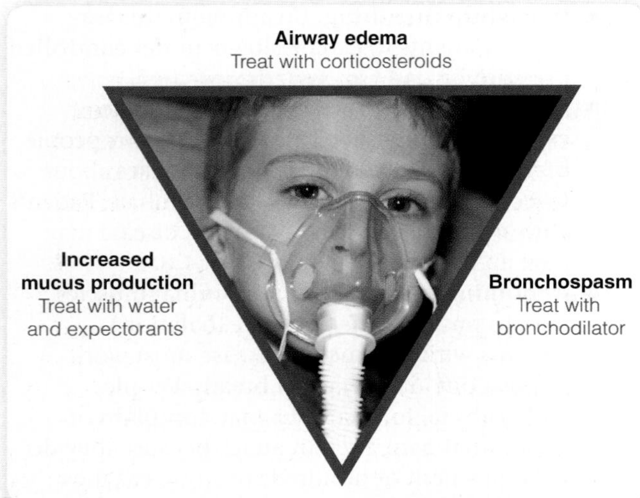

Figure 16-28 The asthma triad consists of the three primary components of asthma and the respective treatments for each. Asthma presents differently in different people, so individual treatment must also vary.

Words of Wisdom

The term *asthma* describes a triad of airway alterations: bronchospasm, increased mucus production, and peripheral airway edema. It may present differently in different people, but it is a common pathologic condition.

According to the Centers for Disease Control and Prevention, more than 24 million people in the United States reported having asthma in 2014[14-16] and the prevalence seems to be increasing. Each year, 2 million people visit an ED because of asthma, and one-fourth of them will be admitted to a medical facility.[17]

The fastest-growing asthma rates are observed in children younger than 5 years. Overall death rates from asthma are also higher in people younger than 35 years.[17] Asthma is more common in men but tends to be more severe in women. African Americans, especially those who live in large urban areas, are three times more likely to be diagnosed with asthma and have death rates that are five times higher than those observed in other racial groups.[4]

Patients who have potentially fatal asthma often have severely compromised ventilation all the time. They are at serious risk if acute bronchospasm is triggered or if they have an infection. A patient with asthma is at high risk of respiratory arrest if his or her history includes any of the factors listed in Table 16-7. Not following the medication regimen and/or having a severe psychiatric disorder also increases the likelihood that a patient with asthma will have a fatal attack. About 10 people per day die of asthma.[4]

Sometimes asthma is referred to as **reactive airway disease**, a label indicating that the patient experiences bronchospasm when exposed to certain triggers, such as dust, cold, or smoke. In addition, edema and inflammation of the airways and increased mucus production can cause significant airway obstruction. Asthma characteristically occurs in acute attacks of variable duration. Between attacks, the person may be relatively asymptomatic.

Table 16-7 Factors Associated With an Increased Risk of Asthma-Related Death

- Previous intubation for respiratory failure or respiratory arrest
- Respiratory acidosis
- Two or more admissions to a medical facility despite oral corticosteroid use
- Two or more episodes of pneumothorax

Status asthmaticus is a severe, prolonged asthmatic attack that cannot be stopped with conventional treatment. *It is a dire medical emergency.* Just as a person with COPD ordinarily does not call for an ambulance unless his or her condition has changed markedly, a person with asthma does not usually dial 9-1-1 unless the attack is much worse than usual. It is reasonable to assume that *any person with asthma who feels sick enough to call 9-1-1 is in status asthmaticus until proved otherwise.*

Assessment

When patients begin wheezing, their inhalers usually help for only a short time before symptoms return. The typical asthma attack that responds to treatment but occurs again in a few hours is sometimes caused by an underlying infection, such as pneumonia or bronchitis, that continually triggers the asthmalike symptoms. The asthma attack will not subside until the trigger is removed or otherwise mitigated. Consider what the triggers might have been for each patient. Does he or she have a fever or chills? Is the patient coughing up colored sputum?

On examination, a patient in status asthmaticus will be desperately struggling to move air through the obstructed airways. You will see prominent use of the accessory muscles of breathing. The chest will be maximally hyperinflated. Breath sounds and wheezes may be entirely inaudible because air movement is negligible, and the patient will usually be exhausted, severely acidotic, and dehydrated.

Bronchospasm. Bronchospasm is caused by the constriction of the smooth muscle that surrounds the larger bronchi in the lungs Figure 16-29. Bronchospasm may be stimulated by an allergen or irritant such as dust, perfume, animal dander, cold air, or other stimuli, such as exercise or stress. When air is forced through the constricted

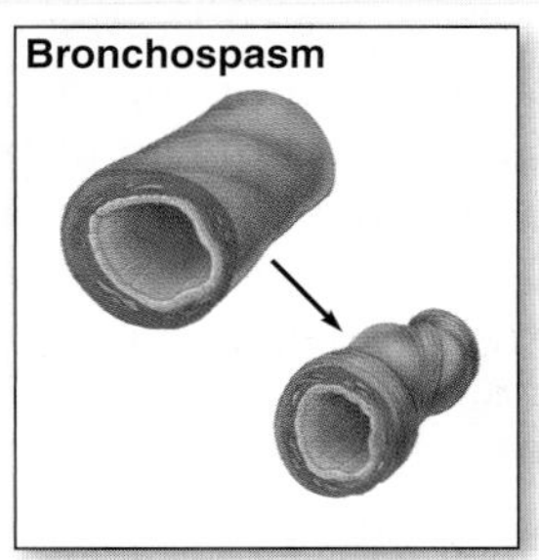

With bronchospasm, the muscle contracts, causing the entire tube to narrow.

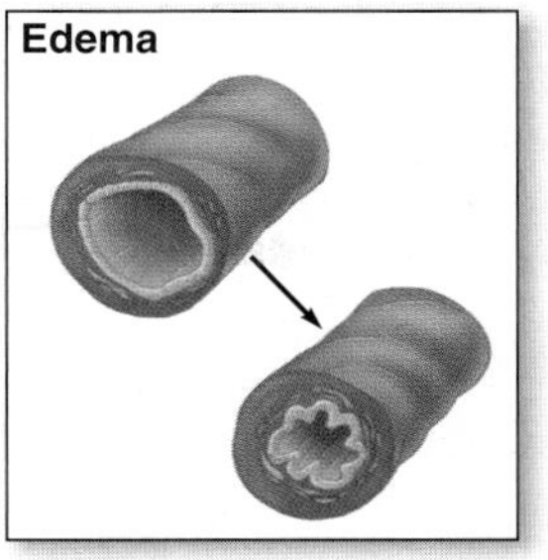

With edema, the wall of the tube swells, causing only the lumen to narrow.

Figure 16-29 Bronchospasm is a constriction or narrowing in the diameter of both the inside and the outside portions of the airway, whereas in bronchial edema, only the diameter of the inside portion (the bronchial lumen) is constricted. Both conditions reduce the functional diameter of the airways.

airways, it causes them to vibrate, which provokes wheezing. Bronchospasm can also reduce the peak expiratory flow by causing turbulent airflow.

Bronchial Edema. Swelling of the bronchi and bronchioles also creates turbulent airflow and air trapping. Bronchodilator medications do little to reduce bronchial edema. If a patient takes such a medication and the peak flow does not dramatically improve, then some degree of bronchial edema is likely.

Increased Mucus Production. Thick secretions may plug the distal airways and contribute to air trapping. People with asthma may be significantly dehydrated as a result of increased fluid loss from tachypnea and inadequate fluid intake. Dehydration makes secretions even thicker, further worsening the air trapping. Taking antihistamine medications may also thicken secretions.

Management

Most people with asthma have a combination of these three pathologic conditions, although their predominance varies among individual patients:

- **Bronchospasm.** Bronchospasm is characterized primarily by bronchoconstriction that tends to respond well to aerosol bronchodilators. The primary treatment for bronchospasm is nebulized bronchodilator medication.
- **Bronchial edema.** Bronchial edema is much less responsive to aerosol bronchodilators and usually shows significant improvement only after corticosteroids have been administered and taken effect. Corticosteroids may or may not be given in the field setting because, unlike bronchodilators, which can improve breathing immediately, corticosteroids take a few hours to reduce inflammation.
- **Excessive mucus secretion.** The primary approach to dealing with secretions in a person with asthma is to improve hydration. Mucolytics, which break down thick mucus, and expectorants, which loosen thick secretions so that they can be coughed out, are also sometimes used, most often in the in-patient setting.

Transport Considerations. Many patients routinely manage their asthma at home and may resist transport to a medical facility once their most acute symptoms have been relieved. Attempt to determine the trigger for an attack. If a patient has an underlying infection, indicated by fever, increased mucus production, or mucus that is green, yellow, or brown, or if the person will be continually exposed to a trigger (such as someone who wears a strong fragrance or smokes), then remove the patient from the environment for additional evaluation. A patient whose wheezing clears but whose peak flow does not improve may need corticosteroids. A patient who is undernourished or dehydrated may need additional IV fluids. If advanced life support assistance is more than a few minutes away, then strongly consider transport to the ED at the closest medical facility.

▶ Chronic Obstructive Pulmonary Disease: Emphysema and Chronic Bronchitis

Pathophysiology

COPD comprises at least two distinct clinical entities: emphysema and chronic bronchitis. Emphysema is thought to damage or destroy the fragile structure of the terminal bronchioles. Groups of alveoli merge into large blebs, or bullae, which are far less efficient than normal lung tissue because they have less surface area for gas exchange. This part of the tracheobronchial tree becomes so weak that its branches collapse during exhalation, trapping air in the alveoli.

Restrictive Disease. Trauma and diseases of the bones and muscles (severe kyphosis and scoliosis Figure 16-30) can significantly impair the ability to move air, causing a group of disorders known as **restrictive lung diseases**, which comprises pathologies that limit the patient's ability to expand the lungs within the chest cavity. These disorders put patients at risk of infection and may severely limit their ability to compensate for any respiratory insult. Restrictive lung diseases by themselves do not generate many calls for EMS response. We mention them for the sake of comparison to obstructive diseases, which you will encounter frequently.

Chronic bronchitis is defined as sputum production most days of the month for 3 or more months out of the year for more than 2 years. The hallmark of this disease is

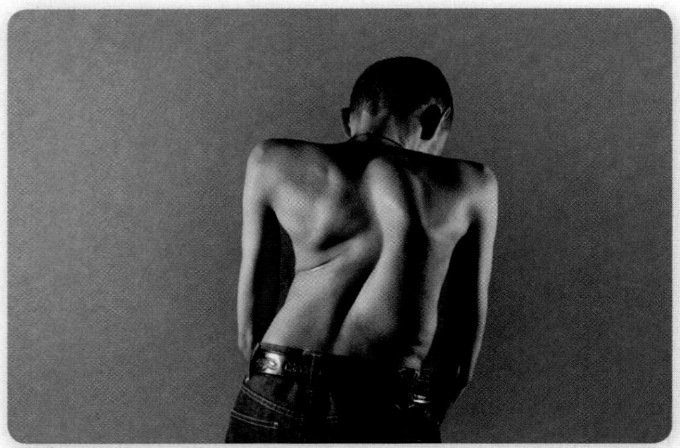

Figure 16-30 Diseases of the bones, such as scoliosis, can impair the patient's ability to move air because of chest compression.

excessive mucus production in the bronchial tree, which is nearly always accompanied by a chronic or recurrent productive cough (a cough that produces phlegm). A typical patient with chronic bronchitis is almost invariably a heavy cigarette smoker. He or she is usually overweight and congested and sometimes has a blue complexion. Blood gas levels tend to be abnormal, with elevated $Paco_2$ (hypercapnia) and decreased Pao_2 (hypoxemia) levels. Often, the patient has associated heart disease and right-sided heart failure (cor pulmonale).

Words of Wisdom

Over the years, people with COPD learn how much exertion they can tolerate, in which position sleep is possible, and so forth. So when a person with COPD calls for an ambulance, it nearly always means something has changed for the worse.

Assessment

Emphysema and chronic bronchitis represent two extremes of the COPD spectrum. In reality, as COPD progresses, most patients fall somewhere between these two clinical extremes, showing signs and symptoms of both disease processes.

Many patients with emphysema have a barrel chest caused by chronic lung hyperinflation. The patients are often tachypneic because they attempt to maintain a normal carbon dioxide level despite their dysfunctional lungs. They often use extreme amounts of energy attempting to breathe, using their own muscle mass for energy in the process.

Among the causes of diffuse wheezing are acute left-sided heart failure ("cardiac asthma"), smoke inhalation, chronic bronchitis, and acute pulmonary embolism. Localized wheezing suggests an obstruction, by foreign body or tumor, in a specific area. Only a careful history and physical examination will reveal the correct diagnosis.

Words of Wisdom

In the 1930s, Chevalier Jackson, renowned laryngoscopist and airway management pioneer, coined the phrase "All that wheezes is not asthma."[18,19] It's particularly important to distinguish the wheezing of asthma from that caused by left-sided heart failure because treatment of the two conditions is markedly different.

The following are some common factors that cause decompensation in a patient with COPD.

Chronic Obstructive Pulmonary Disease With Pneumonia. Because these patients are chronically ill, have poor secretion clearance, and sometimes have excessive mucus production (which acts as a culture medium for pathogenic microorganisms), they often have lung infections. Assessment should ascertain whether fever is present, the color or amount of sputum production has changed, other signs of infection (such as body aches, general malaise, or pain when breathing) are apparent, or auscultated breath sounds (such as localized or one-sided crackles) are consistent with pneumonia. A patient who obviously has COPD might also have another condition, including another respiratory condition.

Chronic Obstructive Pulmonary Disease With Right-Sided Heart Failure. It is a laborious task for the right side of the heart to push thick blood—thick because of polycythemia—through capillaries compressed by hyperinflated alveoli. This situation usually causes right-sided heart failure as a result of lung disease (cor pulmonale). If patients take in too much salt or fluid or do not excrete sufficient amounts of fluid (because of renal failure or not using diuretics as prescribed), then they may have an episode of heart failure. Assessment should look for peripheral edema, jugular venous distention with hepatojugular reflux, end-inspiratory crackles (it's sometimes difficult to differentiate the crackles of heart failure from the crackles always present because of COPD), a progressive increase in dyspnea over several days, a greater-than-usual fluid intake, and improper use of diuretics.

Chronic Obstructive Pulmonary Disease With Left-Sided Heart Failure. Patients with COPD are at high risk of sudden cardiac arrest. Any abrupt left ventricular dysfunction, such as an acute myocardial infarction or a cardiac rhythm disturbance (dysrhythmia), can cause rapid-onset, left-sided heart failure. Do not allow an initial impression of COPD to preclude swift identification of an acute myocardial infarction.

Acute Exacerbation of Chronic Obstructive Pulmonary Disease. In an acute exacerbation, no co-pathologic condition, such as heart failure or pneumonia, clearly accounts for the sudden decompensation. Instead, the patient's condition suddenly becomes worse, often because of some environmental change such as sudden changes in the weather, humidity, or recent seasonal activation of the heating or cooling system. An acute exacerbation can also be prompted by the inhalation of trigger substances, such as dust, mold, animal dander, or fresh paint.

Advances in technology have allowed people with chronic respiratory disease much more freedom to get out of the house and to travel. Paramedics may be called to assist a person who has an acute exacerbation of COPD when an oxygen tank runs dry or a portable ventilator malfunctions, when medications are left at home or packed in checked baggage that is misdirected, or when therapy is deliberately discontinued because the person wants to regain some control over his or her life or does not understand the importance of the therapy.

End-Stage Chronic Obstructive Pulmonary Disease. Patients with severe COPD eventually reach a point at which their lungs can no longer support oxygenation and ventilation. Their calls to 9-1-1 become more frequent as their condition deteriorates. Some will be in hospice care. In the end stages of the disease, it can be difficult to determine whether a patient has an exacerbation that can be resolved or has reached the end of the disease process. Endotracheal intubation may make it impossible for a patient to make his or her wishes known. In addition, the more frequently a patient requires intubation and mechanical ventilation, the more difficult ventilator weaning becomes. Apprehension about these bleak prospects heightens the patient's anxiety, thereby escalating cardiac workload and cardiac oxygen consumption—a potentially lethal series of events for a patient with end-stage COPD.

Each EMS system has its own ways of dealing with do-not-resuscitate orders. It is important to secure documentation of the patient's wishes as the terminal phase of the disease begins. Follow local protocol or contact medical control as needed regarding such matters.

Chronic Obstructive Pulmonary Disease and Trauma. People with COPD are as susceptible to trauma as the rest of the population. However, COPD lessens a person's ability to tolerate trauma. Many patients with COPD must sit up to breathe, so strapping them to a long board can lead to decompensation. Anyone who has performed CPR compressions on a patient with chronic emphysema knows how poorly the chest wall tolerates trauma. Even when a patient with COPD survives the initial trauma, he or she is susceptible to pulmonary emboli and infection during recovery. Patients with COPD rarely have a "normal" oxygen saturation; their normal might be less than 90%. Providing supplemental oxygen in an effort to achieve a saturation of 98% is unrealistic and might be harmful.

Documentation & Communication

Seek guidance from the medical director and observe local protocols when treating a patient with severe COPD or asthma who is in cardiac arrest or near-arrest.

Management

Although little can be done in the field to provide long-term relief for patients with COPD, the associated bronchospasm, edema, fluid, or hypoxia can often be relieved, helping to improve the patient's immediate situation.

Patients with COPD are often debilitated by the disease and have little or no respiratory reserve to help them deal with additional respiratory insults. Paramedics must actively try to determine the circumstances that tipped the precarious balance from relative stability to the state of respiratory insufficiency that prompted the 9-1-1 call. Effective management of COPD requires an understanding of the concepts of hypoxic drive and auto-PEEP (positive end-expiratory pressure).

Hypoxic Drive. **Hypoxic drive** is a state in which a person's stimulus to breathe comes from a decrease in $Pa{O_2}$ rather than from the normal stimulus, an increase in $Pa{CO_2}$. When a patient has chronic hypoventilation, bicarbonate ions (HCO_3^-) migrate into the cerebrospinal fluid, fooling the brain into thinking that acid and base are in balance. The patient's respiratory center might then switch to a hypoxic drive.

This phenomenon affects only a small percentage of patients—those with the most relentless forms of pulmonary disease. It occurs during the end stage of the disease process. You must decide whether the administration of oxygen is appropriate for any given patient. In making this decision, consider the following points:

1. Only a small subset of patients with COPD breathe because of hypoxic drive, but it is impossible to know who they are by just looking at them. Patients on home oxygen at very specific settings (such as 1.5 L/min) should arouse your suspicion.
2. Patients who breathe because of hypoxic drive do not suddenly become apneic after breathing oxygen. High levels of oxygen slowly depress the respiratory drive, and the respiratory rate slowly declines into the single digits before a patient becomes apneic. A paramedic is likely to recognize this phenomenon during a transport; the real concern is for a patient in a medical facility or an extended care facility who is given 100% supplemental oxygen and left alone for a prolonged period.
3. Verbal and physical stimulation can encourage breathing. If the respiratory rate begins to drop, then gently shake the patient and yell "Breathe!" This technique works well in the early stages.

4. If a patient becomes apneic because of increased oxygenation, then his or her skin may still appear perfused.
5. If the patient becomes apneic, then provide artificial ventilation and consider intubation.
6. The decision to intubate a patient with hypoxic drive is often complex. Once intubated, the patient may have to live what is left of his or her life on a ventilator, which is counter to many patients' wishes.
7. Although oxygen saturation (Spo_2) readings may be a valuable adjunct in deciding whether to intubate, Spo_2 values are less useful in cases of COPD because they fail to shed light on the carbon dioxide level.

Supplemental oxygen is integral to therapy for many patients, so it does not make sense to withhold oxygen from someone who needs it for fear of decreasing the respiratory drive in the few patients who might have this complication. Keep in mind that an oxygen saturation of 93% is acceptable, and many patients with COPD routinely have even lower values. It is not necessary or desirable to oxygenate these patients to oxygen saturation levels of 99% or 100%.

Auto-PEEP. Not everyone should be ventilated the same way. When ventilating a patient with severe obstructive disease, such as decompensated asthma or COPD, remember that the person has difficulty exhaling. Complete exhalation must be allowed before the next breath is delivered, or pressure in the thorax will continue to rise. This phenomenon, which is called auto-PEEP, can eventually cause a pneumothorax or cardiac arrest. If the pressure in the chest exceeds the pressure at which blood is returned to the heart, then venous return will be limited and cardiac arrest may occur.

Patients in whom auto-PEEP is a concern should be ventilated at a rate of as little as 4 to 6 breaths/min. Such restraint is difficult, but it is an absolute necessity to avoid the dire consequences of raising the thoracic pressure with each breath. Remember that the standard ventilation rate for adults in cardiac arrest is only 10 breaths/min in patients without COPD.

Pathophysiology, Assessment, and Management of Common Respiratory Conditions

▶ Pulmonary Infections

Pathophysiology

Bacteria, viruses, fungi, protozoa, and a host of other organisms can cause infections. The respiratory tract is particularly vulnerable to a variety of airborne agents and to agents that reside in the nose or throat and may migrate into the lungs.

In general, infectious diseases cause swelling of the respiratory tissues, an increase in mucus production, and the production of pus. Swelling in well-perfused respiratory tissues can be dramatic, particularly in the upper airway. This swelling is problematic because according to the Poiseuille law, the resistance to airflow increases exponentially when the airway diameter is narrowed. Alveoli can also become nonfunctional if they fill with fluid or pus, as occurs in pneumonia (consolidation).

Pneumonia may be caused by any of a variety of bacterial, viral, and fungal agents. Bacterial pneumonia is most often caused by the *Streptococcus pneumoniae* bacterium, for which effective vaccines are now available. (At-risk patients older than 50 years are encouraged to get two different pneumonia vaccines annually.) This type of pneumonia is responsible for about 10% of admissions to medical facilities in the United States and, despite the use of antibiotics, has a mortality rate of 5% to 10%. In many other countries, pneumonia is the leading cause of death.[20]

Older adults, people with chronic illnesses, and people who smoke are at greater risk of pneumonia. Anyone who is not ventilating effectively, who has excessive secretions (such as a person with COPD or asthma, a postoperative patient, or a person who is bedridden or sedentary), or who is immunocompromised (from human immunodeficiency virus, other illnesses, post-transplantation immunosuppression, or chemotherapy) is at risk of developing pneumonia. Patients with acquired immunodeficiency syndrome are particularly susceptible to *Pneumocystis jirovecii* pneumonia; it is a primary cause of morbidity and mortality. All high-risk patients are strongly encouraged to receive pneumonia vaccinations annually.

Another important consideration is that antibiotic-resistant organisms can colonize the respiratory tract. These organisms include, for example, methicillin-resistant *Staphylococcus aureus* and vancomycin-resistant enterococci, discussed in Chapter 26, *Infectious Diseases*. The aerosolization of these organisms when a patient coughs or during advanced airway procedures could be more dangerous to paramedics than when infections caused by these organisms exist in a pressure ulcer covered with a dressing. When presented with a patient in isolation because of an infection with methicillin-resistant *S aureus* (or a similar organism), always ask *where* the organism was found and wear proper respiratory protection if the organism is in the respiratory tract.

Words of Wisdom

Adults sometimes have inflammation and plugging of the bronchioles, resulting in pneumonia distal to the blockages. This condition, bronchiolitis obliterans with organizing pneumonia, is referred to as "BOOP."

Assessment

A patient with pneumonia usually reports several hours to days of weakness, productive cough, fever, and sometimes chest pain worsened by coughing. The illness may have started abruptly, with shaking chills (rigors), or it might have come on more gradually, with progressive weakness. As you obtain the patient's history of recent illness, be particularly attuned to comments such as, "I just got over the flu about a week ago." Pneumonia is often a secondary infection that follows a bout of influenza and is one of the leading causes of death under those circumstances.

Physical examination of a patient with pneumonia often reveals a grievously ill or toxic appearance. The patient may or may not be coughing. Crackles may be heard on auscultation of the chest, and the patient may have increased tactile fremitus and sputum production. Bronchial or bronchovesicular breath sounds may be noted over areas of consolidation; in advanced cases, breath sounds may become diminished or absent. Sputum may be thick (because of dehydration) or purulent. If the infection also causes swelling of the pleural membranes, then the patient may experience significant pain when breathing, especially when taking a deep breath or coughing. A pleural friction rub may be heard over the involved area.

Pneumonia often occurs in the lung bases, typically on only one side. Therefore, patients may have a "coughing fit" when turning from one side to the other. Sometimes patients' oxygen saturation will be significantly lower when they lie on one side versus the other. When the "good lung" is up, respiratory status may seem much better than when that lung is compressed by body weight.

Patients with pneumonia are often dehydrated. Rehydration may temporarily worsen their condition as the thick secretions liquefy and expand in the chest. Supportive care includes oxygenation, secretion management (suctioning), and transport to the closest receiving facility. Bronchodilators will not help the pneumonia itself, but they may slightly improve the patient's ability to ventilate.

Management

Infections of the upper airway may require aggressive airway management approaches. Infections in the lower airway are usually treated with supportive care and by transport to a medical facility.

▶ Atelectasis

Pathophysiology

The alveoli are vulnerable to a number of disorders. They may collapse from obstruction somewhere in the proximal airways or from external pressure produced, for example, by pneumothorax or hemothorax. They may fill with pus in pneumonia, with blood in pulmonary contusion, or with fluid in near-drowning or heart failure. In addition, smoke or toxic gases may displace the fresh air that should be present in the alveoli.

Under normal conditions, most of the air that moves into and out of the lungs (about 79%) is the relatively inert gas nitrogen, which keeps the alveoli open. If a patient is given 100% oxygen, then any alveolus that becomes plugged will collapse once all of the oxygen diffuses out. Patients receiving high concentrations of oxygen are at increased risk of having this type of atelectasis.

The human body has billions of alveoli, and it is common for some of them to collapse from time to time. Humans (and most mammals) periodically sigh, cough, sneeze, and change positions, all actions that are thought to help open closed alveoli and avoid decreased ventilation to any one part of the lung. When people do not use these actions—for example, because they are sedated or in a coma, or because deep breathing or moving causes pain—increasing numbers of alveoli may collapse and not reopen. Like balloons, alveoli are more difficult to blow open once they've completely collapsed; eventually, entire lung segments collapse. This condition is called **atelectasis**, and it increases the chance of pneumonia developing in the affected areas.

Assessment

Although atelectasis can be a significant disease by itself, the larger concern is that the affected areas become breeding grounds for pathogens, resulting in pneumonia. This is a concern in any patient who has a fever in the days following chest or abdominal surgery, particularly if breath sounds are decreased or abnormally colored sputum is produced.

Management

Postsurgical patients are encouraged to cough, deep breathe, and get out of bed with assistance, even if it is painful. Atelectasis may develop in people who cannot get out of bed, and the condition can lead to hypoxia or predispose a patient to lung infections and pneumonia.

At the medical facility, patients are constantly encouraged to take deep breaths. A device called an incentive spirometer helps patients quantify the depth of their breaths **Figure 16-31**. These devices are often sent home with patients for continued use after discharge from the medical facility (such as after rib fracture or chest surgery). Paramedics can reinforce deep breathing in patients who would benefit from it and can be watchful for atelectasis in patients who are sedentary or who take medications with sedative effects, including some analgesics.

▶ Cancer

Pathophysiology

Lung cancer is one of the most common forms of cancer, especially among people who smoke cigarettes and those exposed to occupational lung hazards, such as asbestos, coal dust, or secondhand smoke. According to the American Lung Association, smoking contributes to 90% of new lung

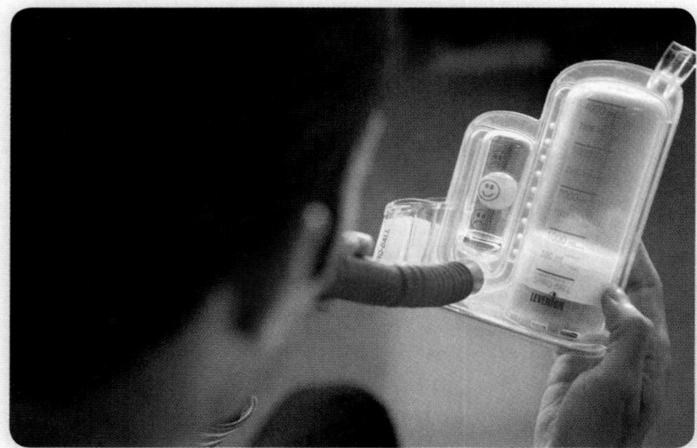

Figure 16-31 An incentive spirometer helps patients quantify how deep their breathing is. It helps them take deep breaths to avoid atelectasis.

cancer cases.[21] Smokers are 13 to 23 times more likely to get lung cancer than are nonsmokers, and nonsmokers have a 30% greater risk of cancer if they are exposed to secondhand smoke at home or at work.[21] Although lung cancer was traditionally considered predominantly a disease of men, today 45% of new cases of lung cancer occur in women, most likely because of the increase in smoking among women.[21]

Assessment

Lung cancer is often identified when tumors in the large airways bleed, causing **hemoptysis** (coughing up blood in the sputum) and uncontrollable coughing. It is frequently accompanied by COPD and impaired lung function. The lung is also a common site for the **metastasis** of cancer from other body sites.

Other types of cancer may invade the lymph nodes in the neck, producing tumors that threaten to occlude the upper airway. Patients with various types of cancer may have pulmonary complications from chemotherapy or radiation therapy. Lung irradiation, for example, may be associated with some degree of pulmonary edema. Tumors or treatment may also cause **pleural effusion**, which can present with rapidly progressing dyspnea.

Management

Paramedics can support oxygenation and ventilation and provide some amount of pain management, but there is little prehospital treatment specific to pleural effusion or hemoptysis other than transport to a medical facility. Paramedics are sometimes called to assist with end-of-life considerations for patients with cancer. Patients in hospice care, for example, may present with depressed respiration caused by the large amounts of narcotics used to relieve pain, anxiety, or other symptoms. In this type of narcotics overdose, titrate naloxone *only* enough to improve respiration; do not completely reverse the patient's primary pain control, or the patient may be plunged abruptly into complete misery. In the past, the respiratory depressant effects of narcotics and antianxiety agents may have been overemphasized, but now these agents are gaining increased popularity in the management of chronic pain, chronic cough, and anxiety in end-of-life scenarios. For example, fentanyl citrate (Sublimaze), a strong narcotic, is sometimes dispensed through an aerosol device to suppress chronic coughing in patients with end-stage lung cancer.

▶ Toxic Inhalations

Pathophysiology

Many potentially toxic substances can be inhaled into the lungs. The type of damage depends largely on the water solubility of the toxic gas. Table 16-8 shows how toxic gases are categorized.

Assessment

Highly water-soluble gases like ammonia will react with the moist mucous membranes of the upper airway, causing swelling and irritation. If the substance gets into the patient's eyes, then the eyes will burn and feel inflamed and irritated.

Less water-soluble gases may get deep into the lower airway, where they may do damage over time. Such toxic gases have been used in war to disable the enemy, because they do not cause immediate distress,

Table 16-8 Categorization of Toxic Gases

Category	Example	Effects
Highly water soluble	Ammonia	Acute upper airway irritation
Moderately water soluble	Chlorine	Effects depend on concentration and amount of exposure and range from coughing, wheezing, and crackles to pulmonary edema and chemical burns
Minimally water soluble	Phosgene	Delayed onset of pulmonary edema

but rather cause pulmonary edema up to 24 hours later. The gases phosgene and nitrogen dioxide behave in this manner.

Some common gases, such as chlorine, are moderately water soluble and produce signs and symptoms somewhere between the extremes of irritation and pulmonary edema. Severe exposure may present with upper airway swelling, whereas lower-level exposure may present with the classic delayed-onset lower airway damage. A common error is pouring household drain cleaner and chlorine bleach into a drain in an attempt to clear a clog, which may produce an irritant chlorine gas that can sicken the person and everyone else in the home or building. Industrial settings often use irritant gas–forming chemicals in large quantities and in higher concentrations than are available for home use, creating the possibility for incidents in which a larger number of people are exposed or a more toxic gas is produced. Paramedics should note industrial settings in their areas that present a high risk for this type of incident.

Management

A patient exposed to such a substance must be immediately removed from contact with the toxic gas and provided with 100% supplemental oxygen or assisted ventilation if breathing is impaired, as evidenced by reduced tidal volume. If the upper airway is compromised, then aggressive airway management (such as intubation or a cricothyrotomy) may be required.

Patients who have been exposed to slightly water-soluble gases may feel fine initially but have acute dyspnea many hours later. When such an exposure is suspected, patients should strongly consider transport to the closest emergency department for observation and further assessment.

▶ Pulmonary Edema

Pathophysiology

Fluid buildup in lung tissue and air spaces occurs when fluid from the blood plasma migrates into the lung parenchyma. This pulmonary edema compromises gas exchange long before overt signs are present.

Pulmonary edema can be classified as high pressure (cardiogenic) or high permeability (noncardiogenic). Cardiogenic pulmonary edema is often called heart failure and can result from dysfunction of the right or left ventricle, chronic hypertension, dysrhythmias such as ventricular tachycardia and supraventricular tachycardia, or cardiac diseases such as myocarditis. (These conditions are discussed in greater detail in Chapter 17, *Cardiovascular Emergencies*.)

Noncardiogenic pulmonary edema occurs in cases of acute hypoxemia, such as when inhaled toxins or near-submersion damages alveolar tissue, causing fluid to seep into the lungs. Toxins or drugs in the bloodstream (such as toxins when a patient is in shock or using heroin) can damage the pulmonary capillaries and have the same effect. Sometimes trauma, severe shock, cardiac arrest, or even altitude changes can damage the alveoli and capillaries, causing acute respiratory distress syndrome or high-altitude pulmonary edema.

Assessment

Some patients present with significant pulmonary edema after a lengthy journey, because they did not take diuretics while traveling. If a patient has been traveling, then ask whether prescribed medications have been taken regularly.

Early in pulmonary edema, few signs are apparent. By the time fine crackles in the bases of the lungs become audible at the end of inspiration, fluid has leaked out of the capillaries, increased the diffusion space between the alveoli and capillaries, swollen the alveolar walls, and begun to seep into the alveoli. This sound is caused by fields of wet alveoli popping open as the lungs reach maximal inflation. Always listen to the lower lobes of the lungs through the patient's back—but never through clothing.

As pulmonary edema worsens, crackles may originate higher in the patient's lung fields—often described as "crackles up to the subscapular level" or "crackles up to the apices." As fluid migrates into the larger airways and mixes with mucus, coarse crackles will become audible during inspiration and exhalation, and tactile fremitus may be identified. Ultimately, the patient will begin to cough up watery sputum that is often tinged pink by the presence of red blood cells. As air is forced into and out of the fluid-filled lungs, the fluid may bubble and foam. Coughing up pink, foamy, or blood-tinged sputum is a classic sign of severe pulmonary edema.

▶ Acute Respiratory Distress Syndrome

Pathophysiology

Acute respiratory distress syndrome (also known as ARDS, shock lung, Da Nang lung, and, in neonates, hyaline membrane disease) is seldom seen in the field. Nevertheless, paramedics may have a vital role in preventing this devastating pathologic condition. This syndrome is caused by diffuse damage to the alveoli, perhaps as a result of shock, aspiration of gastric contents, pulmonary edema, barotrauma (from overly aggressive ventilation), or a hypoxic event. It seems to be worse when there is some direct damage to the lungs, as in trauma patients with severe pulmonary contusions.

Picture the alveoli as a beach surrounded by the sea of the bloodstream. During a near-death crisis, changes in permeability allow the tide to come in and wash over the beach. When the tide goes out, it washes away the surfactant from the alveoli and leaves behind debris, such as dead cells and bacteria, on the shore. The alveoli subsequently become stiff (noncompliant) and difficult to ventilate. Mechanical ventilation under extraordinarily high pressure is ultimately required, which causes even more damage. The delivery of high oxygen concentrations for prolonged periods causes additional destruction.

Assessment

Typically, ARDS is not seen in the field, but paramedics might be asked to transport a patient with ARDS between facilities. The assessment process is similar to that for any patient with a respiratory disorder. Document oxygen saturation, breath sounds, and any sudden change in the patient's condition. Patients with ARDS typically have stiff lungs (that is, low compliance). During manual ventilation, ventilation pressure must be monitored to avoid overventilation and further lung damage. Various lung-protective strategies include low tidal volume, inverse I:E ratio, and permissive hypercapnia.

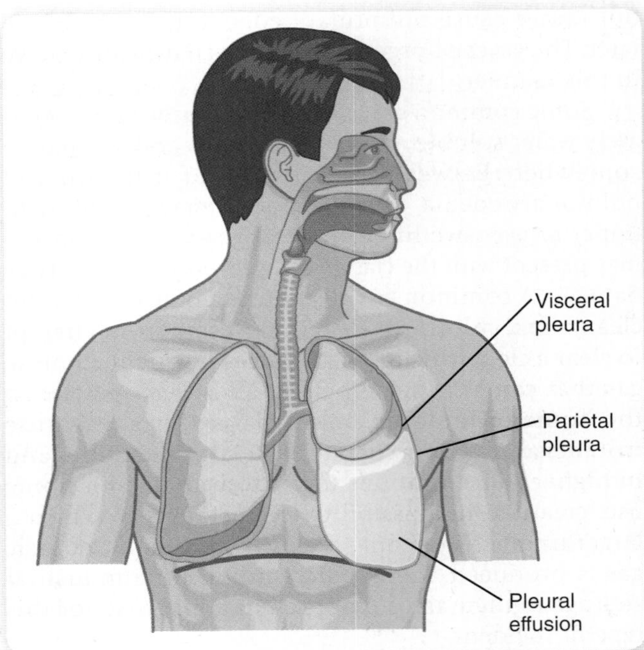

Figure 16-32 A pleural effusion is a buildup of fluid between the visceral pleura and the parietal pleura.
© Jones & Bartlett Learning.

Pathophysiology, Assessment, and Management of Conditions Outside the Lung Parenchyma

▶ Pneumothorax

Pathophysiology

When a patient has a pneumothorax, air typically collects between the visceral pleura and the parietal pleura lining the chest cavity. Some people have blebs in the lung parenchyma that are congenital or that are caused by COPD, and that predispose them to this condition. Blebs are weak spots that can rupture under stress, causing a spontaneous pneumothorax. The stress that ruptures the bleb may be as simple as coughing or as severe as aggressive bag-mask ventilation. People with severe asthma are prone to blebs, as are tall, thin people, especially those who smoke.

Assessment

Some patients who have had multiple simple pneumothoraces previously may actually say, "I'm having another pneumothorax." Patients may describe feeling a sharp pain after coughing, followed by increasing dyspnea during the subsequent minutes or hours.

Management

Most patients will not require acute intervention, such as needle chest decompression, but they must at least receive oxygen and have their respiratory status closely monitored en route to the medical facility.

▶ Pleural Effusion

Pathophysiology

When fluid collects between the visceral pleura and the parietal pleura, it produces a pleural effusion Figure 16-32. The sac of fluid formed is similar to a blister, in which repeated trauma to the tissues causes more fluid to collect. Effusions can be caused by infections, tumors, or trauma.

To visualize how this condition arises, imagine a blister forming at the base of the lung. The tissues rub against each other breath after breath, causing inflammation and fluid accumulation in the space. Some pleural effusions can contain several liters of fluid. A large effusion decreases lung capacity and causes dyspnea.

Assessment

It may be difficult to hear any breath sounds through the effusion. Because the effusion is filled with fluid, the patient's position may affect his or her ability to breathe.

Management

Shifting position may cause significantly more dyspnea, and patients usually resist being placed into anything other than the Fowler position. Supportive care, including proper positioning and aggressive supplemental oxygen administration, should be used until the patient can be transported to a facility at which the effusion can be definitively treated. Large effusions may be drained at the medical facility in a procedure called *thoracentesis*. This procedure frequently provides immediate relief of symptoms.

▶ Pulmonary Embolism

Pathophysiology

The pulmonary circulation may be compromised by a blood clot (embolism), a fat embolism from a broken bone, an amniotic fluid embolism from leakage of amniotic fluid during pregnancy, or an air embolism resulting from air entering the circulation from a laceration in the neck or an IV administration set that was improperly flushed or not flushed. A large embolism, of whatever type, usually lodges in a major branch of the pulmonary artery and prevents blood flow through that branch. Adequate gas exchange in the lungs requires functional alveoli to provide oxygen and take up carbon dioxide, and intact pulmonary vessels to convey oxygen-poor blood to the alveoli. Normal alveoli are of little use if the venous blood cannot reach them, as is the situation in pulmonary embolism.

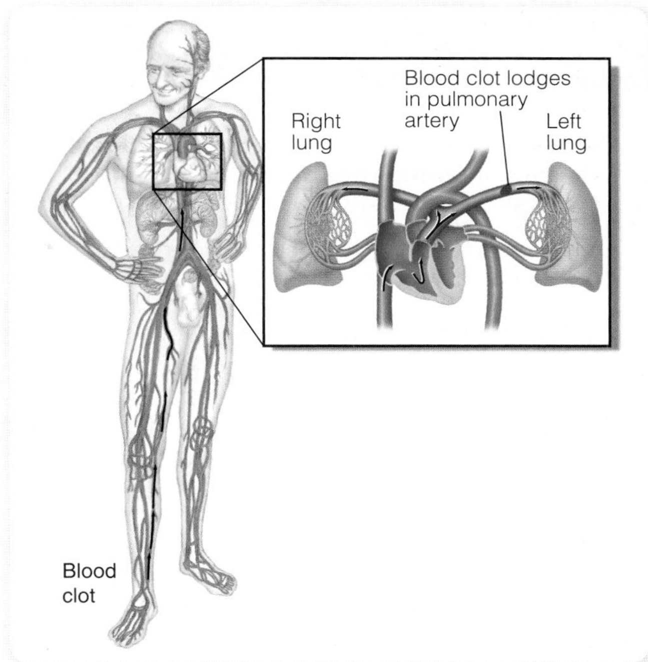

Figure 16-33 Pulmonary emboli are most common in sedentary people, in whom an embolus typically forms in the legs or pelvis. The embolus passes through the right side of the heart and lodges in the pulmonary artery, blocking blood flow to a portion of the lung.

Assessment

Because of its confusing presentation, pulmonary embolism is one of the most frequently misdiagnosed conditions in emergency medicine. The early presentation may reveal normal breath sounds with good peripheral aeration, diverting attention away from a pulmonary pathology. The classic presentation is sudden dyspnea and cyanosis and, perhaps, a sharp pain in the chest. A hallmark of pulmonary embolism is that the cyanosis does not resolve with oxygen therapy.

Pulmonary emboli often originate in the large veins of the leg, particularly the greater saphenous vein, where a clot can form and migrate through the venous circulation, passing through the right side of the heart and into the pulmonary circulation **Figure 16-33**. Patients with thrombophlebitis (inflammation of the veins in the legs) are at high risk for pulmonary embolism. They may have the Homan sign (calf pain during dorsiflexion of the foot caused by thrombophlebitis in the leg).

Clots also tend to form when a person is immobile for a prolonged period, such as during a long car trip or lengthy airplane flight, after removal of a lower extremity cast, or after major surgery.

Management

Bedridden patients are often prescribed anticoagulants, special stockings, or other devices to reduce the formation of blood clots in the legs. Especially for patients with a history of deep venous thrombosis, a physician may insert a **Greenfield filter**. This device, which opens like a mesh umbrella in the main vein that returns blood to the heart, is intended to catch clots that break loose and travel from the legs to the pulmonary circulation. Recent evidence that these devices can erode through the blood vessel wall have caused a shift toward retrievable filters that can be removed when a patient is no longer at high risk of developing a clot.

An exceptionally large pulmonary embolus lodged at the bifurcation of the right and left pulmonary arteries is called a *saddle embolus*, and it may be immediately fatal. Cardiac arrest caused by a large pulmonary embolus is a perilous situation that few patients survive. Patients with such an embolus often have **cape cyanosis**—deep blue pallor of the face, neck, chest, and back—despite good-quality CPR and ventilation with 100% supplemental oxygen. One hallmark of pulmonary embolus, in fact, is cyanosis that does not respond to oxygen. Such patients, as well as those who complain of chest pain, must be transported to the nearest emergency facility.

YOU are the Paramedic SUMMARY

1. What initial, "from the door" findings make you concerned for this patient?

The patient's initial appearance should raise a red flag for you because his ashen-gray skin signals hypoxia. The patient speaking in only one- or two-word sentences indicates that his oxygen saturation is low and he is struggling to take in enough oxygen. Your initial impression of this patient should tell you that he is in serious distress and needs rapid, decisive care.

2. What are your priorities for this patient?

Oxygen is your top priority. Through proper assessment and interviewing techniques, you must also ascertain why the patient is not getting enough oxygen so you can treat the cause. Aggressive airway and breathing care are paramount for this patient.

3. What is your working diagnosis at this time?

Pulmonary edema is the most accurate working diagnosis based on the information you have so far, although the cause of the edema is unclear. Even though you found no medications on the scene, it's possible that the patient is taking or should be taking prescription medications. Acute heart failure can cause pulmonary edema, so you must also rule out a heart attack in this patient.

4. What assessment and treatment steps will you want to accomplish on scene?

This patient's condition is serious, so you do not want to spend a lot of time on the scene; however, certain skills that are difficult to accomplish en route should be performed on scene. You must obtain a 12-lead ECG, for example, before you begin transport, because doing so while moving often produces too much artifact to allow accurate interpretation. In addition, road noise can make it difficult to measure vital signs while driving to the medical facility, so getting a baseline set makes good clinical sense.

5. Does this patient have an airway condition or a breathing disorder?

This is a breathing disorder. The patient is able to speak and move air, although with some difficulty; however, the patient's lungs are not properly exchanging air because they are full of fluid. Diminishing the amount of fluid in the lungs will promote gas exchange and allow oxygen to reach all of the body's cells.

6. Does the absence of chest pain or discomfort indicate the patient is not having a heart attack?

Not necessarily. A patient can be having a heart attack even in the absence of chest pain or discomfort. Never rule out the possibility of a heart attack in the presence of pulmonary edema. A number of diagnostic tests will need to be given at the medical facility to determine if the patient is having a heart attack. At this point, you should contact medical control with a report and request permission to give aspirin.

7. What is the rationale for administering nitroglycerin if the patient has no chest pain or discomfort?

Nitroglycerin has some vasodilatory effects, which aid in eliminating fluid from the patient's lungs and help free the surfaces needed for gas exchange, which, in turn, allows oxygen to reach the cells and tissue. However, expanding the vasculature also lowers the patient's blood pressure and can lower cardiac preload.

YOU are the Paramedic SUMMARY *(continued)*

EMS Patient Care Report (PCR)					
Date: 5-05-18	**Incident No.:** 550		**Nature of Call:** Medical alarm	**Location:** 222 Fifth Street, Apt. 506	
Dispatched: 0900	**En Route:** 0901	**At Scene:** 0903	**Transport:** 0915	**At Hospital:** 0922	**In Service:** 0939
Patient Information					
Age: 74 **Sex:** M **Weight (in kg [lb]):** 100 kg (220 lb)			**Allergies:** None **Medications:** Unknown **Past Medical History:** Unknown **Chief Complaint:** Difficulty breathing		

Vital Signs				
Time: 0908	**BP:** 140/100	**Pulse:** 110	**Respirations:** 34	**Spo_2:** 80%
Time: 0913	**BP:** 130/100	**Pulse:** 100	**Respirations:** 28	**Spo_2:** 85%
Time:	**BP:**	**Pulse:**	**Respirations:**	**Spo_2:**

EMS Treatment (circle all that apply)				
Oxygen @ 15 **L/min via (circle one):** **NC** **(NRM)** **Bag-mask device**		(**Assisted Ventilation:** CPAP)	**Airway Adjunct**	**CPR**
Defibrillation	**Bleeding Control**	**Bandaging**	**Splinting**	(**Other:** Nitroglycerin, aspirin)

Narrative

Arrived to find a 74 yo man in severe breathing distress. Pt states in one- to two-word sentences that he awoke this way and thinks he is going to die. Pt is not able to provide a history owing to severe breathing distress. Pt is in tripod position, skin color is ashen gray, and pt is diaphoretic. Pt given 100% oxygen while breath sounds were obtained. Breath sounds reveal crackles in apices and diminished sounds at bases. Pt denies history of fluid in lungs. Oxygen administration changed to CPAP. Pt becoming more anxious. Monitor showed sinus tachycardia while vital signs were being obtained. Pt not tolerating CPAP and oxygen saturation falling; decision made to assist ventilation with positive pressure bag-mask ventilation. Decision made not to intubate on scene given short transport time to the medical facility. My partner performed ventilations while a 12-lead ECG was obtained. 12-lead shows some ST elevation in chest leads V_2 and V_3, and pt was transported to destination med center. Pt was moved onto stretcher and placed in upright position. Pt given 1 inch (2.5 cm) of nitroglycerin paste and was tolerating assisted ventilation well. Pt was moved into ambulance, vital signs obtained again, and transport begun. Pt had IV established en route. MD 413 contacted at Mercy Medical Center; full report given; requested permission to give additional nitroglycerin paste. MD 413 granted both requests and stated to give pt 324 mg of aspirin. Orders confirmed; 1 inch (2.5 cm) of nitroglycerin paste applied at 0913. Shortly afterward, pt began to feel better and did not need further assistance with ventilation. CPAP resumed and pt able to answer questions appropriately. Oxygen saturation progressively increased with treatment during transport. Arrival at Mercy Medical Center at 0922 and pt admitted to room 5 with report to RN. CPAP maintained until respiratory therapist arrived with device. Pt had significant improvement at time of turnover. IV remained patent; less than 150 mL infused.**End of report**

Prep Kit

▶ Ready for Review

- Respiratory disease is one of the most common pathologic conditions and, consequently, respiratory distress is one of the most common reasons for EMS dispatch.
- The primary components of the respiratory system are like an inverted tree, with the trachea representing the trunk and the alveoli resembling the leaves.
- The trachea bifurcates into the left and right mainstem bronchi of the lungs at a ridgelike projection of tracheal cartilage called the *carina*.
- Pulmonary circulation begins at the right ventricle, where the pulmonary artery branches into increasingly smaller vessels until it reaches the pulmonary capillary bed, which surrounds the alveoli and terminal bronchioles. Gas exchange occurs at the interface of the alveoli and the pulmonary capillaries.
- The respiratory system is closely linked to cardiac regulation and renal function.
- The respiratory system delivers oxygen to the body and removes the primary waste product of metabolism, carbon dioxide. If the lungs are not functioning properly, then either of these vital functions may be impaired. Hypoxia, cell death, and acidosis can then occur.
- Respiratory failure, or hypoventilation, can be caused by a multitude of pathologic conditions, ranging from lung, heart, or neurologic system injury to drug overdose. Care may include administration of supplemental oxygen.
- Impaired ventilation may be caused by upper or lower airway obstructive disease, chest wall impairment, or neuromuscular impairment, among other causes.
- In hyperventilation syndrome, ventilation is excessive. If it continues, then the patient may experience chest pain, carpopedal spasm, and alkalosis.
- Respiratory disease can impair ventilation, diffusion, perfusion, or a combination of the three.
- Certain respiratory diseases have classic presentations. Clues found during the primary survey may lead you to suspect a certain disease.
- Patients with traumatic brain injury may exhibit abnormal respiratory patterns, including agonal gasps; apneustic and ataxic patterns; Biot, Cheyne-Stokes, and Kussmaul respirations; and central neurogenic hyperventilation, bradypnea, hyperpnea, hypopnea, or tachypnea.
- The brain is sensitive to reduced levels of oxygen. Therefore, an altered level of consciousness could represent respiratory compromise.
- It is critical to evaluate how hard a patient is working to breathe by assessing indicators such as respiratory rate and depth and by listening for abnormal breath sounds.
- Assessing a patient's position of comfort and level of difficulty speaking may help in determining the patient's degree of distress. A patient sitting in a Fowler position and speaking only in two- or three-word statements, for example, is probably in considerable distress.
- Patients in respiratory distress tend to seek the tripod position. If a patient in respiratory distress is willing to lie flat, this may indicate that his or her condition is quickly deteriorating. Head bobbing is also an ominous sign.
- Other signs of life-threatening respiratory distress include bony retractions, soft-tissue retractions, nasal flaring, tracheal tugging, paradoxical respiratory movement, pulsus paradoxus, pursed-lip breathing, and grunting.
- Note any audible abnormal respiratory noises. Noisy breathing is obstructed breathing.
- Snoring indicates partial obstruction of the upper airway by the tongue. Stridor indicates narrowing of the upper airway, usually as a result of swelling (laryngeal edema).
- Auscultate the lungs whenever possible. Adventitious breath sounds are the extra noises audible during auscultation; they include wheezing and crackles.
- Crackles are any discontinuous noises heard during auscultation of the lungs. They are caused by the popping open of air spaces and are usually associated with increased fluid in the lungs.
- Wheezes are high-pitched whistling sounds made as air is forced through narrowed airways, making them vibrate. Wheezing may be diffuse in conditions such as asthma and heart failure or localized when caused by a foreign body obstructing a bronchus.
- *Silence means danger!* If breath sounds are inaudible with a stethoscope, then the patient is not moving enough air to ventilate the lungs.
- Irritated airways secrete more mucus, which may be expelled as sputum.
- Assess the patient's mucous membranes for cyanosis (a blue or dusky color), pallor, and moisture.
- Patients with dyspnea are usually transported to the nearest facility.
- Patients with chronic respiratory disease are often knowledgeable about their disease and may have tried several treatment options already. Ask them

Prep Kit (continued)

about these efforts and what results, if any, they produced.

- A patient who has respiratory disease may not be able to talk because he or she is having difficulty breathing. The history may have to be obtained from a family member or from only a few clues.
- Noncompliance with the prescribed medication regimen could trigger an asthma attack. Ask the patient what he or she was doing when the asthma attack began. Ask if the patient took his or her medications today. Ask if movement worsens the dyspnea.
- Onset and duration of distress are important considerations in determining the underlying cause of dyspnea. Find out if the symptoms began suddenly or gradually worsened over time.
- Find out if the patient's condition is a recurrence of a past condition. If so, ask the patient to compare the current situation with other episodes.
- Assessing the level of consciousness is extremely important in dyspneic patients.
- Look for jugular venous distention in the neck, with the patient in a semisitting position. Distended neck veins may be caused by cardiac failure.
- Feel the chest for vibrations as the patient breathes. Check for edema of the ankles and lower back. Check for peripheral cyanosis. Check the pulse, and note the patient's skin temperature. Apply any available monitors.
- A pulse oximeter indicates the percentage of the patient's hemoglobin that has oxygen attached (except in cases of carbon monoxide inhalation). An oxygen saturation level greater than 95% is considered normal.
- The peak flow is the maximum flow rate at which the patient can expel air from the lungs. Normal peak flow ranges from about 350 to 700 L/min. A peak flow of less than 150 L/min is insufficient and signals that the patient is in significant respiratory distress.
- Aerosol nebulizers deliver liquid medications to the respiratory tract in the form of a fine mist. Weigh the potential benefits of aerosol therapy against the lower fraction of inspired oxygen delivered during the treatment.
- Metered-dose inhalers deliver bronchodilators or corticosteroids as an aerosol. Dry-powder inhalers deliver a measured dose of medication in the form of a fine powder. Little or no medication may reach the lungs if improper technique is used.
- Emergency medical care for patients with dyspnea may include securing the airway; decreasing the work of breathing; administering supplemental oxygen, bronchodilators, leukotriene modifiers, electrolytes, inhaled or IV corticosteroids, or vasodilators; restoring fluid balance; administering diuretics; supporting or assisting ventilation; intubating the patient; injecting a beta-adrenergic receptor agonist subcutaneously; and/or instilling medication directly through an ET tube.
- In managing the condition of a patient who is in respiratory distress, begin by establishing and maintaining an open airway. Suction if necessary, and keep the airway optimally positioned. Remove constricting clothing. Reduce the patient's effort to breathe.
- Administration methods that require the patient to inhale the medication may become unreliable or ineffective when the patient's airways are severely compromised. Some cases may warrant administering medications subcutaneously.
- Patients in respiratory failure may ultimately need to be intubated. There are major drawbacks and risks to intubating in the field, but it can also be lifesaving. Weigh these factors along with protocols, medical direction, and the patient's wishes.
- Medications can be instilled directly into the tracheobronchial tree when patients are intubated or have a tracheostomy. Intraosseous access may be a better option if traditional vascular access fails.
- Anatomic or foreign body obstructions of the upper airway, including aspiration of stomach contents, can cause seizures or death. Avoid causing gastric distention when administering bag-mask ventilation, and monitor the patient's ability to protect his or her airway. If the patient cannot protect his or her airway, then he or she must be intubated.
- Common obstructive airway diseases include emphysema, chronic bronchitis, and asthma. Emphysema and chronic bronchitis are collectively classified as COPD.
- Asthma is caused by allergens or irritants and is characterized by widespread, reversible narrowing of the airways (bronchospasm), edema of the airways, and increased mucus production. It can cause significant airway obstruction.
- Status asthmaticus is a severe, prolonged asthmatic attack that cannot be stopped with conventional treatment. *It is a dire medical emergency.* Any person with asthma who feels sick enough to dial 9-1-1 is in status asthmaticus until proved otherwise.
- Primary treatment of bronchospasm is bronchodilator medication. Primary treatment of bronchial edema is corticosteroids; administration of these may or may not be started in the field setting.

Prep Kit (continued)

- Emphysema is a chronic weakening and destruction of the walls of the terminal bronchioles and alveoli. A patient with emphysema classically has a barrel chest, muscle wasting, and pursed-lip breathing. Tachypnea is often present.
- Restrictive lung diseases limit the patient's ability to expand the lungs within the chest cavity, put patients at risk of infection, and may severely limit their ability to compensate for any respiratory insult.
- Chronic bronchitis is characterized by excessive mucus production in the bronchial tree, nearly always accompanied by a chronic or recurrent productive cough. A patient with chronic bronchitis tends to be sedentary and obese, sleep in an upright position, use many tissues, have copious secretions, and be cyanotic.
- In assessing patients who have COPD, search for the cause of a worsened condition that prompted the call to 9-1-1. Look for signs of infection, peripheral edema, jugular venous distention with hepatojugular reflux, and crackles. Find out if the onset of dyspnea was sudden or gradual.
- Hypoxic drive is a phenomenon in which high levels of oxygen decrease the patient's respiratory drive. Nevertheless, supplemental oxygen should not be withheld.
- Not every patient should be ventilated the same way. Allow the patient to exhale completely before delivering the next breath. If the patient is not allowed to do so, then pressure in the thorax will rise, eventually causing pneumothorax or cardiac arrest. This phenomenon is called auto-PEEP. If auto-PEEP is a risk, then ventilation should be given at a rate of 4 to 6 breaths/min. The standard ventilation rate for adults without COPD is 8 to 10 breaths/min.
- Pneumonia may be caused by a variety of bacterial, viral, or fungal agents. A patient with pneumonia usually reports weakness, productive cough, fever, and sometimes chest pain that worsens with coughing. Supportive care includes oxygenation, suctioning, and transport to an appropriate facility.
- Atelectasis is alveolar collapse as a result of proximal airway obstruction, pneumothorax, hemothorax, toxic inhalation, or other causes. It increases the likelihood that pneumonia will develop in the affected lung segment.
- Lung cancer is increasing among women and is one of the most common forms of cancer, especially among people who smoke cigarettes and those exposed to occupational lung hazards.
- Pulmonary edema occurs as fluid migrates into the lungs. A patient expectorating foamy pink secretions probably has severe pulmonary edema.
- Acute respiratory distress syndrome (ARDS) is caused by diffuse alveolar damage as a result of aspiration, pulmonary edema, or some other alveolar insult.
- When a patient has a pneumothorax, air collects between the visceral pleura and the parietal pleura. Administer supplemental oxygen, and monitor the patient's respiratory status closely.
- Pleural effusion will cause dyspnea. Supportive care, including proper positioning and aggressive oxygen administration, should be given.
- A pulmonary embolism occurs when a blood clot breaks off in the circulation and travels to the lung, blocking blood flow and nutrient exchange. It is a frequently misdiagnosed conditions in emergency medicine. The early presentation may reveal normal breath sounds with good peripheral aeration, diverting attention away from a pulmonary pathology. The hallmark of a pulmonary embolus is sudden dyspnea, cyanosis that does not resolve with oxygen therapy, and sometimes chest pain.

▶ Vital Vocabulary

adventitious Refers to abnormal breath sounds or noises that occur in addition to the normal breath sounds; examples are crackles and wheezes.

alveoli (singular, *alveolus*) The saclike units at the end of the bronchioles in which gas exchange takes place.

aspiration The drawing in or out by suction. In the lungs, aspiration of food, liquids, blood, or foreign objects can occur when a patient is unable to protect his or her own airway.

atelectasis Collapse of the alveolar air spaces of the lungs.

beta-2 agonist A pharmacologic agent that stimulates the beta-2 receptor sites found in smooth muscle; includes common bronchodilators such as albuterol and levalbuterol.

botulism Poisoning characterized by severe muscle paralysis and usually caused by eating food containing botulinum toxin.

bronchospasm Severe constriction of smooth muscle surrounding the bronchial tree.

cape cyanosis Deep cyanosis of the face and neck that extends across the chest and back; associated with little or no blood flow; a particularly ominous sign.

carina A ridgelike projection of tracheal cartilage located where the trachea bifurcates into the right and left mainstem bronchi.

Prep Kit *(continued)*

carpopedal spasm Contorted positioning of the hand or foot in which the fingers or toes flex in a clawlike manner; may be caused by hyperventilation.

chronic bronchitis A chronic inflammatory condition affecting the bronchi that is characterized by excessive mucus production as a result of overgrowth of the mucous glands in the airways.

cor pulmonale Heart disease that develops because of chronic lung disease and affects primarily the right side of the heart.

crackles The abnormal breath sounds that have a fine, crackling quality; previously called rales.

croup A common disease of infancy and childhood caused by upper airway obstruction and characterized by stridor, hoarseness, and a barking cough.

diuresis The production of large amounts of urine by the kidney.

emphysema The infiltration of any tissue by air or gas; a chronic obstructive pulmonary disease characterized by distention of the alveoli and destructive changes in the lung parenchyma.

Fowler position A sitting position with the head elevated to a 90° angle. (sitting straight upright).

Greenfield filter A mesh filter placed in the inferior vena cava to catch blood clots in patients who are at high risk of pulmonary embolus.

Guillain-Barré syndrome A disease of unknown cause characterized by progressive paralysis moving from the feet to the head (ascending paralysis); if paralysis reaches the diaphragm, the patient may require respiratory support.

hemoglobin An iron-containing protein within red blood cells that has the ability to combine with oxygen.

hemoptysis Coughing up blood in the sputum.

hepatojugular reflux Engorgement of the jugular veins when the liver is gently pressed; this finding is specific to right-sided heart failure.

hyperoxia An excess of oxygen.

hypoventilate To move inadequate volumes of air into the lungs.

hypoxia A dangerous condition in which the supply of oxygen to the tissues is reduced.

hypoxic drive A state in which the stimulus to breathe comes from a decrease in $Pa{O_2}$, rather than from the normal stimulus, an increase in $Pa{CO_2}$.

jugular venous distention The visible bulging of the jugular veins when a patient is in a semi-Fowler or full Fowler position; indicates inadequate blood movement through the heart and/or lungs.

Kussmaul respirations A respiratory pattern characteristic of diabetic ketoacidosis, with marked hyperpnea and tachypnea; represents the body's attempt to compensate for the acidosis.

laryngotracheobronchitis Inflammation of the larynx, trachea, and bronchi.

lung consolidation Firming of the lungs as a result of fluid accumulation.

metastasis The transfer of a disease from one organ or part of the body to another that is not directly connected to the original site; often used to describe a cancer that has spread to another part of the body.

monophonic The sound of one note during wheezing, caused by the vibration of a single bronchus.

orthopnea Severe dyspnea experienced when recumbent that is relieved by sitting or standing up.

palatine tonsils One of three sets of lymphatic organs that constitute the tonsils; located in the back of the throat, on each side of the posterior opening of the oral cavity; help protect the body from bacteria and other pathogens introduced into the mouth and nose.

parenchyma The functional portions of a gland or solid organ.

paroxysmal nocturnal dyspnea Severe shortness of breath occurring suddenly at night after several hours of recumbency, as fluid pools in the lungs.

pleural effusion Excessive accumulation of fluid in the pleural space.

pneumonia Inflammation of the lung caused by an infectious agent.

pneumonitis Lung inflammation from an irritant, such as a chemical, dust, or radiation, or from aspiration, such as aspiration of gastric contents.

polycythemia The production of too many red blood cells over time, making the blood thick; a characteristic of people with chronic lung disease and chronic hypoxia.

polyphonic The sound of multiple notes during wheezing; caused by the vibrations of multiple bronchi.

pseudomembrane A false membrane formed by a dead tissue layer; seen in the posterior pharynx of patients with diphtheria.

pulsus paradoxus Weakening or loss of a palpable pulse during inspiration; characteristic of conditions that cause profound pressure changes in the thorax, such as cardiac tamponade and severe asthma.

purulent Full of pus; having the character of pus.

Prep Kit (continued)

reactive airway disease A term used to describe any condition that causes hyperreactive bronchioles and bronchospasm in response to certain triggers.

restrictive lung diseases Diseases that limit the ability of the lungs to expand appropriately. Skeletal abnormalities such as kyphosis and scoliosis are common examples of conditions that can cause these diseases.

retractions The drawing in of the intercostal muscles and the muscles above the clavicles that can occur in respiratory distress.

smooth muscle The nonstriated involuntary muscle found in vessel walls, glands, and the gastrointestinal tract.

snoring A noise made during inhalation when the upper airway is partially obstructed by the tongue.

spacer A device that collects medication as it is released from the canister of a metered-dose inhaler, allowing more medication to be delivered to the lungs and less to be lost to the environment.

status asthmaticus A severe, prolonged asthma attack that cannot be stopped with conventional treatment, such as the administration of epinephrine.

stridor A harsh, high-pitched inspiratory sound representing air moving past an obstruction within or immediately above the glottic opening; associated with severe upper airway obstruction, such as that caused by laryngeal edema.

tactile fremitus Vibrations in the chest that can be felt with a hand on the chest as the patient breathes.

tracheostomy The opening created during a tracheotomy procedure.

tuberculosis A chronic bacterial disease caused by *Mycobacterium tuberculosis* that usually affects the lungs but can also affect other organs, such as the brain and kidneys.

ventilation The process of exchanging air between the lungs and the environment; includes inhalation and exhalation.

References

1. National Center for Chronic Disease Prevention and Health Promotion. Chronic diseases overview. Centers for Disease Control and Prevention, U.S. Department of Health and Human Services, website. https://www.cdc.gov/chronicdisease/overview/. Updated February 23, 2016. Accessed January 8, 2017.
2. Office on Smoking and Health, National Center for Chronic Disease Prevention and Health Promotion. Smoking and COPD. Centers for Disease Control and Prevention, U.S. Department of Health and Human Services, website. https://www.cdc.gov/tobacco/campaign/tips/diseases/copd.html. Updated December 28, 2016. Accessed January 8, 2017.
3. Office of Surveillance, Epidemiology and Laboratory Services (OSELS). Asthma in the US. Centers for Disease Control and Prevention, U.S. Department of Health and Human Services, website. https://www.cdc.gov/vitalsigns/asthma/. Updated May 3, 2011. Accessed January 8, 2017.
4. Asthma facts and figures. Asthma and Allergy Foundation of America website. http://www.aafa.org/page/asthma-facts.aspx. Reviewed August 2015. Accessed January 8, 2017.
5. National Center for Immunization and Respiratory Diseases, Division of Bacterial Diseases. Pneumonia can be prevented—vaccines can help. Centers for Disease Control and Prevention, U.S. Department of Health and Human Services, website. https://www.cdc.gov/Features/Pneumonia/. Updated November 2, 2016. Accessed January 8, 2017.
6. Pneumonia. Johns Hopkins Medicine website. http://www.hopkinsmedicine.org/healthlibrary/conditions/respiratory_disorders/pneumonia_85,P01321/. Accessed January 8, 2017.
7. Alpha-1 Foundation website. https://www.alpha1.org/Newly-Diagnosed/Learning-about-Alpha-1/Lung-Disease. Accessed January 8, 2017.
8. Severinghaus JW, Kelleher JF. Recent developments in pulse oximetry. *Anesthesiology*. 1992;76(6):1018-1038.
9. Berg RA, Hemphill R, Abella BS, et al. Part 5: adult basic life support: 2010 American Heart Association Guidelines for Cardiopulmonary Resuscitation and Emergency Cardiovascular Care. *Circulation*. 2010;122(suppl 3):S685-S705.
10. Hale KE, Gavin C, O'Driscoll BR. Audit of oxygen use in emergency ambulances and in a hospital emergency department. *Emerg Med J*. 2008;25:773-776.
11. O'Driscoll BR, Howard LS, Bucknall C, Welham SA, Davison AG. British Thoracic Society emergency oxygen audits. *Thorax*. 2011;66:734-735.
12. Kane B, Decalmer S, O'Driscoll BR. Emergency oxygen therapy: from guideline to implementation. *Breathe*. 2013;9:246-253. European Respiratory Society website. http://breathe.ersjournals.com/content/9/4/246. Accessed January 8, 2017.
13. Web-based Integrated Guidelines for Cardiopulmonary Resuscitation and Emergency Cardiovascular Care. Part 7: Adult Advanced Cardiovascular Life Support. American Heart Association website. https://eccguidelines.heart.org/index.php/circulation/cpr-ecc-guidelines-2/part-7-adult-advanced-cardiovascular-life-support/. Accessed February 9, 2017.

Prep Kit *(continued)*

14. National Center for Environmental Health. Most recent asthma data. Centers for Disease Control and Prevention, U.S. Department of Health and Human Services, website. http://www.cdc.gov/asthma/most_recent_data.htm. Updated April 14, 2016. Accessed August 18, 2016.
15. Global strategy for asthma management and prevention. Global Initiative for Asthma website. http://ginasthma.org/2016-gina-report-global-strategy-for-asthma-management-and-prevention/. Updated 2010. Accessed January 8, 2017.
16. Lopez AD, Shibuya K, Rao C, et al. Chronic obstructive pulmonary disease: current burden and future projections. *Eur Respir J*. 2006;27:397-412.
17. Asthma statistics. American Academy of Asthma, Allergy, and Immunology website. http://www.aaaai.org/about-aaaai/newsroom/asthma-statistics. Accessed January 8, 2017.
18. Taylor RB. *White Coat Tales: Medicine's Heroes, Heritage, and Misadventures*. New York, NY: Springer; 2010.
19. Jackson C. *The Life of Chevalier Jackson: An Autobiography*. New York, NY: The Macmillan Company; 1938.
20. Top 20 pneumonia—2015. American Thoracic Society website. https://www.thoracic.org/patients/patient-resources/resources/top-pneumonia-facts.pdf. Accessed December 23, 2016.
21. Lung cancer fact sheet. American Lung Association website. http://www.lung.org/lung-health-and-diseases/lung-disease-lookup/lung-cancer/learn-about-lung-cancer/lung-cancer-fact-sheet.html?referrer=https://www.google.com/. Accessed January 8, 2016.

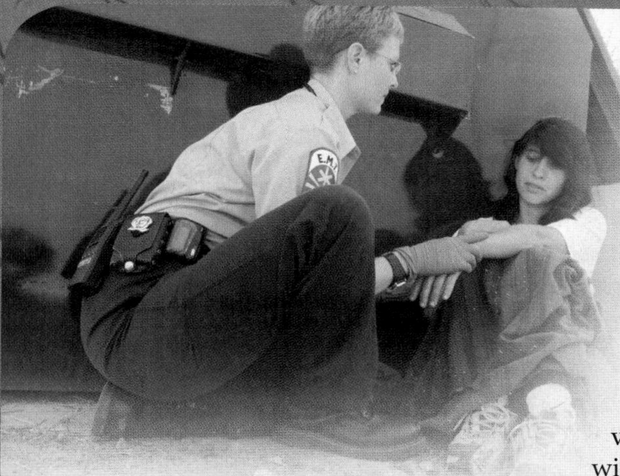

Assessment *in Action*

You are dispatched to a medical clinic for an 18-year-old woman reporting difficulty breathing. According to the nurse on scene, the patient has a history of status asthmaticus but has not had the condition during the past couple of years. You listen to the lungs and hear wheezes in all fields. The patient's vital signs are stable, so you decide to administer a nebulizer with albuterol and ipratropium (Atrovent). The patient says she was mowing her lawn when the breathing difficulty began.

1. Why is asthma considered a reactive airway disease?

- **A.** The patient reacts poorly to asthma.
- **B.** The asthma attack occurs most often when the patient is exposed to a trigger.
- **C.** Asthma interacts with other diseases the patient has.
- **D.** Patients experience asthma only in response to environmental triggers.

2. Which of the following best defines status asthmaticus?

- **A.** A short asthma attack that ends spontaneously
- **B.** A long asthma attack the ends spontaneously
- **C.** A pseudoasthma attack
- **D.** A severe, prolonged asthma attack

Assessment in Action (continued)

3. The breathing treatment you administer is primarily to help:
   - **A.** reduce mucus production.
   - **B.** eliminate the response to a trigger.
   - **C.** reduce bronchospasm.
   - **D.** reduce anxiety.
4. The wheezing you hear during an asthma attack is primarily caused by what?
   - **A.** Air trapped in the lungs
   - **B.** Air forced through constricted tubes, which causes them to vibrate
   - **C.** Air moving normally in lungs
   - **D.** Air moving through mucus in the lungs
5. Because the patient is a woman, you know which of the following is true?
   - **A.** Her asthma attacks are normally self-limiting.
   - **B.** She is more likely than a man to have asthma.
   - **C.** She is at less risk than a man of having a severe attack.
   - **D.** She has a greater risk than a man of having a severe attack.
6. Which other medications may help the patient during the next few hours?
   - **A.** Antibiotics
   - **B.** Corticosteroids
   - **C.** Epinephrine
   - **D.** Oxygen
7. Which of the following changes in the patient's breath sounds would cause you the most concern?
   - **A.** Change from polyphonic to monophonic wheezing
   - **B.** Change from wheezing to clear, vesicular breath sounds
   - **C.** Change from wheezing to a silent chest (no breath sounds)
   - **D.** Change from wheezing to scattered crackles
8. What are some indications the number of people reported to have asthma in the United States is increasing or decreasing?
9. Is administering 100% oxygen to a patient who has had COPD for a long time likely to cause respiratory arrest? Explain why or why not.
10. What conditions would be included in the differential diagnosis for this patient, and how would you rule them in or out?

CHAPTER 17

Cardiovascular Emergencies

National EMS Education Standard Competencies

Medicine

Integrates assessment findings with principles of epidemiology and pathophysiology to formulate a field impression and implement a comprehensive treatment/disposition plan for a patient with a medical complaint.

Cardiovascular

Anatomy, signs, symptoms, and management of

- Chest pain (pp 964-966, 1040-1049)
- Cardiac arrest (pp 1007-1018)

Anatomy, physiology, epidemiology, pathophysiology, psychosocial impact, presentations, prognosis, and management of

- Acute coronary syndrome (pp 1039-1049)
  - Angina pectoris (pp 1040-1049)
  - Myocardial infarction (pp 1041-1049)
- Heart failure (pp 1049-1055)
- Nontraumatic cardiac tamponade (pp 1055-1056)
- Hypertensive emergencies (pp 1057-1060)
- Cardiogenic shock (pp 1056-1057)
- Vascular disorders (pp 1062-1065)
  - Abdominal aortic aneurysm (pp 1062-1064)
  - Arterial occlusion (pp 1064-1065)
  - Venous thrombosis (p 1065)
- Aortic aneurysm/dissection (pp 1062-1064)
- Thromboembolism (pp 1064-1065)
- Cardiac rhythm disturbances (pp 974, 987-1014, 1019-1022)
- Infectious diseases of the heart (pp 1060-1062)
  - Endocarditis (p 1060)
  - Pericarditis (pp 1060-1061)
- Congenital abnormalities (see Chapter 42, *Neonatal Care*)

Shock and Resuscitation

Integrates comprehensive knowledge of causes and pathophysiology into the management of cardiac arrest and peri-arrest states.

Integrates a comprehensive knowledge of the causes and pathophysiology into the management of shock, respiratory failure or arrest with an emphasis on early intervention to prevent arrest.

Knowledge Objectives

1. Review the main structures and functions of the cardiovascular system's anatomy and physiology. (pp 961-963)
2. Summarize the general assessment of a patient with a cardiovascular emergency. (pp 964-968)
3. Explain the phases that comprise the cardiac action potential. (pp 969-970)
4. Identify the structure and course of all divisions and subdivisions of the cardiac conduction system. (pp 971-972)
5. Explain the significance of accessory conduction pathways. (p 972)
6. Recall how the autonomic nervous system influences blood pressure. (pp 972-973)
7. Describe the limitations of 3-lead electrocardiogram (ECG) monitoring. (p 975)
8. Indicate the placement of 12-lead ECG electrodes. (pp 975-981, 1025)
9. Define contiguous leads and precordial leads; include examples of each. (pp 979-981)
10. Indicate the placement of right-sided precordial leads and posterior lead electrodes. (pp 979-981)
11. Indicate the placement of 15- and 18-lead ECG electrodes. (p 981)
12. Identify the components of an ECG rhythm strip. (pp 982-985)
13. Outline a systematic approach to the analysis and interpretation of cardiac dysrhythmias. (pp 985-987)
14. Explain normal sinus rhythm and the ECG characteristics, possible causes, signs and symptoms, and initial emergency care of dysrhythmias originating in the sinoatrial node. (pp 987-993)
15. Explain the emergency medical care for the symptomatic adult patient with bradycardia. (pp 988-991)
16. Explain the ECG characteristics, possible causes, signs and symptoms, and initial emergency medical care for dysrhythmias originating in the atria. (pp 993-1001)

17. Explain the emergency medical care for the symptomatic adult patient with tachycardia. (pp 995-999)
18. Explain the ECG characteristics, possible causes, signs and symptoms, and initial emergency care for dysrhythmias originating in the atrioventricular (AV) junction. (pp 1001-1003)
19. Explain the ECG characteristics, possible causes, signs and symptoms, and initial emergency care for dysrhythmias originating in the ventricles. (pp 1003-1014)
20. Evaluate the dysrhythmias seen in cardiac arrest. (pp 1006-1007, 1014)
21. Compare the indications and procedure for manual defibrillation with the indications and procedure for operating an automated external defibrillator (AED). (pp 1007-1008, 1010-1013)
22. Explain the emergency medical care of the adult patient with cardiac arrest (pp 1007-1018)
23. Describe the components of post–cardiac arrest care. (pp 1017-1018)
24. Explain the ECG characteristics, possible causes, signs and symptoms, and initial emergency care for AV blocks. (pp 1019-1022)
25. Describe the ECG characteristics of artificial pacemaker rhythms. (pp 1022-1023)
26. Give examples of indications for using a 12-lead ECG. (p 1023)
27. Explain a systematic approach to the interpretation of the 12-lead ECG. (pp 1025-1039)
28. Recognize the characteristic ECG changes associated with myocardial ischemia, injury, and infarction. (pp 1029-1034)
29. Explain the etiology, history, physical findings, and management of acute coronary syndromes. (pp 1039-1049)
30. Describe risk factors related to cardiovascular disease. (pp 1039-1041)
31. Explain angina pectoris, including its causes and types. (pp 1040-1049)
32. Explain patient assessment procedures for cardiovascular issues. (pp 1042-1043)
33. Summarize preparation for reperfusion therapy in patients with ST segment elevation myocardial infarction. (pp 1044-1049)
34. Discuss the pathophysiology of heart failure and its signs, symptoms, and treatment. (pp 1049-1055)
35. Discuss the pathophysiology of cardiac tamponade and its signs, symptoms, and treatment. (pp 1055-1056)
36. Discuss the pathophysiology of cardiogenic shock and its signs, symptoms, and treatment. (pp 1056-1057)
37. Discuss the pathophysiology of a hypertensive emergency and its signs, symptoms, and treatment. (pp 1057-1060)
38. Explain the etiology, history, physical findings, and management of endocarditis, pericarditis, and myocarditis, and other infectious diseases of the heart. (pp 1060-1062)
39. Explain the etiology, history, physical findings, and management of aortic aneurysm, acute arterial occlusion, and acute deep vein thrombosis, and other vascular disorders. (pp 1062-1065)

Skills Objectives

1. Demonstrate how to perform cardiac monitoring. (pp 976-977, Skill Drill 17-1)
2. Demonstrate how to provide emergency medical care for the symptomatic adult patient with bradycardia. (pp 988-991)
3. Demonstrate how to perform transcutaneous pacing (TCP). (pp 990-991, Skill Drill 17-2)
4. Demonstrate how to provide emergency medical care for the symptomatic adult patient with tachycardia. (pp 995-999)
5. Demonstrate how to perform synchronized cardioversion. (pp 997-999, Skill Drill 17-3)
6. Demonstrate how to perform manual defibrillation. (pp 1007-1008, 1010-1012, Skill Drill 17-4)
7. Demonstrate how to manage an adult cardiac arrest. (pp 1008-1009, 1014-1017)
8. Demonstrate how to perform defibrillation with an AED. (pp 1012-1013, Skill Drill 17-5)
9. Demonstrate how to perform immediate post–cardiac arrest care. (pp 1017-1018)
10. Demonstrate how to acquire a 12-lead ECG. (pp 1024-1025, Skill Drill 17-6)
11. Demonstrate how to assess and provide emergency medical care for a patient with an acute coronary syndrome. (pp 1044-1046)

Introduction

The job of the paramedic first came into being more than 40 years ago with the purpose of providing early, definitive treatment of patients with acute myocardial infarction. An **acute myocardial infarction (AMI)**—a heart attack—occurs when sudden narrowing or complete occlusion of a coronary artery causes myocardial tissue necrosis. The American Heart Association estimates that one person has an AMI in the United States about every 40 seconds.[1] **Cardiac arrest** is the cessation of cardiac mechanical activity, as confirmed by the absence of signs of circulation. In the United States, emergency medical services (EMS) personnel treat about 60% of out-of-hospital cardiac arrests (OHCAs) each year.[1] It's easy to see why paramedic education continues to put a strong emphasis on recognizing and managing cardiovascular emergencies.

This chapter will prepare you to integrate pathophysiologic principles and assessment findings to formulate a field impression and implement a treatment plan for patients with cardiovascular disease (CVD). After a brief review of the anatomy and function of the cardiovascular system, you'll learn about the electrophysiology of the heart. We'll give considerable emphasis to the interpretation of cardiac **dysrhythmias** (heart rhythm disturbances) and their management within the context of the patient's overall clinical condition. You'll learn about pharmacologic and other treatment modalities surrounding advanced cardiac life support (ACLS). Finally, you'll learn about the pathophysiology, history and physical findings, and how to manage cardiovascular disorders. As part of your study of this chapter, review Chapter 7, *Medical Terminology*, for terminology, acronyms, and abbreviations related to cardiovascular emergencies.

Anatomy and Physiology Review

In Chapter 8, *Anatomy and Physiology*, we discussed the anatomy and physiology of the cardiovascular system. Let's review some key points:

- The cardiovascular system is composed of the heart and blood vessels. Its primary function is to deliver oxygenated blood and nutrients to every cell in the body. The cardiovascular system is also responsible for delivering chemical messengers (hormones) within the body and for transporting the waste products of metabolism from the cells to sites of recycling or disposal.
- The heart has four chambers **Figure 17-1**. The two upper chambers are the right and left atria. The atria have thin walls. The right atrium receives blood low in oxygen from the superior vena cava, inferior vena cava, and the coronary sinus. The coronary sinus is a large vein on the posterior side of the heart that collects blood from the great cardiac vein and several smaller coronary veins and then drains the blood into the right atrium. The left atrium receives freshly oxygenated blood from the lungs by way of the right and left pulmonary veins. Then the atria contract, pumping blood through the atrioventricular (AV) valve into the ventricles.
- The heart's two lower chambers are the right and left ventricles. The walls of the ventricles are much thicker than the atria walls. The right ventricle pumps deoxygenated blood to the lungs. The left ventricle pumps oxygenated blood throughout the body. When the left ventricle contracts, it normally produces an impulse palpable at the apex of the heart (apical impulse). This occurs because as the left ventricle contracts, it rotates forward. In a normal heart, this rotation causes the apex of the left ventricle to strike the chest wall. The apical impulse is also called the **point of maximal impulse (PMI)** because it is the site at which the heartbeat is most strongly felt. The PMI is normally located on the left anterior part of chest, at the fifth intercostal space (ICS) along the midclavicular line.
- An internal wall of connective tissue called a **septum** (plural *septa*) separates the right and left sides of the heart. It's made up of two parts: The

YOU are the Paramedic — PART 1

You and your crew are called to a private residence for a man reporting chest pain. When you arrive, you find a 32-year-old man who reports he's had crushing chest pain for the past 1 to 2 hours. He informs you the pain came on at rest, has steadily become more intense, and is now accompanied by shortness of breath. He rates his current discomfort as 9/10. The patient denies any prior cardiac history.

1. What is your initial impression of this patient's condition?
2. What are some possible causes of the patient's symptoms?
3. Although it's certainly possible, this patient is fairly young to be having an acute myocardial infarction (AMI). What factors might be associated with a cardiac event in a patient of this age?
4. What additional assessment data will be important in evaluating this patient?

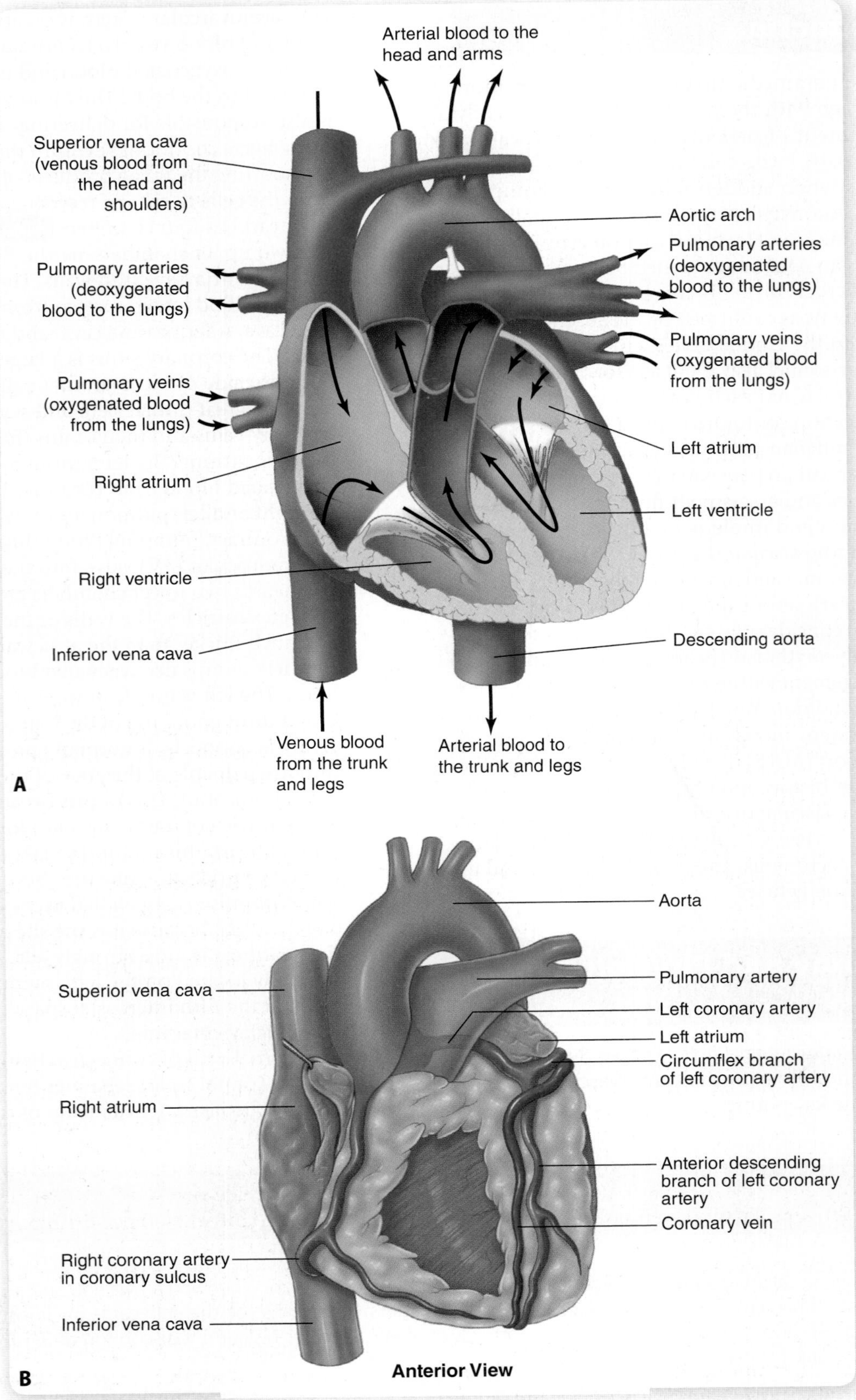

Figure 17-1 A. Blood flow through the heart. **B.** Coronary arteries (anterior view). **C.** Coronary arteries (posterior view).

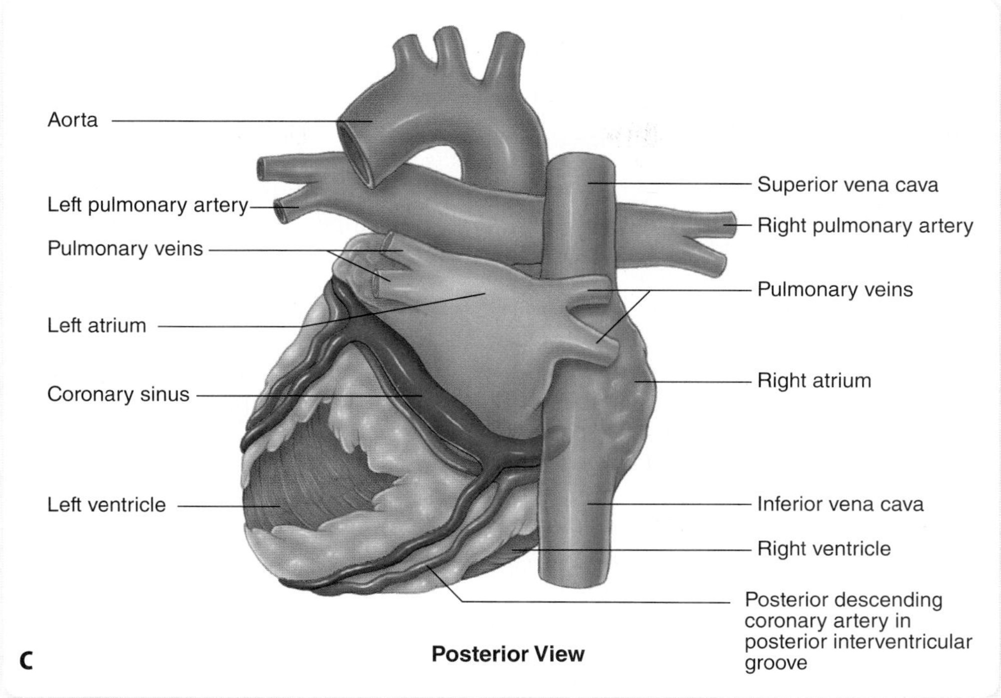

Figure 17-1 *Continued*

interatrial septum separates the right and left atria. The interventricular septum separates the right and left ventricles.

- The septa separate the heart into two functional pumps. The right atrium and right ventricle comprise one pump. The left atrium and left ventricle comprise the other. The right side of the heart (sometimes called the "right heart") is a low-pressure system (pulmonary circulation). The left side of the heart (sometimes called the "left heart") is a high-pressure pump (systemic circulation).
- The myocardium is the middle layer of the heart wall. It is comprised mostly of thick cardiac muscle tissue and is responsible for cardiac contraction and efficient ejection of blood from the heart.
- The **coronary arteries** supply blood to the tissues of the heart. There are two main coronary arteries—left and right. The left main coronary artery (LMCA) is the largest in diameter and shortest of the myocardial blood vessels. It rapidly divides into the **left anterior descending artery (LAD)** and the **circumflex artery (Cx)**. Although the areas supplied by the coronary arteries can differ among patients, the LAD supplies blood to the anterior surface of the left ventricle, part of the lateral surface of the left ventricle, and a portion of the interventricular septum in most patients. The Cx artery supplies the left atrium, part of the lateral surface of the left ventricle, the inferior surface of the left ventricle in about 15% of people, the posterior surface of the left ventricle in 15% of people, the **sinoatrial (SA) node** in about 40% of people, and the AV bundle in 10% to 15% of people. Branches of the **right coronary artery (RCA)** supply blood to the walls of the right atrium and ventricle, a portion of the inferior part of the left ventricle, and portions of the conduction system (the SA node in about 60% of people and the AV bundle in about 85% to 90% of people).
- Cardiac cells have four important properties that help the heart function efficiently: automaticity, excitability, conductivity, and contractility.
- The cardiac conduction system comprises six parts: the SA node, the AV node, the bundle of His, the right and left bundle branches, and the Purkinje fibers.
- Stimulation of sympathetic (accelerator) nerves strengthens the force of contraction and increases the heart rate. Stimulation of parasympathetic (inhibitory) nerve fibers slows the rate of discharge of the SA node, slows conduction through the AV node, weakens the strength of atrial contraction, and can cause a small reduction in the force of ventricular contraction.

Patient Assessment

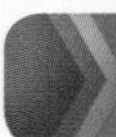

Scene Size-up

A cardiac-related complaint is a common reason a person seeks medical care. A patient with cardiovascular-related symptoms may be a young, middle-aged, or older adult. He or she may be unresponsive, awake and alert, or have an altered mental status. The patient may be stable or unstable and may or may not have a pulse. Regardless of the situation, a systematic approach to patient assessment is important. This approach, including cardiac physical assessment, is discussed in Chapter 11, *Patient Assessment*. When used consistently, this type of approach will help ensure you do not overlook physical findings or important questions pertinent to the treatment plan for your patient. In this section, we will focus on those areas of the assessment that require special attention for the patient who has a cardiovascular complaint or who is experiencing a cardiovascular emergency.

Primary Survey

The order of the steps for performing a primary survey differs depending on the type of cardiac patient. Whereas the order of steps in the primary survey is normally ABCDE (assess airway, breathing, and then circulation, disability, and exposure), if the patient is found unresponsive and is suspected of being in cardiac arrest, the order changes to CABDE (first assess circulation, then airway, breathing, disability, and exposure). In this section, we will assume the patient is conscious and breathing and has a pulse.

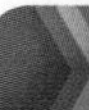

History Taking

Acute coronary syndromes (ACSs) are a series of cardiac conditions that are caused by an abrupt reduction in blood flow through a coronary artery. There are three major ACSs: **unstable angina**, non–ST segment elevation myocardial infarction (NSTEMI), and ST segment elevation myocardial infarction (STEMI). Common chief complaints in the patient experiencing an ACS include chest discomfort, dyspnea, fainting, palpitations, and fatigue.

Chest pain or discomfort is often the presenting symptom in a patient with an ACS. The patient's description of the discomfort is important for assessing its significance. You can use the OPQRST mnemonic (Onset, Provocation/palliation, Quality, Region/radiation, Severity, Timing) to elaborate on the patient's chief complaint.

Some patients may have more than one chief complaint. For example, a patient may report chest pain and difficulty breathing or palpitations and chest pain. If any of these symptoms occur, then ask the patient which symptom started first and which bothers him or her the most. For example, with further questioning of the patient reporting palpitations and chest pain, you may learn that the patient felt his or her heart racing for a few minutes and then began having chest pain.

- **O** What is the *Onset* or origin of the discomfort—that is, how did it begin (suddenly or gradually)? Has anything like this ever happened before? Did a health care provider examine and treat the patient for the symptoms reported? If so, what was the diagnosis? How does the discomfort the patient is feeling right now compare with that?
- **P** What *Provoked* the discomfort—that is, what, if anything, brought it on? Is it exertional or nonexertional? What was the patient doing at the time? Sitting in a chair? Changing a tire? Shoveling snow? Having an argument? **Angina pectoris** is chest discomfort that occurs when the heart muscle does not receive enough oxygen (myocardial **ischemia**). Examples of activities that increase the heart's demand for oxygen include undergoing emotional upset, cigarette smoking, eating a heavy meal, walking up an incline or against a wind, working with the arms over the head, or being exposed to cold weather. An AMI may occur when a patient is at rest, after a serious illness or unusually vigorous exercise, in conjunction with severe emotional stress, or without warning. The circumstances that provoke the patient's symptoms can provide a clue to the cause of the pain or discomfort. For example, pain that worsens with exertion and resolves with rest may be related to myocardial ischemia. Pain that worsens after a meal may have a gastrointestinal cause. Pain that worsens when the patient takes a deep breath may be attributable to a respiratory or musculoskeletal cause. Does anything make it worse? What palliates the pain—that is, does anything make it better? Patients with **coronary artery disease (CAD)** may take nitroglycerin (NTG) for episodes of chest pain. Ask whether the patient took NTG and, if so, how much and did it help?
- **Q** What is the *Quality* of the discomfort—that is, what does it feel like? Get the patient's narrative description. Dull? Sharp? Crushing? Heavy? Squeezing? Note the exact words the patient uses to describe the discomfort, and observe the patient's body language as he or she does so. Try not to lead the patient's responses unless he or she is unable to describe the pain. In these cases, offer alternatives, such as "Is it sharp, dull, or crampy?" Use the word discomfort instead of pain in these questions. Although many patients having a cardiac-related event will tell you they have chest pain, some will not feel true pain. Some patients having a cardiac-related events present with signs and symptoms other than chest pain or discomfort,

such as generalized weakness, sweating, lightheadedness, shortness of breath, back pain, or nausea and vomiting.

R Does the discomfort *Radiate*? From where to where? To the jaw? Down the left arm? Into the back? Chest discomfort associated with myocardial ischemia usually begins in the central or left chest and then radiates to the arm (especially the little finger [ulnar] side of the left arm), wrist, jaw, epigastrium, left shoulder, or between the shoulder blades. A similar pattern may also occur in **pericarditis** (inflammation of the pericardial sac). Severe ischemia may result in radiation to the right chest, right arm, and/or back. The symptoms of a patient having a cardiac-related event, who has epigastric pain, nausea, and vomiting, may be confused with the symptoms of a patient who has a gastrointestinal disorder, such as a peptic ulcer. Aortic **dissection** or enlargement of an **aortic aneurysm** may produce pain that begins in the center of the chest and radiates to the back.

S What is the *Severity* of the discomfort—that is, how bad is it? Assess the patient's discomfort using a 0 to 10 pain rating scale, with 10 being the worst. Although physical signs of pain may be obvious in many patients, some may feel severe pain and not show visible signs of discomfort. Remember, the patient is the authority regarding his or her pain. Using a pain rating scale allows you to evaluate the effectiveness of the emergency care you provide. Document the patient's initial rating of his pain or discomfort. Reassess (and document) the degree of discomfort after each treatment you perform and before transferring care at the receiving facility. If the patient has chronic angina, then ask him or her to compare the pain with the usual angina pain.

T What was the *Timing* of the event—that is, when did it start? How long did it last? What time did it get worse or better? Was it continuous or intermittent? Establishing when the patient's symptoms began is important—particularly if the patient is a candidate for **reperfusion therapy** (ie, medications or procedures used to open a blocked coronary artery. Anginal symptoms usually last less than 20 minutes. Chest discomfort associated with AMI often lasts 20 minutes to several hours. Chest discomfort that lasts for hours may also be seen in patients with pericarditis and aortic dissection.

Another chief complaint among patients with an ACS is dyspnea (difficult or labored breathing). Dyspnea may vary in intensity from simply being aware of one's breathing to severe respiratory distress. Because dyspnea is not a sign but a symptom, assessing its severity is difficult. Ask the patient to rate the severity of his or her breathing difficulty on a scale of 0 to 10.

Dyspnea that develops suddenly suggests **pulmonary embolism**, pneumothorax, acute **pulmonary edema**, pneumonia, or airway obstruction. Dyspnea that occurs on exertion or at rest suggests the presence of chronic obstructive pulmonary disease (COPD) or left ventricular failure. **Left ventricular failure (LVF)** causes fluid to build up in the lungs. In patients who have chronic LVF, dyspnea often develops slowly over weeks or months. Patients who have chronic heart failure may have dyspnea when resting in a horizontal position. This occurs because blood pools in the lungs when the patient lies down. Dyspnea that is relieved by a change in position (either sitting upright or standing) is called **orthopnea**. To avoid dyspnea, patients with orthopnea often sleep on two or more pillows to achieve an upright or semiupright position.

Paroxysmal nocturnal dyspnea (PND) is a sudden onset of difficulty breathing in which the patient suddenly awakens from sleep. PND is often associated with LVF. PND usually begins 2 to 4 hours after the onset of sleep. It is often accompanied by coughing, wheezing, and sweating. The patient may awaken with a feeling of suffocation. The patient's condition usually improves after sitting up or standing for 15 to 30 minutes.

If your patient has a cough, then find out whether it is dry or productive. A dry cough is a nonproductive cough. A productive (or wet) cough clears the airway of mucus (sputum) and foreign material. The characteristics of the sputum produced may be helpful in determining the cause of the cough. For example, pulmonary edema is often accompanied by frothy, pink-tinged sputum. Fainting (**syncope**) is a brief loss of consciousness caused by a temporary decrease in blood flow to the brain. In near syncope (also called presyncope) signs and symptoms of impending syncope occur, including dizziness with or without a blackout (called a gray-out), anxiety, pale skin, sweating, thready pulse, and low blood pressure. Fainting may occur while sitting, standing, walking, and occasionally during exercise. As part of history taking for a patient who has fainted, try to determine whether the patient fainted from cardiac or noncardiac causes. Cardiac causes of syncope include dysrhythmias, increased vagal tone, and heart lesions. Consider a cardiac cause if fainting occurs in a recumbent position, is provoked by exercise, is associated with chest pain, or if a family history of fainting or sudden death is present. Noncardiac causes of syncope are discussed in Chapter 18, *Neurologic Emergencies*.

Patients with cardiac problems may present with a chief complaint of palpitations. Palpitations refer to the sensation of an abnormally fast or irregular heartbeat. Except after extreme exertion, a person normally remains blissfully unaware of his or her heartbeat. Palpitations can be caused by anxiety, lack of sleep, certain medicines, caffeine, stress, cocaine or amphetamine use, heavy cigarette smoking, or metabolic conditions, such as hyperthyroidism. Changes in the heart's rhythm or rate, including fast rhythms (tachycardias) and early beats, may also cause palpitations. A patient may not use the word palpitations but may report feeling his or her heart "skipping beats," "flip-flopping," "fluttering," "racing," or use similar words. In such a case, ask about the onset, frequency, and duration of this symptom and previous episodes of palpitations. Ask about the presence of associated symptoms such as chest discomfort, dizziness, syncope, and dyspnea.

Fatigue is a common complaint in patients with impaired cardiovascular functions. It is also one of the vaguest of all symptoms. Many conditions can cause fatigue. Electrolyte disorders such as an unusually high or low potassium levels, are a common cause of generalized weakness and fatigue. Fatigue may precede or accompany other symptoms associated with ACS. Medications such as beta-blockers, diuretics, or antihypertensives may also cause fatigue. Try to determine when the patient's fatigue began and how long it has been present. Ask about associated symptoms such as chest discomfort, nausea, dyspnea, syncope, or palpitations.

Patients may report a variety of other related symptoms as you explore their history of present illnesses. They may have feelings of impending doom or sense that they will soon experience life-changing events. Some patients report feeling nauseous or vomiting. Listen carefully to patients for indications that trauma may be involved or that their activity levels have been limited due to their conditions. Observe their faces as you listen to them tell their stories. Do you see a look of fear or anguish? Are they holding their chests? Most of the other associated complaints your patients may have are related to hypoxia or poor perfusion resulting from inadequate cardiac output (CO)—for example, decreased level of consciousness, diaphoresis, restlessness and anxiety, headache, behavioral changes, and syncope.

After you explore the patient's chief complaint, inquire briefly about pertinent aspects of the patient's other medical history. History taking is a great opportunity to ask about medications prescribed and whether the patient is taking them as instructed. Ask when the patient last took his or her medications. Ask whether the patient is taking medications prescribed for someone else (borrowed)? Common cardiac medications include the following:

- Antiarrhythmics such as digoxin (Lanoxin), procainamide (Procan, Pronestyl), amiodarone (Cordarone), and verapamil (Calan, Isoptin, Verelan)
- Anticoagulants such as enoxaparin (Lovenox), clopidogrel (Plavix), and warfarin (Coumadin)
- Angiotensin-converting enzyme inhibitors such as captopril (Capoten), enalapril (Vasotec), and lisinopril (Prinivil, Zestril)
- Beta-blockers such as atenolol (Tenormin), metoprolol (Lopressor), and propranolol (Inderal)
- Lipid-lowering agents such as gemfibrozil (Lopid), atorvastatin (Lipitor), fluvastatin (Lescol), lovastatin (Mevacor), pravastatin (Pravachol), rosuvastatin calcium (Crestor), and simvastatin (Zocor)
- Diuretics such as furosemide (Lasix)
- Vasodilators such as nitroglycerin (Nitrostat) or isosorbide (Isordil)

Also ask about any over-the-counter medications or herbal supplements the patient takes. Herbal supplements can cause serious, and even fatal, interactions when taken with certain cardiac medications. It may be appropriate to ask about recreational drug use. Ask the patient whether he or she has taken a phosphodiesterase inhibitor such as sildenafil (Viagra) in the past 24 hours or tadalafil (Cialis), or vardenafil (Levitra) in the past 48 hours. Although you may be uncomfortable asking the question, the patient's response is important and may affect the care you provide. For example, these medications, when taken in combination with vasodilators such as NTG or isosorbide, may cause a sudden and significant drop in blood pressure. Common medications prescribed to patients with cardiovascular conditions are discussed in Chapter 13, *Principles of Pharmacology*.

Ask specifically whether the patient has ever been diagnosed with any of the following:

- Coronary artery disease
- Atherosclerotic heart disease: angina, previous MI, **hypertension** (high blood pressure), heart failure
- Valvular disease
- Aneurysm
- Pulmonary disease
- Diabetes
- Renal disease
- Vascular disease
- Inflammatory cardiac disease
- Previous cardiac surgery (coronary artery bypass graft or valve replacement)
- Congenital anomalies

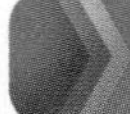

Secondary Assessment

The physical exam during secondary assessment is similar for many medical patients. Nevertheless, certain aspects warrant greater emphasis in the patient whose chief complaint suggests a cardiac problem.

Low CO results in inadequate tissue perfusion. This often results in pale, mottled, or cyanotic skin. The skin of a patient having a heart attack may be cool and sweaty. The skin of a patient in cardiogenic shock may be cold and sweaty. This finding is a sympathetic response in which the blood within peripheral vessels is shunted to the vital organs to maintain adequate perfusion. Flushed, warm skin may be a sign of infection such as pericarditis. Note, the body's response to pain may include restlessness, flushed skin, increased heart rate, increased respiratory rate, and/or elevated blood pressure.

Inspect the neck and tracheal position. Is the trachea midline and mobile to gentle manipulation? Press down with your finger in the patient's suprasternal notch to verify that the trachea is midline. Inspect the neck veins for jugular venous distention (JVD). The external jugular veins reflect the pressure within the patient's systemic circulation. Normally, they are collapsed when a person is sitting or standing and are mildly distended when the patient is supine. Venous pressure rises with a significant increase in blood volume when the right ventricle fails or when increased pressure in the pericardial sac hinders the return of blood to the right atrium. Venous pressure falls when blood volume is decreased significantly or ejection of blood occurs from the left ventricle. To estimate the patient's jugular venous pressure, place the patient in a semi-Fowler position (45° angle) with the head slightly rotated away from the jugular vein you are examining; observe the height of the distended fluid column within the vein, and note how far up the distention extends above the sternal angle.

Continue your assessment by inspecting and palpating the chest. Look for surgical scars that might indicate previous cardiac surgery. Look for other signs that suggest the patient has a history of cardiac disease. For example, the presence of a NTG patch on the patient's skin suggests a history of angina. A slight bulge under the skin of the patient's upper right or left chest or abdominal wall is probably a pacemaker or implantable defibrillator. Is the anterior-posterior diameter of the chest enlarged? This finding, where the expanded chest resembles the shape of a barrel, is called *barrel chest* and may be seen in patients with COPD. Palpating the chest may reveal areas of tenderness or crepitus. For example, costochondritis is a condition that may cause chest pain from inflammation of the cartilage and bones in the chest wall.

Listen carefully to the chest with your stethoscope. Crackles or wheezes may suggest LVF with pulmonary edema. A patient who has pulmonary edema may have foamy, blood-tinged sputum present in the mouth or nose. Inspect and lightly palpate the patient's abdomen for distention and pulsations. Strong pulsations in the epigastric area may be a sign of an abdominal aortic aneurysm. Look at the patient's arms, hands, legs, feet, and ankles for swelling. If the patient is confined to a bed, then check for swelling in the lower back (sacral) area, as swelling occurs in the most dependent body areas. Bilateral pitting edema may be a sign of **right ventricular failure (RVF)**. Pitting edema limited to one side of the body suggests a blockage in a major vein.

When you obtain the vital signs, carefully assess the patient's pulse. A weak, thready pulse suggests a reduction in CO. A pulse that is very rapid (more than 150 beats per minute [beats/min]), very slow (less than 40 beats/min), or irregular may be one of the first indicators of a cardiac dysrhythmia and requires further evaluation. Place any patient who has a cardiac-related symptom on a cardiac monitor. Document the patient's initial rhythm and any changes in the rhythm.

One of the most important and widely used tools you will use as a paramedic is the cardiac monitor-defibrillator. This machine enables you to monitor and record 3-lead electrocardiogram (ECG) tracings, and record 12-lead ECGs in the field. It also enables you to quickly identify suspected AMI, transmit the findings electronically to the receiving facility, and make sound transport decisions with regard to patient destination based on the ECG findings. A monitor-defibrillator also provides you with the ability to treat cardiac dysrhythmias using electrical therapy, such as **defibrillation**, **synchronized cardioversion**, or **transcutaneous pacing (TCP)**, when such procedures are warranted.

While obtaining the vital signs, attach the cardiac monitor, waveform capnography, and pulse oximeter if you have not done so already. Use the ECG and oxygen saturation (Spo_2) measurement just as you do other vital signs—that is, as tools to help you in your assessment and not as the only guide to treatment (treat the patient, not the monitor).

Pulse Findings in Cardiac Patients

Normally, the apical pulse rate is the same as the pulse rate in a peripheral location such as the radial pulse. Assess an apical pulse with a stethoscope. Place the stethoscope over the heart's apex, which is between the fifth and sixth ribs on the left side of the chest in adults. To assess for a pulse deficit, palpate a peripheral pulse while listening to the apical pulse. A difference between the apical pulse and the peripheral pulse rates indicates a pulse deficit. For example, if a patient's apical pulse rate is 100 beats/min and the radial pulse rate is 75 beats/min, a pulse deficit of 25 beats/min is present. Pulse deficit occurs with many abnormal heart rhythms or when the heart's contractions are too weak to propel blood through the peripheral arteries.

When the body is at rest, blood pressure normally fluctuates during the respiratory cycle, falling with inspiration and rising with expiration. The accepted upper limit for a fall in systolic blood pressure with inspiration is 10 mm Hg. Pulsus paradoxus occurs when the systolic blood pressure falls more than 10 mm Hg with inspiration. Cardiac conditions in which this finding may be present include AMI, cardiogenic shock, **cardiac tamponade**, and constrictive pericarditis.

Finally, you might recognize a beat-to-beat difference in the strength of a pulse. This finding is called *pulsus alternans* and may be a sign of severe ventricular failure. It is believed the beat-to-beat changes in pulse strength are a result of a decrease in the number of myocardial cells contracting during alternate beats, resulting in decreased myocardial contractility.

Blood Pressure Findings in Cardiac Patients

In older adults, a systolic blood pressure of more than 140 mm Hg is a much more important risk factor for CVD than the diastolic pressure. Patients with a systolic blood pressure of 120 to 139 mm Hg or a diastolic blood pressure of 80 to 89 mm Hg are considered prehypertensive.

In emergency situations, an elevated blood pressure may reflect the patient's anxiety or pain. A systolic blood pressure of less than 90 mm Hg might suggest serious hypotension and shock, depending on the patient's overall condition and chief complaint. Markedly elevated blood pressures may contribute to aortic dissection, heart failure, or stroke. The pulse pressure reflects stroke volume and the elasticity of the arterial walls. Normal pulse pressure is 30 to 40 mm Hg. A widened (high) pulse pressure (more than 40 mm Hg) may be seen in conditions such as the later stages of shock. A narrowed pulse pressure (less than 30 mm Hg) may be seen in conditions such as tachycardia and cardiac tamponade.

It may be beneficial to obtain blood pressure readings in both arms and compare the readings. Some conditions such as stroke or aortic aneurysm may cause blood pressures to vary from the right to the left side.

Assessment of Heart Sounds

Assessing heart sounds requires a relatively quiet environment. As a result, detailed assessment of heart sounds is usually not always practical in the prehospital setting. However, the ability to recognize normal heart sounds can be useful. The purpose of listening to heart sounds is to identify the "lub-dub" that indicates the cardiac valves are operating properly. Chapter 8, *Anatomy and Physiology,* discusses heart sounds. Chapter 11, *Patient Assessment,* discusses how to auscultate heart sounds.

S_1 heart sounds occur near the beginning of ventricular contraction (systole), when the tricuspid and mitral valves close. The closing of the tricuspid valve can be louder in patients who are experiencing pulmonary hypertension because of the increased pressure that exists past the valve. In patients who have anemia, a fever, or hyperthyroidism, louder S_1 sounds may be heard because of the valves being open when the ventricles contract. A patient who has a stenosed mitral valve will also have a louder S_1. Patients who have mitral valves that are subject to fibrosis or are calcified can have decreased S_1 heart sounds. Other conditions such as obesity, emphysema, and cardiac tamponade (fluid around the heart) can diminish S_1 heart sounds as well. Any delay in the closing of these two valves, heard as a split sound, is considered abnormal.

S_2 heart sounds occur near the end of ventricular contraction (systole), when the pulmonary and aortic valves close. Patients with chronic high blood pressure or pulmonary hypertension may experience a higher closing pressure for these valves, resulting in the aortic valve that makes a louder sound when closing. Patients with hypotension will produce a decreased S_2 sound. The S_2 sound may be split if the patient has a right bundle branch, which results in the delay of the pulmonic valve closing. Left bundle branch blocks may cause a situation where the aortic valve is closing more slowly than the pulmonic valve.

When an S_1, S_2, S_3 sequence is heard in adults, it is called a gallop rhythm because it sounds like a horse galloping. S_3 is heard in early ventricular diastole. It is caused by vibration of the ventricular walls during rapid ventricular filling and is often associated with heart failure.

S_4 is a rare heart sound heard just before S_1. It is caused by turbulent filling of a stiff ventricle as seen in hypertrophy and possibly myocardial infarction.

A murmur is an abnormal whooshing-like sound that is associated with turbulent blood flow through the heart valves. This turbulent blood flow can occur from increased blood flow across a normal valve, flow across an irregular or constricted valve, blood flow into an enlarged chamber of the heart, or blood flow going backward through a compromised valve.

Reassessment

Once the history and vital signs have been obtained and the physical exam has been completed, continue treating the patient and initiate transport. The reassessment is accomplished en route to the hospital. It begins with a repeat of the primary survey (level of consciousness and ABCDEs). Obtain the vital signs every 5 minutes for critical patients or every 15 minutes for patients who are determined to be in stable condition. Repeat the physical exam to see if any changes have occurred or if any conditions were missed in the initial physical exam.

Assess the effectiveness of all interventions implemented. For example, is the intravenous (IV) fluid still flowing or has the pain diminished after NTG administration?

Prepare proper documentation of the call. Notify the receiving facility of any history findings, physical exam findings, and cardiac monitoring or ECG findings. Finally, part of the care of the patient with STEMI should involve transmitting the 12-lead ECG to the catheterization lab to shorten the interval from the arrival time to treatment time. Transmit your findings.

Electrophysiology

The mechanical pumping action of the heart can occur only in response to an electrical stimulus. This impulse causes the heart to beat because of a series of complex chemical changes within the myocardial cells.

Depolarization and Repolarization

Recall, an action potential is a sequence of changes in the membrane potential that occurs when an excitable cell is stimulated. In the heart, **depolarization** is the process of discharging resting cardiac muscle fibers by means of an electrical impulse that stimulates contraction Figure 17-2A.

Like all cells in the body, myocardial cells are bathed in an electrolyte solution. Chemical pumps inside the

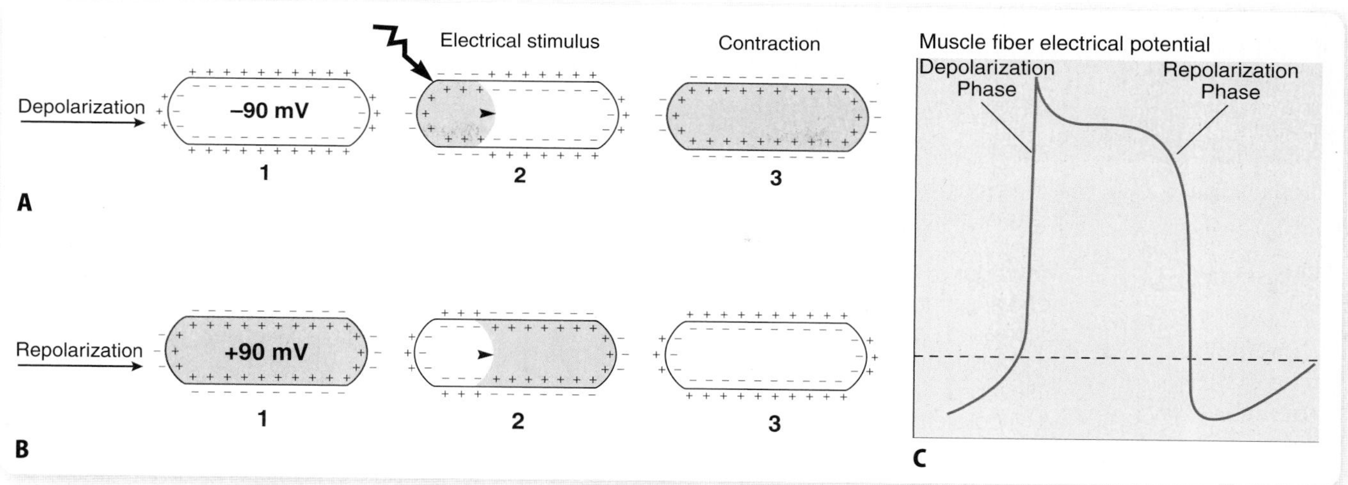

Figure 17-2 Movement of ions to produce a net current flow. **A.** Depolarization. (1) At rest, the cell's interior has a net charge of –90 mV. (2) The wave of depolarization begins as sodium ions pour into the cell. (3) Depolarized cell. **B.** Repolarization. (1) Depolarized cell. (2) The wave of repolarization begins as potassium ions leave the cell. (3) Repolarized cell. **C.** Changes in the electrical potential of muscle fiber associated with contraction.

cell maintain the ion concentration within the cell, creating an electrical gradient across the cell membrane. As a consequence, a resting (polarized) cell normally has a net internal charge of −90 millivolts (mV) relative to the outside of the cell (Figure 17-2, part A1). When a myocardial cell receives a stimulus from the conduction system (Figure 17-2, part A2), the cell wall becomes more permeable as specialized channels open, allowing sodium ions (Na^+) to rush into the cell. Thus, the inside of the cell becomes more positive. Calcium ions (Ca^{+2}) also enter the cell—albeit more slowly and through a different set of specialized channels. These ions help maintain the depolarized state of the cell membrane and allow cardiac muscle tissue to contract. This reversal of the cell's electrical charge begins at one point in the cell wall and spreads in a wave until the cell has been completely depolarized (Figure 17-2, part A3). As the cell depolarizes and calcium ions enter, mechanical contraction occurs.

If the cell remains depolarized, then it can never contract again! However, the cell is able to recover from depolarization through a process called *repolarization* Figure 17-2B. Repolarization begins as the sodium and calcium channels close, halting the rapid inflow of these ions. Next, special potassium channels open, allowing the rapid escape of potassium ions (K^+) from the cell. This helps restore a negative charge inside the cell; the proper electrolyte distribution is then reestablished as sodium ions are pumped out of the cell and potassium ions reenter. After the potassium channels close, this sodium-potassium pump helps move sodium and potassium ions back to their respective locations. For every three sodium ions this pump moves out of the cell, it moves two potassium ions into the cell, thereby maintaining the polarity of the cell membrane.

Table 17-1 summarizes the roles of the various electrolytes in cardiac function.

▶ Cardiac Action Potential

The action potential of a typical myocardial cell can be divided into five phases: phase 0 to phase 4 Figure 17-3:

- **Phase 0.** This phase begins when the cardiac muscle cell receives an impulse. Sodium moves into the cell through sodium channels, causing the interior of the cell to become electrically positive relative to its exterior, resulting in a change in the transmembrane potential (TMP) from −90 mV to about −70 mV. At threshold, still more sodium channels open, allowing a rapid influx of sodium and a rapid rise in membrane voltage to about +30 mV. At the same time, calcium enters more slowly through calcium channels. The influx of calcium causes the sarcoplasmic reticulum to release calcium for muscle contraction. The cell depolarizes and begins to contract. On an ECG, the QRS complex represents phase 0.
- **Phase 1.** During this phase, inward sodium channels close and the cell begins to repolarize. Negatively charged chloride ions enter the cell. Outward potassium channels open briefly, allowing potassium to leave the cell and resulting in a decrease in the TMP.
- **Phase 2.** This phase, called the plateau phase, is the longest phase of the action potential. During this phase, sodium and calcium slowly enter the cell, while potassium flows out of the cell.[2] The presence of calcium prolongs depolarization of

Table 17-1 Role of Electrolytes in Cardiac Function

Electrolyte	Role in Cardiac Function
Sodium (Na^+)	Flows into the cell to initiate depolarization
Potassium (K^+)	Flows out of the cell to initiate repolarization Decreased or increased levels of potassium result in the following: ▪ *Hypo*kalemia → increased myocardial irritability ▪ *Hyper*kalemia → decreased automaticity/conduction
Calcium (Ca^{+2})	Has a critical role in depolarization of pacemaker cells (maintains depolarization) and in myocardial contractility (involved in contraction of heart muscle tissue) Decreased or increased levels of calcium result in the following: ▪ *Hypo*calcemia → decreased contractility and increased myocardial irritability ▪ *Hyper*calcemia → increased contractility
Magnesium (Mg^{+2})	Stabilizes the cell membrane; acts in concert with potassium, and opposes the actions of calcium Decreased or increased levels of magnesium result in the following: ▪ *Hypo*magnesemia → decreased conduction ▪ *Hyper*magnesemia → increased myocardial irritability

the membrane, creating a plateau. Contraction ends when the outward flow of potassium exceeds the inward flow of sodium and calcium. Phase 2 corresponds to the ST segment on the ECG.

- **Phase 3.** This is the final phase of repolarization. Slow calcium channels gradually close and calcium is transported out of the cell. Potassium channels open and the rapid movement of potassium out of the cell causes the TMP to become increasingly negative. By the end of this phase, the membrane potential has been restored to its resting value. With repolarization complete, the cell can now respond to a new stimulus. On an ECG, the T wave represents phase 3.
- **Phase 4.** This phase, called the resting phase, represents the normal working myocardial cell at its resting membrane potential of −90 mV.[2]

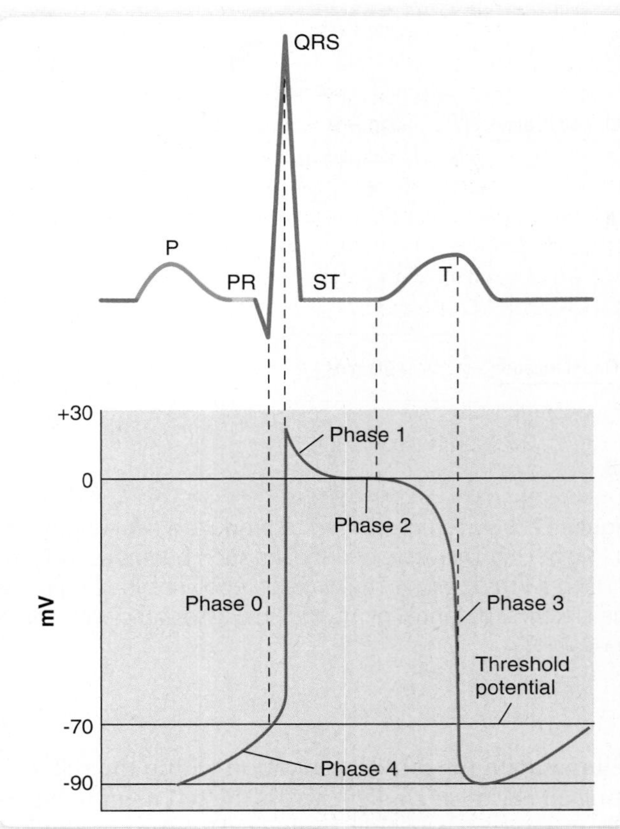

Figure 17-3 The components of an electrocardiogram rhythm correspond to the phases of myocyte stimulation.

Reproduced from *12-Lead ECG: The Art of Interpretation*, courtesy of Tomas B. Garcia, MD.

▶ Refractory Periods

A myocardial cell cannot respond to an electrical stimulus from the conduction system normally unless it is fully polarized. The period during which the cell is depolarized or in the process of repolarizing—the so-called **refractory period (RP)**—consists of two phases. In the **absolute refractory period (ARP)**, cardiac cells are unable to respond to any stimulus. This period lasts from phase 0 to the middle of phase 3 of the cardiac action potential. A helpful analogy is a flushing toilet. If you flush a toilet and then immediately try to flush it again, does the toilet flush? No! Why? Because the tank has not yet filled back up with water.

The **relative refractory period (RRP)** extends from the middle of phase 3 to the beginning of phase 4 of the cardiac action potential. During this time, the heart muscle has been partially repolarized and may depolarize in response to an electrical stimulus. The RRP indicates that some cells have repolarized sufficiently to depolarize again. Let's return to our flushing toilet analogy. If you waited 15 seconds before flushing again, what would happen? You'd get a partial flush, because the tank had refilled with water perhaps halfway. So, during the ARP, nothing can stimulate the ventricles to contract again. During the RRP, however, a strong stimulus can initiate depolarization of those cells that have had enough time to repolarize.

▶ The Conduction System

The network of cardiac tissue that initiates and conducts electrical impulses is called the **electrical conduction system**. The conduction system is composed of specialized pacemaker cells. These cells are found in the tissues of the SA node, internodal conduction pathways, AV node, bundle of His, and Purkinje fibers. The tissue in which the heart's electrical activity arises at any given time, then, is called the pacemaker, because it sets the pace (that is, rate) of cardiac contraction.

Theoretically, any cell within the heart's electrical conduction system can act as a pacemaker. In the normal heart, however, the dominant pacemaker is the SA node Figure 17-4. It normally fires at an intrinsic rate of 60 to 100 times per minute (times/min). The SA node lies at the junction of the superior vena cava and the right atrium, and, in most patients, the RCA supplies it with blood.

In about 0.08 seconds, electrical impulses generated in this node spread across the atria and advance through three **internodal pathways** in the atrial wall:

1. **Anterior internodal pathway.** The Bachmann bundle is the interatrial pathway connecting the right and left atria. A branch of the Bachmann bundle forms a pathway between the SA and AV nodes. This route is called the *anterior internodal pathway.*
2. **Middle internodal tract.** The Wenckebach tract constitutes the middle internodal tract.
3. **Thorel tract.** The Thorel tract is the last of the internodal pathways and is represented by the posterior internodal pathway.

The **atrioventricular (AV) node** is a group of cells located in the floor of the right atrium behind the tricuspid valve, near the opening of the coronary sinus. In most people, its blood supply comes from a branch of the RCA; in others, it comes from a branch of the Cx artery. When the impulse from the SA node enters the AV node, it is delayed for about 0.12 seconds before it is relayed through the rest of the conduction system. This delay allows the atria to empty blood into the ventricles. About 70% to 80% of the blood in the atria fills the ventricles by gravity; the remaining 20% to 30% comes from atrial contraction (atrial kick). The **atrioventricular (AV) junction**, includes the AV node and surrounding tissue, along with the nonbranching portion of the **bundle of His**, also called the *AV bundle*, which conducts impulses from the AV junction to the right and left bundle branches. In the normal heart, the AV junction can be thought of as a gatekeeper because it is the only electrical connection between the atria and ventricles.

Normally, impulses pass through the AV junction into the bundle of His and then move rapidly into the right and left bundle branches on either side of the interventricular septum. If the atrial rate becomes very rapid, then the AV junction can regulate the number of impulses that reach the ventricles. The impulses that do proceed will spread

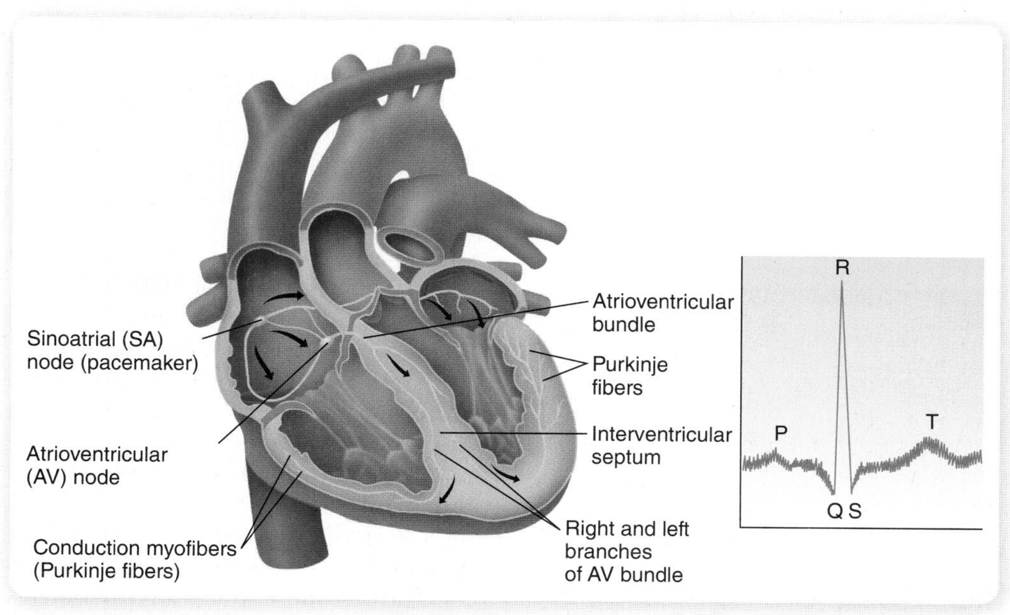

Figure 17-4 The electrical conduction system of the heart.

from the bundle branches to the **Purkinje fibers**, cardiac muscle fibers distributed throughout the inner surfaces of the ventricular walls. It takes about 0.08 seconds for an electric impulse to spread across the ventricles, during which time the ventricles contract.

Secondary Pacemakers

If the SA node is damaged or suppressed, then any component of the conduction system can act as a secondary pacemaker. The farther removed the conduction tissue is from the SA node, however, the slower its intrinsic rate of firing. Suppose the SA node were damaged by ischemia (tissue injury caused by hypoxemia) and consequently could not fire. If the AV node fails to receive an impulse from the SA node, then the AV junction might then begin firing at its own rate of 40 to 60 beats/min. If both the SA node and AV junction fail to initiate an impulse, then the Purkinje fibers will initiate an impulse, generating a ventricular rhythm at a rate of 20 to 40 beats/min Table 17-2.

Accessory Conduction Pathways

Some people are born with extra heart muscle tissue that connects the atria and ventricles, bypassing the AV node. This abnormal tissue is called an *accessory pathway* or a bypass tract:

- **James fibers.** James fibers in the atrial internodal pathways extend into the ventricles while bypassing the AV node.
- **Mahaim fibers.** The AV node, the bundle of His, and the bundle branches contain Mahaim fibers that extend into the ventricles and provide a common pathway for re-entrant dysrhythmias.
- **Bundle of Kent.** The bundle of Kent is an accessory pathway typically located between the left atrium and the left ventricle, although it is sometimes found between the right atrium and the right ventricle. The bundle of Kent enables the depolarization wave to bypass the AV node and trigger early depolarization of a section of ventricular tissue. Simultaneously, depolarization travels through the AV node and bundle of His to the bundle branches. These simultaneous depolarization events create a unique change on the ECG tracing called a **delta wave**.

Table 17-2 Pacemaker Intrinsic Rates

Pacemaker	Rate (beats/min)
SA node	60–100
AV junction	40–60
Purkinje network	20–40

Abbreviations: SA, sinoatrial; AV, atrioventricular

In certain instances, accessory pathways can trigger abnormally fast heart rates (tachydysrhythmias). Medical intervention is often required to terminate such rhythms.

The Autonomic Nervous System and the Heart

Both the sympathetic and parasympathetic divisions of the autonomic nervous system (ANS) affect the heart Figure 17-5. Sympathetic (accelerator) nerves supply specific areas of the heart's electrical system, atrial muscle, and ventricular myocardium. Sympathetic nerves transmit commands by releasing norepinephrine. Norepinephrine travels to the SA node, AV node, and ventricles, spreading the signal from the sympathetic nerves. To prevent a buildup of lactic acid, the heart speeds up, increasing CO and thereby distributing more oxygen and nutrients throughout the body.

An accelerated heart rate shortens all phases of the **cardiac cycle**—the period from one cardiac contraction to the next. When the ventricles have less time to relax, less time is available for these chambers to fill adequately with blood. If the ventricles do not fill completely, then less blood is sent to the coronary arteries, less blood is pumped out of the ventricles, CO decreases, and signs of myocardial ischemia may appear. *Ischemia* is anoxia caused by diminished blood flow to tissue, usually because of narrowing or occlusion of an artery.

Parasympathetic (inhibitory) nerve fibers supply the SA node, atrial muscle, and the AV junction of the heart by way of the vagus nerve. The vagus nerve, also called cranial nerve X (CN X), innervates functional areas ranging from the soft palate to the thoracic organs. It's also responsible for decreasing the heart rate. The vagus can be stimulated in a number of ways, including increasing pressure on the carotid sinus, straining or forced exhalation against a closed glottis (**Valsalva maneuver**), or distention of a hollow organ, such as the bladder or stomach.

When pressure is applied over the carotid sinus or a person is straining during a bowel movement, the brain may sense that the heart should slow its pace. A message in the form of an electrical impulse will travel down the vagus nerve to the point at which the nerve abuts the SA node of the heart Figure 17-6. There, the electrical impulse stimulates the release of acetylcholine (ACh). The ACh then crosses over to the SA node, signaling that the brain is calling for the heart rate to decelerate. To ensure the message is received and acted on, another ACh molecule travels to the AV node. This action, in effect, reminds the SA node to slow down, ensuring no additional impulses get through to the ventricles. Afterward, ACh is escorted away by acetylcholinesterase (AChE). AChE is an enzyme that breaks down ACh so it can be recycled. Atropine is a commonly used parasympathetic blocker that opposes the action of acetylcholine, thereby accelerating the heart rate.

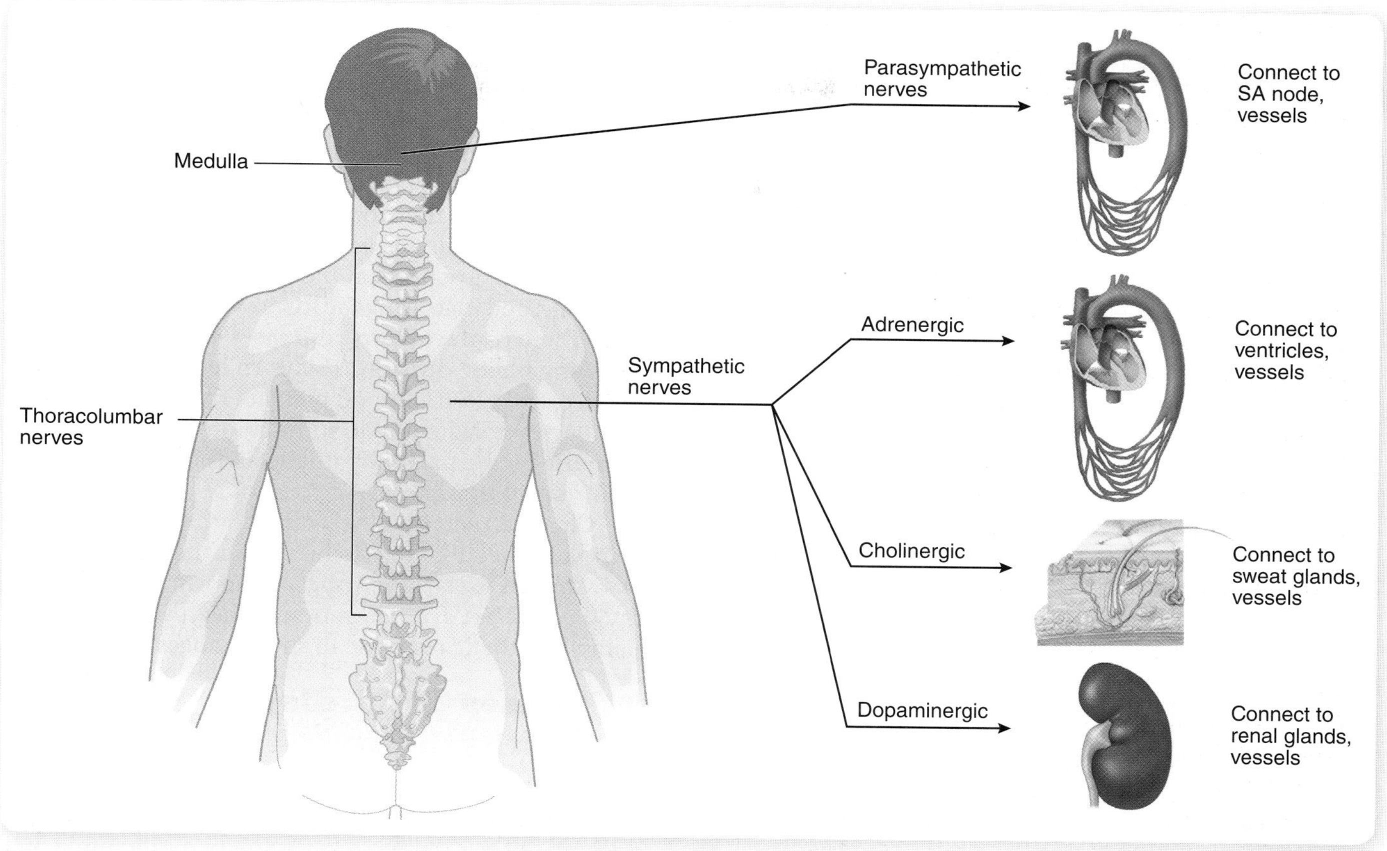

Figure 17-5 Sympathetic and parasympathetic nerve fibers, and their end organs.

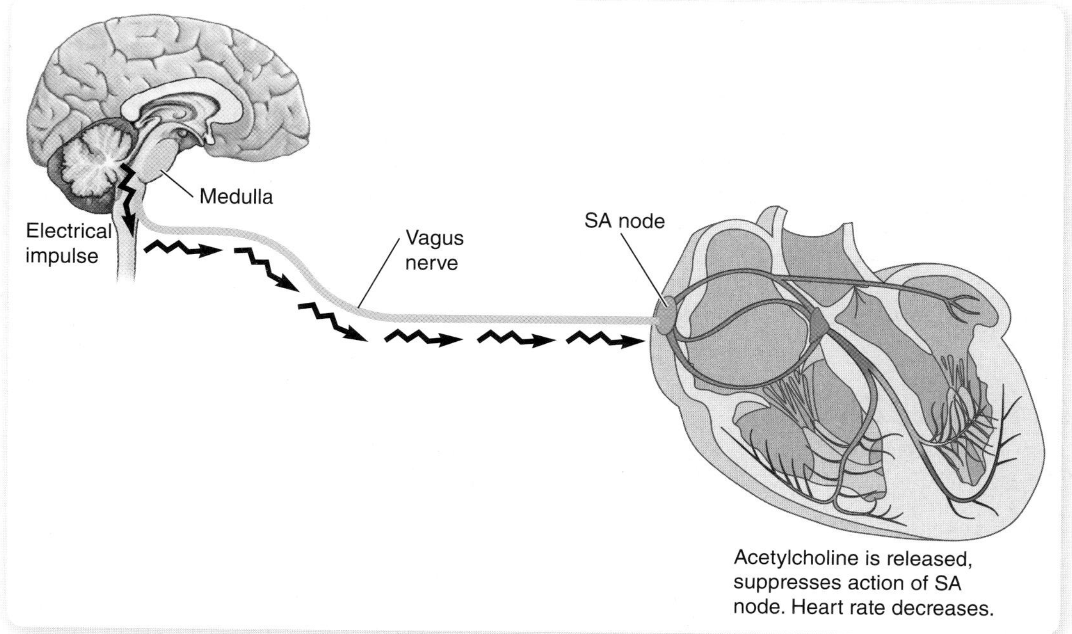

Figure 17-6 Example of an electrical impulse that stimulates the release of a chemical. Here, in this example, an electrical impulse travels from the brain down the vagus nerve, causing the release of acetylcholine (ACh) near the sinoatrial (SA) node. ACh suppresses the action of the SA node, slowing the heart rate.

Words of Wisdom

The below parable, a legacy that originated with Dr. Nancy Caroline, demonstrates the effect of atropine on the parasympathetic nervous system.

"You're firing a little slowly today, aren't you?" says atropine.

"Just following instructions," replies the SA node. "The vagus told me to take it easy."

"Vagus, vagus—why are you always trying to slow everything down?"

"Hey, I'm just following orders from the brain," the vagus nerve explains. "You know a job can't be done well if you rush it."

"Yeah, well, chop chop, SA. We don't have time to slack off around here," says atropine.

"But what about the vagus?" protests the SA node.

"If you keep paying attention to the vagus, before you know it, you'll have slowed down so much that the brain will have to shut down for lack of blood and oxygen! Then where will you be? Take my advice, Bud, and open the gates wide. Let all impulses through, no questions asked."

"Are you sure that's a good idea? The vagus told me . . ."

"Forget about the vagus. He's just an old obstructionist."

"Okay, if you say so," says the SA node, always eager to please when atropine is around. So the SA node speeds up.

Atropine then blocks the vagus nerve so he can't interfere.

"Rats," says the vagus. "I guess I've been overruled."

Baroreceptors and Chemoreceptors

Baroreceptors, or pressoreceptors, are sensors composed of specialized nerve tissue. They are found in the internal carotid arteries and aortic arch. These sensory receptors detect changes in blood pressure. When stimulated, they generate a reflex response in either the sympathetic or parasympathetic division of the ANS. For example, if blood pressure falls, the body will attempt to compensate by constricting peripheral blood vessels, increasing the heart rate, and increasing the force of myocardial contraction. These compensatory responses are orchestrated by the sympathetic division. This is called a *sympathetic* or *adrenergic response*. If blood pressure rises, then the body will decrease sympathetic stimulation and increase the response by the parasympathetic division. This is called a *parasympathetic* or *cholinergic response*.

Chemoreceptors in the internal carotid arteries, aortic arch, and medulla detect changes in the concentration of hydrogen ions (pH), oxygen, and carbon dioxide in the blood. The ANS may mount either a sympathetic or parasympathetic response to such changes.

▶ Causes of Cardiac Dysrhythmia

A cardiac dysrhythmia is a disturbance in the normal cardiac rhythm, which may or may not be clinically significant. Cardiac rhythm disturbance or dysrhythmia may arise from a variety of causes Table 17-3. It is always necessary to evaluate the dysrhythmia in the context of the patient's overall clinical condition. It is the patient's clinical condition—not the lines or tracings on a screen or a

YOU are the Paramedic PART 2

You and your partner begin your assessment. The patient is alert and oriented, but he has pale, diaphoretic skin and is in visible respiratory distress. His initial vital signs are pulse, 150 beats/min; blood pressure, 96/40 mm Hg; respirations, 20 breaths/min and deep; Spo_2 on room air, 91%. The patient denies any recent surgery or trauma.

Recording Time: 5 minutes	
Appearance	Awake; pale, moist skin
Level of consciousness	Alert and oriented × 4
Airway	Open
Breathing	Inadequate; visible respiratory distress
Circulation	Inadequate; tachycardic

5. What interventions should you initiate at this time?

Table 17-3	Causes of Cardiac Dysrhythmias
Acid-base disturbance	
ANS imbalance	
Central nervous system damage	
Certain poisons (eg, organophosphate insecticides)	
Cor pulmonale (right ventricular failure caused by pulmonary disease)	
Distention of cardiac chambers (as in heart failure)	
Drug effects (phenothiazines, tricyclic antidepressants, and drugs used to treat dysrhythmias)	
Electrolyte disturbances, especially those involving potassium, calcium, or magnesium	
Endocrine disorders (hyperthyroidism, hypothyroidism)	
Hypothermia	
Hypoxemia from any cause	
Increased sympathetic output	
Increased vagal (parasympathetic) tone	
Myocardial ischemia or infarction	
Normal variation	
Rheumatic heart disease	
Trauma (eg, cardiac contusion)	

piece of paper—that should ultimately determine whether treatment is necessary. Treat the patient, not the monitor!

▶ The Electrocardiogram

An ECG is a graphic record of the changes in voltage that occur in the heart muscle during depolarization and repolarization. The ECG monitor serves several functions in the prehospital setting **Figure 17-7**. You can use it to monitor the patient's cardiac rhythm continuously during transport, to print out a rhythm strip for interpretation, or to print out a 12-lead ECG for specific disease diagnosis.

Typically, continuous monitoring is performed using three **limb leads**: leads I, II, and III. You can use continuous ECG monitoring during transport to identify any changes in the patient's heart rhythm. When analyzing cardiac monitoring ECGs, the tracing from lead II is usually the most useful.

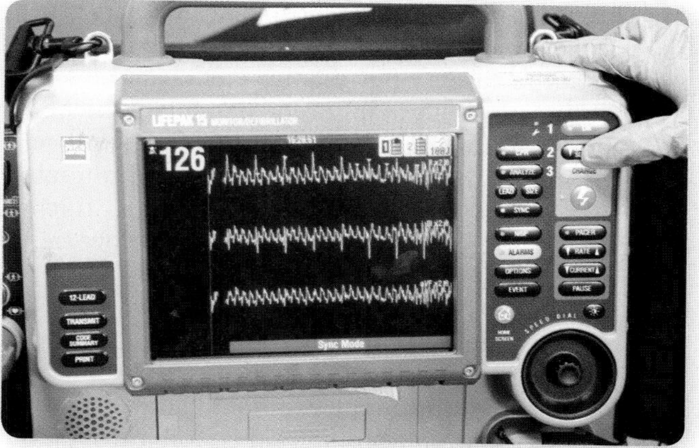

Figure 17-7 A cardiac monitor.

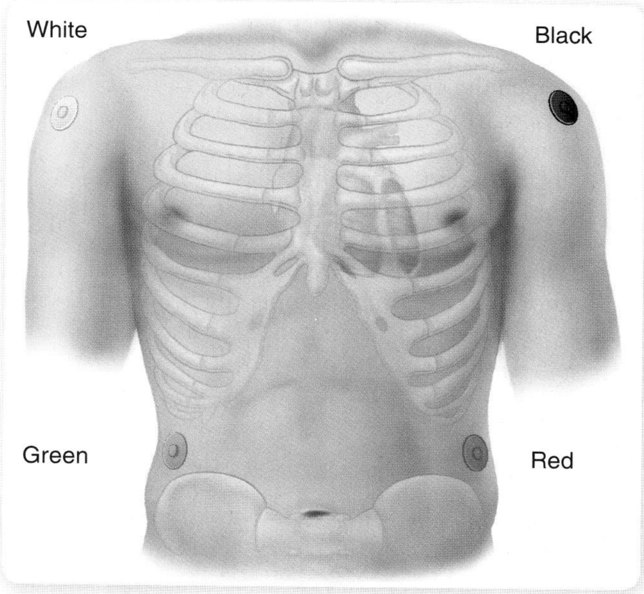

Figure 17-8 Electrode placement for cardiac monitoring.

Because the heart is a 3-dimensional organ, the use of only 3 leads limits the areas of the heart that can be viewed. A 12-lead ECG provides detailed information about the heart's conduction system and records its electrical activity from 12 separate angles. In virtually all cases, when you record a 3-lead ECG, it is because you suspect the patient is experiencing a cardiac event; therefore, a 12-lead ECG should also be captured.

Cardiac monitors are equipped with lead wires that are connected to electrodes, which are placed on the patient. Each **lead** offers an electrical snapshot of a certain part of the heart. The cardiac monitor records an ECG tracing for each lead used; health care professionals trained to interpret the findings can then review the tracings.

Electrode Placement

To obtain a reliable, useful ECG, the electrodes must be placed in consistent, predetermined positions on each patient's body **Figure 17-8**.

Electrodes used in the prehospital setting are generally adhesive and have a gel center to aid in skin contact. Some manufacturers offer diaphoretic electrodes that adhere aggressively to diaphoretic patients. Whichever type you use, following certain basic principles will help in achieving the best skin contact and in minimizing signal distortion. Such distortion of an ECG tracing caused by interference, such as the patient's movement, is called an **artifact.**

- To maintain the correct lead placement, it may be necessary to shave the patient's body hair from the electrode site. Do not be fooled by a hairy chest. It may initially appear that you have good skin contact, but the electrode will peel away from the skin and stick to the hair.
- To remove oil and dead tissue from the surface of the skin, rub the electrode site briskly with a dry gauze pad.
- Attach the electrodes to the ECG cables before placement. Confirm that the electrode now attached to the cable is placed at the correct location on the patient's chest or limbs. Each cable is marked and color coded to indicate the correct location for placement.
- Once all electrodes are in place, switch on the monitor and print a sample rhythm strip. If the strip shows any interference (artifact), then verify that the electrodes are firmly attached to the skin and the monitor cable is plugged in correctly.

Skill Drill 17-1 shows the steps in performing cardiac monitoring.

Words of Wisdom

Artifact on the monitor can be tricky. A wavy baseline resembling ventricular fibrillation may be caused by patient movement or muscle tremor. Before you reach for the defibrillator paddles, look at the patient! If he or she is alert and in no obvious distress, then recheck the leads and equipment. Remember, treat the patient, not the monitor.

The Leads

There are two main groups of leads: the limb leads and the **precordial leads**—that is, the chest leads. Leads I, II, and III are called limb leads, or standard limb leads, and leads aVR, aVL, and aVF are called **augmented limb leads**. The augmented limb leads contain only one true pole; the other is a combination of information from other leads. A standard 12-lead ECG is made up of the three standard limb leads, the three augmented limb leads, and the six precordial leads.

Skill Drill 17-1 Performing Cardiac Monitoring

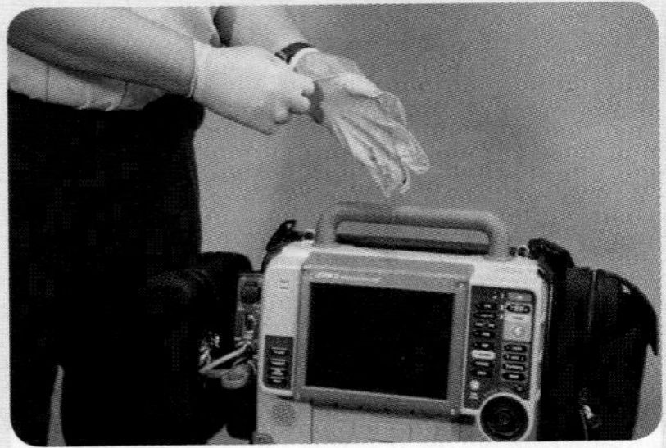

Step 1 Take standard precautions. Check your equipment. Ensure there are no loose pins in the end of the ECG cable and the cable or lead wires are intact. Ensure the monitor has an adequate paper supply. Connect the ECG cable to the machine. Connect the lead wires to the ECG cable (if not already connected). Turn on the power to the monitor. Adjust the screen contrast if necessary.

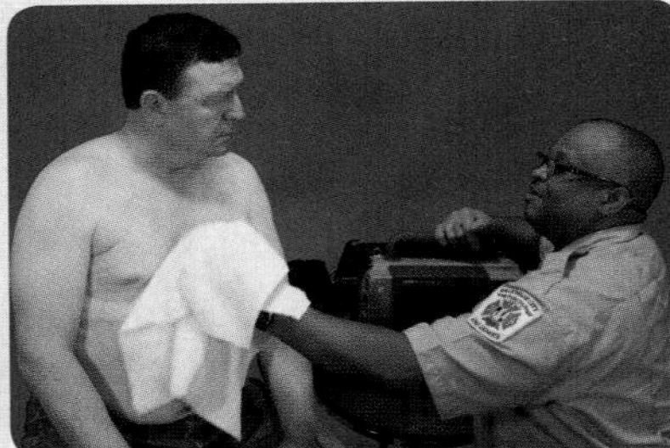

Step 2 Explain the procedure to the patient. To minimize distortion of the ECG tracing, prepare the skin for electrode placement by briskly rubbing it with a dry gauze pad to remove skin oils and improve impulse transmission. If you are applying electrodes to the patient's chest, rather than to his or her limbs, then ensure good contact by shaving small amounts of chest hair if needed.

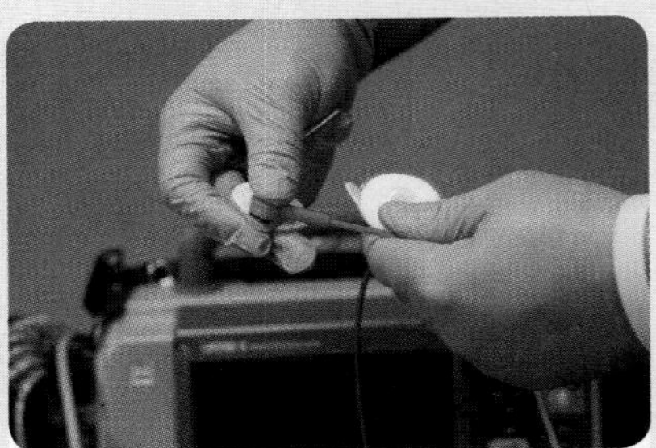

Step 3 Attach the electrodes to the lead wires before placing them on the patient.

Skill Drill 17-1 Performing Cardiac Monitoring *(continued)*

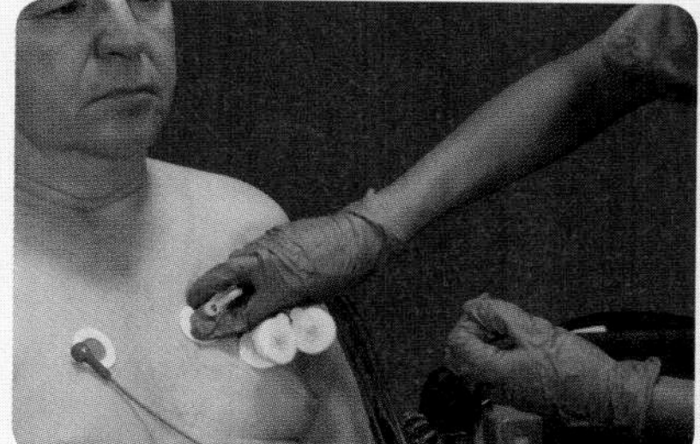

Step 4 One at a time, remove the backing from each electrode and apply it to the patient.

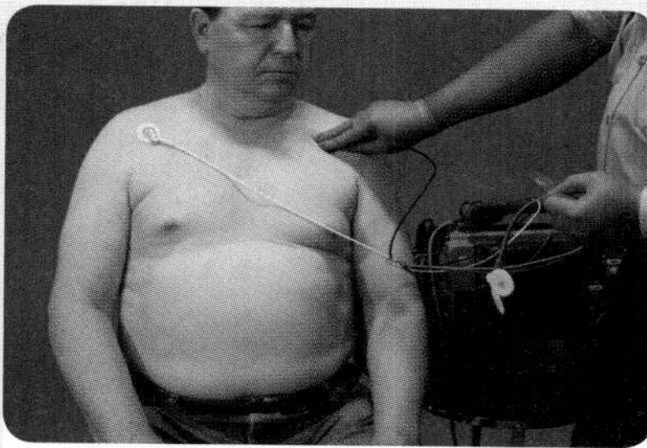

Step 5 If you plan to obtain a 12-lead tracing as well, then place the limb leads. Limb-lead electrodes are usually placed on the wrists and ankles but may be positioned anywhere on the appropriate limb. To reduce muscle tension, ensure the patient's limbs are resting on a supportive surface. Do not apply electrodes over bony areas, broken skin, joints, skin creases, scar tissue, or rashes.

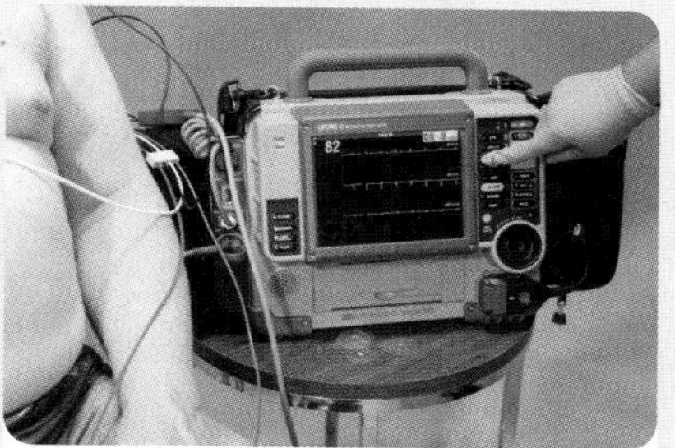

Step 6 Turn on the monitor and select the desired lead, which is typically lead II. Adjust the ECG size if necessary to ensure the machine detects the patient's QRS complexes. Feel the patient's pulse and compare it with the heart rate indicator on the monitor. If not already preset, then set the heart rate alarms on the monitor according to your agency's policy.

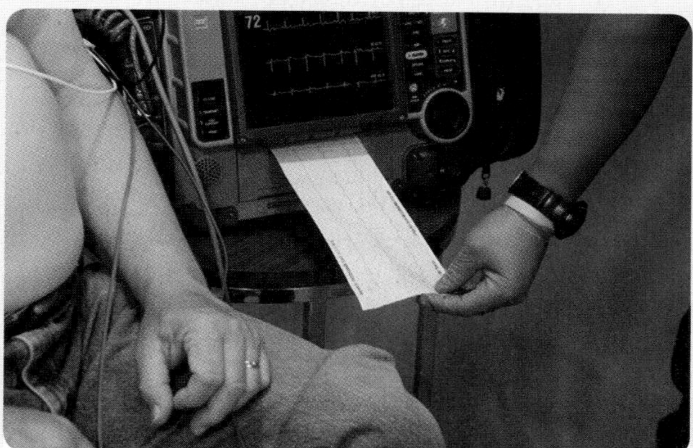

Step 7 Record the tracings.

Step 8 Label each strip.

A lead wire is the electrical cable that attaches an electrode to the ECG monitor. A lead is an image of the heart, taken from a specified vantage point, that measures the difference in electrical potential between two electrodes. An imaginary line joining the positive and negative poles of a lead is called the *lead axis*. The position of the positive electrode determines which area of the heart is viewed by each lead. Suppose you wanted to inspect the condition of a used vehicle you were considering buying. If you needed to know only whether the motor was running, you could stand anywhere near the car and listen. Likewise, you could use any single lead to monitor the cardiac rhythm. However, if you wanted to know the condition of the vehicle's body, you'd have to walk around the vehicle and look at it from all sides. The driver's side might be in mint condition, but the entire doorframe on passenger's side might be caved in from a wreck. Similarly, to localize the site of injury to the heart muscle and to identify other cardiac abnormalities, you must be able to look at the

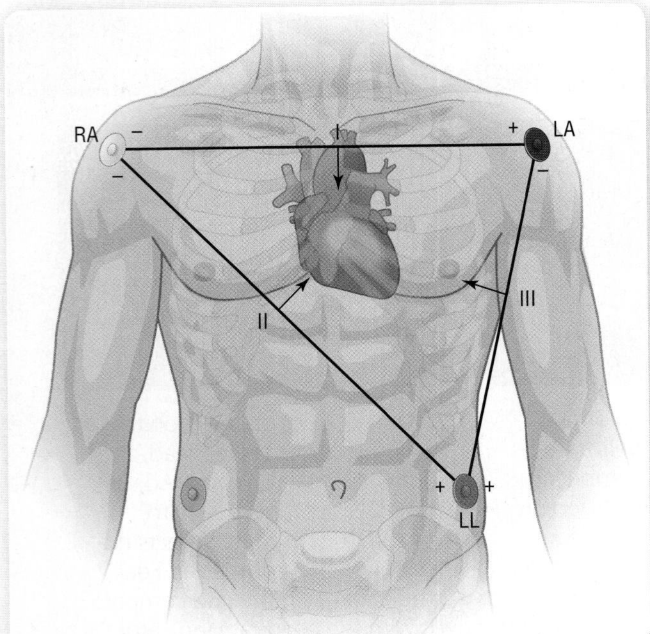

Figure 17-9 The Einthoven triangle. *RA*, right arm; *LA*, left arm; *LL*, left leg.

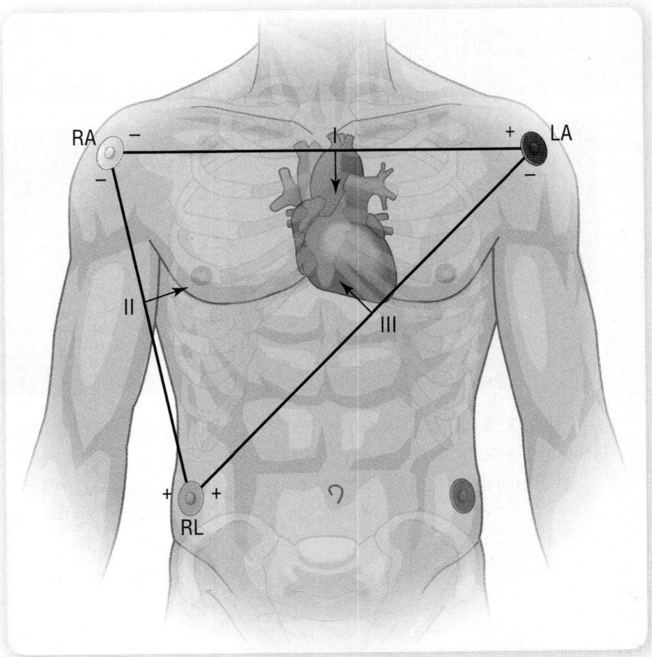

Figure 17-10 Each bipolar lead has a positive end and a negative end.

heart from several angles. One lead may detect major damage that is invisible on another.

Leads I, II, and III view the heart from front of the body; thus, they are called *frontal plane leads.* The precordial leads (V_1 to V_6) are called *unipolar chest leads, anterior leads,* or *V leads.* These leads view the heart in the horizontal plane, so they provide images of the heart from the front (anterior wall of the heart) and from the left side (anterolateral view).

Limb Leads. Willem Einthoven is the physician and physiologist who discovered that every time the heart contracts, it emits a tiny amount of electrical energy that travels across the surface of the skin. Einthoven found that these waves of energy could be recorded and plotted on a piece of grid paper and assigned the letters P, Q, R, S, and T to the ECG deflections he observed. He initially recorded three leads: lead I, attached to the right and left arms, lead II, running between the right arm and left leg, and lead III, running between the left arm and left leg **Figure 17-9**.

Leads I, II, and III are **bipolar leads**. Bipolar leads are those that contain a positive and negative pole. With the standard limb leads, each lead measures the difference in electrical potential between electrodes placed on two extremities.

The left arm electrode is the positive terminal of Lead I. This lead views the lateral surface of the left ventricle. The left leg electrode is the positive terminal of Lead II. The left leg is the positive terminal of Lead III **Figure 17-10**. Leads II and III look at the inferior surface of the left ventricle.

The augmented voltage (aV) leads (leads aVR, aVL, and aVF) are created by combining two of the limb leads, thereby forming a new lead, and using the remaining lead as the other pole. For example, lead aVR is created between the right arm and the combination of the left arm and leg electrodes **Figure 17-11**. The augmented leads are unipolar—that is, they contain one true pole, while the other end of the lead is referenced against a combination of other leads. For example, lead aVR is at the right arm, referenced against a combination of the left arm and the left leg. Lead aVL views the lateral surface of the left ventricle. Lead aVF views the inferior surface of the left ventricle.

If you are performing continuous cardiac monitoring, then place four electrodes on the patient's torso:

White—right upper chest near the shoulder
Black—left upper chest near the shoulder
Red—left lower abdomen
Green—right lower abdomen

If you are acquiring a 12-lead ECG, then place the four electrodes on the patient's limbs:

White—right wrist
Black—left wrist
Red—left ankle
Green—right ankle

Placing these four electrodes on the patient allows the ECG device to record all six limb leads using Einthoven's theory. The green lead serves as a ground in all cases and is electrically neutral.

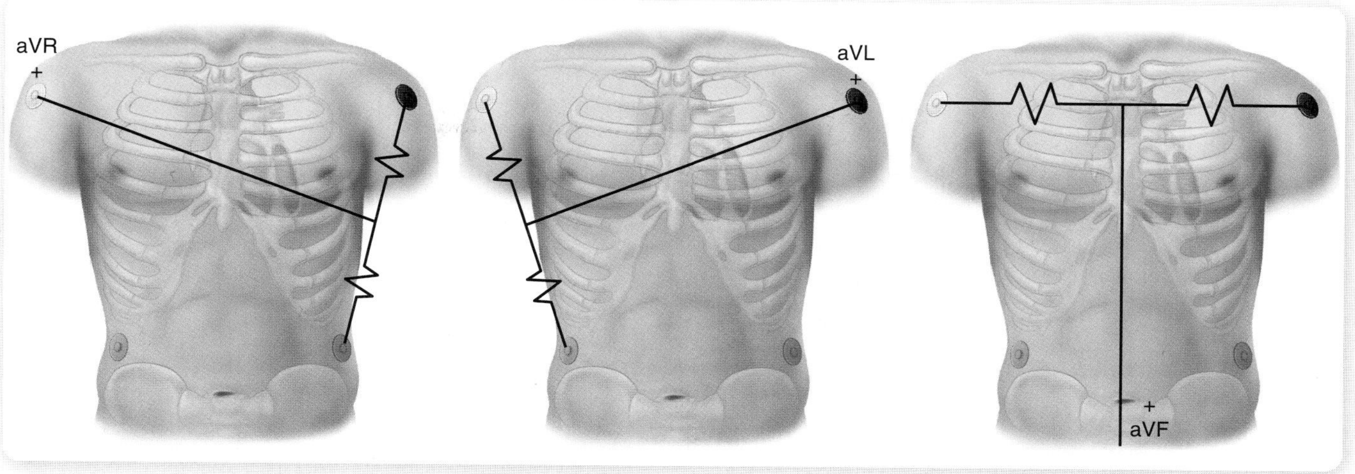

Figure 17-11 Augmented voltage leads analyze the limb leads, taking the data from one lead and synthesizing the information from the other two.

Precordial Leads. The precordial leads V_1 to V_6 are unipolar. These leads are referenced against a calculated point known as *Wilson's central terminal* **Figure 17-12**. Wilson's central terminal is created by bisecting the limb leads in Einthoven's triangle.

The electrode for each unipolar lead is the positive terminal for that lead. Leads V_1 and V_2 view the septum; V_3 and V_4 look at the anterior wall of the left ventricle; and V_5 and V_6 view the lateral wall of the left ventricle.

Correct precordial electrode placement is important to ensure the lead is viewing the heart from the intended angle each time an ECG is recorded. ECGs are often compared with previous ECGs. For this comparison to be reliable in identifying anything out of the ordinary, the precordial lead electrodes must be placed consistently **Figure 17-13 and 17-14**:

1. V_1—Fourth ICS to the right of the sternum
2. V_2—Fourth ICS to the left of the sternum
3. V_3—Directly between leads V_2 and V_4
4. V_4—Fifth ICS at the left midclavicular line
5. V_5—At level of lead V_4 at left anterior axillary line
6. V_6—At level of lead V_4 at left midaxillary line

Contiguous Leads. **Contiguous leads** refer to leads that view geographically similar areas of the myocardium, which can be useful for localizing areas of ischemia, injury, or **infarction**. Leads II, III, and aVF are contiguous. Leads V_1 and V_2, V_2 and V_3, V_3 and V_4, V_4 and V_5, and V_5 and V_6 are pairs of contiguous leads. Leads I and aVL, and aVL and V_5 are also contiguous pairs.

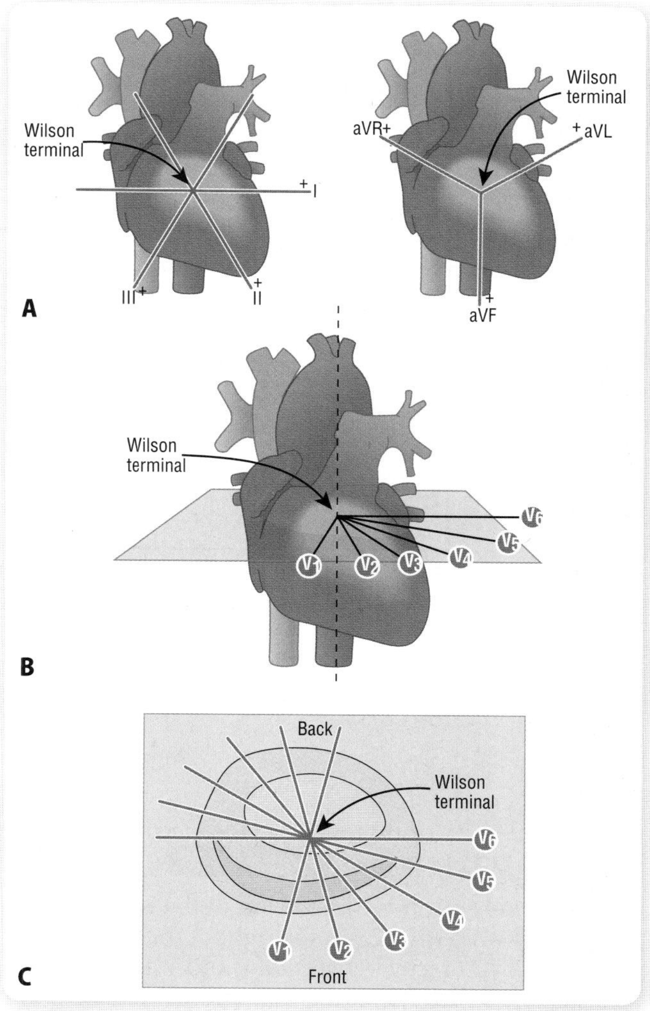

Figure 17-12 The Wilson central terminal, shown in relation to three types of leads: **A.** Bipolar leads. **B.** Augmented unipolar leads. **C.** Precordial leads.

Right-Sided Leads. Certain conditions require that you record a right-sided ECG to evaluate the electrical activity of the right ventricle. In that case, place the precordial leads

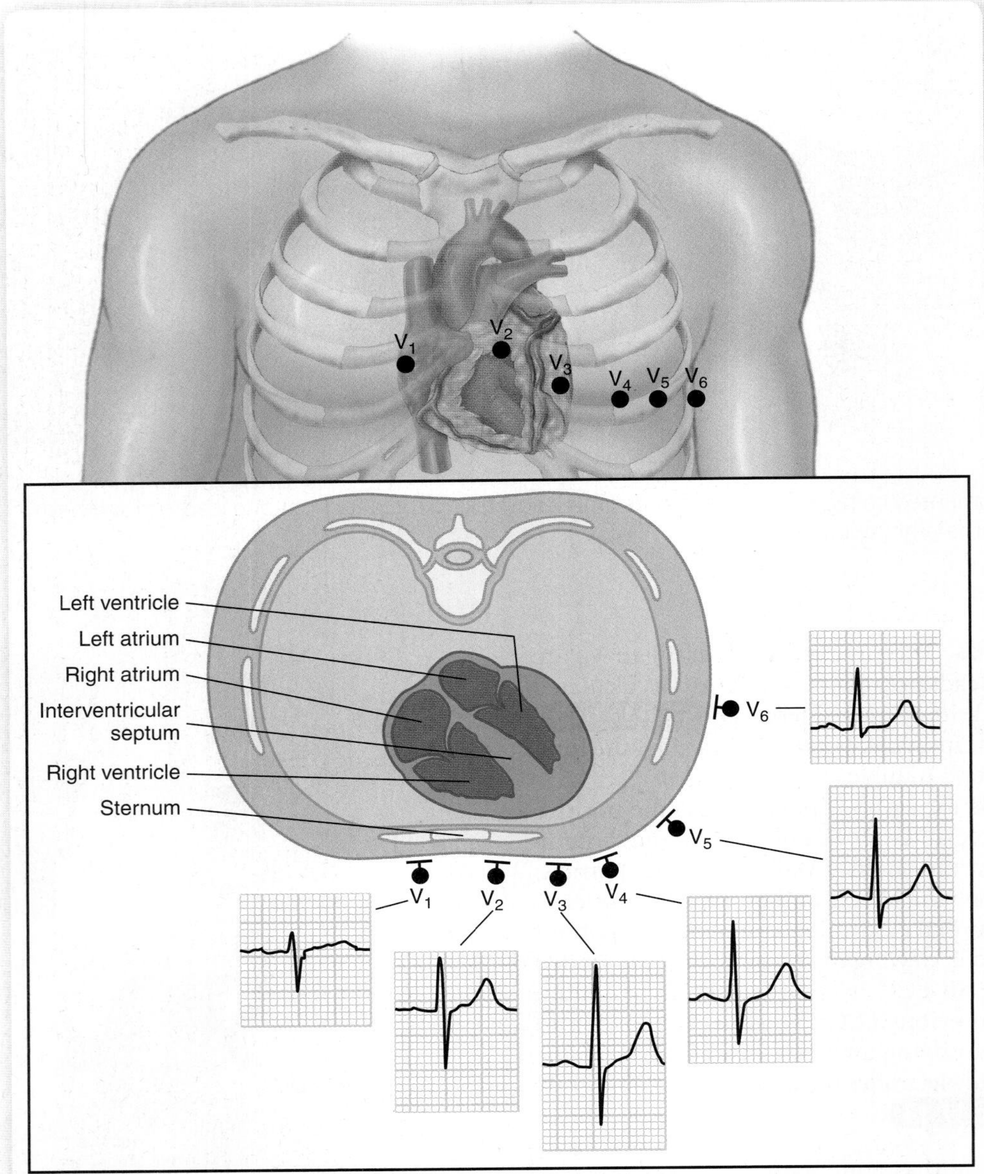

Figure 17-13 Precordial leads (chest leads) depict the heart in the horizontal plane. *Inset:* V_1 and V_2 view at the interventricular septum. V_3 and V_4 view the anterior wall of the left ventricle. V_5 and V_6 represent the low lateral wall. The right ventricle cannot be seen on a standard tracing.

on the right anterior thorax. Place the electrodes for the right-sided ECG as follows Figure 17-15:

1. V_1R—Fourth ICS to the left of the sternum
2. V_2R—Fourth ICS to the right of the sternum
3. V_3R—Directly between V_2R and V_4R
4. V_4R—Fifth ICS at the right midclavicular line
5. V_5R—At level of lead V_4R at right anterior axillary line
6. V_6R—At level of lead V_4R at right midaxillary line

Note: lead V_4R is the most sensitive and specific for right ventricular AMI and is often the only lead recorded on a right-sided ECG.

Posterior Leads. The posterior ECG is used to evaluate the electrical activity of the posterior wall of the left ventricle. In that case, place three of the precordial leads on the left posterior thorax Figure 17-16:

1. V_7—Between V_6 and V_8, fifth ICS
2. V_8—Midscapular, fifth ICS
3. V_9—Just to the left of the spine, fifth ICS

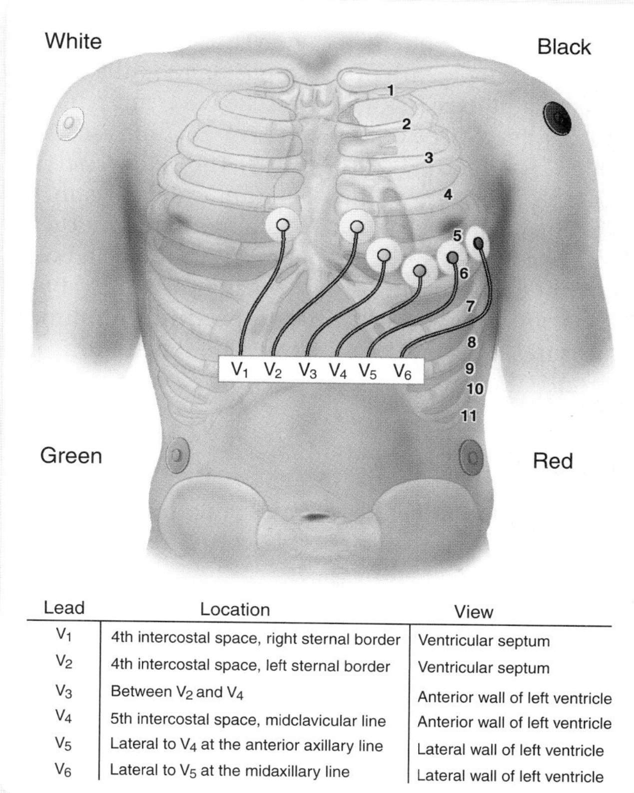

Lead	Location	View
V_1	4th intercostal space, right sternal border	Ventricular septum
V_2	4th intercostal space, left sternal border	Ventricular septum
V_3	Between V_2 and V_4	Anterior wall of left ventricle
V_4	5th intercostal space, midclavicular line	Anterior wall of left ventricle
V_5	Lateral to V_4 at the anterior axillary line	Lateral wall of left ventricle
V_6	Lateral to V_5 at the midaxillary line	Lateral wall of left ventricle

Figure 17-14 Placement of 12-lead electrodes.

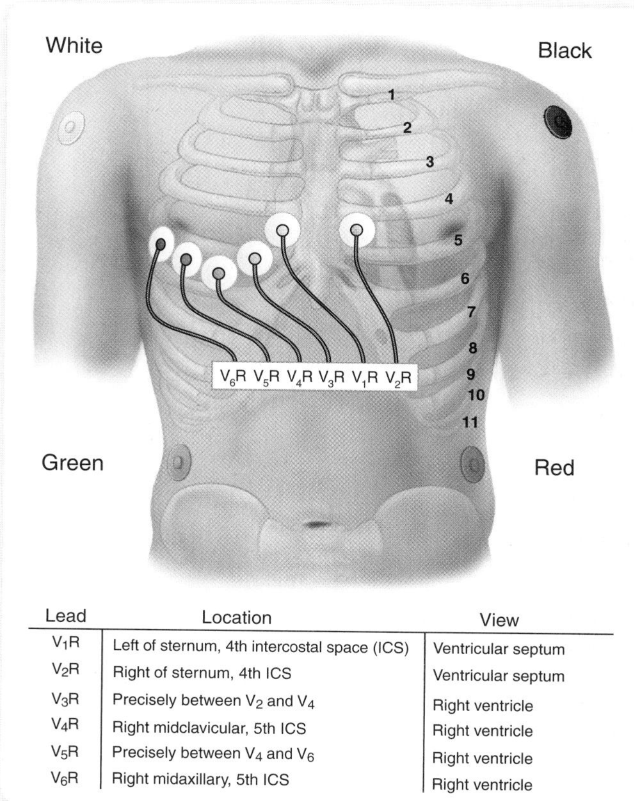

Lead	Location	View
V_1R	Left of sternum, 4th intercostal space (ICS)	Ventricular septum
V_2R	Right of sternum, 4th ICS	Ventricular septum
V_3R	Precisely between V_2 and V_4	Right ventricle
V_4R	Right midclavicular, 5th ICS	Right ventricle
V_5R	Precisely between V_4 and V_6	Right ventricle
V_6R	Right midaxillary, 5th ICS	Right ventricle

Figure 17-15 Placement of right-sided leads.

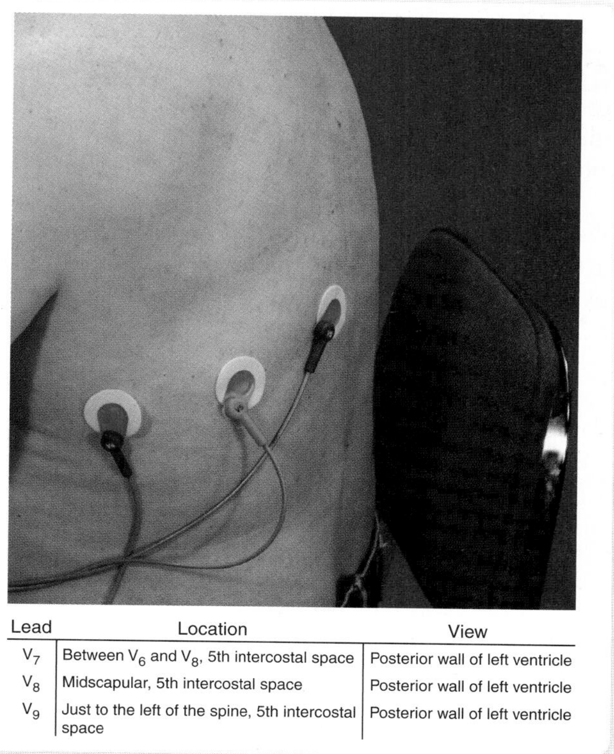

Lead	Location	View
V_7	Between V_6 and V_8, 5th intercostal space	Posterior wall of left ventricle
V_8	Midscapular, 5th intercostal space	Posterior wall of left ventricle
V_9	Just to the left of the spine, 5th intercostal space	Posterior wall of left ventricle

Figure 17-16 Placement of posterior leads.

15- and 18-Lead ECGs. Because a standard 12-lead ECG does not view the right ventricle or the posterior surface of the left ventricle, additional leads are needed to detect ischemia or infarction in those areas. A 15-lead ECG uses the standard 12-lead ECG, plus leads V_4R, V_7, and V_8. Obtaining a 15-lead ECG involves first recording a standard 12-lead and then recording a second tracing containing the additional leads.

An 18-lead ECG uses the standard 12-lead ECG tracing plus leads V_4R through V_6R and V_7 through V_9. To obtain an 18-lead ECG, (1) record a standard 12-lead, (2) record the right-sided precordial leads, and (3) record the posterior leads.

ECG Concepts

As we've mentioned, the ECG uses electrodes placed on the body to detect minute electrical waves traveling across surface of the skin. The ECG baseline is generally a flat, straight, horizontal line that reflects a period of electrical silence in the myocardium **Figure 17-17**. Although the baseline is neither positive nor negative, there is still electrical activity (movement of ions) in the myocardium. Perhaps it would be more accurate to describe the baseline as a period of electrical neutrality. The baseline is also referred to as the **isoelectric line**, *TP segment*, and *isomeric line.*

An electrical impulse moving in the direction of a negative electrode produces a deflection below the baseline.

Conversely, an electrical impulse moving toward a positive electrode produces a deflection above the baseline Figure 17-18. Perpendicular movement of an impulse toward a positive electrode produces either a perfectly flat line or a waveform with both a positive and a negative component. Such waveforms are called *biphasic waves*.

ECG Paper

ECGs are recorded on graph paper that moves past a stylus at a constant speed (25 mm/s). Thus, the horizontal distance on the graph paper represents a given period of time. Specifically, one small (1 mm) box is the equivalent of 0.04 second (1/25th of a second), or 40 milliseconds, and one large box (which consists of five small boxes) is the equivalent of 0.20 second, or 200 milliseconds ($0.04 \times 5 = 0.20$) Figure 17-19. The vertical axis on the graph paper represents the amplitude or "gain" of deflection, expressed in mV. The standard calibration for amplitude is 10 millimeters per mV. A calibration box is printed at the beginning of all 12-lead ECGs. The calibration box informs you of the paper speed and amplitude. It measures 5 mm wide by 10 mm tall, representing the standard 25-mm/s paper speed and 10-mm/mV gain Figure 17-20.

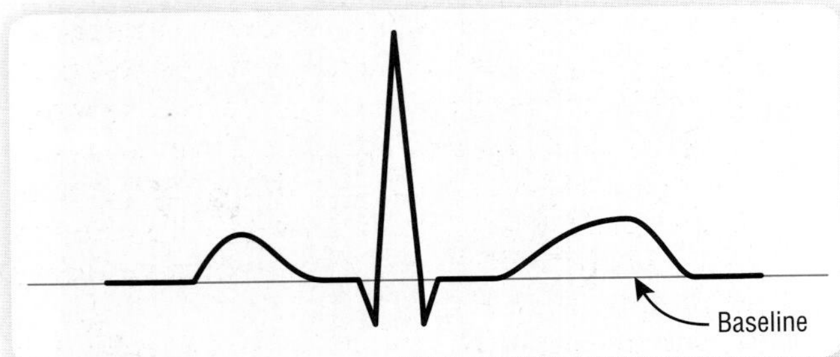

Figure 17-17 The electrocardiogram baseline.

Reproduced from *12-Lead ECG: The Art of Interpretation*, courtesy of Tomas B. Garcia, MD.

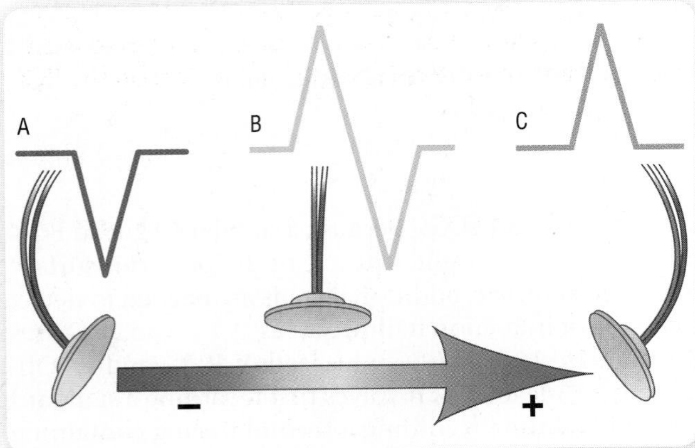

Figure 17-18 Negative, biphasic, and positive waveforms.

Reproduced from *12-Lead ECG: The Art of Interpretation*, courtesy of Tomas B. Garcia, MD.

ECG Components

The electrical conduction events in the heart can be recorded on an ECG as a series of waves, segments, intervals, and complexes Figure 17-21.

P Wave. The **P wave**, the first wave of an ECG complex, represents atrial depolarization and is characterized by a smooth, round, upright shape. The normal duration

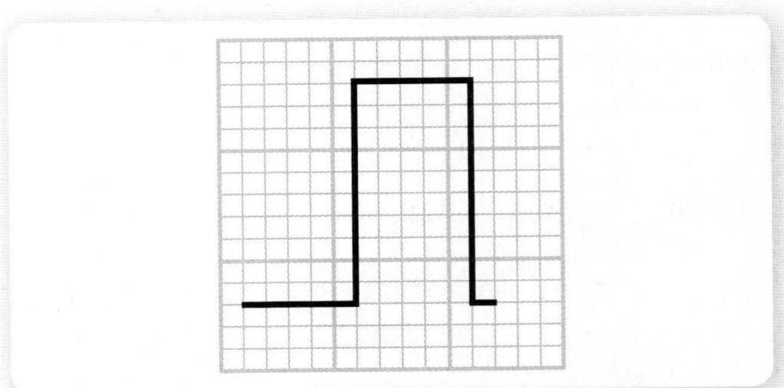

Figure 17-20 Calibration box, normally printed at the beginning of the electrocardiogram.

Reproduced from *12-Lead ECG: The Art of Interpretation*, courtesy of Tomas B. Garcia, MD.

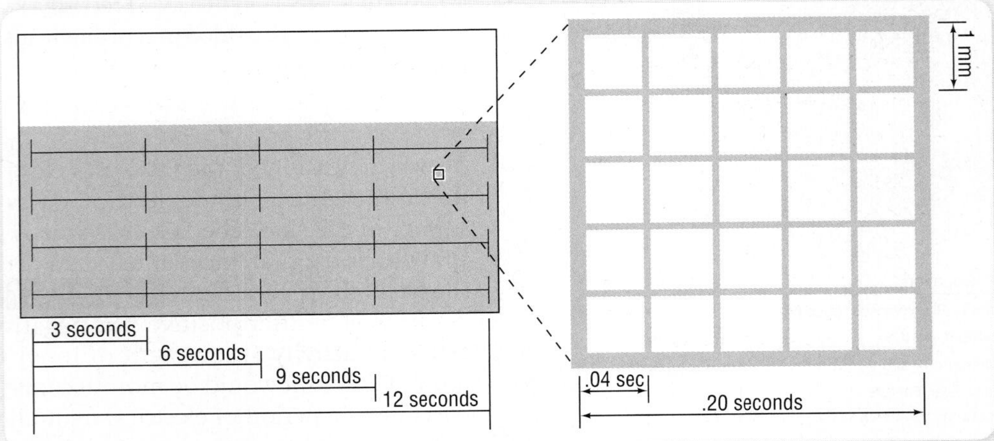

Figure 17-19 Electrocardiogram paper. Height, which indicates amplitude, is measured in millimeters (mm), and width is measured in milliseconds (ms) (0.04 seconds = 40 ms; 0.20 seconds = 200 ms).

Reproduced from *12-Lead ECG: The Art of Interpretation*, courtesy of Tomas B. Garcia, MD.

of a P wave is less than 0.11 seconds (110 milliseconds), and its amplitude is less than 2.5 mm tall.

PR Interval. The **PR interval (PRI)** is the distance from the beginning of the P wave to the beginning of the QRS complex. This distance represents the time required for an impulse to traverse the atria and AV junction, normally a period of 0.12 to 0.20 seconds (120 to 200 milliseconds). That's three to five small boxes on the ECG strip **Figure 17-22**. The PR segment represents the amount of time the AV node delays transmission of atrial activity to the ventricles. The wave produced by repolarization of the atria is too small to be seen on the ECG but occurs during the PR segment. When the AV node is diseased or hypoxic, the PR segment can become elongated **Figure 17-23**. Prolonged PRIs will be discussed later in the chapter, when AV blocks are introduced.

QRS Complex. The **QRS complex**, which consists of three waveforms, represents ventricular depolarization. It is measured from the beginning of the Q wave to the end of the S wave and should follow each P wave consistently.

In healthy adults, the QRS complex is narrow, with a normal duration of 0.11 seconds or less.[3] Such a complex indicates that impulse conduction has proceeded normally from the AV junction, through the bundle of His, left and right bundles, and Purkinje system. If impulse conduction is abnormal, then the complex has a bizarre appearance and a duration of 0.12 seconds (120 milliseconds) or longer.

The first negative deflection in the QRS, the *Q wave*, represents conduction through the interventricular septum. The electrical impulse spreads from right to left through the septum. A normal Q wave should last no more than 0.04 seconds (40 milliseconds) and should be less than one-third the overall height of the QRS complex. Q waves are considered abnormal or pathologic if they are more than 0.04 seconds (40 milliseconds) wide or deeper than one-third the total height (amplitude) of the QRS complex (in lead II). Such a finding is significant because it may indicate an AMI.

The first upward deflection of the QRS is referred to as the *R wave*. The S wave is any downward deflection after the R wave. A second upward deflection is called an R-prime (R′) wave. The R and S waves represent depolarization of the right and left ventricles.

As we discussed earlier, as a current moves toward a lead, it creates a positive (upright) deflection on the ECG

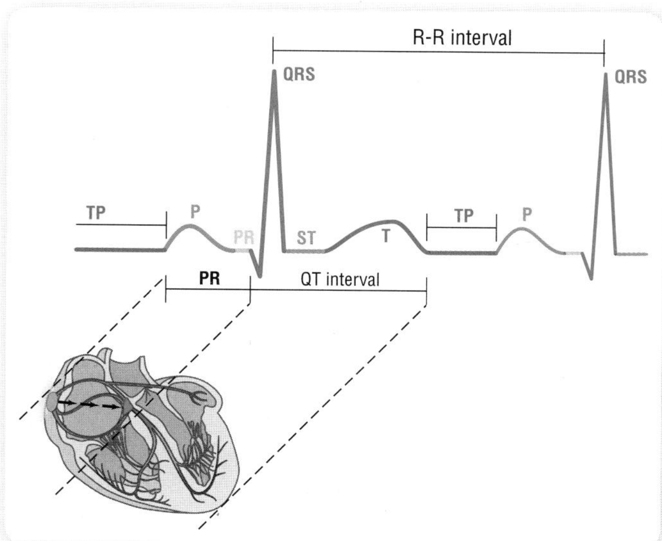

Figure 17-21 The electrocardiogram and cardiac events.

Reproduced from *12-Lead ECG: The Art of Interpretation*, courtesy of Tomas B. Garcia, MD.

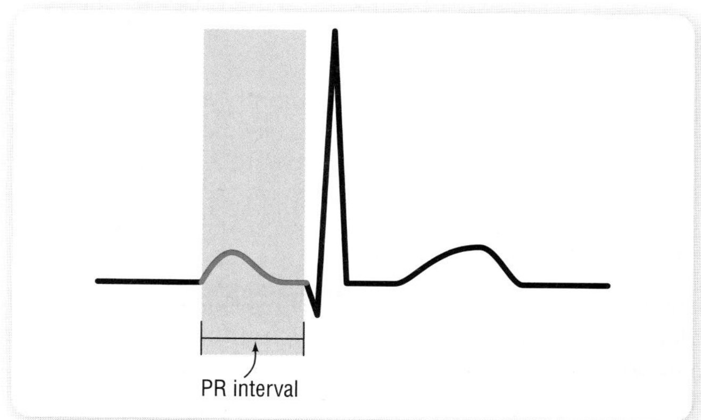

Figure 17-22 The normal PR interval is 0.12 to 0.20 seconds (120 to 200 milliseconds).

Reproduced from *12-Lead ECG: The Art of Interpretation*, courtesy of Tomas B. Garcia, MD.

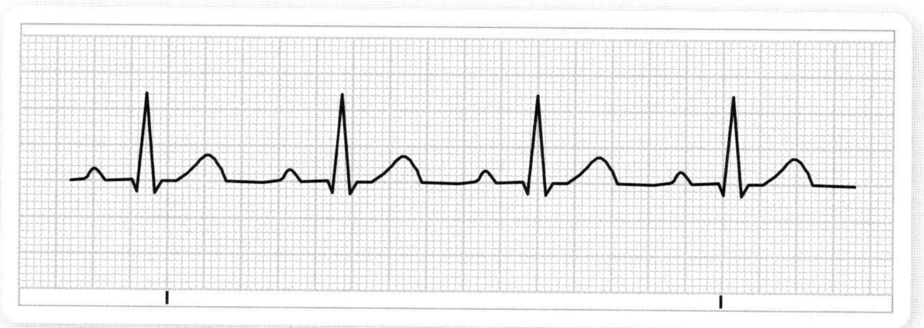

Figure 17-23 A PR interval greater than 0.20 seconds (200 milliseconds) is considered prolonged.

Reproduced from *Arrhythmia Recognition: The Art of Interpretation*, courtesy of Tomas B. Garcia, MD.

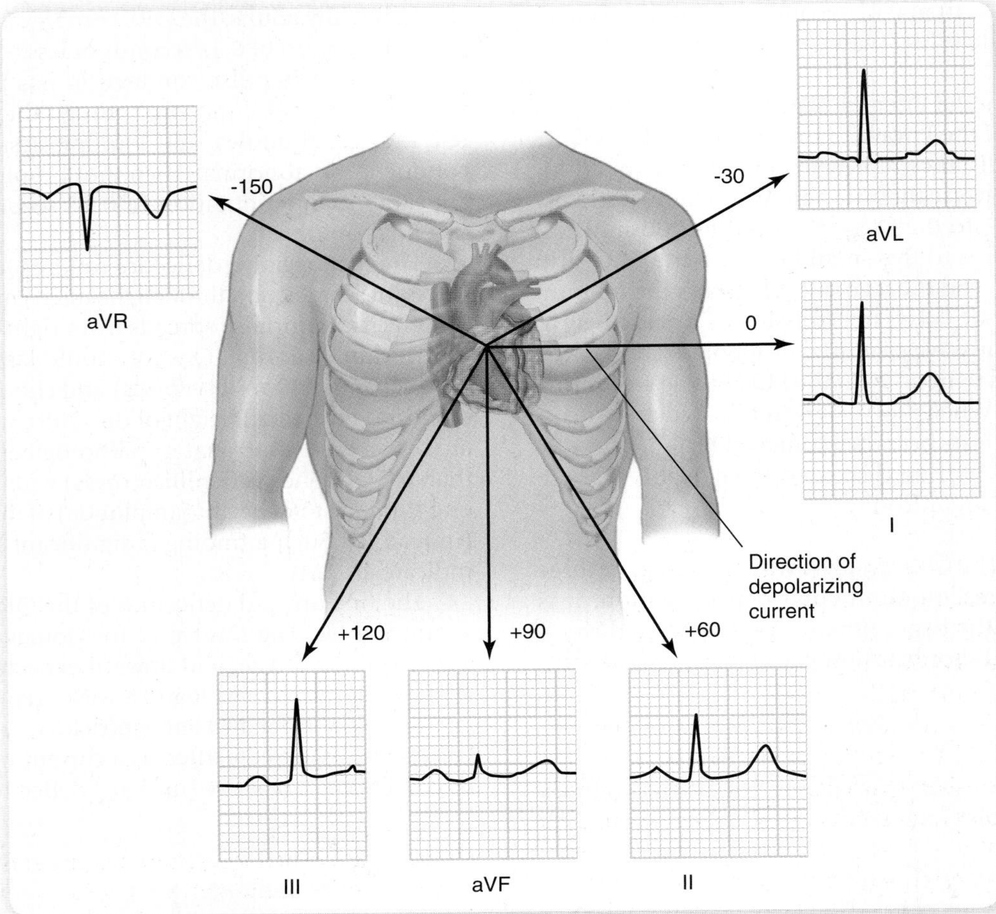

Figure 17-24 The morphology of the QRS complex depends on the lead position and in which direction the electrical impulse is moving within the heart. If the electrical impulse is moving primarily toward lead II, then it will be upright, as shown. However, lead aVR will be inverted because the impulse is moving away from it.

tracing of that lead. Thus, in Figure 17-24, the current depolarizing the ventricles is moving toward lead II, so what you see in lead II is an upright QRS complex. If the depolarizing current is moving toward lead II, then it must be moving away from lead aVR, so you would expect to see a negative deflection in that lead. And, indeed, the QRS complex in aVR reveals a downward deflection. That makes intuitive sense. For example, if you and a friend are standing facing each other at opposite ends of a football field, then a ball thrown toward your friend will appear bigger and bigger as it approaches the friend; however, the same ball will appear smaller and smaller to you. Similarly, leads II and aVR, being nearly opposite each other, will present nearly opposite images of the same wave of electrical depolarization. Like the football, if a depolarizing wave is coming toward lead II, it will be going away from aVR.

J Point. The J point is the point in the ECG at which the QRS complex ends and the ST segment begins Figure 17-25. Thus, it represents the end of depolarization and the apparent beginning of repolarization. The J point is significant because it often becomes depressed or elevated when the myocardium is ischemic. J-point changes are discussed later in this chapter.

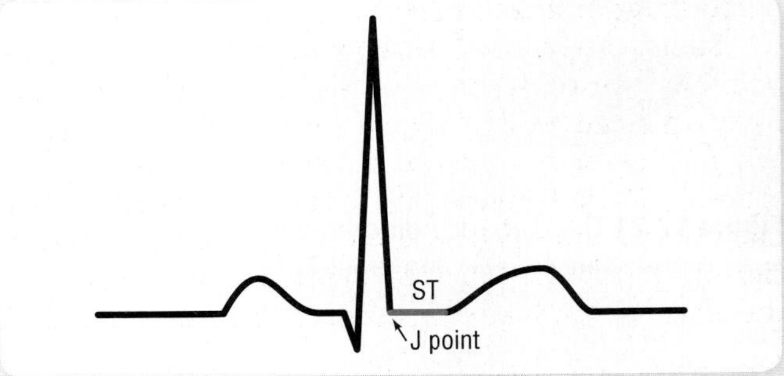

Figure 17-25 The J point.

ST Segment. The **ST segment** begins at the J point and ends at the T wave. The ST segment represents early ventricular repolarization. It can fall below, rise above, or stay at the baseline during a myocardial event. An elevated

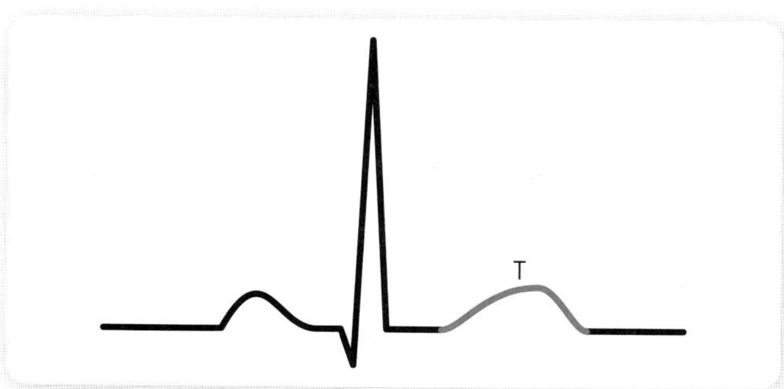

Figure 17-26 The T wave.

Reproduced from *Arrhythmia Recognition: The Art of Interpretation*, courtesy of Tomas B. Garcia, MD

ST segment may indicate myocardial injury. A depressed ST segment may indicate myocardial ischemia.

T Wave. A **T wave** is an upright, flat, or inverted wave following the QRS complex of the ECG, and represents ventricular repolarization. The T wave should be asymmetric, less than half the overall height of the QRS complex, and oriented in the same overall direction **Figure 17-26**. For example, if the QRS complex is predominantly upright, the T wave should be predominantly upright.

The T wave consists of two halves. The first half (closest to the QRS complex) represents the ARP. The second half represents the RRP.

During myocardial ischemia, injury, and infarction, the T wave becomes very large (hyperacute), peaked or tented in shape, symmetric, and broad. It's important to look for these changes on the ECG so you don't miss an ischemic event! Tall, pointed (peaked) T waves may be seen with **hyperkalemia** (an excessive concentration of potassium in the blood). Deeply inverted T waves may be seen with acute CNS events, such as intracranial hemorrhage or massive stroke.[4]

Sometimes, a U wave may be seen after a T wave and before the next P wave. Experts think the U wave most likely represents the final stage of ventricular repolarization. When it's seen, the direction of the U wave is usually the same as that of the preceding T wave in lead II. A U wave taller than 2 mm is considered abnormal and may be a sign of **hypokalemia** (a low concentration of potassium in the blood) or cardiomyopathy, among other conditions.

QT Interval. The QT interval represents all the electrical activity of one complete ventricular cycle (that is, ventricular depolarization and repolarization). It begins at the onset of the Q wave and ends as the T wave comes back to the baseline. If there is no Q wave, then measurement begins with the R wave. The QT interval varies with age, sex, and heart rate. The QT interval is considered short if it is 0.39 seconds (390 milliseconds) or less and prolonged if it is 0.46 seconds (460 milliseconds) or longer in women or 0.45 seconds (450 milliseconds) or longer in men.[5] A long QT interval can lead to ventricular dysrhythmias and sudden cardiac arrest.

Table 17-4 Components of the ECG

ECG Representation	Cardiac Event
P wave	Depolarization of the atria
PRI	Depolarization of the atria and delay at the AV junction
QRS complex	Depolarization of the ventricles
ST segment	Period between ventricular depolarization and beginning of repolarization
T wave	Ventricular repolarization
R-R interval	Time between two successive ventricular depolarizations

Abbreviations: AV, atrioventricular; ECG, electrocardiogram; PRI, PR interval

TP Segment. The TP segment begins at the end of the T wave and ends at the start of the P wave. This portion of the ECG tracing is generally a flat, straight, horizontal line used as the baseline. The baseline is the reference point to which we compare the J point.

R-R Interval. The **R-R interval** is the period between two successive QRS complexes. It represents the interval between two ventricular depolarizations. The R-R interval can be used to calculate the heart rate and to determine the regularity of the patient's cardiac rhythm **Table 17-4**.

▶ Approach to Dysrhythmia Interpretation

Part of your role as a paramedic will be to interpret ECG strips and be alert for dysrhythmias. Here we present a five-step method:

1. Identify the waves (P-QRS-T).
2. Measure the PRI.
3. Measure the QRS duration.
4. Determine rhythm regularity.
5. Measure the heart rate.

It is crucial to follow this method every time so you don't overlook any important findings on the ECG tracing. You'll usually exclusively use lead II for dysrhythmia interpretation.

We've already explained where P, QRS, and T waves appear, defined the PRI, and examined the QRS duration. If you can identify P waves, then note whether they are upright and fall within normal parameters. Is there only one P wave for every QRS complex? Next, we'll outline how to determine rhythm regularity and how to measure the heart rate.

Rhythm Regularity

Heart rhythm can be regular, regularly irregular, or irregularly irregular. Determining rhythm regularity can be as simple as measuring the distance between R waves. If the distance is exactly the same, then the rhythm is regular Figure 17-27. If no two R waves are equidistant, then the rhythm is irregularly irregular Figure 17-28. If the R waves are irregular, but appear to follow a pattern, then the rhythm is regularly irregular Figure 17-29. For example, let's say you obtain the following data when measuring the distance between R waves: 25 mm, 27 mm, 30 mm, 25 mm, 27 mm, and 30 mm. This pattern represents a regularly irregular rhythm. ECG calipers can also be used to measure the distance between R waves, or the edge of a piece of paper may be used as a makeshift ruler.

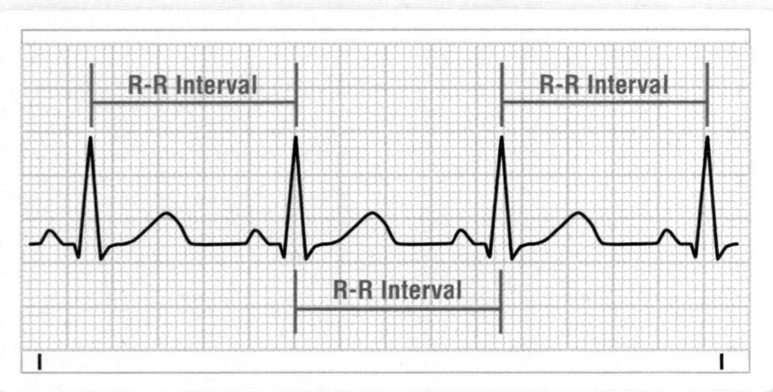

Figure 17-27 When the ventricular rhythm is regular, the R-R intervals are the same.

Reproduced from *Arrhythmia Recognition: The Art of Interpretation*, courtesy of Tomas B. Garcia, MD.

Determining Heart Rate

This section describes some of the more common ways of using a cardiac rhythm strip to determine heart rate.

The 6-Second Method. The 6-second method is the fastest way to measure heart rate from the ECG. Use this method for regular or irregular rhythms. In fact, it's the best method for calculating heart rate when the rhythm is irregular.

- Count the number of QRS complexes in a 6-second strip, and multiply that number by 10 to obtain the rate per minute Figure 17-30.

The Sequence Method. The sequence method Figure 17-31 should be used to determine the heart rate only when the rhythm is regular:

- First, memorize the following sequence: 300, 150, 100, 75, 60, 50.
- Find an R wave on a heavy line (large box), and count off "300, 150, 100, 75, 60, 50" for each large box you land on until you reach the next R wave. (Estimate the rate if the second R wave does not fall exactly on a heavy black line.)

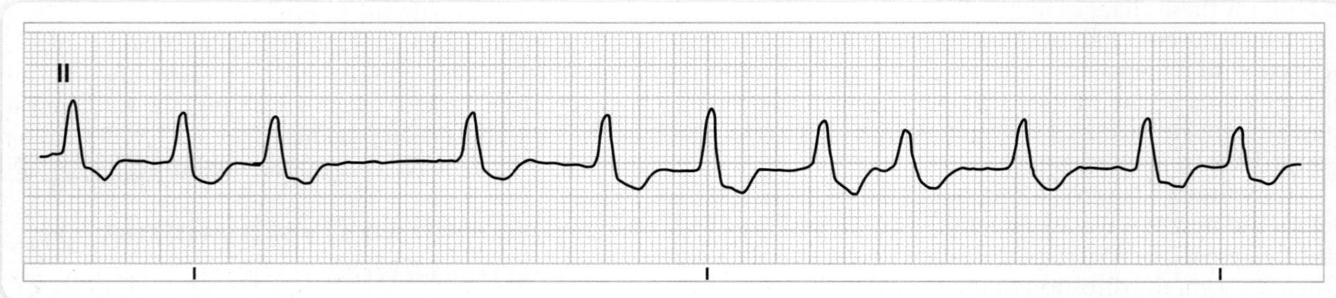

Figure 17-28 In an irregularly irregular rhythm, no two R-R intervals are the same. Note: The "II" in the upper left corner indicates this strip is from lead II.

Reproduced from *Arrhythmia Recognition: The Art of Interpretation*, courtesy of Tomas B. Garcia, MD.

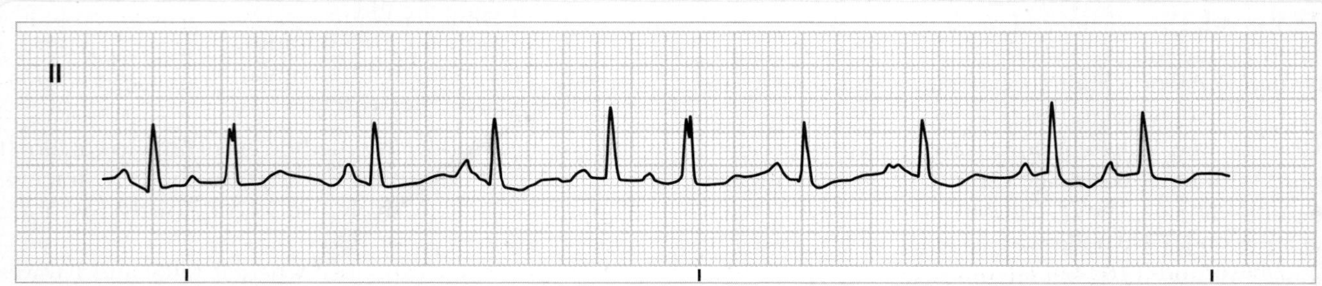

Figure 17-29 In a regularly irregular rhythm, the R-R intervals follow a discernible pattern.

Reproduced from *Arrhythmia Recognition: The Art of Interpretation*, courtesy of Tomas B. Garcia, MD.

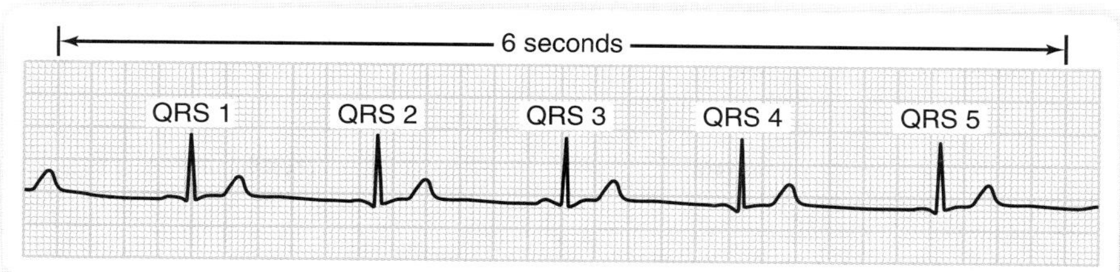

Figure 17-30 Calculation of heart rate. To calculate the rate, count the number of QRS complexes in a 6-second strip and multiply by 10.

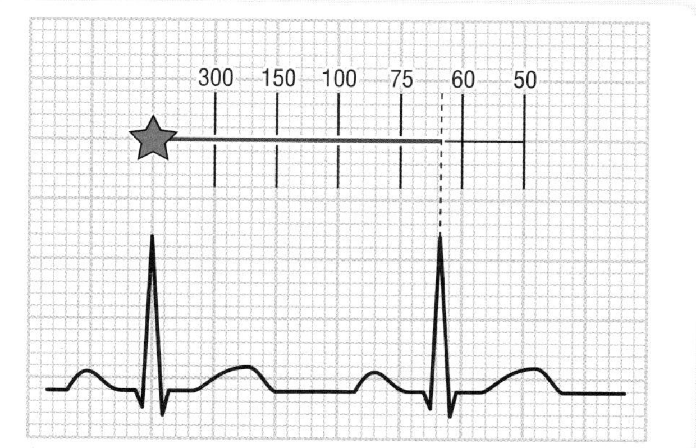

Figure 17-31 The sequence method.

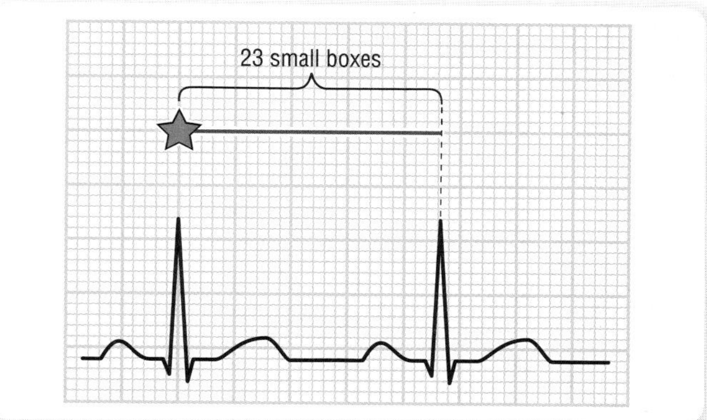

Figure 17-32 The 1500 method.

- If the R-R interval spans fewer than three large boxes, then the rate is greater than 100 (tachycardia). If it covers more than five large boxes, the rate is less than 60 (bradycardia).

The 1500 Method. The 1500 method is the most accurate way to calculate the heart rate from the ECG. It is typically used when the heart rate exceeds 150 beats/min, and only when the rhythm is regular:

- Calculate the rate by counting the number of small boxes between any two QRS complexes (the R-R interval); then divide 1500 by that number.
- In Figure 17-32, for example, there are about 23 small boxes between two successive QRS complexes:

$$1500 \div 23 = 65$$

- This calculation yields a rate of about 65 beats/min.

Specific Cardiac Dysrhythmias

A variety of events can induce cardiac dysrhythmia. Electricity flows differently through damaged or oxygen-deprived tissue from the way it flows through normal, well-oxygenated tissue. This altered flow sometimes appears as an irregularity on the ECG. Many of these irregularities can be traced to ischemia, especially in areas of the heart responsible for conduction. Ischemia often causes spontaneous depolarization, generating a premature complex. These premature complexes interfere with normal impulse conduction and induce dysrhythmia. In other situations, ischemia occurs within the conduction system and is the direct cause of its malfunction.

Many cardiac dysrhythmias are well tolerated and produce no serious symptoms, making it difficult to estimate the number of people affected them. It's well documented, however, that cardiac dysrhythmia is the most common cause of cardiac arrest.

There are nearly as many ways of classifying cardiac dysrhythmias as there are books on the subject. Dysrhythmias can be characterized as disturbances of automaticity or disturbances of conduction. They can be separated into rhythms that are too fast (tachydysrhythmias) or too slow (bradydysrhythmias), or classified as life threatening or non–life threatening. In this section, we have categorized cardiac dysrhythmias according to the site from which they arise (and as they appear in lead II). After looking at a sinus rhythm for comparison, we will cover the dysrhythmias that arise in the SA node, atrial tissue, AV junction, and ventricles. Last, we'll explore paced rhythms.

Rhythms Originating in the SA Node

Normal Sinus Rhythm

The SA node is the primary pacemaker for the heart. A **normal sinus rhythm** Figure 17-33 arises in the SA node,

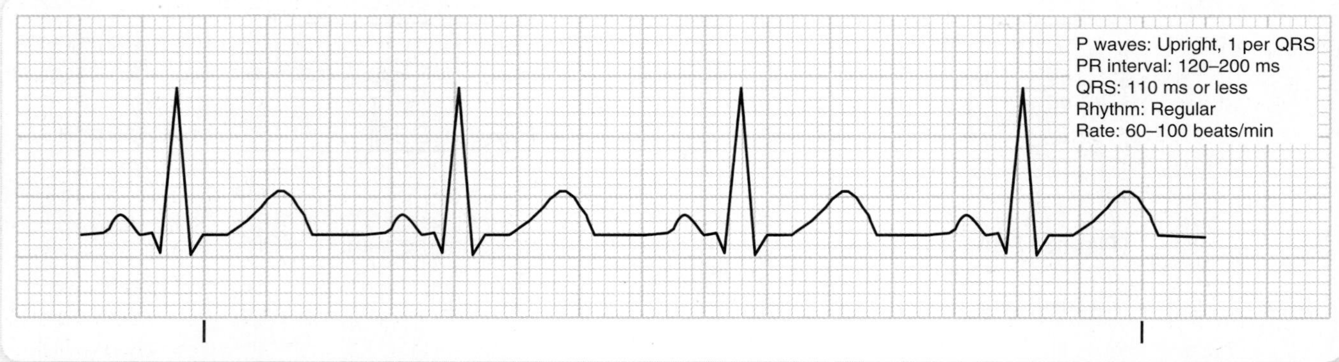

Figure 17-33 Normal sinus rhythm.

Reproduced from *Arrhythmia Recognition: The Art of Interpretation*, courtesy of Tomas B. Garcia, MD.

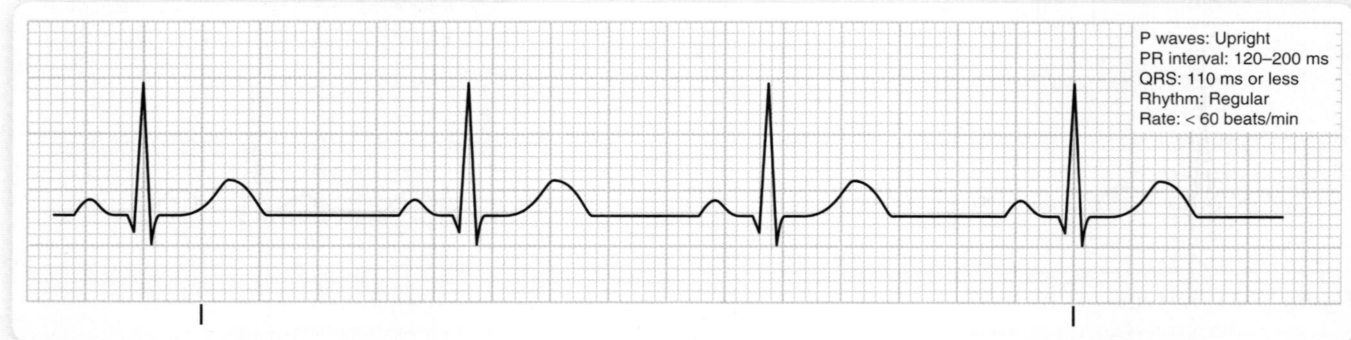

Figure 17-34 Sinus bradycardia.

Reproduced from *Arrhythmia Recognition: The Art of Interpretation*, courtesy of Tomas B. Garcia, MD.

has an intrinsic rate of 60 to 100 beats/min. The rhythm is regular, with minimal variation between R-R intervals. An upright P wave precedes each QRS complex. The PRI measures 0.12 to 0.20 seconds (120 to 200 milliseconds). The QRS complex measures 0.11 seconds (110 milliseconds) or less.

Sinus Bradycardia

In **sinus bradycardia**, the pacemaker is still the SA node, but the rate is less than 60 beats/min **Figure 17-34**. The rhythm is regular, and an upright P wave precedes each QRS complex. The PRI is 0.12 to 0.20 seconds (120 to 200 milliseconds). The QRS complex is 0.11 seconds (110 milliseconds) or less.

A very slow heart rate (usually less than 50 beats/min) leads to inadequate CO and often precipitates electrical instability of the heart. Furthermore, when the sinus rate becomes very slow, ectopic pacemakers in the AV junction or ventricles may fire, producing escape beats to assist in maintaining CO. The term **ectopic** refers to an impulse or rhythm that originates from a site other than the SA node.

In healthy adults, especially conditioned athletes, sinus bradycardia can be an asymptomatic phenomenon and may occur during sleep. In other adults, however, bradycardia can cause altered mental status, ischemic chest discomfort, acute heart failure, or hypotension. Treatment is indicated when these signs and symptoms persist despite an adequate airway and breathing.

Management of Symptomatic Bradycardia. Goals for the emergency medical care of an adult patient with symptomatic bradycardia are listed below:

- Maintain adequate oxygenation, ventilation, and perfusion.
- Correct the rhythm disturbance and restore a stable perfusing rhythm.
- Search for the underlying cause, which may be hypoxia, hypothermia, shock, AMI, AV block, toxin exposure (beta-blockers, calcium channel blockers, organophosphates, digoxin), an electrolyte disorder, increased intracranial pressure, or other factors.

Follow these steps to administer emergency medical care for an adult with symptomatic bradycardia:

1. Maintain an open airway. Assist breathing as necessary. Administer supplemental oxygen as needed to maintain an SpO_2 of 94% or higher.
2. Apply a cardiac monitor, blood pressure monitor, and pulse oximeter. Obtain a 12-lead ECG, but do not delay emergency care.

3. Establish an IV infusion of normal saline. Obtain a finger-stick blood glucose. Treat hypoglycemia if present.
4. Administer atropine IV bolus for symptomatic sinus bradycardia or a conduction block at the level of the AV node. Repeat atropine every 3 to 5 minutes until the desired heart rate is achieved (usually 60 beats/min or faster) or until the dosage limit of 3 mg has been reached. Cardiac-related medications are discussed in detail in Chapter 13, *Principles of Pharmacology*.
5. If atropine is ineffective and the patient's symptoms or hemodynamic instability persist, then consider transcutaneous pacing or the administration of a dopamine or epinephrine infusion.
6. Transport the patient for definitive care.

Recommended treatment guidelines for adult bradycardia are shown in **Figure 17-35**.

Artificial pacemakers deliver repetitive bursts of electrical impulses to the heart. Like the tiny electrical signals generated by natural pacemakers, the current from an artificial pacemaker can depolarize the myocardial tissue. In doing so, the artificial pacemaker can substitute for a blocked or nonfunctional natural pacemaker.

Transcutaneous pacemakers—that is, pacemakers that depolarize the myocardium by delivering electrical energy through the skin of the chest—have come into widespread use. With a TCP, a small electrical charge passes through the patient's skin between one external pacing pad and another, spreading the signal across the heart. The pacer is set for a specific rate, and the energy increases until the heart begins to react to the stimulus. This response, which is termed "capture," is usually associated with ventricular depolarization. It is characterized by a wide QRS complex on the ECG and should result in a corresponding pulse.

In any of the following circumstances, TCP may allow enough time for the patient to reach a medical facility in a state of optimal perfusion, rather than in or near cardiac arrest:

- Patient with a bradydysrhythmia that severely reduces CO and does not respond to atropine

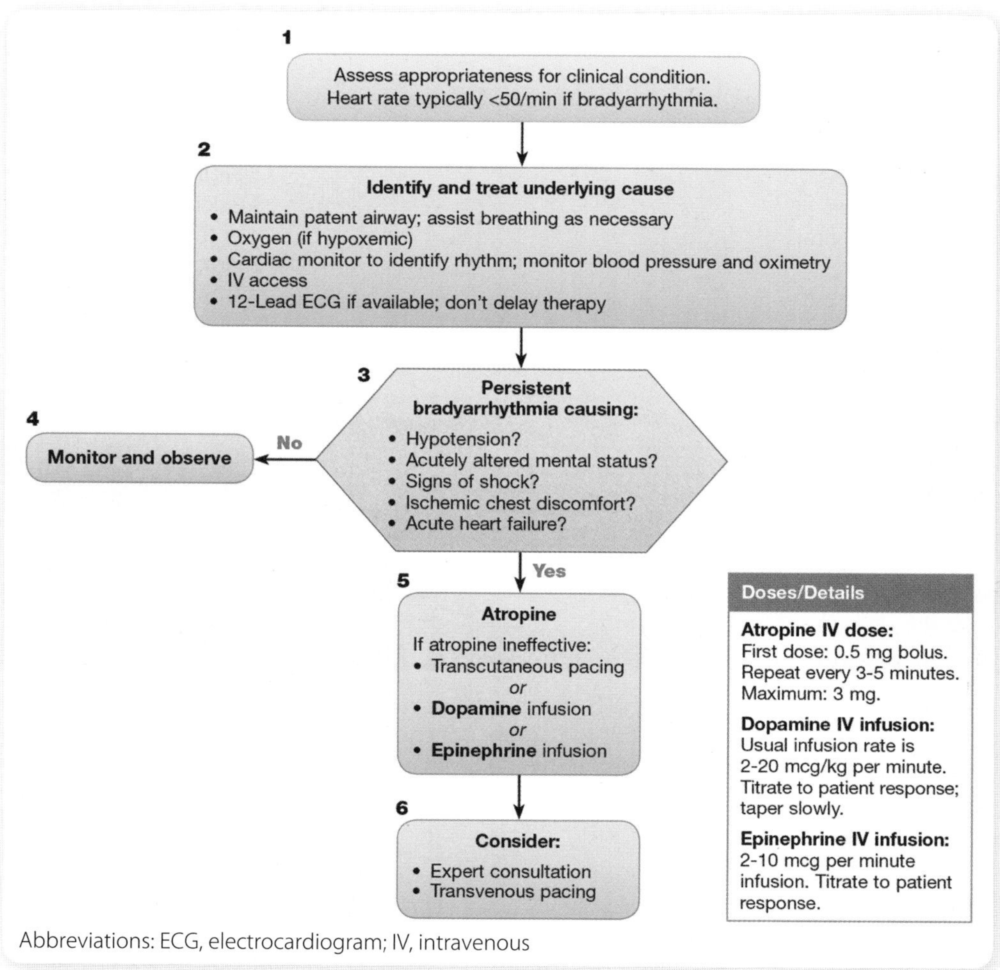

Figure 17-35 Adult bradycardia with a pulse algorithm.

- Patient who requires interhospital transfer for pacemaker implantation
- Symptomatic patient with artificial pacemaker failure

Many brands of TCPs are available, so you must become familiar with the specific device used in your local EMS system. The steps in initiating TCP are shown in Skill Drill 17-2.

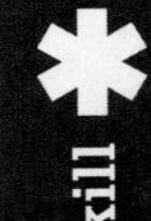

NR Skill

Skill Drill 17-2 Performing Transcutaneous Pacing

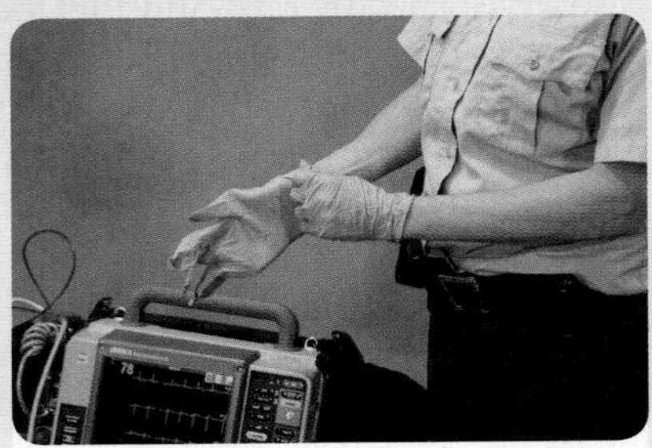

Step 1 Select, check, and assemble all necessary equipment, including a monitor/defibrillator with pacing capability, ECG electrodes, pacing pads, medication for pain or sedation (to be used if necessary), oxygen, and an appropriate oxygen administration device. Take standard precautions. Apply the ECG electrodes and assess the patient's vital signs. Ensure the patient is oxygenated adequately, and establish a patent IV line.

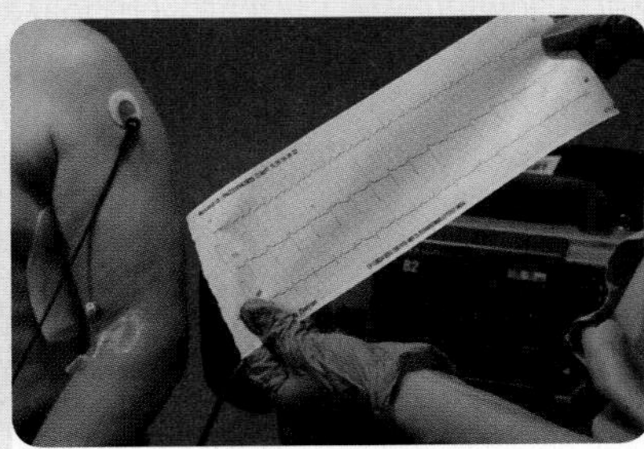

Step 2 Identify the rhythm and confirm TCP is warranted. Obtain a baseline rhythm strip.

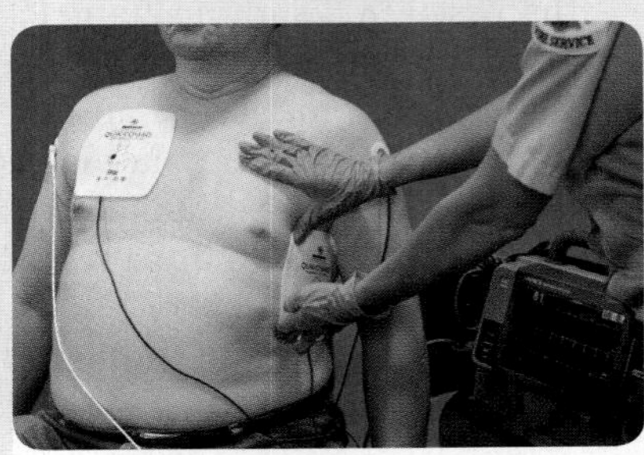

Step 3 Ensure the scene and environment are safe (evaluate the risk of sparks, combustibles, oxygen-rich atmosphere). Explain to the patient and the family the need for the procedure. Apply the pacing pads to the patient according to the manufacturer's recommendations. Sedation or analgesia may be needed to minimize the discomfort associated with this procedure. Ask the patient about any medication allergies before administering medications.

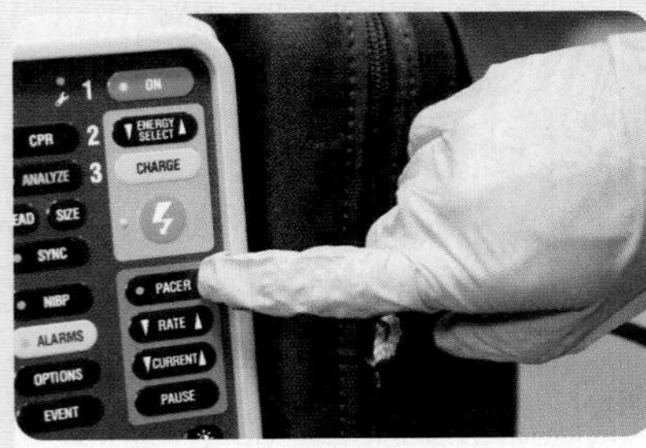

Step 4 Switch on power to the pacer.

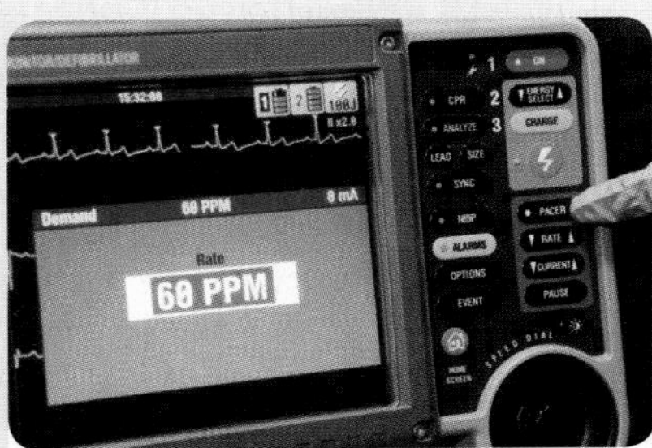

Step 5 Set the pacing rate to the desired number of paced pulses per minute (ppm). A rate between 60 and 80 beats/min is usually selected.

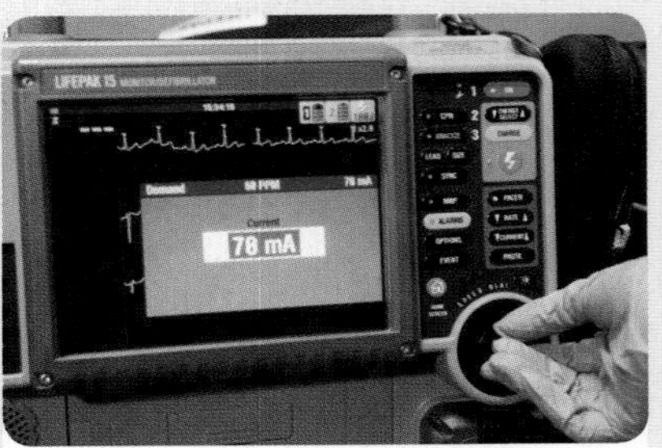

Step 6 Set the current (milliamps) to be delivered to the minimum setting. While watching the monitor screen, slowly but steadily increase the current until you achieve electrical capture (each pacer spike is followed by a wide QRS complex).

Skill Drill 17-2 Performing Transcutaneous Pacing *(continued)*

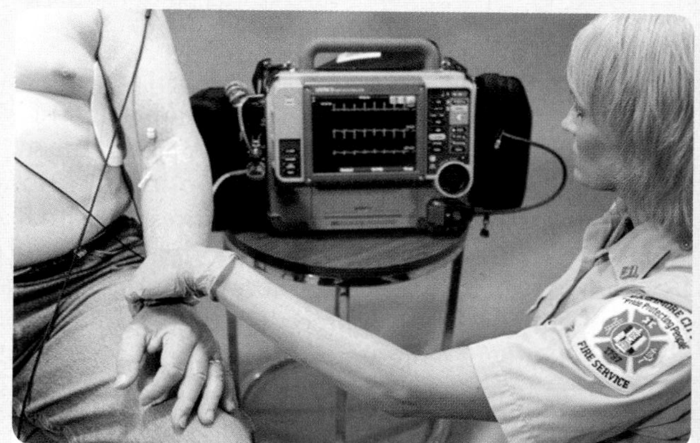

Step 7 Evaluate mechanical capture by assessing the patient's pulse and blood pressure. Reassess the patient's mental status, Spo_2, color, and level of discomfort.

Step 8 Obtain rhythm strips for documentation, and continuously monitor the patient's condition.

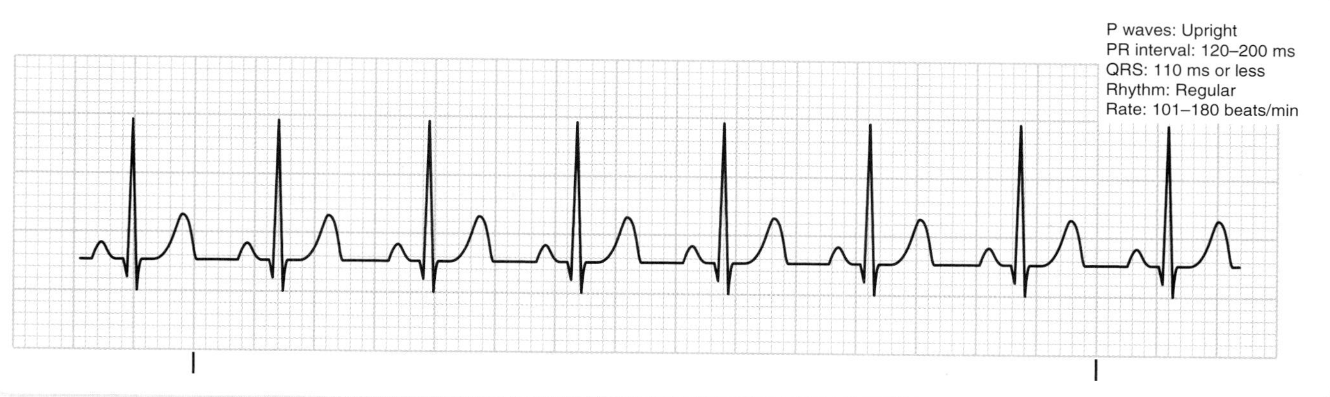

Figure 17-36 Sinus tachycardia.

Reproduced from *Arrhythmia Recognition: The Art of Interpretation*, courtesy of Tomas B. Garcia, MD.

Documentation & Communication

Key documentation elements for the patient with symptomatic bradycardia are as follows:[6]

- Time and dosage of medications given
- Time at which pacing is started (including pulses per minute and energy setting)
- Monitor strips obtained before and during pacing and at time of transfer

Sinus Tachycardia

By definition, a tachycardia has a ventricular rate faster than 100 beats/min. With **sinus tachycardia**, the SA node is still the pacemaker but the heart rate is typically 101 to 180 beats/min in a resting adult **Figure 17-36**. Experts note that the upper rate of sinus tachycardia is age related and can be calculated as approximately 220 beats/min minus the patient's age in years.[7] The rhythm is regular, and an upright P wave precedes each QRS complex (although it is occasionally difficult to see if it is partially buried in the T wave of the beat before it). The PRI is 0.12 to

0.20 seconds (120 to 200 milliseconds). The QRS complex is 0.11 seconds (110 milliseconds) or less.

Sinus tachycardia has a variety of causes, including pain, fever, hypoxia, hypovolemia, exercise, sympathetic nervous system stimulation (caused by stress, fright, or anxiety), AMI, pump failure, or anemia. In addition, caffeine, nicotine, alcohol, and certain other drugs, such as atropine, epinephrine, amphetamine, and cocaine, can cause tachycardia. Hypoxia, metabolic alkalosis, hypokalemia, and **hypocalcemia** can lead to electrical instability, prompting the firing of cells that normally do not generate impulses.

Prolonged tachycardia increases the work of the heart, leading to further ischemia during an AMI. In addition, CO may be significantly reduced when the heart rate exceeds 150 beats/min because the ventricles have inadequate time to fill completely between contractions.

The treatment of sinus tachycardia depends on its underlying cause.

Sinus Dysrhythmia

Sinus dysrhythmia is a slight variation in cycling of a sinus rhythm, usually exceeding 0.12 seconds (120 milliseconds) between the longest and shortest cycles that is often associated with respiratory cycle fluctuations **Figure 17-37**. The rate increases during inspiration and decreases during expiration. The SA node is still the pacemaker, and an upright P wave precedes each QRS complex. The PRI of 0.12 to 0.20 seconds (120 to 200 milliseconds) and the QRS complex of 0.11 seconds (110 milliseconds) or less are the same as in a normal sinus rhythm. Sinus dysrhythmia is often a normal finding in children and young adults and tends to diminish with age.

Sinus Arrest

Sinus arrest occurs when the SA node fails to initiate an impulse, eliminating the P wave, QRS complex, and T wave for one cardiac cycle **Figure 17-38**. After this missed set of waveforms, the SA node resumes normal functioning as if nothing ever happened. In sinus arrest, the atrial and ventricular rates are usually within normal limits and the rhythm is regular except for the absent complexes. P waves are present and upright, preceding every QRS complex, and the PRI, when present, is 0.12 to 0.20 seconds (120 to 200 milliseconds). The QRS complex, when present, is 0.11seconds (110 milliseconds) or less.

Possible causes of sinus arrest include SA node ischemia, increased vagal tone, carotid sinus massage (discussed later in this chapter), and the use of drugs such as digitalis and quinidine. Occasional episodes of sinus arrest are not significant; however, if the heart rate drops below 60 beats/min, CO may fall and an ectopic focus from either the AV junction or the ventricles may take over. In such circumstances, treatment is based on the patient's overall heart rate and tolerance. He or she may benefit from a temporary pacemaker (TCP in the

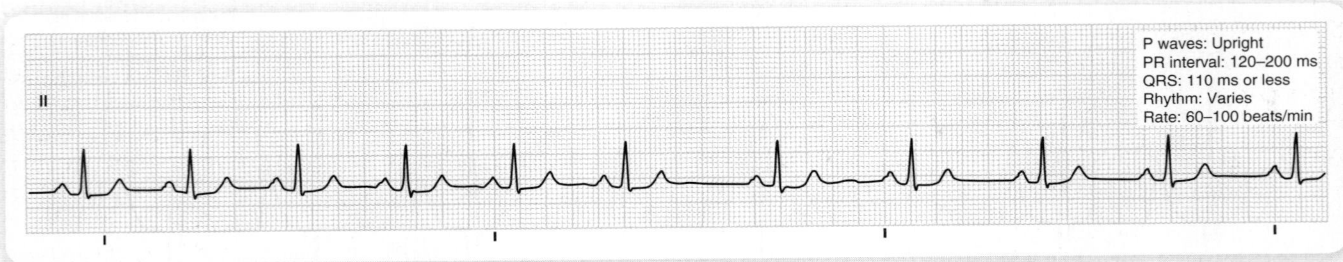

Figure 17-37 Sinus dysrhythmia.

Reproduced from *Arrhythmia Recognition: The Art of Interpretation*, courtesy of Tomas B. Garcia, MD.

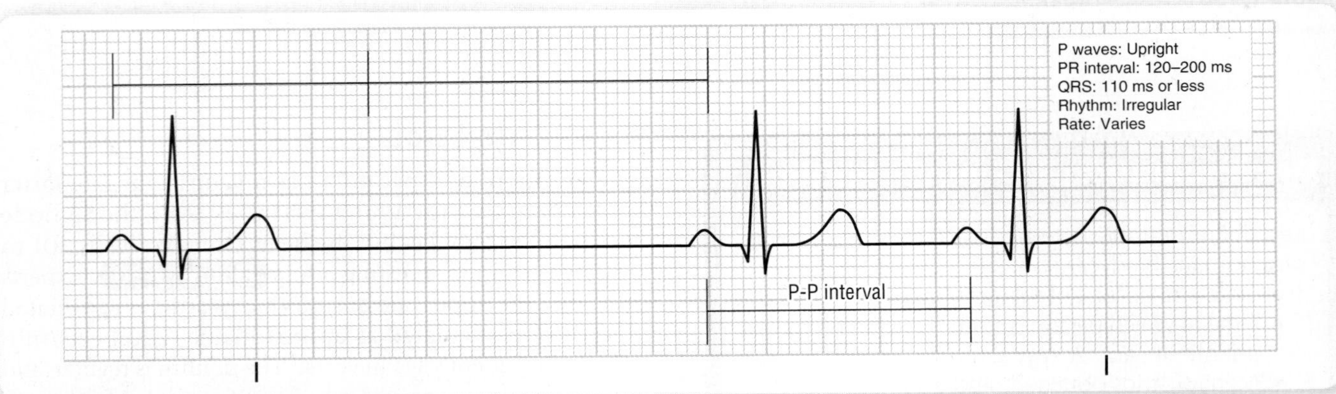

Figure 17-38 With a sinus arrest, at least one PQRST cycle is missing. Because of this, the resulting P-P interval is not an exact multiple of the normal P-P interval.

Modified from *Arrhythmia Recognition: The Art of Interpretation*, courtesy of Tomas B. Garcia, MD.

field) or a permanent pacemaker after admission to the medical facility.

Sick Sinus Syndrome

Sick sinus syndrome (SSS) encompasses a variety of rhythms characterized by a poorly functioning SA node. This condition is common among older adults. Patients may remain asymptomatic, or they may have syncopal or near-syncopal episodes, dizziness, and palpitations. On an ECG, SSS may be evidenced by sinus bradycardia, sinus arrest, SA block, and alternating patterns of extreme bradycardia and tachycardia (bradycardia-tachycardia syndrome).

▶ Rhythms Originating in the Atria

Although the SA node is normally the pacemaker for the heart, any area of the atria can originate an impulse, thereby superseding the pacemaking authority of the SA node. Some rhythms originating from the atria produce upright P waves that precede each QRS complex, but are not as well rounded as those generated by the SA node.

Premature Atrial Complex

A premature atrial complex (PAC) is not, strictly speaking, a dysrhythmia, but rather an ectopic complex that appears within another rhythm Figure 17-39. A PAC occurs earlier than the next expected sinus complex, producing an abnormally short R-R interval between it and the previous complex. The presence of a PAC will make the rhythm irregular. An upright P wave precedes each QRS complex; however, its shape differs from the P waves originating from the SA node, indicating its different site of origin. The PRI measures 0.12 to 0.20 seconds (120 to 200 milliseconds) but may vary slightly based on the origin of the premature complex. The QRS complex measures 0.11 seconds (110 milliseconds).

Premature atrial complexes are not always conducted to the ventricles. A P wave that occurs early on the ECG and is not followed by a QRS complex is called a *nonconducted PAC*. This phenomenon should not be confused with AV block. The two are easily differentiated because, unlike AV block, nonconducted PACs occur infrequently, in no particular pattern, producing a P wave that occurs early on the ECG. If you measure the P-P interval, then the P wave associated with nonconducted PAC will be shorter than the other P-P intervals. However, in AV block, the P-P interval is constant.

PACs are very common and can be caused by stress, stimulants such as caffeine, or conditions such as heart failure or electrolyte imbalance. When PACs are frequent, treatment is focused on correcting the underlying cause.

Supraventricular Tachycardia

Supraventricular tachycardia (SVT) is a rhythm that originates from a site above the ventricles with a ventricular rate faster than 100 beats/min at rest.[8] In patients with normal ventricular function, tachycardia with a rate of less than 150 beats/min rarely causes serious signs and symptoms. However, when the ventricular rate exceeds 150 beats/min, ventricular filling time is reduced, which can in turn reduce CO. When the ventricular rate reaches 150 to 180 beats/min, the P waves (if present) with SVT tend to be completely obscured by the T wave of the preceding beat Figure 17-40, making it impossible to measure the PRI. At a lower heart rate, P waves can be identified. The rhythm is regular, with essentially no variation between R-R intervals. The QRS complexes measure 0.11 seconds (110 milliseconds) or less, indicating that the rhythm originates above the ventricles.

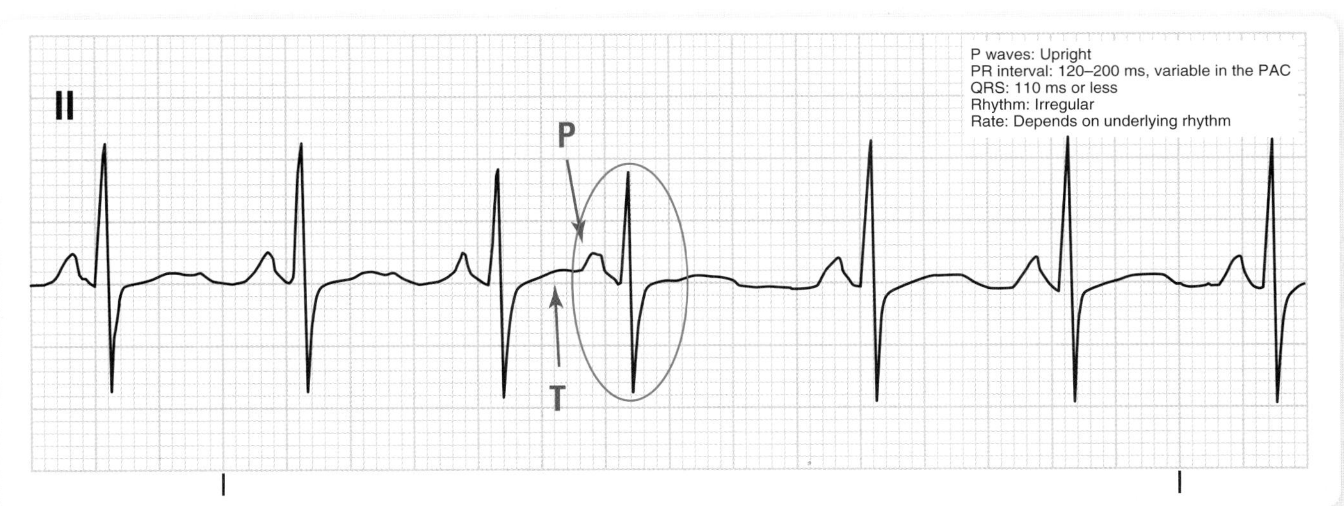

Figure 17-39 Premature atrial complex.

Reproduced from *Arrhythmia Recognition: The Art of Interpretation*, courtesy of Tomas B. Garcia, MD.

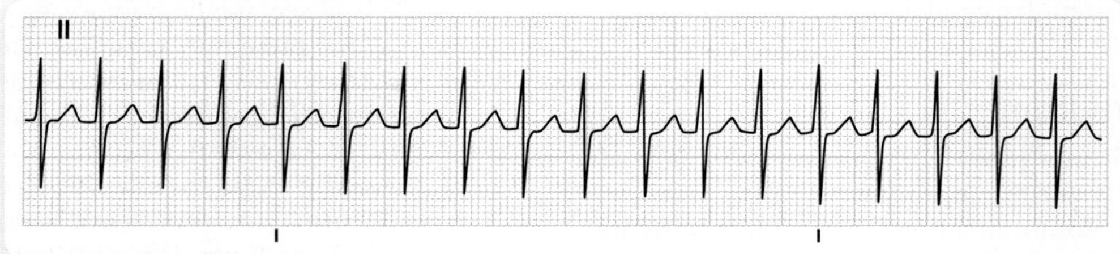

Figure 17-40 Supraventricular tachycardia.

Reproduced from *Arrhythmia Recognition: The Art of Interpretation*, courtesy of Tomas B. Garcia, MD.

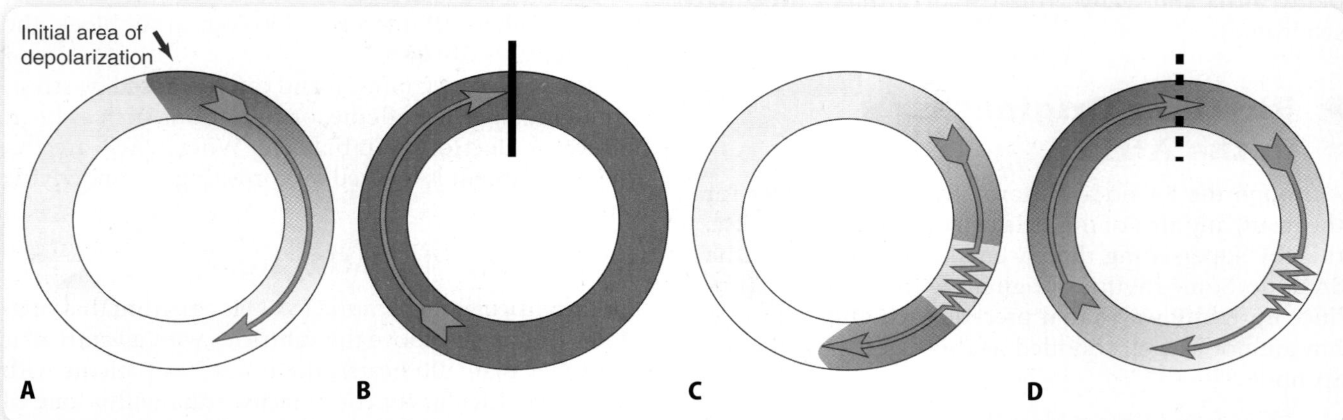

Figure 17-41 Reentry. **A.** The original impulse site fires, triggering a wave of depolarization that spreads over the remaining cells in the direction shown. **B.** When the depolarization wave returns to the original site (represented by the black line) the site is still refractory and cannot respond to the new impulse. The wave essentially subsides at this point. **C.** The yellow portion represents an area of slow conduction. The depolarization wave slows as it traverses this area. **D.** By the time the depolarization wave reaches the original site, represented by the dotted black line, the site is ready to receive a new impulse. The result is a self-perpetuating cyclical movement.

Reproduced from *Arrhythmia Recognition: The Art of Interpretation*, courtesy of Tomas B. Garcia, MD.

Words of Wisdom

As you learn the criteria for cardiac dysrhythmias, you will notice the ventricular rate ranges for various dysrhythmias overlap. Carefully examine the ECG, identifying waveforms and calculating measurements, to aid in correctly identifying the dysrhythmia. When you are unsure about the origin of a rhythm, obtaining a 12-lead ECG can be helpful because you can observe the rhythm in multiple leads.

The most common type of SVT is called *AV nodal reentrant tachycardia.* As its name implies, this type of SVT is associated with **reentry**, which is the spread of an impulse through tissue already stimulated by that same impulse **Figure 17-41**. Under the right conditions, such as when myocardial ischemia is present, a premature impulse can trigger a series of rapid beats. The AV node may be bombarded by more than one impulse, which can block the pathway of one signal and allow another to stimulate cardiac cells that have already depolarized. The danger here comes when these impulses get stuck in a repetitive pattern, generating multiple ectopic beats or a very rapid rhythm.

SVT is sometimes referred to as *paroxysmal SVT (PSVT)*, reflecting its tendency to begin and end abruptly (*paroxysmal* means "occurring in spasms"). Technically, to identify a dysrhythmia as a PSVT, you would need to witness the rhythm acceleration on the ECG.

Patients who present with SVT sometimes have a physical finding known as *cannon "A" waves*. Cannon "A" waves are created when a dissociation between the atria and ventricles occurs. This sign can also occur with right atrial contraction against a closed tricuspid valve. Larger "A" waves can indicate deteriorating functionality of the right ventricle or increasing right ventricular end-diastolic pressure. A corresponding physical sign can be found where the jugular veins are located: during the cannon "A" wave, a depression of the jugular veins occurs, forming an "A."

Symptoms associated with SVT vary. The treatment for SVT depends on the severity of the patient's symptoms and may include medication or electrical therapy to slow the heart rate.

Management of Tachycardia With a Pulse. Treating a patient who presents with or develops tachycardia is more complicated than treating a patient with bradycardia. Tachycardia can originate from a supraventricular pacemaker site or may have a ventricular origin. Generally, wide QRS complexes are presumed to be of ventricular origin, whereas narrow QRS complexes (0.11 seconds [110 milliseconds] or less) are presumed to be of supraventricular origin. VT is discussed later in this chapter. Occasionally, a beat of supraventricular origin will follow an aberrant conduction pathway, making it difficult to determine whether the tachycardia is ventricular or supraventricular. In most cases, the rhythm is ventricular, rather than supraventricular, and should be treated as such.

Goals for emergency medical care of a patient with tachycardia with a pulse include the following:[6]

- Maintain adequate oxygenation, ventilation, and perfusion.
- Correct the rhythm disturbance and restore a sinus rhythm.
- Search for the underlying causes, such as medications (caffeine, diet pills, thyroid agents, or decongestants), illicit drugs (cocaine, amphetamines), heart failure, or a history of dysrhythmia.

Because of the many possible variations among tachycardic patients, you must make several judgments before you begin treatment. First, determine the severity of the patient's signs or symptoms. Determine whether the signs and symptoms were caused by the tachycardia, or whether the tachycardia and its associated signs and symptoms occurred in response to another condition. For example, a patient who is having an MI may be mildly tachycardic, but obviously the MI—not the tachycardia—is responsible for the signs and symptoms. On the other hand, if a patient was previously asymptomatic but develops symptoms after the onset of the tachycardia, it's likely that his or her symptoms can be attributed to the condition. Again, remember to treat the patient, not the monitor.

Conservative therapies, such as vagal maneuvers and medications, are appropriate for a tachycardic adult with stable vital signs who is exhibiting symptoms related to the tachycardia, such as light-headedness or palpitations. However, if a tachycardic adult presents with more serious signs and symptoms such as acutely altered mental status, ischemic chest discomfort, acute heart failure, hypotension, or other signs of shock, then you should consider the patient unstable, and the use of electrical therapy with synchronized cardioversion is recommended.

Follow this procedure for emergency care of an adult who has tachycardia with a pulse:

1. Maintain an open airway. Assist breathing as necessary, and administer supplemental oxygen as needed to maintain an Spo_2 of 94% or higher.
2. Apply a cardiac monitor, blood pressure monitor, and pulse oximeter. Obtain a 12-lead ECG, but do not delay emergency care.
3. Establish an IV infusion of normal saline and obtain a finger-stick blood glucose. Treat hypoglycemia, if present.
4. If the QRS is narrow, the patient is stable, and there are no contraindications, then perform vagal maneuvers. If the rhythm persists, then administer adenosine intravenously. Follow each dose with a 20 mL fluid bolus. Adenosine dosing and administration is discussed in the Appendix, *Emergency Medications*.
5. If the QRS is narrow and the patient is unstable, then consider sedation before performing synchronized cardioversion.
6. Transport the patient for definitive care.

Recommended treatment guidelines for adult tachycardia with a pulse are shown in **Figure 17-42**.

Because vagal maneuvers alone will terminate up to 25% of SVTs caused by reentry, they are attempted for stable patients with narrow-QRS tachycardia before starting medication therapy.[7] Vagal maneuvers stimulate baroreceptors, which in turn signal brainstem centers to stimulate the vagus nerve, thereby slowing the heart rate. Many types of vagal maneuvers exist. Carotid sinus massage, also known as *carotid sinus pressure*, is one such maneuver. You will recall that the carotid sinus is located in the neck **Figure 17-43**. Before performing this procedure, assess for carotid **bruits** by listening to each carotid artery with a stethoscope **Figure 17-44**. A bruit is an abnormal whooshing sound indicating turbulent blood flow within a narrowed vessel. If you hear a bruit, then do not perform the procedure. If you do not hear a bruit and no contraindications are present, then turn the patient's head to one side. Next, locate the carotid pulse and apply firm pressure to the carotid artery for 5 to 10 seconds.[8] Applying pressure to the bifurcation of the carotid artery stretches the wall of the carotid sinus, thereby stimulating baroreceptors.[9] An older adult patient with CAD and high cholesterol would not be a good candidate for carotid massage because of the high risk of **thromboembolism**. Because this procedure has been associated with a number of complications, including stroke, syncope (fainting), and dysrhythmias (including **asystole**), it is not permitted in all EMS systems. Check your local protocol pertaining to this procedure. The Valsalva maneuver is a more commonly used vagal maneuver in which the patient bears down against a closed glottis for 10 to 30 seconds.[8] The patient is often instructed to bear down as if attempting to have a bowel movement.

Words of Wisdom

Never massage the right and left carotid arteries at the same time, as doing so may cause significant bradycardia, cerebrovascular accident, or asystole.

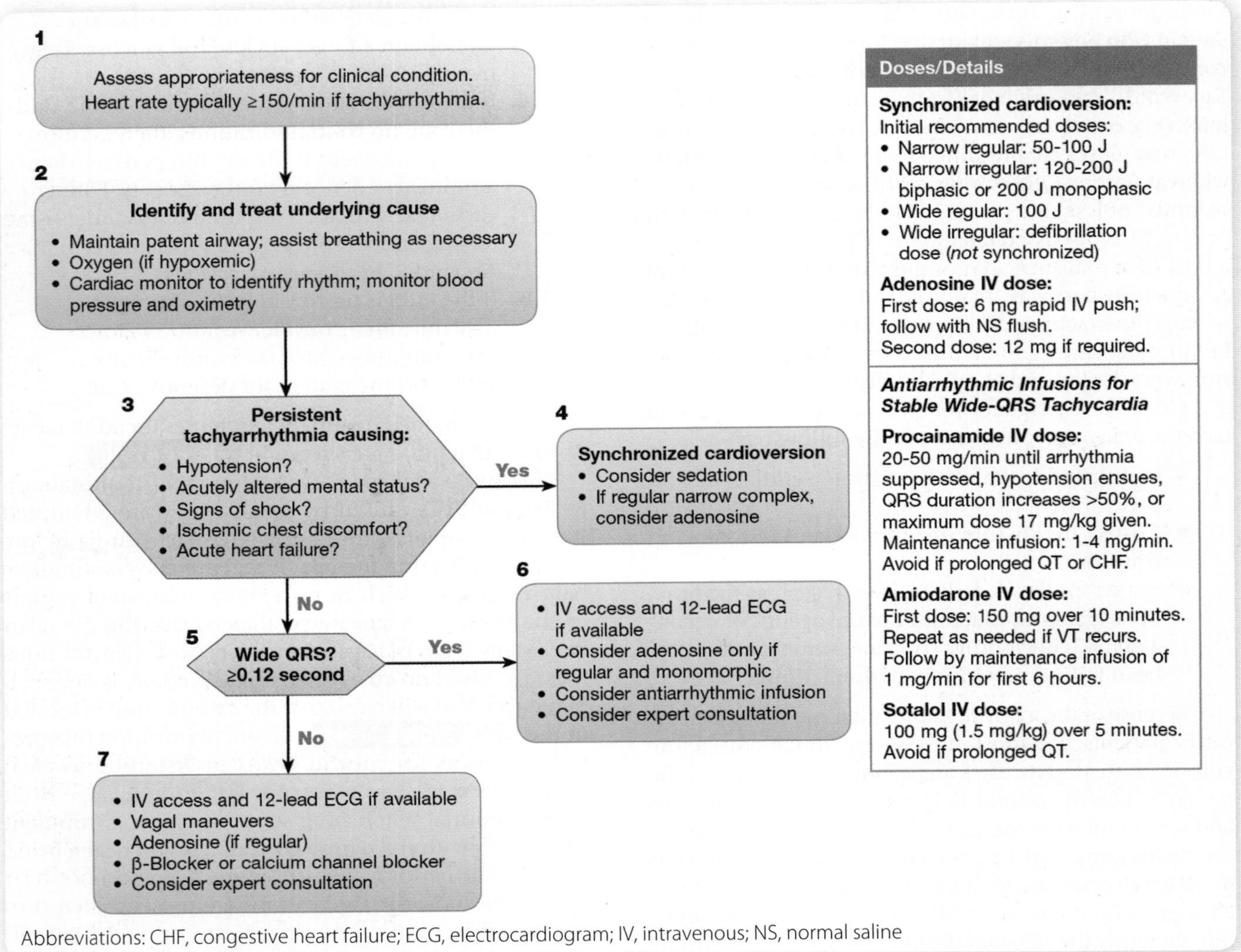

1

Assess appropriateness for clinical condition.
Heart rate typically ≥150/min if tachyarrhythmia.

2

Identify and treat underlying cause

- Maintain patent airway; assist breathing as necessary
- Oxygen (if hypoxemic)
- Cardiac monitor to identify rhythm; monitor blood pressure and oximetry

3

Persistent tachyarrhythmia causing:

- Hypotension?
- Acutely altered mental status?
- Signs of shock?
- Ischemic chest discomfort?
- Acute heart failure?

Yes → 4

4

Synchronized cardioversion

- Consider sedation
- If regular narrow complex, consider adenosine

No → 5

5

Wide QRS? ≥0.12 second

Yes → 6

6

- IV access and 12-lead ECG if available
- Consider adenosine only if regular and monomorphic
- Consider antiarrhythmic infusion
- Consider expert consultation

No → 7

7

- IV access and 12-lead ECG if available
- Vagal maneuvers
- Adenosine (if regular)
- β-Blocker or calcium channel blocker
- Consider expert consultation

Doses/Details

Synchronized cardioversion:
Initial recommended doses:

- Narrow regular: 50-100 J
- Narrow irregular: 120-200 J biphasic or 200 J monophasic
- Wide regular: 100 J
- Wide irregular: defibrillation dose (*not* synchronized)

Adenosine IV dose:
First dose: 6 mg rapid IV push; follow with NS flush.
Second dose: 12 mg if required.

Antiarrhythmic Infusions for Stable Wide-QRS Tachycardia

Procainamide IV dose:
20-50 mg/min until arrhythmia suppressed, hypotension ensues, QRS duration increases >50%, or maximum dose 17 mg/kg given.
Maintenance infusion: 1-4 mg/min.
Avoid if prolonged QT or CHF.

Amiodarone IV dose:
First dose: 150 mg over 10 minutes.
Repeat as needed if VT recurs.
Follow by maintenance infusion of 1 mg/min for first 6 hours.

Sotalol IV dose:
100 mg (1.5 mg/kg) over 5 minutes.
Avoid if prolonged QT.

Abbreviations: CHF, congestive heart failure; ECG, electrocardiogram; IV, intravenous; NS, normal saline

Figure 17-42 Algorithm for adult tachycardia with a pulse.

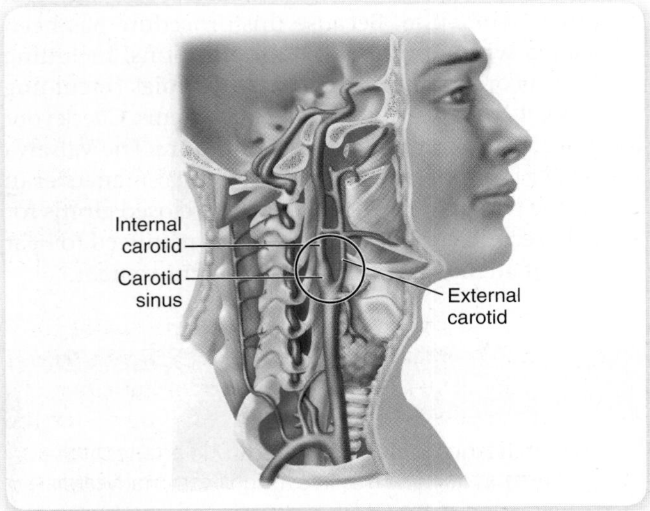

Figure 17-43 Location of the carotid sinus.

If vagal maneuvers are ineffective and the patient with a narrow-QRS tachycardia remains stable, then administer adenosine. It is used to transiently induce AV nodal blockade, interrupting the tachydysrhythmia. Before you begin this treatment, recheck the history for allergies and advise the patient of the possible adverse effects of adenosine administration. Because of the drug's very short half-life, adenosine should be administered at the IV site closest to the patient's heart. After clamping off the IV line above the site, push the adenosine as rapidly as possible, and then follow with a 20-mL flush of normal saline solution as soon as the plunger of the adenosine syringe hits bottom. Be prepared to see a short run of asystole, although this response does not always occur. If the first dose of adenosine is unsuccessful, then administer a double dose of adenosine and administer it again in 1 to 2 minutes. If needed, repeat the dose again in 1 to 2 minutes. If adenosine does not convert the rhythm, rapidly transport the patient to the medical facility.

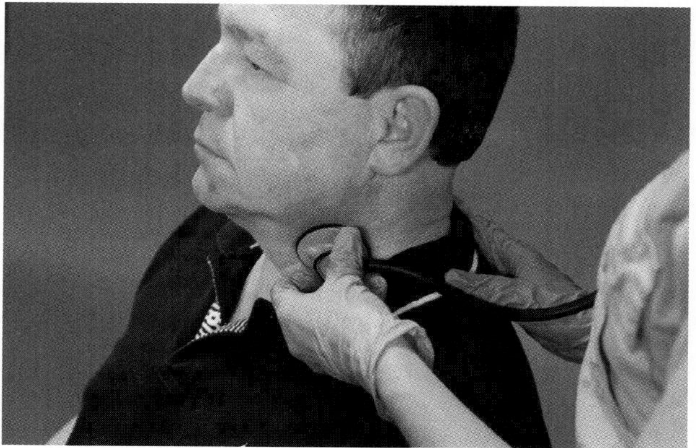

A

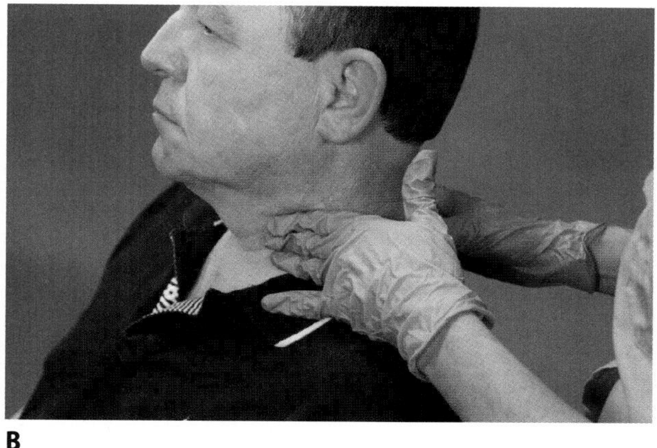

B

Figure 17-44 Carotid sinus pressure. **A.** Listen for bruits. **B.** Apply pressure to the carotid artery for 5 to 10 seconds.

If at any time the condition of a patient with SVT becomes unstable, you should move to the unstable arm of the tachycardia algorithm. A tachycardic patient in unstable condition requires electrical therapy with synchronized cardioversion. Synchronized cardioversion is the use of a defibrillator to terminate a hemodynamically unstable tachydysrhythmia. Unlike defibrillation, a process in which energy may be delivered at any time during the cardiac cycle, synchronized cardioversion delivers timed bursts of electrical energy. The device identifies R waves on the ECG. When you press and hold the shock controls, the machine will discharge with the next detected R wave, avoiding the vulnerable period during the T wave of the cardiac cycle.

Cardioversion is indicated for VT and SVT associated with severely compromised CO. When cardioversion is performed on a responsive patient, the patient *must* be sedated first; cardioversion is a painful and terrifying experience for a patient who is awake. Benzodiazepines, such as diazepam (Valium) and midazolam (Versed), are commonly administered for sedation in these circumstances (follow your protocol).

The procedure for cardioversion is shown in Skill Drill 17-3. Ensure the patient is supine; be prepared for the possibility that the patient could go into cardiac arrest.

Documentation & Communication

Key documentation elements for the adult patient with a tachycardia and a pulse are as follows:[6]

- All rhythm changes
- Time and dose of medications given
- Patient's response to medications
- Patient's response to attempts to cardiovert (including times and energy settings)
- Monitor strips obtained before and after each intervention and at the time of transfer of patient care

Preexcitation

Preexcitation refers to early depolarization of ventricular tissue by means of an accessory pathway between the atria and ventricles. An accessory pathway is an extra bundle of myocardial tissue that forms a connection between the atria and ventricles outside the normal conduction system. Patients with preexcitation syndromes are susceptible to tachydysrhythmias. A reentry SVT involving the AV node and an accessory pathway is called *AV reentrant tachycardia (AVRT)*.

The most common preexcitation disorder is known as **Wolff-Parkinson-White syndrome (WPW)**. WPW syndrome is characterized by a short PRI (that is, a duration of less than 0.12 seconds [120 milliseconds]); nonspecific ST-T wave changes; a widened QRS complex; and the appearance of a *delta wave* on ECG. The delta wave—a slurring of the upstroke of the first part of the QRS complex—indicates an early departure from the PR segment as a result of conduction through the accessory pathway (bundle of Kent) and subsequent early depolarization of ventricular tissue Figure 17-45.

Lown-Ganong-Levine syndrome is another disorder that causes preexcitation of ventricular tissue. The ECG signature of this syndrome is a short PRI and a normal QRS duration. Patients with WPW syndrome and those with Lown-Ganong-Levine syndrome are predisposed to tachydysrhythmias.

Seek the advice of a physician when caring for a symptomatic patient with a preexcitation syndrome. If symptoms are attributable to the rapid ventricular rate, then your treatment will depend on the gravity of the patient's instability, the width of the QRS complex, and the regularity of the ventricular rhythm. Do not administer medication that slows or blocks conduction through the AV node because it may accelerate conduction through the accessory pathway, further increasing the heart rate.

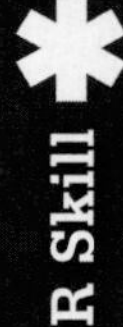
NR Skill

Skill Drill 17-3 Performing Synchronized Cardioversion

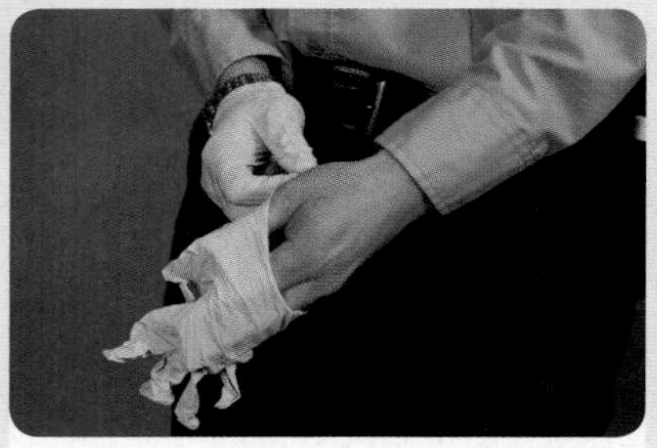

Step 1 Select, check, and assemble all necessary equipment, including a monitor/defibrillator with defibrillation pads, ECG electrodes, medication for pain or sedation (to be used if necessary), oxygen, and an appropriate oxygen administration device. Take standard precautions. Assess the patient's vital signs. Ensure the patient is oxygenated adequately, and establish a patent IV line.

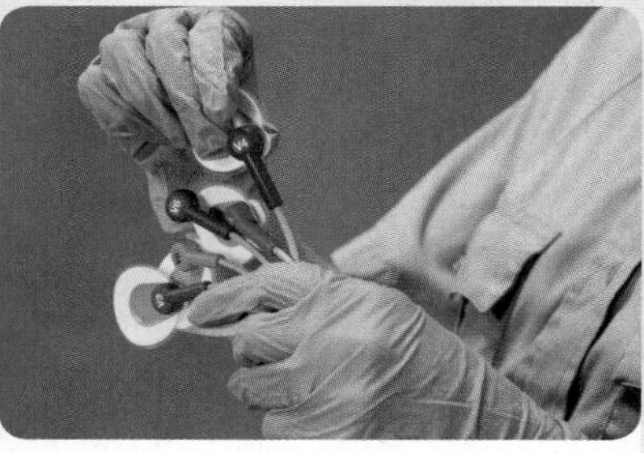

Step 2 Place the ECG electrodes in the same position as you would when performing cardiac monitoring. Obtain a baseline rhythm strip. Identify the rhythm and confirm that cardioversion is warranted. If the patient is responsive, you should consider the appropriate medication to sedate the patient. Ask about medication allergies before administering sedation.

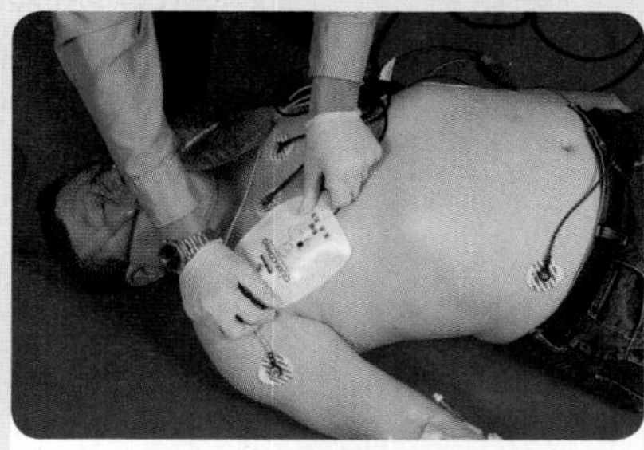

Step 3 Ensure the environment is safe (evaluate the risk of sparks, combustibles, oxygen-rich atmosphere). Explain to the patient and the family the need for the procedure. Apply the defibrillation pads to the patient according to the manufacturer's recommendations. Turn on the power to the defibrillator.

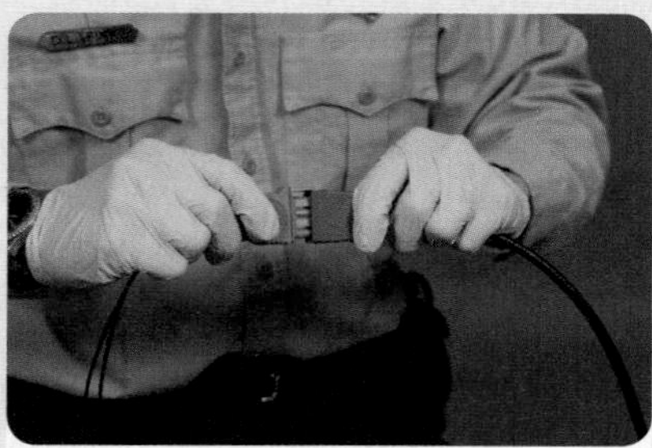

Step 4 Connect the pads to the monitor.

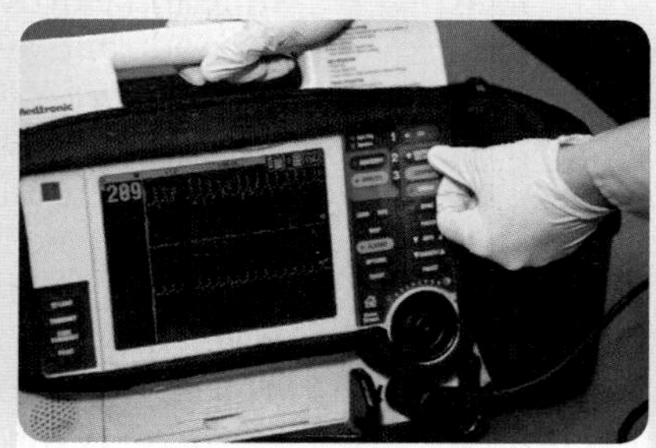

Step 5 Select the appropriate energy setting. Turn the synchronize switch on the machine to the on position.

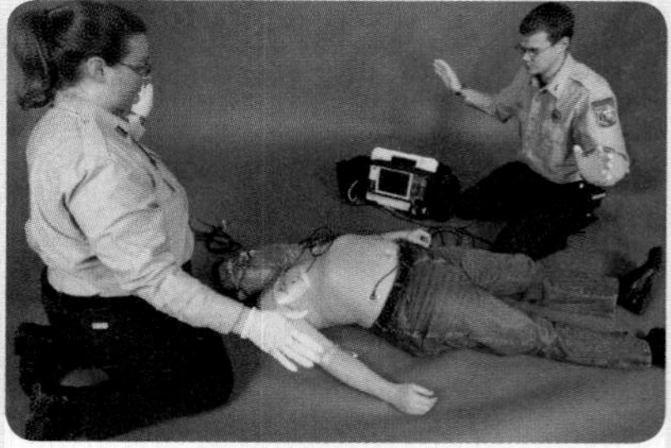

Step 6 Observe the ECG rhythm. Confirm that a sense marker appears near the middle of each QRS complex. If the sense markers are not visible or appear in the wrong location (for example, on the T wave), adjust the ECG size or select another lead until the machine reads the QRS complexes appropriately. Clear the area by announcing, "All clear!" and ensure everyone is clear of the patient.

Skill Drill 17-3 Performing Synchronized Cardioversion *(continued)*

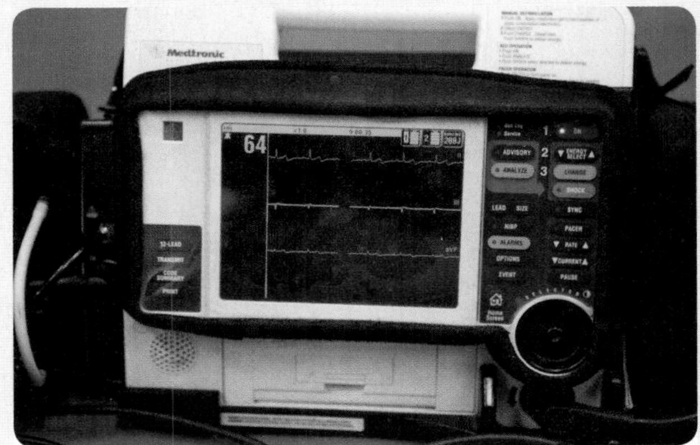

Step 7 Depress the *Shock* button. Keep them depressed until the defibrillator discharges.

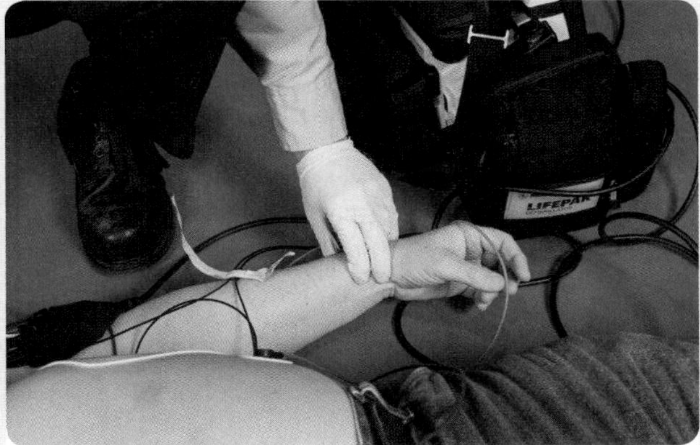

Step 8 Reassess the ECG rhythm and the patient (pulse and blood pressure). If the tachycardia persists, ensure the machine is in sync mode before delivering another shock. If the rhythm changes to ventricular fibrillation, ensure the patient has no pulse. If no pulse is present, ensure the sync control is off and proceed with defibrillation.

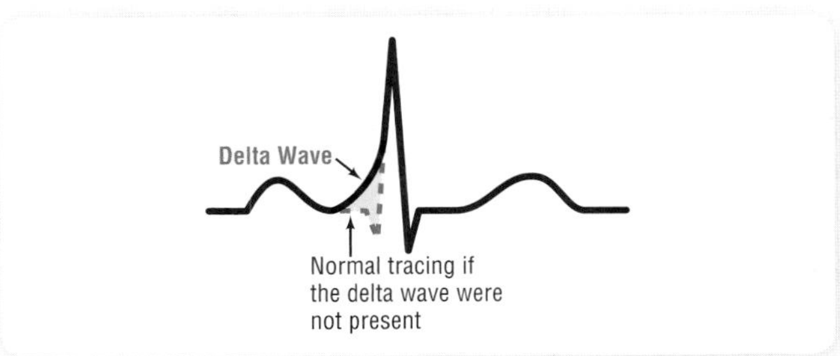

Figure 17-45 Delta wave: Wolff-Parkinson-White syndrome.

Reproduced from *12-Lead ECG: The Art of Interpretation*, courtesy of Tomas B. Garcia, MD.

Atrial Fibrillation

Atrial fibrillation (AF) is a rhythm in which the atria no longer contract but instead fibrillate or quiver, with no organized contraction Figure 17-46. The condition occurs when many different cells in the atria depolarize independently, rather than in response to an SA node impulse. The result of this random depolarization throughout the atria is a fibrillating or chaotic baseline. In AF, there is usually no visible P wave on the ECG strip and, hence, no PRI to measure. Instead, one of the hallmarks of this condition is its irregularly irregular appearance. Because the AV node is bombarded with impulses from the fibrillating atria, it allows impulses to pass on randomly to the ventricles, which produces the highly irregular ventricular rhythm. The QRS complex typically measures 0.11 seconds (110 milliseconds) or less.

AF is a common rhythm among older adult patients. One of the main hazards associated with this dysrhythmia is the blood within the fibrillating atria has a tendency to clot. These clots may become emboli that block circulation elsewhere in the body. Thus, AF increases the risk of stroke. Because of this risk, many older adult patients with AF are prescribed anticoagulant medications such as warfarin (Coumadin). A beta-blocker, calcium channel blocker, or digoxin may also be prescribed to regulate the ventricular response rate. AF accompanied by a rapid ventricular response is considered an irregular tachycardia. If the patient is stable but symptomatic, AF with a rapid ventricular response may be treated with a beta-blocker or calcium channel blocker. Because of the risk of a thromboembolic event, prehospital treatment of AF is uncommon in stable patients. If the patient is unstable, synchronized cardioversion may be necessary.

Atrial Flutter

Atrial flutter is a rhythm in which an atrial impulse fires at a rate much too rapid for the ventricles to keep up Figure 17-47. The atrial complexes in atrial flutter are known as *flutter waves* or *F waves* rather than P waves. F waves have a distinctive sawtooth shape resembling a picket fence.

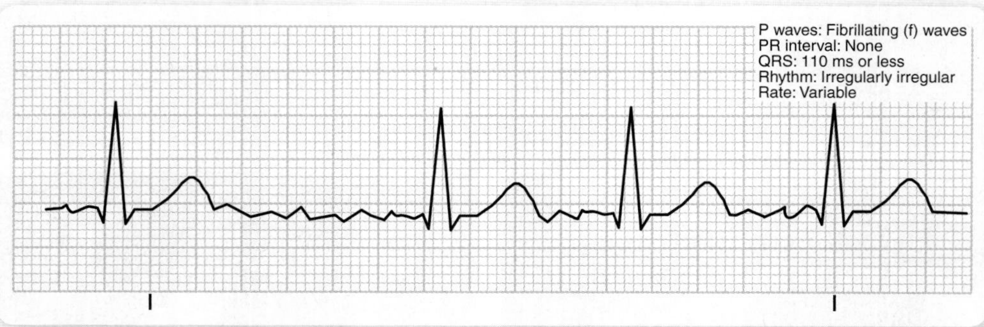

Figure 17-46 Atrial fibrillation.

Reproduced from *Arrhythmia Recognition: The Art of Interpretation*, courtesy of Tomas B. Garcia, MD.

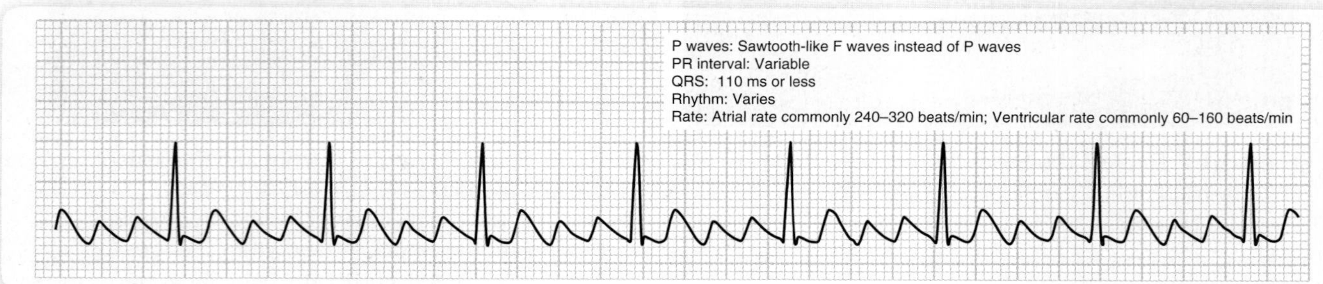

Figure 17-47 Atrial flutter (sawtooth flutter waves).

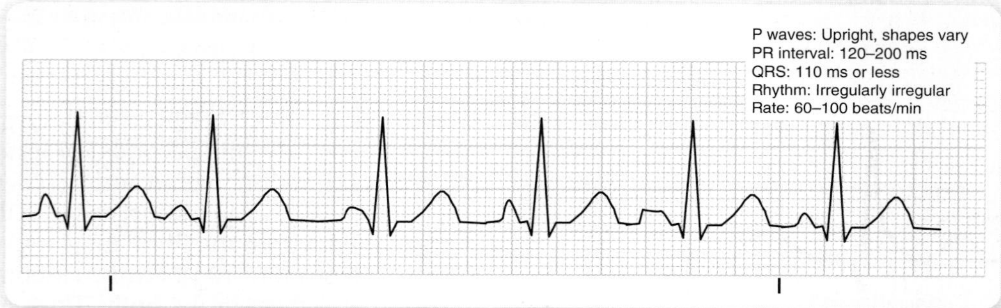

Figure 17-48 Wandering atrial pacemaker.

Reproduced from *Arrhythmia Recognition: The Art of Interpretation*, courtesy of Tomas B. Garcia, MD.

In atrial flutter, one or more of the F waves is blocked by the AV node, generating several flutter waves before each QRS complex. The rhythm is usually regular, with a constant (usually 2:1) conduction. The rhythm can be irregular if the conduction of atrial impulses to the ventricles varies. The QRS complex measures 0.11 seconds (110 milliseconds) or less.

Hypoxia, pneumonia, chronic lung disease, endocrine disorders, ischemic heart disease, valvular heart disease, and other conditions are associated with atrial flutter, which can degenerate into AF. In fact, it is common for atrial flutter and AF to coexist in the same patient.[8] Patients with atrial flutter are often prescribed anticoagulant medications because these patients are thought to have the same risk of thromboembolism as patients with AF.[8]

Like AF, atrial flutter accompanied by a rapid ventricular response is considered an irregular tachycardia. A beta-blocker or calcium channel blocker may be administered if the patient is stable but symptomatic. Synchronized cardioversion may be necessary if the patient is unstable. As with AF, prehospital treatment of atrial flutter is uncommon in stable patients.

Wandering Atrial Pacemaker

In wandering atrial pacemaker, as the name suggests, the pacemaker of the heart **Figure 17-48** moves from the SA node to various areas within the atria or AV junction. Wandering atrial pacemaker usually has a rate of 60 to 100 beats/min. The rhythm is slightly irregular, with R-R intervals that vary depending on the site of the pacemaker for that particular complex. An upright P wave precedes each QRS complex; however, its shape varies, indicating multiple sites of origin. The definition of wandering atrial pacemaker requires the presence of at least three

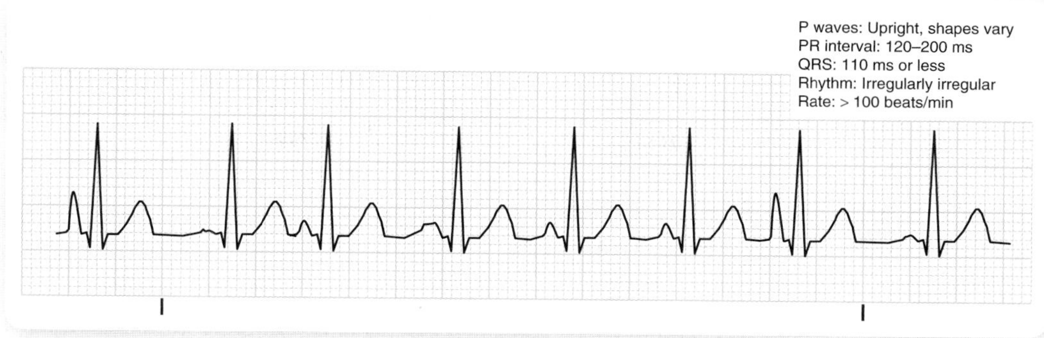

Figure 17-49 Multifocal atrial tachycardia.

Reproduced from *Arrhythmia Recognition: The Art of Interpretation*, courtesy of Tomas B. Garcia, MD.

different shapes of P waves within one ECG strip. The PRI measures 0.12 to 0.20 seconds (120 to 200 milliseconds), but also varies slightly based on the origin of a given complex. The QRS complex measures 0.11 seconds (110 milliseconds) or less.

Wandering atrial pacemaker is most often seen in children, older adults, and athletes. Treatment is usually not indicated in the prehospital setting unless the dysrhythmia is associated with a slow rate and the patient is symptomatic. Under those circumstances, treatment is the same as for symptomatic sinus bradycardia.

Multifocal Atrial Tachycardia

In multifocal atrial tachycardia (MAT), multiple ectopic sites within the atria depolarize at different but rapid rates Figure 17-49. MAT is characterized by a rate of more than 100 beats/min and is, in effect, a tachycardic wandering atrial pacemaker. The rhythm is irregular, with R-R intervals that vary depending on the site of the pacemaker for that particular complex. An upright P wave precedes each QRS complex; however, its shape varies, indicating multiple sites of origin. The PRI measures 0.12 to 0.20 seconds (120 to 200 milliseconds), but also varies slightly based on the origin of a given complex. If the MAT increases to a rate exceeding 150 beats/min, then the P wave may no longer be visible; thus, the only indication of the rhythm may be the irregularity associated with the varying sites of origin within the atria. The QRS complex measures 0.11 seconds (110 milliseconds) or less.

MAT is most often seen in patients with significant lung disease, pulmonary hypertension, coronary disease, and valvular heart disease, and hypomagnesemia, as well as patients undergoing theophylline therapy.[8] Because therapies aimed at correcting SVT are usually ineffective with MAT, treatment is usually deferred until arrival at the emergency department (ED).

▶ Rhythms Originating at the AV Junction

If the SA node—the body's dominant pacemaker—fails to initiate an impulse, then the AV junction should take over as pacemaker of the heart. Because the AV junction is a secondary pacemaker, its intrinsic rate is slower than that of the SA node. As a result, junctional rhythms normally have a rate of 40 to 60 beats/min.

When an impulse is generated in the AV junction, it travels down through the conduction system into the ventricles as if it had come from the SA node, resulting in normal QRS complexes. At the same time, the impulse travels upward, through the atria and the internodal pathways toward the SA node. There are, then, three possible circumstances—none associated with an upright P wave—in which the QRS complex appears normal:

- If the impulse begins moving upward through the atria before the other part of it enters the ventricles, an upside-down P wave will be visible. (It's upside down because the impulse is traveling in the direction opposite of that which generates normal, upright P waves.) This P wave is usually followed immediately by a QRS complex.
- If the impulse moves through the atria at exactly the same time as it travels through the ventricles, the smaller inverted P wave will be buried within the larger QRS complex. As a result, the P wave will appear to be missing—that is, the baseline will remain flat until a normal QRS complex begins.
- The impulse may begin late through the atria, resulting in an inverted P wave that appears after the QRS complex.

Premature Junctional Complex

A premature junctional complex (PJC) is not, strictly speaking, a dysrhythmia (just as PAC is not), but rather an early complex that appears within another rhythm Figure 17-50. PJCs are also known as *ectopic complexes*, meaning they arise from a site other than the SA node.

The rate depends on the underlying rhythm. Because a PJC is, by definition, an early beat, the underlying rhythm is irregular. The P wave, if present, will be inverted and may either precede or follow the QRS complex. The PRI, if present, will measure less than 0.12 seconds (120 milliseconds). The QRS complex measures 0.11 seconds (110 milliseconds) or less.

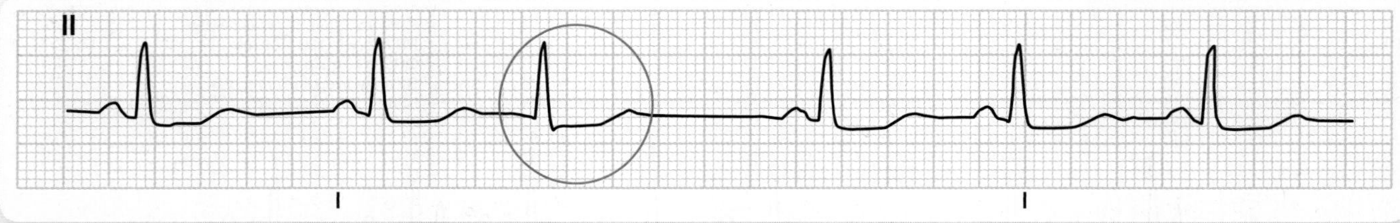

Figure 17-50 Sinus rhythm with a premature junctional complex.

Reproduced from *Arrhythmia Recognition: The Art of Interpretation*, courtesy of Tomas B. Garcia, MD.

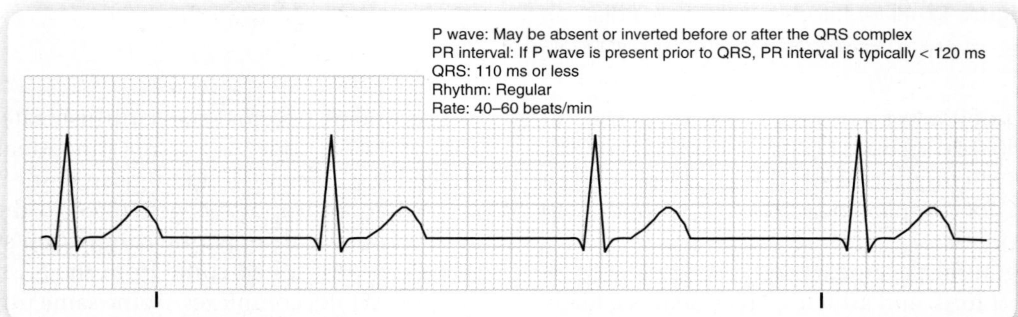

Figure 17-51 Junctional escape rhythm.

Reproduced from *Arrhythmia Recognition: The Art of Interpretation*, courtesy of Tomas B. Garcia, MD.

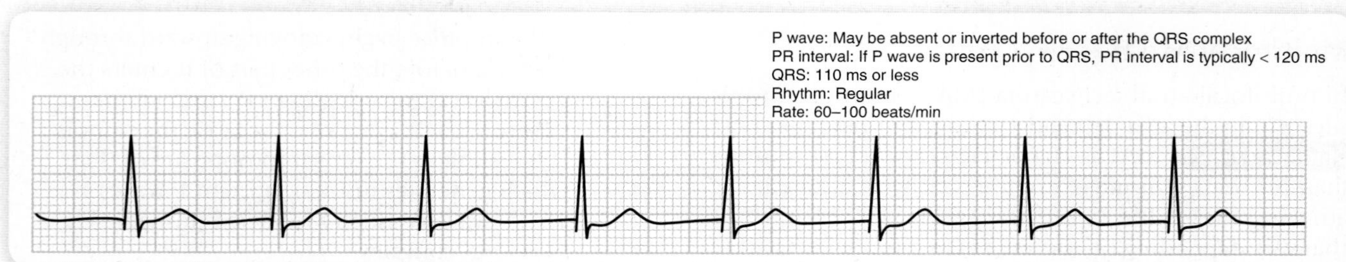

Figure 17-52 Accelerated junctional rhythm.

Reproduced from *Arrhythmia Recognition: The Art of Interpretation*, courtesy of Tomas B. Garcia, MD.

PJCs can be caused by many of the same factors that cause PACs. PJCs do not normally require treatment, since most people with the condition are asymptomatic. Some people with PJCs, however, may perceive skipped beats. Light-headedness, dizziness, and other signs of decreased CO can occur if PJCs occur frequently. Frequent PJCs may be a predictor of future cardiac dysrhythmias.

Junctional Escape Rhythm

A **junctional escape rhythm**, also called a *junctional rhythm*, is a dysrhythmia that occurs when the SA node ceases functioning and the AV junction takes over as the pacemaker of the heart at a rate of 40 to 60 beats/min Figure 17-51. The rhythm is usually regular, with little variation between R-R intervals. The P wave may be absent or inverted before or after the QRS complex. If an inverted P wave is present before the QRS, then the PRI will measure less than 0.12 seconds (120 milliseconds). The QRS complex measures 0.11 seconds (110 milliseconds) or less.

A junctional rhythm often accompanies SA node disease, increased vagal tone, valvular heart disease, inferior wall MI, and other conditions, or it can occur after resuscitation from cardiac arrest. Because of the slow rate, treatment in symptomatic patients depends on the underlying cause and may require a surgically implanted pacemaker. In the field, atropine should be considered and TCP may be necessary if the patient's condition is severely compromised (see Figure 17-35).

Accelerated Junctional Rhythm

Occasionally, a junctional rhythm is accompanied by a rate that exceeds its normal upper rate of 60 beats/min but remains less than 100 beats/min. Such a rhythm is called an *accelerated junctional rhythm*. This rhythm is regular, with little variation between R-R intervals Figure 17-52. The P wave may be absent or, if present, be inverted before or after the QRS complex. The PRI, if an inverted P wave is present before the QRS, measures less than 0.12 seconds (120 milliseconds). The QRS complex measures 0.11 seconds (110 milliseconds) or less.

Accelerated junctional rhythms may be associated with digoxin toxicity (most common cause), hypoxia, inferior wall MI, **rheumatic fever**, recent cardiac surgery, or an electrolyte imbalance, such as hypokalemia. Because the rate is fast enough to maintain a reasonable CO, the patient usually is asymptomatic. Nevertheless, he or she should be closely monitored.

Junctional Tachycardia

Occasionally, a junctional rhythm is accompanied by a rate that exceeds 100 beats/min. Such a rhythm is termed *junctional tachycardia*. Junctional tachycardia is regular, with little variation between R-R intervals **Figure 17-53**. The ECG characteristics of junctional tachycardia are the same as those of an accelerated junctional rhythm but the rate is faster than 100 beats/min.

Junctional tachycardia is uncommon in adults but is associated with acute coronary syndrome, heart failure, theophylline administration, or digoxin toxicity. Because the rate is fast enough to maintain a reasonable CO, it seldom requires treatment in the prehospital setting. However, if the rate exceeds 150 beats/min, CO could suffer. At a rapid ventricular rate, distinguishing junctional tachycardia from other narrow-QRS tachycardias is often difficult. Such a rhythm is referred to as *SVT*. If the patient is symptomatic, then treat in accordance with the tachycardia algorithm (see Figure 17-42).

Rhythms Originating in the Ventricles

If the SA node fails to initiate an impulse, then the AV junction usually takes over as pacemaker. If the AV junction cannot perform this duty, the ventricles may initiate the impulses, becoming the pacemaker of the heart. A missing P wave and wide QRS complex (0.12 seconds [120 milliseconds] or more in duration) are characteristic features of such ventricular beats or rhythms.

Premature Ventricular Complex

A premature ventricular complex (PVC) is not, strictly speaking, a dysrhythmia (just as premature atrial and junctional complexes are not), but rather an early complex that appears within another rhythm **Figure 17-54**. PVCs are ectopic complexes because they originate from a site other than the SA node. A PVC occurs earlier than the next expected sinus complex, producing an irregular ventricular rhythm. There

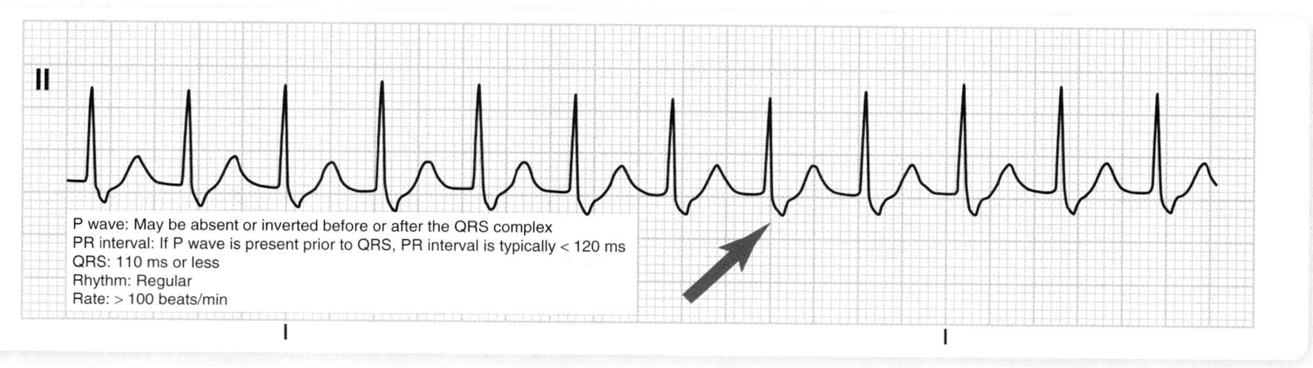

Figure 17-53 Junctional tachycardia. The blue arrow points to an inverted P wave after the QRS complex.

Reproduced from *Arrhythmia Recognition: The Art of Interpretation*, courtesy of Tomas B. Garcia, MD.

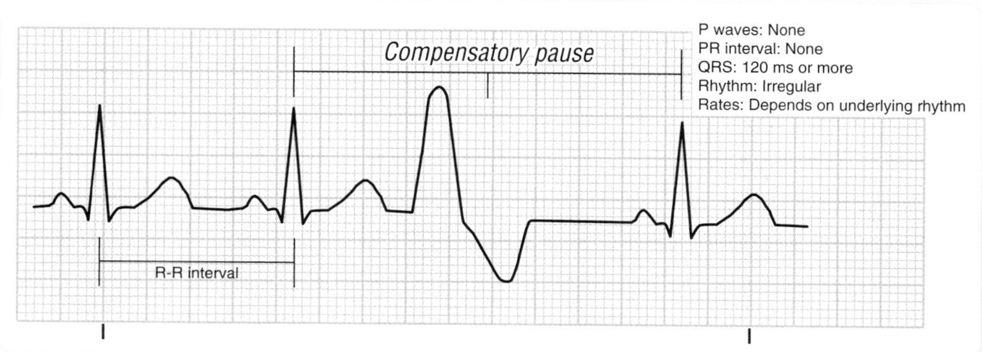

Figure 17-54 Sinus rhythm with a premature ventricular complex (PVC). A full compensatory pause usually follows a PVC. A pause is compensatory if the R-R interval that includes the PVC measures twice that of the underlying rhythm.

Modified from *Arrhythmia Recognition: The Art of Interpretation*, courtesy of Tomas B. Garcia, MD.

is no P wave associated with the PVC, so there is no PRI. The QRS complex associated with the PVC measures 0.12 seconds (120 milliseconds) or more. A full compensatory pause usually follows a PVC. A compensatory pause allows time for restoration of the underlying rhythm (that is, the pause compensates for the PVC). To determine if such a pause is present, measure an R-R interval of the underlying rhythm. Next, measure from the R wave of the QRS complex before the PVC to the R wave of the QRS complex after the PVC. A full compensatory pause has occurred if the R-R interval that includes the PVC measures twice that of the underlying rhythm.

Premature ventricular complexes may be further distinguished as unifocal or multifocal. **Unifocal** PVCs originate from the same area or "focus" within the ventricle and look alike on the ECG Figure 17-55. PVCs with a varied appearance are **multifocal**, meaning that there is more than one focus initiating the ventricular impulses Figure 17-56.

Sometimes two consecutive PVCs occur, with no intervening pause. These paired PVCs constitute a ventricular **couplet** Figure 17-57. The occurrence of three or more PVCs in a row is called a "run" of ventricular tachycardia; these surges are also referred to as *salvos* or

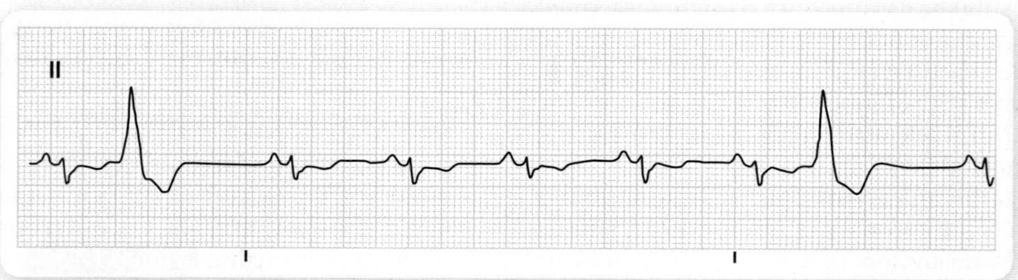

Figure 17-55 Unifocal premature ventricular complexes.

Reproduced from *Arrhythmia Recognition: The Art of Interpretation*, courtesy of Tomas B. Garcia, MD.

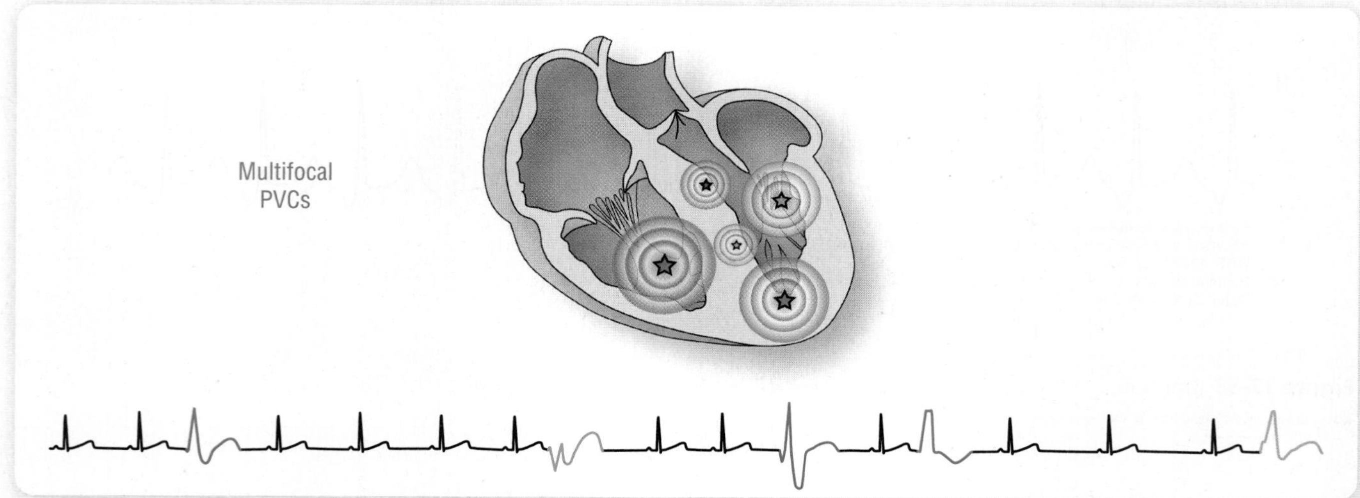

Figure 17-56 Multifocal premature ventricular complexes.

Reproduced from *Arrhythmia Recognition: The Art of Interpretation*, courtesy of Tomas B. Garcia, MD.

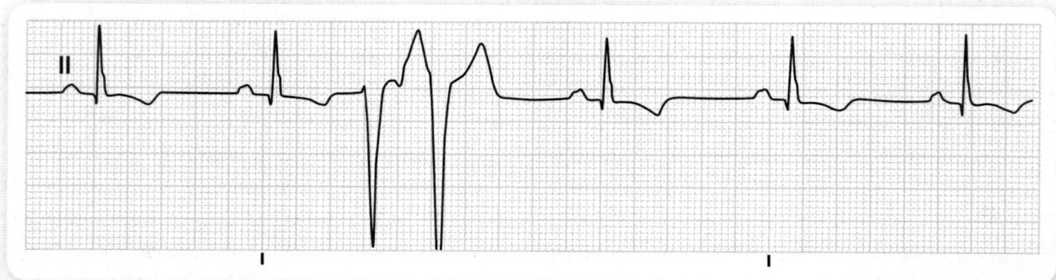

Figure 17-57 Ventricular couplet (paired premature ventricular complexes).

Reproduced from *Arrhythmia Recognition: The Art of Interpretation*, courtesy of Tomas B. Garcia, MD.

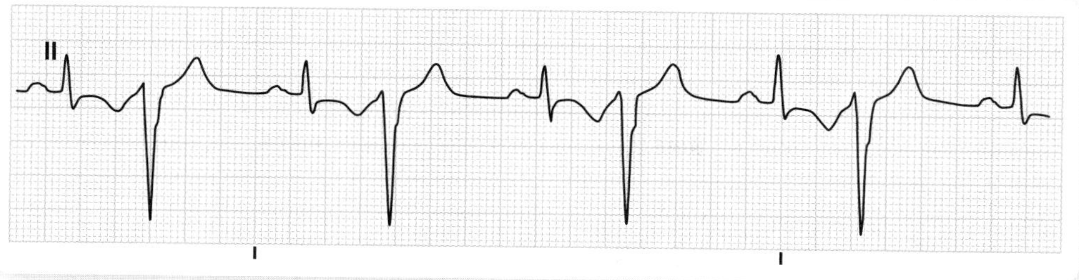

Figure 17-58 Ventricular bigeminy.

Reproduced from *Arrhythmia Recognition: The Art of Interpretation*, courtesy of Tomas B. Garcia, MD.

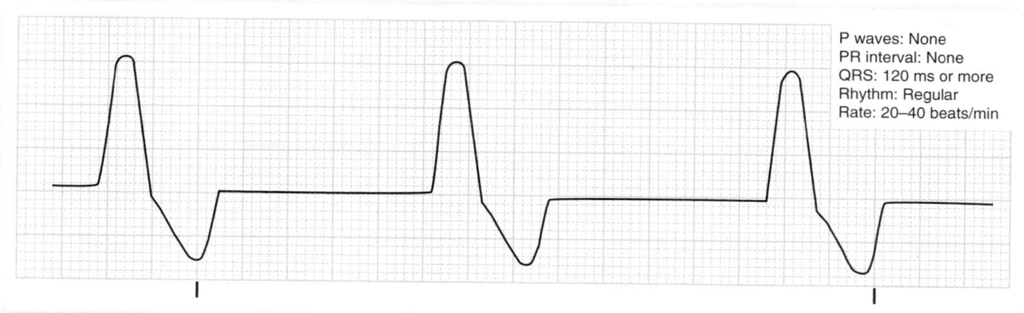

Figure 17-59 Idioventricular rhythm.

Reproduced from *Arrhythmia Recognition; The Art of Interpretation*, courtesy of Tomas B. Garcia, MD.

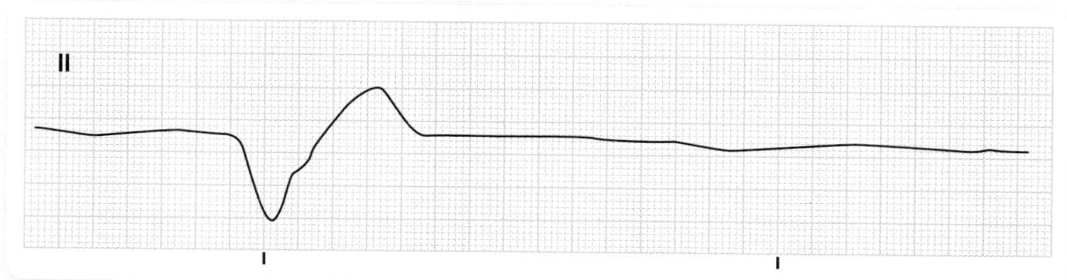

Figure 17-60 Agonal rhythm.

Reproduced from *Arrhythmia Recognition: The Art of Interpretation*, courtesy of Tomas B. Garcia, MD.

bursts. Occasionally, the complexes become so frequent that they begin to alternate with normal complexes, generating a *normal–PVC–normal–PVC* pattern. This pattern is called ventricular **bigeminy** Figure 17-58. If every third beat is a PVC (*normal–normal–PVC*), then the pattern is called ventricular **trigeminy**.

PVCs can arise in many of the same circumstances associated with premature atrial and junctional complexes, but they most often originate from ischemia in the ventricular tissue. They are generally considered more serious than premature atrial or junctional complexes. Multifocal PVCs, couplets, and ventricular bigeminy are considered more serious rhythm disturbances than unifocal PVCs.

One of the principal hazards of PVCs is they might occur before the ventricles have fully repolarized (that is, during the RRP). In other words, the R wave of the PVC occurs during the T wave of the preceding complex. This so-called R-on-T phenomenon can lead to ventricular fibrillation.

Occasional PVCs are common and usually don't require treatment in otherwise healthy patients. PVCs that occur in patients with heart disease require close monitoring and a search for the underlying cause.

Idioventricular Rhythm

The term **idioventricular** means "only the ventricles" or "produced by the ventricles." An idioventricular rhythm (IVR), then, is one that occurs when the SA and AV nodes fail and responsibility for pacing the heart shifts to the ventricles Figure 17-59. An IVR is usually regular, with little variation between R-R intervals. P waves are absent owing to the failure of the SA and AV nodes. Because there is no P wave, there is no PRI. The QRS complex will measure 0.12 seconds (120 milliseconds) or more because it originates in the ventricles. An IVR has a rate of 20 to 40 beats/min, which is the intrinsic rate of the ventricles. When the ventricular rate slows to less than 20 beats/min, the pattern is called an **agonal rhythm** Figure 17-60. **Agonal** means "pertaining to the period of dying."

Because of the slow rate, the patient with an IVR is often symptomatic. IVRs may or may not be

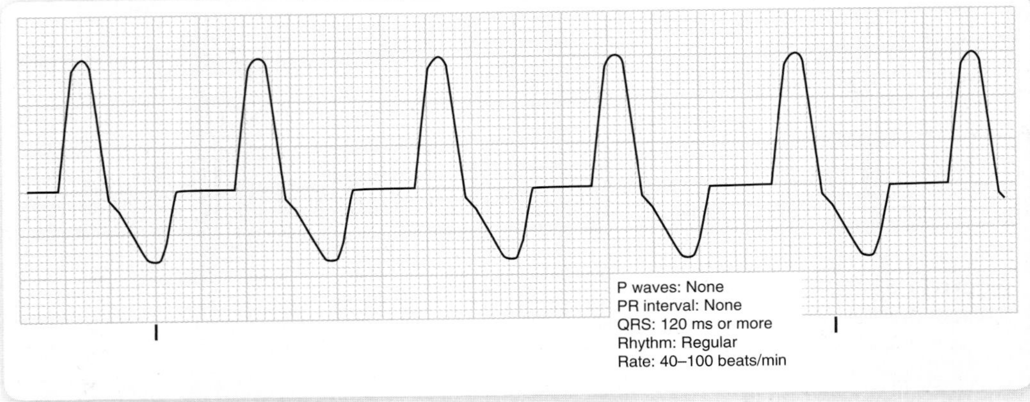

Figure 17-61 Accelerated idioventricular rhythm.

Reproduced from *Arrhythmia Recognition: The Art of Interpretation*, courtesy of Tomas B. Garcia, MD.

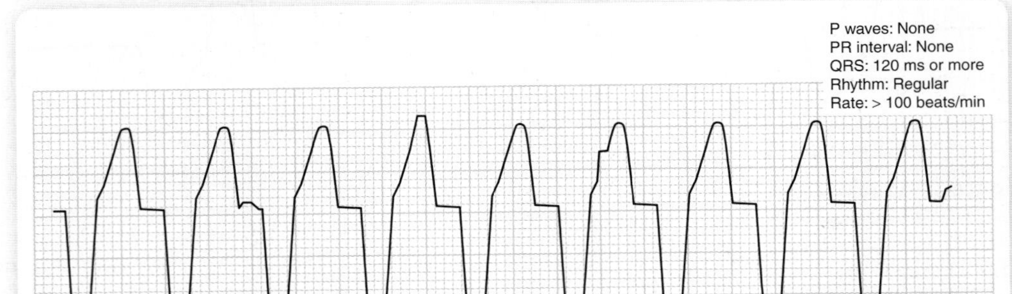

Figure 17-62 Monomorphic ventricular tachycardia.

Reproduced from *Arrhythmia Recognition: The Art of Interpretation*, courtesy of Tomas B. Garcia, MD.

accompanied by a palpable pulse. Treatment is geared toward improving CO by increasing the rate and, if possible, treating the underlying cause. If IVR is associated with a pulse, then treat the rhythm in accordance with the bradycardia algorithm (see Figure 17-35). If there is no pulse associated with IVR, then the patient is in cardiac arrest. Treatment for cardiac arrest is discussed later in this chapter.

Accelerated Idioventricular Rhythm

Occasionally, an IVR exceeds the normal upper limit of 40 beats/min but remains less than 100 beats/min. Because the rate is faster than the intrinsic rate of the ventricles but less than 100 beats/min, it is called *accelerated idioventricular rhythm (AIVR)*.

AIVR is regular, with little variation between R-R intervals. The P waves are absent, so there is no PRI **Figure 17-61**. The QRS complex measures 0.12 seconds (120 milliseconds) or more.

AIVR may be observed during the first 12 hours of an AMI or after reperfusion therapy. Because IVR and AIVR are rhythms generated by the last available internal cardiac pacemaker site, these rhythms should not be suppressed with ventricular antidysrhythmic agents such as amiodarone or lidocaine. These medications are discussed in the Appendix, *Emergency Medications*.

Ventricular Tachycardia

Occasionally, a ventricular rhythm has a rate exceeding 100 beats/min. In this case, the rhythm is termed ventricular tachycardia (VT). VT is regular, with no variation between R-R intervals. The P waves are absent, so the PRI is also absent. Because the QRS complex in VT measures 0.12 seconds (120 milliseconds) or more, VT is considered a wide-QRS tachycardia. When this dysrhythmia presents with QRS complexes that appear uniform, it's referred to as *monomorphic VT*. The word **monomorphic**, meaning a common shape or form, comes from the Greek words *monos* (one) and *morphe* (shape). In this case, the VT is said to be monomorphic because the shape of QRS complex is constant **Figure 17-62**. Occasionally, VT presents with irregular QRS complexes of varied height in an alternating pattern. This type is called polymorphic VT **Figure 17-63**. Polymorphic VT is a wide irregular tachycardia. The American Heart Association (AHA) estimates that polymorphic VT is present in about 25% of all OHCAs involving VT.[1]

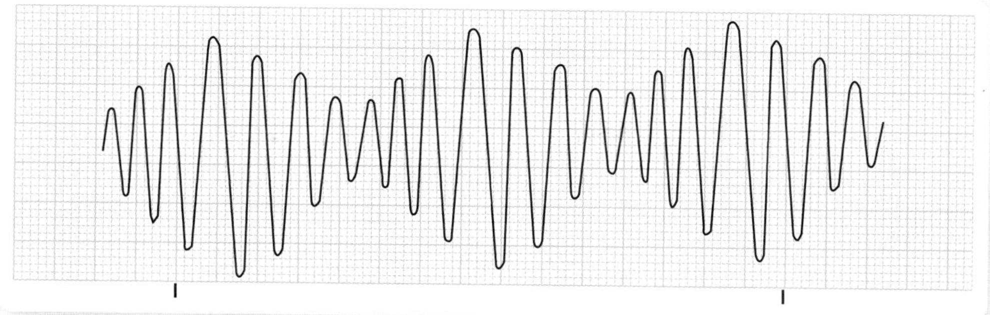

Figure 17-63 Polymorphic ventricular tachycardia.

Reproduced from *Arrhythmia Recognition: The Art of Interpretation*, courtesy of Tomas B. Garcia, MD.

Polymorphic VT with a prolonged QT interval is called *torsades de pointes*. A prolonged QT interval may be congenital or acquired (medication induced). Examples of medications that prolong the QT interval are amiodarone (Cordarone), quinidine (Quinidex, Quinora), procainamide (Pronestyl), sotalol (Betapace), phenothiazines, and tricyclic antidepressants. Polymorphic VT may convert spontaneously to a normal rhythm, or it may degenerate into ventricular fibrillation. Long-QT syndrome is discussed in more detail later in this chapter.

Because the rate is usually too fast to maintain adequate CO, VT is extremely serious and requires treatment. This reduced CO can lead to ventricular failure or fibrillation if not addressed promptly. If the patient is symptomatic but hemodynamically stable, emergency care should focus on treatment with antidysrhythmic medications (see Figure 17-42). If the patient is unstable and the cardiac monitor shows monomorphic VT, electrical therapy using synchronized cardioversion may be necessary. The energy levels used for VT are higher than those for SVT. If the patient is unstable and the cardiac monitor shows polymorphic VT, defibrillation is used because the machine cannot synchronize QRS complexes of varying amplitude. If the cardiac monitor shows VT but the patient is pulseless, then he or she is in cardiac arrest. Pulseless VT is treated the same as ventricular fibrillation.

Words of Wisdom

The calcium channel blocker verapamil may be used to control the rate of a tachydysrhythmia. Verapamil slows conduction of electrical impulses through the AV node, protecting the ventricles from atrial tachydysrhythmias and slowing the overall heart rate. Wide QRS complexes on the ECG may indicate bundle branch block, a ventricular dysrhythmia, or preexcitation. Administering verapamil to a patient with preexcitation can lead to VF or VT and sudden death. Therefore, the agent must be reserved for patients exhibiting narrow–QRS complex tachydysrhythmias and should never be given in wide-complex tachycardias.

Ventricular Fibrillation

Ventricular fibrillation (VF) occurs when many different cells within the ventricles depolarize independently, rather than in response to an SA node impulse. As a result, the ventricles no longer contract, but fibrillate or quiver in no discernible pattern. Indeed, if you were to look at a fibrillating heart, you would see movement resembling that of a bag of energetic worms. The result of this random depolarization is a fibrillating or chaotic baseline with no evidence of organized electrical activity—no P waves, no PRI, no QRS complexes. When fibrillatory waves are greater than 3 mm in amplitude, the dysrhythmia is sometimes referred to as "coarse" VF **Figure 17-64**. When the fibrillatory waves are less than 3 mm in amplitude, the dysrhythmia is sometimes called "fine" VF **Figure 17-65**.

Defibrillation. According to the AHA, 23% of EMS-treated patients with OHCA present with an initial rhythm of VT or VF.[1] VF and pulseless VT are considered shockable cardiac arrest rhythms, which means that they are likely to respond to defibrillation. Defibrillation is the process by which a surge of unsynchronized direct current electrical energy is delivered to the heart to terminate VF. The goal of defibrillation is to administer a current powerful enough to depolarize all of the heart's component muscle cells; ideally, when those cells repolarize after the shock, they will respond to an impulse from the SA node and resume organized depolarization, leading to cardiac contraction. Defibrillation is also called *unsynchronized countershock* or *asynchronous countershock* because, unlike in synchronized cardioversion, the timing of delivery of the current bears no relation to the cardiac cycle. When a shockable rhythm is identified, defibrillation must be carried out as soon as possible because the likelihood of its success declines rapidly.

An **automated external defibrillator (AED)** interprets the cardiac rhythm, determines if defibrillation is needed, and guides the user through the resuscitation. A fully automated AED delivers a shock automatically if defibrillation is necessary. A **manual defibrillator** is a device that requires you, as a trained user, to interpret the cardiac rhythm and determine if defibrillation is needed. Some defibrillators can

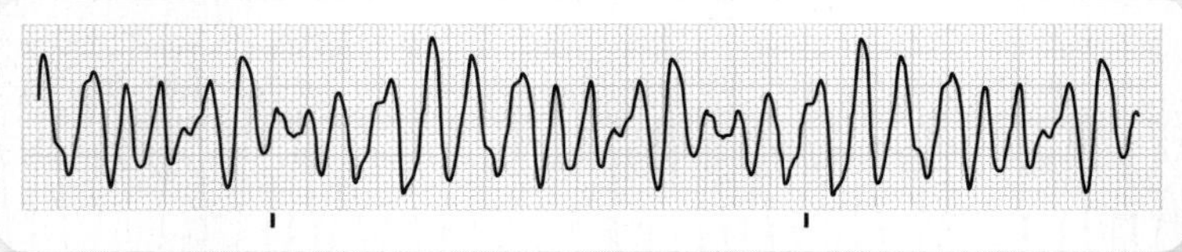

Figure 17-64 Coarse ventricular fibrillation.

Reproduced from *Arrhythmia Recognition: The Art of Interpretation*, courtesy of Tomas B. Garcia, MD.

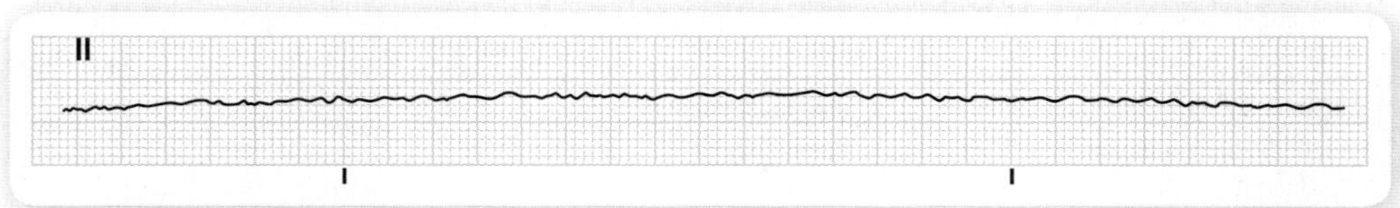

Figure 17-65 Fine ventricular fibrillation.

Reproduced from *Arrhythmia Recognition: The Art of Interpretation*, courtesy of Tomas B. Garcia, MD.

perform defibrillation either manually or automatically, at the user's discretion. Regardless of which type of defibrillator you're using, ensure high-quality CPR is ongoing while the defibrillator is readied for use. If you witness a patient's cardiac arrest, begin CPR starting with chest compressions, and attach the defibrillator as soon as it is available. For adults with an unmonitored cardiac arrest or in situations where a defibrillator is not readily available, current resuscitation guidelines recommend you start CPR while the machine is retrieved and then perform defibrillation, if indicated, as soon as the device is ready for use.[10]

Handheld paddles or adhesive pads are placed on the patient's chest wall to maximize the flow of current through the heart. Paddles consist of a large metal surface that comes into contact with the patient's skin, requiring application of a conductive gel on the paddles' surface to make good electrical contact between the paddles and the skin. Failure to use conductive gel on the paddles often results in burns and ineffective energy delivery to the heart. Apply about 25 lb (11 kg) of pressure to hold the paddles against the chest. Adhesive pads placed on the patient's bare chest and connected to the defibrillator are commonly used today. These pads allow you to quickly assess the patient's cardiac rhythm and deliver an electrical shock, if indicated. Whether using the adhesive pads or handheld paddles, it's crucial to follow the manufacturer's recommended placement on the chest to avoid electrical arcing between the two contact points. From here on, we will use the term *defibrillation pads* to refer to the handheld paddles and adhesive pads used for defibrillation.

Special Populations

Remember to immediately note the patient's age. Use pediatric defibrillation pads when appropriate.

AEDs and manual defibrillators deliver energy in waveforms. Monophasic waveforms, used in older defibrillators, deliver energy through the heart from one defibrillation pad to the other in a single direction. With biphasic waveforms, energy travels through the heart from one defibrillation pad to the other and then reverses direction, flowing back through the heart from one pad to the other. Defibrillator units equipped with biphasic waveforms are superior to monophasic defibrillators because of their greater success in terminating dysrhythmias.[7] It is essential that you know the recommended energy level for the type of defibrillator you're using Figure 17-66.

The same safety measures are used when performing manual defibrillation and when using an AED:

- Ensure no one is touching the patient.
- Do not defibrillate a patient who is in pooled water. There will be some danger to you if you are also in the water. The electricity will diffuse into the water instead of traveling between the defibrillation pads and through the patient's heart; therefore, the heart will not receive enough electricity to cause defibrillation. You can defibrillate a soaking-wet patient, but first try to dry the patient's chest.
- Do not defibrillate someone who is touching metal that others are touching.
- Do not place a defibrillation pad over a medication patch or any metal objects such as jewelry. Doing so could result in burns.
- If the patient has an implanted pacemaker or internal defibrillator, place the defibrillation pad below the device, or place the pads in anterior and posterior positions.

The defibrillator should be inspected at the beginning of each shift, using a checklist to cover all aspects of the device and its gear: defibrillation pads, cables and

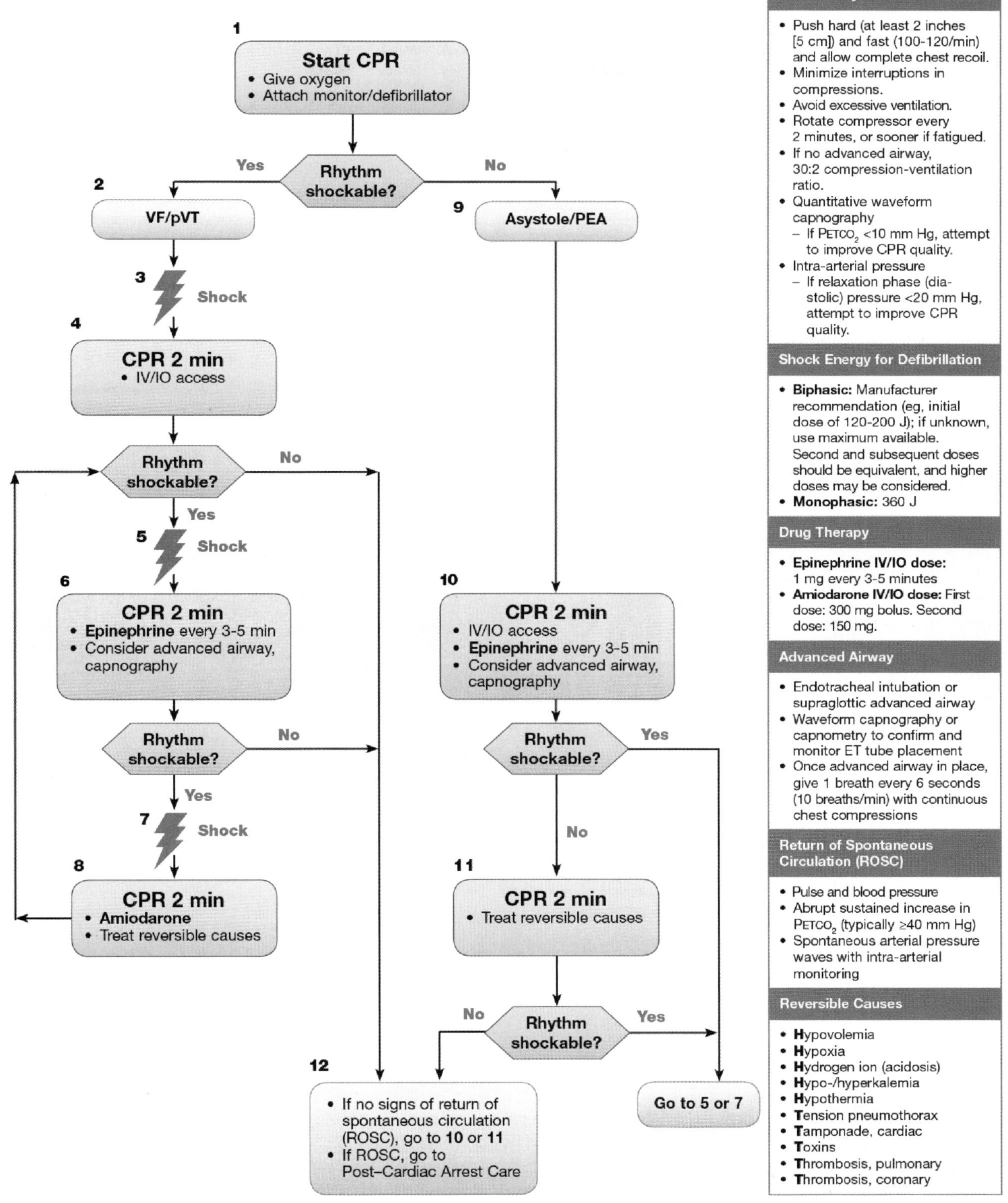

Abbreviations: CPR, cardiopulmonary resuscitation; ET, endotracheal; IO, intraosseous; IV, intravenous; PEA, pulseless electrical activity; $PETCO_2$, end-tidal partial pressure of carbon dioxide; ROSC, return of spontaneous circulation, VF, ventricular fibrillation; pVT, polymorphic ventricular tachycardia

Figure 17-66 Adult cardiac arrest algorithm.

Words of Wisdom

An implanted pacemaker—which you may detect by identifying the pacemaker-produced spikes on the ECG or by noticing the bulge where the pacemaker's battery pack has been implanted under the patient's skin—is *not* a contraindication to defibrillation. Just ensure not to place the defibrillation pads directly over the pacemaker battery.

connectors, power supply, monitor, ECG recorder, and any ancillary supplies, such as electrode gel, pads, and spare battery. The US Food and Drug Administration (FDA) has developed an Operator's Shift Checklist for inspecting defibrillators. Conscientious use of the checklist will significantly reduce the likelihood of defibrillator failure.

Skill Drill 17-4 summarizes the procedures for manual defibrillation.

Although you will usually perform manual defibrillation, you may encounter a scene where law enforcement

Patient Safety

The US FDA Adverse Event Reporting System (FAERS) is a system used to report adverse medication or device malfunctions. For example, if a defibrillator failed to charge or deliver a shock during a call, the provider or agency could report the event directly to the FDA or to the manufacturer. If a manufacturer receives an adverse report, it is required to report it to the FDA.

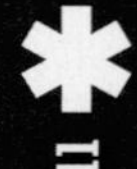

NR Skill

Skill Drill 17-4 Performing Manual Defibrillation

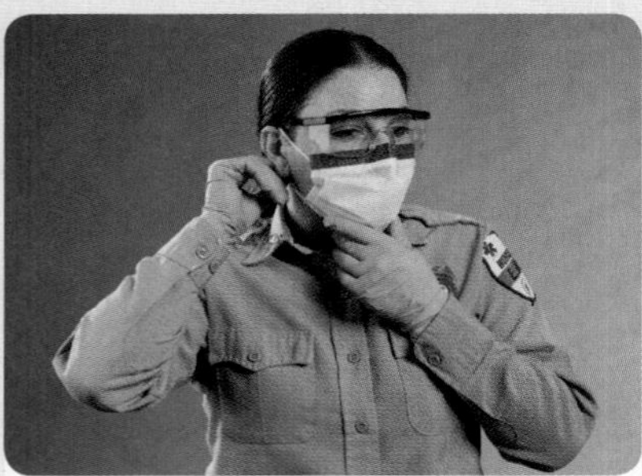

Step 1 Select, check, and assemble all necessary equipment, including a monitor/defibrillator with defibrillation pads, oxygen, and an appropriate oxygen administration device. Take standard precautions and ensure the scene and environment are safe (evaluate the risk of sparks, combustibles, oxygen-rich atmosphere).

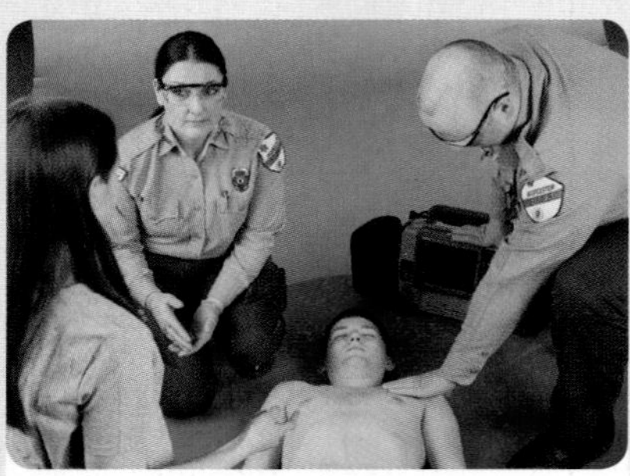

Step 2 If available (and possible without interrupting care), ask bystanders about the events surrounding the arrest. Check responsiveness. Request additional help, if needed.

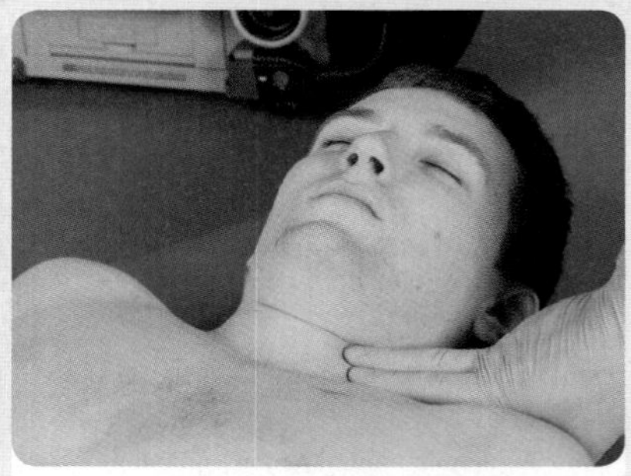

Step 3 Assess the patient for breathing while simultaneously checking for a carotid pulse.

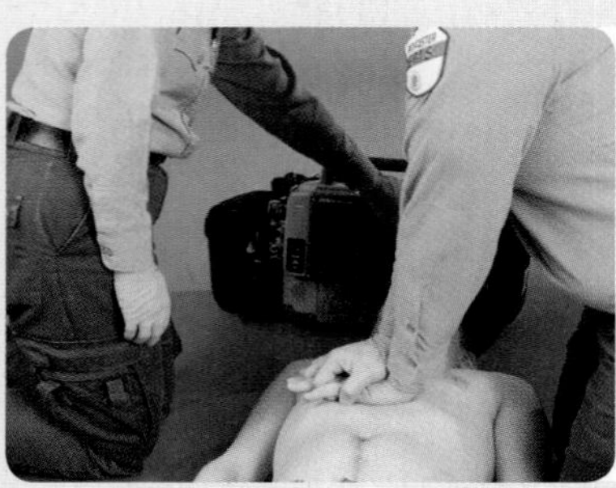

Step 4 Begin chest compressions if the patient is not breathing or is only gasping and has no pulse. Ensure an adequate depth and rate, use the correct compression-to-ventilation ratio, allow the chest to recoil completely, deliver an adequate volume for each breath, and keep interruption of chest compressions to 10 seconds or less throughout the resuscitation effort.

Skill Drill 17-4 Performing Manual Defibrillation (continued)

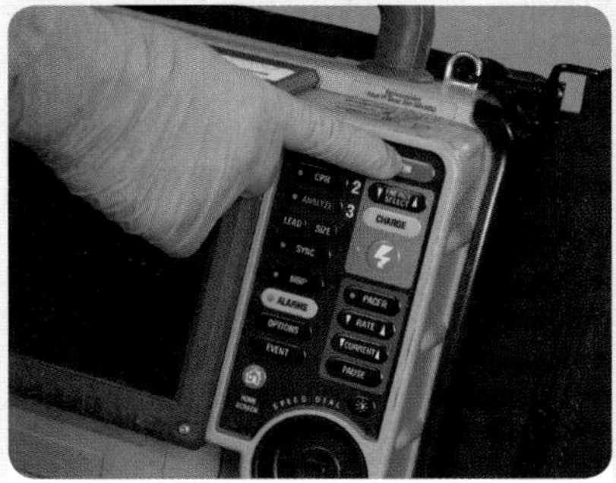

Step 5 Turn on the power to the defibrillator. If EMS providers have been using the machine in AED mode before your arrival, switch the machine to manual mode.

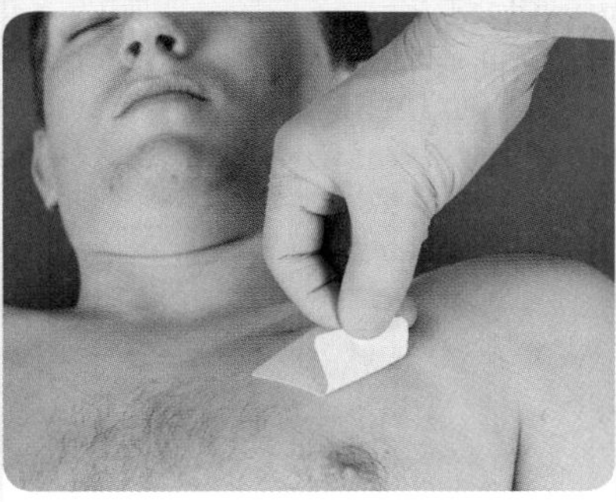

Step 6 Remove the clothing from the patient's upper body. With gloves, remove any medication paste or patches from the patient's chest and wipe away any residue.

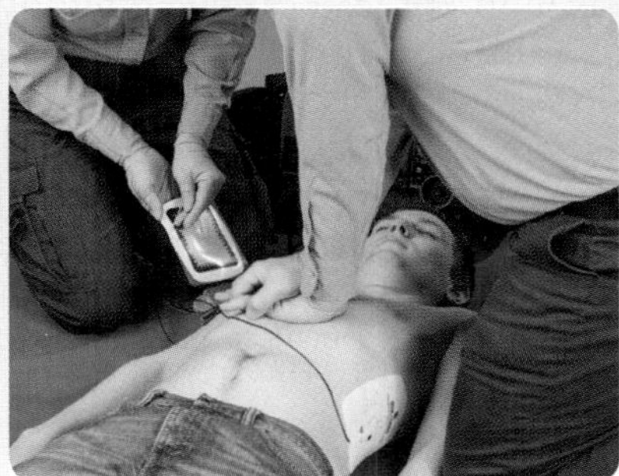

Step 7 If using standard paddles, place pre-gelled defibrillator pads on the patient's chest (or apply defibrillator gel to the electrode surface of the paddles). If using adhesive electrodes, place one electrode just to the right of the sternum just below the clavicle and place the other on the left lower chest area with the top of the pad 2 to 3 inches below the armpit (or position the electrodes according to the manufacturer's instructions). Do not place electrodes on top of breast tissue. If necessary, lift the breast out of the way and place the electrode underneath.

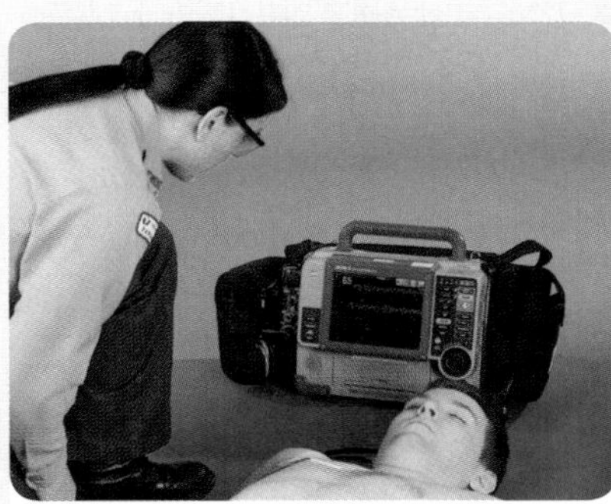

Step 8 Stop CPR, identify the rhythm, and confirm that defibrillation is warranted. After verifying that a shockable rhythm is present, set the defibrillator to the proper energy setting.

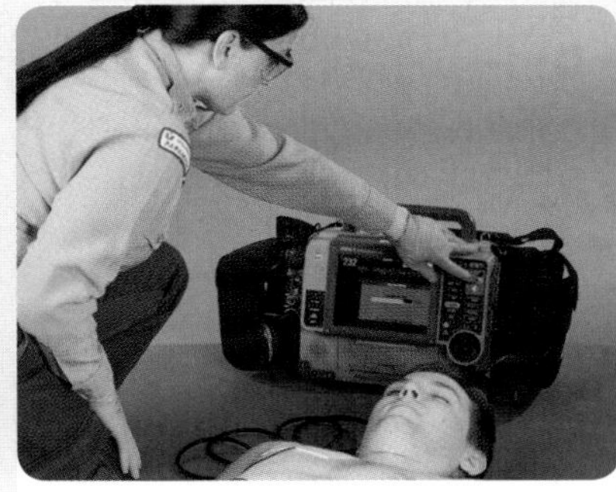

Step 9 Charge the defibrillator.

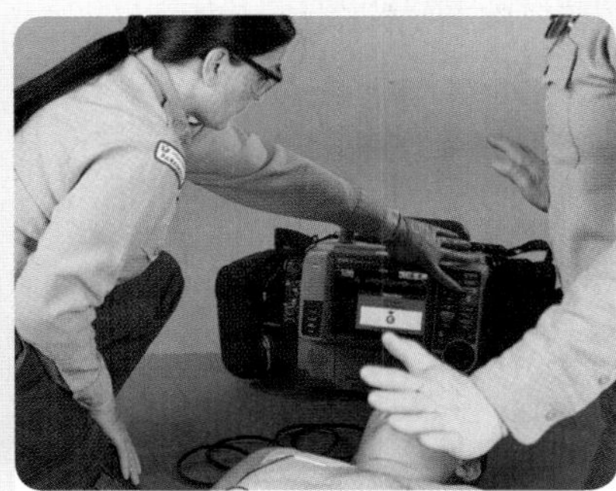

Step 10 Clear the area. Announce, "All clear!" and ensure no one is touching the patient. Press the *Shock* button on the machine if using a hands-free system. If using paddles, depress the *Shock* button on each paddle at the same time, and hold until the defibrillator discharges. Resume CPR immediately.

or other EMS providers have already attached to the patient an AED that is set in AED mode. In such cases, use the AED, but switch it to manual mode. Manual mode allows use of all electrical therapy functions (such as TCP and synchronized cardioversion), as well as multiple-lead cardiac monitoring and 12-lead ECG acquisition. You may also arrive at a scene where an AED is not in use, but the patient then goes into cardiac arrest. In that case, select manual mode on the defibrillator unit. You can then look at the monitor and determine if the rhythm is shockable. If so, proceed with charging the unit and shocking the patient. Doing so saves time, because CPR can continue until the moment the defibrillator is ready to shock; you don't need to wait for the AED mode to analyze the rhythm and make a recommendation. Remember, it is essential to minimize the interruption of chest compressions with patients in cardiac arrest.

A fully automated AED (rarely used) can assess the patient's rhythm and—if VF or VT is present—charge the pads and defibrillate, with no intervention by the rescuer. A semiautomated AED (commonly used), on the other hand, detects VF and VT and uses visual and verbal prompts to indicate when a shock is advised. The rescuer must then depress the *Shock* button to defibrillate the patient. The steps for using an AED are shown in Skill Drill 17-5.

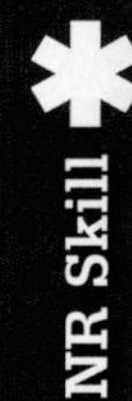

Skill Drill 17-5 Performing Defibrillation With an AED

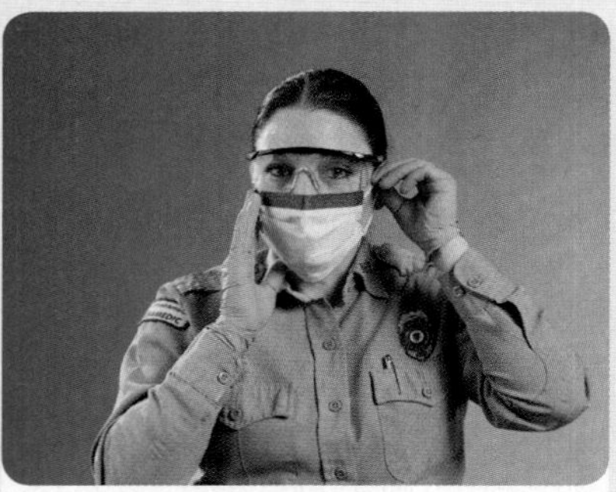

Step 1 Select, check, and assemble all necessary equipment, including an AED, AED pads, oxygen, and an appropriate oxygen administration device. Take standard precautions and ensure the scene and environment are safe (evaluate the risk of sparks, combustibles, oxygen-rich atmosphere).

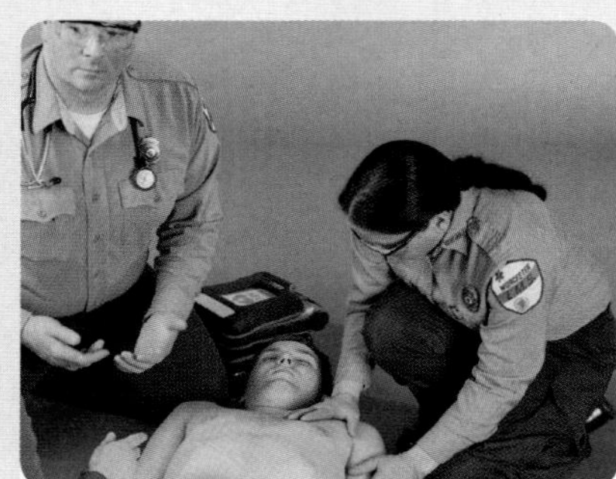

Step 2 If available (and possible without interrupting care), ask bystanders about the events surrounding the arrest. Check responsiveness. Request additional help, if needed.

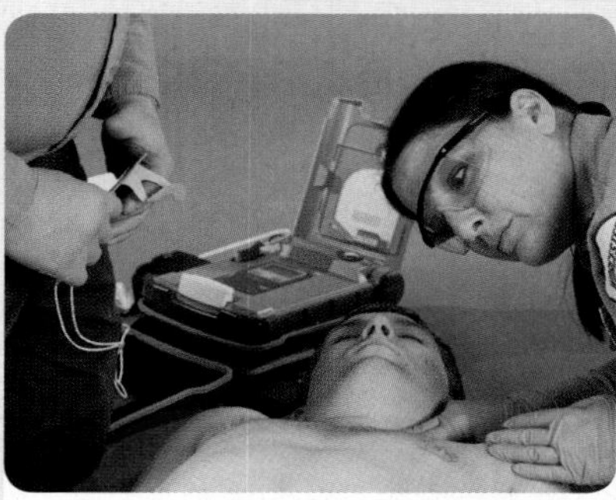

Step 3 Assess the patient for breathing while simultaneously checking for a carotid pulse.

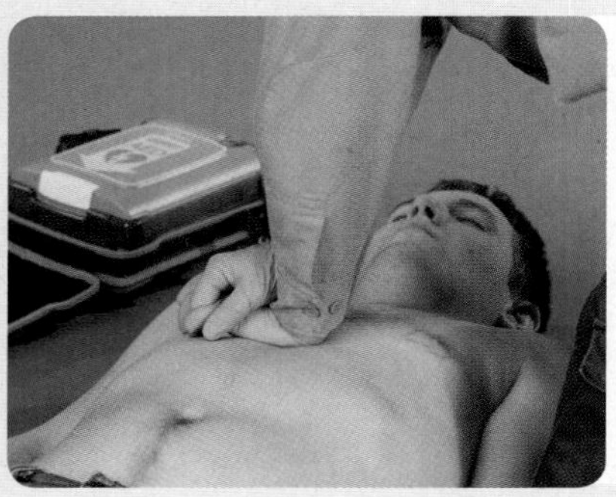

Step 4 If CPR is already in progress, then assess the effectiveness of chest compressions. If the patient is not breathing or is only gasping and has no pulse, and CPR has not been started, then begin chest compressions and rescue breaths. Ensure an adequate depth and rate, use the correct compression-to-ventilation ratio, allow the chest to recoil completely, deliver an adequate volume for each breath, and keep interruption of chest compressions to 10 seconds or less throughout the resuscitation effort. Continue until an AED arrives and is ready for use.

Skill Drill 17-5 Performing Defibrillation With an AED *(continued)*

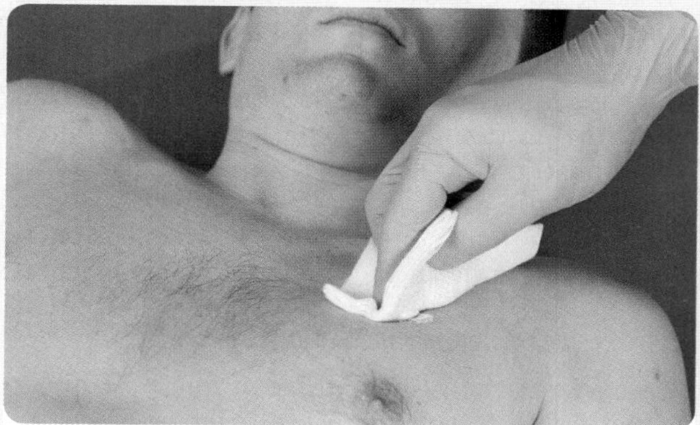

Step 5 Turn on the AED. Remove the clothing from the patient's upper body. With gloves, remove medication paste or patches from the patient's chest, if present, and wipe away any residue.

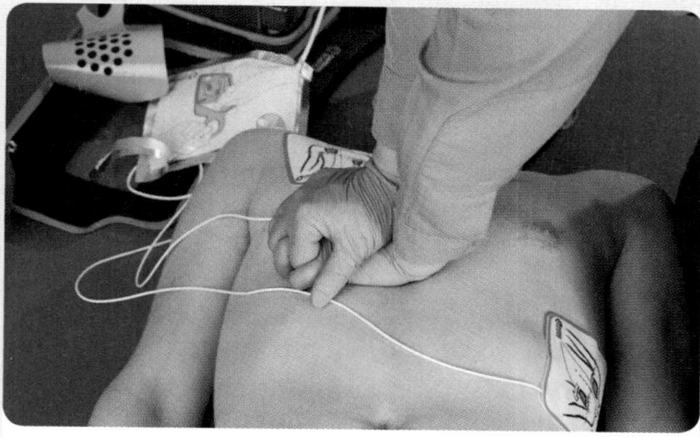

Step 6 Follow the machine's prompts; apply the AED pads to the patient's bare chest according to the manufacturer's recommendations. Attach the pads to the AED.

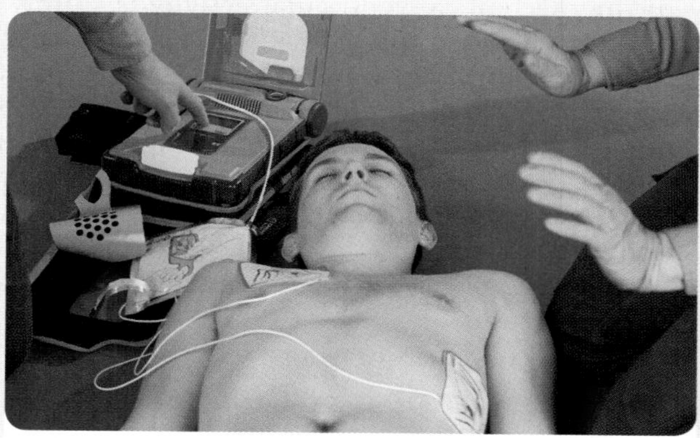

Step 7 Stop CPR and press the *Analyze* button (some AEDs will begin analyzing the patient's rhythm automatically). Ensure everyone is clear of the patient. Wait for the AED to analyze the cardiac rhythm. If no shock is advised, then resume CPR, starting with chest compressions. Perform five cycles (about 2 minutes) of CPR and then reanalyze the cardiac rhythm. If a shock is advised, then recheck that all are clear, and press the *Shock* button.

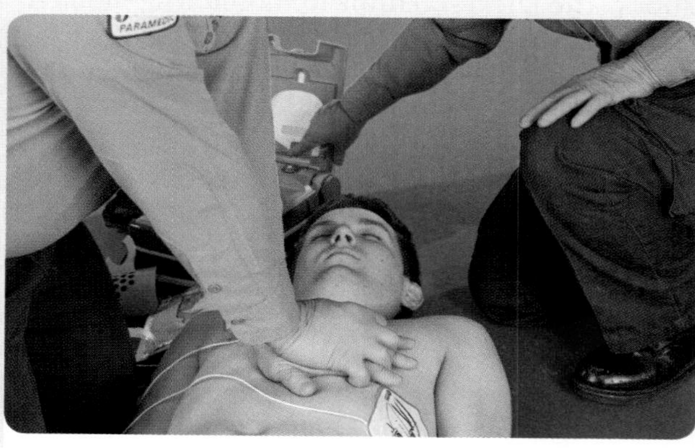

Step 8 After the shock is delivered, immediately resume CPR, beginning with chest compressions. Do not interrupt chest compressions for more than 10 seconds. Do not turn off the AED during CPR. Continue to follow the AED prompts. To reduce the likelihood of rescuer fatigue, rotate the position of the chest compressor and ventilator during the AED's analysis phase.

Care of the patient after the AED delivers a shock depends on your location and EMS system; therefore, you should follow your local protocol. After doing so, one of the following outcomes is likely:

- Pulse is regained.
- Pulse is not regained, and the AED indicates that no shock is advised.
- Pulse is not regained, and the AED indicates that a shock is advised.

For each of these scenarios, the sequence of compressions and defibrillation is the same as we described in the earlier section on manual defibrillation. The only difference is the AED determines whether the rhythm is shockable.

Wearable Cardioverter-Defibrillators. You may encounter a patient with a wearable cardioverter-defibrillator (WCD). This device is designed for patients at risk of sudden cardiac death, but who are not immediate candidates for therapy with an implantable cardioverter-defibrillator.[11] An example of such a device is the LifeVest, manufactured by ZOLL, which was approved for use in 2002 by the FDA. It consists of a lightweight garment with a belt and shoulder straps and a battery-powered monitor-defibrillator. The garment, which is worn under the patient's clothing, houses nonadhesive sensing electrodes and separate defibrillation electrodes. The monitor continuously reads and records the patient's ECG. Patients are instructed to wear the device continuously, except when bathing or showering. When a potential dysrhythmia is detected, the patient is alerted by means of the alarm system consisting of a vibration signal, low- and high-volume sound alarms, and a verbal warning that indicates that a shock is imminent.[12] If the patient is responsive, he or she can respond by pressing two buttons to stop the treatment sequence. If the response buttons are not depressed, the device charges and the defibrillation electrodes exude gel just before delivery of a shock. The LifeVest returns to monitoring mode if a normal rhythm is detected after the shock. If the dysrhythmia persists after the first defibrillation, then the cycle is repeated. Up to five biphasic energy shocks can be delivered for a single event.[12] The overall response time from detection to shock can take between 25 and 60 seconds.[11] Replace the garment and electrodes after a dysrhythmia has been treated.

Asystole

Asystole ("flat line"), the only true **arrhythmia**, is a rhythm in which the heart is no longer contracting and shows no evidence of organized activity **Figure 17-67**. Asystole is also known as *cardiac standstill*. This rhythm presents with a complete absence of ventricular electrical activity. Atrial activity, represented by P waves, may occasionally be seen but, when present, they are not accompanied by QRS complexes or T waves. The term *P-wave asystole, ventricular asystole,* or *ventricular standstill* is used when P waves are observed in the absence of ventricular electrical activity.

A flat line on an ECG monitor may or may not indicate asystole. Thus, one of the first things to do when you see a flat-line ECG is to rule out causes other than asystole. Possible causes of a flat-line ECG include leads that are not connected to the patient, loose leads, leads that are not connected to the monitor-defibrillator, an incorrect monitor setting, very low–voltage VF, and true asystole.

Asystole is considered a nonshockable cardiac arrest rhythm (see Figure 17-66). Recall, the purpose of defibrillation is to deliver a shock of sufficient intensity to depolarize myocardial cells, enabling the SA node to resume pacemaking responsibility when the cells repolarize. In asystole, there is no electrical activity to reset.

Pulseless Electrical Activity

So far we have discussed three of four possible cardiac arrest rhythms: pulseless VT, VF, and asystole. The final cardiac arrest rhythm is **pulseless electrical activity (PEA)**, an organized cardiac rhythm (other than VT) on the monitor that is not accompanied by a detectable pulse. PEA was once called *electromechanical dissociation*. With PEA, there is either no mechanical ventricular activity or the mechanical ventricular activity is simply too weak to produce a palpable pulse. This may occur, for example, in cardiogenic or hypovolemic shock, cardiac tamponade, massive pulmonary embolism, electrolyte imbalance (including hyperkalemia in renal failure), or drug overdose. Providing the appropriate treatment for PEA, then, depends on identifying its cause. PEA is a nonshockable cardiac arrest rhythm (see Figure 17-66). Management of cardiac arrest is discussed in detail in the next section.

▶ Management of Adult Cardiac Arrest

Nothing gets the adrenaline pumping more furiously—in paramedics, if not in patients—than a "code," or cardiac arrest. Although prior heart disease is a major risk factor for cardiac arrest, the condition can also occur secondary to electrocution, a submersion incident, and other traumatic events, or to noncardiac conditions such as

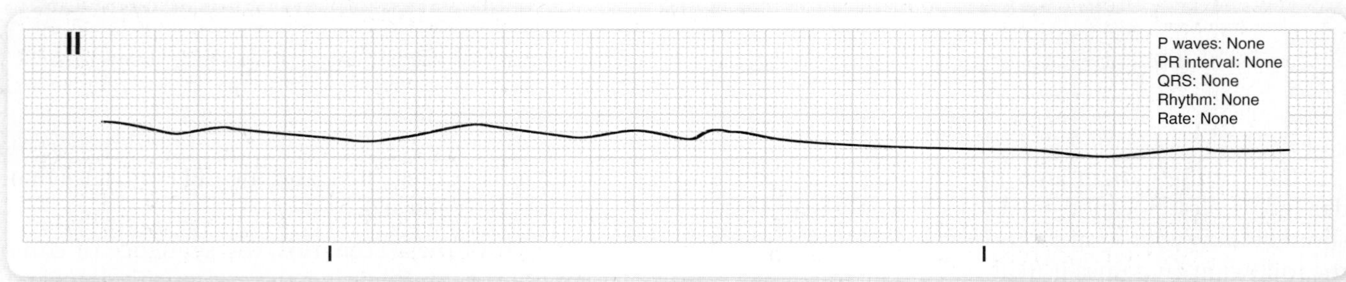

Figure 17-67 Asystole.

Reproduced from *Arrhythmia Recognition: The Art of Interpretation*, courtesy of Tomas B. Garcia, MD.

drug overdose, asthma, or anaphylaxis. Many people who experience cardiac arrest have no warning signs before the event occurs. No matter what the cause, cardiac arrest is stressful for all involved. The best way to reduce the stress among providers and increase the likelihood of returning spontaneous circulation in the patient is to practice, practice, and practice, so your team works like a pit crew. This concept is discussed further in Chapter 39, *Responding to the Field Code*.

Managing a cardiac arrest requires you to deploy many of the advanced life support (ALS) skills you've learned and to do so under circumstances in which minutes may mean the difference between life and death. It is difficult to think clearly in such tense circumstances, especially when there are other distressed and panicky people at the scene (the patient's family, for example). For these reasons, it is absolutely essential for you to follow an orderly, systematic approach to cardiac arrest emergencies. That approach must be rehearsed exhaustively, in a team setting, until it becomes nearly automatic.

Bring the following devices and equipment when you initially approach the scene:

- Defibrillator
- Portable oxygen cylinder
- Airway management equipment, including an intubation kit
- IV equipment
- Drug box

If you're shorthanded, don't spend time carrying every piece of equipment from the emergency vehicle to the patient; you can send someone to the vehicle later to retrieve other equipment, such as the backboard and stretcher.

The goals of emergency medical care of a patient in cardiac arrest include the return of spontaneous circulation (ROSC) and the preservation of neurologic function. The "no flow" phase of a cardiac arrest is the period during which an arrest has occurred but CPR has not begun. To minimize the duration of this phase, begin emergency medical care immediately upon discovering pulselessness.

Although it is expected that emergency care be provided to a person in cardiac arrest, the AHA has identified the following situations in which withholding CPR is considered appropriate:[13]

- Attempts to perform CPR would place rescuers at risk of serious injury or mortal peril, such as exposure to infectious diseases.
- There are obvious clinical signs of irreversible death, such as rigor mortis, dependent lividity, decapitation, transection, or decomposition.
- A valid advance directive, a Physician Order for Life-Sustaining Treatment (POLST) form indicating that resuscitation is not desired, or a valid Do Not Attempt Resuscitation (DNAR) order is presented to rescuers.

Words of Wisdom

Withholding Resuscitative Efforts

In situations in which the patient's status is unclear and the appropriateness of withholding resuscitation efforts uncertain, begin CPR and then contact medical control.[6] When there is a personal physician present at the scene who has an ongoing relationship with the patient, that provider may decide if resuscitation is to be initiated. When there is a registered nurse from a home health care or hospice agency present at the scene who has an ongoing relationship with the patient, and who is operating under orders from the patient's personal physician, that authorized nurse may decide if resuscitation is to be initiated. If the physician or nurse decides that resuscitation is appropriate, follow usual direct medical oversight procedures.

If bystanders have delivered adequate uninterrupted chest compressions before your arrival, or if the arrest is witnessed by EMS personnel, then proceed with rhythm analysis. If compressions have not been provided, or if the arrest was not witnessed by EMS personnel, then begin chest compressions while a second rescuer sets up the AED or defibrillator. Proceed with rhythm analysis. Your initial efforts should focus either on creating a "low flow" state, in which the delivery of high-quality CPR begins and is continued throughout the resuscitation effort, or on creating a "normal flow" state through the ROSC by means of defibrillation or other interventions. Components of high-quality adult CPR include the following:

- Perform chest compressions at a rate of 100/min to 120/min.
- Compress the chest to a depth of at least 2 inches (5 cm).
- Allow full chest recoil after each compression.
- Minimize interruption of compressions.
- Deliver adequate ventilation (2 breaths after 30 compressions).

What you see on the monitor will determine which side of the cardiac arrest algorithm you will now follow (see Figure 17-66). Remember, there are four possible cardiac arrest rhythms: (1) pulseless VT, (2) VF, (3) asystole, and (4) PEA. Pulseless VT and VF are shockable rhythms; asystole and PEA are not. Key points to keep in mind include the following:

- If defibrillation is indicated, then the provider giving chest compressions should continue while a second rescuer charges the defibrillator. Then pause CPR, clear the patient, and deliver the shock. Resume chest compressions immediately, without pausing for a rhythm or pulse check.

- After 2 minutes or five cycles of CPR, pause resuscitation efforts and check the rhythm on the monitor. If a rhythm other than VF or VT appears, then identify the new rhythm and check for a pulse. If there is no pulse, then move down the algorithm to the asystole-PEA pathway and immediately resume CPR. If there is a pulse, then move to the appropriate algorithm for the new rhythm. If the rhythm is VF or VT, then resume CPR while charging the defibrillator. Clear the patient and then defibrillate.
- Minimize rescuer fatigue by switching the CPR compressor and ventilator at the end of each 2-minute session of CPR (while the rhythm and pulse are being checked). Rescuer fatigue can reduce the effectiveness of chest compressions.
- To maximize the number of compressions delivered per minute, interruptions should not exceed 10 seconds.[10]
- Using normal saline, attempt to establish vascular access only after beginning CPR and, when a shockable rhythm is present, attempting defibrillation. If you are unable to establish IV access, then establish intraosseous (IO) access using an adult IO system. Vascular access should be achieved without interrupting chest compressions. As soon as IV or IO access has been established, administer epinephrine. Epinephrine 1 mg (0.1 mg/mL [1:10,000]) is administered IV or IO and is repeated every 3 to 5 minutes until a pulse returns. Whenever you give a medication through a peripheral IV line during CPR, follow it immediately with a 20-mL flush of normal saline IV, and then elevate the extremity for 1 to 2 minutes to facilitate delivery of the medication to the central circulation.
- Several options are available for airway management. A bag-mask device may be used throughout the resuscitation effort. For adults in cardiac arrest without an advanced airway, use a 30:2 compression to ventilation ratio. Ventilate with just enough volume to produce visible chest rise. Deliver each breath over about 1 second. If the decision is made to insert an advanced airway, then verify placement by multiple methods, including waveform capnography, and secure the tube. Deliver 1 breath every 6 seconds (10 breaths/min) without interrupting chest compressions.
- VF or pulseless VT that persists or recurs after one or more shocks is called refractory VF/VT. An antidysrhythmic, such as amiodarone, may be considered for VF/VT that is unresponsive to CPR, defibrillation, and vasopressor therapy.[7] Lidocaine may be considered as an alternative to amiodarone for VF/VT. Antidysrhythmic medications are discussed in more detail in Chapter 13, *Principles of Pharmacology*.
- During the arrest, consider the Hs and Ts to identify possible reversible causes of the arrest and factors that may complicate the resuscitation effort Table 17-5.
- If at any point there is a ROSC, then assess the patient's vital signs, support the airway and breathing, as required, and give medications as indicated for regulating the heart rate, controlling cardiac dysrhythmias, and maintain the blood pressure.

Patients who do not regain a pulse at the scene of a cardiac arrest usually do not survive. Whether and where you transport such patients depends on your EMS system and is dictated by your local protocol.

Administering CPR while a patient is being moved or transported is usually not effective. A patient has the best chance of survival when he or she is resuscitated at the scene, unless the location is unsafe.

If your local protocol allows, begin transport when any of the following occurs:

- The patient regains a pulse.
- Six to nine shocks have been delivered (or as directed by local protocol).
- The device indicates three consecutive messages (separated by 2 minutes of CPR) and no shock is advised (or as directed by local protocol).

If you transport a patient while performing CPR, then you need a plan for managing the patient in the ambulance. Ideally, EMS providers are in the patient compartment while a third provider drives. You may deliver additional shocks at the scene or en route with the approval of medical control. It is not as safe to defibrillate a patient in a moving ambulance; therefore, the vehicle should come to a complete stop if an additional shock is needed. Ensure you follow the local protocol of your EMS system.

Documentation & Communication

EMS systems regularly evaluate the emergency care provided to patients who have had a cardiac arrest. Key elements to document are the following:[6]

- Resuscitation attempts and all interventions performed
- Witnesses of the cardiac arrest
- Location of the cardiac arrest
- First monitored rhythm
- CPR efforts before EMS arrival
- Outcome or disposition (including any ROSC)
- Presumed etiology (presumed cardiac, trauma, submersion, respiratory, other noncardiac, unknown)

Table 17-5 Hs and Ts: Causes and Treatment of Cardiac Arrest Rhythms

Possible Reversible Cause	Clues	Treatment*
Hypovolemia	▪ History ▪ Flat neck veins	Volume replacement
Hypoxemia	▪ Cyanosis ▪ Airway compromise	Ventilation with 100% oxygen; consider advanced airway insertion
Hypothermia	History of exposure to cold	See hypothermia algorithm in Chapter 38, *Environmental Emergencies*, for information on treating hypothermia.
▪ Hyperkalemia ▪ Hypokalemia ▪ Hydrogen ions (acidosis)	▪ History ▪ ECG changes	▪ Immediate transport ▪ Consider sodium bicarbonate if certain of acidosis
Tension pneumothorax	▪ History (trauma, asthma, COPD) ▪ No pulse with CPR ▪ Difficult to ventilate ▪ Unequal breath sounds, with hyperresonance to percussion on affected side	Needle decompression of the affected side of the chest
Cardiac tamponade	▪ History ▪ No pulse with CPR ▪ Jugular venous distention	Immediate transport for pericardiocentesis
▪ Toxins (drug overdose) ▪ Thrombosis (massive MI, pulmonary embolism)	History	▪ Consider immediate transport. ▪ Naloxone (Narcan) for opioid overdose

* Beyond managing the cardiac arrest
Abbreviations: ECG, electrocardiogram; COPD, chronic obstructive pulmonary disease; CPR, cardiopulmonary resuscitation; MI, myocardial infarction.

Special Circumstances in Cardiac Arrest

Some cardiac arrests occur in circumstances that require special considerations, treatments, or procedures beyond those typically applied or provided during a resuscitation effort. For example, you many need to alter certain techniques to accommodate a patient with morbid obesity.

Early, rapid advanced airway management is essential for the patient whose cardiac arrest is the result of anaphylaxis. Planning for advanced airway management, including a surgical airway, is recommended for such patients, and aggressive fluid resuscitation may be required.[14]

Patients with opioid-associated cardiac arrest are managed in accordance with standard ACLS practices; however, you may need to administer naloxone during the post–cardiac arrest period to reverse the effects of long-acting opioids.

When cardiac arrest occurs in a patient with acute asthma and the patient becomes difficult to ventilate, you must watch for and be prepared to treat a tension pneumothorax.

Cardiac arrest associated with severe electrolyte disturbances may require administering medications that you don't routinely give during a resuscitation effort such as sodium bicarbonate, calcium, or magnesium.

Cardiac arrest in pregnant patients is discussed in Chapter 41, *Obstetrics*. Cardiac arrest in pediatric patients is discussed in Chapter 43, *Pediatric Emergencies*.

Post–Cardiac Arrest Care

Post–cardiac arrest care is an important component of overall care of cardiac arrest patients. The goals of post–cardiac arrest care are to optimize cardiopulmonary function and vital organ perfusion. If an effective cardiac rhythm is restored in the field, transport the patient immediately, ideally, to a facility with comprehensive post–cardiac arrest treatment, including acute coronary interventions, advanced neurologic monitoring and care, goal-directed critical care, and **targeted temperature management (TTM)**.

Begin by optimizing oxygenation and ventilation. Assess breath sounds (also known as lung sounds). After ROSC, most patients require ventilatory assistance. Titrate oxygen therapy to achieve and maintain an Spo_2 of 94% or higher. Avoid hyperventilation. Obtain a 12-lead ECG as soon as possible to determine whether acute ST-segment elevation is present.

Perform a neurologic assessment; assess for signs of hypoperfusion. Marked hypotension needs to be corrected rapidly because the brain will not be adequately perfused if the blood pressure is very low. Administer a fluid bolus of 1 to 2 liters (L) normal saline or lactated Ringer solution. If the patient has marked hypotension and the transport time to the medical facility will be prolonged, then consider administering a vasopressor infusion. If the rhythm is bradycardic or tachycardic, then follow the bradycardia or tachycardia algorithm.

To protect the brain and other organs, current resuscitation guidelines recommend you start TTM after cardiac arrests for comatose adult patients with ROSC. This therapy, which is begun in the hospital, involves maintaining a constant target body temperature between 32°C (89.6°F) and 38°C (100.4°F) for at least 24 hours. The prehospital cooling of patients after ROSC with rapid infusion of cold IV fluids is no longer recommended.[15]

Regardless of the cause of a cardiac arrest, the hypoxemia, ischemia, and reperfusion that occurs during the arrest and resuscitation effort may damage multiple organ systems.[15] During the post–cardiac arrest period, patients are often hemodynamically unstable. Many of them will re-arrest. Thus, the post–cardiac arrest patient requires close monitoring. The adult post–cardiac arrest care algorithm is shown in **Figure 17-68**.

When to Stop CPR

The goals of resuscitation are to preserve life, restore health, relieve suffering, limit disability, and respect patients' decisions, rights, and privacy.[13] When the objective of a medical treatment cannot be achieved, the treatment is considered futile.[13]

The AHA recommends rescuers who begin CPR continue until one of the following occurs:[13]

- Effective spontaneous circulation is restored.
- Care is transferred to a team providing advanced life support.
- The rescuer is unable to continue because of exhaustion, because environmental hazards are identified, or because continuing the resuscitative efforts places others in jeopardy.

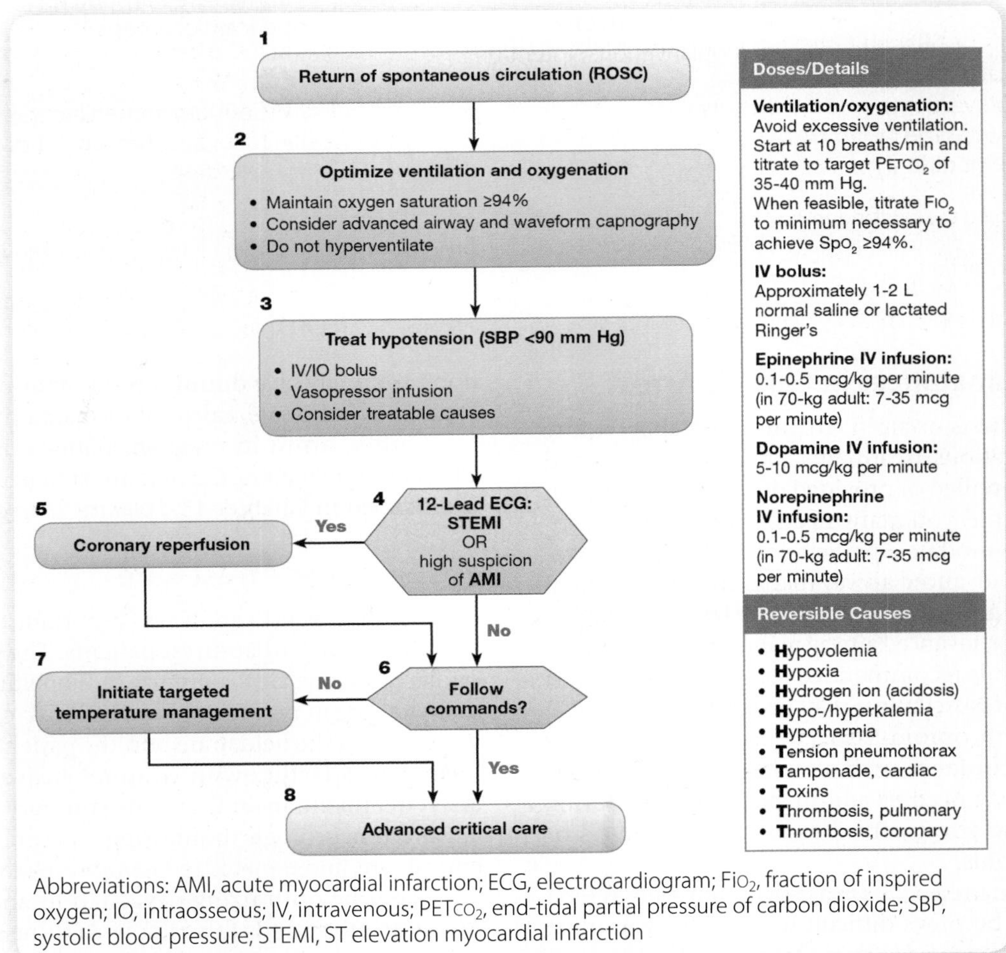

Abbreviations: AMI, acute myocardial infarction; ECG, electrocardiogram; FIO_2, fraction of inspired oxygen; IO, intraosseous; IV, intravenous; $PETCO_2$, end-tidal partial pressure of carbon dioxide; SBP, systolic blood pressure; STEMI, ST elevation myocardial infarction

Figure 17-68 Adult immediate post–cardiac arrest care algorithm.

- Reliable and valid criteria indicating irreversible death have been met, criteria of obvious death have been identified, or criteria for terminating resuscitation have been met.

When the patient does not respond to prehospital cardiac arrest treatment, it is acceptable and often preferable to cease futile resuscitation efforts in the field. There are several reasons for this:[6]

- In most situations, ALS providers are capable of performing an initial resuscitation equivalent to an in-hospital resuscitation attempt, and there are no additional benefits to ED resuscitation.
- CPR performed during patient packaging and transport is much less effective than CPR administered at the scene.
- EMS providers risk physical injury while attempting to perform CPR in a moving ambulance while unrestrained.
- Continuing resuscitation in futile cases places other motorists and pedestrians at risk, increases the amount of time during which the EMS crew is unavailable for other calls, impedes ED care of other patients, and incurs unnecessary charges from the medical facility.

The AHA has published criteria for BLS and ALS termination of resuscitation for adult OHCA (Table 17-6).[13]

In some jurisdictions, state law does not permit paramedics to pronounce death at the scene. If legislation were enacted to permit such pronouncements in these jurisdictions, each EMS system would have to formulate its own criteria for terminating CPR in the prehospital setting.

Receiving permission to stop CPR in the field doesn't necessarily make your life easier. Delicate issues are involved such as the expectations of the patient's family and proper disposition of the body. In addition, you may face enormous pressure from bystanders to continue resuscitative efforts long after there is any medical justification for doing so. Stopping CPR may also be difficult for you; you may not be accustomed to having to explain to a family, that the person has died and nothing more can be done. It's much easier to transport the person to the medical facility and leave the ED staff with the unpleasant task of breaking the bad news.

Many jurisdictions have adopted protocols to help providers decide when resuscitation attempts are futile and should be terminated. If it is legal in your EMS system to terminate CPR in the field, then meet with your medical director to walk through scenarios you may have to face. Role-play exercises can be particularly useful to help you identify, in advance, situations in which you may feel uncomfortable and to help you develop strategies for coping with them.

▶ Atrioventricular Blocks

After the SA node initiates an impulse, it proceeds through the atria and ventricles, resulting in contraction of the heart. When the signal reaches the AV node, it is delayed to allow the atria to contract and fill the ventricles. This delay is a normal function of the AV node and usually causes no signs or symptoms. Occasionally, however, the impulse traveling through the AV node is delayed more than usual or is completely blocked, resulting in an AV block, which is a type of heart block. This prolonged delay or block in impulse conduction can occur at the level of the AV node or below the bundle of His (infranodal), and it may involve one or more of the bundle branches and their fascicles.

AV blocks are classified into different degrees, depending on the seriousness of the block and the amount of myocardial damage. The least serious is a first-degree

Table 17-6 American Heart Association Rules for Terminating Resuscitation in Adults With OHCA

BLS Rule	ALS Rule
Consider terminating BLS resuscitative attempts for adults with OHCA before moving them to the ambulance for transport when *all* of the following criteria are met: **1.** The arrest was not witnessed by an EMS provider or first responder. **2.** No ROSC after 3 full rounds of CPR and AED analysis (before transport). **3.** No AED shocks were delivered before transport.	Consider terminating ALS resuscitative attempts for adults with OHCA before moving them to the ambulance for transport when *all* of the following criteria are met: **1.** The arrest was not witnessed by EMS personnel. **2.** No bystander CPR was provided. **3.** No ROSC after full ALS care in the field before transport. **4.** No AED shocks were delivered before transport.

If *any* criteria are missing, continue resuscitation and transport.

Abbreviations: BLS, basic life support; ALS, advanced life support; OHCA, out-of-hospital cardiac arrest; EMS, emergency medical services; ROSC, return of spontaneous circulation; AED, automated external defibrillator; CPR, cardiopulmonary resuscitation.

Data from: Mancini ME, Diekema DS, Hoadley TA, Kadlec KD, Leveille MH, McGowan JE, Sinz EH. (2015, Oct). *2015 American Heart Association Guidelines for CPR & ECC.* Retrieved Apr 15, 2016, from American Heart Association. Web-based Integrated Guidelines for Cardiopulmonary Resuscitation and Emergency Cardiovascular Care—Part 3: Ethical Issues: www.eccguidelines.heart.org.

AV block; the most serious is a third-degree block. In between, of course, is a second-degree block.

First-Degree AV Block

A **first-degree AV block**, also called *first-degree heart block*, occurs when each impulse reaching the AV node is delayed longer than normal, resulting in a constant PRI that exceeds 0.20 seconds (200 milliseconds). Because each impulse eventually passes through the AV node, generating a QRS complex, AV block is considered the least serious kind of heart block. Nevertheless, it is often the first indication that the AV node has been damaged.

Because first-degree AV block may occur with any rhythm in which a P wave precedes the QRS, the rate associated with it is that of the underlying rhythm Figure 17-69. The rhythm is usually regular, with minimal variation between R-R intervals, but its regularity depends on the underlying rhythm. An upright P wave precedes each QRS complex. Its size and shape may vary, depending on the underlying rhythm. The PRI measures greater than 0.20 seconds (200 milliseconds) and is constant in duration. The QRS complex measure 0.11 seconds (110 milliseconds) or less. The primary difference between first-degree AV block and normal sinus rhythm is the prolonged PRI.

First-degree AV block generally doesn't require treatment in the prehospital setting unless it is associated with a symptomatic bradycardia. In such cases, the bradycardia is treated in accordance with the bradycardia algorithm, which is discussed later in this chapter.

Second-Degree AV Block Type I

A second-degree AV block occurs when an interruption in impulse conduction occurs within the AV node, bundle of His, or His-Purkinje system, preventing the impulse from proceeding to the ventricles and generating a QRS complex. Second-degree AV block type I, also called Mobitz type I second-degree block or Wenckebach, most often occurs because of impaired conduction through the AV node; however, it may infrequently occur below the AV node within the bundle of His or bundle branches.

With second-degree AV block type I, the interval between P waves is regular. An upright P wave precedes most QRS complexes. The ventricular rhythm is irregular, with a prolonged R-R interval between the last QRS complex before the blocked P wave and the QRS complex after the first unblocked P wave Figure 17-70. The PRI starts out within the normal limits of 0.12 to 0.20 seconds (120 to 200 milliseconds) but grows longer with each successive P wave. Finally, a P wave appears that is followed not by a QRS complex, but by another P wave. This P wave is then followed by a QRS complex with a normal PRI. This pattern repeats over and over in this rhythm. The QRS complex measures 0.11 seconds (110 milliseconds) or less.

The keys to recognizing second-degree AV block type I include: (1) observing there are more P waves than QRS complexes, (2) noting the P waves occur at regular intervals, (3) identifying the PRIs associated with the conducted P waves get longer and longer until a P wave appears that is not followed by a QRS complex, and (4) noting the ventricular rhythm is irregular.

Conditions in which second-degree AV block type I may be seen include ischemic heart disease, acute inferior wall or right ventricular MI, increased vagal tone, digoxin toxicity, and certain electrolyte imbalances. Administering amiodarone, beta-blockers, and calcium channel blockers can cause second-degree AV block type I.

The patient with this type of AV block is usually asymptomatic, because the ventricular rate often remains nearly normal and CO is not significantly compromised; however, if the ventricular rate slows and the patient becomes symptomatic because of the slow rate, the bradycardia is treated in accordance with the bradycardia algorithm (see Figure 17-35). When this rhythm occurs in conjunction with AMI, continuously monitor the patient for increasing AV block.

Second-Degree AV Block Type II

Second-degree AV block type II, also called Mobitz type II second-degree block or type II AV block, is more serious than second-degree AV block type I. With AV block

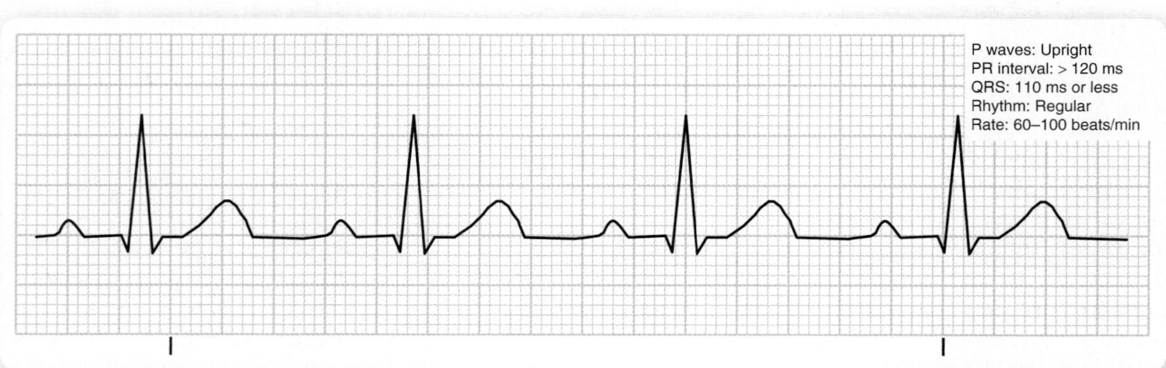

Figure 17-69 Sinus bradycardia with first-degree atrioventricular block.

Reproduced from *Arrhythmia Recognition: The Art of Interpretation*, courtesy of Tomas B. Garcia, MD.

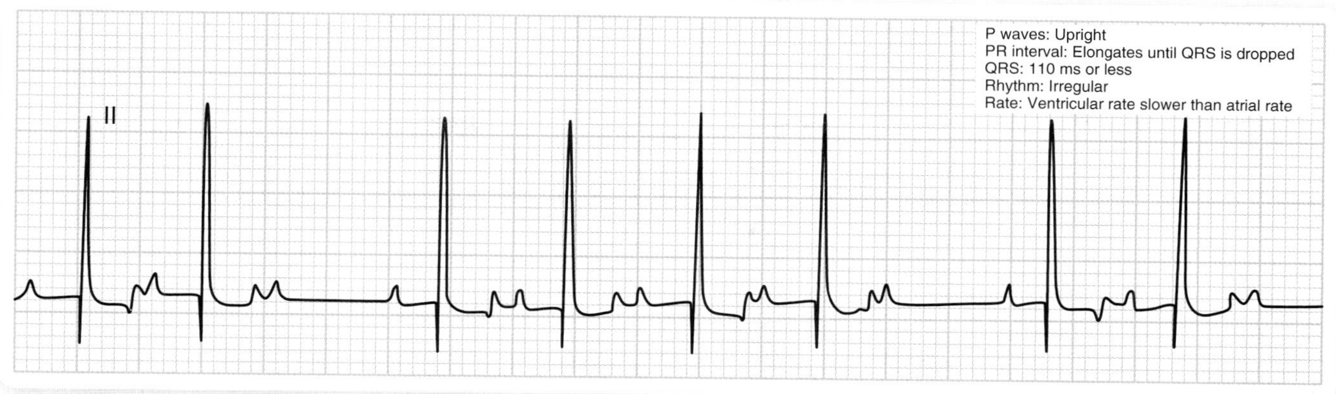

Figure 17-70 Second-degree atrioventricular block type I.

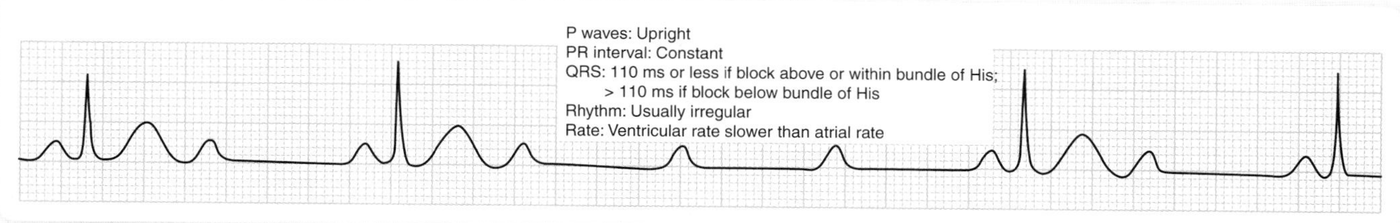

Figure 17-71 Second-degree atrioventricular block type II.

type II, impaired conduction usually occurs within the bundle of His or, more commonly, the bundle branches.

Second-degree AV block type II is an intermittent block characterized by regularly occurring P waves and the abrupt appearance of at least one P wave that is not followed by a QRS complex Figure 17-71. A P wave that occurs without a subsequent QRS complex indicates the SA node impulse was not conducted to the ventricles. The ventricular rhythm is irregular because of the dropped QRS complexes. The PRI is always constant. The QRS will measure 0.11 seconds (110 milliseconds) or less if the block occurs above or within the bundle of His. If the block occurs below the bundle of His, then the QRS will be greater than 0.11 seconds (110 milliseconds).

Causes of second-degree AV block type II include ischemic heart disease, acute anterior wall MI, and infectious heart diseases. It may also occur as a consequence of a cardiac operation. Second-degree type II AV block is often associated with a slow ventricular rate, and significantly reduced CO may be evident. Patients may experience dizziness, fatigue, dyspnea on exertion, or syncope. Because atropine is usually ineffective in reversing this type of block, emergency care may require the use of TCP (see Figure 17-35). Second-degree AV block type II can progress to third-degree AV block without warning. Patient monitoring is critical.

Second-degree AV blocks can occur in patterns. When two P waves appear for each QRS, a 2:1 AV block is present; when three P waves appear for one QRS, a 3:1 AV block is present. In such situations, it can be difficult to determine if the second-degree AV block is type I or type II. Although exceptions do occur, the QRS duration is usually within normal limits in type I blocks, and it is usually longer than normal in type II blocks.

Third-Degree AV Block

A third-degree AV block occurs when all impulses reaching the AV junction are prevented from proceeding to the ventricles and generating a QRS complex. As a consequence, this block is also known as a complete heart block or complete AV block. Because all impulses from the SA node are blocked, a secondary pacemaker (either junctional or ventricular) must assume responsibility for impulse conduction.

The classic way to identify a third-degree AV block is to look for nonconducted P waves and the absence of any relationship between the P waves and the QRS complexes. There is no PRI because the atrial and ventricular rhythms occur independently of each other. The rhythm is usually regular, with consistent P-P and R-R intervals Figure 17-72. The P wave is present and upright. The ventricular rate, which depends on the activity of a secondary pacemaker, is 40 to 60 beats/min if the pacemaker originates in the AV junction and 20 to 40 beats/min if it originates in the ventricles.

The QRS complexes seen in third-degree AV block may be of normal duration if they originate in the AV junction.

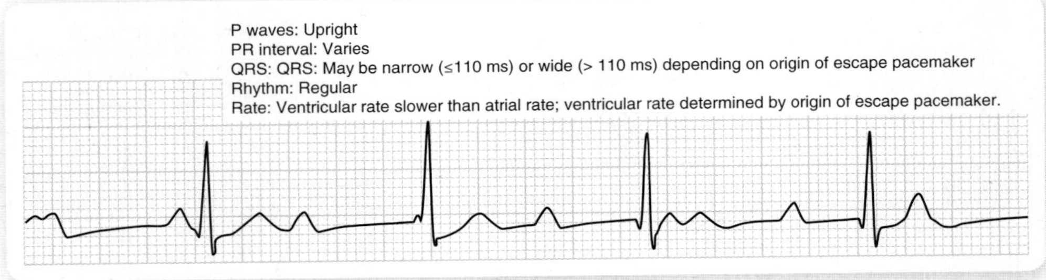

Figure 17-72 Third-degree atrioventricular block.

Reproduced from *Arrhythmia Recognition: The Art of Interpretation*, courtesy of Tomas B. Garcia, MD.

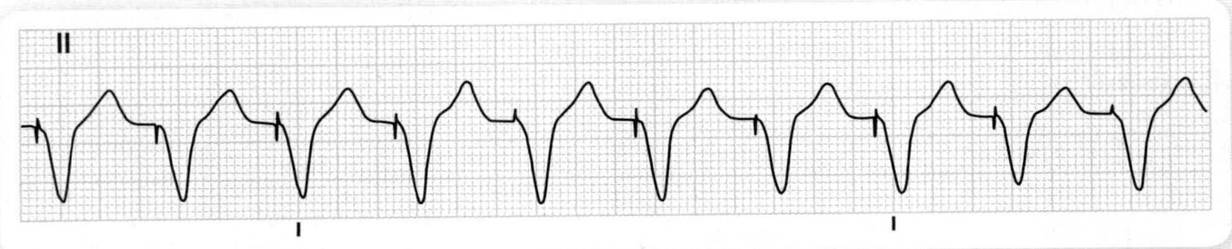

Figure 17-73 Ventricular paced rhythm.

Reproduced from *Arrhythmia Recognition: The Art of Interpretation*, courtesy of Tomas B. Garcia, MD.

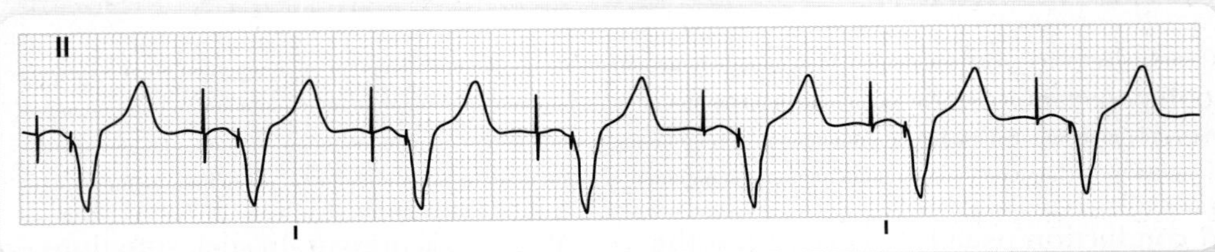

Figure 17-74 Dual-chamber (atrioventricular sequential) pacemaker rhythm.

Reproduced from *Arrhythmia Recognition: The Art of Interpretation*, courtesy of Tomas B. Garcia, MD.

They are generally 0.12 seconds (120 milliseconds) or more if the pacemaker site is in the ventricles.

Third-degree AV blocks can be produced by AMI, ischemic heart disease, hyperkalemia, or too high a dose of certain rate-control medications. Symptoms are related to the location of the block within the conduction system. The patient may be asymptomatic if the site of the block is in the AV node and a junctional rhythm is present, with a reasonable ventricular rate. However, syncope or sudden cardiac death can occur if the site of the block is below the AV node, with a slow or no ventricular escape rhythm.[16] If the patient is symptomatic because of the slow rate, then treat the bradycardia in accordance with the bradycardia algorithm (see Figure 17-35).

▶ Artificial Pacemaker Rhythms

Many of your patients will have experienced cardiac conduction system disorders for which an artificial pacemaker was implanted. An artificial pacemaker consists of a pulse generator, which is the battery-powered energy source, and wire electrodes attached to one or more chambers of the heart. The pulse generator of a permanent pacemaker contains programmable hardware. It is implanted in the subcutaneous tissue of the chest, below the right or left clavicle.

The firing of an artificial pacemaker generates a unique vertical spike on the ECG tracing **Figure 17-73**. A single-chamber pacemaker paces only one cardiac chamber—either the right atrium or the right ventricle. A dual-chamber pacemaker, also called an *AV sequential pacemaker*, paces the right atrium and right ventricle. This type of device produces a pacemaker spike followed by a P wave and another pacemaker spike followed by a wide QRS complex **Figure 17-74**. A biventricular pacemaker, which synchronizes contraction of the right and left ventricles, is used to treat patients with severe or moderately severe heart failure.

Pacemakers are available in two rate types. A fixed-rate pacemaker, which is seldom used today, generates a pacing impulse at a preprogrammed rate. In contrast, a demand pacemaker is equipped with a sensor that detects the rate of spontaneous cardiac depolarization. It generates a paced impulse only when it senses that the patient's heart rate has dropped below a predetermined rate (usually 60 beats/min) **Figure 17-75**.

Implanted Pacemaker Malfunction

Occasionally, a pacemaker fails. If the patient's pacemaker is failing, the pacemaker spikes may still be visible, but

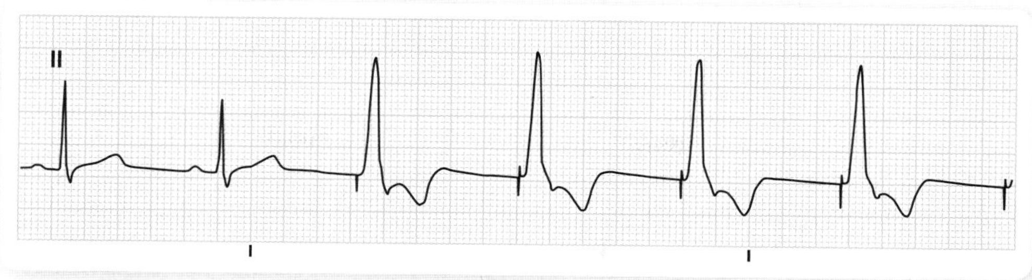

Figure 17-75 Ventricular demand pacemaker rhythm.

Reproduced from *Arrhythmia Recognition: The Art of Interpretation*, courtesy of Tomas B. Garcia, MD.

they will not be followed by a QRS complex. This failure to capture indicates the pacemaker is not operating properly. Failure to capture may occur if the wire connecting the pacemaker to the patient's heart is dislodged. It may also occur because of battery depletion or ventricular perforation.

Failure to pace is a pacemaker malfunction indicated on the ECG by the absence of pacemaker spikes at expected times. Possible causes of failure to pace include pulse generator failure, a broken lead wire or dislodged lead, a disconnected wire or cable, or battery depletion.

Failure to sense is a malfunction in which the pacemaker competes with the patient's own intrinsic rhythm. Pulse generator failure, a broken lead wire or dislodged lead, an excessively high sensitivity setting, or battery depletion can all cause undersensing. Undersensing is indicated on the ECG by the appearance of pacemaker spikes within the P wave, QRS complex, or T wave. Because pacemaker spikes occur inappropriately, this type of pacemaker malfunction poses a threat of VT or VF caused by the occurrence of pacemaker spikes during the vulnerable period of the cardiac cycle.

When oversensing occurs, the pacemaker fails to generate an impulse because it has sensed extraneous signals (often muscular) and misinterpreted them as QRS complexes. It is indicated on the ECG by the occurrence of pacemaker spikes at a rate slower than the pacemaker's preset rate, or by the absence of paced beats even though the pacemaker's preset rate is faster than the patient's rate.

Another type of pacemaker failure is the so-called runaway pacemaker. A runaway pacemaker is indicated by a very tachycardic pacemaker rhythm that must be slowed to preserve the patient's cardiac function. Placing a strong magnet over the pacemaker will usually reset a runaway pacemaker. This recalibration would be done in the ED by a cardiologist.

If any of these malfunctions occurs, the patient's heartbeat will depend on a natural pacemaker (usually the ventricles), causing greatly reduced CO. In such cases, TCP may be required to support CO until the pacemaker can be replaced.

12-Lead ECGs

For rhythm interpretation and identification of lethal rhythms, a single lead—typically lead II—is usually sufficient. However, a 12-lead ECG is useful when you want to see views of the heart from several angles to localize the site of cardiac injury or to identify dysrhythmias and other cardiac abnormalities. Indications for using a 12-lead ECG include the following:

- Chest pain or discomfort
- Electrical injury
- Known or suspected electrolyte imbalance
- Known or suspected medication overdose
- RVF and/or LVF
- Stroke
- Syncope or near-syncope
- Hemodynamic instability of unknown etiology

Devices capable of recording 12-lead ECGs contain interpretation software. This software is a good tool and is generally very accurate in measuring intervals and durations, but it has many limitations. It is best to rely on your own interpretation, not the automated findings, when reading the ECG; think of automated interpretation software as a nudge or hint as to what may be happening in the patient's heart, not a definitive conclusion. Some devices are also capable of transmitting ECGs to the medical facility, allowing ED physicians to review the ECG before your arrival and prepare specialized resources in advance.

Acquisition Modes

The ECG device can record tracings using various electromagnetic frequency ranges in either of two acquisition modes: monitor mode or diagnostic mode. For rhythm interpretation, the ECG is recorded in monitor mode. This mode employs electronic filters to remove artifact and other unwanted information from the tracing. Unfortunately, monitor mode can also skew the shape and location of the ST segment and T wave. Monitor mode captures electrical information within the range of 1 to 30, 40, 100, or 150 hertz (Hz).

Diagnostic mode is the other acquisition mode. It filters out very little electrical information, however, so more artifact may appear on the tracing. A bandwidth of 0.05 to 150 Hz is used for diagnostic ECGs and the 12-lead ECG machine's interpretive analysis is performed using this bandwidth. Diagnostic mode is the default mode used to record a 12-lead ECG, and it cannot be changed. Many devices enable users to record 3-lead ECGs in diagnostic mode as well. However, the 3-lead ECG is usually acquired in the early minutes of patient contact, when there tends to be a lot of movement. This crosstalk can create substantial artifact on the tracing, making it impossible to interpret the rhythm. The frequency range is always printed near the bottom of the ECG tracing **Figure 17-76**.

▶ Lead Placement

The best way to learn how to record a 12-lead ECG is to practice with the actual equipment. When positioning the electrodes, don't allow the patient to become chilled, because shivering will produce artifact in the ECG tracing. **Skill Drill 17-6** outlines the steps in 12-lead ECG acquisition.

Figure 17-76 The electromagnetic frequency range is printed near the bottom of the electrocardiogram (ECG). Diagnostic mode is always used in 12-lead ECG tracings.

NR Skill

Skill Drill 17-6 Acquiring a 12-lead ECG

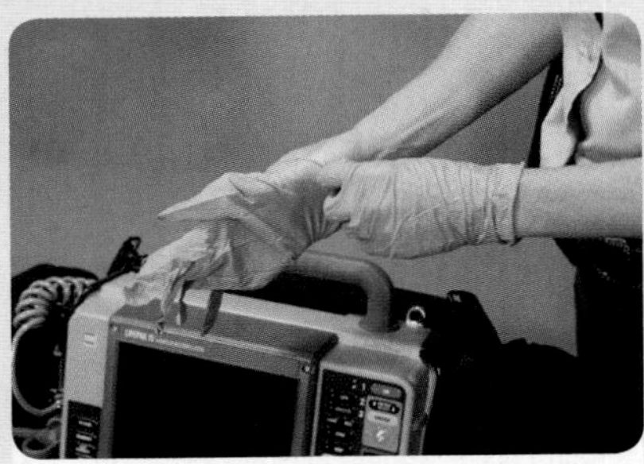

Step 1 Take standard precautions. Check your equipment. Ensure the end of the ECG cable has no loose pins and the cable or lead wires are intact. Ensure the monitor has an adequate paper supply. Connect the ECG cable to the machine. Connect the lead wires to the ECG cable (if not already connected).

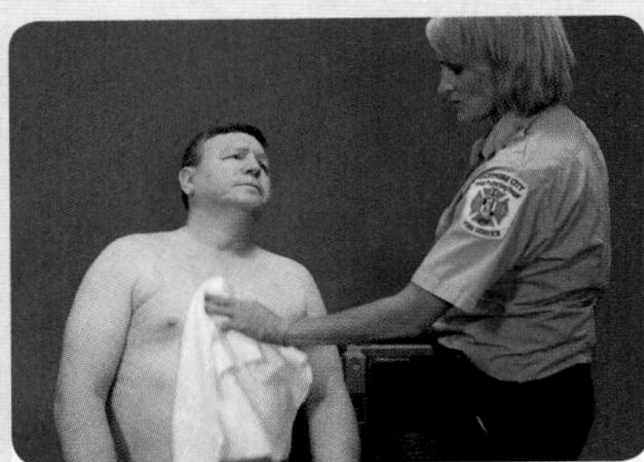

Step 2 Explain the procedure to the patient. Prepare the patient's skin for electrode placement; shave and cleanse the patient's skin as needed before placing the monitoring electrodes.

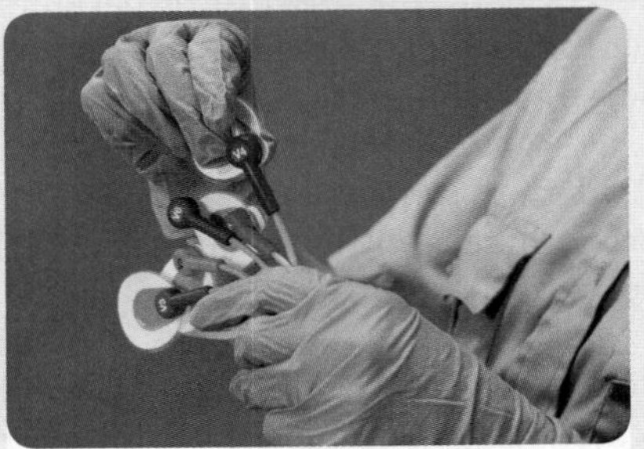

Step 3 Attach the electrodes to the leads before you place them on the patient.

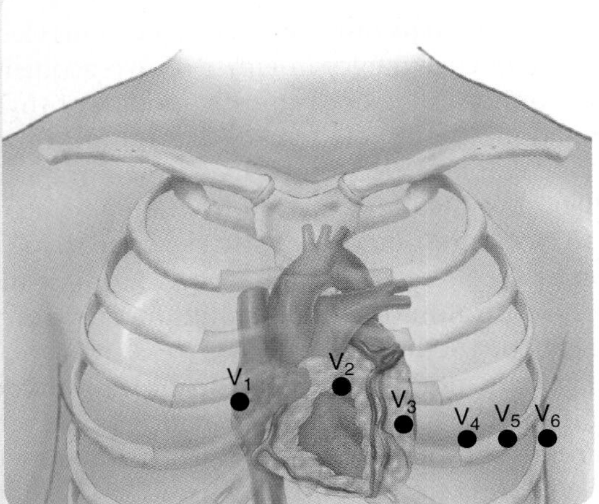

Step 4 Position the electrodes on the patient. Connect the four limb electrodes. Place them on the arms and legs. *Do not* place the electrodes on the trunk of the body, as is sometimes done for ECG monitoring. Double-check to confirm the correct electrode has been positioned on each limb (the LA electrode on the left arm, the RA electrode on the right arm, and so on).

Once the limb electrodes have been secured, connect and apply the electrodes for the precordial leads:

- V_1—Fourth ICS to the right of the sternum
- V_2—Fourth ICS to the left of the sternum
- V_3—Directly between leads V_2 and V_4
- V_4—Fifth ICS at the left midclavicular line
- V_5—At level of lead V_4 at left anterior axillary line
- V_6—At level of lead V_4 at left midaxillary line

Skill Drill 17-6 Acquiring a 12-lead ECG *(continued)*

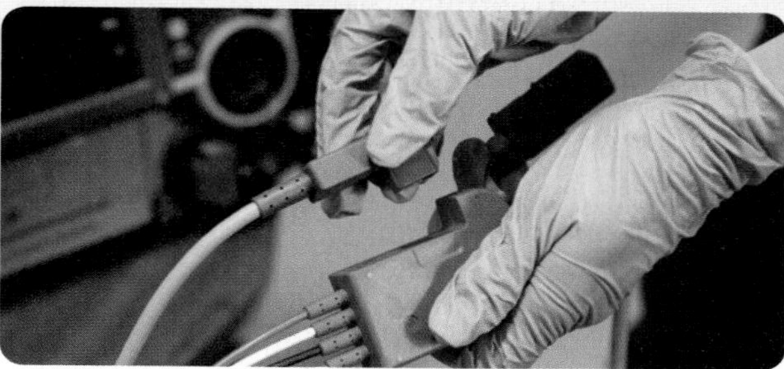

Step 5 Connect the cables to the monitor. Ensure the patient is sitting or lying still, the extremities are not crossed, and he or she is breathing normally and is not talking. Turn on the power to the monitor and adjust the screen contrast if necessary. Ensure all electrodes and cables are still connected and that no error message is displayed.

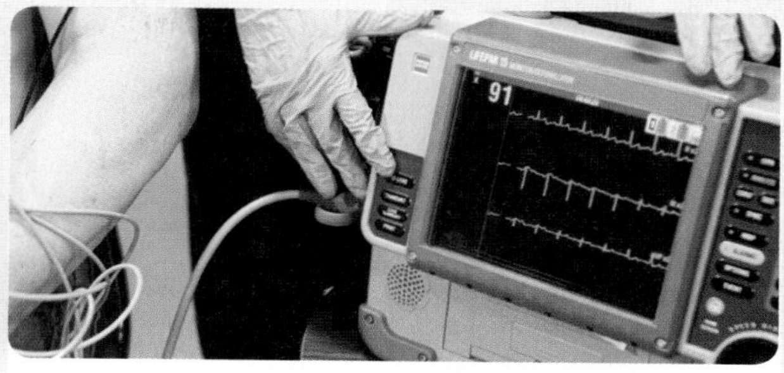

Step 6 Press the *12-Lead Analyze* button.

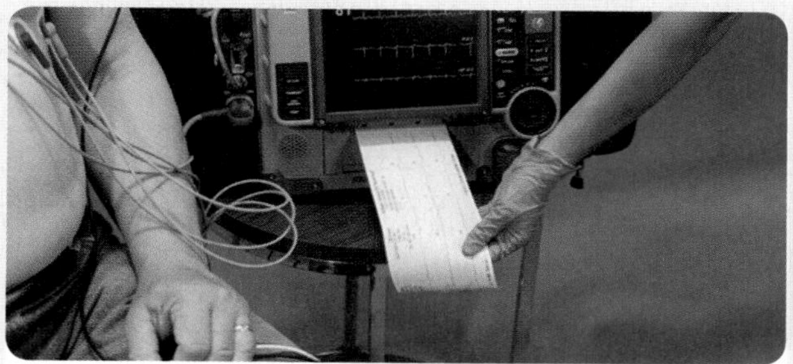

Step 7 Obtain the 12-lead ECG recording.

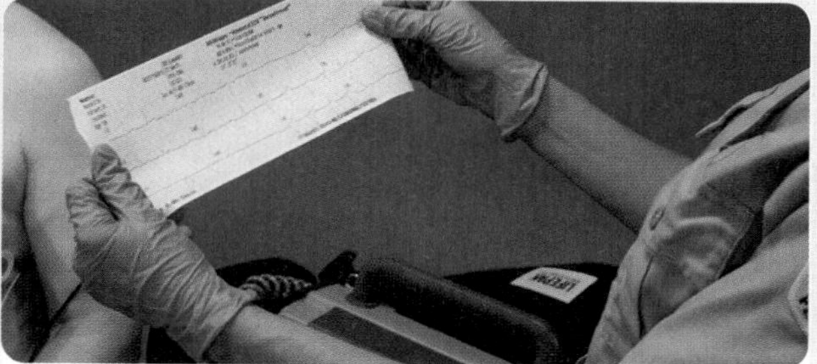

Step 8 Examine the tracing for acceptable quality. Interpret the 12-lead ECG, label it, and determine whether additional views of the right and posterior walls (15- or 18-lead tracings) are needed. Obtain a 12-lead ECG every 5 to 10 minutes in high-risk patients and post treatment.

▶ Approach to 12-Lead ECG Interpretation

Like dysrhythmia interpretation, 12-lead ECG interpretation requires a systemic approach to ensure nothing is missed. A seven-step method to 12-lead ECG interpretation follows:

1. Review the snapshot.
2. Interpret the dysrhythmia.
3. Determine the axis.
4. Identify conduction system disturbances.
5. Evaluate chamber size.
6. Review for zones of ischemia, injury, infarction.
7. Identify noncardiac causes.

Review the Snapshot

First, look at the tracing to see if anything stands out. For example, is the heart rate extremely slow or fast? This step is a quick overall look at the 12-lead ECG to see if all the leads printed, if artifact is present, and if the rate is at either extreme.

Interpret the Dysrhythmia

This is the same five-step process presented earlier in the chapter. Use these rules to identify the underlying rhythm:

1. Identify the waves (P-QRS-T).
2. Measure the PRI.
3. Measure the QRS duration.
4. Determine rhythm regularity.
5. Measure the heart rate.

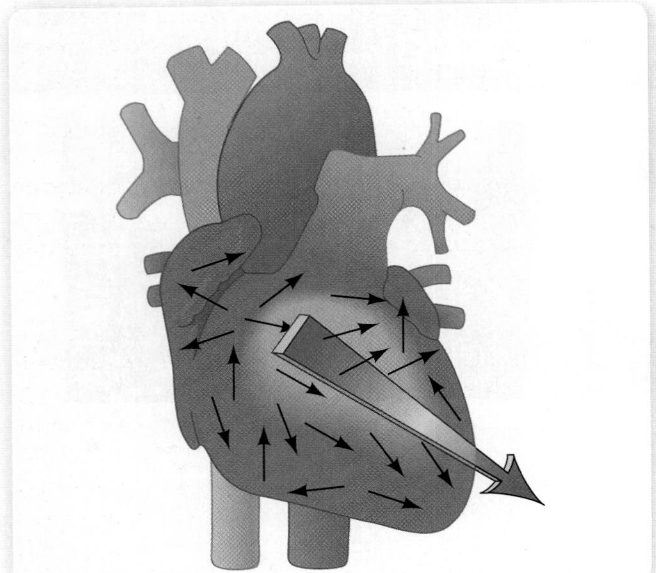

Figure 17-77 The QRS axis is the average of all ventricular vectors.

Reproduced from *Arrhythmia Recognition: The Art of Interpretation*, courtesy of Tomas B. Garcia, MD.

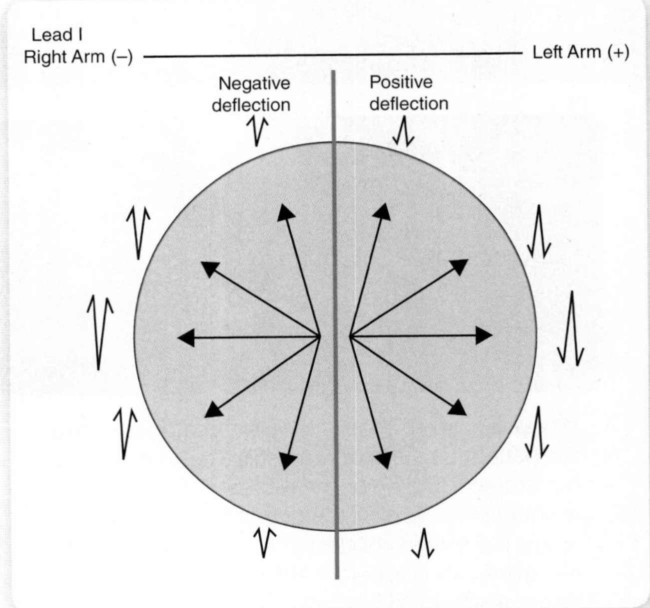

Figure 17-78 Viewed from lead I, the QRS will have a positive deflection if it's heading toward the left arm and a negative deflection if it's heading toward the right arm.

Determine the Axis

Every myocyte emits a small electrical charge when it depolarizes. A vector, often illustrated using an arrow, is a quantity, such as force, that has magnitude and direction. The **QRS axis** is a single vector that represents the mean (or average) of all vectors created by the ventricles during depolarization Figure 17-77.

A positive QRS deflection in lead I means the vector is heading toward the left arm, whereas a negative QRS deflection shows the vector is heading toward the right arm Figure 17-78. A positive QRS deflection in lead aVF means the vector is moving toward the feet, whereas a negative QRS deflection shows the vector is moving toward the head Figure 17-79.

Axis deviation refers to movement of the QRS axis to the right or left of its normal position. Although axis deviation provides an important clue about electrical activity in the heart, it is not sensitive or specific to any particular diagnosis. Rather, clinicians use it with other information to determine what is happening in the heart.

A number of methods can help you determine the QRS axis. The easiest and fastest method entails using the QRS complexes in leads I and aVF. These two leads are used because they are the only perfectly horizontal and vertical leads, respectively. Using these leads, then, you can create a simple quadrant system Figure 17-80. Now you have four quadrants. The center is the point at which the two lines intersect and represents the origin of the impulse. The four quadrants represent the space through which the impulse can travel. To determine the QRS axis, use the direction of the QRS complexes in leads I and aVF.

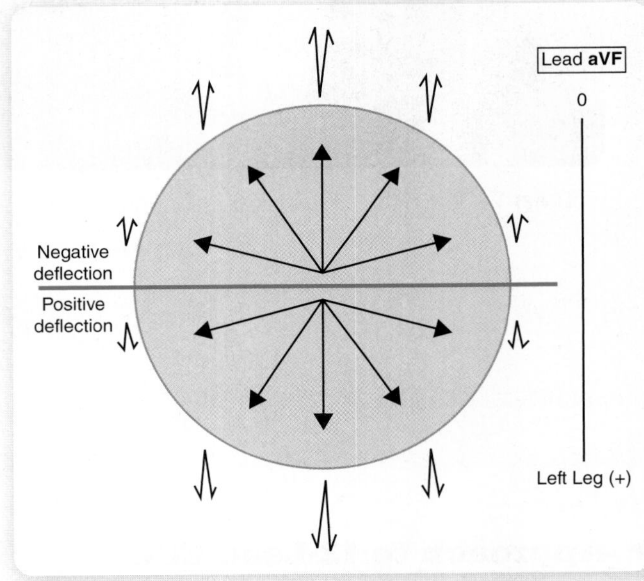

Figure 17-79 Viewed from lead aVF, the QRS will have a positive deflection if it's heading toward the patient's feet and a negative deflection if it's heading toward the patient's head.

First, look at the QRS complex in leads I and aVF, and decide if it is positive or negative. If the QRS complex is positive in leads I and aVF, then the axis falls in quadrant 4 and lies between 0 and 90 degrees. The normal QRS axis ranges from −30 to +90 degrees, not 0 to 90 degrees. This estimate of the QRS axis, however, is close enough. Left axis deviation is present if the QRS

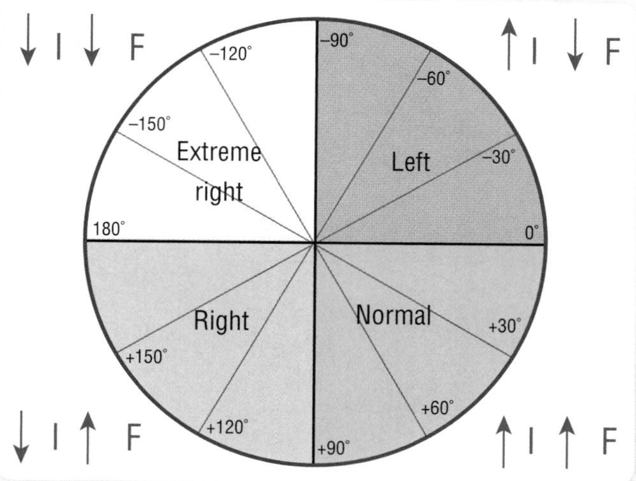

Figure 17-80 The four-quadrant system can be used to determine the overall direction of an electrical vector in the ventricular region of the heart. This system of imaginary reference points helps determine the QRS axis.

Table 17-7 Determining the QRS Axis Using Leads I and aVF

	Lead I		Lead aVF		Position of QRS Axis
If	Positive	*and*	Positive	*then*	Normal axis
If	Positive	*and*	Negative	*then*	Left axis deviation
If	Negative	*and*	Positive	*then*	Right axis deviation
If	Negative	*and*	Negative	*then*	Extreme right axis deviation

complex is positive in lead I and negative in lead aVF. A negative QRS in lead I and a positive QRS in lead aVF suggests right axis deviation. Finally, extreme right axis deviation exists when the QRS complex is negative in leads I and aVF. Table 17-7 summarizes how to determine the QRS axis using leads I and aVF.

Recall, the P wave represents electrical activity in the SA node, whereas the QRS complex indicates ventricular depolarization. Therefore, the direction of the QRS axis, or the axis deviation, corresponds to electrical activity in the ventricles. If one of the ventricles is enlarged (hypertrophic), then it contributes more electrical energy than it normally would and the resulting electrical vector points in the direction of the hypertrophy. Conversely, an infarcted area is composed of dead tissue, which emits no electrical signal. Therefore, if a portion of the ventricle is infarcted, then the vector will point away from it.

Identify Conduction System Disturbances

Next, look for conduction system disturbances on the 12-lead ECG. These include AV blocks and preexcitation, which were discussed earlier in this chapter, the bundle branch blocks, and fascicular or hemiblocks.

Bundle Branch Block. Normally, the right and left ventricles depolarize at the same time. A QRS complex with a bizarre appearance and a duration of 0.12 seconds (120 milliseconds) or more signifies some abnormality in conduction through the ventricles. A **bundle branch block (BBB)** is a type of intraventricular conduction defect involving impaired conduction from the bundle of His to one or more of the bundle branches. A blockage at the level of the bundle branches affects the order in which they are activated, with the blocked bundle being the last to be depolarized.

Right bundle branch block (RBBB) and left bundle branch block (LBBB) are among the most common 12-lead ECG findings. The names of these electrical conduction abnormalities indicate where the electrical impulse is delayed. RBBB is characterized by a duration of 0.12 seconds (120 milliseconds) or more and a terminal R wave in lead V_1 (the second half of the QRS complex terminates in an R wave) Figure 17-81. The QRS complex in lead V_1 typically appears as an rSR′ complex. (The ′ symbol represents an R-prime wave. An R-prime wave is never normal; it indicates trouble in the ventricular conduction system.) A terminal S wave also appears in leads I, aVL, and V_6.

LBBB is characterized by a QRS duration of 0.12 seconds (120 milliseconds) or more and a terminal S wave in lead V_1 (the second half of the QRS complex terminates in an S wave) Figure 17-82. Terminal R waves are also seen in leads I, aVL, and V_6.

The term RBBB or LBBB **aberration** describes the shape of the QRS complex in aberrantly (abnormally) conducted beats. For example, if a particular complex has an rSR′ shape, it is said to have RBBB morphology.

Fascicular Block (Hemiblock). The left bundle branch divides into anterior and posterior fascicles. When these tissues become diseased or ischemic, one or both fascicles become unable to conduct electrical impulses, resulting in a **fascicular block (hemiblock)**. An anterior fascicular block is characterized by rS complexes in leads II, III, and aVF, and qR complexes in leads I and aVL. A posterior fascicular block is rare and requires a diagnosis of exclusion. This kind of block is characterized by qR complexes in leads II, III, and aVF, and rS complexes in lead I.

When RBBB, LBBB, anterior hemiblock, and posterior hemiblock are described, you will often hear the term *bifascicular block*. In a **bifascicular block**, two of the fascicles

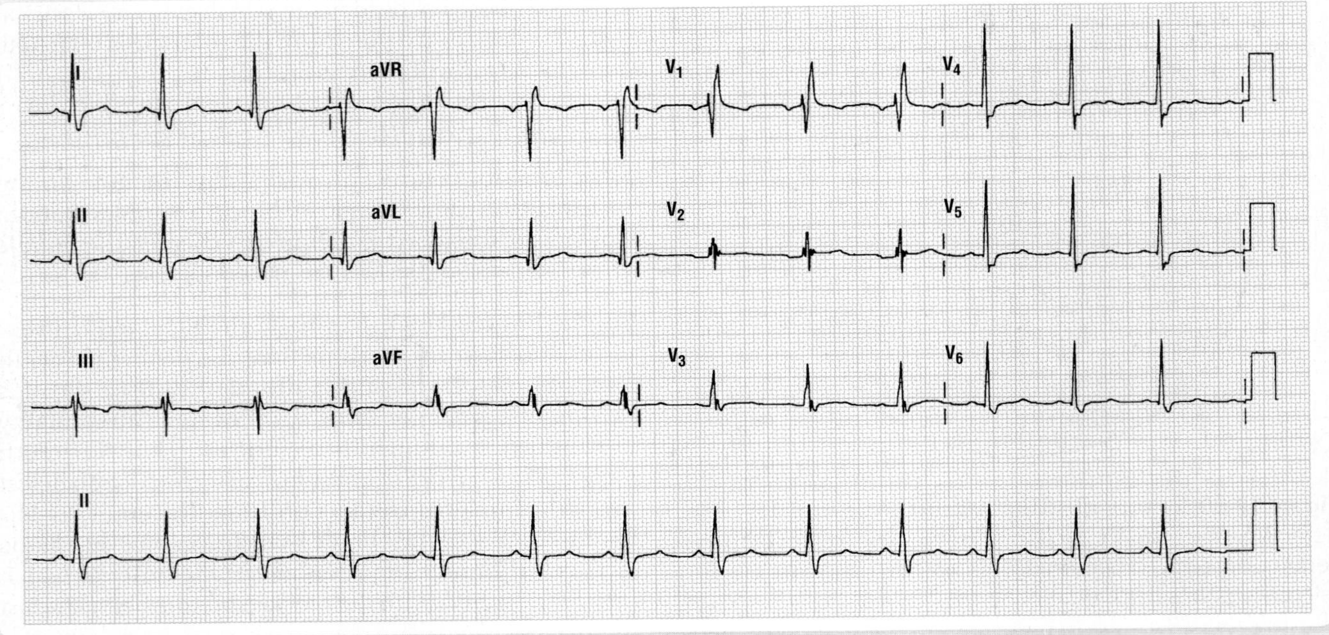

Figure 17-81 A 12-lead electrocardiogram showing right bundle branch block.

Reproduced from *12-Lead ECG: The Art of Interpretation*, courtesy of Tomas B. Garcia, MD.

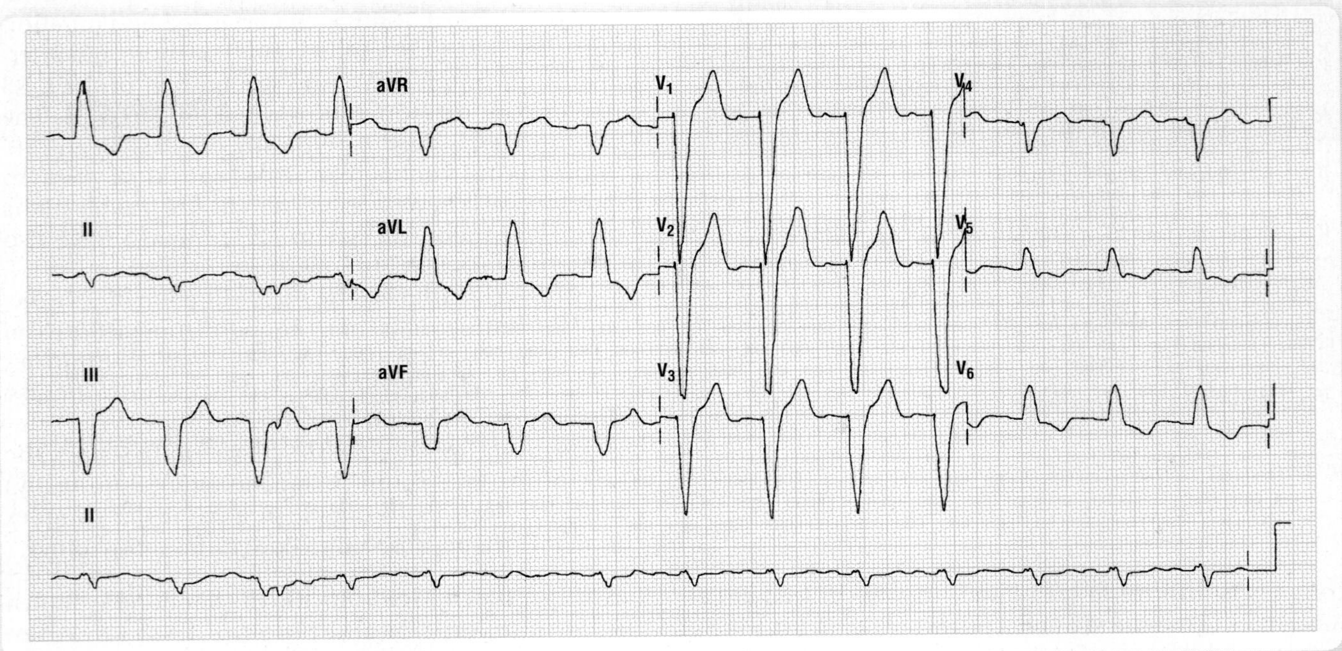

Figure 17-82 A 12-lead electrocardiogram showing left bundle branch block.

Reproduced from *12-Lead ECG: The Art of Interpretation*, courtesy of Tomas B. Garcia, MD.

or conduction pathways are blocked. This combination can vary, producing different effects in different patients. The two blocked pathways might be RBBB with anterior hemiblock, RBBB with posterior hemiblock, or anterior hemiblock and posterior hemiblock (a combination known as *LBBB*). In a **trifascicular block**, all three components of the ventricular conduction system are blocked or impaired, but one still occasionally works to provide AV conduction.

QRS complexes in the precordial leads are said to have a **concordant precordial pattern** when they are all in the same direction. For example, if all the QRS complexes are upright in leads V_1 to V_6, then the QRS complexes exhibit concordance across the precordium. QRS concordance in

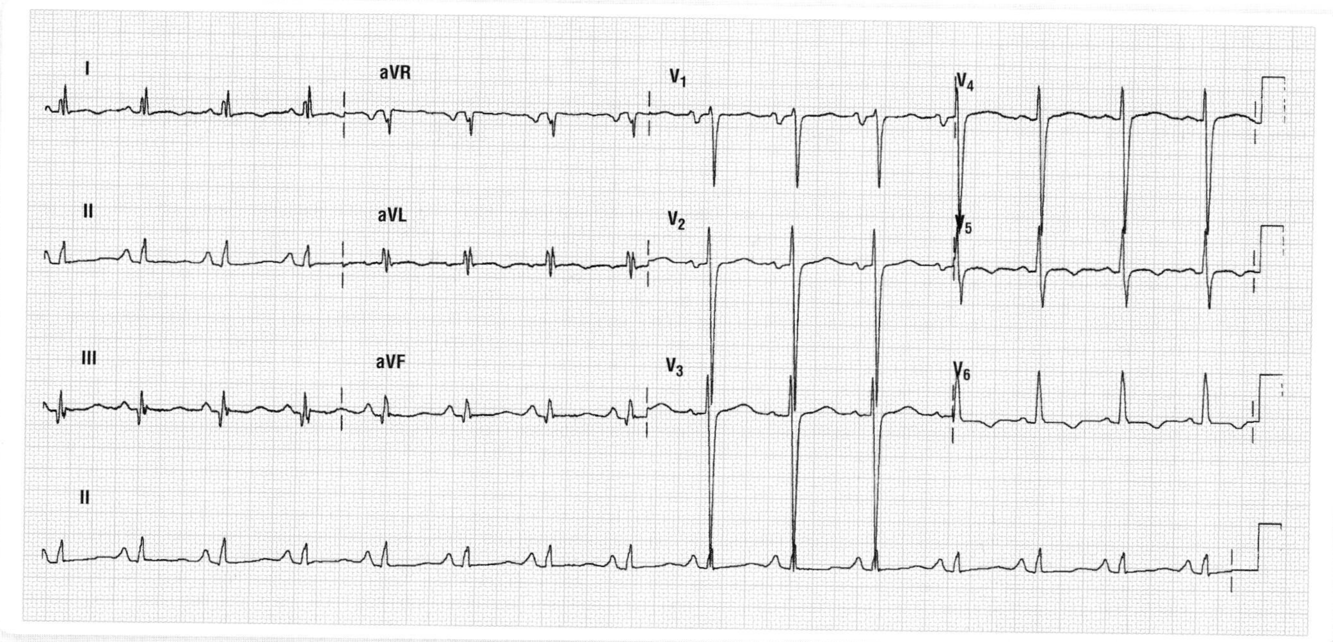

Figure 17-83 A 12-lead electrocardiogram showing right atrial abnormality.

the precordial leads can have several possible explanations, including improper lead placement, anterior wall MI, or VT.

Evaluate Chamber Size

The 12-lead ECG can also reveal the size of the heart's chambers. The right atrium is a small, thin structure designed to function efficiently in a low-pressure environment. If returning venous pressure is elevated, or if pulmonary pressure is high, then the right atrium will dilate. **Right atrial abnormality**, formerly called *right atrial enlargement* or *right atrial hypertrophy*, is often associated with chronic pulmonary disorders. This abnormality is characterized by a P wave with an amplitude higher than 2.5 mm in lead II and/or higher than 1.5 mm in lead V_1 **Figure 17-83**. The duration of the P wave is usually normal.

Left atrial abnormality is characterized by a P wave of normal height but prolonged duration, lasting 0.12 seconds (120 milliseconds) or more in lead II. A widely notched P wave may or may not be present **Figure 17-84**. Lead V_1 may show a biphasic P wave with a small initial positive deflection and a wide, negative terminal deflection. Left atrial abnormality may be seen in patients with valvular heart disease, particularly in those with mitral or aortic valve stenosis, hypertensive heart disease, cardiomyopathy, and CAD. It can also occur in an athletic heart.

In **right ventricular hypertrophy (RVH)**, the right ventricle becomes enlarged. This condition is usually caused by pulmonary hypertension. Normally, the R wave in lead V_1 is smaller than the S wave. An R wave that exceeds the height of the S wave in this lead suggests RVH **Figure 17-85**.

In **left ventricular hypertrophy (LVH)**, the left ventricle becomes enlarged, most often as the result of systemic hypertension, although this condition can also arise with some cardiac abnormalities. The left ventricle becomes enlarged as the left ventricular wall thickens in response to an increased workload. The left ventricle will then lose elasticity and may fail to pump blood effectively, leading to heart failure. ECG criteria for identification of LVH are typically based on QRS voltages. A guideline commonly followed for adults older than 35 years is this: If the sum of the depth of the S wave in lead V_1 and the height of the R wave in either lead V_5 or V_6 exceeds 35 mm, then LVH should be considered **Figure 17-86**. LVH can produce tall R waves in lead aVL. An R wave with an amplitude greater than 11 mm in this lead suggests LVH.

Diagnosis of LVH is made by echocardiogram, not ECG. It is inaccurate to say a patient has LVH if his or her ECG meets the criteria listed previously. It is more precise to say the ECG meets the voltage criteria for LVH.

Review for Zones of Ischemia, Injury, Infarction

Recall, ACSs are cardiac conditions precipitated by abruptly diminished blood flow through a coronary artery. Unstable angina, non–ST segment elevation MI (NSTEMI), and ST segment elevation MI (STEMI) are the three major ACSs.

When a coronary artery becomes narrowed or blocked significantly, the tissue supplied by that vessel is deprived of oxygen and essential nutrients. Cells must resort to anaerobic metabolism, which results in acidosis. If this ischemic process is not interrupted, that is, if adequate blood flow is not restored, then signs of cellular injury

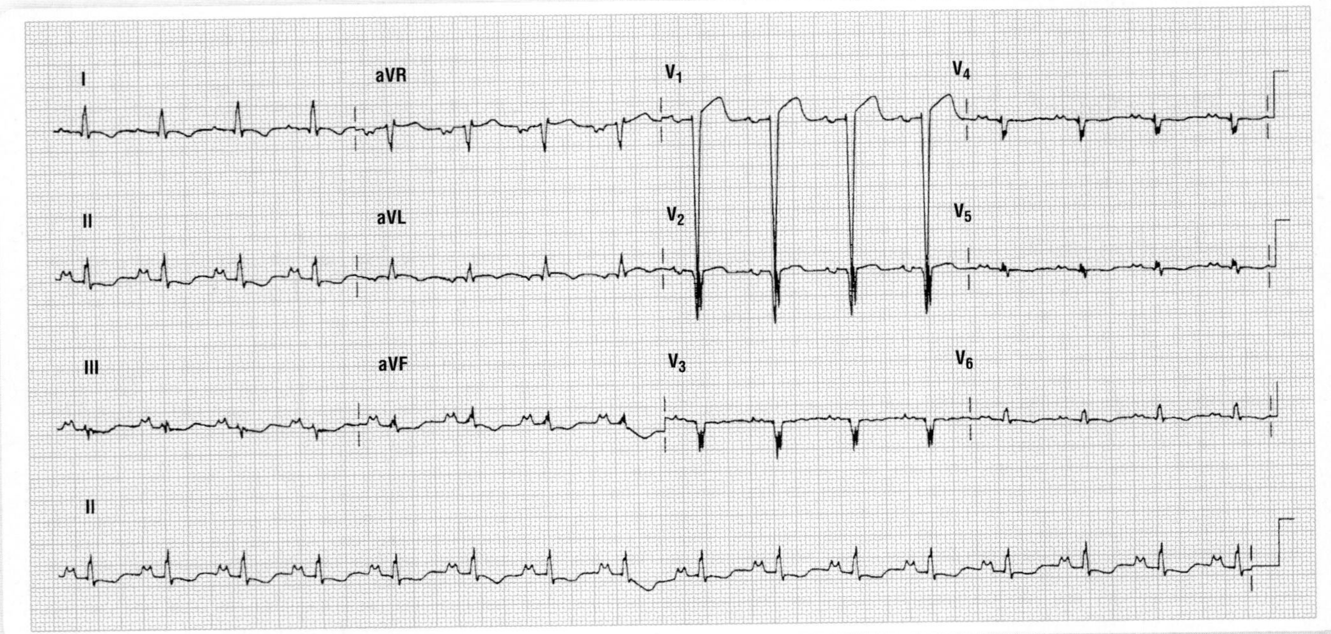

Figure 17-84 A 12-lead electrocardiogram showing left atrial abnormality.

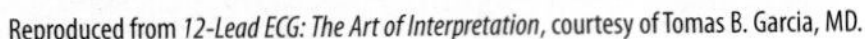
Reproduced from *12-Lead ECG: The Art of Interpretation*, courtesy of Tomas B. Garcia, MD.

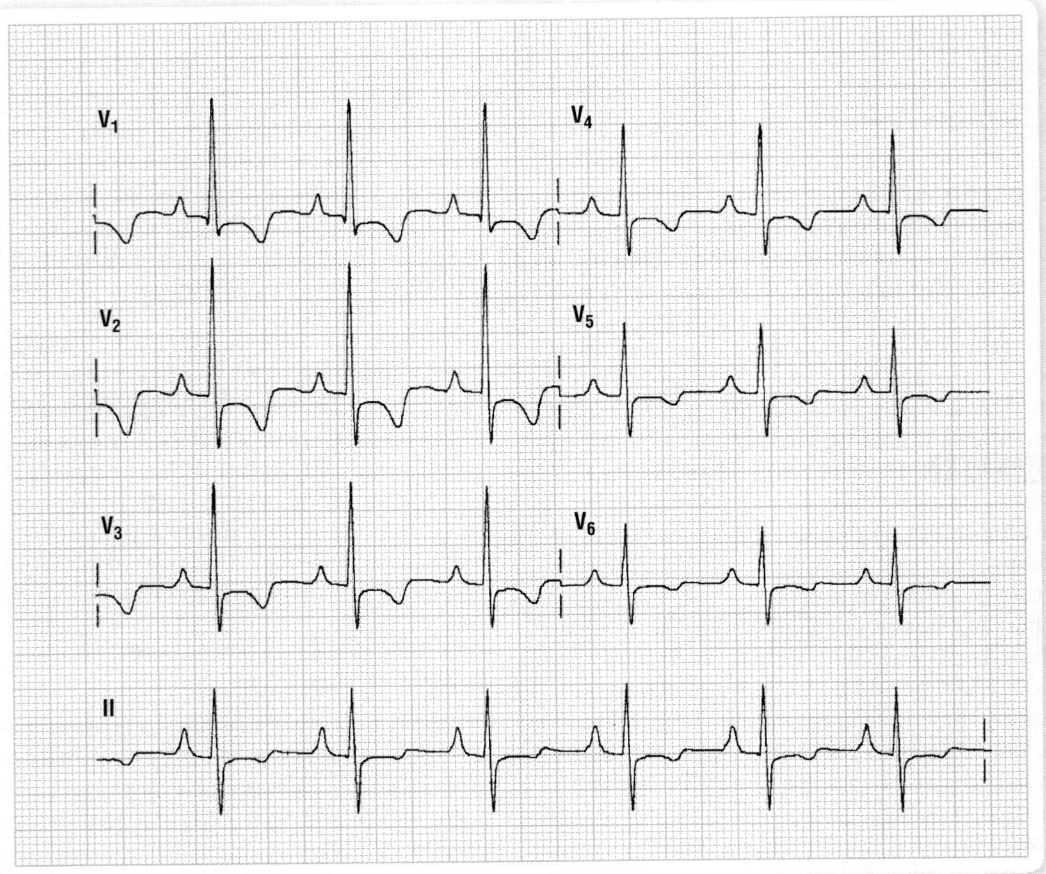

Figure 17-85 A 12-lead electrocardiogram showing right ventricular hypertrophy.

Reproduced from *12-Lead ECG: The Art of Interpretation*, courtesy of Tomas B. Garcia, MD.

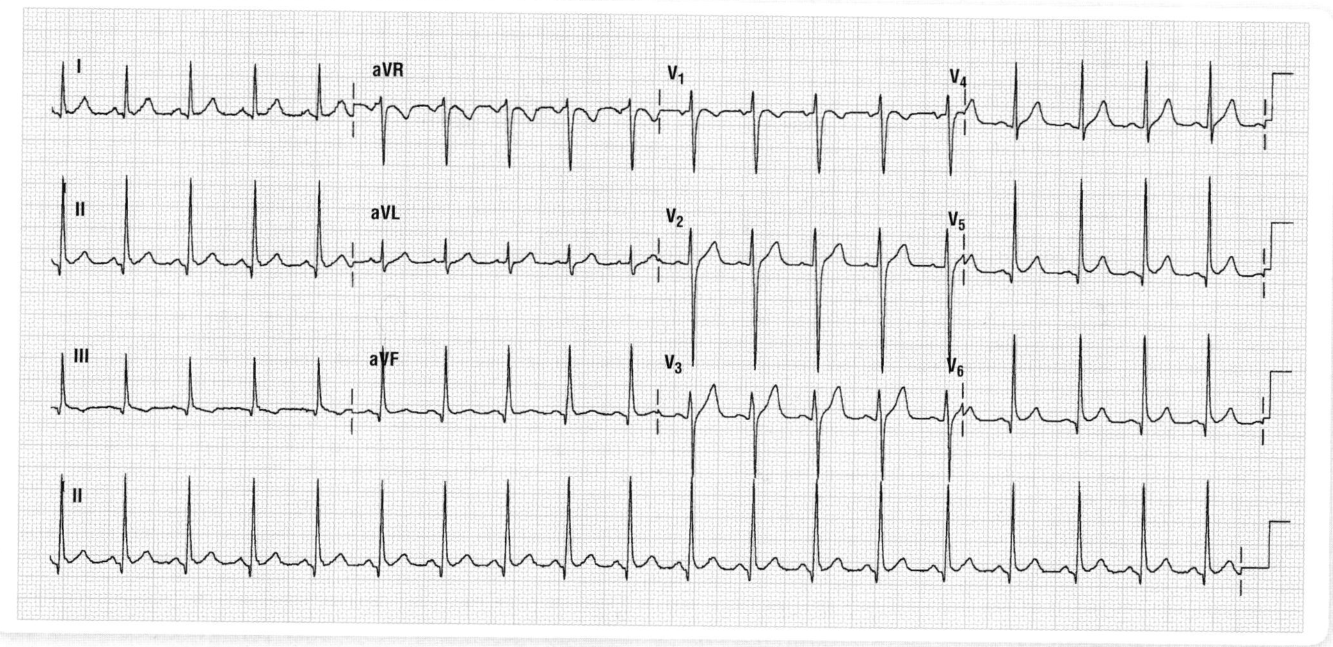

Figure 17-86 A 12-lead electrocardiogram showing left ventricular hypertrophy.

Reproduced from *12-Lead ECG: The Art of Interpretation*, courtesy of Tomas B. Garcia, MD.

will become evident. An *infarction* occurs when this ischemic process is not interrupted, resulting in tissue death. Because ischemia and injury are reversible processes, early recognition of ACS is critical in limiting the loss of heart tissue. Time is muscle.

When a coronary artery is blocked, the tissue it supplies undergoes characteristic changes that appear on the ECG in the leads facing the affected tissue. Ischemia is evidenced by ST-segment depression, and myocardial injury is evidenced by ST-segment elevation. Infarction may or may not be demonstrated by the appearance of pathologic Q waves. Currently, ST-segment depression greater than 0.5 mm in 2 or more contiguous leads in a patient with chest pain or discomfort indicates unstable angina or NSTEMI.[17] For leads V_2 and V_3, STEMI should be suspected if ST-segment elevation is 2 mm or more in men older than 40 years or 1.5 mm or more in women, or if it is elevated 1 mm or more in the other leads.[18] **Figure 17-87** shows the progression of a heart from its normal state to ischemia to injury to infarction. An absence of ST segment changes associated with an ACS presentation is referred to as a *nondiagnostic ECG.* Such a finding does not rule out acute myocardial ischemia, injury, or infarction; it simply means the tracing is nondiagnostic for those events. Serial blood work and additional testing is required.

Early acquisition of a 12-lead ECG in a patient who may have an ACS is essential. You should obtain the first 12-lead ECG within 10 minutes of patient contact.[4] Treatment decisions are made on the basis of the patient's

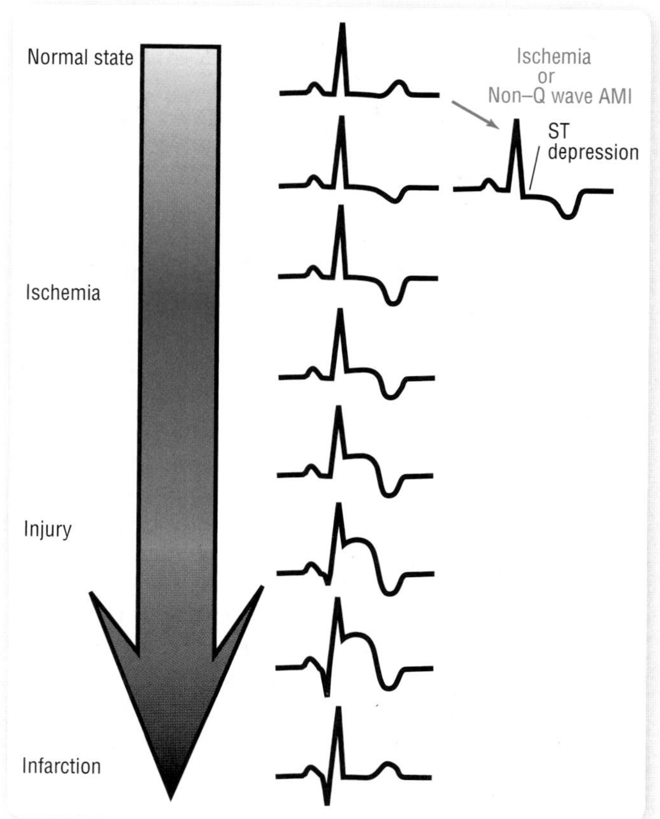

Figure 17-87 Evolutionary pattern of acute myocardial infarction.

Reproduced from *12-Lead ECG: The Art of Interpretation*, courtesy of Tomas B. Garcia, MD.

I	aVR	V_1	V_4
High lateral wall LV Cx		Interventricular septum LAD	Anterior wall LV LAD
II	**aVL**	**V_2**	**V_5**
Inferior wall LV RCA	High lateral wall LV Cx	Interventricular septum LAD	Low lateral wall LV Cx
III	**aVF**	**V_3**	**V_6**
Inferior wall LV RCA	Inferior wall LV RCA	Anterior wall LV LAD	Low lateral wall LV Cx

Abbreviations: Cx, circumflex artery; LAD, left anterior descending artery; LV, left ventricle; RCA, right coronary artery

Figure 17-88 The surfaces of the heart viewed by each lead of a standard 12-lead electrocardiogram. The coronary artery that typically supplies each surface is also listed.

presentation and history, the 12-lead ECG findings, and any laboratory test results (that is, cardiac biomarkers). For example, a patient with chest discomfort whose 12-lead ECG shows ST-segment elevation in two or more contiguous leads may be a candidate for immediate reperfusion therapy.

You must be able to correlate the patient's cardiovascular anatomy, including the areas supplied by each coronary artery, with the heart surface viewed by each ECG lead. Lead groups enable you to localize the areas of the ECG that show changes consistent with ischemia, injury, or infarction. Figure 17-88 shows colors associated with specific leads of the 12-lead ECG. Each color corresponds to a particular heart surface. From this figure, you can see which leads provide views of the same area of the heart. For example, leads II, III, and aVF view the inferior wall. Lead aVR is not used for this purpose, so no color is assigned to it.

Reciprocal changes are another important concept in identifying MI. Reciprocal changes are mirror image J-point, ST-segment, and T-wave changes seen on the ECG during an ACS. These ECG changes represent a location in the chest wall opposite the infarction. For example, if ST-segment elevation is present in a lead, then ST-segment depression and T-wave inversion is often seen in the reciprocal leads. The presence of reciprocal changes is evidence of AMI; however, the absence of such changes is not diagnostic. Table 17-8 summarizes the heart surfaces, the facing leads, the leads likely to show reciprocal changes, and the coronary artery most likely affected.

Figure 17-89 shows an inferior infarction. An example of an anteroseptal infarction is shown in Figure 17-90. Figure 17-91 depicts a lateral infarction, and Figure 17-92 illustrates inferior and right ventricular infarction. Managing patients with an ACS is discussed in detail later in this chapter.

Other Cardiovascular Conditions. Benign early repolarization and pericarditis are two conditions that may produce ST-segment elevation, mimicking AMI. Benign early repolarization is characterized by ST-segment elevation, a J or fishhook appearance at the J point, and concave ST segment morphology Figure 17-93. This pattern is thought to be a normal variant. The diagnosis is almost always a coincidental finding made while recording an

Table 17-8 Facing Leads and Reciprocal Changes

Location	Facing Leads	Reciprocal Leads	Coronary Artery Involved
Inferior wall of the left ventricle	II, III, aVF	I, aVL	RCA or Cx
Septum	V_1 and V_2	None	LAD
Anterior wall of the left ventricle	V_3 and V_4	None	LAD
Lateral wall of the left ventricle	I, aVL, V_5, V_6	II, III, aVF	Cx
Right ventricle	V_4R	None	RCA or Cx
Posterior wall	V_7-V_9	V_1, V_2	RCA or Cx

Abbreviations: RCA, right coronary artery; Cx, circumflex artery; LAD, left anterior descending artery

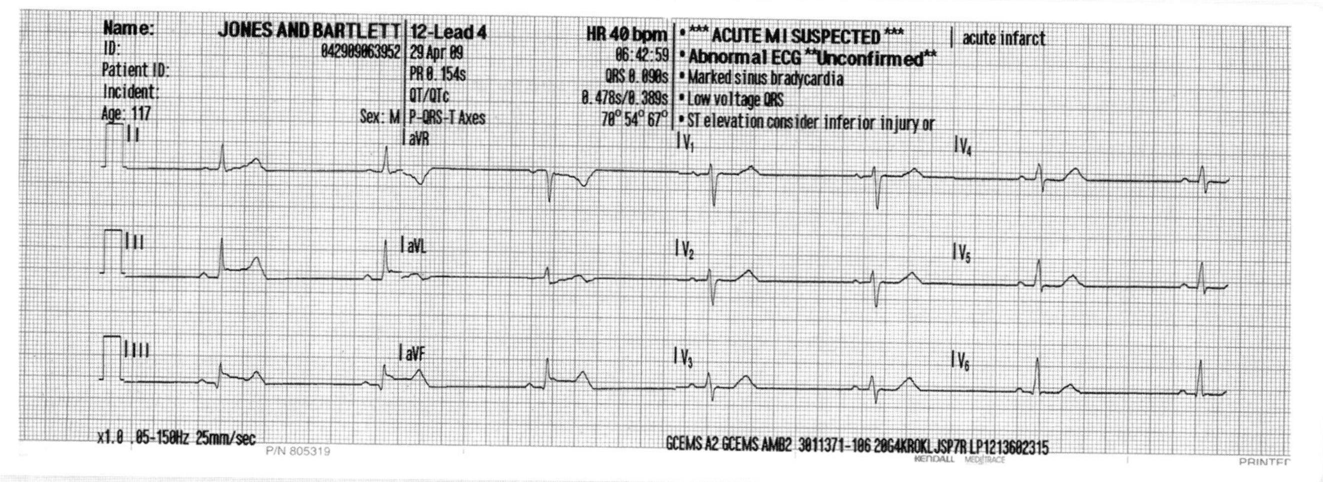

Figure 17-89 Inferior infarction.

Courtesy of Brian J. Williams.

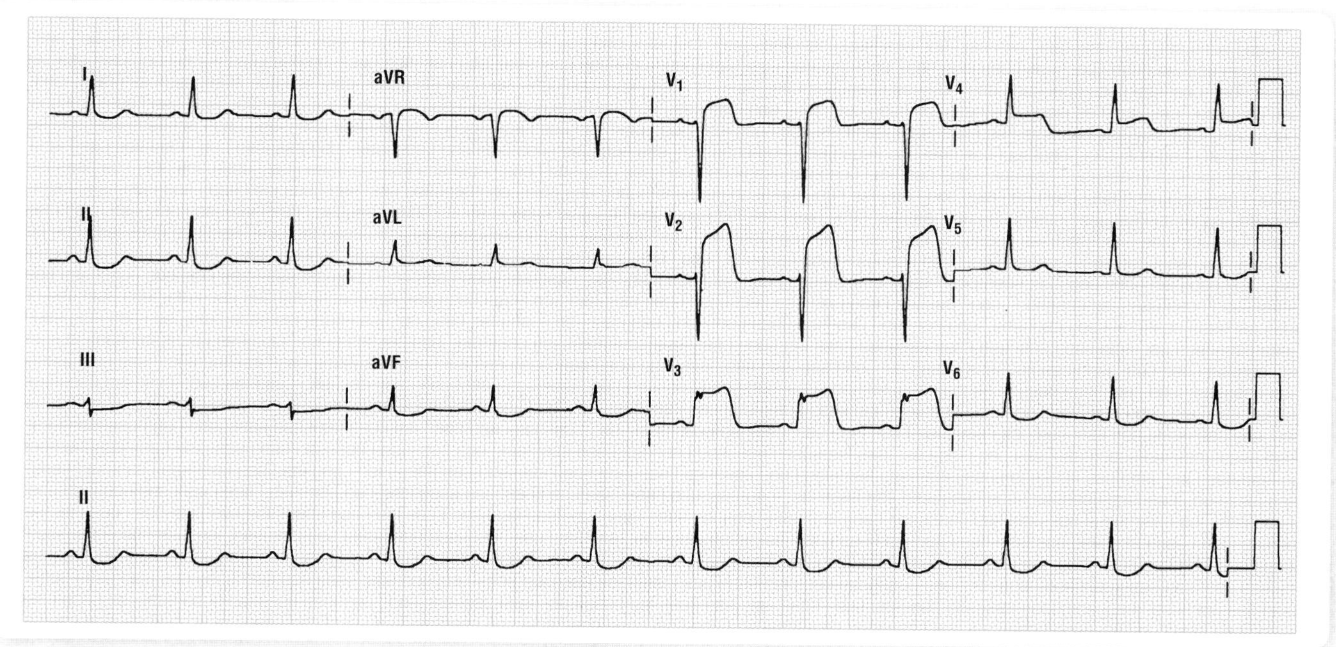

Figure 17-90 Anteroseptal infarction.

Reproduced from *12-Lead ECG: The Art of Interpretation*, courtesy of Tomas B. Garcia, MD.

ECG during a routine physical exam or during testing for an unrelated condition. The changes are often seen exclusively in the left precordial leads (V_4 to V_6) and/or the inferior leads. Reciprocal changes are never seen in benign early repolarization.

Pericarditis is the inflammation of the pericardial sac as a result of an infection (bacterial, viral, or fungal) or trauma. Patients can present with positional chest pain (often alleviated by sitting forward), shortness of breath, and history of recent infection or fever. The condition is characterized by ST-segment elevation (not exceeding 5 mm) that is present in multiple leads, a depressed or down-sloping PR segment **Figure 17-94**, a PR segment that is elevated or up-sloping in lead aVR, and a concave ST segment. Reciprocal ST-segment depression is never seen.

Identify Noncardiac Causes of ECG Abnormalities

The 12-lead ECG can also provide information about noncardiovascular conditions, including pulmonary embolism, acute intracranial hemorrhage, electrolyte abnormalities, and genetic disorders that affect the size or function of the heart.

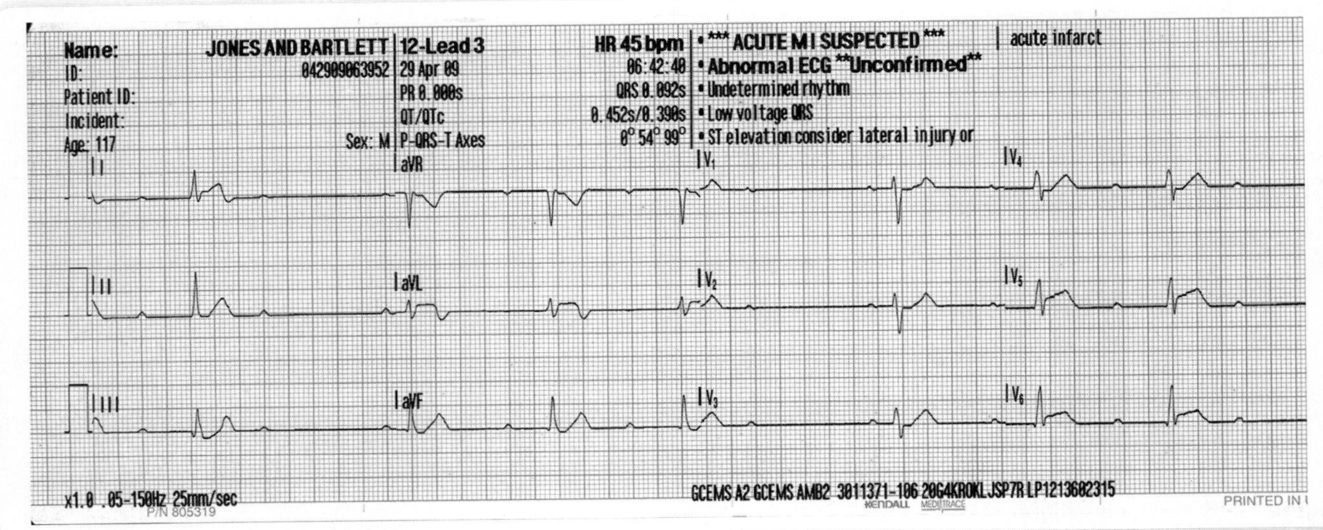

Figure 17-91 Lateral infarction.

Courtesy of Brian J. Williams.

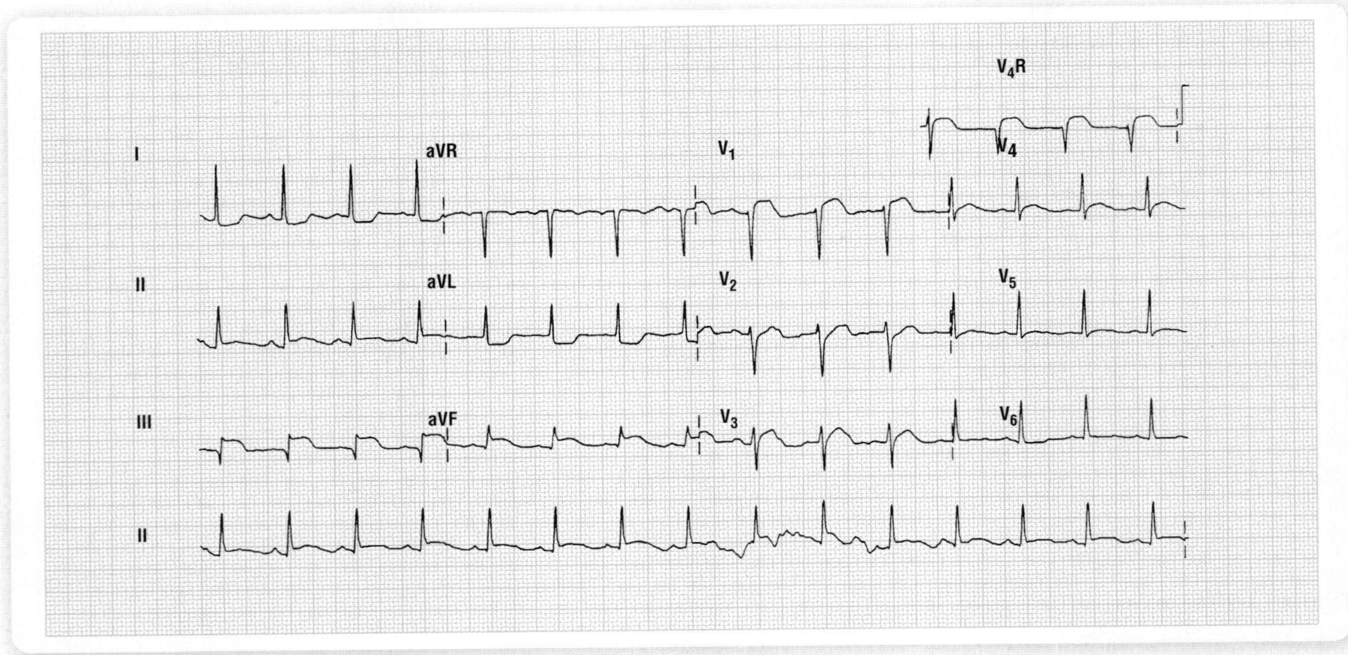

Figure 17-92 Inferior and right ventricular infarction.

Reproduced from *12-Lead ECG: The Art of Interpretation*, courtesy of Tomas B. Garcia, MD.

Pulmonary Embolism. A pulmonary embolism, an obstruction in one or more of the pulmonary arteries, may also be identified on a 12-lead ECG. The criteria for suspecting a pulmonary embolism include the appearance of an S1Q3T3 pattern, new RBBB, and ST-segment depression in leads V_1 to V_3 **Figure 17-95**. The S1Q3T3 pattern refers to a deep S wave in lead I, a deep, narrow Q wave in lead III, and T-wave inversion in lead III. This is also sometimes written as S1Q3⊥3, with the T upside-down to indicate T-wave inversion. Unfortunately, these changes are seen almost exclusively in cases of large pulmonary embolism. Thus, the absence of S1Q3T3 and RBBB on the surface ECG does not rule out pulmonary embolism, and it remains one of the most frequently missed conditions. It is crucial to perform a thorough physical exam and to collect pertinent information about the patient's medical history, including any surgeries or medications, current health status, and family history.

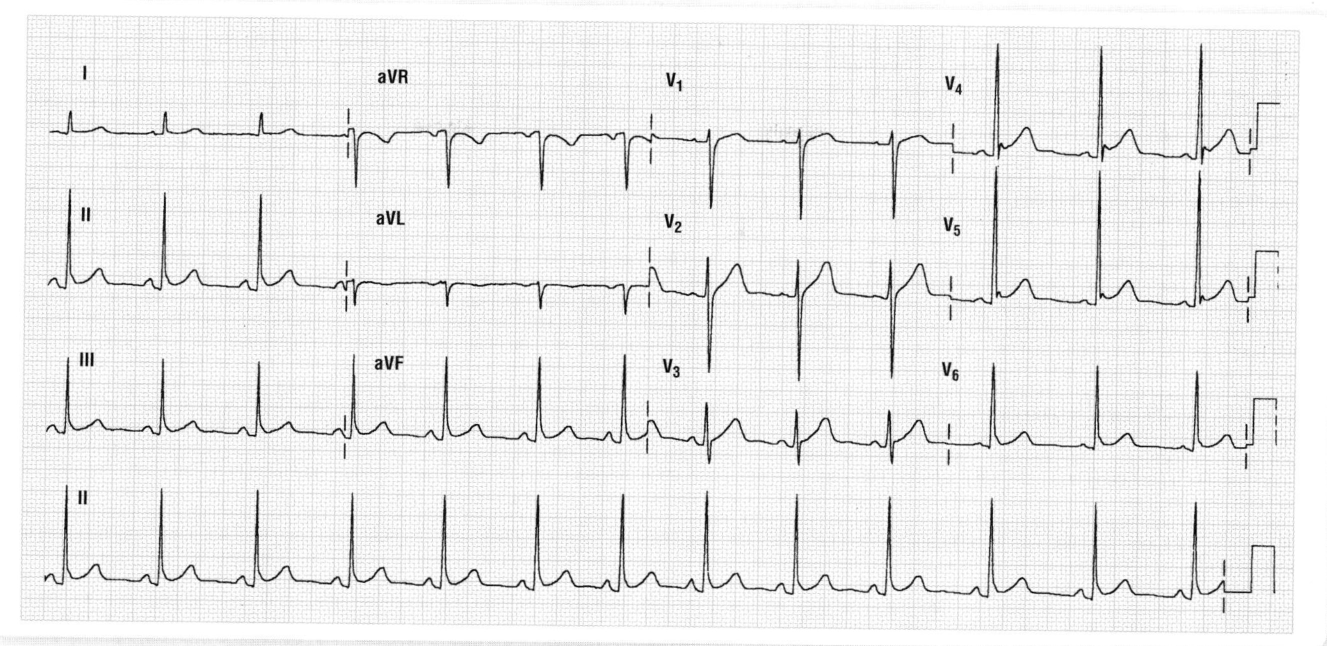

Figure 17-93 A 12-lead electrocardiogram showing benign early repolarization.

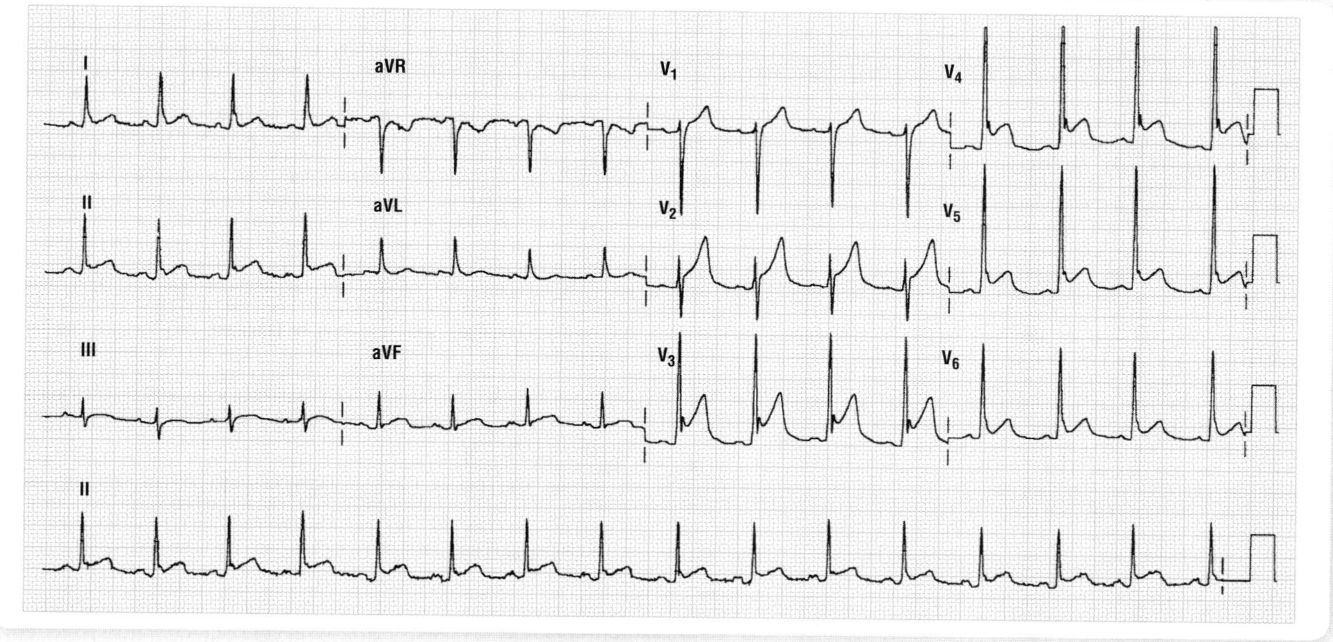

Figure 17-94 A 12-lead electrocardiogram showing pericarditis.

Hypothermia. Patients with severe hypothermia may develop J waves (Osborne) on the ECG. The J wave is often a large, upright wave that appears on the terminal wave of the QRS complex. It may be accompanied by ST-segment depression and T-wave inversion. Generally, the more serious the hypothermia, the larger the J wave. The ECG also typically reveals a bradycardic rhythm and baseline containing artifact from shivering and poor electrode adhesion to cold skin Figure 17-96. Evidence of a J wave is only an indication of hypothermia; it is not enough to make a definitive diagnosis.

Electrolyte Imbalances. Electrolyte imbalances can also cause ECG changes. The two most common electrolyte

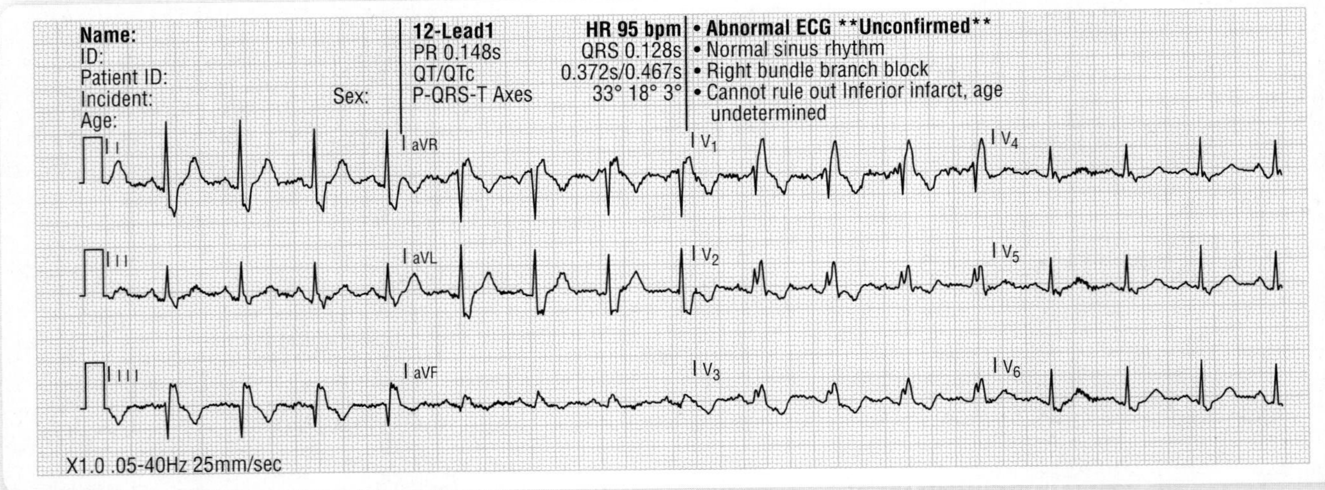

Figure 17-95 A 12-lead electrocardiogram showing pulmonary embolism.

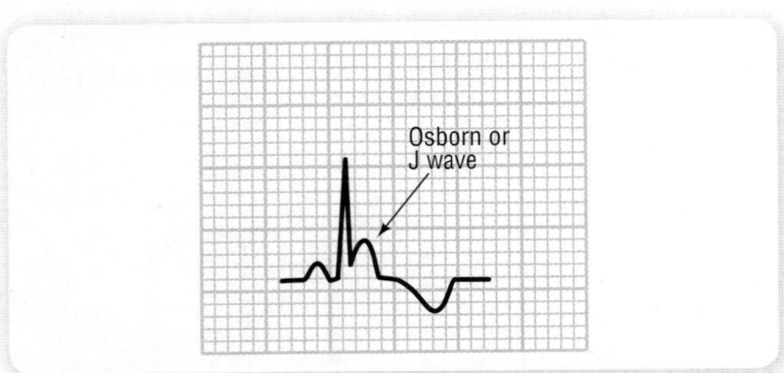

Figure 17-96 Osborne (J) wave.

Reproduced from *12-Lead ECG: The Art of Interpretation*, courtesy of Tomas B. Garcia, MD.

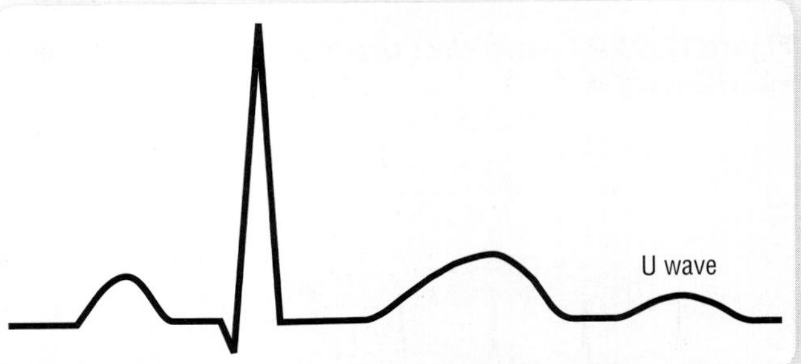

Figure 17-98 Hypokalemia.

Reproduced from *12-Lead ECG: The Art of Interpretation*, courtesy of Tomas B. Garcia, MD.

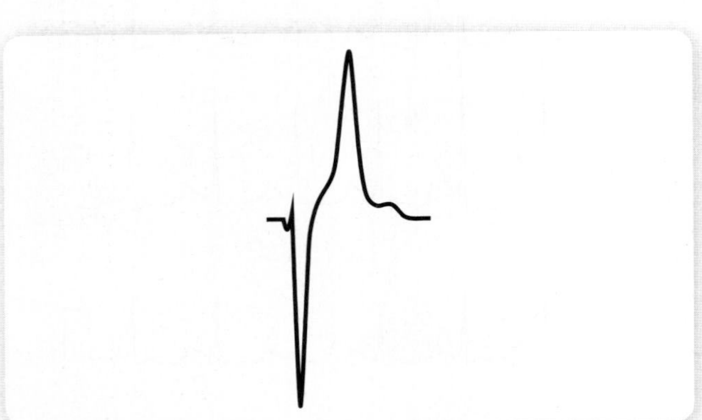

Figure 17-97 Hyperkalemia.

Reproduced from *12-Lead ECG: The Art of Interpretation*, courtesy of Tomas B. Garcia, MD.

imbalances involve potassium and calcium. Hyperkalemia causes specific ECG changes. First, tall, peaked, asymmetric T waves develop. The P waves can become flattened and eventually disappear from the tracing. In severe cases, the QRS complex widens **Figure 17-97**. By contrast, hypokalemia usually presents with flat or apparently absent T waves, as well as a **U wave**. A U wave is even smaller even than a P wave. It occurs after a T wave but before the next P wave. U waves are rare. When they occur, they are often mistaken for extra P waves or are misinterpreted as some other unknown abnormality **Figure 17-98**.

Hypercalcemia may produce a shortened QT interval, for example, whereas hypocalcemia may slightly lengthen the QT interval. The shortening or lengthening of the QT interval in hypercalcemia or hypocalcemia, respectively, is attributable entirely to the change in length of the ST segment. The T wave itself is unaffected by changes in calcium concentration.

Cardiomyopathy. Cardiomyopathy is a disease of the heart muscle. The main types of cardiomyopathy are dilated, hypertrophic, and restrictive—named for the types of muscle damage each causes. With dilated cardiomyopathy, the heart muscle weakens, diminishing its ability to pump enough blood to the rest of the body. The pressure of the blood within the left ventricle causes the heart to enlarge and stretch.

Hypertrophic cardiomyopathy is a genetic condition in which the myocardial wall becomes very thick. The greatest thickening tends to occur in the left ventricle. The thickened heart walls are stiff, impairing ventricular filling. Inadequate filling can lead to left atrial enlargement and pulmonary congestion.

Patients with hypertrophic cardiomyopathy often experience shortness of breath, chest pain, or syncope. Such signs and symptoms are often associated with physical activity. Patients are often diagnosed in their 30s or 40s. In most cases, the disease is inherited. In other cases, the cause is unclear or unknown. On ECG, hypertrophic cardiomyopathy is characterized by deep, narrow Q waves in the inferior leads and high lateral leads, and very tall R waves in the left precordial leads. These changes are similar to those seen in LVH **Figure 17-99**. With restrictive cardiomyopathy, the ventricular walls stiffen because of abnormal substances deposited between heart muscle cells throughout the heart or because the inner surface of the heart is lined with a layer of scar tissue. The rigidity of the ventricular walls hinders ventricular filling, and the heart eventually loses its ability to pump adequately.

Words of Wisdom

Takotsubo cardiomyopathy, also called *broken heart syndrome* or *stress cardiomyopathy*, is a temporary condition that can mimic AMI. Patients often present with chest pain or discomfort, ST-segment elevation, and elevated cardiac biomarkers, consistent with AMI. However, when the patient undergoes cardiac angiography, the coronary arteries are found to be essentially normal. In some patients, weakening and ballooning of the left ventricular apex during systole has been found.

This condition is often, but not always, associated with emotional or physical stress. Examples of triggers that have been identified include the loss of a loved one, financial difficulties, relationship disagreements, earthquakes, lightning strikes, noncardiac surgery, seizures, trauma, anesthesia, and alcohol withdrawal. Although the exact cause is not yet known, possible causes include spasm of multiple coronary arteries or stress-induced catecholamine release, among others. Normal heart function is restored within weeks of supportive therapy.

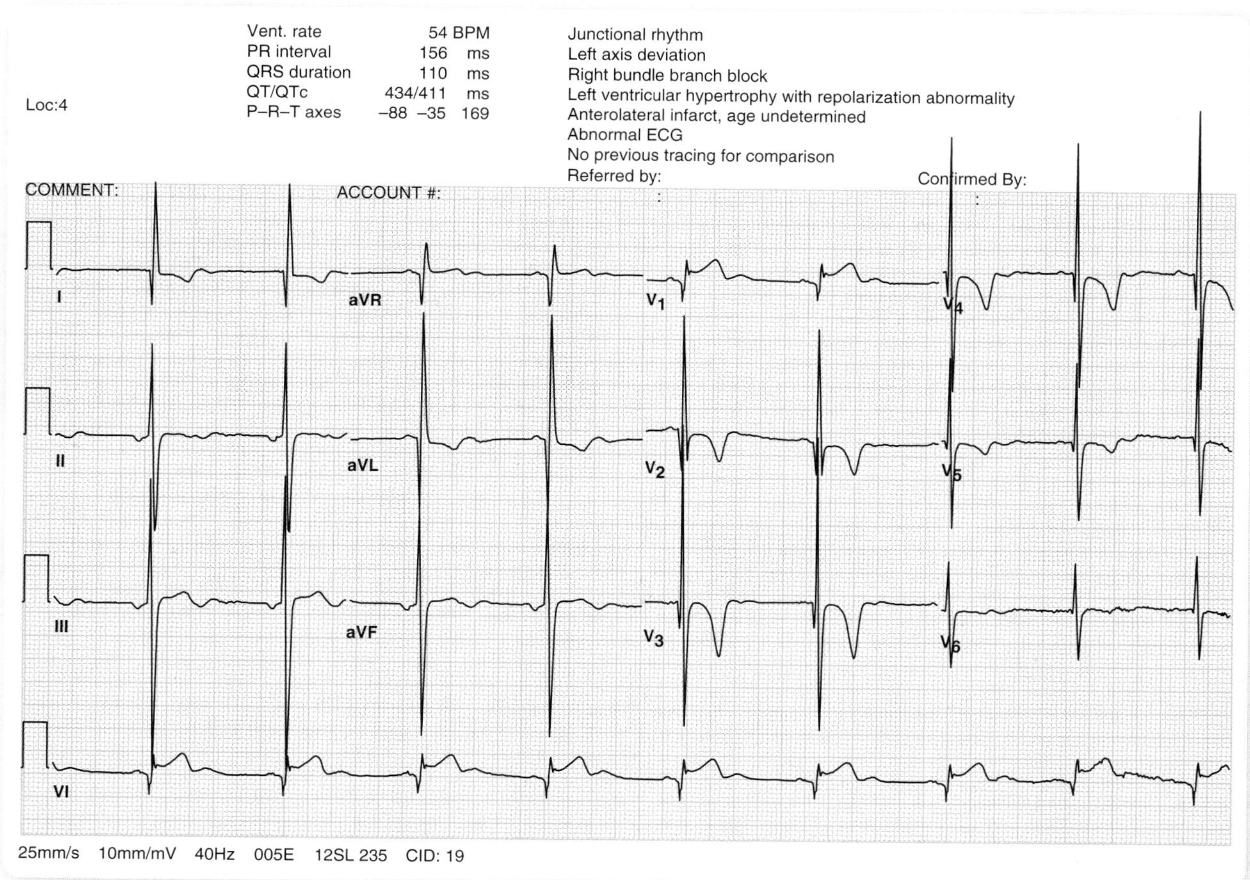

Figure 17-99 A 12-lead electrocardiogram showing evidence of hypertrophic cardiomyopathy.

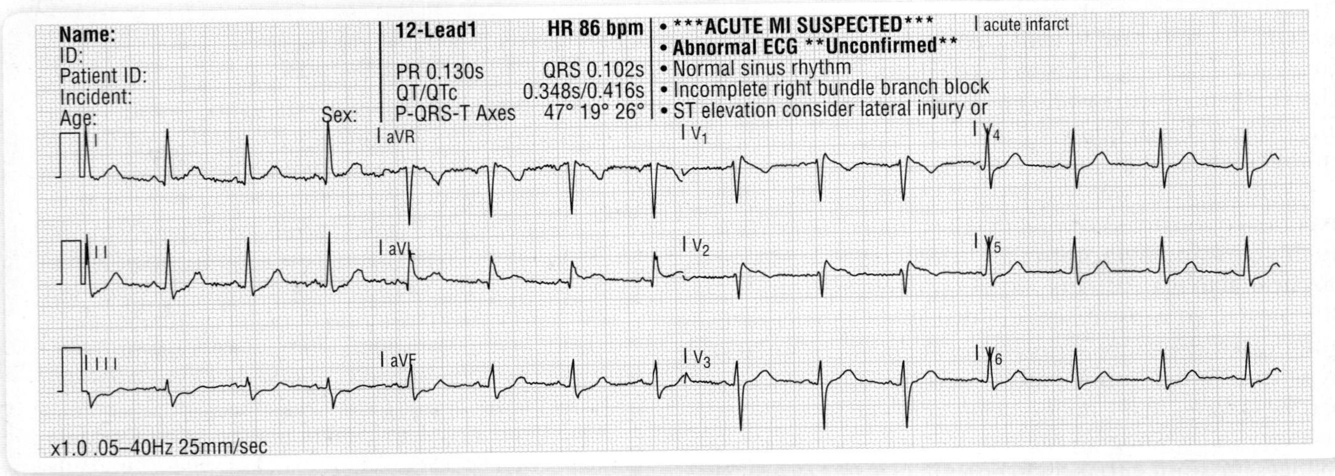

Figure 17-100 A 12-lead electrocardiogram showing evidence of Brugada syndrome.

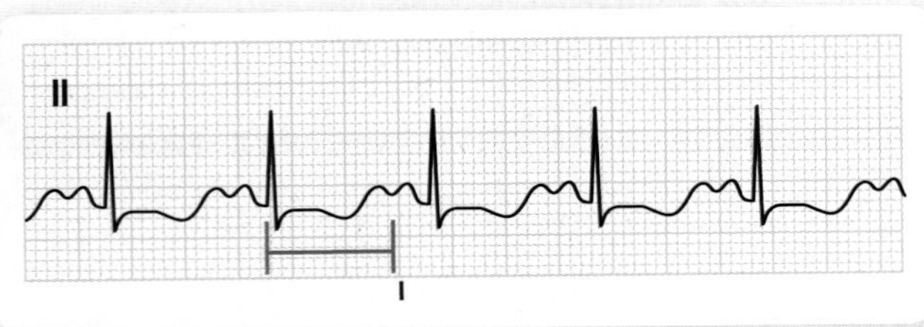

Figure 17-101 A 12-lead electrocardiogram showing long QT syndrome.

Brugada Syndrome. Brugada syndrome is a rare genetic disorder involving sodium channels in the heart. The condition is characterized by incomplete RBBB (rSR pattern in lead V_1 and a QRS duration of less than 140 milliseconds), and ST-segment elevation that returns aggressively to baseline Figure 17-100. These changes are seen in leads V_1 to V_2 (and possibly in V_3). The disease often remains undiagnosed until patients are in their 40s or 50s, when a sudden event, such as syncope or cardiac arrest, prompts the person to seek medical care.

Long QT Syndrome. **Long QT syndrome** is a condition characterized by a QT interval exceeding approximately 0.45 seconds (450 milliseconds) Figure 17-101. A prolonged QT interval (long QT syndrome) indicates that the heart is experiencing an extended RP, predisposing the ventricles to dysrhythmia. Long QT syndrome is a result of mutation of several genes. It is also associated with the administration of certain drugs, such as amiodarone, and with conditions such as hypocalcemia, AMI, and pericarditis. Conversely, the QT interval may be shortened in hypercalcemia and in patients taking digoxin.

The QT interval is age- and gender-specific, so there is no single value for all patients. This condition can be brought on by myocardial ischemia, intracranial hemorrhage, certain congenital disorders, or administration of certain medications. Patients with long-QT syndrome are at increased risk of ventricular dysrhythmias, including torsades de pointes and VF. EMS is often called to treat patients with syncope or palpitations, or they are summoned when sudden death occurs. It is critical to record an ECG on all patients experiencing syncope, including younger patients.

Intracranial Hemorrhage. Intracranial hemorrhage can also cause ECG changes. The mechanism by which the changes appear is not fully understood. Intracranial hemorrhage may cause deeply inverted, symmetric T waves in the precordial leads and a prolonged QT interval Figure 17-102. As a rule, patients with ECG changes resulting from intracranial hemorrhage almost always have neurologic symptoms or are unresponsive.

Pathophysiology, Assessment, and Management of Specific Cardiovascular Conditions

Epidemiology of Cardiovascular Disease

According to the AHA, CVD is the leading global cause of death.[1] Examples of CVD include angina pectoris, AMI, and heart failure. It is estimated that more than 1 in 3 Americans has one or more types of CVD.[1]

Coronary heart disease (CHD) refers to disease of the coronary arteries and its associated signs, symptoms, and complications, such as angina pectoris and AMI. Patients with documented CHD have five to seven times the risk of having a heart attack or dying as the general population.[1] CAD is a pathologic process characterized by atherosclerotic narrowing and eventual blockage of the arteries that supply the heart muscle with blood. The patient with CAD may be asymptomatic, or he or she may present with stable angina pectoris, unstable angina, AMI, or sudden cardiac death.

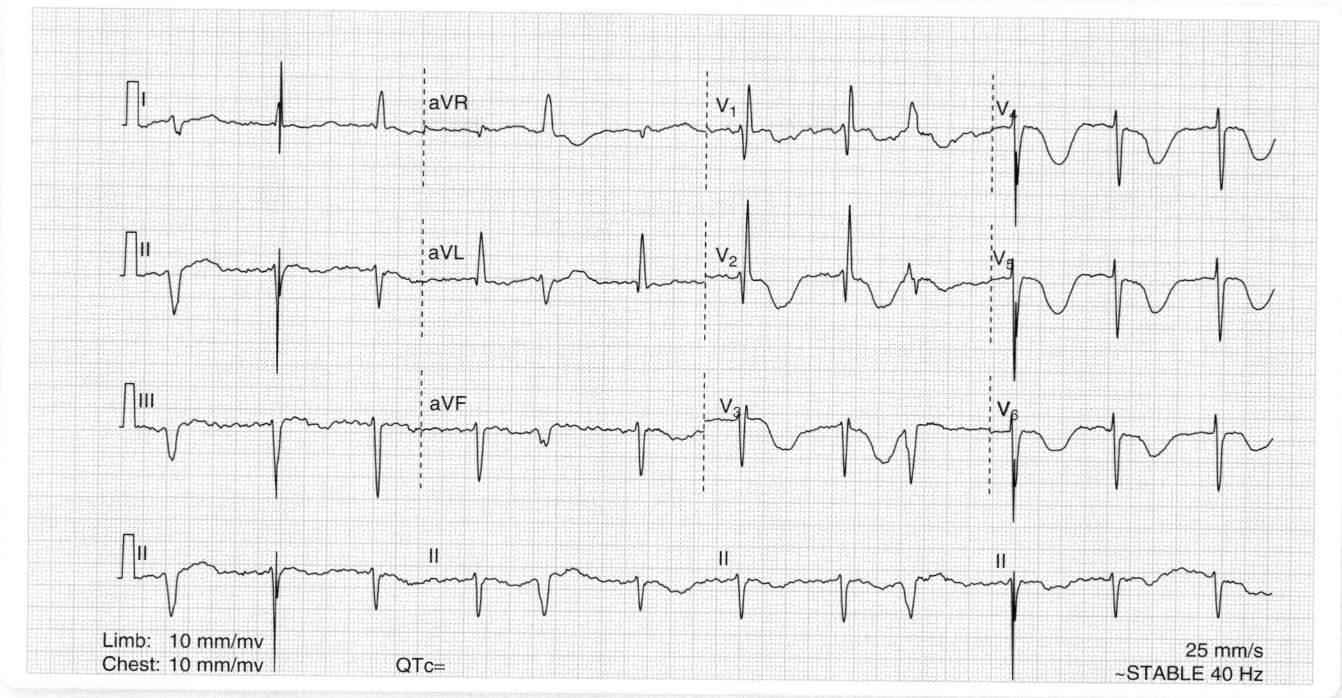

Figure 17-102 A 12-lead electrocardiogram showing deeply inverted T waves in a patient with an intracranial hemorrhage.

▶ Acute Coronary Syndromes

The coronary arteries, of course, supply oxygen and nutrients to the myocardium. Several cardiac conditions, known as ACSs, are characterized by diminished flow through the coronary arteries: coronary artery occlusion by a blood clot (**thrombus**), coronary artery spasm, and reduction of overall blood flow from any cause (such as shock, dysrhythmia, or pulmonary embolism). If one of these blood vessels becomes blocked, then the muscle it supplies will be deprived of oxygen, a condition called ischemia. If the oxygen supply is not restored quickly, then the ischemic area of heart muscle will eventually die. Such tissue death is known as *infarction*.

Etiology

The usual cause of an ACS is the rupture of an atherosclerotic plaque. **Atherosclerosis** is of particular concern because it affects the inner lining of blood vessels, narrowing the vessels and reducing the flow of blood through them. The atherosclerotic process probably begins in childhood, when small amounts of fatty material are deposited along the inner wall (intima) of arteries. This usually occurs at points of turbulent blood flow, such as where the arteries branch or where the arterial wall has been damaged. The streak of fat gradually enlarges, becoming a mass of fatty tissue called an **atheroma** or *atheromatous plaque*. This mass eventually calcifies, hardening into a lesion that infiltrates the arterial wall, diminishing its elasticity. At the same time, the expanding atheroma narrows the artery, decreasing the amount of blood flow through the **lumen**—the hollow interior space within the artery. The narrowed, roughened area of the arterial intima is an ideal site for the formation of a fixed blood clot, or thrombus, which may then obstruct the artery altogether. When such a clot forms in a coronary artery, it's known as a *coronary thrombosis*. In addition, calcium may precipitate from the bloodstream into the arterial walls, causing **arteriosclerosis**, a condition in which thickening and stiffening of the arterial walls greatly reduces the elasticity of the arteries.

Risk Factors for Coronary Heart Disease

Risk factors are traits and lifestyle habits that may increase a person's chance of developing a disease. More than 90% of CAD events occur in people who have at least one risk factor.[19]

Risk factors you cannot control are called *nonmodifiable risk factors*. Examples are age, family history of CHD, sex, and race or ethnicity. Risk factors you can control are called *modifiable risk factors*. Examples are diabetes, excessive alcohol use, high blood cholesterol and triglyceride levels, high blood pressure, obesity, physical inactivity, smoking, stress, and an unhealthy diet Table 17-9.

Although atherosclerosis is widespread in industrialized countries, certain factors increase the risk of developing atherosclerosis and CHD: hypertension (high blood pressure), cigarette smoking, diabetes, high serum cholesterol levels, lack of exercise, obesity, family history of heart disease or stroke, and being a male. Clearly, these risk factors include factors beyond a person's control.

Table 17-9 Risk Factors for CHD

Modifiable Risks	Nonmodifiable Risks
Diabetes	Age
Excessive alcohol use	Family history of CHD
High blood cholesterol and triglyceride levels	Sex
High blood pressure	Race or ethnicity
Obesity	
Physical inactivity	
Smoking	
Stress	
Unhealthy diet	

Abbreviation: CHD, coronary heart disease

You cannot, for example, select your parents and grandparents or choose to be born female. Nevertheless, you can address your modifiable risk factors:

- Diabetes increases the risk of CHD, cerebrovascular disease, peripheral vascular disease, and heart failure.
- Excessive alcohol consumption can raise blood pressure and triglyceride levels. According to the US Centers for Disease Control and Prevention, women should limit alcohol intake to no more than one drink per day and men to no more than two drinks per day.[20]
- High blood pressure is a risk factor for heart disease, stroke, and end-stage renal disease. Hypertension cannot always be prevented or cured, but it can be controlled with diet and medication.
- A diet high in saturated fat, trans fat, and cholesterol increases the risk of atherosclerosis and heart disease. The level of serum cholesterol is at least in part a consequence of dietary intake of saturated fat. In populations with low fat intake, the incidence of CHD is also low. Furthermore, lowering the serum cholesterol level has been shown to reduce the risk of heart attack. Cholesterol may also be controlled with medication, if necessary.
- Obesity is associated with an increased risk of heart disease. Patients with obesity have an increased likelihood of developing other CHD risk factors, including high blood pressure, diabetes, and high cholesterol. Weight reduction, by means of a sensible diet and increased physical activity, can bestow several lifelong and life-extending benefits. Having a healthy body weight can lower the risk of CHD.
- People who are not physically active have a greater risk of CVD than do people who participate in regular physical activity. Such activity improves overall fitness, cardiac reserve, and collateral coronary circulation. It can also help reduce stress.
- A smoker's chance of sudden death is several times greater than that of a nonsmoker. Tobacco use increases the risk of damage to the heart and blood vessels, thereby increasing the risk of atherosclerosis and AMI. The chemicals in cigarettes increase levels of fibrinogen, promoting clotting. Nicotine increases heart rate and blood pressure. The good news is that smokers who quit return rapidly to the same risk level as that of nonsmokers.
- Because every person manages stress differently, researchers aren't sure how stress increases the risk of heart disease. It's clear, though, that hormones such as epinephrine are released during times of stress. The release of epinephrine accelerates the heart rate, raises blood pressure, and increases the body's need for oxygen. Chronic stress exposes the body to persistent levels of epinephrine and increased blood pressure. The body's response to stress can also worsen other risk factors. For example, a person who is stressed may be less active, overeat, start smoking, or smoke more than usual.

Contributing risk factors are thought to increase the risk of heart disease and stroke, but the exact role has not been defined. Education, family income, and employment are examples of contributing risk factors. People in difficult socioeconomic circumstances, who may not have easy access to health care, are more likely to smoke, and are less likely to have a healthy diet. Those who do have access to health care may be less likely to report warning signs of CHD, such as chest discomfort, to their physicians.

Prevention. Education and early recognition are important prevention strategies. Educating people about the risk factors of heart disease may decrease mortality. This is an area of interest for EMS providers involved in community health promotion. Table 17-10 lists methods to reduce CHD risk.

Angina Pectoris

The principal symptom of CAD is angina pectoris (literally "choking in the chest"). Angina is the sudden pain that occurs when the supply of oxygen to the myocardium is insufficient to meet demand. As a result, the cardiac muscle becomes ischemic, switching to anaerobic metabolism. This altered metabolism leads to the buildup of lactic acid and carbon dioxide. Understanding the concept of "supply and demand" is crucial here: At rest, a person with heart disease who remains sedentary may have an adequate supply of oxygen to the myocardium despite

Table 17-10 Factors That Reduce the Risk of Cardiovascular Disease

- Aerobic exercise
- Awareness
- Behavior modification
- Blood pressure control
- Cholesterol management
- Lipid management
- Smoking cessation
- Weight management

some narrowing of the coronary arteries. However, when the same person exercises or experiences some other physiologic stress, blood flow to the myocardium may not be able to satisfy the heart's increased oxygen demand; in that case, angina will result. Clearly, then, the patient with angina at rest, when oxygen needs are minimal, has more severe CAD than a person who reports angina only during vigorous exercise.

Stable Angina. **Stable angina** is episodic chest discomfort caused by myocardial ischemia that usually follows a recurrent pattern: A person with stable angina experiences pain after a certain, predictable amount of exertion, such as climbing one flight of stairs or walking for 3 blocks. The pain has a predictable location, intensity, and duration. The patient may report, for example, "Every time I walk up the hill to the bus stop, I get a squeezing pain under my breast bone, and I have to sit down for 2 or 3 minutes until it goes away."

Patients with chronic, stable angina often take NTG or some other nitrate agent to relieve anginal pain. NTG is supplied as a sublingual tablet or formulated as a liquid that is sprayed under the tongue. It may also be given in a sustained-release capsule taken two or three times a day, as a cream rubbed into the skin (topical agent), or as a patch worn on the skin. Regardless of its form, NTG has a predictable effect in patients with stable angina, relieving symptoms within a few minutes. ST-segment depression or inverted T waves may be observed on the ECG. These ECG changes usually resolve when the heart's oxygen demand is reduced to a level that can be supplied by the coronary artery (such as with rest) or when blood flow is increased by dilating the coronary arteries with NTG.

Unstable Angina. Unstable angina is more serious than stable angina. It is characterized by changes in the frequency, severity, and duration of pain and other symptoms. Other names for unstable angina include *preinfarction angina*, *crescendo angina*, *preocclusive syndrome*, *intermediate coronary syndrome*, and *ACS*. Unlike stable angina, unstable angina often occurs unpredictably. The patient may report that the anginal attacks have become more frequent and severe during the past several days or weeks, or the attacks may awaken him or her from sleep or otherwise occur when at rest. The anginal pain may or may not be relieved by rest or medications. Such attacks are often warning signs of an impending MI.

Prinzmetal Angina. **Prinzmetal angina**, also called *vasospastic angina*, is a type of angina caused by coronary artery vasospasm. It usually occurs at rest, but may be brought on by emotional stress, hyperventilation, exercise, or cold weather.[4] This type of angina can occur in patients with normal coronary arteries as well as in patients with CAD. ST-segment elevation is often seen on the ECG. Symptoms may resolve on their own or with NTG. People with Prinzmetal angina have an increased risk of dysrhythmia, AMI, syncope, and sudden death.[4]

Acute Myocardial Infarction

An AMI, or heart attack, occurs when a portion of the cardiac muscle is deprived of coronary blood flow long enough for portions of the muscle to die—in other words, to undergo **necrosis**, or infarct. The location and size of an MI depend on which coronary artery is blocked and where along its course the blockage occurs. Most infarcts involve the left ventricle. When the anterior, lateral, or septal wall of the left ventricle is infarcted, the source is usually occlusion of the left coronary artery or one of its branches. Inferior wall infarcts are usually the result of RCA occlusion.

When the ischemic process affects only the inner layer of muscle, the infarct is referred to as a **subendocardial myocardial infarction**. When the infarct extends through the entire wall of the ventricle, it is said to be **transmural myocardial infarction**. The infarcted tissue is surrounded by a ring of ischemic tissue—an area that is relatively deprived of oxygen but still viable. That ischemic tissue tends to be electrically unstable and is often the source of cardiac dysrhythmias. The longer a segment of myocardium remains ischemic, the less likelihood of salvaging the tissue and restoring its normal function. The sooner reperfusion therapy can begin after the onset of the blockage, the better the chances for saving the affected distal myocardium.

Patients with STEMI have ECG evidence of ST-segment elevation. As its name implies, NSTEMI produces no sign of myocardial injury (ST-segment elevation) on the patient's ECG. Distinguishing patients with unstable angina from those with AMI may be impossible during initial presentation, because the signs, symptoms, and ECG findings associated with these two conditions may be identical.

Words of Wisdom

For purposes of treatment outside the medical facility, assume the patient with chest pain is having an AMI until proven otherwise.

Assessment

Half of all patients who die of ACS do so before reaching a medical facility.[17] Remember, time is muscle, so you must rapidly and systematically assess the patient with a suspected ACS. Patient care goals include the following:[6]

- Identify quickly whether STEMI is present and, if so, notify the medical facility.
- Determine the time of symptom onset.
- Monitor the patient's cardiac rhythm and vital signs; be prepared to provide CPR and defibrillation, if needed.
- Administer appropriate medications.
- Transport to an appropriate facility.

Symptoms. The most common symptom of an ACS is chest discomfort. Although some patients will have a history of stable angina, ACS will be the initial presentation of CAD in others.[4] A person with an ACS typically feels pain just beneath the sternum, variously described as heavy, squeezing, crushing, or tight. The pain may radiate to the arms (most often the left arm) and into the fingers; it may also radiate to the neck, jaw, upper back, or epigastrium. Ischemic chest discomfort is usually dull, rather than sharp. The pain is unaffected by deep inspiration, movement, or position. It may or may not be relieved by nitrates or rest. To convey the squeezing nature of the discomfort, the patient may clench his or her fist and hold it against the sternum (Levine sign). Occasionally, a patient may mistake the pain of an ACS for indigestion and take antacids in an attempt to relieve the discomfort.

Not every ACS patient has chest discomfort. Some have no chest pain, a phenomenon referred to as "silent MI." Others may present solely with dyspnea or with arm, shoulder, back, jaw, neck, epigastric, or ear discomfort.[4] Symptoms of myocardial ischemia other than chest pain or discomfort are called *anginal equivalents* Table 17-11.

Atypical or unusual symptoms are more common in women, older adults, and patients with diabetes. Women with an ACS often describe the discomfort as aching, tightness, pressure, sharpness, burning, fullness, or tingling. The location of the discomfort is often in the back, shoulder, or neck. Some women have vague chest discomfort that tends to come and go, with no known aggravating factors. Frequent acute symptoms include shortness of breath, weakness, unusual fatigue, cold sweats, dizziness, and nausea or vomiting. Older adults may also have atypical symptoms, such as compromised mental status, generalized weakness, syncope, shortness of breath, fatigue, unexplained nausea, and abdominal or epigastric discomfort. Likewise, patients with diabetes may present atypically, with generalized weakness, syncope, light-headedness, or a diminished mental status.

When obtaining a history from a patient whose chief complaint is chest discomfort, ask the usual SAMPLE (Signs and symptoms, Allergies, Medications, Pertinent past medical history, Last oral intake, Events leading up to the illness or injury) and OPQRST questions to elaborate on the chief complaint. In addition, ask whether the patient has taken anything for the pain and, if so, whether it helped. If the patient reports having taken NTG without relief, then it's important to establish *why* the pain was unrelieved. One of two reasons might explain this failure. It's possible that the patient is, indeed, having an ACS, for which NTG did not provide complete pain relief. The other possibility is the NTG has simply gone stale. To distinguish between the two explanations, ask the patient whether the last few doses of NTG have had the usual effects. Therapeutically active NTG tablets provoke a slight burning sensation under the tongue and may make the patient feel flushed or give him or her a transient throbbing headache. If the patient confirms he or she felt some of those effects but the chest pain still would not go away, then you know there was nothing wrong with the NTG. Nevertheless, there may be something very wrong with the patient.

When you assess the severity of the patient's discomfort, use a pain rating scale. Using a pain scale will allow you to evaluate the effectiveness of your emergency care. Document the patient's initial rating of his or her pain or discomfort. Reassess (and document) the degree of discomfort after each treatment you perform and before transferring care at the receiving facility.

Begin treatment as soon as you elicit a chief complaint of a cardiac nature; the more in-depth history taking and the secondary assessment can wait. For the purpose of discussions in this section, however, we'll proceed through the history and secondary assessment. Besides pain (or sometimes instead of pain), a number of other symptoms are associated with ACSs:

- Diaphoresis (sweating), often profuse, is principally the result of massive discharge by the ANS. The sweat may soak through the patient's clothing, and he or she may report having a cold sweat.
- Dyspnea may be a warning sign of impending LVF.
- Anorexia (loss of appetite), nausea, vomiting, or belching frequently accompanies MI. Hiccups

Table 17-11 Anginal Equivalents
Abdominal pain
Acute change in mental status
Dizziness
Dyspnea
Dysrhythmia
Epigastric pain
Fatigue
Generalized weakness
Indigestion
Isolated arm or jaw pain
Light-headedness
Palpitations
Restlessness
Syncope or near syncope
Unexplained nausea or vomiting

caused by diaphragmatic irritation in an inferior wall MI may occasionally occur as well.

- Weakness may be profound, and the patient may say he or she feels like "a limp dishrag" or something similar.
- If CO is diminished significantly, then the reduced circulation to the brain may cause dizziness.
- Patients with cardiac dysrhythmias sometimes perceive palpitations as a sensation that the heart has skipped a beat.
- A feeling of impending doom is common among patients having an MI. The patient is frightened, appears frightened, and expresses his or her fear to other people—all of which adds to a general atmosphere of panic and dread.

Words of Wisdom

Begin treatment immediately for any patient with chest pain or discomfort or an anginal equivalent.

Signs. Although ACS patients may have abnormalities in the physical exam, many have relatively normal exam findings, and diagnosis in the field depends chiefly on the history and 12-lead ECG findings. Nevertheless, a few specific physical exam findings can help you detect the development of complications of AMI, such as heart failure or cardiogenic shock.

- Pay attention to the patient's general appearance. Does the patient appear anxious? Frightened? In obvious pain? Of course, not all chest pain is caused by ischemia, injury, or infarction. Many other conditions may cause chest pain that can mimic angina or an AMI.
- What is the patient's level of responsiveness? Is he or she fully alert? Confused? Remember: Poor perfusion creates confusion. If the patient does not seem mentally sound, it may be because the heart is giving out and not enough oxygenated blood is reaching the brain.
- Is the skin pale, cold, and clammy? A typical patient with an AMI is apprehensive, with ashen-gray pallor and cold, wet skin.
- Assess the patient's vital signs. Is the pulse strong or weak? Regular or irregular? Is the respiratory rate abnormally rapid? Is the blood pressure abnormally high or low? In a patient with AMI, the pulse rate may be normal, rapid, or slow. The blood pressure may be decreased, reflecting decreased CO from the damaged heart, or it may be elevated from pain and anxiety.
- Are there signs of LVF (wheezes or crackles)? Signs of RVF (distended neck veins, pedal or presacral edema)?

Table 17-12 Differential Diagnosis of Chest Pain and Discomfort

Classification	Possible Diagnoses
Cardiovascular causes	▪ Aneurysm ▪ Aortic dissection ▪ Myocardial ischemia ▪ Myocarditis ▪ Pericarditis
Gastrointestinal causes	▪ Cholecystitis ▪ Esophageal spasm ▪ Gastroesophageal reflux disease ▪ Hiatal hernia ▪ Indigestion ▪ Pancreatitis ▪ Peptic ulcer disease
Musculoskeletal causes	▪ Acromioclavicular disease ▪ Chest wall trauma ▪ Chest wall tumor ▪ Costochondritis ▪ Intercostal muscle cramps
Respiratory causes	▪ Pleurisy ▪ Pneumonia ▪ Pneumothorax ▪ Pulmonary embolism ▪ Respiratory infection
Other causes	▪ Anxiety disorder/panic attack ▪ Herpes zoster (shingles)

It is crucial for you to perform a thorough physical exam, including history taking, to determine whether the cause of the patient's signs and symptoms is likely cardiac in origin. Table 17-12 shows differential diagnoses to consider throughout your assessment.

Words of Wisdom

As a general rule, it's safe to assume any patient who has called for medical assistance because of chest pain has, at the least, unstable angina and perhaps an evolving AMI. Patients with a history of angina rarely call for help unless something has changed—often dramatically—for the worse. Because it is difficult to differentiate between angina and an AMI in the field, the treatment of angina should be the same as for an AMI. It's far better for you to overtreat angina as an AMI than to undertreat an AMI by assuming it's just angina.

Management of Acute Coronary Syndromes

Among patients with an ACS, those with STEMI are most likely to benefit from reperfusion therapy. Several variables affect the efficacy of perfusion therapy, but the most significant is probably the duration from symptom onset to treatment. Because the benefits of reperfusion therapy are time sensitive, start treatment at once on arrival at the scene for any patient with chest discomfort, even before you complete the history and secondary assessment. The ACS algorithm is shown in **Figure 17-103**.

Place the Patient at Physical and Emotional Rest. The stress response triggers a surge of catecholamines (epinephrine and norepinephrine) from the adrenal glands, which in turn can send the damaged heart racing. At the same time, the massive discharge throughout the fight-or-flight system puts the peripheral circulation in a state of severe vasoconstriction; thus, not only is the heart being pushed to go faster, but it must also work harder against the escalating afterload. The heart's need for oxygen, therefore, soars precisely when it is already in a state of marked oxygen deprivation. This cycle can lead quickly to dysrhythmias and death.

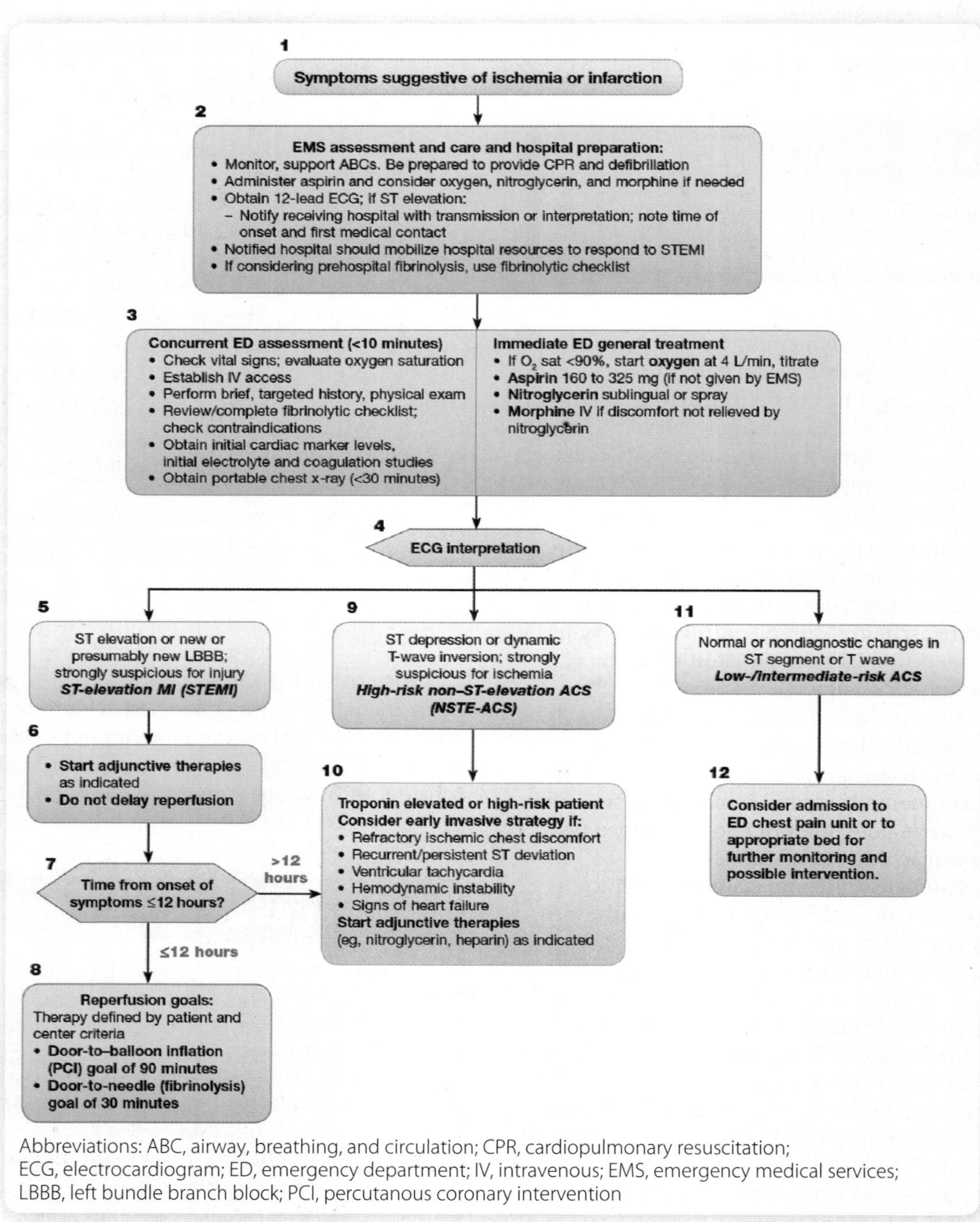

Figure 17-103 Acute coronary syndromes algorithm.

Words of Wisdom

For the patient with an ACS, reperfusion therapy may be delayed at three key points: (1) between onset and the patient's recognition of symptoms, (2) during prehospital care and transport, and (3) during ED evaluation.[17] Delays in prehospital care can occur during response time, on-scene time, and/or travel time to the receiving facility.[21] These delays prolong time to treatment and can ultimately harm the patient's outcome. You can make a difference by working quickly and efficiently when providing emergency care to the patient with a suspected ACS.

One way to limit infarct size is to decrease the amount of work the heart must do, which will immediately begin to decrease the patient's myocardial oxygen requirements. Begin your care by allowing the patient to assume a position of comfort. Most patients prefer a semi-Fowler position. From the time you arrive, the patient must not expend any effort—not even to walk to the stretcher.

Obtain Vital Signs and Perform Cardiac Monitoring. Obtain vital signs, including pulse, respiration, blood pressure, and Spo_2. Measure the blood pressure, and repeat that measurement at least every 5 minutes. Measure the pulse rate. The ECG monitor provides information only about the electrical activity of the heart; it reveals nothing about the heart's mechanical function. Therefore, it is necessary to monitor the patient's pulse to assess peripheral blood flow and the strength of the heartbeat. This is especially important during transport, when vital sign measurements can be difficult to obtain.

Apply the cardiac monitor. Run a strip to document and identify the patient's initial rhythm. Ideally, your monitor should emit an audible tone or beep with each QRS complex (also called a "systole beep"), so you can keep track of the patient's cardiac rhythm even when you have to look away from the monitor to do other things. The ear, in any case, is far more sensitive than the eye in detecting slight rhythm irregularities, so you're more likely to hear the beginning of a cardiac dysrhythmia much sooner than you would see it on the monitor. Keep your drug box handy so you can quickly reach medications if a cardiac dysrhythmia develops. Treat pulseless rhythms, tachycardia, and symptomatic bradycardia in accordance with the algorithm for each respective dysrhythmia. Initiate CPR, defibrillation, or cardioversion, if indicated.

Administer Oxygen and Aspirin. The mnemonic MONA can help you recall the supportive treatments of Morphine, Oxygen, Nitroglycerin, and Aspirin for a patient with an ACS—but do not administer these treatments in that order. Administer MONA in the following order, provided these measures are not contraindicated by hypotension: (1) oxygen, (2) aspirin, (3) NTG, and (4) morphine.

If the patient is dyspneic, hypoxemic, or has obvious signs of heart failure, administer oxygen and titrate therapy to maintain the Spo_2 level at 94% or higher. In most EMS systems, as long as the patient has no aspirin allergy or gastrointestinal bleeding, dispatchers advise patients to chew baby aspirin (160 to 325 mg). If the patient has not already taken aspirin before your arrival, give him or her 160 to 325 mg of non–enteric-coated aspirin to chew.

Obtain a 12-lead ECG. Obtain a 12-lead ECG within 10 minutes of patient contact while another crew member establishes vascular access. One of the most important components in the rapid identification and treatment of a cardiac event is rapid acquisition of the 12-lead ECG. Always perform a 12-lead ECG *before* administering any medication (except possibly aspirin and oxygen). Repeat the 12-lead ECG with each set of vital signs, when symptoms change, and as often as necessary. This is important because the patient's ECG may be normal between episodes of discomfort but show signs of ischemia, injury, or infarction during episodes of discomfort.

In patients whose symptoms suggest ischemia or infarction, the 12-lead ECG allows for rapid stratification into one of three categories: (1) STEMI (ST elevation in two or more contiguous leads, or new or suspected LBBB) **Figure 17-104**, (2) NSTEMI, and (3) normal (nondiagnostic). It is important to remember that a normal ECG does not rule out ischemia, injury, or infarction.

STEMI treatment involves rapid reperfusion of the affected lesion or lesions. *Reperfusion therapy* refers to restoration of blood flow, either by procedural means (such as percutaneous coronary intervention [PCI]), or by administering a fibrinolytic medication to dissolve blood clots (pharmacologic reperfusion). You should know which medical facilities in your area are equipped to administer **fibrinolytic therapy** and/or PCI.

Cardiac catheterization is a minimally invasive procedure performed under fluoroscopy to diagnose and treat blocked coronary arteries. Cardiac catheterization, PCI, and percutaneous transluminal coronary angioplasty (PTCA) are used interchangeably to refer to cardiac catheterization. With this therapy, a balloon, stent, or other device are passed through a peripheral artery catheter to reopen a blocked coronary artery by compressing the plaque against the vessel wall. The success rate is high, and the risks are low. PCI is often used for patients who are not candidates for fibrinolytic therapy. The AHA recommends prehospital notification of the receiving medical facility (if **fibrinolysis** [the process of dissolving blood clots] is the likely reperfusion strategy) and/or prehospital activation of the catheterization laboratory for all patients with a recognized STEMI on the prehospital ECG.[17] Prenotification allows medical facility personnel to assemble and begin preparations while the patient is in transit to the facility.

Most treatment regimens for fibrinolysis rely on one of three agents: alteplase (Activase), streptokinase (Streptase), or reteplase (Retavase). These agents work by converting, in one way or another, the body's clot-dissolving enzyme from its inactive form, plasminogen, to its active form, **plasmin**. Unfortunately, if an agent capable of promoting clot dissolution is given intravenously, its effects cannot be limited to the clot in the coronary artery; the agent can act

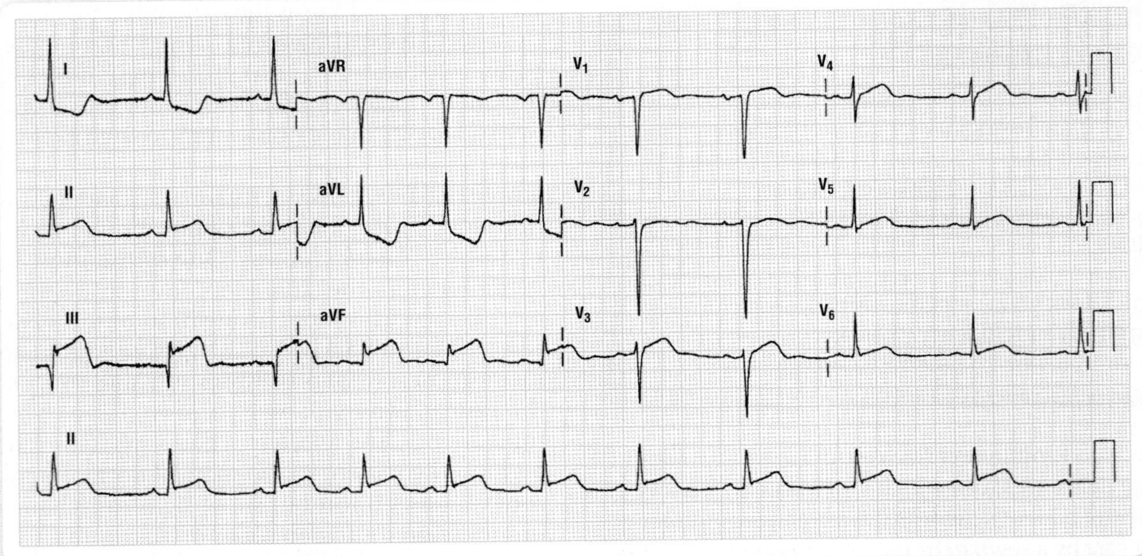

Figure 17-104 ST-segment elevation in leads II, III, and aVF, with ST-segment depression and T-wave inversion in reciprocal leads I and aVL.

anywhere else in the body where clots are being formed and, therefore, may lead to uncontrolled bleeding. Thus, the benefit of fibrinolytic therapy—the possible salvage of myocardial tissue—must always be weighed against its risks—principally, the risk of bleeding.

When discussing STEMI, it is important to understand that it is critical to minimize EMS-to-balloon time, door-to-balloon time, and door-to-needle time. These concepts refer to the time that elapses before the patient receives definitive reperfusion therapy. EMS-to-balloon time starts at the first moment of patient contact by EMS providers and ends when definitive therapy occurs (when a catheter passes through the lesion in the affected coronary vessel). Door-to-balloon time is the interval between patient presentation to the medical facility and definitive therapy. Door-to-needle time begins when the patient arrives at the ED and ends when a fibrinolytic medication is administered.

Evidence-Based Medicine

Up to 20% of patients with STEMI do not present with chest pain or discomfort.[22] Research shows that more than 25% of STEMI patients presenting without chest pain do not receive prehospital ECGs and have significantly longer EMS-to-balloon times.[22] To avoid delays in reperfusion therapy when caring for a patient with a possible ACS, keep in mind the concepts of atypical presentation and anginal equivalents. When in doubt, obtain a 12-lead ECG.

In some areas, prehospital fibrinolysis is available as part of a STEMI system of care. The ideal STEMI system includes the following:

- Well-established protocols
- Comprehensive training
- Fibrinolytic checklist **Figure 17-105**
- 12-lead ECG acquisition and interpretation capability
- Staff experienced in ACLS
- Ability to communicate with the receiving institution
- Medical direction with training and experience in managing STEMI
- Quality assurance[17]

Not all EMS systems are able to support a STEMI system. When a STEMI system of care exists, and transport times are expected to be more than 30 minutes, the AHA considers it reasonable to administer fibrinolytics in the prehospital setting.[17] However, when both prehospital fibrinolysis and direct transport to a PCI center are available, transport may be preferred because fibrinolysis carries a higher risk of intracranial hemorrhage than PCI.[17]

Transport patients with STEMI to a facility capable of performing PCI. Fibrinolysis is contraindicated for patients with unstable angina/NSTEMI.[17] Patients with unstable angina/NSTEMI who are clinically unstable and who have positive cardiac biomarkers may undergo PCI.[17]

Words of Wisdom

Your ability to identify candidates for reperfusion therapy plays a decisive role in helping medical facility personnel begin treatment early enough to make a difference. For this reason, ensure you have a thorough understanding of the principles of reperfusion therapy for ACS. Time is muscle!

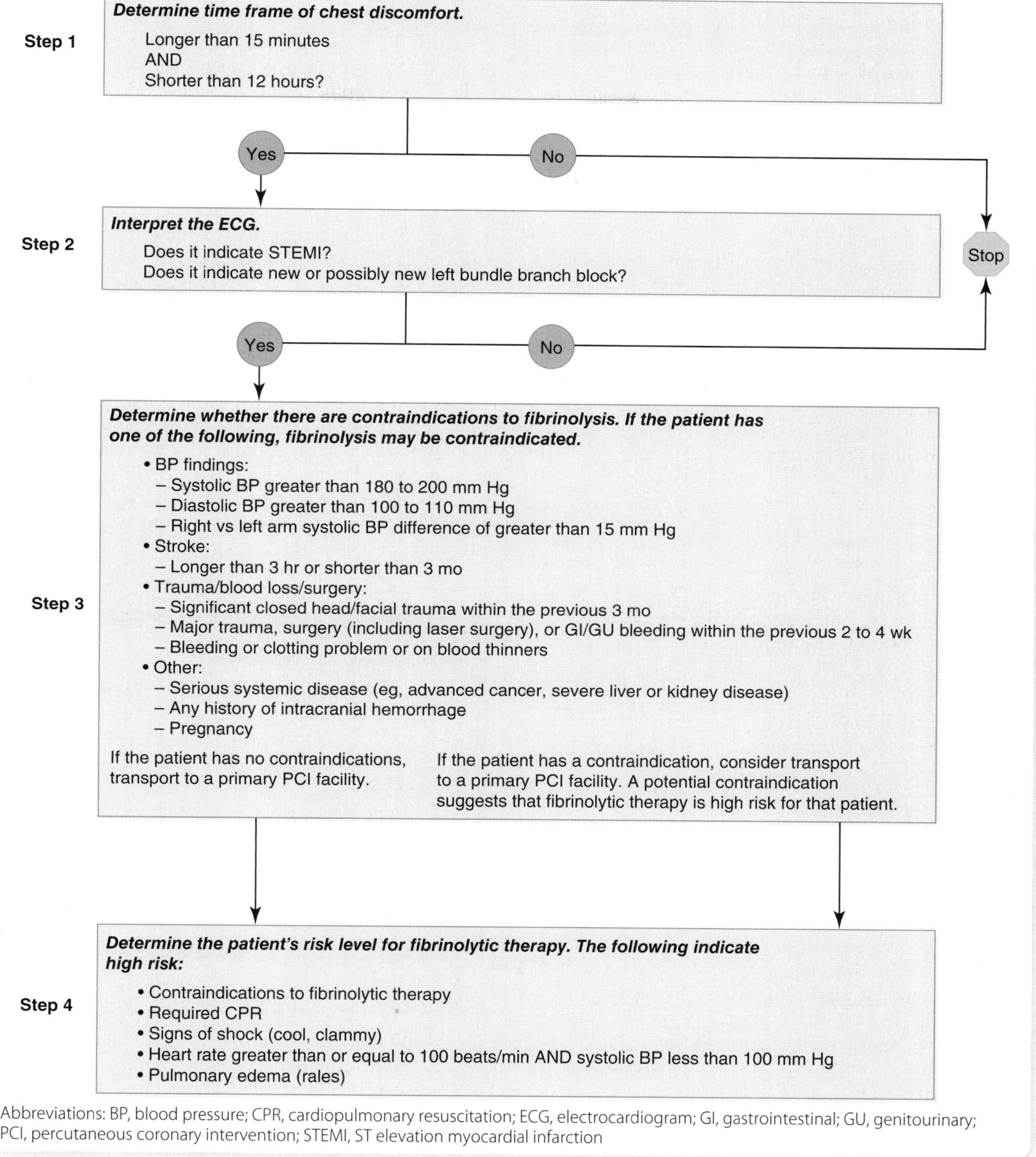

Figure 17-105 Prehospital fibrinolytic checklist.

Provide Pain Relief. Some form of pain relief must be provided, because the severe pain of AMI places enormous stress on the patient's ANS, which may contribute to complications. NTG is a good place to start, but ensure there are no contraindications to its use before you administer it. NTG is contraindicated for patients with an initial systolic blood pressure (SBP) less than 90 mm Hg. Avoid administering NTG if right ventricular infarction (RVI) is suspected. When an infarction involves the right ventricle, the effectiveness of that heart chamber is diminished, and the right heart becomes preload dependent. Hypotension can result if preload is reduced. This occurs with the administration of any medication that decreases preload (NTG, morphine, diuretics). If the 12-lead ECG indicates an inferior MI, then apply right-sided chest leads to assess right ventricular involvement. Do not administer nitrates if the patient has used the phosphodiesterase inhibitor sildenafil (Viagra) in the past 24 hours, or tadalafil (Cialis) or vardenafil (Levitra) in the past 48 hours.

Administer NTG sublingually as a 0.4-mg tablet or metered-dose spray. It may be repeated every 3 to 5 minutes, up to a total of three doses, as long as the patient's condition remains stable.

If the patient's discomfort persists and his or her vital signs remain stable, consider administering morphine sulfate. Morphine is the preferred analgesic for patients with STEMI; however, it may have adverse effects in patients with unstable angina/STEMI.[17] Follow your local protocol regarding its use. For pain not relieved by NTG, fentanyl (Sublimaze) is favored over morphine in some EMS systems, because of its rapid onset, relatively short duration, and fewer side effects.

Take a History and Perform the Secondary Assessment. After you have completed the preceding steps (as appropriate), you should obtain a more detailed history and perform the secondary assessment. Gathering this information should not delay transport to the medical facility. Once you've taken the necessary precautions to stabilize the patient's condition (aspirin, oxygen, IV saline lock, monitor/12-lead ECG, and analgesia), there is no reason to remain at the scene unless a cardiac arrest or dysrhythmia requires immediate treatment. Obtain the rest of the history en route to the medical facility.

Transport the Patient. Once the patient is in stable condition, transport him or her to an appropriate medical facility in a semi-Fowler position (unless the patient is in shock, in which case he or she should be supine). Do all you can to ensure the patient is as relaxed and as comfortable as possible. En route, some additional treatment measures may be worthwhile, especially when the transport time will be lengthy.

Dysrhythmias are common in the first few hours of an infarction. Be prepared to give antidysrhythmics or perform TCP, synchronized cardioversion, or defibrillation. If the patient's condition is stable, transport him or her without lights and siren. Initiate rapid transport if the patient has had no relief of symptoms after your initial care, if signs and symptoms of shock are present, or if there are significant changes in the patient's ECG. Such changes may include the development of a dysrhythmia, changes in the ST segment, or the development of pathologic Q waves.

If STEMI is identified, experts recommend preferential patient transport to a medical facility capable of performing PCI; doing so has been shown to speed reperfusion and improve clinical outcomes.[18] Destination decisions should be based on your local resources and system of care.

You will encounter people who refuse treatment or transport despite having signs and symptoms consistent with an ACS. A person with chest discomfort who refuses care is an example of a "high-risk refusal"—in other words, there is a high risk of legal liability under these circumstances. Calmly and carefully, try to persuade the person to accept the care you wish to provide, including transport. If you believe the patient may be having an MI, communicate in words the patient can easily understand. For example, use the phrase "heart attack" instead of MI. Let the patient know what emergency care you'd like to provide and the benefits of accepting it. Explain the risks of turning away the care you have offered. Because an MI may be fatal, you must present this possible outcome to the patient. The point is not to scare the patient, but you must clearly outline the perils of refusing treatment, including transport. It may be help to contact medical direction in these situations. In some cases, the physician may ask to speak directly to the patient and may be successful in persuading him or her to accept treatment and transport. If you are unable to convince the patient to accept care, carefully document the patient's refusal.

Words of Wisdom

AMI has many possible complications. Familiarize yourself with them. Electrical complications include bradycardia, AV block, bundle branch and fascicular blocks, tachycardia, and sudden cardiac death. Ischemic complications include an extension of the infarction and reinfarction. Mechanical complications can also occur, including LVF, RVF, cardiogenic shock, and ventricular aneurysm. Pericarditis may be an inflammatory complication of AMI. Stroke, deep vein thrombosis (DVT), and pulmonary embolism are possible embolic complications.

Patient and Family Education

The time from symptom onset to emergency care can be shortened if patients, families, and bystanders recognize heart attack symptoms early and activate their EMS system. Teach your patients and their families how to recognize the signs and symptoms of a heart attack. Instruct them to call 9-1-1 within 5 minutes of symptom onset. Explain to them that not all heart attacks are accompanied by sudden, crushing chest pain and a loss of responsiveness. Symptoms may begin gradually or they may come and go. Advise patients who have had a previous heart attack that the signs and symptoms of a second or subsequent cardiac event may differ from those of the first.

Documentation & Communication

EMS systems regularly evaluate the care provided to patients with ACS. Key documentation elements are as follows:[6]

- Time of symptom onset
- Time of arrival on scene
- Time of acquisition of a 12-lead ECG
- Time of identification of STEMI
- Time at which aspirin was administered; or reason why it was not given
- Time of STEMI notification

▶ Heart Failure

Heart failure occurs when the heart is unable, for any reason, to pump powerfully enough or fast enough to empty its chambers; as a result, blood backs up into the systemic circuit, the pulmonary circuit, or both. Heart failure is a syndrome, not a disease, caused by any of several disorders that impair the ability of the ventricles to fill with or eject blood.

Heart failure can be identified based on symptom onset (acute versus chronic) and the ventricle initially involved (left versus right). In acute heart failure, symptoms occur suddenly. In chronic heart failure, symptoms develop more slowly. A person with chronic heart failure can develop acute heart failure. Although failure of either ventricle can occur by itself, they often occur together: RVF is often a result of LVF.

Disorders of the pericardium, myocardium, endocardium, or great vessels may cause heart failure. Examples of these disorders include CAD, valvular heart disease, dysrhythmias, cardiomyopathy, and long-standing high blood pressure. In fact, CAD—with or without MI—is the most common cause of heart failure.

Regardless of its cause, heart failure produces symptoms in most patients because the left ventricle is unable to pump blood effectively. To understand what happens in heart failure, a quick review of the physiology of the normal heart is helpful. Remember, CO is equal to stroke volume multiplied by the heart rate. Three main factors affect stroke volume: preload, afterload, and cardiac contractility. Thus, any condition that impairs preload, afterload, cardiac contractility, or heart rate can cause heart failure.

According to Starling law of the heart, increased venous return augments preload. Heart muscle fibers stretch in response to the expanded volume (preload) before contracting. The stretching of the muscle fibers allows the heart to eject more forcefully the additional volume, thereby boosting stroke volume. So, in the normal heart, the greater the preload, the greater the force of ventricular

YOU are the Paramedic — PART 3

You administer supplemental oxygen and then prepare the patient for transfer into the ambulance for further assessment and transport. As you lift the stretcher into the ambulance, the patient experiences a tonic-clonic seizure lasting 30 to 45 seconds, followed by agonal breathing at a rate of 4 to 6 breaths/min. He is unresponsive. A member of your crew begins bag-mask ventilation while you apply the cardiac monitor. The monitor shows a wide QRS third-degree AV block, with a ventricular rate of 36 beats/min. Before departing for the medical facility, you establish an IV line while another crew member gets a second set of vital signs.

Recording Time: 10 minutes	
Respirations	6 breaths/min; 12 breaths/min with bag-mask ventilation
Pulse	36 beats/min, regular
Skin	Cool, pale, moist
Blood pressure	62/40 mm Hg
Oxygen saturation (Spo_2)	99% with bag-mask ventilation
Pupils	PERRLA

6. Is this patient high priority? Why or why not?
7. Given what you know at this time, what is the most likely cause of the seizure activity?
8. What is this patient's greatest life threat at this time? How will you treat it?
9. How will you manage the cardiac rhythm?

contraction, and the greater the stroke volume, resulting in increased CO.

The heart's normal workload can become overwhelmed if the left ventricle becomes damaged. There are two types of LVF. With systolic failure, the left ventricle doesn't contract normally and has trouble pumping out all the blood in the chamber to the body. With diastolic failure, the left ventricle contracts normally but it has become stiff, impeding its ability to relax and fill with blood between each contraction of the heart. Common causes of LVF are a faulty heart valve, AMI, and cardiomyopathy. Cardiomyopathy is discussed in Chapter 43, *Pediatric Emergencies*. Increased demands on the heart associated with excessive volume or pressure can also cause heart failure. For example, giving a large volume of IV fluid over a short period (as in a runaway IV line) in a patient with a weakened left ventricle can cause volume overload. If a heart valve becomes thickened or narrowed, obstructing the flow of blood through it, pressure overload can occur.

Left Ventricular Failure

When the left ventricle fails, blood backs up behind it, causing a chain reaction Figure 17-106. Blood builds up in the lungs because the left ventricle is unable to eject all the blood within its walls. Consequently, the left atrium

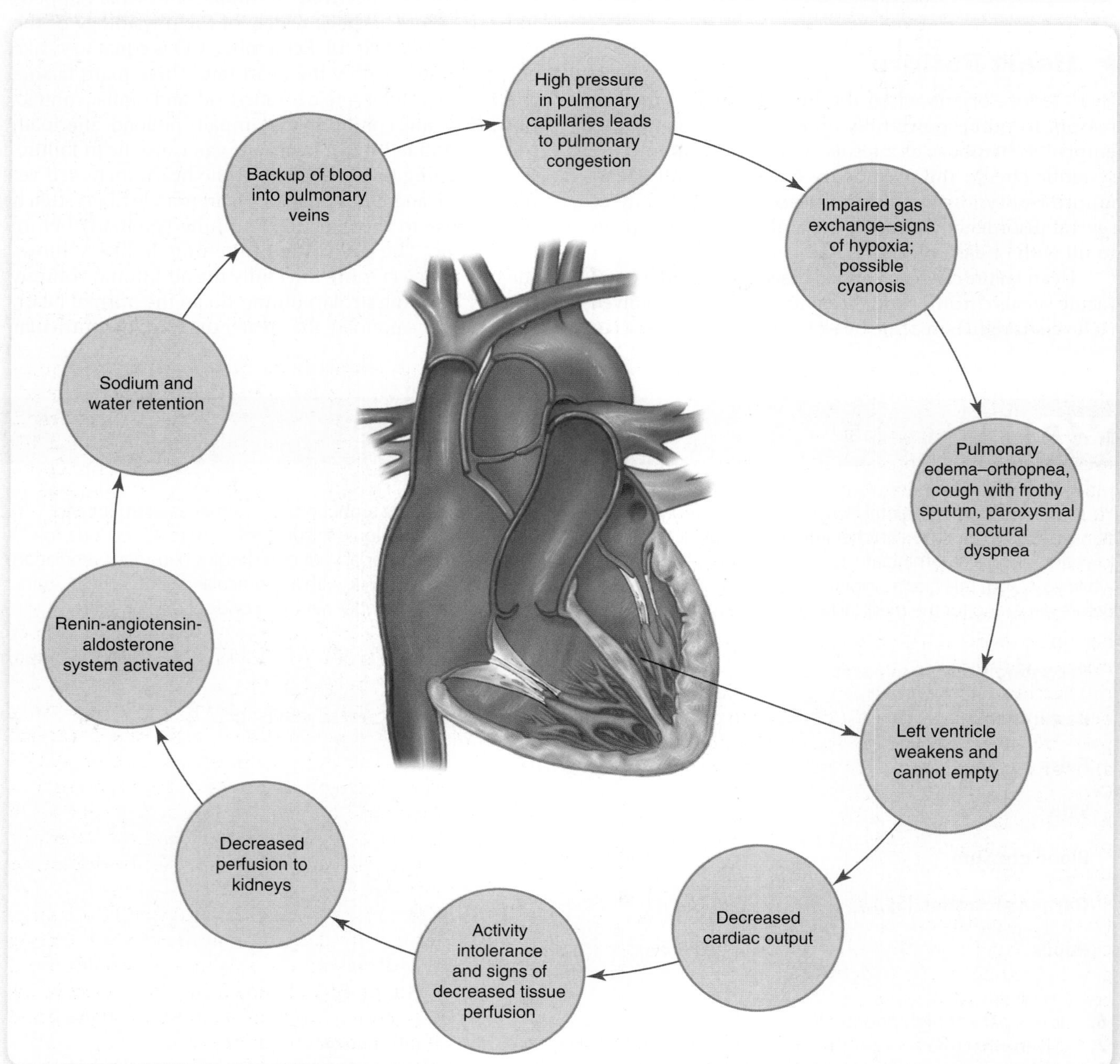

Figure 17-106 Left ventricular failure.

swells with blood because it cannot empty the blood within its walls into the left ventricle. The stretching of the atrial muscle fibers may cause atrial dysrhythmia. Likewise, the pulmonary veins cannot empty the blood from the pulmonary arteries into the left atrium because it is already full. Pressure within the pulmonary vessels increases, forcing fluid from the pulmonary capillaries across the alveolar walls into the alveoli. This causes pulmonary edema. The congestion that can be heard in the lungs is the reason Heart failure is often called *congestive heart failure*. The buildup of fluid widens the gap between the alveoli/capillary membrane, impairing the diffusion of oxygen and carbon dioxide.

Words of Wisdom

Pulmonary edema of cardiac origin is called *cardiogenic pulmonary edema*. Pulmonary edema attributable to climbing or living at a high altitude is called *high-altitude pulmonary edema*. Pulmonary edema can also be caused by other conditions such as toxic inhalation, excessive IV fluids, and some opioid medications. This type of pulmonary edema is called *noncardiogenic pulmonary edema*.

Right Ventricular Failure

To eject the blood within its walls, the right ventricle must overcome high pressure and congestion within the pulmonary vessels. When it cannot keep up with the increased workload, the right ventricle fails **Figure 17-107**. Blood backs up behind the right ventricle, raising the pressure in the right atrium. If the right atrium is unable to eject the blood within its walls, then blood backs up into the superior and inferior venae cavae. The veins become congested with blood because the superior and inferior venae cavae cannot drain into an already full right atrium. Because venous return is delayed, organs become congested with blood. For example, increased pressure in the hepatic veins enlarges the liver (hepatomegaly), making it tender. As venous congestion worsens, rising pressure within the veins forces serous fluid through capillary walls and into body's tissues, producing edema. Peripheral edema is most apparent in dependent areas of the body such as the feet and ankles. Serous fluid may also build up in the abdomen (ascites), pleural cavity (pleural effusion), and/or pericardial cavity (pericardial effusion). As RVF progresses, generalized edema of the entire body may occur. This condition is called *anasarca*.

Cor Pulmonale. RVF may occur by itself (without LVF) in conditions such as RVI, pulmonary embolism, and pulmonary hypertension. Pulmonary hypertension is a disorder in which the pressure in the pulmonary arteries is higher than normal. The right ventricle must work hard to overcome this increased resistance in order to eject blood. Over time, the right ventricle enlarges and eventually fails. RVF caused by pulmonary disease is called *cor pulmonale*. Cor pulmonale is usually the result of COPD.

Compensatory Mechanisms

As the heart begins to fail, the body's compensatory mechanisms attempt to improve CO by manipulating preload, afterload, cardiac contractility, and/or heart rate. Ultimately, compensatory mechanisms may actually worsen heart failure. For example, the sympathetic nervous system boosts the heart rate, increases the force of contraction, and constricts blood vessels. The accelerated heart rate and stronger force of contraction increase the heart's oxygen demand, reduce the amount of time the ventricles have to fill, and decrease time for coronary artery perfusion. Decreased blood flow to the kidneys stimulates the renin-angiotensin-aldosterone system. Angiotensin I forms angiotensin II, promoting more vasoconstriction. Constricted blood vessels (increased afterload) require the heart to work even harder to pump against high pressure. Angiotensin II encourages the release of aldosterone, which encourages sodium and water retention and increased blood volume (increased preload).

These compensatory mechanisms are effective in increasing CO for a time, but eventually heart failure advances. Sodium and water retention enlarges the heart's chambers, thickening the walls of the ventricles and, ultimately, weakening the force of ventricular contraction. As the force of contraction decreases, the weakened heart muscle is unable to handle the increased volume of fluid, and CO decreases.

Assessment

The patient with heart failure may report a sudden onset of shortness of breath, or shortness of breath that has worsened over a period of hours or days. At first, the patient may have difficulty breathing only with activity or when lying down for a while. Respiratory or cardiac disorders can cause these symptoms. However, as LVF worsens, signs and symptoms also become present at rest. The likelihood of a cardiac origin is greater if the patient tells you he has had a previous heart attack or has a history of high blood pressure, valvular disease, or another cardiovascular condition.

The patient may report having had trouble sleeping. The patient may also describe episodes of PND. During these nighttime episodes of shortness of breath, fluid pools in the lungs, literally drowning the patient in his or her own secretions. The patient awakens coughing and feeling as if he or she were suffocating.

In addition to shortness of breath or other breathing difficulties, patients with heart failure often report feeling tired or weak or having no energy. These symptoms,

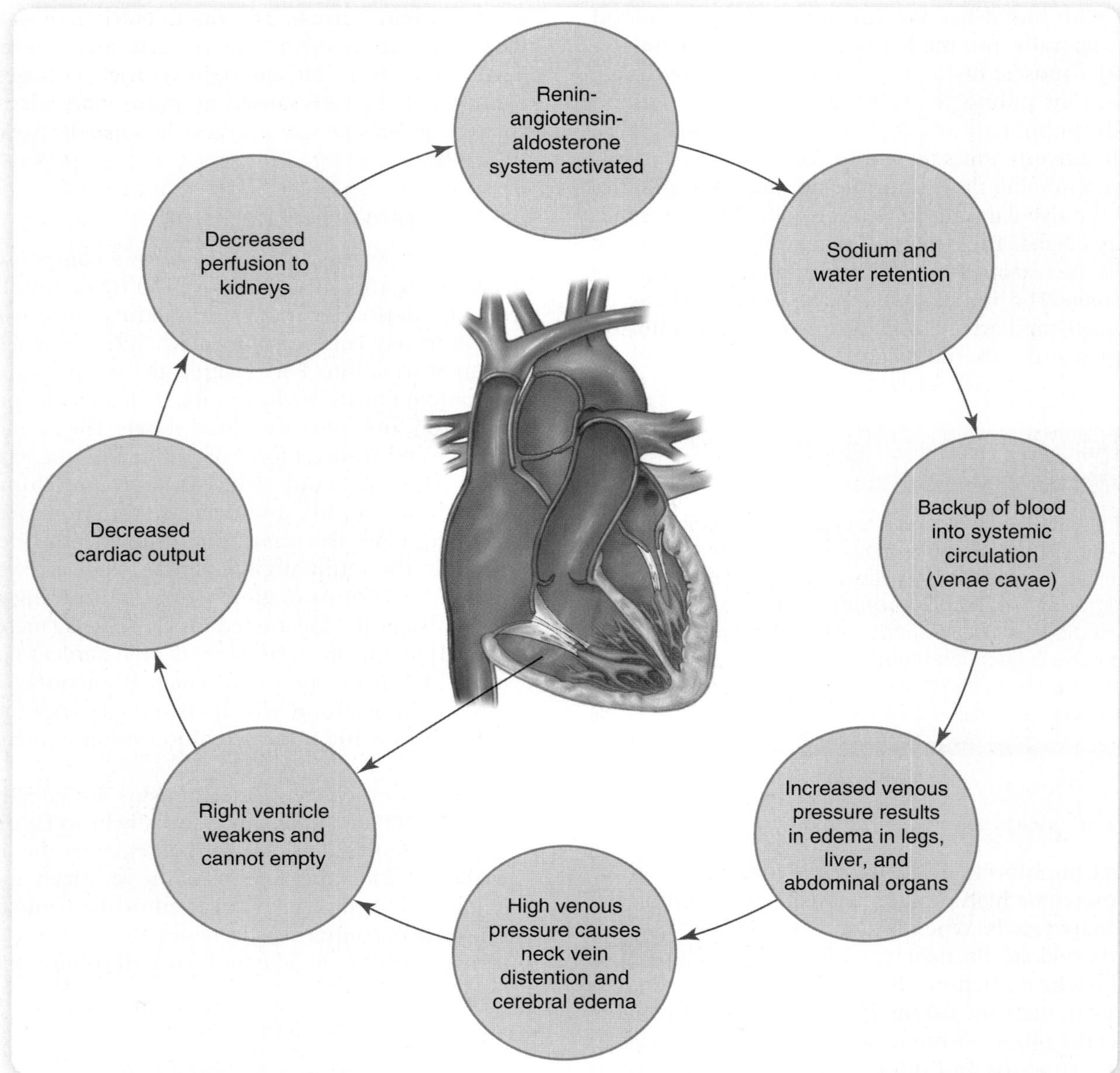

Figure 17-107 Right ventricular failure.

combined with a history of recent weight gain over a short period and/or progressive swelling of the lower extremities, are a red flag for heart failure Table 17-13.

The patient may report having had trouble concentrating recently. This symptom may be the result of hypoxia. The patient may report having had nausea and a loss of appetite. Such symptoms usually arise from congestion of the liver and other abdominal organs. Some patients may describe having had feelings of faintness, palpitations, or an irregular or rapid pulse. Ask the patient about prescribed medications he or she is taking. Specifically, ask whether the patient is taking beta-blockers or calcium channel blockers, because these agents can affect the force with which the heart contracts.

Although obtaining an accurate medical history is important, the patient with heart failure is often too short of breath to answer your questions. While providing emergency care for the patient, you may be able to obtain the patient's history from a family member or neighbor at the scene.

When either side of the heart fails, blood supply to the body's tissues decreases and oxygenation is impaired. Restlessness, anxiety, or unexplained confusion (especially in older adults) may be signs of hypoxia. When talking with the patient, notice if he or she is able to

Table 17-13 Signs and Symptoms of Heart Failure

Left Ventricular Failure	Right Ventricular Failure
Signs	
Restlessness, anxiety	Weight gain
Respiratory rate above normal for age	Dependent edema
Heart rate above normal for age	Ascites
Pulsus alternans	Anasarca
Crackles	Jugular venous distention
Cough with frothy sputum	Liver enlargement (hepatomegaly)
Third heart sound	Spleen enlargement (splenomegaly)
Retractions; accessory muscle use	
Labored breathing; tripod position	
Sweating	
Inability to speak in complete sentences; limited to phrases or words	
Symptoms	
Fatigue	Fatigue
Difficulty breathing	Nausea
Orthopnea	Loss of appetite
Paroxysmal nocturnal dyspnea	Right or left upper abdominal quadrant pain

speak in complete sentences. As heart failure worsens, the patient's shortness of breath will limit speech from sentences to phrases and then only to words. Because keeping the upper body elevated improves breathing (orthopnea), the patient may instinctively assume a tripod position.

The patient's respiratory rate and heart rate are often rapid. The skin may be pale and feel cool. Peripheral pulses may be diminished. These signs represent the sympathetic nervous system's response to hypoxia and the body's compensatory mechanism to maintain CO. You may see signs of increased work of breathing, including retractions and use of accessory muscles.

As hypoxia worsens, the patient may become cyanotic or may cough frequently as fluid irritates the airways. Coughing may produce pink, frothy sputum. As compensatory mechanisms fail, the progressive buildup of fluid in the lungs causes crackles (rales) that do not clear with coughing. This sound may be accompanied by wheezing if bronchospasm occurs. Crackles are heard first at the base of the lungs. As the fluid builds up, you will hear crackles further up the chest. Pulsus paradoxus, pulsus alternans, and a third heart sound may be perceptible. The apical pulse may be displaced as enlargement of the left ventricle displaces the cardiac apex.

If RVF accompanies LVF, then JVD will be visible as the venous system becomes congested. Patients who are able to walk will have swelling of the ankles, feet, calves, or legs. Swelling of the sacral area may occur in patients confined to bed. If edema is present, note (and document) if it is pitting or nonpitting and localized in the ankles, to the mid-calf, or to the knees. Ascites, a buildup of fluid in the peritoneal cavity, may also occur. As the liver and spleen swell, the patient may report upper abdominal quadrant pain.

As the pump continues to fail, the heart rate begins to slow, blood pressure falls, and CO decreases substantially. Cardiogenic shock occurs when heart failure is accompanied by hypotension.

Some of the signs and symptoms that are present with heart failure may also be present with other conditions. Table 17-14 outlines the differential diagnosis of heart failure.

Words of Wisdom

JVD may be present in conditions other than RVF. Listening to breath sounds and heart sounds can help you differentiate the patient's underlying condition. For example, JVD in a patient with cardiac tamponade is usually characterized by clear breath sounds but muffled heart sounds. JVD in a patient with tension pneumothorax is usually characterized by diminished or absent breath sounds on the affected side. JVD in a patient with RVF associated with LVF will usually produce crackles in the lungs. In such patients, fluid administration is often limited and closely monitored. JVD in a patient with RVF associated with RVI usually produces clear breath sounds. A patient with RVI often requires IV fluid boluses to increase preload.

Table 17-14 Differential Diagnosis of Heart Failure

Classification	Possible Diagnoses
Cardiovascular causes	▪ Cardiac tamponade ▪ Cardiogenic pulmonary edema ▪ Cardiogenic shock ▪ High-altitude pulmonary edema ▪ Myocardial ischemia ▪ Myocardial infarction ▪ Noncardiogenic pulmonary edema ▪ Pulmonary embolism
Respiratory causes	▪ Acute respiratory distress syndrome ▪ Asthma ▪ Chronic bronchitis ▪ Chronic obstructive pulmonary disease ▪ Pneumonia ▪ Pneumothorax ▪ Respiratory failure
Other causes	▪ Anaphylaxis ▪ Aspiration ▪ Toxin exposure

Management

Goals when caring for a patient with heart failure include the following:[6]

- Decrease respiratory distress and work of breathing.
- Maintain adequate oxygenation and perfusion.
- Direct supportive efforts toward decreasing the workload of the heart.

A patient who is having difficulty breathing is usually quite anxious. Begin your care by offering the patient reassurance. You will need to work quickly to help relieve the patient's symptoms.

Place him or her in a position of comfort. If pulmonary congestion is present and the patient's blood pressure will tolerate it, place him or her in a sitting position with the feet dangling. This position encourages venous pooling in the legs, which will help decrease venous return, thereby decreasing the work of breathing.

Apply a pulse oximeter and provide supplemental oxygen as needed to maintain the patient's Spo_2 at 94% or higher. Noninvasive positive-pressure ventilation (NIPPV) has been proved an effective tool in managing pulmonary edema associated with heart failure. NIPPV has several benefits:[6]

- Improves oxygenation and perfusion by reducing the work of breathing
- Maintains alveolar inflation
- Improves pulmonary compliance
- Slows respiratory rate, thereby decreasing the work of breathing, heart rate, and SBP
- Facilitates delivery of bronchodilators
- Reduces preload and afterload, improving CO

NIPPV should not be used if the patient has a compromised airway, altered mental status, risk of aspiration, a pneumothorax, or SBP of less than 90 mm Hg. It may be necessary to insert an advanced airway if the patient is in severe distress. Assess breath sounds before and after each intervention. Monitor the patient's respiratory status using waveform capnography. Pulse oximetry will suffice if waveform capnography is unavailable.

Limit the patient's physical activity. Do not allow the patient to walk up or down stairs or to the stretcher. Place the patient on a cardiac monitor and obtain a 12-lead ECG. A dysrhythmia may lead to heart failure. On the other hand, hypoxia and acidosis predispose patients with heart failure to dysrhythmias ranging from tachycardia to bradycardia.

Establish IV access. To help ensure the patient in heart failure does not receive too much IV fluid, use a heparin lock or saline lock. If local protocol require you to use an IV bag and tubing, infuse the fluid at a "to keep open" rate (30 mL/hr). Check and recheck the volume of fluid in the bag while the patient is in your care. Document the amount of fluid in the bag when you start the IV line and the amount of fluid remaining when you transfer patient care at the receiving facility.

Pharmacologic therapy for heart failure may vary slightly by EMS system, so be sure to check your local protocol. Sublingual NTG may be given to reduce both preload and afterload, thereby supporting CO. Ask how much, if any, NTG the patient has already taken.

Furosemide (Lasix) is a diuretic that was used for many years in the prehospital management of heart failure. Currently, it is not recommended for use in treating heart failure and acute pulmonary edema. It carries a risk of inducing hypokalemia, dysrhythmia, or increased systemic vascular resistance by enhancing the renin-angiotensin-aldosterone system. Any of these conditions may be deleterious to the patient with acute heart failure.[6] A misdiagnosis of heart failure and the subsequent inducement of inappropriate diuresis can increase the likelihood of morbidity and mortality.

When preparing to transport the patient, avoid the use of lights and siren, which may increase the patient's anxiety, heart rate, and blood pressure. This response increases the heart's workload and oxygen demand and should be avoided if possible. If the patient's condition is stable, transport without lights and siren. Rapid transport is warranted if the patient's breathing worsens, if he or she has signs and symptoms of shock, or if a life-threatening dysrhythmia develops.

Surgically implanted ventricular assist devices (VADs) may be used in patients who have heart failure. A VAD acts as an artificial ventricle and does not depend on the contractility or electrical conduction of the patient's heart. A VAD can be placed in either the left ventricle (LVAD), the right ventricle (RVAD), or both (biventricular assist device) depending on which ventricle is failing. Because LVF is more common than RVF, the LVAD is the most common type of VAD.

A VAD may be used (1) to allow the heart to "rest" until the patient's heart can recover and resume its pumping function, (2) as a bridge to heart transplantation, and (3) as lifetime therapy, also called destination therapy, to maintain circulatory support in patients who are not candidates for a heart transplant. There are several types of VADs and they typically consist of a blood pump, tubing (an inflow cannula and an outflow cannula), and an external power source that connects to a controller. The controller regulates and monitors the VADs functions. Alarms serve as reminders when the batteries require changing, when a connection is loose, or if the pump is malfunctioning. VADs are categorized according to type of blood flow (eg, continuous, pulsatile), the length of time the device can be used for circulatory support (eg, short-, intermediate-, or long-term), source of driving power (eg, pneumatic or electric), and device location (eg, internal or external). It is important to recognize that continuous-flow VADs deliver flow throughout the cardiac cycle. These patients may not have a palpable pulse, despite adequate perfusion. Obtaining a blood pressure using a manual cuff and stethoscope and obtaining a pulse oximetry reading may be difficult or the results may be inaccurate because of the patient's weak or absent pulse.

With a transcutaneous VAD, both the pump and power source are located externally. A tube from the pump goes through the patient's abdominal wall to the outside of the unit, where it connects to the battery pack. With an implantable VAD, the pump is located inside the body and the power source is located externally. A cable connects the internal VAD to the power source via a small incision in the abdomen. With a LVAD, blood is withdrawn from the left atrium or the apex of the left ventricle through a tube into the LVAD and is then returned to the ascending aorta via a second tube. With a RVAD, blood is withdrawn from the right atrium into the RVAD and is returned to the pulmonary artery.

Complications associated with VADs include device malfunction or failure, thromboemboli (eg, stroke, AMI, pulmonary embolism), bleeding (eg, nasal, gastrointestinal, intracranial), RVF, infection, and sepsis. Because there are differences in VAD designs, methods for troubleshooting device failure are typically unique to each device. The patient with a VAD may be prescribed anticoagulant medications to prevent the development of clots within the VAD and bloodstream.

The patient with a VAD will have a VAD coordinator who can assist you in making treatment and transport destination decisions. Contact the VAD coordinator if the patient with a VAD experiences a cardiac arrest. In this situation, chest compressions are not usually performed because of the possibility of pump dislodgement. If the patient with a VAD requires defibrillation or cardioversion, be careful not to place the pads directly over the pump.

Documentation & Communication

Key documentation elements for the patient with heart failure are as follows:[6]

- Vital signs
- Oxygen saturation
- Time of interventions
- Response to interventions

Cardiac Tamponade

Pathophysiology

A pericardial effusion is an increase in the volume and/or a change in the character of the pericardial fluid—the fluid that surrounds the heart. The pressure within the pericardium increases as pericardial fluid builds up. The volume of blood or fluid in the pericardial space necessary to impair the heart's ability to fill depends on several factors:

- The rate at which the buildup of blood or fluid occurs
- The ability of the pericardium to stretch to accommodate the expanded fluid volume

If excess fluid builds up slowly, the pericardium will gradually expand and make room for a large volume before signs and symptoms appear. If the fluid builds up rapidly, then the pressure within the pericardium significantly increases with a smaller volume of fluid.

Cardiac tamponade occurs when the buildup of pericardial fluid compresses the heart, impairing contraction and restricting ventricular filling. Limited ventricular filling decreases stroke volume and CO, causing signs of shock.

Cardiac tamponade may develop gradually if caused by an infection or tumor. It can develop rapidly when caused by heart surgery, pacemaker or central venous catheter insertion, or cardiac trauma such as a stab wound or gunshot wound. Table 17-15 shows some possible causes of cardiac tamponade.

Assessment

The patient with cardiac tamponade is usually too ill to answer questions pertaining to his or her medical history. The patient is likely anxious and restless, and reports shortness of breath, chest tightness, and/or dizziness. Family members may tell you of a recent invasive procedure, heart attack, chronic illness, or medications the patient is taking that may provide clues as to why the cardiac tamponade developed. Although tension pneumothorax

Table 17-15	Causes of Cardiac Tamponade

- Aortic dissection
- Blunt trauma (including CPR)
- Cardiac rupture after MI
- Heart surgery
- Medical facility procedures (angioplasty, central venous catheter insertion, pacemaker wire insertion)
- Hypothyroidism
- Penetrating trauma
- Pericarditis, pericardial effusion
- Radiation induced (cancer treatment)
- Renal disease

Abbreviations: CPR, cardiopulmonary resuscitation; MI, myocardial infarction

is more common, suspect cardiac tamponade in any patient who has sustained a penetrating wound of the chest or upper abdomen. If the tamponade is not from trauma, the patient may relate a history of a medical illness such as pericarditis or end-stage renal disease. One way to differentiate between a tamponade and tension pneumothorax is to remember that in cardiac tamponade, the breath sounds will be equal and the trachea will be midline because the lungs are not affected.

Signs of injury to the chest wall are usually present if cardiac tamponade occurs as a result of trauma. Cardiac tamponade produces a classic trio of signs known as **Beck triad**: JVD, hypotension, and muffled heart sounds. These signs, however, are present in less than half of all patients with the condition. JVD may be absent if the patient is hypovolemic. Heart sounds may be normal early on, becoming progressively more faint or muffled as the condition worsens. The patient may have other signs of cardiac tamponade:

- Cold, pale, mottled, or cyanotic skin
- Tachycardia
- Weak or absent peripheral pulses
- Narrowing pulse pressure (early sign)
- Pulsus paradoxus (late sign; may be absent if the patient has severe hypotension)
- Signs and symptoms mimicking heart failure (when cardiac tamponade develops slowly):
  - Dyspnea
  - Orthopnea
  - JVD

The ECG is of limited value in identifying cardiac tamponade. Low amplitude QRS complexes and T waves, ST-segment elevation, or nonspecific T-wave changes may occur. Electrical alternans may be observed on the ECG in which the P wave, QRS complex, and T wave alternate in amplitude with every other beat because of the constant motion of the heart within the fluid-filled pericardium.

Words of Wisdom

To identify cardiac tamponade you must perform a thorough assessment. Trends in blood pressure measurements can be recognized only after obtaining at least three values, usually 5 to 10 minutes apart. Muffled heart sounds, pulsus alternans, electrical alternans, and pulsus paradoxus are uncommon signs and, thus, may be easily overlooked.

Management

If trauma is the source of the patient's signs and symptoms, manage him or her as discussed in Chapter 35, *Chest Trauma*. Address any life-threatening hemorrhage. Ensure adequate oxygenation and ventilation. Apply a pulse oximeter and provide supplemental oxygen as needed to maintain the patient's Spo_2 at 94% or higher. Apply the cardiac monitor. Avoid performing additional procedures on the scene that will delay transport to the medical facility.

Establish IV access en route to definitive care. Give IV fluids and medications per local protocol or medical direction. If the patient has no signs of heart failure, then order an IV fluid challenge of normal saline to maintain circulating blood volume. Give IV fluids as a temporizing measure; however, do not delay transport. Check the patient's response by assessing mental status, heart rate, respiratory effort, breath sounds, and blood pressure. Explain all procedures to the patient and provide emotional support to the patient and family.

The definitive treatment for cardiac tamponade is in-hospital pericardiocentesis. Pericardiocentesis is a procedure in which a needle is inserted into the pericardial space to drain (aspirate) excess fluid through the needle. Often, withdrawal of as little as 50 mL of fluid will significantly improve the patient's condition. If scarring is the cause of the tamponade, then surgery may be necessary to remove the affected area of the pericardium. When you are reporting to medical control, ensure you identify all signs and symptoms that led you to believe the patient has cardiac tamponade, so the receiving medical facility will be prepared to perform the pericardiocentesis.

▶ Cardiogenic Shock

Cardiogenic shock is a condition in which heart muscle function is severely impaired, decreasing CO and resulting in inadequate tissue perfusion. The most common cause of cardiogenic shock is AMI.

Pathophysiology

Cardiogenic shock may occur as a complication of shock of any cause. Cardiogenic shock may also occur if myocardial contractility has diminished because of prolonged cardiac surgery, ventricular aneurysm, cardiac arrest, or ventricular wall rupture. When such a rupture occurs, blood leaks into the pericardial space, quickly leading to cardiac tamponade and cardiovascular collapse. Transient cardiogenic shock can occur after resuscitation. Patients recovering from defibrillation for ventricular fibrillation, for example, often have signs of cardiogenic shock.

Assessment

A patient in cardiogenic shock may be unable to provide a medical history. If family members are present, you should ask whether the patient has a history of heart disease. They may be able to describe the signs and symptoms that prompted the call to 9-1-1.

The patient's history often includes cardiomyopathy, congenital heart disease, or a recent MI. Patients with cardiogenic shock who have had a recent MI are more likely to be older adults, to have had a STEMI, to have a history of a previous MI or heart failure, and to have an anterior infarction at the time shock develops.

Mechanical conditions associated with a recent MI often occur several days to a week after the infarction. If a dysrhythmia is associated with the patient's symptoms, the patient may describe recent episodes of palpitations, fainting, or light-headedness.

In compensated cardiogenic shock, the patient's initial mental status may be normal. As cerebral perfusion declines, the patient becomes restless, agitated, and confused. Breath sounds reveal crackles in most patients. However, patients with RVI and those who are hypovolemic may have less evidence of pulmonary congestion. JVD, indicating RVF, may be present. If the patient is hypovolemic, then JVD will be absent. Peripheral pulse is often weak and rapid. However, the pulse may be weak and slow if an AV block is present. The patient's skin is usually pale or mottled. The extremities often feel cool and moist. This finding is attributable to a sympathetic response in which the blood within peripheral vessels is shunted to the vital organs to maintain adequate perfusion. The ECG may show evidence of both old and new infarctions. Right-sided chest leads can detect RVI. Initially, the patient's SBP may be normal, but pulse pressure is usually narrowed. If cardiogenic shock is associated with cardiac tamponade, then it may produce muffled heart sounds.

In decompensated cardiogenic shock, the patient usually has an altered mental status or is unresponsive. Breathing is often rapid and shallow. Breath sounds usually reveal increasing pulmonary congestion and crackles. Peripheral pulses may be absent, and central pulses are often weak and rapid. The patient's skin is usually pale, mottled, or cyanotic. The extremities feel cold and sweaty. As ventricular function worsens and CO falls, the SBP progressively decreases.

Management

Cardiogenic shock treatment is generally focused on strengthening contractility without significantly increasing the heart rate, altering preload and afterload, and controlling any dysrhythmias that are contributing to shock.

Apply a pulse oximeter and administer supplemental oxygen as indicated. Place the patient in a supine position. If pulmonary congestion is present and the patient's blood pressure will tolerate it, then place him or her in a sitting position with the feet dangling. Ensure you limit the patient's physical activity while in your care. This includes making sure the patient does not walk up or down stairs or to the stretcher.

Place the patient on a cardiac monitor and establish IV access. Obtain a 12-lead ECG. Maintain normal body temperature. Give IV fluids and medications per local protocol or medical direction. Order a trial of fluids to help you determine whether the shock has a hypovolemic component. If so, rapidly infuse 100 to 200 mL normal saline, and closely monitor the patient's mental status, breath sounds, pulse, and blood pressure. If the patient's condition deteriorates after fluid administration, or crackles or hepatomegaly develop, then withhold further fluid administration. Vasoactive IV medications to treat cardiogenic shock include dopamine, norepinephrine, and epinephrine, titrated to achieve a minimum SBP of 90 mm Hg or higher. If you are instructed to give a vasoactive medication, be sure to check the IV site often during administration, because these medications can cause significant vasoconstriction. If the IV fluid leaks out of a vein, considerable tissue damage can occur. Check the patient's response to the medication by assessing his mental status, heart rate, respiratory effort, breath sounds, and blood pressure. If the patient does not improve, give additional emergency care as instructed by medical direction. Treat any dysrhythmias that are contributing to shock. Provide emotional support to the patient and family.

Except for correcting a life-threatening dysrhythmia, there are no other measures you can take in the field to stabilize a patient in cardiogenic shock Therefore, you must transport the patient expeditiously to the medical facility. En route, complete a fibrinolytic checklist. Although cardiogenic shock is associated with a high mortality rate, patients who are candidates for reperfusion therapy and receive prompt treatment may have an increased chance of survival.

If the patient refuses care, repeatedly urge him or her to accept your assistance, including transport. Explain to the patient that if his or her condition is not treated, symptoms are likely to worsen and could result in death. Consider contacting medical direction for advice. If you are unable to persuade the patient to accept care, carefully document the patient's refusal and your attempts to persuade the patient to accept help.

▶ Hypertensive Emergencies

A diastolic pressure exceeding 90 mm Hg usually constitutes hypertension. Hypertension has been called the "silent killer" because it usually produces no signs or symptoms, yet damages the heart, brain, eyes, blood vessels, and kidneys.

A person can have it for years without knowing it. Uncontrolled high blood pressure can lead to low vision or blindness and an increased risk of serious health conditions such as stroke, heart attack, heart failure, and kidney failure.

A **hypertensive emergency** is defined as an acute elevation of blood pressure with evidence of end-organ damage. That last phrase is important, because it is the evidence of end-organ dysfunction, not the reading on the sphygmomanometer, which determines the urgency of the situation. Hypertensive emergencies usually occur in patients with a history of hypertension. Failure to take blood pressure medications or other treatments as prescribed is a common cause of such an emergency. A hypertensive emergency may also occur as a result of toxemia of pregnancy.

Hypertensive encephalopathy, also known as an *acute hypertensive crisis*, may complicate any form of hypertension. A hypertensive crisis is usually signaled by a sudden escalation of blood pressure to levels exceeding 200/130 mm Hg.

Pathophysiology

Most hypertension is the result of advanced atherosclerosis or arteriosclerosis, which narrows the lumen of the arteries and reduces their elasticity. The resulting high afterload on the heart expands filling volume and stimulates the Frank-Starling reflex, which raises the pressure at which blood is ejected from the heart.

Hypertension is present when the blood pressure at rest is consistently greater than about 140/90 mm Hg. Many conditions, such as anxiety or pain, can transiently elevate a person's blood pressure (especially the SBP), so a single blood pressure measurement taken during an emergency scarcely constitutes adequate grounds for telling a patient that he or she is hypertensive. Instead, you may say something like this: "Sir, your blood pressure is a little high right now. That may be because of the stress you're under and may not have any real significance. To be safe, though, you should have your blood pressure rechecked a couple of times in the next few months under less stressful circumstances."

Persistent elevation of the diastolic pressure, by contrast, indicates hypertensive disease. If left untreated, hypertension significantly shortens a person's life span and predisposes him or her to a variety of other medical conditions. The most common complications associated with hypertension are renal damage, stroke, and heart failure, which occurs as a result of the left ventricle having to pump for years against a markedly increased afterload.

Hypertensive emergencies require rapid lowering of blood pressure to prevent or limit organ damage. Malignant hypertension is one type of hypertensive emergency.

YOU are the Paramedic PART 4

You continue bag-mask ventilation with high-flow oxygen and then begin transcutaneous pacing, with mechanical capture verified by peripheral pulses. On arrival at the ED, the patient remains unresponsive, with a heart rate of 70 paced pulses/min; blood pressure 100/70 mm Hg; and spontaneous respirations, 0. The patient's wife informs the physician that her husband has been smoking crack cocaine on a regular basis for the past year. His use has escalated during the past 2 months. The physician inserts a temporary pacemaker. The patient's mental status improves, and he is admitted to the ICU. Seven days after placement of a permanent pacemaker, the patient is discharged from the medical facility.

Recording Time: 15 minutes	
Respirations	12 breaths/min with bag-mask ventilation
Pulse	70 paced pulses/min, regular
Skin	Warm, pink, dry
Blood pressure	100/70 mm Hg
Oxygen saturation (Spo_2)	99% with bag-mask ventilation
Pupils	PERRLA

10. Assume the patient remained unresponsive, with an unacceptably low blood pressure despite pacing. What treatment would be appropriate under those circumstances?

11. Given the patient's final disposition, was your treatment appropriate? Why or why not?

It occurs when there is a rapid rise in blood pressure, causing acute and progressive damage to organs such as the heart, brain, and kidneys. The increase in blood pressure damages blood vessels, causing them to become inflamed. Inflamed blood vessels may leak fluid or blood. If untreated, malignant hypertension may cause acute renal failure, MI, stroke, or hypertensive encephalopathy. The determining factor for hypertensive encephalopathy is usually the mean arterial pressure (MAP), which is calculated by adding one-third of the difference between the SBP and the diastolic blood pressure (DBP) to the DBP.

$$MAP = DBP + 1/3\ (SBP - DBP)$$

When the MAP exceeds 150 mm Hg, the pressure breaches the blood-brain barrier and fluid leaks out, increasing intracranial pressure. Usually the first symptoms are a severe headache, nausea, and vomiting, followed by seizures and alterations in mental status ranging from confusion to unresponsiveness. Sometimes patients have focal neurologic signs, such as sudden blindness, aphasia (disturbances in speech production or comprehension), or hemiparesis (weakness on one side of the body). Widespread neuromuscular irritability may be signaled by muscle twitching. If malignant hypertension is untreated, then death may occur within a few hours.

Assessment

Hypertensive emergencies often develop rapidly. The patient is usually quite anxious and may report a severe headache, blurred vision, dizziness, ringing in the ears (tinnitus), dyspnea, chest pain or tightness, nosebleed, muscle cramps, weakness, or palpitations. He or she may describe symptoms of PND and orthopnea.

Ensure you ask the patient about prescribed and over-the-counter medications he or she is taking. Because noncompliance with blood pressure medication is a common cause of malignant hypertension, find out if the patient has been prescribed blood pressure medication and whether he or she takes it as prescribed. Ask the patient about recreational drug use such as amphetamines, cocaine, and other sympathomimetic agents. These drugs can cause severe hypertension.

A patient having a hypertensive emergency appears sick. The patient's mental status may range from responsive to altered or unresponsive. His or her skin may be pale, flushed, or normal and feel dry or moist, warm or cool. Peripheral pulses may feel strong or bounding. Check (and document) the patient's blood pressure in both arms in case aortic dissection has occurred. The patient's DBP is usually higher than 130 mm Hg. The patient may have seizures, signs of heart failure (such as crackles in the lungs), or signs consistent with AMI. Ischemic changes may be seen on the 12-lead ECG. Differential diagnoses to consider for hypertensive emergencies are shown in Table 17-16.

Table 17-16 Differential Diagnosis of Hypertensive Emergencies

Classification	Possible Diagnoses
Cardiovascular	• Aortic dissection
Genitourinary	• Pheochromocytoma • Renal failure • Toxemia of pregnancy
Neurologic	• Epilepsy or postictal state • Head injury • Intracranial mass • Stroke • Subarachnoid hemorrhage
Other causes	• Acute anxiety • Cocaine or amphetamine use • Connective tissue disease • Drug overdose or withdrawal

Management

Prehospital care of hypertensive emergencies includes supportive care. Give oxygen, if indicated, establish an IV line, and apply the cardiac monitor and pulse oximeter. Maintain the Spo_2 at 94% or higher. Avoid performing additional procedures on the scene that will delay transport to the medical facility. If the patient has heart failure or chest discomfort from myocardial ischemia, provide care according to local protocol. Offer reassurance to the patient and family while providing assistance at the scene and during transport to the medical facility.

Paramedics working in rural areas or other circumstances in which long transport times to the medical facility are unavoidable may have to initiate drug therapy for hypertensive encephalopathy in the field. One widely accepted drug for this purpose is labetalol (Normodyne, Trandate), which has alpha- and beta-blocking properties. As an alpha-blocker, it prevents vasoconstriction, thereby decreasing overall peripheral vascular resistance. Meanwhile, its beta-blocking actions prevent the reflex tachycardia that would otherwise occur in response to a drop in blood pressure. As a beta-blocker, however, labetalol is relatively contraindicated in patients with asthma and COPD. Whenever you give a drug to lower a patient's blood pressure, keep the patient supine, and measure the blood pressure at least every 2 to 3 minutes. Document each measurement. When it has fallen to the target level specified by the physician, stop the infusion.

A patient with a hypertensive emergency requires transport to the closest appropriate facility. If the patient refuses care, repeatedly urge him or her to accept your assistance, including transport. Explain to the patient that if his or her condition is not treated, symptoms are likely to worsen and could result in death. Consider contacting medical direction for advice. If you are unable to persuade the patient to accept care, carefully document the patient's refusal and any patient education you provided.

▶ Infectious Diseases of the Heart

Endocarditis

Endocarditis is an infection of the lining of the heart. The condition is characterized by inflammation of the endocardium—that is, the lining of the heart chambers, including the heart valves. It occurs when bacteria in the bloodstream colonize a heart valve or other damaged tissue in the heart and begin to multiply. If left untreated, endocarditis can damage the heart valve, causing it to malfunction.

Endocarditis occurs most often in people with preexisting valvular disease such as mitral or aortic valve disease, or in those with mechanical (prosthetic) heart valves. It can also occur in people with congenital heart disease. Right-sided endocarditis is a type of infective endocarditis that affects the tricuspid and pulmonary valves. This type of endocarditis is seen most often in people who use IV drugs and in patients with infected central venous catheters, dialysis shunts, or transvenous pacing wires.

A variety of different pathogens may cause endocarditis. Most cases are caused by bacterial infection. Most organisms originate from the skin, upper airway, or genitourinary or gastrointestinal tract. The organism may gain access to the body in any of several ways, including minor skin infection, dental procedure, upper respiratory infection, or a major operation. Body piercing and tattooing have also been linked to endocarditis. The severity of the patient's illness often reflects the virulence of the infecting organism. Less virulent organisms cause a low-grade fever and symptoms that usually develop over several weeks to months. Organisms that are more virulent cause high-grade fever and signs of serious illness that develop over days to weeks.

Assessment. The most common symptoms of endocarditis are fever and chills. The patient may also report headache, loss of appetite, weight loss, muscle and joint aches and pains, night sweats, shortness of breath, or cough. Signs of heart failure may be present because of progressive heart valve destruction. If infective endocarditis invades the heart's conduction system, then ECG changes may be seen, including a prolonged PRI, third-degree AV block, or LBBB. Flat, painless, red-to-blue lesions (Janeway lesions) may appear on the palms and soles. Some patients develop small, tender nodules on the pads of the fingers or toes (Osler nodes).

Management. Prehospital care of endocarditis is mainly supportive. Allow the patient to assume a position of comfort, establish an IV line, and apply the cardiac monitor. Apply a pulse oximeter and administer oxygen, if indicated. If the patient has heart failure, then proceed according to your local protocol or instructions from medical direction. The patient will usually receive IV antibiotics at the medical facility. If a prosthetic valve is the site of infection, then an operation may be necessary. Most patients with endocarditis can be transported to the closest appropriate facility without lights and siren.

If the patient refuses care, repeatedly urge him or her to accept your assistance, including transport. Consider contacting medical direction for advice. If you are unable to persuade the patient to accept care, carefully document the patient's refusal.

Words of Wisdom

Blood flow through the heart can be compromised if a valve does not function properly. A malfunctioning heart valve is a type of valvular heart disease, which is classified as follows:

- **Valvular stenosis.** A valve is stenosed if it narrows, stiffens, or thickens. The heart must work harder to pump blood through a stenosed valve.
- **Valve prolapse.** If a valve flap becomes inverted, it is said to prolapse. Prolapse can occur if one valve flap is larger than the other. It can also occur if the chordae tendineae stretch markedly or rupture.
- **Valvular regurgitation.** Blood can flow backward, or regurgitate, if one or more of the heart's valves do not close properly.

Think about what might happen if a papillary muscle in the left ventricle were to tear or rupture. The flaps of the mitral valve may not completely close, and the valve flap may become inverted (prolapse). This may allow blood from the left ventricle to leak into the left atrium (regurgitation) during ventricular contraction. Blood flow to the body (CO) may be diminished as a result.

Pericarditis

Pericarditis is an inflammation of the double-walled sac (pericardium) that envelops the heart. The pericardium helps anchor the heart, preventing excessive movement of the organ in the chest when body position changes, and protecting it from trauma and infection.

Pericarditis is caused by either a viral (most common), bacterial, or, occasionally, fungal infection. Pericarditis may develop days or weeks after a patient has a heart attack. It may also develop after blunt or penetrating chest trauma, open-heart surgery, or procedures such as coronary angioplasty or implantable defibrillator or pacemaker insertion. Radiation therapy may also cause pericarditis. It can develop in patients with kidney failure or inflammatory disorders, such as rheumatoid arthritis and lupus. It can also develop as a result of breast or lung cancer, lymphoma, or leukemia. In many cases, no cause for pericarditis can be identified (idiopathic pericarditis).

Assessment. Ask the patient about recent flulike signs and symptoms. Patients with pericarditis may relate a history of a recent upper respiratory infection. The patient may describe a recent fever with shaking chills, shortness of breath, coughing, skin rash, or weight loss. The patient may have a history of lupus, kidney disease, or recent MI, leukemia, Hodgkin disease, lymphoma, chest trauma, or heart surgery.

Chest discomfort is the most common symptom of pericarditis. The patient usually describes a sharp, stabbing pain, but sometimes it's a steady, constricting pain that radiates to the shoulder and to either or both arms, mimicking the discomfort of an ACS. However, unlike the pain of an ACS, the discomfort associated with pericarditis is usually made worse by deep inspiration, coughing, or lying flat. The discomfort often improves when the patient sits up and leans forward.

The patient's chest discomfort is most often located under the sternum but may be centered in the left anterior chest or epigastrium. It may persist for days. Listening to heart sounds may reveal a pericardial friction rub, although this sign is not always present. A pericardial friction rub is a scratchy or grating sound caused by contact between the visceral and parietal pericardium. It is best heard with the patient leaning forward as you listen at the third to fifth ICS to the left of the sternum. Ask the patient to hold his or her breath while you listen. If you hear a sound that resembles two pieces of dried leather rubbing together, or the sound made when walking on crunchy snow, then pericarditis is the probable cause.

The patient often has a fever, tachycardia, and tachypnea. He or she may look pale, and JVD may or may not be present. If JVD is present, it may indicate pericardial effusion (a buildup of fluid in the pericardial space) resulting from the infection. Breath sounds are usually normal unless another condition, such as heart failure, exists. The ECG often reveals ST-segment elevation in multiple leads. Differential diagnoses to consider for pericarditis are shown in Table 17-17.

Table 17-17 Differential Diagnosis of Pericarditis

Classification	Possible Diagnoses
Cardiovascular	▪ ACS ▪ Aortic dissection ▪ Cardiomyopathy
Respiratory	▪ Pleurisy ▪ Pneumothorax ▪ Pulmonary embolism
Other causes	▪ Costochondritis ▪ Gastroesophageal reflux disease ▪ Lupus

Abbreviation: ACS, acute coronary syndrome

Management. Prehospital care of pericarditis is mainly supportive. Allow the patient to assume a position of comfort, establish an IV line, and apply the cardiac monitor. Apply a pulse oximeter and administer oxygen, if indicated. Obtain a 12-lead ECG. Pericarditis is usually treated with nonsteroidal antiinflammatory drugs. Viral pericarditis usually resolves on its own. Bacterial pericarditis is treated with antibiotics, and fungal pericarditis is treated with antifungal medications. Most patients can be transported to the closest appropriate facility without lights and siren.

If the patient refuses care, repeatedly urge him or her to accept your assistance, including transport. Consider contacting medical direction for advice. If you are unable to persuade the patient to accept care, carefully document the patient's refusal.

Myocarditis

Myocarditis is an inflammation of the thickest layer of the heart, the myocardium. The myocardium, the middle layer of the heart, contains the conduction system and the cardiac muscle fibers that allow the heart to contract. Myocarditis may or may not involve the endocardium or pericardium.

Myocarditis is usually benign and self-limiting. However, if inflammation in the heart muscle becomes widespread, the extensive destruction of heart muscle cells will impair the heart's ability to pump. This can result in RVF and LVF, dysrhythmia, or death. In some cases, myocarditis may lead to dilated cardiomyopathy.

Myocarditis can be caused by many different pathogens, including bacteria, viruses, and parasites. The most common cause of myocarditis is viral infection. Other causes of myocarditis are rheumatic fever and exposure to chemical poisons, such as occurs in chronic alcoholism and as a side effect of radiation therapy for cancer, especially with large doses to the chest. In many cases, the cause of myocarditis is unknown.

Assessment. Most cases of myocarditis are associated with flulike symptoms for which the patient does not seek medical care. The patient may have fatigue, decreased appetite, mild shortness of breath, joint and muscle aches and pains, or fever.

Cardiac symptoms usually appear 10 to 14 days after the initial onset of symptoms, at which time the patient seeks medical attention. Complaints of palpitations are common. Some patients report chest discomfort, often described as a sharp, stabbing pain in the center of the chest. If a patient with myocarditis describes a complaint of squeezing chest discomfort, it may be very difficult in the field to differentiate symptoms from those associated with an ACS.

The patient's physical exam may range from mild or no signs to severe heart failure. Tachycardia and tachypnea are common. The ECG may show low-voltage QRS complexes and/or ST-segment elevation. Atrial or ventricular dysrhythmia is common. Although sinus tachycardia is probably the most common rhythm seen, patients sometimes have a second- or third-degree AV block. LBBB or RBBB also may be seen. JVD, crackles, ascites, and peripheral edema may be seen if heart failure is present. Differential diagnoses to consider for myocarditis include the following:

- ACS
- Aortic dissection
- Esophageal perforation, rupture, or tear
- Heart failure
- Kawasaki disease
- Pneumonia
- Pulmonary disease

Management. Prehospital care for myocarditis is mainly supportive. Allow the patient to assume a position of comfort, establish an IV line, and apply the cardiac monitor. Apply a pulse oximeter and administer oxygen, if indicated. Obtain a 12-lead ECG. Be prepared to treat heart failure and dysrhythmia according to local protocol or instructions from medical direction.

Rheumatic Fever

Rheumatic fever is an inflammatory disease caused by streptococcal bacteria. This disease can cause stenosis of the mitral valve or aortic valve, leading to heart complications. Prehospital care is supportive.

Scarlet Fever

Scarlet fever is a disease caused by the bacterium *Streptococcus pyogenes*. This is the same bacterium responsible for causing strep throat. The disease is characterized by a sore throat, fever, rash, and "strawberry tongue" (a white tongue with red speckles). Patients younger than 1 year are at greatest risk of developing the infection. Scarlet fever is treated with antibiotics, and prehospital care is entirely supportive.

▶ Vascular Disorders

Aortic Aneurysm

Like other arteries, the aorta is composed of three layers: The *adventitia* is the thin outer layer, the *media* is the thick, elastic middle layer, and the *intima* is the thin, innermost layer. The elastic tissue of the aorta's middle layer stretches as blood is forcefully ejected from the left ventricle. The tissue recoils as the heart relaxes. These efficient movements keep blood moving throughout the cardiac cycle.

Even in healthy adults, this ability of the arteries to stretch and recoil diminishes with age. In some people, the constant stress on the wall of the aorta weakens it. As a result, the aorta swells (dilates) gradually. We call this an aortic aneurysm. The word *aneurysm* comes from a Greek word meaning "a widening"; it refers to the dilation or outpouching of a blood vessel (or the wall of a chamber of the heart). The dilated area may leak or rupture if it stretches too far.

If the vessel wall tears, then its layers can separate in a process called dissection. Aortic dissection may begin with a tear in the inner lining of the aorta (the intima) near the weakened portion of the vessel. Blood flows through the tear and between the layers of the vessel wall, exposing the middle layer to blood under high pressure. Blood fills the space between the layers of the vessel, causing them to separate (dissect). With each ventricular systole, a jet of blood is forced into the torn arterial wall, creating a false channel between the intimal and medial layers of the wall. This channel is propagated distally and sometimes proximally along the length of the wall. If the dissection progresses back into the aortic valve, then it may prevent the valve from closing. Blood will then be regurgitated back from the aorta into the left ventricle during systole. Recall, the coronary arteries branch off from the aorta just above the leaflets of the aortic valve; thus, if the valve is affected, coronary blood flow will likely be compromised as well. If the dissection involves the takeoff point of the innominate, left common carotid, or left subclavian artery, then blood flow through the affected artery or arteries will be diminished. Although an aortic dissection may begin anywhere along the aorta, most begin in the ascending aorta within 2 inches (5 cm) of the aortic valve or in the descending thoracic aorta just beyond the origin of the left subclavian artery at the site of the ligamentum arteriosum.

High blood cholesterol, hypertension, and CHD can all cause the arteries to lose elasticity prematurely. Atherosclerosis is the most common cause of aneurysms. The buildup of plaque in the lining of the vessel weakens eventually and erodes the middle (medial) layer.

Aneurysms of the ascending thoracic aorta are usually caused by cystic medial degeneration (formerly called cystic medial necrosis), a connective tissue disease characterized by degeneration of the elastic tissue and smooth muscle fiber of the middle layer of large arteries. The area of the vessel that was previously filled with normal elastic tissue is replaced with cystlike connective tissue.

A mild form of medial degeneration is often present in the aortas of older adults and may occur as a natural consequence of aging. In younger people, medial degeneration of the aorta frequently accompanies Marfan syndrome. Marfan syndrome is an inherited connective tissue disease that causes severe elastic tissue degeneration and increased stiffness of the aortic wall. Aortic aneurysms can also be congenital or traumatic (usually a deceleration injury in a motor vehicle crash), syphilis, infective endocarditis, or other infection.

Assessment. An aneurysm does not always cause symptoms. If it does, the signs and symptoms will depend on the location of the aneurysm. As the aneurysm increases in size, stretching of the aortic wall produces pain. The pressure of a large amount of blood on surrounding organs may produce symptoms. For example, difficulty swallowing (dysphagia) may occur as the esophagus is compressed. Laryngeal nerve compression may cause hoarseness. Heart failure or tracheal or bronchial compression may cause difficulty breathing. The sudden development of new or worsening pain may be a sign of impending aneurysm rupture.

The patient's description of the pain may provide clues to the location of the dissection. When the aorta dissects, almost all patients report the abrupt onset of constant, unbearable pain. The pain may last for hours to days. It is described as tearing or ripping and sharp, stabbing, or knifelike. Common phrases used to describe the pain include "it feels like someone stabbed me in the chest with a knife" or "hit me in the back with an axe." Dissection of the ascending aorta is usually associated with pain that is either substernal or located in the neck, throat, jaw, or face. Descending aortic dissection usually produces flank pain, pain between the shoulder blades, or pain in the back, abdomen, or lower extremities. No matter where it begins, the pain may move as the dissection extends along the aorta. Based on the patient's description, it may be difficult to distinguish the chest pain of a dissecting aneurysm from that of an AMI, but a number of distinctive features may help differentiate it. Table 17-18 compares the clinical presentation of AMI with a dissecting aortic aneurysm.

The patient with an aortic dissection is usually anxious and may describe a feeling of impending doom. Peripheral nerve ischemia may cause pain, weakness, or numbness and tingling in the extremities. Coronary artery compression may produce signs of myocardial ischemia. Although less common, with or without accompanying chest pain, the patient may have signs and symptoms of heart failure, altered mental status, stroke, paraplegia, or cardiac arrest. Sudden death can occur. In some patients, increased vagal tone, hypovolemia, or dysrhythmia can lead to syncope.

In dissections of the ascending aorta, which tend to occur in younger patients previously in good health, one or more of the vessels of the aortic arch is compromised. Disruption of flow through the innominate artery, for example, is likely to produce a difference in blood pressure between the two arms. Pressure differences greater than 20 mm Hg between the arms may indicate the presence of an aortic aneurysm. (If you do not routinely check the blood pressure in both arms of a patient, you'll never pick up that sign!) Suspect dissection if this finding is accompanied by other findings such as acute neurologic changes. Disruption of blood flow into the left common carotid artery may produce signs and symptoms of a stroke. When the dissection extends proximal to the coronary artery ostia, coronary blood flow is likely to be compromised, producing ECG changes characteristic of myocardial ischemia.

Dissection of the descending aorta is more common in older patients, especially in those with a history of hypertension. The pain is likely to be somewhat less severe when the descending aorta is involved. The patient may wait a few days before seeking help. Distal pulses may be hard to feel.

Rupture of a thoracic aneurysm usually occurs into the left intrapleural space or mediastinum or, less commonly, into the esophagus. Signs of a hemothorax may be present if the dissection ruptures into the pleural cavity. Signs of cardiac tamponade may be present if the dissection ruptures into the pericardial cavity.

Rupture of an abdominal aortic aneurysm is usually associated with sudden back pain accompanied by abdominal pain and tenderness. The patient may be hypotensive and have a pulsating abdominal mass between the xiphoid process and umbilicus. An aneurysm is often sensitive to palpation and may be quite tender if it is expanding rapidly or about to rupture. When an abdominal aortic

Table 17-18 Comparison of AMI With Dissecting Aortic Aneurysm

	AMI	Dissecting Aortic Aneurysm
Onset of pain	Gradual, with prodromal symptoms	Abrupt, without prodromal symptoms
Severity of pain	Increases with time	Maximal from the outset
Timing of pain	May wax and wane	Does not abate once it has started
Location of pain	Substernal; back is rarely involved	Back is often involved, between the shoulder blades
Clinical signs	Peripheral pulses equal	Blood pressure discrepancy between arms or a decrease in the femoral or carotid pulse

Abbreviation: AMI, acute myocardial infarction

aneurysm does rupture, distention of the abdominal cavity usually occurs. Massive gastrointestinal hemorrhage may be present if the aneurysm ruptures into the duodenum.

Management. Aortic dissection is a medical emergency. The goal of prehospital management in a suspected dissecting aneurysm is primarily to provide adequate pain relief and rapid transport. Establish an IV line, and apply the cardiac monitor. Apply a pulse oximeter and administer oxygen, if indicated. Give IV fluids and medications per local protocol or medical direction. If the patient's blood pressure can tolerate it, then opioids may be ordered for pain control; however, they may not be strong enough to relieve the patient's pain. Avoid performing any procedures on the scene that may delay transport to the medical facility. Nothing can be done to stabilize the patient's condition in the field. He or she will require aggressive therapy in the intensive care unit and possibly surgery.

Contact medical direction as soon as you suspect the patient has a dissecting aneurysm. Relay this information to the receiving facility to allow the staff time to gather the necessary resources for the patient while you are in transit. En route to the medical facility, reassess the patient at least every 5 minutes. A patient with signs and symptoms of a dissecting aortic aneurysm requires rapid transport to the closest appropriate facility.

In the medical facility, the patient will be given medications to lower his or her blood pressure and reduce myocardial contractility to take some of the hemodynamic load off the aorta. Such therapy would be started in the field only under unusual circumstances, because it requires careful monitoring of intra-arterial pressure.

Acute Arterial Occlusion and Acute Limb Ischemia

An acute arterial occlusion is a sudden disruption of arterial blood flow that occurs because of a thrombus, embolus, tumor, direct trauma to an artery, or an unknown cause. Acute limb (extremity) ischemia results when an arterial occlusion suddenly reduces blood flow to an arm or leg.

In most cases, acute arterial occlusion is caused by an embolus that begins in the heart and travels to the extremities. Any of several conditions may favor origination of an embolus in the heart, including AF, clot formation in the left ventricle after AMI, a rheumatic or prosthetic heart valve, and left ventricular aneurysm.

Arterial emboli can travel to a variety of sites in the body, but most lodge in the femoral artery, compromising lower-extremity circulation. Although less common, arterial emboli can also lodge in the brain, intestines, kidney, spleen, or upper extremities. Most emboli occur in patients with significant underlying heart disease.

A thrombus usually blocks an artery that was previously open but had been narrowed by atherosclerosis. The area distal to the blockage becomes ischemic. When the blockage affects an extremity, blood flow to the muscle is limited. During exercise, blood flow to the area decreases further, and muscle contraction may actually stop blood flow. However, some patients have few symptoms because the process occurs gradually, allowing collateral circulation to develop as atherosclerosis causes the major vessel to narrow. If the patient develops extensive collateral circulation in the extremity, he or she may notice no change or only a mild increase in symptoms when a major atherosclerotic vessel becomes blocked.

Patients with peripheral arterial disease often have intermittent **claudication**, or pain, cramping, muscle tightness, fatigue, or weakness of the legs when walking or during exercise. These symptoms occur as a result of increased oxygen demand during activity. The arteries that supply the muscles of the calves, hips, or buttocks are narrowed or blocked by atherosclerotic plaques that limit blood flow to the tissues. Symptoms disappear within a few minutes, after a brief rest, and the patient can resume activity until the pain recurs.

Direct trauma to an artery may result from an extremity injury or diagnostic procedure such as cardiac catheterization. Less common causes of acute arterial occlusion include dissecting aneurysm, vasospasm (usually attributable to IV drug use), and blockage of a vascular graft.

Assessment. You must gather an accurate history from a patient with acute limb ischemia. If he or she tells you the symptoms began suddenly, then an embolus is the probable cause of the ischemia. If the patient tells you symptoms have gradually worsened, then a thrombus is the more likely cause. Ask the patient whether he or she has ever had similar symptoms. If the answer is yes, find out if the episodes have become more frequent and how long each event lasts.

When obtaining the patient's history and performing the physical exam, keep in mind the five Ps of acute arterial occlusion: Pain, Pulselessness, Pallor, Paresthesia, and Paralysis. Pain associated with acute limb ischemia usually begins distal to the site of obstruction and gradually increases in severity. Ischemia of peripheral nerves in the affected limb causes motor impairment and sensory loss. The patient may report a decrease in pain as sensory loss progresses. Paralysis and paresthesia are signs and symptoms of limb-threatening ischemia.

Find out whether the patient has risk factors for the development of a blood clot, such as a recent extremity injury, IV drug use, heart surgery or AMI, clotting disorder, pulmonary embolism, AF, contraceptive use, hormone replacement therapy, or rheumatic heart disease.

Assessing a patient with acute limb ischemia should include feeling for arterial pulses. Feel the brachial, radial, femoral, posterior tibial, and dorsalis pedis arteries in pairs, and document your findings. The skin of the affected limb usually appears pale or mottled distal to or over the affected area. If arterial blood flow to the limb is severely restricted, then the foot will turn pale when it is raised and very red after 1 minute of placing it at a level lower than the heart. The skin of the affected limb may feel cool and may be either moist or dry.

Because advanced limb ischemia affects motor and sensory functions, assess movement and sensation in all extremities. Sensory deficits over the dorsum of the foot are often an early sign of vascular compromise.

Breath sounds are usually clear. Changes in heart rate and rhythm may occur. Peripheral pulses may be absent or diminished in the affected limb. Check the patient's blood pressure in both arms. Unequal blood pressure readings may indicate a thoracic aneurysm. Listen for a bruit over the affected vessel or vessels. In general, information from the patient's ECG does not contribute significantly to emergency care for this condition.

If the patient has had symptoms of peripheral arterial disease for some time, then signs of chronic limb ischemia may be present. These signs include muscle wasting, with shiny, scaly skin on the affected limb, cessation of hair growth over the dorsum of the toes and foot, and thickening of the toenails. The differential diagnosis of acute arterial occlusion and acute limb ischemia includes the following possible conditions:

- Abdominal aneurysm
- Arthritis
- DVT
- Scleroderma
- Soft-tissue injury
- Systemic lupus erythematosus

Management. Allow the patient to assume a position of comfort. If limb ischemia affects a lower extremity, then place the patient in a sitting position if doing so is not contraindicated. Place the patient's feet lower than the chest to allow gravity to help perfuse the limb. Establish an IV line and apply the cardiac monitor. Apply a pulse oximeter and administer oxygen, if indicated. Give medications as instructed by medical direction. Medications to reduce pain may be ordered. Keep the patient compartment of the ambulance warm to avoid cold-induced vasoconstriction of the skin. Do not apply heat or cold to the affected limb. Ischemic tissue burns at a lower temperature and is more susceptible to frostbite than nonischemic skin. The patient with acute limb ischemia requires rapid transport to the closest appropriate facility. Reassess the patient's condition frequently en route. Monitor the five Ps.

If the patient refuses care, repeatedly urge or her to accept your assistance, including transport. Consider contacting medical direction for advice. If you are unable to persuade the patient to accept care, carefully document the patient's refusal.

Acute Deep Vein Thrombosis

Thrombophlebitis is the development of a blood clot in an inflamed or damaged vein. Superficial thrombophlebitis occurs when a clot develops in a vein near the surface of the skin. If a clot develops in the deep veins of the extremities, then DVT is present. DVT is associated with an increased risk of pulmonary embolism.

Three important factors predispose a person to develop a thrombus:

1. **Venous stasis, or sluggish blood flow.** Venous stasis is present in patients who are pregnant, immobile for long periods, and those with obesity or heart failure.
2. **Damage to the inner lining of the vessel.** Vascular damage can be caused by trauma, inflammation, venipuncture, or the action of agents given during IV therapy.
3. **Blood clotting disorders.** Conditions that promote blood clotting include dehydration, certain types of cancer, and use of oral contraceptives or hormone replacement therapy.

Assessment. The patient with DVT may seek medical care because of swelling, pain, or tenderness in a limb. In some cases, the patient will seek help after the onset of symptoms from a pulmonary embolus. Ask the patient questions to find out if he or she has risk factors for DVT.

Carefully assess the patient's upper and lower extremities. Compare the extremities in pairs. Classic signs of DVT include swelling of the affected limb, with pain or tenderness. However, these findings are present in only about half of patients with DVT. Look for signs of inflammation such as redness and warmth of the skin over the affected vein. Pain and tenderness of the calf muscle on dorsiflexion of the foot (Homan sign) may be present. As you assess the patient, be careful not to rub or massage the affected limb. Such action could dislodge a clot, at which point it would be termed a thromboembolism.

The differential diagnoses for DVT include the following conditions:

- Arthritis
- Cellulitis
- Muscle or soft-tissue injury
- Superficial thrombophlebitis

Management. Prehospital care for DVT is mainly supportive. Allow the patient to assume a position of comfort. Establish an IV line and apply the cardiac monitor. Apply a pulse oximeter and administer oxygen, if indicated. Monitor the patient closely for development of a pulmonary embolism.

Most patients with DVT can be transported to the closest appropriate facility without lights and siren. If the patient refuses care, repeatedly urge him or her to accept assistance, including transport. Consider contacting medical direction for advice. If you are unable to persuade the patient to accept care, carefully document the patient's refusal.

A few other cardiac conditions may lead to emergencies. These include congenital heart disease and cardiomyopathy. Congenital heart disease is discussed in Chapter 42, *Neonatal Care*. Cardiomyopathy is discussed in Chapter 43, *Pediatric Emergencies*.

YOU are the Paramedic SUMMARY

1. What is your initial impression of this patient's condition?

The patient is pale and diaphoretic, with tachycardia and hypotension. These signs together suggest poor cellular perfusion, shock, and increased oxygen demand. The symptoms suggest a cardiac origin, and the onset at rest suggests an unstable condition. You should expedite your evaluation, stabilization, and transport to an appropriate facility.

2. What are some possible causes of the patient's symptoms?

Given the patient's description of the pain (crushing), you should consider a cardiac cause. Other possible causes of chest pain are trauma, pneumothorax, and pneumonia.

3. Although it's certainly possible, this patient is fairly young to be having an MI. What factors might be associated with a cardiac event in a patient of this age?

Although an MI can't be ruled out in a young adult, especially if he or she has a family history, stimulant drugs (cocaine or methamphetamine) are more commonly associated with acute MI in young people. However, your initial management is the same, so don't waste valuable time trying to identify a drug cause.

4. What additional assessment steps will be important in evaluating this patient?

Evaluate and assess the skin and vital signs (to assess CO), the heart and lungs (to look for other causes and signs of heart failure), and the prior medical history. The ECG will also play an important role in evaluating this patient.

5. What interventions should you initiate at this time?

In this case, rapidly administer supplemental oxygen, establish IV access, and evaluate the ECG.

6. Is this patient high priority? Why or why not?

He was high priority before the seizure, and he is very high priority now. In addition to having had a tonic-clonic seizure, the patient has a compromised airway and ventilation, bradycardia, and decreased CO.

7. Given what you know at this time, what is the most likely cause of the seizure activity?

In the absence of other information, the two most likely causes of seizure are hypoxia (caused by a sudden drop in the pulse rate and cerebral perfusion) and stimulant drug use (given the risk for stimulant use related to cardiac symptoms in young people).

8. What is this patient's greatest life threat at this time? How will you treat it?

Shock poses the greatest threat at this point. The sudden drop in the patient's cardiac rate has resulted in a dramatic drop in blood pressure. Overall, the strategy for treating this patient should begin with an attempt to restore normal cardiac rhythm and rate, followed by an effort to improve CO and blood pressure.

9. How will you manage the cardiac rhythm?

Although atropine is the preferred drug for symptomatic bradycardia, it is unlikely to be effective in cases of third-degree AV block. Reasonable alternative treatment options include TCP or a dopamine or epinephrine IV infusion.

10. Assume the patient remained unconscious, with an unacceptably low blood pressure despite pacing. What treatment would be appropriate under those circumstances?

Once the pulse rate has been normalized, several strategies may be used to improve blood pressure, depending on local protocol. If the patient's breath sounds remain clear, then a fluid challenge (usually 250 mL) may be used to increase preload to improve cardiac contractility and output. Dopamine may also be considered to improve contractility and, depending on the dose, increase afterload. A disadvantage of dopamine is it escalates myocardial oxygen demand, which may increase the size and severity of infarction.

11. Given the patient's final disposition, was your treatment appropriate? Why or why not?

Consider two things in answering this question. First, a better choice may have been to attach the patient to the cardiac monitor before preparing him for transfer to the ambulance. Although this may have increased scene time, it could have allowed you to identify a lethal dysrhythmia (we do not know what the preseizure rhythm was). Early recognition and treatment *may have* prevented the onset of third-degree AV block.

YOU are the Paramedic SUMMARY *(continued)*

EMS Patient Care Report (PCR)

Date: 09-09-18	**Incident No.:** 889	**Nature of Call:** Cardiac	**Location:** 220 Halifax Ave		
Dispatched: 0828	**En Route:** 0828	**At Scene:** 0835	**Transport:** 0902	**At Hospital:** 0914	**In Service:** 0928

Patient Information

Age: 32 **Sex:** Male **Weight (in kg [lb]):** 89 kg (195 lb)	**Allergies:** None **Medications:** None **Past Medical History:** None **Chief Complaint:** Chest pain

Vital Signs

Time: 0845	**BP:** 96/40	**Pulse:** 150 reg	**Respirations:** 20, deep	**Spo$_2$:** 91% on room air
Time: 0850	**BP:** 62/40	**Pulse:** 36 irreg	**Respirations:** 6 (12 with bag-mask ventilation)	**Spo$_2$:** 99% with bag-mask ventilation
Time: 0905	**BP:** 100/70	**Pulse:** 70 paced pulses/min; regular	**Respirations:** 12 with bag-mask ventilation	**Spo$_2$:** 99% with bag-mask ventilation

EMS Treatment (circle all that apply)

Oxygen @ 15 **L/min via (circle one):** **NC** **NRM** **(Bag-mask device)**		**(Assisted Ventilation)**	**Airway Adjunct**	**CPR**
Defibrillation	**Bleeding Control**	**Bandaging**	**Splinting**	**(Other:** TCP**)**

Narrative

Arrived to find a 32-year-old male who reports crushing chest pain (rated 9/10) with shortness of breath. Symptoms came on at rest and became more intense over 1 to 2 hours. Pt was initially awake, alert, and oriented, but he experienced a tonic-clonic seizure lasting 30 to 45 seconds while being loaded into the ambulance. Pt unresponsive, with no spontaneous breathing. Bag-mask ventilation begun. Cardiac monitor showed third-degree AV block with wide QRS at 36 beats/min. BP 62/40. Started IV of NS and began TCP. Electrical and mechanical capture achieved at 70 pulses/min with 60 mA. Patient remains unresponsive and apneic; bag-mask ventilation continued. BP 100/70, skin warm, pink, and dry. Report to RMC upon arrival to Susan RN.**End of report**

Prep Kit

▶ Ready for Review

- It is estimated that one person has an AMI in the United States every 40 seconds.[1] Recognizing and managing cardiovascular emergencies is an important part of paramedic education.
- Cardiac rhythm disturbances (dysrhythmias) may arise from a variety of causes, including AMI.
- The cardiovascular system is composed of the heart and blood vessels. Its primary function is to deliver oxygenated blood and nutrients to all of the body's tissues.
- The cardiac action potential of a typical myocardial cell consists of five phases of electrical activity within the heart: phase 0 to phase 4. These phases reflect changes in cardiac cell voltage, which correspond with the waveforms viewed on a rhythm strip.
- The heart's electrical conduction system is composed of pacemaker cells that are found in the tissues of the sinoatrial node, internodal conduction pathways, atrioventricular node, bundle of His, and Purkinje fibers. In some patients, an accessory conduction pathway allows electrical impulses to bypass the AV node and trigger ventricular depolarization.
- The body attempts to maintain a fairly constant blood pressure to ensure perfusion of vital organs. When stimulated, baroreceptors in the internal carotid arteries and aortic arch generate compensatory responses that facilitate blood pressure regulation by the sympathetic division of the autonomic nervous system.
- Assess a patient with a cardiovascular complaint in the same systematic approach used in all emergencies. In patients who are conscious, breathing, and have a pulse, the history and secondary assessment, including ECG acquisition, can greatly help distinguish acute coronary syndromes (ACS), such as non–ST-segment elevation myocardial infarction (NSTEMI), and ST-segment elevation myocardial infarction (STEMI).
- Cardiac monitors consist of lead wires connected to electrodes, which are placed on the patient. Each lead provides an electrical snapshot of a certain part of the heart. The cardiac monitor enables you to monitor and record 3-lead ECG tracings and record 12-lead ECGs.
- One of the most important tasks in the prehospital care of a patient with an AMI is to anticipate, recognize, and treat life-threatening dysrhythmias. In fact, ECG analysis is indicated in any patient who might have a cardiac-related condition.
- The 12-lead ECG enables localization of cardiac ischemia to specific areas of the heart. The 12 leads include three limb leads (I, II, and III), three augmented limb leads (aVR, aVL, and aVF), and six precordial leads (V_1 to V_6).
- Leads that view at the same general area of the heart are called contiguous leads.
- Because a standard 12-lead ECG does not view the right ventricle or the posterior surface of the left ventricle, use additional leads to detect ischemia or infarction in those areas. To analyze the electrical activity of the right ventricle, right-sided precordial leads are positioned in specific locations on the right anterior thorax. If you need to view the posterior wall of the left ventricle, three precordial leads are placed in specific locations on the left posterior thorax.
- A 15-lead ECG uses the standard 12-lead ECG, plus leads V_4R, V_7, and V_8.
- Components of a rhythm strip produced by an ECG include the P wave, PRI, QRS complex, J point, ST segment, T wave, and QT interval.
- A systematic approach to analyzing and interpreting cardiac dysrhythmias includes identifying the P-QRS-T waves, measuring the PRI and QRS, determining rhythm regularity, and measuring the heart rate.
- A normal sinus rhythm arises in the SA node, has an intrinsic rate of 60 to 100 beats/min, a regular rhythm, and minimal variation between R-R intervals.
- Rhythms originating in the SA node include sinus bradycardia, sinus tachycardia, and sinus dysrhythmia. Sinus arrest occurs when the SA node fails to initiate an impulse.
- Treatment of symptomatic bradycardia may include atropine IV bolus (for symptomatic sinus bradycardia or a conduction block at the level of the AV node), transcutaneous pacing, or a dopamine or epinephrine infusion as well as supportive care.
- Transcutaneous pacing is an intervention used to depolarize heart muscle using an external stimulus. Pads placed on the patient's chest deliver electrical energy to the heart, causing muscle contraction. The external pacemaker may serve as a bridge to permanent internal pacemaker implantation.
- Any area of the atria can originate an impulse, thereby superseding the pacemaking authority of the SA node. The resulting rhythms include premature atrial complexes, supraventricular tachycardia, AV reentrant tachycardia (Wolff-Parkinson-White and Lown-Ganong-Levine syndromes), atrial fibrillation and atrial flutter, wandering atrial pacemaker, and multifocal atrial tachycardia.
- Conservative therapies, such as vagal maneuvers and medications, are appropriate for symptomatic

Prep Kit *(continued)*

adults with stable vital signs who are experiencing an SVT. However, if the patient becomes unstable, then electrical therapy using synchronized cardioversion is recommended.

- Synchronized cardioversion is an intervention used to interrupt rapid, organized, hemodynamically unstable rhythms, such as SVT and AF, and allow the SA node to resume the primary pacemaking function. Unlike defibrillation, synchronized cardioversion is timed or synchronized to the patient's cardiac rhythm. After identifying the R waves on the ECG, the machine will discharge with the next detected R wave, avoiding the vulnerable period during the T wave of the cardiac cycle.
- If the SA node fails to initiate an impulse, then the AV junction can take over as pacemaker of the heart, generating premature junctional complexes, junctional escape rhythms, accelerated junctional rhythms, or junctional tachycardia. Treatment in symptomatic patients depends on the underlying cause.
- The ventricles may initiate their own impulses, producing a premature ventricular complex, an idioventricular rhythm or accelerated idioventricular rhythm, or ventricular tachycardia, fibrillation, or flutter. VF and pulseless VT are shockable cardiac arrest rhythms likely to respond to defibrillation.
- Defibrillation is an intervention used to interrupt rapid chaotic rhythms, such as VT and VF. Defibrillation simultaneously depolarizes all cardiac tissue to allow the SA node to resume the function of primary pacemaker. Paramedics most often perform manual defibrillation rather than automated external defibrillation, because they are trained in cardiac rhythm interpretation.
- An automated external defibrillator interprets the cardiac rhythm, determines if defibrillation is needed, and guides the user through the resuscitation effort via voice commands.
- Inspect the defibrillator at the beginning of each shift. Use a checklist to ensure the device and its components—defibrillation pads, cables and connectors, power supply, monitor, ECG recorder, electrode gel, pads, and spare battery—are in good working condition.
- VF and pulseless VT may lead to asystole, a complete absence of ventricular electrical activity, or to pulseless electrical activity, an organized cardiac rhythm (other than VT) on the monitor unaccompanied by a detectable pulse.
- Most adults who experience cardiac arrests have evidence of atherosclerosis or other underlying cardiac disease. However, cardiac arrest can also occur secondary to electrocution, a submersion incident, and other traumatic events, or to non-cardiac conditions such as drug overdose, asthma, or anaphylaxis. Many adults who go into cardiac arrest have no warning before the event occurs.
- Performing a systematic, exhaustively rehearsed assessment approach in cardiac arrest emergencies is essential to achieve a return of spontaneous circulation and to preserve neurologic function. High-quality CPR, defibrillation, airway management, administration of fluid and medications, and rapid transport are all important elements of emergency medical care for cardiac arrest patients.
- The goals of post–cardiac arrest care are to optimize cardiopulmonary function and vital organ perfusion.
- If the impulse traveling through the AV node is delayed more than usual or is completely blocked, an AV block can occur at the level of the AV node or below the bundle of His (infranodal), involving one or more of the bundle branches and the fascicles.
- AV blocks are classified into degrees, from least to most serious: first-degree AV block, second-degree block, and third-degree block.
- A 12-lead ECG is performed before and after electrical therapy (defibrillation, cardioversion, pacing). Other indications include dysrhythmia identification, chest pain or discomfort, electrical injury, electrolyte imbalance, overdose, right or left ventricular failure, stroke, syncope or near-syncope, and hemodynamic instability of unknown etiology.
- Transmitting 12-lead ECG findings to the receiving facility is a crucial step that can lead to a faster STEMI diagnosis, decrease the time from emergency onset to definitive therapy, and decrease mortality.
- A systematic approach to 12-lead ECG interpretation is essential. It includes a snapshot, dysrhythmia interpretation, and analysis of axis, conduction system, chamber size, zones of ischemia, injury, and infarction, and investigating noncardiac causes. 12-lead interpretation is an important paramedic skill. Practice it regularly because, even with transmission capability, equipment failure can occur.
- Injured, ischemic, or infarcted tissue undergoes characteristic changes that appear on the ECG in the facing leads. Ischemia is evidenced by ST-segment depression, and myocardial injury is evidenced by ST-segment elevation.
- Acute coronary syndromes are characterized by diminished flow through the coronary arteries as a result of occlusion by a blood clot (thrombus), coronary artery spasm, or some other cause (such

Prep Kit *(continued)*

as shock, dysrhythmia, or pulmonary embolism). This ischemia will lead to infarction if perfusion is not quickly restored.

- More than 1 in 3 Americans has one or more types of CVD, and it's the leading cause of death among US adults.[1]
- Risk factors for coronary heart disease include nonmodifiable risk factors such as age, family history, sex, and race or ethnicity, and modifiable risk factors such as excessive alcohol use, high blood cholesterol and triglyceride levels, high blood pressure, obesity, physical inactivity, smoking, stress, and an unhealthy diet.
- Patients experience a variety of symptoms when they have a cardiovascular conditions, the most common of which are chest pain, dyspnea, fainting, palpitations, and fatigue.
- Older adults, women, and people with diabetes often have atypical symptoms of CVD. The location or quality of the discomfort or pain may be unusual, and the person may have nausea, mental status changes, weakness, restlessness, or other symptoms that should be viewed as anginal equivalents.
- Rapid, systematic assessment of cardiovascular issues requires quick STEMI identification, determination of symptom onset, close monitoring of cardiac rhythm and the patient's vital signs, CPR and defibrillation if indicated, medication administration if appropriate, and rapid transport.
- Cardiac monitoring and ECG analysis are indicated in any patient who might have a cardiac-related condition. Any patient with chest pain or a history of a heart condition should undergo ECG analysis.
- STEMI treatment involves rapid reperfusion therapy to restore blood flow by means of percutaneous coronary intervention, or a fibrinolytic agent to dissolve blood clots.
- Heart failure occurs when the heart is unable to pump powerfully enough or fast enough to empty its chambers; as a result, blood backs up into the systemic circuit, the pulmonary circuit, or both. Disorders of the pericardium, myocardium, endocardium, or great vessels, such as coronary artery disease, valvular heart disease, dysrhythmias, cardiomyopathy, or long-standing high blood pressure, may cause heart failure.
- Cardiac tamponade occurs when excessive fluid accumulates within the pericardium, limiting the heart's ability to expand fully. This can reduce cardiac filling to the point the heart is unable to circulate blood. Emergent pericardiocentesis is lifesaving in patients with cardiac tamponade and hemodynamic instability. Transport the patient to the closest emergency facility.
- Cardiogenic shock is a condition in which heart muscle function is severely impaired, decreasing cardiac output and resulting in inadequate tissue perfusion. Acute myocardial infarction is the most common cause of cardiogenic shock. Transport the patient expeditiously to the medical facility. Treating life-threatening dysrhythmias is the only out-of-hospital measure you can take to stabilize the condition of a patient in cardiogenic shock, which has a high mortality rate.
- A hypertensive emergency is as an acute elevation of blood pressure with evidence of end-organ dysfunction. It can occur in a woman with toxemia of pregnancy or in a patient who is noncompliant with blood pressure medication. A hypertensive emergency may lead to hypertensive encephalopathy (hypertensive crisis), characterized by a sudden, marked rise in blood pressure to levels exceeding 200/130 mm Hg.
- Treating hypertensive emergencies involves slow, controlled lowering of the patient's blood pressure. Systemic hypertension can be caused by increased intracranial pressure, and it is essential to maintain cerebral perfusion pressure.
- Infectious diseases of the heart include endocarditis, pericarditis, and myocarditis. Endocarditis is an inflammation of the lining of the heart often caused by a bacterial infection. Symptoms range from low-grade fever and chills to high-grade fever and signs of serious illness, such as heart failure, Janeway lesions, and Osler nodes. Pericarditis is an infection of the pericardial sac that envelops the heart caused by a viral, bacterial, or fungal infection. It may cause fever, flulike symptoms, and a pericardial friction rub. Myocarditis is an infection of the myocardium. It is usually benign and self-limiting but it can impair the heart's pumping ability if the myocardial inflammation is extensive.
- Aortic aneurysms—particularly acute dissecting aneurysms of the thoracic aorta and expanding or ruptured aneurysms of the abdominal aorta—are of critical concern to the EMS responder. Patients describe sudden, severe ripping, tearing, or stabbing pain in the neck, throat, jaw, face, back, abdomen, chest, lower extremities, or between the shoulder blades. The pain may last hours or days. The condition

Prep Kit *(continued)*

is often characterized by a discrepancy between the blood pressure in the arms, or a decrease in the femoral or carotid pulse.

▶ Vital Vocabulary

aberration A term describing the shape of the QRS complex in aberrantly (abnormally) conducted beats.

absolute refractory period (ARP) The early phase of cardiac repolarization, wherein the heart muscle cannot be stimulated to depolarize; also known as the effective refractory period.

acute coronary syndromes (ACSs) A series of cardiac conditions caused by an abrupt reduction in coronary artery blood flow.

acute myocardial infarction (AMI) Cardiac ischemia that occurs when sudden narrowing or complete occlusion of a coronary artery leads to death (necrosis) of myocardial tissue.

agonal Pertaining to the period of dying.

agonal rhythm A ventricular rate of less than 20 beats/min; this rhythm is seen just before the heart stops beating altogether.

angina pectoris The sudden pain that occurs when the oxygen supply to the myocardium is insufficient to meet demand, causing ischemic changes in the tissue.

aortic aneurysm An outpouching or bulge in the wall of a portion of the aorta, caused by weakening and dilation of the vessel wall; a ruptured aortic aneurysm is life threatening.

arrhythmia The absence of any cardiac rhythm or organized activity; asystole or ventricular standstill.

arteriosclerosis A pathologic condition in which the thickening and stiffening of the arterial walls makes the arteries less elastic.

artifact An artificial product; in cardiology, used to refer to noise or interference in an ECG tracing.

asystole The absence of ventricular contraction or electrical activity; a straight-line or flat-line ECG.

atheroma A mass of fatty tissue that gradually calcifies, hardening into an atheromatous plaque that infiltrates the arterial wall, diminishing its elasticity.

atherosclerosis An accumulation of fat inside a blood vessel that narrows the diameter of the lumen.

atrioventricular (AV) junction The portion of the conduction system of the heart that consists of the AV node and the nonbranching portion of the bundle of His.

atrioventricular (AV) node A group of cells that slows the electrical impulses from the sinoatrial node before relaying it to the ventricles; located in the floor of the right atrium immediately behind the tricuspid valve and near the opening of the coronary sinus.

augmented limb leads On an ECG, leads aVR, aVL, and aVF. They contain only one true pole; the other is a combination of information from other leads. A standard12-lead ECG consists of the three augmented leads, along with the three standard limb leads and the six precordial leads.

automated external defibrillator (AED) A smart defibrillator that can analyze the patient's ECG rhythm, determine whether a defibrillating shock is needed, and guide the user through the resuscitation effort via voice commands.

axis deviation Movement of the heart's QRS axis to the right or left of its normal position.

Beck triad The classic trio of signs associated with cardiac tamponade: narrowed pulse pressure, muffled heart tones, and jugular vein distention.

bifascicular block Blockage of any two fascicles or conduction pathways: a right bundle branch block (RBBB) with anterior hemiblock, RBBB with posterior hemiblock, or anterior hemiblock and posterior hemiblock (a combination known as LBBB).

bigeminy A dysrhythmia in which every other complex is a premature complex, causing a *normal–early beat–normal–early beat* pattern; can be atrial, junctional, or ventricular.

bipolar leads On an ECG, leads that contain both a positive and a negative pole: leads I, II, and III.

bruits Abnormal whooshing sounds indicating turbulent blood flow within a narrowed vessel; usually heard in the carotid arteries.

bundle branch block (BBB) An intraventricular conduction disturbance involving impedance of electrical impulses from the bundle of His to the right or left bundle branch.

bundle of His The portion of the heart's conduction system located in the upper portion of the interventricular septum that conducts electrical impulses from the atrioventricular junction to the right and left bundle branches; also called the AV bundle.

cardiac arrest The cessation of cardiac mechanical activity, as confirmed by the absence of signs of circulation; also called cardiopulmonary arrest.

Prep Kit *(continued)*

cardiac catheterization A minimally invasive procedure performed under fluoroscopic guidance, a balloon, stent, or other device is advanced through a peripheral artery catheter and into an obstructed coronary vessel to diagnose and treat coronary artery obstruction; also known as percutaneous coronary intervention and percutaneous transluminal coronary angioplasty.

cardiac cycle The period from one cardiac contraction to the next. Each cardiac cycle consists of ventricular contraction (systole) and relaxation (diastole).

cardiac tamponade A pathologic condition characterized by restriction of cardiac contraction, falling cardiac output, and shock as a result of pericardial fluid accumulation.

circumflex artery (Cx) One of the two branches of the left main coronary artery; branches of the Cx supply the left atrium, part of the lateral surface of the left ventricle, the inferior surface of the left ventricle in about 15% of people, the posterior surface of the left ventricle in 15%, the sinoatrial node in about 40%, and the atrioventricular bundle in 10% to 15%.

claudication Pain, cramping, muscle tightness, fatigue, or weakness of the legs during physical activity as a result of increased oxygen demand by the muscle tissue of the legs, hips, and buttocks.

concordant precordial pattern An ECG pattern in which the QRS complexes are all in the same direction in the precordial leads as a result of improper lead placement, anterior wall MI, VT, or other variables.

contiguous leads Leads that view geographically similar areas of the myocardium, such as leads II, III, and aVF; useful for localizing areas of ischemia.

coronary arteries The blood vessels that supply blood to the tissues of the heart.

coronary artery disease (CAD) Pathologic process characterized by progressive atherosclerotic narrowing and eventual obstruction of the coronary arteries.

coronary heart disease (CHD) Disease of the coronary arteries and its associated signs, symptoms, and complications, such as angina pectoris and acute myocardial infarction.

couplet Two consecutive (paired) premature ventricular complexes.

defibrillation The process by which an unsynchronized direct current (DC) electric shock is delivered to the heart to terminate ventricular fibrillation or pulseless ventricular tachycardia.

delta wave The slurring of the upstroke of the first part of the QRS complex that occurs in Wolff-Parkinson-White syndrome.

depolarization The process of discharging resting cardiac muscle fibers by means of an electrical impulse that stimulates contraction.

dissection The process by which the intimal and medial layers of a vessel separate (dissect) after a tear occurs in an aneurysmal portion of the arterial wall. With each ventricular systole, a jet of blood is forced into the torn arterial wall, creating and propagating a false channel.

dysrhythmias Cardiac rhythm disturbances.

ectopic An impulse or rhythm that originates from a site other than the SA node.

electrical conduction system In the heart, the specialized cardiac tissue that initiates and conducts electric impulses; includes the SA node, internodal conduction pathways, atrioventricular node, bundle of His, and the Purkinje network.

endocarditis Inflammation of the endocardium as a result of infection.

fascicular block (hemiblock) Failure of the anterior or posterior fascicles of the heart to conduct electrical impulses because of disease or ischemia.

fibrinolysis The process of dissolving blood clots.

fibrinolytic therapy The use of medications that act to dissolve blood clots.

first-degree AV block A delay in the conduction of the depolarizing impulse from the SA node to the ventricles, prolonging the PR interval; also called first-degree heart block.

heart failure A syndrome that occurs when the heart is unable to pump powerfully enough or fast enough to empty its chambers; as a result, blood backs up into the systemic circuit, the pulmonary circuit, or both.

hyperkalemia A high concentration of potassium in the blood.

hypertension High blood pressure, usually a diastolic pressure of greater than 90 mm Hg.

hypertensive emergency An acute elevation of blood pressure with evidence of end-organ damage.

hypertensive encephalopathy A condition that may complicate any form of hypertension, and which is usually signaled by a sudden, marked rise in blood pressure to levels exceeding 200/130 mm Hg; also known as acute hypertensive crisis.

hypertrophic cardiomyopathy A genetic condition in which the heart muscle wall is unusually thick,

Prep Kit (continued)

requiring the heart to pump harder to eject blood from the left ventricle.

hypocalcemia A low concentration of calcium in the blood.

hypokalemia A low concentration of potassium in the blood.

idioventricular Related to only the ventricles; produced by the ventricles.

infarction Death (necrosis) of a localized area of tissue caused by ischemia.

internodal pathways The three atrial pathways of electrical conduction that transmit impulses from the SA node to the AV node.

ischemia Tissue anoxia caused by diminished blood flow, usually as a result of narrowing or occlusion of an artery.

isoelectric line The baseline of the ECG; isoelectric means neither positive nor negative.

junctional escape rhythm A dysrhythmia arising from the atrioventricular junction with an intrinsic rate of 40 to 60 beats/min; also called junctional rhythm.

lead The electrical potential difference between two points. For example, lead I represents the difference in electrical potential between the right and left arm electrodes.

left anterior descending artery (LAD) One of the two branches of the left main coronary artery; branches of the LAD supply the left ventricle, interventricular septum, and part of the right ventricle.

left atrial abnormality Dilation of the left atrium that can occur in patients with valvular heart disease (particularly mitral or aortic valve stenosis), hypertensive disease, cardiomyopathy, or coronary artery disease; it can also occur in an athlete.

left ventricular failure (LVF) A condition in which the left ventricle must work harder to pump blood throughout the body; with systolic failure, the left ventricle doesn't contract normally and has trouble pumping all the blood in the chamber out to the body; with diastolic failure, the left ventricle contracts normally but it has become stiff, impeding its ability to relax and fill with blood between each contraction of the heart.

left ventricular hypertrophy (LVH) A cardiac condition in which the left ventricle becomes enlarged, most often as a result of hypertension.

limb leads The ECG leads attached to the limbs; together, the standard limb leads (I, II, and III) and augmented limb leads (aVR, aVL, and aVF) form the hexaxial reference system along the frontal plane.

long QT syndrome A condition characterized by a QT interval exceeding approximately 0.45 seconds (450 milliseconds).

Lown-Ganong-Levine syndrome A disorder that causes preexcitation of ventricular tissue and is characterized on ECG by a short PR interval and a normal QRS duration.

lumen The hollow interior space within an artery or other hollow structure.

manual defibrillator A device that requires the paramedic or other trained rescuer to interpret the cardiac rhythm and determine whether defibrillation is needed (rather than the relying on a device to make that determination automatically).

monomorphic Having a common shape.

multifocal Arising from or pertaining to many foci or locations.

myocarditis Inflammation of the myocardium.

necrosis The death of tissue, usually caused by a cessation of its blood supply.

normal sinus rhythm The normal rhythm of the heart that has an intrinsic rate of 60 to 100 beats/min; the rhythm is regular, with minimal variation between R-R intervals, and all measurements are within normal limits.

orthopnea Severe dyspnea experienced when lying down that is relieved by a change in position, such as sitting up or standing.

P wave The first wave of the ECG complex, representing depolarization of the atria.

paroxysmal nocturnal dyspnea (PND) Severe shortness of breath occurring at night after several hours of recumbency, during which fluid pools in the lungs; the person is forced to sit up to breathe; caused by left heart failure or decompensation of chronic obstructive pulmonary disease.

pericarditis Inflammation of the pericardial sac.

plasmin A naturally occurring clot-dissolving enzyme.

point of maximal impulse (PMI) The palpable beat of the apex of the heart against the chest wall during ventricular contraction; normally palpated at the fifth left intercostal space along the midclavicular line.

PR interval (PRI) The distance between the beginning of the P wave (atrial depolarization) and the beginning of the QRS complex (ventricular depolarization), signifying the time required for the atria to depolarize and the excitation impulse to pass through the atrioventricular junction.

precordial leads A term used to describe the chest leads in an ECG.

Prep Kit (continued)

preexcitation Early depolarization of ventricular tissue by means of an accessory pathway between the atria and ventricles.

Prinzmetal angina A type of angina that occurs when a person is at rest, when oxygen needs are minimal; also called vasospastic angina.

pulmonary edema Congestion of the pulmonary air spaces with exudate and foam, often secondary to left ventricular failure.

pulmonary embolism Obstruction in one or more pulmonary arteries by a solid, liquid, or gas that has swept through the right side of the heart into the lungs.

pulseless electrical activity (PEA) An organized cardiac rhythm (other than ventricular tachycardia) on an ECG monitor that is not accompanied by any detectable pulse.

Purkinje fibers A network of cardiac muscle fibers distributed throughout the inner surfaces of the ventricular walls that conducts the excitation impulse from the bundle branches to the ventricular myocardium.

QRS axis A single vector that represents the mean (or average) of all vectors created by the ventricles during depolarization.

QRS complex Deflection of the ECG produced by ventricular depolarization.

reciprocal changes Mirror-image J-point, ST-segment, and T-wave changes seen on the ECG during an ACS.

reentry Spread of an impulse through tissue already stimulated by that same impulse.

refractory period (RP) A short period immediately after depolarization during which the myocytes have not yet repolarized and are unable to fire or conduct an impulse (the absolute refractory period) or have partially repolarized and may depolarize in response to an electrical stimulus (the relative refractory period).

relative refractory period (RRP) The portion of the cardiac action potential that extends from the middle of phase 3 to the beginning of phase 4; during this time, the heart muscle has been partially repolarized and may depolarize in response to an electrical stimulus.

reperfusion therapy Treatment intended to facilitate the resumption of blood flow through a blocked vessel; therapy may be either procedural, such as cardiac catheterization, or pharmacologic, such as administration of a fibrinolytic agent.

rheumatic fever An inflammatory disease caused by streptococcal bacteria; the disease can cause mitral or aortic valve stenosis.

right atrial abnormality Dilation of the right atrium that occurs when returning venous pressure is elevated or pulmonary pressure is high.

right coronary artery (RCA) Artery that provides oxygenated blood to the walls of the right atrium and ventricle, a portion of the inferior part of the left ventricle, and portions of the conduction system.

right ventricular failure (RVF) A condition in which the right side of the heart must work increasingly hard to pump blood into engorged pulmonary vessels; eventually, it is unable to keep up with the increased workload.

right ventricular hypertrophy (RVH) A cardiac condition in which the right ventricle becomes enlarged, usually as a result of pulmonary hypertension.

R-R interval The period between the onset of one QRS complex and the onset of the next QRS complex.

scarlet fever A disease caused by the bacterium *Streptococcus pyogenes* and characterized by a sore throat, fever, rash, and "strawberry tongue."

septum A thick wall that separates the right and left sides of the heart.

sinoatrial (SA) node The dominant pacemaker of the heart, located at the junction of the superior vena cava and the right atrium.

sinus bradycardia A sinus rhythm characterized by a heart rate of less than 60 beats/min.

sinus dysrhythmia A variation of cycling of a sinus rhythm that is often associated with respiratory cycle fluctuations; the rate increases during inspiration and decreases during expiration.

sinus tachycardia A sinus rhythm characterized by a heart rate greater than 100 beats/min.

ST segment The interval between the end of the QRS complex (the J point) and the beginning of the T wave; when there is significant myocardial ischemia or injury, the ST segment is often depressed or elevated with respect to the isoelectric line.

stable angina Angina pectoris characterized by periodic pain with a predictable pattern.

subendocardial myocardial infarction A type of acute myocardial infarction in which the ischemic process affects only the inner layer of muscle.

synchronized cardioversion The use of a synchronized direct current (DC) electric shock to convert a

Prep Kit *(continued)*

tachydysrhythmia (such as supraventricular tachycardia) to a normal sinus rhythm.

syncope Fainting; brief loss of consciousness caused by transiently inadequate blood flow to the brain.

T wave The upright, flat, or inverted wave following the QRS complex of the ECG, representing ventricular repolarization.

targeted temperature management (TTM) The utilization of cool fluids to get the patient to a targeted hypothermic state during various critical conditions.

thromboembolism A blood clot that initially formed within a blood vessel but is now circulating through the bloodstream.

thrombus A fixed blood clot that can obstruct passage of blood flow through an artery.

transcutaneous pacemaker A device that depolarize myocardial tissue by sending a small electrical charge through the skin of the chest between one externally placed pacing pad and another.

transcutaneous pacing (TCP) An intervention used to depolarize heart muscle using an external stimulus; pads placed on the patient's chest deliver electrical energy to the heart, causing muscle contraction.

transmural myocardial infarction A type of acute myocardial infarction in which the infarct extends through the entire wall of the ventricle.

trifascicular block Blockage or impairment of all three components of the ventricular conduction system, with one working occasionally to provide AV conduction.

trigeminy A dysrhythmia in which every third complex is a premature complex, causing a *normal–normal–early beat pattern*; can be atrial, junctional, or ventricular.

U wave A small, flat wave sometimes seen after the T wave and before the next P wave.

unifocal Arising from a single site.

unstable angina Angina pectoris characterized by a variable, unpredictable pattern of pain, which may signal an impending acute myocardial infarction.

Valsalva maneuver Straining or forced exhalation against a closed glottis, the effect of which is to stimulate the vagus nerve, thereby slowing the heart rate.

Wolff-Parkinson-White (WPW) syndrome A preexcitation syndrome characterized by a short PR interval, a delta wave, a widened QRS complex, and nonspecific ST-T wave changes, indicating the presence of an accessory pathway.

▶ References

1. Mozaffarian D, Benjamin EJ, Go AS, et al. Heart disease and stroke statistics—2016 update: a report from the American Heart Association. *Circulation.* 2016;133(4):e38-e360.
2. Grant AO. Cardiac ion channels. *Circ Arrhythm Electrophysiol.* 2009;2(2):185-194.
3. Surawicz B, Childers R, Deal BJ, Gettes LS. AHA/ACCF/HRS recommendations for the standardization and interpretation of the electrocardiogram: part III: intraventricular conduction disturbances: a scientific statement from the American Heart Association Electrocardiography and Arrhythmias Committee, Council on Clinical Cardiology; the American College of Cardiology Foundation; and the Heart Rhythm Society. Endorsed by the International Society for Computerized Electrocardiology. *J Am Coll Cardiol.* 2009;53(11):976-981.
4. Amsterdam EA, Wenger NK, Brindis RG, et al. 2014 AHA/ACC guideline for the management of patients with non-ST-elevation acute coronary syndromes: a report of the American College of Cardiology/American Heart Association Task Force on Practice Guidelines. *J Am Coll Cardiol.* 2014;64(24):e139-e228.
5. Rautaharju PM, Surawicz B, Gettes LS. AHA/ACCF/HRS recommendations for the standardization and interpretation of the electrocardiogram: part IV: the ST segment, T and U waves, and the QT interval: a scientific statement from the American Heart Association Electrocardiography and Arrhythmias Committee, Council on Clinical Cardiology; the American College of Cardiology Foundation; and the Heart Rhythm Society. Endorsed by the International Society for Computerized Electrocardiology *J Am Coll Cardiol.* 2009;53(11):982-991.
6. National Model EMS Clinical Guidelines. National Association of State EMS Officials website. www.nasemso.org. Accessed April 15, 2016.
7. Web-based Integrated Guidelines for Cardiopulmonary Resuscitation and Emergency Cardiovascular Care – Part 7: Adult Advanced Cardiovascular Life Support. The American Heart Association website. https://eccguidelines.heart.org/index.php/circulation/cpr-ecc-guidelines-2/part-7-adult-advanced-cardiovascular-life-support/. Acccessed April 11, 2016.
8. Page RL, Joglar JA, Caldwell MA, et al. 2015 ACC/AHA/HRS guideline for the management of adult patients with supraventricular tachycardia: a report of the American College of Cardiology/American Heart Association Task Force on Clinical Practice Guidelines and the Heart Rhythm Society. *Circulation.* 2016;133:e506-e574.

Prep Kit (continued)

9. Lederer WJ. Cardiac electrophysiology and the electrocardiogram. In: Boron WF, Boulpaep EL, eds. *Medical Physiology: A Cellular and Molecular Approach*. 2nd ed. Philadelphia, PA: Elsevier-Saunders; 2012:504-528.
10. Web-based Integrated Guidelines for Cardiopulmonary Resuscitation and Emergency Cardiovascular Care–Part 5: Adult Basic Life Support and Cardiopulmonary Resuscitation Quality. American Heart Association website. https://eccguidelines.heart.org/index.php/circulation/cpr-ecc-guidelines-2/part-5-adult-basic-life-support-and-cardiopulmonary-resuscitation-quality/. Accessed January 11, 2016.
11. Piccini JP Sr, Allen LA, Kudenchuk PJ, Page RL, Patel MR, Turakhia MP. Wearable cardioverter-defibrillator therapy for the prevention of sudden cardiac death: a scientific statement from the American Heart Association. *Circulation*. 2016;133(17):1715-1727.
12. Adler A, Halkin A, Viskin S. Wearable cardioverter-defibrillators. *Circulation*. 2013;127(7):854-860.
13. Web-based Integrated Guidelines for Cardiopulmonary Resuscitation and Emergency Cardiovascular Care – Part 3: Ethical Issues. American Heart Association website. https://eccguidelines.heart.org/index.php/circulation/cpr-ecc-guidelines-2/part-3-ethical-issues/. Accessed April 15, 2016.
14. Web-based Integrated Guidelines for Cardiopulmonary Resuscitation and Emergency Cardiovascular Care – Part 10: Special Circumstances of Resuscitation. American Heart Association website. https://eccguidelines.heart.org/index.php/circulation/cpr-ecc-guidelines-2/part-10-special-circumstances-of-resuscitation/. Accessed January 11, 2016.
15. Web-based Integrated Guidelines for Cardiopulmonary Resuscitation and Emergency Cardiovascular Care – Part 8: Post–Cardiac Arrest Care. American Heart Association website. https://eccguidelines.heart.org/index.php/circulation/cpr-ecc-guidelines-2/part-8-post-cardiac-arrest-care/. Accessed November 7, 2015.
16. Blank AC, Loh P, Vos MA. Atrioventricular block. In: Zipes DP, Jalife J, eds. *Cardiac Electrophysiology: From Cell to Bedside*. 6th ed. Philadelphia, PA: Elsevier-Saunders; 2014:1043-1049.
17. Web-based Integrated Guidelines for Cardiopulmonary Resuscitation and Emergency Cardiovascular Care – Part 9: Acute Coronary Syndromes. American Heart Association website. https://eccguidelines.heart.org/index.php/circulation/cpr-ecc-guidelines-2/part-9-acute-coronary-syndromes/. Accessed November 20, 2015.
18. O'Gara PT, Kushner FG, Ascheim DD, et al. 2013 ACCF/AHA guideline for the management of ST-elevation myocardial infarction: executive summary: a report of the American College of Cardiology Foundation/American Heart Association Task Force on Practice Guidelines. *J Am Coll Cardiol*. 2013;61(4):485-510.
19. Mack M, Gopal A. Epidemiology, traditional, and novel risk factors in coronary artery disease. *Cardiol Clin*. 2014;32(3):323-332.
20. Heart Disease Behavior. Centers for Disease Control and Prevention. www.cdc.gov/heartdisease/behavior.htm. Accessed April 18, 2016.
21. Golden AP, Odoi A. Emergency medical services transport delays for suspected stroke and myocardial infarction patients. *BMC Emerg Med*. 2015;15(34):1-13.
22. Cannon AR, Lin L, Lytle B, Peterson ED, Cairns CB, Glickman SW. Use of prehospital 12-lead electrocardiography and treatment times among ST-elevation myocardial infarction patients with atypical symptoms. *Acad Emerg Med*. 2014;21(8):892-898.

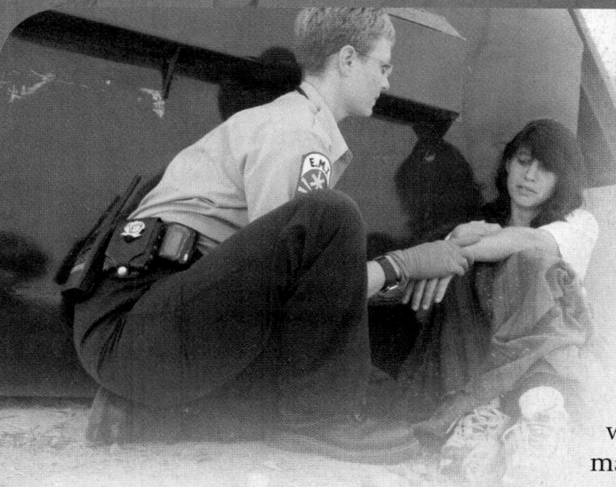

Assessment *in Action*

You and your crew are dispatched to a single-family residence for a person with chest pain. On arrival at the residence, you find a 56-year-old man lying on the sofa in his living room. He tells you he has had a "squeezing" pain in the center of his chest for about 2 hours. It came on suddenly while he was watching television. When describing his pain, the patient makes a fist and places it over his sternum. He rates his pain 10 on a pain rating scale. You note the patient is very anxious, pale, and sweaty. He has no significant past medical history and does not take medications regularly.

1. Which of the reasons below is the most important reason you suspect this patient is having an acute coronary syndrome?

- **A.** The patient's discomfort is located in his chest.
- **B.** The patient is anxious, pale, and sweating.
- **C.** The patient rates his pain 10/10.
- **D.** The patient's chest pain has been present for 2 hours.

2. Which of the following is true of STEMI?

- **A.** Blood flow through one or more coronary arteries is completely blocked, resulting in death of myocardial tissue.
- **B.** Subsequent laboratory tests will reveal normal levels of cardiac biomarkers, indicating no myocardial damage.
- **C.** Most patients with STEMI do not experience chest pain or discomfort.
- **D.** Blood flow through one or more coronary arteries is intermittently blocked because of coronary artery vasospasm.

3. You have obtained vital signs on this patient. They are BP, 96/58 mm Hg; pulse, 82 beats/min; respirations, 16 breaths/min; and Spo_2, 96%. The patient's skin is pale, cool, and diaphoretic. What is the next step in assessing this patient?

- **A.** Obtain a list of his current medications.
- **B.** Obtain an ECG strip of lead aVL.
- **C.** Obtain a 12-lead ECG.
- **D.** Obtain a blood draw for blood chemistry.

4. The 12-lead ECG shows ST changes in leads II, III, and aVF. Which anatomic region of the heart reflects a condition associated with changes in these leads?

- **A.** Anterior
- **B.** Lateral
- **C.** Septal
- **D.** Inferior

5. When ECG changes are observed in leads facing the area of the heart described in the previous question, what action should you take next?

- **A.** Administer nitroglycerin.
- **B.** Administer morphine.
- **C.** Apply right-sided chest leads.
- **D.** Apply posterior chest leads.

Assessment in Action (continued)

6. You have observed ST changes in leads II, III, and aVF. Reciprocal changes may be seen in which of the following leads?

A. V_1 and V_2
B. I and aVL
C. V_3 and V_4
D. V_5 and V_6

7. A member of your crew calls your attention to a rhythm change on the cardiac monitor. The monitor shows an irregular ventricular rhythm, regularly occurring P waves, and PRIs that lengthen before a P wave appears without a subsequent QRS complex. The pattern then starts again. The patient's ventricular rate ranges from 60 to 72 beats/min. What rhythm do you suspect this is?

A. Sinus dysrhythmia
B. Sinus rhythm with premature atrial complexes
C. Third-degree AV block
D. Second-degree AV block type I

8. When leads II, III, and/or aVF show evidence of ischemia, injury, or infarction, which coronary artery is usually involved?

A. Right coronary artery
B. Left anterior descending artery
C. Circumflex artery
D. Left coronary artery

9. Which signs and symptoms are most likely to occur with right ventricular failure?

A. Accessory muscle use, cough with frothy sputum
B. Dependent edema, weight gain, jugular venous distention
C. Orthopnea, speech limited to phrases or words
D. Restlessness, third heart sound, crackles

10. List the intrinsic rates of each of the heart's normal pacemaker sites.

CHAPTER 18

Neurologic Emergencies

National EMS Education Standard Competencies

Medicine

Integrates assessment findings with principles of epidemiology and pathophysiology to formulate a field impression and implement a comprehensive treatment/disposition plan for a patient with a medical complaint.

Neurology

Anatomy, presentations, and management of

- Decreased level of responsiveness (pp 1085-1087, 1109-1113)

Anatomy, physiology, pathophysiology, assessment, and management of

- Stroke/transient ischemic attack (pp 1099-1109)
- Seizure (pp 1113-1116)
- Status epilepticus (pp 1116-1117)
- Headache (pp 1118-1119)

Anatomy, physiology, epidemiology, pathophysiology, psychosocial impact, presentations, prognosis, and management of

- Stroke/intracranial hemorrhage/transient ischemic attack (pp 1099-1109)
- Seizure (pp 1113-1116)
- Status epilepticus (pp 1116-1117)
- Headache (pp 1118-1119)
- Dementia (pp 1119-1120)
- Neoplasms (pp 1119, 1121)
- Demyelinating disorders (pp 1121-1124)
- Parkinson disease (p 1123)
- Cranial nerve disorders (pp 1124-1126)
- Movement disorders (pp 1126-1127)
- Neurologic inflammation/infection (pp 1127-1128)
- Spinal cord compression (p 1121; see Chapter 34, *Head and Spine Trauma*)
- Hydrocephalus (see Chapter 43, *Pediatric Emergencies*)
- Wernicke encephalopathy (pp 1119-1120)

Knowledge Objectives

1. Describe the incidence, morbidity, and mortality of neurologic emergencies. (pp 1080-1081)
2. Review the anatomy and physiology of the organs and structures that make up the nervous system. (pp 1081-1084)
3. Explain the importance of taking standard precautions and ensuring scene safety when caring for a patient with a neurologic illness. (p 1085)
4. Describe how to determine level of consciousness (LOC) when assessing a patient with a neurologic illness. (pp 1085-1087)
5. Compare the characteristics of decorticate and decerebrate posturing, including the likely implications of each for the patient's outcome. (pp 1086-1087)
6. Identify the abnormal respiratory patterns associated with central nervous system illness. (pp 1087-1088)
7. List the signs of increased intracranial pressure. (pp 1088-1089)
8. Compare how to investigate a chief complaint in an unresponsive patient with how you would do so in a responsive patient. (p 1089)
9. Review the components of the physical exam that are unique to a patient with a neurologic illness. (pp 1090-1096)
10. Specify several speech and movement difficulties that can reveal a diminished LOC. (pp 1093-1096)
11. Review the standard guidelines and interventions for treating a patient with a neurologic illness. (pp 1097-1099)
12. Describe the factors that influence the development of multifactorial neurologic conditions. (p 1099)
13. Explain the pathophysiology, assessment, and management of stroke. (pp 1099-1109)
14. Compare the causes, signs, and symptoms of vascular neurologic conditions that occur suddenly with those that develop gradually. (pp 1100-1101)
15. Compare the pathophysiology of ischemic (occlusive) stroke with that of hemorrhagic stroke. (p 1101)
16. Specify how contents of the cranial vault interact to increase intracranial pressure, and the major conditions that result. (pp 1101-1102)

17. Describe several tools used to screen for stroke. (pp 1105-1107)
18. Explain transient ischemic attack as it relates to stroke. (p 1109)
19. Explain the pathophysiology, assessment, and management of seizure, including how to differentiate stroke from seizure. (pp 1113-1116)
20. Compare generalized seizures with partial seizures, including how seizures are further classified. (pp 1113-1115)
21. Explain the pathophysiology, assessment, and management of status epilepticus. (pp 1116-1117)
22. Explain the pathophysiology, assessment, and management of syncope. (pp 1117-1118)
23. Explain the pathophysiology, assessment, and management of the most common types of headaches. (pp 1118-1119)
24. Explain the pathophysiology, assessment, and management of dementia, including the causes, signs and symptoms, and typical course of several common types. (pp 1119-1120)
25. Identify the types of neoplasms that affect the nervous system. (pp 1119, 1121)
26. Analyze the common features of demyelinating conditions. (p 1121)
27. Explain the pathophysiology, assessment, and management of multiple sclerosis. (pp 1121-1122)
28. Explain the pathophysiology, assessment, and management of Guillain-Barré syndrome. (pp 1122-1123)
29. Explain the pathophysiology, assessment, and management of Parkinson disease. (p 1123)
30. Explain the pathophysiology, assessment, and management of amyotrophic lateral sclerosis. (pp 1123-1124)
31. List several cranial nerve disorders, including the shared characteristics. (pp 1124-1126)
32. Explain the pathophysiology, assessment, and management of dystonia. (pp 1126-1127)
33. Describe the types of pathogenic organisms that can infect the nervous system; include the signs and symptoms of a nervous system infection. (pp 1127-1128)
34. Explain the pathophysiology, assessment, and management of an abscess. (p 1129)
35. Explain the pathophysiology, assessment, and management of poliomyelitis. (p 1129)
36. Explain pathophysiology, assessment, and management of peripheral neuropathy. (pp 1129-1130)

Skills Objectives

1. Assess a patient's level of consciousness. (pp 1085-1087)
2. Use several commonly used screening tools to screen a patient suspected of having had a stroke. (pp 1105-1107)

Introduction

The National Center for Health Statistics lists two of the top 10 causes of death in 2015 as neurologic in nature.[1] **Stroke**, a serious medical condition in which blood supply to areas of the brain is interrupted, is the fifth leading cause of death in the United States.[1] The sixth leading cause of death is Alzheimer disease.[1] Table 18-1 shows the occurrence of neurologic disorders throughout the United States. As you consider these statistics, it is important to place them in context. The United States Census Bureau places the US population at 324,700,000 and the world population at 7.3 billion as of October 2016.[2]

YOU are the Paramedic — PART 1

You are dispatched for a stroke. You arrive at a three-story home in an urban setting. The house appears to be well kept. Police arrive with you. You are met by a concerned family member who directs you to the basement, where you find a 49-year-old man sitting on a couch. His wife quickly begins to tell you that she woke up about 15 minutes ago and found her husband sitting on the couch and unable to speak. Your patient is over 6 feet (2 m) tall and weighs approximately 240 pounds (109 kg). He is obviously awake and tracking you with his eyes. He makes no attempt to speak.

1. What are your next questions?
2. What assessment information do you need to gather?

Table 18-1 Neurologic Disorders in the United States

Disorder	Estimated Occurrence
Headache (chronic, recurring)	45 million
Alzheimer disease	5.3 million cases (more than 90% of all cases occur in patients 65 or older)
Neoplasm, spinal	0.5–2.5 cases per 100,000 (primary spinal tumors) 5%–10% of all patients with cancer have metastasis to the spinal cord
Neoplasm, brain	7–19 cases per 100,000 population (primary brain tumors) 200,000 patients with metastatic brain tumors per year
Dystonia	About 300,000 people affected within North America
Peripheral neuropathy	Approximately 14 million people with diabetes who have neuropathy (almost half of all patients with diabetes)
Cerebral palsy	2–2.5 cases per 1,000 live births

Data from: Headache overview, types of headaches. Remedy's Health Communities website. http://www.healthcommunities.com/headache/headache-types-overview.shtml. Updated September 18, 2015. Accessed March 27, 2016; Alzheimer's Disease Information Page: National Institute of Neurological Disorders and Stroke (NINDS). https://www.ninds.nih.gov/Disorders/All-Disorders/Alzheimers-Disease-Information-Page Accessed January 18, 2017; Huff JS. Spinal cord neoplasms. Medscape website. http://emedicine.medscape.com/article/779872-overview. Updated December 7, 2016. Accessed March 27, 2016; Lo BM. Brain neoplasms. Medscape website. http://emedicine.medscape.com/article/779664-overview. Updated November 9, 2015. Accessed March 27, 2016; Forms of dystonia. Dystonia Medical Research Foundation website. https://www.dystonia-foundation.org/what-is-dystonia/forms-of-dystonia. Accessed March 25, 2016; Quan D. Diabetic neuropathy. Medscape website. http://emedicine.medscape.com/article/1170337-overview. Updated July 31, 2015. Accessed March 26, 2016; and Abdel-Hamid HZ. Cerebral palsy. Medscape website. http://emedicine.medscape.com/article/1179555-overview. Updated August 12, 2016. Accessed March 26, 2016.

You may ask, "Why it is important to have this information?" When you assess a patient, the signs and symptoms you record may indicate many possible conditions. However, you must also take into account the likelihood of those conditions to help ground your conclusions. For example, a 10-year-old with chest pain is unlikely to be having a myocardial infarction (MI). Disease occurrence information helps you to expect that the patient with dementia is more likely to have Alzheimer disease than Creutzfeldt-Jakob disease.

Patients with neurologic conditions are vulnerable and can be in danger. Many of the reflexes that protect an awake person can be temporarily inactive when the nervous system is depressed by any cause (for example, a stroke or severe head injury). The eyelids do not blink away dust and irritants. The larynx does not cause gagging and coughing in reaction to secretions oozing down the airway. The body does not seek a more comfortable position in response to compression of a limb in an awkward position. The tongue goes slack. The airway is at risk.

To help you better determine each patient's problem, a brief review of the anatomy and physiology of the nervous system is presented in this chapter. This information will provide the proper foundation on which to begin a discussion of assessment and treatment.

Anatomy and Physiology Review

The basic structures of the nervous system are shown in **Figure 18-1**. Recall from Chapter 8, *Anatomy and Physiology*, that the major structures are divided into the central nervous system (CNS), which is responsible for thought, perception, feeling, and autonomic body functions; and the peripheral nervous system (PNS), which is responsible for transmitting commands from the brain to the body and receiving feedback from the body.

To review the nervous system, consider the example of a child riding a bicycle. This common and seemingly simple activity requires many conscious and unconscious functions. The child has to do many things so that he or she does not fall or ride into a tree.

On a summer morning the rider, Justin, goes to the garage to get his bike. Already the brain is hard at work. As Justin enters the garage, the brain must determine which object is a bike. As Justin scans the garage, the images produced by his eyes are transmitted via the optic nerve to the occipital lobe of the brain. There, the image, which is transmitted upside down, needs to be reoriented. The occipital lobe now scans through tens of thousands of images that are stored to determine whether this image has been seen before.

After the image is recognized, an existing pathway is accessed to the temporal lobe. Here, language and speech are stored. As Justin walks through the garage, he is able to put names to what he sees—car, workbench, bike. When Justin was learning to speak, he often became confused about the correct names of objects. As he practiced, he received reinforcement for the correct names and redirection for the names that were incorrect. In his brain, more and more pathways were laid down between the image of an object with two wheels, a seat, and pedals. These pathways are stored in the occipital lobe as the word "bike."

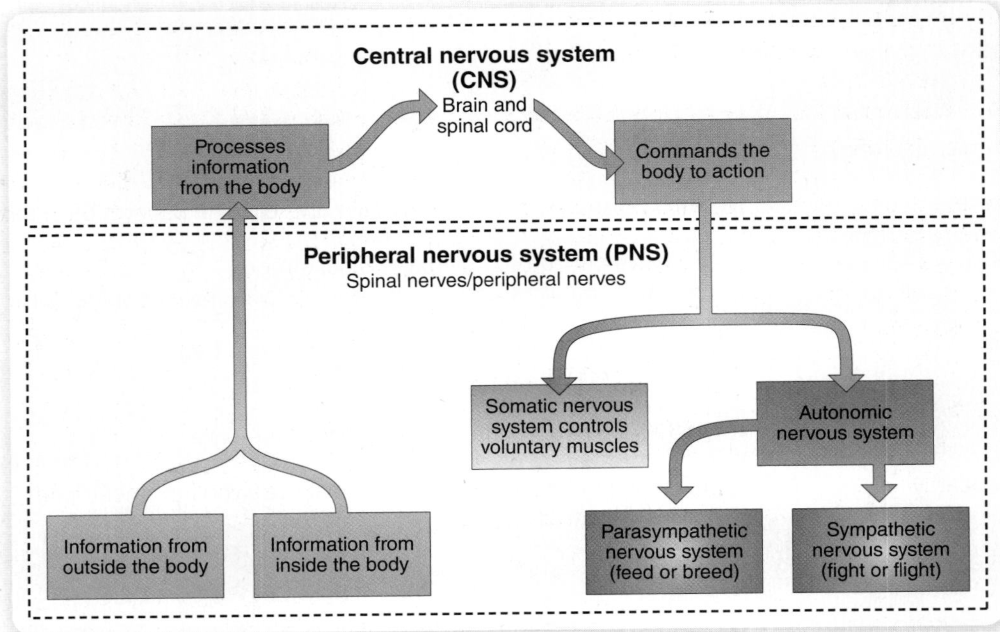

Figure 18-1 Basic organization of the nervous system.

As Justin reaches for his helmet, commands from the frontal lobe of the brain are sent to his arms so that he can pick up the helmet and place it on his head. The frontal lobe, which controls voluntary motion, sends signals out of the CNS to the arms, shoulders, chest, and hands to perform the task of picking up his helmet.

Which way should he apply the helmet? This motor memory is stored within the frontal lobe. The brain is storing memories in the areas that were initially stimulated. While he applies the helmet, Justin needs to make fine adjustments to its position. His brain is receiving impulses from nerves within the skull and muscle of the head.

If the helmet is uncomfortable, then Justin will sense pressure and possibly pain from the improperly placed helmet. Signals of discomfort are sent to the parietal lobe where the body's sense of touch and pain perception

YOU are the Paramedic PART 2

The patient is mute; he neither makes nor attempts any sounds. He does follow commands. You note a slight weakness to his left hand and slight facial droop to the left side of his face. You find no other cranial nerve deficits. The patient is not drooling and is able to swallow easily. You do not observe any evidence of respiratory distress or inability to protect his airway.

Recording Time: 0 Minutes	
Appearance	Awake
Level of consciousness	Alert and following commands, but mute
Airway	Patent
Breathing	Adequate
Circulation	Adequate

3. How can you determine whether the patient is oriented when he will not speak?
4. What vital signs or laboratory values are critical to gather for this patient?
5. What is this patient's Glasgow Coma Scale (GCS) score? Does it accurately depict this patient's acuity?

are found. Signals are sent from the parietal lobe to the frontal lobe to signal the body to adjust the helmet until the pressure signals have stopped.

How does the brain manage a massive amount of information without confusion and misdirection? The information is divided into items that need to be managed consciously and those that can be handled unconsciously. This process is the responsibility of the diencephalon, which filters out unneeded information before it reaches the cerebral cortex. For example, the midbrain portion of the brainstem helps regulate the level of consciousness (LOC). This function needs to occur constantly, but Justin could not ride his bike if he needed to spend time and energy consciously controlling his LOC. The brainstem is one of the portions of the brain that frees the cerebral cortex for higher activities.

Justin now mounts his bike and begins to ride. The smile on his face indicates that he is having a good time. Emotions come from two main areas within the brain: the **limbic system**, where rage and anger are generated, and the hypothalamus, where pleasure, thirst, and hunger are found. All emotions are mediated by the prefrontal cortex so people can choose how they are going to act in response to how they feel.

Justin begins to pick up speed. As he approaches a corner, he must turn or risk crashing into a tree. Justin is able to shift his weight and make the turn successfully due in large part to his cerebellum. This lobe of the brain, located in the posterior, inferior area of the skull, manages complex motor activity unconsciously. When Justin first learned to ride a bike, he had to think about what to do, where to shift his weight, and how to hold his upper body. Over time, and with practice, the frontal lobe of the brain tired of sending the same commands again and again, so this task was transferred to the cerebellum.

Table 18-2 provides a basic reference of various portions of the nervous system.

Table 18-2 Structures and General Functions of the Nervous System

Major Structure	Subdivision	General Functions
CNS		
Brain	Occipital	▪ Vision and storage of visual memories
	Parietal	▪ Sense of touch and texture and storage of tactile memories
	Temporal	▪ Hearing and smell ▪ Language ▪ Storage of sound and odor memories
	Frontal	▪ Motor cortex: Voluntary muscle control and storage of spatial memories ▪ Prefrontal cortex: Judgment and prediction of consequences of a person's actions, abstract intellectual functions
	Limbic system	▪ Basic emotions ▪ Basic reflexes, such as chewing and swallowing
	Diencephalon (thalamus)	▪ Relay center that prioritizes signals to hone in on important messages
	Diencephalon (hypothalamus)	▪ Emotions ▪ Temperature control ▪ Interface with the endocrine system
Brainstem	Midbrain	▪ LOC ▪ Location of the reticular activating system (RAS), which controls arousal and consciousness ▪ Muscle tone and posture
	Pons	▪ Respiratory pattern and depth
	Medulla oblongata	▪ Pulse rate, blood pressure, and respiratory rate

(continued)

Table 18-2 Structures and General Functions of the Nervous System *(Continued)*

Major Structure	Subdivision	General Functions
Spinal cord		▪ Reflexes ▪ Relay of information to and from the body
PNS		
Cranial nerves		▪ Special peripheral nerves that connect directly from the brain to body parts to relay information from the brain
Peripheral nerves		▪ Brain to spinal cord to body part ▪ Receive stimulus from body; send commands to body
CNS and PNS		
Neuron	Cell body	▪ Portion of the neuron where the nucleus resides; site of protein synthesis
	Axon	▪ Projection from the cell body that reaches out to connect with other neurons or target organs; signals are sent away from the cell body ▪ Some axons are covered with insulation called myelin; myelin increases speed of nerve conduction
	Dendrite	▪ Projection from cell body that receives signals from axons of other neurons; most neurons have multiple dendrites
	Synapse	▪ The gap between an axon and a dendrite
	Neurotransmitter	▪ A chemical released into a synapse that helps make the connection between one neuron and another (eg, serotonin, dopamine, and epinephrine)

Abbreviations: CNS, central nervous system; LOC, level of consciousness; PNS, peripheral nervous system

Data from: Bailey R. Neurons. About.com website. http://biology.about.com/od/humananatomybiology/ss/neurons.htm. Updated December 15, 2016. Accessed January 8, 2017.

Patient Assessment

The brain is the most sensitive organ within the body to variable temperatures and fluctuating levels of oxygen and glucose. Even small alterations can impair its function. Conversely, the brain is also surprisingly resilient to internal environmental changes. It does not simply shut down when the oxygen level falls. Assessment of a patient would most likely be easier if the patient were either completely awake or completely asleep. When you are trying to determine whether your patient has a neurologic condition, you need to look for both gross (obvious) changes and also subtle, sometimes hidden changes that can indicate disease.

You will still need to perform all of the general steps of patient assessment, such as scene safety, taking standard precautions, considering the mechanism of injury, and determining whether medications, alcohol, or other substances were taken (and if so, then how much and when). The information in this section will allow you to focus on areas that are unique or important in the patient with a neurologic condition.

A good assessment provides the backbone to excellent patient care. Be curious. Be inquisitive. Be adaptable. Rarely do patients demonstrate textbook disease presentations, showing every sign and symptom, every change in vital sign, and a perfect history of present illness. Use this review of the assessment process to sharpen your focus, but avoid tunnel vision. If the patient you are caring for reports chest pain and is demonstrating new-onset facial droop, then you must assess both the cardiovascular and nervous systems.

Patient Safety

Consider the following scenario in which you need to give a medication to patient with a neurologic disorder. As a first step, you check for medical alert tags and find none. Patients with neurologic disorders may have speech difficulties. Patients may choose the wrong word to answer your question. For example:

You ask, "Do you have any allergies?"

Although the patient may be aware that he has allergies and may intend to say yes, he responds, "No."

Unfortunately, you will often be unable to ascertain this issue in the context of a limited evaluation in the field. To attempt to do so, consider phrasing your question using at least two different formats. For example:

You ask, "Do you have any allergies?"

The patient states, "No."

You say, "Just to make sure, please tell me the names of medications to which you are allergic."

Now compare the patient's answers to questions one and two. If the answers are not the same, then you need to ask more questions to ensure you do not give a medication that could harm the patient. Unfortunately, this approach is not feasible for all patients in the field, and therefore it may not be possible to rely on all the information you receive from a patient with an apparent cognitive or communicative deficit.

Scene Size-up

Take standard precautions. For example, a patient who has a **seizure** (the sudden, erratic firing of neurons) may be incontinent, and a patient with neurologic symptoms may have meningitis.

Your assessment of the physical environment begins at dispatch. The location of a neurologic patient can place you in scenes that may be unsafe. Some patients are unresponsive because of a drug overdose. When people use illegal drugs, weapons and crime are likely to be close at hand. Ensure that no matter what type of event is taking place, you have a way to remove yourself from the scene. If an entire family in the same house is reporting a headache, then consider the possibility of carbon monoxide exposure and understand the house is an unsafe scene.

Finally, if the distance to the nearest stroke center is greater than 1 hour, then request air medical transport early.

Primary Survey

Patients who state, "It hurts right here," provide evidence of a functioning nervous system. Patients found unresponsive should be evaluated as being in an unstable condition with obvious nervous system impairment. The answers to the following questions can give you clues to the overall functioning of the patient's nervous system:

- Where is the patient?
- Does the patient appear to be in distress or pain?
- Is the patient standing, sitting, or lying down?
- Is the patient outside or inside?
- Does the patient have obvious injuries?
- What does the environment look like?
- Do you see evidence of drug paraphernalia?
- What are the living conditions: clean, cluttered, dirty
- Is the patient able to ambulate within his or her home?
- Is the patient awake (aware of his or her surroundings) and alert (responding to his or her surroundings)?
- Is the patient in a stable or unstable condition?

Examining the living conditions can provide insight into the general functioning of the patient's brain. Cluttered or disorganized living conditions may be an indicator of a degenerative nervous system condition. Patients with progressive neurologic disease may initially be able to care for themselves, but it become more difficult over time. With some conditions, such as amyotrophic lateral sclerosis (ALS; discussed later in this chapter), patients experience a loss of motor ability.

Assessing Level of Consciousness

Recall from Chapter 11, *Patient Assessment*, that tools to assess the patient's LOC include the AVPU mnemonic, assessment of orientation, and the Glasgow Coma Scale (GCS). The GCS uses parameters that test a patient's eye opening, best verbal response, and best motor response. The three numeric scores are added together to form a total score that defines the patient's brain function. Refer to Chapter 11, *Patient Assessment*, to review how to perform and calculate the GCS.

This tool is useful in helping you determine how to proceed with patient care, what care you should give, and where to transport the patient. Mildly ill patients need care that conforms to standard care guidelines; usually you can honor the patient's request to be transported to a particular hospital. Patients with moderate conditions require you to make more challenging decisions. They are not critically ill but are considered to be in an unstable condition; therefore, your most appropriate action should be to perform close assessment and provide prompt transport to the closest appropriate facility. Critically ill patients need airway management and prompt transport to the closest appropriate hospital.

Words of Wisdom

Patients may be confused. Confusion may indicate a low blood glucose level, decreased oxygen level, overdose, or even decreased blood pressure (hypotension). Ask questions to which you know the answers if you are trying to determine the level of orientation.

As you determine a patient's level of orientation, examine the speed and intensity at which the patient responds. Generally, patients either undergo excitation or sedation. As you are talking, does the patient appear to be sleepy or sluggish? Is the patient talking quickly and unable to sit still? How many words are in the sentences the patient uses? Do you have to speak loudly at the patient to get a response?

Methods for Measuring Response to Pain

Imagine that you have walked up to a patient and announced yourself, and the patient has not responded. Now, the goal is to elicit pain but not cause harm to the patient. For the patient to respond to pain, he or she needs a functioning brain, an intact spinal cord, and an intact peripheral nervous system. You can evaluate a patient's response to pain in several ways; here are some recommended methods.

The first method is to apply pressure to the fingernail. Take a pen, a penlight, or the handle of a pair of trauma scissors. Hold one of the patient's fingers in your hand and place the finger between your index finger and your thumb. Now place the object between your thumb and the patient's finger. The object should be parallel to the nail bed. You want the object at the most proximal portion of the nail. Now squeeze the object against the nail. The more pressure you apply, the more pain the patient should feel; however, the procedure should not cause trauma. The downside of this pain stimulation technique is that the patient must have an intact spinal cord to feel the pain **Figure 18-2**.

Another assessment technique is to apply pressure to the **supraorbital foramen**. The supraorbital foramen is part of the frontal bone and feels like a notch near the bridge of the nose. Place your thumb in the upper, inner orbit and feel for a notch about 0.5 inch to 1 inch (1 to 2 cm) lateral to the bridge of the nose. With the tip of your thumb, apply pressure in an inward, upward manner over the top of this notch. This action will generate a significant amount of pain. This is another area of the body in which more pressure increases the degree of pain quickly. When this technique is done correctly, no trauma should occur to the patient. This pain response does not require the patient to have an intact spinal cord, so it is ideal pain stimulation for patients with back trauma or spina bifida within the thoracic spine **Figure 18-3**.

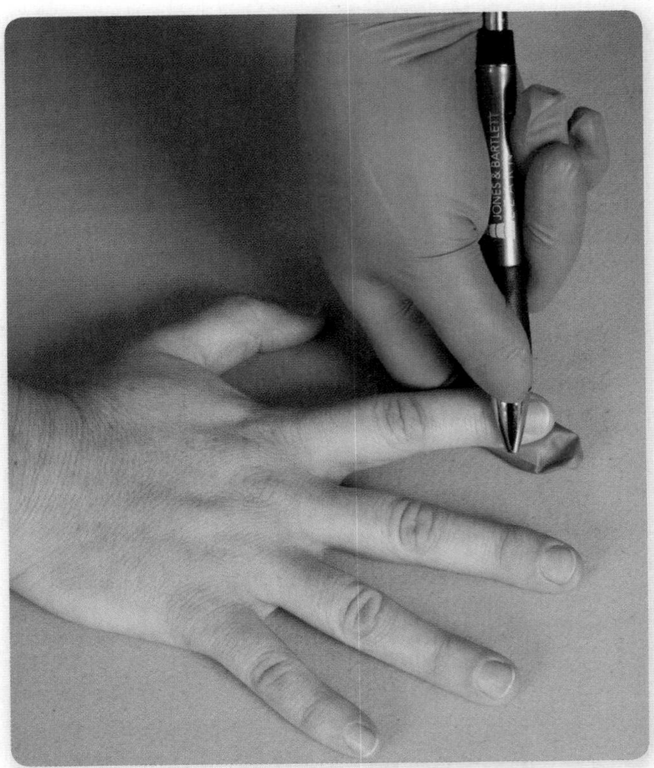

Figure 18-2 Eliciting pain using the nail bed technique.

You must take some precautions with this procedure. First, ensure the patient does not have a facial fracture before you apply pressure to the head. Second, apply pressure only along the upper, inner orbital ridge. Do not apply pressure directly onto the eye. Finally, be aware of your technique when performing this procedure. If your thumb is too far to the left or right of the supraorbital foramen, then the patient will not experience great discomfort. You need to place your thumb directly over the foramen (the notch) to elicit a pain response.

While you generate a pain response from the patient, observe what happens. Does the patient wake up? Does the patient move away from the pain? Does the patient move in an abnormal fashion? Does the patient exhibit one of the two main abnormal postures that occur with any painful stimulation? It is important to understand that abnormal **posturing** (abnormal body positioning that indicates damage to the brain) occurs involuntarily in patients who are otherwise unresponsive. You may notice these postures during the insertion of an intravenous (IV)

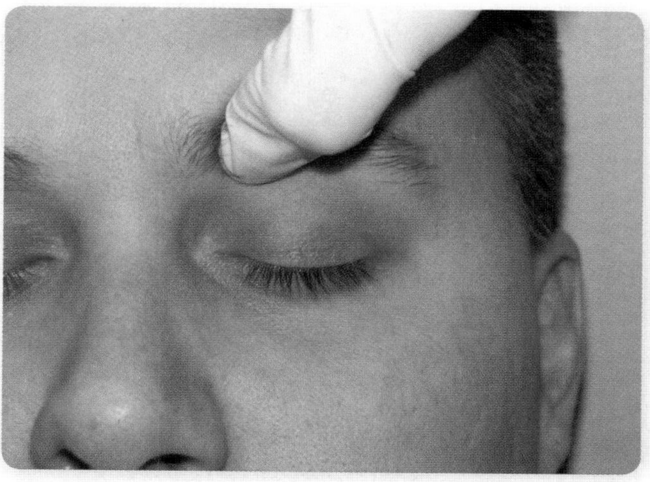

Figure 18-3 Eliciting pain using the supraorbital technique.
Courtesy of Chuck Sowerbrower, MED, NREMT-P.

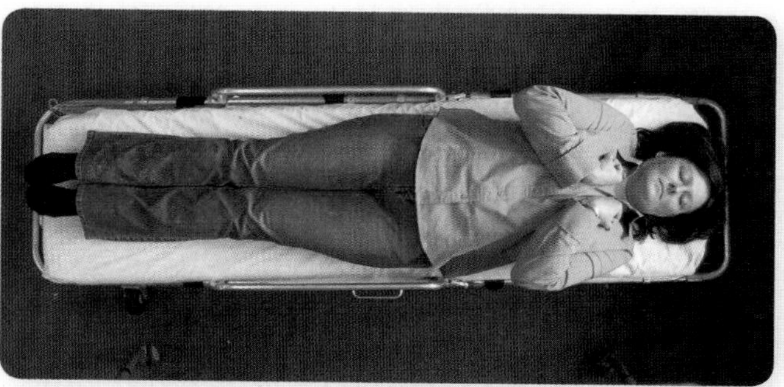

Figure 18-4 Decorticate posturing.
Courtesy of Chuck Sowerbrower, MED, NREMT-P.

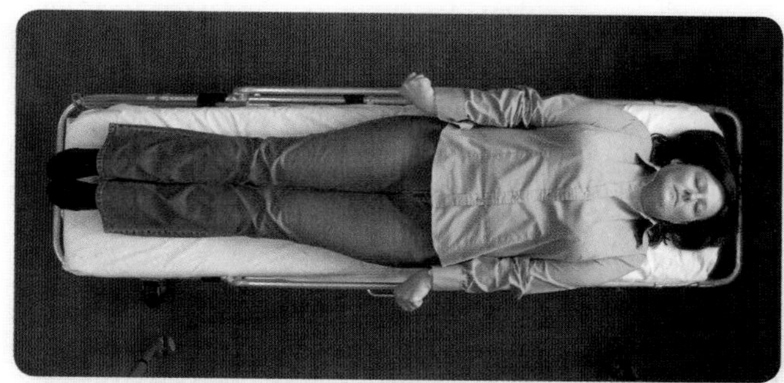

Figure 18-5 Decerebrate posturing.
Courtesy of Chuck Sowerbrower, MED, NREMT-P.

line. The patient may move involuntarily after the painful stimulus occurs. These postures indicate unresponsiveness and if you see either of these postures, then immediately consider your patient to be in critical condition.

The first abnormal posture is **decorticate posturing**, or abnormal flexion. In this posture, patients contract their arms and curl them toward their chests (remember bending the arms toward the "core" of the patient). At the same time, they point their toes. Finally, the wrists are flexed. This posture may indicate damage to the area directly below the cerebral hemispheres Figure 18-4.

The other abnormal posture is called **decerebrate posturing** or abnormal extension. In this posture, patients again point their toes, but now extend their arms outward and rotate the lower arms in a palms-down manner (called **pronation**). The wrists are again flexed. This type of posturing is a more severe finding than decorticate posturing. In decerebrate posturing, the level of damage is within or near the brainstem (diencephalon/pons/midbrain) Figure 18-5.

Airway, Breathing, and Circulation Considerations

The trigeminal, glossopharyngeal, vagus, and hypoglossal nerves are responsible for airway control. These nerves allow for swallowing, controlling the tongue, and ensuring the muscles in the hypopharynx are slightly contracted. Alteration in the signals from these nerves can produce too much relaxation or too much constriction of the airway.

If the patient is not responding to stimuli, then carefully assess the airway. A relatively common presentation is tightly clenched teeth. This state, called **trismus**, can make it difficult to manage the airway. Trismus can occur in either responsive or unresponsive patients. In the unresponsive patient, trismus can indicate a seizure in progress, severe head injury, and/or cerebral hypoxia. In the case of trismus, the patient may need to be sedated/paralyzed to relax the facial muscles causing the clenched teeth, allowing you to better control the airway.

If you note trismus, then initially determine how effectively you can ventilate the patient with a bag-mask device. If ventilation is poor or unsuccessful, then attempt a nasotracheal airway, as long as the patient is still breathing on his or her own. If a nasotracheal airway is unsuccessful, then consider a sedative/paralytic agent to relax the mouth and allow for airway management. If sedative/paralytics are unavailable or contraindicated and you cannot ventilate the patient, then transtracheal airway management is the only remaining option to prevent hypoxia and death. For further information on how to manage the complicated airway, refer to Chapter 15, *Airway Management*.

Remember that routine hyperventilation of neurologic patients can be harmful. Provide hyperventilation only to those patients with documented signs of increased intracranial pressure (ICP) and impending herniation. The management of patients with ICP is discussed later in this chapter. For additional information on rapid sequence intubation or airway obstruction clearance, refer to Chapter 15, *Airway Management*.

Recall that the functions of breathing are controlled by the pons and the medulla oblongata. Check the rate and rhythm of the breathing. Breathing patterns are summarized in Table 18-3. Notice how the rhythms can have subtle changes or can be dramatically different from normal. The greater the deviation from normal, the more severely affected the nervous system is likely to be.

Table 18-3 Respiratory Patterns

Waveform	Pattern	Description	Causes
	Eupnea	Regular rate and pattern; inspiration and expiration are equal	Normal
	Tachypnea	Increased respiratory rate Regular pattern	Stimulants Exercise Excitement
	Bradypnea	Decreased respiratory rate Regular pattern	Narcotics
	Apnea	Absence of breathing	Severe hypoxia Depressants
	Hyperpnea	Rapid, regular, deep respirations	Stimulants Overdose Exercise
	Cheyne-Stokes respirations	Gradual increases and decreases in respirations with periods of apnea	Pre-death pattern Brainstem injury
	Biot/ataxic respirations	Irregular respirations with periods of apnea; unpredictable	Brainstem injury
	Kussmaul respirations	Extreme tachypnea and hyperpnea	Acidosis Diabetic ketoacidosis
	Apneustic respirations	Prolonged inspiratory phase with shortened expiratory phase and bradypnea	Brainstem injury

Signs of Increased Intracranial Pressure

If a patient has increased pressure within the cranium, then the vital signs may change. The blood pressure rises and the pulse rate and respiratory rate fall in the setting of increased ICP Table 18-4. This response is called Cushing reflex, and is indicated by the following signs:

- Decreased pulse rate (bradycardia)
- Decreased/irregular respiratory rate (bradypnea)
- Widened pulse pressure (systolic hypertension)

Cushing reflex is the opposite of what typically occurs in shock, when blood pressure falls and the pulse rate and respiratory rate climb. The hallmarks of increased ICP are as follows:

- Cushing reflex
- Decorticate posturing
- Decerebrate posturing
- Biot respirations
- Apneustic respirations
- Cheyne-Stokes respirations

Table 18-4 Vital Signs for Shock and Increased ICP

	Pulse Rate	Respiratory Rate	Blood Pressure	Pulse Pressure
Shock	↑	↑	↓	Narrowed
Increased ICP	↓	↓	↑	Widened

Abbreviation: ICP, intracranial pressure

- Unresponsive and dilated pupils or **anisocoria** (unequal pupils with greater than 1-mm difference)

As the ICP rises, blood flow to the brain diminishes. To compensate, the medulla oblongata sends signals to the heart to increase the force of contraction. This increase causes systolic pressure to rise. If the ICP continues to increase, then downward forces on the brainstem begin to damage the ability of the medulla to send signals to the body. Diastolic pressure falls as the blood vessels relax or dilate, resulting in a widened pulse pressure. Finally, this pressure also damages the ability to control the respiratory and pulse rates; consequently, they both decrease. Increased ICP is discussed in detail later in this chapter.

Special Populations

In the pediatric population, you must consider the child's developmental stage. A 1-year-old child should cry when you conduct an assessment, because this is considered a normal reaction to strangers. A 5-year-old child who normally talks freely may be quiet with a stranger. Evaluate the child at his or her appropriate developmental level.

When you assess ICP in infants, consider the quality of the baby's cry. As ICP increases, the pitch of the cry rises as well, until it resembles a shriek similar to that of a cat. At the same time, the shape of the pupils can change from round to more oval. These two findings are the basis of the mnemonic related to infants and ICP: "Cat's eyes and cat's cries."

The Rapid Full-Body Scan

When you have completed the primary survey, you now need to decide how to proceed. Is the patient in a stable or unstable condition? Do you suspect a major underlying problem? Consider how to transport this patient. At this point, you have the following two choices:

1. Complete a rapid full-body scan, which would involve a head-to-toe approach, *or*
2. Complete a secondary assessment and evaluate only the area(s) of the patient's chief complaint(s).

Perform a rapid full-body scan on any patient with an abnormal assessment, any patient with a significant MOI/NOI, or any patient who you suspect may have a major problem. Examples would be a patient who is unresponsive, is experiencing a seizure, or has a sudden loss of movement of the body.

If the patient is in stable condition, then it is appropriate to conduct a secondary assessment based on the chief complaint(s). These patients, such as those with headaches or nontraumatic back pain, have a completely normal primary survey, have a minor MOI/NOI, and/or you suspect a localized problem.

Be cautious, though. Just because a patient has a headache does not mean it is the result of a simple cause, such as stress. Patients who have sustained a stroke can also have headaches. If you suspect a more complicated condition, then quickly perform the secondary assessment, covering the entire body. This expanded assessment will ensure you are giving the patient the best possible care.

History Taking

While taking the history, look for signs and symptoms that may indicate the cause of the altered mental status (such as a stroke), as well as any evidence of the patient having had a seizure, such as incontinence or a bitten tongue. Evaluate the patient's speech. Is it slurred? Does the patient make sense? Remember to ask about over-the-counter (OTC) medications.

If you know that the patient has had a seizure and is now in a postictal state, then you will be unable to obtain a history. Look for any obvious explanation for why the patient had a seizure, such as trauma. If the patient has a headache, then try to determine the patient's level of stress, the likelihood of infection, and the patient's history of headaches. If you believe a more complicated condition may be present, then perform a more detailed evaluation.

Special Populations

Age will determine how much interaction the pediatric patient is able to have with you. If the child is able to speak and understands the concept of time, then talk to him or her to gather information. Talk to the parents or caregivers as well.

Try to speak with family or friends who can explain the events leading up to the altered mental status. Remember, time can be critical in a neurologic emergency. As a paramedic in the field, you may be the only person with the opportunity to obtain crucial information about the time of onset.

Documentation & Communication

The patient's family or friends may report the patient was last seen normal when he or she went to bed the night before. If that is the case, then report the time last seen normal was at bedtime, not when the patient awoke with symptoms.

Words of Wisdom

Although a patient who has had a stroke might appear to be unresponsive and is unable to speak, he or she may still be able to hear and understand what is taking place. As with any patient, avoid making any remarks that might cause the patient distress. Reassure the patient that you understand that verbal communication may be difficult at this time, but that you will keep him or her continually informed about what you and your team members are doing. Compassionate communication can help you calm the patient and ease his or her fears, which are undoubtedly intensified by the inability to communicate.

Special Populations

When you apply assessment and history of present illness information to the older adult population, take into account the patient's pertinent past medical history. Patients with a history of dementia (discussed later in this chapter) are complicated to manage. The primary question you need to answer is how much change has occurred in the patient's LOC. Do not evaluate the patient from the point of a normal LOC. Speak to family, friends, or other caregivers to determine the patient's baseline LOC. Document that level clearly using active language.

Medications can also create alterations in the LOC. Explore all medications that the patient is taking. Include prescription, nonprescription, herbal, supplements, homeopathic, and illegal medications. Older adult patients are at a higher risk for having many physicians, many conditions, and many medications (polypharmacy). Combinations of medications can result in unexpected neurologic effects.

Your SAMPLE history (Signs and symptoms, Allergies, Medications, Pertinent past history, Last oral intake, Events leading to injury or illness) should reveal whether the patient has a history of seizures. If so, then it is important to find out what triggers them and whether this episode differs from previous ones. Also find out what medications the patient takes. Phenytoin (Dilantin) and phenobarbital (Solfoton) point strongly toward a seizure disorder. Your history may reveal that the patient has run out of medication, recently adjusted the dosage, or has stopped taking it. You may uncover coexisting conditions, such as diabetes. A patient who has diabetes and has a seizure may use up glucose in his or her body to fuel the seizure.

If a patient with no history of seizures is now experiencing a seizure for the first time, then suspect a grave condition, such as a brain tumor, intracranial bleeding, or a serious infection. Determine whether the patient takes medications that lower the blood glucose level, such as insulin or oral antihyperglycemic agents. Finally, inquire about drug use and exposure to toxins if appropriate.

Secondary Assessment

Chapter 11, *Patient Assessment,* covers how to perform a neurologic exam. The head is the area in which you will spend the most time during a neurologic exam, because you can gather critical information on the functioning of the nervous system. As you perform the assessment, notice the symmetry of the face. Do you observe any obvious facial droop? Look at the eyes. Are the eyelids even bilaterally? Drooping or sagging of the eyelids is called **ptosis**. Ptosis can indicate **Bell palsy** or a stroke. **Figure 18-6** demonstrates facial droop and ptosis.

The following findings during the neurologic exam are notable:

- Nausea and vomiting are common with some types of headaches.
- Urinary and/or fecal incontinence are common findings with seizures and fainting. Incontinence is also a relatively objective marker in determining the severity of illness in the unresponsive patient. Obviously, patients are able to control their bowel and bladder

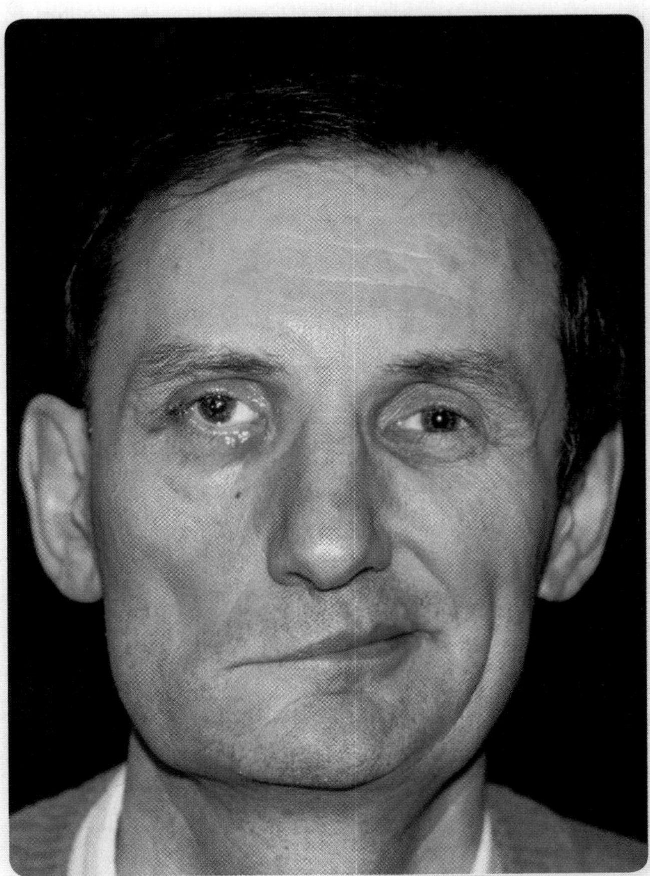

Figure 18-6 Facial droop and ptosis.

functions when they are asleep. If incontinence is present, then the LOC has decreased below that of sleep.
- Signs of recent venipuncture marks which may indicate recent illegal drug use.

Many cardiac dysrhythmias can cause neurologic disorders by decreasing the amount of blood supplied to the brain. Any patient with a sudden loss of consciousness will need a 12-lead ECG.

Level of Consciousness

A patient's LOC can vary widely. To better understand all the variations in LOC, refer to **Figure 18-7**. This figure shows a continuum from what most people would consider normal to a patient who has no responses whatsoever. The point on the extreme right side of the continuum (completely unresponsive to environment) is called coma. **Coma** is a state in which a person does not respond to either verbal or painful stimuli. The points in between are guide markings. Patients do not stop at every point, of course, as the LOC increases or decreases. Nevertheless, these points provide you with an idea of the relationships among various LOCs. Whereas the extremes of the scale are easy to understand, the points in the middle can be more difficult to interpret. The following section explains these questionable areas in more detail.

Common Reality

Some patients experience **hallucinations**, or sensory stimulation that cannot be verified by others. People use their senses to determine what is real. If you see flames, smell smoke, and feel heat, then there must be a fire. But what if all of these sensations exist purely in your mind? One way to determine that the sensations you are experiencing are real is to ask others what they are experiencing. If others also see flames, smell smoke, and feel heat, then the fire is real. **Common reality** is sensory stimulation that can be confirmed by others.

Hallucinations vary. Some patients can hear voices, see snakes, feel insects, smell burning paper, or taste metal. The patient will respond as if the stimulus is real. Keep in mind that hallucinations are vivid. If the patient is afraid of snakes, for example, then he or she will be frightened by the hallucination. Tell the patient that you do not see the snake but you understand that he or she sees it. Do not reinforce the hallucination. Your task is to try to bring the patient back to a common reality, but do not argue if the patient is insistent. Reassure the patient that he or she is safe.

Delusions are similar to hallucinations. Delusions are thoughts, ideas, or perceived abilities that are also not based in a common reality. Examples of delusions include patients who believe they can fly or that everyone is out to get them (paranoia). As with hallucinations, try to redirect patients, but do not argue with them.

As delusions and hallucinations increase, the patient may move farther and farther away from a common reality. Eventually, the amount of shared reality between you and your patient becomes so minimal that the patient can no longer determine what is real and what is inside his or her mind. This state is called **psychosis**.

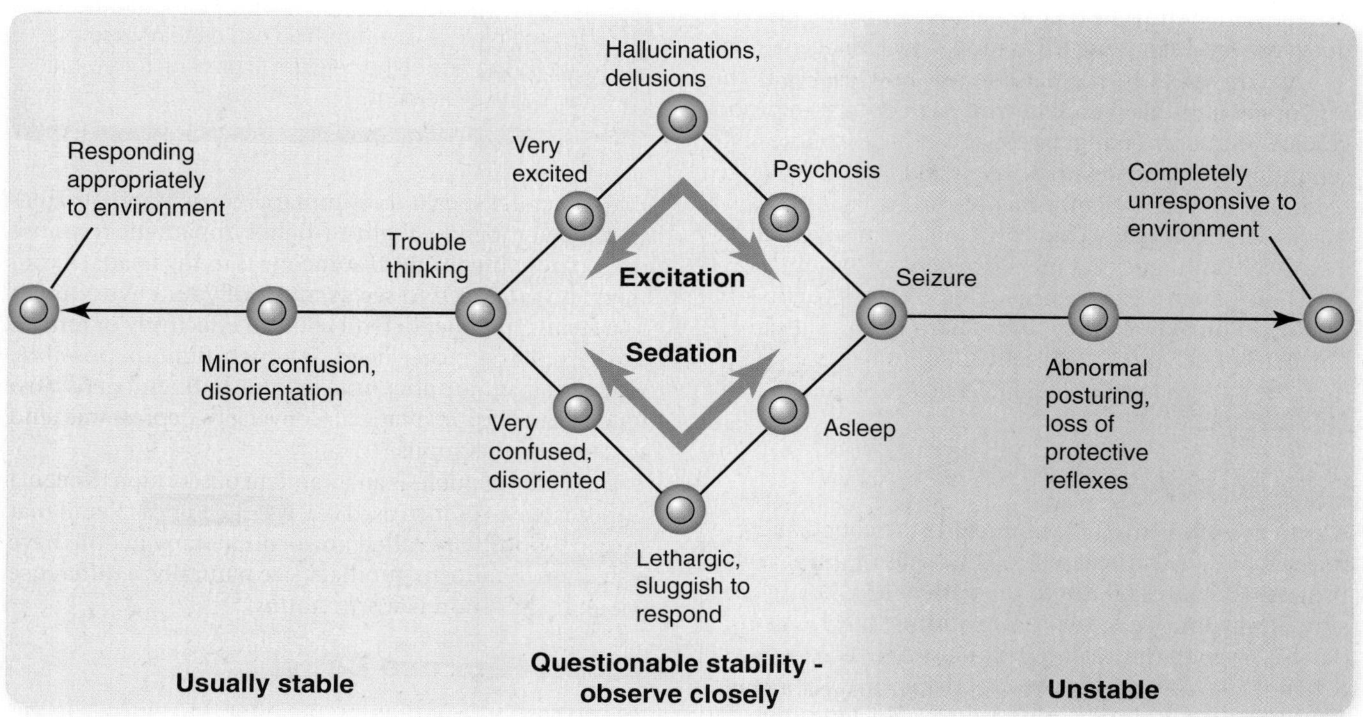

Figure 18-7 Level of consciousness continuum.

Patients with psychosis can be unpredictable. They are responding to a barrage of stimulation that no one else is experiencing. They are struggling to interact with a world in which the rules are constantly changing. Fear, anger, and helplessness are common emotions when a patient is in this state.

When you care for patients who are experiencing psychosis, ensure your safety. Because of the unpredictable nature of patients with psychosis, ensure you are not alone with the patient and have a clear avenue of retreat. Your job is to decrease stimulation as much as possible. Limit the number of people talking to the patient to one person. Give clear, simple commands and be ready to patiently repeat those commands. Do not place the patient in a dimly lit room or ambulance. The patient may interpret the shadows as harmful. The patient may need medication to help manage hallucinations, delusions, and psychosis. For more recommendations on the management of patients with hallucinations, delusions, and/or psychosis, see Chapter 28, *Psychiatric Emergencies*.

Mood and Other Changes

Changes in the patient's mood or the tempo of the nervous system should alert you to changes in the patient's neurologic status. The oxygen level or blood pressure could be falling. Body temperature could be climbing. A psychiatric condition can be escalating. The level of blood glucose could be either critically low or high. Regardless of the underlying cause, this observation of a change requires you to further evaluate the patient to ensure the appropriate level of care. Mood or affect is another attribute that provides insight into the patient. Ask the patient how he or she feels. A low blood glucose or oxygen level can cause frustration, anger, or aggression.

As you speak to the patient, ask how easy it is for him or her to think. A patient who has a decreased blood glucose level or is taking narcotics can have trouble concentrating. Low blood glucose levels and narcotics tend to sedate the nervous system. Patients who are taking cocaine can also have difficulty concentrating, because cocaine is a sympathomimetic that increases nervous system activity. These patients experience mania. Their thoughts can tumble in quickly, so they find it hard to concentrate. If the speed of nervous system activity continues to increase, then the patient may hallucinate, become delusional, or become psychotic.

Corneal Reflex

A patient's protective reflexes include the cough and gag reflexes, and the corneal reflex. The status of the patient's protective reflexes relates to the patient's LOC. A quick, simple way for you to determine indirectly whether the patient's cough and gag reflexes are intact is to assess the **corneal reflex**, which protects the eyes from trauma. This reflex closes the eyelids, pulls the head posteriorly, and constricts the pupils when an object either touches the eyes or eyelids or moves quickly toward the eyes.

To see whether this reflex is present, tap between the patient's eyes. Patients who are asleep or pretending to be unresponsive will blink reflexively with each tap. Even if the eyes are closed tightly, you should see the eyelids twitch.

If you tap lightly between the eyes and the patient does not blink or twitch, then assume that the patient does not have an intact cough or gag reflex and will not be able to protect the airway. Insert an oral airway. If the patient does not cough or gag, then you have confirmed that the airway is unprotected and you must take measures to protect it. The presence of the corneal reflex does not guarantee that the cough and gag reflexes are intact. If you remain doubtful about the patient's ability to protect the airway, then attempt to insert an oral airway.

Pupillary Response

When you assess the patient's eyes, ensure you are eliciting a reaction to light and not movement. To avoid engaging the corneal reflex, take your penlight and approach the eyes from a 45-degree angle. This technique should ensure the pupils react to the light itself, rather than to the approach of the penlight.

Examine the pupils. The pupils should be round, respond quickly to a light by constricting, and be equal in size, shape, and response. Pupillary shape can be changed by trauma, glaucoma, or increased ICP.

Words of Wisdom

Pupil size is measured in millimeters (mm). A quick way to determine size is to imagine how many dimes can be stacked across the pupil. The width (thickness) of a dime is close to 1 mm. You can certainly use the gauge on the side of the penlight (if present) for a more accurate measurement.

Generally speaking, stimulants cause pupillary dilation. Remember the flight-or-fight sympathetic response caused by epinephrine. If someone is trying to attack you, then you will need to see as much of your environment as possible to either defend yourself effectively or retreat. Your eyes, therefore, need as much light as possible. Cocaine, methamphetamines, and hallucinogens also tend to cause pupil dilation. Conversely, depressants tend to constrict the pupils.

Equality of pupils is an important observation. Unequal pupils is a sign of increased ICP **Figure 18-8**. Recall that unequal pupils are called anisocoria. Many people have a slight inequality in pupillary size naturally; a difference greater than 1 mm is worth noting.

Blood Glucose Level

As you assess the patient, remember that glucose is important. Glucose is the fuel that runs the brain. The brain uses glucose faster than any other part of the body and it

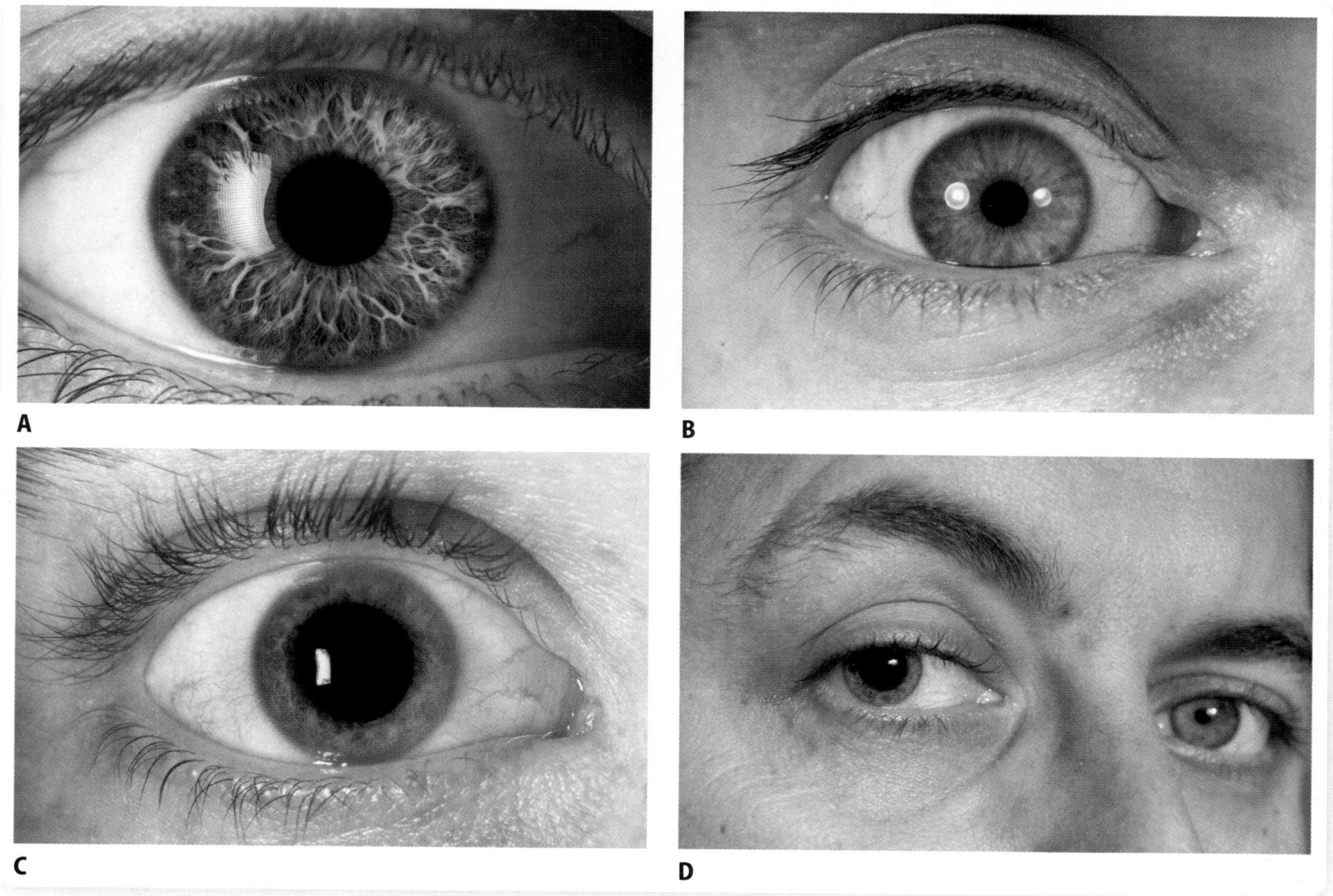

Figure 18-8 Pupillary responses. **A.** Normal. **B.** Constricted. **C.** Dilated. **D.** Unequal (anisocoria).

A: © photoJS/Shutterstock; B: © Biophoto Associates/Science Source; C: © Tim Mainiero/Shutterstock.

has no means to store glucose. All patients with a change in LOC should have their blood glucose level checked. A normal blood glucose reading is 60 to 120 mg/dL. As the glucose level falls, so does the LOC. A high blood glucose level also can affect the patient's LOC; however, the level must increase significantly before the LOC is diminished. A blood glucose level of below 10 mg/dL is incompatible with brain functioning and is usually fatal. Generally, if the level of blood glucose falls below 30 mg/dL or rises above 300 mg/dL, then the patient will become confused or unresponsive. Blood glucose monitoring is now the standard of care for the patient with an altered LOC.

Cranial Nerve Functioning

Assessment of the head includes gathering information on the functioning of the cranial nerves **Table 18-5**. These nerves tend to be bundled as they enter or exit the spinal canal; they control various portions of the body. Refer to Chapter 11, *Patient Assessment*, for more information on how to assess the cranial nerves. When you perform this assessment, look for the patient's ability to respond, strength of response, and symmetry. Patients with stroke, trigeminal neuralgia, **myasthenia gravis**, or other conditions may demonstrate abnormal cranial nerve functioning.

Speech

Listen to the quality of the patient's speech. Is it slurred? Slurring is a classic finding with stroke. It the speech appropriate? You need to focus not only on the quality of the words that are spoken but also on the words a patient chooses. Several situations exist in which speech may be clear but word choice is incorrect. Assess the patient's ability to recognize objects. It is possible for patients to have both slurred speech and object recognition difficulties.

Language can be affected by injury or disease. In aphasia, a person's speech is affected. There are three main forms of aphasia. Depending on the form, the patient may be unable to understand (receive) speech, but able to speak clearly; unable to speak (express him- or herself) clearly, but able to understand speech; or may have a combination of both.

Ask questions to which you and the patient know the answer, such as "Who is the president?" and "What month is it?" This strategy will allow you to verify that the patient understands the questions. Do not ask yes or

Table 18-5 The Cranial Nerves

Cranial Nerve	Function
I. Olfactory	Smell
II. Optic	Vision
III. Oculomotor	Movement of the eye, pupil, and eyelid
IV. Trochlear	Movement of the eye
V. Trigeminal	Chewing Pain Temperature Touch of the mouth and face
VI. Abducens	Movement of the eye
VII. Facial	Movement of the face Tears Salivation and taste
VIII. Auditory	Hearing and balance
IX. Glossopharyngeal and X. Vagus	Glossopharyngeal: Swallowing, taste, and sensations in the mouth and pharynx Vagus: Sensation and movement of the pharynx, larynx, thorax, and GI system
XI. Accessory	Movement of the head and shoulders
XII. Hypoglossal	Movement of the tongue

no questions. Note if the patient speaks clearly but gives you incorrect answers.

Ask the patient to raise his or her arm. If he or she does, the patient can understand you. Then ask for his or her name. Note if the patient does not respond, or provides a slurred response.

Finally, if the patient can neither follow commands nor answer questions, then note these findings in your documentation.

It is important to remember that these patients often can think clearly. They have needs, anxieties, and discomforts, but no way to express them. This dysfunction can be frightening to patients who cannot understand what you are saying and cannot respond to your questions despite being able to formulate the answers in their minds. Be sensitive to this condition and reassure the patient by moving slowly and purposefully, using therapeutic touch, and maintaining good eye contact.

Patients may quickly tire of making the effort to communicate, and become frustrated or emotionally exhausted. Be prepared for patients to shut down—and then gently encourage them to continue to try.

Words of Wisdom

The following approaches can be useful in patients with aphasia:

- **Use a communication board.** This tool can be purchased, handmade, or accessed via a smartphone or tablet in the form of an application. A communication board allows the patient to select pictures or symbols to convey his or her meaning, thus helping you to understand what the patient is thinking. This tool allows you to ask more complicated questions than the yes-or-no method. If the communication board is stored in the ambulance, then you may have to delay its use until the patient is loaded in the ambulance.
- **Writing.** Consider asking the patient to write down his or her response using a pencil and paper, or type it using the keypad of a mobile phone. These tools must be on hand, otherwise you may experience a delay in getting information.

Body Movement

Hemiparesis and Hemiplegia

Patients with strokes can have weakness or paralysis of one side of the body. Weakness of one side of the body is called **hemiparesis**. Paralysis of one side of the body is called **hemiplegia**. At times, you will assess patients who have weakness on one side of the body but facial droop on the other side. In a patient who has had a left cerebral stroke, for example, the patient may have right-sided arm and leg weakness, as well as loss of visual fields in the left eye, because the left side of the brain controls the right side of the body and the left eye.

Have the patient close his or her eyes and hold out the arms in front of the body at the same level. With the eyes closed, the patient's only way to tell where his or her arms are located is from the sensations being processed by the cerebellum. If the patient has had a stroke, then one of the arms may drift away from the other **Figure 18-9**.

Some patients have alterations in their **gait** (walking patterns). **Ataxia** is the term used to describe alteration of a person's ability to perform coordinated motions such as walking. A person's gait can become slow, shuffling, or scissors-like, for example.

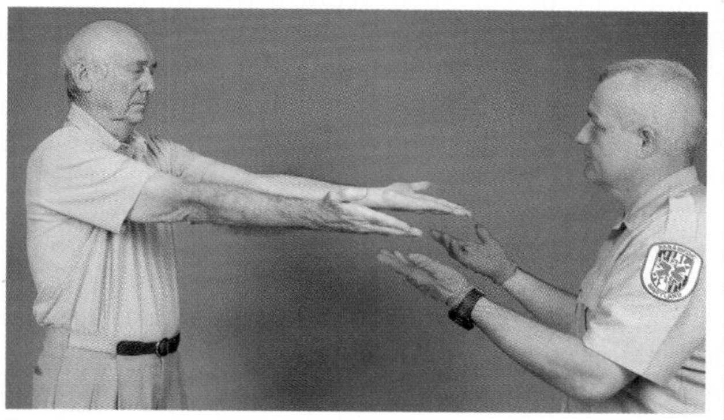

A

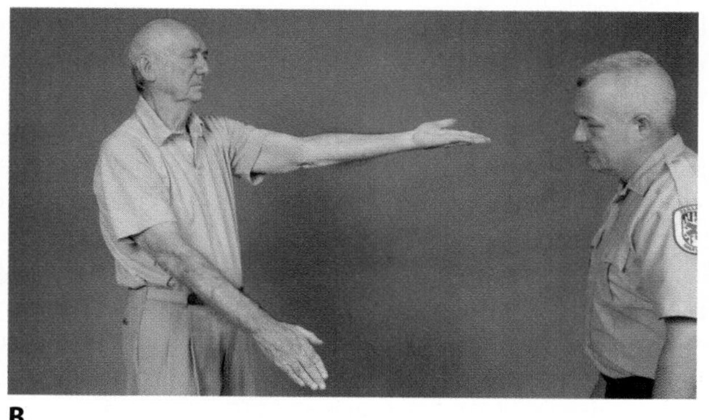

B

Figure 18-9 A. A person who has not had a stroke will be able to hold both arms in front of the body even with his or her eyes closed. **B.** A person who has had a stroke might not be able to maintain this position. One arm will drift down and turn toward the body.

Unless you observe some medical reason to avoid it, have the patient walk for several steps. Assessing gait is another test of activity of the cerebellum. The cerebellum controls the mechanics of walking and allows you to focus on where you want to walk, rather than how to walk. If damage to the cerebellum occurs, then you may observe your patient walking erratically, stumbling, or even experiencing a loss of the ability to walk.

In addition to alterations in gait, a patient's posture may become rigid. Have your patient stand up straight. Place one hand on the patient's chest and your other hand behind the patient's back. Now push on the chest. Normally, as you push backward, the patient compensates quickly by taking a step to keep from falling. In patients with certain disorders, such as **Parkinson disease** (discussed later in this chapter), the patient cannot compensate quickly enough, and you will push the patient over. It is important to have a hand behind the patient to keep the patient from falling.

Bizarre Movement

Patients can exhibit bizarre movement that indicates disruption within the nervous system. **Myoclonus** is a type of rapid, jerky muscle contraction that occurs involuntarily. Most people have experienced myoclonic jerks. A classic example of this phenomenon is the student who is about to fall asleep in class. As the student gets sleepier, the head begins to sag, until the head involuntarily jerks upward and the student wakes up. This startled response is called a myoclonic jerk.

Another form of bizarre movement is called **dystonia**. In this movement, a part of the body contracts and remains contracted. Dystonia is discussed later in this chapter.

Alterations in Smooth Motion

As you assess your patient, does he or she move smoothly? When neurologic structures are functioning correctly, muscle groups alternately contract and relax, allowing the body to move. When this fine balance is upset, patients may have **rigidity** (a condition in which muscles do not contract and relax smoothly, resulting in stiffness of motion).

Tremors are example of an alteration in smooth motion. This fine, oscillating (back and forth) movement usually occurs in the hands and head. Tremors involve the motion of joints. Several types of tremor exist, named for the kind of activity that elicits them:

- **Rest tremor.** Occurs with the patient at rest and not moving.
- **Intention tremor.** Occurs when the patient is asked to reach out and grab an object. It is common for this tremor to increase as the patient gets closer to the object to be grabbed.
- **Postural tremor.** Occurs when a body part is placed in a particular position and required to maintain that position for a long period. Most people have experienced this type of tremor

when working hard for a long time. As fatigue sets in, the body parts being used the most begin to shake. A postural tremor can also occur when a person is standing. The body's muscles are constantly making tiny corrections to maintain posture. The head can oscillate back and forth as the person tries to keep it still.

A type of movement that may appear similar to a tremor is a seizure. Seizures can be classified as either generalized (affecting large portions of the brain) or partial (affecting a limited area of the brain). Whereas a tremor is a fine movement, a generalized or tonic-clonic seizure (formerly called a grand mal seizure) is a larger, less focused type of movement. Generalized seizures are associated with tonic and clonic activity, described as follows:

- **Tonic activity** is a rigid, contracted body posture. The arms, legs, neck, and back can contract so tightly that the body part shakes from the intensity of the contraction.
- **Clonic activity** is characterized by rhythmic contraction and relaxation of muscle groups. Clonic activity can be described as the bizarre, nonpurposeful movement of any body part. Arms and legs may flail, teeth may clench, the head may bob, and the torso may convulse wildly.

Seizures are discussed in more detail later in this chapter.

Sensation

The last area for you to assess is sensation within the body. Many nervous system conditions can alter the ability to feel pain, temperature, pressure, or light touch. A sensation of numbness or tingling is called **paresthesia**. If the patient can feel nothing within a body part, then this is called **anesthesia**.

Vital Signs

In the patient who is having a stroke or seizure, check and document the pulse rate, rhythm, and quality; respiratory rate, rhythm, and quality; blood pressure; skin temperature, color, and condition; and pupil size and reactivity.

During most active seizures, it is impossible to evaluate vital signs, and doing so is not a priority. Unless the situation is unusual, vital signs obtained during the postictal state will be close to normal.

Given the critical importance of normal cerebral perfusion, you must closely monitor blood pressure in any patient with the potential for increased ICP. Frequent reassessment becomes even more essential when the blood pressure has dropped. Ensure the patient maintains a systolic blood pressure of at least 110 to 120 mm Hg. Ensure adequate respiratory rate and pattern, and effective pulse rate and rhythm.

Words of Wisdom

Automatic, noninvasive blood pressure cuffs can be inaccurate if used in moving ambulances. Check your patient's blood pressure manually to have an accurate baseline before relying on automatic systems.

The patient's temperature can be difficult to determine in the prehospital setting. If you suspect hypothermia or hyperthermia, then the standard of care is to use a thermometer to establish the patient's temperature, as discussed in Chapter 11, *Patient Assessment*. Refer to Chapter 38, *Environmental Emergencies*, for guidance in active rewarming and cooling for environmentally induced temperature alterations.

Reassessment

Notify the receiving facility of your patient's chief complaint and your assessment findings. Most designated stroke centers will want you to call a stroke alert for patients you have assessed and found to be having a stroke (check your local protocol). This step will alert the stroke team members at the hospital and give them time to assemble their resources to treat the patient without delay. Be sure to communicate the time that the patient was last seen to be healthy, the findings of your neurologic exam, and the time you anticipate arriving at the hospital.

A key piece of information to document is the time of onset of the patient's signs and symptoms. If the diagnosis is an ischemic stroke, then this information is critical in determining whether the patient is a candidate for treatment with clot-dissolving (fibrinolytic) drugs. It is also important to document your findings from your stroke scale and the score of the GCS, along with any changes you found during your reassessment. As always, document interventions performed, any change in the patient during transport, and the reason for the choice of hospital.

For patients who have had a seizure, give a description of the seizure activity, if known. Include bystanders' comments if they witnessed the seizure. Document the onset and duration of the seizure. Did the patient notice or express noticing an **aura** (visual changes such as flashing lights or blind spots in the field of vision)? Record any evidence of trauma and interventions performed. Document whether this is the patient's first seizure or whether the patient has a history of seizures. If the latter, determine how often he or she has them, and whether the patient has any history of status epilepticus (discussed later in this chapter). When you document your interventions, record the time each intervention was performed, how the patient responded to the intervention, and what the findings of continued reassessments showed.

You may be the only provider to witness some patient activity, so accurate documentation is critical to the continuity of care. Avoid using words that can have multiple meanings, such as "lethargic," "sleepy," "obtunded," and "out of it." Describe the patient using active language, as in the following examples:

"Arrive to find a male patient disoriented to place and time."

"Caring for a 43-year-old man who is slow to respond to verbal or painful stimulation."

Standard Care Guideline for the Neurologic Patient

The focus of care of a neurologic patient is to ensure the body has an adequate internal environment to allow for optimal brain function. Remember, the brain needs oxygen, glucose, and normal temperature to function. The following guidelines serve as the foundation on which additional care for specific neurologic conditions will be built. Through the remainder of this chapter, this guideline will be called the standard care guideline **Table 18-6**.

Administration of Dextrose

Follow your local protocol regarding what blood glucose reading is considered low. One guideline to consider is if the blood glucose level is below 60 mg/dL, then the patient needs glucose. Two medications are available for the prehospital treatment of hypoglycemia: dextrose and glucagon.

Chapter 23, *Endocrine Emergencies,* discusses how to administer dextrose. The effects of dextrose typically begin

Table 18-6 Standard Care Guideline for the Adult Neurologic Patient

Step	Description
Ensure scene safety and take standard precautions.	Ensure you and your partner are safe. Don appropriate personal protective equipment. Use masks and eye protection when managing the airway.
Assess airway and breathing.	Evaluate the airway and effectiveness of breathing. If needed, then secure the airway and provide ventilatory support to ensure oxygen saturation is between 94% and 99%. ▪ Hyperoxygenation (as evidenced by an oxygen saturation level of 100%) may be harmful. ▪ Consider rapid sequence intubation, as appropriate. If respiratory failure or apnea is present, then ventilate the patient at 8 to 12 breaths/min. ▪ Routine hyperventilation may be harmful. Only provide hyperventilation to a patient with documented unresponsiveness *and* signs of increased ICP.
Assess circulation.	Establish IV access. Use your assessment information about the patient's circulatory status as a guide to whether you should use a saline lock or hang a bag of fluids. If fluids are needed, then saline, normosol, or lactated Ringer solution are isotonic choices. ▪ Do not use solutions containing dextrose. Consider drawing blood samples for later analysis at the hospital. Check blood pressure and heart rate. ▪ Correct hypotension with IV fluids or vasopressors based on the cause of hypotension. Ensure continuous ECG monitoring. Perform a 12-lead ECG.

Check blood glucose level.	If <60 mg/dL *and* signs of decreased LOC, then determine:
	▪ Does the patient have a patent airway? Can the patient swallow?
	  • If yes, then consider oral glucose, candy, or orange juice. Closely monitor swallowing.
	  • If no, then administer dextrose, 25 g IVP.
	  • Hyperglycemia can increase the morbidity of patients who have had a stroke.

(continued)

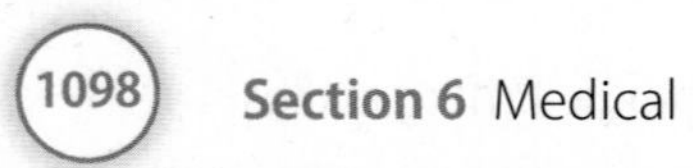

Table 18-6 Standard Care Guideline for the Adult Neurologic Patient *(Continued)*

Step	Description

Assess for increased ICP.	Look for the hallmarks of increased ICP:
	▪ Cushing reflex
	  • Bradycardia
	  • Bradypnea or irregular breathing pattern
	  • Widened pulse pressure (systolic hypertension)
	▪ Other signs
	  • Decorticate posturing
	  • Decerebrate posturing
	  • Anisocoria or dilated and unresponsive pupils
	  • Biot respirations
	  • Apneustic respirations
	  • Cheyne Stokes respirations
	▪ In patients who are unresponsive, have Cushing, reflex *and* demonstrate other signs of increased ICP:
	  • Ensure systolic blood pressure of 110–120 mm Hg. Administer fluids as needed.
	  • Unless you suspect possible cervical spine fracture, elevate the head 30 degrees. This position will cause a slight decrease in ICP.
	  • Provide ventilatory support at 16 to 20 breaths/min. Do not increase the rate any higher than 30 breaths/min. Severe hypocapnia will cause vasoconstriction and decrease perfusion to the brain.
	  • If using end-tidal carbon dioxide ($ETCO_2$) readings, then ventilate to maintain an $ETCO_2$ between high 20s and low 30s mm Hg.
	  • Ensure the airway is clear, but do not vigorously suction. Stimulating the cough and gag reflexes will increase ICP.
	  • Watch for seizures. Be prepared to administer benzodiazepines.
	  • The patient may have bradycardia caused by increased ICP. Atropine and transcutaneous pacing are not indicated due to the systolic hypertension that accompanies the bradycardia.
	  • Notify the hospital.
	  • Provide prompt transport.

Check for drug use.	If you suspect that the patient may have taken a narcotic, then administer naloxone, 0.4–2 mg IV/IN.
Assess for seizures.	If the seizure is prolonged, then administer benzodiazepines.
Evaluate temperature.	If low, then cover the patient, turn on the heat in the patient compartment, and prevent heat loss. If high, then remove clothing and cover the naked patient in a sheet. Turn off the heat in the patient compartment.
Provide emotional support for the patient and family.	Neurologic emergencies can produce feelings of confusion, fear, anger, and helplessness. Provide a therapeutic, gentle touch on the shoulder. Touch can communicate compassion. Use a calm, reassuring voice. Assure the patient and family that you are there to help. If the patient is confused, then try to reorient the patient.

Abbreviations: ECG, electrocardiogram; end-tidal carbon dioxide, $ETCO_2$; ICP, intracranial pressure; IN, intranasal; IV, intravenous; IVP, intravenous push; LOC, level of consciousness

Modified from: National Model EMS Clinical Guidelines. National Association of State EMS Officials. https://www.nasemso.org/Projects/ModelEMSClinicalGuidelines/index.asp. Accessed December 22, 2015.

within 30 seconds to 2 minutes. If the dextrose has no effect or if the patient's blood glucose level remains low, then ensure adequate IV access and administer a second dose.

Words of Wisdom

Cases of dextrose shortages have occurred throughout the country. One solution to this problem is to give two syringes of D_{25} (12.5 g of dextrose per syringe). This option gives the patient twice as much volume but the same amount of dextrose as found in D_{50}. Another option is to give one 250-mL bag of D_{10} (25 g of dextrose per bag). Consider whether it is safe to give the additional fluid volume, especially for pediatric patients or those with head injuries.

If you cannot obtain IV access, then administer 0.5 to 1 mg of glucagon subcutaneously or intramuscularly. This naturally occurring body chemical is responsible for converting the body's stores of glycogen into glucose. You should see an increase in the LOC and blood glucose level within 20 minutes of administration. If the blood glucose level remains low, then repeat the glucagon to a maximum of three doses.

If the blood glucose level is high, then be aware that no safe way to decrease blood glucose in the prehospital setting currently exists. Administration of insulin can be problematic because it is easy to overcorrect the imbalance, resulting in a hypoglycemic state. Ensure adequate support of blood pressure. Patients with hyperglycemia are often dehydrated and may need volume support. Note that rehydration alone in a severely dehydrated patient with hyperglycemia can dramatically lower the patient's blood glucose level.

Finally, be cautious in patients whose blood glucose level cannot be checked. If the patient is unresponsive or has decreased LOC and no blood glucose monitor is available, then administer 12.5 g (one-half syringe) of D_{50} and then reassess the patient for response. Proceed with additional dextrose cautiously, based on responses to previous doses. Hyperglycemia can increase the morbidity of patients who have had a stroke.

▶ Administration of Naloxone

Naloxone (Narcan) is used for the treatment of unresponsive or unknown patients, or those with suspected narcotic overdose. The initial dose is 0.4 to 2 mg via intravenous push (IVP). You may repeat this dose until you reach 10 mg. You may also administer naloxone using a mucosal atomization device. This intranasal (IN) device provides a safe, noninvasive, rapid-acting method of naloxone delivery. Many states allow laypeople to administer naloxone via nasal spray. It is important that you ask bystanders if naloxone has been given. Find out how much and when. For more information regarding naloxone, see Chapter 27, *Toxicology*.

▶ Interventions for Increased Intracranial Pressure

If the patient has signs of increased ICP, then establish vascular access and administer normal saline or lactated Ringer solution as needed. Do not use solutions containing dextrose. Consider drawing blood samples for later analysis at the hospital. Check the patient's blood pressure and pulse rate. If the patient is hypotensive, then support blood pressure to ensure adequate cerebral perfusion pressure (CPP). (Normal CPP is 70 to 90 mm Hg.) The target is a systolic blood pressure of 110 mm Hg to 120 mm Hg. Perform continuous heart monitoring with an electrocardiogram (ECG).

Pathophysiology, Assessment, and Management of Common Neurologic Emergencies

Most diseases or conditions, including neurologic disorders, are caused by more than one factor, so they are said to be *multifactorial*. If diseases had only one cause, then every person exposed to a particular pathogen would become infected. For example, every person with a diet high in saturated fat would develop blocked arteries. But disease susceptibility is often related to a number of causes, such as the following:

- How the body system was created during development of the embryo/fetus
- How effective the body's defense and repair functions are
- How severe or prolonged the body's exposure is to the pathogen, toxin, or other damaging factor

During the following discussion on some common neurologic conditions, keep in mind that the reason for disease development usually cannot be attributed to a single cause.

▶ Stroke

As mentioned previously, a stroke (brain attack) is a serious medical condition in which blood supply to areas of the brain is interrupted, causing ischemia. A stroke is also known as a cerebrovascular accident (CVA). People older than 65 years represent almost 75% of all patients who have strokes.[3] The American Heart Association (AHA) reports that a significant number of patients who have strokes either deny their symptoms or do not understand what their symptoms mean.[4] Many patients fail to activate EMS and consequently delay care. The goal of treatment, as recommended by the AHA, is early recognition and rapid, appropriate intervention. The longer the stroke continues, the less likely the patient will have a promising outcome, because "time is brain." Early recognition begins with an EMS system that can effectively identify potential strokes at dispatch and rapidly request the appropriate resources. As an EMS provider, do not delay your response to a patient with a potential stroke. According to the AHA, one-fifth of patients with an intracranial hemorrhage will have a significant decrease in their LOC between emergency medical care provided by EMS and care upon transfer to the ED. Again, time is brain!

Pathophysiology

Neurologic conditions can have a vascular origin. Vascular emergencies can occur suddenly or gradually. Sudden occurrences are typically the result of emboli or aneurysms Figure 18-10. If a blood vessel is suddenly blocked, as in an embolism, then the cells beyond the blockage can become ischemic. As oxygen and glucose levels drop, brain cells turn to anaerobic metabolism to stay alive. This mechanism, however, is only a stopgap measure. Anaerobic metabolism creates only minuscule amounts

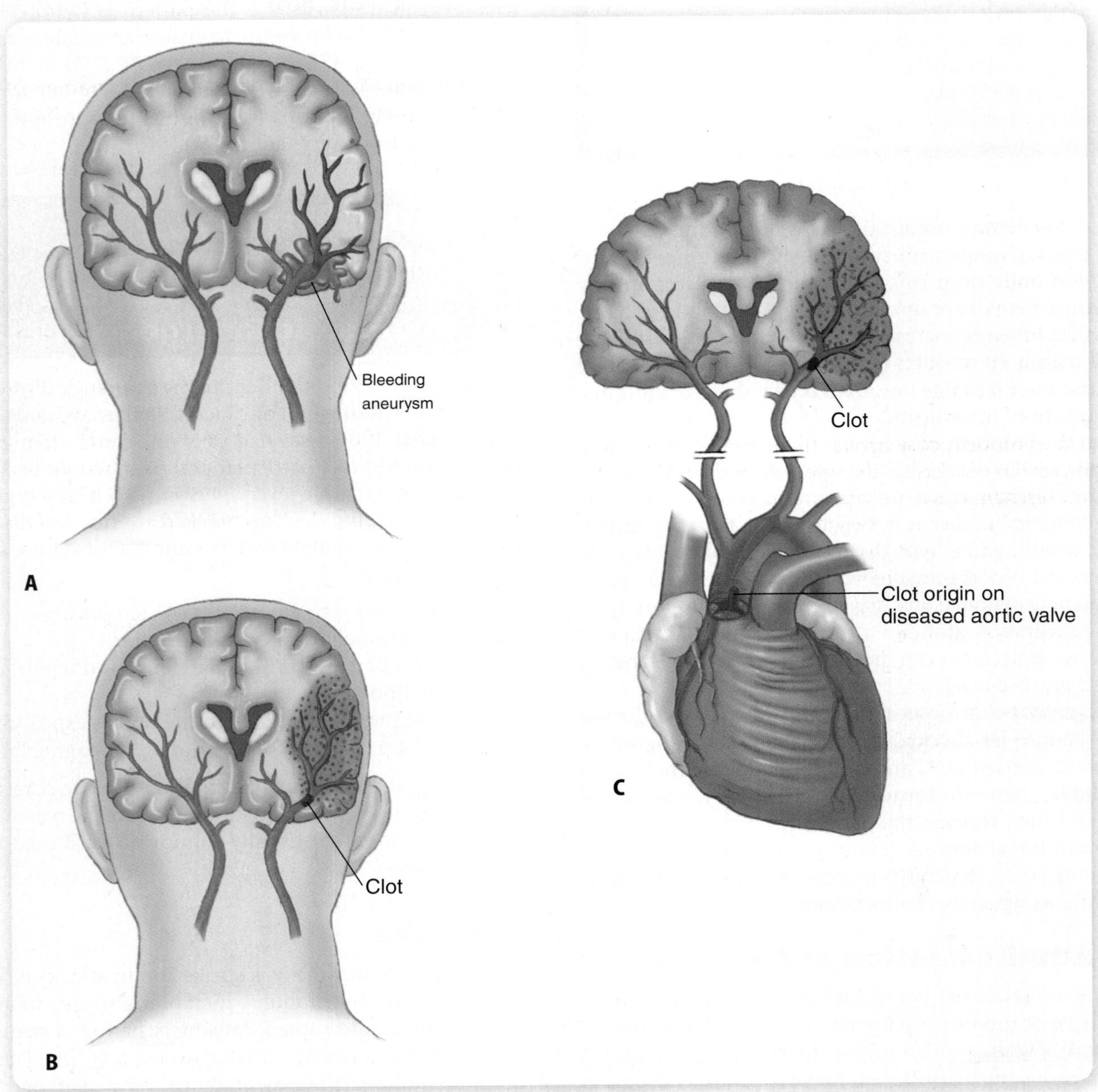

Figure 18-10 Vascular causes of neurologic conditions. **A.** An aneurysm is an area of weakness in the wall of an artery that can bulge out and eventually leak or rupture. **B.** Atherosclerosis can damage the wall of a cerebral artery, narrowing the artery or producing a clot. When the vessel is completely blocked, brain cells begin to die. **C.** An embolus is a blood clot formed elsewhere in the body, often on a diseased heart valve. It can travel through the vascular system and lodge in a cerebral artery, causing a stroke.

of energy for the cell and produces acidic by-products. If circulation is not returned quickly, then the cell will not have enough fuel to survive.

Artery walls consist of three layers of tissue that lie on top of each other. An aneurysm is a weakness in one or more of those layers. The process of aneurysm development is as follows:

1. Small tears or defects occur within the arterial wall.
2. Blood enters between the layers of the artery.
3. Pressure builds up, and the initial small tear increases in size.

If this process continues, then the arterial wall will become so damaged that it can no longer withstand the normal pressure of blood flowing through the artery. The weakened wall will begin to bulge. If the damage is severe, then the bulging artery can leak or the wall can catastrophically fail, causing an intracranial hemorrhage.

Pathophysiology of Stroke. The two basic types of strokes are **ischemic stroke**, which account for 87% according to the AHA, and **hemorrhagic stroke** which account for 13%.[5] Ischemic strokes are also called occlusive strokes because they are caused by an occlusion (blockage). This blockage can be caused by either a thrombus or embolus. These two causes of strokes have presentation patterns that differ. The graph shown in Figure 18-11 provides some insight into the evolution of a stroke. In an ischemic stroke, a blood vessel is blocked so the tissue distal to the blockage becomes ischemic. Eventually that tissue will die if blood flow is not returned. But this pathology is self-limiting. Only the tissue beyond the blockage is affected, so the area or areas of the brain involved are limited.

Notice how the line representing signs and symptoms stops climbing and begins to stabilize. This stabilization does not imply that a patient cannot die from an ischemic stroke. The exact extent of the stroke and its severity are dictated by the artery involved and the portion of the brain being denied oxygen. For example, an ischemic stroke in which blood flow to the brainstem is blocked is certainly life threatening. The plateau indicates that signs and symptoms have reached a peak and leveled off because the area of the brain affected is no longer working.

Hemorrhagic strokes have a different pattern. They tend to get worse over time because of bleeding within the cranium. This bleeding can cause increased ICP and brainstem herniation. One of the hallmarks of a hemorrhagic stroke is a chief complaint of the "worst headache of my life." If the patient reports a severe headache and later cannot speak, becomes difficult to arouse, and finally begins showing signs of increased ICP, then strongly consider a hemorrhagic stroke.

It is important to understand the dynamics of ICP. The skull (cranial vault) is filled with three substances: brain, blood, and cerebrospinal fluid (CSF). These three substances exert pressure against the skull and the skull exerts a reflected pressure Figure 18-12. This exchange is balanced, allowing the brain to fit snugly within with skull. If spaces or voids were present within the skull, then the brain would slam into the skull with only minimal head movement. The pressure of these substances within the skull constitutes ICP. Normally, ICP measures from 1 to 20 mm Hg.[6]

Two difficulties arise when the pressure within the cranial vault begins to climb and remains high. First, the brain may become ischemic because of a lack of blood supply and/or the brain may herniate. Herniation is the movement of a structure from its normal location into another space. Portions of the brain can be pushed into different locations, causing tissue damage and potential death. As ICP rises, the amount of blood available to the brain decreases. CPP, the pressure of blood within the cranial vault, begins to fall. (Recall that normal CPP is 70 to 90 mm Hg.) With a CPP below 50 mm Hg, the brain

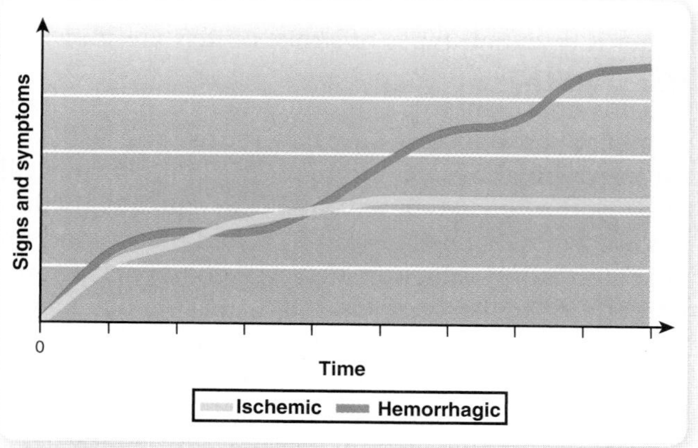

Figure 18-11 Symptom patterns for hemorrhagic compared with ischemic stroke.

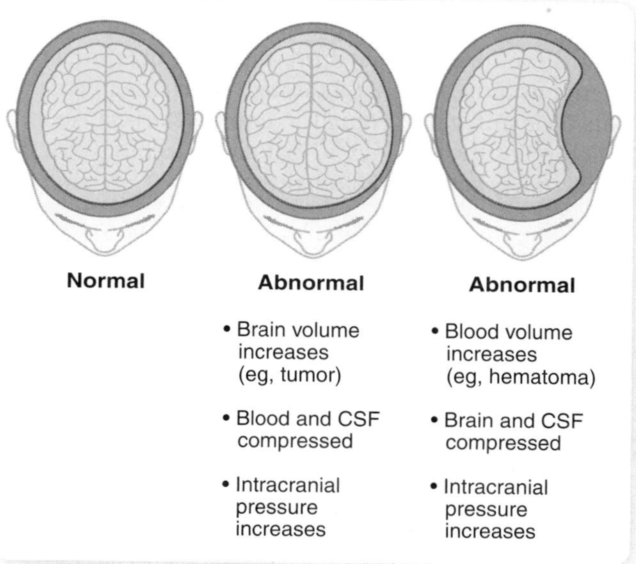

Figure 18-12 Normal and abnormal intracranial pressure.

begins to become ischemic. Use the following equation to calculate CPP:

$$CPP = MAP - ICP$$

The MAP, or mean arterial pressure, is the average (mean) pressure within the blood vessels at any given time. Typically, MAP is about 80 to 90 mm Hg. Many cardiac monitors that have automatic blood pressure readings will display the MAP on the screen.

Consider a patient with the following findings: a MAP of 80 mm Hg and an ICP of 10 mm Hg. These findings indicate that the CPP is 70 mm Hg. However, as ICP rises, CPP falls. An ICP of 15 mm Hg in the same patient will result in a CPP of 65 mm Hg. This condition results in less blood into the brain.

As another example, consider a patient with multisystem trauma. If the patient's blood pressure drops because of bleeding while the ICP is elevated, then severe cerebral ischemia may result. A MAP of 60 mm Hg with an ICP of 15 mm Hg will result in a CPP of 45 mm Hg—which is below the minimum blood flow requirements to keep the brain supplied with oxygen. Refer to Chapter 34, *Head and Spine Trauma*, for an in-depth discussion of this topic.

As with most readings within the body, ICP changes constantly. Coughing, vomiting, or bearing down, for instance, tends to increase ICP. These momentary spikes in ICP are not harmful. If blood, swelling, pus, or a tumor within the cranial vault are present, then ICP will increase and remain high. The volume of the cranial vault is limited and inflexible, so the pressure increases as more and more substances are squeezed into this space. Patients can have life-threating issues when ICP rises sharply and/or blood pressure becomes critically low.

The second possible outcome of increased ICP is herniation; specifically, a shift of the intracranial contents within the cranial vault or displacement of the contents toward the foramen magnum, the large opening at the inferior portion of the skull through which the spinal cord exits. This shift will eventually compress the brainstem, at which point the patient will experience a loss of control of his or her autonomic functions.

Assessment

Stroke causes sudden-onset changes in neurologic status. As mentioned previously, patients can exhibit any combination of the following signs and symptoms:

- **Language effects.** Slurred speech, aphasia, agnosia, and apraxia
- **Movement effects.** Hemiparesis, hemiplegia, arm drifting, facial droop, tongue deviation, swallowing difficulties, ptosis, and ataxia
- **Sensory effects.** Headache (hemorrhagic), sudden blindness, and sudden unilateral paresthesia
- **Cognitive effects.** Decreased LOC, difficulty thinking, seizures, and coma
- **Cardiac effects.** Hypertension

You can also use the FAST mnemonic to assess for a stroke:

- **F:** Facial droop
- **A:** Arm drift
- **S:** Speech impairment
- **T:** Time is critical—call 9-1-1

Vital signs may provide evidence of whether a patient has increased pressure within the cranium. Refer to Table 18-4 to distinguish signs of increased ICP from those of shock. Recall that other signs of increased ICP include posturing, abnormal respiratory patterns, and unequal pupils.

Documentation & Communication

Patients with strokes can present with a wide range of communication difficulties.

- Patients who are multilingual may have a loss of understanding of one language but not another.
- Patients may be able to understand the written word but not the spoken word.
- Patients may not be able to understand any form of communication.

Be open to trying various ways to communicate. Remember, communication challenges do not indicate that the patient is not thinking. The problem is that the patient cannot get you to understand what he or she is thinking.

Management

Management of the neurologic patient begins with the standard care guideline as discussed previously. Because time is brain, prompt evaluation and transport to a stroke center is essential. Types of stroke centers are shown in Table 18-7.

It is important to monitor the patient. A significant number of patients who have had a stroke will also have cardiac dysrhythmias. Continuous ECG monitoring will allow you to quickly intervene if the patient's rhythm destabilizes. Obtain a 12-lead ECG and draw blood for later laboratory evaluation; however, do not delay transport to accomplish these tasks. If the patient has a fever, then contact medical control. You may be ordered to give acetaminophen. Unless the patient is hypoxic, allow the patient to remain supine.[4]

In patients who are unresponsive *and* demonstrate other signs of increased ICP, administer fluids as needed to maintain near-normal systolic blood pressure. Unless you suspect a possible cervical spine injury, elevate the

Table 18-7 Types of Stroke Centers

American Heart Association/ American Stroke Association Designation	Capabilities	Types of Patients
Acute Stroke Ready Hospital (ASRH)	IV thrombolytics with subsequent transfer to PSC/CSC	Uncomplicated stroke
Primary Stroke Center (PSC)	IV thrombolytics; may have microsurgical aneurysm/ carotid artery management and endovascular therapy	Uncomplicated stroke
Comprehensive Stroke Center (CSC)	IV thrombolytics; microsurgical aneurysm/carotid artery management; endovascular therapy	Complicated stroke

Abbreviation: IV, intravenous

Modified from: Stroke Certification Programs – Program Concept Comparison. The Joint Commission website. https://www.jointcommission.org/assets/1/18/StrokeProgramGrid_abbr_AHA-TJC_5-1-15.pdf. Accessed January 7, 2017.

patient's head 30 degrees.[4] Keep the head and neck in neutral alignment without flexing the neck. This position will cause a slight decrease in ICP and allow the patient to better manage any airway secretions. Ensure the airway is clear, but do not vigorously suction because stimulating the cough and gag reflexes will increase ICP. Watch for seizures and be prepared to administer benzodiazepines. The patient may have bradycardia. However, atropine and transcutaneous pacing are not indicated because of the systolic hypertension that accompanies the bradycardia. The ICP is causing the bradycardia, not the other way around. Notify the hospital and provide prompt transport.

It is important for you to monitor blood pressure closely in any patient with a potential problem with ICP. Frequent assessment becomes even more critical when a decrease in blood pressure is also present. For any patient at risk for ICP, ensure the systolic blood pressure remains at least 110 to 120 mm Hg.

Carbon dioxide (CO_2) levels are also important in patients with increased ICP. A high CO_2 level causes vasodilation of the cerebral arteries. This vasodilation allows more blood into the skull, increasing ICP. Alternatively, a diminished level of CO_2 lowers ICP by causing vasoconstriction, decreasing blood supply to the brain. Increasing ventilation, then, decreases ICP (good) by decreasing blood supply (bad). This incompatibility can make decision making difficult because prehospital treatment is simply not effective at decreasing ICP. Provide ventilatory support at a rate of 20 breaths/min.[7] Do not increase the rate any higher than 30 breaths/min. Capnography is the ideal method; using $ETCO_2$ readings, ventilate to maintain a $ETCO_2$ at 30 to 35 mm Hg.[4]

Consider the AHA's algorithm showing goals for the management of patients with suspected stroke **Figure 18-13**. Treatment at the hospital takes different paths of care for each type of stroke. One feature, however, is common to both: Time is essential. For ischemic strokes, fibrinolytics need to be administered within 3 to 4.5 hours of onset. This time limit may be extended, depending on how the fibrinolytics are administered. In hemorrhagic strokes, the more the patient bleeds into the cranium, the greater the potential for increased ICP and herniation.

Evidence-Based Medicine

The National Model EMS Clinical Guidelines from the National Association of State EMS Officials indicate the following considerations regarding head injury[8]:

- Moderate to severe head injury: Continuous waveform capnography and $ETCO_2$ measurement, if available
- Supraglottic airway or endotracheal intubation only if bag-mask ventilation is inadequate to maintain adequate oxygenation. Target $ETCO_2$ level is 35 to 40 mm Hg.
- Severe head injury with signs of herniation: Hyperventilation to target $ETCO_2$ level of 30 to 35 mm Hg. This is a short-term option, and it is only indicated for patients with severe head injury (GCS is ≤ 8 or U [unresponsive] on the AVPU scale) with signs of herniation.

Hyperventilation is defined by the Brain Trauma Foundation as follows[7]:

- 20 breaths/min in an adult
- 25 breaths/min in a child
- 30 breaths/min in an infant (younger than 1 year)

The goal of hyperventilation is an $ETCO_2$ level of 30 to 35 mm Hg. Capnography is the preferred method for monitoring ventilation. If capnography is unavailable, then ventilate the patient to 20 breaths/min until signs of herniation either subside or diminish.

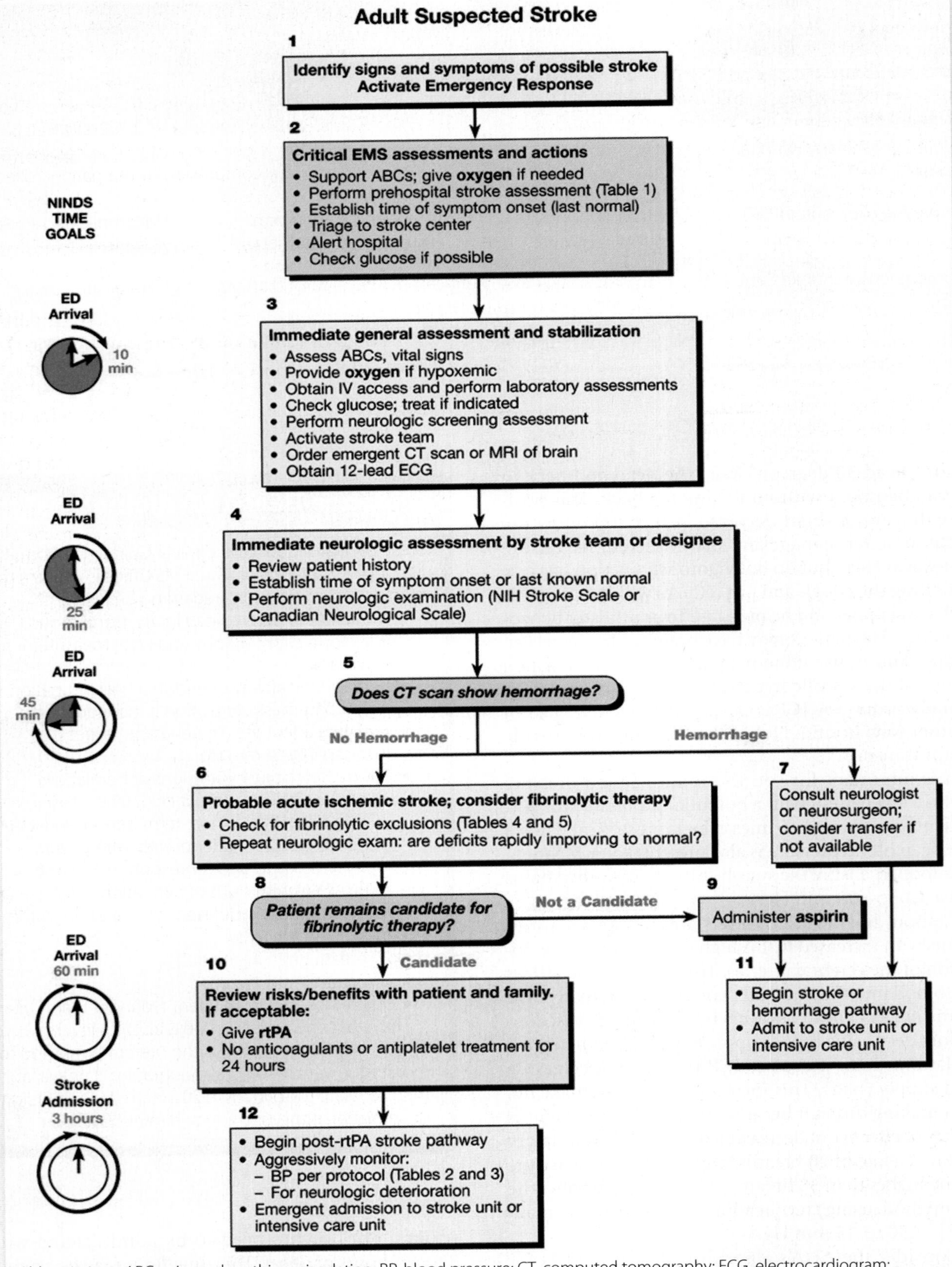

Figure 18-13 The Adult Suspected Stroke Algorithm from the American Heart Association.

The AHA and the American Stroke Association (ASA) recommend a comprehensive approach to the emergency medical care of the patient experiencing a stroke. The general public needs to be educated as to the signs and symptoms of stroke. The public then needs to call 9-1-1 so trained dispatchers can summon the appropriate prehospital resources. As an EMS provider, you need to have adequate training in the delivery of care to patients with strokes, including which patients would benefit from a stroke center. After the patient arrives in the ED, a coordinated and comprehensive approach to care is essential. Some patients will benefit from fibrinolytics, some need intra-arterial clot removal, and others may need neurosurgery. After care has been delivered and the stroke mitigated, appropriate rehabilitation needs to be considered to ensure the patient returns to the highest quality of life possible.

All EMS providers need to be involved in educating the community about stroke signs and symptoms, the effects of strokes, and how to activate EMS. Too many patients deny their symptoms or drive themselves to EDs. Patients need to understand that immediately on discovering stroke symptoms, they must call EMS for assistance.

In addition, all levels of EMS providers should be trained to recognize stroke signs and symptoms. Rapid identification is imperative. Time is brain, and IV fibrinolytic agents must be administered within 3 to 4.5 hours of stroke onset. The checklist presented in Table 18-8 will help you focus on gathering the information that the ED physician will need before fibrinolytics can be considered. Patients who receive fibrinolytic therapy need to be evaluated to determine whether the medication will be helpful. Talk quickly with the family or caregivers to gather medical history, discharge instructions, all medications, allergy information, transfer orders, etc. During the assessment phase, use a standard stroke assessment tool, such as the Cincinnati Prehospital Stroke Scale Table 18-9 to increase the accuracy of your field impressions. You may also use the Los Angeles Prehospital Stroke Screen Table 18-10.

Documentation & Communication

Neurologic emergencies can produce feelings of confusion, fear, anger, and helplessness. Therefore, you need to provide emotional support for the patient and family. A therapeutic, gentle touch on the shoulder can communicate your compassion to the patient. Use a calm, reassuring voice to reorient the patient and tell him or her that you are there to help.

YOU are the Paramedic PART 3

Your patient is calm, but you have to make multiple requests before he complies. You ask him if he has a headache he shakes his head "no." He also denies chest pain, shortness of breath, and abdominal pain. After many yes or no questions, you determine that he awoke about 2 hours ago. He has been unable to speak since that time. The patient's wife gave him 325 mg of aspirin before your arrival. His wife states that he had an episode of left-sided weakness about a year ago. The cause was unclear, but his physician did not think he had experienced a stroke.

Recording Time: 5 Minutes	
Respirations	16 breaths/min, calm
Pulse	112 beats/min, regular
Skin	Warm, pink, dry
Blood pressure	142/96 mm Hg
Oxygen saturation (Spo_2)	98% on room air
Pupils	PERRLA
Blood glucose level	164 mg/dL

6. Which portion of the neurologic assessment is inconsistent with the remainder of the exam?
7. If this patient is having a stroke, then how will the aspirin affect him?

Table 18-8 Sample Prehospital Fibrinolytic Checklist for Stroke

Use this checklist for all patients suspected of having a stroke.		
DATE: ________ TIME: ________		Time signs and symptoms began (record time). If unknown, answer the next question.
DATE: ________ TIME: ________		Time patient was last seen to be normal (record time)
________ mg/dL		Blood glucose level (record number)
_____/_____ Manual Automatic Right arm Left arm		Blood pressure (record readings, circle method and location)
Yes	No	(Check Yes or No for each item.)
❑	❑	Facial droop?
❑	❑	Slurred speech?
❑	❑	Arm drift (eyes closed and held for 10 seconds)?
❑	❑	In the past 7 days, has the patient had a procedure in which an artery was punctured?
❑	❑	In the past 14 days, has the patient had a major operation or serious trauma?
❑	❑	In the past 21 days, has the patient had any bleeding from the gastrointestinal or urinary tract?
❑	❑	In the past 3 months, has the patient experienced an MI, stroke, or head trauma?
❑	❑	When the signs and symptoms began, did the patient have a seizure?
❑	❑	Are current bleeding or clotting problems evident?
❑	❑	Is the patient taking anticoagulant medication?
❑	❑	Does the patient have intracranial bleeding either now or in the past?
❑	❑	Are the patient's signs and symptoms of stroke rapidly improving?

Standard stroke care includes titrating oxygen therapy to the patient's need. Evaluate the patient's pulse oximetry to maintain a Spo_2 level of 94% to 99%.[4] Ensure your Spo_2 reading is accurate. Use other assessment techniques to ensure your patient does not need large amounts of oxygen. From a respiratory point of view, if the patient is in stable condition, then the nasal cannula is probably sufficient.

Evidence-Based Medicine

According to age-old wisdom, "Oxygen is good and more oxygen is better." Oxygen is needed for cellular activity, but for patients in whom cells are being damaged and destroyed, more oxygen is not always better. After the cell membrane fails, cellular materials that were contained within that cell are able to move into the interstitial space. Some of these materials are chemicals (free radicals) that can cause damage to neighboring cells. In an oxygen-rich environment, these free radicals can increase their reactivity and "burn" hotter, causing damage or death to more neighboring cells.

As research continues into this concept, you can expect that conventional wisdom will continue to be challenged. The AHA/ASA report that patients who start with normal Spo_2 levels and receive high concentrations of oxygen have similar outcomes compared with patients with normal Spo_2 levels who receive no supplemental oxygen when experiencing strokes.[4]

Table 18-9 Cincinnati Prehospital Stroke Scale

Assessment	Normal	Abnormal
Facial Droop		
Ask the patient to smile and show his or her teeth.	Both sides of the face move equally.	One side of the face does not move as well as the other side.
Arm Drift		
Ask the patient to close the eyes and hold the arms out with palms up for 10 seconds.	Both arms move the same or neither arm moves. (If neither arm moves, then this may indicate the patient did not understand the instructions. Perform the test again.)	One arm does not move, or one arm drifts down compared with the other.
Speech		
Ask patient to say, "The sky is blue in Cincinnati."	The patient uses correct words with no slurring.	Patient slurs words, uses inappropriate words, or is unable to speak.

Interpretation: If any one item is abnormal, then the probability of a stroke is 72%.

Table 18-10 Los Angeles Prehospital Stroke Screen

Criteria	Yes	Unknown	No
1. Age >45	❑	❑	❑
2. History of seizures or epilepsy absent	❑	❑	❑
3. Symptoms <24 hours	❑	❑	❑
4. At baseline, patient does not use a wheelchair or is not bedridden.	❑	❑	❑
5. Blood glucose level between 60 and 400 mg/dL	❑	❑	❑
6. Obvious asymmetry (right vs. left) in any of the following three exam categories (must be unilateral):	❑	❑	❑
	Equal	**Right Weak**	**Left Weak**
Facial smile/grimace	❑	❑ Droop	❑ Droop
Grip	❑	❑ Weak grip ❑ No grip	❑ Weak grip ❑ No grip
Arm strength	❑	❑ Drifts down ❑ Falls rapidly	❑ Drifts down ❑ Fall rapidly

Interpretation: If criteria 1–6 are marked yes, then the probability of a stroke is 97%.

Currently, no AHA/ASA guideline exists for the prehospital control of hypertension. Do not administer aspirin. As discussed previously, aspirin is helpful in patients with ischemic stroke but is harmful in patients with hemorrhagic stroke. Therefore, you should administer it only after obtaining a computerized tomography (CT) or magnetic resonance imaging (MRI) scan. Because neurologic patients may be unable to feel or move their arms or legs, make sure to protect them from injury.

Complete a fibrinolytic checklist, focusing on when the signs and symptoms began or when the patient was last seen normal. Recall that it can be difficult to pin down the exact time the stroke began. If possible, then transport a family member or significant other who can speak to medical personnel in the ED.

Transport Decisions. Determine an appropriate facility for transport. You should transport patients with strokes to designated stroke centers (facilities with medical teams

Words of Wisdom

Protocols are the beginning of patient care, not the totality of care.

The chronic medical patient is arguably the most complicated type of patient you will encounter. Often, these patients have many diseases to manage and may take numerous different medications. Your protocols are treatment guidelines that provide you with a beginning framework to effectively care for your patient. To be an effective paramedic, you must think critically and adapt to your specific patient. For example, the patient who has had a stroke who also has a history of chronic obstructive pulmonary disease will complicate care. If your patient does not fit well into your protocol, then you need to reach out to your supervisor, your partner, or medical control. These resources can help you deliver safe and effective care to your patient.

Controversies

Imagine the following scenario: You are unsure whether your patient is having an ischemic stroke or a hemorrhagic stroke. The patient wants to go to General Hospital, which does not handle hemorrhagic strokes. Regional Hospital handles both types of strokes but is located 45 minutes away. To make the best decision, you need to determine which type of stroke is present.

In some parts of the country, EMS agencies are using an innovative system to answer this question.[9] Mobile stroke units—ambulances specially equipped with a CT scanner—are typically operated by a paramedic, a critical care nurse, a CT technologist, and an EMS vehicle operator **Figure 18-14**. When a dispatch occurs for a patient with a possible stroke, the portable CT unit is also dispatched. The team arrives, evaluates the patient, and then takes the patient, on the cot, into the mobile stroke unit. A quick scan is performed. This CT scan is transmitted to the hospital, where a neurosurgeon evaluates it to determine if the patient is having a hemorrhagic or ischemic stroke. At the same time, a paramedic and critical care nurse perform a detailed assessment, including blood work. If appropriate, then thrombolytics can be initiated while en route to the closest stroke center.

This novel approach to stroke care prompts many questions, such as the following:

- Does this system decrease the time from initial EMS contact to the administration of thrombolytics?
- Are patients better triaged to the facilities that can best care for them?
- Does this system decrease the amount of neurologic deficit caused by strokes?
- What is the additional cost to the patient for this service?
- Which factors that affect stroke can best be mitigated using this system?

The only way for medicine to advance is to try something new and learn from the experience. This high-tech approach has many attractive aspects. Obviously, time is a major contributor to the devastating effects related to stroke. How long until EMS arrives? How long until a physician evaluates the patient? How long until a CT is done? How long until fibrinolytics are administered? However, this intervention cannot help answer the critical question, "When was the patient last seen normal?"

The AHA/ASA report that fewer than half of all stroke patients who call 9-1-1 did so within 1 hour of the onset of signs and symptoms.[4] If the patient waited several hours before calling 9-1-1, then all the technology in the world may be unable to prevent permanent neurologic damage. So, the real question may be: Is it better to spend money on ways to more quickly get medical care to patients who have had a stroke, or is it better to educate people about strokes so they call 9-1-1 sooner?

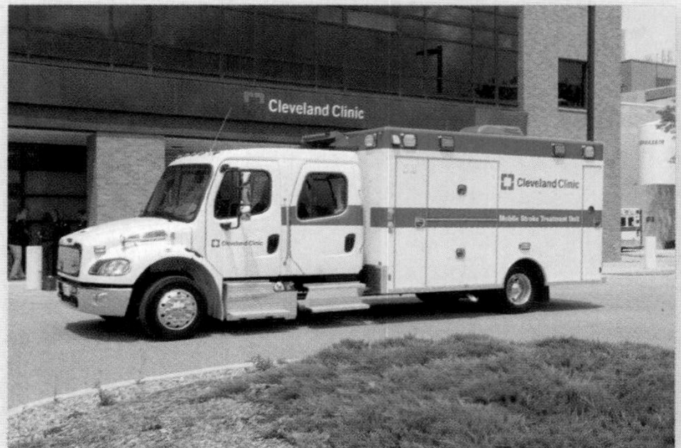

Figure 18-14 A mobile stroke unit.

who are trained in the administration of fibrinolytics and in the diagnosis and management of various types of strokes). If you are more than 1 hour away from a stroke center, then consider air medical transportation. Contact the facility to ensure their CT/MRI capabilities are operational. Some facilities will need to contact scan technicians who are on call during night hours or weekends. Early hospital notification to the ED can decrease the time that elapses before the patient receives a CT/MRI scan. Many facilities now allow ambulance patients to be transported directly to the CT scanner. This initial bypass of the ED can save valuable time, so call ahead to alert the ED. Typically, members of the ED team will meet you and guide you to the CT scanner. While you walk to the scanner, you will be asked to give your verbal report.

If the patient is rapidly decompensating or you suspect a hemorrhagic stroke, then consider transporting the patient to a facility that can perform neurosurgery. Again, call ahead to alert the hospital of the need for rapid evaluation.

▶ Transient Ischemic Attacks

Pathophysiology

Transient ischemic attacks (TIAs) are episodes of cerebral ischemia without any permanent damage. Any of the typical presentations associated with a stroke can occur with TIAs. What makes these different from a stroke is the resolution of signs and symptoms. According to the AHA/ASA, many TIAs resolve completely within 1 hour—which can mean you are dispatched for stroke, but arrive to find a patient who appears perfectly normal.[10]

No residual damage to brain tissue occurs, and no signs and symptoms appear after the episode ends. However, these mini-strokes are often signs of a serious vascular condition that requires medical evaluation. The National Institute of Neurological Disorders and Stroke reports that about one-third of patients with TIAs will have an acute stroke sometime in the future.[11] Think of the relationship between TIA and stroke as the equivalent of the relationship between angina and MI.

Assessment

Any of the signs and symptoms of strokes can occur with a TIA. Your assessment of the patient will therefore be the same whether the patient is experiencing a stroke or a TIA.

Management

To manage TIAs, follow the stroke management guidelines discussed earlier. Close neurologic assessment is needed. Patients may experience a multitude of TIAs, coming and going. Strongly encourage the patient to be transported. If the patient refuses transportation, then appeal to the patient's family for assistance. If the patient still refuses, then encourage him or her to seek medical care soon. It is important to reinforce with the patient that this TIA was a warning sign of a serious and potentially deadly problem with the blood vessels within the brain. Hypertension is the number one preventable cause of strokes and TIAs. Encourage the patient to talk with his or her physician about blood pressure control and to take antihypertensive medications as prescribed.

▶ Coma

Pathophysiology

The call for the unresponsive person is common. One way to remember the most common causes of a decreased LOC is to use the mnemonic AEIOUTIPS Table 18-11. This memory aid will help you focus on general groups of causes. Note that each grouping has a different onset of signs and symptoms.

As with most medical complaints, the history of present illness is vital to determining the underlying cause of the patient's complaints. It would be exceedingly unusual for a person to be absolutely healthy one minute and unresponsive because of an infection the next. A seizure, however, is an example of a condition that can cause unresponsiveness almost instantly.

Assessment

Determine when the patient was last seen functioning normally. Evaluate the speed of onset of the patient's altered LOC. Again, the onset will help to distinguish one cause from another.

The common signs and symptoms of diminished LOC and imminent coma are as follows:

- **Cognitive effects.** Decreasing LOC, confusion, hallucinations, delusions, psychosis, difficulty thinking, and sleepiness
- **Speech effects.** Slurred speech, agnosia, apraxia, and aphasia
- **Movement effects.** Ataxia, aphagia, seizures, and posturing
- **General CNS effects.** Total unresponsiveness (coma)

It can be difficult to determine the cause of an altered LOC. However, finding the cause will allow you to more effectively treat the patient and focus your care. See Figure 18-15 for an algorithm based on AEIOUTIPS, which may help you to progress to the correct area of your protocol.

Management

The focus of care for patients who are comatose occurs in two stages. First, support vital functions. Following the standard care guideline should allow you to secure and maintain the ABCs effectively. The second goal is to gather information about the possible cause of the altered LOC or coma. Gather past medical history, evaluate medications, look for signs of trauma, and determine the history of the present illness. This information will help you direct your

Table 18-11 AEIOUTIPS: Altered Mental Status Causes

Letter	Name	Onset	Signs and Symptoms	Treatment Focus
A	Alcohol	Acute (hours) Chronic (days)	Intoxication; slurred speech; ataxia; odor of alcohol on breath; tremors; hallucinations	Ensure oxygen, glucose, and temperature for proper brain functioning. Consider thiamine with dextrose.
	Acidosis	Acute (hours)	Multiple causes; tachypnea and hyperpnea are common	Ventilation Sodium bicarbonate
E	Epilepsy (seizure)	Sudden (seconds)	Aura; hypertonic, tonic-clonic activity; postictal state	If prolonged, then diazepam (Valium) or lorazepam (Ativan)
	Endocrine	Chronic (days to weeks)	For thyroid conditions, increased metabolism (hyperthermia, hypertension, tachypnea, tachycardia) OR decreased metabolism (hypothermia, bradycardia, bradypnea, and hypotension)	Supportive care. See Chapter 23, *Endocrine Emergencies,* for more information.
	Electrolytes	Acute (hours) Chronic (days)	Dehydration; renal failure; liver failure; ECG changes, etc	Ensure adequate circulating volume; monitor ECG
I	Insulin	Acute (hours)	Diaphoresis; tachycardia; tremors; ataxia	Dextrose or glucagon
O	Opiates	Acute (minutes to hours)	Constricted pupils; decreased LOC; bradypnea; cyanosis	Naloxone (Narcan). Be prepared to administer additional doses as needed.
	Other drugs	Acute to gradual (hours to days, depending on agent)	Varies depending on agent involved; track marks; drug paraphernalia	Administration of selected drugs; consider naloxone (Narcan).
U	**Uremia** (kidney failure)	Gradual (days to weeks)	Nausea/vomiting; uremic frost; muscle cramping; dysrhythmias; pulmonary edema	Ensure oxygen, glucose, and temperature for proper brain functioning.
T	Trauma	Sudden (seconds)	Generally, hypotension causes altered LOC or direct head injury.	Consider manual in-line-stabilization; ensure adequate blood pressure.
	Temperature	Acute to gradual (hours to days, depending on mechanism)	Hyperthermia (exertional, environmental, or endocrine); hypothermia (environmental, endocrine, situational [eg, immobile person lying on floor for days])	Stop cooling or heating process—get patient inside, take off wet clothing, get off cold floor. Assess for trauma and other medical conditions. See Chapter 23, *Endocrine Emergencies,* and Chapter 38, *Environmental Emergencies,* for more information.

Letter	Name	Onset	Signs and Symptoms	Treatment Focus
I	Infection	Gradual (hours to days)	Fever; rash; malaise; tachycardia; tachypnea; skin may be cold or warm depending on degree of infection	Ensure adequate blood pressure.
P	Poisoning	Acute to gradual (hours to days, depending on agent)	Varies depending on agent involved; empty pill bottles; chemical odors within a child's mouth; broken leaves of plants, open containers of pesticide	Supportive care based on the suspected agent involved. See Chapter 27, *Toxicology*, for more information.
	Psychogenic causes	Sudden (seconds) History of mental illness or substance abuse is typical	Delusions; hallucinations; disorganization; bizarre behavior or posture	Ensure oxygen, glucose, and temperature for proper brain functioning; restraints and sedation may be needed.
S	Shock	Acute to gradual (hours to days, depending on mechanism)	Decreased blood pressure and other signs of poor perfusion	Ensure adequate circulating volume; administer vasopressors if needed.
	Stroke	Sudden (seconds to hours)	Facial droop; slurred speech; ataxia; abnormal/irregular respiratory pattern; potential bradycardia	Ensure oxygen, glucose, and temperature for proper brain functioning.
	Syncope	Acute onset	Prodrome of weakness or loss of peripheral vision, then LOC which resolves quickly.	Ensure adequate circulating volume, oxygenation and cardiac rhythm. Check for trauma that may have occurred during fall.
	Space-occupying lesion	Gradual, subtle changes	Headache; new onset seizures; stroke-like symptoms	Treat for stroke/seizure
	Subarachnoid hemorrhage	Acute (minutes to hours)	Thunderclap headache; worst headache of life; signs and symptoms of stroke; seizures	Treat for stroke/seizure

Abbreviations: ECG, electrocardiogram; LOC, level of consciousness

care to the most likely cause. As always, a good assessment is the foundation of excellent patient care.

It is not uncommon to have too little information to determine a cause. This fact should not deter you from looking for one. Is the patient wearing medical identification tags? How was the patient acting before you were called? Do you see drug paraphernalia near the patient? This information can be crucial to providing the continued, quality care this patient will need to return to health. If you suspect that the patient may have taken a narcotic, then administer naloxone, 0.4 to 2 mg IVP, as discussed in Chapter 27, *Toxicology*.

Finally, do not think you are a poor paramedic if you cannot find the cause of the patient's altered LOC. In such a case, report to the ED staff that you do not know what is wrong with the patient, and then report what is *not* wrong. For example, advise that you have checked the patient's blood glucose level, given naloxone, and gathered a large amount of information, and the patient does not appear to have had a stroke. The cause of the patient's condition may

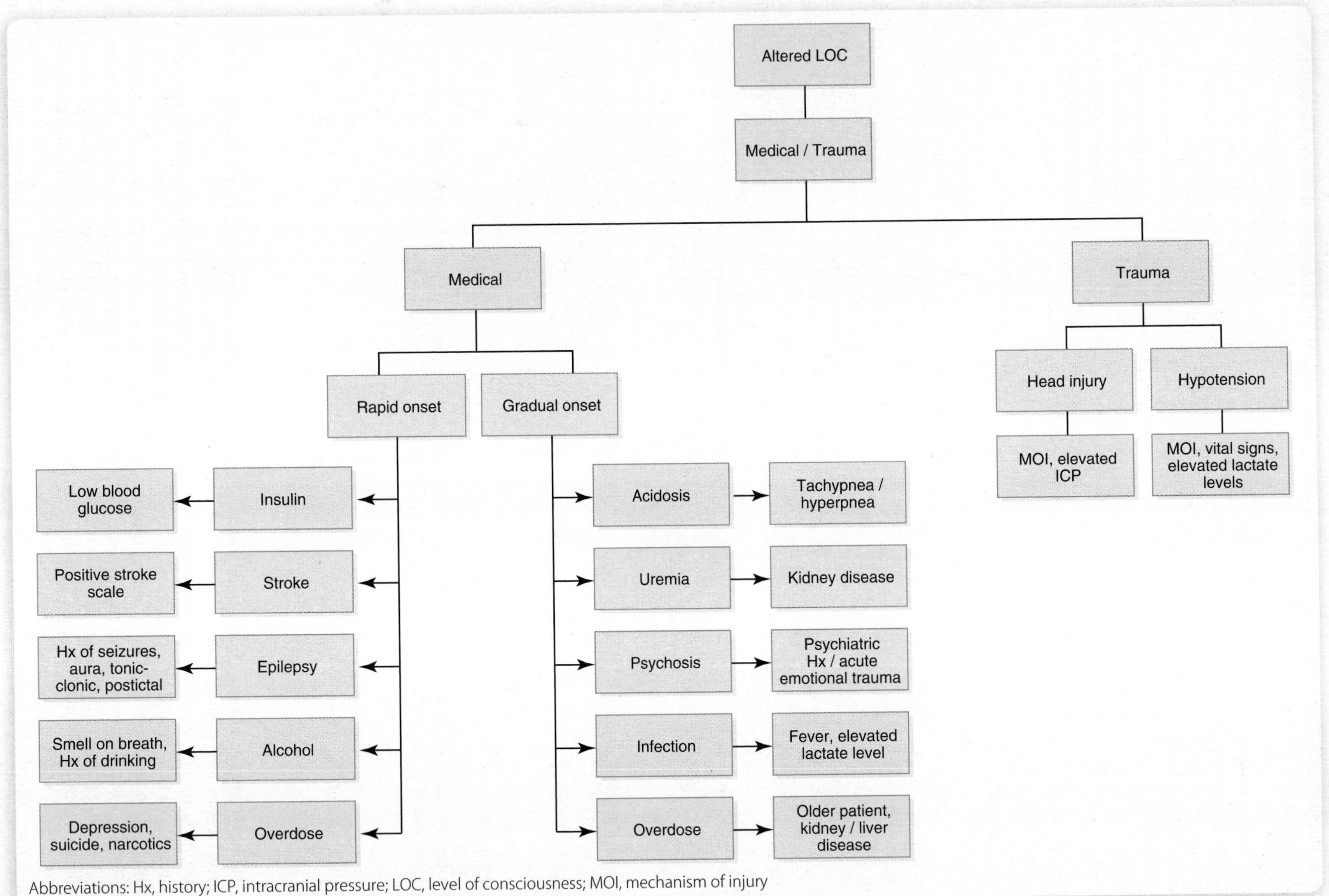

Figure 18-15 Altered level of consciousness algorithm.

be unclear, but you can still provide excellent emergency medical care while you diligently attempt to determine the cause. The practice of medicine is sometimes more a process of ruling out conditions than ruling them in.

In-hospital care will focus on supporting the ABCs, and attempting to discover or confirm a diagnosis. Patients will routinely need urine and blood analysis, conventional radiography, and CT/MRI scans.

▶ Seizures

Pathophysiology

Recall that a seizure is the sudden, erratic firing of neurons. Patients can experience a wide array of signs and symptoms when having seizures, such as muscle spasms, increased secretions, diaphoresis, and cyanosis. A seizure can be limited to the shaking of one hand or a metallic taste in the mouth, or it can involve the movement of every limb or the complete loss of consciousness. Patients may be aware of the seizure or wake up afterwards not knowing what happened. Each of these experiences is defined as a seizure if it is brought on by the random firing of neurons.

If a seizure continues for a long period, then profound changes occur within the brain and body. Cerebral glucose and oxygen supplies can be depleted. Systemic (body-wide) hypoxia, hypercapnia, blood pressure changes, and hyperthermia can occur. A single, short duration seizure is typically not a major life-threatening concern. However, if seizures group together and/or last for long periods, then these complications can cause serious long-term effects to the patient, including death. It is also not uncommon for EMS personnel to be dispatched for a seizure patient, only to arrive and find a patient in cardiac arrest. What happened? The patient experienced a lethal dysrhythmia, blood pressure dropped, blood flow to the brain dropped, and subsequently, the patient seized.

As with most medical patients, try to determine the cause of the problem—in this case, the seizure. Ask about medication compliance. Phenytoin (Dilantin), lorazepam (Ativan), carbamazepine (Tegretol), and valproic acid (Depakene) are common anticonvulsant medications. For various reasons, however, patients may have taken an insufficient amount of medication to prevent seizures. Patients may stop taking their medication because they have not had a seizure in several months and believe they are cured. Children can outgrow the dosage of their anticonvulsant medication. Older adults may be unable to afford the medication entirely.

In infants, a common cause of seizure is fever (febrile seizure). Febrile seizures will be covered in Chapter 43, *Pediatric Emergencies*. Seizure may also occur in people with diabetes who have a low blood glucose level. Knowing the cause of the seizure will help you direct management. Some common causes of seizure are listed in Table 18-12.

Generalized Seizures. Recall that seizures can be classified as either generalized (affecting large portions of the brain) or partial (affecting a limited area of the brain).

YOU are the Paramedic — PART 4

The patient's condition does not change during transport to the hospital. Because you called ahead to the closest stroke center, a stroke team is awaiting your arrival. You are advised to take the patient directly to the CT scanner. You give your report to the emergency physician while you assist in transferring the patient from your cot onto the CT scanner. You then write your patient care report. As you leave, the emergency physician tells you the CT scan was unremarkable, with no sign of stroke or bleeding. She is beginning to consider nonstroke causes of this patient's muteness and other symptoms. The ED staff will continue to monitor the patient for several hours.

Recording Time: 15 Minutes	
Respirations	20 breaths/min
Pulse	116 beats/min, regular
Skin	Warm, dry, normal
Blood pressure	146/96 mm Hg
Oxygen saturation (Spo_2)	98% on room air
Pupils	PERRLA

8. What are other possible causes of stroke-like presentations?
9. Were you correct to treat this patient as if he had experienced a stroke?

Table 18-12 Common Causes of Seizures

- **Abscess**
- Alcohol
- Birth anomaly
- Brain infections (meningitis, encephalitis)
- Brain trauma
- Diabetes mellitus
- Fever (rapid rate of rise)
- Hypertension during pregnancy (eclampsia)
- **Idiopathic** (of no known cause)
- Inappropriate medication dosage
- Organic brain syndromes
- Recreational drug use (cocaine)
- Stroke or TIA
- Systemic infection
- Tumor
- Uremia (kidney failure)

Abbreviation: TIA, transient ischemic attack

The two types of generalized seizures are tonic-clonic and absence seizures.

Tonic-Clonic Seizures. Tonic-clonic seizures, formerly called grand mal seizures, present you with the greatest assessment challenges.[12] This type of seizure has a peculiar pattern. Most tonic-clonic seizures proceed through each of the following steps in sequence (however, some patients may not experience every step):

1. Loss of consciousness
2. Tonic phase: Systemic rigidity
3. Hypertonic phase: Arched back and rigidity
4. Clonic phase: Intermittent contractions of major muscle groups: arms, legs, head movement, lip smacking, biting, clenching teeth. Contractions are chaotic, disorganized, and of small amplitude. Imagine ventricular fibrillation (VF) of the brain—that is what a seizure is electrically.
5. Postseizure: Major muscles relax, and **nystagmus** (an involuntary, rhythmic eye movement) may still be occurring. Eyes may be looking posterior (at back of head).
6. **Postictal** phase: Reset period of the brain. It can take several minutes to hours before the patient gradually returns to his or her pre-seizure LOC. During this time, the patient may display the following signs:
   - Initially aphasic (unable to speak)
   - Confused or unable to follow commands
   - Emotional
   - Tired
   - Headache
   - Gradual return of normal brain function

Words of Wisdom

Tonic-clonic seizures are very difficult to mimic or fake. If you care for a patient who is demonstrating coordinated seizure activity, then suspect a pseudoseizure. The patient may also be faking the seizure. Report your findings to the ED before administering any benzodiazepines.

Tonic-clonic seizures are disconcerting for both family and health care providers to watch. During the seizure process, respiration may become erratic, loud, and obviously abnormal. Alternatively, the patient may stop breathing and become cyanotic. These periods of apnea are usually short lived and do not require intervention. If the patient is apneic for more than 30 seconds, then immediately begin ventilatory assistance. Another disconcerting aspect of seizures, particularly for the patient, is incontinence.

Pseudoseizures. Pseudoseizures, or psychogenic nonepileptic seizures, are a generalized neurologic event. Symptomatically, you may not notice any difference from a tonic-clonic seizure. Tonic-clonic motion, loss of consciousness, and a postictal phase are all present during these events. The difference is that in pseudoseizures, the root cause is of psychiatric origin. It is important to understand that in most cases of pseudoseizure, the patient is not intentionally causing this behavior.

Patients with pseudoseizures present with loss of consciousness, which is usually triggered by some emotional event, stress, lights, or pain. Pseudoseizures conspicuously occur with witnesses. This fact may lead health care providers to believe pseudoseizures are contrived. Motion that occurs during the seizure is relatively organized—side-to-side movement of the head, pedaling movements of the legs (like riding a bicycle), weeping, or stuttering. These patients often have a psychiatric history and/or other medical history, such as fibromyalgia, chronic pain, or chronic fatigue.

Absence Seizures. In contrast to tonic-clonic seizures, absence seizures (formerly called petit mal seizures) present with little or no movement. The typical patient with absence seizures is a child. Classically, the child will simply stop—stop walking, stop speaking mid-sentence, or stop playing and freeze with a toy in the hand. The child rarely falls. Absence seizures usually last no more than several seconds, with no postictal period and no confusion. Flashing lights or hyperventilation may bring on this type of seizure.

Partial Seizures. Partial seizures affect a limited portion of the brain and can be further divided into either simple partial or complex partial seizures. Partial seizures can be localized to just one spot within the brain, or they can begin in one spot and spread to other locations. Like dropping a pebble in a still pond, this wavelike movement is called a **Jacksonian march**.

Simple partial seizures involve either movement of one part of the body (frontal lobe) or sensations in one part of the body (parietal lobe). An example of a Jacksonian march in a simple partial seizure is shaking of the left hand, which moves to the left arm, then shoulder, then head, then right arm, then right hand, and finally moves out of the body. Complex partial seizures involve subtle changes in LOC. Here the patient can become confused or less alert, have hallucinations, or become unable to speak. Some small movements of the head or eyes may occur. Patients typically do not become unresponsive.

Patients with partial seizures tend to experience an aura before the seizure occurs. It might be a muscle twitch, a funny taste, or the perception of seeing lights or hearing a high-pitched noise.

The classification of seizures is summarized in Table 18-13.

Assessment

Whether they are generalized or partial, most seizures are self-limiting and all you need to do is monitor and protect patients from injuring themselves. Other important characteristics of your assessment of a patient with a seizure are listed below:

- How long did the seizure last? What did it look like to bystanders or family?
- Describe the seizure as best as possible (unique body motions, regions of the body involved, body positions, etc).
- Does the patient have a history of seizures?
  - How many seizures does the patient normally have in a day or week? How long do they last? What do they look like?
  - Is the patient taking antiseizure medication as prescribed?
  - Have any recent changes to medications occurred?
  - Were any medications administered by bystanders?
- Does the patient have a recent history of head trauma, overdose, pregnancy, diabetes, hypoglycemia, or heat exposure?
- Was the patient incontinent or apneic during the seizure?
- Does the patient have a fever?
- Was the patient apneic, cyanotic, and/or vomiting?
- Did the patient experience bowel or bladder incontinence?

Together with your thorough assessment, the answers to these questions will help the ED staff determine the cause of the seizure.

Management

To manage a seizure, begin with the standard care guideline for the neurologic patient. Quickly determine whether trauma is a concern. Where was the patient before the seizure? What was the patient doing before the seizure? How did the patient get to his or her current position? If trauma is unclear or confirmed, then perform manual in-line stabilization.

If you arrive during the seizure, then do not restrain or try to stop the seizing movement. Remain calm and prevent the patient from striking objects and becoming injured. Do not place anything in the patient's mouth while the patient is seizing. If bystanders have placed objects in the patient's mouth (for example, a spoon or a butter knife inserted sideways), then remove them. If you believe the event is a pseudoseizure, then treat it like any other seizure. Do not dismiss this behavior as a patient acting out. Correct hypoglycemia by giving IV glucose as needed; otherwise, most seizures are self-limiting. You may need to provide ventilatory assistance if the patient's seizure or apnea is prolonged, but it is difficult to ventilate a patient who is actively having a seizure. It is next to impossible to

Table 18-13 Classification of Seizures

Grouping	Type	Presentation
Generalized	Tonic-clonic (formerly grand mal) Absence (formerly petit mal) Pseudoseizures	Full-body, violent jerking movements Freezing or staring Tonic-clonic but caused by a psychiatric mechanism (the patient is not faking the seizure)
Partial	Simple partial	Shaking of one area of the body Sensation in one area of the body
	Complex partial	Subtle alterations in LOC

Abbreviation: LOC, level of consciousness

perform oral or nasotracheal intubation during a seizure (see the discussion of status epilepticus).

After the seizure, it is important that you provide emotional support. Provide privacy for the patient and speak calmly and slowly. Be prepared to repeat yourself. Reorient the patient to place and time. If the seizure was febrile, then encourage the patient or parents or caregivers to administer medications for fever reduction (acetaminophen or ibuprofen). Consult your protocols for the appropriate administration of OTC medications to patients.

Unless a clear and easily reversible cause for the seizure is found, transport all patients. Seizures can be a warning sign of more serious nervous system condition such as stroke, brain tumor, or severe metabolic imbalance. If the patient has a known history of seizures, then he or she may not wish to go to the hospital. Advise the patient to follow up with his or her physician within 24 hours. The patient with diabetes who is awakened after administration of glucose may also not wish to be transported. Advise the patient to eat a good meal and follow up with his or her physician.

It may be difficult to differentiate a seizure from a stroke. Consider your assessment findings and the past medical history. Patients with a history of seizures can have similar seizure patterns over time. Family can therefore anticipate what will happen. When a patient has a seizure caused by a stroke, however, it is unlikely that the pattern will be the same as that of the patient's baseline seizure. That difference can be a clue. Talk to the patient's family members and friends and determine whether the current seizure is the same as his or her typical seizure. Table 18-14 provides additional guidelines for differentiating between a seizure and a stroke.

If you are concerned that a patient may have a seizure during transport, then establish vascular access so you are prepared to administer diazepam (Valium), lorazepam (Ativan), or midazolam (Versed), the drugs of choice to stop seizures.[8] Place blankets over the rails of the ambulance cot and over any hard surfaces near the patient. Ensure the patient's cot straps are not too tight.

In-hospital management involves determining the cause of the seizure. Hematologic studies, electrolyte level analysis, drug level and blood glucose level, will be ordered. The patient may also need CT and/or MRI scans.

Table 18-14 Differentiating Stroke From Seizure

Characteristic	Stroke	Seizure
Prodromal signs and symptoms	May have a headache	May have an odd taste in the mouth Seeing lights or hearing sounds Twitching
Activity during event	Muscle weakness that is often lateralized (one side)	Generalized body movement that will stop typically within 1-2 min
Response after event	May completely resolve (eg, TIA) May have no change in muscle weakness May progress to worsening symptoms	Slow return of orientation

Abbreviation: TIA, transient ischemic attack

Status Epilepticus

Pathophysiology

Status epilepticus can be defined as a seizure that lasts longer than 4 to 5 minutes or consecutive seizures without a return to consciousness between seizures. This time frame is arbitrary. Some authors suggest status epilepticus does not occur until 30 minutes of uninterrupted seizure activity. Refer to your local protocols for guidelines related to how long a seizure can continue before you should intervene. Status epilepticus is a life-threatening neurologic disorder and it should not be taken lightly. The authors of a 2015 study report that the mortality rate for patients in refractory status epilepticus was 70%.[13]

During a seizure, neurons are in a hypermetabolic state (using large amounts of glucose and producing lactic acid). For a short period, this state does not produce long-term damage. If the seizure continues, then the body becomes unable to remove the waste products effectively or to ensure adequate glucose supplies. Status epilepticus can result in neurons being damaged or killed. The goal of prehospital care is to stop the seizure and to ensure adequate ABCs.

Assessment

Assessment of the patient with status epilepticus is the same as that of the patient experiencing a seizure. The only difference is the length of time that the seizure lasts. In patients with status epilepticus, it is important to ask bystanders or family if any antiseizure medication was administered before you arrived. Epileptic patients may have implanted IV access ports to allow for the administration of benzodiazepines. You may need to adjust your dose of antiseizure medication based on recent dose or doses given by the family.

Management

Follow the standard care guideline for the neurologic patient. Ensure the patient does not have hypoglycemia, and administer a benzodiazepine. These medications may be administered via several routes depending on the drug, although rectal administration is no longer recommended. See Table 18-15 for more information about antiseizure medications. Generally speaking, if two doses of a benzodiazepine have not stopped the seizure, then contact medical control. This guideline applies to all doses, whether they were administered by family or EMS providers.

Be prepared to control airway and ventilation completely because benzodiazepines can cause respiratory depression or arrest. Continue to use airway positioning and bag-mask ventilations until the medication has stopped the seizure. If the seizure cannot be quickly controlled by benzodiazepines and the patient cannot be ventilated, then sedative/paralytics may be needed to allow for adequate airway management.

A subset of patients with tonic-clonic seizures will need a different medication; pregnant patients who are experiencing eclampsia need to be managed with magnesium. More information about eclampsia and its treatment can be found in Chapter 41, *Obstetrics*.

Table 18-15 Antiseizure Medications

Antiseizure Medication	Routes	Administration Considerations
Diazepam (Valium)	IM, IV, IO	IV/IO slowly (over 2 min). IV push into closest port. Do not administer into solutions containing dextrose or lactated Ringer solution.
Midazolam (Versed)	IM, IV, IO, IN	IV/IO slowly (over 2 min).
Lorazepam (Ativan)	IM, IV, IO	IV/IO slowly (over 2 min).

Abbreviations: IM, intramuscular; IO, intraosseous; IV, intravenous; IN, intranasal

Data from: Diazepam injection. Drugs.com website. https://www.drugs.com/pro/diazepam-injection.html. Updated October 2016. Accessed April 9, 2016; Midazolam injection. Drugs.com website. https://www.drugs.com/pro/midazolam-injection.html. Updated November 2016. Accessed April 9, 2016; and Lorazepam injection. Drugs.com website. http://www.drugs.com/pro/lorazepam-injection.html. Updated November 2016. Accessed April 9, 2016.

Syncope

Pathophysiology

Syncope (fainting) is the sudden and temporary loss of consciousness with accompanying loss of postural tone. Syncope can be a sign of life-threatening cardiac dysrhythmia, stroke, or other serious medical condition. Syncope accounts for 1% to 3% of all ED visits.[14] The brain uses glucose at an astounding rate and has no ability to store glucose, so even a 3- to 5-second interruption in blood flow causes loss of consciousness. This interruption in blood flow is the typical underlying reason for syncope. The question is, what caused the sudden decrease in cerebral perfusion? Table 18-16 provides the common causes of syncope.

Assessment

Classically, the patient with syncope is in a standing position when the event occurs. In younger adults, the pattern is usually one of vasovagal syncope. The adult experiences fear, emotional stress, or pain. The person then suddenly experiences a spinning sensation and passes out (which is why you should seat the patient before drawing blood

Table 18-16 Common Causes of Syncope

General Cause	Specific Cause
Cardiac rhythm disturbances	Bradycardia of any type Sick sinus syndrome Supraventricular tachycardia Pacemaker malfunction Torsades de pointes Transient asystole Transient VF Ventricular tachycardia (VT)
Other cardiac causes	Cardiomyopathy MI Cardiac medications (beta-blockers, alpha-blockers, nitrates, digitalis, diuretics) Cardiac valvular insufficiency
Noncardiac causes	Dehydration Hypoglycemia Vasovagal response Pulmonary embolism Situational (during urination, swallowing, or coughing) Other medications (alcohol, cocaine, opioid analgesics, tricyclic antidepressants)

Abbreviations: MI, myocardial infarction; VF, ventricular fibrillation or starting an IV line). In older adults, the more typical cause of syncope is a cardiac dysrhythmia. The patient experiences sudden VT, the blood pressure drops, and the patient falls to the floor. The rhythm terminates, blood pressure rises, and the patient feels fine. In either case, the whole process takes less than 60 seconds.

Patients with syncope usually experience a **prodrome**. Prodromes are the signs or symptoms that precede a disease or condition. For syncope, the prodromal signs and symptoms include feelings of dizziness, weakness, shortness of breath, chest pain, a headache, or the patient stating his or her vision went black. Incontinence is possible with syncope. Gathering information about the situation can also help ED staff to diagnose the cause of syncope. Was the patient hot? Was he or she standing for a long period? Was he or she performing a strenuous activity? Did the patient need to bear down while lifting something heavy? Was alcohol involved? The history of present illness is often invaluable when managing the patient with syncope.

Seizures and syncope can be difficult to differentiate if they are not witnessed. Table 18-17 offers some guidance.

Management

The first step in managing syncope is determining possible trauma during the patient's fall and whether spinal stabilization is needed. Next, focus on blood pressure and cardiac causes. Continuous ECG monitoring and 12-lead ECG evaluation are important. Evaluate the blood glucose level and oxygen saturation level, and obtain orthostatic vital signs. If the patient's blood pressure remains low, then provide fluids or vasopressors as appropriate, based on the cause of the hypotension. Provide emotional support; syncope can be embarrassing. Because you will not know the exact cause of the syncope, it is important to transport any patient with syncope to the hospital.

Table 18-17 Differentiating Syncope from Seizure

Characteristic	Syncope	Seizure
Position of patient before event	Standing	Any position
Prodromal signs and symptoms	Dizziness, visual changes, shortness of breath, weakness	Odd taste in the mouth Seeing lights or hearing sounds (hallucinations) Twitching
Activity during event	Relaxed	Generalized body movement
Response after event	Quick return of orientation	Slow return of orientation

▶ Headache

Everyone has had a headache at one time or another. What exactly is hurting? The brain and skull do not have pain receptors. Headaches originate from the nerves within the scalp, face, blood vessels, and muscles of the neck and head. The most common types of headaches are discussed in the next section. Other types of headaches are rare, but they may be caused by tumor, inflammation of the temporal artery, stroke, CNS infection, or hypertension. Presentation varies, depending on the underlying cause.

Pathophysiology and Assessment of Muscle Tension Headaches

Muscle tension headaches may be caused by stress, altered cortisol levels, and/or depression, which causes residual muscle contractions (tension) within the face and head. The majority of headaches are this type. The pain tends to be perceived on both sides of head, traveling from back to front, and can be characterized as a dull ache or a squeezing pain. The jaw, neck, or shoulders may also be stiff or sore.

Pathophysiology and Assessment of Migraine Headaches

A migraine headache is a complex condition thought to be caused by minor instability within certain clusters of neurons and also changes in the size of blood vessels at the base of the brain. The patient may report seeing an aura. The pain tends to be unilateral and focused, becoming more diffuse as the migraine headache progresses. The patient often describes throbbing, pounding, pulsating pain and may have nausea and vomiting. He or she may prefer to remain in a dark (photophobia) and quiet environment. A migraine headache can last several days.

Pathophysiology and Assessment of Cluster Headaches

A cluster headache is a rare vascular headache that begins in the face as a minor pain around one eye. The pain—described as sharp and excruciating, or as if someone is pushing the eyeball out—quickly intensifies and spreads to one side of the face. These headaches occur in groups, or clusters, and last 30 to 45 minutes each. However, a person may have several cluster headaches per day. The headaches can recur for days and then stop entirely. They may return at the same time the following month or the same time the next day. It is unclear what triggers these headaches, but serotonin and histamine may play a role. The headaches are often accompanied by anxiety.

Pathophysiology and Assessment of Sinus Headaches

Sinus headaches are caused by inflammation or infection within the sinus cavities of the face. The pain is located in the superior portions of the face and increases when the patient bends over. Sinus headache pain is often worst on waking. This kind of headache may be accompanied by postnasal drip, a sore throat, and nasal discharge.

Management

When you care for a patient with a headache, be cautious because headaches can indicate a more serious condition. If other signs indicate that a stroke may be in progress, then treat the patient for stroke. Remember, a patient who reports the worst headache of his or her life may be having a stroke.

Ask what medications the patient has taken, such as ibuprofen, acetaminophen, and aspirin. Determine how much the patient took and when the last dose or doses were taken.

Medications for pain management might include ketorolac tromethamine (Toradol IM; 30 mg IVP), meperidine (Demerol; 25 mg slow IVP), fentanyl (50 mcg), and morphine (2 to 4 mg slow IVP). Most patients, however, do not require narcotics. Also consider promethazine (Phenergan; 12.5 to 25 mg IVP) or ondansetron (Zofran; 4 mg IVP/orally disintegrating tablet) for nausea and vomiting. In-hospital management includes administering analgesics and ruling out serious medical conditions.

▶ Dementia

Pathophysiology

Dementia is the chronic deterioration of memory, personality, language skills, perception, reasoning, or judgment, with no loss of consciousness. These changes can occur over weeks to years and can be subtle. The reasons for these neurologic changes are dramatically different. Wernicke encephalopathy presents with dementia and is caused by a vitamin B_1 deficiency. This condition occurs in patients who are chronically malnourished. The classic patient is a patient with chronic alcoholism who ingests a diet mostly consisting of simple sugars. Without vitamin B_1, brain neurochemistry will not work correctly.

Compare Wernicke encephalopathy to **Alzheimer disease**, the most common form of dementia. Alzheimer disease is a progressive, organic condition in which neurons die. When the affected brain tissue is examined under a microscope, it appears to be riddled with tangles and clumps of damaged tissue.

Do not confuse dementia with delirium. Delirium is a sudden state of confusion or disorientation. By definition, delirium is reversible, whereas many dementias are irreversible. If you have ever been to a bar and seen someone drunk, then you have witnessed delirium.

Assessment

The initial demonstration of the disease can be dismissed as forgetfulness or so-called old age. However, Alzheimer disease is not a natural part of aging. As the disease progresses, it becomes obvious that this is not simple memory loss when patients cannot remember names, addresses, directions, or how to perform tasks. Patients can become aggressive and violent because the disease damages their judgment centers. Confusion is the hallmark sign. Eventually, the damage involves the ability to swallow. See Table 18-18 for a comparison of selected types of dementia.

Management

Prehospital management follows the standard care guideline. Ensure no reversible cause is present. Check the blood glucose level, oxygen level, and blood chemistry. Changes in any of these levels can cause confusion. You need to be compassionate and ready to repeat yourself. Dementia-related conditions can be frustrating for the patient. In the early stages, patients realize that they are not able to think as efficiently as in the past. Depression and withdrawal are common.

Wernicke encephalopathy bears special mention. In this condition, the confusion and dementia are partially reversible. Remember that the brain needs vitamin B_1 to metabolize sugars, so in patients suspected of being malnourished, you should administer thiamine, 100 to 200 mg IVP, before any glucose is given. In patients with a vitamin B_1 deficit, giving glucose can actually cause confusion or worsen the patient's presentation if thiamine is not present.

Patients with dementia may have other malnutrition concerns, including hypomagnesemia, hypokalemia, and hyponatremia. It would be prudent to perform ECG monitoring and obtain blood chemistries.

In-hospital care of patients with dementia begins with diagnosis. CT/MRI scans, neurologic functioning tests, electroencephalograms, and blood work are done to determine the cause. In many dementias, no definitive treatment exists for the destroyed neurons.

▶ Neoplasms

Pathophysiology

Neoplasm is the medical term for growths within the body that serve no useful purpose and are caused by errors that occur during cellular reproduction. Recall the discussion of neoplasm in Chapter 9, *Pathophysiology*. Within the context of the neurologic system, a neoplasm is a cancer of the brain or spinal cord.

Tumors can be classified according to whether they represent primary or metastatic disease. Primary neoplasms of the neurologic system are cancers that arise within the nervous system. Because mature neurons no longer divide, however, they rarely become cancerous. Primary CNS tumors, then, are usually caused by errors

Table 18-18 Comparison of Selected Types of Dementia

Disease	Cause	Presentation	Typical Course of Disease
Alzheimer disease	Multifactorial: Gradual buildup of plaques within the brain, which cause neuronal death. Eventual decrease in brain mass. Process begins 10 to 20 yr before signs and symptoms appear.	Chronic, insidious memory loss is the earliest finding. In moderate disease, a decrease in attention, judgment, and language functions (people get lost, cannot balance a checkbook, repeat questions). In severe disease, cannot recognize people; eventually cannot communicate and become bedridden.	3 to 10 yr
Pick disease	Unknown. Disease has a genetic aspect. Disease has its roots in damage to neurons in the frontal and temporal lobes.	Occurs in people between ages 55 and 65 years, with insidious presentation of socially inappropriate behavior, such as stealing and obsessive behaviors. Patient may be apathetic, depressed, or inappropriately elated. Additionally, rest tremors, difficulty naming common objects (anomia), and incontinence may be present.	6 yr
Huntington disease (Huntington chorea)	An adult-onset genetic disorder marked by severe loss of neurons.	Initially fidgetiness, abnormal eye movements, tics, myoclonus, irritability, and loss of interest. As the disease progresses, bradykinesia, difficulty standing, ataxia, slowing of thinking, and memory loss occur.	19 yr
Creutzfeldt-Jakob disease	Prions (proteins) clump together with resultant death of neurons.	Myoclonic jerking, major cognitive deterioration, visual impairment, unstable gait (ataxia). Disease is always fatal.	8 mo
Wernicke encephalopathy	Thiamine (vitamin B_1) deficiency. Occurs in patients with longstanding malnutrition, such as those with chronic alcoholism.	Ataxia, confusion, agitation, memory loss, nystagmus, generalized weakness, foot drop, and peripheral neuropathy	Variable, depending on cause and extent of malnutrition
AIDS dementia	Infection with HIV and subsequent destruction of nervous system cells	Blunted affect, impaired memory loss or slowed verbal response, and difficulty concentrating; will progress to partial paralysis of the lower extremities, mutism, and eventually a vegetative state	Untreated: 3–6 mo Treated: approximately 3 yr

Abbreviations: AIDS, acquired immune deficiency syndrome; HIV, human immunodeficiency virus

Data from: Alzheimer's Disease Information Page: National Institute of Neurological Disorders and Stroke (NINDS). https://www.ninds.nih.gov/Disorders/All-Disorders/Alzheimers-Disease-Information-Page Accessed January 18, 2017; Lakhan SE. Alzheimer disease. Medscape website. http://emedicine.medscape.com/article/1134817-overview. Updated September 28, 2016. Accessed March 13, 2016; Barrett AM. Pick disease. Medscape website. http://emedicine.medscape.com/article/1135504-overview. Updated June 6, 2014. Accessed March 13, 2016; Revilla FJ. Huntington disease. Medscape website. http://emedicine.medscape.com/article/1150165-overview. Updated July 8, 2016. Accessed March 13, 2016; Creutzfeldt-Jakob disease fact sheet. National Institute of Neurological Disorders and Stroke website. http://www.ninds.nih.gov/disorders/cjd/detail_cjd.htm. Updated February 2, 2016. Accessed March 13, 2016; Salen PN. Wernicke encephalopathy. Medscape website. http://emedicine.medscape.com/article/794583-overview. Updated October 28, 2015. Accessed March 13, 2016; and Thomas FP. HIV encephalopathy and AIDS dementia complex. Medscape website. http://emedicine.medscape.com/article/1166894-overview. Updated February 23, 2016. Accessed March 13, 2016.

in mitosis within the support structures of the CNS, such as a meningioma.

The process by which cancerous cells move to sites distant from their site of origin is called **metastasis**. Metastatic neoplasms of the neurologic system are tumors that arise elsewhere in the body, travel through the bloodstream or lymphatic system, and take up residence within nervous system tissues. Lung and breast cancers are the two most common types of cancer to metastasize to the CNS.

Assessment

Headache, nausea and vomiting, seizures, ataxia, change in mental status, and stroke-like signs and symptoms are common in patients with brain tumors. The rate and intensity of these signs and symptoms depends on how quickly the cancer is growing and its location. Patients may have months of headaches or suddenly have a seizure without any prior signs or symptoms. Middle-aged to older adults with new onset seizures should receive CT/MRI scans for possible brain tumors.

Patients with spinal tumors have signs and symptoms related to compression of the spinal cord. Back pain is the most common symptom. Patients may also experience weakness, ataxia, loss of sensation in a limb, incontinence, and a deformity along the spine. Other symptoms related to compression of the spinal cord are discussed in Chapter 34, *Head and Spine Trauma*.

Management

Prehospital management is supportive. Watch for status epilepticus. If needed, then administer diazepam (Valium). These patients can have elevated ICP. All patients with new onset seizures or chronic headaches that cannot be managed need medical evaluation. If the patient has a spinal tumor, then be prepared to protect the limbs from injury. In-hospital management is complex depending on the type of cancer and location.

Pathophysiology, Assessment, and Management of Demyelinating, Degenerating, and Motor Neuron Disorders

The three types of neurologic conditions discussed in this section—demyelinating, degenerating, and motor neuron disorders—have similar presentations. Demyelinating conditions occur after damage is done to the myelin sheath surrounding the neuron, which prevents smooth signal transmission from neuron to neuron. Degenerating conditions are incurable and the major characteristics are progressive damage and/or death of neurons. Motor neuron diseases are a grouping of conditions that feature destruction of the motor neuron. These tend to be progressive conditions in which patients experience difficulties with speech, ambulation, and general movement.

Multiple Sclerosis

Pathophysiology

Multiple sclerosis (MS) is an autoimmune condition in which the body attacks the myelin of the brain and spinal cord **Figure 18-16**. This results in demyelination, or destruction of the myelin. The resulting areas of scarring led to the name *multiple sclerosis* (from the Greek word *skleros,* meaning "hard"). As discussed in Chapter 9, *Pathophysiology,* the body has the ability to determine which proteins are "self" and which are "non-self." In an autoimmune disorder, the body begins to attack its own cells. The immune system is no longer able to distinguish friend from foe.

Consider the normal neuron. Myelin coats the axons of most nerve cells and allows for smooth transmission of signals to their target cell. In MS, the body believes that the proteins making up this insulation are foreign. It subsequently attacks that myelin, creating gaps in the insulation. These gaps cause characteristic signs and symptoms. It is believed that some unknown environmental trigger, such as a virus, begins to focus the attention of the immune system on the myelin.

Assessment

The presentation of MS follows a pattern of episodes and remissions. In the initial episode, double vision and blurred vision are common symptoms. The patient may have nystagmus.

The episodes can vary in intensity and remissions can vary in length. Patients experience muscle weakness; impairment of pain, temperature, and touch senses; pain (moderate to severe); ataxia; intention tremors; speech and vision disturbances; vertigo; bladder and bowel dysfunction; sexual dysfunction; depression; euphoria; cognitive abnormalities; and fatigue during episodes **Figure 18-17**. Patients may also experience a strange

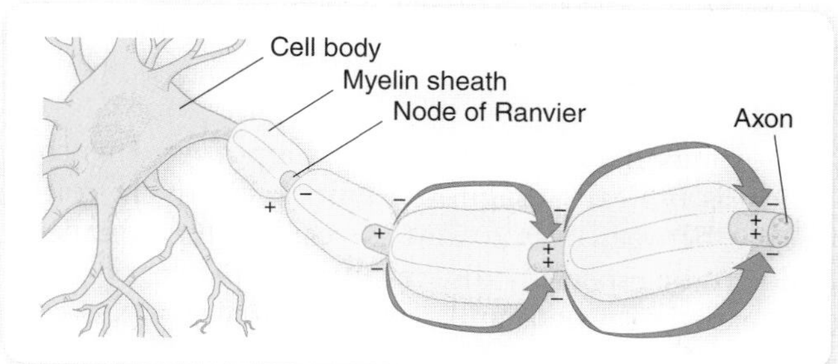

Figure 18-16 The myelin sheath insulates the axon, allowing impulses to jump from node to node, which accelerates the rate of signal transmission. In MS and other demyelinating conditions, this protective sheath is destroyed by inflammation and signals can no longer be transmitted smoothly.

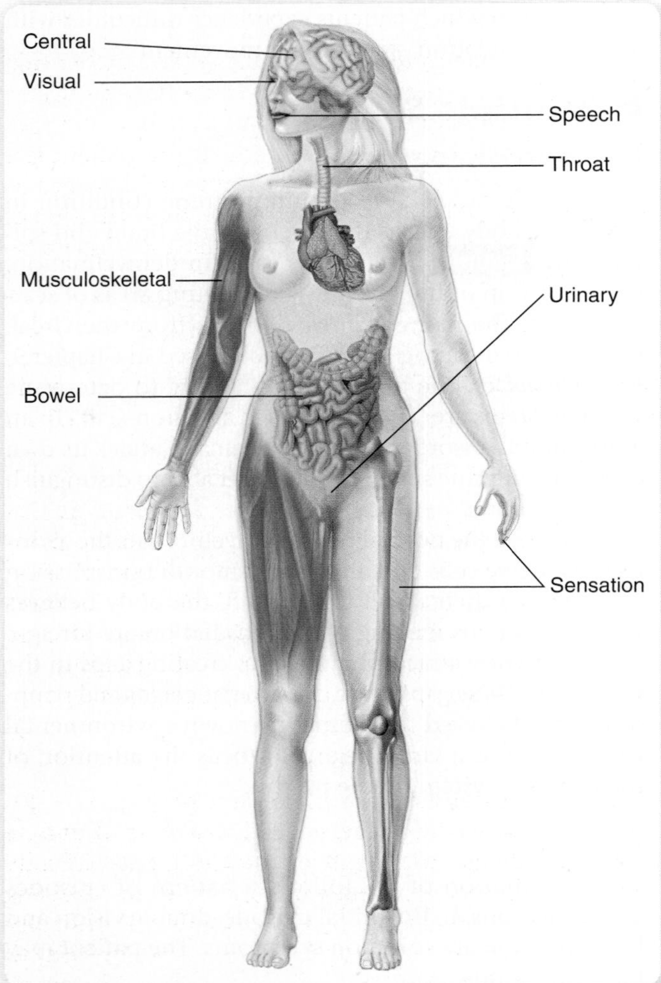

Figure 18-17 Areas of the body affected by the signs and symptoms of multiple sclerosis.

electric sensation down the spine or extremities when the head is flexed forward (Lhermitte sign). Episodes may be brief in nature, with little pattern to either frequency or intensity. Subsequent episodes may involve other locations of the body.

Management

Prehospital management of MS is supportive. This condition is typically diagnosed among relatively young people, between ages 20 and 50 years, so the initial episode can be especially disconcerting. A patient with MS may experience signs and symptoms that progress over several hours, from a sense of weakness to the inability to stand. Be prepared for possible trauma related to a fall. Additionally, the patient may have true confusion and anxiety—not because of some brain malfunction, but because this previously healthy person is trying to understand what is happening.

In-hospital management is directed at controlling the symptoms. Administration of anti-inflammatory medications may be used to decrease the length of the attack. Currently, no cure exists for MS.

▶ Guillain-Barré Syndrome

Pathophysiology

Guillain-Barré syndrome is a rare disease in which the immune system attacks portions of the nervous system. The cause of the condition is unclear, although some degree of immune response appears to be present. Patients report having a minor respiratory or gastrointestinal infection prior to the beginning of the weakness. One theory is that an infectious agent attacks the body. The agent has a protein structure that is similar to that of myelin. As the body attacks the invading organism, it confuses normal myelin with the invader. Once triggered, the immune system attacks and damages the myelin, and therefore it is a demyelinating condition. Signals being transmitted along the axon are impaired.

The reversal of Guillain-Barré syndrome can be almost as dramatic as its onset. Some patients recover completely without residual weakness in as little as several weeks.[15] Around one-third of all of these patients will need respiratory support at some point. Of patients who survive Guillain-Barré syndrome, 15% to 20% have motor weakness.[15]

Assessment

This rare condition is frightening for most patients. It begins as weakness and tingling sensations in the legs. This weakness moves up the legs and begins to affect the thorax and arms. The weakness can become severe and may lead to paralysis. This transition from being able to walk and speak to needing a ventilator to breathe can take as little as several hours. Most patients experience maximum muscle weakness or paralysis within 2 weeks of the onset of the disease. In addition to the peripheral motor neuron involvement, the autoregulatory systems can be involved. Patients are prone to severe swings in pulse rate and blood pressure.

Management

Prehospital management includes close assessment of the ability of the patient to effectively protect the airway and ventilate. Monitor the patient closely with ECG and repeat vital signs. Continuous $ETCO_2$ readings can provide evidence of impending respiratory failure. Be prepared to administer IV fluids to maintain blood pressure and treat hemodynamically significant bradycardia following AHA guidelines. Patients may experience terror as the condition progresses; therefore, use a comforting voice and a therapeutic touch as you care for the patient.

Upwards of 10% of Guillain-Barré patients have residual weakness. This weakness can be profound, requiring ventilatory support. Be prepared to manage a transport ventilator and assist with ambulation or other activities in these chronic patients. These patients do not experience subsequent attacks as occurs in MS. In-hospital management includes plasmapheresis (exchanging the plasma within the blood) and immunoglobulin injections. These therapies decrease the patient's recovery time.

▶ Parkinson Disease

Pathophysiology

Parkinson disease is a neurologic condition in which environmental and genetic factors can place patients at risk for damage to certain neurons. A portion of the brain, the substantia nigra, is responsible for production of dopamine. If this section is damaged or overused, then Parkinson disease can result. In some patients, the damage can be linked to past injuries, whereas in other patients, the damage is unexplainable. Dopamine is a neurotransmitter that, among other things, is needed for muscles to contract smoothly.

Assessment

A gradual onset of symptoms over months to years is typical. The initial signs are often unilateral tremors. Over time, as the dopamine level falls, more areas of the body are involved. Genetics play an important role. Parkinson-like activity can be observed in patients with head injuries and some patients who have overdosed.

The classic presentation of Parkinson disease involves the following four characteristics:

1. **Tremor.** Rest tremors and postural tremors are common among patients with Parkinson disease.
2. **Postural instability.** Patients have a stiff posture in which they are stooped over, and the disease alters their gait. This stiffness, together with increased response times, makes these patients unsteady when walking. Therefore, they are at an increased risk of falling.
3. **Rigidity.** Rigidity causes the patient to move in fits and starts.
4. **Bradykinesia.** Patients have a classic type of gait. They tend to shuffle in a straight line, with their feet close together. When asked to turn, they take small steps until the turn is complete. This is called **bradykinesia**, the slowing down of routine motions. Bradykinesia may also be demonstrated in slow blinking, a soft voice, or decreased facial expressions.

Other symptoms of Parkinson disease include depression, dementia, difficulty swallowing (aphagia), speech impairment, fatigue, and dystonia. Foot and leg contractions, in which the leg is arched, or the adduction of the arm into a posture where the arm is flexed across the chest or abdomen, are commonly seen. Prognosis is poor as the condition advances. Patients in later stages are at a much greater risk of death from aspiration, pneumonia, falls, or complications due to immobility.

Management

Prehospital management is supportive. Remember that these patients may be depressed or even have some degree of dementia. Reorient the patient if needed. A compassionate gesture can be very helpful. If the patient has trauma, then those injuries will need to be managed as well. In-hospital management includes administration of levodopa, which helps to temporarily restore dopamine levels. Other medications, surgery, and modification of diet and exercise are other options.

▶ Amyotrophic Lateral Sclerosis

Pathophysiology

Amyotrophic lateral sclerosis (ALS), also known as Lou Gehrig disease, is a disease that strikes the voluntary motor neurons. It is unclear exactly what causes the death of the motor neurons. One theory is that the body's immune system selectively attacks and kills them. Some evidence suggest that genetics may play a role. The condition is more common in middle-aged men of any race.

Assessment

Initially this condition is subtle and progresses without being noticed. Fatigue, general weakness of muscle groups, fasciculations (muscle twitching), and difficulty doing routine activities like eating, writing, and dressing will develop. Patients may also experience difficulty speaking. As the condition progresses, a loss of ability to walk, move the arms, eat, and speak occurs. The speed of progression is different for every patient. Because this condition impacts the motor neuron only, the patient is completely aware of his or her surroundings and the inability to move.

The average person diagnosed with this condition dies within 3 to 5 years. As the destruction of motor neurons continues, eventually patients are unable to breathe effectively without ventilatory assistance. Patients die from respiratory infections or other complications related to immobility.

Management

Prehospital treatment for these patients follows the standard care guideline. Assess the patient's ability to swallow and monitor the airway closely. Patients may rely on a variety of home medical technologies, including feeding pumps, IV pumps, long-term IV access ports, and ventilators. It can become complicated to transport such patients. Ask for guidance from the family or home health care provider to operate any unfamiliar devices. If needed, then disconnect the patient from the technology after consulting medical control and then transport.

In-hospital care for patients with ALS is geared toward supporting vital functions. Patients undergo physical therapy to help strengthen remaining neurons and muscles. Medications can be given to mitigate some of the symptoms; however, this condition has no cure.

▶ Cranial Nerve Disorders

Pathophysiology

This portion of the chapter will discuss relatively rare disorders. Understand that some neurologic disorders can mimic other conditions.

Someone with severe facial pain or sudden-onset facial paralysis is not necessarily having a stroke. Not everyone with chest pain is having an MI. Cranial nerve disorders are no different: They may not be as clear-cut as they first appear. The key to understanding these disorders is good assessment and detailed history-taking skills.

All of these conditions involve one or more of the cranial nerves, typically of the facial region. Table 18-19 provides an overview of these disorders.

Assessment

Conduct the neurologic assessment described earlier in this chapter. Additionally, test for vertigo. However, this test can only be done in patients who are at no risk of cervical spine trauma or other neck disease. Have the patient lie supine. Place your hands on either side of the head and move the head rapidly from side to side once. Then return the head to the neutral position. This maneuver causes the liquid within the inner ear to move. Next, look at the patient's eyes. If the patient has vertigo, then you should see nystagmus. Also, the motion of the head will typically increase the patient's sensation of vertigo.

Documentation & Communication

When you consider cranial nerve disorders, it is important to make a clear distinction between vertigo and dizziness. Vertigo, which involves the cranial nerves, is the sensation that you are moving when you are not, like the feeling you had as a child rolling down a hill. It is typically caused by inner ear disease. Vertigo is not the same as dizziness. Dizziness is a sensation of lightheadedness typically related to low blood pressure in the brain. So how can you differentiate the two? Talk with the patient. Ask him or her to describe the sensation without using the word "dizzy." Listen carefully to the words the patient chooses. Words and phrases like "spinning," "whirling," and "off balance" point toward vertigo, whereas descriptors such as "fuzzy" and "blackout" suggest dizziness. Good communication with your patient can help you draw accurate conclusions.

Management

Prehospital management of cranial nerve disorders is mainly supportive. Patients may need promethazine (Phenergan; 12.5 to 25 mg IVP) or ondansetron (Zofran; 4 mg IVP/orally

Table 18-19 Cranial Nerve Disorders

Disorder	Cause/Cranial Nerve Involved	Presentation	Treatment
Acoustic neuroma	Neoplasm (tumor) at the base of the brain. As the tumor grows, it can apply pressure to nerves, prevent movement of CSF, or compress blood vessels, causing ischemia. This process takes years because this tumor grows slowly. Affects cranial nerve VIII or VII (vestibulocochlear and facial nerves).	Unilateral hearing loss, headache, tinnitus, facial numbness, and balance disorders. Hearing loss may be gradual or intermittent.	Provide supportive care. To prevent falls, ensure you walk with the patient due to balance disorders. Speak clearly and look directly at the patient.
Bell palsy	Minor infection of the facial nerve, cranial nerve VII.	The episode is sudden and can easily be confused with a stroke. Signs and symptoms are eyelid ptosis, facial droop or weakness, excessive salivation, loss of the ability to taste. Episodes can last up to 2 weeks.	Consider CVA. If Bell palsy is known, then apply dressing to the closed eyelid. This step will help to prevent drying of the eye.

Disorder	Cause/Cranial Nerve Involved	Presentation	Treatment
Glossopharyngeal neuralgia	Irritation of the glossopharyngeal nerve (cranial nerve IX). Cause of irritation is unknown.	Episodes of severe, sharp unilateral pain in the tongue, at the back of the throat, in the middle ear, and in the tonsil area. Pain can last from seconds to several minutes, with multiple episodes possible in one day. Swallowing, eating cold food or drinks, sneezing, or coughing can trigger attacks.	Provide supportive care.
Hemifacial spasm	Dilated blood vessels irritate the facial nerve. Involves cranial nerve VII.	Involuntary unilateral facial movements. Tics, myoclonic contractions, jaw distortion, and facial tremors. No pain is associated with this condition.	Provide supportive care.
Ménière disease	Cause is unclear but the disease is believed to be related to an increase in fluid pressure within the inner ear. This pressure stimulates the VIII cranial nerve (vestibulocochlear nerve).	Recurrent and spontaneous unilateral tinnitus, dizziness, hearing loss, and a sensation of fullness in the ear. Episodes tend to last 2 to 4 hours. Repeated attacks can cause permanent deafness.	Provide supportive care. To prevent falls, ensure you walk with the patient due to balance disorders. Speak clearly and look directly at the patient.
Trigeminal neuralgia Also called *tic douloureux* (tik' doo-loo-roo')	The usual cause is irritation by an artery lying too close to the nerve. Over time, as the artery changes diameter to meet blood supply needs, this motion can grate the myelin sheath off of the nerve. With the insulation partially gone, the nerve can "short out," causing pain without trauma to the area. Involves the trigeminal nerve (cranial nerve V).	Severe, shock-like, or stabbing pain, usually on one side of the face. Episodes typically last several minutes and occur with a frequency of less than one per day to hundreds per day. Pain abates between attacks. Episodes are triggered by touching the face, speaking, brushing teeth, eating, putting on clothing, the wind—essentially any activity in which the face is stimulated.	Minimize touching while assessing the face. If small amounts of oxygen are needed for other reasons, then consider administering via blow-by technique directed at the unaffected side of the face. Masks or nasal cannula may trigger episodes. Episodes are severe but short lived. Opiate therapy is not typically needed.

Abbreviations: CSF, cerebrospinal fluid; CVA, cerebrovascular accident

Data from: Kutz JW Jr. Acoustic neuroma. Medscape website. http://emedicine.medscape.com/article/882876-overview#a6. Updated May 13, 2016. Accessed March 10, 2016; Taylor, DC. Bell palsy. Medscape website. http://emedicine.medscape.com/article/1146903-overview. Updated July 8, 2016. Accessed March 10, 2016; Glossopharyngeal neuralgia. MedlinePlus website. https://medlineplus.gov/ency/article/001636.htm. Updated September 28, 2016. Accessed March 10, 2016; Singh PM, Manpreet K, Trikha A. An uncommonly common: glossopharyngeal neuralgia. *Ann Indian Acad Neurol.* 2013;16(1):1-8. https://www.ncbi.nlm.nih.gov/pmc/articles/PMC3644765/. Accessed March 10, 2016; Gulevich S. Hemifacial spasm. Medscape website. http://emedicine.medscape.com/article/1170722-overview. Updated May 16, 2016. Accessed March 10, 2016; Hemifacial spasm. Health Communities website. http://www.healthcommunities.com/hemifacial-spasm/hemifacial-spasm-overview.shtml. Published January 1, 2002. Updated September 18, 2015. Accessed March 10, 2016; Hemifacial spasm information page. National Institute of Neurological Disorders and Stroke website. https://www.ninds.nih.gov/Disorders/All-Disorders/Hemifacial-Spasm-Information-Page. Accessed January 19, 2017; Li JC. Meniere disease (idiopathic endolymphatic hydrops). Medscape website. http://emedicine.medscape.com/article/1159069-overview. Updated December 22, 2015. Accessed March 10, 2016; and Singh MK. Trigeminal neuralgia. Medscape website. http://emedicine.medscape.com/article/1145144-overview. Updated October 22, 2015. Accessed March 10, 2016.

disintegrating tablet) for the nausea and vomiting that may be present with some cranial nerve disorders. Benzodiazepines such as diazepam (Valium) may provide some relief from the vertigo. In most cases, NSAIDs and opiates have limited benefit in managing pain caused by cranial nerve disorders.

In-hospital management of these conditions is related to the specific condition and its cause. Care is focused on ensuring that a serious condition, such as a brain tumor, is not present. Therapy is then directed at making the patient comfortable and treating the underlying cause. Carbamazepine (Tegretol) and gabapentin (Neurontin) are often used to treat these conditions. Antivirals and corticosteroid medications may also be used.

▶ Dystonia

Pathophysiology

Dystonias are severe, abnormal muscle spasms that cause bizarre contortions, repetitive motions, or postures. Dystonia can be either a sign (occurring within another condition) or a condition in itself. Consider a patient with a headache. The headache could be a sign of a CVA, or the patient could simply have a headache. Patients with dystonia have normal intelligence, are able to think clearly, and are not experiencing a seizure. Dystonia does not impact the patient's LOC.

Primary dystonias occur for an unknown reason. A defect in the body's ability to process neurotransmitters is thought to be at the core of the problem. In these patients, dystonia would correctly be referred to as a condition. Some patients who take antipsychotic medications may have sudden onset of bizarre contortions of the face or body. This finding would be a secondary dystonia and would more appropriately be considered a sign rather than a condition.

Spasmodic torticollis Figure 18-18, in which the neck muscles contract, twisting the head to one side and usually pulling it forward or backward, is a common example of a dystonia. The head then remains painfully frozen in that position. Facial dystonia can take several forms.

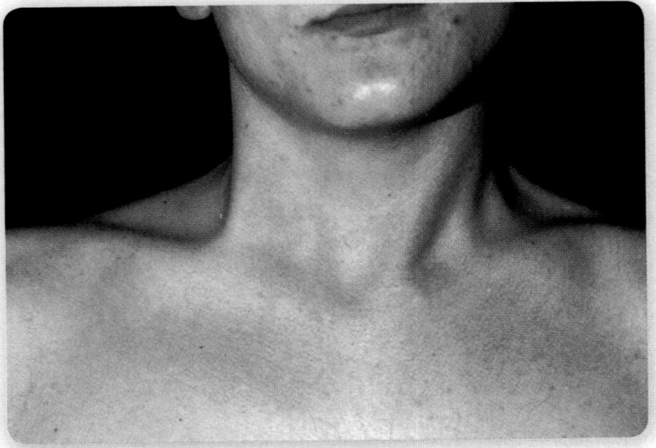

Figure 18-18 Example of torticollis or "wry neck" dystonia.

Assessment

Spasms due to dystonia are involuntary and are often painful. Table 18-20 describes a wide variety of dystonias.

Words of Wisdom

Regardless of the underlying cause, dystonias are socially upsetting because patients suddenly twist and writhe uncontrollably. It is critical that you provide compassionate care.

Table 18-20 Types of Dystonias

Type	Presentation
Cervical dystonia (torticollis)	Most common form of focal dystonia; intermittent, patterned, repetitive, spasmodic motion of the head in a twisting, flexing, extending, or tilting manner; can involve more than one motion type
Oculogyric crisis	Deviation of the eyes in any direction, usually with eyes strained towards the top of the head
Oromandibular	Forceful contractions of the face, which can involve the tongue darting in and out of the mouth
Blepharospasm	Eyelid spasms or uncontrollable blinking
Athetosis	Slow, writhing motions commonly involving the face and distal extremities
Upper limb dystonia	Cramping of the hands, elbows, and arms (eg, graphospasm [writer's cramp])
Choreiform movements	Quick, jerky, irregular, and unpredictable movements; often found in the face, arms, and hands
Spasmodic dysphonia	Involuntary contraction of the vocal cords, interrupting speech

Management

Prehospital management is focused on ruling out other conditions, such as seizures, strokes, or reactions to psychiatric medications. If you suspect a dystonic reaction to an antipsychotic medication, then diphenhydramine (Benadryl; 25 mg IVP) is the drug of choice to stop the contraction within 10 to 30 minutes. Dystonias tend to occur within 5 days of either starting a new psychotropic medication or changing dosage. Dystonic reactions secondary to psychiatric medications are not considered to be allergic in nature. Diphenhydramine is effective for this type of dystonia because of its anticholinergic properties.

Unfortunately, diphenhydramine is ineffective in primary dystonias. Regardless of the cause, dystonias can be very unnerving and even painful. Pain management may be appropriate. Talk with your patient and let him or her know you are trying to help. Be calm and reassuring. In-hospital management involves a variety of medication options to control the condition.

▶ Central Nervous System Infections and Inflammation

Pathophysiology

To begin the discussion on CNS infections and inflammation, it is important for you to understand some fundamental definitions. Encephalitis is inflammation of the brain. Meningitis is the inflammation of the meninges, the outer covering of the central nervous system. Clinically, these conditions are difficult, if not impossible, to distinguish in the prehospital setting. Both conditions can result from a variety of causes, including infectious, chemical, and/or metabolic causes. Infectious pathology is the most common form for both conditions when it presents in the acute phase.

Infectious causes for encephalitis and meningitis are the result of bacteria, viruses, fungi, or prions gaining access to the body, which then reproduce and cause damage. These organisms have a basic goal—to continue to live. To do so, all organisms need food and must reproduce. As the organism begins to attack the body, it is looking for fuel with which to create the next generation of bacteria, viruses, or other pathogens. The damage that these organisms create occurs due to several mechanisms. Either the damage is caused by the body's reaction to the infection or by the activities of the attacking organisms.

A common sign of infectious disease is the presence of a fever. Many pathogenic organisms prefer to grow within a narrow temperature range, so even a 2° to 3°F (1.2° to 1.8°C) climb in body temperature can slow the reproduction of some viruses or bacteria. This increase in temperature allows the immune system to gain control, providing valuable time for neutrophils (the body's defenses) to find and kill the invading organisms. It also signals the rest of the body that an attack is underway. More white blood cells are produced and chemical mediators are released to improve the body's effectiveness at finding and eliminating the organisms. In this regard, fevers are good.

If the temperature of the body becomes too high, then the brain can be affected. Remember the last time you felt ill and had a fever. The increased temperature made your thinking dull, it was difficult to concentrate, and you may have had a headache. These effects are common with fevers. Neurons are sensitive to temperature changes. As the temperature rises, the effects on the neurons can become more profound. Eventually, a person may hallucinate, become delusional, or experience a LOC. Another possibility is the random firing of neurons, which in this case would be referred to as a febrile seizure.

Another mechanism by which infectious agents can cause damage to the body is through destruction of cells. Organisms can produce **endotoxins** or **exotoxins** that can damage nearby living cells, thus providing the bacterium with a source of food. Endotoxins are proteins that are released by gram-negative bacteria when they die. *Neisseria meningitidis* is a type of bacteria that releases endotoxins; it is associated with meningitis.

Clostridium tetani is another bacterium that releases an exotoxin. *C tetani* causes tetanus (lockjaw), in which patients experience muscle contractions, stiff neck, difficulty moving the jaw, and dysphagia. Fortunately, this once-common condition is rare today because of the efforts of public health professionals and immunization.

Assessment

Table 18-21 shows that the presentation of encephalitis and meningitis is similar. Both illnesses begin with flulike symptoms. As the organism reproduces and causes more damage, a stiff neck, photophobia, lethargy, an altered LOC, and seizures are possible. Kernig sign or Brudzinski sign Figure 18-19 may be elicited in meningitis.

Management

Prehospital management of these conditions is mainly supportive. For patients with suspected meningitis, place a mask over their mouths to limit the spread of organisms. Also wear a mask if the patient is coughing. Be prepared for seizures and treat accordingly. One of the risks of these conditions, particularly for bacterial meningitis, is increased ICP. Another risk is septicemia, which indicates the infection is now present within the bloodstream. Septicemia can cause ruptures of capillaries and loss of vasomotor control of blood vessels. See Chapter 26, *Infectious Diseases*, for more information on septicemia.

Encephalitis is not particularly contagious from person to person, but meningitis can be. As a paramedic, your follow-up care may involve preventive antibiotic treatment for possible bacterial meningitis. It is important for you (or your supervisor) to stay in contact with the infection control officer from the hospital to which the patient was transported. In-hospital management is directed at decreasing swelling in the brain and spinal cord, fighting the infection, and supporting the patient's vital signs.

Table 18-21 Comparison of Encephalitis and Meningitis

Condition	Organisms Usually Responsible	Presentation	Timeline
Encephalitis	Herpes simplex virus: Most common sporadic form. Arboviruses: Most common episodic form. These viruses are transmitted by vectors and cause outbreaks of illnesses. Examples include West Nile virus, rabies, and Japanese virus encephalitis.	First signs and symptoms are fever, headache, nausea/vomiting, and general malaise. As the condition progresses, changes in LOC occur, including behavioral and personality changes, nuchal rigidity (stiff neck), photophobia, lethargy, confusion, and seizure.	Several days, depending on the specific virus involved
Bacterial meningitis	Neonates: *Group B Streptococci* and *Escherichia coli.* Infants/children: *Haemophilus influenzae* (more common in children), *Streptococcus pneumoniae*, and *N meningitidis.* Adults: *S pneumoniae, N meningitidis* (more common in young adults), and *Listeria monocytogenes.*	First signs and symptoms are upper respiratory infection (runny nose, cough, malaise). As the condition progresses, the patient may have headache, nuchal rigidity, fever (the classic triad of symptoms). Chills, photophobia, vomiting, seizures, confusion, Kernig sign, and Brudzinski sign may also occur. Patients can experience life-threatening issues with increased ICP. Infants are irritable when held, and have a high-pitched cry (cat's cry) and bulging fontanelles.	Bacterial pathogen: presentation within 24 h
Viral meningitis	Non-polio enterovirus is the most common viral type. Examples include echovirus and coxsackievirus.	Signs and symptoms are similar to bacterial meningitis. Viral meningitis does not cause increased ICP.	Viral pathogen: presentation in 1 d to 7 d

Abbreviations: ICP, intracranial pressure; LOC, level of consciousness

Data from: Hasbun R. Meningitis. Medscape website. http://emedicine.medscape.com/article/232915-overview#a5. Updated February 16, 2016. Accessed March 26, 2016; Howes DS. Encephalitis. Medscape website. http://emedicine.medscape.com/article/791896-overview. Updated April 13, 2016. Accessed March 26, 2016; and Bacterial meningitis. Centers for Disease Control and Prevention website. www.cdc.gov/meningitis/bacterial.html. Updated June 15, 2016. Accessed March 26, 2016.

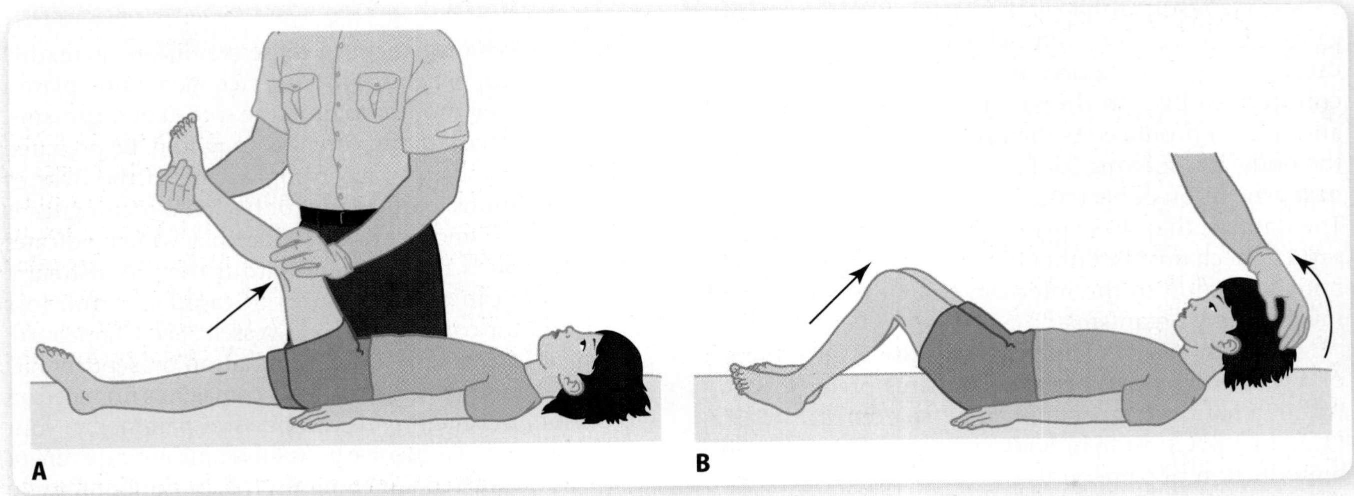

Figure 18-19 A. Kernig sign. Meningeal irritation results in pain when attempting to straighten the knee with the hips flexed. **B.** Brudzinski sign. Meningeal irritation results in an involuntary flexion of the knees when the head is flexed toward the chest. These classic signs do not occur frequently.

▶ Abscesses

Pathophysiology

Abscesses are caused by an infectious agent within the brain or spinal cord. When an infectious agent attacks brain or spinal cord cells and destroys tissue, the immune system responds by attempting to kill the pathogen. If it cannot, then the body's second line of defense is to erect a "wall" to prevent the pathogen from spreading. This capsule envelops the infectious agent, as well as dead or dying brain or spinal cord cells, dead white blood cells, and white blood cells that are still fighting the infection. Over time, with continued tissue destruction and immune system response, swelling can occur. The result is an abscess.

The underlying reason for an infection within the brain or spinal cord is varied. Such an infection is often preceded by an infection of the sinuses, throat, gums, or ear. The pathogenic organism can also be introduced to the brain when head or spinal cord trauma occurs.

Assessment

The two main consequences of the infection are damage to an area of the brain or spinal cord and the presence of an abscess within the cranial vault or spinal cord. These two factors dictate the presentation of a patient with a CNS abscess. Look for a low- or high-grade fever, persistent headache, drowsiness, confusion, generalized or focal seizures, nausea and vomiting, focal motor or sensory impairments, nuchal rigidity, and hemiparesis.

Management

Follow the standard care guideline. Pay close attention for evidence of increased ICP. Take seizure precautions. Evaluate temperature. If it is high, then remove the patient's clothing, cover the patient with a sheet, and turn off the heat in the patient compartment of the ambulance. These patients may be critically ill and require prompt transport.

In-hospital management involves antibiotics, seizure precautions, and sometimes surgical removal of the abscess.

▶ Poliomyelitis and Postpolio Syndrome

Pathophysiology

Poliomyelitis is a viral infection transmitted by the fecal–oral route. Its incidence peaked in the United States in the 1950s. Since then, an effective vaccine has been developed. No cases of wild polio within the United States have occurred since 1979. In the United States, people who contract the disease typically have not been immunized.

Assessment

Signs and symptoms for those people who become infected begin in as little as 1 week after exposure. In the most severe cases, they include sore throat, nausea, vomiting, diarrhea, stiff neck, and muscle weakness or paralysis.

Management

In-hospital care for patients with the acute illness is directed at hydration, ventilation, and calorie support until the infection has been managed by the immune system. The way the virus damages the nervous system places patients at risk for problems decades after the initial infection. The virus attacks motor neurons within the brain and brainstem, thereby causing the classic signs of weakness and paralysis. The remaining neurons now begin to send out new axons to try to compensate for this loss. This process allows the patient to regain function.

Over time, these motor neurons are doing more work than they are accustomed and they can begin to break down and die. This process creates **postpolio syndrome**. Patients who had polio in the early- to mid-20th century may now have difficulty swallowing, weakness, fatigue, or breathing conditions. Typically, the muscle groups affected by the post-polio syndrome are the same as those affected by the original polio infection, but at a milder level of weakness.

Prehospital management emphasizes managing possible airway obstruction due to swallowing difficulties. Remember, polio will present in older patients who contracted polio decades ago. Patients within extended care facilities may have this condition as a past medical history. Although postpolio syndrome does not specifically modify care for other conditions, it can affect the speed in which a patient decompensates. Consider a patient with congestive heart disease. As the patient struggles with fluid buildup in the alveoli, he or she has difficulty breathing. When coupled with decreased respiratory muscle strength due to postpolio syndrome, this patient may more quickly move into respiratory failure. Consider a patient's past medical history and medications when delivering emergency medical care.

In-hospital treatment for postpolio syndrome includes physical therapy and some experimental medications.

▶ Peripheral Neuropathy

Pathophysiology

Peripheral neuropathy is a group of conditions in which the nerves leaving the spinal cord are damaged. The signals moving to or from the brain become distorted. The many causes for this group of conditions include trauma, toxins, tumors, autoimmune attacks, and metabolic disorders. Trigeminal neuralgia and Guillain-Barré syndrome are examples. The remainder of this discussion will be limited to the most common form of peripheral neuropathy, which is diabetic neuropathy.

Assessment

As the blood glucose level rises, damage can occur to the peripheral nerves. The result is misfiring and shorting of signals. Patients may have sensory or motor impairment. Loss of sensation, numbness, burning, pain, paresthesia, and muscle weakness are common. Patients may eventually have a loss of the ability to feel their feet or other areas. The condition is progressive and is accelerated by high blood glucose levels.

Management

Management in the prehospital setting is supportive. In-hospital management includes pain medication and helping the patient gain better control over his or her blood glucose levels. The use of antidepressants and anticonvulsants seems to have a positive effect on calming the peripheral nerves.

Special Populations

Neurologic conditions with special relevance to pediatric patients include hydrocephalus, spina bifida, and cerebral palsy.[16,17] These diseases are covered in Chapter 43, *Pediatric Emergencies*. You can also find information about patients with neurologic conditions requiring long-term care in Chapter 45, *Patients With Special Challenges*.

YOU are the Paramedic SUMMARY

1. What are your next questions?

It is paramount that you assess scene safety. This patient is physically imposing, but is he a potential safety risk? It is important to understand that his mere presence does not make him a threat. You need to make a more conscientious evaluation of the scene. A scene size-up involves more than simply listing the available risks. It also involves some degree of situational awareness—how likely is a certain risk to become a real threat?

In this scenario, the following questions can help you assess the level of risk:

- How would you describe the patient's mood?
- How would you describe his posture? Is he sitting or standing?
- What is his facial expression? Could you appropriately interpret it if he were having a stroke?
- Do you notice signs that he may be upset (eg, quick head movements, clenched fists, inability to sit still, etc)?
- If you determine that the patient presents a real threat, then do you have enough help available? Are police officers present in the room with you?

As a paramedic, you cannot remove all risks from a situation. Your job is to use situational awareness to ensure you are constantly thinking about potential risks, weighing the probabilities, and then acting in the best interest of the patient while you keep yourself and your team safe.

2. What assessment information do you need to gather?

Initially, stroke should be high on the differential diagnosis list. Determine when the patient was last seen normal. Does the patient report a headache? A detailed neurologic assessment is appropriate.

3. How can you determine whether the patient is oriented when he will not speak?

To determine whether this patient is oriented, you can ask yes or no questions to which you know the answers; use a communication board; or ask the patient to either write down his or her responses using a pencil and paper, or type it using the keypad of a mobile phone.

4. What vital signs or laboratory values are critical to gather for this patient?

Obtain a full set of vital signs, including pulse oximetry. A blood glucose level is needed to ensure hypoglycemia is not present. Focus on ensuring your blood pressure reading is accurate. A lactate level would be of limited value in this patient, as would hemoglobin and hematocrit levels. If this patient were experiencing a hemorrhagic stroke, then the amount of blood loss would not be dramatic. The patient would have clear signs and symptoms of increased ICP long before a significant drop occurred in his hemoglobin and hematocrit levels. If you suspect a stroke, then transport the patient quickly.

5. What is this patient's Glasgow Coma Scale (GCS) score? Does it accurately depict this patient's acuity?

This patient's GCS score is 11. This score implies a diminished LOC. However, the only reason that this patient's score is 11 is that he cannot or will not speak.

6. Which portion of the neurologic assessment is inconsistent with the remainder of the exam?

The patient's inability to make any sound is inconsistent. The creation and processing of speech is complicated, and it involves multiples areas within the brain. The temporal lobe plays a major role in speech. Essentially, speech production can be broken down into a two-sided system: one that processes the auditory information coming in, and one that adjusts the vocal cords, breathing pattern, and mouth to create words. The latter side is impaired with this patient. His complete absence of sound generation is compelling. If this patient were having a stroke so severe as to completely impair his ability to make any

YOU are the Paramedic SUMMARY (continued)

sounds, you would expect him to have a decreased LOC. You would also expect an impaired ability to maintain the airway, such as swallowing difficulties. However, the patient appears to be functioning normally with the exception of his inability to make any sounds. His condition has removed his ability to make any sounds, yet it is not affecting his airway or LOC.

7. If this patient is having a stroke, then how will the aspirin affect him?

The three possible outcomes of aspirin administration are as follows:

1. If the patient is having an ischemic stroke, then the aspirin may be beneficial.
2. If the patient is having a hemorrhagic stroke, then the aspirin may be harmful. As the patient bleeds into his head, the body will attempt to form a clot. This clotting can limit the bleeding and, therefore, limit the intracranial pressure. However, the presence of the aspirin can diminish the effectiveness of this clotting, therefore increase the amount of bleeding. This process could result in a more significant hemorrhagic stroke.
3. If the patient is not having a stroke, then the effect of the aspirin is unpredictable. If he is having is bleeding-related event, then the same problem described above could occur.

8. What are other possible causes of stroke-like presentations?

Bell palsy can cause facial paralysis. Headaches can be caused by tension (stress), clusters, or migraine. Medications can cause changes in LOC. A psychiatric condition called a conversion reaction can cause muteness.

9. Were you correct to treat this patient as if he had experienced a stroke?

Even though the presentation is not textbook, the patient should still be treated as having a potential stroke. It is important to contact the closest stroke center and initiate a stroke alert. Because of the risk of brain damage if this patient is having a stroke, a CT/MRI scan is needed after he arrives at the ED.

YOU are the Paramedic SUMMARY *(continued)*

EMS Patient Care Report (PCR)					
Date: 11-06-18	**Incident No.:** 3986		**Nature of Call:** Stroke	**Location:** 1070 First St	
Dispatched: 0853	**En Route:** 0854	**At Scene:** 0858	**Transport:** 0916	**At Hospital:** 0923	**In Service:** 0940

Patient Information	
Age: 49 **Sex:** M **Weight (in kg [lb]):** 109 kg (240 lb)	**Allergies:** No known drug allergies **Medications:** Hydrochlorothiazide, exercise supplements **Past Medical History:** 1 year ago had an episode of left-sided weakness that was not diagnosed as a stroke. Completely resolved. No diagnosis known. HTN. **Chief Complaint:** Unable to speak

Vital Signs				
Time: 0903	**BP:** 142/96	**Pulse:** 112	**Respirations:** 16	**Spo$_2$:** 98% RA
Time: 0914	**BP:** 146/96	**Pulse:** 116	**Respirations:** 20	**Spo$_2$:** 98% RA
Time:	**BP:**	**Pulse:**	**Respirations:**	**Spo$_2$:**

EMS Treatment (circle all that apply)				
Oxygen @ _______ L/min via (circle one): **NC NRM Bag-mask device**		**Assisted Ventilation**	**Airway Adjunct**	**CPR**
Defibrillation	**Bleeding Control**	**Bandaging**	**Splinting**	**Other:** IV started (circled)

Narrative

Dispatched: Stroke
CC: None stated by patient
HPI: Pt was discovered by his wife this morning unable to speak. She administered 325 mg of aspirin. Pt admits to awaking this morning about 2 hours ago and not being able to speak. He did alert his family.
PMH: HTN, 1 year ago had left-sided weakness that completely resolved. Was not diagnosed as a stroke.
Meds: Hydrochlorothiazide
Allergies: NKDA
Physical Exam
General impression—Male patient sitting on couch in basement of home with family in attendance. Pt has adequate hygiene and house is clean and organized.
Neuro—Awake, alert and appears to be oriented. Will answer yes/no questions by nodding. Slight facial droop noted to left face, neg ptosis, PERRLA, slight weakness noted to left arm. Able to stand and ambulate with minor assistance. Neg c/o headache. Cranial nerves II-XII are grossly intact unless otherwise noted, pt is able to swallow without difficulty, neg drooling noted, pt is mute without any sound generation or attempts at making words.
Cardiovascular—Skin is warm, dry, and nonpale. Heart with regular rhythm, monitor shows sinus tach without obvious ST changes or ectopy noted, 12-lead shows no acute changes, neg c/o chest pain.
Respiratory—Lungs CTA bilaterally, neg use of accessory muscles, neg retractions noted, acyanotic, neg c/o difficulty breathing.
Gastrointestinal—Abd soft and non-tender without obvious masses or pulsation noted. Neg c/o nausea, neg vomiting noted.
Genitourinary—Stable pelvis to ambulation, neg overt incontinence noted.
Extr—Without obvious trauma, edema, or venipuncture marks noted.
Disposition—Transported pt to ABS hospital without incident, no change in patient condition or vital signs upon arrival at hospital. Pt taken directly to CT scanner. Report to ED physician. Medic 123 available.
Impression—Potential stroke.**End of report**

Prep Kit

▶ Ready for Review

- Neurologic disorders can be dangerous because depressed reflexes leave the airway and other body systems vulnerable.
- A variety of disease processes can cause neurologic dysfunction, including cancer, degenerative conditions, developmental anomalies, infectious diseases, and vascular conditions. Most neurologic diseases are thought to be multifactorial—that is, a number of factors combine to induce vulnerability to a particular disease process.
- ICP is determined by the volume of the intracranial contents: the brain, blood, and cerebrospinal fluid.
- The primary dangers of ICP are ischemia and brain herniation.
- The neurologic assessment identifies small alterations that can impair nervous system function.
- Investigating the neurologic patient's chief complaint requires taking a history to determine the MOI or the NOI. This task is more difficult when the patient is unresponsive, but environmental clues and the reports of family, friends, and bystanders can be helpful.
- It is critical to determine when the patient was last seen normal because the amount of time elapsed since the onset of symptoms will dictate the treatments available.
- LOC can be evaluated using the GCS, the AVPU mnemonic, a test of corneal reflex or pupillary response, evaluation of cranial nerve functioning, assessment of the patient's orientation and alertness, assessment of the patient's speech and ability to recognize and name objects, evaluation of the patient's movement, testing of the patient's sensory perceptual abilities, testing of the blood glucose level, and measurement of the vital signs.
- Following the standard care guideline can help you address common neurologic disorders in a systematic way.
- Stroke is a condition in which the blood supply to the brain is interrupted. In ischemic stroke, the blood supply may be blocked by a clot (thrombus or embolus). In hemorrhagic stroke, a damaged artery bleeds into the brain.
- Stroke causes sudden-onset changes in neurologic status, including effects on language, movement, sensation, LOC, and blood pressure.
- Time is brain. Fibrinolytic (clot-busting) agents need to be administered within 3 to 4.5 hours of the onset of a stroke for the agents to be effective. To achieve this target, a stroke must be recognized and EMS dispatched quickly, and the patient must be transported promptly to a stroke center (if available in your region).
- TIAs are episodes of cerebral ischemia that resolve within 24 hours, leaving no permanent damage. They may, however, signal an underlying vascular problem that can lead to a stroke. Prompt medical evaluation is essential.
- A diminished LOC is marked by increasing deficits in cognition and speech and changes in movement and posture. The patient may become comatose without timely medical intervention.
- Seizures are cause by the sudden, erratic firing of neurons; they have a wide range of causes, from drug use to tumors.
- Status epilepticus can be defined as a seizure that lasts longer than 4 to 5 minutes or consecutive seizures without a return to consciousness between seizures. Lengthy seizures can have devastating effects on the brain and body and may even be life threatening.
- Seizures are classified as either generalized (affecting large portions of the brain) or partial (affecting only a limited area of the brain).
- Generalized seizures are divided into tonic-clonic (formerly grand mal) seizures, which follow a particular sequence; absence (formerly petit mal) seizures, which are characterized by the absence of movement; and pseudoseizures, which have a psychiatric origin.
- Simple partial seizures involve either movement of one part of the body (frontal lobe) or sensations in one part of the body (parietal lobe). Complex partial seizures subtly diminish the LOC, causing confusion, a lack of alertness, or an inability to speak.
- Syncope (fainting) is caused by a brief interruption in cerebral blood flow that can be traced to cardiac rhythm disturbances, other cardiac causes, or noncardiac causes.
- Headaches can be classified as muscle tension, migraine, cluster, or sinus headaches. Each has a different cause and a different presentation. Other types of headache may occur as well.
- Dementia is not a single illness, but a chronic process that can take many forms. It is characterized by deterioration of memory, personality, language skills, perception, reasoning, or judgment, with no loss of consciousness. Management is similar for the various dementias and is primarily supportive.
- Tumors of the neurologic system affect the brain and spinal cord and are classified as either primary or metastatic disease.

Prep Kit (continued)

- Demyelinating conditions attack the insulating sheath that surrounds and protects the axon, so that nerve impulses can no longer travel smoothly.
- MS is an autoimmune condition in which episodes are followed by periods of remission. Patients with MS can have a range of neurologic deficits, from incontinence to significant sensory impairments.
- ALS (Lou Gehrig disease) is a disease that strikes the voluntary motor neurons, causing progressive paralysis and death.
- Parkinson disease damages the substantia nigra, the portion of the brain that produces dopamine, which is needed for muscle contraction.
- Cranial nerve disorders have a range of signs and symptoms and are often mistaken for other disorders.
- Dystonias are severe, abnormal muscle spasms that cause bizarre contortions, repetitive motions, or postures. They can affect the neck, face, jaw, or other muscles, and they are often painful.
- Encephalitis and meningitis are CNS infections that cause inflammation of the brain and meninges, respectively.
- Abscesses indicate the presence of an infectious agent within the brain or spinal cord.
- Polio is a viral infection that can cause long-term damage to the brain and brainstem (postpolio syndrome), leading to muscle weakness and paralysis.
- Peripheral neuropathy is a group of conditions in which the nerves leaving the spinal cord are damaged by trauma, toxins, tumors, autoimmune attack, and metabolic disorders, or other processes. Diabetic neuropathy is the most common form.

▶ Vital Vocabulary

abscess An area in the brain or spinal cord in which cells have been attacked, typically by an infectious agent. To prevent the spread of infection, the immune system "walls off" the area. Pus can collect in this pocket.

Alzheimer disease A progressive, organic condition in which neurons in the brain die, causing dementia.

amyotrophic lateral sclerosis (ALS) A condition that strikes the voluntary motor neurons, causing their death. The disease is characterized by fatigue and general weakness of muscle groups; eventually the patient becomes unable to walk, eat, or speak; also known as Lou Gehrig disease.

anesthesia Lack of feeling within a body part.

anisocoria Unequal pupils with a greater than 1-mm difference.

ataxia Alteration in the ability to perform coordinated motions such as walking.

aura Sensations commonly experienced before a seizure or migraine headache occurs; may include visual changes in addition to hallucinations.

Bell palsy A temporary paralysis of the facial nerve (cranial nerve VII), which controls the muscles on each side of the face.

bradykinesia The slowing down of voluntary body movements; found in patients with Parkinson disease.

clonic activity Type of seizure movement involving the contraction and relaxation of muscle groups.

coma A state in which a person does not respond to either verbal or painful stimuli.

common reality Sensory stimulation that can be verified by others.

corneal reflex A protective movement that results in blinking, moving the head posteriorly, and pupillary constriction.

decerebrate posturing Abnormal extension of the arms with rotation of the wrists along with the toes pointed; this finding indicates brainstem damage.

decorticate posturing Abnormal flexion of the arms toward the chest with the toes pointed; this finding indicates lower cerebral damage.

delusions Thoughts, ideas, or perceived abilities that have no basis in common reality.

dementia The slow, progressive onset of disorientation, shortened attention span, and loss of cognitive function.

dystonia Contractions of body into bizarre positions.

endotoxin A toxin released by some bacteria when they die.

exotoxin A toxin secreted by living cells to aid in the death and digestion of other cells.

gait Patterns of walking or ambulating.

Guillain-Barré syndrome A rare condition that begins as a sensation of weakness and tingling in the legs, moving to the arms and thorax; the disorder can lead to paralysis within 2 weeks.

hallucinations Sensory stimulation that cannot be verified by others.

hemiparesis Weakness of one side of the body.

hemiplegia Paralysis of one side of the body.

Prep Kit *(continued)*

hemorrhagic stroke One of the two main types of stroke; occurs as a result of bleeding inside the brain.

idiopathic Of no known cause.

intention tremor A tremor that occurs when trying to accomplish a task.

ischemic stroke One of the two main types of stroke, also called an occlusive stroke; occurs when blood flow to a particular part of the brain is cut off by a blockage, such as a blood clot, within an artery.

Jacksonian march The wavelike movement of a seizure from a point of focus to other areas of the brain.

limbic system Structures within the cerebrum and diencephalon that influence emotions, motivation, mood, and sensations of pain and pleasure.

metastasis The process by which cells from a malignant neoplasm break away from the site of origin, such as the lung, and move through the bloodstream or lymphatic system to other body sites, such as the brain.

multiple sclerosis (MS) An autoimmune condition in which the body attacks the myelin that insulates the brain and spinal cord, causing scarring.

myasthenia gravis A condition in which the body generates antibodies against its own acetylcholine receptors, causing muscle weakness, often in the face.

myoclonus Involuntary jerking motions of the body.

neoplasm A tumor.

nystagmus Involuntary, rhythmic shaking of the eyes.

paresthesia Sensation of tingling or numbness in a body part.

Parkinson disease A neurologic condition in which the portion of the brain responsible for production of dopamine has been damaged or overused, resulting in tremors.

peripheral neuropathy A group of conditions in which the nerves that exit the spinal cord are damaged, distorting signals to or from the brain. One type is caused by diabetes; peripheral nerves are damaged as the blood glucose level rises, resulting in lack of sensation, numbness, burning, pain, paresthesia, and muscle weakness.

poliomyelitis A now-rare viral infection that attacks and destroys nerve axons, especially motor axons; the disease can cause weakness, paralysis, and respiratory arrest.

postictal The period after a seizure in which the brain is reorganizing activity.

postpolio syndrome The death of nerve fibers as a late consequence of poliomyelitis; characterized by swallowing difficulties, weakness, fatigue, and breathing problems.

postural tremor A tremor that occurs as the person holds a body part still.

posturing Abnormal body positioning that indicates damage to the brain.

prodrome An early sign or symptom that occurs before a disease or condition fully appears (eg, dizziness before fainting).

pronation Rotation of the lower arms in a palms-down manner.

psychosis Breaking with common reality and existing mainly within an internal world.

ptosis Prolapse of a body part; often refers to drooping of the eyelid.

rest tremor A tremor that occurs when the body part is not in motion.

rigidity A condition in which muscles do not contract and relax smoothly, resulting in stiffness of motion; found in patients with Parkinson disease.

seizure The sudden, erratic firing of neurons; a neurologic episode caused by a surge of electric activity in the brain; can be a convulsion characterized by generalized, uncoordinated muscular activity, and may be associated with loss of consciousness.

status epilepticus A condition in which seizures recur every few minutes, or consecutive seizures without a return to consciousness between seizures.

stroke An interruption of blood flow to the brain that results in the loss of brain function; also called a cerebrovascular accident.

supraorbital foramen A small notch located on the frontal bone near the inner, upper area of each orbit.

syncope A fainting spell or transient loss of consciousness.

tonic activity A type of seizure movement involving the constant contraction and trembling of muscle groups.

transient ischemic attack (TIA) A disorder in which brain cells temporarily stop working because of insufficient oxygen, causing stroke-like symptoms that resolve completely within 24 hours of onset.

tremors Fine involuntary, rhythmic movements, usually involving the hands or head.

trismus The involuntary contraction of the mouth resulting in clenched teeth; occurs during seizures and head injuries.

uremia Severe renal failure resulting in the buildup of waste products within the blood; eventually impairs brain function.

Prep Kit *(continued)*

References

1. Deaths and mortality. Centers for Disease Control and Prevention website. http://www.cdc.gov/nchs/fastats/deaths.htm. Published October 7, 2016. Accessed January 2, 2017.
2. Census Bureau projects U.S. and world populations on New Year's Day [press release]. Washington, DC: United States Census Bureau; December 28, 2016. https://www.census.gov/newsroom/press-releases/2016/cb16-tps158.html.
3. Jauch EC. Ischemic stroke. Medscape website. http://emedicine.medscape.com/article/1916852-overview. Updated November 23, 2015. Accessed March 31, 2016.
4. Jauch EC, Saver JL, Adams HP Jr, Bruno A, Connors JJ, Demaerschalk BM, Khatri P, McMullan PW Jr, Qureshi AI, Rosenfield K, Scott PA, Summers DR, Wang DZ, Wintermark M, Yonas H; on behalf of the American Heart Association Stroke Council, Council on Cardiovascular Nursing, Council on Peripheral Vascular Disease, and Council on Clinical Cardiology. Guidelines for the early management of patients with acute ischemic stroke: a guideline for healthcare professionals from the American Heart Association/American Stroke Association. *Stroke*. 2013;44:870–947.
5. Mozaffarian D, Benjamin EJ, Go AS, Arnett DK, Blaha MJ, Cushman M, Das SR, de Ferranti S, Després J-P, Fullerton HJ, Howard VJ, Huffman MD, Isasi CR, Jiménez MC, Judd SE, Kissela BM, Lichtman JH, Lisabeth LD, Liu S, Mackey RH, Magid DJ, McGuire DK, Mohler ER III, Moy CS, Muntner P, Mussolino ME, Nasir K, Neumar RW, Nichol G, Palaniappan L, Pandey DK, Reeves MJ, Rodriguez CJ, Rosamond W, Sorlie PD, Stein J, Towfighi A, Turan TN, Virani SS, Woo D, Yeh RW, Turner MB; on behalf of the American Heart Association Statistics Committee and Stroke Statistics Subcommittee. Heart disease and stroke statistics—2016 update: a report from the American Heart Association. *Circulation*. 2016;133:000-000.
6. Intracranial pressure monitoring. MedlinePlus website. https://medlineplus.gov/ency/article/003411.htm. Updated June 1, 2015. Accessed September 26, 2016.
7. Badjatia N, Carney N, Crocco T, et al. Guidelines for prehospital management of traumatic brain injury, 2nd edition. *Prehosp Emerg Care.* 2008;12 Suppl 1: S1-S52.
8. National Model EMS Clinical Guidelines. National Association of State EMS Officials. https://www.nasemso.org/Projects/ModelEMSClinicalGuidelines/index.asp. Accessed December 22, 2015.
9. Mobile stroke unit. Cleveland Clinic website. http://my.clevelandclinic.org/services/neurological_institute/cerebrovascular-center/treatment-services/mobile-stroke-unit. Accessed April 3, 2016.
10. Sacco RL, Kasner SE, Broderick JP, Caplan LR, Connors JJ, Culebras A, Elkind MSV, George MG, Hamdan AD, Higashida RT, Hoh BL, Janis LS, Kase CS, Kleindorfer DO, Lee J-M, Moseley ME, Peterson ED, Turan TN, Valderrama AL, Vinters HV; on behalf of the American Heart Association Stroke Council, Council on Cardiovascular Surgery and Anesthesia, Council on Cardiovascular Radiology and Intervention, Council on Cardiovascular and Stroke Nursing, Council on Epidemiology and Prevention, Council on Peripheral Vascular Disease, and Council on Nutrition, Physical Activity and Metabolism. An updated definition of stroke for the 21st century: a statement for healthcare professionals from the American Heart Association/American Stroke Association. Stroke. 2013;44:2064-2089.
11. Transient Ischemic Attack Information Page: National Institute of Neurological Disorders and Stroke (NINDS). https://www.ninds.nih.gov/Disorders/All-Disorders/Transient-Ischemic-Attack-Information-Page. Accessed January 18, 2017.
12. Ko DY. Epilepsy and seizures. Medscape website. http://emedicine.medscape.com/article/1184846-overview. Updated July 12, 2016. Accessed April 8, 2016.
13. Moghaddasi M, Joodat R, Ataei E. Evaluation of short-term mortality of status epilepticus and its risk factors. *J Epilepsy Res*. 2015;5(1):13-16. https://www.ncbi.nlm.nih.gov/pmc/articles/PMC4494989/. Accessed January 7, 2017.
14. Morag R. Syncope. Medscape website.http://emedicine.medscape.com/article/811669-overview. Updated December 7, 2015. Accessed April 8, 2016.
15. Andary MT. Guillain-Barré syndrome. Medscape website. http://emedicine.medscape.com/article/315632-overview. Updated February 12, 2016. Accessed March 27, 2016.
16. Foster MR. Spina bifida. Medscape website. http://emedicine.medscape.com/article/311113-overview. Updated September 22, 2016. Accessed March 26, 2016.
17. Nelson SL, Jr. Hydrocephalus. Medscape website. http://emedicine.medscape.com/article/1135286-overview. Updated April 13, 2016. Accessed March 26, 2016.

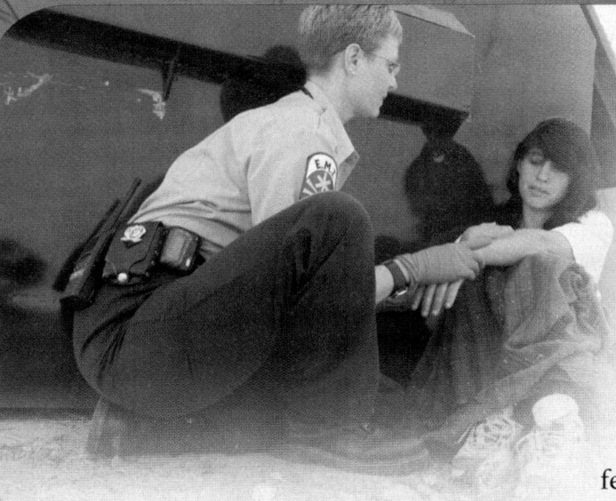

Assessment *in Action*

You arrive at a mobile home and are directed to the master bedroom in the rear of the home. You find a middle-aged man lying in bed and not moving. The patient's wife tells you he laid down for a nap about 3 hours ago and has not woken up. He was feeling tired and weak for the past several weeks. The wife is concerned and cooperative. She states she feels well.

1. Based on the scene size-up, which patient moving equipment is most likely to be needed?

A. Stokes basket
B. Ambulance cot
C. Flexible stretcher
D. Scoop stretcher

2. Which common causes of unresponsiveness can you rule out based on the information you have gathered?

A. Trauma
B. Overdose
C. Uremia
D. Altered glucose levels

At this point in the call, your patient has been moved into the ambulance. His skin is cool and clammy. His heart rate is 124 beats/min, his respiratory rate is 140 breaths/min, and his blood pressure level is 74/52 mm Hg. When you established IV access, he moaned. He has not opened his eyes or moved. You examine his eyes and note they are twitching with pupils at 3 mm and equal bilaterally.

3. What is this patient's GCS score?

A. 3
B. 4
C. 5
D. 6

4. Based on the information you have gathered, which $ETCO_2$ level should you anticipate?

A. 15 mm Hg
B. 25 mm Hg
C. 35 mm Hg
D. 45 mm Hg

5. Which term is the MOST appropriate to describe the twitching of this patient's eyes?

A. Anisocoria
B. Presbyopia
C. Nystagmus
D. Miosis

6. Which laboratory value is the MOST important to gather regarding this patient?

A. Potassium level
B. Lactate level
C. Carbon monoxide level
D. Glucose level

7. What assessment information would be MOST valuable in determining the cause of this patient's altered LOC?

A. Tactile fremitus
B. Doll eye test
C. Percussion findings on the chest
D. Body temperature

Assessment *in Action* *(continued)*

You are dispatched to a nursing home for an unresponsive patient having a seizure. You find a man having a sustained tonic seizure. The nursing staff states the patient is normally awake and alert, but began feeling poorly today. His blood glucose level is 183 mg/dL and his blood pressure is 134/80 mm Hg. The seizure started at least 5 minutes earlier and has been tonic the entire time. The patient has not awoken.

The GCS score is 3. His skin is warm, dry, and pink. Heart rhythm is regular and rapid with a wide complex at a rate of 170 beats/min. This rhythm spontaneously resolves after about 3 minutes to sinus tachycardia with narrow QRS.

8. Which diagnostic tests should be performed on this patient?

9. Why has a sudden change occurred in this patient's cardiac rhythm?

10. How should this patient be managed?

CHAPTER 19

Diseases of the Eyes, Ears, Nose, and Throat

National EMS Education Standard Competencies

Medicine

Integrates assessment findings with principles of epidemiology and pathophysiology to formulate a field impression and implement a comprehensive treatment/disposition plan for a patient with a medical complaint.

Diseases of the Eyes, Ears, Nose, and Throat

Knowledge of the anatomy, physiology, epidemiology, pathophysiology, psychosocial impact, presentations, prognosis, and management of

- Common or major diseases of the eyes, ears, nose, and throat, including nose bleed (pp 1144-1163)

Knowledge Objectives

1. Explain facial anatomy and relate physiology to facial disorders. (pp 1140-1141, 1149, 1154, 1157-1159)
2. Relate assessment findings associated with eye disorders to pathophysiology. (pp 1141-1145)
3. Describe assessment, treatment, and management of specific eye conditions. (pp 1144-1149)
4. Relate assessment findings associated with ear disorders to pathophysiology. (pp 1149-1151)
5. Describe assessment, treatment, and management of specific ear conditions. (pp 1150-1153)
6. Relate assessment findings associated with nose disorders to pathophysiology. (p 1154)
7. Describe assessment, treatment, and management of specific nose conditions. (pp 1154-1157)
8. Relate assessment findings associated with throat and mouth disorders to pathophysiology. (p 1158)
9. Describe assessment, treatment, and management of specific throat and mouth conditions. (pp 1158-1163)

Skills Objectives

1. Use an ophthalmoscope to examine a patient's eyes. (pp 1144-1145, Skill Drill 19-1)
2. Use an otoscope to examine a patient's ears. (pp 1150-1151, Skill Drill 19-2)

Introduction

Disorders of the eye, ear, nose, and throat (EENT) are a common focus of concern for paramedics who are treating medical patients. Understanding of the basics of EENT diseases and injuries is an essential piece of the paramedic's medical assessment and treatment knowledge base.

A significant number of calls for emergency medical services (EMS) involving EENT structures are a result of trauma; such injuries are discussed in detail in Chapter 33, *Face and Neck Trauma*. This chapter covers medical conditions that could result in a call to 9-1-1, or that you could notice when you are assessing a patient who called 9-1-1 for an unrelated reason. During such calls, familiarity with EENT conditions will help you during assessment of the patient. Knowledge of these conditions also enables you to educate the patient about prevention of or potential care for a condition that the patient may have.

Oftentimes, when you encounter a patient with an EENT disorder, it makes sense to transport the patient, possibly to an emergency department with access to an eye specialist or an ear, nose, and throat specialist for further evaluation. For example, whenever an object is lodged in the eye, ear, nose, or throat, the patient must be transported to the hospital. Patients with eye injuries should be transported to a Level 1 or 2 trauma center that has ophthalmology services available.

This chapter begins by discussing general considerations when you are assessing a patient with a complaint related to a condition of the eyes, ears, nose, and throat. You will also learn about specific conditions and their field treatment, if any.

The Eye

The American College of Ophthalmology reports more than 2.4 million Americans have eye emergencies each year.[1] Examples of eye disease emergencies include **glaucoma**, macular degeneration, and **diabetic retinopathy**. Patients with these diseases have a long-standing history of an underlying condition that then predisposes them to the eye disorder (comorbidity). Mortality from eye disease is quite low, however.

Anatomy and Physiology Review

The eye is the body's window to the world. It is connected to the brain by two nerves. The **oculomotor nerve** (third cranial nerve) innervates the muscles that cause eye movement as well as the parasympathetic nerve fibers that

Special Populations

According to the United States Centers for Disease Control and Prevention (CDC), vision disability is one of the top 10 disabilities among children.[2]

In the geriatric population, you are likely to encounter patients who have undergone laser-assisted eye surgery (Lasik surgery), a procedure that can reduce the need for corrective lenses. Traditional Lasik surgery uses a special laser to slice a flap in the cornea and adjust the shape of the middle section of the cornea (stroma); the latest techniques manipulate the stroma without creating the "flap" in the cornea. Immediately following the surgery and for the next few weeks, patients are instructed to not let air blow directly into their eyes and to wear goggles while they sleep so they do not scratch their cornea. Geriatric patients are also more likely to undergo **cataract** surgery and eye surgery for glaucoma.

Older people may also experience eye injuries from falls. Eye conditions and problems are among the many different comorbid conditions often found in the geriatric population.

Diabetes is the leading cause of new cases of blindness in adults, according to the CDC.[3] One in three adults with diabetes who is older than 40 years has diabetic retinopathy, a disease that affects the small blood vessels in the retina. Vision disturbances associated with this condition can include blurred vision, floaters and flashes of light, blind spots, or blindness. Currently, vision-threatening retinopathy affects approximately 899,000 Americans.[3] According to the CDC, the prevalence of diabetic retinopathy is expected to increase from 2.5 million cases (all levels of severity) in 2005 to 9.9 million cases by 2050 among Americans 65 years or older.[4]

YOU are the Paramedic — PART 1

You are dispatched to a local acute care rehabilitation center for a 62-year-old woman recovering from left-side weakness after a stroke who is experiencing a severe nose bleed. It is a blustery winter day outside. When you arrive on scene, you are directed to the dining area, where you find the patient seated at a table, with staff helping her hold a towel to her nose. Blood is visible on the table in front of the patient as well as on the towel. The patient is sitting upright and leaning slightly forward, breathing through her mouth, and looks pale. The staff advises you that the patient was eating lunch when suddenly her nose began to bleed.

1. What is your primary concern after scene safety is established?
2. Do you have concerns other than the nose bleed?

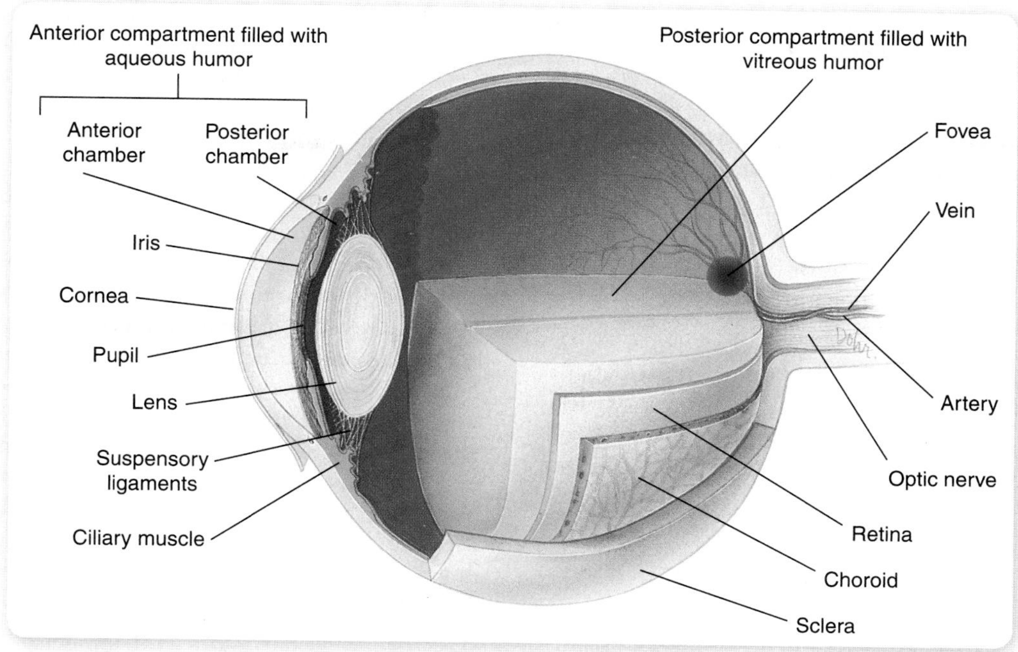

Figure 19-1 A review of the structures of the eye.

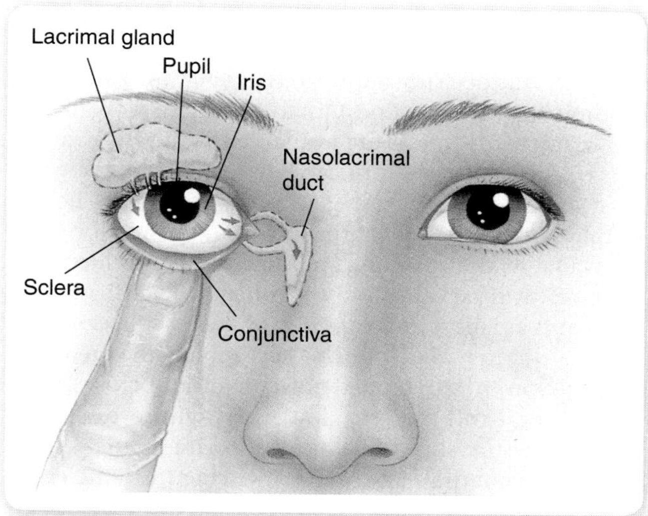

Figure 19-2 The lacrimal system of tear glands and ducts.

cause constriction of the pupil and accommodation of the lens. The optic nerve (second cranial nerve) provides the sense of vision. **Figure 19-1** and **Figure 19-2** depict the anatomy of the eye and the lacrimal system.

▶ Patient Assessment

Keeping your team safe from the often hidden dangers at medical scenes should be the first item on your priority list. In patients with eye disorders, fear and panic from loss of vision can sometimes trigger dangerous and bizarre behavior. Keep the patient calm. The scene size-up is an opportunity to discover clues to the cause of the complaint, while avoiding potential hazards.

As you form a general impression of the patient, note environmental clues at the scene, the approximate age and sex of the patient, and his or her degree of distress. Do not let the high degree of distress or concern over the potential visual impairment sidetrack your observations of the scene and cause you to miss the hazards that may have caused an injury or condition.

Do not become distracted by a swollen, irritated, or deformed eye to the extent that you bypass the highest-priority aspects of the patient's care. You must ensure the patient has an open and adequate airway, that the patient is breathing, that there are no threats to ventilation, that the patient has an adequate pulse, and that no life threats to the patient's circulation need your immediate attention.

Depending on the severity of the eye condition, an early transport decision to the right facility can improve outcomes. Level 1 trauma centers have the skilled services necessary to treat a serious eye problem.

Covering both eyes can limit damage to the affected eye. Consider pain management and, if necessary, mild sedation during transport for patients with eye emergencies. Cardiac monitoring is recommended in these patients as well. Ocular pressure can stimulate the vagus nerve, leading to a vagal response in the patient. Eye drops and eye medication can cause side effects such as low or high blood pressure.

As a paramedic, your demeanor should be supportive and calm. Remember, a patient facing potential long-term vision loss will need emotional care as well; this can be a life-changing event for the patient.

Obtain the chief complaint from the patient and begin to elaborate on it using the OPQRST (Onset, Provocation/palliation, Quality, Region/radiation, Severity, Timing) mnemonic. When you are obtaining the history, determine how and when the symptoms began, and which symptoms the patient is experiencing. Are both eyes affected? Does the patient have any underlying diseases or conditions of the eye (such as glaucoma)? Does the patient take medications for his or her eyes?

A variety of symptoms may indicate a serious ocular condition:

- *Visual loss* that does not improve when the patient blinks is an important symptom. It may indicate damage to the globe or to the optic nerve.
- *Double vision* usually points to trauma involving the extraocular muscles, such as a fracture of the orbit.
- *Severe eye pain* is a symptom of a significant eye injury.
- A *foreign body sensation* usually indicates superficial injury to the cornea or the presence of a foreign object trapped behind the eyelids.

Assessment of specific eye conditions begins with a thorough examination to determine the extent and nature of the situation. Always perform your examination while maintaining standard precautions, taking great care to avoid aggravating the affected area. Assess for pain or tenderness, swelling, abnormal or loss of movement, sensation changes, circulatory changes, deformity, visual changes, and airway compromise.

Physical examination of the eyes includes assessment of the visible ocular structures, as well as ocular function. This evaluation is described in Chapter 11, *Patient Assessment*. Assess the ocular structures for the following findings:

- **Orbital rim.** Assess for ecchymosis, swelling, lacerations, and tenderness.
- **Eyelids.** Assess for ecchymosis, swelling, lacerations, and any abnormalities.
- **Corneas.** Assess for foreign bodies.
- **Conjunctivae.** Assess for redness, pus, inflammation, and foreign bodies.
- **Globes.** Assess for redness, abnormal pigmentation, and lacerations. Inspect the eye surface for growths, discoloration, and differences between the eyes.
- **Pupils.** Assess for PERRLA (pupils equal, round, reactive to light and accommodation). Note whether the pupils are symmetric.

When you are assessing ocular function, perform the following tests:

- **Visual acuity.** Assess the patient's ability to see large and small letters—for example, by reading the writing on a prescription bottle, or by using a hand-held visual acuity chart such as the Snellen chart (shown in Chapter 11, *Patient Assessment*). Test each eye separately and document the results.
- **Peripheral vision.** Evaluate the patient's peripheral vision by testing the ability to recognize an object entering the extremes of the visual field (confrontation).
- **Ocular motility.** Check the patient's ability to move the eyes in all directions. Check for paralysis of gaze or discoordination between the movements of the two eyes (**dysconjugate gaze**).

In addition to the physical examination, you should obtain a full set of baseline vital signs during the secondary assessment. During reassessment, vital signs should be monitored every 5 to 15 minutes, depending on the severity of the patient's condition. Continuing assessment allows you to track any trends in these indicators.

Note that a patient may experience adverse effects if he or she uses multiple eye medications. Also, if a patient uses too much of one or several medications, he or she may experience both local and systemic adverse effects; the systemic effects are possible because the medication can enter the bloodstream via the nasolacrimal system, which drains tears from the eyes.

Ask the patient how he or she administered the eye medications. Sometimes part of the problem is that the patient did not follow the instructions for the specific medication. For example, it is usually recommended to wait approximately 5 minutes between administering the first and second drops of an eye medication. Of course, this 5-minute rule does not apply to emergency measures such as administering tetracaine prior to inserting a Morgan lens.

Many medications are available to address a variety of eye problems. Eye drops can be used for **conjunctivitis**, dry eyes, red eyes, eye pain, glaucoma, eye surgery, herpes simplex, itchy eyes, and corneal abrasions. Eye lubricants are available for protecting eyes that do not produce tears (as a result of seventh nerve damage). Eye drops and lubricants are most often applied by gently squeezing the lower eyelid to make a pouch and applying the medicine into the lower lid. The patient then should close his or her eyes and roll the eyes downward with eyes closed. Gentle pressure should be applied to the corner of the eyes to prevent drainage of the medicine from the eye.

Always ask patients which medications they have taken prior to your arrival on the scene. For the paramedic, administration of eye medications in the prehospital setting is usually limited to tetracaine (Pontocaine, Dicaine) for pain relief, or emergency irrigation for removal of a damaging or irritating substance from the eyes. As the population of geriatric patients—who are more vulnerable to eye conditions such as glaucoma—increases, however, the scope of practice for the paramedic may change to include limited eye care.

Irrigation of the eyes may be necessary for chemical burns or thermal burns. Such treatment consists of application of sterile water or isotonic saline solution to the eye, with the liquid being flushed from the inside corner to the outside of the eye, except when a Morgan lens is being used (described later in this chapter).

Eye injuries should be seen in the emergency department. Children with eye emergencies may need to be treated under anesthesia, and many patients with eye injuries will need a topical anesthetic and antibiotic. These medications are not generally administered by a paramedic, but rather by hospital personnel.

Words of Wisdom

Anisocoria, a condition in which the pupils are not of equal size, is a significant finding in patients with ocular injuries or closed head trauma. However, simple or physiologic anisocoria occurs in approximately 20% of the population, according to the American Academy of Ophthalmology.[5] In other words, approximately one person out of five has some degree of difference in the sizes of the pupils. Usually, the patient's pupils differ in size by less than 1 mm; however, approximately 4% of people have pupils that vary in size by more than 1 mm. This is not a clinically significant finding.

Unilateral cataract surgery may also cause inequality of pupil size. The pupil of the eye affected by the cataract will be nonreactive to light.

Eye injuries may be irreversible, and patients may or may not be aware of the seriousness of the event. Patients may exhibit denial, anger, fear, hysteria, and depression in response to the potential loss of vision. Communication is key to keeping the patient calm and informed. Remember that early decisions to transport to the appropriate facility can improve outcomes in some patients, and early communication with a medical control physician can help direct your care and inform transport decisions.

Patients Wearing Contact Lenses

You may encounter patients who wear contact lenses. In general, if the eye is injured, you should not attempt to remove contact lenses because you may further aggravate the injury. The only indication for removing contact lenses in the prehospital setting is a chemical burn of the eye (discussed in Chapter 33, *Face and Neck Trauma*). In this situation, the lens can trap the offending chemical and make irrigation difficult, thereby worsening the injury.

There are three types of contact lenses: hard, rigid gas-permeable, and soft (hydrophilic). Small, hard contact lenses usually are tinted, making them relatively easy to see. Large, soft contact lenses are clear and can be difficult to see, especially if they "float" up or down under an eyelid.

To remove a hard contact lens, use a small suction cup, moistening the end with saline **Figure 19-3A**. To remove soft lenses, place one to two drops of saline in the eye **Figure 19-3B**, gently pinch the lens between your gloved thumb and index finger, and lift it off the surface of the eye **Figure 19-3C**. Place the contact lens

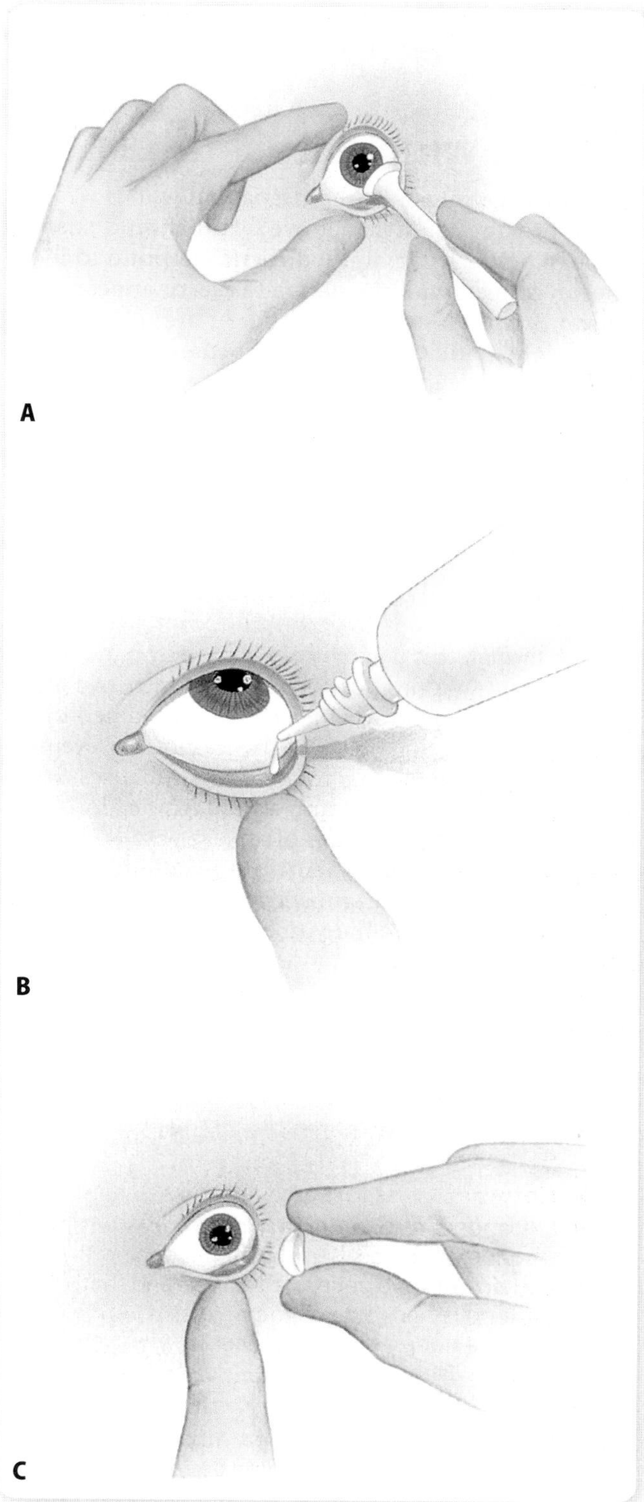

Figure 19-3 Removal of contact lenses should be limited to patients with chemical burns to the eye. **A.** To remove hard contact lenses, use a specialized suction cup moistened with sterile saline solution. **B.** Step 1: To remove soft contact lenses, instill 1 or 2 drops of saline or irrigating solution. **C.** Step 2: Pinch off the lens with your gloved thumb and index fingers.

in a container with sterile saline solution. Always advise emergency department staff if a patient is wearing contact lenses.

Patients With an Eye Prosthesis

Occasionally, you may care for a patient who is wearing an eye prosthesis (artificial eye). You should suspect an eye of being artificial if it does not respond to light, move in concert with the opposite eye, or appear quite the same as the opposite eye. If you are unsure as to whether the patient has an eye prosthesis, ask the patient. No harm will be done if you care for an artificial eye as you would a normal one; however, you should make every attempt to accurately determine the patient's eye function.

Use of an Ophthalmoscope

In the hospital and physician's office, practitioners may use an **ophthalmoscope** to perform a thorough eye examination, though this device is rarely used by paramedics. The ophthalmoscope consists of a concave mirror and a battery-powered light, which is usually contained in the device's handle **Figure 19-4**. The monocular eyepiece is usually equipped with a rotating disk of lenses; selection of a lens allows the depth and magnification to be adjusted. Effective evaluation of the eye with this device requires dilation of the patient's pupil with medication, as well as significant diagnostic expertise to be able to accurately determine what you are looking at and how to interpret it clinically.

The steps in **Skill Drill 19-1** show how to examine the eye with an ophthalmoscope.

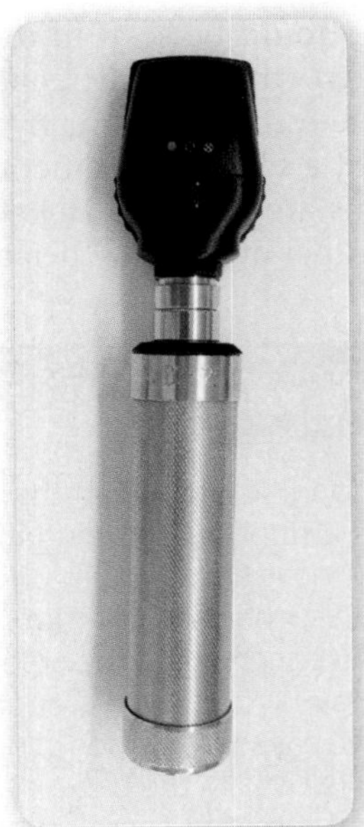

Figure 19-4 Ophthalmoscope.

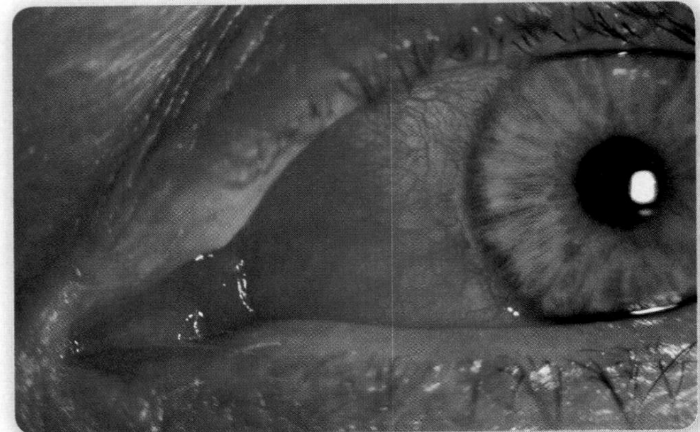

Figure 19-5 Conjunctivitis is inflammation of the eye. It may be associated with the presence of a foreign object in the eye.

Words of Wisdom

When patients ask you what you think is wrong, remember that you are serving them. Remind them that you do not have definitive answers and that you are not a physician, but tell them what you think is going on. Be honest and sincere about what you are telling them, with the goal of keeping patients both informed and calm.

▶ Pathophysiology, Assessment, and Management of Specific Eye Conditions

This section covers specific eye conditions. Eye trauma (ie, adnexa, burns of the eye, corneal abrasion, foreign body in the eye, hyphema, and retinal detachment and defect) is covered in Chapter 33, *Face and Neck Trauma*.

Conjunctivitis

Conjunctivitis, also known as "pink eye," is a condition in which the conjunctiva becomes inflamed and red **Figure 19-5**. The conjunctiva is a thin layer that lines the inside of the eyelids and the white part of the eye. Inflammation causes the white part of the eye to take on a red or pink tint.

Conjunctivitis most often starts in one eye and spreads to the other eye. Most often, this condition is caused by bacteria, viruses, allergies, chemicals, or foreign bodies present in the eye. The viral and bacterial forms are highly contagious and can become an epidemic. In fact, conjunctivitis accounts for a significant number of absences in daycare and school settings.[6] Viral conjunctivitis is often associated with an upper respiratory virus or cold, whereas bacterial conjunctivitis is caused by various bacterial infections. Allergic conjunctivitis is caused by a trigger or irritating

Skill Drill 19-1 Examining the Eye With an Ophthalmoscope

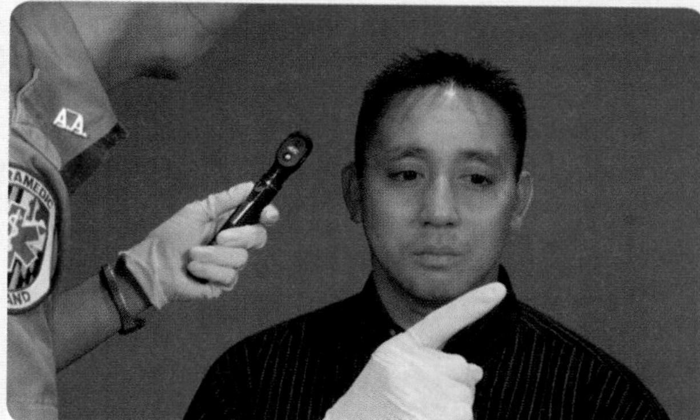

Step 1 Darken the environment as much as possible. Ask the patient to look straight ahead and focus on a distant object.

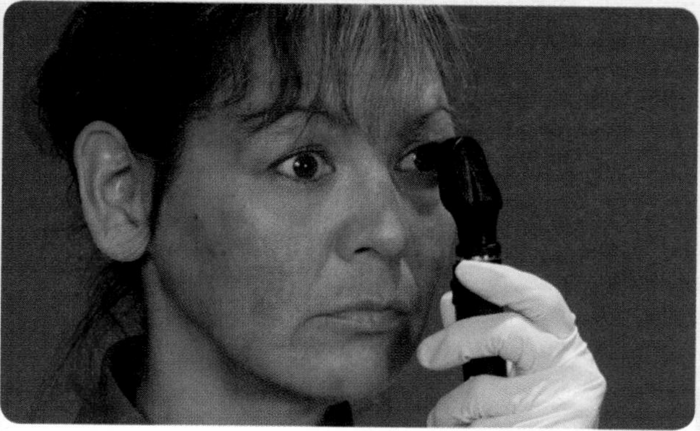

Step 2 Set the light on the ophthalmoscope to a setting no brighter than necessary and the lens to 0, unless another setting works better for your eyes. Use your right hand and eye to examine the patient's right eye; use your left hand and eye to examine the patient's left eye.

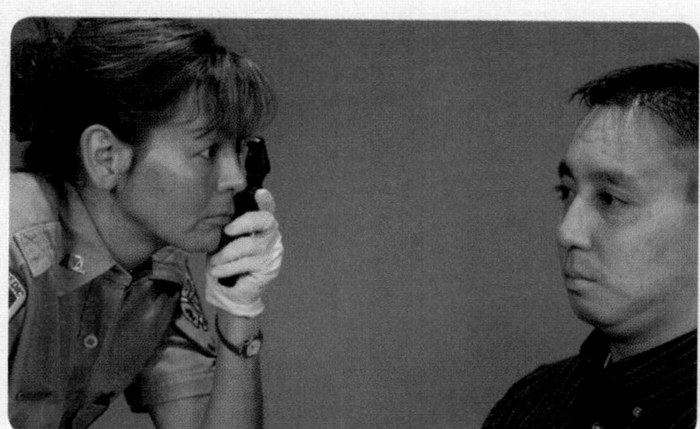

Step 3 Place the scope to your eye and look into the patient's pupil from 10 to 20 inches (25 to 51 cm) away at a 45° angle to the eye. You should see the retina as a "red reflex," or a bright orange glow. Slowly move toward the patient to appreciate the structures of the fundus. Adjust the lens as needed to improve the focus. Locate a blood vessel and follow it back to the disk. Use this blood vessel as a point of reference.

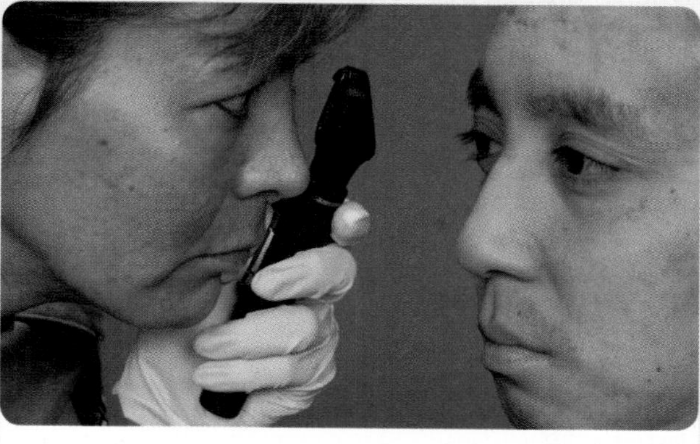

Step 4 Inspect for the size, color, and clarity of the disk. Note the integrity of the blood vessels and any lesions present on the retina. Move nasally to observe the macula. Repeat the process with the other eye.

allergen, such as pollen. Chlorine in swimming pools and air pollution are potential causes of chemical conjunctivitis. If conjunctivitis is due to a foreign body, the eye will begin to produce tears in an attempt to flush out the object.

Assessment and Management. When conjunctivitis is suspected, general assessment of the patient's vision should be performed, including assessment of visual acuity, assessment of the external eye, assessment of the pupils, assessment of peripheral vision, and assessment of eye movement.

Viral conjunctivitis normally resolves on its own. It can last up to 2 weeks but usually reaches a peak in 3 to 5 days. Bacterial conjunctivitis requires a topical antibiotic to eliminate the infection. Severe cases of allergic conjunctivitis may require nonsteroidal anti-inflammatory drugs (NSAIDs), antihistamines, and topical steroid eye drops prescribed by the physician in the emergency department.

Inflammation of the Eyelid (Chalazion and Hordeolum)

The eyelid contains oil glands and oil ducts that provide a protective film across the eye. A **chalazion** is a small, usually painless lump or pustule on the external eyelid that appears red and swollen, and that forms because of blockage and swelling of an oil gland in the eyelid **Figure 19-6**. A chalazion is often confused with a **hordeolum**. A hordeolum **Figure 19-7** is an infection of an oil gland in the eyelid that produces a red, swollen, painful lump in the eyelid or at the lid margin. It may be either internal (rare) or external. An external hordeolum is commonly called a stye.

Assessment and Management. A thorough assessment of vital signs, history, and transport for physician evaluation is warranted when a patient has an inflammation of the eyelid. The patient will usually be asked to apply warm compresses for 5 to 10 minutes several times a day to help soften the hardened oil that is blocking the ducts, thereby allowing the duct to drain. Topical or oral antibiotics may be prescribed.

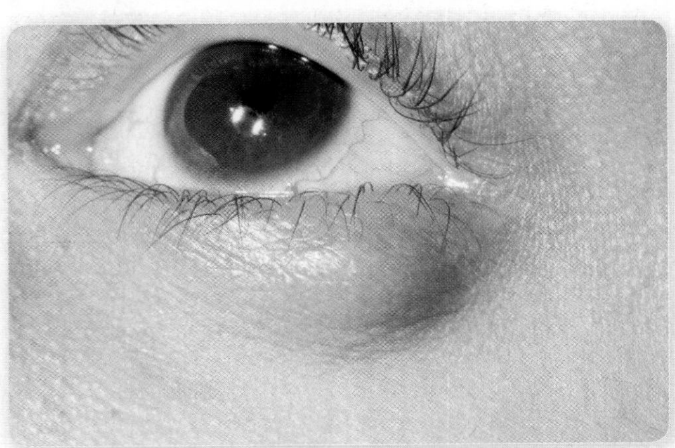

Figure 19-6 A chalazion is a small lump or pustule on the external eyelid.

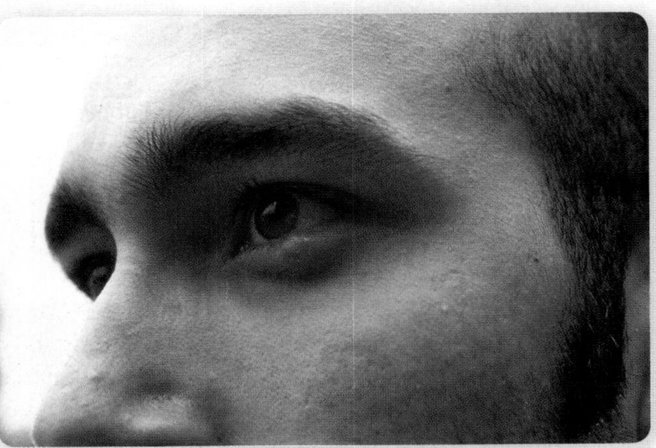

Figure 19-7 An external hordeolum, or stye, is a red, tender lump in the eyelid or at the lid margin.

YOU are the Paramedic PART 2

The patient seems tired and weak. While your partner is obtaining her vital signs, you ask the patient and care staff what happened. The patient states that she sat down to eat lunch and blood started gushing out of her nose. She is coughing and spitting up some blood as well.

Recording Time: 0 Minutes	
Appearance	Awake
Level of consciousness	Alert (oriented to person, place, time, and event)
Airway	Open
Breathing	Coughing; some gurgling in mouth as patient spits blood
Circulation	Adequate, epistaxis noted

3. What do you need to know about the patient's history?
4. What is the priority in managing this patient?

Glaucoma

Glaucoma is a group of conditions that lead to increased intraocular pressure. It is one of the leading causes of blindness.

Recall from Chapter 8, *Anatomy and Physiology*, the aqueous humor is a clear, watery fluid that fills the eye's anterior chamber. It maintains intraocular pressure, provides nutrients to the inner surface of the eye, and helps to bend light.[7] The aqueous humor circulates through the pupil and drains into the venous system by the canal of Schlemm, which is a thin-walled vein that extends around the eye.

Several types of glaucoma are distinguished. In *open-angle glaucoma*, the aqueous fluid drains too slowly. Over time, pressure builds up within the eye (intraocular pressure) and damages the optic nerve. This is the most common type of glaucoma. *Normal-tension glaucoma* is a type of glaucoma that can cause vision changes with no increase in intraocular pressure. In *narrow-angle glaucoma* (also called angle-closure glaucoma), access to the drainage channel is narrowed, which prevents proper drainage of aqueous fluid. Pressure builds up in the posterior chamber of the eye, which pushes the lens forward. The lens then pushes the iris into the drainage channel, completely blocking it.

Secondary glaucoma occurs as a result of conditions that damage the drainage channel in the eye. Examples of these conditions include diabetes, eye injuries, leukemia, sickle cell anemia, some types of arthritis, and cataracts.

The incidence of glaucoma increases with age, so that it is more common among older adults. Nevertheless, this condition can occur at any time from birth onward. Glaucoma is usually treated with eye drops to reduce the ocular pressure.

Assessment and Management. Glaucoma usually affects a person's peripheral vision first. Eventually, the patient develops tunnel vision, in which he or she can see only what is directly ahead. With chronic glaucoma, the patient may have no symptoms until vision loss occurs.

A patient who has an acute attack of narrow-angle glaucoma may report severe eye pain, headache, photophobia, nausea, and vomiting. The cornea may look cloudy. The patient may report blurred vision and halos around lights because of corneal swelling. The pupils often have irregular margins and can be fixed in mid-position and dilated. An attack may be triggered by pupil dilation, such as eye drops given during an eye examination or dim lighting. Acute narrow-angle glaucoma is a medical emergency—the patient needs evaluation by a physician. If intraocular pressure is not reduced, permanent vision loss can occur.

Assessment should rule out any trauma or physical injury to the eye. You should perform a general eye assessment as described earlier, evaluating vision, motility, and any abnormalities of the external eye or anterior surface. Document any pertinent negatives and all abnormal findings. An ophthalmologist will later perform a much more comprehensive exam, assessing the intraocular pressure, the shape and color of the optic nerve viewed through a dilated pupil, the angle in the eye where the iris meets the cornea, and the thickness of the cornea. This physician will also perform a test to assess the complete field of vision. Because paramedics are not normally trained to conduct this kind of comprehensive eye exam, all patients with eye injuries or conditions should be transported to the emergency department for evaluation.

Central Retinal Artery Occlusion

Central retinal artery occlusion is a condition in which the blood supply to the retina becomes blocked because of a clot or embolus in the central retinal artery or one of its branches. Possible causes of central retinal artery occlusion include an embolus from the carotid artery, valvular heart disease, drug abuse, fat emboli, arterial spasm, and oral contraceptive use. Central retinal artery occlusion may cause partial blindness, which may be temporary or permanent.

Assessment and Management. The patient with central retinal artery occlusion usually seeks medical assistance because of a sudden, painless loss of vision in one eye. If the central retinal artery is blocked, then the patient is likely to experience a complete loss of vision in one eye. If a branch of the central retinal artery is blocked, then the patient will likely develop partial loss of vision in one eye. In some patients, symptoms may be preceded by flickering or a transient loss of vision weeks or months before the acute event.

Vision loss in central retinal *vein* occlusion is not as sudden as that of central retinal artery occlusion. Instead, this vision loss progresses over 30 to 120 minutes, with the end result being very reduced vision in the affected eye.[8]

A situation involving a rapid loss of vision is an emergency. Retinal damage begins within minutes of the cessation of blood flow, which can lead to permanent visual deficits. Immediately transport the patient to the closest appropriate facility and provide supportive care en route.

Iritis

Iritis, also known as anterior uveitis, involves inflammation of the iris Figure 19-8. Uveitis is the third leading preventable cause of blindness.

Iritis can be acute or chronic. When acute, it can be caused by trauma or irritants, and usually affects only one eye. Autoimmune diseases, different types of arthritis, irritable bowel disease, and Crohn disease can predispose patients to developing iritis. Infectious causes include Lyme disease, tuberculosis, and sexually transmitted diseases.

Assessment and Management. Iritis presents as a red area surrounding the iris, cloudy vision, or an unusually shaped pupil. The assessment should focus on history.

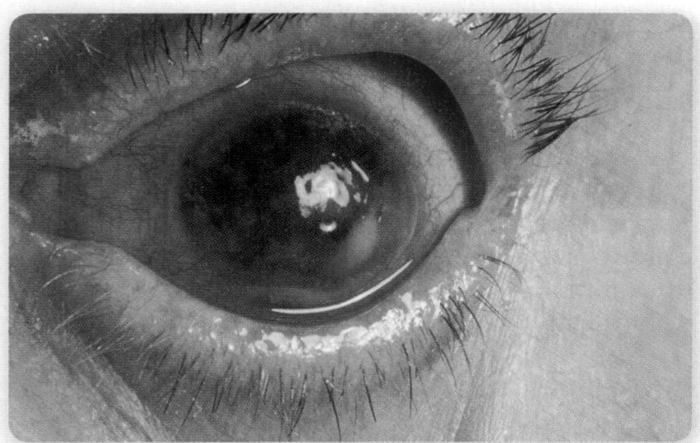

Figure 19-8 Iritis is inflammation of the iris.

Because many ophthalmologists are not trained to recognize iritis, patients suspected of having this condition should be directed to a uveitis specialist or an ocular immunologist.

Acute iritis usually responds well to topical corticosteroids as long as the cause is not fungal, viral, or bacterial. According to the Iritis Organization, more than 90 different pathogens or autoimmune processes have a relationship to chronic or recurrent iritis.[9] Patients with this condition should be referred to a specialist. Failure to treat iritis can result in permanent disability.

Papilledema

Papilledema results from swelling or inflammation of the optic nerve at the rear part of the eye. The optic nerve communicates between the eyes and the brain. When it is affected, patients may experience headaches, nausea with possible vomiting, temporary vision loss, or narrowing vision fields. They may also experience a "graying" in their field of vision.

The increased pressure in the brain that causes optic nerve swelling and inflammation may have several different causes. Space-occupying lesions such as abscesses and tumors can create increased intracranial pressure. An inner ear infection, lung infection, or dental infection can lead to pus accumulation in the brain, causing an abscess that presses on the optic nerve. Meningitis, fever, brain tumors, hypertensive crisis, chronic high blood pressure, and other diseases such as Guillain-Barré syndrome may all result in an increase in cerebrospinal fluid (CSF) pressures, leading to papilledema.

Assessment and Management. The diagnosis of papilledema is made by an ophthalmologist, or an emergency department physician, who has been trained to examine the patient's retina with an ophthalmoscope. Paramedics who have an expanded scope of practice that includes use of an ophthalmoscope should receive further training in the use of this device from their medical director. If swelling is present, red spots will also indicate the presence of bleeding.

Prehospital management consists of treating the symptoms and transporting the patient. As always, assess the ABCDEs to ensure that there are no life threats. Depending on the severity of anxiousness or pain, the patient may benefit from analgesics or a mild sedative. Vision loss can become permanent if treatment of papilledema does not begin within a few days of this condition's onset; therefore, immediate treatment should be encouraged. Treatment is aimed at remedying the underlying cause of the intracranial pressure increase.

Cellulitis of the Orbit: Periorbital and Orbital Cellulitis

Periorbital and orbital cellulitis are most commonly caused by *Staphylococcus* and *Streptococcus* bacterial infections. The location of the infection determines which type is diagnosed.

Periorbital cellulitis is more prevalent in children than adults. Also known as preseptal cellulitis or eyelid cellulitis, it presents as a painful, red, swollen eyelid. Fever may also be a symptom, along with redness of the white part of the eyes (conjunctivitis). Insect bites, upper respiratory disorders, and trauma increase the patient's risk of developing periorbital cellulitis.

Orbital cellulitis is an infection within the eye socket that is considered a medical emergency because it can lead to permanent vision problems and blindness. The goal of treatment is to avoid the formation of an abscess. Risk factors that predispose individuals to develop orbital cellulitis include **sinusitis**, tooth infections, facial or middle ear infections, trauma, and sinus infections.

Assessment and Management. Prehospital management of cellulitis of the orbit is directed at ruling out life threats, taking a thorough history, and transporting the patient to an appropriate care site. Treatment of children usually consists of intravenous (IV) antibiotics for both forms of cellulitis. Adults are treated with oral antibiotics; however, if symptoms are severe, IV antibiotics may be used for adults as well.

Corneal Abrasion or Ulcer

Recall, the cornea is the transparent outer covering of the eye. It is susceptible to injury and infection because of its location. A corneal abrasion is a common eye injury typically caused by direct trauma, foreign bodies, contact lenses, or exposure to ultraviolet radiation.[10] For example, traumatic corneal abrasions may be the result of fingernails, makeup applicators, tree branches, hand tools, sports injuries, or deployed air bags. Construction workers and mechanics are prone to corneal abrasions from foreign bodies such as pieces of metal, wood, glass, plastic, or fiberglass. Improperly fitted or maintained contact lenses can also cause a corneal abrasion. An ulcer can develop if an abrasion is not treated promptly. A corneal ulcer is always a medical emergency because it can cause blindness if left untreated.

Assessment and Management. Although some patients who have a corneal abrasion will be able to tell you precisely when the event occurred, other patients will be unable to do so because symptoms may not occur until hours after the injury. Signs and symptoms of corneal abrasion and ulcer include pain with extraocular movement, redness, and excessive tearing. The patient may describe a sensation of having something foreign in the eye, blurred vision or loss of vision, photophobia, and headache.

Prehospital management of is directed at ruling out life threats, taking a thorough history, and transporting the patient promptly for definitive care.

The Ear

The ear is the primary structure for hearing and balance, but is also integral to self-protection. When you think of ear problems, you most likely think of hearing loss. In reality, hearing is not all the ear affects: The ear also plays in important part in balance and orientation. Disorders and injury to the ear can leave a person unable to communicate, react, and maintain equilibrium. For example, scuba divers are susceptible to **vertigo** (dizziness) from cold water moving into the ear canal during pressure equalization. Changes in air pressure when at higher levels above sea level (eg, in the mountains) as well as when flying can also cause ear discomfort. A tumor that grows on the eighth cranial nerve (acoustic neuroma) can affect the inner ear and balance. Such a tumor is usually slow growing, but if it grows larger, other cranial nerves can be affected, including the fifth, sixth, and seventh cranial nerves. This kind of damage can affect facial sensation, eye movement, facial movement, taste, and hearing.

Loss of hearing is a major health problem for adults, most likely associated with occupational noise injury. Hearing loss can affect a child's ability to develop communication, language, and social skills. The earlier children with hearing loss start receiving services, the more likely they are to reach their full potential.

Anatomy and Physiology Review

The ear is divided into three anatomic parts: external, middle, and inner **Figure 19-9**. Sound waves travel through the ear, and then the internal ear structures form nerve impulses that travel to the brain via the auditory nerve. The brain then converts these impulses into sound.

Special Populations

Hearing loss is a common problem in the older population. With age, changes in the structures of the ear result in loss of high-frequency hearing, or even deafness. If an older patient uses a hearing aid for everyday activity, it is best to keep this device in place to provide for better communication during transport to the hospital.

Consider learning American Sign Language so that you can better communicate with patients who are deaf.

Patient Assessment

Conditions affecting the ears may be due to either trauma (covered in Chapter 33, *Face and Neck Trauma*) or medical causes.

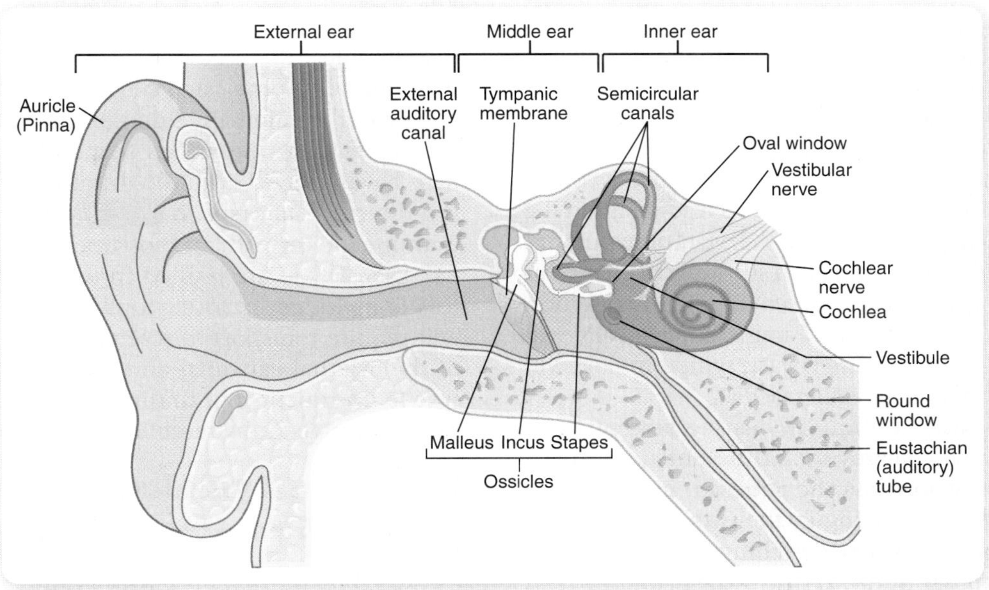

Figure 19-9 The structures of the ear.

Foreign objects forced into the auditory canal can damage the eardrum. Ear infections may cause the eardrum to blister and bleed, and inner ear infections can cause excessive pressures behind the eardrum. With rapidly changing altitudes, equalizing pressures can be difficult if the eustachian tubes are clogged from a cold, allergy, or inflammation. When a person moves to a higher altitude, expanding air needs to be released from the inner ear; swallowing and plugging the nose and blowing against a closed glottis can relieve this pressure. Blast pressure waves can burst the eardrum. If the ear damage is due to a blast injury, then special consideration is warranted as to approach, staging, and scene safety; these issues are discussed in Chapter 29, *Trauma Systems and Mechanism of Injury*.

As you approach the patient with an ear condition, aside from determining the approximate age, sex, environmental conditions, and degree of distress, note whether the patient has a hearing aid. Sometimes patients do not sleep with their hearing aid in, and they may seem confused until you are told by someone else that the patient cannot hear you!

Assessment and management of the patient with an ear condition begins by ensuring airway patency, breathing adequacy, and circulation, and managing any threats to life. Although patients with ear conditions may be in pain or have a hearing deficit, they generally are not considered the highest priority in a triage situation, nor does an ear condition represent a life threat that needs to be immediately dealt with. Typically, medical conditions involving the ears are not life threats unless the ear condition is a symptom of a much more serious problem (eg, ear damage from a blast injury or head trauma). These patients may be very uncomfortable, but their condition cannot be resolved in the field. Instead, you should transport these patients to the emergency department, where they can receive the appropriate physical examination, diagnosis, and treatment.

Take a complete history and find out if the patient has had this condition before. Observe the ears for drainage, excess **cerumen** (earwax), and inflammation or swelling. If the patient has pain, quantify it on a pain scale and identify it by region and cause. When asking OPQRST assessment questions, "P" (provocation) should include pertinent negatives, such as "Does it hurt when you swallow, sneeze, cough, or bend over?" The history of the events leading up to the complaint can help provide clues to the onset of symptoms. The patient may describe unusual pressure changes with "ear popping," itching in the ears, a recent respiratory infection or cold, or a scuba diving trip. Paramedics generally will treat only the discomfort caused by the symptoms and will pass on the history to the treating facility.

Assess for new aberrations in hearing perception. If hearing is affected, changes should be noted and reassessed during transport. Ask the patient if he or she has experienced **tinnitus** (ringing in the ears) or dizziness. Inspect and palpate for wounds, swelling, or drainage (pus, blood, cerebrospinal fluid). Often the mastoid process of the skull, which is palpated immediately posterior to the auricle, is assessed for discoloration and tenderness (**Battle sign**).

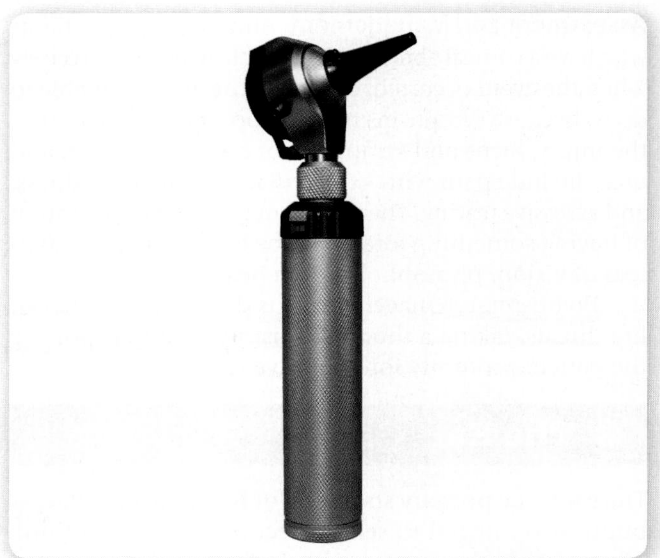

Figure 19-10 Otoscope.

Use of an Otoscope

Abnormalities of the external canal and tympanic membrane are visualized by use of an **otoscope** Figure 19-10. This instrument consists of a head and a handle. The head contains an electric light source and a low-power magnifying lens; the front of the headpiece has an attachment for a disposable plastic earpiece (speculum). The examiner inserts the speculum into the ear and looks through a lens on the rear of the headpiece. Some otoscopes include a sliding rear window that permits insertion of an additional instrument (ie, to remove earwax). Most have an insertion point for a bulb used to push air into the ear canal, allowing the examiner to visualize movement of the tympanic membrane. The rechargeable batteries are located in the handle unless the otoscope is a wall-mounted unit, like that found in a physician's office.

Typically paramedics do not use an otoscope unless they work in an expanded scope of practice in which they have received additional training from their medical director. The steps in Skill Drill 19-2 show how to examine the ear with an otoscope.

Even if you are trained in use of an otoscope and this is included in your scope of practice, the patient will require transport to receive a complete assessment of the external ear canal and middle ear. As always, be sure to document your findings and communicate them as appropriate to the receiving facility.

▶ Pathophysiology, Assessment, and Management of Specific Ear Conditions

This section covers specific ear conditions. Ear trauma (specifically, perforated tympanic membrane and foreign body in the ear) is covered in Chapter 33, *Face and Neck Trauma*.

Skill Drill 19-2 Examining the Ear With an Otoscope

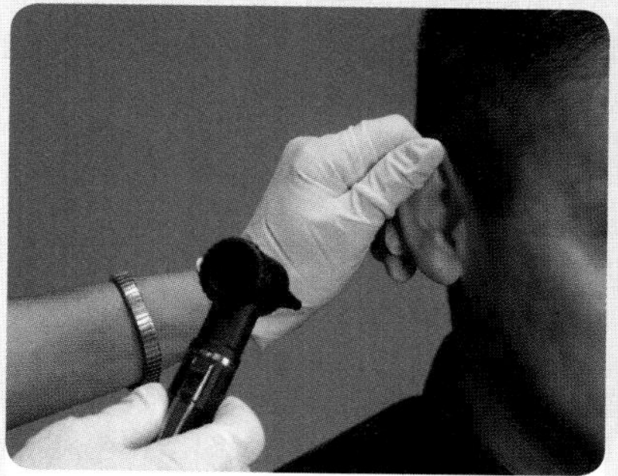

Step 1 Select an appropriately sized speculum. Dim the lights as much as possible. Ensure the ear is free of foreign bodies. Place your hand firmly against the patient's head, and gently grasp the auricle. Move the ear to best visualize the canal, usually upward and backward in an adult patient.

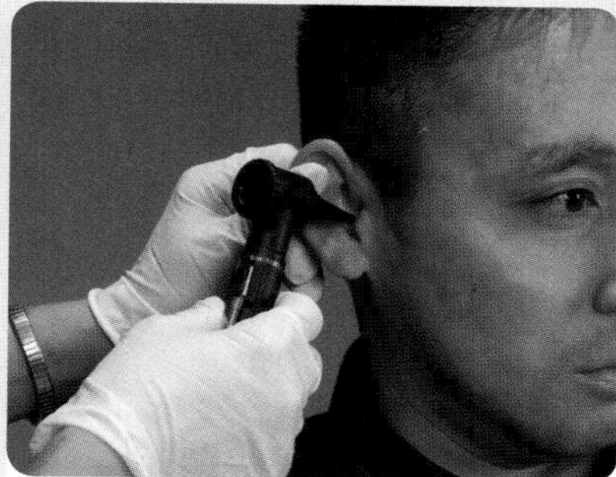

Step 2 To avoid damaging the ear, instruct the patient not to move during the exam. Turn on the otoscope and insert the speculum into the ear. Do not insert the speculum deeply into the canal.

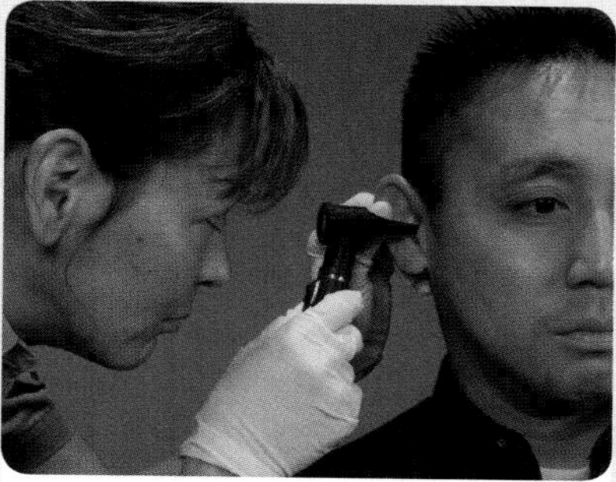

Step 3 Inspect the canal for any lesions or discharge. A small amount of cerumen (earwax) is normal. Visualize the tympanic membrane (eardrum), and inspect it for integrity and color. It should be translucent or a pearly gray color. Note any signs of inflammation, including swelling or discoloration (a pink-tinged or red ear canal or tympanic membrane).

Words of Wisdom

Ear pain is a common problem experienced by airplane travelers. It occurs when pressure builds on the eardrum as a result of changes in atmospheric pressure, which occur with increases or decreases in altitude. The pressure is different in the middle ear than outside the ear.

Ear pain can also occur when diving deep under water. Patients often complain of pressure, feeling as if their ear is going to pop, or loss of hearing.

Patients can usually self-manage these feelings by sucking or swallowing (a reflex that is easily activated by chewing gum), which directs airflow from the nose to the eustachian tube of the ear and helps balance the pressure. A patient can also be directed to perform a Valsalva maneuver (pinch the nose, blow out with the mouth closed), which helps force air into the eustachian tube. In rare cases, if the symptoms do not resolve and the patient is still experiencing severe pain, transport may be needed to the emergency department for physician evaluation.

Impacted Cerumen

Cerumen is the yellowish, oily substance found in the outer ear canal. It helps prevent dirt and water from entering the middle ear canal and may protect the ear from invasion by bacteria or fungi. Cerumen may present as "wet," which is a sticky brown color, or "dry," which consists of a grayish flaky substance. Commonly known as "earwax," cerumen can become impacted and cause pressure against the eardrum. Impaction occurs when too much cerumen builds up and gets stuck in the outer ear canal.

Normally cerumen flows outward, toward the outer ear, and gets washed away. This process helps remove dead skin cells from the ear canal. Cerumen impaction is more common in older adults, in whom hearing aids may block the normal flow. Older adults also tend to produce cerumen that is dry and, therefore, more prone to buildup. Other risk factors for impaction include abnormal ear canal shape and diseases that cause more production of cerumen, such as keratosis. Improper use of cotton swabs and other hygiene tools or objects can block the flow and cause a cerumen plug.

Assessment and Management. Symptoms of impacted cerumen include sensation of pressure or fullness in the ear, dizziness, ringing in the ears, loss of hearing, and pain or itching in the ear. Prehospital treatment should include a thorough history and visual inspection of the ear canal. Because an older adult may have many different medical conditions, it may be difficult to rule out other serious problems.

Treatment is aimed at removing the excess cerumen. Do not attempt to extract the material yourself. Rather, a physician will use an otoscope to identify the problem; the physician will then use specially designed tools to remove the wax. Suction and eardrops such as wax softeners may also be used. If left untreated, then cerumen impaction can cause infection and irritation that can potentially damage the eardrum and hearing. The process of removing cerumen may also cause injury, so follow-up is necessary after the procedure.

Labyrinthitis

Labyrinthitis is most commonly recognized as the feeling of vertigo or loss of balance after an ear infection or upper respiratory infection. In this condition, irritation and swelling in the inner ear affect the nerves of the inner ear and produce a loss of balance. Other symptoms include ringing in the ears (tinnitus), dizziness, temporary loss of hearing, nausea, and vomiting. Permanent hearing loss can occur as well.

Assessment and Management. Severe symptoms of labyrinthitis usually resolve within a week. Prehospital treatment is directed toward reducing the severity of the nausea and vomiting and transporting the patient in a position of comfort. The differential diagnoses for vertigo with associated nausea include neurologic disorders such as Meniere disease and acoustic neuroma. These serious disorders will need to be ruled out by a computed tomography (CT) scan and magnetic resonance imaging (MRI). You should be able to recognize the serious implications of the symptoms, however, and suggest the patient be seen at the emergency department.

Hospital treatment of labyrinthitis includes an antiemetic for nausea and vomiting, an antihistamine to reduce swelling, antivertigo medicine, and diazepam (Valium) as a sedative/muscle relaxant. Prompt treatment of respiratory and ear infections can reduce the risk of labyrinthitis.

Meniere Disease

Meniere disease is a chronic condition of the inner ear disorder characterized by four symptoms that may or may not occur at the same time: (1) dizziness described as spinning vertigo, (2) low-frequency hearing loss, (3) tinnitus, and (4) a feeling of fullness in the affected ear.[11] It usually affects adults older than 50 years, although it can affect young children and older adults.

Meniere disease involves the overproduction and defective absorption of endolymphatic fluid, which increases the volume and pressure within the labyrinth of the inner ear until distention results in rupture and mixing of the endolymph and perilymph fluids.[12] This mixture disrupts the balance of fluid and electrolytes within the labyrinth and damages the vestibular and cochlear hair cells. What causes the excessive fluid production is unclear; allergies, viral and bacterial infections, head trauma, metabolic disorders, and chronic stress have been suggested as potential causes.

In the early stages of this disease, attacks last less than 2 hours, although altered balance may last up to two days. Hearing loss fluctuates, returning to normal between episodes after the rupture heals. As the disease progresses, symptoms last hours to days, the episodes occur with less warning and become more disabling, recovery between attacks is incomplete, and permanent tinnitus, moderate to severe hearing loss, and chronic unsteadiness may result.[12]

Assessment and Management. The symptoms of hearing loss, ear pressure, vertigo, dizziness, nausea, and vomiting have a number of causes, including viral, bacterial, and neurologic causes, among others. In the prehospital setting, care is focused on treating the nausea and vomiting with an antiemetic. In the clinical setting, antiemetics and anticholinergics may be administered during an acute episode to manage symptoms. After diagnosis of Meniere disease, the physician may prescribe diuretics to reduce the volume of endolymph and restore fluid balance in the inner ear. Some surgical procedures have had limited success in treating this condition.

Otitis Externa and Media

Otitis is an infection that results from bacterial growth in the ear canal. It can be categorized as either otitis externa or otitis media—infection of the outer and middle ear cavity, respectively. Otitis is more common in children than in adults partially because as humans grow, the angle of the eustachian tube becomes more vertical, allowing it to drain more easily. By comparison, the angle of the eustachian tube in some children is almost horizontal, preventing the tube from properly draining and allowing infective material to collect there. In children younger than 5 years, otitis media is the most common affliction requiring medical intervention.

Otitis externa and otitis media are most commonly bacterial infections. Nevertheless, otitis externa can also be an allergic or fungal reaction, and otitis media can be virally induced, developing when sinusitis or **rhinitis** spreads along the eustachian tubes. Also, auditory canal blockage from excessive cerumen or lack of enough cerumen can lead to bacterial growth that can cause infection.

Assessment and Management. Both otitis externa and otitis media are painful conditions. Allergic or fungal otitis externa may be accompanied by itching, and examination of the external ear canal will show edema and erythema. Patients with otitis media may experience diminished hearing acuity, and examination with an otoscope will reveal an inflamed, bulging tympanic membrane (eardrum). Both disorders are common in children. Prior to language development, children will often indicate such ear pain by pulling at or rubbing the infected ear. In severe cases the tympanic membrane may tear or rupture, revealing blood in the external ear canal. Untreated infections can cause permanent hearing loss.

Prehospital treatment should be directed at relieving unbearable symptoms. The physician will treat the patient with topical antibiotics and possibly corticosteroids to reduce inflammation. The paramedic should monitor the patient's condition and administer pain medication when necessary. In the hospital setting, if the symptoms are tolerated, the patient's condition is monitored. If no improvement occurs, antibiotics are administered. When the physician can see a bulging tympanic membrane from excess fluid buildup in the middle ear, additional antibiotics may be administered. when several trials of antibiotics have been unsuccessful, such as in children who have immune deficiencies, the physician will perform tympanocentesis (needle aspiration). The middle ear fluid that has been aspirated is cultured; the results of the culture will indicate the type of bacteria present and aid in determining the treatment necessary.

The Nose

The nose is subject to increased rates of injury because of its prominent location on the human face. The nose is a filter, humidifier, and heater for the air that enters the body. Allergens, particles, and chemicals can all cause inflammation, infection, and injury to this structure. Because the sinus cavities are located in the forehead and face, and drain to the back of the throat, complications from nasal disorders are common. Sinus headaches from pressure, scratchy throat from drainage, and respiratory infection from the aspiration of draining, infected material may all lead to other manifestations and systemic infections. You may encounter a myriad of symptoms that began as a nasal infection.

The inside of the nose is extremely vascular. Although this characteristic can cause it to bleed, it also makes intranasal administration an excellent route for giving some medicines. The intranasal route is also commonly used for delivering drugs of abuse such as cocaine; some abusers literally burn a hole in their nasal septum over time. In addition, the nasal mucosa offers a short route to the brain. The blood-brain barrier can be bypassed through the nasal mucosa, with substances passing through this mucosa and then entering the spinal fluid. Consequently, drug delivery via the intranasal route may proceed more rapidly than intravenous administration of some medicines.

Another major function of the nose is the ability to smell. Loss of smelling sensation may have many different causes, including aging, smoking, allergies, rhinitis, polyps, the flu, medications, and traumatic brain injury (damage to cranial nerve I [the olfactory nerve]). Types of smelling disorders include anosmia (total loss of sense of smell), dysosmia (distorted sense of smell, in which the person perceives unpleasant odors when the odors do not exist), hyperosmia (increased sensitivity to smell), hyposmia (decreased sense of smell), and presbyosmia (loss of smell from normal aging). Loss of smell also affects a person's sense of taste.

YOU are the Paramedic PART 3

You ask the patient, "Ma'am, what is your medical history? Are you taking any medications? Do you have any allergies?" Instead of answering your answers, she starts coughing up blood. This finding suggests some blood has flowed from the back of her nose into her oropharynx; it could put her at risk for aspiration if the bleeding is not stopped. The staff explains the patient has a history of ischemic stroke, high cholesterol, and high blood pressure. She takes Pradaxa (dabigatran etexilate), Prinivil (lisinopril), Microzide (hydrochlorothiazide), and Lipitor (atorvastatin calcium). Her only known allergy is penicillin.

Recording Time: 3 Minutes	
Respirations	18 breaths/min
Pulse	115 beats/min
Skin	Warm, pale
Blood pressure	98/70 mm Hg
Oxygen saturation (Spo_2)	95% room air
Pupils	PERRLA

5. What do you suspect is wrong with the patient?
6. Do you have additional concerns other than stopping the bleeding?

Anatomy and Physiology Review

The nose is one of the two primary entry points for oxygen-rich air to enter the body (the mouth is the other entry point). The nose warms and humidifies air as it enters the body. It also contains bony structures Figure 19-11 and is connected with the sinuses Figure 19-12.

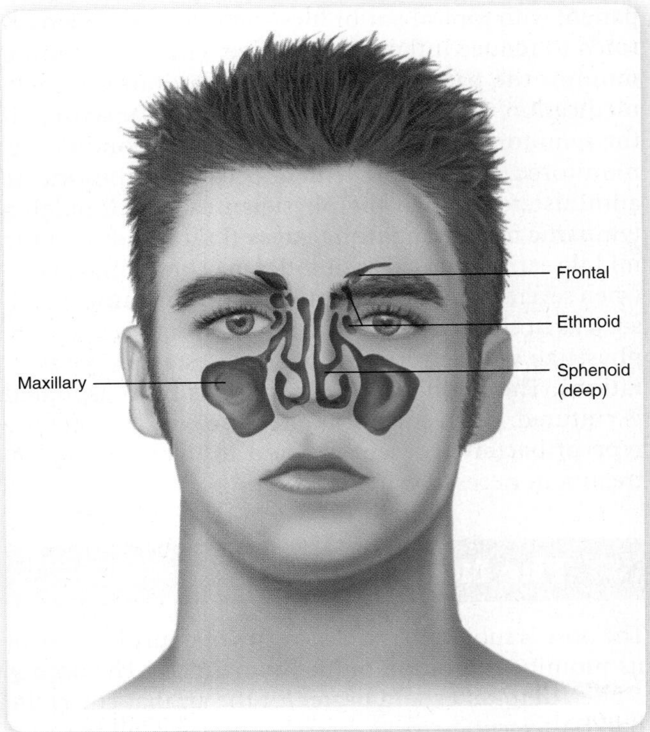

Figure 19-12 The paranasal sinuses.

Patient Assessment

A complaint related to the nose that is severe enough to warrant calling an ambulance could have several etiologies. The condition of the residence as you approach can give clues to exposure. A factory spewing toxins, the scent of cleaning agents in the hallway, or other unpleasant odors can alert the paramedic to possible dangers to the crew. Until the seriousness of the problem is known, standard precautions are key to limiting the spread of respiratory infections.

When the scene is determined to be safe for the crew to respond, the first impression of the patient can tell you if airway and breathing are sufficient, and you can note the amount of distress the patient is experiencing. Environmental clues, as well as your own nose, can identify possible irritants. Remember—a sneezing, sniffling, coughing patient easily spreads airborne germs in water droplets.

The vascular nature of the nasal cavities make them susceptible to bleeding. A severe nosebleed or condition that blocks the airway with swelling or blood is a life-threatening condition. In such a case, you must be able to determine whether the patient has a general medical condition or if the condition is or could become life threatening.

Insert an airway adjunct as needed to maintain airway patency. However, *do not insert a nasopharyngeal airway or attempt nasotracheal intubation in any patient with suspected nasal fractures or in patients with CSF or blood leakage from the nose.* After establishing and maintaining a patent airway, assess the patient's breathing and intervene appropriately.

Inquire about a previous history of nose conditions or bleeding that needed to be packed and quartered in the emergency department. Always consider hypertensive crisis when an older person has a nosebleed.

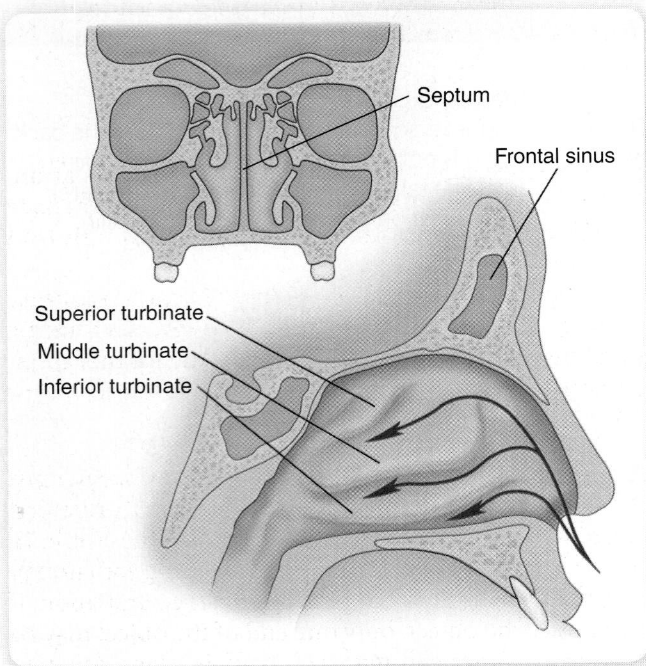

Figure 19-11 The nose has two chambers, which are divided by the septum.

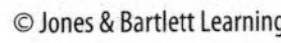

Pathophysiology, Assessment, and Management of Specific Nose Conditions

Epistaxis

Epistaxis, or nosebleed, is a common problem that can occur spontaneously or from trauma. One of the most common causes of nosebleeds is digital trauma (picking the nose with a finger); other causes include dryness and hypertension. Nosebleeds are further classified into anterior and posterior epistaxis. Anterior nosebleeds are the most common, most typically occurring in the Kiesselbach plexus.[13] This plexus, which is formed by the convergence of branches of the external and internal carotid arteries, supplies an area on the anterior-inferior nasal septum known as Little's area, the most common site for epistaxis.[13]

Anterior nosebleeds usually bleed fairly slowly, are usually self-limiting, and resolve quickly. Posterior nosebleeds are usually more severe and often cause blood to drain into the patient's throat, causing nausea and vomiting.

Words of Wisdom

Blood or CSF drainage from the nose (**cerebrospinal rhinorrhea**) suggests a skull fracture. *Do not make any attempt to control this bleeding*; doing so may increase intracranial pressure (ICP) if the patient has a concomitant brain injury. Furthermore, the insertion of nasal airway adjuncts and nasotracheal intubation should be avoided in patients with suspected nasal fractures, especially if rhinorrhea is present. A nasally inserted airway device could enter the cranial vault through an occult fracture (such as a cribriform plate fracture) and penetrate the brain, further worsening the situation.

Assessment and Management. Try to estimate the amount of blood loss and relay this information to the staff at the receiving facility. For example, ask the patient if he or she has lost enough blood to soak a handkerchief, facecloth, or towel and over which period of time the blood loss occurred.[14] With a nontrauma patient who is bleeding from the nose, you should place the patient in a sitting position, leaning forward with the mouth open over a container so that further blood loss can be estimated, and apply constant, firm pressure over the lower (nonbony) part of the nose for 20 minutes.[14] Alternatively, you may place pressure on the upper gums under the nose, or use a commercial nasal compression clip, if available **Figure 19-13**.[14] Direct the patient not to sniffle or blow his or her nose or to release pressure too soon to check whether the bleeding has stopped. For a detailed discussion of the care for epistaxis in the context of trauma, see Chapter 30, *Bleeding*.

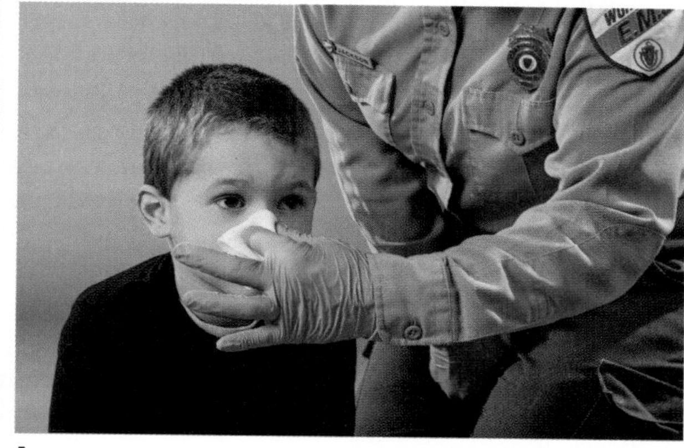

A

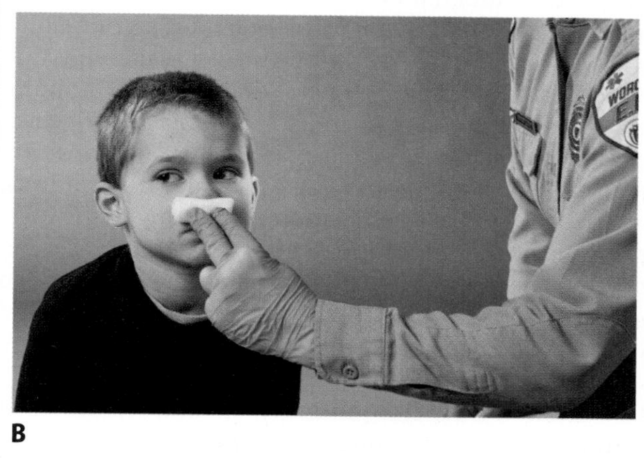

B

Figure 19-13 Control bleeding from the nose by one of the following methods: Either pinch the nostrils together **(A)** or apply pressure on the upper gums, beneath the nose, with gloved fingers and gauze **(B)**. Alternatively, you may control bleeding with a commercial nasal compression clip.

Foreign Body

Foreign bodies in the nose are most likely to be seen in the pediatric population; these items are commonly solid objects, such as beads, stones, marbles, or small pieces of food. Young children have the greatest incidence of exploring their nasal cavities with foreign objects. At age 9 months, a child's grip is sufficient to grasp an object and direct it up one or both nares. Food, toys, rocks, and beads may become lodged or travel to the mouth through the nasal pharyngeal cavity. Those objects that make it to the mouth become a risk for inhalation or may become lodged in the esophagus if swallowed. Sometimes these objects can be in place for several days before someone realizes something is wrong; by then, the drainage and smell may have become significant. Objects lodged in the nose can cause other complications as well. For example, pressure in the delicate nasal passage can cause tissue necrosis, inflammation, and swelling; the inflammatory process can cause tissue ulceration and epistaxis; and nasal blockage can lead to sinusitis.

Rhinotillexomania (nose picking) in adults is a cause of nasal infections and may introduce irritants into the nasal mucosa. There is even limited evidence that spontaneous epistaxis from nose picking has led to motor vehicle crashes!

Assessment and Management. In all patients, you must determine if the foreign body presents a life-threatening condition. Nasal foreign bodies are usually visible in the anterior nares, but some may be tucked far enough into the nares as to not be seen on visual examination. If you do see the object, only one end of the object may be visible; the other end may be lodged in place. Any persistent, foul-smelling, purulent discharge from the nares should lead to suspicion of a foreign body. If you note a discharge from the nose, let it drain, treat it as potentially infective material, and transport the patient. Remember to always use standard precautions.

Transport the patient in the position of comfort, with an emphasis on limiting the ability of gravity to introduce the object farther into the cavity. Preventing aspiration is a priority. Where the object is an extreme irritant, pain management may be necessary. Sedation may be necessary in rare cases. Consultation with medical control is advised.

Rhinitis

Rhinitis, or inflammation of the nasal cavity, is a common nasal disorder that may be caused by bacterial or viral infection, allergens, medications, or changes in environmental temperature. Acute rhinitis most commonly occurs as a result of a viral infection and is accompanied by symptoms of the "common cold:" nasal congestion and obstruction, increased nasal drainage, and a diminished sense of smell.[15] Allergic rhinitis may be triggered by allergens such as pollen, grasses, dust mites, or animal dander. Some patients, particularly older adults, experience rhinitis in association with eating or a change in the weather.[15] Rhinitis can also be caused by certain medications (eg, antihypertensive medications), foreign bodies, irritants in the air (eg, smoke, chemicals), and hormonal changes in pregnancy.

Assessment and Management. Signs and symptoms of rhinitis include nasal congestion, sneezing, itchy runny nose, itchy eyes, postnasal drip (which may feel like a tickle in the throat), and possibly cough. Prehospital care for rhinitis is primarily supportive. Keep the patient in Fowler position and provide transport. Physician-directed treatment is aimed at treating the cause of the rhinitis.

Sinusitis

Sinusitis (sinus inflammation) occurs when drainage from one of more of the sinuses (most often the paranasal sinuses) becomes disrupted, blocking drainage into the nasal cavity. The sinuses, which are normally sterile, then become colonized with nasal bacteria, and infection results.[16] As mucus builds up inside the sinus cavity and thickens, pressure increases, causing facial pressure and pain. Sinusitis may be accompanied by a sore throat, nasal congestion, toothache (maxillary sinus), headache (ethmoid sinus), fever, chills, and muscle aches and pains.

Sinusitis affects 29.3 million adult Americans per year, or approximately 12% of the US population, according to the CDC.[17] Young children are especially susceptible to this disease due to their greater frequency of colds. Their smaller nasal air passages easily become clogged, providing the supportive environment necessary for bacterial growth. Older adults are also relatively more likely to experience sinusitis due to their dry nasal passages. Their weaker immune systems, coupled with a diminished cough and gag reflex, make them generally more prone to respiratory infections.

YOU are the Paramedic PART 4

Your partner places some gauze and an epistaxis nose clip on the patient, but she pulls on it and says it hurts. You explain that the clip will help control her bleeding, and attempt to calm her down. The patient insists that she cannot breathe with the nose clip on. You suction the patient's mouth and encourage her to breathe through her mouth. You encourage her to breathe through her mouth.

Recording Time: 8 Minutes	
Respirations	24 breaths/min
Pulse	125 beats/min
Skin	Warm, pale
Blood pressure	99/75 mm Hg
Oxygen saturation (Spo_2)	95% on room air
Pupils	PERRLA

7. Does this patient require any additional airway management?
8. Should you consider starting an IV line on this patient?

Assessment and Management. The duration of the symptoms determines whether sinusitis is characterized as chronic, acute, or recurrent. Prehospital management should include treatment of any respiratory compromise and transport for physician evaluation. Treatment is aimed at reducing inflammation and draining the sinuses. Mild to moderate symptoms lasting 7 to 10 days can be treated with a saline rinse and a decongestant. Note that decongestants can dry the nasal passages and delay healing if they are overused. Antibiotics are usually prescribed only after the sinusitis has persisted for 7 to 10 days without relief.

The Throat

Disorders of the pharynx and larynx may represent acute inflammation and infections, chronic inflammation, or abnormal growths. Specific disorders include vocal cord polyps and nodules, contact ulcers, vocal cord paralysis, laryngoceles, laryngeal papillomas, and cancer.

Throat infections (pharyngitis) are particularly common among children, although adults may be affected as well. Causes, symptoms, and treatment are similar in both groups, except that in adults and sexually abused children, gonorrhea—a sexually transmitted infection—may affect the throat.

Throat problems can be exacerbated by swallowing problems (**dysphagia**). Cranial nerves VI, VII, IX, and XII all play a role in swallowing. Neurologic problems associated with stroke or trauma can cause swallowing difficulty. Facial nerve paralysis (cranial nerve VII) can cause unilateral facial and gag reflex paralysis. People who have swallowing difficulty are at increased risk of aspiration pneumonia. This type of pneumonia may occur following the aspiration of vomitus in a patient with an altered mental status resulting from a seizure, drugs, alcohol, anesthesia, acute infection, or shock. It may also occur after the aspiration of a foreign body, or after aspiration of caustic substances such as gasoline. Prehospital care includes maintaining a patent airway, ensuring adequate breathing, close monitoring of vital signs, and prompt transport for definitive care.

Esophageal disorders can also affect the throat. The valve at the end of the esophagus (lower esophageal sphincter) keeps the acidic stomach contents from coming back up the throat after swallowing. In the case of esophageal reflux, the valve only partially closes or, alternatively, opens too often. Symptoms of this condition include a burning sensation in the chest and indigestion. If the stomach acids come up the throat and reach the vocal cords, voice tone may change from inflammation and swelling. This phenomenon can cause a precancerous condition from tissue scarring in the esophagus.

Anatomy and Physiology Review

Your assessment of the throat will begin at the opening of the mouth with the teeth **Figure 19-14**. The hypoglossal, glossopharyngeal, trigeminal, and facial nerves supply the mouth and its structures **Figure 19-15**.

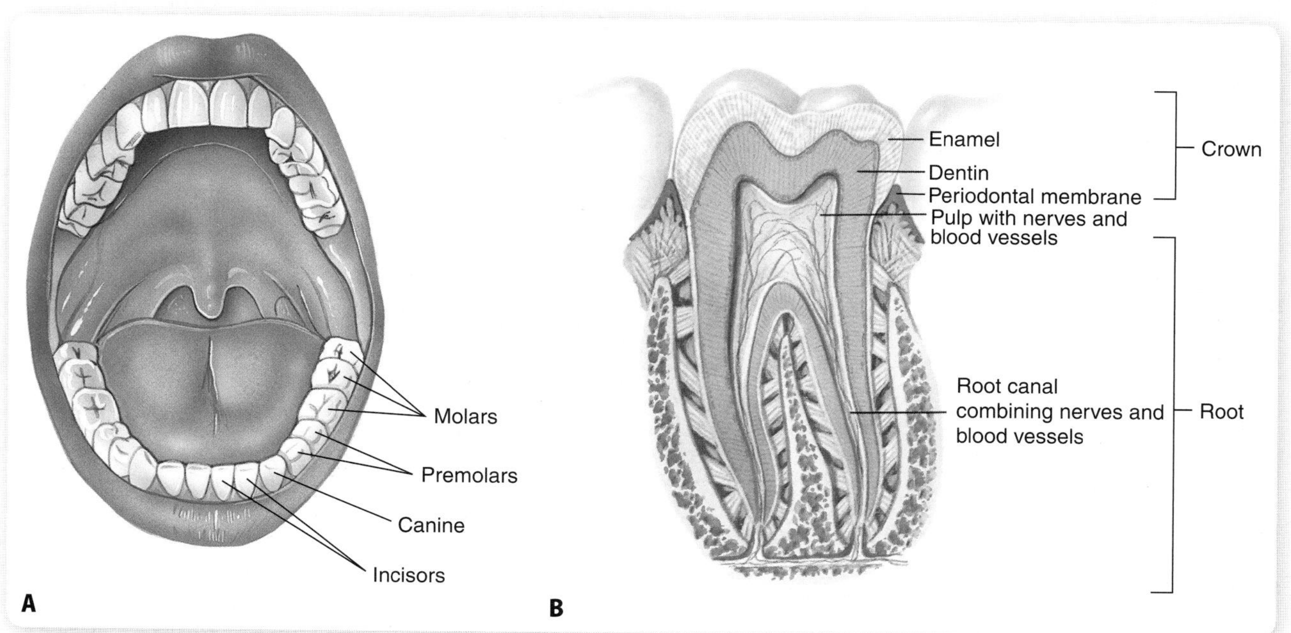

Figure 19-14 The teeth of the adult mouth. **A.** The incisors are used for biting. The canines are used for tearing food. The premolars and molars are used for grinding and crushing. **B.** Each tooth contains nerves and blood vessels.

The Neck

The principal structures of the anterior part of the neck include the thyroid and cricoid cartilage, trachea, and numerous muscles and nerves Figure 19-16. The major blood vessels in this area are the internal and external carotid arteries Figure 19-17 and the internal and external jugular veins Figure 19-18. The vertebral arteries run laterally to the cervical vertebrae in the posterior part of the neck.

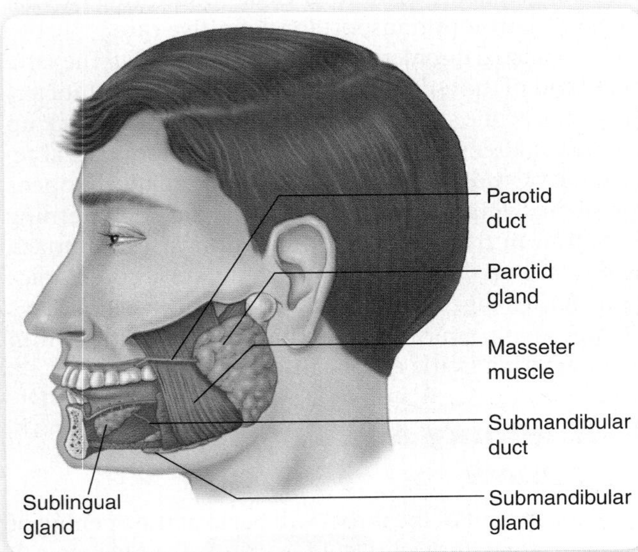

Figure 19-15 The glands and muscles of the mouth.

▶ Patient Assessment

Patients with swallowing abnormalities or copious mucus production should be placed in a position to allow drainage. A lateral recumbent position or recovery position will allow mouth drainage and help protect the airway. Patients who have experienced a stroke may not be able to swallow as a result of neurologic deficit. Assessing these patients must include early recognition of threats to their airway. When patients cannot protect their airways and are at risk for aspiration into the lungs, intubation should be considered.

Medical problems of the mouth, neck, and throat can seriously affect breathing. Assessments should consider **epiglottitis** if the patient's symptoms include sore throat, fever, drooling, and a head that is hung forward.

▶ Pathophysiology, Assessment, and Management of Specific Throat Conditions

This section covers specific throat conditions. Throat trauma (specifically, foreign body in the throat) is covered in Chapter 33, *Face and Neck Trauma*.

Dentalgia and Dental Abscess

Dentalgia or "toothache" can be the starting point for the development of a dental abscess. A cavity in a tooth harbors bacteria, resulting in rapid decay of the tooth. Eventually the integrity of the tooth is compromised, giving access to the tooth root and nerve. This can cause inflammation, swelling, and intense pain.

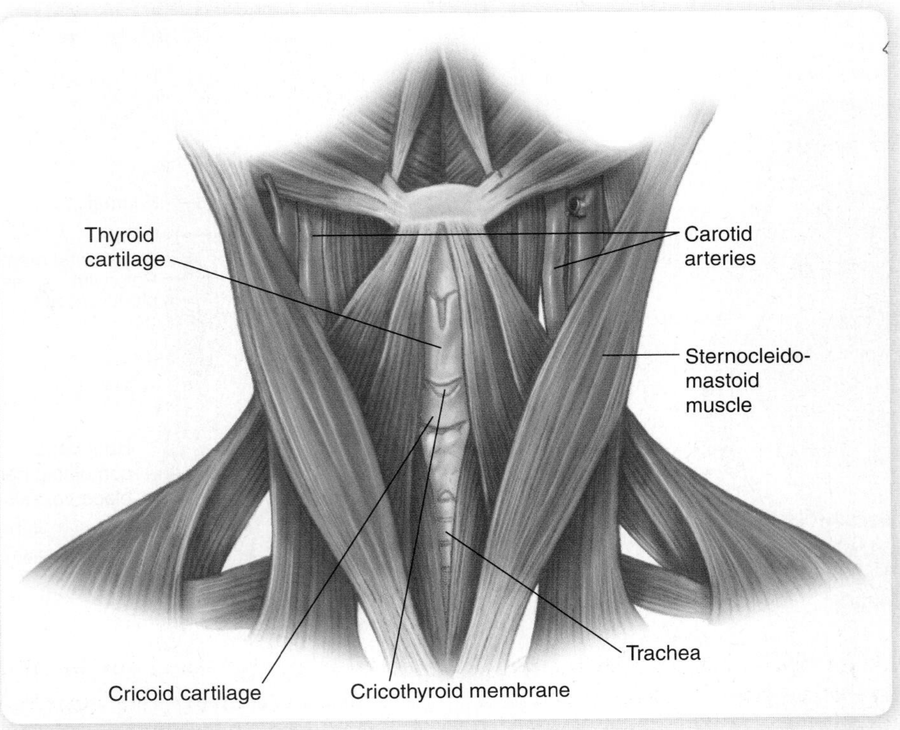

Figure 19-16 Anatomy of the anterior part of the neck.

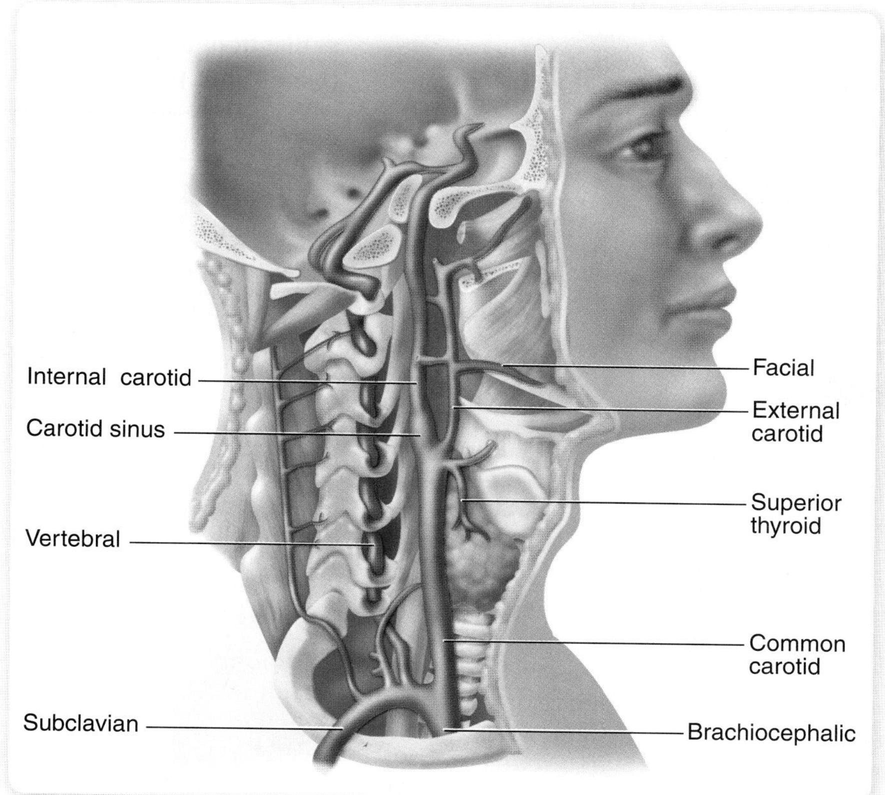

Figure 19-17 The arteries of the neck.

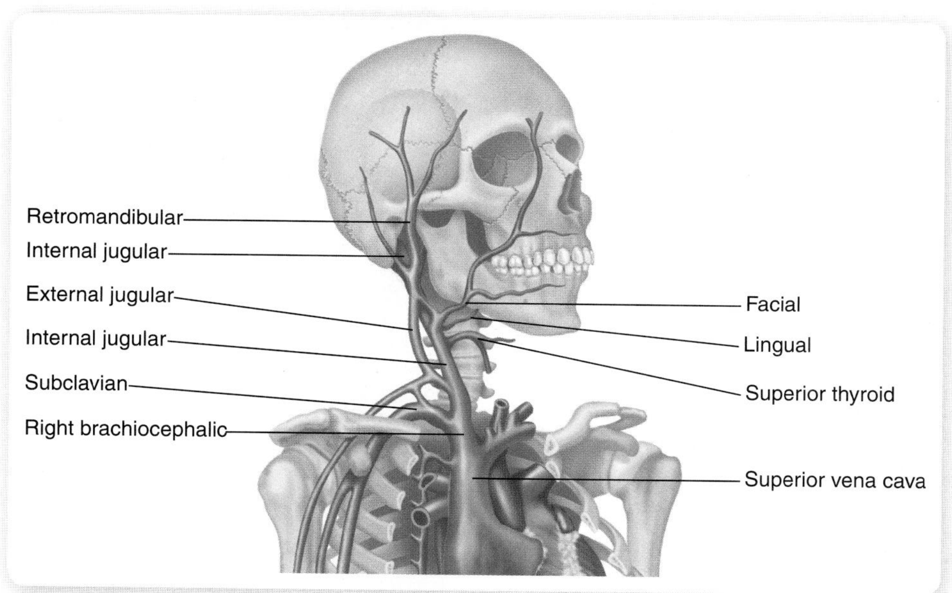

Figure 19-18 The veins of the neck.

A **dental abscess** occurs when the bacteria growth spreads directly from the cavity into the gums, facial tissue, bones, and/or neck Figure 19-19. The pain is relieved somewhat when the abscess ruptures and drains pus, reducing the swelling. An abscess may have to be drained surgically.

Assessment and Management. If fever, chills, nausea, and vomiting are part of the symptoms accompanying the dental abscess, the infection may have become systemic. In this case, a physician will prescribe antibiotics. An abscess in the throat, in the neck, or under the tongue can affect

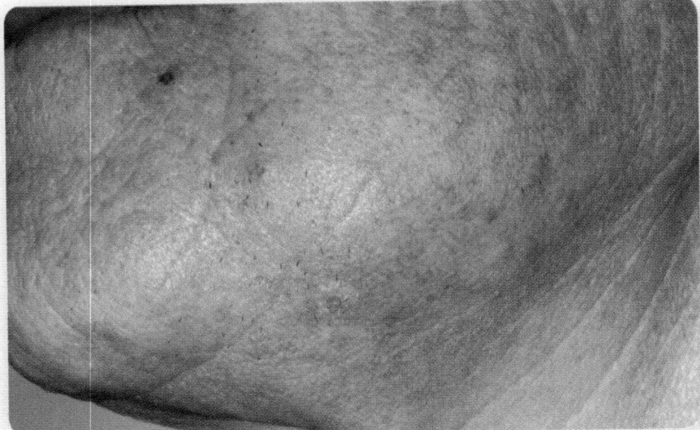

Figure 19-19 A dental abscess.

the ability to breathe—a condition that is a true emergency. Depending on the location of the abscess, it may have to be surgically drained under anesthesia in the operating room.

Prehospital treatment of a dental abscess or dentalgia is mostly aimed at relieving the symptoms. For example, the patient may take over-the-counter NSAIDs for relief of pain and inflammation. Any rupture and drainage of an abscess into the mouth should be rinsed with warm water.

Progression of the infection into bone and surrounding tissue can have serious complications. For this reason, you should encourage patients to accept transport to an appropriate facility for further treatment.

Diseases of Oral Soft Tissue

Diseases of the soft tissues of the mouth can be the root causes of other health problems. For example, gum disease has been linked to heart disease, stroke, diabetes, osteoporosis, and low–birth-weight babies. Infective endocarditis, which affects the lining of the heart and heart valves, can be linked directly to tooth infection and gum disease. The condition of the mouth reflects the condition of the human body. Indeed, many of the diseases affecting the human body may have oral manifestations, and a good dental examination may find these potential diseases in their early stages.[18] For example, diabetes, leukemia, cancer, heart disease, and kidney disease may manifest with mouth ulcers, swollen gums, and dry mouth. Poor oral health also affects the digestive system and may be a cause of irritable bowel syndrome.

Common mouth disorders include the following conditions:

- **Cold sores.** Painful sores on the lips and around the mouth caused by a type of herpesvirus.
- **Canker sores.** Shallow, painful ulcers in the mouth caused by stress or trauma (eg, braces, hot food, rough denture).
- **Oral candidiasis (thrush).** A yeast infection that causes white patches on the oral mucosa involving the mouth, tongue, palate, gums, and sometimes the throat (discussed further in Chapter 26, *Infectious Diseases*).
- **Leukoplakia.** Excess cell growth in the mouth, cheek, or gums that presents as white patches; it usually results from chronic irritation such as that from tobacco smoke, chewing tobacco, cheek biting, or ill-fitting dentures.
- **Gingivitis.** Red swollen gums that bleed easily during brushing.
- **Bad breath.** Usually linked to impacted plaque and poor oral hygiene. Bacteria release sulfur compounds that account for the foul smell. Fruity breath odor can be linked to diabetes and high blood glucose levels. Breath that smells like feces can be caused by a bowel obstruction. Breath odor that smells of urine or that smells "fishy" may be caused by chronic renal failure.

Assessment and Management. Sores and diseases of the mouth can be embarrassing to the patient. Consequently, the patient may not want to tell you about them. Be sure to rule out urticaria and allergic reactions when you are assessing lumps and sores of the mouth.

Oral Candidiasis

More commonly called "thrush," **oral candidiasis** is a condition in which the fungus *Candida albicans* accumulates on the lining of the mouth. When a patient has oral thrush, he or she will have creamy white lesions on the tongue and inner cheeks that can spread to the roof of the mouth, gums, tonsils, or posterior pharynx **Figure 19-20**. These lesions may be painful and bleed if they are rubbed or scraped.

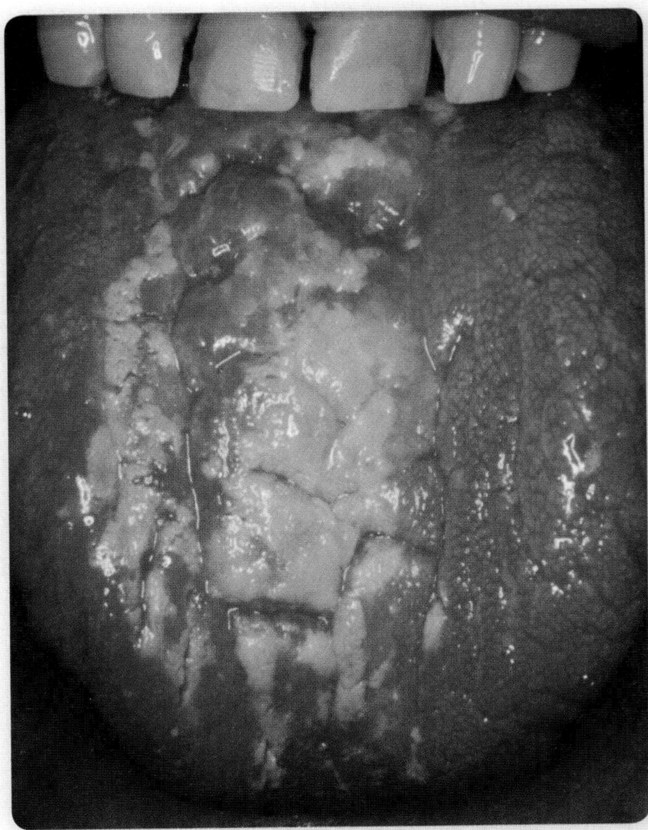

Figure 19-20 Oral candidiasis.

Assessment and Management. Thrush is most likely to be found in babies, patients with compromised immune systems, patients who wear dentures, and patients who use inhaled corticosteroids (eg, prednisone). In addition to the white lesions and slight bleeding, signs and symptoms of thrush include pain, cracking and redness at the corners of the mouth, and a loss of taste. Patients often describe a "cottony" feeling in the mouth. In severe cases, the lesions can spread down the esophagus, causing the sensation that food is getting stuck in the throat when swallowing. Patients with a medical history of HIV/AIDS, cancer, diabetes, and vaginal yeast infections are more prone to develop thrush.

Oral candidiasis is not a condition that requires paramedic care aside from treating higher priorities, making the patient comfortable, and encouraging the patient to follow up with a physician. You are likely to come across patients with thrush when treating or transporting immune-deficient patients under physician care for the conditions already mentioned. Always use standard precautions when managing a patient with thrush.

Ludwig Angina

Ludwig angina is a type of cellulitis caused by bacteria from an infected tooth root (tooth abscess) or mouth injury. It occurs on the floor of the mouth under the tongue. Because of the swelling associated with this infection, which may have a rapid onset, an airway obstruction may occur. A physical exam may show redness and swelling of the neck or under the chin. The tongue may also be swollen. In severe cases, the swelling caused by Ludwig angina is a potential life threat. You may have to provide an airway through the nasal passages to avoid the affected and swollen tissue, and a tracheostomy may have to be surgically performed to adequately ventilate these patients. The abscess may also have to be surgically drained.

Assessment and Management. Symptoms of Ludwig angina may include difficulty breathing, difficulty swallowing, neck pain, neck swelling, fever, drooling, and altered speech sounds. Prehospital treatment requires aggressive management of the patient's airway in severe cases. Early treatment with steroids may slow the inflammatory process and reduce swelling. Early contact with a medical control physician is important to determine your management options. Treatment may include dental surgery to repair the source of the infection at the tooth root.

Ludwig angina is painful and frightening for the patient because symptoms may develop rapidly. You should remain calm and organized as you attend to the ABCs while formulating a plan for aggressive airway management. Pay careful attention to the patient's condition and smells originating in the mouth to alert you to other disease processes that may be in progress.

Epiglottitis

Epiglottitis is an inflammation of the epiglottis (the flap at the base of the tongue that covers the trachea). As the epiglottis swells, it may begin to block the trachea and obstruct the airway. In the past, epiglottitis most commonly arose in pediatric patients (age 1 to 5 years), but today it is occurring more often in adults who did not receive inoculation for this disease. Because it often results from infection with the *Haemophilus influenzae* type b virus, this disease's incidence has decreased over time with widespread adoption of the Hib vaccine.

Assessment and Management. Patients with epiglottitis experience fever, sore throat, painful swallowing (dysphagia), stridor, and respiratory distress. A patient with epiglottitis looks sick and will be anxious, will sit upright in the classic "tripod" position or in the sniffing position with the chin thrust forward to allow for maximal air entry, and is often drooling because of an inability to swallow secretions. Work of breathing is increased, and pallor or cyanosis may be evident.

Transport a patient with suspected epiglottitis to an appropriate hospital while maintaining the patient's airway. Because this rapidly progressive disease carries a risk for acute airway obstruction and respiratory arrest, you should minimize your on-scene time and not attempt procedures that might agitate the patient. Remember not to attempt to look in the mouth—this step can precipitate complete airway obstruction. Alert personnel at the receiving facility to the suspected diagnosis and the patient's condition because they will need to mobilize a team for the management of this difficult airway.

Laryngitis

Swelling and inflammation of the larynx are associated with hoarseness or loss of voice. These conditions can be the result of overuse, such that the vocal cords and larynx become inflamed, causing hoarseness. The most common form of **laryngitis** is caused by a virus, similar to the cold or flu. This condition can also be caused by pneumonia, irritants and chemicals, gastroesophageal reflux disease (GERD), bronchitis, allergies, and bacterial infection. Typically laryngitis is not serious unless it leads to epiglottitis or croup; these serious diseases are covered in further depth in Chapter 43, *Pediatric Emergencies*.

Assessment and Management. A patient with laryngitis will present with fever, hoarseness, and swollen lymph nodes or glands in the neck. Obtain a good history to rule out evolving upper airway obstruction or an allergic reaction. If the patient speaks in a quiet tone and has a raspy voice, he or she may have sustained a hyoid bone fracture from a blow to the anterior neck. Otherwise, laryngitis is typically a symptom of an ongoing upper respiratory infection and the patient should follow up with a physician.

Tracheitis

Tracheitis is a bacterial infection of the trachea that is caused by the bacterium *Staphylococcus aureus*. Tracheitis frequently occurs in young children following a recent viral upper respiratory infection. In small children, the trachea is easily blocked by swelling, so this can be a life-threatening condition.

Assessment and Management. The symptoms of tracheitis include a deep "croup-like" (barking) cough, difficulty breathing, high fever, and high-pitched stridor with breathing. As the illness progresses, the child may exhibit tripod positioning and intercostal retractions. This condition can proceed from respiratory distress to respiratory failure if not managed quickly.

Prehospital care is supportive, minimizing stress to the child and administering 100% oxygen. Use pulse oximetry and monitor vital signs en route. Be prepared for a difficult intubation and have the correct size of endotracheal (ET) tube as well as the next smaller size available based on your length-based tape measurement of the child (Broselow tape). Transport the child as soon as possible to a facility capable of handling critically ill children.

In the critical care setting, many of these children will be managed with ET tube placement and administration of IV antibiotics.

Tonsillitis

Tonsillitis is swelling and inflammation of the tonsils, which are the two oval-shaped pads of tissue at the back of the throat Figure 19-21. Most cases of tonsillitis are caused by viral infections, although this condition has been known to be caused by bacteria. As the tonsils become inflamed, they swell and cause difficulty swallowing.

Assessment and Management. The symptoms of tonsillitis include swollen tonsils, a sore throat, and difficulty swallowing. Patients will have red, swollen tonsils; white or yellow coating or patches on the tonsils; a fever; and a sore throat. Patients may also present with pain when swallowing, enlarged and tender lymph nodes in the neck, bad breath, headache, and a stiff neck. In severe cases, drooling indicates difficulty swallowing.

Surgery to remove the tonsils used to be a common treatment for tonsillitis, but today this procedure is reserved for patients who have frequent bouts of tonsillitis that do not respond to drugs. Serious cases involving partial airway obstruction are also an indication for surgery. You should transport all patients with suspected tonsillitis to the emergency department for further evaluation.

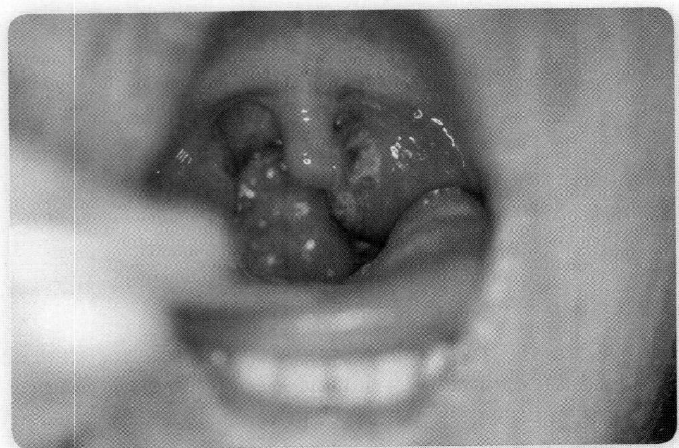

Figure 19-21 Tonsillitis.

Pharyngitis

Pharyngitis is an inflammation of the pharynx, which is the back of the throat between the tonsils and the larynx Figure 19-22. Pharyngitis is often due to a rapid onset of sore throat with discomfort or pain on swallowing.

Assessment and Management. Symptoms of pharyngitis also include a fever; pharyngeal erythema; headache; purulent, patchy yellow, gray, or white exudate; nasal congestion; hoarseness; cough; and ulcers on the soft palate.

The treatment involves follow-up in the emergency department so the patient can be examined, with cultures obtained to assess for streptococcal infection; a decision will also be made as to the usefulness of antibiotics. As a paramedic, your major prehospital concern is assessment for partial airway obstruction in severe cases with difficulty swallowing.

Peritonsillar Abscess

Peritonsillar abscess is a collection of infected material around the tonsils Figure 19-23. A complication of tonsillitis, it is most often caused by bacterial infection.

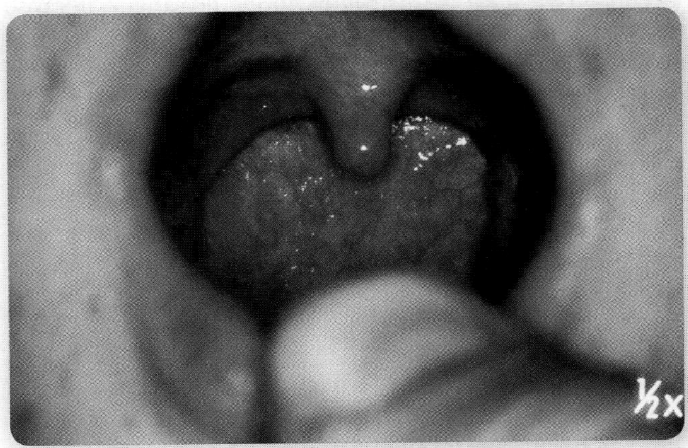

Figure 19-22 Pharyngitis.

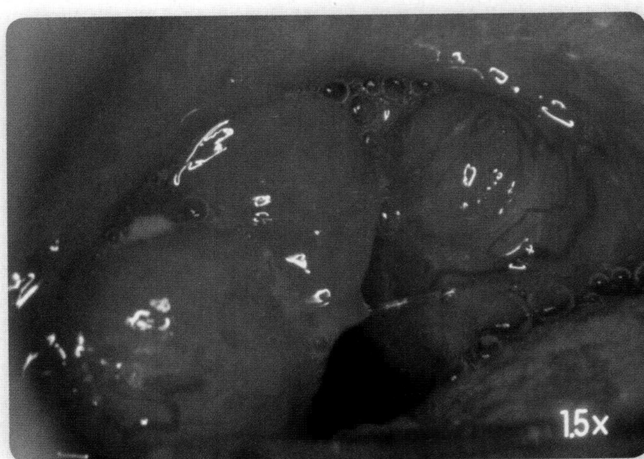

Figure 19-23 Peritonsillar abscess.

Although this condition is usually found in older children and young adults, it has become relatively rare today due to the use of antibiotics to treat tonsillitis.

Assessment and Management. With peritonsillar abscess, one or both tonsils are infected. The roof of the mouth and the neck or chest may be infected as well. The patient may have chills, difficulty opening the mouth, and pain when opening the mouth. He or she may develop facial swelling, fever, drooling or inability to swallow saliva, headache, muffled voice, sore throat (usually on one side), and tender glands of the jaw and throat.

Treatment involves administering antibiotics and draining the abscess. It may also include a tonsillectomy, so it is important to take these patients to the hospital. In some cases, peritonsillar abscess could be life threatening if the swollen tissues block the airway.

Temporomandibular Joint Disorders

The mandible is the large bone that forms the lower jaw and contains the lower teeth. Numerous muscles of chewing attach to the mandible and its rami. The posterior condyle of the mandible articulates with the temporal bone at the temporomandibular joint (TMJ), allowing movement of the mandible **Figure 19-24**. The actions of the TMJ allow a person to talk, chew, and yawn. When patients report jaw pain, clicking when they "jut" their jaw, or headaches, they often have been diagnosed, or may soon be, with a **temporomandibular joint (TMJ) disorder**.

Causes of TMJ disorders include arthritis-related damage to the joint's cartilage, jaw injury, and jaw muscle fatigue from grinding or clenching of the teeth, especially during sleep. The disk can erode or move out of its proper alignment, leading to TMJ disorder.

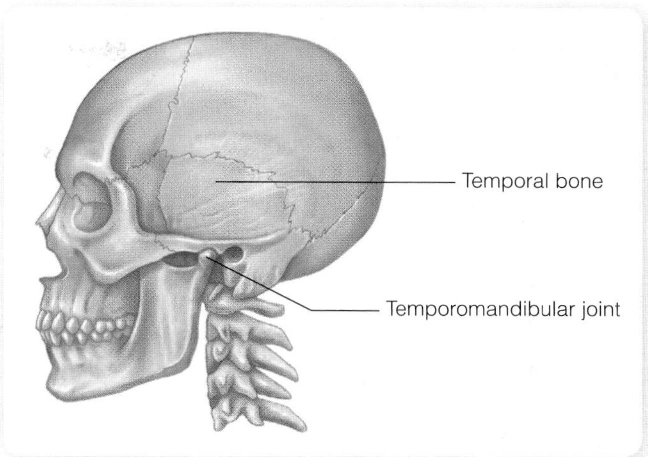

Figure 19-24 The temporomandibular joint articulates with the temporal bone.

Assessment and Management. The symptoms of TMJ disorders include headache, jaw pain, aching around the ear, an uneven or painful bite, difficulty chewing, and locking of the joint that causes difficulty either opening or closing the mouth. The symptoms are usually managed by over-the-counter pain medications. In severe cases, TMJ disorders may require dental or surgical intervention. As a paramedic, you should be aware of TMJ disorders, the symptoms they cause, and the fact that these conditions are usually managed by the patient's physician or dentist.

YOU are the Paramedic SUMMARY

1. What is your primary concern after scene safety is established?

The patient appears ill. She is bleeding profusely from the nose, and the bleeding needs to be controlled.

2. Do you have concerns other than the nose bleed?

Because the nose is part of the airway system, concern must be given to ensure the bleeding is not affecting the patient's ability to maintain a patent airway and breathe adequately. Remember the "A" (airway) and "B" (breathing) components of the ABCDEs, even though the bleeding is the most obvious sign.

3. What do you need to know about the patient's history?

Immediate thoughts about the patient's medical history should include questions about whether she has a history of nose bleeds, and if so, how the current incident compares to previous episodes. You should also seek to determine whether she has any associated medical conditions or takes any medications that could cause epistaxis or make it worse.

4. What is the priority in managing this patient?

In this patient, the priorities are managing the ABCs. Exerting immediate pressure by squeezing the nose and instructing the patient to lean forward to help reduce blood from going backward down into her mouth and near her airway are important. Other important priorities include continual assessment of the airway and suctioning to remove any blood from the mouth. In addition, assessment of lung sounds and breathing to ensure the patient is not aspirating blood is important.

5. What do you suspect is wrong with the patient?

This patient has classic signs of epistaxis. While the cause appears to be nontraumatic and unknown, the fact that the patient is on a blood thinner (Pradaxa) will make it

YOU are the Paramedic SUMMARY (continued)

more challenging to stop the bleeding in the field. In the emergency department, the patient may require medications or procedures to control the bleeding. Your efforts should focus on reducing the bleeding and protecting the patient's airway and breathing from aspiration.

6. Do you have additional concerns other than stopping the bleeding?

The primary concern with this patient, in tandem with stopping the bleeding, will be suctioning and protecting the airway from aspiration of blood. History of hypertension and a history of taking Pradaxa, which can cause bleeding, are additional concerns in a patient who is now borderline hypotensive. Given the amount of blood loss and ongoing bleeding, you should also continue to assess the patient's vital signs, monitor for any signs or symptoms of hemorrhagic shock, and treat the patient accordingly if needed.

7. Does this patient require any additional airway management?

This scenario does not clearly warrant any advanced airway procedures given what you know here. As long as you can get the patient to lean forward and you are able to control the bleeding by pinching the patient's nose, keeping suction available and using it as needed, along with (perhaps) administering blow-by oxygen, should be sufficient. However, if the patient becomes unable to sit or loses consciousness, rapid-sequence intubation might be appropriate as a means to protect the airway from aspiration of blood.

8. Should you consider starting an IV on this patient?

If you are able to stop the bleeding and the patient's systolic blood pressure remains greater than 90 mm Hg, an IV line is probably not necessary unless other signs and symptoms of shock are present. Any risk of shock or a decline in blood pressure would indicate the need for an IV line and fluid bolus. Establishing a saline lock as a precaution would be appropriate, as permitted by protocol. If you decide a fluid bolus is necessary to maintain a perfusing blood pressure, then keep in mind that letting the pressure rise too high may inhibit your ability to stop the bleeding or may cause any clots that have formed to dissolve or dislodge, such that the bleeding will continue.

EMS Patient Care Report (PCR)					
Date: 11-10-18	**Incident No.:** 99722		**Nature of Call:** Epistaxis		**Location:** Sunshine Acute Rehab Center
Dispatched: 1218	**En Route:** 1220	**At Scene:** 1230	**Transport:** 1245	**At Hospital:** 1250	**In Service:** 1305
Patient Information					
Age: 62 **Sex:** F **Weight (in kg [lb]):** 69 kg (150 lb)			**Allergies:** Penicillin **Medications:** Lisinopril, hydrochlorothiazide, Pradaxa, and Lipitor **Past Medical History:** HTN, high cholesterol, and history of ischemic stroke **Chief Complaint:** Severe nose bleed		

Vital Signs				
Time: 1233	**BP:** 98/70	**Pulse:** 115	**Respirations:** 18	**Spo_2:** 95% RA
Time: 1238	**BP:** 99/75	**Pulse:** 125	**Respirations:** 24	**Spo_2:** 95% RA
Time: 1247	**BP:** 102/85	**Pulse:** 120	**Respirations:** 20	**Spo_2:** 95% RA
EMS Treatment (circle all that apply)				
Oxygen @ _______ L/min via (circle one): **NC NRM Bag-mask device**		**Assisted Ventilation**	**Airway Adjunct**	**CPR**
Defibrillation	**Bleeding Control**	**Bandaging**	**Splinting**	**Other:**

YOU are the Paramedic SUMMARY (continued)

Narrative
Arrived to find 62 F sitting at a lunch table in extended-care facility dining room with severe epistaxis. Blood was noted on table as well as patient's clothing. ECF staff was applying a towel to the patient's nose. We took over care and applied gauze and pinched patient's nose closed and instructed her to learn forward. Patient's oral cavity was suctioned and breathing assessed. Patient vitals and medical history obtained as noted. Patient assisted to cot and placed in upright position and moved to truck. IV saline lock placed in patient's left forearm. Continued to assess airway, breathing, circulation, and vitals as noted en route. Report called to University Medical Center. Pt had no change during transport. Report and care transferred to Betty, RN, on arrival and patient left in ED bed 15.**End of report**

Prep Kit

▶ Ready for Review

- A patient may call emergency medical services with an emergency related to a disorder of the eye, ear, nose, or throat (EENT), or paramedics may encounter patients with these disorders while assessing an unrelated emergency. Paramedics should be familiar with these important structures and diseases that affect them.
- Be sure to assess patients' eyes for pain or tenderness, swelling, abnormal or loss of movement, sensation changes, circulatory changes, deformity, and visual changes. Obtain a thorough history of eye conditions, including when the problem began, whether both eyes are affected, and what the symptoms are.
- An early transport decision to the right facility can improve the outcome for a patient with eye disease. Consider transport to a facility that has the skilled services necessary to treat a serious eye problem. Consider pain management and mild sedation during transport.
- Remember to provide emotional care to patients with eye conditions. Fear and panic from loss of vision can cause dangerous and bizarre behavior, which may be alleviated if you practice good, calming communication skills.
- Specific medical conditions of the eye include conjunctivitis, inflammation, glaucoma, central retinal artery occlusion, iritis, papilledema, cellulitis of the orbit, and corneal abrasion. Become familiar with these conditions so that you can recognize them in the field and transport the patient as needed.
- The ear is the primary structure for hearing and balance. Disorders of the ear can leave a person unable to communicate, react, and maintain equilibrium.
- Assessment of the external ear canal and middle ear can be conducted with an otoscope. The treatment for an ear condition is to transport the patient so that he or she can be further evaluated at the receiving facility.
- Specific medical conditions of the ear include impacted cerumen, labyrinthitis, Meniere disease, and otitis.
- The nose is a highly vascular structure, which contains nasal mucosa that provides a short route to the brain.
- Never insert a nasopharyngeal airway or attempt nasotracheal intubation in any patient with suspected nasal fractures or in a patient with cerebrospinal fluid or blood leakage from the nose. The airway or tube could penetrate the brain and cause further damage.
- Specific medical problems related to the nose include epistaxis, foreign body obstruction, rhinitis, and

Prep Kit (continued)

sinusitis. Treatment of epistaxis focuses on controlling the bleeding. Treatment for foreign body obstruction is to transport the patient.

- Disorders of the throat (pharynx and larynx) may represent acute inflammation and infections, chronic inflammation, or abnormal growths. Throat infections are particularly common among children.
- When you are assessing a patient with a throat complaint, note whether the patient is able to swallow. If not, position the patient to allow drainage. Be sure to assess for threats to the airway and breathing.
- Specific medical disorders related to the throat include dentalgia, dental abscess, diseases of oral soft tissue, oral candidiasis, Ludwig angina, epiglottitis, laryngitis, tracheitis, pharyngitis/tonsillitis, peritonsillar abscess, and temporomandibular joint disorders.

▶ Vital Vocabulary

anisocoria A condition in which the pupils are not of equal size.

Battle sign Bruising over the mastoid bone behind the ear, commonly seen following a basilar skull fracture; also called retroauricular ecchymosis.

cataract A clouding of the lens of the eye that is normally a result of aging.

cerebrospinal rhinorrhea Cerebrospinal fluid drainage from the nose.

cerumen Earwax.

chalazion A small, swollen bump or pustule on the external eyelid, which arises when the eyelid's oil glands or ducts become blocked.

conjunctivitis An inflammation of the conjunctivae of the eye that usually is caused by bacteria, viruses, allergies, or foreign bodies; it should be considered highly contagious. Also called pink eye.

dental abscess A collection of pus that forms in the gums, facial tissue, bones, and/or neck.

dentalgia Toothache.

diabetic retinopathy A condition associated with diabetes, in which the small blood vessels of the retina are affected; it can eventually lead to blindness.

dysconjugate gaze Paralysis of gaze or lack of coordination between the movements of the two eyes.

dysphagia Pain, discomfort, or difficulty in swallowing.

epiglottitis An inflammation of the epiglottis.

epistaxis Nosebleed.

glaucoma A group of conditions that lead to increased intraocular pressure, causing damage to the optic nerve; a leading cause of blindness.

hordeolum A red tender lump in the eyelid or at the lid margin; commonly known as a stye.

iritis Inflammation of the iris; also called anterior uveitis.

labyrinthitis Irritation and swelling in the inner ear that produces a loss of balance and possibly tinnitus, dizziness, loss of hearing, nausea, and vomiting.

laryngitis Swelling and inflammation of the larynx that is associated with hoarseness or loss of voice.

Ludwig angina A type of cellulitis that occurs on the floor of the mouth under the tongue; it is caused by bacteria from an infected tooth root (tooth abscess) or mouth injury.

Meniere disease An inner ear disorder in which endolymphatic rupture creates increased pressure in the cochlear duct, which then leads to damage to the organ of Corti and the semicircular canal; symptoms include severe vertigo, tinnitus, and sensorineuronal hearing loss.

oculomotor nerve Third cranial nerve; it innervates the muscles that cause motion of the eyeballs and upper eyelid.

ophthalmoscope A device used to examine the fundus of the eye.

optic nerve Either of the second cranial nerves that enter the eyeball posteriorly, through the optic foramen.

oral candidiasis A condition that presents as white lesions on the tongue and inner cheeks, caused by the fungus *Candida albicans*; also called thrush.

orbital cellulitis An infection within the eye socket.

otitis An infection of either the outer or middle ear cavity.

otoscope A device used to examine the inside of the ears.

papilledema An eye condition that results from increased pressure on the optic nerve at the rear part of the eye; symptoms include headaches, nausea with possible vomiting, temporary vision loss, or narrowing vision fields.

periorbital cellulitis An infection of the eyelid; also known as preseptal cellulitis or eyelid cellulitis.

peritonsillar abscess A collection of infected material around the tonsils.

pharyngitis Inflammation of the pharynx.

Prep Kit *(continued)*

rhinitis A nasal disorder generally caused by allergens, which, once inhaled, result in production of chemicals that can cause inflammation.

sinusitis An infection of the sinuses, characterized by thick nasal discharge, sinus and facial pressure, headache, and fever.

temporomandibular joint (TMJ) disorders A collection of disorders that present with jaw pain, and that occur when the connection between the temporal bone and the TMJ erodes or moves out of proper alignment.

tinnitus The perception of sound in the inner ear with no external environmental cause; often reported as "ringing" in the ears, but may be roaring, buzzing, or clicking.

tonsillitis Inflammation of the tonsils.

tracheitis Bacterial infection of the trachea.

vertigo A type of dizziness in which a person experiences the sensation of movement when standing still or of the environment moving around himself or herself; often due to an inner ear disorder.

► References

1. American Academy of Ophthalmology. Eye health statistics. https://www.aao.org/newsroom/eye-health-statistics. Accessed December 7, 2016.
2. Fast facts. Centers for Disease Control and Prevention, Vision Health Initiative website. https://www.cdc.gov/visionhealth/basics/ced/fastfacts.htm. Accessed December 6, 2016.
3. Common eye disorders. Centers for Disease Control and Prevention, Vision Health Initiative website. http://www.cdc.gov/visionhealth/basics/ced/index.html. Accessed December 6, 2016.
4. Centers for Disease Control and Prevention, Vision Health Initiative. Projection of diabetic retinopathy and other major eye diseases among people with diabetes mellitus, United States, 2005–2050. http://www.cdc.gov/visionhealth/publications/diabetic_retinopathy.htm. Accessed March 8, 2017.
5. What is anisocoria? American Academy of Ophthalmology website. https://www.aao.org/eye-health/diseases/what-is-anisocoria. Accessed December 7, 2016.
6. Patel PB, Diaz MC, Bennett JE, Attia MW. Clinical features of bacterial conjunctivitis in children. *Acad Emerg Med.* 2007;14:1-5.
7. Rizzo DC. The nervous system: the brain, cranial nerves, autonomic nervous system, and the special senses. In: *Fundamentals of Anatomy and Physiology*. 4th ed. Boston, MA: Cengage Learning; 2016:250-277.
8. Haine CL. The ophthalmic case historian. In: Benjamin WJ, ed. *Borish's Clinical Refraction*. 2nd ed. St. Louis, MO: Butterworth Heinemann; 2006:195-216.
9. About the Iritis Organization. Iritis Organization website. http://www.iritis.org/about-iritis-organization/. Accessed December 7, 2016.
10. Chang JS, Banta JT. Corneal surface defects and ocular surface foreign bodies. In: Buttaro TM, Trybulski J, Bailey PP, Sandberg-Cook J, eds. *Primary Care: A Collaborative Practice*. 4th ed. St. Louis, MO: Mosby; 2013:330-332.
11. Boodley CA, Buttaro TM. Inner ear disturbances. In: Buttaro TM, Trybulski J, Bailey PP, Sandberg-Cook J, eds. *Primary Care: A Collaborative Practice*. 4th ed. St. Louis, MO: Mosby; 2013:353-357.
12. Barnett TO. Problems of the ear. In: Monahan FD, Neighbors M, Sands JK, Marek JF, Green CJ, eds. *Phipps' Medical–Surgical Nursing: Health and Illness Perspectives*. 8th ed. St. Louis, MO: Mosby; 2007:1845-1857.
13. Connelly A, Ramakrishnan VR. Epistaxis. In: Scholes MA, Ramakrishnan VR, eds. *ENT Secrets*. 4th ed. Philadelphia, PA: Elsevier; 2016:161-166.
14. Simmen DB, Jones NS. Epistaxis. In: Flint PW, Haughey BH, Lund V, Niparko JK, Robbins T, Thomas JR, Lesperance MM, eds. *Cummings Otolaryngology*. 6th ed. Philadelphia, PA: Saunders; 2015:678-690.
15. Courey MS, Pletcher SD. Upper airway disorders. In: Broaddus VC, Mason RJ, Ernst JD, King TE, Lazaarus SC, Murray JF, Gotway MB, eds. *Murray and Nadel's Textbook of Respiratory Medicine*. 6th ed. Philadelphia, PA: Saunders; 2016:877-896.
16. Wang EJ. Infections of the head and neck. In: Benjamin IJ, Griggs RC, Wing EJ, Fitz JG, eds. *Andreoli and Carpenter's Cecil Essentials of Medicine*. 9th ed. Philadelphia, PA: Saunders; 2016:867-871.
17. Centers for Disease Control and Prevention. Summary health statistics: National Health Interview Survey, 2014. Table C-2a. Age-adjusted percentages (with standard errors) of hay fever, respiratory allergies, food allergies, and skin allergies in the past 12 months for children under age 18 years, by selected characteristics: United States, 2014. https://ftp.cdc.gov/pub/Health_Statistics/NCHS/NHIS/SHS/2014_SHS_Table_A-2.pdf. Accessed December 7, 2016.
18. Babu NC, Gomes AJ. Systemic manifestations of oral diseases. *J Oral Maxillofac Pathol.* 2011;15(2):144-147. https://www.ncbi.nlm.nih.gov/pmc/articles/PMC3329699/. Accessed March 8, 2017.

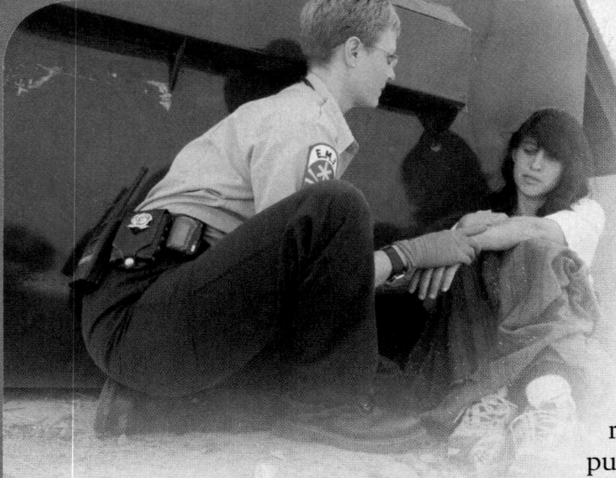

Assessment in Action

You are responding to a call at a local childcare center for a 4-year-old child with an eye problem. On arrival, you find a young child with very pink-red eyes complaining of eye irritation. The patient also appears to have difficulty fully opening one eye. A staff member reports the child has been rubbing his eyes all morning. The child says that he did not put anything in his eye. The parents have been contacted at work; they advised that the patient had the symptoms this morning before going to the childcare center and authorized any medical evaluation or treatment needed. They are en route.

1. What is the first step you should take in the care of this patient?

A. Assess the eye and apply a bandage.
B. Ensure the patient can maintain his airway.
C. Clean the patient's eyes with normal saline.
D. Pack the nose with gauze.

2. What is the likely diagnosis for this patient?

A. Corneal abrasion
B. Glaucoma
C. Eye cancer
D. Conjunctivitis

3. Does this patient require emergent treatment?

A. The patient should be taken to the emergency department immediately.
B. This patient needs assessment and treatment and should be transported—either by EMS or by his parents.
C. This patient needs to go to a Level 1 trauma center.
D. This patient should rest at home.

4. What is another common name for conjunctivitis?

A. Cataract
B. Epistaxis
C. Pink eye
D. Anisocoria

5. What is conjunctivitis?

A. An acute infection of the eye, which may be either viral or bacterial in origin
B. Elevated intracranial pressure
C. Elevated blood pressure in the eye
D. A blown blood vessel in the eye

6. Is this condition contagious?

A. Yes, but only if you make direct eye contact.
B. Yes, and it spreads easily among children when they are playing.
C. Yes, it is highly infectious and dangerous; assume the need for full standard precautions.
D. No.

7. What is the best way to protect yourself from contracting pink eye from your patient?

A. Wear gloves and wash your hands.
B. Wear goggles.
C. Wear a full gown and observe standard precautions.
D. No precautions are needed.

8. What would you recommend as first-line treatment for someone complaining of ear pain after just getting off an airplane?

9. How would you manage a patient with suspected epiglottitis?

10. How should you treat a patient who calls you complaining of a tooth infection?

CHAPTER 20

Abdominal and Gastrointestinal Emergencies

National EMS Education Standard Competencies

Medicine

Integrates assessment findings with principles of epidemiology and pathophysiology to formulate a field impression and implement a comprehensive treatment/disposition plan for a patient with a medical complaint.

Abdominal and Gastrointestinal Disorders

Anatomy, presentations, and management of shock associated with abdominal emergencies

- Gastrointestinal bleeding (pp 1183-1187)

Anatomy, physiology, epidemiology, pathophysiology, psychosocial impact, presentations, prognosis, and management of

- Acute and chronic gastrointestinal hemorrhage (pp 1183-1187)
- Liver disorders (pp 1197-1198)
- Peritonitis (pp 1189-1190)
- Ulcerative diseases (pp 1185-1186, 1194)
- Irritable bowel syndrome (p 1195)
- Inflammatory disorders (pp 1194-1195)
- Pancreatitis (pp 1193-1194)
- Bowel obstruction (pp 1198-1200)
- Hernias (pp 1186, 1200-1201)
- Infectious disorders (pp 1196-1197)
- Gall bladder and biliary tract disorders (pp 1190-1191)
- Rectal abscess (p 1197)
- Rectal foreign body obstruction (pp 1201-1202)
- Mesenteric ischemia (pp 1202-1203)

Knowledge Objectives

1. Describe the incidence, morbidity, and mortality of gastrointestinal emergencies. (p 1171)
2. Identify the primary risk factors for gastrointestinal disease. (pp 1171-1172)
3. Discuss the anatomy and physiology of the organs and structures of the gastrointestinal system. (pp 1172-1175)
4. Explain how to size up scene safety when responding to a patient with a gastrointestinal emergency. (p 1175)
5. List the personal protective equipment that is likely to be necessary during a call in response to a patient with a gastrointestinal emergency. (p 1175)
6. Explain how to integrate pathophysiologic principles and assessment findings to formulate a field impression and implement a treatment plan for the patient with a gastrointestinal emergency. (pp 1175-1180)
7. Evaluate the mechanisms by which airway patency might be compromised in the patient with a gastrointestinal emergency. (p 1175)
8. Summarize assessment of breathing and circulation in a patient with a gastrointestinal emergency. (pp 1175-1176)
9. Indicate the considerations that go into making a transport decision for the patient with a gastrointestinal emergency. (p 1176)
10. Explore ways of investigating the chief complaint and taking the history of a patient with a gastrointestinal disorder. (p 1176)
11. Describe the technique for performing a comprehensive physical examination on a patient with abdominal pain, including percussion and auscultation of bowel sounds and palpation to evaluate for pain and masses. (pp 1176-1179)
12. Discuss how orthostatic vital signs can help assess the extent of abdominal bleeding. (p 1179)
13. Consider the proper extent of pain management for the patient with an abdominal emergency. (pp 1180-1181)
14. Discuss the pathophysiologic mechanisms that can cause hypovolemia. (p 1182)
15. Compare the pathophysiology, assessment, and management of upper gastrointestinal bleeding with that of lower gastrointestinal bleeding. (pp 1183-1187)
16. Discuss the pathophysiology, assessment, and management of esophagogastric varices. (pp 1183-1184)

17. Discuss the pathophysiology, assessment, and management of Mallory-Weiss syndrome and Boerhaave syndrome. (pp 1184-1185)
18. Discuss the pathophysiology, assessment, and management of peptic ulcer disease and gastritis. (pp 1185-1186)
19. Discuss the pathophysiology, assessment, and management of gastroesophageal reflux disease and hiatal hernia. (p 1186)
20. Discuss the pathophysiology, assessment, and management of hemorrhoids. (pp 1186-1187)
21. Discuss the pathophysiology, assessment, and management of anal fissures. (p 1187)
22. Discuss the pathophysiology, assessment, and management of esophageal pathologies, including esophagitis, tracheoesophageal fistula, and esophageal stricture (or stenosis). (pp 1187-1189)
23. Explain how the immune system responds to acute and chronic inflammation within the gastrointestinal tract. (p 1189)
24. Discuss the pathophysiology, assessment, and management of peritonitis. (pp 1189-1190)
25. Discuss the pathophysiology, assessment, and management of cholecystitis. (pp 1190-1191)
26. Discuss the pathophysiology, assessment, and management of appendicitis. (pp 1191-1192)
27. Discuss the pathophysiology, assessment, and management of diverticulitis. (pp 1192-1193)
28. Discuss the pathophysiology, assessment, and management of pancreatitis. (pp 1193-1194)
29. Discuss the pathophysiology, assessment, and management of ulcerative colitis. (p 1194)
30. Discuss the pathophysiology, assessment, and management of Crohn disease. (pp 1194-1195)
31. Discuss the pathophysiology, assessment, and management of irritable bowel syndrome. (p 1195)
32. Explain why the gastrointestinal system is vulnerable to infection and how the immune system reacts to infection within the gastrointestinal tract. (pp 1195-1196)
33. Discuss the pathophysiology, assessment, and management of acute gastroenteritis. (pp 1196-1197)
34. Discuss the pathophysiology, assessment, and management of rectal abscess. (p 1197)
35. Discuss the pathophysiology, assessment, and management of cirrhosis. (pp 1197-1198)
36. Discuss the pathophysiology, assessment, and management of hepatic encephalopathy. (p 1198)
37. Discuss the pathophysiology, assessment, and management of esophageal obstruction. (p 1199)
38. Discuss the pathophysiology, assessment, and management of small- and large-bowel obstruction. (pp 1199-1200)
39. Discuss the pathophysiology, assessment, and management of gastrointestinal hernias. (pp 1200-1201)
40. Compare the four types of abdominal hernias: reducible, incarcerated, strangulated, and incisional. (p 1201)
41. Compare rectal foreign body obstructions caused by swallowed objects with obstructions caused by inserted objects. (pp 1201-1202)
42. Discuss the pathophysiology, assessment, and management of rectal foreign body obstructions. (pp 1201-1202)
43. Discuss the pathophysiology, assessment, and management of ischemic and neoplastic disorders, including mesenteric ischemia and tumors of the colon, pancreas, and liver. (pp 1202-1204)
44. Describe lifestyle changes that reduce the likelihood of developing gastrointestinal disease. (p 1204)

Skills Objectives

1. Demonstrate how to auscultate the abdomen to assess for diminished, absent, or abnormal bowel sounds. (pp 1177-1178)
2. Demonstrate how to palpate the abdomen to assess for pain, rebound tenderness, and masses. (pp 1178-1179)
3. Demonstrate how to palpate the right upper quadrant to assess for Murphy sign, indicating cholecystitis. (p 1190)

Introduction

Gastrointestinal (GI) conditions can become life threatening because systemic consequences can result from untreated or undertreated disorders of the GI system. For example, the appendix, a small, inconsequential portion of the intestine, has no known function. Yet when this small, fleshy pouch becomes infected, the consequences can be deadly.

This chapter will review the structures that perform **digestion** and their functions and locations. After a brief review of the general assessment process for a patient with an **acute abdomen** (sudden onset of abdominal pain) or other abdominal emergency, the pathophysiology, assessment, and management of common GI conditions will be discussed. To begin, you need to gain an appreciation for the scope of GI emergencies.

At one time or another, everyone has had abdominal pain or a case of GI distress. **Diarrhea**, nausea, and vomiting are the undesirable signs and symptoms of such an illness. They might cause intense discomfort and indicate an underlying condition. In other words, they cannot themselves be considered conditions or illnesses.

The number of disorders responsible for causing abdominal pain, diarrhea, and nausea is impressive. GI disorders account for 246,000 deaths per year, and 21.7 million hospitalizations per year.[1] Fortunately, most GI disorders are not deadly. With the exception of **septicemia** (a generalized infection of the bloodstream that could be caused by a GI disorder), GI disorders are not among the top 10 diseases that cause death within the United States.

According to estimates by the US Census Bureau, in September of 2016 the population of the United States was over 320 million.[2] Twenty-five to forty percent have **gastroesophageal reflux disease (GERD)**.[3] This certainly accounts for the number of advertisements for heartburn relief medications on television, in magazines, and on health-related websites. The National Institute of Diabetes and Digestive and Kidney Diseases, a segment of the National Institutes of Health, reports that 60 to 70 million people are affected by digestive diseases.[1] It is clear that paramedics will be called on frequently to treat patients with GI disorders. As you explore these conditions, knowing which behaviors and characteristics may predispose patients to GI disorders can assist you with the care or prevention of future GI disorders. Two known behavioral risk factors are smoking and excessive alcohol consumption. Both nicotine and alcohol increase the release of gastric acid in the stomach. This is why a small amount of wine or a beer taken before a meal is known as an aperitif, from a French word meaning "to open": it primes the stomach for the forthcoming meal. Smoking or chronic alcohol consumption, however, increases the acidity of the stomach beyond the ability of the mucosal lining to protect it. The result is an increased risk for ulcers of the upper GI tract.

Other activities that place patients at increased risk are listed in **Table 20-1**. You can use this information to help educate patients about ways in which they can decrease or even eliminate their GI discomfort.

Anatomy and Physiology Review

The anatomy and physiology of the GI system are covered in detail in Chapter 8, *Anatomy and Physiology*. **Figure 20-1** reviews the anatomy of the abdomen. The entire journey of food from mouth to anus, summarized in **Table 20-2**, takes 8 to 72 hours and involves the liver, pancreas, stomach, intestines, and other structures. At this pace, a normal number of bowel movements is between three per day and one every 3 days. Of course, this number varies according to the types of food you eat, the amount of water you consume, the amount of exercise you get, and how much stress your body is under.

Digestion begins with chewing, during which molars crush and grind the food. Saliva is added to lubricate the food, allowing it to be more easily swallowed. Changing

YOU are the Paramedic — PART 1

Your unit is dispatched for an unresponsive person at a local residence. The dispatcher tells you the patient is a 64-year-old woman who became unresponsive in her bathroom. You arrive at the residence and are met at the door by the patient's husband. The husband leads you to the upstairs bathroom where you find the patient lying next to the toilet. There is a foul odor in the room and you notice about 0.5 pint (250 mL) of melanotic stool covering the patient's clothing and around the floor near her buttocks. The patient is responsive when you approach. The husband explains that his wife had been sleeping, woke up, and asked him to help her to the bathroom because she had to have a bowel movement. He said when they reached the bathroom she passed out so he helped her to the floor next to the toilet. The patient said the last thing she remembers is walking to the bathroom with her husband. The patient has been feeling ill with stomach cramps for the past several days.

1. What is melena?
2. What part of the GI system do you believe might be affected?

the consistency of food into a smooth bolus helps to prevent aspiration of food into the lungs. Saliva also contains enzymes that begin the chemical breakdown of starches, or complex carbohydrates, so the body can more easily absorb them.

Swallowed food is moved to the esophagus. The esophagus, a hollow tube, lies in a collapsed position, which discourages air from entering it during breathing. However, during bag-mask ventilation, air can be pushed into the esophagus as well as the lungs, causing

Table 20-1 Behaviors and Corresponding Risk Factors for GI Disease

Behavior	Risk Factor
Smoking	Stomach/esophageal disease
Ingestion of caustic agents (acids or alkali agents that burn the tissue within the stomach or esophagus)	Stomach/esophageal disease
Low-fiber diet	Colon disease/constipation
Alcohol	Stomach/esophageal/liver disease
Ingestion of certain medications: acetylsalicylic acid, nonsteroidal anti-inflammatory drugs (NSAIDs), anticoagulants	Stomach/esophageal disease
Stress	Disease throughout the GI tract

Abbreviation: GI, gastrointestinal

Data from: Nordqvist C. Esophagitis: causes, symptoms, and treatments. Medical News Today website. http://www.medicalnewstoday.com/articles/9274.php. Updated November 27, 2015. Accessed March 24, 2017; and Wedro B. Esophageal cancer (cancer of the esophagus). MedicineNet website. http://www.medicinenet.com/esophageal_cancer/page3.htm. Reviewed November 30, 2016. Accessed March 24, 2017.

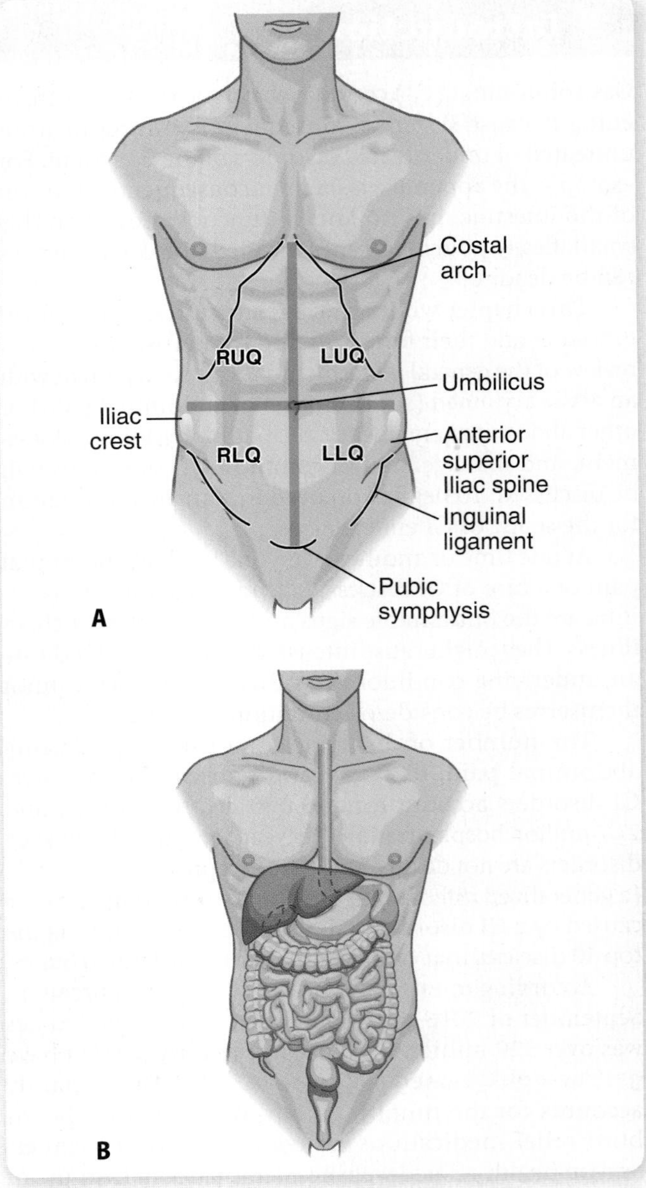

Figure 20-1 The anatomy of the abdomen. **A.** The four quadrants of the abdomen. **B.** Abdominal organs can lie in more than one quadrant. Although the kidneys are located in the abdomen (behind the structures shown here), they are considered part of the genitourinary system.

Table 20-2 Location and Functions of the GI System–Related Organs

Organ/Structure	Location	Function
Mouth	Head	Mechanically breaks down food; begins chemical breakdown of food with saliva
Esophagus	Substernal, **epigastric**	Tube that moves food from the mouth to the stomach (muscular and vascular structure)
Stomach	Left upper quadrant, epigastric	Performs mechanical and chemical breakdown of food (food in, chyme out)

Organ/Structure	Location	Function
Liver	Upper abdomen. Mainly right with central upper abdomen.	Produces bile; assists with carbohydrate, protein, and fat metabolism; vitamin storage and manufacture; blood detoxification; waste elimination
Pancreas	Posterior to the stomach	
Exocrine		Produces enzymes for protein, carbohydrate, and fat breakdown within the duodenum
Endocrine		Produces insulin, somatostatin, and glucagon
Gallbladder	Inferior surface of the liver	Storage of bile
Spleen	Left upper abdomen	Filtering of blood; recycling of dead red blood cells
Aorta	Central upper abdomen	Main artery supplying blood to the lower body
Bladder	Suprapubic area	Storage of urine
Uterus	Suprapubic area	Reproduction
Iliac arteries	Central abdomen and lower right/left quadrants	Supply blood to the legs and pelvis
Small Intestine		
Duodenum	Central, upper **umbilical**	Major site for chemical breakdown of food; major site of water, fat, protein, carbohydrate, and vitamin absorption
Jejunum	Central, umbilical	Moves chyme forward, absorbs nutrients
Ileum	Central, hypogastric to lower right abdomen	Moves chyme forward, absorbs nutrients
Large Intestine		
Ascending colon	Right lower quadrant, hypogastric into epigastric	Water reabsorption, formation of feces, bacterial digestion of food
Transverse colon	Right to left upper quadrant, epigastric	Water reabsorption, formation of feces, bacterial digestion of food
Descending colon	Left upper and lower quadrant, epigastric to umbilical	Water reabsorption, formation of feces, bacterial digestion of food
Sigmoid colon	Left lower quadrant, hypogastric	Water reabsorption, formation of feces, bacterial digestion of food
Rectum	Suprapubic, hypogastric	Stores feces for later release
Anus	Most inferior portion of the large intestine	Sphincter to control release of feces
Peritoneum		
Parietal peritoneum	The lining or bag that contains abdominal organs	Protects and supports the organs within the abdomen
Visceral peritoneum	The lining that covers organs	
Peritoneal cavity	The space between the parietal and visceral peritoneum	

Abbreviation: GI, gastrointestinal

gastric distention. Using a wavelike muscular contraction called peristalsis, the food is moved inferiorly towards the stomach.

Words of Wisdom

If the pressure of ventilation is too great, the esophagus will dilate. Air follows the path of least resistance. Given the choice of moving through a broad tube into a large open space—the stomach—or winding its way down through a series of progressively smaller tubes, from the trachea into the bronchi, the air will flow into the stomach. This causes gastric distention that can impede lung expansion and cause regurgitation.

In the stomach, hydrochloric acid is added to the food. As the stomach contracts, it mixes the food and acid together. The acid begins the breakdown of food to transform it into chyme. Some absorption occurs in the stomach. Substances that are of small molecular size are absorbed, such as water, alcohol, caffeine, and some medications. Chyme exits the pyloric sphincter and enters the duodenum, the first part of the small intestine. Here the pancreas, liver, and gallbladder connect to the digestive system.

The main function of the GI system is to absorb the products of digestion to fuel the cells within the body. The real workhorse of the digestive system is the small intestine, where 90% of all absorption occurs. It would be difficult to stay properly nourished if a section of your small intestine had to be removed because of **Crohn disease**, cancer, or some other disease process. The exocrine portion of the pancreas secretes several enzymes into the duodenum. These enzymes assist with digestion of fats, proteins, and carbohydrates. Additionally, pancreatic juice, as it is called, helps to neutralize gastric acid.

The liver produces bile, which is stored in the gallbladder. Bile is an enzyme used by the body to help break down fats. Bile is released into the duodenum, where it helps to dissolve fats. The liver also promotes carbohydrate metabolism. If the blood glucose level falls, the liver can convert glycogen into glucose. Dramatic decreases in glucose stores will prompt the liver to convert fats and proteins into glucose. Remember, your brain cells can burn only one fuel source—glucose. As blood flows through the liver, fat and protein metabolism continues. Without a functioning liver, you would be dead in a few days because your body would not be able to use any of the proteins absorbed through the GI system. Finally, the liver detoxifies drugs, completes the breakdown of dead red and white blood cells, and stores vitamins and minerals.

Recall that the portal vein transports venous blood from the GI tract to the liver. For a variety of reasons, blood flow through the liver can be slow. The veins surrounding the stomach and esophagus can become dilated if blood backs up. Even a small amount of pressure can cause leaking or rupture of these vessels. This bleeding can be minor or severe. This problem will be discussed later in the pathology section for each condition.

YOU are the Paramedic PART 2

The patient states she has been ill for several days with dark, smelly stools twice every day for the past 3 days. She denies any vomiting but reports pain throughout her entire abdomen. She states the pain can be bad enough to wake her. She did not go to the hospital because she thought this was just a case of a stomach virus.

You obtain a set of orthostatic vital signs. As the patient sits up with your assistance, she reports being dizzy. Assessment of the abdomen reveals normal bowel sounds. The abdomen is soft, but tender in all four quadrants.

Recording Time: 0 Minutes	
Appearance	Awake, lying on bathroom floor
Level of consciousness	Alert and oriented to person, place, time, and event
Airway	Open
Breathing	Adequate
Circulation	Adequate

3. What do orthostatic vital signs indicate?
4. Do you expect the patient's blood pressure and pulse rate to increase or decrease when the patient is moved?

The large intestine, or colon, contains the remaining waste products, called feces. The main role of the large intestine is to complete the reabsorption of water. Most water is reabsorbed in the small intestine. This osmotic function of the colon helps to solidify the stool. Failure of this bowel function results in **soft stool**, or diarrhea. The colon is also the site of bacterial digestion. Bacteria normally found in the colon help to complete the breakdown of chyme. This process produces gas as a by-product. Flatulence may be considered impolite, but it is certainly normal.

Finally, the appendix is a small, saclike outcropping of the colon. The appendix has no known function, but may become infected with retained fecal material. Appendicitis is discussed in detail later in this chapter.

Patient Assessment

You have probably heard this a hundred times, but it is true: Good assessment is the foundation of good patient care. GI system emergencies often result from a medical condition rather than trauma. This means that one of the most important areas of the assessment is the history of present illness. Ask the patient about dietary habits, discharge from the body, and types of pain.

Scene Size-up

Assessment of the GI system begins with the scene size-up. Standard precautions are particularly important when treating a patient with a GI emergency because of the high likelihood of contact with infectious agents. When you may come into contact with vomitus, diarrhea, blood, and soiled patient clothing, additional personal protective equipment (PPE) may be necessary. Gowns can be helpful when dealing with patients who have become incontinent. Masks can help with noxious odors. Cleaning the patient helps provide some degree of dignity to a person humiliated by the circumstances of his or her disease.

Words of Wisdom

When responding to a patient with abdominal pain and diarrhea in a nursing home, suspect *Clostridium difficile*. Wear proper PPE—gloves, gown, and mask.

Primary Survey

As you begin to form your general impression of the patient, closely examine where he or she is found. The patient's body posture or position can give you hints as to what happened. Was the patient walking to the bathroom when he or she passed out? Has the patient been in bed sick for several days? Was the patient at work when a sudden bout of pain caused him or her to double over? Look to the environment for clues as to the length and degree of illness the patient is experiencing.

One aspect of the general impression of the patient with a GI emergency is odor. What is the smell of the room or location of the patient? Few conditions create such a noxious odor as upper GI bleeding. The foul-smelling stool often present during these calls can make even experienced emergency medical services (EMS) providers nauseated.

A tip when dealing with these strong odors is to hold your ground. The sense of smell is the most acute for about 1 minute. After that time, more than 50% of the intensity of an odor is lost due to the olfactory nerve becoming tired of sending the same signal. If you are faced with a strong odor on a call, stay in the environment. After about 2 to 5 minutes, your nose will tire of sending the same odor signal, and the smell may be hardly noticeable.

Airway patency becomes more pertinent in a patient with a GI condition. A patient who is vomiting has a greater chance of aspiration.

Closely inspect the airway for foreign bodies. Remove or suction obstructions within the airway. While evaluating the airway, take note of any unusual odors from the mouth. Patients who have extremely advanced bowel obstructions can have breath smelling of stool.

For the patient with a GI condition, airway concerns include possible aspiration or obstruction of the airway because of the presence of vomit or blood. Although rare, these situations do pose real concerns for the paramedic.

- Place the patient so as to ensure adequate drainage of material out of the mouth. If trauma is considered, be prepared to tilt the long backboard. This means the patient must be secured and padded well so spinal movement is minimized when the backboard is moved.
- Portable suction should be part of every department's "first in" equipment.
- Management of GI bleeding may require the use of a nasogastric tube. This tube, placed in the stomach, allows stomach contents to be removed via suctioning. Its use can be beneficial in patients with severe upper GI bleeding or to decompress the stomach.

Breathing is rarely directly affected by a GI condition. If a patient is having trouble breathing, it typically stems from a severe complication. If the patient has aspirated, the ability to oxygenate and ventilate can be impaired. Monitoring the patient's capnography can assist with ensuring an effective respiratory pattern. Breathing management includes:

- **Administer high-concentration oxygen.** Do not rely on oxygen saturation readings as evidence that oxygen is not needed. A patient who has been bleeding internally may have a severely decreased level of hemoglobin. The oxygen saturation may read 96%, but if the hemoglobin level is low, oxygen is still needed.

- **Prevent aspiration.** Oxygen masks can cause some patients to experience a sense of confinement. This is problematic with patients who are experiencing nausea. Monitor patients using a mask to ensure they are able to remove it quickly if they need to vomit.
- **Auscultate lung sounds.** Obtain baseline information and continue to monitor lung sounds to ensure the safe administration of fluids.

Assessment of the circulatory system is essential in understanding the impact of GI disease on the body. As with all patients, assess skin color, temperature, and moisture. Note findings that would be consistent with shock. Determine the pulse rate. Evaluate the peripheral pulses and how they compare with central pulses.

Words of Wisdom

When you are treating a patient who has had significant bleeding, remember that pulse oximetry reads the percentage of circulating hemoglobin that is saturated (typically with oxygen). If the patient's hemoglobin is 7 g/dL, the oxygen saturation may read 100%. This indicates that 100% of the available hemoglobin is saturated; however, if the patient has lost half of his or her blood supply, he or she would have half the normal amount of hemoglobin. This reading, then, is dangerously misleading.

When making your transport decision, integrate the information gathered from the primary survey. If the patient has positive orthostatic vital signs (vital signs vary with a change in position), give close consideration to how the patient will be moved. Can the patient sit up in a stair chair or will this cause the patient to pass out? Be cautious when transporting any patient in severe pain because syncope, simply from increased pain, is a real possibility. Transportation of the patient with GI disease rarely requires lights and sirens.

History Taking

The mnemonic SAMPLE (Signs and symptoms, Allergies, Medications, Pertinent past medical history, Last oral intake, Events leading up to the illness or injury) helps you gather information about the history of present illness and past medical history. Many people with GI emergencies have long-standing medical conditions, so the information provided can help you to determine an appropriate field impression. Many GI disorders can quickly increase in intensity after months of minimal signs and symptoms. Ask if this emergency has ever occurred before. When asking the patient about his or her symptoms, you might need to discuss subjects that do not often come up in everyday conversation. It is important that you and your patient have a common frame of reference. For example, one person's diarrhea is another person's soft stool. Table 20-3 presents standardized language you can use so that the health care providers taking over care from you will have the same understanding of the patient's condition as you do.

Be sure to ask whether the patient has had a recent change in bowel habits or in the color or quality of his or her stool. Find out if the patient has had a recent onset of diarrhea, constipation, or nausea and vomiting. Ask about any recent weight loss. Finally, ask about the patient's last meal. Some types of meals are associated with particular conditions. When a patient has cholecystitis, a flare-up of this condition is often associated with a fatty meal that was eaten several hours before the pain occurred. Ask the patient how he or she has been tolerating meals. Does nausea occur after eating? Any abnormal symptoms? Ask the patient if these signs and symptoms have been occurring at greater frequencies than usual. The signs and symptoms may be related to food intolerance or can be an indication of a more significant condition.

Documentation & Communication

When you are recording information about the patient's body substances, be as accurate as possible. Describe the substances in detail. Saying a patient had feces covering his legs is adequate if melena is not present. If you see diarrhea, use terms to describe how liquid it is. This information can help to determine the degree of dehydration the patient may be experiencing.

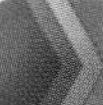

Secondary Assessment

For patients whose conditions are unstable, the physical exam gives you ample opportunity to discover clues to the condition or conditions. There should be no major changes within the examination of the head, neck, or chest that directly relate to GI concerns. The major effects from GI disease on the nervous, cardiovascular, or respiratory systems result from pain, hypovolemia, and/or infection. If a patient has an esophageal pathology, throat pain is possible.

Examining the abdomen requires more detail. This examination sometimes can be embarrassing for both you and the patient. Be professional and talk calmly as you proceed with the examination in a quick and compassionate manner. Use the examination principles described in Chapter 11, *Patient Assessment*. Place a pillow under the patient's knees if the patient is stable. Make sure your hands are warm before you touch the abdomen. Look at the skin for irregularities. Are there scars indicating

Table 20-3 Body Substances Originating in the GI Tract

Substance	Description	Possible Cause
Vomitus	Food and partially digested food; strong acidic odor mixed with the odor of food	Influenza, food intolerance
Hematemesis or "coffee grounds" emesis	Black or very dark red granular material; this slurry may contain food, but the food and blood are indistinguishable	Blood from the mouth, esophagus, or stomach that has been digested by stomach acids and then vomited
Vomitus with gross blood	Vomitus in which red blood is obvious; food and blood are distinguishable	Bleeding from the mouth or esophagus that has not been exposed to stomach acids
Diarrhea	Frequent liquid stool with the consistency of water; it can range in color from clear to dark brown	Intestinal infections, bowel obstructions; usually associated with small intestinal disorders; is always considered abnormal
Acholic stools	Tan-colored, formed stools; may be softer than typical	Liver disease: the liver releases bile into the small intestine; bile gives stool its normally dark color
Steatorrhea	Foamy, foul-smelling, mushy, yellow to gray stools; these oily stools usually float within water	Liver or pancreas disease causing excessive excretion of fat within the stool
Soft stool	Bowel movement that is the consistency of soft-serve ice cream; can range in color from tan to dark brown	Normal variant for some people; caused by new foods or a rapid change in diet
Hematochezia	Stool and blood that are incorporated together into the same substance, yet are easily distinguished from each other	Bleeding from the lower GI tract
Melena	Black, tarry, sticky, and very odorous stool and blood blended together into one substance; blood cannot be distinguished from stool	Bleeding from the upper GI tract

Abbreviation: GI, gastrointestinal

trauma or past surgery? Do you notice stretch marks, also called **striae** Figure 20-2? These indicate a change in the size of the abdomen over a short period of time, such as increases or decreases in weight, pregnancy, or severe abdominal edema.

Is the abdomen symmetric? Tumors, hernia, enlarged or distended organs, pregnancy, and other masses can cause asymmetry.

What is the appearance of the abdomen Figure 20-3? Is it flat, distended, or **scaphoid** (concave)? A scaphoid abdomen is the result of decreased abdominal volume, such as that associated with diaphragmatic hernia.

Auscultate the abdomen as appropriate given the time and noise level in your surroundings. Normal bowel sounds sound like gurgles and clicks. These sounds occur between 5 and 30 times per minute. You are merely listening for the presence or absence of these sounds. Sometimes you will hear loud, prolonged sounds. This

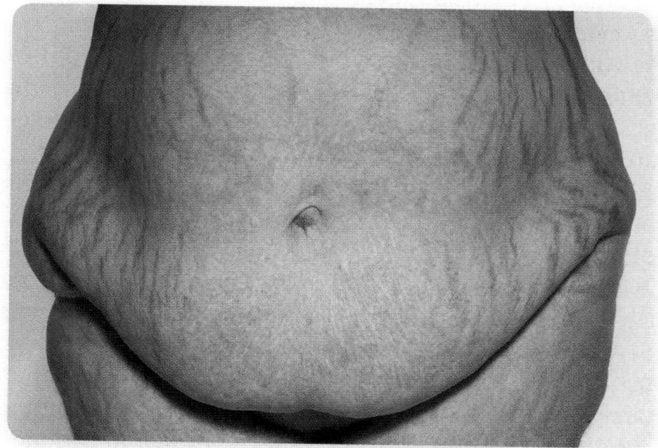

Figure 20-2 Striae. These vertical lines usually indicate a relatively rapid change in weight or a large amount of fluid accumulation in the abdomen.

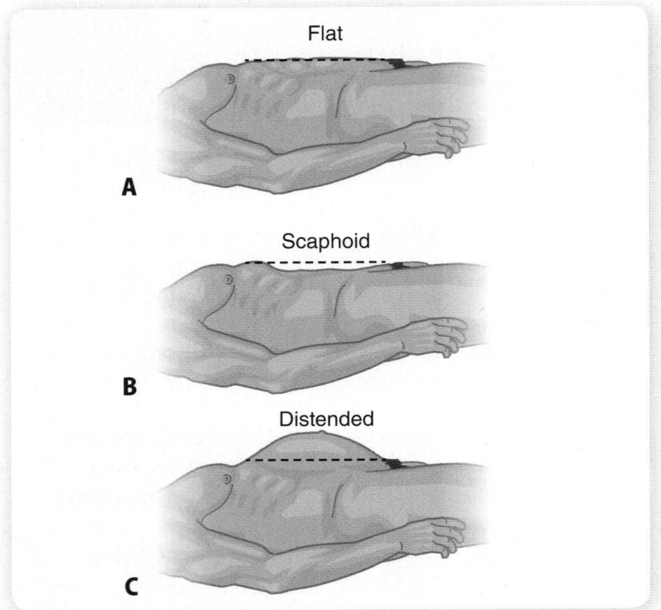

Figure 20-3 Appearance of abdomen. **A.** Flat. **B.** Scaphoid. **C.** Distended.

"stomach growling" is called **borborygmi**. It indicates strong contractions of the intestines. This can be normal or be present with diarrhea. Interestingly, increased activity in the bowel (**hyperperistalsis**) can also be present in patients with early bowel obstruction. In this case, the bowel is contracting forcefully to try to overcome the obstruction.

Decreased bowel sounds can indicate decreased peristalsis of the intestines (**hypoperistalsis**). This lack of movement can lead to bowel obstruction. Absent bowel sounds may be difficult to note in the prehospital setting. These are characterized by no sounds heard for 2 minutes. The absence of bowel sounds indicates the intestines are not contracting; therefore, any material within them is not in motion. Bowel sounds are summarized in Table 20-4.

Percussion of the abdomen can reveal information about its contents. Typically, the abdomen should be **tympanic** (empty sounding) to percussion, due to the gas in the abdominal cavity. A duller sound is generated around the upper left and upper right quadrants, due to the location of the spleen and liver, respectively. Percussion of the epigastrium may reveal tympany (empty stomach) or dullness (full stomach).

Unfortunately, the intestines often mask or augment any of these findings based on their contents. Use the results of your percussion as just one more piece of information: no more or less important than any other. Remember, rarely does one assessment finding have any true meaning. You should continue to gather information and compare assessment findings, looking for trends and associations. This is how to determine the correct field impression.

Palpation of the abdomen can reveal important information. Recall the palpation principles discussed in

Table 20-4 Bowel Sounds

Name	Description	Possible Causes
Normal	Soft gurgles or clicks occurring at 5–30 per min	Normal movement of material through the intestines
Borborygmi	Loud gurgles, often heard without a stethoscope often occurring at greater than 30 per min	Hyperperistalsis Can be normal If prolonged, can indicate increased intestinal contractions, as with diarrhea of any cause
Decreased	Quiet sounds occurring at less than 1 sound per 15–20 seconds	Hypoperistalsis Can indicate impending intestinal obstruction
Absent	No sounds after 2 min of continuous listening	Bowel obstruction/ intestinal paralysis

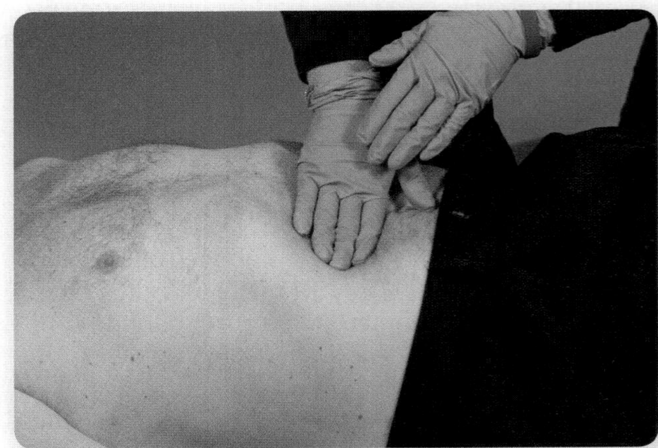

Figure 20-4 Palpating the four quadrants of the abdomen.

Chapter 11, *Patient Assessment*. As you palpate the abdomen, it should be soft and nontender Figure 20-4. A rigid abdomen can indicate hemorrhage or infection. Pain is often an important finding in patients with abdominal emergencies. It can indicate trauma, hemorrhage, infection, obstruction, or other serious conditions. As blood volume begins to drop, the body compensates by releasing catecholamines (ie, epinephrine and norepinephrine)

Table 20-5 Types of Abdominal Pain

Type	Origin	Description	Cause
Visceral pain	Hollow organs	Difficult to localize Described as burning, cramping, gnawing, or aching Usually felt superficially	Organ contracts too forcefully or is distended (stretched)
Parietal pain/ Rebound pain	Peritoneum	Steady, achy pain Easier to localize than visceral pain Pain increases with movement	Inflammation of the peritoneum (caused by bleeding or infection)
Somatic pain	Peripheral nerve tracts	Localized pain, usually felt deeply	Irritation of or injury to tissue, causing activation of peripheral nerve tracts
Referred pain	Peripheral nerve tracts	Pain originating in the abdomen and causing the perception of pain in distant locations Attributable to similar paths for the peripheral nerves of the abdomen and those in the distant location	Usually occurs after an initial visceral, parietal, or somatic pain

to vasoconstrict the periphery, increase the pulse rate, and increase the force of left ventricular contraction. Pain stimulates similar body responses. Both pain and hemorrhage can cause tachycardia, diminished peripheral pulses, diaphoresis, and pale, cool, clammy skin in the patient. Types of abdominal pain include visceral, parietal, somatic, and referred pain Table 20-5.

Rebound tenderness, or **parietal pain**, can sometimes accompany abdominal pain. Rebound tenderness occurs when the peritoneum is irritated because of either hemorrhage or infection, and it suggests serious and possibly life-threatening pathology. As mentioned in Chapter 11, *Patient Assessment*, it is not common for rebound tenderness to be checked in the field.

As you palpate the abdomen, note the presence of any masses. These will feel like areas of increased density compared with the soft surrounding tissue. A mass may indicate an engorged liver, bowel distention, aortic aneurysm, or a cancerous tumor.

It is helpful to obtain the patient's orthostatic vital signs to gauge the extent of any bleeding. Normally, there should be little variation in the blood pressure or pulse rate with this change in position. When a patient has a significant loss of fluid within the vascular space, however, you will note a 20-mm Hg drop in systolic blood pressure, a 10-mm Hg increase in diastolic pressure (a narrowing pulse pressure), or a 20-beat increase in the pulse rate. Any of these findings indicates a significant volume loss.

Ultrasonography is an additional tool that may be available to the EMS provider; however, limited evidence has been found of improved patient outcomes in the small number of departments that are using this technology.[4] Ultrasonography is more typically seen in the critical care transport setting. The information gathered can be used to effectively triage patients to the correct medical facility, avoiding interfacility transfers. Patients are also able to receive the definitive care they need more quickly.

Reassessment

The purpose of the reassessment is to monitor your patient for changes. Routine monitoring should include pulse rate, electrocardiogram, blood pressure, respiratory rate, and pulse oximetry. If the patient has GI bleeding, it is important to continue to assess for signs of shock. Remember that capnography can provide some insight into the patient's degree of shock. It is equally important to know the effects of your treatment on the patient. Before giving additional fluid boluses, for example, it is a good habit to auscultate lung sounds. In the prehospital setting, this is valuable information in determining if the patient is deteriorating into heart failure.

Many patients with abdominal pain are given pain medication. How effective was your treatment? Does the patient need more medication? How is his or her blood pressure and respiratory rate? These findings will help you evaluate the effectiveness of your treatment and form the foundation of future treatments.

Talk with the patient during your initial care and transport. Patient care is more than just administering medications and watching intravenous (IV) line rates. Patients with GI disorders are often upset and embarrassed. Be kind and treat the patient with respect. When creating your documentation, try to be objective about your visual findings. Avoid terms like "covered in blood" when describing your visual findings of the patient and/or scene. It is best for you to use more descriptive sentences like, "Blood noted on the floor, toilet, and patient's clothing." "Patient's clothing saturated with blood" also helps the reader to understand the quantity that was seen.

Emergency Medical Care

If there is a sudden dramatic change in the patient's condition, repeat the assessments as if you were assessing a new patient. Starting from the beginning will give you the best chance of modifying your care to adequately manage any worrisome new developments.

Often there is little you can do about the GI disease itself, but you are able to care for the effects of the disease. Patients may have severe pain; they may be experiencing severe dehydration, hypotension, or extreme nausea. The patient may be thirsty, but you must inform the patient that he or she cannot have anything to eat or drink at this time. GI emergencies can result in the need for surgery, and ingestion of food or drink could delay needed medical treatment. Your main goals are observation of standard precautions, maintenance of airway, breathing, and circulation (ABCs), and management of pain and nausea.

Pain Management

When you are providing pain management for GI conditions, the goal should be to make the patient more comfortable, not to abolish the pain. Enough medication to completely remove the pain may result in severe hemodynamic compromise. The following five medications provide you with tools to manage abdominal pain, and may be administered via the IV, intraosseous, and intramuscular routes. These and other medications, as well as dosages, are covered in the Appendix, *Emergency Medications*.

- **Meperidine hydrochloride (Demerol).** This is a synthetic narcotic that is often given with hydroxyzine to decrease nausea.
- **Morphine.** This narcotic can cause hypotension and respiratory depression.
- **Ketorolac (Toradol).** This medication is a non-narcotic and therefore does not tend to cause hypotension and respiratory depression. It should be given with caution in patients with renal disease or patients who are bleeding.
- **Nalbuphine (Nubain).** This is a synthetic narcotic and therefore can cause hypotension and respiratory depression.
- **Fentanyl (Sublimaze).** This is a commonly used opioid agonist. It is very potent, rapid acting, and has a short half-life. This narcotic can cause hypotension and respiratory depression.

YOU are the Paramedic PART 3

Your patient has a past medical history for diabetes, hypertension, and atrial fibrillation. She is currently taking propranolol, diltiazem, warfarin, and glyburide. She has no allergies to medications. She has also been taking an over-the-counter bismuth solution (Pepto Bismol) hoping to relieve the pain.

Recording Time: 5 Minutes	
Respirations	20 breaths/min
Pulse	120 beats/min, lying down; 136 beats/min sitting
Skin	Cool, pale, moist
Blood pressure	106/82 mm Hg, lying down; 92/78 mm Hg, sitting
Oxygen saturation (Spo_2)	98% with oxygen at 15 L/min via nonrebreathing mask
Pupils	PERRLA

5. On the basis of the patient's orthostatic vital signs, what is your suggested treatment?
6. Which of the patient's medications most concerns you?

The following medications may be administered to address nausea:

- **Ondansetron (Zofran).** This medication may cause damage to the developing fetus; therefore, it is not recommended as first-line agent for nausea and vomiting in pregnant patients.
- **Diphenhydramine (Benadryl).** This medication is typically used for allergic reactions, but also has antiemetic properties. Be cautious when using this medication because it can cause drowsiness and a drop in blood pressure.
- **Hydroxyzine (Vistaril).** Be cautious when administering this medication to patients who have taken any medication that has central nervous system (CNS) depressive effects. Hydroxyzine increases the CNS depressive effects of other medications.
- **Promethazine (Phenergan).** Be cautious when administering this medication to patients who have taken any medication that has CNS depressive effects. Like hydroxyzine, promethazine increases the CNS depressive effects of other medications. Also, this medication tends to cause a marked burning sensation during injection. Administer slowly.

Controversies

Should paramedics provide pain relief for patients with abdominal pain? This question may provoke some debate. In the past, surgeons relied on the location, quality, and intensity of abdominal pain to guide them during exploratory surgery. In medicine today, technologies such as computed tomography (CT) and ultrasonography allow abdominal tissues to be viewed more clearly. The images provided by these technologies show incredibly detailed information about disease.

One reason often given for withholding pain medication from a patient is the risk of addiction. The specter of drug addiction can be a powerful force that must be weighed when considering alleviation of pain. Now, however, pain management can be provided without the risk of addiction because of the availability of non-narcotic medications.

With all of these advances, it is most humane to make a patient in pain more comfortable. Administer analgesia and antiemetics per local medical control.

Fluid Resuscitation

Dehydration is also a concern. In patients who are dehydrated, the overall goal of treatment is to refill the cellular space. The degree of hemodynamic stability will dictate whether to use a hypotonic or isotonic solution. A patient in stable condition should receive a hypotonic solution. This will effectively move fluids from the vascular space into the interstitial and finally into the intracellular space, refilling the cells. In these patients, an infusion rate of 125 mL/h is usually sufficient to slowly rehydrate cells without causing dramatic swings in either fluid volume or electrolyte balance.

If the patient is more profoundly dehydrated, isotonic fluid would be needed to reexpand the vascular space first. Though the cells in this setting are dehydrated, the resultant decrease in blood volume can be life threatening, so refilling the vascular space takes priority over rehydrating the cells. This step is essential to ensuring adequate perfusion to the vital organs of the body. The guidelines for emergent filling of the vascular space and refilling the vascular space due to hemorrhage are the same.

As with the severely dehydrated patient, care for the patient with hemorrhaging is directed at maintaining perfusion of vital organs. This can be a rather controversial subject. Internal hemorrhaging falls into the category of hemorrhaging that cannot be controlled. Volume replacement is critical to ensuring adequate circulation to the vital organs. However, very aggressive volume replacement can result in dramatic hemodilution (dilution of the blood). Without an adequate supply of blood, its oxygen supply, and clotting capabilities, the patient will die. As blood pressure falls, the amount of bleeding decreases; therefore, the body actually retains more blood. Low pressure equals decreased perfusion, but retention of clotting factors and hemoglobin. Titrate fluids to a blood pressure of 90 to 100 mm Hg; do not normalize the blood pressure.

If the blood pressure cannot be maintained at adequate levels to maintain peripheral perfusion, then you may need to consider the use of vasoactive medications. Dopamine and epinephrine are the two medications commonly used in the prehospital setting for blood pressure support through vasoconstriction. These medications should only be used in circumstances where it has been determined that the patient has sufficient fluid volume to squeeze against. Fluid resuscitation should be accomplished before these medications are considered.

Once the patient arrives at the hospital, blood administration will be critical to stabilization. If you are assisting with an interfacility transfer, be prepared to manage blood products. Patients with GI bleeding often require blood replacement.

Pathophysiology, Assessment, and Management of Specific Abdominal and Gastrointestinal Emergencies

The paramedic must have an understanding of many conditions to care effectively for the patient with an abdominal condition. Some of these conditions are difficult, if not impossible, to differentiate from one another in the prehospital setting. In addition, many of the conditions cannot be treated in the field. However, you must learn about each of them because EMS is changing, as are the demands being placed on paramedics.

In some EMS systems, paramedics are asked to help online medical directors decide if the patient should be transported to a hospital, to a family physician, or to a clinic or pharmacy, for example. The sophistication with which you assess patients must increase if you are to meet the demands of this new role. Another reason to change is economics. It is less expensive to have a paramedic safely triage a patient to a family physician or a clinic than to transport every patient to the emergency department.

The other main reason that you need to know about these conditions is patient education. How the body is maintained and how it functions are often key factors that affect whether a disease is well controlled or life threatening. GI conditions are no different. Patients make choices that can increase or diminish the severity of their diseases.

Consider patients with **cholecystitis** (inflammation of the gallbladder). Medical experts would agree that such patients should closely monitor the types of food they eat. If these patients eat very fatty meals, they are more likely to have an attack of pain and discomfort. Patients may need to try small amounts of fatty food to see which ones they should avoid. This education is essential to improving the well-being of patients with cholecystitis. By learning about GI diseases, you may be able to help patients make better choices so they can stay healthy.

Remember to consider hypovolemia when managing a GI emergency. Hypovolemia is caused by either dehydration or hemorrhage. Dehydration occurs from vomiting and/or diarrhea. As the patient loses fluid, the body continues to shift water from inside the cells to interstitial space and finally into the vascular space to maintain adequate fluid volume in the blood vessels, until the patient has reached the limits of effectively moving fluid.

During this process, electrolyte levels are also affected. Although persistent vomiting decreases the amount of food ingested, diarrhea causes more dramatic swings in the levels of electrolytes. The main electrolytes affected by diarrhea are sodium and potassium. Diarrhea can either increase or decrease electrolytes, depending on the water content of the diarrhea. Table 20-6 outlines the effects of electrolyte imbalances on the body.

The second cause of hypovolemia in GI patients is hemorrhage. Bleeding in the GI system typically occurs from either the rupture or the destruction of a structure. The GI system is well supplied with blood. This fact is essential to the underlying function of getting nutrients out of what is eaten and then transporting the nutrients to the cells that need replenishing. Without blood, the entire process of digestion would accomplish very little. This close proximity to the blood supply, however, makes damage to the GI system more likely to cause severe hemorrhage.

Table 20-6 Electrolyte Imbalances Due to Diarrhea

Condition	Effects	Signs and Symptoms
Hyponatremia: Low sodium	Swelling of cells	Muscle weakness, cramps, coma, convulsions
Hypernatremia: High sodium	Shrinking of cells caused by excessive water loss	Coma, convulsions
Hypokalemia: Low potassium	More stimulation needed to fire nerve/muscle cells	Muscle cramps, weakness, paralysis, heart failure, dysrhythmias, flattened T waves, possible U waves
Hyperkalemia: High potassium	Less stimulation needed to fire nerve/muscle cells	Muscle weakness and cramps, dysrhythmias, tall T waves

Trauma is an obvious mechanism for bleeding in the GI system. Other mechanisms include erosion of the protective mucosal layers, chemical destruction of tissue, and dilation of blood vessels. It is possible to experience a fatal hemorrhage from GI bleeding. The bleeding can occur slowly, over several days or weeks, or it can be sudden, with a large volume of blood loss. In either case, assessment is the key to correctly identifying and treating these patients.

In patients with diarrhea or hemorrhage, an absolute loss of volume occurs. Consequently, classic signs and symptoms of shock are typically present. The brain is the first organ to show the effects of shock, and the patient becomes anxious and restless. Pale, cool, clammy skin and tachycardia are common. The pulse pressure is usually narrowed because the epinephrine released into the bloodstream causes vasoconstriction. The respiratory rate increases. All of these changes occur with a near-normal blood pressure. A drop in the patient's blood pressure indicates that a significant volume of blood has been lost, and the body's efforts to compensate have failed. Such a patient is critically ill. See the management section of each condition for advice on how to manage these problems.

Pathophysiology, Assessment, and Management of Gastrointestinal Bleeding

Bleeding in the GI tract is a symptom of another disease, not a disease itself. Causes of GI bleeding are shown in Table 20-7. The presentation differences between upper and lower GI bleeding are predominately related to the consistency and characteristics of the vomit and stool that may be present. Upper GI bleeding is far more common than lower GI bleeding.

Table 20-7 GI Bleeding by Organ and Cause

Organ	Causes	Symptoms
Esophagus	Inflammation (esophagitis) Varices Tear (Mallory-Weiss syndrome) Cancer Dilated veins (cirrhosis, liver disease) GERD	Melena, hematemesis, vomitus with gross blood
Stomach	Ulcers Cancer Inflammation (gastritis)	Melena, hematemesis, vomitus with gross blood
Small intestine	Ulcer (duodenal) Cancer Inflammation (irritable bowel disease)	Melena, hematemesis, vomitus with gross blood
Large intestine	Infections Inflammation (ulcerative colitis) Colorectal polyps Colorectal cancer Diverticular disease	Hematochezia
Rectum	Hemorrhoids	Hematochezia, gross bleeding

Abbreviations: GERD, gastroesophageal reflux disease; GI, gastrointestinal

Generally speaking, upper GI bleeding causes **melena** (dark, tarry stool) and lower GI bleeding causes **hematochezia** (bright red blood in the stool). However, you must also consider the speed at which the blood is moving through the GI tract. If a patient is bleeding from a gastric ulcer and transit time of the blood to the rectum is short, instead of melena, the patient will have hematochezia. Copious bleeding can also have a similar effect.

Presentation of GI bleeding is variable. Each of the many conditions that can cause GI bleeding has its own pattern of disease progression. For example, diverticular disease has a rather gradual onset and tends to affect people in their 50s, 60s, or older. Mallory-Weiss syndrome has a sudden onset and affects people of any age. Gathering the information about how the patient moved from being healthy to needing an ambulance is critical in determining the correct field impression.

The patient's past medical history and other possible events of abdominal pain or bleeding from the GI tract are also important. Find out the medications the patient is taking. As previously mentioned, several medications can cause irritation to the GI tract, precipitating bleeding. Question the patient about the length of time he or she has been experiencing bleeding. Ask whether the patient is taking any medications that affect coagulation. This will help you to estimate how easily the bleeding can be controlled. Aspirin, warfarin (Coumadin), clopidogrel (Plavix), and rivaroxaban (Xarelto) are examples of medications that affect bleeding.

Treatment for patients with GI bleeding consists of several general management guidelines. Fluid resuscitation is common. In most patients, even those with stable vital signs, it is prudent to establish an IV line, providing 1,000 mL of normal saline solution or lactated Ringer solution using a macrodrip tubing. This will allow you to quickly resuscitate the patient with fluids should conditions change. Specific conditions that cause GI bleeding will be discussed next.

Upper Gastrointestinal Bleeding: Esophagogastric Varices

Pathophysiology

Esophagogastric varices are caused by pressure increases in the blood vessels that surround the esophagus and stomach. These esophageal blood vessels drain into the portal system. However, if the liver is damaged and blood cannot flow through it easily, the blood will begin to back up into the portal vessels, which can ultimately lead to rupture of the vessels. In the Westernized world, alcohol used to be the main cause of **portal hypertension**. Today, hepatitis C is the primary cause.

Assessment

Presentation of esophagogastric varices has a two-fold appearance. Initially, the patient exhibits signs of liver disease. Examples include fatigue, weight loss, jaundice, anorexia, an edematous abdomen, **pruritus**, abdominal pain, nausea, and vomiting. The disease process is gradual, taking months to years to reach a state of extreme discomfort.

Rupture of the varices is far more sudden. The patient will report an abrupt onset of discomfort in the throat. He or she may have severe dysphagia, vomiting of bright red blood, hypotension, and signs of shock. If the bleeding is less dramatic, **hematemesis** (vomit with blood) and melena are likely. Regardless of the speed of bleeding, damage to these vessels can be life threatening. The patient's hemoglobin level and hematocrit value will drop. These laboratory results can help determine the severity of the hemorrhaging. As with any patient who has liver disease, elevated levels of liver enzymes (alanine aminotransferase [ALT] and aspartate aminotransferase [AST]) should be expected.

Management

Treatment for these patients in the prehospital setting includes use of the general management guidelines. As with any GI bleeding disorder, accurate assessment of the degree of blood loss is critical. Be prepared for a hemodynamically unstable patient needing volume resuscitation and aggressive suctioning of the airway. If the patient's level of consciousness (LOC) begins to decrease, consider securing the airway to prevent aspiration.

In-hospital treatment involves stopping the bleeding and aggressive fluid resuscitation. It may be necessary to perform an **endoscopy**. In this procedure, an endoscope is advanced into the esophagus and a flexible fiberoptic tube is advanced into the stomach. Internal structures can then be seen, and specimens can be taken. The physician will then attempt to control the bleeding directly at the site of hemorrhage by either using chemicals to cauterize the bleeding veins or a type of rubber band to constrict them. Once bleeding has been controlled, surgical management may be an option. If the primary problem is liver failure, the only real cure for this condition may be liver transplantation.

▶ Upper Gastrointestinal Bleeding: Mallory-Weiss Syndrome and Boerhaave Syndrome

Pathophysiology

Mallory-Weiss syndrome is a special type of esophageal condition in which severe hemorrhage can occur. In this condition, the junction between the esophagus and the stomach tears, causing severe bleeding and potentially death. The reason for the tearing is that during the act of vomiting, pressure in the stomach can increase so greatly that it causes a failure of the structure of the esophagus. The tear that occurs is within the mucosal lining and does not travel entirely through the wall of the esophagus. Mallory-Weiss syndrome occurs in men more often than women.[5] Mallory-Weiss syndrome has a mortality rate of as high as 8.6%.[5]

Similar to Mallory-Weiss syndrome, **Boerhaave syndrome** occurs during vomiting. In this case, the esophagus tears longitudinally and the tear travels entirely through the wall of the esophagus. This creates a passage for blood, air, and food out of the esophagus into the mediastinum. Occurring more often in men, Boerhaave syndrome typically presents after a large meal that included alcohol consumption. If this condition is not treated within 2 days, mortality is approximately 90%.[6]

To summarize, forceful vomiting that results in a tear in the esophagus near the stomach that *does not* go entirely through the esophageal wall is Mallory-Weiss syndrome. Forceful vomiting that results in a tear in the esophagus that extends entirely through the esophageal wall, creating a hole, is Boerhaave syndrome.

Assessment

Both conditions have a presentation linked to vomiting. In women, the vomiting may be associated with hyperemesis gravidarum, a condition of severe vomiting related to pregnancy. In men more often than in women, the vomiting is associated with alcohol consumption. Mallory-Weiss syndrome classically presents with bleeding. The extent of the bleeding can be small, resulting in little blood loss to severe bleeding and extreme hypovolemia. In extreme cases, patients will have signs and symptoms of shock, epigastric abdominal pain, hematemesis, and melena.

In contrast, Boerhaave syndrome presents with vomiting that is suddenly accompanied by upper chest pain. Swallowing often exacerbates the pain. There is little bleeding noted in this condition because any bleeding can travel into the newly created hole in the esophagus. This hole allows nonsterile materials, such as food and liquid, to enter into a sterile environment. The result is septicemia, pneumomediastinum (air in the mediastinum), mediastinitis (inflammation), empyema (a pocket of pus, in this case within the chest), or subcutaneous emphysema. Patients can have fever, sepsis (infection in the bloodstream), difficulty breathing, subcutaneous emphysema in the upper chest and neck region, and chest pain.

The time between when the tear occurs and when medical care is sought will determine the extent of the signs and symptoms. Mallory-Weiss syndrome's classical presentation is very difficult to ignore: vomiting blood. Therefore, most people will seek medical care immediately after the tear occurs. Boerhaave syndrome, although a much more critical tear of the esophagus, has the unfortunate classical characteristic of causing chest pain after vomiting. This symptom is more easily ignored, especially by a man who has consumed an excessive amount of alcohol. Often the patient will find a position of comfort and wait to feel better. He may drink some water or milk. This liquid is now deposited into his chest where it begins to cause infection. As he breathes, small amounts of air can be trapped in the chest cavity. The longer he waits, the sicker he becomes and the more likely he will die from this condition.

Management

Management for Mallory-Weiss syndrome is the same as for esophagogastric varices and is directed at determining the extent of blood loss. In this case, the patient may be dehydrated from the repeated vomiting so blood loss can be exaggerated in its effects. In-hospital management may include volume resuscitation as needed, endoscopy to visualize the extent of the damage, and possibly an attempt to repair the tear. However, in most patients with Mallory-Weiss syndrome, the tears will resolve spontaneously.

Boerhaave syndrome requires management related to the potential for sepsis. Complicating this presentation is the symptom of chest pain. Because this condition tends to occur in men age 50 to 70 years, the possibility of myocardial infarction (MI) is a reasonable conclusion.[6] The patient should be managed as if he had experienced an MI until proven otherwise. Be comfortable contacting medical control to help with these patients. Aspirin therapy is not desirable. In the hospital, patients with Boerhaave syndrome will require endoscopy to repair the tear and antibiotics to manage the infection.

▶ Upper Gastrointestinal Bleeding: Peptic Ulcer Disease and Gastritis

Pathophysiology

The stomach and duodenum are subjected to high levels of acidity. To help prevent damage, protective mucous layers line both organs. In **peptic ulcer disease (PUD)**, the protective layer has been eroded, allowing the acid to eat into the organ itself. This erosion typically occurs over weeks, months, or even years. Gastritis is caused by the same imbalance between stomach acid and the protective layers. **Gastritis** is a pre-ulcerative state where the stomach is inflamed, but erosions have not yet occurred.

PUD and gastritis, which affect men and women equally, are now known to have a variety of causes.[7] PUD was thought to be related to eating a highly spiced diet; however, the most common cause is an infection of the stomach with the bacterium *Helicobacter pylori*. Another major cause is erosive gastritis. Chronic use of NSAIDs is the most frequent cause of this condition, in which the mucosal lining of the stomach slowly erodes and ulcerates. Patients who have sustained severe burns or other types of trauma also are susceptible to this disease. These extreme stress states increase gastric acid production. Ulcers caused by the stress related to burns are called Curling ulcers. Those caused by head injuries or brain tumors are called Cushing ulcers. Remember the Cushing triad related to increased intracranial pressure? This is the same Cushing. Alcohol and smoking can also affect the severity of PUD by increasing gastric acidity.

All of the cited factors for PUD can also cause gastritis. Foodborne infections and food allergies also can cause inflammation of the stomach.

Special Populations

Older adults are more vulnerable to the primary and secondary causes of PUD. As a result, PUD tends to affect an older population. As people age, the immune system's ability to fight infection decreases, making infection with *Helicobacter pylori* more likely. In addition, older adults frequently use NSAIDs for arthritis and other musculoskeletal conditions. Thus, older adults are more likely to develop erosive gastritis; it occurs more often in people older than 60 years.[8]

Assessment

In both conditions, patients will experience a classic sequence of pain in the epigastrium that subsides or diminishes immediately after eating and then reemerges 2 to 3 hours later. The pain is described as burning or gnawing. Nausea, vomiting, belching, and heartburn are common. In PUD, if the erosion is severe, gastric bleeding can occur with the result of hematemesis and melena. Both groups of patients may experience dyspepsia (belching, bloating, and fatty food intolerance), fatigue, and anemia.

In PUD, if the erosion has eaten through the wall of the stomach or duodenum, the ulcer is said to have *perforated*. The result is a sudden increase in the severity and quality of pain. What was epigastric now becomes more diffuse abdominal pain where any motion exacerbates the pain. Now, stomach contents have access to the sterile peritoneum and infection easily can occur. **Peritonitis** (inflammation of the peritoneum) is the result, with rebound tenderness and potential hypotension due to sepsis.

Management

The major focus for prehospital management is for you to accurately assess the degree of blood loss and prepare to manage any hypotension that is present. Orthostatic vital signs are critical in determining fluid needs and transportation/packaging issues. Sudden vomiting of blood can occur with a change in position. Therefore, take the patient down stairs in a stair chair rather than having him or her stand up.

IV fluids may be needed based on the degree of blood loss. Also, if you suspect a perforated gastric ulcer, then sepsis is of real concern. Management for gastritis is supportive. Consider antiemetics in patients with PUD and gastritis.

In-hospital management will include acid neutralization and reduction therapies. Antibiotic therapy is often effective at stopping any new erosion. Management for erosion of the GI tract will be tailored to the degree of damage to the GI tract. Patients will often undergo endoscopy of the upper GI system. The stomach wall can then be directly assessed for damage. Surgical repair of the damaged stomach lining in concert with medication therapy is often effective.

▶ Upper Gastrointestinal Bleeding: Gastroesophageal Reflux Disease and Hiatal Hernia

Pathophysiology

Gastroesophageal reflux disease (GERD) is a condition in which the **lower esophageal sphincter (LES)**—the sphincter between the esophagus and the stomach, also called the cardiac sphincter—opens and allows stomach acid to move superiorly. This condition, also referred to as acid reflux disease, can cause a burning sensation within the chest (heartburn). Various factors can make some people more prone to this condition. Smoking, obesity, and pregnancy all increase the chances of GERD. Eating fatty fried foods, drinking alcohol, and eating citrus fruits are also factors that are associated with GERD. If the reflux continues over a long period of time, damage can occur to the esophageal wall. This damage could result in weakened portions that are more prone to bleeding.

A **hiatal hernia** is a protrusion of a portion of the stomach through the diaphragm. If there is a weakness in the wall of the diaphragm (through which the esophagus normally traverses), a portion of the stomach can be trapped superiorly to the diaphragm. This creates a small pocket in which the superior "door" is the LES and the inferior "door" is the diaphragm **Figure 20-5**. Food and acid can become temporarily trapped in this space, leading to GERD-like symptoms. In actuality, most hiatal hernias are asymptomatic. Hiatal hernias are caused by increased intra-abdominal pressure.

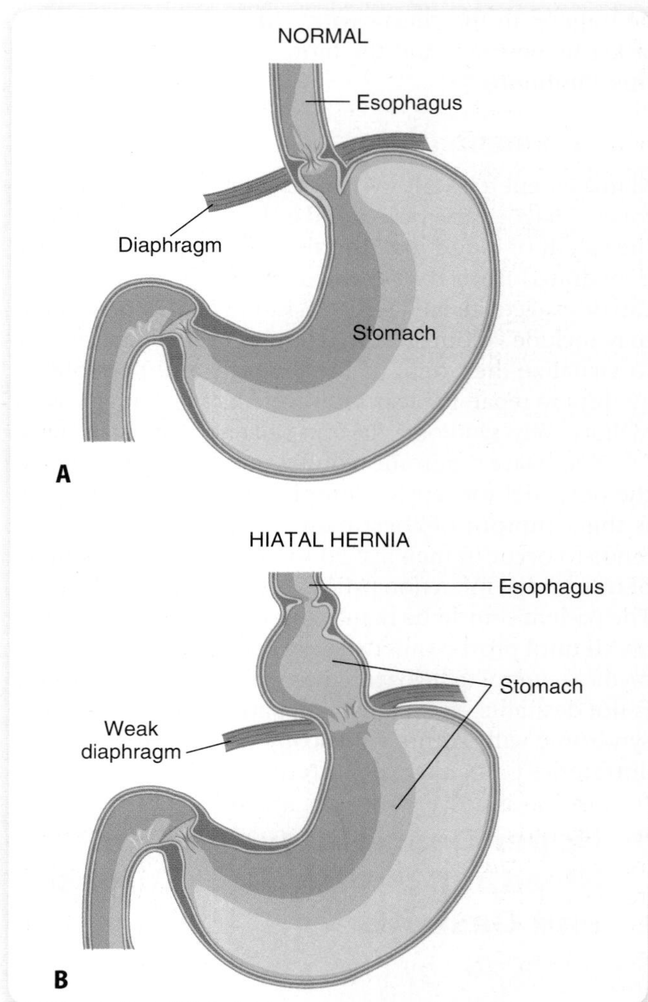

Figure 20-5 A. Normal configuration. **B.** Hiatal hernia.

Assessment

Heartburn is the predominant clinical finding for GERD. The pain may increase with positional changes—sitting upright is preferred whereas lying flat makes the condition worse. Some patients may not have pain, but experience coughing or have difficulty swallowing. Bleeding can occur if the damage is long term, resulting in hematemesis and melena. Hiatal hernias typically do not become symptomatic unless food and acid cannot be flushed efficiently from the pocket. The retained acid can cause erosion of the herniated stomach wall, causing bleeding and pain.

Management

Prehospital treatment for both conditions is supportive in nature. Medical treatment is focused on decreasing the acidity of the material within the esophagus by neutralizing it or preventing the acid from being produced. Antacids, proton pump inhibitors, and H_2 blockers are the common classifications of medications used for this condition. If these medications fail to control the discomfort, then surgical repair may be needed.

One confounding circumstance that can occur is when the patient with a history of GERD begins to have an MI. Such a patient may confuse the pain in his or her chest with GERD. Patients may begin to self-medicate, taking large amounts of antacid to try to control the pain. If you have a patient who reports chest pain and has a white "milk moustache," the coating around his or her mouth may be an antacid. Ask how much antacid the patient has taken. Large amounts of antacid can cause metabolic alkalosis.

▶ Lower Gastrointestinal Bleeding: Hemorrhoids

Pathophysiology

A number of conditions can cause lower GI bleeding. Hemorrhoids are a swelling and inflammation of the vascular cushions surrounding the rectum that can result in lower GI bleeding. These vascular cushions, or sinusoids, are made up of connections between arteries and veins along with their supportive muscle and connective tissue. It is a common problem. At some point in their lives, nearly 75% of all people have experienced or continue to experience problems from hemorrhoids.[9] These can either be caused by conditions that increase pressure on the rectum or cause irritation of the rectum. Pregnancy, straining at stool, and chronic constipation cause increased pressure. Anal intercourse and diarrhea can cause irritation and lower GI bleeding.

Hemorrhoids are divided into two types: internal and external. Internal hemorrhoids are painless, however they can prolapse (protrude from the anal canal). External hemorrhoids are painful and tend to have an area of swelling and clot formation.[10]

Assessment

Hemorrhoids present with bright red blood during defecation. This hematochezia, or frank bleeding, tends to be minimal and is easily controlled. Additionally, patients may experience itching and a small mass on the rectum. Typically this mass is a clot formed in response to the mild bleeding.

Management

Prehospital management is supportive. In isolation, hemorrhoids are more of an inconvenience than they are a life-threatening condition. Some patients may be at greater risk for serious consequences. Cautiously assess the patient who has any bleeding disorder or is taking anticoagulants. In this setting, even a minor bleeding disorder can become life threatening. To ensure the patient is hemodynamically stable, obtain orthostatic vital signs.

In-hospital management may include creams to help shrink the inflamed tissues. If the condition becomes chronic, surgical removal is a possibility. The best management for hemorrhoids is prevention, which includes eating a high-fiber diet and exercise.

▶ Lower Gastrointestinal Bleeding: Anal Fissures

Pathophysiology

Another cause of lower GI bleeding is **anal fissures**, linear tears to the mucosal lining in and near the anus. The exact reason why a fissure is created near the anus is unclear. It is thought to be precipitated by the passage of large, hard stools. Patients who have diets that are low in raw fruits and vegetables are at highest risk. Crohn disease, human immunodeficiency virus infection, trauma, and anorectal cancer are other causes of this painful condition.

Assessment

Patients present with painful defecation. There may be a small amount of bright red blood noted on the toilet paper, but rarely do these fissures cause significant blood loss. The pain persists for several minutes to several hours after the bowel movement. Any time this area is stretched, the fissure stretches, causing pain and more tearing. Pain is common with every bowel movement.

This pain creates a vicious cycle. Because it hurts to have a bowel movement, patients delay as long as possible. This delay causes the feces to become larger and harder, thus making them more difficult to pass. Eventually, when the movement is inevitable, the large stool causes more stretching, more tearing, and consequently more pain. This painful bowel movement precipitates an even greater reluctance to have a bowel movement.

Management

Treatment of anal fissures is the same as for hemorrhoids: supportive care. To facilitate patient comfort, a 5-inch × 9-inch dressing can be placed over the patient's anus to help pad the area. Do not under any circumstances pack dressings into the fissure or the anus. Remember, bleeding for this condition, as with hemorrhoids, is typically minimal and non–life threatening.

In-hospital treatment is conservative. Patients are encouraged to modify their diet, use analgesics if needed, take stool softeners, and apply warm water after bowel movements. Most anal fissures heal without surgical intervention.

The next sections will discuss acute inflammatory conditions and chronic inflammatory conditions.

Pathophysiology, Assessment, and Management of Esophageal Pathologies

▶ Esophagitis

Pathophysiology

As its name suggests, **esophagitis** is an inflammation of the esophagus. This can be caused by an infectious process or by reflux of gastric secretions into the esophagus. Additionally, some medications can be irritating, as can chemotherapy or radiation therapy. Esophagitis also is associated with eosinophils, a type of white blood cell.

Regardless of the underlying cause, the effects are irritation and swelling. Generally speaking, patients will present with either dyspepsia (heartburn or choking as their primary complaint.

Assessment

Due to the irritation, patients experience dyspepsia and upper abdominal and lower chest pain. This pain tends to increase with bending over or lying supine. Water brash, the bitter taste of gastric acid in the mouth, may also occur. These symptoms are common with esophagitis caused by GERD. Other symptoms include dysphagia, odynophagia (painful dysphagia), and potential food impaction within the esophagus. These later symptoms are more common in eosinophilic, medication-related, and infectious esophagitis. There are few physical signs that are directly related to this condition.

Management

Care for esophagitis is supportive in nature. One of the potentially confusing components of this condition is related to the symptom of chest pain. It can be difficult, if not impossible, to determine the exact cause of the chest pain. Be cautious. If your patient presents with chest pain, consider myocardial infarction as the cause and treat accordingly. For patients who present with dyspepsia, see the section on GERD for management options. For patients with dysphagia, see the section on esophageal stricture for management options.

▶ Tracheoesophageal Fistula

Pathophysiology

The trachea and the esophagus lie next to each other as they move inferiorly into the thorax. These two structures touch, which explains why patients frequently report coughing when they have something stuck in their esophagus. An opening between two portions of the body or between a body part and the outside of the body is called a **fistula**. The fistula allows communication of material between the two spaces. If a connection is made between the esophagus and the trachea, it is referred to as a **tracheoesophageal fistula (TEF)**.

Patients are either born with this unnatural connection or it is acquired. Common methods of acquiring TEF are through cancer, trauma, or iatrogenic (caused by a medical procedure such as endotracheal [ET] intubation) means. The cuff on the ET tube is used to isolate the trachea from secretions moving inferiorly and also to improve ventilation of the lungs. To perform its job, the cuff must have enough air pressure to seal around the circumference of the trachea. When you press your thumb against a hard surface you squeeze the blood out, as evidenced by the blanching that occurs. Similarly, the pressure used to seal the ET tube can squeeze blood away from an area of the tracheal wall. Over many days, this area may become ischemic and can eventually die. An opening may be created through the weakened area of the trachea and the anterior portion of the esophagus. Similarly, a tumor within the esophagus or trachea can erode a hole between the two structures. A penetrating wound also can create an opening.

TEF allows food to move from the esophagus into the trachea and eventually into the lungs. Pneumonia and sepsis are two possible serious consequences of TEF. If left uncorrected, the patient can die. Fortunately, it takes many days to cause that degree of damage to the tracheal wall. This is the reason why patients are not intubated for longer than 10 to 14 days. To prevent TEF, patients receive a tracheotomy, which limits, but does not eliminate, the risk of TEF.

Assessment

If TEF is due to cancer, the patient will present with cough, fever, and aspiration. He or she may report excessive gas in the stomach and increased oral secretions. Patients who are intubated or have undergone a tracheostomy are more complicated. These patients may have a decreased LOC or may be fed via gastrostomy tubes. In these cases, the main presentation is fever and sepsis of unknown origin. Coughing may still be present.

Management

The main focus of the acute care of TEF patients is ensuring adequate ventilation and managing potential sepsis. You may need to suction the patient due to increased oral secretions. If the patient needs ET intubation, it should be accomplished meticulously. Ensure proper tube placement and then reconfirm. Waveform capnography should provide early evidence of a misplaced tube. The fistula could allow the ET tube to be accidentally placed within the esophagus. If appropriate, elevating the head of the cot can help the patient manage secretions. IV fluids and appropriate vasopressors may be needed if the patient is septic. Ultimately, this condition will need surgical repair.

▶ Esophageal Stricture or Stenosis

Pathophysiology

A **stricture** (or stenosis) is an abnormal narrowing of a structure. The esophagus can become narrowed as a result of inflammation, tumors, infection, and acid reflux. As the diameter of the esophagus diminishes, it becomes more difficult for the person to swallow **Figure 20-6**.

Assessment

Most patients with this condition have a history of multiple episodes of choking. They may have volumes of secretions and the sensation of choking, with spitting up or gagging on a large quantity of saliva. They commonly will report not being able to move a piece of food they just swallowed. This dysphagia can progress to odynophagia. There may be accompanying difficulty in breathing, but cyanosis is rare, as the obstruction is in the esophagus. In the middle of an obstructive event, the patient may not be able to speak. Difficulty in managing oral secretions may also be present.

Management

As you might expect, the main concern with esophageal strictures is airway compromise. The patient may aspirate or have an obstruction that interferes significantly with airflow. Ensure the patient has a stable airway. If the airway is stable, then aggressive attempts at removal of the obstruction are not needed. If the patient is unable to move air effectively, then treat the situation as an airway obstruction and manage it appropriately.

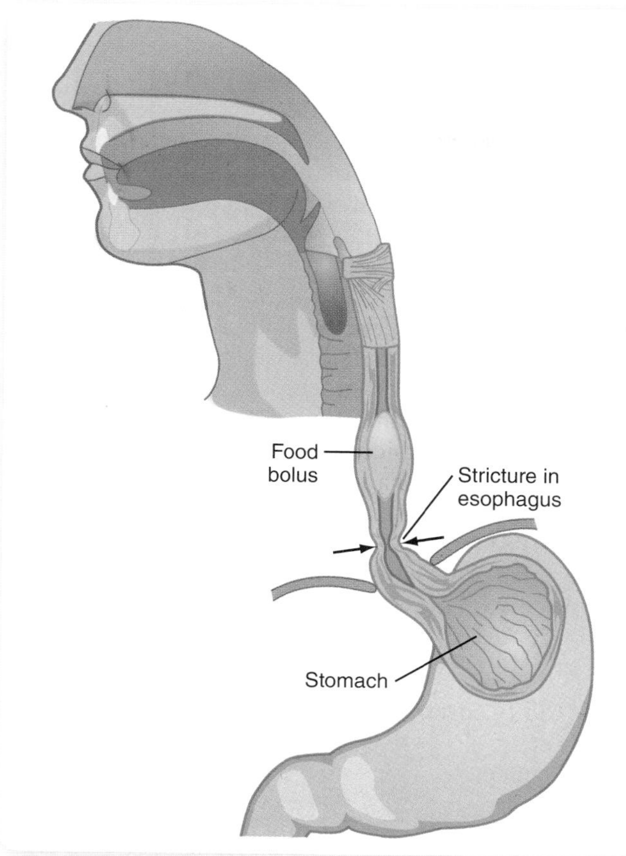

Figure 20-6 Esophageal stricture.

Glucagon can be considered in patients with esophageal obstruction. This medication causes dilation of the esophagus and hopefully will allow the obstruction to pass into the stomach. Glucagon has a limited effect on strictures. Contact online medical direction to use this medication for this purpose. Have the patient sit upright and be prepared to assist with oral secretions. If you arrive and the patient has already cleared the obstruction, encourage the patient to go to the emergency department.

Ultimately, patients will need to have diagnostic imaging to determine the location and extent of the narrowing. Many patients find improvement with dilation of their esophagus through endoscopy.

Pathophysiology, Assessment, and Management of Acute Inflammatory Conditions

Inflammation is a natural response to injury. If the body is attacked by one of the infectious agents discussed in the previous section, then vasodilation, mobilization of white blood cells, and changes in cellular metabolic processes will result. All of these effects allow the cell to move from a normal operating mode into one of being under siege. The purpose of inflammation is to assist the white blood cells in either destroying the invading agent or, at the least, seal it off so it cannot spread.

The redness, swelling, and tenderness that occur during an infection are the result of inflammation. The change in vascular permeability and vasodilation will cause redness and swelling. Swelling can cause pressure, which causes pain. Vasodilation and increased capillary permeability enable white blood cells to more effectively get to the area of damage.

Inflammation in the GI system can occur at many levels. Localized inflammation will cause localized signs and symptoms. For example, patients with **hepatitis**, an inflammation of the liver, can experience pain in the right upper quadrant of the abdomen. This pain can be due to mild swelling of the liver. In peritonitis, inflammation and irritation occurs to the peritoneum throughout the abdomen, so the patient may experience generalized pain that is rebound in nature. If an infectious agent causes the inflammation, the peritonitis can be a sign of movement of bacteria into the abdomen and eventually into the bloodstream (sepsis).

The body will respond to sepsis with a more generalized inflammatory response. One of the severe consequences of sepsis is the depletion of resources to manage the infection. In sepsis, infection is almost literally everywhere in the body. The body is trying to fight many battles but does not have adequate white blood cells, histamine, blood, and energy. Soon the battles being fought are inadequate, resulting in possible detriment to the patient. If a balance between resource demand and supply cannot soon be restored, death will occur.

Many of the diseases of the GI system are caused by inflammation. The difference is there is no defined reason for the inflammation. The body is attacking and killing its own cells. This is referred to as an autoimmune condition.

There are a variety of reasons postulated for this misdirected attack, but no conclusive cause and effect relationship has been found. One theory is that the patient ingests some type of food with a little-known antigen present. This protein substance is identified as foreign and antibodies are created. Another speculation is the patient comes in contact with a virus that triggers an immune response. White blood cells begin to destroy a portion of the GI system, causing damage. The body works to rebuild the damaged areas, but scarred portions of the GI tract may result.

Peritonitis

Pathophysiology

Recall that the peritoneum is the thin membrane that forms a sac containing all of the organs and structures within the abdominal cavity. This region is sterile. If an infectious agent is able to gain access, this lining can become inflamed. The two main ways that infections occur are through the rupture of an internal organ or the movement of bacteria out of the intestines. In **appendicitis**, if the appendix ruptures, purulent (containing pus) material can leak into the peritoneal space, thus irritating the peritoneum. This can also happen with a ruptured bowel.

Spontaneous bacterial peritonitis refers to a condition where bacteria migrate out of the intestine and enter the peritoneal space. **Ascites**, or abdominal edema, is associated with this condition in most adults. In these cases, there is no failure of an internal organ. The presence of excess fluid within the peritoneal space changes the permeability of the intestinal walls, allowing bacteria to exit.

In either case, the bacteria are able to flourish. It does not take long until sepsis can occur. Uncomplicated peritonitis has a mortality rate of about 5%; however, if sepsis, acute respiratory distress syndrome, and multiorgan failure occur, the mortality rate jumps to nearly 70%.[11]

Assessment

Peritoneal irritation is displayed through abdominal pain. This pain tends to be diffuse, with a focal point over the area of greatest irritation. For bowel rupture, the pain may be focused over the left upper quadrant if the transverse colon has failed. In appendicitis, the right lower quadrant of the abdomen will have greatest pain. A ruptured **diverticulum** will most commonly have the focal point in the left lower quadrant. Pain will often increase with coughing (Dunphy sign) and pain will be rebound in nature. Patients tend to have board-hard abdomens and will not want to lie flat.

Pain can be dull to severe. Patients will often be febrile and want to lie in a fetal position. This position relieves stress on the abdominal wall. Tachycardia, anorexia, nausea, vomiting, and dehydration also occur. These patients are at risk for both hypovolemic shock and septic shock. If in septic shock, lactate levels will be elevated, indicating unusually high amounts of anaerobic metabolism.

Management

Patients with peritonitis are critically ill. Management is directed at supporting vital signs. Treat the patient for shock. Be prepared to administer several fluid boluses to maintain blood pressure. Norepinephrine may be indicated if sepsis is present. Measuring the patient's lactate level can help to determine the state of generalized body perfusion. A high lactate level, regardless of the patient's blood pressure, indicates poor perfusion, greater anaerobic metabolism, and generally portends a poorer outcome.

Managing these patients' pain is often tricky. Antiemetics are certainly indicated. Many of the analgesics carried by paramedics also cause vasodilation. In cases of sepsis, this side effect is greatly undesirable. In-hospital management involves surgery to drain the infection and to identify and repair the primary cause of the infection, then treating it with antibiotics, and supporting vital signs.

▶ Cholecystitis and Biliary Tract Disorders

Pathophysiology

Biliary tract disorders involve inflammation of the gallbladder. Biliary tract disorders are a group of conditions including **cholangitis**, an inflammation of the bile duct; **cholelithiasis**, the presence of stones within the gallbladder; choledocholithiasis (the presence of at least one of the gallstones within the common bile duct), cholecystitis, inflammation of the gallbladder; and acalculous cholecystitis, inflammation of the gallbladder without the presence of gallstones. Cholangitis can cause acalculous cholecystitis. These conditions have similar presentation patterns and so they will be discussed as a group.

It is unclear why gallstones are formed; it is believed to be either due to increased production of bile or decreased emptying of the gallbladder. Other causes of gallbladder inflammation arise from decreased flow of biliary materials. These include major trauma, sepsis, sickle cell disease, and prolonged fasting.

Women have cholecystitis two to three times more often than men. Pregnancy is also associated with an increased risk.[12] Caucasians have a higher prevalence than do African Americans.[13] Other persons at risk are older people and people who are overweight or obese or have had a recent extreme weight loss.[13] Remember the "five Fs" of cholecystitis related to people who have this condition most often.

- Fair (Caucasian)
- Fat
- Female
- Fertile
- Forty to fifty

The gallbladder's function is to store bile, an enzyme used to break down fat, and then contract, releasing the bile. When fatty foods are present in the duodenum, the gallbladder contracts, but if a blockage is present, extreme pain in the right upper quadrant, radiating to the right shoulder, will occur.

Assessment

The presentation of this condition also takes on a pattern. The classic pattern is for the patient to have no pain until a fatty meal is eaten. Two to three hours later the patient begins to develop severe upper right quadrant abdominal pain. This pattern is not absolute. The variability in presentation is based on the consistency of the food that is eaten. A fatty steak will remain in the stomach longer than a cheesy casserole. The faster the food is emptied from the stomach, the sooner the pain begins after the meal.

The abdominal pain can be quite severe. In addition to the pain, the patient may demonstrate a positive Murphy sign. Ask the patient to breathe out. Then take the tips of your fingers and palpate deeply along the intercostal margin of the right upper quadrant. You are now applying pressure to the liver and subsequently to the gallbladder.

Next, ask the patient to inhale deeply. As inspiration continues, the diaphragm will drop and eventually come into contact with the gallbladder. If the patient has cholecystitis, he or she may suddenly stop inspiring because of a sharp increase in pain—a positive Murphy sign. Although not specific for cholecystitis, Murphy sign, along with additional assessment information, can help to provide valuable information.

Nausea, vomiting, fever, jaundice, and tachycardia are also often present with this disease. Charcot triad—fever, right upper quadrant pain, and jaundice—may indicate an inflammation of the common bile duct in 50% to 70% of patients.[14]

Management

Prehospital treatment for this condition is directed at making the patient comfortable. Rarely is this condition life threatening, though the pain from cholecystitis can cause the patient to experience vasovagal stimulation.

Medications to control pain include opiates. Nausea should be controlled using the medications listed earlier. IV fluids are also indicated because the patient is often vomiting.

In-hospital treatment will include antibiotics, pain medication, ultrasound, and potential removal of the gallbladder through surgery.

▶ Appendicitis

Pathophysiology

Appendicitis is a condition most people are familiar with and it is a frequent cause of acute abdomen. The condition occurs when fecal matter or other material accumulates in the appendix. When the organ can no longer flush out this material normally, pressure builds. This pressure decreases the flow of blood and lymph fluid, hindering the body's ability to fight infection. The combination of bacteria in the feces and diminished ability to combat local infection creates an ideal environment for the uncontrolled reproduction of bacteria. If left unchecked, overpressurization of the appendix will eventually cause it to rupture, resulting in peritonitis, sepsis, and death.

Appendicitis occurs in every age group. The peak time for the occurrence of this condition is during adolescence. Though the elderly experience appendicitis less often, they have a higher mortality rate. Men are slightly more prone to appendicitis than women.

Assessment

Appendicitis can be difficult to diagnose. The classic presentation of appendicitis can be divided into three stages: early, ripe, and rupture.

- **Early.** Periumbilical pain, nausea, vomiting, low-grade fever, loss of appetite
- **Ripe.** Pain in lower right quadrant (McBurney point)
- **Rupture.** Decrease in pain (decreased pressure), generalized pain, rebound tenderness

In early stages, patients classically present with poorly defined periumbilical pain. Nausea, vomiting, anorexia, and a low-grade fever are typically present. The vomiting tends to occur after the pain starts and not before. Over several hours, the appendix will swell and eventually pressure will increase. This takes approximately 48 hours. The patient is now in the ripe stage. During this time, the pain will migrate to localized right lower quadrant pain and become more severe. If the appendix ruptures, the rupture stage is entered.

In this stage, at first there may be a sudden decrease of pain with a sense of relief because of the sudden decreased pressure. Now the infectious material has access to the entire abdominal cavity. During this stage the pain becomes generalized throughout the abdomen. Rebound tenderness is a sign of perforation of the appendix with resultant peritonitis. Dunphy sign, severe abdominal pain in the right lower quadrant with coughing, is another way for you to evaluate the patient for peritonitis. Another indication is Rovsing sign. Here, you deeply palpate the *left* lower abdominal quadrant. When you do so, the patient has *right* lower abdominal quadrant pain.

Words of Wisdom

The average age at which a person experiences appendicitis is 22 years.[15] How old are you?

EMS can be a stressful, emotionally demanding career, and often our dietary choices are guided by these emotions—the desire for "comfort" foods and "rewards" that are high in sugar and saturated fat, for energy boosts that contain sugar and caffeine, maybe even for a couple alcoholic beverages after our shift to "unwind." Furthermore, paramedics are often pressed for time. Running from call to call does not make it easy to eat well. What do you choose for lunch when you have only a few free minutes? Often, something unhealthy from a drive-thru or convenience store seems like the only option.

Did you know that the rate of appendicitis is higher in the United States than in Asia or Africa.[15] Why? Fiber, fiber, fiber. People who live in those regions have diets that are higher in fiber. Fiber decreases the transit time of stool through the bowel, thus flushing the appendix. Thus, one of the easiest ways to prevent appendicitis is to eat a high-fiber diet.

You don't have to become a vegan, but eating a whole apple, having a salad instead of a burger, or adding baked beans to a dinner can go a long way to increasing your fiber intake.

Broccoli or barbeque? Why not both—better for your heart and better for your appendix!

Special Populations

As mentioned, appendicitis can be difficult to diagnosis. Consider that appendicitis occurs most often in young people, even young women who are pregnant. As the uterus expands to accommodate the growing fetus, it moves the appendix out of its normal position. A woman in her third trimester of pregnancy will more likely present with right upper quadrant or right flank pain instead of right lower quadrant pain if she has appendicitis. Even the most attentive paramedic will have difficulty determining if this pain is appendicitis, cholecystitis, or renal calculi.

Additional diagnostic information can be obtained through blood work and imaging studies. Patients with appendicitis will have an elevated white blood cell count and C-reactive protein levels. C-reactive protein is a chemical created by the liver in response to infection or inflammation. Ultrasonography and CT provide the physician with images of the abdomen and are valuable in diagnosing appendicitis.

Management

Prehospital management of appendicitis should include a cautious assessment for septicemia. If this blood infection is present, septic shock can occur. Volume resuscitation may not be adequate to restore blood pressure. Be prepared to use norepinephrine if crystalloids are not effective. Administration of pain and antinausea medications are clearly indicated with these patients.

In-hospital treatment includes antibiotics and typically surgical removal of the appendix.

▶ Diverticulitis

Pathophysiology

To understand **diverticulitis**, you must first know what a diverticulum is—a weak area in the colon that begins to have small outcroppings that turn into pouches. These pockets are called diverticula (the plural of diverticulum). The condition of having diverticula is referred to as diverticulosis. When these diverticula become inflamed, it is called diverticulitis.

What causes these pouches is unclear, but research has shown that people in the Western world tend to get diverticulitis at higher rates than people from Africa and Asia. The disease was first recognized around 1900, when the type of foods people were eating began to dramatically change. The amount of fiber in the American diet plummeted as the amount of processed foods increased.

What is believed is that as the amount of fiber in a person's diet decreases, the consistency of the normal stool becomes more solid. This hard stool takes more contractions to move and subsequently increases colon pressure. In this environment, small defects in the colonic wall that would otherwise never pose a problem now fail, resulting in bulges in the wall.

The next step is similar to appendicitis. As feces travel through the colon, some may be trapped in the pouch. Bacteria can grow and cause localized inflammation and infection. As the body attempts to manage this infection, scarring, adhesions, and even fistulas can develop. A fistula is an abnormal connection between two cavities. The common location for fistulas in diverticulitis is between the colon and the bladder. Significant infections can develop from having feces in the bladder.

The typical patient is older than age 60 years. More important than sex or race is the amount of fiber in the patient's diet. Decreased amounts of fiber increase the patient's risk for this disease.

Assessment

Presentation of diverticulitis is abdominal pain that tends to be localized to the left side of the lower abdomen. Classic signs of infection include: fever, malaise, body aches, chills, nausea, and vomiting. Bleeding is rare with this condition. Patients can have either diarrhea

YOU are the Paramedic PART 4

You establish an IV line and administer a 250-mL fluid challenge after listening to lung sounds in all fields. The patient continues to report abdominal pain, which she describes as an 8 on a scale of 0 to 10. The patient is still unable to sit up and appears restless.

Recording Time: 10 Minutes	
Respirations	18 breaths/min
Pulse	110 beats/min, lying down
Skin	Cool, pale, moist
Blood pressure	110/86 mm Hg, lying down
Oxygen saturation (Spo_2)	98% with oxygen at 15 L/min via nonrebreathing mask
Pupils	PERRLA

7. Knowing that your patient has postural vital signs, how are you going to move the patient downstairs?
8. Should you administer a pain medication to make your patient more comfortable?

or constipation. Because of the local infections of these pouches, adhesions can develop, thus narrowing the diameter of the colon. This can result in constipation, and potentially bowel obstruction. Though this condition typically results in left-sided pain, it can occur anywhere within the colon. Thus, diverticulitis can look like many other abdominal pain conditions.

Management

Management of this condition is directed at making the patient comfortable. Examine the patient closely to ensure severe infection is not present. Sepsis can occur easily in patients with fistulas to the urinary bladder. These patients may need large amounts of fluids and/or norepinephrine to maintain blood pressure. The general management guidelines will assist in helping the patient's comfort. In-hospital treatment will include antibiotics, allowing the GI tract to rest by giving the patient a liquid diet, and possibly surgery to remove the pouches and repair any fistulas.

▶ Pancreatitis

Pathophysiology

The enzymes the pancreas creates are designed to break down the food into substances that can be absorbed by the intestines. If the tube carrying these enzymes becomes blocked, the enzymes will perform their chemical process on the protein and fat of the pancreas itself. This is referred to as autodigestion of the pancreas.

Autodigestion leads to inflammation of the pancreas, or **pancreatitis**. This process can occur suddenly or over many months. Patients can have single attacks or episodic attacks and remissions for a long time. Men tend to have this condition more commonly than women. It also occurs more often in African Americans aged 35 to 64 years. The main causes of this condition are increased alcohol consumption and gallstones. Other causes include medication reactions, trauma, cancer, and high triglyceride levels.

Assessment

The pain of this condition tends to be localized to the epigastric area. It can be sharp and may be quite severe. Radiation of the pain to the back is not uncommon. In addition to the pain, the patient may experience nausea, vomiting, fever, tachycardia, hypotension, and muscle spasms in the extremities. This condition tends to cause hypocalcemia, low blood calcium, which can lead to muscle spasms.

The most alarming concern of this condition is internal hemorrhage. If autodigestion is advanced, blood vessels in and near the pancreas can be compromised. Severe and uncontrolled hemorrhage can ensue. In these patients, hemodynamic instability can be present. In addition, Cullen sign (bruising around the umbilicus) **Figure 20-7** or Grey Turner sign (bruising in the flanks) **Figure 20-8** may be present, indicating severe internal bleeding.

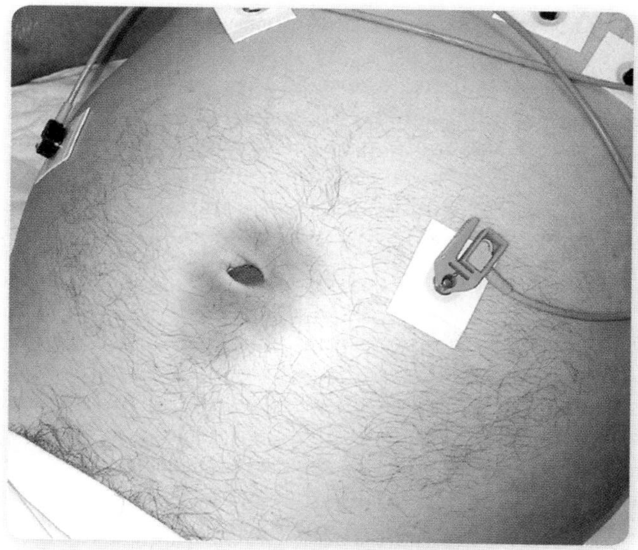

Figure 20-7 Periumbilical ecchymosis, or Cullen sign, indicating intraperitoneal hemorrhage.

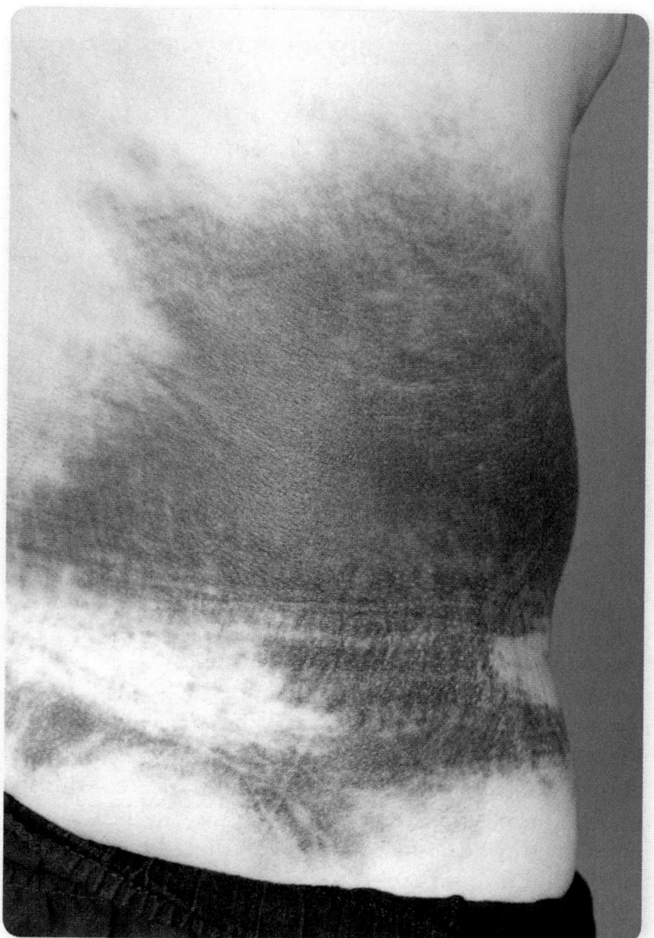

Figure 20-8 Flank ecchymosis, or Grey Turner sign, indicating retroperitoneal hemorrhage.

Laboratory findings of importance with this condition include lipase and amylase levels. These levels are indicative of pancreatic damage: the higher the levels the more severe the damage. Hemoglobin and hematocrit levels are also important to determine the extent of any potential hemorrhage. Patients with pancreatitis have a 10% to 15% mortality rate.[16] Sepsis and hemorrhage are the main causes of death.

Management

Treatment for the prehospital patient with pancreatitis should be directed by general management guidelines. Pay special attention to assessing the patient for signs of severe hemorrhage. If present, begin fluid resuscitation. Because some of these patients will also have gallstones, the most conservative choice for the management of abdominal pain is meperidine. Morphine may cause spasms of the gallbladder, thus increasing the patient's pain.

In-hospital management includes GI rest and fluid resuscitation. In some patients, antibiotics and surgery can be helpful. Though the pancreas cannot be removed unless it is immediately replaced (ie, during transplantation), surgery can be done to control bleeding or manage the gallstones and subsequent blockage of bile from the liver.

Pathophysiology, Assessment, and Management of Chronic Inflammatory Conditions

Patients who have chronic inflammation of all or part of the GI tract are said to have **inflammatory bowel disease (IBD)**. This broad definition covers both ulcerative colitis and Crohn disease. In both conditions, this inflammation causes damage to the wall of the GI tract and places patients at greater risk for cancer. A similar sounding condition, irritable bowel syndrome (IBS), is different. Though symptomatically similar, IBS does not cause structural changes to the walls of the GI tract.

▶ Ulcerative Colitis

Pathophysiology

Ulcerative colitis is caused by inflammation of the colon. The inflammation is generalized and does not occur in patches, as in Crohn disease. It is unclear what causes the chronic inflammation, though genetics, stress, and autoimmunity have been speculated. In this condition, the inflammation causes a thinning of the wall of the intestine, resulting in a weakened, dilated rectum. This damaged lining of the colon is now prone to infections by bacteria and bleeding. These two states establish the foundation on which the signs and symptoms develop. In the typical patient with ulcerative colitis, the disease peaks between ages 15 and 25 years and then again between 55 and 65 years.[17] It occurs more often in women than men.[17] There is a strong family history component for this disease with 1 in 6 patients reporting a family member with this disease.[17] This fact reinforces that genetics plays some role in this disease. The disease is more prevalent among Caucasians.[17]

Assessment

The presentation of this condition is gradual onset of bloody diarrhea, discharge of mucus via the rectum, hematochezia, and mild to severe abdominal pain. Patients may also report a feeling of rectal fullness, known as *tenesmus*. Other signs and symptoms can be joint pain and skin lesions. These effects lend credence to the idea of an autoimmune component to the disease. Finally, the patient can experience fever, fatigue, and loss of appetite from the infection.

Management

Management consists of determining the degree of hemodynamic instability. Look for signs of shock. If the diarrhea and bleeding have caused sufficient volume loss to make the patient's condition unstable, administer fluids to return the patient to a near-normal volume balance. Otherwise, care is supportive. Follow the general management guidelines.

In-hospital care for these patients will include anti-inflammatory medications, antibiotics, antidiarrheals, and potentially surgical removal of the diseased sections of the colon. This is a long-term disease where many people have periods of diarrhea and abdominal pain for years. A large number of these patients will have part of their colon removed.

▶ Crohn Disease

Pathophysiology

Crohn disease is similar to ulcerative colitis; however, the entire GI tract can be involved. The main part of the GI tract that tends to be involved is the ileum. This is the last portion of the small intestine before it joins the large intestine. There are several theories as to the cause, though no definitive cause has been identified.

Typical patients are between 15 and 30 years and then again between 60 and 70 years.[18] Men and women are diagnosed equally often.[18] African Americans tend not to have this condition whereas people of Jewish descent have an increased incidence.[18]

Of interest with Crohn disease and colitis is the presence of signs and symptoms outside the GI system. This evidence helps to support the theory that an autoimmune component is operating within this disease. It is unclear what is causing this immune reaction. Does the presence of antigens in the GI tract trigger an immune response? Is the immune system itself not working correctly? Another theory is that the immune system creates antibodies for an antigen that does not exist, thus creating a cascade of reactions to a nonexistent invader.

Family history and genetics play a role with this disease. Medical researchers are discovering that how the body is made and how it is able to function are important characteristics in whether a person gets a disease and how that disease progresses. The fact that many of the people with Crohn disease have family members who have some type of bowel disease suggests a familial or genetic component. Crohn disease helps prove most conditions are both nature and nurture.

Regardless of the underlying reason, the result is a series of attacks by the immune system on the GI tract. This activity of white blood cells damages all layers of the portion of GI tract involved. The result is most often a scarred, narrowed, stiff, and weakened portion of the small intestine. This patch of damage is found among areas of intestine that are normal. This narrowing can cause bowel obstruction.

Assessment

Patients with Crohn disease present with chronic abdominal pain, often in the lower right area. This pain corresponds to the location of the ileum. Rectal bleeding, weight loss, diarrhea, arthritis, skin problems, and fever may also be present with this condition. Bleeding tends to occur in small amounts over a long period of time. Acute severe hemorrhage is rare, but chronic bleeding resulting in anemia and hypotension does occur. Patients can have episodes of mild to severe signs and symptoms. One of the key symptoms that provide support for the autoimmune theory is coincidence with arthritis and arthralgia—patients tend to report hip, knee, and ankle pain.

Management

Management in the prehospital setting is focused on the general management guidelines. Volume resuscitation may be needed if diarrhea and chronic hemorrhage are occurring. Patients with Crohn disease commonly require control of nausea and pain. In-hospital care will focus on stopping the inflammation, correcting any fluid imbalances that are present, managing infections, and creating an environment where the GI tract can heal itself. The damage to the intestines can at times be so severe that surgical removal of portions is needed. New medications are working well to control this chronic condition and allow patients to live near-normal lives.

▶ Irritable Bowel Syndrome

Pathophysiology

Irritable bowel syndrome (IBS) is a condition in which patients have abdominal pain and changes in their bowel habits. One diagnostic criterion is that patients have pain at least 3 days a month for at least 3 months with accompanying changes in bowel habits. The pathology of the disease is unclear. A new theory is that the normal bacteria found within the small bowel begin to overgrow. This causes pain, distention, and changes in bowel habits.

The following three main factors are prevalent in patients with IBS.

- **Hypersensitivity of bowel pain receptors.** Normal stretching of the bowel can cause pain in these patients.
- **Hyperresponsiveness of the smooth muscles in the bowel.** This produces the cramping sensations and diarrhea.
- **Psychiatric disorder connection and irritable bowel syndrome.** It is unclear if the bowel disorder causes the psychiatric disorder or vice versa.

Hyperresponsiveness of the bowel in IBS can cause areas of spasm. These spasms can stop fecal movement, creating constipation and bloating. Conversely, if the spasms are more wavelike than localized, the patient can experience diarrhea as the feces are moved quickly through the bowel.

Patients typically begin to have problems with bowel habits during childhood. In Western countries, women are more prone to this disease. Interestingly, in the Indian subcontinent, the typical patient is a man. This condition strikes most cultures evenly. This condition can be triggered by stress and is often associated with eating.

Assessment

IBS is a chronic condition. Prehospital presentations will typically involve a flare-up of the condition. Signs and symptoms tend to be individualized. Patients may present with abdominal pain or discomfort. The pain tends to be diffuse and nonradiating. This pain is relieved by a bowel movement. When the pain starts, there is usually a change in the frequency and consistency of bowel movements. Patients may experience diarrhea, **steatorrhea**, or constipation. They may also feel bloated.

Management

Management of these patients is supportive. The paramedic must understand that a coexisting psychiatric condition may be present. Be kind and compassionate. Do not minimize the patient's pain or discomfort. Your assessment must include the patient's mood and thought content. Consider whether the patient is severely depressed. If depression and/or suicide are noted, treat those accordingly. Analgesia may be needed in patients with irritable bowel syndrome.

Pathophysiology, Assessment, and Management of Acute Infectious Conditions

Many foods are teeming with bacteria, viruses, and fungi. These microorganisms are present throughout the food chain. Infections in the GI system typically occur either when contaminated food is ingested or when the GI tract ruptures. For a person to become ill, either the number or complexity of the organisms overwhelms the immune system, or the immune system is weakened and cannot effectively defend the body.

Most people who become ill have stomachaches, vomiting, or diarrhea. According to the Centers for Disease Control and Prevention, in the United States, it is estimated that 48 million people will contract a foodborne illness every year.[19] Of this group, 3,000 will die; in other words, only 0.006% of those who become ill die.[19] So what makes that small group different from the vast majority? People who are immunocompromised, very old, and very young generally have a more difficult time combating an infection of any type. Types of patients who are immunocompromised would include people with acquired immunodeficiency syndrome or certain types of cancers, people undergoing chemotherapy, and transplant patients.

In the United States, the food chain is very clean. Compared with other countries, the number of people who fall ill or die of foodborne disease is low. Traveling to other countries can place patients at greater risk for food intolerances or foodborne infections. Traveler's diarrhea can occur in as many as 33% of all people who travel to countries where food cleanliness is less than adequate as reported by the Centers for Disease Control and Prevention.[20] Travel within North America and Europe is generally safer than travel throughout South America, Asia, and Africa in terms of the risk of foodborne illness.[20]

Damage to the GI system is another way infection can occur. A breach in the container allows GI contents filled with organisms to move into the surrounding tissues. In appendicitis, feces moving through the intestines become trapped in the appendix. The normal flushing of this structure is now prevented and fecal bacteria multiply. Pus and gas—by-products of bacterial activity—can cause pressure on the appendix. If the pressure is too high, the structure will fail, spilling material laden with pus and feces into the peritoneum. This can cause peritonitis, or inflammation of the protective lining of the abdominal cavity. Sepsis can also occur. Sepsis and its hemodynamic complications are discussed in Chapter 26, *Infectious Diseases*.

▶ Acute Gastroenteritis

Pathophysiology

Acute gastroenteritis is a family of conditions all revolving around a central theme of infection with fever, abdominal pain, diarrhea, nausea, and vomiting. These illnesses can be caused by a wide variety of organisms, as shown in Table 20-8. These agents typically enter the body via the fecal-oral route through contaminated food or water.

Cholera, relatively unknown in the United States, is common in other parts of the world. The norovirus is responsible for most cases of acute viral gastroenteritis in adults, whereas rotavirus causes the same condition in children. Various parasites may be contracted by swimming in or drinking contaminated water. The majority of patients who die from gastroenteritis are infected with either *Norovirus* or *Clostridium difficile*.[21] These patients tend to be older than 65 years.[21]

Table 20-8 Gastroenteritis: Causative Organisms

Type of Organism	Organism
Viruses	*Norovirus*: Norwalk virus *Rotavirus*
Parasites	*Giardia lamblia* (protozoan) *Cryptosporidium parvum* *Cyclospora cayetanensis*
Bacteria	*Escherichia coli* *Klebsiella pneumoniae* *Enterobacter* *Campylobacter jejuni* *Vibrio cholera* *Shigella* *Salmonella* *Clostridium difficile*

Assessment

Depending on the organism involved, patients may begin to experience GI upset and diarrhea in as little as hours or days after contact with the contaminated food or water. The disease can run its course in 2 to 3 days or continue for several weeks.

The presentation involves diarrhea of various types. Patients can experience large dumping-type diarrhea or frequent small liquid stools. The diarrhea can contain blood and/or pus, and it may have a foul odor or be odorless. Abdominal cramping is frequent as hyperperistalsis continues. Nausea and vomiting, fever, and anorexia are also present. The vomiting can occur quite suddenly. Sudden vomiting is typical in norovirus infections.

If the diarrhea continues, dehydration and hemodynamic instability will result. As the volume of fluid loss increases, the likelihood of potassium and sodium imbalance also increases. You should be watching for changes in LOC and other profound signs of shock, which clearly indicate a critical volume loss. Severely dehydrated patients can demonstrate skin tenting, weight loss, tachycardia, orthostatic hypotension, and dry mucous membranes.

Management

Prehospital management is directed by the general management guidelines. Special attention should be paid to determining the degree of fluid deficit the patient is experiencing. If the patient's condition is stable, one-half normal saline solution may be indicated to begin rehydration.

Additionally, patients often feel markedly better after rehydration. Fluid resuscitation may be needed; therefore, obtain orthostatic vital signs to best determine the need for isotonic fluids. Performing cardiac monitoring is reasonable due to the risk of hypokalemia. Analgesic and antiemetic medications are also indicated for these patients. One of the most critical issues in managing this condition is patient education. You need to instruct patients about safe food and water use to prevent future infections.

As you are caring for these patients, consider your risk of being contaminated by vomit or stool. Gloves, gowns, and masks are appropriate when treating patients who are actively vomiting or have uncontrolled diarrhea.

In-hospital care is directed at rehydration, control of vomiting and diarrhea, identification of the organism involved, antibiotic therapy, and stabilization of electrolyte imbalances.

▶ Rectal Abscess

Pathophysiology

The rectum creates mucus to lubricate feces during defecation. If the ducts through which this mucus travels are blocked, a **rectal abscess** can result. This area has large amounts of bacteria present. The blockage can allow bacteria to grow and spread around the anus. Men are twice as likely to have this condition as women. The most common age groups are people in their 30s and 40s.

Assessment

Patients present with rectal pain that increases with defecation and then diminishes. The pain will continue between defecations. Fever, itching (pruritus), and rectal drainage are also common findings. Bleeding is typically not a problem. Patients may become constipated and unwilling to defecate because of increased pain.

Management

Management in the prehospital setting involves keeping the patient comfortable. Transport the patient in a position of comfort. The lateral position may be preferable to supine or Fowler position. In the hospital, patients will typically need surgery to explore the exact extent of this abscess. Drainage, repair, and antibiotics typically follow.

▶ Liver Disease: Cirrhosis

Pathophysiology

The liver is a very resilient and important organ. Beyond its role in the metabolism of fats, proteins, and glucose, the liver is responsible for detoxifying the blood, creating coagulation factors, recycling dead red blood cells, storing vitamins, and creating hormones needed in growth. Damage to this organ can result in severe imbalances in the body. Few portions of the body are able to operate normally without a functioning liver.

When the liver is damaged by infection, it is referred to as hepatitis. This disease will be discussed in Chapter 26, *Infectious Diseases*. Other ways to damage the liver are from direct trauma, toxic ingestion, and autoimmune disorders. Regardless of the cause, if the damage to the liver is severe, the patient will experience the beginning stages of liver failure. Early failure is referred to as **cirrhosis**.

As the liver is damaged, it works to rebuild itself. The liver is so resilient it is possible for adults to donate a portion of the liver to someone else. The donated portion will grow to normal size and the remaining portion will return to normal size and function. During the regeneration process, fibrotic tissue can result. This dense material will prevent proper filtering and flow of blood. Consequently, the hallmarks of cirrhosis are portal hypertension (discussed earlier in this chapter), deficiencies with coagulation, and diminished detoxification, which can result in hepatic encephalopathy.

Assessment

Clinically, the disease has two phases. In the first phase, patients experience joint aches, weakness, fatigue, nausea, vomiting, anorexia, **urticaria**, and pruritus (itching). During this phase, the patient may be misdiagnosed as having influenza or gastroenteritis.

The second clinical phase involves sufficient damage to the liver. The damage must reach a point where liver failure results. It is characterized by **acholic stools**, darkening of the urine, jaundice, **icteric** conjunctiva (yellow eyes) Figure 20-9, and ascites. Abdominal pain found in the right upper quadrant, along with an enlarged liver, are also present at this time. Patients may also have dilation of blood vessels on the surface of the abdomen. The term *caput medusa* refers to dilated blood vessels around the umbilicus. The literal translation is "head of Medusa." This term reflects the snake-like appearance of the dilated blood vessels.

Laboratory findings may reveal abnormal liver functions. Aminotransferases (ALT and AST), alkaline phosphatase, albumin, and bilirubin are common blood tests used to gauge liver function. Additionally, coagulation studies are needed to determine the effect of the liver failure on coagulation.

Management

The prehospital management for cirrhosis is supportive. Follow the general management guidelines for the patient with GI conditions. Some important areas of focus involve bleeding control and medication administration. With the damaged liver, the ability for blood clotting may be impaired. Be cautious with all venipunctures.

Because of the liver's detoxification functions, any drug that is given will remain active in the body far longer than anticipated when the liver is compromised. When administering medications to patients with signs of liver failure, use the lower ends of the normal dose range. Give

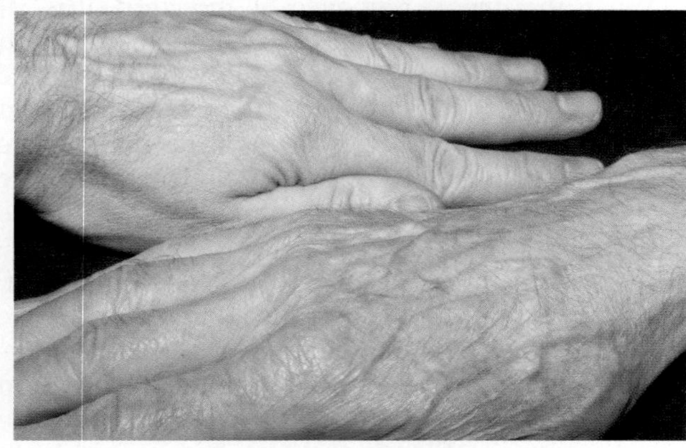
A

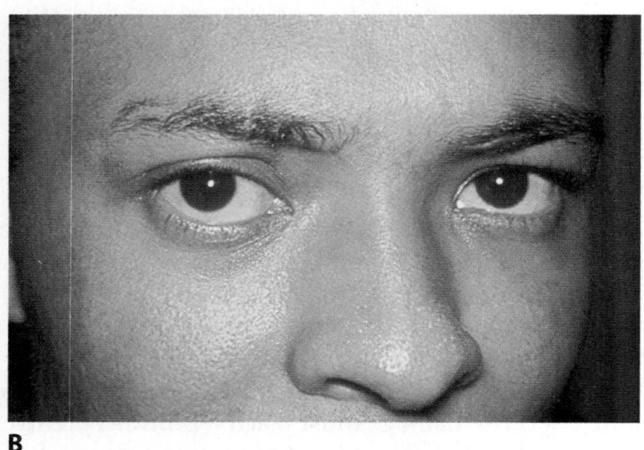
B

Figure 20-9 Jaundiced skin **(A)** and icteric sclera **(B)** caused by the buildup of bilirubin in the skin and conjunctiva.

medications at longer intervals and watch for signs of cumulative effects.

In-hospital management is directed at supporting liver function. There is no artificial liver available and without a functioning liver, death is days away. In extreme cases, liver transplantation is the only viable treatment.

▶ Liver Disease: Hepatic Encephalopathy

Pathophysiology

As the functions of the liver continue to diminish, eventually brain function will be impaired. This is called **hepatic encephalopathy**. There are several theories as to the underlying cause of the brain dysfunction. Ammonia levels tend to rise as liver functions fail. Ammonia can affect neurons by changing the flow of materials across the semipermeable membrane. Diminished functions of the nervous system may be due to simply diminished cellular energy supplies. The liver has a pivotal role in providing cellular substrates necessary for metabolism. Diminished liver function equals diminished metabolism. The decrease in function may also be caused by a change in the blood-brain barrier permeability. If this barrier could be easily breached, neurotoxins could cause cellular damage resulting in an altered LOC. Regardless of the underlying cause, the brain is affected.

Assessment

The mental status of a patient with hepatic encephalopathy can range from mild loss of memory to coma. Patients may present with attention deficits, inability to concentrate, and impaired complex reasoning. These subtle changes can progress to disorientation, impaired behavior, and incomprehensible speech. Other signs and symptoms include bradykinesia, shuffling gait, and tremor. These last signs are reminiscent of Parkinson disease.

The patient's clinical findings are more important than laboratory results. Most patients will have ammonia levels checked, but these results are not always a good indicator of the severity of brain impairment. The results of CT and magnetic resonance imaging are inconclusive for this disease. Patients may have the encephalopathy precipitated by an infection, renal failure, GI bleeding, or constipation. Opiates, benzodiazepines, and psychotropic medications can worsen the presentation.

Management

Treatment is primarily supportive. One of the most important issues is for you to ensure that some other reversible cause for an altered LOC is not present. Check the patient's blood glucose level and vital signs. Assess for trauma and overdose. These patients will typically have a significant past medical history for cirrhosis. Gather detailed information about the history of present illness. What is normal for this patient? How long has the patient been sick? Focus on infections, renal function, bleeding, and constipation because these issues can precipitate hepatic encephalopathy.

In-hospital treatment is geared towards decreasing ammonia levels and managing the altered LOC. There is no definitive treatment for hepatic encephalopathy other than liver transplantation.

Pathophysiology, Assessment, and Management of Obstructive Conditions

Obstructions within the GI system can occur anywhere from the oropharynx to the rectum. The reasons for these obstructions vary depending on the location. Rectal obstructions tend to occur in young men and the obstruction is a foreign body. Esophageal obstructions also tend to be caused by foreign bodies, but the population tends to be children.

The cardinal sign of bowel obstruction is decreased intestinal motility, a condition in which the intestines become unable to move material through the digestive tract. Two main reasons for this condition are paralysis of the intestines or a change in the diameter of their lumen. Paralysis can be caused by infection, kidney disease, impaired blood flow to the intestines, or medications. Narcotics and anesthetics are specific types of medications that can paralyze the intestinal muscles. This is why patients who have major surgery often will not be released from the hospital until they have had at least one bowel movement.

Intestinal lumen diameter compromise can be caused by neoplasms, tumors of the intestines, objects that the patient has swallowed, or strictures (narrowing of the lumen due to damage in the intestinal wall). Other causes include hernia (intestine trapped and compressed), **intussusception** (telescoping of the intestines into themselves), or **volvulus** (twisting of the intestines). The end result is that the diameter of the intestines is narrowed or blocked.

▶ Esophageal Obstruction

Pathophysiology

Contractions of smooth muscles within the walls of the esophagus rhythmically move the food ingested. But, imagine a tube of toothpaste—as you squeeze the center, toothpaste moves in both directions: out toward the end of the tube and back deeper into the tube. Similarly, the esophagus has to manage both desired and undesired food motion resulting from its muscular contractions.

The upper esophageal sphincter (UES) is located at the superior end of the esophagus. As this ring of muscles tightens, it closes the superior portion of the esophagus to prevent food from moving superiorly back into the hypopharynx. As discussed earlier in the section on hiatal hernia, the LES closes to prevent food from exiting the stomach when the stomach contracts. It is undesirable to have food squeezed out of the stomach back into the esophagus. To prevent this reflux, the LES closes.

Obstructions within the esophagus typically occur at either the upper or lower sphincter. When young children explore new objects, they like to place them in their mouth. This is one way for children to learn about their world. Unsupervised, a child can accidentally swallow an object. In these cases the child is typically age 18 to 48 months; the object is a coin, toy piece, button, or marble; and the location of entrapment is at the UES. Adults, on the other hand, tend to have entrapment at the LES, and the object can be almost anything that can fit in the mouth. Ingestion in adults is either accidental—a fruit pit or a denture plate—or intentional. Prisoners or psychiatric patients may swallow objects to hide or transport them. In 90% of cases, if the object reaches the stomach, it will pass through the remainder of the GI tract.[22]

Assessment

Dysphagia is the primary symptom in these patients. How this is demonstrated will be markedly different if your patient is a 2-year-old child who swallowed a battery, a 28-year-old man who is trying to conceal a key, or a 69-year-old woman who had some alcohol with dinner and swallowed her dentures. The UES is located close to the cricoid cartilage. The cricoid is the only cartilage within the trachea that forms a complete 360° ring. This prevents severe impingement from the esophagus in the event of obstruction.

Depending on the location of the object and its shape, it can generate a minor to severe sense of difficulty in breathing. If the object is inferior to the cricoid, it can impinge on the posterior wall of the trachea (which has no cartilage), and the patient will feel a strong sense of choking. Drooling, inability to swallow, pain, vomiting, and gagging can occur. In approximately one-third of children, there are no symptoms until they try to eat.

Management

Airway patency is the primary concern for these patients. Allow the patient to sit in a high Fowler position. Be prepared to manage oral sections with suction and have an emesis basin ready. Eye protection, mask, and gowns will be needed if there is a reasonable risk of vomiting. Simply looking into the mouth to see if the object can easily be removed is reasonable. However, do not fight the patient to remove the object. It is better to keep the patient calm and allow the emergency department to remove it.

If the patient has obvious airway compromise as evidenced by hypoxia, cyanosis, and altered LOC, then a more aggressive investigation of the hypopharynx is indicated. Refer to Chapter 15, *Airway Management*, to review use of Magill forceps and foreign body removal from the airway.

Glucagon can be considered in patients with esophageal obstruction. Due to its smooth muscle relaxation properties, this medication can potentially relax the LES. This may allow the object to pass into the stomach, relieving the patient of pain and dysphagia. Contact online medical direction or medical control to use this medication for this purpose.

Within the emergency department, a variety of methods can be used to remove the object. Radiographs and other scans can determine the exact location of the object. Removal of the object can be accomplished using Magill forceps, a Foley catheter (the catheter is inserted beyond the object, the balloon is inflated, and the catheter is removed, dragging the object with it), or endoscopy. Sedation and pain management are an integral part of these procedures.

Encourage patients to seek medical care even if the object is cleared when you arrive. Esophageal laceration and aspiration or pneumonia are risks, so medical follow-up is important.

▶ Small-Bowel Obstruction

Pathophysiology

In the small intestine, postoperative adhesions are the most common cause of obstruction. When a patient undergoes a surgical procedure that requires opening the abdomen, the resulting inflammation results in scarring as the body heals. These weblike bands of tissue, called adhesions, can constrict the diameter of the intestine or decrease the ability of the intestine to dilate. Other causes of small-bowel obstruction include cancer, Crohn disease, hernias, and foreign bodies (objects that have been swallowed).[23]

Assessment

The presentation of a small-bowel obstruction begins with abdominal pain. The pain tends to be crampy and intermittent. Patients will initially experience diarrhea, nausea, and vomiting because of the increased pressure on the intestine. As the patient continues to eat, some food is able to advance beyond the blockage. This causes increased intestinal pressure. The result is the increased peristalsis to try to move the blockage. Constipation will eventually occur because limited food will be able to get beyond the blockage. This will yield hyperactive bowel sounds in the early stages of the obstruction and hypoactive bowel sounds in late stages of the obstruction.

The material that is vomited may be **feculent**, having the smell of feces. Fever and tachycardia are also associated with small-bowel obstruction, and can indicate infection within the abdominal cavity. Untreated, this can lead to sepsis. Ask your patient if he or she has a history of abdominal surgery; if the patient is unresponsive or unreliable, look for a scar that could indicate such surgery. Patients can experience a small-bowel obstruction decades after undergoing abdominal surgery. Due to the vomiting and decreased ability to obtain nutrients, there may be changes in electrolytes.

A blockage of the small intestines can cause several localized changes. The area involved becomes irritated; therefore, swelling occurs. This further complicates the blockage. If the bowel becomes twisted or for any other reason blood supply is compromised, ischemia can occur. This is referred to as a strangulated obstruction. Mortality in the untreated strangulated obstruction is near 100%.[23] If treated early, the mortality rate is markedly lower.

Management

Treatment is supportive. As with most conditions involving the GI tract, there is a concern related to sepsis. Monitor blood pressure and be prepared for volume resuscitation and administration of dopamine as needed. A nasogastric tube may be used to decompress the stomach of any material. Antiemetics are clearly indicated with small-bowel obstruction. Based on the length of time the patient has had the obstruction, IV fluids may be needed due to dehydration.

In-hospital management will include antibiotic therapy. Imaging studies will be done to help determine the cause of the obstruction. If needed, surgery will be performed to help ensure adequate blood supply and a restoration of bowel movement.

▶ Large-Bowel Obstruction

Pathophysiology

As with small-bowel obstructions, large-bowel obstructions are caused by either mechanical obstruction or constricture of the colon resulting in decreased internal diameter. In the case of mechanical obstruction, the most common causes are colon cancer and diverticulitis. Both of these conditions are more closely associated with older patients; therefore, large-bowel obstructions are more common in that age group. Another cause is a volvulus, or twisting of the bowel until a kink occurs, blocking flow. In pediatric populations, intussusception is a more common diagnosis than in adults.[24]

Imaging studies are used to determine the location and extent of the obstruction. Finding the exact cause will direct eventual hospital treatment. Once located, many obstructions can be easily treated. Untreated, the mortality can be high if cancer is the cause of the obstruction. In addition, the blockage can lead to increased permeability of the intestinal wall, which allows intestinal bacteria to gain access to the bloodstream, and septicemia can occur.

If the condition is caused by cancer, an erosion of the bowel into adjacent cavities can occur. These fistulas can allow feces into the vagina or bladder. This results in patients with either feculent discharge from the vagina or fecaluria (feces in the bladder being discharged with the urine).

Assessment

Assessment reveals a patient with abdominal pain. Nausea and vomiting are also common. The abdomen is distended and typically bowel sounds are absent. Percussion of the abdomen should reveal hyperresonance. If the obstruction has ruptured into the peritoneum, the classic signs of peritonitis (fever, tachycardia, and pain) will be present. Gather information about the patient's recent bowel habits and weight. If the obstruction is related to cancer, recent unexplained weight loss and gradually increasing difficulty in having bowel movements tend to occur.

Management

The treatment for large-bowel obstruction is the same as that for small-bowel obstruction. As a result of the elastic properties of the colon, a patient may be obstructed for a longer period of time with large-bowel obstructions versus small-bowel obstructions. This can lead to a greater degree of dehydration and need for fluid resuscitation.

▶ Abdominal Wall Hernia

Pathophysiology

A **hernia** is a protrusion of an organ or structure into an adjacent cavity. During a physical examination, a physician

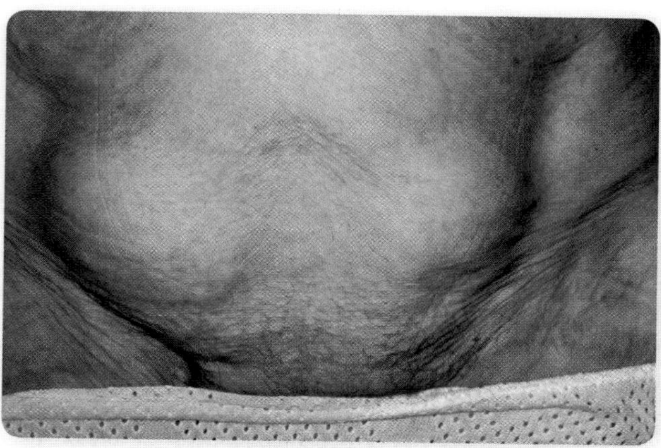

Figure 20-10 An inguinal hernia.

will often place his or her fingers on the wall of the lower abdomen as the patient is instructed to cough. Coughing increases intra-abdominal pressure. If there is a weakness in the wall of the abdomen, it can be felt as bulging during the cough. This procedure is done to check for an inguinal hernia. *Inguinal* simply refers to the location of the protrusion Figure 20-10. In this case, the intestines are typically the protruding organ. Over 1 million hernia repairs are done each year in the United States, with the inguinal hernia being the most common form.[25] Abdominal wall hernias are seven times more common in men than in women.[25]

Any condition or state that increases intra-abdominal pressure can facilitate the creation of a hernia. Obesity, standing for long periods, heavy lifting, straining during a bowel movement, or chronic obstructive pulmonary disease can precipitate this condition. Chronic obstructive pulmonary disease is associated with hernias because of the increased work of breathing and subsequent use of the abdominal muscles.

Assessment

In the abdomen there are four types of hernias and several common locations Figure 20-11. The common assessment finding is a bulging of the area where the hernia is present.

- **Reducible.** A hernia that will return to its normal location either spontaneously or by manual manipulation. The patient typically experiences little discomfort unless he or she has increasing intra-abdominal pressure. The patient may perceive a fullness or swelling, or report achiness at the hernia site.
- **Incarcerated.** Consider the nonmedical meaning of the word *incarcerate*: to place in jail. In this type of hernia, the organ is trapped in the new location. The most common cause of this condition is bowel obstruction. Incarcerated hernias are more painful as a result of the obstruction.
- **Strangulated.** A strangulated hernia is one in which the intestine is trapped and squeezed to the point that blood supply to the area is diminished. Consequently, this kind of hernia is considered an emergency. Patients experience severe pain and sepsis and require urgent transport.
- **Incisional.** In another type of hernia, called an incisional hernia, patients who are recovering from abdominal surgery will have intestinal contents herniate through the incision. This is similar to the trauma condition known as evisceration.

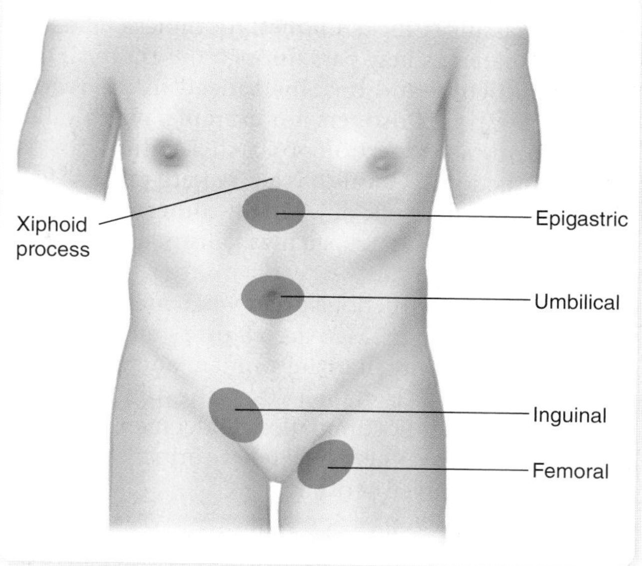

Figure 20-11 Common locations of abdominal hernias.

Management

Prehospital treatment for hernias is supportive with care directed at pain management. Place the patient in a comfortable position. Lying supine will probably not be comfortable because this stretches the abdominal wall. Closely assess the patient for sepsis. Though minimally to moderately painful, unless strangulated, a hernia is not a life-threatening emergency. In the hospital, reduction of the hernia may be attempted in the emergency department. If unsuccessful or not appropriate, surgical repair will be explored.

▶ Rectal Foreign Body Obstruction

Pathophysiology

A foreign body in the rectum interferes with defecation. Objects can be introduced from the upper GI tract or by anal insertion. Indigestible swallowed objects may have difficulty passing. Chicken bones, toothpicks, and various other materials may pass through the entire GI tract without difficulty and become lodged in the rectum during defecation. Prisoners, for example, may swallow objects during an inspection or search. Fecaliths can also cause obstructions. A fecalith is a very hard piece of feces (*fecal* = feces, *lith* = stone). Finally, other objects that pass through the GI tract, such as gallstones, can cause obstructions.

Most rectal obstructions occur when an object is inserted into the rectum. Men are 28 times more likely to engage in this activity than are women, and the average age of these patients is in their 20s.[26] The primary reason for the activity is erotic stimulation. Older men may insert objects into their rectum to help relieve urinary difficulties caused by an enlarged prostate.

Assessment

These two types of causes create two very different patient presentations. If the obstruction originated from the upper GI tract, the patient will present with a sudden onset of rectal pain with defecation. Rarely is bleeding or abdominal pain noted in the acute phase. If the object has perforated the rectum, peritonitis is possible. Peritonitis would in turn lead to fever, diffuse abdominal pain, and possible sepsis.

Most patients who have rectal obstructions seek medical care for removal of an intentionally placed object. Knowing what type of object was inserted and whether the patient has attempted to remove the object can be important. This information can help you determine whether the patient's rectum is perforated. During your history taking, ensure that the patient was not assaulted. Rectal insertion during an assault can cause severe and possibly life-threatening internal damage.

In either case, physical findings may be limited to the patient's report of rectal pain. If perforation has occurred, peritonitis and consequent sepsis may be present. Depending on the size and shape of the object, it may be apparent on physical examination.

Management

Even when the inserted object is visible on physical examination, you should not attempt to remove it. Treatment in the prehospital setting should be limited to ensuring that the patient is comfortable. Allow the patient to sit laterally, if possible, in order to reduce the pressure on the rectum. If the patient is in pain, analgesia is indicated. As with other abdominal emergencies in which peritonitis is a possibility, close monitoring of vital signs is important. Keep in mind that these patients are often horribly embarrassed. Be compassionate and nonjudgmental. It took courage for the patient to seek medical care.

Pathophysiology, Assessment, and Management of Ischemic and Neoplastic Disorders

▶ Mesenteric Ischemia

Pathophysiology

Mesenteric ischemia is a condition in which the blood supply to the mesentery is interrupted. There are four main causes of this condition:

- **Acute arterial embolism.** These emboli tend to come from a cardiac thrombus (MI, atrial fibrillation, mitral stenosis, etc).
- **Acute arterial thrombosis.** These patients have underlying thrombotic disease in the mesenteric arteries. Plaque buildup narrows the lumen, which can suddenly close off. This process is very similar to how most MIs occur.
- **Profound vasospasm.** This can occur with the use of cocaine, with ergot poisoning, norepinephrine, or in severe shock.
- **Mesenteric venous thrombosis.** Here a thrombus forms in one of the mesenteric veins. This prevents blood from leaving the intestinal veins. Blood begins to pool. This creates back pressure that prevents fresh blood from entering the area. Tissues are starved of oxygen.

Mesenteric ischemia occurs in both sexes and is more prevalent among older patients.[27] It is a rare but serious condition, with a mortality rate of 50% to 80%.[27]

Assessment

Depending on the exact cause of the abdominal pain, it may have a gradual or sudden onset. The location of the pain within the abdomen tends to be ill defined and is severe. Nausea, vomiting, and diarrhea are also common. Blood may be present in the stool. The disease is difficult to diagnose. Its cardinal presentation includes severe abdominal pain with normal abdominal examination results. A thorough history is needed. If the patient has ingested something, this information will dramatically change the in-hospital therapy. Discovering the cause of the ischemia is essential to offering correct life-saving therapy in the hospital.

Management

Treatment for these patients requires rapid transportation. Monitor these patients closely, checking vital signs for evidence of sepsis. If shock is present, fluid resuscitation should be initiated. If sepsis is the cause of hypotension, be prepared to use vasopressors to stabilize blood pressure; these are warranted only after initial fluid therapy and, preferably, in consultation with medical direction or per local protocols. Analgesics may be indicated. In-hospital treatment will include imaging studies, possibly thrombolytics, anticoagulants, and antibiotics. Depending on the cause, surgery or vasodilators will be used.

▶ Neoplasms

Neoplasm is the medical term for growths or tumors within the body that serve no purpose and are caused by errors that occur during cellular reproduction. When an altered cell reproduces, it copies the error to its own daughter cells. The new cells may grow more rapidly and aggressively than normal surrounding cells. Neoplasms can be categorized as either benign or malignant and primary or metastatic. Any portion of the GI system can develop a neoplasm or cancer. The most common forms are discussed in this section.

▶ Tumors of the Colon

Pathophysiology

Colon, or colorectal, cancer is the third leading cause of cancer and the third leading cause of deaths related to cancer. It is the most common form of cancer within the GI system. As with many cancers, the cause is multifactorial. People with diets high in red meat and low in fiber and people who smoke are at greater risk of developing this cancer. There is a strong correlation between heredity and colorectal cancer. One specific gene mutation that imparts a near-100% chance of developing colon cancer by age 40 has been identified.[28] Inflammatory bowel diseases, ulcerative colitis, and Crohn disease are also associated with increased risk for colorectal cancer.[28]

Assessment

Abdominal pain, rectal bleeding, and changes in bowel habits are the most common signs. Fortunately, colorectal screening catches many cancers before symptoms begin. If the cancer is found on the right side of the colon, patients more commonly have bleeding and diarrhea. Left-sided tumors tend to cause obstruction.

Management

Care is supportive. Many patients will require some degree of resection of the colon. This is currently the only curative measure for this cancer. Depending on the location and extent of the cancer, patients may require a colostomy. If caught early, this cancer has a survival rate of nearly 95%.[28]

▶ Pancreatic Tumors

Pathophysiology

Pancreatic cancer is the fourth leading cause of death from cancer.[29] Remember, the pancreas is located centrally in the upper abdomen and comprises both exocrine and endocrine cells. The vast majority of malignancies in this organ occur in the exocrine cells.[29] Of all pancreatic cancers, 40% are sporadic in nature with little evidence pointing to a direct cause.[29] Smoking causes 30%, diet causes 20%, and 10% are related to heredity.[29] Patients with diabetes may have an increased risk of pancreatic cancer.[29] This condition affects males more often than females and is also more prevalent in African Americans. The most common age for onset is the mid 60s.[29]

Assessment

Symptomatically, pancreatic cancer has a gradual, insidious presentation that is often mistaken for other benign conditions. Patients experience malaise, fatigue, nausea, vomiting, midepigastric pain, or back pain. As the cancer continues, anorexia and weight loss become apparent. It is rare that a patient with new onset diabetes will have an occult pancreatic cancer.[29]

If the cancer is on the head of the pancreas, it can cause obstruction of bile flow from the gallbladder. The common bile duct travels through the pancreas and then interconnects with the pancreatic duct. A growing tumor can block this structure, preventing bile from reaching the duodenum. This will result in darkening of the urine, pale-colored stool, and steatorrhea. Interestingly, depression is more common in pancreatic cancer than any other abdominal cancer. Men with pancreatic cancer have an 11 times higher risk of suicide.[29] Patients may have increased depression due to the poor prognosis of this disease, the fact that many patients are not diagnosed with this disease until the cancer is well established, or because they do not feel well.

If the cancer has metastasized, it can lead to hepatic cancer and resultant liver failure.

Management

Care for these patients will be supportive in nature. This cancer is particularly fatal. It has a 1-year survival rate of only 28% and a 5-year survival rate of 7%.[29] Many of these patients will have a living will, do not resuscitate (DNR) order, or will be on hospice, so it is important to understand the wishes of the patient and family.

▶ Hepatic Tumors

Pathophysiology

Cancer of the liver is rare. Due to the liver's outstanding regenerative properties, it is able to repair most damage or cellular errors. Primary liver cancer accounts for only 2% of all reported cancers.[30] When it is present, liver cancer is more common among men.[30] In fact, 75% of cases involve men.[30] Frequently (approximately 75% of the time), primary liver cancers within the United States are associated with cirrhosis.[30] Alcohol consumption and hepatitis B and C are known factors that increase risk of liver cancer.[30]

Assessment

Patients will be sick. This is not a condition that occurs overnight. The patient will likely have already been diagnosed prior to EMS involvement. You can expect a patient with pruritus, jaundice, splenomegaly, cachexia (profound malnutrition and weight loss), ascites, and abdominal pain. Patients may also experience all of the signs and symptoms related to cirrhosis and hepatic encephalopathy.

Management

EMS care is directed at supporting vital signs and can be quite complicated. These patients will often have major fluid and electrolyte imbalances. This can create cardiac rhythm disturbances that may be lethal; therefore, ECG monitoring is critical. Check potassium levels if possible. The patient will often have a severely altered LOC, so airway protection may be needed. Respiratory distress from pulmonary edema may require positive pressure ventilation with positive end-expiratory pressure. To complicate matters, because of damage to the liver, most medications that you administer will not be metabolized normally. This may lead to potential medication toxicity issues. Generally speaking, if medications need to be administered, choose the lower end of the accepted range or increase the time between doses. Only about 5% of liver cancer patients are candidates for liver resectioning (removal of a portion of the liver).[30] This means that a large number of these patients are terminal. Talk with the patient and his or her family to determine whether there is an advance directive. Ask to see the appropriate documentation (living will/DNR/medical power of attorney).

In-hospital care is also directed at supporting the patient's vital signs. Liver transplantation is the only way to cure a patient with this disease.

Prevention Strategies

As EMS evolves, it becomes more important for paramedics to consider the prevention of diseases. EMS is moving from a service that is strictly related to the delivery of 9-1-1 services to a system that augments nonemergency aspects of health care. There are many patient behaviors that can limit the intensity or entirely prevent the onset of many GI diseases. Table 20-9 lists some of the behaviors and the diseases that can be affected.

Table 20-9 Prevention of Selected GI Conditions

Condition	Prevention Strategy
Constipation	Increase fiber and fluid content in diet Exercise Chew food fully
Diverticulitis	Increase fiber and fluid content in diet Exercise Chew food fully
Gallstones	Most gallstones cannot be prevented, but a lower-fat diet may provide some protection
Heartburn	Avoid smoking Avoid eating close to bedtime Avoid chocolate, peppermint, caffeine
Hemorrhoids	Increase fiber and fluid content in diet
Liver disease	Limit alcohol Avoid high doses of vitamins unless prescribed Follow directions on cleaning supplies (ventilation/gloves/masks)
Peptic ulcers	Manage stress well Limit caffeine Limit alcohol

Abbreviation: GI, gastrointestinal

Following a healthy diet is one of the best ways to prevent GI disorders. A diet that is high in fiber and low in fat will facilitate movement of materials through the GI tract. Good sources of dietary fiber are listed in Table 20-10. Not only does such a diet help improve bowel health, but it also has a strong connection to heart health. Another heart-healthy behavior that has a positive effect on the GI system is to eliminate smoking and to control the amount of alcohol consumed. Finally, the connection between stress and disease is clear. Meditating, exercising, and practicing relaxation techniques can have a profound effect on a person's quality and quantity of life.

Table 20-10 Selected Sources of Dietary Fiber

Fruits	Vegetables	Other Good Fiber Choices
Artichokes	Beans (navy, black, lima, pinto)	Barley
Apples, pears (with skin)	Broccoli	Bread, muffins (whole wheat, bran)
Berries (blackberries, blueberries, raspberries)	Chickpeas	Cereals (bran flakes, bran, oatmeal, shredded wheat)
Dates	Lentils	Coconut
Figs	Parsnips	Crackers (rye, whole wheat)
Prunes	Peas	Nuts (almonds, Brazil, peanuts, pecans, walnuts)
	Pumpkin	Rice (brown)
	Rutabaga	Seeds (pumpkin, sunflower)
	Squash (winter)	

YOU are the Paramedic SUMMARY

1. What is melena?

Melena is black, tarry, sticky, and very odorous stool and blood blended together into one substance. You are unable to distinguish blood from stool.

2. What part of the GI system do you believe might be affected?

Melena is common when there is bleeding from the esophagus, stomach, or proximal small intestine.

3. What do orthostatic vital signs indicate?

Orthostatic vital signs will help you to determine the extent of bleeding that has occurred. Normally, there should be little change in the blood pressure or pulse rate with this change.

4. Do you expect the blood pressure and pulse rate to increase or decrease when the patient is moved?

When a patient has a significant loss of fluid within the vascular space, there will be a 10-beat increase in the pulse rate and/or a 10-mm Hg drop in blood pressure. Either finding indicates a significant volume loss.

5. On the basis of the patient's orthostatic vital signs, what is your suggested treatment?

The patient's vital signs indicate that she is hypovolemic. The patient should be given IV fluids as long as no findings are present that would contraindicate it. You should also attempt to keep the patient lying as flat as possible to minimize the postural effects.

6. Which of the patient's medications most concerns you?

You should be concerned with the warfarin because it is an anticoagulant. Volume replacement is still your treatment of choice, but warfarin should increase your suspicion of substantial bleeding somewhere in the GI tract. Bismuth solutions (Pepto Bismol) will also color stools black without any bleeding.

YOU are the Paramedic SUMMARY *(continued)*

7. Knowing that your patient has postural vital signs, how are you going to move the patient downstairs?

The best method to help the patient's comfort level would be to maintain a lying position if at all possible. A stair chair would not be a good choice for this patient. A Reeves device or a scoop stretcher may be your best choice.

8. Should you administer a pain medication to make your patient more comfortable?

Because this patient is already hemodynamically compromised, fentanyl or tramadol may be a better choice than morphine or meperidine (which cause vascular pooling), if your local protocols allow. Consult medical control regarding the best choice.

EMS Patient Care Report (PCR)

Date: 08-10-18	**Incident No.:** 73542	**Nature of Call:** Unresponsive	**Location:** 215 Brooks Street		
Dispatched: 0115	**En Route:** 0116	**At Scene:** 0121	**Transport:** 0146	**At Hospital:** 0153	**In Service:** 0211

Patient Information

Age: 64 **Sex:** F **Weight (in kg [lb]):** 91 kg (200 lb)	**Allergies:** No known drug allergies **Medications:** Propranolol, diltiazem, warfarin, glyburide, bismuth OTC **Past Medical History:** Diabetic, HTN, AFib **Chief Complaint:** GI bleeding

Vital Signs

Time: 0126	**BP:** 106/82 lying, 92/78 sitting	**Pulse:** 120 lying, 136 sitting	**Respirations:** 20	**Spo_2:** 98% on 15 L/min
Time: 0134	**BP:** 110/86 lying	**Pulse:** 110 lying	**Respirations:** 18	**Spo_2:** 98% on 15 L/min
Time:	**BP:**	**Pulse:**	**Respirations:**	**Spo_2:**

EMS Treatment (circle all that apply)

Oxygen @ 15 **L/min via (circle one):** **NC** **(NRM)** **Bag-mask device**		**Assisted Ventilation**	**Airway Adjunct**	**CPR**
Defibrillation	**Bleeding Control**	**Bandaging**	**Splinting**	**Other:**

Narrative

Arrived to find 64-year-old woman in an upstairs bathroom at her residence. Husband states the pt has been feeling ill for a few days. Pt awoke and he assisted her to the bathroom when she became syncopal. The husband helped her down to the floor and she did not fall. Pt has approx. 250 mL of melena on the floor near her position. Pt reports abdominal pain an 8 on 1:10 scale. Pt denies any vomiting. Abd assessment equals soft, tender in all quads.
Pt orthostatic vital signs show postural changes. IV established and 250-mL challenge administered. Pt lifted off floor with a scoop stretcher and carried down stairs to ambulance. Pt had no change during transport to Charity Hospital. Report given to charge nurse on arrival.**End of report**

Prep Kit

▶ Ready for Review

- Gastrointestinal conditions alone are rarely life threatening. This fact does not minimize the systemic disorders that can erupt from untreated or undertreated diseases of the GI system.
- The structures and functions of the GI system perform digestion, which begins in the mouth, and continues through a multitude of organs and structures: the esophagus, portal vein, stomach, duodenum, pancreas, liver, gallbladder, small intestine, large intestine, appendix, and anus.
- During calls for patients with suspected abdominal or GI emergencies, it is likely you will come into contact with blood, vomitus, urine, or feces. A complete size-up of scene safety requires a survey of the personal protective equipment required for protection against infectious agents.
- You form your general impression of the patient with a suspected abdominal or GI emergency by observing the patient's posture, his or her environment, any foul odors present, and the patient's level of consciousness.
- Airway patency and adequate circulation must be maintained, and you must assess the extent of any bleeding by obtaining the patient's orthostatic vital signs.
- The transport decision is made by evaluating the patient's stability; use of rapid transport with lights and sirens is rarely necessary for abdominal emergencies.
- Your field impression of the patient and the information you gather about the patient's medications, allergies, past medical history, and precipitating events can provide information about the cause of the patient's chief complaint.
- Secondary assessment is accomplished with a comprehensive physical examination in which you pay special attention to the appearance of the shape, size, color, and other characteristics of the abdomen, auscultate bowel sounds, and perform percussion and palpation to assess for dullness, rigidity, guarding, pain or discomfort, rebound tenderness, fluid accumulation, and masses.
- When taking a patient's orthostatic vital signs, a 20-beat increase in the pulse rate or a 20-mm Hg drop in blood pressure indicates a significant volume loss caused by uncontrolled bleeding.
- Reassessment includes monitoring for changes in pulse rate, ECG readings, blood pressure, respiratory rate, oxygen saturation, or signs of shock.
- Advances in technology allow pain relief to be offered to most patients with abdominal or GI emergencies. It is also important to manage nausea and, by extension, vomiting.
- Talking with patients and their families to keep them calm and informed is the foundation of compassionate, high-quality care. Documenting your observations and the results of all assessments, examinations, and tests is also essential to delivering excellent patient care.
- Sudden, worrisome changes in a patient's condition warrant performing comprehensive and detailed new assessments and examinations.
- Airway management includes delivery of high-concentration oxygen, prevention of aspiration, and auscultation of lung sounds, as dictated by the patient's condition.
- Circulation may be compromised in a patient with a GI emergency by dehydration or hemorrhage. Fluid resuscitation to replace volume and maintain perfusion may be a life-saving intervention.
- You must learn about individual GI diseases to keep pace with the rising stature of the EMS field and the increasing level of responsibility paramedics must be prepared to assume. Such knowledge is also necessary to educate patients about their own or a loved one's disease.
- Four major conditions are responsible for abdominal and GI emergencies:
  - Hypovolemia caused by dehydration or hemorrhage
  - Acute or chronic inflammation
  - Infection
  - Obstruction
- Bleeding within the GI tract is a symptom of another disease, not a disease itself. Presentation of GI bleeding is variable because it can reflect the presence of a number of diseases. Each of these conditions has its own pattern of disease progression.
- Following a healthy diet, eliminating smoking, and reducing stress are all ways to prevent GI disorders. A diet that is high in fiber and low in fat will facilitate movement of materials through the GI tract.

▶ Vital Vocabulary

acholic stools Light, clay-colored stools indicative of liver failure.

acute abdomen A condition of sudden onset of pain within the abdomen, usually indicating peritonitis; demands immediate medical or surgical treatment.

Prep Kit (continued)

acute gastroenteritis A family of conditions that revolve around a central theme of infection with fever, abdominal pain, diarrhea, nausea, and vomiting.

anal fissures Linear tears to the mucosal lining in and near the anus, possibly caused by the passage of large, hard stools; a cause of lower gastrointestinal bleeding.

appendicitis Inflammation of the appendix.

ascites Abdominal edema typically signaling liver failure.

biliary tract disorders A group of disorders that involve inflammation of the gallbladder; these include cholangitis, cholelithiasis, cholecystitis, and acalculous cholecystitis.

Boerhaave syndrome Forceful vomiting that results in a tear in the esophagus that extends entirely through the esophageal wall, creating a hole.

borborygmi A bowel sound characterized by increased activity within the bowel; also called hyperperistalsis.

cholangitis Inflammation of the bile duct.

cholelithiasis The presence of stones within the gallbladder.

cholecystitis Inflammation of the gallbladder.

cirrhosis Early failure of the liver; characterized by portal hypertension, coagulation deficiencies, and diminished detoxification.

Crohn disease Inflammation of the ileum and possibly other portions of the gastrointestinal tract, in which the immune system attacks portions of the intestinal walls, causing them to become scarred, narrowed, stiff, and weakened.

diarrhea Liquid stool.

digestion The mechanical and chemical breakdown of the large molecules in food into small molecules that can be absorbed in the gastrointestinal tract and converted to energy for cellular function.

diverticulitis Inflammation of pouches in the colon; these pouches form as a result of difficulty moving feces through the colon. Bacteria can become trapped in the pouches, leading to inflammation and infection.

diverticulum A weak area in the colon that begins to have small outcroppings that turn into pouches; plural is diverticula.

endoscopy Insertion of a flexible fiberoptic tube into the esophagus to visualize, remove, or repair damaged or diseased tissue.

epigastric The region of the abdomen directly inferior to the xiphoid process and superior to the umbilicus.

esophagitis An inflammation of the esophagus.

esophagogastric varices Dilated blood vessels of the esophagus, commonly caused by difficulty in blood flow through the liver; the presence of these can lead to vessel rupture.

feculent Smelling of feces.

fistula An abnormal connection between two cavities.

gastritis A preulcerative state where the stomach is inflamed, but erosions have not yet occurred.

gastroesophageal reflux disease (GERD) A condition in which the sphincter between the esophagus and the stomach opens, allowing stomach acid to move superiorly; can cause a burning sensation within the chest (heartburn); also called acid reflux disease.

hematemesis Vomit with blood; can either look like coffee grounds, indicating the presence of partially digested blood, or contain bright-red blood, indicating active bleeding.

hematochezia The passage of stool in which bright red blood can be distinguished; caused by lower gastrointestinal bleeding.

hepatic encephalopathy Impairment of brain function resulting from failure of the liver.

hepatitis Inflammation of the liver, usually caused by a virus, that causes fever, loss of appetite, jaundice, fatigue, and altered liver function.

hernia The protrusion of a loop of an organ or tissue through an abnormal body opening.

hiatal hernia A protrusion of a portion of the stomach through the diaphragm.

hyperperistalsis Increased activity within the bowel; also called borborygmi.

hypoperistalsis Decreased activity in the bowel.

icteric Yellowish coloration of the conjunctiva (the whites of the eyes) caused by the buildup of bilirubin in the blood during liver failure.

incarcerated A type of hernia in which an organ is trapped in the new location; most commonly obstructs the bowel.

incisional A type of hernia in which intestinal contents herniate through an incision, for example after abdominal surgery.

Prep Kit (continued)

inflammatory bowel disease (IBD) Chronic inflammation of all or part of the gastrointestinal tract.

intussusception Telescoping of the intestines into themselves.

irritable bowel syndrome (IBS) A condition in which patients have abdominal pain and changes in their bowel habits; generally the pain and accompanying changes in bowel habits must be present for at least 3 days a month for at least 3 months to be considered this disease.

lower esophageal sphincter (LES) The sphincter between the esophagus and the stomach; controls the amount of food that moves up the esophagus; also called the cardiac sphincter.

Mallory-Weiss syndrome A condition in which the junction between the esophagus and the stomach tears, causing severe bleeding and, potentially, death.

melena Dark, tarry, malodorous stools caused by upper gastrointestinal bleeding.

mesenteric ischemia An interruption of the blood supply to the mesentery.

neoplasm A mass of tissue produced by abnormal cell growth and division that may be malignant (cancerous) or benign.

pancreatitis Inflammation of the pancreas.

parietal pain Pain caused by inflammation of the parietal peritoneum that is generally described as steady, aching, and aggravated by movement.

peptic ulcer disease (PUD) A disease in which the mucous lining of the stomach and duodenum have been eroded, allowing the acid to eat into these organs.

peritonitis Inflammation of the peritoneum, the protective membrane that lines the abdominal and pelvic cavities.

portal hypertension Increased pressure in the portal veins; caused by the inability of blood to flow normally through the liver; can lead to rupture of these vessels.

pruritus Itching.

rebound tenderness Pain that the patient feels when pressure is released as opposed to when pressure is applied; characteristic of appendicitis.

rectal abscess An infection involving a collection of pus in the rectal walls that results from blockage of the rectal mucous ducts.

reducible A type of hernia that will return to its normal location either spontaneously or by manual manipulation.

scaphoid A concave shape of the abdomen; can be caused by evisceration.

septicemia A generalized infection of the bloodstream.

soft stool A bowel movement that is the consistency of soft-serve ice cream; can range in color from tan to dark brown.

steatorrhea Foamy, fatty stools associated with liver failure or gallbladder conditions.

strangulated A type of hernia that causes complete obstruction of blood circulation in a given organ as a result of compression or entrapment; an emergency situation causing death of tissue.

striae Vertical stretch marks that occur when a person loses or gains weight rapidly.

stricture An abnormal narrowing of a structure; also called stenosis.

tracheoesophageal fistula (TEF) A connection between the esophagus and the trachea.

tympanic A loud, high-pitched sound, similar to the sound of a drum, heard on percussion of a hollow space (eg, the empty stomach or a puffed out cheek).

ulcerative colitis Generalized inflammation of the colon that results in a weakened, dilated rectum, making it prone to infection and bleeding.

umbilical The region of the abdomen surrounding the umbilicus.

urticaria An itching rash.

volvulus Twisting of the bowel until a kink occurs; results in blocked flow.

▶ References

1. Digestive diseases statistics for the United States. National Institute of Diabetes and Digestive and Kidney Diseases website. http://www.niddk.nih.gov/health-information/health-statistics/pages/digestive-diseases-statistics-for-the-united-states.aspx. Published November 2014. Accessed April 23, 2016.
2. US Census Bureau. US Census Bureau website. http://www.census.gov/. Published September 11, 2016. Accessed September 11, 2016.
3. Patti MG. Gastroesophageal reflux disease: practice essentials, background, anatomy. Medscape website. http://emedicine.medscape.com/article/176595-overview. Updated May 2, 2016. Accessed May 8, 2016.

Prep Kit (continued)

4. Taylor J, McLaughlin K, MacRae A, Lang E, Anton A. Use of prehospital ultrasound in North America: a survey of emergency medical services medical directors. *BMC Emergency Medicine*. 2014;14(6). http://bmcemergmed.biomedcentral.com/articles/10.1186/1471-227X-14-6. Accessed May 15, 2016.
5. Wong Kee Song LM. Mallory-Weiss tear overview of Mallory-Weiss syndrome. Medscape website. http://emedicine.medscape.com/article/187134-overview. Updated June 25, 2015. Accessed April 23, 2016.
6. Roy PK. Boerhaave syndrome: background, pathophysiology, epidemiology. Medscape website. http://emedicine.medscape.com/article/171683-overview. Updated July 6, 2015. Accessed April 23, 2016.
7. Anand BS. Peptic ulcer disease: background, anatomy, pathophysiology. Medscape website. http://emedicine.medscape.com/article/181753-overview. Updated January 29, 2017. Accessed March 17, 2017.
8. Wehbi M. Acute gastritis: background, pathophysiology, etiology. Medscape website. http://emedicine.medscape.com/article/175909-overview. Updated February 25, 2016. Accessed May 8, 2016.
9. Hemorrhoids overview. Remedy's Health Communities website. http://www.healthcommunities.com/hemorrhoids/hemorrhoids-overview.shtml. Updated February 21, 2013. Accessed October 11, 2016.
10. Wedro B. Hemorrhoids: facts, symptoms, signs, itch & home remedies for pain. eMedicineHealth website. http://www.emedicinehealth.com/hemorrhoids/article_em.htm. Published February 26, 2015. Accessed May 3, 2016.
11. Daley B. Peritonitis and abdominal sepsis: background, anatomy, pathophysiology. Medscape website. http://emedicine.medscape.com/article/180234-overview. Updated January 11, 2017. Accessed March 17, 2017.
12. Brooks DC. Gallstones in pregnancy. UpToDate website. http://www.uptodate.com/contents/gallstones-in-pregnancy. Updated January 25, 2017. Accessed March 17, 2017.
13. Heuman DM. Gallstones (cholelithiasis): practice essentials, background, pathophysiology. Medscape website. http://emedicine.medscape.com/article/175667-overview. Updated April 14, 2016. Accessed May 2, 2016.
14. Scott TM. Acute cholangitis clinical presentation. Medscape website. http://emedicine.medscape.com/article/774245-clinical#showall. Updated November 21, 2016. Accessed March 17, 2017.
15. Craig S. Appendicitis: practice essentials, background, anatomy. Medscape website. http://emedicine.medscape.com/article/773895-overview. Updated January 19, 2017. Accessed March 28, 2017.
16. Tang JCF. Acute pancreatitis: practice essentials, background, pathophysiology. Medscape website. http://emedicine.medscape.com/article/181364-overview. Updated February 14, 2017. Accessed March 17, 2017.
17. Basson MD. Ulcerative colitis: practice essentials, background, anatomy. Medscape website. http://emedicine.medscape.com/article/183084-overview. Updated February 14, 2017. Accessed March 17, 2017.
18. Ghazi LJ. Crohn disease: practice essentials, background, pathophysiology. Medscape website. http://emedicine.medscape.com/article/172940-overview. Updated January 6, 2017. Accessed March 17, 2017.
19. Estimates of foodborne illness in the United States. Centers for Disease Control and Prevention website. http://www.cdc.gov/foodborneburden/index.html. Updated August 19, 2016. Accessed March 17, 2017.
20. Traveler's health: traveler's diarrhea. Centers for Disease Control and Prevention website. http://wwwnc.cdc.gov/travel/yellowbook/2016/the-pre-travel-consultation/travelers-diarrhea. Updated July 10, 2015. Accessed October 11, 2016.
21. Diskin A. Emergent treatment of gastroenteritis: background, pathophysiology, epidemiology. Medscape website. http://emedicine.medscape.com/article/775277-overview. Updated February 10, 2017. Accessed March 17, 2017.
22. Munter DW. Gastrointestinal foreign bodies: background, pathophysiology, epidemiology. Medscape website. http://emedicine.medscape.com/article/776566-overview. Updated February 20, 2014. Accessed May 8, 2016.
23. Nobie BA. Small-bowel obstruction: practice essentials, background, pathophysiology. Medscape website. http://emedicine.medscape.com/article/774140-overview. Updated January 20, 2015. Accessed May 3, 2016.
24. Hopkins C. Large-bowel obstruction: practice essentials, background, pathophysiology. Medscape website. http://emedicine.medscape.com/article/774045-overview. Updated December 9, 2015. Accessed May 3, 2016.
25. Rather AA. Abdominal hernias: practice essentials, background, anatomy. Medscape website. http://emedicine.medscape.com/article/189563-overview. Updated December 22, 2016. Accessed March 17, 2017.
26. Munter DW. Rectal foreign bodies: background, etiology, epidemiology. Medscape website. http://emedicine.medscape.com/article/776795-overview. Updated December 28, 2015. Accessed October 11, 2016.

Prep Kit *(continued)*

27. Dang CV. Acute mesenteric ischemia: background, anatomy, pathophysiology. Medscape website. http://emedicine.medscape.com/article/189146-overview. Updated December 27, 2016. Accessed March 17, 2017.
28. Dragovich T. Colon cancer: practice essentials, background, pathophysiology. Medscape website. http://emedicine.medscape.com/article/277496-overview. Updated March 1, 2017. Accessed March 17, 2017.
29. Dragovich T. Pancreatic cancer: practice essentials, background, pathophysiology. Medscape website. http://emedicine.medscape.com/article/280605-overview. Updated January 11, 2016. Accessed May 1, 2016.
30. Stuart KE. Primary hepatic carcinoma: background, pathophysiology, epidemiology. http://emedicine.medscape.com/article/282814-overview. Updated April 16, 2015. Accessed April 30, 2016.

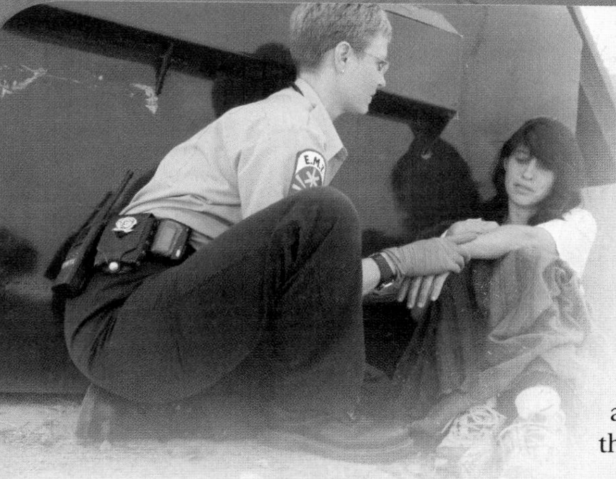

Assessment *in Action*

Your unit is dispatched to a local park for a man down. Law enforcement has cleared the scene so it is safe to enter. You find a man who is unresponsive on a park bench. There is copious blood coming from his mouth. You recognize him as a frequent patient who has alcoholism and who stays at the local mission.

You have transported the man before for conditions related to cirrhosis of the liver resulting from his chronic alcoholism. The physician who treated him last time told the patient he had the beginning stages of varices. As you approach the patient, you find he is incontinent of urine and feces. There is a dark, tarry look to the fecal matter.

1. What does the portal vein do?

A. Transports blood to the lungs
B. Transports blood to the liver
C. Transports blood to the legs
D. Transports blood to the brain

2. An increase in hepatic pressure through the portal vein can cause leaking of blood in the esophagus. This is called:

A. esophageal erosion.
B. esophagogastric varices.
C. cholecystitis.
D. gastroenteritis.

3. Because you suspect this patient has upper GI bleeding, which sign would you not expect to see?

A. Hematemesis
B. Melena
C. Hematochezia
D. Bright red stools

4. Because this patient may be bleeding from ruptured esophagogastric varices, which is the most important step in management of his airway?

A. Suction
B. Oxygen via a nonrebreathing mask
C. Insertion of a dual-lumen airway device
D. Endotracheal intubation

Assessment *in Action* *(continued)*

5. A sharp pain on inspiration when pressure is applied to the right upper quadrant is called:

A. Biot sign.
B. hematemesis.
C. Beck sign.
D. Murphy sign.

6. Autodigestion of the pancreas results in:

A. Mallory-Weiss syndrome.
B. pancreatitis.
C. autoimmune disorder.
D. diabetes.

7. Which portion of the body will give the best evidence of poor perfusion?

A. Palms
B. Arms
C. Face
D. Lips

8. How does alcohol affect this patient's ability to manage his hemorrhage? Alcohol:

A. decreases the amount of urine production.
B. causes bradycardia.
C. prevents the spleen from contracting.
D. impairs the ability to form clots.

9. You are dispatched to a private residence for a person with abdominal pain. When you arrive on scene, the patient is doubled over in pain and reports point tenderness to the upper right quadrant. The patient's vital signs are: pulse rate, 108 beats/min with sinus tachycardia; blood pressure, 110/70 mm Hg; respiratory rate, 24 breaths/min; and pulse oximetry, 100% on room air. What management is required for this patient?

10. You are caring for a 14-year-old girl who reports abdominal pain. She is awake, alert, and oriented and her condition appears to be stable. Her skin is warm and non-pale. The patient's vital signs are: pulse rate 104 beats/min; respiratory rate, 16 breaths/min, and quiet.

Consider this patient's age and sex. What are the assessment implications for this patient?

CHAPTER 21

Genitourinary and Renal Emergencies

National EMS Education Standard Competencies

Medicine

Integrates assessment findings with principles of epidemiology and pathophysiology to formulate a field impression and implement a comprehensive treatment/disposition plan for a patient with a medical complaint.

Genitourinary/Renal

- Blood pressure assessment in hemodialysis patients (p 1228)

Anatomy, physiology, pathophysiology, assessment, and management of

- Complications related to
  - Renal dialysis (pp 1227-1229)
  - Urinary catheter management (not insertion) (p 1221)
- Kidney stones (pp 1221-1223)

Anatomy, physiology, epidemiology, pathophysiology, psychosocial impact, presentations, prognosis, and management of

- Complications of
  - Acute renal failure (pp 1223-1225)
  - Chronic renal failure (pp 1225-1226)
  - Dialysis (pp 1227-1229)
- Renal calculi (pp 1221-1223)
- Acid-base disturbances (pp 1223-1224)
- Fluid and electrolytes (pp 1225, 1227-1228)
- Infection (pp 1220-1221)
- Male genital tract conditions (pp 1229-1230)

Knowledge Objectives

1. Describe the anatomy and physiology of the male and female urinary systems: kidneys, ureters, urinary bladder, and urethra. (pp 1214-1216)
2. Describe the primary survey and secondary assessment processes for patients with renal and genitourinary emergencies. (pp 1217-1219)
3. Specify factors that influence transport decisions for patients with renal and genitourinary emergencies. (p 1217)
4. Discuss the questions that must be asked to obtain thorough historical information from a patient. (pp 1217-1218)
5. Specify best practices for documenting renal and genitourinary emergencies and communicating with the receiving facility. (pp 1217, 1219)
6. Compare visceral pain with referred pain. (p 1218)
7. Explain how visceral pain and referred pain each contribute to the field diagnosis. (p 1218)
8. Indicate the components of the physical exam for a patient with a renal or genitourinary emergency. (pp 1218-1219)
9. Name the components of an effective treatment plan. (p 1219)
10. Outline the pathophysiology, assessment, and management of common diseases and conditions of the renal and genitourinary systems, including urinary tract infections, kidney stones, acute kidney injury, chronic kidney disease, and end-stage renal disease. (pp 1220-1226)
11. Discuss the purpose and types of renal dialysis. (p 1227)
12. Identify the possible complications of dialysis and the prehospital interventions associated with each. (pp 1227-1229)
13. Discuss the pathophysiology, assessment, and management of conditions related to the male genital tract, including epididymitis, orchitis, Fournier gangrene, priapism, phimosis, paraphimosis, benign prostate hypertrophy, testicular masses, and testicular torsion. (pp 1229-1230)

Skills Objectives

There are no skills objectives for this chapter.

Introduction

The urinary system performs the essential jobs of filtering the blood and removing metabolic wastes. In addition, the urinary system manages concentrations of electrolytes and maintains acid-base balance in the bloodstream. It also regulates fluid volume and blood pressure.

Kidney disease affects more than 26 million Americans, and approximately 47,000 Americans die of kidney disease each year, with more than 468,000 requiring dialysis.[1] The most common acute renal disease is nephrolithiasis (kidney stones or renal calculi), which affects roughly 10% of the US population.[1] Common urinary tract diseases include **urinary tract infections (UTIs)**, which occur in more than 50% of women, and noncancerous enlargement of the prostate, which 60% of men will develop by age 50 years.[1]

Anatomy and Physiology Review

The urinary system Figure 21-1 consists of the **kidneys**, which filter the blood and produce **urine**; the paired **ureters**, which transport urine from the kidneys to the bladder; the **urinary bladder**, which stores the urine until it is released from the body; and the **urethra**, the route by which urine leaves the bladder and exits the body. In females, the urethra is significantly shorter than in males, which increases susceptibility to infections.

The internal anatomy of the kidney can be divided into three distinct regions: the cortex, the medulla, and the pelvis, which drains urine into the ureter. **Nephrons** Figure 21-2, found in the cortex, are the structural and functional units of the kidney that form urine. Each nephron is composed of the glomerulus; the **glomerular (Bowman) capsule**, which surrounds the glomerulus; the **proximal convoluted tubule (PCT)**; the **loop of Henle**; and the **distal convoluted tubule (DCT)**, which connects with the kidney's collecting tubules.

The male genital system Figure 21-3 is closely related to the urinary system, sharing the urethra as a conduit for urine as well as for semen and other secretions. The prostate gland surrounds the urethra and, along with the seminal vesicles, secretes fluids into the urethra during ejaculation. The testes are located in the scrotum and create spermatozoa, which are stored in the epididymis for maturation. During ejaculation, the sperm travels from the epididymis into the vas deferens and through the ejaculatory ducts where it mixes with fluid from the seminal vesicles, bulbourethral glands, and prostate to form semen. It then enters the urethra through which it exits the body. The female genital system is discussed in detail in Chapter 22, *Gynecologic Emergencies*.

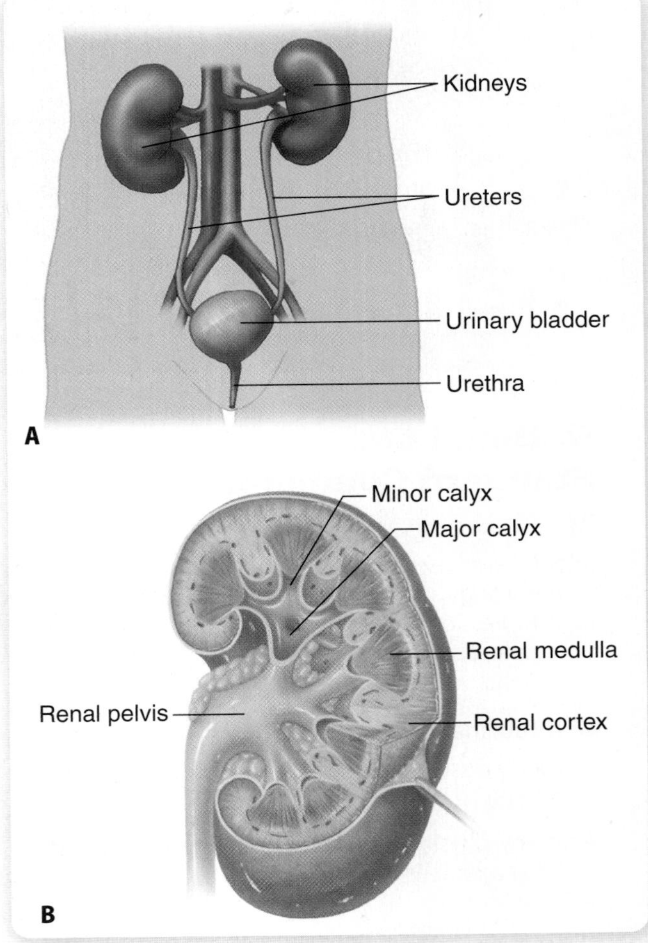

Figure 21-1 The urinary system. **A.** Anterior view showing the relationship of the kidneys, ureters, urinary bladder, and urethra. **B.** Cross section of the human kidney showing the renal cortex, renal medulla, and renal pelvis.

YOU are the Paramedic PART 1

At about 0600 hours you are dispatched to 327 West Main Street for a woman reporting back pain. You arrive to find a slender, gray-haired man waiting for you at the front door of the turn-of-the-century residence. He motions for you and says, "It's my daughter. She's very sick. I would have taken her to the hospital myself, but I can't carry her. She's in the upstairs bedroom." The stairway is dark and narrow. As you walk up the steps, you hear a young woman say, "Dad, I'm going to be sick again."

1. What concerns may you have about the scene?
2. Although you have not seen your patient yet, what information do you already know that is part of the primary survey?

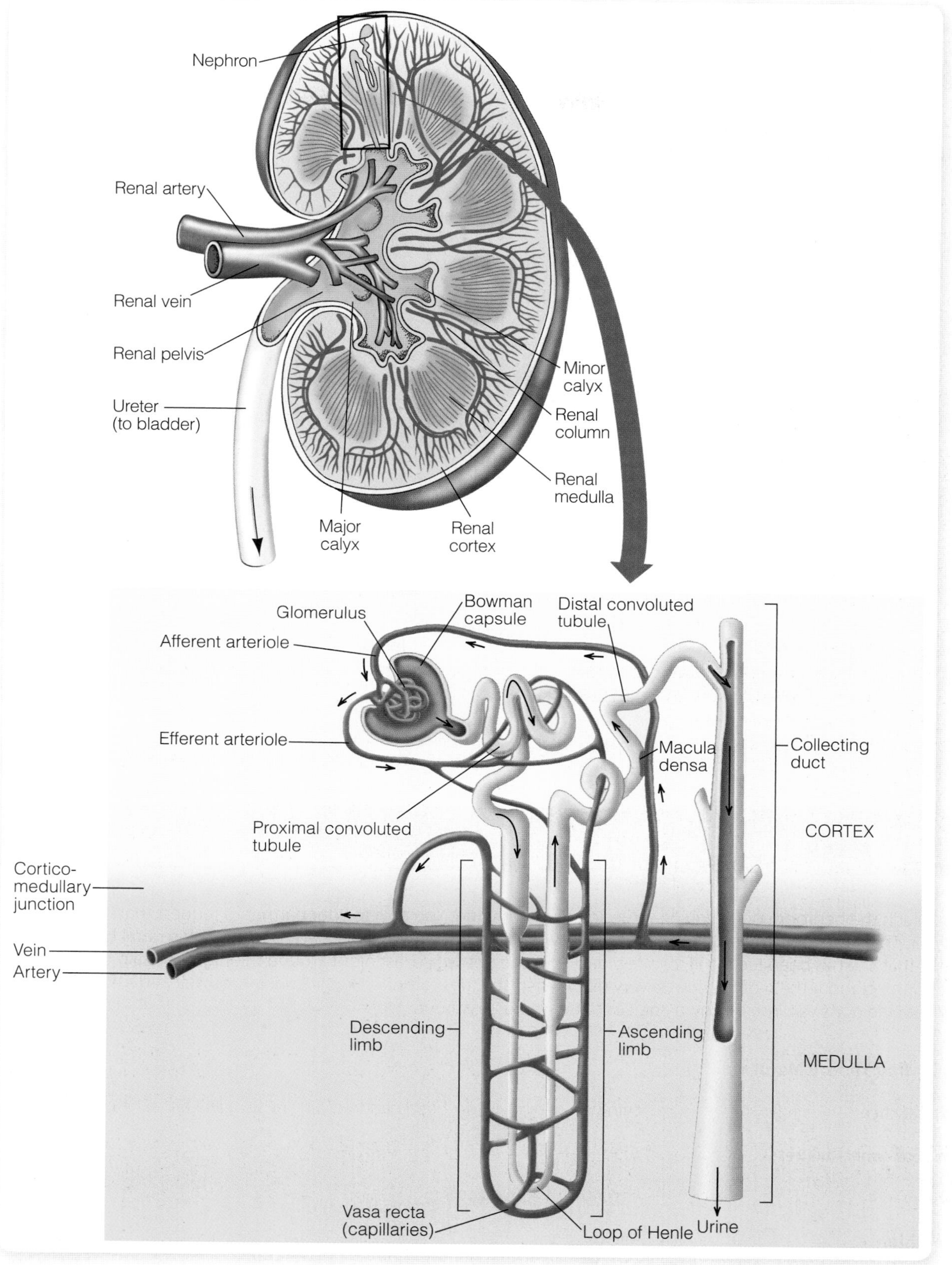

Figure 21-2 The nephrons of the kidney. Part of the nephron is located in the cortex, and part is located in the medulla.

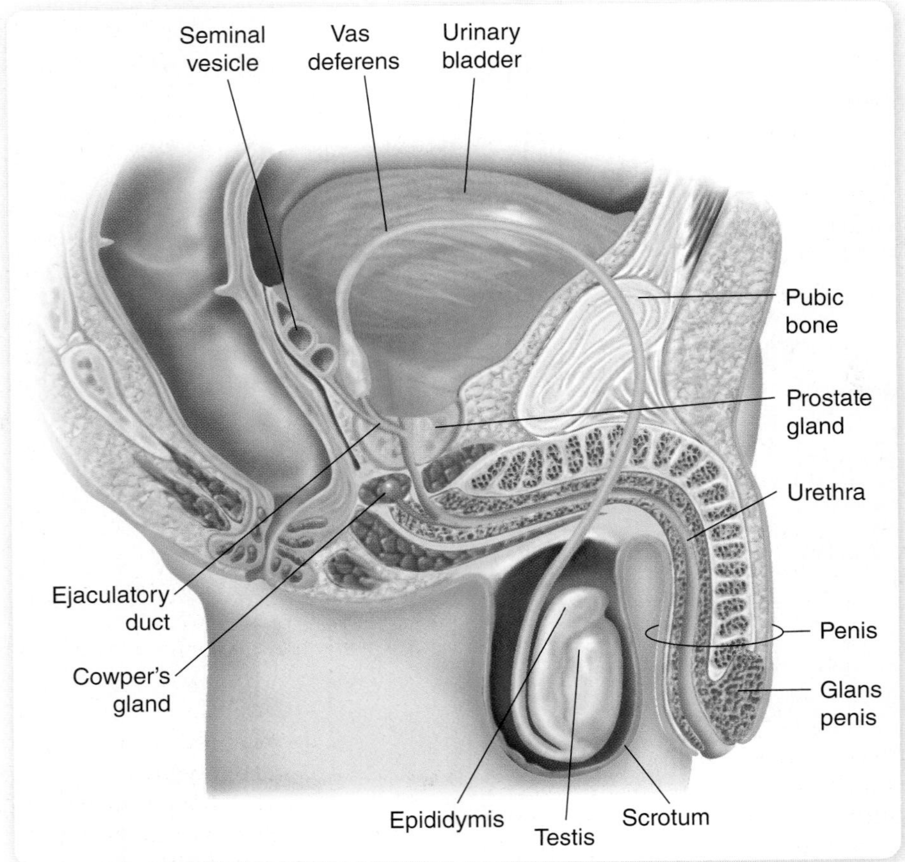

Figure 21-3 The male genital anatomy.

YOU are the Paramedic PART 2

As you reach the bedroom door, you hear the sound of vomiting. You turn to your partner to request that he retrieve the stair chair. The father opens the door, and you see a woman in her early 20s in a bed covered with several blankets. The father tells you that she has been feeling ill for a few days, but she got worse last night around midnight. He said that she has been vomiting throughout the night and feels very dizzy when she tries to stand. You introduce yourself and ask if you can take her vital signs. She nods yes. You sit down and continue your assessment.

Recording Time: 0 Minutes	
Appearance	Lying on her right side, head hanging off the bed over a trash can
Level of consciousness	Alert
Airway	Patent with active vomiting
Breathing	Rapid
Circulation	Flushed, sweaty skin

3. What concerns do you have about her history, signs, and symptoms?
4. What should be done with the emesis?

Patient Assessment

Assessment of a patient with a renal and genitourinary emergency is the same as for any other medical patient. Begin with the scene size-up, perform a primary survey, obtain a history, perform a secondary assessment including physical exam, form a field impression, make a treatment decision, and reassess the patient continuously en route to the hospital.

Scene Size-up

In the scene size-up, you should not only ensure that the scene is safe for you and your fellow providers, but also consider the mechanism of injury, assess for hazards and the need for additional help, and determine the number of patients. Remember that urine is a body fluid and that, as always, you must take standard precautions to avoid contact.

Patients who are experiencing renal or genital conditions may exhibit many of the same symptoms as a patient with other abdominal conditions—nausea and vomiting, constipation or diarrhea, flank pain, and abdominal pain.

Because pain is a common symptom in both abdominal and genitourinary ailments, it is often difficult to determine the source of the pain. Genitourinary pain can have many origins—eg, bacterial infection, extension of the ureter by a kidney stone, or distention of the bladder because of prostate enlargement. Your assessment should be intended to detect and prevent life threats and provide supportive care for the patient. Be sure to keep a wide differential diagnosis as you progress through your evaluation.

Primary Survey

In the primary survey, you form a general impression of the patient and check for life-threatening conditions. A patient with a genitourinary or renal condition may exhibit extremes of activity. Is the patient changing position constantly in an attempt to find a comfortable position ("the kidney stone dance")? Or is the patient sitting very still with the knees drawn up to the chest? Is the patient in obvious pain? Does he or she appear pale or jaundiced? What is the patient's level of consciousness? Your observation of the patient's body movements, posture, skin color, breathing pattern, mental acuity, and other factors will give you a good overall sense of the severity of the patient's condition.

Check for life threats by assessing the patient's mental status and airway, breathing, and circulation (ABCs). Begin by observing the patient's breathing and ensure that the airway is patent. Look for signs of respiratory distress. Clear the airway and provide treatment as indicated by the patient's respiratory status.

Documentation & Communication

Establish and document your baseline impression early in the assessment process. Document any changes in mental status or level of consciousness as you reevaluate the patient, and note how he or she responds to administration of supplemental oxygen, fluids, pain medication, and other interventions. Stay in close contact with medical control, and notify the receiving facility as soon as possible if life threats are apparent. Record the findings of your serial assessments in your report to the receiving facility, concluding with your overall impression of the patient's condition at the time of transfer.

Next, assess skin color, heart rate, and blood pressure. Look for signs of shock, such as a rapid heart rate and low blood pressure. Is the abdomen distended or rigid? If you discover any life-threatening conditions, take immediate steps to correct them and provide urgent transport to an appropriately equipped receiving facility. Advise the facility en route to begin mobilizing resources and staff so that they will be on standby at the time of transfer.

When making your transport decision, integrate the information you obtained in the primary survey. Determine as quickly as possible whether urgent transport is warranted for life threats such as **uremia** (excessive amounts of urea and other waste products in the blood), hyperkalemia, or testicular torsion. Consider how you will move the patient, especially if doing so is likely to cause a drop in blood pressure with the change of position. Take into account any special equipment needed to handle the patient, such as a bariatric stretcher. Also keep in mind which receiving facility has the diagnostic or treatment equipment that will be necessary after transfer, such as dialysis or a urologist on staff.

Ensure that the ride during transport is as gentle as possible for the patient. Drive smoothly and steadily. Rapid driving can result in increased vehicle movement, potentially aggravating and possibly worsening the patient's pain.

History Taking

In genitourinary patients, the history and physical exam will provide the information you need to successfully manage the patient. Because so many medical diagnoses are based on the patient's history, it is imperative that you ask the right questions during this exam. Determining that the patient's pain actually started in the flank, for example, and not in its present location in the lower right quadrant, could mean the difference between a correct field diagnosis of a kidney stone and an incorrect field diagnosis of appendicitis. Similarly, determining that the patient has a history of diabetes and hypertension along with signs of uremia can help confirm your impression of chronic kidney failure.

The SAMPLE mnemonic (Signs and symptoms, Allergies, Medications, Pertinent past medical history, Last oral intake, Events leading up to the injury or illness) can guide you in obtaining pertinent historical information from the patient. For example, a patient who reports flank pain (S); who has had two previous kidney stone attacks (P); who had bacon, eggs, and coffee for breakfast 7 hours ago (L); and who has been working in the sun all day (E) has presented a history that would lead you to suspect kidney stones. Before proceeding with treatment, you would also want to assess allergies (A) and any medications (M) the patient has taken.

Pain

Diseases and conditions of the renal and urologic systems range from mild (UTIs) to emergent (acute kidney injury). Although the prehospital care for many urologic diseases is supportive, your ability to recognize the signs and symptoms of these conditions, especially when they are genuine emergencies, is critical to providing your patients with the best chance of a positive outcome.

Understanding the pathophysiology of pain, particularly referred pain (pain that feels as if it is originating from a body part other than the site being stimulated), is key to determining its origin. Visceral pain (deep pain caused by activation of pain receptors in internal areas of the body enclosed within a cavity)—the type of pain most commonly associated with urologic conditions—usually occurs when receptors in the hollow structures, such as the ureters, urinary bladder, and urethra, are stimulated. Pinpointing the source of such pain is challenging because only a few nerve fibers may be involved in the pain transmission. Because many different nerve fibers travel to the brain through the spinal cord, pain that originates in one area of the body (eg, the urinary bladder) may be perceived by the brain as coming from a different area of the body (eg, the neck or shoulder). This is called referred pain.

Pain Assessment Findings

The OPQRST (Onset, Provocation, Quality, Region/radiation/referral, Severity, Timing) mnemonic is used to evaluate the type and severity of pain. *Onset* involves questions about when the pain started and what the patient was doing at the time. The patient may describe visceral pain, such as that caused by a kidney stone, as a crampy or aching sensation deep within the body. It often begins as a vague discomfort and then gradually increases. Next, determine what, if anything, *provokes* the pain (eg, the kidney stone dance or statue stillness). To help rule out other abdominal causes of pain, take note of any relationship between food consumption and the pain.

After determining the onset and provocation, assess the *quality* of the pain. As stated earlier, pain from a kidney stone usually begins as vague discomfort that becomes extremely sharp pain within an hour. The *R* stands for *region (location)*, *radiation*, or *referral*; for example, the pain from a kidney stone moves from the flank anteriorly, toward the groin. The fact that the pain has moved also suggests that a kidney stone is passing through the system.

Special Populations

Older adults generally underreport pain for a variety of reasons.[2] Even mild atraumatic abdominal, back, or flank pain in an older patient should be taken seriously.

To evaluate the *severity* of the pain, ask the patient, "On a scale of 0 to 10, with 10 being the worst pain you have ever experienced, how would you rate the pain?" Although this number is helpful, by itself it tells you very little. The severity of the pain may not be consistent with the severity of the condition. It is important to repeat the pain severity assessment to look for trends or to verify the efficacy of treatment.

The final pain evaluation is to inquire about the *timing* of the pain. Did the pain come on suddenly, or more gradually? Has it been constant, or does it come and go? In the case of a kidney stone, you would expect fairly constant pain that varies in severity and moves as the stone travels through the system.

Secondary Assessment

The physical exam may be focused or you may move from head to toe, depending on the presentation of signs and symptoms. The abdominal region is divided into either four quadrants overlying the internal organs Figure 21-4A or nine anatomic segments Figure 21-4B. A more detailed physical exam may be performed en route if one is not done at the scene. Be sure to assess for flank tenderness, which could imply kidney infection or distention. If a male patient reports lower abdominal pain without other clear cause, visually inspect the genitalia for signs of infection, swelling, or torsion.

Monitoring the patient's vital signs is part of the physical exam. You should obtain serial vital signs at least every 5 minutes if renal failure is suspected. Take prompt action if you note any deterioration in the patient's vital signs or level of consciousness.

Special Populations

Abnormal vital signs in an older adult patient may be particularly worrisome. An older adult patient with a fever, for instance, should receive especially close scrutiny for other signs of infection. A UTI in an older adult can cause a recrudescence (return of signs and symptoms of a past disease that had resolved) of past stroke symptoms and significant mental status changes. Abdominal pain in the older patient is a serious complaint that carries a high mortality rate; older patients require thorough evaluation in the emergency department (ED).[3]

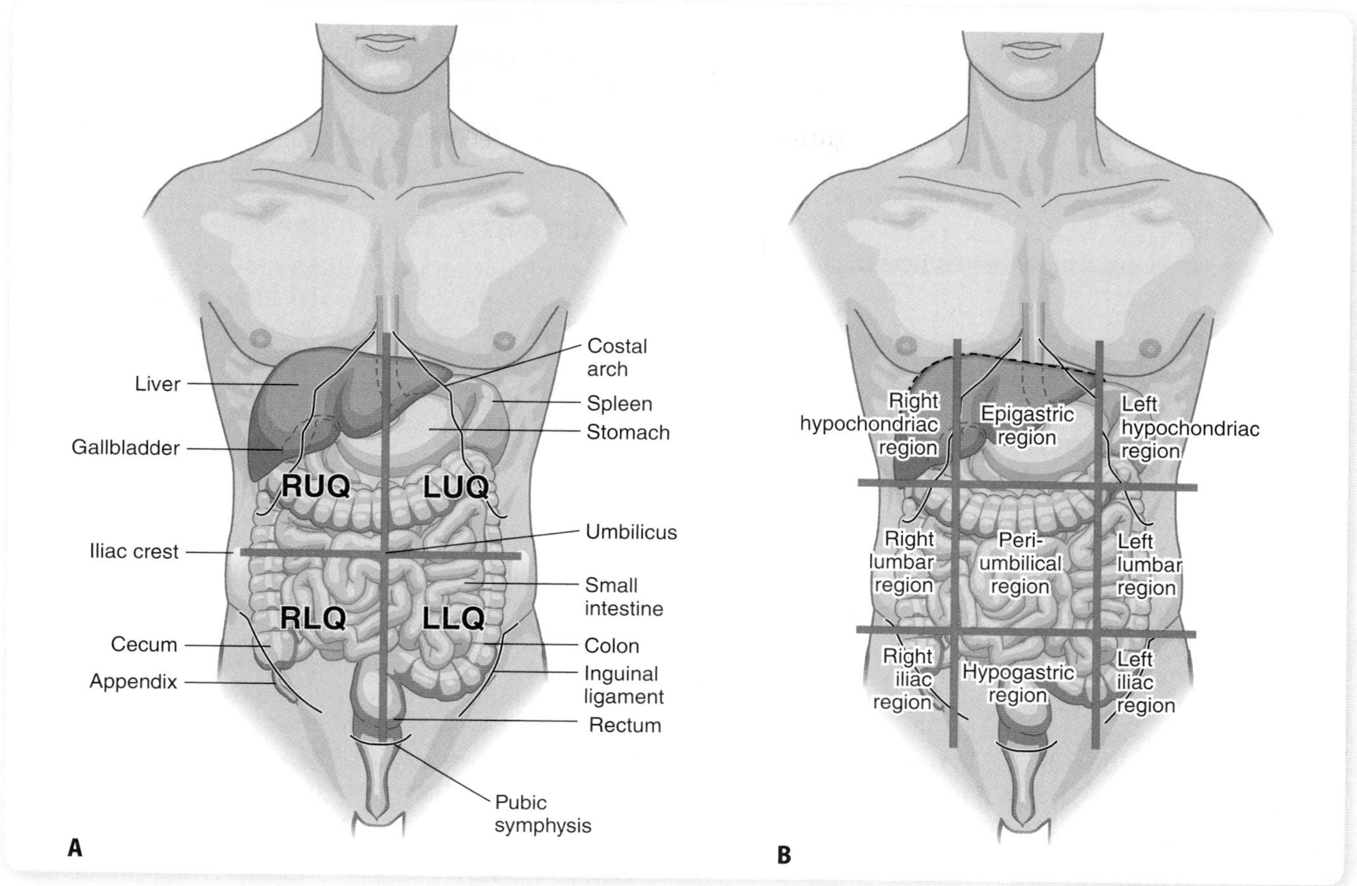

Figure 21-4 A. The four-quadrant system. **B.** Abdominal region mapping in nine sections.

Finally, consider the link between abnormal vital signs and the patient's history. For example, a diuretic or other medication might be responsible for a patient's low blood pressure. Diabetes, chronic obstructive pulmonary disease, or another chronic condition noted in the patient's history might explain other abnormal findings and provide clues to the patient's current genitourinary diagnosis.

Electrocardiogram (ECG) monitoring is extremely important in any patient with a suspected urologic emergency because of the possibility of electrolyte imbalances that may affect the heart.

Reassessment

Patients with urologic emergencies, especially those with signs and symptoms of renal failure, require frequent reassessment. The electrolyte imbalances caused by the buildup of toxins can cause rapid deterioration in the functioning of the body's organs. The heart is particularly susceptible to electrolyte changes, so cardiac monitoring should be established for every renal patient.

The information obtained from the history and physical exam is used to formulate a more nuanced field impression and to select a treatment plan. The interventions might be as simple as monitoring the ABCs and providing circulatory support to a patient with a UTI, or as complex as adjusting medications and providing support (with medical consultation and direction) for a patient with renal failure, identified on the basis of ECG changes. The treatment plan includes the transport decision, which may be made at any time during the assessment process. If the disease process requires immediate medical procedures (ie, removal of a urinary catheter, adjustment of a fistula or shunt, etc) that may go beyond the scope of the prehospital provider, perform the primary survey and transport, reassessing the patient en route to the hospital.

Serial vital signs should be obtained and documented on the patient care report. Note any trends in the vital signs and level of consciousness because they can be indicators of disease progression. Patients with a possible genitourinary disease should not be given anything by mouth because this may induce vomiting or complicate anesthesia administration for any necessary surgical procedures. Document all vital signs and report any apparent trends to the receiving facility.

Words of Wisdom

Patients with renal failure who miss their dialysis treatments are prone to hyperkalemia, among other conditions. You should suspect hyperkalemia if the patient has muscle weakness and tall, peaked T waves appear on the ECG.

Emergency Medical Care

Pain Management

Once you have checked and established adequate ABCs, allow the patient to assume a position of comfort. Patients in severe pain may have nausea and vomiting, so be prepared to suction as needed. Establish an IV line if the patient has nausea or severe pain, and consider administering an antiemetic. If there are signs of dehydration or hemodynamic instability, administer an IV bolus of crystalloid fluid. Analgesia should be provided as necessary. Although historically providers may have been concerned with reducing ED diagnostic accuracy by masking symptoms, this is not a reason to withhold pain control. Further, evidence has shown that the administration of pain medication does not reduce later diagnostic accuracy.[4]

Pathophysiology, Assessment, and Management of Specific Emergencies

Urinary Tract Infections

UTIs result in over two million ED visits per year.[5] They are most common in females after infancy. After the age of 50, there is an increase in UTIs in men because of obstruction of the urethra by the prostate. Definitive treatment requires antibiotics. Mild cases respond well to oral antibiotics, whereas severe cases may require IV administration.

Pathophysiology

UTIs usually develop in the lower urinary tract (urethra and bladder) when normal flora (bacteria that naturally populate the skin) enter the urethra and grow. These infections are more common in women because of the relatively short urethra and its close proximity to the vagina and rectum. UTIs in the upper urinary tract occur most often when lower UTIs go untreated. Upper UTIs can lead to **pyelonephritis** (inflammation of the kidney linings) and even a perinephric abscess (a collection of pus around the kidney), which may lead to sepsis and become life threatening.

YOU are the Paramedic — PART 3

Your partner returns with the stair chair and you ask him to obtain the patient's temperature while you finish obtaining the SAMPLE history and assemble your supplies to start an intravenous (IV) line. The patient tells you that she has had burning with urination for a few days and that she has had urinary tract infections in the past. At one point, her physician put her on prophylactic ciprofloxacin (Cipro). She decided that was not a good idea, and now just takes herbal supplements containing cranberry when she feels an infection is starting.

Recording Time: 5 Minutes	
Respirations	24 breaths/min
Pulse	110 beats/min
Skin	Flushed, sweaty
Blood pressure	108/60 mm Hg; lying down
Oxygen saturation (Spo_2)	98%
Pupils	PERRLA

5. What additional assessment techniques might you use?
6. Why is assessing her body temperature important?

Assessment

Patients with UTIs display a classic triad of symptoms: painful urination, frequent urges to urinate, and difficulty in urination. The pain usually begins as a visceral discomfort, but soon becomes an extreme, burning pain, especially during urination. The pain, which remains localized in the pelvis, is often perceived as bladder pain in women and as prostate pain in men. Sometimes the pain is referred to the shoulder or neck. In addition, the urine may have a foul odor or cloudy appearance or may contain blood.

Patients with UTIs frequently appear to be restless and uncomfortable. Patients with a simple UTI will appear well with normal vital signs. They may have suprapubic tenderness. In contrast, a patient with pyelonephritis or a perinephric abscess will present as ill, have flank tenderness, generally have a fever, and may have unstable vital signs. UTIs are a common cause of sepsis in older adults and should be considered in any older patient with fever, shock, or unexplained mental status changes.

Management

Management of patients with UTIs consists mainly of supportive care of the ABCs. Allow the patient to ride in a position of comfort, but be prepared for nausea and vomiting. Patients with pyelonephritis or sepsis will require more aggressive care, including IV fluids, antiemetics, and pain control. Transport the patient to the nearest appropriate facility for evaluation.

▶ Urinary Catheters

Many patients who are hospitalized for a urinary condition or other medical disease receive catheterization with a Foley catheter. Bladder catheterization involves introducing a latex or plastic tube through the urethra and into the bladder. The tube is connected to a drainage bag, which is attached to the bed frame or wheelchair at a level below the bladder. The catheter allows a continuous outflow of urine and provides a means of measuring urine output in a hemodynamically unstable patient.

When you are transporting a catheterized patient, urine backflow is a concern. If the drainage bag is raised above the level of the patient's bladder, urine can flow back into the bladder, increasing the chance of infection. Care should also be taken not to inadvertently pull out the catheter or kink it, obstructing flow. In the event that a Foley catheter must be removed, ensure that the internal balloon is deflated.

▶ Urinary Obstruction and Incontinence

Many conditions discussed in this section can cause **urinary retention**, which is defined as incomplete emptying of the bladder or a complete inability to empty the bladder. Conditions that may cause urinary retention are listed in Table 21-1. Patients with these conditions may present with extreme discomfort and should be transported to the nearest facility for urinary catheter placement.

Table 21-1 Conditions That May Cause Urinary Retention
Kidney stones (renal calculi)
Acute kidney injury
Benign prostate hypertrophy
Urethral obstructions
Urinary tract infections
Nerve damage

Urinary incontinence is loss of bladder control—the inability to control the release of urine from the bladder. Whereas urinary incontinence can occur in anyone (for example from sneezing or a forceful cough), it may be a sign of a medical condition if it falls into one of the following two categories:

- **Urge incontinence.** This is a sudden, intense urge to urinate followed within seconds to minutes by involuntary urine loss. Urination is frequent—for example, throughout the night. Urge incontinence has many potential medical causes, including UTI, medications, bladder irritants (eg, caffeine, carbonated drinks), bowel conditions, Parkinson disease, Alzheimer disease, stroke, cancers of the uterus and the urinary system, or nervous system damage associated with multiple sclerosis.
- **Overflow incontinence.** This is a constant, continual slow flow of urine. Overflow incontinence can have medical causes, such as a damaged bladder, blocked urethra, or nerve damage from diabetes, and prostate gland conditions in men.[6]

▶ Kidney Stones (Renal Calculi)

Pathophysiology

Kidney stones are extremely common and originate in the renal pelvis. They form when an excess of insoluble salts or uric acid crystallizes in the urine Figure 21-5. In the United States, roughly 1 in 11 people will experience a kidney stone, and men are affected more often than women.[7] The cause of kidney stones varies by type. Certain risk factors have been identified, including diet and hydration. General risk factors include a personal or family history of kidney stones, as well as hypertension.

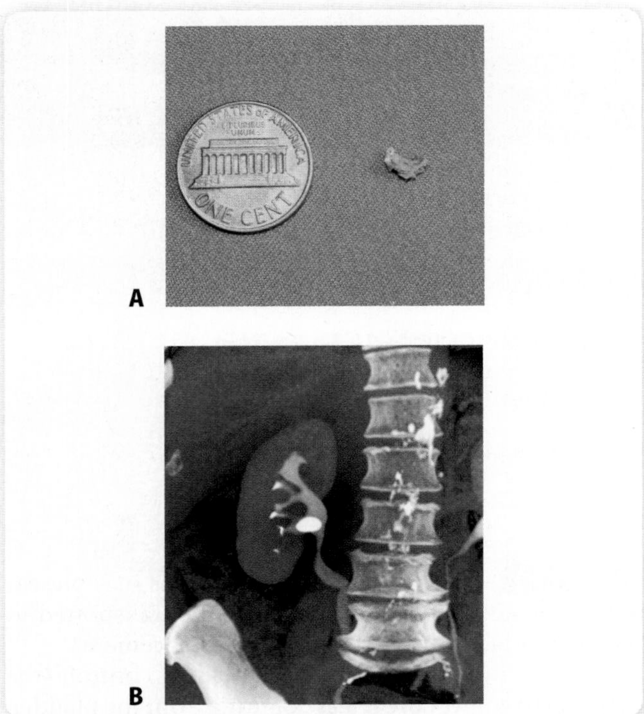

Figure 21-5 A. A kidney stone. **B.** A computed tomography (CT) scan of a kidney stone.

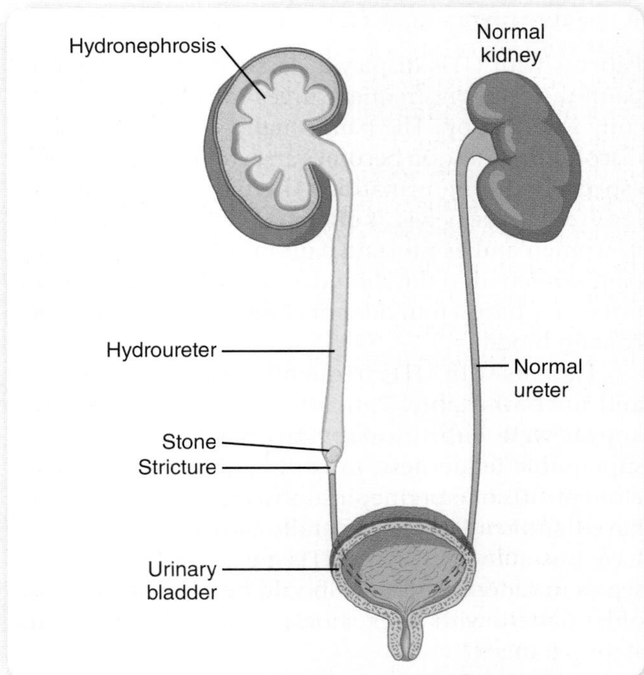

Figure 21-6 When a kidney stone obstructs the flow of urine, the patient may have blood in the urine (hematuria) and flank tenderness.

The most common types of stones are calcium oxalate and calcium phosphate, accounting for up to 80% of kidney stones.[8] It is thought that they form when the concentration of calcium oxalate or phosphate becomes too high in the urine, although other theories exist. Their formation may have a hereditary component, and risk is increased in people with a history of gout, gastric bypass surgery, and certain metabolic disorders. Struvite stones are more common in women and are associated with chronic UTIs or frequent catheterization. Uric acid stones are most common in those with a history of gout and are more common in dry and arid regions of the United States. Cystine stones are associated with a condition that causes large amounts of amino acids and proteins to be excreted in the urine.

Assessment

Patients who have kidney stones are almost always in pain. It usually starts in the flank but may migrate forward, toward the groin, as the stone passes through the system. The patient may feel vague discomfort that progresses to intense pain within 30 to 60 minutes. Kidney stone pain can be severe, and it is frequently described as the worst pain of a person's life. Be sure to obtain a detailed patient and family history, as this can supply clues to the cause of the stone.

Some patients appear agitated and restless, pacing and moving about in an attempt to relieve the pain. Other patients try to remain motionless to guard the abdomen. Either behavior makes palpation of the abdomen difficult. Vital signs vary according to the severity of pain. The greater the pain, the higher the patient's blood pressure and pulse will be. Patients often present with **hematuria**, and if the stone is obstructing urine flow in the ureter Figure 21-6, with flank tenderness.

> **Words of Wisdom**
>
> Patients with kidney stones usually have severe, nearly unbearable pain, and should be given aggressive pain control, such as narcotic analgesics (ie, morphine, fentanyl). Because higher-than-usual doses are often required, naloxone (Narcan) must be readily available in the event that central nervous system depression occurs. Follow local protocols or contact medical control as needed regarding pain relief for these patients.

Management

The prehospital management of kidney stones centers on pain relief. After ensuring the ABCs, allow the patient to assume a position of comfort. Administer analgesia; if your local protocols do not allow for this, contact medical control regarding pain relief options. Nitrous oxide is an alternative treatment to narcotics. Establish an IV line and administer IV fluids to hydrate the patient and antiemetics as needed.

Some kidney stones can be treated without surgery and will pass on their own. Management is focused on supporting the patient with hydration, pain control, and antiemetics. In addition, an alpha (α)-blocker such as tamsulosin (Flomax) is often used to relax smooth muscle in the bladder neck to allow increased urine flow. When a UTI is present along with an obstructing kidney stone, the patient may have signs and symptoms of a UTI and can become quite ill and septic; this is an emergency requiring urologic intervention. The treatment approach for persistent stones depends on the size, consistency, and location of the stones. Treatment options include the following:

- **Extracorporeal lithotripsy.** High-energy shock waves break up stones from outside the body, resulting in much smaller stone fragments and dust that can pass easily.
- **Cystoscopy with stent placement.** Cystoscopy is the direct visualization of the ureter and urinary collection system. Visualization is accomplished by inserting a small camera through the urethra and into the ureter. A stent can be placed to enlarge the diameter of the ureter and allow for stone passage.
- **Percutaneous nephrostomy (PCN) tube placement.** A PCN tube is a small catheter that is placed from the outside of the body into the kidney to allow for the drainage of material that is obstructed by a stone. This method is frequently used to decompress the kidney when there is an infection associated with a stone.

Table 21-2 Signs and Symptoms of Acute Kidney Injury

Type of Acute Kidney Injury	Signs and Symptoms
Prerenal	Hypotension Tachycardia Dizziness Thirst
Intrarenal	Flank pain Joint pain Oliguria Hypertension Headache Confusion Seizure
Postrenal	Pain in lower flank, abdomen, groin, and genitalia Oliguria Distended bladder Hematuria Peripheral edema

Acute Kidney Injury

Acute kidney injury (AKI) is a sudden decrease in the rate of filtration through the glomeruli, causing toxins to accumulate in the blood. This loss of function may occur over a period of several days. AKI is most often secondary to another disease process and is found in 1% of patients admitted to hospitals, rising to 5% during the course of hospital admission. Up to 20% of critically ill patients develop AKI, and the mortality for these patients has been reported to be as high as 70%.[9]

Urine output of less than 500 mL/day is called **oliguria**. Complete cessation of urine production is called **anuria**. Whenever AKI occurs, the patient may experience generalized edema, acid buildup, and high levels of nitrogenous and metabolic wastes in the blood. If left untreated, AKI can lead to life-threatening volume overload, hyperkalemia, uremia, and metabolic acidosis.

AKI is classified into three types, based on the area in which the failure occurs: prerenal, intrarenal, and postrenal. The signs and symptoms of each type are summarized in Table 21-2.

Pathophysiology

The toxic buildup of nitrogenous wastes and salts in the blood associated with AKI causes impaired mentation, fluid retention, tachycardia, acid-base imbalances, and increased PR and QT intervals associated with hyperkalemia.

Prerenal acute kidney injury is caused by hypoperfusion of the kidneys. In other words, not enough blood passes into the glomeruli for them to produce filtrate. The most common causes of prerenal AKI are hypovolemia (low blood volume caused by hemorrhage or dehydration), trauma, shock, sepsis, and heart failure. Prerenal AKI is often reversible if the underlying condition can be treated and perfusion restored to the kidney. Hepatorenal syndrome is a specific type of AKI that occurs in patients with advanced liver disease, in which renal perfusion is severely decreased due to portal hypertension. The prognosis of patients with hepatorenal syndrome is linked to their recovery from the inciting liver disease, and as such is much worse than for other forms of AKI.[10]

Intrarenal acute kidney injury (IAKI) involves damage to one of three areas in the kidney: the glomeruli capillaries and small blood vessels, the cells of the kidney tubules, or the renal parenchyma (the interstitial cells around the nephrons). Damage to the small vessels and glomeruli hinders blood flow through these vital parts of the nephrons. This damage is often caused by immune-mediated diseases (eg, type 1 diabetes mellitus). Tubule damage can be caused by hypoperfusion leading to acute tubular necrosis or toxins (eg, heavy metals). Rhabdomyolysis is another cause of IAKI, in which the released myoglobin damages the tubules. Chronic inflammation of the interstitial cells surrounding the nephrons (**interstitial nephritis**) can also produce IAKI. This type of renal failure may be caused by medications such as antibiotics, anticancer drugs, alcohol, and drugs of abuse (eg, cocaine).

Postrenal acute kidney injury is caused by obstruction of urine flow from the kidneys. The source of this obstruction is often a blockage of the urethra by an enlarged prostate, kidney stones, blood clots, or strictures. This blockage raises pressure in the nephrons, which eventually shuts them down.

Regardless of the mechanism, all forms of AKI lead to a common ending: the inability of the kidneys to carry out their cleansing functions. This can lead to the development of hyperkalemia (an increase in the blood potassium level), metabolic acidosis (an increase in the hydrogen ion content of the blood), and uremia (an increase of urea in the blood). These conditions are life-threatening emergencies that can lead to fatal cardiac dysrhythmias secondary to hyperkalemia and acidosis, hypotension secondary to acidosis, and mental status changes secondary to uremia.

Assessment

The presentation of the patient with AKI will vary based on the cause. Patients with prerenal AKI will generally appear dehydrated or in shock with pale, cool, and moist skin. Frequently, a decreased urine output or darkening of the urine will be reported. Flank pain may also be present, particularly in the patient with intrarenal AKI. In patients with postrenal AKI, there usually will be pain in the suprapubic area related to bladder distention or in the penis from obstruction. More severe cases of AKI may present with altered mental status or signs of heart failure.

During the physical exam, you should fully evaluate the abdomen for other causes of discomfort or the presence of ascites. Assess flank tenderness. Perform an ECG to evaluate for dysrhythmias or signs of hyperkalemia. Evaluate for signs of infection, such as a fever or dysuria, and closely monitor vital signs for signs of shock.

Management

Because the metabolic changes caused by AKI can be life threatening, it is imperative that the treatment plan support and manage the ABCs as needed. Consider administering an IV bolus if the patient exhibits signs of shock, but use caution to prevent pulmonary edema. Patients with concern for rhabdomyolysis may benefit from IV fluid boluses. If signs of hyperkalemia are present on the ECG, discuss with medical control, and consider treating with IV calcium and bicarbonate.

YOU are the Paramedic PART 4

You explain to your patient that her condition requires that blood be drawn, and that it is necessary to establish an IV line to perform the blood draw and to administer fluids. Your partner has assembled the stair chair, listened to lung sounds, and placed her on the cardiac monitor. After you initiate the IV line and draw blood samples, you tell her, "We are going to put you in this chair with wheels to take you down the stairs." Her father tells you that is probably not a good idea because she "doesn't do well sitting up."

Recording Time: 10 Minutes	
Respirations	24 breaths/min
Pulse	112 beats/min
Skin	Flushed, sweaty
Blood pressure	108/60 mm Hg; lying down
Oxygen saturation (Spo_2)	98%
Pupils	PERRLA
Blood glucose level	96 mg/dL

7. What should you consider with regard to moving the patient to the ambulance based on the father's comment?
8. What other questions may you have for the patient?

The increase of metabolites in patients with AKI may be toxic to the kidneys. Many medications can be nephrotoxic (toxic to the kidneys), including many analgesics and antibiotics. Consult medical control if you suspect AKI and are transporting a patient with antibiotic or analgesic drips. Many patients with AKI have other comorbid diseases that also may need to be addressed.

▶ Chronic Kidney Disease

As mentioned earlier, in the United States, over 468,000 people are on long-term dialysis.[1] In the population age 65 years and older, the incidence of chronic kidney disease is growing rapidly, and it doubled from 2000 to 2008. In the United States, over 20 million people have some form of this condition.[11]

Pathophysiology

Chronic kidney disease (CKD) is progressive and irreversible inadequate kidney function that is the result of permanent loss of nephrons. This disease develops over months or years. More than half of all cases are a consequence of systemic disease, such as diabetes or hypertension. CKD can also be caused by congenital disorders or prolonged pyelonephritis.

As the damaged nephrons cease to function, scarring occurs in the kidneys. The tissue begins to shrink and waste away as the scarring progresses, leading to a loss of nephrons and renal mass. As kidney function diminishes, waste products and fluid build up in the blood. Uremia (an increased concentration of urea and other waste products in the blood) and **azotemia** (an increased level of nitrogenous wastes in the blood) develop, leading to systemic complications such as hypertension, heart failure, anemia, and electrolyte imbalances.

Assessment

Patients with CKD may have an altered level of consciousness caused by electrolyte imbalances and their effects on transmission of nerve impulses in the brain. Patients may also present with lethargy, nausea, headaches, cramps, signs of anemia, weakness, vomiting, anorexia, increased thirst, pruritus, and hypertension. Ask if the patient still produces urine, and ask the patient to describe the appearance of any urine. Urine volume may have decreased or the urine may appear rusty brown.

> **Documentation & Communication**
>
> In patients with CKD, frequently assess mental status, noting any apparent decline or improvement. Document your findings and include them in your report to the receiving facility.

In a patient with CKD, the skin is pale, cool, and moist, and the patient may appear jaundiced because of the buildup of nitrogenous wastes. A powdery accumulation of uric acid called **uremic frost** may also be present, especially on the face. The skin may have bruises from coagulopathy, and muscle twitching may be present.

Patients with CKD exhibit edema in the extremities and face because of fluid imbalances; they can also be hypotensive and tachycardic if dehydrated or infected. If hyperkalemia develops, alterations in the waveforms and intervals can be seen on the ECG. Pericarditis and pulmonary edema are also common in patients with CKD and should be evaluated during auscultation of the chest.

Management

Because CKD is a chronic condition, management of a patient with CKD is generally not acutely performed in the field. However, there are some special considerations when treating a patient with CKD for other complaints. Patients with CKD may be at higher risk for pulmonary edema because they may not have the full ability to regulate their fluid balance; this possibility should be taken into consideration if a fluid bolus is planned. Patients with CKD have an increased risk of cardiac disease; any complaint of chest pain should be taken seriously.

> **Words of Wisdom**
>
> Do not give medications to patients with chronic kidney disease unless specifically instructed to do so by medical control.

Transport should be undertaken in a calm manner; talk quietly and confidently with the patient. If the patient has an altered mental status, be sure to assess his or her orientation frequently and record any changes.

▶ End-Stage Renal Disease

Pathophysiology

If left untreated, acute or chronic kidney disease will progress to **end-stage renal disease (ESRD)**. In a patient with ESRD, the kidneys are unable to function and toxic waste materials build up in the patient's blood. ESRD is fatal unless treated by dialysis or renal transplant. At the end of 2015, over 661,000 people in the United States were undergoing treatment for ESRD.

Assessment

The patient with ESRD is chronically ill, and assessment findings can change based on the amount of time from the last dialysis. After dialysis, patients can appear well, but occasionally they will be weak or dehydrated. If a patient has missed dialysis, he or she will frequently present with signs of volume overload: shortness of breath and peripheral edema. If toxins have accumulated, the patient may have uremic frost, confusion, and muscle twitching. Most patients with ESRD will have some form of coagulopathy, and easy bruising may be apparent. Weakness and easy fatigue can be chronic and pronounced, and most patients with ESRD will be anemic. Evaluate the ECG for signs of hyperkalemia, particularly if dialysis was missed. As with patients with CKD, any chest pain should be taken seriously, and a full cardiac assessment should be performed. Patients with ESRD are more prone to infections and pericarditis as well as pericardial effusions: consider these in your differential diagnosis based on the complaint. If a patient with ESRD has been untreated for some time, significant confusion, seizures, and even coma can occur.

Words of Wisdom

Patients with ESRD who are on hemodialysis will sometimes require ambulance transportation between their home and the dialysis facility. These transports may become routine for prehospital providers; however, it is important that you always complete a full assessment and be alert for changes in mental status or vital signs that could suggest an acute condition.

Management

Definitive treatment for patients with ESRD is limited to renal dialysis or kidney transplant. When managing a patient with ESRD, ensure ABC stability and provide supportive care as needed. If a patient appears to have volume overload, consider use of a diuretic if urine is still produced. If a patient appears dehydrated or in shock, carefully administer a fluid bolus and closely monitor for signs of pulmonary edema. If there is chest pain or signs of cardiac ischemia, treat with nitroglycerin and aspirin per local protocol. If a patient has missed dialysis, be alert for hyperkalemia and treat with calcium and bicarbonate as directed by local protocol. Any time a patient with ESRD is found in cardiac arrest, strongly consider hyperkalemia as the cause.

YOU are the Paramedic PART 5

Because family members serve as invaluable sources of information, you thank the patient's father. You explain that it is necessary to move her in order to treat her properly, but that you will handle her very gently and you will prepare for changes in her condition. As you help the patient slowly sit up, she reports some dizziness, but seems to tolerate the position. You buckle her into the stair chair and explain how she will be moved down the stairs. You reach the front door, transfer her to the gurney, and cover her with blankets. You reassess her in the ambulance, and she tells you she feels better lying down. You note that her orthostatic vital signs are positive for change. After contacting medical control, you are advised to administer another 500-mL bolus of normal saline. You are further advised to administer ondansetron (Zofran), 4 mg, and to begin transport.

Recording Time: 15 Minutes	
Respirations	24 breaths/min
Pulse	120 beats/min
Skin	Flushed, sweaty
Blood pressure	100/50 mm Hg; lying down
Oxygen saturation (Spo_2)	98%
Pupils	PERRLA
IV fluids	500 mL normal saline (NS); repeated

9. What may you consider requesting from medical control in addition to antiemetics?
10. How will her condition affect transport?

Renal Dialysis

Although not truly a urologic disorder, **renal dialysis** and associated problems may require prehospital interventions. Renal dialysis is a technique for filtering toxic wastes from the blood, removing excess fluid, and restoring the normal balance of electrolytes Figure 21-7.

There are two types of dialysis—peritoneal dialysis and hemodialysis. In peritoneal dialysis, large amounts of specially formulated dialysis fluid are infused into (and then drained from) the abdominal cavity. This fluid remains in the cavity for 1 to 2 hours, allowing equilibrium to occur as waste diffuses across the peritoneal membrane and into the fluid. Peritoneal dialysis is very effective but carries a high risk of peritonitis; consequently, aseptic technique is essential. With proper training, however, peritoneal dialysis can be performed in the home.

In hemodialysis, the patient's blood circulates through a dialysis machine that functions in much the same way (albeit not as elegantly) as a normal kidney. Hemodialysis involves vascular access through either a fistula or an arteriovenous (AV) shunt, or in emergencies, a central venous catheter. A **fistula**, **shunt**, or **arteriovenous graft** is a surgically created arterial-to-venous vessel anastomosis tunneled through the subcutaneous tissue. It is usually located in the forearm or upper arm Figure 21-8. The patient is connected to the dialysis machine using this shunt, which allows blood to flow from the body into the dialysis machine and back into the body.

In patients with cardiac or respiratory arrest, when intraosseous access is difficult or impossible, the fistula or shunt may be used for IV access; the procedure should be performed only in accordance with local protocols. In all other instances, an IV site in the opposite arm should be selected. AV shunts should not be used for routine blood draws, and blood pressure readings should be taken using the opposite arm.

The only time you are likely to see a dialysis machine is if your service transports patients to and from dialysis centers. If there is a dialysis machine in a private residence, treatments will most likely be performed by a trained dialysis technician or possibly by the patient or family members.

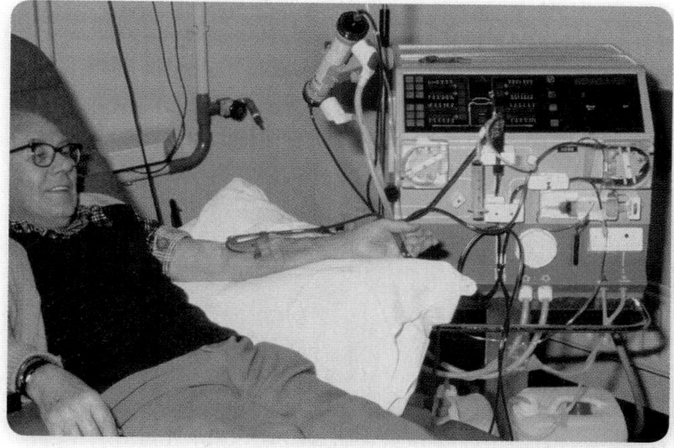

Figure 21-7 A patient undergoing dialysis.

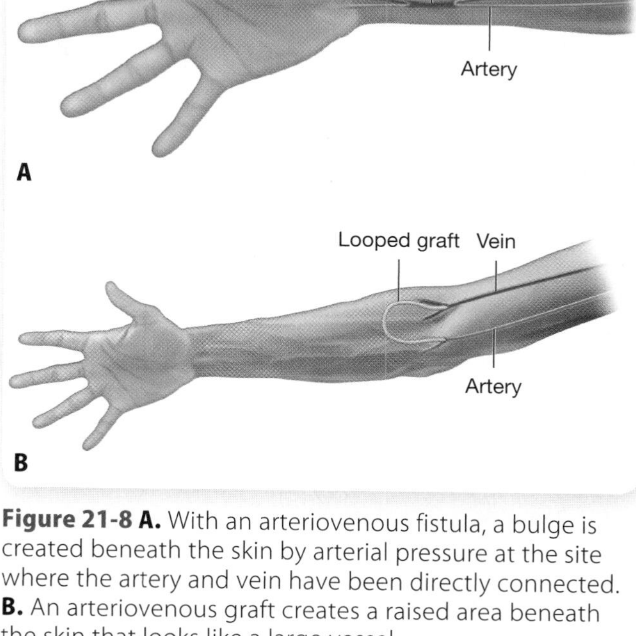

Figure 21-8 A. With an arteriovenous fistula, a bulge is created beneath the skin by arterial pressure at the site where the artery and vein have been directly connected. **B.** An arteriovenous graft creates a raised area beneath the skin that looks like a large vessel.

Patients requiring chronic dialysis usually undergo the process every 2 or 3 days for 3 to 5 hours. Many receive dialysis in the hospital or in community dialysis facilities, but a significant number have home dialysis units. Patients undergoing dialysis at home usually have extensive training in the procedures, and often someone else in the home has also been trained. If a problem with the machine occurs, the patient or family member may know more about it than you do, so always ask what the patient has done prior to your arrival.

Whereas patients undergoing chronic dialysis can experience the same spectrum of illnesses and injuries as other patients, they are particularly vulnerable to certain problems, either because of the dialysis itself or because of the underlying renal failure. Problems associated with dialysis may result from accidental disconnection from the machine, bleeding from a fistula or shunt, malfunction of the machine, or rapid shifts in fluids and electrolytes that produce hypotension, potassium imbalances, and disequilibrium syndrome. The management of medical emergencies resulting from dialysis is summarized in Table 21-3.

People who miss dialysis treatments will often present with signs of electrolyte imbalance, including weakness

Table 21-3 Medical Emergencies in Dialysis Patients

Problem	Prehospital Management
Problems related to dialysis itself:	
Hypotension	Administer 50 mL of normal saline intravenously.
Hemorrhage from the fistula or shunt	If the shunt cannot be reconnected, clamp it off; apply direct pressure to control bleeding; check for signs of shock.
Potassium imbalance	For hypokalemia: treat bradycardia with atropine. For hyperkalemia: calcium and bicarbonate may be considered in the event that a lab value was obtained at a sending facility.
Disequilibrium syndrome	Provide only supportive treatment.
Air embolism	Position the patient in the left lateral recumbent position with about 10° of head-down tilt.
Machine dysfunction	Turn off machine; clamp ends of shunt; disconnect patient from machine; transport.
Problems to which dialysis patients are more vulnerable:	
Heart failure	Administer oxygen; place in sitting position; administer diuretic if the patient is producing urine; provide rapid transport to dialysis-capable facility.
Myocardial infarction and cardiac dysrhythmias	Treat as any other patient, but use caution in administering any medications.
Hypertension	Transport; provide supportive care.
Pericardial tamponade	Provide emergency transport as soon as detected.
Uremic pericarditis	Administer oxygen; allow patient to assume position of comfort; transport.

of muscles, cramping, pulmonary edema, and uremic frost. Other general complications of dialysis include muscle cramps, nausea and vomiting, and infections at the fistula or shunt site.

Hypotension and Shock

A sudden drop in blood pressure is not uncommon during or immediately after a patient undergoes dialysis, but it can lead to cardiac arrest if not promptly detected and treated.

Words of Wisdom

When you measure the blood pressure in a dialysis patient, use the arm that does not have the shunt.

The patient may feel light-headed or become confused, and often he or she yawns more than usual. Because dialysis alters the blood's chemistry, the patient may experience an electrolyte imbalance. For this reason, you should always monitor dialysis patients for cardiac dysrhythmias. Shock secondary to bleeding is also possible from any number of causes, such as hypovolemia resulting from fluid shifts or bleeding due to less functional platelets. Bleeding may also occur at the site of the dialysis cannula and should be controlled with direct pressure.

Potassium Imbalance

One consequence of renal impairment is the inability to excrete ingested potassium. As a consequence, CKD patients are prone to the development of hyperkalemia. ECG changes to intervals and waveforms may be seen.

Hypokalemia may also occur as a consequence of overaggressive dialysis. The potassium level is most likely to fall during or immediately after a dialysis cycle. The patient may be hypotensive, and cardiac dysrhythmias may be present. Treat the dysrhythmia if it is hemodynamically significant or persistently symptomatic (see Chapter 17, *Cardiovascular Emergencies*).

Disequilibrium Syndrome

Dialysis rapidly lowers the concentration of urea in the blood, whereas the concentration of solutes in the cerebrospinal fluid (CSF) remains high. Water, of course, moves by osmosis from a solution of lower concentration into a solution of higher concentration. Thus, as a consequence of dialysis, water initially shifts from the bloodstream into the CSF, thereby mildly increasing intracranial pressure. When this occurs, the patient may experience **disequilibrium syndrome**, a condition characterized by nausea, vomiting, headache, and confusion. After a few hours, the fluid will re-equilibrate between the blood and CSF, and the patient's symptoms will improve.

Words of Wisdom

In the field, it may be impossible to distinguish between disequilibrium syndrome and stroke or subdural hematoma, other conditions to which dialysis patients are particularly vulnerable. In such a case, transport the patient to the hospital immediately for a full neurologic evaluation.

Air Embolism

If any of the fittings and connections in the dialysis system are loose, air may enter the system, producing an **air embolism** in the patient. Symptoms of an air embolism include sudden dyspnea, hypotension, and cyanosis. If you suspect an air embolism, disconnect the patient from the dialysis machine, place him or her in the left lateral recumbent position with about 10° of head-down tilt, and transport immediately.

▶ Male Genital Tract Conditions

Epididymitis and Orchitis

One possible complication of male UTI is **epididymitis**, an infection that causes inflammation of the epididymis along the posterior border of the testis. When one or both testes become infected, this is called **orchitis**. With orchitis, the infection causes one or both testes to become enlarged and tender, causing pain and swelling in the scrotum. Swelling may occur in the groin on the affected side. The pain may increase during bowel movements. The patient frequently will have a fever, and the urine will have a foul odor.

Prehospital management of these conditions is supportive. Because the patient likely is in pain, consider administering analgesics.

Fournier Gangrene

If bacteria enter the scrotum or perineum, **Fournier gangrene** may occur. This infection causes necrosis of the subcutaneous tissue and muscle in the scrotum. The patient will be febrile and the scrotum and perineum will be tender, warm, and erythematous. Purulent drainage may be present, and if unchecked, skin in the area may become gray-black. This is a true emergency and prompt transport to the hospital is indicated. These patients can rapidly become septic and unstable, and will require aggressive treatment with IV fluids.

Priapism

Priapism, a painful, tender, persistent erection, can result from sickle cell disease, leukemia, spinal cord injury, and certain medications, such as antidepressants, anticonvulsants, and those used to treat erectile dysfunction. This condition is discussed in more detail in Chapter 36, *Abdominal and Genitourinary Trauma*. Be sure to maintain the patient's privacy and do not make assumptions about the cause of the condition. Whatever the cause, treat all patients with respect, and administer analgesics for pain. If a spinal cord injury is suspected, use proper immobilization techniques.

Words of Wisdom

A patient who sustained blunt renal trauma often presents with flank pain and hematuria (blood in the urine) that usually goes undetected until evaluation in the ED. Obvious hematomas or ecchymoses over the upper abdomen, middle back, or lower rib cage may also suggest renal injuries. Keep this in mind when assessing a patient with a urologic emergency (discussed in detail in Chapter 36, *Abdominal and Genitourinary Trauma*).

Phimosis and Paraphimosis

Phimosis is the inability to retract the distal foreskin over the glans penis **Figure 21-9A**. This condition can be congenital or acquired, generally from poor hygiene or recurrent infections and scarring of the foreskin. Prehospital treatment includes cold compresses and transport.

Paraphimosis results when the foreskin is retracted over the glans penis and becomes entrapped **Figure 21-9B**. The tightness of the foreskin causes the glans to swell even further, making it even harder to slide the foreskin back into the normal position. Paraphimosis can occur after

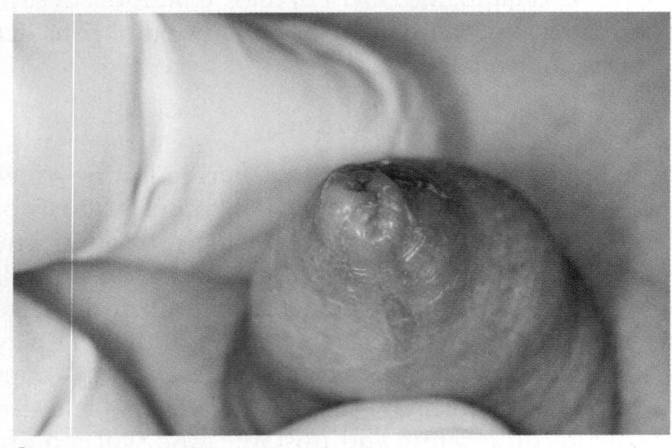
A

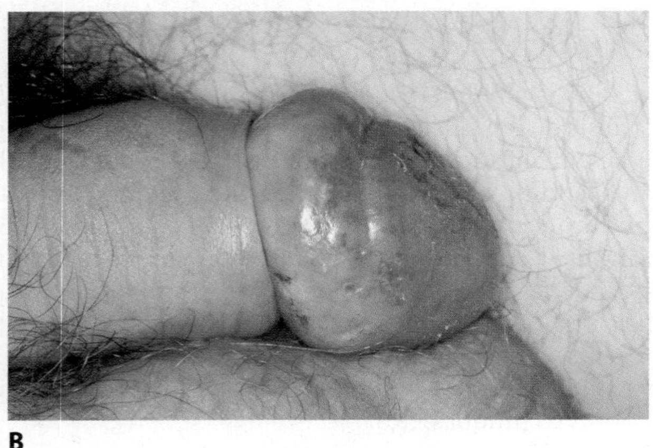
B

Figure 21-9 A. Phimosis. **B.** Paraphimosis.

manual retraction of the foreskin, such as when a Foley catheter is placed. It can also occur after phimosis retraction or after piercings of the glans penis. Paraphimosis is a true emergency. Failure to relieve the paraphimosis can result in necrosis of the glans.

Benign Prostate Hypertrophy

Benign prostate hypertrophy (BPH) is an age-related nonmalignant (noncancerous) enlargement of the prostate gland. It occurs in about 50% of men older than age 50 years and continues to increase with age beyond that.[12] It may be asymptomatic, or it may lead to difficulty starting urine flow, a slow, weak urine flow once started, incomplete emptying of the bladder, increased urination at night, and urinary retention. If the prostate becomes infected, a condition called **prostatitis** occurs, which can present with symptoms similar to a UTI as well as with fever, tremors, or urinary obstruction.

Testicular Masses

Testicular masses rarely require prehospital treatment. They may be painful or painless, and if painful, the pain may radiate up the spermatic cord or be localized to a specific scrotal point. Most are benign cystic masses or a varicocele—a painless mass of dilated veins posterior to the testicle. Testicular cancer usually presents as a painless solid lump on the testicle.

Testicular Torsion

Testicular torsion is a twisting of the testicle on the spermatic cord, from which it is suspended. This condition is associated with the sudden onset of scrotal pain and swelling. It is a medical emergency if the twisting of the vessels reduces blood flow to the testis. The torsion is usually unilateral, occurring in only one testis at a time. Torsions may occur with or without blunt trauma, a testicular lump, infection, or blood in the semen. Patients should be carefully and promptly transported and allowed to assume the position of greatest comfort. Analgesics may be given for pain control.

YOU are the Paramedic SUMMARY

1. What concerns may you have about the scene?

Performing a scene assessment is essential to ensure the safety of you and your crew. Knowing this is an older home with a narrow stairwell and the patient is on the second floor should prompt you to consider requesting additional personnel if needed for safe moving and lifting.

2. Although you have not seen your patient yet, what information do you already know that is part of the primary survey?

Because you heard your patient call out for her father telling him she was about to "be sick again," you know that she is alert, has a patent airway, and is breathing. This information may change rapidly, but you have gathered a lot of information before seeing her.

3. What concerns do you have about her history, signs, and symptoms?

More information is needed to narrow your differential diagnosis. Causes for concern include her skin signs, which point to fever/infection, as well as dizziness while standing. She is likely to have positive orthostatic vital signs and be significantly dehydrated because of the vomiting.

4. What should be done with the emesis?

Do not forget to look at the emesis for any signs of blood. Follow local protocols regarding transport of specimens to the hospital.

5. What additional assessment techniques might you use?

One technique used to assess for kidney infection or pyelonephritis is to place your fist over the flank and gently tap with the other hand. If the kidney is infected, this will elicit a painful response; therefore, you should use this technique with caution.

6. Why is assessing her body temperature important?

Assessing body temperature is important and should not be forgotten in the prehospital setting. Having appropriate thermometers can provide a wealth of information in hypothermic and hyperthermic patients. Assessing this patient's temperature, along with other assessment findings, can assist you in treating and documenting infection.

7. What should you consider with regard to moving the patient to the ambulance based on the father's comment?

You should be prepared for neurologic symptoms including syncope. You may have to adjust your method of moving her to the ambulance. Prehospital providers have a wide range of moving and lifting options to accommodate patient needs, and access/egress challenges. In this scenario, moving the patient via a Reeves sleeve may be another option if she becomes too symptomatic while sitting up in a stair chair.

8. What other questions may you have for the patient?

Because she is a woman of childbearing age, you should ask her questions about her last menstrual cycle. Also ask about urination—color, frequency, odor, the presence of blood, or other symptoms.

9. What may you consider requesting from medical control in addition to antiemetics?

Pain management in the patient with a kidney emergency is an important part of patient care. Many protocols will specifically address pain associated with kidney stones. Follow local protocols.

10. How will her condition affect transport?

This patient is not demonstrating signs and symptoms of a life-threatening renal emergency. Therefore, she should be transported in a position of comfort with minimal jostling and slow, careful driving to avoid excessive bumps, sudden acceleration, deceleration, or turns.

YOU are the Paramedic SUMMARY *(continued)*

<table>
<tr><th colspan="6">EMS Patient Care Report (PCR)</th></tr>
<tr><td>Date: 04-11-18</td><td colspan="2">Incident No.: 20227</td><td colspan="2">Nature of Call: Medical</td><td>Location: 327 West Main Street</td></tr>
<tr><td>Dispatched: 0600</td><td>En Route: 0603</td><td>At Scene: 0608</td><td>Transport: 0632</td><td>At Hospital: 0645</td><td>In Service: 0655</td></tr>
<tr><th colspan="6">Patient Information</th></tr>
<tr><td colspan="3">Age: 23
Sex: F
Weight (in kg [lb]): 70 kg (154 lb)</td><td colspan="3">Allergies: No known drug allergies
Medications: Cipro, OTC cranberry supplement
Past Medical History: UTIs
Chief Complaint: Lower back pain</td></tr>
</table>

<table>
<tr><th colspan="5">Vital Signs</th></tr>
<tr><td>Time: 0613</td><td>BP: 108/60</td><td>Pulse: 110</td><td>Respirations: 24</td><td>Spo_2: 98%</td></tr>
<tr><td>Time: 0618</td><td>BP: 108/60</td><td>Pulse: 112</td><td>Respirations: 24</td><td>Spo_2: 98%</td></tr>
<tr><td>Time: 0623</td><td>BP: 100/50</td><td>Pulse: 120</td><td>Respirations: 24</td><td>Spo_2: 98%</td></tr>
<tr><th colspan="5">EMS Treatment (circle all that apply)</th></tr>
<tr><td colspan="2">Oxygen @ _______ L/min via (circle one):
NC NRM Bag-mask device</td><td>Assisted Ventilation</td><td>Airway Adjunct</td><td>CPR</td></tr>
<tr><td>Defibrillation</td><td>Bleeding Control</td><td>Bandaging</td><td>Splinting</td><td>Other:</td></tr>
<tr><th colspan="5">Narrative</th></tr>
</table>

Dispatched to female reporting lower back pain at 327 West Main Street. Pt 23 yo female lying on her right side in bed, vomiting into trash can. Alert, skin diaphoretic, very warm, flushed. Pt reporting lower back pain, stated she's been "feeling ill" for the past 2–3 days including burning with urination and n/v since last night around midnight. Urinating makes the pain worse. Pt describes lower back pain as "achy" radiating from flank to pubic bone. Pt rates severity as 4 on scale of 0 to 10 with 10 being the worst. Pt last ate yesterday 2100 hours.
Vital signs lying down as noted above. Temp 38.3°C, blood glucose level 96 mg/dL, PERRLA, HEENT atraumatic, breath sounds clear and equal bilaterally. Abd has overactive bowel tones, soft, diffuse tenderness in all 4 quadrants with increased tenderness of both lower, right flank pain, p/m/s/X4. Suspect possible pyelonephritis.
Established IV 18g NS 500-mL bolus. ECG ST w/o further ectopy. Moved pt with stair chair. Transported to WWMC. Contacted MCC for instructions to administer additional 500-mL bolus NS. Continued to monitor en route w/o changes. Arrived at ED transfer of care to J. Smith, RN.**End of report**

Prep Kit

Ready for Review

- Chronic kidney disease is the most common renal disorder. Kidney stones and urinary tract infections also affect many people.
- The genitourinary system includes the kidneys, urinary bladder, ureters, urethra, male and female reproductive organs, and specific structures within the kidneys.
- Urine forms in the nephrons. The nephrons are composed of the glomerulus, the glomerular capsule, the proximal convoluted tubule, the loop of Henle, and the distal convoluted tubule.
- The anatomy of the urethra is different in males and females. The female urethra is shorter and, therefore, more prone to urinary tract infections.
- Visceral pain is the type most often associated with genitourinary conditions. Referred pain originates in one organ or tissue but is perceived by the patient to be located in a different area of the body.
- The OPQRST (Onset, Provocation, Quality, Region/radiation/referral, Severity, Timing) mnemonic is used during the primary survey and secondary assessments to evaluate and reevaluate the type and severity of pain.
- In the physical exam, use the four-quadrant system and abdominal region mapping. Perform cardiac monitoring, and do not give patients with a possible genitourinary disease anything by mouth.
- Pain is managed with patient positioning, analgesics, and fluids as indicated, and supportive care.
- Symptoms of urinary tract infection include painful urination, frequent urges to urinate, difficulty urinating, and possibly referred pain in the shoulder or neck. The urine may have a foul odor and be cloudy. Management of patients with UTIs consists mainly of supportive care of the ABCs, allowing the patient to remain in a position of comfort, and possibly administering analgesics.
- Catheterization of the bladder allows a continuous outflow of urine and provides a means of measuring urine output in hemodynamically unstable patients. To avoid backflow of urine, the drainage bag should not be lifted above the level of the patient's bladder.
- Kidney stones result when an excess of insoluble salts or uric acid crystallizes in the urine. Symptoms include severe flank pain that may migrate to the groin. The pain may produce a spike in blood pressure and pulse rate.
- Acute kidney injury is a sudden decrease in filtration through the glomeruli, resulting in a buildup of toxins in the blood. The three types of acute kidney injury are prerenal, intrarenal, and postrenal. Signs and symptoms range from hypotension, tachycardia, dizziness, and thirst, to pain, oliguria, distended bladder, hematuria, and peripheral edema.
- Chronic kidney disease is progressive and results in irreversible inadequate kidney function. Nephrons become damaged, losing their functionality and causing a buildup of wastes and fluid in the blood. Signs and symptoms can include an altered level of consciousness, lethargy, nausea, headaches, cramps, anemia, bruised skin, edema in the extremities and face, hypotension, and tachycardia.
- Patients with acute or chronic kidney disease require support of airway, breathing, and circulation; possibly administration of medications to regulate acidosis, electrolyte imbalances, and fluid volume; and calm transport with emotional support.
- If left untreated, acute or chronic kidney disease will progress to end-stage renal disease, meaning that the kidneys are unable to function. Toxic waste materials build up in the patient's blood, leading to a multitude of potential signs and symptoms and possibly dysrhythmias. Prehospital care is supportive, including treating for shock and, under medical direction, regulating fluid imbalances, electrolyte abnormalities, and cardiovascular function.
- Renal dialysis is a procedure for removing toxic wastes and excess fluid from the blood. Dialysis patients usually have a fistula or shunt through which they are connected to the dialysis machine. Such patients are vulnerable to problems such as hypotension, potassium imbalance, disequilibrium syndrome, and air embolism.
- Always monitor dialysis patients for cardiac dysrhythmias. Shock secondary to bleeding is also possible from any number of causes. Watch for peaked T waves on the ECG, a classic sign of hyperkalemia.
- Specific conditions that may occur in the male genital tract include epididymitis, Fournier gangrene, priapism, phimosis, paraphimosis, benign prostate hypertrophy, testicular masses, and testicular torsion. Prehospital management for most of these conditions is supportive. Because the patient likely is in pain, consider administering analgesics, and transport gently.

Vital Vocabulary

acute kidney injury (AKI) A sudden decrease in filtration through the glomeruli.

air embolism The presence of air in the venous circulation, which forms a gas bubble that can block the outflow of blood from the right ventricle to

Prep Kit (continued)

the lung; can lead to cardiac arrest, shock, or other life-threatening complications.

anuria A complete cessation of urine production.

arteriovenous graft A surgical connection between an artery and a vein.

azotemia Increased nitrogenous wastes in the blood.

benign prostate hypertrophy (BPH) Age-related nonmalignant (noncancerous) enlargement of the prostate gland.

chronic kidney disease (CKD) Progressive and irreversible inadequate kidney function caused by the permanent loss of nephrons.

disequilibrium syndrome A condition characterized by nausea, vomiting, headache, and confusion, which results when, as a consequence of dialysis, water initially shifts from the bloodstream into the cerebrospinal fluid, mildly increasing intracranial pressure.

distal convoluted tubule (DCT) Connects with the kidney's collecting tubules.

end-stage renal disease (ESRD) A condition in which the kidneys are unable to function, and toxic waste materials build up in the patient's blood; occurs after acute or chronic kidney injury.

epididymitis An infection that causes inflammation of the epididymis along the posterior border of the testis; a possible complication of male urinary tract infection.

fistula A surgically created connection between an artery and a vein, usually in the arm, for dialysis access.

Fournier gangrene A condition that results from bacteria entering the skin of the scrotum or perineum, causing infection and subsequent necrosis of the subcutaneal tissue and muscle in the scrotum.

glomerular (Bowman) capsule A double-layered cup with the inner layer infiltrating and surrounding the capillaries of the glomerulus.

hematuria The presence of blood in the urine.

interstitial nephritis A chronic inflammation of the interstitial cells surrounding the nephrons.

intrarenal acute kidney injury (IAKI) A type of acute kidney injury characterized by damage in the kidney itself, often caused by immune-mediated diseases, prerenal acute kidney injury, toxins, heavy metals, some medications, or some organic compounds.

kidneys Solid, bean-shaped organs housed in the retroperitoneal space that filter blood and excrete body wastes in the form of urine.

kidney stones Solid crystalline masses formed in the kidney, resulting from an excess of insoluble salts or uric acid crystallizing in the urine; may become trapped anywhere along the urinary tract. Also called renal calculi.

loop of Henle The U-shaped portion of the renal tubule that extends from the proximal to the distal convoluted tubule; concentrates the filtrate and converts it to urine.

nephrons The structural and functional units of the kidney that form urine; composed of the glomerulus, the glomerular (Bowman) capsule, the proximal convoluted tubule, the loop of Henle, and the distal convoluted tubule.

oliguria Urine output of less than 500 mL/day.

orchitis A complication of a male urinary tract infection in which one or both testes become infected, enlarged, and tender, causing pain and swelling in the scrotum.

paraphimosis A condition that results when the foreskin is retracted over the glans penis and becomes entrapped; constriction of the glans causes it to swell even further.

phimosis Inability to retract the distal foreskin over the glans penis.

postrenal acute kidney injury A type of acute kidney injury caused by obstruction of urine flow from the kidneys, commonly caused by a blockage of the urethra by an enlarged prostate gland, blood clots, or strictures.

prerenal acute kidney injury A type of acute kidney injury that is caused by hypoperfusion of the kidneys, resulting from hypovolemia (hemorrhage, dehydration), trauma, shock, sepsis, and heart failure (secondary to myocardial infarction); often reversible if the underlying condition can be found and perfusion restored to the kidney.

priapism A painful, tender, persistent erection of the penis; can result from spinal cord injury, erectile dysfunction drugs, or sickle cell disease.

prostatitis Inflammation of the prostate gland.

proximal convoluted tubule (PCT) One of two complex sections of the nephron, the proximal convoluted tubule includes an enlargement at the end called the glomerular capsule.

pyelonephritis An upper urinary tract infection in which the kidneys are involved.

renal dialysis A technique for filtering the blood of its toxic wastes, removing excess fluids, and restoring the normal balance of electrolytes.

Prep Kit *(continued)*

shunt A connection between the arterial and venous system in which no gas exchange occurs.

testicular torsion Twisting of the testicle on the spermatic cord, from which it is suspended; associated with scrotal pain and swelling, and is a medical emergency.

uremia The presence of excessive amounts of urea and other waste products in the blood.

uremic frost A powdery buildup of uric acid, especially on the skin of the face.

ureters A pair of thick-walled, hollow tubes that transport urine from the kidneys to the bladder.

urethra A hollow tubular structure that drains urine from the bladder, expelling it from the body.

urinary bladder A hollow muscular sac in the midline of the lower abdominal area that stores urine until it is released from the body.

urinary incontinence The inability to control the release of urine from the bladder; loss of bladder control.

urinary retention Incomplete emptying of the bladder, or a complete lack of ability to empty the bladder.

urinary tract infections (UTIs) Infections, usually of the lower urinary tract (urethra and bladder), that occur when normal flora (bacteria that naturally populate the skin) enter the urethra and multiply.

urine Liquid waste products filtered out of the body by the urinary system.

▶ References

1. Newsroom. National Kidney Foundation website. https://www.kidney.org/news/newsroom/factsheets/FastFacts. Accessed February 13, 2017.
2. Lyon C, Clark DC. Diagnosis of acute abdominal pain in older patients. *Am Fam Physician.* 2006; 74(9):1537-1544.
3. Martel JW, Ownbey M, Simmons C. Stroke mimics: a clinical dilemma. *Emerg Med Rep.* 2015 Sept 20.
4. Manterola C, Vial M, Moraga J, Astudillo P. Analgesia in patients with acute abdominal pain. *Cochrane Database Syst Rev.* 2011 Jan 19; (1):CD005660.
5. Rui P, Kang K, Albert M. National Hospital Ambulatory Medical Care Survey: 2013 emergency department summary tables. U.S. Department of Health and Human Services, Centers for Disease Control and Prevention, National Center for Health Statistics. https://www.cdc.gov/nchs/data/ahcd/nhamcs_emergency/2013_ed_web_tables.pdf. Accessed February 20, 2017.
6. Khandelwal C, Kistler C. Diagnosis of urinary incontinence. *Am Fam Physician.* 2013 Apr 15; 87(8):543-550.
7. Scales CD, Smith AC, Hanley JM, Saigal CS. Urologic Diseases in America Project. Prevalence of kidney stones in the United States. *Eur Urol.* 2012;62(1):160-165.
8. Kirkali Z, Rasooly R, Star RA, Rodgers GP. Urinary stone disease: progress, status, and needs. *Urology.* 2015;86(4):651-653.
9. Lewington A, Kanagasundaram S. Clinical practice guidelines: acute kidney injury. The Renal Association website. www.renal.org/guidelines. Accessed May 6, 2016.
10. Karvellas CJ, Durand F, Nadim MK. Acute kidney injury in cirrhosis. *Crit Care Clin.* 2015 Oct;31(4):737-750.
11. Kidney disease statistics for the United States. National Institute of Diabetes and Digestive and Kidney Diseases website. htttps://www.niddk.nih.gov/health-information/health-statistics/Pages/kidney-disease-statistics-united-states.aspx. Accessed May 6, 2016.
12. Vuichoud C, Loughlin KR. Benign prostatic hyperplasia: epidemiology, economics and evaluation. *Urol Clin North Am.* 2009;36(4):403-415.

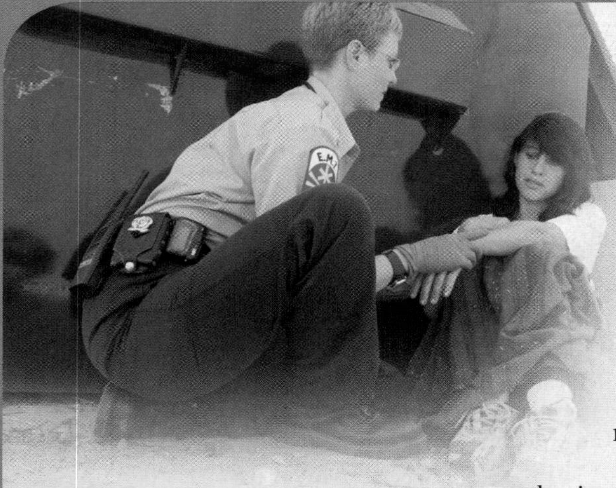

Assessment *in Action*

It is a beautiful sunny summer day. You and your partner are called to an apartment building for a boy reporting groin pain. On arrival, you first encounter the patient's mother, who states that her 15-year-old son has been experiencing severe on-and-off pain in his scrotum since he woke up this morning. He was reportedly fine and without any pain last night.

You move into a back bedroom where you meet the patient who is curled up in pain. He states that the pain is sharp and severe and has been getting worse with each episode. The current episode has been ongoing for almost an hour.

1. What is your chief concern?

- **A.** Duty to act
- **B.** Expectations of family
- **C.** Calling 9-1-1
- **D.** Scene safety

2. According to your differential diagnosis, you would expect this patient to experience:

- **A.** sudden, severe pain.
- **B.** intermittent pain.
- **C.** no pain.
- **D.** referred pain.

3. As you enter the bedroom, you see the patient is lying on the bed in the fetal position. Of the following injuries, which would be considered a true emergency?

- **A.** Urinary tract infection
- **B.** Testicular torsion
- **C.** Benign prostatic hypertrophy
- **D.** End-stage renal disease

4. From your choice in the preceding question, what treatment will be required?

- **A.** Antibiotics
- **B.** Surgical intervention
- **C.** Rest, ice, compression, elevation
- **D.** Steroids

5. How should you examine this patient's genital area?

- **A.** Never examine the genital area in the field.
- **B.** Ask the mother to remain present and explain to the patient the need for visual exam.
- **C.** Ask the mother to leave to ensure the patient's privacy.
- **D.** Ask the patient whether he would like his mother to be present for the exam.

6. How should this patient be treated in the field?

- **A.** Oxygen
- **B.** Immobilization
- **C.** Bandaging
- **D.** Analgesic

7. What is the feared complication of this diagnosis?

- **A.** Infertility
- **B.** Sepsis
- **C.** Cancer
- **D.** Chronic pain

8. What other conditions could be causing this pain?

9. How can you best ensure patient modesty while performing a genital exam?

10. What other issues or questions may arise from this diagnosis?

CHAPTER 22

Gynecologic Emergencies

National EMS Education Standard Competencies

Medicine

Integrates assessment findings with principles of epidemiology and pathophysiology to formulate a field impression and implement a comprehensive treatment/disposition plan for a patient with a medical complaint.

Gynecology

Recognition and management of shock associated with

- Vaginal bleeding (pp 1241-1242, 1246-1247)

Anatomy, physiology, assessment findings, and management of

- Vaginal bleeding (pp 1241-1242, 1245-1247)
- Sexual assault (to include appropriate emotional support) (pp 1248-1249)
- Infections (pp 1242-1244)

Anatomy, physiology, epidemiology, pathophysiology, psychosocial impact, presentations, prognosis, and management of common or major gynecologic diseases and/or emergencies

- Vaginal bleeding (pp 1241-1242, 1245-1247)
- Sexual assault (pp 1248-1249)
- Infections (pp 1242-1244)
- Pelvic inflammatory disease (pp 1242-1243)
- Ovarian cysts (p 1244)
- Dysfunctional uterine bleeding (pp 1245-1246)
- Vaginal foreign body (pp 1249-1250)

Knowledge Objectives

1. Recall the anatomy and physiology of the female reproductive system. (pp 1238-1240)
2. Identify the normal events of the menstrual cycle. (p 1239)
3. Describe the assessment process for patients with gynecologic emergencies. (pp 1239-1242)
4. Discuss the importance of history taking when assessing a patient with a gynecologic emergency. (pp 1240-1241)
5. Describe how to treat a patient with significant vaginal bleeding. (pp 1241-1242, 1245-1247)
6. Discuss the general management of a patient with a gynecologic emergency. (p 1242)
7. Discuss the management of a patient with gynecologic trauma. (p 1242)
8. Discuss the pathophysiology, assessment, and management of infections related to the gynecologic system. (pp 1242-1244)
9. Discuss the pathophysiology, assessment, and management of ovarian disorders. (p 1244)
10. Discuss the pathophysiology, assessment, and management of uterine disorders. (p 1245)
11. Discuss the pathophysiology, assessment, and management of ectopic pregnancy. (pp 1246-1248)
12. Discuss special concerns, assessment, and management, when caring for a suspected sexual assault patient. (pp 1248-1249)

Skills Objectives

There are no skills objectives for this chapter.

Introduction

Gynecology is the branch of medicine that deals with the diseases and routine physical care of the female reproductive system. This chapter first reviews the female anatomy and physiology, and then outlines issues that are unique to female patients, including conditions that may be encountered in the emergency setting. The chapter covers the gynecologic causes of abdominal pain and looks in detail at life-threatening conditions. Also discussed are the topics of vaginal bleeding and sexual assault, and how these two emergencies should be managed in the field.

Anatomy and Physiology Review

The female reproductive structures include the external female genitalia, uterus, vagina, cervix, fallopian tubes, ovaries, and the mammary glands Figure 22-1. The **ovaries** are a pair of organs that release eggs, or ova (singular, ovum), as well as reproductive hormones. The egg travels down the adjacent **fallopian tube** into the uterus.

The **uterus** is a pear-shaped organ where the **embryo**, or fertilized egg, implants and grows. The upper, convex portion of the uterus is called the fundus and internally, has a uterine cavity. The uterine wall consists of a muscular layer, called the myometrium, and the **endometrium**, or nutrient-rich inner layer, which is shed during **menstruation**, the monthly flow of blood. If the egg is fertilized (which usually occurs within the fallopian tube), it travels to the uterine cavity and implants into the endometrium, where it will grow and mature. The neck of the uterus, called the **cervix**, inserts into the **vagina**, which leads to the outside of the body. Together, the lower part of the uterus, the cervix, and the vagina are referred to as the birth canal. The **perineum** refers to the tissue between the vaginal opening and the anus.

The external female genitalia Figure 22-2, or vulva, include the **mons pubis**, a hair-covered fat pad overlying the symphysis pubis; the **labia majora**, rounded folds of

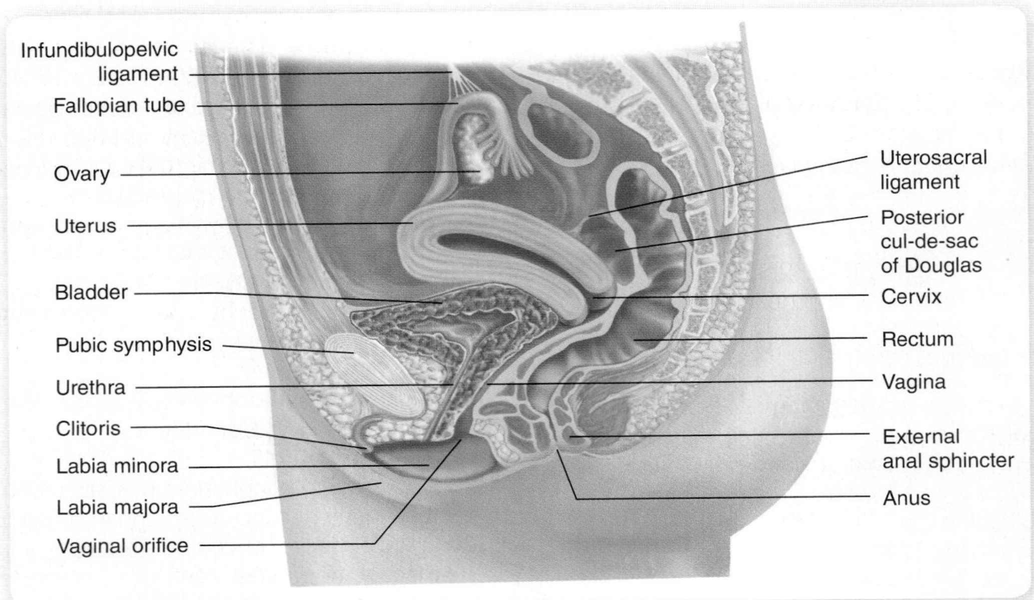

Figure 22-1 Anatomy of the female genital tract and pelvis.

YOU are the Paramedic PART 1

Your unit is dispatched for a patient with abdominal pain. While en route, the dispatcher tells you the patient is a 24-year-old woman who is reporting lower abdominal pain and vaginal bleeding. When you arrive at the residence, the patient's husband meets you. He tells you that his wife has had "problems with her period for months." He called 9-1-1 because she is in a lot of pain today.

1. What are you looking for in your scene size-up?
2. What are you looking for in your primary survey?

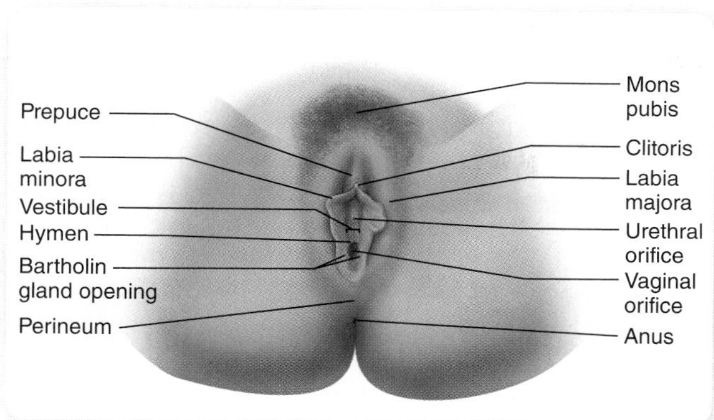

Figure 22-2 Anatomy of the external female genitalia.

external adipose tissue; and the **labia minora**, thinner, pink-red folds that extend anteriorly to form the **clitoris**, the region of sexual stimulation. Coarse, dark hair normally appears on the mons pubis in early puberty, becoming sparser later in life with the advent of menopause. The urethral meatus opens into the area between the clitoris and the vagina. Below the urethral meatus lies the opening to the vagina. This vaginal orifice is protected by the **hymen**. This membrane forms a border around the vaginal orifice, partially enclosing it. The hymen ruptures during the first intercourse, or may be ruptured before first intercourse by trauma or by events such as horseback riding, gymnastics, or other sports. Pain and vaginal bleeding will generally be present in such an event.

In some cases, the hymen may completely cover the vaginal orifice, a condition called *imperforate hymen*. If it remains undetected until puberty, this condition will block the flow of first menses, resulting in relatively acute pain, with severe constipation and low back pain. Such a condition may lead to endometriosis or cause other secondary painful effects as well. Imperforate hymen can also be caused by childhood sexual abuse, in which the imperforation results from scarring from digital or penile penetration.

▶ Menstruation

Menstruation, also called the menses, period, or menstrual cycle, is the normal discharge of blood, epithelial cells, mucus, and tissue from the uterine cavity. **Menarche** is the onset of the first menses, when a girl reaches childbearing age. **Menopause**, also called the female climacteric, is the cessation of ovarian function and of the menstrual cycle.

The menstrual cycle is divided into two phases: the ovarian cycle (ovarian changes) and the uterine cycle (changes in the uterus). The ovarian cycle is divided into the follicular phase (days 1 to 13) and the luteal phase (days 14 to 28). The uterine cycle is divided into the proliferative phase (days 5 to 14) and the secretory phase (days 15 to 28).

Ovulation occurs when an ovum, or egg, is released from an ovarian follicle. This usually occurs 14 days after the start of the previous menstrual period. In case of fertilization, the endometrium is prepared to receive the fertilized ovum. If the ovum is not fertilized, menstruation ensues with discharge of the endometrial lining. Menstruation lasts 4 to 6 days, with blood loss of approximately 25 to 65 mL. The menstrual cycle, and the hormones released during each of its phases, is discussed in more detail in Chapter 8, *Anatomy and Physiology*.

Some women may experience abdominal pain and cramping in the middle of the menstrual cycle. This pain and its accompanying symptoms result from the physiologic rupture of an ovarian follicle and are collectively called *mittelschmerz* (pronounced "MITT-ul-shmurz"; German for "middle pain"). In most cases, the pain is not severe; it may last only a few minutes or as long as 48 hours (average, 6 to 8 hours). Signs and symptoms include sharp, cramping pain in the lower abdomen, localized to one side, beginning mid-cycle, with a history of similar pain episodes during previous periods. The pain may also be reported as "switching sides" from month to month. The condition itself is not serious, and the pain can often be relieved by over-the-counter analgesics.

Amenorrhea is the absence or cessation of menses. This condition may be caused by a number of factors, but the most common cause is pregnancy. Exercise-induced amenorrhea is common in female athletes, particularly those who participate in physically intense sports. Amenorrhea may occur when a woman's body fat drops below a certain percentage. Amenorrhea can also be caused by emotional problems or extreme stress. In an adolescent or young adult, the condition may have its origination in anorexia nervosa; in this case, it is a symptom of the patient's malnutrition and emotional state.

Words of Wisdom

The most common cause of amenorrhea is pregnancy.

Patient Assessment

Women have many of the same conditions that cause abdominal pain in men—for example, renal colic, ulcers, gastroenteritis, cholecystitis, diverticulitis, pancreatitis, appendicitis, and dissecting aneurysm. In addition, there are numerous gynecologic causes of abdominal pain. Gynecologic emergencies are usually associated with one or more of the following signs or symptoms: vaginal bleeding, abdominal pain or tenderness, vomiting, fever, tachycardia, hypotension, diaphoresis, syncope, changes in stool pattern, dyspareunia (pain during intercourse), or urinary symptoms Figure 22-3.

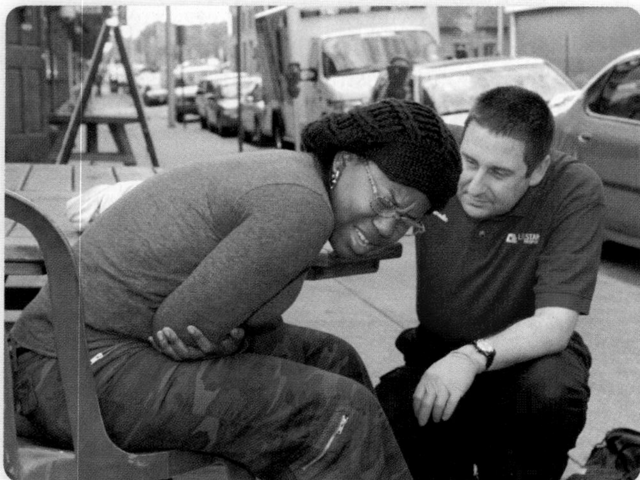

Figure 22-3 A patient experiencing a gynecologic emergency may be uncomfortable discussing her symptoms. Be professional and respectful so you can obtain the information needed to provide appropriate care.

Words of Wisdom

Any patient of childbearing years with abdominal pain should be considered to have a gynecologic emergency until proven otherwise.

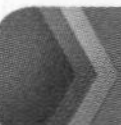

Scene Size-up

As always, begin with a thorough scene size-up. Is the scene safe? Will you need assistance? Gynecologic emergencies can involve large amounts of blood and body fluids that can be contaminated with communicable diseases.

All information you obtain will contribute to your assessment of the patient's overall health and the safety of the scene. In case of a crime scene, you may also be required to testify in court regarding the conditions at the scene.

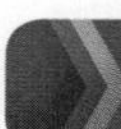

Primary Survey

When evaluating a patient with a potential gynecologic emergency, assess the ABCDEs (Airway, Breathing, Circulation, Disability, and Exposure), and manage life threats. Provide pain management and fluid resuscitation as indicated by the patient's condition. Even if bleeding from the vagina is significant, do not pack any dressings inside the vagina. Make note of the amount, color, and type of discharge or bleeding, including the presence of clots or tissue. Transport these patients to a hospital for further evaluation. If the patient passed any clots or tissue before or during transport, bring these with the patient to the hospital in a sealed container if possible.

Words of Wisdom

In the woman with abdominal pain, the most important things to look for are signs of shock.

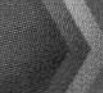

History Taking

A complete gynecologic history should include the chief complaint as well as associated symptoms. If vaginal bleeding has occurred, try to quantify this in pads per hour or in comparison with the patient's normal menstrual period. Ask about the date of the last normal menstrual period, regularity of menstrual cycles, whether a current pregnancy exists, number of previous pregnancies, number of pregnancies carried to term, number of miscarriages or abortions, history of prior gynecologic problems or surgeries, current sexual activity, type of birth control, and history of sexually transmitted diseases **Table 22-1**. (Sexually transmitted diseases are covered in Chapter 26, *Infectious Diseases*.)

Gynecologic emergencies can be highly embarrassing for the patient, and many women may be extremely uncomfortable about discussing their sexual history in front of strangers or even close family members. A teenage or

Table 22-1 Elements of the Gynecologic History
Current symptoms: Vaginal bleeding? Amount? Any tissue passed?
Current symptoms: Abdominal pain? Onset, duration, character, location, radiation, severity?
Current symptoms: Vaginal discharge? Color, amount, odor, itching?
Currently pregnant?
Current sexual activity? Birth control?
Last menstrual period (LMP)
Prior pregnancies (gravidity)
Prior births (parity)
Prior pregnancy complications or losses?
Prior cesarean sections or other abdominal surgery?
Other past medical history, medications, allergies
Prior or current sexually transmitted diseases

adolescent girl may want to keep her sexual history from her parents, and few women are comfortable with having their genitals exposed to a crowd of family, neighbors, paramedics, police officers, or firefighters. Protect the patient's modesty at all times while obtaining your history and conducting your assessment.

Obtaining an accurate and detailed patient assessment is of utmost importance when dealing with gynecologic issues. You may not be able to make a specific diagnosis in the field, but a thorough assessment and patient history will help determine whether the patient is experiencing a life-threatening emergency.

Documentation & Communication

Your attempts to obtain accurate, truthful information from the patient may be hindered by the presence of family members, loved ones, or bystanders. Removing nonessential personnel from the area will increase the likelihood that you obtain accurate information from the patient.

Secondary Assessment

When possible, the paramedic performing the physical examination should be the same gender as the patient. Limit the crowd to personnel required to perform the necessary tasks, and show the patient you respect her by being the advocate for her modesty. You also serve as a role model for other EMS providers when you act this way.

You should examine and assess the patient's abdomen. Inspect the abdomen for signs of abuse, such as bruising. Also note bruising in other areas, which could indicate possible abuse. The abdomen is a favorite target of abusers, especially if a woman is pregnant. Because clothing hides the evidence, the abdomen is also a favorite injection spot for chronic drug abusers. Look for a positive *Cullen sign* (ecchymosis at the umbilicus) or *Grey Turner sign* (ecchymosis at the flanks); either is indicative of internal bleeding.

Palpate the abdomen, starting at the quadrant farthest from the pain and working toward the quadrant where the pain is located. Examine this quadrant last. Is the abdomen rigid (possibly indicative of internal bleeding)? Is there point tenderness? Does the palpation elicit more pain? Is rebound tenderness present (indicative of infection, such as may be associated with appendicitis)? Are there masses present? If yes, are they pulsating (abdominal aortic aneurysm)?

What are the patient's vital signs? Is the blood pressure normal, low, or elevated? Check the pressure in sitting and standing positions, provided the patient is not dizzy. Are there significant orthostatic changes? If yes, the patient must be presumed to be in shock.

Words of Wisdom

Vaginal bleeding is a sign of internal bleeding and should not be taken lightly. Apply a pad over the vaginal area, and transport all used pads with the patient to the hospital.

YOU are the Paramedic PART 2

Your patient is lying on the sofa and is conscious, alert, and cooperative. The patient tells you she has been having lower back and pelvic pain for at least 3 months. She has had a very heavy menstrual flow with spotting between periods. She adamantly denies any possibility she could be pregnant.

Recording Time: 0 Minutes	
Appearance	Awake
Level of consciousness	Alert and oriented to person, place, time, and event
Airway	Open
Breathing	Adequate
Circulation	Adequate

3. Which gynecologic emergencies present with pain?
4. What steps will you take in your further assessment of this patient?

Reassessment

En route to the hospital, recheck your interventions and remember to obtain serial vital signs. Pay specific attention to the needs of your patient, and accommodate her desire for conversation or silence.

Communication and documentation are important, but in gynecologic cases, do not focus on your documentation during the call. Your main focus must be on the patient, including providing emotional care. You are caring for a human being—documentation can wait until the patient has been delivered to the receiving facility.

Emergency Medical Care

Primary management of a gynecologic patient is directed at mitigating life threats, being supportive and compassionate, and protecting the patient's modesty. In most gynecologic emergencies, your role will be primarily investigatory. The more accurate and detailed the history and examination are, the better you will be at differentiating gynecologic and non-gynecologic pathology. For all patients, assess and supply the appropriate oxygen needs. Obtain vital signs, and continue to monitor vital signs throughout your patient care.

Initiate fluid therapy, providing for pharmacologic interventions (pain management) or volume replacement as necessary. General management of abdominal or pelvic pain is primarily supportive. Local protocols may allow for pain management medications, including narcotics. Consider gaining IV access in any woman of childbearing age with abdominal pain. Pain-free or reduced pain during transport will greatly reduce your patient's anxiety.

Provide transport. Protect the patient's modesty, and provide emotional care with a supportive attitude.

> **Words of Wisdom**
>
> You do not carry the necessary supplies and equipment for a definitive diagnosis of a gynecologic problem in the field. Look for life threats, treat for shock, and transport in a position of comfort.

Management of Gynecologic Trauma

The female genital area is highly vascular and very susceptible to trauma. Motor vehicle crashes, sporting events, assault, and even consensual sex are common mechanisms of injury. Bleeding from genital trauma may be profuse (and very painful), and, if the patient is currently having her period, trying to differentiate between menstrual blood and trauma-related blood can be difficult.

Applying simple external pressure over the area of the laceration is usually sufficient to control bleeding. Bleeding from the internal genitalia, by contrast, can be massive and very difficult to control. Blindly packing the vagina is dangerous and is not recommended or even useful. A woman with exsanguinating vaginal hemorrhage must be treated as any other injured patient with exsanguinating hemorrhage—that is, she must be treated for shock and rapidly transported to the hospital, preferably one with obstetric and gynecologic services.

Do *not* perform an internal vaginal examination. Examination of the external genitalia is only warranted in the presence of genital trauma.

Pathophysiology, Assessment, and Management of Specific Emergencies

Infections

Pelvic Inflammatory Disease

Pelvic inflammatory disease (PID) is an infection of a woman's reproductive organs. Although PID is a complication often caused by a sexually transmitted disease (STD), such as chlamydia or gonorrhea, other infections that are not sexually transmitted can also cause PID.[1] Many women who have PID have no signs or symptoms or have symptoms but do not seek treatment. The disease is most prevalent in sexually active women who are age 25 years or younger.[1]

With PID, disease-causing organisms enter the vagina, generally by the process of sexual activity, and migrate through the opening of the cervix and into the uterine cavity, where they invade the mucosa. The infection may then expand to the fallopian tubes, where the tubal walls swell and the lumen of the tube fills with purulent fluid that obstructs the tube. The purulent fluid drips out of the tube and onto the ovary and surrounding tissue. Peritonitis may develop and pelvic abscesses may form as the inflammatory response attempts to contain the infection. Sepsis may result if the infection spreads. Because PID can affect the fallopian tubes and ovaries, long-term complications of PID include infertility and an increased risk of ectopic pregnancy.

If a patient with PID has symptoms, she may report pain that generally starts during or after normal menstruation, so eliciting the LMP is an important component of the history. The pain is typically diffuse and is spread over both quadrants of the lower abdomen. It may be described as "achy," and the patient may volunteer that the pain is made worse by walking or by sexual intercourse. The latter revelation usually indicates cervical involvement in the infective process. Pain localized to the right upper quadrant is indicative of infection that has spread to the abdominal cavity. Associated symptoms may include

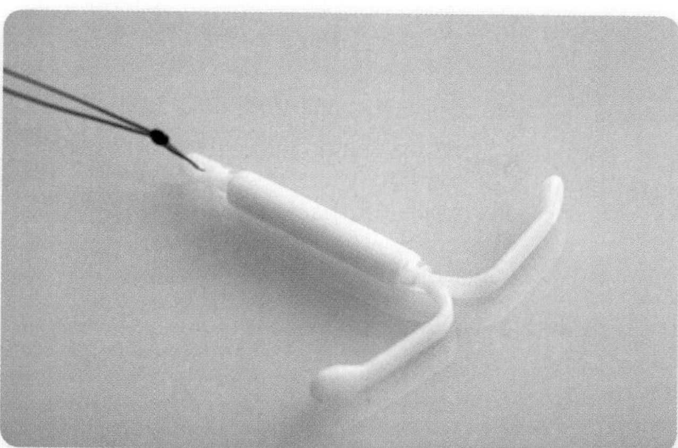

Figure 22-4 Insertion of an intrauterine device can increase a woman's risk of developing pelvic inflammatory disease for a brief time after insertion.

vaginal discharge, fever and chills, and pain or burning on urination (dysuria).

Risk factors for PID include an untreated sexually transmitted disease, sexual activity with multiple partners, douching, and a history of previous PID. PID may be associated with abortion, childbirth, or the insertion of an intrauterine device (IUD), which is used to prevent pregnancy, or other instrument contaminated by organisms from the lower reproductive tract or other source. With regard to IUD use, the increased risk of PID is mostly limited to the first 3 weeks after placement of the IUD **Figure 22-4**.[1]

Any woman with PID who feels sick enough to seek medical assistance probably has a severe infection and is likely to present as febrile and look sick. Physical examination findings may be sparse or may include the entire textbook profile. Be alert for signs of peritoneal irritation (that is, the patient winces on palpation of the abdomen or every time the ambulance hits a bump). Be very gentle should you decide to palpate this patient's abdomen as part of the examination.

PID generally requires administration of an appropriate antibiotic for 10 to 14 days. Prehospital care is primarily supportive, but may require the administration of supplemental oxygen, intravenous fluids, or both, depending on the patient's presentation. Make the patient as comfortable as possible and transport with as gentle a ride as can be managed.

Bartholin Abscess

Just inside the lower vagina are two small ducts, one on each side, that lead to the **Bartholin glands**. These glands secrete mucus that acts as a lubricant during intercourse. A cyst may form if one of these ducts becomes blocked, causing the duct and gland to swell. A Bartholin abscess can develop if the cyst or the gland itself becomes infected.

A Bartholin cyst is typically small. A large cyst or a cyst that becomes infected can cause symptoms including vulvar pain, pain with intercourse, and a painful lump in the vulvar area. A Bartholin abscess may be unilateral or bilateral.[2] If a cyst is infected or if an abscess is present, a surgical incision to drain the infected gland is usually required. Prehospital care is primarily supportive.

Vaginitis

Vaginitis, by definition, is an inflammation of the vagina that is caused by an infection. Vaginitis can spread upward to the cervix, uterus, fallopian tubes, and ovaries to cause PID. Although some patients may be asymptomatic, common symptoms include itching, irritation, discharge, odor, painful intercourse, and lower abdominal pain. Vaginal foreign bodies such as retained tampons, condoms, or other devices may predispose to vaginitis. A physician can usually remove them easily. There are several different types of vaginitis, including vaginal yeast infections.

Vaginal yeast infections are typically caused by the *Candida albicans* fungus. Yeasts are tiny organisms that normally live in small numbers inside the vagina and on the skin. The normal acidic environment of the vagina helps keep yeast from growing. If the vagina becomes less acidic, however, the yeast population may increase dramatically and result in infection. Conditions that may alter the acidic balance of the vagina include the use of oral contraceptives, menstruation, pregnancy, diabetes, some antibiotics, deodorant tampons, and the excessive use of vaginal sprays or douches.[3] Moisture and irritation of the vagina also seem to encourage yeast growth. Stress from lack of sleep, illness, or poor diet are other contributing factors. Women with immunosuppressive diseases such as human immunodeficiency virus infection or diabetes are also at increased risk. Symptoms may include itching, burning, soreness in the vagina and around the vulva, and vulvar swelling. Some women may report a thick, white vaginal discharge ("cottage cheese" appearance), pain during sexual intercourse, and burning on urination.

Vulvovaginitis is an inflammation of the external vulva. Symptoms of vulvovaginitis include redness, pain, swelling, discharge, burning, and itching. A physician should evaluate patients with this condition.

If not treated, vaginitis can lead to infertility, preterm birth, endometritis, PID, and an increased risk for STDs. Antibiotics are required for definitive treatment. Prehospital management is generally limited to a supportive role. Treatment of vulvovaginitis includes antibiotics and topical creams.

Cystitis

Cystitis (bladder infection) is usually caused by bacteria that ascend from the perineum through the genital tract into the urethral opening. Infection is isolated in the bladder. Patients often present with suprapubic pain, cloudy urine, urinary frequency, hematuria, and dysuria. If untreated, it may lead to **pyelonephritis**, or infection of the kidneys. Pyelonephritis is more serious, and patients may be severely ill, with fevers, chills, and vomiting. Treatment of cystitis and pyelonephritis includes antibiotics and pain relief.

▶ Ovarian Disorders

An **ovarian cyst** is a fluid-filled sac on or within an ovary. Ovarian cysts are common, developing in both ruptured and unruptured ovarian follicles.[4] Cysts may be solitary or multiple and they can occur unilaterally or bilaterally.[5] Most ovarian cysts are asymptomatic, generally lasting about 8 to 12 weeks before disappearing on their own without complications.[4]

Sometimes, a cyst will become large enough to cause pelvic discomfort, urinary retention or urinary frequency, or menstrual irregularities.[4] Symptom onset is usually gradual and the patient may report a feeling of heaviness in the pelvis. An ovarian cyst may rupture spontaneously or after mild abdominal injury, intercourse, or exercise. If rupture occurs, the patient may have no symptoms, mild symptoms, or severe symptoms. The patient may report a sudden onset of moderate to severe lower abdominal discomfort, which may radiate to the back. If internal bleeding is severe, the patient may experience light-headedness, accompanied by hypotension and tachycardia. Patients also may have a small amount of vaginal bleeding. Possible assessment findings of a **ruptured ovarian cyst** are shown in Table 22-2.

Table 22-2 Ruptured Ovarian Cyst: Assessment Findings

- Possible sudden onset of moderate to severe lower abdominal discomfort
- Typically affects one side, pain may radiate to back
- Possible vaginal bleeding

Ovarian torsion, or twisting of the ovary such that its blood supply is interrupted, must be considered if lower abdominal pain is severe or symptoms worsen. Ovarian torsion is more common in patients with a history of ovarian cysts, as a cyst may make the ovary more prone to twisting on its axis. Torsion is a surgical emergency and can lead to permanent damage to the ovary. The pain associated with this condition is an acute onset of moderate to severe unilateral pain in the lower abdomen that increases over a period of hours. The pain may be intermittent and may radiate to the back, pelvis, or thigh. Nausea and vomiting is common with ovarian torsion; unfortunately, however, this is a nonspecific finding. The affected side will be tender to palpation, and often a mass may be felt. However, the absence of these findings does not rule out the possibility of ovarian torsion. Prehospital treatment for a ruptured ovarian cyst and for suspected ovarian torsion involves recognition, quick transport to the emergency department, and treatment of any symptoms.

YOU are the Paramedic — PART 3

Your partner begins assessing her vital signs. The patient states she is not under a physician's care for this problem because it seemed normal at first. She tells you that she has been taking ibuprofen in an attempt to alleviate the pain but it has not been working. She describes the pain as a constant dull ache in her pelvis and lower back.

Recording Time: 5 Minutes	
Respirations	18 breaths/min
Pulse	80 beats/min
Skin	Pink, warm, and dry
Blood pressure	128/60 mm Hg
Oxygen saturation (Spo_2)	98% on room air
Pupils	PERRLA

5. What is the next question you should ask this patient?

Uterine Disorders

Endometritis is an inflammation of the endometrium (uterine lining) that often is associated with a bacterial infection. Women are more likely to have endometritis after having a baby or after a miscarriage. In most cases, the signs and symptoms of endometritis occur within 36 hours after childbirth.[6] Signs and symptoms of endometritis may include fever, chills, vomiting, tachycardia, lower abdominal or pelvic pain and cramping, and a foul-smelling vaginal discharge. Reassure your patient and transport in a position of comfort. If necessary, start an IV line and titrate to the patient's vital signs. Left untreated, severe infection and sepsis may result. Most patients fully recover after antibiotic treatment.

Endometriosis is the presence of tissue outside the uterus that resembles the endometrium in both structure and function. This tissue is usually found on pelvic structures around the uterus such as the ovaries, fallopian tubes, bowel, or rectum. This condition can be extremely painful, or there may be no symptoms. Many women do not even realize they have endometriosis until they encounter difficulties trying to get pregnant. In women who experience symptoms, the most common complaint is pain (sometimes chronic pain), generally localized in the lower back, pelvic, and abdominal regions. The pain is often described as constant and deep; it may be unilateral or bilateral, and either sharp or dull.[6] Other symptoms include heavy or prolonged menstrual flow, extremely painful and escalating menstrual cramping, pain with intercourse, sensations of rectal pressure or urgency, and fatigue (perhaps leading to misdiagnosis as chronic fatigue syndrome). Patients may also experience bleeding between periods or report premenstrual spotting. Prehospital care for endometriosis is based on the patient's signs and symptoms. If the patient reports severe pain, provide pain relief with analgesics if allowed in your protocol. Let the patient position herself so she is as comfortable as possible. Use dressings or towels as needed to absorb any significant vaginal bleeding.

Fascia, muscles, tendons, and ligaments support the pelvic organs. If these structures weaken, they may no longer be able to hold an organ in place. **Uterine prolapse** is the protrusion of part, or all, of the uterus outside the vagina. Uterine prolapse is classified as first degree if the cervix drops but remains within the vagina, second degree if the cervix lies at the opening to the vagina and the body of the uterus is in the vagina, and third degree if the uterus and cervix protrude through the vaginal opening.[5] In addition to genetics, factors predisposing patients to this condition include obesity, weakening of pelvic support because of decreased estrogen, increased intra-abdominal pressure related to pregnancy, and difficult childbirth including prolonged labor, multiple births, birth of a large baby, and repeated pregnancies separated by short intervals.[4] Although the early stages of uterine prolapse may be asymptomatic, more advanced stages can cause a feeling of pelvic heaviness or fullness, fatigue, and low back pain. Symptoms typically become worse after prolonged standing and they are relieved when lying down. If vaginal tissue is visibly prolapsed outside the vaginal orifice, cover it with sterile, moist gauze and transport the patient to the closest appropriate facility for further care. Assessment findings associated with uterine disorders are listed in Table 22-3.

Vaginal Bleeding

Although vaginal bleeding is a normal part of the monthly menstrual cycle, it may at times be quite heavy or irregular. It also may be accompanied by severe, cramping pain. Vaginal bleeding in a non-pregnant patient is not usually life threatening. However, a woman may not yet realize she is pregnant if the bleeding occurs early in the pregnancy.

Dysfunctional Uterine Bleeding

Dysfunctional uterine bleeding is uterine bleeding that is abnormal in amount or frequency (more than every 21 days). A diagnosis of dysfunctional uterine bleeding is made after ruling out anatomic or systemic conditions such as medication therapy or disease.[7] Dysfunctional uterine bleeding occurs when the hormonal events responsible for the balance of the menstrual cycle are interrupted. This occurs most often at the beginning or

Table 22-3 Uterine Disorders: Assessment Findings

Endometritis	Endometriosis	Uterine Prolapse
▪ Fever ▪ Chills ▪ Vomiting ▪ Tachycardia ▪ Lower abdominal or pelvic pain and cramping ▪ Foul-smelling vaginal discharge	▪ Constant and deep pain generally localized in the lower back, pelvic, and abdominal regions ▪ Heavy or prolonged menstrual flow ▪ Extremely painful and escalating menstrual cramping ▪ Pain with intercourse ▪ Sensations of rectal pressure or urgency ▪ Fatigue	▪ Protrusion of tissue ▪ Feeling of pelvic heaviness or fullness ▪ Fatigue ▪ Low back pain

end of a woman's reproductive years—when ovulation is becoming established or when it is becoming irregular at or after menopause.[7] Risk factors associated with dysfunctional uterine bleeding include extreme weight loss or gain, age over 40 years, high stress levels, polycystic ovary disease, long-term medication use (eg, oral contraceptives), excessive exercise, and anatomic abnormalities such as uterine fibroids.[7] A woman with dysfunctional uterine bleeding may require hormone therapy or, if she does not respond to medical management, surgery. Prehospital care for the patient with dysfunctional uterine bleeding is supportive. Allow the patient to assume a position of comfort. If necessary, use dressings or towels to absorb any significant vaginal bleeding.

Words of Wisdom

Assume that any woman of childbearing age with vaginal bleeding has a potentially life-threatening condition until proven otherwise.

Traumatic Vaginal Bleeding

Traumatic vaginal bleeding is not uncommon after vigorous voluntary intercourse, although violent involuntary sexual activity should be considered. Other causes of traumatic vaginal bleeding are shown in Table 22-4. The posterior vaginal wall behind the cervix is most commonly injured, although all pelvic organs can be involved. Complications include bleeding, organ rupture, and hypovolemic shock.

Treat these patients as you would any other patient with the potential for hemorrhagic shock. Keep the patient warm, give oxygen, obtain IV access, and give IV fluids if indicated. Carefully monitor vital signs and give this patient high priority for transport and treatment.

Ectopic Pregnancy

An **ectopic pregnancy** occurs outside the uterus. Ectopic pregnancies are often called *tubal pregnancies* because most are located in the fallopian tube Figure 22-5. Other possible sites, although much less common, include the abdominal cavity, on an ovary, or on the cervix.

An ectopic pregnancy is a life-threatening cause of vaginal bleeding in early pregnancy. Risk factors include anything that may promote scarring or inflammation in the pelvis, such as previous surgical adhesions or ectopic pregnancies, PID, tubal ligation, and use of an IUD to prevent pregnancy. This is because the IUD prevents pregnancy by interfering with implantation of a fertilized ovum in the uterine cavity. By interfering with implantation in the uterine cavity, the IUD increases the probability of implantation in the fallopian tube.

Table 22-4 Possible Causes of Traumatic Vaginal Bleeding

- Vigorous intercourse
- Straddle-type injury
- Pelvic fracture
- Direct blow to perineum
- Blunt force to lower abdomen from assault or seat belt
- Foreign body inserted into vagina
- Abortion attempts

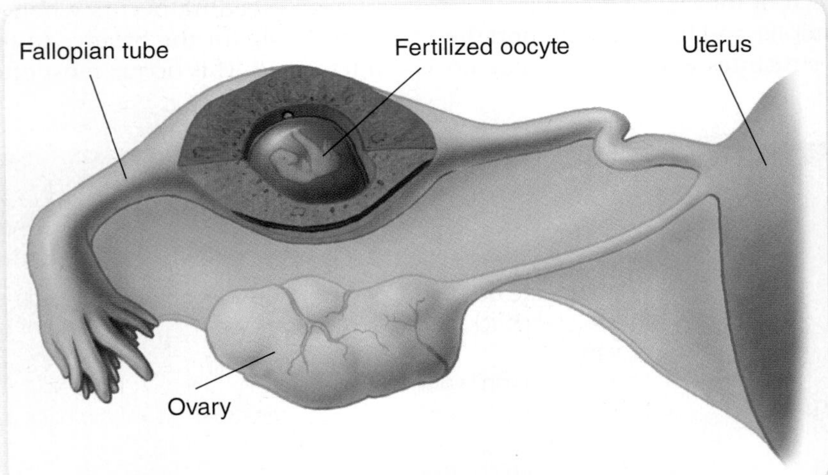

Figure 22-5 In an ectopic pregnancy, a fertilized oocyte implants somewhere other than the uterus. Here it is implanted in one of the fallopian tubes.

If the fertilized oocyte implants in the fallopian tube instead of the uterus, it stretches the tube as it grows. The fallopian tube, lacking the expansive muscle capacity of the uterus, has little stretching ability, so the developing embryo will soon run out of growing room. When this occurs, the tube is likely to rupture, causing pain and possible life-threatening bleeding.

When the site of oocyte implantation is a fallopian tube, most cases are diagnosed before rupture on the basis of three classic findings: (1) abdominal pain, (2) delayed menses, and (3) abnormal vaginal bleeding (spotting) that occurs about 6 to 8 weeks after the last normal menstrual period.[8] Most patients with an ectopic pregnancy will report abdominal pain. If the tube is unruptured, the pain begins as a dull, lower quadrant pain on one side. As the tube stretches, the pain changes to a colicky pain, then a sharp, stabbing pain, and, with tube rupture, to a sudden, excruciating pain that is felt throughout the lower abdomen. Referred shoulder pain is possible as the abdomen fills with blood. Most women report having a period that is delayed 1 to 2 weeks, a period that is lighter than usual, or an irregular period. Up to 80% of women experience mild to moderate dark red or brown intermittent vaginal bleeding.[8]

Words of Wisdom

In ectopic pregnancy, bleeding usually occurs after the onset of pain.

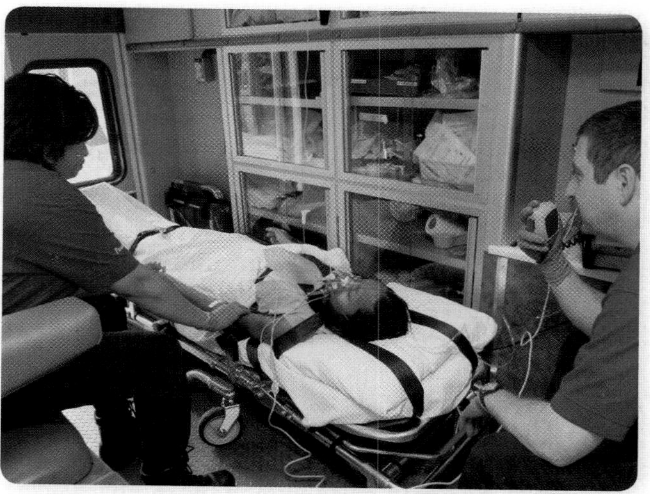

Figure 22-6 Always treat for shock in any woman with abdominal pain and vaginal bleeding.

Follow these steps in the management of a patient with a suspected ectopic pregnancy **Figure 22-6**:

- Ensure an adequate airway and administer supplemental oxygen if indicated. Give nothing by mouth, including water.
- Keep the patient left laterally recumbent, even if unconscious and intubated.
- Initiate IV fluid therapy with an 18-gauge IV line following local protocol.

YOU are the Paramedic PART 4

The patient tells you her last menstrual period was 7 days ago. The flow was very heavy and she was in a great deal of pain. She is still having the pain, but now she is also spotting. You determine the hospital of choice for the patient and she agrees to transport. Prior to placing the patient on your stretcher, you have your partner assess her vital signs, which show no change. En route, the patient rests comfortably with no change in signs or symptoms.

Recording Time: 10 Minutes	
Respirations	18 breaths/min
Pulse	80 beats/min, lying; 82 beats/min, sitting
Skin	Pink, warm, dry
Blood pressure	128/60 mm Hg, lying; 128/60 mm Hg, sitting
Oxygen saturation (Spo_2)	98% on room air
Pupils	PERRLA

6. What is the general patient care for this patient?
7. Can you accurately diagnose a difference between a gynecologic and abdominal problem in the field?

- Anticipate vomiting. Have an emesis bag and suction within arm's reach.
- Keep the patient warm.
- Place the patient on a cardiac monitor.
- Transport the patient to the nearest facility with surgical capabilities. Notify the receiving hospital of the patient's suspected diagnosis, her condition, and your estimated time of arrival.
- Recheck vital signs frequently during transport.

▶ Sexual Assault

The US Department of Justice defines **sexual assault** as any type of sexual contact or behavior that occurs without the explicit consent of the recipient.[9] The Centers for Disease Control and Prevention defines sexual violence as a sexual act that is committed or attempted by another person without freely given consent of the victim or against someone who is unable to consent or refuse.[10,11] Although definitions vary by state, the National Institute of Justice observes that most statutes define **rape** as nonconsensual oral, anal, or vaginal penetration of the victim by body parts or objects using force or threats of bodily harm, or by taking advantage of a victim who is incapacitated or otherwise incapable of giving consent.[12]

Unfortunately, sexual assault and rape are all too common. EMS providers called to treat a victim of sexual assault, sexual abuse, or actual or alleged rape face many complex issues, ranging from obvious medical conditions to serious psychological and legal issues. You may be the first person the victim has contact with after the encounter. How you manage the situation from first contact throughout treatment and transport may have a lasting effect for the patient and you. Being professional, respectful, and sensitive is very important.

Both men and women can be victims of sexual assault. A rape victim has just experienced a purposeful "major vehicle crash" of his or her mind and body. The act was most likely perpetrated by someone he or she knew and trusted. The last thing the victim wants to do is give a concise, detailed report of what he or she has just experienced, and attempting to elicit information in this manner most likely will cause the victim to shut down. Whenever possible, a female rape victim should be given the option of being treated by a female paramedic because the patient may be experiencing ambivalent feelings toward men in general; these feelings will hinder assessment and the patient's well-being.

Because sexual assault and rape are crimes, you can expect law enforcement to be involved early in the situation. In many cases, EMS may be called by law enforcement. Police officers usually have basic medical training but their primary focus is on criminal investigation, not patient care.

It is the job of law enforcement officers to solve the crime, arrest the perpetrator, and see justice served. The job of paramedics is to manage the medical aspects of the case and to act as the patient advocate. In this capacity, it is important for you to focus on several key issues.

> **Words of Wisdom**
>
> Work with law enforcement to preserve the scene whenever possible. However, your primary responsibility is to attend to the physical and emotional needs of your patient.

Assessment

Begin your assessment by asking the patient if he or she would be more comfortable with a female or male paramedic, and make every effort to fulfill this request.

Limit any physical examination to a brief survey for life-threatening injuries. Expose and examine the vaginal area only if there is evidence of bleeding that needs to be treated. Do everything possible to protect the patient's privacy and give some sense of control back to the patient. Examine and interview the patient with a minimum of people present, moving him or her to the ambulance if necessary.

The first issue is the medical treatment of the patient. Is the patient physically injured? Are any life-threatening injuries present? Does the patient complain of any pain?

The second issue is your emotional care of the patient. Do not cross-examine or attempt to elicit information for the benefit of the police. These issues will be handled later in the emergency department. Do not pass judgment on the patient, and protect the patient from the judgment of others on the scene. Many victims report feeling "re-raped" when subjected to interrogation, criticism, or incredulity.

When performing your assessment, be aware of information suggesting the potential use of date rape or *club* drugs. The patient may or may not be aware of the use of drugs in the assault, but an inability to remember the event should create suspicion. Flunitrazepam (Rohypnol; roofies), gamma-hydroxybutyrate (GHB; liquid E or liquid ecstasy), ketamine (Special K), clonazepam (Klonopin), alprazolam (Xanax), and alcohol are drugs that are typically used during sexual assault and rape for the intended purpose of incapacitating a person. These drugs can be put into a person's drink and may go undetected because they often do not have a color, smell, or taste. The effects may be immediate and are made more active with alcohol. The patient may become weak and confused and may even have a loss of consciousness. These drugs cause muscle relaxation and loss of muscle compliance, which may make the victim more compliant during a sexual assault. If the drugs are still in the patient's system during your assessment, you may see hypotension, bradycardia, difficulty breathing, seizures, coma, and even death.

Management

Remember that you are at a crime scene. Although your job is to treat the medical aspects of the incident and not collect evidence, you still have a responsibility to preserve evidence. Do not cut through any clothing or throw away anything from the scene. Place bloodstained articles in separate paper (not plastic) bags. Obtain evidentiary bags from the police if necessary. Paper bags allow wet items to dry naturally, whereas plastic allows mold to grow and may destroy biologic evidence.

It may also be necessary to gently persuade the patient to not clean up. This will be a natural desire on the part of the patient, stemming from the desire to "wash away" the humiliation and embarrassment of the assault. Valuable evidence can be destroyed in this process. The patient also needs to be discouraged from using hand sanitizer, urinating, changing clothes, having a bowel movement, or rinsing out his or her mouth. Respect the patient's feelings.

Some patients may refuse transport. For adults who are mentally competent, this is the patient's right. In such cases, follow your system's refusal of treatment policy or procedure for sexual assault victims without judging or being condescending to the patient. In no instance should you simply accept the patient's refusal and leave. Offer to call the local rape crisis center for the patient. Many communities have rape crisis centers, with victim advocates on-call. Getting a professional advocate to the scene may help the patient deal with the trauma, and the advocate can better explain the necessities of evidence preservation in more compassionate detail. Many victim advocates are rape-trauma survivors themselves. Most rape victims are photographed and examined by nurses or physicians trained in sexual assault examination and management (sometimes called Sexual Assault Nurse Examiners, or SANE nurses).

Follow your protocol concerning this type of call. Some EMS systems may consider administering a sedative to a patient in this situation.

The patient care report is a legal document and, should the case result in an arrest and subsequent trial, may be subpoenaed. Keep the report concise, and record only what the patient stated in his or her own words. Use quotation marks to indicate that you are reporting the patient's version of events. Do not insert your own opinion as to whether the patient was raped or offer any conclusions that would validate or invalidate the patient's account of the event. Focus on the facts. Record your observations during the physical examination—the patient's emotional state, the condition of his or her clothing, and any obvious injuries. Bear in mind that rape is a legal diagnosis, not a medical diagnosis. The medical team can only establish whether sexual intercourse occurred; a court must decide whether intercourse was inflicted forcibly on the victim.

Documentation & Communication

Just as you might be uncomfortable talking about your last sexual encounter to a total stranger, so your patient might feel a mix of emotions, including shame and frustration after being assaulted. A calm, nonjudgmental approach from a same-gender paramedic will be helpful.

Intimate Partner Violence

Intimate partner violence refers to physical, sexual, or psychological harm by a current or former partner or spouse. This type of violence can occur among heterosexual or same-sex couples and does not require sexual intimacy.[13] As the first member of the health care team to contact the patient outside the hospital or at his or her home, you may be able to gather valuable information not available to hospital personnel. If you arrive at an uncontrolled scene where you suspect intimate partner violence has occurred, avoid confronting those involved. Your priority is safety—yours and your patient's.

► Sexual Practices and Vaginal Foreign Bodies

There is a variety of ways that men and women engage in sexual acts. Your exposure to these practices will most likely occur when these private sexual practices go bad, resulting in an embarrassing call to 9-1-1.

The most common sexual gynecologic emergency you may encounter is simply a foreign object (a soda pop or beer bottle or a sex toy) that has become stuck in the vagina or anus. For example, a bottle may develop a vacuum inside of the body and stick to an interior structure. Attempts at removal by the patient may result in intense pain or even vaginal bleeding as internal structures tear. Bleeding and pain cause the patient to panic. With this type of call, keep the patient calm, protect his or her dignity as much as possible, and transport. Do not attempt to remove any foreign objects from the vagina or anus. If at all possible, do not let the patient walk. Overpenetration of any item may lead to internal injury, and should be managed as such.

Some cases of bottle insertion may be associated with rape, so bear in mind that the patient may be an assault victim. Some gangs have been known to insert beer bottles in a woman's vagina after rape, then take turns punching the woman in the lower abdomen until the bottle breaks. If this is the case, use extreme care and do not move the patient more than necessary to prevent even more internal damage.

Among some of the more bizarre practices you may encounter includes a technique known as "fisting," which involves placing the closed fist and wrist into a body orifice (vagina or rectum) for sexual stimulation. Whether the patient is male or female, organ rupture (rectum, vagina) is likely. Life-threatening peritonitis may result. Another sexual practice is the insertion of live animals into the vagina, including fish, eels, snakes, worms, and hamsters. The patient becomes alarmed when the animal goes in but does not come out.

Assessment

Assessment in this situation is sensitive. Maintain your patient's privacy. Depending on the circumstances, you may need to inspect the genital area for bleeding, wounds, or objects that may need to be stabilized. Avoid focusing on only one part of your patient; you still need to conduct a thorough patient assessment including vital signs and history.

Management

Treat such a case as you would with any other foreign object, remain nonjudgmental, and transport. Do not attempt to retrieve the object, even if it is an animal, from inside the vagina. Transport the patient in a knees-flexed, legs-together position.

YOU are the Paramedic SUMMARY

1. What are you looking for in your scene size-up?

Look for the elements of scene size-up, as you would for any call: scene safety, need for additional resources, initial impression (medical, trauma, or both), and number of patients. Take standard precautions. Note the conditions at the scene; this information may be helpful should you be asked to testify in court.

2. What are you looking for in your primary survey?

Answer the following questions during your primary survey: What is the overall presentation of the patient? Does your rapid scan reveal any obvious life threats? Is she conscious? Does she have obvious breathing difficulty or evidence of injury? Does she appear pale, cyanotic, red, or gray? Is she alert and oriented or confused? Is she calm or distraught? What is her emotional state? What is her physical appearance—well kempt or dirty? Do you find the patient sitting up, lying down, prone, supine, in the fetal position, in the tripod position, in the bathtub, or on all fours?

Once you have answered these basic questions and treated any immediate threats to airway, breathing, or circulation, you can proceed with a secondary assessment and obtain more history of the present illness.

3. Which gynecologic emergencies present with pain?

Most gynecologic emergencies can present with pain (eg, abdominal pain, pelvic pain, low back pain, pain during intercourse, cramping). Ectopic pregnancy and ruptured ovarian cyst are two conditions that are potentially life threatening. Although other gynecologic causes of pain may not be life threatening, any manifestation of pain will naturally be worrisome to the patient.

4. What steps will you take in your further assessment of this patient?

What is the patient's chief complaint? If it is excessive bleeding, you can move on to obtaining the gynecologic history. If the chief complaint is abdominal pain, you need to find out more about the pain itself, using the OPQRST method (Onset; Provoking factors; Quality of pain; Region of pain and whether it radiates or refers; Severity; and Time [duration]).

5. What is the next question you should ask this patient?

Proceed to obtain a gynecologic history. Probably the single most important question to ask is, "When did you have your last menstrual period (LMP)?" If the patient is certain, record the beginning and ending dates of the LMP. If she is unsure, record the approximate dates. Ask the patient whether she noticed anything unusual about the LMP.

6. What is the general patient care for this patient?

The management of a gynecologic patient is generally supportive because definitive care cannot be provided in the field. Primary management will be directed at mitigating life threats, being supportive and compassionate, and protecting the patient's modesty. Assess and supply the appropriate oxygen needs. Obtain the patient's vital signs, and continue to monitor her vital signs throughout her care.

7. Can you accurately diagnose a difference between a gynecologic and abdominal problem in the field?

No. Gynecologic emergencies often have the same signs and symptoms as emergencies involving other abdominal organs. Assess the patient carefully to determine the nature and extent of the problem. Be sure to follow the SAMPLE (Signs and symptoms, Allergies, Medications, Pertinent past medical history, Last oral intake, Events leading up to the illness or injury) mnemonic. What, if any, associated signs and symptoms are noted: fever, diaphoresis, syncope, diarrhea, constipation, and dysuria? Other medical problems may present as an abdominal problem. For example, cardiac pain may be misinterpreted as epigastric pain.

YOU are the Paramedic SUMMARY *(continued)*

<table>
<tr><th colspan="6">EMS Patient Care Report (PCR)</th></tr>
<tr><td>Date: 05-31-18</td><td colspan="2">Incident No.: 78865</td><td colspan="2">Nature of Call: Abdominal pain</td><td>Location: 1065 Meadow Lane</td></tr>
<tr><td>Dispatched: 1005</td><td>En Route: 1005</td><td>At Scene: 1010</td><td>Transport: 1040</td><td>At Hospital: 1047</td><td>In Service: 1058</td></tr>
<tr><th colspan="6">Patient Information</th></tr>
<tr><td colspan="3">Age: 24
Sex: F
Weight (in kg [lb]): 91 kg (200 lb)</td><td colspan="3">Allergies: No known drug allergies
Medications: OTC ibuprofen
Past Medical History: Denies
Chief Complaint: Abdominal/pelvic pain</td></tr>
</table>

<table>
<tr><th colspan="5">Vital Signs</th></tr>
<tr><td>Time: 1015</td><td>BP: 128/60</td><td>Pulse: 80</td><td>Respirations: 18</td><td>Spo$_2$: 98%</td></tr>
<tr><td>Time: 1020</td><td>BP: 128/60 lying/sitting</td><td>Pulse: 88 lying, 82 sitting</td><td>Respirations: 18</td><td>Spo$_2$: 98%</td></tr>
<tr><td>Time: 1030</td><td>BP: 125/62 lying/sitting</td><td>Pulse: 86 lying</td><td>Respirations: 18</td><td>Spo$_2$: 98%</td></tr>
<tr><th colspan="5">EMS Treatment (circle all that apply)</th></tr>
<tr><td colspan="2">Oxygen @ _______ L/min via (circle one):
NC NRM Bag-mask device</td><td>Assisted Ventilation</td><td>Airway Adjunct</td><td>CPR</td></tr>
<tr><td>Defibrillation</td><td>Bleeding Control</td><td>Bandaging</td><td>Splinting</td><td>Other:</td></tr>
<tr><th colspan="5">Narrative</th></tr>
<tr><td colspan="5">Arrived to find 24-year-old woman complaining of abdominal and pelvic pain. Pt states the pain is a dull ache located in her pelvis and lower back that has been present for 3 months. Pt also complains of increased menstrual flow with spotting between periods. Pt states LMP was 7 days ago. Pt states pain is constant and does not change with movement or OTC medication. Pt is not under a doctor's care for same. Pt states she is not pregnant. Orthostatic vital signs assessed, which show no change. Pt agreed to transport to Community Hospital. Pt rested comfortably during transport with no change in condition noted. Report to Dr. Sullivan on arrival in ED bed 4.
End of report</td></tr>
</table>

Prep Kit

▶ Ready for Review

- Gynecology is the study and care of diseases of the female reproductive system.
- The internal female genitalia include the ovaries, fallopian tubes, uterus, cervix, and vagina. The external female genitalia include the mons pubis, labia majora, labia minora, perineum, and clitoris.
- Menstruation is the cyclical shedding of the endometrial lining from the uterine cavity. Menarche refers to the onset of the first menses, when a girl reaches childbearing age. Menopause is the period when a woman's reproductive cycle ceases.
- Ovulation occurs when an ovum, or egg, is released from an ovarian follicle. This usually occurs 14 days after the start of the previous menstrual period. Some women experience abdominal pain and cramping (mittelschmerz) in the middle of the menstrual cycle.
- Amenorrhea is the absence or cessation of menses. The most common cause is pregnancy. Amenorrhea can also occur in athletes, and in people with anorexia nervosa, emotional problems, extreme stress, or low body fat.
- Signs and symptoms of gynecologic emergencies generally include one or more of the following: vaginal bleeding, abdominal pain, vomiting, fever, tachycardia, hypotension, diaphoresis, syncope, changes in stool pattern, dyspareunia (pain during intercourse), or urinary symptoms.
- When assessing a patient with a gynecologic emergency, begin by focusing on the ABCDEs and assessing for shock. Additional care includes obtaining intravenous (IV) access, monitoring vital signs, providing pain management and fluid resuscitation as indicated by the patient's condition, and transport.
- While taking the patient's history, determine when the patient had her last menstrual period, if it is unusual in any way, whether she could be pregnant, and whether she uses contraception. Also note any previous pregnancies, miscarriages, or abortions. If the patient has a vaginal discharge, ask about the color, amount, and whether there is any odor.
- General management for gynecologic emergencies is supportive, including addressing life threats, providing emotional support, and protecting the patient's modesty. When possible, the paramedic performing the physical examination should be the same gender as the patient.
- The female genital area is highly vascular and very susceptible to trauma. If the patient has sustained trauma to the external genitalia, apply pressure to control bleeding. Do not perform an interior vaginal examination.
- Pelvic inflammatory disease (PID) is an infection of a woman's female reproductive organs. Because PID can affect the fallopian tubes and ovaries, long-term complications of PID include infertility and a high risk of ectopic pregnancy.
- A patient with a large Bartholin cyst or abscess may report vulvar pain, pain with intercourse, or a painful lump in the vulvar area. If the cyst is infected or if an abscess is present, a surgical incision to drain the infected gland is usually required. Prehospital care is primarily supportive.
- Vaginitis and vulvovaginitis are inflammations of the vaginal tissues and external vulva caused by an infection. Symptoms include itching, irritation, discharge, odor, painful intercourse, and lower abdominal pain. Both of these common conditions are treated with antibiotics.
- Ovarian disorders include ovarian cysts and ovarian torsion. If an ovarian cyst ruptures, the patient may have no symptoms, mild symptoms, or severe symptoms. If internal bleeding is severe, the patient may experience light-headedness, accompanied by hypotension and tachycardia. Ovarian torsion must be considered if lower abdominal pain is severe or symptoms worsen. Torsion is a surgical emergency and can lead to permanent damage to the ovary. Prehospital treatment for a ruptured ovarian cyst and for suspected ovarian torsion involves recognition, quick transport to the emergency department, and treatment of any symptoms.
- Uterine disorders include endometritis, endometriosis, and uterine prolapse. Endometritis is inflammation of the endometrium. Signs and symptoms of endometritis may include fever, chills, vomiting, tachycardia, lower abdominal or pelvic pain and cramping, and a foul-smelling vaginal discharge. Endometriosis is the presence of tissue outside the uterus that resembles the endometrium in both structure and function. It can cause infertility. In women who experience symptoms, the most common complaint is pain (sometimes chronic pain), generally localized in the lower back, pelvic, and abdominal regions. Uterine prolapse is the protrusion of part or all of the uterus outside the vagina. If vaginal tissue is visibly prolapsed outside the vaginal orifice, cover it with sterile, moist gauze and transport the patient.
- Vaginal bleeding that does not occur during the course of regular menstruation is cause for concern. Consider whether there is a mechanism of injury. Dysfunctional uterine bleeding is uterine bleeding

Prep Kit *(continued)*

that is abnormal in amount or frequency (more than every 21 days). Treat these patients as if they have the potential for hemorrhagic shock.

- In ectopic pregnancy, a fertilized oocyte implants somewhere other than the uterus, usually in a fallopian tube, which can lead to rupture of the fallopian tube. This can be life threatening. Treat the patient for shock, and transport.
- In sexual assault, sexual violence, and rape cases, your professionalism, respect, and sensitivity are of the utmost importance.
- It may be difficult to obtain a history from a victim of rape. Have a same-gender paramedic treat the patient when possible.
- Remember that your job is to medically treat the patient. Ask only medical questions, and do not judge the patient. Limit the physical examination to addressing life-threatening injuries.
- Preserve evidence when possible. Try to persuade the rape victim not to clean up.
- Document cases of sexual assault properly and professionally. On your patient care report, report the patient's words in quotation marks. Record facts obtained from the physical examination. Document any information suggesting the potential use of date rape or club drugs.
- In scenes involving intimate partner violence, do not confront those involved. Remember that safety is your priority.
- Sexual emergencies may involve foreign objects stuck in the vagina or anus, which may potentially lead to internal injury. Do not remove the object. Remain professional, and transport the patient.

▶ Vital Vocabulary

amenorrhea Absence of menstruation.

Bartholin glands The glands that secrete mucus for sexual lubrication.

cervix The narrowest portion (lower third of the neck) of the uterus that opens into the vagina.

clitoris A small, cylindrical mass of erectile tissue and nerves located at the anterior junction of the labia minora, similar to the glans penis of the male.

cystitis Infection caused by bacteria that travel from the perineum, through the genital tract, into the urethral opening; also called bladder infection.

dysfunctional uterine bleeding Uterine bleeding that is abnormal in amount or frequency (more than every 21 days).

ectopic pregnancy A pregnancy in which the fertilized oocyte implants somewhere other than the uterus.

embryo A fertilized egg.

endometriosis The presence of tissue outside the uterus that resembles the endometrium in both structure and function.

endometritis An inflammation of the endometrium that often is associated with a bacterial infection.

endometrium The inner layer of the uterine wall.

fallopian tube The anatomic structure that connects each ovary with the uterus and provides a passageway for the ova.

hymen A membrane that protects the vaginal orifice before first intercourse.

labia majora A pair of prominent, rounded folds of skin covered with pubic hair that protect the vagina.

labia minora A pair of skin folds devoid of pubic hair that protect the vagina.

menarche The first menstrual cycle; the onset of menses.

menopause The period when a woman's reproductive cycle ceases; also called the female climacteric.

menstruation Cyclical shedding of the endometrial lining from the uterine cavity.

mons pubis A rounded pad of fatty tissue that overlies the symphysis pubis and is anterior to the urethral and vaginal openings.

ovarian cyst A fluid-filled sac that forms on or within an ovary.

ovarian torsion A painful condition in which the ovary becomes twisted.

ovaries A pair of female reproductive organs that release eggs (ova) that, if fertilized, will develop into a fetus.

ovulation Midcycle release of an egg (ovum) during the menstrual cycle.

pelvic inflammatory disease (PID) An infection of the female reproductive organs.

perineum The area between the vaginal opening and the anus.

pyelonephritis Kidney infection.

rape Nonconsensual oral, anal, or vaginal penetration of the victim by body parts or objects using force, threats of bodily harm, or by taking advantage of a victim who is incapacitated or otherwise incapable of giving consent.

ruptured ovarian cyst A fluid-filled sac within the ovary that bursts from internal pressure.

sexual assault Any type of sexual contact or behavior that occurs without the explicit consent of the recipient.

Prep Kit *(continued)*

uterine prolapse A condition in which the uterus moves or drops into the vagina.

uterus The muscular inverted pear-shaped organ where the fetus grows.

vagina The genital canal in the female that serves as a passageway for the elimination of menstrual fluids, receives the penis during sexual intercourse, holds the spermatozoa before their passage into the uterus, and serves as the passageway for childbirth.

vaginal yeast infection An infection caused by the fungus, *Candida albicans*, in which fungi overpopulate the vagina.

vaginitis An inflammation of the vagina that is caused by an infection.

vulvovaginitis An inflammation of the external vulva.

▶ References

1. Pelvic inflammatory disease (PID) – CDC fact sheet. Centers for Disease Control and Prevention website. https://www.cdc.gov/std/PID/STDFact-PID.htm. Updated May 23, 2016. Accessed March 7, 2017.
2. Harkreader H, Hogan MA, Thobaben M. Physical assessment. In: Harkreader H, Hogan MA, Thobaben, M. *Fundamentals of Nursing: Caring and Clinical Judgment*. 3rd ed. St. Louis, MO: Saunders; 2007:138-187.
3. Leifer G. Reproductive anatomy and physiology. In: Leifer G. *Maternity Nursing: An Introductory Text*. 11th ed. St. Louis, MO: Saunders; 2012:16-28.
4. VanMeter KC, Hubert RJ. Reproductive system disorders. In: VanMeter KC, Hubert RJ. *Gould's Pathophysiology for the Health Professions*. 5th ed. St. Louis, MO: Saunders; 2014:516-546.
5. Wilson SF, Giddens JF. Reproductive system and the perineum. In: Wilson SF, Giddens, JF. *Health Assessment for Nursing Practice*. 5th ed. St. Louis, MO: Mosby; 2013:386-438.
6. Murray SS, McKinney ES. Postpartum maternal complications. In: Murray SS, McKinney ES. *Foundations of Maternal-Newborn and Women's Health Nursing*. 6th ed. St. Louis, MO: Saunders; 2014:598-620.
7. Ignatavicius DD. Care of patients with gynecologic problems. In: Ignatavicius DD, Workman ML, eds. *Medical-Surgical Nursing: Patient-Centered Collaborative Care*. 7th ed. St. Louis, MO: Saunders; 2013:1611-1628.
8. Cashion K. Hemorrhagic disorders. In: Lowdermilk DL, Perry SE, Cashion K, Alden KR, eds. *Maternity & Women's Health Care*. 11th ed. St. Louis, MO: Elsevier; 2016:669-686.
9. Sexual assault. The United States Department of Justice website. https://www.justice.gov/ovw/sexual-assault. Updated April 1, 2016. Accessed March 8, 2017.
10. Basile KC, Smith SG, Breiding MJ, Black MC, Mahendra R. *Sexual Violence Surveillance: Uniform Definitions and Recommended Data Elements, Version 2.0*. Atlanta, GA: National Center for Injury Prevention and Control, Centers for Disease Control and Prevention; 2014. https://www.cdc.gov/violenceprevention/pdf/sv_surveillance_definitionsl-2009-a.pdf. Accessed March 8, 2017.
11. Sexual violence. Centers for Disease Control and Prevention website. https://www.cdc.gov/violenceprevention/sexualviolence/index.html. Updated February 14, 2017. Accessed March 7, 2017.
12. Rape and sexual violence. National Institute of Justice website. https://www.nij.gov/topics/crime/rape-sexual-violence/Pages/welcome.aspx. Modified January 18, 2017. Accessed March 8, 2017.
13. Intimate partner violence. Centers for Disease Control and Prevention website. https://www.cdc.gov/violenceprevention/intimatepartnerviolence/index.html. Updated May 3, 2016. Accessed March 8, 2017.

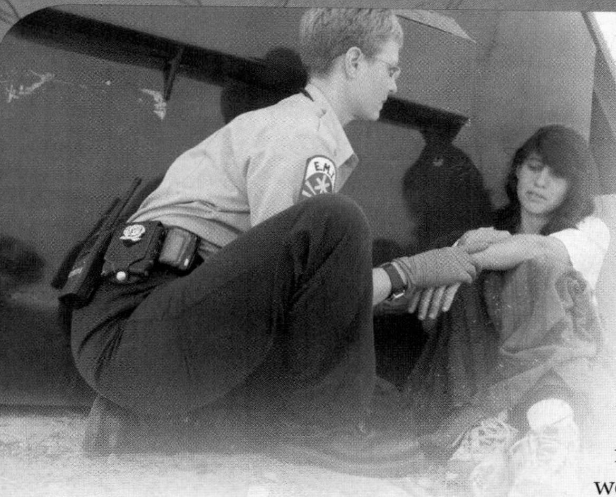

Assessment *in Action*

Your unit is dispatched for a patient with abdominal pain. While en route, the dispatcher tells you the patient is a 24-year-old woman who is complaining of severe abdominal pain and vaginal bleeding. When you arrive on scene, you find that the patient looks very ill. She is pale, lying in a fetal position on the floor, and in severe pain. Her pants are wet with blood in the vaginal area. The patient tells you that she has been trying to get pregnant, but she knows something is terribly wrong.

1. On the basis of the information provided, which of the following is the most important to determine when obtaining this patient's gynecologic history?

- **A.** Current sexual activity
- **B.** The number of previous pregnancies
- **C.** History of sexually transmitted diseases
- **D.** Amount of vaginal bleeding in pads per hour

2. Cullen sign is:

- **A.** discoloration over the pelvic bone.
- **B.** discoloration of the periumbilical skin.
- **C.** a change in blood pressure.
- **D.** a change in the pulse rate.

3. Bleeding followed by pelvic pain in a patient who is less than 20 weeks' pregnant may be caused by:

- **A.** a spontaneous abortion.
- **B.** an ectopic pregnancy.
- **C.** Braxton-Hicks contractions.
- **D.** pelvic inflammatory disease.

4. Which of the following is a predisposing factor in the development of an ectopic pregnancy?

- **A.** Uterine prolapse
- **B.** Pelvic inflammatory disease
- **C.** Mittelschmerz
- **D.** Ovarian cyst

5. Which of the following reflects typical findings associated with an ectopic pregnancy?

- **A.** Headache, lower abdominal pain, and vaginal bleeding
- **B.** Sudden high fever, diarrhea, and abdominal tenderness
- **C.** Syncope, dizziness, and no abdominal pain
- **D.** Abdominal pain, delayed menses, and abnormal vaginal bleeding

6. The site of implantation for most ectopic pregnancies is:

- **A.** on an ovary.
- **B.** on the cervix.
- **C.** in a fallopian tube.
- **D.** in the abdominal cavity.

7. The primary focus in the care of this patient is:

- **A.** treatment for pain.
- **B.** treatment for shock.
- **C.** treatment for abdominal pain.
- **D.** treatment depending on the severity of the signs and symptoms.

Assessment *in Action* *(continued)*

8. You are called for a 48-year-old woman reporting abdominal cramping and vaginal bleeding. She states that her periods have become irregular over the past 6 months with her last period occurring 2 weeks ago. Her symptoms have recurred today with blood flow that is much heavier than usual. You suspect:

   A. vaginitis.
   B. ovarian torsion.
   C. pelvic inflammatory disease.
   D. dysfunctional uterine bleeding.

9. A 41-year-old woman has called you for what she describes as "something falling out of my vagina." Her symptoms began after a lengthy shopping excursion. She proudly reports that she exercises regularly, adheres to a healthy diet, and is the mother of six children. You suspect:

   A. endometriosis.
   B. uterine prolapse.
   C. ectopic pregnancy.
   D. ruptured ovarian cyst.

10. The primary concern for the treatment of a victim of sexual assault is medical treatment based on any injuries. What is the secondary concern in this situation?

CHAPTER 23

Endocrine Emergencies

National EMS Education Standard Competencies

Medicine

Integrates assessment findings with principles of epidemiology and pathophysiology to formulate a field impression and implement a comprehensive treatment/ disposition plan for a patient with a medical complaint.

Endocrine Disorders

Awareness that

- Diabetic emergencies cause altered mental status (pp 1261-1262, 1267, 1270)

Anatomy, physiology, pathophysiology, assessment, and management of

- Acute diabetic emergencies (pp 1264-1278)

Anatomy, physiology, epidemiology, pathophysiology, psychosocial impact, presentations, prognosis, and management of

- Acute diabetic emergencies (pp 1264-1278)
- Diabetes (pp 1264-1270)
- Adrenal disease (pp 1279-1281)
- Pituitary and thyroid disorders (pp 1281-1284)

Knowledge Objectives

1. Review the anatomy and physiology of the organs and structures of the endocrine system. (pp 1258-1260)
2. Discuss the role of glucose as a major source of energy for the body, including the relationship of glucose to insulin. (pp 1260, 1265)
3. Describe the patient assessment process for a broad range of endocrine disorders. (pp 1261-1264)
4. Specify how to manage airway, breathing, and circulation in patients with endocrine system emergencies. (p 1261)
5. Define the term diabetes. (pp 1261, 1264)
6. Describe the factors that lead to glucose metabolic derangements. (p 1264)
7. Describe the incidence, morbidity, and mortality of diabetic emergencies. (pp 1265-1266, 1268, 1270, 1274)
8. Identify the common characteristics of the various types of diabetes. (p 1265)
9. Describe the chronic and acute complications associated with diabetes mellitus. (pp 1265-1266)
10. Explain some age-related considerations to keep in mind when treating an older adult patient who is thought to have undiagnosed diabetes. (p 1267)
11. Compare the pathophysiology, assessment, and management of type 1 diabetes mellitus with that of type 2 diabetes. (pp 1267-1269)
12. Identify risk factors associated with prediabetes, including the role of hemoglobin A1c blood tests, in distinguishing prediabetes from diabetes. (pp 1269-1270)
13. Explain how to diagnose and manage gestational diabetes. (p 1270)
14. Compare hyperglycemic and hypoglycemic diabetic emergencies, including their pathophysiology, assessment, and management. (pp 1270-1277)
15. Describe the interventions for providing emergency medical care during a hypoglycemic crisis to conscious and unconscious patients who have a history of diabetes. (pp 1272-1274)
16. Provide the generic and trade names, form, dose, indications, contraindications, and procedure for administering 50% dextrose to a patient with hypoglycemia. (pp 1272-1274)
17. Define hyperglycemia and discuss its pathophysiology, assessment, and management. (pp 1274-1277)
18. Describe the relationship between DKA and hyperglycemia. (pp 1274-1276)
19. List the signs and symptoms of diabetic ketoacidosis (DKA). (pp 1275-1276)
20. Describe the interventions for providing emergency medical care during a hyperglycemic crisis to conscious and unconscious patients who have a history of diabetes. (pp 1276-1277)
21. Define hyperosmolar hyperglycemic syndrome/ hyperosmolar nonketotic coma (HHS/HONK) and the findings characteristic of this condition. (pp 1277-1278)
22. Describe the pathophysiology, assessment, and management of pancreatitis. (pp 1278-1279)
23. Compare primary and secondary adrenal insufficiency, including their incidence, morbidity and mortality, pathophysiology, assessment, and management. (pp 1279-1281)

24. Identify addisonian crisis, what triggers this emergency, its chief clinical manifestation and other signs and symptoms, and its management. (pp 1279-1280)
25. Identify Cushing syndrome, the physical manifestations characteristic of the disorder, and its pathophysiology, assessment, and management. (p 1281)
26. Discuss the clinical presentation of a patient with an adrenal gland tumor. (p 1281)
27. Compare the effects of hypothyroidism and hyperthyroidism on the body. (pp 1281-1282)
28. Explain the pathophysiology of Graves disease, including the characteristic signs and symptoms of the disease. (pp 1281-1282)
29. Explain the pathophysiology of Hashimoto disease, including how it compares with Graves disease. (p 1282)
30. Outline the characteristic signs and symptoms of myxedema coma, as well as its management. (pp 1282-1283)
31. Describe thyrotoxicosis and thyroid storm, and their relationship to hyperthyroidism. (p 1283)
32. Describe hyperparathyroidism, including its pathophysiology, presentation, and management. (p 1283)
33. Differentiate between diabetes insipidus and syndrome of inappropriate antidiuretic hormone secretion (SIADH). (p 1284)

Skills Objectives

1. Demonstrate the assessment and care of a patient with hypoglycemia and a decreased level of consciousness. (pp 1271-1274)
2. Demonstrate how to administer glucose to a patient with an altered mental status. (pp 1272-1273)
3. Demonstrate how to administer dextrose to a patient with hypoglycemia. (pp 1273-1274)
4. Demonstrate how to administer glucagon to a patient with hypoglycemia. (p 1274)

Introduction

Few other systems in the body share the level of responsibility assigned to the endocrine system. This system directly or indirectly influences almost every cell, organ, and function of the body. Consequently, patients with an endocrine disorder often have a broad range of signs and symptoms, necessitating a thorough assessment and immediate treatment to avert life-threatening emergencies.

Anatomy and Physiology Review

As discussed in Chapter 8, *Anatomy and Physiology*, the endocrine system is responsible for the control and regulation of all systems of the body.

Many diseases are a result of hormone imbalances. Disease occurs when normal cell signaling is interrupted, resulting in positive feedback. As a consequence, the system

YOU are the Paramedic — PART 1

You are dispatched to a local grocery store for a woman "sitting in the butter." When you arrive, you are greeted by an older man, who tells you there is a large woman sitting in one of the refrigerated sections of the store. The man points down the dairy aisle and says, "There she is. We found her like that. She was shaking all over and is very hot to the touch. I tried to help her, but now I have to go."

From a distance, you see an obese woman with a ruddy complexion casually sitting on top of a refrigerated dairy case. As you approach, you notice her bulging eyes and that she is diaphoretic. There are numerous large white tablets scattered on the aisle floor and what appears to be a food wrapper next to her feet. There is emesis on the floor nearby. When you call out to her, she does not respond.

1. Which key information is provided from the dispatch and scene size-up?
2. Which types of medical conditions can cause an altered mental status?

stops providing the critical negative feedback required to regulate function. Cell signaling is covered in more detail in Chapter 9, *Pathophysiology*.

▶ Components of the Endocrine System

The major components of the endocrine system include the hypothalamus; the pineal gland, pituitary gland, thyroid gland, thymus gland, parathyroid gland, and adrenal glands; the pancreas; and the gonads, including the ovaries and testes. The pancreas has a role in hormone production as well as in digestion.

Hormones are chemical messengers that are secreted into the bloodstream by endocrine glands. Hormones circulate throughout the body and target organs to maintain homeostasis. The action triggered by a hormone depends on the specific organ affected. Chapter 8, *Anatomy and Physiology*, discusses the hormones produced by the endocrine system.

Hypothalamus

The hypothalamus is not a gland, but rather a small region of the brain that contains several control centers for body functions and emotions. It is the primary link between the endocrine system and the nervous system.

The hypothalamus also produces regulatory (releasing and inhibitory) hormones, which control the release of hormones by the pituitary gland. The hypothalamus and pituitary gland are intimately related through the vascular system. The hypothalamic–pituitary system controls the function of multiple peripheral endocrine organs (eg, thyroid, adrenal cortex, gonads, and breasts).

Some of the hormones produced by the hypothalamus have physiologic effects that depend on their concentration. For example, a decrease in the body's water content triggers the release of **antidiuretic hormone (ADH)**. The hypothalamus senses the concentration of salt in body fluids and signals the posterior pituitary gland to increase ADH secretion. Increased levels of ADH stimulate the renal tubules to reabsorb sodium and water. At the same time, ADH acts as a vasopressor.

Pituitary Gland

Located at the base of the brain, the pituitary gland is divided into anterior and posterior regions.

Six of the hormones secreted by the pituitary gland stimulate other endocrine glands and are referred to as "tropic" (from the Greek *tropos*, meaning "to turn" or "change") hormones. These include **adrenocorticotropic hormone (ACTH)**, follicle-stimulating hormone, growth hormone, **luteinizing hormone**, prolactin, and **thyroid-stimulating hormone**. The other two hormones, ADH and oxytocin, control other body functions.

During times of stress, the hypothalamus secretes a hormone that stimulates the anterior pituitary to release ACTH. ACTH targets the adrenal cortex and causes it to secrete **cortisol** (a glucocorticoid and adrenocorticoid). Cortisol stimulates most body cells to increase their energy production.

Thyroid Gland

Thyroid hormones, which affect metabolism, are secreted in response to the stimulation of the thyroid gland by the anterior pituitary gland. The anterior pituitary gland secretes thyroid-stimulating hormone (TSH) in response to the hypothalamus's secretion of thyrotropin-releasing hormone (TRH).

The thyroid gland secretes **thyroxine (T_4)** when the body's metabolic rate decreases. Thyroxine, the body's major metabolic hormone, stimulates energy production in cells, which increases the rate at which cells consume oxygen and use carbohydrates, fats, and proteins. Without the proper intake level of dietary iodine, thyroxine cannot be produced, and the patient's physical and mental growth are diminished.

The thyroid gland also secretes **calcitonin**, which helps maintain normal calcium levels in the blood. This hormone is secreted when the thyroid detects high levels of calcium. Calcitonin travels to the bones, where it stimulates the bone-building cells to absorb the excess calcium. It also stimulates the kidneys to absorb and excrete excess calcium.

Parathyroid Glands

The parathyroid glands assist in the regulation of calcium. However, the **parathyroid hormone**, when secreted by the parathyroid, acts as an antagonist to calcitonin. Parathyroid hormone is secreted when calcium blood levels are low. It stimulates the bone-dissolving cells to break down bone and release calcium into the bloodstream. In the kidneys, parathyroid hormone decreases the amount of calcium released in the urine.

Thymus Gland

The function of the thymus gland, or *thymus*, is to help the immune system identify and destroy foreign intruders. In studies involving organ transplantation in baby mice that had their thymus removed, the organ that was transplanted was not rejected; however, the mice became highly susceptible to disease-causing pathogens and to various pathogenic processes such as cancer.

Controversies

Although it has long been thought that as we age, the immune system does not function as well and infections are more likely, current research does not appear to support this theory. However, increased morbidity and mortality secondary to infection do occur. Anatomic and functional deterioration of systems is thought to be the reason for this trend. For example, urinary retention leads to an increase in urinary tract infections.

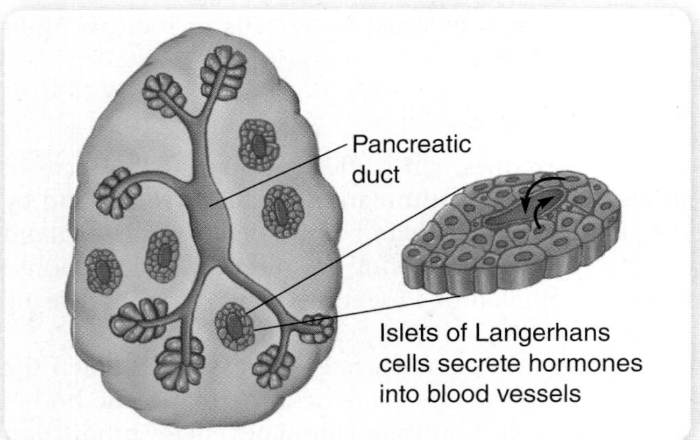

Figure 23-1 The islets of Langerhans secrete hormones into blood vessels.

Pancreas

The pancreas is considered both an endocrine gland and an exocrine gland. The exocrine component secretes digestive enzymes into the duodenum via the pancreatic duct. The endocrine component secretes three hormones from cell groups called the **islets of Langerhans**. These cell groups within the pancreas act like "an organ within an organ," secreting **glucagon** from alpha cells, **insulin** from beta cells, and **somatostatin** from delta cells.

Somatostatin is responsible for the inhibition of insulin and glucagon secretion **Figure 23-1**.

In a healthy patient, the body regulates blood glucose levels using both insulin and glucagon. When the body's blood glucose level falls, glucagon is secreted to raise the glucose level. When it enters the bloodstream, glucagon stimulates the liver to convert glycogen into sugar and secrete it into the bloodstream, where cells can use it for energy.

When blood glucose levels are elevated, the islets of Langerhans secrete insulin, which is carried by the bloodstream to the cells. Cell membrane permeability is increased by insulin, allowing the movement of glucose into the cells. The cells then take in more glucose and use it to produce energy. Insulin also stimulates the liver to take in more glucose and store it as glycogen for later use by the body.

Insulin is the *only* hormone that decreases the blood glucose levels. It is essential for glucose to enter and nourish the cells. Once the blood glucose levels have returned to normal, the islets of Langerhans discontinue the secretion of insulin.

Adrenal Glands

The adrenal glands, located on each side of the body on the superior aspect of each kidney, are divided into two distinct sections, the adrenal cortex and the adrenal medulla. The adrenal cortex completely surrounds the inner adrenal medulla.

If the body experiences a drop in blood pressure or volume, a decrease in sodium level, or an increase in the potassium level, the adrenal cortex is stimulated to secrete **aldosterone** (a mineralocorticoid). Aldosterone stimulates the kidneys to reabsorb sodium from the urine and excrete potassium by altering the osmotic gradient in the blood. When sodium is reabsorbed into the blood, water follows; this action increases both blood volume and blood pressure. Aldosterone also reduces the amount of salt and water lost through the sweat and salivary glands.

When the hypothalamus is stimulated as part of the "fight or flight" response, the adrenal medulla secretes small amounts of **norepinephrine** and large amounts of **epinephrine**. Norepinephrine raises blood pressure by causing contraction of the smooth muscle that lines the arterioles and relaxation of the smooth muscle that lines the bronchioles. Epinephrine stimulates sympathetic nervous system receptors throughout the body. In addition, it stimulates the liver to convert glycogen to glucose for use as energy in the cells. The actions of both hormones result in increased levels of oxygen and glucose in the blood and faster circulation of blood to the brain, heart, and muscles, which in turn enables the body to respond to the short-term emergency situation.

Gonads

In both men and women the primary functions of the gonads are to promote sexual maturation to puberty and fulfill any subsequent reproductive needs; the gonads are the main source of sex hormones.

In men, the interstitial cells of the testes produce male hormones known as **androgens**. Androgens regulate body changes associated with sexual development (puberty), including growth spurts, deepening of the voice, growth of facial and pubic hair, and muscle growth and strength. The most prominent of these hormones is **testosterone**. Testosterone promotes healthy sperm production, determines secondary male sex characteristics such as hair production, and stimulates growth. Testosterone is responsible for male secondary characteristics such as increased muscle and bone mass as well as aggressive behavior.

In women, the gonads are the ovaries. The anterior pituitary gland directs the actions of the ovaries through the follicle-stimulating hormone (FSH) and luteinizing hormone (LH). The ovaries release the eggs and secrete the hormones **estrogen** and **progesterone**, along with a small amount of testosterone. Estrogen signals the anterior pituitary gland to secrete LH when an egg is developing in an ovarian follicle. Estrogen and progesterone also assist in the regulation of the menstrual cycle. At puberty, estrogen also supports development of the secondary sex characteristics: enlargement of the breasts, uterine enlargement, fat deposits in the hips and thighs, and development of hair under the arms and in the pubic area. Progesterone prepares the uterus for implantation of the fertilized egg. During pregnancy, progesterone ensures that the uterine wall maintains functionality and prepares the mammary glands for activity.

Words of Wisdom

Although specific pathophysiology varies for each disease, endocrine emergencies are usually caused by the following:

- Failure of normal hormone production
- Excessive hormone production
- Failure of feedback inhibition systems involving the hypothalamus, pituitary gland, endocrine gland, and the target organ

Patient Assessment

The difficult part of assessing patients with endocrine emergencies is that their problems tend to affect many organ systems and the seriousness of their presentations varies greatly. Many of the patients will have had their conditions for some time and may already be receiving treatment. These patients or their family members will likely share with you that there is a history of an endocrine problem; this information, in addition to the common signs and symptoms associated with each endocrine emergency, should help you determine the cause of the current problem. In any event, do not take these calls lightly because poor outcomes can result quickly.

Scene Size-up

Scene safety should always be a primary concern as you arrive on scene. Make sure that all hazards are addressed and that you take standard precautions.

Your observations of the scene can also give valuable information regarding what might have happened. Check bureau tops, bedside tables, and medicine cabinets for medications that might give a clue as to the patient's underlying illness. Also, check the refrigerator for insulin.

Primary Survey

The primary survey begins with the basics: airway, breathing, circulation, disability, and exposure (ABCDE). Patients experiencing an endocrine emergency may be in serious distress, so it is essential that you identify and manage any life threats immediately. In patients with an altered mental status, check for a medical identification bracelet or necklace that may list allergies or known conditions.

Your general impression combined with a thorough physical assessment and patient history is essential in helping you to identify the causes of your patient's distress. Endocrine diseases present with signs and symptoms that depend on the hormone production or secretion that is affected. Is the patient alert, or is there a change in the normal mental status? An unresponsive patient is obviously in a critical state and may be experiencing an endocrine crisis, such as **hypoglycemia** (abnormally low blood glucose level), **hyperglycemia** (abnormally high blood glucose level), or a **myxedema coma** (a rare condition that can occur in patients who have severe, untreated hypothyroidism) with severe thyroid deficiency. Diaphoresis is usually a sign of severe distress and is present in **thyrotoxicosis** (a toxic condition caused by excessive levels of circulating thyroid hormone), along with pulmonary edema.

Your general impression can assist you in initiating the process of forming a field impression. A "buffalo hump," "moon face," and acne are telltale signs of **Cushing syndrome**, discussed later in this chapter. Mottled skin may be associated with pancreatitis. Enlarged or abnormal-appearing body parts may occur with conditions such as edema with **syndrome of inappropriate antidiuretic hormone secretion (SIADH)** (an endocrine disorder in which an excess of ADH results in decreased urinary output and, therefore, systemic fluid overload) or anasarca (extreme, generalized edema) with myxedema coma. Underweight or overweight patients may indicate an endocrine dysfunction such as hypothyroidism, hyperthyroidism, or **diabetes**—a group of complex metabolic disorders with many causes. **Exophthalmos** (protruding eyeballs) is present in **Graves disease**, an autoimmune disorder that causes thyroid gland hypertrophy and severe hyperthyroidism. Children with **panhypopituitarism** (inadequate production or absence of the pituitary hormones) may have abnormal development.

Check the patient's airway to ensure that it is patent and there are no obstructions. When patients present with an altered level of consciousness, they may be unable to protect their airway. Also, many will be very ill and have chronic episodes of vomiting. Maintain the airway as needed through patient positioning, suctioning, or basic airways.

Patients with endocrine emergencies may present with varied levels of breathing rate, rhythm, quality, and effort. You should immediately assess the patient's effort of breathing—breathing should be effortless—and administer supplemental oxygen as necessary.

Assess the color, moisture, and temperature of the patient's skin, and obtain the patient's blood pressure. Skin condition can assist you in determining the patient's medical status. A patient with pale, cool, moist skin may be in shock or have hypoglycemia, whereas a patient with hot, dry skin may have a fever or hyperglycemia. A patient in hypoglycemic crisis will have a rapid, weak pulse. Because endocrine emergencies may affect the body's compensating systems, intravenous (IV) fluid administration may be necessary. Follow your local protocols.

Many patients with endocrine disorders are being treated by specialists, and they should be transported to a facility that specializes in these conditions. If the patient's condition is unstable or shows signs of becoming unstable, such as a diminished level of consciousness, transport the patient rapidly to the closest facility for stabilization first.

History Taking

Particularly in diabetic emergencies, the family history can provide important information. Because diabetes is a genetic disease (passed down through family members), learning that a parent or grandparent has a history of diabetes is a major clue and can prove to be invaluable in your treatment decision. This is especially true if the patient is a child and has a new onset of altered mental status.

Investigate the chief complaint or the history of the present illness. While you are assessing the chief complaint, you should consider the patient's signs and symptoms and any pertinent negatives.

If a patient is unresponsive, obtain a blood glucose level and manage any abnormalities appropriately. Do not assume that because a patient does not have a history of diabetes he or she does not have a new onset of the disease.

Follow the SAMPLE mnemonic (Signs and symptoms, Allergies, Medications, Pertinent past medical history, Last oral intake, Events leading up to the illness or injury). Gather as much information as possible from the scene and any family members or bystanders present.

Observe the patient for any signs that may assist you in confirming the patient's reported symptoms. Signs and symptoms of endocrine disorders include those mentioned earlier, as well as many symptoms such as polyphagia, polyuria, and polydipsia in patients with undiagnosed or poorly managed diabetes. Tachycardia, premature ventricular contractions, premature atrial contractions, and atrial dysrhythmias all can occur with hyperthyroidism and thyrotoxicosis.

It is essential to ascertain any allergies the patient may have prior to medication administration. Document all medications the patient is currently taking on a regular basis and whether the patient has been compliant with the regimen. Is the patient taking medications associated with diabetes (such as insulin)? Is the patient undergoing thyroid hormone replacement therapy for hypothyroidism or using glucocorticoids to manage Cushing syndrome?

Pertinent past medical history is important when diagnosing and managing the patient with an endocrine condition. Many conditions will have been diagnosed prior to your arrival and the patient may have a substantial amount of information regarding his or her condition. Family members also are often well informed in these conditions.

In addition to inquiring about last oral intake, ask women of childbearing age about their last menstrual period. This information may be important, for example, for patients with hypothyroidism who have a history of light or absent periods.

The patient, family members, or bystanders may be able to give additional information regarding anything that happened prior to the current situation. For example, a patient with diabetes may not have eaten that day or may have been under a high level of emotional stress or physical activity.

YOU are the Paramedic PART 2

As you introduce yourself and ask the patient what is wrong, you see she has chocolate all over her mouth and an ice cream sandwich melting in her hand. She does not respond to you until you pinch the back of her hand. She then pushes your hand away.

Recording Time: 0 Minutes	
Appearance	Sitting upright with a blank stare
Level of consciousness	P (responsive to painful stimulus)
Airway	Open
Breathing	Adequate chest rise and volume
Circulation	Weak, rapid radial pulse

3. Although the patient is cooperative, what do you need to consider when you treat any patient with an altered mental status?
4. What could be the cause of the patient's reported shaking?

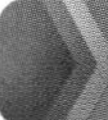

Secondary Assessment

Begin the physical exam by observing the patient's general appearance. Decorticate or decerebrate posturing should also be noted, if present; both are signs of serious illness.

Your physical exam should be geared toward identifying as many atypical findings as possible. Unless the patient had an endocrine emergency that caused some form of trauma, a focused exam is usually not necessary. In this situation, a full-body exam is more appropriate, although life threats always should be managed first.

The physical exam will reveal the finer abnormalities that will help determine your treatment. For example, the condition of the patient's skin provides important information. Cold, clammy skin is a classic sign of shock but may also signal severe hypoglycemia, as from an insulin reaction and the body's response to catecholamine release. Cold, dry skin can indicate an overdose of sedative drugs or alcohol intoxication. Hot, dry skin suggests hyperglycemia, fever, or possibly heat stroke.

The goals of the physical exam in the comatose patient are twofold. First, you want to determine the patient's level of consciousness with precision so that later assessments can readily determine whether the patient's condition is improving or deteriorating. Second, you should look for signs that might provide clues to the source of the coma.

When you check the patient's vital signs, look for the combination of hypertension and bradycardia, which suggests increased intracranial pressure. Be alert for abnormal respiratory patterns. Cheyne-Stokes breathing usually points to a nonneurologic source of the coma. Kussmaul respirations are often present in patients experiencing **diabetic ketoacidosis (DKA)** (a form of acidosis in uncontrolled diabetes in which certain acids accumulate when insulin is not available); such respirations are one of the body's compensatory mechanisms to "blow off" the excess acid that is produced in this condition.

More worrisome are other abnormal breathing patterns, such as central neurogenic ventilation or huffing and puffing that do not seem to move much air. Look for respiratory-related motions such as sneezing and yawning. An intact brainstem is required to produce a sneeze or a yawn, so both of those actions have positive prognostic importance. Hiccupping and coughing, by contrast, can indicate brainstem damage.

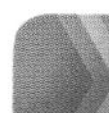

Reassessment

After you have initiated your treatment plan, continually reassess the patient to check for obvious and subtle changes. For every action you take, there should be a response. No response *is* a response. Document your findings along the way.

YOU are the Paramedic PART 3

Your protocol requires obtaining a blood glucose reading for any patient with a decreased level of consciousness. You record this patient's blood glucose level as 30 mg/dL. You obtain IV access and prepare to administer dextrose 50%. A bystander comes up to you and says, "Is she going to be okay? When another shopper and I found her there, I called 9-1-1. An older gentleman said she was probably diabetic, so he tried to shove ice cream in her mouth, but it didn't seem to help."

Recording Time: 5 Minutes	
Respirations	24 breaths/min
Pulse	100 beats/min, weak, and regular
Skin	Cool, pale, and diaphoretic
Blood pressure	160/94 mm Hg
Oxygen saturation (Spo_2)	97% on room air
Pupils	PERRLA

5. What concerns you about the bystander's statement?
6. If your partner was unable to obtain IV access, which additional treatment options exist for correcting the patient's blood glucose level?

The ABCs should be managed during the primary survey. Remember that a patient whose gag reflex is absent cannot protect his or her own airway from aspiration, so you should be prepared to suction the airway in an unresponsive patient. If the patient does not regain consciousness with treatment (eg, a hypoglycemic patient receives glucose and remains unresponsive), intubation should be considered. Be sure to obtain blood specimens early in patients with diabetes, because any administration of prehospital dextrose or other medications will substantially change the chemical makeup of subsequent blood samples.

An important aspect of patient care is to address the patient's emotional needs. Diabetes can be a stressful condition to manage, and patients who are diabetic have an increased risk of depression. Be empathetic and responsive to the patient's needs and provide emotional support as needed.

Monitor the cardiac rhythm of every comatose patient. During neurologic assessment, the most important consideration is not one measurement obtained at a single time but rather the *trend* shown by several measurements you obtained. Recheck the patient's vital signs, pupils, and level of consciousness (every 5 minutes in unstable patients and every 15 minutes in stable patients) and *record your findings* immediately. Every patient you transport should have at least two sets of vital signs documented regardless of the length of the transport.

Documentation & Communication

Communication with hospital staff is important for the continuity of care. Hospital personnel need to be informed about the patient's history, the present situation, assessment findings, and your interventions and the results. Your PCR is the only legal document in which you have to say that appropriate care was provided. Document your assessment findings clearly as the basis for your treatment. Patients who refuse transport because you "cured" them with oral glucose may require even more thorough documentation. Follow your local protocols for patients who refuse treatment or transport.

Emergency Medical Care

If the patient has an altered mental status, establish an IV line with 0.9% normal saline (NS) or a saline lock. Measure the blood glucose level immediately and initiate treatment if the reading is less than 60 mg/dL. Give 12.5 to 25 g of D_{50} (50 g of dextrose per every 100 mL, or 50% concentration); this dose will reverse most cases of hypoglycemia. Some EMS systems no longer carry D_{50} and may use glucagon or D_{10} (10% dextrose concentration). Glucagon is administered 1 g intramuscularly (IM), with a greatly increased recovery time as compared with IV D_{50} or D_{10}. D_{10} is a lesser concentration and is not hypertonic. The decreased osmolarity in D_{10} is less caustic to the veins and tissues. D_{50} also causes greater fluctuations in blood glucose levels after administration.

If the patient's condition does not improve after a dose of dextrose, and if you have reason to suspect a narcotic overdose (based on signs of pinpoint pupils, needle tracks on the arms, depressed respirations), consider administering naloxone (Narcan).

Transport the comatose patient *supine* with a cervical collar in place if the patient is intubated to decrease the risk of unintentional extubation during transport; otherwise, you can transport the patient in the lateral recumbent or recovery position (unless any injuries preclude that position). If there are indications of increasing intracranial pressure such as the Cushing reflex (slowing pulse, rising blood pressure, and an erratic respiratory pattern), posturing, or unequal pupils, transport with the head elevated to a 30° to 45° angle and the head midline to assist in venous return and minimize intracranial pressure. Always keep the mouth and pharynx suctioned free of secretions, vomitus, and blood.

Pathophysiology, Assessment, and Management of Glucose Metabolic Derangements

Endocrine disorders are caused by either hypersecretion or insufficient secretion of a gland. Hypersecretion presents as overactivity of the target organ regulated by the gland. Insufficient secretion results in underactivity of the organ controlled by the gland. The effects of a disturbance of endocrine gland function are determined by the degree of dysfunction of the gland and by the age and sex of the patient.

Glucose metabolic derangements, or disorders, are caused by dysfunction of the pancreas, which impairs the body's ability to metabolize glucose. Pancreatic dysfunction can range from barely detectable to extreme. Most glucose derangements and other clinically important endocrine emergencies result in compromise of the ABCs, improper fluid balance, deteriorating mental status, and abnormal vital signs and blood glucose levels.

▶ Diabetes Mellitus

Diabetes is a metabolic disorder that is now considered to encompass a group of complex diseases with many causes (ie, **diabetes mellitus** [a disease characterized by the body's inability to sufficiently metabolize glucose], **gestational diabetes** [diabetes that develops during pregnancy in women who did not have diabetes before pregnancy], hypoglycemia/hyperglycemia, diabetic ketoacidosis, hyperosmolar hyperglycemic syndrome). These pathologic conditions reflect a flaw in the production or function of insulin, or both. Insulin, a hormone produced in the pancreas, assists in the metabolism of carbohydrates and the transport of glucose into the cells. The end result of diabetes is hyperglycemia, also known as high blood sugar. Medically, the term *diabetes* refers to a metabolic disorder in which the body's ability to metabolize simple carbohydrates (glucose) is impaired. It is characterized by the following symptoms:

- **Polyphagia**, an increased appetite caused by the inability of glucose to be transported across the cell membrane.
- **Polydipsia**, a significant thirst caused by dehydration brought about by an increase in **diuresis** (the production of large amounts of urine by the kidney).
- **Polyuria**, the passage of large quantities of urine. In diabetes, excess glucose is excreted the urine (**glycosuria**) and attracts water, resulting in excessive diuresis.

Glucose (also known as *dextrose*) is one of the basic sugars in the body and, along with oxygen, is the primary fuel for cellular metabolism. *Diabetes mellitus* is characterized by the body's inability to sufficiently metabolize glucose. *Mellitus*, from the Greek word for honeybee, means "sweet"—a reference to the presence of glucose in the urine. In people with this disease, the pancreas does not produce enough insulin or the body's cells do not respond to the effects of the insulin that is produced. In either case, the result is the same: an elevated level of glucose in both the blood and the urine. Glucose builds up in the blood, overflows into the urine, and flows out of the body. Thus, cells can "starve," or be deprived of glucose, even when the blood contains large amounts of glucose **Figure 23-2**.

According to the 2014 National Diabetes Statistics Report, 29.1 million people in the United States (approximately 9.3% of the population) have diabetes; of these, 8.1 million remain undiagnosed. Thus, one in four people with diabetes is unaware of his or her disease status.[1,2]

In 2013, diabetes was the seventh leading cause of death in United States, although the US Centers for Disease Control and Prevention (CDC) suggest diabetes may be underreported as a source of mortality.[1] In 2012, the estimated total cost of diabetes in the United States was $245 billion.[2] Direct medical costs are approximately 2.3 times higher for people with diabetes than for those without diabetes and were estimated to be $176 billion in 2012.[2] The indirect costs of diabetes, which include disability, work loss, and premature death, were estimated to be $69 billion.[2]

Diabetes mellitus is responsible for myriad life-altering complications, some of which are listed here:

- **Kidneys.** Diabetes is the principal cause of kidney failure, accounting for 44% of new cases in 2011.[2] The glomeruli of the kidney become sclerotic, causing necrosis of the papillary tissue and leading to nephropathy (end-stage renal disease) and renal failure. High levels of glucose in the blood cause the kidneys to work harder than normal and can result in decreased kidney function over time.
- **Heart.** Adults with diabetes are approximately two times more likely to die of heart disease or to have a stroke than those who do not have diabetes.[2] When diabetes is poorly controlled, the process of **lipolysis** (from *lipo-*, meaning "fat," and *-lysis*, meaning "breakdown") raises the level of fat in the blood. As a result of the raised fat level (**dyslipidemia**), the risk of

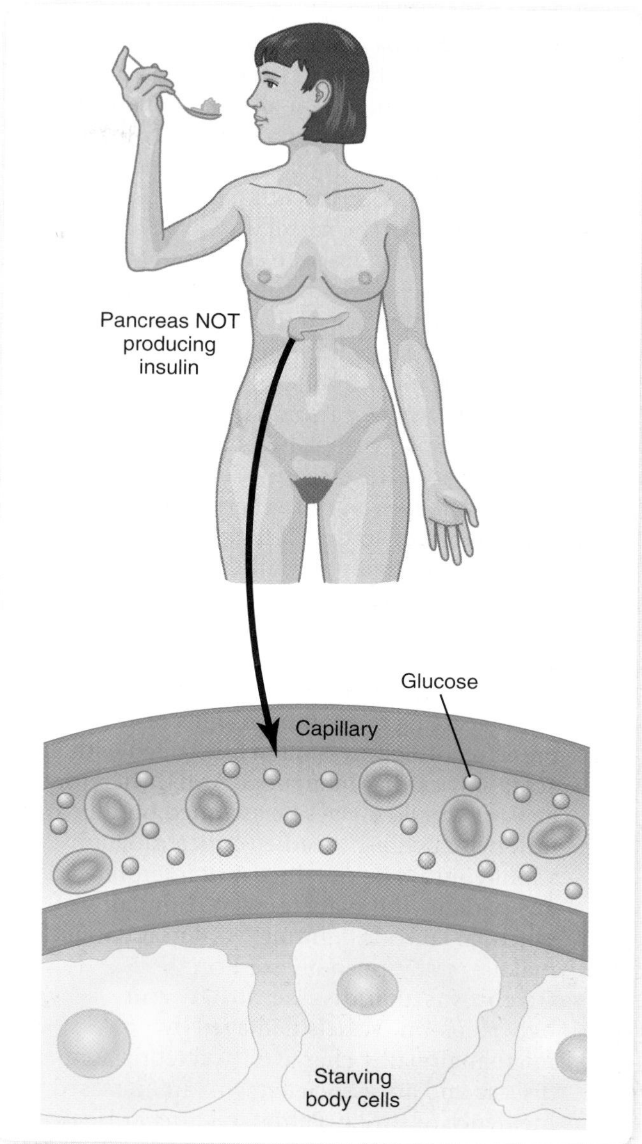

Figure 23-2 Diabetes is defined as a lack of or ineffective action of insulin. Without insulin, cells begin to "starve" because insulin is needed to allow glucose to enter and nourish the cells.

atherosclerosis and coronary artery disease increases. The fat circulating through the bloodstream adheres to the vessel walls, eventually causing them to be stiff and brittle. In addition, glucose crystals are sharp and their frequent elevation in blood glucose levels can damage the blood vessels. The microscopic deterioration of the vessel walls, called **microangiopathy**, leads to swelling of basement membrane cells, which then restricts the flow of blood to organs and tissues. Inadequate blood flow (ischemia) causes necrosis, or tissue death. Chronic heart failure develops over a period of several years and is twice as prevalent among people with diabetes than among those without the disease.[2] Central nervous system damage can cause cardiac dysrhythmias, which can lead to cardiac arrest and sudden death. Microangiopathy and neuropathy both contribute to an increased risk for a *silent* myocardial infarction to be experienced by a patient with diabetes. These pathologies combine and result in the patient with diabetes not perceiving the common signs of chest pain, pressure, or tightness often associated with an acute myocardial infarction (AMI). Therefore, an AMI should always be assumed until proved otherwise and a 12-lead electrocardiogram should always be obtained and interpreted for any patient with diabetes who complains of a syncopal episode, fainting, weakness, fatigue, malaise, or dyspnea on exertion.

- **Cerebrovascular disease, stroke, and hypertension.** Vessels damaged by microangiopathy characterize cerebrovascular disease and are associated with an increased incidence of stroke. Peripheral artery disease is also common in people with diabetes and impairs circulation to the lower extremities. Hypertension is present in 71% of people with diabetes.[2] Hypertension is associated with an increased risk of heart disease, stroke, kidney disease, and blindness.
- **Eyes.** In adults age 20 to 74 years, diabetes is the chief cause of new cases of blindness as a result of retinopathy. High glucose levels in the blood damage the vessels of the eye, causing swelling, wall weakness, and obstruction. Scar tissue can form that causes a pulling of the retina from the eye, or retinal detachment. Cataracts are a cloudy film that forms when fructose and sorbitol are deposited in the lens of the eye.
- **Neuropathy.** Neuropathy is nerve damage that results in a loss of sensation and function in the area innervated by the affected nerves. Such damage can cause sexual impotence, neurogenic bladder, constipation, or diarrhea. Neuropathy associated with diabetes often affects peripheral nerves, causing diminished sensation and function in the extremities. Patients with peripheral neuropathy often have paresthesia, a pinprick sensation in the hands, feet, arms, or legs. Paresthesia and dysesthesia—the absence of sensation—can blunt pain perception, making it possible for foot ulcers to go unnoticed until they become seriously infected. Because many of these patients also have poor circulation in the extremities, gangrene can develop in adjacent tissues and infection may spread to the bone. In fact, more than 60% of nontraumatic lower limb amputations can be attributed to diabetes.[2]

Because of the widespread effect of diabetes on all systems of the body, any preexisting condition will be more complex to manage after diabetes develops in the patient. The more closely patients adhere to the recommended management of their diabetes, the better the outcome of their other conditions will be. Conditions that develop subsequent to the onset of diabetes will respond more effectively when diabetes is managed appropriately. Many conditions associated with the presence of diabetes can be delayed or prevented with appropriate lifestyle changes and continued management of diabetes. Conversely, any kind of distress can have a negative effect on the patient and result in a 9-1-1 call because blood glucose levels are more difficult to control in the setting of increased physical activity or emotional stress.

Both chronic and acute complications are associated with diabetes mellitus. Although these complications are present in both forms of the disease (type 1 and type 2), they tend to be more severe in people with diabetes who require insulin. Left untreated, diabetes leads to organ system dysfunction, wasting of body tissues, and death. Even with excellent medical care, some patients with particularly aggressive forms of diabetes will die at a relatively young age from complications of the disease. The severity of diabetic complications correlates with the average blood glucose level and the age of onset. Although most patients with well-controlled diabetes have a normal life span, they must be willing to adjust their lives to the demands of the disease, especially their eating habits and physical activity levels. There is no cure for the disease, so treatment focuses on maintaining the level of blood glucose within the patient's normal range.

Two forms of diabetes mellitus exist: type 1 (formerly known as juvenile-onset diabetes) and type 2 (formerly known as adult-onset diabetes). The age of onset of the patient's symptoms is less important than whether the patient requires insulin to survive. Both types of diabetes mellitus are serious conditions that affect many tissues and functions other than the glucose-regulating mechanism, and both require lifelong medical management. In addition, the condition known as **prediabetes** is now recognized as a warning sign that may precede the development of **type 2 diabetes**, and is discussed later in this chapter.

The Diabetes Control and Complications Trial (DCCT) and its follow-up study, Epidemiology of Diabetes Interventions and Complications (EDIC), both of which were funded by the National Institute of Diabetes and Digestive and Kidney Diseases, have emphasized the need for intensive control of diabetes to prevent and minimize long-term complications from this disease.[3] The initial study noted that patients who maintained intensive diabetes control had a significant reduction in nephropathy, neuropathy, and retinopathy.[3] The follow-up study demonstrated a significant reduction in the incidence of cardiovascular disease in patients who implemented intensive glucose control.[3]

Special Populations

You might encounter an older adult patient who has undiagnosed diabetes. These patients report that they have not been feeling well for a while but have not seen a physician. A patient with undiagnosed diabetes or one who is in denial or ignores the advice of his or her physician may call 9-1-1 when the signs and symptoms get worse. Nonhealing wounds, blindness, renal failure, and other complications are associated with poorly controlled or uncontrolled diabetes. It is important that you recognize the signs and symptoms of diabetes because you might be the first health care provider to suggest medical treatment to an older adult patient who might otherwise ignore the condition.

Older adult patients and those with diabetes commonly present atypically with an AMI. They often do not present with classic crushing substernal chest pain or pressure because of the neuropathy associated with increasing age and diabetes. Older adults also generally have a higher pain tolerance compared with younger patients. Other causes of an altered perception of pain can include impaired cognition or slowed nerve conduction. You should maintain a high index of suspicion when these populations experience a syncopal episode, fatigue, shortness of breath, or nausea and diaphoresis.

Older adult patients are also more susceptible to dehydration and infections. As we age, our bodies tend to lose approximately 10% of the total body fluid.[4] Older adult patients may not become thirsty or react to thirst until they are extremely dehydrated. Medications can also cause an increase in diuresis, compounding the problem.

Type 1 Diabetes Mellitus

Pathophysiology. **Type 1 diabetes** has historically been referred to as insulin-dependent diabetes mellitus (IDDM) or juvenile-onset diabetes because it generally affects children. Although type 1 diabetes has a hereditary predisposition, it is believed that environmental factors may play a role—for example, with an infection that triggers an autoimmune disorder. With type I diabetes, the body develops autoantibodies that incorrectly identify the body's own tissues or substances as foreign invaders to be destroyed. Contributing to pancreatic destruction are autoantibodies to the insulin-secreting beta cells in the islets of Langerhans, to insulin, and to other pancreatic substances. The rate of beta-cell destruction is variable, occurring rapidly in some patients (mainly children) and slowly in others (mainly adults).[5] Eventually, the pancreatic beta cells become incapable of secreting insulin and regulating intracellular glucose. Because beta cells are the only source of insulin, it must then be administered by injection or with a pump when the cells are destroyed.

Latent autoimmune diabetes in adults is a variant of type 1 diabetes that occurs in adults older than 30 years. The pathophysiology is the same as that of young-onset diabetes, with the body's immune system destroying the beta cells. Thus, patients with latent autoimmune diabetes in adults will ultimately require insulin therapy.

When the endocrine system (or pancreas) fails to produce insulin (as is the case in most patients with type 1 diabetes), people require daily injections of supplementary, synthetic insulin throughout their lives to control their blood glucose levels. In addition to daily insulin injections, strict dietary control must be observed, which can be difficult to achieve with young children. Increased activity and alcohol consumption can lead to low blood glucose levels (alcohol depletes glycogen stores in the liver). Therefore, in adults with type 1 diabetes, alcohol consumption also must be controlled.

Assessment. Assessment of a patient with a history of diabetes will be similar to your assessment of any other medical patient; however, there are some considerations you will want to keep in mind. Determine whether the patient is compliant with the management of his or her disease.

If the patient has an altered mental status, you should suspect a low blood glucose level. Hypoglycemia is a potentially life-threatening event. Patients with diabetes also potentially may have other chronic conditions such as renal failure, congestive heart failure, coronary artery disease, hypertension, and vision and hearing impairment. Because patients may have an altered perception of pain, particularly in their extremities, it is important to assess for any signs of sores or infections. It is also important to ask about tingling, numbness, or swelling of the extremities. Patients with long-standing diabetes may have undergone amputation, and their residual limb may become infected or septic.

Ask the patient about any vision changes, headaches, dizziness, bleeding, or sores in the mouth. Also ask whether there has been a recent change in the patient's bowel movements or eating habits.

Evidence-Based Medicine

Research suggests that lethal cardiac dysrhythmias may be triggered by hypoglycemia and may lead to the sudden death of patients with type 1 diabetes who experience hypoglycemia.[6]

Management. Type 1 diabetes always requires the use of insulin that is administered by injection or an insulin pump, also called continuous subcutaneous insulin infusion therapy. Insulin cannot be ingested orally because the digestive process will render it inactive.

You will likely encounter patients with diabetes who use insulin pumps to treat their disease. An alternative to multiple daily injections of insulin, insulin pumps provide improved control of blood glucose levels and better quality of life for many patients. These small devices consist of an infusion set, a reservoir for insulin, and the pump itself. The pump is approximately the size of a deck of cards, weighs approximately 3 ounces, and can be worn on a belt or carried in a pocket **Figure 23-3**. Insulin is administered through a catheter under the skin. The pump is often set to deliver a basal amount of insulin continuously throughout the day. Alternatively, the pump can be set to deliver a bolus of insulin at specific times such as mealtimes, when blood glucose levels are high.

Currently, several different types of insulin are available in the United States: rapid-acting insulin, regular or short-acting insulin, intermediate-acting insulin, and long-acting insulin. The various types of insulin differ in their onset of action, duration, and peak time. All of the US versions of insulin are synthetic; however, animal insulin can be imported.

Type 2 Diabetes Mellitus

Pathophysiology. The most common form of diabetes is *type 2 diabetes*, a condition in which blood glucose levels are elevated because the body cannot produce enough insulin to compensate for the inability to utilize insulin effectively. In many people with type 2 diabetes, the pancreas actually produces enough insulin; however, for reasons not fully understood, the body cannot effectively use it—a condition known as **insulin resistance**. One possible explanation is that the insulin receptor cells located on the target cells have changed in some way and are no longer able to receive the insulin when it arrives at the target cell.

In some cases, an abnormal increase in the production of glucose by the liver causes an increase in blood glucose levels. Normally, when blood glucose and insulin levels are low, the pancreas releases glucagon and stimulates the liver to produce and release glucose into the blood. In some people, however, the levels of glucagon stay high. When glucagon levels remain high, excess amounts of glucose are produced, leading to high blood glucose levels. Metformin, the medication most commonly prescribed for the management of type 2 diabetes, causes a decrease in glucose production.

According to the World Health Organization, approximately 8.5% of the world's population is affected by diabetes, mostly type 2, making it a global health concern.[7] Approximately 90% of all people with diabetes in the United States have type 2 diabetes, which typically develops in middle-aged adult patients.[8] The development of type 2 diabetes has been associated with obesity and physical inactivity, two characteristics becoming more common in today's younger population. Type 2 diabetes may also be related to *metabolic syndrome*, a cluster of characteristics including excessive fat in the abdominal area, elevated blood pressure, and high levels of blood lipids. Risk factors for developing metabolic syndrome include excess weight, lack of physical activity, and genetic factors.

Assessment. Symptoms of type 2 diabetes may include the following:

- Fatigue
- Nausea
- Frequent urination

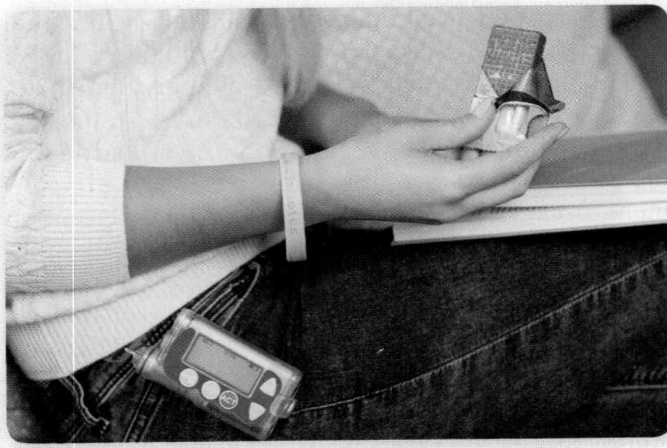

Figure 23-3 An insulin pump is a small electronic device that automatically delivers insulin to maintain the desired blood glucose level.

Evidence-Based Medicine

According to the National Institutes of Health, most of the genetic risk for type 2 diabetes can be attributed to common, shared genetic variants—each contributing a small amount to a patient's overall risk of the disease—rather than to many rare variants unique to a single patient.[7] This multifactorial nature resolves a question about the genetics of type 2 diabetes that has puzzled researchers for decades. It suggests the need to account for both environmental factors and the patient's genetic profile when developing a plan of treatment or prevention.[9]

- Thirst
- Unexplained weight loss
- Blurred vision
- Frequent infections and slow healing of wounds
- Being cranky, confused, or shaky
- Unresponsiveness
- Seizure

These symptoms tend to develop gradually and usually become noticeable in middle age. In fact, the onset of type 2 diabetes may be so insidious that patients may not realize they have the disease. In some instances, the symptoms can develop over several years in overweight adults older than 40 years. A small percentage of patients do not display any symptoms.

Words of Wisdom

New-onset weakness in a patient known to have diabetes must be considered a myocardial infarction until proved otherwise. Many patients with either type 1 or type 2 diabetes have an acquired dysfunction in the peripheral nervous system (neuropathy). Also, increased insulin levels result in increased blood lipid levels. This combination often leads to an earlier onset of coronary artery disease. People with diabetes do not always have typical clinical symptoms of acute coronary syndrome because of an alteration in sensation. They are more likely to present with general body weakness.

Management. Weight loss is an important factor in helping to control type 2 diabetes. Exercise and a well-balanced, nutritious diet are key components in combating the complications of diabetes. To maintain glucose levels within the normal range, food intake must be spread throughout the day in coordination with daily medications/insulin injections. You can help patients by reinforcing this message to the patient and by helping the family understand how to reduce the patient's risk of diabetic complications.

Oral medications used to manage type 2 diabetes can be used alone or in combination because they exhibit different mechanisms of action. As with all medications, there is always the risk of interaction with other medications. A physician or pharmacist should be consulted prior to the addition of any medication, whether an over-the-counter or prescription agent. These oral medications can be divided into six classes, as shown in Table 23-1.

Prediabetes

Prediabetes is a condition identified in people who have certain risk factors associated with type 2 diabetes and exists when blood glucose levels or hemoglobin A1c levels are above normal levels, yet not high enough to be diagnosed as diabetes. The A1c blood test reveals information regarding the patient's blood glucose levels over the previous 3 months. A normal A1c level is less than 5.7%, prediabetes is diagnosed with an A1c level between 5.7% and 6.4%, and type 2 diabetes is diagnosed at with an A1c level greater than 6.4%.

Table 23-1 Oral Agents Used to Treat Type 2 Diabetes Mellitus

Medication Class	Function	Examples
Sulfonylureas	Stimulate beta cells to produce more insulin	Chlorpropamide (Diabinese) Glipizide (Glucotrol, Glucotrol XL) Glyburide (Micronase, Glynase, DiaBeta) Glimepiride (Amaryl)
Meglitinides	Stimulate beta cells to produce more insulin	Repaglinide (Prandin) Nateglinide (Starlix)
Biguanides	Decrease the amount of glucose produced by the liver	Metformin (Glucophage)
Thiazolidinediones	Increase insulin effectiveness in the muscle and decrease liver glucose production	Rosiglitazone (Avandia) Pioglitazone (ACTOS)
Alpha-glucosidase inhibitors	Prevent the breakdown of starches	Acarbose (Precose) Miglitol (Glyset)
DPP-4 inhibitors	Inhibit the breakdown of GLP-1, a naturally occurring compound in the body that reduces blood glucose levels	Sitagliptin (Januvia) Saxagliptin (Onglyza)

Words of Wisdom

The hemoglobin A1c test does not require fasting and can be performed at any time of the day. Unfortunately, it can be inaccurate in people of African, Mediterranean, or Southeast Asian descent or those with a family history of sickle cell anemia. People with kidney or liver failure may also have inaccurate A1c results.

According to the CDC, prediabetes affects 1 out of 3 adults in the United States, or approximately 86 million people, and 90% are unaware of their status. Within 5 years and with no intervention, 15% to 30% of people with prediabetes will develop type 2 diabetes. Risk factors for experiencing this disease course include the following characteristics:[10]

- Older than 45 years
- Being overweight
- A family history of diabetes—specifically, a parent or sibling who has been diagnosed as having type 2 diabetes
- Being of African American, Hispanic/Latino, American Indian, Pacific Islander, and some Asian American racial or ethnic backgrounds
- Gestational diabetes or having given birth to a baby who weighed more than 9 pounds (4 kg)
- Being physically active fewer than 3 times per week

Although some of the risk factors affecting the pathway from prediabetes to type 2 diabetes cannot be altered, others can. According to the CDC, interventions affecting two specific factors can help prevent or delay the onset of type 2 diabetes by 58%, specifically, losing 5% to 7% of the patient's body weight and getting at least 150 minutes of physical activity per week.[11]

▶ Gestational Diabetes

Pathophysiology

Gestational diabetes does not have a pancreatic component, but rather is a form of glucose intolerance that can occur during pregnancy. This condition has been identified more often in African American, Hispanic/Latino, and Native American populations, as well as in women with obesity or who have a family history of diabetes. Women who experience gestational diabetes during pregnancy have a 40% to 60% increased risk of developing type 2 diabetes within one decade.[12,13] For most women, gestational diabetes will resolve before delivery. In a few women, however, diabetes will not resolve or type 2 diabetes will develop.

Blood glucose crosses the placental barrier. When a pregnant woman is hyperglycemic, high levels of glucose enter the fetus, causing increased production of insulin by the fetus in an attempt to normalize blood glucose levels. The extra glucose is converted into fat in the fetus, such that women experiencing gestational diabetes often deliver large babies (macrosomia) and may encounter difficult deliveries. Often, cesarean sections are required.

Gestational diabetes is usually diagnosed at 28 weeks' gestation and peaks in the third trimester of pregnancy. It is thought that two hormones produced by the placenta, progesterone and estrogen, result in increased sensitivity to insulin. Because this condition does not occur until later in pregnancy, it does not produce birth defects. Infants of mothers in whom gestational diabetes developed are at higher risk for obesity and diabetes in their lifetime.

Assessment

The oral glucose tolerance test is used to diagnose gestational diabetes. This test should be used until the pregnant woman is within 12 weeks of delivery. The hemoglobin A1c test can be used during the first pregnancy visit to identify the presence of preexisting diabetes or prediabetes.

Management

Management of gestational diabetes should be initiated as soon as possible to stabilize blood glucose levels and minimize potential complications to both mother and baby. Management includes diet modification, exercise, and blood glucose testing. Oral medications are not prescribed for this form of diabetes, and insulin injections may be required.

▶ Hypoglycemia

Normal blood glucose levels range from approximately 60 to 120 mg/dL; *hypoglycemia* (a low blood glucose level) occurs when blood glucose levels drop to 45 mg/dL or less. Hypoglycemia is a common problem experienced by both patients with type 1 and type 2 diabetes. These patients must closely monitor and intensively control their diabetes to prevent long-term complications. According to the CDC, approximately 282,000 US emergency department visits made by adults 18 years or older in 2011 involved hypoglycemia as the diagnosis.[2]

Hypoglycemia is relatively common and, although not completely preventable, can be treated easily. This condition can be detected with regular blood glucose monitoring and rarely results in complications for the patient.

In contrast, severe hypoglycemia, resulting in loss of consciousness or altered mental status, is a more common reason for a call to 9-1-1, and requires intervention and treatment. As an EMS professional, you will need to promptly provide treatment to these patients. If untreated or not detected, serious hypoglycemia can lead to coma or death.

Pathophysiology

Hypoglycemia in people with type 1 diabetes often is the result of having taken too much insulin, too little food, or both. The tissues of the central nervous system (including the brain), unlike other tissues that can usually metabolize fat or protein in addition to sugar, depend entirely on glucose as their source of energy. If the glucose level in the blood drops dramatically, the brain is literally starved.

Counterregulation is the body's natural defensive ability to maintain blood glucose at an appropriate level. An understanding of this concept is critical, as it will help you treat (and ideally prevent) severe hypoglycemia.

The body's first line of defense against low blood glucose is to reduce insulin production by the pancreas and to increase glucagon production by the alpha cells. The body's second line of defense is the secretion of catecholamines—including epinephrine and norepinephrine—by the adrenal gland. The effects of this catecholamine release can be seen in the hypoglycemic patient as tachycardia and diaphoresis. This second line of defense also includes cortisol, an adrenocorticoid (ie, a steroid produced in the adrenal gland). Cortisol release leads to an increase in blood glucose levels, which in turn counteracts insulin's actions. Other hormones produced by the intestine and growth hormone produced by the pituitary gland also increase blood glucose levels.

Last, stimulation of the autonomic nervous system generates signals that allow production of counterregulatory hormones to increase. The same stimulation also triggers symptoms telling the body that the blood glucose level is low; ideally, the affected patient will recognize these symptoms and consume a source of sugar to remedy the imbalance. In response to the action of these hormones, the body mobilizes fatty acids and amino acids from adipose and muscle, respectively. The liver uses these products to make new glucose for the body in a process called *gluconeogenesis*.

In patients with type 1 diabetes, the islets of Langerhans do not make insulin. As a result, the body's first line of defense against hypoglycemia is lost because the ability to decrease insulin levels via this mechanism is not possible. Often, a low blood glucose level in a patient with diabetes is caused by an elevated level of exogenous insulin from inaccurate dosing, intentional overdose, or perhaps a mismatch with carbohydrate intake and exogenous insulin intake. In addition, increased use of glucose, such as what occurs during exercise, causes the blood glucose level to drop sharply, resulting in hypoglycemia.

In patients with type 2 diabetes, the pancreas can generate insulin, so these patients can suppress insulin production from within their own bodies. However, their bodies may be resistant to the effects of insulin, or they may not make enough insulin over time to lower the blood glucose level adequately. Medications given to treat type 2 diabetes act by either stimulating the body's ability to secrete insulin or by improving insulin's actions. These medications also tend to contribute to hypoglycemia, especially in certain groups of patients such as older adults and those who are not metabolizing these medications properly because of liver or kidney disease. Often, if the hypoglycemia is caused by excessive insulin dosing by the patient or by the prolonged or exaggerated effects of oral diabetes medications, the low blood glucose level will have a prolonged effect and more long-term treatment may be needed.

Some patients who have had type 1 diabetes for many years, and to a lesser degree, patients who have had type 2 diabetes for many years, may not have a glucagon release from the pancreas in response to hypoglycemia.[14] Lack of glucagon response makes the body more dependent on epinephrine to overcome the effects of hypoglycemia, yet there may be some lack of responsiveness to epinephrine in diabetes as well.[15,16] Prolonged disease can also decrease a patient's ability to recognize having a low blood glucose level (a state called *hypoglycemic unawareness*), preventing him or her from taking the necessary measures of self treatment.

Assessment

A patient with hypoglycemia will tremble, have a rapid pulse rate, sweat, and feel hungry. The brain is highly sensitive to glucose levels, so the signs and symptoms associated with this condition reflect the disordered function of the brain cells and the alarm reaction (sympathetic nervous system discharge) set off by the brain's distress signals. If hypoglycemia persists, cerebral dysfunction progresses quickly to permanent brain damage.

Some of the most common signs and symptoms of hypoglycemia include:

- Blood glucose level less than 60 mg/dL
- Hunger
- Agitation, irritability, or combative behavior that cannot be explained
- Altered mentation or confusion
- Nausea
- Weakness
- Tachycardia (poor cardiac output)
- Cool, clammy skin

Additional signs and symptoms associated with hypoglycemia include headache, memory loss, incoordination, slurred speech, dilated pupils, and seizures and coma in severe cases.

Hypoglycemia develops *very rapidly*, over a period ranging from minutes to a few hours, and should be suspected in any patient with diabetes who presents with bizarre behavior, neurologic signs, or coma. Often the hypoglycemic patient appears intoxicated because of slurred speech and lack of coordination and may be paranoid, hostile, and aggressive.

Of course, people with diabetes are not the only ones who are likely to have episodes of hypoglycemia. Patients with alcoholism, patients who have ingested certain poisons or overdosed with certain drugs (notably aspirin), and patients with certain cancers, liver disease, kidney disease, and some other conditions may also experience hypoglycemic episodes. Do not discount the possibility of hypoglycemia in a comatose patient just because the patient is not known to have diabetes. Conversely, do not let a known diagnosis of diabetes prevent you from considering other causes of coma. People with diabetes can also experience head injury, stroke, seizures, meningitis, and other traumatic injuries or conditions. Keep an open mind and assess the patient thoroughly.

Words of Wisdom

The longer a patient remains unconscious from hypoglycemia, the more likely permanent brain damage will occur! If more than 20 to 30 minutes pass, toxic compounds (free radicals) in the brain are produced that can cause permanent neuronal damage. Therefore once you have determined that a patient has a low blood glucose level, you must fix it right away. Do not wait until after you have moved the patient to the ambulance, or until en route to the ED.

Patient Safety

A patient experiencing a hypoglycemic event may be confused with a patient having a cerebrovascular accident (CVA). D_{50} is *contraindicated* in CVA in the presence of normal blood glucose levels. Thus, the blood glucose level should be assessed and verified carefully in patients with signs associated with CVA prior to administering D_{50}. The hypertonic properties of D_{50} may result in increased cerebral edema in the event of a cerebrovascular event.

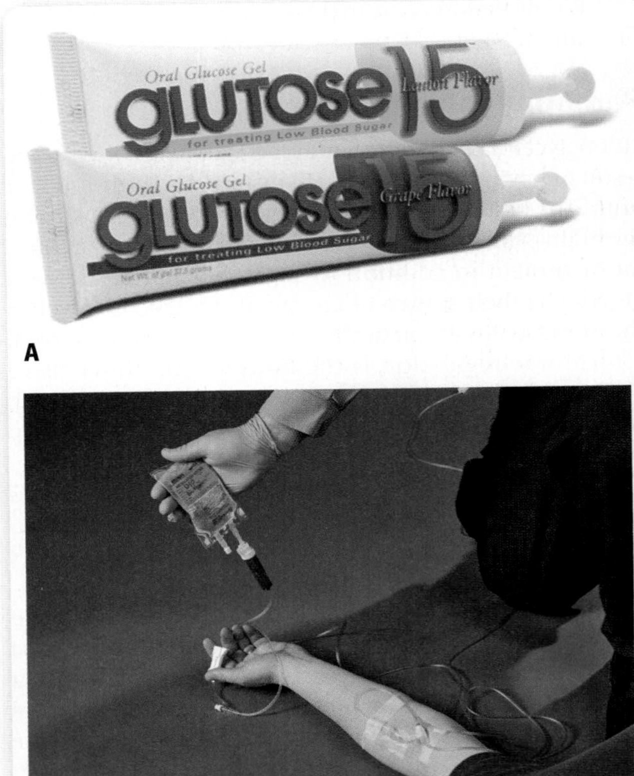

Figure 23-4 Administering glucose is appropriate in diabetic emergencies unless you have a reliable blood glucose measurement indicating normal or high blood glucose levels. Available forms include oral glucose paste **(A)** and glucose solution for intravenous infusion **(B)**.

Courtesy of Paddock Laboratories, Inc.

Management

Management of hypoglycemia includes immediately increasing blood glucose levels, with the precise treatment depending on several factors. It is always preferable to provide the least invasive method of treatment possible that will successfully address the condition.

Measure the patient's blood glucose level, especially if you are treating an older adult or a patient whose clinical history suggests that the problem may be stroke—administration of concentrated glucose solutions in a situation of suspected stroke may exacerbate cerebral damage Figure 23-4. When the comatose patient is older than 55 years or the family gives a history of recent transient ischemic attacks, perform a field glucose test to rule out hypoglycemia. A field glucose test involves obtaining a small amount of blood and using a blood glucose monitor to determine the patient's blood glucose level. This test is summarized here and discussed in detail in Chapter 11, *Patient Assessment*.

1. Take appropriate infection control precautions.
2. Verify the device is calibrated appropriately.
3. Clean the site to be punctured with alcohol.
4. Allow the patient's arm to hang briefly to allow blood to flow to the fingertips.
5. Grasp the finger near the area to be pricked (the side of the finger is less painful to prick than the top) and squeeze for 3 seconds.
6. Use a sterile lancet device and quickly prick the side of the fingertip. Apply adequate pressure to puncture the skin.
7. Properly dispose of the lancet.
8. Keep the hand down, and squeeze gently until you obtain a drop of blood. Be careful not to squeeze too hard.
9. Place a sterile dressing on the wound as needed.

10. Apply the blood to the test strips according to the manufacturer's instructions.
11. Accurately read and document the results.

If the patient is alert, able to swallow, and has an intact gag reflex, encourage him or her to take glucose tablets. You can provide 15 to 30 g of oral glucose. If glucose tablets are not available, household sources of glucose may be used. For example, you may administer sugar by mouth. Provide a candy bar, a glass of warm water to which a few teaspoons of sugar have been added, or a non-diet cola drink—any of those should improve the patient's condition. An unresponsive patient should *never* be given oral glucose or anything by mouth because of the risk of choking and aspiration.

Patient Safety

Before you give a conscious patient glucose tablets, anything to eat or drink, or instant glucose, you must ensure that there is no danger of aspiration. One rule of thumb: If patients can lift the cup or squirt the glucose into their own mouths, they are most likely not in danger of aspiration. Watch them carefully!

If the patient has an altered level of consciousness or you are potentially unable to manage the airway, aspiration may result with administration of oral substances. In that case, you will need to manage the airway and breathing as you would with any patient with an altered level of consciousness. An advanced airway should be avoided until the patient has received dextrose. If the patient remains unresponsive, an advanced airway can be considered.

The steps for performing an IV infusion are covered in Chapter 14, *Medication Administration*. To administer dextrose to a patient with altered level of consciousness, follow these steps:

1. Insert an IV line and ensure it is patent. An 18-gauge catheter is preferable in a large vein due to the viscosity of dextrose. If you are using D_{50}, note that it is hypertonic and acidic, so any extravasation may lead to tissue necrosis.
2. Administer a 0.9% NS flush of 10 to 20 mL to confirm patency of the IV line.
3. Administer 12.5 to 25 g of dextrose (milliliter-based regimens: 50 mL of 50% dextrose [D_{50}], 100 mL of 25% dextrose, 250 mL of 10% dextrose [D_{10}]) over a minimum of 3 minutes, while continuously assessing patient response.

YOU are the Paramedic — PART 4

As you administer dextrose, you notice the patient begins to look around. After a few minutes, she says, "Oh! That one snuck up on me!" She tells you that she has type 1 diabetes, and she felt her blood glucose level dropping. She tried to open her package of glucose tablets, and that was the last thing she remembers. You assist her up out of the refrigerator case and reassess her vital signs, including her blood glucose level. Her blood glucose level is now 120 mg/dL.

The patient's 21-year-old son arrives. The patient tells you, "Thanks very much. I'll be fine now." After discussing the case with medical control and receiving their agreement to leave the patient with her son, you inform dispatch the patient refused further treatment and transport and your medic unit is available for calls. You assist your patient to the food court, where she orders a hamburger and fries.

Recording Time: 10 Minutes	
Respirations	20 breaths/min; regular
Pulse	90 beats/min, regular
Skin	Slightly cool, pale, diaphoretic
Blood pressure	156/92 mm Hg
Oxygen saturation (Spo_2)	98% on room air
Pupils	PERRLA

7. Which challenges often occur on calls such as this one?
8. How would you document this patient contact?

4. If the coma is caused by hypoglycemia, the patient will often awaken rapidly. In cases of severe hypoglycemia, another 25 g of D_{50} may be required to restore a normal level of consciousness.

If the patient has a decreased level of consciousness and you are unable to obtain a patent IV line, administer glucagon 1 mg IM in adults. Hypoglycemia is a life-threatening event, and glucose administration should not be delayed if an IV line cannot be established.

Glucagon increases blood glucose levels and relaxes the smooth muscle located in the gastrointestinal tract if administered parenterally. Patients with type 1 diabetes may not experience as great an increase in blood glucose levels as those with stable type 2 diabetes. Therefore, patients with type 1 diabetes require immediate access to oral carbohydrates or additional glucose administration. See the Appendix, *Emergency Medications*, for more information on glucagon.

▶ Hyperglycemia and Diabetic Ketoacidosis

According to the CDC, approximately 175,000 US emergency department visits for adults in 2011 involved a hyperglycemic crisis.[17] In 2010, hyperglycemic crisis resulted in the deaths of 2,361 adults age 20 years and older.[17]

Pathophysiology

Hyperglycemia (a high blood glucose level) is one of the classic symptoms of diabetes mellitus. Common early signs include frequent and excessive thirst accompanied by frequent and excessive urination. Hyperglycemia occurs when blood glucose levels exceed the normal range (60 to 120 mg/dL). In patients with diabetes, physicians try to maintain glucose levels at less than 160 mg/dL. Hyperglycemia can be caused by excessive food intake, insufficient insulin dosages, infection or illness, injury, surgery, and emotional stress. Reassess the patient frequently for the presence of these underlying causes so that definitive treatment can be given. Onset may be rapid (within minutes) or gradual (hours to days), depending on the cause. For example, excessive food intake may cause blood glucose to rise quickly, whereas an infection or illness will result in hyperglycemia over the course of several days.

Other causes of hyperglycemia include the *dawn phenomenon* and the *Somogyi effect*. The dawn phenomenon occurs in the hours before waking. As the body prepares for a new day, it releases hormones such as cortisol and catecholamines. These hormones trigger a release of glucose from the liver, resulting in hyperglycemia. Alternatively, the Somogyi effect occurs when a low blood glucose level generates a release of hormones that initiate a release of glucose from the liver, causing hyperglycemia.

Some patients with type 2 diabetes can go undiagnosed for several years. Over time, however, repeated episodes of hyperglycemia will cause several physiologic changes that have detrimental long-term effects. Largely because of the increased hyperosmolarity it causes, hyperglycemia puts undue strain on the cardiovascular system, kidneys, and other end organs that are sensitive to increased serum viscosity and the subsequent pressures exerted by the thicker serum. The eventual result is increased incidence of disorders such as renal failure, congestive heart failure, retinopathy, coronary artery disease, and neuropathy.

When serum glucose levels rise above tolerable levels, other physiologic changes occur. These changes represent actual pathologic conditions called diabetic ketoacidosis (blood glucose level greater than approximately 350 mg/dL) and **hyperosmolar hyperglycemic syndrome (HHS)** (blood glucose level greater than approximately 600 mg/dL). DKA is associated predominately with people with type 1 diabetes. A life-threatening condition, DKA occurs when certain acids accumulate in the body because insulin is not available **Figure 23-5**. Common causes of DKA include infection, injury, alcohol use, emotional distress, and illness such as stroke or myocardial infarction. Patients who have this condition tend to be young—teenagers and young adults.

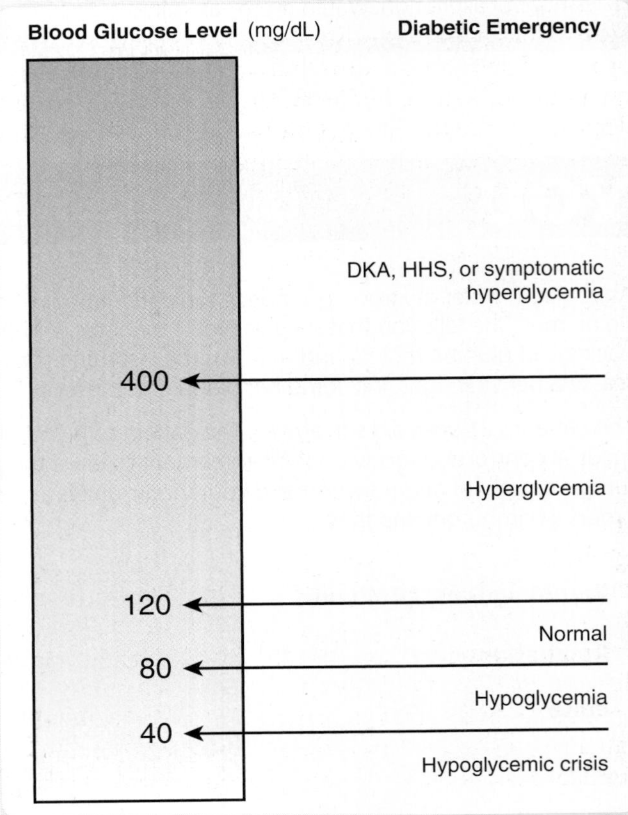

Figure 23-5 The two most common diabetic emergencies, diabetic ketoacidosis and hypoglycemic crisis, occur when the patient has too much or too little glucose in the blood, respectively. The left column illustrates blood glucose levels; the right column illustrates the conditions associated with that particular level of blood glucose. Notice that the normal range is rather small in comparison to the other ranges.

In patients with DKA, hyperglycemia continues—that is, glucose continues to accumulate in the blood. Eventually, the patient undergoes massive osmotic diuresis (passing large amounts of urine because of the high solute concentration of the blood); this, together with vomiting, causes dehydration and even shock.

In DKA, the deficiency of insulin prevents cells from taking up the extra glucose. The cells are starving, and a distress signal goes out over the sympathetic nervous system, causing the release of various stress hormones. Because the body cannot use glucose, it turns instead to other sources of energy—principally, fat. The metabolism of fat generates *acids* and *ketones* as waste products. (The ketone bodies give the characteristic fruity odor to the breath of a patent in DKA, but not all providers are able to detect this odor.) Because glucose must be excreted in the urine in solution, the body loses excessive amounts of water and electrolytes (sodium and potassium), which may lead to disturbances in water balance and acid-base balance. (Disturbances in acid-base balance and the compensatory role of the kidneys are covered in more detail in Chapter 9, *Pathophysiology*.)

Fatty acids are broken down primarily by the mitochondria in liver cells. As part of this process, ketone bodies are released into the bloodstream. Ketone bodies consist of acetoacetate, beta-hydroxybutyrate, and acetone. Large quantities of ketone bodies in the bloodstream cause a decrease in the blood's pH and result in acidosis. This acidosis triggers the body's attempts to buffer the acidity with bicarbonate (HCO_3^-), and the blood pH decreases because of the inability to keep up with the ongoing acidity. In addition to fat tissue breaking down its stores of energy, muscle tissue mobilizes its stores in an effort to create more glucose for the body. This process creates amino acids that may be used by the liver to make glucose (gluconeogenesis). In addition, lactate increases in the bloodstream and contributes to lowering the body's pH.

In patients with type 2 diabetes, DKA is rare because insulin is still present, at least early in the course of the disease. Despite the elevated blood glucose levels, the level of insulin is sufficient to prevent uncontrolled breakdown of glycogen, adipose tissue, and muscle. In all patients with type 2 diabetes, regardless of the duration of the disease, ketone bodies can be found in the urine when the patient experiences hyperglycemia. With increased duration of type 2 diabetes, a loss of pancreatic insulin production may occur. In fact, patients can develop elevated serum ketone levels, reduced blood pH, and DKA similar to those patients with type 1 diabetes.

Assessment

A hyperglycemic condition without other classic symptoms is not conclusive evidence of the presence of diabetes mellitus; hyperglycemia is also an independent medical condition with other causes.

The signs and symptoms of hypoglycemia and hyperglycemia can be similar **Table 23-2**. The signs and symptoms of simple hyperglycemia are usually mild, if present at all. They can include blurred vision, polyuria, polydipsia, polyphagia, orthostatic syncope, frequent infections, and skin ulcerations. If you encounter a patient with simple hyperglycemia who has not progressed to a more serious syndrome, treatment should include supportive care and transport.

Hyperglycemia usually progresses slowly, over a period of 12 to 48 hours, with the patient's level of consciousness deteriorating only gradually. The load of glucose present within the kidneys during hyperglycemia results in glucose spilling into the urine, causing the body to become hyperosmotic. As the kidneys remove excess glucose, water is removed via increased urination, leading to dehydration. The kidneys also help clear ketone bodies from the blood. As part of the substantial amount of water lost through diuresis, patients lose excessive amounts of sodium, potassium, and phosphates in the urine. This combination of effects leads to both dehydration and metabolic acidosis with associated electrolyte imbalances.

The resulting signs and symptoms manifest these etiologic factors:

- Polyuria (excessive urine output), because of osmotic diuresis
- Polydipsia (excessive thirst), because of dehydration
- Polyphagia (excessive eating), probably related to inefficient utilization of nutrients
- Nausea and vomiting, the latter worsening the patient's dehydration
- Tachycardia as a consequence of dehydration
- Deep, rapid respirations (Kussmaul respirations)—the body's attempt to compensate for acidosis by blowing off carbon dioxide (CO_2)
- Warm, dry skin and dry mucous membranes, also reflecting dehydration
- Fruity odor of ketones (acetone smell) on the breath
- Abdominal pain
- Sometimes fever

Patients usually appear thin or dehydrated and have warm, dry skin. Patients also may exhibit orthostatic hypotension, supine hypotension, fatigue, altered mental status, and, with time, weight loss from the hypermetabolic state. However, patients in DKA are seldom deeply comatose, so if the patient is totally unresponsive, look for another source of the coma such as head injury, stroke, or drug overdose.

The respiratory rate is usually elevated and the tidal volume is increased (Kussmaul respirations) because of **ketonemia** (excess amounts of ketone bodies in the blood), acidosis, and the body's attempt to relieve itself of the excessive burden of CO_2. These respiratory changes result in hypocapnia, which is recognized by lower than normal end-tidal CO_2 levels. Because end-tidal CO_2 levels are affected, capnography is another tool you can use to confirm your diagnosis. DKA results in both Kussmaul respirations and metabolic acidosis; a capnography value less than 25 mm Hg corroborates your suspicions.[18]

Table 23-2 Comparison of Hypoglycemia and Hyperglycemia

	Hypoglycemia	Hyperglycemia: Diabetic Ketoacidosis[a]	Hyperglycemia: HHS[b]
Food intake	Insufficient	Excessive	Excessive
Insulin dosage	Excessive	Insufficient	Insufficient
Onset	Rapid, within minutes	Gradual—hours to days	Gradual—days to weeks
Skin	Pale and moist	Warm and dry	Warm and dry
Infection	Uncommon	Common	Usual
Thirst	Absent	Intense	Very intense
Hunger	Intense	Excessive	Excessive
Vomiting	Uncommon	Common	Uncommon
Breathing	Normal or rapid	Rapid, deep (Kussmaul respirations)	Tachycardia
Odor of breath	Normal	Sweet, fruity (nail polish remover/acetone smell)	No ketone bodies are produced; therefore, there is no fruity odor
Blood pressure	Low	Normal to low	Hypotension
Pulse	Rapid, weak	Normal or rapid and full	Rapid, weak
Level of consciousness	Irritability, confusion, seizure, or coma	Restless merging to coma	Restless merging to coma
Urine: Sugar	Absent	Present	Present
Urine: Acetone	Absent	Present	Absent
Blood glucose level (mg/dL)	<60	>250	>600
Response to treatment	Immediately after administration of glucose	Gradual, within 6 to 12 hours following medical treatment	

Abbreviation: HHS, hyperosmolar hyperglycemic syndrome

[a] Usually associated with type 1 diabetes

[b] Usually associated with type 2 diabetes

There is no predictable correlation between the increase in a patient's blood glucose level and the degree of ketoacidosis in the blood. Rely on the patient's clinical presentation rather than on test results.

Management

The treatment of DKA in the field depends on making the correct diagnosis. If the patient's history and physical exam are consistent with DKA and your field measurement of the patient's glucose level reveals that it is markedly elevated (more than 250 mg/dL), the physician will probably order treatment for DKA. The goals of prehospital treatment are to begin rehydration and to correct the patient's electrolyte and acid-base abnormalities. In most instances, specific treatment with insulin should await the patient's arrival at the hospital, where therapy can be closely monitored with laboratory determinations of blood glucose and ketone levels.

Follow the procedure for any comatose patient with regard to airway maintenance and oxygen. Be particularly alert for *vomiting*, and have suction ready.

- Start an IV line and infuse up to 1 L of NS during the first half-hour or at the rate suggested by protocol or online medical control. Remember, a patient in DKA is severely dehydrated, often to the point of shock, and needs volume, usually at a rate of about 1 L/h for at least the first few hours. (See Chapter 43, *Pediatric Emergencies*, for information specific to treatment of pediatric patients.)
- If the patient is hypotensive, rapidly administer isotonic fluids until the systolic pressure is 80 mm Hg, then slow the infusion. As with any patient in whom fluid boluses are being administered, closely monitor the patient for the development of pulmonary edema.
- Monitor cardiac rhythm. Changes in serum potassium caused by DKA can lead to marked myocardial instability. Note the contour of the T waves on the rhythm strip; if they are sharply peaked, the patient's potassium level may be dangerously high, and you may need to administer sodium bicarbonate ($NaHCO_3$). As potassium levels rise, the QRS complex will widen and may blend with the T wave, and the heart rate may become bradycardic. At this point, management with calcium chloride or gluconate may be indicated to antagonize potassium at the receptor site. If ordered to do so, proceed with caution—even a slight excess can cause serious problems or death.

Controversies

The administration of $NaHCO_3$ as part of the management of metabolic acidosis in DKA remains controversial. $NaHCO_3$ is generally not considered unless the patient's pH is less than 7.0. $NaHCO_3$ should not be used in a prehospital setting and must be deemed necessary by the medical team. Arbitrary administration of $NaHCO_3$ can cause a paradoxical acidosis in the cerebrospinal fluid as well as several other complications that worsen the patient's condition and outcome. The patient's vital signs should be closely monitored, including blood pressure, heart rate, respiratory rate, and assessment of neurologic status.[19,20]

Hypomagnesemia (a low level of magnesium in the blood) is commonly associated with DKA as a result of the loss of magnesium through the urine. This electrolyte imbalance can worsen vomiting, cause alterations in mental status, induce other electrolyte abnormalities, and lead to potentially fatal cardiac dysrhythmias. Magnesium deficiency from DKA is generally not treated in the prehospital setting.

Complications of DKA are frequently associated with its management. The infusion of insulin can lead to hypoglycemia, so blood glucose levels should be monitored continuously. Hypokalemia may result when insulin shifts potassium into cells, lowering blood serum levels; therefore, management of hyperkalemia should be considered cautiously. Cerebral edema may occur if blood glucose levels shift too rapidly; however, this complication is more prevalent in pediatric patients, particularly newborns and premature infants. Children are less likely to have cardiovascular complications secondary to hyperkalemia.

Hyperosmolar Hyperglycemic Syndrome

Pathophysiology

HHS, which stands for hyperosmolar hyperglycemic syndrome and is also called **hyperosmolar nonketotic coma (HONK)**, is a metabolic derangement that occurs principally in patients with type 2 diabetes.[21-24] This condition is characterized by hyperglycemia, hyperosmolarity, and an absence of significant ketosis. The term *hyperosmolarity* describes highly concentrated blood as a result of relative dehydration. Key signs and symptoms of HHS include:

- Hyperglycemia
- Altered mental status, drowsiness, and lethargy
- Severe dehydration, thirst, and dark urine
- Visual or sensory deficits
- Partial paralysis or muscle weakness
- Seizures

Oddly enough, fewer than 20% of patients present in a comatose state.[25] Instead, most patients have severe dehydration and focal or global neurologic deficits. In addition, AMI is frequently associated with HHS/HONK. The clinical features of HHS/HONK and DKA tend to overlap and are often observed simultaneously.

HHS/HONK often develops in patients with diabetes who have a secondary illness that leads to reduced fluid intake. Although infection (in particular, pneumonia and urinary tract infection) is the most common cause, many other conditions can cause altered mentation or dehydration. In most cases, the secondary illness is not identified.

Words of Wisdom

Certain medications—including diuretics, beta-blockers, histamine-2 (H_2) blockers, dialysis, total parenteral nutrition, and dextrose-containing fluids—may contribute to the development of HHS/HONK by raising serum glucose levels, inhibiting insulin, or causing dehydration. Hyperglycemia and hyperosmolarity lead to osmotic diuresis and an osmotic shift of fluid to the intravascular space, resulting in further intracellular dehydration.

Assessment

Unlike patients with DKA, patients with HHS/HONK do not experience ketoacidosis. The onset of DKA can occur in as little as a few hours, whereas HHS/HONK can take up to weeks to develop. Blood glucose levels tend to be substantially higher in HHS/HONK as compared to DKA Table 23-3. Although most patients diagnosed as having HHS/HONK have a known history of diabetes (usually type 2), approximately 30% do not have a prior diagnosis of diabetes. The stress response to any acute illness tends to increase hormones that favor elevated glucose levels; cortisol, catecholamines (epinephrine and norepinephrine), glucagon, and many other hormones have effects that tend to counter those of insulin. Various neurologic changes may be found, including drowsiness and lethargy, delirium and coma, focal or generalized seizures, visual disturbances, hemiparesis, and sensory deficits.

Not all patients with increased blood glucose levels have DKA or HHS/HONK. Many people have glucose intolerance and hyperglycemia with no symptoms. To determine the precise condition, look at the patient, not at the number.

Management

The treatment of HHS/HONK in the prehospital setting follows the pathway for dehydration and altered mental status. Airway management is the top priority because the comatose patient often is unable to maintain and protect his or her airway. For this reason, advanced airway management may be indicated and should be completed as early as possible. Cervical spine immobilization should be used for all unresponsive patients found lying down, unless witnesses can validate that no fall occurred. Large-bore IV access should be gained as soon as possible, but do not delay transfer while initiating the IV line. If necessary, obtain IV access during transport to the emergency department. Also, obtain a blood glucose level as soon as possible.

After you have initiated the IV line, a bolus of 500 mL 0.9% NS is appropriate for almost all adults who are clinically dehydrated. In patients with a history of congestive heart failure and/or renal insufficiency, a 250-mL bolus may be a more appropriate starting point. Fluid deficits in patients with HHS/HONK may amount to 10 L or more. These patients may receive 1 to 2 L of fluids within the first hour of treatment.

Table 23-3 Comparison of Hyperglycemic Conditions

	HHS/HONK	Diabetic Ketoacidosis
Glucose	>600 mg/dL	>250 mg/dL
Arterial pH	>7.3	<7.3
Ketone bodies	Absent	Present
Type of diabetes mellitus	Type 2	Type 1

Abbreviations: HHS, hyperosmolar hyperglycemic syndrome; HONK, hyperosmolar nonketotic coma

Data from: Hyperosmolar Hyperglycemic Nonketotic Syndrome (HHNS). American Diabetes Association website. http://www.diabetes.org/living-with-diabetes/complications/hyperosmolar-hyperglycemic.html. Updated December 6, 2013. Accessed March 23, 2017; Hemphill RR. Hyperosmolar Hyperglycemic State. Medscape website. http://emedicine.medscape.com/article/1914705-overview. Updated August 3, 2016. Accessed March 23, 2017; Westerberg DP. Diabetic ketoacidosis: Evaluation and treatment. *Am Fam Physician*. 2013 Mar 1;87(5):337-346; Gosmanov AR, Gosmanova EO, Cannon ED. Management of adult diabetic ketoacidosis. *Diabetes Metab Syndr Obes*. 2014;7:255-264; and Chiasson JL, Aris-Jilwan N, Bélanger R, et al. Diagnosis and treatment of diabetic ketoacidosis and the hyperglycemic hyperosmolar state. *CMAJ*. 2003 Apr 1; 168(7):859–866.

Pathophysiology, Assessment, and Management of Other Disorders of the Pancreas

▶ Pancreatitis

Pathophysiology

Pancreatitis is an inflammation of the pancreas, can occur as either an acute or a chronic condition, and is more common in men. Acute pancreatitis is a medical emergency and can lead to dehydration and hypotension. The most common causes of pancreatitis are gallstones, which cause bile duct obstruction, and chronic alcohol abuse. As in acute pancreatitis, years of alcohol abuse is the most common cause of chronic pancreatitis. These two etiologies account for 60% to 80% of acute pancreatitis cases, with alcohol abuse being more common in younger patients and obstruction more common in older adults.[26,27] Other potential causes of pancreatitis include the use of certain medications, trauma, pancreatic cancer, and genetic predisposition.

Chronic pancreatitis refers to a progressive disease that destroys the pancreas, eventually leading to the loss of all endocrine and exocrine functions. It often causes chronic pain. Computed tomography is used to diagnosis the presence of this condition.

Assessment

Patients with acute pancreatitis present with what is described as a constant dull, boring flank and/or epigastric pain that worsens if the patient is placed in a supine position. Tachycardia, fever, and jaundice also can be present. Typically, a pancreatic attack is a result of a large, heavy meal or excessive drinking. Symptoms include nausea and vomiting, abdominal distention or muscle spasms, and less frequently, necrosis and organ failure. Laboratory tests used to diagnose acute pancreatitis include determinations of serum amylase, lipase, and trypsin, if available.

Management

After pancreatitis has been diagnosed, most patients are treated with supportive care. Patients should not eat until nausea and vomiting have subsided. The patients should be transported and pain management can be considered, although it is not always effective with pancreatitis. Endoscopic retrograde cholangiopancreatography is used for patients who have cholelithiasis. No other treatments have been shown to decrease pain or hospital stay length.

For patients with chronic pancreatitis, lifestyle changes, including changes in diet and the termination of alcohol and tobacco use, are critical to treatment. Analgesics are used to control pain, pancreatic enzymes assist with steatorrhea (excessive fat in the stool) and malabsorption, and finally, surgical intervention may be considered. Patients should be monitored for pancreatic cancer because there is a higher incidence of this disease noted in patients who have chronic pancreatitis.

Words of Wisdom

Adenocarcinoma is a type of cancer that affects the epithelial cells lining glandular tissue. This type of cancer can affect the pancreas. Pancreatic cancer is a common cause of cancer death in the United States. Signs and symptoms are vague and nondifferential and include pain, weight loss, and jaundice. These manifestations usually are not present in the early stages of pancreatic cancer, making diagnosis uncommon.

Cystadenoma refers to benign cysts that are present in glandular tissue and can affect the pancreas. Secretion function is maintained; however, it may result in more cysts.

Neuroendocrine tumors have an effect on the endocrine and nervous systems and begin in the endocrine-secreting cells. This can be found anywhere in the body; however, gasteroenteropancreatic endocrine tumors affect the gastrointestinal tract and the pancreas. These tumors are rare and slow growing.

Pathophysiology, Assessment, and Management of Adrenal Insufficiency

Adrenal insufficiency is characterized by decreased function of the adrenal cortex and consequent underproduction of cortisol and aldosterone. A decrease in either of these adrenal hormones will result in weakness, dehydration, and an inability of the body to maintain adequate blood pressure or to properly respond to stress.

Cortisol affects almost every organ and tissue in the body. Although its primary role is to assist with the body's response to stress, this adrenal hormone also helps maintain blood pressure and cardiovascular function; regulates the metabolism of carbohydrates, proteins, and fats; modulates glucose levels in the blood by balancing the effects of insulin; and functions as an anti-inflammatory agent by slowing the inflammatory response.

Secretion of aldosterone is regulated chiefly by the renin-angiotensin system, but also is stimulated by increased serum potassium concentrations. Abnormal adrenal cortical function produces abnormalities in the metabolism of carbohydrates and protein as well as disturbances in salt and water metabolism.

Adrenal insufficiency is usually well tolerated unless the clinical picture is complicated by coexisting factors such as infection or stress. It affects approximately 4 people per 100,000 in the United States, occurs equally in men and women, and is found in patients of all races and ages. Adrenal insufficiency is classified as either primary or secondary.

▶ Primary Adrenal Insufficiency

Pathophysiology

Primary adrenal insufficiency (also known as Addison disease) is caused by atrophy or destruction of both adrenal glands, leading to deficiency of all steroid hormones produced by these glands. A rare disease (occurring in approximately 1 per 100,000 people in the United States), primary adrenal insufficiency is usually the result of idiopathic atrophy, an autoimmune process in which the immune system creates antibodies that attack the adrenal cortex, leading to its gradual destruction.[28] This phenomenon accounts for approximately 70% of cases of Addison disease in the United States.[28] Adrenal insufficiency occurs when at least 90% of the adrenal cortex has been destroyed. Less commonly (approximately 30% of cases), the adrenal destruction is caused by tuberculosis; a bacterial, viral, or fungal infection; adrenal hemorrhage; or cancer of the adrenal glands.[28] Patients with Addison disease who undergo treatment have a normal life expectancy.

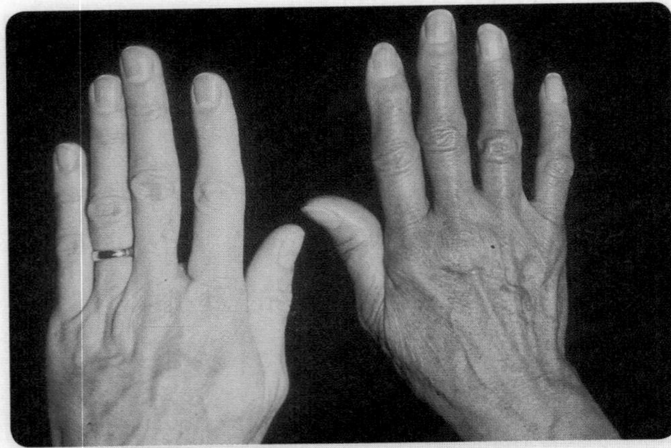

Figure 23-6 The hand of a patient with Addison disease (right) compared with the hand of a normal subject (left).

Assessment

Signs of chronic adrenal insufficiency include unexplained weight loss, fatigue, vomiting, diarrhea, anorexia, salt craving, muscle and joint pain, abdominal pain, postural dizziness, and increased pigmentation in the extensor surfaces, palmar creases, and oral mucosa Figure 23-6. In patients with Addison disease, the body improperly regulates the content of sodium, potassium, and water in body fluids. Blood volume and blood pressure fall, as does the sodium concentration of the blood; blood potassium level rises. The blood volume may become so reduced that the circulation can no longer be maintained efficiently.

Management

Treatment of patients experiencing an adrenal crisis includes the assessment and management of the ABCs. If needed, use the coma protocol of glucose, thiamine, and naloxone as indicated. Aggressive fluid replacement using 5% dextrose in normal saline should be initiated. Hydrocortisone, 100 mg IV, is indicated in the acute management of a crisis. Electrolyte imbalances are common and may not be obvious in the prehospital environment.

▶ Secondary Adrenal Insufficiency

Pathophysiology

Secondary adrenal insufficiency is a relatively common condition characterized by a lack of adrenocorticotropic hormone (ACTH) secretion from the pituitary gland. ACTH, a pituitary messenger, stimulates the adrenal cortex to manufacture and secrete cortisol. If ACTH secretion is insufficient, cortisol production is not stimulated. Patients who abruptly stop taking **corticosteroids** (eg, prednisone) may also experience secondary adrenal insufficiency. Corticosteroid treatments suppress natural cortical production; however, aldosterone production is usually not affected in this form of adrenal insufficiency.

> **Words of Wisdom**
>
> Although oral corticosteroid therapy is the most common cause of exogenous adrenal suppression, inhaled corticosteroids (used for asthma or chronic obstructive pulmonary disease) also may have a similar effect.

Assessment

Signs and symptoms of acute adrenal insufficiency can appear suddenly, which is called an **addisonian crisis**. An addisonian crisis may be triggered by an acute exacerbation of chronic insufficiency, usually brought on by stress, trauma, surgery, or severe infection. Corticosteroid withdrawal is the most common cause.

Although most patients with acute adrenal insufficiency have symptoms severe enough to prompt them to seek medical treatment before a crisis occurs, approximately 25% of patients first experience symptoms during an addisonian crisis.[28] The chief clinical manifestation of adrenal crisis is shock. Patients also may manifest nonspecific symptoms, including weakness; lethargy; confusion or loss of consciousness; low blood pressure (vascular collapse); elevated temperature; severe pain in the lower back, legs, or abdomen; and severe vomiting and diarrhea that leads to dehydration.

Management

An unrecognized, untreated episode of acute adrenal insufficiency can be fatal. Death usually is attributable to hypotension or cardiac dysrhythmias caused by hyperkalemia. Treatment is based on the patient's clinical presentation and findings and is geared toward maintaining the ABCs until arrival at the emergency department. Regarding airway maintenance and supplemental oxygen, follow the procedure for a patient who has altered mental status or is comatose. Be alert for vomiting and have suction ready.

Other goals of prehospital treatment are to begin rehydrating the patient and to correct the electrolyte and acid-base abnormalities. Start an IV line and infuse up to 1 L of 0.9% NS. If the patient is hypotensive, administer an NS bolus at 20 mL/kg. Remember, a patient in adrenal insufficiency may be severely dehydrated, often to the point of shock, and needs fluid volume replenishment.

Check the patient's blood glucose level. Administer 25 to 50 g of D_{50} to correct the hypoglycemia. D_5NS is the preferred IV fluid, but is not often carried in the field. Administering D_5W through a second IV can help maintain the patient's blood glucose level. Monitor cardiac rhythm because changes in serum electrolytes can lead to marked myocardial instability.

Pathophysiology, Assessment, and Management of Other Adrenal Emergencies

Cushing Syndrome

Pathophysiology

Cushing syndrome is caused by an excess of cortisol production by the adrenal glands or by excessive use of cortisol or other similar corticosteroid (glucocorticoid) hormones. Tumors of the pituitary gland or adrenal cortex can stimulate the production of excess hormone, for example, and lead to Cushing syndrome. Administration of large amounts of cortisol or other glucocorticoid hormones (eg, hydrocortisone, prednisone, methylprednisolone, or dexamethasone) for the treatment of life-threatening illnesses, such as asthma, rheumatoid arthritis, systemic lupus, inflammatory bowel disease, and some allergies, can also cause this syndrome.

Regardless of the cause, excess cortisol causes characteristic changes in many body systems. Metabolism of carbohydrates, proteins, and fats is disturbed such that the blood glucose level rises. Protein synthesis is impaired so that body proteins are broken down, which leads to loss of muscle fibers and muscle weakness. Bones become weaker and more susceptible to fracture.

Assessment

Other common signs and symptoms related to excess cortisol include the following:

- Weakness and fatigue
- Depression and mood swings
- Increased thirst and urination
- High blood glucose level
- Weight gain, especially on the abdomen, face ("moon face"), neck, and upper back ("buffalo hump")
- Thinning of the skin, with easy bruising and pink or purple stretch marks (striae) on the abdomen, thighs, breasts, and shoulders
- Increased acne, facial hair growth, and scalp hair loss in women, and cessation of menstrual periods
- Darkening of skin (acanthosis) on the neck
- Obesity and poor growth in height in children

Management

Management is designed to decrease the level of cortisol in the body, which is difficult in the prehospital environment. Assess and manage the patient's ABCs and treat any life-threatening conditions immediately. Prehospital treatment is generally supportive. Obtain a blood glucose level.

Adrenal Gland Tumor

Pheochromocytoma is a rare condition of the adrenal gland in which a tumor, usually in the medulla, causes excessive release of the hormones epinephrine and norepinephrine. Approximately 10% of such tumors are malignant (cancerous).[29]

The tumors can occur at any age, but they are most common in young adult to mid-adult life. A common clinical presentation is a combination of symptoms (ie, hypertension, anxiety, chest pain, abdominal pain, fatigue, weight loss, vision problems, and sometimes seizures) that may be frequent but sporadic, and may increase in frequency, duration, and severity.

Pathophysiology, Assessment, and Management of Thyroid, Parathyroid, and Pituitary Gland Disorders

Growth Hormone Pathologies

The anterior pituitary gland secrets growth hormone. Problems associated with growth hormone secretion include both oversecretion or undersecretion, are rare, and usually are the result of a tumor. Oversecretion results in *acromegaly*, a condition usually diagnosed in young adulthood. This disease results in gigantism and abnormally large hands and face, as well as facial characteristics: enlarged jaw, and brow and teeth that are abnormally widely spaced.[30] Undersecretion of growth hormone is a rare event and is characterized by delayed development and growth. A lack of treatment may lead to *dwarfism*.[31] Proportionate dwarfism presents with normal body proportions and mental functions.

Hypothyroidism and Hyperthyroidism

Approximately 20 million people in the United States have some kind thyroid disorder, and many of them will be unaware of their condition. Graves disease is the most common type of hyperthyroidism and increases metabolism. In contrast, hypothyroidism, often a result of autoimmune disease, decreases metabolism. Table 23-4 summarizes the major effects of hypothyroidism and hyperthyroidism.

Patients with hyperthyroidism and hypothyroidism are likely to require supplemental oxygen. Hyperthyroid metabolic activity increases oxygen demand. Hypothyroid conditions may lead to diminished respiratory effort that may require positive-pressure ventilation.

Graves Disease

The most severe and common cause of hyperthyroidism is Graves disease. This disorder is 10 times more common

Table 23-4 Comparison of the Major Effects of Hypothyroidism and Hyperthyroidism

	Hypothyroidism	Hyperthyroidism
Cardiovascular effects	Slow pulse, reduced cardiac output	Rapid pulse, increased cardiac output
Metabolic effects	Decreased metabolism, cold skin, weight gain	Increased metabolism, skin hot and flushed, weight loss
Neuromuscular effects	Weakness, sluggish reflexes	Tremor, hyperactive reflexes
Mental, emotional effects	Mental processes sluggish, personality placid	Restlessness, irritability, emotional lability
Gastrointestinal effects	Constipated	Diarrhea
General somatic effects	Cold, dry skin	Warm, moist skin

in women than in men; the overall incidence in women is 0.4 cases per 1,000.[32] Graves disease tends to follow a chronic course of remission and relapse. If left untreated, it can be fatal.

Graves disease is an autoimmune disorder in which the thyroid gland hypertrophies, or enlarges, as its activity increases. The hypertrophied thyroid gland produces a visible mass called a **goiter** in the anterior part of the neck. The overactive gland secretes an excessive amount of thyroxine, causing the hyperthyroidism that characterizes Graves disease. In addition to having a goiter, signs and symptoms of the condition include a substantially increased appetite with marked weight loss that may progress to cachexia (wasting of muscle and tissue). Patients also have polydipsia as a result of dehydration caused by diarrhea and excessive sweating. They also may present with exophthalmos. This condition is caused by edema of the tissue behind the eyes. Another sign of Graves disease is **pretibial myxedema**, an "orange peel" appearance and nonpitting edema of the skin on the anterior part of the leg below the knee. Finally, the hypermetabolism that accompanies Graves disease increases stress on the heart and may lead to heart failure.

Hashimoto Disease

Hashimoto disease is another cause of hyperthyroidism that is also more common in women. The thyroid gland is enlarged as a result of the infiltration of T lymphocytes and plasma cells. Like Graves disease, Hashimoto disease is an autoimmune disorder that affects the TSH receptors; however, it is milder than Graves disease. The hyperthyroidism is transient, with a subsequent hypothyroidism after antibodies destroy the follicles.

Myxedema Coma

Thyroid hormones are critical for cell metabolism and organ function. If their supply becomes inadequate, organ tissues do not grow or mature (due to the decreased metabolic rate), energy production declines (a cause of the decreased metabolic rate), and the actions of other hormones are affected.

Adult hypothyroidism is sometimes called *myxedema*. Frequently, patients have localized accumulations of mucinous material in the skin, which gives the disease its name (the prefix *myx-* refers to "mucin," and *edema* means "swelling") Figure 23-7. The condition is manifested by a general slowing of the body's metabolic processes due to the reduction or absence of thyroid hormone. All organ systems may exhibit symptoms of the disorder, and the severity of the symptoms will be consistent with the degree of the hormone deficiency.

Symptoms of hypothyroidism include fatigue, feeling cold, weight gain, dry skin, and sleepiness. Because these symptoms are often subtle and can be mistaken for other conditions, the disease may go undiagnosed. Continued decrease of the hormone levels may lead to myxedema coma, an extreme manifestation of untreated hypothyroidism that is accompanied by physiologic decompensation. When hypothyroidism is long-standing,

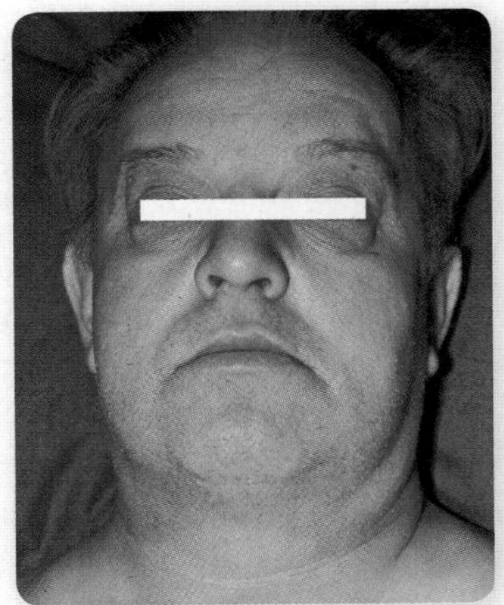

Figure 23-7 Localized accumulations of mucinous material in the neck of a hypothyroid patient.

physiologic adaptations occur, such as reduced metabolic rate and decreased oxygen consumption, which in turn lead to peripheral vasoconstriction. Triggers such as infection (especially pulmonary and urinary tract infections), exposure to cold, trauma, surgery, and certain medications are often precipitating factors in the progression to myxedema coma.

The hallmark of myxedema coma is deterioration of the patient's mental status. Although family members may not be overly concerned about more subtle changes, such as apathy or decreased intellectual function, more obvious changes, such as confusion, psychosis, and coma, will most certainly elicit a call for emergency assistance.

Most cases of myxedema coma occur during the winter in women older than 60 years. It is more common in women than in men. Just as the incidence of hypothyroidism increases with age, myxedema coma occurs primarily in older adult patients. One consistent finding is hypothermia, and you may need to use a thermometer that records temperatures less than 90°F in cases of myxedema coma. Thus, absence of fever in the presence of infection is a common finding.

Hypothyroidism decreases intestinal motility, and the decreased metabolic rate associated with this condition can lead to drug toxicity, especially in older adults. A slower metabolic rate causes the levels of medications, especially those that affect the central nervous system, to rise to toxic levels in the blood. This accidental overdose in the hypothyroid patient can actually precipitate myxedema coma.

Myxedema coma is a metabolic and cardiovascular emergency. If not diagnosed and treated immediately, mortality rates are estimated to be as high as 40%.[33] Thus, the patient's condition must be stabilized as soon as possible.

Administer supplemental oxygen therapy to correct hypoxia. Intubation and ventilation are indicated for patients with diminished respiratory drive or those who are unable to protect their airway; these measures will help prevent respiratory failure.

Monitor the patient's cardiac status. Hypotension may respond to crystalloid therapy, and vasopressive agents may be necessary (eg, dopamine). Administer 25 to 50 g of D_{50} if blood glucose levels are less than 60 mg/dL.

Treat hypothermia with passive rewarming methods because aggressive rewarming may lead to vasodilation and hypotension. Hemodynamically unstable patients with profound hypothermia, however, will require active rewarming. Avoid sedatives, narcotics, and anesthetics because of the delayed metabolism.

▶ Thyrotoxicosis

Thyrotoxicosis is a toxic condition caused by excessive levels of circulating thyroid hormone. Although hyperthyroidism can cause thyrotoxicosis in some patients, the two conditions are not identical. Thyrotoxicosis also may be caused by goiters, autoimmune disorders such as Graves disease, or thyroid cancer.

Thyroid storm is a rare, life-threatening condition that may occur in patients with thyrotoxicosis. The condition is usually triggered by a stressful event or increased volume of thyroid hormones in the circulation. In addition to the normal signs and symptoms of hyperthyroidism, patients may present with fever, severe tachycardia, nausea, vomiting, altered mental status, and possibly heart failure.

Words of Wisdom

Both hyperthyroidism and hypothyroidism can adversely affect the electrical status of the myocardium. Application of the cardiac monitor may reveal tachydysrhythmias in hyperthyroidism or bradydysrhythmias in hypothyroidism. Treat all dysrhythmias according to local protocol, while keeping in mind that these dysrhythmias may be difficult to correct without first fixing the underlying disorder.

▶ Hyperparathyroidism

The increased parathyroid hormone level that occurs in hyperparathyroidism will result in increased levels of blood calcium, hypercalcemia, and decreased phosphate blood levels. Causes of hyperparathyroidism can be divided between primary and secondary causes. Primary causes are those that result from the gland itself, while secondary causes occur elsewhere in the body and affect gland secretion. The most common cause of hyperparathyroidism is a benign neoplasia on the gland called an adenoma.

Signs and symptoms of this disorder can be vague, as in many endocrine conditions. Fatigue, weakness, nausea, vomiting, and confusion may be present. Occasionally, pathologic fractures can occur secondary to thinning bones or kidney stones can occur due to an increase in calcium and phosphorus in the urine. Surgery to remove the enlarged gland is definitive management and has a 95% success rate.[34] Patients with mild forms of the disease require monitoring of calcium blood levels. Prehospital management involves the management of ABCs and supportive care as indicated.

▶ Panhypopituitarism

Panhypopituitarism is the inadequate production or absence of the pituitary hormones, including adrenocorticotropic hormone, cortisol, thyroxine, LH, FSH, growth hormone, and ADH. The anterior pituitary gland is responsible for the production of several different hormones; therefore, clinical presentation varies depending on the hormone or hormones that are lacking. **Figure 23-8** summarizes these hormones and the symptoms associated with each deficiency.

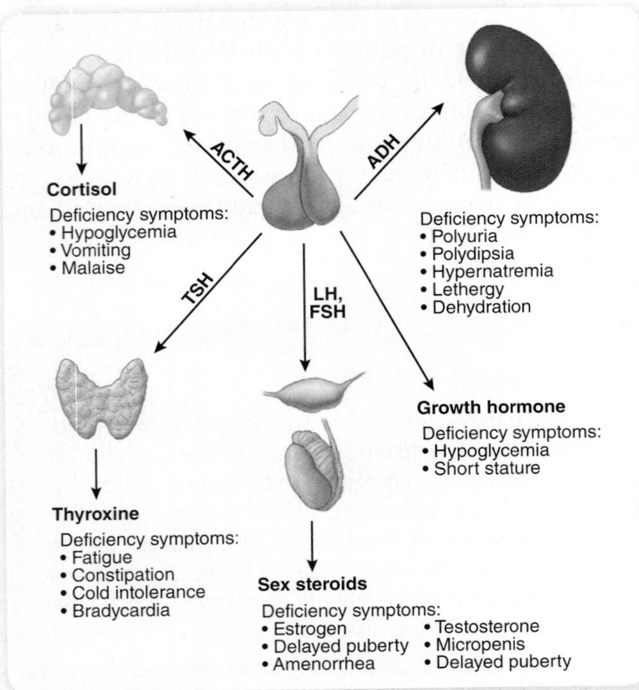

Figure 23-8 Panhypopituitarism.

Courtesy of Leonard Crowley.

▶ Diabetes Insipidus and SIADH

Diabetes insipidus (DI) has some of the same characteristics as diabetes mellitus, such as polyuria and polydipsia. Diabetes insipidus is a relatively uncommon disorder; however, unlike diabetes mellitus, this is not a pancreatic pathology. In diabetes insipidus, the body is unable to regulate fluid owing to a lack of ADH (central diabetes insipidus) or the kidneys are unable to respond appropriately (nephrogenic diabetes insipidus). ADH causes the kidneys to retain water; therefore, a lack of ADH will cause increased urination (polyuria), like that seen in diabetes mellitus. One difference between diabetes insipidus and diabetes mellitus is the amount of glucose present in the urine. In diabetes insipidus, the urine is very dilute; in contrast, excessive glucose is present in the urine of patients with diabetes mellitus. It seems obvious that dehydration and electrolyte imbalances may occur in diabetes insipidus, but there is also the risk of water intoxication as well and hyponatremia. In extreme cases, hypotension can occur. Management may include synthetic ADH.

In SIADH (syndrome of inappropriate antidiuretic hormone secretion), an excess of ADH results in a decrease in urinary output and, therefore, systemic fluid overload. This condition may cause hypertension, tachycardia, hyponatremia, seizures, and confusion. Management may include loop diuretics and hypertonic fluids. Table 23-5 compares diabetes insipidus and SIADH.

Table 23-5 Comparison of Diabetes Insipidus and SIADH Secretion

Diabetes Insipidus	Syndrome of Inappropriate ADH Secretion
Decreased levels of ADH	Increased levels of ADH
Polyuria	Oliguria
Dehydration, hypotension	Systemic fluid overload

Abbreviations: ADH, antidiuretic hormone; SIADH, syndrome of inappropriate antidiuretic hormone

YOU are the Paramedic SUMMARY

1. Which key information is provided from the dispatch and scene size-up?

The dispatch information indicated unusual circumstances or bizarre behavior. Your scene size-up has confirmed a patient with an altered mental status. The presence of medication and an ice cream wrapper lead you to suspect the patient could have hypoglycemia.

2. Which types of medical conditions can cause an altered mental status?

Numerous medical emergencies can cause an altered mental status, including seizure, stroke, or drug overdose.

3. Although the patient is cooperative, what do you need to consider when you treat any patient with an altered mental status?

Patients with an altered mental status can become combative, particularly those experiencing hypoglycemia. Some patients may stare off into space, whereas others may curse and exhibit bizarre or sometimes violent behavior. When you are in doubt about scene safety, wait until police officers declare the scene safe before you begin treatment.

4. What could be the cause of the patient's reported shaking?

In addition to epilepsy, the patient could be having a seizure from an extremely low blood glucose level or simply be shivering from sitting on a refrigeration unit. Look for a medical identification bracelet for additional information and perform a thorough assessment, noting the presence or absence of incontinence. Seizures due to hypoglycemia are an ominous sign.

5. What concerns you about the bystander's statement?

Often, laypeople are well intentioned but do not know what to do. Patients with an altered mental status frequently have airway problems and sometimes require airway management. It is possible that in addition to hypoglycemia, the patient has aspirated food into his or her lungs.

6. If your partner were unable to obtain IV access, which additional treatment options exist for correcting the patient's blood glucose level?

Patients with diabetes often have fragile veins. Also, this patient is obese, and obtaining IV access could be difficult. Another treatment option is to administer glucagon IM. The typical dosage of glucagon IM requires the patient to have adequate glycogen stores in the liver to be effective.

7. Which challenges often occur on calls such as this one?

Often, patients with diabetes do not wish to be transported. It is vitally important that the patient eat a meal as soon as possible. Administration of IV dextrose is only a temporary measure. If the patient does not eat a meal containing complex carbohydrates, his or her blood glucose level will likely drop again, and another 9-1-1 call will be necessary.

8. How would you document this patient contact?

It is imperative to thoroughly document not only the patient assessment findings and interventions provided, but also the consequences of refusal of treatment and/or transport to document that the patient refusal was an informed decision. Document the contact and discussion with medical control in which you obtained authorization to refuse transport (or treatment). Also document that you left the patient in the care of her son, with instructions to call back if needed.

YOU are the Paramedic SUMMARY *(continued)*

EMS Patient Care Report (PCR)

Date: 05-30-18	**Incident No.:** 53011	**Nature of Call:** Altered mental status	**Location:** Walt's Grocery		
Dispatched: 0900	**En Route:** 0901	**At Scene:** 0903	**Transport:** N/A	**At Hospital:** N/A	**In Service:** 0930

Patient Information

Age: 40 **Sex:** F **Weight (in kg [lb]):** 160 kg (353 lb)	**Allergies:** Penicillin **Medications:** Insulin **Past Medical History:** IDDM **Chief Complaint:** Hunger

Vital Signs

Time: 0908	**BP:** 160/94	**Pulse:** 100	**Respirations:** 24	**Spo_2:** 97% on room air
Time: 0913	**BP:** 156/92	**Pulse:** 90	**Respirations:** 20	**Spo_2:** 98% on room air
Time:	**BP:**	**Pulse:**	**Respirations:**	**Spo_2:**

EMS Treatment (circle all that apply)

Oxygen @ _______ L/min via (circle one): **NC NRM Bag-mask device**		**Assisted Ventilation**	**Airway Adjunct**	**CPR**
Defibrillation	**Bleeding Control**	**Bandaging**	**Splinting**	**Other:**

Narrative

Dispatched to "woman sitting in the butter" at a grocery store. Pt, a 40-year-old woman, was found sitting in the refrigerated section by a man bystander. Man reported the pt was "shaking all over." On arrival, pt was found sitting upright in the dairy section with chocolate all over her face and an ice cream sandwich melting in her hand. Medication tablets were on the floor. Airway was open and breathing adequate. Weak, rapid radial pulse present. Pt was responsive to pain (a pinch to the back of her hand); skin was cool, pale, and diaphoretic; no trauma noted to head, eyes, ears, nose, or throat; PERRLA; chest rise and volume adequate, no apparent trauma and bilateral breath sounds present/no adventitious lung sounds; no trauma noted to abdomen. Pt had an altered mental status secondary to hypoglycemia. Blood glucose level was 30 mg/dL, IV line started with 18-gauge R AC, normal saline to keep the vein open. Pt administered 25 g of dextrose 50. Pt's blood glucose level increased to 120 mg/dL. Pt's 21-year-old son arrived. Pt refused transport; IV and oxygen discontinued. Pt advised IV dextrose will not prevent glucose level from dropping again and she could have aspirated food into her lungs. Pt assisted to food court where she ordered a hamburger and fries. Signature obtained for refusal of care; advised pt she could call back if she changed her mind. Pt released to self and left in care of 21-year-old son; notified dispatch, contacted medical control and obtained approval.**End of report**

Prep Kit

▶ Ready for Review

- The endocrine system directly or indirectly influences almost every cell, organ, and function of the body.
- The endocrine system comprises a network of glands that produce and secrete hormones. The main function of the endocrine system and its hormonal messengers is to maintain homeostasis and promote permanent structural changes in the body.
- The major components of the endocrine system are the hypothalamus, pituitary, pineal gland, thyroid, parathyroid, thymus, pancreas, adrenal glands, and reproductive organs (gonads).
- Endocrine emergencies can be difficult to assess because they affect many organ systems and the seriousness of their presentations varies greatly. Do not take these calls lightly because poor outcomes can result quickly.
- Management of an endocrine emergency may require intubation, administration of supplemental oxygen, infusion of dextrose, or other measures. All findings must be thoroughly documented.
- Endocrine disorders are caused either by hypersecretion or insufficient secretion of a gland. Hypersecretion presents as overactivity of the target organ regulated by the gland; insufficient secretion results in underactivity of the organ controlled by the gland.
- Diabetes is a metabolic disorder that encompasses a group of complex diseases with many causes (ie, diabetes mellitus, gestational diabetes, hypoglycemia/hyperglycemia, diabetic ketoacidosis, hyperosmolar hyperglycemic syndrome); in all cases, the body's ability to metabolize glucose is impaired. It is characterized by the passage of large quantities of urine containing glucose, significant thirst, and deterioration of body function.
- In type 1 diabetes mellitus, the beta cells in the islets of Langerhans have been destroyed and no longer produce insulin. Patients with this type of diabetes require close monitoring of blood glucose and at least daily administration of insulin by injection or pump.
- The most common form of diabetes is type 2 diabetes, in which the blood glucose level is elevated because the body cannot produce enough insulin to compensate for the inability to utilize insulin effectively.
- Prediabetes is a condition in which blood glucose levels or hemoglobin A1c levels are above normal levels, yet not high enough to be diagnosed as diabetes. Prediabetes is often a precursor condition to type 2 diabetes.
- Gestational diabetes is a form of glucose intolerance that usually manifests itself late in pregnancy.
- Hypoglycemia (abnormally low blood glucose level) in a patient with insulin-dependent diabetes is often the result of having taken too much insulin, eaten too little food, or both. As a result of the actions of epinephrine, the patient will tremble, have a rapid pulse rate, sweat, and feel hungry.
- Hyperglycemia (abnormally high blood glucose level) is one of the classic symptoms of diabetes mellitus. Common early signs include frequent and excessive thirst accompanied by frequent and excessive urination.
- If left untreated, hyperglycemia may progress to the life-threatening condition known as DKA. DKA occurs when certain acids accumulate in the body because insulin is not available.
- HHS/HONK is a metabolic derangement that occurs principally in patients with type 2 diabetes. This condition is characterized by hyperglycemia, hyperosmolarity, and an absence of substantial ketosis.
- Acute pancreatitis is a medical emergency and can lead to dehydration and hypotension. By comparison, chronic pancreatitis is a progressive disease that destroys the pancreas, eventually leading to the loss of all endocrine and exocrine functions, and often causing chronic pain.
- Adrenal insufficiency is characterized by underproduction of cortisol and aldosterone, which leads to weakness, dehydration, and the body's inability to maintain adequate blood pressure or to respond properly to stress.
- Primary adrenal insufficiency (Addison disease) is caused by atrophy or destruction of both adrenal glands, leading to deficiency of all the steroid hormones produced by these glands.
- Secondary adrenal insufficiency is defined as a lack of ACTH secretion from the pituitary gland.
- Acute adrenal insufficiency, referred to as addisonian crisis, may result from an acute exacerbation of chronic adrenal insufficiency, usually brought on by a period of stress, trauma, surgery, or severe infection.
- Cushing syndrome is caused by an excess of cortisol production by the adrenal glands or by excessive use of cortisol or other similar corticosteroid (glucocorticoid) hormones.
- Pheochromocytoma is generally a nonmalignant tumor of the adrenal gland, usually in the medulla, that causes excessive release of the hormones epinephrine and norepinephrine.

Prep Kit *(continued)*

- Graves disease is the most severe and common cause of hyperthyroidism. This disease can produce goiter, exophthalmos, and pretibial myxedema.
- Hashimoto disease, another cause of hyperthyroidism, is an autoimmune disease in which the thyroid gland is enlarged as a result of the infiltration of T lymphocytes and plasma cells.
- Symptoms of hypothyroidism include feeling fatigued, feeling cold, gaining weight, having dry skin, and being sleepy. Continued decrease of thyroid hormone levels may lead to myxedema coma, a condition in which a general slowing of the body's metabolic processes occurs in the setting of reduced or absent thyroid hormone.
- Thyrotoxicosis is a toxic condition caused by excessive levels of circulating thyroid hormone. Thyroid storm is a rare, life-threatening condition that may occur in patients with thyrotoxicosis.
- In hyperparathyroidism, blood calcium levels increase, resulting in hypercalcemia and decreased phosphate blood levels.
- Panhypopituitarism is the inadequate production or absence of the pituitary hormones.
- Diabetes insipidus is a result of decreased levels of ADH, which leads to polyuria and dehydration.
- SIADH is caused by increased levels of ADH, which leads to retention of fluid and systemic fluid overload.

▶ Vital Vocabulary

addisonian crisis Acute adrenal insufficiency.

adrenocorticotropic hormone (ACTH) Hormone that targets the adrenal cortex to secrete cortisol (a glucocorticoid).

aldosterone Hormone that stimulates the kidneys to reabsorb sodium from the urine and excrete potassium by altering the osmotic gradient in the blood.

androgens Male sex hormones that regulate body changes associated with sexual development (puberty), including growth spurts, deepening of the voice, growth of facial and pubic hair, and muscle growth and strength.

antidiuretic hormone (ADH) A hormone secreted by the posterior pituitary lobe of the pituitary gland, ADH constricts blood vessels and raises the blood pressure; also called *vasopressin.*

calcitonin The hormone secreted by the thyroid gland that helps maintain normal calcium levels in the blood.

corticosteroids Hormones that regulate the body's metabolism, the balance of salt and water in the body, the immune system, and sexual function.

cortisol Hormone that stimulates most body cells to increase their energy production.

Cushing syndrome A condition caused by an excess of cortisol production by the adrenal glands or by excessive use of cortisol or other similar corticosteroid (glucocorticoid) hormones.

diabetes A group of complex metabolic disorders with many causes. These disorders include diabetes mellitus, gestational diabetes, hypoglycemia/hyperglycemia, diabetic ketoacidosis, and hyperosmolar hyperglycemic syndrome.

diabetes insipidus (DI) A relatively uncommon disorder that has some of the same characteristics as diabetes, such as polyuria and polydipsia, in which the body is unable to regulate fluid owing to a lack of antidiuretic hormone (central diabetes insipidus) or the kidneys are unable to respond appropriately (nephrogenic diabetes insipidus).

diabetes mellitus Disease characterized by the body's inability to sufficiently metabolize glucose. The condition occurs either because the pancreas does not produce enough insulin or because the cells do not respond to the effects of the insulin that is produced.

diabetic ketoacidosis (DKA) A form of acidosis in uncontrolled diabetes in which certain acids accumulate when insulin is not available.

diuresis The production of large amounts of urine by the kidney.

dyslipidemia An excessive level of lipids (fats) circulating in the blood, increasing the risk of atherosclerosis and coronary artery disease.

epinephrine Hormone produced by the adrenal medulla that plays a vital role in the function of the sympathetic nervous system.

estrogen One of the three major female hormones. At puberty, estrogen brings about the secondary sex characteristics.

exophthalmos Protrusion of the eyes from the normal position within the socket.

gestational diabetes Diabetes that develops during pregnancy in women who did not have diabetes before pregnancy.

glucagon Hormone produced by the pancreas that is vital to the control of the body's metabolism and blood glucose level. Glucagon stimulates the breakdown of glycogen to glucose.

Prep Kit *(continued)*

glycosuria The passage of large quantities of urine containing glucose.

goiter A visible mass in the anterior part of the neck caused by enlargement of the thyroid gland.

Graves disease An autoimmune disorder that causes thyroid gland hypertrophy and severe hyperthyroidism.

Hashimoto disease A type of hyperthyroidism in which the thyroid gland becomes enlarged as it is infiltrated by T lymphocytes and plasma cells.

hyperglycemia Abnormally high blood glucose level.

hyperosmolar hyperglycemic syndrome (HHS) A metabolic derangement that occurs principally in patients with type 2 diabetes; it is characterized by hyperglycemia, hyperosmolarity, and an absence of significant ketosis. Also known as hyperosmolar nonketotic coma (HONK).

hyperosmolar nonketotic coma (HONK) See *hyperosmolar hyperglycemic syndrome (HHS)*.

hypoglycemia Abnormally low blood glucose level.

insulin Hormone produced by the pancreas that is vital to the control of the body's metabolism and blood glucose level. Insulin causes sugar, fatty acids, and amino acids to be absorbed and metabolized by cells.

insulin resistance Condition in which the pancreas produces enough insulin but the body cannot effectively use it.

islets of Langerhans A specialized group of cells in the pancreas in which insulin and glucagon are produced.

ketonemia Excess amounts of ketone bodies in the blood.

lipolysis The metabolism (breakdown or destruction) of stored fat that has been released into the circulation.

luteinizing hormone (LH) Hormone that regulates the production of both eggs and sperm, as well as production of reproductive hormones.

microangiopathy Microscopic deterioration of vessel walls caused primarily by adherence of blood lipids to vessel walls.

myxedema coma A rare condition that can occur in patients who have severe, untreated hypothyroidism.

norepinephrine Hormone produced by the adrenal glands that is vital in the function of the sympathetic nervous system.

panhypopituitarism The inadequate production or absence of the pituitary hormones, including adrenocorticotropic hormone (ACTH), cortisol, thyroxine, luteinizing hormone (LH), follicle-stimulating hormone (FSH), estrogen, testosterone, growth hormone, and antidiuretic hormone (ADH).

parathyroid hormone A hormone secreted by the parathyroids that acts as an antagonist to calcitonin; secreted when calcium blood levels are low.

pheochromocytoma A tumor of the adrenal gland, usually in the medulla, that causes excessive release of the hormones epinephrine and norepinephrine.

polydipsia Significant thirst.

polyphagia Increased appetite.

polyuria Frequent and plentiful urination.

prediabetes A condition identified in people who have certain risk factors associated with type 2 diabetes and exists when blood glucose levels or hemoglobin A1c levels are above normal levels, yet not high enough to be diagnosed as diabetes.

pretibial myxedema An "orange peel" appearance and nonpitting edema of the skin on the anterior part of the leg below the knee.

primary adrenal insufficiency Also known as Addison disease. A rare condition in which the adrenal glands produce an insufficient amount of adrenal hormones.

progesterone One of the three major female hormones.

secondary adrenal insufficiency A common condition characterized by a lack of adrenocorticotropic hormone (also called corticotrophin) secretion from the pituitary gland.

somatostatin A hormone that inhibits insulin and glucagon secretion by the pancreas.

syndrome of inappropriate antidiuretic hormone secretion (SIADH) An endocrine disorder in which an excess of antidiuretic hormone results in a decrease in urinary output and, therefore, systemic fluid overload.

testosterone The most important androgen in men.

thyroid-stimulating hormone (TSH) Hormone that controls the release of thyroid hormone from the thyroid gland.

thyroid storm A rare, life-threatening condition that may occur in patients with thyrotoxicosis. The condition is usually triggered by a stressful event or increased volume of thyroid hormones in the circulation.

thyrotoxicosis A toxic condition caused by excessive levels of circulating thyroid hormone.

thyroxine (T_4) The body's major metabolic hormone. Thyroxine stimulates energy production in cells, which increases the rate at which the cells consume oxygen and use carbohydrates, fats, and proteins.

Prep Kit *(continued)*

type 1 diabetes The type of diabetic disease that usually starts in childhood and requires daily injections of supplemental synthetic insulin to control blood glucose; formerly called juvenile diabetes *or* juvenile-onset diabetes.

type 2 diabetes The type of diabetic disease that usually starts in later life and often can be controlled through diet and oral medications; formerly called adult-onset diabetes.

▶ References

1. Diabetes. Centers for Disease Control and Prevention website. https://www.cdc.gov/chronicdisease/resources/publications/aag/diabetes.htm. Updated July 25, 2016. Accessed March 6, 2017.
2. Statistics About Diabetes. American Diabetes Association. http://www.diabetes.org/diabetes-basics/statistics/. Last edited December 12, 2016. Accessed March 6, 2017.
3. Nathan DM, Cleary PA, Backlund JY, et al. Diabetes Control and Complications Trial/Epidemiology of Diabetes Interventions and Complications (DCCT/EDIC) Study Research Group. Intensive diabetes treatment and cardiovascular disease in patients with type 1 diabetes. *N Engl J Med.* 2005;353:2643–2653.
4. Health Information for Older Adults. Centers for Disease Control and Prevention website. https://www.cdc.gov/aging/aginginfo/index.htm. Updated January 31, 2017. Accessed March 6, 2017.
5. Lough ME. Endocrine disorders and therapeutic management. In: Urden LD, Stacy KM, Lough ME, eds. *Critical Care Nursing: Diagnosis and Management.* 7th ed. St. Louis, MO: Mosby; 2014:809-848.
6. Reno CM, Daphna-Iken D, Chen S, et al. Severe hypoglycemia-induced lethal cardiac arrhythmias are mediated by sympathoadrenal activation. *Diabetes.* 2013;62(10):3570-3581.
7. Diabetes Fact Sheet. World Health Organization website. http://www.who.int/mediacentre/factsheets/fs312/en/. Reviewed November 2016. Accessed March 8, 2017.
8. NIH Fact Sheets—Diabetes, Type 2. National Institutes of Health website. https://www.report.nih.gov/nihfactsheets/ViewFactSheet.aspx?csid=121. Updated March 29, 2013. Accessed March 6, 2017.
9. Fuchsberger C, Flannick J, Teslovich TM, et al. The genetic architecture of type 2 diabetes. *Nature.* 2016;536;41-47.
10. About Prediabetes & Type 2 Diabetes. Centers for Disease Control and Prevention website. http://www.cdc.gov/diabetes/prevention/prediabetes-type2/index.html. Updated July 19, 2016. Accessed March 8, 2017.
11. National Diabetes Prevention Program. Centers for Disease Control and Prevention website. https://www.cdc.gov/diabetes/prevention/prediabetes-type2/preventing.html. Updated January 14, 2016. Accessed March 8, 2017.
12. Gestational Diabetes and Pregnancy. Centers for Disease Control and Prevention website. https://www.cdc.gov/pregnancy/diabetes-gestational.html. Updated September 16, 2015. Accessed March 6, 2017.
13. Diabetes and Pregnancy: Gestational Diabetes. Centers for Disease Control and Prevention website. https://www.cdc.gov/pregnancy/documents/Diabetes_and_Pregnancy508.pdf. Accessed March 6, 2017.
14. Gerich JE, Langlois M, Noacco C, et al. Lack of glucagon response to hypoglycemia in diabetes: evidence for an intrinsic pancreatic alpha cell defect. *Science*. 1973 Oct 12; 182(4108):171-3.
15. Sandoval DA, Guy DL, Richardson MA, et al. Effects of low and moderate antecedent exercise on counterregulatory responses to subsequent hypoglycemia in type 1 diabetes. *Diabetes*. 2004 July; 53(7):1798-806.
16. Cryer P. Hypoglycemia during therapy of diabetes. In: DeGroot LJ, Chrousos G, Dungan K, et al, eds. *Endotext [Internet]*. South Dartmouth, MA: MDText.com, Inc.;2000. https://www.ncbi.nlm.nih.gov/books/NBK279100/. Updated May 28, 2015. Accessed March 23, 2017.
17. 2014 National Diabetes Statistics Report. Centers for Disease Control and Prevention website. https://www.cdc.gov/diabetes/data/statistics/2014statisticsreport.html. Updated May 15, 2015. Accessed March 6, 2017.
18. Soleimanpour H, Taghizadieh A, Niafar M, et al. Predictive value of capnography for suspected diabetic ketoacidosis in the emergency department. *West J Emerg Med.* 2013;14(6):590-594.
19. Sabatini S, Kurtzman NA. Bicarbonate therapy in severe metabolic acidosis. *J Am Soc Nephrol.* 2008;20(4):692-695.
20. Umpierrez GE, Kitabchi AE. Diabetic ketoacidosis. *Treat Endocrinol.* 2003;2(2):95-108.
21. Diabetic hyperglycemic hyperosmolar syndrome. U.S. National Library of Medicine Medline website. https://medlineplus.gov/ency/article/000304.htm. Updated April 4, 2017. Accessed May 1, 2017.
22. Crandall J, Shamoon H. Diabetes mellitus. In: Goldman L, Schafer AI, eds. *Goldman-Cecil Medicine.* 25th ed. Philadelphia, PA: Saunders; 2016:1527-1548.
23. Cydulka RK, Maloney GE. Diabetes mellitus and disorders of glucose homeostasis. In: Marx JA, Hockberger RS, Walls RM, eds. *Rosen's Emergency Medicine*. 8th ed. Philadelphia, PA: Saunders; 2014:1652-1666.
24. Whitlatch HB. Hyperosmolar hyperglycemic syndrome. In: Ferri FF, ed. *Ferri's Clinical Advisor 2017*. Philadelphia, PA: Elsevier; 2017:632-633.

Prep Kit (continued)

25. Collopy K, Kivlehan S, Snyder S. Prehospital Treatment of Hyperglycemia. 2013 (September 1). http://www.emsworld.com/article/11112993/prehospital-treatment-of-hyperglycemia. Accessed March 6, 2017.
26. Forsmark CE, Vaillie J, AGA Institute Clinical Practice and Economics Committee, AGA institute Governing Board. AGA Institute technical review on acute pancreatitis. *Gastroenterology*. 2007 May;132(5):2022-44.
27. Yang AL, Vadhavkar S, Singh G, Omary MB. Epidemiology of alcohol-related liver and pancreatic disease in the United States. *Arch Intern Med*. 2008 Mar 24;168(6) 649-56.
28. Corrigan EK. Adrenal Insufficiency (Addison's Disease). Pituitary Network Association website. https://pituitary.org/knowledge-base/disorders/adrenal-insuffieciency-addison-s-disease. Accessed March 06, 2017.
29. Scholz T, Eisenhofer G, Pacak K, et al. Clinical review: current treatment of malignant pheochromocytoma. *J Clin Endocrinol Metab*. 2007 Apr;92(4):1217–25.
30. Acromegaly. National Institutes of Diabetes and Digestive and Kidney Diseases website. https://www.niddk.nih.gov/health-information/endocrine-diseases/acromegaly. Published April 2012. Accessed March 6, 2017.
31. Growth Hormone Deficiency. National Organization of Rare Diseases website. https://rarediseases.org/rare-diseases/growth-hormone-deficiency/. Accessed March 6, 2017.
32. Vanderpump MPJ. The epidemiology of thyroid disease. *Br Med Bull*. 2011 Sept;99(1):39-51.
33. Beynon J, Akhtar S, Kearney T. Predictors of outcome in myxoedema coma. *Crit Care*. 2008;12(1):111.
34. Silverberg SJ, Bilezikian JP. Primary hyperparathyroidism. In: Jameson JL, DeGroot LJ, sr eds. *Endocrinology: Adult and Pediatric*. 6th ed. (online version). Philadelphia: Saunders; 2010.

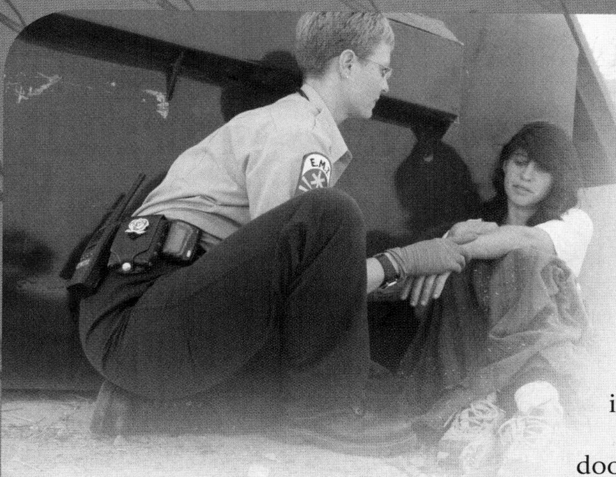

Assessment *in Action*

Your response area includes a large number of low-income families, and many people in the area do not receive medical care. Although your agency does not have a high call volume, when you are dispatched, it is often for extremely ill or substantially injured patients.

One morning, you hear frantic knocking on the station door. You open it to find a frightened teenager who tells you, "My mom needs help! She's not acting right, and can't stop throwing up. We were evicted from our apartment a few days ago. Please help us." As you have your partner pull the ambulance out and notify dispatch, you approach the vehicle to find an approximately 30-year-old woman in the passenger seat. She is confused and febrile to the touch. Her radial pulse is very rapid, weak, and irregular. When you assess her pupils, you notice her eyes are bulging.

1. What is your primary concern regarding this patient's condition?

- **A.** Decreased level of consciousness
- **B.** Fast, irregular pulse rate
- **C.** Fever
- **D.** Bulging eyes

2. Which interventions may be required?

- **A.** Epinephrine
- **B.** Atropine
- **C.** Beta-blockers
- **D.** Nitrous oxide

Assessment in Action *(continued)*

3. This condition is often precipitated by which type of event?

- **A.** Sudden, transient loss of consciousness
- **B.** Stressful event
- **C.** Severe abdominal pain
- **D.** Sudden blindness

4. Given the patient's condition, what is the most likely cause?

- **A.** Narcotic overdose
- **B.** Thyroid storm
- **C.** Malignant hypothermia
- **D.** Addisonian crisis

5. Which additional signs and symptoms could have been experienced by the patient prior to this event?

- **A.** Palpitations
- **B.** Slow pulse rate
- **C.** Weight gain
- **D.** Hair growth

6. All conditions may cause these signs and symptoms EXCEPT:

- **A.** Thyroid cancer
- **B.** Goiter
- **C.** Graves disease
- **D.** Myxedema

7. Which procedure is required to diagnose this condition?

- **A.** Chest radiograph
- **B.** Skin biopsy
- **C.** Thyroidectomy
- **D.** Blood testing

8. When you are forming a general impression, why is it important to make note of a patient's vital statistics, dress/grooming and hygiene, and breath or body odors?

9. Why is it important to perform a rapid full-body scan?

10. Why is it important to be aware of endocrine-related diseases and their signs and symptoms in prehospital care?

CHAPTER 24

Hematologic Emergencies

National EMS Education Standard Competencies

Medicine

Integrates assessment findings with principles of epidemiology and pathophysiology to formulate a field impression and implement a comprehensive treatment/disposition plan for a patient with a medical complaint.

Hematology

Anatomy, physiology, pathophysiology, assessment, and management of

- Sickle cell crisis (pp 1301-1303)
- Clotting disorders (pp 1297-1298, 1306-1307)

Anatomy, physiology, epidemiology, pathophysiology, psychosocial impact, presentations, prognosis, and management of common or major hematological diseases and/or emergencies

- Sickle cell crisis (pp 1301-1303)
- Blood transfusion complications (pp 1307-1309)
- Hemostatic disorders (pp 1306-1307)
- Lymphomas (p 1305)
- Red blood cell disorders (pp 1301-1303, 1305-1306)
- White blood cell disorders (pp 1304-1305)
- Coagulopathies (pp 1306-1307)

Knowledge Objectives

1. Discuss the composition and functions of blood's essential components. (pp 1294-1298)
2. Summarize the role of white blood cells in the normal inflammatory process. (p 1296)
3. Define hemostasis and the mechanisms essential to its maintenance in the body. (pp 1297-1298)
4. Outline the steps in the primary survey and management of a patient with a hematologic disorder. (p 1299)
5. Summarize general emergency care for a patient with a hematologic disorder. (pp 1300-1301)
6. Describe the pathophysiology, assessment, and management of sickle cell disease. (pp 1301-1303)
7. Describe three types of sickle cell crisis. (pp 1301-1302)
8. Outline the pathophysiology, assessment, and management of other common diseases and conditions of the blood, including anemia, leukopenia, thrombocytopenia, leukemia, lymphomas, polycythemia, disseminated intravascular coagulation, hemophilia, and multiple myeloma. (pp 1303-1307)
9. Discuss the causes, symptoms, assessment, and management of blood transfusion complications. (pp 1307-1309)

Skills Objectives

There are no skills objectives for this chapter.

YOU are the Paramedic PART 1

Your unit is dispatched to a private residence for a "general medical" complaint. The dispatcher informs you that the patient is a 73-year-old man with a history of leukemia who is feeling "poorly." When you arrive on scene, you find a man who appears frail. Family members confirm the patient was diagnosed with leukemia years ago. A family member states the patient has a fever (temperature of 102°F [39°C]) and is feeling pain all over. You notice bruising on the patient's arms.

1. Why is a fever significant in this patient?
2. What do you need to know about this patient's status?

Introduction

Hematology is, by definition, simply the study of blood; however, it addresses not only the blood, but also the ways in which its constituent parts are involved in health and disease. These components include red blood cells (RBCs), white blood cells (WBCs), platelets, and other proteins involved in the bleeding and clotting cascades, as well as the **hematopoietic system**—that is, organs and tissues involved in the production of blood components (primarily bone marrow, spleen, and lymph nodes). Most emergency medical services (EMS) systems rarely respond to hematologic emergencies.

The blanket term **hematologic disorder** refers to any disorder of the blood. Within this general category, **hemolytic disorders** refer to disease processes that cause the breakdown of RBCs, and **hemostatic disorders** refer to bleeding and clotting abnormalities. These disorders can be complex, difficult to assess, and challenging to treat in the prehospital setting.

As a paramedic, you should have a basic understanding of the hematopoietic system and hematologic disorders, and know how to respond to these kinds of emergencies appropriately. Although you may be able to provide only limited interventions in the field for patients with hematologic disorders, your actions may not just offer support, but actually save the patient's life.

Anatomy and Physiology Review

Blood and Plasma

Blood is a connective tissue. It is composed of cells and cell fragments, which are suspended in **plasma**, the liquid portion of blood. In the adult body, blood accounts for approximately 8% of the total body weight, or approximately 5 to 6 L. The primary functions of blood are as follows:

- Supply oxygen and nutrients to the cells.
- Transport carbon dioxide and nitrogenous wastes from the tissues to the lungs and kidneys, where the wastes can be removed from the body.
- Carry hormones from the endocrine glands to the target tissues.
- Regulate body temperature.
- Regulate pH through the buffering components in the blood.
- Keep fluid and electrolytes balanced through sodium and plasma proteins.
- Regulate the immune system through the actions of WBCs and antibodies.
- Form clots through the action of platelets.

Blood consists of two main components: plasma and formed elements (cells). Plasma is 92% water, with the remaining 8% of plasma being made up of various solutes, including proteins, electrolytes, clotting factors, and glucose. Plasma accounts for 55% of the total blood volume, and the formed elements account for the remaining 45%. The formed elements include RBCs, or **erythrocytes**; WBCs, or **leukocytes**; and platelets, or **thrombocytes**. Most of these elements (99%) are RBCs Figure 24-1.

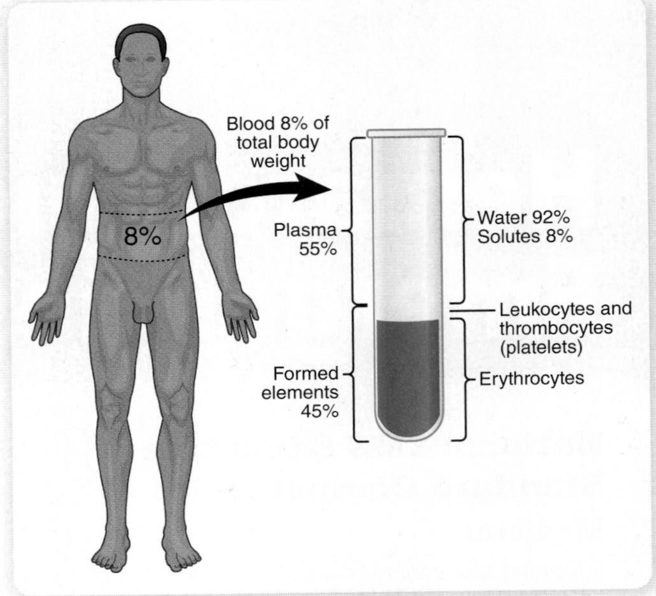

Figure 24-1 Components of a spun-down blood sample.

Figure 24-2 shows the development of the cells of the hematologic system. The production of RBCs occurs within **stem cells**, or cells that develop into other types of cells in the body; this production is stimulated by a protein (called erythropoietin) that is secreted by the kidneys in response to circulatory need. The RBCs may take as long as 5 days to mature and have an average life of 120 days. Within the RBCs, iron-rich **hemoglobin** is responsible for carrying oxygen to the tissues. Oxygen attached to hemoglobin gives blood its characteristic red color, although many other factors can change the color of blood (such as carbon monoxide poisoning, which changes the blood's color to bright red). When the oxygen-rich RBCs encounter an environment that contains higher concentrations of carbon dioxide (and, therefore, is more acidotic), they release the oxygen there. This physiologic phenomenon is called the Bohr effect.

Three laboratory tests are commonly performed on blood: RBC counts, hemoglobin levels, and hematocrit measurements. The RBC count measures the number of RBCs in a sample of blood, whereas the hemoglobin level identifies the amount of hemoglobin found within the RBCs. The measurement of **hematocrit** gives the overall proportion of RBCs in the blood. The patient's blood is considered balanced (even if the numbers are too high or low) if the hemoglobin level is one-third of the hematocrit value and the RBC count is one-third of the hemoglobin level. Table 24-1 describes these tests in more detail.

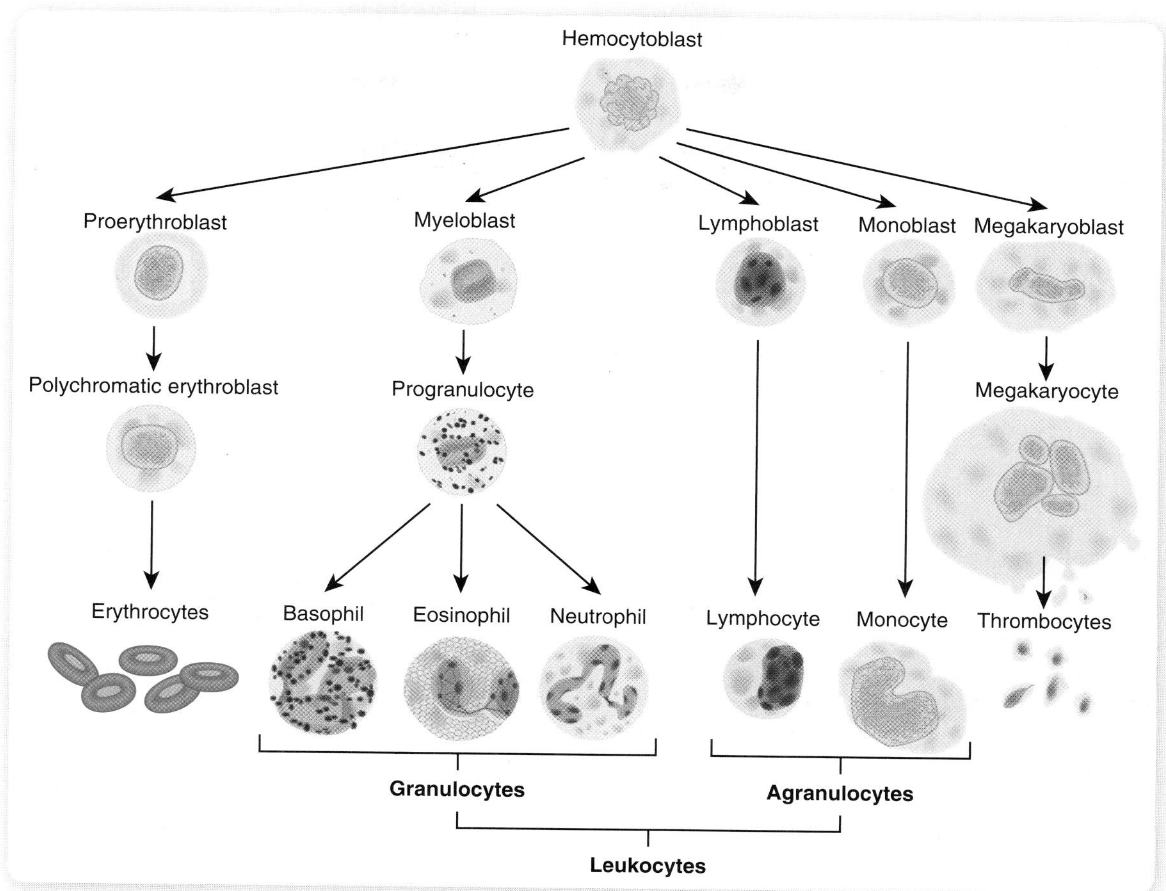

Figure 24-2 Development of the cells of the hematologic system.

Table 24-1 RBC and Platelet Counts

Name	Normal Values[a]	Examples of Conditions Associated With Low Readings	Examples of Conditions Associated With High Readings
RBC count (× 10^6/mcL)	4.5–6.0 in adults; 3.3–5.5 in children	Anemia, hemorrhage, certain leukemias, overhydration, chronic infections	Polycythemia, cardiovascular disease, hemoconcentration, dehydration
Hemoglobin (g/dL)	12.0–16.0 in females; 14.0–18.0 in males; 10.7–17.1 in children	Anemia, hyperthyroidism, liver disease, hemorrhage, hemolytic reactions	COPD, HF, polycythemia, high-altitude sickness
Hematocrit (%)	35–45 in females; 40–50 in males; 32–55 in children	Same as for RBCs and hemoglobin, including leukemia, lupus, endocarditis, rheumatic fever, nutritional disorders	Polycythemia and usually anything that produces severe dehydration
Thrombocytes (platelets)	150,000–400,000 cells/mcL	Thrombocytopenia, certain cancers, certain leukemias, sickle cell disease, systemic lupus erythematosus	Pulmonary embolism, polycythemia, acute hemorrhage, metastatic cancer, surgical stress

Abbreviations: COPD, chronic obstructive pulmonary disease; HF, heart failure; RBC, red blood cell

[a] The normal ranges provided are not intended to be definitive. Each laboratory determines its own values, and normal ranges are method dependent.

The WBCs, which are larger than RBCs, provide the body with immunity against "foreign invaders." Just like RBCs, they are derived from stem cells. Several types of WBCs exist, each of which performs a specific task in relation to maintaining the immune system; Table 24-2 summarizes the components of the WBC count and differential. Certain disease processes are also specific to the differential WBCs. For example, **neutropenia** is an abnormally low number of neutrophils, which make up the majority of the circulating WBCs.

Recall from Chapter 9, *Pathophysiology*, that immune system responses can be categorized into humoral immunity and cell-mediated immunity. *Humoral immunity* refers to the secretion of antibodies called immunoglobulins, which recognize a specific antigen. In *cell-mediated immunity*, macrophages and T cells attack and destroy pathogens or foreign substances.

Words of Wisdom

The life cycle of a WBC begins when the bone marrow releases cells called granulocytes. Granulocytes remain in the circulation for 6 to 12 hours. If these cells travel to tissues, then they live for a few more days. At the end of their lives, WBCs are recycled by the **reticuloendothelial system**, as are RBCs.

Table 24-2 WBC Count and Differential

Name	Normal Values	Examples of Conditions Associated With Low Readings	Examples of Conditions Associated With High Readings
WBC count	4,500–10,000 cells/mm^3 in adults; 4,500–15,500 cells/mm^3 in children; 9,400–34,000 cells/mm^3 in infants	Viral infections, bone marrow diseases or disorders, leukemia, radiation, late-stage AIDS	Viral and bacterial infections, hemorrhage, traumatic tissue injuries, leukemia, cigarette smoking
Neutrophils (segmented and unsegmented)	50%–60%;[a] 2,500–8,000 cells/mm^3	Leukemia, infections, rheumatoid arthritis, vitamin B_{12} deficiency, enlarged spleen	Bacterial infections, tissue breakdown, hemolytic reactions, tumors, MI, surgical stress, cancer
Basophils (also known as mast cells)	0.5%–1%[a]; 25–100 cells/mm^3	Allergic reactions, hyperthyroidism, MI, bleeding ulcers, stress	Certain leukemias, inflammations, allergy, polycythemia, hemolytic anemia
Eosinophils	1%–4%[a]; 50–500 cells/mm^3	Mononucleosis, HF, Cushing disease	Addison disease, tumors, skin infections, allergies
Lymphocytes	20%–40%[a]; 1,000–4,000 cells/mm^3	Hodgkin disease, burns, trauma, lupus, Cushing disease, immunodeficiency states	Numerous bacterial and viral infections, hepatitis, leukemia, toxoplasmosis, Graves disease
Monocytes	2%–6%[a]; 100–700 cells/mm^3	Corticosteroid use, infections, rheumatoid arthritis, HIV	Numerous bacterial and parasitic infections, recovery of acute infections, TB, hematologic disorders

Abbreviations: AIDS, acquired immunodeficiency syndrome; HF, heart failure; HIV, human immunodeficiency; MI, myocardial infarction, TB, tuberculosis; WBC, white blood cell

Note: The normal ranges provided are not intended to be definitive. Each laboratory determines its own values, and normal ranges are method dependent.

[a] Percentage of the total WBC count. Example: If the WBC is 5,000, then neutrophils should account for 2,500 to 3,000 of this count.

Words of Wisdom

In a normal adult, the WBC count initially increases in response to infection. As the infection continues, the WBC count may drop as the WBCs are exhausted faster than they can regenerate. Thus a low WBC count does not necessarily indicate absence of infection.

Platelets are the smallest of the formed elements. They are derived from stem cells and have an average life span of approximately 7 to 10 days. Approximately two-thirds of the platelets circulate throughout the blood; the rest are stored in the spleen.

Platelets are responsible for the clotting of the blood. These cells form the initial plug following vascular injury; the clotting proteins then toughen and complete the blood clot. Without platelets, our bodies would not be able to stop bleeding. There can be too much of a good thing with platelets, however: Conditions such as **thrombocytosis**, in which the body produces too many platelets, can lead to other dangerous medical conditions, such as coagulation or clotting of blood inside of a blood vessel, called **thrombosis**.

Hemostasis is a highly complex process that allows the body to stop bleeding through vascular spasm, coagulation, and platelet plugging. The opposite of hemostasis is hemorrhage.

Clots themselves are made up of fibrin. When injury is detected, thrombin converts fibrinogen to fibrin, and the clotting process begins. Calcium acts as a binding agent, holding fibrin fibers close together to form the meshwork of the clot.

The **clotting cascade**—that is, the process by which clotting factors work together to ultimately form fibrin, also called the coagulation cascade—can be initiated through either an intrinsic or an extrinsic pathway **Figure 24-3**. Any process that interferes with the activation or continuation of the clotting cascade or hemostasis is known as a **coagulopathy**. Coagulopathies can lead to heavy or prolonged bleeding. One such bleeding disorder is **von Willebrand disease**, in which the blood's ability to clot

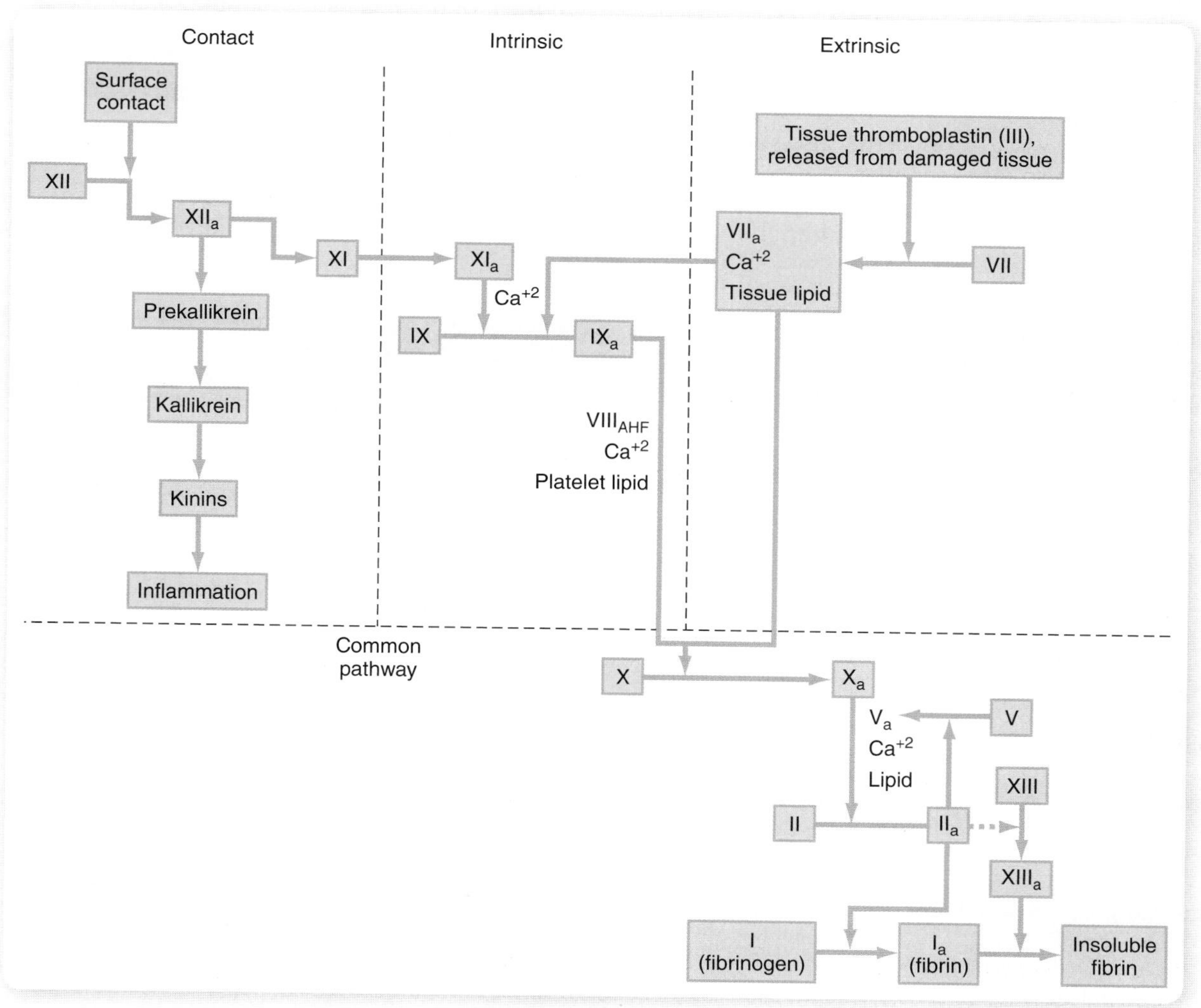

Figure 24-3 The clotting cascade.

is decreased due to the absence of a key protein, von Willebrand factor, that is necessary for platelet adhesion.

Words of Wisdom

"Clot busters" (fibrinolytic therapy given in cases of acute myocardial infarction and stroke) activate the body's fibrinolytic system, resulting in clot decomposition (also known as lysis). Such therapy must be monitored closely in patients with hematologic disorders, because clot busters may cause excess bleeding in these patients.

Blood-Forming Organs and RBC Production

Although many parts and organs of the human body can alter or affect the hematologic system, the major players are the bone marrow, liver, and spleen Figure 24-4.

The bone marrow is the primary site for cell production within the human body. It is found in most of the long bones plus the pelvis, skull, and vertebrae.

The liver produces the **clotting factors** found in the blood. This organ filters the blood, removing toxins, and is essential to normal metabolism and homeostasis. As old RBCs enter the liver, they are broken down into bile. The liver is a highly vascular organ that also stores blood.

The spleen is also quite vascular. It is involved with the filtering and breakdown of RBCs, assists with the production of lymphocytes, and has an important role in providing homeostasis and infection control. The spleen stores about one-third of the platelets. If the spleen is removed, then the platelets formed after that time remain in the blood throughout their life span.

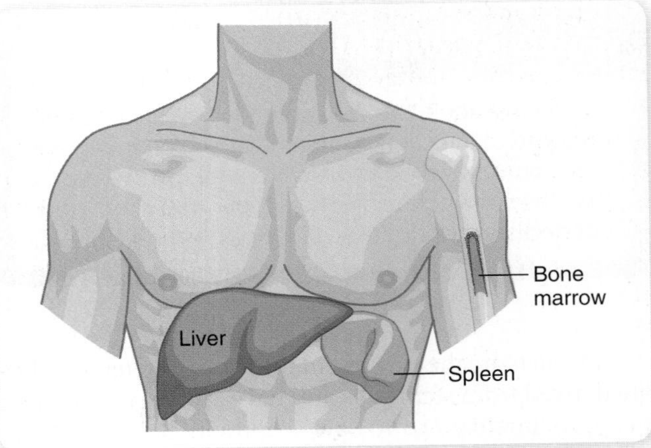

Figure 24-4 The bone marrow, liver, and spleen are major organs responsible for producing and regulating the blood and its components.

Patient Assessment

Assessment of a patient suspected of having a hematologic disorder should be no different from assessment of any other patient, with a few additional items to consider and questions to ask. During the primary survey, note

YOU are the Paramedic PART 2

You begin your assessment of the patient while your partner obtains more information from the family. The patient is alert and cooperative with your questioning. You ask the patient what he is experiencing right now. The patient states, "My bones hurt, and I do not feel well." The patient also tells you that he takes chemotherapy and his most recent treatment was 4 days ago. You notice numerous used facial tissues that appear to have blood on them.

Recording Time: 0 Minutes	
Appearance	Awake, frail
Level of consciousness	Alert and oriented
Airway	Open
Breathing	Adequate
Circulation	Adequate

3. Which signs or symptoms is the patient showing that could indicate thrombocytopenia?
4. How will a patient with leukemia typically present?

any signs and symptoms that may be immediately life threatening. Unusual bleeding or apparently uncontrolled hemorrhage can indicate an underlying pathology. A major purpose of taking a history and performing the secondary assessment is to clearly and thoroughly understanding the chief complaint, which requires asking in-depth and relevant questions about the patient's history and SAMPLE (Signs and symptoms, Allergies, Medications, Pertinent past history, Last oral intake, Events leading to injury or illness) history and following up on the responses to questions. Because some patients with a blood disorder may be unwilling to disclose their conditions for fear of being treated differently from people without the disorder, a nonjudgmental approach is essential.

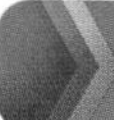

Scene Size-up

As always, ensure the scene is safe for entry, consider the mechanism of injury, determine the number of patients, and assess for hazards and the need for additional help. Standard precautions should consist of gloves and eye protection at a minimum. Remember to evaluate each situation quickly and make sure the necessary personal protective equipment is readily available.

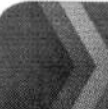

Primary Survey

Perform cervical spine stabilization, if necessary. It is important that you not dismiss a pain complaint of the spine simply because it could be a manifestation of a current disease state. For example, even though a person has a history of **sickle cell disease**, sickle cell disease may not be causing the current problem; trauma or another type of medical emergency may be the cause. For this reason, you must always perform a thorough, careful primary survey, paying attention to assess the ABCDEs (Airway, Breathing, Circulation, Disability, and Exposure), and must immediately correct any life-threatening issues.

Perform a rapid full-body scan of the patient to form an initial general impression. How does the patient look? Does the patient appear anxious, restless, or listless? Is the patient apathetic or irritable? Determine the patient's level of consciousness.

As you are forming your general impression, assess the patient's airway and breathing. Patients showing signs of inadequate breathing or altered mental status should receive appropriate oxygen therapy. Depending on the severity of the patient's condition, this may be accomplished with a nasal cannula, nonrebreathing mask, or even ventilation via bag-mask device as needed. Should you need to provide additional airway support with suctioning and/or basic or advanced airways, be aware that even minor trauma during these procedures can lead to bleeding into the airway and increase the risk of airway compromise.

Once you have assessed the airway and breathing and have performed the necessary interventions, check the patient's circulatory status. An increased pulse rate may indicate a compensatory mechanism. Look for signs of shock, such as a rapid pulse rate and low blood pressure. If you find any life-threatening conditions, then take immediate steps to manage them and provide urgent transport to an appropriately equipped receiving facility.

In patients with suspected **hemophilia**, be alert for signs of acute blood loss such as pallor, a weak pulse, and hypotension. Note any bleeding of unknown origin, such as nosebleeds, bloody sputum, and blood in the urine or stool. Owing to blood loss, patients with hemophilia may exhibit signs of hypoxia or shock. Fluid resuscitation may be necessary for these patients; however, it must be administered with care so as not to "wash out" the clots that are forming.

Whether you decide to rapidly transport the patient will depend on the severity of the patient's condition and the patient's wishes. Transport to the closest, most appropriate facility should always be recommended for any patient who is experiencing a **sickle cell crisis** or uncontrolled bleeding.

History Taking

It is extremely important to understand the chief complaint; to do so, you may need to be overly inquisitive about the patient's history and SAMPLE history. When you are obtaining the patient's history, keep in mind that hematologic disorders may also present with multiple symptoms that at first glance may seem unrelated, such as pneumonia in a patient with sickle cell disease or abdominal pain in a patient with **polycythemia**. It is important that you put these pieces together to get a complete picture of the patient.

During history taking, look for changes in level of consciousness and symptoms such as vertigo, feelings of fatigue, and syncopal episodes. Has the patient had dyspnea, chest pain, changes in pulse rate and rhythm, or coughing up of blood? Has the patient experienced visual disturbances, muscle pain, or stiffness? Are these complaints related as part of a larger disease process, or are they simply multiple unrelated complaints?

If the patient has a complaint of pain, then ascertain whether the pain is isolated to a single location or whether it is felt throughout the entire body. Has the patient experienced skin changes such as color changes, burning, or itching? Bleeding from the nose, gums, and ulcers, or blood in the urine or stool? Be alert for signs of acute blood loss (pallor, weak pulse, and hypotension). Does the patient have an history of liver problems or pain for unknown reasons? Problems with the genitourinary system? Is the patient experiencing any gastrointestinal problems, such as nausea, vomiting, or abdominal cramping?

Documentation & Communication

Many anti-inflammatory medications (such as aspirin and ibuprofen) and some herbal products (such as ginkgo, garlic, ginger, ginseng, and feverfew) decrease platelet aggregation. Although this effect may be beneficial (as in the prevention of myocardial infarction and stroke), these medications may also increase the tendency to bleed. Always ask patients about medications, including over-the-counter and herbal medications.

Secondary Assessment

The secondary assessment may be performed on scene, en route to the emergency department, or not at all. This decision will depend on the transport time and the patient's condition.

When treating a patient with a known or suspected blood disorder, you will need to perform a physical exam. In such cases, it is important to have a basic understanding of some of the common findings in blood disorders 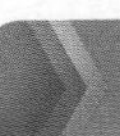 Table 24-3.

Systematically examine the patient, starting at the head and working your way down. You can see from Table 24-3 how your secondary assessment needs to dig a little deeper. For example, instead of just checking the patient's pupils, you need to assess for visual disturbances. During your physical exam, obtain the patient's baseline vital signs, including lung sounds and oxygen saturation level. However, keep in mind that the oxygen saturation reading you obtain may be inaccurate as a result of the patient's anemic state.

Reassessment

It is important to reassess the patient frequently to identify any changes in his or her condition. For example, has the patient's mental status changed? Are the ABCs still intact? How is the patient responding to the interventions performed? Should you adjust or change the interventions? In many patients, you will note marked improvement with appropriate treatment.

Communication with hospital staff is important to ensure continuity of care. Hospital personnel need to be informed about the patient's history, the present situation, your assessment findings, and your interventions and their results.

Be sure to thoroughly document each assessment, your findings, any treatments administered, the time of the interventions, and any changes in the patient's condition. Follow your local protocols for patients who refuse treatment or transport.

Table 24-3 Common Findings With Blood Disorders

System	Examples of Common Findings
Level of consciousness	Alterations in level of consciousness, ranging from excitability, agitation, and combativeness, to complete unresponsiveness
Skin	Uncontrolled bleeding, unexplained or chronic bruising, itching, pallor, or jaundice (yellow appearance usually indicates liver problems)
Visual disturbances	Visual disturbances, including blurred vision, decreased vision, tunnel vision, and seeing black or gray spots
Gastrointestinal	Epistaxis (bloody nose), bleeding or infected gums, ulcers, melena (blood in the stool), and liver failure (causes jaundice)
Skeletal	Chronic joint or bone pain or rigidity
Cardiovascular	Dyspnea, tachycardia, chest pain, hemoptysis (coughing up blood)
Genitourinary	Hematuria, menorrhagia, chronic or recurring infections

Emergency Medical Care

Emergency medical care for any patient with problems related to a blood disorder should include the following measures:

- **Oxygen.** The amount needed and how it is given (that is, via nasal cannula, nonrebreathing mask, or bag-mask ventilation) depend on the severity of the patient's condition and respiratory status.
- **Fluids.** Initiate intravenous (IV) fluid replacement as indicated for the specific disorder or chief complaint.
- **Electrocardiogram (ECG).** Monitor and treat symptomatic cardiac rhythm disturbances as needed.
- **Transport.** Transport the patient to the closest, most appropriate facility.
- **Comfort.** Place the patient in a position of comfort, and cover the patient to maintain his or her body temperature.

- **Pharmacology.** Pain management is often necessary, especially in a sickle cell crisis.
- **Psychological support.** Be supportive of and communicate therapeutically with the patient.

Pathophysiology, Assessment, and Management of Specific Emergencies

The aforementioned general steps in emergency medical care apply to all patients with an emergency related to a blood disorder. Depending on the specific blood disorder, you will also need to refine your assessment and management of the patient, as discussed in the next sections. While not the most common complaints encountered by prehospital care providers, hematologic disorders are serious and often life threatening.

▶ Sickle Cell Crisis

Pathophysiology

Sickle cell disease is—by far—the most common inherited blood disorder. Although it primarily affects African American, Puerto Rican, and European populations, it can occur in anyone. As of 2016, approximately 100,000 people in the United States had sickle cell disease.[1] Mortality at younger ages is common, with the average life expectancy being 42 years for men with sickle cell anemia and 48 years for females with this disorder.[2]

Sickle cell disease starts with a gene defect of the adult-type hemoglobin (HbA). This mutation can be inherited from both parents (HbSS) or from just one parent (HbS). When the gene is inherited from both parents, there is a high probability that their offspring will be prone to sickle cells (ie, the person actually has the disease) or the sickle cell trait (ie, the person is a carrier of the mutation).

The defective RBCs have an oblong shape instead of a smooth, round shape **Figure 24-5**. This shape makes the RBC a poor oxygen carrier, which means a patient with this disease is highly susceptible to hypoxia. Because sickle cells also have a much shorter life span than normal RBCs, the patient is more prone to developing **anemia**.

Sickle cell disease may lead to either an **aplastic crisis** or a **hemolytic crisis**. In an aplastic crisis, the body temporarily stops RBC production, causing the patient to become easily tired, anemic, pale, and short of breath. In contrast, a hemolytic crisis arises when acute RBC destruction leads to jaundice. In both cases, the patient may have rapidly evolving anemia, **leukocytosis**, and fever. The odd shape of the RBCs may also cause these cells to become lodged in small blood vessels, leading to thrombosis. A sickle cell crisis may manifest in several ways:

- **Vasoocclusive crisis** occurs when blood flow to an organ becomes restricted, causing pain, ischemia, and often organ damage. Most vasoocclusive crises last between 5 and 7 days. Frequently, circulation to the spleen becomes

YOU are the Paramedic PART 3

Your partner returns and tells you the family was unsure of what to do. A home health care agency that has been assisting with the patient's supportive care was contacted, and general comforting methods were described for the patient. The patient has a DNR (do not resuscitate) order, and documents show supportive measures should be undertaken as required. The family is concerned that the patient is not responding well to "supportive measures" and wants the patient transported to the Downtown Hospital oncology unit.

Recording Time: 5 Minutes	
Respirations	20 breaths/min
Pulse	100 beats/min
Skin	Cool, pale, and moist
Blood pressure	100/60 mm Hg
Oxygen saturation (Spo_2)	97% while breathing room air
Pupils	PERRLA

5. Are you concerned with the patient's vital signs at this point?
6. What are "supportive measures" for this patient?

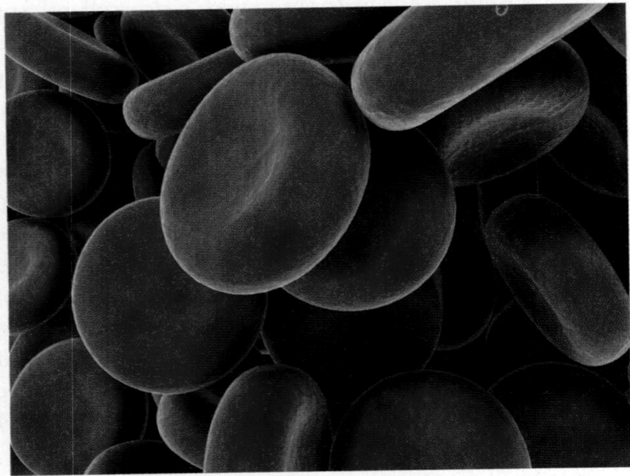

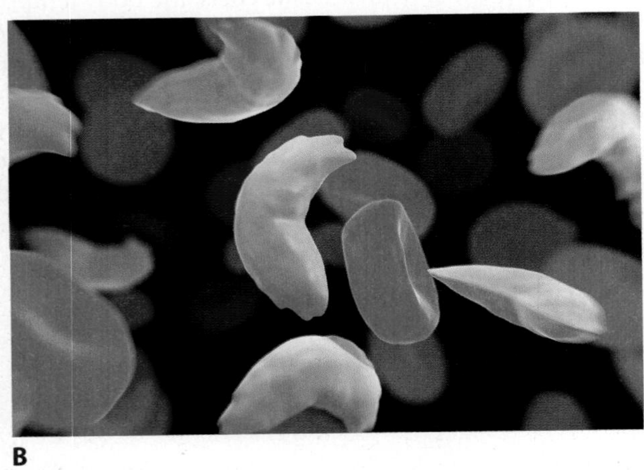

Figure 24-5 A. Normal red blood cells. **B.** Sickle cells.

obstructed as a result of this organ's narrow vessels and function of removing damaged RBCs. The spleen may swell to the point of rupture—an event that can lead to death.

- **Acute chest syndrome** is a vasoocclusive crisis that can be associated with pneumonia. Common signs and symptoms include chest pain, fever, and cough. Vasoocclusion in the brain may result in a cerebrovascular accident (stroke).
- **Splenic sequestration crisis** is caused by sickle cells within the spleen blocking blood from leaving the spleen, which results in painful, acute enlargement of the spleen and a hard and bloated abdomen. **Acute splenic sequestration syndrome** is a life-threatening complication in which RBCs become trapped in the spleen, causing a dramatic decline in the amount of hemoglobin available in the circulation. Patients present not only with a painful, acute abdomen, but also with sudden weakness, pallor, tachypnea, and tachycardia. Acute splenic sequestration syndrome usually occurs in infants or toddlers.

Assessment

Do not take a call for a person having a sickle cell crisis lightly. These patients are often in life-threatening crises, characterized by shortness of breath and signs of pneumonia. Their skin will show signs of inadequate perfusion, accompanied by hypotension. They may display signs of jaundice and yellowing in the eye (icteric sclera). Signs of mild dehydration and many other complaints are often present as well.

In acute crises, patients may have significant pain resulting from congested blood vessels that do not allow the passage of oxygen and nutrients into their tissues and joints. Patients may report multiple system involvement, including chest, abdominal, and arthritic-type pain, although some may report only fatigue or achiness along with fever. Pediatric patients will typically present with initial pain in the hands and feet, whereas adult patients will report back and proximal extremity pain.

Words of Wisdom

Sickle cell disease may mimic appendicitis or opiate withdrawal.

Management

Administer high levels of oxygen to prevent further destruction of the RBCs due to hypoxia, and rapidly transport the patient to an appropriate facility. You may also need to give IV fluid therapy to counter the patient's dehydration and flush damaged RBCs from the organs and peripheral tissues. It is important to maintain the patient's body temperature; cold can contribute to sickling of the cells, whereas warm compresses may reduce further sickling. Patients may have lived with the disease for a long time and, therefore, may have a very high pain threshold. As a consequence, they often require a higher level of analgesia due to a developed tolerance. Recommend that the patient rest as much as possible during transport.

Supplemental oxygen should be administered via nonrebreathing mask in an attempt to hypersaturate the remaining hemoglobin and increase the level of perfusion that has been decreased by the sickled cells or hemophilia. Ventilation should be provided if the patient's respirations are insufficient.

Place the patient in a position of comfort and cover to maintain body temperature. Administer IV fluid for hydration and nitrous oxide for pain as allowed by local protocol. Once the patient has arrived at the hospital, care for sickle cell disease may include analgesics for pain, penicillin to prevent infection, and, depending on the severity of the crisis, a blood transfusion.

Distinguishing a true sickle cell crisis from other nonspecific causes of pain can be difficult. In these situations, perform a thorough assessment and seek medical direction to help sort out the patient's signs and symptoms, to help problem-solve the situation, and to provide guidance on how to manage the patient.

▶ Anemia

Pathophysiology

Anemia is defined as a hemoglobin or RBC level that is lower than normal. Usually this condition is associated with some type of underlying disease process. Anemia may also result from acute or chronic blood loss, or from a decrease in production or an increase in destruction of erythrocytes. Anemia may be an outcome of a preexisting hemolytic disorder (a disorder related to the breakdown of RBCs).

Iron-deficiency anemia is the most common type of anemia. Typical causes include gastrointestinal blood loss, menstrual bleeding (the most common cause in US women, affecting primarily African American women), and blood loss due to frequent donations or diagnostic tests for patients hospitalized for long periods. In children, it is most often related to premature birth or low birth weight.

Anemia may sometimes be caused by an inherited hemolytic disorder, such as sickle cell disease or **thalassemia**. In these disorders, when the RBCs are first developing their membranes, they become rigid and deformed. The RBCs may then become lodged in small blood vessels, leading to a thrombosis (blood clot).

Anemia may also be caused by hematologic disorders resulting from a deficiency of an enzyme known as glucose-6-phosphate dehydrogenase. This enzyme helps protect RBCs during infections. When levels of this enzyme are low, cells can become damaged. Although glucose-6-phosphate dehydrogenase deficiency is most commonly seen in African Americans, it can occur in people of any race.

The most common type of acquired anemia develops when the flow of RBCs is disrupted owing to problems with blood vessel linings (such as aneurysms and weaknesses) or blood clots. In autoimmune disorders, RBCs are destroyed by the body's own antibodies, which erroneously perceive the normal blood cells as foreign invaders. RBCs can also be destroyed by microorganisms in the blood.

Anemia can also have serious consequences for people who travel to high-altitude areas. The combination of a smaller number of RBCs and the reduced partial pressure of oxygen in the atmosphere can lead to serious conditions that a healthy person would not experience, such as hypoxia, difficulty breathing, and chest pain.

Assessment

Your basic assessment should be the same for all patients, although you may want to ask some specific questions when anemia is suspected. Most commonly, patients with anemia will complain of feeling worn down, having no energy, or feeling as if they have overexerted themselves. Patients may also report that they "can't catch their breath." Owing to the reduction in their hemoglobin level, some may have anginal-type chest pain related to decreased oxygen availability to the heart muscle. The reduction in functional RBCs can also result in pale skin signs. Subtle variations may be seen by assessing the conjunctiva of the eyes, the inside of the lips, and the creases of the palms of the hand. These areas can be instrumental in identifying pallor, especially in patients with darker skin. Other conditions that are common in patients with anemia include **leukopenia** (reduction in WBCs) and **thrombocytopenia** (reduction in platelets); both conditions can induce more frequent infections, fevers, cutaneous bleeding, and nosebleeds.

Words of Wisdom

When abnormalities of the blood cells are suspected, note the following:

- Anemia commonly results in complaints of fatigue, lethargy, and dyspnea.
- Low WBC counts (leukopenia) often lead to infection and fever.
- Low platelet counts (thrombocytopenia) often cause cutaneous bleeding (including petechiae) and bleeding from mucous membranes (such as nosebleeds and rectal bleeding).

Management

In cases of anemia, check and monitor the airway and the patient's breathing closely, administering high-flow oxygen when necessary. The patient's oxygen-carrying capacity is limited, so you want to make sure that the RBCs that are present are being maximized. Check vital signs frequently. In cases of chest pain, apply a cardiac monitor and closely watch the rhythm. A 12-lead ECG may also be warranted to confirm that the chest pain is not related to an acute coronary syndrome. Blood pressure management may be needed as well, along with fluid replacement therapy. Monitor patients closely during fluid replacement—IV fluids do not contain RBCs or blood components, so they may induce unwanted or unexpected bleeding. Do not be surprised if you have to control significant nosebleeds in any patient with anemia.

Allow the patient to assume a position of comfort, and transport him or her to the closest, most appropriate facility. In most cases, a gentle, easy transport is appropriate. However, if the patient experiences an abrupt change in the level of consciousness, hypotension develops, or other significant perfusion inadequacies arise, consider rapid transport.

Leukemia

Pathophysiology

Leukemia is a disease that develops in the **lymphoid system**. In this type of cancer, blood cells—particularly WBCs—develop abnormally and/or excessively. Leukemia can cause anemia, thrombocytopenia (decrease in platelets), and leukocytosis (increased WBCs). The chemotherapy used to treat leukemia typically leads to leukopenia (decreased WBCs). Patients with leukemia experience frequent bleeding, bruising, infections, and fever **Figure 24-6**.

Leukemia can be classified as acute or chronic. In most situations, but especially in chronic cases, the disease tends to develop more frequently in older adults (65 years or older). In acute leukemia, bone marrow is replaced with abnormal **lymphoblasts**. In chronic leukemia, abnormal mature lymphoid cells accumulate in the bone marrow, lymph nodes, spleen, and peripheral blood. This form of leukemia is typically found by chance during routine blood tests; suspicions are raised when the tests reveal a high lymphocyte count.

Survival of a person with leukemia depends on factors such as the stage at which the disease is detected, the patient's underlying medical condition, and the response to treatment. Acute and chronic leukemia are treated with chemotherapy and radiation therapy. In most cases, treatment results in remission, especially when the condition was identified early. According to the National Cancer Institute, children with acute lymphocytic leukemia have a 5-year survival rate of more than 85%.[3]

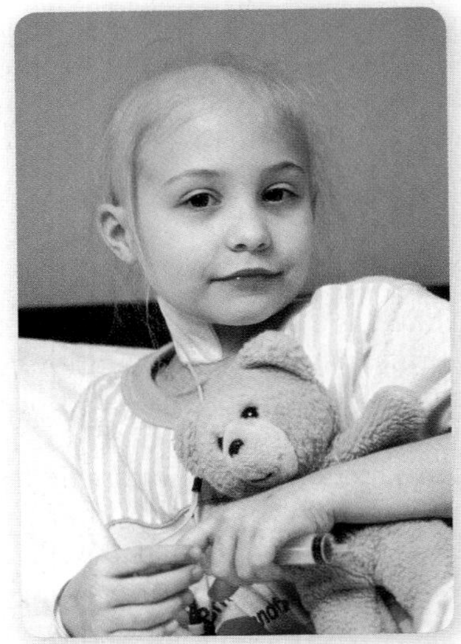

Figure 24-6 People with leukemia may have frequent bleeding, bruising, infections, and fever.

Assessment

Assessment starts with appropriate standard precautions, including gloves and a mask. The patient with leukemia may be immunocompromised, so that even your small cold could be enough to lead to a fatal outcome.

How patients with leukemia present depends on the stage of the leukemia and the patient's current treatment. Patients typically complain of fatigue, headaches,

YOU are the Paramedic PART 4

Your partner administers oxygen to the patient at 4 L/min via nasal cannula and looks for a location to insert an IV line. The patient is agreeable to being transported to the hospital for evaluation. The patient is still feeling considerable pain throughout his body. You lift the patient to the stretcher and move the patient to the ambulance for transport.

Recording Time: 10 Minutes	
Respirations	20 breaths/min
Pulse	100 beats/min
Skin	Cool, pale, and moist
Blood pressure	98/60 mm Hg
Oxygen saturation (Spo_2)	97% on room air
Pupils	PERRLA

7. Do you think the patient's family has called you unnecessarily?
8. Would you classify this patient as having acute or chronic leukemia?
9. If this patient were 7 years old instead of 73, what would be different about the course of the disease process?

or dyspnea and may have signs of neurologic defects. During the physical exam, fever, bone pain, and diaphoresis may be found. Patients may report feeling full, soreness in the midpart of the chest, and unexplained bleeding. You should monitor all basic vital signs (blood pressure, pulse, respirations, temperature, and pulse oximetry) and the cardiac rhythm. Hypotension and tachycardia are often present; therefore, vital signs may be consistent with signs of shock.

Management

Management of leukemia includes providing airway support and oxygen therapy as appropriate. IV fluid therapy and analgesics for comfort may be needed as well. Patients typically need constant positive support because many have a negative outlook on their condition. The patient's loved ones may be quite concerned, especially during advanced stages of the disease; be supportive of them as well. In some cases, you may be called because the patient's condition has deteriorated and the family is uncertain about what to do. In such a scenario, your assessment may indicate normal findings for the patient. The patient or family may change their minds about transport, or they may not have wanted transport at all, but rather professional insight and support. Discuss this situation with medical control, document all findings before leaving, and get a refusal and/or release form signed if the patient or family member decides against transport.

Few calls for patients with leukemia require extreme measures or rapid transport; however, you should be alert to rapid changes in the patient's condition. If you transport the patient, then be aware that he or she could go into arrest. Make sure you find out the patient's and family's wishes about what to do in this situation.

▶ Lymphomas

Pathophysiology

Lymphomas are a group of malignant diseases that arise within the lymphoid system. They are classified into two categories: non-Hodgkin lymphoma (which accounts for the majority of cases) and Hodgkin lymphoma.

Non-Hodgkin lymphoma can occur at any age in any person and can be hereditary. Furthermore, these types of cancer may be characterized based on the progression of the disease: indolent, aggressive, or highly aggressive. With very slow (indolent) progression, the disease may never leave the lymphoid system. In the highly aggressive form, the disease may affect multiple organs in a relatively short period, usually within several months. How well the disease responds to treatment depends on the specific type of non-Hodgkin lymphoma and how early it is recognized and classified.

Hodgkin lymphoma is a painless, progressive enlargement of the lymphoid glands, most commonly affecting the spleen and the lymph nodes. A highly rare form of lymphoma, it is suspected to have some hereditary components. The incidence of Hodgkin lymphoma has two peaks: a first peak between 10 and 35 years of age and a second peak in late life.[4] Patients may not show any symptoms for many years, with the disease being found only after patients complain of night sweats, chills, persistent cough, and swelling of various lymph nodes (usually in the neck first). They may also note loss of appetite for an unknown reason, significant weight loss, generalized itching, fatigue, and bone pain. According to the American Cancer Society, with treatment, symptoms may disappear for long periods; 65% to 90% of patients may actually be cured, increasing the 5-year survival rate.[5]

Assessment

Generally speaking, lymphomas require specialized levels of treatment involving some form of chemotherapy or radiation therapy. How well the disease responds to these treatments depends on the stage of the disease and its classification. As a rule, lymphomas respond well to chemotherapy; in fact, aggressive lymphomas respond better than indolent ones. Even if an indolent lymphoma is not cured with chemotherapy, many patients may survive as long as 10 years.

When you are assessing patients with lymphoma, ask specific questions such as "Which type of lymphoma (cancer) do you have?" and "Which type of treatment are you receiving?" As you perform your assessment, you will usually note pallor. The patient's airway will usually be patent and the breathing adequate, although sometimes you may note some congestion in the lower lung fields. The patient may describe being first hot and then cold, or even both hot and cold in different areas of the body. Signs of inadequate perfusion are common, including low blood pressure accompanied by an elevated pulse rate. Abnormal ECG rhythms may also be evident.

Management

Patients with lymphoma may be in constant, extreme pain; therefore, if pain management is needed and available, it may have to be aggressive because the patient will likely already be receiving a high-dose analgesic regimen. Treat inadequate perfusion with fluid therapy, and provide supplemental oxygen **Figure 24-7**. If necessary, then treat abnormal heart rhythms. If the patient's condition does not improve or even deteriorates following these measures, then initiate rapid transport to the closest facility. As in cases involving patients with leukemia, you may be called to offer support but no transport. Be supportive, discuss your findings with medical control, explain the options to the patient and family, and allow them to make a decision.

▶ Polycythemia

Pathophysiology

Polycythemia is characterized by an overabundance or overproduction of RBCs, resulting in increased blood viscosity and volume. This hyperviscosity and hypervolemia can

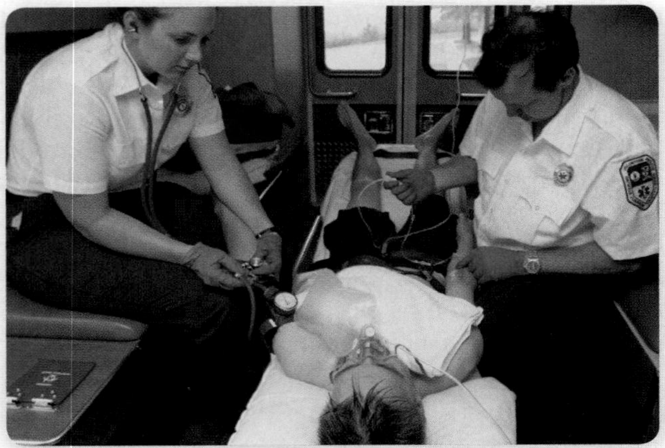

Figure 24-7 Patients with lymphoma who are in extreme pain should receive fluid therapy, oxygen, and analgesics.

result in congestion of tissues and organs. Hyperviscosity of the blood increases the risk of thrombus formation. The increased RBC production can be caused by a rare disorder originating in a single stem cell or by an existing disease, such as heart failure or hypertension. Polycythemia can also arise in people who live in high-altitude areas for long periods.

The overabundance of the blood components associated with polycythemia may lead to many other conditions, such as strokes, transient ischemic attacks, deep vein thrombosis, pulmonary embolism, myocardial infarction, headaches, and abdominal pain (usually associated with an enlarged spleen). Many times this disease is found incidentally when blood cell counts are performed after a patient reports frequent episodes of signs and symptoms associated with hematologic diseases.

Clinical treatment usually includes phlebotomy to try to maintain hematocrit levels at less than 45% in men and less than 42% in women. Other treatments have included cancer-type therapy intended to slow the production of new RBCs within the bone marrow.

Assessment

Owing to the nature of polycythemia and its plethora of symptoms, assessment findings may vary widely in patients with this disease. Altered level of consciousness may be evident due to stroke or transient ischemic attack–like events; hypoxia may occur due to poor circulation. Respiratory distress can occur, as can changes in peripheral pulses, pulse rate, and skin color. Tachycardia is the most common change in heart rhythm. Patients with polycythemia also tend to have purplish skin with red hands and feet.

As you assess the patient, note the extent and duration of dyspnea. Has the patient experienced uncontrolled itching (pruritus) or noted changes in skin temperature? Make sure to obtain a thorough medical history in cases of known or suspected polycythemia. In fact, it may be your assessment, treatment, and transport that helps lead to the correct diagnosis: Some patients may have called for the previously mentioned complaints and have yet to receive a diagnosis of polycythemia.

Management

Prehospital treatment should initially focus on the chief complaint. Although the underlying pathology may be polycythemia, the patient may now be experiencing a different medical emergency, such as a stroke or cardiac event. Otherwise, treatment largely consists of supportive care and transporting the patient to an appropriate facility. Administer oxygen as needed. Establish IV access for possible pharmacologic interventions for pain as appropriate. Be supportive of the patient and family.

▶ Disseminated Intravascular Coagulation

Pathophysiology

Disseminated intravascular coagulation (DIC) may result from any number of life-threatening conditions, including massive injury and hypotension due to trauma. Sepsis and obstetric complications also may cause DIC.

This condition progresses in two stages. First, free thrombin and fibrin deposits in the blood increase, and platelets begin to aggregate. In this stage, defibrination, or a breakdown of the fibrin clots, occurs owing to excessive bleeding, massive blood loss, or tissue injury. Second, uncontrolled hemorrhage results from the severe reduction in clotting factors.

The mortality rate for patients with DIC is quite high, especially in acute cases; some studies have shown it to be 60% to 65%.[6] The primary causes of death relate to uncontrolled bleeding, hypotension, and shock.

> **Words of Wisdom**
>
> Patients with DIC experience the failure of multiple organs (such as kidneys, lungs, and heart) at once, accompanied by bleeding from IV sites, bleeding into joints, and, possibly, intracranial hemorrhage.

Assessment

As you assess and care for critically injured or ill patients, keep in mind the issues that may lead to DIC. Your goal is to identify signs and symptoms commonly associated with DIC or progression toward this coagulopathy. In cases involving severe trauma, patients may have episodes of respiratory difficulty, signs of shock, and skin changes ranging from cold and clammy to pallor to small black-and-blue marks (purpura) on the chest and abdomen.

Management

It is important to identify the underlying cause of the patient's presenting condition and establish treatment early, while not delaying transport to an appropriate facility. Maintain the patient's airway, administer supplemental oxygen, and treat the patient for shock (keep the patient warm, control bleeding, administer IV fluids for hypotension) per local protocol. Pharmacologic interventions may entail pain management and treatment for abnormal heart rhythms, although treatment for altered heart rhythms should come last. Patients who have DIC due to severe trauma have a poor survival rate; they and their family members need strong support. Be optimistic but honest with patients and family, and do not give false hope regarding survival.

Hemophilia

Pathophysiology

Hemophilia is a bleeding disorder in which clotting does not occur or occurs insufficiently (as in von Willebrand disease). It is usually associated with an X-linked recessive inheritance pattern, albeit one that is poorly understood. This disease is classified into two primary types: type A, which is due to low levels of factor VIII (antihemophilic globulin and antihemophilic factor), and type B, which is associated with a deficiency of factor IX (plasma thromboplastin component, also known as the Christmas factor). Hemophilia primarily affects males. The levels of factors VIII and IX determine the severity of the disease.

Both type A and type B hemophilia have the same signs and symptoms. Acute and chronic bleeding can occur at any time and may or may not be life threatening. Any injury or illness that can cause bleeding should not be taken lightly in a person with hemophilia. Spontaneous intracranial bleeding is common in patients with hemophilia and is a major cause of death. Patients with significant acute bleeding episodes require hospitalization for transfusion and often require infusion of factors VIII and IX.

Assessment

When you are obtaining the patient's history, you may learn that the patient has a history of conditions associated with hemophilia. In addition to managing the ABCs, be alert for signs of acute blood loss (pallor, weak pulse, and hypotension). Note any bleeding of unknown origin, such as nosebleeds, bloody sputum, and blood in the urine or stool (melena). Owing to blood loss, patients may exhibit signs of hypoxia due to the reduction in oxygen-carrying capacity.

Management

Any patient who complains of respiratory problems should receive high-flow oxygen. Note the ECG findings, and treat symptomatic dysrhythmias as appropriate. Prehospital care for a patient with hemophilia may include IV therapy to treat hypotension. Understand, however, that these patients actually need a transfusion of blood or plasma, which will occur at the hospital. Some patients will have significant pain, so analgesics may be appropriate. Cover patients to maintain their body temperatures. Although you may be called to treat someone with bleeding of unknown cause, only to find that the bleeding stopped before you arrived on scene, you should suggest that the patient get immediate hospital or physician follow-up.

Multiple Myeloma

Pathophysiology

In **multiple myeloma**, the number of plasma cells (B cells that form antibodies) in the bone marrow increases abnormally, leading to the formation of tumors in the bone. These tumors impair the ability of the bone marrow to function normally, which in turn decreases RBC, WBC, and platelet formation. Anemia and susceptibility to infection result. Neoplastic (cancerous) cells may also accelerate protein development in the bloodstream, leading to organ failure (primarily the kidneys) and eventually death. Multiple myeloma rarely occurs early in life—most patients are older than 40 years. Men have this disease more frequently than do women.

As the disease progresses further and tumors grow or become more numerous, patients may have weakness in the bones, resulting in spontaneous fractures. Pain in the bones and back is also common. In advanced cases of myeloma, chemotherapy and other anticancer-type treatment may be given but may not cure the disease. Morbidity and mortality primarily depend on the extent of the disease and any underlying medical conditions.

Assessment

Because of their susceptibility to infection, you need to be vigilant about adhering to the appropriate standard precautions, including wearing a mask and gloves, to help keep patients with multiple myeloma safe. Findings during your assessment and management of patients with multiple myeloma will depend on the stage of the disease. Early-stage complaints may be as simple as fatigue or mild pain. Later-stage disease may be evidenced by unexplained hemorrhage and significant weight loss, frequent bone fractures, and pain in any number of locations.

Management

Management of patients with multiple myeloma is similar to that for patients with other blood disorders: IV fluid therapy, pain management, and supportive care. Do not assume that the patient is ready to or going to die; he or she may be having a complication of the myeloma. Definitive care at an appropriate facility may improve the patient's condition.

Transfusion Reactions

Pathophysiology

Emergency care may be required in response to a patient's reaction to a blood transfusion. **Transfusion reactions** occur in approximately 0.2% to 10% of blood transfusions.[7]

Transfusion reactions are similar to an anaphylactic reaction—they occur rapidly and can cause severe circulatory collapse and even death. When a patient receives a blood transfusion, it is important to monitor the individual very closely for the first 30 to 60 minutes because transfusion reactions typically begin within this time frame.

It is important to determine the patient's blood type and the type of blood received. When a patient receives blood or plasma that matches his or her blood type (eg, A+ given to an A+ patient) or the universal donor blood type (O), problems rarely arise. However, if a patient receives a blood type that is different from his or her own—for example, if a patient with type A receives type B blood—a transfusion reaction will occur. Also, if a patient with A− blood receives an A+ transfusion, a transfusion reaction could occur. Such reactions are rare, however, because the response to the Rh factor (indicated by the "+" or "−" after the blood type) is not as prevalent and the reaction is not as significant. Table 24-4 summarizes the ABO and Rh compatibility rules.

Assessment

Signs and symptoms of transfusion reactions are generally easy to spot in a responsive patient, but they may be more subtle in an unresponsive or intubated patient. In an acute reaction, the patient experiences a rapid onset of chills, fever, back pain, vomiting, tachycardia, and hypotension. Transfusion reactions may also be delayed up to 7 days after the transfusion, although these events tend to be less severe than the typical acute reaction.

Table 24-4 ABO Rh Type and Preferred and Alternative Donor Types

Recipient Blood Type	Preferred Donor Type	Additional Permissible Types
A+	A+	A−, O+, O−
A−	A−	O−
AB+	AB+	AB−, A+, A−, B+, B−, O+, O−
AB−	AB−	A−, B−, O−
B+	B+	B−, O+, O−
B−	B−	O−
O+	O+	O−
O−	O−	None

Data from: Applegate EJ. *The Anatomy and Physiology Learning System.* 4th ed. Philadelphia, PA: Saunders; 2011.

Complications generally fall into the following categories:

- **Hemolytic reaction.** An acute hemolytic reaction is the greatest threat to the patient during blood transfusion. The primary cause is incompatibility between the recipient and the donor blood. The recipient's immune system is activated by the donor blood, with the new RBCs being destroyed as a result of this reaction. Not only does this outcome return the patient to the state in which he or she needed the transfusion, but the patient's body has the added burden of managing and clearing all of the destroyed RBCs. Careful screening of the patient and the blood product can typically prevent a hemolytic reaction from occurring.
- **Febrile reaction.** A simple febrile reaction is the most common transfusion complication. It is usually benign, and is treated with an antipyretic and observation.
- **Allergic reaction.** In addition to the transfusion reaction, a patient may experience an anaphylactic reaction to preservatives or other agents in the product being transfused. This allergic reaction typically begins within the first few minutes of transfusion and is accompanied by classic signs and symptoms of an anaphylactic state, adding to the already compromised state of the patient.
- **Transfusion-related lung injury.** Transfusion-related lung injury is a noncardiogenic pulmonary edema caused by increased capillary permeability post transfusion. Treatment of this condition focuses on supporting the ABCs. Because this type of lung injury is not a cardiac failure or fluid overload issue, diuretics are generally not effective.
- **Circulatory overload.** The rapid infusion of blood products can lead to circulatory overload, mimicking congestive heart failure. This type of reaction typically occurs in patient populations with preexisting cardiomyopathy or ventricular dysfunction. Treatment consists of relieving the system of its excess fluids through diuresis, and with the use of oxygen, nitrates, and morphine.
- **Bacterial infection.** Bacterial infection is typically a result of poor blood product handling, or contamination during the infusion process. It occurs most commonly with platelet transfusions, because platelets are kept at room temperature. This kind of infection can lead to full systemic sepsis, requiring antibiotic administration and supportive care.

Management

In general, the severity of the transfusion reaction is directly correlated to the amount of blood volume transfused. There is no specific antidote or remedy for a transfusion reaction; instead, care centers on immediately stopping the transfusion, providing hemodynamic supportive care to counteract shock, and maximizing kidney perfusion.

In a patient in hemodynamically unstable condition, early invasive monitoring, vasopressors, and the promotion of diuresis with isotonic fluids and a loop diuretic (furosemide) are indicated. Dopamine in a renal dose regimen (2 to 4 mcg/kg/min) may be helpful. Other treatments, such as steroids, mannitol, or heparin, are controversial due to the inconclusive results of studies investigating their use.

High-flow oxygen should be administered, and administration of epinephrine and diphenhydramine should be considered to counteract the reactive process. Epinephrine and diphenhydramine are essential components of any anaphylactic treatment regimen, and should be administered according to local protocol.

YOU are the Paramedic SUMMARY

1. Why is a fever in this patient significant?

With the development of abnormally functioning WBCs, the body is more susceptible to infections. This patient's fever indicates that in addition to leukemia, he now has an infection of some sort. The excessive production of the abnormal WBCs can also interfere with the production of the other blood cells, resulting in additional hematologic complications.

2. What do you need to know about this patient's status?

The family and patient should be prepared to provide you with written documentation concerning the patient's status. This documentation should include information such as the patient's "code" status and what care should be provided to the patient. Many states have standard forms that are designed for use by medical care providers. Make sure you know the legal requirements for documentation of patients receiving home care in your area.

3. Which signs or symptoms is the patient showing that could indicate thrombocytopenia?

The clearest sign is the presence of the bloody tissues. Under normal conditions, blowing the nose does not cause bleeding. If bleeding starts, then the formation of a platelet plug early in the cascade triggers a number of other biochemical reactions. However, in this patient, the decreased number of circulating platelets results in not only less clotting, but also reduced signaling in the rest of the cascade to follow.

4. How will a patient with leukemia typically present?

Patients with leukemia experience frequent bleeding, bruising, infections, and fever.

5. Are you concerned with the patient's vital signs at this point?

Although the vital signs obtained in this case would commonly indicate shock or impending shock, they may be "normal" for this patient. Anemia can lead to an increased pulse rate and respirations as the body tries to compensate for the inadequate number of RBCs, which carry the hemoglobin, the oxygen-carrying component of blood. It is essential to carefully observe the patient's vital signs throughout your care and to contact medical control for advice about analgesic doses. Nevertheless, unless there is a substantial or sudden change in the patient's condition, symptomatic treatment—such as oxygen, IV fluids, and analgesics—is sufficient.

6. What are "supportive measures" for this patient?

Management of this patient includes providing airway support and oxygen therapy as appropriate. IV fluid therapy and analgesics for comfort may be needed as well. Also, provide positive support; the patient may feel discouraged about his condition. Be honest and do not give false hope.

7. Do you think the patient's family has called you unnecessarily?

You should not think the call for service was unwarranted. The patient's loved ones are concerned, especially because the patient is in the advanced stages of the disease; be supportive of the family members as well as the patient. In some cases, you may be called because the patient's condition has deteriorated and the family is uncertain about what to do.

YOU are the Paramedic SUMMARY (continued)

8. Would you classify this patient as having acute or chronic leukemia?

Based on the age of the patient and the family's comment that he was "diagnosed years ago," this case appears to involve chronic leukemia.

9. If this patient were 7 years old instead of 73, what would be different about the course of the disease process?

A 7-year-old would typically be experiencing acute leukemia, whereas this patient likely has chronic leukemia. Although the symptoms are the same, acute leukemia can result in remission and even a cure if treatment is initiated early; by comparison, the cure rate for chronic leukemia is lower.

EMS Patient Care Report (PCR)					
Date: 11-06-18	**Incident No.:** 9875		**Nature of Call:** General medical	**Location:** 11384 Castle Rock Road	
Dispatched: 1840	**En Route:** 1841	**At Scene:** 1845	**Transport:** 1908	**At Hospital:** 1918	**In Service:** 1940
Patient Information					
Age: 73 **Sex:** M **Weight (in kg [lb]):** 59 kg (130 lb)			**Allergies:** No known drug allergies **Medications:** Numerous, see list **Past Medical History:** Leukemia **Chief Complaint:** Fever/body pain		
Vital Signs					
Time: 1850	**BP:** 100/60	**Pulse:** 100	**Respirations:** 20	**Spo_2:** 97%, room air	
Time: 1855	**BP:** 98/60	**Pulse:** 100	**Respirations:** 20	**Spo_2:** 97%, room air	
Time:	**BP:**	**Pulse:**	**Respirations:**	**Spo_2:**	
EMS Treatment (circle all that apply)					
Oxygen @ ______ L/min via (circle one): **NC NRM Bag-mask device**		**Assisted Ventilation**	**Airway Adjunct**	**CPR**	
Defibrillation	**Bleeding Control**	**Bandaging**	**Splinting**	**Other:**	
Narrative					
This unit dispatched to this address for a 73-year-old man with a history of leukemia. Pt is experiencing general body pain and a temperature of 102°F. Pt is receiving chemotherapy and had last treatment on 11-02-18. Pt is under home health agency care and has advance directive for supportive care only. Family presented appropriate written documentation verifying same. Family contacted home health agency and received instructions to reduce fever and manage pt's pain. Family stated they became concerned when these measures were not effective and called 9-1-1 for response. Pt is responsive, alert, oriented, and cooperative. IV established TKO. Pt agreed to transport to Downtown Hospital. Medical control contacted concerning administration of analgesic for pain, B/P is low. Medical control advised to administer 1 mg of morphine sulfate IV titrated to effect. Pain decreased, and pt rested comfortably during transport. Report to charge nurse on arrival.**End of report**					

Prep Kit

▶ Ready for Review

- Most EMS systems rarely respond to hematologic emergencies.
- Blood performs respiratory, nutritional, excretory, regulatory, and defensive functions.
- Blood is made up of plasma and formed elements, or cells, including red blood cells, white blood cells, and platelets.
- Laboratory tests commonly performed on blood include red blood cell counts, hemoglobin levels, and hematocrit measurements.
- During the primary survey of a patient with a hematologic disorder, it is important to note any signs and symptoms that may be immediately life threatening.
- While taking a history and during the secondary assessment, look for changes in the level of consciousness such as vertigo, feelings of fatigue, or syncopal episodes.
- General management for any patient with problems related to a blood disorder should include the following elements: oxygen, fluids, ECG, transport, medications, and psychological support.
- Hematologic disorders include sickle cell crisis, anemia, leukopenia, thrombocytopenia, leukemia, lymphomas, polycythemia, disseminated intravascular coagulation, hemophilia, multiple myeloma, and complications of blood transfusions.
- A patient experiencing a sickle cell crisis will experience significant pain due to congested vessels and may have a serious infection that can lead to sepsis and death.
- A patient with anemia has a hemoglobin or red blood cell level that is lower than normal. Anemia may be caused by an underlying hematologic or hemolytic disorder.
- Leukopenia is a reduction in the number of white blood cells; thrombocytopenia is a reduction in the number of platelets. Both of these conditions are often seen in patients with anemia or leukemia.
- Leukemia is a type of cancer that affects the production of white blood cells. Patients often experience bleeding, bruising, infections, and fever.
- Lymphomas are a group of malignant disorders that arise within the lymphoid system. The two types distinguished are non-Hodgkin (making up the majority of cases) and Hodgkin lymphoma.
- Polycythemia is characterized by an overabundance or overproduction of red blood cells, which leads to hyperviscosity of the circulatory system.
- Disseminated intravascular coagulation may result from a massive injury, sepsis, or obstetric complications. In the first stage, too much blood clotting results from an overactivated coagulation system. In the second stage, the body's natural reaction to break up these clots causes uncontrolled hemorrhage.
- Hemophilia is a bleeding disorder found primarily in males, in which clotting does not occur or occurs insufficiently. Type A hemophilia is due to a low level of factor VIII; type B hemophilia is due to a deficiency in factor IX.
- Multiple myeloma is a cancer of the bone marrow caused by malignant plasma cells.
- Complications of blood transfusions are similar to anaphylactic reactions; they are caused by a mismatch of the patient's blood type to that received or an allergic reaction to preservatives or agents in the transfused product.

▶ Vital Vocabulary

acute chest syndrome A vasoocclusive crisis that can be associated with pneumonia; common signs and symptoms include chest pain, fever, and cough; associated with sickle cell disease.

acute splenic sequestration syndrome A condition in which red blood cells become trapped in the spleen, causing a dramatic fall in hemoglobin available in the circulation; it usually occurs in infants or toddlers.

anemia A lower than normal hemoglobin or erythrocyte level.

aplastic crisis A temporary halt in the production of red blood cells; it may occur as a result of sickle cell disease.

clotting cascade The process by which clotting factors work together to ultimately form fibrin.

clotting factors Substances in the blood that are necessary for clotting; also called coagulation factors.

coagulopathy Any type of bleeding disorder that interferes with the activation or continuation of the clotting cascade or hemostasis.

disseminated intravascular coagulation (DIC) A condition that begins with widespread activation of the clotting cascade, which depletes the clotting factors and platelets, and eventually results in uncontrolled hemorrhage.

erythrocytes Red blood cells.

hematocrit The proportion of red blood cells in the total blood volume.

hematologic disorder Any disorder of the blood.

Prep Kit (continued)

hematology The study of the physiology of blood.

hematopoietic system The system that includes all blood components and the organs involved in their development and production.

hemoglobin The iron-rich protein in the blood that carries oxygen.

hemolytic crisis A condition in which red blood cells break down quickly; it may occur as a result of sickle cell disease.

hemolytic disorder A disorder relating to the breakdown of red blood cells.

hemophilia A bleeding disorder that is primarily hereditary, in which clotting does not occur or occurs insufficiently.

hemostasis The body's natural blood-clotting mechanism.

hemostatic disorder A bleeding and clotting abnormality.

iron-deficiency anemia The most common type of anemia, in which iron stores are low or lacking and the serum iron concentration is low.

leukemia A cancer or malignancy of the blood-forming organs that particularly affects the white blood cells, which develop abnormally and/or excessively at the expense of normal blood cells.

leukocytes White blood cells.

leukocytosis An increase in the total number of white blood cells.

leukopenia A reduction in the number of white blood cells.

lymphoblasts Lymphocytes that have been transformed because of stimulation by an antigen.

lymphoid system The system primarily made up of the bone marrow, lymph nodes, and spleen, which participates in formation of lymphocytes and immune responses.

lymphomas Malignant diseases that arise within the lymphoid system; they include non-Hodgkin and Hodgkin lymphomas.

multiple myeloma A disease in which the number of plasma cells in the bone marrow increases abnormally, causing tumors to form in the bones.

neutropenia An abnormally low number of neutrophils.

plasma A component of blood, made of 92% water, 6% to 7% proteins, and electrolytes, clotting factors, and glucose; plasma accounts for 55% of the total blood volume.

polycythemia An overabundance or overproduction of red blood cells, white blood cells, and platelets.

reticuloendothelial system The system in the body that is primarily used to defend against infection.

sickle cell crisis A condition in which a patient with sickle cell disease experiences significant pain due to insufficient passage of oxygen and nutrients into tissues and joints because of vessel congestion.

sickle cell disease A disease that causes the red blood cells to be misshapen, resulting in poor oxygen-carrying capability and potentially resulting in lodging of the red blood cells in blood vessels or the spleen.

splenic sequestration crisis An acute, painful enlargement of the spleen caused by sickle cell disease.

stem cells Cells that can develop into other types of cells in the body.

thalassemia A type of anemia in which either not enough hemoglobin is produced or the hemoglobin is defective.

thrombocytes Platelets.

thrombocytopenia A reduction in the number of platelets.

thrombocytosis A condition in which the body produces too many platelets.

thrombosis Coagulation or clotting of blood in a blood vessel.

transfusion reaction A physiologic response that is similar to an anaphylactic reaction, in which the body reacts to the infusion of blood; it occurs rapidly and can cause severe circulatory collapse and death.

transfusion-related lung injury A transfusion reaction characterized by increased pulmonary capillary permeability, resulting in noncardiogenic pulmonary edema.

vasoocclusive crisis Ischemia and pain caused by sickle-shaped red blood cells that obstruct blood flow to a portion of the body.

von Willebrand disease A bleeding disorder in which the patient is missing the von Willebrand factor (a protein essential for platelet adhesion), preventing the blood from clotting well.

▶ References

1. Sickle cell disease (SCD). Centers for Disease Control and Prevention website. https://www.cdc.gov/ncbddd/sicklecell/data.html. Updated August 31, 2016. Accessed March 13, 2017.
2. Platt OS, Brambilla DJ, Rosse WF, et al. Mortality in sickle cell disease: life expectancy and risk factors for early death. *N Engl J Med.* 1994;330:1639-1644.

Prep Kit *(continued)*

http://www.nejm.org/doi/full/10.1056/NEJM199406093302303#t=article. Accessed March 13, 2017.

3. Adult acute lymphoblastic leukemia treatment (PDQ®)—health professional version. National Cancer Institute website. https://www.cancer.gov/types/leukemia/hp/adult-all-treatment-pdq. Updated January 19, 2017. Accessed March 13, 2017.
4. Harris NL. Hodgkin's lymphomas: classification, diagnosis, and grading. *Semin Hematol.* 1996;36(3):220-232.
5. Survival rates for Hodgkin disease by stage. American Cancer Society website. https://www.cancer.org/cancer/hodgkin-lymphoma/detection-diagnosis-staging/survival-rates.html. Revised May 23, 2016. Accessed March 13, 2017.
6. Lee JH, Song JW, Song KS. Diagnosis of overt disseminated intravascular coagulation: a comparative study using criteria from the International Society versus the Korean Society on Thrombosis and Hemostasis. *Yonsei Med J.* 2007;48(4):595-600. https://www.ncbi.nlm.nih.gov/pmc/articles/PMC2628057/. Accessed March 13, 2017.
7. Kumar R, Gupta M, Gupta V, et al. Acute transfusion reactions (ATRs) in intensive care unit (ICU): a retrospective study. *J Clin Diagn Res.* 2014;8(2):127-129. https://www.ncbi.nlm.nih.gov/pmc/articles/PMC3972528/. Accessed March 13, 2017.

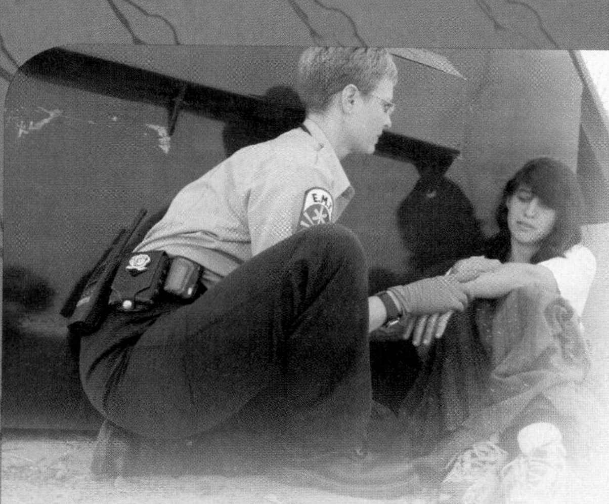

Assessment *in Action*

Your unit is transporting a patient on an interfacility transfer. The unresponsive patient had a reaction to a blood transfusion. The patient was given the transfusion 6 hours ago during elective surgery.

1. When you are assessing a patient whom you suspect is having a reaction to a blood transfusion, the signs and symptoms will be similar to those associated with:

A. asthma.
B. anaphylaxis.
C. acute myocardial infarction.
D. overdose.

2. What are the three goals of treatment for a transfusion reaction?

A. Stop the transfusion, counteract shock, provide cardioversion.
B. Stop the transfusion, counteract shock, provide kidney perfusion.
C. Stop the transfusion, counteract shock, provide liver perfusion.
D. Stop the transfusion, counteract shock, provide peripheral perfusion.

Assessment *in Action* *(continued)*

3. What is the renal dose of dopamine for a patient with a transfusion reaction?

A. 2 to 4 mcg/kg/min
B. 4 to 10 mcg/kg/min
C. 10 to 20 mcg/kg/min
D. More than 20 mcg/kg/min

4. A hemolytic blood transfusion reaction is the result of:

A. decreased RBC production.
B. contamination of the blood product.
C. antibodies reacting against donor WBCs.
D. incompatible ABO or Rh blood type.

5. Which blood type is the universal donor?

A. Type O
B. Type A
C. Type B
D. Type AB

6. What is the most common type of transfusion reaction?

A. Hemolytic
B. Febrile
C. Allergic
D. Transfusion-related lung injury

7. Which of the standard treatments for infusion reactions is NOT beneficial for a patient experiencing transfusion-related lung injury?

A. Diuretics
B. Oxygen
C. Vasopressors
D. Diphenhydramine

8. Is it true that sickle cell disease affects only the African American population?

9. How should you address analgesia with patients who have lymphoma?

10. What is the progression of disseminated intravascular coagulation in the patient with massive trauma and subsequent hypotension?

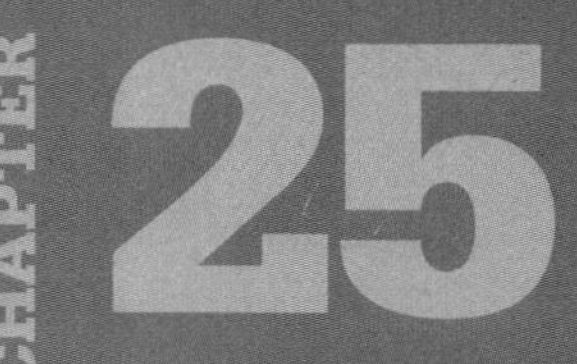

Immunologic Emergencies

National EMS Education Standard Competencies

Medicine

Integrate assessment findings with principles of epidemiology and pathophysiology to formulate a field impression and implement a comprehensive treatment/disposition plan for a patient with a medical complaint.

Immunology

Recognition and management of shock and difficulty breathing related to

- Anaphylactic reactions (pp 1323-1325, 1327-1331)

Anatomy, physiology, pathophysiology, assessment, and management of hypersensitivity disorders and/or emergencies

- Allergic and anaphylactic reactions (pp 1320-1331)

Anatomy, physiology, epidemiology, pathophysiology, psychosocial impact, presentations, prognosis, and management of common or major immunologic system disorders and/or emergencies

- Hypersensitivity (p 1317)
- Allergic and anaphylactic reactions (pp 1320-1331)
- Anaphylactoid reactions (pp 1317, 1320-1331)
- Collagen vascular diseases (pp 1331-1333, 1335)
- Transplant-related problems (pp 1332, 1334-1336)

Knowledge Objectives

1. Describe the purpose of the immune system. (p 1316)
2. Define the terms allergic reaction, anaphylaxis, biphasic reaction, prolonged (persistent) reaction, and anaphylactoid reaction. (pp 1316-1317)
3. Explain the difference between a local and a systemic response to allergens. (p 1317)
4. Discuss the process that begins when a foreign substance is detected in the body (primary response). (pp 1320-1322)
5. Describe the process that occurs when the body undergoes a secondary response. (pp 1320-1322)
6. Explain the role of basophils and mast cells in the immune response process. (pp 1320-1321)
7. Explain the roles of chemical mediators, including histamines and leukotrienes, in the immune response process. (pp 1320-1322, 1326-1327)
8. Describe the assessment process for a patient with an allergic reaction. (pp 1321-1326)
9. Explain the importance of managing the care of a patient who is having an allergic reaction. (p 1322)
10. Compare the signs and symptoms of an allergic reaction with those of anaphylaxis. (pp 1327-1328)
11. Review the process for providing emergency medical care to a patient who is experiencing an allergic reaction. (pp 1328-1331)
12. Describe the administration of epinephrine to a patient who is having an allergic reaction, including different forms of epinephrine. (pp 1329-1330)
13. Explain the various treatment options and pharmacologic interventions used to manage anaphylaxis. (pp 1329-1330)
14. Explain the factors involved when making a transport decision for a patient having an allergic reaction. (pp 1330-1331)
15. Discuss autoimmune disorders and collagen vascular diseases, including systemic lupus erythematosus and scleroderma. (pp 1331-1333)
16. Describe the principles of organ transplantation and disorders related to organ transplants. (pp 1332, 1334-1335)
17. Explain the importance of patient education in the management of anaphylaxis and allergic reactions. (pp 1335-1336)

Skills Objectives

1. Demonstrate how to remove a stinger from a bee sting and proper patient management following its removal. (p 1329)
2. Demonstrate how to administer epinephrine using an auto-injector. (pp 1329-1330)

Introduction

"Please respond to an allergic reaction." Hearing this request from dispatch tends to make emergency medical services (EMS) providers uncomfortable. It is not the care of the patient's **allergic reaction**, rather it is the potential for a life-threatening anaphylactic reaction that causes concern. The good news about **anaphylaxis** is that the incidence is relatively low. Based on survey results by Wood et al, less than 6% of the US population has experienced an anaphylactic reaction.[1] The majority of the anaphylaxis incidents were due to medications, followed by foods, and then insect stings **Figure 25-1**.[1] The bad news is that the incidence of anaphylactic reactions has been increasing.[2,3] One study found that the greatest incidence of increase was in children and young adults, and that food allergies were the most frequently cited causes.[2] Of the anaphylaxis deaths studied, the risk of drug-related anaphylactic deaths was higher in the older adult and African-American populations.[4]

In dealing with allergy-related emergencies, you must prepare for the possibility of acute airway obstruction and cardiovascular collapse. Because allergic reactions and anaphylaxis often begin similarly, you must be able to distinguish between the body's natural response to a sting or bite, an allergic reaction, and a severe anaphylactic reaction. It is crucial to identify an anaphylactic reaction and be prepared to administer epinephrine. Your ability to recognize and manage anaphylactic reactions may be the only thing standing between life and imminent death for a patient.

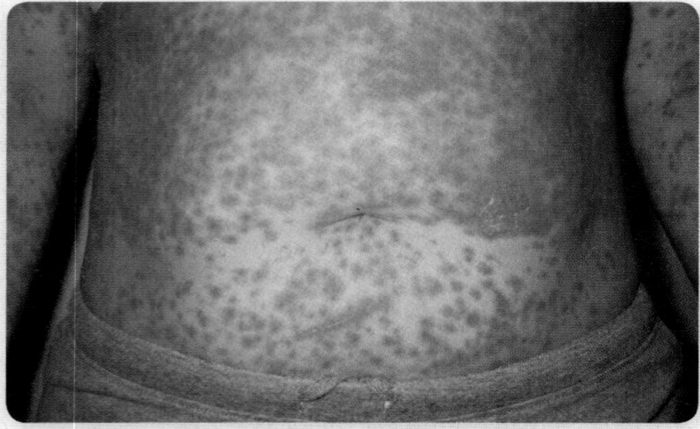

Figure 25-1 A severe allergic reaction to medication. This patient was allergic to penicillin and most other antibiotics.

Courtesy of Carol B. Guerrero.

This chapter begins by reviewing the physiology of the body's immune response and the pathophysiology of an allergic reaction—how an immune response can become a potentially life-threatening event. You will explore hypersensitivity, allergic reactions, anaphylaxis, biphasic allergic reactions, anaphylactoid reactions, collagen vascular diseases, and transplant-related disorders.

Anatomy and Physiology Review

The immune system protects the human body from substances and organisms that are considered foreign. Without the immune system for protection, life as it is now would not exist. The body would be under constant attack from any bacterium, virus, or other type of exposure. Luckily, for the majority of the population, the body is equipped with an amazing immune system that is on patrol 24 hours a day, 7 days a week, to detect unauthorized visits or invading attacks by foreign substances.

As discussed in Chapter 9, *Pathophysiology*, the body protects itself via two types of systems: cell-mediated immunity and humoral immunity. In cell-mediated immunity, also called *cellular immunity*, the body produces special white blood cells called T cells that attack and destroy invaders. In humoral immunity, B cell lymphocytes produce antibodies that dissolve in the plasma and lymph to wage war on invading organisms. The cells producing immunity are located throughout the body in the lymph nodes, spleen, and gastrointestinal tract. The goal is to intercept foreign forces as they enter the body, thereby limiting the spread and damage of invaders.

YOU are the Paramedic — PART 1

Your unit is dispatched to a local clinic for a 70-year-old man with an altered mental status and difficulty speaking. The dispatcher tells you the patient was initially seen for an upper respiratory infection, but there is no further information because the call was made from the front desk. When you enter the clinic, you are directed to an examination room and find an older African-American man lying on the exam table. The head of the bed is elevated. The patient's wife, a nurse, and a physician's assistant (PA) are present. When you look at the man, his mouth looks swollen. He is responsive but does not focus on you as you address him.

1. What is your first impression of this patient?
2. Do you need to take any immediate actions?
3. What differential diagnoses are you considering?

Immune Response

There are many terms associated with the various immune system reactions. An **allergen** is a foreign substance that produces allergic symptoms in a patient. Most allergens are usually harmless substances that do not pose a threat to other people—for example, eggs, peanuts, antibiotics, and insect venom. An **antibody** is a protein the body produces in response to an **antigen**. This protein (globulin) is found in the plasma—hence, its other name *immunoglobulin* (Ig). The IgE antibody is the primary antibody responsible for allergic reactions. (An in-depth discussion of globulins can be found in Chapter 9, *Pathophysiology*.)

When the body is exposed to a foreign substance, the immune system responds, resulting in a localized or systemic reaction. In a **local reaction**, the body limits its response to a specific area after being exposed to a foreign substance; the swelling around an insect bite is an example. A **systemic reaction** occurs throughout the body, possibly affecting multiple body systems. An example of this type of reaction is seen when a person who is allergic to strawberries develops swelling and hives all over his or her body after eating strawberry shortcake. **Hypersensitivity** occurs when a person's immune system reacts with exaggerated or inappropriate symptoms after coming into contact with a substance perceived by the body to be harmful. Hypersensitivity is typically divided into four types.

1. **Allergic reaction.** An abnormal immune response that the body develops when the person has been previously exposed or sensitized to a substance or allergen. In most people, exposure to this substance would produce no reaction or a minor reaction; in a person who is sensitive to the allergen, a significant local or systemic reaction may occur.
2. **Anaphylaxis.** An extreme systemic form of an allergic reaction involving a single, two, or more body systems. In anaphylactic reactions, life-threatening effects are the greatest concern.
3. **Biphasic reaction.** A two-phase allergic reaction in which the patient's symptoms improve and then reappear without exposure to the trigger (allergen) a second time. The symptoms can resurface up to 8 or more hours after the initial incident. The literature reports a wide variance in incidence of biphasic reactions—anywhere from less than 1% to up to 23%.[5–8]
4. **Prolonged (persistent) reactions.** Anaphylaxis symptoms that continue over time, with time frames anywhere from 5 to 72 hours.[9] Once again, there is an inconsistent report of incidence, from uncommon to up to 23% to 28%.[9]

Anaphylaxis is classified as a response mediated by IgE antibodies, while an **anaphylactoid reaction** is a response that does not involve IgE antibody mediation. The exact mechanism is unknown, but an anaphylactoid event may occur without the patient being previously exposed to the offending agent. Examples of causes of anaphylactic reactions are nuts, fish, and latex. Causes of anaphylactoid reactions include some contrasts given before radiography, morphine-derivative medications, and aspirin. Even though the process that causes the reaction is different, the patient presentation is the same.

Words of Wisdom

Anaphylactic and anaphylactoid responses are clinically indistinguishable and should be treated in the same manner because both can be life threatening.

Words of Wisdom

The term *anaphylaxis* is not really accurate; the fundamental problem in an anaphylactic reaction is not a lack of protection but rather overprotection. That is, anaphylaxis is a form of allergy—a very extreme and devastating form—it represents the body's protective immune system gone overboard. The term was first used in 1902, when Portier and Richet were experimenting with vaccinating dogs with sea anemone toxin. After the second dose of the toxin, one of the dogs died due to a severe allergic response. Because this response was against protection, it was referred to as anaphylaxis (meaning "without protection").

Routes of Entry for Allergens

Substances can enter and invade the body through the skin, the respiratory tract, or the gastrointestinal tract. Invasion through the skin may come in the form of injection or absorption. In **injection**, the invading substance pierces the skin and deposits foreign material into the skin. Bees and hornets are often the cause of this type of invasion. Intravenous or parenteral administration of medications are other examples. **Absorption** occurs when foreign material is deposited on and absorbed through the skin. Absorption can also occur through the vaginal wall. Instances of anaphylactic response to seminal fluid have been documented, so asking about recent sexual activity may be necessary.[10] Invasion by allergens does not stop at the skin; substances may also enter the respiratory tract as the patient quietly breathes. This is referred to as an **inhalation** exposure. The foreign substance advances through the respiratory system and launches its attack from the lungs. Cat hair and dander, peanuts, and many plants are involved in this type of exposure. The final way allergens enter the body is through the gastrointestinal tract via **ingestion**. Foods such as strawberry shortcake, a mushroom and cheese omelet, or peanut butter pie can cause an allergic reaction.

Although it is estimated that millions of Americans are at risk for anaphylaxis, no exact cause or route of exposure or entry for this life-threatening event can be determined in up to two-thirds of patients.[1] Furthermore, no one route of exposure is identified as having a greater risk of anaphylaxis. It is important to note that people with high sensitivity can be at risk to routes of exposure not commonly associated with an antigen. For example, you would suspect someone with a peanut allergy to have a reaction from ingesting peanuts or peanut-containing foods. However, these patients may have a reaction simply by being present where peanuts are being served and may experience an inhalation exposure.

To anticipate anaphylaxis, of course, it would be useful to be able to identify people at greatest risk. Neither race nor sex seems to affect the incidence of anaphylaxis; however, certain ages and sexes tend to have a greater incidence of anaphylaxis associated with specific types of exposure.[11] The incidence of anaphylaxis from insect stings tends to be higher in men.[12] Women have a greater incidence of anaphylactic reactions to latex, aspirin, and IV muscle relaxants.[12,13] Anaphylactic reactions have been documented in children as young as 4 months and in the geriatric population as well.[4,14] Children are more likely to have severe food allergies, whereas adults tend to have anaphylactic reactions to insect stings, anesthetics, radiocontrast media, and medications. Table 25-1 lists the common substances associated with anaphylaxis.

Table 25-1 Causes of Anaphylactic Reactions

Antigen, General Category	Comments
Foods	▪ Most common prehospital cause of anaphylactic reactions; associated with high incidence of fatalities ▪ Peanuts: As little as 100 mcg can cause reaction ▪ Peanuts, tree nuts, and shellfish allergies: common to all ages ▪ Cow's milk, wheat, soy, eggs: common in children ▪ Eggs: formerly a contraindication for receiving the flu vaccine (now encouraged to receive a single dose of influenza vaccine)
Medications	▪ Penicillin, beta-lactam antibiotics, and cephalosporins are the most common causes of anaphylactic reactions • Penicillin-allergy more likely to have a reaction when administered cephalosporins (especially with cephalothin, cephalexin, cefadroxil, or cefazolin) ♦ May have a higher incidence of allergies to other medications ▪ Other medications that can cause reactions: • Antibiotics: ampicillin and sulfa drugs (sulfonamide, sulfisoxazole) • Muscle relaxants: Neuromuscular blocking agents are most common cause (50% to 70%) of anaphylaxis during anesthesia • Induction agents: Barbiturates may cause IgE response; allergies to soy and eggs are contraindications to propofol use • Opioids: IV administration of opioids is often associated with flushing and **urticaria**. Slowing IV administration usually decreases the effect • Plasma expanders: dextran, hydroxyethyl starch. If expander is gelatin based, reaction is possible with gelatin sensitivity • Insulin isophane suspension (NPH) (Humulin N, Novolin N) may increase anaphylaxis potential • Salicylates and NSAIDs: Aspirin and NSAIDs are common causes of anaphylactic reactions; cross allergies may occur • Local anesthetics • Enzymes: Examples include chymotrypsin, penicillinase • Biologic extracts: Examples include insulin and heparin • Vaccines: Monitor the patient for reactions
Latex (gloves, supplies, or materials containing latex)	▪ Use latex-free supplies. Some moulage/simulation supplies contain latex ▪ Rate of incidence is decreasing ▪ Cross-reactions may occur with banana, kiwi, strawberry allergies ▪ Risk factors: patients with frequent exposure to latex, sensitized health care workers

Antigen, General Category	Comments
Blood transfusions (mismatched)	▪ Administering A+ blood to a B− recipient ▪ IV immunoglobulin or animal antiserum
Hymenoptera stings (bees, yellow jackets, hornets, wasps, and fire ants)	▪ Systemic reactions occur in 0.5%–3% of people after being stung. ▪ Adults who develop generalized urticaria are at greater risk for anaphylactic reactions. ▪ Localized reactions are not considered risk factors for anaphylaxis.
Animals	▪ Dander (long-haired animals) ▪ Animal serum products: Examples include horse serum and gamma globulins
Seminal fluid	▪ Incidences of anaphylactic reactions to seminal fluid have been reported.
Allergen-specific SCIT (allergy injections and skin testing)	▪ Common cause of anaphylaxis, but rarely cause fatal reactions ▪ Risk factors: poorly controlled asthma, concurrent use of beta-blockers, high allergen dose, errors in administration, and lack of a sufficient observation period following the injection, atopic disease history
Chlorhexidine (antiseptic)	▪ Used in dental rinses and for a surgical scrub
Anti-cancer drugs	▪ Chemotherapy • Encountered more often • Platinum-containing medications are more commonly associated with reactions. ▪ Monoclonal antibodies • Omalizumab often results in a delayed and prolonged reaction. Monitor for 3 hours after the first three injections and for 30 minutes after subsequent injections.
RCM (iodinated radiocontrast dyes used in taking radiographs)	▪ Both anaphylactic and anaphylactoid reactions have been reported. ▪ Risk factors for more severe reactions: patients with asthma, beta-blocker use, cardiovascular disease ▪ No evidence that seafood or iodine-containing solutions applied topically are related to anaphylactoid RCM reactions
Other	▪ Rare incidences of anaphylaxis coinciding with menstruation have been reported. ▪ Exercise-induced physical activity has been reported to cause anaphylaxis. • Risk factors or co-triggers: Ingestion of foods (may be specific foods or general ingestion); NSAID use, especially aspirin; high pollen count (rare) • Reactions/incidents do not consistently recur with similar incidents.
Idiopathic (unknown cause)	▪ Patient may experience anaphylaxis without an identifiable cause. ▪ Treatment should be initiated; a cause can be determined later. ▪ Patients may have multiple episodes of idiopathic anaphylaxis per year.

Abbreviations: IgE, immunoglobulin E; IV, intravenous; NPH, neutral protamine Hagedorn; NSAID, nonsteroidal anti-inflammatory drug; SCIT, subcutaneous immunotherapy; RCM, radio contrast media

Data from: Mustafa S. Anaphylaxis. Medscape website. http://emedicine.medscape.com/article/135065-overview#a4. Updated February 22, 2017. Accessed March 31, 2017; and Peroni DG, Sansotta N, Bernardini R, et al. Muscle relaxants allergy. *Int J Immunopathol Pharmacol*. 2011;24(suppl 3):S35-46. Pub Med Abstract. https://www.ncbi.nlm.nih.gov/pubmed/22014924. Accessed January 17, 2017.

Patient Safety

EMS providers are required to be prepared for latex allergies in the field and to consider a latex-free or latex-safe environment. The National Institute for Occupational Safety and Health offers publications on preventing allergic reactions to latex in the workplace.

Diseases related to allergies, also referred to as atopic diseases, include allergic rhinitis, asthma, and atopic dermatitis. The presence of atopic diseases increases the potential for anaphylactic reactions. Anaphylaxis recurrence has a higher incidence in patients with atopic diseases.[15]

It is important to note the route of exposure, though a severe reaction can occur by any route. The time between exposures to a substance also should be noted, because the greater the time between exposures, the less likely a severe anaphylactic reaction will occur. This is thought to be due to the decreased production of the specific immunoglobulin (Ig) or antibody cells in the body over time. This is *not* the case for anaphylactoid reactions, so being prepared for intervention is key as it may not be possible to differentiate between the two reactions in the field.

Words of Wisdom

The severity of a future allergic reaction cannot be predicted based on the severity of a past reaction. A mild allergic reaction can be followed by a life-threatening reaction.[16]

▶ Physiology of Immune Response

Once a foreign substance enters the body, the body initiates a series of responses. The first encounter with the foreign substance begins the **primary response**. Cells (macrophages) immediately confront and engulf the foreign substances to determine if they are allowed in the body. If the body is unable to identify the substance, it uses immune cells to record the salient features of the outside substance. These cells record one or two of the proteins on the surface of the invading substance and then design specific proteins to match each substance. These proteins—called antibodies—are intended to match up with the antigen and inactivate it.

Through the primary response, the body develops **sensitivity**—that is, the ability to recognize the antigen the next time it is encountered. To determine whether the substance is "one of us," the body records enough details to assist in future identification of the substance and production of antibodies to perfectly fit the invading antigen. The **secondary response** occurs with reexposure to a foreign substance.

The **basophils** and **mast cells** produce the body's **chemical mediators** Table 25-2. These cells contain granules filled with a host of powerful substances that are ready to be released to fight invading antigens. As long as the body is not invaded by one of the previously identified foreign substances, the granules are kept encapsulated in their protective walls and remain inactive. If an antigen invades the body and combines with one of the antibodies, however, the granules are ejected from the mast cells and the chemical mediators are then released into the

YOU are the Paramedic PART 2

While your partner sets up the oxygen equipment to start treating the patient, you ask what happened. The PA shares that the patient came to the clinic for an upper respiratory infection. The patient was diagnosed with an ear and sinus infection and was administered penicillin and given an albuterol inhaler for bronchitis. You ask if the patient has ever had this type of reaction before. The nurse replies, "no," and adds "he has an allergy to aspirin, but not to penicillin." The wife agrees with these statements. She says they were in the waiting room after her husband got his shot, when he started having trouble talking and started acting funny. She called the nurse, and the nurse called you. The nurse also states the patient has a history of hypertension and takes an angiotensin-converting enzyme (ACE) inhibitor. The staff administered Benadryl and 0.3 mg of epinephrine via the intramuscular (IM) route before your arrival. You ask your partner to attach the patient to the cardiac monitor.

Recording Time: 0 Minutes	
Appearance	Awake
Level of consciousness	Not alert
Airway	Open with swelling of the lips
Breathing	Audible stridor and wheezing without stethoscope, developing as you are applying oxygen and collecting an initial report.
Circulation	Weak, rapid radial pulse

4. Can this be an allergic reaction if the patient has not had a previous reaction?
5. What are the implications of a history of hypertension and taking an ACE inhibitor for this case?
6. Was the administration route and dose of epinephrine appropriate, and should you allow them to administer a second dose? Defend your decision.

Table 25-2 Chemical Mediators

Mediator	Physiologic Effects
Histamine	▪ Systemic vasodilation ▪ Increased permeability of blood vessels ▪ Decreased cardiac contractility ▪ Decreased coronary blood flow ▪ Dysrhythmias ▪ Bronchoconstriction ▪ Pulmonary vasoconstriction
Eosinophil chemotactic factor	▪ Attracts eosinophils and neutrophils
Arachidonic acid (precursor of the following): Prostaglandin Leukotrienes (SRS-A)	These factors act to produce other inflammatory mediators: ▪ Smooth muscle contraction ▪ Vascular permeability ▪ Bronchoconstriction ▪ Decreased force of cardiac contraction ▪ Decreased coronary blood flow ▪ Dysrhythmias • More potent than histamine (thousands of times) • React more slowly than histamine
Platelet-activating factor	▪ Platelet aggregation ▪ Causes histamine release
Serotonin	▪ Pulmonary vasoconstriction ▪ Bronchoconstriction
Proteoglycans	
Heparin Chondroitin sulfate	▪ Control the release of histamine. These mediators as a whole work to activate the kinin system and are thought to contribute to prolonged and biphasic reactions.
Chemokines Cytokines	▪ These mediators trigger inflammatory pathways and increase the recruitment of inflammatory cells.
Kinins	▪ Bradykinin is one of the stronger kinins and is responsible for increased vascular permeability.

Abbreviation: SRS-A, slow-reacting substance of anaphylaxis

surrounding tissue and the bloodstream **Figure 25-2**. (An in-depth review of the immune system is included in Chapter 9, *Pathophysiology*.)

Patient Assessment

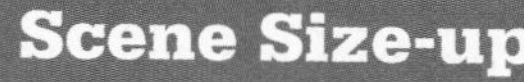

Scene Size-up

Assess the scene for safety issues—an angry swarm of bees may put you, your crew, and the patient at risk. Once you have ensured that the scene is safe, determine the nature of the illness by observing for any potential exposure problems. For example, if the patient was gardening, a bee sting might be a cause of the problem. Dinner at a seafood restaurant should make you suspicious of the shellfish menu items or food fried in peanut oil. Because anaphylaxis is a life-threatening event, taking the time to survey the scene for potential hazards for anaphylaxis is important.

Patient Safety

Before applying latex gloves, check if the patient has a latex allergy. Ensure that patients receiving any sterile techniques are not allergic to latex, since most sterile kits contain latex gloves. Some states require latex-free kits on all ambulances.

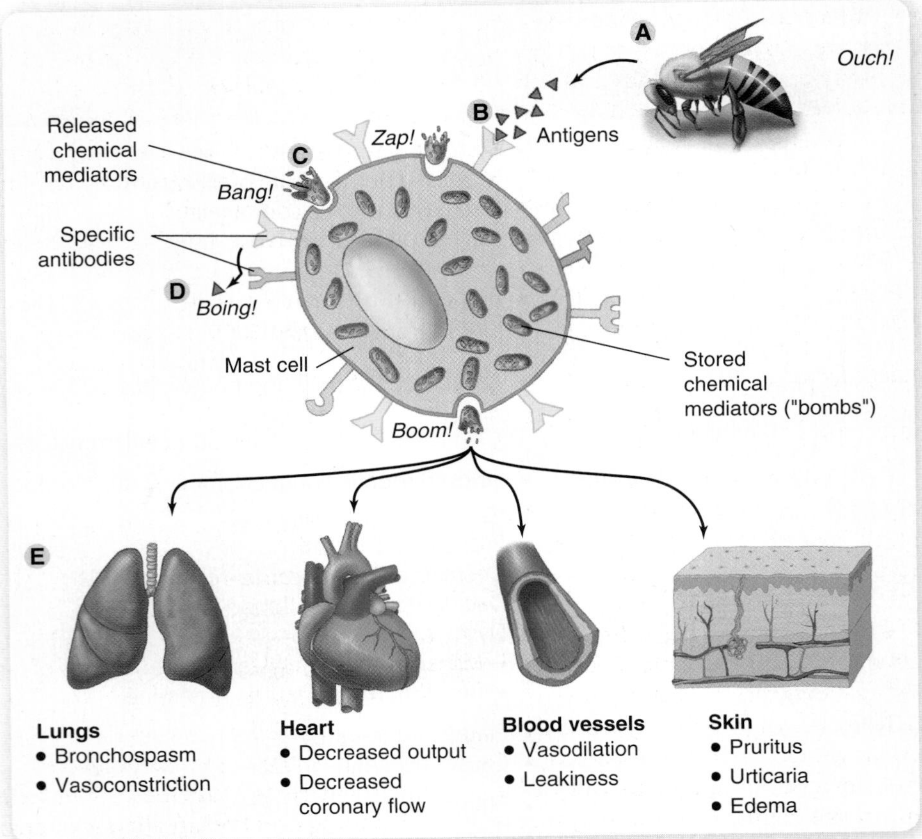

Figure 25-2 The sequence of events in anaphylaxis. **A.** The antigen is introduced into the body. **B.** The antigen–antibody reaction at the surface of a mast cell. **C.** Release of mast cell chemical mediators. **D.** Specific antibody reacts with its corresponding antigen. **E.** Chemical mediators exert their effects on end organs.

Primary Survey

Assessment of a patient with an allergic or anaphylactic reaction can be highly challenging. To save the patient's life you may have to simultaneously assess the patient, identify the problem, and intervene within seconds of arriving on the scene. Index of suspicion for anaphylaxis must be high on your list if any of the symptoms discussed previously are present. You may not have a second opportunity because the patient's condition may deteriorate before your eyes.

Allergic symptoms are almost as varied as the allergens themselves. A patient may have bite or sting marks that may accompany other signs and symptoms of an allergic reaction. Your assessment of a patient experiencing an allergic reaction should include evaluations of the level of consciousness, the respiratory system, the circulatory system, mental status, and the skin. As mentioned earlier, allergic reactions can range from local to systemic. They can be categorized as mild, moderate, or severe. Mild reactions affect a local area of the body and do not spread to other areas. Itchy, watery eyes or a rash are examples of a mild reaction. Slight congestion would also be considered a mild reaction. Moderate reactions begin as mild reactions, but the symptoms do spread to other parts of the body. For example, your patient initially reports itchy, watery eyes and then develops tightness in the chest with trouble breathing. Severe reactions are considered anaphylactic reactions, and they result in potentially life-threatening emergencies. Severe reactions are systemic; for example, the patient may report congestion that progresses to respiratory distress, and hypotension. Onset may be sudden and affect the entire body.

Observe the patient to form a general impression. The patient's presentation will give you an indication of the severity of the problem. If the patient is unable to speak, edema may be impacting the vocal cords. level of consciousness is an indicator of the patient's severity and a reflection of the patient's oxygenation and circulatory status. Restlessness, confusion, anxiety, and combativeness are common signs of hypoxia. Any change in mental status in an anaphylactic patient should direct you to immediate epinephrine administration and airway evaluation and management.

Part of determining a general impression involves evaluating the airway and breathing. A noisy upper airway is a concern in any patient, but even more so in an anaphylactic patient, because it may be an early sign of impending airway occlusion due to swelling. Listen for stridor and hoarseness. In addition, the patient may report a tight feeling or a "lump in the throat." Observe the patient for difficulty speaking, noisy airway, tachypnea, labored breathing, accessory muscle use, abnormal retractions, and prolonged expiration. The severity of these findings predicts the stability of the patient's condition. Breath sounds are also a predictor of severity. Initially, you will hear wheezing. As the patient's condition deteriorates and the lungs become tighter and less ventilated (hypoventilation), the diminished lung sounds will be present and the chest may become silent. A silent chest is an ominous finding and requires immediate intervention. Early intervention is key in these patients. Not all patients will have respiratory issues, so keep your index of suspicion high.

Monitor closely for changes in circulation. Evaluate the skin for erythema, rashes, edema, moisture, **pruritus** (itching), and urticaria (hives or reddened elevated patches on the skin). these symptoms are more commonly associated with an anaphylactic reaction due to histamine release; however, anaphylaxis can occur without these common skin signs. Pallor and cyanosis may be present as well. A weak, thready, or absent radial pulse is indicative of potential cardiovascular collapse. Recall that anaphylaxis can present with hypotension alone or that hypotension may not be present even in life-threatening cases. Do not wait for the signs of shock to develop. Early recognition and initiation of immediate treatment is a priority.

As you are completing the primary survey, you should be making transport decisions. You must decide whether to remain on the scene, load the patient and initiate treatment during transport, or even call for air transport. In addition, you should determine which facility the patient should be transported to based on the patient's need for services.

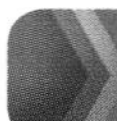

History Taking

The patient history should include investigation of the chief complaint, SAMPLE (Signs and symptoms, Allergies, Medications, Pertinent past history, Last oral intake, Events leading to injury or illness), and OPQRST (Onset, Provocation/palliation, Quality, Region/radiation, Severity, Timing). The history should be specifically directed at this incident. Some steps may be skipped or collected later if a life threat exists. Does the patient have any allergies? Has the patient ever had an allergic or anaphylactic reaction?

YOU are the Paramedic — PART 3

You elect to administer a second dose of epinephrine IM. Your partner administers oxygen to the patient, who is starting to focus and is complaining of trouble breathing. Stridor can be heard clearly. Wheezing is still present on auscultation. The PA recommends sitting the patient upright to assist with his breathing. Your partner recommends initiation of albuterol via nebulizer while you start an intravenous (IV) line.

Recording Time: 5 Minutes	
Respirations	26 breaths/min, very shallow
Pulse	120 beats/min
Skin	Urticaria forming across the chest and arms, warm, dry
Blood pressure	90/58 mm Hg
Oxygen saturation (Spo_2)	92% on room air, 94% on oxygen via NRM
Pupils	PERRLA

7. Are there concerns with allowing this patient to sit upright, and would you position the patient in an upright position?
8. What effect can you expect the albuterol to have on this patient?
9. What type of fluid should you administer, and how much fluid is indicated? Are there any concerns with fluid administration for this patient?

If so, how severe was the incident and how rapidly did it progress? Comparing it to this incident by asking how severe this incident is and how rapidly it is progressing is a useful tool as well.

> **Words of Wisdom**
>
> In patients with high sensitivity to an allergen, always ask about less traditional routes of exposure as you collect the history. For example, ask about inhalation exposure with a peanut allergy.

Ask whether any interventions have been taken. Interview the patient to determine whether he or she had a previous exposure to the antigen; for example, if the patient just ate peanuts, asking about previous ingestions may be useful. A severe reaction may occur at the first or second exposure to an antigen, so the patient might not know about the allergy. Asking about medications, in particular new medications, may help identify the antigen. In addition, ask questions regarding risk factors for severe anaphylaxis, such as the following:[17]

- Peanut and tree nut allergy history (especially in adolescents)
- Preexisting respiratory or cardiovascular disease
- Asthma
- Delayed administration of epinephrine
- Previous biphasic anaphylactic reactions
- Advanced age
- Mast cell disease

In some anaphylactoid (non-IgE) reactions, a previous exposure may not be present. Additionally, there will be cases in which you cannot identify the offending antigen. In the presence of a severe reaction, intervention takes precedence over identifying the antigen. To help determine where the patient is in the reaction process, ask when the symptoms began. Direct your assessment to potential signs of life threats, such as feelings of tightness in the throat, feelings of dyspnea, syncopal events, or signs of hypotension.

Also determine whether the patient or first responders have administered any treatment before your arrival. This may include using an EpiPen, taking diphenhydramine (Benadryl), or using an inhaler with a beta-agonist (such as albuterol or metaproterenol) or aerosolized epinephrine (such as Primatene Mist or racemic epinephrine) **Figure 25-3**. If the patient has an EpiPen or has used one, be aware that some EpiPens come with two doses. Do not discard the second dose.

Ask about the less common causes of anaphylaxis such as exercise-induced reactions. In the rare case of seminal fluid reactions, ask about recent sexual activity. Do not delay treatment to find the cause. Patients may have idiopathic anaphylaxis, so you may not be able to identify the cause. **Table 25-3** shows a guideline for identifying anaphylaxis.

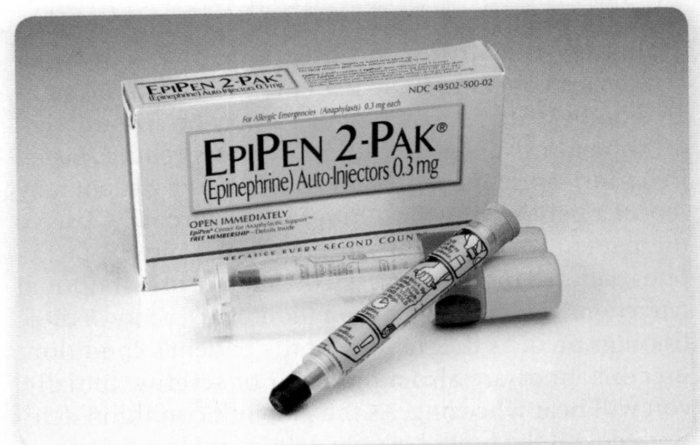

Figure 25-3 Patients who experience severe allergic reactions often carry prescription epinephrine, which comes predosed in an auto-injector or a prefilled syringe.

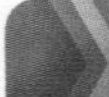

Secondary Assessment

As time and conditions allow, perform a physical examination. The classic presentation of anaphylaxis includes respiratory symptoms and hypotension. Gastrointestinal symptoms such as abnormal cramping, nausea, vomiting, and diarrhea may be present. If the patient is identified as having a life-threatening condition, a physical examination should be performed; however, it should be done after life threats are addressed and you are en route to the hospital.

The secondary assessment may help direct treatment. As in all emergencies, your assessment of a patient experiencing an allergic reaction should include a systematic head-to-toe or focused assessment to determine hidden trauma or other unrelated medical conditions.

Perform evaluations of the respiratory system. Thoroughly assess the airway and breathing, including stridor, increased work of breathing, use of accessory muscles, head bobbing, tripod positioning, nostril flaring, and grunting. Carefully auscultate the trachea and the chest.

Stridor and wheezing may be present during an allergic reaction. Stridor occurs when swelling in the upper airway closes off the airway and can lead to total obstruction. Wheezing occurs because excessive fluid and mucus are secreted into the bronchial passages, and muscles around these passages tighten in response to the release of histamines and leukotrienes induced by the allergen. Exhalation, normally the passive, relaxed phase of breathing, becomes increasingly difficult as the patient tries to cough up the secretions or move air past the constricted airways. The combination of fluid in the air passages and the constricted bronchi produce the wheezing

Table 25-3 Diagnosis of Anaphylaxis

Anaphylaxis is likely when any one of the three criteria is fulfilled.

Criterion 1 Acute onset of an illness (minutes to several hours) with involvement of:	**Criterion 2** *Two or more* of the following that occur rapidly after exposure to a likely allergen for that patient:	**Criterion 3** After exposure to a known allergen for that patient (minutes to several hours):
Skin and/or mucosa: ▪ Pruritus ▪ Flushing ▪ Hives ▪ Angioedema *And either:* Respiratory compromise: ▪ Dyspnea ▪ Wheeze-bronchospasm ▪ Decreased peak expiratory flow ▪ Stridor ▪ Hypoxemia *Or:* Decreased blood pressure or end-organ dysfunction: ▪ Collapse ▪ Syncope ▪ Incontinence	Skin and/or mucosa: ▪ Pruritus ▪ Flushing ▪ Hives ▪ Angioedema Respiratory compromise: ▪ Dyspnea ▪ Wheeze-bronchospasm ▪ Decreased peak expiratory flow ▪ Stridor ▪ Hypoxemia Decreased blood pressure or end-organ dysfunction: ▪ Collapse ▪ Syncope ▪ Incontinence Persistent GI symptoms: ▪ Vomiting ▪ Crampy abdominal pain ▪ Diarrhea	Decreased blood pressure

Abbreviation: GI, gastrointestinal

Modified from: Manivannan, V., Decker, W.W., Stead, L.G. et al. Int J Emerg Med (2009) 2: 3. doi:10.1007/s12245-009-0093-z. https://link.springer.com/article/10.1007%2Fs12245-009-0093-z. Accessed January 23, 2017.

sound. Breathing rapidly becomes more difficult, and the patient may even stop breathing. Prolonged respiratory difficulty can cause a rapid heartbeat (tachycardia), shock, respiratory failure, and death.

Assess the circulatory system. Monitor for signs of hemodynamic compromise, including blood pressure, pulse rate, cardiac monitoring, and pulse oximetry. Remember, the presence of hypoperfusion (shock) or respiratory distress indicates that the patient's reaction is severe and may result in death.

Carefully assess the skin for swelling, rash, hives, and signs of the source of the reaction: bite, sting, or contact marks. A rapidly spreading rash can be concerning because it may indicate a systemic reaction and may quickly proceed to anaphylaxis. Red, hot skin may also indicate a systemic reaction as the blood vessels lose their ability to constrict and blood moves to the extremities. If this reaction continues, the body will have difficulty supplying blood and oxygen to the vital organs, and one of the first signs will be altered mental status as the organs are deprived of oxygen and glucose.

Words of Wisdom

Even though cutaneous signs such as urticaria and flushing are common in anaphylaxis, it is important to remember that rapid and severe cardiovascular collapse may occur without cutaneous signs being present.

Vital signs help determine whether the body is compensating for stress. Assess baseline vital signs, including pulse, respirations, blood pressure, skin, pupils, and oxygen saturation. Rapid, labored breathing indicates airway compromise. Rapid respiratory and pulse rates may indicate respiratory distress or systemic shock. Fast pulse rates and hypotension are ominous signs, indicating systemic vascular collapse and shock. Skin signs may not be consistent with signs of hypoperfusion because of rashes and swelling.

Utilize monitoring devices to confirm the patient's status. Use tools such as a cardiac monitor in your assessment because dysrhythmias may be associated with anaphylaxis. Consider a 12-lead ECG to monitor for cardiac ischemia. This is even more important in patients with a history of cardiovascular or pulmonary disease. End-tidal carbon dioxide levels may be elevated in anaphylaxis. watch for a "shark fin" waveform on the $ETCO_2$ monitor, which is indicative of bronchoconstriction. $ETCO_2$ may be decreased with hypoperfusion and should improve as the pressure and hemodynamic status improve. Monitoring pulse oximetry may alert you to low oxygen saturation, which will assist in identifying the degree of respiratory distress. Oxygen administration should be considered for patients with signs of anaphylaxis, cardiovascular, or respiratory compromise, whether respiratory distress is present or not.

Reassessment

Reassessment typically is conducted en route to the emergency department. Be vigilant in monitoring a patient experiencing a suspected allergic reaction because deterioration of the patient's condition can be rapid and fatal. Give special attention to any signs of airway compromise, including increasing work of breathing, stridor, and wheezing. Monitor the patient's anxiety level because increased anxiety is a good indication that the reaction may be progressing. Watch the skin for signs of shock, including pallor and diaphoresis, as well as for flushing. Serial vital signs are an important resource when evaluating your patient's status. Note any increase in the respiratory or pulse rate or decrease in blood pressure. Continue to reassess the chief complaint.

Once you have performed interventions, recheck them. If you administered epinephrine, what was the effect? Is the patient's condition improving? Do you need to consider a second dose? You may need to give more than one injection of epinephrine or consider an infusion if you note that the patient has decreasing mental status, increased breathing difficulty, or a decreasing blood pressure. Be sure to consult medical control or your protocols first. Identify and treat changes in the patient's condition.

Remember, with a severe condition, the more time you can give the staff at the facility to prepare for the patient, the better. Communicate and document the patient's status, interventions completed, and the patient's response.

Emergency Medical Care

To treat allergic reactions, you must first identify how much distress the patient is experiencing. Some allergic reactions will produce severe signs and symptoms in a matter of minutes and threaten the patient's life. Early epinephrine administration is a priority in care of the patient experiencing an anaphylactic reaction. Ventilatory support and/or fluid resuscitation are required for severe reactions. Other allergic reactions have a slower onset, cause less severe distress, and may resolve without intervention. Milder reactions, without respiratory or cardiovascular distress, may require only supportive care, such as oxygen. In either situation, the patient should be transported to a medical facility for further evaluation.

Pathophysiology, Assessment, and Management of Specific Emergencies

Anaphylactic Reactions

Pathophysiology

As discussed earlier, an overzealous immune system can result in problems that range in severity along the spectrum from a simple annoyance to a life-threatening crisis. The immune cells of the allergic person are more sensitive than the immune cells of a person without allergies. Although these cells are able to recognize and react to dangerous invaders, such as bacteria and viruses, they also identify harmless substances as posing a threat.

When the invading substance enters the body, the mast cells recognize it as potentially harmful and begin releasing chemical mediators. Histamine, one of the primary chemical weapons, causes the blood vessels in the local area to dilate and the capillaries to leak. Leukotrienes, which are even more powerful, are released and cause additional dilation and leaking. White blood cells are called to the area to help engulf and destroy the enemy, and platelets begin to collect and clump together. In most cases, this overreaction to harmless invaders is restricted to the local area being invaded. The runny, itchy nose and swollen eyes associated with hay fever are examples of a local allergic reaction.

In the case of anaphylaxis, the person is not so lucky. chemical mediators are released, and the effect involves more than one system throughout the body. An initial effect may be seen from the histamine release, with secondary effects following a few hours later when additional chemicals are released.

Histamine release causes immediate vasodilation, which often presents as erythematous skin and hypotension. It also increases vascular permeability, which results in edema, fluid secretion, and fluid loss. The edema can present as urticaria Figure 25-4, airway constriction, and increased fluids in the airway. Histamine likewise causes smooth muscle contraction, especially in the respiratory system and gastrointestinal system. This results in laryngospasm or bronchospasm and abdominal cramping. Finally, histamine decreases the inotropic effects of the heart. When this effect is coupled with vasodilation, the person may experience profound hypotension. Dysrhythmias due to hypoperfusion and hypoxia are also common.

Later responses from the much more powerful leukotrienes compound the effects of histamine. The person's respiratory status will become even more dire as these

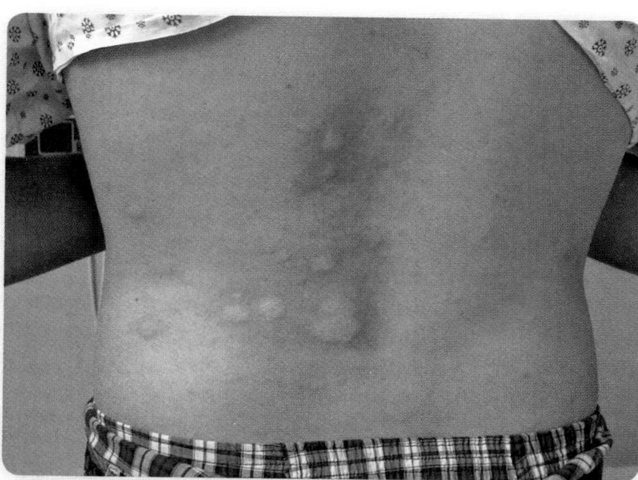

Figure 25-4 Urticaria, or hives, may appear following a sting and are characterized by multiple, small, raised areas on the skin.

highly potent bronchoconstrictors are released. In addition, leukotriene release causes coronary vasoconstriction, which contributes to a worsening cardiac condition and myocardial irritability. Leukotrienes are also associated with increased vascular permeability, contributing to a further state of hypoperfusion.

The remaining chemical mediators continue to worsen the situation as they undertake what they see as steps to protect the body from this foreign invader. As a result of these activities, when the body undergoes an anaphylactic reaction, it may not survive without immediate intervention. (For a more in-depth discussion see Chapter 9, *Pathophysiology.*)

Clinical Symptoms of Anaphylaxis

The skin is the body's first line of defense against would-be invaders, so skin symptoms are often the first indications of anaphylaxis. Initially, the person may be aware of feeling warm and flushed. Pruritus is another early sign that is due to vasodilation and capillary leaking. The area around the eyes is often susceptible to this effect, which causes swollen, red eyes. Swelling of the face and tongue (angioedema) may contribute to airway compromise. Edema of the hands and feet may also be noted. Histamine is responsible for the urticaria (hives) experienced by the patient with anaphylaxis.

Common complaints include respiratory symptoms, which often present as shortness of breath or dyspnea and tightness in the throat and chest. Stridor and/or hoarseness may also be noted. These signs and symptoms are often due to upper airway swelling in the laryngeal and epiglottic areas. Affected patients may report a lump in the throat or have difficulty speaking. The lower airway is often involved as well. Bronchoconstriction and increased secretions may result in wheezes and crackles (rales). It is not uncommon for the patient to cough or sneeze as the body tries to clear the airway. These symptoms may progress slowly or alarmingly fast. You may have only 1 to 3 minutes to halt this rapid, life-threatening process.

Cardiovascular symptoms are serious complications of anaphylaxis. As noted earlier, histamine and leukotrienes work directly on the heart to decrease its contractility. The resulting decrease in cardiac output is complicated by vasodilation and increased capillary permeability, which further decrease the amount of fluid returned to the heart. As cardiac output declines, perfusion decreases, leading to ischemia and bringing the potential for cardiac dysrhythmias. As the fluid leaks out of the capillaries, the intravascular system is left short on fluid. (As much as 50% of the vascular volume can be shifted to the extravascular space within 10 minutes of exposure to an antigen.[18] This is like having 3 L of blood in a 6-L container.) Instead of responding normally to the fluid loss and constricting, the blood vessels do just the opposite: they dilate. The already low vascular volume becomes totally inadequate, and hypotension reigns. In response to the low blood pressure, the heart rate increases, putting stress on an already compromised heart. In this situation, tachycardia, flushed skin, and hypotension are synonymous with anaphylactic shock.

Gastrointestinal symptoms may also be part of an anaphylactic response, particularly if the offending antigen has been ingested. Abdominal cramping is a common presentation, but nausea, bloating, vomiting, abdominal distention, and profuse, watery diarrhea may also be present.

Patients may present with central nervous system symptoms in response to decreased cerebral perfusion and hypoxia. These symptoms include headache, dizziness, confusion, syncopal event, and anxiety. A sense of "impending doom" aptly represents the patient's sense of being near death. A patient who expresses a sense of impending doom requires rapid assessment and treatment.

Table 25-4 summarizes the signs and symptoms of anaphylaxis. Anaphylaxis may present as affecting any two or more of these body systems, so the picture can be confusing at times. Think of a patient with anaphylaxis as experiencing three types of shock: (1) cardiogenic shock due to decreased cardiac output, (2) hypovolemic shock due to fluids leaking into the tissues, and (3) neurogenic shock due to inability of the blood vessels to constrict. You will need to use your assessment skills to identify the potential for anaphylaxis and take aggressive action to manage the patient and stop the anaphylactic process as rapidly as possible.

Assessment

You will need to rapidly differentiate between anaphylaxis and other conditions with similar symptoms. Questioning the patient for allergy history and exposure to triggers is

Table 25-4 Signs and Symptoms of Anaphylaxis*

System	Signs and Symptoms
Skin	▪ Warm ▪ Flushed ▪ Itching (pruritus) ▪ Swollen, red eyes ▪ Swelling of the face and tongue ▪ Swelling of the hands and feet ▪ Hives (urticaria)
Respiratory	▪ Dyspnea ▪ Tightness in the throat and chest ▪ Stridor ▪ Hoarseness ▪ Lump in throat ▪ Wheezes ▪ Crackles ▪ Coughing ▪ Sneezing
Cardiovascular	▪ Dysrhythmias ▪ Hypotension
Gastrointestinal	▪ Abdominal cramping ▪ Nausea ▪ Bloating ▪ Vomiting ▪ Abdominal distention ▪ Profuse, watery diarrhea
Central nervous	▪ Headache ▪ Dizziness ▪ Confusion ▪ Anxiety and restlessness ▪ Sense of impending doom ▪ Altered mental status ▪ Syncope

*Dyspnea, hypotension, and tachycardia are considered key indicators.

the key to identifying the diagnosis of anaphylaxis. Time is of the essence, so be familiar with the other possibilities, such the following:

- **Syncope.** Consider vasovagal incidents or other causes of syncope or shock.
- **Flushing.** Ask about a history of cancer or mast cell disease.
- **Red man syndrome.** Ask about vancomycin infusions as they can cause this condition, a flushing pruritus and a rash to the upper body.
- **Severe anxiety and respiratory distress.** This can be associated with panic attacks.
- **Wheezing and respiratory distress.** Ask about chronic obstructive pulmonary disease, foreign body aspiration, and asthma history, and whether current symptoms are different than usual.
- **Monosodium glutamate poisoning.** This condition should also be considered. Signs and symptoms include headache, hives, numbness around the mouth, sweating, and upset stomach. With high doses, palpitations, chest pain, and shortness of breath may be present.
- **Scombroid fish poisoning.** This condition can mimic food-induced anaphylactic reactions. The bacteria found in the spoiled fish release enzymes that are capable of mast cell degranulation.
- **Transfusion-related acute lung injury.** This may occur up to 6 hours after administration and presents with hypoxia, shortness of breath, and hypotension.
- **ACE inhibitor angioedema may be confused with anaphylaxis.** Angioedema is a common side effect of ACE inhibitor use and is more common in the African-American population.[19] Swelling of the tongue, lips, and face is common. Bronchoconstriction is not commonly seen in ACE inhibitor angioedema. Most patients respond to antihistamine administration and discontinuation of the medication.[19] Close monitoring and preparation for airway management is essential in these patients.

If you are unable to determine another cause of the symptoms and the patient continues to present with anaphylactic symptoms, do not delay treatment for a more complete diagnosis.

Management

People having allergic reactions are separated into two groups for management purposes. The first group includes patients who have signs of an allergic reaction—for example, urticaria—but no respiratory distress or dyspnea. The drug of choice is diphenhydramine (Benadryl). Continue to monitor for changes in the patient's condition, but most patients in this group will recover with no further problems.

The second group includes patients who are not stable initially, are deteriorating, or have a history of deterioration. These are the patients with anaphylaxis or the potential to develop anaphylaxis.

Remove the offending agent. When possible, remove the patient from the situation involving the antigen or the antigen from the patient. For example, if the patient is allergic to peanuts and is being exposed to peanuts through inspiration, you may need to remove the patient from the room, because you may not be able to eliminate

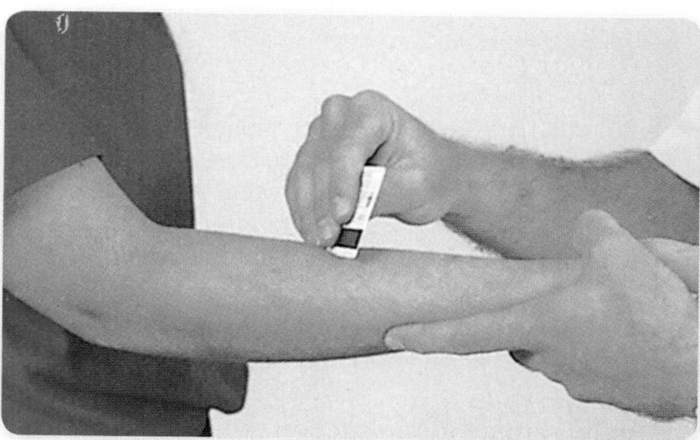

Figure 25-5 To remove the stinger of a honeybee, gently scrape the skin with the edge of a sharp, stiff object such as a credit card.

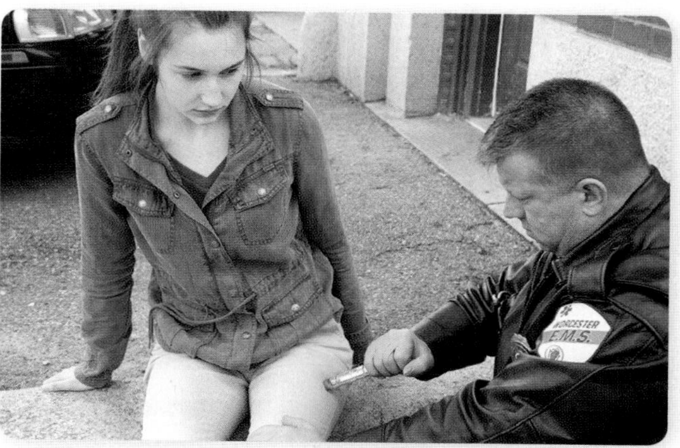

Figure 25-6 Administration of epinephrine with an auto-injector.

the peanut allergen from the air. If the patient has a stinger from a bee sting still in place, you need to remove the stinger. Remember to scrape the stinger off because you can inject more venom into the patient if you pinch or squeeze the stinger **Figure 25-5**.

Maintain the airway. The airway is always a priority in every situation. Be prepared to assist breathing as needed. Assessing for the presence of stridor and hoarseness should indicate the severity of the airway compromise. Be cautious in changing the position of an anaphylactic patient from a supine to an upright or standing position. Upright positions have been associated with an increased mortality rate.[17] Use an appropriate oxygen device for supplemental oxygen administration, and consider early transport. *Early administration of epinephrine should be a priority.*

Words of Wisdom

Intramuscular administration of epinephrine is preferred over subcutaneous administration of epinephrine because it provides more rapid absorption. Additionally, the anterolateral thigh site is preferred over the deltoid site for more rapid absorption. If the patient does not respond to IM administration, IV or intraosseous (IO) infusion of epinephrine is recommended.[20]

Administer epinephrine. IM administration of epinephrine in the anterolateral thigh is the drug and route of choice for anaphylaxis and must be considered early. Do not delay administration of epinephrine; delay is considered the major contributing factor to fatalities.[16] Many patients will require more than one dose of epinephrine to reverse the reaction. Additional IM doses may be repeated every 5 to 15 minutes as needed. If there is no response to the IM doses, an IV infusion of epinephrine should be administered in conjunction with an IV fluid bolus to support the hemodynamic status as needed. IV or IO boluses are only recommended if you are unable to quickly deliver infusions of epinephrine, for impending cardiovascular collapse, or if initial infusions are not effective. Endotracheal administration may be considered if other routes are not available.

Epinephrine is the drug of choice for anaphylactic reactions because it stops the process of mast cell degranulation. The action of epinephrine is immediate; it can rapidly reverse the effects of anaphylaxis. In addition, epinephrine reverses the effects of the chemical mediators released via degranulation. Its alpha-adrenergic properties cause the blood vessels to constrict, which reverses vasodilation and hypotension. This, in turn, elevates the diastolic pressure and improves coronary blood flow. The beta-1 adrenergic effects increase cardiac contractility, reversing the depressing effects on the heart and improving the strength of cardiac contractions. The beta-2 adrenergic effects cause bronchodilation, relieving bronchospasm in the lungs.

Many patients and EMTs carry epinephrine in the form of an EpiPen, and they may have administered a dose before your arrival. The patient may have taken other medications as well, so it is important to obtain a medication history. See the Appendix, *Emergency Medications*, for recommended epinephrine doses. The adult EpiPen delivers 0.3 mg of epinephrine intramuscularly and is used for patients approximately 66 pounds or greater (30 kg) **Figure 25-6**.[21] The EpiPen Jr, which delivers 0.15 mg of epinephrine, is used for children who weigh 33 to 66 pounds (15 to 30 kg).[21] Administration of epinephrine with an auto-injector involves firmly stabilizing the leg prior to and during administration (particularly in young children), pushing the auto-injector firmly against the anterolateral aspect of the thigh, and holding the injector in place for approximately 3 seconds until the medication is injected. This will reduce the chance of harm to the leg should the patient move his or her leg during the injection process.[21]

Evidence-Based Medicine

Take steps to ensure the patient's leg does not move during administration of epinephrine with an auto-injector. The injection time (the time the device is held against the leg) is 3 seconds, reduced from the formerly recommended 10 seconds. Both of these actions (the act of ensuring the patient's leg does not move, and the reduced injection time) are recommended to decrease the chance of patient harm during the administration process.[21]

Maintain circulation. Insert at least one 18-gauge IV catheter to administer an isotonic solution (lactated Ringer or normal saline). Ideally, you should place two IV lines en route to the emergency department. If IV access is not available, utilize IO access. This step is crucial, especially if the patient is hypotensive and does not respond to the epinephrine. Initially, administer 20 mL/kg of isotonic fluid (normal saline or lactated Ringer) rapidly over 15 minutes IV or IO, repeating as needed.[22] If there is no response, consider administering a vasopressor in conjunction with fluid administration. Take caution to avoid fluid overload, especially in the cardiac patient.

Initiate pharmacologic therapy. Administer high-flow oxygen, epinephrine, antihistamines, anti-inflammatory and immunosuppressant agents, and a vasopressor.

Special Populations

According to one source, "Complications associated with parenteral administration of epinephrine, other than IV administration are very rare."[17] Administering epinephrine to treat anaphylaxis has been associated with myocardial infarction and acute coronary syndrome. However, the incidence is infrequent, and it has been questioned whether the epinephrine contributed to the condition.[16]

There are mast cells in the human heart, and in the case of anaphylaxis, the mast cells cause coronary artery vasospasm and thus myocardial infarction. Still, there are no absolute contraindications to administration of epinephrine. This is true for older adult patients or patients with a cardiac history, so you need to weigh the risks and benefits of administration and consult medical control or local protocols. Epinephrine can stress the heart, so it is important to closely monitor patients for cardiac conditions or hypertension; however, it may not be a reason to delay or withhold epinephrine administration.

Controversies

Although there is no absolute contraindication to epinephrine administration, when you have a patient with cardiovascular disease, you must weigh the risks versus benefits when choosing to administer epinephrine. Usually the administration of epinephrine is indicated, but the patient must be monitored closely.

Antihistamine administration should be considered only in the patient with a mild reaction, or after epinephrine has been administered. Antihistamines block the histamine 1 (H_1) and histamine 2 (H_2) receptor sites. diphenhydramine (Benadryl) is commonly used in the prehospital setting following the administration of epinephrine. This medication does not prevent histamine release, but rather blocks histamine effects at the H_1 receptor sites. The typical dose of diphenhydramine (Benadryl) is 25 to 50 mg administered slowly via the IM or IV route. H_2 blockers such as cimetidine (Tagamet) and ranitidine (Zantac) are also indicated but are more commonly used in the hospital setting. It is recommended that H_1 and H_2 blockers be administered until the anaphylactic symptoms resolve.

Corticosteroids have been used for anaphylaxis. The time of onset after administration is 4 to 6 hours. Corticosteroid use may be indicated in select situations such as prevention of idiopathic reactions or recurrent anaphylactic reactions to radiocontrast media.

Inhaled beta-adrenergic agents such as albuterol (Ventolin) may also be included as part of the care regimen if bronchospasm is present. Many patients will benefit with the addition of albuterol in conjunction with the administration of epinephrine. Maintain a supine position for patients in anaphylaxis with hypotension. With respiratory distress, reassess the patient's lung sounds and consider slight elevation of the head, but avoid an upright position.

Emotional support is a crucial component of management. Anaphylaxis can progress rapidly and has the potential to be a life-threatening event. Patients and their families will need reassurance as you perform the necessary interventions. Many of the patients have experienced similar events and may recognize how serious their conditions have become. For others, this may be a first-time event. You need to be professional and reassuring and focus on early intervention and transport.

Initiate early transport if the patient needs resources beyond your capabilities. Even if you are able to stop the reaction and the patient begins to recover, it is recommended that patients be observed in a medical facility. As many as 20% of patients will have a recurrence of the symptoms within the next 8 hours, even if they have been free of symptoms for a time.[23] Once the patient has been symptom-free for 4 hours, he or she can be released from the facility but should be instructed to return or call an ambulance if the symptoms recur.

▶ Autoimmune Disorders and Collagen Vascular Diseases

In anaphylactic and allergic reactions, the body responds to a foreign invader as the enemy, but not so with autoimmune disorders. In an autoimmune disorder, the immune system inappropriately attacks its own host tissue. Many disorders and conditions are considered to be autoimmune, as listed in Table 25-5; those that are not discussed in this section are discussed in other chapters.

Collagen vascular diseases are considered autoimmune diseases, which means that the body perceives its own tissues or cells—in this case collagen tissue—as a dangerous invader and attacks that tissue. The attack can be chronic, causing long-term inflammation, or severe enough to result in death. The next sections address two collagen vascular diseases: systemic lupus erythematosus and scleroderma.

Systemic lupus erythematosus (SLE or lupus) is a multisystem autoimmune disease that occurs more commonly in women than in men. In the United States, it affects an estimated 1.5 million Americans.[24] African-American women are four times more likely to have lupus than Caucasian women, and Asian women also have a higher incidence of lupus than Caucasian women.[24] Lupus is most often diagnosed in young women, particularly young African-American women of childbearing age, and it can be a debilitating and life-threatening problem.[25] In

Table 25-5 Autoimmune Disorders and Conditions

- Addison disease
- Cardiomyopathy
- Celiac disease (also called *gluten-sensitive enteropathy* or *nontropical sprue*)
- Chronic active hepatitis
- Chronic persistent hepatitis
- Crohn disease
- Demyelinating neuropathies
- Endometriosis
- Glomerulonephritis
- Graves disease
- Guillain-Barré syndrome
- Hemolytic anemia
- Lyme disease
- Meniere disease
- Multiple sclerosis
- Myasthenia gravis
- Myositis
- Narcolepsy
- Neutropenia
- Peripheral neuropathy
- Psoriasis
- Raynaud phenomenon
- Restless legs syndrome
- Rheumatic fever
- Rheumatoid arthritis
- Thrombocytopenic purpura (TTP)
- Ulcerative colitis
- Scleroderma
- Systemic lupus erythematosus
- Type 1 diabetes mellitus
- Vasculitis

Data from: Autoimmune and Autoimmune-related diseases. American Autoimmune Related Diseases Association website. https://www.aarda.org/autoimmune-information/list-of-diseases/. Accessed April 7, 2017.

YOU are the Paramedic PART 4

The patient indicates his breathing is slightly better. The PA recommends another dose of epinephrine, either via IV push or infusion. You agree that additional epinephrine may be indicated if there has been no improvement in the blood pressure after administering a fluid bolus of 20 mL/kg. You agree to initiate an epinephrine infusion en route if needed. The patient stabilizes.

Recording Time: 10 Minutes	
Respirations	20 breaths/min. Wheezes continue.
Pulse	126 beats/min
Skin	Urticaria on upper body and arms resolving, warm, dry
Blood pressure	122/76 mm Hg
Oxygen saturation (Spo_2)	98% on oxygen via NRM
Pupils	PERRLA

10. If the patient deteriorates, how would you mix and administer the epinephrine drip?

lupus, multiple systems are under attack—dermatologic, renal, neurologic, cardiac, pulmonary, gastrointestinal, and hematologic—and the disease may also result in rheumatologic problems. Patients with lupus tend to die of infections and complications of the disease or as the result of a cardiovascular disease, pulmonary hypertension, and renal failure.[25] You should assess for these life threats when caring for patients with lupus.

Scleroderma (*sclero* meaning hard and *derma* meaning skin) is an autoimmune connective tissue disease that causes fibrotic (scar tissue–like) changes to the skin, blood vessels, muscles, and internal organs. Women have a higher incidence of scleroderma than do men.[26] The life-threatening complications of scleroderma involve the lungs, heart, and kidneys, so assessment should focus on these systems.

Pathophysiology

Systemic Lupus Erythematosus. Systemic lupus erythematosus should be suspected in women of childbearing age who present with fever, rash, and joint pain. It is not your job to diagnose lupus, but awareness of the signs, symptoms, and life threats associated with lupus are important. Lupus is a multisystem autoimmune disease, and the effects on the various body systems are outlined in Table 25-6.

Lupus affects the entire body. The priority of care should be directed at monitoring for life threats should the patient present with any change in his or her normal presentation. Because these patients may be on medications to suppress their immune system, slight changes such as fever, cough, or an increase in pain should alert you to be prepared to treat these patients aggressively as their conditions warrant.

Scleroderma. Patients with scleroderma present with tightening, thickening, and scarring of the skin. Patients will often have symptoms of Raynaud phenomenon (pain, blanching, cyanosis or redness of the fingers and toes when stress occurs or when exposed to the cold). Pulmonary presentations are due to the stiffness of the lungs and blood vessels resulting in pulmonary fibrosis and pulmonary hypertension. Renal damage from scleroderma may result in hypertension and renal crisis. One of the major complications of scleroderma is damage to the heart muscle. Assessment for dysrhythmias, palpitations, and heart failure is a priority when caring for these patients. Pulmonary complications are the most common cause of death in scleroderma patients. Renal crisis is a major concern as well.[26]

Assessment

Assessment of patients with lupus or scleroderma should focus on ruling out life threats. These patients may have extensive multisystem problems, so avoid attributing their complaints to their chronic conditions until life threats can be ruled out.

Management

With lupus and scleroderma, the patient's condition stems from the body attacking itself because of an overactive immune system. Treatment may include the administration of medications to *suppress* the immune system and decrease the attack.

Management should be directed at treating any life threats. Monitor patients for signs of infection. Because each patient may present with different system involvement, you will need to determine the patient's care according to the affected system.

▶ Organ Transplant Disorders

Pathophysiology

When a patient's organs are severely damaged, a transplant may be performed. The problem with a transplant is that the body sees the replacement organ as foreign, and even though the body could not survive without the new organ, the immune system will work to eliminate or "reject" the organ. To prevent the rejection, patients are placed on medications that prevent the immune system from attacking the new organs. These medications, however, place the person at greater risk for infection. The medications cause the body's self-defense mechanism to either not recognize other threats or to shut down portions of its function, putting them at risk for infection and/or sepsis.

As a paramedic, you will encounter patients who have undergone organ transplants. The organs most likely transplanted include the heart, liver, kidney, pancreas, and lungs. As you care for these patients, it is important to address the priorities in caring for the specific organ that has been transplanted.

Heart Transplant. Approximately 2,000 heart transplants are performed in the United States each year.[27] In the most common procedure used, the recipient's heart is removed and replaced by the donor heart. On the ECG, you may notice an increase in heart rate or a tachycardia at the rate of 100 to 110 beats/min due to denervation of the vagus nerve. Chest pain is uncommon because the denervated heart cannot generate angina-like pain. Therefore, a patient with ischemia tends to present with signs of heart failure or dysrhythmias rather than angina. Atropine is not indicated for bradycardia or heart blocks (a delay or disruption of the normal electrical signals that cause the heart to beat). Because the implanted heart does not have vagus nerve innervation, the heart would not respond to the vagolytic action of atropine. Sympathomimetic drugs tend to work well for heart transplant patients. If hypertension occurs, antihypertensive medications tend to work even in crisis situations. Norepinephrine and isoproterenol (Isuprel) may have a slightly increased response in heart transplant patients.

The majority of rejections occur in the first 3 months post transplant.[28] Fifty to eighty percent of patients will

Table 25-6 Signs, Symptoms, and Prehospital Implications of Lupus		
System	**Signs and Symptoms**	**Prehospital Implications**
Cutaneous	▪ Rash that is aggravated by sunlight ▪ Butterfly-like rash across the cheeks and nose ▪ Sores or lesions in the mouth ▪ Hair loss ▪ Bruising	▪ Patients are sensitive to the sun; protect them from prolonged exposure to the sun.
Musculoskeletal	▪ Joint pain and swelling ▪ Muscle aches and pain ▪ Inflammation of the hands causing symmetric hand pain ▪ Lesions on the extremities that result in gangrene	▪ Do not let the complaints of joint and muscle pain distract you from assessing for a life threat. ▪ Assess potential for infection.
Pleural	▪ Pleurisy, pleural effusions, or pleural rub ▪ Pulmonary hemorrhage with hemoptysis ▪ Pneumonia ▪ Pulmonary emboli ▪ Pulmonary hypertension	▪ Assess for any of these conditions if a patient reports fever, tachypnea, cough, or worsening of chest pain.
Pericardial	▪ Pericarditis (most common) ▪ Myocardial infarction ▪ Pericardial effusion ▪ Hypertension ▪ Endocarditis ▪ Myocarditis ▪ Vasculitis ▪ Valvular heart disease	▪ Obtain a 12-lead ECG and assess for signs of pericarditis or ischemia. ▪ Patients with lupus have an increased risk of AMI and post-AMI mortality.
Neurologic	▪ Stroke ▪ Seizures ▪ Behavioral changes ▪ Psychosis ▪ Migraines ▪ Peripheral neuropathies ▪ Meningitis	▪ Monitor for stroke and initiate seizure precautions when neurologic symptoms are present.
Renal	▪ Nephritis ▪ Proteinuria ▪ Renal failure that may require dialysis ▪ Urinary tract infection ▪ Fluid and electrolyte imbalance ▪ Edema	▪ Assess for history of renal failure and electrolyte imbalance. ▪ Assess for urinary tract infections.
Hematologic	▪ Anemia ▪ Decreased white blood cell count ▪ Thrombocytopenia	▪ Recognize potential for hypoxia due to anemia, risk for infection and bleeding (usually not severe).
Gastrointestinal	▪ Oral ulcers ▪ Abdominal cramping ▪ Pseudo-obstruction ▪ Pancreatitis ▪ Vasculitis that may result in perforation ▪ Gangrene and peritonitis	▪ Collect a history to include bloody stools. ▪ Maintain a high index of suspicion.

Abbreviations: ECG, electrocardiogram; AMI, acute myocardial infarction

Data from: Lin C-Y, Shih C-C, Yeh C-C, et al. Increased risk of acute myocardial infarction and mortality in patients with systemic lupus erythematosus: two nationwide retrospective cohort studies, *Intl J Cardiology*, 2014;176(3):847-851.

experience one episode of rejection, but additional episodes are possible.[28] The signs and symptoms may be subtle and require a biopsy for confirmation. Dysrhythmias have also been associated with rejection. Common problems include sepsis and pneumonia. Paramedics should assess for fever, shortness of breath, hypoxia, hypotension pressure, poorly controlled hypertension, or the development of a new dysrhythmia, as these are indicators of infection.

Liver Transplant. Liver transplants are the second most common solid organ procedure. If rejection occurs, the loss of function results in rapid deterioration of the patient and possibly death. Infection, in particular opportunistic infection, is a problem for liver transplant patients. Observe for jaundice and palpate for tenderness over the site. Patients may present with symptoms that are anywhere from vague to full fulminate hepatic failure. Monitor for hyperkalemia caused by immunosuppressive drugs.

Kidney Transplant. Kidney transplants are the most common type of transplant in the United States and are extremely successful. Infection is one of the major concerns for these patients as with all transplants. These patients also have a tendency to develop hepatitis C and later liver disease. Rejection of the graft presents as fever, with tenderness and swelling over the implanted kidney, which is located in the anterior area of the retroperitoneal pelvis. Monitor for hypovolemia because hypotension is a common complication. Up to 50% of these patients have hypertension, so ask about their normal blood pressure as part of your assessment.[29] When dealing with a renal transplant patient, it is important to understand that many of these patients are extremely knowledgeable about their condition and can provide you with valuable information. Your assessment should include observation of the site for infection, auscultation for the development of a bruit, and evaluation for other signs of infection. Ask whether the patient has had the spleen removed, because this increases the risk for infection progressing more rapidly.

Lung Transplant. Lung transplants are performed alone or in conjunction with a heart transplant. Three types of lung transplants are performed: bilateral, unilateral, and lobar. In the case of single-lung transplants, unequal breath sounds are a common finding. Adhesions may be present that may complicate the placement of the chest tube on the side of the lung transplant. Hemothorax is an early complication of lung transplant. Signs of rejection include cough, dyspnea, vomiting, fever, crackles, rhonchi, and a decrease in oxygenation. Infection presents similar to the signs of rejection and requires immediate intervention.

Pancreas Transplant. Pancreas transplants have a high rate of complications and a lower survival rate than the other single-organ transplants at 1 year. Most pancreas transplants are for diabetic patients and are often performed along with kidney transplants. The pancreas has an exocrine function, so a route to drain the exocrine component must be placed. The secretions may be drained into the intestine or the bladder. When drained into the bladder, monitor for urinary tract signs and symptoms such as infections and hematuria. In addition, these patients have a chronic non-anion gap acidosis because the bicarbonate the pancreas produces is drained directly into the bladder for excretion. Remember this when evaluating the patient and the patient's arterial blood gases, to avoid confusing it with lactic acidosis. These patients take oral bicarbonate supplements. Assess for compliance with these medications, as well as other medications. They are also at risk for dehydration and may present with orthostatic hypotension. Infection and rejection are common problems for patients with pancreas transplants.

Assessment

Assessment of the patient who has had an organ transplant requires an awareness of subtle signs and symptoms. Keep a high index of suspicion for infection and rejection. Signs and symptoms of organ rejection vary depending on the organ; for example, rejection of a transplanted kidney may cause the patient to excrete less urine. Patients who are experiencing organ transplant rejection will usually have general discomfort and feel ill. Remember that if a transplant patient calls for EMS, the condition is usually serious. Consider contacting the patient's transplant center if you have any questions regarding the assessment or findings in these patients. Monitor the cardiac rhythm for indications of hyperkalemia caused by the antirejection drugs and for dysrhythmias in general, particularly in the heart transplant patient.

Management

The priorities of care for transplant patients are focused on the organ transplanted, the medications, recognition of infection or rejection, and transport to the most appropriate facility. Care for patients with transplants varies depending on the organ that is transplanted. It is therefore essential that you familiarize yourself with the priorities of patient care with each type of transplant. Before you administer medication, make sure you know how the medication will interact with the medications the patient is taking and how the medication will be metabolized to ensure that toxicity will not develop. Because patients who have undergone transplants may be immunosuppressed, monitor them for signs and symptoms of infection or organ rejection. Remember, missing even one dose of their immunosuppressive medications is an emergency. Finally, consider transporting the patient to a transplant facility when possible, or consulting the facility about care when transport to the facility is not possible.

Patients who have had organ transplants receive immunosuppressant medications. Suppression of the immune system is key to the survival of these patients. Solid organ transplants include the heart, liver, kidney, pancreas, and lungs. No matter what type of transplant the patient has received, you must understand the anatomic considerations, and you must be prepared to identify signs of rejection, infection, and medication toxicity.

When the body receives a new organ, the organ comes without its previous connections and message-relaying ability. This means that the organ may not behave "normally" when it is having problems. Pain is a symptom; however, the organ cannot relay this information to its new host, so pain, such as angina, is not as reliable an indicator of problems as it may be normally. In addition, the new organs will be tethered to the structures in the body such as blood vessels, other organs, and tissues. Knowing where and how an organ is placed and attached may also be useful in identifying problems.

With any organ transplant, infection is the greatest threat to survival, so you must be constantly alert of the potential for infection. Rejection of the organ immediately after the surgery is less common than in the past because of improved donor-recipient matching. It is essential that patients take their immunosuppressant medications. The failure to take even one dose may result in rejection of the organ. Drug toxicity is also a problem for transplant patients.

Patient Education

Anaphylaxis

The best management of anaphylaxis and allergic reactions is to educate patients about prevention and self-preservation. At a minimum, discuss the following topics:

- **Avoid the antigen.** Review information on the offending item. For example, if the patient is allergic to penicillin, he or she should be provided with a list of drugs that include penicillin and the alternative names for penicillin. Drugs that may produce a cross-reaction should also be discussed. Remind patients that remaining at the facility for monitoring for at least 30 minutes or longer is indicated for parenterally administered medications. Food allergies can be even more difficult to avoid. Peanuts are an example of a food that may be a problem. Peanut oil may be used to prepare foods that do not actually contain peanuts, and peanut butter may be an ingredient in various foods. Some patients are so allergic to peanuts that just using the same devices to process non–peanut-containing foods can cause a reaction. Patients must be educated to avoid the allergen, read labels, and ask about how food is prepared to avoid exposure. When traveling outside of the United States, do not assume food standards are the same. Latex allergies are also a concern, so advising patients to notify care providers of latex allergies is essential. Many services are latex-free, but not all of them, so patients must inform providers of their allergies so exposures can be avoided.
- **Notify all health personnel of the allergy.** Review the need to alert health personnel to the allergy. This is important because people often think only a physician would need this information, not an EMS provider.
- **Wear identification tags or bracelets.** These items notify health care providers of allergies in case the patient is unable to do so.
- **Carry an anaphylaxis kit.** A reaction may happen rapidly or worsen before help can arrive. Many anaphylactic reactions require more than one dose of epinephrine, so patients should consider carrying two kits or a kit with more than one dose. Make sure the patients and their families know how to use the kit.
- **Report symptoms early.** Ideally, intervention should begin before the situation becomes life threatening. The patient should recognize that reactions can occur more rapidly and with greater severity with repeated exposures. Additionally, remind patients that the severity of the previous incident may not predict the severity of the next incident.
- **Biphasic reactions.** Explain to patients that they may develop a biphasic reaction, so monitoring for up to 4 to 8 hours after an anaphylactic incident is recommended.

Collagen Vascular Diseases

Education for patients with collagen vascular diseases should include the following topics:

- **Encourage self-monitoring.** Encourage patients to monitor themselves for signs of infection and take these signs seriously.
- **Consult a physician before taking a new medication.** Emphasize the fact that patients should not take any new medications without consulting their physician.
- **Comply with the immunosuppressive regimen.** Encourage patients to always take their oral dose of immunosuppressive medications. Missing even one dose is an emergency; their physician or contact should be notified if this occurs.
- **Know the signs of life-threatening concerns.** Advise patients of signs and symptoms that may be life threatening. Emphasize signs and symptoms of pulmonary, cardiac, and neurologic presentations as well as signs of infection.

Organ Transplants

Education for patients with organ transplants should include the following topics:

- **Encourage self-monitoring.** Encourage patients to monitor themselves for signs of infection or rejection and take these signs seriously.

- **Consult a physician before taking a new medication.** Emphasize the fact that patients should not take any new medications without consulting their physician.
- **Comply with the immunosuppressive regimen.** Encourage patients to always take their oral dose of immunosuppressive medications. Missing even one dose is an emergency; their physician or contact should be notified if this occurs.
- **Know who to contact.** Patients should know to call the transplant facility to seek prehospital care, as directed by their physician or transplant contact. If traveling, encourage patients to know how to contact a transplant center where they will be traveling.

YOU are the Paramedic SUMMARY

1. What is your first impression of this patient?

Looking at the patient can give you an indication of the severity of the problem. In this situation, the patient has been having trouble speaking, and although he is responsive, he is not following you with his eyes. This suggests that his level of consciousness is beginning to decrease.

2. Do you need to take any immediate actions?

Due to the swelling of the patient's lips, the recent receipt of an antibiotic, and the change in level of consciousness, you need to act quickly to address possible airway compromise and determine the cause of this patient's condition. Because he just received an antibiotic, is older, and is African-American, anaphylaxis is a concern as drug-related anaphylactic reactions occur at a higher incidence in this population.

3. What differential diagnoses are you considering?

Besides anaphylaxis, you should also consider angioedema because he is on an ACE inhibitor. The difficulty speaking should make you evaluate this patient for a possible stroke, and cardiac issues altering his level of consciousness cannot be ruled out because he is older and has a history of hypertension.

4. Can this be an allergic reaction if the patient has not had a previous reaction?

Yes, although patients may need to be sensitized to the allergen before an anaphylactic reaction will occur, in some cases of anaphylaxis or anaphylactoid reactions, previous sensitization may not be present.

5. What are the implications of a history of hypertension and taking an ACE inhibitor for this case?

The swelling of the patient's lips and possible angioedema due to ACE inhibitor ingestion are a concern; however, this appears to be an anaphylactic issue and care should be focused on anaphylaxis treatment. This patient will need close cardiac monitoring due to concerns about his cardiovascular history.

6. Was the administration route and dose of epinephrine appropriate, and should you allow them to administer a second dose? Defend your decision.

The intramuscular route into the lateral thigh is the recommended route for initial epinephrine administration. The benefits are rapid access and rapid and more reliable absorption.

7. Are there concerns with allowing this patient to sit upright, and would you position the patient in an upright position?

Yes, an increase in mortality has occurred in patients who have been moved to an upright position. Sitting patients upright or standing patients in anaphylaxis is not recommended. The supine position is the position of choice, but slight elevation of the head for ventilation may be considered.

8. What effect can you expect the albuterol to have on this patient?

The beta-2 effect of the albuterol decreases the bronchospasm in most patients and typically relieves respiratory distress. It does not affect the angioedema or hypotension, so epinephrine administration is still indicated.

9. What type of fluid should you administer, and how much fluid is indicated? Are there any concerns with fluid administration for this patient?

This patient should receive an isotonic crystalloid. A bolus of 20 mL/kg should be administered to address the hypotension. Due to this patient's possible cardiovascular history, close monitoring for possible fluid overload is necessary especially if additional fluids are needed. If necessary, administering epinephrine via IV infusion is

YOU are the Paramedic SUMMARY (continued)

preferred. Intravenous bolus administration is associated with dysrhythmias, which may be a concern for this patient. The patient was beginning to improve and you had time to mix the infusion, so the infusion was preferred over the bolus, but close cardiac monitoring is still necessary due to his history.

10. If the patient deteriorates, how would you mix and administer the epinephrine drip?

The infusion or drip would be prepared by adding 1 mg/1 mL (1:1,000) epinephrine concentration to 1,000 mL of D_5W or normal saline. This produces a 1 mcg/mL concentration.

<table>
<tr><th colspan="6">EMS Patient Care Report (PCR)</th></tr>
<tr><td>Date: 06-30-18</td><td colspan="2">Incident No.: 4563</td><td colspan="2">Nature of Call: Altered mental status</td><td>Location: Main Street Clinic, 100 N. Main Street</td></tr>
<tr><td>Dispatched: 1810</td><td>En Route: 1810</td><td>At Scene: 1818</td><td>Transport: 1832</td><td>At Hospital: 1841</td><td>In Service: 1856</td></tr>
<tr><th colspan="6">Patient Information</th></tr>
<tr><td colspan="3">Age: 70
Sex: M
Weight (in kg [lb]): 78 kg (172 lb)</td><td colspan="3">Allergies: Aspirin
Medications: ACE inhibitor
Past Medical History: Hypertension, upper airway infection
Chief Complaint: Altered mental status with difficulty speaking</td></tr>
<tr><th colspan="6">Vital Signs</th></tr>
<tr><td>Time: 1823</td><td>BP: 90/58</td><td>Pulse: 120</td><td>Respirations: 26</td><td colspan="2">Spo₂: 92% on room air</td></tr>
<tr><td>Time: 1828</td><td>BP: 122/76</td><td>Pulse: 126</td><td>Respirations: 20</td><td colspan="2">Spo₂: 98% O₂</td></tr>
<tr><td>Time:</td><td>BP:</td><td>Pulse:</td><td>Respirations:</td><td colspan="2">Spo₂:</td></tr>
<tr><th colspan="6">EMS Treatment (circle all that apply)</th></tr>
<tr><td colspan="2">Oxygen @ 15 L/min via (circle one):
NC (NRM) Bag-mask device</td><td>Assisted Ventilation</td><td>Airway Adjunct</td><td colspan="2">CPR</td></tr>
<tr><td>Defibrillation</td><td>Bleeding Control</td><td>Bandaging</td><td>Splinting</td><td colspan="2">Other:</td></tr>
<tr><th colspan="6">Narrative</th></tr>
<tr><td colspan="6">Arrived at the Main Street Clinic for a reported altered mental status. Upon arrival, we found a 70-year-old man lying on an exam table with his head slightly elevated. PA, nurse and pt's wife are present. The medical personnel report the pt was being seen for an upper respiratory infection and bronchitis, and was administered penicillin and albuterol. During his observation period, he started to have difficulty speaking and his LOC changed. The patient is allergic to aspirin, but no other known allergies. He takes an ACE inhibitor for hypertension. The staff administered 0.3 mg of epinephrine intramuscularly. Attached pt to cardiac monitor which shows sinus tachycardia. The pt has edema around the lips and does not respond to verbal stimuli. His skin was warm and dry initially and then developed urticaria. Wheezing presented but began to reverse after a second dose of epinephrine 0.3 mg IM. Patient's mental status improved and he reported improved breathing. Albuterol nebulizer was administered with an improvement in respiratory status. Wheezing continued. IV with an 18-gauge catheter in the left forearm was obtained and a 20 mL/kg fluid bolus of normal saline was administered en route. Continued improvement noted until arrival at ED. Report to Dr. Morrison on arrival.**End of report**</td></tr>
</table>

Prep Kit

▶ Ready for Review

- An antigen is a substance the body recognizes as foreign. This recognition causes the body to produce antibodies to destroy the foreign substance.
- The immune system protects the human body from substances and organisms that are considered foreign.
- An allergic response occurs when the body produces an antigen–antibody reaction when exposed to a substance that is usually harmless. An allergic response is usually limited to one body system or a local area.
- Hypersensitivity occurs when a person's immune system reacts with exaggerated or inappropriate symptoms after coming into contact with a substance perceived by the body to be harmful. Hypersensitivity is typically divided into four types: allergic reaction, anaphylaxis, biphasic reaction, and prolonged (persistent) reactions.
- Most often a person has been sensitized to an antigen before an allergic or anaphylactic reaction occurs; however, patients may present with anaphylaxis without prior exposure.
- Anaphylaxis is an extreme form of systemic allergic response typically involving two or more body systems. However it may present in a single system, such as respiratory.
- An anaphylactoid reaction may occur without the patient being previously exposed to the offending agent.
- The routes of exposure to an antigen include injection, absorption, inhalation, and ingestion.
- Assess for nontraditional causes of anaphylaxis, such as seminal fluid exposure, exercise induced, or idiopathic.
- Mast cells release chemical mediators to stimulate the allergic reaction.
- Chemical mediators produce signs and symptoms through their effects on the skin, cardiovascular, respiratory, neurologic, and gastrointestinal systems.
- Skin effects include erythema, urticaria, and pruritus. Cyanosis and pallor may also be present.
- Cardiovascular effects include vasodilation, hypotension, decreased cardiac output, cardiac ischemia, and dysrhythmias.
- Respiratory effects include upper airway edema and stridor, hoarseness, bronchoconstriction, increased bronchial secretions, wheezes, and hypoxia.
- Neurologic symptoms include syncope, altered level of consciousness, anxiety, restlessness, combativeness, and unresponsiveness.
- Gastrointestinal symptoms include nausea, vomiting, diarrhea, and cramping.
- As part of your assessment, you should evaluate the scene, patient history, level of consciousness, upper airway, lower airway, skin, and vital signs.
- Treatment of anaphylaxis includes removing the offending agent; maintaining the airway; administering medications such as epinephrine, antihistamines (diphenhydramine, cimetidine, ranitidine), corticosteroids, inhaled beta-adrenergic agents, and vasopressors; resuscitating with IV fluids; and initiating rapid transport.
- Intramuscular epinephrine is first-line drug therapy for anaphylaxis.
- Patient education to prevent reexposure, to understand symptoms, and to understand the need to use an anaphylaxis kit is essential.
- Collagen vascular diseases and other autoimmune diseases may require treatment that involves administering medications to suppress the immune system and decrease the attack.
- Organ transplant disorders can present a multitude of problems in patients. It is important to know the treatment priorities when you care for patients who have undergone organ transplants.

▶ Vital Vocabulary

absorption In allergic reactions, when foreign material is deposited on and moves into the skin.

allergen A substance that produces allergic symptoms in a patient.

allergic reaction An abnormal immune response the body develops when reexposed to a substance or allergen.

anaphylactoid reaction An extreme allergic response that does not involve IgE antibody mediation. The exact mechanism is unknown, but an event of this type may occur without the patient being previously exposed to the offending agent.

anaphylaxis An extreme systemic form of an allergic reaction involving one, two, or more body systems.

antibody A protein the body produces in response to an antigen; an immunoglobulin.

antigen An agent that, when taken into the body, stimulates the formation of specific protective proteins called antibodies.

Prep Kit *(continued)*

basophils White blood cells that work to produce chemical mediators during an immune response.

biphasic reaction A two-phase allergic reaction in which the patient's symptoms improve and then reappear without being exposed to the trigger (allergen) a second time; the symptoms can resurface up to 8 or more hours after the initial incident.

chemical mediators Chemicals that work to cause the immune or allergic response; for example, histamine.

collagen vascular diseases A group of autoimmune disorders that affect the collagen in tendons, bones, and connective tissues.

histamine A chemical found in mast cells that, when released, causes vasodilation, capillary leaking, and bronchiole constriction.

hypersensitivity Occurs when a patient reacts with exaggerated or inappropriate allergic symptoms after coming into contact with a substance the body perceives as harmful.

ingestion Eating or drinking materials for absorption through the gastrointestinal tract.

inhalation In allergic reactions, foreign substances are breathed in through the respiratory system.

injection In allergic reactions, when the skin is pierced, and foreign material is deposited into the skin.

local reaction When the body limits a response to a specific area after being exposed to a foreign substance.

mast cells Basophils that are located in the tissues.

primary response The first encounter with the foreign substance to begin the immune response.

prolonged (persistent) reaction Anaphylaxis symptoms that continue over time, with time frames anywhere from 5 to 32 hours.

pruritus Itching.

scleroderma An autoimmune connective tissue disease that causes fibrotic (scar tissue–like) changes to the skin, blood vessels, muscles, and internal organs.

secondary response The body's reaction when it is exposed to an antigen for which it already has antibodies, in which it responds by killing the invading substance.

sensitivity The ability to recognize a foreign substance the next time it is encountered.

systemic lupus erythematosus A multisystem autoimmune disease.

systemic reaction A reaction that occurs throughout the body, possibly affecting multiple body systems.

urticaria Hives or reddened elevated patches on the skin.

▶ References

1. Wood RA, Camargo CA, Lieberman P, et al. Anaphylaxis in America: the prevalence and characteristics of anaphylaxis in the United States. *J Allergy Clin Immunol.* 2014;133(2)461-467.
2. Lin RY, Anderson AS, Shah SN, et al. Increasing anaphylaxis hospitalizations in the first 2 decades of life: New York State, 1990-2006. *Ann Allergy Asthma Immunol.* 2008;101(4):387-393.
3. Mulla ZD, Lin RY, Simon MR. Perspectives on anaphylaxis epidemiology in the United States with new data and analyses. *Curr Allergy Asthma Rep.* 2001;11(1):37-44.
4. Jerschow E, Lin RY, Scaperotti MM, et al. Fatal anaphylaxis in the United States, 1999-2010: temporal patterns and demographic associations. *J Allergy Clin Immunol.* 2014;134(6):1318-1328.
5. Mustafa S. Anaphylaxis. Medscape website. http://emedicine.medscape.com/article/135065-overview#a4. Updated February 22, 2017. Accessed March 31, 2017.
6. Grunau BE, Li J, Stenstrom R, et al. Incidence of clinically important biphasic reactions in emergency department patients with allergic reactions or anaphylaxis. *Ann Emerg Med.* 2014;63(6):736-744.
7. Tole JW, Lieberman P. Biphasic anaphylaxis: review of incidence, clinical predictors, and observation recommendations. *Immunol Allergy Clin North Am.* 2007;27(2):309-326.
8. Scranton SE, Gonzalez EG, Waibel KH. Incidence and characteristics of biphasic reactions after allergen immunotherapy. *J Allergy Clin Immunol.* 2009;123(2):493-498.
9. Johnson RF, Peebles RS. Anaphylactic shock: pathophysiology, recognition, and treatment. Medscape website. http://www.medscape.com/viewarticle/497498_8. Accessed April 4, 2017.
10. Bernstein DI. Allergic reactions to seminal plasma. UpToDate website. http://www.uptodate.com/contents/allergic-reactions-to-seminal-plasma. Updated December 9, 2015. Accessed April 1, 2017.

Prep Kit *(continued)*

11. Allergy facts and figures. Asthma and Allergy Foundation website. http://www.aafa.org/page/allergy-facts.aspx. Accessed April 5, 2017.
12. Hsieh F. Anaphylaxis. Cleveland Clinic Center for Continuing Education website. Published December 2013. Accessed April 4, 2017.
13. Peroni DG, Sansotta N, Bernardini R, et al. Muscle relaxants allergy. *Int J Immunopathol Pharmacol.* 2011;24(suppl 3):S35-46.
14. Dosanjh A. Infant anaphylaxis: the importance of early recognition. *J Asthma Allergy*. 2013; 6:103-107.
15. Alonso T, Moro Moro M, García M. Epidemiology of anaphylaxis. *Clin Exp Allergy*. 2015;45(6): 1027-1039.
16. Lieberman P, Nicklas RA, Randolph C, et al. Anaphylaxis—a practice parameter update 2015. *Ann Allergy Asthma Immunol.* 2015;115:348. https://www.aaaai.org/Aaaai/media/MediaLibrary/PDF%20Documents/Practice%20and%20Parameters/2015-Anaphylaxis-PP-Update.pdf. Accessed January 30, 2017.
17. Campbell RL, Li JT, Nicklas RA, et al. Emergency department diagnosis and treatment of anaphylaxis: a practice parameter. *Ann Allergy Asthma Immunol.* 2014;113:603.
18. Kaplan MS. Anaphylaxis. *Perm J.* 2007;11(3):53-56.
19. Sica DA, Black HR. ACE inhibitor-related angioedema: can angiotensin-receptor blockers be safely used? MedScape website. http://www.medscape.com/viewarticle/443226. Accessed April 7, 2017.
20. Campbell RL, Li JT, Nicklas RA, et al. Emergency department diagnosis and treatment of anaphylaxis: a practice parameter. *Ann Allergy Asthma Immunol.* 2014;113:602.
21. EPIPEN – epinephrine injection, EPIPEN JR – epinephrine injection. DailyMed U.S. National Library of Medicine website. https://dailymed.nlm.nih.gov/dailymed/fda/fdaDrugXsl.cfm?setid=7560c201-9246-487c-a13b-6295db04274a&type=display. Revised May 2016. Accessed April 5, 2017.
22. National Model EMS Clinical Guidelines. National Association of State EMS Officials. V.08-16:49-52. https://www.nasemso.org/Projects/ModelEMSClinicalGuidelines/index.asp. Revised September 15, 2014. Accessed April 7, 2017.
23. Campbell RL, Li JT, Nicklas RA, et al. Emergency department diagnosis and treatment of anaphylaxis: a practice parameter. *Ann Allergy Asthma Immunol.* 2014;113:606.
24. Lupus facts and statistics. Lupus Foundation of American website. http://www.resources.lupus.org/entry/facts-and-statistics. Accessed April 5, 2017.
25. Lupus detailed fact sheet. Centers for Disease Control and Prevention website. https://www.cdc.gov/lupus/facts/detailed.html. Updated January 30, 2017. Accessed April 5, 2017.
26. Jimenez SA. Scleroderma. Medscape website. http://emedicine.medscape.com/article/331864-overview#a5. Updated November 22, 2016. Accessed April 5, 2017.
27. Everly MJ. Cardiac transplantation in the United States: an analysis of the UNOS registry. *Clin Transpl.* 2008:35-43.
28. Eisen HJ. Patient education: Heart transplantation (Beyond the Basics). UpToDate website. https://www.uptodate.com/contents/heart-transplantation-beyond-the-basics. Updated February 16, 2016. Accessed April 5, 2017.
29. Kaufman DB. Assessment and management of the renal transplant patient. Medscape website. http://emedicine.medscape.com/article/429314-overview#a1. Updated July 21, 2015. Accessed January 23, 2017.

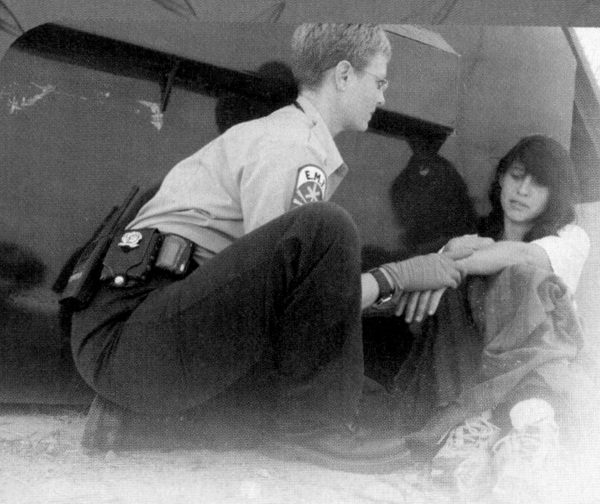

Assessment *in Action*

Your unit is dispatched to an apartment building. Dispatch tells you the patient is 48 years old and is having difficulty breathing. When you arrive on the scene, the patient has slightly labored breathing and informs you she has a history of lupus. It is a cold, windy day outside.

1. What type of disease is systemic lupus erythematosus (SLE)?

A. Cardiac
B. Endocrine
C. Autoimmune
D. Respiratory

2. Which of the following is a common finding in the early diagnosis of lupus?

A. Tightening of the skin
B. Butterfly rash to the face
C. Cardiac dysrhythmias
D. Bronchospasms

3. As you assess the patient, she tells you she has problems with her joints. Which of the following joint problems would you anticipate in a patient with lupus?

A. Immobility and rigidity
B. Joints that easily dislocate
C. Pain and swelling
D. Rash and redness over the joints

4. As you move this patient to the ambulance you notice her fingers are turning blue and she tells you they are very painful. Which of the following is most likely the cause of her complaint?

A. Her respiratory condition is worsening.
B. She developed a pulmonary embolism.
C. She has Raynaud phenomenon.
D. Her cardiovascular status is unstable.

5. What actions are most likely indicated for this patient?

A. Administer high-flow oxygen.
B. Place her hands under a blanket.
C. Administer corticosteroids and pain medication.
D. Reassure her and initiate rapid transport.

6. As you collect a history, which of the following medication classes would you anticipate this patient is taking?

A. Bronchodilators, steroids, cough suppressants
B. Beta-blockers, ACE inhibitors, diuretics
C. Narcotics, cholinergics, anticoagulants
D. Steroids, NSAIDs, and immunosuppressants

7. You auscultate the lungs and obtain a pulse oximetry reading. Which of the following should be the next priority in your assessment?

A. Collect a thorough history regarding any recent bleeding.
B. Question her regarding her urine output and the color of the urine.
C. Obtain a blood glucose level and ask about recent seizure history.
D. Place her on a cardiac monitor and obtain a 12-lead ECG.

Assessment in Action (continued)

8. As you are completing your assessment, you notice this patient has small bruises in various stages of healing. Which of the following is most likely the cause?

A. The lupus is affecting her platelets.
B. She takes an anticoagulant.
C. The lupus is affecting her liver.
D. She is the victim of abuse.

9. Why are immunosuppressant drugs prescribed to patients who already have a malfunctioning immune system?

10. Which life threats are most common in the patient with SLE and what is the implication for EMS providers?

CHAPTER 26

Infectious Diseases

National EMS Education Standard Competencies

Medicine

Integrates assessment findings with principles of epidemiology and pathophysiology to formulate a field impression and implement a comprehensive treatment/disposition plan for a patient with a medical complaint.

Infectious Diseases

Awareness, assessment, and management of

- A patient who may have an infectious disease (pp 1346-1347, 1354-1355)
- How to decontaminate equipment after treating a patient (p 1346)

Assessment and management of

- How to decontaminate the ambulance and equipment after treating a patient (p 1346)
- A patient who may be infected with a bloodborne pathogen (pp 1348-1350, 1354-1355, 1370-1374)
  - Human immunodeficiency virus (HIV) (pp 1372-1374)
  - Hepatitis B (pp 1370-1371)
- Antibiotic-resistant infections (pp 1381-1384)
- Current infectious diseases prevalent in the community (pp 1346-1351, 1354-1355)

Anatomy, physiology, epidemiology, pathophysiology, psychosocial impact, presentations, prognosis, and management of

- HIV-related disease (pp 1372-1374)
- Hepatitis (pp 1370-1372, 1375-1376)
- Pneumonia (see Chapter 16, *Respiratory Emergencies*)
- Meningococcal meningitis (pp 1357-1358)
- Tuberculosis (pp 1361-1362)
- Tetanus (p 1381)
- Viral diseases (pp 1357-1360, 1362-1365, 1370-1378, 1379-1381, 1384-1385, see also Chapter 16, *Respiratory Emergencies,* and Chapter 43, *Pediatric Emergencies*)
- Sexually transmitted diseases (pp 1365-1368)
- Gastroenteritis (p 1375)
- Fungal infections (pp 1368-1369)
- Rabies (p 1380)
- Scabies and lice (pp 1367-1368)
- Lyme disease (pp 1378-1379)
- Rocky Mountain spotted fever (p 1379)
- Antibiotic-resistant infections (pp 1381-1384)

Knowledge Objectives

1. Define communicable disease. (p 1345)
2. Outline the functions of the agencies responsible for protecting the public health in the United States at the national, state, and local levels. (p 1345)
3. Describe the paramedic's obligation to protect the public from infection and what steps the paramedic can take to meet it. (pp 1345-1346)
4. Describe how communicable diseases are transmitted by direct and indirect contact, droplet transmission, and airborne transmission. (pp 1346-1347)
5. Discuss transmission-based precautions. (pp 1347-1348)
6. Recall the standard precautions the paramedic must take to prevent exposure during patient care activities. (pp 1347-1348)
7. List the personal protective equipment (PPE) a paramedic may need in specific circumstances to prevent exposure to communicable and other infectious diseases. (pp 1348-1350)
8. Describe the steps to take for personal protection from airborne and bloodborne pathogens. (pp 1348-1350)
9. Describe how to remove PPE properly. (pp 1350-1351)
10. Explain proper follow-up after exposure to a patient's blood or other potentially infectious materials (OPIM), including documentation of the event and communication with a designated infection control officer and public health authorities. (pp 1350, 1352-1354)
11. List the general assessment and management principles for a patient with a communicable disease. (pp 1354-1355)
12. Discuss the importance of obtaining travel histories on all patients. (pp 1354-1355, 1374)
13. List the general management principles when caring for a patient with a suspected communicable disease. (p 1355)
14. Describe the cycle of infection, including factors that affect susceptibility to communicable diseases. (pp 1355-1357)

15. Discuss the pathophysiology, assessment, and management of a patient with sepsis. (p 1357)
16. Discuss the pathophysiology, assessment, and management of a patient with meningitis. (pp 1357-1358)
17. Discuss the pathophysiology, assessment, and management of a patient with influenza. (p 1359)
18. Discuss the pathophysiology, assessment, and management of a patient with pertussis, mumps, or rubella. (pp 1359-1360)
19. Discuss the pathophysiology, assessment, and management of a patient with tuberculosis. (pp 1361-1362)
20. Discuss precautions paramedics should take to protect themselves from exposure to tuberculosis. (p 1362)
21. Discuss the pathophysiology, assessment, and management of a patient with chickenpox. (pp 1362-1363)
22. Discuss the pathophysiology, assessment, and management of a patient with measles. (pp 1363-1364)
23. Discuss the pathophysiology, assessment, and management of a patient with mononucleosis. (pp 1364-1365)
24. Discuss general principles of assessment and management for a patient with a possible sexually transmitted disease. (p 1365)
25. Discuss the pathophysiology, assessment, and management of patients with gonorrhea, syphilis, genital herpes, and chlamydia. (pp 1365-1367)
26. Describe the risk factors, incidence, pathophysiology, assessment, and management of scabies and lice infestation. (pp 1367-1368)
27. Discuss other sexually transmitted diseases and conditions. (p 1368)
28. Discuss the pathophysiology, assessment, and management of a patient with a fungal skin infection. (pp 1368-1369)
29. Compare the types of viral hepatitis, including general assessment findings and management principles for the patient with hepatitis. (pp 1370-1372)
30. Discuss precautions paramedics should take to protect themselves from exposure to hepatitis, and postexposure follow-up. (pp 1371-1372)
31. Discuss the pathophysiology, assessment, and management of a patient with human immunodeficiency virus/acquired immunodeficiency syndrome (HIV/AIDS). (pp 1372-1374)
32. Discuss precautions paramedics should take to protect themselves from exposure to HIV, and postexposure follow-up. (pp 1373-1374)
33. Discuss the pathophysiology, assessment, and management of a patient with suspected Ebola. (pp 1374-1375)
34. Discuss precautions paramedics should take to protect themselves from exposure to Ebola, and postexposure follow-up. (p 1375)
35. Discuss the pathophysiology, assessment, and management of a patient with gastroenteritis. (p 1375)
36. Discuss the pathophysiology, assessment, and management of patients with non-bloodborne hepatitis viruses. (pp 1375-1376)
37. Discuss the pathophysiology, assessment, and management of patients with West Nile virus, dengue fever, chikungunya fever, and zika virus. (pp 1377-1378)
38. Discuss the pathophysiology, assessment, and management of patients with Lyme disease, Rocky Mountain spotted fever, hantavirus, rabies, Middle East respiratory syndrome (MERS), and tetanus. (pp 1378-1381)
39. Compare the most common antibiotic-resistant organisms and multidrug resistant organisms (MDROs), including what steps paramedics and patients can take to curb their spread. (pp 1381-1384)
40. Discuss general principles of assessment and management for patients with severe acute respiratory syndrome (SARS) and avian flu. (pp 1384-1385)

Skills Objectives

1. Demonstrate how to clean and disinfect the ambulance interior and equipment. (p 1346)

YOU are the Paramedic PART 1

Your unit is dispatched to an assisted care facility for a patient who is vomiting and has had diarrhea for a few days. While you are en route, the dispatcher states that the nurse on scene says the patient has watery diarrhea, low-grade fever, and nausea. When you arrive on scene, staff members meet you at the door. As they are guiding you to the room, one of the nurses tells you that the staff physician thinks the patient may have *Clostridium difficile (C diff)* due to antibiotic treatment.

1. What is your first concern at this scene?
2. What is *C diff* and what precautions should you put in place for transport?

Introduction

In 1913, Randolph Borne said, "We can become as much slaves to precaution as we can to fear." This statement is particularly relevant to EMS care today because many health care providers are fearful when caring for patients who have or are suspected of having a **communicable disease**—that is, an **infectious disease** that can be passed from one person to another. A paramedic who does not understand how communicable diseases are transmitted and how to take sensible precautions will be hesitant in caring for some patients, no matter what the cause of their illness. This chapter explores the ways in which such diseases are transmitted and outlines some measures a paramedic can take to protect against them. The communicable diseases that paramedics are most likely to encounter in the course of their work are examined, as are the illnesses that create the greatest anxiety among EMS personnel and the public at large.

Protecting Public Health

Responsibilities of Public Health Agencies

A number of government agencies are responsible for protecting the health of the general public. Agencies at the national level include the Occupational Health and Safety Administration (OSHA), which has promulgated rules and regulations designed to protect the employees of public and private organizations. This chapter refers to several OSHA regulations, for example, CFR 1910.1030, commonly known as the Bloodborne Pathogen Standard (Recall, **bloodborne pathogens** are pathogenic microorganisms that are present in human blood and can cause disease in humans.) OSHA is now enforcing several of the Centers for Disease Control and Prevention (CDC) Guidelines using the General Duty Clause. These will be identified in this chapter. Data on the numbers of patients infected and research and guidance for health care providers and the general public are available from the CDC. Another federal law, the Ryan White Comprehensive AIDS Resources Emergency (CARE) Act, Part G, requires that medical facilities notify emergency response personnel of airborne and droplet-transmitted disease involving patients they transported. This notification must happen as soon as possible, and no longer than 48 hours from the time they have a "suspect" case. The diseases listed in the original act include human immunodeficiency virus, hepatitis B, tuberculosis, meningococcal disease, diphtheria, pneumonic plague, viral hemorrhagic fevers, and rabies. In August 2011, the CDC published an expanded list of diseases covered under this mandate. The diseases added include hepatitis C, measles, rubella, severe acute respiratory syndrome coronavirus (SARS-CoV), pertussis, cutaneous anthrax, chickenpox, mumps, vaccinia, novel influenza A viruses, and potentially life-threatening diseases caused by biologic agents.[1] Now, there is much broader coverage for emergency responders to be notified and followed for exposures.

On the state and local levels, state and county public health departments bear the responsibility for protection of the public from disease, prevention of epidemics, and management of outbreaks. Although paramedics may not believe that supervision of water quality, cleanliness of restaurants, and routine immunization and vaccination programs relate directly to emergency care, it is beneficial for emergency medical services (EMS) agencies to know their local public health officials and to work with them. When potential threats to a community's health exist—such as the aftermath from Hurricane Katrina, the anthrax and smallpox scares, avian flu, H1N1, and Zika virus—a close working relationship between EMS providers and public health agencies is essential. If you do not know the public health professionals and officials in your county or parish, reach out to them and learn who they are.

State and local public health departments are responsible for many activities related to infectious/communicable diseases, including collecting data on the incidence of diseases, performing contact follow-up, and running tuberculosis (TB) and immunization clinics. The public health department monitors reportable disease weekly, monthly, and annually. This surveillance helps public health officials identify any upswing in the incidence of a particular disease. If the incidence of cases of a specific disease in a particular geographic area remains steady over time, that figure is said to be the **endemic** number of cases for that area. A rising caseload may signal the beginning of an **epidemic**. When a disease infects large numbers of people and spreads all over the world, it is considered a **pandemic**. Public health departments have a major role in investigating epidemics and pandemics.

The public health department collects all disease statistics for each locality and shares the information with the state health department, which then sends the state totals to the CDC.

Responsibilities of Paramedics

Paramedics have an obligation to protect patients from **health care–associated infection** (infection acquired from a health care setting). Health care–associated infections occur in all types of care settings and can be associated with procedures and the devices used in medical procedures, such as catheters.[2] One way to protect patients is by participating in protective vaccine and immunization programs; another is by complying with work restriction guidelines: Reporting for work when you have a sore throat or the flu is *not* in the best interest of your patients, your coworkers, or yourself. OSHA's General Duty Clause is being used to enforce the CDC work restriction guidelines. In Section 5(a)(1) the General Duty Clause states that each employer is required to furnish to each of its employees a workplace that is free from recognized hazards that are causing or likely to cause death or serious physical harm. Most of us are familiar with this employer responsibility. But part (b) of this clause addresses employee responsibilities. Section 5(b) of the General Duty Clause states, "Each employee shall comply with occupational safety and health standards and all rules, regulations, and orders issued pursuant to this Act which are applicable to his own actions and conduct." It is important to remember that infection control is for patient protection as well as care provider protection.

Another way to protect patients from health care–associated infections is to keep the ambulance interior and its equipment clean and disinfected. When cleaning and disinfecting equipment, select cleaning solutions to fit the equipment category:

- **Critical equipment.** Items that come in contact with mucous membranes: for example, laryngoscope blades and endotracheal tubes. High-level disinfection (that is, use of Environmental Protection Agency [EPA]-registered chemical "sterilants" is the minimum level for this equipment.
- **Semicritical equipment.** Items that come in direct contact with intact skin: for example, stethoscopes, blood pressure cuffs, splints, uniforms, and personal protection equipment (PPE). Clean with solutions that have a label claiming to kill hepatitis B virus (HBV). Bleach and water at a 1:100 dilution fits this requirement.
- **Noncritical equipment.** Cleaning surfaces, floors, ambulance seats, and work surfaces: For this equipment, a mixture of EPA-registered hospital-grade cleaner or bleach and water is effective at a 1:100 dilution (1/4 cup (62 mL) bleach to one gallon (4 L) of water.

General cleaning routines need to be listed in the department's exposure control plan. A basic rule of thumb is to follow the steps below after *every* call:

1. Strip used linens from the stretcher immediately after use, and place them in a plastic bag or the designated receptacle in the emergency department.
2. In an appropriate receptacle, discard all disposable equipment used for care of a patient that meets your state's definition of medical waste. Most items will be considered general trash. Refer to your state law definitions on medical waste disposal.
3. Wash contaminated areas with soap and water. For disinfection to be effective, cleaning must be done first.
4. Disinfect all nondisposable equipment used in the care of a patient. For example, disassemble the bag-mask device, and place the components in a liquid sterilization solution as recommended by the manufacturer.
5. Clean the stretcher with an EPA-registered germicidal-virucidal solution or bleach and water at a 1:100 dilution. Wear heavy-duty utility gloves for all cleaning activities. This is an OSHA requirement.
6. If any spillage or other contamination occurred in the ambulance, clean it up with the same germicidal-virucidal or bleach-water solution.
7. Create a schedule for routine full cleaning for the vehicle, as required by the exposure control plan. Name the brands of solution to be used.
8. Have a written policy and procedure for cleaning each piece of equipment. Refer to the manufacturer's recommendations as a guide.
9. Cleaning should focus on "high touch" items—what was used for patient care and items with which the patient was in contact.

Words of Wisdom

OSHA has a waiver clause to the use of PPE, to the effect of do not delay the provision of health care or public safety services if you do not have your PPE (OSHA Regulation 1910.1030 under use of PPE and CPL 02-02.069.)

Protecting Health Care Providers

Although the risk of contracting a communicable disease is real, it should not be exaggerated and certainly should not be a source of fear and stress. Fear comes from lack of proper education and training, and there is no reason a paramedic should not be properly educated about disease transmission. Measurable risk rates have been determined by the National Institute for Occupational Safety and Health, the CDC, and the World Health Organization (WHO).[3] Data reveals that there is low risk for providers to contract these diseases.

Communicable Disease Transmission

By the very nature of their work, health care providers come in contact with sick people; a certain proportion of the sick people have communicable diseases. Communicable diseases are diseases that can be transmitted from one person to another under certain conditions. These conditions are listed in the formula for infection and are dependent on dose, virulence, mode of entry, and the health status of the host. Infectious diseases cause illness in the patient but do not always pose a risk to the health care provider.

To understand the principles of prevention, you must first understand how diseases are spread. Infectious diseases are caused by pathogenic microorganisms—usually

bacteria or **viruses**, but sometimes **fungi** and **parasites**. They spread from person to person by several specific mechanisms:

- **Contact transmission**. Direct contact with an infected person may be brief, such as touching a patient. Most cases of the common cold are thought to be transmitted through casual direct contact. Venereal diseases, such as syphilis and gonorrhea, are transmitted principally by direct sexual contact and are, therefore, referred to as sexually transmitted diseases (STDs).

  Direct contact also includes puncture by a contaminated needle or other sharp instrument. Punctures may occur if a health care provider is not using needle-safe or needleless devices.

  Direct contact may also occur by transfusion of contaminated blood products from one patient to another. Screening tests for bloodborne disease have vastly reduced the risks of contracting illnesses from contaminated blood. However, donated blood is not 100% safe from bloodborne pathogens.

  Indirect contact occurs by touching or handling an infected object or by coming into contact with a person who is contaminated with pathogens from an infected person or his or her secretions. For example, a paramedic can become infected by touching a bloody stretcher railing with an open cut or sore on his or her hand or by not washing his or her hands after touching a contaminated surface. Objects that harbor microorganisms and can transmit them to others, such as the stretcher railing in the preceding example, are called **fomites**.
- **Droplet transmission**. Droplet transmission occurs with inhalation of infected droplets, such as those released into the surroundings when a person with influenza coughs or sneezes. With these diseases, there is generally a 3-foot (1-m) rule. Droplets fall after traveling 3 feet (1 m).
- **Airborne transmission**. Pathogens transmitted by the airborne route are carried in microscopic particles that become aerosolized when an infected person coughs or sneezes. These infectious particles can remain suspended in the air for some period of time. Airborne particles travel up to 6 feet (2 m) and then fall.

Disease transmission can also occur by means other than person-to-person transmission. A **vector** is an organism that harbors pathogens that are harmless to the organism but cause disease when transmitted to a human host. For example, a mosquito infected with West Nile virus or Zika virus that bites a susceptible person may transmit the disease.

Once it is established how a disease is transmitted, it is easy to know what PPE is needed when rendering care. This concept is termed **transmission-based precautions**.

Transmission-Based Precautions

Standard Precautions

The term **standard precautions** describes infection control practices that reduce the opportunity for an exposure to occur in the daily care of patients. It replaces the older terms *universal precautions* and *body substance isolation (BSI)*. BSI precautions have been taught to EMS providers for the past decade; this approach assumes that all blood and body fluids are infectious. Standard precautions add another element: protection from moist body substances that may transmit other bacterial or viral infections. For example, a paramedic with a cut on a finger who suctions a patient with oral herpes lesions and does not wear a glove could become infected with herpes whitlow. Standard precautions apply to all body substances *except* sweat.

In addition to standard precautions, three other categories have been added: airborne, droplet, and contact. Some diseases may require a combination of precautions. An example would be Ebola. For care of an Ebola patient, the recommendations for care include standard, contact, and droplet precautions.

Words of Wisdom

Standard precautions are used with all transmission-based categories.

Airborne Precautions

In the context of EMS, **airborne precautions** apply to diseases that can travel a distance of 6 feet (2 m) before dropping to the floor, and are large-particle. Examples of when airborne precautions apply include when working with a patient suspected of or diagnosed with tuberculosis, chickenpox, or measles. Airborne precautions involve the use of a surgical mask on the patient and airflow in the vehicle (exhaust system). Opening windows or using the recycle function on a heating or air-conditioning unit is also a preventive measure. If the patient cannot wear the mask, the health care provider should wear a surgical mask. It is not necessary for both the patient and the health care provider to be masked; masking one suffices.

Words of Wisdom

According to the CDC, respirators are not needed for EMS care and transport of patients with TB.[4,5]

Droplet Precautions

Droplet precautions apply to diseases that involve medium- to large-sized particles that travel 3 feet (1 m) and then drop to the floor. Such diseases include influenza, meningitis, pertussis (whooping cough), mumps, rubella (German measles), and Ebola. EMS providers should place a surgical mask on the patient.[6] Basic infection control is to contain at the source. As with airborne precautions, use the airflow system in the vehicle.

Contact Precautions

Contact precautions are appropriate with all patients presenting with draining wounds, multidrug resistant infection, lice, norovirus, and Ebola. Contact precautions include the use of gloves, a gown if clothing could be contaminated, and cleaning of high-touch items. High-touch items include areas the patient was in contact with, and equipment used to care for the patient.

▶ Personal Protective Equipment and Practices—Task Based

PPE serves as a secondary protective barrier beyond what your body provides. The selection and use of PPE depends on the task and procedure at hand or, as mentioned, on how the disease is transmitted (transmission-based precautions). Your department's exposure control plan should contain a listing of its risk procedures and the recommended use of PPE. The CDC has also developed guidelines for PPE Table 26-1.

Table 26-1 Recommended Personal Protective Equipment for Preventing Transmission of Human Immunodeficiency Virus and Hepatitis B Virus in the Prehospital Setting

Task or Activity	Disposable Gloves	Gown	Mask	Protective Eyewear
Bleeding control with spurting blood	Yes	Yes	Yes	Yes
Bleeding control with minimal bleeding	Yes	No	No	No
Emergency childbirth	Yes	Yes	Yes, if spatter is likely	Yes, if spatter is likely
Drawing blood samples	Yes	No	No	No
Inserting an IV line	Yes	No	No	No
Advanced airway insertion (eg, endotracheal intubation, laryngeal mask airway, Combitube)	Yes	No	No, unless spatter is likely[a]	No, unless spatter is likely[a]
Oral/nasal suctioning, manually cleaning airway	Yes	No	No, unless spatter is likely[a]	No, unless spatter is likely[a]
Handling and cleaning instruments with microbial contamination	Yes	No, unless soiling is likely	No	No
Measuring blood pressure	No	No	No	No
Measuring temperature	No	No	No	No
Giving an injection	No	No	No	No

[a]Splashing is often likely, so use personal protective equipment accordingly.
Abbreviation: IV, intravenous

Data from: Centers for Disease Control and Prevention (CDC): Guidelines for prevention of transmission of human immunodeficiency virus and hepatitis B virus to health-care and public-safety workers: a response to P.L. 100-607 The Health Omnibus Programs Extention Act of 1988. *MMWR*. 1989;38(S-6):Table 4, (d)(3)(ix)(A)-(C). http://wonder.cdc.gov/wonder/prevguid/p0000114/p0000114.asp. Accessed November 10, 2011; Ask the expert: gloves for injections. HCPro OSHA Heathcare Advisor website. http://blogs.hcpro.com/osha/2012/01/ask-the-expert-gloves-for-injections/; and Standard interpretations. United States Department of Labor, OSHA website. https://www.osha.gov/pls/oshaweb/owadisp.show_document?p_table=INTERPRETATIONS&p_id=20819

Hand hygiene, including handwashing, is your major protective measure. The current standard for handwashing is to use antimicrobial, alcohol-based foams or gels, and to scrub vigorously for at least 20 seconds before rinsing with clean water.[7] Use of antibacterial products is not recommended. The friction used to get alcohol-based foams and gels to evaporate removes surface organisms and kills viruses but leaves the normal protective flora intact.

Evidence-Based Medicine

Several studies on handwashing compliance in EMS reveal that this important practice has a low compliance rate for EMS providers.[8,9]

Words of Wisdom

Wash your hands before and after every call—and after glove removal!

According to the CDC, OSHA, and National Fire Protection Association (NFPA) 1581, *Standard on Fire Department Infection Control Program*, health care providers who have open cuts or sores on their hands should cover the area with a dressing.[10-12] If the area is too large to cover, the provider should not perform high-risk tasks and procedures. Tattoos are considered an open area anywhere from one week to about a month. The health care provider should be placed on work restriction until the areas have healed. Health care providers are not permitted to wear artificial nails or nail extensions. Studies reported in the CDC Hand Hygiene Guidelines document the transmission of bacterial and fungal infections from health care workers to patients wearing these nails.[13]

PPE should include, but not be limited to, disposable gloves, protective eyewear, cover gowns, surgical masks, N95 respirators (or N100 respirators required in California under certain circumstances), waterless handwashing alcohol-based foam or gel, needle-safe or needleless devices, biohazard bags, and resuscitative equipment.

A particulate respirator filters particles that come in through the mask. Never place a respirator on a patient. A full respiratory protection program that complies with the OSHA respiratory protection program 1910.134 must be in place if N95 or P100 respirators are on EMS vehicles.[11]

Gloves are not needed for intramuscular or subcutaneous injections or contact with sweat. However, according to the CDC and OSHA, they are recommended for starting IV lines, suctioning, intubation, or use of advanced airway, contact with blood or **other potentially infectious materials (OPIM)**, and contact with patient mucous membranes or

Evidence-Based Medicine

Surgical masks protect against spatter into the mouth or nose. Patients thought to have airborne or droplet-transmitted diseases may be asked to wear them because they filter what goes out through the mask. According to the CDC, N95 or P100 respirators are indicated for emergency intubation and open suctioning.[14] Some health officials suggest that such procedures generate aerosols that could transmit airborne/droplet particles. No evidence-based studies support the assertion that using an N95 or P100 respirator offers more protection than wearing a surgical mask in most cases. In fact, well-controlled studies indicate that surgical masks are as effective as respirators in protecting against infection.[15-18] For more information, review the CDC guidelines "Prevention Strategies for Seasonal Influenza in Healthcare Settings" (September 2010).

The CDC also downgraded from N95s for Ebola to surgical masks in December 2014.[19] Ebola is not airborne, but rather is droplet transmitted.

nonintact skin.[20] OPIM includes cerebrospinal fluid (CSF), pericardial fluid, amniotic fluid, synovial fluid, peritoneal fluid, and any fluid containing visible blood. For cleaning activities, OSHA requires the use of utility-style gloves (dishwashing gloves). These are washable and reusable as long as they are free of tears and holes **Figure 26-1**. Hands should be washed *after* glove removal because gloves are not a primary protection. Many gloves contain holes and absorb viruses and bacteria; this is termed *viral penetration*.

Words of Wisdom

Blood is not the only fluid that poses a threat of infection. Other potentially infectious materials (OPIM; an OSHA term), include semen, vaginal secretions, cerebrospinal fluid, synovial fluid, pleural fluid, pericardial fluid, peritoneal fluid, amniotic fluid, saliva in dental procedures, any body fluid that is visibly contaminated with blood, and all body fluids in situations where it is difficult or impossible to differentiate between body fluids.[21]

According to the CDC and OSHA, tears, sweat, saliva, stool, urine, vomitus, nasal secretions, and sputum *do not* pose a risk for transmission of HIV, HBV, or hepatitis C virus (HCV) unless they contain visible blood.[22]

Protective eyewear blocks spatter into the eye. Prescription eyeglasses may be worn with disposable or reusable side shields. Goggles should not be worn over prescription eyeglasses because vision may be distorted **Figure 26-2**.

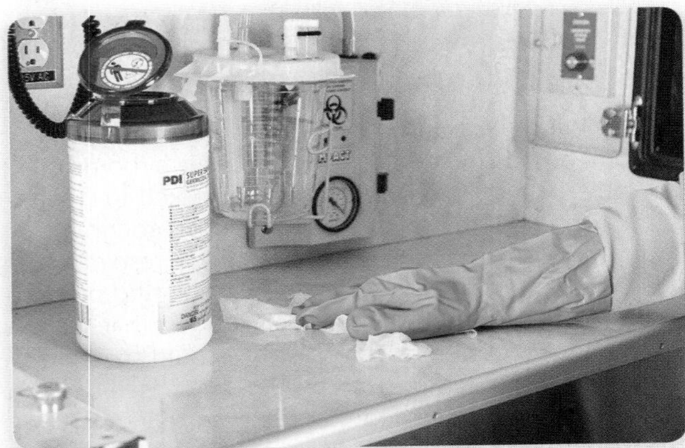

Figure 26-1 Utility-style gloves are washable and reusable as long as they are free of tears and holes.

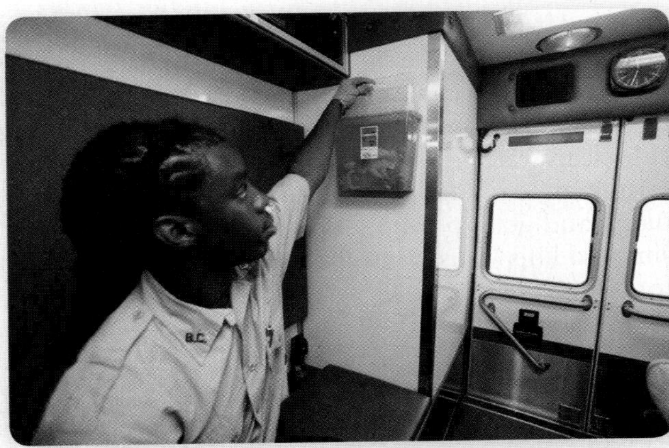

Figure 26-3 For proper disposal, all sharps must be placed in containers that are puncture-resistant, closable, leakproof, and that bear the biohazard symbol.

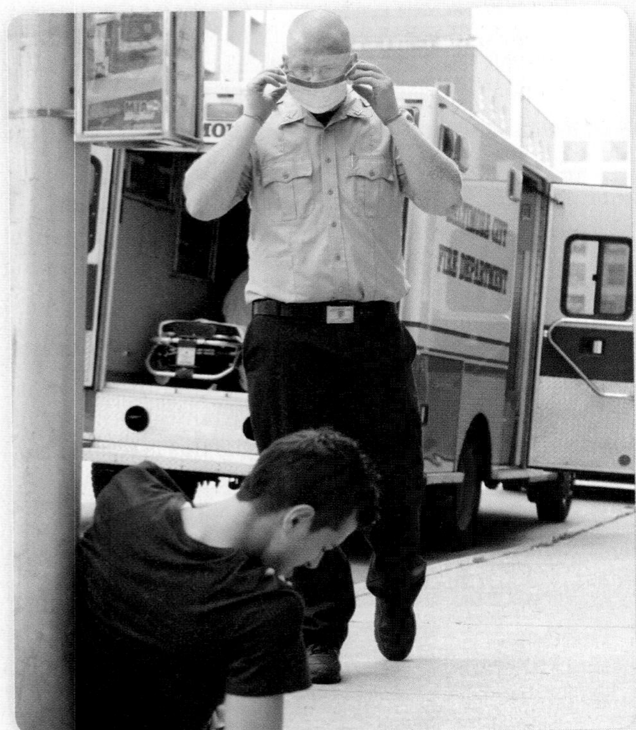

Figure 26-2 Wear eye protection and a mask to prevent blood and oral secretions from spattering into your eyes, nose, and mouth.

Cover garments are recommended for large-splatter situations. These garments could be washable or disposable jackets or gowns. Uniforms may also serve as PPE if the employer purchases, maintains, and launders them. Booties and hair covers are not routinely needed in the prehospital setting. Pocket masks and/or respiratory assistive devices (for example, bag-mask devices) must be readily available.

According to the CDC, a sharps injury is a penetrating stab wound from a needle, scalpel, or other sharp object that may result in exposure to blood or other body fluids.[23] In 2000, Congress passed the Needlestick Safety and Prevention Act, which required that all sharps be needle-safe or **needleless systems**.[24] The systems that have adopted needle-safe and needleless devices have reported no sharps injuries. All sharps must be placed into sharps containers that are puncture-resistant, closable, leakproof, and contain the biohazard symbol Figure 26-3. Sharps containers must be located at the site of use.

▶ Removal of PPE

No matter how high tech PPE may be, it is only effective if proper removal techniques are employed. Figure 26-4 shows the proper removal of PPE according to the CDC. PPE removal for pathogens is different than the procedure for removal of hazardous material (hazmat) PPE. Remember, handwashing after glove removal is always important!

▶ Postexposure Medical Follow-up

Postexposure medical follow-up is your third line of defense against the effects of communicable diseases.

Designated Infection Control Officer

The federal Ryan White CARE Act, Part G, requires that every emergency response agency have a **designated infection control officer (DICO)**. This person is charged with ensuring that proper postexposure medical treatment and counseling are provided to the exposed employee or volunteer.

Postexposure medical treatment is offered to reduce the chances that an exposed health care provider might contract the disease to which he or she was exposed. Treatment should be offered within 24 to 48 hours following an exposure, with the actual time frame based on the diagnosis. Exposure to bacterial meningitis, for example, would require treatment within 24 hours.

HOW TO SAFELY REMOVE PERSONAL PROTECTIVE EQUIPMENT (PPE) EXAMPLE 1

There are a variety of ways to safely remove PPE without contaminating your clothing, skin, or mucous membranes with potentially infectious materials. Here is one example. **Remove all PPE before exiting the patient room** except a respirator, if worn. Remove the respirator **after** leaving the patient room and closing the door. Remove PPE in the following sequence:

1. GLOVES

- Outside of gloves are contaminated!
- If your hands get contaminated during glove removal, immediately wash your hands or use an alcohol-based hand sanitizer
- Using a gloved hand, grasp the palm area of the other gloved hand and peel off first glove
- Hold removed glove in gloved hand
- Slide fingers of ungloved hand under remaining glove at wrist and peel off second glove over first glove
- Discard gloves in a waste container

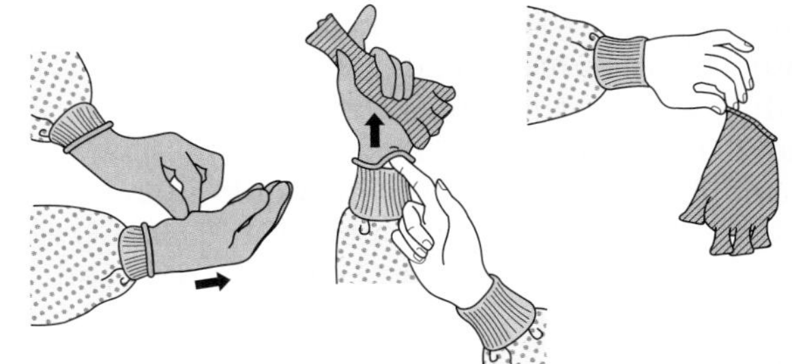

2. GOGGLES OR FACE SHIELD

- Outside of goggles or face shield are contaminated!
- If your hands get contaminated during goggle or face shield removal, immediately wash your hands or use an alcohol-based hand sanitizer
- Remove goggles or face shield from the back by lifting head band or ear pieces
- If the item is reusable, place in designated receptacle for reprocessing. Otherwise, discard in a waste container

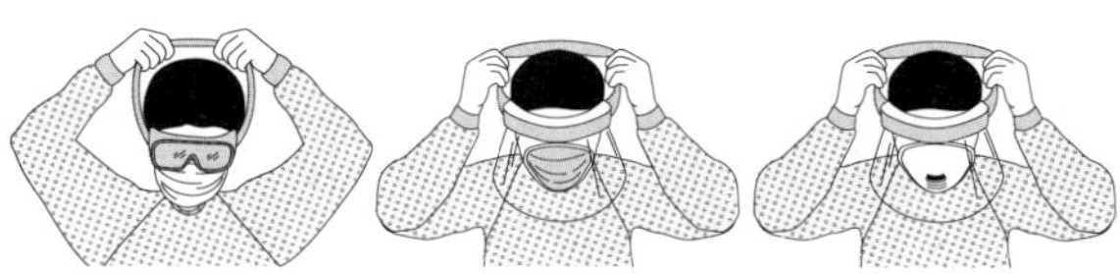

3. GOWN

- Gown front and sleeves are contaminated!
- If your hands get contaminated during gown removal, immediately wash your hands or use an alcohol-based hand sanitizer
- Unfasten gown ties, taking care that sleeves don't contact your body when reaching for ties
- Pull gown away from neck and shoulders, touching inside of gown only
- Turn gown inside out
- Fold or roll into a bundle and discard in a waste container

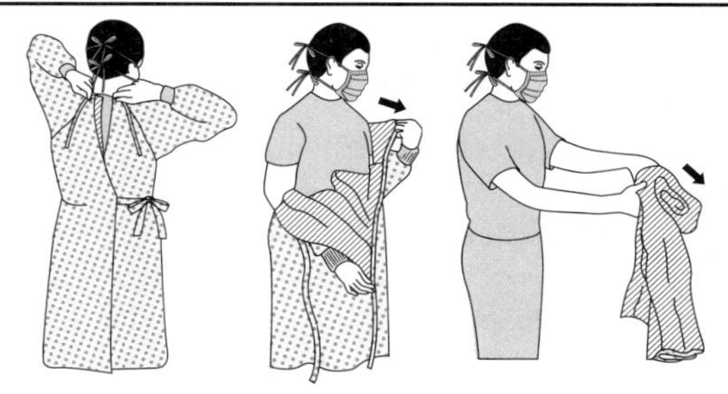

4. MASK OR RESPIRATOR

- Front of mask/respirator is contaminated — DO NOT TOUCH!
- If your hands get contaminated during mask/respirator removal, immediately wash your hands or use an alcohol-based hand sanitizer
- Grasp bottom ties or elastics of the mask/respirator, then the ones at the top, and remove without touching the front
- Discard in a waste container

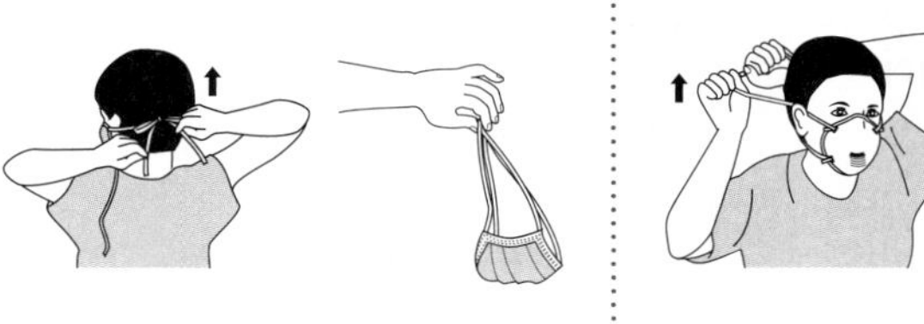

5. WASH HANDS OR USE AN ALCOHOL-BASED HAND SANITIZER IMMEDIATELY AFTER REMOVING ALL PPE

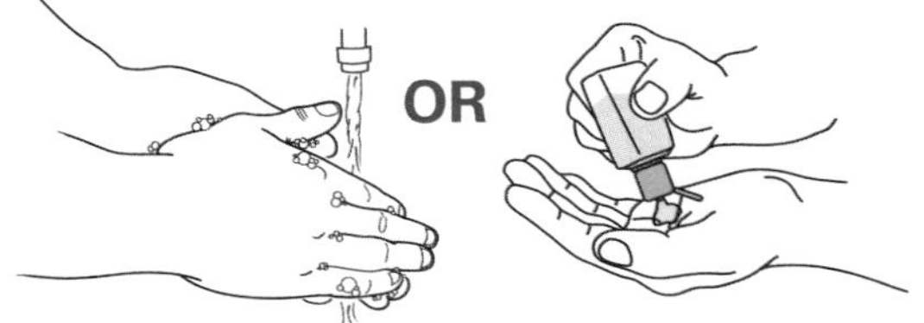

PERFORM HAND HYGIENE BETWEEN STEPS IF HANDS BECOME CONTAMINATED AND IMMEDIATELY AFTER REMOVING ALL PPE

Figure 26-4 Centers for Disease Control and Prevention chart on proper removal of personal protective equipment. Note that for incidents involving hazardous materials, the sequence is different than that shown here.

Modified from Centers for Disease Control and Prevention.

The DICO tracks and monitors compliance with the correct time frames, serves as a liaison between the exposed employee and the medical facility, ensures that confidentiality is maintained, and ensures that documentation adheres to guidelines. This role of the DICO is important for workers' compensation issues.

The communication network for exposure reporting involves three people: the exposed paramedic, the DICO, and the treating physician. A paramedic who believes an exposure has occurred should call the DICO directly. It is the DICO's job to determine whether an actual exposure occurred. Each department must have a reporting system that complies with the Ryan White notification law and the OSHA-required exposure control plan. The DICO must be available 24 hours per day, 7 days per week and, for confidentiality reasons, must work outside of the normal chain of command.

The public health department acts as a backup for exposure notification and determination of the need for medical follow-up treatment. Under the Ryan White notification law, the local public health department must know the identity of the DICO for each EMS department. The public health department director serves as a liaison for problems that may arise regarding exposure notification by the medical facility and the sharing of source-patient testing results.

The Process When an Exposure Occurs

If an exposure occurs, the DICO will ensure the source patient is tested. If the test is positive, you will receive proper postexposure medical treatment, including counseling, to reduce your chances of developing the disease to which you were exposed. Postexposure medical prophylaxis (prevention) is available for many communicable diseases, except HCV infection. If HCV is acquired, it can often be cured.

Exposure to bloodborne pathogens can occur in a number of different ways:

- A contaminated needlestick injury (sharp has been in the patient's body)
- Blood or OPIM spattered into the eye, nose, or mouth
- Blood or OPIM in contact with an open area of the skin (a fresh cut, an abrasion, an area of dermatitis)
- Cuts with a sharp object covered with blood or OPIM
- Human bites involving blood exposure (The source is the person who is bleeding, not the biter.) Recent data show no bloodborne pathogen diseases have been transmitted this way.[25]

Words of Wisdom

If you are bitten and blood is drawn, it is not an exposure, because that is your blood. Unless the biter has blood in his or her mouth, no exposure has occurred.

If any of these events occurs, you should immediately contact your DICO. This is important, because the DICO determines whether an exposure has occurred.

Evidence-Based Medicine

Research shows that bloodborne pathogen transmission as a result of human bites is rare. According to a paper published in the Journal of the National Medical Association, no bite-related transmission occurred in one institution between 1993 and 2011.[26]

For airborne- and/or droplet-transmissible diseases, the DICO receives notice from the medical facility and reviews the following criteria: the organism involved, the amount of time spent with the patient, the provider's distance from the patient, the procedure or task being performed, and the ventilation present.

Words of Wisdom

An ambulance has an air exchange rate of every 2 minutes. Does your vehicle require that this be turned on, or is it automatic? This risk reduction is built in per the KKK ambulance specifications, which were developed by the US General Services Administration in the 1970s.

Postexposure medical management includes identification of the **source individual**.[27] The source is the key to identifying whether there is risk. Employee baseline testing is only needed if the source tests positive. According to the OSHA Compliance Directive for Bloodborne Pathogens, employers must pay for all costs related to exposure events, including testing the source individual.[28]

Bloodwork for the source patient should include the following: rapid HIV testing, testing for HB surface antigen, rapid HCV antibody and, if the HIV or HCV test is positive, syphilis testing. The HIV and HCV results should be available in less than 1 hour, and HB surface antigen results usually are available by the following day. Because most health care providers have been vaccinated against some diseases already, however, the time frame is not a major concern. Testing for HIV requires patient consent in roughly half the states in the United States, but state law often makes exceptions for occupational exposure of health care providers. In the other states, there is "deemed consent"—that is, the state assumes consent to be tested. Each EMS department should be aware of the state testing law.

Under the Ryan White CARE Act (otherwise known as the Ryan White notification law), the medical facility must release the source patient's test results to the DICO; this release is not considered a violation of privacy under the Health Insurance Portability and Accountability Act. The Ryan White CARE Act, Part G, also requires medical facilities to notify the DICO if a patient who is suspected of having or is known to have an airborne- or droplet-transmitted disease is transported.[1]

This information is shared with the exposed employee, and if the source patient tests positive, proper care and counseling begin. The baseline blood work that is done on an exposed paramedic does not yield information on the exposure that just occurred; rather, it documents whether the paramedic already has one of these diseases. As mentioned, postexposure medical counseling and treatment should begin within 24 to 48 hours, unless testing of the source patient yields information that necessitates more rapid follow-up.

CDC-Recommended Immunizations and Vaccinations

Vaccines are suspensions of whole (live or inactivated) or fractionated bacteria or viruses that have been rendered nonpathogenic; they bring about immunity by causing the immune system to produce antibodies. Vaccines are now being made using DNA technology, which removes the risks of a person experiencing an allergic reaction or developing Guillain-Barré syndrome (GBS). GBS is a temporary paralysis that usually resolves over time. Keeping current with recommended **vaccinations** boosts host resistance and the immune response.

In 1999, OSHA began enforcing the CDC guidelines on immunization of health care personnel. In 2011, the CDC published an updated **immunization** schedule for health care providers. A **tetanus**, diphtheria, and pertussis (Tdap) booster is required because of the increasing incidence of pertussis (whooping cough) in the United States. Table 26-2 lists the CDC recommendations for health care providers.

Each employer must offer the CDC-recommended vaccinations to staff and pay for them. This includes volunteer departments, because the CDC defines health care personnel as "all paid and unpaid persons." Individual paramedics have the right to decline being vaccinated but will be required to sign a declination form.[12]

Table 26-2 Recommended Vaccinations for Health Care Providers
Hepatitis B
Measles, mumps, rubella (MMR)
Varicella (chickenpox)
Tuberculosis (TB) testing
Tetanus, diphtheria, and pertussis (Tdap): one-time dose [a]
Influenza (annually)

[a]Td boosters are needed every 10 years. It has not yet been determined when pertussis boosters are needed.

Data from: Healthcare Personnel Vaccination Recommendations. Atlanta, GA: Centers for Disease Control and Prevention. March 2011.

YOU are the Paramedic PART 2

You and your partner arrive at the patient's room, which is shared with another resident. Your patient is an 86-year-old woman who appears very ill. She is pale and appears weak but is alert and able to answer questions. The staff member tells you the patient has been vomiting and having watery, nonbloody diarrhea for 2 days. The patient leans forward to vomit into a basin, and nothing comes up. The staff member, who is not wearing gloves, takes a tissue from a container, wipes the patient's mouth, and discards the tissue in the trash can.

Recording Time: 1 Minute	
Appearance	Awake
Level of consciousness	Alert (oriented to person, place, time, and event)
Airway	Open
Breathing	Adequate
Circulation	Adequate

3. What can you determine about the patient's condition now?
4. Because a diagnosis of *C diff* infection has not been confirmed for this patient, are you concerned about exposure?

It is important for each new employee and volunteer to obtain his or her vaccination records. These records can be obtained from a personal physician, high school, college, training program, or previous employer. Current staff members also need to obtain these records. To comply with privacy regulations, records must be requested by the employee or volunteer from one of the aforementioned sources.

Department Responsibilities

Under the OSHA mandate and the Ryan White CARE Act, Part G, to protect staff from exposure to bloodborne pathogens and airborne and droplet diseases, each EMS department is required to have a comprehensive exposure control plan. This document lays out the specifics of how the department plans to reduce the risk of exposure to infectious agents and provide postexposure medical follow-up, if needed. Key elements of the exposure control plan include proper education and training related to bloodborne pathogens and airborne and droplet diseases, and establishment of postexposure medical follow-up procedures Table 26-3.

Another key component of the plan is compliance monitoring. Management must make spot checks to ensure that staff members are following the exposure control plan and that the plan is working effectively. Although management is responsible for developing and implementing the plan, OSHA has made it clear that the employees are required to follow the plan. This is addressed in the General Duty Clause (b) which states, "Each employee shall comply with occupational safety and health standards and all rules, regulations, and orders issued pursuant to this Act which are applicable to his own actions and conduct."

A part of the exposure control plan that benefits department personnel and patients is the work restriction guidelines. These guidelines, which were published by the CDC and are enforced by OSHA, indicate when employees with various illnesses may or may not be at work and when they may not care for high-risk patients. Work restriction guidelines require employees to use sick time unless the illness is the result of an occupational exposure, in which case it is covered under workers' compensation. Following work restriction guidelines is of particular importance during the flu (respiratory influenza) season.

Infection is defined as the invasion of a host or host tissue by pathogenic organisms such as bacteria, viruses, or parasites that produces illness that may or may not have clinical manifestations. It is important to distinguish between contamination and infection. An object that has microorganisms on or in it is **contaminated**. This term applies to water, food, dressing materials, linens, sharps, equipment, and even the ambulance. A person is not infected, however, unless the microorganisms actually produce an illness. With some diseases, such as HBV or HCV infection, a person may have the disease and not be aware of it; there are no signs or symptoms, and the person is not ill. However, such **carriers** can pass the disease to others through their blood and through sexual contact.

Table 26-3 Exposure Control Plan Components
Exposure determination
Education and training
Hepatitis B vaccine program
Tuberculosis testing program
Expanded vaccine program: MMR, chickenpox vaccine, Tdap booster
Personal protective equipment
Engineering controls and work practices
Postexposure management
Medical waste management
Compliance monitoring
Record keeping

Abbreviations: MMR, measles, mumps, rubella; Tdap, tetanus, diphtheria, and pertussis

Patient Assessment

The assessment of a patient suspected of having a communicable disease should be approached much like that of any other medical patient. First, the scene must be sized up and standard precautions taken. Once you have ensured that the scene is safe (there is no threatening person or animal), proceed with the primary survey by following the ABCDE process—assess the patient's airway, breathing, circulation, disability, and exposure—to identify all injuries. Include mental status assessment, and prioritize treatment of the patient. With most patients who have a potentially communicable disease and are being seen in the prehospital setting, the next step is to take the patient's history, using OPQRST (onset, provocation/palliation, quality, radiation, severity, time of onset) to elaborate on the chief complaint. Typical chief complaints include fever, nausea, rash, pleuritic chest pain, and difficulty breathing. Be sure to obtain a SAMPLE (Signs and symptoms, Allergies, Medications, Pertinent past history, Last oral intake, Events leading to injury or illness) history and a set of baseline vital signs, paying particular attention to medications the patient is currently taking, the events leading up to the patient's problem today, and whether the patient has recently traveled. The importance of travel history has been demonstrated with SARS, Ebola, H1N1, and Zika infections and should be a routine assessment question. Always show respect for the feelings of patients, family, and others at the scene. Then proceed to the secondary assessment, including the physical exam.

General Management Principles

The general management of a patient with a suspected communicable disease first focuses on any life-threatening conditions that were identified in the primary survey (airway maintenance, oxygen and ventilatory assistance, bleeding control, and circulatory support). Remember to be empathetic. Because most patients with a communicable disease will have a fever of an unexplained origin or mild breathing problems, place the patient in a position of comfort on the stretcher and keep him or her warm. If the patient has early signs of dehydration, a preliminary IV line and a fluid infusion of normal saline or lactated Ringer solution may be appropriate. Remember to take standard precautions and to properly dispose of sharps, even needle-safe devices.[5] Always follow your agency's exposure control plan for cleaning the suction unit and any reusable equipment, and properly discard any disposable supplies and linens.

Chain of Infection

Infection involves a chain of events through which the communicable disease spreads. In some cases, solving the puzzle of why a specific disease developed in a particular person or group of people may be as simple as retracing steps to find the source of exposure. In other cases, the puzzle is more difficult to solve, with infectious disease experts taking years to find a pattern in the spread of a disease and then plan a strategy to break the chain of the infection. The study of communicable diseases takes into consideration population demographics that can affect the spread of a disease, such as age distributions; genetic factors; income levels; ethnic groups; workplaces and schools; geographic boundaries; and the expansion, decline, or movement of the disease.

Here is a scenario that illustrates how easily disease may spread. In a local hospital pediatric unit, a visitor brought a box of candy for a child. Because of the "no food" rule, an attentive nurse placed the candy at the nurses' station. Another nurse had emptied a bedpan of stool from a child admitted for a hepatitis A infection but was in such a rush that she forgot to wash her hands. She then noticed the box of candy, poked at a few selections with her fingernails, and finally found one she wanted to eat. The candy was consumed throughout the morning. Subsequently, another nurse came down with hepatitis A, a disease that is typically spread by the oral-fecal route. The chain of infection in this scenario could have been broken by handwashing.

Exposure and the Risk of Infection

Several factors determine a person's risk of contracting an infection following an exposure. An organism's mere presence presents a risk. However, other factors influence the level of risk, including the dose of the organism, the virulence of the organism, its mode of entry, and the host resistance of the exposed person.

Type of Organism

Pathogenic organisms include bacteria, viruses, fungi, and parasites. They differ in the ways in which they infect the host, grow and reproduce within host tissues, and cause illness. Table 26-4 compares these organisms.

Dose of the Organism

A certain number of organisms must be present for infection to occur. For example, the laboratory report on a urine specimen sent for culture may note "greater than 100,000 colonies of bacteria per milliliter" of urine indicating infection. A value of equal to or less than 100,000 is considered as not indicating infection. When you are establishing risk for transmission of HIV, colonies of the virus greater than 1,500 per milliliter of blood would be significant.

Virulence of the Organism

Virulence is the ability of an organism to invade and create disease in a host. It also encompasses the organism's ability to survive outside the living host. For example, HIV does not pose a risk outside the human body because it dies when it is exposed to light and air. A bacterium like *Salmonella* can multiply every 15 to 20 minutes in the presence of the right temperature and nutrients.

Mode of Entry

If the organism does not enter the body by the "correct" route, infection cannot occur. For example, a respiratory virus that enters the body through a cut will not cause a respiratory infection and likely will not cause any infection. On the other hand, an inhaled respiratory droplet could cause respiratory illness. Thus, if you apply a mask to a patient who might have a communicable respiratory disease, you will not inhale the droplets.

Host Resistance

The healthier you are, the less susceptible you are to infection. Your ability to fight off infection is called **host resistance**. Your immune system will help protect you from acquiring disease even though all of the other risk factors may be present. Wellness programs and immunization programs serve to boost host resistance.

Once a susceptible person has been exposed to an organism, it takes time for the organism to multiply within the body and produce symptoms. That period between exposure to the organism and the first symptoms of illness

Table 26-4 Comparison of Selected Pathogenic Organisms

Organism	Life Cycle	Effect on Host	Example
Bacteria	Grow and reproduce outside the human cell in an environment characterized by the appropriate temperature and nutrients	Cause disease when they invade and multiply within the host's tissues	*Salmonella* bacteria can multiply in potato salad that has been unrefrigerated, leading to human illness when the food is eaten
Viruses	Much smaller than bacteria and can multiply only inside a host; die when exposed to the environment	Cause disease when they invade and multiply within the host's tissues	HIV does not multiply or maintain its infectiousness outside a living host
Fungi	Similar to bacteria in that they can grow rapidly in the presence of nutrients and organic material	Most infections acquired from contact with decaying organic matter or airborne spores in the environment; often cause opportunistic infections in people with compromised immune systems	Range from relatively harmless infections of the skin, such as athlete's foot (*Tinea pedis*), to life-threatening systemic infections, such as pneumonia (*Pneumocystis jirovecii*, formerly known as *Pneumocystis carinii*) in people with AIDS
Parasites	Live in or on another living creature	Take advantage of their host by feeding off the host cells and tissues	Scabies and lice **Protozoa**: single-celled, usually microscopic, eukaryotic organisms such as amoebas, ciliates, flagellates, and sporozoans. *Entamoeba histolytica*, for example, causes dysentery Helminths (commonly called worms): invertebrates with long, flexible, rounded, or flattened bodies; *Ascaris lumbricoides*, for example, causes hookworm

Abbreviations: AIDS, acquired immunodeficiency syndrome; HIV, human immunodeficiency virus

is called the **incubation period**. For example, it usually takes 12 to 26 days from a susceptible person's exposure to the mumps virus until the person begins to feel feverish and ill. The incubation period for the influenza virus is much shorter—usually 24 to 72 hours.

Most communicable diseases are contagious only during a portion of the illness. A person may be sick with chickenpox for 2 to 3 weeks but is capable of transmitting the virus to another person for only about 1 week—from 1 day before the **vesicles** appear on the skin to about 6 days after. The period during which a person can transmit the illness to someone else is called the **communicable period**.

In the context of communicable disease, a **reservoir** is a place where organisms may live and multiply. In institutional settings, for example, air-conditioning systems and showerheads have been identified as reservoirs for the bacterium that causes Legionnaires' disease. In ambulances, the oxygen humidifier is commonly implicated as a reservoir for infection. Health care personnel are responsible not only for protecting themselves from contracting communicable diseases, but also ensuring, to the extent possible, that they and their equipment do not transmit illness to others. This is very important; if a patient with Medicare or Medicaid insurance acquires an infection after being cared for by EMS and is hospitalized, the government may not reimburse the cost of that infection. Medical facilities are monitoring EMS as a possible source for some patient infections.

Host Defense Mechanisms

The human body provides built-in protection from pathogenic organisms with several defenses that protect against infection. Skin, which covers the entire exterior of the body, offers a primary protective barrier blocking pathogens' ability to enter through the intact surface. The normal secretions of the skin also provide an antibacterial property that protects against pathogen entry. Antibacterial handwashing solutions should not be used because they kill all bacteria on the skin, including normal flora.

Mucous membranes offer another protective barrier. For example, the eyes produce tears that dilute and remove foreign substances. The mucous membranes that line the urinary, respiratory, and gastrointestinal (GI) tracts also trap and remove organisms. Cells that line the respiratory tract secrete lysozymes that destroy bacteria, while macrophages trap and destroy bacteria; thus, these mucous membranes serve as a first line of defense against airborne and droplet-transmitted diseases. Goblet cells lining the GI tract produce highly acidic and alkaline secretions, which form barriers that prevent penetration by bacteria and some viruses.

The immune system contains proteins that kill viruses. Immune response ignites the production of antibodies that are directed against specific invading organisms. B cells and T cells work together to fight infection.

Infection and Sepsis

The CDC is working to raise awareness on **sepsis**. Their report published in August 2016 stated that 80% of patients with sepsis developed the infection that lead to sepsis in a setting outside the hospital, and that 7 of 10 patients diagnosed with sepsis had received recent health care services or had a chronic disease that required frequent medical care visits.[29]

Part 1 of the report suggests the importance of EMS providers recognizing sepsis and alerting the receiving facility when a patient with possible sepsis is being transported is key in improving patient outcomes. The definitions of sepsis and **septic shock** were revised by an international task force and were presented at the Society of Critical Care Medicine 45th Critical Care Congress. A Surviving Sepsis Campaign (SSC) has been established to improve the diagnosis and management of sepsis.[30] Also, evidence-based interventions called bundles have been developed as an approach to increasing patient survival. One bundle addresses resuscitation and one addresses management of care.

Pathophysiology

Sepsis is the body's overreaction to an infection or virus that can progress to shock. Sepsis is a medical emergency and requires rapid treatment to prevent tissue damage, organ failure, and death. People identified as being at risk for sepsis include those 65 and older, infants younger than 1 year, people with compromised immune systems, and those with chronic medical conditions such as diabetes.

Assessment

Perform a primary survey and obtain a focused history and appropriate physical exam. Signs and symptoms of sepsis include one or more of the following:

- Shivering, fever or feeling very cold
- Extreme pain or discomfort
- Clammy or discolored skin
- Confusion or disorientation
- Shortness of breath
- Elevated heart rates

You have learned that definitive care and optimum patient outcome are time-sensitive for patients experiencing trauma, myocardial infarction, and stroke. Similarly, the early identification of patients with sepsis and the prompt emergency care in the initial hours after sepsis develops improves outcomes.[30] The quick Sepsis-related Organ Failure Assessment (qSOFA) is a rapid scoring system that can be used to identify patients who have an infection and may be at risk of dying from sepsis. The objective of early identification of sepsis is to begin treatment before the syndrome worsens. The qSOFA score is easy to calculate because it only has three components, each of which are easily identified: (1) Respiratory rate (≥22 breaths/min), (2) altered mentation (Glasgow Coma Scale score <15), and (3) systolic blood pressure (≤100 mm Hg).[31] The score ranges from 0 to 3 points. One point is assigned for each component. A score of 2 or more is associated with poor outcomes due to sepsis.

Management

If you suspect sepsis or septic shock, initiate pulse oximetry and cardiac and blood pressure monitoring. Give supplemental oxygen if indicated. Bag-mask ventilation may be necessary if breathing is inadequate.

Obtain vascular access and begin fluid resuscitation. If sepsis-induced hypoperfusion is present, the Surviving Sepsis Campaign recommends the administration of at least 30 mL/kg of IV crystalloid within the first 3 hours.[30] In addition to monitoring the patient's oxygen saturation, heart rate, and blood pressure, carefully monitor him or her for increased work of breathing or the development of crackles. If hypotension persists despite fluid administration, consult medical direction for advice with regard to giving additional fluids versus the use of vasopressors. Transport the patient to the closest appropriate facility.

Pathophysiology, Assessment, and Management of Droplet-Transmitted Diseases

Meningitis

Meningitis is an inflammation of the membranes that cover the brain and spinal cord, called the *meninges*. Two types of meningitis are distinguished: bacterial and viral. The bacterial form is communicable, and the viral form is not. More than 90% of meningitis cases in the United States are viral and do not pose a risk to health care providers.[32] Meningitis is droplet-transmitted. Transmission is by direct contact with a patient's oral or nasal secretions. The most common bacterial organisms implicated in meningitis are *Neisseria meningitidis, Streptococcus pneumoniae, Haemophilus influenzae*, group B *Streptococcus*, and *Listeria monocytogenes*.

The most common type of meningitis is **meningococcal meningitis**, which is caused by *N meningitidis*. In the past, sporadic cases of meningococcal meningitis occurred most frequently during winter and spring, especially when people lived together in crowded conditions, such as in college dorms, homeless shelters, or military barracks. Currently, all pre-teens, high school students, and college students entering dormitory living are vaccinated against the primary types of meningitis. This has resulted in a decrease in cases on a national level.

Pathophysiology

Transmission occurs following direct contact with the nasopharyngeal secretions of an infected person (mouth-to-mouth, suctioning, or intubation with spraying of secretions) or prolonged contact time of 8 or more hours. The incubation period for meningococcal meningitis is between 2 and 10 days. The communicable period is variable; it lasts as long as meningococcal bacteria are present in the patient's nasal and oral secretions. The microorganisms generally disappear from the patient's upper respiratory tract within 24 hours after antibiotic treatment begins.

Words of Wisdom

Meningitis is not transmitted by airborne means. Viral meningitis is infectious but not communicable.

Assessment

The classic signs and symptoms of meningitis are the same for the viral and bacterial forms: sudden-onset fever, severe headache, stiff neck, Kernig sign (the patient cannot extend his or her leg at the knee when the thigh is flexed because of stiffness in the hamstrings), Brudzinski sign (passive flexion of the leg on one side causes a similar movement in the opposite leg), photosensitivity, and a pink rash that becomes purple. The patient almost always experiences changes in mental status, ranging from apathy to delirium. Projectile vomiting is common. Diagnosis is made by Gram stain, a simple test in which CSF (obtained by a procedure known as a lumbar puncture) is placed on a slide, crystal violet stain is added to the CSF, and there is an initial identification of whether a bacterium is present. A Gram stain gives a quick result and can help distinguish viral from bacterial infection often in just a few minutes after a CSF sample is obtained.

Management

When you are treating a patient with meningitis, ask the patient to wear a surgical mask or a nonrebreathing mask. If this is not possible, you should wear a surgical mask. Routine standard precautions, including gloves and good handwashing technique, are also important. Diagnosis is not made until a lumbar puncture is performed, so precautions must be maintained throughout your interactions with the patient.

Special Populations

Meningitis in infants and children has decreased in incidence and mortality with the development and administration of vaccines. Vaccines protect against *Haemophilus influenzae* type b, *Streptococcus pneumoniae*, and *Neisseria meningitidis*. Vaccine administration is started at age 2 months. However, in a child who has not been vaccinated, meningitis remains a major emergency that requires antibiotic treatment.

The health care provider must assess the patient for signs and symptoms suggestive of meningitis, which include fever, vomiting, irritability, and lethargy. In infants, a bulging fontanelle may also be noted. The paramedic should assess the patient for respiratory distress, which may indicate the need for intubation en route, oxygen administration, and rapid transport.

Additional treatment will be added based on symptoms. Patient needs may include oxygen, airway management, and ventilation support. Medical control may order IV fluids based on the patient's signs and symptoms, and medications may be ordered en route if seizures occur or the patient shows signs of shock. Only patients with severe signs and symptoms require rapid transport to a medical facility.

Transmission from patient to health care provider is rare. Postexposure treatment typically includes ciprofloxacin (one dose given orally) or rifampin for 2 days. This treatment is not appropriate if the person is taking birth control pills, and it should not be offered to pregnant patients. Ceftriaxone (Rocephin) is the drug of choice if an exposed health care provider is pregnant. The meningitis vaccine is not recommended for any health care provider group; it is recommended for college students entering dormitory living for the first time, military recruits, and middle school and high school students. Ciprofloxacin-resistant bacterial meningitis has now been documented in at least three states within the United States. It is important to offer postexposure treatment only when an actual exposure has occurred.

▶ Respiratory Conditions

A number of respiratory conditions may (or may not) be associated with a fever and may (or may not) be infectious. These conditions run the gamut from mildly annoying symptoms to potentially life-threatening conditions.

Respiratory syncytial virus is the leading cause of lower respiratory tract infections in infants, older adults, and immunocompromised people. It and other communicable diseases relevant to the pediatric population (such as bronchiolitis and croup) are discussed in Chapter 43, *Pediatric Emergencies*.

▶ Seasonal Influenza

Influenza (flu) viruses cause acute respiratory illnesses generally presenting as winter epidemics. In the United States, the flu causes approximately 36,000 deaths each year.[16]

nH1N1 (novel H1N1) influenza began in California and was first believed to be poised to cause a major pandemic. Fortunately, however, it proved to be a new seasonal flu virus that did not result in a significant number of deaths worldwide.[33,34] The comparison to the number of deaths in the United States each year from normal seasonal flu makes this very clear. For nH1N1 worldwide, the WHO reported fewer than 19,000 deaths. It is now called H1N1.

> **Special Populations**
>
> Infection rates are high in children, but the most deaths occur among adults older than 65 years, especially people with medical conditions such as chronic pulmonary or heart disease.
>
> Death is preventable with vaccination.

Pathophysiology

For this droplet-transmitted disease, transmission was thought to be airborne. However, further research has shown transmission to be hand-to-nose-to-mouth-to-eye. The incubation period is about 1 to 4 days following exposure. The communicable period in adults lasts from the day before symptoms begin until about 5 days after the onset of the illness.

Assessment

Signs and symptoms of influenza include systemic fever, shaking chills, headache, muscle pain, malaise, and loss of appetite. Respiratory symptoms include dry, often protracted coughing; hoarseness; and nasal discharge. The duration of illness is about 3 to 4 days, and complications may include viral or bacterial pneumonia.

Management

Prevention of influenza, which has been a mild disease during the past 4 years, involves placing a surgical mask or nonrebreathing mask on the patient. Very few patients have required IV fluids for dehydration or ventilation assistance during transport. The key preventive measure, however, is an annual flu shot. Each year, a new vaccine is developed based on the anticipated strains for that year. The injectable form of the vaccine does not contain live virus, so you cannot get the disease from the flu shot. An alternative to the injectable form is the nasal spray, which contains live attenuated virus. However, in 2015/2016 there was a low response to the nasal spray and it was not offered in 2016/2017. A vaccine is also available for people who have egg, mercury, and antibiotic allergies. An effort is under way to make seasonal flu vaccination mandatory for all health care providers as a patient safety issue. Medical facilities have made flu shots a condition of employment for their employees. If you do not take a flu shot, you must sign a declination form. This provision is set forth by OSHA, NFPA 1581, and the CDC, and wear a mask whenever working around patients. If EMS providers decline the flu shot, they will be required to wear a mask when entering the medical facility.

If you have not been vaccinated and have an exposure, antiviral drugs may be offered within 48 hours to reduce the severity of the flu should you contract it.

▶ Pertussis (Whooping Cough)

Pertussis is a disease caused by the *Bordetella pertussis* bacteria. Cases have been increasing in the United States over the past several years because of unvaccinated children and waning protection for adults. Currently, pertussis is the disease with the largest case number in this country. The CDC recommends that all health care providers receive a booster for pertussis.[35]

Pathophysiology

Pertussis is a large-droplet–transmitted disease (3-foot [1-m] rule). It is considered to be highly contagious. The incubation period is 7 to 10 days following an exposure. All pregnant women are given Tdap boosters.

Assessment

The patient presents with fever, thick nasal discharge, and a cough that progresses to coughing spasms. The patient is not able to take a breath. Children often develop black eyes from the coughing. When the patient can finally take a breath, a "whoop" sound is heard. Vomiting generally follows.

Management

Pertussis in children must be treated quickly. This illness also must be reported to the public health department to prevent additional cases. Patients are considered to be infectious at the time of presentation of the runny nose, sneezing, and low-grade fever. This is referred to as the catarrhal stage. The second stage (paroxysms) is when the coughing attacks occur.

The recommended treatment is azithromycin, but other antibiotics may be prescribed, such as erythromycin. In 2013, the Food and Drug Administration published a warning that azithromycin could cause abnormal changes in cardiac electrical activity. Another drug should be considered for people with known cardiac disease.

For health care providers, protection via the recommended Tdap booster is important.

▶ Mumps

Mumps (infectious parotitis) is a droplet-transmitted disease. Before a vaccine was available in 1967, many children sustained permanent deafness, encephalitis, and death from mumps. About 186,000 cases were reported each year in the United States.[10] Many health care providers are unaware of the complications of childhood diseases. There have been several recent outbreaks in colleges, corporations, and even the National Hockey League (2015). Outbreaks are related to people not being vaccinated or not receiving two doses of mumps vaccine. Case numbers began to decrease in 2015 with more people, including health care providers, being vaccinated. However, data from the CDC for 2016 are showing an increase in cases. This is especially important because 20% to 40% of infected people may not show signs or symptoms of this disease.

Pathophysiology

Mumps virus multiplies in the upper respiratory tract and is transmitted through direct contact with saliva or respiratory secretions. Mumps virus can also be transmitted by fomites. The incubation period for this illness is 16 to 18 days following exposure.

Complications from acquiring mumps occur in adults more often than in children. According to the CDC,[36] the most common complication is orchitis (inflammation of one testis). This can occur in 3% to 10% of males. Other complications in adults include deafness, meningitis, encephalitis, and pancreatitis. These complications have occurred in less than 1% of cases in recent US outbreaks. For women who acquire mumps when pregnant, complications may also occur.

Assessment

Mumps presents with fever, headache, muscle aches, loss of appetite, and swelling of the salivary glands under the ears. This can be on one side or bilateral.

Management

Treatment is supportive. Age-appropriate pain management and cold packs may offer some relief. This is a reportable disease to the public health department. Vaccination is the key to protection. If no history of mumps or confirmation of receipt of two doses of the measles, mumps, rubella (MMR) vaccine can be produced, the person should be considered nonimmune and offered the vaccine. Titers (tests that detect the presence and measure the amount of antibodies within a person's blood) do not need to be done unless it is deemed cost effective. Generally, titers cost more than the vaccine.[10] Vaccination before an exposure occurs is important. The vaccine is *not* effective post exposure. If an exposure occurs in a nonimmune person, he or she will be placed on work restriction from days 12 to 25 following the exposure event.

▶ Rubella (German Measles)

Rubella is a caused by a virus. It is also called the German measles, but it is caused by a different virus than measles. It was thought that rubella had been eliminated from the United States in 2004. Although it is no longer endemic (constantly present) in the United States, it is being brought into the United States from other countries.

The rubella vaccination program started in 1969. During the last major rubella epidemic in the United States from 1964 to 1965, an estimated 12.5 million people acquired rubella, 11,000 pregnant women miscarried, 2,100 newborns died, and 20,000 babies were born with congenital rubella syndrome.[37] The birth defects seen in congenital rubella syndrome are very much like those seen with Zika virus infection. Once the vaccine became widely used, the number of people infected with rubella in the United States dropped significantly.

Pathophysiology

Rubella is droplet transmitted and spreads when an infected person coughs or sneezes. An individual with rubella may spread the disease to others up to 1 week before the rash appears. The incubation period is from 12 to 23 days following an exposure event. An infected person can remain contagious up to 7 days after the rash appears. About 25% to 50% of people infected with rubella do not develop a rash or have any symptoms.[38,39] This makes vaccination an important factor for exposure protection.

Assessment

People infected with rubella will present with a rash that usually begins on the face and then spreads to the rest of the body. This is generally a mild disease. Additional signs and symptoms include headache, mild pink eye, swollen and enlarged lymph nodes, cough, and a runny nose.

Management

There is no specific treatment for rubella.

Words of Wisdom

Prevention is important. Know your childhood disease history and if you are not protected, get vaccinated. If you are not protected, put a surgical mask on the patient. If you are not able to mask the patient, then you should wear the surgical mask.

Pathophysiology, Assessment, and Management of Airborne-Transmitted Diseases

Tuberculosis

Tuberculosis (TB) has been an important cause of disability and death in much of the developing world. This disease was once widespread in the United States, but no longer. In 2014, the lowest incidence of TB in US history was documented. Since 2014, reported cases have been less than 10,000 per year in the US, which is approximately 320 million people (or approximately 1 case per 32,000 people. Four states (California, Texas, New York, and Florida), representing about one third of the US population, accounted for half of all TB cases reported in 2014.[40] The WHO and the CDC are working together to eliminate this disease worldwide. The goal was to achieve this by 2015, but that was not met due to medication shortages and wars in areas where disease cases are the highest. This goal has now been reset for 2035.

Pathophysiology

TB is *not* a highly communicable disease. Three types of TB exist: *typical*, which is communicable, and *atypical* and *extrapulmonary* (TB of the bone, kidney, lymph glands, and so on), which are not communicable. All types of TB are counted as one number. People at risk for contracting TB include people born in Asia and Africa and incarcerated people. The rate is high in the incarcerated population due to overcrowded conditions and poor health care. Immunocompromised people, homeless people, and residents in long-term care facilities are also at risk. In the United States, the highest rate of cases for TB is in the Asian population.[41]

> **Words of Wisdom**
>
> The classic presentation of tuberculosis (TB) includes sudden weight loss, night sweats, fever, and cough with blood-tinged sputum. This clinical presentation should raise a red flag. The best protection against TB is good airflow through your environment. Do not let a patient cough in your face, and keep the rear windows of the ambulance open, weather permitting. Consider using an oxygen mask on the patient instead of a nasal cannula. You can administer the same fraction of inspired oxygen while limiting the spread of droplets when the patient coughs. Place a surgical mask on the patient. If you are unable to do this, you should wear the surgical mask. Use the exhaust fan to exchange the air!

TB infection (latent TB) means that a person has tested positive for exposure to TB but does not have, and may never develop, active disease. People with TB infection do not pose a risk to others. *TB disease* means that the person has active TB disease verified by laboratory testing and a positive chest radiograph.

Drug-resistant TB can occur with misuse or mismanagement of the medications used to treat TB. Multidrug-resistant TB (MDR TB) means that the bacterium is resistant to two or more of the first-line medications (of several available) used to treat TB. Extensively drug-resistant TB (XDR TB) is an uncommon type of TB that is resistant to two of the first-line oral medications and at least one of three injectable second-line medications.[42] MDR TB and XDR TB are treatable diseases.

> **Words of Wisdom**
>
> Noncompliance has been addressed by "direct observed therapy," in which health nurses ensure patients take their medications.
>
> TB patients are now cared for while living in their own homes with family members.

Transmission occurs by large, airborne particles from a person with active untreated disease. In general, that type of spread occurs among people who have prolonged contact or intimate exposure to the infected person (primarily people living in the same household). For paramedics, such intense exposure is likely to occur only when mouth-to-mouth ventilation is given to a patient with active untreated TB or intubation and suctioning without PPE.

The incubation period for TB is 4 to 12 weeks. The disease is communicable only when an active lesion develops in the lungs and bacteria are expelled into the air by coughing. Of patients who are treated, 10% are no longer communicable after 2 days of treatment. After 14 days of treatment, virtually all patients are no longer communicable.

> **Words of Wisdom**
>
> Notify your DICO if you believe you may have been exposed to TB. The medical facility is required to notify the DICO if a patient you have transported may have or is suspected of having TB.

Early infection with TB can be detected by a **tuberculin skin test** or by the **tuberculosis blood test**. There are two in the marketplace: QuantiFERON-TB Gold blood test and T-spot TB.

The TB blood test is a one-time blood draw with very accurate results available in 2 days. Health departments and fire/EMS agencies across the country are now using the TB blood test, because it is reliable and convenient. All health care providers, including paramedics, should have a tuberculin test at the beginning of employment and periodically based on the TB risk assessment for the department. The TB risk assessment is based on the number of patients with active-untreated TB the department transported in the previous 12 months, not on the number of patients in the community served. The CDC TB guidelines have a chart that guides this process.[43] If a known positive history is present when a person is hired, a questionnaire must be completed by the employee. The designated physician then reviews the questionnaire. As mentioned, TB develops in only 10% of persons with a positive TB test. Disease activation would depend on the overall health status of the person later in life. A chest radiograph is indicated only for a first positive test.

Assessment

Signs and symptoms of TB include a persistent cough for more than 3 weeks plus one or more of the following: night sweats, headache, fever, fatigue, weight loss, hemoptysis, hoarseness, or chest pain.

Management

As a preventive measure, place a surgical mask on a patient suspected of having TB. If the patient cannot be masked, place a surgical mask on yourself to block transmission of TB. According to the CDC 2005 TB Guidelines and OSHA enforcement of those, N95 or HEPA respirators are not needed or required for EMS transport of a patient with suspected TB.[44] The patient may require high-concentration oxygen administration and/or airway or ventilation support based on assessment. If preventive measures were not taken, report the incident to your DICO. Given that the incubation period for TB is 4 to 12 weeks, a paramedic who suspects he or she has been exposed to TB should work with the department DICO to assess the need for baseline testing and then be retested in 8 to 10 weeks. If the test has become positive at that time, the paramedic needs to have a chest radiograph to rule out infection and usually will be offered a 12-week course of antibiotic therapy (2012).[45] This short course of therapy was adopted by the WHO and the CDC. Because these drugs are toxic to the liver, the paramedic should not consume alcohol while taking the drugs, and liver function tests should be conducted monthly.

No special measures are required after transporting a patient suspected of having active TB. The vehicle should be cleaned as usual. No airing is required.

▶ Varicella Zoster (Chickenpox)

Varicella zoster (chickenpox) is a highly contagious disease. Varicella zoster virus (VZV) is a member of the herpes virus family. Reactivation of latent infection causes herpes zoster (shingles). Chickenpox cases have been on the increase in the United States over the past several years. Chickenpox vaccine became available in 1995. Fewer outbreaks have been reported since the inception of a two-dose chickenpox vaccination program, which is very effective at preventing severe cases.[46] People who take the vaccine are also protected from developing shingles later in life.

Pathophysiology

After the primary infection, VZV stays in the body (in the sensory nerve ganglia) as a latent infection. Primary infection with VZV causes varicella. Transmission can occur in two ways: via direct contact or by inhalation of aerosols from the lesions. Respiratory secretions can also transmit this disease. The incubation period is 14 to 16 days after exposure, but the average time frame is between 10 and 21 days.

Assessment

People who had chickenpox develop lifelong immunity. Establish a history if the patient presents with rash beginning on the abdomen that spreads to other parts of the body, or has a fever and photosensitivity (wants to be in the dark) **Figure 26-5**.

Management

Use airborne precautions and contact precautions when caring for a patient diagnosed with or suspected of having chickenpox. There is no specific treatment for chickenpox. Antipuretic agents may assist in relieving the itching. The patient should be observed for signs of secondary infection of the lesions.

Exposure to chickenpox is defined as greater than 5 minutes to 1 hour in the same room (indoors) or face-to-face contact. If an unprotected exposure occurs, contact the DICO. Vaccine may be administered within 72 hours to prevent infection from occurring in a nonimmune health care provider. However, if the exposed health care provider is pregnant or immunocompromised, the vaccine cannot be given. A special immunoglobulin (varicella zoster immune

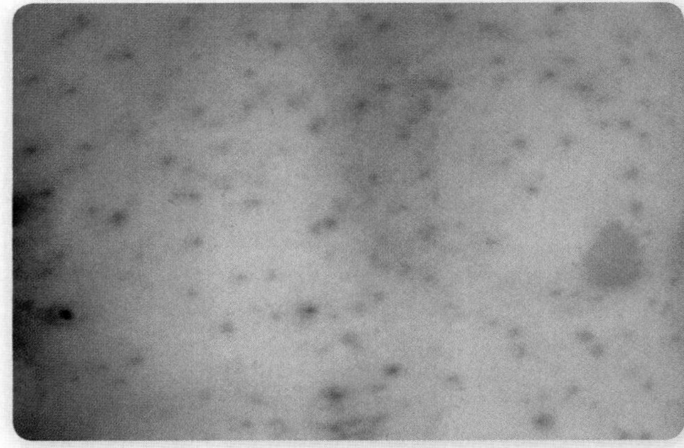

Figure 26-5 The distinctive rash produced by chickenpox is composed of small, blisterlike vesicles that arise in clusters.

Courtesy of Centers for Disease Control and Prevention.

globulin), VariZig, must be ordered for protection to be achieved. Work restriction will need to be implemented as well for 18 days following the exposure event. This illustrates the importance of vaccine administration to a nonimmune person before an exposure occurs.

▶ Measles

Measles (rubeola, not to be confused with German measles [rubella]) is considered highly communicable. Outbreaks have occurred in many states over the years. The vaccine became available in 1963, but before it was available, about 500,000 cases were documented each year. Of that 500,000, about 500 deaths occurred, 48,000 were hospitalized, and about 1,000 people sustained brain damage as the result of encephalitis. Outbreaks still occur; in 2015 several were documented.[47] From 2001 to 2008, 557 cases were reported in the United States. In 2015, over 800 cases were reported.

Pathophysiology

Measles is caused by a virus that is transmitted when an infected person coughs or sneezes. This is an airborne transmissible disease, so it has a 6-foot (2-m) rule; particles can travel up to 6 feet (2 m) and then fall to the ground.

Assessment

Measles in the early (prodromal) phase is characterized by fever, conjunctivitis, and coryza (acute rhinitis). Onset of coughing, a blotchy red rash (which often starts on the head), and white-gray spots on the buccal (mouth) mucosa (known as Koplik spots) follow **Figure 26-6**. The rash spreads from the head to the trunk to the lower extremities. Patients are considered to be contagious from 4 days before to 4 days after the rash appears.

Common complications from measles include otitis media, bronchopneumonia, laryngotracheobronchitis, and diarrhea.

Management

Care of a patient with measles is supportive. There is no treatment for measles other than reducing fever and

Figure 26-6 A blotchy red rash is characteristic of measles.

Courtesy of Dr. Heinz F. Eichenwald/CDC.

YOU are the Paramedic PART 3

You begin your assessment of the patient. When asked, she says that she has been nauseated and having diarrhea for a few days. She also says she is too weak to stand and has not been able to keep water down. When your partner feels for the patient's pulse, there is obvious tenting when the skin on her forearm is pinched.

Recording Time: 5 Minutes	
Respirations	18 breaths/min
Pulse	106 beats/min
Skin	Pale, cool, dry; tenting noted
Blood pressure	98/58 mm Hg
Oxygen saturation (Spo_2)	97% on room air
Pupils	PERRLA

5. What is your first choice of treatment for this patient?
6. Are there any notifications you should make concerning the scene?

maintaining comfort. Although placing a mask on the patient may prevent droplet transmission, the only certain protection against measles is immunity. Exposure is defined as transport of a patient or being in the same room as the patient, so the patient should remain isolated, though this may not be realistic when transporting a patient in an ambulance.

Words of Wisdom

The incubation period for measles is 7 to 18 days following an exposure event. The measles virus can remain in the air for at least 2 hours. This shows the importance of using the exhaust feature of your vehicle.

Words of Wisdom

People who were vaccinated between 1963 and 1967 need to be revaccinated with the live measles vaccine. From 1963 to 1967, a killed virus vaccine was used and has shown not to be protective.

People who were born during or after 1957 who do not have evidence of immunity against measles should get at least one dose of the MMR vaccine.[48]

Special Populations

Because of their relatively immature immune systems, infants and young children are especially susceptible to infectious diseases. Pediatric immunizations prevent disease in children who receive them and protect those who come into contact with unvaccinated people. Although the incidence of vaccine-preventable diseases has decreased in the United States, the viruses and bacteria that cause them still exist. According to the CDC, the following immunizations are recommended for all children:[49]

- Diphtheria, pertussis, and tetanus
- *Haemophilus influenzae* type b
- Hepatitis A
- Hepatitis B
- Human papillomavirus
- Inactivated polio virus
- Measles, mumps, and rubella
- Meningococcal ACWY
- Meningococcal B
- Pneumococcal conjugate
- Pneumococcal polysaccharide
- Rotavirus
- Influenza
- Varicella

Prevention is by vaccination. All health care workers should receive measles vaccinations. Anyone who has had measles or who received two doses of live virus measles vaccine after 1968 should be able to document immunity to measles. If you received a vaccine between 1963 and 1967, you need to be revaccinated with a live measles vaccine. It is important that the immunity status of all fire department and EMS employees be assessed. Postexposure treatment includes vaccination if you are not immune. If an unprotected exposure occurs, MMR can be given within 72 hours of the exposure event.

No special disinfection measures are required for the ambulance after transporting a patient known to have measles. Simply washing patient contact areas and laundering any soiled linens are sufficient.

Words of Wisdom

Cases of pneumococcal pneumonia are decreasing due to the pneumonia vaccine. The key to influencing cases of pneumonia is vaccination for people in the recommend age groups. Pneumococcal conjugate vaccine (PCV13) is recommended for all children younger than 5 years, all adults older than 65 years, and people 6 years or older with certain risk factors. Pneumococcal polysaccharide vaccine (PPSV23) is recommended for all adults 65 years or older. Vaccine programs are geared toward reducing or eliminating vaccine-preventable diseases.

Pneumonia is discussed in Chapter 16, *Respiratory Emergencies.*

Other Infections of the Respiratory Tract

▶ Mononucleosis

Pathophysiology

Mononucleosis (mono) is caused by the Epstein-Barr virus (EBV). This virus is also suspected of causing a related disease, chronic fatigue syndrome. The virus grows in the epithelium of the oropharynx and sheds into saliva—hence the name kissing disease. In most cases of mononucleosis there are no symptoms, which means the EBV infection is subclinical. At least one in every four teens and young adults who acquire EBV become infected with mono.[50] This illness is not reportable in all states.

Transmission occurs via direct contact with the saliva of an infected person. Some cases have also been linked to contaminated blood transfusions. The incubation period is 4 to 6 weeks following exposure, with a prolonged communicable period. Most cases resolve in 2 to 4 weeks.

Assessment

Signs and symptoms of mononucleosis include sore throat, fever, secretions from the pharynx, swollen lymph glands (especially the posterior cervical glands), malaise, anorexia, headache, rash, muscle pain, and an enlarged liver and/or spleen. Pharyngeal secretions may persist for 1 year or more after infection. In severe cases, complications may include anemia, dehydration, spleen rupture, seizures, or pneumonia.

Management

Prevention of mononucleosis involves the use of gloves and good handwashing techniques when in direct contact with a patient's oral secretions (standard precautions). No special cleaning solutions are required following transport of a patient.

Words of Wisdom

A paramedic with a cold or flu can be extremely hazardous to a patient who is immunocompromised.

Pathophysiology, Assessment, and Management of Sexually Transmitted Diseases

As the name implies, **sexually transmitted diseases (STDs)** are usually acquired by sexual contact. Although the term *STD* ordinarily conjures up diagnoses such as gonorrhea or syphilis, the range of diseases transmitted sexually is wide and includes such conditions as herpes, hepatitis, and HIV infection. Hepatitis, HIV infection, and AIDS are considered separately in this chapter. The latter are more commonly known as bloodborne diseases. This section reviews the features of gonorrhea, syphilis, scabies, and genital herpes infections, as well as STDs. In most cases, you will not know that a patient has an STD; therefore, standard precautions and good handwashing are appropriate.

In general, there is no specific prehospital treatment for STDs. Protect your patient's privacy and modesty. Your assessment will reveal the signs and symptoms that require treatment. The most common signs and symptoms that require treatment include pain, nausea and vomiting, bleeding, and fever. If indicated, start an IV line (titrate to vital signs), and administer analgesics and antiemetics.

▶ Gonorrhea

Pathophysiology

Gonorrhea is an infection caused by the gonococcal bacteria, *Neisseria gonorrhoeae*. Gonorrhea is especially common in people aged 15 to 24 years. Transmission occurs sexually, by contact with the pus-containing fluid from mucous membranes of infected people. Therefore, anyone who engages in unprotected sexual contact is at risk. The incubation period is usually 2 to 7 days but may be longer. This infection is communicable for months if not treated. If treated, the disease is noncommunicable within hours.

Assessment

Signs and symptoms of gonorrhea differ between males and females. Males usually experience a pus-containing discharge from the urethra and often report pain on urination (dysuria) starting a few days after exposure. In women, the initial inflammation of the urethra or cervix may be so mild that it passes unnoticed, and the illness may progress to pelvic inflammatory disease (PID), with signs and symptoms of an acute abdomen. Depending on the patient's sexual practices, gonorrheal infection may also involve the anus and throat.

Management

The risk of acquiring any STD through a route other than sexual contact is remote. Prevention (standard precautions) includes glove use if touching drainage from the genital area and thorough handwashing. Providing care for a person with gonorrhea would not be considered an occupational health risk.

▶ Syphilis

Pathophysiology

Syphilis is caused by the spiral-shaped bacterium *Treponema pallidum*. Because the disease progresses in three stages, it is considered to be an acute and a chronic disease. Its incidence has been increasing in the United States for the past 7 years. In 2016, the CDC reported that there were about 24,000 cases reported in the United States.[51] The groups with the highest incidence rates are people aged 20 to 35 years. High numbers of cases are also reported in urban areas. This disease has been increasing in major areas: California, Texas, Florida, and New York City. The listing of these states has not changed in the past 7 years. Generally, men who have sex with men have a high incidence rate, but in Florida the highest rate was noted in a large retirement community. The high incidence rate in this age group has been identified across the country and senior communities have been added to the high-risk-group listing. Many states have written plans to eliminate syphilis, but it does not appear that all are following their plans. The CDC initially published a plan to eliminate this disease in the United States by 2010. However, due to new STD guidelines, this was reset. The new target is 2020. The CDC broadened testing recommendations in the 2015 updated version of the STD guidelines.

Transmission occurs by direct contact with the infectious fluids of the primary lesion or chancre. The bacteria can be transmitted across the placenta from an infected mother to her fetus, by sexual contact, or through blood transfusion. The incubation period is 10 days to 3 months; the communicable period is variable. If treated with penicillin, the person is considered noncontagious within 48 hours.

Assessment

The primary infection with syphilis produces an ulcerative lesion, called a **chancre**, of the skin or mucous membrane at the site of infection. Chancres are most commonly located in the genital region. *Secondary infection* is the term used to describe the presence of skin rash, patchy hair loss, and swollen lymph glands. Complications of syphilis in the tertiary (third) stage can include cardiac, ophthalmic, auditory, and central nervous system complications and lesions of the tissues and bone.

Management

Prevention measures include taking standard precautions—gloves and good handwashing techniques. No special cleaning precautions are required. The occupational risk for transmission to a health care provider would be a contaminated needlestick injury. If a contaminated needlestick injury occurs, notify your DICO. Treatment is available with procaine penicillin G. If you are allergic to penicillin, tetracycline or doxycycline are available. Syphilis is a common co-infection in HIV-infected persons.

▶ Genital Herpes

Pathophysiology

Genital herpes is a chronic, recurrent illness produced by infection with the herpes simplex virus. The herpes simplex virus is further classified into two types: type 1 is generally transmitted via contact with oral secretions, and type 2 is spread through sexual contact. All sexually active persons are at risk for this infection. Cases of genital herpes do not have to be reported to the CDC, so data on incidence are not available. Herpes simplex type 1 infection is usually activated from a dormant status by stress and febrile illness. It causes a blister-like sore, usually on the lips or inside the mouth. Infants may become infected if delivered through the birth canal of a woman with active disease.

The incubation period is 2 to 12 days. Secretion of the virus in saliva has been noted to persist for up to 7 weeks following the appearance of a lesion. Genital lesions are infectious for 4 to 7 days. This disease is elusive; it can suddenly become reactivated, often repeatedly, over many years. Outbreaks are often stress-related.

Paramedics need to use basic standard precautions—gloves and good handwashing practices if they come in contact with the lesions.

Assessment

Genital herpes is characterized by vesicular lesions **Figure 26-7**. In women, the vesicles occur initially on the cervix; during recurrent infections, vesicles may also appear around the vulva, legs, and buttocks. In men, lesions commonly occur on the penis, as well as around the anus, depending on sexual practices. Herpes type 1 oral lesions may be present on the patient's mouth. If a paramedic has an open cut on the hand or finger and is in contact with the drainage from a herpes type 1 oral lesion, the paramedic may develop herpetic whitlow (herpes infection of the finger), which is considered an occupational risk. To avoid such risks, use of gloves is important when suctioning or intubating a patient with oral lesions. There is no postexposure treatment for this infection.

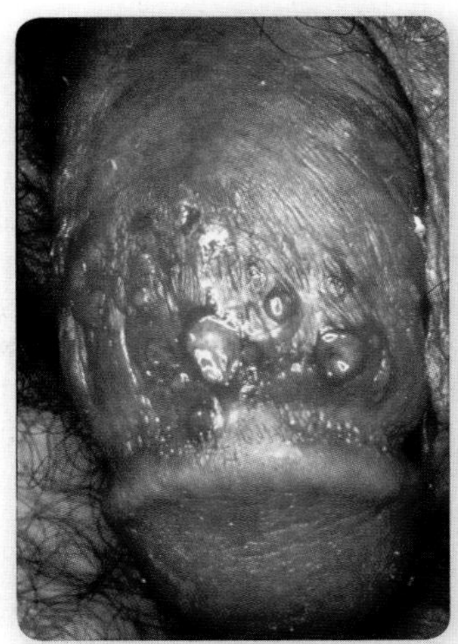

Figure 26-7 Genital herpes.

Courtesy of Dr. N.J. Fumara and Dr. Gavin Hart/CDC.

Management

There is no cure for genital herpes. However, it can be treated with acyclovir, valacyclovir, or famciclovir for 7 to 10 days to reduce outbreaks. Preventive measures include standard precautions—the use of gloves when touching drainage from lesions and good handwashing techniques. No special cleaning precautions are necessary.

Genital herpes is not an occupational health risk. Herpetic whitlow is considered an occupational health risk.

▶ Chlamydia

Pathophysiology

Chlamydia infections are the most frequently reported bacterial sexually transmitted infection in the United States.[52] In 2015, more than 1.5 million cases were reported to the CDC; the growth in this number is believed to be the result of the availability of more sensitive screening tests and the trend toward routine screening.

Transmission occurs through sexual contact. Perinatal infections may result in premature rupture of membranes, premature birth, or stillbirth. The incubation period is believed to be 7 to 14 days or longer. The communicable period is unknown.

Assessment

In most women with chlamydia, the infection initially remains asymptomatic. However, in many women infected with *Chlamydia trachomatis*, PID eventually develops. In men, infection may lead to epididymitis, prostatitis, proctitis, and proctocolitis.

Signs and symptoms include inflammation of the urethra, epididymis, cervix, and fallopian tubes when the infection is acquired through sexual transmission. Urethral discharge may be gray or white. The amount of discharge is variable.

Management

Chlamydia infection is treated with antibiotics. Preventive measures include wearing gloves when in contact with discharge from the genital area and using good handwashing techniques. There are no special cleaning requirements for the EMS vehicle or linens.

▶ Scabies

Pathophysiology

Scabies is caused by infection with *Sarcoptes scabiei*, a parasite. The incidence of this disease has been increasing during the past few years in the United States and Europe. This infection commonly affects families, children, sexual partners, chronically ill patients, and people in group homes. People of every race and social class are vulnerable to scabies infection.

Transmission occurs via direct skin-to-skin contact, such as through wrestling, sexual contact, and by sharing undergarments, towels, and linens. The incubation period is 4 to 6 weeks for people with no prior exposure to the pathogen. A second or subsequent infestation may appear in as little as a few days. The communicable period lasts until the mites and eggs are destroyed by treatment. The female mite can live on a human host for several weeks. Without a host, the parasite dies in 2 to 4 days. Transmission generally requires direct prolonged contact.

Assessment

Signs and symptoms of scabies include a rash of small, raised red bumps where the mite has burrowed into the skin, causing intense itching, especially at night. The rash appears on the hands, flexor aspects of the wrists, axillary folds, ankles, toes, genital area, buttocks, and abdomen **Figure 26-8**. The patient may develop sores from scratching the rash.

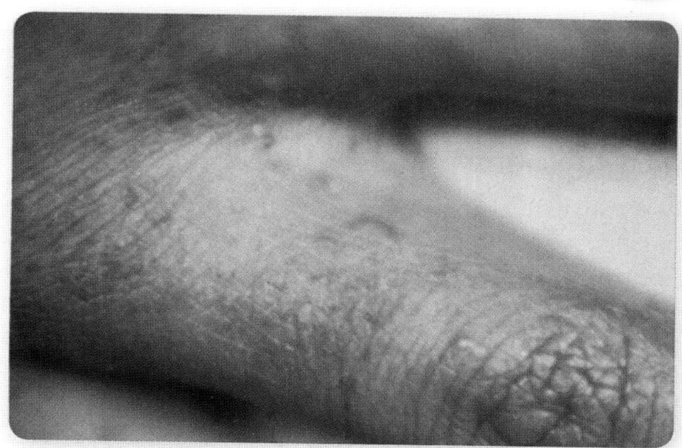

Figure 26-8 Rash produced by scabies.

Courtesy of Centers for Disease Control and Prevention.

Management

Prevention—standard precautions—consists of wearing gloves and practicing good handwashing techniques. Vehicle linens require only routine washing in hot water, with routine cleaning of the vehicle after patient transport. Products used to treat scabies are called *scabicides* because they kill scabies mites; some also kill mite eggs. These medications require a prescription. No treatment cream or lotion should be applied on a routine basis because of reports of toxicity. In case of documented exposure, treatment will be undertaken and work restrictions from patient care may be ordered.

This would be considered an occupational health risk. Exposure should be reported to the DICO.

▶ Lice

Pathophysiology

Lice are small insects that crawl through the hair and feed on blood through the skin. They cannot hop or fly. There are three types of lice: the head louse *(Pediculus humanus capitis)*, body louse *(Pediculus humanus corporis)*, and pubic louse *(Phthirus pubis)*.

All types of lice are acquired through direct contact with an infested person. Head and body lice can also be acquired from objects such as hats, combs, or clothes infested with lice. Lice eggs look like small white or tan dots on the skin. The eggs hatch after about 1 week, and the new lice mature in 1 to 2 weeks. Thereafter, an adult will begin to reproduce and will lay eggs over the next 28 days. Head lice can be found in the hair and in other hairy areas of the head, such as eyebrows, eyelashes, mustaches, and beards. Body lice are usually found in the seams of clothing and can transfer certain diseases.

When discussing lice as an STD, the focus is on pubic or crab lice. *Phthirus pubis* is a parasite that is usually gray in color. Lice are common in people with poor hygiene, people living in group homes, and people with multiple sexual partners.

Transmission of pubic lice occurs through intimate physical or sexual contact. The incubation period lasts approximately 8 to 10 days after the eggs hatch. The communicable period ends when all lice and eggs are destroyed by treatment.

Assessment

Signs and symptoms of pubic lice include slight to severe itching and irritation and, possibly, sores. Nits (eggs) can be seen clinging to the pubic, perianal, or perineal hair. Pubic lice can also infest eyelashes, eyebrows, axillae, scalp, and other body hairs.

Management

Preventive measures include standard precautions: wearing gloves and practicing good handwashing techniques. Routine cleaning of the vehicle after transport is sufficient. In case of documented exposure, treatment with permethrin cream may be prescribed, and restrictions from patient care may be indicated until the paramedic is free of lice.

This would be considered an occupational health risk. Exposure should be reported to the DICO.

▶ Other Sexually Transmitted Diseases and Related Conditions

Genital Warts and Human Papillomavirus

Genital warts (also called condylomata acuminata and venereal warts) are caused by the **human papillomavirus (HPV)**. Of the more than 100 types of HPV that have been identified (most are harmless), about 30 types are spread through sexual contact. HPV is the most common STD, with millions of new cases being reported every year. Sources estimate that 75% to 80% of all people in the United States will be infected with HPV at some time in their lives.[53] Some people infected with HPV have no symptoms. In others, multiple growths develop in the genital areas—that is, the vagina, vulva, cervix, or rectum, or the penis and scrotum in men. HPV has been identified as a causative agent in cervical, vulvar, and anal cancers. In pregnant women, warts may develop that become large enough to impede urination or obstruct the birth canal. If the virus is passed to the fetus, the child may develop *laryngeal papillomatosis* (throat warts that block the airway), a potentially life-threatening condition.

Chancroid

Chancroid is caused by infection with the bacterium *Haemophilus ducreyi*. This is a highly contagious yet curable disease. Chancroid is known to facilitate the transmission of HIV. This disease causes painful sores (ulcers), usually of the genitals. Swollen, painful lymph glands or inguinal buboes in the groin area may be present as well. Women may be asymptomatic and, thus, unaware they have the disease. Prehospital treatment is supportive only.

Trichomoniasis

Trichomoniasis, a parasitic infection caused by *Trichomonas vaginalis*, is a single-cell parasite that is transmitted through sexual contact. According to the CDC,[54] in men, the urethra is the most commonly infected body part; in women, the lower genital tract (eg, vulva, vagina, cervix, urethra) are most commonly infected. About 70% of infected people are asymptomatic. When present, symptoms usually appear within 5 to 28 days of exposure but can occur much later after exposure. In men, signs and symptoms may include a feeling of itching or irritation inside the penis, frequent urination, burning after urination or ejaculation, and, possibly, a purulent discharge from the penis. In women, signs and symptoms may include a foul-smelling vaginal discharge that is clear, white, yellow, gray, or green in color. She may complain of vaginal itching and tenderness, frequent urination, and spotting. Trichomoniasis can be treated with oral medication. Left untreated, the infection can lead to low birth weight or premature birth in pregnant women and to increased susceptibility to HIV infection.

Bacterial Vaginosis

Bacterial vaginosis is one of the most common conditions to afflict women. In this infection, normal bacteria in the vagina are replaced by an overgrowth of other bacterial forms. Symptoms may include itching, burning, or pain and may be accompanied by a fishy, foul-smelling discharge. Left untreated, bacterial vaginosis can lead to premature birth or low birth weight in cases of pregnancy, make the patient more susceptible to more serious infections, and result in PID. It is treated with metronidazole, an antibiotic. If the patient consumes alcohol while taking this therapy, severe nausea and vomiting may develop.

Candidiasis

Candidiasis or *thrush* can develop after having sex with someone who is also infected. It is not technically defined as a sexually transmitted infection. More commonly known as a yeast infection, candidiasis occurs in pregnant and nonpregnant females, although it seems to be more common during pregnancy due to the chemical changes in the vagina (increased glycogen facilitates growth). Risk factors include poorly controlled diabetes and gestational diabetes, taking antibiotics, wearing tight-fitting clothing (increases warmth and decreases airflow), menstruation, excessive use of vaginal sprays or douches, and other activities as insignificant as a bubble bath that can cause an irritation that leads to an infection.[55]

Treatment involves the use of prescription creams and over-the-counter medications. In the context of pregnancy, the fetus will not be affected by this infection while in utero. There is a chance an infant may develop thrush in the mouth after delivery if the infection is active during a vaginal delivery or if the woman breastfeeds.

Fungal Skin Infections

▶ Dermatophyte Infections

Pathophysiology

Fungal infections of the skin are common and usually superficial. They most commonly result from a group of

Table 26-5 Tinea Infection Sites		
Name	**Location**	**Appearance**
Tinea capitis	Head, scalp	Round, scaly area where no hair is growing; diffuse scaling
Tinea corporis	Body	Round lesion appears in a small area; ringworm
Tinea cruris	Groin, genitalia	Sharply demarcated area with elevated scaling, geographic borders
Tinea pedis	Feet	Thinning of tissue between the toes, scaling on soles or sides of the foot, sometimes vesicles and/or pustules Figure 26-9
Tinea manuum	Hands	Dry, diffuse scaling, usually on palm
Tinea unguium	On or under fingernails or toenails	Dark debris under nails
Tinea versicolor	Trunk	Pink, tan, or white patches with scaly skin areas

fungal infections called *dermatophytes.* Most fungal infections are superficial and are identified by the word *tinea* and then followed with a term that denotes the location of the lesion. Table 26-5 lists the most common tinea infections and their locations.

Assessment

The history and physical findings vary with the types of tinea. In most cases the patient has a scaly rash and associated itching. The differential diagnosis varies with the type of tinea (see Table 26-5). Other types of dermatitis may mimic tinea.

Management

Because most dermatophyte infections involve limited areas, they respond well to topical antifungal agents. Complications are rare.[56]

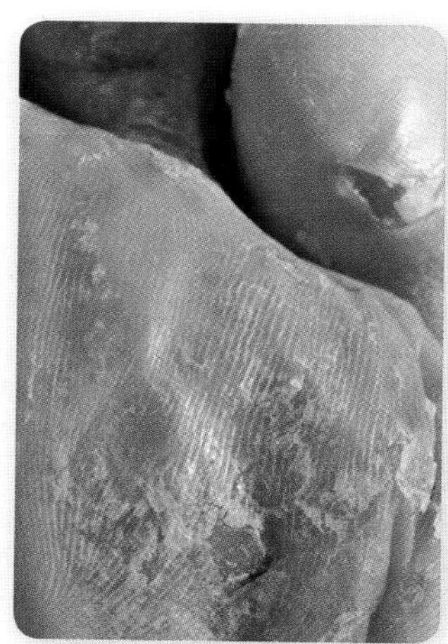

Figure 26-9 Tinea pedis.

Helminths

A helminth is a worm classified as a parasite that lives in human beings. Helminth eggs can contaminate pets, livestock, and water. Human beings can contract helminths by touching contaminated water or an animal and not washing their hands afterwards. They then ingest the eggs, which hatch in the intestine. Common symptoms include fatigue, weight loss, abdominal cramps, nausea, and vomiting. Treatment includes medications such as albendazole, ivermectin, mebendazole, and pyrantel pamoate. The toxicity of these medications varies but may include gastrointestinal distress, headache, weakness, tachycardia, and hypotension.

Hookworm

Ancylostoma duodenale and *Necator americanus* are two human hookworms. The larva (immature worms) of these parasites penetrate intact skin, enters the circulation, travels to the lungs, and is coughed up, swallowed, and develops to adulthood in the small intestine.[57] Adult worms lay eggs, which are released into the feces. Egg laying begins 4 to 8 weeks after exposure and can last as long as 5 years. The primary method of transmission occurs by walking barefoot on contaminated soil. Ancylostoma duodenalecan also be transmitted through the ingestion of larvae.[58] Although some people may have no symptoms, possible early signs of infection include itching and a localized rash. As the infection worsens, the patient may have abdominal pain, diarrhea, loss of appetite, weight loss, and fatigue. The diagnosis is made by stool examination for ova and parasites.

Pinworm

Pinworm infection, caused by a small roundworm called *Enterobius vermicularis,* is common in crowded conditions such as daycare centers, schools, and mental institutions.[57] Pinworm infection is spread by the fecal-oral route. Larvae hatch in the small intestine and travel to the large intestine, where they mature in 2 to 6 weeks. During sleep, female pinworms leave the intestine through the anus and deposit their eggs on the surrounding skin.[59] These egg deposits can cause itching and may be transmitted from hand to mouth when the infected person scratches the inflamed area. Pinworms can survive long periods in the dust that builds up over doors, on windowsills, and under beds in the rooms of infected people. Indirect transmission can occur when handling contaminated clothing, bedding, food, or play objects. Diagnosis is usually made by the tape test in which transparent tape is applied to the skin around the anus. The tape is then examined for eggs using a microscope. Pinworm can be treated with over-the-counter or prescription medication.

Parasitic Insects

Bedbugs

Bedbugs are small, red-brown insects about the size of a tick that feed on the blood of humans as well as other warm-blooded animals such as dogs, cats, birds, and rodents. They hide in the cracks and crevices of beds, particularly along mattress seams, and in luggage, overnight bags, folded clothing, and furniture. Bedbug infestations generally occur around the areas where people sleep including suburban homes, apartments, hotels, and dormitories. They sometimes appear in movie theaters, health care facilities, and office buildings. Bedbugs typically bite humans at night during sleep and crawl to a secluded area to digest their meal after feeding. Bites are usually found on the face, neck, shoulder, back, arms, and legs. Because a bedbug injects an anesthetic and an anticoagulant when biting, a person may not realize they have been bitten. Although some people develop a red, itchy welt within a day or so of the bite, others have little or no reaction. Topical corticosteroids are used to treat bites. Bedbugs can harbor various pathogens, but disease transmission to humans has not been proven.[60] Eradicating bedbugs can be accomplished using a spray bottle and 90% alcohol, which can be purchased at a hardware store or local pharmacy. The bugs are killed on contact when sprayed. Heavy extermination, which is sometimes necessary, involves washing and drying of all bedding on a hot setting, and placing the mattress and box spring in a zippered plastic case.

Pathophysiology, Assessment, and Management of Common Bloodborne Diseases

Types of Viral Hepatitis

Viral hepatitis is an inflammation of the liver produced by a virus. Five distinct forms of viral hepatitis (A, B, C, D, and E) exist. They are produced by different viruses and vary somewhat in their means of transmission. However, all types present with the same signs and symptoms, so the type causing illness is ultimately determined by blood testing. Hepatitis A and hepatitis E are discussed as enteric (intestinal) diseases in this chapter, because they are not bloodborne infections. Hepatitis E is not generally present in the United States.

Hepatitis B Virus Infection

Hepatitis type B virus (HBV), also known as **serum hepatitis**, is transmitted through infectious blood, semen, and other body fluids primarily through sexual contact, blood transfusion, or puncture of the skin with contaminated needles or other contaminated sharp instruments.[61] In the United States, the rate of new HBV infections has declined by about 82% since 1991, when a national immunization program to eliminate HBV infection was implemented.[62] Until immunization programs began in the United States, health care providers, especially those involved in surgery, dentistry, and emergency medicine, were deemed to have a particularly high risk of contracting hepatitis through accidental needlestick injuries. There is no recommendation for routine titer testing or boosters.

Pathophysiology

Needles, including those used for tattooing and acupuncture, and occasionally other objects, such as shared razors, have been implicated in transmission of HBV. Type B hepatitis is particularly common among intravenous (IV) drug users who share needles.

Limited data suggest that the HBV can survive outside the body in the medium of dried blood for as long as 7 days; for example, in the presence of dried blood on stainless steel in a hemodialysis center. The incubation period for HBV varies widely—from 60 to 150 days, with symptom onset beginning an average of 90 days after exposure to HBV. In 2016, according to WHO,[63] an estimate of less than 5% of all people infected with HBV will become chronic carriers; 20% to 30% of people chronically infected with HBV will experience cirrhosis of the liver and/or liver cancer.

Assessment

Signs and symptoms of HBV infection include loss of appetite, nausea, vomiting, general fatigue and malaise, low-grade fever, vague abdominal discomfort, and, sometimes, aching in the joints. The very smell of food may provoke nausea, and smokers often notice a sudden distaste for cigarettes. At this point, signs and symptoms subside for 50% to 60% of infected persons, which explains why many infected people never know that they have acquired the disease. For people whose disease progresses into the second phase, their urine begins to turn dark. A day or two later, **jaundice**, a yellowing of the skin, and scleral **icterus**, a yellowing of the sclera (the whites of the eyes),

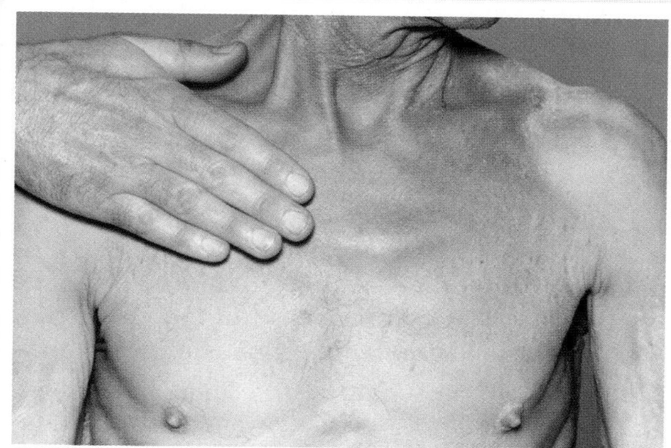
A

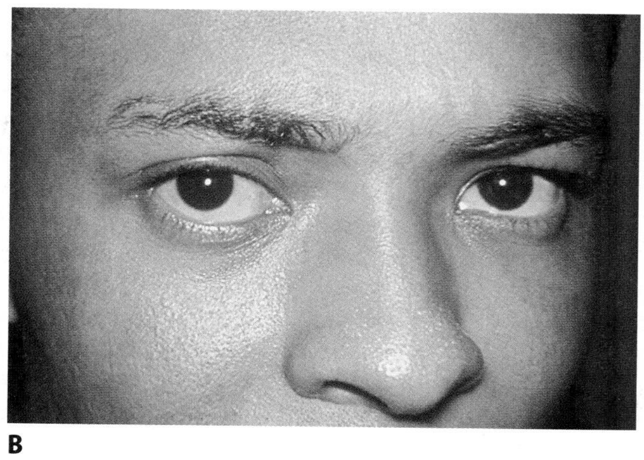
B

Figure 26-10 Signs of infection caused by hepatitis type B virus. **A.** Jaundice. **B.** Scleral icterus.

develop in the patient Figure 26-10. Type B hepatitis usually lasts several weeks, although complete recovery may take 3 to 4 months.

Management

Prevention of HBV transmission focuses on practicing standard precautions—using gloves when handling blood, OPIM, or materials containing visible blood. Good handwashing technique is also essential. Paramedics should be immunized against HBV when hired, if not previously vaccinated. Vaccination, which is safe and effective, protects against HBV for life; it also protects indirectly against hepatitis D virus (HDV) infection, because a person must be infected with type B to acquire type D.

OSHA requires that employers of health care workers offer the HBV immunization at no cost to at-risk staff members. If you are allergic to yeast or mercury (thimerosal), notify the vaccine administrator, and arrangements will be made to obtain the proper vaccine to meet your needs. The vaccine is administered in a three-dose series over a 6-month time frame Table 26-6. When the series has been completed, you should have a blood test (titer) performed 1 to 2 months later to ensure that your immune system responded. Periodic titer testing is neither required nor recommended. It is important to complete all three doses to achieve protection.

Table 26-6 Hepatitis B Vaccination Series
Initial dose
Second dose: 4 weeks after first dose
Third dose: 6 months after first dose
Titer: 1 to 2 months after completion of the three-dose series

Practice routine standard precautions. If you are exposed, notify your DICO. The DICO will verify the source patient's test results. If you have a positive titer on file, no follow-up treatment is needed. If you do not have a titer report on file and the patient is positive for HBV infection, a titer test will be ordered for you. Treatment will depend on the results of the titer testing. If you have not been vaccinated and the patient is positive for HBV, you will be offered hepatitis B immune globulin and the vaccine series.

▶ Hepatitis C Virus Infection

Hepatitis type C virus is spread primarily through contact with the blood of an infected person. A hepatitis C infection can be acute or chronic. An acute HCV infection occurs within the first 6 months after exposure to the HCV. An acute infection often leads to a chronic infection; in fact, it is estimated that about 75% to 85% of people who become infected with HCV will experience chronic infection.[64] Chronic HCV occurs when HCV remains in a person's body. It can lead to serious liver problems, including cirrhosis (scarring of the liver) or liver cancer. HCV is the leading cause of liver transplantation in the United States, Europe, and Japan.[65]

About 15% to 25% of hepatitis C infections resolve on their own.[66] New testing methods and new treatment medications have changed diagnosis and treatment options for hepatitis C infection. Hepatitis C infection can now be cured. This includes all six genotypes of the virus.

Pathophysiology

Transmission of HCV most often occurs by sharing needles, syringes, or other equipment to inject drugs; needlestick injuries in health care settings; and being born to a mother who has Hepatitis C. HCV was once commonly spread through the transfusion of blood and blood products and organ transplants. This method of HCV transmission is now rare in the United States because of blood screening for HCV that became available in 1992. HCV is less commonly spread by sharing personal care items that may have come in contact with another person's blood, such as razors or toothbrushes, or having sexual contact with a person infected with HCV.

A few cases of HCV transmission via blood splash to the eye have been reported.[67] Studies have not shown Hepatitis C to be spread through licensed, commercial tattooing facilities; however, transmission of HCV (and other infectious diseases) is possible when poor infection-control practices are used during tattooing or piercing.[68]

This virus can survive on environmental surfaces for up to 3 weeks at room temperature if not properly cleaned.

Assessment

It is estimated that 70% to 80% of people with acute HCV do not have any symptoms.[69] When signs and symptoms do occur, they generally appear within 6 to 7 weeks after exposure, with an average time of 4 to 12 weeks. Signs and symptoms are the same as those for HBV infection: lack of appetite, nausea and vomiting, low-grade fever, abdominal distress, joint discomfort, dark urine, clay-colored bowel movements, jaundice, and a general feeling of illness and listlessness. The diagnosis is established by testing for HCV antibody.

Management

To prevent HCV transmission, take standard precautions—gloves when in direct contact with blood or OPIM, and use needle-safe or needleless devices. Any blood spills, including dried blood, should be cleaned using a dilution of one part household bleach to 100 parts water.[70]

If you have sustained an exposure, testing will begin with the source patient; permission to test for hepatitis C is not required. Rapid HCV testing should be performed on the source with results in 1 hour. If the source is HCV positive, you will have a baseline HCV antibody test and liver function test. You should have an HCV-RNA test (test for the virus) 3 weeks or later following the exposure event.[71,72] If it is negative, you did not acquire HCV from the exposure. If it is positive, you will be offered 8 to 12 weeks of treatment.

Treatment is available that is highly successful in curing this infection. However, there is currently no medication to offer after exposure to prevent infection. A vaccine for prevention of HCV infection is currently in human clinical trials in Sweden. In some cases, it is being offered to people with newly diagnosed HCV infection as part of the trials. This is currently a therapeutic vaccine because it is only given to newly diagnosed persons.

▶ Hepatitis D Virus Infection

Hepatitis type D, also called delta hepatitis, requires that the host be infected with hepatitis B for HDV infection to occur. For this reason, HDV is considered a parasite for HBV. There are three known genotypes of HDV. Genotype 1 has a worldwide distribution; genotype 2 exists in Taiwan, Japan, and northern Asia; and genotype 3 is found in South America. This viral infection is rare in the United States.

Pathophysiology

Transmission is generally by percutaneous exposure, because HDV is not effectively transmitted through sexual contact. Perinatal transmission is rare. The incubation period for HDV infection ranges from 30 to 180 days. Blood is considered to be infectious during all phases of the illness.

Assessment

Signs and symptoms are the same as those associated with HBV infection.

Management

To protect against HDV transmission, take standard precautions: use gloves when in contact with blood or OPIM, use needle-safe or needleless devices, and perform routine cleaning of the vehicle following patient transport. Do not go through the pockets of known IV drug users who are found unconscious because they may contain contaminated sharps. If a documented exposure occurs, notify your DICO. Testing begins with the source patient in accordance with state testing laws. If the source is positive for HDV and you are protected against HBV, no further treatment is indicated.

▶ Human Immunodeficiency Virus Infection and Acquired Immunodeficiency Syndrome

Human immunodeficiency virus (HIV), type 1, has existed in the United States since at least the mid to late 1970s. In 2015, the CDC reported that there were about 40,000 newly diagnosed cases of HIV infection in the United States.[73] Worldwide, there were about 2.1 million new cases of HIV in 2015.[74] Reporting HIV infection to public health authorities is not legally mandated in all states in the United States. Because of testing and treatment, persons with HIV and AIDS are living 50 years after diagnosis as productive members of society.[75]

Special Populations

HIV infection is a bloodborne disease that can be transmitted from mother to infant in the birthing process. In the United States, all pregnant women who receive prenatal care are tested for HIV infection. In the United States, the rate of infection from mother to child is only 1% to 2% because infected mothers are treated with antiretroviral drugs beginning in the second trimester of pregnancy.[76]

Pathophysiology

In addition to other means of transmission by contact with blood and/or OPIM, including sexual transmission, HIV can be transmitted through blood transfusions. Although all blood donated is tested, it is not 100% safe. Such transmission has occurred at a very low rate, however, since the initiation of testing for the presence of P24 (a protein present from the beginning of the HIV life cycle) in donated blood. With P24 testing of donated blood, the virus can now be detected 1 to 6 days after infection.

HIV is not transmitted through casual or even household contact. Even among people who routinely share eating utensils, toothbrushes, and razors with HIV-infected patients, there is no evidence of an increased rate of HIV infection. This disease is not transmitted by airborne or droplet means.

The HIV pathogen envelops infected cells and attacks the immune system and other body organs. As a result, the immune system is unable to assist in protecting an infected person from other diseases. It takes about 7 days for the virus to envelop a cell, and this process may occur 4 to 6 weeks after the exposure event. The communicable period is unknown but is believed to span from the onset of infection until about 48 weeks after the start of medications. After 48 weeks of treatment, replicated studies show there is no circulating virus, therefore, no risk for disease transmission.[77] This also reduces the incidence of progression to **acquired immunodeficiency syndrome (AIDS)**, the end-stage disease process.

A patient with AIDS is extremely vulnerable to numerous **opportunistic infections** that would not affect a person with an intact immune system. Patients who respond to the cocktail drug treatment render the virus unable to multiply, and thus 96% cannot transmit the disease. This means that there is prevention through treatment.

The incubation period of AIDS spans the time between documented infection (that is, becoming HIV-positive) and development of the end-stage disease; it is determined by the CD4 cell count and the presence of opportunistic infections. The Ryan White CARE Act (1990) makes HIV drugs available to all people in the United States with or without the ability to pay.

Assessment

Signs and symptoms may include acute febrile illness, malaise, swollen lymph glands, headache, and, possibly, rash. Following initial infection with HIV, most people present with enlargement of the lymph nodes but appear otherwise healthy. However, if the infection is left untreated, the number of T-helper lymphocytes (CD4 cells) gradually declines. T-helper cells are essential components of the immune system that mediate cellular and humoral immunity. Seroconversion, meaning that antibodies can be detected in the blood, occurs, usually within the first 3 months following exposure. However, new testing (rapid) can detect two proteins that are present in the beginning of the life cycle of this virus. People who are **seropositive** for HIV are prescribed antiretroviral drug treatment (triple drug treatment).

The development of specific opportunistic bacterial, viral, and fungal infections defines the transition from HIV infection to AIDS. The conditions are known accordingly as *AIDS-defining* or *AIDS-related conditions*. They include *Pneumocystis carinii* pneumonia in infants or people with compromised immune systems; cytomegalovirus, which can cause blindness; reddish or purple skin cancers known as Kaposi sarcoma; atypical TB; and cryptococcal meningitis.

Management

Prevention focuses on standard precautions—use of gloves when in direct contact with patient blood or OPIM, the use of needle-safe or needleless devices, good handwashing technique, and routine cleaning of the vehicle after transport.

The risk for acquiring HIV infection for health care providers is related to handling and disposal of sharps. As of December 2013, documented occupationally acquired HIV infection had developed in 58 health care providers; none were fire or EMS personnel.[78] Of these occupational infections, 50 were the result of a needlestick injury exposure. A needlestick exposure to HIV includes *all* of the following: a deep stick with a large-gauge hollow-bore needle, visible blood on the device, an HIV-positive patient with a high viral load, and a device that had been in the patient's vein or artery. Following this type of exposure, the risk of transmission is 0.3% for exposure to the mucous membrane of the eye and 0.09% for nonintact skin (only one case has been reported and documented).

Prevention of AIDS transmission involves taking standard precautions. Wear gloves when in contact with blood or OPIM, use needle-safe or needleless devices, and perform routine cleaning of the vehicle and equipment. There is no need to restrict pregnant health care providers from contact with patients with known HIV infection or AIDS.

If an exposure occurs, notify your DICO. The source patient will be tested in accordance with state law, ideally using the rapid HIV testing method. Its results are accurate and available in less than 1 hour. If the test is negative, no further testing is indicated. If the source is positive, a blood sample is sent for assessment of viral load and the paramedic may be offered antiretroviral drugs for a period of 4 weeks. However, with the new data on viral load, the need for these drugs postexposure has diminished. The CDC publishes the criteria for use of these drugs; they are not given automatically. OSHA enforces the CDC guidelines for postexposure prophylaxis under the bloodborne pathogens regulation (CFR 1910.1030). The CDC recommends that a physician knowledgeable in the use of these drugs be consulted. If one is not available, then the physician should contact the 24-hour Post-Exposure Prophylaxis (PEP) Hotline at 1-888-448-4911 before prescribing these drugs. The PEP hotline is staffed by infectious disease physicians who will determine if PEP is appropriate.[79,80]

Words of Wisdom

Unless they contain visible blood, the following body fluids do not transmit bloodborne disease: saliva, tears, sweat, urine, stool, vomitus, nasal secretions, and sputum.

New antiretroviral medications offer protection from transmission through treatment. Antiretroviral drugs are toxic, so careful and complete counseling should be provided to exposed health care providers. Before initiating antiretroviral therapy, baseline laboratory testing should be done—complete blood count and liver and kidney function tests. For a female of childbearing age, pregnancy testing is appropriate. These tests should be repeated every 2 weeks during drug therapy.

Words of Wisdom

Diseases acquired through contact with bloodborne pathogens are considered protected handicaps under the Americans with Disabilities Act.

Words of Wisdom

Some diseases require a combination of precautions based on how the disease is transmitted. For example, Ebola requires taking standard precautions, droplet precautions, and contact precautions.

Ebola

Ebola is a disease that falls in two categories for precautions: contact and droplet. Ebola is not a new disease. Health care workers have been dealing with Ebola for more than 40 years, but its presence has been limited to West Africa for most of the outbreaks. Where this virus hides between outbreaks has not been determined, but now it is known that the African fruit bat plays a significant role in its transmission. In the past, outbreaks were limited to one local area, but the last outbreak in 2013 to 2014 occurred on the border between three countries, which was problematic. In December 2015, the latest Ebola outbreak was pronounced over. In 2016 there were about six new cases. An Ebola vaccine has been expedited and is being administered to contacts of the six new cases. Thus far, the vaccine has been proven to be very effective.

The Ebola virus is an enveloped virus, which means it is very susceptible to killing with many common EPA-registered agents. This virus dies after a few hours on surfaces.

Pathophysiology

Ebola virus can be spread to others through direct contact through nonintact skin or mucous membranes. The incubation period is 2 to 21 days following exposure. Sources are listed in Table 26-7.

People coming from West Africa into the United States enter through only four airports. These airports are close to medical facilities that are designated to treat patients with Ebola. Transport of patients suspected of having Ebola is by designated transport crews linked to the designated medical facilities. This lessens the number of people in possible contact with the virus.

Assessment

Travel history is important for Ebola and many other diseases. Determine whether the patient has come from West Africa or been in contact with a person with Ebola. Assess for fever. Initial symptoms include a sudden onset of fever (101.5°F [38.6°C]), intense weakness, muscle pain, headaches, and sore throat. As the disease progresses, the patient often experiences profuse diarrhea and vomiting, rash, and impaired kidney and liver function. Some infected people experience internal and external bleeding.

Words of Wisdom

Travel history should be a routine part of patient assessment—we live in a global society.

Table 26-7 Methods of Ebola Transmission

- Direct contact through nonintact skin or mucous membranes
- Infected fruit bats or primates (apes and monkeys) when butchered and used as food
- Blood or body fluids (including but not limited to urine, saliva, sweat, feces, vomit, breast milk, and semen) of a person who is sick with or has died from Ebola
- Needles and syringes that have been contaminated with body fluids of a person who is sick with Ebola
- The body of a person who has died from Ebola
- Contact with contaminated surfaces

Data from: Ebola virus disease, World Health Organization. www.who.int/mediacertre/factsheet/fs103/en. Interim Guidance for Emergency Medical Services (EMS) System and 9-1-1 Public Safety Answering Points (PSAPs) for Management of Patients Who Present with Possible Ebola Virus Disease in the United States, Centers for Disease Control and Prevention, December 2, 2014; http://www.cdc.gov.vhf/ebola/hep/interim-guidance-emergency-medical-services-systems.

▶ Management

Follow EMS guidelines, not hospital guidelines, for patient care on transport. Limit the use of sharps, and limit invasive procedures. Keep a list of names of people involved in patient care for contact follow-up, if needed.

There is no specific treatment for Ebola. Treatment is supportive: rehydration, balance of fluids and electrolytes, and maintenance of oxygen and blood pressure status. The CDC recommends taking standard, droplet, and contact precautions when within 3 feet (1 m) of the patient.[81] Use a surgical mask. A surgical mask should be placed on the patient when possible, otherwise the health care provider should wear a surgical mask. A cover gown and protective eyewear should be worn. Shoe covers and double gloves are only needed if there is profuse vomiting and diarrhea. If the patient is vomiting, give him or her a biohazard bag to contain any emesis. If the patient has profuse diarrhea, consider wrapping the patient in an impermeable sheet to reduce contamination of other surfaces. When transporting a patient with suspected EBV, notify the receiving facility in advance, so that proper infection control precautions are prepared at the facility before arrival.

Care should be taken when removing contaminated PPE. No special cleaning solution is needed for Ebola. Ebola virus can be killed with many common chemical agents. Household bleach is an acceptable cleaning agent. There are no special laundry requirements. Follow state medical waste regulations for disposal of medical waste.

Words of Wisdom

PPE is only as effective as its proper removal. PPE removal for pathogens is different than the procedure for removal of hazmat PPE.

Handwashing after glove removal is always important!

Should an exposure event such as contaminated needlestick injury or mucous membrane contact with body fluids occur, perform first aid and notify your DICO. Work restriction may need to be addressed for up to 21 days.

Pathophysiology, Assessment, and Management of Enteric (Intestinal) Diseases

▶ Norovirus Infection

Pathophysiology

Previously termed Norwalk agent, norovirus causes about 90% of epidemic nonbacterial outbreaks of **gastroenteritis** in the world. Norovirus may be responsible for up to 50% of all foodborne outbreaks in the United States. This virus affects people of all ages. Noroviruses are classified into six genogroups, three of which cause human disease (GI, GII, and GIV).[82] This is a spore-forming organism.

When norovirus enters the body, it begins to multiply in the small intestines. Transmission can be person-to-person, by ingestion of food or water that has been contaminated by infected feces (the fecal-oral route), or by contaminated surfaces. Symptoms may appear within 1 to 2 days. Acute symptoms usually begin in 24 to 28 hours and may last 24 to 60 hours. The virus can be shed for weeks after infection.

Assessment

Patients will present with nausea, forceful vomiting, watery diarrhea, abdominal pain, weakness, and low-grade fever; they are rarely admitted to the hospital.

Management

Standard precautions include wearing gloves and practicing good handwashing technique using soap and warm water. Alcohol sanitizers are not considered effective against norovirus. Spore-forming organisms required a chlorine-based product to kill the spores. Therefore, cleaning after transport will require the use of a chlorine-based product such as bleach diluted with water.

Pathophysiology, Assessment, and Management of Non-Bloodborne Hepatitis Viruses

▶ Hepatitis A Virus Infection

Pathophysiology

Hepatitis type A (HAV), or **infectious hepatitis**, was formerly one of the most common types of hepatitis in the United States. In the past, outbreaks of this disease have been reported in several states. Transmission is by the fecal-oral route. Epidemic outbreaks are most often traced to contaminated drinking water, milk, sliced meats, and undercooked shellfish. The incidence has been declining; however, and no cases related to flood water have been reported since the early 1980s. As a result of programs focused on vaccination of children against all vaccine-preventable diseases, case numbers are falling each year.

Infection with HAV is often described as a benign disease because acquiring it provides lifelong immunity to it. Since 2000, children in the United States have been immunized to protect them from contracting this disease. The vaccine is usually administered at age 12 months (between 12 and 23 months of age). Children who have not been vaccinated by 2 years of age should be vaccinated as soon as possible.

The incubation period is usually about 2 to 4 weeks, although it can range from 15 to 50 days after ingestion of the virus. The communicable period probably starts toward the end of the incubation period and continues for a few days after the patient becomes jaundiced.

Assessment

Signs and symptoms in phase 1 include fatigue, loss of appetite, fever, nausea, and abdominal pain; smokers lose their interest in smoking. In phase 2, patients have jaundice, dark-colored urine, and pale, clay-colored stools.

Depending on the type of hepatitis contracted, chronic liver disease or liver cancer may develop. This is true for HBV and HCV. Hepatitis A, however, is not associated with long-term disease and is considered a "mild" disease because it resolves after several weeks.

Management

Prevention includes taking standard precautions: good handwashing technique, and, if in contact with patient stool, gloves. No special cleaning of the vehicle is needed. Hepatitis A vaccine is recommended for Federal Emergency Management Agency response team members who may respond *outside* the United States, but not for any other health care provider groups or emergency response teams who respond inside the United States.

▶ Hepatitis E Virus Infection

Pathophysiology

Hepatitis E virus (HEV) is also referred to as enterically transmitted non-A, non-B hepatitis. HEV is most common in developing countries with an inadequate water supply and poor environmental sanitation. When symptomatic hepatitis E does occur in the United States, it is usually the result of travel to a developing country where hepatitis E is endemic. Sporadic hepatitis E cases not associated with travel have been identified in developed countries.[83] For nontravel-related domestically acquired cases, no clear exposure was found.

Transmission typically occurs via the fecal-oral route by ingestion of fecally contaminated drinking water. There is a possibility that HEV can be spread by animals; some cases of HEV have occurred after eating uncooked or undercooked pork or deer meat.

This disease has an incubation period of about 15 to 60 days, with an average of 40 days after exposure. The communicable period has not been determined.

Assessment

Signs and symptoms of HEV infection are the same as for other forms of hepatitis.

Management

Hepatitis E usually requires only symptomatic treatment and resolves on its own. Patients are typically asked to maintain adequate nutrition and fluids, avoid alcohol, and obtain the advice of their physicians before taking any medications that can damage the liver, especially acetaminophen. Prevention includes the use of gloves when in contact with stool, good handwashing technique, and cleaning contaminated equipment.

YOU are the Paramedic PART 4

You move the patient to your unit for transport after starting an IV line and administering fluid. The transport is uneventful, and you report to the receiving facility staff on arrival. The patient's blood pressure improves slightly in response to the fluid administration. After you transfer your patient to the hospital bed, you notice the sheets on your stretcher are wet.

Recording Time: 10 Minutes	
Respirations	18 breaths/min
Pulse	96 beats/min
Skin	Cool, pale, and dry
Blood pressure	102/60 mm Hg
Oxygen saturation (Spo_2)	97% on room air
Pupils	PERRLA

7. What decontamination measures should you use for your stretcher?
8. What measures should you use for handwashing?

Pathophysiology, Assessment, and Management of Vector-borne and Zoonotic (Animal-borne) Diseases

Introduction

Diseases that are transmitted through a vector (vector-borne diseases) are usually transmitted by ticks or mosquitoes and include diseases such as Rocky Mountain spotted fever, Lyme disease, West Nile virus, dengue fever, and now, Zika. These diseases may also be referred to as **zoonotic** diseases.

Mosquito-Borne Diseases

West Nile Virus

West Nile virus (WNV) has been present in the United States for several years. The virus was first discovered in Uganda in the 1930s and was first detected in North America in 1999. In the United States, the only states that have not reported cases of WNV are Alaska and Hawaii.

Pathophysiology. Tranmission of WNV most often occurs via a bite from a mosquito carrying the virus after feeding on infected birds; however, a small number of human infections have been documented following blood transfusions, organ transplants, exposure in a laboratory setting, and from mother to baby during pregnancy, delivery, or breastfeeding.[84] This infection is not transmitted from person to person, so there is no period of communicability. The incubation period is usually 2 to 6 days but ranges from 2 to 14 days after transmission.

Assessment. In most cases, this disease is mild and uneventful; 70% to 80% of people who acquire WNV infection remain unaware that they have it.[85] Many cases are identified when an individual goes to donate blood. Those who are symptomatic exhibit a fever with symptoms such as headache, fatigue, weakness, joint pain, vomiting, diarrhea, or rash. Mild symptoms appear in older people and immunocompromised people. In healthy people, the immune system fights off the disease. Serious neurologic illness, such as encephalitis or meningitis, develops in less than 1% of people who are infected.[86]

Management. Use needle-safe devices to avoid a contaminated sharps injury when WNV infection is suspected. If you sustain a contaminated sharps injury involving a patient with WNV, notify your DICO. There is no recommended medical follow-up treatment. No special cleaning of the vehicle is needed or recommended.

Dengue Fever

Dengue is transmitted between people by the mosquitoes *Aedes aegypti* and *Aedes albopictus*, which are found throughout the world. This mosquito is also a vector for chikungunya and the Zika virus. There are four dengue viruses (DENV-1, -2, -3, and -4). If one is contracted, you have acquired immunity, but only to the one you contracted, not the other three. The CDC reports that nearly all dengue cases reported in the 48 continental states were acquired elsewhere by travelers or immigrants.[87]

Pathophysiology. Transmission is usually by the bite of a mosquito. One week or 8 to 12 days after a mosquito becomes infected, it can transmit the virus by biting a healthy person. This is its incubation period. Although a mosquito bite is the most common method of dengue transmission, there are reports of transmission in organ transplants, blood transfusions from infected donors, and there is evidence of transmission from an infected pregnant woman to her fetus.

Assessment. Signs and symptoms begin about 4 to 7 days after the mosquito bite and usually last 3 to 10 days. The primary signs and symptoms of dengue are a high fever that is accompanied by two or more of the following: severe headache, severe pain behind the eyes, joint pain, muscle and/or bone pain, rash, or mild bleeding (eg, bleeding from nose or gums, petechiae, easy bruising).

In some patients, dengue fever may progress to dengue hemorrhagic fever. Warning signs may develop as the patient's fever declines, heralding the start of a 24- to 48-hour period when capillaries become leaky, allowing fluid to escape from the blood vessels into the peritoneum (causing ascites) and into the pleural cavity (leading to pleural effusions). This may lead to hemorrhage, hypovolemic shock, and possibly death without prompt, appropriate treatment.

Management. There is no specific treatment for dengue fever. There is no occupational health risk for health care providers caring for a patient with dengue fever. A vaccine is close to being developed and will be expedited when available.

Chikungunya Fever

Chikungunya virus appears to have originated in Africa. It made its most recent appearance in 2013 after almost 200 years. In Cuba, it was called dengue, but the two viruses have been differentiated. The mosquito that transmits dengue fever, the *Aedes aegypti* mosquito, also transmits chikungunya virus. The *Aedes* mosquitoes that transmit chikungunya virus breed in rain-filled containers commonly found around homes and workplaces, such as water storage containers, saucers under potted plants, and drinking bowls for domestic animals, as well as discarded tires, birdbaths, and food containers.

Pathophysiology. Transmission is by the bite of the *Aedes aegypti* mosquito. It is rarely life threatening.

Assessment. Complaints include fever that typically lasts from 5 to 7 days, and severe, possibly incapacitating joint pain. The patient may not be aware of a mosquito bite.

Management. There is no specific treatment for the disease but analgesics and nonsteroidal anti-inflammatory medication may be used to reduce the pain and swelling. Aspirin should be avoided.

This is not an occupational health risk related to patient care. Because this virus is very similar to dengue, the vaccine for dengue may influence a vaccine for this disease as well.

Zika Virus

Zika virus is new to the United States. It first appeared in mid-2015. Thus far, cases have been related to travel to areas where this infection is prevalent. This is a mosquito-borne infection that is transmitted by the bite of the *Aedes aegypti* mosquito. This mosquito is known for biting more often in the daylight hours than in the evening hours. Most cases in the United States have been acquired elsewhere; however, cases have been acquired in the Miami, Florida, area.

Transmission from an infected mother to her fetus, resulting in microcephaly, difficulty swallowing, and learning disabilities has been documented. Also, sexual transmission from an infected male to his sexual partners has been documented. There has also been a well-documented correlation between Zika virus and the onset of GBS, which has been described earlier.

There have been no cases of Zika virus transmission through blood transfusions. People who have traveled to areas where Zika is found are not to donate blood for 28 days after returning to the United States. Currently, all donated blood in the United States is tested for Zika virus.

Pathophysiology. The incubation period is 3 to 14 days following the mosquito bite. The virus is present in urine, saliva, and semen. There is an approved test for Zika. It is believed that urine testing is the most accurate.

Assessment. Many people infected with Zika virus are are asymptomic.[88] For those who have symptoms, the most common are fever, rash, joint pain, conjunctivitis (no drainage), muscle pain, and headache. Note any travel history to areas where Zika virus is prevalent.

Management. Care is supportive—rest, fluids, analgesics, and antipyretics. Take standard precautions for patient care. There are currently no recommendations for special protective equipment for medical personnel, except to prevent person-to-person transmission through blood or body fluids. Routine standard precautions are all that is needed or recommended. If wounds and skin sites have been exposed to blood or body fluids, they should be washed promptly with soap and water. Mucous membranes should be flushed with copious amounts of clean water.

> **Words of Wisdom**
>
> Mosquito control is an essential part of risk reduction. Remove standing pools of water. Wear clothing to cover exposed areas of the body and use insect repellent.

Standard precautions should be used when caring for a patient with suspected Zika. Occupational risk may be related to a contaminated sharps injury. Report all sharps injuries directly to the DICO.

▶ Tick-borne Diseases

Lyme Disease

Lyme disease is named for Lyme, Connecticut, the town where the disease was first identified. It is the most common tick-borne disease in the United States. The deer tick can be a vector for the bacterium *Borrelia burgdorferi*. The tick's bite injects the pathogen into the bloodstream of a human host. In 1982, a national reporting system was established for this infection. The highest prevalence of Lyme disease is found along the Atlantic coast, in the upper Midwest, and along the Pacific coast. The peak season is between June and August; incidence rates decrease in the early fall. Each year there are about 30,000 cases reported in the United States—the most commonly reported vector-borne illness in this country. In 2014, it was the fifth most common Nationally Notifiable disease (each state has a list of diseases that the Public Health Department requires to be reported); however, this disease does *not* occur nationwide and is concentrated heavily in the northeast and upper midwest.[75]

Pathophysiology. Lyme disease occurs more often in children younger than 10 years and in middle-aged adults. It is not transmitted from person to person. The incubation period ranges from 3 to 32 days.

Assessment. Lyme disease primarily affects the skin, heart, joints, and nervous system. Some patients remain asymptomatic. For patients in whom signs and symptoms develop, the disease is usually divided into three stages: early localized, early disseminated, and late manifestations:

1. **Early localized stage.** The early stage is characterized by a round, red skin lesion. This bull's-eye rash (so called because it extends outward with a ring in the center) is most common in the area of the groin, thigh, or axilla Figure 26-11. If present, it is warm to the touch and may blister or scab.
2. **Early disseminated stage.** In the early disseminated stage, secondary lesions may develop within days, and the patient may

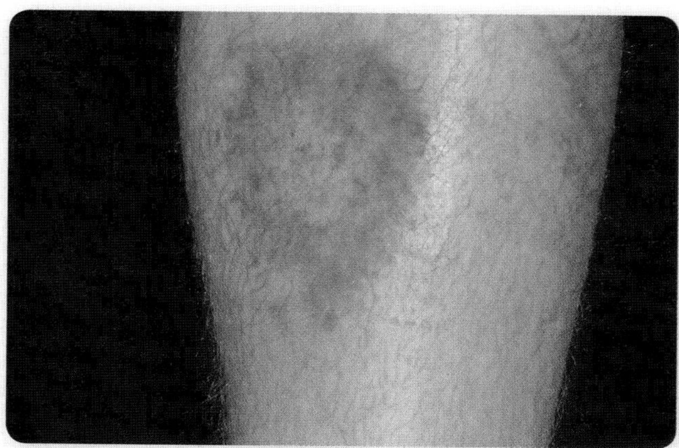

Figure 26-11 The bull's-eye rash of Lyme disease is most common in the area of the groin, thigh, or axilla.

report flulike symptoms—fever, chills, headache, malaise, and muscle pain. Nonproductive cough, testicular swelling, sore throat, enlarged spleen, and enlarged lymph nodes may be present. Neurologic involvement, including meningoencephalitis and cranial and peripheral neuropathy, occurs in untreated patients within 2 to 8 weeks. Cardiac involvement, including pericarditis, myocarditis, and atrioventricular conduction difficulties, occurs in untreated patients.

3. **Late manifestations.** In the third stage of the illness, arthritis may occur in untreated patients, beginning days to years after the initial infection. Intermittent joint pain may affect patients and lasts from days to months. Chronic neurologic symptoms are uncommon. In the United States, memory impairment, depressed mood, and severe fatigue are the most common symptoms of Lyme disease.

Management. Prevention includes wearing long sleeves and pants when in tick-infested areas, and using insecticides that contain carabaril, diazinon, chlorpyrifos, or cyfluthrin. If you sustain a tick bite, use proper technique for removing ticks. Postexposure treatment with antibiotics is not warranted or recommended.

Rocky Mountain Spotted Fever

Rocky Mountain spotted fever (RMSF) is a tick-borne disease caused by the bacterium *Rickettsia rickettsii*. This organism is a cause of potentially fatal human illness in North and South America. Transmission to humans occurs by the bite of infected tick species. In the United States, these include the American dog tick (*Dermacentor variabilis*), Rocky Mountain wood tick (*Dermacentor andersoni*), and brown dog tick (*Rhipicephalus sanguineus*). There were approximately 1,985 cases in 2010 but only 156 were confirmed, with the highest incidence in Missouri and Tennessee.[75]

Pathophysiology. RMSF can be a severe or even fatal illness if not treated in the first few days of symptoms. Patients who had a particularly severe infection requiring prolonged hospitalization may have long-term health problems caused by this disease.

Assessment. Typical symptoms include fever, headache, abdominal pain, vomiting, and muscle pain. A rash may also develop, but is often absent in the first few days, and in some patients a rash never develops.

The initial diagnosis is made based on clinical signs and symptoms and medical history and can later be confirmed by using specialized laboratory tests. RMSF and other tick-borne diseases can be prevented.

Management. Doxycycline is the first-line treatment for adults and children of all ages, and it is most effective if started before the fifth day of symptoms.

RMSF is not a communicable disease. It is not transmitted from patient to health care provider. To be exposed, a person needs to be bitten by the tick.

▶ Hantavirus Infection

Hantavirus infection, also known as *hemorrhagic fever with pulmonary syndrome*, is associated with the deer mouse, white-footed mouse, and cotton rat. Hantavirus pulmonary syndrome may also occur and is characterized by flulike symptoms that can progress rapidly to potentially life-threatening breathing problems. It has also been found in rats in urban areas. This disease was first identified in Korea in the early 1950s and in the southwestern United States in 1993. According to the CDC,[89] by 2016, about 690 cases had been reported in the United States. In 2015, 18 cases of hantavirus infection were diagnosed in the United States. In Canada and the United States, the deer mouse, which carries the Sin Nombre hantavirus, is responsible for the majority of cases of hantavirus.

Pathophysiology

Hantavirus is found in the urine, feces, and saliva of chronically infected rodents. Transmission occurs via direct contact with rodent waste matter, often through aerosol inhalation, which can occur when cleaning up infested areas such as households, barns, and sheds. The incubation period usually lasts 12 to 16 days following exposure but has been noted to range from 5 to 42 days. This disease is not transmitted from person to person, so there is no period of communicability.

Assessment

Signs and symptoms of hantavirus infection begin with the sudden onset of fever, which lasts 3 to 8 days. It is accompanied by headache, abdominal pain, loss of appetite, and vomiting. For pulmonary syndrome, signs and symptoms present in two stages. In stage 1, complaints may include fever, chills, headaches, muscle aches, vomiting, diarrhea, and abdominal pain. In stage 2, the patient may present with a cough that produces secretions, shortness of breath, and fluid accumulation within the lungs. Low blood pressure and cardiac insufficiency may also be noted.

Management

Prevention focuses on standard precautions. Routine cleaning of the vehicle is all that is indicated. Depending on the stage of illness and presenting symptoms, other supportive measures may be needed. Assisted respiration, through advanced airway management or mechanical ventilation, may be indicated. Oxygen therapy may also be needed. Rapid transport is paramount, as a diagnosis will be made at the medical facility following antibody testing for hantavirus.

This is not an occupationally acquired disease because it is not transmitted person to person.

▶ Rabies

Rabies (hydrophobia) is found worldwide. In the United States, human cases have been declining since rabies control programs began in the 1940s. Deaths from rabies reported in the United States have declined from more than 100 per year to 1 or 2 per year.[90] The vaccination of domestic animals and the development of a vaccine and rabies immunoglobulin have greatly reduced the number of deaths in humans who contract rabies.

Pathophysiology

Transmission of rabies is primarily related to the direct bite of an infected animal. The virus is shed in the saliva of the infected animal from the time it becomes infected. Animals most commonly identified to have rabies include raccoons, skunks, foxes, coyotes, and insectivorous bats. Other (rare) routes of transmission include contamination of mucous membranes (ie, eyes, nose, mouth), aerosol transmission, and corneal and organ transplantations. In general, however, nonbite exposures to rabies—scratches, abrasions, open wounds, or mucous membranes contaminated with saliva or other potentially infectious material from a rabid animal—are rare. There are no documented cases of human-to-human transmission of rabies. The incubation period is usually 2 to 8 weeks but varies depending on the severity of the bite and the location of the wound.

Assessment

Signs and symptoms in human infection are generally nonspecific, much like signs of the flu: fever, chills, sore throat, malaise, headache, and weakness. Paresthesia (tingling skin sensation with no apparent cause) may develop at or near the site of exposure. Following these initial signs, the neurologic phase of the disease begins—hyperactivity, seizures, bizarre behavior, and hydrophobia. Patients may also have fear of the sight of water or while drinking it as a result of severe spasms of the throat and masseter (chewing) muscles. As the disease progresses, paralysis may develop and mental status may deteriorate, leading to coma. Although rabies is generally viewed as a fatal disease, several cases of survival have been reported recently even after symptoms had appeared.

Management

For prevention, take standard precautions for patient care and cleaning of the vehicle. If you are bitten or scratched by a suspect animal, you will be offered an injection of human immunoglobulin and started on human rabies vaccine if deemed appropriate. The CDC does not recommend rabies vaccination for EMS personnel on a routine basis. Follow-up would include wound care. Remember, first aid always comes before reporting to your DICO.

▶ Middle East Respiratory Syndrome

Middle East respiratory syndrome (MERS) is a viral disease that presents a very low risk to health care providers and the general public in the United States. In May 2014, two cases of MERS were identified and treated in the United States. One case was in Florida and the other in Indiana. Both cases involved health care providers who worked and lived in Saudi Arabia. They acquired this disease in Saudi Arabia, were diagnosed and treated, and then discharged in the United States.

Pathophysiology

MERSCoV is a coronavirus. Coronavirus has been associated with patients developing severe acute respiratory illness. Studies have linked this disease to the nasal secretions of camels. Transmission occurs through close contact with an infected person even in the health care setting. Research has not documented any ongoing transmission in communities. Infected people have, for the most part, shown symptoms much like the common cold. People with underlying medical conditions have experienced pneumonia or kidney failure. The incubation period appears to be 5 to 6 days but can be as long as up to 14 days.

A reduced level of lymphocytes in the blood (lymphopenia) has been noted in most patients infected with MERS-CoV, as was also noted in SARS infections.

Laboratory testing for MERS-CoV is not routinely available, although polymerase chain reaction for MERS-CoV is available at state health departments, the CDC, and some international laboratories.

Assessment

Obtain a travel history to identify travel to or from the Arabian Peninsula and possible contact with camels (urine or nasal secretions), camel milk, or meat. Assess for fever, cough, and shortness of breath. GI disturbances, including nausea and vomiting, may also be reported. People who develop severe disease may require ventilation assistance for acute respiratory distress syndrome.

Management

No specific antiviral treatment exists for MERS-CoV. Medical care is focused on relief of symptoms. Health care providers should take standard precautions, contact precautions, and airborne precautions. Airborne precautions for EMS involve the use of the air exchange system and a surgical mask.

If an unprotected exposure occurs, notify your DICO directly. No vaccine currently exists for MERS, and no specific treatment has been recommended. Current treatment is supportive.

▶ Tetanus

According to the CDC,[91] reported tetanus cases have declined more than 95%, and deaths from tetanus have declined more than 99% in the United States since 1947, when the disease became reportable nationally. Tetanus is more common in agricultural areas and in underdeveloped areas, where contact with animal waste is common and immunization is inadequate. This is a vaccine-preventable disease. Vaccination is given at ages 2 months, 4 months, 6 months, and 18 months, followed by doses at 4 and 6 years of age. A booster is recommended for children between ages 11 and 12; thereafter a booster should be given every 10 years. Occasional cases of tetanus continue to occur in adults, especially in those who were not vaccinated in childhood or did not remain current on their 10-year booster shots.

Pathophysiology

The tetanus bacillus is found in the intestines of horses and other animals, but some cases have been linked to use of IV drugs.

Transmission occurs when tetanus spores enter the body by either of two means: (1) a puncture wound contaminated with animal feces, street dust, or soil; or (2) contaminated street drugs. Tetanus is not transmitted from person to person. Occasionally, cases have occurred postoperatively or following seemingly minor injuries.

The incubation period is usually about 14 days from the exposure but has been documented to be as short as 3 days. The cases that have short incubation periods tend to have a higher level of contamination.

Assessment

Signs and symptoms begin at the site of the wound, followed by painful muscle contractions or rigidity (tetany) in the neck, face, jaw, and trunk muscles. The key sign that suggests tetanus, particularly in children, is abdominal rigidity, although this rigidity may be confined to the location of the injury. Dysphagia, hydrophobia, drooling, and respiratory distress may also occur.

Management

Prevention involves taking standard precautions: gloves when treating any patient wounds and management of drainage. A patient with tetanus may require airway and ventilation support en route. Oxygen may be ordered along with IV fluids. Tetanus immune globulin is recommended for treatment of tetanus. A single intramuscular dose of 3,000 to 5,000 units is generally recommended for children and adults, with part of the dose infiltrated around the wound if it can be identified. Paramedics should be offered tetanus booster doses every 10 years for protection. No special cleaning routines are necessary after transport of a patient with tetanus.

Pathophysiology, Assessment, and Management of Infection With Antibiotic-Resistant Organisms and Multidrug-Resistant Organisms

The overuse and misuse of antibiotics have led some pathogens to develop resistance to the antibiotic drugs commonly prescribed to eradicate them. The medical community has been concerned that some infections would soon be untreatable. This situation has now occurred. Currently, no new antibiotics are under development. As a consequence, medical facility pharmacies and the CDC now restrict the use of many antibiotics.

Patients infected with some types of antibiotic-resistant organisms, particularly vancomycin-resistant *enterococci* (VRE) and methicillin-resistant *Staphylococcus aureus* (MRSA), may be protected by the Americans with Disabilities Act (infection with these organisms is discussed in the sections that follow), depending on the definition of "disability" in state law. It is important not to use more PPE than is reasonably required when treating patients with such infections because doing so may be considered discrimination.

▶ Methicillin-Resistant *Staphylococcus aureus*

Staphylococcus aureus (S aureus) became resistant to penicillin in the late 1950s. The drug methicillin became available in the early 1960s to treat infections with *S aureus*. By the mid 1970s, MRSA was present in US hospitals; it has since moved into the community. Today, most cases are community-acquired MRSA. The number of health care–associated cases of MRSA is starting to decline with the increased focus on infection control. In 2010, encouraging results from a CDC study showed that life-threatening MRSA infections in health care settings are declining.[92] MRSA infections that began in hospitals declined 54% between 2005 and 2011, with 30,800 fewer severe MRSA cases.[93] Decreases in infection rates were even greater for patients with bloodstream infections.

Strains of MRSA are also resistant to some other antibiotics, including cephalosporins, erythromycins, clindamycin (Cleocin), tetracyclines, and aminoglycosides. Although vancomycin (Vancocin) has been shown to treat MRSA effectively, some mild strains are showing resistance to this drug as well. Other drugs used to treat MRSA include a quinupristin-dalfopristin combination (Synercid), linezolid (Zyvox), and daptomycin (Cubicin).

Special Populations

Community-acquired MRSA infection with clone USA300 is a major cause of infectious diseases in children. It presents primarily as a superficial soft-tissue infection and can be easily treated by incision and drainage without the use of antibiotics.

Pathophysiology

In health care settings, it is believed that MRSA is transmitted from patient to patient via the unwashed hands of health care providers. Studies have shown that 33% of people carry staph in their nose and 2 in 100 people carry MRSA.[94] The pathogen can subsequently be transferred to skin and other areas of the body through a break in the skin, causing infection **Figure 26-12**. Surfaces contaminated with MRSA do not seem to be important in transmission. The presence of MRSA in ambulances and fire stations has been documented, which suggests that cleaning routines and good handwashing techniques are not being followed. Factors that increase the risk for developing MRSA include antibiotic therapy, prolonged hospital stays, a stay in an intensive care or a burn unit, and exposure to an infected patient. Many patients who contract MRSA live in long-term care facilities.

Assessment

Patients with MRSA may be **colonized** with this organism or infected. The incubation period seems to be between 5 and 45 days. The communicable period varies; patients who have active infection may carry MRSA for months. In community-acquired cases, MRSA results in soft-tissue infections. Manifestations of MRSA may include localized skin abscesses and cellulitis, empyemas, and endocarditis. Sepsis is found in older patients with *S aureus* infections. After bloodstream infection with MRSA, secondary infections

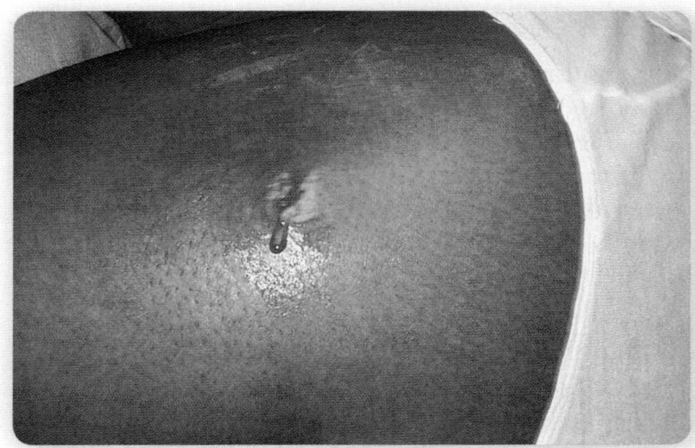

Figure 26-12 A draining, purulent skin abscess on the thigh caused by methicillin-resistant *Staphylococcus aureus*. Consider any drainage from a wound to be potentially infectious and use appropriate precautions.

Courtesy of Bruno Coignard, M.D./Jeff Hageman, M.H.S/CDC.

such as osteomyelitis and septic arthritis may develop at sites other than the initial site of MRSA infection.

Management

Patients will undergo incision and drainage for soft-tissue infections. No antibiotics need to be prescribed. This treatment is in accordance with the guidelines published by the Infectious Disease Society of America. Most MRSA soft-tissue infections will clear following incision and drainage alone. To prevent MRSA transmission, take standard precautions (gloves and good handwashing technique) when in contact with wounds and nonintact skin. If you are in direct contact with wound drainage but your skin is intact, no exposure will occur. No special cleaning is required and normal laundry of linens is appropriate. If you have a true exposure, notify your DICO. No post-exposure treatment is recommended.

▶ Vancomycin-Resistant *Staphylococcus aureus*

Vancomycin is one of the leading drugs for treating *Staphylococcus* infections. However, once the organism has become resistant to this drug, it is no longer effective in treating the infections. Like MRSA, vancomycin-resistant *Staphylococcus aureus* (VRSA) infections present as pimples, boils, and other skin conditions. VRSA infections can become severe, resulting in sepsis, a dangerous systemic bloodstream infection; however, the incidence of infection is rare in the United States.

Pathophysiology

People at risk for the development of VRSA infections include those with several underlying health conditions (such as diabetes and kidney disease), previous infections with MRSA, indwelling catheters (such as indwelling urinary catheters), recent hospitalizations, and recent exposure to vancomycin or other antimicrobial agents.

Assessment

Signs and symptoms may include localized skin abscesses and cellulites, pneumonia, bloodstream infections, meningitis, or osteomyelitis. Fever, chills, or body weakness and pain, cough, chest pain, and trouble breathing are commonly present, but other signs and symptoms will depend on the location of the infection.

Management

This form of infection is currently treatable with antibiotics. Standard precautions and routine cleaning of the vehicle and patient care equipment after each call are important, as is routine handwashing. Make sure all open cuts on your skin are covered. No postexposure treatment is recommended, but if you are exposed, notify your DICO.

▶ Vancomycin-Resistant Enterococci

Enterococcus is a common, normal organism of the GI tract, urinary tract, and genitourinary tract. More than 450 species of enterococci exist, many of which are resistant to antimicrobial agents. These organisms grow under reduced oxygen and oxygenated conditions. When they become resistant to the main drug used for treating enterococcal infection, vancomycin, the patient is said to have VRE.

According to recent National Nosocomial Infections Surveillance surveys,[95] enterococci remain in the top three most common pathogens that cause health care–associated infections in the United States. These infections have occurred in the general hospitalized population. There are an estimated 20,000 to 85,000 cases of VRE each year in US hospitals.

Pathophysiology

Infection with VRE is primarily a health care-associated infection. Patients identified with VRE infections outside the hospital setting typically reside in nursing homes or visit hemodialysis centers. In fact, people are not susceptible to VRE infection unless they are already ill or immunocompromised. Patients in the ICU and transplant recipients are especially vulnerable.

VRE may be found in urinary tract infections (UTIs) and bloodstream infections; it has also been identified in livestock stool, uncooked chicken, and people who work at farms or processing plants. The infectious organisms can live on surfaces for long periods, so transmission may occur by direct contact with contaminated surfaces or equipment.

A person can be colonized or infected with VRE, but only infected patients can transmit the organism. Thus, transmission may occur when you have direct contact with wound drainage and an open cut or sore allows entry of the organism. Infection with VRE can be treated with a new synthetic antibiotic, linezolid.

Assessment

VRE can cause UTIs, particularly in patients who have urinary catheters. Other kinds of catheters, such as central lines, can serve as a port of entry for VRE, causing bacteremia that sometimes evolves into sepsis. Surgical wounds, especially in patients who have had abdominal or chest surgery, may also become infected with VRE.

Management

Prevention relies on taking standard precautions, wearing gloves, and practicing good handwashing technique when in contact with wound drainage. A cover gown is necessary only if your uniform may come in contact with wound drainage. Post-transport cleaning of all areas that came in contact with the patient is important, but no special cleaning solution is required. If you sustain direct contact with an open wound and body fluids from a patient with a VRE infection, notify your DICO and complete an exposure report. No postexposure medical treatment is indicated.

▶ *Clostridium difficile*

Clostridium difficile (commonly referred to as *C diff*) is not a multidrug-resistant organism but is being treated like one. It can occur after antibiotic treatment because some antibiotics can destroy the normal bacteria in the intestine, and the *C diff* organisms take over. Infections with *C diff* were generally related to a stay in a health care facility, but now are mainly found in the community setting. *C diff* is now most prevalent in the community setting because of issues with antibiotic prescribing.

Pathophysiology

The spore-forming bacterium *C diff* produces two endotoxins that cause watery diarrhea, the chief symptom of infection. Transmission occurs by contact with surfaces contaminated with feces. The bacterium can be transmitted to patients by contact with the unwashed hands of health care providers. Diagnosis is usually made by stool culture. Illness resolves 2 to 3 days after discontinuing antibiotics. Recurrence is common, especially in people 65 years and older.

Assessment

Infection with *C diff* causes frequent watery, green, foul-smelling diarrhea; nausea and vomiting; fever; loss of appetite; and abdominal discomfort. Diseases associated with *C diff* infection include pseudomembranous colitis, sepsis, and colonic perforation. For patients presenting with these signs and symptoms, a paramedic should ask about the patient's medications, especially any antibiotics he or she is taking.

Management

Standard precautions for *C diff* include wearing gloves and using good handwashing technique. In addition, cleaning of contaminated surfaces with an appropriate cleaning agent is important in managing *C diff*. Because

C diff is a spore-forming agent, a chlorine-based cleaning solution is required. Also, alcohol-based foams and gels for handwashing will not kill spores, so soap and warm water should be used. Report contamination of open skin areas to your DICO. No medical follow-up is recommended.

Carbapenem-Resistant Enterobacteriaceae

Carbapenem-resistant enterobacteriaceae (CRE) are bacteria that are highly resistant to most antibiotics. This includes the carbapenem class of antibiotics, which are used as a last resort for treating infections. This organism came to the United States via medical tourism (people leaving the United States for health care at a lower cost). It is believed that CRE originated in India. Again, this makes travel history very important. The question to ask is: "Have you been hospitalized overnight outside the United States in the past 6 months?" The death rate from this infection is about 40% and could be higher.[96]

Pathophysiology

Enterobacteriaceae are bacteria normally found in the GI and vaginal tracts. These organisms have acquired the ability to counteract antibiotics. These bacteria, either *Klebsiella* or *E coli*, develop resistance due to antibiotic treatment. Transmission is through unwashed hands and contaminated surfaces. It has not been determined how long CRE can live on a surface. CRE is a spore-forming organism. This affects the selection of cleaning product and the product for handwashing.

Assessment

Symptoms may vary from patient to patient depending on the location of the bacteria. Observe for signs of sepsis and an indwelling device (IV catheter, indwelling urinary catheter, ventilators). Patients may present with fever, UTI, fatigue, chills, and sepsis. Also ask about the use of over-the-counter antibiotic treatments that were used for open sores. Assess if the patient has been on long-term antibiotic treatment.

Management

Take standard precautions and contact precautions if there are draining wounds. Use soap and warm water for handwashing; alcohol-based cleaners do not kill spores. Use a chlorine-based cleaning solution for vehicles and equipment used for patient care.

> **Words of Wisdom**
>
> The most important action for you to take if you believe you have been exposed is to wash your hands immediately and to clean any contaminated equipment or clothing. Report the incident to your DICO.There is no medical follow up needed or recommended.

Pathophysiology, Assessment, and Management of Newly Recognized Diseases

In the past, a disease would "jump" from animals to humans every 20 to 30 years. Today, this transmission occurs much more frequently. Recent examples include HIV infection, monkeypox, severe acute respiratory syndrome (SARS), and avian flu. The latter two are discussed here.

Severe Acute Respiratory Syndrome

Severe acute respiratory syndrome (SARS) is a new disease that arose from the merger of two viruses, one from mammals and one from birds. The source of this virus has been identified as bats found in Hong Kong. SARS was first reported in Asia in February 2003. Within a few months, the disease had spread from Asia to Canada, South America, and Europe. By spring 2003, the WHO reported a total of 8,098 cases worldwide and 774 deaths. In the United States, there were eight confirmed cases (all mild) and no deaths; all of the US cases involved people who had traveled to areas where SARS cases had been reported. The last cases of SARS were reported in April 2004 in China and resulted from a laboratory accident. In the United States, no health care providers have contracted SARS.

Pathophysiology

Transmission of SARS is by close personal contact—that is, living with and caring for a person with the disease or having direct contact with respiratory secretions or body fluids of an infected person (for example, kissing or hugging, sharing eating utensils, or standing within 3 feet (1 m) of an infected person who is talking). The incubation period is about 10 days from the date of exposure; the communicable period has not been well defined.

Assessment

Signs and symptoms include a fever of greater than 100.4°F (38°C), headache, overall feeling of discomfort, and body aches. Initially, SARS resembles any general flulike illness; however, after 2 to 7 days, a dry cough appears, and severe cases may progress to pneumonia; patients may need respiratory support.

Management

Caring for a person suspected of having SARS consists of using adequate PPE, notifying the DICO, completing an exposure form, and perhaps being placed on a 10-day quarantine.

▶ Avian Flu

The first cases of **avian (bird) flu** in humans were reported in Hong Kong in 1997; 18 people became infected and 6 died in this outbreak.[97] There have been two cases of avian flu in Canada. Patients acquired it from their flocks, but recovered and no additional transmission was reported. A new strain has been identified in China and is a concern to the World Health Organization and the United Nations. Sustained person-to-person transmission has not been noted.

Pathophysiology

Avian flu is caused by a virus that occurs naturally in the bird population. This virus is carried in the intestinal tract of wild birds and does not usually cause illness. However, in domestic bird populations (eg, chickens, ducks, and turkeys), it is very contagious. Birds acquire the illness from contact with contaminated excretions or surfaces that are contaminated with excretions. If an infected bird is used for food and is cooked, it does not pose a risk to the people who eat it.

No rapidly spread human-to-human cases of this disease have been reported. Instead, the cases occurring in humans have involved close contact with infected birds. The transmission risk for humans is quite low.

Some concern exists that someone infected with a regular type A flu virus may become coinfected with avian flu, allowing the two to merge and form a new virus. In August 2011, the United Nations stated that it appeared that the avian flu was once again on the rise in Asia. In 2013 there was an outbreak in China and this presented a new strain of the virus. Another outbreak occurred in China in 2016/2017.

Assessment

Obtain a travel history. Signs and symptoms of avian flu include fever, sore throat, cough, and muscle aches; some eye infections have also been noted. Illness may eventually progress to pneumonia and severe respiratory distress.

Management

Preventive measures include placing a surgical mask on the patient to contain secretions. If the patient's condition does not permit this action, you can wear a surgical mask for protection. Follow current CDC guidelines regarding protection for health care providers. Under the current information-sharing system, the medical facility is required to notify the DICO if a patient transported is later given a diagnosis of avian flu. If an exposure is documented, an antiviral drug may be offered within 48 hours of exposure. Antiviral drugs do not prevent the flu, but rather reduce the severity of the illness. It is also important to get an annual flu shot to ensure protection from type A viruses. Finally, a vaccine for avian flu is currently available.

Words of Wisdom

The lead agency for responding to potential pandemic diseases in the United States is the Department of Health and Human Services. The CDC is part of this agency.

YOU are the Paramedic SUMMARY

1. What is your first concern at this scene?

Because *C diff* is a possibility, you should immediately don gloves during this call.

2. What is *C diff* and what precautions should you put in place for transport?

C diff is a bacterium that is shed in feces. To prevent contamination with *C diff*, use good handwashing technique with soap and warm water, and clean contaminated surfaces with a chlorine-based cleaning solution. Use contact precautions in addition to standard precautions.

3. What can you determine about the patient's condition now?

Staff members have advised that the patient has been ill for a few days and has been vomiting and having diarrhea. You witnessed the patient attempt to vomit, and nothing was produced. This information, along with the tenting of the skin on the forearm, should lead you to believe that substantial dehydration exists.

4. Because a diagnosis of *C diff* has not actually been made for this patient, are you concerned about exposure?

Yes, you should be concerned about exposure. However, it is important to note that no postexposure treatment is recommended. Gastroenteritis, also known as the stomach flu, comprises many types of infections and irritations of the gastrointestinal tract, including those caused by norovirus. Patients experience symptoms such as nausea and vomiting, fever, abdominal cramps, and diarrhea. In healthy people, gastroenteritis is usually not serious. In children, older adults, and patients with chronic illness, severe complications such as dehydration may develop. Some of the viral strains are extremely contagious.

5. What is your first choice of treatment for this patient?

You should be working on fluid replacement because of the evidence of dehydration. You should consider a fluid challenge after assessing lung sounds. Consider starting at

YOU are the Paramedic SUMMARY (continued)

250 mL and repeating until the desired effect is reached or whatever is appropriate in your protocol.

6. Are there any notifications you should make concerning the scene?

The federal Ryan White Law, Part G (2009), requires that every emergency response agency have a designated infection control officer (DICO). This person is charged with ensuring that proper postexposure medical treatment and counseling are provided to exposed employees and volunteers. Postexposure medical treatment is offered to prevent an exposed health care provider from contracting the disease to which he or she was exposed. Treatment should be offered within 24 to 48 hours following an exposure, with the actual time frame based on the diagnosis. Exposure to bacterial meningitis, for example, would require treatment within 24 hours.

7. What decontamination measures should you use for your stretcher?

Strip used linens from the stretcher immediately after use, and place them in a plastic bag or in the designated receptacle in the emergency department. Clean the stretcher with an EPA–registered germicidal/virucidal solution or bleach and water at 1:100 bleach/water solution.

8. What measures should you use for handwashing?

You should have already been using standard precautions. These precautions apply to all body substances except sweat. You should also wash your hands well, using warm water and soap. Alcohol-based handwashing solutions do not kill a spore-forming organism. If your uniform was contaminated, you should change into a clean uniform and wash exposed skin. If you have a significant exposure, notify your DICO or follow your company policy.

EMS Patient Care Report (PCR)					
Date: 07-30-18	**Incident No.:** 9678		**Nature of Call:** Vomiting		**Location:** 550 Health Care Blvd
Dispatched: 0950	**En Route:** 0950	**At Scene:** 0955	**Transport:** 1015	**At Hospital:** 1020	**In Service:** 1040
Patient Information					
Age: 86 **Sex:** F **Weight (in kg [lb]):** 54 kg (120 lb)			**Allergies:** Denies **Medications:** Diltiazem (Cardizem) **Past Medical History:** Heart disease, diabetes **Chief Complaint:** Nausea and vomiting for 48 h		
Vital Signs					
Time: 1000	**BP:** 98/58	**Pulse:** 106	**Respirations:** 18	**Spo_2:** 97% on room air	
Time: 1005	**BP:** 102/60	**Pulse:** 96	**Respirations:** 18	**Spo_2:** 97% on room air	
EMS Treatment (circle all that apply)					
Oxygen @ ______ L/min via (circle one): **NC NRM Bag-mask device**		**Assisted Ventilation**	**Airway Adjunct**	**CPR**	
Defibrillation	**Bleeding Control**	**Bandaging**	**Splinting**	**Other:** IV established, 250-mL (circled)	
Narrative					
Arrived at The Springs assisted living facility for an 86-year-old woman reporting nausea and vomiting for 48 h. Staff member reports a staff physician believes the patient may have *C diff.* Pt appears weak and reports she is unable to stand because of weakness. Pt attempted to vomit, but nothing was produced. Assessment reveals tenting of skin on the pt's forearm. IV established with a 250-mL challenge per protocol. Lung sounds are clear in all fields before and after challenge. Pt has slight improvement in vital signs during transport to receiving hospital.**End of report**					

Prep Kit

▶ Ready for Review

- Government agencies such as the Occupational Safety and Health Administration (OSHA), the Centers for Disease Control and Prevention (CDC), and state and county public health departments bear the responsibility for protection of the public health, prevention of epidemics, and management of outbreaks.
- Clean and disinfect the ambulance and your equipment to protect patients from infection.
- Communicable diseases can be transmitted from one person to another under certain conditions.
- Transmission-based precautions refer to infection control practices that reduce the opportunity for an exposure to occur in the daily care of patients. Standard precautions add the element of protection from moist body substances that may transmit bacterial or viral infections.
- It is critical to remove personal protective equipment (PPE) properly. Handwashing after glove removal is always important.
- Protection against and reduction of the occurrence of communicable diseases involve the designated infection control officer (DICO), the public health department, standard precautions, immunizations and vaccinations, PPE, postexposure medical follow-up, and an exposure control plan.
- A patient suspected of having an infectious disease is assessed like any other medical patient.
- Infection involves a typical chain of events through which a communicable disease spreads.
- General management principles for a patient with a suspected communicable disease include taking standard precautions, treating life-threatening conditions, placing the patient in the position of comfort, administering IV fluid if needed, and treating the patient with empathy. The risk of infection depends on the type and dose of the organism, its virulence, its mode of entry, and the host's resistance.
- The human body offers several defenses to protect against infection, such as skin, the mucous membranes, and the immune system.
- Droplet-transmitted diseases include meningitis, various respiratory conditions, seasonal influenza, pertussis, mumps, and rubella. Droplet precautions include placing a surgical mask on the patient, basic infection control measures, and use of the ambulance's airflow system.
- Airborne-transmitted diseases include tuberculosis, chickenpox, measles, and mononucleosis. Airborne precautions include placing a surgical mask on the patient and using the ambulance's airflow system. Airborne diseases are large particles and travel 6 feet (2 m) and drop to the ground. Droplet diseases are medium to large particles and travel 3 feet (1 m) before dropping to the ground.
- Sexually transmitted diseases (STDs) are usually acquired by sexual contact and are caused by a wide range of organisms.
- Common bloodborne diseases include viral hepatitis and human immunodeficiency virus (HIV).
- Ebola virus requires both contact and droplet precautions. Contact precautions include the use of a cover gown if clothing may become soiled and taking standard precautions.
- Enteric diseases are infectious diseases that affect the gastrointestinal tract. The organisms that cause enteric infections include rotaviruses, parasites, and bacteria.
- Non-bloodborne hepatitis viruses include the hepatitis A and E viruses.
- A vector is a living organism such as an insect or rodent that carries a disease-causing human pathogen. This pathogen does not harm the organism itself, but it can be transmitted to humans by means of a bite, inhalation of contaminated animal feces, or other means.
- Mosquito-borne diseases include West Nile virus, dengue fever, chikungunya fever, and zika virus.
- Tick-borne diseases include Lyme disease, Rocky Mountain spotted fever, hantavirus, rabies, Middle East respiratory syndrome, and tetanus.
- The overuse and misuse of antibiotics has made some pathogens resistant to the antibiotic drugs commonly prescribed to eradicate them.

▶ Vital Vocabulary

acquired immunodeficiency syndrome (AIDS) The end-stage disease process caused by the human immunodeficiency virus; results in extreme vulnerability to numerous opportunistic bacterial, viral, and fungal infections that would not affect a person with an intact immune system.

airborne precautions The use of a surgical mask on the patient and the use of airflow measures to prevent airborne transmission; apply to diseases that are large particle and can travel a distance of 6 feet (2 m), then drop to the floor.

airborne transmission The transmission of an infectious agent by inhalation of small particles that become aerosolized when the infected person coughs, sneezes, talks, or exhales; particles remain suspended in this vapor and can be carried a short distance, usually 3 feet (1 m) to 6 feet (2 m).

Prep Kit *(continued)*

avian (bird) flu A disease caused by a virus that occurs naturally in the bird population; signs and symptoms include fever, sore throat, cough, and muscle aches.

bacteria Small organisms that can grow and reproduce outside the human cell in the presence of the needed temperature and nutrients and cause disease by invading and multiplying in the tissues of the host.

bacterial vaginosis An overgrowth of bacteria in the vagina, characterized by itching, burning, or pain, and possibly a fishy smelling discharge.

bloodborne pathogens Pathogenic microorganisms that are present in human blood and can cause disease in humans. These pathogens include, but are not limited to, hepatitis B virus, human immunodeficiency virus, hepatitis C virus, and syphilis.

candidiasis A vaginal infection that is not technically a sexually transmitted infection, and that can occur in a pregnant or nonpregnant female, but is more common in pregnancy; also called thrush or a yeast infection.

carriers People who harbor an infectious agent and, although not personally ill, can transmit the infection to other people.

chancre The primary hard lesion or ulcer of syphilis that occurs at the entry site of the infection.

chancroid A highly contagious sexually transmitted disease caused by the bacteria *Haemophilus ducreyi*, which causes painful sores (ulcers), usually of the genitals.

chikungunya A virus that originated in Africa and is transmitted by the *Aedes aegypti* mosquito; signs and symptoms include fever that typically lasts from 5 to 7 days, and possibly incapacitating joint pain.

chlamydia A sexually transmitted disease caused by the bacterium *Chlamydia trachomatis*; has the highest incidence in sexually transmitted diseases; signs and symptoms include inflammation of the urethra, epididymis, cervix, and fallopian tubes, and discharge from the urethra.

colonized A pathogen is present but has produced no illness in the host; often progresses to active infection; a colonized host is often called a *carrier* because he or she can transmit the pathogen to others.

communicable disease An infectious disease that can be transmitted from one person to another by direct contact or by indirect contact through a vector or fomite; also called contagious disease.

communicable period The period during which an infected person can transmit a communicable disease to someone else.

contact precautions The use of precautions (gloves, gown, good handwashing, and cleaning of high-touch items) to prevent contact transmission; used for patients presenting with draining wounds, multidrug resistant infection, lice, norovirus, and Ebola.

contact transmission The transmission of an infectious agent by means of direct or indirect contact with the infected persons, such as skin-to-skin contact or contact with the patient's environment and/or equipment.

contaminated The presence of blood or other potentially infectious materials on an item or surface.

dengue A virus transmitted by the mosquitos *Aedes aegypti* and *Aedes albopictus*, found throughout the world, in which the majority of people are asymptomatic; if the severe form develops, it is characterized by hypovolemic shock, hemorrhage, and potentially death.

designated infection control officer (DICO) A person trained to ensure that proper postexposure medical treatment and counseling are provided to an exposed employee or volunteer.

droplet precautions Use of a surgical mask on the patient and airflow measures to prevent droplet transmission; used for patients with possible influenza, meningitis, pertussis (whooping cough), mumps, rubella (German measles), and Ebola.

droplet transmission The transmission of an infectious agent by inhalation of relatively large particles generated when an infected person coughs or sneezes; these particles travel a short distance through the air before falling to the ground.

Ebola A virus formerly limited to West Africa, spread through direct contact through nonintact skin or mucous membranes, and whose initial symptoms include fever, intense weakness, muscle pain, headaches, and sore throat; both contact and droplet precautions are needed with this disease; approximately 10% of infected people experience internal or external bleeding.

endemic Consistently present or prevalent in a population or geographic area.

epidemic An outbreak of disease that substantially exceeds what is expected based on recent experience.

Enterococcus A common, normal organism of the gastrointestinal tract, urinary tract, and genitourinary

Prep Kit *(continued)*

tract that can be pathogenic and become resistant to vancomycin.

fomites Inanimate objects contaminated with microorganisms that serve as a means of transmitting an illness.

fungi Small organisms that can grow rapidly in the presence of the needed nutrients and organic material and can cause infection related to contact with decaying organic matter or from airborne spores in the environment such as molds; singular term, fungus.

gastroenteritis A term that comprises many types of infections and irritations of the gastrointestinal tract; symptoms include nausea and vomiting, fever, abdominal cramps, and diarrhea; also called stomach flu.

genital warts Warts caused by the human papillomavirus, a sexually transmitted disease; also called condylomata acuminata or venereal warts.

gonorrhea A sexually transmitted disease that results in infection caused by the gonococcal bacteria *Neisseria gonorrhea*; signs and symptoms include pus-containing discharge from the urethra and painful urination in males, and signs and symptoms of an acute abdomen in females.

hantavirus A type of virus found in wild rodents, which can also cause disease in humans, characterized by fever, headache, abdominal pain, loss of appetite, and vomiting; diseases caused are hemorrhagic fever with renal syndrome and hantavirus pulmonary syndrome.

health care–associated infection An infection acquired 2 days after admission to a health care setting or 30 days after discharge from one.

host resistance One's ability to fight off infection.

human immunodeficiency virus (HIV) The virus that may lead to acquired immunodeficiency syndrome; cells in the immune system are killed or damaged so that the body is unable to fight infections and certain cancers.

human papilloma virus (HPV) The most common sexually transmitted disease that can cause genital warts and some types of cancer.

icterus Jaundice; the yellow appearance of the skin and other tissues caused by an accumulation of bile pigments.

immunization The process of producing widespread immunity to a specific infectious disease among a targeted group by inoculating individual members of the population; can also refer to a set of vaccinations given together or on a recommended schedule.

incubation period The period between exposure to an organism and the first symptoms of illness, during which the organism multiplies within the body and starts to produce symptoms. This period is when the disease can be transmitted to another person.

infection The invasion of a host or host tissue by pathogenic organisms such as bacteria, viruses, or parasites that produces illness that may or may not have clinical manifestations.

infectious disease A disease caused by pathogenic organisms.

infectious hepatitis Another name for hepatitis A; an inflammation from a virus that causes mild fatigue, loss of appetite, fever, nausea, abdominal pain, and, eventually, jaundice, dark-colored urine, and pale, clay-colored stools.

influenza The flu, a respiratory infection caused by a variety of viruses; differs from the common cold in that the flu involves a fever, headache, and extreme exhaustion.

jaundice The presence of excessive bile pigments in the bloodstream that give the skin, mucous membranes, and eyes a distinct yellow color; often associated with liver disease.

lice Tiny, wingless, parasitic insects that feed on blood; an infestation is easily spread through close personal contact; types include head, body, and pubic lice.

Lyme disease A tick-borne disease that primarily affects the skin, heart, joints, and nervous system and is characterized by a round, red lesion or bull's-eye rash.

measles An infectious viral disease that occurs most often in late winter and spring; begins with a fever followed by a cough, running nose, and pink eye; a rash spreads from the face and neck down the back and trunk.

meningitis An inflammation of the meningeal coverings of the brain and spinal cord; usually caused by a virus or bacterium; the viral type is not communicable and is less severe than the bacterial type, which can result in brain damage, hearing loss, learning disability, or death.

meningococcal meningitis A type of meningitis caused by the meningococcal bacterium, *Neisseria meningitidis*.

Middle East respiratory syndrome (MERS) A disease originating from the Arabian peninsula, transmitted by close contact with camel urine or nasal secretions.

Prep Kit (continued)

Symptoms include fever, cough, and shortness of breath, and gastrointestinal disturbances; there is very low risk to health care providers and the general public in the United States.

mononucleosis Infectious mononucleosis or mono (glandular fever); caused by the Epstein-Barr virus, is often called the kissing disease; also spread by coughing or sneezing.

mumps A viral infection that primarily affects the parotid glands, which are one of the three pairs of salivary glands, causing swelling in front of the ears.

needleless systems Devices that do not use needles for the collection of body fluids or withdrawal of body fluids after initial venous or arterial access is established, the administration of medication or fluids, or any other procedure involving the potential for occupational exposure to bloodborne pathogens by percutaneous injuries from contaminated sharps.

opportunistic infections The infections in which an organism thrives when the immune system has been compromised by illness, chemotherapeutic medications, or antirejection drugs in an organ transplant recipient. These fungi, bacteria, viruses, and parasites are normally held in check by a healthy immune system.

other potentially infectious materials (OPIM) Cerebrospinal fluid, pericardial fluid, amniotic fluid, synovial fluid, peritoneal fluid, and any fluid containing visible blood.

pandemic An outbreak of disease that occurs on a global scale.

parasites Any living organisms in or on any other living creature; take advantage of the host by feeding off cells and tissues.

pertussis An acute communicable disease characterized by a catarrhal stage, followed by a paroxysmal cough that ends in a whooping inspiration; also called whooping cough.

protozoa Single-celled, usually microscopic, eukaryotic organisms such as amoebas, ciliates, flagellates, and sporozoans; a type of parasite.

rabies A fatal infection of the central nervous system caused by a bite from an animal that has been infected with the rabies virus.

reservoir In the context of communicable disease, a place where organisms may live and multiply.

rubella A viral disease similar to measles, best known by the distinctive red rash on the skin; not nearly as infectious or severe as measles.

scabies An infestation of the skin with the mite *Sarcoptes scabiei*; spreads rapidly with skin-to-skin contact.

sepsis Life-threatening organ dysfunction caused by a dysregulated host response to infection.

septic shock Sepsis with circulatory and cellular/metabolic abnormalities profound enough to substantially increase mortality.

seropositive Having a positive blood test for an infectious agent, such as human immunodeficiency virus or hepatitis B or C virus.

serum hepatitis Infection with the hepatitis B virus, which is transmitted through sexual contact, blood transfusion, or puncture of the skin with contaminated needles; signs and symptoms include loss of appetite, nausea, vomiting, general fatigue and malaise, low-grade fever, vague abdominal discomfort, and sometimes aching in the joints; eventually, jaundice occurs.

severe acute respiratory syndrome (SARS) A potentially life-threatening viral infection that usually starts with flulike symptoms.

sexually transmitted diseases (STDs) A group of diseases usually acquired by sexual contact and that include gonorrhea, syphilis, chlamydia, scabies, pubic lice, herpes, hepatitis, and human immunodeficiency virus infection.

source individual Any person, living or dead, whose blood or other potentially infectious materials may be a source of occupational exposure to another person; examples include but are not limited to, hospital and clinic patients; clients in institutions for the developmentally disabled; trauma victims; clients of drug and alcohol treatment facilities; residents of hospices and nursing homes; human remains; and people who donate or sell blood or blood components.

standard precautions The term currently used to describe the infection control practices that will reduce the opportunity for exposure of providers in the daily care of patients; considers all body fluids, except sweat, to present a possible risk.

Staphylococcus aureus (S aureus) A strain of bacteria that became resistant to the drug methicillin, creating a new strain; symptoms include infection and possibly localized skin abscesses and cellulites, empyemas, and endocarditis.

syphilis A sexually transmitted disease caused by the spiral-shaped bacteria *Treponema pallidum* with signs and symptoms that include an ulcerative lesion or chancre of the skin or mucous membrane at the site of infection, commonly in the genital region.

Prep Kit *(continued)*

tetanus A disease caused by spores that enter the body through a puncture wound contaminated with animal feces, street dust, or soil or that can enter through contaminated street drugs; signs and symptoms include pain at the wound site and painful muscle contractions in the neck and trunk muscles.

transmission-based precautions Precautions beyond standard precautions designed to interrupt specific disease transmission routes. There are three types: airborne, droplet, and contact. Can be used alone or in combination; always used in conjunction with standard precautions.

trichomoniasis A parasitic infection caused by a single-cell parasite that is transmitted through sexual contact.

tuberculin skin test A test to determine if a person has ever been infected with tuberculosis.

tuberculosis (TB) An infection that can progress to a disease characterized by a persistent cough lasting longer than 3 weeks plus night sweats, headache, weight loss, hemoptysis, and/or chest pain.

tuberculosis blood test Measurement via interferon-gamma release assays of how the immune system reacts to the bacteria that cause tuberculosis; also called blood analysis mycobacteria tuberculosis.

vaccinations Inoculations with a vaccine, usually by injection or inhalation, to bring about immunity to a specific disease in a person.

vaccines The products formulated to bring about immunity by introducing into the body a killed or weakened virus to which the immune system produces antibodies.

varicella zoster A very contagious disease caused by the varicella zoster virus, which is part of the herpes virus family, occurring most often in the winter and early spring; also called chickenpox

vector An animal or insect that carries a disease-causing organism and transmits it to a human host, without itself becoming ill.

vesicles Tiny fluid-filled sacs; small blisters.

viral hepatitis An inflammation of the liver produced by one of five distinct forms of hepatitis virus—A, B, C, D, and E. The types differ in transmission but present with the same signs and symptoms.

virulence The ability of an organism to invade and create disease in a host; also refers to the ability of an organism to survive outside the living host.

viruses Small organisms that can multiply only inside a host, such as a human, and cause disease.

West Nile virus (WNV) A type of virus that is transmitted by mosquitos, and usually causes only mild disease in humans but can cause encephalitis, meningitis, and death; symptoms, if any, include fever, headache, body rash, and swollen lymph glands.

Zika A type of virus that is transmitted by the *Aedes aegypti* mosquito in which the majority of infected persons are asymptomatic; transmission can occur from an infected mother to her fetus, and from an infected male to his sexual partners; related to onset of Guillain-Barré syndrome.

zoonotic Refers to infectious diseases of animals that can be transmitted to humans and cause disease.

▶ References

1. Infectious diseases and circumstances relevant to notification requirements. US Government Printing Office website. https://www.gpo.gov/fdsys/search/pagedetails.action?collectionCode=FR&browsePath=2011%2F11%2F11-02%5C%2F4%2FCenters+for+Disease+Control+and+Prevention&isCollapsed=false&leafLevelBrowse=true&packageId=FR-2011-11-02&isDocumentResults=true&ycord=552. Accessed March 22, 2017.
2. Healthcare-associated infections. Office of Disease Prevention and Health Promotion website. https://www.healthypeople.gov/2020/topics-objectives/topic/healthcare-associated-infections. Accessed March 24, 2017.
3. Centers for Disease Control and Prevention. Notes from the field: occupationally acquired HIV infection among health care workers—United States, 1985-2013. *MMWR.* 2015;63(53):1245-1246.
4. Centers for Disease Control and Prevention. Guidelines for preventing the transmission of *Mycobacterium tuberculosis* in health-care settings, 2005. *MMWR.* 2005;54(17):26.
5. Occupational Safety and Health Administration. CPL 02-02.078, Enforcement Procedures and Scheduling of Occupational Exposure to Tuberculosis, Occupational Safety and Health Administraton, Washington, DC. June 30, 2015.
6. Interim guidance for emergency medical services (EMS) system and 9-1-1 public safety answering points (PSAPs) for management of patients who present with possible Ebola virus disease in the United States. Centers for Disease Control and Prevention website. http://www.cdc.gov.vhf/ebola/hep/interim-guidance-emergency-medical-services-systems. Updated September 10, 2015. Accessed March 22, 2017.
7. Handwashing: clean hands save lives. Centers for Disease Control and Prevention website. http://www.cdc.gov/handwashing/when-how-handwashing.html. Updated September 4, 2015. Accessed October 14, 2016.

Prep Kit (continued)

8. Bucher J, Donovan C, Ohman-Strickland P, McCoy J. Hand washing practices among emergency medical services providers. *Western J Emerg Med*. 2015;16(5):727-735. doi:10.5811/westjem.2015.7.25917.
9. Teter J, Millin MG, Bissell R. Hand hygiene in emergency medical services. *Prehosp Emerg Care*. 2015 Apr-Jun;19(2):313-9. doi:10.3109/10903127.2014.967427.
10. Centers for Disease Control and Prevention. Immunization of health-care personnel: recommendations of the Advisory Committee on Immunization Practices (ACIP), 2011. *MMWR*. 2011;60(7):1-72.
11. OSHA Act 1970 General Duty Clause. US Department of Labor, OSHA website. https://www.osha.gov/pls/oshaweb/owadisp.show_document?p_table=OSHACT&p_id=3359. Accessed March 21, 2017.
12. National Fire Protection Association. *NFPA 1581: Standard on Fire Department Infection Control Program*. Quincy, MA: National Fire Protection Association, 2010.
13. Hand hygiene guidelines. Centers for Disease Control and Prevention website. http://www.cdc.gov/handhygiene/providers/guideline.html. Accessed March 24, 2017.
14. N95 respirators and surgical masks. Centers for Disease Control and Prevention website. https://blogs.cdc.gov/niosh-science-blog/2009/10/14/n95. Accessed March 24, 2017.
15. Ang B, Fong Poh B, Win Kyaw M, Chow A. Surgical masks for protection of health care personnel against pandemic novel swine-origin influenza A (H1N1)–2009: results from an observational study. *Clin Infect Dis*. 2010;50(7):1011-1014.
16. Influenza (flu): prevention strategies for seasonal influenza in healthcare settings. Centers for Disease Control and Prevention website. http://www.cdc.gov/flu/professionals/infectioncontrol/healthcaresettings.htm. Accessed March 29, 2017.
17. Diaz K, Smaldone GC. Quantifying exposure risk: surgical mask and respirators, *Am J Infect Control*. 2010;38(7):501-508. doi:10.1016/j.ajic.2010.06.002.
18. Loeb M, Dafoe N, Mahoney J, et al. Surgical mask vs N95 respirator for preventing influenza among health care workers. *JAMA*. 2009;302(17):1865-1871. doi:10.1001/jama.2009.1466.
19. Interim guidance for emergency medical services (EMS) system and 9-1-1 public safety answering points (PSAPs) for management of patients who present with possible Ebola virus disease in the United States. Centers for Disease Control and Prevention website. http://www.cdc.gov.vhf/ebola/hep/interim-guidance-emergency-medical-services-systems. Accessed October 16, 2016.
20. Standard interpretations. US Department of Labor, Occupational Safety and Health Administration website. https://www.osha.gov/pls/oshaweb/owadisp.show_document?p_table=INTERPRETATIONS&p_id=20819. Accessed March 29, 2017.
21. Oral care. Centers for Disease Control and Prevention website. https://www.cdc.gov/oralhealth/infectioncontrol/glossary.htm#O. Accessed March 23, 2017.
22. Occupational and safety health standards. US Department of Labor, Occupational Safety and Health Administration website. https://www.osha.gov/pls/oshaweb/owadisp.show_document?p_id=10051&p_table=STANDARDS. Accessed March 24, 2017.
23. Stop sticks campaign. Centers for Disease Control and Prevention website. https://www.cdc.gov/niosh/stopsticks/sharpsinjuries.html. Accessed March 24, 2017.
24. PL 106-430 – Needlestick Safety and Prevention Act. US Government Publishing Office website. https://www.gpo.gov/fdsys/pkg/PLAW-106publ430/content-detail.html. Accessed March 29, 2017.
25. Oral health: infection control. Centers for Disease Control and Prevention website. https://www.cdc.gov/oralhealth/infectioncontrol/faq/bloodborne_exposures.htm. Accessed March 29, 2017.
26. Lohiya G-S, Tan-Figueroa L, Lohiya S, Lohiya S. Human bites: bloodborne pathogen risk and postexposure follow-up algorithm. *J Natl Med Assoc*. 2013;105(1):92-95.
27. Bloodborne pathogen exposure incidents. US Department of Labor, Occupational Safety and Health Administration website. https://www.osha.gov/OshDoc/data_BloodborneFacts/bbfact04.html. Accessed March 24, 2017.
28. Enforcement procedures for the occupational exposure to bloodborne pathogens US Department of Labor, Occupational Safety and Health Administration website. CPL 02-02.069: November 27, 2001; paragraph (d)(3)(ii). https://www.osha.gov/pls/oshaweb/owadisp.show_document?p_table=directives&p_id=2570. Accessed March 24, 2017.
29. Centers for Disease Control and Prevention. Vital signs: epidemiology of sepsis. Prevalence of health care factors and opportunities for prevention. *MMWR*. 2016;65(33):864–869.
30. Rhodes A, Evans L, Alhazzani W, et al. Surviving sepsis campaign: international guidelines for

Prep Kit *(continued)*

management of sepsis and septic shock: 2016. *Critical Care Med*. 2017;45(3):486-552.

31. Lamontagne F, Harrison DA, Rowan KM. qSOFA for identifying sepsis among patients with infection. *JAMA*. 2017;317(3):267-268. doi:10.1001/jama.2016.19684.
32. Centers for Disease Control and Prevention. Prevention and control of meningococcal disease: recommendations of the advisory committee on immunization practices (ACIP). *MMWR*. 2013;62(2):1-22.
33. The 2009 H1N1 Pandemic: summary highlights, April 2009-April 2010. Centers for Disease Control and Prevention website. https://cdc.gov/h1n1flu/cdcresponse.htm. Accessed March 22, 2017.
34. Estimating seasonal influenza-associated deaths in the United States: questions and answers. Centers for Disease Control and Prevention website. https://www.cdc.gov/flu/about/disease/us_flu-related_deaths.htm. Accessed March 22, 2017.
35. Pertussis: summary of vaccine recommendations. Centers for Disease Control and Prevention website. https://www.cdc.gov/vaccines/vpd/pertussis/recs-summary.html. Accessed March 21, 2017.
36. Mumps. Centers for Disease Control and Prevention website. https://www.cdc.gov/mumps/hcp.html. Accessed March 21, 2017.
37. Rubella: fact sheet. World Health Organization website. http://www.who.int/mediacentre/factsheets/fs367/en/. Accessed March 3, 2016.
38. Rubella: signs and symptoms. Centers for Disease Control and Prevention website. https://www.cdc.gov/rubella/about/symptoms.html. Accessed March 23, 2017.
39. Rubella: for healthcare professionals. Centers for Disease Control and Prevention website. https://www.cdc.gov/rubella/hcp.html. Accessed March 23, 2017.
40. Centers for Disease Control and Prevention. Tuberculosis trends—United States, 2014. *MMWR*. 2015;64(10):265-269.
41. Health disparities in HIV/AIDS, viral hepatitis, STDs, and TB. Centers for Disease Control and Prevention website. https://www.cdc.gov/nchhstp/health disparities/asians.html. Accessed March 23, 2017.
42. Tuberculosis: drug-resistant TB. Centers for Disease Control and Prevention website. https://www.cdc.gov/tb/topic/drtb/default.htm. Accessed March 23, 2017.
43. Centers for Disease Control and Prevention. Guidelines for preventing the transmission of *Mycobacterium tuberculosis* in health-care settings, 2005. *MMWR*. 2005;54(17):1-141.
44. Enforcement procedures and scheduling for occupational exposure to tuberculosis. US Department of Labor, Occupational Safety and Health Administration website. https://www.osha.gov/OshDoc/Directive_pdf/CPL_02-02-078.pdf. Accessed March 30, 2017.
45. TB elimination: treatment options for latent tuberculosis infection. Centers for Disease Control and Prevention website. https://www.cdc.gov/tb/publications/factsheets/treatment/ltbitreatmentoptions.pdf. Accessed March 21, 2017.
46. Chickenpox: outbreaks. Centers for Disease Controland Prevention website. http://www.cdc.gov/chickenpox/outbreaks.html. Accessed February 16, 2017.
47. Centers for Disease Control and Prevention. Measles—United States, January 4–April 2, 2015. *MMWR*. 2015;64(14):373-376.
48. Vaccines and preventable diseases: measles, mumps, rubella (MMR) vaccination—what everyone should know. Centers for Disease Control and Prevention website. https://www.cdc.gov/vaccines/vpd/mmr/public/index.html. Accessed February 16, 2017.
49. Immunization schedules: child and adolescent schedule. Centers for Disease Control and Prevention. https://www.cdc.gov/vaccines/schedules/hcp/imz/child-adolescent.html. Accessed March 21, 2017.
50. Epstein-Barr virus and infectious mononucleosis: about infectious mononucleosis. Centers for Disease Control and Prevention website. https://www.cdc.gov/Epstein-barr/about-mono.html. Accessed March 21, 2017.
51. 2015 STD Surveillance Report Press Release. Centers for Disease Control and Prevention website. https://www.cdc.gov/nchhstp/newsroom/2016/std-surveillance-report-2015-press-release.html. Updated October 19, 2016. Accessed April 17, 2017.
52. Chlamydia: chlamydia—CDC fact sheet. Centers for Disease Control and Prevention website. https://www.cdc.gov/std/chlamydia/stdfact-chlamydia-detailed.htm. Accessed March 15, 2017.
53. Centers for Disease Control and Prevention. Sexually transmitted diseases treatment guidelines, 2015: recommendations and reports. *MMWR*. 2015;64(3):1-137.
54. Trichomoniasis: trichomoniaisis—CDC fact sheet. Centers for Disease Control and Prevention website. https://www.cdc.gov/std/trichomonas/stdfact-trichomoniasis.htm. Accessed March 16, 2017.
55. Leifer G. Reproductive anatomy and physiology. In: *Maternity Nursing: An Introductory Text,* 11th ed. St. Louis, MO: Saunders; 2012:16-28.

Prep Kit *(continued)*

56. Lookingbill DP, Marks JG. *Principles of Dermatology.* 3rd ed. Philadelphia, PA: Saunders; 2000.
57. Nematodes. In: Murray PR, Rosenthal KS, Pfaller MA, eds. *Medical Microbiology,* 6th ed. St. Louis, MO: Mosby; 2009:853-870.
58. Parasites—hookworm: hookworm FAQs. Centers for Disease Control and Prevention website. https://www.cdc.gov/parasites/hookworm/gen_info/faqs.html. Accessed March 24, 2017.
59. Parasites—enterobiasis (also known as pinworm infection): pinworm infection FAQs. Centers for Disease Control and Prevention website. https://www.cdc.gov/parasites/pinworm/gen_info/faqs.html. Accessed March 24, 2017.
60. Parasites—bed bugs: bed bugs FAQs. Centers for Disease Control and Prevention website. https://www.cdc.gov/parasites/bedbugs/faqs.html. Accessed March 24, 2017.
61. Viral hepatitis—hepatitis B information: the ABCs of hepatitis fact sheet. Centers for Disease Control and Prevention website. https://www.cdc.gov/hepatitis/hbv/profresourcesb.htm. Accessed March 24, 2017.
62. Viral hepatitis—hepatitis B information: hepatitis B FAQs for health professionals. Centers for Disease Control and Prevention website. https://www.cdc.gov/hepatitis/hbv/hbvfaq.htm#overview. Accessed March 24, 2017.
63. Hepatitis B: fact sheet updated July 2016. World Health Organization website. www.who.int/mediacentre/factsheets/fs204/en/. Accessed March 24, 2107.
64. Viral hepatitis—hepatitis C information: hepatitis C FAQs for the public. Centers for Disease Control and Prevention website. https://www.cdc.gov/hepatitis/hcv/cfaq.htm. Accessed March 24, 2017.
65. Tsoulfas G, Goulis I, Giakoustidis D, et al. Hepatitis C and liver transplantation. *Hippokratia.* 2009;13(4):211-215.
66. Centers for Disease Control and Prevention. Recommendations for prevention and control of hepatitis C virus (HCV) infection and HCV-related chronic disease. *MMWR.* 1998;47(19):1-39.
67. Hosoqlu S, Celen MK, Akalin S, et al. Transmission of hepatitis C by blood splash into conjunctiva in a nurse. *Am J Infect Control.* 2003;31(8):502-504.
68. Hepatitis C and tattoos. Hepatitis Central website. www.hepatitiscentral.com/hcv/hepatitis/tattoos/. Accessed March 29, 2017.
69. Viral hepatitis—hepatitis C information: overview and statistics. Centers for Disease Control and Prevention website. https://www.cdc.gov/hepatitis/hcv/cfaq.htm. Accessed March 29, 2017.
70. Healthcare infection control practices advisory committee (HICPAC). Guideline for disinfection and sterilization in healthcare facilities, 2008. Centers for Disease Control and Prevention website. https://www.cdc.gov/hicpac/disinfection_sterilization/6_0disinfection.html. Accessed March 29, 2017.
71. Information for healthcare personnel potentially exposed to hepatitis C virus (HCV). Centers for Disease Control and Prevention website. https://www.cdc.gov/hepatitis/pdfs/testing-followup-exposed-hc-personnel.pdf. February 2017. Accessed April 17, 2017.
72. Viral hepatitis. U.S. Department of Veterans Affairs website. https://www.hepatitis.va.gov/patient/hcv/testing/time-required-to-test-positive.asp. Updated August 25, 2016. Accessed April 5, 2017.
73. HIV/AIDS: basic statistics. Centers for Disease Control and Prevention website. https://www.cdc.gov/hiv/basics/statistics.html. Accessed March 29, 2017.
74. Fact sheet November 2016: global HIV statistics. UNAIDS website. www.unaids.org/en/resources/fact-sheet. Accessed March 30, 2017.
75. Centers for Disease Control and Prevention. Final 2015 reports of nationally notifiable infectious diseases and conditions. *MMWR.* 2016;65(46):1306-1321.
76. Centers for Disease Control and Prevention. Revised recommendations for HIV screening of pregnant women. *MMWR.* 2001;50(19)59-86.
77. Guidelines for the use of antiretroviral agents in HIV-1-infected adults and adolescents. AIDSinfo website. https://aidsinfo.nih.gov/guidelines/html/1/adult-and-adolescent-treatment-guidelines/0/. Accessed March 29, 2017.
78. Centers for Disease Control and Prevention. Notes from the field: occupationally acquired HIV infection among health care workers—United States, 1985-2013. *MMWR.* 2015;63(53):1245-1246.
79. Centers for Disease Control and Prevention. Updated US Public Health Service guidelines for the management of occupational exposures to HBV, HCV, and HIV and recommendations for postexposure prophylaxis. *MMWR.* 2001;50(11):1-42.
80. Centers for Disease Control and Prevention. Updated US Public Health Service guidelines for the management of occupational exposures to HIV and recommendations for postexposure prophylaxis. Chicago, IL: University of Chicago Press, September, 2013.

Prep Kit *(continued)*

81. Ebola—Ebola virus disease: interim guidance for emergency medical services (EMS) systems and 9-1-1 public safety answering points (PSAPs) for management of patients under investigation (PUIs) for Ebola virus disease (EVD) in the United States. Centers for Disease Control and Prevention website. https://www.cdc.gov/vhf/ebola/healthcare-us/emergency-services/ems-systems.html. Accessed March 24, 2017.
82. Rooney BL, Pettipas J, Grudeski E, et al. Detection of circulating norovirus genotypes: hitting a moving target. *Virol J.* 2014;11:129. doi:10.1186/1743-422X-11-129.
83. Viral hepatitis—hepatitis E information: hepatitis E FAQs for health professionals. CDC website. Centers for Disease Control and Prevention website. https://www.cdc.gov/hepatitis/hev/hevfaq.htm. Accessed March 24, 2017.
84. West Nile virus: transmission. Centers for Disease Control and Prevention website. https://www.cdc.gov/westnile/transmission/index.html. Accessed March 24, 2017.
85. West Nile virus: general questions about West Nile virus. Centers for Disease Control and Prevention website. https://www.cdc.gov/westnile/faq/genQuestions.html. Accessed March 24, 2017.
86. CDC Features: West Nile virus. Centers for Disease Control and Prevention website. https://www.cdc.gov/features/westnilevirus/. Accessed March 24, 2017.
87. Dengue: epidemiology. Centers for Disease Control and Prevention website. https://www.cdc.gov/dengue/epidemiology/index.html. Accessed March 24, 2017.
88. Zika virus: symptoms. Centers for Disease Control and Prevention website. https://www.cdc.gov/zika/symptoms/symptoms.html. Accessed March 24, 2017.
89. Hantavirus: reported cases of HPS. Centers for Disease Control and Prevention website. https://www.cdc.gov/hantavirus/surveillance/. Accessed March 24, 2017.
90. Rabies: Rabies in the US. Centers for Disease Control and Prevention website. https://www.cdc.gov/rabies/location/usa/index.html. Accessed March 24, 2017.
91. Tetanus: surveillance. Centers for Disease Control and Prevention website. https://www.cdc.gov/tetanus/surveillance.html. Accessed March 24, 2017.
92. Malani PN. National burden of invasive methicillin-resistant *Staphylococcus aureus* infection. *JAMA.* 2014;311(14):1438-1439. doi:10.1001/jama.2014.1666.
93. Methicillin-resistant *Staphylococcus aureus* (MRSA): MRSA tracking. Centers for Disease Control and Prevention website. https://www.cdc.gov/mrsa/tracking/index.html. Accessed March 26, 2017.
94. Methicillin-resistant *Staphylococcus aureus* (MRSA): general information about MRSA in healthcare settings. Centers for Disease Control and Prevention website. https://www.cdc.gov/mrsa/healthcare/index.html. Accessed March 26, 2017.
95. VRE has a domino effect among regional hospitals. Infection Control Today website. https://www.infectioncontroltoday.com/news/2013/07/vre-has-a-domino-effect-among-regional-hospitals.aspx. Accessed March 26, 2017.
96. New carbapenem-resistant enterobacteriaceae warrant additional action by healthcare providers. Infectious Diseases Society of America website. http://www.idsociety.org/CDCHAN341.htm. February 14, 2013. Accessed May 3, 2017.
97. Outbreaks of avian flu in North America. Centers for Disease Control and Prevention website. www.cdc.gov/flu/avianflu/outbreaks.htm. Accessed March 26, 2017.

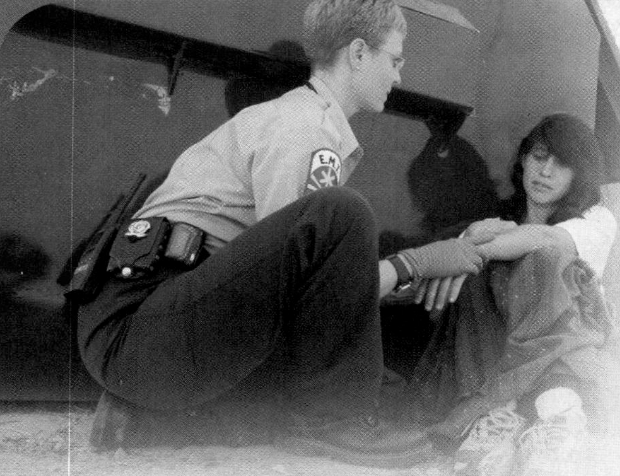

Assessment *in Action*

You are called to a local rehab center for a person vomiting. When you arrive, the staff nurse tells you the patient has a history of hepatitis. The patient has been vomiting most of the day, has a fever, and is very weak. When you enter the patient's room, you notice the patient's skin appears yellow.

1. Before you physically assess this patient, what type of precautions should be taken?

A. Standard precautions
B. Special precautions
C. Barrier precautions
D. Cutaneous precautions

2. The yellow coloring to the patient's skin is caused by:

A. a decrease in the red blood cell count.
B. an increase in the bilirubin level in the blood.
C. a decrease in the bilirubin level in the blood.
D. an increase in the red blood cell count.

3. The most common chronic bloodborne infection and the leading reason for liver transplantation in the United States is:

A. hepatitis A.
B. hepatitis B.
C. hepatitis C.
D. hepatitis D.

4. If you had a positive exposure to confirmed HBV while treating this patient and you have a positive titer test on file, what follow-up treatment is recommended?

A. A follow-up titer test to make sure of immunity
B. None because you show immunity to HBV
C. Precautionary antibiotics as soon as possible
D. Repeating the three-vaccination series

5. Which of the following types of hepatitis is enteric?

A. A
B. B
C. C
D. D

6. The ability of an organism to invade and create disease in a host is called:

A. indirect transmission.
B. direct transmission.
C. vector transmission.
D. virulence.

7. What are key facts to know when caring for a patient with norovirus infection?

A. Norovirus quickly multiplies in the lungs after entering the body.
B. Norovirus is spread by respiratory droplets.
C. Alcohol sanitizers are preferred for handwashing.
D. A bleach-based cleaning solution is required.

8. What are the requirements for the designated infection control officer (DICO)?

9. What is the role of the public health department in infectious disease outbreaks?

10. What is the major protective measure that your vehicle offers for the care and transport of patients with airborne- or droplet-transmitted diseases?

CHAPTER 27

Toxicology

National EMS Education Standard Competencies

Medicine

Integrates assessment findings with principles of epidemiology and pathophysiology to formulate a field impression and implement a comprehensive treatment/disposition plan for a patient with a medical complaint.

Toxicology

Recognition and management of
- Carbon monoxide poisoning (pp 1425-1426)
- Nerve agent poisoning (pp 1424-1425)

How and when to contact a poison control center (p 1400)
Anatomy, physiology, pathophysiology, assessment, and management of
- Inhaled poisons (pp 1401-1402, 1412-1417, 1424-1430, 1432-1435)
- Ingested poisons (pp 1400-1401, 1409-1425, 1427-1444)
- Injected poisons (pp 1402-1403, 1421-1423)
- Absorbed poisons (pp 1403, 1424-1425, 1427-1430, 1434)
- Alcohol intoxication and withdrawal (pp 1409-1412)
- Opiate toxidrome (pp 1404, 1421-1423)

Anatomy, physiology, epidemiology, pathophysiology, psychosocial impact, presentations, prognosis, and management of the following toxidromes and poisonings:
- Cholinergics (pp 1404, 1441-1442)
- Anticholinergics (pp 1404, 1435-1436, 1441)
- Sympathomimetics (pp 1413-1419)
- Sedative-hypnotics (pp 1419-1420)
- Opiates (pp 1421-1423)
- Alcohol intoxication and withdrawal (pp 1409-1412)
- Over-the-counter and prescription medications (pp 1412, 1414, 1419-1420, 1422-1424, 1430, 1435-1438)
- Carbon monoxide (pp 1425-1426)
- Illegal drugs (pp 1412-1418, 1421-1423, 1431)
- Herbal preparations (pp 1399, 1444)

Knowledge Objectives

1. Define toxicology, poison, and overdose. (p 1398)
2. Describe routes of entry of toxic substances into the body, including ingestion, inhalation, injection, and absorption. (pp 1400-1403)
3. Explain the appropriate use of activated charcoal, including situations when it may be most beneficial to the patient. (p 1401)
4. Explain the importance of situational awareness and an accurate scene size-up when responding to a toxicologic emergency. (pp 1401, 1406)
5. Discuss the major toxidromes and their use in the assessment and management of toxicologic emergencies. (pp 1403-1404)
6. Identify the common signs and symptoms of poisoning. (pp 1403, 1405)
7. Discuss substance abuse and concepts associated with it. (pp 1403-1404, 1406)
8. Describe the assessment and management of the patient with suspected poisoning or overdose. (pp 1406-1409)
9. Recognize the role of airway management in the patient with suspected poisoning or overdose. (p 1407)
10. Identify the main types of specific poisons and their effects. (pp 1409-1444)
11. Discuss emergencies related to severe intoxication, including alcoholism. (pp 1409-1412)
12. Describe the assessment and management of the patient with suspected plant or mushroom poisoning. (pp 1440-1443)
13. Describe the assessment and management of the patient with suspected food poisoning. (pp 1443-1444)

Skills Objectives

1. Demonstrate the steps in the assessment and management of the patient with suspected poisoning. (pp 1406-1409)
2. Demonstrate the steps in the assessment and management of the patient with suspected overdose. (pp 1406-1409)

Introduction

Toxicologic emergencies are some of the most challenging situations you will face as a paramedic. Toxicologic emergencies require you to think critically to identify the substances involved, determine your differential diagnosis, and formulate your treatment based on the anticipated clinical course of your patient. **Licit** (legal) or **illicit** (illegal) drugs will frequently play a role in situations you encounter in the field **Figure 27-1**, even when drug use is not the primary reason for the 9-1-1 call. One of the cornerstones of prehospital emergency medicine is a solid understanding of various substances and medications, as well as pharmacokinetics (the activity of drugs in the body over time, including the processes of absorption, distribution, and elimination). In this chapter, you will form a working knowledge of common substances to which patients may have been exposed and the resulting effects on the patient. This foundation will allow you to initiate appropriate treatment of patients with poisoning or drug overdose. Although illicit drugs such as heroin and methamphetamine are still common on the streets, waves of new, chemically engineered drugs may be finding their way into your local community as well.

To begin, it is important to define some key terms. **Toxicology** is the study of toxic or poisonous substances. A **poison** is a substance whose chemical action could damage structures or impair function when introduced into the body. Even a small amount of poison may cause serious symptoms and possible death. By contrast, a **drug** is a substance that has some therapeutic effect (such as reducing inflammation, fighting bacteria, or producing euphoria) when given in the appropriate circumstances and in the appropriate dose. A **toxin** is a poison or harmful substance produced by bacteria, animals, or plants. An **overdose** occurs when a drug (either licit or illicit) is taken in excess. An overdose can be a true medical emergency because of the profound effects of the overwhelming presence of the drug in the body. To put it concisely, a poison is always a poison, whereas a licit or illicit substance may poison a person if it is taken to excess.

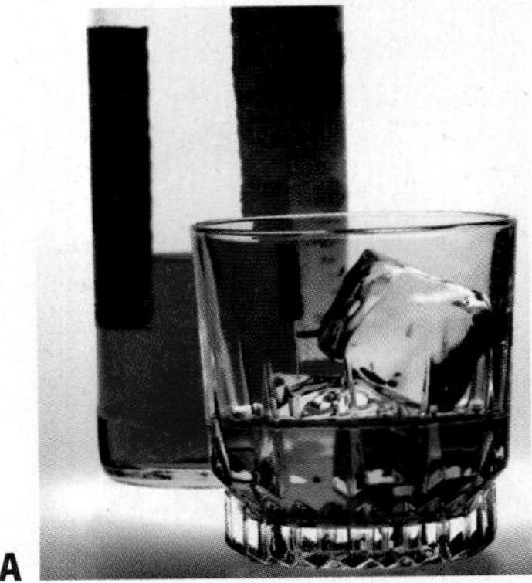
A

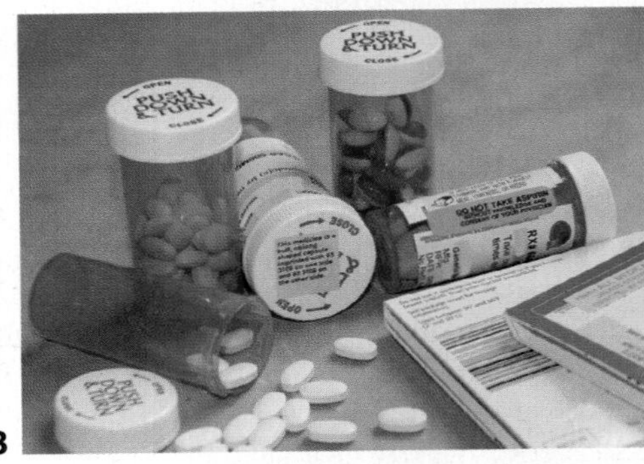

B

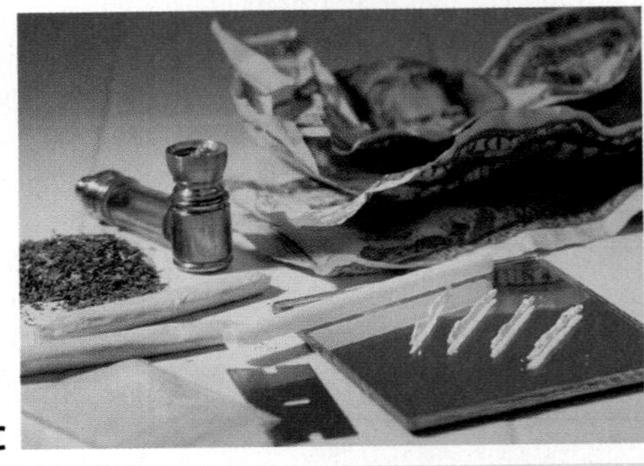
C

Figure 27-1 A. Alcohol is a legal substance that is a drug. **B.** Medications are legal substances that can be abused. **C.** Illegal drugs can also be abused.

YOU are the Paramedic PART 1

At 1430 hours, your unit is dispatched to single-family residence. The dispatcher tells you that a woman was found unresponsive by family members. Fire department personnel are responding with you, but no law enforcement officers have been dispatched. When you arrive, you find a middle-aged woman lying supine in bed. The room is neat and well-kept. Nothing looks obviously out of place or suspicious. Your primary survey reveals that the patient is barely breathing but has a strong pulse. The family reports that the patient had back surgery 4 days earlier. The family says she was last seen normal about 6 hours earlier when she laid down for a nap. The patient had trouble sleeping during the previous night because of pain in her back.

1. What is your first impression of this patient?
2. What is your priority for patient care?

Bioavailability describes the percentage of unchanged substance that is present in the systemic circulation. *Half-life* describes the amount of time needed for the average person to metabolize or eliminate 50% of a substance in the plasma. The half-life of a drug is commonly expressed in minutes, but it is possible for the half-life to last for hours or even days. Lastly, *excretion* is used to describe how a drug is removed from the body.

Types of Toxicologic Emergencies

Toxicologic emergencies usually fall under one of two general headings: intentional and unintentional. According to the National Capital Poison Center, 79.4% of all poison exposures reported in 2014 were unintentional. It was also noted that intentional exposures were 32 times more likely to have serious outcomes (ie, major or fatal effects) than unintentional exposures.[1] Intentional toxicologic emergencies frequently involve a person who is depressed and may be attempting to die by suicide. The patient may have ingested several different substances, so you need to be thorough in your interview and assessment. Emergency medical services (EMS) providers have also seen an increase in chemical suicides in recent years (discussed later in this chapter). Such situations may pose a significant threat to you and other responders who are unaware of the presence of toxic gases in enclosed spaces.

Intentional overdoses may also play a role in criminal activities. Historically, drugs such as flunitrazepam (Rohypnol) have been used to facilitate sexual assault. Flunitrazepam may cause both antegrade and retrograde amnesia, so the patient's ability to recall the events surrounding the assault may be significantly impaired. Flunitrazepam is discussed later in this chapter. Finally, another type of intentional poisoning is that caused by chemical warfare, which is covered in Chapter 50, *Terrorism Response*.

An unintentional toxicologic emergency can occur in many ways, such as neglect, oversight, an idiosyncratic reaction (discussed in Chapter 13, *Principles of Pharmacology*), or confusion about one's drug regimen. For example, consider an older adult man who forgets that he has already taken his daily dose of the prescription beta-blocker used to control his hypertension. He then takes a second dose, which leaves the patient feeling weak and dizzy as his heart rate and blood pressure drop in response to the increased level of the medication in his system.

You must be able to decipher the patient's list of medications while paying particular attention to any new medications or changes to the dosage. If your patient has multiple physicians, then check to see if the patient is taking multiple medications prescribed by different physicians for the same indication. The patient may not understand that two similar medications with different trade names, such as the beta-blockers carvedilol (Coreg) and metoprolol (Toprol XL), could result in a dangerous drug interaction if mixed. Recent changes in pharmacy policies and procedures have attempted to prevent such a situation. You will also want to consider over-the-counter medications, home remedies, and herbal therapies to obtain a complete picture of what the patient has been taking. The potential for a polypharmacy overdose (involving multiple medications) should be considered with any toxicologic emergency.

Patient Safety

To avoid creating an unintentional overdose in patients, you must be diligent in the administration of all medications. A simple miscalculation in volume or dose can cause you to give 10 mg of morphine to a pediatric patient instead of the 1 mg that you had planned to administer. This error can be the difference between therapeutic relief of pain and quickly scrambling for a bag-mask device to support the patient with acute respiratory depression.

Unintentional toxic exposures commonly occur with children. Anyone who has spent any length of time around young children knows they explore the world using their mouths, which may result in unintentional ingestions Figure 27-2. From holly berries around the holidays to brightly colored prenatal gummy vitamins, an innocent toddler may become seriously ill after deciding to taste his or her newfound treasure.

Finally, unintentional toxicologic emergencies can also occur in the workplace. For example, employees at an airplane assembly plant may work in several areas during their daily duties that contain chemicals, including hydrocarbons and hydrofluoric acid. A patient experiencing shortness of breath could have been exposed to either chemical, so a thorough scene size-up and history taking would be prudent to help identify the specific toxins to which the patient may have been exposed.

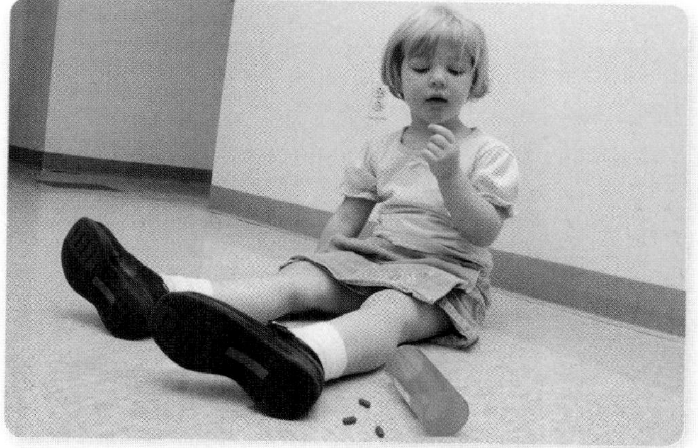

Figure 27-2 A toddler may mistake brightly colored pills for candy. This unintentional exposure can lead to devastating illness, even with very small amounts of the substance.

Poison Centers

Given the variety of illicit drugs and the continued growth of prescription drug abuse, even veteran paramedics may find it difficult to keep current with the myriad drugs sold in the streets today. For this reason, the American Association of Poison Control Centers (AAPCC) may be an indispensable aid. The AAPCC supports the nation's poison centers in their efforts to prevent and treat poison exposures. The phone number for the Poison Control hotline is 1-800-222-1222 (available 24 hours a day, 7 days a week). Some mobile device apps, such as Epocrates, can assist with pill identification. If you input basic information about the pills (size, shape, color, or markings), then the software may help to narrow down the list of potential medications. The National Capital Poison Center has an online tool and mobile device app called webPOISONCONTROL that can be used by laypeople or health care providers.

Suppose you are called to a home in which a frantic mother is hovering over a toddler who sits beside an empty packet that contained the dog's flea medication. Is the medication poisonous? How poisonous? Is an **antidote** (something to counteract the effect of the poison) available? In such a scenario, you can call the poison center and get a fast rundown on the ingestion, its toxic potential, and steps to negate its effects. With this information in hand, you can initiate proper patient care while contacting online medical control, if needed, for specific orders or instructions if they go beyond the range of your standing orders.

Poison centers are a virtual goldmine of information that you should add to your paramedic toolbox. Never hesitate to tap these resources when you are confronted with any toxin for which you have limited or no familiarity. When in doubt, call!

At the same time, your call helps the center's staff to collect data on poisonings in your region. These data may be analyzed to help detect trends, spot developing public health problems, and evaluate current treatment protocols for different poisonings.

Words of Wisdom

The National Capital Poison Center was founded in 1980 to help prevent poisonings, limit injuries from poisonings, and save lives. The organization is accredited by the AAPCC and offers 24-hour guidance for poisoning by certified specialists in poison information. Board-certified physician toxicologists back up the team of specialists and help manage each case.

In addition to knowing how to reach the National Capital Poison Center, familiarize yourself with information on poisoning available at the Centers for Disease Control and Prevention (CDC) website. The website documents recent trends and current statistics to help health care providers stay informed.

Words of Wisdom

In toxicology, it is important to observe and record all of the patient's symptoms and clinical signs. Do not dismiss subtle changes or seemingly benign symptoms that the patient may report. Thorough documentation may be the key in determining the substances to which the patient has been exposed.

Pathophysiology

Routes of Entry

To have an effect, a substance must first enter the body. The four primary methods of entry are ingestion, inhalation, injection, and absorption. The rate at which the toxin is absorbed into the body varies based on the route of entry. After a toxin has entered the body, the combination of the amount of toxin and the relative speed at which it is metabolized affect both the bioavailability of the toxin and the excretion rate.

Poisoning by Ingestion

Ingested poisons may produce immediate damage to tissues, or the toxic effects may be delayed for several hours. Damage can occur rapidly when a caustic substance is ingested. A household cleaner that contains a strong acid or alkali substance will immediately cause significant damage to local tissues. Although personal care products and cleaning products remain the most common ingestions for pediatric patients, analgesics account for the majority of ingestions for patients older than 20 years.[1]

When you are faced with a patient who has ingested a toxic substance, you must consider all possibilities regarding the substance and whether the ingestion was intentional or unintentional. Consider, for example, the curious child who eats a liquid laundry detergent capsule after mistakenly thinking it is candy **Figure 27-3**. Now consider a person who is taking prescription medication for pain relief following a surgical procedure. In an effort to control his or her pain levels, the patient may take several doses of more than one medication that contains opiates. Both of these scenarios are considered unintentional ingestions.

Assessment clues pointing toward ingestion can be as obvious as a plant with partially chewed leaves or a section of plant with berries missing. Look for stained fingers, lips, or tongues. Any patient reporting the sudden onset of stomach cramps with or without nausea, vomiting, or diarrhea may have an ingestion-related condition. Prescription and over-the-counter (OTC) pill bottles can provide you with valuable information in your assessment of the patient and the scene. Pay particular attention to the date when the prescriptions were filled. Does it make sense that the pill bottle is empty 6 weeks

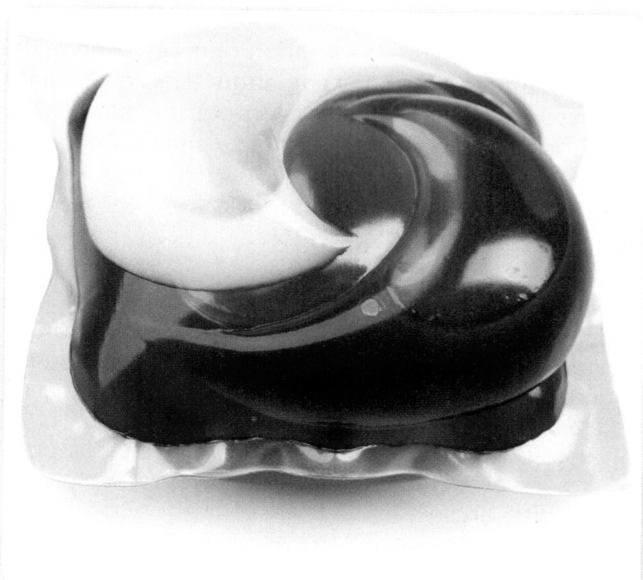

Figure 27-3 Although companies have attempted to repackage laundry detergent capsules to make them less visually appealing to children, unintentional ingestions can still occur.

after being filled? Possibly. What if the prescription was filled only 2 days earlier? These clues can paint vastly different pictures.

After a substance is ingested, the amount of time that it spends in the stomach may vary from person to person. Because little absorption occurs in the stomach, you have time to work on identifying the ingested substance. The goal of treatment is to develop a plan to either remove or neutralize the toxin before it has a chance to enter the small intestine, where most absorption takes place. The practice of forced vomiting via administration of ipecac is not indicated in any patient. Activated charcoal with sorbitol may be appropriate, depending on the substance, because it helps prevent the body from absorbing the poison. Activated charcoal is most effective when given close to the time of ingestion, and it may be more beneficial when treating an ingestion of extended release capsules. Activated charcoal will not bind to certain substances, such as alcohols, and, therefore, it should not be administered for ingestions of those substances. Gastric decontamination may occur at the hospital after an accurate clinical assessment and anticipated course of treatment has been determined.

Poisoning by Inhalation

A person can be poisoned by inhalation when the toxic agent is present in the surrounding atmosphere. This situation also poses a high risk to you as a responder. Similar to ingestion, poisoning by inhalation can be either unintentional or intentional. Your scene size-up should include extra precautions when dealing with the possibility of an inhaled toxin. If the patient remains in the potentially hazardous environment, then any responder who attempts to move the patient should be fitted with an appropriate self-contained breathing apparatus. Do not make the mistake of rushing to the patient's aid only to become a patient yourself.

Even if an inhaled toxin was not included in your initial dispatch information, you must remain alert that it may be the cause of your patient's symptoms. For example, you are called to assess a man who has passed out at a swimming pool. En route, you may be thinking that the patient could have heat exhaustion or a cardiac condition. When you arrive, the fire department personnel inform you that they found two other people who have passed out behind a building next to the pool. At this point, warning sirens should be going off inside your head, and you should immediately reevaluate the safety of the scene. If you do not include the possibility of an inhaled poison, then you run the risk of missing this critical decision point. If you do not think about it, then you cannot catch it.

Also be aware of an emerging method of suicide in the United States that places EMS, fire, and law enforcement officers at risk.[2] **Chemical suicide**, also called detergent suicide, is a method that involves mixing certain household chemicals in an enclosed space to create toxic gases (such as hydrogen sulfide and hydrogen cyanide), which are then inhaled.

The resulting chemical vapors are often colorless and may or may not have a recognizable odor. Emergency responders are at risk of serious injury when attempting to access the vehicle, area, or patient after observing an unresponsive person inside. In some instances, the suicidal person has left a note, warning bystanders and emergency responders of the presence of toxic chemicals. Therefore, maintain your situational awareness and, before opening any door, be sure to read any note you come across. In other instances, bystanders attempting to render aid and emergency responders have been exposed to extremely hazardous chemicals while trying to access and assess a person who is already dead. According to the Agency for Toxic Substances and Disease Registry's National Toxic Substance Incidents Program, eight responders were injured while responding to a chemical suicide between 2011 to 2013.[3]

Words of Wisdom

Your diagnostic equipment is only one piece of the puzzle. Be aware that CO and cyanide poisoning may result in falsely high pulse oximeter readings. CO binds to hemoglobin and does not let go, and cyanide impairs the offloading of oxygen at the cellular level. Therefore, do not get a false sense of security from an oxygen saturation reading of 100% in an acutely ill patient. If a patient is acutely short of breath following an exposure or suspected exposure, then administer a high concentration of oxygen.

From the physiologic perspective, inhaled toxins are quick to produce signs and symptoms. The toxin enters the body through the respiratory tract and rapidly reaches the alveoli. From there, simple diffusion allows the toxin to cross the alveolar-capillary membrane where the toxin can be readily transported through the cardiovascular system. Carbon monoxide (CO) is an example of an inhaled toxin. It has a high affinity for hemoglobin and severe CO poisoning is often fatal. Rapid systemic distribution of CO can occur with an equally rapid onset of signs and symptoms. For this reason, the window of opportunity for problem identification and subsequent treatment is limited. CO poisoning is discussed later in this chapter.

When you are dealing with an inhalation incident, the first general management consideration is that of scene safety. Only personnel fitted with the appropriate breathing apparatus should consider removing the patient or patients to a safe environment before beginning any assessment or treatment.

Words of Wisdom

Scene safety is your primary concern when you are called to an inhalation incident. Be suspicious of some form of poisoning whenever you have multiple patients with similar complaints. It is your critical thinking that will save you; do not rely on your sense of sight or smell alone. Toxic fumes may be odorless and colorless, and they do not discriminate between responders and patients.

After you have identified the possibility of an inhalation incident, do not allow your emotions to cloud your ability to make sound decisions regarding your own personal safety and that of your fellow responders. You cannot help your patient if you become a patient yourself.

Inhaled toxins produce a wide range of signs and symptoms, many of which are unique to the toxin involved. It is critical to use all of the information available to you to determine the toxins involved. For residential calls, rely on your suspicions and gut instincts. Ask appropriate questions regarding recent events and the potential substances involved. If you are in an industrial environment or a large workplace, then search for clues such as a safety data sheet (SDS), a shipping manifest, a bill of lading, or transportation placards. The National Library of Medicine has developed the Wireless Information System for Emergency Responders (WISER). WISER is available for download via personal computers, as well as smartphone applications. WISER provides information about hazardous chemicals and other substances, including human health and treatment information.[4] Talk to the patient's coworkers about substances that may be located in the patient's work area or stored at the facility. That information, coupled with the assistance of the poison center and direction from the medical control physician, will drive your treatment plan. Correction of hypoxia is a must; deliver a high concentration of oxygen and make sure to support adequate ventilation, if needed. Establish vascular access, apply an electrocardiogram (ECG) monitor, and perform pulse oximetry and capnography.

Words of Wisdom

Because e-cigarettes are becoming more popular due to their cost, flavor options, and their ability to be used indoors, they are becoming a rare but emerging poisoning. The liquid nicotine contained in the e-cigarette is often the offending agent. The most common route of exposure is inhalation, but there are also reported cases of ingestion and absorption through the eyes. Nausea, vomiting, and eye irritation are common symptoms following an exposure.[5]

Poisoning by Injection

Injected poisons usually gain access to the body as the result of stings or bites from a variety of insects and animals. Depending on your geographic location, possibilities for poisoning by injection frequently exist in the environment. Snakebites and scorpion stings are more prevalent in the southwestern United States, whereas people in coastal areas are more likely to be stung by jellyfish, Portuguese man-of-wars, sea urchins, or sea anemones. Wasps, yellow jackets, and hornets have a wider geographic distribution.

Some of these injected poisons produce localized or systemic reactions, whereas others may be neurotoxic. When a bite or sting hits a blood vessel, it results in a toxin immediately entering the bloodstream. The outcome is much more dangerous than when the same toxin enters a muscle mass, from which the toxin has a much slower rate of absorption and distribution.

When you assess bites and stings, physical findings will usually provide the most obvious clues, especially local reactions such as pain at the wound site. Depending on the specific toxin, the patient's signs and symptoms can vary. Occasionally, the patient may be able to identify the culprit, greatly simplifying the assessment process. Chapter 38, *Environmental Emergencies*, discusses bites and stings in detail.

Patient Safety

All tools used to inject substances or puncture the skin should be considered biohazards. These needles, blades, or injection devices may have been shared with drug users and may carry the human immunodeficiency virus, hepatitis, or other pathogens. Make sure you do your part in disposing of hazardous materials and place all sharps into a sharps container.

Abuse of intravenously administered drugs such as heroin, cocaine, amphetamines may prompt a call for EMS. *Speedballing* refers to the simultaneous use of heroin and cocaine. Although the patient or bystanders may not be forthcoming with information about the substances involved, you can focus your attention on the physical assessment, signs, and symptoms to help with possible identification. The patient's presentation will likely help to guide you in identifying the type of drug involved. Drugs that are injected directly into the bloodstream will have a more rapid onset than those injected into the muscle or subcutaneous tissue.

Poisoning by Absorption

Some poisons gain access to the body by being absorbed through the skin. When you consider the time from exposure to the emergence of symptoms, remember that substances that are absorbed through the skin have a longer time of onset than ones that are inhaled or injected. Of the poisonings that occur by absorption, those caused by pesticides such as organophosphates and similar substances are often the most serious. Because of the highly toxic nature of organophosphates, scene safety remains paramount. These patients may need to be decontaminated. Follow your agency's decontamination protocols, which may include using a hazmat team. Organophosphates are discussed in detail later in this chapter.

Words of Wisdom

Absorption of toxic substances through the skin is a common problem in the agriculture and manufacturing industries. Most solvents, insecticides, herbicides, and pesticides are toxic and can be readily absorbed through the skin.

▶ Understanding and Using Toxidromes

You may feel overwhelmed when you first consider the growing list of thousands of potentially harmful substances, OTC drugs, and prescription medications. Fortunately, many different drugs react in a similar fashion after they enter the body. While you perform a thorough patient assessment, you may be able to note a pattern in the signs and symptoms. For example, consider the category of stimulants. Regardless of whether the stimulant is a natural product derived from a coca plant (cocaine) or a synthetic compound created in a makeshift laboratory (methamphetamine), all drugs in this group work in a similar manner by stimulating the central nervous system (CNS), and thereby produce similar signs and symptoms. The syndrome-like symptoms of a class or group of similar poisonous agents are termed a toxic syndrome, or **toxidrome**. Knowledge of common toxidromes can help guide you through the assessment and management of different substances that fall under the same clinical umbrella. Five major toxidromes exist: narcotic, sympathomimetic, sedative-hypnotic, cholinergic, and anticholinergic Table 27-1.

Common signs and symptoms of poisoning are listed in Table 27-2. If you look at the patient history and physical exam findings in conjunction with the vital signs, more often than not you can develop a working diagnosis that will allow you to provide appropriate emergency medical care until you can deliver the patient to the receiving facility. For example, imagine that your patient has respiratory depression, bradycardia, hypotension, and constricted pupils. Using Table 27-1, you could see that narcotics produce all of those signs and symptoms. Now imagine that a similar patient presents with all of the same symptoms, but the patient has dilated pupils. Would that finding change your working diagnosis for the patient? If yes, which causative agent would be a better fit? Consider a barbiturate as the offending agent.

▶ Overview of Substance Abuse

During your career as a paramedic, you will undoubtedly come into contact with patients who have a problem with substance abuse. Apart from the physical effects of substance abuse, addiction carries a social stigma than can lead to feelings of isolation, paranoia, and depression. In addition, innovative methods of synthesizing new drugs or altering existing drugs are constantly being developed with the aim of improving their effects. Because of the sheer number of drugs available today, scientists and researchers are faced with the never-ending task of documenting the effects of each substance and the potential for abuse.

In recent years, one of the most interesting discussions regarding the definition of substance abuse involves marijuana. For centuries, this drug was used recreationally for its euphoric and psychoactive properties. However, recent research has demonstrated medicinal uses for marijuana. One example involves an extract called cannabidiol that can be effective at controlling seizure activity. It is important to note that this specific type of marijuana has been designed to have a high cannabidiol content and a low tetrahydrocannabinol (THC; the psychoactive component of marijuana) content. Ongoing debate continues about whether its use for medical conditions outweighs potential negatives associated with recreational use.

Another component of the discussion around substance abuse points out that the societal definition of abuse may have little relation to the potential harm from the abused substance. For example, other than defining a legal age to purchase tobacco, our culture places no restrictions on the long-term and compulsive use of this substance, even though it is a major contributor to cardiovascular

Table 27-1 Major Toxidromes

Toxidrome	Drug Examples	Signs and Symptoms
Narcotic (opiate and opioid)	Morphine, codeine, heroin, methadone, opium, morphine, hydromorphone, fentanyl, oxycodone and aspirin combination	Hypoventilation, respiratory arrest, constricted (pinpoint) pupils, bradycardia, hypotension, track marks (intravenous [IV] drug abusers), drowsiness, stupor, coma
Sympathomimetic	Pseudoephedrine, phenylephrine, phenylpropanolamine, amphetamine, methamphetamine, cocaine, caffeine, nasal decongestants, synthetic cathinones (bath salts)	Hypertension, diaphoresis, tachycardia, tachypnea, dilated pupils (mydriasis), agitation, seizures, hyperthermia, paranoia
Sedative-hypnotic	Phenobarbital, secobarbital, diazepam, thiopental, midazolam, lorazepam, propofol, ethanol, flunitrazepam, zolpidem tartrate	Hypoventilation, respiratory arrest, drowsiness, disinhibition, ataxia, slurred speech, mental confusion, respiratory depression, progressive CNS depression, hypotension
Cholinergic	Organophosphates, acephate, diazinon, malathion, parathion, sarin, tabun, V agent	**DUMBELS**: (Diarrhea, Urination, Miosis [constriction of the pupils]/muscle weakness, Bradycardia/Bronchospasm/Bronchorrhea [discharge of mucus from the lungs], Emesis [vomiting], Lacrimation [excessive tearing of the eyes], Seizures/Salivation/Sweating); respiratory depression; apnea; coma; tachycardia can occur early with bradycardia developing as toxicity progresses
Anticholinergic	Atropine, scopolamine, antihistamines, diphenhydramine, chlorpheniramine, tricyclic antidepressants, antipsychotics, jimson weed	Agitation, dry mucous membranes, flushed skin, hyperthermia, tachycardia, dilated pupils, blurred vision, mild hallucinations, dramatic delirium

Abbreviation: CNS, central nervous system

and respiratory disease Figure 27-4. By comparison, use of marijuana, which has less damaging effects than tobacco, is often punishable by fines or imprisonment.

Words of Wisdom

Drug abuse is not limited to members of the younger generation or to any particular section of society. It occurs in all age groups and at all social levels.

The following list defines some basic terms and concepts related to substance abuse:

- **Drug abuse.** Any use of a drug that causes physical, psychological, economic, legal, or social harm to the user or others affected by the user's behavior.
- **Habituation.** A physical and psychological dependence on a drug.
- **Physical dependence.** A physiologic state of adaptation to a drug caused by chronic use, usually characterized by tolerance to the effects of the drug and withdrawal if use of the drug is stopped (especially abruptly).
- **Psychological dependence.** The emotional state of craving a drug to maintain a feeling of well-being.
- **Tolerance.** Physiologic adaptation to the effects of a drug such that increasingly larger doses of the drug are required to achieve the same effect.
- **Withdrawal syndrome.** A predictable set of signs and symptoms, usually involving altered CNS activity, that occurs after the abrupt cessation of a drug or after a rapid decrease in the usual dosage of a drug.
- **Drug addiction.** A chronic disorder characterized by the compulsive use of a substance that results in physical, psychological, economic, legal, or social harm to the user; the user continues to use the substance despite the harm.

Table 27-2 Common Signs and Symptoms of Poisoning

Sign or Symptom	Type	Possible Causative Agents
Odor	Bitter almonds	Cyanide
	Garlic	Arsenic, organophosphates, phosphorus
	Acetone	Methyl alcohol, isopropyl alcohol, aspirin, acetone, diabetes
	Wintergreen	Methyl salicylate
	Pears	Chloral hydrate
	Violets	Turpentine
	Camphor	Camphor
	Alcohol	Alcohol
Pupils	Constricted	Narcotics, organophosphates, jimson weed, nutmeg, propoxyphene (Darvon)
	Dilated	Barbiturates, atropine, amphetamine, glutethimide (Doriden), lysergic acid diethylamide (LSD), cyanide, CO
Mouth	Salivation	Organophosphates, arsenic, strychnine, mercury, salicylates
	Dry mouth	Atropine (belladonna), amphetamines, diphenhydramine (Benadryl), narcotics
	Burns in mouth	Formaldehyde, iodine, lye, toxic plants, phenols, phosphorous, pine oil, silver nitrate, acids
Skin	Pruritus	Jimson weed, belladonna, boric acid
	Dry, hot skin	Atropine (in belladonna), botulism, nutmeg
	Sweating	Organophosphates, arsenic, aspirin, amphetamines, barbiturates, mushrooms, naphthalene
Respiratory	Depressed respirations	Narcotics, alcohol, propoxyphene, CO, barbiturates
	Increased respirations	Aspirin, amphetamines, boric acid, cyanide, kerosene, methyl alcohol, nicotine
	Pulmonary edema	Organophosphates, petroleum products, narcotics, CO
Cardiovascular	Tachycardia	Alcohol, amphetamines, arsenic, atropine, aspirin, cocaine, some antiasthma drugs
	Bradycardia	Digitalis, gasoline, nicotine, mushrooms, narcotics, cyanide, mistletoe, rhododendron
	Hypertension	Amphetamines, lead, nicotine, antiasthma drugs
	Hypotension	Barbiturates, narcotics, tranquilizers, house plants, mistletoe, nitroglycerin, antifreeze
CNS	Seizures	Amphetamines, camphor, cocaine, strychnine, arsenic, CO, petroleum products, scorpion sting
	Coma	All depressant drugs (such as narcotics, barbiturates, tranquilizers, alcohol), CO, cyanide
	Hallucinations	Atropine, LSD, mushrooms, organic solvents, PCP, nutmeg
	Headache	CO, alcohol, disulfiram (Antabuse)
	Tremors	Organophosphates, CO, amphetamine, tranquilizers, poisonous marine animals
	Weakness or paralysis	Organophosphates, botulism, eel, hemlock, puffer fish, pine oil, rhododendron
GI	Cramps, nausea, vomiting, and/or diarrhea	Many, if not most, ingested poisons

Abbreviations: CNS, central nervous system; CO, carbon monoxide; GI, gastrointestinal; LSD, lysergic acid diethylamide; PCP, phencyclidine

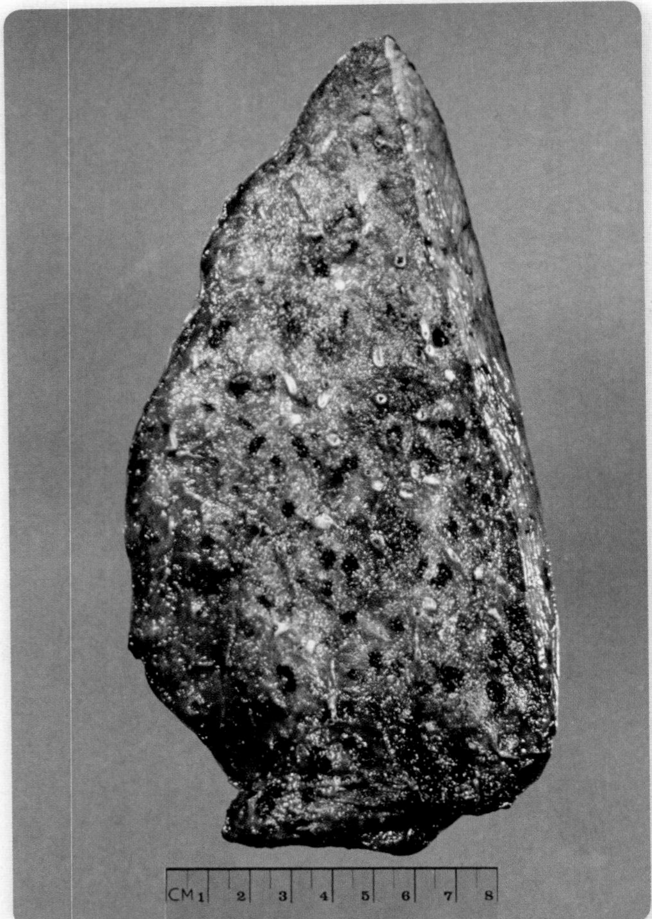

Figure 27-4 A diseased lung as a result of frequent tobacco use.

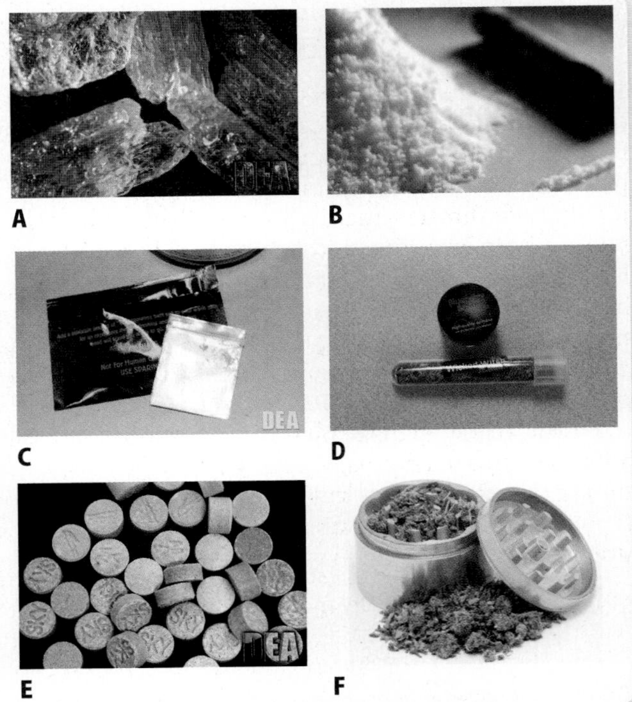

Figure 27-5 Abused substances include a wide and ever-evolving range of street drugs such as methamphetamine **(A)**, cocaine **(B)**, bath salts (Flakka) **(C)**, synthetic cannabinoids (Spice) **(D)**, Ecstasy **(E)**, and marijuana **(F)**.

- **Antagonist.** A molecule that blocks the ability of a given chemical to bind to its receptor, preventing a biologic response.
- **Potentiation.** The enhancement of the effect of one drug by another drug.
- **Synergism.** The action of two substances such as drugs, in which the total effects are greater than the sum of the independent effects of the two substances.

Patient Assessment

The general assessment approach is the same for all patients: scene size-up, primary survey, history taking, secondary assessment, and reassessment. If the mental status is altered, then diligently monitor the patient's airway and breathing to ensure he or she does not aspirate and has adequate minute ventilation. Prepare your suction equipment. Ensure you get a good overall clinical picture of the patient. Is the patient able to maintain his or her own airway, or is the patient struggling to swallow and clear secretions? If the patient is unresponsive, then obtain vital signs and complete a rapid full-body scan; obtain the patient history from bystanders and family members, if possible. If the patient is responsive, then use the OPQRST mnemonic (Onset, Provocation/palliation, Quality, Region/radiation, Severity, Timing) to elaborate on the chief complaint. Next, obtain the patient's vital signs and a SAMPLE history (Signs and symptoms, Allergies, Medications, Pertinent past history, Last oral intake, Events leading up to the illness or injury). Then perform a rapid full-body scan before moving on to a thorough physical exam.

Do not forget that patients with toxicologic emergencies may also have sustained traumatic injuries prior to your arrival.

Scene Size-up

Scene safety is paramount with toxicologic emergencies. Continually reevaluate your surroundings from the moment you arrive at the scene. As you approach the patient, look for clues such as pill bottles, household cleaners, or handwritten notes that may be useful to you Figure 27-5. Be aware that patients who have taken an overdose may be extremely dangerous. If necessary, call for law enforcement backup or a crisis unit to minimize potential for injury to you and your team.

Primary Survey

The primary survey of a patient who has overdosed on drugs or has been poisoned begins with forming your general impression. It can be as simple as "an adult woman lying prone on the bed." The primary survey seeks to rapidly identify life threats—that is, any concerns with mental status, airway, breathing, and circulation that require rapid intervention. By the end of your primary survey, you should be able to identify the nature of the illness (NOI) or possible mechanism of injury (MOI). Based on your findings, you can determine the severity of the patient's condition and begin to establish your priorities for the rest of the call.

Basic airway management is a crucial skill that will allow you time to obtain the information needed to make the appropriate decisions regarding the patient's treatment. If you can ventilate the patient effectively, then you have time to decide what needs to be done for him or her.

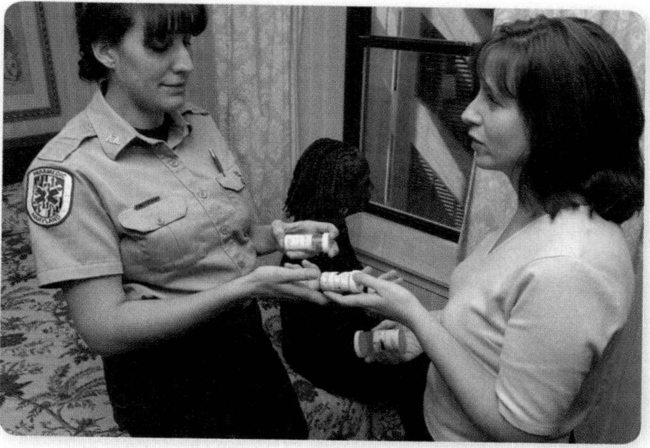

Figure 27-6 If the patient has overdosed on a prescription drug, then bring the medication container and its remaining contents to the emergency department.

History Taking

Toxicologic emergencies frequently involve symptomatic patients, so you need to elaborate on the chief complaint using the OPQRST mnemonic as part of history taking. Work to establish a rapport while you obtain a SAMPLE history directly from the patient. If the patient is unable or unwilling to speak, then obtain the OPQRST and SAMPLE history from bystanders and family members, if possible. Obtain as much information as you can early in the call, because acute changes may occur to the patient's mental status that may keep you from gathering additional information later.

To choose the appropriate course of action in a toxicologic emergency, obtain the following specific information at a minimum:

- **What is the substance?** If the patient has overdosed on a prescription drug, then bring the pill bottle and the remaining pills to the emergency department (ED) with the patient Figure 27-6. Consider taking the SDS if available. You may also copy or photograph the drug label information for review by hospital staff if you cannot safely transport the container. If the patient ingested a plant, then find out what part (roots, leaves, stem, flower, or fruit) and take a sample of the plant to the ED for identification. If you suspect an unintentional drug overdose, then ask questions about any medications, OTC drugs, or home remedies the patient may have been taking.
- **When was the substance ingested, injected, absorbed, or inhaled?** Time often works against you when treating a patient who has been exposed to a toxic substance. The longer the toxin is inside the body, the more time it has to cause an effect. It is important to obtain an accurate timeline for the poisoning. As a general rule, acute-onset symptoms often indicate a more serious patient scenario than delayed-onset symptoms—for example, if the patient immediately began to have crushing chest pain after he or she smoked crack cocaine.
- **How much was taken, injected, absorbed, or inhaled?** In almost all cases, the dosage of the toxin is directly proportional to its toxic effects on the body. An unintentional overdose commonly involves taking too much of a medication. It may be more difficult for you to determine the quantity that was taken in an intentional overdose. The patient may be unwilling or unable to tell you how much he or she took, so you must rely on your observational skills. Observe the drug label to determine how much of the medication would have been in the container when it was full, and compare that amount with the amount that remains.
- **What else was taken?** A majority of intentional self-poisonings (suicide attempts) or illicit drug overdoses involve polydrug ingestions, often with alcohol as one of the drugs. The patient may also have tried to take an antidote. This information can be invaluable to ED staff when deciding which laboratory tests to order.
- **Has the patient vomited or aspirated?** If so, then how soon after the ingestion or exposure? How much? Inspect the vomitus for pill fragments. If the patient vomited into a clear emesis bag, then consider transporting the contents to the ED.
- **Why was the substance taken?** Ask this question of every patient. Do not make assumptions. The patient may have taken the substance mistakenly, or it could be a suicide attempt caused by severe depression. Whenever possible, use quotation marks to record the patient's own words in your patient care report.

Documentation & Communication

When you document the contents of any medication bottle, be specific about the number and type of pills that you counted, even if several different types of pills are present in one bottle. Consider having another individual, such as a nurse at the ED, count the pills on your arrival at the hospital. This practice will help to account for all of the medications that were present when you delivered the patient to the hospital. Include the details of this count (including who was present) in your documentation. This step is considered a best practice and will help mitigate any claims in the event that medications are missing.

Documentation & Communication

Remember, you are the only reliable link between the emergency scene and the hospital. The hospital staff will look to you to provide them with relevant information from the scene. Ensure you have obtained all of the pertinent details about the substance involved in a poisoning while you are on scene. Write down the type and amount of substances involved. Finally, ensure your verbal and written reports are complete and thorough.

Secondary Assessment

After completing the primary survey, begin the secondary assessment. Toxicologic emergencies are often medical emergencies only. Complete the appropriate secondary assessment for every patient. Remember, the secondary assessment is a systematic scan that allows you to observe any abnormalities that may be present. Toxins can either target a single body system or result in a critical systemic event. You must be able to appreciate the subtle differences that may be present based on the interactions of the toxin with the body. These interactions may range from subtle tachypnea to obvious organophosphate poisoning with abnormal findings in almost every body system. Do not hesitate to use the five major toxidromes (see Table 27-1) or mnemonics to help you remember the wide variety of abnormal presentations associated with toxicologic emergencies.

Patients with a toxicologic emergency may have alterations in mental status and may be prone to nausea and vomiting. Nausea and vomiting may lead to a critical airway problem, so be sure to perform a thorough assessment and develop a plan of action based on your findings.

In the event that trauma is also present, perform the appropriate trauma assessment (rapid full-body scan or focused exam) based on whether the patient has a significant MOI. Because some patients with a toxicologic emergency may have gruesome self-inflicted injuries (for example, self-evisceration), focus on completing your entire exam. You must be able to properly prioritize your treatment and interventions.

YOU are the Paramedic PART 2

You check the patient's carotid pulse and note it is strong and regular at a rate of 100 beats/min. The patient is breathing at a rate of about 4 breaths/min, so you ask your partner to place a nasopharyngeal airway and assist the patient's respirations with a bag-mask device connected to supplemental oxygen. While you consider a list of differential diagnoses, you turn to the family members to ask questions about the events leading up to the 9-1-1 call.

Recording Time: 2 Minutes	
Appearance	Unconscious
Level of consciousness	Unresponsive
Airway	Open
Breathing	Very slow
Circulation	Adequate

3. If this patient has overdosed, then which drug classification would be your focus?
4. Give some examples of drugs that would meet this classification.

Special Populations

In an unintentional overdose or poisoning, an older adult patient may have become confused about his or her drug regimen. The person may have forgotten that he or she already took the medication and may repeat the dose one or more times. The patient may also have forgotten the physician's instructions to discard leftover medication and might have taken both the current medication and the older drug, resulting in increased effects or unwanted drug interactions.

Controversies

If a pediatric patient is in stable condition and has a history of a single, small ingestion of a low-risk agent, then some EMS systems allow the transport to be canceled after agreement from medical control. Although this approach may be medically sound, it eliminates an opportunity for assessment of psychosocial and risk factors in the ED.

Reassessment

Reassessment focuses on monitoring the patient's condition, reprioritizing the patient's status if necessary, and checking the effectiveness of interventions provided. Reassessment is typically done in the ambulance while en route to the ED. Continually monitor all patients who have ingested, injected, absorbed, or inhaled a poisonous substance.

Emergency Medical Care

From a management perspective, advanced life support (ALS) care for toxicologic emergencies builds on the following basics:

- Ensure the scene is safe for access and egress.
- Maintain the airway.
- Ensure breathing is adequate.
- Ensure circulation is not compromised (that is, either by hypoperfusion or a dysrhythmia).
- Administer high-concentration supplemental oxygen to maintain saturation levels of 94% or higher.
- Establish vascular access.
- Consider administration of an antidote or mitigating medication, if available.
- Prepare to manage shock, coma, seizures, and dysrhythmias.
- Transport the patient as soon as possible. If any risk of vomiting exists, then place the patient in the left lateral recumbent position to reduce the risk of aspiration.

Pathophysiology, Assessment, and Management of Abuse of and Overdose With Specific Substances

Alcohol

The form of alcohol consumed by humans in alcoholic beverages is ethyl alcohol (or ethanol). It is not conventionally recognized as a poison, even though it has many properties of a poison when ingested in sufficient quantities. Alcohol is undeniably part of human society. People commonly drink alcohol to relax, socialize, and celebrate. According to a 2015 study by the National Institute on Alcohol Abuse and Alcoholism (NIAAA), approximately 87% of people age 18 years or older have consumed alcohol at some point in their lives. Furthermore, almost 27% of people age 18 years or older reported that they had engaged in binge drinking (occasional heavy use) within the past month.[6] With increased alcohol use comes an increased risk of developing **alcoholism**, a disorder characterized by a physical and psychological addiction to ethanol.

From million-dollar gated communities to low-income housing developments, alcoholism occurs in all social strata and in almost every culture. The American Psychiatric Association publishes the *Diagnostic and Statistical Manual of Mental Disorders, Fifth Edition,* which outlines criteria that are used to diagnose someone with an alcohol use disorder. Common warning signs include the following:[7]

- Consuming alcohol in large quantities or over a long period
- Spending considerable time in activities necessary to obtain alcohol, use alcohol, or recover from its effects
- Causing or exacerbating social or interpersonal problems due to alcohol use
- Reducing social, occupational, or recreational activities due to alcohol use
- Continuing to use alcohol even after acknowledging the physical or psychological problems that are caused or exacerbated by alcohol use

Pathophysiology

As mentioned previously, psychological dependence on alcohol involves drinking to function "normally" and feel good. Alcohol acts as a depressant in the frontal lobe and can alter the decision-making process and/or decrease a person's inhibitions. Because of the disinhibition and euphoria that can accompany alcohol consumption, people often use it as a "social lubricant" to feel more comfortable in social situations. In some people, the perception of social acceptance or increased social ease may influence them to drink more. People may feel as though they can escape their worries or become more likeable while they are under the influence of alcohol. The psychological dependence may escalate to a point where people feel they require alcohol to survive socially or emotionally.

Physical dependence results from the regular consumption of large quantities of alcohol. At this level of dependence, should a person abruptly stop consuming alcohol, withdrawal symptoms will result. The severity of the withdrawal can vary according to the severity of the dependence. Minor withdrawal is characterized by restlessness, anxiousness, difficulty sleeping, agitation, and tremors. For those with a more serious physical dependence, sudden abstinence can cause significant symptoms, such as hypertension, tachycardia, vomiting, hallucinations, and delirium tremens (discussed later in this chapter).

It is important to understand that people with severe dependence may go to extreme lengths to obtain alcohol. People with chronic alcoholism (or those without the financial means to afford alcoholic beverages) may resort to drinking mouthwash, hand sanitizer, and other hazardous products with alcohol content. When you treat a patient who has ingested a toxic substance just for the alcohol content, always consider the other ingredients of those substances.

Words of Wisdom

You will commonly encounter patients who have consumed alcohol. When you assess a patient with an altered mental status and a history of recent alcohol consumption, never assume that he or she is "just drunk." Perform the appropriate assessments and remember to consider other possible causes for the altered mental status.

A person with alcoholism is prone to a number of serious illnesses and injuries Table 27-3 . Alcohol has profound effects on the neurologic, cardiovascular, and GI systems.

The CNS is particularly vulnerable to alcohol abuse. From neurotransmitter imbalances to structural breakdown of the cells, the body will experience slower cognitive and motor function capabilities. The effect of alcohol on neurotransmitters (such as glutamate) is the reason you

YOU are the Paramedic PART 3

Your partner has placed a nasopharyngeal airway and is assisting ventilations with a bag-mask device and supplemental oxygen while you finish your rapid full-body scan. You note the patient is unresponsive with respiratory depression and pinpoint pupils. The pulse oximeter reading was initially 90%, but it has been steadily rising. The family members report that the patient was prescribed 10 mg of hydrocodone for pain control after her surgical procedure. The prescription was filled 4 days earlier, and only two tablets are missing from the bottle. You wonder if two tablets could have produced such a dramatic patient presentation.

Recording Time: 5 Minutes	
Respirations	Assisted via bag-mask device
Pulse	100 beats/min
Skin	Cyanosis around lips; dry and cool
Blood pressure	92/58 mm Hg
Oxygen saturation (Spo_2)	90% room air
Pupils	Pinpoint, nonreactive

5. Should you intubate this patient?
6. What is your next step in treating this patient after the airway is controlled?

Table 27-3 Medical Conditions to Which People With Alcoholism Are Particularly Susceptible

Condition	Contributing Factors
Subdural hematoma	Frequent falls; impaired clotting mechanisms; brain atrophy allows for significant movement during impact
GI bleeding	Irritation of stomach lining (leading to gastritis); impaired clotting mechanisms; cirrhosis (excess scar tissue) of the liver, leading to engorgement of esophageal veins (esophageal varices)
Pancreatitis	Secretion of enzymes, causing inflammation
Hypoglycemia	Damage to the liver; impairs gluconeogenesis
Pneumonia	Aspiration of vomitus occurring during intoxication and coma; suppression of immune system by alcohol
Burns	Risky behaviors during intoxication; decreased pain sensitivity during intoxication
Hypothermia	Insensitivity to extremes of temperatures while intoxicated; falling asleep outside in the cold; impaired thermoregulation
Seizures	Effect of withdrawal from alcohol; neurotransmitter or electrolyte imbalance
Dysrhythmias (atrial fibrillation or ventricular tachycardia)	Toxic effects of alcohol on the heart; hypertension; electrolyte imbalance
Cancer	Products of alcohol metabolized by the liver are toxic to cells; may cause alterations in normal cellular pathways
Esophageal varices	Develop when normal blood flow to the liver is blocked and blood backs up into smaller, more fragile blood vessels in the esophagus

Abbreviation: GI, gastrointestinal

may note slurred speech, memory loss, and an unsteady gait in a severely intoxicated patient.

As alcohol travels through the digestive system, it irritates tissue and can damage the lining of the stomach by causing acid imbalances, inflammation, and acute gastric distress. Often, the result is gastritis (an inflamed stomach), gastric esophageal reflux disease, or heartburn. The more frequently someone drinks, the more likely it is that the GI system will be irritated. Alcohol abuse is also a risk factor for some cancers, specifically cancer of the mouth and esophagus. The National Cancer Institute reports that people who consume 3.5 or more drinks per day have a two to three times greater risk of developing mouth or throat cancer.[8]

The toxic effects of alcohol on the liver produce a variety of complications, such as coagulopathies (easy bleeding and poor clotting ability), hypoglycemia, and GI bleeding. From fatty liver disease to cirrhosis, alcohol can significantly impact the body's ability to metabolize and filter harmful substances. This impairment also causes a fluid backup and may lead to elevated pressures in the hepatic system. As pressures continue to rise, smaller vessels leading into the liver can become engorged with blood and swell. This swelling is the pathology behind esophageal varices, which can rupture and cause bleeding into the esophagus and oropharynx. This condition requires rapid suctioning and effective airway management.

Acute Alcohol Intoxication

Alcohol is known to suppress excitatory neurotransmitters and, thus, acts as a CNS depressant. When you consider the amount of alcohol that someone has consumed, you must also take into account his or her size. For example, a 240-pound (109-kg) man may consume three drinks and have a blood alcohol content (BAC) of 0.07% (note that most states define legal intoxication as a BAC of 0.08% or more). However, a smaller woman weighing 140 pounds (64 kg) may consume the same three drinks and have a BAC of 0.14%. Always look at the entire clinical picture. Keep in mind the concept of proportion.[9] Symptoms usually progress proportionately to blood alcohol content. Death from alcohol intoxication can occur with blood alcohol levels of 0.40% (400 mg/dL).[10]

One of the most significant risks to an acutely intoxicated person is from respiratory depression and/or aspiration of vomitus, secondary to the inability to protect his or her own airway. If an intoxicated patient is unconscious, then treat him or her as you would any unconscious patient. Assess the patency of the airway. Is the patient able to maintain his or her own airway? Is the patient swallowing spontaneously? Are secretions pooled in the oropharynx (a clear indicator of a markedly depressed or absent gag reflex)? Because of the high risk for aspiration, consider advanced airway management if the patient is unable to maintain his or her own airway. Always have suction equipment prepared and ready to use.

In addition, provide supplemental oxygen to maintain adequate oxygen saturation levels. Assist ventilations as needed. Do not use excessive force when ventilating your patient. Gastric insufflation may cause vomiting and further complicate airway management if you ventilate with excessive force or too quickly. Establish vascular access. Monitor the ECG rhythm. Assess the patient's blood glucose level, and treat hypoglycemia if it is found. Local protocols or online medical control may direct the administration of 100 mg of IV thiamine to prevent Wernicke-Korsakoff syndrome (acute onset of confusion and delirium secondary to thiamine deficiency). Finally, transport the patient to an appropriate facility.

Words of Wisdom

Alcohol may be one small piece of the clinical puzzle. Although the odor of alcohol on the breath of an intoxicated patient may be one of the most obvious signs during your assessment, remember alcohol is often used in conjunction with other substances in both unintentional and intentional overdoses.

Withdrawal Seizures

A person who has been drinking heavily for an extended period and suddenly stops drinking may experience a variety of withdrawal phenomena. Seizures usually occur within about 12 to 48 hours, but may occur as quickly as 6 hours after the last drink. The approach to a patient with withdrawal seizures should be similar to your treatment of an intoxicated patient. Short, isolated seizures do not require treatment, but medical control may direct the administration of a benzodiazepine as prophylaxis against another seizure. Prolonged seizures usually respond to lorazepam (1.0 to 3.0 mg). Keep in mind that patients with chronic alcoholism may have cross-tolerance to medications used to treat withdrawal or seizure activity.[10]

Delirium Tremens

One of the most serious and lethal complications of alcohol withdrawal is **delirium tremens (DTs)**. Symptoms usually start 48 to 72 hours after the last alcohol intake, although the onset could be delayed by several days. Signs and symptoms include confusion, tremors, restlessness, fever, diaphoresis, tachycardia, and hypotension, often secondary to dehydration. The patient with DTs is susceptible to vivid hallucinations and is extremely responsive to external stimuli. Cognitive function often decreases as the heart rate and temperature increase. The condition may result in increased mortality if the patient is not treated aggressively.

The treatment of a patient with DTs is aimed at protecting the patient from injury and supporting the cardiovascular system. Try to keep the patient calm. Minimize external stimuli if possible. Do not position yourself in a dark area because the patient may confuse you for something else (such as a threat) during the hallucinations. Follow local protocols for benzodiazepine administration if the patient is agitated or combative. Physical restraints may cause additional agitation and could worsen the patient's condition, but always consider your safety first. Consider contacting online medical control to discuss aggressive benzodiazepine use. In addition, administer supplemental oxygen and establish vascular access. Manage hypotension with an infusion of normal saline; this administration may also help to manage increasing body temperature. Maintain an ongoing dialogue with the patient throughout transport to help orient and reassure the patient.

▶ Stimulants

Stimulants, in both licit and illicit forms, can have devastating effects on those who abuse them. From smokable cocaine (crack) and methamphetamine to prescription diet aids and medications for attention deficit disorder, you will at some point care for a patient who is under the influence of stimulants.

Stimulants have various forms that allow for absorption by ingestion, inhalation, or injection. Most stimulants work to enhance the release of catecholamines, which stimulate the CNS (specifically, alpha and beta receptors). This CNS stimulation can increase alertness and create a sense of euphoria. Increased catecholamine release can also lead to agitation, hyperthermia, tachycardia, hypertension, and seizures.

Taking the adverse effects into account, try to get a visual picture of a patient who uses or abuses stimulants. CNS excitation can create agitation, anxiousness, delirium, and dilated pupils. The patient may struggle to sit still and may fidget frequently. Hyperthermia and tachycardia will cause the patient to be hypermetabolic. You may note profuse sweating while assessing the skin. The body is constantly running at a faster rate, so the energy stores will be depleted, creating an overall thin appearance. You may observe signs of drug abuse, such as track marks from IV injection or burns to the fingers from a crack cocaine pipe. Remember that patients who use or abuse stimulants may be sleep deprived, anxious, and even paranoid. Always maintain your situational awareness to ensure a safe environment for you and your partner.

Patient Safety

While treating a patient experiencing the effects of a potent sympathomimetic, sedatives may be used to help safely treat and transport the patient. Do not allow the agitation or combativeness of your patient to distract you while calculating an appropriate dose for the patient. Take the time to double check your dose and the volume that you are preparing to administer. Prior to administration, communicate the dose to your partner. This step could help prevent a serious medication error.

Cocaine

Cocaine is a naturally occurring alkaloid that is extracted from the leaves of the *Erythroxylon coca* plant that grows in South America. After the leaves are processed into cocaine hydrochloride, the active ingredient in the leaves increases in potency. In the 19th and early 20th centuries, elixirs often contained cocaine as an active ingredient to treat various illnesses. Ear, nose, and throat physicians once used cocaine as a local anesthetic. The euphoria and addictive qualities of cocaine have contributed to its demand on the streets.

The results of a National Survey of Drug Use and Health from the National Institute on Drug Abuse (NIDA) have identified trends in the prevalence of various drugs from 2013 to 2015. These trends show that cocaine use has declined slightly for people ages 12 to 25 years, but the overall use for people age 26 and older has increased.[11] The amount of biologically active cocaine may vary from one form to another. Some variance may exist based on the amount of filler (potentially toxic adulterants) used to dilute or "cut" the drug. The higher the purity of the cocaine, the more severe the potential dependence becomes. People who occasionally use a less pure solution of the drug will not be as psychologically or physiologically dependent as someone who is using a purer solution. Cocaine users with serious dependence problems may have significant health conditions as well as social and psychological challenges.

Pathophysiology. Cocaine is a local anesthetic and a nervous system stimulant. It enhances the release and activity of neurotransmitters in the body, including norepinephrine, dopamine, and serotonin. The enhanced dopamine activity is responsible for the euphoria that features enhanced alertness and a tremendous sense of well-being. Collectively, this constellation of effects makes cocaine one of—if not the most—psychologically addictive drugs available. The enhanced norepinephrine activity results in the stimulation of the sympathetic nervous system. The physical manifestation of this stimulation accounts for many of the common adverse effects related to cocaine use, such as tachycardia, hypertension, and hyperthermia. This sympathetic nervous system stimulation can place every organ system at risk due to significant vasoconstriction, along with increased metabolic and oxygen demands from the cells.

One chemical form of cocaine, water-soluble hydrochloride salt, is quickly absorbed across all mucosal membranes, allowing it to be applied topically, insufflated (snorted), swallowed, or injected intravenously. Another form of cocaine, crack cocaine, is simply cocaine mixed with two inexpensive ingredients, baking soda and water. After the ingredients are mixed together into a paste-like slurry and cooked or baked, the end result is smokable cocaine.

When cocaine is snorted nasally, the patient may begin to feel high within 1 to 5 minutes. When crack cocaine is smoked and the alveoli are bathed in cocaine-laden smoke, the onset of effects is much more rapid (in the 8- to 10-second range). Injection of cocaine has a similar rapid onset as it enters cerebral circulation. Smoking and injecting cocaine are known to produce a rush followed by a high.[12] The duration of the effects will depend on the patient's tolerance level and purity of the drug. People who have a high tolerance level or commonly use higher purity cocaine may seek to repeat their doses more frequently due to the body's dependence on higher levels of the drug.

When the effects of cocaine wear off, the user experiences a so-called crash, which is characterized by depression, irritability, and exhaustion. Depending on the amount and length of cocaine use, the person may experience a cascade of adverse effects collectively referred to as *cocaine washout syndrome*. This syndrome presents as a hypoactive state related to a lack of synaptic neurotransmitters. While the user is experiencing the high, he or she has large quantities of neurotransmitters interacting with the central and peripheral nervous systems. After the effects of cocaine wear off, all of those neurotransmitters become less active or unavailable for use by the body.

The patient who is experiencing cocaine washout syndrome may be difficult to assess. Signs of hyperactivity may have already dissipated. The patient may be on the downward slope of his or her high, so the patient may be hypoactive. Remember to assess for other pathology during your assessment. Consider other potential—and far more ominous—causes of the patient's hypoactive state, such as stroke or myocardial infarction (MI) with profound shock.

Adding to the problem, a person with cocaine addiction who is trying to avoid the unpleasant effects of a crash may take more cocaine or a sedative (such as diazepam [Valium], alcohol, or heroin). The patient may have several types of drugs in his or her system when he or she requires assistance from EMS. People with heroin addiction may use cocaine to withdraw or detoxify themselves from heroin by gradually decreasing the amounts of heroin taken while increasing the amounts of cocaine used.

Assessment. A person who has overdosed on cocaine may exhibit any of the signs and symptoms for stimulant abuse, including chest pain, shortness of breath, diaphoresis, and psychosis. Cardiac effects may be observed with ventricular dysrhythmias, MI, or sudden cardiac arrest. Because of the sodium channel–blocking properties of cocaine, you may observe a widened QRS complex or prolonged QT interval on an ECG tracing. Chronic users may exhibit significant left ventricular hypertrophy.

As mentioned earlier, the significant vasoconstriction created by cocaine use can cause the drug to impact any organ system. During your assessment, be alert for signs of neurologic insult and renal failure. Always assess your patient based on his or her clinical presentation and symptoms.

Amphetamine, Methamphetamine, and Amphetamine-like Drugs

Amphetamines are structurally similar to the derivatives of phenylethylamine and include methamphetamine (crank or ice), methylenedioxyamphetamine (MDA, Adam), and methylenedioxymethamphetamine (MDMA, Eve, Ecstasy). Amphetamine and amphetamine-like drugs have a number of legitimate clinical applications including nasal decongestants, and treatment of narcolepsy, attention-deficit disorder, and attention-deficit/hyperactivity disorder **Figure 27-7**. Increased amphetamine abuse has been noted in schools. Adolescents with attentional disorders may be prescribed amphetamines for increased alertness and focus. However, the possibility exists for the person to abuse his or her own prescription medication and/or to participate in drug diversion (the process of transferring a prescription medication from the person from whom it was prescribed to another person) for financial gain.

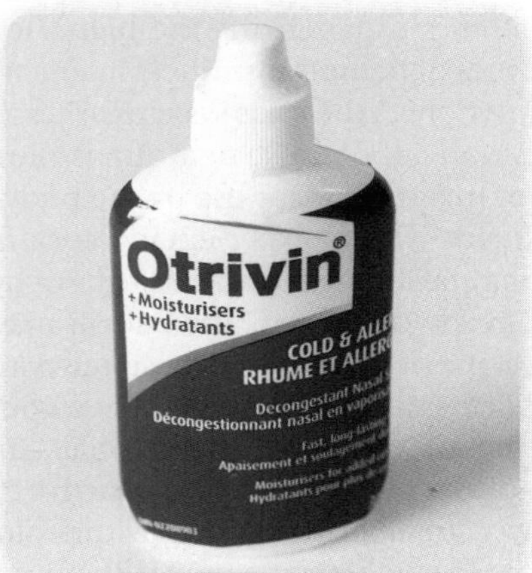

Figure 27-7 Drugs such as nasal decongestants and diet pills generally fall into the category of amphetamines.

Molly, the "chemically pure" crystal powder form of MDMA, has been appearing on the streets. This drug is highly desired on the streets because of its incredible high, but most drug users fail to realize the substance may be tainted with other additives that could produce adverse effects and significant medical conditions. Research has shown that its actual prevalence is underreported because of confusion or lack of awareness that this is a type of MDMA.[13]

Methamphetamine is a low-cost, long-acting stimulant that is extremely addictive. The ingredients required to manufacture methamphetamine can be purchased in stores, although federal regulations are intended to make obtaining large quantities of the pseudophedrine and other required ingredients more difficult to obtain. The process of manufacturing methamphetamine involves the use of hazardous chemicals that could present a health and safety hazard to you and your fellow responders. Remember scene safety when you are assessing a patient who may have been involved in the manufacturing process.

The clinical presentation of the patient abusing amphetamine or methamphetamine is almost identical to that of a person abusing cocaine, with the primary exception that the effects of amphetamines last longer than those of cocaine. Never forget about the potential emotional and psychological instability seen in drug abusers, particularly in patients who have been on a binge. With each passing day of no sleep and little or no food, they become increasingly paranoid. Their behavior can quickly become violent, so always be mindful of your exit strategy when on scene. Do not hesitate to ask for law enforcement support if the scene seems likely to destabilize.

Synthetic Cathinones (Bath Salts)

Synthetic cathinones, also known as bath salts, refer to an emerging group of drugs similar to MDMA. Synthetic cathinones are psychoactive substances related to the chemical compound derived from the khat plant, which is native to East Africa. Khat leaves are traditionally chewed for a stimulant and euphoric effect. Synthetic cathinones are chemically engineered to have a higher potency than the natural compound. However, bath salts should not be confused with bathing products such as Epsom salt (magnesium sulfate).

Several of the chemical components used in synthetic cathinones enter the United States from countries such as China. In early 2015, three to four people were hospitalized every day in areas of South Florida following use of a synthetic cathinone called Flakka. International pressure for governments to ban the substances used to make synthetic cathinones have curbed some of the production, and, therefore, the frequency with which the drug appears on the street.[14] However, people have found replacement substances and ingredients that are chemically similar to synthetic cathinones. Synthetic cathinones are popular because they offer effects similar to stimulants such as cocaine and amphetamines, but usually cost less. Bath salts are sometimes sold as plant food or cleaners, and are labeled as "not for human consumption." Synthetic cathinones often have a white or brown crystal-like appearance and come in foil packages with names like Flakka, Cloud Nine, or White Lightning. They may be sold in convenience stores or gas stations, making them more accessible than other illicit drugs. It is difficult to identify new psychoactive substances and their unique characteristics; therefore, creating huge challenges in recognizing and treating patients appropriately.

Similar to other stimulants, synthetic cathinones can be ingested, insufflated, smoked, or injected. The speed of onset depends on the route of absorption. According to the NIDA, the two routes associated with the highest mortality rates are insufflation and needle injection.[15] Synthetic cathinone use has been associated with significant paranoia, hallucinations, incredible strength, excited delirium, and other bizarre behaviors. Tachycardia, diaphoresis, nausea, and hyperthermia may also be present.

Management of Stimulant Abuse

The most life-threatening presentations of stimulant abuse include dysrhythmias, vascular events, hypertension, hyperthermia, seizures, and agitation. Treatment of stimulant abuse and toxicity includes supportive care, maintaining oxygenation, proper monitoring, and assessing the need for appropriate intervention with IV fluids and/or medications, as follows:

- Establish and maintain the airway. Consider an advanced airway as needed.
- Provide supplemental oxygen to maintain saturation levels of greater than 94%.
- Establish vascular access.
- Apply the ECG monitor, pulse oximeter, and capnometer.
- To control anxiety and seizures, administer benzodiazepines per local protocols.
- Manage hypotension with serial fluid infusions of normal saline.
- For violent behavior, follow local protocols or contact medical control for sedation.
- Transport to the appropriate facility.

Fluid resuscitation may be required for patients with signs of hypoperfusion. Assess the patient for cardiac dysrhythmias that may require treatment. Treat chest pain as acute coronary syndrome and consider other symptoms (such as respiratory distress) as an atypical presentation of acute coronary syndrome. Vasospasm may be causing some of the patient's symptoms. Administer sublingual nitroglycerin every 3 minutes as long as systolic blood pressure is greater than 100 mm Hg and until pain resolves. Local protocols may allow administration of benzodiazepines for chest pain, tachycardia, hypertension, sedation, and seizures. Medical control is always a viable option if you believe that the patient has a true stimulant overdose. Hypertension that does not respond to benzodiazepines may be treated with nitrates, such as nitroprusside—although its use in the prehospital environment remains controversial.

Severe agitation and excited delirium are thought to be linked to stimulant overdose. If the patient exhibits bizarre behavior, is found naked, or has a history of noncompliance with psychiatric medications, then this finding may elevate the suspicion of stimulant overdose and excited delirium. Chemical restraints and sedation may be indicated to keep the patient and yourself safe. Local protocols may dictate which agent you use. Antipsychotics, benzodiazepines, and dissociative agents are commonly used in the field. As an example, ketamine can be given intravenously (2 mg/kg) or intramuscularly (4 mg/kg) based on the needs of the patient and scene dynamics.

Aggressive cooling may be indicated if the patient is hyperthermic and signs of delirium or severe agitation are present. Consider external cooling packs on the groin, axilla, and forearms. Cooled fluids may be administered per local protocol. Throughout the resuscitation process, it is essential to maintain urine output with aggressive fluid therapy.

If the patient has a seizure, then benzodiazepines remain the treatment of choice. Haloperidol (Haldol) is another choice because it can be given intramuscularly without having to gain vascular access. Should the situation worsen into status epilepticus, phenobarbital (Luminal) or IV or rectal diazepam (Valium) may be administered. Consider other routes for administration to help keep you and your partner safe around an actively seizing patient. Local protocol may allow for intranasal administration of medications. In addition, neuromuscular blockade may be needed to control motor activity to avoid hyperthermia, acidosis, and, potentially, **rhabdomyolysis** (the destruction of muscle tissue leading to a release of potassium and myoglobin). Online medical control will usually be required before reaching this step in your treatment algorithm.

▶ Marijuana and Cannabis Compounds

When the leaves and flower buds of the *Cannabis sativa* plant are harvested and dried, the end product is referred to as **marijuana** (also known as weed, pot, dope, and bud) Figure 27-8. The resin produced by the maturing flower tops can also be harvested and used to produce hashish (also known as hash). Over the past decade, some states have begun to legalize marijuana and some of its compounds for medical use; other states have made it legal for any use. This has created many controversial discussions about marijuana use. According to results from the National Survey on Drug Use and Health from the NIDA, marijuana remains the most commonly used illicit drug in the United States with approximately 32% of people ages 18 to 25 years using marijuana within the past year.[11] For these reasons, it is important to have

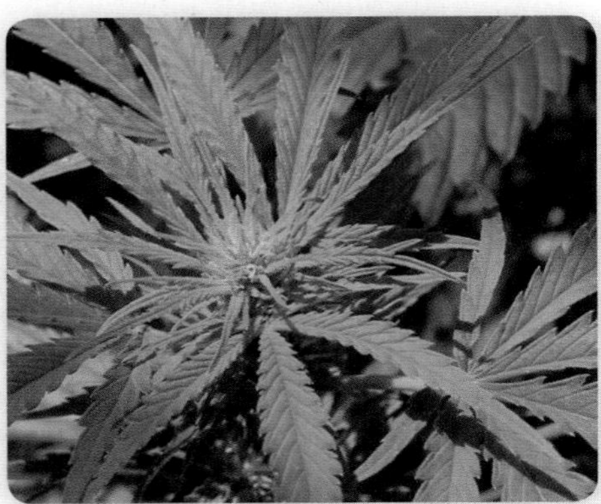

Figure 27-8 A marijuana plant.

a thorough understanding of marijuana and cannabis compounds.

Marijuana contains a number of cannabis compounds, which may have different therapeutic effects. Cannabidiol (CBD) is one of the main active chemical compounds. Recent preclinical research has demonstrated CBD may have significant therapeutic effects, including antiseizure, neuroprotective, analgesia, and antitumor properties. CBD does not have the euphoric or intoxicating effects of THC, and it has served as the driving force for some states to enact laws to allow access to cannabidiol oil or high-CBD strains of marijuana.

Pathophysiology

The primary psychoactive ingredient in marijuana and hashish is delta 9-tetrahydrocannabinol, or THC, as mentioned earlier. THC binds to cannabinoid receptors throughout the brain. Marijuana may cause the user to have enhanced sensory perception and euphoria. These unusual effects may cause anxiety or panic. Common short-term effects of marijuana include tachycardia, balance and coordination problems, increased appetite, conjunctival injection, dry mouth, and possible memory loss. Drowsiness and relaxation may also occur following use of the drug. Chronic use of marijuana may result in pulmonary symptoms without developing obstructive airway disease as is seen with tobacco use.[16]

Smoking marijuana usually causes euphoria and relaxation that can last as long as 4 to 6 hours. Fine motor skills, concentration, and depth perception can be altered for up to 24 hours. Marijuana products may also be ingested, insufflated, vaporized, and applied topically to the skin.

Assessment and Management

When you assess the patient who has used marijuana or cannabis compounds, know that intoxication and withdrawal from marijuana are not life threatening. Novice users may become panicked or anxious due to the euphoria, spatial disorientation, and altered sense of reality that can occur. Emotional support and supportive care is often all that is required. Benzodiazepines may be considered for sedation if the patient is significantly anxious. If the patient has severe or life-threatening signs and symptoms, then consider that another substance or drug may be at work as you continue your assessment and search for other causes.

You need to understand that patients may be unaware of their exposure, such as when someone has unknowingly ingested marijuana in a brownie. Pediatric patients may experience more serious signs and symptoms after ingestion of an edible food source that has been adulterated with marijuana (eg, lollipops, brownies, or gummy bears). Contact poison control and provide prompt transport to the hospital as the child may likely require hospitalization based on their symptoms.[17]

Occasionally, you may encounter a patient with cannabinoid hyperemesis syndrome. This syndrome involves cyclic episodes of nausea and vomiting in chronic cannabis users. IV fluids and antiemetics are indicated during transport to the appropriate facility.[16]

Spice

Similar to synthetic cathinones, **spice** is a synthetic cannabinoid that falls into the category of new psychoactive substances. Because the cannabinoids act on the same cellular receptors as THC, spice is often marketed as synthetic marijuana. However, the active substance is a blend of chemicals that is either sprayed onto plantlike material for smoking, or sold as a liquid for vaporizing in electronic cigarettes. Some users report euphoria similar to marijuana use; however, these chemicals can be much more dangerous than marijuana. Adverse effects of spice use include psychosis, hallucinations, tachycardia, vomiting, renal conditions, and seizures.

As with synthetic cathinones, it can be challenging to obtain a good assessment and form a treatment plan for someone who has used spice. Remember that various chemicals may have been used in the spice, so patient presentations may vary. Supportive care with fluids and antiemetics is often appropriate. If the patient is experiencing a seizure, then benzodiazepines are the medication of choice.

▶ Hallucinogens

A **hallucinogen** is a substance that can impair judgment, alter the user's perception of reality, and create a realistic sensation of images or sounds that are not actually present. Experiences with hallucinogens are unpredictable and can vary markedly from person to person. The overall drug experience is affected by the user's previous drug experience, the dose taken, and the social setting. Keep this information in mind when you move the patient into an environment that may have bright lights, loud sirens, and significant bumps and vibrations, such as the ambulance.

Hallucinogenic substances can be classified into two categories: synthetic and naturally occurring. The synthetic class of hallucinogens includes phencyclidine

(PCP) and ketamine. Naturally occurring hallucinogens include mescaline, psilocybin mushrooms, and the seeds of the jimson weed plant.

LSD

Lysergic acid diethylamide (LSD) is derived from a fungus that contaminates rye flour and wheat. It is usually ingested orally and is sold on the street in tablets, capsules, or liquid form. Small, colorful squares of paper may also be dipped in LSD and then placed on the tongue. A single dose is represented by one square of paper. The onset is usually 30 to 60 minutes. The duration of the effects can last up to 24 hours. LSD is considered a non–habit-forming drug, although tolerance can occur if it is taken for several days in a row.

Pathophysiology. LSD is a serotonin receptor agonist. LSD has the ability to distort reality, change a person's mood, or alter perceptions and/or reality. LSD may also result in the user experiencing synesthesias. Synesthesias, a crossing of the senses, often prompt a user to respond to the question, "What were you doing?" with a bizarre reply such as, "I was tasting the colors shining from that traffic light." Users may experiment with LSD for self-exploration or for religious reasons.

Because of the potency of LSD, even small doses may create a significant experience for the first-time user. Higher doses may lead to a longer duration or more intense experience. Tolerance can develop to LSD, requiring chronic users to take higher doses, but almost no evidence exists of a physical dependence or withdrawal syndrome if the user stops using the drug.

From a physiologic perspective, the effects of LSD are mostly sympathomimetic, often consisting of mild tachycardia, palpitations, mydriasis, and sweating. In a "bad trip," the user has a vivid, frightening experience similar to a nightmare, resulting in an acute anxiety attack and the physical effects secondary to increased anxiety. The bad trip does not end until the drug wears off.

Assessment and Management. The treatment of a patient using LSD is primarily supportive, focusing on the psychological aspects of the drug experience. Follow local protocols when considering anxiolytics for patients with severe anxiety.

During transport of a patient who has taken LSD, try to limit sensory stimulation as much as possible—for example, by avoiding the use of the emergency lights and siren. Routine transport to the appropriate facility and providing emotional support are usually all that is required for these patients.

Phencyclidine

Phencyclidine (PCP), also called angel dust or rocket fuel, is a dissociative anesthetic that has hallucinogenic properties. It was developed for use in the 1950s as an IV anesthetic, but patients experienced significant delirium following its administration. It is no longer used for any medical purpose in the United States. Although it is commonly sold in powder, crystal, or tablet form, some users dip marijuana cigarettes in PCP (known as wets or super grass). PCP is commonly added to other illicit drugs to create a more intense high. This practice can occur without the user's knowledge. Users may believe they are going to relax after smoking a marijuana joint (rolled cigarette), only to find that it has been laced with PCP.

Pathophysiology. Phencyclidine works at the N-methyl-D-aspartate (NMDA) receptors. As a dissociative drug, PCP has the ability to distort sight and sound and make the user feel separated from his or her own body. It is typically smoked or snorted, although it can be injected. Doses of 5 to 10 mg can produce signs and symptoms of intoxication in an adult. Slurred speech, staggering gait, tachycardia, hypertension, staring blankly for extended periods, and horizontal nystagmus (involuntary, rhythmic movement of the eyes) are common with PCP use. Users may also display extraordinary strength, have a sense of invincibility, or seem to lack awareness of pain, continuing to function despite significant orthopaedic injuries. A small, thin man on PCP may be able to successfully attack several larger people despite sustaining injuries—which can become a significant issue when considering scene safety and management of a combative patient.

Assessment and Management. PCP can cause some of the most violent and difficult behavior you will encounter in the field. The patient may rapidly change moods and attack without warning. For that reason, the safety of the EMS team is a continuous concern when responding to calls involving PCP users. Emergency medical care focuses on trying to calm the patient and addressing any wounds. Intramuscular (IM) sedatives may be considered for an aggressive or combative patient. Coordinate your efforts with your fellow responders to ensure that everyone knows the plan before moving to administer the medication. It may be feasible to obtain IV access after the patient has initially been sedated. Administer high-flow oxygen, monitor vital signs, and provide safe transport to an appropriate facility.

Ketamine

Ketamine (special K, vitamin K) is another dissociative anesthetic (discussed further in Chapter 28, *Psychiatric Emergencies*). Ketamine is relatively short-acting and has clinical uses in the veterinary and medical fields. As a paramedic, you may even carry this drug for specific prehospital indications, such as pain control or management of aggressive patients. Ketamine is at risk for drug diversion from veterinary clinics or hospitals, and a significant amount of illicit ketamine has been smuggled into the United States from Mexico. Ketamine is sometimes added to other illicit drugs to produce a more intense experience for the user.

Pathophysiology. Like PCP, ketamine works at the NMDA receptors. It also binds to mu-opioid receptors, giving it analgesic properties. At low doses, a user presents with mild inebriation, euphoria, and increased sociability. At higher doses, a patient may have pronounced nausea, difficulty moving, and significant hallucinations.

Assessment and Management. Although violent outbreaks in patients are much less likely with ketamine than with PCP, the principles of management are the same for patients who have used either drug. Secure the patient well, assess the ABCDEs and manage any life threats, provide oxygen therapy, establish vascular access if the patient is receptive, and provide safe transport to the appropriate facility. Keep a close eye on the patient, because violent behavior can occur suddenly. Benzodiazepines may be helpful in calming an agitated patient who is experiencing significant delirium.

Peyote and Mescaline

Native tribes in the southwestern United States and Mexico have been using hallucinogens for thousands of years, primarily for religious purposes, with mescaline as the substance of choice. Mescaline is the hallucinogenic agent found in the small peyote cactus. Peyote and mescaline are Schedule I substances with a high potential for abuse and no currently accepted medical use in the United States.

Pathophysiology. The exact mechanism of action for mescaline has not been determined. The dried flower "buttons" may be ingested or soaked in water to produce a liquid infused with mescaline Figure 27-9 . The buttons have a bitter taste and are a potent gastric irritant, with profound vomiting occurring shortly after ingestion. The psychedelic experience then typically begins with feelings of increased sensitivity to sensory stimulation. Flashes of color, commonly in geometric patterns, are noted. Similar to other hallucinogens, the experience may be guided by the social environment of the user; reports of hallucinations involving talking animals and vivid nature-based experiences are common. Users experience a distortion of time and space, and out-of-body experiences are commonly reported.

Structurally, mescaline looks more like amphetamine, which accounts for its physical effects: dilated pupils, increased pulse rate, mild hypertension, and increased body temperature.

Assessment and Management. Emergency medical care in the field setting is primarily supportive. Administer supplemental oxygen, monitor vital signs, provide positive emotional support, and arrange safe transport to the receiving facility. Consider fluids and antiemetics if the patient has nausea and intense vomiting.

Psilocybin Mushrooms

Certain mushrooms contain the hallucinogenic substances psilocybin and psilocyn Figure 27-10 . In the United States, the most commonly abused mushrooms are *Psilocybe mexicana* and *Psilocybe cyaescens*, but several varieties are also indigenous to tropical and subtropical climates in North, Central, and South America. The typical dose is estimated to be 4 to 10 mg (approximately 2 to 4 mushrooms). These mushrooms typically have a bitter taste, and they may be combined with other liquids or foods to disguise the foul flavor.

Pathophysiology. The onset of symptoms and hallucinogenic effects (similar to LSD but less intense) is within 30 minutes of ingestion, and effects usually last 4 to 6 hours. Signs and symptoms include muscle weakness, drowsiness, nausea and vomiting, mydriasis, mild tachycardia, and mild hypertension. The likelihood of serious adverse effects is low, although the literature describes seizures and hyperthermia in some patients.

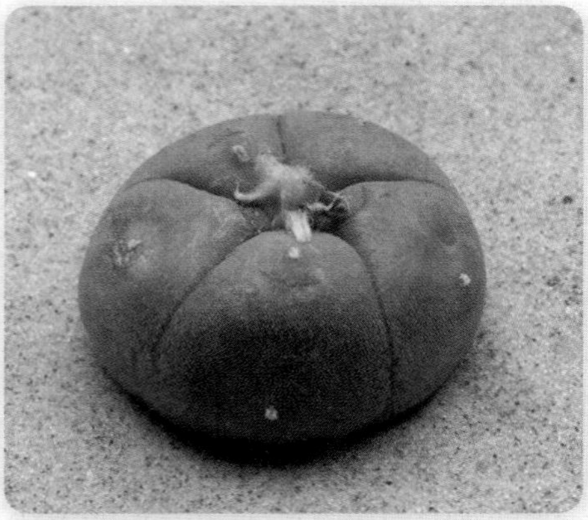

Figure 27-9 Dried flower buttons of the peyote cactus contain mescaline and produce a hallucinogenic effect if ingested.

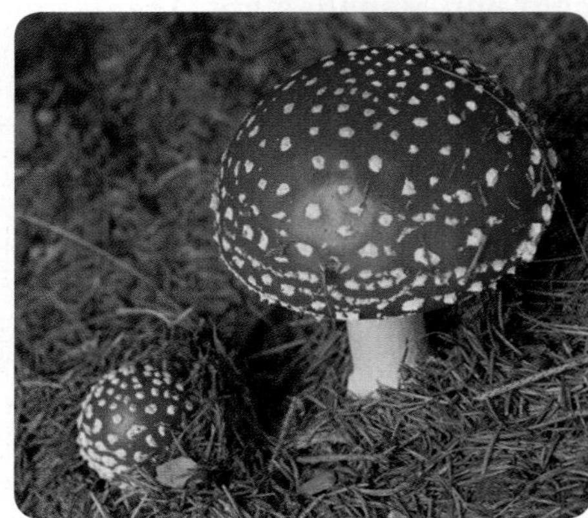

Figure 27-10 Mushrooms containing psilocybin are hallucinogenic if ingested.

Assessment and Management. Treat the patient with supportive care. Hallucinations are likely to subside quickly if the patient is in a secure, safe environment. Managing the ABCs and monitoring vital signs are usually all that is required, along with safe transport to the appropriate facility. If time and circumstances allow, then establish vascular access to facilitate seizure control with benzodiazepines, if necessary.

Sedatives and Hypnotics

The drugs in the sedative-hypnotic category have a wide range of applications with well-established therapeutic benefits. These drugs work as CNS depressants and can produce a range of effects, from light sedation to total anesthesia. Drugs with sedative qualities are used to reduce anxiety and to calm agitated patients. Drugs with hypnotic qualities are used as sleep aids, helping to produce drowsiness and sleep. Because of the effectiveness of sedative and hypnotic medications, they have a high potential for abuse and are at high risk for drug diversion in the medical field.

Barbiturates

Barbiturates are a class of medications that act as a CNS depressant. As such, they have established therapeutic uses as anxiolytics, anticonvulsants, and hypnotics. Analgesic effects are associated with barbiturate use, but these effects are often minimal. Clinically speaking, barbiturates are similar to alcohol in terms of dependence and withdrawal symptoms.

The frequent combination of alcohol and barbiturates as a suicide mechanism, coupled with the high incidence of unintentional overdoses, pushed researchers to develop sedative-hypnotic drugs that had fewer depressive effects on the respiratory system and were less lethal. Today, the likelihood of death after the ingestion of a single-entity sedative-hypnotic such as diazepam (Valium) is small.

Pathophysiology. Barbiturates potentiate gamma-aminobutyric acid (GABA) at specific receptors to inhibit cellular excitation. As the dose increases, barbiturates bind to other receptor sites and cause more widespread CNS depression. Barbiturates come in four basic configurations: long-acting, intermediate-acting, short-acting, and ultra–short-acting. Ultra–short acting barbiturates are highly lipid-soluble and have a rapid onset because they quickly cross the blood-brain barrier. These substances are preferred when time is of the essence, such as with airway management or stopping an active seizure. Long-acting barbiturates are less lipid-soluble; therefore, they have a delayed onset of action and are preferred when a sustained therapeutic level of a medication is required over a long period. The liver metabolizes most barbiturates into inactive waste products, although barbiturates that bind less tightly to proteins tend to be excreted unchanged in the urine.

Assessment. Your assessment findings will reflect the dosing and the configuration of the barbiturate. Mild to moderate barbiturate intoxication is similar to alcohol intoxication; symptoms include decreased alertness, nystagmus, ataxia, mental confusion, and slurred speech. As the dose increases, the patient moves further down the scale of CNS depression, becoming increasingly lethargic and eventually unresponsive. Be aware of the potential for respiratory depression.

Management. With barbiturate overdose, pay particular attention to the patient's airway status. Because some degree of CNS depression is likely, perform a thorough airway assessment. These patients are often at risk for vomiting and aspiration. Get a good clinical picture of the patient. If the patient is unable to protect his or her own airway, then move to secure the airway. Proper oxygenation and proper ventilation should be monitored with pulse oximetry and capnometry.

If signs of shock are evident, then administer fluid support in 250-mL increments (up to 2 L) of crystalloids. Perform a frequent reevaluation of breath sounds to ensure pulmonary edema is not developing. If the patient has received adequate fluid replacement but hypotension persists, then administer a vasopressor such as dopamine (Intropin). Remember to ensure the "tank is full" before adding a vasopressor.

If you are treating a conscious patient within 1 hour of ingestion, then consider administration of activated charcoal. Ensure the patient can maintain his or her own airway prior to administration. Activated charcoal may prove more beneficial for overdoses involving long-acting barbiturates.

Evidence-Based Medicine

Administration of activated charcoal for barbiturate overdose has not shown any decrease in overall morbidity and mortality.[18] Historically, the process of gastric lavage (or gastric emptying) was regularly practiced in emergency medicine. This practice may have been considered for substances that were ingested several hours earlier or were unable to be bound by activated charcoal. Recent research has failed to demonstrate the benefits of gastric lavage for gastric decontamination.[19]

If the substance is a long-acting barbiturate, then consider consulting online medical control regarding administration of sodium bicarbonate to assist with urine alkalinization to trap the drug in its ionized form. This practice may allow the drug to be more rapidly excreted through the urine before the substance can have a profound effect on the body. Recommended dosing ranges from 1 to 2 mEq/kg in 1 L of 5% dextrose in water (D_5W) infused over 1 hour.[18]

> **Words of Wisdom**
>
> Activated charcoal can be a messy drug to administer. Consider covering the cup and providing a straw through which the patient may drink the solution. Often, the patient will not continue to drink the solution after he or she sees or smells it. Keep an emesis bag or large receptacle handy for the patient to use should he or she vomit during or following administration.

Barbiturate abusers quickly develop tolerance and require ever-larger doses to produce the desired effects. Long-term use results in physical addiction. Abrupt cessation in a long-term barbiturate abuser will produce typical signs and symptoms of withdrawal syndrome in approximately 24 hours. In the case of minor withdrawal, the patient may present with symptoms similar to those observed in a patient with alcohol withdrawal: restlessness, tremulousness, insomnia, diaphoresis, abdominal cramping, and nausea and vomiting. With patients in severe withdrawal, you may also see delirium, hallucinations, psychosis, hyperthermia, and cardiovascular collapse. Life-threatening withdrawal, similar to DTs, is possible with abrupt cessation of large doses of barbiturates.

If you encounter barbiturate withdrawal syndrome in the prehospital setting, then focus your treatment efforts on preventing seizures (IV benzodiazepines are a common choice) and cardiovascular collapse (serial fluid boluses). Rapid transport to an ED, with subsequent intensive care, will be required to best manage the patient over the long-term.

> **Words of Wisdom**
>
> Consider the possibility of a drug-related condition in any patient presenting with unexplained behavioral changes, stupor, coma, or seizures.

Benzodiazepines

Benzodiazepines are also members of the sedative-hypnotic family. They are most commonly used to treat anxiety, seizures, and withdrawal symptoms. In recent years, the use of fast-acting benzodiazepines, such as zolpidem tartrate (Ambien) for treatment of insomnia, has grown rapidly. These drugs are often readily available on the Internet or from people selling their own prescription medications to seek financial gain.

Pathophysiology. Similar to barbiturates, benzodiazepines exert their effects by stimulating the GABA pathways, resulting in sedation and reduced anxiety. When taken orally, these medications are readily absorbed from the GI tract. IV administration allows for more rapid onset of action and more controlled dosing. IM injections may have a variable rate of absorption. These drugs are metabolized primarily by the liver.

Assessment. In a single-entity overdose, benzodiazepines have a relatively low rate of morbidity and mortality. The most common clinical effects of benzodiazepine overdose include altered mentation, drowsiness, confusion, slurred speech, ataxia, and general loss of coordination. Overdose of benzodiazepine rarely causes hypotension and has not been known to cause dysrhythmias. If either condition is present, then search for another cause.[18] In the case of intentional overdose, it is likely that multiple substances have been taken. Use your investigative skills and assessment to guide clinical management of the patient. On occasion, extrapyramidal reactions may occur in tandem with hepatotoxic or hematologic reactions.

Withdrawal from benzodiazepines may include tachycardia, tremulousness, confusion, and possibly seizures. Withdrawal is rarely a life-threatening event, but it can be complicated by withdrawal from other substances, such as alcohol.

Management. A reversal agent is available for the management of a benzodiazepine overdose. Flumazenil (Romazicon) is a benzodiazepine receptor antagonist. It is indicated for respiratory depression secondary to benzodiazepine overdose. Contraindications for flumazenil include long-term benzodiazepine use, concomitant epileptogenic overdose (tricyclic antidepressants), and underlying seizure disorders. Because of the difficulty of determining this information in the field, flumazenil is not frequently given in the prehospital environment. Consider flumazenil for a known, single-substance overdose involving a benzodiazepine. An example of this situation would be a patient who has been unintentionally overdosed by a medical provider treating a condition. Administration may precipitate seizure activity. Additional treatment of benzodiazepine overdose is relatively straightforward:

- Assess and manage the airway.
- Administer supplemental oxygen.
- Establish vascular access.
- Apply the ECG monitor, pulse oximeter, and capnometer.
- Consider administering flumazenil (a benzodiazepine antagonist) via slow IV push (0.2 mg IV/min) up to a total of 3 mg.
- Consider activated charcoal administration (in consultation with poison control or medical control), especially with extended release medications.
- Transport to the appropriate facility.

▶ Narcotics (Opiates and Opioids)

Narcotics are drugs that act as CNS depressants and produce insensibility or stupor. Historically, narcotics have been classified into two major divisions: opiates and opioids. The term **opiate** is used to describe various alkaloids derived from the opium or poppy plant (such as morphine and codeine). The term **opioid** refers to a synthetic narcotic with sedative properties that is not derived from opium (such as oxycodone, hydrocodone, tramadol, and fentanyl). In this textbook, *opioid* is used to describe licit therapeutic agents and illicit substances in this group. In recent years, incredibly potent drugs such as carfentanil and desomorphine have increased in use on the streets. Carfentanil is an animal tranquilizer used for large mammals, such as elephants. It is far more potent than morphine or fentanyl, and its use by abusers seeking a quick opioid high can be fatal.

Prehospital providers have seen a significant increase in the number of opioid overdoses since 2000. The *Morbidity and Mortality Weekly Report* from the CDC noted that in 2014, approximately 1.5 times more drug overdose deaths occurred in the United States than deaths from motor vehicle collisions. Prescription opioids and heroin are the primary drugs associated with these overdose deaths.[20] The medical community has responded to these alarming statistics with changes regarding the use of opioid medications. In 2016, the FDA published a special report which outlined a multifaceted approach to help combat this epidemic. The FDA's approach works to address the issues of individual needs and societal risks. It creates clear guidelines for opioid use, addresses the lack of nonopioid alternatives for pain management, addresses guidelines for writing opioid prescriptions, and creates a better evidence base to guide the use of opioid medications.[21]

In recent years, the FDA has approved an auto-injector device that delivers an IM or subcutaneous injection of naloxone (Narcan) to reverse opioid overdose. The FDA has also approved intranasal devices, allowing for rapid administration to treat overdose. Local pharmacies may sell naloxone to people with or without a prescription. Law enforcement officers may administer naloxone prior to EMS arrival. Always ask whether naloxone has been administered by family members, bystanders, or other responders. Expanded access to naloxone is one approach to deal with the deadly opioid epidemic.

As a paramedic, what role do you play in this epidemic? The rapid recognition of opioid overdose followed by appropriate treatment is critical. Patient education and the identification of those who are at high risk for abusing opioids is important. This risk of addiction or abuse should not, however, influence your decision to treat acute pain in the prehospital environment. A significant portion of the opioid abuse epidemic is caused by abuse of prescription pain medication. For the treatment of severe pain in an emergency situation, opioid administration is currently the most common option in the field. However, many EMS agencies have developed protocols using ketamine (a non-opioid) for the treatment of severe pain.

Never forget the basics in terms of splinting, positioning, and supportive care, but do not withhold opioid pain medication due to concerns about making the patient susceptible to addiction. Consider your options when choosing how to treat a patient's pain. Does the patient have a stubbed toe that may be best treated with an ice pack? Or, does the patient have an open femur fracture with severe pain? Conduct a thorough exam and attempt to relieve the pain with basic maneuvers before considering opioid administration.

Pathophysiology

Opioids produce major effects on the CNS by binding with three main opioid receptor sites: delta, kappa, and mu. These receptor sites can produce analgesia and a euphoric sensation. The highest concentrations of receptor sites are found in the limbic system, frontal and temporal cortices, thalamus, hypothalamus, midbrain, and spinal cord.

Opioids can be ingested, insufflated, inhaled, and injected. As with other substances, the route of absorption will help determine the speed of onset and duration of effect. When taken orally, the effects of these drugs are lessened owing to their significant first-pass metabolism through the liver compared with their effects when given parenterally. Opioids can also be absorbed through the skin via transdermal patches. It is important to remember that a dose of naloxone may not permanently reverse the effects of the opioid, and the patient may lapse into unconsciousness due to the shorter half-life of the naloxone.

Morphine and fentanyl are two commonly used analgesics in the prehospital setting. Fentanyl is a far more potent drug than morphine. This potency does not mean that fentanyl is a stronger or better medication; it simply takes less of the medication to create a therapeutic effect. Morphine has some vasodilatory properties due to histamine release, and fentanyl has a shorter half-life. Based on the clinical situation, one of these medications may be more appropriate for the patient than the other.

Assessment

The classic presentation of opioid use features euphoria, hypotension, respiratory depression, and pinpoint pupils. Depending on the particular agent, nausea, vomiting, and constipation may occur as well. With increased doses, coma, seizures (usually secondary to hypoxia), and cardiac arrest (usually secondary to respiratory arrest) are common.

Morphine and heroin produce a dreamlike state. Shortly after injecting heroin, a user will appear to pass out. However, the user is typically lucid and remains acutely aware of what is being done or said even though he or she appears to have dozed off.

Patient Safety

Remember the importance of a rapid full-body scan on patients who have overdosed on opioids. Recall that people may use multiple routes of administration when abusing opioids. In particular, look for transdermal patches. Missing a fentanyl patch that was covered by clothing could lead to the patient lapsing back into respiratory arrest. If you have not found and removed the patch, then you may not be successful in treating the life-threatening overdose.

Management

Because of the CNS depressant effects, patient management initially focuses on establishing and maintaining a patent airway and providing adequate ventilation. A patient who has overdosed on opioids is almost always hypoventilating with slow and shallow respirations. Hypoventilation will create increased carbon dioxide retention (hypercapnia) and respiratory acidosis. Rather than moving immediately to intubation, place a nasopharyngeal or oropharyngeal airway and provide bag-mask ventilation with 15 L/min of supplemental oxygen.

Next, establish vascular access and administer 0.4 to 2 mg of naloxone. Remember that naloxone is given to improve the patient's spontaneous respiratory effort. You can titrate IV naloxone to improve the respiratory status without bringing the patient back to a fully conscious and alert state. Adverse effects of rapid naloxone administration include projectile vomiting and potential agitation associated with the patient regaining consciousness. IM naloxone is a valid option for administration if IV access is unavailable. Intranasal naloxone may be given; divide administration of the dose equally between the nostrils to a maximum of 1 mL of solution per nostril.

Sometimes the patient may not respond to the initial dose of naloxone, and may remain unconscious. It is possible that the patient is under the influence of a very potent and/or large dose of the opioid. Follow local protocols or consider contacting medical control if you believe the patient may require higher doses of naloxone. Alternatively, the coma may be from another source altogether, such as a cerebrovascular accident or an overdose caused by polypharmacy. In either scenario, you should insert an advanced airway, provide supportive care as needed, and transport the patient to an appropriate facility.

Because of the nature of opioid overdose, you may find the patient in cardiac arrest in your primary survey. Structure your resuscitation around high-quality chest compressions and providing ventilations at the proper rate. Early administration of naloxone is indicated if you have a high index of suspicion that opioid poisoning may have precipitated the cardiac arrest **Figure 27-11**.

▶ Cardiac Medications

Pathophysiology

Cardiac medications can be beneficial to patients with chronic cardiovascular disorders involving blood pressure, heart rate, or dysrhythmias. As a paramedic, you also have the ability to treat life-threatening events with appropriate doses of these medications. However, these medications can produce severe effects on the body when they reach toxic levels. The major classes of cardiac drugs include antidysrhythmics, beta-blockers, calcium channel blockers, cardiac glycosides, and angiotensin-converting enzyme inhibitors. These medications are classified using the Vaughan-Williams system. Medications that have similar mechanisms of action are grouped as Class I, Class II, Class III, or Class IV, as discussed in Chapter 13, *Principles of Pharmacology*.

Overdoses of cardiac medications are usually unintentional. For example, an older adult may forget that he or she has already taken the daily dose and may take a second dose. A patient who is starting a new medication for heart rate control may not know he or she already takes two similar medications. Both scenarios may result in toxic levels of the medications. A single pill or tablet of many of these cardiac medications can cause serious effects or death in small children and infants who unintentionally ingest them.

Assessment and Management

Because of the wide variety of presentations associated with the different classes of antidysrhythmics, use the patient's history and list of medications to help guide you in identifying what substances are involved in the overdose. Identification is key because many standard treatments may be ineffective due to the toxic levels of the medication. Work to minimize the negative effects of the overdose while determining if an antidote is available. As with all emergencies, ensure a patent airway, provide adequate ventilation, and administer high-flow supplemental oxygen.

With most cardiac medications, you should contact poison control or medical control early in your management of the patient. You may receive an order from medical control to administer activated charcoal without sorbitol at a dose of 1 g/kg if the patient is within the first hour of ingestion. If you are able to identify that an extended release medication has been ingested, then this information may create additional consideration for activated charcoal. Do not administer activated charcoal if the patient is at risk for a rapidly declining mental status.

For sodium channel blocker toxicity, overdoses can cause QRS prolongation, QT prolongation, hypotension secondary to depressed myocardial contractility, and ventricular dysrhythmias. You may consider atropine sulfate for the bradycardic patient who is symptomatic. In certain instances, you may use IV sodium bicarbonate

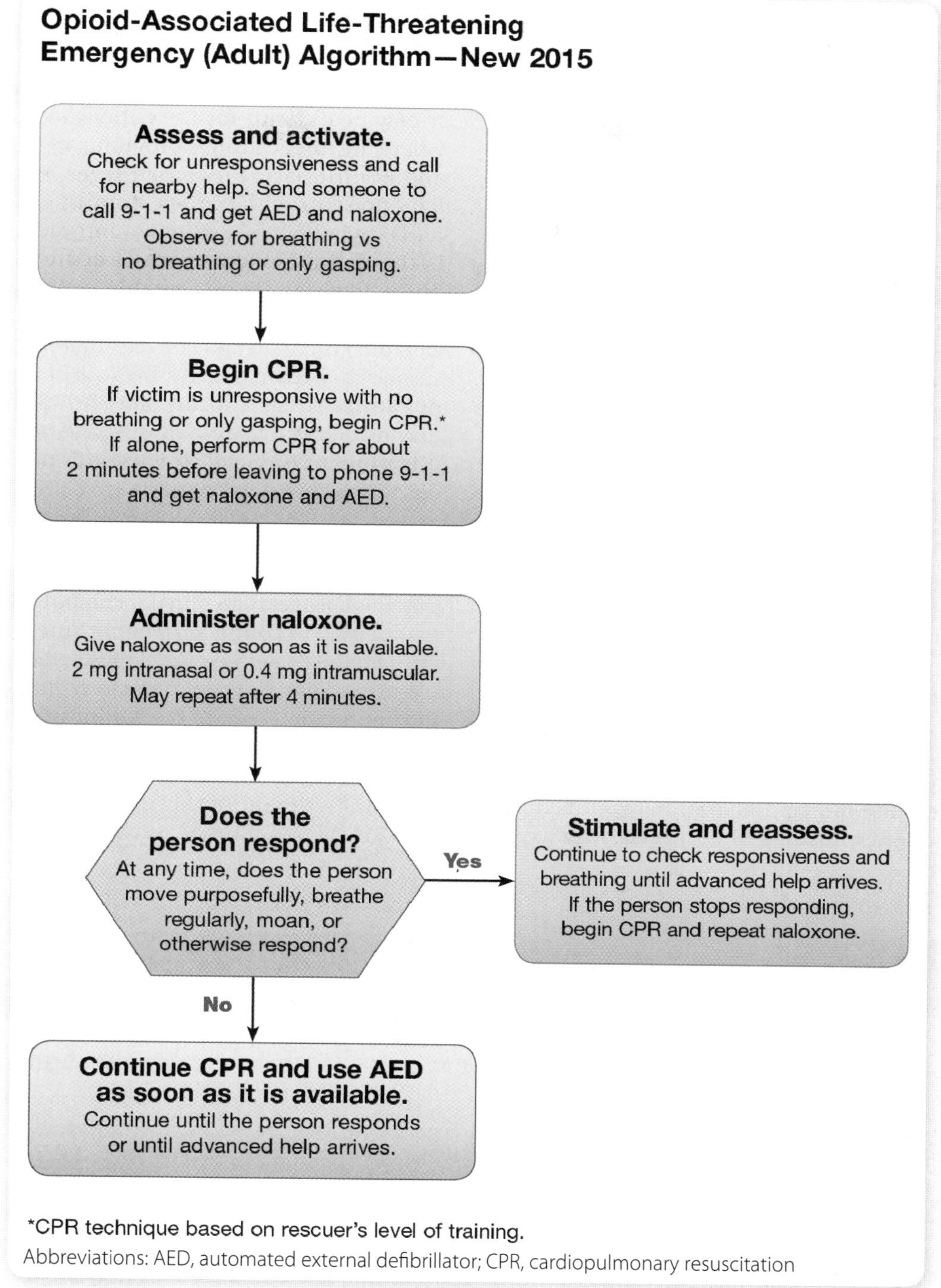

Figure 27-11 The American Heart Association's algorithm for life-threatening opioid overdose.

to treat slowed impulse conduction (widening QRS), bradycardia, and hypotension by reversing the inhibition of fast sodium channels within cardiac cells.

Patients with beta-adrenergic blocker toxicity typically present with hypotension, bradycardia, or related symptoms such as lethargy, weakness, shortness of breath, and possible seizures. Hypoglycemia can also occur following an overdose of beta-adrenergic blocking medications, especially in pediatric patients. Bronchospasm is possible following beta-adrenergic blocker overdose in patients with reactive airway disease.

Consider atropine sulfate for symptomatic bradycardia, but it may only be useful in mild overdoses. Consider fluid boluses for hypotension. IV glucagon is the antidote to beta-adrenergic blocker toxicity. Administer 1 mg of IV glucagon every 5 minutes. The patient may not respond until at least 6 mg have been given. The ED may administer a glucagon infusion after the bolus has been initiated. This infusion usually requires more glucagon than is generally available on most ALS ambulances. Utilize normal saline or sterile water to reconstitute the glucagon, minimizing the risk of phenol toxicity. Additionally, be aware of the risk of increased vomiting from the glucagon administration. You can mitigate this risk by lowering the dose, lengthening the time of administration, or administering antiemetics. Vasopressor infusions (norepinephrine or dopamine) after adequate fluid resuscitation and cardiac pacing may be required in severe overdose situations. If the patient experiences seizure activity, then midazolam is the medication of choice.

Acute toxicity from potassium channel blockers may present as hypotension, bradycardia, or certain ventricular dysrhythmias. One of the predominant effects observed on the ECG is a prolonged QT interval. The treatment of acute potassium channel blocker toxicity is primarily supportive, although you may use IV magnesium sulfate to treat torsades de pointes.

Calcium channel blocker toxicity causes a decrease in pulse rate, decreased AV nodal conduction, decreased myocardial contractility, and vasodilation. Calcium channel blockers may also cause nausea and vomiting, altered mental status, and metabolic acidosis. IV calcium chloride or calcium gluconate is the initial treatment of calcium channel blocker toxicity. IV glucagon may improve both the pulse rate and myocardial contractility. Standard crystalloid infusions of 20 mL/kg may assist with hypotension. Recommended vasopressors after fluid resuscitation include norepinephrine and dopamine.

Cardiac glycosides (such as digoxin) are particularly problematic to maintain within a therapeutic range. It may be difficult for the patient to remain at a level where the medication is providing its therapeutic effect and not increasing to a toxic level. Acute digoxin toxicity presents with nausea, vomiting, GI distress, and lethal hyperkalemia. Digoxin immune fab (Digibind) is the definitive treatment of acute digoxin toxicity, but is likely to be unavailable in the prehospital environment. Supportive care and the consideration of calcium gluconate may be reasonable in a patient with suspected digoxin toxicity. Because of the sophistication of cardiac drugs and the likelihood that the patient may be taking multiple cardiac and other medications, it is prudent to make contact with medical control to consult with a physician.

▶ Organophosphates

Organophosphates are a major component in many insecticides used in commercial agriculture and in the home. Organophosphates were developed in the early 1900s when German scientists were trying to reduce dependence on the importation of food by creating new insecticides. The people exposed to these insecticides experienced serious adverse effects, and the role of organophosphates as a chemical weapon quickly arose. Organophosphates fit into the classification of acetylcholinesterase inhibitors.

YOU are the Paramedic — PART 4

You place the patient on the cardiac monitor and you see a rhythm of sinus tachycardia. You wonder whether any other drugs could be present in the patient's system, so you ask the family to search the bathroom again. As you place a constricting band on the patient's arm to assess for a site to initiate IV access, you feel something underneath the patient's shirt. You log roll the patient to discover that her entire back is covered with fentanyl patches.

Recording Time: 10 Minutes	
Respirations	Assisted
Pulse	100 beats/min
Skin	Cyanosis is resolving
Blood pressure	98/56 mm Hg
Oxygen saturation (Spo_2)	96% (assisted with bag-mask device and 100% oxygen)
Pupils	Pinpoint and nonreactive

7. What is your medication choice and dosage to treat this patient?
8. What should you do if this medication does not correct the overdose?

This classification also includes acephate (Orthene), diazinon (Spectracide), malathion (Cythion), carbamates, and nerve agents (sarin, soman, V agent).

Suicide attempts account for a considerable share of organophosphate poisonings, with ingestions accounting for the majority of these exposures.[22] Unintentional agricultural exposure is another common cause of organophosphate poisoning, and people involved in the manufacture of organophosphates and similar compounds are also at risk. For example, farmers who distribute or transport pesticides may be exposed to a large amount of organophosphates very quickly and sustain an acute exposure, or they could be exposed to a small amount over days or weeks and build up a toxic level over time.

Pathophysiology

Organophosphates exert toxic effects at junctions (synapses) of the nerve cells of the autonomic nervous system. The conduction of an impulse from one nerve to another occurs through the release of acetylcholine (ACh) at the synapse. ACh works as a chemical messenger, crossing the synapse to depolarize the nerve on the other side of the junction. Organophosphates and carbamates are potent inhibitors of acetylcholinesterase, which serves to terminate synaptic transmissions. This termination creates an abundance of ACh in the CNS and peripheral nervous system. When the muscarinic and nicotinic receptors are overstimulated, a predictable response occurs in the body.

The symptoms of organophosphate poisoning are fundamentally the same, regardless of whether the poison was ingested, inhaled, or absorbed. Patients who have ingested an organophosphate may have a delayed onset of the symptoms, whereas vapor exposure will cause nearly immediate symptoms. The predictable response is the basis for the toxidrome represented by the mnemonic DUMBELS **Table 27-4**. In patients with moderate to severe organophosphate poisoning, the following symptoms may also be present: muscle fasciculations, severe respiratory distress, seizures, and flaccid paralysis.

Table 27-4 The DUMBELS Mnemonic

- Diarrhea
- Urination
- Miosis (constriction of the pupils), muscle weakness
- Bradycardia, bronchospasm, bronchorrhea (discharge of mucus from the lungs)
- Emesis (vomiting)
- Lacrimation (excessive tearing of the eyes)
- Seizures, salivation, sweating

Assessment and Management

The first component to patient assessment and management is decontamination, which is likely performed by a hazmat crew according to local protocol. If possible, position the non-ambulatory patient in a lateral recumbent position to allow for passive drainage of oral secretions, and help prevent unintentional aspiration. After proper decontamination, the patient may be assessed. Consider the following measures for a patient with organophosphate poisoning:

- Establish and maintain the airway. Consider an advanced airway as needed.
- Suction as needed.
- Administer high-flow oxygen to maintain saturation levels of greater than 94%.
- Establish vascular access (IV or IO), if possible without delay.
- Administer 1.0 mg atropine IV/IO push or by auto-injector, and repeat the dose every 3 to 5 minutes until easing of ventilation and reduction of secretions (atropinization) occurs.
- Administer up to three pralidoxime (2-PAM) auto-injectors (600 mg/each) in the first hour. Multiple doses may be required for patients with severe exposure.
- Apply the ECG monitor, pulse oximeter, and capnometer.
- Notify the receiving hospital early, and transport to the appropriate facility.

Atropine is the primary antidote for acetylcholinesterase inhibitor poisoning. Liberally administer repeat doses to symptomatic patients. Relief of bronchospasm and lessening of bronchorrhea indicate clinical improvement. Do not rely on the patient's pupillary response or heart rate to determine the clinical end point of atropine administration. The patient's heart rate may be low, normal, or elevated during the exposure. Treat seizures with benzodiazepines at appropriate dosages. Intranasal midazolam may be a preferred route of administration; however, extensive nasal discharge may hinder its absorption.

▶ Carbon Monoxide

As mentioned previously, CO is one of the most common fatal poisonings. CO is produced during the incomplete combustion of organic fuels, such as in a motor vehicle engine or a home-heating device. CO poisoning may occur more frequently in colder climates as a result of the use of gas-powered heaters in poorly ventilated areas.[23] A motor vehicle running in a closed garage can quickly generate a lethal concentration of CO, making CO inhalation a common method of suicide. For these patients, remember that suicidal people often take other substances (alcohol, pills, etc) prior to attempted CO poisoning. CO is also a major contributor to death in house fires.

Pathophysiology

CO is a colorless, odorless, tasteless gas, so people exposed to this toxin have no idea that they are inhaling a toxic substance until it is too late. CO displaces oxygen from the hemoglobin molecule in red blood cells because of its greater affinity for binding to hemoglobin. Even relatively small concentrations of CO in the atmosphere can convert a significant proportion of hemoglobin into carboxyhemoglobin (COHb)—hemoglobin combined with CO—making it ineffective as an oxygen carrier.

Any increase in the body's metabolic or oxygen demands, such as fever, tachycardia, or exertion, will increase the severity of the poisoning. Children, whose metabolic rates are intrinsically higher than those of adults, tend to have more severe symptoms at any given level of exposure. According to one study that assessed data from 1999 to 2012, approximately 439 deaths occur each year from unintentional, non–fire-related CO poisoning.[24]

Assessment

CO poisoning can be difficult to diagnose in the field. Consider the patient's environment. Was adequate ventilation available? Was a source of combustion present (eg, gasoline engines)? The signs and symptoms of CO poisoning are highly variable and vague, often resembling early onset of the flu—for example, headache, nausea, and vomiting. With acute CO poisoning, the patient may experience headache, fatigue, nausea, tachypnea, tachycardia, and confusion. The cherry red color that can be seen in light-skinned people is a late sign of CO poisoning—that is, seen in the morgue.

Given the difficulty in detection, many EMS organizations have placed CO detectors on portable equipment carried into emergency scenes to alert the crew of the hazard.

Words of Wisdom

CO can be hazardous to responders. If you have multiple patients from the same residence who are sick, then warning bells should be going off in your head. Consider evacuating everyone to a safe location. Allow fire department personnel equipped with self-contained breathing apparatus to check the air quality of that location.

Recent developments in technology have given paramedics the ability to perform noninvasive identification of CO poisoning (SpCO) in the field (similar to pulse oximetry), which helps address the problem of delayed diagnosis. A high reading on a CO oximeter may help confirm suspicions of CO poisoning; however, do not allow a low reading to exclude CO poisoning from your differential diagnosis. Research is still ongoing to determine the correlation between CO oximeter readings and COHb values in a blood sample.

Note that pulse oximetry will not provide a true assessment of arterial oxygenation under these circumstances because the device cannot determine whether it is CO or oxygen that is bound to the hemoglobin. Therefore, do not trust an SpO_2 level of 99% in a symptomatic patient suspected of CO poisoning.

Management

Treatment of CO poisoning in the field is aimed at providing the highest concentration of oxygen possible to attempt to displace CO molecules from the hemoglobin. For patients with mild symptoms, such as headache, nausea, and flulike symptoms, the elimination half-life of COHb is roughly 4 hours. By comparison, if the patient is breathing 100% oxygen, then the half-time can be reduced to about 1.5 hours. Hyperbaric oxygen therapy at 2.5 atmospheres of pressure can further reduce the elimination time to 15 to 20 minutes. Note that pregnant women suspected of CO poisoning may be more likely to receive hyperbaric oxygen therapy due to difficulties with estimating fetal levels of COHb.

If you suspect CO poisoning, then take the following actions:

- Remove the patient from the exposure environment.
- Establish and maintain the airway, inserting an advanced airway as needed.
- Administer high-flow supplemental oxygen by a tight-fitting nonrebreathing mask.
- Establish vascular access.
- Keep the patient calm and at rest to minimize oxygen demand.
- Monitor the ECG rhythm and level of consciousness.
- Transport to the appropriate facility. If the patient is unresponsive or has signs of serious CO poisoning, then direct transport to a facility capable of providing hyperbaric medicine is preferred.
- For patients with injuries or illness from a structural or vehicular fire, consider the possibility of combined CO/cyanide poisoning, especially if the patient has signs of shock or altered mental status. Contact medical control for an order to administer hydroxocobalamin or sodium thiosulfate, if available.

CO poisoning can be reversed if it is diagnosed and treated in time. You can have a significant impact on the patient's recovery with early recognition and early intervention. However, even if the patient recovers, acute CO poisoning may result in permanent damage to vital organs and lead to mild to severe neurologic deficits.

▶ Chlorine Gas

Incidents involving chlorine gas are relatively common because of the widespread use of chlorine compounds in the home and occupational settings. Household exposures can occur when someone mixes a cleaning agent containing sodium hypochlorite (such as bleach) with a strong acid or with ammonia in an overzealous attempt at cleaning or disinfecting. The resulting chemical reaction releases chlorine gas, often in concentrations high enough to be toxic. Household ingestions can occur if chlorine-containing solutions are kept in unlabeled containers. Most cases of chlorine gas exposure occur outside the home, however. Acute exposures are often caused by faulty industrial valves or pumps that dump large amounts of gas into the environment, possibly exposing many people. Leakage of chlorine gas from an industrial storage tank, truck, or rail car can also result in a mass-casualty incident.

Pathophysiology

The signs and symptoms of chlorine gas exposure depend on the concentration of the inhaled gas and the duration of exposure. Chlorine gas is extremely irritating to all mucous membranes. When it comes in contact with the moisture on those surfaces, it can form hydrochloric acid and other substances that are damaging to human tissue. With a minor exposure, the patient will experience burning sensations in the eyes, nose, and throat along with a slight cough. More intense exposure to chlorine gas causes chest tightness, choking, paroxysmal cough, headache, nausea and vomiting, and diffuse wheezing. Patients with more severe exposures may also develop cyanosis, pulmonary edema shock, seizures, and loss of consciousness.

Assessment and Management

When you treat patients who have been exposed to chlorine gas, your first priority is to remove them from the area of exposure. Take the same precautions that would apply in a hazmat situation when you choose where to position your vehicle and what PPE is needed.

After you have moved the patients to a safe environment, quickly triage the patients (triage is discussed in Chapter 47, *Incident Management and Mass-Casualty Incidents*). Irrigate burning or itching eyes with water, as well as any areas of the skin that have come in contact with the chlorine gas. People with dyspnea, wheezing, severe cough, or other signs of respiratory distress are priority patients and should ideally receive high-concentration, humidified oxygen by mask. Nebulized bronchodilators (ie, albuterol) may ease wheezing. Patients with a significant exposure may develop noncardiogenic pulmonary edema. The use of continuous positive airway pressure/bilevel positive airway pressure may benefit these patients. The administration of approximately 4% nebulized sodium bicarbonate solution (2 mL 8.4% $NaHCO_3^+$ and 2 mL sterile water) may be ordered in confirmed symptomatic chlorine exposures and can provide symptomatic relief. Also consider intubation and rapid sequence intubation (RSI) for patients who are fatigued and can no longer compensate. If patients are exposed to very high concentrations of chlorine gas, then laryngospasm and edema may also complicate your airway management. As in all poisonings, the effects and onsets are dose dependent.

▶ Cyanide

Cyanide is a chemical substance that is a byproduct of the combustion of synthetic materials that contain carbon and nitrogen. The combustion of household goods—insulation, carpeting, upholstery, plastic, and synthetic rubber—can release a significant amount of cyanide. In gaseous form (hydrogen cyanide), it is often colorless with occasional reports of a "bitter almond" scent. Cyanide may also be found in chemicals used in manufacturing plastic, paper, and textiles and also in the process of electroplating. Some plants and seeds contain cyanide in small amounts. Cyanide poisoning has been used as a method of execution, genocide, and suicide.

Pathophysiology

Cyanide is one of the most rapid-acting and deadly poisons. It is considered a mitochondrial toxin that does its damage by combining with a crucial cellular enzyme, cytochrome oxidase, which in turn blocks the utilization of oxygen at the cellular level. Cellular hypoxia can rapidly develop throughout the body, causing cardiovascular collapse and death.

Assessment

Depending on its form, cyanide can enter the body through inhalation, ingestion, or absorption through the skin. Physical exam of a patient who has been poisoned with cyanide may reveal an altered mental status. If awake enough to answer questions, then the patient may report a headache, nausea, vomiting, anxiety, vertigo, weakness, and dyspnea. Patients who have either inhaled or ingested cyanide may have the most dramatic presentations, with rapid decompensation toward either respiratory or cardiac arrest. Respirations are usually rapid and labored early on; as the poisoning progresses, respirations become slow and gasping. The patient may have an elevated blood pressure, initially followed by profound hypotension. The pulse is usually rapid and thready. The patient's venous blood and sometimes the patient's body may be bright red—even though oxygen is available in the bloodstream, it is not being taken up by the tissues. Cyanide impairs the body's ability to properly offload the oxygen molecules at a cellular level, which means the pulse oximeter reading may be high despite true hypoxia at a cellular level.

Management

Cyanide poisoning may be unusual to encounter on the streets, but it is a dire emergency. You must initiate treatment as fast as possible, involving the administration of 100% oxygen via nonrebreathing mask or bag-mask-assisted ventilations. The aim of treatment is to displace the cyanide from the cytochrome oxidase by introducing another chemical that will "attract" the cyanide and bind to it. Several medications may be considered; check with your local service to see what is available on the ambulance or in any specially equipped hazmat response vehicles.

One of the most common treatments is amyl nitrite. Commercial kits containing amyl nitrite may be available depending on your service. Take a gauze pad soaked in amyl nitrite and hold it over the patient's nose for about 20 seconds, and then remove it to allow the patient to breathe high-concentration oxygen for about 40 seconds. Keep switching between the amyl nitrite and the oxygen while maintaining this ratio. While you are administering the amyl nitrite, your partner should establish vascular access. (Note that amyl nitrite is not recommended for use in conjunction with CO poisoning.)

Anticipate hypotension as a consequence of amyl nitrite therapy, and keep the patient supine with the legs elevated. If the systolic blood pressure falls below 80 mm Hg, then consult medical control about whether to administer an IV vasopressor. Monitor the ECG rhythm carefully. Notify the receiving hospital of the probable diagnosis so that staff can begin preparation of sodium thiosulfate. Transport the patient without delay to an appropriate facility.

Sodium nitrite is another medication to consider for cyanide poisoning. If you do not suspect CO poisoning, then administer a dose of 300 mg IV over 2 to 4 minutes.

Words of Wisdom

The most important aspect of treatment in toxic inhalations is to remove the patient from the toxic environment. You cannot help the patient if you become ill yourself, so always ensure the rescue is performed by someone using an appropriate self-contained breathing apparatus.

Hydroxocobalamin. One of the most common treatments for cyanide poisoning is the administration of hydroxocobalamin, a member of the vitamin B_{12} family. Consider hydroxocobalamin, if available, for patients who are hypotensive, have an altered mental status, or are in cardiac arrest after being removed from a house fire. Some EMS agency kits with hydroxocobalamin are available, and they include blood tubes to obtain a sample (if feasible). Hydroxocobalamin is known to skew laboratory findings, so obtain the blood sample before administering the drug. An adult dose of 5 g IV/IO may be given over 15 minutes. Consider contacting medical control for guidance on additional dosing.

Hydroxocobalamin is considered a relatively safe antidote, with allergy/anaphylaxis as the primary concern. Patients will also experience some temporary effects such as redness of the skin, eyes, and urine, as well as itching after hydroxocobalamin administration.

Methylene Blue. Methylene blue is an antidote used to treat methemoglobinemia (an alteration of the structure of hemoglobin) that may occur during the treatment of cyanide poisoning with sodium nitrite. In patients with severe cyanide poisoning, methemoglobinemia is induced by the administration of amyl nitrite and sodium nitrite. In mild cases of cyanide poisoning, methemoglobinemia may cause its own severe or fatal toxicity and should be avoided. Methylene blue is typically administered in acute health care settings under the guidance of expert consultation. You may transport patients who have received methylene blue as treatment of methemoglobinemia as a result of treatment of cyanide poisoning, or from another unrelated cause.

▶ Caustics

Caustics include strong acids ($pH < 2.0$) and strong alkalis ($pH > 12.0$). Both types of chemicals are commonly used in industry, agriculture (anhydrous ammonia), and the home as cleaning agents Table 27-5 and

Table 27-5 Common Caustic Substances

Substance	Example	Source
Acids	Hydrochloric acid	Toilet bowl cleaners, swimming pool cleaners
	Sulfuric acid	Battery acid, toilet bowl cleaners (such as bisulfate)
	Others	Bleach disinfectants, slate cleaners
Alkalis	Lye (sodium or potassium hydroxide)	Paint removers, washing powders, drain cleaners (such as Drano, Liquid-Plumr, Plunge), button-shaped batteries, Clinitest tablets
	Sodium hypochlorite	Bleach (Clorox)
	Sodium carbonate	Bleach (Purex), nonphosphate detergents
	Ammonia	Hair dyes, jewelry cleaners, metal cleaners or polishes, antirust agents
	Potassium permanganate	Electric dishwasher detergents

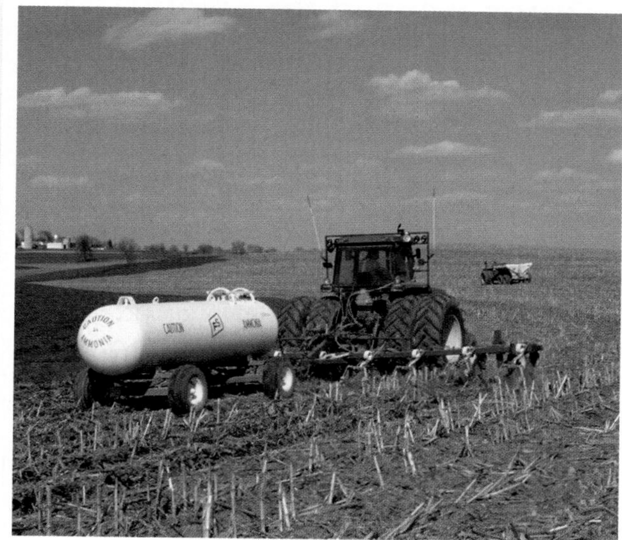

A

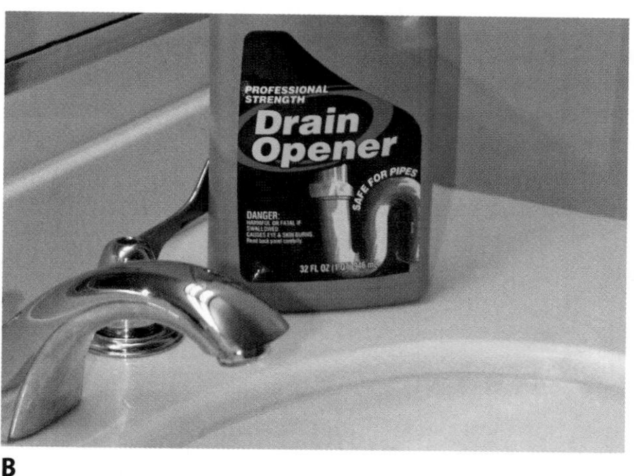

B

Figure 27-12 Caustic chemicals are commonly used in industry. **A.** Anhydrous ammonia tank used in agriculture. **B.** Plumbing agents used in the home.

Figure 27-12. According to the 2014 Annual Report of the AAPCC's National Poison Data System, over 118,000 exposures involving cleaning agents occurred in pediatric patients and over 64,000 exposures occurred in adults.[25] As mentioned previously in this chapter, pediatric ingestions are generally unintentional. If the patient is an adult, then oral ingestion of caustics is usually an intentional suicide attempt.

Pathophysiology

Caustic substances cause direct chemical injury to the tissues they contact. Acids cause coagulation necrosis. Normally, a layer of eschar (leathery scar tissue) forms and contains the damaged tissue. Alkalis cause liquefaction necrosis, a breakdown of tissue to pus and the liquid contents of the involved cells. Dilution or neutralization is usually required to slow or stop the damage process. Signs and symptoms of a caustic exposure include drooling, burns, difficulty talking or swallowing (with oral ingestions), and hypoperfusion or shock (rarely, usually secondary to internal bleeding).

In the home, caustic liquids may start to leak from the original containers and the homeowner may choose to store the product in a plastic soda bottle, or to keep small amount in an open plastic cup while using it. These practices increase the likelihood that someone may unintentionally drink from the container and ingest a caustic substance. As the liquid enters the mouth and begins to burn, the patient may simultaneously remove the bottle and turn the head, resulting in burns to the mouth, tongue, face, and neck.

As noted earlier, the intentional mixing of different household chemicals may also result in the release of toxic vapors (ie, chlorine, chloramine).

Assessment and Management

Most patients who have swallowed caustic substances present with severe pain in the mouth, throat, or chest. Respiratory distress, if present, is most probably due to soft-tissue swelling in the larynx, epiglottis, or vocal cords, which means that the patient is in immediate danger of complete airway obstruction. Identify the specific substance and call the poison center or contact online medical control. For a caustic ingestion, dilution with milk or water is only useful in the minutes immediately following the exposure. Gastric tube placement is contraindicated because it can cause further damage to tissue. Establish vascular access, usually en route, because prompt transport to the ED is indicated.

Words of Wisdom

If a patient who swallowed a caustic agent is in respiratory distress, then provide prompt transport to the hospital. Coughing, tachypnea, and stridor are ominous signs. Significant hypopharyngeal edema may develop and require consideration of a surgical airway.

With dermal exposure to a strong acid, the result is immediate and excruciating pain. For a strong alkali, the onset of pain is somewhat delayed, allowing more time before the patient reacts and increasing the severity of the burn. In such an injury, diluting and flushing away the caustic substance is the main goal of field treatment. Acids tend to be more water-soluble than alkalis, so they can often be diluted relatively quickly. With alkalis, it is more important to keep water continually flowing because it usually takes much longer to rinse away the substance.

Words of Wisdom

Some chemicals react vigorously with water, so be sure to check the relevant warnings or placard for information. When you decontaminate a patient with water, do your best to avoid secondary exposures to surrounding tissues while the substances are washed from the primary point of contact.

For an eye exposure, cut off the prong section of a nasal cannula, place it on the bridge of the patient's nose, plug in a macrodrip IV administration set, and run it wide open to provide continuous irrigation. This practice also frees you up to perform other tasks. You may also use a Morgan lens after the initial gross flushing has been accomplished. Use of a Morgan lens is covered in Chapter 19, *Diseases of the Eyes, Ears, Nose, and Throat*.

One of the most common caustic exposures in the agricultural setting involves anhydrous ammonia. The exposure usually occurs during the hook-up or disconnection of a tank. Eye exposure to anhydrous ammonia can cause devastating damage in less than a minute, resulting in cataracts or blindness. Inhalation exposure can create respiratory distress secondary to pulmonary edema. After the patient has been appropriately decontaminated, start appropriate airway management and supportive care.

Keep the following points in mind for patients with caustic ingestions:

- *Do not* give any "neutralizing substances" orally. Now-outdated recommendations incorrectly advised the administration of an acid after an alkali ingestion, or vice versa. Mixing an acid and an alkali may produce an *exothermic reaction*, adding a thermal injury to the chemical injury.
- *Do not* induce vomiting. Re-exposure with a caustic substance will worsen the damage.
- *Do not* perform gastric lavage.
- *Do not* give activated charcoal. It is ineffective in acid or alkali ingestion, and it may interfere with the patient's subsequent medical care by blackening the field of vision when an endoscope is used to inspect the esophagus and stomach for damage.

▶ Common Household Items

From a toxicologic perspective, the average home is full of dangerous substances—from colorful plants to sweet-smelling cleaning products. Identification of the substance involved is the most important part of the history of the ingestion. It is not possible within the scope of this chapter to discuss all of the possibilities when it comes to household poisonings. As always, keep in mind that the poison center is an invaluable resource.

▶ Drugs Abused for Sexual Purposes

Drugs that are abused for sexual purposes include those that increase sexual gratification and those that are used to facilitate sexual assault.

Drugs That Increase Sexual Gratification

Phosphodiesterase type 5 (PDE5) inhibitors (ie, sildenafil, tadalafil, and vardenafil) are among the most commonly prescribed drugs used to treat erectile dysfunction. Unintentional toxic levels are usually the result of aggressive dosing to achieve maximum sexual performance. Occasionally, the patient may have unknowingly received a dose of a PDE5 inhibitor as a prank. Elevated levels may produce hypotension, tachycardia, ischemic chest pain, tachydysrhythmias, and prolonged priapism requiring urologic evaluation. Supportive care is usually all that is required for overdose of PDE5 inhibitors. If you are treating a patient with acute coronary syndrome, then avoid nitrates because they may cause significant hypotension.

Cocaine and other stimulant drugs (such as amphetamines and methamphetamine) are popular choices for people seeking a more intense sexual experience. Treatment is identical to the treatment detailed earlier in this chapter regarding stimulant abuse. Be aware that the stimulant may have been laced with another drug to intensify the patient's response.

Another drug that increases sexual gratification is amyl nitrite (also known as poppers, rush, and happy snaps). This organic nitrate drug can be crushed and inhaled to produce an intense sexual experience. As mentioned earlier, use may cause methemoglobinemia, affecting the oxygen-carrying ability of blood, and result in the associated ischemic effects. As with any nitrate, hypotension may result from blood pooling in the periphery owing to the vasodilatory effects of the drug.

One of the most unique drugs in this group is MDMA (Ecstasy, Adam), as mentioned earlier in the section on stimulants. MDMA is an analog of methamphetamine, and it may have similar toxic effects on a smaller scale. The release of serotonin, a sensation of euphoria, and disinhibition are the effects associated with its use to enhance a person's sexual experience. More significant adverse effects (such as hyperthermia) and electrolyte abnormalities (such as hyponatremia) may also result. Supportive care is appropriate during transport.

Dextromethorphan (DXM), which is found in several OTC cough suppressants, can produce a euphoric floating sensation or out-of-body experience. Structurally related to codeine, DXM produces a mild stimulant effect that may enhance a sexual experience. Consuming large quantities of DXM can lead to hallucinations, psychedelic visions, loss of motor control, confusion, blurred vision, dreamlike euphoria, and out-of-body sensations.

Drugs Used to Facilitate Sexual Assault

Drugs used to facilitate sexual assault are often administered to an unsuspecting person, frequently dissolved in an alcoholic drink. Sexual predators use these substances to incapacitate others, which explains why they are called "date rape" drugs. They are discussed further in Chapter 22, *Gynecologic Emergencies*.

GHB. Gamma-hydroxybutyrate (GHB) is an endogenous metabolite of gamma-aminobutyric acid that causes intoxication similar to alcohol use. In the late 1980s, GHB gained popularity with young people as a club drug, earning the name "Liquid Ecstasy" from its euphoric effects at raves (all-night dance parties). By the mid 1990s, GHB became increasingly associated with sexual assaults. In 1990, the FDA banned this drug from OTC sales.

GHB is a colorless and odorless liquid that may go undetected when placed in a drink. Once ingested, GHB quickly crosses the blood-brain barrier, exerting its effects within 30 to 60 minutes. Ingestion may produce disinhibition, severe passivity (that is, a lack of the will to resist), and antegrade amnesia. Associated use with alcohol increases the risk of respiratory depression, coma, and death. GHB also has a withdrawal presentation similar to that of alcohol or benzodiazepine use.[26]

Treatment of GHB intoxication focuses on supportive care. The patient may be unable to protect the airway. First, establish and maintain the airway, inserting an advanced airway as needed. Monitor oxygenation and ventilation. Administer supplemental oxygen as needed. Establish vascular access. Apply the ECG monitor, pulse oximeter, and capnometer. Finally, provide rapid transport to the ED.

Flunitrazepam (Rohypnol). Also known as roofies, this drug is a potent benzodiazepine that is also used to facilitate sexual assault. When combined with another drug that works to depress the CNS, flunitrazepam may cause the patient to experience profound effects including unconsciousness, respiratory depression, and death. This drug is illegal to make or distribute, so most of the supply found in the United States enters the country from Mexico.

▶ Poisonous Alcohols

As mentioned previously, the form of alcohol consumed by humans in alcoholic beverages (ethanol) is not conventionally recognized as a poison. Instead, poisonous alcohols are generally considered to encompass alcohols manufactured for industrial or nongastronomic purposes, such as methyl alcohol and ethylene glycol.

Methyl Alcohol

Methyl alcohol (also known as wood alcohol or methanol) is present in paints, paint remover, windshield washer fluids, varnishes, antifreeze, and canned fuels such as Sterno **Figure 27-13**. Methanol may be a popular substitute for ethanol among people with alcoholism when they do not have the means to obtain ethanol. This colorless liquid has a unique odor. Ingestion of as little as 60 to 250 mL in adults or 8 to 10 mL in children is associated with severe toxicity.

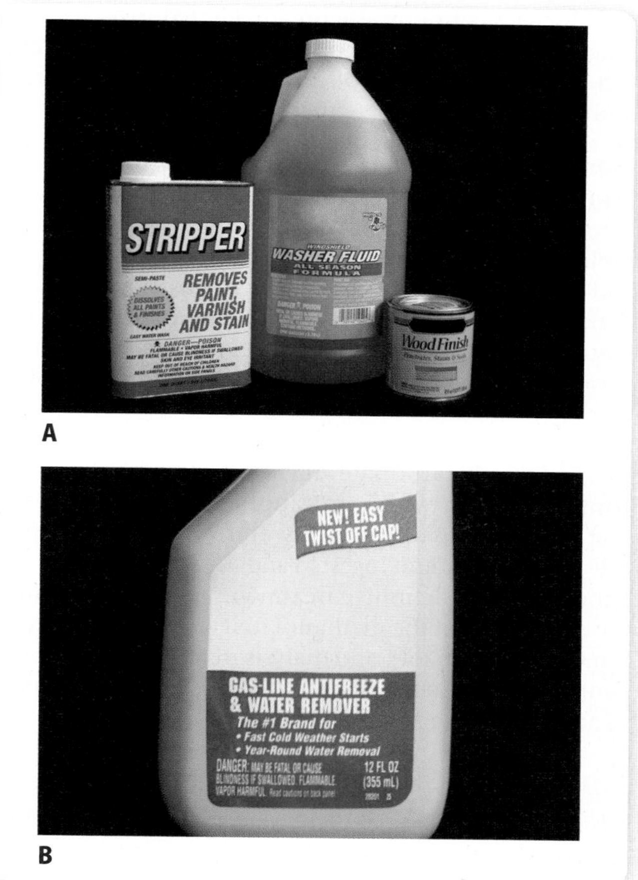

Figure 27-13 Methyl alcohol is present in paints, paint remover, windshield washer fluids, and varnishes **(A)** and in antifreeze and canned fuels **(B)**.

Pathophysiology. When methanol is ingested, its metabolic breakdown products (formaldehyde and formic acid) are responsible for the characteristic signs and symptoms of methanol poisoning. Once ingested, methanol is quickly absorbed from the GI tract, with peak blood levels attained within 30 to 90 minutes. In mild toxicity, the half-life of methanol is 14 to 20 hours. As toxicity increases, the half-life increases to 24 to 30 hours. The liver eliminates 90% to 95% of the methanol.

Assessment. The symptoms of methanol poisoning do not usually appear immediately but begin from 12 to 18 hours, occasionally up to 72 hours, after ingestion. Because of this latency period, it may be difficult to determine the source of the symptoms. Be thorough in your history taking and assessment. Patient complaints include nausea and vomiting (in almost 50% of cases), headache or vertigo, abdominal pain (often from pancreatitis), and blurred vision (the patient may say, "It looks like a snowstorm"). Findings on the physical exam may include an odor of alcohol on the breath, altered mental status ranging from agitation to coma, mydriasis, hyperpnea and tachypnea (from metabolic acidosis), and bradycardia and hypotension as a late presentation.

Management. Field care for methanol poisoning is primarily supportive. Establish and manage the airway, considering advanced airway placement as needed. Establish vascular access. Assess the blood glucose level, and administer glucose if the patient has hypoglycemia. Activated charcoal does not bind well to alcohol, and methanol is rapidly absorbed in the stomach. For these reasons, activated charcoal is often contraindicated unless you have identified other substances that were ingested for which activated charcoal may be beneficial.

Sodium bicarbonate may be ordered by medical control to assist with ion trapping and counteracting metabolic acidosis. Morbidity and mortality are often driven by the amount ingested and the speed at which the patient receives definitive treatment. Ethanol (to reduce the conversion of the methanol to its toxic metabolites), fomepizole (Antizol), and dialysis may be part of the patient's treatment at the hospital. Provide prompt transport to an appropriate facility.[27]

Ethylene Glycol

Ethylene glycol is a colorless, odorless liquid found in a variety of commercial products, including antifreeze, coolant, deicers, polishes, and paints. Similar to methanol, it may be used by people with alcoholism who are unable to obtain ethanol. The lethal dose of ethylene glycol is estimated to be 2 mL/kg, or as little as 150 mL in the average-size adult.

Pathophysiology. Ethylene glycol is water-soluble. With oral intake, it is absorbed rapidly, with peak blood levels attained within 1 to 4 hours after ingestion. The liver and kidneys metabolize ethylene glycol into a number of toxic metabolites, including aldehydes, lactate, oxalate, and glycolate. In turn, these metabolites inhibit cellular respiration and glucose metabolism, and impair cellular function through an anion gap metabolic acidosis.

Assessment. Toxicity from ethylene glycol occurs in three stages, so the signs and symptoms vary depending on when you encounter the patient relative to the time of ingestion:

- **Stage 1.** CNS depression is the hallmark of the initial stage. The patient may appear intoxicated, as evidenced by slurred speech and ataxia, without the obvious odor of alcohol present. These symptoms progress to include nausea, vomiting, seizures, or coma as metabolites begin to accumulate in the body. Stage 1 begins soon after ingestion and can last up to 12 hours.
- **Stage 2.** Cardiopulmonary symptoms begin to appear as the patient enters the second stage. The patient may exhibit hypertension, hypotension, or tachycardia. Pulmonary injury may present as pulmonary edema, pneumonitis, or acute respiratory distress syndrome. The patient may have hypocalcemia due to calcium oxalate precipitation. Stage 2 may develop between 12 and 24 hours after ingestion.
- **Stage 3.** Flank pain, anuria, and hematuria often characterize the third stage. The kidneys are injured, and acute renal failure may develop. Stage 3 may develop 24 to 72 hours after ingestion.

Management. The treatment plan for a patient with suspected ethylene glycol poisoning is the same as for methanol poisoning, with the exception of possibly getting an order from medical control to administer 10 mL of 10% calcium gluconate via slow IV push to treat the hypocalcemia that accompanies ethylene glycol toxicity. This medication is usually ordered only after good urine flow is established and after the IV line is flushed clear of sodium bicarbonate. After the patient arrives at the hospital, medical care focuses on correction of acidosis, administration of fomepizole or ethanol, and renal dialysis.

▶ Hydrocarbons

Hydrocarbons are structurally simple organic molecules comprised of only hydrogen and carbon. Hydrocarbons are found in a variety of products around the home, including natural gas (such as methane, butane, and propane), cleaning agents, petroleum distillates (such as gasoline, lamp oil, and paint thinner), and fluorocarbons (used as propellants in aerosols). While you focus on memorizing illicit drugs, do not forget about the harmful substances that can be purchased at the local hardware or office supply store.

Hydrocarbon Inhalation

Because of the widespread availability of products containing hydrocarbons, inhalation is often the route of exposure for users who may not have access to, or funds to purchase, illicit drugs. Recreational abuse of hydrocarbons may be seen in both pediatric and adult populations. The three common methods for inhalation are huffing, sniffing, and bagging. Huffing usually involves soaking a cloth in a substance and then holding the saturated cloth over the mouth and nose. Sniffing involves inhaling the substance directly from an open container. Bagging refers to the process of inhaling fumes from a plastic bag into which the substance was sprayed. Low viscosity hydrocarbons can cover a large surface area in the lungs and produce a rapid onset of action.

Hydrocarbon inhalation can produce a euphoric high, creating a high abuse potential from those seeking a "cheap buzz." The signs and symptoms of inhalation involve the cardiopulmonary and central nervous systems. Altered mental status, seizures, tachycardia, dyspnea, and

Table 27-6 Compounds Commonly Abused by Huffing, Sniffing, and Bagging

Example	Sources	Signs and Symptoms of Toxicity
Halogenated Hydrocarbons		
1,1,1-Trichloroethane (methylchloroform)	Cleaning solvents, typewriter correction fluid, aerosol propellant	Eye irritation, light-headedness, incoordination, CNS depression, respiratory failure, cardiac dysrhythmias, sudden death
Trichloroethylene	Degreasing solvent, aerosol propellant, rubber cement, plastic cement	Euphoria, anesthesia, weakness, vomiting, abdominal cramps, loss of coordination, neuropathy, blindness, cardiac dysrhythmias, "degreaser's flush" (flushed face, neck, and shoulders when taken along with alcohol)
Tetrachloroethylene (perchloroethylene)	Solvent, dry cleaning agent	Drunken behavior, dizziness, light-headedness, difficulty walking, numbness, sleepiness, visual disturbances, memory impairment, eye irritation, cutaneous flushing, sudden death
Methylene chloride (dichloromethane)	Refrigerant, paint remover, aerosol propellant	Fatigue, weakness, chills, sleepiness, nausea, dizziness, incoordination, pulmonary edema
Carbon tetrachloride	Cleaning fluid	Narcosis, sudden death
Petroleum Hydrocarbons		
Benzene	Cable cleaner, industrial solvents, rubber cement	Delirium, agitation, seizures, sudden death
Toluene	Spray paint, model and plastic cements, lacquer thinner	Narcosis, hallucinations, mania; loss of fine motor skills; impulsive, destructive, accident-prone behavior; sudden death
Gasoline	Gasoline tank/portable gasoline can	Sudden death

Abbreviation: CNS, central nervous system

ventricular dysrhythmias may occur with toxic inhalations of hydrocarbons. Table 27-6 lists commonly abused inhaled compounds.

When you care for a patient who has inhaled hydrocarbons, the primary goals focus on removal from the noxious environment, administering high-concentration supplemental oxygen, and prompt transport to the appropriate facility.

Hydrocarbon Ingestion

Pathophysiology. Hydrocarbons represent an ingestion hazard because many common household items contain hydrocarbons. Even when stored appropriately in labeled containers, hydrocarbons may be mistakenly ingested by a child looking for a drink. Adult ingestion of hydrocarbons is likely to be intentional with the intent of causing self-harm. Hydrocarbons with a high viscosity, such as motor oil, are less likely to be aspirated. However, low viscosity hydrocarbons, such as gasoline, may easily be aspirated when the patient coughs or vomits after the ingestion. Patients who develop symptoms or signs of respiratory distress within a few minutes of ingestion are likely to have aspirated and need immediate attention.

Low viscosity also facilitates the uptake of hydrocarbons by tissues of the CNS and, therefore, its anesthetic effects. At first, the patient may experience excitement and euphoria, followed by loss of fine motor skills, drowsiness, confusion, and coma. Cardiac dysrhythmias may also be present during monitoring.

Many hydrocarbon products cause gastric irritation, which results in severe abdominal pain, diarrhea, and belching, sometimes lasting for hours after the incident. Conversely, just a single hydrocarbon substance exposure may cause life-threatening toxicity.

Assessment and Management. Asymptomatic patients may not wish to be transported to the hospital. Contact local medical control for advice. Promptly transport all symptomatic patients who are suspected of ingesting a hydrocarbon product—especially patients with respiratory symptoms—to the ED. Management should include the following measures:

- Ensure the patient with contaminated skin or clothing has been decontaminated prior to treatment, because the vapors can be harmful to others (including health care providers).
- Establish and maintain the airway, and ensure adequate ventilation.
- Administer high-flow supplemental oxygen to maintain blood saturation levels of greater than 94%.
- Establish vascular access.
- Continuously monitor the ECG rhythm; consider running a 12-lead ECG.
- Administer sequential bolus infusions of normal saline to treat hypotension.
- Transport the patient to the most appropriate facility.

▶ Hydrofluoric Acid/Hydrogen Fluoride

Pathophysiology

Hydrofluoric acid is hydrogen fluoride (HF) that has been placed into an aqueous solution. This potent caustic substance can cause devastating local and systemic toxicity from exposure to an extremely small amount of concentrated liquid. HF is primarily used in industrial settings as a cleaning product to remove impurities from steel, automotive parts, glass, and porcelain, though exposures have occurred in glass etching hobbyists. The fluoride in HF leaches calcium and magnesium from body tissues, resulting in profound, often lethal hypocalcemia and hypomagnesemia. These electrolyte alterations also prompt development of hyperkalemia following a massive release of sequestered potassium into the systemic circulation. Systemic effects from HF poisoning are primarily related to electrolyte imbalance. Dysrhythmias, tremors, seizures, CNS depression, acidemia, and renal failure are common with exposures to large amounts of HF.

Dermal exposure usually has a latent period during which the patient is pain free and may not realize an exposure has occurred. As the HF penetrates into the skin, significant local tissue damage, necrosis, and persistent pain quickly develop, often without obvious dermal injury.

HF may cause throat discomfort, bronchospasm, stridor, and local airway injury following inhalation. Lung auscultation reveals wheezes, rhonchi, or crackles (formerly called rales). Serious inhalation exposures can cause delayed chemical pneumonitis or pulmonary edema.

Ingestion of HF may cause vomiting, abdominal pain, and gastritis, in addition to profound systemic toxicity. Ingestions of large amounts or concentrated solutions of HF are often lethal.

Assessment and Management

Patients exposed to HF may deteriorate rapidly; careful monitoring is critical. As always, manage the ABCs. For ingestion exposure, consider dilution with milk or water. Calcium gluconate may be utilized for HF exposure. A paste of water-soluble lubricant and 10% calcium gluconate may be applied to local burns. IV administration of 10% calcium gluconate may be allowed by local protocols or online medical control in the presence of cardiac irritability.

▶ Hydrogen Sulfide

Pathophysiology

A highly toxic, colorless gas, hydrogen sulfide (H_2S) is usually identified by its distinctive rotten-egg odor. Poisoning by H_2S usually occurs by inhalation. This gas affects all organs, but has the most impact on the lungs and CNS.

Workers in industrial settings may be exposed to low levels over a long period. Low-level exposures cause eye, nose, and throat irritation, as well as headaches and bronchitis. Workers in confined spaces (especially containing fish, sewage, or manure) are at high risk of H_2S exposure. When patients are exposed to high concentrations of the gas, they present with nausea and vomiting, confusion, dyspnea, and often, immediate loss of consciousness. Frequently, coworkers without adequate respiratory protection are subsequently killed in their attempt to rescue the initial patient. Seizures, shock, coma, and cardiopulmonary arrest may result from exposure to very high concentrations.

Assessment and Management

No proven antidote exists for H_2S poisoning. Therefore, quickly remove the patient from the contaminated area. After the patient has been moved to a safe area, management is largely supportive. Monitor and assist the patient's respiratory and cardiovascular functions.

▶ Oxides of Nitrogen

The group of gases known as nitrogen oxides includes nitric oxide and nitrogen dioxide. These gases form as a byproduct of fuel combustion. Nitric oxide is colorless or brown at room temperature and has a sweet smell. Nitrogen dioxide is also normally colorless or brown and is generally described as having a harsh odor. Patients may be exposed to very high concentrations from kerosene heaters in their homes or in an occupational setting in facilities that produce nitric acid.

Pathophysiology

Exposure to oxides of nitrogen can result in irritation of the throat and upper respiratory tract, pulmonary edema, difficulty breathing, and weakness. Symptoms may be delayed unless the patient encountered very high levels of the substance in the environment.

Assessment and Management

Take precautions, including a self-contained breathing apparatus, before entering the scene. Prehospital treatment includes immediately removing the patient from the environment. Provide supportive care, gain IV access, and be prepared to manage the patient's airway.

▶ Psychiatric Medications

Psychiatric medications are designed to alter dysfunctions of mood and affect (most commonly depression) and of thought, orientation, or perception; thus, they are sophisticated pharmacologic agents. According to the AAPCC's National Poison Data System, antidepressants accounted for over 75,000 adult exposures and were the fourth most common pharmaceutical involved in fatal exposures in 2014.[25] As with other toxicologic emergencies, ingestion may have been intentional. Search for other substances that may have been used in a polypharmacy overdose. The various mechanisms of action of different psychiatric medications will create a challenging situation for you to manage.

Tricyclic Antidepressants

Pathophysiology. **Tricyclic antidepressants (TCAs)** are medications that were frequently prescribed for depression in the past, and you may see them prescribed for insomnia, eating disorders, and personality disorders. This class of medications has a very narrow therapeutic window that causes difficulty for the patient who is noncompliant with his or her treatment regimen. Common TCAs include amitriptyline, doxepin, nortriptyline, trimipramine, and clomipramine.

TCAs are absorbed by the body within the first couple of hours after ingestion, and they easily cross the blood-brain barrier. They work as norepinephrine and serotonin reuptake inhibitors. Overdose can cause sympathomimetic and serotonergic effects. Some of the cardiac effects are a result of the fast sodium channel and potassium channel blockade. TCAs can also cause muscarinic and histamine blockade.

Assessment. TCAs affect the body through several mechanisms, so be alert for different types of presentations with a tricyclic overdose. Patients with toxic ingestions are likely to present with tachycardia, tachypnea, hypotension, and hyperthermia due to the sympathomimetic response. The antimuscarinic qualities may produce signs and symptoms similar to the anticholinergic toxidrome; that is, "hot as a hare, blind as a bat, dry as a bone, red as a beet, and mad as a hatter." In other words, the patient will exhibit hyperthermia, dilated pupils, dry skin and mucous membranes, reddened skin, and agitation or delirium. Because of the sodium channel and potassium channel blockade, be alert for ECG changes to include a prolonged PR interval, tachycardia, widening QRS, a terminal R wave greater than 3 mm in aVR, and a prolonged QT interval **Figure 27-14**. Altered mental status, delirium, and seizures are also possible with toxic ingestion of TCAs.

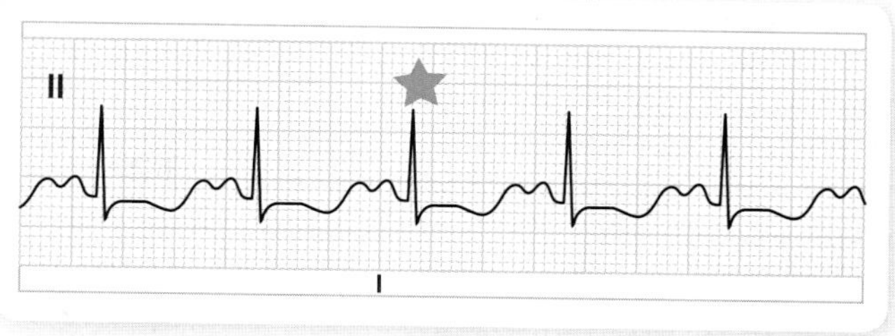

Figure 27-14 QT prolongation.

Reproduced from *Arrhythmia Recognition: The Art of Interpretation*, courtesy of Tomas B. Garcia, MD.

A significant number of the drug overdoses involving TCAs also involve other drugs and frequently alcohol, which contributes to increased morbidity and mortality. A patient who presents with serious signs and symptoms within 6 hours of the ingestion should be considered to be in critical condition.

Management. Management of patients with a TCA overdose includes the following measures:

- Maintain the airway. If the patient's mental status suddenly deteriorates (as is often the case), then insert an advanced airway.
- Administer high-flow supplemental oxygen to maintain blood saturation levels of greater than 94%.
- Establish vascular access.
- Provide continuous ECG monitoring (watch for widening of the QRS).
- Administer activated charcoal per medical control orders.
- Consult with medical control to consider sodium bicarbonate administration (if ECG abnormalities are noted).
- Manage hypotension with sequential boluses of normal saline. Be alert to the possibility of pulmonary edema; it occurs frequently in patients with TCA overdose.
- Assess blood glucose levels. Administer IV dextrose if the patient is hypoglycemic.
- Be alert for agitation or violence. Provide reassurance and administer benzodiazepines, if needed.
- *Do not give* flumazenil (Romazicon; may cause seizures) or physostigmine (Eserine, Antilirium).
- Treat seizures with benzodiazepines.
- Provide rapid transport to the appropriate facility.

Monoamine Oxidase Inhibitors

Pathophysiology. **Monoamine oxidase inhibitors (MAOIs)** are used primarily to treat atypical depression. Norepinephrine, serotonin, and dopamine are the primary neurotransmitters that assist with improving mood and affect with their presence in certain cells and circuits in the brain. Monoamine oxidase (MAO) is an enzyme that removes these neurotransmitters from the brain. MAOIs prevent the regular removal of the neurotransmitters, resulting in increased levels in circulation. In toxic levels, MAOIs can block these enzymes for a short or long duration based on the medication. Some ingestions may require days before a new series of enzymes can be synthesized by the body. Examples of MAOIs include phenelzine and tranylcypromine.

Assessment. Symptoms of MAOI toxicity are often delayed, occurring 6 to 12 hours after ingestion. Cardiovascular effects of MAOI toxicity include hypertension, tachycardia, palpitations, chest pain, diaphoresis, and atrial dysrhythmias. Marked hyperthermia, muscle rigidity, respiratory failure, delirium, and seizures may occur in severe toxicity. After signs and symptoms begin to appear, you should prepare to manage a life-threatening event. When death occurs from an MAOI overdose, it is usually secondary to multiple-system organ failure.

Management. Unfortunately, no antidote is available for an MAOI overdose. With any suspected MAOI overdose, establish and maintain the airway, inserting an advanced airway as needed. In addition, administer high-flow supplemental oxygen. If RSI is required, then the use of a nondepolarizing paralytic such as rocuronium is recommended because MAOIs may enhance the actions of succinylcholine. Establish large-bore vascular access. Monitor the ECG rhythm, staying alert for changes indicative of hyperkalemia. After consultation with medical control, you may administer a single dose of activated charcoal.

With a patient in deteriorating condition, treat hypotension with sequential fluid boluses of normal saline. If seizures occur, then treat them with benzodiazepines per local protocol because persistent seizures may contribute to the combined problems of metabolic acidosis, hyperkalemia, and rhabdomyolysis. If the patient is hyperthermic, then you may consider the administration of midazolam. A dose of 0.1 mg/kg in 2-mg increments over 1 to 2 minutes is appropriate for both adult and pediatric patients.

Selective Serotonin Reuptake Inhibitors

Pathophysiology. A larger therapeutic window has helped make **selective serotonin reuptake inhibitors (SSRIs)** a common choice for managing depression. SSRIs work by enhancing serotonergic neurotransmission and inhibiting the breakdown of serotonin. SSRIs have few cardiac effects or anticholinergic effects, so they are a safer option for the management of depression compared to TCAs. Popular SSRIs include fluoxetine (Prozac), paroxetine (Paxil), citalopram (Celexa), and sertraline (Zoloft).

Assessment. As many as 50% of adult patients may be asymptomatic with an SSRI overdose. When SSRIs are taken in conjunction with alcohol, look for tachycardia, mild hypotension, and lethargy as the most common signs and symptoms. Other symptoms include nausea, vomiting, and tremors. Dilated pupils, agitation, hypotension or hypertension, seizures, and hallucinations may be less commonly noted. Dysrhythmias are also rare but may include QT prolongation and torsades de pointes.

Management. A pure SSRI overdose with no other drugs or alcohol involved usually produces limited toxic effects, with the exception of seizures or serotonin syndrome (discussed later in this section). As such, management of an SSRI overdose follows the general approach for poisoned patients:

- Establish and maintain the airway.
- Administer high-flow supplemental oxygen to maintain blood saturation levels of greater than 94%.
- Establish vascular access.
- Provide continuous ECG monitoring.
- Consider a single dose of activated charcoal per medical control orders.
- Treat seizure activity with benzodiazepines per local protocol.
- Should widening of the QRS occur, consult with medical control for consideration of sodium bicarbonate administration.
- Transport to the appropriate facility.

Serotonin Syndrome. **Serotonin syndrome** is an idiosyncratic complication that occasionally occurs with antidepressant therapy. This condition is not limited to patients taking SSRIs, but can also occur when patients take any combination of drugs that increase central serotonin neurotransmission. Drugs that can cause serotonin syndrome include MAOIs, SSRIs, TCAs, lithium, stimulants, and opioids. The presentation can vary widely in severity and may be complicated by consideration of single or multiple substance toxicity versus serotonin syndrome. The onset of serotonin syndrome is commonly within 6 hours of ingestion (and possibly the result of something as simple as an increased dosage of a medication). Signs and symptoms of serotonin syndrome include delirium, tachycardia, hypertension, diaphoresis, diarrhea, muscle rigidity, myoclonus, hyperreflexia, and trismus. Prehospital treatment is supportive, and you may consider cooling if hyperthermia is present. If the patient is diagnosed with serotonin syndrome, then cyproheptadine may be administered at the hospital. Symptoms may persist beyond 24 hours in severe cases or if extended release medications are involved.

Lithium

Despite the major advances made in many areas of psychiatric medicine, **lithium** remains a common mood stabilizer used in the treatment of bipolar disorder. In 1949, lithium salts made their debut for the treatment of mania. Eventually, they were found to be much more efficacious for the treatment of bipolar disorder, and they retain their position as the main treatment of this condition. Lithium assists with dampening mood swings rather than affecting the normal mood.

Pathophysiology. Lithium is almost completely absorbed in the GI tract roughly 8 hours after ingestion. Bioelimination occurs relatively slowly, with approximately one-third of the dose remaining for roughly 2 weeks after administration. Given its small therapeutic window and slow excretion process, the threat of toxic levels and overdosing is ever present.

Assessment. Early signs and symptoms of lithium overdose include nausea, vomiting, headache, hand tremors, excessive thirst, and slurred speech. With increased toxicity come increased neurologic symptoms: ataxia, muscle weakness and incoordination, abnormal thermoregulation, blurred vision, and hyperreflexia (twitching). Eventually, the patient may have seizures and become comatose.

Management. Management of a patient suspected of a lithium overdose is mostly supportive. Establish and maintain the airway, inserting an advanced airway as needed. Provide high-concentration supplemental oxygen, and establish vascular access. If the patient experiences hypotension, then administer serial boluses of normal saline. Maintain continuous ECG monitoring, being alert for AV blocks and ventricular dysrhythmias. Finally, transport the patient to an appropriate facility. Hemodialysis and continuous renal replacement therapy may be indicated at the hospital, so consider these possibilities in your transport disposition.

▶ Nonprescription Pain Medications

Medications used for pain management make up a large part of the OTC drug market. In the OTC and prescription drug markets, nonsteroidal anti-inflammatory drugs (NSAIDs) are some of the most popular options for pain relief, fever control, and anti-inflammatory action. Their convenient dosing schemes and large therapeutic windows, coupled with their safe track records relative to acute ingestion and overdose, enhance their popularity.

Pathophysiology

NSAIDs are rapidly absorbed from the GI tract before being eliminated from the body in urine and feces. The half-lives of these agents vary widely, ranging from 2 to 4 hours for ibuprofen, to approximately 15 hours for selective cyclooxygenase-2 inhibitors, to 50 hours for some long-acting agents. Patients who take lithium and NSAIDs have slowed renal clearance of the lithium, increasing the likelihood that they will inadvertently reach a toxic lithium level.

Most of the conditions associated with NSAID use involve long-term use; patients may experience GI bleeding and kidney dysfunction. Acute ingestion and overdoses are rare, with ibuprofen being the NSAID most commonly encountered in the acute setting.

Assessment

Many NSAID overdoses remain asymptomatic. Very large doses are usually required before any signs or symptoms of toxicity occur. At toxic levels, the signs and symptoms of NSAID overdose may include nausea with vomiting and abdominal pain. Metabolic acidosis can occur with severe NSAID toxicity.

Management

For symptomatic patients, emergency medical care is usually supportive. Establish and maintain the airway, inserting an advanced airway as needed. Administer high-concentration supplemental oxygen, and establish vascular access. Administer crystalloid fluid boluses for hypotensive patients. Treat seizures with benzodiazepines per local protocol. Finally, transport the patient to an appropriate facility.

A unique adverse effect of NSAID use is aseptic meningitis, in which a patient presents with reports of a stiff neck, headache, and fever within several hours after taking an NSAID. Discontinuing the NSAID therapy generally resolves the condition, but patients must be evaluated at the hospital to rule out other causes.

Salicylates

Although aspirin (acetylsalicylic acid, or ASA) can be involved in a toxic event, it is more typical for OTC products containing **salicylates** to cause unintentional toxicity. For example, a single 30-mL dose of bismuth subsalicylate (Pepto-Bismol) contains 261 mg of salicylate (two-thirds the total dose of one aspirin). Aggressive dosing of salicylates for analgesia or fever control may lead to toxic levels of the substance.

Pathophysiology. Ingestion of 150 mg/kg or less will usually result in mild toxicity. At this level, chief complaints are usually nausea, vomiting, and abdominal pain. With a dosing range of 150 to 300 mg/kg, signs and symptoms may include ringing in the ears (tinnitus), pulmonary edema, and acid-base disturbances. At levels of 300 mg/kg, severe toxicity may produce metabolic acidosis. Although you may be unable to analyze an actual blood gas level in the field, you may note that the patient has tachypnea and hyperpnea—the body's compensatory mechanism for correcting metabolic acidosis.

An acute salicylate event with an adult usually involves an intentional overdose, with a common patient profile being young women with a history of drug abuse or psychiatric conditions. A fatal event is possible if an adult with suspected salicylate overdose is unresponsive during the primary survey and presents with a high fever, seizures, or cardiac dysrhythmias.

Assessment and Management. No salicylate antidote or antagonist is available, so field management is primarily supportive. Establish and maintain the airway, inserting an advanced airway as needed. Provide high-concentration supplemental oxygen and monitor carbon dioxide levels with capnometry. If you are ventilating the patient, then you may consider not immediately correcting hypocapnia. The patient was compensating by breathing fast. Failing to provide a rate similar to his or her compensatory rate may result in rising carbon dioxide levels that worsen the acidosis. Obtain vascular access. If hypotension develops, then administer serial boluses of normal saline. Following consultation with medical control, administer one dose of activated charcoal. In addition, consult with medical control regarding urine alkalinization with sodium bicarbonate. Finally, transport the patient to an appropriate facility.

Acetaminophen

Acetaminophen is a well-tolerated OTC drug with few adverse effects. These characteristics have made this drug one of the best-selling analgesics in the United States—and a common culprit in toxic exposures. Similar to NSAIDs, many OTC medications have acetaminophen as an active ingredient. Unintentional overdoses may occur when several medications containing acetaminophen are taken together. These unintentional overdoses may occur several times throughout the course of a day or several days, and the patient may unknowingly build up a toxic level.

Pathophysiology. After it is ingested, acetaminophen is rapidly absorbed from the GI tract, producing peak serum levels in 30 to 120 minutes. Absorption slows when the drug is combined with diphenhydramine (Tylenol PM) or with propoxyphene (Darvocet). One unique aspect of acetaminophen toxicity is that the signs and symptoms appear in four distinct stages (Table 27-7).

Table 27-7 Signs and Symptoms of Acetaminophen Toxicity

Stage	Time Frame	Signs and Symptoms
I	<24 h	Nausea, vomiting, loss of appetite, pallor, malaise
II	24–72 h	Right upper quadrant abdominal pain; abdomen tender to palpation
III	72–96 h	Metabolic acidosis, renal failure, coagulopathies, recurring GI symptoms
IV	4–14 d (or longer)	Recovery slowly begins, or liver failure progresses and the patient dies

Abbreviation: GI, gastrointestinal

Assessment and Management. It is important for you to try to accurately estimate the time of ingestion because this information drives the decision-making process for patient care in the field and the hospital. An antidote for acetaminophen toxicity exists—acetylcysteine (Acetadote). Ideally, this drug should be given less than 8 hours after the ingestion. Typically, however, it is administered based on the patient's laboratory results; as such, it is not a field intervention.

Management of the patient in the field first focuses on establishing and maintaining the airway, with an advanced airway being inserted as needed. Establish vascular access. For recent ingestions, administer activated charcoal after consulting with medical control. Finally, transport the patient to an appropriate facility.

▶ Metals and Metalloids

Although acute metal and metalloid toxic exposures are relatively rare, when they occur, they can produce devastating results, usually because of delayed diagnosis or misdiagnosis. Asymptomatic patients or patients who have vague, nonspecific symptoms can be difficult to diagnose. The difficulty reaching the correct diagnosis may contribute to increased mortality or morbidity because of delayed or inadequate treatment. Toxic exposures involving metals or metalloids usually manifest by affecting four body systems: neurologic, hematologic, renal, and GI.

Lead

Lead is a toxic metal that can accumulate in the body and affect the cardiovascular, GI, hematologic, neurologic, and renal systems. Most toxic ingestions of lead are unintentional and are the result of environmental contamination. According to the 2014 Annual Report of the AAPCC's National Poison Data System, lead poisoning remains the most common heavy metal involved in a toxic ingestion.[25]

Pathophysiology. With inorganic lead, absorption usually occurs via the respiratory or GI tract. Once in the body, approximately 90% of the lead is stored in bone. Inorganic lead can also cross the placental barrier and negatively affect fetal development. In pediatric patients, elevated blood lead levels can cause adverse neurologic development that may significantly impair cognitive function. Its excretion from the body is incredibly slow, with the half-life of lead in bone estimated at 30 years.

Most organic lead (tetraethyl lead) exposures occur in the occupational setting, although they can also occur from gas sniffing where leaded gasoline is available. Once

Table 27-8	Systems Affected by Lead Poisoning
System	**Signs and Symptoms**
CNS	Altered mentation, including irritability, mood changes; weakness; tremors; headache; seizures; ataxia
GI	Abdominal pain, constipation, diarrhea, anorexia
Renal	Renal insufficiency, hypertension, gout
Hematologic	Anemia

Abbreviations: CNS, central nervous system; GI, gastrointestinal

in the body, tetraethyl lead is metabolized to inorganic lead and triethyl lead, with triethyl lead being the primary cause of CNS toxicity.

Assessment and Management. Lead poisoning is associated with a long list of signs and symptoms Table 27-8. In particular, encephalopathy is a major cause of mortality and morbidity from lead poisoning.

In the field, you have few treatment options for lead poisoning. Your most helpful move may be identification of the source of the lead, which can assist the appropriate government agency to prevent more occurrences by removing the toxin. When you are managing the patient, first establish and maintain the airway, inserting an advanced airway as needed. Administer high-flow supplemental oxygen. Establish vascular access with a saline or heparin lock. Cautious fluid administration is required to avoid worsening any cerebral edema. Transport the patient to an appropriate facility.

Iron

Although only a small amount of iron is required as part of a healthy diet, many adult and pediatric multivitamins contain iron. Children younger than 6 years have frequent iron exposures, usually secondary to ingesting chewable vitamins. Many chewable vitamins are marketed to look and taste like candy. Prenatal vitamins are a common source for lethal pediatric iron ingestions. By comparison, most toxic exposures in adults are intentional.

Pathophysiology. In the average 155-pound (70-kg) adult, the body's entire iron supply consists of only about 4 g. Of that total, roughly 65% is found in hemoglobin. Excessive amounts of iron in the body can speed up the formation of oxygen free radicals, creating a metabolic acidosis. It may also have an effect on the coagulation cascade and the liver, causing significant coagulopathy.

From a practical perspective, the toxic effects of an iron exposure reflect the amount of elemental iron ingested. With ingestion of 20 to 60 mg/kg, mild to moderate toxicity should be expected. With dosing of more than 60 mg/kg, severe and potentially lethal toxicity is a possibility.

Assessment and Management. From the time of ingestion, iron poisoning will usually cause symptoms within the first 6 hours. If the patient does not have symptoms during this time, then it is unlikely they will have a serious toxicity. Early stages of iron poisoning may include vomiting, diarrhea, abdominal pain, hematemesis, tachycardia, hypotension, and altered mental status. Patients are commonly in metabolic acidosis and become tachypneic as the body attempts to correct the pH by increasing the elimination of carbon dioxide. A patient in the later stages of iron poisoning will present with profound shock, seizures, hyperthermia, liver failure, and coagulopathy.

Unfortunately, you can do little in the field for iron poisoning, other than provide attention to the ABCs and transport the patient to the hospital for further evaluation and laboratory studies. Provide supportive care directed at maintaining adequate perfusion and oxygenation. Activated charcoal does not adsorb iron and should not be used unless other toxins were ingested.

Mercury

Mercury exists in a variety of organic and inorganic forms. In the human body, all forms produce toxic effects. Although unintentional exposures to mercury often occur in the occupational setting, mercury can be found in the home in thermometers and in some switches used in heating and air conditioning.

Pathophysiology. Organic mercury is lipid-soluble and quickly accumulates in the liver, CNS, and kidneys. It can also cross the placental membrane into the fetus.

Assessment. Mercury poisoning can present differently depending on the type of mercury and its route of entry into the body. Most signs and symptoms involve the GI and renal systems. CNS alterations may include anxiety, depression, irritability, sleep disturbances, and memory loss. In addition, tremors, ataxia, paresthesias, muscle weakness or rigidity, and excessive drooling may develop. The patient may have abdominal pain, vomiting, flank pain, anuria, or uremia.

Management. In the occupational setting, safe removal of the patient from the exposure source is the primary intervention. In all patients with suspected mercury poisoning, your management is supportive and includes basic attention to the ABCs and transport to the hospital. In the hospital setting, the patient may undergo aggressive GI decontamination and receive succimer (DMSA), a medication used in chelation therapy. Hemodialysis may be required for renal failure.

Arsenic

In 2014, the AAPCC reported that arsenic (not contained in pesticides) was involved in approximately 8% of all heavy metal poisonings.[25] This metal is used in a variety of industries and appears in a variety of compounds, so it is often the source of unintentional exposures. Intentional exposures include the use of arsenic in homicide and suicide.

Pathophysiology. Arsenic can enter the body by ingestion, inhalation, and absorption and dermally through a wound. It is eliminated from the body through the kidneys.

Assessment. The clinical presentation of arsenic poisoning depends on the type, amount, and concentration of arsenic that enters the body and the rate of absorption and elimination. In general, symptoms appear within 30 minutes to several hours of arsenic ingestion. Arsenic poisoning should be suspected with patients who present with hypotension of unknown cause following a bout of severe gastroenteritis.

Signs and symptoms of arsenic poisoning include severe abdominal pain, nausea, explosive diarrhea, "metallic taste" in the mouth, dysphagia, general malaise, weakness, hypotension, pulmonary edema, rhabdomyolysis, metabolic acidosis, and renal failure. ECG changes and dysrhythmias (usually SVTs) may be apparent, but nonspecific ST-segment and T-wave changes are also possible, as is QT prolongation. Ventricular tachycardia and torsades de pointes can occur as well.

Management. A patient with acute arsenic toxicity is in critical condition and requires aggressive interventions. Establish and maintain the airway, inserting an advanced airway as needed. Administer high-flow supplemental oxygen, and establish vascular access. For hypotension, administer sequential boluses of normal saline. If the hypotension proves refractory to fluid therapy, then administer a vasopressor (dopamine [Inotropin] or dobutamine [Dobutrex]). Continuously monitor the ECG, and follow advanced cardiac life support algorithms for dysrhythmias. Finally, provide rapid transport to an appropriate facility.

▶ Poisonous Plants

Of the thousands of plant varieties, only a few are poisonous Figure 27-15. Oddly enough, poisonous plants represent some of the most common ornamental garden shrubs and houseplants. Perhaps for that reason, approximately 65% of plant-related exposures involve children age 5 years or younger. In the AAPCC's 2014 Annual Report, plant ingestions were in the top 25 substance categories most frequently involved in human exposures and in the top 10 substances for pediatric exposures.[25]

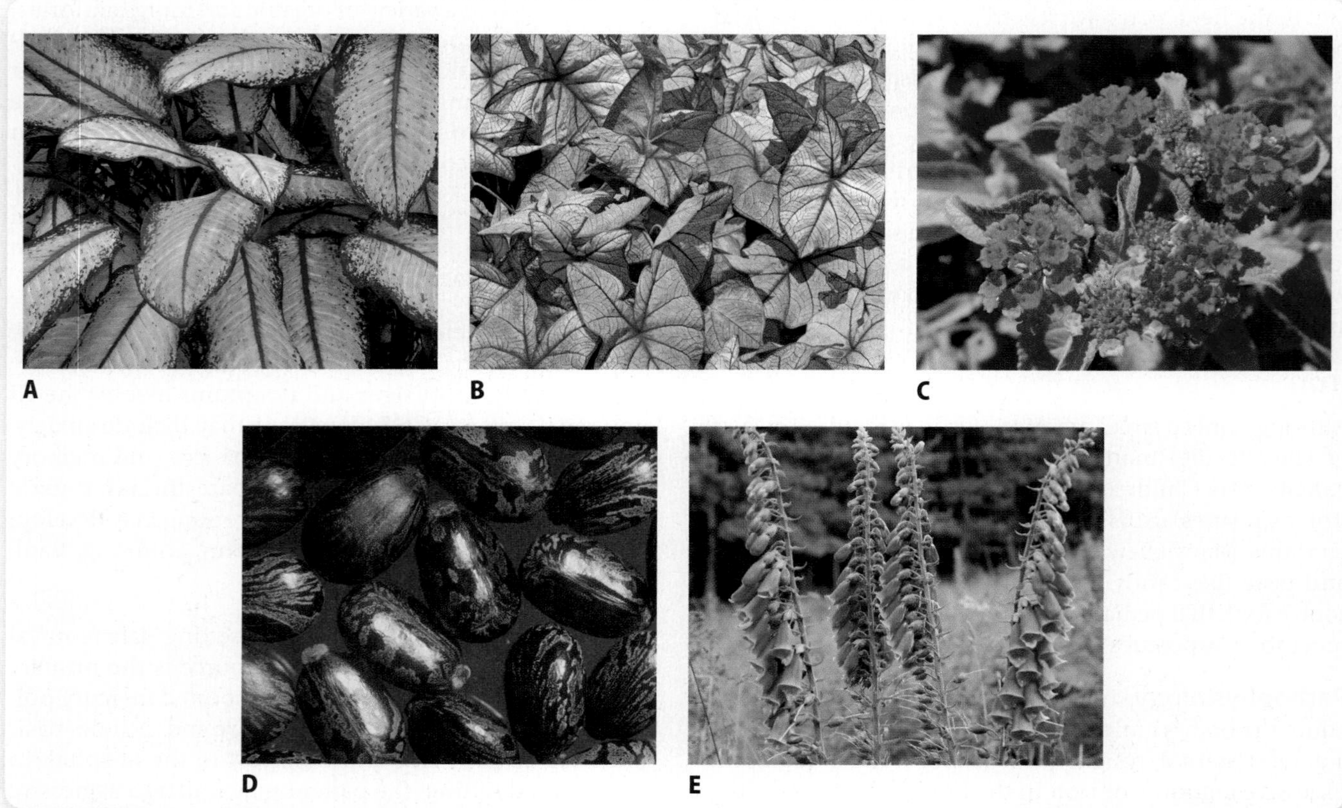

Figure 27-15 Poisonous plants. **A.** Dieffenbachia. **B.** Caladium. **C.** Lantana. **D.** Castor beans. **E.** Foxglove.

Thankfully, deaths from plant ingestions are rare; in 2014, only four fatal ingestions were reported in over 44,000 reported cases. Most plant ingestions result in minimal symptoms unless a large amount is ingested or the substance has been concentrated in a tea or paste. **Table 27-9** lists plants that can cause toxic results and, in some cases, death.

Pathophysiology

The ubiquitous **dieffenbachia** is a lovely green plant with broad, variegated leaves. It is nicknamed "dumb cane," because eating dieffenbachia can result in a person being unable to speak. All parts of the dieffenbachia plant—leaves, stems, and roots—contain sharp calcium oxalate

Table 27-9 Poisons in Some Common Plants

Plant	Poisonous Part	Poison	Signs and Symptoms of Poisoning
Apricot	Seeds	Cyanide	Headache, dizziness, weakness, nausea, vomiting, coma, seizures, metabolic acidosis
Autumn crocus	Entire plant	Colchicine	Delayed cramps, nausea, diarrhea, dehydration, coagulopathy, multiple organ failure
Azalea	Entire plant	Grayanotoxin	Nausea, salivation, vomiting, dizziness, dyspnea, cholinergic symptoms
Bloodroot	Root	Sanguinarine	Cramps, diarrhea, dizziness, paralysis, coma
Buttercup	Entire plant	Protoanemonin	Gastroenteritis, seizures
Caladium	Leaves and roots	Calcium oxalate	Burning of mucous membranes, swelling of the tongue and throat, salivation, gastroenteritis
Cherry tree	Bark, leaves, seed	Amygdalin	Stupor, vocal cord paralysis, seizures, coma
Chinaberry	Berry; leaves and bark to a lesser extent	Tetranortriterpenoid neurotoxins	Vomiting, diarrhea, sometimes excitement or depression
Daffodil	Bulb	Multiple	Gastroenteritis
Deadly nightshade	Berry, leaf, root	Atropine	Hyperthermia, seizures, hallucinations, anticholinergic symptoms
Dieffenbachia	Leaves and roots	Calcium oxalate	Mucosal damage similar to caladium
Elderberry	Leaf, shoot, bark	Sambunigrin	Gastroenteritis
Holly	Berries	Ilicin	Gastroenteritis, coma
Hyacinth	Bulb	Multiple	Severe gastroenteritis
Jack-in-the-pulpit	All parts	Calcium oxalate	Severe gastroenteritis
Jimson weed	All parts	Atropine	Dry mouth; hot, red skin; headache; hallucinations; tachycardia; hypertension; delirium; seizures
Laurel	All parts	Andromedotoxin	Salivation, lacrimation, rhinorrhea, vomiting, seizures, bradycardia, hypotension, paralysis
Lily of the valley	Leaf, flowers	Glycosides	Hyperkalemia, cardiac dysrhythmias, gastroenteritis, altered mental status

(continued)

Table 27-9 Poisons in Some Common Plants (Continued)			
Plant	**Poisonous Part**	**Poison**	**Signs and Symptoms of Poisoning**
Mistletoe	All parts	Tyramine	Bradycardia, gastroenteritis, hypertension, dyspnea, delirium, sweating, shock
Morning glory	Seeds	LSD	Hallucinations
Narcissus	Bulb	Multiple	Gastroenteritis
Oleander	Entire plant	Oleanin	Cramps, bradycardia, dilated pupils, bloody diarrhea, coma, apnea (one leaf is lethal)
Philodendron	Entire plant	Calcium oxalate	Edema of tongue, throat
Poinsettia	Leaves, stem, sap	Multiple	Contact dermatitis, gastroenteritis
Potato	Green tubers, new sprouts	Solanine	Severe gastroenteritis, headache, apnea, shock
Rhododendron	Entire plant	Grayanotoxin	Nausea, salivation, vomiting, dizziness, dyspnea, cholinergic symptoms
Rhubarb	Leaves only	Oxalic acid	Cramps, nausea, vomiting, anuria
Wisteria	Pods	Glycoside	Severe gastroenteritis, shock

Abbreviation: LSD, lysergic acid diethylamide

crystals. When ingested, the crystals cause burns of the mouth and tongue and, sometimes, paralysis of the vocal cords. In severe cases, edema of the tongue and larynx may lead to airway compromise. **Caladium**, with its stunning multicolored leaves, is another hazardous plant that has a similar presentation to dieffenbachia.

Azaleas and rhododendrons have a similar mechanism of toxicity based on grayanotoxins that are present in the plants. Ingestion of the leaves or flowers of the plants, as well as the nectar of honey made by the bees that feed on them, can cause cholinergic symptoms.[28]

Lantana (also known as red sage or wild sage) is a perennial flowering shrub with clusters of little red berries. These berries—particularly when ripe—can lead to serious poisoning. Even when still green, the berries contain lantadene A, a poison that causes GI upset, muscle weakness, shock, and sometimes death.

Another dangerous plant is the **castor bean**. The seeds of this attractive shrub are highly poisonous—chewing on just a few seeds (and, in some cases, just one) can kill a child. Ricin, the poison in castor beans, causes a variety of toxic effects: burning of the mouth and throat; nausea, vomiting, diarrhea, and severe stomach pains; prostration; failing vision; and kidney failure (the usual cause of death).

Foxglove, which has beautiful trumpet-like flowers, contains cardiac glycosides and is used in making the drug digitalis. Along with nausea, vomiting, diarrhea, and abdominal cramps, ingestion of foxglove can produce hyperkalemia and cardiac dysrhythmias, usually bradydysrhythmias.

Assessment

When you encounter a pediatric patient with plant poisoning, get all the information you can from the parent and/or caregiver, and then consult your regional poison center for advice, as follows:

- **When was the plant ingested?** If it was more than 12 hours ago and the patient is still asymptomatic, it is likely that the patient will not experience any medical emergencies. Most plant poisonings produce signs and symptoms of toxicity, if they are going to do so, within 4 hours of ingestion. One notable exception is the castor bean, for which symptoms may not appear until 1 to 3 days after ingestion.
- **What, exactly, did the child eat?** Try to find out not just which type of plant, but also which parts of the plant (leaves, root, stem, flower, or fruit) were eaten. If possible, then estimate how much was ingested (such as a bite or two from a leaf, or three or four leaves). If you transport the child to the hospital, then take the offending plant—or whatever is left of it—with you.
- **What signs or symptoms, if any, does the child have?**

Management

If the patient is symptomatic, then treat this ingestion like any other and initiate transport to the most appropriate facility. However, it is important to remember that most plant-related exposures require no treatment—a decision that can be made after consulting with the poison center and medical control per local protocol. If a responsible adult is present who can keep a close eye on the child for at least 4 to 6 hours after the ingestion, then there is no need to transport the child to the hospital.

▶ Poisonous Mushrooms

Four groups of people are most likely to experience poisoning related to mushroom ingestion: wild mushroom pickers, people looking for hallucinogenic mushrooms to get high, people attempting suicide or homicide, and young children who eat them by accident. Even among educated people who like to gather their own mushrooms in the wild, mistakes can happen. In 2014, poison centers received over 6,400 calls related to mushroom ingestions, with 55% of ingestions occurring in children younger than 6 years. Thankfully, most of these events result in limited or no toxic effects; only three fatal ingestions were reported.[25]

Pathophysiology

A variety of factors determine whether a mushroom ingestion will produce toxic results: the age of the mushroom, the season in which it was gathered, the amount ingested, and the preparation method. Toxic effects vary from mild GI signs and symptoms to severe cytotoxic—even lethal—effects. In the United States, deaths from mushroom ingestion usually involve the *Amanita* species (*Amanita phalloides, Amanita virosa,* and *Amanita verna*) **Figure 27-16**.

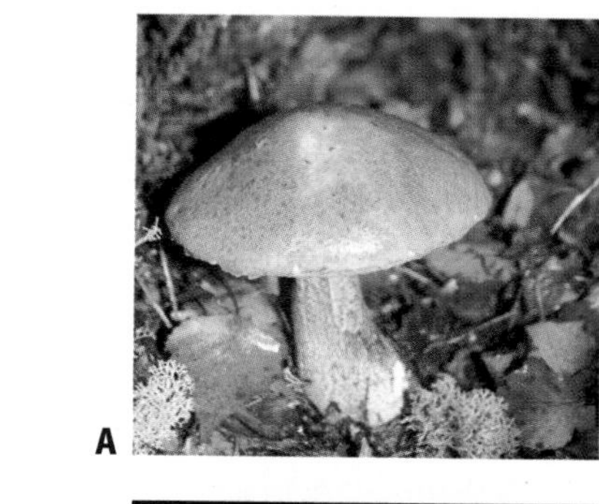
A

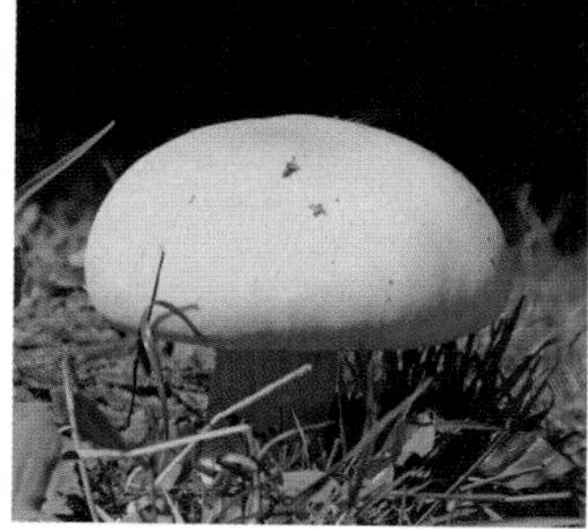
B

Figure 27-16 A. The deadly *Amanita* mushroom.
B. A nonpoisonous, edible mushroom.

Mushrooms are classified according to the toxins they produce. These classifications include cyclopeptides (amatoxins), gyromitrin, orellanine, muscarine, muscimol, coprine, psilocybin, and GI irritants.

Assessment

Time of symptom onset can serve as a predictor of potential severity. If the patient presents with symptoms within approximately 2 hours of ingestion, then the event is most likely to be non–life-threatening. By comparison, if symptom onset occurs 6 hours or later, a much greater likelihood exists that the event will be serious and potentially fatal. The most common patient complaints involve abdominal pain, diarrhea, vomiting, GI bleeding, anuria, and headache. Depending on the toxins involved, multiple organ failure may occur approximately 24 hours after ingestion. Hemodialysis may be required following kidney failure.

Management

Management for a symptomatic patient with a toxic mushroom ingestion includes supportive measures. Establish and maintain the airway, and establish vascular access. For hypotension secondary to vomiting and diarrhea, administer fluid boluses of normal saline. Contact the poison center and medical control per local protocol. Finally, transport the patient to an appropriate facility.

▶ Food Poisoning

Whenever you encounter two or more people sick at the same time and at the same scene with similar symptoms, think food poisoning or CO poisoning—your hunch will likely be correct. You also may be asked to evaluate patients who have grown concerned after being notified of food recalls by local grocery stores or restaurant chains.

Pathophysiology

Three toxins—*Salmonella, Listeria,* and *Toxoplasma*—are frequently associated with food-related deaths. Poisoning with *Clostridium botulinum,* an extremely deadly toxin, is usually the result of improper food storage or canning. In addition, the toxins produced by dinoflagellates in "red tides" may contaminate bivalve shellfish such as oysters, clams, and mussels and produce life-threatening or fatal paralytic shellfish poisoning. Cooking does not kill these toxins.

Assessment

Depending on the toxin, onset of signs and symptoms can range from several hours after ingestion to days or weeks. This delayed onset may make it difficult to isolate the offending agent while interviewing the patient. GI complaints are the most common and include abdominal pain, cramping, nausea, vomiting, and diarrhea. With prolonged episodes of vomiting or diarrhea, hypotension secondary to fluid loss and electrolyte imbalance becomes likely. Respiratory distress or arrest can occur with toxins such as *C botulinum* or those found in paralytic shellfish poisoning.

Management

Management for patients with food poisoning is usually supportive because most cases you encounter will not be life threatening, and the signs and symptoms of acute gastroenteritis are typically self-limiting. Manage the patient's airway or support his or her respiratory status with supplemental oxygen as needed. Establish vascular access and treat hypotension secondary to fluid loss with fluid boluses of normal saline. Consider administration of antiemetics, per local protocol. For patients with facial flushing (most likely secondary to histamine release), consider administration of diphenhydramine per local protocol. Finally, transport the patient to an appropriate facility.

Words of Wisdom

Herbal preparations can cause potentially serious interactions with traditional medications. Cases of overdose that involved herbal preparations have been reported. Be sure to determine all medications the patient may have taken, including herbal medications or supplements.

YOU are the Paramedic SUMMARY

1. What is your first impression of this patient?

The patient is in critical condition. As you begin your assessment and interview, you will likely have several thoughts regarding the possible cause of her condition. Stroke, hypoglycemia, sepsis, and overdose could be among the possible causes. After you have determined that the patient is acutely ill, begin setting priorities for patient care and searching for any reversible causes.

2. What is your priority for patient care?

The patient has a strong carotid pulse with respiratory depression. Take appropriate measures to maintain a patent airway while ensuring a proper ventilatory rate and tidal volume. Have suction prepared and ready at the patient's side. Placement of a nasopharyngeal or an oropharyngeal airway would be appropriate based on the patient's clinical presentation.

3. If this patient has overdosed, then which drug classification would be your focus?

The patient's most critical issue is the hypoventilation and respiratory depression. These issues are components of two major toxidromes: narcotic (opioid) and sedative-hypnotic. You can refine your differential diagnosis based on additional physical findings or by performing a thorough patient interview and scene survey to determine what drugs or medications may be present in the home.

4. Give some examples of drugs that would meet this classification.

Narcotic agents include morphine, codeine, heroin, fentanyl (Sublimaze), oxycodone (OxyContin), meperidine (Demerol), propoxyphene (Darvon), and dextromethorphan. Opioids are used primarily in clinical medicine for analgesia, whereas the illicit drug heroin is abused for the unique euphoria it produces. Sedative-hypnotics include barbiturates and benzodiazepines.

5. Should you intubate this patient?

Advanced airway management may be in this patient's future, but start with the basics first. Your initial action should be to provide supplemental oxygen and assisted ventilations with a bag-mask device. The patient has hypoventilation and hypercapnia. The elevated carbon dioxide levels may cause the patient to have an altered mental status. First correct the issues that you can have an immediate effect on, and then determine your next step after evaluating the patient's response to the treatment.

6. What is your next step in treating this patient after the airway is controlled?

As a paramedic, you should always be moving with purpose and trying to anticipate the future needs of the patient. Ensure the patient is connected to all of the appropriate monitoring equipment, including the cardiac monitor, noninvasive blood pressure monitor, pulse oximeter, and carbon dioxide detector (sidestream or connected to the bag-mask device). Obtain IV access and continue to search for the underlying cause of the patient's condition. While you will have a list of priorities for treatment, always be thinking: "If it is not this, then next I will search for that." Seizure, stroke, hypoglycemia, sepsis, and toxins should all be in your mind while treating this patient.

7. What is your medication choice and dosage to treat this patient?

Administer 0.4 to 2 mg of naloxone (Narcan). The best approach is to draw up 2 mg of naloxone in a 10-mL syringe and fill the rest of the syringe with normal saline. Administer the naloxone just to the point that the patient's respirations improve. You do not have to "wake the patient

YOU are the Paramedic SUMMARY (continued)

up" all the way; you simply need to improve the patient's respiratory status. Pushing too large of a dose or even an appropriate dose too rapidly may cause the patient to vomit or experience withdrawal. Both situations could harm the patient.

8. What should you do if this medication does not correct the overdose?

Sometimes the patient may not respond to naloxone, and some opioids may require higher doses of naloxone to combat the respiratory depression. This situation may also be a mixed overdose in which more than one drug was taken. If allowed by protocol, then repeat the naloxone dose or call for orders to increase the dose. Remember that basic airway maneuvers and successful bag-mask ventilation allow you more time to determine your next course of action. This patient may require advanced airway management. If the patient remains at high risk for aspiration, then protect the patient's airway and perform endotracheal intubation.

EMS Patient Care Report (PCR)					
Date: 08-10-18	**Incident No.:** 4563		**Nature of Call:** OD	**Location:** Edenvale Rd	
Dispatched: 1430	**En Route:** 1431	**At Scene:** 1438	**Transport:** 1450	**At Hospital:** 1510	**In Service:** 1530
Patient Information					
Age: 45 **Sex:** F **Weight (in kg [lb]):** 70 kg (154 lb)			**Allergies:** Unknown **Medications:** Hydrocodone **Past Medical History:** Back surgery **Chief Complaint:** Possible overdose		

Vital Signs				
Time: 1443	**BP:** 92/58	**Pulse:** 100	**Respirations:** 4	**Spo$_2$:** 90% on room air
Time: 1448	**BP:** 98/56	**Pulse:** 100	**Respirations:** Assisted	**Spo$_2$:** 96% O_2
Time: 1454	**BP:** 100/60	**Pulse:** 98	**Respirations:** 12	**Spo$_2$:** 97% O_2
Time: 1505	**BP:** 112/64	**Pulse:** 94	**Respirations:** 12	**Spo$_2$:** 98% O_2
Time: 1510	**BP:** 108/84	**Pulse:** 92	**Respirations:** 14	**Spo$_2$:** 98% O_2

EMS Treatment (circle all that apply)				
Oxygen @ 15 **L/min via (circle one):** **NC NRM (Bag-mask device)** (circled)		**Assisted Ventilation** (circled)	**Airway Adjunct:** NPA (circled)	**CPR**
Defibrillation	**Bleeding Control**	**Bandaging**	**Splinting**	**Other:**

Narrative
Arrived on scene to find female pt lying supine in bed. Pt has PMH of recent back surgery and prescription narcotic use (hydrocodone 10 mg). Last seen normal time @ 0800 this morning. Pt is unconscious with a resp of 4 per min. The pt has a strong carotid pulse. Airway maintained with NPA and bag-mask device at 15 L/min assisted to a rate of 12 breaths/min. Sinus tachycardia on the monitor. IV established, BGL is 120 mg/dL. Found fentanyl patches on pt's back and removed. Naloxone (Narcan) administered at 0.4 mg IVP without change. Dose repeated × 2 per protocol with an increase in respiratory effort noted. Pt responds to painful stimuli post Narcan and is able to maintain airway. Pt transported emergency to regional hospital. Report to Dr. Phillips on arrival.**End of report**

Prep Kit

▶ Ready for Review

- Toxicologic emergencies can be categorized as either unintentional or intentional.
- Both licit and illicit drugs are constantly evolving. You may also encounter patients with complex presentations involving multiple substances that have different pharmacokinetics. For these reasons, poison centers may be an indispensable aid.
- The four primary methods whereby a toxin commonly enters the body are ingestion, inhalation, injection, and absorption.
- Toxidromes can help you work toward identifying the toxic substance in situations where that information is not readily available. After you conduct your assessment and have identified the presentation, you can proceed with a focused treatment plan.
- As a paramedic, you will encounter patients involved in substance abuse. The physiologic and societal effects of alcohol abuse are well known and thoroughly documented. Effects of new drugs and new variations are more difficult to know and document due to their continual evolution.
- Generally, patients with toxicologic emergencies are considered medical patients, although toxicologic emergencies may lead to trauma, too.
- Maintain a high level of situational awareness when responding to toxicologic emergencies. Patients who have taken an overdose may be extremely dangerous.
- Basic airway management is important in these patients and is a mainstay of the primary survey.
- Obtain as much information about the substance as possible, early in the call.
- Management for toxicologic emergencies includes ALS care built on the basics:
  - Ensure the scene is safe for access and egress.
  - Maintain the airway; secure it as needed.
  - Ensure that breathing is adequate.
  - Ensure that circulation is not compromised (by hypoperfusion or dysrhythmia).
  - Maintain adequate blood/oxygen saturation levels (95%).
  - Establish vascular access.
  - Consider administration of an antidote, if available.
  - Be prepared to manage shock, coma, seizures, and dysrhythmias.
  - Transport the patient as soon as possible. Place the patient in the left lateral recumbent position if any risk of vomiting exists to reduce the risk of aspiration.
- Additional management for stimulant abuse includes obtaining an ECG, pulse oximetry level, and capnography reading; administering benzodiazepines per local protocol for anxiety and seizures; and managing hypotension with fluid resuscitation.
- Marijuana use is legal in some states for medical purposes and in other states for any purpose. Management of these patients is primarily supportive and may include benzodiazepines for sedation.
- Hallucinogens include LSD, PCP, and ketamine. Emergency medical care is primarily supportive, with scene safety remaining a concern; IM sedatives may be necessary. Benzodiazepines may be helpful in calming a patient who is delirious as a result of ketamine use.
- Sedative hypnotics include barbiturates and benzodiazepines. In patients who have used barbiturates, CNS depression is likely, making airway management critical. Benzodiazepines, while also a prehospital agent for sedation, are also a potential substance of abuse. A reversal agent is available for benzodiazepine overdose.
- Opioids have become the driving cause of most overdose deaths. Management of a patient with narcotic, opiate, and opioid overdose focuses on airway management. Naloxone (Narcan) may be administered to improve the patient's spontaneous respiratory effort. Follow the American Heart Association algorithm for management of a life-threatening opioid overdose.
- An additional step when a patient has organophosphate poisoning is to perform decontamination prior to assessment and management. Specific medications such as atropine and pralidoxime may be required. Also perform pulse oximetry, capnometry, and ECG monitoring.
- If a patient has carbon monoxide poisoning, then remove the patient from the exposure environment, provide the highest concentration of oxygen possible, establish IV access, and perform ECG monitoring.
- For a caustic ingestion, identify the specific substance and contact the poison control center or online medical control for further instructions.
- Contact medical control regarding use of activated charcoal; it is often contraindicated when the exact ingested substance(s) is unknown. It typically may be used with 1 hour of ingestion in the following overdoses: known long-acting barbiturate, tricyclic antidepressant, selective serotonin reuptake inhibitor, salicylate, or acetaminophen. It also may be used with most cardiac medication overdoses. The patient must be able to maintain his or her own airway prior to and during administration.

Prep Kit *(continued)*

- Hydrocarbons may be inhaled or ingested. The primary treatment goal for a patient who has inhaled hydrocarbons is removal from the exposure environment, administration of high-concentration oxygen, and prompt transport. The primary treatment goal for a patient how has ingested hydrocarbons is decontamination, high-flow oxygen administration, ECG monitoring, and fluid resuscitation if hypotension is present.
- Most ingested plant poisonings are treated like any other ingestion. Most plant-related exposures require no treatment, but this decision should be determined by poison control.

▶ Vital Vocabulary

alcoholism A disorder characterized by a physical and psychological addiction to ethanol.

amphetamines A class of drugs that increase alertness and excitation (stimulants); includes methamphetamine (crank or ice), methylenedioxyamphetamine (MDA, Adam), and methylenedioxymethamphetamine (MDMA, Eve, Ecstasy).

antagonist A molecule that blocks the ability of a given chemical to bind to its receptor, preventing a biologic response.

antidote Something to counteract the effect of a poison.

barbiturates Potent sedative-hypnotics historically used as sleep aids, antianxiety drugs, and as part of the regimen for seizure control; include drugs such as thiopental (Pentothal, Trapanal) and methohexital (Brevital).

benzodiazepines The family of sedative-hypnotics that provide muscle relaxation and mild sedation; most commonly used to treat anxiety, seizures, and alcohol withdrawal; include drugs such as diazepam (Valium) and midazolam (Versed).

caladium A common houseplant that contains calcium oxalate crystals; ingestion leads to nausea, vomiting, and diarrhea.

castor bean A seed that contains the poison ricin; causes a variety of toxic effects: burning of the mouth and throat; nausea, vomiting, diarrhea, and severe stomach pains; prostration; failing vision; and kidney failure, which is the usual cause of death.

caustics Chemicals that are acids or alkalis; cause direct chemical injury to the tissues they contact.

chemical suicide A method of suicide that involves mixing certain household chemicals in an enclosed space to create toxic gases, such as hydrogen sulfide and hydrogen cyanide, as the chemicals combine; also called detergent suicide.

cocaine A stimulant; a naturally occurring alkaloid that is extracted from the *Erythroxylon coca* plant leaves found in South America.

delirium tremens (DTs) A severe withdrawal syndrome seen in people with alcoholism who are deprived of ethyl alcohol; characterized by restlessness, fever, sweating, disorientation, agitation, and seizures; can be fatal if untreated.

dieffenbachia A common houseplant that is also called dumb cane; ingestion leads to burns of the mouth and tongue and, possibly, paralysis of the vocal cords and nausea and vomiting; in severe cases, edema of the tongue and larynx, leading to airway compromise.

drug Substance that has some therapeutic effect (such as reducing inflammation, fighting bacteria, or producing euphoria) when given in the appropriate circumstances and in the appropriate dose.

drug abuse Any use of drugs that causes physical, psychological, economic, legal, or social harm to the user or others affected by the user's behavior.

drug addiction A chronic disorder characterized by the compulsive use of a substance that results in physical, psychological, or social harm to the user who continues to use the substance despite the harm.

DUMBELS An acronym that represents the symptoms of organophosphate poisoning: diarrhea, urination, miosis, bradycardia, bronchospasm, bronchorrhea, emesis, lacrimation, seizures, salivation, and sweating.

foxglove A plant that contains cardiac glycosides used in making digitalis; ingestion of leaves causes nausea, vomiting, diarrhea, abdominal cramps, hyperkalemia, and a variety of dysrhythmias.

habituation A physical tolerance and psychological dependence on a drug or drugs.

hallucinogen An agent that produces false perceptions in any one of the five senses.

hydrocarbons Compounds made up principally of hydrogen and carbon atoms mostly obtained from the distillation of petroleum.

illicit In relation to drugs, illegal drugs such as marijuana, cocaine, and lysergic acid diethylamide.

lantana A perennial flowering shrub with clusters of red berries that can lead to serious and even fatal poisoning. Also known as red sage or wild sage; ingestion causes stomach upsets, muscle weakness, shock, and, sometimes, death.

Prep Kit (continued)

licit In relation to drugs, legalized drugs such as coffee, alcohol, and tobacco.

lithium A common mood stabilizer used in the treatment of bipolar disorder.

marijuana The dried leaves and flower buds of the *Cannabis sativa* plant that are smoked to achieve a high.

methamphetamine A highly addictive drug in the amphetamine family.

monoamine oxidase inhibitors (MAOIs) Psychiatric medication used primarily to treat atypical depression by increasing norepinephrine and serotonin levels in the central nervous system.

narcotic The generic term for opiates and opioids, drugs that act as a central nervous system depressant and produce insensibility or stupor.

opiate Various alkaloids derived from the opium or poppy plant.

opioid A synthetic narcotic not derived from opium, with sedative properties; examples are fentanyl (Sublimaze) and alfentanil (Alfenta); also called narcotics.

organophosphates A class of chemical found in many insecticides used in agriculture and in the home.

overdose A condition that occurs when a drug (either licit or illicit) is taken in excess; can have toxic or lethal consequences.

physical dependence A physiologic state of adaptation to a drug, usually characterized by tolerance to the effects of the drug and a withdrawal syndrome if use of the drug is stopped, especially abruptly.

poison A substance whose chemical action could damage structures or impair function when introduced into the body.

potentiation Enhancement of the effect of one drug by another drug.

psychological dependence The emotional state of craving a drug to maintain a feeling of well-being.

rhabdomyolysis The destruction of muscle tissue leading to a release of potassium and myoglobin.

salicylates Chemicals found in plants and a primary ingredient in aspirin.

sedative-hypnotic A drug used to reduce anxiety, calm agitated patients, and help produce drowsiness and sleep (central nervous system depressants).

selective serotonin reuptake inhibitors (SSRIs) A class of antidepressants that inhibit the reuptake of serotonin.

serotonin syndrome An idiosyncratic complication that occurs with antidepressant therapy in which patients have lower extremity muscle rigidity, confusion or disorientation, and/or agitation.

spice An illicit drug consisting of a blend of synthetic cannabinoids; it can produce delirium and short- and long-term psychotic effects.

synergism The action of two substances such as drugs, in which the total effects are greater than the sum of the independent effects of the two substances.

tolerance Physiologic adaptation to the effects of a drug such that increasingly larger doses of the drug are required to achieve the same effect.

toxicologic emergencies Medical emergencies caused by toxic agents such as poison; may be intentional or unintentional.

toxicology The study of toxic or poisonous substances.

toxidrome The syndrome-like symptoms of any given class or group of poisonous agents.

toxin A poison or harmful substance produced by bacteria, animals, or plants.

tricyclic antidepressants (TCAs) A group of drugs used to treat severe depression and manage pain; minimal dosing errors can cause toxic results.

withdrawal syndrome A predictable set of signs and symptoms, usually involving altered central nervous system activity that occurs after the abrupt cessation of a drug or after rapidly decreasing the usual dosage of a drug.

▶ References

1. Poison statistics: national data 2014. National Capital Poison Center website. http://www.poison.org/poison-statistics-national. Accessed May 21, 2016.
2. Chemical suicides: the risk to emergency responders. Chemical Hazards Emergency Medical Management website. https://chemm.nlm.nih.gov/chemicalsuicide.htm. Published November 14, 2014. Accessed March 1, 2017.
3. Anderson A. Chemical suicides and the adverse impact on responders and bystanders. November 22, 2016. http://www.physiciansnewsnetwork.com/westjem/article_845ddf32-b10e-11e6-b114-f75c56b76600.html. Accessed March 1, 2017.
4. WebWISER home. U.S. National Library of Medicine. National Institutes of Health, Health & Human Services. https://webwiser.nlm.nih.gov. Accessed December 16, 2016.
5. New CDC study finds dramatic increase in e-cigarette-related calls to poison centers. Centers for Disease Control and Prevention website. https://www.cdc.gov/media/releases/2014/p0403-e-cigarette-poison.html. Published April 3, 2014. Accessed March 1, 2017.

Prep Kit *(continued)*

6. Alcohol facts and statistics. National Institute on Alcohol Abuse and Alcoholism (NIAAA) website. http://www.niaaa.nih.gov/alcohol-health/overview-alcohol-consumption/alcohol-facts-and-statistics. Published January 2016. Accessed May 30, 2016.
7. American Psychiatric Association. *Diagnostic and Statistical Manual of Mental Disorders,* 5th ed. Washington, DC: APA; 2013.
8. Alcohol and cancer risk. National Cancer Institute website. http://www.cancer.gov/about-cancer/causes-prevention/risk/alcohol/alcohol-fact-sheet. Published June 24, 2013. Accessed May 30, 2016.
9. State of California Department of Motor Vehicles. *California Driver Handbook - Alcohol and Drugs.* https://www.dmv.ca.gov/portal/dmv/detail/pubs/hdbk/actions_drink. Accessed March 1, 2017.
10. O'Malley GF, O'Malley R. Alcohol toxicity and withdrawal. *Merck Manuals Professional Edition.* https://www.merckmanuals.com/professional/special-subjects/recreational-drugs-and-intoxicants/alcohol-toxicity-and-withdrawal. Published January 2016. Accessed June 27, 2016.
11. National survey of drug use and health. National Institute on Drug Abuse (NIDA) website. https://www.drugabuse.gov/national-survey-drug-use-health. Accessed June 4, 2016.
12. Cocaine overview: pharmacology. MethOIDE - methamphetamine and other illicit drug education website http://methoide.fcm.arizona.edu/infocenter/index.cfm?stid=170. Accessed March 1, 2017.
13. Communications NYU. Rolling on Molly: US high school seniors underreport ecstasy use when not asked about Molly. http://www.nyu.edu/about/news-publications/news/2016/june/rolling-on-molly-us-high-school-seniors-underreport-ecstasy-use-when-not-asked-about-molly.html. Published June 9, 2016. Accessed March 1, 2017.
14. Stores C. Is flakka gone for good? http://www.cnn.com/2016/04/18/health/flakka-drug-disappearance/. Published April 18, 2016. Accessed March 1, 2017.
15. Synthetic cathinones ("bath salts"). National Institute on Drug Abuse (NIDA) website. DrugFacts: https://www.drugabuse.gov/publications/drugfacts/synthetic-cathinones-bath-salts. Published January 2016. Accessed June 4, 2016.
16. O'Malley GF, O'Malley R. Marijuana (cannabis). *Merck Manuals Professional Edition.* https://www.merckmanuals.com/professional/special-subjects/recreational-drugs-and-intoxicants/marijuana-cannabis. Published January 2016. Accessed June 4, 2016.
17. Acute marijuana intoxication. Children's Hospital Colorado website. https://www.childrenscolorado.org/conditions-and-advice/conditions-and-symptoms/conditions/acute-marijuana-intoxication/. Accessed March 4, 2017.
18. O'Malley GF, O'Malley R. Anxiolytics and sedatives. *Merck Manuals Professional Edition.* http://www.merckmanuals.com/professional/special-subjects/recreational-drugs-and-intoxicants/anxiolytics-and-sedatives. Published January 2016. Accessed June 5, 2016.
19. Benson BE, Hoppu K, Troutman WG, et al. Position paper update: gastric lavage for gastrointestinal decontamination. *Clin Toxicol.* 2013;51(3):140-146.
20. Rudd RA, Aleshire N, Zibbell JE, Gladden RM. Increases in drug and opioid overdose deaths—United States, 2000–2014. *Morb Mortal Wkly Rep.* 2016;64(50-51):1378-1382.
21. Cliff RM, Woodcock J, Ostroff S. A proactive response to prescription opioid abuse. http://www.nejm.org/doi/pdf/10.1056/nejmsr1601307. Published February 4, 2016. Accessed June 5, 2016.
22. Bertolote JM, Fleischmann A, Eddleston M, Gunnell D. Deaths from pesticide poisoning: are we lacking a global response? *Br J Psychiatry.* 2006;189:201-203. https://www.ncbi.nlm.nih.gov/pmc/articles/PMC2493385/. Published September 2006. Accessed March 2, 2017.
23. Preventing carbon monoxide poisoning after an emergency. Centers for Disease Control and Prevention website. https://www.cdc.gov/disasters/cofacts.html. Updated June 20, 2014. Accessed February 27, 2017.
24. Sircar K, Clower J, Shin M-K, Bailey C, King M, Yip F. Carbon monoxide poisoning deaths in the United States, 1999 to 2012. *Am J Emerg Med.* http://www.sciencedirect.com/science/article/pii/S0735675715003800. Published May 7, 2015. Accessed December 4, 2016.
25. Mowry JB, Spyker DA, Brooks DE, McMillan N, Schauben JL. 2014 Annual Report of the American Association of Poison Control Centers' National Poison Data System (NPDS): 32nd Annual Report. *Clin Toxicol.* 2015;53(10):962-1146.
26. O'Malley GF, O'Malley R. Gamma hydroxybutyrate. *Merck Manuals Professional Edition.* https://www.merckmanuals.com/professional/special-subjects/recreational-drugs-and-intoxicants/gamma-hydroxybutyrate. Published January 2016. Accessed June 14, 2016.
27. O'Malley GF, O'Malley R. Specific poisons. *Merck Manuals Professional Edition.* http://www.merckmanuals.com/professional/injuries-poisoning/poisoning/specific-poisons. Published May 2015. Accessed June 15, 2016.
28. Mekonnen S. Azaleas and rhododendrons. http://www.poison.org/articles/2015-mar/azaleas-and-rhododendrons. Accessed June 27, 2016.

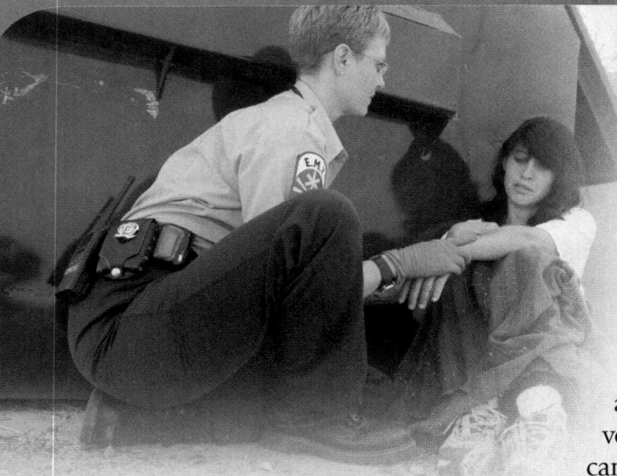

Assessment *in Action*

You respond to reports of a patient experiencing a psychiatric emergency who is "high on something." Local law enforcement officers have detained a man who is approximately 25 years old. As you approach this patient, you hear him shouting loudly and observe him banging his head on the window of the police vehicle. The man is naked with his arms restrained behind him. You can see he has an obvious forearm fracture of his left arm. Despite the fracture, the man is still swinging his arms violently behind him.

1. The officers report that the man was found wandering through traffic without any clothes on and with an obviously deformed left arm. When they attempted to detain the man, he became aggressive, and it took six officers to detain the subject. If this patient has used illicit drugs, then which of the following classification would fit his presentation?

A. Sedatives
B. Narcotics
C. Sympathomimetics
D. Hallucinogens

2. Which of the following statements does NOT increase your index of suspicion that the patient is under the influence of some type of illicit substance?

A. He was found naked and wandering through traffic.
B. He is in handcuffs.
C. It took six law enforcement officers to restrain him.
D. Despite an obvious forearm fracture, he remains combative.

3. Which consideration should be at the forefront of your mind regarding your approach to this patient?

A. Closest hospital
B. Scene safety and proper PPE
C. Proper sedative medication
D. Need for more physical restraints

4. You note that the patient is potentially experiencing a stimulant overdose. Which other symptom fits for the sympathomimetic toxidrome?

A. Dry skin
B. Diaphoresis
C. Bradycardia
D. Constricted pupils

5. What is the primary treatment of the patient in this scenario?

A. Chemical sedation with benzodiazepines
B. Nitroprusside administration to decrease his blood pressure
C. Rapid cooling with cold fluids
D. Rapid sequence intubation

6. Which other differential diagnosis should you have for this patient?

A. Psychotic episode
B. Excited delirium
C. Heatstroke
D. Alcohol intoxication

7. In a patient with suspected excited delirium, what would you expect to happen regarding the patient's core temperature?

A. Elevated
B. Decreased
C. Variable
D. No change

8. As you prepare for transport, which of the following positions is NOT indicated for this patient?

A. Supine
B. Trendelenburg
C. Semi-Fowler
D. Hogtied

9. What does the DUMBELS mnemonic stand for, and which type of chemical exposure causes it?

10. Why do patients who experience a tricyclic antidepressant overdose develop a widened QRS complex?

CHAPTER 28

Psychiatric Emergencies

National EMS Education Standard Competencies

Medicine

Integrates assessment findings with principles of epidemiology and pathophysiology to formulate a field impression and implement a comprehensive treatment/disposition plan for a patient with a medical complaint.

Psychiatric

Recognition of

- Behaviors that pose a risk to the EMS provider, patient, or others (pp 1452, 1457-1458, 1471-1472)

Assessment and management of

- Basic principles of the mental health system (p 1452)
- Suicidal/risk (pp 1470-1471)

Anatomy, physiology, epidemiology, pathophysiology, psychosocial impact, presentations, assessment, prognosis, and management of

- Acute psychosis (pp 1467-1469)
- Agitated delirium (pp 1469-1470)
- Cognitive disorders (pp 1469-1470)
- Thought disorders (pp 1467-1469)
- Mood disorders (pp 1472-1474)
- Neurotic disorders (pp 1474-1476)
- Substance-related disorders/addictive behavior (p 1476)
- Somatoform disorders (p 1476)
- Factitious disorders (pp 1476-1477)
- Personality disorders (pp 1477-1478)
- Patterns of violence/abuse/neglect (pp 1471-1472)
- Organic psychoses (p 1454)

Knowledge Objectives

1. Discuss the possible causes of behavioral emergencies, including drug overdoses, violent behavior, and mental illness. (p 1452)
2. Define normal, abnormal, overt, and covert behavior. (p 1452)
3. Identify the prevalence of mental illness in the United States. (p 1453)
4. Discuss medicolegal considerations and its role in psychiatric emergencies. (pp 1453-1454)
5. Discuss the organic and environmental causes of abnormal behavior. (pp 1454-1455)
6. Explain how psychiatric signs and symptoms are categorized. (pp 1455-1456)
7. Describe the assessment process for patients with psychiatric emergencies, including safety guidelines and specific questions to ask. (pp 1455-1460)
8. Discuss the importance of history taking in assessing a patient with a psychiatric emergency. (p 1459)
9. Identify strategies for communicating with patients during behavioral crises. (pp 1460-1462)
10. Discuss general management of a patient with a psychiatric emergency. (pp 1460-1462)
11. Compare physical restraint with chemical restraint, including examples of when each might be used and situations in which the use of restraint might be justified. (pp 1463-1466)
12. Describe the emergency medical care of a patient with psychosis. (pp 1467-1469)
13. Describe the emergency medical care of a patient with agitated delirium. (p 1470)
14. Explain how to recognize the behavior of a patient at risk of suicide, including the management of such a patient. (pp 1470-1471)
15. Discuss factors indicating that a patient is at risk of becoming violent. (pp 1471-1472)
16. Explain the safe management of a potentially violent patient. (p 1472)
17. List specific psychiatric disorders that can be characterized by a state of acute psychosis or agitated delirium. (pp 1472-1478)
18. Discuss assessment and management of specific psychiatric emergencies, including those related to mood disorders, schizophrenia, neurotic disorders, substance abuse, somatoform disorders, factitious disorders, impulse control disorders, and personality disorders. (pp 1472-1478)
19. Discuss medications used to treat psychiatric disorders and manage behavioral emergencies. (pp 1478-1481)
20. Recognize issues specific to posttraumatic stress disorder and the returning combat veteran. (pp 1481-1482)

Skills Objectives

1. Demonstrate the technique used to perform four-point physical restraint of a patient. (pp 1463-1465, Skill Drill 28-1)

Introduction

The mind and the body are not separate entities; they are inseparable parts of a whole human being. When a person becomes ill with any disease, that illness will inevitably affect the person's behavior, often making the person anxious or depressed. Similarly, changes in mental state affect the body's physical health. A person with depression, for example, may lose his or her appetite or become more susceptible to bodily disease. Thus, whenever you examine a patient, you must view the patient as a whole person. Try to learn both the physical and the mental factors that contribute to the patient's distress.

As a paramedic, you can expect to care for patients undergoing a psychological or behavioral crisis. This chapter covers various kinds of behavioral emergencies. These emergencies can involve overdoses, violent behavior, and mental illness. This chapter will also cover legal concerns in the emergency medical care of patients who are disturbed.

Definition of Behavioral Emergency

The concept of **behavior** has been debated over the years, with most experts defining it as the way people act or perform, such as the way they respond to a situation. Behavior includes all the things people do and the reasons they do those things. Who defines abnormal and normal behavior is a source of debate. These concepts can be defined by society in general, a particular community or social group, a parent, a boss, a friend, or even a stranger. Both normal and abnormal behavior may be overt. **Overt behaviors** are open and generally understood by those around the person. **Covert behaviors** are those that have hidden meanings or intentions that only the person with the behavior understands.

Abnormal behavior in itself may not be a medical condition and is hardly cause for alarm. The real questions are, "When does abnormal behavior require medical intervention?" and "When does it require emergency medical services (EMS)?" Almost all disordered behavior represents the person's effort to adapt to some stress, whether internal or external. The disruptive behavior usually is temporary, fading when the person has managed to mobilize his or her psychological defense mechanisms.

Behavioral emergencies are situations in which the patient's presenting problem is some disorder of mood, thought, or behavior that interferes with his or her **activities of daily living (ADLs)**. ADLs are normal, everyday activities such as getting dressed and taking out the garbage. When a person becomes so depressed that he or she cannot get up in the morning, shower, and make breakfast, or when someone has **delusions** (false beliefs) or **hallucinations** (sense perceptions not founded on objective reality) that prohibit holding a job, the condition becomes a behavioral emergency.

A **psychiatric emergency** occurs when the abnormal behavior threatens a person's health and safety or the health and safety of another person. In the most extreme cases, a person has a suicidal, homicidal, or psychotic episode. In a psychotic episode, a person often experiences delusions or hallucinations and illusions (errors in perception) that result in loss of contact with reality. For example, a patient who has taken illicit drugs may experience an alteration of reality—a "bad trip." Psychotic episodes can be dangerous for the patient, bystanders, and you because the patient may display violent behavior, usually from exaggerated fear or paranoia.

Regardless of how textbooks define a psychiatric emergency, the operative definition of a behavioral or psychiatric emergency is given by the person who dials 9-1-1. A behavioral or psychiatric emergency often becomes an "emergency" because of panic on the part of the patient, the family, bystanders, or all of these parties. That panic, in turn, may translate into a demand for action on your part, and you may therefore face intense pressure to do something. For example, you may be pressured to transport the patient to an emergency department (ED). Paradoxically, it's precisely in this

YOU are the Paramedic — PART 1

A call dispatches you to the third floor of an apartment building for a 44-year-old man who says he fears for his life. You learn that police have been on scene with this patient for 20 minutes, and the patient won't leave his apartment. The apartment building is known to house residents with psychiatric disorders. As you arrive at the building, a police officer directs you to the elevator and tells you that the patient is not armed, but officers are remaining on scene in case he becomes violent.

You go to the third floor, where another officer meets you. He informs you that the police were called to the scene by the patient, who had stated that someone was trying to kill him. He told officers that he had overheard information that was not meant for him, and now someone is planning to kill him. The door to the apartment is open, and the patient is visible. He doesn't appear to have a weapon but refuses to leave the apartment or let anyone in.

1. What are the initial components of the assessment for this patient?
2. What are your safety concerns in dealing with this patient?

situation—when the patient is behaving strangely and bystanders are clamoring for action—that you may feel least able to do something.

You may have difficulty performing to the best of your ability when you're trying to understand the confused and frayed feelings that the patient often presents during a psychiatric emergency. Some paramedics may feel more comfortable dealing with straightforward problems such as fractures of the legs, cardiac dysrhythmias, or narcotic overdoses. Paramedics tend to be action-oriented people who like to see tangible results, such as a patient with hypoglycemia improving after a bolus of glucose, or a clinically dead patient restored to life by cardiopulmonary resuscitation and defibrillation. What tangible rewards can you gain in escorting a confused, hallucinating patient to a medical facility, or caring for a belligerent and violent patient who is screaming obscenities?

In fact, prehospital behavioral intervention *is* possible and often critical in these emergencies. You can make a difference in the life of a patient who is disturbed, and you can learn these skills just like any other skill. Indeed, these skills you learn for dealing with abnormal behavior ultimately may be much more important to your work than more tangible skills such as endotracheal intubation. How many of your calls require you to place an advanced airway? Many more calls require you to care for people who are angry, depressed, agitated, panicky, or out of control. Clearly, you'll benefit greatly by learning how to take an organized and systematic approach to emergencies that involve abnormal behavior.

Prevalence

According to the Centers for Disease Control and Prevention (CDC), the average number of mentally unhealthy days (those including stress, **depression**, and problems with emotions) for Americans has increased. In 1993, Americans reported an average of 2.9 mentally unhealthy days per month, but by 2008, this number had increased to 3.4 days, where it remains today.[1]

According to a 2014 study published by the US Department of Health and Human Services, an estimated 43.5 million adults age 18 years or older were estimated to have had a mental illness in the past year.[2] This figure represents 18.1% of all adults in the United States.[2] Almost 10 million adults age 18 years or older, representing 4.1% of the American population, are estimated to have had a serious mental illness within the past year. Serious mental illness was generally defined as a diagnosis of a psychiatric disorder, for example, with serious functional impairment.[2] The prevalence of serious mental illness among specific age groups and ethnicities is shown in Table 28-1. Results from the same survey showed that 39.8 million Americans, age 18 years or older, an estimated 16.6% of the population, are considered current illicit drug users, a compounding factor in many mental illnesses.[2]

Table 28-1 Prevalence of Serious Mental Illness in Selected US Population Subgroups

Population	Prevalence of Serious Mental Illness (% of population)
Sex	
Women, 18 years or older	5.0
Men, 18 years or older	3.1
Employment	
Unemployed adults	6.7
Employed adults, part-time	4.2
Employed adults, full-time	2.9
Race	
Caucasian	4.4
Native American or Alaska Native	4.0
Hispanic	3.5
African American	3.1
Asian	2.4

Data from: Center for Behavioral Health Statistics and Quality. *2014 National Survey on Drug Use and Health: Mental Health Detailed Tables*. Rockville, MD: Substance Abuse and Mental Health Services Administration; 2015. https://www.samhsa.gov/data/sites/default/files/NSDUH-MHDetTabs2014/NSDUH-MHDetTabs2014.pdf. Accessed March 13, 2017.

Medicolegal Considerations

Every call has potential legal complications, especially calls for behavioral emergencies. When a patient's behavior, speech, and thoughts are erratic and disorganized, you may encounter difficulty in communicating clearly and understanding the situation. Be prepared to spend time with the patient. Don't be in a hurry; rather, convey the message that you have the time and concern to learn what is bothering the patient. Obtain consent as with any other patient when possible. If the patient refuses to engage with you, then continue to talk with him or her about the situation. Explain your responsibilities now that you have been called to the scene and have responded.

If the patient refuses transportation, then follow your local protocols and standing orders for providing transport against the patient's will. You will often need help from law enforcement personnel. In most jurisdictions, paramedics (and others) are not allowed to restrain or transport people against their will except possibly at the express order of a county mental health physician.

Be clear in explaining the treatments and medications you will administer. Don't assume that the patient is unable to understand what you're doing, regardless of the patient's state of mind. As always, include the patient in his or her own care as much as possible. As you take more time to assess and manage a patient with mental health concerns, you must take extra time to thoroughly record the call. Be objective and factual, and include comments the patient makes. Communicating well, following standards and protocols, and having patience will be your best protection against legal action.

Pathophysiology

Causes of Abnormal Behavior

Abnormal behavior typically results from a complex interaction of biologic or organic causes, developmental factors, psychological stressors, emotional stimuli, and sociocultural influences. These causes can be classified into four broad categories: (1) causes that are biologic or organic, (2) causes resulting from the person's environment, (3) causes resulting from acute injury or illness, and (4) causes that are substance-related.

Biologic or Organic Causes

Many patients who present with psychiatric symptoms are actually affected by biologic or organic factors that interfere with normal cerebral function. Such patients were previously described as having **organic brain syndrome**. This term encompassed disorders that were due to organic or physiologic causes as opposed to purely psychiatric causes. The distinction was somewhat arbitrary, however; we now know that many people with what were previously thought to be nonorganic abnormalities actually do have physiologic dysfunction in the brain causing their psychiatric illness. Examples of biologic or organic causes of abnormal behavior include conditions such as chronic hypoxia, seizure, traumatic brain injury, chronic alcohol and drug abuse, and brain tumors (Table 28-2). These conditions alter the normal functioning of the brain and may cause derangements in behavior. The most common offenders are probably alcohol and drugs, but you also should consider dementia and delirium.

Table 28-2 Selected Disease States That May Produce Psychotic Symptoms

Disease State	Psychotic Symptoms
Toxic and deficiency states	Drug-induced psychoses, especially from: ▪ Digitalis ▪ Steroids ▪ Disulfiram ▪ Amphetamines ▪ LSD, PCP, and other psychedelics Nutrition disorders: ▪ Alcohol abuse ▪ Vitamin deficiencies Poisoning with bromide or other heavy metals: ▪ Kidney failure ▪ Liver failure
Infections	▪ Syphilis ▪ Parasites ▪ Viral encephalitis (eg, after measles) ▪ Brain abscess
Neurologic disease	▪ Seizure disorders (especially temporal lobe seizures) ▪ Primary and metastatic tumors of the brain ▪ Dementia ▪ Stroke ▪ Closed head injury
Cardiovascular disorders	▪ Low cardiac output (eg, in heart failure)
Endocrine disorders	▪ Thyroid hyperfunction (thyrotoxicosis) ▪ Adrenal hyperfunction (Cushing syndrome)
Metabolic disorders	▪ Electrolyte imbalances (eg, after severe diarrhea) ▪ Hypoglycemia ▪ Diabetic ketoacidosis

Abbreviations: LSD, lysergic acid diethylamide; PCP, phencyclidine

Environmental Causes

A person's environment exerts a tremendous influence on behavior. Typically, that environment includes both psychosocial and sociocultural influences on behavior.

When people are consistently exposed to stressful psychosocial events (eg, childhood trauma) or developmental influences (eg, parents who deprived them of love, caring, support, and encouragement), they may develop abnormal reactions. When a person's basic needs are threatened, that person faces a crisis. A person in crisis has two alternatives for dealing with this threat: (1) cope with it, finding ways to alter the situation or his or her perception of it so that it's no longer as stressful, or (2) attempt to alleviate the discomfort by escaping from the stress. Escape may take many forms, including alcohol, drugs, psychiatric symptoms, and even suicide (discussed later in this chapter).

Humans are social, preferring to live in groups. Thus, it's not surprising that sociocultural factors directly affect biology, behavior, and responses to the stress of emergencies. For example, assault, rape, racial violence, or the death of a loved one may produce significant changes in a person's behavior.

Injury and Illness as Causes

Acute illness can overwhelm a person, causing changes in behavior. Medical conditions such as severe infections, electrolyte abnormalities, and many types of metabolic disorders stress coping mechanisms and can cause abnormal behaviors.

Traumatic events occurring in the general population have increased in both frequency and intensity in recent years. An acutely traumatic situation creates a great deal of stress for the person experiencing the trauma as well as those around that person. You are not immune to this stress. **Posttraumatic stress disorder (PTSD)** is a severe form of anxiety that stems from a traumatic experience. In this condition, the individual relives the stress of the original situation. Causes of PTSD can include military combat, terrorist attacks, car crashes, and sexual assault **Figure 28-1**. PTSD is discussed in more detail later in this chapter.

Substance-Related Causes

Substance-related disorders include the use of alcohol, cigarettes, illicit drugs, and other substances to change the way a person feels, behaves, or thinks. These disorders cost thousands of lives and billions of dollars annually. Substance-related disorders are recognized as a complex biologic and psychological problem rather than a sign of moral weakness.

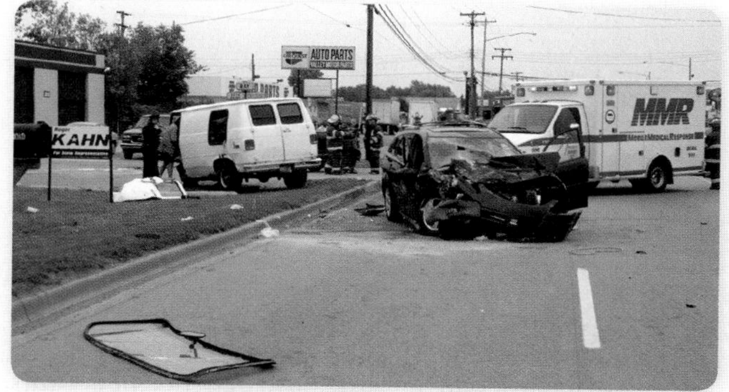

Figure 28-1 Posttraumatic stress disorder can be caused by a traumatic event such as a fatal car crash.

Courtesy of Captain David Jackson, Saginaw Township Fire Department.

▶ Psychiatric Signs and Symptoms

When a person's physical health is challenged, the human body mobilizes various defenses to correct the abnormality. The patient experiences the effects of those abnormalities and corrective measures as symptoms, and you observe these effects as signs. Physical symptoms and signs reveal the body's attempt to maintain its balance in the face of physical stress. When a person's mental health is challenged, similar psychological mechanisms or behaviors mobilize to help return the person's mental state to homeostasis. These defense mechanisms present as various types of psychiatric signs, symptoms, or behaviors that you may observe.

Like the symptoms and signs of physical illness, psychiatric symptoms and signs can be grouped according to the "systems" they affect. Here, however, the focus is on systems of psychological (rather than physiologic) functioning. The psychological functions that can be affected are consciousness, motor activity, speech, thought, **affect** (the outward expression of a person's inner feelings, such as happy, sad, angry, fearful, withdrawn), memory, orientation, and perception. Psychiatric signs and symptoms include these areas, as well as changes in thought progression, thought content, mood, and intelligence. The signs and symptoms of these disorders are listed in **Table 28-3**.

Patient Assessment

Your assessment of the patient with a psychiatric emergency differs in at least two ways from the typical methods of patient assessment you have studied so far. First, when you assess the patient with trauma or acute illness, you use a variety of diagnostic instruments to measure vital functions and detect abnormalities, such as a stethoscope to evaluate breath sounds and a sphygmomanometer to measure blood pressure. When you assess a patient who is disturbed, however, *you* are the diagnostic instrument. You must use your thinking processes to evaluate someone else's thinking processes, your perceptions to test the validity of someone else's perceptions, and your feelings to measure someone else's feelings. This skill takes practice, because most EMS providers are not accustomed to using their feelings in this way. For example, if you feel angry at something someone says, your natural instinct may be to respond angrily to him or her. In working an emergency call, however, a more useful paradigm is, "I feel infuriated with that patient, so it's likely he is paranoid, because paranoid patients often elicit anger in others."

A second way the assessment in a behavioral emergency differs from assessment in acute illness or trauma is that the assessment is part of the treatment. As soon

Table 28-3 Classification of Psychiatric Signs and Symptoms

Function Affected	Psychiatric Signs and Symptoms
Consciousness	▪ Distractibility and inattention ▪ Confusion ▪ Delirium ▪ Stupor and coma
Motor activity	▪ Restlessness ▪ **Stereotyped movements** (repetition of movements that don't seem to serve any useful purpose) ▪ **Compulsions** (repetitive actions that are carried out to relieve the anxiety of obsessive thoughts) ▪ Slow movements
Speech	▪ Slow speech ▪ Acceleration or **pressure of speech** (the pouring out of words like water escaping under pressure) ▪ **Neologisms** (words the patient invents) ▪ **Echolalia** (the patient echoes words he or she hears) ▪ **Mutism** (the patient does not speak at all)
Thought progression	▪ **Flight of ideas** (accelerated thinking in which the mind skips very rapidly from one thought to the next) ▪ Slowness of thought ▪ **Perseveration** (repetition of the same idea over and over again) ▪ **Circumstantial thinking** (the inclusion of many irrelevant details)
Thought content	▪ Delusions ▪ Obsessions ▪ **Phobias** (obsessive, irrational fears of specific things or situations, such as fear of heights, fear of open places, fear of confined spaces, or fear of certain animals)
Mood and affect	▪ Anxiety ▪ Euphoria ▪ Depression ▪ **Inappropriate affect** (emotion that is out of sync with the situation; eg, wearing a smile while discussing a parent's death) ▪ **Flat affect** (the absence of emotion; appearing to feel no emotion at all)
Memory	▪ Amnesia ▪ **Confabulation** (inventing experiences to fill gaps in memory)
Orientation	▪ Disorientation to person, place, and time
Perception	▪ Illusions ▪ Hallucinations
Intelligence	▪ Difficulty learning

as you speak to the patient, your voice and manner will affect his or her condition, for better or worse. Your process of listening to the patient describe the issue at hand can also mitigate it.

Assess the patient at the site of the emergency. Do not immediately rush the patient to the medical facility because the medical facility is likely to be a strange, intimidating place for the patient. Your haste to get to a medical facility may reinforce the patient's belief that something is terribly wrong. Let the patient attempt to recover his or her bearings in familiar surroundings when medically possible.

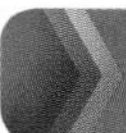

Scene Size-up

The safety concerns at a behavioral emergency may not appear as threatening as a hazardous chemical spill or a motor vehicle crash on a busy highway. However, a situation involving a distraught person with severe depression or a person with a drug addiction experiencing an acute psychotic break poses its own unique threats. Although every situation you encounter has the potential for surprises, situations with a strong behavioral component are those most likely to present surprises. At first look, these calls may appear to be simple "injury with bleeding" or "breathing difficulty" calls, but the superficial problem may be the result of the patient's own erratic behavior. Follow the general guidelines listed in Table 28-4 to ensure your safety at the scene of a behavioral emergency.

Assessing the environment can give you clues to the patient's condition or the cause of the emergency. In a behavioral crisis, it's especially important to look for clues from the patient's social history; general living conditions; availability of social and family support; activity level; medications; overall appearance with respect to nutrition, general health, cleanliness, and personal hygiene; and attitude and mental well-being.

Finally, consider the mechanism of injury and/or nature of illness. For example, a patient with diabetes may have an altered mental status because of a low blood glucose level.

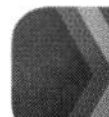

Primary Survey

Identify yourself clearly. Tell the patient who you are and what you're trying to do. If the patient is confused or delusional, then you may have to explain who you are at frequent intervals. Do so in a nonargumentative, emotionally neutral tone of voice. ("No, Mr. Jones, I'm not from the Central Intelligence Agency. I'm a paramedic with the city ambulance service, and I'm here to help you.")

The patient's overall condition and the nature of his or her psychiatric emergency will determine how much of the assessment you can perform. A patient who is disturbed may prefer not to be touched. You must respect that wish unless a compelling medical reason exists for doing otherwise (eg, profuse bleeding from slashed wrists or a decreased level of consciousness from an overdose). At the very least, you should be able to assess the patient's general appearance, such as the patient's dress, cleanliness, and grooming. All of these factors are clues

YOU are the Paramedic PART 2

As you approach the apartment, you note the patient is pacing back and forth just inside the doorway. He is clenching and unclenching his fists. You hear him repeating, "They're coming for me," in a low voice. Speaking calmly, you ask the patient his name and tell him that you're with emergency medical services and are here to help him. He stops pacing, turns to you, and tells you his name. He tells you that you cannot help him because "they" are going to kill him.

You repeat that you want to help him, and ask him to tell you why he feels this way. He looks around nervously and says he must whisper because "they" can hear him. He continues to refuse to come into the hall because he says he'd be an easier target there. You ask if you can come in and sit with him. He allows you in and you sit in a chair near the door so that your access to the exit is not blocked. The apartment appears neat. No visible evidence of alcohol in the kitchen or living area is present. The patient is fully dressed in wrinkled clothes that appear clean. You don't notice any unusual odors. You are limited to a visual assessment of the patient at this time.

Recording Time: 0 Minutes	
Appearance	Agitated, anxious
Level of consciousness	Alert and oriented to person and place; distracted by delusions
Airway	Patent
Breathing	Appears adequate; occasionally rapid
Circulation	Skin color appears normal

3. What is your initial impression of this patient? What factors, signs, or symptoms lead you to this conclusion?
4. Does this patient need to be evaluated at a medical facility?

Table 28-4 Safety Guidelines for Behavioral Emergencies
Assess the scene. If the patient is armed or has potentially harmful objects in his or her possession, then have law enforcement personnel remove these objects before you provide emergency medical care.
Be prepared to spend extra time. You may need more time than usual to assess, listen to, and prepare the patient for transport.
Have a definitive plan of action. Decide who will do what. If restraint is needed, then how will it be implemented?
Know where the exits are. Identify your exit strategy in case the situation becomes volatile. Never let a patient get between you and the door! Park your ambulance in a location that gives you a safe and easy way out should it become necessary for you to leave the scene.
Don personal protective equipment. An agitated patient may try to spit on you or worse. Anticipate such a threat by wearing the necessary PPE.
Urgently de-escalate the patient's level of agitation. It's critical to keep a high-pressure situation from erupting into violence.
Identify yourself calmly. Try to gain the patient's confidence. If you begin shouting, then the patient is likely to shout louder or become more excited. Maintain a calm voice and demeanor to ensure a quieting influence.
Be direct. State your intentions and what you expect of the patient.
Stay with the patient. *Do not let the patient leave the area, and do not leave the area yourself unless law enforcement personnel can and will stay with the patient.* Otherwise, the patient may go to another room and obtain weapons, lock himself or herself in the bathroom, or take pills.
Encourage purposeful movement. Help the patient get dressed and gather appropriate belongings to take to the medical facility.
Express interest in the patient's story. Let the patient tell you in his or her own words what happened or what is going on now. However, don't play along with auditory or visual disturbances, as doing so may reinforce the patient's delusion or hallucination.
Keep a safe distance from the patient. Everyone needs personal space. Be sure you can move quickly if the patient becomes violent or tries to run away. Don't physically talk down to or directly confront the patient. A squatting, 45-degree angle approach is usually not confrontational, but may hinder your movements. Do not allow the patient to get between you and the exit.
Avoid arguing or fighting with the patient. Do not get into a power struggle. Remember, the patient is not responding to you in a normal manner; he or she may be wrestling with internal forces over which neither of you has control. You and others may be unknowingly stimulating these inner forces. If you can respond with understanding to the feeling that the patient is expressing, whether this is anger, fear, or desperation, then you may be able to gain his or her cooperation. If you must use force, then ensure that you have adequate help and move toward the patient quietly and with assured firmness.
Be honest and reassuring. If the patient asks whether he or she has to go to the medical facility, then your answer should be, "Yes, that is where you can receive medical help."
Don't judge. You may see behavior that you dislike. Set those feelings aside and concentrate on providing emergency medical care.

Abbreviation: PPE, personal protective equipment

to the way the patient perceives himself or herself. Note the patient's posture. Does the patient appear frustrated, angry, grief-stricken, or **catatonic** (lacking expression or movement, or appearing rigid)?

You must also carefully assess the pupils because they may indicate other causes of altered mental status. For example, constricted pupils may indicate opiate ingestion, or unequal pupils may indicate cerebral trauma.

When performing your assessment, limit the number of people around the patient. Remember to stay alert to potential danger. A patient in unstable condition may become violent at any time. Watch for signs of agitation or aggression. Separate the patient from bystanders or family members who seem to be worsening the patient's condition. You may ask them to step into another room and speak to your partner, or you may take your patient to the ambulance before beginning your primary survey, if appropriate.

Attend first to priority problems (ie, airway, breathing, and circulation [the ABCs]). Assess the airway to make sure it is patent and adequate. Next, evaluate the patient's breathing. Provide appropriate interventions based on your assessment findings. In most patients with behavioral emergencies, however, the problem will be more psychiatric than physiologic. During your assessment, look for signs and symptoms of abnormal functioning or behavior and remain alert for threatening gestures.

Assess the patient's pulse rate, quality, and rhythm. Obtain the systolic and diastolic blood pressures when possible. Evaluate for the presence of shock and bleeding. Assess the patient's perfusion level by evaluating skin color, temperature, condition, and capillary refill time.

Patients who are seriously disturbed should be seen by a physician and evaluated for possible hospitalization. Many such patients will consent to be transported to the medical facility. Others won't want your help and will try to prevent you from taking them to a medical facility. Because transporting patients against their will deprives them of their civil liberties, you must never make this decision lightly. Even an experienced psychiatrist may have difficulty defining behavior that justifies removal from society or that constitutes so-called dangerous behavior. Furthermore, laws vary from region to region, so know the legal requirements in your community.

As a general rule, a conscious adult must consent to be taken to a medical facility. If the patient withholds this consent, then the patient may be taken against his or her will only at the express request of the police or the county mental health physician (in many jurisdictions). The same policy applies to the use of forcible restraint. If such measures are deemed necessary, then summon law enforcement officers.

In addition, every ambulance service should have clearly defined protocols, drawn up with legal advice, for dealing with patients who require involuntary commitment. Follow those protocols to the letter and consult medical command as necessary.

History Taking

The **mental status exam (MSE)** is a key part of your assessment of a patient who is experiencing an acute psychiatric emergency. To conduct the MSE, you must check each of the "systems" of mental function in order. A useful mnemonic for the elements of the MSE is COASTMAP:

- **Consciousness.** Determine the patient's level of consciousness (alert, confused, responds to pain, unresponsive). Note the patient's ability to pay attention to a discussion and concentrate. Is the patient easily distracted, or can he or she focus on the events at hand?
- **Orientation.** Ask the patient the current year or month. Ask the patient to state his or her location—country, state, town, or specific location. If the patient is not sure, then have the patient make a best guess.
- **Activity.** Examine the patient's behavior. Is the patient restless and agitated, pacing up and down? Experiencing tremors? Sitting still, scarcely moving at all? Making any strange or repetitive movements (scanning of the environment, odd or repetitive gestures)?
- **Speech.** Identify the form, rather than the content, of the patient's speech. Note the rate, volume, flow, articulation, and intonation of speech. Is it too fast or too slow? Too loud or too soft? Is the speech garbled or slurred (dysarthria)? Is the patient stuttering or mumbling? Using any strange words?
- **Thought.** Listen to the patient's story. What is on his or her mind? Is the patient making sense? Is anything unusual about his or her reasoning? Is the patient expressing apparently false ideas (delusions), such as a belief that someone is after him or her? Is the patient experiencing any false sensory impressions (hallucinations), such as hearing voices? Is the patient experiencing a flight of ideas (rapid shifting of ideas)?
- **Memory.** Develop a general impression of the patient's memory, including recent, remote, and immediate. If the patient has memory loss, then determine whether it's constant or variable. Some patients may create memories to take the place of things they cannot recall (confabulation).
- **Affect and mood.** The patient's mood may be objectively noted via body language. Is the mood euphoric or sad? Is it **labile**? Does the affect seem appropriate to the situation or is it animated, angry, flat, or withdrawn?
- **Perception.** Detecting disorders of perception may be difficult, because patients often hesitate to answer direct questions about hallucinations or illusions. Sometimes it's helpful to ask the patient, "Do you ever hear things that other people cannot hear?"

You can conduct nearly all of the MSE just by watching and listening (and knowing what to watch and listen for). Only the assessment of memory, orientation, and perhaps perception requires you to ask some direct questions.

Words of Wisdom

Practice being an observer. As you sit in a restaurant, eavesdrop on the waitress talking to other customers and systematically go through the COASTMAP sequence to evaluate her mental status. Get into the habit of noticing how other people talk, move, and express their feelings, and practice describing those elements to your partner.

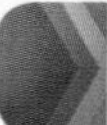

Secondary Assessment

While much of your assessment focuses on interviewing the patient about psychiatric history and performing the MSE, you must also look for signs of an organic cause of the patient's behavior:

- Obtain the vital signs to identify fever or indications of increased intracranial pressure.
- Examine the skin temperature and moisture, and note any prominent tattoos. Scars may indicate self-mutilation in **borderline personality disorders**.
- Inspect the head for evidence of trauma.
- Check the pupils for size, equality, and reaction to light. Pupillary abnormalities may indicate a toxic ingestion or an intracranial process as the source of the patient's behavior.
- Note any unusual odors on the patient's breath such as poisons, alcohol, or ketones from diabetic ketoacidosis.
- As you examine the extremities, check for needle tracks, tremors, and unilateral weakness or loss of sensation.

Reassessment

Reassess the patient during transport. This is a good time to further explore your patient's mental status or confirm findings you have already obtained.

Patients with abnormal behavior often settle down physically by the time you start your assessment. However, their minds may still be in a state of flux, and this could lead to impulsive behavior. Monitor patients vigilantly for sudden changes in thought or behavior, particularly in transit as you near the medical facility. If patients don't want help, then they may try to jump from the ambulance or hurt themselves in an attempt to complete a suicide before arriving at the medical facility. They may even turn that aggressive and impulsive behavior toward you.

Your radio report to the medical facility should include your usual report of medical and mental health history, medications prescribed, and assessment findings based on local protocols and guidelines. Be sure to include pertinent information from the mental status exam to create a clear picture of your patient.

Discuss with the medical facility the need for restraints or medications to control behavior before instituting these interventions when possible. If such measures already have been used or other standing orders have been instituted to protect the patient and providers, then inform the medical facility staff.

If your patient is aggressive or potentially violent, then give the ED staff advance notice to so they can mobilize security or additional help before your arrival.

Emergency Medical Care

Management of the patient with a psychiatric emergency follows the approach used throughout this text. Ensure scene safety and focus on life-threatening conditions. If the erratic behavior might be caused by a medical disorder (eg, hypoglycemia, overdose, or hypoxia), then treat the patient for the medical disorder before assuming that the patient's behavior has an emotional or psychiatric cause. These measures may include oxygen therapy, testing of the blood glucose level, and administration of dextrose, as well as general interventions for hypothermia or shock management.

Communication Techniques

As always, good communication with the patient is part of the treatment of a patient with a psychiatric emergency.

When you evaluate a trauma patient, you can generally obtain enough information to select appropriate initial treatment based only on the physical exam findings, even if the patient is unresponsive and cannot provide a history. On the other hand, when you evaluate a patient with a behavioral emergency, virtually all of the diagnostic information, and much of the therapeutic benefit, comes from your communication with the patient. Your skill in interviewing a patient with a behavioral crisis, therefore, is central to treating psychiatric emergencies.

Set some ground rules for your interview. Let the patient know what you expect, and what he or she may expect of you. ("It's okay to cry or even scream, but we aren't going to let you hurt yourself or anyone else.") Allow the patient to tell the story in his or her own way. Don't attempt to direct the conversation, but allow the patient to vent his or her feelings. Following are some communication guidelines:

- **Begin with an open-ended question.** An open-ended question does not give the patient possible answers, but rather allows the patient to form his or her own answer. For example, you may say, "It's clear you've been feeling bad. Tell me something about the kind of troubles you've been having." (You may begin with more direct questioning when you must obtain specific information quickly, such as, "What kind of pills did you take? How many?")

- **Let the patient talk and tell the story in his or her own way, even if it takes a little more time.** Letting patients talk allows them to gain some control over themselves and their situations. At the same time, it enables you to assess the patient's speech, affect, and thought processes.
- **Listen, and show that you are listening.** Your facial expression, posture, eye contact, an occasional nod—all of these things can show the patient that you're paying close attention to what he or she is saying Figure 28-2.
- **Don't be afraid of silent pauses, even if they seem intolerably long.** Maintain an attentive and relaxed attitude until the patient takes up the story again. It's especially important to be silent when the patient stops speaking because of overwhelming emotion. Avoid the temptation to jump into the silence to comfort the patient or to forestall expressions of emotion, such as crying. The expression of feelings is often therapeutic in itself, and the patient will probably be better able to express him- or herself after this emotional release.
- **Acknowledge and label the patient's feelings.** The patient who is disturbed may feel overwhelmed by intense and chaotic feelings. Identifying those feelings and giving them a name (eg, "You seem angry") can help the patient gain control over them.
- **Don't argue.** If the patient misperceives reality, then make note of the misperceptions, but don't try to talk the patient out of them. When a misperception frightens or distresses the patient, you may try once to make a simple and factual statement, in a neutral tone of voice ("Yes, that does look a lot like a snake, but actually it's just a shadow."). But don't get into a dispute on the nature of reality.
- **Facilitate communication.** Facilitation is a technique used to encourage the patient to communicate by using gestures or noncommittal words, such as a nod of the head or a phrase such as, "Go on," "I see," or "What happened after that?" You can also use facilitation to return the patient to a topic on which you would like some elaboration. For example, a patient may have made a passing reference to suicidal thoughts and then moved on to another subject. When the patient finishes, you might comment, "You say you've had thoughts of suicide?" This remark tells the patient that you have been paying attention to the story and would like to learn more.
- **Direct the patient's attention.** Confrontation means pointing out something of interest in the patient's conversation or behavior, thereby directing the patient's attention to something he or she may not have noticed. Confrontations describe the way the patient appears to the interviewer and are based on observations, *not* judgments. For example, you might remark, "You seem worried," or "You look sad." Such comments often elicit a freer expression of feelings from the patient. Confrontations must be carefully phrased so that they don't sound nagging or condescending.
- **Ask questions.** When the patient finishes giving the initial account of the problem, you'll want to ask questions. Keep them as open ended as possible. Avoid asking questions that can be answered with a yes or no ("Are you angry?") or asking leading questions ("Do you think that your husband is a part of the problem?"). Instead, pose open-ended *how* and *what* questions ("How did you feel when that happened?" "What factors have contributed to how you're feeling right now?").
- **Adjust your approach as needed.** Some patients have difficulty with the lack of structure in open-ended questioning and may become anxious during silences. This reaction is especially common among adolescents, patients with severe depression, and patients who are

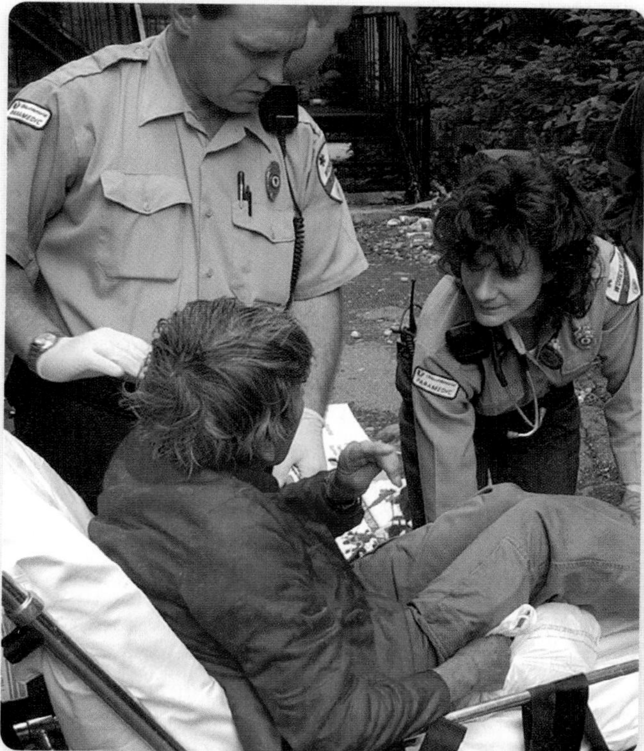

Figure 28-2 Making eye contact with a patient can yield useful clues about the patient's emotional state. Be careful, though, not to stare at the patient.

confused or disorganized. When your open-ended questions meet with uncomprehending silence, try another approach and perform a more structured interview.

▶ Crisis Intervention Skills

The following guidelines apply to the care of any patient with a psychiatric emergency:

- **Be as calm and direct as possible.** Patients who are disturbed are often afraid of losing self-control. Your behavior should show that you have confidence in the patient's ability to maintain control. One of the main purposes of the interview is to help the patient reestablish some self-mastery. If you show anxiety or panic, then you merely affirm the patient's conviction that the situation is overwhelming.
- **Exclude disruptive people.** In most cases, you should interview the patient alone. Relatives and bystanders should wait in another room, where your partner can interview them. Some patients, however, become anxious if separated from an important person, such as a parent or a friend. If another person has a calming effect on the patient, then ask that person to remain present.
- **Sit down.** Sit down to interview the patient, preferably at a 45° angle from the patient so you don't encroach on the patient's personal space Figure 28-3.
- **Maintain a nonjudgmental attitude.** Accept the patient's right to have his or her own feelings about things, and don't blame, judge, or criticize the patient for those feelings.
- **Give honest reassurance.** Give supportive, truthful information. You might say, "Many people go through periods of hopelessness like you're having, but today we have effective treatments for those feelings." Avoid excessive reassurances, such as "Everything's going to be all right." Such statements merely convince patients that you don't understand how bad things are for them.
- **Develop a plan of action.** After the patient has finished telling his or her story and you have concluded your assessment, you develop a specific plan of action. This step gives the patient the feeling that something is being done to help, which in turn relieves anxiety. In addition, people in crisis need direction. Don't give the patient an array of choices (eg, "Do you want to go to the medical facility, or would you rather stay at home and call your physician tomorrow?"). Rather, state what you think is the best course of action ("I think it's important for you to go to the medical facility. There are physicians there who can help you."). When the plan has been determined and you have begun to carry it out, allow the patient to make choices and thereby exercise some control over the situation. You might ask the patient, for example, whether he or she prefers to be carried on a stretcher or to walk to the ambulance on his or her own. These small decisions may seem minor, but they allow the patient to attain a measure of autonomy and self-respect.
- **Encourage some motor activity.** Moving about can help ease anxiety. If you're taking the patient to the medical facility, then accompany the patient while he or she gathers the things he or she wants to bring. Let patients do as much for themselves as possible to reinforce the feeling that you expect them to improve.
- **Stay with the patient at all times.** When you have responded to the emergency, the patient's safety becomes your responsibility. Do not allow the patient to leave you. For example, allowing the patient to go to the bathroom alone might allow the patient to swallow the contents of a bottle of pills.
- **Bring all of the patient's medications to the medical facility.** If the patient is currently receiving treatment for psychiatric emergencies, then knowing the medications that already have been prescribed can help physicians identify the condition for which the patient has been treated. Medications for other medical conditions may cause adverse effects or unusual interactions that alter behavior.
- **Never assume that it's impossible to talk with any patient until you have tried to do so.** Even if the patient sits silently and appears unaware of your presence, assume that he or she can hear and understand everything you say.

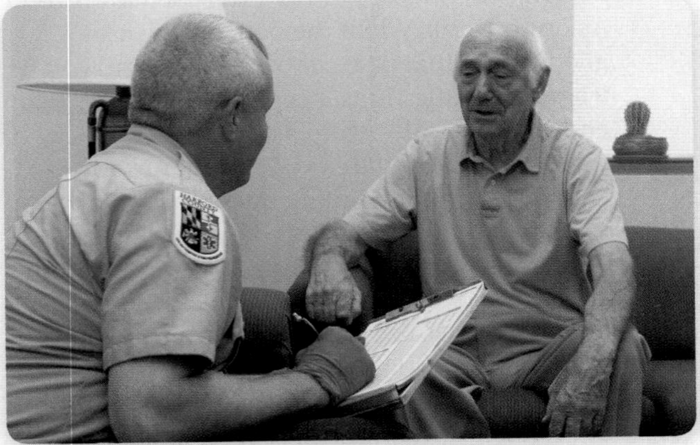

Figure 28-3 When interviewing the patient, sitting at a 45° angle is one way to avoid encroaching on the patient's personal space.

▶ Use of Force and Types of Restraint

When verbal interventions fail to reduce severe agitation in a patient, consider the use of physical or chemical restraint.

Physical Restraint

Some devices used for physical restraint may be improvised from materials on the ambulance; others are commercially made from leather or nylon that is padded for comfort and safety. Most commercial restraints are applied to the wrists and ankles to prevent movement of the arms and legs. Some are placed around the waist to restrict movement of the torso.

Vest-type restraints are applied from the front of the patient and may include sleeves to prevent the arms from moving. Make sure you're familiar with the restraints used by your agency before you need to use them.

Before you attempt to restrain the patient, make sure you have enough personnel to overpower and restrain the patient. You must have overwhelming force to apply a physical restraint, which means a minimum of five trained, able-bodied people—one for each limb and one for the head. Assign a specific limb in advance to each emergency responder. Appoint one leader to direct the team and maintain verbal contact with the patient.

Before you begin, discuss the plan of action. Law enforcement personnel are often trained in both verbal and physical techniques used to subdue violent people. They should be included in any plan to physically restrain a violent patient. They can also offer an objective view of the situation. However, law enforcement personnel will sometimes refuse to help restrain a patient in the absence of a warrant for the subject's arrest or evidence that he or she is an immediate threat to others. Paramedics must be prepared to physically restrain patients on their own when necessary and practice these techniques regularly.

When subduing a patient who is disturbed, use the minimum force necessary. Avoid acts of physical force that may injure the patient. Do not move toward the patient immediately; give him or her a chance to choose a nonviolent alternative behavior.

If the show of force does not calm the patient, then emergency responders must prepare to restrain the patient. Remove any equipment or jewelry from your own body that could be used as a weapon (eg, name badge, scissors

YOU are the Paramedic PART 3

The patient agrees to sit in a chair opposite you. You ask the patient if he knows what day it is. He replies with the correct day of the week. You use the COASTMAP method to continue your mental status assessment of this patient. The patient is restless in his seat. He is gripping the edge of the chair and rocking back and forth. You ask the patient if he has any medical conditions. He tells you that he sees his physician regularly because he has schizophrenia. He is supposed to take medication every day, but he has not taken any for the past week. He says he overheard "them" at the drug store when he was refilling his prescriptions. When he realized that they knew he overheard them, he stopped taking his medications because they were poisoned. He explains to you that he wanted to take the medications but he is afraid. He says he cannot go out to get more.

You ask the patient if your partner can check his vital signs while you look at the medications he takes. He consents and directs you to a basket on the table with medicine bottles. You locate two new bottles. The patient should take thioridazine (Mellaril), 200 mg twice daily, and mesoridazine (Serentil), 50 mg twice daily. The bottles indicate they are for treatment of schizophrenia.

Recording Time: 8 Minutes	
Respirations	20 breaths/min
Pulse	110 beats/min
Skin	Warm, pink, dry
Blood pressure	130/84 mm Hg
Oxygen saturation (Spo_2)	99% on room air
Pupils	PERRLA

5. What conclusions might you make about medication compliance and the patient's medical history?
6. If the patient refuses to be transported, then what options should you, as a paramedic, consider?

worn on the belt, key chain, earrings). Make sure you have adequate restraining devices—preferably padded leather or nylon restraints—immediately available.

The best position in which to secure the patient to the stretcher is the supine position, with both legs and both arms secured to one side of the stretcher, with the patient's head turned to the side. This position prevents aspiration in case of vomiting. Never place your patient facedown because you cannot adequately monitor the patient in this position. This position also may inhibit the breathing of an impaired or exhausted patient. Be careful not to place restraints in a way that compromises the patient's respirations. Never tie the patient's ankles and wrists together as one; this type of restraint has been known to result in death. Never "hobble tie" a patient (tying just the feet together). Placing a patient facedown in a Reeves stretcher also can be dangerous and can lead to positional asphyxia or aspiration.

Throughout the process, someone, preferably you or your partner, should talk with the patient. Remember to treat the patient with dignity and sensitivity at all times. Keeping the patient informed in a calm, respectful manner reduces the amount of stimuli the patient experiences. After the restraints are in place, do not remove them. Don't negotiate or make deals.

Words of Wisdom

During the process of restraining an agitated patient, the patient may try to bite you or spit at you. Take appropriate precautions to avoid either action. A surgical mask may be used to protect against spitting.

Continuously monitor the patient for clear airway and breathing, vomiting, airway obstruction, and cardiovascular stability. Drug or alcohol intoxication initially may cause violent behavior but then can lead to physical problems such as vomiting and aspiration or respiratory depression.

Check the patient's peripheral circulation every few minutes to ensure that the restraints are not too tight Figure 28-4. Check the radial pulses in the arms and the dorsalis pedis pulses in the feet.

Be careful if a combative patient suddenly becomes calm and cooperative. This is not the time to relax; continue to remain vigilant. The patient may suddenly become combative again and injure someone.

Document everything in the patient's chart. This information should include the reasons for using restraints. Be specific, giving examples of the patient's behavior and the indications of the violence potential; the number of people used to subdue the patient; the restraining devices used; and the status of the patient's airway, breathing, and peripheral circulation after restraints were applied. Remember that you may use reasonable force to defend yourself against an attack by a patient who is emotionally disturbed. Having witnesses in attendance, even during transport, and documenting their presence, may be extremely helpful in protecting you from false accusations.

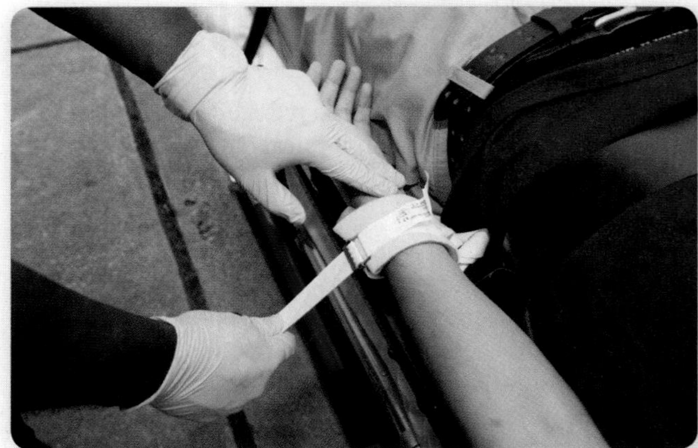

Figure 28-4 Assess circulation frequently while a patient is restrained.

Proper use of the four-point physical restraint technique is shown in Skill Drill 28-1.

A two-point restraint technique is an option if allowed per local protocols. This technique is performed in the same way as four-point restraint, except instead of restraining all four extremities to the stationary frame of the stretcher, one arm is placed upward toward the head and the other is placed downward toward the waist.

Chemical Restraint

Physical restraint of a patient for aggressive and psychotic behavior can be complicated and dangerous for you and for patients. One alternative to physical restraint is **chemical restraint**—the use of medication to subdue a patient. This option should be used only with approval from medical control and by following clearly established local protocols and guidelines.

Chemical restraint is not always easier than physical restraint, and it has its own hazards. Combinations of sedative medications may produce unexpected drug interactions and should be avoided. Use physical and/or chemical restraint only after verbal attempts to de-escalate a patient with excited delirium have failed. Giving the patient a blanket or pillow, or otherwise trying to make him or her comfortable, may help to reduce the anxiety that often accompanies **psychosis** (a state of delusion in which a person is out of touch with reality). Both excited delirium and psychosis are discussed later in this chapter.

The medications used most often for chemical restraint include short-acting benzodiazepines, antipsychotics, dissociative agents, and antihistamines. Many of these medications have not been approved by the FDA for chemical restraint. In addition, the FDA has issued black box warnings for some of these medications. A black box warning indicates that the drug may be associated with serious adverse effects.

Skill Drill 28-1 Restraining a Patient

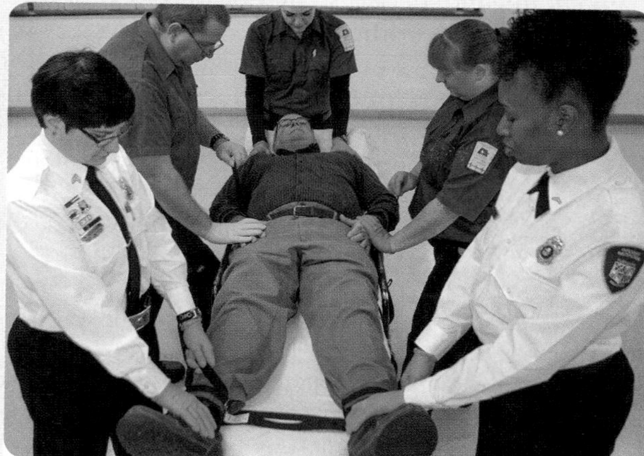

Step 1 Make sure you have enough personnel to perform this skill (five trained, able-bodied responders). Bring down the patient into the prone position. Then, acting at the same time, secure the patient in the supine or left lateral position with wrist and ankle restraints. Some services require the use of the backboard for restraint so a patient who becomes unconscious or who vomits can be turned onto his or her side quickly to manage the airway.

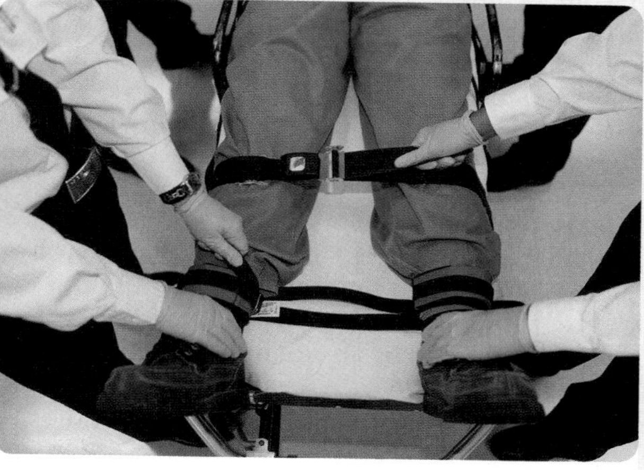

Step 2 Use stretcher straps or sheets to secure the patient's legs.

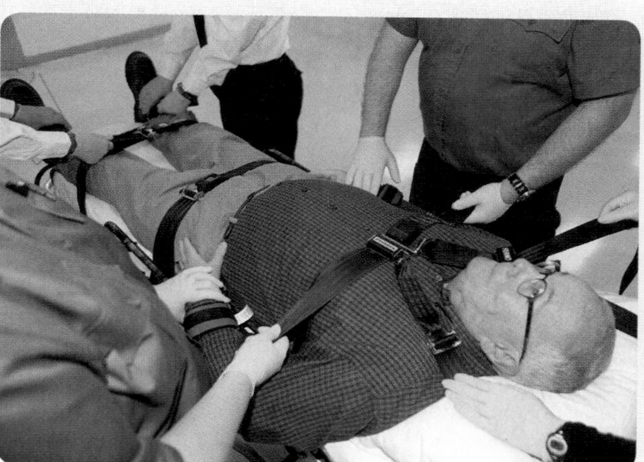

Step 3 Fasten the remaining stretcher straps.

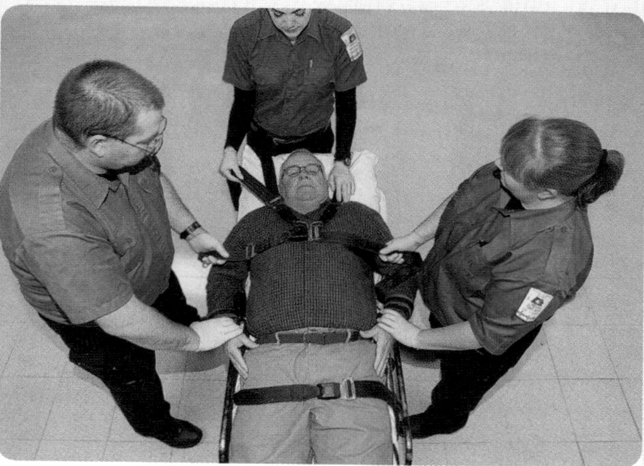

Step 4 Continue to verbally reassure and calm the patient following physical restraint. Regularly check circulation to the extremities.

Patient Safety

When you administer psychiatric medications to older patients, you should begin with lower doses (as with any medication). Repeat the dose based on the advice of medical control.

Benzodiazepines. Benzodiazepines such as diazepam (Valium), lorazepam (Ativan), and midazolam (Versed) can be given as either intramuscular (IM) or intravenous (IV) injections. However, only midazolam and lorazepam have reliable IM absorption. The adverse effects of benzodiazepines are usually mild and easily treated. Drowsiness, decreased mental alertness, sedation, and ataxia are the most common adverse effects.

However, respiratory depression is possible. Although infrequent, paradoxical responses to benzodiazepines, such as insomnia and agitation, are more common among older adults.

Because aggressive and dangerous behaviors are often caused by the use of illicit drugs (eg, cocaine, methamphetamines, PCP), benzodiazepines are usually a safer and more effective form of chemical restraint when compared with other medications.

Benzodiazepines that are shorter acting, such as midazolam, may be given intranasally, such as through a mucosal atomizer device. This method provides easy preparation and quick administration with less risk to health care providers than IM or IV injections. When you deliver midazolam by an atomizer device, administer half the total dose in each nostril. Consider a more concentrated solution because of the limited volume of medication the nares can reliably absorb.

The onset of action for the various benzodiazepines varies depending on the route of administration and the dose. Diazepam, lorazepam, and midazolam can be administered to pediatric or adult patients. Doses for these and the other medications discussed in this section are listed in the Appendix, *Emergency Medications*.

Antipsychotic Medications. You may use antipsychotic medications, such as droperidol (Inapsine), haloperidol (Haldol), and ziprasidone (Geodon), in the treatment of agitated patients. The FDA has issued a black box warning for droperidol because of its association with prolonged QT syndromes.[3] Higher doses and IV administration of haloperidol, a typical antipsychotic agent, also appears to be associated with a higher risk of QT prolongation and torsades de pointes.

Patient Safety

Exercise caution with droperidol and haloperidol in patients with suspected electrolyte imbalances or known cardiac abnormalities, or patients who are taking drugs that affect the QT interval. When either medication is administered intravenously, electrocardiographic (ECG) monitoring is recommended.

Although the FDA has not approved haloperidol for IV administration, it is commonly administered using this route. Do not administer haloperidol to patients younger than 14 years, those with a suspected head injury, or those who may be pregnant. Haloperidol has not been approved for the treatment of patients with dementia-related psychosis.

Typical antipsychotics, including droperidol and haloperidol, may cause seizures or a wide array of extrapyramidal symptoms, including involuntary movements, tremors, rigidity, muscle contractions, restlessness, and changes in breathing and pulse rate. Newer atypical antipsychotics such as olanzapine (Zyprexa) and ziprasidone have fewer extrapyramidal symptoms. The incidence of anticholinergic effects also may be lower. Combined use with alcohol and other central nervous system (CNS) suppressants may worsen CNS depression. Monitor for hypotension, bradycardia, and glucose levels in patients receiving atypical antipsychotics.

Special Populations

Exercise caution when administering antipsychotics to pediatric patients. Droperidol is not routinely recommended, but haloperidol may be used in pediatric patients. Limited data is available about the use of olanzapine and ziprasidone in pediatric patients.

Older patients with dementia-related psychosis treated with antipsychotic medications have an increased risk of death.[4,5] Administration of parenteral olanzapine and a benzodiazepine to the same patient can lead to severe orthostatic hypotension, as well as cardiac or respiratory depression. Avoid this combination of medications in geriatric patients.

Evidence-Based Medicine

Ketamine, an N-methyl-D-aspartate receptor antagonist, falls in the dissociative class of medications often used for procedural sedation in a medical facility environment. It's emerging as an effective treatment for managing acute psychosis in prehospital situations.[6] Some research shows that ketamine produces an adequate level of sedation in patients with excited delirium more effectively and faster than haloperidol does. However, ketamine has been associated with a higher rate of complications (ie, hypersalivation, emergence reaction, vomiting, dystonia, and laryngospasm) than haloperidol, including during intubation after arrival at the medical facility.[7] Ketamine, although not currently approved by the FDA for chemical restraint in a prehospital environment, illustrates the need for constant consideration of risk versus benefits in the administration of any medication.

Antihistamines. Antihistamines, specifically diphenhydramine (Benadryl), have been used for many years in the treatment of psychiatric patients. Although diphenhydramine is best known for its sedative properties, it also produces an anticholinergic effect that has some effect on neurotransmitters in the brain that affect behavior. It can be used for both adult and pediatric patients.

Controversies

Many law enforcement agencies use an electroshock device (eg, a TASER) to immobilize people who are behaving in a violent or aggressive manner Figure 28-5. Electroshock devices were designed as an alternative to more violent immobilization methods. The use of these weapons in custody is controversial. Some data support the assertion that they have been associated with, but not causally related to, deaths in custody.[8] In other words, a person on whom a TASER had recently been discharged died while in custody, but the electrical discharge was unrelated to the cause of death. The risk of death seems to be greatest in patients experiencing excited delirium.[8]

Be aware that many patients subjected to a TASER exposure are at high risk for medical complications resulting from an underlying condition. You must identify these underlying conditions and ensure appropriate emergency medical care. Such conditions include drug overdose syndromes, excited delirium, acute psychiatric decompensation, hypoglycemia, heatstroke, hepatic encephalopathy, seizure disorders, dementia, and encephalitis. Police officers are not routinely trained to recognize these conditions. They rely on you to make appropriate medical decisions at the scene.

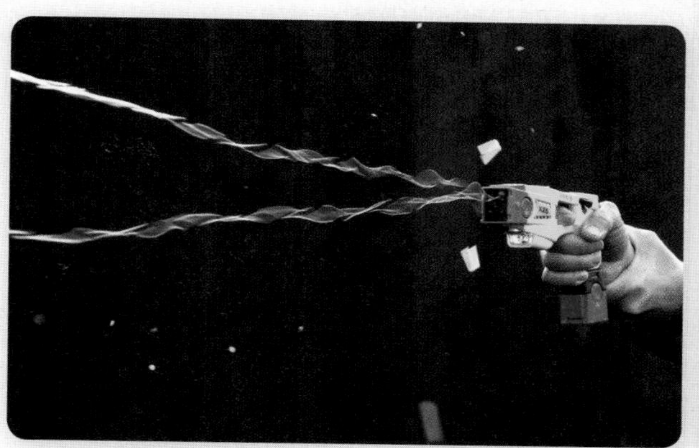

Figure 28-5 TASER X26P. When deployed, compressed nitrogen projects two small probes up to 25 feet (7.6 meters), delivering a 5-second electric shock as the probes make contact with the body or clothing. This shock results in an immediate but temporary incapacitation with minimal risk of injury.

Pathophysiology, Assessment, and Management of Specific Emergencies

Many factors contribute to behavior disturbances. Some of these influences are easily identified and treated, but others may never be clearly understood. The causes, signs, symptoms, and management of abnormal behavior can be grouped into several common areas, shown in Table 28-5. The areas most relevant to paramedicine are acute psychosis, agitated delirium, suicide, and patterns of violence, abuse, and neglect. Finally, we will discuss specific psychiatric disorders.

▶ Acute Psychosis

Pathophysiology

Recall that psychosis is a state of delusion in which a person is out of touch with reality. Affected people are tuned into their own internal reality of ideas and feelings, which they mistake for the reality of the external world. To the person experiencing an acute psychotic episode, the line differentiating reality from fantasy is blurred, rather than distinct, as it is in people without psychoses. That internal reality may make patients belligerent and angry toward others. Alternatively, these patients may become mute and withdrawn as they give all their attention to the voices and feelings within.

Psychoses or psychotic episodes result from many causes. These causes may be biologic or organic, or may result from mental illness or drug abuse. The use of mind-altering substances is one of the most common causes, and that psychotic episode may be limited to the time that the substance is being metabolized within the body. Other causes may be more related to the patient's environment or mental illness. These causes can include intense stress, delusional disorders, and, more often, schizophrenia (discussed later in this chapter). Some psychotic episodes last for brief periods; others last a lifetime.

Disorganization and **disorientation** are not diagnoses, but rather ways in which various conditions such as schizophrenia or organic brain syndromes may present themselves. These presentations account for many ambulance calls, particularly for older people. Although you need not make a specific diagnosis in such cases, you do need to know how to manage these patients in the field.

Assessment

The most characteristic feature of psychosis is a profound thought disorder, often accompanied by disturbances in mood and perception. Patients are usually incoherent or rambling in their speech, although they may be oriented to person and place. These patients often are found wandering aimlessly down a street, dressed oddly, and uttering meaningless words and sentences. A thorough exam of the patient is rarely possible, and your principal objective is to transport the patient to the medical facility without trauma.

Table 28-5 Categorization of Psychiatric Disorders	
Type of Disorder	**Specific Disorder**
Cognitive	▪ Agitated delirium
Thought	▪ Schizophrenia ▪ Acute psychosis
Mood	▪ Bipolar mood disorder ▪ Manic behavior ▪ Depression
Neurotic	▪ Generalized anxiety disorder ▪ Phobias ▪ Panic disorder
Substance-related disorders and addictive behavior	▪ Substance use ▪ Substance intoxication ▪ Substance abuse ▪ Substance dependence ▪ Eating disorders (bulimia nervosa, anorexia nervosa)
Somatoform	▪ Hypochondriasis ▪ Conversion disorder (physical problem that has no identifiable pathophysiology; results from a psychological conflict)
Factitious	Condition in which a person acts as if he or she has an illness by deliberately producing or feigning symptoms ▪ Münchausen syndrome (most severe type of factitious disorder; most symptoms are physical) ▪ Münchausen syndrome by proxy (mental illness in which caregiver makes up or produces illness or injury in a person under his or her care; eg, a parent intentionally makes his or her child sick; also called factitious disorder by proxy)
Impulse control	▪ Intermittent explosive disorder (acting on aggressive impulses involving the destruction of property) ▪ Kleptomania (acting on the urge to steal things) ▪ Pyromania (acting on the urge to set fires) ▪ Pathologic gambling
Personality	▪ Odd or eccentric disorders ▪ Dramatic, erratic, or emotional disorders ▪ Anxious or fearful disorders

The following list, using the COASTMAP mnemonic, describes the common signs and symptoms of the patient with psychosis.

- **Consciousness.** The patient with psychosis is awake and alert, but may be easily distracted, especially if paying attention to hallucinations. If the level of consciousness is fluctuating, then suspect an organic brain syndrome.
- **Orientation.** Disturbances in orientation are more common in organic disorders than in psychoses, but the patient with severe psychosis may be disoriented as to time and place.
- **Activity.** Activity is most often accelerated, with agitation and hyperactivity, but it also may be reduced. Bizarre, stereotyped movements are common.
- **Speech.** Speech may be pressured or sound strange because of unusual words that the patient has invented (neologisms).
- **Thought.** Thought is disturbed in progression and content and may show any of the following disorders:
  - Flight of ideas, with the patient's mind plunging from one thought to another.

- **Loosening of associations**, in which the logical connection between one idea and the next becomes obscure, at least to the listener. In extreme cases, the patient's speech may be entirely incomprehensible.
- Delusions, especially of persecution.
- **Thought broadcasting** (the belief that thoughts are broadcast aloud and can be heard by others).
- **Thought insertion** (the belief that thoughts are being thrust into his or her mind by another person) and **thought withdrawal** (the belief that thoughts are being removed).

- **Memory.** Memory can be relatively or entirely intact in psychosis. You may encounter difficulty in obtaining the patient's cooperation for formal memory testing.
- **Affect and mood.** Mood is likely to be disturbed in psychosis. The disturbance may take the form of euphoria, sadness, or wide swings in mood; affect may reflect those inner states or be flat.
- **Perception.** Auditory hallucinations are common in psychosis. Patients hear voices commenting on their behavior or telling them what to do. Suspect that patients are hearing such voices when they seem to be attending a conversation other than yours or talking to themselves.

Management

Dealing with a patient with acute psychosis is difficult. The usual methods of reasoning with a patient are unlikely to be effective because the person has his or her own rules of logic. These rules may be very different from those that govern nonpsychotic thinking.

In addition, you're likely to feel uncomfortable in the presence of a person with psychosis. Those uncomfortable feelings are one of your built-in diagnostic instruments. They are elicited by the fear, suspicion, and hostility that the patient is broadcasting through body language. Use your uncomfortable feelings to help make a tentative diagnosis of a psychotic problem.

The patient experiencing disorganization needs structure. Explain in plain language what you're doing and what the patient's role is. Directions should be simple, consistent, and firm. It may be impossible to obtain a detailed history—a name and address may be the only information you can obtain. Explain to such patients that they need to be seen by a physician, and that you will take them to the medical facility to get help.

In managing the patient experiencing disorientation, the key is to keep orienting the patient to time, place, and the people in the environment. Tell the patient who you are and explain what you're doing. You may have to repeat that information several times en route. Reassure the patient and point out landmarks to help orient the patient.

Words of Wisdom

Be forewarned! The patient who hears voices that command him to hurt himself or others must be considered dangerous.

When a patient's behavior becomes so excited that it threatens his or her own well-being or the safety of others, you must take more aggressive steps to prevent injury. These steps can include either physical or chemical restraint and, at times, both. When evaluating the need for restraint, also consider calling law enforcement personnel if you haven't already contacted them.

Special Populations

Some communities have crisis intervention teams (CIT) staffed by law enforcement officers with specialized training in recognizing and managing people experiencing a mental health crisis. The primary role of the CIT is to keep patients from revolving through the criminal justice system and the medical facility. Rather, the program seeks to establish long-term care and other solutions for people with chronic and persistent mental health conditions. These patients might otherwise lack the resources or support to get that help.

People experiencing a psychotic episode often do not comply with treatments, especially medication administration. Such patients often leave before an IV line can be started and a sedative agent administered. These patients might have the delusion that you're injecting them with something harmful. You should employ nonpharmacologic interventions first, as discussed earlier. Developing trust is an important therapy, but doing so may be difficult to achieve with a patient in an acutely agitated state.

When these methods fail, safely restraining the patient and administering a medication to treat the behavior may be appropriate. If safe administration is possible, then an antianxiety medication such as a benzodiazepine (eg, midazolam) given intranasally, or an antipsychotic medication such as haloperidol given intramuscularly, should help calm the patient. Follow your medical control direction and standing orders when using medications to control behavior.

▶ Agitated Delirium

Pathophysiology

Agitated delirium, also called excited delirium, is a state of global cognitive impairment that is acute in onset and associated with fluctuations in mental status and behavior, inattention, disorganized thinking, and an altered level of consciousness. Toxic and metabolic conditions or infections are the usual causes. **Dementia** is a more chronic process that produces severe deficits in memory, abstract thinking, and judgment.

People experiencing delirium may become agitated and violent when stressors overwhelm them or they cannot maintain homeostasis. The result is similar to that in a patient who is experiencing an acute psychotic state. Common risk factors for delirium include medical histories of hypertension, chronic obstructive pulmonary disease, alcohol abuse, and smoking.

Assessment

Depending on the level of impairment, you should first try to reorient patients to their surroundings and circumstances. Perform a thorough assessment, including past medical history and medications, to help differentiate delirium from dementia or identify other causes.

Management

Identifying the stressor or metabolic condition may help identify possible treatments (eg, reducing fevers, administering glucose for hypoglycemia, treating dysrhythmias to improve hypoperfusion).

▶ Suicidal Ideation

Pathophysiology

Suicide is any willful act designed to end one's own life. It's the second-leading cause of death among people ages 10 to 34 years.[9] For those between ages 35 and 54 years, suicide is the fourth-leading cause of death.[9] Suicide is more common among men, especially those who are Caucasian and single, widowed, or divorced. Patients with depression are at higher risk of suicide. Alcoholism is another important risk factor. It is estimated that for every 12 acts of self-harm, 1 person commits suicide.[10] Though many suicide attempts are not reported, it is estimated that at least one million people in the United States intentionally harm themselves each year.[10] Table 28-6 summarizes the risk factors for suicide.

Suicide attempts typically occur when the person feels that close emotional attachments are endangered or when the person has lost someone or something important in his or her life. The person who is suicidal also may have feelings characteristic of depression—feelings of worthlessness, lack of self-esteem, and a sense of being unable to manage his or her life.

Table 28-6 Risk Factors for Suicide

- Depression, or sudden improvement in depression
- Male sex, age <55 years
- Single, widowed, or divorced
- Alcohol or other drug abuse
- Recent loss of spouse or significant relationship
- Chronic, debilitating illness
- Schizophrenia
- Expresses suicidal thoughts and concrete plans for carrying them out
- Caucasian
- Social isolation
- Previous suicide attempt(s)
- Financial setback or job loss
- Family history of suicide

Assessment

Your assessment of *every* patient with depression must include an evaluation of suicide risk. Many paramedics are reluctant to ask a patient directly about suicidal thoughts because they fear that they might put ideas into the patient's head. Remember, however, that suicide is not an original idea, and that a patient with depression will have thought of it. Most patients with depression, in fact, are relieved when you bring up the topic because it gives them "permission" to talk about their suicidal ideas.

You and the patient may find the subject easier to broach using a stepwise approach. You might start by asking, "Have you ever thought that life wasn't worth living?" From there, you may proceed by degrees by asking the following questions:

- Did you ever feel that you would be better off dead?
- Have you ever thought of harming yourself? Do you feel that way now?
- Do you have a plan for going about it? Do you have the things you need to carry out the plan?
- Has anyone in your family ever died by suicide?
- Have you ever tried to kill yourself before?

Patients who have made previous attempts, those who have fashioned detailed, concrete plans for suicide, and those with a history of suicide among close relatives are at higher risk and must be evaluated at a medical facility.

Many patients make last-minute efforts to communicate their suicidal intentions. When a person telephones to threaten suicide, someone should stay on the line until the rescue squad has reached the scene. On arrival, quickly survey the area for any implements that the patient might use for self-injury and discreetly remove them. Be sure to protect your own safety. Encourage the patient to discuss his or her feelings. Ask about the patient's suicidal ideas and plans.

Management

Whenever you find a patient with severe depression or you have another reason to suspect that a patient is at risk of suicide, follow these guidelines:

- **Do not leave the patient alone.** The patient's well-being is your responsibility until he or she is transferred to the care of another medical professional.

- **Collect implements.** Bring any implements of potential self-destruction you may have found at the scene (pill bottles, weapons) to the medical facility.
- **Acknowledge the patient's feelings.** Don't argue with his or her wish to die, but provide honest reassurance. For example, "It's not unusual for a person to feel like you do after losing someone close to them. Sometimes it helps to talk about it."
- **Encourage transport.** If the patient refuses transport, then try to get the people who are close to the patient to help the patient cooperate. If the patient continues to resist, then you may need to call for assistance from law enforcement.

When a person has attempted suicide, medical treatment takes priority. The patient who has taken an overdose of sedative or depressant drugs must be managed for possible respiratory depression or circulatory collapse. The patient who has slashed his or her wrists must be treated to control bleeding and restore circulating volume. Nonetheless, if the patient is still conscious, then try to establish communication and ask the patient to talk about the situation.

A person who attempts suicide is in enormous distress. One of the most important skills you can acquire is the ability to see beyond a person's behavior to his or her underlying distress. When called to treat a person who has attempted suicide, say something to communicate empathy to the patient, such as, "Life must have seemed unbearable for you to do something like this. It's time to get some help." Such a statement is also a good reminder to yourself to be compassionate in such situations.

▶ Patterns of Violence, Abuse, and Neglect

Few situations are as difficult as dealing with a hostile, angry patient, or a person who has been abused or neglected. You'll need a great deal of maturity and experience to understand your own feelings, remain professional and positive, and provide the best possible emergency medical care to all parties.

Abuse and Neglect

Perpetrators of violence and abuse or their targets may themselves have a mental illness that contributes to the situation. As an astute paramedic, you must assess not only the patient, but also his or her environment and other involved people. Look for indications of abuse, neglect, or violence. Document your findings so that they can be used to support a legal charge of neglect or abuse. Report your concerns about possible abuse or neglect according to your local protocols. Your priorities in these situations are safety and management of acute medical and trauma conditions.

Violence

Anger may be a response to illness. The patient may use aggressive behavior to deal with feelings of helplessness, as if to say, "There's something wrong with me, and you're not doing everything possible to help." You may be tempted to respond with anger, but doing so rarely serves any useful purpose.

You can calm most angry patients by conveying an attitude of confidence that the patient will behave well. You may find it helpful to ask the patient directly about his or her anger: "Can you explain why you're angry with me?" Giving the patient a chance to talk about these feelings often enables him or her to overcome them.

One of the most difficult challenges you'll face is a patient who is violent or threatening violence. You must prepare yourself beforehand, both psychologically and tactically, to deal with hostile or violent behavior. An encounter with a violent patient always carries the risk that someone will get hurt, including the patient, a bystander, the paramedics, or all of the above.

Assessing the potential for violence is not just an academic exercise. Most paramedics are exposed to some form of violence during their careers. This violence can include verbal intimidation, verbal abuse, physical abuse, sexual harassment, or sexual assault. Stay alert for possible violent encounters and take measures to prevent them.

Identifying Situations With the Potential for Violence

Begin your preventive action by psychologically preparing for a possible violent encounter. Be aware of that possibility during your response to every call. Don't rely completely on the information your dispatcher gives you.

Being psychologically prepared for violence does *not* mean becoming paranoid or treating every patient with distrust. It does mean developing a "nose for danger," also known as survival awareness.

Risk Factors for Violence

Scenarios in which violence is more likely include:

- Situations where alcohol or illicit drugs are being consumed (eg, tavern, party)
- Incidents involving large crowds
- Incidents in which violence has already occurred (eg, shooting, stabbing, domestic disturbances)

People who are more likely to be violent include those who are intoxicated with alcohol or drugs (especially PCP, LSD, amphetamines, and cocaine), experiencing withdrawal from alcohol or drugs, experiencing psychosis (especially manic and paranoid types), or experiencing delirium from any cause (eg, hypoglycemia, sepsis).

The most important clues to the patient's potential for violence are found in the person's behavior and body language. Look for the following warning signals:

- **Posture:** the patient who sits tensely at the edge of the chair or grips at the armrest

- **Speech:** loud, critical, threatening, full of profanity
- **Motor activity:** Inability to sit still; pacing back and forth or in circles; easily startled
- **Other body language:** clenched fists, avoidance of eye contact, turning away when spoken to
- **Your own feelings:** your own "gut" response to the patient. If your instinct tells you that you're in danger, then pay attention!

Management of the Violent Patient

After you have concluded, for any reason, that a situation carries a potential for violence, you must act quickly.

Assess the entire situation. Are factors in the surroundings contributing to the escalation of violence (eg, friends who are encouraging the patient's behavior)? Can those factors be removed? Does evidence suggest drug use, alcohol use, or head injury? Can any bystanders give you some background information? For example, did the patient's behavior come on gradually or suddenly? Does he or she have a history of violent behavior? Are there any known medical conditions, such as diabetes?

Observe your surroundings. Make sure you have an escape route. Place yourself between the patient and the door, but do not move behind an agitated patient. Do not turn your back on the patient, even for a moment. Note any furniture or other potential barriers. Scan the area for anything that could be used as a weapon (eg, heavy or sharp objects) if the level of violence escalates.

If a violent patient is armed with a weapon, then don't try to deal with the situation yourself. Back off and notify law enforcement. Make sure that others at the scene are not endangered while you await the arrival of the police.

Even if the patient is unarmed, you should maintain a safe distance. Moving too close to a potentially violent patient is likely to increase his or her anxiety level. Maintain a safety zone of two arm lengths. If the patient is backing away from you, then you're too close. Let the patient find a comfortable distance. Don't position yourself directly face-to-face with the patient but rather slightly to the side at a 45° angle, with your escape route unobstructed.

Try verbal interventions first. Anger and aggressive behavior are often responses to illness or feelings of helplessness. Simply talking to the angry person in a calm, sympathetic way may defuse some of the anger. Consider the following guidelines:

- Take a moment to concentrate your own thoughts so that you can convey an impression of calmness and self-control to the patient.
- Identify yourself as a medical professional who is there to help. Keep your voice low—that technique forces the patient to stop what he or she is doing to focus on what you're saying.
- Acknowledge the patient's behavior, and restate your willingness to help. ("You look upset. How can we help you?")
- Encourage the patient to talk about what is bothering him or her. Listen to what is said, and show that you're listening by paraphrasing the words back to the patient. ("I think I understand. Are you saying that . . .?")
- Ask the patient specifically if he or she might lose control or is carrying any sort of weapon.
- Define your expectations of the patient's behavior. Acknowledge his or her potential to do harm ("You could really hurt someone with that crowbar . . ."), but emphasize to the patient that he or she will not be permitted to lose control.
- If verbal de-escalation is not working, then back off and get help. ("Sir, I think we need to take a break to see if you can get hold of yourself, but I'm not leaving. We'll try talking again in a few minutes. If that doesn't work, then I'm going to have some people with me to keep you from hurting anyone.")

▶ Specific Psychiatric Disorders

As a paramedic, you won't diagnose the following disorders, but you should be familiar with them as possible causes of acute psychosis or agitated delirium. Assessment and treatment of patients with these conditions follow the general principles discussed earlier in this chapter.

Mood Disorders

Mood disorders, formally known as affective disorders, are among the most common psychiatric disorders. As much as 10% of the US population will experience a mood disorder, such as a **manic-depressive illness** or a major depression, at some point in their lives.[11] As many as 45% of these disorders are classified as severe.[11] Although feelings such as depression and joy are universal, mood disorders differ from normal bouts of sadness or happiness. In mood disorders, the changes in affect are accompanied by other symptoms, and the net effect is to cause a major disturbance in the person's ability to function. Patients who experience either depression or mania have a unipolar mood disorder. That is, their mood remains at only one pole of the depression-mania continuum. Patients who alternate between mania and depression (both poles of the continuum) have **bipolar mood disorder**. Most patients with a unipolar mood disorder have depression. Unipolar mania is relatively rare.

Manic Behavior. **Mania** is one of the most striking psychiatric conditions. The patient is unlikely to believe that anything is wrong. Thus, it's typically a bystander or family member who calls for an ambulance. To the contrary, the patient with mania is apt to report being "on top of the world—I've never felt better in my life." People experiencing mania typically have an exaggerated perception of happiness, joy, or euphoria, with hyperactivity and insomnia.

Patients with mania are typically awake and alert but are easily distracted. They are also often markedly hyperactive and may report being unable to concentrate. Almost all patients with mania report a significantly decreased need for sleep, and they may go for days without sleeping.

In conversation, people experiencing mania are talkative, with pressured and rapid speech. Flight of ideas (rapid shifting of thoughts) and delusions of grandeur (inflated belief with regard to one's own fame, wealth, power, or intelligence) make it difficult for them to focus on one thing. Patients may report that their thoughts are racing. Their monologues may demonstrate **tangential thinking**, which is characterized by skipping rapidly from one topic to another. (Tangential thinking differs from circumstantial thinking, which refers to including many irrelevant details.) Their ideas are often grandiose. For example, they may have unrealistic plans to embark on a large business venture or to run for high public office. Patients may also believe that they have special powers or are famous and wealthy.

The memory of a patient with mania is usually intact but may be distorted by underlying delusions. The affect is elated (the hallmark of mania). The patient seems to be on a "high," and is unusually and infectiously cheerful. The good cheer may be fragile; however, and the person may quickly become irritable, sarcastic, and hostile with little provocation. A person having an acute manic episode may show psychotic symptoms such as hallucinations.

People experiencing acute manic episodes often get themselves into trouble of one sort or another. They may go on wild spending sprees, make foolish business investments, drive recklessly, commit sexual indiscretions, or pick fights. Generally, the ambulance is summoned when the person has gotten into some sort of trouble, or when his or her behavior has become intolerably disruptive.

Because patients with mania are unlikely to consider themselves ill, they may not agree that they need treatment. When dealing with the patient, be calm, firm, and patient. Don't argue or get into a power struggle. Minimize external stimulation. Talk to the patient in a quiet place, away from other people. Meanwhile, have your partner obtain the medical history separately from relatives or bystanders. When you transport the patient, do not use sirens.

If the patient refuses transport, then consult medical control. Obtain assistance from law enforcement for transport if your medical director indicates that medical facility evaluation is necessary.

Depression. In 2015, an estimated 16.1 million adults age 18 years or older in the United States reported that they'd had at least one major depressive episode in the past year.[12] That number represents 6.7% of all adults in the United States.[12] The patient with depression is often readily identified by a sad expression, bouts of crying, and listless or apathetic behavior. He or she expresses feelings of worthlessness, guilt, and pessimism. These patients may want to be left alone, asserting that no one understands or cares about them and that their problems are hopeless.

Depression may occur in episodes with a sudden onset and limited duration. This finding is common in major depressive disorder, in which the patient feels substantial suffering and pain that interfere with social or occupational functioning. In other patients, depression may be subtle in onset and chronic in nature. When a person experiences signs and symptoms of depression for most days over at least 2 years, he or she may be experiencing a chronic form of depression known as dysthymic disorder. The signs and symptoms of dysthymic disorder cause social and occupational distress but rarely require hospitalization unless the person becomes suicidal.

The diagnostic features of depression are most easily remembered by the mnemonic GAS PIPES:

- **Guilt and self-reproach are characteristic features of depression.** One way to explore the

YOU are the Paramedic PART 4

The patient appears to have tolerated having his vital signs taken, but he continues to glance nervously at the police officers outside his apartment. You explain to the patient that you can help him by transporting him to the medical facility. He can obtain safe medication and treatment. You explain that he needs to continue taking his medication to treat his illness. You offer to drive him in the ambulance where he'll be safe. He appears to consider this option but continues to be apprehensive.

The patient becomes more agitated and refuses transport to the medical facility. He tells you that it's dangerous for him to leave his apartment. The officers express concern about allowing him to refuse transport because of the potential for harm to himself or others should his condition worsen.

You consider your options and contact medical control for recommendations. The physician orders administration of haloperidol (Haldol) 5 mg IM. You're concerned about how the patient may react to this decision, but you explain to the patient that the physician at the medical facility feels he should be evaluated and treated for his condition and has ordered some medications to help him relax.

7. What are your considerations and concerns about administering this medication to an uncooperative patient?
8. What are some legal implications of taking this patient to the medical facility without his consent?

patient's guilt feelings is to ask a question such as, "Are you down on yourself?" or "Do you ever feel as if you're worthless?"

- **Appetite is abnormal in depression.** Usually it is decreased, but a minority of patients with depression may report increased appetite.
- **Sleep disturbance usually takes the form of insomnia.** The typical patient with depression reports that he or she awakens at 0300 or 0400 hours and cannot get back to sleep.
- **Paying attention.** The patient with depression has an impaired ability to concentrate. The impairment is sometimes severe. Ask the patient, "When you're reading a book or a newspaper, can you get all the way through what you're reading, or does your mind start to wander after a couple of minutes?"
- **Interest.** The patient with depression loses interest in things that were once important. He or she can no longer summon enthusiasm for work or hobbies. You might ask the patient, "Are you a [local team name] fan?" If the answer is yes, then ask, "How are they doing this season?" The patient will tell you, "Well, I haven't really been following them lately."
- **Psychomotor abnormalities.** In the patient with depression, psychomotor abilities can be either increased (from agitation) or slowed. Although many patients seem to do everything in slow motion, a significant percentage of patients with depression show agitated behavior, such as pacing, wringing their hands, or picking at themselves.
- **Energy.** People with depression have no energy. They are tired all the time and don't feel like doing anything.
- **Suicidal thoughts.** Most worrisome, people with depression tend to have pervasive and recurrent thoughts of suicide.

Schizophrenia

Schizophrenia is a complex disorder that is neither easily defined nor readily treated, yet has a dramatic effect on society. One in 100 people will be affected by schizophrenia in their lifetimes.[13] An estimated 0.2% to 1.5% of the world's population has schizophrenia.[13] The typical onset occurs during early adulthood, with dysfunctional symptoms becoming more prominent over time.

Some people diagnosed with schizophrenia display signs during early childhood. Their disease may be associated with brain damage sustained early in life. Other influences thought to contribute to this disorder include genetics, neurobiologic influences, and psychological and social influences.

People with schizophrenia may experience delusions, hallucinations, apathy, mutism, a flat affect, a lack of interest in pleasure, erratic speech, overly emotional responses, and extreme motor behavior (either a lack of motor behavior or excessive motor behavior).

Neurotic Disorders

Neurotic disorders are a collection of psychiatric disorders without psychotic symptoms and lacking the intense psychopathology of other mood disorders. These disorders cause many problems for people, their families, and society in general. Treating neurotic disorders carries a large price; however, the cost to society of not treating these disorders (in terms of lost production and lost efficiency) is probably higher.

The neurotic category of conditions includes **anxiety disorders**, mental disorders in which the dominant moods are fear and apprehension. Everyone experiences anxiety occasionally, and a certain amount of anxiety helps people adapt constructively to stress. Patients with anxiety disorders, however, experience persistent, incapacitating anxiety in the absence of external threat. In the United States, the prevalence of adults with any anxiety disorder in the last 12 months is 18.1%.[14] Several types of anxiety disorders, including generalized anxiety disorder, phobias, and panic disorder, are likely to elicit a call for an ambulance or affect your delivery of prehospital care.

Generalized Anxiety Disorder. Although some anxiety in everyday life is normal, when a person worries about everything for no particular reason, or if that worrying is unproductive and the person cannot decide what to do about an upcoming situation, the person may be experiencing **generalized anxiety disorder (GAD)**. A diagnosis of GAD requires that symptoms (anxiety and worry) must be present more days than not for a period of at least 6 months, and the worry must be difficult to turn off or control. GAD is one of the most common anxiety disorders. Patients experiencing GAD are often treated with both pharmacologic agents and counseling. The acute symptoms of anxiety and worry can become overwhelming in GAD, however, prompting a family member or coworker to call for an ambulance.

When dealing with a patient with GAD, identify yourself in a calm, confident manner. Listen attentively to the patient and talk with the person generally about his or her feelings.

Phobias. **Phobic disorders** are an unreasonable fear, apprehension, or dread of a specific situation or thing. The patient with a **simple phobia** focuses all his or her anxieties onto one class of objects (eg, mice, spiders, dogs) or situations (eg, high places, darkness, flying). Research suggests that about 7% of Americans are affected by social anxiety disorder or social phobia.[15] People with social phobias have a fear of everyday social situations, such as fear of going to parties, meeting new people, speaking, or eating in public.

When confronted with the feared object or situation, the person experiences intolerable anxiety and all of the autonomic symptoms that anxiety brings. The patient

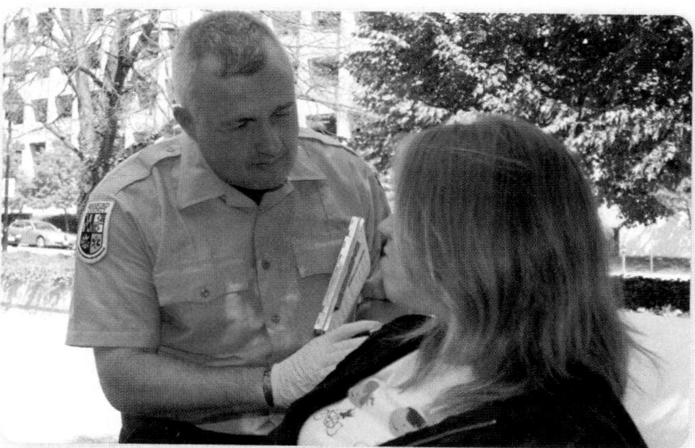

Figure 28-6 When caring for a patient with a phobia, explain each step of treatment in detail before carrying it out.

usually recognizes that the fear is unreasonable but cannot do anything about it.

When you manage a patient with a phobia, explain each step of treatment in detail before you carry it out **Figure 28-6**: "First we'll give you oxygen to help you breathe. Then we're going to move you onto the stretcher, so that we can carry you downstairs."

Panic Disorder. **Panic disorder** is characterized by sudden, usually unexpected, and overwhelming feelings of fear and dread, accompanied by a variety of other symptoms produced by a massive activation of the autonomic nervous system. Women are more likely to be affected by this condition than men.[16]

The attacks usually begin when the patient is in his or her 20s. Most affected people can identify a stressful event that preceded their first attack, such as an illness or loss of a loved one. Thereafter, the attacks may come "out of the blue," without any apparent precipitating stressor. If allowed to continue, then panic attacks may severely limit the patient's lifestyle. The person becomes afraid to go to work, to go shopping, or to leave the house at all, out of fear that an attack will occur away from home. The fear of going into public places is called **agoraphobia** (literally, "fear of the marketplace").

The classic signs and symptoms of panic disorder are summarized in **Table 28-7**. A large percentage of the signs and symptoms, such as palpitations and sweating, are a consequence of autonomic nervous system discharge, while others (chest discomfort, paresthesias) may reflect hyperventilation. The symptoms usually peak in intensity within about 10 minutes and last about an hour.

Table 28-7 Signs and Symptoms of a Panic Attack	
▪ Shortness of breath or a sensation of being smothered ▪ Palpitations or tachycardia ▪ Sweating ▪ Nausea or abdominal distress ▪ Chills or hot flashes ▪ Fear of dying ▪ Feelings of unreality or of being detached from oneself	▪ Feeling dizzy, unsteady, light-headed, or faint ▪ Trembling or shaking ▪ Feeling of choking ▪ Paresthesias ▪ Chest pain or discomfort ▪ Fear of losing control or going crazy

Data from: American Psychiatric Association. *Diagnostic and Statistical Manual of Mental Disorders. 5th ed.* Washington, DC: American Psychiatric Association; 2013.

By the time you arrive at the scene, the patient having a panic attack may be surrounded by many anxious and excited people, who may themselves contribute to the problem. Accordingly, you must take the following steps to control the situation quickly:

- **Separate the patient from panicky bystanders.** However, if you can find a calm friend or member of the patient's family, then having this person present may be helpful.
- **Create a calm environment.** The environment should be as calm as possible as you transport the patient to the medical facility.
- **Tolerate the patient's disability.** The patient having an anxiety attack may not be able to cooperate or answer questions at first because of intense fear and distress. Your manner must convey that everything is under control.
- **Reassure the patient that he or she is safe.** The word *safe* can often reduce symptoms to a more manageable level: "We're going to take you down these stairs on the stretcher. It's going to be okay. We'll go slowly and be careful to keep you safe while we move you."
- **Give the patient's symptoms a name.** After you've checked the patient's vital signs and the ECG, reassure the patient that he or she is not in immediate danger of dying: "I know that the sense of panic you're feeling is distressing, but it's not life-threatening."
- **Help the patient regain control.** Encourage the patient to do things for himself or herself to the extent that he or she can, to help regain a sense of control.

A panic attack may mimic a range of physical disorders in its presentation. Conversely, symptoms of anxiety may be the presenting complaint in medical conditions such as cardiac dysrhythmias, withdrawal states, anaphylaxis, hyperthyroidism, and certain tumors. Therefore, any patient experiencing a panic attack, especially a first-time panic attack, should be fully evaluated in the medical facility. Hyperventilating patients should not be treated with "paper bag therapy." If you use a paper bag, then patients whose anxiety results from an unsuspected pulmonary embolism or cardiac problem may experience serious complications and even die of hypoxemia. You can best manage hyperventilation by coaching patients to slow their breathing until they regain control.

Substance-Related Disorders and Addictive Behavior

Disorders of substance use, addiction, and personal control generally evolve over a relatively long time. Because of the chronic nature of these problems, EMS typically will be called when an underlying problem becomes acutely exacerbated. For example, a patient with bulimia may experience electrolyte imbalances that produce a sudden onset of weakness, dizziness, cardiac or respiratory problems, or seizures, or when an alcoholic experiences respiratory depression from binge drinking. Emergency management of these patients typically focuses on treating symptomatic complaints and the presenting signs and symptoms.

Substance-Related Disorders. Substance-related disorders include psychological disorders associated with the use of alcohol, tobacco, illicit drugs, and other substances that change the way a person feels, behaves, or thinks. These disorders cost thousands of lives and billions of dollars annually.[17–19] An estimated 9.7% of the US population used illicit drugs in 2014.[20]

Substance-related disorders are grouped into four levels. In **substance use**, a person may use moderate amounts of a substance without seriously affecting ADLs (eg, a social drinker).

Substance intoxication describes use that results in impaired thinking and motor function (eg, a drunk driver).

Substance abuse describes the use of a substance that disrupts ADLs (eg, a person has difficulty with work, school, or relationships).

Substance dependence describes an addiction to a substance. The person is physiologically dependent and requires increasingly larger amounts to produce the same effect. An addict may display drug-seeking behaviors. Examples include the repeated use of the substance, taking desperate measures to ingest more of the substance, stealing money, or standing out in the cold to smoke a cigarette.

Determining the most effective treatment for substance-related disorders requires an integrative approach of examining the social, biologic, cultural, cognitive, and psychological dimensions of the problem. As a paramedic, you may be unable to explore all these areas during a short transport to the medical facility, particularly because much of your time will be devoted to ensuring the safety of your crew and managing the patient's ABCs. Understanding the complex nature of substance-related disorders is your first step in providing professional, competent, and compassionate care to all affected people, from the homeless drug addict to the substance-dependent businessperson.

Eating Disorders. The reported incidence of eating disorders began to increase rapidly in the 1950s and 1960s. Today, eating disorders are common in the developed world and are emerging as a problem in developing countries. Some countries are experiencing a fourfold increase in eating disorders.[21] Those most likely to be affected by these disorders are women between the ages of 12 and 25 years.[22]

The two major types of eating disorders are **bulimia nervosa** and **anorexia nervosa**. In both forms, severe electrolyte imbalances may occur, leading to cardiac conditions, seizures, and renal failure, as well as erosion of dental enamel and salivary gland enlargement. Anxiety, depression, and substance abuse disorders are often present in those diagnosed with eating disorders.[23]

Bulimia nervosa is characterized by consumption of large amounts of food, typically more junk food than fruits and vegetables. Many people with this disorder describe their eating as "out of control." Most patients compensate for the binge eating by purging through vomiting, laxatives, diuretics, or excessive exercise. Those with bulimia feel humiliated by both the problem and the lack of control.

People with anorexia differ from those with bulimia in one important way: they lose so much weight that they jeopardize their health and even their lives. They may even binge, albeit on smaller quantities of food. People with anorexia lose weight by exerting extraordinary control over their food consumption. The typical person with anorexia has low body weight for age and height, and demonstrates an intense fear of obesity despite being underweight. If the person with an eating disorder is a woman of child-bearing age, then she may experience amenorrhea (the absence of menstruation).

Somatoform Disorders

People who are overly concerned with their physical health and appearance may have a **somatoform disorder** if their preoccupation dominates their lives. Hypochondriasis is the classic example of a somatoform disorder. In hypochondriasis, patients have extreme anxiety or fear that they may have a serious disease. They are so convinced that they are ill that even a physician will be unable to convince them otherwise. Although the problem in hypochondriasis is anxiety, the person is preoccupied with other imagined symptoms. With somatization disorder, patients also have multiple complaints, but they are more concerned with the symptoms than with their meaning.

In conversion disorders, a physical condition (eg, paralysis, blindness, or seizures) has no identifiable pathophysiology but results from malingering or faking a physical disorder.

Factitious Disorders

A **factitious disorder**, also called Münchausen syndrome, is a condition in which a person intentionally produces or feigns physical or psychological signs or symptoms. In such cases, the patient wishes to be sick. Patients can have various motives for such behavior, such as avoiding legal responsibility or gaining attention. The symptoms the patient is experiencing are under voluntary control, and no obvious physiologic cause of the symptoms is present.

The symptoms the patient experiences may be physical, psychological, or both; are usually dramatic; and indicate an immediate need for medical care. Patients will typically present at night or on weekends in hopes of finding less skilled health care providers or of preventing their insurance or medical records from being found.

One type of factitious disorder is factitious disorder by proxy, also called Münchausen syndrome by proxy. In this condition, a parent or caregiver intentionally makes a child sick to garner attention and pity. This condition is an atypical form of child abuse.

Impulse Control Disorders

People who have **impulse control disorders** lack the ability to resist a temptation or cannot avoid acting on a drive. Examples of impulse control disorders include intermittent explosive disorder, kleptomania, pyromania, and pathologic gambling.

Of course, not every arsonist has pyromania, and not everyone who steals has kleptomania. Impulse control disorders are typically associated with other disorders, such as depression, antisocial or borderline personality disorders, and Alzheimer disease. This group of disorders is rare.

Treatment of impulse control disorders at a medical facility relies on cognitive and behavioral interventions to identify underlying triggers and influences.

Personality Disorders

According to the American Psychiatric Association, **personality disorders** are "a way of thinking, feeling, and behaving that deviates from the expectations of the culture, causes distress or problems functioning, and lasts over time."[24] Common definitions of personality include an individual's distinctive character. How people think or behave in the world and with others may be suspicious, outgoing,

YOU are the Paramedic — PART 5

The patient attempts to rise and move past you as you prepare the medication. Your partner has already explained the medication that has been ordered to the police officers. The officers quickly move to restrain the patient to the chair. They continue to secure him while you administer the medication to a site on the rectus femoris muscle through his slacks.

You expect to see changes in the patient within 10 minutes, so the officers continue to restrain the patient to the chair while your partner prepares the stretcher and you obtain another set of vital signs, including a blood glucose level. You continue to tell the patient what's happening, and you collect his medications and identification. The patient has become much more relaxed and is secured to the stretcher.

You and your partner move him to the ambulance with the assistance of two officers. During transport, you reassess the patient's vital signs every 5 minutes, watching for adverse effects from the medication. On arrival, you give your report to the receiving nurse and place the patient in the psychiatric treatment area of the ED. You complete your patient care report, understanding the importance of good documentation for the patient with a behavioral emergency.

Recording Time: 20 Minutes	
Respirations	14 breaths/min
Pulse	88 beats/min
Skin	Warm, pink, and dry
Blood pressure	118/78 mm Hg
Oxygen saturation (Spo_2)	98% on room air
Pupils	PERRLA
Blood glucose level	96 mg/dL

9. Why must you check blood glucose levels in a patient with a behavioral emergency?
10. What is the most common adverse effect of haloperidol, and how do you treat it?
11. What are some important elements of documentation for a patient having a behavioral emergency that you should include in your report?

fearful, or overly dramatic. When these ways of relating to others become dysfunctional or cause distress to other people, that person is considered to have a personality disorder. The person with the personality disorder often does not feel any subjective distress, and others feel such distress acutely.

True personality disorders are rare in the general population. When a person does have a personality disorder, the person is likely to have another psychiatric illness at the same time. Such patients tend to do poorly during treatment. For example, patients who are depressed in addition to having a personality disorder usually have more difficulty managing the depression when compared with patients who have no personality disorder.

You may have difficulty treating personality disorders over the long term because of your limited interaction with patients. Nevertheless, you must understand these abnormal behaviors so that you can respond appropriately when you encounter them. For example, a patient with an antisocial personality will not hesitate to hurt you if agitated, and a patient with a histrionic personality may be demanding and dictate the level of emergency medical care. Be calm and professional in your interactions with patients exhibiting these traits.

Medications for Psychiatric Disorders and Behavioral Emergencies

Patients with psychiatric emergencies may be taking any of several types of **psychotropic medications**. These medications affect mood, thought, or behavior. During your assessment, identify the medications that have been prescribed for your patient and determine whether the patient is actually taking them.

Refer to Chapter 27, *Toxicology*, for coverage of psychiatric medications as well as other psychiatric-related topics such as substance abuse, street drugs, and withdrawal symptoms.

Words of Wisdom

Psychotropic medications target the autonomic nervous system by either inhibiting or stimulating the sympathetic or parasympathetic nervous systems. You must thoroughly understand these two systems and know how the medications in your paramedic's kit might interact with psychotropic medications.

Psychiatric Medication Types

Antidepressants

Antidepressants are prescribed to combat the symptoms of depressive illness (Table 28-8). The main types of antidepressants are selective serotonin reuptake inhibitors (SSRIs), serotonin-norepinephrine reuptake inhibitors (SNRIs), tricyclic antidepressants (TCAs), and monoamine oxidase inhibitors (MAOIs).

The mechanism of action for most antidepressants is in the ability to alter levels of neurotransmitters (eg, serotonin, norepinephrine, or dopamine) in the autonomic nervous system.

The most commonly prescribed antidepressant in the United States is citalopram (Celexa), an SSRI.[25] Other SSRIs include fluoxetine, sertraline and paroxetine. SSRIs are primarily used to treat major depressive episodes but are also useful in anxiety disorders. These

Table 28-8 Depression Medications

Class	Generic Name	Trade Name
SSRIs	Fluoxetine Citalopram Paroxetine Escitalopram oxalate Sertraline	Prozac Celexa Paxil Lexapro Zoloft
SNRIs	Duloxetine Venlafaxine	Cymbalta Effexor
Heterocyclic (tricyclic and tetracyclic) antidepressants and related medications	Amitriptyline Amoxapine Desipramine Doxepin Imipramine Nortriptyline	Amitril, Endep, Elavil Asendin Norpramin, Pertofrane Adapin, Sinequan Imavate, Janimine, Pramine, Presamine, Tofranil Aventyl, Pamelor
MAOIs	Isocarboxazid Phenelzine Tranylcypromine	Marplan Nardil Parnate
Miscellaneous	Trazodone Bupropion Mirtazapine	Desyrel Wellbutrin Remeron

Abbreviations: SNRIs, serotonin-norepinephrine reuptake inhibitors; SSRIs, selective serotonin reuptake inhibitors; MAOIs, monoamine oxidase inhibitors

Data from: Mancano MA, Gallagher JC. *Frequently Prescribed Medications: Drugs You Need to Know*. 2nd ed. Burlington, MA: Jones & Bartlett Learning; 2014; and Videbeck SL. *Psychiatric Mental Health Nursing*. 6th ed. Hagerstown, MD: Wolters Kluwer Health/Lippincott Williams & Wilkins; 2014.

can include generalized anxiety disorder, panic disorder, and obsessive-compulsive disorder. Adverse effects are minimal, and because the SSRIs lack the anticholinergic and cardiac effects typical of other antidepressants, overdose of SSRIs does relatively little harm. Adverse effects include symptomatic bradycardia with fluoxetine. Other more common adverse effects are headaches, dizziness, sexual dysfunction, nausea, diarrhea, insomnia, and agitation.

Heterocyclic (tricyclic and tetracyclic) antidepressants are a group of medications, some in use since the 1950s, that have been primarily used for major depression but also may be effective for panic disorder, agoraphobia, obsessive-compulsive disorder, enuresis, and school phobia. Examples include amitriptyline, desipramine, imipramine, and nortriptyline.

Adverse effects of heterocyclic antidepressants are common and often occur even when serum levels are within the designated therapeutic range. Most adverse effects are either anticholinergic (dry mouth, metallic taste, blurred vision, constipation, sedation, mydriasis, agitation, and delirium) or cardiotoxic (eg, nonspecific T-wave changes, prolonged QT interval, varying degrees of atrioventricular block, and atrial and ventricular dysrhythmias). Orthostatic hypotension is common in the older adult. Heterocyclic antidepressants are not often prescribed today because of these serious adverse effects.

A third class of antidepressant, MAOIs, are recommended for atypical major depressive episodes. MAOIs also are sometimes useful in selected cases of heterocyclic-refractory major depression and panic disorder. One potential adverse effect is orthostatic hypotension, which, although occasionally severe, usually responds to supportive therapy. Other adverse effects include CNS irritability, including agitation, motor restlessness, and insomnia.

Benzodiazepines

Several classes of medications are effective in the treatment of anxiety disorders, including many antidepressants Table 28-9.

Benzodiazepines are not a substitute for more formal therapy, but a physician may prescribe benzodiazepines for a person experiencing severe emotional distress, even if the patient does not have psychosis or is not an imminent threat to himself or herself or others. Short-term medication therapy may help the anxious patient experiencing crisis or acute panic reactions.

Other uses of benzodiazepines include muscle relaxation; control of seizures; and treatment of alcohol, sedative, or hypnotic withdrawal.

Benzodiazepines are contraindicated in patients with known hypersensitivity to benzodiazepines and in patients with acute, narrow-angle glaucoma. Pregnancy, particularly in the first trimester, is a relative contraindication. Some benzodiazepines have long half-lives, gradually accumulate in the body, and, thus, have a greater potential for causing sedation and confusion, particularly in the older adult.

Table 28-9 Anxiety Medications

Class	Generic Name	Trade Name
Antidepressants		
SSRIs	Citalopram Escitalopram Fluoxetine Fluvoxamine Paroxetine Sertraline	Celexa Lexapro Prozac Luvox Paxil Zoloft
MAOIs	Phenelzine	Nardil
SNRIs	Venlafaxine	Effexor
Anxiolytics		
Benzodiazepines	Alprazolam Chlordiazepoxide Clonazepam Clorazepate Diazepam Lorazepam	Xanax Librium Klonopin Tranxene Valium Ativan
Nonbenzodiazepines	Buspirone	BuSpar
Other Classes		
Antihistamines	Hydroxyzine	Atarax, Vistaril
Beta-blockers	Propranolol	Inderal
Anticonvulsants	Carbamazepine Gabapentin Valproic acid	Tegretol Neurontin Depakote

Abbreviations: SNRIs, serotonin-norepinephrine reuptake inhibitors; SSRIs, selective serotonin reuptake inhibitors; MAOIs, monoamine oxidase inhibitors

Antipsychotics

Antipsychotic medications were introduced in the 1950s to treat mental health illnesses such as schizophrenia and other psychoses. They revolutionized the management of these types of disorders with their effect on the patient's neurologic function, which led to the name *neuroleptics*. These older medications, while still in use today, are known to have varying degrees of adverse effects. Newer antipsychotic medications have less risk of adverse effects and are more effective at treating the

Table 28-10 Antipsychotic Medications

Type	Generic Name	Trade Name
AAP agents	Aripiprazole	Abilify
	Clozapine	Clozaril
	Olanzapine	Zyprexa
	Quetiapine	Seroquel
	Risperidone	Risperdal
	Ziprasidone	Geodon
Traditional antipsychotics	Chlorpromazine	Thorazine
	Chlorprothixene	Taractan
	Fluphenazine	Prolixin, Permitil
	Haloperidol	Haldol
	Loxapine	Loxitane, Daxolin
	Mesoridazine	Serentil
	Molindone	Moban
	Perphenazine	Trilafon
	Thioridazine	Mellaril
	Thiothixene	Navane
	Trifluoperazine	Stelazine

Abbreviation: AAP, atypical antipsychotic

cognitive dysfunction associated with psychoses. This new class of antipsychotics is known as atypical antipsychotic (AAP) drugs. The original, older medications are called typical antipsychotic drugs. The pharmacokinetics of all antipsychotic medications are similar. Table 28-10 lists antipsychotic medications.

The AAP agents often are used as first-line therapy because they not only relieve symptoms such as delusions and hallucinations, but also improve the patient's quality of life by reducing the affective symptoms of anxiety and depression and reducing suicidal tendencies. However, the AAP medications may cause adverse metabolic effects such as glucose deregulation, hypercholesterolemia, and hypertension.

The cardiovascular effects of both typical and atypical antipsychotics depend on the specific medication. They directly affect the heart and blood vessels and indirectly act through CNS and autonomic reflexes to produce other cardiovascular changes. The results are as varied as simple orthostatic hypotension and as complex as ECG changes.

A subcategory of traditional antipsychotics, known as phenothiazines, may reduce contractility of the heart. Haloperidol, commonly used in paramedicine for treatment of acute psychosis, is found in this class. ECG changes include prolongation of the QT and PR intervals, blunting of T waves, and depression of the ST segment.

Patients taking antipsychotic agents may occasionally experience an **acute dystonic reaction** in which the patient develops muscle spasms of the neck, face, and back within a few days of starting treatment with the medication. You can rapidly correct an acute dystonic reaction by giving diphenhydramine (Benadryl), 25 to 50 mg IV. However, the muscle spasms are likely to recur after the diphenhydramine wears off.

Typical antipsychotic medications also have **atropine-like effects** (anticholinergic effects), so patients taking antipsychotic medications may experience the adverse effects associated with atropine use, such as dry mouth, blurred vision, urinary retention, and cardiac dysrhythmias.

Amphetamines

Amphetamines are powerful CNS and parasympathetic nervous system (PNS) stimulants similar to other sympathomimetic medications (eg, epinephrine). Amphetamines (eg, Adderall) are prescribed to help with attention deficit disorder with hyperactivity in both adults and children. They also are used to treat narcolepsy in adults. They raise both systolic and diastolic blood pressure while often slowing the pulse rate. Cardiac dysrhythmias may occur with large doses. The psychological effects depend on the dose, mental state, and personality of the patient. The results are alertness, reduced sense of fatigue, elevated mood, increased concentration, euphoria, and increased motor and speech activities.

▶ Problems Associated With Medication Noncompliance

Most psychotropic medications are designed to alter a patient's mental state, most often to sedate or calm the patient. Dulling of the senses and slowing of thinking are common reasons patients choose not to comply (not stay on their medications).

Another factor in **medication noncompliance** may be the cost of the medications. For example, patients who have been prescribed amphetamines but who cannot afford them or don't have health insurance may consume energy drinks with high doses of caffeine or herbal supplements containing ephedra (ma huang) to compensate. This medication noncompliance often results in frequent conflict with others when abnormal behaviors develop.

Changes in behavior are not always a result of drug abuse. Behavior changes may also result from noncompliance with medications prescribed and dispensed to treat mental health symptoms.

Noncompliance with medications combined with substance abuse increases the risk that a person with a severe mental illness will commit a violent act. When obtaining the patient's medication history, always include previously prescribed medications and missed doses.

▶ Emergency Use of Medications

To some degree, every call you handle has a behavioral component in addition to the patient's trauma or medical problem. For example, the businessman having a heart attack may appear calm and collected, but he is still anxious.

In a behavioral crisis likely to escalate, such as an acute psychotic episode, the threat to the patient, bystanders, and health care professionals may be too great not to intervene, and emergency use of medications may be indicated. The intensity of the situation, the patient's response to you, and your protocols will determine whether verbal, physical, or chemical intervention is necessary.

Before you decide to use medications to control behavior, carry out a complete assessment. Be sure you thoroughly understand the patient's chief complaint, allergies, and medical and medication history. Administration of antipsychotics or benzodiazepines may be beneficial in situations involving aggression, but you must weigh the risks against the possible benefit.

The specific concerns and approaches to managing behavioral or psychiatric emergencies in pediatric and geriatric patients are discussed in Chapter 43, *Pediatric Emergencies*, and Chapter 44, *Geriatric Emergencies*.

The Psychological Effect of War: Returning Combat Veterans

One final topic warrants attention in this chapter. Stressful events such as divorce, failure, rejection, and financial setback are often part of the human experience. These experiences help to shape who we are and what our behavior will be like. In 1980, the third edition of the *Diagnostic and Statistical Manual of Mental Disorders*, introduced the concept that traumatic stressful events outside of an individual's control, such as war, torture, sexual assault, natural disasters, airplane crashes, or factory explosions, can lead to trauma of a psychological nature, not just a physical nature.[26]

Military personnel who experienced combat have a high incidence of PTSD. PTSD occurred in up to 20% of veterans of the Iraq and Afghanistan Wars, 10% of Gulf War veterans, and 30% of Vietnam veterans.[27,28] Reminders of their experiences in the military, such as news coverage or gatherings of veterans, can also be emotional triggers.

A 2008 study explored the effects of war on servicemen and servicewomen deployed for Operation Enduring Freedom in Afghanistan and Operation Iraqi Freedom in Iraq.[29] The study results focus on PTSD, major depression, and traumatic brain injury, and are important not only because of high-level policy interest, but also because—unlike the physical wounds of war—these conditions are often unrecognized and unacknowledged by other service members, family members, and society in general.[29] All three conditions affect mood, thoughts, and behavior.[29]

According to the US Department of Veterans Affairs (VA), PTSD can occur after someone goes through a traumatic event such as combat, assault, or disaster.[30] According to data about VA health care utilization from 2002 through 2015, the three most frequent diagnoses of veterans were (1) musculoskeletal ailments (principally joint and back disorders), (2) mental disorders, and (3) symptoms, signs, and ill-defined conditions.[31] On average, 57% of these patient encounters were for mental health disorders, of which PTSD and depressive disorders were number one and two on the list, respectively.[31]

Symptoms of PTSD vary in severity but are usually based in four categories:[32]

- **Intrusive thoughts**, such as distressing dreams, flashbacks, or nightmares. These thoughts may include a feeling of reliving the experience.
- **Avoiding reminders** of the event, including people, places, objects, situations, etc. The patient may refuse to talk about the event or how he or she is feeling related to it.
- **Negative thoughts and feelings**, such as fear, anger, guilt, and shame, or a feeling of detachment from others.
- **Arousal and reactive symptoms** related to the event that cause problems sleeping or focusing on activities, or even self-destructive behaviors.

People experiencing intense distress will often develop symptoms within days of the event. This condition is known as *acute stress disorder*. The diagnosis of acute stress disorder is made within the first month of the appearance of symptoms.[33] The symptoms differ from those of PTSD in that they are dissociative symptoms, such as amnesia, depersonalization, or a feeling of emotional numbness.[33] Acute stress disorder is considered a precursor to PTSD; if symptoms continue beyond 1 month, further evaluation may lead to a diagnosis of PTSD.[33]

Onset of symptoms of PTSD can develop within several months of the event, but the onset of symptoms may be delayed even longer. PTSD causes significant problems functioning or the inability to respond normally to everyday situations, which is why you may be called to a situation as a paramedic.

Developing military cultural competency is a specific skill that assists you in identifying sometimes-subtle indicators of discharged military personnel. Military culture, beliefs, and ideals of defending a nation or national identity are influenced by courage, loyalty, sacrifice above self (also known as *selfless service*), and a commitment to society. These beliefs can be a source of strength during stressful situations, but they can also cause distress when a sense of failure or injustice challenges their military values. When you encounter military servicemen and servicewomen experiencing acute medical or behavioral problems, use the same compassion, understanding, and protocols as you would use with civilians, but be cognizant of their cultural background.[34]

Words of Wisdom

A hope box is a small container physically kept with a person. It may be a shoe box, envelope, or plastic bag that holds meaningful pictures, quotes, or mementos of happy times and pleasant memories. Hope boxes are used to provide encouragement and hope when a veteran is feeling anxious or stressed. It may provide distraction from more negative behaviors.

A hope box application is available for smartphones. Like a physical hope box, a virtual hope box can assist the patient in shifting distressing thoughts or behaviors. Examples of items that can be included in a virtual hope box include videos, sound recordings, photos, or games.

When working with a combat veteran, ask the patient if he or she has a hope box or virtual hope box to bring with them to the hospital. The hope box can be a useful tool when working with this population.[35]

YOU are the Paramedic SUMMARY

1. What are the initial components of the assessment for this patient?

Provider safety is essential. Carefully assess the scene for hazards or weapons. Forming your general impression of the scene is important to identifying clues to the patient's condition/behavior. Form a general impression of the patient, including his or her behavior, personal hygiene, and posture. Visually assess the patient for life threats, such as signs of alteration in breathing, inadequate circulation, or obvious hemorrhage.

2. What are your safety concerns in dealing with this patient?

This patient is exhibiting behaviors suggestive of an acute psychotic episode. He is experiencing delusions and has an altered perception of reality. He is exhibiting signs of risk for violence, such as refusal to allow the police officers in his apartment, refusal to come out of his apartment, delusions of violence against himself, and low socioeconomic status/potential for history of psychiatric illness based on his residence.

3. What is your initial impression of this patient? What factors, signs, or symptoms would lead you to this conclusion?

The patient appears to be having an acute psychotic episode, possibly schizophrenic. He appears agitated, which is demonstrated by his pacing. He is exhibiting repetitive behavior by clenching and unclenching his fists. He is having paranoid delusions of people wanting to kill him. His mood appears anxious, and he is wary of strangers.

4. Does this patient need to be evaluated at a medical facility?

This patient needs to be evaluated at a medical facility because he is having an acute episode. Because of his delusions, he may be a threat to himself or others. He may not be competent to refuse treatment and transport in his current condition.

5. What conclusions might you make about medication compliance and the patient's medical history?

Based on the fact that the patient is aware of his illness, states that he sees a physician regularly, and filled his prescription recently, it's likely the patient is normally compliant with his medications. Similar to results seen in medication noncompliance, the patient's current episode of psychotic behavior is probably a result of not taking medications for about 1 week. Therapeutic levels may have fallen to a degree that this patient's condition has worsened or behavior has become abnormal.

6. If the patient refuses to be transported, then what options should you, as a paramedic, consider?

You may have local protocols that address the use of restraint or law enforcement intervention in this situation. Local statutes may require that law enforcement personnel intervene out of concern for the patient and the safety of others based on his condition. Consider the legal implications, including the competence of the patient to make decisions. Medical control is an excellent resource. Medical control may grant orders to apply physical restraints or administer medications for the purposes of chemical restraint.

YOU are the Paramedic SUMMARY *(continued)*

7. What are your considerations and concerns for administration of this medication to an uncooperative patient?

Benzodiazepines are typically considered to be the safest class of medication for this purpose because of their ability to be administered intranasally. Administering a medication such as haloperidol IM means that you will expose a large needle. If the patient is unrestrained or restrained ineffectively, then you could be harmed during the administration attempt. The patient may view any medication administered as dangerous or a threat to his person. All medications have risks of adverse effects. A potential advantage of this course is that you may administer haloperidol through clothing in this type of situation.

8. What are some legal implications of taking this patient to the medical facility without his consent?

The patient may be determined to be competent later, and your actions may constitute a violation of his rights. Adverse outcomes may generate other potential for litigation as well as harm to the patient.

9. Why must you check blood glucose levels in a patient with a behavioral emergency?

You can obtain blood glucose levels easily and thereby rule out a medical disorder such as hypoglycemia as a cause for the abnormal behavior. Patients experiencing psychiatric disturbances may not be maintaining adequate nutrition; hypoglycemia may be present and may contribute to the patient's condition.

10. What is the most common adverse effect of haloperidol, and how do you treat it?

The most common adverse effect is extrapyramidal symptoms. If such symptoms occur, then you may administer diphenhydramine hydrochloride in a dose of 25 to 50 mg, depending on local protocols. Because of the risk of this adverse effect, and assuming protocols allow diphenhydramine hydrochloride, you should have this medication readily available after you administer haloperidol (Haldol).

11. What are some important elements of documentation for a patient having a behavioral emergency that you should include in your report?

Take extra care and time to complete a thorough patient care report. Document all assessment findings. Be objective in your findings and factual in your statements. Use direct quotes to incorporate any comments the patient makes. Identify all personnel who cared for the patient, including the name of the physician giving any orders. Document all efforts to convince the patient to consent to treatment and/or transport.

YOU are the Paramedic SUMMARY *(continued)*

EMS Patient Care Report (PCR)					
Date: 08-14-18	**Incident No.:** 201035684		**Nature of Call:** Psychiatric emergency		**Location:** 906 Abbott Street, Apt 312
Dispatched: 1528	**En Route:** 1529	**At Scene:** 1535	**Transport:** 1604	**At Hospital:** 1610	**In Service:** 1630

Patient Information

Age: 44 **Sex:** M **Weight (in kg [lb]):** 76.4 kg (168 lb)	**Allergies:** No known drug allergies **Medications:** Mellaril 200 mg twice daily, Serentil 50 mg twice daily **Past Medical History:** Schizophrenia **Chief Complaint:** Paranoid delusions

Vital Signs

Time: 1543	**BP:** 130/84	**Pulse:** 110	**Respirations:** 20	**Spo_2:** 99%
Time: 1555	**BP:** 118/78	**Pulse:** 88	**Respirations:** 14	**Spo_2:** 98%
Time:	**BP:**	**Pulse:**	**Respirations:**	**Spo_2:**

EMS Treatment (circle all that apply)

Oxygen @ _______ L/min via (circle one): **NC NRM Bag-mask device**		**Assisted Ventilation**	**Airway Adjunct**	**CPR**
Defibrillation	**Bleeding Control**	**Bandaging**	**Splinting**	**Other:** 5 mg haloperidol (circled)

Narrative

EMS requested to above location for a man fearing for his life. On arrival, pt found inside apartment, anxious and agitated, pacing in the living area. Multiple officers on scene in the hallway. Pt refused to leave apartment. Pt stating repeatedly, "They're coming for me." EMS allowed into apartment by pt. Pt sat in chair continuing to clench hands and appear restless. Pt reported he has a history of schizophrenia but has not taken his medications for approximately 1 week because he "knows it's poisoned." EMS advised pt of need for transport to medical facility for evaluation and treatment. Pt refused transport. Medical direction contacted. Dr. Jones ordered administration of 5 mg haloperidol IM for agitation and transport to City Memorial Medical Center for further evaluation and treatment. 5 mg haloperidol IM was given as ordered. Pt placed on stretcher and loaded into ambulance for nonemergent transport. Blood glucose level was 96 mg/dL. Pt became more relaxed and was calm during transport. Pt reassessed en route without changes. Report called to ED before arrival, which included pt's current condition and ETA. On arrival, pt was placed on the ED stretcher, rails up both sides, and report given to RN. Physician signature obtained for medication order.**End of report**

Prep Kit

▶ Ready for Review

- Behavioral emergencies such as drug overdoses, violent behavior, and mental illness can present unique challenges in patient management. Panic by the patient, the family, bystanders, or all of these parties may create a demand for action on your part. Focus on reducing the patient's stress without exposing yourself to unnecessary risks.
- A behavioral or psychiatric emergency is any reaction to events that interferes with ADLs. A person who is no longer able to respond appropriately to the environment and whose abnormal behavior threatens the health and safety of himself or herself or another may be having a true psychiatric emergency.
- Not all behavioral emergencies involve a mental health problem. Some emergencies are a temporary response to a traumatic event.
- Calls for behavioral emergencies have special medical and legal considerations. These considerations can include the need to obtain consent, to follow local guidelines and standing orders for transporting against the patient's will, and to obtain law enforcement assistance when appropriate to do so.
- You have limited legal authority to require a patient to undergo emergency medical care in the absence of a life-threatening emergency. Most states have provisions allowing law enforcement personnel to place mentally impaired people in custody so that such care can be provided. Always involve law enforcement personnel any time you're called to assist a patient with a severe behavioral or psychiatric crisis.
- If a patient poses an immediate threat, then leave the area until law enforcement personnel secure the scene. Always consult medical control and contact law enforcement for help.
- Underlying causes of behavioral emergencies fall into four broad categories: biologic (organic) causes, causes resulting from the person's environment, causes resulting from acute injury or illness, and causes that are substance related.
- Psychiatric signs and symptoms occur when a person's mental health is challenged and psychological mechanisms or behaviors mobilize to help return the person's mental state to homeostasis. Psychiatric signs and symptoms can be grouped according to the systems of psychological (rather than physiologic) functioning they affect: consciousness, motor activity, speech, thought, affect, memory, orientation, and perception.
- Assessing a patient with a behavioral emergency differs from other methods of patient assessment in that with the patient who is disturbed, you are the diagnostic instrument, using your thinking processes, perceptions, and feelings to evaluate and measure the patient. With a behavioral emergency, assessment is also part of the treatment because your voice and manner affect the patient's response.
- In providing emergency medical care to a patient having a behavioral emergency, be direct, honest, and calm; have a definitive plan of action; stay with the patient at all times, but do not get too close; and express interest in the patient's story, but don't judge his or her behavior. Always treat patients with respect.
- When you are assessing the scene, pay special attention to potential dangers and threats (objects that may be used as weapons, hazardous chemicals, and the like). Remove potentially harmful objects. Situations with a strong behavioral component have great potential for sudden and unexpected turns of events, so follow established safety guidelines when responding.
- Primary survey of a behavioral emergency includes identifying yourself clearly, forming a general impression of the patient's overall condition and the nature of the psychiatric emergency, performing the primary survey, making a decision about transport, and taking a history via the MSE. A useful mnemonic for the exam is COASTMAP: consciousness, orientation, activity, speech, thought, memory, affect/mood, and perception.
- Secondary assessment includes looking for signs of an organic cause of the patient's behavioral emergency. This includes inspecting the patient for head trauma, checking pupil size, noting any unusual odors on the patient's breath, and examining the extremities for needle tracks, tremors, or unilateral weakness/loss of sensation.
- Management of the patient with a behavioral emergency focuses on ensuring scene safety and maintaining awareness of life-threatening conditions, while treating the patient for any medical disorders before assuming an emotional or psychiatric cause for the problem.
- Effective communication techniques for a behavioral emergency include beginning with an open-ended question, allowing the patient to talk, showing that you are listening, allowing silence when appropriate, acknowledging and labeling the patient's feelings, avoiding argument, facilitating communication, directing the patient's attention, asking questions, and adjusting your approach as needed.
- Crisis intervention skills include staying calm and being as direct as possible, excluding any disruptive people from the scene, sitting down to interview the patient, maintaining a nonjudgmental attitude,

Prep Kit (continued)

providing honest reassurance, developing a plan of action, encouraging some motor activity, staying with the patient at all times, bringing all of the patient's medications to the medical facility, and assuming that the patient can hear and understand everything you say.

- Use of physical or chemical restraints is reserved for times when verbal intervention fails to reduce severe agitation. Be familiar with the type of restraints and medications used by your agency before you encounter a situation in which they are needed. If restraints are required, then use the minimum force necessary. Assess the ABCs often while the patient is restrained, and maintain a constant dialogue with the patient throughout the restraining process. Maintain constant vigilance to protect safety and document everything that is done.
- Pathophysiologic factors that contribute to behavioral disturbances include cognitive impairment (agitated delirium), thought disorders (including schizophrenia and psychosis), mood disorders (bipolar mood disorder, manic behavior, and depression), neurotic disorders (generalized anxiety disorder, phobias, and panic disorder), substance-related disorders and addictive behavior, somatoform disorders (hypochondriasis and conversion disorder), factitious disorders, impulse control disorders, and personality disorders. Each condition has its own unique pathophysiology as well as standards for assessment and management, so be familiar with each.
- You may encounter patients with psychosis, a thought disorder characterized by a state of delusion in which the person is out of touch with reality. Patients may be belligerent and angry, or silent and withdrawn. The usual methods of reasoning with a patient are unlikely to be effective with patients with psychoses, so be sure to learn the guidelines in caring for a patient with psychosis. These guidelines include being calm, direct, straightforward, and nonconfrontational.
- You may also encounter patients with agitated delirium. This is impairment of cognitive function that can present with disorientation, hallucinations, or delusions, and is characterized by restless and irregular physical activity. One of the most important factors to consider when caring for these patients is your personal safety. Use careful interviewing techniques and refrain from upsetting the patient further.
- The threat of suicide requires immediate intervention. Depression is the most significant risk factor for suicide. Other risk factors include personal or family history of suicide attempts, chronic debilitating illness, financial setback, and severe mental illness. Guidelines for managing the suicidal patient include never leaving the patient alone, collecting any implements of self-destruction, acknowledging the patient's feelings, and providing transport.
- Situations involving violence, abuse, and neglect can present a particular challenge for you because of their potential for escalation and possibility of evoking emotional responses in you. Violent patients make up only a small percentage of those undergoing a behavioral or psychiatric crisis, but you must assess for risk factors for such a patient. These risk factors for violence include history, posture, the scene, speech patterns and other vocal activity, agitation, depression, and physical activity. Managing the violent patient requires you to assess the entire situation, observe your surroundings, maintain a safe distance, try verbal interventions first, and of course request law enforcement personnel if they are not already present.
- Patients with psychiatric emergencies may be taking any of several types of psychotropic medications. During assessment, you must identify the medications the patient has been prescribed and whether he or she is actually taking them. Types of psychiatric medications include antidepressants, benzodiazepines, antipsychotics, and amphetamines. The patient's medication noncompliance often results in abnormal behaviors and confrontational behavior toward others.
- Returning combat veterans have a high incidence of PTSD. Develop military cultural competency, and treat these patients with compassion and understanding.

▶ Vital Vocabulary

activities of daily living (ADLs) The basic activities a person usually accomplishes during a normal day, such as eating, dressing, and washing.

acute dystonic reaction A syndrome that may occur in patients taking typical antipsychotic agents. The patient develops muscle spasms of the neck, face, and back within a few days of starting treatment with the medication.

affect The outward expression of a person's inner feelings (eg, happy, sad, angry, fearful, withdrawn).

agitated delirium An acute confrontational state characterized by global impairment of thinking, perception, judgment, and memory.

Prep Kit *(continued)*

agoraphobia Literally, "fear of the marketplace"; fear of entering a public place from which escape may be impeded.

anorexia nervosa An eating disorder in which a person diets by exerting extraordinary control over his or her eating, and loses weight to the point of jeopardizing his or her health and life.

anxiety disorder A mental disorder in which the dominant mood is fear and apprehension.

atropine-like effects Results of some antipsychotic medications that include adverse effects similar to atropine, resulting in dry mouth, blurred vision, urinary retention, and cardiac dysrhythmias.

behavior How a person functions or acts in response to his or her environment.

behavioral emergency The point at which a person's reactions to events interfere with activities of daily living; becomes a psychiatric emergency when it causes a major life interruption, such as attempted suicide.

bipolar mood disorder A disorder in which a person alternates between mania and depression.

borderline personality disorder A disorder characterized by disordered images of self, impulsive and unpredictable behavior, marked shifts in mood, and instability in relationships with others.

bulimia nervosa An eating disorder characterized by consumption of large amounts of food, for which the patient often compensates by using purging techniques.

catatonic Lacking expression or movement, or appearing rigid.

chemical restraint The use of medication to subdue a patient.

circumstantial thinking Situation in which the patient includes many irrelevant details in his or her account of things.

compulsions Repetitive actions carried out to relieve the anxiety of obsessive thoughts.

confabulation The invention of experiences to cover gaps in memory, seen in patients with certain organic brain syndromes.

confrontation Act of pointing out something of interest in the patient's conversation or behavior, thereby directing the patient's attention to something of which he or she may have been unaware.

covert behavior Behavior that has a hidden meaning or intention that only the person understands.

delusion A fixed belief that is not shared by others of a person's culture or background and that cannot be changed by reasonable argument; a false belief.

dementia The slow onset of progressive disorientation, shortened attention span, and loss of cognitive function.

depression A mental health disorder characterized by a persistent mood of sadness, despair, and discouragement; it may be a symptom of many different mental and physical disorders, or it may be a disorder on its own.

disorganization A condition in which a person is characterized by uncontrolled and disconnected thought, is usually incoherent or rambling in speech, and may or may not be oriented to person and place.

disorientation A condition in which a person may be confused about his or her identity, the location, and the time of day; one of the ways in which various conditions such as schizophrenia or organic brain syndrome may present.

echolalia Meaningless echoing of the interviewer's words by the patient.

factitious disorder A disorder in which a person wishes to be sick and intentionally produces or feigns physical or psychological signs or symptoms. Symptoms are under voluntary control, with no obvious physiologic reason.

flat affect The absence of emotion; appearing to feel no emotion at all.

flight of ideas Accelerated thinking in which the mind skips very rapidly from one thought to the next.

generalized anxiety disorder (GAD) A disorder in which a person worries about everything for no particular reason, or in which the worrying is unproductive and the person cannot decide what to do about an upcoming situation.

hallucination A sense perception not founded on objective reality; a false perception.

impulse control disorder A condition in which a person lacks the ability to resist a temptation or cannot stop acting on a drive.

inappropriate affect Emotion that is out of sync with the situation (eg, wearing a smile while discussing a parent's death).

labile Rapidly shifting among different emotional states.

loosening of associations A situation in which the logical connection between one idea and the next becomes obscure, at least to the listener.

mania A mental disorder characterized by abnormally exaggerated happiness, joy, or euphoria with hyperactivity, insomnia, and grandiose ideas.

manic-depressive illness A bipolar disorder in which mood fluctuates between depression and mania. The alterations in mood are usually episodic and recurrent.

Prep Kit *(continued)*

medication noncompliance A situation in which a patient chooses not to take his or her medications as prescribed, for reasons that may include undesirable adverse effects or prohibitive cost.

mental status exam (MSE) A tool for measuring the "mental vital signs" in a patient who is disturbed. The mnemonic COASTMAP can be used to conduct this exam, assessing consciousness, orientation, activity, speech, thought, memory, affect and mood, and perception.

mood disorder A group of disorders in which the disturbance of mood is accompanied by full or partial manic or depressive syndrome.

mutism The absence of speech.

neologism An invented word that has meaning only to its inventor.

neurotic disorders A collection of psychiatric disorders without psychotic symptoms and lacking the intense psychopathology of other mood disorders; includes anxiety disorders, phobias, and panic disorder.

organic brain syndrome Temporary or permanent dysfunction of the brain, caused by a disturbance in the physical or physiologic functioning of brain tissue.

overt behavior Behavior that is open and generally understood by those around the person.

panic disorder A disorder characterized by sudden, usually unexpected, and overwhelming feelings of fear and dread, accompanied by a variety of other symptoms produced by a massive activation of the autonomic nervous system.

perseveration Repeating the same idea over and over again.

personality disorder The condition in which a person behaves or thinks in a way that is dysfunctional or causes distress to other people.

phobia An abnormal and persistent dread of a specific object or situation.

phobic disorders Disorders involving an unreasonable fear, apprehension, or dread of a specific situation or thing.

posttraumatic stress disorder (PTSD) A severe form of anxiety that stems from a traumatic experience; characterized by the reliving of the stress and nightmares of the original situation.

pressure of speech Speech in which words seem to tumble out under immense emotional pressure.

psychiatric emergency An emergency in which abnormal behavior threatens a person's health and safety or the health and safety of another person, such as with a person who becomes suicidal or homicidal, or who has a psychotic episode.

psychosis A mental disorder characterized by a loss of contact with reality.

psychotropic medications Medications that affect mood, thought, or behavior.

schizophrenia A complex mental disorder that is difficult to identify and whose typical onset is during early adulthood. Dysfunctional symptoms typically become more prominent over time and include delusions, hallucinations, apathy, mutism, flat affect, lack of interest in pleasure, erratic speech, dysfunctional emotional responses, and dysfunctional motor behavior.

simple phobia A fear that is focused on one class of objects (eg, mice, spiders, dogs) or situations (eg, high places, darkness, flying).

somatoform disorder A condition in which a person is overly concerned with physical health and appearance to the point that it dominates his or her life (eg, hypochondria).

stereotyped movements Repetitive movements that don't appear to serve any purpose.

substance abuse Use of a substance that disrupts activities of daily living.

substance dependence Use of a substance that results in addiction and physiologic dependence on the substance.

substance intoxication Use of a substance that results in impaired thinking and motor function.

substance use Use of moderate amounts of a substance without seriously affecting activities of daily living.

tangential thinking A tendency to leave the current topic in conversation to talk about something else, thereby inhibiting interpersonal communication.

thought broadcasting The belief that thoughts are broadcast aloud and can be heard by others.

thought insertion The belief that thoughts are being thrust into one's mind by another person.

thought withdrawal The belief that thoughts are being removed from one's mind.

▶ References

1. Non-specific psychological distress. Centers for Disease Control and Prevention website. https://www.cdc.gov/mentalhealth/data_stats/nspd.htm. Updated October 4, 2013. Accessed March 7, 2017.

Prep Kit *(continued)*

2. Center for Behavioral Health Statistics and Quality. *2014 National Survey on Drug Use and Health: Mental Health Detailed Tables*. Rockville, MD: Substance Abuse and Mental Health Services Administration; 2015. https://www.samhsa.gov/data/sites/default/files/NSDUH-MHDetTabs2014/NSDUH-MHDetTabs2014.pdf. Accessed March 13, 2017.
3. Inapsine (droperidol) dear healthcare professional letter Dec 2001. US Food and Drug Administration website. https://www.fda.gov/safety/medwatch/safetyinformation/safetyalertsforhumanmedicalproducts/ucm173778.htm. Updated July 27, 2009. Accessed March 6, 2017.
4. Antipsychotics, conventional and atypical. US Food and Drug Administration website. https://www.fda.gov/Safety/MedWatch/SafetyInformation/SafetyAlertsforHumanMedicalProducts/ucm110212.htm. Updated August 28, 2013. Accessed March 12, 2017.
5. Seroquel (quetiapine fumarate) tablets August 2008. US Food and Drug Administration website. https://www.fda.gov/Safety/MedWatch/SafetyInformation/Safety-RelatedDrugLabelingChanges/ucm123259.htm. Updated June 19, 2009. Accessed March 12, 2017.
6. Scheppke KA, Braghiroli J, Shalaby M, Chait R. Prehospital use of IM ketamine for sedation of violent and agitated patients. *West J Emerg Med*. 2014;15(7):736-741.
7. Cole JB, Moore JC, Nystrom PC, et al. A prospective study of ketamine versus haloperidol for severe prehospital agitation. *Clin Toxicol*. 2016;54(7):556-562.
8. Strote J, Hutson HR. Taser use in restraint-related deaths. *Prehosp Emerg Care*. 2006;10(4):447-450.
9. National Center for Injury Prevention and Control. Leading causes of death reports, national and regional, 1999-2015. Centers for Disease Control and Prevention website. https://webappa.cdc.gov/sasweb/ncipc/leadcaus10_us.html. Updated June 24, 2015. Accessed November 21, 2016.
10. Suicide statistics. American Foundation for Suicide Prevention website. https://afsp.org/about-suicide/suicide-statistics/. Accessed March 13, 2017.
11. Any mood disorder among adults. National Institute of Mental Health website. https://www.nimh.nih.gov/health/statistics/prevalence/any-mood-disorder-among-adults.shtml. Accessed March 13, 2017.
12. Center for Behavioral Health Statistics and Quality. *Key Substance Use and Mental Health Indicators in the United States: Results From the 2015 National Survey on Drug Use and Health* (HHS Publication No. SMA 16-4984, NSDUH Series H-51). Washington, DC: Department of Health and Human Services; 2016.
13. Schizophrenia. National Institute of Mental Health website. https://www.nimh.nih.gov/health/statistics/prevalence/schizophrenia.shtml. Accessed March 13, 2017.
14. Any anxiety disorder among adults. National Institute of Mental Health website. https://www.nimh.nih.gov/health/statistics/prevalence/any-anxiety-disorder-among-adults.shtml. Accessed November 21, 2016.
15. Social anxiety disorder: more than just shyness. National Institute of Mental Health website. https://www.nimh.nih.gov/health/publications/social-anxiety-disorder-more-than-just-shyness/index.shtml. Accessed March 12, 2017.
16. Anxiety disorders. National Institute of Mental Health website. https://www.nimh.nih.gov/health/topics/anxiety-disorders/index.shtml. Updated March 2016. Accessed March 13, 2017.
17. National Drug Intelligence Center. *The Economic Impact of Illicit Drug Use on American Society*. Washington, DC: US Department of Justice; April 2011.
18. Excessive drinking costs US $223.5 billion. Centers for Disease Control and Prevention website. https://www.cdc.gov/features/alcoholconsumption/. Updated April 17, 2014. Accessed March 7, 2017.
19. US Department of Health and Human Services. *The Health Consequences of Smoking—50 Years of Progress. A Report of the Surgeon General*. Atlanta, GA: US Department of Health and Human Services, Centers for Disease Control and Prevention, National Center for Chronic Disease Prevention and Health Promotion, Office on Smoking and Health; 2014. Printed with corrections, January 2014.
20. Center for Behavioral Statistics and Quality. *2013–2014 National Survey on Drug Use and Health: Model-Based Prevalence Estimates (50 States and the District of Columbia)*. Rockville, MD: Substance Abuse and Mental Health Services Administration [undated report]. https://www.samhsa.gov/data/sites/default/files/NSDUHsaePercents2014.pdf. Accessed November 21, 2016.
21. Pike KM, Dunne PE. The rise of eating disorders in Asia: a review. *J Eat Disord*. 2015;3:33.
22. Child and Adolescent Eating Disorders Program. Anorexia nervosa. University of Rochester Medicine Golisano Children's Hospital website. https://www.urmc.rochester.edu/childrens-hospital/adolescent/eating-disorders/teens/anorexia-nervosa.aspx. Accessed March 10, 2017.
23. Eating Disorders. Anxiety and Depression Association of America website. https://www.adaa.org/understanding-anxiety/related-illnesses/eating-disorders. Accessed March 13, 2017.

Prep Kit *(continued)*

24. American Psychiatric Association. *Diagnostic and Statistical Manual of Mental Disorders.* 5th ed. Washington, DC: American Psychiatric Association; 2013.
25. Coupland C. Antidepressant use and risk of suicide and attempted suicide or self harm in people aged 20 to 64: cohort study using a primary care database. *Brit Med J.* 2015;350:h517. http://www.bmj.com/content/350/bmj.h517. Accessed March 7, 2017.
26. Friedman MJ. PTSD history and overview. US Department of Veterans Affairs website. http://www.ptsd.va.gov/professional/PTSD-overview/ptsd-overview.asp. Accessed March 7, 2017.
27. How common is PTSD? US Department of Veterans Affairs website. http://www.ptsd.va.gov/public/PTSD-overview/basics/how-common-is-ptsd.asp. Updated October 3, 2016. Accessed February 3, 2017.
28. Gradus JL. Epidemiology of PTSD. US Department of Veterans Affairs website. http://www.ptsd.va.gov/professional/PTSD-overview/epidemiological-facts-ptsd.asp. Updated October 3, 2016. Accessed February 3, 2017.
29. Tanielian T, Jaycox LH, Adamson DM, et al. Invisible wounds of war: Psychological and cognitive injuries, their consequences, and services to assist recovery. RAND Corporation website. http://www.rand.org/pubs/monographs/MG720.html. Accessed March 7, 2017.
30. PTSD overview. US Department of Veterans Affairs website. http://www.ptsd.va.gov/professional/PTSD-overview/index.asp. Accessed March 7, 2017.
31. Epidemiology Program, Post-Deployment Health Group, Office of Patient Care Services, Veterans Health Administration, Department of Veterans Affairs. (2017). *Analysis of VA Health Care Utilization Among Operation Enduring Freedom (OEF), Operation Iraqi Freedom (OIF), and Operation New Dawn (OND) Veterans: Cumulative From 1st Qtr FY 2002 Through 3rd Qtr FY 2015.* Washington, DC: US Department of Veterans Affairs; 2017. http://www.publichealth.va.gov/docs/epidemiology/healthcare-utilization-report-fy2015-qtr3.pdf. Accessed March 7, 2017.
32. What is posttraumatic stress disorder? American Psychiatric Association website. https://www.psychiatry.org/patients-families/ptsd/what-is-ptsd?_ga=1.133267214.1055821636.1488863540. Accessed March 7, 2017.
33. Gibson LE. Acute stress disorder. US Department of Veterans Affairs website. http://www.ptsd.va.gov/professional/treatment/early/acute-stress-disorder.asp. Last updated February 23, 2016. Accessed March 13, 2017.
34. Convoy S, Westphal RJ. The importance of developing military cultural competence. *J Emerg Nurs.* 2013 Nov;39(6):591-594.
35. Virtual "hope box" could help reduce suicidal thoughts. US Department of Veterans Affairs website. https://www.va.gov/health/NewsFeatures/20121102a.asp. Accessed March 7, 2017.

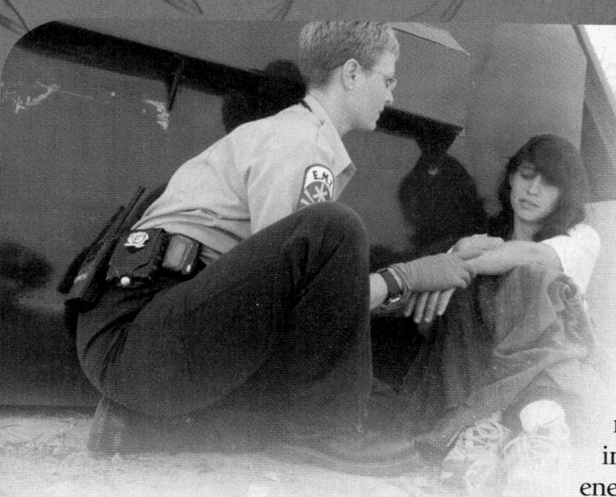

Assessment in Action

At 1100 hours, you are the paramedic on a unit dispatched to an assisted-living facility. Dispatch information shows that you are responding to a 72-year-old woman whom staff describe as having aggressive behavior and mood swings. On arrival at the reception area of the facility, you are greeted by a social worker who informs you that the patient refuses to leave her room, has threatened staff, and has refused all meals and medications since breakfast. The social worker leads you through the facility to a room down the hall.

On arrival at the patient's room, you note that the door is open and that the patient is seated on a chair in a living area just inside the small apartment. She is rubbing a pillow in her lap and watching the doorway as you enter. She appears anxious. You introduce yourself and ask her name. She correctly provides her name but then asks if you know where her husband is. You look to the social worker who says that he is recently deceased. You ask the patient if you may sit with her and talk. She allows this but again asks if you know where her husband is. You calmly explain that he has died recently and ask if she remembers this. She becomes angry and informs you that he is being kept from her and is not dead. You notice that she becomes rigid in her seat and squeezes the pillow tightly.

1. Which of the four causes of behavioral emergencies fits this patient?

A. Biologic or organic
B. Environment
C. Acute injury or illness
D. Substance-related

2. What is always your first step in the assessment and treatment of the patient having a behavioral emergency?

A. Determine the patient's mental status.
B. Obtain vital signs, including a blood glucose level to rule out a medical cause.
C. Assess the scene carefully.
D. Contact medical control for orders to apply chemical or physical restraints in case the patient becomes violent.

3. Which term best describes a state of delusion in which the person is out of touch with reality?

A. Depression
B. Panic disorder
C. Organic brain syndrome
D. Psychosis

4. Which is the safest type of medication to use for chemical restraint?

A. Antipsychotics
B. Benzodiazepines
C. Opiates
D. Antidepressants

5. Which of the following is NOT typically a cause of agitated delirium?

A. Alzheimer disease
B. Drug toxicity
C. Sepsis
D. Metabolic disorders

6. Which of the following is the most appropriate way to respond to this patient's impaired perception of reality?

A. Agree with the patient's belief that she is being kept apart from her husband, and make up a reason this is happening.
B. Ignore her questions and avoid addressing the concern because it clearly upsets her.
C. Continue to attempt to reorient her to reality, and remind her that her husband is deceased while you provide reassurance.
D. Tell her that the people at the medical facility are waiting to take her to her husband so she will agree to be transported.

7. Which interview technique would NOT be appropriate to use with a patient experiencing a behavioral emergency?

A. Ask open-ended questions.
B. Don't argue with the patient.
C. Allow silence.
D. Ask closed-ended questions.

Assessment *in Action* *(continued)*

8. Which of the following is a false assumption about the legal considerations concerning the patient with a behavioral emergency?
   - **A.** You should include the patient in the assessment and treatment as much as possible.
   - **B.** You should spend time with the patient and avoid rushing into treatment and/or transport.
   - **C.** You should remove the patient from the environment as soon as possible to prevent the patient from becoming violent.
   - **D.** You should thoroughly document all aspects of your assessment of the scene and patient, including quoting the patient's specific comments.

9. Why is it important to conduct a thorough physical assessment of the patient having a behavioral emergency?

10. If physical restraints are necessary to transport this patient, then what factors should be considered as you plan and prepare for restraint?

APPENDIX

Emergency Medications

National EMS Education Standard Competencies

Pharmacology

Integrates comprehensive knowledge of pharmacology to formulate a treatment plan intended to mitigate emergencies and improve the overall health of the patient.

Emergency Medications

- Names (pp 1495-1536)
- Effects (pp 1495-1536)
- Indications (pp 1495-1536)
- Routes of administration (pp 1495-1536)
- Dosages for the medications administered (pp 1495-1536)
- Actions (pp 1495-1536)
- Contraindications (pp 1495-1536)
- Complications (pp 1495-1536)
- Side effects (pp 1495-1536)
- Interactions (pp 1495-1536)

Knowledge Objectives

1. Give the generic and trade names, actions, indications, contraindications, routes of administration, adverse effects, interactions, and doses of medications and intravenous (IV) fluids that may be administered by the paramedic as dictated by state protocols and local medical direction. (pp 1495-1536)

Skills Objectives

There are no skills objectives for this chapter.

Pharmacology Formulary

This formulary reflects the most current recommendations from various resources,[1-3] including the 2015 International Liaison Committee on Resuscitation (ILCOR) Guidelines for emergency cardiac care,[4] the National Model EMS Clinical Guidelines,[5] the 2016 Surviving Sepsis Campaign,[6] and the 2016 Tactical Combat Casualty Care guidelines.[7] It is important to remember that state and regional emergency medical services (EMS) systems have the right to include medications and that indications for these medications may not be covered in this formulary. Always follow your local protocols.

A breakdown of the drug profile format utilized within this formulary is provided here, and abbreviations used in the drug profiles are listed in Table A-1. Medications are broken down into the following components, listed in this order. The goal of this formulary is to provide a reference for paramedic students as they progress through their education.

Generic Name (Trade Name[s])
Class
Mechanism of action
Indications
Contraindications
Adverse reactions/side effects
Drug interactions
Dosage and administration *Adult:* ____
Pediatric: ______
Duration of action *Onset:* ________
*Peak effect:*______ *Duration:*______
Special considerations

Table A-1 Abbreviations Used in Formulary Drug Profiles

Abbreviation	Term	Abbreviation	Term
ACS	acute coronary syndrome	MDI	metered-dose inhaler
AF	atrial fibrillation	MI	myocardial infarction
AMI	acute myocardial infarction	NG	nasogastric
ARDS	acute respiratory distress syndrome	NSAID	nonsteroidal anti-inflammatory drug
AV	atrioventricular	NSTEMI	non–ST segment elevation myocardial infarction
BP	blood pressure	NTG	nitroglycerin
CAD	coronary artery disease	PAC	premature atrial complex
CNS	central nervous system	PCI	percutaneous coronary intervention
COPD	chronic obstructive pulmonary disease	PE	pulmonary embolism, phenytoin equivalents
CPR	cardiopulmonary resuscitation	PEA	pulseless electrical activity
CVA	cerebrovascular accident	PO	oral (from the Latin, *per os*)
DVT	deep venous thrombosis	PSVT	paroxysmal supraventricular tachycardia
ECG	electrocardiogram	PTCA	percutaneous transluminal coronary angioplasty
ET	endotracheal	PVC	premature ventricular complex
FDA	US Food and Drug Administration	RSI	rapid sequence intubation
GABA	gamma-amino butyric acid	RV	right ventricular
GERD	gastroesophageal reflux disease	SL	sublingual
GI	gastrointestinal	SNRI	selective norepinephrine reuptake inhibitor
HAPE	high-altitude pulmonary edema	SSRI	selective serotonin reuptake inhibitor
HIV	human immunodeficiency virus	STEMI	ST segment elevation myocardial infarction
ICP	intracranial pressure	SVT	supraventricular tachycardia
IM	intramuscular	TKO	to keep open
IN	intranasal	TTP	thrombotic thrombocytopenic purpura
IO	intraosseous	VF	ventricular fibrillation
IV	intravenous	VT	ventricular tachycardia
MAOI	monoamine oxidase inhibitor		

Drug Profiles

Recall from Chapter 13, *Principles of Pharmacology*, that "tall man" lettering is sometimes used to avoid confusion of medications with similar spellings.[8] With tall man lettering, capitalized letters highlight the area that differentiates the medication from others with similar names. Use of tall man lettering is intended to help reduce medication-related errors. Tall man lettering is used throughout this Appendix.

AcetaZOLAMIDE (Diamox Sequels)

Class Anticonvulsant, antiglaucoma, diuretic, carbonic anhydrase inhibitor.

Mechanism of action Inhibits hydrogen ion excretion in renal tubule, increasing sodium, potassium, bicarbonate, and water excretion and producing alkaline diuresis.

Indications Acute mountain sickness (treatment and prophylaxis), adjunctive therapy for glaucoma, edema, epilepsy, drug-induced edema or edema due to heart failure.

Contraindications Hypersensitivity, hypokalemia, hyponatremia, renal dysfunction, liver dysfunction.

Adverse reactions/side effects Acidosis, thrombocytopenia, flushing.

Drug interactions Methenamine sulfonamides, droperidol, digitalis, and amphetamines. Use caution with diuretics, other anticonvulsants, metformin.

Dosage and administration *Adult*: Acute mountain sickness: 500 to 1,000 mg/day in divided doses PO. Adjunctive glaucoma therapy: 250 to 1,000 mg PO. Epilepsy: 8 to 30 mg/kg/day in divided doses PO. Edema: 5 g/kg IV or 250 to 375 mg PO. *Pediatric*: Safety and efficacy is not established in patients under the age of 12.

Duration of action *Onset*: 2 to 90 minutes. *Peak effect*: *PO* 2 to 4 hours, IV: 15 minutes. *Duration*: 4 to 12 hours.

Special considerations Pregnancy safety: Category C. IV is less common. Prominent within wilderness EMS and may be present in some mobile integrated health care settings. IM administration is not recommended.

Acetic Acid (VoSol, Borofair)

Class Antibacterial.

Mechanism of action Provides an acidic medium during irrigation of the ear that minimizes bacterial and fungal promulgation.

Indications Otitis externa.

Contraindications Hypersensitivity, perforated tympanic membranes.

Adverse reactions/side effects Skin irritation, sensitivity, stinging sensation.

Drug interactions None currently identified.

Dosage and administration *Adult and pediatric*: 3 to 5 drops topically to the affected area every 4 to 6 hours.

Duration of action *Onset*: 5 minutes. *Peak effect*: 45 to 90 minutes. *Duration*: 2 to 3 hours.

Special considerations Pregnancy safety: Category C. May be seen in the mobile integrated health care setting or prescribed to patients.

Acetylcysteine (Mucomyst, Acetadote)

Class Acetaminophen antidote, amino acid, mucolytic agent.

Mechanism of action Lowers mucus viscosity, restores glutathione concentrations within the liver.

Indications Acetaminophen overdose, atelectasis, bronchopulmonary disease, tracheostomy care.

Contraindications Hypersensitivity, acute asthma.

Adverse reactions/side effects Diarrhea, nausea, vomiting, decreased cardiac function, hypervolemia, seizures, bronchospasm, respiratory distress, flushing, tachycardia, rash, itching.

Drug interactions Nitroglycerin.

Dosage and administration *Adult and Pediatric*: Overdose: 300 mg/kg total IV dose divided into 3 portions and given sequentially as a continuous infusion (a loading dose of 150 mg/kg IV is infused over 1 hour; a second dose, 50 mg/kg IV, is infused over 4 hours; a third dose, 100 mg/kg IV, is infused over 16 hours). Respiratory: 1 to 10 mL of 10% or 20% solution by nebulizer.

Duration of action *Onset*: 1 minute. *Peak effect*: 5 to 15 minutes. *Duration*: 100 minutes.

Special considerations IV infusion is mixed with 5% dextrose solution. Pregnancy safety: Category B. Use cautiously in pregnant and breastfeeding women and only if clearly indicated.

When given IV, acetylcysteine can cause allergic reactions (eg, rash, itching, angioedema, bronchospasm, hypotension), usually following the first dose. Reactions can be minimized by ensuring that the medication is infused over a 1-hour period. Acetylcysteine smells like rotten eggs because of its sulfur content.

▶ *Activated Charcoal (EZ-Char, Actidose, Liqui-Char)

Class Adsorbent, antidote.

Mechanism of action Adsorbs toxic substances from the GI tract.

Indications Most oral poisonings and medication overdoses; can be used after evacuation of poisons.

Contraindications Oral administration to comatose patients; after ingestion of corrosives, caustics, petroleum distillates (ineffective and may induce vomiting); simultaneous administration with other oral drugs. Use caution in patients experiencing abdominal pain of unknown origin or known GI obstruction.

Adverse reactions/side effects If aspirated, can induce fatal form of pneumonitis; constipation, black stools, diarrhea, vomiting, bowel obstruction.

Drug interactions Bonds with and generally inactivates whatever it is mixed with (eg, syrup of ipecac).

Dosage and administration *Adult*: 1 to 2 g/kg PO or NG tube. *Pediatric*: 1 to 2 g/kg PO or NG tube.

Duration of action *Onset*: Immediate. *Peak effect*: Depends on GI function. *Duration*: Will act until excreted.

Special considerations Pregnancy safety: Category C. Often used in conjunction with magnesium citrate. Must be stored in a closed container. Be sure to mix contents well before administration due to separation while being stored. Does not absorb cyanide, lithium, iron, lead, or arsenic. Activated charcoal is no longer used in some EMS systems, but paramedics may still encounter it.

▶ Adenosine (Adenocard)

Class Antidysrhythmic.

Mechanism of action Slows conduction through the AV node; can interrupt reentrant AV nodal pathways.

Indications Conversion of narrow-complex regular tachycardia to sinus rhythm. May convert reentry SVT due to Wolff-Parkinson-White syndrome. Can be used diagnostically for stable, regular, monomorphic wide-complex tachycardia. Adenosine may treat the VT or it may help diagnose the underlying rhythm.

Contraindications Known hypersensitivity. Second- or third-degree AV block or sick sinus syndrome or other sinus node disease unless a functioning artificial pacemaker is present; bronchoconstrictive or bronchospastic lung disease (asthma, COPD); poison- or drug-induced tachycardia.

Adverse reactions/side effects Generally short duration and mild; headache, dizziness, dyspnea, bronchospasm, dysrhythmias, palpitations, hypotension, chest pain, facial flushing, cardiac arrest, nausea, metallic taste, pain in the head or neck, paresthesia, diaphoresis.

Drug interactions Methylxanthines (theophylline-like drugs) antagonize the effects of adenosine. Dipyridamole (Persantine) potentiates the effect of adenosine. Carbamazepine (Tegretol) may potentiate the AV node blocking effect of adenosine.

Dosage and administration *Adult*: 6-mg rapid IV bolus over 1 to 3 seconds, followed by a 20-mL saline flush and elevate the extremity. If no response after 1 to 2 minutes, administer second dose of 12-mg rapid IV bolus over 1 to 3 seconds. *Pediatric*: Initial dose 0.1 mg/kg rapid IV/IO push (maximum first dose, 6 mg), followed by a 5- to 10-mL saline flush. Second dose 0.2 mg/kg rapid IV/IO push (maximum second dose, 12 mg), followed by a 5- to 10-mL saline flush.

Duration of action *Onset*: Seconds. *Peak effect*: Seconds. *Duration*: 12 seconds.

Special considerations Pregnancy safety: Category C. Use only in pregnant women if clearly indicated. Not effective in converting AF or atrial flutter or VT. Short half-life limits adverse effects in most patients. A brief period of most any dysrhythmia, including asystole may occur during pharmacologic conversion. Reduce the dose by one-half in patients on dipyridamole (Persantine), carbamazepine (Tegretol), those with transplanted hearts, or if given via a central IV line.[9]

▶ Albuterol (Proventil, Ventolin)

Class Sympathomimetic, bronchodilator.

Mechanism of action Selective beta-2 agonist that stimulates adrenergic receptors of the sympathomimetic nervous system. Results in smooth-muscle relaxation in the bronchial tree and peripheral vasculature.

Indications Treatment of bronchospasm in patients with reversible obstructive airway disease (COPD/asthma). Prevention of exercise-induced bronchospasm.

Contraindications Known prior hypersensitivity reactions to albuterol. Tachycardia, dysrhythmias, especially those caused by digitalis. Synergistic with other sympathomimetics.

Adverse reactions/side effects Often dose-related and include headache, fatigue, light-headedness, irritability, restlessness, aggressive behavior, pulmonary edema, hoarseness, nasal congestion, increased sputum, hypertension, tachycardia, dysrhythmias, chest pain, palpitations, nausea/vomiting, dry mouth, epigastric pain, and tremors.

Drug interactions Tricyclic antidepressants may potentiate vasculature effects. Beta-blockers are antagonistic and may block pulmonary effects. May potentiate hypokalemia caused by diuretics.

Dosage and administration *Adult*: Administer 2.5 mg. Dilute in 0.5 mL of 0.5% solution for inhalation with 2.5 mL normal saline in nebulizer and administer over 10 to 15 minutes. MDI: 1 to 2 inhalations (90 to 180 mcg); wait 5 minutes between inhalations. *Pediatric*: <20 kg: 1.25 mg/dose via handheld nebulizer or mask over 20 minutes. >20 kg: 2.5 mg/dose via handheld nebulizer or mask over 20 minutes. Repeat once in 20 minutes.

Duration of action *Onset*: 5 to 15 minutes. *Peak effect*: 30 minutes to 2 hours. *Duration*: 3 to 4 hours.

Special considerations Pregnancy safety: Category C. May precipitate angina pectoris and dysrhythmias. In prehospital emergency care, albuterol should be administered only via inhalation. Patients may need to be coached on proper use of MDI, particularly with spacer.

Alteplase (Recombinant Tissue Plasminogen Activator [rTPA], Activase)

Class Fibrinolytic.

Mechanism of action The enzyme binds to the fibrin-bound plasminogen at the clot site, converting plasminogen to plasmin. Plasmin digests the fibrin strands of the clot, restoring perfusion.

Indications AMI, STEMI, massive PE, acute ischemic CVA.

Contraindications Known hypersensitivity. See fibrinolytic checklist in Chapter 17, *Cardiovascular Emergencies.*

Adverse reactions/side effects Intracranial bleeding, headache, reperfusion dysrhythmias, chest pain, hypotension, GI bleeding, nausea, vomiting, abdominal pain.

Drug interactions The risk of bleeding is increased by any medication that affects blood clotting (eg, aspirin, heparin, warfarin), and any medication that inhibits platelet aggregation (eg, clopidogrel, dipyridamole, glycoprotein IIb/IIIa antagonists).

Dosage and administration *Adult*: 15-mg IV bolus over 2 minutes; then 0.75 mg/kg over 30 minutes (not to exceed 50 mg); then 0.50 mg/kg over 60 minutes; maximum total dose of 100 mg (other doses may be prescribed by medical direction). Acute ischemic stroke: 0.9 mg/kg IV (not to exceed 90 mg) infused over 60 minutes; administer 10% of total dose in 1 minute and the rest over the next 60 minutes. *Pediatric*: Safety not established.

Duration of action *Onset*: 30 minutes. *Peak effect*: 60 minutes. *Duration*: Variable.

Special considerations Pregnancy safety: Category C. There are no adequate and well-controlled studies in pregnant women; alteplase should be given to a pregnant patient only if the potential benefits justify the potential risks. Closely monitor vital signs and observe for bleeding. Only administer with an infusion pump. Due to severe spontaneous bleeding risk, invasive procedures (eg, IV starts, injections, NG tube, or nasotracheal intubation) should be avoided. Sites used for invasive procedures already performed should be assessed regularly.

Amiodarone (Cordarone, Pacerone)[10]

Class Antidysrhythmic (Class III).

Mechanism of action Blocks sodium, potassium, and calcium channels; prolongs the action potential and repolarization; decreases AV conduction and sinoatrial (SA) node function.

Indications Stable, regular narrow complex tachycardia if the rhythm persists despite vagal maneuvers or adenosine or the tachycardia is recurrent; to control the ventricular rate in stable, irregular narrow complex tachycardia (ie, AF); to control the ventricular rate in preexcited atrial dysrhythmias with conduction over an accessory pathway; stable monomorphic VT; polymorphic VT with a normal QT interval; cardiac arrest resulting from VF or pulseless VT after CPR, defibrillation, and a vasopressor.

Contraindications Known hypersensitivity, cardiogenic shock, second- or third-degree AV block or sick sinus syndrome or other sinus node disease unless a functioning artificial pacemaker is present.[11]

Adverse reactions/side effects Dizziness, fatigue, malaise, tremor, ataxia, lack of coordination, ARDS, pulmonary edema, cough, progressive dyspnea, heart failure, bradycardia, hypotension, worsening of dysrhythmias, prolonged QT interval, nausea, vomiting, burning at IV site, Stevens-Johnson syndrome.

Drug interactions Use with digoxin may cause digitalis toxicity. Beta-blockers and calcium channel blockers may potentiate bradycardia, sinus arrest, and AV blocks.

Dosage and administration *Adult*: VF/pulseless VT: 300 mg IV/IO push. Initial dose can be followed once in 3 to 5 minutes at 150 mg IV/IO push. Other indications: Loading dose of 150 mg IV/IO over 10 minutes; may repeat every 10 minutes if needed. After conversion, follow with a 1-mg/min infusion for 6 hours and then a 0.5-mg/min maintenance infusion over 18 hours. Maximum cumulative dose: 2.2 g IV/IO per 24 hours. *Pediatric*: Refractory VF/pulseless VT: 5 mg/kg IV/IO bolus. Can repeat the 5-mg/kg IV/IO bolus up to a total dose of 15 mg/kg per 24 hours (2.2 g in adolescents). Maximum single dose: 300 mg. Perfusing ventricular or atrial dysrhythmias: Loading dose 5 mg/kg IV/IO over 20 to 60 minutes (maximum single dose of 300 mg). Can repeat to maximum dose of 15 mg/kg per day (2.2 g in adolescents).

Duration of action *Onset*: 2 hours. *Peak effect*: 3 to 7 hours. *Duration*: Unknown.

Special considerations Pregnancy safety: Category D. Drug may cause fetal harm. Fetal risk and maternal benefit should be considered in the emergency setting. Lactating women should not breastfeed following use. May worsen or precipitate new dysrhythmias. Monitor the patient for hypotension and increasing PR and QT intervals. Dosage may change in accordance with the most current ILCOR recommendations.

▶ Amyl Nitrite[12]

Class Antidote, cyanide poisoning adjunct, nitrate.

Mechanism of action Converts hemoglobin to methemoglobin, which reacts with cyanide and chemically binds with it, preventing any toxic effects.

Indications Cyanide poisoning.

Contraindications None in the emergency setting.

Adverse reactions/side effects Headache, dizziness, weakness, increased ICP, shortness of breath, orthostatic hypotension, tachycardia, syncope, cyanosis of the lips, fingernails, or palms (signs of methemoglobinemia).

Drug interactions Increased hypotensive effects with antihypertensives, alcohol ingestion, phenothiazines, or beta-blockers.

Dosage and administration *Adult*: 1 to 2 ampules crushed and inhaled for 30 seconds of each minute until sodium nitrite is prepared or administer for 30 to 60 seconds every 5 minutes until patient is conscious. *Pediatric*: 1 ampule crushed and inhaled for 30 seconds of each minute until sodium nitrite is prepared or administer for 30 to 60 seconds every 5 minutes until patient is conscious.

Duration of action *Onset*: 30 seconds to 5 minutes. *Peak effect*: Varies. *Duration*: 5 to 10 minutes.

Special considerations Pregnancy safety: Category X. May cause fetal harm by reducing maternal BP and decreasing placental blood supply. Highly flammable: Avoid exposure to heat or flame. Patient should remain seated or supine during and after administration due to hypotensive effects of this medication. Use caution in administering to patients with cerebral hemorrhage, increased ICP, or hypotension. This is the first step in a three-step treatment for cyanide poisoning followed by sodium nitrite and then sodium thiosulfate.

▶ Aspirin (Acetylsalicylic Acid [ASA])

Class Platelet inhibitor, anti-inflammatory agent.

Mechanism of action Prevents the formation of thromboxane A_2, which causes platelets to clump together (aggregate) and form plugs that cause obstruction or constriction; has antipyretic and analgesic properties.

Indications New onset chest discomfort suggestive of ACS.

Contraindications Hypersensitivity. Relatively contraindicated in patients with active ulcer disease or asthma.

Adverse reactions/side effects Bronchospasm, anaphylaxis, wheezing in allergic patients, prolonged bleeding, GI bleeding, epigastric distress, nausea, vomiting, heartburn, Reye syndrome.

Drug interactions Use with caution in patients allergic to NSAIDs.

Dosage and administration *Adult*: 160 mg to 325 mg PO. Chewing is preferable to swallowing. *Pediatric*: Not recommended.

Duration of action *Onset*: 5 to 30 minutes. *Peak effect*: 1 to 3 hours. *Duration*: 3 to 6 hours.

Special considerations Pregnancy safety: Category D. Use cautiously during pregnancy, weighing risks and benefits. If there are no contraindications, non–enteric-coated, chewable aspirin should be given as soon as possible to all patients with a suspected ACS as soon as possible after symptom onset.

▶ Atenolol (Tenormin)

Class Beta-blocker (beta-1 selective), antihypertensive.

Mechanism of action Decreases heart rate, myocardial contractility, and myocardial oxygen demand. Inhibits dilation of bronchial smooth muscle.

Indications To decrease heart rate, the force of myocardial contraction, and myocardial oxygen demand in a patient experiencing an ACS; hypertension; stable narrow-QRS tachycardias if the rhythm persists despite vagal maneuvers or adenosine or if the tachycardia is recurrent; for ventricular rate control in AF and atrial flutter if no signs of heart failure; may be used in the treatment of specific forms of polymorphic VT.

Contraindications Heart failure, cardiogenic shock, bradycardia, lung disease, hypotension, second- or third-degree heart block.

Adverse reactions/side effects Dizziness, bronchospasm, bradycardia, AV conduction delays, hypotension, myocardial infarction, heart failure.

Drug interactions May potentiate antihypertensive effects when given to patients taking calcium channel blockers or MAOIs. Catecholamine-depleting drugs may potentiate hypotension. Sympathomimetic drugs may be antagonized. Signs of hypoglycemia may be masked.

Dosage and administration *Adult*: 5 mg slow IV (over 5 minutes). Wait 10 minutes. If the dysrhythmia persists or recurs, give second dose of 5 mg over 5 minutes. *Pediatric*: Not recommended.

Duration of action *Onset*: Within 5 minutes. *Peak effect*: 10 minutes. *Duration*: 2 to 4 hours.

Special considerations Pregnancy safety: Category D. Should not be taken by pregnant women or women suspected of being pregnant, or during breastfeeding. Concurrent administration with IV calcium channel blockers such as verapamil or dilTIAZem can cause severe hypotension. Atenolol should be used with caution in patients with asthma, obstructive airway disease, decompensated heart failure, and pre-excited AF or atrial flutter. Carefully monitor the patient's BP, heart rate, and cardiac rhythm after administration.

Atropine Sulfate

Class Anticholinergic agent.

Mechanism of action Inhibits the action of acetylcholine at postganglionic parasympathetic neuroeffector sites. Increases heart rate in symptomatic bradydysrhythmias.

Indications Hemodynamically unstable bradycardia, organophosphate poisoning, nerve agent exposure, RSI in pediatrics, beta-blocker or calcium channel blocker overdose.

Contraindications Tachycardia, hypersensitivity, unstable cardiovascular status in acute hemorrhage with myocardial ischemia, narrow-angle glaucoma, hypothermic bradycardia.

Adverse reactions/side effects Drowsiness, confusion, headache, tachycardia, palpitations, dysrhythmias, nausea, vomiting, pupil dilation, dry mouth/nose/skin, blurred vision, urinary retention, constipation, flushed, hot, dry skin; paradoxical bradycardia when pushed too slowly or when given at low doses.

Drug interactions Potential adverse effects when administered with digitalis, cholinergics, physostigmine. Effects enhanced by antihistamines, procainamide, quinidine, antipsychotics, benzodiazepines, and antidepressants.

Dosage and administration *Adult*: Unstable bradycardia: 0.5 mg IV/IO every 3 to 5 minutes as needed; maximum total dose 3 mg total. Use shorter dosing interval (3 minutes) and higher doses in severe clinical conditions. Organophosphate poisoning: Extremely large doses (2 to 4 mg or higher) may be needed. *Pediatric*: Unstable bradycardia: 0.02 mg/kg IV/IO (minimum dose: 0.1 mg). May repeat once. Maximum single dose: Child: 0.5 mg. Adolescent: 1 mg. Maximum total dose: Child: 1 mg. Adolescent: 3 mg. ET dose: 0.04 to 0.06 mg/kg.

Duration of action *Onset*: Immediate. *Peak effect*: 2 to 4 minutes. *Duration*: 4 to 6 hours.

Special considerations Pregnancy safety: Category C. Moderate doses may cause pupillary dilation. Paradoxical bradycardia can occur with doses lower than 0.1 mg. May be ineffective in patients who have had a heart transplant or in infranodal AV blocks.

Azithromycin (Zithromax, Zmax)

Class Antibiotic, macrolide.

Mechanism of action Binds to susceptible microorganisms and interferes with the ability to process protein.

Indications Gram-positive infections in the respiratory system, integumentary system, urinary system, gynecologic system, and patients with HIV.

Contraindications Hypersensitivity, liver dysfunction.

Adverse reactions/side effects Prolonged QT interval, liver damage, and myasthenia crisis.

Drug interactions Extensive. QTc prolonging agents, agents metabolized by cytochrome P450 system.

Dosage and administration *Adult*: 250 to 2,000 mg IV, PO. *Pediatric*: 10 to 30 mg/kg IV (maximum 500 mg daily).

Duration of action *Onset*: Rapid. *Peak effect*: 2.5 to 3.5 hours. *Duration*: 24 hours.

Special considerations Pregnancy safety: Category B. Paramedics may encounter this medication during interfacility transports or in the mobile integrated health care environment. When given IV, must be infused over at least 1 hour.

▶ Benzocaine Spray (Hurricane)

Class Topical anesthetic.
Mechanism of action Stabilizes neuronal membrane, which blocks the initiation and conduction of nerve impulses.
Indications Used as a topical anesthetic to facilitate passage of diagnostic and treatment devices. Suppresses the pharyngeal and tracheal gag reflex.
Contraindications Hypersensitivity.
Adverse reactions/side effects Methemoglobinemia has been reported on extremely rare occasions following the use of benzocaine.
Drug interactions None currently identified.
Dosage and administration *Adult*: 0.5 to 1 second spray, repeat as needed. *Pediatric*: 0.25 to 0.5 second spray, repeat as needed.
Duration of action *Onset*: Immediate. *Peak effect*: Less than 5 minutes. *Duration*: 15 to 45 minutes.
Special considerations Pregnancy safety: Category C. Topical use only; not for ocular use or injection.

▶ Bumetanide (Bumex)

Class Loop diuretic.
Mechanism of action A potent loop diuretic with a rapid onset and short duration of action. Inhibits the reabsorption of sodium and chloride in the ascending limb of the loop of Henle.
Indications Pulmonary edema, heart failure.
Contraindications Hypersensitivity to bumetanide or sulfonamides, hypovolemia, anuria, electrolyte deficiencies, hepatic coma. Use caution: hepatic cirrhosis, ascites, diabetes, hypersensitivity to furosemide.
Adverse reactions/side effects Dizziness, headache, orthostatic hypotension, ECG changes due to electrolyte depletion, nausea/vomiting, diarrhea, muscle cramps, metabolic alkalosis, hypovolemia, dehydration.
Drug interactions NSAIDs reduce diuretic effect. May increase blood levels of lithium, increasing risk of lithium poisoning. Antihypertensives and diuretics can cause further hypotension and fluid depletion.
Dosage and administration *Adult*: 0.5 to 1 mg IV slowly over 1 to 2 minutes, or IM. *Pediatric*: Safety and effectiveness in pediatric patients is not established.
Duration of action *Onset*: Immediate. *Peak effect*: 15 to 30 minutes. *Duration*: 3 to 6 hours.
Special considerations Pregnancy safety: Category C. Use cautiously in pregnant women. Not recommended for use by breastfeeding women. Bumetanide does not have the vasodilatory effects of furosemide. 1 mg bumetanide = 40 mg furosemide. May precipitate hypokalemia-induced digoxin toxicity.

▶ Calcium Chloride

Class Electrolyte (anion).
Mechanism of action Increases cardiac contractile state (positive inotropic effect). May enhance ventricular automaticity.
Indications Hypocalcemia, hyperkalemia, hypermagnesemia, beta-blocker and calcium channel blocker toxicity.
Contraindications Hypercalcemia, VF (relative), digitalis toxicity.
Adverse reactions/side effects Syncope, cardiac arrest, dysrhythmia, bradycardia, hypotension, asystole, peripheral vasodilation, nausea, vomiting, metallic taste, tissue necrosis at injection site, coronary and cerebral artery spasm.
Drug interactions May cause severe bradycardia in patients taking digitalis. Potentiated by thiazide diuretics. May antagonize the effects of calcium channel blockers. Incompatible with most all medications; flush IV/IO line before and after administration.
Dosage and administration *Adult*: Calcium channel blocker overdose and hyperkalemia: 500 mg to 1,000 mg (5 to 10 mL of 10% solution) IV push. May repeat as needed. *Pediatric*: Calcium channel blocker overdose and hyperkalemia: 20 mg/kg (0.2 mL/kg) slow IV push. Maximum 1-g dose; may repeat in 10 minutes.
Duration of action *Onset*: 1 to 3 minutes. *Peak effect*: Variable. *Duration*: 20 to 30 minutes, but may persist for 4 hours (dose dependent).
Special considerations Pregnancy safety: Category C. Do not use routinely in cardiac arrest unless the underlying cause of the arrest is an indication. Three times more potent than calcium gluconate.[13] Central venous administration is the preferred route in pediatrics, if available. Monitor IV site carefully; local infiltration can result in severe tissue necrosis and sloughing. Because this medication is highly irritating, do not administer by either the IM or subcutaneous routes.

▶ Calcium Gluconate

Class Electrolyte.
Mechanism of action Counteracts the toxicity of hyperkalemia by stabilizing the membranes of the cardiac cells, reducing the likelihood of fibrillation.

Indications Hyperkalemia, hypocalcemia, hypermagnesemia, beta-blocker and calcium channel blocker overdose.

Contraindications VF, digitalis toxicity, hypercalcemia.

Adverse reactions/side effects Syncope, cardiac arrest, dysrhythmia, bradycardia, hypotension, asystole, peripheral vasodilation, nausea, vomiting, metallic taste, tissue necrosis at injection site, coronary and cerebral artery spasm.

Drug interactions May cause severe bradycardia in patients taking digitalis. May antagonize the effects of calcium channel blockers. Do not mix or infuse immediately before or after sodium bicarbonate without intervening flush.

Dosage and administration *Adult*: Hyperkalemia: 500 to 1,000 mg slow IV/IO push (1 to 1.5 mL/minute) to maximum of 3 g. Beta-blocker and calcium channel blocker overdose: 3 to 6 g (30 to 60 mL) IV/IO followed by a continuous hourly infusion of the same dose. *Pediatric*: Hyperkalemia: 60 to 100 mg/kg IV/IO slowly over 5 to 10 minutes to a maximum of 3 g. Beta-blocker and calcium channel blocker overdose: 60 mg/kg (0.6 mL/kg) IV/IO followed by a continuous hourly infusion of the same dose.

Duration of action *Onset*: Immediate. *Peak effect*: Immediate. *Duration*: 30 minutes to 2 hours.

Special considerations Pregnancy safety: Category C. Monitor IV site carefully; local infiltration can result in severe tissue necrosis and sloughing. Because this medication is highly irritating, do not administer by either the IM or subcutaneous routes.

▶ Cimetidine (Tagamet)

Class Antiulcer, H_2 blocker.

Mechanism of action Blocks the effects of histamine at H_2 receptors of gastric parietal cells, leading to a reduction of gastric acid volume and gastric acidity.

Indications Gastric or duodenal ulcers, GERD, as an adjunct in the treatment of urticaria and/or pruritus in patients experiencing an allergic reaction, suspected upper GI bleeding, acute gastritis.

Contraindications Hypersensitivity.

Adverse reactions/side effects Gynecomastia, seizures, psychotic disorders, and cardiac arrest, headache, dizziness.

Drug interactions Use caution with medications that metabolize in the liver (cytochrome P450 system), SSRIs/SNRIs, benzodiazepines, beta-blockers, calcium channel blockers, antihyperglycemics, tricyclic antidepressants, and antacids.

Dosage and administration *Adult and pediatric*: 300 to 1,600 mg PO.

Duration of action *Onset*: 60 minutes. *Peak effect*: 45 to 90 minutes. *Duration*: 4 to 5 hours.

Special considerations Pregnancy safety: Category B. Paramedics may encounter cimetidine during interfacility transports.

▶ Clindamycin (Cleocin, Clindagel)

Class Antibacterial.

Mechanism of action Mitigates protein synthesis of susceptible bacteria, ultimately complicating the peptide chain initiation.

Indications Sepsis, respiratory infections, integumentary infections, endocarditis and other cardiac infections, gynecologic infections, abdominal infections, osteomyelitis.

Contraindications Hypersensitivity, history of associated colitis or enteritis.

Adverse reactions/side effects Dry skin, erythema, *Clostridium difficile*, hemorrhagic diarrhea, enterocolitis, agranulocytosis, liver dysfunction, metallic taste (IV), thrombophlebitis (IV).

Drug interactions This medication has been shown to exhibit neuromuscular blocking action; it can enhance the effects of opiate agonists if used simultaneously, enhancing respiratory depressant effects, rifampin, erythromycin, drugs metabolized by cytochrome P450 system.

Dosage and administration *Adult*: 600 to 2,700 mg/day in divided doses IV, 150 to 450 mg PO. *Pediatric*: 20 to 40 mg/kg per day in divided doses IV, 8 to 40 mg/kg per day in divided doses PO.

Duration of action *Onset*: Rapid. *Peak effect*: End of the infusion. *Duration*: 6 to 8 hours.

Special considerations Pregnancy safety: Category B. Patients may experience a benign bitter taste during the infusion.

▶ Clopidogrel (Plavix)

Class Thienopyridine antiplatelet.

Mechanism of action Inhibits platelet aggregation by blocking activation of the glycoprotein IIb/IIIa complex.

Indications STEMI, moderate- to high-risk NSTEMI, ACS, substitute for aspirin in patients unable to take aspirin.

Contraindications Active GI bleeding, intracranial hemorrhage, known hypersensitivity.

Adverse reactions/side effects Severe neutropenia, TTP, GI hemorrhage, cerebral hemorrhage, angioedema, Stevens-Johnson syndrome, rash, flulike symptoms.

Drug interactions Use with caution in patients taking other medications that affect bleeding (eg, warfarin, heparin, enoxaparin, streptokinase, aspirin, NSAIDs).

Dosage and administration *Adult*: Loading dose of 300 to 600 mg PO. *Pediatric*: Not recommended.

Duration of action *Onset*: Rapid. *Peak effect*: 1 hour. *Duration*: 7 to 10 days.

Special considerations Pregnancy safety: Category B. Often given with other anticoagulants (heparin, eptifibatide) in ACS. No reversal agent is currently available. If excessive bleeding is encountered in a patient on clopidogrel, prompt platelet transfusions are indicated.

▶ Dexamethasone Sodium Phosphate (Decadron)

Class Corticosteroid, adrenal glucocorticoid.

Mechanism of action Suppresses acute and chronic inflammation; immunosuppressive effects.

Indications Anaphylaxis, asthma, altitude illness, spinal cord injury, croup, elevated ICP (prevention and treatment), as an adjunct in the treatment of shock.

Contraindications Hypersensitivity, use caution in suspected systemic sepsis.

Adverse reactions/side effects Headache, restlessness, euphoria, psychoses, pulmonary tuberculosis, hypertension, peptic ulcer, nausea, vomiting, GI bleeding, edema, hyperglycemia, immunosuppression, sodium and water retention. None from single dose.

Drug interactions Calcium, metaraminol.

Dosage and administration (Dosage varies depending on the indication for its use; for example in altitude illness 8 mg IM, IV, or PO followed by 4 mg IM, IV, or PO every 6 hours until symptoms resolve.[14] Always consult medical direction.) *Adult*: 10 to 100 mg IV (1 mg/kg slow IV bolus). *Pediatric*: 0.25 to 1 mg/kg IV/IO/IM. Given one time with maximum dose of 16 mg.

Duration of action *Onset*: Hours. *Peak effect*: 8 to 12 hours. *Duration*: 24 to 72 hours.

Special considerations Pregnancy safety: Category C. Use cautiously in breastfeeding women. Protect medication from heat. Toxicity and side effects with long-term use.

▶ Dextrose

Class Carbohydrate, antihypoglycemic.

Mechanism of action Rapidly increases serum glucose levels. Short-term osmotic diuresis.

Indications Hypoglycemia, altered level of consciousness, coma of unknown origin, seizure of unknown origin, status epilepticus.

Contraindications Intracranial hemorrhage.

Adverse reactions/side effects Extravasation leads to tissue necrosis. Cerebral hemorrhage; cerebral ischemia; pulmonary edema; warmth, pain, burning from IV infusion; hyperglycemia.

Drug interactions Sodium bicarbonate, warfarin (Coumadin).

Dosage and administration *Adult*: 25 g slow IV push 50% dextrose (D_{50}), or infuse 10% dextrose (250 mL).[15] May be repeated as necessary. *Pediatric*: 1 year and older; 0.5 to 1 g/kg of 25% dextrose (D_{25}) slow IV/IO push. May be repeated as necessary. *Neonates and infants*: 200 to 500 mg/kg slow IV push (see below). May be repeated as necessary. Maximum concentration of 12.5% (vasculature extremely sensitive to high concentrations).

Duration of action *Onset*: Less than 1 minute. *Peak effect*: Variable. *Duration*: Variable.

Special considerations Pregnancy safety: Category C. Draw blood to determine glucose level before administering. Do not administer to patients with known CVA unless hypoglycemia documented. Due to potential medication shortages, this may not be available in a bolus form. If needed, it can be administered via infusion, likely with a 10% dextrose solution.

▶ DiazePAM (Valium and others)

Class Benzodiazepine, long-acting; sedative-hypnotic; anticonvulsant; schedule IV drug.

Mechanism of action Potentiates effects of inhibitory neurotransmitters. Raises the seizure threshold. Induces amnesia and sedation.

Indications Acute anxiety states and agitation, acute alcohol withdrawal, muscle relaxant, seizure activity, sedation for medical procedures (eg, intubation, ventilated patients, cardioversion), chemical restraint, may be helpful in acute symptomatic cocaine overdose.

Contraindications Hypersensitivity, narrow-angle glaucoma, myasthenia gravis, respiratory depression, coma, head injury.

Adverse reactions/side effects Dizziness, drowsiness, confusion, headache, respiratory depression, hypotension, reflex tachycardia, nausea, vomiting, muscle weakness, tissue necrosis, ataxia, thrombosis, phlebitis.

Drug interactions Incompatible with most drugs, and fluids.

Dosage and administration *Adult*: Seizure activity: 5 mg IV over 5 minutes or 10 mg IM.[16] Anxiety: 2 to 10 mg IM/IV. Premedication for cardioversion: 5 to 15 mg IV over 5 to 10 minutes prior to cardioversion. *Pediatric*:

Seizure activity: 0.05 to 0.1 mg/kg slow IV or 0.1 to 2 mg/kg IM.[16]

Duration of action *Onset*: 2 to 5 minutes IV; 15 to 30 minutes IM.[16] *Peak effect*: 15 to 30 minutes (IV). *Duration*: 20 to 50 minutes.

Special considerations Pregnancy safety: Category D. Contraindicated in pregnancy especially during the first trimester. Rectal administration of anticonvulsants is no longer recommended.[17]

Digoxin (Lanoxin)

Class Inotropic agent, cardiac glycoside, antidysrhythmic.

Mechanism of action Rapid-acting cardiac glycoside with direct and indirect effects: Increases force of myocardial contraction, increases refractory period of AV node, and increases total peripheral resistance.

Indications Heart failure, reentry SVTs, ventricular rate control in atrial flutter and AF.

Contraindications VF, VT, digitalis toxicity, hypersensitivity to digoxin. Hypokalemia, hypomagnesemia, and hypercalcemia potentiate digitalis toxicity.

Adverse reactions/side effects Fatigue, headache, blurred yellow or green vision, seizures, confusion, bradycardia, dysrhythmia, nausea, vomiting, anorexia, skin rash.

Drug interactions Amiodarone, verapamil, and quinidine may increase serum digoxin concentrations. Concurrent use of digoxin and verapamil may lead to severe AV block. Diuretics may potentiate cardiac toxicity.

Dosage and administration *Adult*: Loading dose: 4 to 6 mcg/kg over 5 minutes. Second and third: boluses of 2 to 3 mcg/kg to follow at 4 to 8 hour intervals. *Pediatric*: Not recommended in prehospital setting.

Duration of action *Onset*: 5 to 30 minutes. *Peak effect*: 30 to 120 minutes. *Duration*: Several days.

Special considerations Pregnancy safety: Category C. Reduced doses may be indicated in advanced heart failure, myocardial infarction, severe carditis, or severe pulmonary disease. Many medications can alter the effects of digoxin and require adjustments to the dosages listed here. Digoxin can prolong the PR interval and cause ST-segment changes on the ECG; careful cardiac monitoring is essential. Calcium channel blockers or beta blockers are generally preferred for rate control in patients with AF; adenosine is preferred to treat reentry SVT. Use in patients with an accessory AV pathway (eg, Wolff-Parkinson-White syndrome) increases the risk of VF and is not recommended.[13]

DilTIAZem (Cardizem)

Class Calcium channel blocker, antidysrhythmic (Class IV).

Mechanism of action Inhibits extracellular calcium ion influx across membranes of myocardial cells and vascular smooth muscle cells, resulting in inhibition of cardiac and vascular smooth muscle contraction and thereby dilating main coronary and systemic arteries; no effect on serum calcium concentrations; substantial inhibitory effects on the cardiac conduction system, acting principally at the AV node, with some effects at the SA node.[18]

Indications Stable narrow-QRS tachycardia if the rhythm persists despite vagal maneuvers or adenosine or if the tachycardia is recurrent; to control the ventricular rate in patients with AF or atrial flutter.

Contraindications Hypersensitivity, hypotension, cardiogenic shock, wide-complex tachycardia (may lead to hemodynamic deterioration and VF), second- or third-degree AV block or sick sinus syndrome or other sinus node disease unless a functioning artificial pacemaker is present, poison- or drug-induced tachycardia, AF or atrial flutter when associated with an accessory bypass tract (eg, Wolff-Parkinson-White syndrome).

Adverse reactions/side effects Dizziness, weakness, headache, dyspnea, cough, dysrhythmias, heart failure, peripheral edema, bradycardia, hypotension, AV blocks, syncope, VF, VT, cardiac arrest, chest pain, nausea, vomiting, dry mouth.

Drug interactions Caution in patients using medications that affect cardiac contractility. Should not be administered within 2 to 4 hours of IV beta-blockers; doing so may result in decreased cardiac contractility, bradycardia (including AV blocks), and hypotension.

Dosage and administration *Adult*: Initial dose: 0.25 mg/kg IV over 2 minutes. If inadequate response, may re-bolus in 15 minutes with 0.35 mg/kg IV over 2 minutes. Maintenance infusion of 5 to 15 mg/h titrated to physiologically appropriate heart rate. *Pediatric*: Not recommended.

Duration of action *Onset*: 2 to 5 minutes. *Peak effect*: Variable; usually within 7 minutes. *Duration*: 1 to 3 hours.

Special considerations Pregnancy safety: Category C. Use with caution in patients with renal or hepatic dysfunction. Carefully monitor BP, heart rate, and ECG before, during, and after administration. Dysrhythmias may be present during pharmacologic conversion of PSVT to sinus rhythm.

▶ DiphenhydrAMINE (Benadryl)

Class Antihistamine (H_1 blocker).
Mechanism of action Blocks H_1 histamine receptors in the respiratory tract, blood vessels, and GI smooth muscle; decreases motion sickness. Reverses extrapyramidal reactions.
Indications Symptomatic relief of allergies, allergic reactions, and anaphylaxis. Blood administration reactions; used for motion sickness and relief of acute dystonic reactions caused by phenothiazines; may be useful in phenothiazine overdoses.
Contraindications Hypersensitivity to antihistamines, newborns or premature infants, breastfeeding. Use with caution in infants, children, and older adults and in patients with asthma, narrow-angle glaucoma, or patients taking MAOIs.
Adverse reactions/side effects Drowsiness, sedation, seizures, dizziness, headache, blurred vision, wheezing, thickening of bronchial secretions, palpitations, hypotension, dysrhythmias, dry mouth, diarrhea, nausea, vomiting. Hallucinations, confusion, and paradoxical CNS excitation can occur in children.
Drug interactions Potentiates effects of alcohol and other CNS depressants. MAOIs prolong and intensify the anticholinergic (drying) effects of diphenhydrAMINE.
Dosage and administration *Adult*: 25 to 50 mg IM, IV, PO. *Pediatric*: 1 to 2 mg/kg IV, IO slowly, or IM. If PO: 5 mg/kg per 24 hours.
Duration of action *Onset*: 15 to 30 minutes. *Peak effect*: 1 hour. *Duration*: 3 to 12 hours.
Special considerations Pregnancy safety: Category B. DiphenhydrAMINE increases the effectiveness of EPINEPHrine and is often used in conjunction with it, as in anaphylaxis.

▶ DOBUTamine Hydrochloride (Dobutrex)

Class Adrenergic, inotropic agent.
Mechanism of action Synthetic catecholamine that primarily stimulates beta-1 receptors, with minor stimulation of beta-2 and alpha-1 receptors. Increases myocardial contractility and, stroke volume, resulting in increased cardiac output with modest chronotropic effects. Increases renal blood flow secondary to increased cardiac output.
Indications Cardiogenic shock, heart failure; often used in conjunction with other drugs.
Contraindications Hypersensitivity, shock without adequate fluid replacement, idiopathic hypertrophic subaortic stenosis, suspected or known poison/drug-induced shock.
Adverse reactions/side effects Headache, dyspnea, tachycardia, hypertension, chest pain, dysrhythmias, nausea, vomiting.
Drug interactions Incompatible with sodium bicarbonate and furosemide. Beta-blockers may blunt inotropic effects.
Dosage and administration *Adult*: IV infusion at 2 to 20 mcg/kg per minute titrated to desired effect. Initial dose of 5 to 10 mcg/kg per minute may be used in severe cardiogenic shock or immediately post cardiac arrest management. Maximum dose: 40 mcg/kg per minute. *Pediatric*: IV infusion at 2 to 20 mcg/kg per minute titrated to desired effect.
Duration of action *Onset*: 2 minutes. *Peak effect*: 10 minutes. *Duration*: 1 to 2 minutes after infusion discontinued.
Special considerations Pregnancy safety: Category B. Monitor BP closely. Titrate dose to maintain a heart rate increase of no greater than 10% of baseline. May increase infarct size in patients with MI. Older patients may have a significantly decreased response. Patients may become hypotensive from vasodilatory effect.

▶ Dolasetron (Anzemet)

Class Serotonin receptor antagonist, antiemetic.
Mechanism of action Selectively blocks the action of serotonin, a natural substance that causes nausea and vomiting.
Indications For the prevention and control of nausea or vomiting. Used in-hospital for patients undergoing chemotherapy or surgical procedures.
Contraindications Known hypersensitivity to dolasetron or other 5-HT3 receptor antagonists; use caution in patients with cardiac dysrhythmias or electrolyte abnormalities.
Adverse reactions/side effects ECG changes (prolonged PR interval and QT interval, widened QRS), dysrhythmias, anaphylactic reaction, headache, hypotension, dyspepsia, fever, dizziness, headache, constipation.
Drug interactions Use with phenothiazines, verapamil, haloperidol, dilTIAZem, digoxin, beta-blockers, and Class III antidysrhythmics can have increased cardiac side effects.
Dosage and administration *Adult*: 12.5 mg IV one time, 100 mg PO one time. *Pediatric*: Age 2 to 16 years: 0.35 mg/kg IV one time to a maximum of 12.5 mg/dose, 1.2 mg/kg PO one time to a maximum of 100 mg/dose. Safety and effectiveness in children younger than age 2 years not established.

Duration of action *Onset*: 30 minutes. *Peak effect*: 60 minutes. *Duration*: 4 to 9 hours.

Special considerations Pregnancy safety: Category B. Use cautiously in breastfeeding women. Injectable form should no longer be used in any patient with chemotherapy-induced nausea and vomiting. Generally has no effect when symptoms are due to motion sickness.

DOPamine Hydrochloride (Intropin)

Class Adrenergic, vasopressor, inotropic agent.

Mechanism of action Immediate metabolic precursor to norepinephrine. Produces positive inotropic and chronotropic effects. Constricts systemic vasculature, increasing BP and preload. Increases myocardial contractility and stroke volume.

Indications Cardiogenic and septic shock, hypotension with low cardiac output states, distributive shock, second-line drug for symptomatic bradycardia.

Contraindications Hypersensitivity, hypovolemic shock, pheochromocytoma, uncorrected tachydysrhythmias, VF.

Adverse reactions/side effects Extravasation may cause tissue necrosis. Headache, anxiety, dyspnea, dysrhythmias, hypotension, hypertension, palpitations, chest pain, increased myocardial oxygen demand, nausea, vomiting.

Drug interactions Incompatible with alkaline solutions (sodium bicarbonate). MAOIs will enhance the effect of DOPamine. When administered with phenytoin, may cause hypotension, bradycardia, and seizures.

Dosage and administration *Adult*: IV/IO infusion at 5 to 20 mcg/kg per minute, slowly titrated to patient response. *Pediatric*: IV/IO infusion at 5 to 20 mcg/kg per minute, slowly titrated to patient response.

Duration of action *Onset*: 1 to 4 minutes. *Peak effect*: 5 to 10 minutes. *Duration*: Effects cease almost immediately after infusion is discontinued.

Special considerations Pregnancy safety: Category C. Use caution with pregnant and breastfeeding women. Effects are dose-dependent. Beta-adrenergic response: 5 to 10 mcg/kg per minute: positive chronotropic and inotropic effects. Alpha-adrenergic response: 10 to 20 mcg/kg per minute: vasoconstriction and increase in BP. Greater than 20 mcg/kg per minute: alpha effects predominate and may compromise circulation in the limbs. Should be administered by infusion pump.

Droperidol (Inapsine)[19]

Class Antiemetic, typical antipsychotic.

Mechanism of action Reduces motor activity, anxiety, and causes sedation; also possesses adrenergic-blocking, antifibrillatory, antihistaminic, and anticonvulsive properties.[20]

Indications Significant nausea and vomiting, acute delirium or psychosis, chemical restraint.

Contraindications Hypersensitivity, prolonged QT interval. Use with caution in patients with bradycardia, cardiac disease, concurrent MAOI therapy, Class I and Class III antidysrhythmics or other drugs that prolong the QT interval and cause electrolyte disturbances because of its adverse cardiovascular effects (ie, QT prolongation, hypotension, tachycardia, and torsades de pointes).[20]

Adverse reactions/side effects Hypotension, tachycardia, somnolence, anxiety, dysphoric mood, prolonged QT interval, cardiac arrest.

Drug interactions Antihypertensives, nitrates, CNS depressants, antihistamines, alcohol, opiates, antidepressants, other sedatives.

Dosage and administration *Adult*: 2.5 to 10 mg IV; 5 to 10 mg IM.[16] *Pediatric*: 0.1 mg/kg IV/IM.

Duration of action *Onset*: 3 to 10 minutes IV/IM. *Peak effect*: 30 minutes. *Duration*: 2 to 4 hours.

Special considerations Pregnancy safety: Category C. Use cautiously in pregnant women, weighing fetal risk and maternal benefit. Should not be used in breastfeeding women. Usually reserved for patients with postoperative nausea and vomiting or from chemotherapy. Closely monitor vital signs and ECG.

Enoxaparin (Lovenox)

Class Anticoagulant, low-molecular-weight heparin.

Mechanism of action Contains anti-Factor Xa and IIa, which are responsible for the antithrombotic process.

Indications Prophylaxis and treatment of DVT, PE; treatment of AMI.

Contraindications Hypersensitivity, major bleeding, and thrombocytopenia.

Adverse reactions/side effects Diarrhea, nausea, anemia, AF, heart failure, intracranial hemorrhage, pneumonia.

Drug interactions Drugs that affect platelet function or coagulation, NSAIDs, some penicillins.

Dosage and administration *Adult*: Prophylaxis: 30 to 40 mg subcutaneous. Treatment: 1 to 1.5 mg/kg per dose subcutaneous. *Pediatric*: 0.5 to 1 mg/kg subcutaneous.

Duration of action *Onset*: Unknown. *Peak effect*: 3 to 5 hours. *Duration*: 12 hours.

Special considerations Pregnancy safety: Category B. Use cautiously in pregnant women with threatened abortion and monitor all pregnant women for potential bleeding. Do not administer medication from multidose vial to pregnant women due to benzyl alcohol content. Dose adjustments are needed in renal dysfunction.

EPINEPHrine (Adrenalin)

Class Sympathomimetic.

Mechanism of action Direct-acting alpha and beta agonist. Alpha: vasoconstriction. Beta-1: positive inotropic, chronotropic, and dromotropic effects. Beta-2: bronchial smooth muscle relaxation and dilation of skeletal vasculature. Blocks histamine receptors.

Indications Cardiac arrest (asystole, PEA, VF, and pulseless VT), symptomatic bradycardia as an alternative infusion to DOPamine, hypotension from shock other than hypovolemia, allergic reaction, anaphylaxis, asthma.

Contraindications None in the emergency setting. Relative contraindications include hypertension, hypothermia, pulmonary edema, myocardial ischemia, hypovolemic shock.

Adverse reactions/side effects Nervousness, restlessness, headache, tremor, pulmonary edema, dysrhythmias, chest pain, hypertension, tachycardia, nausea, vomiting.

Drug interactions Potentiates other sympathomimetics. Deactivated by alkaline solutions. MAOIs may potentiate effect. Beta-blockers may blunt effects.

Dosage and administration *Adult*: Allergic reactions and asthma: 0.3 to 0.5 mg (0.3 to 0.5 mL of 1 mg/mL [1:1,000]) IM. Cardiac arrest: IV/IO: 1 mg (10 mL of 0.1 mg/mL [1:10,000 solution]) 3 to 5 minutes during resuscitation. Follow each dose with a 20-mL flush and elevate arm for 10 to 20 seconds after dose. ET: 2 to 2.5 mg diluted in 10 mL normal saline. Continuous infusion: Add 1 mg to 250 mL normal saline or 5% dextrose in water (D_5W; 4 mcg/mL). Profound bradycardia or hypotension: 2 to 10 mcg/min titrated to patient response. Higher dose: up to 0.2 mg/kg may be used for specific indications, such as beta-blocker or calcium channel blocker overdose. *Pediatric*: Anaphylaxis/severe status asthmaticus: 0.01 mg/kg (0.01 mL/kg) IM of a 1 mg/mL (1:1,000) solution (maximum single dose: 0.3 mg).[21] Cardiac arrest: IV/IO dose: 0.01 mg/kg (0.1 mL/kg) of a 0.1-mg/mL (1:10,000) solution every 3 to 5 minutes during arrest. ET: 0.1 mg/kg (0.1 mL/kg) of a 1-mg/mL (1:1,000) solution mixed in 3 to 5 mL of saline until IV/IO access is achieved. Maximum single dose 1 mg IV/IO 2.5 mg ET.[22] Stridor at rest: 0.25 to 0.5 mg/kg of a 1-mg/mL (1:1,000) solution (maximum of 5 mg per dose); this can be diluted with normal saline to bring the volume to 3 mL. Administer L-EPINEPHrine via handheld nebulizer. Symptomatic bradycardia: IV/IO: 0.01 mg/kg (0.1 mL/kg) of a 0.1-mg/mL (1:10,000) solution. ET: 0.1 mg/kg (0.1 mL/kg) of a 1-mg/mL (1:1,000) solution.[22] Continuous IV/IO infusion: 0.1 to 1 mcg/kg per minute.[22] *Neonates*: Bradycardia: 0.01 to 0.03 mg/kg of 0.1 mg/mL (1:10,000) EPINEPHrine (equal to 0.1 to 0.3 mL/kg) IV, followed by 0.5-mL to 1-mL normal saline flush to clear the line[23,24]; 0.05 to 0.1 mg/kg of 0.1 mg/mL (1:10,000) ET until IV access can be obtained, but absorption is less reliable via this route.[23,25] If IV access is not yet established, consider starting with the higher dose of 0.3 up to 1 mL/kg of 0.1 mg/mL (1:10,000) EPINEPHrine given via the ET tube. Dosing may be repeated every 3 to 5 minutes when there is persistent bradycardia.

Duration of action *Onset*: Immediate. *Peak effect*: Minutes. *Duration*: Several minutes.

Special considerations Pregnancy safety: Category C. Contraindicated for patients in active labor. May cause syncope in asthmatic children. May increase myocardial oxygen demand.

EPINEPHrine Racemic (MicroNefrin)

Class Sympathomimetic.

Mechanism of action Stimulates beta-2 receptors in lungs: bronchodilation with relaxation of bronchial smooth muscles. Reduces airway resistance. Useful in treating laryngeal edema; inhibits histamine release.

Indications Bronchial asthma, prevention of bronchospasm, croup, laryngeal edema.

Contraindications Hypertension, underlying cardiovascular disease, epiglottitis.

Adverse reactions/side effects Headache, anxiety, fear, nervousness, respiratory weakness, palpitations, tachycardia, dysrhythmias, nausea, vomiting.

Drug interactions MAOIs and bretylium may potentiate effect. Beta-blockers may blunt effects.

Dosage and administration *Adult*: Dilute 5 mL (1%) in 5 mL saline, administer over 15 minutes. *Pediatric*: Children age 4 or younger: 0.25 mL of racemic EPINEPHrine 2.25% inhalation solution mixed in 3 mL NS *or* 0.5 mL/kg of 1 mg/mL (1:1,000) EPINEPHrine mixed in 3 mL NS (maximum dose 2.5 mL).

Children older than 4 years: Up to 0.5 mL of racemic EPINEPHrine 2.25% inhalation solution mixed in 3 mL NS *or* 0.5 mL/kg of 1 mg/mL (1:1,000) EPINEPHrine mixed in 3 mL NS (maximum dose 5 mL).[26] Administer via handheld nebulizer over 15 minutes.

Duration of action *Onset*: Within 5 minutes. *Peak effect*: 5 to 15 minutes. *Duration*: 1 to 3 hours.

Special considerations Pregnancy safety: Category C. May cause tachycardia and other dysrhythmias. Monitor vital signs. Excessive use may cause bronchospasm. May have a strong rebound effect after drug wears off.

Eptifibatide (Integrilin)

Class Glycoprotein IIb/IIIa inhibitor, platelet aggregation inhibitor.

Mechanism of action Prevents the aggregation of platelets by binding to the glycoprotein IIb/IIIa receptor, preventing the binding of fibrinogen and von Willebrand factors.

Indications Unstable angina and NSTEMI being managed medically. Patients undergoing percutaneous coronary intervention.

Contraindications Any prior intracranial hemorrhage, known malignant intracranial neoplasm, suspected aortic dissection, significant closed head trauma or facial trauma within 3 months, ischemic stroke within 3 months except if acute within 3 hours, active internal bleeding or bleeding disorder in past 30 days, surgical procedure or trauma within preceding 6 weeks, platelet count $<150,000 \times 10^3$/mcL, hypersensitivity to and concomitant use of another glycoprotein IIb/IIIa inhibitor, severe uncontrolled hypertension (systolic BP >200 mm Hg or diastolic BP >110 mm Hg), renal dialysis, recent stroke.

Adverse reactions/side effects Cerebral hemorrhage, pulmonary hemorrhage, hypotension, GI bleeding, internal bleeding, anaphylactic shock, thrombocytopenia.

Drug interactions Thrombolytics, oral anticoagulants, aspirin, other antiplatelet medications, NSAIDs, dipyridamole, ticlopidine, and clopidogrel increase effect. Incompatible in the same IV line with furosemide.

Dosage and administration *Adult*: Medical management: 180 mcg/kg IV bolus over 1 to 2 minutes, followed by a 2-mcg/kg infusion for 72 to 96 hours. Percutaneous coronary intervention/percutaneous transluminal coronary angioplasty: 180-mcg/kg IV bolus over 1 to 2 minutes followed by a 2-mcg/kg infusion, then repeat bolus in 10 minutes. Maximum dose: (based on a 121 kg patient). PCI: 22.6-mg bolus, 15-mg/h infusion, infusion duration 18 to 24 hours after procedure. *Pediatric*: Not recommended.

Duration of action *Onset*: Immediate. *Peak effect*: 30 minutes to 4 hours. *Duration*: Platelet function recovers within 4 to 8 hours after discontinuation.

Special considerations Pregnancy safety: Category B. Must be administered only with an infusion pump direct from bottle with a vented IV set. Due to severe spontaneous bleeding risk, invasive procedures (eg, IV starts, injections, NG tube, or nasotracheal intubation) should be avoided.

Erythromycin

Class Antibiotic, macrolide.

Mechanism of action Inhibits bacterial protein synthesis.

Indications Susceptible bacterial infections, surgical prophylaxis for colorectal procedures, bacteremia, acne, Legionnaire disease.

Contraindications Hypersensitivity to macrolide antibiotics, concomitant use with lovastatin.

Adverse reactions/side effects Anaphylaxis, QT segment prolongation, skin rash.

Drug interactions Statins.

Dosage and administration *Adult*: 250 to 500 mg PO every 6 to 12 hours. 15 to 20 mg/kg IV per day divided into doses every 6 hours. Maximum 4,000 mg per day. *Pediatric*: 30 to 50 mg/kg PO per day with maximum 2,000 mg daily. 15 to 20 mg/kg IV per day divided every 6 hours. Maximum 4,000 mg daily.

Duration of action *Onset*: PO: 1 hour. IV: Rapid. *Peak effect*: PO: 1 to 4 hours. IV: End of infusion. *Duration*: PO and IV: 6 to 12 hours.

Special considerations Pregnancy safety: Category B. Use with caution in breastfeeding women.

Esmolol (Brevibloc)

Class Beta-blocker, antidysrhythmic (Class II).

Mechanism of action As a short-acting adrenergic receptor blocker, it blocks beta-1 and beta-2 receptors, reducing heart rate and causing vasodilation.

Indications Treatment of SVT, AF and atrial flutter, tachycardia, hypertension, AMI. Off-label indications: abdominal aortic aneurysm, thyroid storm.

Contraindications Hypersensitivity, cardiogenic shock, heart failure, pulmonary hypertension, second- or third-degree heart blocks, severe bradycardia, sick sinus syndrome.

Adverse reactions/side effects Hypotension, bradycardia, AMI, seizures, bronchospasm.

Drug interactions Extensive list including alpha blockers, alpha/beta agonists, calcium channel antagonists, antipsychotics, amiodarone.

Dosage and administration *Adult*: Bolus of 0.5 mg/kg over 1 minute IV, followed by 50 mcg/kg per minute infusion. Within 5 to 10 minutes, another bolus can be administered followed by an increased infusion of 100 mcg/kg per minute. This pattern is either titrated to therapeutic effect or maximum infusion dose of 200 mcg/kg per minute. *Pediatric*: Not indicated.

Duration of action *Onset*: 2 to 10 minutes. *Peak effect*: Unknown. *Duration*: 1 to 20 minutes.

Special considerations Pregnancy safety: Category C. Lower doses affect the beta-1 receptor. Higher doses also affect the beta-2 receptor. Carefully monitor the patient's BP, heart rate, and cardiac rhythm after administration.

▶ Etomidate (Amidate)[27]

Class Nonbarbiturate hypnotic, anesthesia induction agent.

Mechanism of action Short-acting hypnotic that acts at the level of the reticular activating system.

Indications Premedication for medication-facilitated intubation or procedural sedation.

Contraindications Hypersensitivity, labor/delivery, or septic shock (particularly in children).

Adverse reactions/side effects Apnea of short duration, respiratory depression, hypoventilation, hyperventilation, dysrhythmias, hypotension, hypertension, nausea, vomiting, involuntary muscle movement, pain at injection site.

Drug interactions Effects may be enhanced when given with other CNS depressants.

Dosage and administration *Adult*: 0.2 to 0.6 mg/kg IV over 30 to 60 seconds (typical adult dose is 20 mg). *Pediatric*: 0.2 to 0.4 mg/kg IV/IO over 30 to 60 seconds for RSI (older than 10 years), one time only. Maximum dose: 20 mg.

Duration of action *Onset*: Less than 1 minute. *Peak effect*: 1 minute. *Duration*: 5 to 10 minutes.

Special considerations Pregnancy safety: Category C. Use caution weighing fetal risk and maternal benefit in pregnant and breastfeeding women. Carefully monitor vital signs. Etomidate can suppress adrenal gland production of steroid hormones and cortisol, which can temporarily cause gland failure. Consider decreasing dose in older patients and patients with cardiac conditions.

▶ Famotidine (Pepcid)

Class Antiulcer, histamine H_2 antagonist.

Mechanism of action Inhibits the volume and concentration of gastric secretions.

Indications GI ulcer, suspected upper GI bleeding, GERD.

Contraindications Hypersensitivity.

Adverse reactions/side effects Constipation, diarrhea, rhabdomyolysis, seizures, pneumonia, agitation, vomiting, headache, dizziness.

Drug interactions Ketoconazole, itraconazole.

Dosage and administration *Adult*: 20 mg IV, 20 to 40 mg PO. *Pediatric*: 0.25 to 0.5 mg/kg IV, 0.5 mg/kg PO.

Duration of action *Onset*: 60 minutes. *Peak effect*: 0.5 to 3 hours. *Duration*: 8 to 15 hours.

Special considerations Pregnancy safety: Category B.

▶ FentaNYL Citrate (Sublimaze)

Class Opioid analgesic; schedule II drug.

Mechanism of action Binds to opiate receptors, producing analgesia and euphoria.

Indications Pain management, anesthesia adjunct.

Contraindications Known hypersensitivity. Use with caution in traumatic brain injury.

Adverse reactions/side effects Confusion, paradoxical excitation, delirium, drowsiness, CNS depression, sedation, respiratory depression, apnea, dyspnea, dysrhythmias, bradycardia, tachycardia, hypotension, syncope, nausea, vomiting, abdominal pain, dehydration, fatigue.

Drug interactions Increased respiratory effects when given with other CNS depressants.

Dosage and administration *Adult*: 50 to 100 mcg (1 mcg/kg) IM and IV slow push (over 1 to 2 minutes) to maximum of 150 mcg. IN is rapid push. *Pediatric*: 1 to 2 mcg/kg IM, IV, or IN slow push (over 1 to 2 minutes). The safety and efficacy in children younger than age 2 years has not been established.

Duration of action *Onset*: 1 to 3 minutes. *Peak effect*: 3 to 5 minutes. *Duration*: 30 to 60 minutes.

Special considerations Pregnancy safety: Category C. Chest wall rigidity possible with a high-dose rapid infusion. A dose of 100 mcg of fentaNYL citrate is equivalent to 10 mg of morphine or 75 mg of meperidine.

▶ Flumazenil (Romazicon)

Class Benzodiazepine antagonist, antidote.

Mechanism of action Antagonizes the action of benzodiazepines on the CNS, reversing the sedative effects.

Indications Reversal of respiratory depression and sedative effects from pure benzodiazepine overdose.

Contraindications Hypersensitivity, tricyclic antidepressant overdose, seizure-prone patients, coma of unknown etiology.
Adverse reactions/side effects Seizures, dizziness, agitation, confusion, headache, visual disturbances, dysrhythmias, chest pain, hypertension, nausea, vomiting, hiccups, rigors, shivering, pain at the injection site.
Drug interactions Toxic effects of mixed drug overdose (especially tricyclics).
Dosage and administration *Adult*: First dose: 0.2 mg IV/IO over 15 seconds. Second dose: 0.3 mg may be given over 30 seconds; if no response, give third dose. Third dose: 0.5 mg IV/IO over 30 seconds; if no response, repeat once every minute until adequate response or total of 3 mg is given. *Pediatric*: Not recommended.
Duration of action *Onset*: 1 to 2 minutes. *Peak effect*: Related to plasma concentration of benzodiazepines. *Duration*: Related to plasma concentration of benzodiazepines.
Special considerations Pregnancy safety: Category C. Use cautiously in pregnant women weighing fetal risk and maternal benefit. Use in breastfeeding women is not recommended. Be prepared to manage seizures in patients who are physically dependent on benzodiazepines or who have ingested larger doses of other drugs. Flumazenil may precipitate withdrawal syndromes in patients dependent on benzodiazepines. Monitor patients for re-sedation and respiratory depression; be prepared to assist ventilations. Not recommended in combined drug overdoses, especially with TCAs; may result in death. Controversial use in unknown overdose or polysubstance overdose.

Fosphenytoin (Cerebyx)

Class Hydantoin anticonvulsant.
Mechanism of action Modulates voltage-dependent sodium and calcium channels of neurons, inhibits calcium flux across neuronal membranes. Also selectively elevates the excitability threshold of the cell, reducing its response to stimuli.
Indications Status epilepticus, seizure disorder.
Contraindications Bradycardia, Adams-Stokes syndrome, second- or third-degree AV blocks, SA blocks, known hypersensitivity to fosphenytoin, phenytoin, or other hydantoins.
Adverse reactions/side effects Severe hypotension, bradycardia, dysrhythmias, Stevens-Johnson syndrome, cardiovascular collapse, nystagmus, dizziness, headache, nausea, somnolence, rash, and tremor.
Drug interactions DOPamine may cause severe hypotension. Reacts with many medications, decreasing their effect and increasing the risk of fosphenytoin toxicity. Additive effect with other CNS depressants.
Dosage and administration *Adult*: Loading dose: 10 to 20 mg phenytoin equivalents per kg IM, IV one time to a maximum of 150 mg phenytoin equivalents per minute IV. *Pediatric*: Loading dose: 10 to 20 mg phenytoin equivalents per kg IM, IV one time to a maximum of 3 mg phenytoin equivalents per kg per minute up to 150 mg phenytoin equivalents per minute IV.
Duration of action *Onset*: 10 minutes. *Peak effect*: 30 minutes. *Duration*: 12 to 28 hours.
Special considerations Pregnancy safety: Category D. Contraindicated for use in pregnant or lactating women. Use with caution in patients with hepatic and renal impairment and diabetic, older, and debilitated patients. Fosphenytoin dosing is expressed as phenytoin equivalents to avoid the need for dose conversion between products. Each vial contains 75 mg/mL, which is equivalent to 50 mg/mL of phenytoin.

Furosemide (Lasix)

Class Loop diuretic.
Mechanism of action Blocks the absorption of sodium and chloride at the distal and proximal tubules and the loop of Henle, causing increased urine output.
Indications Heart failure, pulmonary edema, hypertensive crisis.
Contraindications Hypovolemia, anuria, hypotension (relative contraindication), hypersensitivity, hepatic coma, suspected electrolyte imbalances.
Adverse reactions/side effects Dizziness, headache, ECG changes, weakness, orthostatic hypotension, dysrhythmias, nausea, vomiting, diarrhea, dry mouth, may exacerbate hypovolemia and hypokalemia, hyperglycemia (due to hemoconcentration).
Drug interactions Lithium toxicity may be potentiated because of sodium depletion. Digitalis toxicity may be potentiated by potassium depletion.
Dosage and administration *Adult*: 0.5 to 1 mg/kg IV over 1 to 2 minutes. If no response, double the dose to 2 mg/kg slowly over 1 to 2 minutes. *Pediatric*: 1 mg/kg IV/IO.
Duration of action *Onset*: 5 minutes. *Peak effect*: 20 to 60 minutes. *Duration*: 4 to 6 hours.
Special considerations Pregnancy safety: Category C. Should only be used during pregnancy if maternal benefit outweighs fetal risk. Ototoxicity, deafness, and projectile

vomiting can occur with rapid administration. Should be protected from light. Vasodilatory effects within 5 minutes; diuretic effects within 30 minutes. Expect a 10 to 12 mm Hg systolic and a 5 to 7 mm Hg diastolic drop in BP. Being phased out due to nephrotoxic side effects. Furosemide administration has decreased with the advent of CPAP.

Glucagon (GlucaGen)[28]

Class Hyperglycemic agent, pancreatic hormone, insulin antagonist.

Mechanism of action Increases blood glucose level by stimulating glycogenolysis. Unknown mechanism of stabilizing cardiac rhythm in beta-blocker overdose. Minimal positive inotropic and chronotropic response. Decreases GI motility and secretions.

Indications Altered level of consciousness when hypoglycemia is suspected. May be used as a reversal agent in beta-blocker and calcium channel blocker overdoses.

Contraindications Hyperglycemia, hypersensitivity.

Adverse reactions/side effects Dizziness, headache, hypertension, tachycardia, nausea, vomiting, rebound hypoglycemia.

Drug interactions Incompatible in solution with most other substances. No significant drug interactions with other emergency medications.

Dosage and administration *Adult*: Hypoglycemia: 1 mg IM/IN, may repeat in 7 to 10 minutes. Calcium channel blocker or beta-blocker overdose: 3 to 10 mg IV slowly over 3 to 5 minutes initially, followed by a 3 to 5 mg/h infusion as necessary. *Pediatric*: Hypoglycemia: 1 mg IM/IN if 20 kg or greater (or 5 years or more); 0.5 mg IM/IN if less than 20 kg or younger than 5 years.[15] Calcium channel blocker or beta-blocker toxicity: 0.05 to 0.15 mg/kg IV/IO over 3 to 5 minutes initially, followed by a 0.05- to 0.10-mg/kg per hour infusion as necessary.

Duration of action *Onset*: 1 minute. *Peak effect*: 5 to 20 minutes. *Duration*: 60 to 90 minutes.

Special considerations Pregnancy safety: Category B. Use in pregnancy only if clearly indicated. Not recommended for use in lactating women. Ineffective if glycogen stores depleted. Should always be used in conjunction with D_{50} whenever possible. If patient does not respond to second dose of glucagon, D_{50} must be administered. Requires reconstitution with the supplied solution.

Haloperidol Lactate (Haldol)

Class Tranquilizer, antipsychotic.

Mechanism of action Inhibits CNS catecholamine receptors: strong antidopaminergic and weak anticholinergic. Acts on CNS to depress subcortical areas, midbrain, and ascending reticular activating system in the brain.

Indications Acute psychotic episodes.

Contraindications Parkinson disease, depressed mental status, agitation secondary to shock and hypoxia, hypersensitivity.

Adverse reactions/side effects Seizures, sedation, confusion, restlessness, extrapyramidal reactions, dystonia, respiratory depression, hypotension, tachycardia, orthostatic hypotension, QT prolongation, sudden cardiac death, constipation, dry mouth, nausea, vomiting, drooling, blurred vision.

Drug interactions Enhanced CNS depression and hypotension in combination with alcohol. Antagonized amphetamines and EPINEPHrine. Other CNS depressants may potentiate effects.

Dosage and administration *Adult*: 2 to 5 mg IM only every 30 to 60 minutes until sedation is achieved. *Pediatric*: Not recommended.

Duration of action *Onset*: 10 minutes. *Peak effect*: 30 to 45 minutes. *Duration*: Variable (generally 12 to 24 hours).

Special considerations Pregnancy safety: Category C. Use during pregnancy only if maternal benefit outweighs fetal risk, especially during the third trimester. Treat hypotension secondary to haloperidol with fluids and norepinephrine, not EPINEPHrine. Patient may also be taking benztropine mesylate (Cogentin) if on long-term therapy with haloperidol.

Heparin Sodium

Class Anticoagulant.

Mechanism of action Prevents conversion of fibrogen to fibrin. Affects clotting factors IX, XI, XII, plasmin. Does not lyse existing clots.

Indications AMI, prophylaxis and treatment of thromboembolic disorders (eg, PE and DVT).

Contraindications Hypersensitivity, active bleeding, recent intracranial, intraspinal, or eye surgery, severe hypertension, bleeding tendencies, severe thrombocytopenia.

Adverse reactions/side effects Pain, anaphylaxis, shock, hematuria, GI bleeding, hemorrhage, thrombocytopenia, bruising.

Drug interactions Salicylates, ibuprofen, dipyridamole, and hydroxychloroquine may increase risk of bleeding.

Dosage and administration *Adult*: If used with fibrinolytic therapy, always obtain a blood sample for control of partial thromboplastin time before heparin administration. Heparin is given as an IV bolus of 60 units/kg. Maximum dose 4,000 units (weight adjusted). A continuous infusion is given following the bolus at a rate of 12 units/kg per hour rounded to the nearest 50 (maximum: 4,000 units or 1,000 units/h). Follow medical direction and local protocol. *Pediatric*: Not recommended.
Duration of action *Onset*: IV: immediate; subcutaneous: 20 to 60 minutes. *Peak effect*: Variable. *Duration*: 4 to 8 hours.
Special considerations Pregnancy safety: Category C. Use cautiously in pregnant women with threatened abortion and avoid using heparin vials containing benzyl alcohol. Heparin does not lyse existing clots. Heparin along with aspirin is part of the antithrombotic package. If the patient experiences uncontrollable bleeding, the reversal agent is protamine.

HydrALAZINE (Apresoline)

Class Antihypertensive, vasodilator.
Mechanism of action The exact mechanism is unknown, but it reduces the patient's BP through peripheral vasodilation.
Indications Pregnancy-induced hypertension, heart failure.
Contraindications Hypersensitivity, CAD, heart valve complications.
Adverse reactions/side effects Angina, pulmonary edema, palpitations, diarrhea, nausea, vomiting, headache.
Drug interactions MAOIs, NSAIDs, beta-blockers.
Dosage and administration *Adult*: 5 to 10 mg IV, 10 to 50 mg PO. *Pediatric*: 0.1 to 0.2 mg/kg IV, 0.75 mg/kg per day in divided doses PO.
Duration of action *Onset*: 5 to 80 minutes. *Peak effect*: 15 to 30 minutes. *Duration*: 2 to 12 hours.
Special considerations Pregnancy safety: Category C. Not recommended for long-term use during pregnancy.

Hydrocortisone Sodium Succinate (Solu-Cortef)

Class Adrenal glucocorticoid.
Mechanism of action Anti-inflammatory; immunosuppressive with salt-retaining actions.
Indications Shock due to acute adrenocortical insufficiency, anaphylaxis, asthma, and COPD.
Contraindications Systemic fungal infections, premature infants (contains benzyl alcohol, which is associated with "fatal gasping syndrome," characterized by CNS depression, metabolic acidosis, and gasping respirations), known hypersensitivity.
Adverse reactions/side effects Headache, vertigo, pulmonary tuberculosis, heart failure, hypertension, fluid retention, nausea.
Drugs interactions Incompatible with heparin and metaraminol.
Dosage and administration *Adult*: 4 mg/kg slow IV bolus. *Pediatric*: 2 mg/kg slow IV bolus. Maximum dose: 100 mg.
Duration of action *Onset*: 1 hour. *Peak effect*: Variable. *Duration*: 8 to 12 hours.
Special considerations Pregnancy safety: Category C. Use with caution in pregnant and breastfeeding women. May be used in status asthmaticus as a second-line drug.

HYDROmorphone (Dilaudid)

Class Analgesic; schedule II drug.
Mechanism of action Binds to the opioid receptors in the CNS.
Indications Moderate to severe pain.
Contraindications Hypersensitivity, GI obstruction, respiratory depression.
Adverse reactions/side effects Hypotension, syncope, increased intracranial pressure, apnea.
Drug interactions MAOIs, SSRIs, sedatives.
Dosage and administration *Adult*: 1 to 2 mg IM, 0.2 to 1 mg IV, 2 to 8 mg every 4 to 6 hours PO. *Pediatric*: 0.8 to 2 mg IM, 0.2 to 0.6 mg IV.
Duration of action *Onset*: IM, variable; 5 minutes IV, 15 to 30 minutes PO. *Peak effect*: IM, variable; 10 to 20 minutes IV, 30 to 60 minutes PO. *Duration*: 2 to 3 hours.
Special considerations Pregnancy safety: Category C. Use with caution during pregnancy, weighing fetal risk and maternal benefit. Respiratory depression from HYDROmorphone administration is managed with naloxone.

Hydroxocobalamin (Cyanokit)[29]

Class Antidote, cyanide poisoning adjunct.
Mechanism of action Binds with cyanide to form nontoxic cyanocobalamin, preventing its toxic effects; excreted renally.
Indications Treatment of known or suspected cyanide poisoning.
Contraindications None in the emergency setting.
Adverse reactions/side effects Hypertension, allergic reactions, GI bleeding, nausea, vomiting, dyspepsia, dyspnea, dizziness, headache, injection site reactions.

Drug interactions Do not administer in the same IV line with diazePAM, DOBUTamine, DOPamine, fentaNYL, NTG, propofol, sodium nitrite, and sodium thiosulfate.

Dosage and administration *Adult*: 5 g IV infusion over 15 minutes at a rate of 15 mL/min, one time, may be repeated one time at the same dose. Maximum of 10 g. *Pediatric*: 70 mg/kg IV one time, may be repeated one time at the same dose.

Duration of action *Onset*: Rapid. *Peak effect*: 8 to 10 minutes. *Duration*: Varies.

Special considerations Pregnancy safety: Category C. May cause fetal harm although risk from cyanide poisoning may outweigh fetal risk. Breastfeeding should be ceased following medication administration. Make sure to reassess the patient's airway, oxygenation, and hydration during administration. The patient may become hypertensive during treatment (BP greater than 180 mm Hg systolic and 110 mm Hg diastolic are not uncommon) and will return to baseline within 4 hours.

▶ HydrOXYzine (Atarax, Vistaril)

Class Antihistamine, antiemetic, antianxiety agent, anxiolytic.

Mechanism of action Potentiates effects of analgesics. Calming effect without impairing mental alertness. Rapid-acting true ataraxic with probable action of suppressing activity in key locations of the CNS's subcortical area. Exerts bronchodilating, antispasmodic, antihistaminic, analgesic, and antiemetic effects.

Indications Potentiates the effects of analgesics. Controls nausea and vomiting in anxiety reactions and motion sickness; preoperative and postoperative sedation.

Contraindications Hypersensitivity, early pregnancy.

Adverse reactions/side effects Drowsiness, agitation, ataxia, dizziness, headache, weakness, wheezing, chest tightness, urinary retention, dry mouth, constipation, pain at injection site.

Drug interactions Potentiates the effects of CNS depressants such as narcotics, barbiturates, and alcohol.

Dosage and administration *Adult*: 25 to 100 mg IM only. *Pediatric*: 0.5 to 1 mg/kg per dose IM only.

Duration of action *Onset*: 15 to 30 minutes. *Peak effect*: 45 to 90 minutes. *Duration*: 4 to 6 hours.

Special considerations Pregnancy safety: Category C. Contraindicated in pregnancy and for breastfeeding women. Should be administered by IM injection only. Localized burning at the injection site is commonly reported.

▶ Insulin

Class Antidiabetic, hormone.

Mechanism of action Allows glucose transport into cells of all tissues; converts glycogen to fat; produces intracellular shift of potassium and magnesium to reduce elevated serum levels of these electrolytes.

Indications Not used in emergency prehospital setting but may be administered by paramedics during interfacility transports. Diabetic ketoacidosis or other hyperglycemic state, hyperkalemia (insulin and D_{50} used together to lower hyperkalemic state), nonketotic hyperosmolar coma.

Contraindications Hypoglycemia, hypokalemia.

Adverse reactions/side effects Weakness, fatigue, confusion, headache, seizure, coma, tachycardia, nausea, hypokalemia, hypoglycemia, diaphoresis, itching, swelling, redness.

Drug interactions Incompatible in solution with all other drugs. Corticosteroids, DOBUTamine, EPINEPHrine, and thiazide diuretics decrease the hypoglycemic effects of insulin. Alcohol and salicylates may potentiate the effects of insulin.

Dosage and administration Dosages vary widely depending on the patient's blood glucose level and the indication.

Duration of action *Onset*: Minutes. *Peak effect*: Approximately 1 hour (short-acting); 3 to 6 hours (intermediate-acting); 5 to 8 hours (long-acting). *Duration*: Approximately 6 to 8 hours (short-acting); 24 hours (intermediate-acting); 36 hours (long-acting).

Special considerations Pregnancy safety: Category B. Use with caution during pregnancy. Insulin is the drug of choice for control of diabetes in pregnancy. Usually requires refrigeration. Most rapid absorption if injected in abdominal wall; next most rapid absorption if injected in the arm; slowest absorption if injected into the thigh.

▶ Ipratropium (Atrovent)

Class Anticholinergic, bronchodilator.

Mechanism of action Inhibits interaction of acetylcholine at receptor sites of bronchial smooth muscle, resulting in decreased cyclic guanosine monophosphate and bronchodilation.

Indications Persistent bronchospasm, COPD exacerbation.

Contraindications Hypersensitivity to ipratropium, atropine, alkaloids, peanuts.

Adverse reactions/side effects Headache, dizziness, nervousness, fatigue, tremor, blurred vision, cough, dyspnea, worsening COPD

symptoms, tachycardia, palpitations, flushing, MI, dry mouth, nausea, vomiting, GI distress.
Drug interactions None reported.
Dosage and administration *Adult and pediatric*: 250 to 500 mcg via inhalation with handheld nebulizer every 20 minutes up to 3 times.
Duration of action *Onset*: 1 to 3 minutes. *Peak effect*: 90 to 120 minutes. *Duration*: 4 to 6 hours.
Special considerations Pregnancy safety: Category B. Note: When used in combination with beta-agonists (eg, metaproterenol and albuterol), the beta-agonist is always administered first with a 5-minute wait before administering ipratropium. Shake well before use. Use with caution in patients with urinary retention.

Isoetharine (Bronchosol, Bronkometer)

Class Sympathomimetic.
Mechanism of action Beta-2 agonist; relaxes smooth muscle of the bronchioles.
Indications Acute bronchial asthma, bronchospasm (especially in COPD patients).
Contraindications Use with caution in patients with diabetes, hyperthyroidism, cardiovascular disease, and cerebrovascular disease.
Adverse reactions/side effects Nervousness, dose-related tachycardia, palpitations, nausea, tremors. Multiple doses can cause paradoxical bronchoconstriction.
Drug interactions Additive adverse effects if given with other beta-2 agonist drugs.
Dosage and administration *Adult*: 1 to 2 inhalations with MDI. COPD: 2.5 to 5 mg (2.5 to 0.5 mL) diluted in 3 mL normal saline and nebulized. *Pediatric*: 0.01 mg/kg. Maximum dose: 0.5 mL in 3 mL normal saline and nebulized.
Duration of action *Onset*: Immediate. *Peak effect*: 5 to 15 minutes. *Duration*: 1 to 4 hours.
Special considerations None.

Ketamine (Ketalar)[30]

Class Sedative, analgesic dissociative anesthetic.
Mechanism of action Blocks pain receptors and minimizes spinal cord activity, affecting the association pathways of the brain between the thalamus and limbic system.
Indications Excited delirium, pain management, procedural sedation.
Contraindications Hypersensitivity, conditions where hypertension would be hazardous to the patient's care.
Adverse reactions/side effects Hypertension, dysrhythmia, bronchodilation, respiratory depression.
Drug interactions Ketamine increases the effects of opiates, barbiturates, and nondepolarizing neuromuscular blockers.
Dosage and administration *Adult and pediatric*: 1 to 2 mg/kg IV push over 1 to 2 minutes.
Duration of action *Onset*: 30 seconds. *Peak effect*: Unknown. *Duration*: 5 to 10 minutes.
Special considerations Pregnancy safety: Category is not assigned by the FDA for ketamine. Contraindicated for use during pregnancy or by breastfeeding women. Patients may experience excessive drooling. Some patients may experience an emergence reaction after the full duration of the medication's effect.

Ketorolac Tromethamine (Toradol)

Class NSAID analgesic.
Mechanism of action Potent analgesic that does not possess any sedative or anxiolytic activities by inhibiting prostaglandin synthesis.
Indications Short-term management of moderate to severe pain.
Contraindications Allergy to salicylates or other NSAIDs. Patients with history of asthma, bleeding disorders (especially GI related, such as peptic ulcer disease), renal failure.
Adverse reactions/side effects Drowsiness, dizziness, headache, sedation, bronchospasm, dyspnea, edema, vasodilation, hypotension, hypertension, GI bleeding, diarrhea, dyspepsia, nausea.
Drug interactions May increase bleeding time in patients taking anticoagulants.
Dosage and administration *Adult*: 30 to 60 mg IM, 15 to 30 mg IV. *Pediatric*: Not recommended.
Duration of action *Onset*: 10 minutes. *Peak effect*: 1 to 2 hours. *Duration*: 2 to 6 hours.
Special considerations Pregnancy safety: Category C. Contraindicated for use during pregnancy. Use with caution in older patients due to higher risk of renal and fatal GI adverse reactions. Because it is a salicylate derivative, it is important to use caution if pain is possibly from a traumatic source.

Labetalol (Normodyne, Trandate)

Class Selective alpha and nonselective beta-adrenergic blocker, antihypertensive.
Mechanism of action BP reduction without reflex tachycardia; total peripheral resistance

reduced without significant alteration in cardiac output.

Indications Moderate to severe hypertension.

Contraindications Bronchial asthma, heart failure, cardiogenic shock, second- and third-degree heart block, bradycardia.

Adverse reactions/side effects Fatigue, weakness, depression, headache, dizziness, bronchospasm, wheezing, dyspnea, bradycardia, heart failure, pulmonary edema, orthostatic hypotension, ventricular dysrhythmias, nausea, vomiting, diarrhea.

Drug interactions Labetalol may block bronchodilator effects of beta-adrenergic agonists. NTG may augment hypotensive effects.

Dosage and administration *Adult*: 10 mg IV push over 1 to 2 minutes. May repeat or double every 10 minutes to a maximum dose of 150 mg. Infusion: 2 to 8 mg/min, titrated to supine BP. *Pediatric*: Not recommended.

Duration of action *Onset*: Less than 5 minutes. *Peak effect*: Variable. *Duration*: 3 to 6 hours.

Special considerations Pregnancy safety: Category C. BP, pulse rate, and ECG should be monitored continuously. Observe for signs of heart failure, bradycardia, and bronchospasm. Should only be administered with patient in the supine position.

▶ Lansoprazole (Prevacid)

Class Antiulcer, proton pump inhibitor.

Mechanism of action Binds to sulfhydryl group of ATP during the final phases of the gastric acid secretion pathway, reducing the overall production.

Indications Gastric ulcers, upper GI bleeding, GERD.

Contraindications Hypersensitivity.

Adverse reactions/side effects Abdominal pain, constipation, diarrhea, nausea, headache, dizziness.

Drug interactions Use with caution in patients on antiplatelet drugs, iron salts, or digoxin.

Dosage and administration *Adult and pediatric*: 15 to 30 mg PO.

Duration of action *Onset*: 1 to 3 hours. *Peak effect*: 1.5 to 2 hours. *Duration*: 24 hours.

Special considerations Pregnancy safety: Category B. Contraindicated in breastfeeding women.

▶ Levalbuterol (Xopenex)

Class Sympathomimetic, bronchodilator.

Mechanism of action Stimulates beta-2 receptors resulting in smooth muscle relaxation of bronchial tree and peripheral vasculature.

Indications Treatment of acute bronchospasm in patients with reversible obstructive airway disease (COPD/asthma). Bronchospasm prophylaxis in asthma patients.

Contraindications Known hypersensitivity to the drug and other sympathomimetics. Angioedema, tachydysrhythmias, and severe cardiac disease. Avoid use in patients taking phenothiazines; may cause prolonged QT interval and dysrhythmias. Avoid use in patients on sotalol; may decrease bronchodilating effects and cause bronchospasm, prolonged QT interval, and dysrhythmias.

Adverse reactions/side effects Headache, anxiety, dizziness, restlessness, hallucinations, throat irritation, tachycardia, hypertension, hypotension, dysrhythmias, angina, nausea, vomiting, dyspepsia, tremors, hypokalemia, hyperglycemia.

Drug interactions Increased actions of bronchodilators, tricyclic antidepressants, MAOIs, and other adrenergic drugs.

Dosage and administration *Adult*: 1.25 mg to 2.5 mg in 3 mL administered by nebulizer every 20 minutes to a maximum of 3 doses. *Pediatric*: 0.075 mg/kg (minimum of 1.25 mg) administered by nebulizer every 20 minutes to a maximum of 3 doses.

Duration of action *Onset*: 5 to 15 minutes. *Peak effect*: 60 to 90 minutes. *Duration*: 6 to 8 hours.

Special considerations Pregnancy safety: Category C. Use with caution in patients with cardiac dysrhythmias and cardiovascular disorders.

▶ LevoFLOXacin (Levaquin)

Class Antibiotic.

Mechanism of action Inhibits the DNA of bacteria from replicating or repairing itself.

Indications Gram-positive infections of the urinary system, respiratory system, and integumentary system.

Contraindications Hypersensitivity to quinolone antibiotics.

Adverse reactions/side effects Diarrhea, nausea, dizziness, headaches, aortic damage, prolonged hypoglycemia, anemia, thrombocytopenia, liver damage, lethal ventricular dysrhythmias, cardiac arrest.

Drug interactions Class Ia and Class III antidysrhythmics, QTc prolonging agents, anticoagulants, iron salts, zinc salts, corticosteroids, multivitamins.

Dosage and administration *Adult*: 250 to 700 mg IV/PO. *Pediatric*: 8 mg/kg IV.

Duration of action *Onset*: Rapid. *Peak effect*: End of infusion. *Duration*: 24 hours.

Special considerations Pregnancy safety: Category C. Use with caution in pregnant and breastfeeding women. Adjustment needed in renal dysfunction.

Lidocaine Hydrochloride (Xylocaine)

Class Antidysrhythmic (Class Ib), anesthetic.

Mechanism of action *Cardiac*: Decreases automaticity by slowing the rate of spontaneous phase 4 depolarization. *Local anesthetic*: Inhibits transport of ions across the neuronal membrane, blocking conduction of normal nerve impulses.

Indications Alternative to amiodarone in cardiac arrest from VT, VF, stable wide-complex tachycardia (poly- or monomorphic) with normal baseline QT interval. Also used as a local anesthetic for various procedures, including intubation and IO infusions.

Contraindications Hypersensitivity, second- or third-degree AV block in the absence of an artificial pacemaker, Stokes-Adams syndrome, prophylactic use in AMI, wide-complex ventricular escape beats with bradycardia.

Adverse reactions/side effects Anxiety, drowsiness, confusion, seizures, slurred speech, respiratory arrest, hypotension, bradycardia, dysrhythmias, cardiac arrest, AV block, nausea, vomiting.

Drug interactions Apnea induced with succinylcholine may be prolonged with high doses of lidocaine. Cardiac depression may occur in conjunction with IV phenytoin. Procainamide may exacerbate CNS effect. Metabolic clearance is decreased in patients with liver disease or in patients taking beta-blockers.

Dosage and administration *Adult*: Cardiac arrest/pulseless VT/VF: Initial dose: 1 to 1.5 mg/kg IV/IO. Repeat dose: 0.5 to 0.75 mg/kg IV/IO repeated in 5 to 10 minutes. Maximum total dose: 3 mg/kg. Stable VT, and wide-complex tachycardia of unknown etiology: Maintenance infusion: 1 to 4 mg/min (30 to 50 mcg/kg per minute); can dilute in D_5W or normal saline. Local anesthetic dose varies depending on procedure and location. *Pediatric*: IV/IO dose: 1 mg/kg rapid IV/IO push. Maximum dose 100 mg. Continuous IV/IO infusion: 20 to 50 mcg/kg per minute. Repeat bolus dose (1 mg/kg) when infusion is initiated if bolus has not been given within previous 15 minutes. Local anesthetic dose varies depending on procedure and location.

Duration of action *Onset*: 1 to 5 minutes. *Peak effect*: 5 to 10 minutes. *Duration*: Variable (15 minutes to 2 hours).

Special considerations Pregnancy safety: Category B. Reduce maintenance infusion by 50% if patient is older than age 70 years, has liver or renal disease, is in heart failure, or is in shock. A 75- to 100-mg bolus maintains blood levels for only 20 minutes (if not in shock). Exceedingly high doses of lidocaine can result in death and coma. Cross-reactivity with other forms of local anesthetics.

LORazepam (Ativan)

Class Benzodiazepine, short/intermediate acting; sedative, anticonvulsant; schedule IV drug.

Mechanism of action Anxiolytic, anticonvulsant, and sedative effect; suppresses propagation of seizure activity produced by foci in cortex, thalamus, and limbic areas.

Indications Initial control of status epilepticus or severe recurrent seizures, severe anxiety, sedation, chemical restraint.

Contraindications Acute narrow-angle glaucoma, coma, shock, suspected drug abuse.

Adverse reactions/side effects Dizziness, drowsiness, CNS depression, headache, sedation, respiratory depression, apnea, hypotension, bradycardia.

Drug interactions May precipitate CNS depression if already taking CNS depressant medications.

Dosage and administration Note: When given IV/IO, must be diluted with equal volume of sterile water or sterile saline. When given IM, LORazepam is not diluted. *Adult*: Anxiety/sedation: 2 mg IV; 4 mg IM. Seizures: 0.1 mg/kg IV, maximum dose 4 mg.[16] *Pediatric*: 0.05 mg/kg IV or IM.[31]

Duration of action *Onset*: 2 to 5 minutes IV; 15 to 30 minutes IM. *Peak effect*: Variable. *Duration*: 6 to 8 hours.

Special considerations Pregnancy safety: Category D. Contraindicated in pregnant or breastfeeding women. Fetal risk and maternal benefit should be considered prior to using in emergency setting. Monitor respiratory rate and BP during administration. Have advanced airway equipment readily available. Inadvertent arterial injection may result in vasospasm and gangrene. LORazepam expires in 6 weeks when not refrigerated.

Magnesium Sulfate

Class Electrolyte, anti-inflammatory.

Mechanism of action Reduces striated muscle contractions and blocks peripheral neuromuscular transmission by reducing acetylcholine release at the myoneural junction. Manages seizures in toxemia of pregnancy. Induces uterine relaxation. Can cause bronchodilation after beta-agonists and anticholinergics have been administered.

Indications Seizures of eclampsia (toxemia of pregnancy), torsades de pointes, hypomagnesemia, VF/pulseless VT that is refractory to amiodarone, life-threatening dysrhythmias due to digitalis toxicity, severe status asthmaticus, and severe bronchoconstriction with impending respiratory failure.[32]

Contraindications Heart block, myocardial damage.

Adverse reactions/side effects Drowsiness, CNS depression, respiratory depression, respiratory tract paralysis, abnormal ECG, AV block, hypotension, vasodilation, hyporeflexia.

Drug interactions May enhance effects of other CNS depressants. Serious changes in overall cardiac function may occur with cardiac glycosides.

Dosage and administration *Adult*: Seizure activity associated with pregnancy: 1 to 4 g of a 10% solution IV/IO over 3 minutes. Maximum dose 30 to 40 g/day. Cardiac arrest due to hypomagnesemia or torsades de pointes: 1 to 2 g of 10% solution IV/IO over 5 to 20 minutes. Torsades de pointes with pulse: Loading dose of 1 to 2 g in 50 to 100 mL of D_5W over 5 to 60 minutes IV. Follow with 0.5 to 1 g/h IV (titrate dose to control torsades). Status asthmaticus: 1 to 2 g IV over 15 to 30 minutes. Severe bronchoconstriction/impending respiratory failure: 40 mg/kg IV, maximum dose is 2 g.[21] *Pediatric*: Pulseless VT with torsades de pointes: 25 to 50 mg/kg IV/IO bolus of a 10% solution. Maximum dose 2 g. Torsades de pointes with pulses or hypomagnesemia: 25 to 50 mg/kg IV/IO of a 10% solution over 10 to 20 minutes. Maximum dose 2 g. Status asthmaticus: 30 to 60 mg/kg IV/IO of a 10% solution over 15 to 30 minutes. Maximum dose 2 g.

Duration of action *Onset*: IV/IO: immediate. *Peak effect*: Variable. *Duration*: IV/IO: 30 minutes.

Special considerations Pregnancy safety: Category D. Due to confirmed evidence of human fetal risk, must be used cautiously although administration may be justified. Recommended that the drug not be administered in the 2 hours before delivery, if possible. IV calcium gluconate or calcium chloride should be available as an antagonist to magnesium if needed. Use with caution in patients with renal failure.

▶ Mannitol (Osmitrol)

Class Osmotic diuretic.

Mechanism of action Promotes the movement of fluid from the intracellular space to the extracellular space. Decreases cerebral edema and ICP. Promotes urinary excretion of toxins.

Indications Cerebral edema, reduce ICP for certain cause (space-occupying lesions), rhabdomyolysis (myoglobinuria), blood transfusion reactions.

Contraindications Hypotension, pulmonary edema, severe dehydration, intracranial bleeding, heart failure.

Adverse reactions/side effects Headache, confusion, seizures, pulmonary edema, tachycardia, chest pain, heart failure, hypotension, hypertension, edema, nausea, vomiting, dehydration.

Drug interactions May precipitate digitalis toxicity when given concurrently.

Dosage and administration *Adult*: 0.5 to 1 g/kg IV infusion over 30 minutes. Additional doses of 0.25 to 2 g/kg can be given every 4 to 6 hours as needed. *Pediatric*: 0.5 to 1g/kg per dose IV, IO infusion over 30 to 60 minutes; may repeat after 30 minutes if no effect.

Duration of action *Onset*: 1 to 3 hours for diuretic effect; 15 minutes for reduction of ICP. *Peak effect*: Variable. *Duration*: 4 to 6 hours for diuretic effect; 3 to 8 hours for reduction of ICP.

Special considerations Pregnancy safety: Category C. May crystallize at low temperatures; store at room temperature. In-line filter should always be used. Effectiveness depends on large doses and an intact blood-brain barrier. Usage and dosages in emergency care are controversial. Be sure to have ventilatory support available.

▶ Meperidine Hydrochloride (Demerol)

Class Opioid analgesic; schedule II drug.

Mechanism of action Synthetic opioid analgesic whose effects on the CNS and smooth muscle organs are similar to morphine, primarily acting as an analgesic and a sedative.

Indications Analgesia for moderate to severe pain.

Contraindications Hypersensitivity to narcotics, diarrhea caused by poisoning, patients taking MAOIs, during labor or delivery of a premature infant, undiagnosed abdominal pain or head injury.

Adverse reactions/side effects Seizures, confusion, sedation, dysphoria, headache, hallucinations, increased ICP, respiratory depression, apnea, hypotension, orthostatic hypotension, syncope, bradycardia, dysrhythmias, nausea, vomiting, constipation, sweating.

Drug interactions Do not give concurrently with MAOIs (even with a dose in the last 14 days). Exacerbates CNS depression when given with other CNS depressants.

Dosage and administration *Adult*: 50 to 100 mg IM, subcutaneous. 25 to 50 mg slowly IV. *Pediatric*: 1 to 2 mg/kg per dose IV, IO, IM, subcutaneous.

Duration of action *Onset*: IM: 10 to 45 minutes; IV: immediate. *Peak effect*: 30 to 60 minutes. *Duration*: 2 to 4 hours.

Special considerations Pregnancy safety: Category C. Use with caution in patients with asthma and COPD. May aggravate seizures in patients with known convulsive disorders. Naloxone should be readily available as an antagonist.

Metaproterenol Sulfate (Alupent)[33]

Class Nonselective beta-2 adrenergic agonist, bronchodilator.

Mechanism of action Acts directly on bronchial smooth muscle causing relaxation of the bronchial tree and peripheral vasculature.

Indications Bronchial asthma, reversible bronchospasm secondary to bronchitis, COPD.

Contraindications Tachydysrhythmia, hypersensitivity, tachycardia caused by digitalis toxicity.

Adverse reactions/side effects Nervousness, tremor, headache, anxiety, cough, paradoxical bronchospasm, hypertension, chest pain, tachydysrhythmias, palpitations, cardiac arrest, diarrhea, nausea, vomiting, backache, skin reactions, sweating.

Drug interactions Other sympathomimetics may exacerbate cardiovascular effects. MAOIs may potentiate hypotensive effects. Beta-blockers may antagonize metaproterenol.

Dosage and administration *Adult*: Inhalation 0.2 to 0.3 mL of a 5% solution diluted in 2.5 mL saline. *Pediatric*: Age 6 to 12 years: 0.1 to 0.2 mL of a 5% solution diluted in 3 mL saline.

Duration of action *Onset*: 1 minute after inhalation. *Peak effect*: 45 minutes. *Duration*: 3 to 6 hours.

Special considerations Pregnancy safety: Category C. Use with caution in pregnant and breastfeeding women, weighing potential risks and benefits. Monitor for hypotension and tachycardia. Use with caution in patients with CAD, seizures, hypertension, and diabetes mellitus.

MethylPREDNISolone Sodium Succinate (Solu-Medrol)

Class Corticosteroid.

Mechanism of action Highly potent synthetic glucocorticoid that suppresses acute and chronic inflammation; potentiates vascular smooth muscle relaxation by beta-adrenergic agonists.

Indications Anaphylaxis, bronchodilator for unresponsive asthma.

Contraindications Premature infants, systemic fungal infections, use with caution in patients with GI bleeding.

Adverse reactions/side effects Depression, euphoria, headache, restlessness, seizure, increased ICP, pulmonary tuberculosis, hypertension, heart failure, nausea, vomiting, peptic ulcer, fluid retention, hypernatremia, hyperkalemia.

Drug interactions Hypoglycemic responses to insulin and hypoglycemic agents may be blunted.

Dosage and administration *Adult and pediatric*: Asthma, COPD, anaphylaxis: 1 to 2 mg/kg IV. Status asthmaticus/anaphylaxis: 2 mg/kg per dose IV/IO/IM to a maximum dose of 60 mg/24 hours.

Duration of action *Onset*: 1 to 2 hours. *Peak effect*: Variable. *Duration*: 8 to 24 hours.

Special considerations Pregnancy safety: Category C. Crosses the placenta and may cause fetal harm. Use with caution in pregnant and breastfeeding women, weighing potential risks and benefits.

Metoclopramide (Reglan)

Class Antiemetic, prokinetic GI agent.

Mechanism of action Encourages upper GI motility by reducing biliary, gastric, and pancreatic secretions.

Indications Nausea, vomiting, GERD.

Contraindications Hypersensitivity, epilepsy, GI bleeding or obstruction, heart failure, liver disease, Parkinson disease, pheochromocytoma, renal failure, seizure disorder.

Adverse reactions/side effects Fluid retention, nausea, vomiting, headache, fatigue, somnolence, dystonic reaction, dizziness, headache, confusion, AV block, bradycardia.

Drug interactions CNS depressants, antihistamines, anticholinergics, MAOIs.

Dosage and administration *Adult*: 10 mg IV over 1 to 2 minutes, 10 mg PO. *Pediatric*: 0.1 mg/kg over 1 to 2 minutes (maximum 10 mg/dose IV).

Duration of action *Onset*: IV: 1 to 3 minutes, PO: 30 to 60 minutes. *Peak effect*: Immediate. *Duration*: 1 to 2 hours.

Special considerations Pregnancy safety: Category B.

▶ Metoprolol Tartrate (Lopressor)

Class Beta-blocker, beta-1 selective; antihypertensive, antidysrhythmic.

Mechanism of action Decreases heart rate, conduction velocity, myocardial contractility, and cardiac output. Used to control ventricular response in SVT (PSVT, AF, atrial flutter). Considered second-line agent after adenosine, dilTIAZem, or digitalis derivative.

Indications PSVT, atrial flutter, AF, reduces myocardial ischemia and damage in patients with AMI.

Contraindications Heart failure, second- or third-degree AV block, first-degree heart block (if PR interval is equal to or greater than 0.24 seconds), sick sinus syndrome, cardiogenic shock, bradycardia.

Adverse reactions/side effects Weakness, dizziness, depression, bronchospasm, wheezing, dyspnea, bradycardia, pulmonary edema, heart failure, AV blocks, hypotension, nausea, indigestion.

Drug interactions Metoprolol may potentiate antihypertensive effects when given to patients taking calcium channel blockers or MAOIs. Catecholamine-depleting drugs may potentiate hypotension. Sympathomimetic effects may be antagonized. Signs of hypoglycemia may be masked.

Dosage and administration *Adult*: 5 mg IV over 1 to 2 minutes. May repeat as needed every 5 minutes for a total of three doses.[34] *Pediatric*: Safety not established.

Duration of action *Onset*: 1 to 2 minutes. *Peak effect*: 5 to 10 minutes. *Duration*: 3 to 4 hours.

Special considerations Pregnancy safety: Category C. Contraindicated for use in breastfeeding women. Metoprolol must be given slow IV over 5 minutes. Concurrent IV administration with IV calcium channel blocker such as verapamil or dilTIAZem can cause severe hypotension. Metoprolol should be used with caution in patients with liver or renal dysfunction, hypotension, and COPD.

▶ Midazolam Hydrochloride (Versed)

Class Benzodiazepine, short/intermediate acting; schedule IV drug.

Mechanism of action Reversibly interacts with GABA receptors in the CNS causing sedative, anxiolytic, amnesic, and hypnotic effects.

Indications Seizures, sedation for medical procedures (eg, intubation, ventilated patients, cardioversion), chemical restraint.

Contraindications Acute narrow-angle glaucoma, shock, coma, alcohol intoxication, overdose, depressed vital signs. Concomitant use with barbiturates, alcohol, narcotics, or other CNS depressants.

Adverse reactions/side effects Headache, somnolence, respiratory depression, respiratory arrest, apnea, hypotension, cardiac arrest, nausea, vomiting, pain at the injection site.

Drug interactions Should not be used in patients who have taken CNS depressants.

Dosage and administration *Adult*: Seizures: 0.2 mg/kg IM or IN, maximum dose is 10 mg; 0.1 mg/kg IV, maximum dose is 4 mg.[17] Procedural sedation: 0.5 to 2.5 mg IV. May be repeated to total maximum: 0.1 mg/kg. Chemical restraint: 5 mg IV or IN; 5 mg IM.[31] *Pediatric*: Seizure: 0.1 to 0.3 mg/kg IV/IM (maximum single dose: 10 mg), 0.2 mg/kg IN. Procedural sedation: 0.05 to 0.5 mg/kg IV. Chemical restraint: 0.05 to 0.1 mg/kg IV; 0.1 to 0.15 mg/kg IM; 0.3 mg/kg IN.[31]

Duration of action *Onset*: 1 to 3 minutes, IV and dose dependent. *Peak effect*: Variable. *Duration*: 2 to 6 hours, dose dependent.

Special considerations Pregnancy safety: Category D. Fetal risk and maternal benefit should be considered prior to emergent administration. Breastfeeding women should not continue breastfeeding following administration. Administer immediately prior to intubation procedure. Requires continuous monitoring of respiratory and cardiac function. Decrease dose by 50% in older patients and in patients with hepatic and renal dysfunction. IM or IN routes control seizures faster than IV if vascular access has not been obtained.

▶ Milrinone (Primacor)

Class Inotrope.

Mechanism of action By increasing the intracellular ionized calcium, the contractile strength of cardiac muscle is improved.

Indications Heart failure, decreased cardiac output.

Contraindications Hypersensitivity.

Adverse reactions/side effects Headache, hypotension, hypokalemia, thrombocytopenia, bronchospasm, SVT, ventricular dysrhythmias.

Drug interactions Anagrelide.

Dosage and administration *Adult*: 50 mcg/kg IV bolus over 10 minutes followed by an infusion of 0.375 to 0.75 mcg/kg per minute. *Pediatric*: 50 mcg/kg IV bolus over 10 minutes followed by an infusion of 0.25 to 0.75 mcg/kg per minute.

Duration of action *Onset*: 5 to 15 minutes. *Peak effect*: Unknown. *Duration*: 3 to 6 hours.

Special considerations Pregnancy safety: Category C. Utilized commonly in the pediatric ICU setting and it may be seen during interfacility transports. Dose adjustment needed in renal dysfunction.

Morphine Sulfate (Roxanol, MS Contin)

Class Opioid analgesic; schedule II drug.

Mechanism of action Alleviates pain through CNS action. Suppresses fear and anxiety centers in the brain. Depresses brainstem respiratory centers. Increases peripheral venous capacitance and decreases venous return. Decreases preload and afterload, which decreases myocardial oxygen demand.

Indications Severe heart failure, acute cardiogenic pulmonary edema, chest pain associated with AMI, analgesia for moderate to severe acute and chronic pain.

Contraindications Head injury, exacerbated COPD, depressed respiratory drive, hypotension, undiagnosed abdominal pain, decreased level of consciousness, suspected hypovolemia, patients who have taken MAOIs within 14 days.

Adverse reactions/side effects Confusion, sedation, headache, CNS depression, respiratory depression, apnea, bronchospasm, dyspnea, hypotension, orthostatic hypotension, syncope, bradycardia, tachycardia, nausea, vomiting, dry mouth.

Drug interactions Potentiates sedative effects of phenothiazines. CNS depressants may potentiate effects of morphine. MAOIs may cause paradoxical excitation.

Dosage and administration *Adult*: STEMI: Initial dose: 2 to 4 mg slow IV (over 1 to 5 minutes). Repeat dose: 2 to 8 mg at 5 to 15 minute intervals. NSTEMI/unstable angina: 1 to 5 mg IV push if symptoms not relieved by nitrates, use with caution. *Pediatric*: 0.1 to 0.2 mg/kg per dose IV, IO, IM, subcutaneous. Maximum dose: 5 mg.

Duration of action *Onset*: Immediate. *Peak effect*: 20 minutes. *Duration*: 2 to 7 hours.

Special considerations Pregnancy safety: Category C. Use caution weighing risks and benefits during pregnancy. Use cautiously in breastfeeding women. Morphine rapidly crosses the placenta. Safety in neonates has not been established. Use with caution in older patients, those with asthma, and in those susceptible to CNS depression. Vagotonic effect in patients with acute inferior MI (bradycardia, heart block). Naloxone hydrochloride (Narcan) should be readily available as an antidote.

Nalbuphine Hydrochloride (Nubain)

Class Synthetic opioid agonist/antagonist.

Mechanism of action Activates opiate receptor in limbic system of the CNS. Analgesic similar to morphine on a milligram-for-milligram basis. Agonist and antagonist properties. May be preferred for chest pain in setting of acute MI because it reduces the myocardial oxygen demand without reducing the BP.

Indications Chest pain associated with AMI, moderate to severe acute pain.

Contraindications Head injury, undiagnosed abdominal pain, diarrhea caused by poison, hypovolemia, hypotension.

Adverse reactions/side effects Headache, dizziness, vertigo, seizure, CNS depression, paradoxical CNS stimulation, respiratory depression, pulmonary edema, hypotension, hypertension, palpitations, bradycardia, nausea, vomiting, dry mouth.

Drug interactions CNS depressants may potentiate effects.

Dosage and administration *Adult*: 2 to 5 mg slowly IV. May repeat 2 mg doses PRN to a maximum dose of 10 mg. *Pediatric*: Not recommended.

Duration of action *Onset*: 2 to 3 minutes. *Peak effect*: Variable. *Duration*: 3 to 6 hours.

Special considerations Pregnancy safety: Category B. Use with caution in patients with impaired respiratory function. May precipitate withdrawal syndromes in narcotic-dependent patients. Naloxone should be readily available.

Naloxone Hydrochloride (Narcan)[35]

Class Opioid antagonist, antidote.

Mechanism of action Competitive inhibition at narcotic receptor sites. Reverses respiratory depression secondary to opiate drugs. Completely inhibits the effect of morphine.

Indications Opiate overdose, complete or partial reversal of CNS and respiratory depression induced by opioids, decreased level of consciousness, coma of unknown origin. Narcotic agonist for the following: morphine sulfate, heroin, HYDROmorphone (Dilaudid), methadone, meperidine (Demerol), paregoric, fentaNYL (Sublimaze), oxycodone (Percodan), codeine, propoxyphene (Darvon). Narcotic agonist and antagonist for the following: butorphanol (Stadol), pentazocine (Talwin), nalbuphine (Nubain).

Contraindications Use with caution in narcotic-dependent patients. Use with caution in neonates of narcotic-addicted mothers.

Adverse reactions/side effects Restlessness, seizures, dyspnea, pulmonary edema, tachycardia, hypertension, dysrhythmias, cardiac arrest, nausea, vomiting, withdrawal symptoms in opioid-addicted patients, diaphoresis.

Drug interactions Incompatible with bisulfite and alkaline solutions.

Dosage and administration *Adult*: 0.4 to 2 mg IM/IV/IO/subcutaneous/ET/IN (diluted); minimum single dose recommended: 2 mg. Repeat at 5-minute intervals to a maximum total dose of 10 mg (medical control may request higher amounts). For IN route, administer half the dose in each nostril; maximum dose is 1 mL per nostril.[36] *Pediatric*: 0.1 mg/kg per dose IV/IO/IM/ET every 2 minutes as needed. Maximum total dose of 2 mg. If no response in 10 minutes, administer an additional 0.1 mg/kg per dose.

Duration of action *Onset*: Less than 2 minutes. *Peak effect*: Variable. *Duration*: 30 to 60 minutes.

Special considerations Pregnancy safety: Category C. Any use during pregnancy. Use in breastfeeding women should be clearly indicated. Assist ventilations prior to administration to avoid sympathetic stimulation. Seizures without causal relationship have been reported. May not reverse hypotension. Use caution when administering to narcotic addicts (potential violent behavior). Half-life of naloxone is often shorter than the half-life of narcotics; repeat dosing may be required. In cardiac arrest, naloxone is generally not beneficial.

▶ NiCARdipine (Cardene)

Class Antihypertensive, calcium channel blocker.

Mechanism of action Selectively reduces the amount of calcium ions moving into the myocardium and coronary vascular smooth muscles.

Indications CVA, hypertension, stable angina, subarachnoid hemorrhage.

Contraindications Hypersensitivity, aortic stenosis.

Adverse reactions/side effects Hypotension, nausea, vomiting, tachydysrhythmias, myocardial ischemia, flushing, pedal edema, palpitations.

Drug interactions Other antihypertensives, nitrates, NSAIDs, beta-blockers, digoxin, quinidine.

Dosage and administration *Adult*: Initiate infusion at 5 mg/h. Increase by 2.5 mg/h every 5 minutes, titrating to target BP. Maximum dose 15 mg/h. *Pediatric*: Safety and efficacy have not been established.

Duration of action *Onset*: Minutes. *Peak effect*: 45 minutes. *Duration*: 50 hours after discontinuation of the infusion.

Special considerations Pregnancy safety: Category C. Contraindicated in pregnant women. Breastfeeding infants should be monitored closely. Evaluate BP every 5 minutes because changes happen rapidly.

▶ NIFEdipine (Procardia, Adalat)

Class Calcium channel blocker.

Mechanism of action Inhibits movement of calcium ions across cell membranes; calcium channel blocker; arterial and venous vasodilator; reduces preload and afterload; prevents coronary artery spasm and decreases total peripheral resistance; reduces myocardial oxygen demands; does not prolong AV nodal conduction.

Indications Hypertensive crisis, angina pectoris, HAPE.[37]

Contraindications Compensatory hypertension, hypotension, cardiogenic shock.

Adverse reactions/side effects Headache, dizziness, nervousness, weakness, mood changes, dyspnea, cough, wheezing, heart failure, MI, ventricular dysrhythmias, hypotension, syncope, nausea, abdominal discomfort, diarrhea.

Drug interactions Beta-blockers may potentiate effects. Effects of theophylline may be increased. Antihypertensives may potentiate hypotensive effects.

Dosage and administration *Adult*: 10 mg SL or buccal (puncture end of capsule with needle and squeeze or have patient bite and swallow). May repeat in 30 minutes. HAPE: 60 mg sustained-release PO once daily (as adjunct to descent from altitude).[37] *Pediatric*: Not recommended.

Duration of action *Onset*: 15 to 30 minutes. *Peak effect*: 1 to 3 hours. *Duration*: 6 to 8 hours.

Special considerations Pregnancy safety: Category C. Does not slow AV nodal activity. Have beta-blocker available for control of reflex tachycardia. Use with caution in geriatric population. Hypotension and angina pectoris may occur.

Nitroglycerin (Nitrostat, Nitro-Bid, Tridil)

Class Vasodilator.
Mechanism of action Smooth muscle relaxant acting on vasculature, bronchial, uterine, intestinal smooth muscle. Dilation of arterioles and veins in the periphery. Reduces preload and afterload, decreasing workload of the heart and thereby myocardial oxygen demand.
Indications Acute angina pectoris, ischemic chest pain, hypertension, heart failure, pulmonary edema.
Contraindications Hypotension, hypovolemia, intracranial bleeding or head injury, pericardial tamponade, severe bradycardia or tachycardia, RV infarction, previous administration in the last 24 hours: sildenafil (Viagra) or 48 hours: vardenafil (Levitra) or tadalafil (Cialis).[38]
Adverse reactions/side effects Headache, dizziness, weakness, reflex tachycardia, syncope, hypotension, nausea, vomiting, dry mouth, muscle twitching, diaphoresis.
Drug interactions Additive effects with other vasodilators. Incompatible with other drugs IV.
Dosage and administration *Adult*: 0.4 mg SL; may repeat in 3 to 5 minutes to maximum of 3 doses.[39] NTG IV infusion: Begin at 10 mcg/min; increase by 10 mcg/min every 3 to 5 minutes until desired effect. Maximum dose 200 mcg/min. *Pediatric*: Not recommended.
Duration of action *Onset*: 1 to 3 minutes. *Peak effect*: 5 to 10 minutes. *Duration*: SL: 20 to 30 minutes. IV: 1 to 10 minutes after discontinuation of infusion.
Special considerations Pregnancy safety: Category C. Has been used safely during pregnancy. Use caution with breastfeeding women and monitor infants for adverse effects. Hypotension more common in older patients. If 12-lead ECG shows inferior wall infarct, rule out RV infarction via right-sided 12-lead ECG prior to administering NTG. NTG decomposes when exposed to light or heat, must be kept in airtight containers. Must be administered only with an infusion pump direct from bottle with a vented IV set and non-PVC tubing. Active ingredient may have stinging effect when administered.

Nitropaste (Nitro-Bid Ointment)

Class Vasodilator.
Mechanism of action Smooth muscle relaxant acting on vasculature, bronchial, uterine, intestinal smooth muscle. Dilation of arterioles and veins in the periphery. Reduces preload and afterload, decreasing workload of the heart and thereby myocardial oxygen demand.
Indications Acute angina pectoris, chest pain associated with AMI, hypertension, heart failure, pulmonary edema.
Contraindications Hypotension, hypovolemia, intracranial bleeding or head injury, previous administration in the last 24 hours of vardenafil (Levitra), sildenafil (Viagra) or in the last 48 hours of tadalafil (Cialis).
Adverse reactions/side effects Headache, dizziness, weakness, reflex tachycardia, syncope, hypotension, nausea, vomiting, dry mouth, muscle twitching, diaphoresis.
Drug interactions Additive effects with other vasodilators.
Dosage and administration *Adult*: Paste: Apply a ½- to ¾-inch (1 to 2 cm) line (15 to 30 mg), cover with wrap, and secure with tape. Maximum: 5-inch (12.5 cm) line (75 mg) per application. Transdermal: Apply unit to intact skin (usually chest wall) in varying doses. *Pediatric*: Not recommended.
Duration of action *Onset*: 30 minutes. *Peak effect*: Variable. *Duration*: 18 to 24 hours.
Special considerations Pregnancy safety: Category C. Has been used safely during pregnancy. Use caution with breastfeeding women and monitor infants for adverse effects. Not a great value in prehospital arena. Wear gloves when applying paste. Store paste in a cool place with tube tightly capped. Erratic absorption rates quite common.

Nitroprusside (Nitropress)

Class Antihypertensive, vasodilator.
Mechanism of action Relaxes smooth muscles of blood vessels and dilates peripheral arteries.
Indications Heart failure and hypertension.
Contraindications Hypersensitivity, hypotension, heart failure with reduced peripheral vascular resistance.
Adverse reactions/side effects Dysrhythmias, hypotension, decreased platelet aggregation, metabolic acidosis, bowel obstruction, methemoglobinemia, increased ICP.
Drug interactions Ganglionic blocking agents, general anesthetics, other antihypertensives, sympathomimetics.
Dosage and administration *Adult and pediatric*: 0.3 to 10 mcg/kg per minute.
Duration of action *Onset*: Immediate. *Peak effect*: Rapid. *Duration*: 1 to 10 minutes.

Special considerations Pregnancy safety: Category C. Use caution during pregnancy. Contraindicated for use in breastfeeding women. Keep the infusion fluid protected from light.

► Nitrous Oxide 50:50 (Nitronox)

Class Gaseous analgesic and anesthetic.

Mechanism of action Exact mechanism unknown; affects CNS phospholipids.

Indications Moderate to severe pain, anxiety, apprehension.

Contraindications Impaired level of consciousness, head injury, inability to follow or comply with instructions, decompression sickness (nitrogen narcosis, air embolism, and air transport), undiagnosed abdominal pain or marked distention, bowel obstruction, hypotension, shock, COPD, cyanosis, chest trauma with pneumothorax.

Adverse reactions/side effects Light-headedness, drowsiness, respiratory depression, apnea, nausea, vomiting, malignant hyperthermia.

Drug interactions None of significance.

Dosage and administration *Adult*: Instruct the patient to inhale deeply through demand valve and mask or mouthpiece. *Pediatric*: Same as adult.

Duration of action *Onset*: 2 to 5 minutes. *Peak effect*: Variable. *Duration*: 2 to 5 minutes.

Special considerations Pregnancy safety: Category C. Nitrous oxide increases the incidence of spontaneous abortion. Ventilate patient care area during use. Nitrous oxide is nonflammable and nonexplosive. Nitrous oxide is ineffective in 20% of the population.

► Norepinephrine Bitartrate (Levophed)

Class Sympathomimetic, vasopressor.

Mechanism of action Potent alpha-agonist resulting in intense peripheral vasoconstriction, positive chronotropic and increased inotropic effect (from 10% beta effect) with increased cardiac output. Alpha-adrenergic activity resulting in peripheral vasoconstriction and beta-adrenergic activity leading to inotropic stimulation of the heart and coronary artery vasodilation.

Indications Cardiogenic shock, unresponsive to fluid resuscitation, significant hypotensive (<70 mm Hg) states, first-line vasopressor in septic shock.

Contraindications Hypotensive patients with hypovolemia, pregnancy (relative).

Adverse reactions/side effects Headache, anxiety, dizziness, restlessness, dyspnea, bradycardia, hypertension, dysrhythmias, chest pain, peripheral cyanosis, cardiac arrest, nausea, vomiting, urinary retention, renal failure, decreased blood flow to the GI tract, kidneys, skeletal muscle, and skin, tissue necrosis from extravasation.

Drug interactions Can be deactivated by alkaline solutions. Sympathomimetic and phosphodiesterase inhibitors may exacerbate dysrhythmias. Bretylium may potentiate the effects of catecholamines.

Dosage and administration *Adult*: 0.1 to 0.5 mcg/kg per minute (in 70-kg adult, 7 to 35 mcg/min).[40] *Pediatric*: Begin at 0.1 to 2 mcg/kg per minute IV infusion, adjust rate to achieve desired change in BP and systemic perfusion. Titrated to patient response.

Duration of action *Onset*: 1 to 3 minutes. *Peak effect*: Variable. *Duration*: 5 to 10 minutes, lasts only 1 minute after infusion discontinued.

Special considerations Pregnancy safety: Category C. Use cautiously during pregnancy and while breastfeeding. May cause fetal anoxia when used in pregnancy. Infuse norepinephrine through a large, stable vein to avoid extravasation and tissue necrosis. Often used with low-dose DOPamine to spare decreased renal and mesenteric blood flow. Drug or poison-induced hypotension may require higher doses to achieve adequate perfusion.

► Ondansetron Hydrochloride (Zofran)

Class Serotonin receptor antagonist, antiemetic.

Mechanism of action Blocks action of serotonin, a natural substance that causes nausea and vomiting.

Indications Prevention and control of nausea or vomiting. Used in hospitals for patients undergoing chemotherapy or surgical procedures.

Contraindications Known allergy to ondansetron or other 5-HT3 receptor antagonists.

Adverse reactions/side effects Headache, malaise, wheezing, bronchospasm, AF, abnormal ECG, prolonged QT interval, ST segment depression, second-degree AV block, constipation, diarrhea, hives, skin rash.

Drug interactions Not recommended if the patient is taking apomorphine, mesoridazine, pimozide, or thioridazine.

Dosage and administration *Adult*: 4 mg IV/IM/PO/SL, may repeat once in 10 minutes.[41]

Acute mountain sickness: 4 mg IV/PO/SL every 6 hours.[14] *Pediatric*: between age 6 months and 14 years: 0.15 mg/kg IV/PO; maximum dose is 4 mg.[41]

Duration of action *Onset*: 30 minutes. *Peak effect*: 2 hours. *Duration*: 3 to 6 hours.

Special considerations Pregnancy safety: Category B. Use with caution during pregnancy and while breastfeeding.

Oral Glucose (Insta-Glucose)

Class Hyperglycemic, carbohydrate.

Mechanism of action After absorption in the GI tract, glucose is distributed to the tissues providing an increase in circulating blood glucose levels.

Indications Conscious patients with suspected hypoglycemia.

Contraindications Decreased level of consciousness, nausea, vomiting.

Adverse reactions/side effects Nausea, vomiting.

Drug interactions None.

Dosage and administration *Adult*: 25 g PO in patients with intact gag reflex and ability to manage their own secretions.[42] *Pediatric*: 0.5 to 1 g PO in patients with intact gag reflex and ability to manage their own secretions.[15]

Duration of action *Onset*: 10 minutes. *Peak effect*: Variable. *Duration*: Variable.

Special considerations Must be swallowed. Glucose is not absorbed sublingually or buccally. Check a glucometer reading before administering oral glucose and repeat at least 10 minutes after.

Oxygen

Class Naturally occurring atmospheric gas.

Mechanism of action Reverses hypoxemia.

Indications Confirmed or expected hypoxemia, ischemic chest pain, respiratory insufficiency, prophylactically during air transport, confirmed or suspected carbon monoxide poisoning, all other causes of decreased tissue oxygenation, decreased level of consciousness.

Contraindications Certain patients with COPD will not tolerate oxygen concentrations over 35%, hyperventilation.

Adverse reactions/side effects Decreased level of consciousness (COPD patients), decreased respiratory drive in COPD patients, dry mucous membranes.

Drug interactions None.

Dosage and administration *Adult*: Cardiac arrest and carbon monoxide poisoning: 100%. Hypoxemia: 10 to 15 L/min via nonrebreathing mask. COPD: 0 to 2 L/min via nasal cannula or 28% to 35% Venturi mask. Be prepared to provide ventilatory support if higher concentrations of oxygen are needed. *Pediatric*: Same as for adult with exception of premature infant.

Duration of action *Onset*: Immediate. *Peak effect*: Not applicable. *Duration*: Less than 2 minutes.

Special considerations Be familiar with liter flow rates and each type of delivery device used. Supports combustion.

Oxymetazoline (Zicam)

Class Vasoconstrictor.

Mechanism of action Alpha-adrenergic receptor stimulator in the arterioles of the nasal mucosa to produce vasoconstriction.

Indications Epistaxis, relief of nasal congestion.

Contraindications Hypersensitivity.

Adverse reactions/side effects Rebound nasal congestion, nasal mucosa irritation.

Drug interactions May diminish the vasoconstricting effect of alpha 1-agonists. May enhance the hypertensive effect of sympathomimetics.

Dosage and administration *Adult*: 2 to 3 sprays each nare. *Pediatric*: 1 to 2 sprays each nare.

Duration of action *Onset*: Immediate. *Peak effect*: 5 minutes. *Duration*: Up to 5 hours.

Special considerations Pregnancy safety: Category B.

Oxytocin (Pitocin)

Class Pituitary hormone.

Mechanism of action Increases uterine contractions.

Indications Postpartum hemorrhage after infant and placental delivery.

Contraindications Presence of second fetus, unfavorable fetal position.

Adverse reactions/side effects Coma, seizures, anxiety, subarachnoid hemorrhage, hypotension, tachycardia, dysrhythmias, chest pain, nausea, vomiting, painful uterine contractions, uterine rupture.

Drug interactions Other vasopressors may potentiate hypotension.

Dosage and administration *Adult*: IM administration: 10 units IM following delivery of placenta. IV administration: Mix 10 to 40 units in 1,000 mL of nonhydrating diluent, infused at 20 to 40 milliunits/min. Titrated to severity of bleeding and uterine response. *Pediatric*: Not applicable.

Duration of action *Onset*: IM: 3 to 5 minutes, IV: immediate. *Peak effect*: Variable. *Duration*: IM: 30 to 60 minutes, IV: 20 minutes after infusion is stopped.

Special considerations Pregnancy safety: Category C. Monitor vital signs including fetal heart rate and uterine tone closely.

Pancuronium Bromide (Pavulon)

Class Nondepolarizing neuromuscular blocker/paralytic.

Mechanism of action Binds to the receptor for acetylcholine at the neuromuscular junction.

Indications Induction or maintenance of paralysis after intubation to assist ventilations.

Contraindications Hypersensitivity, inability to control airway and/or support ventilations with oxygen and positive pressure, neuromuscular disease (eg, myasthenia gravis), hepatic or renal failure.

Adverse reactions/side effects Weakness, prolonged neuromuscular block, bronchospasm, apnea, respiratory failure, tachydysrhythmias, transient hypotension, hypertension, PVCs, salivation.

Drug interactions Positive chronotropic drugs may potentiate tachycardia.

Dosage and administration *Adult*: 0.06 to 0.1 mg/kg slow IV. Repeat every 30 to 60 minutes as needed. *Pediatric*: 0.04 to 0.1 mg/kg slow IV/IO.

Duration of action *Onset*: 30 seconds. *Peak effect*: Paralysis in 3 to 5 minutes. *Duration*: 45 to 60 minutes.

Special considerations Pregnancy safety: Category C. If patient is conscious, explain the effect of the medication before administration and always sedate the patient before administering pancuronium. Intubation and ventilatory support must be readily available; monitor the patient carefully. Pancuronium has no effect on consciousness or pain. Will not stop neuronal seizure activity. Heart rate and cardiac output will be increased. Use decreased doses for patients with renal impairment or myasthenia gravis.

PHENobarbital (Luminal)[43]

Class Barbiturate, long-acting; anticonvulsant; schedule IV drug.

Mechanism of action Generally unknown but believed to reduce neuronal excitability by increasing the motor cortex threshold to electrical stimulation.

Indications Prevention and treatment of seizure activity, status epilepticus.

Contraindications Patients with porphyria, history of sedative or hypnotic addiction, severe liver or respiratory disease.

Adverse reactions/side effects Coma, drowsiness, headache, vertigo, paradoxic excitation, CNS depression, ataxia, bronchospasm, laryngospasm, respiratory depression, hypotension, bradycardia, syncope, nausea, vomiting.

Drug interactions Effects potentiated by other CNS depressants, anticonvulsants, and MAOIs. Incompatible with all other drugs. Flush line before and after use.

Dosage and administration *Adult*: 100 to 250 mg slow IV or IM. May repeat as needed in 20 to 30 minutes. *Pediatric*: 10 to 20 mg/kg slow IV/IO/IM. Repeat as needed in 20 to 30 minutes.

Duration of action *Onset*: 3 to 30 minutes. *Peak effect*: 30 minutes. *Duration*: 4 to 6 hours.

Special considerations Pregnancy safety: Category D. Weigh fetal risk and maternal benefit prior to use. Contraindicated in breastfeeding women. Potential for abuse. Carefully monitor vital signs. Use with caution in patients with pulmonary, cardiovascular, hepatic, or renal insufficiency. Older patients more likely to experience side effects; consider decreasing dose to 75% of the usual dose. Use large, stable vein for injection.

Phenylephrine (Neo-Synephrine)

Class Adrenergic, alpha-agonist, vasopressor.

Mechanism of action Stimulates adrenergic receptors causing peripheral vasoconstriction.

Indications Transient hypotension and hypotension related to shock.

Contraindications Hypersensitivity, hypertension, glaucoma, VT.

Adverse reactions/side effects Ocular pain, necrosis, angina, dysrhythmias, heart failure, hypertension

Drug interactions MAOIs, alpha-adrenergic antagonists.

Dosage and administration *Adult*: IV push-dose pressor: 50 to 200 mcg every 2 to 5 minutes. IV infusion: 10 to 200 mcg/min, titrated to effect. *Pediatric*: IV push-dose pressor: 5 to 20 mcg/kg per minute every 5 minutes. IV infusion: 0.1 to 0.5 mcg/kg per minute, titrated to effect.

Duration of action *Onset*: Immediate. *Peak effect*: Unknown. *Duration*: 15 to 20 minutes.

Special considerations Pregnancy safety: Category C. Regularly assess peripheral circulation due to possibility of profound vasoconstriction.

Phenytoin (Dilantin)

Class Anticonvulsant.

Mechanism of action Promotes sodium efflux from neurons, thereby stabilizing the neuron's threshold against the excitability caused by excess stimulation. In similar fashion, decreases abnormal ventricular automaticity and decreases the refractory period in the myocardial conduction system.

Indications Prophylaxis and treatment of major motor seizures, digitalis-induced dysrhythmias.

Contraindications Hypersensitivity, bradycardia, second- and third-degree heart block.

Adverse reactions/side effects Ataxia, agitation, dizziness, headache, drowsiness, CNS depression, respiratory depression, hypotension, tachycardia, vasodilation, heart blocks, dysrhythmias, nausea, vomiting, hepatitis, altered taste, rash, Stevens-Johnson syndrome, nystagmus, pain at injection site.

Drug interactions Serum phenytoin levels increased by anticoagulants, cimetidine (Tagamet), sulfonamides, and salicylates. Metabolism increased by chronic alcohol use. Cardiac depressant effects increased by lidocaine, propranolol, and other beta-blockers. Precipitation may occur when mixed with D_5W. Incompatible with many solutions and medications.

Dosage and administration *Adult*: Seizures: 10 to 20 mg/kg slow IV, not to exceed 1 g or rate of 50 mg/min. Dysrhythmias: 50 to 100 mg (diluted) slow IV every 5 to 15 minutes PRN. Maximum 1 g. *Pediatric*: Seizures: 10 to 20 mg/kg slow IV (1 to 3 mg/kg per minute). Dysrhythmias: 5 mg/kg slow IV. Maximum 1 g loading dose.

Duration of action *Onset*: 20 to 30 minutes. *Peak effect*: 1 to 3 hours. *Duration*: 18 to 24 hours but as long as 15 days reported.

Special considerations Pregnancy safety: Category D. Contraindicated in pregnant and breastfeeding women. Carefully monitor vital signs. Venous irritation may occur (use large, stable vein).

Potassium Chloride (K-Tab)

Class Electrolyte.

Mechanism of action Replenishes potassium in the body.

Indications Hypokalemia or hypokalemia prophylaxis.

Contraindications Hypersensitivity, hyperkalemia.

Adverse reactions/side effects Diarrhea, flatulence, nausea, vomiting, abdominal pain, GI ulcers, ECG changes, cardiac arrest.

Drug interactions Potassium-sparing diuretics, ACE inhibitors, angiotensin II receptor antagonists, anticholinergics.

Dosage and administration *Adult*: 10 to 40 mEq IV infusion over 2 to 3 hours. *Pediatric*: 0.3 to 1 mEq/kg per hour IV infusion.

Duration of action *Onset*: Rapid. *Peak effect*: End of infusion. *Duration*: Unknown.

Special considerations Pregnancy safety: Category C. Closely monitor patients while infusing potassium. Watch for T wave changes that may indicate fluctuations in the patient's potassium level. Dilution or slowing rate can help alleviate burning sensation during infusion.

Pralidoxime (2-PAM, Protopam)

Class Cholinesterase reactivator, antidote.

Mechanism of action Reactivates cholinesterase to effectively act as an antidote to organophosphate and pesticide poisonings. This action allows for destruction of accumulated acetylcholine at the neuromuscular junction resulting in reversal of respiratory paralysis and paralysis of skeletal muscle.

Indications Antidote in the treatment of poisoning by organophosphate pesticides and chemicals, anticholinesterase overdoses.

Contraindications Reduce dose in patients with impaired renal function, patients with myasthenia gravis, and inorganic phosphate poisoning.

Adverse reactions/side effects Dizziness, drowsiness, headache, neuromuscular blockade, seizure, laryngospasm, hyperventilation, apnea, tachycardia, cardiac arrest, nausea, muscle rigidity, muscle weakness, rash, pain at injection site.

Drug interactions Avoid use of pralidoxime concurrently with succinylcholine, morphine, aminophylline, theophylline, and other respiratory depressants to include barbiturates, narcotic analgesics, and sedative hypnotics.

Dosage and administration Consult with medical direction; dosage recommendations vary depending on the degree of exposure and patient age and weight. Commercially available autoinjectors contain 600 mg of pralidoxime chloride. Because of the rapidity of onset of signs, symptoms, and potential death from acetylcholinesterase inhibitors (carbamates, nerve agents, organophosphates) IM administration is highly recommended to eliminate the inherent delay associated with establishing IV access.[44]

Duration of action *Onset*: Minutes. *Peak effect*: Variable. *Duration*: Variable.

Special considerations Pregnancy safety: Category C. Slow IV infusion prevents tachycardia, laryngospasm, and muscle rigidity. Consider drawing a blood sample prior to administration for hospital to run pretreatment levels. Treatment will be most effective if given within a few hours after poisoning. Cardiac monitoring should be considered in all cases of severe organophosphate poisoning.

▶ PredniSONE (Rayos)

Class Adrenal glucocorticoid, corticosteroid.

Mechanism of action Suppresses inflammation and normal immune responses.

Indications Asthma, COPD.

Contraindications Hypersensitivity, fungal infections.

Adverse reactions/side effects Fluid retention, GI perforation, pancreatitis, thromboembolic disorders, pulmonary edema, electrolyte imbalances, myocardial damage, heart failure, shock, syncope, cardiac arrest, increased blood glucose, weight gain.

Drug interactions Thiazides, NSAIDs, digoxin.

Dosage and administration *Adult*: 20 to 60 mg PO. *Pediatric*: 1 to 2 mg/kg PO.

Duration of action *Onset*: Hours. *Peak effect*: Unknown. *Duration*: 1.25 to 1.5 days.

Special considerations Pregnancy safety: Category C. Use caution in breastfeeding women. Pediatric formulation is often a suspension, prednisoLONE.

▶ Procainamide Hydrochloride (Pronestyl)

Class Antidysrhythmic.

Mechanism of action Suppresses phase 4 depolarization in normal ventricular muscle and Purkinje fibers, reducing ectopic pacemaker's automaticity; suppresses intraventricular conduction.

Indications Stable monomorphic VT with normal QT interval, reentry SVT uncontrolled by vagal maneuvers and adenosine, stable wide-complex tachycardia of unknown origin, AF with rapid ventricular rate in patients with Wolff-Parkinson-White syndrome.

Contraindications Torsades de pointes, second- and third-degree heart AV block (without functioning artificial pacemaker), preexisting QT prolongation, digitalis toxicity, tricyclic antidepressant overdose.

Adverse reactions/side effects Confusion, seizures, hypotension, bradycardia, reflex tachycardia, ventricular dysrhythmias, AV blocks, asystole, widening of PR, QRS, and QT intervals, nausea, vomiting.

Drug interactions Increases plasma levels of amiodarone and quinidine.

Dosage and administration *Adult*: Recurrent VF/pulseless VT: 20 mg/min slow IV infusion until the dysrhythmia is suppressed. Maximum dose: 17 mg/kg. In urgent situations, up to 50 mg/min may be administered. Maximum dose: 17 mg/kg. Other indications: 20 mg/min slow IV infusion until any one of the following occurs: dysrhythmia suppression, hypotension, QRS widens by >50% of its pretreatment width, or total dose of 17 mg/kg has been given. Maintenance infusion: 1 to 4 mg/min (diluted in D_5W or normal saline). Reduce dose in presence of renal insufficiency. *Pediatric*: Loading dose 15 mg/kg IV/IO over 30 to 60 minutes.

Duration of action *Onset*: 10 to 30 minutes. *Peak effect*: Variable. *Duration*: 3 to 6 hours.

Special considerations Pregnancy safety: Category C. Potent vasodilation and negative inotropic effects. Hypotension may occur with rapid infusion. Administer cautiously to patients with cardiac, hepatic, or renal insufficiency. Administer cautiously to patients with asthma or digitalis-induced dysrhythmias.

▶ Prochlorperazine (Compazine)

Class Antiemetic, typical antipsychotic.

Mechanism of action By depressing the chemoreceptor trigger zone, severe nausea and vomiting is reduced.

Indications Nausea and vomiting.

Contraindications Hypersensitivity, altered level of consciousness, children under 20 pounds (9 kg) or age 2 years.

Adverse reactions/side effects Aspiration, seizures, prolonged QT interval, extrapyramidal reactions.

Drug interactions CNS depressants, antihistamines, antipsychotics.

Dosage and administration *Adult*: 5 to 10 mg IV/IM/PO.[41] *Pediatric*: Over age 2 or greater than 9 kg: 0.1 mg/kg slow IV or deep IM; maximum dose is 10 mg.

Duration of action *Onset*: Rapid. *Peak effect*: 10 to 30 minutes. *Duration*: 3 to 4 hours.

Special considerations Pregnancy safety: Category C. Use during pregnancy only if potential maternal benefit outweighs fetal risk. Contraindicated for use in breastfeeding women.

▶ Promethazine Hydrochloride (Phenergan)

Class Phenothiazine, antiemetic, antihistamine.
Mechanism of action H-1 receptor antagonist; blocks action of histamine; possesses sedative, anti-motion, antiemetic, and anticholinergic activity; potentiates the effects of narcotics to induce analgesia.
Indications Nausea/vomiting, motion sickness, sedation for patients in labor, potentiates the analgesic effects of narcotics.
Contraindications Coma, CNS depression from alcohol, barbiturates, or narcotics, Reye syndrome, lower respiratory symptoms (eg, asthma).
Adverse reactions/side effects Headache, dizziness, drowsiness, confusion, restlessness, wheezing, chest tightness, thickening of bronchial secretions, palpitations, bradycardia, reflex tachycardia, QT prolongation, postural hypotension, diarrhea, nausea, vomiting.
Drug interactions Additive with other CNS depressants, increased extrapyramidal effects with MAOIs.
Dosage and administration *Adult*: 12.5 to 25 mg IV, deep IM, PO, PR. *Pediatric (older than age 2 years)*: 0.25 to 0.5 mg/kg deep IM.
Duration of action *Onset*: IV: Immediate. *Peak effect*: 30 to 60 minutes. *Duration*: 4 to 6 hours.
Special considerations Pregnancy safety: Category C. Use with caution in pregnant women. Contraindicated for use in breastfeeding women. Convulsions and sudden death when used with children. Use caution in patients with asthma, peptic ulcer, and bone marrow suppression. Do not use in children with vomiting of unknown etiology. Avoid intra-arterial injection. Warn patients of impending burning sensation. Some systems have removed IM administration because of reported pain and potential for tissue necrosis.

▶ Propofol (Diprivan)

Class Sedative hypnotic, short-acting.
Mechanism of action Produces rapid and brief state of general anesthesia.
Indications Anesthesia induction, anesthesia maintenance, sedation for mechanically ventilated patients.
Contraindications Hypovolemia, known sensitivity including soybean oil, peanuts, and eggs.
Adverse reactions/side effects Seizure, apnea, dysrhythmias, asystole, hypotension, hypertension, nausea, vomiting, involuntary muscle movement, acute renal failure.
Drug interactions Avoid mixing with medications that cannot pass through lipids. In pediatric patients when used with fentaNYL, propofol can cause profound bradycardia.
Dosage and administration *Adult*: Induction dose: 1.5 to 3 mg/kg IV, IO. Maintenance infusion: 25 to 75 mcg/kg per minute IV, IO. *Pediatric*: Induction dose: 2.5 to 3.5 mg/kg IV, IO. Maintenance infusion: 125 to 300 mcg/kg per minute IV, IO.
Duration of action *Onset*: Less than 1 minute. *Peak effect*: 1 minute. *Duration*: As long as infusion is running.
Special considerations Pregnancy safety: Category B. Contraindicated in pregnant and breastfeeding women due to potential fetal and infant respiratory depression. Avoid rapid administration in older patients to avoid hypotension and airway obstruction. Continue to monitor vital signs and oxygenation. Use large, stable vein to avoid injection site pain. Avoid in pregnancy due to neonatal respiratory depression. Infusions may need to be increased during transport because noxious stimuli may arouse patients.

▶ Propranolol Hydrochloride (Inderal)

Class Beta-adrenergic blocker.
Mechanism of action Nonselective beta-adrenergic blocker that reduces chronotropic, inotropic, and vasodilator response to beta-adrenergic stimulation.
Indications Hypertension, angina pectoris, VT, VF refractory to lidocaine, selected SVT.
Contraindications Sinus bradycardia (if no pacemaker present), second- or third-degree AV block (if no pacemaker present), bronchial asthma, sick sinus syndrome (if no pacemaker present), cardiogenic shock, heart failure, and acute pulmonary edema.
Adverse reactions/side effects Weakness, depression, fatigue, anxiety, dizziness, bronchospasm, wheezing, hypotension, bradycardia, heart failure, AV blocks, nausea, vomiting, diarrhea, hypoglycemia, hyperglycemia.
Drug interactions Verapamil may worsen AV conduction abnormalities. Succinylcholine effects may be enhanced. Effects may be reversed by isoproterenol, norepinephrine, DOPamine (Intropin).

Dosage and administration *Adult*: Dilute 1 to 3 mg in 10 to 30 mL of D_5W. Administer slowly IV at rate of 1 mg/min. Maximum dose: 5 mg. *Pediatric*: 0.01 to 0.05 mg/kg per dose slow IV over 10 minutes. Maximum dose: 3 mg.

Duration of action *Onset*: 15 to 60 minutes. *Peak effect*: Variable. *Duration*: 6 to 12 hours.

Special considerations Pregnancy safety: Category C. Use cautiously in pregnant women due to potential placental and congenital anomalies. Closely monitor patient during administration. Use with caution in older patients. Atropine should be readily available.

RaNITIdine (Zantac)

Class Antiulcer, H_2 antihistamine.

Mechanism of action By blocking H_2 receptors it reduces the volume and concentration of gastric acid.

Indications Gastric ulcers, GERD, upper GI bleeding.

Contraindications Hypersensitivity.

Adverse reactions/side effects Abdominal pain, diarrhea, constipation, rebound gastric hypersecretion, impaired liver function, cardiac dysrhythmias, cardiac arrest.

Drug interactions Increases the effects of warfarin, drugs metabolized by cytochrome P450 system.

Dosage and administration *Adult*: 50 mg IV/IM, 150 to 300 mg PO. *Pediatric*: 2 to 4 mg/kg IV infusion.

Duration of action *Onset*: Unknown. *Peak effect*: 15 minutes. *Duration*: 8 to 12 hours.

Special considerations Pregnancy safety: Category B.

Rocuronium Bromide (Zemuron)

Class Nondepolarizing neuromuscular blocker.

Mechanism of action Antagonizes acetylcholine at the motor end plate producing skeletal muscle paralysis.

Indications RSI.

Contraindications Known sensitivity to bromides; use with caution in heart and liver disease.

Adverse reactions/side effects Bronchospasm, wheezing, rhonchi, respiratory depression, apnea, dysrhythmias, tachycardia, transient hypotension and hypertension, nausea, vomiting.

Drug interactions Use of inhalation anesthetics will enhance neuromuscular blockade.

Dosage and administration *Adult*: 0.6 to 1.2 mg/kg IV, IO. *Pediatric (older than 3 months)*: 0.6 to 1.2 mg/kg IV, IO.

Duration of action *Onset*: 1 to 2 minutes. *Peak effect*: Varies. *Duration*: 45 to 120 minutes.

Special considerations Pregnancy safety: Category B. If patient is conscious, explain the effect of the medication before administration and always sedate the patient before using rocuronium. Intubation and ventilatory support must be readily available. Monitor the patient carefully. Rocuronium has no effect on consciousness or pain. Will not stop neuronal seizure activity. Pulse rate and cardiac output are increased. Decrease doses for patients with renal disease.

Sodium Bicarbonate

Class Systemic hydrogen ion buffer, alkalizing agent.

Mechanism of action Buffers metabolic acidosis and lactic acid buildup in the body caused by anaerobic metabolism secondary to severe hypoxia by reacting with hydrogen ions to form water and carbon dioxide.

Indications Metabolic acidosis during cardiac arrest, tricyclic antidepressant, aspirin, and PHENobarbital overdose, hyperkalemia, crush injuries.

Contraindications Metabolic and respiratory alkalosis, hypokalemia, electrolyte imbalance due to severe vomiting or diarrhea.

Adverse reactions/side effects Hypernatremia, metabolic alkalosis, tissue sloughing, cellulitis, necrosis at injection site, seizures, fluid retention, hypokalemia, electrolyte imbalance, tetany, sodium retention, peripheral edema.

Drug interactions Increases the effects of amphetamines. Decreases the effects of benzodiazepines, tricyclic antidepressants. May deactivate sympathomimetics (DOPamine, EPINEPHrine, norepinephrine).

Dosage and administration *Adult*: 1 mEq/kg slow IV, IO push, may repeat at 0.5 mEq/kg every 10 minutes. *Pediatric*: 1 mEq/kg slow IV, IO push (dilute in small children to 4.2%).

Duration of action *Onset*: Seconds. *Peak effect*: 1 to 2 minutes. *Duration*: 10 minutes.

Special considerations Pregnancy safety: Category C. Repeat as needed in tricyclic antidepressant overdose until QRS narrows. Must be used in conjunction with effective ventilation and chest compressions in cardiac arrest. Avoid contact with other medications; may precipitate or inactivate them. Always flush IV line well before and after injecting. Use with caution in patients with heart failure and renal disease due to high sodium concentration. Monitor patient closely for signs and symptoms of fluid overload.

Sodium Nitrite

Class Antidote cyanide poisoning adjunct.
Mechanism of action Reacts with hemoglobin to form methemoglobin, which reacts with cyanide and chemically binds with it to prevent toxic effect.
Indications Cyanide poisoning.
Contraindications None in the emergency setting.
Adverse reactions/side effects Hypotension, tachycardia, fainting, nausea, vomiting.
Drug interactions None in the emergency setting.
Dosage and administration *Adult*: 300 mg (10 mL of 3% solution) slow IV push over 5 minutes or dilute 300 mg in 100 mL saline and infuse slowly. *Pediatric*: 10 mg/kg (0.33 mL/kg of 10% solution) IV, IO over 3 to 5 minutes.
Duration of action *Onset*: 2 to 10 minutes. *Peak effect*: Varies. *Duration*: 30 minutes to 2 hours.
Special considerations Pregnancy safety: Category C. Weigh potential fetal risk and maternal benefit prior to administration. Women who have been breastfeeding should discontinue doing so. Potent vasodilator causes significant hypotension if given too rapidly. Monitor BP closely. Look for signs of methemoglobinemia (eg, cyanosis, vomiting, shock, and coma).

Sodium Thiosulfate

Class Cyanide antidote.
Mechanism of action Converts cyanide to the less toxic thiocyanate, which is then excreted in the urine.
Indications Cyanide poisoning.
Contraindications None in the emergency setting.
Adverse reactions/side effects Diarrhea.
Drug interactions None.
Dosage and administration *Adult*: 12.5 g (50 mL of 25% solution) IV/IO slow push over 10 minutes. *Pediatric*: 0.5 g/kg IV (2 mL/kg of 25% solution).[45]
Duration of action *Onset*: 2 to 10 minutes. *Peak effect*: Varies. *Duration*: 30 minutes to 2 hours.
Special considerations Pregnancy safety: Category C. Weigh potential fetal risk and maternal benefit prior to administration. Women who have been breastfeeding should discontinue doing so. If response to treatment is inadequate, repeat sodium nitrite and sodium thiosulfate; administer a second dose of each at half the original dose 30 minutes after the first dose. This is the third step in a three-step treatment preceded by amyl nitrite and sodium nitrite.

Streptokinase (Streptase)[46]

Class Thrombolytic.
Mechanism of action Combines with plasminogen to produce an activator complex that converts free plasminogen to the proteolytic enzyme, plasmin. Plasmin degrades fibrin threads and fibrinogen, causing clot lysis.
Indications Acute evolving myocardial infarction, massive PE, arterial thrombosis and embolism, to clear intraventricular cannula.
Contraindications Hypersensitivity, active bleeding, recent cerebral vascular accident, prolonged CPR, intracranial or intraspinal neoplasm, arteriovenous malformation, recent surgery or significant trauma (particularly head trauma), severe uncontrolled hypertension.
Adverse reactions/side effects Intracranial hemorrhage, bronchospastic hemoptysis, acute respiratory distress syndrome, reperfusion dysrhythmias, hypotension, MI, GI bleeding, hematuria, abdominal pain, bleeding from other sites, allergic reactions.
Drug interactions Aspirin, heparin, and other anticoagulants may increase risk of bleeding as well as improve outcome.
Dosage and administration Note: Reconstitute by slowly adding 5 mL of sodium chloride or D_5W, directing stream to side of vial instead of into powder. Gently roll and tilt vial for reconstitution; dilute slowly to 45 mL total. *Adult*: 500,000 to 1,500,000 international units diluted to 45 mL IV over 1 hour. *Pediatric*: Safety not established.
Duration of action *Onset*: 10 to 20 minutes (fibrinolysis, 10 to 20 minutes; clot lysis, 60 to 90 minutes). *Peak effect*: Variable. *Duration*: 3 to 4 hours (prolonged bleeding times up to 24 hours).
Special considerations Pregnancy safety: Category C. Fetal risk should be considered during first 18 weeks of pregnancy; use must be clearly indicated. Use with caution in breastfeeding women. Thin transparent fibers may occur after reconstitution; they do not interfere with safe use. Do not administer IM injections to patients receiving fibrinolytics. Obtain blood sample for coagulation studies prior to administration. Carefully monitor vital signs. Observe patient for bleeding.

Succinylcholine Chloride (Anectine)

Class Neuromuscular blocker, depolarizing; skeletal muscle relaxant.

Mechanism of action Ultra-short-acting depolarizing skeletal muscle relaxant that mimics acetylcholine as it binds with the cholinergic receptors on the motor end plate, producing a phase 1 block as manifested by fasciculations.

Indications RSI.

Contraindications Acute narrow-angle glaucoma, penetrating eye injuries, malignant hyperthermia; acute injury after multisystem trauma, major burns, or extensive muscle injury that may result in hyperkalemia.

Adverse reactions/side effects Apnea, respiratory depression, bradydysrhythmia, tachydysrhythmia, dysrhythmia, cardiac arrest, salivation, prolonged muscle rigidity, rhabdomyolysis, malignant hyperthermia, increased intraocular pressure, hyperkalemia (trauma patients).

Drug interactions Oxytocin, beta-blockers, and organophosphates may potentiate effects. DiazePAM may reduce duration of action.

Dosage and administration *Adult and pediatric*: 1 to 2 mg/kg rapid IV. Repeat once if needed.

Duration of action *Onset*: 1 minute. *Peak effect*: 1 to 3 minutes. *Duration*: 5 to 10 minutes.

Special considerations Pregnancy safety: Category C. If the patient is conscious, explain the effects of the drug before administration. Appropriate sedation and analgesia should be used in any conscious patient before undergoing neuromuscular blockade. Time management is crucial. Postintubation sedation and analgesia should be readily available.

Tenecteplase (TNKase)

Class Thrombolytic.

Mechanism of action Binds to fibrin and converts it to plasmin, reducing circulating fibrinogen.

Indications STEMI.

Contraindications Internal bleeding, risk or history of recent CVA, uncontrolled hypertension.

Adverse reactions/side effects Cardiac dysrhythmias, GI bleeding, intracranial hemorrhage.

Drug interactions Antiplatelet medications, NSAIDs, dabigatran.

Dosage and administration *Adult*: All IV boluses given over 5 seconds. Patients <60 kg: 30-mg IV bolus. Patients 60 to 69 kg: 35-mg IV bolus. Patients 70 to 79 kg: 40-mg IV bolus. Patients 80 to 89 kg: 45-mg IV bolus. Patients 90 kg or greater: 50-mg IV bolus. *Pediatric*: Not indicated.

Duration of action *Onset*: Rapid. *Peak effect*: Unknown. *Duration*: Unknown.

Special considerations Pregnancy safety: Category C. Use with caution in pregnant and breastfeeding women. Use caution in patients with systolic BP >180 mm Hg or diastolic BP >110 mm Hg.

Terbutaline Sulfate (Brethine)

Class Beta-2 adrenergic agonist, bronchodilator, tocolytic.

Mechanism of action Selective beta-2 adrenergic receptor activity resulting in relaxation of smooth muscle of the bronchial tree and peripheral vasculature with minimal cardiac effects.

Indications Bronchial asthma, reversible bronchospasm associated with exercise, chronic bronchitis, emphysema, premature contractions.

Contraindications Hypersensitivity, tachydysrhythmias.

Adverse reactions/side effects CNS stimulation, headache, seizure, restlessness, apprehension, wheezing, coughing, bronchospasm, bradycardia, tachycardia, ST wave changes, PVCs, PACs, chest pain.

Drug interactions Cardiovascular effects exacerbated by other sympathomimetics. MAOIs may potentiate dysrhythmias. Beta-blockers may antagonize terbutaline.

Dosage and administration *Adult*: 0.25 mg subcutaneous, may repeat in 15 to 30 minutes. Maximum dose 0.5 mg in a 4-hour period. *Pediatric*: Not recommended for children younger than age 12 years.

Duration of action *Onset*: 5 to 10 minutes. *Peak effect*: Variable. *Duration*: 1.5 to 4 hours.

Special considerations Pregnancy safety: Category B. Contraindicated in prevention of or prolonged treatment for preterm labor. Carefully monitor vital signs. Use with caution in patients with cardiovascular disease, seizure disorder, hypertension, and diabetes. Patient should receive oxygen before and during administration.

Tirofiban Hydrochloride (Aggrastat)

Class Glycoprotein IIb/IIIa inhibitor, platelet aggregation inhibitor.

Mechanism of action Inhibits aggregation of platelets by reversibly antagonizing fibrinogen binding to the glycoprotein IIb/IIIa receptor.

Indications ACS, patients undergoing PTCA or atherectomy.

Contraindications Trauma or major surgery within the past 30 days, hemorrhagic stroke, intracranial neoplasm, arteriovenous malformation, aneurysm, evidence of aortic dissection, severe uncontrolled hypertension (systolic BP >180 mm Hg, diastolic BP >110 mm Hg), concomitant use of another glycoprotein IIb/IIIa inhibitor, acute pericarditis.

Adverse reactions/side effects Dizziness, pain, sweating, intracranial bleeding, CVA, bradydysrhythmia, dissecting coronary artery aneurysm, GI bleeding, severe bleeding.

Drug interactions Other medications that affect hemostasis: thrombolytics, oral anticoagulants, aspirin and other NSAIDs, dipyridamole, ticlopidine, and clopidogrel.

Dose and administration *Adult*: Loading dose: 0.4 mcg/kg per minute IV for 30 minutes. Infusion: 0.1 mcg/kg per minute for 18 to 24 hours post-angioplasty. *Pediatric*: Not recommended.

Duration of action *Onset*: Minutes. *Peak effect*: Early peak in less than 30 minutes, infusion at a steady rate will peak in approximately 6 hours. *Duration*: Platelet function restored 4 to 8 hours after infusion discontinued.

Special considerations Pregnancy safety: Category B. Must be administered only with an infusion pump direct from bottle with a vented IV set. Due to severe spontaneous bleeding risk, invasive procedures (eg, IV starts, injections, NG tube, or nasotracheal intubation) should be avoided.

Tranexamic Acid (Cyklokapron, Lysteda)[47]

Class Hemostatic agent, antifibrinolytic, plasminogen inactivator.

Mechanism of action Reduces plasminogen activation, mitigating conversion to plasmin.

Indications Blunt or penetrating trauma less than 3 hours from onset with hemodynamic compromise, bleeding.

Contraindications Hypersensitivity; MOI greater than 3 hours; subarachnoid hemorrhage; history of PE, DVT, or other thromboembolic disorder.

Adverse reactions/side effects Fatigue, headache, abdominal pain, anemia, DVT, PE, other thromboembolic disorder. Rapid infusion may cause hypotension.

Drug interactions Hormonal contraceptives, clotting factor complexes.

Dosage and administration *Adult*: 1 g IV infusion over 10 minutes. *Pediatric*: Not recommended.

Duration of action *Onset*: Unknown. *Peak effect*: Unknown. *Duration*: 7 to 8 hours.

Special considerations Pregnancy safety: Category C. Use in pregnant and breastfeeding women should be clearly indicated. Must be mixed into an infusion bag, typically 100 mL of NaCl.

Vancomycin (Vancocin)

Class Antibiotic.

Mechanism of action Inhibits cell wall synthesis, cell membrane permeability, and RNA synthesis of gram-positive bacteria.

Indications Staphylococcal infections, *Clostridium difficile*, endocarditis, meningitis, osteomyelitis, pneumonia, soft-tissue infections.

Contraindications Hypersensitivity, allergy to corn or corn products, heart failure, renal disease or failure, ulcerative colitis.

Adverse reactions/side effects Chills, dizziness, abdominal pain, nausea, vomiting, diarrhea, hypokalemia, hypotension, tinnitus, ototoxicity, nephrotoxicity/renal failure, urticaria, wheezing.

Drug interactions May enhance neuromuscular blockade with nondepolarizing muscle relaxants (eg, pancuronium); combined use with aminoglycosides may increase the risk of ototoxicity and nephrotoxicity.

Dosage and administration *Adult*: 7.5 mg/kg or 500 mg every 6 hours or 15 mg/kg or 1 g every 12 hours for 7 to 10 days IV infusion. *Pediatric*: 40 mg/kg of body weight/24 hr equally divided and given every 6, 8, or 12 hours (10 mg/kg every 6 hours, 13.33 mg/kg every 8 hours, or 20 mg/kg every 12 hours) for 7 to 10 days IV infusion.

Duration of action *Onset*: Rapid. *Peak effect*: End of the infusion. *Duration*: 12 to 24 hours.

Special considerations Pregnancy safety: Category C. Often administered to patients with penicillin allergies. Dose reduction required for patients with impaired renal function. Rapid infusion can cause histamine release resulting in "red man syndrome" that is characterized by flushing of the face, neck, upper body, arms, and/or back.[48] Symptoms usually resolve within 20 minutes but sometimes last for several hours. Stopping or slowing the infusion rate may reduce the severity of the reaction.

Vasopressin (Pitressin)[49]

Class Vasopressor.

Mechanism of action Stimulation of smooth muscle receptors; potent vasoconstrictor when given in high doses.

Indications Vasodilatory shock.

Contraindications Use with caution in patients with CAD, epilepsy, or heart failure.

Adverse reactions/side effects Dizziness, headache, bronchial constriction, MI, chest pain, angina, cardiac dysrhythmia, decreased cardiac output, abdominal cramps, diarrhea, nausea, vomiting, paleness, sweating.

Drug interactions None reported.

Dosage and administration *Adult*: 0.02 to 0.07 unit/min IV infusion. *Pediatric*: Safety and efficacy not established.

Duration of action *Onset*: Unknown. *Peak effect*: Unknown. *Duration*: 30 to 60 minutes.

Special considerations Pregnancy safety: Category C. Use with caution during pregnancy. Breastfeeding women should pump and discard breast milk for 1.5 hours after drug administration. May increase peripheral vascular resistance and provoke cardiac ischemia and angina.

▶ Vecuronium Bromide (Norcuron)

Class Neuromuscular blocker, nondepolarizing.

Mechanism of action Neuromuscular agent with intermediate duration of action that competes with acetylcholine for receptors at the motor end plate, resulting in neuromuscular blockade.

Indications RSI.

Contraindications Acute narrow-angle glaucoma, penetrating eye injuries, inability to control airway or support ventilations with oxygen and positive pressure, newborns, myasthenia gravis, hepatic or renal failure.

Adverse reactions/side effects Weakness, prolonged neuromuscular block, bronchospasm, apnea, dysrhythmias, bradycardia, tachycardia, PVCs, transient hypotension, cardiac arrest, excessive salivation.

Drug interactions Use of inhalation anesthetics will enhance neuromuscular blockade.

Dosage and administration *Adult*: 0.1 to 0.2 mg/kg IV push. Maintenance dose within 45 to 60 minutes: 0.8 to 1.2 mg/kg IV push. *Pediatric*: 0.1 to 0.3 mg/kg IV/IO. Maintenance dose within 20 to 40 minutes: 0.01 to 0.015 mg/kg IV push.

Duration of action *Onset*: 1 to 3 minutes. *Peak effect*: Varies. *Duration*: 45 to 90 minutes.

Special considerations Pregnancy safety: Category C. If patient is conscious, explain the effect of the medication before administration and always sedate the patient before using vecuronium. Intubation and ventilatory support must be readily available. Monitor the patient carefully. Vecuronium has no effect on consciousness or pain. Will not stop neuronal seizure activity. Pulse rate and cardiac output are increased. Decrease doses for patients with renal disease.

▶ Verapamil Hydrochloride (Isoptin, Calan)

Class Calcium channel blocker.

Mechanism of action Slow calcium channel blocker that selectively blocks the transmembrane influx of calcium ions into arterial smooth muscles and myocardial cells, prolongs AV nodal refractory period, reduces systemic vascular resistance and selective vasodilation of peripheral arteries, and dilates coronary arteries and arterioles.

Indications PSVT, atrial flutter, and AF with rapid ventricular response, reentry SVT.

Contraindications Wolff-Parkinson-White syndrome, Lown-Ganong-Levine syndrome, second- or third-degree AV block or sick sinus syndrome or other sinus node disease unless a functioning artificial pacemaker is present, hypotension, cardiogenic shock, severe left ventricular dysfunction (ejection fraction less than 30%), wide-complex tachycardias, children younger than age 12 months, AF.

Adverse reactions/side effects Dizziness, headache, pulmonary edema, sinus arrest, asystole, AV blocks, bradycardia, hypotension, nausea, vomiting, constipation.

Drug interactions Increases the serum concentration of digoxin. Beta-adrenergic blockers may have additive negative inotropic and chronotropic effects. Antihypertensives may potentiate hypotensive effects.

Dosage and administration *Adult*: 2.5 to 5 mg IV bolus over 2 minutes (3 minutes in older patients). Repeat dose of 5 to 10 mg may be given every 15 to 30 minutes. Maximum dose 20 mg. *Pediatric*: 0.01 to 0.02 mg/kg per dose IV, IO push over 2 minutes. Repeat dose in 30 minutes if not effective. Note: Not to be used in children younger than age 12 months.

Duration of action *Onset*: 2 to 5 minutes. *Peak effect*: Variable. *Duration*: 30 to 60 minutes.

Special considerations Pregnancy safety: Category C. Carefully monitor BP, heart rate, and ECG before, during, and after administration. AV block or asystole may occur because of slowed AV conduction.

▶ Ziprasidone (Geodon)

Class Atypical antipsychotic.

Mechanism of action Blocks synaptic reuptake of serotonin and norepinephrine, binds to alpha-adrenergic receptors, dopamine receptors, and serotonin receptors.

Indications Agitation; violence or excited delirium associated with schizophrenia, acute mania, bipolar disorder.

Contraindications Hypersensitivity, heart failure, AMI, prolonged QT interval.

Adverse reactions/side effects Dizziness, suicide attempt, bradycardia, prolonged QT-interval, dystonia.

Drug interactions Antidysrhythmics, droperidol, quinolones.

Dosage and administration *Adult*: 10 to 20 mg IM. *Pediatric*: Safety and efficacy not established.

Duration of action *Onset*: Rapid. *Peak effect*: 60 minutes. *Duration*: Unknown.

Special considerations Pregnancy safety: Category C. Use during third trimester is associated with extrapyramidal symptoms in fetus. Use during pregnancy should be clearly indicated after weighing fetal risk and maternal benefits.

IV Solutions (Colloids and Crystalloids)

Colloids expand plasma volume by colloidal osmotic pressure. Colloids are most often used in hypovolemic shock states. Crystalloids are substances in solution that can diffuse through the intravascular compartment. Crystalloid solutions are used for electrolyte replacement, as a route for medication, and for short-term intravascular volume expansion.

▶ Albumin (Albumarc, Albutein, Flexbumin)

Class Colloid, blood modifier agent, volume expander.

Mechanism of action Oncotically similar to human plasma, it causes the body to shift approximately 3.5 times the amount administered into the intravascular space.

Indications Hypovolemia.

Contraindications Hypersensitivity, patients at risk of hypervolemia.

Adverse reactions/side effects Possible urticaria from hypersensitivity, use caution in patients with renal insufficiency or anemia.

Drug interactions None currently identified.

Dosage and administration *Adult*: 12.5 to 25 g IV. *Pediatric*: 0.5 to 1 g/kg IV.

Duration of action *Onset*: 15 to 30 minutes. *Peak effect*: Unknown. *Duration*: 24 hours.

Special considerations Pregnancy safety: Category C. Administered with 0.9% NaCl, D_5W, or sodium lactate.

▶ Bacteriostatic Water

Class Diluent or solvent.

Mechanism of action Works as a solvent or dilutional agent.

Indications Used for diluting or dissolving drugs for IV, IM, or subcutaneous injections based on drug manufacturer recommendations.

Contraindications Hypersensitivity to benzyl alcohol due to use as preservative.

Adverse reactions/side effects None noted if used according to manufacturer recommendations.

Drug interactions None noted.

Dosage and administration According to drug manufacturer recommendations.

Duration of action Not applicable.

Special considerations Pregnancy category: C. Due to benzyl alcohol additive, other dilutional agents should be used if available. Solution should be made approximately isotonic prior to use.

▶ Dextran

Class Artificial colloid.

Mechanism of action Dextran is a sugar-containing colloid used as an intravascular volume expander. It remains in the intravascular compartment for approximately 12 hours. It increases intravascular volume by attracting water from other fluid compartments by virtue of its colloid osmotic pressure.

Indications Hypovolemic shock.

Contraindications Dextran should not be administered to patients who have a known hypersensitivity to the drug. It should not be administered to patients with heart failure, renal failure, or known bleeding disorders.

Adverse reactions/side effects Rash, itching, dyspnea, chest tightness, mild hypotension. The incidence of these side effects is very low, and reactions are generally mild. Increased bleeding time has also been reported with dextran use due to its interference with platelet function.

Drug interactions Dextran should not be administered to patients who are receiving anticoagulants because it significantly retards blood clotting.

Dosage and administration The dosage of dextran is titrated according to the patient's physiologic response.

Duration of action 8 to 12 hours.

Special considerations In the management of burn shock, it is especially important to follow standard fluid resuscitation regimens to prevent possible circulatory overload.

▶ Hetastarch (Hespan)

Class Artificial colloid.

Mechanism of action Hetastarch is a starch-containing colloid used as an intravascular volume expander. Following administration, the plasma volume is expanded slightly in excess of the volume of hetastarch administered. This effect has been observed for up to 24 to 36 hours. Hetastarch increases intravascular volume by virtue of its colloid osmotic pressure.

Indications Hypovolemic shock, especially burn shock; septic shock.

Contraindications There are no major contraindications to hetastarch when used in the management of life-threatening hypovolemic states.

Adverse reactions/side effects Nausea, vomiting, mild febrile reactions, chills, itching, urticaria; rare severe anaphylactic reactions have been reported.

Drug interactions Hetastarch should not be administered to patients who are receiving anticoagulants.

Dosage and administration The dosage of hetastarch is titrated according to the patient's physiologic response.

Duration of action 24 to 36 hours.

Special considerations Pregnancy safety: Category C. Patients allergic to corn may be allergic to hetastarch.

▶ Lactated Ringer (Hartmann) Solution

Class Isotonic crystalloid solution.

Mechanism of action Lactated Ringer solution replaces water and electrolytes.

Indications Hypovolemic shock; keep open IV, hypoperfusion.

Contraindications Lactated Ringer solution should not be used in patients with heart failure or renal failure.

Adverse reactions/side effects Rare in therapeutic dosages.

Drug interactions Few in the emergency setting.

Dosage and administration Hypovolemic shock; titrate according to patient's physiologic response. Hypoperfusion: 20 mL/kg IV/IO over 15 minutes.[50] *Neonates*: Fluid bolus: 10 mL/kg IV given over 5 to 10 minutes; multiple boluses may be administered if the patient remains clinically hypovolemic.

Duration of action Short-term therapy.

Special considerations None.

▶ Plasma Protein Fraction (Plasmanate)

Class Natural colloid.

Mechanism of action Plasmanate is a protein-containing colloid that remains in the intravascular compartment. It increases intravascular volume by attracting water from other fluid compartments by virtue of its colloid osmotic pressure.

Indications Hypovolemic shock, especially burn shock; hypoproteinemia (low-protein states).

Contraindications There are no major contraindications to plasma protein fraction when used in the treatment of life-threatening hypovolemic states.

Adverse reactions/side effects Chills, fever, urticaria (hives), nausea, vomiting.

Drug interactions Solutions should not be mixed with or administered through the same administration sets as other IV fluids.

Dosage and administration The plasma protein fraction infusion rate should be titrated according to the patient's hemodynamic response. In the management of shock secondary to bums, the physician's orders regarding the rate of administration must be closely followed. Standard formulas for IV fluid administration have been developed. The medical control physician will use these in judging the correct rate of IV administration.

Duration of action 24 to 36 hours.

Special considerations Do not use if the solution is cloudy or if you see sedimentation.

▶ Total Parenteral Nutrition (TPN; varies based on mixture)

Class Electrolyte, nutrition.

Mechanism of action Replenishes electrolytes and nutrients.

Indications Ordered and customized to each patient based on needs identified from lab work.

Contraindications Varies based on the specific mixture.

Adverse reactions/side effects Varies based on the specific mixture.

Drug interactions Varies based on the specific mixture.

Dosage and administration Varies based on the specific mixture.

5% Dextrose in Water

Class Hypotonic dextrose-containing solution.
Mechanism of action D_5W provides nutrients in the form of dextrose as well as free water.
Indications IV access for emergency drugs; for dilution of concentrated drugs for IV infusion.
Contraindications D_5W should not be used as a fluid replacement for hypovolemic states.
Adverse reactions/side effects Rare in therapeutic dosages.
Drug interactions D_5W should not be used with phenytoin (Dilantin) or amrinone (Inocor).
Dosage and administration D_5W is usually administered through a minidrip (60 drops/mL) set at a TKO rate.
Duration of action Short-term therapy.
Special considerations None.

10% Dextrose in Water

Class Hypertonic dextrose-containing solution.
Mechanism of action 10% dextrose in water ($D_{10}W$) provides nutrients in the form of dextrose as well as free water.
Indications Neonatal resuscitation, hypoglycemia.
Contraindications $D_{10}W$ should not be used as a fluid replacement for hypovolemic states.
Adverse reactions/side effects Rare in therapeutic dosages.
Drug interactions Should not be used with phenytoin (Dilantin) or amrinone (Inocor).
Dosage and administration The administration rate of $D_{10}W$ will usually be dependent on the patient's condition. *Neonates*: A 10% dextrose solution may be given as an IV bolus (2 mL/kg) if the newborn's blood glucose level is less than 40 mg/dL and the infant is symptomatic, with a recheck of the blood glucose level in about 30 minutes.[51,52] IV administration of dextrose often needs to be followed by a 10% dextrose infusion run at 60 to 100 mL/kg/d. Infusion of dextrose is based on the newborn's gestational age (60 mL/kg per day for a full-term newborn; adjusted upward based on the recommendations of the referring hospital for premature newborns).
Duration of action Short-term therapy.
Special considerations None.

0.9% Sodium Chloride (Normal Saline)

Class Isotonic crystalloid solution.
Mechanism of action Normal saline replaces water and electrolytes.
Indications Heat-related problems (heat exhaustion, heatstroke), freshwater drowning, hypovolemia, diabetic ketoacidosis, keep open IV.
Contraindications The use of 0.9% sodium chloride should not be considered in patients with heart failure because circulatory overload can be easily induced.
Adverse reactions/side effects Rare in therapeutic dosages.
Drug interactions Few in the emergency setting.
Dosage and administration The specific situation being treated will dictate the rate at which normal saline will be administered. In severe heatstroke, diabetic ketoacidosis, and freshwater drowning, it is likely that you will be called on to administer the fluid quite rapidly. In other cases, it is advisable to administer the fluid at a moderate rate (for example, 100 mL/h). *Neonates*: Fluid bolus: 10 mL/kg IV given over 5 to 10 minutes; multiple boluses may be administered if the patient remains clinically hypovolemic. In a neonate, a 10-mL/kg normal saline bolus may aid in improved perfusion and clearance of acid.
Duration of action Short-term therapy.
Special considerations None.

0.45% Sodium Chloride

Class Hypotonic crystalloid solution.
Mechanism of action 0.45% sodium chloride (one-half normal saline) replaces free water and electrolytes.
Indications Patients with diminished renal or cardiovascular function for which rapid rehydration is not indicated.
Contraindications Cases in which rapid rehydration is indicated.
Adverse reactions/side effects Rare in therapeutic dosages.
Drug interactions Few in the emergency setting.
Dosage and administration The specific situation and patient condition will dictate the rate at which one-half normal saline is administered.
Duration of action Short-term therapy.
Special considerations None.

3% Sodium Chloride (Hypertonic Saline)

Class Hypertonic crystalloid solution.
Mechanism of action The osmotic effect allows fluid to cross the blood-brain barrier, reducing the amount of fluid in the cranial cavity and reducing ICP.
Indications Traumatic brain injuries, fluid resuscitation in severe sepsis, hyponatremia.

Contraindications Hypotension.
Adverse reactions/side effects Increases sodium levels, seizures, neurologic deficits.
Drug interactions None currently identified.
Dosage and administration *Adult*: 250 to 500 mL IV infusion. *Pediatric*: 1 to 6 mL/kg over 30 minutes. Maximum 500 mL IV infusion.
Duration of action *Onset*: Rapid. *Peak effect*: Unknown. *Duration*: Unknown.
Special considerations Use caution in pediatric patients because their sodium levels shift rapidly. Rapid increases can cause significant neurologic complications. Should be administered through central line due to high osmolarity and tonicity.

5% Dextrose in 0.45% Sodium Chloride

Class Hypertonic dextrose-containing crystalloid solution.
Mechanism of action 5% dextrose in 0.45% sodium chloride (D_5½NS) replaces free water and electrolytes and provides nutrients in the form of dextrose.
Indications Heat exhaustion, diabetic disorders; for use as a way to keep open solution in patients with impaired renal or cardiovascular function.
Contraindications D_5½NS should not be used when rapid fluid resuscitation is indicated.
Adverse reactions/side effects Rare in therapeutic dosages.
Drug interactions D_5½NS should not be used with phenytoin (Dilantin) or amrinone (Inocor).
Dosage and administration The specific situation and patient condition will dictate the rate at which D_5½NS should be administered.
Duration of action Short-term therapy.
Special considerations None.

5% Dextrose in 0.9% Sodium Chloride

Class Hypertonic dextrose-containing crystalloid solution.
Mechanism of action 5% dextrose in 0.9% sodium chloride (D_5NS) replaces free water and electrolytes and provides nutrients in the form of dextrose.
Indications Heat-related disorders, freshwater drowning, hypovolemia, peritonitis.
Contraindications D_5NS should not be administered to patients with impaired cardiac or renal function.
Adverse reactions/side effects Rare in therapeutic dosages.
Drug interactions D_5NS should not be used with phenytoin (Dilantin) or amrinone (Inocor).
Dosage and administration The specific situation and patient condition will dictate the rate at which D_5NS is given.
Duration of action Short-term therapy.
Special considerations None.

5% Dextrose in Lactated Ringer Solution

Class Hypertonic dextrose-containing crystalloid solution.
Mechanism of action 5% dextrose in lactated Ringer solution (D_5LR) replaces water and electrolytes and provides nutrients in the form of dextrose.
Indications Hypovolemic shock, hemorrhagic shock, certain cases of acidosis.
Contraindications D_5LR should not be administered to patients with decreased renal or cardiovascular function.
Adverse reactions/side effects Rare in therapeutic dosages.
Drug interactions D_5LR should not be used with phenytoin (Dilantin) or amrinone (Inocor).
Dosage and administration In severe hypovolemic shock, D_5LR should be infused through a large-bore catheter (18-gauge). This infusion should be administered "wide open" until a BP of 100 mm Hg is achieved. When the BP is attained, infusions should be reduced to 100 mL/h. In other cases, the specific situation and patient condition will dictate the rate of administration.
Duration of action Short-term therapy.
Special considerations None.

References

1. Hazard Vallerand A, Sanoski CA. *Davis' Drug Guide for Nurses*. 14th ed. Philadelphia, PA: FA Davis Company; 2016.
2. Truven Health Analytics. Micromedex database. http://www.micromedexsolutions.com/. Accessed February 29, 2017.
3. Lexi-Comp website. online.lexi.com. Accessed April 2017.
4. American Heart Association. 2015 American Heart Association Guidelines for CPR and ECC. https://eccguidelines.heart.org/index.php/circulation/cpr-ecc-guidelines-2/. Accessed February 29, 2017.
5. National Model EMS Clinical Guidelines. National Association of State EMS Officials. V.08-16. https://www.nasemso.org/Projects/ModelEMSClinicalGuidelines/index.asp. Accessed April 7, 2017.

6. Society of Critical Care Medicine. Surviving Sepsis Campaign. http://www.survivingsepsis.org/Pages/default.aspx. Accessed February 29, 2017.
7. National Association of Emergency Medical Technicians (NAEMT). Tactical Combat Casualty Care Guidelines for Medical Personnel. http://www.naemt.org/education/TCCC/guidelines_curriculum. Published June 3, 2016. Accessed February 29, 2017.
8. FDA and ISMP Lists of Look-Alike Drug Names and Recommended Tall Man Letters. Institute for Safe Medication Practices. 2016:1-6.
9. Page RL, Joglar JA, Caldwell MA, et al. 2015 ACC/AHA/HRS guideline for the management of adult patients with supraventricular tachycardia: a report of the American College of Cardiology/American Heart Association Task Force on Clinical Practice Guidelines and the Heart Rhythm Society. *Circulation*. 2016;133:e506-e574.
10. Cordarone—amiodarone hydrochloride tablet. Wyeth Pharmaceuticals Inc. website. http://labeling.pfizer.com/showlabeling.aspx?id=93. Revised December 2016. Accessed March 29, 2017.
11. Brouse SD, Philips SM. Amiodarone use in patients with documented allergy to iodine-containing compounds. *Pharmacotherapy*. 2005;25(3):429-434.
12. Amyl nitrite—medical countermeasures database. Chemical Hazards Emergency Medical Management U.S. Department of Health & Human Services website. https://chemm.nlm.nih.gov/countermeasure_amyl-nitrite.htm#adv. Updated January 2, 2013. Accessed March 29, 2017.
13. Gahart BL, Nazareno AR, Ortega MQ. *2017 Intravenous Medications: A Handbook for Nurses and Health Professionals*. 33rd ed. St. Louis, MO: Elsevier; 2017.
14. Altitude Illness. In: *National Model EMS Clinical Guidelines*. National Association of State EMS Officials. V.08-16:236. https://www.nasemso.org/Projects/ModelEMSClinicalGuidelines/index.asp. Accessed April 7, 2017.
15. Hypoglycemia/Hyperglycemia. In: *National Model EMS Clinical Guidelines*. National Association of State EMS Officials. V.08-16:58. https://www.nasemso.org/Projects/ModelEMSClinicalGuidelines/index.asp. Accessed April 7, 2017.
16. Agitated or Violent Patient/Behavioral Emergency. In: *National Model EMS Clinical Guidelines*. National Association of State EMS Officials. V.08-16:44. https://www.nasemso.org/Projects/ModelEMSClinicalGuidelines/index.asp. Accessed April 7, 2017.
17. Seizures. In: *National Model EMS Clinical Guidelines*. National Association of State EMS Officials. V.08-16:68. https://www.nasemso.org/Projects/ModelEMSClinicalGuidelines/index.asp. Accessed April 7, 2017.
18. Medications. In: *National Model EMS Clinical Guidelines*. National Association of State EMS Officials. V.08-16:262. https://www.nasemso.org/Projects/ModelEMSClinicalGuidelines/index.asp. Accessed April 7, 2017.
19. Inapsine—droperidol injection. Dailymed U.S. National Library of Medicine website. https://dailymed.nlm.nih.gov/dailymed/archives/fdaDrugInfo.cfm?archiveid=236184. Revised December 2011. Accessed March 29, 2017.
20. Medications. In: *National Model EMS Clinical Guidelines*. National Association of State EMS Officials. V.08-16:263. https://www.nasemso.org/Projects/ModelEMSClinicalGuidelines/index.asp. Accessed April 7, 2017.
21. Bronchospasm (due to Asthma and Obstructive Lung Disease). In: *National Model EMS Clinical Guidelines*. National Association of State EMS Officials. V.08-16:135. https://www.nasemso.org/Projects/ModelEMSClinicalGuidelines/index.asp. Accessed April 7, 2017.
22. Web-based Integrated 2010 & 2015 American Heart Association Guidelines for Cardiopulmonary Resuscitation and Emergency Cardiovascular Care—Part 12: Pediatric Advanced Life Support. The American Heart Association website. https://eccguidelines.heart.org/index.php/circulation/cpr-ecc-guidelines-2/part-12-pediatric-advanced-life-support/. Accessed April 11, 2017.
23. Wyckoff MH, Aziz K, Escobedo MB, et al. Part 13: neonatal resuscitation: 2015 American Heart Association Guidelines Update for Cardiopulmonary Resuscitation and Emergency Cardiovascular Care. *Circulation*. 2015;132(suppl 2):S549.
24. Weiner GM, Zaichkin J. Lesson 7: medications. In: *Textbook of Neonatal Resuscitation (NRP)*. 7th ed. Elk Grove Village, IL: American Academy of Pediatrics; 2016:188.
25. Weiner GM, Zaichkin J. Lesson 3: initial steps of newborn care. In: *Textbook of Neonatal Resuscitation (NRP)*. 7th ed. Elk Grove Village, IL: American Academy of Pediatrics; 2016:187.
26. Hospital TH. *Harriet Lane Handbook*. 20th ed. St. Louis, MO: Mosby; 2015.
27. Amidate—etomidate injection, solution. Pfizer website. http://labeling.pfizer.com/ShowLabeling.aspx?id=4444. Revised November 2015. Accessed March 29, 2017.
28. Glucagon for injection. Lilly USA, LLC website. http://pi.lilly.com/us/rglucagon-pi.pdf. Revised September 19, 2012. Accessed March 29, 2017.
29. Cyanokit® Package Insert. Meridian Medical Technologies website. http://www.cyanokit.com/sites/default/files/Single_5-g_Vial_PI.pdf. Revised February 2016. Accessed March 29, 2017.
30. Ketamine hydrochloride. Hospira, Inc. website. http://labeling.pfizer.com/ShowLabeling.aspx?id=4485. Revised January 2013. Accessed March 29, 2017.
31. Agitated or Violent Patient/Behavioral Emergency. In: *National Model EMS Clinical Guidelines*. National Association of State EMS Officials. V.08-16:45. https://www.nasemso.org/Projects/ModelEMSClinicalGuidelines/index.asp. Accessed April 7, 2017.
32. Medications. In: *National Model EMS Clinical Guidelines*. National Association of State EMS Officials. V.08-16:267. https://www.nasemso.org/Projects/ModelEMSClinicalGuidelines/index.asp. Accessed April 7, 2017.

33. Metaproterenol sulfate. MedLibrary website. http://medlibrary.org/lib/rx/meds/metaproterenol-sulfate/. Revised September 14, 2006. Accessed March 29, 2017.
34. Tachycardia with a Pulse. In: *National Model EMS Clinical Guidelines*. National Association of State EMS Officials. V.08-16:31,32. https://www.nasemso.org/Projects/ModelEMSClinicalGuidelines/index.asp. Accessed April 7, 2017.
35. Naloxone hydrochloride. Hospira, Inc. website. http://labeling.pfizer.com/ShowLabeling.aspx?id=4542. Revised January 2007. Accessed March 29, 2017.
36. Opioid Poisoning/Overdose. In: *National Model EMS Clinical Guidelines*. National Association of State EMS Officials. V.08-16:217. https://www.nasemso.org/Projects/ModelEMSClinicalGuidelines/index.asp. Accessed April 7, 2017.
37. Altitude Illness. In: *National Model EMS Clinical Guidelines*. National Association of State EMS Officials. V.08-16:237. https://www.nasemso.org/Projects/ModelEMSClinicalGuidelines/index.asp. Accessed April 7, 2017.
38. Pulmonary Edema. In: *National Model EMS Clinical Guidelines*. National Association of State EMS Officials. V.08-16:143. https://www.nasemso.org/Projects/ModelEMSClinicalGuidelines/index.asp. Accessed April 7, 2017.
39. Pulmonary Edema. In: *National Model EMS Clinical Guidelines*. National Association of State EMS Officials. V.08-16:141. https://www.nasemso.org/Projects/ModelEMSClinicalGuidelines/index.asp. Accessed April 7, 2017.
40. Web-based Integrated 2010 & 2015 American Heart Association Guidelines for Cardiopulmonary Resuscitation and Emergency Cardiovascular Care—Part 8: Post-Cardiac Arrest Care. The American Heart Association website. https://eccguidelines.heart.org/index.php/circulation/cpr-ecc-guidelines-2/part-8-post-cardiac-arrest-care/. Accessed April 11, 2017.
41. Nausea/Vomiting. In: *National Model EMS Clinical Guidelines*. National Association of State EMS Officials. V.08-16:120. https://www.nasemso.org/Projects/ModelEMSClinicalGuidelines/index.asp. Accessed April 7, 2017.
42. Hypoglycemia/Hyperglycemia. In: *National Model EMS Clinical Guidelines*. National Association of State EMS Officials. V.08-16:57. https://www.nasemso.org/Projects/ModelEMSClinicalGuidelines/index.asp. Accessed April 7, 2017.
43. Phenobarbital sodium. DailyMed U.S. National Library of Medicine website. https://dailymed.nlm.nih.gov/dailymed/drugInfo.cfm?setid=ffcaa218-ed6a-4557-9645-b9a91128a214. Updated August 8, 2011. Accessed March 29, 2017.
44. Acetylcholinesterase Inhibitors (Carbamates, Nerve Agents, Organophosphates) Exposure. In: *National Model EMS Clinical Guidelines*. National Association of State EMS Officials. V.08-16:182,184,185,187. https://www.nasemso.org/Projects/ModelEMSClinicalGuidelines/index.asp. Accessed April 7, 2017.
45. Cyanide Exposure. In: *National Model EMS Clinical Guidelines*. National Association of State EMS Officials. V.08-16:201. https://www.nasemso.org/Projects/ModelEMSClinicalGuidelines/index.asp. Accessed April 7, 2017.
46. Streptase. https://www.old.health.gov.il/units/pharmacy/trufot/alonim/Streptase_dr_1358152899014.pdf. Accessed March 29, 2017.
47. Cyklokapron—tranexamic acid injection, solution. Pharmacia and Upjohn Company LLC website. http://labeling.pfizer.com/ShowLabeling.aspx?id=556. Revised July 2016. Accessed March 29, 2017.
48. Sivagnanam S, Deleu D. Red man syndrome. *Crit Care*. 2003;7(2):119-120.
49. Highlights of Prescribing Information—Vasostrict (vasopressin injection) for intravenous use. Par Pharmaceutical Companies, Inc. website. https://www.accessdata.fda.gov/drugsatfda_docs/label/2014/204485Orig1s000lbl.pdf. Revised April 2014. Accessed March 29, 2017.
50. Anaphylaxis and Allergic Reaction. In: *National Model EMS Clinical Guidelines*. National Association of State EMS Officials. V.08-16:50. https://www.nasemso.org/Projects/ModelEMSClinicalGuidelines/index.asp. Accessed April 7, 2017.
51. Kliegman RM, Stanton BF, St. Geme JW, Schor NF. Chapter 92: hypoglycemia. In: *Nelson Textbook of Pediatrics.* 20th ed. Philadelphia, PA: Elsevier; 2016:787.
52. Kliegman RM, Stanton BF, St. Geme JW, Schor NF. Chapter 107: the endocrine system. In: *Nelson Textbook of Pediatrics.* 20th ed. Philadelphia, PA: Elsevier; 2016:898.

Glossary: Volume 1

3-3-2 rule A method used to predict difficult intubation. A mouth opening of less than three fingerbreadths, a mandible length of less than three fingerbreadths, and a distance from hyoid bone to thyroid notch of less than two fingerbreadths indicate a possibly difficult airway.

abandonment Termination of medical care for the patient without giving the patient sufficient opportunity to find another suitable health care professional to take over his or her medical treatment; in the context of abuse and neglect, a type of child maltreatment in which a parent or guardian physically leaves a child without regard to the child's health, safety, or welfare.

abdominal thrust maneuver Abdominal thrusts performed to relieve a foreign body airway obstruction.

abduction Movement of a limb away from the midline.

aberration A term describing the shape of the QRS complex in aberrantly (abnormally) conducted beats.

ABO system The commonly used blood classification system, based on the antigens present or absent in the blood.

abscess An area in the brain or spinal cord in which cells have been attacked, typically by an infectious agent. To prevent the spread of infection, the immune system "walls off" the area. Pus can collect in this pocket.

absolute refractory period (ARP) The early phase of cardiac repolarization, wherein the heart muscle cannot be stimulated to depolarize; also known as the effective refractory period.

absorption The process by which the molecules of a substance are moved from the site of entry or administration into systemic circulation; in the context of decontamination, a type of decontamination that is done with large pads that the hazardous materials team uses to soak up liquid and remove it from the patient.

access port A sealed hub on an administration set designed for sterile access to the IV fluid.

accessory muscles The muscles not normally used during normal breathing; include the sternocleidomastoid muscles of the neck, the pectoralis major muscles of the chest, and the abdominal muscles.

accommodation The ability of the lens of the eye to change its shape to focus on a close object.

acetabulum The socket formed by the coxal (hip) bone into which the ball-shaped femoral head fits snugly.

acetylcholine (ACh) A neurotransmitter released at synapses within the autonomic nervous system and by motor neurons to stimulate skeletal muscle contraction.

acetylcholinesterase An enzyme found in the central nervous system, in red blood cells, and in motor endplates of skeletal muscle that causes the decomposition of acetylcholine.

acholic stools Light, clay-colored stools indicative of liver failure.

acid Any molecule that can give up a hydrogen ion, and therefore increases the concentration of hydrogen ions in a water solution.

acidosis A pathologic condition resulting from the accumulation of acids (increase in extracellular H^+ ions) in the body; a blood pH of less than 7.35.

acquired immunity The immunity that occurs when the body is exposed to a foreign substance or disease and produces antibodies to the invader.

acquired immunodeficiency syndrome (AIDS) The end-stage disease process caused by the human immunodeficiency virus; results in extreme vulnerability to numerous opportunistic bacterial, viral, and fungal infections that would not affect a person with an intact immune system.

acromion process The tip of the shoulder and the site of attachment for the clavicle and various shoulder muscles.

actin A contractile protein found in the thin filaments of skeletal muscle cells.

action potential Sequence of changes in the membrane potential that occurs when an excitable cell (neuron or muscle) is stimulated.

activation Mediators of inflammation trigger the appearance of molecules known as selectins and integrins on the surfaces of endothelial cells and polymorphonuclear neutrophils, respectively.

active metabolite A medication that has undergone biotransformation and is able to alter a cellular process or body function.

active transport A method used to move compounds across a cell membrane to create or maintain an imbalance of charges, usually against a concentration gradient and requiring the expenditure of energy.

activities of daily living (ADLs) The basic activities a person usually accomplishes during a normal day, such as eating, dressing, and washing.

acute abdomen A condition of sudden onset of pain within the abdomen, usually indicating peritonitis; demands immediate medical or surgical treatment.

acute chest syndrome A vasoocclusive crisis that can be associated with pneumonia; common signs and symptoms include chest pain, fever, and cough; associated with sickle cell disease.

acute coronary syndromes (ACSs) A series of cardiac conditions caused by an abrupt reduction in coronary artery blood flow.

acute dystonic reaction A syndrome that may occur in patients taking typical antipsychotic agents. The patient develops muscle spasms of the neck, face, and back within a few days of starting treatment with the medication.

acute gastroenteritis A family of conditions that revolve around a central theme of infection with fever, abdominal pain, diarrhea, nausea, and vomiting.

acute kidney injury (AKI) A sudden decrease in filtration through the glomeruli.

acute myocardial infarction (AMI) Cardiac ischemia that occurs when sudden narrowing or complete occlusion of a coronary artery leads to death (necrosis) of myocardial tissue.

acute splenic sequestration syndrome A condition in which red blood cells become trapped in the spleen, causing a dramatic fall in hemoglobin available in the circulation; it usually occurs in infants or toddlers.

acute stress reaction A reaction to stress that occurs during a stressful situation.

adaptation The temporary or permanent reduction of sensitivity to a particular stimulus.

addisonian crisis Acute adrenal insufficiency.

adduction Movement of a limb toward the midline.

adenosine triphosphate (ATP) The nucleotide formed from the metabolism of nutrients in the cell; involved in energy metabolism; used to store energy.

adhesion The attachment of polymorphonuclear neutrophils to endothelial cells, mediated by selectins and integrins.

administration set Tubing that connects to the IV bag access port and the catheter to deliver IV fluid.

adolescents People who are 13 to 18 years of age.

adrenal cortex The outer layer of the adrenal gland; it produces hormones that are important in regulating the water and salt balance of the body.

adrenal glands Paired endocrine glands located on top of the kidneys that release epinephrine and norepinephrine when stimulated by the sympathetic nervous system; each adrenal gland consists of an inner adrenal medulla and an adrenal cortex.

adrenergic Having the characteristics of the sympathetic division of the autonomic nervous system.

adrenocorticotropic hormone (ACTH) A hormone that targets the adrenal cortex to secrete cortisol (a glucocorticoid).

advance directive A written document or oral statement that expresses the wants, needs, and desires of a patient in reference to future medical care; examples include living wills, do not resuscitate orders, and organ donation orders.

adventitious Abnormal.

adventitious breath sounds Abnormal breath sounds, such as wheezing, rhonchi, crackles, stridor, and pleural friction rubs.

adverse effect Abnormal or harmful effect to an organism caused by exposure to a chemical. It is indicated by some result such as death, a change in food or water consumption, altered body and organ weights, altered enzyme levels, or visible illness.

aerobic metabolism Metabolism that can proceed only in the presence of oxygen.

affect The outward, physical expression of a person's inner feelings (eg, happy, sad, angry, fearful, withdrawn).

affinity The ability of a medication to bind with a particular receptor site.

afterimage The perception that a stimulus is still present after the stimulus has been removed.

afterload The pressure gradient in the aorta against which the left ventricle of the heart must pump; an increase in this pressure can decrease cardiac output.

agitated delirium An acute confrontational state characterized by global impairment of thinking, perception, judgment, and memory.

agonal Pertaining to the period of dying.

agonal gasps Slow, shallow, irregular respirations or occasional gasping breaths that result from cerebral anoxia.

agonal rhythm A ventricular rate of less than 20 beats/min; this rhythm is seen just before the heart stops beating altogether.

agonist medications The group of medications that initiates or alters a cellular activity by attaching to receptor sites, prompting a cellular response.

agoraphobia Literally, "fear of the marketplace"; fear of entering a public place from which escape may be impeded.

air embolism The presence of air in the venous circulation, which forms a gas bubble that can block the outflow of blood from the right ventricle to the lung; can lead to cardiac arrest, shock, or other life-threatening complications.

airborne precautions The use of a surgical mask on the patient and the use of airflow measures to prevent airborne transmission; apply to diseases that are large particle and can travel a distance of 6 feet (2 m), then drop to the floor.

airborne transmission The transmission of an organism or infectious agent in aerosol form, such as droplets or dust; transmission occurs by inhalation of small particles that become aerosolized when the infected person coughs, sneezes, talks, or exhales; particles remain suspended in this vapor and can be carried a short distance, usually 3 feet (1 m) to 6 feet (2 m).

albumins The smallest of plasma proteins; they make up around 60% of the plasma proteins and are responsible for the oncotic pressure in the vasculature, thereby controlling the movement of water into and out of the circulation.

alcoholic ketoacidosis The metabolic acidotic state that manifests because of the inadequate nutritional habits associated with chronic alcohol abuse. The liver and body experience inadequate fuel reserves of glycogen and, thus, have to switch to fatty acid metabolism.

alcoholism A disorder characterized by a physical and psychological addiction to ethanol.

aldosterone A hormone that stimulates the kidneys to reabsorb sodium and water from the urine and excrete potassium by altering the osmotic gradient in the blood.

alert and oriented (A × O) A determination made when assessing mental status by looking at whether the patient is oriented in four areas: person, place, time, and the event itself. Each element provides information about different aspects of the patient's memory.

alkalosis A pathologic condition resulting from the accumulation of bases (decrease in extracellular H^+ ions) in the body; a blood pH of greater than 7.45.

alleles Variant forms of a gene, which can be identical or slightly different in a sequence of deoxyribonucleic acid.

allergen A substance that produces allergic symptoms or a hypersensitivity reaction in a patient.

allergic reaction An abnormal immune response the body develops when reexposed to a substance or allergen.

allergy A hypersensitivity reaction to the presence of an agent (allergen) that is intrinsically harmless.

alternative time sampling Time parameters that are set during a research project.

alveoli The air sacs at the end of the bronchioles in the lungs, in which the exchange of oxygen and carbon dioxide takes place; also, small pits or cavities, such as the bony sockets for the teeth that reside in the mandible and maxilla; (singular, *alveolus*).

Alzheimer disease A progressive, organic condition in which neurons in the brain die, causing dementia.

amenorrhea Absence of menstruation.

amphetamines A class of drugs that increase alertness and excitation (stimulants); includes methamphetamine (crank or ice), methylenedioxyamphetamine (MDA, Adam), and methylenedioxymethamphetamine (MDMA, Eve, Ecstasy).

ampules Small glass containers that are sealed and the contents sterilized.

amyotrophic lateral sclerosis (ALS) A condition that strikes the voluntary motor neurons, causing their death. The disease is characterized by fatigue and general weakness of muscle groups; eventually the patient becomes unable to walk, eat, or speak; also known as Lou Gehrig disease.

anabolism The building of larger substances from smaller substances, such as the building of proteins from amino acids.

anaerobic metabolism Metabolism that occurs in the absence of oxygen.

anal fissures Linear tears to the mucosal lining in and near the anus, possibly caused by the passage of large, hard stools; a cause of lower gastrointestinal bleeding.

analgesia The state of being insensible to pain while still conscious.

anaphylactic shock A severe hypersensitivity reaction that involves bronchoconstriction and cardiovascular collapse.

anaphylactoid reaction An extreme allergic response that does not involve IgE antibody mediation. The exact mechanism is unknown, but an event of this type may occur without the patient being previously exposed to the offending agent.

anaphylaxis An extreme systemic form of an allergic reaction involving one, two, or more body systems.

anatomic position The position of reference, in which the patient stands facing you, arms at the side, with the palms of the hands facing forward.

anatomy The study of the structure of an organism and its parts.

androgens Male sex hormones that regulate body changes associated with sexual development (puberty), including growth spurts, deepening of the voice, growth of facial and pubic hair, and muscle growth and strength.

anemia A lower than normal hemoglobin or erythrocyte level.

anesthesia Lack of feeling within a body part.

anesthetic A medication that causes the inability to feel sensation.

aneurysm A swelling or enlargement of part of a blood vessel, resulting from weakening of the vessel wall.

angina pectoris The sudden pain that occurs when the oxygen supply to the myocardium is insufficient to meet demand, causing ischemic changes in the tissue.

angiogenesis The growth of new blood vessels.

angle of Louis A prominence of the sternum that indicates the point where the second rib joins the sternum; also called the sternal angle or manubriosternal junction.

anisocoria Unequal pupils with a greater than 1-mm difference.

anorexia nervosa An eating disorder in which a person diets by exerting extraordinary control over his or her eating, and loses weight to the point of jeopardizing his or her health and life.

anoxia An absence of oxygen.

antagonist A molecule that blocks the ability of a given chemical to bind to its receptor, preventing a biologic response.

antagonist medications The group of medications that prevent endogenous or exogenous agonist chemicals from reaching cell receptor sites and initiating or altering a particular cellular activity.

antecubital The anterior aspect of the elbow.

anterior The front surface of the body; the side facing you in the anatomic position.

anterograde (posttraumatic) amnesia Loss of memory of events that occurred after an injury.

anteroposterior axis The axis that runs perpendicular to the coronal plane.

antibiotics The medications used to fight infection by killing the microorganisms or preventing their multiplication to allow the body's immune system to overcome them.

antibody A protein secreted by certain immune cells in response to an antigen, which binds antigens to make them more visible to the immune system; an immunoglobulin.

anticoagulant A substance that prevents blood from clotting.

antidiuretic hormone (ADH) A hormone secreted by the posterior pituitary lobe of the pituitary gland, ADH constricts blood vessels and raises the blood pressure; also called *vasopressin*.

antidote Something to counteract the effect of a poison.

antifungals The medications used to treat fungal infections.

antigens Proteins, polysaccharides, glycoproteins, or glycolipids commonly found on the surfaces of red blood cells that stimulate an immune system response and cause formation of antibodies; cells learn to recognize these as either "self" or "nonself" (foreign).

antimicrobials The medications used to kill or suppress the growth of microorganisms.

antiseptics Chemicals used to cleanse an area before performing an invasive procedure, such as starting an IV line; not toxic to living tissues; examples include isopropyl alcohol and iodine.

antonyms Pairs of word roots, prefixes, or suffixes that have opposite meanings.

anuria A complete cessation of urine production.

anxiety disorder A mental disorder in which the dominant mood is fear and apprehension.

anxious avoidant attachment A bond between an infant and his or her parent or caregiver in which the infant is repeatedly rejected and develops an isolated lifestyle that does not depend on the support and care of others.

aorta The principal artery leaving the left side of the heart and carrying freshly oxygenated blood to the body; the largest artery in the body.

aortic aneurysm An outpouching or bulge in the wall of a portion of the aorta, caused by weakening and dilation of the vessel wall; a ruptured aortic aneurysm is life threatening.

aortic valve The semilunar valve that regulates blood flow from the left ventricle to the aorta.

apex (plural apices or apexes) The pointed extremity of a conical structure.

aphasia The language impairment that affects the production or understanding of speech and the ability to read or write.

aphonia The inability to speak.

aplastic crisis A temporary halt in the production of red blood cells; it may occur as a result of sickle cell disease.

apneic oxygenation The continued alveolar uptake of oxygen, even when the patient is apneic; can be facilitated by administering oxygen via nasal cannula during intubation.

apneustic center A portion of the pons that is thought to work with the pontine respiratory group to regulate the length and depth of inspiration.

apneustic respirations Prolonged gasping inspirations followed by extremely short, ineffective expirations; associated with brainstem insult.

apoptosis Normal, genetically programmed cell death.

apparent life-threatening event (ALTE) An episode characterized by some combination of apnea (central or obstructive), color change (cyanotic, pallid, erythematous, or plethoric) change in muscle tone (usually diminished), and choking or gagging.

appendicitis Inflammation of the appendix.

appendicular skeleton The portion of the skeletal system made up of the upper extremities, shoulder girdle, pelvic girdle, and lower extremities.

aqueous humor Watery fluid filling the anterior eye cavity; the quantity determines the intraocular pressure, which is critical to sight.

areolar tissue A type of loose connective tissue that binds skin to underlying organs and fills in spaces between muscles.

arrhythmia The absence of any cardiac rhythm or organized activity; asystole or ventricular standstill.

arteriosclerosis A pathologic condition in which the thickening and stiffening of the arterial walls makes the arteries less elastic.

arteriovenous graft A surgical connection between an artery and a vein.

artifact An artificial product; in cardiology, used to refer to noise or interference in an ECG tracing.

arytenoid cartilages Six paired cartilages stacked on top of each other in the larynx.

ascites Abnormal accumulation of fluid in the peritoneal cavity; typically signals liver failure.

aseptic technique A method of cleansing used to prevent contamination of a site when you are performing an invasive procedure, such as starting an IV line.

aspiration The entry of fluids or solids into the trachea, bronchi, and lungs; the act of drawing material in or out by suction; can occur when a patient is unable to protect his or her own airway.

assault To create in another person a fear of immediate bodily harm or invasion of bodily security (including loss of freedom).

asthma A chronic inflammatory lower airway condition resulting in intermittent wheezing and excess mucus production.

astigmatism Condition where parts of the image are out of focus and others are in focus; caused by irregularities in the shape of the eye lens.

asymmetric chest wall movement Unequal movement of the two sides of the chest; indicates decreased airflow into one lung.

asystole The absence of ventricular contraction or electrical activity; a straight-line or flat-line ECG.

ataxia Alteration in the ability to perform coordinated motions such as walking.

atelectasis Collapse of the alveolar air spaces of the lungs.

atheroma A mass of fatty tissue that gradually calcifies, hardening into an atheromatous plaque that infiltrates the arterial wall, diminishing its elasticity.

atherosclerosis A disorder in which cholesterol and calcium build up inside the walls of the blood vessels, forming plaque, which eventually leads to partial or complete blockage of blood flow.

atlas The first cervical vertebra (C1), which provides support for the head.

atopic An allergic tendency.

atria The two upper chambers of the heart (singular, atrium).

atrial natriuretic peptide A hormone produced by the atria when they are distended by increased blood volume; it inhibits the absorption of water and sodium in the renal tubules, thereby increasing the elimination of water.

atrioventricular (AV) junction The portion of the conduction system of the heart that consists of the AV node and the nonbranching portion of the bundle of His.

atrioventricular (AV) node A group of cells that conduct an electrical impulse through the heart, slowing the impulses from the sinoatrial node before relaying them to the ventricles; located in the floor of the right atrium immediately behind the tricuspid valve and near the opening of the coronary sinus.

atrioventricular (AV) valves The mitral and tricuspid valves through which blood flows from the atria to the ventricles.

atrophy A decrease in cell size due to a loss of subcellular components.

atropine-like effects Results of some antipsychotic medications that include adverse effects similar to atropine, resulting in dry mouth, blurred vision, urinary retention, and cardiac dysrhythmias.

augmented limb leads On an ECG, leads aVR, aVL, and aVF. They contain only one true pole; the other is a combination of information from other leads. A standard12-lead ECG consists of the three of these leads, along with the three standard limb leads and the six precordial leads.

aura Sensations commonly experienced before a seizure or migraine headache occurs; may include visual changes in addition to hallucinations.

aural Pertaining to the ear.

auscultation The act of using a stethoscope to listen to sounds within the body.

authoritarian A parenting style that demands absolute obedience.

authoritative A parenting style that balances parental authority with the child's freedom by setting and enforcing rules, but also allowing the child to have some freedom.

autoantibodies Antibodies directed against the person's own proteins.

autoimmunity The production of antibodies or T cells that work against the tissues of a person's body, producing autoimmune disease or a hypersensitivity reaction.

automated external defibrillator (AED) A defibrillator that can analyze the patient's heart rhythm and determine whether a defibrillating shock is needed to terminate ventricular fibrillation or ventricular tachycardia, and which can guide the user through the resuscitation effort via voice commands.

automatic crash notification (ACN) On-board computer systems in motor vehicles that automatically send telemetry data to a monitoring service in the event of a crash, which then relays the data to emergency responders; also called advanced automatic crash notification.

automatic transport ventilator (ATV) A portable mechanical ventilator attached to a control box that allows the variables of ventilation (such as rate and tidal volume) to be set.

automaticity A state in which cardiac cells are at rest, waiting for the generation of a spontaneous impulse from within; the ability of cardiac pacemaker cells to initiate an electrical impulse spontaneously without being stimulated from another source (such as a nerve).

autonomic nervous system (ANS) A subdivision of the nervous system that controls primarily involuntary body functions; comprised of the sympathetic and parasympathetic nervous systems.

autosomal dominant A pattern of inheritance that involves genes that are located on autosomes or the nonsex chromosomes. Inheritance of only one copy of a particular form of a gene is needed to show the trait.

autosomal recessive A pattern of inheritance that involves genes located on autosomes or the nonsex chromosomes. Inheritance of two copies of a particular form of a gene is needed to show the trait.

autosomes The chromosomes that do not carry genes that determine sex.

avian (bird) flu A disease caused by a virus that occurs naturally in the bird population; signs and symptoms include fever, sore throat, cough, and muscle aches.

AVPU A method of assessing mental status by determining whether a patient is Awake and alert, responsive to Verbal stimuli or Pain, or Unresponsive; used principally in the primary survey.

axial skeleton The portion of the skeleton made up of the skull, spinal column, and thoracic cage.

axis Imaginary line joining the positive and negative electrodes of a lead; also the second cervical vertebra.

axis deviation Movement of the heart's QRS axis to the right or left of its normal position.

axon A long, slender extension of a neuron (nerve cell) that conducts electrical impulses away from the nerve cell body to adjacent cells.

azotemia Increased nitrogenous wastes in the blood.

B lymphocytes Lymphocytes that exist in the blood, and are abundant in the lymph nodes, bone marrow, intestinal lining, and spleen; also called B cells.

bacteria Small organisms that can grow and reproduce outside the human cell in the presence of the needed temperature and nutrients and cause disease by invading and multiplying in the tissues of the host.

bacterial vaginosis An overgrowth of bacteria in the vagina, characterized by itching, burning, or pain, and possibly a fishy smelling discharge.

bag-mask device A manual ventilation device that consists of a bag, mask, reservoir, and oxygen inlet; capable of delivering up to 100% oxygen.

barbiturates Potent sedative-hypnotics historically used as sleep aids, antianxiety drugs, and as part of the regimen for seizure control; include drugs such as thiopental (Pentothal, Trapanal) and methohexital (Brevital).

baroreceptors Nerve endings that are stimulated by pressure changes, including increased arterial blood pressure; they are located in the aortic arch and carotid sinuses.

barotrauma Injury resulting from pressure disequilibrium (too much pressure) across body surfaces, for example in the lungs.

Bartholin glands The glands that secrete mucus for sexual lubrication.

basal ganglia Structures located deep within the cerebrum, diencephalon, and midbrain that have an important role in coordination of motor movements and posture.

basal metabolic rate (BMR) The heat energy produced at rest from normal body metabolic reactions; the rate at which nutrients are consumed in the body; determined mostly by the liver and skeletal muscles.

base station A radio at a fixed location (such as a hospital or dispatch center) consisting of a transmitter, receiver, and antenna.

basophils White blood cells that contain histamine granules and other substances that are released during inflammatory and allergic responses.

battery The unlawful physical acting upon a threat—the use of force against another, resulting in harmful, offensive, or sexual contact.

Battle sign Bruising over the mastoid bone behind the ear, which may indicate a basilar skull fracture; also called retroauricular ecchymosis or raccoon eyes.

Beck triad The combination of a narrowed pulse pressure, muffled heart tones, and jugular venous distention associated with cardiac tamponade; usually caused by penetrating chest trauma.

behavior How a person functions or acts in response to his or her environment.

behavioral emergency The point at which a person's reactions to events interfere with activities of daily living; becomes a psychiatric emergency when it causes a major life interruption, such as attempted suicide.

Bell palsy A temporary paralysis of the facial nerve (cranial nerve VII), which controls the muscles on each side of the face.

benign prostate hypertrophy (BPH) Age-related nonmalignant (noncancerous) enlargement of the prostate gland.

benzodiazepines The family of sedative-hypnotics that provide muscle relaxation and mild sedation; most commonly used to treat anxiety, seizures, and alcohol withdrawal; include drugs such as diazepam (Valium) and midazolam (Versed).

beta-2 agonist A pharmacologic agent that stimulates the beta-2 receptor sites found in smooth muscle; includes common bronchodilators such as albuterol and levalbuterol.

bifascicular block Blockage of any two fascicles or conduction pathways: a right bundle branch block (RBBB) with anterior hemiblock, RBBB with posterior hemiblock, or anterior hemiblock and posterior hemiblock (a combination known as LBBB).

bigeminy A dysrhythmia in which every other complex is a premature complex, causing a *normal–early beat–normal–early beat* pattern; can be atrial, junctional, or ventricular.

bilateral In anatomy, a body part or condition that appears on both sides of the midline.

bilevel positive airway pressure (BPAP) A form of noninvasive positive pressure ventilation that delivers two pressures (a higher inspiratory positive airway pressure, and a lower expiratory positive airway pressure).

biliary tract disorders A group of disorders that involve inflammation of the gallbladder; these include cholangitis, cholelithiasis, cholecystitis, and acalculous cholecystitis.

bilirubin A waste product of red blood cell destruction that undergoes further metabolism in the liver.

bimanual laryngoscopy An effective technique to improve laryngoscopic view of the vocal cords by external manipulation of the larynx.

binocular vision The merging of two images into one.

bioavailability The percentage of the unchanged medication that reaches systemic circulation.

Biot (ataxic) respirations Irregular pattern, rate, and depth of respirations with intermittent periods of apnea; result from increased intracranial pressure.

biotelemetry Transmission of physiologic data, such as an electrocardiogram, from the patient to a distant point of reception (commonly referred to in emergency medical services as telemetry).

biotransformation A process with four possible effects on a medication absorbed into the body: (1) An inactive substance can become active, capable of producing desired or unwanted clinical effects. (2) An active medication can be changed into another active medication. (3) An active medication may be completely or partially inactivated. (4) A medication is transformed into a substance (active or inactive) that is easier for the body to eliminate.

biphasic reaction A two-phase allergic reaction in which the patient's symptoms improve and then reappear without being exposed to the trigger (allergen) a second time; the symptoms can resurface up to 8 or more hours after the initial incident.

bipolar leads On an ECG, leads that contain both a positive and a negative pole: leads I, II, and III.

bipolar mood disorder A disorder in which a person alternates between mania and depression.

blind panic A fear reaction in which a person's judgment seems to disappear entirely; it is particularly dangerous because it may cause mass panic among others.

blinding The method of not giving the specifics of a project to the people participating in a research or study.

bloodborne pathogens Pathogenic microorganisms that are present in human blood and can cause disease in humans; include, but are not limited to, hepatitis B virus, human immunodeficiency virus, hepatitis C virus, and syphilis.

blood-brain barrier A layer of tightly-adhered cells that protects the brain and spinal cord from exposure to medications, toxins, and infectious particles.

blood pressure (BP) The measurement of the force exerted against the walls of the blood vessels as the heart contracts and relaxes; it is calculated as the product of cardiac output and peripheral vascular resistance.

blood tubing A special type of macrodrip administration set designed to facilitate rapid fluid replacement by manual infusion of multiple IV bags or IV–blood replacement combinations.

Boerhaave syndrome Forceful vomiting that results in a tear in the esophagus that extends entirely through the esophageal wall, creating a hole.

bolus A term used to describe "in one mass"; in medication administration, a single dose given by the intravenous or intraosseous route; may be a small or large quantity of the drug.

bonding The formation of a close, personal relationship.

Bone Injection Gun (BIG) A spring-loaded device that is used for inserting an intraosseous needle into the proximal tibia in adult and pediatric patients.

bone marrow Soft tissue that fills the inside of bones and is the site of production of red blood cells, platelets, and most white blood cells.

bony labyrinth The collection of hollows in the bone of the inner ear that provide protection to the structures of the inner ear from damage and from extraneous stimulation.

borborygmi A bowel sound characterized by increased activity within the bowel; also called hyperperistalsis.

borderline personality disorder A disorder characterized by disordered images of self, impulsive and unpredictable behavior, marked shifts in mood, and instability in relationships with others.

borrowed servant doctrine A principle which absolves an institution of liability when one of its members acts beyond his or her scope of certification or training by following someone else's orders.

botulism Poisoning characterized by severe muscle paralysis and usually caused by eating food containing botulinum toxin.

Bourdon-gauge flowmeter An oxygen flowmeter that is commonly used because it is not affected by gravity and can be placed in any position.

Boyle's law A gas law that demonstrates that as pressure increases, volume decreases; at a constant temperature, the volume of a gas is inversely proportional to its pressure (if the pressure on a gas is doubled, then its volume is halved); written as $PV = K$, where P = pressure, V = volume, and K = a constant.

bradykinesia The slowing down of voluntary body movements; found in patients with Parkinson disease.

bradypnea A slow respiratory rate.

brain The part of the central nervous system located within the cranium; contains billions of neurons that serve a variety of functions including consciousness, perception, control of reactions to the environment, emotional responses, and judgment.

brainstem The area of the brain between the spinal cord and cerebrum that contains the midbrain, pons, and medulla; controls functions that are necessary for life, such as breathing.

bronchial sounds Hollow, tubular, lower-pitched sounds heard over the trachea.

bronchoconstriction Narrowing of the bronchial tubes.

bronchodilation Widening of the bronchial tubes.

bronchophony A test of decreased breath sounds performed by placing the diaphragm of the stethoscope over the area in question while the patient says "ninety-nine;" a loud, clear sound indicates lung consolidation.

bronchospasm Severe constriction of smooth muscle surrounding the bronchial tree.

bronchovesicular sounds A combination of the tracheal and vesicular breath sounds; heard where airways and alveoli are found, in the upper part of the sternum and between the scapulae.

bruit An abnormal whooshing sound of turbulent blood flow moving through a narrowed artery; usually heard in the carotid arteries.

buccal Between the cheek and gums.

buffer system Fast-acting defenses for acid-base changes, providing almost immediate protection against changes in the hydrogen ion concentration of extracellular fluid.

bulimia nervosa An eating disorder characterized by consumption of large amounts of food, for which the patient often compensates by using purging techniques.

bundle branch block (BBB) An intraventricular conduction disturbance involving impedance of electrical impulses from the bundle of His to the right or left bundle branch.

bundle of His The portion of the heart's conduction system located in the upper portion of the interventricular septum that conducts electrical impulses from the atrioventricular junction to the right and left bundle branches; also called the AV bundle.

burnout The exhaustion of physical or emotional strength.

BURP maneuver The backward, upward, and rightward pressure used during intubation to improve the laryngoscopic view of the glottic opening and vocal cords; also called external laryngeal manipulation.

bursa A small, padlike sac or cavity filled with a small amount of synovial fluid that helps reduce the amount of friction between a tendon and a bone or between a tendon and a ligament, usually located near a joint.

butterfly catheter A rigid, hollow, venous cannulation device identified by its plastic "wings" that act as anchoring points for securing the catheter.

caladium A common houseplant that contains calcium oxalate crystals; ingestion leads to nausea, vomiting, and diarrhea.

calcaneus The heel bone; the largest of the tarsal bones.

calcitonin The hormone secreted by the thyroid gland that helps maintain normal calcium levels in the blood.

calorie The amount of heat needed to raise the temperature of a gram of water by 33°F (1°C); the amount of energy that can be obtained from the nutrients you eat; also called a kilocalorie.

candidiasis A vaginal infection that is not technically a sexually transmitted infection, and that can occur in a pregnant or nonpregnant female, but is more common in pregnancy; also called thrush or a yeast infection.

cannulation The insertion of a catheter, such as into a vein to allow for fluid flow.

cape cyanosis Deep cyanosis of the face and neck that extends across the chest and back; associated with little or no blood flow; a particularly ominous sign.

capillary refill time A test performed on the fingernails or toenails that involves briefly squeezing the toenail or fingernail and evaluating the time it takes for the color to return.

capnographer A device that attaches between the endotracheal tube and ventilation device; provides graphic information about the presence of exhaled carbon dioxide.

capnography The use of a noninvasive diagnostic tool that can quickly and efficiently provide information on a patient's ventilatory and circulatory status with a graphic and digital depiction similar to an electrocardiogram.

capnometer A device that performs the same function and attaches in the same way as a capnographer but provides a digital reading of the exhaled carbon dioxide.

capnometry The use of a capnometer, which is a monitoring device used to measure the amount of expired carbon dioxide. The reading is usually given as a digital reading.

carbohydrates Substances (including sugars and starches) that provide much of the energy required by the body's cells, as well as helping to build cell structures.

carbon monoxide oximeter A device that measures absorption at several wavelengths to distinguish oxyhemoglobin from carboxyhemoglobin.

carboxyhemoglobin (COHb) Hemoglobin loaded with carbon monoxide.

cardiac arrest The cessation of cardiac mechanical activity, as confirmed by the absence of signs of circulation; also called cardiopulmonary arrest.

cardiac catheterization A minimally invasive procedure performed under fluoroscopic guidance, a balloon, stent, or other device is advanced through a peripheral artery catheter and into an obstructed coronary vessel to diagnose and treat coronary artery obstruction; also known as percutaneous coronary intervention and percutaneous transluminal coronary angioplasty.

cardiac cycle The period from one cardiac contraction to the next. Each cardiac cycle consists of ventricular contraction (systole) and relaxation (diastole).

cardiac tamponade A pathologic condition characterized by restriction of cardiac contraction, falling cardiac output, and shock as a result of pericardial fluid accumulation.

cardiogenic shock A condition caused by loss of 40% or more of the functioning myocardium; the heart is no longer able to circulate sufficient blood to maintain adequate oxygen delivery.

carina A ridgelike projection of tracheal cartilage located where the trachea bifurcates into the right and left mainstem bronchi.

carpal bones The eight small bones of the wrist.

carpopedal spasm A contorted position of the hand or foot in which the fingers or toes flex in a clawlike manner; may result from hyperventilation or hypocalcemia.

carriers People who harbor an infectious agent and, although not personally ill, can transmit the infection to other people.

cartilaginous joints Those connected by hyaline cartilage, or fibrocartilage, such as the joints that separate the vertebrae.

case study A type of research in which a single case is investigated and documented over a period of time.

castor bean A seed that contains the poison ricin; causes a variety of toxic effects: burning of the mouth and throat; nausea, vomiting, diarrhea, and severe stomach pains; prostration; failing vision; and kidney failure, which is the usual cause of death.

catabolism The breakdown of larger molecules into smaller ones.

cataract A clouding of the lens of the eye or its surrounding transparent membrane, which is normally a result of aging.

catatonic Lacking expression or movement, or appearing rigid.

catecholamines Amine substances such as dopamine, epinephrine, and norepinephrine that function as neurotransmitters, hormones, or both.

catheter shear Occurs when a needle is reinserted into the catheter, and it slices through the catheter, creating a free-floating segment.

caustics Chemicals that are acids or alkalis; cause direct chemical injury to the tissues they contact.

cell-mediated immunity The immune process by which T-cell lymphocytes recognize antigens and then secrete cytokines (specifically lymphokines) that attract other cells or stimulate the production of cytotoxic cells that kill the infected cells.

cell membrane The cell wall; a selectively permeable layer of cells that surround intracellular contents and control movement of substances into and out of the cell; also called the cytoplasmic membrane or plasma membrane.

cell phones Wireless telephones that communicate via radio waves with the telephone system through an interconnected network of repeater stations called cells.

cellular respiration A biochemical process resulting in the production of energy in the form of adenosine triphosphate.

Celsius scale A scale for measuring temperature where water freezes at 0° and boils at 100°.

central nervous system (CNS) The brain and spinal cord.

central shock A type of shock caused by central pump failure, including cardiogenic shock and obstructive shock (Weil-Shubin classification).

cerebellum Area of the brain involved in fine and gross muscle coordination; responsible for interpretation of actual movement and correction of any movements that interfere with coordination and the body's position.

cerebral cortex The largest portion of the cerebrum; outer covering of gray matter that covers the cerebral hemispheres; regulates voluntary skeletal movement and plays an important role in one's level of awareness.

cerebral perfusion pressure (CPP) The pressure inside the cerebral arteries and an indicator of brain perfusion; calculated by subtracting intracranial pressure from mean arterial pressure.

cerebrospinal fluid (CSF) Fluid produced in the ventricles of the brain that flows in the subarachnoid space and bathes the meninges.

cerebrospinal rhinorrhea Cerebrospinal fluid drainage from the nose.

cerebrum The largest part of the brain, responsible for higher functions, such as reasoning; made up of several lobes that control movement, hearing, balance, speech, visual perception, emotions, and personality; divided into right and left hemispheres; also called gray matter.

certification A process in which a person, an institution, or a program is evaluated and recognized as meeting certain predetermined standards to provide safe and ethical care.

cerumen Ear wax.

cervical canal The interior of the cervix.

cervix The narrowest portion (lower third of the neck) of the uterus that opens into the vagina.

chalazion A small, swollen bump or pustule on the external eyelid, which arises when the eyelid's oil glands or ducts become blocked.

chancre The primary hard lesion or ulcer of syphilis that occurs at the entry site of the infection.

chancroid A highly contagious sexually transmitted disease caused by the bacteria *Haemophilus ducreyi*, which causes painful sores (ulcers), usually of the genitals.

CHARTE method A narrative writing method that allows the narrative to be broken down into logical sections similar to the steps of the patient assessment; components include chief complaint, history, assessment, treatment, transport, and exceptions.

chelating agents Medications that bind with heavy metals in the body and create a compound that can be eliminated; used in cases of ingestion or poisoning.

chemical mediators Chemicals that work to cause the immune or allergic response; for example, histamine.

chemical restraint The use of medication to subdue a patient.

chemical suicide A method of suicide that involves mixing certain household chemicals in an enclosed space to create toxic gases, such as hydrogen sulfide and hydrogen cyanide, as the chemicals combine; also called detergent suicide.

chemoreceptors Sense organs that monitor the levels of oxygen and carbon dioxide and the pH of cerebrospinal fluid and blood and provide feedback to the respiratory centers to modify the rate and depth of breathing based on the body's needs at any given time.

chemotaxins Components of the activated complement system that attract leukocytes from the circulation to help fight infections.

chemotaxis The movement of additional white blood cells to an area of inflammation in response to the release of chemical mediators, such as neutrophils, injured tissue, and monocytes.

Cheyne-Stokes respirations A gradually increasing rate and depth of respirations followed by a gradual decrease with intermittent periods of apnea; associated with brainstem insult.

chief complaint The reason the patient is seeking help.

chikungunya A virus that originated in Africa and is transmitted by the *Aedes aegypti* mosquito; signs and symptoms include fever that typically lasts from 5 to 7 days, and possibly incapacitating joint pain.

chlamydia A sexually transmitted disease caused by the bacterium *Chlamydia trachomatis*; has the highest incidence in sexually transmitted diseases; signs and symptoms include inflammation of the urethra, epididymis, cervix, and fallopian tubes, and discharge from the urethra.

cholangitis Inflammation of the bile duct.

cholecystitis Inflammation of the gallbladder.

cholelithiasis The presence of stones within the gallbladder.

cholinergic Having the characteristics of the parasympathetic division of the autonomic nervous system; also refers to other structures or functions that are related to acetylcholine.

chordae tendineae Thin bands of fibrous tissue that attach to the atrioventricular valves in the heart and prevent them from inverting.

choroid The vascular, pigmented middle layer of the eye wall.

choroid plexus Group of specialized cells in the ventricles of the brain; filters blood through cerebral capillaries to create cerebrospinal fluid.

chromosomes Structures formed from condensed fibers and protein of deoxyribonucleic acid; they are threadlike, and are contained within the nucleus of the cells.

chronic bronchitis A chronic inflammatory condition affecting the bronchi that is characterized by excessive mucus production as a result of overgrowth of the mucous glands in the airways.

chronic kidney disease (CKD) Progressive and irreversible inadequate kidney function caused by the permanent loss of nephrons.

chronotropic effect Related to the effect of the rate of contraction of the heart.

ciliary body The structure associated with the choroid layer of the eye that secretes aqueous humor and contains the ciliary muscle.

circulatory system The complex arrangement of connected tubes, including the arteries, arterioles, capillaries, venules, and veins, that moves blood, oxygen, nutrients, carbon dioxide, and cellular waste throughout the body.

circumflex artery (Cx) One of the two branches of the left main coronary artery; branches of the Cx supply the left atrium, part of the lateral surface of the left ventricle, the inferior surface of the left ventricle in about 15% of people, the posterior surface of the left ventricle in 15%, the sinoatrial node in about 40%, and the atrioventricular bundle in 10% to 15%.

circumflex coronary artery One of two branches of the left main coronary artery.

circumstantial thinking Situation in which the patient includes many irrelevant details in his or her account of things.

cirrhosis Early failure of the liver; characterized by portal hypertension, coagulation deficiencies, and diminished detoxification.

citric acid cycle A sequence of enzymatic reactions involving the metabolism of carbon chains of glucose, fatty acids, and amino acids to yield carbon dioxide, water, and high-energy phosphate bonds; also known as the Krebs cycle or tricarboxylic acid cycle.

civil lawsuit An action instituted by a person or entity against another person or entity.

class The grouping to which a medication belongs. Medications are grouped according to their characteristics, traits, or primary components.

claudication Pain, cramping, muscle tightness, fatigue, or weakness of the legs during physical activity as a result of increased oxygen demand by the muscle tissue of the legs, hips, and buttocks.

clear text Using regular language (plain English) and accepted terms to enhance clarity of communication, rather than using ten-codes or other code systems.

clitoris A small, cylindrical mass of erectile tissue and nerves located at the anterior junction of the labia minora, similar to the glans penis of the male.

clonic activity Type of seizure movement involving the contraction and relaxation of muscle groups.

closed-ended question A question that is specific and focused, requiring either a yes or no answer, or an answer chosen from specific options.

clotting cascade A set of interactions that lead to the formation of a fibrin clot; also called the coagulation cascade.

clotting factors Substances in the blood that are necessary for clotting; also called coagulation factors.

coagulation system The system that forms blood clots in the body and facilitates repairs to the vascular tree.

coagulopathy Any type of bleeding disorder that interferes with the activation or continuation of the clotting cascade or hemostasis.

Cobra perilaryngeal airway (CobraPLA) A supraglottic airway device with a shape that allows the device to slide easily along the hard palate and to hold the soft tissue away from the laryngeal inlet.

cocaine A stimulant; a naturally occurring alkaloid that is extracted from the *Erythroxylon coca* plant leaves found in South America.

cochlea The portion of the inner ear that has hearing receptors.

cohort research A type of research that examines patterns of change, a sequence of events, or trends over time within a certain population of study subjects.

collagen vascular diseases A group of autoimmune disorders that affect the collagen in tendons, bones, and connective tissues.

colloid solutions Solutions that contain molecules (usually proteins) that are too large to pass out of the capillary membranes and, therefore, remain in the vascular compartment.

colonized A pathogen is present but has produced no illness in the host; often progresses to active infection; a colonized host is often called a *carrier* because he or she can transmit the pathogen to others.

colorimetric carbon dioxide detector A device that attaches between the endotracheal tube and ventilation device; uses special paper that should turn from purple to yellow during exhalation, indicating the presence of exhaled carbon dioxide.

coma A state in which a person does not respond to either verbal or painful stimuli.

combining form A word root followed by a vowel.

combining vowel The vowel used to combine two word roots or a word root and a prefix or suffix.

Combitube A multilumen airway device that consists of a single tube with two lumens, two balloons, and two ventilation ports; an alternative device if endotracheal intubation is not possible or has failed.

Commission on Accreditation for Pre-Hospital Continuing Education (CAPCE) An organization that develops continuing education standards and is involved in setting accreditation standards for prehospital providers; formerly called the Continuing Education Coordinating Board for Emergency Medical Service (CECBEMS).

common law A decision that has been made by a judge through a court case based on his or her interpretation of the statutes and constitutions; can be overturned either by another court with a higher authority or the issuing court at a later time; also called case law.

common reality Sensory stimulation that can be verified by others.

communicable disease An infectious disease that can be transmitted from one person to another by direct contact or by indirect contact through a vector or fomite; also called contagious disease.

communicable period The period during which an infected person can transmit a communicable disease to someone else.

comorbidity The existence of two or more chronic diseases or conditions in a patient.

competitive antagonists Medications that temporarily bind with cellular receptor sites, displacing agonist chemicals.

competitive depolarizing A term used to describe paralytic agents that act at the neuromuscular junction by binding with nicotinic receptors on muscles, causing fasciculations and preventing additional activation by acetylcholine.

complement system A group of plasma proteins whose function is to do one of three things: attract leukocytes to sites of inflammation, activate leukocytes, and directly destroy cells.

compound A substance that can be broken down into the two or more elements contained within it.

compound word A word containing more than one word root.

compulsions Repetitive actions carried out to relieve the anxiety of obsessive thoughts.

computer assisted dispatch (CAD) Linked dispatch center computer consoles and vehicle-mounted mobile data terminals

concentration The total weight of a drug contained in a specific volume of liquid.

concept formation Pattern of understanding based on initially obtained information; the first stage of the critical thinking process in prehospital care.

concordant precordial pattern An ECG pattern in which the QRS complexes are all in the same direction in the precordial leads as a result of improper lead placement, anterior wall MI, VT, or other variables.

conductivity The property that allows a cardiac cell to receive an electrical impulse and pass it on to an adjoining cardiac cell.

cones One of two photoreceptors of the retina that can distinguish colors, but requires a greater amount of light to activate and create an image.

confabulation The invention of experiences to cover gaps in memory, seen in patients with certain organic brain syndromes.

confrontation Act of pointing out something of interest in the patient's conversation or behavior, thereby directing the patient's attention to something of which he or she may have been unaware.

conjunctiva The membranous covering on the anterior surface of the eye that also lines the eyelids.

conjunctivitis An inflammation of the conjunctivae that usually is caused by bacteria, viruses, allergies, or foreign bodies; should be considered highly contagious if infectious in origin; also called pinkeye.

connective tissues Tissues that bind, support, protect, frame, and fill body structures; they also store fat, produce blood cells, repair tissues, and protect against infection.

consent Agreement by the patient to accept a medical intervention.

contact precautions The use of precautions (gloves, gown, good handwashing, and cleaning of high-touch items) to prevent contact transmission; used for patients presenting with draining wounds, multidrug resistant infection, lice, norovirus, and Ebola.

contact transmission The transmission of an infectious agent by means of direct or indirect contact with the infected persons, such as skin-to-skin contact or contact with the patient's environment and/or equipment.

contaminated The presence of blood or other potentially infectious materials on an item or surface.

contaminated stick The puncturing of an emergency care provider's skin with a needle or catheter that was used on a patient.

contiguous leads Leads that view geographically similar areas of the myocardium, such as leads II, III, and aVF; useful for localizing areas of ischemia.

continuous positive airway pressure (CPAP) A method of ventilation that delivers a single pressure, used primarily in the treatment of critically ill patients with respiratory distress; can prevent the need for endotracheal intubation.

continuous quality improvement (CQI) A system of internal and external reviews and audits of all aspects of an EMS system.

contractility The ability of myocardial cells to shorten in response to an impulse, which results in contraction.

contraindication Any condition, especially any condition of disease, that renders some particular line of treatment improper or undesirable.

contralateral On the opposite side of the body.

contributory negligence Act(s) committed by plaintiff that contributes to adverse outcomes.

convenience sampling A type of research in which subjects are manually assigned to a specific person or crew, rather than being randomly assigned; the least-preferred component of research.

conventional reasoning A type of reasoning in which a child looks for approval from peers and society.

conversion hysteria A reaction in which a person subconsciously transforms his or her anxiety into a bodily dysfunction; the person may be unable to see or hear or may become partially paralyzed.

cookbook medicine Blindly following a protocol or algorithm without thinking about what is being done and whether or not it is working.

cor pulmonale Heart disease that develops because of chronic lung disease and affects primarily the right side of the heart.

Cormack-Lehane classification A system used to predict intubation difficulty based on the airway structures observed during laryngoscopy.

cornea The transparent anterior portion of the eye that overlies the iris and pupil.

corneal reflex A protective movement that results in blinking, moving the head posteriorly, and pupillary constriction.

coronal plane An imaginary plane in which the body is cut into front and back portions.

coronary arteries The blood vessels that supply blood to the tissues of the heart.

coronary artery disease (CAD) Pathologic process characterized by progressive atherosclerotic narrowing and eventual obstruction of the coronary arteries.

coronary heart disease (CHD) Disease of the coronary arteries and its associated signs, symptoms, and complications, such as angina pectoris and acute myocardial infarction.

coronary sinus Venous drain for the coronary circulation into the right atrium.

corpus callosum A deep bridge of nerve fibers connecting the brain hemispheres.

corticosteroids Hormones secreted by the adrenal gland, that regulate the body's metabolism, the balance of salt and water in the body, the immune system, and sexual function.

cortisol Hormone that stimulates most body cells to increase their energy production; produced by the middle adrenal cortex, and influences protein and fat metabolism; a glucocorticoid that stimulates glucose to be synthesized from noncarbohydrates.

couplet Two consecutive (paired) premature ventricular complexes.

covert behavior Behavior that has a hidden meaning or intention that only the person understands.

crackles The breath sounds produced as fluid-filled alveoli pop open under increasing inspiratory pressure; can be fine or coarse; formerly called *rales*.

cranial nerves The 12 pairs of nerves that arise from the base of the brain.

cranial vault The bones that encase and protect the brain, including the parietal, temporal, frontal, occipital, sphenoid, and ethmoid bones; the roof of the skull (cranium).

cranium The area of the head above the ears and eyes; the part of the skull that houses the brain.

crepitus A grating, grinding, or crackling sensation made when two pieces of broken bone rub together or subcutaneous emphysema is palpated.

crew resource management (CRM) An operational practice designed to enhance communication and teamwork, and to thereby reduce preventable errors.

cribriform plate A horizontal bone perforated with numerous openings for the passage of the olfactory nerve filaments from the nasal cavity.

cricoid cartilage A firm ridge of cartilage that forms the lower part of the larynx; the first ring of the trachea and the only upper airway structure that forms a complete ring; also called the cricoid ring.

cricothyroid membrane A thin sheet of fascia located between the thyroid and cricoid cartilage that is relatively avascular and contains few nerves; the site for emergency access to the airway.

criminal prosecution An action instituted by the government against a person for violation of criminal law.

critical incident An event that overwhelms the ability to cope with the experience, either at the scene or later.

critical incident stress management (CISM) A process which utilizes trained counselors who confront responses to critical incidents and help to defuse them, directing emergency services personnel toward physical and emotional equilibrium.

Crohn disease Inflammation of the ileum and possibly other portions of the gastrointestinal tract, in which the immune system attacks portions of the intestinal walls, causing them to become scarred, narrowed, stiff, and weakened.

cross section The product of slicing an object crosswise, perpendicular to its long axis.

cross-sectional design A data collection method in which all data at one point in time is collected, essentially serving as a "snapshot" of events and information.

cross-tolerance A process in which repeated exposure to a medication within a particular class causes a tolerance that may be "transferred" to other medications in the same class.

croup A common disease of infancy and childhood caused by upper airway obstruction and characterized by stridor, hoarseness, and a barking cough.

crystalloid solutions Solutions of dissolved crystals (for example, salts or sugars) in water; contain compounds that quickly dissociate in solution.

cultural competence An understanding of the predominant cultures that exist in the geographic area in which the paramedic provides patient care.

culture The system of beliefs, attitudes, and behaviors that are learned and shared by members of a group.

cumulative action Several smaller doses of a particular medication capable of producing the same clinical effects as a single larger dose of that same medication.

cumulative stress reaction Prolonged or excessive stress.

current health status A composite picture of a number of factors in a patient's life, such as dietary habits, current medications, allergies, exercise, alcohol or tobacco use, recreational drug use, sleep patterns and disorders, and immunizations.

curved laryngoscope blade A blade designed to fit into the vallecula, indirectly lifting the epiglottis and exposing the vocal cords; also called the Macintosh blade.

Cushing reflex The combination of a slowing pulse, rising blood pressure, and an erratic respiratory pattern; a grave sign for patients with head trauma or cerebrovascular accident.

Cushing syndrome A condition caused by an excess of cortisol production by the adrenal glands or by excessive use of cortisol or other similar corticosteroid (glucocorticoid) hormones.

cyanosis A blue-gray skin color that is caused by inadequate levels of oxygen in the blood.

cystitis Infection caused by bacteria that travel from the perineum, through the genital tract, into the urethral opening; also called bladder infection.

cytochrome P-450 system A hemoprotein involved in the detoxification of many drugs.

cytokines The products of cells that affect the function of other cells.

cytoplasm The gel-like material that fills out a cell; it makes up most of the volume of the cell, and suspends the organelles of the cell.

D_5W An intravenous solution made up of 5% dextrose in water.

damages Compensation for injury awarded by a court.

data interpretation The process of reaching conclusions based on comparing the patient's presentation with information from your training, education, and past experiences; the second stage of the critical thinking process in prehospital care.

decerebrate (extensor) posturing Abnormal posture of the arms and legs, in which the arms are extended with rotation of the wrists and the toes are pointed; indicates pressure on the brainstem.

decision-making capacity The patient's ability to understand and process the information given to him or her and the proposed treatment plan.

decorticate (flexor) posturing Abnormal posture of the arms and legs, in which the arms are flexed toward the chest the toes are pointed; this finding indicates lower cerebral damage.

deep Farther inside the body and away from the skin.

deep fascia A dense layer of fibrous tissue below the subcutaneous tissue; composed of tough bands of tissue that surround muscles and other internal structures.

defamation Intentionally making a false statement, through written or verbal communication, which injures a person's good name or reputation.

defendant In a civil lawsuit, the person against whom a legal action is brought.

defense mechanisms Psychological ways to relieve stress; they are usually automatic or subconscious; they include denial, regression, projection, and displacement.

defibrillation The use of an unsynchronized direct current electric shock to terminate ventricular fibrillation or pulseless ventricular tachycardia.

dehydration Depletion of the body's systemic fluid volume.

delayed sequence intubation (DSI) A procedure in which a patient is sedated for the purpose of preoxygenation prior to the administration of a paralytic and intubation.

delayed stress reaction Reaction to stress that occurs after a stressful situation.

delirium An acute confusional state characterized by global impairment of thinking, perception, judgment, and memory.

delirium tremens (DTs) A severe withdrawal syndrome seen in people with alcoholism who are deprived of ethyl alcohol; characterized by restlessness, fever, sweating, disorientation, agitation, and seizures; can be fatal if untreated.

delta wave The slurring of the upstroke of the first part of the QRS complex that occurs in Wolff-Parkinson-White syndrome.

delusion A fixed belief that is not shared by others of a person's culture or background and that cannot be changed by reasonable argument; a false belief.

dementia The slow, progressive onset of disorientation, shortened attention span, and loss of cognitive function.

dendrites Branchlike projections of nerve cells that receive impulses or sensory information from nearby cells and conduct impulses toward the nerve cell body.

dengue A virus transmitted by the mosquitos *Aedes aegypti* and *Aedes albopictus*, found throughout the world, in which the majority of people are asymptomatic; if the severe form develops, it is characterized by hypovolemic shock, hemorrhage, and potentially death.

denial An early response to a serious medical emergency, in which the severity of the emergency is diminished or minimized; the first coping mechanism for people who believe they are going to die.

denitrogenation The process of replacing nitrogen in the lungs with oxygen to maintain a normal oxygen saturation level during intubation.

dental abscess A collection of pus that forms in the gums, facial tissue, bones, and/or neck.

dentalgia Toothache.

deoxyribonucleic acid (DNA) Specialized structure within the cell that carries genetic material for reproduction.

dependence The physical, behavioral, or emotional need for a medication or chemical to maintain "normal" physiologic function.

depolarization The process of discharging resting cardiac muscle fibers by an electric impulse that causes them to contract; the rapid movement of electrolytes across a cell membrane changes the overall charge of the cell, and is the main catalyst for muscle contraction and neural transmissions.

depolarizing neuromuscular blocker A drug that competitively binds with the acetylcholine receptor sites but is not affected as quickly by acetylcholinesterase; an example is succinylcholine chloride.

depressant A chemical or medication that decreases the performance of the central nervous system or sympathetic nervous system.

depression A mental health disorder characterized by a persistent mood of sadness, despair, and discouragement; it may be a symptom of many different mental and physical disorders, or it may be a disorder on its own.

dermatome An area of the skin supplied by a specific sensory spinal nerve.

descending aorta The portion of the aorta that extends through the thorax and abdomen into the pelvis.

descriptive A research format in which an observation of an event is made, but without attempts to alter or change it.

designated infection control officer (DICO) A person trained to ensure that proper postexposure medical treatment and counseling are provided to an exposed employee or volunteer.

desired dose The amount of a drug that the physician orders for a patient; the drug order.

despair phase The second phase of an infant's response to a situational crisis; characterized by monotonous wailing.

diabetes A group of complex metabolic disorders with many causes. These disorders include diabetes mellitus, gestational diabetes, hypoglycemia/hyperglycemia, diabetic ketoacidosis, and hyperosmolar hyperglycemic syndrome.

diabetes insipidus (DI) A relatively uncommon disorder that has some of the same characteristics as diabetes, such as polyuria and polydipsia, in which the body is unable to regulate fluid owing to a lack of antidiuretic hormone (central diabetes insipidus) or the kidneys are unable to respond appropriately (nephrogenic diabetes insipidus).

diabetes mellitus Disease characterized by the body's inability to sufficiently metabolize glucose. The condition occurs either because the pancreas does not produce enough insulin or because the cells do not respond to the effects of the insulin that is produced.

diabetic ketoacidosis (DKA) A form of acidosis in uncontrolled diabetes in which certain acids accumulate when insulin is not available.

diabetic retinopathy A condition associated with diabetes, in which the small blood vessels of the retina are affected; it can eventually lead to blindness.

diapedesis A process whereby leukocytes move through the wall of a capillary and out to the tissues where they are needed most.

diaphoresis Excessive sweating; it is often associated with shock.

diaphragm Large skeletal muscle that plays a major role in breathing and separates the chest cavity from the abdominal cavity.

diaphysis The shaft of a long bone.

diarrhea Liquid stool.

diastole Phase of the cardiac cycle in which the atria and ventricles relax between contractions and blood enters these chambers.

diastolic pressure The result of residual pressure in the circulatory system while the left ventricle is relaxing (ie, in diastole).

dieffenbachia A common houseplant that is also called dumb cane; ingestion leads to burns of the mouth and tongue and, possibly, paralysis of the vocal cords and nausea and vomiting; in severe cases, edema of the tongue and larynx, leading to airway compromise.

diencephalon Portion of the brain between the brainstem and cerebrum; contains the epithalamus, the thalamus, the hypothalamus, and the subthalamus.

differential diagnosis The process of weighing the probability of one disease versus other diseases by comparing clinical findings that could account for a patient's illness; also refers to the list of possible conditions considered based on the patient's signs and symptoms.

differentiation The process of specialization of a cell.

diffusion The process of particles moving from an area of higher concentration to an area of lower concentration along a concentration gradient until equilibrium is achieved.

digestion The mechanical and chemical breakdown of the large molecules in food into small molecules that can be absorbed in the gastrointestinal tract and converted to energy for cellular function.

digital intubation A method of intubation that involves directly palpating the glottic structures and elevating the epiglottis with the middle finger while guiding the endotracheal tube into the trachea by using the sense of touch.

digitalis preparation A drug used in the treatment of heart failure and certain atrial dysrhythmias.

digital radio The transmission of information via radio waves using native digital (computer) data or analog (voice) signals that have been converted to a digital signal and compressed.

diluent A solution (usually water or normal saline) used for diluting a medication.

diploid cells Cells that carry two of each of the 23 chromosomes—one from the father and one from the mother.

diplopia Double vision.

direct contact Exposure to or transmission of a communicable disease from one person to another by physical contact.

direct laryngoscopy Visualization of the airway with a laryngoscope.

disequilibrium syndrome A condition characterized by nausea, vomiting, headache, and confusion, which results when, as a consequence of dialysis, water initially shifts from the bloodstream into the cerebrospinal fluid, mildly increasing intracranial pressure.

disinfectants Chemicals used on nonliving objects to kill organisms; toxic to living tissues.

disorganization A condition in which a person is characterized by uncontrolled and disconnected thought, is usually incoherent or rambling in speech, and may or may not be oriented to person and place.

disorientation A condition in which a person may be confused about his or her identity, the location, and the time of day; one of the ways in which various conditions such as schizophrenia or organic brain syndrome may present.

dispatch To send to a specific destination or to send on a task.

displacement A defense mechanism characterized by the redirection of an emotion from one person to another.

dissection The process by which the intimal and medial layers of a vessel separate (dissect) after a tear occurs in an aneurysmal portion of the arterial wall. With each ventricular systole, a jet of blood is forced into the torn arterial wall, creating and propagating a false channel.

disseminated intravascular coagulation (DIC) A condition that begins with widespread activation of the clotting cascade, which depletes the clotting factors and platelets, and eventually results in uncontrolled hemorrhage.

dissociative anesthetic A medication that distorts perception of sight and sound and induces a feeling of detachment from environment and self.

distal Farther from the trunk and nearer to the free end of the extremity.

distal convoluted tubule (DCT) Connects with the kidney's collecting tubules.

distal traction Gentle downward or lateral traction on the skin.

distribution The movement and transportation of a medication throughout the bloodstream to tissues and cells and, ultimately, to its target receptor.

distributive shock The type of shock caused by widespread dilation of the resistance vessels (small arterioles), the capacitance vessels (small venules), or both.

diuresis The production of large amounts of urine by the kidney.

diuretic A chemical that increases urinary output.

diverticulitis Inflammation of pouches in the colon; these pouches form as a result of difficulty moving feces through the colon. Bacteria can become trapped in the pouches, leading to inflammation and infection.

diverticulum A weak area in the colon that begins to have small outcroppings that turn into pouches; plural is diverticula.

do not resuscitate (DNR) order A type of advance directive that describes which life-sustaining procedures should be performed in the event of a sudden deterioration in a patient's medical condition.

dorsal The posterior surface of the body, including the back of the hand.

dorsal respiratory group (DRG) A portion of the medulla oblongata that functions as an respiratory integration center; it receives input from several sources including the pontine respiratory group, sensory input through the glossopharyngeal and vagus nerves, central chemoreceptors in the medulla, and peripheral chemoreceptors.

dose-response curve A graphic illustration of the response of a drug according to the dose administered.

dosing The specified amount of a medication to be given at specific intervals.

down-regulation The process in which a mechanism reducing available cell receptors for a particular medication results in tolerance.

drip chamber The area of the administration set where fluid accumulates so that the tubing remains filled with fluid.

droplet precautions Use of a surgical mask on the patient and airflow measures to prevent droplet transmission; used for patients with possible influenza, meningitis, pertussis (whooping cough), mumps, rubella (German measles), and Ebola.

droplet transmission The transmission of an infectious agent by inhalation of relatively large particles generated when an infected person coughs or sneezes; these particles travel a short distance through the air before falling to the ground.

drug A substance that has some therapeutic effect (such as reducing inflammation, fighting bacteria, or producing euphoria) when given in the appropriate circumstances and in the appropriate dose.

drug abuse Any use of drugs that causes physical, psychological, economic, legal, or social harm to the user or others affected by the user's behavior.

drug addiction A chronic disorder characterized by the compulsive use of a substance that results in physical, psychological, or social harm to the user who continues to use the substance despite the harm.

drug reconstitution Injecting sterile water or saline from one vial into another vial containing a powdered form of the drug.

due process A right to a fair procedure for a legal action against a person or agency; has two components: Notice and Opportunity to be Heard.

DUMBELS A mnemonic that stands for diarrhea, urination, miosis/muscle weakness, bradycardia/bronchospasm/bronchorrhea, emesis, lacrimation, seizures/salivation/sweating, which are the signs and symptoms that can be produced by exposure to organophosphate and carbamate pesticides or other nerve-stimulating agents.

duplex Radio system using paired frequencies to permit the use of remote repeaters or simultaneous transmission and reception.

dura mater The outermost layer of the three meninges that enclose the brain and spinal cord; the toughest meningeal layer.

duration (of action) In a pharmacologic context, the time a medication concentration can be expected to remain above the minimum level needed to provide the intended action.

duty Legal obligation of public and certain other ambulance services to respond to a call for help in their jurisdiction.

dysconjugate gaze Paralysis of gaze or lack of coordination between the movements of the two eyes.

dysfunctional uterine bleeding Uterine bleeding that is abnormal in amount or frequency (more than every 21 days).

dyslipidemia An excessive level of lipids (fats) circulating in the blood, increasing the risk of atherosclerosis and coronary artery disease.

dysphagia Pain, discomfort, or difficulty in swallowing.

dysphonia Difficulty speaking.

dysplasia An alteration in the size, shape, and organization of cells.

dyspnea Difficult or labored breathing.

dysrhythmias Cardiac rhythm disturbances.

dystonia Contractions of body into bizarre positions.

dystonic Pertaining to voluntary muscle movements that are distorted or impaired because of abnormal muscle tone.

early adults People who are 18 to 40 years of age.

Ebola A virus formerly limited to West Africa, spread through direct contact through nonintact skin or mucous membranes, and whose initial symptoms include fever, intense weakness, muscle pain, headaches, and sore throat; both contact and droplet precautions are needed with this disease; approximately 10% of infected people experience internal or external bleeding.

ecchymosis Localized bruising or collection of blood within or under the skin.

echolalia Meaningless echoing of the interviewer's words by the patient.

ectopic An impulse or rhythm that originates from a site other than the SA node.

ectopic foci Sites of generation of electrical impulses other than normal pacemaker cells.

ectopic pregnancy A pregnancy in which the fertilized oocyte implants somewhere other than the uterus, typically in a fallopian tube.

edema Swelling caused by excessive fluid trapped in the body tissues

efficacy In a pharmacologic context, the ability of a medication to produce the desired effect.

egophony A test of decreased breath sounds performed by placing the diaphragm of the stethoscope over the area in question while the patient saying a drawn-out "ee;" an "A" sound indicates lung consolidation.

electrical conduction system In the heart, the specialized cardiac tissue that initiates and conducts electric impulses; includes the SA node, internodal conduction pathways, atrioventricular node, bundle of His, and the Purkinje network.

electrolytes Salt or acid substances that become ionic conductors when dissolved in a solvent (such as water); chemicals dissolved in the blood.

elimination In a pharmacologic context, the removal of a medication or its by-products from the body.

emancipated minor A person who is under the legal age (generally 18 years) in a given state, but is legally considered an adult because of other circumstances.

embryo A fertilized egg.

emergency medical dispatch (EMD) A program specifically designed to meet the unique needs of emergency medical services response and of callers reporting a medical emergency, including first aid instructions given by specially trained dispatchers to callers over the telephone while an ambulance is en route to the call.

emergency medical services (EMS) A health care system designed to bring immediate on-scene care to those in need along with transport to a definitive medical care facility.

Emergency Medical Treatment and Active Labor Act (EMTALA) A federal law enacted in 1986 to combat the practice of patient dumping (hospitals refusing to admit seriously ill patients or women in labor who could not pay, forcing emergency medical services providers to dump the patients at another hospital). Issues are regulated by the Centers for Medicare and Medicaid Services and the law carries severe monetary penalties—up to and including loss of Medicare funding—for hospitals and physicians that fail to comply.

emphysema The infiltration of any tissue by air or gas; a chronic obstructive pulmonary disease characterized by distention of the alveoli and destructive changes in the lung parenchyma.

employee assistance program (EAP) A counseling program to help with situations that may affect the health and well-being of emergency medical services professionals.

encoded radio signals An embedded signal that permits controlled access to the radio transmission.

endemic Consistently present or prevalent in a population or geographic area.

endocarditis Inflammation of the endocardium as a result of infection.

endocardium The thin membrane lining the inside of the heart.

endocrine glands Glands that have no ducts and secrete directly into tissue fluid or blood.

endocrine system The complex message and control system that integrates many body functions, including the release of hormones.

endogenous Originating from within the organism (body).

endolymph The fluid containing nerve receptors that resides inside the membranous labyrinth. Sound waves converted into pressure waves are transmitted through this fluid to the auditory nerves.

endometriosis The presence of tissue outside the uterus that resembles the endometrium in both structure and function.

endometritis An inflammation of the endometrium that often is associated with a bacterial infection.

endometrium The inner layer of the uterine wall.

endoscopy Insertion of a flexible fiberoptic tube into the esophagus to visualize, remove, or repair damaged or diseased tissue.

endotoxin A toxin released by some bacteria when they die.

endotracheal (ET) intubation Inserting an endotracheal tube through the glottic opening and sealing the tube with a cuff inflated against the tracheal wall.

endotracheal (ET) tube A tube that is inserted into the trachea for definitive airway maintenance; equipped with a distal cuff, proximal inflation port, a 15/22-mm adapter, and centimeter markings on the side.

end-stage renal disease (ESRD) A condition in which the kidneys are unable to function, and toxic waste materials build up in the patient's blood; occurs after acute or chronic kidney injury.

end-tidal carbon dioxide ($ETCO_2$) monitors Devices that detect the presence of carbon dioxide in exhaled air.

enema A fluid solution, possibly containing supplemental medications, that can be administered rectally to aid in a variety of gastrointestinal complications.

enhanced 9-1-1 system An emergency communications system that collects information about 9-1-1 calls from the telephone network, such as the phone number and location of the caller, and displays this information on the dispatcher's computer terminal.

enteral medications Medication administration that involves the medication passing through a portion of the gastrointestinal tract.

enteric nervous system (ENS) A subdivision of the autonomic nervous system that controls the digestive system.

Enterococcus A common, normal organism of the gastrointestinal tract, urinary tract, and genitourinary tract that can be pathogenic and become resistant to vancomycin.

enzymes Substances designed to speed up the rate of specific biochemical reactions.

eosinophil A leukocyte that may play a role following infection in various areas in the body.

epicardium The layer of the serous pericardium that lies closely against the heart; also called the visceral pericardium.

epidemic An illness or disease that affects or tends to affect a disproportionately large number of people within a specific population, community, or region at the same time.

epidemiologist Public health professional who investigates patterns and causes of disease and injury in a given population, and seeks to reduce the risk, occurrence, and negative impacts of these threats through research, public education, and legislative change.

epidemiology The study of the causes, patterns, prevalence, and control of disease in groups of people.

epididymitis An infection that causes inflammation of the epididymis along the posterior border of the testis; a possible complication of male urinary tract infection.

epigastric The region of the abdomen directly inferior to the xiphoid process and superior to the umbilicus.

epiglottis A leaf-shaped cartilaginous structure that closes over the trachea during swallowing.

epiglottitis Inflammation of the epiglottis.

epinephrine A hormone produced by the adrenal medulla that has a vital role in the function of the sympathetic division of the autonomic nervous system; mediates the fight-or-flight response; also called adrenaline.

epiphyseal plate The growth plate of a long bone; a major site of bone development during childhood; also called the physis.

epiphyses The ends of a long bone.

epistaxis Nosebleed.

epithelial tissues Body tissues that cover organs, form the inner lining of cavities, and line hollow organs.

eponym The name of a disease, device, procedure, or drug that is based on the person who invented, discovered, or first described it.

erythrocytes Red blood cells.

esophageal detector device A bulb or syringe that is attached to the proximal end of the endotracheal tube; a device used to confirm proper endotracheal tube placement.

esophagitis An inflammation of the esophagus.

esophagogastric varices Dilated blood vessels of the esophagus, commonly caused by difficulty in blood flow through the liver; the presence of these can lead to vessel rupture.

estrogen A hormone released from the ovaries that stimulates the uterine lining during the menstrual cycle; at puberty, it brings about the secondary sex characteristics.

ethical A behavior expected by a person or group following a set of rules.

ethics A set of values in society that differentiates right from wrong.

ethnocentrism Viewing other cultures based solely upon the standards and values of one's own culture; a belief in the inherent superiority of one's own cultural or ethnic group.

eustachian tube A branch of the internal auditory canal that connects the middle ear to the oropharynx.

evaluation Collection of the methods, skills, and activities necessary to determine whether a service or program is needed, likely to be used, conducted as planned, and actually helps people.

evidence-based practice The use of practices that have been proven to be effective in improving patient outcomes.

excitability The ability of cardiac muscle cells to respond to an electrical, chemical, or mechanical stimulus.

exhalation The passive part of the breathing process in which the diaphragm and the intercostal muscles relax, forcing air out of the lungs.

exocrine glands Glands that secrete chemicals into ducts that open onto a surface for elimination.

exogenous Originating outside the organism (body).

exophthalmos Protrusion of the eyes from the normal position within the socket.

exotoxin A toxin secreted by living cells to aid in the death and digestion of other cells.

expiratory reserve volume The amount of air that can be exhaled following a normal exhalation; average volume is about 1,200 mL.

expressed consent A type of informed consent that occurs when the patient does something, either through words (verbal or written) or by taking some sort of action, that demonstrates permission to provide emergency medical care.

extension The straightening of a joint.

external jugular (EJ) vein Large neck vein that is lateral to the carotid artery.

external rotation Rotating an extremity at its joint away from the midline.

extracellular fluid (ECF) Fluid outside of the cell, in which most of the body's supply of sodium is contained; accounts for 15% to 20% of body weight.

extravasation Seepage of blood and medication into the tissue surrounding the blood vessel.

extrinsic muscles Referring to the eye; six muscles that attach to the exterior of the globe and are controlled by the cranial nerves.

extubation The process of removing the endotracheal tube from an intubated patient.

EZ-IO A handheld, battery-powered driver to which a special intraosseous needle is attached; used for insertion of the intraosseous needle into the proximal tibia of children and adults.

face-to-face intubation Performing intubation at the same level as the patient's face; used when the standard position is not possible. In this position, the laryngoscope is held in the provider's right hand and the endotracheal tube in the left.

facilitated diffusion The process of medication molecules binding with carrier proteins when no energy is expended.

factitious disorder A disorder in which a person wishes to be sick and intentionally produces or feigns physical or psychological signs or symptoms. Symptoms are under voluntary control, with no obvious physiologic reason.

Fahrenheit scale A scale for measuring temperature where water freezes at 32° and boils at 212°.

fallopian tube The anatomic structure that connects each ovary with the uterus and provides a passageway for the ova.

false imprisonment Intentionally or unjustifiably detaining a person against his or her will. Some examples include transporting a patient without his or her consent, or using restraints in a wrongful manner.

fascia A sheet or band of tough fibrous connective tissue that covers, supports, and separates muscles, and which also covers arteries, veins, tendons, and ligaments.

fascicular block (hemiblock) Failure of the anterior or posterior fascicles of the heart to conduct electrical impulses because of disease or ischemia.

fasciculation Brief, uncoordinated, visible twitching of small muscle groups in the face, neck, trunk, and extremities; may be caused by the administration of a depolarizing neuromuscular blocking agent (namely, succinylcholine chloride).

feculent Smelling of feces.

Federal Communications Commission (FCC) The independent government agency that regulates interstate and international communications by radio, television, wire, satellite and cable in all 50 states, the District of Columbia, and US territories.

fibrin A white, insoluble, filamentous protein formed by the action of thrombin on fibrinogen during the blood clotting process; bonds to form the fibrous component of a blood clot.

fibrinogen A plasma protein that is important for blood clotting.

fibrinolysis The process of dissolving blood clots.

fibrinolysis cascade The breakdown of fibrin in blood clots and the prevention of the polymerization of fibrin into new clots.

fibrinolytic therapy The use of medications that act to dissolve blood clots.

fibrous joints Joints that lie between bones that closely contact each other, joined by thin, dense connective tissue.

field impression A field conclusion of the patient's problem based on the clinical presentation and the exclusion of other possible causes through considering the differential diagnoses.

fight-or-flight response A physiologic response to a profound stressor that helps a person deal with the situation at hand; features increased sympathetic tone and results in dilation of the pupils, increased heart rate, dilation of the bronchi, mobilization of glucose, shunting of blood away from the gastrointestinal tract and cerebrum, and increased blood flow to the skeletal muscles.

filtration The movement of fluid from intravascular fluid under high pressure to interstitial fluid, which is generally under lower pressure, through a semipermeable membrane.

First Access for Shock Trauma (FAST) devices Manual sternal intraosseous devices used in patients age 12 and older; include an infusion tube, subcutaneous portal, an introducer, a target/strain relief patch, and a protective dome.

first-degree AV block A delay in the conduction of the depolarizing impulse from the SA node to the ventricles, prolonging the PR interval; also called first-degree heart block.

first-order elimination The process in which the rate of elimination is directly influenced by plasma levels of a substance.

first-pass effect The alteration of a medication via metabolism within the gastrointestinal tract before it reaches systemic circulation.

fistula A surgically created connection between an artery and a vein, usually in the arm, for dialysis access; an abnormal connection between two cavities.

flash chamber The area of an IV catheter that fills with blood to help indicate when a vein is cannulated.

flat affect The absence of emotion; appearing to feel no emotion at all.

flexion The bending of a joint.

flight of ideas Accelerated thinking in which the mind skips very rapidly from one thought to the next.

fluid balance The process of maintaining homeostasis through equal intake (water taken into the body) and output (water excreted from the body) of fluids.

focused exam A type of physical exam that is typically performed on responsive patients who have sustained an isolated injury. This type of exam is based on the chief complaint and focuses on one body system or part.

fomites Inanimate objects contaminated with microorganisms that serve as a means of transmitting an illness.

fontanelles Areas where the infant's skull has not fused together; usually disappear at approximately 18 months of age; also called soft spots.

Fournier gangrene A condition that results from bacteria entering the skin of the scrotum or perineum, causing infection and subsequent necrosis of the subcutaneal tissue and muscle in the scrotum.

Fowler position A sitting position with the head elevated to a 90° angle (sitting straight upright).

foxglove A plant that contains cardiac glycosides used in making digitalis; ingestion of leaves causes nausea, vomiting, diarrhea, abdominal cramps, hyperkalemia, and a variety of dysrhythmias.

fraction of inspired oxygen (FiO_2) The percentage of oxygen in inhaled air.

free radicals A molecule that is missing one electron in its outer shell.

frequency The number of cycles (oscillations) per second of a radio signal.

full-body exam A systematic head-to-toe exam performed during the secondary assessment of a patient who has sustained a significant mechanism of injury, is unresponsive, or is in critical condition.

fungi Small organisms that can grow rapidly in the presence of the needed nutrients and organic material and can cause infection related to contact with decaying organic matter or from airborne spores in the environment such as molds; singular term, fungus.

gag reflex A normal neural reflex elicited by touching the soft palate or posterior pharynx, that helps protect the lower airway from aspiration; the responses are symmetric elevation of the palate, retraction of the tongue, and contraction of the pharyngeal muscles.

gait Patterns of walking or ambulating.

gastric distention The enlargement or expansion of the stomach, often with air; can be a complication of ventilating the esophagus instead of the trachea.

gastric tubes Tubes that are commonly inserted in patients in the prehospital setting to decompress the stomach; can also be used to administer certain enteral medications.

gastritis A preulcerative state where the stomach is inflamed, but erosions have not yet occurred.

gastroenteritis A term that comprises many types of infections and irritations of the gastrointestinal tract; symptoms include nausea and vomiting, fever, abdominal cramps, and diarrhea; also called stomach flu.

gastroesophageal reflux disease (GERD) A condition in which the sphincter between the esophagus and the stomach opens, allowing stomach acid to move superiorly; can cause a burning sensation within the chest (heartburn); also called acid reflux disease.

gauge The internal diameter of an IV catheter or needle.

general adaptation syndrome A three-stage description of the body's short- and long-term reactions to stress.

general impression The overall initial impression that determines the priority of patient care; based on the patient's surroundings, the mechanism of injury, signs and symptoms, and the chief complaint.

generalized anxiety disorder (GAD) A disorder in which a person worries about everything for no particular reason, or in which the worrying is unproductive and the person cannot decide what to do about an upcoming situation.

general senses Sensations monitored throughout the body by receptors scattered throughout many different tissues.

genital warts Warts caused by the human papillomavirus, a sexually transmitted disease; also called condylomata acuminata or venereal warts.

genotype The arrangement of a person's genes and their characteristics is based on the combination of alleles, for one gene or many.

geographic information system (GIS) Technology that uses global positioning system and other data to map the locations of objects and events.

gestational diabetes Diabetes that develops during pregnancy in women who did not have diabetes before pregnancy.

Glasgow Coma Scale (GCS) An evaluation tool used to determine level of consciousness by evaluating and assigning point values (scores) for eye opening, verbal response, and motor response, which are then totaled; effective in helping predict patient outcomes.

glaucoma A disease of the eye caused by an increase in intraocular pressure; when severe enough, this may damage the optic nerve and potentially cause permanent loss of vision.

globulins Antibodies made by the liver or lymphatic tissues that make up around 36% of the plasma proteins.

glomerular (Bowman) capsule A double-layered cup with the inner layer infiltrating and surrounding the capillaries of the glomerulus.

glottis The true vocal cords and the opening between them.

glucagon Hormone produced by the pancreas that is vital to the control of the body's metabolism and blood glucose level. Glucagon stimulates the breakdown of glycogen to glucose.

gluconeogenesis A process that stimulates both the liver and the kidneys to produce glucose from noncarbohydrate molecules.

glycogen A long polymer from which glucose is converted in the liver (animal starch).

glycogenolysis The breakdown of glycogen to glucose.

glycolysis Process by which glucose and other sugars are broken down to yield lactic acid (anaerobic glycolysis) or pyruvic acid (aerobic glycolysis). The breakdown releases energy in the form of adenosine triphosphate.

glycosuria The passage of large quantities of urine containing glucose.

goiter A visible mass in the anterior part of the neck caused by enlargement of the thyroid gland.

gonorrhea A sexually transmitted disease that results in infection caused by the gonococcal bacteria *Neisseria gonorrhea*; signs and symptoms include pus-containing discharge from the urethra and painful urination in males, and signs and symptoms of an acute abdomen in females.

Good Samaritan law A statute providing limited immunity from liability to people responding voluntarily and in good faith to the aid of an injured person outside the hospital.

gram-negative A reaction of bacteria to a Gram stain in which the bacteria do not retain the dark purple stain; this type of bacteria has cell walls that consist largely of lipids, and have pathogenic qualities that make them especially problematic for humans.

gram-positive A reaction of bacteria to a Gram stain in which the bacteria retain the dark purple stain; this type of bacteria has thick cell walls composed of many layers.

Graves disease An autoimmune disorder that causes thyroid gland hypertrophy and severe hyperthyroidism.

Greenfield filter A mesh filter placed in the inferior vena cava to catch blood clots in patients who are at high risk of pulmonary embolus.

gross negligence Negligence that is willful, wanton, intentional, or reckless; a serious departure from the accepted standards.

growth plates Structures located on either end of an infant's bone that aid in lengthening bones as the child grows.

gtt A unit of measure that indicates drops.

guarding Contraction of the abdominal muscles indicating peritoneal irritation.

Guillain-Barré syndrome A rare disease of unknown cause characterized by progressive paralysis moving from the feet to the head (ascending paralysis); if paralysis reaches the diaphragm, the patient may require respiratory support; can lead to paralysis within 2 weeks.

gum elastic bougie A flexible device that is inserted between the glottis under direct laryngoscopy; the endotracheal tube is threaded over the device, facilitating its entry into the trachea. Also called a tracheal tube introducer.

habituation A physical tolerance and psychological dependence on a drug or drugs.

Haddon matrix A framework developed by William Haddon, Jr, MD, as a method to generate ideas about injury prevention that address the host, agent, and environment and their impact in the pre-event, event, and post-event phases of the injury process.

half-life The time needed in an average person for metabolism or elimination of 50% of a substance in the plasma.

hallucination A sense perception not founded on objective reality; a false perception.

hallucinogen An agent that produces false perceptions in any one of the five senses.

hantavirus A type of virus found in wild rodents, which can also cause disease in humans, characterized by fever, headache, abdominal pain, loss of appetite, and vomiting; diseases caused are hemorrhagic fever with renal syndrome and hantavirus pulmonary syndrome.

haploid cells Cells that carry genetic instructions via 23 individual chromosomes.

hapten A substance that normally does not stimulate an immune response but can be combined with an antigen and at a later point initiate an antibody response.

hard palate The bony anterior part of the palate that is supported by bone (primarily maxillary bone) and forms the roof of the mouth.

Hashimoto disease A type of hyperthyroidism in which the thyroid gland becomes enlarged as it is infiltrated by T lymphocytes and plasma cells.

head tilt–chin lift maneuver Manual airway maneuver that involves tilting the head back while lifting up on the chin; used to open the airway of an unresponsive nontrauma patient.

health care–associated infection An infection acquired 2 days after admission to a health care setting or 30 days after discharge from one.

health care power of attorney A legal document that allows another person to make health care decisions for the patient, including withdrawal or withholding of care, when the patient is incapacitated.

health care professional A person who follows specific professional attributes that are outlined in this profession.

Health Insurance Portability and Accountability Act (HIPAA) The law enacted in 1996 that provides for criminal sanctions as well as for civil penalties for releasing a patient's protected health information in a way not authorized by the patient.

heart failure A syndrome that occurs when the heart is unable to pump powerfully enough or fast enough to empty its chambers; as a result, blood backs up into the systemic circuit, the pulmonary circuit, or both.

heave The perception that the heart is beating very strongly; felt upon palpation of the chest wall, this finding suggests hypertrophy; also called a lift.

helper T cells A type of T lymphocyte that is involved in cell-mediated and antibody-mediated immune responses. It secretes cytokines that stimulate the B cells and other T cells.

hematemesis Vomit with blood; can either look like coffee grounds, indicating the presence of partially digested blood, or contain bright-red blood, indicating active bleeding.

hematochezia The passage of stool in which bright red blood can be distinguished; caused by lower gastrointestinal bleeding.

hematocrit The proportion of red blood cells in the total blood volume.

hematologic disorder Any disorder of the blood.

hematology The study of the physiology of blood.

hematoma A mass of blood in the soft tissues beneath the skin; it indicates bleeding into soft tissues and may be the result of a minor or a severe injury; a potential complication of IV therapy..

hematopoietic system The system that includes all blood components and the organs involved in their development and production.

hematuria The presence of blood in the urine.

hemiparesis Weakness of one side of the body.

hemiplegia Paralysis of one side of the body.

hemochromatosis An inherited disease in which the body absorbs more iron than it needs and stores it in the liver, kidneys, and pancreas.

hemoglobin An iron-containing pigment found in red blood cells that carries oxygen to the cells from the lungs and carbon dioxide away from the cells to the lungs.

hemolysis The destruction of red blood cells by disruption of the cell membrane.

hemolytic anemia A disease characterized by increased destruction of the red blood cells. It can occur from an Rh factor reaction (primarily in Rh-positive neonates born to sensitized Rh-negative mothers), exposure to chemicals, or a disorder of the immune system.

hemolytic crisis A condition in which red blood cells break down quickly; it may occur as a result of sickle cell disease.

hemolytic disorder A disorder relating to the breakdown of red blood cells.

hemophilia A bleeding disorder that is primarily hereditary, in which clotting does not occur or occurs insufficiently.

hemoptysis Coughing up blood in the sputum.

hemorrhagic stroke One of the two main types of stroke; occurs as a result of bleeding inside the brain.

hemostasis The body's natural blood-clotting mechanism; involves the steps of blood vessel spasm, platelet plug formation, and blood clotting.

hemostatic disorder A bleeding and clotting abnormality.

Henry's law A law of gas that states that the amount of a gas in a solution varies directly with the partial pressure of a gas over a solution.

hepatic encephalopathy Impairment of brain function resulting from failure of the liver.

hepatic portal system A specialized part of the venous system that carries blood from the digestive tract to the liver and then to the inferior vena cava.

hepatitis Inflammation of the liver, usually caused by a virus, that causes fever, loss of appetite, jaundice, fatigue, and altered liver function.

hepatojugular reflux Engorgement of the jugular veins when the liver is gently pressed; this finding is specific to right-sided heart failure.

Hering-Breuer reflex A protective mechanism that terminates inhalation, thus preventing overexpansion of the lungs.

hernia The protrusion of a loop of an organ or tissue through an abnormal body opening.

hertz (Hz) Unit of measure of a frequency equal to 1 cycle per second; 1 million Hz equals one megahertz and 1,000 megahertz equals one gigahertz.

hiatal hernia A protrusion of a portion of the stomach through the diaphragm.

histamine A chemical found in mast cells that, when released, causes vasodilation, capillary leaking, and bronchiole constriction; found in large amounts in basophils; increases tissue inflammation.

history of the present illness A narrative detail of the symptoms that a patient is experiencing, usually obtained using the OPQRST mnemonic.

homeostasis A tendency to constancy or stability in the body's internal environment; processes that balance the supply and demand of the body's needs.

homologous chromosome A chromosome of the same numbered pair from the opposite parent.

homonyms Words that sound alike but are spelled differently and have different meanings.

hordeolum A red tender lump in the eyelid or at the lid margin; commonly known as a stye.

horizontal axis The axis that runs perpendicular to the sagittal plane; also called the mediolateral axis.

hormone A substance that is produced in one tissue or organ and is released into the blood and carried to other (target) organs, where it acts to produce a specific response.

host resistance One's ability to fight off infection.

hostile environment Situation in which an employer or an employer's agent either creates or allows to continue an offensive practice related to sex that makes it uncomfortable or impossible for an employee to continue working.

human immunodeficiency virus (HIV) The virus that may lead to acquired immunodeficiency syndrome; cells in the immune system are killed or damaged so that the body is unable to fight infections and certain cancers.

human papilloma virus (HPV) The most common sexually transmitted disease that can cause genital warts and some types of cancer.

humoral immunity A type of immunity in which B-cell lymphocytes produce antibodies called immunoglobulins which recognize a specific antigen and then react with it.

hydrocarbons Compounds made up principally of hydrogen and carbon atoms mostly obtained from the distillation of petroleum.

hydrophilic Attracted to water molecules.

hydrostatic pressure The pressure of water against the walls of its container.

hymen A membrane that protects the vaginal orifice before first intercourse.

hyoid bone A bone at the base of the tongue that supports the tongue and its muscles.

hypercalcemia An elevated blood calcium level.

hypercapnia Increased carbon dioxide levels in arterial blood.

hypercholesterolemia An elevated blood cholesterol level.

hyperextension Extension of a limb or other body part beyond its usual range of motion.

hyperflexion Maximum flexion or flexion beyond the normal range of motion.

hyperglycemia Abnormally high blood glucose level.

hyperkalemia An abnormally elevated level of potassium in the blood.

hypermagnesemia An increased serum magnesium level.

hypernatremia A serum sodium level greater than or equal to 143 mEq/L.

hyperopia Farsighted; the ability to see distant objects with difficulty focusing on objects close.

hyperosmolar hyperglycemic syndrome (HHS) A metabolic derangement that occurs principally in patients with type 2 diabetes; it is characterized by hyperglycemia, hyperosmolarity, and an absence of significant ketosis. Also known as hyperosmolar nonketotic coma (HONK).

hyperosmolar nonketotic coma (HONK) *See* hyperosmolar hyperglycemic syndrome (HHS).

hyperoxia An excess of oxygen.

hyperperistalsis Increased activity within the bowel; also called borborygmi.

hyperphosphatemia An abnormally elevated level of phosphate in the blood; often associated with decreased calcium. Normal levels are between 0.81 and 1.45 mmol/L.

hyperplasia An increase in the actual number of cells in an organ or tissue, usually resulting in an increase in the size of the organ or tissue.

hypersensitivity A generic term for responses of the body to a substance to which a patient has increased sensitivity; occurs when a patient reacts with exaggerated or inappropriate allergic symptoms after coming into contact with a substance the body perceives as harmful.

hypertension High blood pressure, usually a diastolic pressure of greater than 90 mm Hg.

hypertensive emergency An acute elevation of blood pressure with evidence of end-organ damage.

hypertensive encephalopathy A condition that may complicate any form of hypertension, and which is usually signaled by a sudden, marked rise in blood pressure to levels exceeding 200/130 mm Hg; also known as acute hypertensive crisis.

hypertonic Concentration of solute is higher compared with another solution.

hypertonic solution A solution that has a greater concentration of sodium than does the cell; the increased osmotic pressure can draw out water from the cell and cause it to collapse.

hypertrophic cardiomyopathy A condition in which the heart muscle wall is unusually thick, requiring the heart to pump harder to eject blood from the left ventricle.

hypertrophy An increase in the size of the cells due to synthesis of more subcellular components, leading to an increase in tissue and organ size.

hyperventilation A condition in which an increased amount of air enters the alveoli; carbon dioxide elimination exceeds carbon dioxide production.

hypocalcemia A low concentration of calcium in the blood.

hypocapnia Decreased carbon dioxide content in arterial blood.

hypoglycemia Abnormally low blood glucose level.

hypokalemia A low concentration of potassium in the blood.

hypomagnesemia A decreased serum magnesium level.

hyponatremia A serum sodium level that is less than or equal to 135 mEq/L.

hypoperfusion A condition that occurs when the level of tissue perfusion decreases below that needed to maintain normal cellular functions; also called shock.

hypoperistalsis Decreased activity in the bowel.

hypophosphatemia A decreased serum phosphate level.

hypothalamic-pituitary-adrenal axis A major part of the neuroendocrine system that controls reactions to stress. It is the mechanism for a set of interactions among glands, hormones, and parts of the midbrain that mediate the general adaptation syndrome.

hypothalamus An area of the diencephalon that is the primary link between the endocrine system and the nervous system; responsible for control of many body functions, including heart rate, digestion, sexual development, temperature regulation, emotion, hunger, thirst, and regulation of the sleep cycle.

hypotonic Concentration of solute is lower compared with another solution.

hypotonic solution A solution that has a lower concentration of sodium than does the cell; the increased osmotic pressure lets water flow into the cell, causing it to swell and possibly burst.

hypoventilate To move inadequate volumes of air into the lungs.

hypoventilation A condition in which a decreased amount of air enters the alveoli; carbon dioxide production exceeds the body's ability to eliminate it by ventilation.

hypovolemic shock A condition that occurs when the circulating blood volume is inadequate to deliver adequate oxygen and nutrients to the body; also referred to as *burn shock,* the shock or hypoperfusion caused by a burn injury and the tremendous loss of fluids; capillaries leak, resulting in intravascular fluid volume oozing out of the circulation and into the interstitial spaces, and cells take in increased amounts of salt and water.

hypoxemia A decrease in arterial oxygen level.

hypoxia A dangerous condition in which the supply of oxygen to the tissues is reduced.

hypoxic drive A state in which the stimulus to breathe comes from a decrease in Pa_{O_2}, rather than from the normal stimulus, an increase in Pa_{CO_2}.

iatrogenic Related to a side effect or complication of medications or other medical treatment.

icteric Yellow coloration of the conjunctiva (the whites of the eyes) caused by the buildup of bilirubin in the blood during liver failure.

icterus Jaundice; the yellow appearance of the skin and other tissues caused by an accumulation of bile pigments.

idiopathic Of no known cause.

idiosyncratic In a pharmacologic context, abnormal susceptibility to a medication, possibly due to genetic traits or dysfunction of a metabolic enzyme, that is peculiar to an individual patient (and usually unexplained).

idioventricular Related to only the ventricles; produced by the ventricles.

i-gel A supraglottic airway device that uses a noninflatable, gel-like mask to isolate the larynx and facilitate ventilation.

illicit In relation to drugs, illegal drugs such as marijuana, cocaine, and lysergic acid diethylamide.

immune response The body's defense reaction to any substance that is recognized as foreign.

immune system The body system that includes all of the structures and processes designed to mount a defense against foreign substances and disease-causing agents.

immunity The body's ability to protect itself from acquiring a disease; in the context of law, legal protection from penalties that could normally be incurred under the law.

immunization The process of producing widespread immunity to a specific infectious disease among a targeted group by inoculating individual members of the population; can also refer to a set of vaccinations given together or on a recommended schedule.

immunodeficiency An abnormal condition in which some part of the body's immune system is inadequate, and, consequently, resistance to infectious disease is decreased.

immunogen An antigen that is capable of generating an immune response.

immunoglobulins Antibodies secreted by the B cells.

implanted vascular access devices Devices that are implanted in surgery, sutured under the skin, for the purpose of long-term medication administration, total parenteral nutrition, chemotherapy, blood product administration, and venous blood sampling; an arteriovenous fistula is an example.

implied consent Assumption on behalf of a person unable to give consent that he or she would have done so.

impulse control disorder A condition in which a person lacks the ability to resist a temptation or cannot stop acting on a drive.

in loco parentis Phrase meaning "in the place of the parent" that is used to describe situations in which a designated authority figure makes medical treatment and transport decisions for a minor child when a parent or guardian is unavailable.

inactive metabolite A medication that has undergone biotransformation and is no longer able to alter a cell process or body function; not pharmacologically active.

inappropriate affect Emotion that is out of sync with the situation (eg, wearing a smile while discussing a parent's death).

incarcerated A type of hernia in which an organ is trapped in the new location; most commonly obstructs the bowel.

incidence The number of new cases of a disease in a population.

incisional A type of hernia in which intestinal contents herniate through an incision, for example after abdominal surgery.

incubation period The period between exposure to an organism and the first symptoms of illness, during which the organism multiplies within the body and starts to produce symptoms. This period is when the disease can be transmitted to another person.

indication A circumstance that points to or shows the cause, pathology, treatment, or issue of an attack of disease; that which points out; that which serves as a guide or warning.

indirect contact Exposure or transmission of disease from one person to another by contact with a contaminated, inanimate object.

infants People who are 1 month to 1 year of age.

infarction Death (necrosis) of a localized area of tissue caused by ischemia.

infection The invasion of a host or host tissue by pathogenic organisms such as bacteria, viruses, or parasites that produces illness that may or may not have clinical manifestations.

infection control Procedures to reduce transmission of infection among patients and health care personnel.

infectious disease A disease that is caused by the growth and spread of small, harmful organisms within the body. or one that is capable of being transmitted with or without direct contact.

infectious hepatitis Another name for hepatitis A; an inflammation from a virus that causes mild fatigue, loss of appetite, fever, nausea, abdominal pain, and, eventually, jaundice, dark-colored urine, and pale, clay-colored stools.

inferential A research format that uses a hypothesis to prove one finding from another.

inferior Below or closer to the feet.

infiltration The escape of fluid into the surrounding tissue; the result of vein perforation during intravenous cannulation.

inflammatory bowel disease (IBD) Chronic inflammation of all or part of the gastrointestinal tract.

inflammatory response A reaction by tissues of the body to irritation or injury, characterized by pain, swelling, redness, and heat.

influenza The flu, a respiratory infection caused by a variety of viruses; differs from the common cold in that the flu involves a fever, headache, and extreme exhaustion.

informed consent A patient's voluntary agreement to be treated after being told about the nature of the disease, the risks and benefits of the proposed treatment, alternative treatments, or the choice of no treatment at all.

infusion pump A mechanical device that infuses a precise intravenous volume programmed by the clinician.

ingestion Eating or drinking materials for absorption through the gastrointestinal tract.

inhalation The active process of moving air into the lungs; also called inspiration; also a route of medication delivery. In allergic reactions, foreign substances enter this way through the respiratory system.

injection In allergic reactions, when the skin is pierced, and foreign material is deposited into the skin.

inotropic effect The effect on the contractility of muscle tissue, especially cardiac muscle.

insertion A moveable part of the body to which a skeletal muscle is fastened at a moveable joint; its action opposes that of an origin.

inspection Looking at the patient, either in general or at a specific area (ie, a patient's overall appearance from the doorway, versus looking specifically at the chest wall for abnormalities/deformities).

inspiratory/expiratory (I/E) ratio An expression for comparing the length of inspiration with that of expiration, normally 1:2, meaning that expiration is twice as long as inspiration (not measured in seconds).

inspiratory reserve volume The additional amount of air that can be inhaled after the normal tidal volume has been reached.

institutional review board (IRB) A group or institution that follows a set of requirements for review that were devised by the US Public Health Service.

insulin Hormone produced by the pancreas that is vital to the control of the body's metabolism and blood glucose level. Insulin causes sugar, fatty acids, and amino acids to be absorbed and metabolized by cells.

insulin resistance Condition in which the pancreas produces enough insulin but the body cannot effectively use it.

integumentary system The largest organ system in the body, consisting of the skin and accessory structures (eg, hair, nails, glands).

intention tremor A tremor that occurs when trying to accomplish a task.

intentional injuries Injuries that are purposefully inflicted by a person on himself or herself or on another person; examples include suicide or attempted suicide, homicide, rape, assault, domestic abuse, elder abuse, and child abuse.

interference One medication or chemical taken by a patient that undermines the effectiveness of another medication taken by or administered to a patient.

interferon A protein produced by cells in response to viral invasion that is released into the bloodstream or intercellular fluid to induce healthy cells to manufacture an enzyme that counters the infection.

interleukins Chemical substances that attract white blood cells to the sites of injury and bacterial invasions.

internal rotation Rotating the anterior surface of an extremity toward the midline.

internodal pathways The three atrial pathways of electrical conduction that transmit impulses from the SA node to the AV node.

interoperability Public safety communications systems which are compatible across all local, tribal, state, and federal agencies.

interstitial fluid The fluid located outside of the blood vessels in the spaces between the body's cells.

interstitial nephritis A chronic inflammation of the interstitial cells surrounding the nephrons.

interstitial space The space in between the cells.

interventions In the context of prevention, specific measures or activities designed to meet a program objective; categories include education/behavior change, enforcement/legislation, engineering/technology, and economic incentives.

intracellular fluid (ICF) Fluid within cells in which most of the body's supply of potassium is contained; accounts for 40% to 45% of body weight.

intradermal The layer of the dermis, just beneath the epidermis; a medication delivery route.

intramuscular (IM) Into a muscle; a medication delivery route.

intranasal Within the nose.

intraosseous (IO) Within the bone.

intraosseous infusion A technique of administering fluids, blood and blood products, and medications into the intraosseous space of a long bone, usually the proximal tibia.

intraosseous space The spongy cancellous bone of the epiphyses and the medullary cavity of the diaphysis, collectively.

intrapulmonary shunting Bypassing of oxygen-poor blood past nonfunctional alveoli.

intrarenal acute kidney injury (IAKI) A type of acute kidney injury characterized by damage in the kidney itself, often caused by immune-mediated diseases, prerenal acute kidney injury, toxins, heavy metals, some medications, or some organic compounds.

intravascular fluid Fluid outside cells but inside the circulatory system; the majority of it is plasma, which is the fluid component of blood.

intravenous (IV) Within a vein.

intravenous therapy Cannulation of a vein with an IV catheter to access the patient's vascular system.

intussusception An event where one part of the intestine folds into another part of the intestines leading to a blockage.

involuntary consent An oxymoron, because consent is never involuntary; often used to describe a figure of authority dictating medical care be given to someone in custody, incapacitated, or a minor.

ionic bond A chemical bond where oppositely charged ions attract each other.

ionic concentration The amount of charged particles found in a particular area.

ions Atoms that have become positively or negatively charged, either by giving up or acquiring an electron.

ipsilateral On the same side of the body.

iritis Inflammation of the iris; also called anterior uveitis.

iron-deficiency anemia The most common type of anemia, in which iron stores are low or lacking and the serum iron concentration is low.

irritable bowel syndrome (IBS) A condition in which patients have abdominal pain and changes in their bowel habits; generally the pain and accompanying changes in bowel habits must be present for at least 3 days a month for at least 3 months to be considered this disease.

ischemia Tissue anoxia caused by diminished blood flow, usually as a result of narrowing or occlusion of an artery.

ischemic stroke One of the two main types of stroke, also called an occlusive stroke; occurs when blood flow to a particular part of the brain is cut off by a blockage, such as a blood clot, within an artery.

islets of Langerhans Groups of specialized cells located in the pancreas that produce insulin, glucagon, somatostatin, and pancreatic polypeptide.

isoelectric line The baseline of the ECG; isoelectric means neither positive nor negative.

isoimmunity The formation of antibodies or T cells that are directed against antigens or another person's cells.

isotonic crystalloid solutions Intravenous solution that does not cause a fluid shift into or out of the cell; examples include normal saline and lactated Ringer solutions.

isotonic solution A solution in which there is an equal concentration of solutes and water on either side of a semipermeable membrane. In this case, water does not shift, and no change in cell shape occurs.

Jacksonian march The wavelike movement of a seizure from a point of focus to other areas of the brain.

jaundice The presence of excessive bile pigments in the bloodstream that give the skin, mucous membranes, and eyes a distinct yellow color; often associated with liver disease.

jaw-thrust maneuver A technique to open the airway by placing the fingers behind the angle of the jaw and bringing the jaw forward; used when a patient may have a cervical spine injury.

joint capsule A saclike envelope that encloses the cavity of a synovial joint.

jugular venous distention (JVD) The visible bulging of the jugular veins when a patient is in semi-Fowler or full Fowler position, due to increased volume or increased pressure within the central venous system or the thoracic cavity; indicates inadequate blood movement through the heart and/or lungs.

junctional escape rhythm A dysrhythmia arising from the atrioventricular junction with an intrinsic rate of 40 to 60 beats/min; also called junctional rhythm.

ketoacidosis An acidotic state created by the production of ketones via fat metabolism.

ketonemia Excess amounts of ketone bodies in the blood.

ketones Acidic by-products of fat metabolism.

kidneys Solid, bean-shaped organs housed in the retroperitoneal space that filter blood and excrete body wastes in the form of urine.

kidney stones Solid crystalline masses formed in the kidney, resulting from an excess of insoluble salts or uric acid crystallizing in the urine; may become trapped anywhere along the urinary tract. Also called renal calculi.

killer T cells The cells released during a type IV allergic reaction that kill antigen-bearing target cells.

kilocalorie The amount of heat needed to raise the temperature of a gram of water by 33°F (1°C); the amount of energy that can be obtained from the nutrients you eat; also known as a calorie.

King LT airway A single-lumen airway that is blindly inserted into the esophagus; when properly placed in the esophagus, one cuff seals the esophagus, and the other seals the oropharynx.

kinin system A group of polypeptides that mediate inflammatory responses by stimulating visceral smooth muscle and relaxing vascular smooth muscle to produce vasodilation.

Korotkoff sounds Sounds related to blood pressure measurement that are heard by stethoscope.

Kussmaul respirations A respiratory pattern characteristic of diabetic ketoacidosis, with marked hyperpnea and tachypnea; represents the body's attempt to compensate for the acidosis.

kyphosis Outward curve of the thoracic spine.

labia majora A pair of prominent, rounded folds of skin of the female external genitalia, covered with pubic hair, that protect the vagina.

labia minora A pair of skin folds of the female external genitalia that border the vestibule, are devoid of pubic hair, and protect the vagina.

labile Rapidly shifting among different emotional states.

labyrinthitis Irritation and swelling in the inner ear that produces a loss of balance and possibly tinnitus, dizziness, loss of hearing, nausea, and vomiting.

lacrimal glands The glands that produce fluids to keep the eye moist; also called tear glands.

lactated Ringer (LR) solution A sterile isotonic crystalloid IV solution of specified amounts of calcium chloride, potassium chloride, sodium chloride, and sodium lactate in water.

lactic acid A metabolic end product of the breakdown of glucose that accumulates when metabolism proceeds in the absence of oxygen.

lactic acidosis Anaerobic cellular respiration due to hypoperfusion of tissues and organs.

landline Communications system linked by wires, usually in reference to a conventional telephone system.

lantana A perennial flowering shrub with clusters of red berries that can lead to serious and even fatal poisoning. Also known as red sage or wild sage; ingestion causes stomach upsets, muscle weakness, shock, and, sometimes, death.

laryngeal mask airway (LMA) A device that surrounds the opening of the larynx with an inflatable silicone cuff positioned in the hypopharynx; an alternative to bag-mask ventilation.

laryngectomy A surgical procedure in which the larynx is removed.

laryngitis Swelling and inflammation of the larynx that is associated with hoarseness or loss of voice.

laryngoscope A device that is used in conjunction with a laryngoscope blade to perform direct laryngoscopy.

laryngotracheobronchitis Inflammation of the larynx, trachea, and bronchi.

larynx A complete structure formed by the epiglottis, thyroid cartilage, cricoid cartilage, arytenoid cartilage, corniculate cartilage, and cuneiform cartilage; also called the voice box.

late adults People who are 61 years of age or older.

lateral In anatomy, parts of the body that lie farther from the midline.

lead The electrical potential difference between two points. For example, lead I represents the difference in electrical potential between the right and left arm electrodes.

left anterior descending artery (LAD) One of the two branches of the left main coronary artery; branches of the LAD supply the left ventricle, interventricular septum, and part of the right ventricle.

left atrial abnormality Dilation of the left atrium that can occur in patients with valvular heart disease (particularly mitral or aortic valve stenosis), hypertensive disease, cardiomyopathy, or coronary artery disease; it can also occur in an athlete.

left ventricular failure (LVF) A condition in which the left ventricle must work harder to pump blood throughout the body; with systolic failure, the left ventricle doesn't contract normally and has trouble pumping all the blood in the chamber out to the body; with diastolic failure, the left ventricle contracts normally but it has become stiff, impeding its ability to relax and fill with blood between each contraction of the heart.

left ventricular hypertrophy (LVH) A cardiac condition in which the left ventricle becomes enlarged, most often as a result of hypertension.

legal obligation A duty that is enforceable in a court of law.

lens The transparent disc within the eye that refracts light to focus images on the retina.

lesions Localized areas of the skin that do not resemble the area surrounding it.

leukemia A cancer or malignancy of the blood-forming organs that particularly affects the white blood cells, which develop abnormally and/or excessively at the expense of normal blood cells.

leukocytes White blood cells.

leukocytosis An elevated white blood cell count, often due to inflammation.

leukopenia A reduction in the number of white blood cells.

leukotrienes Arachidonic acid metabolites that function as chemical mediators of inflammation; also known as slow-reacting substances of anaphylaxis.

liability A finding in civil cases that the majority of the evidence shows the defendant was responsible for the plaintiff's injuries.

libel A false statement in written form that defames a person's good name.

lice Tiny, wingless, parasitic insects that feed on blood; an infestation is easily spread through close personal contact; types include head, body, and pubic lice.

licensure The process whereby a state allows qualified people to perform a regulated act.

licit In relation to drugs, legalized drugs such as coffee, alcohol, and tobacco.

life expectancy The average amount of years a person can be expected to live.

lift A sensation felt upon palpation of the chest wall, in which the heart beats extremely strongly; suggests hypertrophy; also called a heave.

limb leads The ECG leads attached to the limbs; together, the standard limb leads (I, II, and III) and augmented limb leads (aVR, aVL, and aVF) form the hexaxial reference system along the frontal plane.

limbic system Structures within the cerebrum and diencephalon that influence emotions, motivation, mood, and sensations of pain and pleasure.

lipids Fats, fatlike substances (cholesterol and phospholipids), and oils that supply energy for body processes and building of certain structures.

lipolysis The metabolism (breakdown or destruction) of stored fat that has been released into the circulation.

lipophilic Attracted to fats and lipids.

literature review A form of research in which the existing literature is reviewed, and the researcher analyzes the collection of research to draw a conclusion.

lithium A common mood stabilizer used in the treatment of bipolar disorder.

living will A type of advance directive, generally requiring a precondition for withholding resuscitation when the patient is incapacitated.

local reactions Reactions that occur in a localized area, for example after being exposed to a foreign substance; also a potential complication of intravenous therapy.

long QT syndrome A condition characterized by a QT interval exceeding approximately 0.45 seconds (450 milliseconds).

longitudinal axis The axis that runs perpendicular to the transverse plane.

longitudinal design A data collection method in which information is collected at various set time intervals, and not just at one time.

longitudinal section The view of an object cut along its long axis.

loop of Henle The U-shaped portion of the renal tubule that extends from the proximal to the distal convoluted tubule; concentrates the filtrate and converts it to urine.

loosening of associations A situation in which the logical connection between one idea and the next becomes obscure, at least to the listener.

lordosis Inward curve of the lumbar spine just above the buttocks. An exaggerated form results in the condition known as swayback.

lower esophageal sphincter (LES) The sphincter between the esophagus and the stomach; controls the amount of food that moves up the esophagus; also called the cardiac sphincter.

Lown-Ganong-Levine syndrome A disorder that causes preexcitation of ventricular tissue and is characterized on ECG by a short PR interval and a normal QRS duration.

Ludwig angina A type of cellulitis that occurs on the floor of the mouth under the tongue; it is caused by bacteria from an infected tooth root (tooth abscess) or mouth injury.

lumen The hollow interior space within an artery or other hollow structure.

lung compliance The ability of the alveoli to expand when air is drawn into the lungs during negative pressure ventilation or positive pressure ventilation.

lung consolidation Firming of the lungs as a result of fluid accumulation.

luteinizing hormone (LH) Hormone that regulates the production of both eggs and sperm, as well as production of reproductive hormones.

Lyme disease A tick-borne disease that primarily affects the skin, heart, joints, and nervous system and is characterized by a round, red lesion or bull's-eye rash.

lymph A thin liquid formed from interstitial fluid that flows through the lymphatic vessels and lymph nodes and aids in immune response and debris removal.

lymph nodes Round or bean-shaped structures interspersed along the course of the lymph vessels, which filter the lymph and serve as a source of lymphocytes.

lymph vessels Unidirectional, thin-walled vessels through which lymph circulates through the body; they travel close to the major veins.

lymphatic system A network of capillaries, vessels, ducts, nodes, and organs that helps to maintain the fluid environment of the body by producing lymph and transporting it through the body.

lymphoblasts Lymphocytes that have been transformed because of stimulation by an antigen.

lymphocytes A type of white blood cell that has an important role in immunity.

lymphoid system The system primarily made up of the bone marrow, lymph nodes, and spleen, which participates in formation of lymphocytes and immune responses.

lymphokines Cytokines released by lymphocytes, including many of the interleukins, gamma interferon, tumor necrosis factor beta, and chemokines.

lymphomas Malignant diseases that arise within the lymphoid system; they include non-Hodgkin and Hodgkin lymphomas.

macrodrip sets Administration sets named for the large orifice between the piercing spike and the drip chamber; allow for rapid fluid flow into the vascular system; allow 10 or 15 gtt/mL, depending on the manufacturer.

macrophages Large cells, usually derived from monocytes, that are specialized for phagocytosis; they kill pathogens, absorb foreign materials, and slow infections and infectious agents.

macula A yellow depression in the retina where acute vision arises; also known as the macula lutea.

Magill forceps A special type of forceps that is curved, thus allowing paramedics to maneuver it in the airway.

malfeasance Unauthorized act committed outside the scope of medical practice defined by law.

Mallampati classification A system for predicting the relative difficulty of intubation based on the amount of oropharyngeal structures visible in an upright, seated patient who is fully able to open his or her mouth.

Mallory-Weiss syndrome A condition in which the junction between the esophagus and the stomach tears, causing severe bleeding and, potentially, death.

mania A mental disorder characterized by abnormally exaggerated happiness, joy, or euphoria with hyperactivity, insomnia, and grandiose ideas.

manic-depressive illness A bipolar disorder in which mood fluctuates between depression and mania. The alterations in mood are usually episodic and recurrent.

manual defibrillator A device that requires the paramedic or other trained rescuer to interpret the cardiac rhythm and determine whether defibrillation is needed (rather than the relying on a device to make that determination automatically).

margination The loss of fluid from the blood vessels into the tissue, causing the blood left in the vessels to have increased viscosity, which in turn slows the flow of blood and produces stasis.

marijuana The dried leaves and flower buds of the *Cannabis sativa* plant that are smoked to achieve a high.

mast cells Basophil cells located in connective tissues to which antibodies, formed in response to allergens, attach, bursting the cells and releasing chemical mediators in response to an antigen-antibody reaction.

measles An infectious viral disease that occurs most often in late winter and spring; begins with a fever followed by a cough, running nose, and pink eye; a rash spreads from the face and neck down the back and trunk.

mechanism of action The way in which a medication produces the intended response.

mechanism of injury (MOI) The series of events that result in traumatic injuries; the forces that act on the body to cause injury.

medial Closer to the midline.

median effective dose (ED_{50}) The weight-based dose of a medication that was effective in 50% of the humans and animals tested.

median lethal dose (LD_{50}) The weight-based dose of a medication that caused death in 50% of the animals tested.

median toxic dose (TD_{50}) The weight-based dose of a medication that demonstrated toxicity in 50% of the animals tested.

mediastinum The space between the lungs, in the center of the chest, that contains the heart, great vessels, part of the esophagus, lymphatic channels, trachea, primary bronchi, and paired vagus and phrenic nerves.

medical ambiguity Vague or unclear aspects of medicine.

medical asepsis A term applied to the practice of preventing contamination of the patient by using aseptic technique.

medical direction Direction given to an EMS system or provider by a physician.

medical necessity A standard used by Medicare to determine whether a patient's condition requires ambulance transport in a particular situation.

Medical Practice Act An act that usually defines the minimum qualifications of those who may perform various health services, defines the skills that each type of practitioner is legally permitted to use, and establishes a means of licensure or certification for different categories of health care professionals.

medical priority dispatch system (MPDS) A dispatch system using a specific format to indicate the nature of the emergency and its priority.

medication A substance used to treat an illness or condition.

medication monograph A document that gives detailed information about drugs, such as the indications and uses, dosing information, precautions, contraindications, and adverse effects.

medication noncompliance A situation in which a patient chooses not to take his or her medications as prescribed, for reasons that may include undesirable adverse effects or prohibitive cost.

medication sensitivity A mild to severe reaction after the first exposure to a medication or other substance, often with many of the same signs and symptoms as an immune-mediated reaction.

medulla oblongata Inferior part of the brainstem that is continuous inferiorly with the spinal cord; serves as a conduction pathway for ascending and descending nerve tracts; responsible for maintenance of basic life functions, such as heart rate and breathing.

meiosis A type of cell division that occurs in the production of eggs and sperm.

melanin The pigment that gives skin its color.

melena Dark, tarry, malodorous stools caused by upper gastrointestinal bleeding.

membrane attack complex Molecules that insert themselves into the bacterial membrane, leading to weakened areas in the membrane.

menarche The first menstrual cycle; the onset of menses.

Meniere disease An inner ear disorder in which endolymphatic rupture creates increased pressure in the cochlear duct, which then leads to damage to the organ of Corti and the semicircular canal; symptoms include severe vertigo, tinnitus, and sensorineuronal hearing loss.

meninges A set of three tough membranes—the dura mater, arachnoid, and pia mater—that encloses the entire brain and spinal cord.

meningitis An inflammation of the meningeal coverings of the brain and spinal cord; usually caused by a virus or bacterium; the viral type is not communicable and is less severe than the bacterial type, which can result in brain damage, hearing loss, learning disability, or death.

meningococcal meningitis A type of meningitis caused by the meningococcal bacterium, *Neisseria meningitidis*.

menopause The cessation of menstruation, which begins in a woman's late 40s or early 50s, and which marks the end of the reproductive years; also called the female climacteric.

menstruation Cyclical shedding of the endometrial lining from the uterine cavity.

mental status exam (MSE) A tool for measuring the "mental vital signs" in a patient who is disturbed. The mnemonic COASTMAP can be used to conduct this exam, assessing consciousness, orientation, activity, speech, thought, memory, affect and mood, and perception.

mesenteric ischemia An interruption of the blood supply to the mesentery.

metabolic acidosis A pathologic condition characterized by a blood pH of less than 7.35 and caused by an accumulation of acids in the body from a metabolic cause.

metabolic alkalosis A pathologic condition characterized by a blood pH of greater than 7.45 and caused by an accumulation of bases in the body from a metabolic cause.

metabolism The chemical processes that provide the cells with energy from nutrients.

metacarpals The five bones that form the palm and back of the hand.

metaplasia A reversible, cellular adaptation in which one adult cell type is replaced by another adult cell type.

metastasis The transfer of a disease from one organ or part of the body to another that is not directly connected to the original site; often used to describe a cancer that has spread to another part of the body.

metered-dose inhaler (MDI) A pressurized canister that delivers a specific dose of a medication; commonly used for beta-agonist bronchodilators.

methamphetamine A highly addictive drug in the amphetamine family.

methemoglobin (metHb) A compound formed by oxidation of the iron on hemoglobin.

metric system A decimal system based on tens for the measurement of length, weight, and volume.

microangiopathy Microscopic deterioration of vessel walls caused primarily by adherence of blood lipids to vessel walls.

microdrip sets Administration sets named for the small needlelike orifice between the piercing spike and the drip chamber; allow for carefully controlled fluid flow and are ideally suited for medication administration; allow for 60 gtt/mL.

midbrain The most superior portion of the brainstem; it works with the pons to route information from higher within the brain to the spinal cord and vice versa.

middle adults People who are 41 to 60 years of age.

Middle East respiratory syndrome (MERS) A disease originating from the Arabian peninsula, transmitted by close contact with camel urine or nasal secretions. Symptoms include fever, cough, and shortness of breath, and gastrointestinal disturbances; there is very low risk to health care providers and the general public in the United States.

midsagittal plane (midline) An imaginary vertical line drawn from the middle of the forehead through the nose and the umbilicus (navel) to the floor.

mineral An inorganic element essential for human metabolism.

minimum data set The mandatory clinical assessment standard information that must be documented on every emergency call as set by Medicare and Medicaid, and per the National Highway Traffic Safety Administration for the purpose of the national data system.

minute volume The amount of air that moves in and out of the lungs per minute minus the dead space; also called minute ventilation.

misfeasance Appropriate act performed in an improper manner, such as a medication administered at the wrong dose.

mitosis The division of chromosomes in a cell nucleus.

mitral valve The atrioventricular valve in the heart that separates the left atrium from the left ventricle.

Mix-o-Vial A single vial divided into two compartments by a rubber stopper; methylprednisolone sodium succinate (Solu-Medrol) is stored this way.

mobile intensive care units (MICUs) An early title given to an ambulance-style unit.

monoamine oxidase inhibitors (MAOIs) Psychiatric medication used primarily to treat atypical depression by increasing norepinephrine and serotonin levels in the central nervous system.

monocytes White blood cells that mature in the blood and then travel to the tissues, where they differentiate into macrophages; these function primarily as scavengers for the tissues.

monomorphic Having a common shape.

mononucleosis Infectious mononucleosis or mono (glandular fever); caused by the Epstein-Barr virus, is often called the kissing disease; also spread by coughing or sneezing.

monophonic The sound of one note during wheezing, caused by the vibration of a single bronchus.

monosaccharides The simplest carbohydrate molecule.

mons pubis A rounded pad of fatty tissue that overlies the symphysis pubis and is anterior to the urethral and vaginal openings.

mood disorder A group of disorders in which the disturbance of mood is accompanied by full or partial manic or depressive syndrome.

morality Pertaining to conscience, conduct, and character.

morbid obesity An excessively unhealthy accumulation of body fat, defined as a body mass index of greater than or equal to 40 kg/m^2.

morbidity Number of nonfatally injured or disabled people; usually expressed as a rate, meaning the number of nonfatal injuries in a certain population in a given time period divided by the size of the population.

Moro reflex An infant reflex in which, when caught off guard, the infant opens his or her arms wide, spreads the fingers, and seems to grab at things.

mortality Deaths caused by injury and disease; usually expressed as a rate, meaning the number of deaths in a certain population in a given time period divided by the size of the population.

motor nerve Nerve that carries information from the central nervous system to the muscles of the body.

motor neurons Nerve cells that transmit instructions from the central nervous system to the end organs; also known as efferent neurons.

mottling A blotchy pattern on the skin, caused by vasoconstriction or inadequate perfusion; a typical finding in states of severe protracted hypoperfusion and shock.

mucosal atomizer device (MAD) A device that attaches to the end of a syringe that is used to spray (atomize) certain medications via the intranasal route.

mucous membranes The lining of body cavities and passages that communicate directly or indirectly with the environment outside the body.

mucus The opaque, sticky secretion of the mucous membranes that lubricates the body openings.

multifocal Arising from or pertaining to many foci or locations.

multilumen airway Airway device with a single long tube that can be used for esophageal obturation or endotracheal tube ventilation, depending on where the device comes to rest following blind positioning.

multiple myeloma A disease in which the number of plasma cells in the bone marrow increases abnormally, causing tumors to form in the bones.

multiple organ dysfunction syndrome (MODS) A grave but sometimes reversible condition in an acutely ill patient characterized by the progressive dysfunction of two or more organs or organ systems not affected by the patient's initial illness or injury.

multiple sclerosis (MS) An autoimmune condition in which the body attacks the myelin that insulates the brain and spinal cord, causing scarring.

multiplex Simultaneous transmission of multiple data streams, most often voice and electrocardiogram signals.

mumps A viral infection that primarily affects the parotid glands, which are one of the three pairs of salivary glands, causing swelling in front of the ears.

murmur An abnormal *whooshing* sound heard over the heart that indicates turbulent blood flow around a cardiac valve.

Murphy eye An opening on the side of an endotracheal tube at its distal tip that permits ventilation to occur even if the tip becomes occluded by blood, mucus, or the tracheal wall.

muscle tissue Contractile tissue consisting of filaments of actin and myosin, which slide past each other, shortening cells.

musculoskeletal The bones and voluntary muscles of the body.

mutism The absence of speech.

mutual aid Assistance to other nearby agencies when local resources are overwhelmed.

myasthenia gravis A condition in which the body generates antibodies against its own acetylcholine receptors, causing muscle weakness, often in the face.

myocarditis Inflammation of the myocardium.

myocardium The middle and thickest layer of the heart; it contains the cardiac muscle fibers that cause contraction of the heart, as well as the conduction system and blood supply.

myoclonus Involuntary jerking motions of the body.

myoglobin A pigment synthesized in the muscles to give skeletal muscles their red-brown color.

myopia Nearsighted; the ability to see objects close with difficulty seeing objects far away.

myosin A contractile protein found in the thick filaments of skeletal muscle cells.

myxedema coma A rare condition that can occur in patients who have severe, untreated hypothyroidism.

narcotic The generic term for opiates and opioids, drugs that act as a central nervous system depressant and produce insensibility or stupor.

narrow band Reassignment of frequencies by the Federal Communications Commission to a 12.5 megahertz spacing, now required for all emergency medical services and public safety radio systems.

nasal cannula A device that delivers oxygen via two small prongs that fit into the patient's nostrils; with an oxygen flow rate of 1 to 6 L/min, an oxygen concentration of 24% to 44% can be delivered.

nasogastric (NG) tube A gastric tube is inserted into the stomach through the nose.

nasopharyngeal (nasal) airway A soft rubber tube about 6 inches (15 cm) long that is inserted through the nose into the posterior pharynx behind the tongue, thereby allowing passage of air from the nose to the lower airway.

nasopharynx The part of the pharynx that lies above the level of the palate.

nasotracheal intubation Insertion of an endotracheal tube into the trachea through the nose.

natural immunity A nonspecific cellular and humoral response that operates as the body's first line of defense against pathogens; also called native immunity.

nature of illness (NOI) The general type of illness a patient is apparently experiencing.

nebulizer A device for producing a fine spray or mist that is used to deliver inhaled medications.

necrosis The death of tissue, usually caused by a cessation of its blood supply.

needle cricothyrotomy Insertion of a 14- to 16-gauge over-the-needle intravenous catheter (such as an Angiocath) through the cricothyroid membrane and into the trachea.

needleless systems Devices that do not use needles for the collection of body fluids or withdrawal of body fluids after initial venous or arterial access is established, the administration of medication or fluids, or any other procedure involving the potential for occupational exposure to bloodborne pathogens by percutaneous injuries from contaminated sharps.

negative feedback The concept that once the desired effect of a process has been achieved, further action is inhibited until it is needed again; also called feedback inhibition.

negative pressure ventilation Drawing of air into the lungs; airflow from a region of higher pressure (outside the body) to a region of lower pressure (the lungs); occurs during normal (unassisted) breathing.

negligence Professional action or inaction on the part of the health care practitioner that does not meet the standard of ordinary care expected of similarly trained and prudent health care practitioners and that results in injury to the patient.

negligence per se Inexcusable violation of a statute, such as practicing paramedicine without a valid license or certification.

neologism An invented word that has meaning only to its inventor.

neoplasm A mass of tissue produced by abnormal cell growth and division that may be malignant (cancerous) or benign; a tumor.

nephrons The structural and functional units of the kidney that form urine; composed of the glomerulus, the glomerular (Bowman) capsule, the proximal convoluted tubule, the loop of Henle, and the distal convoluted tubule.

nervous system The system that controls virtually all activities of the body, both voluntary and involuntary.

nervous tissue Composed of neurons and neuroglia.

neurogenic shock A type of shock in which circulatory failure is caused by paralysis of the nerves that control the size of the blood vessels, leading to widespread dilation; seen in patients with spinal cord injuries.

neuroglia Supporting cells that provide a supporting skeleton for neural tissue, isolate and protect the cell membranes of neurons, regulate the composition of interstitial fluid, defend neural tissue from pathogens, and aid in the repair of injury.

neuromuscular junction The connection between a motor neuron and a muscle fiber.

neurons The basic nerve cells of the nervous system, containing a nucleus within a cell body and extending one or more processes; they exist in masses to form nervous tissue.

neurotic disorders A collection of psychiatric disorders without psychotic symptoms and lacking the intense psychopathology of other mood disorders; includes anxiety disorders, phobias, and panic disorder.

neurotransmitter A chemical released from one nerve that crosses the synaptic cleft to reach a receptor.

neutropenia An abnormally low number of neutrophils.

neutrophils One of the three types of granulocytes; they have multi-lobed nuclei that resemble a string of baseballs held together by a thin strand of thread; they destroy bacteria, antigen-antibody complexes, and foreign matter.

New Intraosseous (NIO) device A spring-loaded device that contains neither drill nor battery, used for inserting an intraosseous needle into the proximal tibia of an adult patient.

noise Interference in a radio signal.

noncompetitive antagonists Medications that permanently bind with receptor sites and prevent activation by agonist chemicals.

nondepolarizing A term used to describe drugs that produce muscle relaxation by interfering with impulses between the nerve ending and muscle receptor.

nondepolarizing neuromuscular blockers Drugs that bind to acetylcholine receptor sites; they do not cause depolarization of the muscle fiber; examples are vecuronium (Norcuron) and pancuronium (Pavulon); also called paralytics.

nonfeasance Failing to perform a required or expected act.

nonionic Uncharged.

nonrebreathing mask A combination mask and reservoir bag system in which oxygen fills a reservoir bag attached to the mask by a one-way valve permitting a patient to inhale from the reservoir bag but not to exhale into it; at a flow rate of 15 L/min, it can deliver 90% to 100% inspired oxygen.

non-tunneling devices Devices that have been inserted by direct venipuncture through the skin directly into a selected vein, for the purpose of long-term medication administration, total parenteral nutrition, chemotherapy, and venous blood sampling; peripheral inserted central catheters and central venous catheters are examples.

norepinephrine A naturally occurring catecholamine that functions as a neurotransmitter and adrenal hormone; it is synthesized by the adrenal medulla, the peripheral sympathetic nerves, and the central nervous system. It is also available as a drug sometimes used in the treatment of severe hypotension; produces vasoconstriction through its alpha-stimulator properties.

normal saline A solution of 0.9% sodium chloride; an isotonic crystalloid.

normal sinus rhythm The normal rhythm of the heart that has an intrinsic rate of 60 to 100 beats/min; the rhythm is regular, with minimal variation between R-R intervals, and all measurements are within normal limits.

nucleic acids Large organic molecules, or macromolecules, that carry genetic information or form structures within cells, and include deoxyribonucleic acid and ribonucleic acid.

nucleus In the context of the cell, a cellular organelle that contains the genetic information; controls the function and structure of a cell. In the context of an atom, the central portion of an atom that contains protons and neutrons.

nutrients Substances that provide nourishment for growth such as carbohydrates, lipids, proteins, vitamins, minerals, and water.

nystagmus Involuntary, rhythmic shaking of the eyes.

obesity A condition in which a person's body mass index is greater than 30 kilograms per meters squared (kg/m^2).
objective information Information that is observable and measurable, such as a patient's blood pressure.
obstructive shock The type of shock that occurs when there is a block to blood flow in the heart or great vessels, causing an insufficient blood supply to the body's tissues.
occlusion Blockage, usually of a tubular structure such as a blood vessel or IV catheter.
ocular Pertaining to the eye.
oculomotor nerve Third cranial nerve; it innervates the muscles that cause motion of the eyeballs and upper eyelid.
off-line (indirect) medical control Patient care orders in the form of protocols, policies, or standing orders that do not require direct contact with the medical control physician.
oligosaccharide A simple sugar composed of 2 to 10 monosaccharides.
oliguria Decreased urine output; urine output of less than 500 mL/day.
oncotic pressure The pressure of water to move, typically into the capillary, as the result of the presence of plasma proteins.
online (direct) medical control Patient care orders provided directly to the paramedic by the medical control physician by radio or telephone.
onset The time needed for the concentration of the medication at the target tissue to reach the minimum effective level.
oocyte Immature female sex cell produced in the ovary that may develop by meiosis into an ovum (egg).
oogenesis The process of egg cell formation, which begins at puberty.
open cricothyrotomy An emergency incision of the cricothyroid membrane with a scalpel and insertion of an endotracheal or a tracheostomy tube directly into the subglottic area of the trachea; also called surgical cricothyrotomy.
open-ended question A question that does not have a yes or no answer, and that does not give the patient specific options from which to choose.
ophthalmoscope An instrument used to examine the fundus of the eye and view the retina and aqueous fluid; consists of a concave mirror and a battery-powered light that is usually contained in the handle.
opiate Various alkaloids derived from the opium or poppy plant.
opioid A synthetic, potent narcotic analgesic not derived from opium, with sedative properties; examples are fentanyl (Sublimaze) and alfentanil (Alfenta); also called narcotics.
opportunistic infections The infections in which an organism thrives when the immune system has been compromised by illness, chemotherapeutic medications, or antirejection drugs in an organ transplant recipient. These fungi, bacteria, viruses, and parasites are normally held in check by a healthy immune system.
opsonization The process by which an antibody coats an antigen to facilitate its recognition by immune cells.
optic chiasm Location where approximately half of the nerve fibers from each eye cross over to the opposite side of the brain.
optic nerve Either of the second cranial nerves that enter the eyeball posteriorly, through the optic foramen.
oral candidiasis A condition that presents as white lesions on the tongue and inner cheeks, caused by the fungus *Candida albicans*; also called thrush.
orbit An eye socket of the skull.
orbital cellulitis An infection within the eye socket.
orchitis A complication of a male urinary tract infection in which one or both testes become infected, enlarged, and tender, causing pain and swelling in the scrotum.
ordinary negligence Negligence that is a failure to act, or a simple mistake that causes harm to a patient.
organ of Corti The organ that is the primary receptor for sound, and is made up of thousands of individual cilia, each with their own associated nerve.
organelles Structures within cells that have specialized functions.
organic brain syndrome Temporary or permanent dysfunction of the brain, caused by a disturbance in the physical or physiologic functioning of brain tissue.
organophosphates A class of chemical found in many insecticides used in agriculture and in the home.
origin A relatively immovable part of the body where a skeletal muscle is fastened at a moveable joint; its action opposes that of an insertion.
orogastric (OG) tube A gastric tube inserted into the stomach through the mouth.
oropharyngeal (oral) airway A hard plastic device that is curved so that it fits over the back of the tongue with the tip in the posterior pharynx.
oropharynx A tubular structure that extends vertically from the back of the mouth to the esophagus and trachea.
orotracheal intubation Insertion of an endotracheal tube into the trachea through the mouth.
orthopnea Severe dyspnea experienced when lying down that is relieved by a change in position, such as sitting up or standing.
orthostatic hypotension A fall in blood pressure that occurs when moving from a recumbent to a sitting or standing position.
orthostatic vital signs Multiple sets of vital signs taken from the patient in different positions. (for example, in the supine and sitting or standing positions) to determine the degree of hypovolemia; also called a tilt test.
osmolarity The ability to influence the movement of water across a semipermeable membrane.
osmosis The movement of a solvent, such as water, from an area of low solute concentration to one of high concentration through a selectively permeable membrane to equalize concentrations of a solute on both sides of the membrane.
osmotic Characterized by the movement of a solvent, such as water, across a semipermeable membrane (eg, the cell wall) from an area of lower solute concentration to one of higher concentration.
osmotic pressure The pressure exerted by the concentration of the solutes in a given space to stop the flow of solvent across a semipermeable membrane.
ossification The formation of bone by osteoblasts.
osteoblasts Cells involved in the formation of bony tissue.

osteoclasts Macrophages of the bone surface that dissolve the matrix and return minerals to the extracellular fluid.

osteocytes Mature bone cells.

osteogenesis imperfecta A congenital bone disease that results in fragile bones.

osteomyelitis Inflammation of the bone and muscle caused by infection.

other potentially infectious materials (OPIM) Cerebrospinal fluid, pericardial fluid, amniotic fluid, synovial fluid, peritoneal fluid, and any fluid containing visible blood.

otitis An infection of either the outer or middle ear cavity.

otoliths A pair of fluid-filled sacs within the inner ear that are used by the central nervous system to collect information about movement and orientation in space.

otoscope An instrument used to examine the inside of the ears; consists of a head and a handle. The head contains an electric light source and a low-power magnifying lens.

outcome (impact) objectives State the intended effect of the program on participants or on the community in such terms as the participants' increased knowledge, changed behaviors or attitudes, or decreased injury rates.

oval window The opening between the stapes and inner ear.

ovarian cyst A fluid-filled sac that forms on or within an ovary.

ovarian torsion A painful condition in which the ovary becomes twisted.

ovaries A pair of female reproductive organs that produce sex hormones and release eggs (ova) that, if fertilized, will develop into a fetus.

overdose A condition that occurs when a drug (either licit or illicit) is taken in excess; can have toxic or lethal consequences.

overhydration An increase in the body's systemic fluid volume.

overt behavior Behavior that is open and generally understood by those around the person.

over-the-needle catheter A Teflon (plastic) catheter inserted over a hollow needle.

overweight An unhealthy accumulation of body fat, defined as a body mass index of 25 to 29.9 kg/m^2.

ovulation Midcycle release of an egg (ovum) during the menstrual cycle.

oxygen humidifier A small bottle of water through which the oxygen leaving the cylinder is moisturized before it reaches the patient.

oxygenation The process of loading oxygen molecules onto hemoglobin molecules in the bloodstream.

oxyhemoglobin (Hbo_2) Hemoglobin that has oxygen molecules bound to it.

P wave The first wave of the ECG complex, representing depolarization of the atria.

palate The roof of the nasal cavity; it separates the nasal cavity from the oral cavity.

palatine tonsils One of three sets of lymphatic organs that constitute the tonsils; located in the back of the throat, on each side of the posterior opening of the oral cavity; help protect the body from bacteria and other pathogens introduced into the mouth and nose.

palliative care A type of medical care intended to provide comfort and relief from pain, for example in terminally ill patients.

pallor Paleness.

palmar The forward-facing part of the hand in the anatomic position.

palmar grasp An infant reflex that occurs when something is placed in the infant's palm; the infant grasps the object.

palpation Physical touching for the purpose of obtaining information (for example, to detect tenderness).

pancreas An organ with both endocrine and exocrine functions; it is a major source of digestive enzymes and produces the hormone insulin.

pancreatitis Inflammation of the pancreas.

pancuronium A nondepolarizing neuromuscular blocking agent; used to maintain paralysis following succinylcholine-facilitated intubation.

pandemic An illness or disease that affects a high proportion of the population over a broad or potentially worldwide geographic area.

panhypopituitarism The inadequate production or absence of the pituitary hormones, including adrenocorticotropic hormone, cortisol, thyroxine, luteinizing hormone, follicle-stimulating hormone, estrogen, testosterone, growth hormone, and antidiuretic hormone.

panic disorder A disorder characterized by sudden, usually unexpected, and overwhelming feelings of fear and dread, accompanied by a variety of other symptoms produced by a massive activation of the autonomic nervous system.

papillary muscles Muscles attached to the chordae tendineae of the atrioventricular heart valves and the ventricular muscle of the heart.

papilledema An eye condition that results from increased pressure on the optic nerve at the rear part of the eye; symptoms include headaches, nausea with possible vomiting, temporary vision loss, or narrowing vision fields.

paradoxical Opposite from expected.

paradoxical motion The inward movement of the chest during inhalation and outward movement during exhalation; the opposite of normal chest wall movement during breathing.

paralytics Drugs that paralyze skeletal muscles; used in emergency situations to facilitate intubation; also called neuromuscular blocking agents.

parameters Outlined measures that may be difficult to obtain in a research project.

paranasal sinuses The sinuses, or hollowed sections of bone in the front of the head, which are lined with mucous membrane and drain into the nasal cavity; the frontal, ethmoid, sphenoid, and maxillary sinuses.

paraphimosis A condition that results when the foreskin is retracted over the glans penis and becomes entrapped; constriction of the glans causes it to swell even further.

parasites Any living organisms in or on any other living creature; take advantage of the host by feeding off cells and tissues.

parathyroid glands Four glands that are embedded in the posterior portion of each lobe of the thyroid; they produce and secrete parathyroid hormone.

parathyroid hormone (PTH) A hormone produced and secreted by the parathyroid glands that acts as an antagonist to calcitonin, secreted when calcium blood levels are low; it maintains normal levels of calcium in the blood and normal neuromuscular function.

parenchyma The functional portions of a gland or solid organ.

parenteral route A route of medication administration that involves any route other than the gastrointestinal tract.

paresthesia An abnormal sensation such as burning, numbness, or tingling.

parietal pain Pain caused by inflammation of the parietal peritoneum that is generally described as steady, aching, and aggravated by movement.

parietal pleura The lining of the pleural cavity attached tightly to the interior of the chest cage.

Parkinson disease A neurologic condition in which the portion of the brain responsible for production of dopamine has been damaged or overused, resulting in tremors.

paroxysmal nocturnal dyspnea (PND) Severe shortness of breath occurring at night after several hours of recumbency, during which fluid pools in the lungs; the person is forced to sit up to breathe; caused by left heart failure or decompensation of chronic obstructive pulmonary disease.

partial agonist A chemical that binds to the receptor site but does not initiate as much cellular activity or change as other agonists do; lowers the efficacy of other agonist chemicals present at the cells.

partial laryngectomy Surgical removal of a portion of the larynx.

partial pressure The amount of the total pressure contributed by various gases in solution.

partial rebreathing mask A mask similar to the nonrebreathing mask but without a one-way valve between the mask and the reservoir; room air is not drawn in with inspiration; residual expired air is mixed in the mask and rebreathed.

passive interventions Something that offers automatic protection from injury or illness, often without requiring any conscious change of behavior by the person; child-resistant bottles and airbags are examples.

past medical history Information obtained during the history-taking process, such as the patient's general state of health, childhood and adult diseases, surgeries and hospitalizations, psychiatric and mental illnesses, or traumatic injuries, which may relate to the patient's current condition.

patent Open.

pathologic fracture A fracture that occurs when normal forces are applied to abnormal bone structures, such as a weakened bone.

pathophysiology The study of the physiology of altered functioning in the presence of disease.

patient autonomy The right to direct one's own medical care, and to decide how end-of-life medical care should be provided.

patient care report (PCR) A legal document used to record all patient care activities during an incident; a handwritten or electronic report that describes the nature of the patient's injuries or illness at the scene and the treatment provided; also known as the prehospital care report.

patient history Information about the patient's chief complaint, present symptoms, and previous illnesses.

peak In a pharmacologic context, the point of maximum effect of a drug.

peak expiratory flow An approximation of the extent of bronchoconstriction; used to determine whether therapy (such as with inhaled bronchodilators) is effective.

peer review The process used by medical magazines, journals, and other publications to ensure the quality and validity of an article before it is published, and which involves sending the article to subject matter experts for review of the content and research methods.

pelvic inflammatory disease (PID) An infection of the female reproductive organs.

pelvis The attachment of the lower extremities to the body, consisting of the sacrum and two pelvic bones.

penis The cylindrical male sex organ; it conveys urine and semen through the urethra.

Penrose drain A type of surgical drain often used as a constricting band.

peptic ulcer disease (PUD) A disease in which the mucous lining of the stomach and duodenum have been eroded, allowing the acid to eat into these organs.

peptide Protein molecule consisting of amino acids held together by peptide bonds.

perception Becoming aware of or understanding something using the senses.

percussion Gently striking the surface of the body, typically overlying various body cavities, to detect changes in the densities of the underlying structures.

percutaneous Through the skin or mucous membrane.

perfusion The delivery of oxygen and nutrients to the cells, organs, and tissues of the body; also involves the removal of wastes.

pericardial tamponade The impairment of diastolic filling of the right ventricle due to significant amounts of fluid in the pericardial sac surrounding the heart, leading to a decrease in the cardiac output.

pericarditis Inflammation of the pericardial sac.

pericardium A thin, double-layered membrane made up of the fibrous pericardium and serous pericardium.

perilymph Fluid within the bony labyrinth that surrounds and protects the membranous labyrinth while allowing transmission of pressure waves caused by sound.

perineum The area between the vaginal opening and the anus.

periorbital cellulitis An infection of the eyelid; also known as preseptal cellulitis or eyelid cellulitis.

peripheral nervous system (PNS) The part of the nervous system that consists of 31 pairs of spinal nerves and 12 pairs of cranial nerves that are responsible for communication between the central nervous system and the rest of the body. These may be sensory nerves, motor nerves, or connecting nerves.

peripheral neuropathy A group of conditions in which the nerves that exit the spinal cord are damaged, distorting signals to or from the brain. One type is caused by diabetes; peripheral nerves are damaged as the blood glucose level rises, resulting in lack of sensation, numbness, burning, pain, paresthesia, and muscle weakness.

peripheral shock Shock caused by peripheral circulatory abnormalities; includes hypovolemic shock and distributive shock (Weil-Shubin classification).

peripheral vein cannulation A technique in which a cannula (tube) is inserted into veins of the peripheral areas, that is, veins that can be seen and/or palpated. Examples of peripheral veins include those of the hand, arm, and lower extremity and the external jugular vein.

peristalsis The wavelike contraction of smooth muscle by which the ureters or other tubular organs propel their contents.

peritoneum A double-layered serous membrane that lines the abdominal cavity, encasing the liver, spleen, diaphragm, stomach, and transverse colon.

peritonitis Inflammation of the peritoneum, the protective membrane that lines the abdominal and pelvic cavities.

peritonsillar abscess A collection of infected material around the tonsils.

permissive A parenting style in which the parent does not impose many rules, if any, on the child; two subcategories include indifferent and indulgent.

perseveration Repeating the same idea over and over again.

personality disorder The condition in which a person behaves or thinks in a way that is dysfunctional or causes distress to other people.

pertinent negatives The absence of certain signs and symptoms normally expected of specific illnesses or conditions; these findings warrant no medical care or intervention, but demonstrate the thoroughness of the patient exam and history.

pertussis An acute communicable, infectious disease characterized by a catarrhal stage, followed by a paroxysmal cough that ends in a whooping inspiration; also called whooping cough.

pervasive developmental disorders (PDDs) A group of disorders that cause delays in many areas of childhood development, such as the development of skills to communicate and interact socially, and may include repetitive body movements and difficulty with changes in routine; includes autism and Asperger syndrome, among others.

pH The measure of acidity or alkalinity of a solution.

phagocytes The cells that engulf and consume foreign material such as microorganisms and debris.

phagocytosis The process in which one cell "eats" or engulfs a foreign substance to destroy it; a form of endocytosis.

phantom pain A sensation of pain in a part of the body that is no longer present.

pharmacodynamics The biochemical and physiologic effects and mechanism of action of a medication in the body.

pharmacokinetics The activity of medications in the body over time, such as absorption, distribution, and elimination.

pharmacology The scientific study of how various substances interact with or alter the function of living organisms.

pharyngitis Inflammation of the pharynx.

pharynx The area between the nasal cavity and the larynx and posterior to the oral cavity; the throat.

phenotype The appearance, health condition, or other characteristics associated with a particular genotype.

pheochromocytoma A tumor of the adrenal gland, usually in the medulla, that causes excessive release of the hormones epinephrine and norepinephrine.

phimosis Inability to retract the distal foreskin over the glans penis.

phobia An abnormal and persistent dread of a specific object or situation.

phobic disorders Disorders involving an unreasonable fear, apprehension, or dread of a specific situation or thing.

phospholipid A type of lipid molecule that comprises the cell membrane.

physical dependence A physiologic state of adaptation to a drug, usually characterized by tolerance to the effects of the drug and a withdrawal syndrome if use of the drug is stopped, especially abruptly.

physiology The study of the processes and functions of the living organism.

pia mater The innermost and thinnest of the three meninges that enclose the brain and spinal cord; rests directly on the brain and spinal cord.

piercing spike The hard, sharpened plastic spike on the end of the administration set designed to pierce the sterile membrane of the IV bag.

pineal gland A gland in the brain that synthesizes and secretes melatonin, a hormone that affects patterns of sleep and wakefulness.

pinna A formation of cartilage within the inner ear that protects the ear and collects sounds into the ear canal, while allowing some perception of the direction from which the sound comes; also called the auricle.

pinocytosis A form of endocytosis in which cells ingest extracellular fluid and its contents; in this process, in which the cell membrane sinks inward and ingests droplets of extracellular fluid.

pituitary gland An endocrine gland responsible for directly or indirectly affecting all body functions; also called the hypophysis.

placebo effect In a pharmacologic context, the positive and negative effects of an inactive medication on a person that are related to the person's expectations and other factors.

plaintiff In a civil lawsuit, the person who brings a legal action against another person.

plantar The sole or bottom surface of the foot.

plasma A component of blood, made of 92% water, 6% to 7% proteins, and electrolytes, clotting factors, and glucose; plasma accounts for 55% of the total blood volume; this watery, yellow fluid carries the blood cells and nutrients and transports cellular waste material to the organs of excretion.

plasma cells Cells that produce antibodies (immunoglobulins) to destroy antigens or antigen-containing particles; formed from divided and differentiated B cells.

plasma protein binding A process in which medication molecules temporarily attach to proteins in the blood plasma, significantly altering medication distribution in the body.

plasmin A naturally occurring enzyme that dissolves the fibrin fibers in blood clots; usually present in the body in its inactive form, plasminogen.

platelets Formed elements of the blood that function in blood clotting; also called thrombocytes.

pleura The serous membranes covering the lungs and lining the thoracic cavity.

pleural effusion Excessive accumulation of fluid in the pleural space.

pleural friction rubs Squeaking or grating sounds that occur when the pleural linings rub together, which may be heard on inspiration, expiration, or both; commonly caused by inflammation of the pleura.

pleural space The potential space between the parietal pleura and the visceral pleura.

plexus A cluster of nerve roots that permits peripheral nerve roots to rejoin and function as a group.

pneumonia An inflammation of the lungs caused by bacterial, viral, or fungal infections or infections with other microorganisms.

pneumonitis Lung inflammation from an irritant, such as a chemical, dust, or radiation, or from aspiration, such as aspiration of gastric contents.

point of maximal impulse (PMI) The palpable beat of the apex of the heart against the chest wall during ventricular contraction; normally palpated at the fifth left intercostal space along the midclavicular line.

poison A substance whose chemical action could damage structures or impair function when introduced into the body.

polarized When a cell is at rest, ions are actively transported into and out of the cell to create an electrochemical gradient across the cell membrane.

poliomyelitis A viral infection that attacks and destroys nerve axons, especially motor axons; the disease can cause weakness, paralysis, and respiratory arrest; the development of an effective vaccine has made its incidence rare.

polycythemia An overabundance or overproduction of red blood cells, white blood cells, and platelets, making the blood thick; a characteristic of people with chronic lung disease and chronic hypoxia.

polydipsia Significant thirst.

polymorphonuclear neutrophils (PMNs) The type of white blood cells formed by bone marrow tissue that have a nucleus consisting of several parts or lobes connected by fine strands.

polypeptide Formed from many amino acids bound into a chain. When this has more than 100 molecules, it is considered to be a protein. Certain protein molecules have more than one.

polyphagia Increased appetite.

polyphonic The sound of multiple notes during wheezing; caused by the vibrations of multiple bronchi.

polysaccharides Complex carbohydrates that contain many simple joined sugar units, such as plant starch. Some, such as cellulose, cannot be broken down for nutrition in humans but play important roles in digestion.

polyuria Frequent and plentiful urination.

pons Area of the brainstem that contains the sleep and respiratory centers for the body, which along with the medulla, control breathing.

pontine respiratory group (PRG) A portion of the pons that communicates information to both the ventral and dorsal respiratory groups; it is thought to smooth the transition between each phase of the ventilatory cycle and alter breathing by making each breath shorter and shallower or longer and deeper, depending on the body's needs.

portal hypertension Increased pressure in the portal veins; caused by the inability of blood to flow normally through the liver; can lead to rupture of these vessels.

positive end-expiratory pressure (PEEP) Mechanical maintenance of pressure in the airway at the end of expiration to increase the volume of gas remaining in the lungs.

positive pressure ventilation Forcing of air into the lungs.

postconventional reasoning A type of reasoning in which a child bases decisions on his or her conscience.

posterior In anatomy, the back surface of the body; the side away from you in the standard anatomic position.

postictal The period after a seizure in which the brain is reorganizing activity.

postpolio syndrome The death of nerve fibers as a late consequence of poliomyelitis; characterized by swallowing difficulties, weakness, fatigue, and breathing problems.

postrenal acute kidney injury A type of acute kidney injury caused by obstruction of urine flow from the kidneys, commonly caused by a blockage of the urethra by an enlarged prostate gland, blood clots, or strictures.

posttraumatic stress disorder (PTSD) A severe form of anxiety or delayed stress reaction that stems from a traumatic experience; characterized by the reliving of the stress and nightmares of the original situation.

postural tremor A tremor that occurs as the person holds a body part still.

posturing Abnormal body positioning that indicates damage to the brain.

potency The relationship between the desired response of a medication and the dose required to achieve the response.

potentiation Enhancement of the effect of one drug by another drug.

PR interval (PRI) The distance between the beginning of the P wave (atrial depolarization) and the beginning of the QRS complex (ventricular depolarization), signifying the time required for the atria to depolarize and the excitation impulse to pass through the atrioventricular junction.

precapillary sphincters Smooth muscle located at the entrances to the capillaries; responsive to local tissue needs.

preconventional reasoning A type of reasoning in which a child acts almost purely to avoid punishment and to get what he or she wants.

precordial leads A term used to describe the chest leads in an ECG.

prediabetes A condition identified in people who have certain risk factors associated with type 2 diabetes and exists when blood glucose levels or hemoglobin A1c levels are above normal levels, yet not high enough to be diagnosed as diabetes.

preexcitation Early depolarization of ventricular tissue by means of an accessory pathway between the atria and ventricles.

prefilled syringes Medication syringes that are prepackaged and prepared with a specific concentration.

prefix Part of a term that appears before a word root, changing the meaning of the term.

preload The precontraction pressure in the heart, which increases as the volume of blood builds up, stretching the cardiac muscle; the pressure of blood that is returned to the heart (venous return).

prerenal acute kidney injury A type of acute kidney injury that is caused by hypoperfusion of the kidneys, resulting from hypovolemia (hemorrhage, dehydration), trauma, shock, sepsis, and heart failure (secondary to myocardial infarction); often reversible if the underlying condition can be found and perfusion restored to the kidney.

presbyopia The increased difficulty in focusing on objects that occurs with aging.

preschoolers People who are 3 to 5 years of age.

pressure-compensated flowmeter An oxygen flowmeter that incorporates a float ball in a tapered calibrated tube; the float rises or falls according to the gas flow in the tube; is affected by gravity and must remain in an upright position for an accurate reading.

pressure infuser device A sleeve that is placed around the IV bag and inflated to force fluid to flow from the IV bag and into the tubing.

pressure of speech Speech in which words seem to tumble out under immense emotional pressure.

pretibial myxedema An "orange peel" appearance and nonpitting edema of the skin on the anterior part of the leg below the knee.

prevalence The number of cases of a disease in a specific population within a given period.

priapism A painful, tender, persistent erection of the penis; can result from spinal cord injury, erectile dysfunction drugs, or sickle cell disease.

primary adrenal insufficiency Also known as Addison disease. A rare condition in which the adrenal glands produce an insufficient amount of adrenal hormones.

primary prevention Keeping an injury or illness from occurring.

primary response The first encounter with the foreign substance to begin the immune response.

primary survey The part of the assessment process that focuses on identifying immediate or potential life-threatening conditions so you can initiate lifesaving care.

primitive reflexes Reflex reactions such as Babinski, grasping, and sucking signs normally found in infants.

Prinzmetal angina A type of angina that occurs when a person is at rest, when oxygen needs are minimal; also called vasospastic angina.

process objectives State how a program will be implemented, describing the service to be provided, the nature of the service, and to whom it will be directed.

prodrome An early sign or symptom that occurs before a disease or condition fully appears (eg, dizziness before fainting).

profession A specialized set of knowledge, skills, and/or expertise.

progesterone A female hormone released from the ovaries that promotes changes in the uterus during the reproductive cycle, affects the mammary glands, and helps regulate gonadotropin secretion.

projection A defense mechanism characterized by blaming unacceptable feelings, motives, or desires on others.

prolonged (persistent) reaction Anaphylaxis symptoms that continue over time, with time frames anywhere from 5 to 32 hours.

pronation Turning the palms downward (toward the ground).

pronator drift The drifting of one arm downward toward a patient's feet while he or she holds out his or her arms, palm side up, with his or her eyes shut; can be a sign of a stroke.

prone Lying flat, face down.

proprioception The ability to perceive the position and movement of one's body or limbs.

prospective research A type of research that gathers information as events occur in real time.

prostaglandins Lipids that act as chemical messengers, made from arachidonic acid that usually act more locally than hormones, are very potent, stimulate hormone secretions, and help to regulate blood pressure.

prostatitis Inflammation of the prostate gland.

proteins Created from amino acids, they include enzymes, plasma proteins, muscle components (actin and myosin), hormones, and antibodies.

protest phase An infant's initial response to a situational crisis; characterized by loud crying.

prothrombin A protein made in the liver and released into the blood where it is converted into thrombin during the process of blood clotting.

protocol A treatment plan developed for a specific illness or injury.

protozoa Single-celled, usually microscopic, eukaryotic organisms such as amoebas, ciliates, flagellates, and sporozoans; a type of parasite.

proximal Closer to the trunk.

proximal convoluted tubule (PCT) One of two complex sections of the nephron, the proximal convoluted tubule includes an enlargement at the end called the glomerular capsule.

proximate cause The specific reason that an injury occurred; one of the items that must be proven in order for a paramedic to be held liable for negligence.

pruritus Itching.

pseudomembrane A false membrane formed by a dead tissue layer; seen in the posterior pharynx of patients with diphtheria.

psychiatric emergency An emergency in which abnormal behavior threatens a person's health and safety or the health and safety of another person, such as with a person who becomes suicidal or homicidal, or who has a psychotic episode.

psychological dependence The emotional state of craving a drug to maintain a feeling of well-being.

psychosis A mental disorder characterized by a loss of contact with reality.

psychotropic medications Medications that affect mood, thought, or behavior.

ptosis Prolapse of a body part; often refers to drooping of the eyelid.

public health An industry whose mission is to prevent disease and promote good health within groups of people.

public safety answering point (PSAP) The location to which 9-1-1 calls are routed, which may or may not serve as the dispatch center.

pulmonary artery One of two arteries that carry deoxygenated blood from the right ventricle to the lungs.

pulmonary circulation The flow of blood from the right ventricle through the pulmonary arteries and all of their branches and capillaries in the lungs and back to the left atrium through the venules and pulmonary veins; also called the lesser circulation.

pulmonary edema Congestion of the pulmonary air spaces with exudate and foam, often secondary to left ventricular failure.

pulmonary embolism Obstruction of a pulmonary artery or arteries by solid, liquid, or gaseous material, such as a blood clot or foreign matter, which is swept through the right side of the heart into the lungs and becomes trapped within the pulmonary circulation.

pulmonary veins The four veins that return oxygenated blood from the lungs to the left atrium of the heart.

pulmonic valve The semilunar valve that regulates blood flow between the right ventricle and the pulmonary artery; also called the pulmonary semilunar valve.

pulse The wave of pressure created as the heart contracts and forces blood out the left ventricle and into the major arteries; palpated at a point where an artery passes close to a bone.

pulse oximeter A device that measures oxygen saturation level (Spo_2).

pulse oximetry An assessment tool used to measure oxygen saturation of hemoglobin in the capillary beds.

pulse pressure The difference between the systolic and diastolic pressures.

pulseless electrical activity (PEA) An organized cardiac rhythm (other than ventricular tachycardia) on an ECG monitor that is not accompanied by any detectable pulse.

pulsus paradoxus A drop in the systolic blood pressure of 10 mm Hg more during inspiration; characteristic of conditions that cause profound pressure changes in the thorax; commonly seen in patients with cardiac tamponade or severe asthma.

punitive damages Compensation, usually monetary, awarded to a plaintiff for intentional or reckless acts committed by the defendant.

Purkinje fibers A network of cardiac muscle fibers distributed throughout the inner surfaces of the ventricular walls that conducts the excitation impulse from the bundle branches to the ventricular myocardium.

purulent Full of pus; having the character of pus.

pyelonephritis An upper urinary tract infection in which the kidneys are involved.

pyrogenic reaction A reaction characterized by an abrupt temperature elevation (as high as 106°F [41°C]) with severe chills, backache, headache, weakness, nausea, and vomiting; a potential complication of intravenous or intraosseous therapy.

pyrogens Chemicals or proteins that travel to the brain and affect the hypothalamus and stimulate a rise in the body's core temperature.

QRS axis A single vector that represents the mean (or average) of all vectors created by the ventricles during depolarization.

QRS complex Deflection of the ECG produced by ventricular depolarization.

quadrants The four sections of the abdominal cavity shown by two imaginary lines intersecting at the umbilicus, dividing the abdomen into four equal areas.

qualified immunity Protection in which the paramedic is only held liable when the plaintiff can show that the paramedic violated clearly established law of which he or she should have known.

qualitative A type of descriptive statistic in research that does not use numeric information.

quality control The responsibility of the medical director to ensure the appropriate medical care standards are met by EMS personnel on each call.

quantitative A type of measurement in research that uses a mean, median, and mode.

quid pro quo Circumstance in which a person in authority attempts to exchange some work-related benefit, such as a raise or promotion, for an inappropriate employee action (eg, sexual favors); literal translation from Latin is "this for that."

rabies A fatal infection of the central nervous system caused by a bite from an animal that has been infected with the rabies virus.

radio dead spots Areas where mobile or portable radios are unable to communicate with a repeater.

radiopaque Feature of an IV catheter (or any other object) that allows it to appear on a radiograph.

range of motion (ROM) The arc of movement of an extremity at a joint in a particular direction; the full distance that a joint can be moved.

rape Nonconsensual oral, anal, or vaginal penetration of the victim by body parts or objects using force, threats of bodily harm, or by taking advantage of a victim who is incapacitated or otherwise incapable of giving consent.

rapid full-body scan A 60- to 90-second nonsystematic review and palpation of the patient's body to identify injuries that must be managed or protected immediately; also called the rapid full-body sweep.

rapid sequence intubation (RSI) A specific set of procedures, combined in rapid succession, to induce sedation and paralysis and intubate a patient quickly.

reactive airway disease A term used to describe any condition that causes hyperreactive bronchioles and bronchospasm in response to certain triggers.

reassessment The portion of the assessment process in which a patient's condition is reevaluated and responses to treatment is assessed.

rebound tenderness Pain that the patient feels when pressure is released as opposed to when pressure is applied; characteristic of appendicitis.

receptor A specialized area in tissues that initiates certain actions after specific stimulation.

reciprocal changes Mirror-image J-point, ST-segment, and T-wave changes seen on the ECG during an ACS.

reciprocity The process of granting licensure or certification to a provider from another state or agency.

recovery position Left lateral recumbent position; used in all unresponsive nontrauma patients who are able to maintain their own airway spontaneously and are breathing adequately.

rectal abscess An infection involving a collection of pus in the rectal walls that results from blockage of the rectal mucous ducts.

reduced hemoglobin The hemoglobin after the oxygen has been released to the cells.

reducible A type of hernia that will return to its normal location either spontaneously or by manual manipulation.

reemergence phenomenon The occurrence of dreams, nightmares, or delirium that can take place during the end of the half-life of ketamine.

reentry Spread of an impulse through tissue already stimulated by that same impulse.

referred pain Pain that feels as if it is originating from a body part other than the site being stimulated.

reflex arc A sensory message that reaches the spinal cord and meets with a motor nerve to cause an action; the reflex action occurs without the message first having to reach the brain to voluntarily cause the action.

reflexes Involuntary motor responses to specific sensory stimuli, such as a tap on the knee or stroking the eyelash.

refracting system A series of transparent structures within the eye that redirect light as it passes through mediums of different densities.

refractory period (RP) A short period immediately after depolarization during which the myocytes have not yet repolarized and are unable to fire or conduct an impulse (the absolute refractory period) or have partially repolarized and may depolarize in response to an electrical stimulus (the relative refractory period).

registration Providing information to an entity that stores it in some form of record book. In the context of EMS, records of your education, state or local licensure, and recertification are held by a recognized board.

regression A defense mechanism characterized by a return to more childlike behavior while under stress.

relative refractory period (RRP) The portion of the cardiac action potential that extends from the middle of phase 3 to the beginning of phase 4; during this time, the heart muscle has been partially repolarized and may depolarize in response to an electrical stimulus.

remote terminal A terminal that receives transmissions of telemetry and voice from the field and transmits messages back, usually through the base station.

renal corpuscle The initial blood-filtering component of the nephron.

renal cortex The outer portion of each kidney; it forms renal columns and has tiny tubules associated with the nephrons.

renal dialysis A technique for filtering the blood of its toxic wastes, removing excess fluids, and restoring the normal balance of electrolytes.

renal medulla The inner portion of each kidney; it is made of conical renal pyramids, and has striations.

renal pelvis A cone-shaped collecting area that connects the ureter and the kidney.

renal tubule The portion of the nephron containing the tubular fluid filtered through the glomerulus.

renin A hormone produced by cells in the juxtaglomerular apparatus when the blood pressure is low.

repeater Remote radio transceiver that receives radio signals and rebroadcasts them at a higher power, extending the range of a radio communications system.

reperfusion therapy Treatment intended to facilitate the resumption of blood flow through a blocked vessel; therapy may be either procedural, such as cardiac catheterization, or pharmacologic, such as administration of a fibrinolytic agent.

repolarization The process by which ions are moved across the cell membrane to return to a polarized state.

reproductive system The system in males and females that controls the reproductive processes via organs and glands that create sex cells and transport them to areas where fertilization can occur.

res ipsa loquitur Theory of negligence that assumes an injury can only occur when a negligent act occurs.

research agenda The specific questions that a study aims to answer, and the precise methods in which the data will be gathered.

research consortium A group of agencies working together to study a particular topic.

research domain The area (clinical, basic science, systems, or education) that will be impacted by a study.

reservoir In the context of communicable disease, a place where organisms may live and multiply.

residual volume The amount of air remaining in the lungs and airway passages that is unable to be expelled after a maximal forced exhalation.

respiration The exchange of gases between a living organism and its environment.

respiratory acidosis A pathologic condition characterized by a blood pH of less than 7.35 and caused by an accumulation of acids in the body from a respiratory cause.

respiratory alkalosis A pathologic condition characterized by a blood pH of greater than 7.45 and resulting from the accumulation of bases in the body from a respiratory cause.

respiratory membrane Where gas exchange takes place; oxygen is picked up in the bloodstream and carbon dioxide is eliminated through the lungs.

respiratory system All the structures of the body that contribute to the process of breathing, consisting of the upper and lower airways and their component parts.

restrictive lung diseases Diseases that limit the ability of the lungs to expand appropriately. Skeletal abnormalities such as kyphosis and scoliosis are common examples of conditions that can cause these diseases.

rest tremor A tremor that occurs when the body part is not in motion.

reticular activating system (RAS) Group of specialized neurons in the brainstem; involved in sleep and wake cycles; maintains consciousness, specifically one's level of arousal.

reticuloendothelial system The system in the body that is primarily used to defend against infection.

retina A delicate 10-layered structure of nervous tissue located in the rear of the interior of the globe of the eye; it receives light and generates nerve signals that are transmitted to the brain through the optic nerve; the inner layer of the eye wall, including the visual receptors.

retractions A sign of respiratory distress characterized by skin pulling inward between and around the ribs and clavicles during inhalation.

retrograde intubation A technique in which a wire is placed through the trachea and into the mouth with a needle via the cricoid membrane; the endotracheal tube is then placed over the wire and guided into the trachea.

retrospective research Research performed from current available information.

Rh factor An antigen found on the red blood cells of most people; when a woman without this protein is impregnated by a man with this protein, the woman's body can create antibodies against the protein and attack future pregnancies.

rhabdomyolysis The destruction of muscle tissue leading to a release of potassium and myoglobin.

rheumatic fever An inflammatory disease caused by streptococcal bacteria; the disease can cause mitral or aortic valve stenosis.

rhinitis A nasal disorder generally caused by allergens, which, once inhaled, result in production of chemicals that can cause inflammation.

rhonchi Coarse, low-pitched breath sounds heard in patients with chronic mucus or fluid in the upper or larger lower airways.

right atrial abnormality Dilation of the right atrium that occurs when returning venous pressure is elevated or pulmonary pressure is high.

right coronary artery (RCA) Artery that provides oxygenated blood to the walls of the right atrium and ventricle, a portion of the inferior part of the left ventricle, and portions of the conduction system.

right ventricular failure (RVF) A condition in which the right side of the heart must work increasingly hard to pump blood into engorged pulmonary vessels; eventually, it is unable to keep up with the increased workload.

right ventricular hypertrophy (RVH) A cardiac condition in which the right ventricle becomes enlarged, usually as a result of pulmonary hypertension.

rigidity A clinically important sign characterized by marked peritoneal irritation and guarding, indicating an injury or illness for which urgent surgical intervention may be required; in the context of Parkinson disease, a condition in which muscles do not contract and relax smoothly, resulting in stiffness of motion.

risk A potentially hazardous situation that puts people in a position in which they could be harmed.

risk factors Characteristics of people, behaviors, or environments that increase the chances of disease or injury; some examples are alcohol use, poverty, smoking, or gender.

rocuronium A nondepolarizing neuromuscular blocking agent; used to maintain paralysis following succinylcholine-facilitated intubation.

rods One of two photoreceptors of the retina sensitive to light, but does not discriminate colors, producing a picture that is somewhat less focused and essentially black and white.

rooting reflex An infant reflex that occurs when something touches an infant's cheek, and the infant instinctively turns his or her head toward the touch.

R-R interval The period between the onset of one QRS complex and the onset of the next QRS complex.

rubella A viral disease similar to measles, best known by the distinctive red rash on the skin; not nearly as infectious or severe as measles.

rubor Redness; one of the classic signs of inflammation.

ruptured ovarian cyst A fluid-filled sac within the ovary that bursts from internal pressure.

sacroiliac joint The point of attachment of the ilium to the sacrum.

saddle joint Two saddle-shaped articulating surfaces oriented at right angles to each other so that complementary surfaces articulate with each other, such as is the case with the thumb.

safe residual pressure The pressure at which an oxygen cylinder should be replaced with a full one; often is 200 psi.

safety culture In an EMS organization, a system of beliefs and practices that: (1) acknowledge that organizations engage in high-risk activities, (2) determine the importance of consistent safe operations to counteract these activities, (3) support a blame-free environment where errors can be reported without fear of punishment, and (4) maintain organizational commitment to address reported errors and safety concerns.

sagittal (lateral) plane A plane of the body that passes vertically from front to back, dividing the body into left and right portions.

salicylates Chemicals found in plants and a primary ingredient in aspirin.

saline locks Special types of IV devices that eliminate the need to hang a bag of IV fluid; also called a buff cap or INT (intermittent); commonly used for patients who do not require fluid boluses but may require medication therapy.

sampling errors Expected errors that occur in the sampling phase of research.

scabies An infestation of the skin with the mite *Sarcoptes scabiei*; spreads rapidly with skin-to-skin contact.

scaffolding An instructional technique that builds on what has already been learned.

scaphoid A concave shape of the abdomen; can be caused by evisceration; in the context of anatomy, the wrist bone that is found just beyond the most distal portion of the radius.

scarlet fever A disease caused by the bacterium *Streptococcus pyogenes* and characterized by a sore throat, fever, rash, and "strawberry tongue."

scene size-up A step in the patient assessment process involving a quick assessment of the scene and its surroundings to gather information about the overall safety and stability of the scene and the mechanism of injury or nature of illness. This process is carried out before you enter and begin patient care.

schizophrenia A complex mental disorder that is difficult to identify and whose typical onset is during early adulthood. Dysfunctional symptoms typically become more prominent over time and include delusions, hallucinations, apathy, mutism, flat affect, lack of interest in pleasure, erratic speech, dysfunctional emotional responses, and dysfunctional motor behavior.

school-age children People who are 6 to 12 years of age.

Schwann cells Neuroglial cells in the peripheral nervous system that form a myelin sheath around axons.

sclera The white, fibrous outer layer of the eyeball.

scleroderma An autoimmune connective tissue disease that causes fibrotic (scar tissue–like) changes to the skin, blood vessels, muscles, and internal organs.

scoliosis Sideways curvature of the spine.

scope of practice Describes what a state permits a paramedic practicing under a license or certification to do.

scrotum A pouch of skin and subcutaneous tissue hanging from the lower abdominal region, posterior to the penis.

sebaceous glands Glands that produce an oily substance called sebum, which discharges along the shafts of the hairs.

secondary adrenal insufficiency A common condition characterized by a lack of adrenocorticotropic hormone (also called corticotrophin) secretion from the pituitary gland.

secondary assessment The process by which more detailed, quantifiable, objective information is obtained from the patient about his or her overall state of health.

secondary prevention Reducing the effects of an injury or illness that has already happened.

secondary response The body's reaction when it is exposed to an antigen for which it already has antibodies, in which it responds by killing the invading substance.

secure attachment A bond between an infant and his or her parent or caregiver, in which the infant understands that parents and/or caregivers will be responsive to his or her needs and provide care when help is needed.

sedation The reduction of a patient's anxiety, induction of amnesia, and suppression of the gag reflex, usually by pharmacologic means.

sedative-hypnotic A drug used to reduce anxiety, calm agitated patients, and help produce drowsiness and sleep (central nervous system depressants).

seizure The sudden, erratic firing of neurons; a neurologic episode caused by a surge of electric activity in the brain; can be a convulsion characterized by generalized, uncoordinated muscular activity, and may be associated with loss of consciousness.

selective serotonin reuptake inhibitors (SSRIs) A class of antidepressants that inhibit the reuptake of serotonin.

self-concept A person's perception of himself or herself.

self-esteem How a person feels about himself or herself, and how a person feels about how he or she fits in with peers.

semilunar (SL) valves The two valves, the aortic and pulmonic valves, that are shaped like half-moons and separate the heart from the aorta and pulmonary arteries.

semipermeable Property of the cell membrane that describes the ability to allow certain elements to pass through while not allowing others to do so.

sensitivity The ability to recognize a foreign substance the next time it is encountered.

sensory nerves The nerves that carry sensations of touch, taste, heat, cold, pain, and other modalities from the body to the central nervous system.

sensory receptors Structures located in the dermis that initiate nerve impulses that can reach one's conscious awareness.

sepsis A disease state of life-threatening organ dysfunction that results from the presence of invading microorganisms or their toxic products in the bloodstream; usually occurs in a febrile patient.

septic shock The type of shock that occurs as a result of widespread infection, usually bacterial; untreated, the result is multiple organ dysfunction syndrome and often death.

septicemia A generalized infection of the bloodstream.

septum A thick wall that separates the right and left sides of the heart.

seropositive Having a positive blood test for an infectious agent, such as human immunodeficiency virus or hepatitis B or C virus.

serotonin A vasoactive amine that increases vascular permeability to cause vasodilation.

serotonin syndrome An idiosyncratic complication that occurs with antidepressant therapy in which patients have lower extremity muscle rigidity, confusion or disorientation, and/or agitation.

serum hepatitis Infection with the hepatitis B virus, which is transmitted through sexual contact, blood transfusion, or puncture of the skin with contaminated needles; signs and symptoms include loss of appetite, nausea, vomiting, general fatigue and malaise, low-grade fever, vague abdominal discomfort, and sometimes aching in the joints; eventually, jaundice occurs.

serum sickness A condition in which antigen-antibody complexes formed in the bloodstream deposit in sites around the body, most notably the kidneys, with resultant inflammatory reactions.

severe acute respiratory syndrome (SARS) A potentially life-threatening viral infection that usually starts with flulike symptoms.

sex chromosomes The X and Y chromosomes, which determine sex.

sexual assault Any type of sexual contact or behavior that occurs without the explicit consent of the recipient.

sexually transmitted diseases (STDs) A group of diseases usually acquired by sexual contact and that include gonorrhea, syphilis, chlamydia, scabies, pubic lice, herpes, hepatitis, and human immunodeficiency virus infection.

sharps Any contaminated item that can cause injury; includes IV needles and catheters, broken ampules or vials, or anything else that can penetrate or lacerate the skin.

shunt A connection between the arterial and venous system in which no gas exchange occurs.

sickle cell crisis A condition in which a patient with sickle cell disease experiences significant pain due to insufficient passage of oxygen and nutrients into tissues and joints because of vessel congestion.

sickle cell disease A disease that causes the red blood cells to be misshapen, resulting in poor oxygen-carrying capability and potentially resulting in lodging of the red blood cells in blood vessels or the spleen.

signs Objective observations that can be seen, heard, felt, smelled, or measured.

simple phobia A fear that is focused on one class of objects (eg, mice, spiders, dogs) or situations (eg, high places, darkness, flying).

simplex Radio communication using a single frequency.

sinoatrial (SA) node The normal site of the origin of electrical impulses; located high in the right atrium at the junction of the superior vena cava and the right atrium; the natural pacemaker of the heart.

sinus bradycardia A sinus rhythm characterized by a heart rate of less than 60 beats/min.

sinus dysrhythmia A variation of cycling of a sinus rhythm that is often associated with respiratory cycle fluctuations; the rate increases during inspiration and decreases during expiration.

sinus tachycardia A sinus rhythm characterized by a heart rate greater than 100 beats/min.

sinuses Cavities formed by the cranial bones that trap contaminants from entering the respiratory tract and act as tributaries for fluid to and from the eustachian tubes and tear ducts.

sinusitis An infection of the sinuses, characterized by thick nasal discharge, sinus and facial pressure, headache, and fever.

situation, background, assessment, and recommendation (SBAR) A structured patient report format designed to convey important information in a concise manner.

situational crisis A crisis caused by a specific set of circumstances.

skeletal muscle tissue Voluntary muscle tissue attached to bones and composed of long, threadlike cells that have light and dark striations.

slander A false verbal statement that injures a person's good name.

sliding filament theory A method of action of muscle contraction involving how sarcomeres shorten, with thick and thin filaments sliding past each other toward the center of the sarcomere from both ends.

smooth muscle The nonstriated involuntary muscle found in vessel walls, glands, and the gastrointestinal tract.

snoring A noise made during inhalation when the upper airway is partially obstructed by the tongue.

SOAP method A narrative writing method in which information is organized into four categories: Subjective information, Objective information, Assessment, and Plan (for treatment).

social history A subsection of the patient history that provides valuable information regarding the patient's overall health status and helps to identify risk factors for various disease processes; includes items such as tobacco use, alcohol and drug use, sexual behavior, diet, travel history, living environment, and occupation.

sodium-potassium pump The mechanism by which the cell brings in two potassium ions and releases three sodium ions.

soft palate The posterior portion of the palate that is made up of mucous membrane, muscular fibers, and mucous glands; it is so named because it has no bony support.

soft stool A bowel movement that is the consistency of soft-serve ice cream; can range in color from tan to dark brown.

solute The dissolved particles contained in a solvent.

solution A mixture of a solvent and a solute.

solvent The fluid that dissolves a solute, or the substance in which a solute is dissolved or mixed.

somatic nervous system The part of the nervous system that regulates activities over which there is voluntary control.

somatic pain Pain caused by the activation of pain receptors in the body's superficial tissues, such as the skin, bones, muscles, and joints, usually felt deeply, that represents irritation or injury to tissue; in contrast to visceral pain, this is generally more intense and more precisely localized.

somatoform disorder A condition in which a person is overly concerned with physical health and appearance to the point that it dominates his or her life (eg, hypochondria).

somatostatin A hormone that inhibits insulin and glucagon secretion by the pancreas.

source individual Any person, living or dead, whose blood or other potentially infectious materials may be a source of occupational exposure to another person; examples include but are not limited to, hospital and clinic patients; clients in institutions for the developmentally disabled; trauma victims; clients of drug and alcohol treatment facilities; residents of hospices and nursing homes; human remains; and people who donate or sell blood or blood components.

spacer A device that collects medication as it is released from the canister of a metered-dose inhaler, allowing more medication to be delivered to the lungs and less to be lost to the environment.

spermatogenesis The process by which sperm cells are formed.

sphincters Muscles arranged in circles that are able to decrease the diameter of tubes. Examples are found within the rectum, bladder, and blood vessels.

sphygmomanometer A blood pressure cuff.

spice An illicit drug consisting of a blend of synthetic cannabinoids; it can produce delirium and short- and long-term psychotic effects.

spinal nerves 31 pairs of nerves that originate from the spinal cord and exit the spine on either side between vertebrae; each has a sensory root and a motor root and is responsible for sending and receiving sensory and motor messages to and from the central nervous system from a portion of the body.

splenic sequestration crisis An acute, painful enlargement of the spleen caused by sickle cell disease.

splitting In the context of heart sounds, a situation in which events on the right side of heart occur slightly later than those on the left side, and create two discernible sounds rather than one heart sound.

squelch Filtering system to block background noise when a radio is on but not receiving a signal.

stable angina Angina pectoris characterized by periodic pain with a predictable pattern.

standard deviation A measure of the range of scores in a set of data relative to the mean score.

standard of care Describes what a reasonable paramedic with training would do in the same or a similar situation.

standard precautions Protective measures that have traditionally been developed by the Centers for Disease Control and Prevention for use in dealing with objects, blood, body fluids, or other potential exposure risks of communicable disease; considers all body fluids, except sweat, to present a possible risk.

standing order A type of protocol that is a written document signed by the EMS system's medical director that outlines specific directions, permissions, and sometimes prohibitions regarding patient care that is rendered prior to contacting medical control.

Staphylococcus aureus (S aureus) A strain of bacteria that became resistant to the drug methicillin, creating a new strain; symptoms include infection and possibly localized skin abscesses and cellulites, empyemas, and endocarditis.

status asthmaticus A severe, prolonged asthma attack that cannot be stopped with conventional treatment, such as the administration of epinephrine.

status epilepticus A condition in which a seizure lasts longer than 4 to 5 minutes, or consecutive seizures without a return to consciousness between seizures.

statutes of limitations Laws that limit the time period within which a lawsuit may be filed.

steatorrhea Foamy, fatty stools associated with liver failure or gallbladder conditions.

stem cells Cells that can develop into other types of cells in the body; they retain the ability to divide repeatedly without specializing, and allow for continual growth and renewal.

stenosis A narrowing, such as of a blood vessel or stoma.

stereotyped movements Repetitive movements that don't appear to serve any purpose.

sterile The destruction of all living organisms; achieved by using heat, gas, or chemicals.

Stevens-Johnson syndrome A severe, possibly fatal reaction that mimics a burn; may be due to a medication.

stimulant A medication or chemical that temporarily enhances central nervous system and sympathetic nervous system functioning.

stoma In the context of the airway, the resultant orifice of a tracheostomy that connects the trachea to the outside air; located in the midline of the anterior part of the neck.

strabismus Loss of perception of depth and overlapping or doubled images.

straight laryngoscope blade A blade designed to lift the epiglottis and expose the vocal cords; also called the Miller blade.

strangulated A type of hernia that causes complete obstruction of blood circulation in a given organ as a result of compression or entrapment; an emergency situation causing death of tissue.

stratum corneum The outermost or dead layer of the skin.

stress A reaction of the body to any agent or situation that requires the person to adapt.

stressor Any agent or situation that causes stress, whether good or bad.

striae Vertical stretch marks that occur when a person loses or gains weight rapidly.

stricture An abnormal narrowing of a structure; also called stenosis.

stridor A harsh, high-pitched respiratory sound produced as air moves past an obstruction within or immediately above the glottic opening; associated with severe upper airway obstruction, such as that caused by laryngeal edema.

stroke An interruption of blood flow to the brain that results in the loss of brain function; also called a cerebrovascular accident.

stroke volume (SV) The amount of blood that the left ventricle ejects into the aorta per contraction.

ST segment The interval between the end of the QRS complex (the J point) and the beginning of the T wave; when there is significant myocardial ischemia or injury, it is often depressed or elevated with respect to the isoelectric line.

stylet In the context of intubation, a semirigid wire inserted into an endotracheal tube to mold and maintain the shape of the tube.

subarachnoid space The space located between the pia mater and the arachnoid membrane.

subcutaneous Into the tissue between the skin and muscle; a medication delivery route.

subendocardial myocardial infarction A type of acute myocardial infarction in which the ischemic process affects only the inner layer of muscle.

subjective information Information that is obtained from the patient, but which cannot be seen, such as the symptoms a patient describes.

sublingual Under the tongue; a medication delivery route.

substance abuse Use of a substance that disrupts activities of daily living.

substance dependence Use of a substance that results in addiction and physiologic dependence on the substance.

substance intoxication Use of a substance that results in impaired thinking and motor function.

substance use Use of moderate amounts of a substance without seriously affecting activities of daily living.

succinylcholine chloride A depolarizing neuromuscular blocker frequently used as the initial paralytic during rapid sequence intubation; causes muscle fasciculations.

sucking reflex An infant reflex in which the infant starts sucking when his or her lips are stroked.

suffix The part of a term that comes after the word root, at the end of the term.

superficial Closer to or on the surface of the skin.

superior Above or closer to the head.

supination Turning the palms upward (toward the sky).

supine Lying face up.

suppository A drug mixed in a firm base that melts at body temperature and is shaped to fit the rectum.

supraorbital foramen A small notch located on the frontal bone near the inner, upper area of each orbit.

suprasternal notch The indentation formed by the superior border of the manubrium and the clavicles, often used as a landmark for procedures such as subclavian vein access; also known as the jugular notch.

surfactant A liquid protein substance that coats the alveoli in the lungs, decreases alveolar surface tension, and keeps the alveoli expanded; a low level in a premature infant contributes to respiratory distress syndrome.

surrogate decision maker A person legally authorized to make health care decisions on behalf of a patient who is incapable of making or communicating the decision on his or her own.

surveillance The ongoing systematic collection, analysis, and interpretation of injury data essential to the planning, implementation, and evaluation of public health practice.

sutures Seams that occur only between the bones of the skull; they are a type of fibrous joint.

sweat glands The glands that secrete sweat, located in the dermal layer of the skin.

sympathomimetics Medications administered to stimulate the sympathetic nervous system.

symptoms Subjective information the patient feels, such as pain, discomfort, or other abnormality.

synapse A functional connection where neurons communicate with other cells.

synaptic cleft The space between neurons; also called the synaptic gap.

synaptic vesicles Small sacs that contain neurotransmitters.

synchronized cardioversion The use of a synchronized direct current (DC) electric shock to convert a tachydysrhythmia (such as atrial fibrillation or supraventricular tachycardia) to a normal sinus rhythm.

syncopal episodes Fainting; brief losses of consciousness caused by transiently inadequate blood flow to the brain.

syncope Fainting; brief loss of consciousness caused by transiently inadequate blood flow to the brain.

syndrome of inappropriate antidiuretic hormone secretion (SIADH) An endocrine disorder in which an excess of antidiuretic hormone results in a decrease in urinary output and, therefore, systemic fluid overload.

syndromic surveillance The monitoring, usually by local or state health departments, of the number and nature of medical cases against the expected volume of these cases at a given time and place in the community; can include the recording of EMS call volume, and the monitoring of the use of over-the-counter medications.

synergism The action of two substances such as drugs, in which the total effects are greater than the sum of the independent effects of the two substances.

synonyms Pairs of word roots, prefixes, or suffixes that have the same or almost the same meaning.

synovial fluid The fluid secreted by synovial membranes that lubricates synovial joints.

synovial joints Complex joints that allow free movement of the component bones and are lubricated with synovial fluid.

synovial membrane The lining of a joint that secretes synovial fluid into the joint space.

syphilis A sexually transmitted disease caused by the spiral-shaped bacteria *Treponema pallidum* with signs and symptoms that include an ulcerative lesion or chancre of the skin or mucous membrane at the site of infection, commonly in the genital region.

systematic sampling A computer-generated list of subjects or groups for research.

systemic complications Reactions that affect systems of the body.

systemic lupus erythematosus A multisystem autoimmune disease.

systemic reaction A reaction that occurs throughout the body, possibly affecting multiple body systems.

systemic vascular resistance The resistance that blood must overcome to be able to move within the blood vessels; related to the amount of dilation or constriction in the blood vessel; present in all blood vessels except the pulmonary vessels.

systolic pressure Blood pressure created by the left ventricle as it contracts (that is, in systole).

T lymphocytes Lymphocytes that interact directly with antigens, producing the cellular immune response; they also stimulate the B lymphocytes to produce antibodies; also called T cells.

T wave The upright, flat, or inverted wave following the QRS complex of the ECG, representing ventricular repolarization.

tachyphylaxis A condition in which repeated doses of medication within a short period rapidly cause tolerance, making the medication virtually ineffective.

tactile fremitus Vibrations in the chest that can be felt with a hand on the chest as the patient breathes.

tangential thinking A tendency to leave the current topic in conversation to talk about something else, thereby inhibiting interpersonal communication.

targeted temperature management (TTM) A procedure intended to lower body temperature in patients who are in a coma after return of spontaneous circulation; ideally performed in the hospital setting; formerly called therapeutic hypothermia.

telemedicine Computer-based system permitting real-time two-way audio, video, and data communication between the paramedic and medical control physician.

temporomandibular joint (TMJ) disorders A collection of disorders that present with jaw pain, and that occur when the connection between the temporal bone and the TMJ erodes or moves out of proper alignment.

ten-code A radio code system using the number 10 plus another number. No longer used in many emergency medical services systems.

tenting A condition in which the skin slowly retracts after being pinched and pulled away slightly from the body; a sign of dehydration.

tentorium A horizontal projection of the dura that separates the cerebellum from the cerebrum.

terminal drop hypothesis The theory that a person's mental function declines in the last 5 years of life.

testicular torsion Twisting of the testicle on the spermatic cord, from which it is suspended; associated with scrotal pain and swelling, and is a medical emergency.

testosterone The most important male sex hormone (androgen).

tetanus A disease caused by spores that enter the body through a puncture wound contaminated with animal feces, street dust, or soil or that can enter through contaminated street drugs; signs and symptoms include pain at the wound site and painful muscle contractions in the neck and trunk muscles.

thalamus Structure of the diencephalon that is the sensory switchboard of the brain, through which almost all signals travel on their way in or out of the brain.

thalassemia A type of anemia in which either not enough hemoglobin is produced or the hemoglobin is defective.

therapeutic communication Communicating with the patient using specific strategies to encourage the patient to express ideas and feelings, and to convey respect and acceptance.

therapeutic index The relationship between the median effective dose and the median lethal dose or median toxic dose; also known as the therapeutic ratio.

therapy regulator A device that attaches to the stem of the oxygen cylinder and reduces the high pressure of gas to a safe range (about 50 psi).

thermoregulation The process by which the body maintains temperature through a combination of heat gain by metabolic processes and muscular movement and heat loss through breathing, evaporation, conduction, convection, and perspiration.

third spacing The shifting of fluid into the tissues, creating edema.

thoracic duct One of two great lymph vessels; it empties into the superior vena cava.

thought broadcasting The belief that thoughts are broadcast aloud and can be heard by others.

thought insertion The belief that thoughts are being thrust into one's mind by another person.

thought withdrawal The belief that thoughts are being removed from one's mind.

threshold level In a pharmacologic context, the concentration of medication at which initiation or alteration of cellular activity begins.

thrill A humming vibration that can be palpated through the chest wall, suggesting an underlying bruit or murmur.

thrombin An enzyme that causes the conversion of fibrinogen to fibrin, which binds to a platelet plug, forming a final mature clot.

thrombocytes Platelets.

thrombocytopenia A reduction in the number of platelets in the blood.

thrombocytosis A condition in which the body produces too many platelets.

thromboembolism A blood clot that initially formed within a blood vessel but is now circulating through the bloodstream.

thrombophlebitis Inflammation of a vein.

thromboplastin A chemical that stimulates blood clotting.

thrombosis The development of a blood clot.

thrombus A fixed blood clot that can obstruct passage of blood flow through an artery.

thymus A lymphatic organ located in the thorax that is important in early immunity; it shrinks with age and is eventually replaced by other types of tissue.

thyroid cartilage A firm prominence of cartilage that forms the upper part of the larynx; the Adam's apple.

thyroid gland A large endocrine gland that is located at the base of the neck and produces and excretes hormones that influence growth, development, and metabolism.

thyroid-stimulating hormone (TSH) Hormone that controls the release of thyroid hormone from the thyroid gland.

thyroid storm A rare, life-threatening condition that may occur in patients with thyrotoxicosis. The condition is usually triggered by a stressful event or increased volume of thyroid hormones in the circulation.

thyrotoxicosis A toxic condition caused by excessive levels of circulating thyroid hormone.

thyroxine (T_4) The body's major metabolic hormone. Thyroxine stimulates energy production in cells, which increases the rate at which the cells consume oxygen and use carbohydrates, fats, and proteins.

tidal volume The amount of air moved in and out of the lungs in one relaxed breath; about 500 mL for an adult.

tinnitus The perception of sound in the inner ear with no external environmental cause; often reported as "ringing" in the ears, but may be roaring, buzzing, or clicking.

tissue A group of cells that are similar in structure and function.

titin A noncontractile protein found in sarcomeres of cardiac and skeletal muscle.

toddlers People who are 1 to 3 years of age.

tolerance Physiologic adaptation to the effects of a drug such that increasingly larger doses of the drug are required to achieve the same effect.

tongue-jaw lift maneuver A manual maneuver that involves grasping the tongue and jaw and lifting; commonly used to suction the airway and to place certain airway devices.

tonic activity A type of seizure movement involving the constant contraction and trembling of muscle groups.

tonsillitis Inflammation of the tonsils.

tonsil-tip catheter A hard or rigid suction catheter; also called a Yankauer catheter.

topographic anatomy Superficial landmarks of the body that serve as guides to the structures that lie beneath them.

tort A wrongful act that gives rise to a civil lawsuit.

total body water (TBW) Total amount of fluid in the human body; accounts for about 60% of the weight of a healthy adult male; divided into various compartments.

total laryngectomy Surgical removal of the entire larynx.

toxicologic emergencies Medical emergencies caused by toxic agents such as poison; may be intentional or unintentional.

toxicology The study of toxic or poisonous substances.

toxidrome The syndrome-like symptoms of any given class or group of poisonous agents.

toxin A poison or harmful substance produced by bacteria, animals, or plants.

tracheal breath sounds Breath sounds heard by placing the stethoscope diaphragm over the trachea or sternum; also called bronchial breath sounds.

tracheitis Bacterial infection of the trachea.

tracheobronchial suctioning Inserting a suction catheter into the endotracheal tube to remove pulmonary secretions.

tracheoesophageal fistula (TEF) A connection between the esophagus and the trachea.

tracheostomy A surgical opening into the trachea, created during a tracheotomy procedure.

tracheostomy tube A plastic tube placed within the tracheostomy site (stoma).

track marks The visible scars from repeated cannulation of a vein; commonly associated with illicit drug use.

transceiver A radio containing both a transmitter and a receiver, a two-way radio.

transcellular fluid Fluid classified as extracellular but distinct because it is formed from the transport activities of cells. Examples include cerebrospinal fluid, bladder urine, the aqueous humor, and the synovial fluid of the joints.

transcutaneous pacemaker A device that depolarize myocardial tissue by sending a small electrical charge through the skin of the chest between one externally placed pacing pad and another.

transcutaneous pacing (TCP) An intervention used to depolarize heart muscle using an external stimulus; pads placed on the patient's chest deliver electrical energy to the heart, causing muscle contraction.

transdermal Across the skin; a medication delivery route.

transfusion reaction A physiologic response that is similar to an anaphylactic reaction, in which the body reacts to the infusion of blood; it occurs rapidly and can cause severe circulatory collapse and death.

transfusion-related lung injury A transfusion reaction characterized by increased pulmonary capillary permeability, resulting in noncardiogenic pulmonary edema.

transient ischemic attack (TIA) A disorder in which brain cells temporarily stop working because of insufficient oxygen, causing stroke-like symptoms that resolve completely within 24 hours of onset.

transillumination intubation A method of intubation that uses a lighted stylet to guide the endotracheal tube into the trachea.

translaryngeal catheter ventilation A method used in conjunction with needle cricothyrotomy to ventilate a patient; requires a high-pressure jet ventilator.

transmigration (diapedesis) The polymorphonuclear neutrophils permeate through the vessel wall, moving into the interstitial space.

transmission The way in which an infectious agent is spread: contact (direct or indirect), airborne, foodborne, or vector-borne.

transmission-based precautions Precautions beyond standard precautions designed to interrupt specific disease transmission routes. There are three types: airborne, droplet, and contact. Can be used alone or in combination; always used in conjunction with standard precautions.

transmural myocardial infarction A type of acute myocardial infarction in which the infarct extends through the entire wall of the ventricle.

transverse (axial) plane An imaginary plane passing horizontally through the body at the waist, dividing it into top and bottom halves.

trauma systems The collaboration of prehospital and in-hospital medicine that focuses on optimizing the use of resources and assets of each with a primary goal of reducing the mortality and morbidity of trauma patients.

traumatic fracture A fracture that occurs when abnormal forces are applied to normal bone structures.

tremors Fine involuntary, rhythmic movements, usually involving the hands or head.

trichomoniasis A parasitic infection caused by a single-cell parasite that is transmitted through sexual contact.

tricuspid valve The atrioventricular valve that separates the right atrium from the right ventricle.

tricyclic antidepressants (TCAs) A group of drugs used to treat severe depression and manage pain; minimal dosing errors can cause toxic results.

trifascicular block Blockage or impairment of all three components of the ventricular conduction system, with one working occasionally to provide AV conduction.

trigeminy A dysrhythmia in which every third complex is a premature complex, causing a *normal–normal–early beat pattern*; can be atrial, junctional, or ventricular.

trismus The involuntary contraction of the mouth resulting in clenched teeth; occurs during seizures and head injuries.

trocar A solid boring needle.

tropomyosin An actin-binding protein that regulates muscle contraction and other actin-related mechanical functions of the body.

troponin A regulatory protein in the actin filaments of skeletal and cardiac muscle that attaches to tropomyosin.

trunked radio system Computerized sharing of radio frequencies by multiple units, agencies, or systems.

trust and mistrust A phrase that refers to a stage of development from birth to approximately 18 months of age, during which infants gain trust of their parents and/or caregivers if their world is planned, organized, and routine.

tuberculin skin test A test to determine if a person has ever been infected with tuberculosis.

tuberculosis (TB) An infection caused by *Mycobacterium tuberculosis* that can progress to a chronic bacterial disease that usually affects the lungs but can also affect other organs, such as the brain and kidneys; characterized by a persistent cough lasting longer than 3 weeks plus night sweats, headache, weight loss, hemoptysis, and/or chest pain.

tuberculosis blood test Measurement via interferon-gamma release assays of how the immune system reacts to the bacteria that cause tuberculosis; also called blood analysis mycobacteria tuberculosis.

tubular reabsorption The process that moves substances from the tubular fluid into the blood, within the peritubular capillary.

tubular secretion The process that moves substances from the blood in the peritubular capillary into the renal tubule.

tunica adventitia The outer layer of tissue of a blood vessel wall, composed of elastic and fibrous connective tissue.

tunica intima The smooth, thin, inner lining of a blood vessel.

tunica media The middle and thickest layer of tissue of a blood vessel wall, composed of elastic tissue and smooth muscle cells that allow the vessel to expand or contract in response to changes in blood pressure and tissue demand.

tunnel vision A situation in which a paramedic becomes so completely involved with patient care that he or she fails to see the possibility of physical harm to the patient or other care providers; focusing on or considering only one aspect of a situation without first taking into account all possibilities.

turgor Loss of skin elasticity.

tympanic A loud, high-pitched sound, similar to the sound of a drum, heard on percussion of a hollow space (eg, the empty stomach or a puffed out cheek).

type 1 diabetes The type of diabetic disease that usually starts in childhood and requires daily injections of supplemental synthetic insulin to control blood glucose; formerly called juvenile diabetes *or* juvenile-onset diabetes.

type 2 diabetes The type of diabetic disease that usually starts in later life and often can be controlled through diet and oral medications; formerly called adult-onset diabetes.

ulcerative colitis Generalized inflammation of the colon that results in a weakened, dilated rectum, making it prone to infection and bleeding.

ultra high frequency (UHF) band The portion of the radio frequency spectrum between 300 and 3,000 megahertz.

umbilical The region of the abdomen surrounding the umbilicus.

unblinded study A type of study in which the subjects are advised of all aspects of the study.

unifocal Arising from a single site.

unilateral Occurring or appearing on only one side of the body.

unintentional injuries Injuries that occur without intent to harm (commonly called accidents); some examples are motor vehicle collisions, poisonings, drownings, falls, and most burns.

universal timeout A planned pause before the beginning of a procedure that improves communication among all personnel involved and reduces preventable errors.

unstable angina Angina pectoris characterized by a variable, unpredictable pattern of pain, which may signal an impending acute myocardial infarction.

untoward effect A clinical change caused by a medication that causes harm or discomfort to a patient; also known as adverse effect.

uremia The presence of excessive amounts of urea and other waste products in the blood; caused by severe renal failure; eventually impairs brain function.

uremic frost A powdery buildup of uric acid, especially on the skin of the face.

ureters A pair of thick-walled, hollow tubes that transport urine from the kidneys to the bladder.

urethra A hollow tubular structure that drains urine from the bladder, expelling it from the body.

urinary bladder A hollow sac made of smooth muscle in the midline of the lower abdominal area that stores urine until it is released from the body.

urinary incontinence The inability to control the release of urine from the bladder; loss of bladder control.

urinary retention Incomplete emptying of the bladder, or a complete lack of ability to empty the bladder.

urinary system The organs that control the discharge of certain waste materials filtered from the blood and excreted as urine.

urinary tract infections (UTIs) Infections, usually of the lower urinary tract (urethra and bladder), that occur when normal flora (bacteria that naturally populate the skin) enter the urethra and multiply.

urine Liquid waste products filtered out of the body by the urinary system.

urticaria Multiple small, raised areas on the skin that may be one of the warning signs of impending anaphylaxis; also known as hives.

uterine prolapse A condition in which the uterus moves or drops into the vagina.

uterus The muscular, inverted pear-shaped organ where the fetus grows.

U wave A small, flat wave sometimes seen after the T wave and before the next P wave.

vaccinations Inoculations with a vaccine, usually by injection or inhalation, to bring about immunity to a specific disease in a person.

vaccines The products formulated to bring about immunity by introducing into the body a killed or weakened virus to which the immune system produces antibodies.

Vacutainer A cylindrical device that attaches to an 18- or 20-gauge sampling needle; accommodates self-sealing blood tubes when blood samples are being obtained.

vagina The genital canal in the female that serves as a passageway for the elimination of menstrual fluids, receives the penis during sexual intercourse, holds the spermatozoa before their passage into the uterus, and serves as the passageway for childbirth.

vaginal yeast infection An infection caused by the fungus, *Candida albicans*, in which fungi overpopulate the vagina.

vaginitis An inflammation of the vagina that is caused by an infection.

Valsalva maneuver Straining or forced exhalation against a closed glottis, the effect of which is to stimulate the vagus nerve, thereby slowing the heart rate.

varicella zoster A very contagious disease caused by the varicella zoster virus, which is part of the herpes virus family, occurring most often in the winter and early spring; also called chickenpox

varicose veins Veins on the leg that are large, twisted, and ropelike and can cause pain, swelling, or itching.

vasculitis An inflammation of the blood vessels.

vasoactive amines Substances such as histamine and serotonin that increase vascular permeability.

vasoconstriction Narrowing of the diameter of a blood vessel.

vasodilation Widening of the diameter of a blood vessel.

vasoocclusive crisis Ischemia and pain caused by sickle-shaped red blood cells that obstruct blood flow to a portion of the body.

Vaughan-Williams classification A classification scheme based on the mechanism of action rather than on specific medication groups.

vector An animal or insect that carries a disease-causing organism and transmits it to a human host, without itself becoming ill.

vecuronium A nondepolarizing neuromuscular blocking agent; used to maintain paralysis following succinylcholine-facilitated intubation.

venous thrombosis The development of a stationary blood clot in the venous circulation.

ventilation The mechanical process of moving air into and out of the lungs in two separate phases: inhalation (inspiration) and exhalation (expiration).

ventral The anterior surface of the body.

ventral respiratory group (VRG) An area of the medulla oblongata that can cause inspiration or expiration depending on which motor neurons are stimulated.

Venturi mask A mask with a number of interchangeable adapters that draws room air into the mask along with the oxygen flow; allows for the administration of highly specific oxygen concentrations.

vertigo A type of dizziness in which a person experiences the sensation of movement when standing still or of the environment moving around himself or herself; often due to an inner ear disorder.

very high frequency (VHF) band The portion of the radio frequency spectrum between 30 and 300 megahertz.

vesicles Tiny fluid-filled sacs; small blisters.

vesicular breath sounds Soft, muffled breath sounds in which the expiratory phase is barely audible.

vesicular sounds Normal breath sounds made by air moving in and out of the alveoli.

vestibule The structure into which the vagina opens posteriorly, and the female urethra opens into in the midline; also the central part of the labyrinth of the ear, behind the cochlea and in front of the semicircular canals.

vials Small glass or plastic bottles that contain medication; may contain single or multiple doses.

video laryngoscopy Visualization of the epiglottis and vocal cords through a video monitor that is attached to a laryngoscope.

viral hepatitis An inflammation of the liver produced by one of five distinct forms of hepatitis virus—A, B, C, D, and E. The types differ in transmission but present with the same signs and symptoms.

virulence The ability of an organism to invade and create disease in a host; also refers to the ability of an organism to survive outside the living host.

viruses Small organisms that can multiply only inside a host, such as a human, and cause disease.

visceral pain Crampy, aching, deep pain caused by activation of pain receptors in internal areas of the body that are enclosed within a cavity, such as the chest, abdomen, or pelvis; common with genitourinary problems.

visceral pleura Lining of the pleural cavity that adheres tightly to the surface of the lung.

visual acuity Determined by the ability or inability to see, and by how far.

vital capacity The amount of air moved in and out of the lungs with maximum inspiration and exhalation.

vitamins Organic compounds required for normal metabolism.

vitreous humor A jellylike substance found in the posterior compartment of the eye between the lens and the retina; helps the globe maintain its shape without distorting light.

volume of distribution The extent to which a medication will spread within the body.

volume on hand The amount of fluid you have on hand, such as the amount of fluid in an IV bag or the amount of fluid in a vial of medication.

Volutrol A special type of microdrip set that features a 100- or 200-mL calibrated drip chamber; used for fluid regulation in patients prone to circulatory overload, such as pediatric and older patients; also called a Buretrol.

volvulus Twisting of the bowel until a kink occurs; results in blocked flow.

von Willebrand disease A bleeding disorder in which the patient is missing the von Willebrand factor (a protein essential for platelet adhesion), preventing the blood from clotting well.

$\dot{V}/\dot{Q}$ mismatch An imbalance between the anatomic portions of the lung being ventilated (V) and the anatomic portions being perfused (Q).

vulvovaginitis An inflammation of the external vulva.

water soluble A property that indicates a material can be dissolved in water.

waveform capnography A waveform display of exhaled carbon dioxide shown on a portable cardiac monitor/defibrillator.

West Nile virus (WNV) A type of virus that is transmitted by mosquitos, and usually causes only mild disease in humans but can cause encephalitis, meningitis, and death; symptoms, if any, include fever, headache, body rash, and swollen lymph glands.

wheezing A high-pitched whistling sound that may be heard on inspiration, expiration, or both; indicates air movement through a constricted lower airway, such as with asthma.

whispered pectoriloquy A test of decreased breath sounds performed by placing the diaphragm of the stethoscope over the area in question as the patient whispers "ninety-nine;" a loud, clear sound indicates lung consolidation.

whistle-tip catheters Soft plastic, nonrigid catheters; also called French catheters.

white matter Bundles of myelinated nerves.

withdrawal In the context of infant behavior, the final phase of an infant's response to a situational crisis; characterized by apathy and boredom.

withdrawal syndrome A predictable set of signs and symptoms, usually involving altered central nervous system activity that occurs after the abrupt cessation of a drug or after rapidly decreasing the usual dosage of a drug.

Wolff-Parkinson-White (WPW) syndrome A preexcitation syndrome characterized by a short PR interval, a delta wave, a widened QRS complex, and nonspecific ST-T wave changes, indicating the presence of an accessory pathway.

word root The foundation of a word; establishes the basic meaning of a word.

working diagnosis The one diagnosis from a differential list used to base the patient's treatment plan.

years of potential life lost (YPLL) A way of measuring and comparing the overall impact of deaths resulting from different causes; calculated based on a fixed age minus the age at death.

zero-order elimination A process in which a fixed amount of a substance is removed during a certain period, regardless of the total amount in the body.

Zika A type of virus that is transmitted by the *Aedes aegypti* mosquito in which the majority of infected persons are asymptomatic; transmission can occur from an infected mother to her fetus, and from an infected male to his sexual partners; related to onset of Guillain-Barré syndrome.

zoonotic Refers to infectious diseases of animals that can be transmitted to humans and cause disease.

Index: Volume 1

Figures and tables are indicated with *f* and *t* following the page numbers.

A

B

C

D

G

H

I

M

O

P

S

W

X

Y

Z